ANA* SCREENING GUIDELINES   Adult Preventive Care Time Line

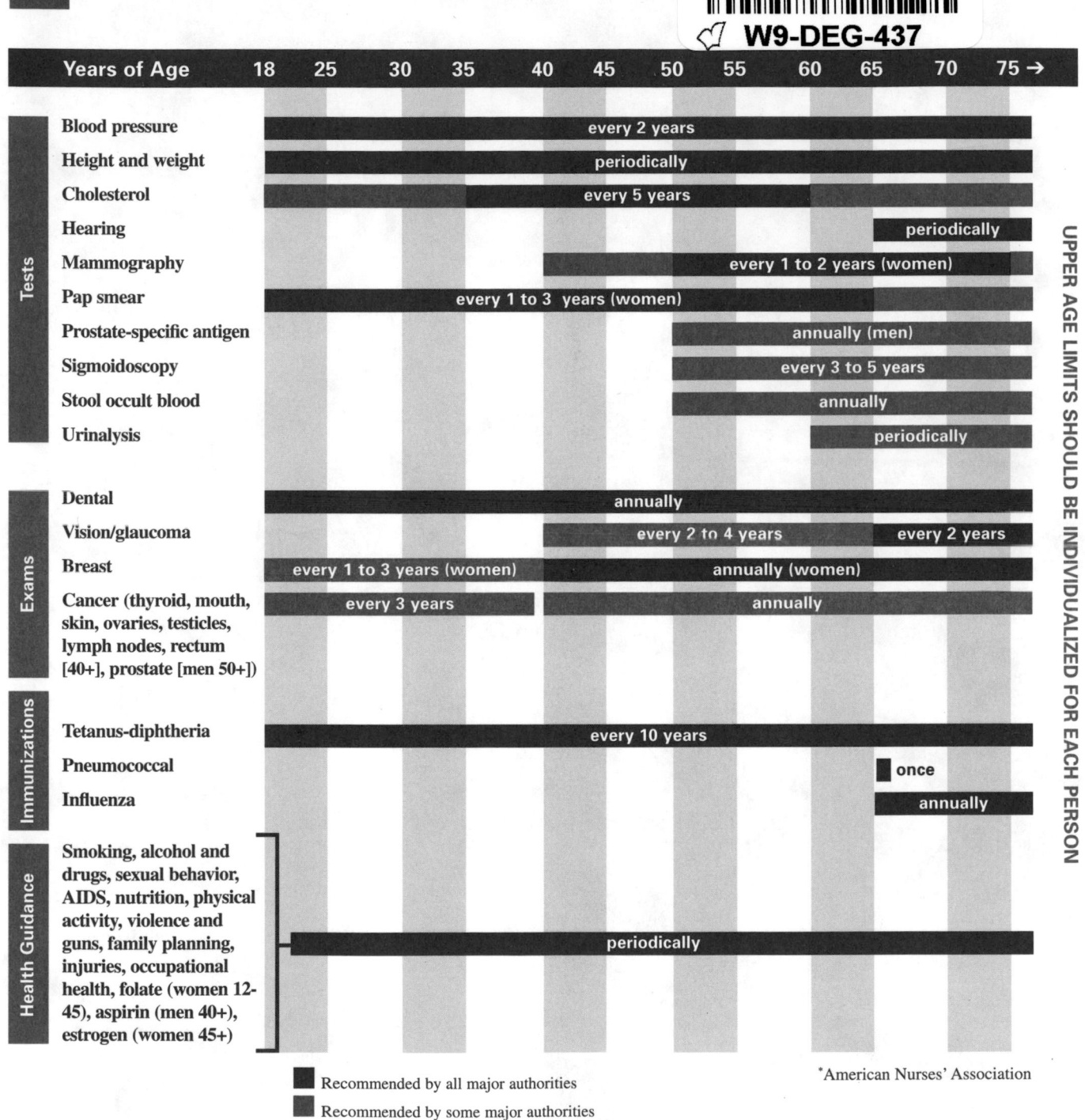

Years of Age	18	25	30	35	40	45	50	55	60	65	70	75 →

Tests

- Blood pressure — every 2 years
- Height and weight — periodically
- Cholesterol — every 5 years
- Hearing — periodically
- Mammography — every 1 to 2 years (women)
- Pap smear — every 1 to 3 years (women)
- Prostate-specific antigen — annually (men)
- Sigmoidoscopy — every 3 to 5 years
- Stool occult blood — annually
- Urinalysis — periodically

Exams

- Dental — annually
- Vision/glaucoma — every 2 to 4 years; every 2 years
- Breast — every 1 to 3 years (women); annually (women)
- Cancer (thyroid, mouth, skin, ovaries, testicles, lymph nodes, rectum [40+], prostate [men 50+]) — every 3 years; annually

Immunizations

- Tetanus-diphtheria — every 10 years
- Pneumococcal — once
- Influenza — annually

Health Guidance

- Smoking, alcohol and drugs, sexual behavior, AIDS, nutrition, physical activity, violence and guns, family planning, injuries, occupational health, folate (women 12-45), aspirin (men 40+), estrogen (women 45+) — periodically

UPPER AGE LIMITS SHOULD BE INDIVIDUALIZED FOR EACH PERSON

■ Recommended by all major authorities
■ Recommended by some major authorities

*American Nurses' Association

Checkup visits with a physician or other health care provider are important for good health. Most authorities recommend these visits every 1 to 3 years until age 65 and yearly thereafter. Each individual should speak with a physician or other health care provider about the proper schedule of checkup visits. This chart shows the different types of preventive care that are needed at each age.

Please note: Recommended intervals for each type of preventive care may vary among authorities. Individuals with special risk factors may need more frequent and additional types of preventive care. Some examples:

Risk factor	Preventive service(s) needed
Diabetes	Eye, foot examinations, urine test
Drug abuse	AIDS, TB tests, hepatitis immunization
Alcoholism	Influenza, pneumococcal immunizations, TB test
Overweight	Blood sugar test
Homeless, recent refugee or immigrant	TB test
High-risk sexual behavior	AIDS, syphilis, gonorrhea, chlamydia tests

Mosby's
Clinical
Nursing

Mosby's Clinical Nursing

Fourth Edition

June M. Thompson, R.N., Dr.P.H.
Director of Nursing Research, Education, and Standards,
University Hospital,
University of New Mexico Health Sciences Center,
Albuquerque, New Mexico

Gertrude K. McFarland, R.N., D.N.Sc., F.A.A.N.
Health Scientist Administrator,
Nursing Research Study Section,
Division of Research Grants,
National Institutes of Health,
Bethesda, Maryland

Jane E. Hirsch, R.N., M.S.
Director of Nursing,
The Medical Center at UCSF,
University of California,
San Francisco, California

Susan M. Tucker, R.N., M.S.N., P.H.N., C.N.A.A.
Patient Care Services Director,
Kaiser Permanente Medical Center,
Walnut Creek, California

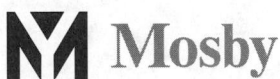

St. Louis Baltimore Boston Carlsbad Chicago Naples New York Philadelphia Portland
London Madrid Mexico City Singapore Sydney Tokyo Toronto Wiesbaden

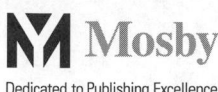

Dedicated to Publishing Excellence

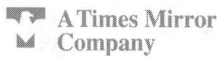

A Times Mirror
Company

Vice President and Publisher: Nancy L. Coon
Senior Editor: Sally Schrefer
Developmental Editor: Gail Brower
Project Manager: Mark Spann
Production Editor: Steve Hetager
Book Design Manager: Judi Lang
Manufacturing Manager: Betty Mueller

Fourth Edition

Printed in the United States of America
Editing and production by Graphic World Publishing Services
Composition by Graphic World, Inc.
Printing/binding by Rand McNally

Mosby–Year Book, Inc.
11830 Westline Industrial Drive
St. Louis, Missouri 63146

Library of Congress Cataloging in Publication Data
Mosby's clinical nursing / June M. Thompson . . . [et al.]. -- 4th ed.
     p.   cm.
    Includes bibliographical references and index.
    ISBN 0-8151-8893-5
    1. Nursing.   I. Thompson, June M., 1946-   .
    [DNLM: 1. Nursing Care.   2. Nursing Process.   WY 100 M89448 1997]
RT41.C65   1997
610.73--dc21
DNLM/DLC
for Library of Congress
                                                  97-4331
                                                  CIP

97 98 99 00 01 / 9 8 7 6 5 4 3 2 1

Contributors

Anne Elizabeth Belcher, R.N., Ph.D., F.A.A.N.
Associate Professor and Chair,
Department of Acute and Long-Term Care,
University of Maryland School of Nursing,
Baltimore, Maryland

Kathleen Calitri Brown, R.N., M.N., C.E.T.N.
Enterostomal Therapy Nurse Coordinator,
Faculty, Enterostomal Therapy Nursing Education Program,
Emory Clinic/Egleston Hospital for Children at Emory,
Atlanta, Georgia

Dorothy J. Brundage, R.N., Ph.D., F.A.A.N.
Associate Professor,
Duke University School of Nursing,
Durham, North Carolina

Ann Wolbert Burgess, R.N., C.S., D.N.Sc., F.A.A.N.
van Ameringen Professor of Psychiatric Mental Health Nursing,
University of Pennsylvania,
School of Nursing,
Philadelphia, Pennsylvania

Joan M. Caley, R.N., M.S., C.S., C.N.A.A.*
Associate Chief Nurse,
Department of Veterans Affairs,
Medical Center/Vancouver Division,
Portland, Oregon

Victor G. Campbell, R.N., Ph.D.
Senior Director, Patient Care,
Director, Education,
Columbus Community Hospital,
Columbus, Ohio

Mary M. Canobbio, R.N., M.N., F.A.A.N.
Cardiovascular Clinical Nurse Specialist,
Assistant Clinical Professor,
UCLA School of Nursing,
Los Angeles, California

Shelley A. Carroll, R.N., M.S.N., C.N.O.R.
Clinical Nurse III,
The Medical Center at UCSF,
University of California,
San Francisco, California

Ann Crowley, R.N., C.R.N.A., M.S.
Department of Anesthesia,
San Francisco General Hospital,
San Francisco, California

Joyce E. Dains, R.N., Dr.P.H., J.D., F.N.P., C.S.
Assistant Professor,
Department of Family Medicine,
Baylor College of Medicine,
Houston, Texas

Kathleen D. Davis, R.N., M.B.A.
Director, Specialty Services,
Lovelace Health Systems,
Albuquerque, New Mexico

Jacqueline Dienemann, R.N., Ph.D., C.N.A.A., F.A.A.N.
Associate Professor,
School of Nursing,
The Johns Hopkins University,
Baltimore, Maryland

Janice A. Drass, R.N., M.A., C.D.E.*
Clinical Nurse IV,
National Institutes for Health, Clinical Center,
Nursing Department,
Bethesda, Maryland

Richard J. Fehring, R.N., D.N.Sc
Associate Professor,
Marquette University,
College of Nursing,
Milwaukee, Wisconsin

Margie L. French, R.N., M.S., C.S.*
Clinical Nurse Specialist, Clinical Manager,
Comprehensive Rehabilitation Unit,
Department of Veterans Affairs Medical Center,
Vancouver Division,
Portland, Oregon

*The opinions expressed herein are those of the authors and do not necessarily reflect those of the U.S. Department of Health and Human Services; the National Institutes of Health; the U.S. Department of Veterans Affairs; Uniformed Services University of the Health Sciences; or Walter Reed Army Medical Center.

Elizabeth Kelchner Gerety, R.N., M.S., C.S., F.A.A.N.*
Clinical Nurse Specialist, Psychiatry,
Psychiatry Consultation Service,
Portland Veterans Affairs Medical Center,
Portland, Oregon;
Instructor, Department of Mental Health Nursing,
School of Nursing,
Oregon Health Sciences University,
Portland, Oregon

Mikel Gray, R.N., Ph.D., P.N.P., C.U.R.N., F.A.A.N.
Nurse Practitioner,
University of Virginia;
Associate Professor of Nursing and Urology,
University of Virginia,
School of Nursing and School of Medicine,
Charlottesville, Virginia;
Adjunct Professor,
Lansing School of Nursing,
Bellarmine College,
Louisville, Kentucky

Deanna E. Grimes, R.N., Dr.P.H., M.S.N., R.N.C.S.
Associate Professor,
University of Texas, Houston,
Health Science Center, School of Nursing,
Houston, Texas

Kevin A. Grimes, B.S.
Clinical Trials Research Coordinator,
Division of Infectious Diseases,
University of Texas, Houston,
Health Science Center, Medical School,
Houston, Texas

Kathleen E. Gunta, R.N., M.S.N., O.N.C.
Clinical Nurse Specialist,
St. Luke's Medical Center,
Milwaukee, Wisconsin

Debra A. Hagler, R.N., M.S., C.S., C.C.R.N.
Clinical Associate Professor,
College of Nursing,
Arizona State University,
Tempe, Arizona

Janice C. Hallal, R.N., D.N.Sc.
Associate Professor,
School of Nursing,
The Catholic University of America,
Washington, D.C.

Maureen P. Hanlon, R.N.
Division of Plastic and Reconstructive Surgery,
University of California, San Francisco,
San Francisco, California

Carol R. Hartman, R.N., C.S., D.N.Sc.
Professor Emeritus,
Boston College,
School of Nursing,
Chesnut Hill, Massachusetts

Joan Mesch Heather, R.N., M.S.*
Consultant,
DBJ Enterprises,
Vancouver, Washington

Jane E. Hirsch, R.N., M.S.
Director of Nursing,
The Medical Center at UCSF,
University of California,
San Francisco, California

Mary G. Hirsch, R.N., M.S.N., C.E.T.N.
Director, Medical Services,
St. Louis Medical Supply Company,
St. Louis, Missouri

Lois M. Hoskins, R.N., Ph.D., F.A.A.N.*
Associate Professor,
School of Nursing,
The Catholic University of America,
Washington, D.C.

Elizabeth A. Howey, R.N., M.N.
Instructor,
Camosun College,
Department of Nursing,
Victoria, British Columbia,
Canada

Karen E. Inaba, R.N., M.S., C.S., P.M.H.N.P.*
Psychiatric Mental Health Nurse Practitioner,
Emergency Care Unit,
Portland Veterans Affairs Medical Center,
Portland, Oregon

Jacqueline L. Kartman, R.N., M.S.N., C.S., A.P.N.P.
Advanced Practice Nurse,
Cardiothoracic Surgery,
Gundersen Lutheran Medical Center,
La Crosse, Wisconsin

Carol Kupperberg, R.N., M.S.N.
Nurse Coordinator,
Montgomery County Infants and Toddlers Program,
Rockville, Maryland

Rae W. Langford, R.N., Ed.D.
Rehabilitation Nurse Consultant,
Private Practice,
Houston, Texas

Teresa Choate Loriaux, R.N., M.S.N.
Managing Editor,
The Endocrinologist,
West Linn, Oregon

---

*The opinions expressed herein are those of the authors and do not necessarily reflect those of the U.S. Department of Health and Human Services; the National Institutes of Health; the U.S. Department of Veterans Affairs; Uniformed Services University of the Health Sciences; or Walter Reed Army Medical Center.

Gertrude K. McFarland, R.N., D.N.Sc., F.A.A.N.*
Health Scientist Administrator,
Nursing Research Study Section,
Division of Research Grants,
National Institutes of Health,
Bethesda, Maryland

Elizabeth A. McFarlane, R.N., D.N.Sc, F.A.A.N.
Associate Professor,
School of Nursing,
The Catholic University of America,
Washington, D.C.

Audrey M. McLane, R.N., Ph.D.
Professor Emeritus,
College of Nursing,
Marquette University,
Milwaukee, Wisconsin

Ruth E. McShane, R.N., Ph.D.
Assistant Professor,
University of Wisconsin—Milwaukee,
Milwaukee, Wisconsin

Karen A. McWhorter, R.N., M.N., C.S.*
Clinical Nurse Specialist,
Adult Day Health Care,
Department of Veterans Affairs Medical Center,
Vancouver Division,
Portland, Oregon

Christine Miaskowski, R.N., Ph.D., F.A.A.N.
Associate Professor and Chair,
Department of Physiological Nursing,
University of California School of Nursing,
San Francisco, California

Marsha A. Miller, R.N., M.Ed., C.N.O.R.
Nurse Manager,
The Medical Center at UCSF,
University of California,
San Francisco, California

Pamela D. Miner, R.N., M.N.
Cardiovascular Clinical Nurse Specialist,
UCLA Medical Center,
Los Angeles, California

Victoria L. Mock, R.N., D.N.Sc., O.C.N.
Director, Oncology Nursing Research,
The Johns Hopkins Hospital,
Baltimore, Maryland

Viola Morofka, Ph.D., R.N.C.S.
Professor Emeritus of Nursing,
School of Nursing,
Kent State University,
Kent, Ohio

Martha M. Morris-Day, R.N., Ed.D.
Associate Professor,
St. Louis University School of Nursing,
St. Louis, Missouri

Leona A. Mourad, R.N., M.S., O.N.C.
Nursing Consultant,
Mourad Consultant Associates,
Dublin, Ohio;
Associate Professor Emeritus,
Ohio State University,
Columbus, Ohio

Charlotte E. Naschinski, R.N., M.S.*
Deputy Director,
Continuing Education for Health Professionals,
Uniformed Services University of the Health Sciences,
Bethesda, Maryland

Anne M. O'Connor, R.N., Ph.D.
Associate Professor,
School of Nursing,
University of Ottawa,
Ottawa, Ontario,
Canada

Ann M. O'Mara, R.N., Ph.D.
Assistant Professor,
University of Maryland School of Nursing,
Baltimore, Maryland

Barbara K. Redman, R.N., Ph.D., F.A.A.N.
Dean and Professor,
University of Connecticut, School of Nursing,
Storrs, Connecticut

M. Gaie Rubenfeld, R.N., M.S.*
Associate Professor,
Department of Nursing Education,
Eastern Michigan University,
Ypsilanti, Michigan

Marlene F. Schwartz, R.N., M.S.N., Ph.D.
Nurse Licensed Psychologist,
Psychiatric Consultation Associates,
Milwaukee, Wisconsin

Kathleen C. Sheppard, R.N., Ph.D.
Director of Nursing,
University of Texas,
M.D. Anderson Cancer Center,
Houston, Texas

Barbara A. Sigler, R.N., M.N.Ed., C.O.R.L.N.
Technical Publications Editor,
Oncology Nursing Press, Inc.,
Oncology Nursing Society,
Pittsburgh, Pennsylvania

---

*The opinions expressed herein are those of the authors and do not necessarily reflect those of the U.S. Department of Health and Human Services; the National Institutes of Health; the U.S. Department of Veterans Affairs; Uniformed Services University of the Health Sciences; or Walter Reed Army Medical Center.

Sarah C. Smith, M.A., C.R.N.D.
Educational Associate,
University of Iowa,
Department of Ophthalmology,
Iowa City, Iowa

Barbara L. Barrat Solomon, R.N., M.S., D.N.Sc.*
Nurse Researcher,
Endocrine Metabolic Service,
Walter Reed Army Medical Center,
Washington, D.C.

Ann D. Sprengel, R.N., Ed.D.
Associate Professor,
Department of Nursing,
Southeast Missouri State University,
Cape Girardeau, Missouri

Sylvia Rae Stevens, R.N., M.S., C.S.
Private Practice of Psychotherapy,
Assistant Professor of Nursing,
The Catholic University of America,
Washington, D.C.

June M. Thompson, R.N., Dr.P.H.
Director of Nursing Research, Education, and Standards,
University Hospital,
University of New Mexico Health Sciences Center,
Albuquerque, New Mexico

Gayle A. Traver, R.N., M.S.N.
Clinical Assistant Professor of Medicine,
Associate Professor of Nursing,
College of Nursing,
University of Arizona,
Tucson, Arizona

Jean O. Trotter, R.N., M.S., C.
Instructor,
School of Nursing,
The Johns Hopkins University,
Baltimore, Maryland

Susan M. Tucker, R.N., M.S.N., P.H.N., C.N.A.A.
Patient Care Services Director,
Kaiser Permanente Medical Center,
Walnut Creek, California

Kerry Twite, R.N., M.S.N., A.O.C.N.
Clinical Nurse Specialist,
St. Luke's Medical Center,
Milwaukee, Wisconsin

Evelyn L. Wasli, R.N., D.N.Sc.
Chief Nurse,
Emergency Psychiatric Response Unit,
D.C. Commission on Mental Health Service,
Washington, D.C.

Janet R. Weber, R.N., M.S.N., Ed.D.
Associate Professor,
Department of Nursing,
Southeast Missouri State University,
Cape Girardeau, Missouri

Susan Fickertt Wilson, R.N., Ph.D., F.N.P.
Associate Professor,
Harris College of Nursing,
Fort Worth, Texas;
Family Nurse Practitioner,
Medical Center at Riverside,
Grand Prairie, Texas

*The opinions expressed herein are those of the authors and do not necessarily reflect those of the U.S. Department of Health and Human Services; the National Institutes of Health; the U.S. Department of Veterans Affairs; Uniformed Services University of the Health Sciences; or Walter Reed Army Medical Center.

Consultants

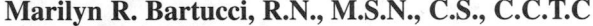

Marilyn R. Bartucci, R.N., M.S.N., C.S., C.C.T.C
Head Nurse Manager, Transplant Center,
Medical-Surgical Nursing,
University Hospital of Cleveland;
Case Western Reserve University—FPB,
Cleveland, Ohio

Wanda C. Dubisson, B.S.N., M.N.
Assistant Professor,
Department of Nursing,
University of Southern Mississippi,
Hattiesburg, Mississippi

Sheila Dunn, M.S.N., C.S.
Adjunct Instructor,
Department of Nursing,
St. Louis University,
St. Louis, Missouri

Jane F. Marek, R.N., M.S.N.
Clinical Instructor, Research Nurse,
Medical-Surgical Department,
Meridia Huron Hospital School of Nursing,
Cleveland, Ohio

Edwina A. McConnell, R.N., Ph.D., F.R.N.C.A.
Professor,
Texas Tech University School of Nursing,
Lubbock, Texas;
Independent Nurse Consultant,
Madison, Wisconsin;
Staff Nurse,
Meriter Hospital,
Madison, Wisconsin

Suzanne B. Millar, Pharm. D.*
Clinical Pharmacist Specialist,
Veterans Administration Medical Center,
Portland, Oregon;
Assistant Professor of Clinical Pharmacy,
Oregon State University, College of Pharmacy,
Portland Campus at Oregon Health Sciences University

Martha M. Morris-Day, R.N., Ed.D.
Associate Professor,
St. Louis University School of Nursing,
St. Louis, Missouri

Hildy M. Schell, R.N., M.S.
Clinical Nurse Specialist, Critical Care
The Medical Center at UCSF
San Francisco, California

Marlene F. Schwartz, R.N., M.S.N., Ph.D.
Nurse Licensed Psychologist,
Psychiatric Consultation Associates,
Milwaukee, Wisconsin

David M. Smith, M.D.
Psychiatrist,
Portland, Oregon

Pamela Becker Weilitz, M.S.N. (R.), C.S.
Director of Nursing Practice,
Department of Nursing Practice,
Barnes-Jewish Hospital,
St. Louis, Missouri

---

*The opinions expressed herein are those of the authors and do not necessarily reflect those of the U.S. Department of Health and Human Services; the National Institutes of Health; the U.S. Department of Veterans Affairs; Uniformed Services University of the Health Sciences; or Walter Reed Army Medical Center.

Preface

Are you riding the whitewater of change into the twenty-first century? Well, climb on board. This book can help you. Health care is fraught with change, and it's not going to stop. The flurry of change initiatives in the clinical setting include redesign, reengineering, guidelines for disease management, timeline care plans or clinical pathways, new utilization guidelines, shorter inpatient hospital stays, dramatic shifts away from acute care services to ambulatory care, capitation plans, case managers, hospital-based physicians, more unlicensed assistive personnel, and much more. There is no escape. Change is permanent. The professional nurse often has less time to spend on direct care, coordination of care, interdisciplinary collaboration, teaching, and providing comfort measures.

The public is beginning to realize that being admitted to a hospital is not without risk and that the professional nurse is its most important ally and advocate. As health care organizations are going over troubled water, you can, however, build your ship while sailing it over turbulent seas. Just consider *Mosby's Clinical Nursing* your anchor!

Mosby's Clinical Nursing was designed exclusively for your evolving and challenging clinical nursing practice in caring for the adult patient. Each chapter in *Part One* relates the anatomy, physiology, and associated pathophysiology according to body system in the adult. Normal adult findings are described, which can be used in assessing the patient. The normal laboratory data and diagnostic studies are clustered together in *Part Three* so that there is just one place to look for this information. You won't need all of it every time you take care of a patient, but when you do you will appreciate having the most accurate, comprehensive, and up-to-date information in one place.

Health problems related to the specific body system are presented in *Part One* using a systematic format for each condition, disease, disorder, and surgical procedure. The comprehensive information is presented in a practical manner, with a description, epidemiologic factors, and pathophysiology in a narrative format. This provides the theory base for the student as well as the practicing professional nurse. Diagnostic studies with anticipated findings are included, followed by a multidisciplinary plan of care based on the therapies prescribed by other members of the health care team. The use of the nursing process has been the foundation for the nursing care component, which consists of assessment criteria, nursing diagnoses, interventions with selected rationales in italics (to help the stu-

dent or those who need a refresher), patient education/home care planning, and evaluation. This information is presented in a readily retrievable outline-type format and can be used as a quick reference for the nurse on the go. Color shading helps you to quickly identify nursing care as well as patient education and home care planning. Sharing this information with patients and families recognizes their role as partners in achieving high-quality outcomes. In addition, there are emergency alert boxes in many sections to expedite your retrieval of lifesaving information.

Part Two is devoted to perioperative nursing, and if you are at all involved in caring for patients having a surgical procedure and anesthesia, this is for you. The preoperative nursing assessment and care section applies to nurses who are involved in preparing the patient for surgery, with a focus on the immediate preoperative period. Following the discussion of asepsis and positioning the patient, there is a detailed discussion of anesthesia, postoperative complications, and nursing care for the postanesthesia patient. In addition to being informative for the perioperative nurse, the content is important to all nurses caring for patients in the post-recovery period.

Part Three relates everything you would want and need to know about laboratory studies and diagnostic procedures. Information on conscious sedation has been added to this section to ensure that you comply with regulatory and accreditation agencies.

Part Four provides nursing care information for NANDA (North American Nursing Diagnosis Association) nursing diagnoses and guides the provision of care to those patients who may or may not have a medical diagnosis or those who may not be ill. There is a near-exhaustive list of outcome-driven nursing interventions, so if you can't find exactly the intervention your specific patient needs under the condition, disease, or disorder in *Part One,* you'll find it here.

Mosby's Clinical Nursing is written for *you,* whether you are a nurse practicing in an inpatient or outpatient setting, a case manager or discharge planner, educator, or student. This text contains the theoretical, didactic, and scientific information that you need to enhance the art and science of your nursing practice. The information will expand your knowledge base and broaden your horizons, and you have it all in a user-friendly format to get at the information you need to guide the clinical care of your patients.

Mosby's Clinical Nursing is written by nurses: scholars, practitioners, clinicians, educators, and experts. We are pleased that so many of you have chosen *Mosby's Clinical Nursing* as your primary source for clinical practice to facilitate the patient's progression through the health care continuum. This book is your ally; it provides the most comprehensive theory- and research-based nursing to meet your patients' needs. It has been updated to provide you with state-of-the-art information.

During these turbulent times in health care, there *is* something you can depend on—*Mosby's Clinical Nursing.* Our patients are counting on us.

June M. Thompson
Gertrude K. McFarland
Jane E. Hirsch
Susan M. Tucker

How to Use This Book

Mosby's Clinical Nursing was designed to blend the traditional body system–disease approach with contemporary theory-based nursing practice. The text is divided into four major parts. Part One, "Clinical Nursing Practice," is organized by body system and consists of 18 chapters. Part Two, "Perioperative Nursing," is an illustrated overview of care of the surgical patient. Part Three, "Diagnostic and Laboratory Procedures," includes common and not-so-common diagnostic studies. Part Four, "Nursing Diagnoses and Interventions," includes 11 functional health patterns subsuming all of the currently accepted nursing diagnoses, including the new diagnoses approved in 1996.

Part One: Clinical Nursing Practice

Part One is organized by body system for easy reference. The description of each body system is divided into three sections:

Overview   The overview presents the system in terms of its importance and functioning. Presented in detail are:

Normal anatomy and physiology of the system

Normal clinical assessment findings for the system

Conditions, diseases, and disorders   Health problems related to the specific body system are presented using a systematic format:

Definition of the condition, disease, or disorder

Pathophysiology of the problem

Diagnostic studies with anticipated findings

Multidisciplinary plan, including general management, medications, and surgery

Assessment criteria

Nursing diagnoses

Nursing interventions and selected rationales

Patient education/Home care planning

Evaluation based on patient outcome criteria

Medical interventions and related nursing care   Major therapeutic interventions are presented and discussed thoroughly:

Overview of intervention, including description and rationale

Contraindications and cautions

Preprocedural nursing care

Medical plan

Assessment criteria

Nursing diagnoses

Nursing interventions and selected rationales

Patient education/Home care planning

Evaluation

Part Two: Perioperative Nursing

Part Two defines the general principles used to guide the care of patients during the perioperative phase of their hospitalization. Care of the surgical patient is discussed from preoperative assessment to postoperative evaluation, and responsibilities of the operating room nurse are detailed. An extensive section of anesthesia is also included.

Part Three: Diagnostic and Laboratory Procedures

Part Three presents more than 225 diagnostic tests within 20 categories for easy reference. A description, contraindications, complications, and nursing care are presented for each diagnostic test. This new edition also includes guidelines for conscious sedation of patients during diagnostic and therapeutic procedures.

Part Four: Nursing Diagnoses and Interventions

Part Four is organized into the 11 functional health patterns. It contains all of the nursing diagnoses accepted by the North American Nursing Diagnosis Association (NANDA), including new diagnoses approved in 1996. Each diagnosis includes the following information:

Definition and brief description of the nursing diagnosis

Related or risk factors and defining characteristics, including those accepted by NANDA and other research- or clinically based factors and characteristics determined by the authors

Expected patient outcomes along with outcome criteria

Nursing interventions

Principles and rationales for nursing interventions

Evaluation based on patient outcome criteria

In addition to the four major parts of the text, an appendix provides conversion factors to International System of Units (SI units). In May 1977 the Thirtieth World Health Assembly recommended that SI units be used in medicine. Although health care agencies in the United States continue to use the metric system, many health care systems throughout the world have adopted SI units.

Parts One, Two, Three, and Four can be used independently or interdependently. The nurse can look up a particular disease in Part One and find virtually all the information needed to provide optimal care for the patient. In particular, care of the surgical patient is detailed in Part Two. The operating room nurse's responsibilities are discussed, and information on anesthesia is provided. The nurse can consult Part Three for additional information related to tests the patient may be undergoing. Part Three will be especially helpful in planning care for a patient whose disease has not yet been diagnosed by a physician. The nurse can consult Part Four for a specific nursing diagnosis and can use the related or risk factors, defining characteristics, expected patient outcomes and outcome criteria, and nursing intervention sections presented to implement a plan of care. Part Four can also be used in planning nursing care for people when a medical diagnosis is inappropriate, such as for well patients.

Although the nurse is concerned with medical diagnoses and nursing diagnoses as separate entities, the two should be integrated to deliver high-quality nursing care. Parts One and Four of this book facilitate this integration. The nurse can look up a particular disorder in Part One. Within that discussion, in the section "Nursing Dx & Intervention," are the details the nurse needs to provide nursing care for a patient with the disorder. In addition, many times cross-references are provided to specific nursing diagnoses discussed in Part Four. The expanded discussions in Parts Three and Four will help the nurse consider additional strategies of care.

The interrelationship of the four parts of the text provides the nurse with complete information that can be used to develop an effective plan of care. This book offers all the information the nurse needs to determine, implement, and evaluate an individual plan of nursing care.

Contents in Brief

Detailed Contents

PART ONE Clinical Nursing Practice

CHAPTER 13 **Infectious Diseases, 1071**
Deanna E. Grimes, Kevin A. Grimes

Overview, 1071

Conditions, Diseases, and Disorders, 1079

Medical Interventions and Related Nursing Care, 1162

CHAPTER 14 **Immunologic System, 1171**
Christine Miaskowski

Overview, 1171

Conditions, Diseases, and Disorders, 1180

Medical Interventions and Related Nursing Care, 1234

PART TWO   Perioperative Nursing

Marsha A. Miller, Shelley A. Carroll, Ann Crowley, Maureen P. Hanlon

PART THREE   Diagnostic and Laboratory Procedures

Jane E. Hirsch

PART FOUR   Nursing Diagnoses and Interventions

Mosby's
Clinical
Nursing

PART ONE

Clinical Nursing Practice

Cardiovascular System

1

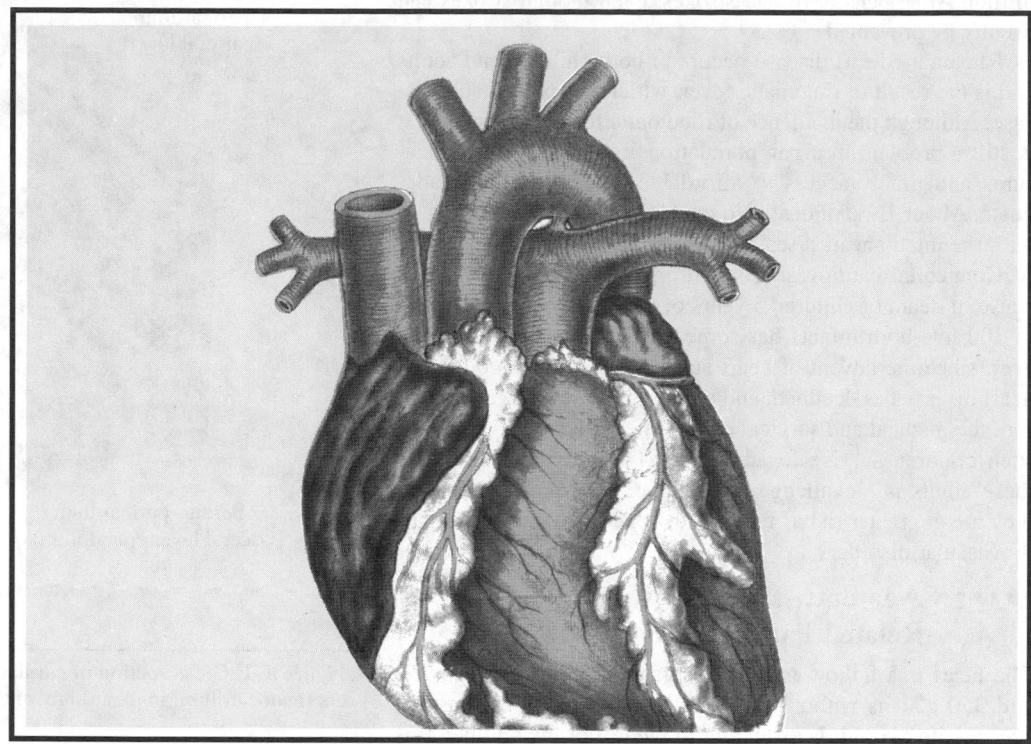

OVERVIEW

Despite recent advances in medicine and surgery, cardiovascular disorders continue to be a principal cause of morbidity and mortality in the United States. In the day-to-day care of patients, nurses deal with cardiovascular disorders in terms of their physical signs and symptoms and appropriate therapeutic interventions. However, they must also consider the socioeconomic and emotional effect of these disorders on the patient and family.

During the past 30 years, progress has been made in prevention, diagnosis, treatment, and rehabilitation. Yet, despite a demonstrated decrease in cardiac mortality, more people die from cardiovascular disease than from all other causes of death combined. More than 60 million Americans have some form of cardiovascular disease, at an estimated cost of $1 billion.[1] Additional costs incurred through job-related losses are difficult to determine.

Cardiac diseases can be divided into those acquired during life and congenital defects.

Major acquired cardiovascular disorders, which cause approximately 1 million deaths per year, include hypertension (high blood pressure), myocardial infarction (heart attacks), congestive heart failure, cerebrovascular accident (stroke), and rheumatic heart disease.

High blood pressure, known as the silent killer, is a major factor contributing to heart attacks and strokes. Studies have estimated that one in four adults has high blood pressure.[3] Among African-Americans the prevalence is 30% or greater. Research is now focusing on early detection because studies have identified high blood pressure in children as young as 4 years of age.[3]

Heart attacks are the number one cause of death in the United States.[3] About 6 million Americans are treated for heart attacks, or angina pectoris, each year. Major research has been undertaken to identify factors, such as occupation, sex, age, dietary habits, serum lipoprotein levels, and activity levels, that may be linked to many underlying diseases that contribute to death by heart attack.[46] In recent years health professionals and community organizations have made major efforts to inform the public about risk factors and early warning signals of heart attacks and strokes. Because fewer than half of cardiac deaths occur in hospitals, organizations such as the American Heart Association and the American Red Cross have initiated programs to teach the public the basic techniques of cardiopulmonary resuscitation (CPR). An encouraging shift in mortality may be credited to increased public awareness and education; the death rate from heart attack declined 31.4% from 1982 to 1992.[2,3]

Congestive heart failure is a consequence of a myocardial dysfunction. Although often controllable with drugs, it remains the major form of chronic cardiac disability. It is also one of the most expensive in terms of medical and nursing services, repeated hospital and nursing home services, drug costs, and job disability.

Stroke, which is the third leading cause of death, occurs most often as a result of high blood pressure. Approximately 3 million Americans have had strokes, even though strokes can usually be prevented.[3]

Rheumatic heart disease occurs in both children and adults and is the result of rheumatic fever, which is a preventable disease. Although the incidence of rheumatic fever has declined, it is still a problem in urban populations where preventive measures and timely access to affordable health care are inadequate. About 1.9% of deaths in the United States are associated with rheumatic heart disease.[3]

Congenital cardiovascular malformations are the principal cause of death of children 5 years of age and younger. About 1 in 300 live-born infants has some form of heart defect. However, since the advent of heart surgery, death from congenital heart disease has declined, and although the severity and therefore the medical and surgical care of these disorders vary, most such children survive to adulthood. The growing number of these adults is a challenge to caregivers, particularly because they are at greater risk if faced with concomitant acquired cardiovascular disorders.

•••••• Anatomy, Physiology, and Related Pathophysiology

The heart is a hollow muscular organ weighing between 250 and 350 g. It is within the thoracic cavity in the mediastinal space, with two thirds extending to the left of the midline. It is flanked by the lungs and protected anteriorly by the sternum and ribs and posteriorly by the vertebral column.

Layers of the Heart

Cardiac muscle has three layers (Figure 1-1). The epicardium, the outer layer, covers the surface of the heart and extends to the great vessels. The myocardium, the middle layer, is responsible for the major pumping action of the ventricles. The endocardium, the innermost layer, is a thin layer of endothelium and a thin layer of underlying connective tissue. The endocardium lines the inner chambers of the heart, valves, chordae tendineae, and papillary muscles. It is continuous with the blood vessels that enter and leave the heart. Cardiac muscle cells are made of striated muscle fibrils consisting of contractile elements known as myofibrils. The fibrils are grouped together in a band and are arranged in parallel rows extending from one end of a cell to the other (Figure 1-2). A membrane junction, the intercalated disc, connects cell to cell.

Pericardium

The heart is enclosed in a double-walled fibroserous sac, the pericardium. The inner layer (visceral pericardium), made of fibrous elastic connective tissue, covers the entire surface of the heart and is the outermost layer of the heart wall (epicardium) (see Figure 1-1).

The outer layer (parietal pericardium) is made of strong, elastic, fibrous connective tissue lined with smooth, translucent serous membrane. It is attached inferiorly to the diaphragm and laterally to the pleura of the lung. Superiorly the parietal pericardium attaches to the larger blood vessels (aorta, pulmonary

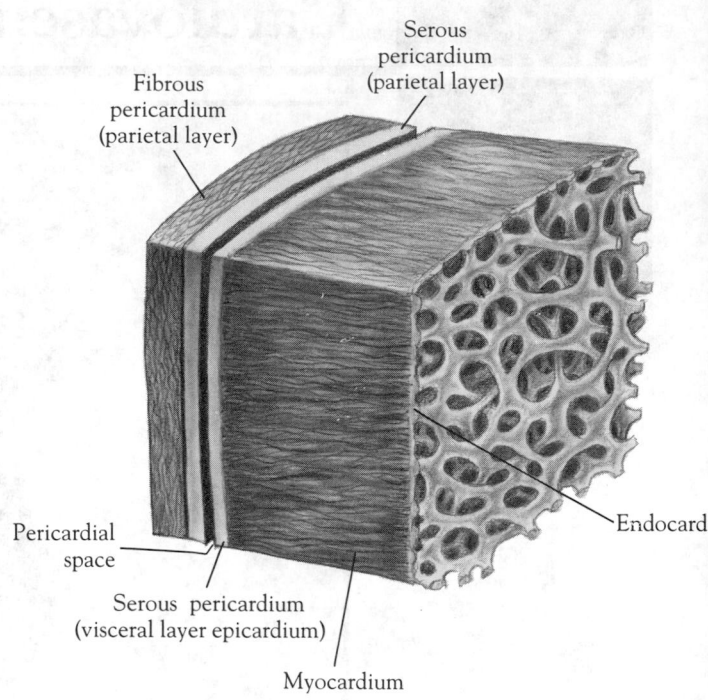

Figure 1-1 Cross section of cardiac muscle showing its three layers (endocardium, myocardium, and epicardium) and pericardium.

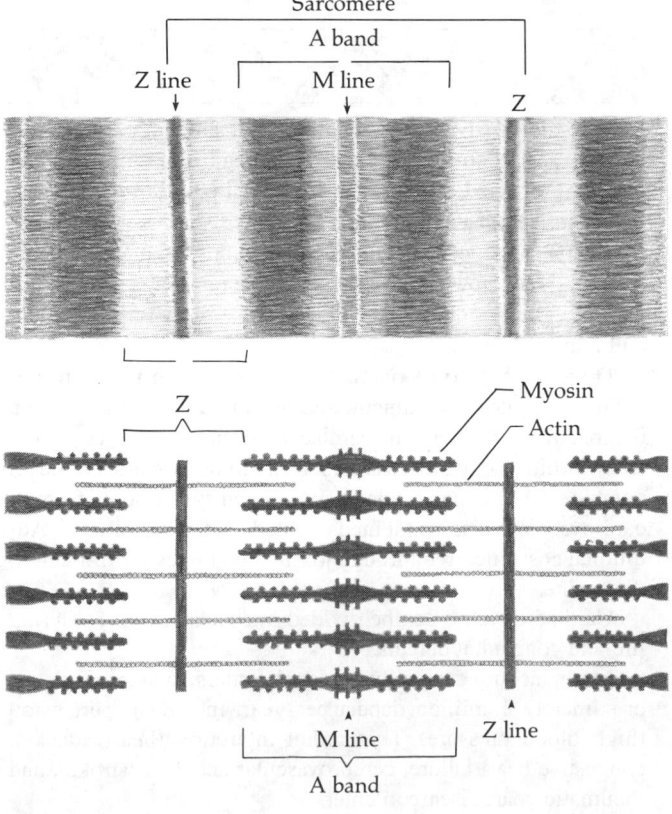

Figure 1-2 Histologic representation of myocardial tissue showing arrangement of myofibrils in relaxed state.

artery, and superior vena cava) but not to the heart itself. This results in a potential space known as the pericardial cavity.

The space between the visceral and parietal layers contains 10 to 30 ml of clear, lymphlike fluid that helps maintain the smooth, easy motion of the heart during contraction and expansion. The pericardial cavity can hold 300 ml of fluid without interference in cardiac function. It can hold up to 1 L in some chronic disease states. The degree to which pericardial fluid compromises cardiac function depends more on the rate of rise in intrapericardial volume than on the amount. During rapid filling, as little as 100 ml may cause acute tamponade,[10] but patients who have slowly developing pericardial effusions can hold up to 1 L of fluid without hampering heart function. The rate of filling is also more important than the amount in the relationship between intrapericardial fluid volume and intrapericardial pressure. Normal pressure is −2 to −5 mm Hg. A sudden increase in pressure may occur with rapid filling of fluid in the pericardial space, regardless of the amount of fluid.

The pericardium shields against infection and trauma and aids cardiac function by helping with the free pumping motion of the heart.

Chambers of the Heart

The heart is a four-chambered organ but functions as a two-sided pump (Figure 1-3). The right side is a low-pressure system pumping venous or deoxygenated blood to the lung. The left side is a higher-pressure system pumping arterial or oxygenated blood to the systemic circulation.

Right atrium   The right atrium (RA) is a thin-walled muscle that acts as a receiving chamber. It receives systemic venous blood from the superior vena cava (SVC), which drains the upper part of the body, and from the inferior vena cava (IVC), which drains blood from the lower extremities.

The coronary sinus, which drains venous blood from myocardial circulation, also empties into the RA just above the tricuspid valve. The pressure exerted during normal filling of the RA is 0 to 7 mm Hg and varies with respiration. During inspiration, RA pressure drops below the pressure in veins outside the chest cavity. Because blood flows from an area of high pressure to an area of lower pressure, blood flow to the RA occurs mainly during inspiration.

Oxygen saturation of blood in the RA varies depending on the place of entry into the RA (IVC, 80%; SVC, 70%; coronary sinus, 30%), but the combined oxygen saturation of RA mixed venous blood is about 75%, or 40 mm Hg.

Right ventricle   The right ventricle (RV) is normally the most anterior chamber of the heart, lying directly beneath the sternum. The RV functions as both an inflow and an outflow tract. The inflow tract includes the tricuspid area and the criss-cross muscular bands (trabeculations) that make up the inner surface of the ventricle. The outflow tract is commonly referred to as the infundibulum.

During diastole, blood enters the RV through the tricuspid valve and is ejected into pulmonary circulation through the pulmonic valve. Because of low pulmonary resistance, systolic or ejection pressures of the RV are also low. RV pressures are 20 to 25/0 to 5 mm Hg. RV oxygen saturation is similar to that in the RA.

Left atrium   The left atrium (LA), the most posterior cardiac structure, receives oxygenated blood from the lungs via the right and left pulmonary veins. The wall of the LA is slightly thicker than that of the RA and exerts a filling pressure of 5 to 10 mm Hg with little breathing variation. The arterial oxygen saturation is 98% (95 mm Hg).

Left ventricle   The left ventricle (LV) lies posterior to and to the left of the RV. It is ellipsoid, with a wall made of thick muscular tissue measuring 8 to 16 mm, two to three times thicker than that of the RV. This increased muscle mass is necessary to generate enough pressure to move blood into circulation. LV pressure is normally 100 to 120/0 to 10 mm Hg with oxygen saturation of 95%. The inflow tract is funnel shaped, formed by the mitral anulus, the two mitral leaflets, and the chordae tendineae. The outflow tract is surrounded by the anterior mitral leaflet, the interventricular septum, and the left ventricular free wall. During systole, blood is propelled above and to the right across the aortic valve.

Cardiac Valves

The heart's efficiency as a pump depends on the integrity of the cardiac valves (Figure 1-4). Their sole purpose is to ensure the one-way, forward blood flow.

Atrioventricular valves   The two atrioventricular (A-V) valves are similar in function but differ in several anatomic details. They are positioned along the atrioventricular groove, which separates the atria from the ventricles.

The tricuspid (right side) and mitral (left side) apparatus is composed of the anulus fibrosus, the valvular tissue (leaflets) to

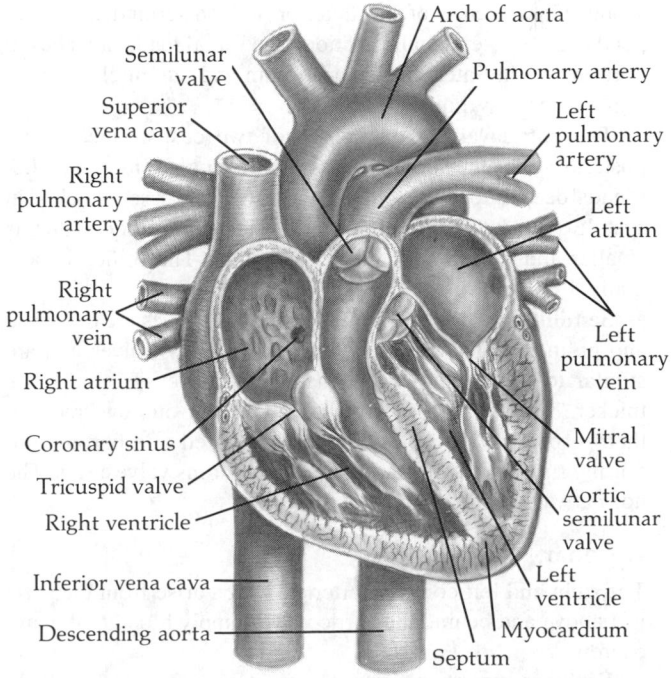

Figure 1-3 Frontal schematic view of heart.

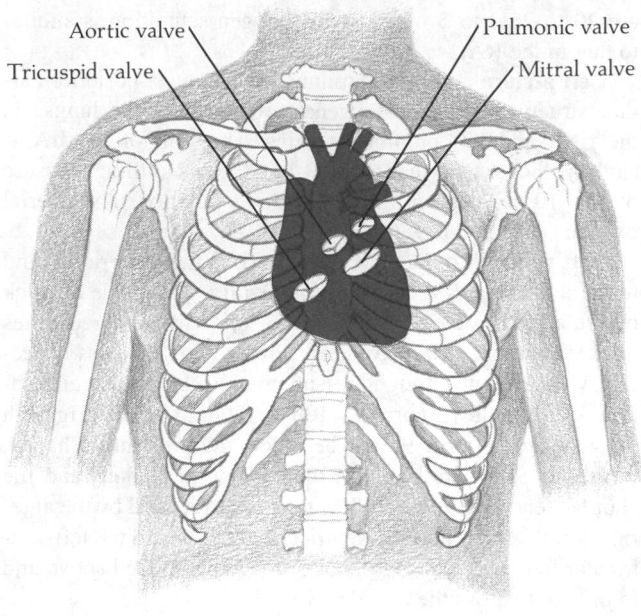

Aortic valve
Tricuspid valve
Pulmonic valve
Mitral valve

Figure 1-4 Anatomic position of cardiac valves.

which the chordae tendineae are attached, and the papillary muscles connecting the chordae to the floor of the ventricular wall. This arrangement allows the leaflets to balloon upward during ventricular systole, but it prevents eversion of the cusps into the atria. These components are considered as a single unit because disruption of any one element can result in serious hemodynamic dysfunction.

The tricuspid valve is larger and thinner than the mitral valve and has three separate leaflets: anterior, posterior, and septal. Competence of the anterior and posterior leaflets depends on RV lateral wall function. The septal leaflet attaches to portions of the interventricular septum and sits in close proximity to the A-V node.

The mitral valve is composed of two cusps: anterior and posterior. The anterior leaflet has a wide range of motion. It descends deep into the LV during diastole and rises quickly in systole to meet the posterior leaflet. The posterior leaflet is smaller and more restricted in its motion. The orifice is normally 4 to 6 cm² in adults.

Semilunar valves   The two semilunar valves are the aortic and pulmonic. They are smaller than the A-V valves and are similar to each other except that the aortic cusps tend to be thicker. The semilunar valves sit above the outflow tracts of their respective ventricles. Each is composed of a fibrous supporting ring called the anulus and three fibrous valve cusps. The normal valve orifice is 2.6 to 3.5 cm².

Coronary Circulation

The right and left coronary arteries, which arise from the aorta just above and behind the aortic valve, supply blood to the myocardium.

Right coronary artery   The right coronary artery (RCA) arises from the right aortic sinus of Valsalva and branches out

along the atrioventricular groove to supply the anterior portion of the right ventricle. In 90% of persons, the RCA curves posteriorly within the interventricular groove and supplies the posterior septum, the posterior left papillary muscle, and the sinus and A-V nodes.

Left coronary artery   The left coronary artery (LCA) arises from the left aortic sinus of Valsalva. It begins as a common artery referred to as the left main and then divides into the left anterior descending (LAD) artery and the circumflex artery. The LAD artery descends along the anterior intraventricular groove to nourish a large portion of the anterior left ventricular wall, including the anterior septum, the anterior papillary muscle, and the apical portion of the myocardium.

The circumflex artery extends from the left main coronary artery along a groove between the LA and LV. In some persons the circumflex artery supplies the inferior and posterior portions of the LV. This is known as left coronary dominance.

Cardiac veins   Three main divisions of cardiac veins comprise the venous circulation and closely parallel the coronary arteries. These include the thebesian veins, most of which empty into the atria; the anterior cardiac veins, which empty into the RA; and the coronary sinus, a short vein lying on the posterior side of the heart. Most venous circulation drains into the coronary sinus, which receives blood from the deeper myocardium and empties into the RA at the coronary sinus ostium between the tricuspid valve and the opening of the inferior vena cava.

Conduction

A special system transmits and coordinates electrical impulses throughout the heart. It consists of atypical muscle fibers and has the following characteristics.

Impulse formation   The sinoatrial (S-A), or sinus, node gives rise to a self-generating impulse known as the heartbeat. The S-A node is at the border of the superior vena cava and the right atrium. It is the primary pacemaker of the heart and can generate electrical impulses at a rate of 60 to 100 beats per minute (Figure 1-5, *A*).

The S-A node is supplied primarily by the proximal RCA (60%) and the left circumflex artery and is innervated by sympathetic and parasympathetic nerve fibers. If the sinus node is depressed, escape ectopic beats from other inherent pacemakers in the A-V node or ventricle appear and can assume pacemaker function. In addition, rapid impulses in other areas of the heart may produce atrial, junctional, or ventricular tachycardias. These can occur when an ischemic myocardium causes an alteration in the heart's conductivity, producing what are called reentry pathways.

Conduction pathways   The normal sinus impulse is transmitted through the heart by a highly specialized network of fibers known as the conduction system. When the impulse reaches the ventricles, stimulation of the myocardium causes depolarization of the cells, and contraction occurs.

The conduction system is made up of the A-V node, bundle of His, and right and left bundle branches. The A-V node filters atrial impulses as they pass through to the ventricles. It can ini-

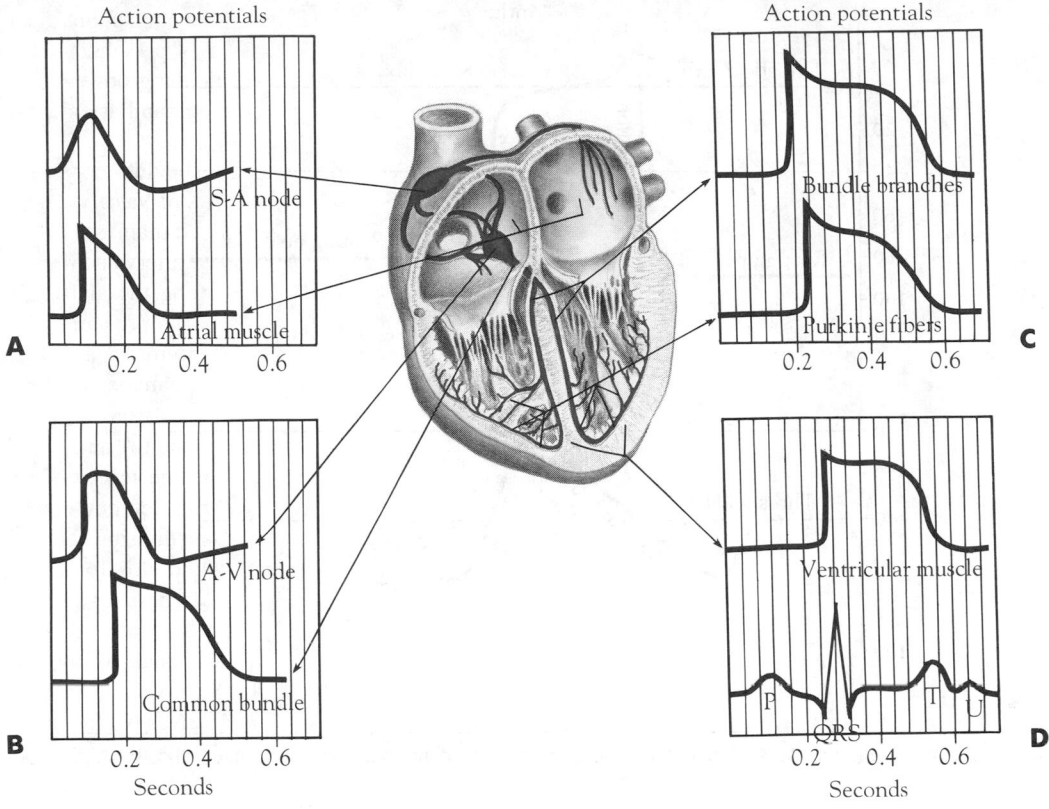

Action potentials

A   0.2   0.4   0.6

S-A node

Atrial muscle

B   0.2   0.4   0.6
Seconds

A-V node

Common bundle

Action potentials

C   0.2   0.4   0.6

Bundle branches

Purkinje fibers

D   0.2   0.4   0.6
Seconds

Ventricular muscle

P   QRS   T   U

Figure 1-5 Heart with normal conduction pathways and transmembrane action potential of **A,** S-A node, **B,** A-V node, **C,** bundle branches, and **D,** ventricular muscle.

tiate its own impulse, but usually at lower rates (40 to 60 beats per minute). It is generally supplied by the RCA and is also innervated by the autonomic nervous system (Figure 1-5, *B*).

The bundle of His provides infranodal conduction traversing the two sides of the intraventricular system, where it divides into the right and left bundle branches. The bundle branches end in a fine network of conductive tissue called the Purkinje fibers. These fibers extend to the papillary muscles and lateral walls of the ventricles. The His bundle and its branches are supplied by the proximal branches of the LAD coronary artery (Figure 1-5, *C*).

Electrophysiology Transmission of the electrical impulse or action potential of the myocardium is preceded by a series of sequential ionic changes across the cardiac cell membrane, which results in depolarization and subsequent contraction of the myocardium. These events correspond in time to the mechanical events described below. After depolarization the cells return for recovery to a resting state called repolarization, diastole, or relaxation.

A resting (polarized) cell has a net charge of −90 mV. Potassium is the predominant intracellular cation, and sodium is the predominant extracellular cation. The difference in concentrations of these ions results in a resting state of electrical potential commonly referred to as the resting membrane potential (RMP).

On initiation of an electrical stimulus, sodium ions move across the cell membrane, converting the net electrical force within the cell to a positive charge. The cell is then depolarized, resulting in a shortening of the cell.

The electrical potential created by this ionic movement progresses through adjacent regions of the cell membrane and is referred to as the action potential. Figure 1-6 illustrates the five phases of the cardiac action potential and its relationship to the electrocardiogram.

Phase 0 represents the depolarization of the cell with the rapid influx of sodium causing a reversal of the ionic charge (the inner surface of the cell becomes positive). This is depicted by the upstroke of the action potential curve (see Figure 1-6, *A*).

Phase 1 is the brief rapid change toward the repolarization process, during which the membrane potential returns to 0 mV.

Phase 2 is a plateau or stabilization period caused by the slow influx of sodium and the slow exit of potassium. During this period, calcium ions enter the cell through slow calcium channels, triggering the release of large quantities of calcium. Calcium functions in the process of cellular contraction.

Phase 3 represents sudden acceleration in repolarization as potassium leaves rapidly, causing the inside of the cell to move toward a more negative state.

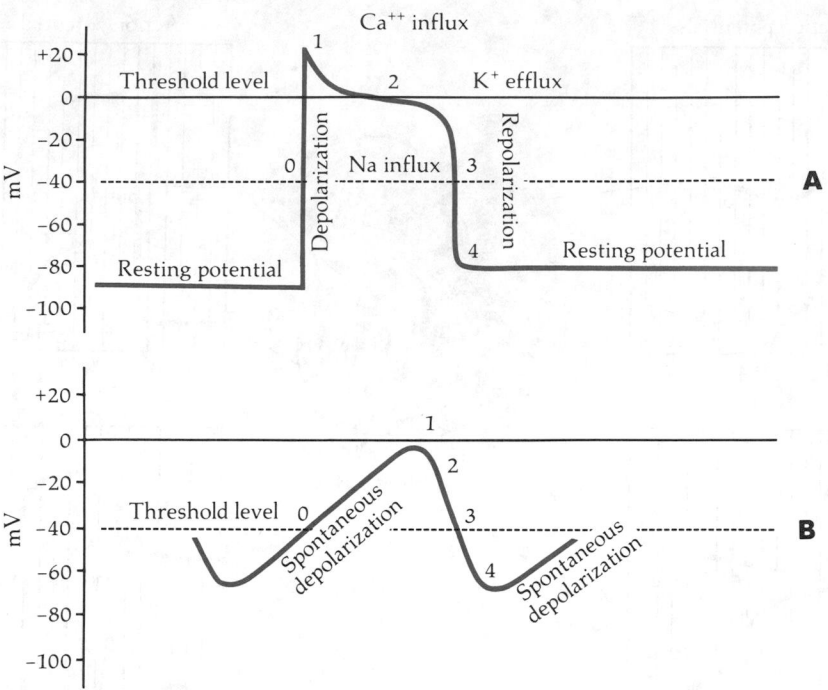

Figure 1-6 Cardiac action potentials. **A,** Action potential phases 0 to 4 of nonpacemaker cardiac cells. **B,** Action potential of pacemaker cell.

Phase 4 represents the return to the resting phase during which the intracellular charge is once again electronegative, leading to the initiation of the action potential (phase 0). Any excess sodium is eliminated from the cell in exchange for potassium that left the cell during phases 2 and 3.

Throughout these phases the cardiac cell goes through a series of refractory periods during which the cell is incapable of accepting another stimulus and responding with a full action potential. An *absolute refractory period* occurs during depolarization and at the beginning of repolarization (phases 0, 1, and 2). During this period, excitation of the cardiac cell will not result in another impulse no matter how strong the stimulus. The *relative refractory period* represents the time when the cell is once again electronegative. A stronger-than-threshold stimulus can initiate another impulse. A *vulnerable* or *supernormal period* occurs as phase 4 begins and the cell is returning to its resting potential. During this time a weaker-than-threshold stimulus can initiate an action potential.

Electrocardiogram.   The electromechanical events of the heart can be recorded and interpreted on an electrocardiogram (ECG). The various waveforms in Figure 1-7 have been correlated with the normal conduction sequence. Any deviation from normal indicates dysrhythmia.

The cardiac cycle includes the following waveforms and time intervals:

P wave—the electrical activity associated with the sinus node impulse and its depolarization of the atria

PR interval—the time the impulse takes to travel through the atria to the A-V node, the bundle of His and bundle

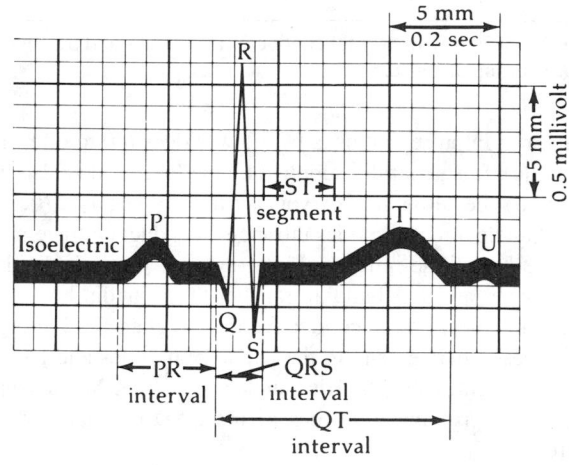

Figure 1-7 Normal electrocardiographic waveform. (From Tucker.[89])

branches, and the ventricles; normal duration is 0.12 to 0.20 seconds

QRS complex—electrical depolarization and contraction of the ventricles

ST segment—the period between the completion of depolarization and the repolarization of the ventricles

T wave—the recovery or repolarization phase of the ventricles

Intervals between these waveforms reflect the time an impulse takes to travel through the heart.

Identification of rhythms, normal or otherwise, requires a careful systematic approach to interpretation. One method is described in box at right.

Cardiac Cycle

The cardiac cycle is divided into two phases, systole and diastole. Systole is the time interval during which blood is ejected from the ventricles. Diastole is the time interval during which the ventricles are relaxed and filling with blood from the atria. Diastole is discussed first because filling pressures often predict the effectiveness of systolic ejection.

As described previously, the atria are reservoirs for blood entering the heart. During diastole the semilunar valves are closed, the ventricles are at rest, and the A-V valves are forced open, allowing blood to flow from the atria into the ventricles. During the initial phase of diastole, approximately 70% of the blood flows rapidly into the ventricles. In the second half of diastole, blood flow slows until atrial contraction is accelerated, forcing the remainder of the blood into the ventricles. This added atrial thrust completes diastolic filling of the ventricle and is reflected as the a wave on the atrial pressure tracing (Fig-

ure 1-8). The blood present in the ventricles at the end of diastole is the end-diastolic volume.

With filling of the ventricles complete, isovolumetric contraction begins. During this initial phase, systolic pressures begin to rise, forcing the closure of the A-V valves, The deceleration of blood associated with the closure of the A-V valves is

---

SYSTEMATIC APPROACH TO ECG INTERPRETATION

1. Calculate the heart rate. Calculate atrial (P waves) rate. Calculate ventricular (QRS complexes) rate.
2. Determine rhythm regularity.
3. Determine whether P waves are present. Determine the position of P waves with relation to the QRS complex.
4. Measure the PR interval.
5. Measure the QRS interval.
6. Identify and examine the ST segment and T wave.
7. Determine the origin of the rhythm. Is it of sinus, atrial, junctional, or ventricular origin?

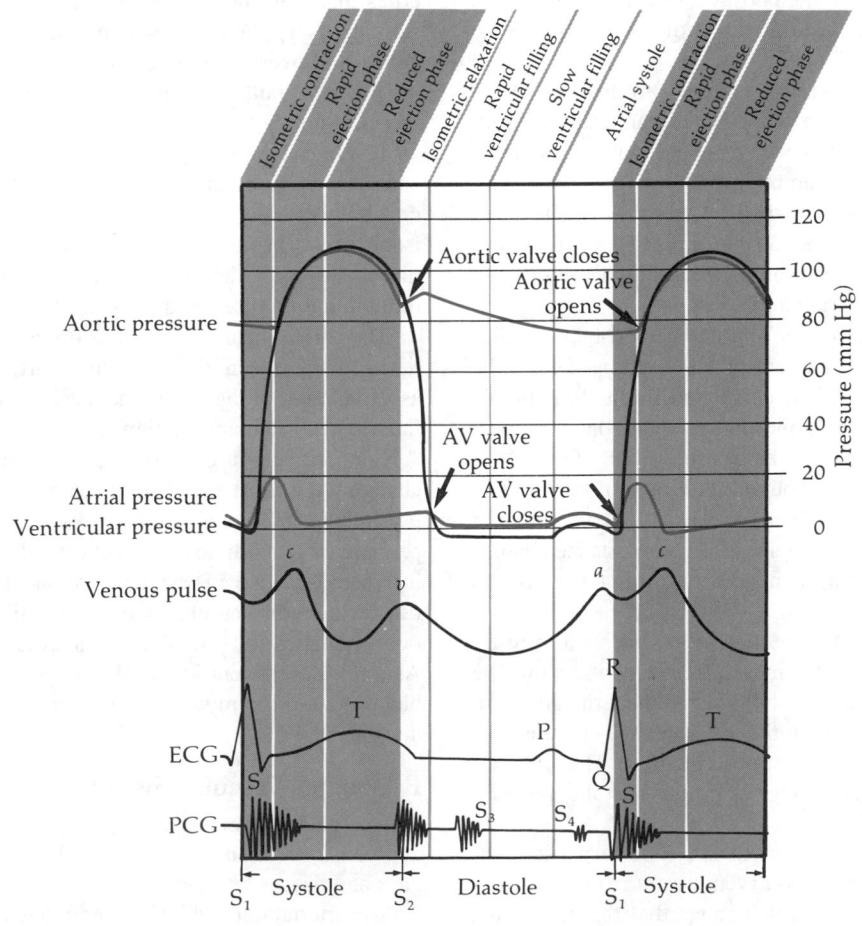

Figure 1-8 Left ventricular pressure pulses correlated in time with ventricular volume, heart sounds, and electrocardiogram. (From Guzzetta.[40])

the source of the first heart sound (S_1) (see Figure 1-8). Isovolumetric contraction continues until ventricular pressure exceeds aortic pressure, forcing open the semilunar valves. Blood is ejected rapidly into the pulmonary artery and aorta on the left side.

As the ejection phase ends, the ventricular muscle relaxes. This decreases intraventricular pressures and causes reversal of blood flow in the aorta, which forces the semilunar valves to close. Ventricular relaxation with the closure of the semilunar valves is the source of the second heart sound (S_2), reflected by a dicrotic notch on the pressure waveform of the aorta (see Figure 1-8).

After the semilunar valves close, ventricular wall tension or pressure falls rapidly. On the atrial pressure tracing, the **v** wave reflects this period in which the ventricles are relaxing and blood is entering the atrium. The downsloping after the **v** wave is the signal that ventricular relaxation is complete. As ventricular pressure falls below atrial pressure, the A-V valves once again open and the cycle is repeated.

Factors Affecting Cardiac Function

A basic function of the heart is to transport oxygen and other nutrients to various parts of the body via circulation and to return carbon dioxide and waste products of metabolism to the lungs for excretion.

The circulating volume varies according to the need of tissue cells. Any increase in the work of the cells causes an increase in blood flow and thus increases the work of the heart and myocardial oxygen consumption (MVO_2).

The heart's function is governed by the closely integrated working of three major factors: intrinsic properties of the heart; extrinsic factors, including nervous system, blood volume, and venous return; and peripheral circulation.

Cardiac function is based on the adequacy of the cardiac output (CO), which is the amount of blood pumped from the left ventricle per minute. CO is calculated by multiplying the amount of blood ejected from one ventricle with one heart beat (stroke volume, or SV) by the heart rate (HR): CO = SV × HR. In a normal 70 kg (150-pound) adult at rest, the CO is 5 L/minute. The main factors affecting CO are preload (filling of the heart during diastole), afterload (the resistance against which the heart must pump), contractility of the heart muscle, and heart rate.

Preload is the degree of fiber stretch that occurs as a result of load or tension placed on the muscle before contraction. The term *load* refers to the quantity of blood and the term *tension* to the pressure the blood exerts in the left ventricle at the end of diastole (filling) just before systole (ejection). This is commonly referred to as left ventricular end-diastolic pressure (LVEDP).

The ability of the muscle fibers to stretch in response to increasing loads of incoming blood (venous return) is related to the Frank-Starling principle, which states that the greater the presystolic fiber stretch (within physiologic limits), the stronger the ventricular contraction. In other words, the more

the ventricle fills with blood during diastole, the greater the quantity of blood it will pump during systole. Preload is a major determinant of myocardial oxygen consumption.

Afterload is the resistance to blood flow as it leaves the ventricles. Afterload is a function of both arterial pressure and left ventricular size. Any increase in vascular resistance (pressure against which the heart is forced to pump) will cause ventricular contractility to increase in an attempt to maintain stroke volume and cardiac output.

The principle factors causing impedance or resistance to left ventricular outflow are the peripheral vascular resistance and the compliance and distensibility of the aorta and large arteries. Arterial pressure is a major factor offering resistance to blood flow from the ventricles. As arterial pressure increases, more energy is required to generate enough pressure to eject blood. As more energy is required for ventricular systole, the myocardial oxygen demand increases. Conditions that increase afterload include those causing obstruction to ventricular outflow (such as aortic stenosis) and those causing high peripheral vascular resistance (such as hypertension).

Contractility is the force of muscle contraction. The myocardium is a unique muscle because it has some specific properties that contribute to its effective pumping action. When a stimulus is applied to heart muscle, the myofibrils slide together and overlap, and contraction occurs. During relaxation the filaments pull away from each other and return to their former positions.

The rate (chronotropic force) and force (inotropic force) of contraction can be increased by sympathetic nerve stimulation or administration of drugs with inotropic properties, such as isoproterenol, epinephrine, and dopamine. Depressed contractility is generally the result of a loss of contractile muscle mass through injury, disease, dysrhythmias, or drugs.

The normal heart rate is 60 to 100 beats per minute. It is initiated by the S-A node within the heart, but other factors such as stimulation of the autonomic nervous system can greatly influence heart rate and rhythm.

Cardiac output can be depressed or increased, directly changing the heart rate. With a heart rate of less than 40 beats per minute, the cardiac output often falls, impairing cardiac performance. With low rates the tendency for dysrhythmias increases because of the uncoordinated myocardial contraction, which further depresses contractility. With rapid pulse rates the length of time that the heart is in diastole is reduced. As a result, left ventricular filling is decreased, as is coronary blood flow to the myocardium, which occurs primarily during diastole.

Peripheral Vascular System

The vascular system is composed of the arteries, capillaries, and veins. Its main function is to distribute blood to body organs and tissues.

The arterial tree, which carries oxygenated blood to all body tissues, is made up of arteries, arterioles, and capillaries. Arteries are easily distended, high-pressure conduits (Figure 1-9)

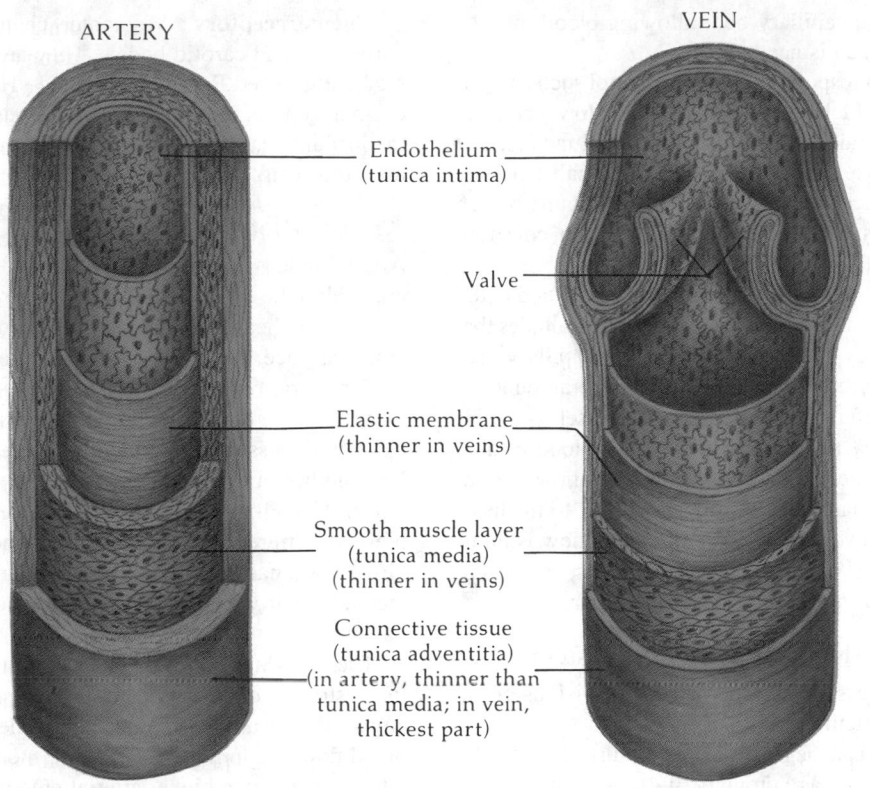

Figure 1-9 Cross sections of artery and vein showing the three layers: tunica intima, tunica media, and tunica adventitia. Note difference in wall thickness between artery and vein.

known as resistance vessels. They have a high elastic fiber content that can support high pressure and hold large volumes of blood. About 20% of the total circulating blood is contained within the arteries. Arterioles are smaller branches whose walls contain less elastic tissue and more smooth muscle. Constriction or dilation of the lumens of the arterioles is the major control of pressure and blood flow. By changing the diameter of the blood vessels, the volume of blood supplied to the tissues may be increased or decreased.

Arteries and arterioles respond to the autonomic nervous system and to chemical stimulation. Nerve impulses from reflex centers in the brain may constrict or dilate the vessels. Chemical substances may alter the size of a blood vessel by acting directly on the vessel or by stimulating sensory receptors, thus beginning reflex control. Temperature can also alter the size of the blood vessels.

Capillaries are microscopic (>1 mm), inelastic endothelial vessels. The large capillary bed is permeable to the molecules that are exchanged between blood cells and tissue cells (Figure 1-10). The vital exchange of oxygen, nutrients, and metabolic waste products between blood and interstitial fluid occurs here. Blood flow through the capillaries is regulated by the demand for oxygen by cells. The precapillary sphincter helps control

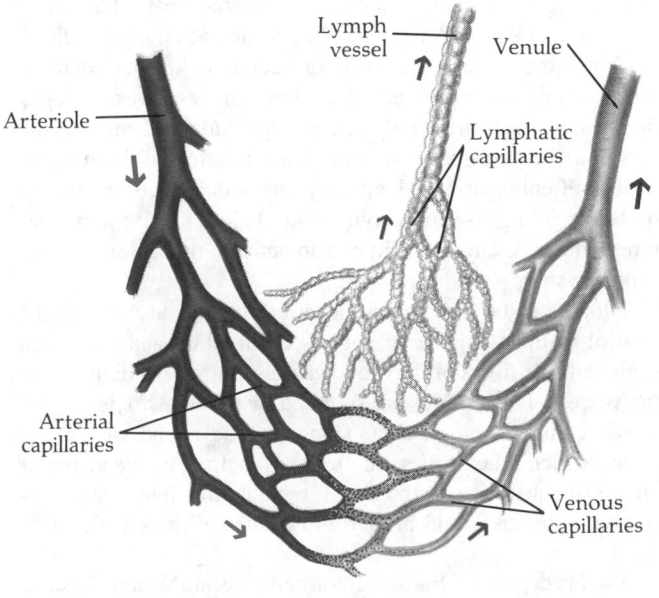

Figure 1-10 Microcirculation involving blood, interstitial fluid, oxygen, and nutrients.

blood flow through the capillary bed, allowing blood into the tissue when more oxygen is needed.

The capillaries also respond to nervous control such as sympathetic stimulation, which causes constriction. However, local capillary response is mainly the result of humoral factors, that is, chemicals from tissue metabolism or chemical substances in the blood. Such chemical substances include histamine, which dilates, and hormones such as epinephrine, which constrict. Oxygen and pH can also influence local blood flow.

The venous system of venules and veins returns blood to the heart. Venules, the exchange vessels, are small, thin tubules that join to form veins. They collect blood from the capillary bed. Veins are thin, elastic vessels that can store large amounts of blood. Thus they are referred to as capacitance vessels (see Figure 1-9). They hold 60% to 70% of a body's total blood volume and change as tissue needs change. Veins contain valves at varying intervals that maintain forward blood flow to the heart (venous return) and prevent reflux. Venous blood flow is influenced by arterial flow, skeletal muscle contractions, changes in thoracic and abdominal pressure, and right atrial pressure.

Neural Control of the Cardiovascular System

The heart and blood vessels are innervated by divisions of the autonomic nervous system.

Heart   The heart can begin its own impulse through the S-A node. This is known as automaticity. It is influenced by both divisions of the autonomic nervous system. Sympathetic fibers innervate the heart through nerves arising from the cervical and upper thoracic ganglia of the sympathetic trunks and by the parasympathetic fibers arising in the vagal branches. Combined, they form the cardiac plexuses located close to the arch of the aorta.[86] From these plexuses, nerve fibers accompany the right and left coronary arteries to enter the heart. The fibers then extend to the S-A node, A-V node, and atrial myocardium.

Sympathetic cardiac nerves, or acclerator nerves, increase the heart rate when activated. Parasympathetic nerves, or vagus fibers, slow the heart rate by decreasing conduction through the A-V node. Sympathetic system action is effected through the release of epinephrine. The parasympathetic effects are caused by the vagal release of acetylcholine. Pain, exercise, temperature, emotions, and drugs may also activate this autonomic receptor system.

Blood vessels   Arteries and arterioles are also under the control of the sympathetic nerves. Contraction and relaxation of the muscle fibers of the blood vessels control the diameter of the vessels. The muscles are supplied by vasoconstrictor fibers, which constrict the vascular smooth muscle, and vasodilator fibers, which relax it. Vascular reflexes, helped by the action of chemical substances in the blood, regulate the diameter of vessels to distribute blood properly to tissues in response to their needs.

Baroreceptors   Baroreceptor cells are in the carotid sinus and aortic arch. Stimulation by stretch or pressure slows the vasomotor center, resulting in vasodilation. As more impulses go to the heart, stimulating parasympathetic fibers, the heartbeat slows and the arterioles and venules dilate.

Chemoreceptors   Vasomotor chemoreceptors are in the aortic arch and carotid bodies. They are very sensitive to lowered Pao_2, raised Pco_2, and lowered pH. When stimulated, the chemoreceptors send impulses to the vasoconstrictor centers in the medulla, causing vasoconstriction of arterioles and the venous reservoir.

Arterial Blood Pressure

Arterial blood pressure is a measure of the pressure blood exerts within the blood vessels. This pressure depends largely on work of the heart (cardiac output), blood volume, and peripheral resistance, including the elasticity of arterial walls.

Peripheral resistance is the resistance to blood flow caused by the force created by the aorta, arteries, and arterioles. The amount of pressure on the blood is highest in the aorta (120 mm Hg) and becomes lower in arteries (80 mm Hg), arterioles (55 mm Hg), capillaries (30 mm Hg), and veins (20 mm Hg).[39] This pressure difference (gradient) determines blood flow because blood flows naturally from high pressure to low. Other factors include blood viscosity and the size and patency of the vessel lumen.

The vascular tone of the arteries and arterioles allows them to constrict or dilate, influencing the resistance to flow. For example, the greater the resistance in the arteriole, the less the blood flow to capillaries. Therefore more blood remains in the arteries, creating a higher arterial pressure.

Blood viscosity depends on red blood cells and protein molecules in the blood. Greater pressure is needed to propel viscous, or thick, fluid. Altered blood protein levels or reduced red cell levels, as in anemia or hemorrhage, reduce peripheral resistance and arterial pressure.

Measurement of arterial pressure   Arterial pressure may be measured directly or indirectly. Direct measurement is done by placing a catheter, attached to a recording monitor, into the artery. Indirect measurement is performed with a stethoscope and a blood pressure cuff.

Fetal Development

From the onset of gestation the developing embryo undergoes rapid cellular diffusion, forming tissues that will later become the heart. By the third week a primitive single-tubular structure made up of two layers of germ cells is formed. The mesoderm contributes to the pericardial wall (epicardium) and myocardium, and within this layer a single longitudinal tube is formed that will eventually become the endocardium.

The tube's position permits it to accommodate rapid growth. During the first 28 days the primitive cardiac tube grows and bends to the side, twisting into a loop. At this stage the cardiac structures are developing and identifiable: the sinuatrium, which connects the atria with the primitive ventricle; the conus cordis, which will later become the outflow tract for the ventricles; and the truncus arteriosus, which later divides into the aorta and pulmonary artery.

From the fourth through the eighth weeks, transition to a four-chambered heart occurs. A midline groove forms at the apex of the ventricular loop, beginning the division between the

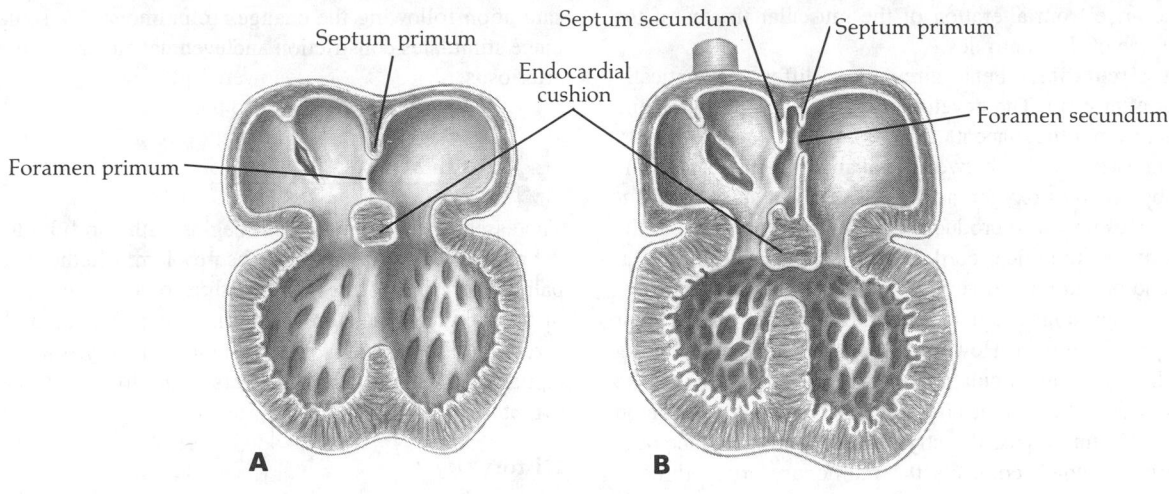

Figure 1-11 Chamber development showing atrial and ventricular septation.

right and left sides. Blood flow remains undivided and continuously enters the atria and sinus venosus and leaves via the truncus arteriosus.

Atria Atrial development begins from the common atrioventricular (A-V) canal. Two tissue bundles, the endocardial cushions, arise from the A-V canal, forming a dorsal (back) and ventral side. By the sixth week these tissues merge in the center of the heart, dividing the A-V canal into left and right channels and developing what will later be the tricuspid and mitral valves.

Atrial septation develops from the septum primum, which grows toward the A-V canal and endocardial cushions. An intercommunication between the left and right atria called the foramen primum remains (Figure 1-11, *A*). As atrial division continues, a second atrial septum (septum secundum) is established in the center and to the right of the septum primum. The septum primum continues to fuse with the endocardial cushions, obliterating the foramen primum (Figure 1-11, *B*). However, the lower portion remains as a flap valve that prevents blood flow from reversing to flow from left to right. Throughout fetal life, blood flow is directed right to left through the foramen ovale, supplying oxygen to the left side of the heart and fetal structures (Figure 1-12). The foramen ovale closes shortly after birth.

Ventricles Septation of the ventricles takes place during the second month of fetal development. Rapid growth occurs from the apex of the common ventricle upward toward the expanding endocardial cushions and A-V canal. This upward-growing muscular tissue does not merge with the cushions. Thus an interventricular communication is created that exists until the tissues from the endocardial cushion and conus ridges of the truncus arteriosus grow downward and eventually obliterate it. The upper portion of the septum thins out into a fibrous sheet referred to as the membranous portion of the septum, while the lower portion remains muscular.

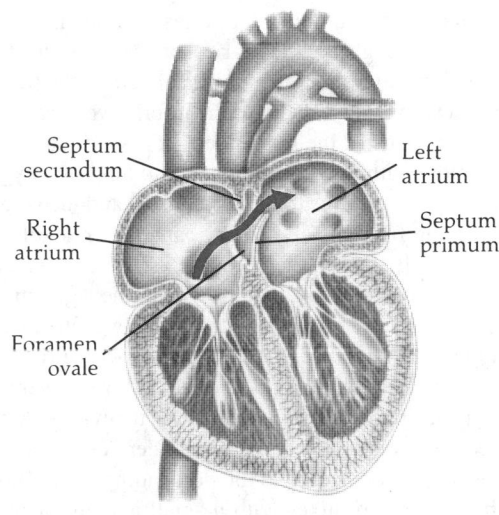

Figure 1-12 Blood flow being directed through foramen ovale.

Great vessels and cardiac valves The truncus arteriosus, which is initially a single undivided tubular structure, undergoes its own partitioning process. The conus ridges in the ventricular septum fuse and divide the truncus into a left and a right side, forming the aorta and pulmonary artery. These vessels continue to develop in a spiral fashion, so the aorta receives blood from the left ventricle, and the pulmonary artery receives blood from the right ventricle.

Embryonic connective tissue grows outward from the endocardial tissue of each conus ridge to form the three cusps of the aortic and pulmonic valves. Meanwhile, the mitral and tricuspid valves are being formed by the proliferation and thinning of the tissues that project from the endocardial tissues and outer walls of the A-V canal. The papillary muscles and chordae tendineae arise from alteration of the muscular tissues of the inner surface of the ventricles.

Fetal circulation   Fetal circulation differs dramatically from that after birth. The developing fetus secures oxygen and nutrients through the placenta, where an interchange of gases, foods, and wastes occurs between fetal and maternal blood. The fetal blood receives oxygen and nutritive substances by diffusion and gives up waste products. The fetus is connected to the placenta by the umbilical cord, which contains two umbilical arteries and one umbilical vein.

Because the lungs are nonfunctional during fetal life, their blood supply is limited. However, three structures exist during the fetal life to ensure circulation within the heart. These are the foramen ovale in the interatrial septum, which allows the blood in the right atrium to pass directly into the left atrium; the ductus arteriosus, which connects the pulmonary artery directly with the aorta; and the ductus venosus, which allows blood to pass directly to the inferior vena cava.

The heart begins to beat in about the fourth week of fetal life. Fetal circulation of blood is similar to that in adults with the exception of the heart, lungs, and placenta. Blood reaches the placenta via the umbilical arteries. Within the placenta, blood passes through the capillaries of the villi and then returns to the fetus by way of the umbilical vein to the liver. Most of the blood is shunted directly to the inferior vena cava by way of the ductus venosus; the remainder is directed into the liver.

Circulation within the heart is a mixture of oxygenated blood received from the ductus venosus and deoxygenated blood returning from the alimentary canal, liver, and lower extremities, as well as from the coronary arteries, upper extremities, and superior vena cava. Blood enters the right atrium via the inferior vena cava and is shunted directly to the left atrium through the foramen ovale, bypassing most of the right ventricle and lungs. Blood that does enter the right ventricle is pumped to the pulmonary artery where it divides. A portion goes directly to the lung, and the remainder is shunted through the narrow ductus arteriosus to the descending aorta. Blood entering the left atrium mixes with a small amount of blood received from the pulmonary veins and passes into the left ventricle. From there it is pumped through the aorta and into the general circulation.

Circulatory changes at birth   With the first inspiration at birth, the lungs expand and begin functioning. Placental circulation ceases, and the connection with the placenta ends with the cutting of the umbilical cord, causing several major changes. During fetal life the lungs have a high vascular resistance. As a result, the blood ejected from the right ventricle into the pulmonary artery is shunted via the ductus arteriosus into the descending aorta. With the first breath the alveoli expand, the pulmonary vascular resistance drops rapidly, and pulmonary blood flow increases. Simultaneously, the loss of placental blood flow causes the right atrial pressure to drop. The combination of decreased pulmonary vascular resistance, increased pulmonary blood flow, and decreased right atrial pressure causes the left atrial pressure to rise above right atrial pressure. The foramen ovale then closes, and the increase in oxygen saturation following the changes in pulmonary vascular resistance stimulates constriction and eventual closure of the ductus arteriosus.

NORMAL FINDINGS

The assessment of any patient begins with careful attention to the patient's chief complaint. The problem, whether chest pain, palpitations, or shortness of breath, should guide the direction of questioning. Questions regarding the problem may be organized into seven categories: location, quality, quantity, precipitating or aggravating factors, duration, and associated symptoms.

History

Cardiovascular risk factor profile (see p. 29)

Past medical history and general health status   Congenital heart disease; childhood disease (rheumatic fever, scarlet fever); coronary artery disease; vascular disorders; bleeding disorders; hypertension; kidney disease; diabetes; hyperlipidemia; heart murmurs; allergies; genetic disorders (e.g., Marfan's syndrome)

Family history   Age, sex, and health of parents, siblings, and children, and cause of death for deceased members; data regarding history of hypertension, heart disease, diabetes, elevated lipid levels, sudden deaths

Sociocultural   Culture, ethnicity, and religion; alcohol consumption; economic situation

Occupation   Type of employment; physical and emotional demands; environmental or occupational hazards (actual, potential) (e.g., chemical exposures, dust)

Activity level   Exercise: amount, frequency, intensity; sexual: frequency, recent changes, problems or presence of symptoms (e.g., chest pain, shortness of breath during or after intercourse); sports: type (e.g., competitive versus leisure), contact (e.g., football, soccer)

Sleep   Number of pillows used; presence of paroxysmal nocturnal dyspnea; number of times up to urinate

Nutrition   Fluid and dietary restriction; any recent weight increases or decreases

Dental history   Major problems; last dental visit; knowledge regarding antibiotic prophylaxis if pertinent

Medications   Prescription and nonprescription drugs; contraceptives; regular use of street drugs (e.g., cocaine, crack)

Smoking history   Type: cigarettes, cigars, pipe, chewing tobacco, snuff; duration; frequency

Female history   Birth control measures: intrauterine devices, diaphragm, sponge/foam, male contraception; hormone therapy: type and years used; pregnancies: para, gravida, any related complications; menopause: age, types of hormone replacement therapy

Psychosocial   Perception of illness; response to health problems; patterns of coping or adaptation; understanding of current and past health problems

Support system   Marital status; primary support system

Physical Examination

General appearance Level of consciousness (alert, oriented); respiratory rate and pattern (passive breathing 12 to 20 respirations per minute, respiratory/pulse rate ratio 1:4, no shortness of breath or dyspnea); nutritional state (well nourished); weight and height normal

Blood pressure Systolic 100 to 140 mm Hg (tends to be 5 to 15 mm Hg higher in right arm); diastolic 60 to 90 mm Hg; pulse pressure 30 to 40 mm Hg; *older adult:* maximum systolic pressure 160 mm Hg; with standing, there may be systolic drop of 10 to 15 mm Hg and diastolic drop of 5 mm Hg

Arterial pulse (heart rate) 60 to 90 beats per minute; *older adult:* slows with age because of increase in vagal tone; wide range (40 to 100 beats per minute), occasional ectopic beats may be felt, rhythm (regular); amplitude and contour (upstroke full, strong, rounded, brisk); symmetric response (equal on right and left); timing (equal for all arterial pulsations, e.g., brachial, femoral); auscultation (no murmurs or bruits); amplitude:

4+ = strong, bounding (normal)
3+ = easily palpable
2+ = difficult to palpate
1+ = diminished, weak, thready
0 = absent

Older adult: amplitude and contour (upstroke more rapid, smooth)

Jugular venous pressure (JVP) (Figure 1-13) Should not exceed 3 cm (1 inch) above level of sternal angle (see Figure 1-13) with head of client elevated to 30 to 45 degrees

Jugular pulsations Undulations; movement with inspiration; increase or decrease with change in body position

Wave pulsations (see Figure 1-8)

a wave

First positive wave visualized; coincides with S_1; represents right atrial contraction and retrograde transmission of pressure pulse to jugular veins

x descent

First negative "trough" undulation; occurs between S_1 and S_2; results from right atrial diastole, plus the effects of the tricuspid valve being pulled down during ventricular systole

v wave

Third positive wave; coincides with S_2; continued atrial filling

y descent

Represents fall in right atrial pressure from peak of v wave following tricuspid valve opening and occurs during period of rapid atrial emptying in early diastole

Precordium (Figure 1-14) Point of maximum impulse (PMI) 5 to 7 cm left of midsternal border at fifth intercostal space (ICS) and 1 to 2 cm ($\frac{1}{3}$ to $\frac{1}{2}$ inch) in diameter; palpable areas: aortic area—at second ICS to right of sternal border, pulmonic area—at second ICS to left of sternal border, apex—at fifth ICS 5 to 7 cm to left of sternal border; precordial motion symmetric, even with respiration

Heart sounds (see Figure 1-8) First heart sound (S_1) closing of A-V valves; components are tricuspid first heart sound (T_1), located at fifth intercostal space (ICS) and left lower sternal border (LLSB), and mitral (M_1), located in apical area at fifth ICS and 5 to 7 cm left of sternal border; loudest at apical area; normal splitting heard LLSB at fifth ICS; S_2 closure of semilunar valves; components are aortic (A_2), located at second ICS to right of sternal border, and pulmonic (P_2), located at second ICS to left of sternal border; loudest at base; normal splitting heard at P_2

CONDITIONS, DISEASES, AND DISORDERS

CARDIAC DISEASES

■ CARDIAC DYSRHYTHMIAS

A dysrhythmia is a disorder of the heart rate and rhythm caused by a conduction system disturbance (Figure 1-15).

Cardiac dysrhythmias can cause sudden death resulting from electromechanical failure (as in ventricular fibrillation) or from impaired cardiac function.

Early recognition and treatment are needed because dysrhythmias such as premature ventricular ectopic beats may spontaneously become frequent or multifocal. For example, in a patient with myocardial ischemia the ectopic beat may convert to ventricular tachycardia or ventricular fibrillation without warning. About 60% of deaths from acute myocardial infarction occur within the first hour, generally before the victim can reach a hospital.

Careful continuous ECG monitoring now enables early detection and prompt treatment of potentially serious

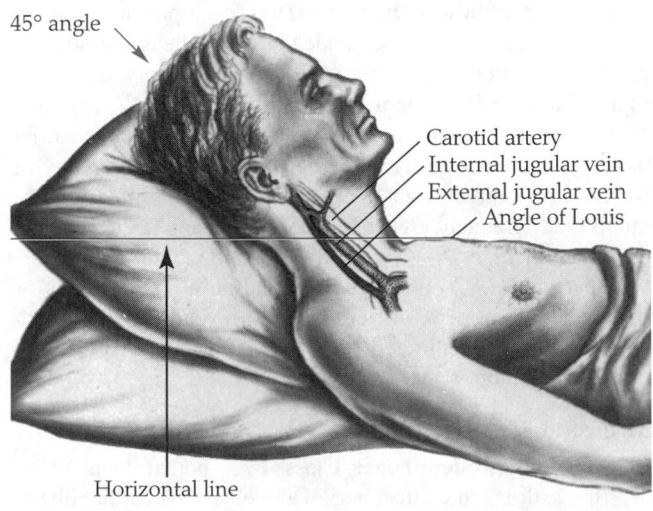

45° angle

Carotid artery
Internal jugular vein
External jugular vein
Angle of Louis

Horizontal line

Figure 1-13 Inspection of external jugular venous pressure.

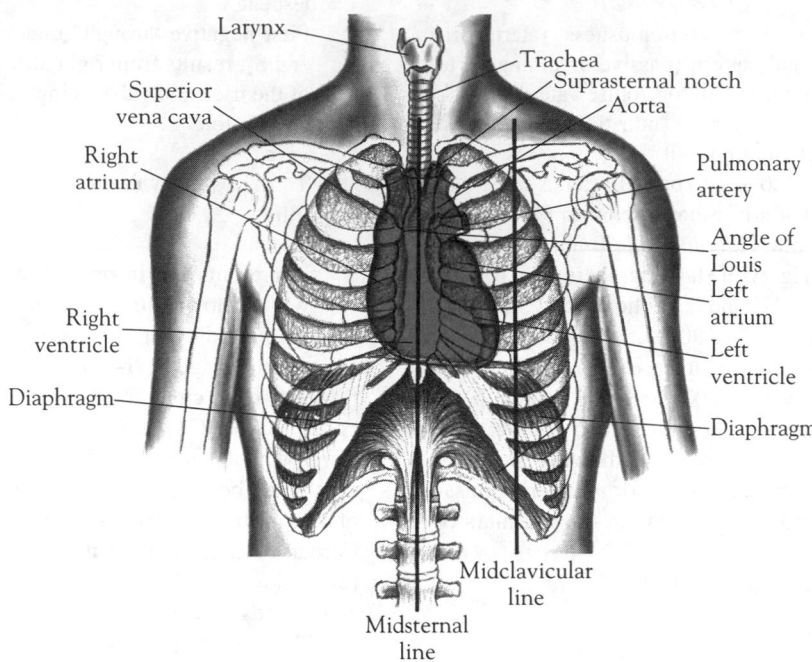

Larynx

Trachea
Suprasternal notch
Aorta

Superior
vena cava

Right
atrium

Pulmonary
artery

Angle of
Louis

Left
atrium

Left
ventricle

Right
ventricle

Diaphragm

Diaphragm

Midclavicular
line

Midsternal
line

Figure 1-14 Chest wall landmarks for inspection, percussion, and palpation.

dysrhythmias. However, proper treatment involves diagnosis and a thorough understanding of the underlying etiologic factors.

•••••• Pathophysiology

Cardiac dysrhythmias may be classified into abnormalities of impulse formation (sinus, atrial, ventricular), impulse conduction, or a combination.[8] Dysrhythmias may also be described on the basis of rate (bradydysrhythmia, tachydysrhythmia) or seriousness (minor, life threatening). Dysrhythmias may occur as a result of a primary cardiac disorder, as a secondary response to a systemic problem, or as a complication of drug toxicity or electrolyte imbalance.

Each of the major dysrhythmias is described in the section on nursing assessment.

•••••• Diagnostic Studies and Findings

Electrocardiogram (ECG)
See Table 1-1
24-Hour ambulatory ECG
Cardiac event recorder
Exercise electrocardiogram
Tilt table
Electrophysiologic (EP) studies

•••••• Multidisciplinary Plan

Surgery

Surgical ablation, or resection, is a specialized procedure performed by direct visualization in the operating room. It is performed only on patients with highly refractory ventricular

tachycardia. The surgical objective is to excise, isolate, or interrupt heart tissue that is responsible for the tachycardia. Cardiac sympathectomy, a radical treatment that alters adrenergic influences to the heart, has been effective in some patients with ventricular tachycardia with a long QT syndrome. Surgical correction for tachydysrhythmias through an accessory pathway (Wolff-Parkinson-White syndrome) may be performed during surgical repair for an associated structural defect (e.g., Ebstein's anomaly of the tricuspid valve).

Interventional Therapy

Catheter ablation therapy The development of better energy delivery systems has made the 1990s the era of nonsurgical interventional procedures for drug-refractory tachydysrhythmias, especially supraventricular tachycardia.[47] The object of catheter ablation is to destroy arrhythmogenic myocardial tissue and conduction tissue by delivering electrical energy in the form of a direct high-energy current shock or, more commonly, radiofrequency energy. The refined application of this technique includes A-V junctional ablation, ablation of accessory pathways, A-V nodal reentry, and atrial tachycardias or flutters.[24,82] Treatment of ventricular tachycardias (VT) with catheter ablation is limited only to those patients with focal-origin VT without structural heart disease.

Medications

Antidysrhythmic drugs: Class I-A—potent local anesthetic drugs that affect nerves as well as myocardial fibers; decrease conduction velocity by retarding influx of sodium and reduce maximum rate of depolarizing action potential

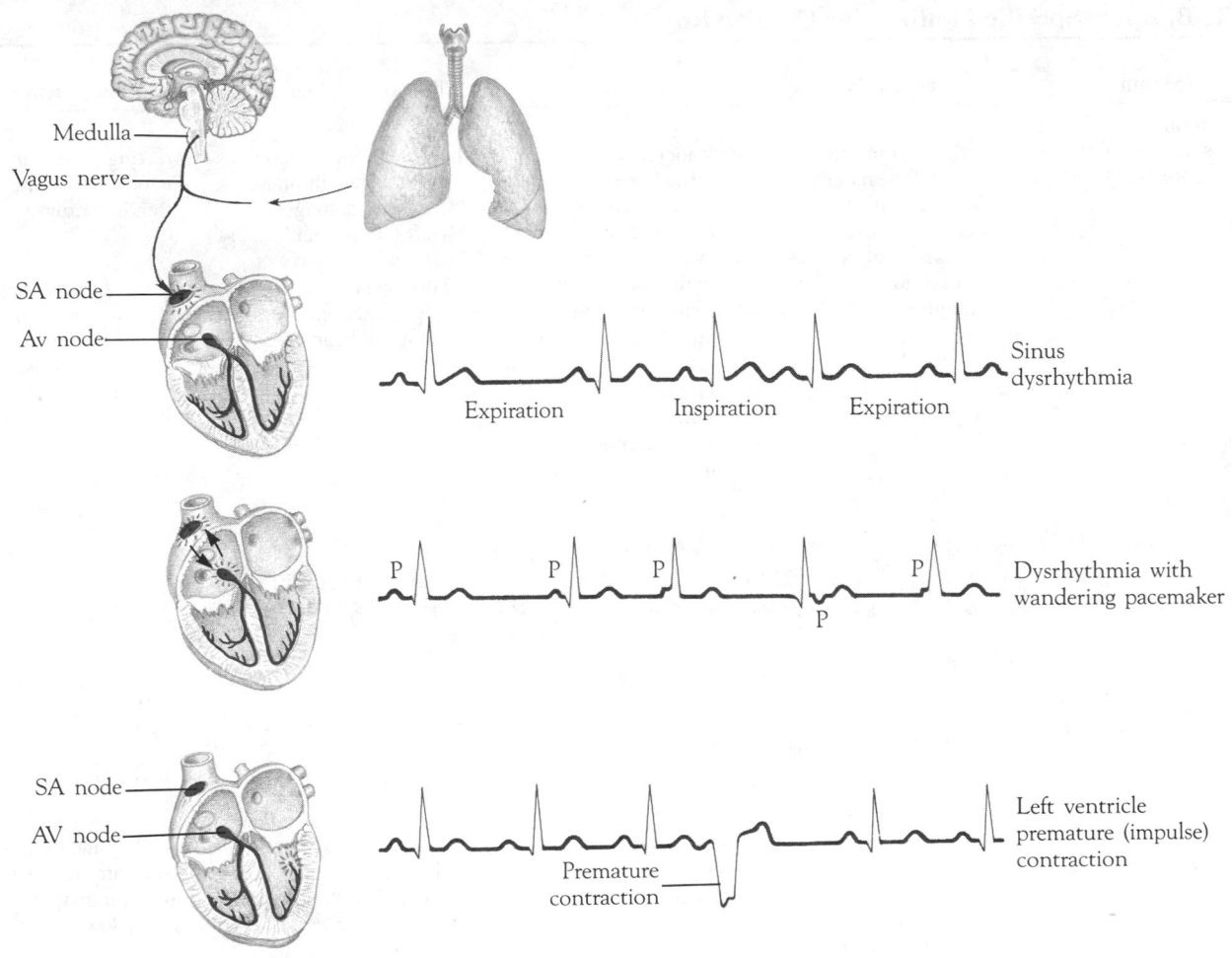

Figure 1-15 Cardiac dysrhythmias. (From Canobbio.[13])

Quinidine

Indications: Suppresses atrial, junctional, or ventricular ectopy, ventricular tachycardia, and paroxysmal atrial tachycardia; may be used to convert atrial fibrillation or flutter to sinus rhythm or to maintain sinus rhythm after cardioversion

Usual dosage: 200-400 mg po q4-6h

Onset of action: 15 min with peak activity in 2-4 h

Therapeutic blood levels: 2-6 mg/ml

Toxic signs: Widened QRS, prolonged QT bundle branch block, complete heart block, ventricular tachycardia, asystole

Sustained-release preparations: Quinidex, 300 mg q8-12h; Quinaglute, 324 mg q8-12h; Cardioquin, 275 mg q6h

Procainamide (Pronestyl)

Indications: Similar to quinidine; suppresses ventricular ectopy; may be less effective in controlling atrial dysrhythmias

Usual dosage: 250-750 mg po q4-6h; 100 mg q5-15 min for total of 1 g IV

Peak action: Within 30 min

Therapeutic blood levels: 4-8 mg/ml

Sustained-release preparations: Procan SR, 500-1000 mg q6h

Disopyramide phosphate (Norpace)

Indications: Suppresses or prevents ventricular dysrhythmias; not particularly effective in treating atrial dysrhythmias

Usual dosage: 400-800 mg/day po in four doses with loading dose of 200 mg

Peak action: 2-4 h

Therapeutic blood levels: 2-4 mg/ml

Antidysrhythmic agents: Class I-B—reduce rapid upstroke and shorten action potential duration

Lidocaine (Xylocaine)

Indications and actions: Controls ventricular dysrhythmias by depressing automaticity in Purkinje network and increasing excitability threshold of ventricles

Usual dosage: 50-100 mg (1-2 mg/kg) by IV bolus followed by 1.5-4 mg/min

Text continued on p. 26.

TABLE 1-1 Specific Findings for Cardiac Rhythms

Rhythm	Characteristics	Etiology	Clinical Significance	Management
Sinus origin Sinus tachycardia (Figure 1-16)	Regular rhythm; rate 100-180 beats/min (higher in infants); normal P wave; normal segment of electrocardiogram (QRS) complex	Rate increase may be normal response to exercise, emotion, or abnormal stressors such as pain, fever, pump failure, hyperthyroidism, and certain pharmacologic agents, including caffeine, nitrates, atropine, epinephrine, isoproterenol, and nicotine	May have hemodynamic consequence in patient with damaged heart that is unable to sustain increased workloads brought on by persistent increases in heart rate	Correcting underlying factors; discontinuing offending drugs

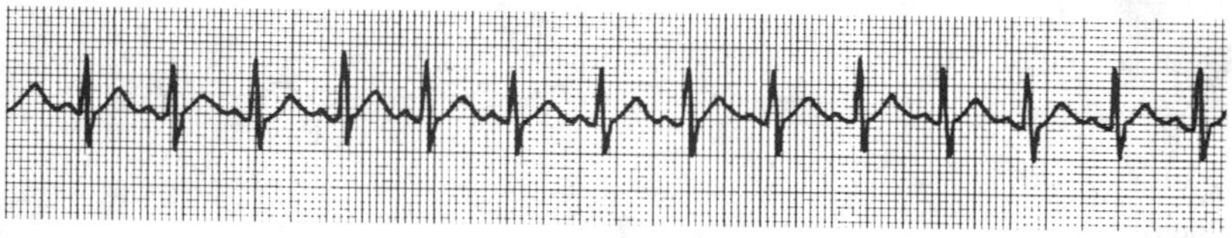

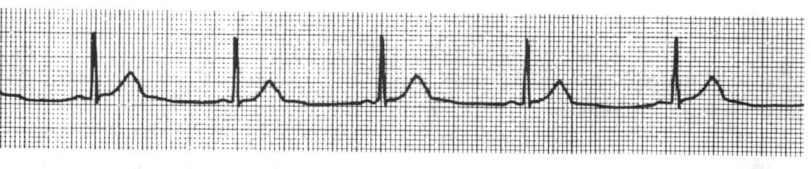

Figure 1-16 Sinus tachycardia. (From Andreoli.[4])

Sinus bradycardia (Figure 1-17)	Regular rhythm; rate less than 60 beats/min; normal P wave; normal PR interval; normal QRS complex	Rate decrease may be normal response to sleep or in well-conditioned athlete; abnormal drops in rate may be caused by diminished blood flow to S-A node, vagal stimulation, hypothyroidism, increased intracranial pressure, or pharmacologic agents such as digoxin, propranolol, quinidine, or procainamide	None unless associated with signs of impaired cardiac output; symptoms: dizziness, syncope, chest pain	Correcting underlying cause; atropine 0.5-1 mg IV; transvenous pacemaker

Figure 1-17 Sinus bradycardia. (From Andreoli.[4])

■ TABLE 1-1 Specific Findings for Cardiac Rhythms—cont'd

Rhythm	Characteristics	Etiology	Clinical Significance	Management
Sinus dysrhythmia (Figure 1-18)	Irregular rhythm; may be phasic with respiration, slowing during inspiration and increasing with expiration; rate 60-100 beats/min; normal PR interval; normal QRS complex	Sinus rhythm with cyclic variation caused by vagal impulses that influence rhythm during respiration; occurs commonly in children, young adults, and the elderly; usually disappears as heart rate increases	None unless heart rate decreases; symptoms: dizziness with decreased rate	None indicated unless heart rate decreases and symptoms occur

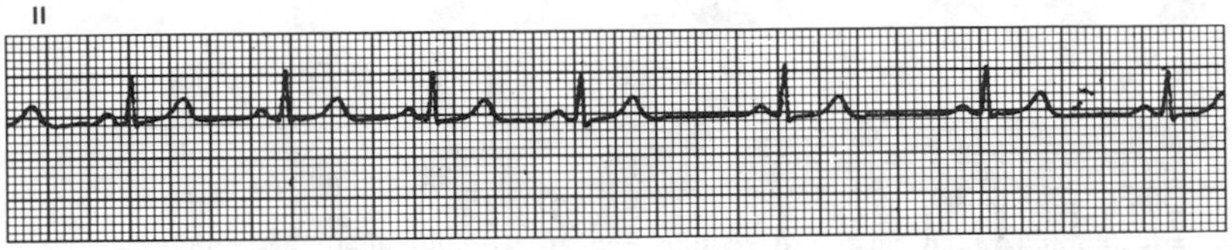

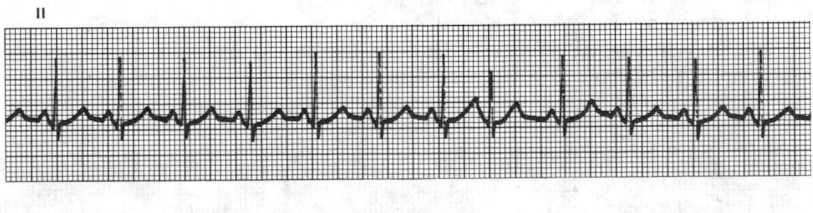

Figure 1-18 Sinus dysrhythmia. (From Conover.[17])

Rhythm	Characteristics	Etiology	Clinical Significance	Management
Atrial origin Atrial premature contractions (APCs, PACs) (Figure 1-19)	Irregular rhythm owing to ectopic beats followed by incomplete compensatory pause; rate normal or increased depending on number of ectopic beats; P wave present but different from normal underlying sinus beat; PR interval may be shorter or longer than normal sinus beat; normal QRS complex	May be precipitated in healthy persons by anxiety, fatigue, caffeine, smoking, and alcohol; observed in patients with ischemia or organic heart disease and those receiving digoxin	May indicate atrial strain or hypoxia; frequent PACs (more than 6/min) reflect atrial irritability and often mark onset of atrial fibrillation	Correcting underlying cause; for frequent PACs, class 1-A antidysrhythmic drugs

Figure 1-19 Atrial premature contractions. (From Conover.[19])

Continued.

■ **TABLE 1-1 Specific Findings for Cardiac Rhythms—cont'd**

Rhythm	Characteristics	Etiology	Clinical Significance	Management
Paroxysmal supraventricular tachycardia (PSVT) (Figure 1-20)	Sudden, rapid onset of tachycardia with stimulus originating above A-V node; regular rhythm; rate 150-250 beats/min; P wave uniform, may or may not be buried in preceding T wave; PR interval may vary, often difficult to measure; normal QRS complex	May begin and end spontaneously or be precipitated by excitement, fatigue, caffeine, smoking, or alcohol	Usually no significant impairment; patient complains of palpitations and shortness of breath; if persistent or occurring in patients with preexisting organic heart disease, may cause decrease in cardiac output and/or blood pressure resulting in pump failure or shock	Performing vagal stimulation with carotid sinus massage; using Valsalva maneuver to stimulate baroreceptors (may be used in conjunction with carotid sinus massage); decreasing ventricular response with medication to block A-V conduction; sedation to reduce sympathetic stimulation; adenosine 6-12 mg IV push rapidly; verapamil 5-10 mg IV push; propanolol (Inderal) slowly IV in 1 mg increments up to 4 mg (contraindicated in patients with heart failure); cardioversion if resistant to preceding; for chronic control of recurrent PSVT: disopyramide, flecainide, propafenone, sotalol hydrochloride

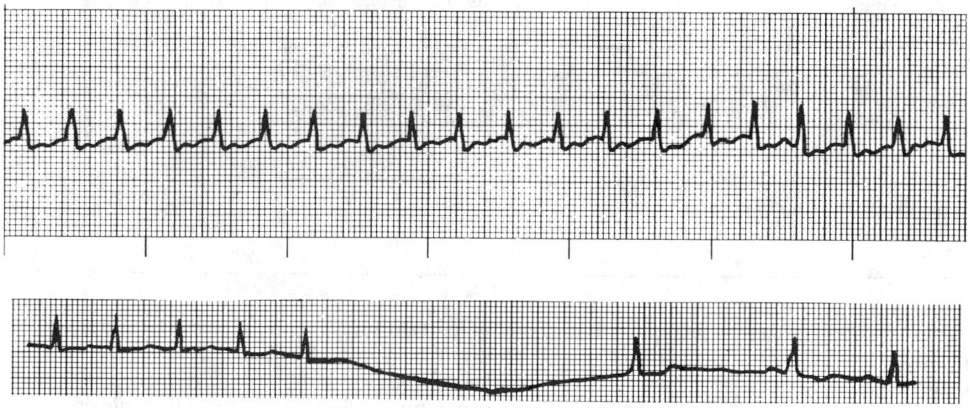

Figure 1-20 Paroxysmal supraventricular tachycardia (PSVT). (From Andreoli.[4])

Rhythm	Characteristics	Etiology	Clinical Significance	Management
Atrial flutter (AF) (Figure 1-21)	Rhythm may be regular or irregular; rate: atrial 250-350 beats/min, characterized by sawtooth flutter waves; ventricular depends on A-V conduction, may occur at 2:1, 3:1, or 4:1 ratio; PR interval not measurable; normal QRS complex	Results from rapidly firing ectopic atrial focus; most likely underlying mechanism is localized atrial reentry phenomenon; seen in patients with organic heart disorders such as coronary heart disease and valvular heart disease	Patient complains of palpitations, which may be associated with heart failure, and chest pain, particularly in presence of rapid ventricular rates	Cardioversion; digoxin if cardioversion is not used or is unsuccessful; quinidine or procainamide in acute phase; for chronic control of recurrent AF may also use disopyramide flecainide

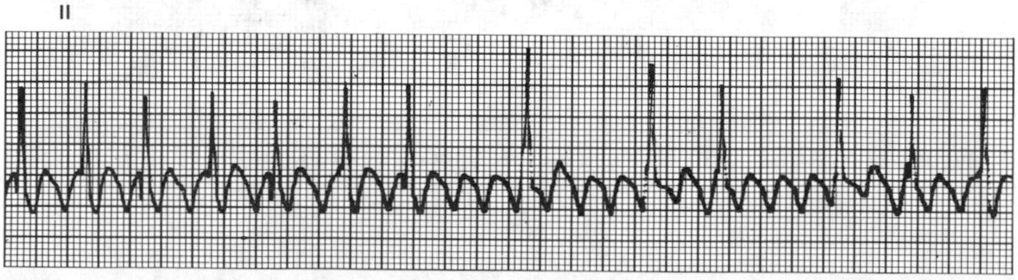

Figure 1-21 Atrial flutter (AF). (From Conover.[19])

■ **TABLE 1-1 Specific Findings for Cardiac Rhythms—cont'd**

Rhythm	Characteristics	Etiology	Clinical Significance	Management
Atrial fibrillation (Figure 1-22)	Rhythm irregular; rate: atrial more than 350 beats/min; absence of uniform atrial depolarization produces undulations (f waves); ventricular varies according to A-V conduction; may range between 50 and 150 beats/min	Results from multiple atrial foci discharging almost simultaneously; atria never uniformly depolarize; reflects organic heart disease; may also occur with digitalis toxicity	With rapid ventricular rates, cardiac output may be impaired, resulting in heart failure, angina, and shock	Determination of underlying cause and whether acute or chronic; cardioversion for rapid ventricular response; digoxin if cardioversion is not used; quinidine; procainamide; verapamil in acute phase; for chronic management of recurrent atrial fibrillation: disopyramide, propafenone, sotalol, amiodarone

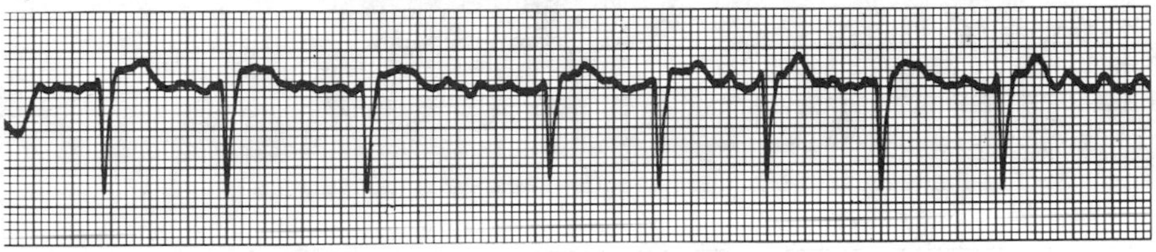

V₁

Figure 1-22 Atrial fibrillation. (From Conover.[19])

Rhythm	Characteristics	Etiology	Clinical Significance	Management
Junctional rhythms Junctional escape rhythm (nodal) (Figure 1-23)	Regular rhythm; rate 40-60 beats/min; P wave abnormal, may occur before, during, or after QRS complex, may be inverted in leads II, III, and augmented V lead (aVF); QRS complex usually normal	Occurs when sinus node is suppressed and atria fail to depolarize A-V junction; may be the result of digitalis toxicity, vagal stimulation, or ischemic damage to S-A node	Usually none; transient; if condition persists, slow rates may allow foci with rapid rates to take over; may also produce symptoms of diminished cardiac output	Treatment or correction of underlying cause if persistent or if symptoms occur; atropine IV; pacemaker may be indicated

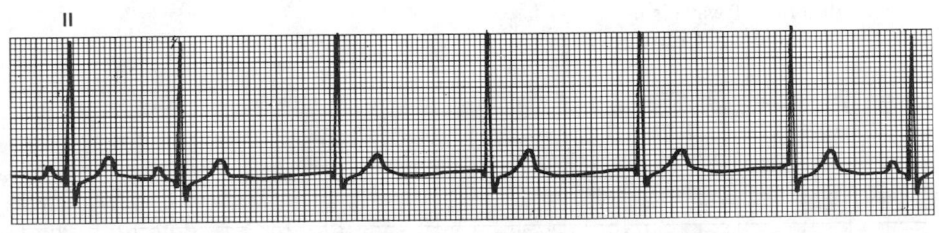

II

Figure 1-23 Junctional escape rhythm (nodal). (From Conover.[19])

Continued.

■ **TABLE 1-1 Specific Findings for Cardiac Rhythms—cont'd**

Rhythm	Characteristics	Etiology	Clinical Significance	Management
Premature junctional contractions (Figure 1-24)	Rhythm regular except for junctional beat; rate normal; P wave as described for junctional escape rhythm; PR interval shortened when P wave precedes QRS complex; QRS complex usually normal	Results from increased automaticity of A-V junction, causing ectopic focus in A-V node to discharge before onset of impulse from sinus node; cause of ectopic beats: ischemia or digitalis toxicity	Usually none; frequency reflects junctional irritability	None indicated if infrequent; if frequent, quinidine

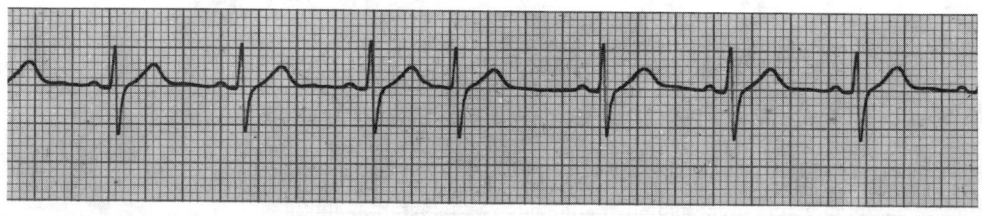

Figure 1-24 Premature junctional contractions. (From Conover.[19])

Ventricular
dysrhythmias

Premature ventricular contractions (PVCs) (Figure 1-25)	Rhythm irregular owing to ectopic beats followed by full compensatory pause; rate normal or increased depending on number of ectopic beats; P wave absent in ectopic beat; PR interval absent; QRS complex widened and distorted; T wave is in opposition to R wave	Caused by irritable focus within ventricle, commonly associated with myocardial infarction; other causes include hypoxia, hypocalcemia, and acidosis	PVCs occurring frequently (more than 6/min) or in pairs indicate increased ventricular irritability	Aimed at suppression of PVCs; if frequent, IV bolus of lidocaine (50-100 mg) followed by continuous IV infusion; additional antidysrhythmic agents in classes I and II may be given

V_1

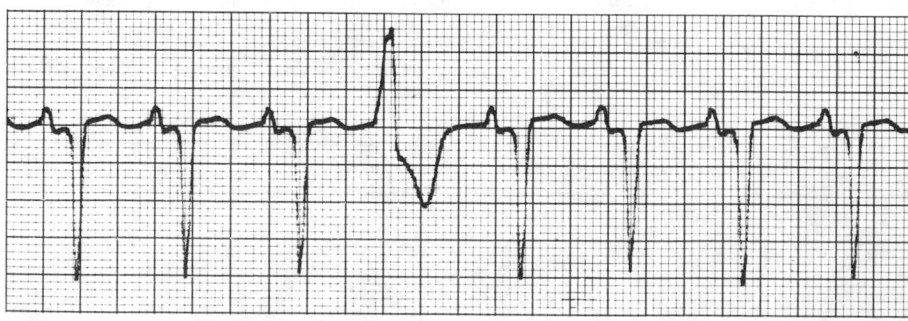

Figure 1-25 Left ventricular PVC. (From Conover.[19])

TABLE 1-1 Specific Findings for Cardiac Rhythms—cont'd

Rhythm	Characteristics	Etiology	Clinical Significance	Management
Ventricular tachycardia (Figure 1-26)	Rhythm slightly irregular; rate 100-200 beats/min; P wave absent; PR interval absent; QRS complex wide and bizarre, greater than 0.12 sec	Caused by irritable ventricular foci firing repetitively; commonly caused by myocardial infarction	Often a forerunner of ventricular fibrillation; if persistent and rapid, causes decreased cardiac output owing to decreased ventricular filling time	Most episodes terminate abruptly without treatment; lidocaine bolus 75-100 mg IV followed by continuous IV drip; defibrillation; alternatives: procainamide, bretylium tosylate for acute management; chronic control of recurrent VT: sotalol, propafenone, amiodarone HCl

Figure 1-26 Ventricular tachycardia. (From Conover.[19])

| Torsades de pointes (polymorphous ventricular tachycardia) (Figure 1-27) | Atypical ventricular tachycardia occurring in setting of delayed repolarization (prolonged QT interval); rhythm regular or irregular; ventricular rate, 150-300 beats/min; PR interval not measurable; QRS complex wide and bizarre in configuration lasting >0.12 sec; amplitude and direction of QRS complex vary; QT interval during baseline rhythm >0.46 sec-ond or >33% of baseline; T wave during baseline rhythm very broad and flat | Drug toxicity (e.g., quinidine, procainamide, amiodarone HCl); electrolyte imbalance (e.g., hypokalemia, hypomagnesemia) | Palpitations, which may lead to faintness, syncope; often forerunner of ventricular fibrillation and sudden death | Treatment initiated only if QT prolonged; if present, temporary overdrive ventricular or atrial pacing; IV magnesium sulfate: IV push 2 g over 1-2 min, IV infusion 1-2 g for 4-6 h |

Figure 1-27 Torsade de pointes. **A,** Sinus rhythm. T waves are flat, and QT interval is prolonged. Patient's serum potassium level was 3.1 mEq/L. **B,** Taken next day, characteristic torsade. (Courtesy Dr. Daniel H. Schwartz, South Fallsburg, N.Y. From Goldberger.[38])

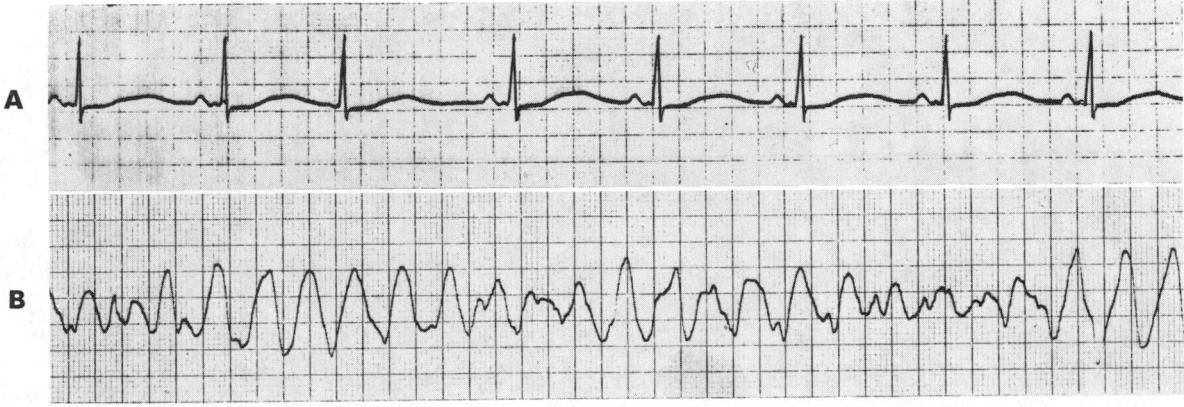

Continued.

■ TABLE 1-1 Specific Findings for Cardiac Rhythms—cont'd

Rhythm	Characteristics	Etiology	Clinical Significance	Management
Ventricular fibrillation (Figure 1-28)	Rhythm irregular; rate: rapid repetitive waves or undulations that have no uniformity and are coarse or fine; P wave, QRS complex, and T wave cannot be identified	Lethal dysrhythmia resulting from electrical stimulation of ventricular muscle; leads to abrupt cessation of effective blood flow; occurs in severely damaged hearts as with ischemia, drug toxicity, trauma, or contact with high-voltage electricity	Loss of consciousness; decreases in blood pressure and peripheral pulse owing to loss of cardiac output	Cardiopulmonary resuscitation; defibrillation

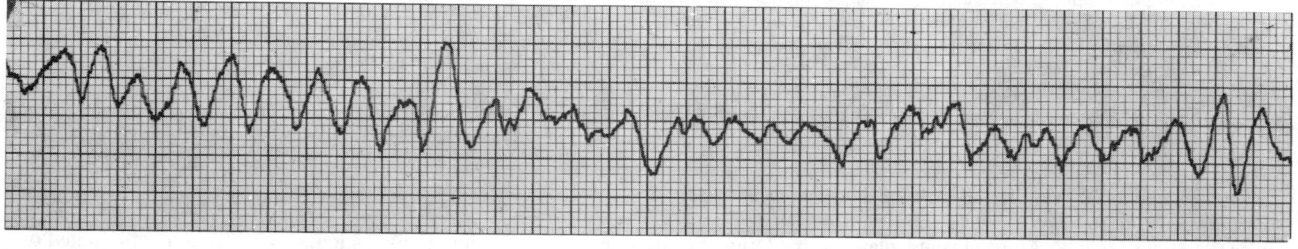

Figure 1-28 Ventricular fibrillation. (From Conover.[19])

Conduction disturbances First-dgree A-V heart block (Figure 1-29)	Rhythm regular; rate normal; P wave normal; PR interval prolonged to greater than 0.2 sec; QRS complex normal	Represents delay in impulse conduction through A-V node; occurs as result of increased vagal tone, digoxin administration, or congenital anomalies	No associated symptoms	None indicated; digitalis discontinued if causative factor; observation for development of further A-V block

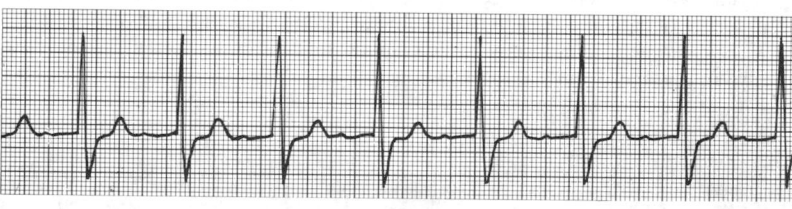

Figure 1-29 First-degree A-V block. (From Conover.[19])

■ TABLE 1-1 Specific Findings for Cardiac Rhythms—cont'd

Rhythm	Characteristics	Etiology	Clinical Significance	Management
Second-degree A-V heart block Mobitz type I (Wenckebach phenomenon) (Figure 1-30)	Rhythm: atrial regular, ventricular irregular; rate: atrial greater than ventricular; P wave: multiple P waves before QRS complex; PR interval: progressive prolongation of PR interval until one impulse is completely blocked; QRS complex normal: RR interval becomes progressively shortened until one QRS complex is dropped	Represents progressive decrease in conduction velocity involving A-V node and proximal bundle of His; occurs as result of coronary artery disease, digitalis toxicity, rheumatic fever, viral infections, or inferior wall myocardial infarction	No associated symptoms if ventricular rate is adequately maintained	None usually indicated; elimination or correction of underlying cause; observation for progression to higher degree of block

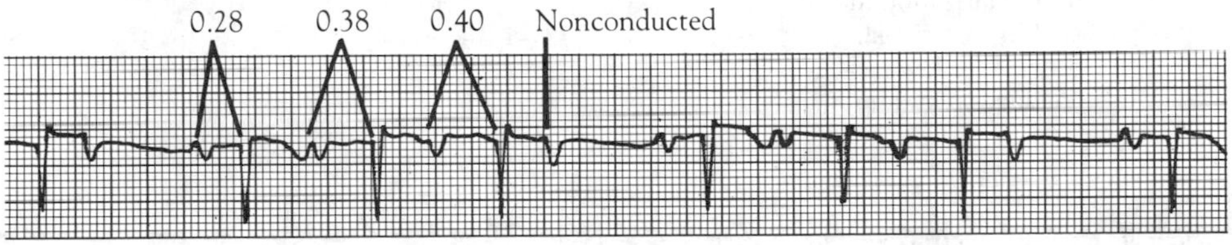

0.28   0.38   0.40   Nonconducted

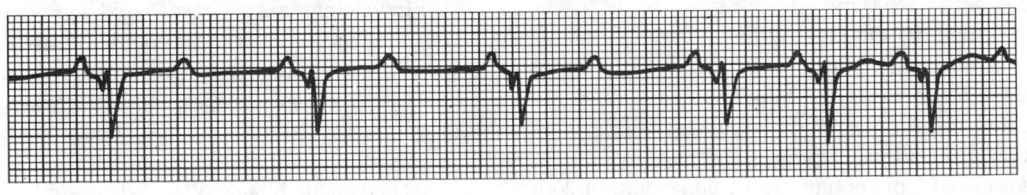

Figure 1-30 Mobitz type I. (From Conover.[19])

Mobitz type II (Figure 1-31)	Rhythm: atrial regular, ventricular varies; rate: atrial slow to normal, ventricular may be slow, usually half or one-third atrial rate; P wave normal, occurring in multiples before QRS complex; PR interval normal or slightly prolonged, always constant; QRS complex normal or slightly prolonged	Represents block of impulse below level of A-V node and within His-Purkinje system; occurs as result of ischemia, digitalis or quinidine toxicity, anterior wall myocardial infarction	No associated symptoms if ventricular rate is adequately maintained; if rate is slow, cardiac output may be impaired, causing dizziness and weakness	Correction or elimination of underlying cause; tends to be recurrent, may progress to complete heart block; transvenous demand pacing may be required

Figure 1-31 Mobitz type II. (From Conover.[19])

Continued.

■ TABLE 1-1 Specific Findings for Cardiac Rhythms—cont'd

Rhythm	Characteristics	Etiology	Clinical Significance	Management
Third-degree A-V block (complete heart block) (Figure 1-32)	Rhythm: atrial and ventricular regular but act independent of each other; rate: atrial 60-90 beats/min, ventricular 30-40 beats/min; P wave normal but occurs in greater frequency than QRS complex; PR interval: no relationship with QRS complex, therefore never constant; QRS complex normal if ventricular depolarization initiated by junctional escape pacemaker, widened if depolarization initiated by ventricular pacemaker low in conduction system	Represents failure of A-V node to conduct impulse to ventricles; block may occur at any point in conduction system at or below level of A-V node; occurs as result of coronary artery disease, degenerative fibrosis of conduction system, congenital anomalies, myocarditis, drug toxicity (digitalis, quinidine, procainamide, verapamil), trauma	Symptoms associated with low cardiac output owing to slow ventricular rates; include syncope and signs of ventricular failure	Transvenous demand pacing; while awaiting pacemaker insertion, isoproterenol infusion to accelerate ventricular rate

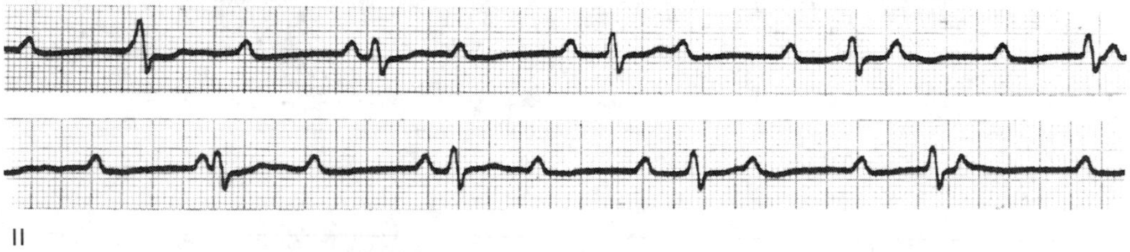

II

Figure 1-32 Third-degree A-V block. (From Andreoli.[4])

Antidysrhythmic agents: Class I-C—significantly reduces rapid upstroke, primarily slows conduction and minimally prolongs refractoriness (e.g., Flecainide)

Flecainide (Tambocar)
   Indications: Ventricular arrhythmias, supraventricular tachycardia
   Usual dosage: 100-200 mg q12h
Propafenone (Rhythmol)
   Indications: Ventricular tachycardia
   Usual dosage: 150-300 mg tid
   Onset of action: 45-90 sec
   Duration of action: 20 min
   Therapeutic blood levels: 1.5-5 mg/ml
Phenytoin (Dilantin)
   Indications and actions: Depresses automaticity
   Usual dosage: 100 mg q6h po with loading dose of 200 mg or 50-100 mg IV over 5-10 min up to 1 g
   Onset of action: Slow and variable
   Therapeutic blood levels: 10-15 mg/ml
Mexiletine

   Indications: Local anesthetic whose electrophysiologic properties closely resemble those of lidocaine; used in management of ventricular dysrhythmias
   Usual dosage: IV loading 10-15 mg/min (200-300 mg over 30 min), maintenance 250-500 mg q12h; po loading 100-400 mg, maintenance 200-300 mg q8h
   Onset of action: IV <5 min; po 1-2 h
   Therapeutic blood levels: 0.5-2 μg/ml
Tocainide (Tonocard)
   Indications and actions: Class I antidysrhythmic similar to lidocaine given for control of ventricular dysrhythmias; decreases excitability of myocardial cells
   Usual dosage: Loading 400-600 mg po q8h, maintenance 1200-1800 mg, in divided doses over 8 h
   Onset of action: $1\frac{1}{2}$ h
   Therapeutic blood levels: 6-12 μg/ml
Antidysrhythmic drugs: Class II—control dysrhythmias by blocking sympathetic stimulation, which shortens phase 4 depolarization of action potential
Propranolol (Inderal)

Indications and actions: Controls supraventricular tachycardia resulting from reentry mechanism; used to control ventricular response to atrial fibrillation and flutter by depressing A-V nodal conduction

Usual dosage: 10-80 mg po qid; 0.5-1 mg IV push slowly to control heart rate

Onset of action: 1-1½ h (po)

Therapeutic blood levels: Not determined

Atenolol

Usual dosage: 50-100 mg/d

Pindolol

Usual dosage: 10-60 mg bid

Sotalol

Indications: Nonselective beta-blocker with some class IV qualities; used in treatment of ventricular arrhythmias and atrial tachycardia

Usual dosage: 80-160 mg bid

Antidysrhythmic drugs: Class III—act directly on myocardium, prolonging action potential

Bretylium tosylate (Bretylol)

Indications: Life-threatening ventricular dysrhythmias; not recommended to treat asymptomatic ventricular ectopic beats

Usual dosage: 5-10 mg/kg IV push up to total of 30 mg/kg; may repeat in 15-30 min; slow continuous infusion 5-10 mg/kg q6-8h

Amiodarone

Indications: Effective in treatment and prevention of wide variety of atrial and ventricular dysrhythmias

Usual dosage: 200-800 mg/d; loading dose 800-1200 mg/d for 1 wk

Onset of action: 4-8 h

Antidysrhythmic drugs: Class IV—inhibit calcium transport into cells, depress activity of the S-A and A-V nodes, prolong conduction in A-V node, and increase A-V node refractoriness

Verapamil (Calan, Isoptin)

Indications: Reentrant paroxysmal supraventricular tachydysrhythmias; suppresses A-V junctional tachycardia and controls ventricular response to atrial fibrillation and flutter

Usual dosage: 5-10 mg (0.1 mg/kg) IV or 40-80 mg po q6-8h

Peak action: IV 3-5 min; po 3-4 h

Diltiazem (Cardizem)

Indications: Same as verapamil

Usual dosage: 0.25 mg/kg bolus over 2 min (approx. 20 mg); infusion rate at 10 mg/hr for 24 hours

Other agents: New generation, which may exert combined effects from more than one class: adenosine, sotolol

General Management

Cardiac monitoring—continuous electrocardiographic monitoring provides most efficient and reliable method of detection of dysrhythmias

Electrical countershock—often treatment of choice for tachydysrhythmias that are life threatening or producing a decrease in cardiac output and are resistant to pharmacologic interventions

Cardioversion—synchronized discharge of electrical impulse used to convert atrial fibrillation, atrial flutter, or supraventricular tachycardia to sinus rhythm

Defibrillation—emergency procedure that is unsynchronized; used in treatment of ventricular fibrillation

Cardiac pacemakers—battery-operated electrical devices used to initiate and control heart rate; may be used as temporary assistive devices or implanted permanently; have variety of modalities that are selected on basis of rhythm disturbance; most common indication for pacemaker implantation is bradydysrhythmias, but recent advances in technology have broadened their use to treatment of suppressing supraventricular dysrhythmias otherwise resistant to drug therapy (see p. 108 for further discussion)

Automatic implantable cardioverter defibrillator (AICD)—device capable of detecting the presence of ventricular tachydysrhythmias, and then delivering electrical countershock via cardioversion or defibrillation within 15 to 20 seconds (further discussion on p. 93)

Manage contributing factors—control or treat underlying causes of dysrhythmia, including thyroid imbalance, adrenal abnormality, recent cardiac surgery, fever, anxiety disorder (panic attacks)

Diet—restrictions usually directed to underlying disease process; patients with diagnosed supraventricular tachydysrhythmias instructed to avoid using stimulants such as caffeine, which is found in coffee, certain teas, soft drinks, and chocolate

Smoking—use of nicotine contraindicated because of its effect on ventricular threshold, which may be basis for dysrhythmias that could precipitate fatal rhythms

Activity—restrictions based on inducibility characteristics of dysrhythmia (usually ventricular) determined by exercise stress testing

NURSING CARE

Nursing Assessment

General Complaints

- Palpitations, dizziness, light-headedness, chest pain, syncope

Physical Examination

- Skin: pallor, diaphoresis
- Arterial pulse: normal with ectopy, tachycardia, bradycardia
- Rhythm: normal, irregular
- Hypotension
- Mental status: confusion, agitation, anxiety

Drug History

- Names, dosages of current antidysrhythmic agents
- Laboratory values: electrolyte imbalance; therapeutic levels of drug, thyroid imbalance
- Use of artificial stimulants: caffeine, nicotine, diet pills, decongestants, illicit drugs

Nursing Dx & Intervention

Anxiety related to threat of death secondary to sympathetic stimulation and altered heart action

- Assess degree of anxiety, level of understanding, and fears associated with dysrhythmias and treatment *to determine source of anxiety.*
- Provide continual explanations for the various monitoring devices in use; use short, simple explanations.
- Offer reassurance during periods of heightened anxiety.
- Administer sedation as ordered *to reduce anxiety and to promote rest.*
- Provide referrals for continued supportive counseling to deal with fears and anxieties.

Decreased cardiac output related to electrical factors (alteration in rate, rhythm, and conduction)

- Assess and monitor patient continuously *to determine cardiac rate, rhythm, and level of consciousness.*
- Monitor vital signs frequently, according to policy and patient's condition.
- Initiate prompt treatment of life-threatening dysrhythmias per protocol: cardiopulmonary resuscitation (CPR), electrical cardioversion, appropriate drug therapy, and preparation for pacemaker insertion.
- Monitor and record changes in ECG tracings to use as baseline.
- Notify physician promptly if any decrease in cardiac output occurs as evidenced by disturbance in rate, respirations, blood pressure, or mental status.
- Administer antidysrhythmic agents as ordered; monitor serum blood levels as guide for dosage *to maintain therapeutic drug levels and avoid drug toxicity;* use caution to avoid drug interactions.
- Administer oxygen therapy *to increase cardiac oxygenation.*

Patient Education/Home Care Planning

Instruction for a patient with a cardiac dysrhythmia begins with the initial phase of care, whether in a coronary care unit or in an outpatient setting. The following points should be included:

1. Brief description of the disease etiology, rhythm disturbances, and associated symptoms
2. Explanation of any diagnostic or therapeutic procedures that are planned
3. Explanation of monitoring equipment that may be used
4. Dietary restrictions that may be prescribed: need to avoid caffeine, nicotine, over-the-counter diet pills and decongestants
5. Instructions regarding drug therapy and its purpose, desired effects, dosage, and side effects to report to the physician
6. Explanation and method of taking pulse
7. Emphasize need for follow-up care: pacemaker check, AICD check, drug levels
8. Provide documentation of dysrhythmia (ECG strip) for patient to carry and Medic Alert card describing medications, device, etc. in case of emergency
9. Advise family to learn CPR for high-risk dysrhythmias

Evaluation

Anxiety level is reduced Patient demonstrates decreased anxiety. Patient appears relaxed, with decreased tension. Patient verbalizes fears and asks questions.

Heart returns to baseline rhythm ECG tracing reflects baseline rhythm. Blood pressure and heart rate are within normal limits. There is no ectopy.

Cardiac output is adequate to maintain cerebral perfusion Patient is alert and has no dizziness, syncopal episodes, or chest pains. Vital signs are stable. Peripheral perfusion is good.

■ CORONARY ARTERY DISEASE

Coronary artery disease (CAD) is a disorder of the coronary arteries that disrupts blood supply to the myocardium. Permanent disruption of blood flow causes myocardial dysfunction and necrosis, which may lead to a cascade of complications including sudden death (Figure 1-33).

The rate and severity of CAD vary considerably among world populations. Serious study of the natural history of CAD began in 1950 with the Framingham study and other projects.[46] The data collected in these early studies established certain factors related to the incidence and progression of coronary atherosclerotic disease. These include age, sex, hypertension, lipid levels, obesity, smoking, sedentary lifestyle, diabetes, and psychosocial factors (see box on p. 29).

Age and sex Men have a higher incidence of CAD than women. Deaths are reported to be five times as frequent for men as for women in the 35- to 40-year-old age group. After menopause women approach the same risk of CAD as men. About four out of five people who die of heart attacks are age 65 or older. Much attention is now focused on women to determine factors that may affect their risks for CAD (lifestyle, stress, estrogens, smoking, contraceptives). CAD in persons younger than 30 is usually linked to hyperlipidemia, hypertension, and smoking.

Hypertension   Although systolic hypertension is closely linked to cardiovascular disease, elevated systolic and diastolic pressures are associated with ischemic heart disease. Systolic pressures greater than 140 mm Hg or diastolic pressures greater than 90 mm Hg are considered a high risk factor for heart attacks, particularly in younger persons.[45]

Lipid levels   Of the various types of circulating lipoproteins, cholesterol and triglycerides are most commonly linked to CAD. Increased levels of blood cholesterol, a by-product of metabolism, raise the risk of CAD. In the presence of other risk factors (e.g., high blood pressure or smoking), the risk rises even more. Serum concentrations of 200 mg/dl in middle-aged adults indicate a relatively low risk of CAD; rates of 200 to 240 mg/dl indicate moderate and increasing risk; and levels of

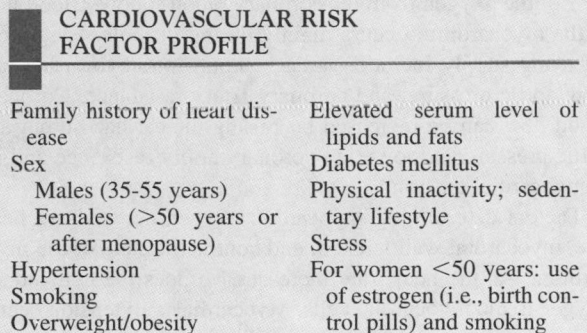

CARDIOVASCULAR RISK FACTOR PROFILE

Family history of heart disease	Elevated serum level of lipids and fats
Sex	Diabetes mellitus
Males (35-55 years)	Physical inactivity; sedentary lifestyle
Females (>50 years or after menopause)	Stress
Hypertension	For women <50 years: use of estrogen (i.e., birth control pills) and smoking
Smoking	
Overweight/obesity	

From Tucker.[89]

 EMERGENCY ALERT

CHEST PAIN WITH MYOCARDIAL INFARCTION

Pain described as crushing, sharp, heavy, or burning, may localize in the substernal area into the jaw and the left arm, and may last from minutes to several weeks. Myocardial infarction is localized ischemic necrosis of an area of the heart muscle caused by narrowing of one or more of the coronary arteries.

Assessment

- Possible nausea, vomiting, or hiccups
- Possible decrease in blood pressure, shortness of breath
- Possible jugular venous distention
- Diaphoresis
- Elevated temperature
- Increased pulse
- Anxiety
- PQRST pain assessment
  - P—provoking
  - Q—quality
  - R—radiating
  - S—severity
  - T—time

Interventions

- Place patient in comfortable position.
- Administer oxygen by nasal cannula (3 to 5 L).
- Obtain 12-lead ECG.
- Administer nitroglycerin (sublingual or IV as ordered).
- Establish IV at keep-open rate.
- Obtain blood samples.
- Monitor oxygen saturation.
- Administer morphine sulfate for pain as ordered.

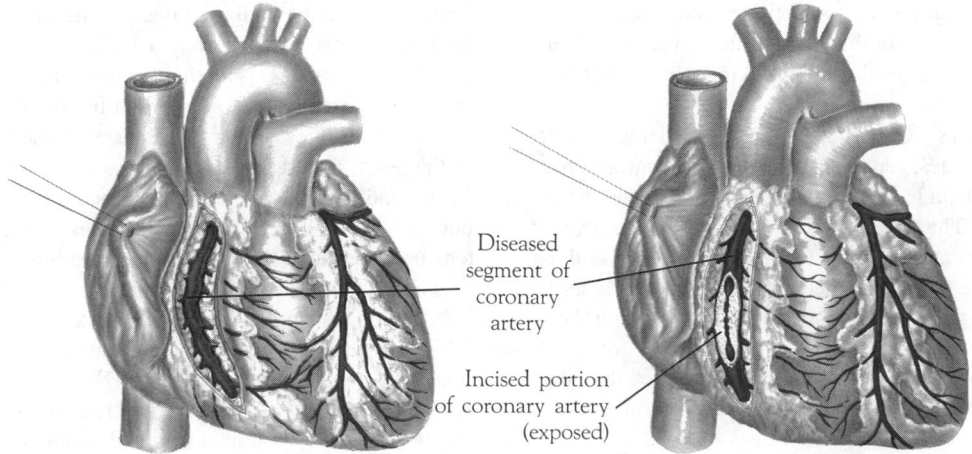

Diseased segment of coronary artery

Incised portion of coronary artery (exposed)

Figure 1-33 Coronary artery disease. (From Canobbio.[13])

greater than 240 mg/dl double the risk.[5] It is estimated that more than 27% of the U.S. population falls into this category.

Hyperlipidemia may be a primary disorder or may occur as a result of diabetes, myxedema, or alcoholism. Lipoproteins are broken down and measured separately to determine levels of those that are atherogenic. Low-density lipids (LDLs) carry a high percentage of cholesterol in plasma, and in high levels help produce atheromas. High-density lipids (HDLs), however, are mostly protein and carry a smaller percentage of cholesterol, thereby helping to remove lipids from the cell through liver metabolism. Studies show that the ratio of HDLs to LDLs is lower in patients with CAD and that a high ratio of HDLs help reduce vascular disease. HDLs are formed through exercise, fat-controlled diets, and estrogens.[8]

Obesity   Studies have shown that obese people (those who are more than 30% over their ideal weight) are more likely to develop CAD because obesity influences blood pressure and blood cholesterol. Obesity also can lead to diabetes.[3]

Smoking   Cigarette smoking is now clearly linked to heart disease. New studies show that smokers' risk of heart attack is more than twice that of nonsmokers.[3] Primarily through adrenergic stimulation, nicotine contributes to increases in heart rate, stroke volume, cardiac output, and blood pressure. Nicotine also causes peripheral vasoconstriction and in persons with decreased blood flow enhances ischemic changes. Cigarette smoking has also been demonstrated to have adverse effects on the lipid profile. Smoking decreases the threshold for ventricular fibrillation because it interferes with oxygen binding with hemoglobin, thus slowing the diffusion of oxygen into mitochondria. Nonsmokers may be exposed to increased risk of CAD by passive, or secondhand, smoke.

Sedentary lifestyle   Although the positive effects of exercise on the risk of CAD are difficult to assess, studies show that people who exercise heavily are at a decreased risk of having CAD. Inactivity is associated with decreases in HDLs.

Psychosocial factors   A type A personality is more characteristic of persons in whom CAD will develop. This type of person is usually aggressive, competitive, and rushed. When the type A personality is combined with other risk factors such as older age, high lipid levels, and smoking, the risk of heart disease may increase.

Other risk factors   Other factors that have also been linked to CAD include diabetes, genetic factors, and oral contraceptives.

For reasons not understood, patients with diabetes have a high risk of CAD. The role of heredity is also unclear. Apparently a tendency toward hypertension, hyperlipidemia, and diabetes exists in some families. Whether the tendency is inherited or simply the result of lifestyle patterns is unknown. Oral contraceptives have been linked to CAD when taken by women 45 years or younger. This finding results from studies that show high serum cholesterol and triglyceride levels in women taking oral contraceptives.[26]

•••••• Pathophysiology

Atherosclerosis, the basic underlying disease affecting coronary lumen size, is marked by changes in the intimal lining of the arteries. It begins as an irregular thickening process producing fatty streaks. This becomes a more severe form combining large amounts of lipids with collagen to produce fibroblasts that lead to fibrous atherosclerotic plaques.

The severity of the disease is measured by the degree of obstruction within each artery and the number of vessels involved. Obstructions of more than 75% of the lumen of one or more of the three coronary arteries increase the risk of death. The annual death rate of persons with one-vessel disease is 1% to 3%. Three-vessel disease increases the risk to 10% to 15%. Among people with 75% obstruction of the left main artery, however, the annual death rate is 30% to 40%.

Myocardial Perfusion

The basic physiologic changes resulting from the atherosclerotic process are problems of myocardial oxygen supply and demand. When myocardial oxygen demand exceeds the supply provided by the coronary arteries, ischemia results. Myocardial metabolism is oxygen dependent (aerobic), extracting up to 80% of the oxygen from the coronary blood supply. Blood flow to the myocardium occurs mainly during diastole. Factors influencing supply include cardiac output, intramyocardial tension, aortic pressure, and coronary artery resistance. Coronary blood flow can be increased by raising the cardiac output and aortic pressure and lowering coronary artery resistance and intramyocardial tension.

Factors determining myocardial oxygen demand are heart rate, myocardial wall tension, and contractile state of the myocardium. As the heart rate increases, so does the demand for oxygen to the myocardial cells. Myocardial wall tension occurs during contraction and is influenced by ventricular and systolic (arterial) pressure. Myocardial contractility is stimulated by the release of catecholamines or sympathetic stimulation. These increase wall tension and thus energy or oxygen demands.

Myocardial ischemia is the result of impaired myocardial perfusion. Coronary atherosclerotic heart disease is the most common cause of myocardial ischemia. Obstruction varies in degree and may be well tolerated as long as myocardial oxygen demand is low. As the demand increases and the obstruction persists or advances, ischemic changes result. Coronary blood vessel distribution is also important in providing oxygen to the myocardium. The coronary arteries sit on the epicardial surface of the heart. Blood travels in toward the endocardium. The inner subendocardial layers of the myocardium therefore are particularly at risk for ischemia. Increases in heart rate and wall tension can reduce flow to the endocardium.

The coronary arteries also supply major conduction structures within the myocardium. The RCA supplies the sinus node in 55% to 60% of persons. In the remainder it is supplied by a branch of the circumflex artery. The RCA also supplies the A-V node in 85% of persons. The remaining 15% is supplied by the LCA. The septum is supplied mainly by the LAD artery, although part of the posterior wall is supplied by the RCA. An obstruction of any of the major arteries or their branches results in ischemia to the portion of myocardium supplied by that vessel. Obstruction of the LAD results in ischemic changes of the anterior wall of the ventricle. RCA obstruction results in infarction and ischemia of the right ventricle. The degree of obstruction and number of coronary arteries involved influence how serious the disease will be. CAD is described in single-, double-, or triple-vessel disease. When a major obstruction occurs in the first branch of the LCA or the left main artery before bifurcation, the risk for a major infarction and death rises. This is called left main disease.

The major signs of ischemia are chest pain and ECG changes. Other symptoms result from compromised cardiac function.

Angina Pectoris

The term *angina pectoris,* which means chest pain, is used to describe pain as a symptom of myocardial ischemia. Myocardial ischemia is the result of an imbalance between myocardial oxygen supply and demand. It occurs most often with coronary atherosclerosis but can also occur in patients with normal coronary arteries. For example, patients with aortic stenosis, hypertension, and hypertrophic cardiomyopathy may have symptoms of angina pectoris. In these patients myocardial work is increased, but perfusion of the hypertrophied muscle is inadequate. This results in myocardial ischemia despite normal coronary arteries.

Various terms have been used to describe the many syndromes linked to myocardial ischemia. The following describe chest pain that is transient and linked to myocardial ischemia.

Stable angina pectoris is marked by chest discomfort caused by effort, with or without radiation, that lasts from a few seconds to 15 minutes. It is generally relieved by rest and the removal of provoking factors or by sublingual vasodilators.

Unstable angina pectoris is marked by pain that lasts longer, occurs more often, and may be caused by factors other than effort. Various names used to describe this syndrome include crescendo angina, preinfarction angina, angina decubitus, and nocturnal angina.

Variant (Prinzmetal's) angina is marked by chest pain that occurs at rest and is often linked to ST elevations on the ECG. The underlying cause is thought to be coronary artery spasm. Unlike angina pectoris, variant angina is caused by a sudden reduction in coronary blood flow brought on by the spasm and not by an increase in myocardial oxygen demand. The decrease in oxygen consumption occurring during sleep or rest may lead to coronary artery vasoconstriction and may be the cause of the spasm.[8]

Some have suggested a link between the spasm and stimulation of α (vasoconstriction) and β (vasodilation) adrenergic receptors.[8] Others have suggested various mechanisms involved in the case of spasm, including parasympathetic nervous system activity and possibly local abnormalities of vascular smooth muscle.

Myocardial Infarction

Myocardial infarction (MI) is the development of ischemia and necrosis of myocardial tissue. It results from a sudden decrease in coronary perfusion or an increase in myocardial oxygen demand without adequate coronary perfusion.

Two types of infarction have been described. Subendocardial infarction is generally confined to small areas of myocardium. It is usually within the subendocardial wall of the left ventricle, the ventricular septum, and papillary muscles. Transmural, or full-thickness, infarction is widespread myocardial necrosis, extending from the endocardium to the epicardium (Figure 1-34).

Myocardial tissue death is usually preceded by sudden occlusion of a major coronary artery. Coronary thrombosis is the most common cause of infarction, but other factors may be responsible. These include coronary artery spasm, platelet aggregation and embolism from a mural thrombus, a thrombus on a prosthetic mitral or aortic valve, or a dislodged calcium plaque from a calcified aortic or mitral valve.

Persistent cellular ischemia interferes with myocardial tissue metabolism, causing a rapid development of permanent cell damage. At first there are three zones of tissue damage. The first is a central area of necrotic myocardial cells, capillaries, and connective tissue. Surrounding this tissue is a second zone of "injured" cells that are potentially viable if enough circulation is quickly restored. The third zone, characterized by ischemia, is also viable and can be expected to recover unless the ischemia persists or worsens. The severity or extension of a myocardial infarction often depends on the fate of the injured and ischemic zones. Ischemia may progress to necrosis if untreated. Because the infarction process may take up to 6 hours to complete, restoration of adequate myocardial perfusion is important to limit necrosis.

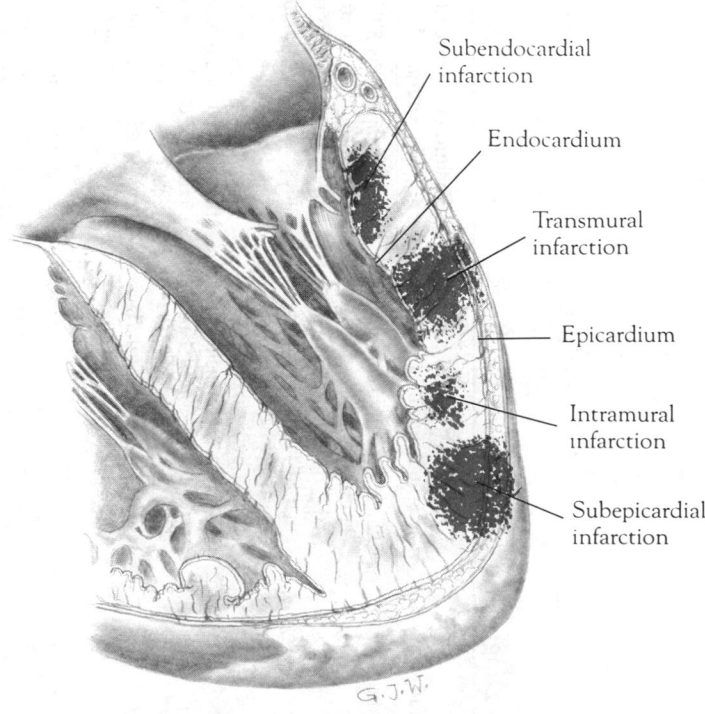

Figure 1-34 Location of infarctions in ventricle wall. (From Thelan.[85])

•••••• Diagnostic Studies and Findings

Study	Stable Angina Pectoris	Variant (Prinzmetal's) Angina	Unstable Angina Pectoris	Myocardial Infarction
Electrocardiogram (ECG)	Changes usually seen during anginal episodes; 50%-70% of patients have normal ECG during pain-free episodes; ischemia determined by horizontal ST segment or downsloping with depression of 1 mm; T wave inversion represents impaired repolarization caused by ischemia	Ischemia appears as ST elevation during anginal attack but regresses as pain subsides; ECG changes may be seen before patient complains of chest pain or may be recorded in absence of pain; A-V conduction defects may occur, particularly when RCA is involved, and include Mobitz type II and complete A-V block; ventricular irritability such as premature ventricular contractions, ventricular tachycardia, or fibrillation can occur, particularly during ischemic attack	Ischemia determined by horizontal ST segment or downsloping with depression of 1 mm; T wave inversion represents impaired repolarization caused by ischemia; ventricular irritability such as premature ventricular contractions, ventricular tachycardia, or fibrillation	Changes are evolutionary and indicate progression of infarction; in acute stage, ST elevations with subsequent T wave inversion and Q wave formation; Q waves indicate necrosis and are considered pathologic if they are 0.04 sec or greater in duration, 0.4 mm or greater in depth, or present in leads that do not normally have Q waves; ST elevations reflect myocardial injury that interferes with polarization of cells are seen in leads facing injured area, and return to normal (isoelectric) within days; ST elevations beyond 4-6 weeks should raise suspicion of ventricular aneurysm; infarction location determined by identifying leads that demonstrate characteristic ECG changes; such leads are those with positive terminals that face injured site of heart; reciprocal changes, seen in leads that face *opposite* surface of damaged heart, are absence of Q wave, increase in R wave amplitude, depressed ST segment, upright tall T wave. RV myocardial infarction (RVMI): ST elevation in right precordial leads (V_3R to V_6R); V_4R may be most sensitive and predictive

	Onset	*Peak*	*Return to normal*
SGOT	6-12 hours	36 hours	5-7 days
CPK-MB	4-12 hours	24 hours	3-4 days
LDH (isoenzyme)	24-48 hours	3-6 days	8-14 days

Laboratory tests

Study	Stable Angina Pectoris	Variant (Prinzmetal's) Angina	Unstable Angina Pectoris	Myocardial Infarction
Enzymes	No elevation; checked to rule out MI	No elevation; checked to rule out MI	No elevation; checked to rule out MI	
Complete blood count (CBC)	No elevation; checked to rule out anemia-induced angina	No elevation; checked to rule out anemia-induced angina	No elevation; checked to rule out anemia-induced angina	Elevated white count (WBC) and erythrocyte sedimentation rate (ESR) reflect myocardial damage

••••••• Diagnostic Studies and Findings—cont'd

Study	Stable Angina Pectoris	Variant (Prinzmetal's) Angina	Unstable Angina Pectoris	Myocardial Infarction
Glucose	No elevation	No elevation	No elevation	Transiently elevated owing to adrenergic response
Lipid levels (triglycerides, cholesterol, high- and low-density lipids)	Checked to determine any lipoprotein abnormalities	Checked to rule out presence of atherosclerotic process	Checked to determine any lipoprotein abnormalities	Checked to determine any lipoprotein abnormalities
Exercise stress test (EST)	Chest pain; horizontal ST segment or downsloping of 1 mm or more; failure of systolic blood pressure to rise or drop; ST elevations	Normal stress test done to differentiate between variant and classic angina; ST elevation with or without associated chest pain occasionally develops	As in stable angina pectoris; should not be done until patient has been stable and pain free for 24 hours	Not done in presence of documented myocardial infarction; low-level test may be performed before discharge from hospital
Thallium-201 scintigraphy	Ischemic areas appear as "cold" areas, reflecting reduced thallium uptake; when ischemia relieved, "cold" areas show normal thallium uptake		Similar to stable angina pectoris	Similar to stable angina pectoris; used to confirm diagnosis; with decreased blood flow an area of decreased activity is visualized
Radionuclide blood pool imaging with technetium 99m				Confirms myocardial damage by localizing and permitting estimation of size of transmural infarction; must be done within 2-6 days after acute infarction; determines wall motion abnormalities; permits estimation of ventricular function by determining ejection fractions
Cardiac catheterization and coronary angiography	Determines number and location of obstructive lesions, "graftability" of artery distal to obstructive lesion, and ventricular function	Distinguishes spasm in normal coronary arteries from those with severe obstructive lesions; intravenous injection or ergonovine maleate provokes coronary artery spasm in patients with variant angina	As in stable angina pectoris	Generally not performed as diagnostic procedure during acute period; procedures used in the administration of thrombolysis or percutaneous angioplasty

••••• Multidisciplinary Plan

Surgery

Coronary artery bypass grafting (CABG)—only direct method of increasing myocardial coronary blood flow; provides symptomatic relief in 80% of patients with significant angina and has low operative mortality

Indications: Disabling angina that is refractory to medical therapy, significantly abnormal ECG response to exercise, 50% or greater obstruction of left main coronary artery, and significant obstructive lesions in all three coronary arteries (p. 95 describes care of patients undergoing open-heart surgery)

Interventional Therapy

Percutaneous transluminal coronary angioplasty (PTCA)—alternative approach to coronary artery bypass surgery in selected patients; attempts to restore luminal patency by compressing atheromatous plaques with balloon inflation

Atherectomy—interventional devices to revascularize stenotic coronary arteries: directional atherectomy, rotational atherectomy, laser angioplasty, and coronary artery stenting. These devices may be used alone or in combination with balloon angioplasty for access to more complex lesions and prevention of restenosis (see p. 111)

Medications

Thrombolytic therapy (intracoronary or intravenous thrombolysis)—nonsurgical reperfusion procedure used in treatment of acute transmural myocardial infarction; purpose is to interrupt evolution of myocardial ischemia to necrosis and to limit infarction size; improvement of ischemic area can be achieved if therapy is initiated within 4 to 6 hours of onset of infarction (p. 114 describes care of patients undergoing thrombolytic therapy)

Indications: Chest pain not relieved by nitroglycerin, 4 hours from onset of chest pain, and ST elevations with reciprocal ECG changes

Vasodilators

Nitrates

Short-acting nitrates: Sublingual nitroglycerin (0.4-0.6 mg; isosorbide dinitrate (5 mg)

Duration of action: ½-2 h

Long-acting oral nitrates: Isosorbide dinitrate (10-20 mg qid)

Topical 2% nitroglycerin ointment (1-2 inches q4-6h)

Duration of action: Up to 6 h or longer

β-Adrenergic blocking agents

Propranolol (Inderal)

Usual dosage: 10-20 mg po tid or qid; IV 1 mg/min not exceeding 3-5 mg

Metoprolol (Lopressor)

Indication: Early treatment for MI

Usual dose: IV bolus 5 mg q2min × 3, then 50 mg po q6h × 48 h, maintenance dose 100 mg bid

Nadolol (Corgard)

Indications: Treatment of angina and hypertension

Usual dosage: 40-80 mg po up to 240 mg/d as necessary

Duration of action: About 20-24 h

Timolol (Blocadren)

Indications: Reduction of mortality and reinfarction after myocardial infarctions; hypertension

Usual dosage: 20-60 mg bid

Atenolol (Tenormin)

Indications: Approved for use of hypertension but may have potential use in treating angina and reducing infarction size

Usual dosage: 50-100 mg/d

Angiotensin-converting enzyme (ACE) inhibitors—reduces mortality after myocardial infarction by preventing progressive ventricular enlargement, thereby preventing complications such as congestive heart failure; also thought to prevent future infarctions

Captopril (Capoten)

Usual dosage: 6.25-100 mg tid

Enalapril maleate (Vasotec)

Usual dosage: 2.5-20 mg bid

Calcium antagonists

Nifedipine (Procardia)

Indications: Angina pectoris caused by coronary artery spasm, chronic stable angina pectoris

Usual dosage: 10 mg po; sublingual 10-40 mg q8h (not to exceed 180 mg); IV 5-15 mg/kg

Verapamil (Calan, Isoptin)

Indications: Treatment of angina pectoris and coronary artery spasm

Usual dosage: 80-160 mg q8h (not to exceed 480 mg/d); IV 0.075-0.15 mg/kg (not to exceed 15 mg/30 min)

Diltiazem (Cardizem)

Indications: Treatment of variant angina

Usual dosage: Initially 30 mg po qid, increasing gradually to 80 mg tid (total 240 mg/d)

Antihyperlipidemic agents—interfere with reabsorption of cholesterol and lower triglyceride levels

Simvastatin (Zocor)

Usual dosage: 5-40 mg qPM

Pravastatin (Lipostat)

Usual dosage: 10-40 mg qPM

Lovastatin (Mevacor)

Usual dosage: 20 mg po bid

Cholestyramine (Questran)

Usual dosage: 8-12 g bid

Neomycin sulfate

Usual dosage: 0.5-2 g/d

Clofibrate (Atromid-S)

Usual dosage: 0.5 g tid

Gemfibrozil (Lopid)

Usual dosage: 0.6 g bid

Niacin (nicotinic acid)

Usual dosage: 0.5-1 g tid

Anticoagulation

Heparin

Indications: Used in acute-setting MI to aid lysis of existing clot and prevent thrombus formation

Usual dosage: 5000 U IV initial dose followed by continuous infusion to maintain control, PTT 1.5-2 times

Antiplatelet agents

Aspirin (acetylsalicylic acid, ASA)

Indications: Used in setting of coronary artery thrombosis and in the prevention of further atherogenesis; because of possible beneficial effects, may be used in patients with unstable angina syndrome and myocardial infarction

Usual dosage: 325-1300 mg/d

Dipyridamole (Persantine, Persantin)

Indications: Used in combination with aspirin to maintain patency of saphenous vein coronary artery bypass grafts

Usual dosage: 100 mg tid 1 h before meals (with ASA, 325 mg tid after meals)

Magnesium sulfate

Indications: Cardioprotective properties include limiting progression of ischemic to infarcted myocardium, reduces risk of arrhythmia

Usual dosage: Used experimentally to date via IV route for 48 h after acute MI

General Management

Cardiovascular monitoring—used to assess and monitor for signs of life-threatening complications associated with severe myocardial ischemia and necrosis, including dysrhythmias, heart failure, extension of MI, cardiogenic shock (p. 102), ventricular or papillary muscle rupture, and ventricular aneurysm; complications occur within first 5 days in half of patients with acute MI; early detection depends on careful and frequent continuous monitoring of various hemodynamic parameters and clinical status that reflect left ventricular function: arterial pressure, pulmonary artery pressure (PAP), pulmonary capillary wedge pressure (PCWP)

Electrocardiogram (ECG)—used to detect changes in heart rhythms and to determine serial changes reflective of myocardial ischemia, injury, or extension of MI

Intraaortic balloon counterpulsation (IABP)—used mainly in patients with acute MI to protect ischemic myocardium by decreasing preload, afterload, and myocardial oxygen demand; diastolic pressure is supported, thus improving coronary perfusion and cardiac output; most successful in patients who are treated less than 6 hours after infarction, are undergoing their first MI, and have no aortic insufficiency (p. 106 describes specific care)

Admission to coronary care unit (CCU) or coronary observation unit—indicated for patients with acute chest pain for evaluation, surveillance, and management

---

NURSING CARE

Nursing Assessment

Area of Concern	Stable Angina Pectoris	Variant (Prinzmetal's) Angina	Unstable Angina Pectoris	Myocardial Infarction
Chest pain				
Quality	Aching, sharp, tingling, or burning sensation or pressure	Similar to stable angina pectoris	Similar to stable angina pectoris but may be more severe	Crushing, squeezing, stabbing, oppressive sensation or as if heavy object is sitting on chest
Location and radiation	Substernal with radiation to left shoulder, down inner aspect of left arm or both arms; neck, jaw, and scapula may be additional sites of radiation	Similar to stable angina pectoris	Similar to stable angina pectoris	Retrosternal and left precordial radiating down left arm and to neck, jaws, teeth, epigastric area, and back
Precipitating factors	Onset classically associated with exercise or activities that increase myocardial oxygen demand, e.g., physical exercise, heavy lifting, emotional stress, cold temperatures	Onset at rest; pain is cyclic, often occurring during sleep	Pain may be brought on with less than usual exertion; may occur at rest	May occur at rest or during exertion
Duration and alleviating factors	3-15 min; relieved by rest, stopping pain-inducing activities, taking sublingual nitroglycerin (NTG) tablet	Characteristically, pain intensifies quickly, tends to last longer than angina, and subsides with exercise	Prolonged and not usually as quickly relieved by rest or taking NTG	Described as continuous, lasting more than 30 minutes, unrelieved by rest, position change, or taking NTG tablets

Continued.

Area of Concern	Stable Angina Pectoris	Variant (Prinzmetal's) Angina	Unstable Angina Pectoris	Myocardial Infarction
Associated signs and symptoms	During anginal attack, dyspnea, anxiety, diaphoresis, cool clammy skin	Similar to stable angina pectoris	Similar to stable angina pectoris but symptoms may be more prominent and may persist; may be associated with nausea	Anxiety, restlessness, weakness, associated profuse diaphoresis, dyspnea, dizziness; signs of vasomotor response including nausea, vomiting, faintness, and cold clammy skin; hiccups and other gastrointestinal distress may be present; low-grade temperature elevations common for first 24-48 hours but may last several days (this is inflammatory response to myocardial tissue damage)
Physical examination	Normal during asymptomatic periods; during anginal attacks, increased heart rate, pulsus alternans, and transient abnormal findings including precordial bulge and atrial and ventricular gallops (S_3, S_4)	Similar to stable angina pectoris	Similar to stable angina pectoris; may also demonstrate irregular pulse, hypotension, or signs of left ventricular dysfunction	May be unremarkable unless signs of ventricular failure or cardiogenic shock are present; blood pressure normal, elevated, or decreased (initially elevated when pain is present but usually decreases for first few days); respirations: Cheyne-Stokes respiration owing to central nervous system hypoperfusion or opiate therapy; initial tachypnea returns to normal once pain subsides; heart sounds: S_3, S_4 gallops indicative of ventricular dysfunction; systolic murmurs reflecting papillary muscle dysfunction; diminished heart sounds and pericardial friction rub may occur; with left ventricular dysfunction: pulmonary rales, decreased urine output, increased amplitude of "a" wave in jugular vein; with right ventricular dysfunction: increased jugular venous distention, peripheral edema, liver tenderness; pulse often within normal limits; bradycardia present with inferior wall myocardial infarction; tachycardia with rates greater than 100 beats/min may reflect compromised ventricle

Diet

Admission diet—depends on clinical status; during acute phase, patient may be permitted nothing by mouth (NPO) or receive clear liquids progressing to 1500-calorie, soft, low-fat, no-added-salt diet; iced beverages limited to 600 to 800 ml[52]; caffeine, a cardiac stimulant, restricted because it lowers threshold for certain dysrhythmias[75]

Discharge diet—depends on several factors including cholesterol and triglyceride levels, total body weight, and clinical status; American Heart Association suggests diet of reduced saturated fats and cholesterol, restriction of sodium, and limiting total caloric consumption to maintain ideal body weight[4]

Activity—bedrest with bedside commode for 24 to 36 hrs for uncomplicated MI, progressing to monitored activity

Oxygenation—patients evaluated early for hypoxemia, which may result from ventilation-perfusion abnormalities; providing additional inspired oxygen to patient in absence of hypoxemia does not ensure increased oxygen delivery to myocardium and may rarely increase systemic vascular resistance and arterial pressure, causing subsequent decrease in cardiac output and oxygen delivery to tissues; arterial oxygen saturation by pulse oximetry should be measured on admission to coronary care unit; if normal, oxygen therapy may be omitted; hypoxemic patients should receive oxygen therapy as required; continuous pulse oximetry and arterial blood gas determinations as indicated by clinical picture to monitor effectiveness of therapy

Nursing Dx & Intervention

Pain: chest, related to imbalance of myocardial oxygen supply and demand

Acute care
- Assess and record description of pain and activity *to determine etiology* or possible extension of infarction.
- Stop angina-inducing activity.
- Maintain bed rest *to reduce myocardial oxygen demand.*
- Administer drug therapy as ordered *to relieve pain;* assess and record response.
- Administer oxygen therapy as ordered *to increase oxygen supply to myocardium.*
- Obtain 12-lead ECG *to document ischemia during chest pain episode.*
- Monitor vital signs frequently throughout episode of chest pain.
- Avoid activities and stimulants that increase vasoconstriction.

 EMERGENCY ALERT

CARDIAC ARREST

Complete cessation of systemic circulation; patient is unconscious, apneic, pale, or cyanotic, and pulses are absent in major arteries (carotid or femoral).

Assessment
- Airway patency
- Breathing effectiveness, chest rise and fall, spontaneous respiration
- Circulation—are femoral or carotid pulses present?

Interventions
- Perform basic life support.
- Call emergency medical services (EMS).
- Clear airway using jaw-thrust or chin-lift maneuver.
- Suction patient and remove foreign body if present.
- Assist ventilation using mouth-to-mouth or bag-valve mask assistance.
- Administer high-flow oxygen by mask (10-15 L).
- Perform external cardiac compressions, 80 to 100 per minute, 15:2 compression:breath ratio.

- Limit offerings of hot or cold beverages.
- Avoid offering caffeine beverage such as coffee, tea, or colas.

Convalescent care
- Administer long-acting nitrates as ordered.
- Encourage limitation of activities as needed *to prevent pain.*

Decreased cardiac output (risk for) related to loss of myocardial contractility

Acute care
- Assess and report signs of decreased cardiac output: decreased blood pressure, increased heart rate, decreased urine output, fatigue, and cool clammy skin.
- Maintain bed rest *to reduce myocardial oxygen demand.*
- Monitor ECG for dysrhythmias and alterations.
- Maintain IV as ordered with 5% glucose in water for drug administration.
- Auscultate breath sounds and heart tones every 1 to 4 hours.
- Administer drug therapy as ordered.
- Monitor vital signs and hemodynamic parameters as indicated: arterial pressure, PA, pulmonary capillary wedge pressure (PCWP), and central venous pressure (CVP) *to detect signs and symptoms of myocardial dysfunction.*

Convalescent care
- Monitor for early complications: hypotension, dysrhythmias, heart failure, and heart rupture.
- Begin progressive ambulation as patient's condition stabilizes.
- Restrict sodium intake as ordered.
- Monitor intake and output closely *to detect and prevent circulatory overload.*
- Provide IV fluids as ordered if patient is unable to eat because of nausea or vomiting.

Anxiety related to perceived or actual threat to biologic integrity

- Assess for signs and symptoms of fear and anxiety: verbalizations, restlessness, insomnia, irritability, facial expressions, and noncompliance.
- Offer reassurance during episodes of pain.
- Initiate comfort measures such as a quiet, restful environment and relaxation techniques.
- Administer sedation as ordered.
- Stay with patient as much as possible.
- Use a calm, reassuring voice.
- Allow family members to assist patient if possible.
- Explain all procedures and routine care as they occur.
- Encourage expression of feelings.
- Permit crying.

Activity intolerance related to imbalance of oxygen supply and demand

Acute care
- Maintain bed rest *to reduce myocardial workload and increase oxygenation.*

- Increase activities as ordered, using ECG changes, heart rate, blood pressure, and patient's clinical status (e.g., complicated versus uncomplicated myocardial infarction) as guidelines. Bed or tub baths cause *fewer hemodynamic and postural changes than showers.* Backrubs may have a soothing effect.
- Allow patient out of bed for toileting because this does not seem to have adverse effects.
- Perform passive range of motion (ROM) exercise to prevent thromboembolism, progressing to active ROM exercises.

Convalescent care

- Begin phase I rehabilitation shown in the box below.
- Teach necessity for increasing activity gradually at home while continuing periods of rest.

Patient Education/Home Care Planning

1. Explain the disease process, risk factors involved, methods of modification, associated symptoms, and actions to take when the symptoms occur. Associated complications are irregular heartbeats, chest pain, and shortness of breath.
2. Explain the name, purpose, side effects, and method of administration of all drugs.
3. Explain activity allowances and limitations, including the patient's return to work, resumption of sexual activity, and need to avoid or modify activity after heavy meals and alcohol consumption and in periods of emotional stress or extremes of temperatures.
4. Refer the patient to a rehabilitation program to assist with progressive increase in activity levels.
5. Teach the patient to avoid foods high in sodium, saturated fats, and triglycerides. Teach good nutritional habits and alternative ways of seasoning food to avoid cooking with salt and salt products.
6. Explain importance of controlling any coexisting condition that may aggravate recovery, such as hypertension, obesity, and diabetes.

Evaluation

Patient is free from chest pain Patient verbalizes absence of pain. Blood pressure and heart rate are within normal limits. Patient engages in hospital routines and activities without pain. Patient appears relaxed and expresses a sense of calm.

Cardiac output is improved or maintained ECG, vital signs, and urine output are within normal limits.

Anxiety level is reduced Patient appears relaxed.

Activity level is improved Patient verbalizes ability to perform activities of daily living (ADL) without difficulty; ECG, blood pressure (BP), and heart rate (HR) are within acceptable limits.

CONGESTIVE HEART FAILURE

Congestive heart failure (CHF) is a complex clinical syndrome that results from the heart's inability to increase cardiac output sufficiently to meet the body's metabolic demands (Figure 1-35).

Congestive heart failure occurs as a result of myocardial damage. It is estimated that 3 million Americans suffer from CHF and that up to 35,000 will die from this chronic disorder.[1]

•••••• Pathophysiology

The underlying causes of CHF vary, but it ultimately results in the heart's inability to act as an effective pump.

Decreased myocardial contractility may result from a primary disorder or an excessive workload placed on the heart such as systemic hypertension or a valvular disorder. Causes of primary myocardial disorders and disorders that increase the heart's workload are summarized as follows:

Causes of decreased myocardial contractility
- Coronary artery disease
- Myocarditis
- Cardiomyopathies
    Dilated
    Restrictive
    Hypertrophic

■ PHASES OF CARDIAC REHABILITATION

Phase I: Inpatient activities; anywhere from 4 to 16 stages; patient should be at 3 to 5 metabolic equivalents of tasks (METs) at discharge

Phase II: Begins with discharge and continues until healing has been completed; patient is evaluated with a stress test that is symptom limited

Phase III: Begins 4 to 6 weeks after myocardial infarction or surgery; training phase; patient exercises two to five times a week under supervision for usually 12 weeks; patient should be able to perform at 10 METs or greater at the end of this phase

Phase IV: A maintenance phase of indefinite length; begins at the end of the training phase and continues for another 3 to 6 months (some believe it continues for the patient's lifetime); patient maintains level of training by exercising two or three times a week; stress tests usually done at yearly intervals to measure effectiveness and amend exercise prescription

Modified from Guzzetta.[40]

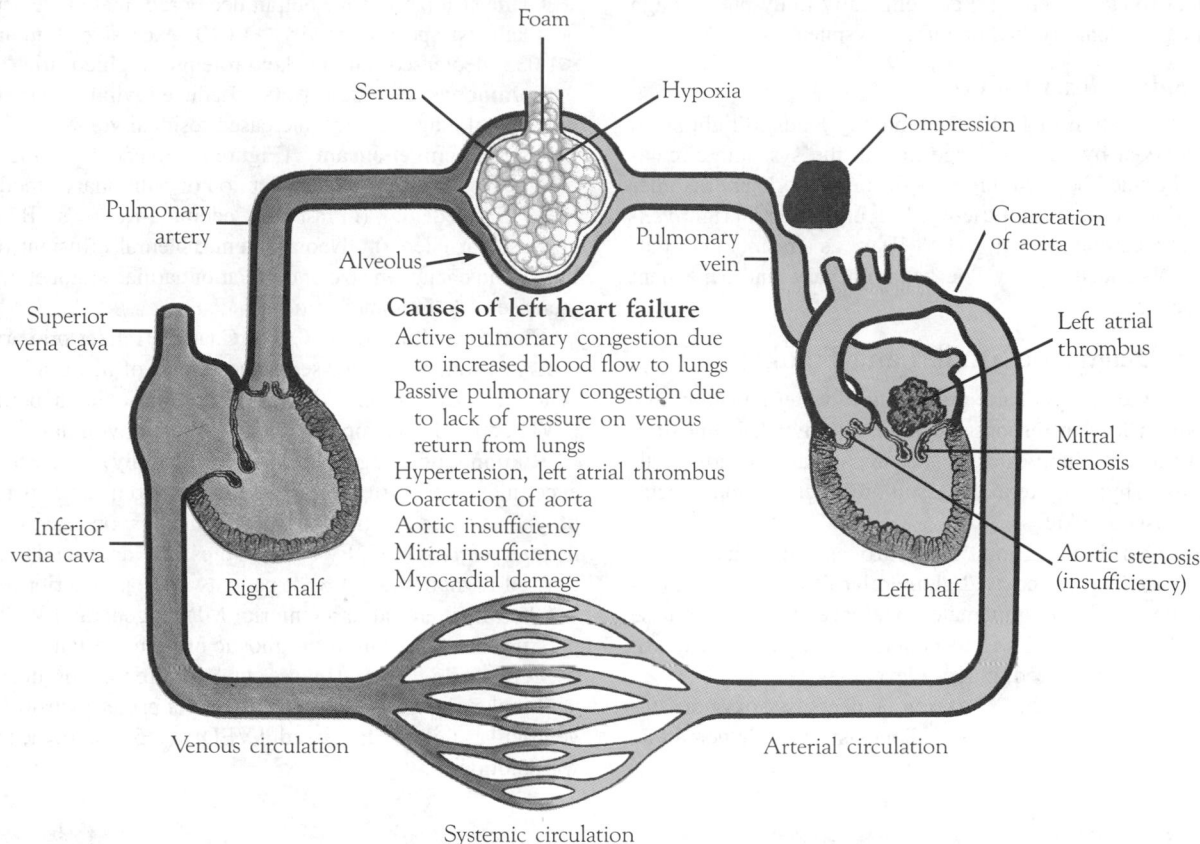

Figure 1-35 Congestive heart failure. (From Canobbio.[13])

- Infiltrative diseases
  - Amyloidosis
  - Tumors
  - Sarcoidosis
- Collagen-vascular diseases
  - Systemic lupus erythematosus
  - Scleroderma
- Iatrogenic factors
  - Drugs such as β-blockers; calcium antagonists, alcohol

Causes of increased myocardial workload
- Hypertension
- Pulmonary hypertension
- Valvular heart disease
  - Aortic or pulmonic stenosis
  - Mitral, tricuspid, or aortic insufficiency
- Intracardiac shunting
- High-output states
  - Anemia
  - Hyperthyroidism
  - Beriberi
  - Arteriovenous fistula

Disorders that interfere with the normal stretch of the ventricle, thereby decreasing ventricular filling, cause a drop in cardiac output. Pericardial tamponade and constrictive pericarditis are examples.

Persistent tachydysrhythmias reduce ventricular filling time, and marked bradydysrhythmias greatly reduce cardiac output because the ventricles cannot augment the stroke volume.

Loss of coordinated atrial contraction, as occurs in atrial fibrillation, can decrease cardiac output, probably because of loss of the atrial "booster pump" that contributes to normal ventricular filling.

The primary dysfunction in CHF is decreased myocardial contractility. However, secondary changes in preload and afterload also contribute to the heart failure.

Heart failure can be divided into left- and right-sided failure; they can occur independently or together.

Left-Sided Heart Failure

Any sustained elevation in left ventricular end-diastolic pressure (LVEDP) increases left atrial pressure. This is transmitted to the pulmonary vascular bed and is manifest as an increase in pulmonary capillary wedge pressure (PCWP). If the PCWP exceeds the colloid osmotic pressure of the pulmonary capillaries, transudation of fluid into the interstitial spaces and eventually into alveolar spaces will occur. This leads to hypoxia (resulting from poor oxygen exchange) and clinically to dyspnea, cough orthopnea, and paroxysmal nocturnal dyspnea.

Right-Sided Heart Failure

Persistent elevation of LVEDP eventually leads to right-sided failure marked by venous congestion in the systemic circulation. Right-sided heart failure may occur as a primary disorder of the right ventricle as in tricuspid regurgitation, in right ventricular myocardial infarction (RVMI), or as a result of cor pulmonale. Distended neck veins, hepatomegaly, and dependent edema occur.

•••••• Diagnostic Studies and Findings

Electrolytes Hyponatremia owing to water retention; urinary sodium loss in response to diuretics; hypokalemia from excessive use of diuretics or as secondary manifestation of aldosteronism; hypochloremia as result of diuretic therapy; metabolic acidosis or alkalosis

Blood chemistry Blood urea nitrogen (BUN) and creatinine increased with decreased glomerular filtration; liver function values (serum glutamate oxaloacetate transaminase [SGOT], bilirubin, alkaline phosphatase) mildly increased; prothrombin time prolonged; glucose level elevated

Arterial blood gases Hypoxemia; decreased oxygen saturation; (early) mild respiratory alkalosis; (late) hypercarbia, hypoxia

Urine studies Urine output decreased; metabolic acidosis or alkalosis; specific gravity >1.010: excessive fluid intake, <1.035: decreased fluid intake; proteinuria; glucosuria

Pulmonary function tests Reduced vital capacity; reduced total lung capacity; increased residual volume

Chest roentgenogram (Figures 1-36 and 1-37) Increased pulmonary congestion: redistribution of pulmonary blood flow, interstitial edema (intraseptal edema—Kerley's B lines; perivascular edema), alveolar edema, pleural effusion; (early) little or no change in size or contour of cardiac silhouette; (late) increased cardiothoracic ratio

Electrocardiogram (ECG) Changes reflect primary disorders as well as chronic sedentary effects of heart failure: left ventricular hypertrophy (LVH), right ventricular hypertrophy (RVH), atrial hypertrophy, tachycardia, dysrhythmias

Radionuclide angiography (scintigraphy) Detects presence and severity of ventricular dysfunction; used to predict prognosis based on etiology or determine response to therapeutic interventions (e.g., LV ejection pressures are found to be depressed in more than 90% of patients after an anterior MI and in 50% of patients after an inferior MI); in general, LV ejection pressure of <0.30 mm is prognostic of high mortality

Echocardiogram (Figure 1-38) Increased or decreased ventricular chambers or structures reflect primary disorder; left ventricular failure: increased LVEDP (>5.6 cm), decreased wall motion

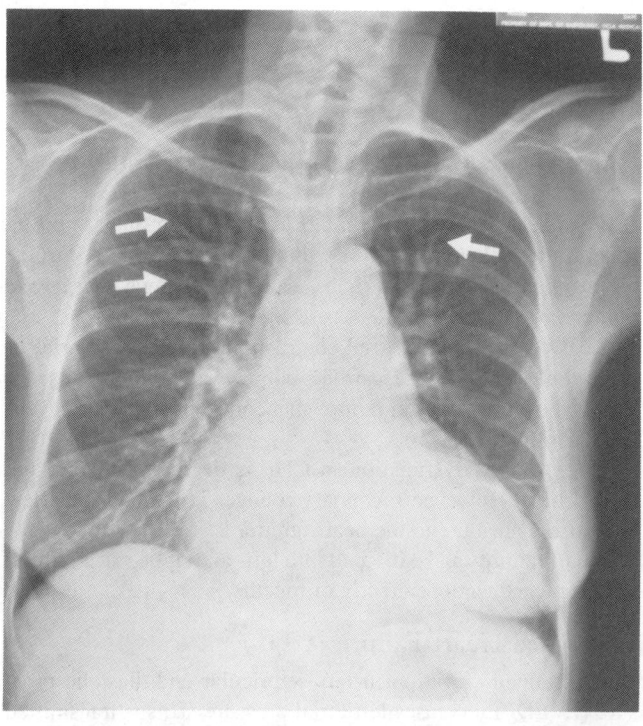

Figure 1-36 Pulmonary congestion. Upper lobe distention *(arrows)*. Enlarged cardiac silhouette. (Courtesy Batra P, Department of Radiology, UCLA School of Medicine, Los Angeles. From Michaelson CR, editor: *Congestive heart failure,* St Louis, 1983, Mosby.)

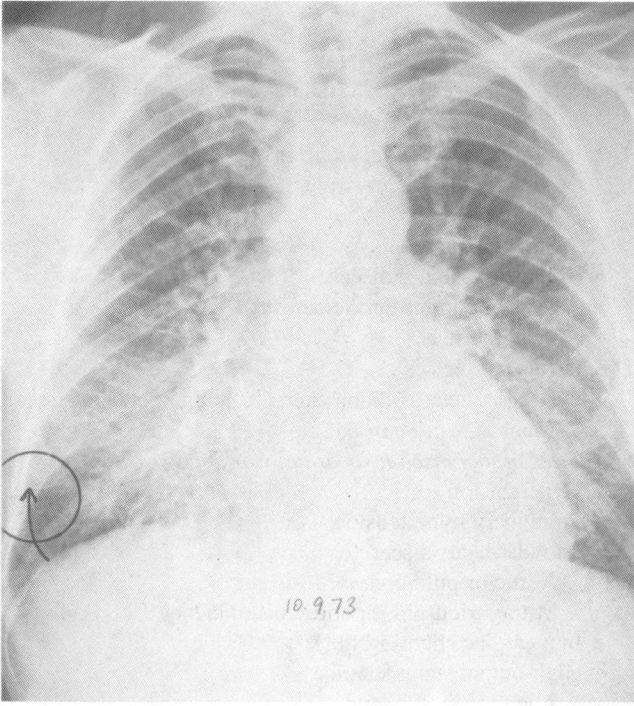

Figure 1-37 Interstitial edema. Hilar areas are blurred and hazy. Cardiac silhouette is enlarged. Fluid collected within intralobular septa of lungs is visible as Kerley-B lines *(arrow)*. (Courtesy Batra P, Department of Radiology, UCLA School of Medicine, Los Angeles.)

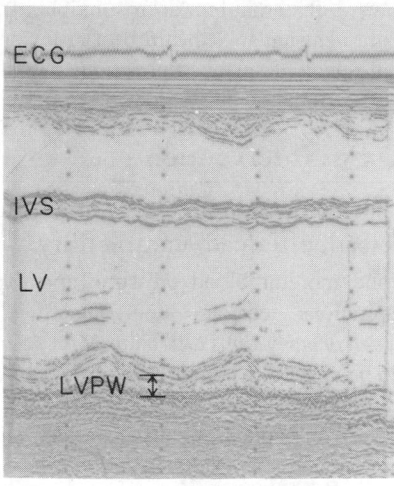

Figure 1-38 Patient with dilated left ventricle (6.7 cm) and normal intraventricular septum (1 cm). (Courtesy Non Invasive Labs, Division of Cardiology, UCLA School of Medicine, Los Angeles.)

Hemodynamic monitoring (right heart catheterization)
Left ventricular failure: elevated PCWP and pulmonary artery diastolic pressure (PADP), decreased CO, decreased ejection fractions; right ventricular failure: elevated pulmonary artery pressure (PAP), right ventricular pressure, and right atrial pressure (RAP)

•••••• Multidisciplinary Plan

Surgery

Directed by underlying condition; mortality is greater among patients with left ventricular dysfunction
Coronary revascularization
Dynamic cardiomyoplasty
Cardiac transplantation may be considered as an option for end-stage myocardial dysfunction

Medications

Diuretics—reduce sodium retention by inhibiting the reabsorption of sodium or chloride at specific sites in the renal tubules
Thiazide diuretics (hydrochlorothiazide)—may be used for mild volume overload; usual dosage 25-50 mg
Loop diuretics—used for more severe volume overload or persistent edema despite thiazide diuretics
Usual dosage: Furosemide (Lasix) 10-40 mg qd to 240 mg bid
  Bumetanide (Bumex) 0.5-1.0 mg qd to 10 mg qd
  Ethacrynic acid (Edecrin) 50 mg qd to 200 mg bid
Potassium-sparing diuretics—may be more effective than oral potassium supplements at maintaining total body potassium stores

Usual dosage: Spironolactone (Aldactone): 25 mg qd to 100 mg bid
  Amiloride (Midamor): 5-40 mg qd
Thiazide-related diuretic (metolazone)—potent diuretic used for refractory volume overload despite increased doses of loop diuretics
Usual dosage: 2.5-10 mg qd
Angiotensin-converting enzyme (ACE) inhibitors—should be used in patients with left ventricular dysfunction as primary afterload-reducing agent; shown to reduce mortality and improve functional class
Usual dosage: Captopril (Capoten) 6.25-100 mg tid
  Enalapril (Vasotec) 2.5-20 mg bid
  Lisinopril (Prinivil) 5-40 mg qd
  Quinapril (Accupril) 5-20 mg bid
Side effects: hypotension, hyperkalemia, renal insufficiency, cough
Digoxin—increased cardiac contractility and cardiac output; shown to improve physical function and decrease symptoms of heart failure in some studies
Usual dosage: 0.125-0.25 mg qd
Hydralazine/isosorbide dinitrate—alternative in patients with contraindications or intolerance of ACE inhibitors, or refractory hypertension or CHF
Usual dosage: Hydralazine 10-100 mg tid
  Side effects: headache, nausea, dizziness, lupuslike syndrome
Usual dosage: Isosorbide dinitrate 10-80 mg tid
  Side effects: Headache, hypotension, flushing
Beta-blocker therapy—studies are currently evaluating the efficacy of beta blockade in improving the functional status and natural history in patients with heart failure. Although still experimental, this form of therapy in combination with ACE inhibition in stabilized heart failure patients looks promising
Intravenous inotropic therapy—to increase renal blood flow and facilitate diuresis in patients with severe heart failure
Dobutamine—increases contractility, cardiac output
  Usual dosage: 2-15 μg/kg/min; in stable patient, may be used in home care setting infused through a long-term central venous port as a bridge to cardiac transplantation
Dopamine—increases systemic vascular resistance
  Usual dosage: 2-10 μg/kg/min
Amrinone lactate—phosphodiesterase inhibitor; increases contractility and peripheral vasodilation
  Usual dosage: 5-10 μg/kg/min
Milrinone—similar to amrinone
  Usual dosage: 0.375-0.75 μg/kg/min
Vesnarinone—mild phosphodiesterase inhibitor activity, slows heart rate, antidysrhythmic effects; still experimental, studies are promising at dose levels of 60 mg/d

General Management

Intraaortic balloon pump (IABP)—counterpulsation device that assists failing heart by decreasing afterload and increasing coronary artery perfusion (p. 106 gives further discussion)

Hemodynamic monitoring (PAP, PCWP, SVR, CO/CI)—initiated as a direct means of assessing hemodynamic status of heart and effectiveness of treatment; also assists in direction of therapy

Ventricular assist devices (VAD), right or left—mechanical devices that decrease work of the myocardium while maintaining systemic pressure. Positioned outside the body or implanted into the abdomen, VAD works as an artificial pump to maintain circulation so the heart can rest and recover

Electrocardiogram—used to assess for drug-induced dysrhythmias and for dysrhythmias induced by an underlying disorder

Bed rest—head of bed elevated to 45 degrees to reduce myocardial oxygen demand and decrease circulating volume returning to the heart

Restriction of sodium and water; weighing daily to monitor fluid retention

Sodium-restricted diet—4 g is "no added salt," 2 g is all salt eliminated from cooking

Oxygen therapy—initiated if patient is hypoxic

NURSING CARE

Nursing Assessment

General Complaints

- Dyspnea owing to increased pulmonary venous and interstitial pressures; variations; dyspnea on exertion (DOE), orthopnea, paroxysmal nocturnal dyspnea (PND)
- Fatigue: moderate to severe owing to diminished cardiac output
- Skin: pallor, diaphoresis
- Gastrointestinal symptoms resulting from splanchnic congestion: anorexia, nausea, vomiting, abdominal distention, right upper quadrant pain

Physical Examination

- Decreased cardiac output: fatigue, tachycardia, pulsus alternans, weak thready pulse, hypotension, narrowed pulse pressure, pallor, diaphoresis, cool and clammy skin, altered mental status, dizziness, syncope, decreased urine output
- Increased pulmonary capillary pressure: rapid labored respiration, cough, frothy or blood-tinged sputum, moist rales on pulmonary auscultation, left ventricular S_3 and systolic murmur at apex on cardiac auscultation, precordial movement—displaced apical impulse and palpable thrills
- Increased right atrial pressure: weight gain, elevated jugular venous pressure (rise in a and v waves), hepatojugular reflex, precordial movement (right ventricular impulse along lower left sternal border or subxiphoid), on auscultation right ventricular S_3 heard best at lower left sternal border; presence of systolic murmur, hepatomegaly, splenomegaly, peripheral edema, dilation of peripheral veins

Nursing Dx & Intervention

Decreased cardiac output related to mechanical factors (preload, afterload, contractility)

- Assess and monitor blood pressure, apical pulse, heart rate, respirations, heart and lung sounds q4h *or as indicated to detect early signs and symptoms of decreased CO.*
- Maintain bed rest *to conserve energy and decrease oxygen demand.* Elevate head of bed 30 to 60 degrees. Lean patient forward on padded over-bed table *to facilitate ventilation and decrease workload of breathing.*
- Monitor hemodynamic parameters as ordered *to evaluate patient's clinical status and response to therapy.* Blood pressure and arterial pressures reflect tissue perfusion. Pulmonary artery pressure, pulmonary capillary wedge pressure, and cardiac output reflect LVEDP and myocardial contractility.
- Administer drug therapy as ordered. Monitor for signs of drug toxicity.
- Monitor ECG rate and rhythm *to detect early dysrhythmias.*
- Limit IV fluids as ordered *to prevent circulatory overload.*
- Restrict activities as indicated. Plan care *to prevent fatigue, which increases oxygen demand.* Provide rest periods between procedures.

Impaired gas exchange related to elevated alveolar-capillary membrane changes caused by increased pulmonary capillary pressure

- Assess and monitor for changes in respiratory function *to detect signs and symptoms of impaired ventilation or perfusion:* restlessness, confusion, somnolence, hypoxia, and hypercapnia.
- Monitor arterial blood gas *to identify hypoxemia and hypercapnia.*
- Administer oxygen therapy as ordered, via nasal prongs, mask, or positive-pressure device.
- Administer morphine sulfate IV per protocol *to reduce hyperventilation.*
- Elevate head of bed *to enhance ventilation.*
- Auscultate breath sounds every hour *to detect increases in congestion and determine adequacy of ventilatory effort.*
- Prepare for intubation and assisted ventilation if required.
- Explain all procedures and modalities briefly to patient *to prevent hyperventilation resulting from fear or anxiety.*

Fluid volume excess related to increased systemic venous congestion or right ventricular failure

- Assess and monitor increased or decreased jugular venous distention; assess and monitor intake and output *to detect signs of fluid retention.*

- Auscultate heart sounds and breath sounds every 1 to 2 hours *to detect increased congestion and response to treatment.*
- Maintain patent IV for drug administration.
- Administer rapid-acting diuretics as ordered *to decrease circulating volume.*
- Restrict sodium and fluid intake *to control sodium reabsorption.*
- Weigh patient daily (same time of day, same amount of clothing) *to determine fluid loss or retention.*
- Monitor intake and output; report output of less than 30 ml/h.
- Monitor serum electrolytes, especially sodium and potassium.

Altered nutrition: less than body requirements, related to impaired absorption of nutrients, secondary to low cardiac output; to increased catabolic rate, secondary to increased myocardial demands

- Observe daily for signs of malnutrition: dry body weight 20% less than ideal weight for age, height, and body size; decreased triceps skinfold measurements; stomatitis; anorexia; increasing fatigue and weakness; decreased serum albumin, transferrin, and BUN levels.
- Weigh patient daily: upon rising, after voiding, with same clothing *to obtain consistent and accurate body weight.*
- Maintain diet as ordered. Do not force patient to eat, but offer small frequent meals, tempt appetite with food preferences compatible with diet restrictions and cultural values, and supplement with high-caloric feedings as indicated *to maintain minimum required caloric intake.*
- Administer antiemetics and analgesics before meals *to ensure patient's comfort and improve appetite.*
- Initiate caloric count if patient's nutritional status fails to improve. Obtain dietary consultation *to evaluate nutritional status and assist patient in selection of foods.*

Impaired skin integrity related to altered circulation, metabolic state, and immobility

- Assess skin integrity, noting color, texture, temperature, and signs of redness, scaling, breaks, or ulcerations.
- If patient is on bed rest, turn and reposition every 2 to 4 hours *to relieve pressure areas and improve circulation, muscle tone, and joint mobility.*
- Administer skin care daily. Massage bony pressure areas *to increase tissue perfusion to affected areas. To avoid causing skin excoriations,* do not massage reddened areas.
- Anticipate and initiate preventive measures for a patient considered at high risk for skin breakdown: a cachectic, debilitated, or edematous patient who is immobile.
- Use alternative preventive measures *to ensure skin integrity as indicated:* air pressure bed, alternating pressure mattress, sheepskin.

- Prevent and eliminate pressure and friction. Position pillows or other supports between pressure areas *to prevent friction, abrasions, and rubbing of two skin areas.*
- Keep skin dry when diaphoretic *because moisture contributes to skin breakdown and infection.*
- Initiate aggressive decubitus care at first sign of reddened areas, tissue breakdown, or ulceration *because decubiti can develop in a matter of hours.*

Activity intolerance related to weakness secondary to decreased CO

- Assess and monitor for signs of activity intolerance.
- Check BP, HR, and respiration before and after activity because *orthostatic hypotension can result from prolonged periods of bed rest.*
- Identify factors known to cause fatigue. Restrict or limit activities as indicated *to promote energy conservation.*
- Space treatment and procedures to allow for periods of uninterrupted rest *to ensure periods of complete rest.*
- Implement measures that will improve activity tolerance by minimizing fatigue *to limit or reduce energy expenditure.*

Patient Education/Home Care Planning

Instruction is directed toward long-term maintenance of the therapeutic program.
1. Describe the disease process, the underlying cause, and any precipitating factors.
2. Discuss with the patient the need to report symptoms of increased failure to physician: dyspnea on exertion, cough, paroxysmal nocturnal dyspnea, and decreased exercise tolerance.
3. Explain to the patient the need to limit strenuous physical activity and avoid fatigue.
4. Explain to the patient the need to limit the intake of salt in the diet and avoid foods that have a high sodium content; instruct the patient in label reading. Provide information about alternative ways to season food.
5. Discuss with the patient the need to weigh daily in the morning before the first meal with the same scale and wearing the same clothing and to report weight gain of more than 2 pounds in 24 hours.
6. Ensure that the patient can name and describe methods of administering drugs and their potential side effects.
7. Instruct the patient to avoid alcoholic beverages and refrain from inhaling passive cigarette smoke.
8. Emphasize and reevaluate patient compliance to medical regimen as an important variable for future referral for cardiac transplantation.
9. Perform home care monitoring as indicated, especially for outpatient IV inotropic support.

Evaluation

Ventricular function is improved   Heart rate and pulmonary capillary wedge pressure (PCWP) are decreased. Cardiac output is increased. Mental status is improved. Urine output is increased.

Fluid overload is decreased   Patient loses weight. Jugular venous distention is decreased. Breath sounds are improved. Peripheral edema is decreased.

Gas exchange is improved   Lung sounds are clear. Anxiety level is diminished. Orthopnea and dyspnea are reduced. Hypoxemia and hypercarbia are absent. Respirations are improved.

Knowledge level is increased   Patient verbalizes knowledge regarding importance of daily weight, taking prescribed medication, activity allowances and limitations, and dietary restrictions.

Anxiety level is decreased   Patient appears relaxed. Patient demonstrates ability to rest and sleep without complaints. Patient verbalizes fears regarding disease process, asking appropriate questions.

Skin integrity is maintained   Skin: intact, warm, dry; signs of healing over areas of breakdown.

Nutritional status is improved   Dry body weight normal or improved for age and body build.

SHOCK (HYPOVOLEMIC, VASOGENIC, CARDIOGENIC)

Shock is an abnormal physical state that is the first phase of the body's alarm reaction to stress (Figure 1-39).

Shock occurs most commonly as an extreme syndrome linked to abnormal cellular metabolism, which in most cases is caused by inadequate tissue perfusion. If shock is untreated, circulatory collapse and impaired cellular metabolism develop, eventually leading to death.

•••••• **Pathophysiology**

Various methods of classifying shock have been used. The following four categories based on causes are commonly used in the clinical setting:

Hypovolemic
   Loss of blood volume (hemorrhage)
   Loss of plasma volume (dehydration)
Vasogenic
   Sepsis
   Immune mediated (anaphylaxis)
   Deep anesthesia effects

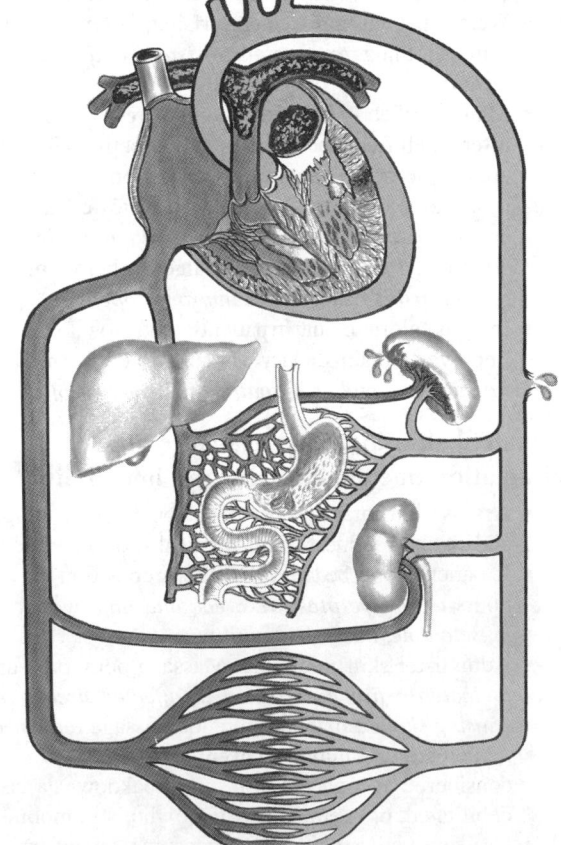

Figure 1-39 Shock.
From Canobbio.[17]

Primary insufficiency of cardiac output	Hypovolemia
A. Infarction	A. Hemorrhagic loss of blood
Myocarditis	Loss of plasma
Rupture of valve cusps	Burns
Rupture of chordae tendineae	Dehydration
B. Pericardial tamponade	Heat exhaustion
Embolism	B. Severe infection
Obstruction by thrombus	Anaphylaxis
Tachycardias	Pain
Dysrhythmias (severe)	Heat stroke

Figure 1-39 Shock. (From Canobbio.[13])

Cardiogenic
  Acute myocardial infarction
  Other causes (pulmonary emboli, cardiac surgery, tamponade)

Hypovolemic Shock

Hypovolemic shock, or "cold" shock, results from a decrease in intravascular volume and generally occurs when there is also a deficit involving at least 15% of the total blood volume. Hypovolemia is the most common cause of hypotension in critically ill patients, particularly in the postoperative phase.

Hypovolemic shock may be caused by excessive loss of plasma volume as occurs in burns or pancreatitis when extracellular fluid is sequestered in injured or inflamed tissue cells. Severe dehydration and hypovolemia may also be caused by diabetic ketoacidosis, extreme vomiting, or diarrhea. The most common cause of hypovolemic shock, however, is excessive blood loss through damage to a major blood vessel or organ such as the kidney, spleen, or liver; through injury or disease of the gastrointestinal system, such as rupture of esophageal varices; or through ruptured aneurysms.

The severity of hypovolemic shock is related to the amount and rate of volume loss. If volume is replaced quickly, the shock state can be easily reversed. If low aortic pressures last longer than 60 minutes, the process may be irreversible.

The major hemodynamic changes linked to fluid loss are low cardiac output, increased systemic vascular resistance, and decreased central venous pressure. The patient usually has cool clammy skin, increased heart and respiratory rates, and decreased urine output, owing to compensatory vasoconstriction. The blood pressure may be normal or low, particularly in the early phase of cold shock.

Vasogenic Shock

Unlike hypovolemic shock, which leads to vasoconstriction, vasogenic shock results in massive vasodilation from an increase in total vascular capacity. Circulating volume is lost because of venous pooling, increased capillary permeability, and third spacing of fluid. If intravascular volume is not replaced, hypovolemia occurs. Whereas a patient with hypovolemia has cold extremities as a result of vasoconstriction, a patient with vasogenic shock has warm extremities, giving rise to the term *warm shock*. Warm shock is present in 30% to 50% of patients in the early phase of septic shock.

Sepsis is the most common form of vasogenic shock, but it may also occur as a result of other factors, including food allergies and anaphylactic reactions to drugs and insect stings.

Septic shock is commonly related to the release of bacterial endotoxins after a gram-negative bacterial infection. The organisms most often found in septic shock are the gram-negative bacteria *Escherichia coli, Klebsiella, Enterobacter, Pseudomonas, Serratia, Proteus,* and *Bacteroides fragilis;* the gram-positive bacteria *Staphylococcus, Pneumococcus,* and α- or β-*Streptococcus;* and the fungus *Candida.* Many are a part of the natural body flora or are commonly present in hospitals. The microbes linked to the highest death rate are *Proteus, Pseudomonas, Candida,* and *B. fragilis.* Although patients in critical care units are the most likely to acquire infections in the hospital, patients in general hospital units are also vulnerable. Patients particularly susceptible to septic shock are the elderly, immunosuppressed patients, patients who have indwelling catheters (urinary, intravenous, or intracardiac) or urinary tract infection, patients who have had surgery of the digestive tract or urinary tract, and patients who have undergone manipulative instrumentation.

Although deaths from septic shock have decreased since the 1960s, the death rate continues to be as high as 50%. This is the result of several factors, the most striking of which are the changing pattern of microbial resistance to antimicrobial agents[10] and the rapidly changing nature of microbes.

Certain hemodynamic changes have been recognized as probable causes of septic shock. In early phases a hyperdynamic state exists in which the cardiac output, stroke volume, and heart rate are increased and the systemic vascular resistance and central venous pressure are decreased. The patient appears warm, dry, and flushed because of generalized vasodilation and venous pooling. This state is probably caused by the effects of various substances released by exotoxins or from the injured or infected tissue.

The circulatory changes combined with the decreased systemic vascular resistance may stimulate a sympathetic response. This causes the increased heart rate and maintenance of normal blood pressure that occur during this warm shock phase.

If hyperdynamic shock continues, the continued increase in capillary leaking increases hypovolemia to the point that the process converts to a hypodynamic phase known as the cold phase of septic shock. In this state the systemic vascular resistance increases, cardiac output drops, and the patient appears cold, pale, and clammy. The cause of this change is related to ineffective circulating blood volume, sympathetic vasoconstriction, and pump failure.

In *anaphylactic reactions* from drugs, insect stings, or food allergies, the mechanism involved is an antibody-antigen interaction that provokes the release of chemicals such as histamine. These mediators act mainly on the vascular membranes and smooth muscles. Histamine release causes veins and arterioles to dilate, decreasing cardiac output and arterial pressure. Histamine also increases capillary permeability, causing fluid to escape from the intravascular compartment into the interstitial space. The result is volume depletion; however, while plasma water is removed from the capillaries, the red cells remain and the hemoglobin levels and hematocrit values rise. The immediate reactions in anaphylaxis are pharyngeal and laryngeal edema, probably because of the effects of histamines, and bronchoconstriction with the immediate threat of death from asphyxiation.

Deep anesthesia can cause severe depression of the vasomotor centers of the brain, which may result in vasomotor collapse and venous pooling. These responses decrease venous return to the heart and diminish cardiac output.

Cardiogenic Shock

Cardiogenic shock occurs when the heart cannot maintain enough output to meet the body's demands (Figure 1-40).

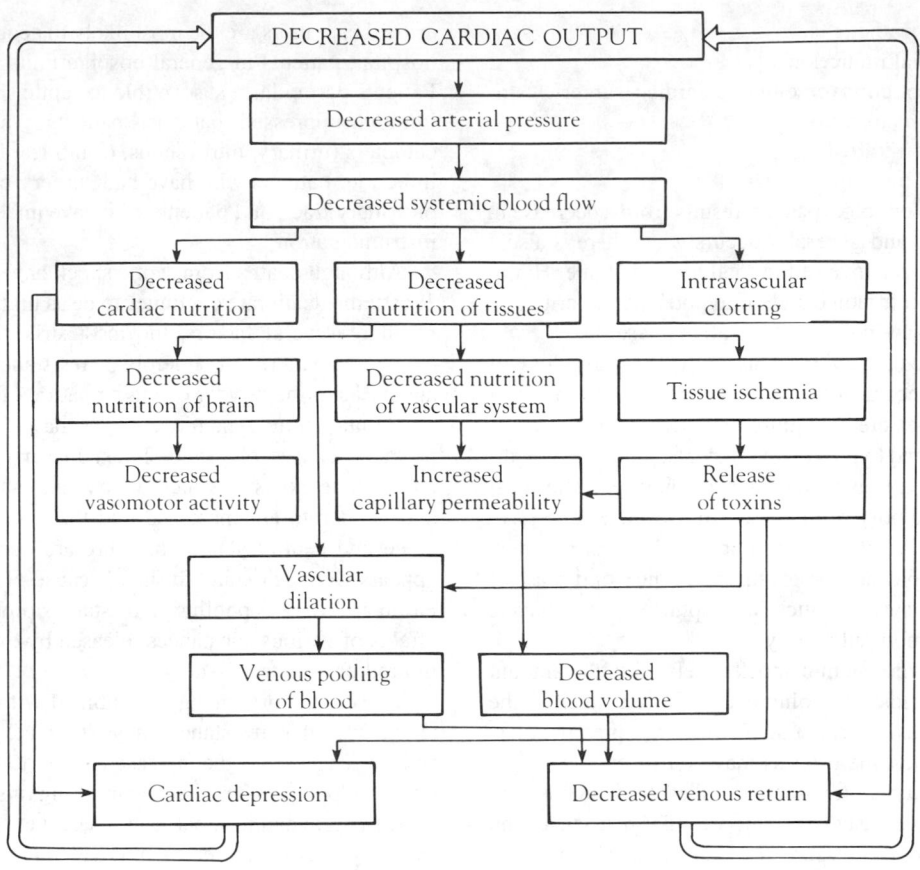

Figure 1-40 Different types of feedback that can lead to progression of shock. (Modified by Guyton.[39])

Myocardial infarction is the most common cause of cardiogenic shock, but it also may be the result of a variety of other cardiac disorders: acute myocarditis, end-stage cardiomyopathy (dilated, hypertrophic, or restrictive), valvular heart disease (ruptured papillary muscle), cardiac tamponade, acute ventricular septal defect, and prolonged cardiopulmonary bypass. Other causes include pulmonary embolism and tension pneumothorax. The major feature of cardiogenic shock is inadequate tissue perfusion and oxygen delivery resulting from a severely impaired ventricle.

The incidence of cardiogenic shock resulting from myocardial infarction is 10% to 15%, with a mortality rate exceeding 80%. The higher mortality rates are seen in hospitals without facilities for intraaortic balloon pumping, high-risk angioplasty, and surgical revascularization. Accordingly, current therapies focus on early aggressive intervention to reduce ischemia and limit permanent myocardial damage.

In patients with myocardial infarction, shock develops as a result of abnormal reflexes arising from the ischemic myocardium. The inability to increase systemic vascular resistance makes it difficult to maintain an adequate arterial pressure. This leads to hypoperfusion to an already ischemic myocardium, causing further insufficiency of the pumping action of the left ventricle. Failure of the left ventricle to generate enough energy to pump blood into the systemic circulation further decreases perfusion and myocardial oxygen supply.

Cardiogenic shock has been linked to the destruction of 40% or more of left ventricular muscle. The mechanism of cardiogenic shock is complex, with a vicious cycle of changes that lead rapidly to further deterioration of cardiac function. If left untreated, the reduction in tissue blood flow and oxygen delivery to the myocardium results in circulatory collapse, impaired cellular metabolism, and eventual death.

Compensatory Mechanisms of Shock

A number of compensatory mechanisms are activated when arterial pressure and tissue perfusion are reduced. These mechanisms are controlled by the sympathetic nervous system and the release of endogenous vasoconstrictors and hormonal substances.[71]

Baroreceptors   A reduction in mean arterial pressure and pulse pressure is sensed by baroreceptors in the carotid sinus and aortic arch. By secreting epinephrine and norepinephrine, they produce a generalized sympathetic stimulation, resulting in increased peripheral vascular resistance, arterial pressure, and myocardial contractility.

Fluid shifts   The major endogenous vasoactive substances released during shock are catecholamines and vasopressin, which augment sympathetic activity when activated further. The release of these substances also reduces vascular capacity, which eases the osmotic movement of interstitial fluid into the vascular compartments to restore blood volume.

Renin-angiotensin-aldosterone system When renal ischemia occurs, the renin-angiotensin-aldosterone system is activated to help maintain blood pressure and intravascular volume. Reducing renal perfusion pressure results in the release of renin, which in time is converted to angiotensin II, a powerful vasoconstrictor. Angiotensin II stimulates the release of aldosterone, which enhances sodium and water reabsorption by the renal tubules to help maintain intravascular volume.

Antidiuretic hormone The release of antidiuretic hormone (ADH) from the posterior pituitary gland in response to hypotension plays a role in volume regulation during circulatory shock. ADH enhances reabsorption of sodium and water by increasing permeability of the renal tubules.

Progressive Shock

If the compensatory mechanisms cannot restore effective perfusion to vital organs, circulatory function deteriorates further, leading to a cycle of changes that decrease cardiac output. Figure 1-40 illustrates some of the changes that contribute to decreased cardiac output and circulatory collapse.

Cell deterioration As shock becomes severe, local changes in cellular metabolism occur. Prolonged tissue ischemia results in incomplete oxidation at the cellular level, diminishing mitochondrial activity. Adenosine triphosphate (ATP) stores then begin to be used, and the cells resort to anaerobic metabolism of glucose to provide energy. This process of glycolysis produces lactic acid, which builds up in the blood. The effects of an acidic pH include depressed myocardial function and a decreased vascular response to epinephrine and norepinephrine, leading to vasomotor collapse late in shock.[8,25]

Another significant cellular change resulting from continued ischemia is the release of vasoactive metabolites into the circulation. Substances such as bradykinin, histamine, serotonin, and prostaglandins, along with decreased vascular tone, lead to increases in venous pooling and capillary permeability. Excessive vasodilation then decreases venous return and cardiac filling. The increased permeability of the capillaries allows large quantities of fluid to escape into the interstitial spaces.

Organ and Tissue Changes

As the shock syndrome becomes severe, generalized organ deterioration begins.

Renal function Although reduced renal perfusion activates certain compensatory mechanisms, in the early phases of shock, prolonged decreased renal blood flow leads to ischemia and acute tubular necrosis. This is marked by fluid, electrolyte, and metabolic disturbances.

Pulmonary function Ischemia to the pulmonary circulation in the early phases of shock can damage pulmonary function to cause adult respiratory distress syndrome. Damage to the pulmonary capillary endothelial cells increases capillary permeability. This leads to interstitial and alveolar edema that impairs gas exchange. The resulting hypoxemia and respiratory acidosis further reduce tissue oxygen delivery and organ function.

Gastrointestinal function Ischemic damage to the digestive tract causes a loss of the protective mucosal covering in the intestine. This can lead to intestinal damage and necrosis by digestive enzymes. It may also account for the release of bacteria and toxins into the bloodstream, causing sepsis and further circulatory problems.

The reticuloendothelial system may also be damaged during shock, impairing the patient's ability to withstand infection.

Intravascular clotting As the products of cell deterioration begin to accumulate in the capillaries and vasodilation occurs, blood flow becomes sluggish. The stagnation, along with local chemical changes in the capillaries, leads to blood aggregation and intravascular clotting. The formation of microemboli enhances tissue ischemia by further decreasing blood flow through the capillaries. This hypercoagulability response may occur as an early compensatory mechanism, particularly with hemorrhage. In the late stages of shock, however, a reversal in clotting occurs, leading to a hypocoagulability state. This results from loss in clotting factors through bleeding or decreased production caused by poor tissue perfusion. It may also be the result of a consumption of clotting factors that occurs in disseminated intravascular coagulation.

Myocardial depression Except with cardiogenic shock, the major cardiac effects of shock occur in the late stage and are by far the most important factor in the deterioration caused by shock. As arterial pressure continues to drop, so does coronary blood flow. This leads to depressed myocardial function and a further reduction in cardiac output. Myocardial contractility is depressed further by the combined effects of toxins, acidosis, and tissue hypoxia that results from cell deterioration. Thus circulatory failure is a syndrome that involves all systems, and it is usually the deterioration of heart function that makes shock irreversible.

•••••• Diagnostic Studies and Findings

Hematocrit Decreased; however, in hypovolemia, may be increased because of intravascular fluid shift

Hemoglobin Decreased in hemorrhage

White blood cell count with differential Increased; leukopenia in gram-negative sepsis; leukocytosis with increased neutrophils in all forms of shock

Erythrocyte sedimentation rate Increase in response to tissue injury

Cultures (blood [obtain two to four cultures before initiation of antibiotic therapy], urine, sputum); positive growth of an organism

Serum electrolytes Sodium: increased during diuretic phase of acute tubular necrosis, decreased with administration of hypotonic fluid after fluid loss; potassium: increased with cellular death during oliguric phase, in acidosis, and after transfusion reactions

Serum chemistry BUN, creatinine: increased, reflecting impaired renal function; lactate levels: increased; glucose levels: increased in early shock, reflecting release of liver glycogen stores in response to catecholamines

Prothrombin time (PT), partial thromboplastin time (PTT)   Prolonged

Arterial blood gases   Respiratory alkalosis; metabolic acidosis

Urine studies   Specific gravity: increased in response to action of ADH and during oliguric phase; osmolality: high during oliguric phase; sodium: decreased

Electrocardiogram (ECG) (12-lead continuous monitoring)   To determine changes in heart rate and rhythm and ischemic changes

Chest x-ray   To determine pulmonary status and rule out other causes of shock state: early—normal; late—shows signs of pulmonary congestion

Hemodynamic monitoring (pulmonary artery pressure, pulmonary capillary wedge pressure, cardiac output)   To provide information regarding serial changes in left ventricular function in response to specific treatments, such as fluid replacement and vasoactive agents

Echocardiography   Noninvasive method of sorting out etiology of shock; also provides information on regional and global systolic wall function, valvular integrity, and presence or absence of pericardial effusion

•••••• Multidisciplinary Plan

Medications

Fluid-volume regulation   Except with patients in cardiogenic shock, restoration of intravascular volume is the most significant therapeutic intervention, particularly in the early phases of therapy.

Volume replacement should be initiated rapidly with 3 to 5 L of saline or other volume expanders over a 30- to 60-minute period. Ringer's lactate provides effective intravascular expansion and is the usual fluid of choice; however, a buffered solution with lactate may be used for severe shock.

Regulation of fluids should be based on hemodynamic response to the rapid fluid infusion. Careful monitoring of mean arterial pressure, pulmonary capillary wedge pressure (PCWP), pulmonary artery end-diastolic pressure (PAEDP), or central venous pressure (CVP), and urine output is used to guide fluid replacement.

Blood plasma expanders should be given after the initial volume deficit is corrected. In cases of massive hemorrhage, replacement should be with whole blood if the hematocrit value is less than 30%. If the hematocrit value is greater than 30%, plasma expanders may be given. Packed cells are used if the right atrial pressure or PCWP is elevated and in cases such as cardiogenic shock in which myocardial dysfunction limits the amount and speed of fluid replacement.

In a patient in shock after acute myocardial infarction, volume deficits may occur and fluid replacement may be necessary to restore a depressed cardiac output to normal. Continuous monitoring of the PCWP is the most precise method of determining volume deficits. If the PCWP is below the desired level of 15 to 18 mm Hg, fluid replacement may be given to increase cardiac output (Starling's law). The PCWP should be kept below 18 mm Hg to prevent pulmonary congestion.

If the PCWP of a patient in shock is elevated, fluid replacement is contraindicated and diuretics may be necessary to return the PCWP to therapeutic range. Diuretics are generally given only to patients in cardiogenic shock with an elevated PCWP. They reduce preload through their effect on venous capacitance and decrease total circulating fluid.

Maintenance of adequate hemodynamic state   In shock, myocardial dysfunction develops as a result of workload, limited coronary blood flow, and decreased myocardial oxygenation. Sympathomimetic agents are used to maintain an adequate hemodynamic state. The effects of these agents are mediated through the action of α- and β-adrenergic receptors. α-Receptors in the smooth muscle of the vascular bed cause vasoconstriction, thereby increasing peripheral resistance and venous return. By contrast, β_1-receptors are located in the myocardium, arteries, and lungs. Myocardial β_1-receptors act to increase heart rate and contractility, whereas activation of β_2-receptors causes vasodilation.

The various adrenergic drugs differ with respect to their relative α (peripheral) and β (peripheral, myocardial) effects. The rationale for selecting any drug depends on the specific vascular bed on which the drug acts and the desired cardiovascular effect. In cardiogenic shock, for example, drugs with positive inotropic and vasoconstrictor properties are used to increase cardiac output by augmenting myocardial contractility and to improve blood flow to vital organs by increasing total vascular resistance. Dopamine, norepinephrine, and epinephrine, which have both constrictor and inotropic properties, are commonly used in treatment of cardiogenic shock.

The following agents are most commonly used in the treatment of patients with shock.

Adrenergic drugs.   Dopamine (Intropin) is one of the most widely used drugs in the treatment of shock. Its effects depend on the dose used. In low doses (2 to 5 μg/kg/min) it produces dilation of renal, mesenteric, coronary, and cerebral blood vessels. In higher doses (6 to 15 μg/kg/min) it improves cardiac output by increasing contractility (β effect) but has no effect on blood pressure. At therapeutic levels (10 to 15 μg/kg/min) dopamine increases cardiac output and blood pressure with little change or reduction in pulmonary vascular resistance. The increase in blood pressure is due primarily to an enhanced cardiac output. In addition, the vasodilator effect on renal blood vessels increases renal blood flow, which improves urine output. In very high doses (>20 μg/kg/min) dopamine causes generalized vasoconstriction (α effect), which opposes the desired vasodilator effect obtained with lower doses. Infusions should be started with low doses (3 to 5 μg/kg/min), increasing slowly until optimum arterial pressure is achieved.

Dobutamine (Dobutrex) is used primarily for its inotropic effect. It stimulates β_1-receptors to increase myocardial contractility and stroke volume, resulting in improved cardiac output. Because dobutamine has minimal β_2 and α effects, it produces little change in blood pressure and heart rate; however, systolic blood pressure may be increased because of increased cardiac output. Coronary blood flow and myocardial oxygen consumption (MVo_2) are also increased because of increased myocardial contractility. Infusions begin at 2 to 4 µg/kg/min, with therapeutic doses between 2.5 and 10 µg/kg/min.

Amrinone is a nonglycoside that also is used primarily for its inotropic effect. It inhibits phosphodiesterase (PDE) II activity, which increases myocardial contractility and vasodilation. Infusion begins at 0.75 mg/kg as a bolus over 2 to 3 minutes, with a maintenance infusion of 5 to 10 mg/kg/min.

Epinephrine is a potent β- and α-catecholamine causing vasoconstriction of the splanchnic and renal beds. Although it does increase cardiac output, its effects on peripheral resistance do not favor redistribution of blood flow to vital organs. It is also considered less advantageous than other adrenergic drugs because it increases automaticity, which can initiate serious dysrhythmias.

Norepinephrine has both α and β actions. It increases myocardial contractility by stimulating β_1-receptors and causes arteriovenous constriction by stimulating α-receptors. Thus norepinephrine increases systemic arterial pressure by increasing the cardiac output and peripheral vascular resistance. Once again the actual hemodynamic effects depend on the dose employed. With small doses a β effect predominates, causing slight increases in blood pressure and cardiac output. With very high doses norepinephrine produces significant vasoconstriction, causing an increased systemic resistance and blood pressure. However, the cardiac output may fall despite the positive inotropic effect. The usual starting dose is 2 to 8 µg per minute. Norepinephrine should be administered through an indwelling catheter placed in a large vein because it is known to cause tissue necrosis with extravasation. The disadvantage of this drug is its vasoconstricting effect on the kidneys, which can result in impaired renal perfusion and oliguria.

Isoproterenol (Isuprel) acts as a peripheral dilator through β_2 stimulation. More important is the β_1 effect, which augments myocardial contractility and heart rate, thereby improving cardiac output. However, it may cause a substantial increase in myocardial oxygen demand, which can exacerbate myocardial ischemia in a patient with cardiogenic shock.

Cardiac glycosides. The role of digitalis in the treatment of shock is being questioned. It has been noted that inotropic drugs such as digoxin become less effective as the degree of left ventricular failure increases. As an inotropic agent for treatment of severe or cardiogenic shock, digitalis is relatively weak when compared with the sympathomimetic drugs. In addition, it could be hemodynamically detrimental because of the increased maximum venous oxygen produced by the increased contractility, as well as by the decrease in afterload associated with it. Furthermore, because of the impaired renal function, acidosis, and hypoxia occurring in shock states, the patient is predisposed to digitalis-induced dysrhythmias.[25]

Vasodilators. Vasodilator therapy is generally limited to patients with failing ventricular function and is still debated in the routine treatment of cardiogenic shock. However, it may be of use in patients with severe hypotension whose severe vasoconstriction continues despite volume replacement. Excessive

vasoconstriction, which occurs initially as a compensatory response to hypoperfusion, can reduce blood flow and oxygen delivery, as well as cause such a loss of intravascular volume that it leads to further reduction of cardiac output. The rationale for using vasodilator therapy in shock is to break this progressive positive-feedback cycle.

Vasodilator agents improve left ventricular function by decreasing myocardial oxygen demand through the reduction of preload and afterload. These drugs have no direct inotropic action on the heart. The increased cardiac output produced by vasodilators is caused by the changes in preload and afterload.

Arterial vasodilators are used to decrease peripheral vascular resistance, which then decreases resistance to left ventricular ejection and therefore afterload. Venodilators are used to increase venous capacitance, causing a decrease in venous return that decreases PCWP and preload.

The potential role of vasodilator therapy in cardiogenic shock merits further study. Although inappropriate as a single form of therapy, the use of vasodilators combined with external counterpulsation and other inotropic agents appears to be effective in providing efficient ventricular function. Nitroprusside and phentolamine are the vasodilator agents most commonly used in the treatment of cardiogenic shock.

Antihypertensive agents. Nitroprusside (Nipride, Nitropress) causes both arterial and venous dilation, thereby decreasing venous return and left ventricular filling (decreased preload), as well as resistance to left ventricular ejection (decreased afterload). The drug is administered intravenously with an initial dose of 0.5 to 10 µg/kg/min, which is increased in increments of 5 to 10 µg/kg/min every 5 minutes or until an improvement in hemodynamics is observed. Fluid replacement may be required if filling pressures drop excessively. Fluid volumes should be determined before administration of these agents. In hypovolemic patients, massive vasodilation only worsens the clinical picture by further decreasing venous return.

α-Adrenergic blocking agents. Phentolamine mesylate (Regitine) inhibits vasoconstriction by blocking α-adrenergic receptors. It lowers arterial pressure, thereby decreasing afterload. The drug is given intravenously at a dosage of 0.1 to 2 mg/min.

General Management

Intraaortic balloon pump (IABP) Counterpulsation is the most frequently used method of mechanically assisting circulation after profound cardiovascular collapse. Counterpulsation augments aortic pressure during diastole with subsequent reduction of afterload, thus effectively reducing the work of the myocardium and improving coronary blood flow.

The intraaortic balloon pump (IABP) is the most widely used counterpulsation technique. A catheter with a 10 to 50 cc balloon is inserted into the femoral artery and positioned in the thoracic aorta just distal to the left subclavian artery. With the ECG used for synchronization, the balloon is inflated during diastole and deflated during systole.

Ventricular assist device (VAD) VADs support failing left, right, or both ventricles. VADs approximate normal hemodynamic parameters, supporting circulation for several days.

NURSING CARE

Nursing Assessment

Area of Concern	Hypovolemic Shock	Cardiogenic Shock	Vasogenic Shock
General appearance	Anxiety, restlessness	Anxiety, restlessness	Anxiety, vertigo, restlessness
Level of consciousness	Lethargy, stupor, or coma	Lethargy, stupor, or coma	Lethargy, stupor, or coma
Temperature	Increased or decreased	Increased	Increased or decreased
Heart rate	Increased, pulse thready	Increased, pulse thready	Increased, pulse thready
Auscultation		S_3, S_4; murmurs	
Blood pressure			
Early	Pulse pressure decreased; diastolic pressure increased	Pulse pressure decreased; diastolic pressure increased	Normal; pulse pressure decreased
Late	Systolic pressure decreased	Systolic pressure decreased	Systolic pressure decreased
Skin temperature and texture	Cool, moist, clammy, pale	Cool, moist, clammy, pale, cyanosis	Early: warm, dry; late: cool, moist, clammy; color: pale, cyanosis (late)
Capillary refill time	Decreased	Decreased	Decreased
Peripheral pulses	Absent or diminished	Absent or diminished	Absent or diminished (late)
Jugular venous distention	Absent or flat	Elevated	
Hemodynamic findings			
Central venous pressure	Decreased	Increased	Decreased
Pulmonary capillary wedge pressure	Decreased	Increased	Decreased
Cardiac output	Decreased	Decreased	Increased or decreased
Peripheral vascular resistance	Decreased	Increased	Decreased or normal; late: increased
Pulmonary function			
Respiratory rate	Increased; shallow or Cheyne-Stokes respirations	Increased; late: Cheyne-Stokes respirations, apnea	Increased; late: Cheyne-Stokes respirations
Auscultation	Early: clear; late: rales	Rales	Early: clear; late: rales
Acid-base changes			
Early	Respiratory alkalosis	Respiratory alkalosis	Respiratory alkalosis
Late	Metabolic (lactic) acidosis	Metabolic (lactic) acidosis	Metabolic (lactic) acidosis
Urine output			
Early	Decreased (<20 ml/mm)	Decreased (<20 ml/mm)	Decreased (<20 ml/mm)
Late	Anuria	Anuria	Anuria
Urine sodium concentration	Decreased	Decreased	Decreased
Urine osmolality	Increased	Increased	Increased

Oxygenation   Ventilation/perfusion ratios should be determined early to ensure adequate ventilation. Oxygen exchange may be impaired in patients with shock, especially if cardiac output is decreased. Oxygen therapy should be given from the onset of treatment to maintain an arterial Po_2 of at least 80 mm Hg. Intubation may be indicated if arterial blood gases show worsening hypoxemia despite high oxygen concentrations. The indications for mechanical ventilation are a Pao_2 of less than 50 mm Hg while the patient is receiving oxygen concentrations of 50%, a vital capacity of less than 15 ml/kg body weight, a Pco_2 of greater than 45 mm Hg, and an arterial pH of less than 7.25.

Hemodynamic monitoring   For diagnostic information and evaluation of ongoing therapy, arterial pressures, pulmonary artery pressure (PAP), pulmonary artery diastolic pressures (PAD), and PCWP should be monitored initially every 5 to 10 minutes. A cardiac index of less than 2 L per minute is reflective of a shock state.

Nutrition   Patients in shock should receive nothing by mouth, but care must be taken to provide nutrition, preferably with total parenteral nutrition.

Acid-base balance   Frequent monitoring of acid-base balance is necessary to avert profound acidosis. Intravenous administration of sodium bicarbonate may be necessary to maintain or correct the pH to 7.35.

Renal function   Hourly urine output measurements with frequent checks are necessary to determine adequate kidney perfusion. Urine output of less than 30 ml per hour reflects inadequate renal perfusion. Elevated serum BUN and creatinine levels reflect renal dysfunction.

Activity   Efforts should be made to minimize energy expenditure. The patient should be maintained on complete bed rest in a supine position, with legs elevated to 45 degrees.

EMERGENCY ALERT

CARDIOGENIC SHOCK

Cardiogenic shock occurs when systolic blood pressure falls below 90 mm Hg during an acute myocardial infarction; this leads to pump failure. The heart cannot contract effectively and is unable to pump enough blood. Cardiogenic shock occurs in about 15% of patients with acute MI; 85% to 90% of these patients do not survive.

Assessment

- Signs of MI
- Decreased peripheral pulses
- Increased but shallow respirations
- Decreased blood pressure
- Altered level of consciousness, anxiety, or restlessness
- Clammy skin
- Decreased urinary output
- Acute metabolic acidosis
- ECG changes

Interventions

- Administer high-flow oxygen (10 to 15 L).
- Obtain IV access.
- Prepare to administer inotropic agents and vasodilators.

Nursing Dx & Intervention

Altered tissue perfusion (renal, cerebral, cardiopulmonary, and peripheral) related to decreased cardiac output (CO)

- Assess for signs and symptoms indicative of altered tissue perfusion: cool skin temperature, pale or cyanotic color, decreased arterial pulsations, altered mental status, decreased blood pressure, tachycardia, decreased urine output, thirst.
- Maintain complete bed rest *to minimize metabolic needs.*
- Maintain flat position or position that *facilitates or improves circulation.*
- Keep patient warm *to minimize metabolic needs.*
- Measure intake and output every 1 to 2 hours or as indicated *to evaluate renal function.*
- Administer parenteral therapy as ordered: whole blood, Plasmanate, and volume expanders.
- Check blood pressure and peripheral pulses every 1 to 2 hours as ordered *to assess tissue perfusion.*
- Apply support measures to control bleeding as indicated: pressure dressings, shock trousers.

Decreased cardiac output related to mechanical factors (preload, afterload, contractility)

- Assess and monitor for signs and symptoms indicative of decreased cardiac output: fatigue, skin pallor, diaphoresis, oliguria, anuria, hypotension, tachycardia.
- Maintain bed rest *to conserve energy and decrease oxygen demand.*

- Monitor hemodynamic parameters as ordered *to evaluate patient's clinical status and response to therapy:* blood pressure, arterial pressure, PAP, PCWP.
- Monitor and calculate cardiac output (CO) and cardiac index (CI) *to evaluate cardiac function.*
- Calculate systemic vascular resistance as ordered *to determine LV afterload.*
- Frequently assess cardiovascular response to drug therapy.
- Adjust flow and dosage according to blood pressure and heart rate response.
- Administer sympathomimetic and vasodilator drugs as ordered *to increase myocardial contractility and reduce peripheral vascular resistance (PVR).*
- Administer plasma volume expanders as ordered.
- Adjust flow rate according to PAP and PCWP readings.
- Restrict activities as indicated.
- Plan care *to prevent fatigue,* which increases oxygen demand.
- Initiate intraaortic balloon pumping (IABP) or ventricular assist device (VAD) as ordered *to decrease cardiac workload and increase coronary perfusion.*
- Measure intake and output every 1 to 2 hours.
- Monitor indices of renal function: BUN and creatinine levels.

Fluid volume deficit related to hemorrhage and fluid loss

- Assess for signs and symptoms of fluid volume deficit: hypotension and decreased venous filling, pulse volume, and pressure.
- Assess skin for increased temperature, color, and turgor.
- Administer fluids as ordered.
- Monitor hemodynamic parameters, including pulmonary capillary wedge pressure, heart rate, urine output, and central venous pressure.
- Maintain patient's core temperature by covering patient with blankets as needed.
- Maintain accurate intake and output record.
- Monitor electrolytes.
- Measure all body fluid loss; estimate loss in dressings.

Impaired gas exchange related to perceived threat to or change in health status

- Assess and monitor respiratory pattern, noting rate, rhythm, and use of accessory muscles.
- Monitor arterial blood gas levels, and venous oxygen saturation (Svo_2) if pulmonary artery (PA) catheter is in place.
- Report if Svo_2 is less than 60%.
- Administer oxygen as ordered via mask or through endotracheal tube.
- Auscultate breath sounds every hour *for increasing pulmonary congestion and atelectasis.*
- Prepare for intubation and assisted ventilation as indicated.

- Review serial chest roentgenograms as ordered.
- Assess for signs of increased congestion.

Altered nutrition: less than body requirements related to depleted glycogen stores

- Record weight on admission to establish baseline.
- Weigh daily at same time of day, using same scale.
- Begin tube feedings, intralipids, and total parenteral nutrition as ordered.
- Assess signs of early malnutrition; monitor laboratory values daily.

Anxiety related to increased pulmonary capillary permeability

- Assess for signs of fear and anxiety; determine source of fears.
- Explain all procedures and treatments.
- Remain with patient *to offer reassurance.*
- Maintain as quiet and calm an atmosphere as possible.
- Allow family to be with patient as condition permits.
- Encourage expressions of feelings, such as crying.
- Maintain calm and reassuring manner; stay with patient *to provide sense of security.*

Risk for infection related to sepsis and impaired immune response

- Assess for signs and symptoms of systemic infection.
- Maintain strict asepsis of all invasive lines, changing wound dressings and lines daily.
- Administer antibiotics as ordered.

Other related nursing diagnosis High risk for impaired skin integrity.

Patient Education/Home Care Planning

1. Explain all procedures and treatments as they occur. Refer to the primary disorder for specific teaching protocol.

Evaluation

Tissue perfusion is improved Patient is alert, oriented, and normotensive; urine output is normal; skin is warm and dry; peripheral pulses >2+.

Cardiac output is improved Patient is normotensive. Cardiac output is 4 to 5 L per minute. PCWP is 10 to 15 mm Hg. Skin is warm and dry. Patient is resting quietly.

Fluid volume is restored Patient is normotensive. PCWP is 10 to 15 mm Hg. Urine output is increased.

Gas exchange is improved Pao_2 is 80 to 100 mm Hg. Pco_2 is 35 to 45 mm Hg. Lungs are clear. Patient verbalizes that breathing is easier.

Nutritional status is maintained or improved Weight remains stable or increases. Albumin, transferrins are within normal limits. Nitrogen balance is maintained.

Anxiety is decreased Patient verbalizes fears and asks questions. Patient appears relaxed and is resting quietly.

CARDIOMYOPATHY

The term *cardiomyopathy* is applied to diseases that affect the myocardium, resulting in enlargement or ventricular dysfunction (Figure 1-41).

In the past three decades great advances in the understanding of this complex disorder have been made. There are three main types of cardiomyopathy, classified according to the pathophysiologic process resulting in myocardial dysfunction: dilated, hypertrophic, and restrictive. The etiologic factors contributing to cardiomyopathy are frequently unknown (idiopathic) but can be summarized in the following categories:

Primary myocardial disease
  Ischemic (coronary artery disease)
Endocardial fibroelastosis
Familial cardiomyopathies
  Metabolic storage diseases
    Pompe's disease (glycogen)
    Fabry's disease (glycolipid)
  Muscular dystrophies
  Friedreich's ataxia
  Sickle cell anemia
Inflammatory
  Infectious
    Viral (such as coxsackievirus, rubella, HIV)
    Rickettsial (typhus, Q fever)
    Bacterial (streptococcal)
    Spirochetal (leptospirosis, syphilis)
    Fungal (histoplasmosis, coccidioidomycosis)
    Parasitic (Chagas' disease, schistosomiasis)
  Noninfectious (collagen)
    Rheumatic heart disease
    Scleroderma
    Systemic lupus erythematosus
    Polyarteritis
    Löffler's disease
    Dermatomyositis
Infiltrative
  Sarcoidosis
  Amyloidosis
  Neoplastic disease
Metabolic
  Endocrine disorders
    Thyrotoxicosis
    Myxedema
  Nutritional
    Starvation, malnutrition
    Beriberi
Toxic
  Alcohol
  Carbon monoxide
  Arsenic

SYSTOLE DIASTOLE

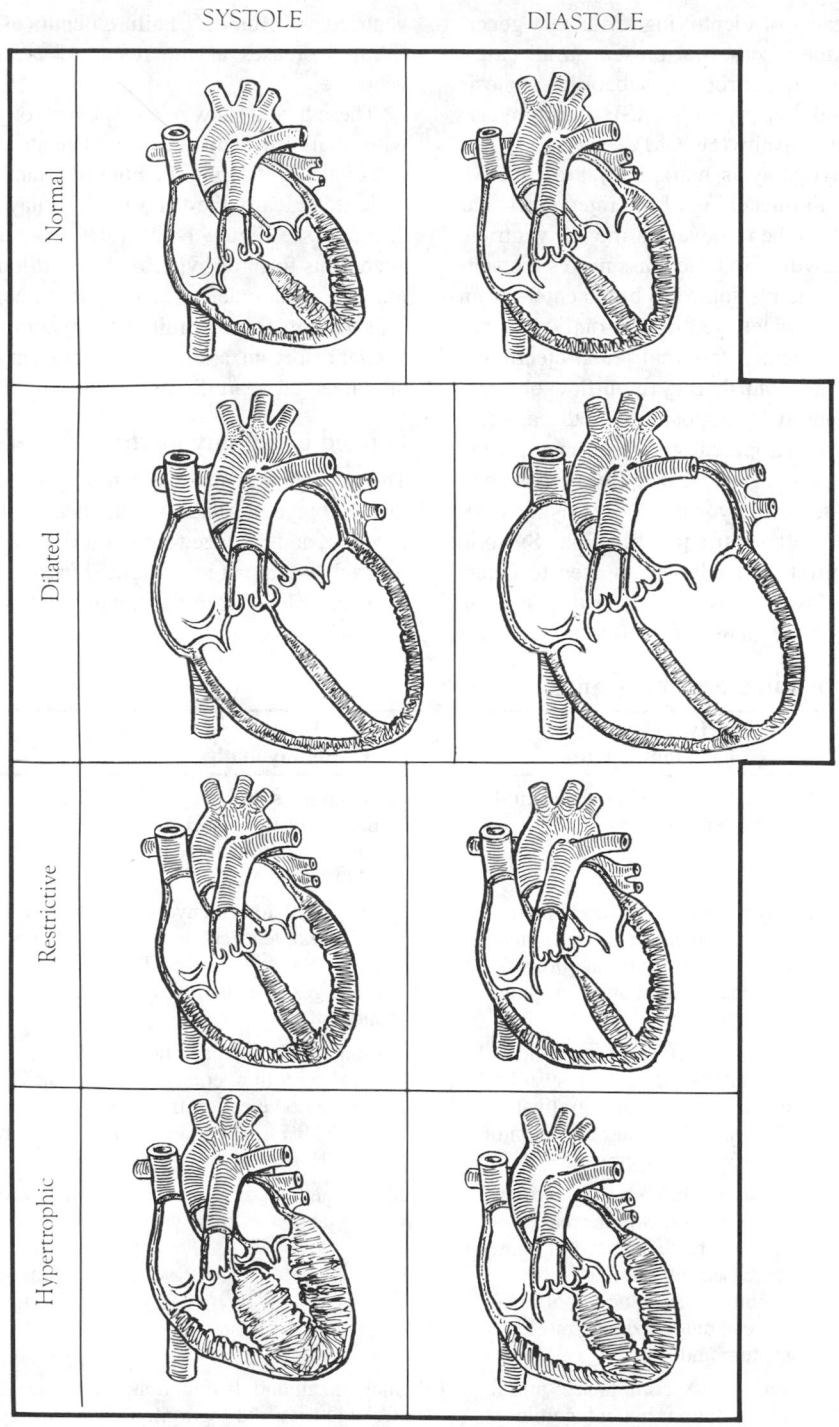

Figure 1-41 Types of cardiomyopathies. (From Thelan.[85])

Immunosuppressive drugs (doxorubicin)
  Emetine
  Cocaine
Miscellaneous
  Postpartum
  Radiation

•••••• **Pathophysiology**

Hypertrophic Cardiomyopathy

Hypertrophic cardiomyopathy (HCM) is the form of myocardial disease whose pathophysiologic, etiologic, and clinical features continue to receive the widest attention. As a result it has acquired an extensive list of identifying terms that generally describe features of the disease not present in all cases. These include idiopathic hypertrophic subaortic stenosis (IHSS), asymmetric septal hypertrophy (ASH), and hypertrophic obstructive cardiomyopathy (HOCM).

Hypertrophic cardiomyopathy is marked by a distinctive pattern of hypertrophy, with thickening of the interventricular septum when compared with the free wall of the left ventricle (Figure 1-42). The overgrowth of muscle mass makes the ventricular walls rigid, increasing resistance as blood enters from the left atrium. Obstruction of left ventricular outflow is another characteristic. Consequently, left ventricular ejection is impeded throughout systole. Contributing to outflow obstruction is the obstruction caused by apposition of the anterior mitral leaflet against the hypertrophied septum during midsystole. Left ventricular function in HCM is usually supranormal, but later in the disease extensive myocardial fibrosis may occur, resulting in impaired left ventricular function. Systolic motion of the anterior mitral leaflet has been used to determine the severity of outflow obstruction.[8] Elevated systolic pressure gradients occur in the range of 70% to 90% of left

ventricular volumes.[61] Failure occurs as resistance to diastolic filling increases as the result of a stiff, noncompliant left ventricle.

These hearts show massive overgrowth of myocardial tissue with small ventricular cavities. The atria are also hypertrophied and dilated, reflecting the high resistance to ventricular filling.

Histologically the heart muscle may show myocardial fiber disarray (see Figure 1-42). First described in 1958 by Donald Teare, this form of hypertrophic cardiomyopathy is thought to reflect a genetic defect that results in abnormal heart structure. This feature is not limited to hypertrophic cardiomyopathy; similar disorganization has been seen in some cases of acquired or congenital heart disease.

Dilated Cardiomyopathy

The second and most common form of cardiomyopathy is marked by gross dilation of the heart, interference with systolic function, and damage to myofibrils. Dilated cardiomyopathy is marked by impaired systolic function (ejection fractions of 15% to 20% are common), which leads to increased end-diastolic and end-systolic volumes.

•••••• Diagnostic Studies and Findings

Study	Hypertrophic Cardiomyopathy	Dilated Cardiomyopathy	Restrictive Cardiomyopathy
Chest x-ray	Enlarged cardiac silhouette (mild to moderate)	Enlarged cardiac silhouette; prominence of left ventricle (LV) (moderate to marked); pleural effusions	Cardiac enlargement (mild)
Electrocardiogram (ECG) (24-hour ambulatory monitor)	LV hypertrophy; ST segment and T wave changes; Q waves may be seen in inferior and precordial leads; atrial and ventricular dysrhythmias	LV hypertrophy; sinus tachycardia; atrial and ventricular dysrhythmias; ST segment and T wave changes; conduction disturbances	Low-voltage; conduction disturbances
Echocardiogram	Narrow LV outflow tract; abnormal thickened septum; systolic anterior motion of mitral valve; decreased internal dimension of LV; LV hypertrophy	LV dilation; abnormal diastolic mitral valve motion; enlarged atria; decreased ejection fraction (15%-20%)	Increased LV wall thickness and mass; small or normal LV cavity; normal systolic function; pericardial effusion
Radionuclide studies	Hyperdynamic systolic function; technetium shows decreased LV volume; thallium-201 shows increased muscle mass, ischemia; gated blood pool imaging evaluates size and motion of septum and LV	LV dilation and hypokinesis; decreased ejection fraction	Myocardial infiltration; small or normal LV cavity; normal systolic function; computed tomography and MRI define pericardial thickness
Cardiac catheterization	Decreased LV compliance; mitral regurgitation; hyperdynamic systolic function; LV outflow obstruction	LV enlargement and dysfunction; mitral and tricuspid regurgitation; elevated diastolic filling pressures; decreased cardiac output	Decreased LV compliance; normal systolic function; elevated diastolic filling process
Endomyocardial biopsy		To identify specific etiologies (i.e., sarcoidosis, myocarditis)	To detect eosinophil infiltration

The heart has a globular shape with enlargement and dilation of all four chambers (Figure 1-43). Although the heart may weigh up to 700 g (normal 350 g), the wall thickness may be normal or decreased. Left ventricular filling pressures are generally higher as a result of poor contractile function. The cardiac valves are basically normal, as are the coronary arteries. Endocardial thrombi are common, particularly in the ventricular apex.

Histologic examination reveals nonspecific changes including cell hypertrophy and extensive interstitial and perivascular fibrosis.

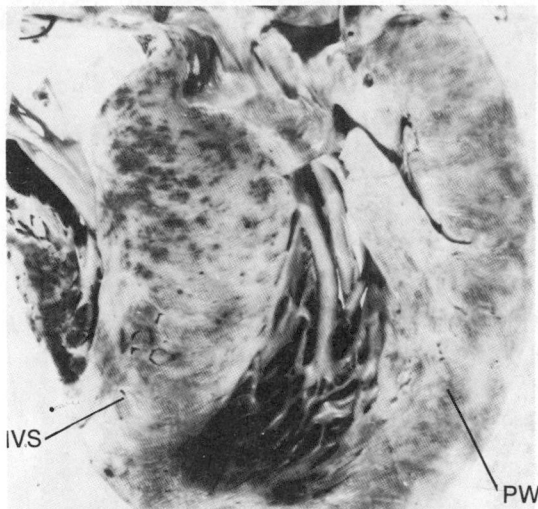

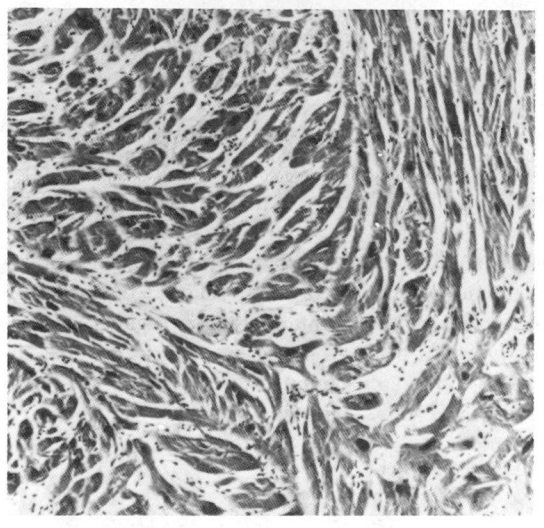

Figure 1-42 Heart with hypertrophic cardiomyopathy. Interventricular septum, *IVS,* is thicker than posterior wall, *PW.* Histologic section (lower illustration) shows marked disorganization of myocardium that is especially prominent in septum. (Hematoxylin and eosin, × 50.) (From Bulkley BH: Advances in cardiac pathology. In Hurst JW, editor: *The heart, update I,* New York, 1979, McGraw-Hill.)

The cause of this disorder is not clear, but it has been linked to various factors that predispose to the development of cardiomyopathy, including alcohol, pregnancy, infections, and toxic agents.

Restrictive Cardiomyopathy

A less common form of cardiomyopathy, restrictive cardiomyopathy, is marked by abnormal diastolic (filling) function and excessively rigid ventricular walls. Contractility is relatively unimpaired with normal systolic emptying of the ventricles. Hemodynamically, this group of cardiomyopathies resembles constrictive pericarditis.

The abnormal diastolic filling occurs as a result of infiltration of the endocardium or myocardium with fibroelastic tissue similar to that seen in Löffler's endocarditis, endomyocardial fibrosis, and amyloidosis.

••••• Multidisciplinary Plan

Surgery

Septalmyotomy-myectomy—for patient with hypertrophic cardiomyopathy who has intractable symptoms and severe obstruction; hypertrophied septum is excised, which diminishes left ventricular gradient and mitral regurgitation; procedure improves symptoms but has not been reported to prolong life

Excision of fibrotic endocardium—successful in limited number of cases of restrictive cardiomyopathy; procedure apparently decreases ventricular filling pressures and increases cardiac output

Cardiac transplantation—increasingly becoming the treatment of choice for dilated cardiomyopathy refractory to medical therapy, but requires careful evaluation of patient and family (p. 99 describes care of patient after transplantation)

Other surgical interventions—essentially nonexistent; valve replacement considered in individual cases but generally not favored

Medications

Hypertrophic cardiomyopathy—goals of drug therapy are to decrease ventricular contractility and increase ventricular volume and left ventricular outflow without vasodilation

Type IA antidysrhythmic

Disopyramide (Norpace)

Indications: negative inotropic drug demonstrated to significantly decrease left ventricular pressure gradient; currently drug of choice in treatment of obstructive HCM

Usual dosage: 600 to 800 mg/d

β-Adrenergic blocking agents: propranolol (Inderal)

Indications: negative inotropic effects on myocardial contractility and thus is believed to prevent increase in outflow obstruction, decrease myocardial oxygen consumption, and exert antidysrhythmic actions; may be used in combination with Norpace for optimizing therapy

Calcium channel blockers: verapamil (Calan)

Indications: has been shown to decrease left ventricular outflow obstruction and increase exercise tolerance; however, the vasodilatory effects may lead to worsening obstruction, thus should be used with caution.

Usual dosage: 80 to 160 mg q8h (not to exceed 480 mg/d)

Dilated cardiomyopathy—cannot be halted or reversed by any pharmacologic agent; pharmacologic interventions directed largely by symptoms of congestive heart failure or dysrhythmias

Restrictive cardiomyopathy—pharmacologic agents directed by underlying disorder; digitalis and diuretics often employed to treat dysrhythmias and signs of failure, but their effectiveness is limited

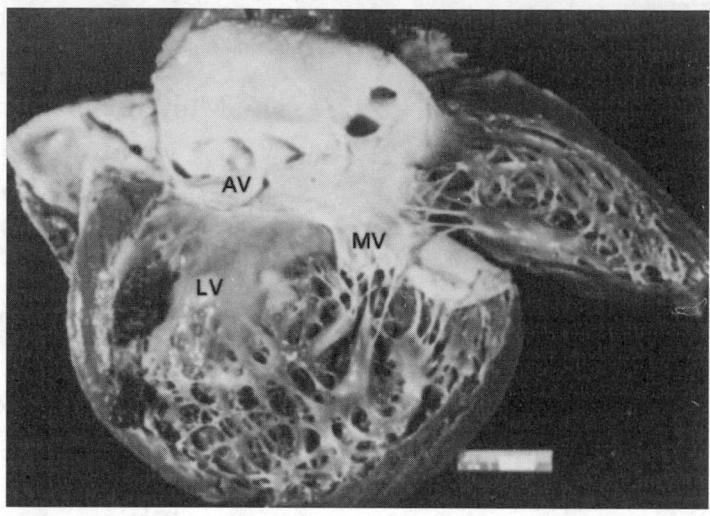

Figure 1-43 Heart with idiopathic dilated congestive cardiomyopathy. Opened left ventricle, *LV*, has dilated and globular configuration. Aortic valves, *AV*, and mitral valves, *MV*, are normal. (From Kaye.[48])

General Management

Hemodynamic monitoring—initiated as means of assessing left ventricular function and cardiac output

Intraaortic balloon pumping—used to sustain severely depressed ventricular function

Ventricular assist device—bridge to cardiac transplantation for end-stage ventricular failure

Atrioventricular sequential pacing—capable of reducing or abolishing obstructive pressure gradient in HCM by pacing right side of ventricular septum, widening left ventricular outflow tract

Automatic implantable cardiac defibrillator (AICD)—may be used in HCM with ventricular tachycardia or fibrillation

Cardiac monitoring—used to determine presence of atrial or ventricular dysrhythmias or conduction defects and to assess effectiveness of antidysrhythmic agents

Cardioversion—used in treatment of atrial fibrillation with rapid ventricular response

Restriction of sodium and fluid intake

Oxygen therapy

NURSING CARE

Nursing Assessment

Area of Concern	Hypertrophic Cardiomyopathy	Dilated Cardiomyopathy	Restrictive Cardiomyopathy
General complaints	Dyspnea; shortness of breath; angina pectoris; fatigue; palpitations; syncope (may be exertional)	Dyspnea; fatigue; complaints associated with biventricular failure; palpitations	Dyspnea; fatigue; complaints associated with right ventricular failure
Arterial pressure		Normal or low systolic; narrowed pulse pressure	Narrowed pulse pressure
Arterial pulse	Brisk carotid upstroke; pulsus bisferiens	Low amplitude and volume; pulsus alternans	
Jugular venous pressure	Dominant a wave	Distended; prominent a and v waves	Distended
Palpation	Apical systolic thrill and heave	Apical impulse displaced laterally; parasternal impulses and heaves; pulsatile liver	Apical impulse difficult to palpate
Auscultation	Systolic murmur heard best at apex and at lower left sternal border, increasing in intensity with Valsalva maneuver; S_4 gallop	Murmurs of mitral and tricuspid regurgitation; S_3 and S_4 gallops; pulmonary crackles	Murmurs of mitral regurgitation; S_3 and S_4 gallops; heart sounds distant

Nursing Dx & Intervention

Decreased cardiac output related to mechanical factors (preload, afterload, or contractility)

- Observe for signs and symptoms of decreased left ventricular functioning: chest pain, syncope, peripheral constriction, and cyanosis.
- Encourage bed rest.
- Limit self-care activities *to conserve energy and decrease oxygen demand.*
- Monitor arterial pressure, PCWP, cardiac output, and ECG as indicated.
- Administer drugs as ordered.
- Limit and monitor IV fluids as ordered.

Convalescent care

- Progressively increase activity level as indicated by improvement in patient status.
- Monitor vital signs and report any changes in heart rate or blood pressure.
- Teach patient and family the importance of monitoring vital signs and how to check blood pressure and pulse accurately.

Ineffective individual coping related to inability to deal with multiple stressors and progressive deterioration of health status

- Determine baseline knowledge of disease.
- Answer all questions about disease and future health.
- Encourage discussion of feelings of hopelessness and fears.
- Assist patient to participate in decision-making process with regard to any adjustments in lifestyle.
- Provide patient education and instructions for home care.
- Include family or significant other in care.
- Encourage family to learn cardiopulmonary resuscitation.

Activity intolerance related to diminished cardiac reserve

- Assess and monitor patient's tolerance to activities, noting which activities aggravate symptoms.
- Check BP, HR, and respiration before and after each activity to observe for orthostatic changes and *to identify signs of unmet oxygen demand.*
- Coordinate care to promote rest and *to ensure periods of uninterrupted rest.*
- Increase activities gradually; assist as necessary.
- Instruct patient in energy conservation methods *to limit or reduce energy expenditure.*

Fluid volume excess related to increased levels of aldosterone, sodium retention, and antidiuretic hormone (secondary to right or left ventricular dysfunction)

- Observe for signs of decreased ventricular function and fluid retention: increased adventitious lung sounds, presence of S_3, shortness of breath, cough, peripheral edema, increased venous filling.
- Maintain patent IV line for drug administration.
- Administer diuretics as ordered *to decrease circulating volume.*
- Restrict sodium and fluid intake.
- Weigh patient daily (same time of day, same amount of clothing) *to determine fluid loss or retention.*
- Monitor intake and output.
- Monitor serum electrolytes, especially sodium and potassium.
- Inspect for increased or decreased jugular venous distention.
- Auscultate heart tones and breath sounds every 1 to 2 hours for increased congestion.

Other related nursing diagnoses Impaired gas exchange related to elevated pulmonary capillary pressure; altered nutrition: less than body requirements related to impaired absorption of nutrients; pain: chest related to myocardial ischemia.

Patient Education/Home Care Planning

1. Describe the nature and type of cardiomyopathy.
2. Explain the prognosis and the limitations of the disease on lifestyle, especially important because many patients were considered "healthy" before diagnosis was made.
3. Explain the signs and symptoms to report to the physician.
4. Describe activity allowances and limitations; explain the importance of avoiding isometric exercises; explain the importance of resting when feeling fatigued.
5. Explain dietary and fluid restrictions.
6. Explain the name, purpose, dosage, and side effects of prescribed medications; warn against the effects of abruptly stopping propranolol.
7. Explain the need for daily weighing when ordered and reporting increase of more than 2 lb in a 24-hour period.
8. Discuss the importance of follow-up appointment.
9. Provide referrals for community support services.

Evaluation

Ventricular volume is increased; outflow obstruction is decreased Cardiac output is increased and left ventricular end-diastolic pressure (LVEDP) is decreased. Fatigue, dyspnea, and angina are relieved.

LV diastolic volume is decreased; ventricular contractility is improved LVEDP is decreased. Stroke volume is improved. Patient loses excess fluid weight. Dyspnea and shortness of breath are relieved.

Patient copes effectively with diagnosis Patient follows up with medical therapy. Patient reports taking medications. Patient verbalizes feeling less anxious and fearful.

Patient exhibits tolerance to ADL and to an increasing level of activity Patient is normotensive; HR is within 10 to 20 beats per minute (BPM) of resting rate; reports no symptoms of activity intolerance.

VALVULAR HEART DISEASE

Valvular heart disease (VHD) is an acquired or congenital disorder of a cardiac valve, marked by stenosis and obstructed blood flow or by valvular breakdown and regurgitation of blood (Figure 1-44).

With the introduction of antibiotic therapy and with improved diagnostic procedures, the incidence of VHD has declined over the past three decades. It is most commonly a chronic illness, and symptoms requiring therapy may take years to develop. VHD may also occur as an acute illness after trauma, myocardial infarction, or endocarditis.

•••••• Pathophysiology

The etiology of VHD can be classified into congenital and acquired disorders.

Congenital disorders include bicuspid aortic valve and pulmonary stenosis. Although not usually classified as VHD, tricuspid and pulmonary atresia, mitral valve prolapse, and Ebstein's anomaly are all defects involving valve function.

Rheumatic fever and endocarditis account for the greatest number of cases of acquired VHD.[3,8] Other disorders such as Marfan's syndrome, cardiomyopathy, myocardial infarction, myxomatous degeneration of the mitral valve, and trauma can also lead to valve dysfunction.

Cardiac valves are unidirectional, ensuring efficient flow of blood throughout the heart and the pulmonary and systemic circulation. Valve disorders occur when the integrity of the valve leaflets or the surrounding structures are disrupted.

Two basic valve abnormalities exist: stenosis and regurgitation. In stenosis the valve opening narrows as a result of thickening and rigidity of the valve leaflets. Stenosis blocks the flow of blood across the valve, increasing the pressure gradient. In regurgitation (insufficiency, incompetency), calcification, scarring, and retraction of the leaflets or adjacent structures lead to an incomplete valve closure that results in reversed blood flow.

Mixed lesions producing both stenosis and regurgitation can occur. In addition, more than one valve may be affected.

Mitral Stenosis

The most common cause of mitral stenosis is rheumatic valvulitis that leads to fibrotic thickening and fusion of the valve commissures. Scarring of the free margins of the leaflets occurs with shortening and thickening of the chordae tendineae, which may lead to regurgitation often seen with mitral stenosis.

The normal mitral valve opening is 4 to 6 cm². When this opening is reduced, flow across the valve is blocked, increasing the pressure gradient needed to eject blood from the left atrium to the left ventricle. The pressure gradient rises to maintain cardiac output. When the mitral orifice is decreased to 2 cm², cardiac output drops and symptoms appear with exertion. As the disease progresses, the mean left atrial pressure rises, causing the left atrial chamber to enlarge. The increased left atrial pressure is reflected in the pulmonary capillaries and pulmonary artery. As pulmonary capillary pressure rises, fluid flows back across the alveolar membrane, eventually exceeding oncotic pressure of the plasma proteins in the blood and forcing fluid out of the capillaries into the lung. If this fluid cannot be removed by drainage, pulmonary edema develops.

Mitral Regurgitation

Rheumatic fever, the usual cause of mitral regurgitation, causes thickening, scarring, rigidity, and calcification of the valve leaflets. The commissures become fused with the chordae tendineae, causing the leaflets to shorten and retract, which prevents them from complete closure during systole. A nonrheumatic cause of mitral regurgitation is myocardial infarction, which causes dilation of the left ventricle and displacement of the papillary muscles. Papillary muscle dysfunction may also occur as a result of rupture or fibrosis caused by ischemia, infarction, and ventricular aneurysm at the base of a papillary muscle. In addition, annu-

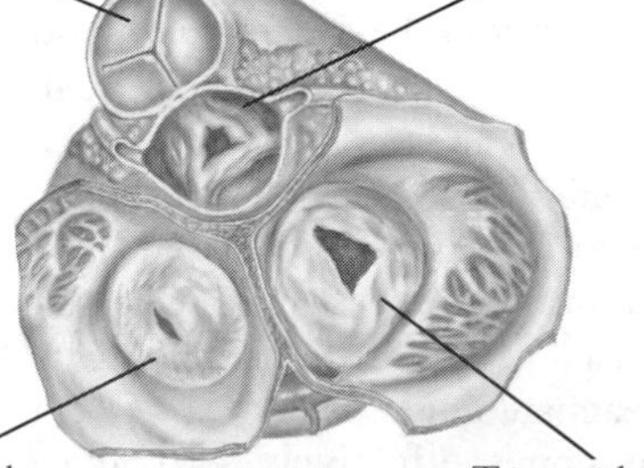

Figure 1-44 Valvular heart disease. (From Canobbio.[13])

Pulmonic valve (normal)
Aortic valve (stenotic, fused cusps)
Mitral valve ("slitlike" stenotic orifice)
Tricuspid valve (triangular, fixed, stenotic orifice)

MITRAL VALVE PROLAPSE

Mitral valve prolapse (MVP) is the superior systolic displacement of the mitral leaflets. It has become one of the most commonly found disorders involving the mitral valve. It is reported that as many as 15% of otherwise healthy young persons will demonstrate some normal superior systolic displacement of the mitral leaflets. However, excessive valvuloventricular disproportion reflects a primary connective tissue abnormality of the mitral leaflets, the annulus, and chordae tendineae. This abnormality is referred to as MVP (Figure 1-45).

Clinical findings depend on the degree to which the leaflets prolapse in the atrium. If the mitral leaflets prolapse to such an extent that the contact between the two leaflets is impaired, mitral regurgitation will result.

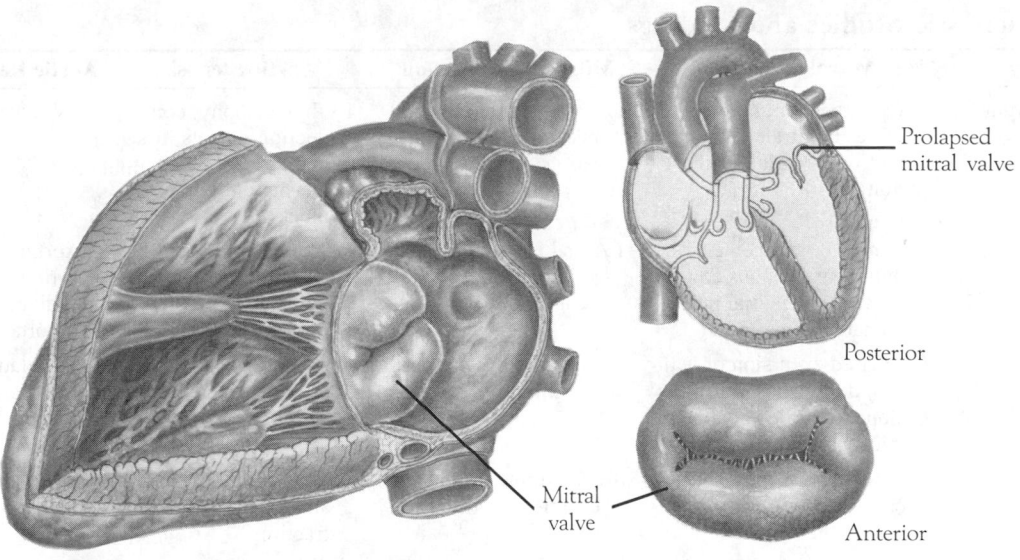

Figure 1-45 Mitral valve prolapse. (From Canobbio.[13])

lar dilation may lead to an incomplete mitral apparatus. The most common cause is left ventricular dilation resulting from aortic regurgitation, coronary artery disease, or dilated cardiomyopathy.

As the mitral valve disorder progresses, the reverse flow to the left atrium causes left atrial pressure to rise. This pressure is reflected in the pulmonary veins, leading to leakage of fluid into the lungs.

The increase in left atrial pressure causes atrial dilation and enlargement. The left ventricle becomes hypertrophied because it must deal with the larger volume of blood that is lost to the left atrium during systole.

Aortic Stenosis

The most common cause of aortic stenosis is congenital bicuspid valve. This defect occurs in 1% of the population, more often in males (3:1).

The normal aortic valve opening measures 2.6 to 3.5 cm². Valve narrowing results from calcification of the leaflets. Calcification may extend into the aortic wall or onto the anterior leaflet of the mitral valve, which accounts for the mitral disease commonly occurring with aortic stenosis. Calcification may also extend into the conduction system, leading to conduction defects. As the disease progresses, calcification makes the valve inflexible, reducing the opening to a small slit.

As the aortic valve opening decreases, left ventricular pressure rises to create enough pressure to eject a normal stroke volume and propel flow across the valve into the aorta. This obstruction to left ventricular outflow leads to a pressure gradient between the aorta and left ventricle during systole. To maintain flow across the narrowed opening, wall thickness gradually increases in the pressure-overloaded left ventricle, leading to hypertrophy. In time the flow across the valve be-

comes fixed and cardiac output does not increase in response to demand. During exercise the increased flow to extremities with fixed cardiac output causes a decreased cerebral and coronary blood flow, resulting in dizziness or syncope and chest pain.

Left atrial hypertrophy occurs in an attempt to increase cardiac output. To produce a forceful atrial contraction, left ventricular end-diastolic pressure (LVEDP) rises, which in turn increases the myocardial fiber stretch and leads to increased contraction and improved stroke volume.

The course of aortic stenosis depends on the size of the valve opening and the left ventricle. When myocardial contractility falls, the left ventricle dilates, causing diastolic and left atrial pressure to increase further.

The onset of symptoms of heart failure indicates moderate to severe disease, and death often occurs less than 5 years after symptoms appear. Sudden death is linked to severe aortic stenosis (0.5 to 0.6 cm²).

Aortic Regurgitation

Rheumatic fever, syphilis, connective tissue disorder, and infective endocarditis are common causes of aortic valve disorders.

The basic hemodynamic problem in aortic regurgitation is a volume-overloaded left ventricle. Blood ejected during normal systole reenters the left ventricle in diastole. To compensate for this volume, the left ventricle must produce a higher stroke volume by increasing the systolic pressure, resulting in eventual hypertrophy of the left ventricle.

With time, LVEDP and left atrial pressure increase. As myocardial contractility diminishes and failure takes place, mitral regurgitation may occur as a result of the malpositioning of papillary muscles.

•••••• Diagnostic Studies and Findings

Study	Mitral Stenosis	Mitral Regurgitation	Aortic Stenosis	Aortic Regurgitation
Electrocardiogram (ECG)	LA enlargement; notched P wave (P mitrale); RV hypertrophy; atrial fibrillation (in 40%-50% of cases)	LA enlargement; LV hypertrophy; atrial fibrillation	LV hypertrophy; conduction defects; first-degree A-V block, left bundle-branch block	LV hypertrophy
Chest x-ray	LA and RV enlargement; pulmonary venous congestion; interstitial pulmonary edema	LA and LV enlargement; pulmonary vascular congestion	Poststenotic aortic dilation; aortic valve calcification	Aortic valve calcification; LV enlargement; dilation of ascending aorta
Echocardiogram	Decreased excursion of leaflets; diminished E to F slope; stenotic valve is thickened	LA enlargement; hyperdynamic LV	Nonrestricted movement of aortic valve; thickening of LV wall	LV dilation; diastolic fluttering of anterior leaflet
Radionuclide studies	To determine resting and exercise ejection fraction	To determine resting and exercise ejection fraction	To determine resting and exercise ejection fraction	To determine resting and exercise ejection fraction
Cardiac catheterization	Pressure across mitral valve increased; LA pressure increased; PCWP increased; low cardiac output	LVEDP increased; LAP increased; angiography with contrast media performed to quantify regurgitation	Pressure gradient in systole across aortic valve; LVEDP increased	Pulse pressure increased; LVEDP increased; LAP increased; angiography with contrast media performed to quantify regurgitation

•••••• Multidisciplinary Plan

Surgery

Indicated when medical therapy no longer alleviates clinical symptoms or when there is diagnostic evidence of progressive myocardial dysfunction (such as progressive enlargement of heart)

Valvotomy—surgical splitting of fused commissures or thickened leaflets

Valvular annuloplasty—reparative procedure of valve ring, chordae, or papillary muscle performed primarily for mitral and tricuspid regurgitation

Valve replacement—replacement of stenotic or incompetent valve with bioprosthetic or mechanical valve; commonly used valves include pynolite tilting disks, porcine heterografts, homografts, autografts, pericardial valves, and ball-in-cage valves

Medications

Guided by patient's clinical signs and symptoms or echocardiographic evidence of increasing left atrial or left ventricular size or increased regurgitation

ACE inhibitors, afterload reduction for a volume-loaded left atrium or left ventricle (MR or AR)

Digitalis and diuretics for heart failure (see p. 41)

Dysrhythmia management (see p. 16)

Anticoagulants for patients in atrial fibrillation who are at risk for systemic or pulmonary embolization; warfarin sodium (Coumadin) in doses titrated to maintain prothrombin time at two times control or International Normalized Ratio (INR) of 1.5 to 2.5

Antibiotic prophylaxis before any procedure that increases risk of endocarditis (Table 1-2)

General Management

Cardioversion—indicated for patients with mitral stenosis in atrial fibrillation to decrease risk of emboli

Dictated by severity of valvular disorder (see pp. 16 and 41 for supportive care of patients in heart failure or with dysrhythmias)

Diet therapy—sodium restriction for patients with mild to moderate signs of pulmonary congestion

Balloon valvuloplasty—nonsurgical procedure used in treatment of calcific valvular stenosis, the procedure involves passing a balloon-tipped catheter under fluoroscopy across the stenotic valve; once in place the balloon is inflated repeatedly until the valve gradient is relieved; currently the procedure is limited to patients who may be at some risk for valve surgery, including children, the elderly, and women of childbearing age

■ TABLE 1-2 Recommended Antibiotic Coverage for Endocarditis Prophylaxis

Drug	Dosing Regimen†‡§
Recommended Standard Prophylactic Regimen for Dental, Oral, or Upper Respiratory Tract Procedures in Patients Who Are at Risk*	
Standard Regimen†	
Amoxicillin	3.0 g orally 1 h before procedure; then 1.5 g 6 h after initial dose
Amoxicillin/Penicillin–Allergic Patients	
Erythromycin	Erythromycin ethylsuccinate, 600 mg, or erythromycin stearate, 1.0 g orally 2 h before procedure; then half the dose 6 h after initial dose
Clindamycin	300 mg orally 1 h before procedure and 150 mg 6 h after initial dose
Alternate Prophylactic Regimens for Dental, Oral, or Upper Respiratory Tract Procedures in Patients Who Are at Risk‡	
Patients Unable to Take Oral Medications	
Ampicillin	Intravenous or intramuscular administration of ampicillin, 2.0 g 30 min before procedure; then intravenous or intramuscular administration of ampicillin, 1.0 g, or oral administration of amoxicillin, 1.5 g 6 h after initial dose
Ampicillin/Amoxicillin/Penicillin–Allergic Patients Unable to Take Oral Medications	
Clindamycin	Intravenous administration of 300 mg 30 min before procedure and an intravenous or oral administration of 150 mg 6 h after initial dose
Patients Considered High Risk and Not Candidates for Standard Regimen	
Ampicillin, gentamicin, and amoxicillin	Intravenous or intramuscular administration of ampicillin, 2.0 g, plus gentamicin, 1.5 mg/kg (not to exceed 80 mg) 30 min before procedure; followed by amoxicillin, 1.5 g orally 6 h after initial dose; alternatively, the parenteral regimen may be repeated 8 h after initial dose
Ampicillin/Amoxicillin/Penicillin–Allergic Patients Considered High Risk	
Vancomycin	Intravenous administration of 1.0 g over 1 h, starting 1 h before procedure; no repeated dose necessary
Regimen for Genitourinary/Gastrointestinal Procedures§	
Standard Regimen	
Ampicillin, gentamicin, and amoxicillin	Intravenous or intramuscular administration of ampicillin, 2.0 g, plus gentamicin, 1.5 mg/kg (not to exceed 80 mg) 30 min before procedure; followed by amoxicillin, 1.5 g orally 6 h after initial dose; alternatively, the parenteral regimen may be repeated once 8 h after initial dose
Ampicillin/Amoxicillin/Penicillin–Allergic Patient Regimen	
Vancomycin and gentamicin	Intravenous administration of vancomycin, 1.0 g over 1 h plus intravenous or intramuscular administration of gentamicin, 1.5 mg/kg (not to exceed 80 mg) 1 h before procedure; may be repeated once 8 h after initial dose
Alternate Low-Risk Patient Regimen	
Amoxicillin	3.0 g orally 1 h before procedure; then 1.5 6 h after initial dose

Data from American Heart Association. *JAMA* 264:2918-2922, 1990, American Medical Association.

*Includes those with prosthetic heart valves and other high risk patients.

†Initial pediatric doses are as follows: amoxicillin, 50 mg/kg; erythromycin ethylsuccinate or erythromycin stearate, 20 mg/kg; and clindamycin, 10 mg/kg. Follow-up doses should be one half the initial dose. *Total pediatric dose should not exceed total adult dose.* The following weight ranges may also be used for the initial pediatric dose of amoxicillin: <15 kg, 750 mg; 15 to 30 kg, 1500 mgl and >3000 mg, full adult dose.

‡Initial pediatric doses are as follows: ampicillin, 50 mg/kg; clindamycin, 10 mg/kg; gentamicin, 2.0 mg/kg; and vancomycin, 20 mg/kg. Follow-up doses should be one half the initial dose. *Total pediatric dose should not exceed total adult dose.* No initial dose is recommended in this table for amoxicillin (25 mg/kg is the follow-up dose).

§Initial pediatric doses are as follows: ampicillin, 50 mg/kg; amoxicillin, 50 mg/kg; gentamicin, 2.0 mg/kg; and vancomycin, 20 mg/kg. Follow-up doses should be half the initial dose. *Total pediatric dose should not exceed total adult dose.*

NURSING CARE

Nursing Assessment

Area of Concern	Mitral Stenosis	Mitral Regurgitation	Aortic Stenosis	Aortic Regurgitation
General complaints	Fatigue; dyspnea on exertion; palpitations; hemoptysis; hoarseness; orthopnea; paroxysmal nocturnal dyspnea	Dyspnea; fatigue; exercise intolerance; orthopnea; palpitations	Fatigue; dyspnea; orthopnea; angina pectoris; dizziness; syncope	Dyspnea on exertion; palpitations; orthopnea; exertional chest pain
Physical examination	Resting tachycardia; irregular pulse; jugular venous distention increased in presence of RV failure; prominent a wave in presence of pulmonary hypertension (absent in atrial fibrillation)	Irregular pulse; sharp upstroke of arterial pulse; jugular venous distention increased in presence of RV failure; prominent a wave in presence of increased RV pressure	Early: normal blood pressure; late: systolic pressure decreased; narrow pulse pressure; carotid pulse slow with small pulse volume	Arterial pulsations; bounding pulse with rapid rise and fall (water-hammer pulse); widened pulse pressure; head bobbing (Musset's sign); skin warm, damp, and flushed
Palpation	Diastolic thrill at apex	Apical impulse forceful and displaced downward and to left	Systolic thrill palpable at base of heart; apical pulse strong and sustained throughout systole	Diastolic thrill along left sternal border; laterally displaced apical impulse; systolic thrill in jugular notch and along carotid arteries
Auscultation (Figure 1-46)	Loud S_1; opening snap; low snap; low-pitched, rumbling diastolic murmur	Diminished or absent S_1; wide splitting of S_2; S_3, S_4 heard in severe regurgitation; holosystolic murmur heard best at apex	Diminished or absent A_2; crescendo-decrescendo harsh systolic murmur heard best at base (second intercostal space to right of sternum); aortic ejection sound	Decrescendo diastolic murmur (blowing), high pitched and heard best at base (second intercostal space to right of sternum); systolic ejection murmur heard best at base

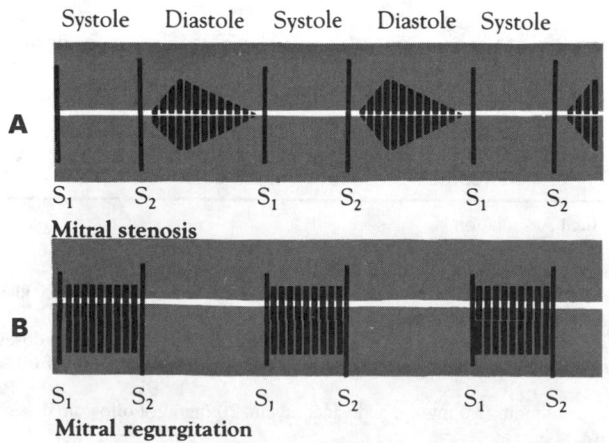

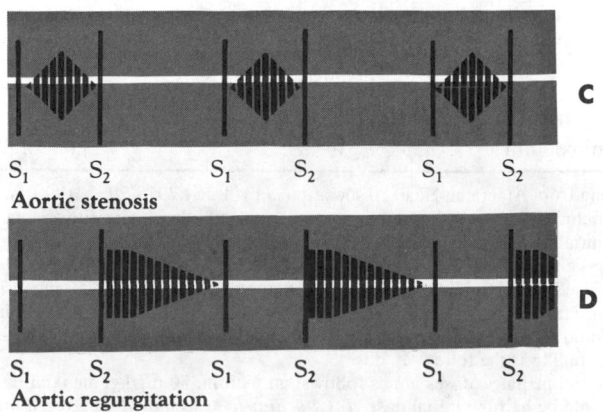

Figure 1-46 Auscultation of valvular heart disease murmurs. **A,** Mitral stenosis. **B,** Mitral regurgitation. **C,** Aortic stenosis. **D,** Aortic regurgitation. (From Guzzetta.[40])

Nursing Dx & Intervention

Decreased cardiac output related to mechanical factors (preload, afterload)

- Establish baseline assessment of cardiovascular status *to evaluate disease process and response to therapy.*
- Monitor vital signs every 4 to 8 hours or as indicated.
- Administer medications as ordered.
- Limit or modify activities during acute phase to conserve energy and decrease myocardial oxygen demand.
- Monitor and record ECG rate and rhythm; observe and record dysrhythmia.
- Auscultate heart sounds every 4 to 8 hours as indicated; record quality of murmurs.

Fluid volume excess (risk for) related to cardiac decompensation

- Assess for signs and symptoms of fluid volume excess: weight gain, increased jugular venous pressure, lung congestion.
- Administer diuretic and vasodilator therapy as ordered.
- Auscultate lung sounds every 8 hours.
- Monitor nutrition with dietary sodium and fluid restrictions.
- Weigh patient daily (same time of day, same amount of clothing) *to detect fluid retention.*
- Monitor intake and output *to determine response to therapy.*
- Monitor electrolyte levels, blood chemistry findings, hemoglobin level, and hematocrit.

Other related nursing diagnoses High risk for altered cerebral tissue perfusion related to interruption of arterial blood flow secondary to embolism; activity intolerance related to cardiac decompensation; anxiety related to altered heart action.

Patient Education/Home Care Planning

1. Assess the patient's level of knowledge and teach the patient about the disease, including etiology, medications, diet restrictions, exercise levels, and possible complications.
2. Assist the patient during diagnostic workup and assist with the decision for medical or surgical treatment.
3. Include the patient's family in the teaching and decision-making process.
4. Ensure that the patient knows the name, dosage, and purpose of medications.
5. Discuss with the patient the disease process and associated symptoms to report to the physician.
6. Discuss activity allowances and limitations.
7. Explain diet and fluid restrictions.
8. Explain to the patient antibiotic prophylaxis to prevent infectious endocarditis (see Table 1-2, p. 61).
9. Explain the importance of notifying the dentist, urologist, and gynecologist of valvular heart disease.
10. Provide a female patient with instruction regarding contraception and risk associated with pregnancy.
11. Discuss with the patient the need to maintain good oral hygiene, daily care, and regular visits to dentist.
12. Discuss importance of ongoing medical care.

Evaluation

Cardiac output is maintained Lungs are clear. Patient reports improvement of symptoms. Heart rate is within acceptable limits.

Fluid balance is regained Baseline weight is achieved. There is no peripheral edema or sign of fluid overload.

PERICARDITIS

Pericarditis is an inflammatory process involving the parietal and visceral layers of the pericardium and outer myocardium (Figure 1-47).

Pericarditis may occur by itself or as a complication of another disease. Acute pericarditis, which can occur within 2 weeks of the offending condition, lasts up to 6 weeks. There may be effusion or tamponade (see box on p. 66). Chronic pericarditis may follow acute pericarditis and may last up to 6 months.

•••••• Pathophysiology

Because of the closeness of the pericardium to the pleura, lung, sternum, diaphragm, and myocardium, pericarditis may be the result of a number of disease states. The most common cause is probably viral, which generally has a good prognosis. The causes of pericarditis can be summarized as follows:

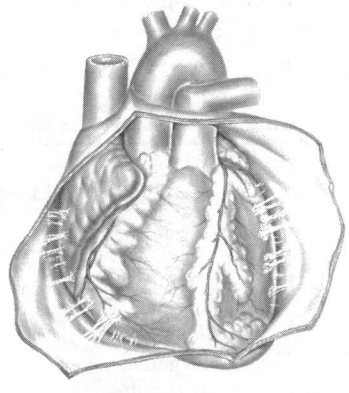

Figure 1-47 Pericarditis. (From Canobbio.[13])

Viral (idiopathic)—organism may never be isolated
Infectious
    Bacterial
    Tuberculous
    Fungal
Following myocardial infarction
    Dressler's syndrome
    Postmyocardial infarction syndrome
Following cardiac surgery (postpericardiotomy syndrome or
    Dressler's syndrome)
Neoplastic diseases
Chemotherapy
Radiotherapy
Uremia
Trauma, blunt or penetrating
Connective tissue diseases
    Systemic lupus erythematosus
    Rheumatoid arthritis
    Scleroderma
    Dermatomyositis

Inflammation may occur by direct extension or by irritation. Under normal conditions the pericardial sac contains up to 50 ml of clear, serouslike fluid. When an injury occurs, an exudate of fibrin, white blood cells, and endothelial cells is released, covering the parietal and visceral layers of pericardium. Friction between the layers causes irritation and inflammation of the surrounding pleura and tissues. This may remain in one region of the heart or be widespread. Acute pericarditis may be "dry" and fibrinous or obstruct the heart's venous and lymphatic drainage, causing seepage into the pericardial sac, which creates pericardial effusion.[8]

Serofibrinous exudates occur in varying amounts from 100 ml to 3 L and may appear straw colored or turbid with fibrin strands. The exudate of pyrogenic pericarditis is purulent. The characteristics of pericardial exudate fluid are summarized in Table 1-3.

A slowly developing effusion of a moderate amount (350 to 500 ml) may not alter the cardiovascular dynamics. However, a rapidly accumulating effusion, regardless of amount, can interfere with diastolic filling and lead to cardiac tamponade (Figure 1-48).

Chronic pericarditis can occur in a variety of forms, including chronic pericardial effusion and constrictive or adhesive pericarditis. Chronic effusion may lead to constrictive effusion.

Constrictive pericarditis is marked by pericardial thickening and scarring of the parietal or visceral pericardium. The layers adhere to each other, blocking out the pericardial space. This eventually involves the surface of the myocardium, causing the pericardium to become useless. In some cases the pericardium calcifies.

As the pericardium becomes scarred and rigid, normal diastolic filling of the heart is impeded. In severe cases, left ventricular end-diastolic volume may be less than stroke volume. This causes the stroke volume to be reduced with a subsequent drop in cardiac output. The normal tachycardia is unable to improve the cardiac output because of the constriction of the myocardium.

Constrictive pericarditis usually occurs in all four chambers but may be limited to certain areas such as the right ventricle, pulmonary artery, or aortic root. When all chambers are involved, left and right ventricular diastolic pressure and atrial pressures become equal. As stroke volume diminishes, left and right filling pressures rise. When this is combined with reduced cardiac output, systemic and pulmonary congestion results.

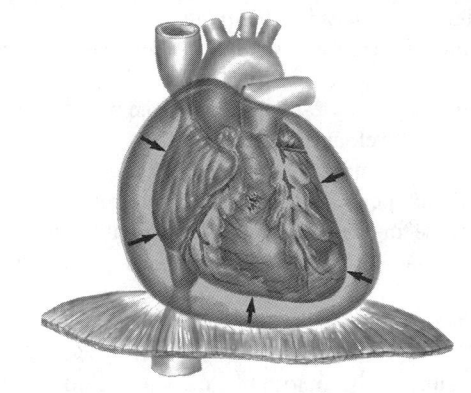

Figure 1-48 Hemopericardium and cardiac tamponade. (From Canobbio.[13])

TABLE 1-3 **Characteristics of Pericardial Fluid**

Characteristic	Normal Fluid	Exudate Effusion
Appearance	Clear	Clear or turbid with fibrin shreds; straw or amber color; may appear hemorrhagic because of RBCs; may be purulent
Volume	50 ml	>100 ml (up to 3 L)
Specific gravity	<1.015	>1.015 (usually 1.017)
Total protein	<2 g/dl	>3 g/dl
Seromucin clot	Negative	Positive
Coagulation	Uncommon	Usual
Cells	Few	Few
Glucose	Nearly equal to plasma glucose	Nearly equal to plasma glucose
Culture	Negative	Negative

•••••• Diagnostic Studies and Findings

Blood studies   Elevated WBC, ESR

Viral serology studies; elevated titers   Performed during acute and convalescent periods

Blood and urine cultures   Identification of organism in infectious process

Electrocardiogram (ECG)

Acute pericarditis

Stage 1 (Figure 1-49)   ST-T segment elevation in left ventricular leads V_5, V_6, I, II, aV_L, and a V_F during first few days; PR interval depression

Stage II   Return of ST segment to baseline; PR interval depression may persist

Stage III   T wave inversions

Stage IV   Normalization of T waves

Low-voltage QRS complexes in presence of pericardial effusion

Atrial dysrhythmias

Constrictive pericarditis

Wide P wave in leads I, II, and V_6; Q waves deep and wide; T waves flattened or inverted; low QRS voltage

Chest x-ray

Cardiac silhouette

Enlargement depends on underlying disease or amount of pericardial effusion (enlarges with 250 ml or more of accumulated fluid) (Figure 1-50)

Acute pericarditis

Normal if pericardial fluid less than 250 ml

Constrictive pericarditis

Normal or small; enlargement occurs as result of pericardial thickening or effusion; calcification of pericardium; pleural effusion

Echocardiogram   Confirms accumulation of free fluid in pericardial sac: as fluid accumulates, separation of pericardial and epicardial echoes occurs, resulting in echo-free space; minimum of 20 ml detected; evaluates ventricular function; in constrictive pericarditis demonstrates reduced motion of posterior wall of LV; abnormal movement of interventricular septum characterized by flattening in systole and paradoxic movement in diastole; two separate echoes representing visceral and parietal pericardium separated by clear space of 1 mm throughout cardiac cycle

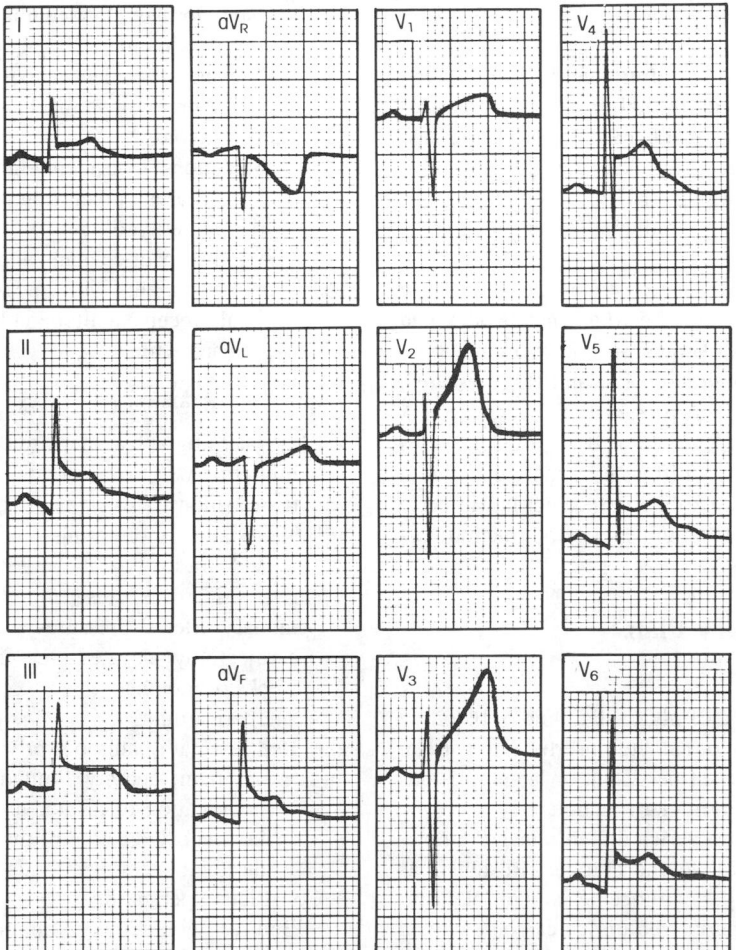

Figure 1-49 In acute pericarditis, ST segment elevation is typically upward and concave in leads I, II, aV_F, and V_4 to V_6. (From Guzzetta.[40])

CARDIAC TAMPONADE

Cardiac tamponade is an acute cardiac compression caused when fluid accumulates within the pericardial sac and exerts increased pressure around the heart (Figure 1-49). Normally the sac holds 30 to 50 ml of fluid. Fluid or blood can fill the pericardial space slowly or rapidly, depending on inflammatory vs. traumatic etiologies. Ultimately, the result of this excessive extracardiac volume is restricted blood flow in and out of the ventricles causing decreased cardiac output. Pulsus paradoxus, an important hemodynamic feature of tamponade, is a measurable fall in systemic blood pressure of 10 mm Hg or more during inspiration. Hypotension and shock are the inevitable manifestations of severe tamponade. Medical management of this life-threatening problem is frequently emergent and occasionally resuscitative. Needle aspiration of pericardial fluid or blood (pericardiocentesis) is the only nonsurgical method to rapidly decompress the pericardial space. Hemodynamic improvement is immediate. Subsequently, medical care must be directed at the inciting cause of fluid accumulation (e.g., postoperative bleeding, traumatic injury, pericarditis, malignancy).

Radionuclide blood pool scanning (technetium-labeled macroaggregated albumin and thallium) Demonstrates shadow of pericardial effusion outside cardiac chambers; seen as abnormal space between heart and liver or heart and lungs

Magnetic resonance imaging (MRI) Visualizes pericardium; can define thickened pericardium differentiating acute vs. chronic

Cardiac catheterization Demonstrates characteristic pericardial shadow outside opacified cardiac chambers, which are increased by pericardial thickening or fluid accumulation

Constrictive pericarditis: Increased LA and RA pressures; loss of respiratory variation of RA pressure curve; elevated PA systolic pressure (35 to 40 mm Hg); elevated diastolic pressures equal in all four chambers, rarely differing by more than 5 mm Hg at rest or during exercise; cardiac output normal in early stages, later decreased (<2.3 L/min/m²); ejection fraction normal or decreased

•••••• Multidisciplinary Plan

Surgery

Pericardiocentesis—removal of pericardial fluid or blood by aspiration through needle or catheter inserted into parietal pericardium; indicated when persistent or large effusions are compromising left ventricular function

Pericardial window—open pericardial drainage implemented for acute suppurative and chronic effusions: has certain advantages over pericardiocentesis: multiple aspirations can be avoided, pericardial tissue can be obtained for culture, pericardium can be visualized, and clots and fibrin deposits can be removed

Pericardiectomy—surgical removal of visceral and parietal pericardium; has excellent long-term benefits; operative mortality of about 10%; best results when myocardial fibrosis and ventricular atrophy are not far advanced and when total or near-total pericardiectomy is performed; if hemodynamic improvement is not seen immediately, elevated pressures and abnormal waveforms continue for several weeks owing to atrophy of ventricles that have been immobilized for long periods—thus early pericardiectomy is encouraged before dense fibrosis and myocardial atrophy occur; postoperative care similar to that of any cardiac surgical patient (p. 96)

Medications

Acute pericarditis

Antiinflammatory agents for symptomatic relief of chest pain, fever, and malaise in absence of clinical signs of cardiac tamponade

Analgesic-antipyretics: aspirin

Usual dosage: 600-900 mg qid

Nonsteroidal antiinflammatory agents: indomethacin (Indocin)

Usual dosage: Divided doses beginning with 25 mg qid to maximum of 200 mg/d

Precautions: Patients should be instructed to take medicine on a full stomach

Corticosteroids

Indications: Considered in treatment of moderate to severe cases in recurring pericarditis and effusion

Constrictive pericarditis

Chemotherapeutic agents aimed at specific cause; for example, patients with known or suspected tuberculosis should receive antituberculous therapy before and after pericardiectomy

General Management

Electrocardiography—performed to rule out myocardial infarction when cardiac tamponade is suspected and if patient demonstrates signs of cardiac decompensation

Hemodynamic monitoring—indicated if cardiac tamponade is evident (see box above left); for patients with constrictive pericarditis, closer monitoring of right atrial and pulmonary arterial pressures and cardiac output; after pericardiectomy, elevated pressures may continue for several weeks or months

Acute pericarditis

Bed rest with bathroom privileges during period of fever and pain; activity limited during acute period, with modification of all activities for 2 weeks to allow inflammatory reaction of the pericardium to resolve; regular diet; encourage fluids during febrile period

Constrictive pericarditis

Bed rest with activity limitations before pericardiectomy; extent of limitation dictated by degree of hemodynamic compromise and symptoms

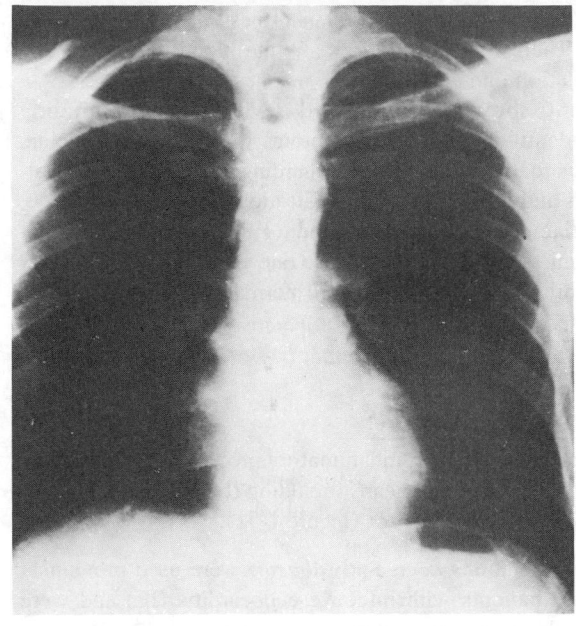
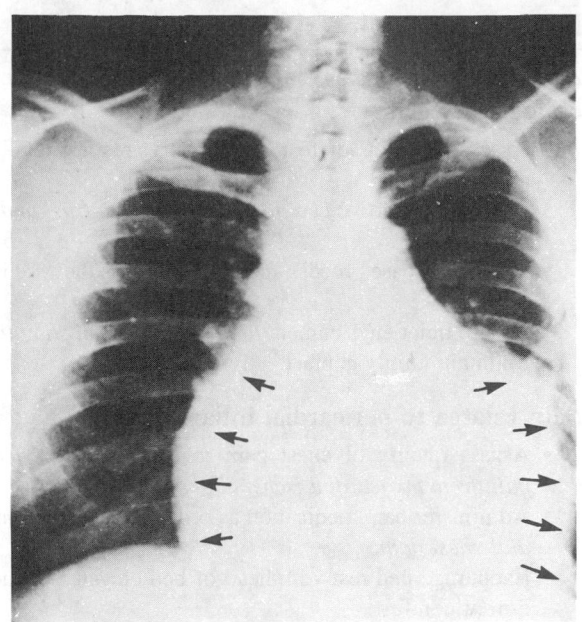

Figure 1-50 A, Normal chest x-ray. **B,** With pericardial effusion, cardiac silhouette is enlarged and has globular shape *(arrows)*. (From Guzzetta.[40])

NURSING CARE

Nursing Assessment

Area of Concern	Acute Pericarditis	Constrictive Pericarditis
General complaints	Chest pain: location retrosternal or precordial radiating to neck and back, sudden pleuritic-like pain that worsens with deep inspiration, movement, or lying down and is relieved by sitting up or leaning forward; sharp, deep, persistent ache; tachypnea; shallow breathing; dyspnea in presence of pleural effusion or owing to impaired cardiac filling from compression of heart; restlessness; anxiety; malaise; dysphagia	Exertional dyspnea; fatigue; orthopnea; palpitations; paroxysmal nocturnal dyspnea; cough; pericardial edema
Physical examination	Low-grade temperature (30°C [102°F]); may be associated with diaphoresis and chills; auscultation: pericardial friction rub—best heard with patient leaning forward, heard in second, third, or fourth intercostal space to left of sternal border or at apex, loudest during inspiration, varies in intensity (grade 4 to 5), may be transient, triphasic consisting of presystolic, systolic, and diastolic components, scratchy, grating	Afebrile; elevated jugular venous pressure with presence of Kussmaul's sign (increased distention during inspiration); arterial pressure normal or slightly reduced; diffuse precordial movement; decreased amplitude; absence of localized apical impulse; paradoxic pulse (rarely exceeds 15 mm Hg); auscultation: quiet, distant heart sounds, pericardial knock—early diastolic sound, accentuated with inspiration and heard best along lower left sternal border; clinical signs of elevated venous pressure: peripheral edema, hepatomegaly, ascites

Nursing Dx & Intervention

Anxiety related to actual or perceived threat to biologic integrity

- Assess for signs of fear and anxiety: restlessness, facial expressions.
- Provide supportive care *to ensure sense of trust and comfort.*
- Explain disease process and procedures as they are implemented.
- Ensure quiet environment *to reduce external stimuli.*
- Maintain family contact.

Pain related to pericardial inflammation

- Assess quality of chest pain *to distinguish pericardial pain from myocardial ischemia.*
- Administer pain medication as ordered *to relieve pericardial chest pain.*
- Encourage bed rest with head of bed elevated or in position of comfort.
- Instruct patient to lean forward on over-bed table *to reduce pain.*

Decreased cardiac output high risk for related to reduced ventricular pressure

- Assess for signs of cardiac tamponade (p. 66); narrowing pulse pressure and pulsus paradoxus *to detect early signs of increasing intrapericardial pressure and development of tamponade.*
- Monitor vital signs *to detect signs of ventricular decompensation.*
- Prepare for pericardiocentesis or pericardiectomy as indicated by clinical status.
- Place on cardiac monitor, checking rhythm every 1 to 2 hours.
- Auscultate heart sounds for presence of pericardial friction rub (may be distant).

Patient Education/Home Care Planning

1. Explain the underlying cause and disease process.
2. Explain signs and symptoms of recurring inflammation to the patient, and tell the patient to notify the physician if they occur.
3. Explain the purpose, method of administration, and side effects of medications.

Evaluation

Patient demonstrates decreased anxiety   Patient verbalizes relief of pain. Patient demonstrates ability to rest and sleep without complaint. Patient appears relaxed.

Patient is free of chest pain   Patient verbalizes no chest discomfort. Patient tolerates routine activities and procedures without complaining of pain or shortness of breath. ECG is normal. There is no friction rub. White blood cell count and sedimentation rate are normal.

Patient shows an increased level of understanding   Patient identifies signs and symptoms to report to physician. Patient verbalizes knowledge regarding disease, activity allowances and limitations, and medications.

Cardiac output is maintained   Patient demonstrates hemodynamic stability; BP and pulse rate are maintained at baseline. Heart and breath sounds are normal. Absence of pulsus paradoxus.

ENDOCARDITIS

Endocarditis is an inflammatory process involving the endothelial layer of the heart, including the cardiac valves and septal defects, if present (Figure 1-51).

The designations *acute* and *subacute* were used previously to classify patients with infective endocarditis (IE) and were based on the progression of untreated infection.

The incidence of IE is not known. In one report the frequency was about 0.16 to 5.4 cases per 1000 hospital admissions.[8] Endocarditis primarily involves older adults, with a mean age of 55 years. Men are affected more often by a ratio of 2:1 to 5:1 in several series.[20]

Persons at risk for IE include patients who have a history of rheumatic heart disease, valvular heart disease, or congenital heart defects or who have prosthetic heart valves, arteriovenous shunts for dialysis, or who are intravenous drug users. Previously, rheumatic valvular heart disease was the most common predisposing factor; now mitral valve prolapse (MVP) with regurgitation is the most common underlying cardiac defect predisposing to IE.

Immunosuppressed patients are susceptible to transient bacteremia. The fatality rate remains at 20% to 30%, but among elderly patients, mortality may be as high as 70%. Congestive heart failure is the major cause of death.

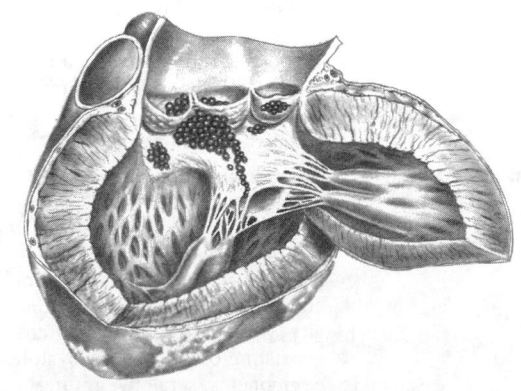

Figure 1-51 Endocarditis. (From Canobbio.[13])

••••• Pathophysiology

Endocarditis can be linked to a number of organisms. Diagnosis and treatment depend on isolating the organism.

Streptococcal strains account for 50% to 60% of all subacute bacterial endocarditis (SBE) cases. These low-virulence bacteria generally affect already damaged valves. *S. viridans,* the most commonly implicated α-hemolytic organism, is found in the mouth and upper respiratory tract.

Staphylococcus aureus, which affects normal valves, is responsible for 25% of cases of IE. It is associated with a mortality rate ranging from 45% to 73%. Less common enterococcal strains *(S. faecalis)* have increasingly been seen in IE. *Enterococcus* is found in the gastrointestinal and genitourinary tracts and the oral cavity. It occurs often in elderly patients, particularly men undergoing urologic procedures, and has been reported in women of childbearing age. *S. epidermidis* is commonly seen in endocarditis after prosthetic valve replacement.

Other known pathogens linked to endocarditis include gram-negative organisms, fungi, and yeast. Endocarditis caused by gram-negative cocci and bacilli *(Serratia marcescens, Klebsiella, Pseudomonas)* occurs in the elderly and in mainline drug abusers. The increase in incidence of endocarditis caused by fungi *(Candida, Aspergillus)* may be linked to the increase in IV drug abuse and the widespread use of antimicrobial and corticosteroid therapies. Fungal vegetations tend to be large and to embolize in major blood vessels, particularly in the legs.

Endocarditis generally begins as a transient bacteremia (or fungemia) introduced into the circulation through several portals of entry (Table 1-4). Bacteria more commonly settle on cardiac structures that have already been damaged. The valves are especially susceptible. Unrepaired ventricular septal defects, coarctation of aorta, patent ductus arteriosus, and unrepaired tetralogy of Fallot are also susceptible. Infected structures are often those in which turbulent blood flow is forced across an area of high pressure to low pressure. Trauma to the endothelial surface of the low-pressure side of the damaged site causes local clotting. As a result, an aggregation of platelets and fibrin thrombi forms on the injured structure. During the active phase of the infection these thrombi can foster the growth of microorganisms.

The pathogenesis of endocarditis is related to the adherence of infected thrombi to cardiac structures, which in the case of the valves can lead to scarring and retraction of the leaflets. The destruction may be sufficient to cause erosion of the leaflets and perforation leading to valvular insufficiency. The infectious process may also spread to the anulus, creating abscesses, or rupture the chordae tendineae. Mycotic aneurysms may result from septic embolization, which develops in the aorta, cerebral arteries, sinus of Valsalva, ligated ductus arteriosus, and smaller arterial vessels (of the lung, kidney, or spleen).

•••••• Diagnostic Studies and Findings

Complete blood count (CBC) Anemia; elevated sedimentation rate; leukocytosis; thrombocytopenia

TABLE 1-4 Possible Ports of Entry and Factors Predisposing to Bacteremia

Port of Entry	Infecting Organism
Oral cavity Extractions, teeth cleaning, periodontal disease (abscesses), periodontal operations, use of unwaxed dental floss, oral irrigation, bridgework	*Streptococcus, Staphylococcus epidermidis*
Upper respiratory tract Tonsilloadenoidectomy, orotracheal intubation, bronchoscopy (rigid tubes), pneumonia	*Staphylococcus aureus, Streptococcus, Haemophilus* species, *Streptococcus pneumoniae, S. epidermidis*
Gastrointestinal tract Barium enema, sigmoidoscopy, colonscopy, percutaneous biopsy of liver	Gram-negative rods, *Enterobacter, Escherichia coli, Klebsiella*
Genitourinary system Catheterization, urethrotomy, transurethral prostatectomy, retropubic prostatectomy, cystoscopy	*E. coli,* gram-negative bacilli, *Enterococcus*
Female reproductive system Delivery, abortion (therapeutic, illegal), intrauterine devices	*E. coli*
Skin Furuncles, acne (infected, squeezed), skin piercing, tattoos, acupuncture	*S. aureus, S. epidermidis*
Other sources of infection Pacemaker (transvenous), prolonged use of polyethylene catheter (atrial), hemodialysis (arteriovenous cannulas), infection (hematogenous osteomyelitis, Q fever, meningococcemia)	

Blood cultures (four to six cultures from different venipuncture sites within 6 to 72 hours before therapy started) Identification of causative organism

Urine Proteinuria; red cell or leukocyte casts; microhematuria

Rheumatoid factor Positive in 50% of patients with infection of 6 weeks' duration

Blood chemistry Elevated BUN and creatinine values in patients with renal complications

Echocardiogram (Transesophageal Echocardiogram) Presence of vegetations or abscesses; involvement or damage of cardiac valves; ventricular function; hemodynamic changes such as regurgitation

Electrocardiogram (ECG) Early infection—normal; Late infection—conduction defects; atrial fibrillation, flutter

Radionuclide studies   Gallium 67 citrate may accumulate in areas of inflammation

•••••• Multidisciplinary Plan

Surgery

Valvuloplasty by debridement or valvectomy with or without valve replacement; surgical removal of vegetations and thrombi not indicated unless uncontrollable sepsis occurs, and then combined with long-term antimicrobial therapy; if infectious process is fulminant and resistant to antimicrobial therapy, excision of vegetations, unroofing of abscesses, and valve replacement recommended; presence of congestive heart failure is a major indication for surgery, reducing the high mortality rate to a range of 9% to 14%[8]

Medications

Antibiotics—long-term IV antibiotic therapy inhibits bacterial growth; because appropriate therapy depends on isolation of infecting organism, serial blood cultures are required *before* initiation of therapy; initiation of antibiotic therapy is guided by patients' clinical state: for patients who have been ill for weeks or months, delaying therapy until culture results are available will not endanger patient, but treatment for an acutely ill patient should begin immediately; therapy usually continues 4 to 6 weeks with parenteral administration as recommended route; culture-negative endocarditis is uncom-mon (5%), and most often occurs in patients who have recently received broad-spectrum antibiotics. For these patients and those with fulminating acute IE a combination of IV vancomycin and low-dose gentamycin should be instituted

Analgesic-antipyretics (salicylates) given for elevated temperature

Other agents dictated by presence of complications
    Cardiac
        Abscesses
        Valvular dysfunction (p. 60)
        Heart failure (p. 41)
        Myocarditis
    Embolization
        Cerebral
        Renal
        Splenic
        Coronary
    Mycotic aneurysms

General Management

Rest—encouraged during acute phase; patient may require prolonged hospitalization or home intravenous therapy lasting several weeks

Vital signs—checked every 4 to 8 hours, decreasing frequency as indicated by improved clinical condition

Diet—regular; patient may require high-caloric supplemental feedings; force fluids during periods of elevated temperature provided there is no ventricular failure

Monitor parenteral therapy for rate and amount of infusion; check regularly for localized signs of inflammation, phlebitis; assess antibiotic drug levels to avoid toxic effects, while optimizing treatment; evaluate patient's aptitude for home parenteral antibiotic therapy

NURSING CARE

Nursing Assessment

General Complaints

- Acute: high-grade fever (39° to 40°C [102° to 104°F])
- Chronic: low-grade fever (less than 39.4° C [103° F]), weakness, malaise, weight loss, anorexia, arthralgia, sweats, headache, dyspnea

Signs of Embolization (Peripheral, Cerebral, Systemic)

- Petechiae in conjunctivae, palate, buccal mucosa, and extremities; splinter hemorrhages (linear, dark-red streaks on nail beds); Osler's nodes (small, tender, raised nodules frequently found on finger and toe pads); Janeway's lesions (nontender, flat, erythematous, maculae on palms and soles); splenomegaly; Roth's spots (retinal hemorrhages with white centers); neurologic changes (behavioral changes, aphasia, paralysis, seizures)

Auscultation

- Murmurs not present in early phase of infection may become apparent if valvular damage occurs, or existing murmurs may change in intensity

Nursing Dx & Intervention

Altered nutrition: less than body requirements related to biologic factors (fever, infection)

- Assess patient for signs of progressive weight loss or malnutrition: dry weight below normal for age and height, fatigue, decreased triceps skinfold measurements.
- Weigh patient daily *to determine weight loss and need for supplemental feedings.* Decrease frequency as weight stabilizes.
- Monitor daily caloric intake as indicated by patient's appetite and food intake.
- Offer high-caloric, high-protein supplemental feedings *to ensure adequate intake of daily nutrients during anorexic periods.*
- Ensure patient comfort during mealtime *to stimulate appetite.*
- Encourage patient participation in food selections.

Risk for altered tissue perfusion related to embolism

- Assess for signs of embolization each shift and as needed.
- Report any changes to physician immediately.

- Administer anticoagulant therapy as ordered.
- Instruct patient about need to continue with anticoagulants, if ordered, *to prevent further embolic episodes.*

Cerebral
- Perform neurologic checks every shift or as indicated by condition.

Splenic
- Assess for splenomegaly; report signs and symptoms as indicated by tender or painful abdomen.

Renal
- Monitor intake and output every 8 hours or as indicated by condition.
- A decrease in urine output may reflect embolism or infarction.

Pulmonary
- Auscultate lung sounds every 4 to 8 hours or as indicated
- Obtain and monitor arterial blood gases as ordered.

Hyperthermia (elevated body temperature) related to infectious process
- Assess for dehydration; diaphoresis, poor skin turgor, dry mucous membranes; monitor laboratory reports.
- Obtain temperature every 4 to 8 hours as indicated.
- Monitor fluid intake and output, noting water loss through perspiration.
- Encourage fluid intake as tolerated to maintain fluid balance.
- Administer antipyretics as ordered.

Patient Education/Home Care Planning

1. Provide instruction regarding the disease process and the purpose and method of treatment.
2. Coordinate outpatient parenteral antibiotic management with home care nurse, home care pharmacy, and infectious disease specialist.
3. Teach patient care of long-term intravenous (IV) antibiotic therapy; review care of IV site and signs of infection and inflammation to report to nurse or physician; discuss care of antibiotics infusion; permit time for return demonstration.
4. Explain precipitating risk factors that can lead to bacteremia and reinfection: poor oral hygiene, dental work (gum cleaning or treatment, extractions), gastrointestinal or genitourinary procedures, vaginal deliveries, furuncles, staphylococcal infections, surgical procedures.
5. Encourage regular follow-up care with a physician.
6. Explain to the patient the need for good oral hygiene and regular dental care.
7. Explain and reinforce the need for antibiotic prophylaxis before procedures that predispose to bacteremia (see Table 1-2, p. 61 for specific recommendations).

Evaluation

There is absence of inflammatory processes Temperature, blood cultures, white cell count, and other laboratory findings are normal. Patient's sense of well-being is improved. Patient reports feeling less fatigued, improved appetite, weight gain, and absence of sweats and headache.

Nutritional status is improved and maintained Baseline or normal body weight is regained. Patient demonstrates improved appetite.

Activity is resumed Patient is referred for outpatient management as appropriate. Resumption of work and family role occurs.

Tissue perfusion is maintained Patient is alert and oriented. No signs of embolism present. Lung sounds are clear and urine output is normal.

MYOCARDITIS
Myocarditis is an inflammatory process of the heart caused by an infectious agent.

Endocarditis and pericarditis are also inflammatory diseases of the heart, but myocarditis specifically involves the myocytes, interstitium, and vascular elements. The prevalence and incidence of viral myocarditis in the general population are unknown, but approximately 5% of a population infected with a virus (e.g., influenza) may experience some form of cardiac involvement associated with the acute illness.

Pathophysiology
Myocarditis characteristically develops after a period of several weeks following the initial systemic infection, suggesting involvement of an immunologic mechanism. The physiologic end point of severe myocarditis is dilated cardiomyopathy, presumably a consequence of viral-mediated immunologic cardiac damage.[8] Virtually any infectious agent may produce cardiac inflammation, viruses being the most common (see box on p. 72). Myocarditis may also be caused by allergic reactions and pharmacologic agents.

The clinical consequences of myocarditis depend on the size and number of myocardial lesions, which are usually randomly distributed in the heart. Clinical expression ranges from often asymptomatic and unrecognized cases to acute, and sometimes fatal, congestive heart failure. Dysrhythmias, particularly ventricular, may be the only sign of otherwise unrecognized myocarditis. Specifically, 17% to 21% of sudden deaths not attributed to accidents or violence can be linked to myocarditis.

Signs and symptoms of cardiovascular disease are usually absent but, depending on the severity of disease, may include fatigue, dyspnea, palpitations, chest pain, and tachycardia. Histologic findings are usually nonspecific, but the hallmark of myocarditis is an inflammatory myocardial infiltrate with associated evidence of myocardial damage.[8]

Diagnostic Studies and Findings
Electrocardiogram (ECG) ST-segment and T wave abnormalities

Chest x-ray Enlarged cardiac silhouette; pulmonary congestion in severe cases

---

■ ETIOLOGIES OF MYOCARDITIS
■

Viral	Protozoal and metazoal
Coxsackievirus (A and B)	Trypanosomiasis
Influenza	Toxoplasmosis
Cytomegalovirus	Malaria
Hepatitis	Schistosomiasis
Mumps	Trichinosis
Herpes simplex	Bacterial
Rabies	Diphtheria
Epstein-Barr virus	Tuberculosis
Human immunodefi-	*Legionella*
ciency virus	*Brucella*
Echovirus	Clostridium
Rickettsial	*Salmonella/Shigella*
Q fever	Meningococcus
Rocky Mountain spotted	*Yersinia*
fever	Spirochetal
Scrub typhus	*Borrelia* (Lyme disease)
Fungal	
Cryptococcus	
Candidiasis	
Histoplasmosis	
Aspergillus	

Echocardiogram Left ventricular wall motion abnormalities; increased wall thickness or late stage dilation; left ventricular thrombi

Radionuclide scanning Inflammatory and necrotic changes characteristic of myocarditis

Viral serology studies Culture stool, throat, blood, myocardium, pericardial fluid; distinct increase in virus-neutralizing antibody, complement fixation, and hemagglutination inhibition titers

Endomyocardial biopsy To confirm diagnosis; however, a negative biopsy does not exclude myocarditis

• • • • • • Multidisciplinary Plan

Surgery

None for primary disease; cardiac transplant for end-stage dilated cardiomyopathy

Medications

Diuretics, digoxin, ACE inhibitors for heart failure management
Antidysrhythmic therapy
Immunosuppressant therapy (use in acute disease is controversial)
  Corticosteroids
  Cyclosporine
  Nonsteroidal antiinflammatory drugs (NSAIDs)
Anticoagulation (with caution in setting of thrombus)

General Management

Focus on systemic manifestations (heart failure, dysrhythmias)

Bed rest: restrict activity during acute phase of disease because exercise may intensify myocardial damage

Nursing Dx & Intervention

Alteration in cardiac tissue perfusion related to inflammatory myocardial lesions, dysrhythmias

- Assess for signs of congestive heart failure and dysrhythmia frequently during acute phase.
- Maintain bed rest.

Anxiety/fear related to sick role restriction/risk of death in previously healthy individual

- Provide for quiet environment, access to significant others, rest time.
- Explain procedures, changes, medications to enhance self-control.

Denial related to absence of disabling symptoms and lack of cardiovascular disease

- Explain risks associated with sudden death during exertional activity.
- Outline long-term consequences of myocardial damage if not recognized early.

Patient Education/Home Care Planning

1. Monitor patient's cardiac status, medication tolerance, compliance.
2. Perform cardiac rehabilitation if patient's preillness activity level has been compromised by prolonged bed rest, symptoms.
3. Monitor medication regimen/heart failure management routine by phone.
4. Assess patient and family for cardiac transplant candidacy.

Evaluation

Cardiac output is maintained Vital signs are stable. Urine output is adequate. Dysrhythmia is under control.

Patient's anxiety is minimized in acute care environment Patient verbalizes understanding of procedures, medications. Patient seeks support of significant others.

Patient shows increased level of cooperation Patient arranges follow-up appointments and takes medications as prescribed. Patient makes arrangements to modify work responsibilities and defer athletic activity.

■ CONGENITAL HEART DISEASE
■

A congenital heart disorder is any structural or functional abnormality or defect of the heart or great vessels existing from birth.

Congenital heart disease is a specialty of pediatrics. However, because of advances in medical and surgical management, persons with congenital defects are now living longer and are being treated as adults. Although the incidence of congenital heart disease has decreased over the decades, it continues to occur at a rate of 5 to 8 per 1000 live births.[3]

•••••• Pathophysiology

In most cases the cause for the congenital defect cannot be determined. However, various factors are believed to contribute to these malformations.

Genetics Several studies have demonstrated prevalence rates among siblings and blood relatives to be 1.5% to 5%,[70] suggesting a genetic link in the etiology of cardiac malformations. This genetic link could become important as more children with congenital heart disease reach adulthood and are therefore capable of bearing offspring. This growing population of procreating adults with congenital heart disease offers geneticists a closer look at inheritance of heart defects. Certain chromosomal abnormalities, including Turner's syndrome and Down syndrome, have been linked to heart defects.

Environmental factors Although difficult to prove as isolated causes, environmental factors along with genetic factors have been linked to heart defects. Factors include pollution, smoking, and alcohol use by the mother.

Teratogens Use of certain drugs such as alcohol and warfarin and exposure to viruses such as rubella during fetal development have been shown to cause not only heart defects but also widespread injury to the embryo.

Altitude Altitude may cause the ductus arteriosus to fail to close after birth.

Common Defects in Which Prolonged Survival Occurs

Patent ductus arteriosus (Figure 1-52) The ductus arteriosus is a vascular connection that during fetal life directs blood flow from the pulmonary artery to the aorta, bypassing the lungs. Functional closure of the ductus arteriosus occurs after birth. In some cases it takes 6 months to several years before complete closure. If the ductus remains patent, the direction of blood flow is reversed from left to right because of high systemic pressure in the aorta. Blood is shunted through the ductus arteriosus to the pulmonary artery during both systole and diastole. This raises pressure in the pulmonary circulation and increases the pressure against which the right ventricle must work. Consequently, a large ductus arteriosus with unrestricted flow could eventually lead to pulmonary vascular disease and Eisenmenger's complex (see the box on p. 74).

Survival into adulthood is possible. Patent ductus arteriosus occurs more often in girls and can be linked to other defects such as ventricular septal defect and coarctation of the aorta.

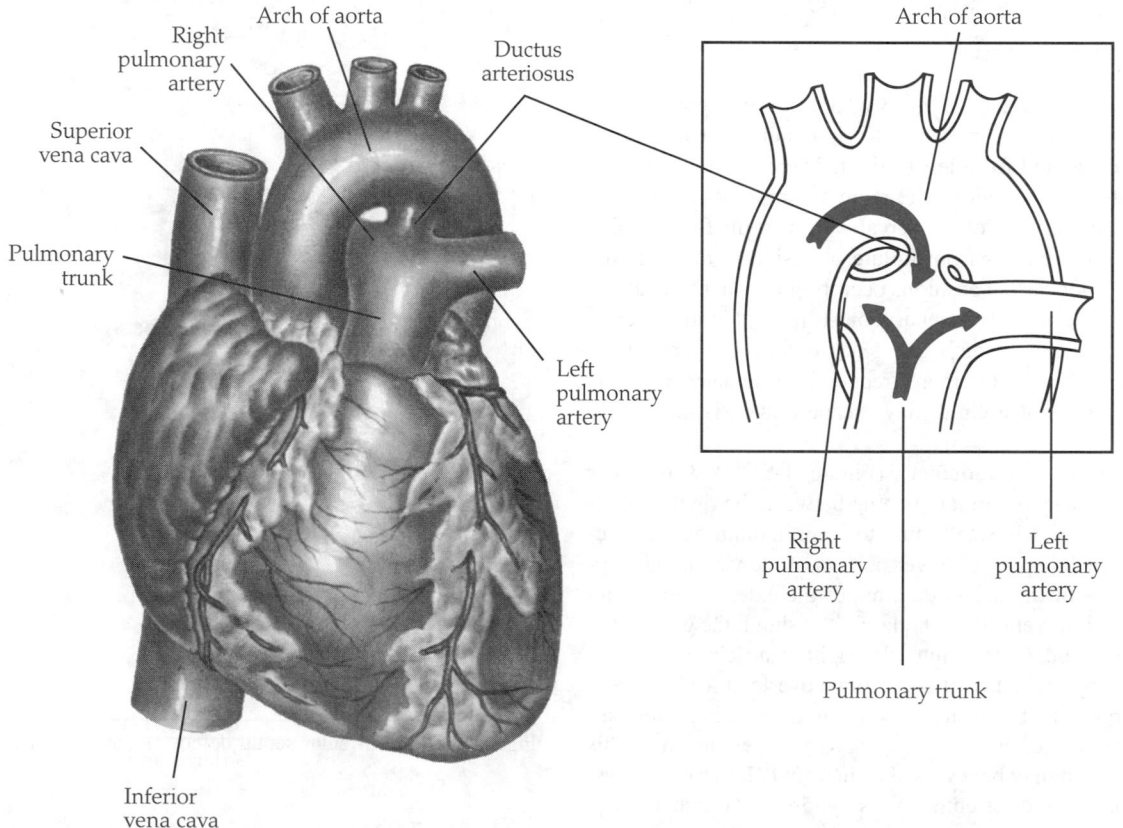

Figure 1-52 Patent ductus arteriosus. (From Canobbio.[13])

■ EISENMENGER'S REACTION

Eisenmenger's reaction is a complication that results from the development of high pulmonary vascular resistance (PVR) that is greater than 800 dynes-sec/cm^{-5}. PVR rises in response to chronic unrestricted systemic blood flow into the pulmonary circuit. As a result, reversed or bidirectional shunts occur at the aorticopulmonary, ventricular, or atrial levels, allowing unoxygenated venous blood to cross the defect and enter the systemic arterial circulation. PVR is associated with decreased oxygen saturation, cyanosis, and polycythemia.

The term *Eisenmenger's reaction* applies to a number of shunting defects, such as VSD and ASD, which are similar because of the presence of pulmonary hypertension and an associated right to left shunt. It usually occurs as a result of delayed operation and may be undiagnosed until adolescence or adulthood, when surgical correction is no longer possible.

Clinically, the most common complaint is effort intolerance, probably because of decreased arterial oxygen saturation. In later stages, symptoms are more commonly caused by right ventricular failure. Other common features include cyanosis, with clubbing, and polycythemia.

Most patients survive and live reasonably active lives throughout the fourth and fifth decades. Sudden death, presumably from dysrhythmias, is the most common cause of death. Other causes of death include heart failure and pulmonary infarction from arterial thrombosis.

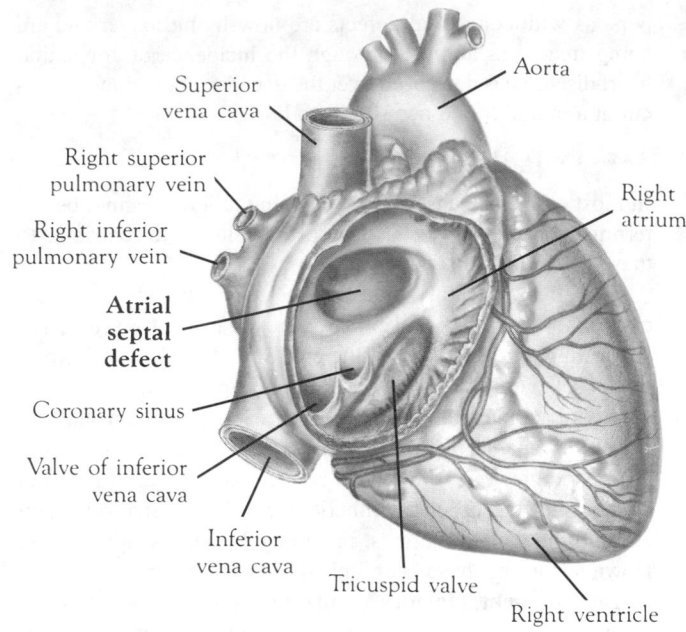

Figure 1-53 Atrial septal defect. (From Canobbio.[13])

Atrial septal defect   (Figure 1-53) An atrial septal defect is an abnormal opening between the right and left atria causing blood to be shunted from left to right. There are two common forms. In ostium secundum, the more common of the two, the defect is in the middle of the septal wall near the fossa ovalis. Ostium primum results from failure of fusion of the left portions of the endocardial cushions occurring low in the atrial position. An associated cleft (separation) is present in the anterior mitral valve leaflet, which can lead to mitral regurgitation. Again, this defect occurs more frequently in females, and it is not uncommon that a child may escape diagnosis until early adult life.

Ventricular septal defect   (Figure 1-54) A ventricular septal defect is an abnormal opening between the right and left ventricles. It varies in size (7 mm to 3 cm in diameter) and occurs in either the upper or lower portion of the ventricular septum. The size of the defect determines the extent of the shunt from left to right ventricle. The larger the shunt, the greater the volume of blood ejected into the right ventricle and lungs. Therefore large defects cause a volume overload for both ventricles. Large defects can also lead to an increase in pulmonary vascular resistance, producing pulmonary hypertension. If this occurs the shunt may be reversed from right to left, causing systemic cyanosis and Eisenmenger's syndrome, which renders the patient inoperable.

Tetralogy of Fallot   (Figure 1-55) Tetralogy of Fallot is an anomaly marked by four defects: ventricular septal defect, right

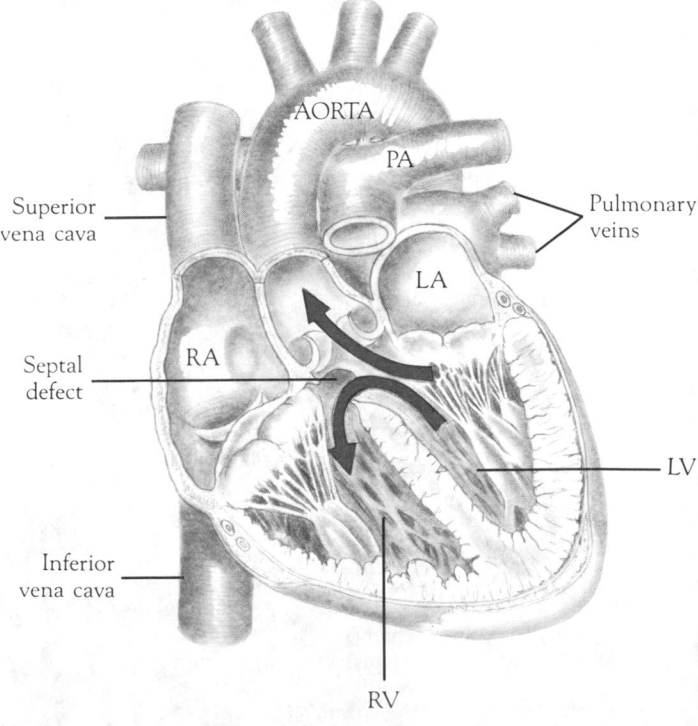

Figure 1-54 Ventricular septal defect. (From Canobbio.[13])

ventricular outflow obstruction (pulmonic stenosis), deviation (dextroposition) of the aorta so it overrides the ventricular septum, and right ventricular hypertrophy. It is the most com-

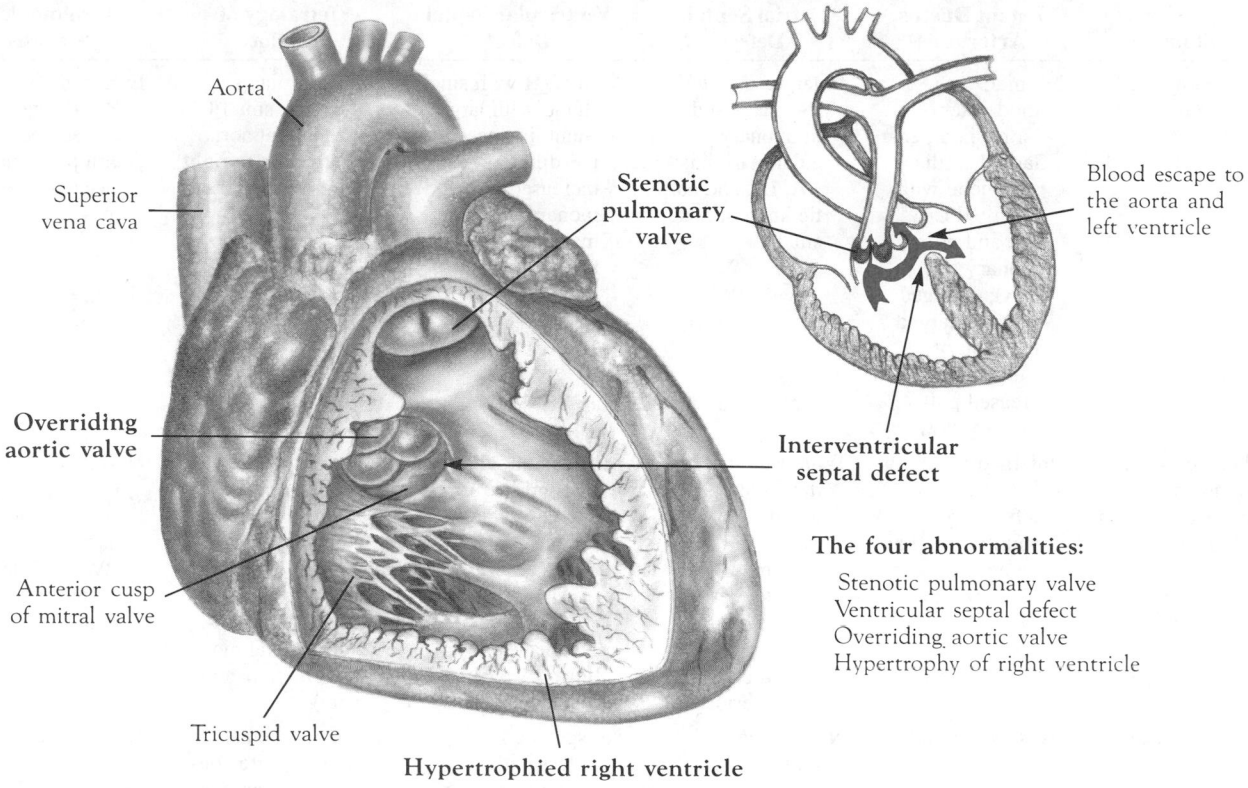

Aorta

Superior
vena cava

**Stenotic
pulmonary
valve**

Blood escape to
the aorta and
left ventricle

**Overriding
aortic valve**

**Interventricular
septal defect**

Anterior cusp
of mitral valve

The four abnormalities:

Stenotic pulmonary valve
Ventricular septal defect
Overriding aortic valve
Hypertrophy of right ventricle

Tricuspid valve

Hypertrophied right ventricle

Figure 1-55 Tetralogy of Fallot. (From Canobbio.[13])

mon cyanotic lesion in which survival to adulthood is expected. The severity of symptoms depends on the size of the ventricular septal defect, degree of pulmonic stenosis, and position of the aorta. Right ventricular outflow is obstructed, resulting in hypertrophy of the right ventricle and a right-to-left shunt. This produces a decrease in systemic arterial oxygen saturation, cyanosis, reduced pulmonary blood flow, and in some cases a hypoplastic pulmonary artery.

Pulmonic valvular stenosis (Figure 1-56) Congenital pulmonic valvular stenosis may occur by itself, with other defects such as atrial or ventricular septal defect, or as part of tetralogy of Fallot. If it occurs by itself, the chance of survival to adulthood is good. Pulmonic stenosis may occur as one of three types: valvular, subvalvular (infundibular), or supravalvular. The degree of right ventricular hypertrophy varies with the degree of obstruction.

•••••• Diagnostic Studies and Findings

Study	Patent Ductus Arteriosus	Atrial Septal Defect	Ventricular Septal Defect	Tetralogy of Fallot	Pulmonic Stenosis
Electrocardiogram (ECG)	Normal (small ductus); left ventricular hypertrophy (LVH); PR interval may be prolonged; atrial fibrillation in adults	Normal; right ventricular hypertrophy (RVH); right bundle-branch block; PR interval may be prolonged; left axis deviation (ostium primum); normal or right axis (ostium secundum)	Normal if defect is small; if moderate to large, LVH; LVH/RVH in presence of pulmonary hypertension	RVH	Normal if stenosis is mild; if moderate to severe, RVH and right axis deviation; if severe, right atrial hypertrophy (RAH)

Continued.

Study	Patent Ductus Arteriosus	Atrial Septal Defect	Ventricular Septal Defect	Tetralogy of Fallot	Pulmonic Stenosis
Chest x-ray	Normal; with moderate to large shunt, enlarged cardiac silhouette with enlarged LA, LV, and pulmonary artery (PA); enlarged aorta; enlarged pulmonary trunk and increased pulmonary flow	Enlarged RA, RV, PA; increased pulmonary vascular markings; LA, LV, and aortic knob may be small	Mild LVH with small shunt; with large shunt, increased LV, dilation of PA, increased pulmonary vascular markings, enlarged LA	Small cardiac silhouette; small PA; prominent aorta (may arch to right in 25% of cases)	Enlarged RV and PA; if severe, decreased peripheral pulmonary vascular markings
Echocardiogram/ transesophogeal echocardiogram (TEE)	Enlarged LA and LV owing to left-to-right shunt; TEE may be necessary to visualize ductus	With ostium secundum, enlarged RV, paradoxic movement of septum during systole; with ostium primum, mitral valve displaced inferiorly and anteriorly	Large shunt; enlarged RA and RV; for smaller defects, bubble contrast through peripheral IV can be visualized crossing defect, especially during Valsalva's maneuver	Overriding aorta visualized; pulmonary stenosis visualized with degree of obstruction; enlarged ventricular septum (septal motion remains normal)	Normal if stenosis is mild; if moderate to severe, enlarged RA and RV, possible tricuspid regurgitation
Laboratory tests	No specific findings	No specific findings	No specific findings unless patient is cyanotic, then increased hematocrit value and hemoglobin level and decreased arterial oxygen saturation	Increased hematocrit value; degree depends on amount of deoxygenated systemic blood	No specific findings
Cardiac catheterization	Left-to-right shunt; increased pulmonary blood flow; increased oxygen saturation in PA; intracardiac pressures normal; RV and PA pressures may be slightly elevated	Left-to-right shunt at atrial level; increased oxygen saturation in RA; RA pressure usually normal; mitral regurgitation	Left-to-right shunt (LV to RV); study determines degree of shunt; increased pulmonary blood flow, oxygen saturation in RV, and systolic pressure in RV and PA	RV outflow obstruction; increased RV pressure; RV to LV shunt; decreased PA pressure as catheter crosses obstruction	Increased RA pressure, which determines systolic pressure gradient between RV and PA
Magnetic resonance imaging (MRI)/angiography	Angiography capability to image anatomy of ductus and flow without contrast			Images anatomy of pulmonary arteries without contrast of invasive catheter	

•••••• Multidisciplinary Plan

Surgery

Patent ductus arteriosus
  Ligation of ductus
Atrial septal defect
  Direct closure by suturing or placement of Dacron or pericardial patch across defect
Correction of mitral regurgitation by valvuloplasty or replacement (depends on degree of regurgitation)
Ventricular septal defect
  Direct closure by suturing or with placement of Dacron or pericardial patch across defect
Tetralogy of Fallot
  Palliative procedures performed on infants to enhance blood flow to lungs, thereby reducing hypoxia

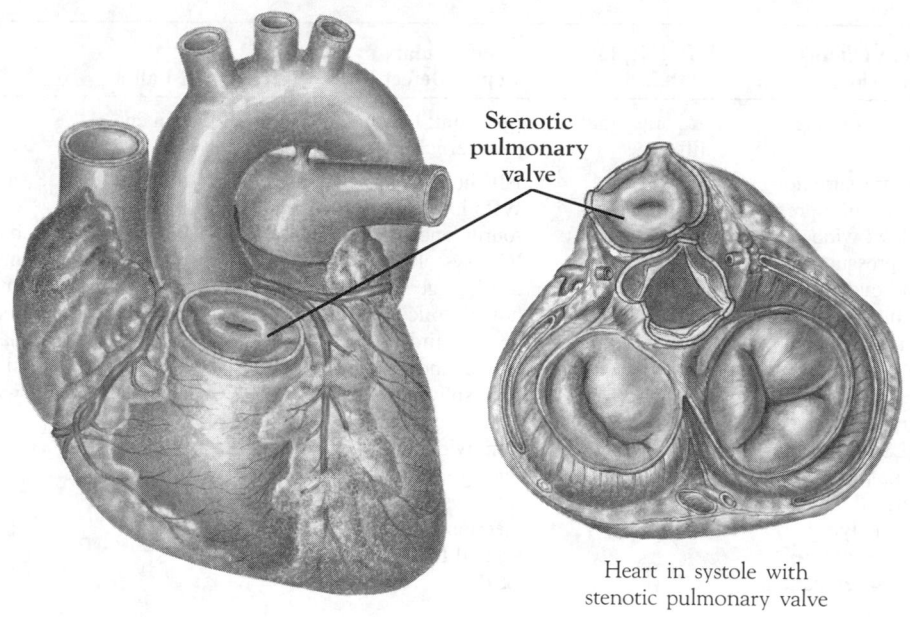

Stenotic pulmonary valve

Heart in systole with stenotic pulmonary valve

Figure 1-56 Pulmonic valvular stenosis. (From Canobbio.[13])

Blalock-Taussig procedure—anastomosis between sub-clavian artery and pulmonary artery

Potts' anastomosis—side-to-side anastomosis of left pulmonary artery to descending aorta

Waterston-Cooley procedure—anastomosis of right pulmonary artery to ascending aorta

Pulmonic stenosis

Valvotomy; resection of excess infundibular muscle; valve replacement

Corrective surgery—intracardiac repair of ventricular septal defect and pulmonic stenosis; contraindicated if pulmonary artery is hypoplastic

Medications

Dictated by patient's clinical picture and presence of ventricular failure and dysrhythmias; with few exceptions, antibiotic prophylaxis for infective endocarditis is given for dental and other invasive procedures

General Management

Nonspecific unless indicated by complications such as heart failure, dysrhythmias, or effects of polycythemia in cyanotic patient

NURSING CARE

Nursing Assessment

Area of Concern	Patent Ductus Arteriosus	Atrial Septal Defect	Ventricular Septal Defect	Tetralogy of Fallot	Pulmonic Stenosis
Physical examination	Small shunt: asymptomatic, increased respiratory infections, small for age; large shunt: exertional dyspnea, decreased exercise tolerance	Small shunt: asymptomatic; moderate to large shunt: exertional dyspnea, decreased exercise tolerance, palpitations	Small to moderate shunt: asymptomatic, exertional dyspnea; large shunt: failure **in infancy,** growth failure, feeding difficulties	**In infancy:** paroxysmal attacks of dyspnea with loss of consciousness ("blue" spells), small for age; **in later childhood:** cyanosis with clubbing of fingers and toes; **in adulthood** (after palliation): exertional dyspnea, cyanosis with clubbing	Asymptomatic during childhood; exertional dyspnea; decreased exercise tolerance

Continued.

Area of Concern	Patent Ductus Arteriosus	Atrial Septal Defect	Ventricular Septal Defect	Tetralogy of Fallot	Pulmonic Stenosis
Palpation	Neck vessels dilated and pulsating	Left parasternal lift	Large shunt: left parasternal lift	Precordial prominence; parasternal heave	Left parasternal heave; subxiphoid pulsation
Auscultation	Systolic pressure normal; diastolic pressure low; wide pulse pressure; harsh, loud, continuous murmur in first, second, and third intercostal spaces (ICS) at lower sternal border (LSB); machinery-like murmur best heard when patient is lying down, becoming fainter when patient is standing	Soft blowing systolic murmur at second ICS at LSB	Small shunt: holosystolic at third, fourth, and fifth ICS, systolic thrill; large shunt: holosystolic murmur at third, fourth, and fifth ICS, splitting of S_2 during expiration, widening during inspiration, systolic ejection sound at second ICS at LSB	Single S_2; systolic ejection murmur at third ICS, may radiate upward to left side of neck	S_1 normal; early systolic ejection click heard at base; midsystolic murmur at second and third ICS at LSB, radiates to suprasternal notch and to left side of neck; S_2 widely split

Nursing Dx & Intervention

Knowledge deficit related to lack of understanding or information misinterpretation

- Instruct patient and family on type of defect and how to manage at home; provide referral services for assistance with home care.
- For adult patients, provide detailed explanation of defect, surgical interventions, and treatments as dictated by defect.

Anxiety related to actual or perceived threat to biologic integrity

- Assess level of anxiety: determine primary cause to identify any misconceptions, fears, and concerns.
- Encourage verbalization of feelings.
- Elicit questions and concerns of patient.
- Assess usual coping mechanisms for dealing with stress to determine if they are adequate to control anxiety.
- Assist the patient to deal realistically with anxiety, providing alternative methods for dealing with anxiety.
- Refer the patient to long-term counseling if necessary.

Activity intolerance, high risk for related to lack of mobility or progressive decrease in cardiac reserve

- Assess usual level of activity; determine if appropriate for medical condition. May be overly restricted, inappropriate to degree of cardiac impairment by parental overprotectiveness or patient's own fears.
- Assess and monitor response to activity, noting type of activity, intensity, frequency, and type of symptoms that develop.

Patient Education/Home Care Planning

1. Instruct the patient and family about the primary defect and any surgical procedures that have occurred. Explain the associated signs and symptoms and describe what is normal and abnormal.
2. Explain activity allowances and limitations, including schooling, sports, and occupation.
3. For adolescents and adults provide counseling on issues concerning genetics, marriage, contraception, and child-bearing.
4. Explain dietary restrictions as indicated.
5. Explain the need to prevent endocarditis (p. 71).

Evaluation

Level of knowledge is increased   Patient and family verbalize knowledge regarding defect, prescribed care, medication, need for return visits, and endocarditis prophylaxis.

Anxiety is decreased   Patient and family verbalize reduction in anxiety level and demonstrate appropriate behavior in self-care management.

Optimum level of activity is maintained   Patient engages in activities appropriate to clinical status; verbalizes absence of fatigue, weakness.

VASCULAR DISEASES

■ SYSTEMIC HYPERTENSION

■ An intermittent or sustained elevation in systolic or diastolic blood pressure, hypertension is a major cause of cerebrovascular accident (stroke), cardiac disease, and renal failure (Figure 1-57).

It is estimated that 60 million Americans have hypertension, and an additional 25 million have borderline hypertension. Half of those affected are unaware of it. Among African-Americans hypertension is estimated to be higher than in whites, appears earlier, and results in higher risks of mortality and morbidity from stroke and heart failure. Death rates from cardiovascular disease are 45% higher for black men than for white men and 67% higher for black women than for white women.[3,66]

Hypertension is now defined as a blood pressure greater than 140/90 mm Hg. Current guidelines define persons with blood pressures less than 130/85 as normal; those with systolic blood pressure (SBP) between 130 and 139 and diastolic blood pressure (DBP) 85 to 89 are defined as high normal (Table 1-5).

In the elderly, systolic hypertension results from a loss of arterial compliance, reduced cardiac output and left ventricular ejection rate, and an increase in resistance of the larger arteries.[99] After age 50, systemic vascular resistance is noted to increase at the rate of 1% per year.[90,99] For persons aged 65 to 74 years, isolated systolic hypertension (SBP >140 mm Hg and DPB <90 mm Hg) has been reported to affect 10.3% of the male population and 11.8% of the female population. The results of clinical trials demonstrate significant cardiovascular benefit in treating hypertension.[93]

Although there is no way of predicting in whom high blood pressure will develop, hypertension can be detected easily.

Therefore the major emphasis in the control of hypertension should be on early detection and effective treatment.

••••• Pathophysiology

Primary (essential) hypertension is the most common form, accounting for 90% of all cases. It is an abnormal state in which excessive neurohumoral stimulation results in increased arterial tone. The cause is unknown, but certain risk factors have been identified. These include family history, age group, race, obesity, stress, cigarette smoking, and a diet high in salt and saturated fats.

Secondary hypertension refers to elevated blood pressure that is related to some underlying disease. The most common causes include the following:

Renal parenchymal disorders
   Pyelonephritis
   Glomerulonephritis
   Hydronephrosis
   Polycystic kidney
   Juxtaglomerular (renin-producing) tumors
   Following kidney transplant
Renal artery disease
   Atherosclerosis
   Arthritis
   Embolism
   Aneurysm
   Diabetic nephrosclerosis
Endocrine and metabolic disorders
   Pheochromocytoma
   Cushing's syndrome
   Aldosteronism (primary)
   Hypercalcemia
   Acromegaly
   Myxedema
   Oral contraceptives
   Chronic licorice use
Central nervous system disorders
   Increased intracranial pressure

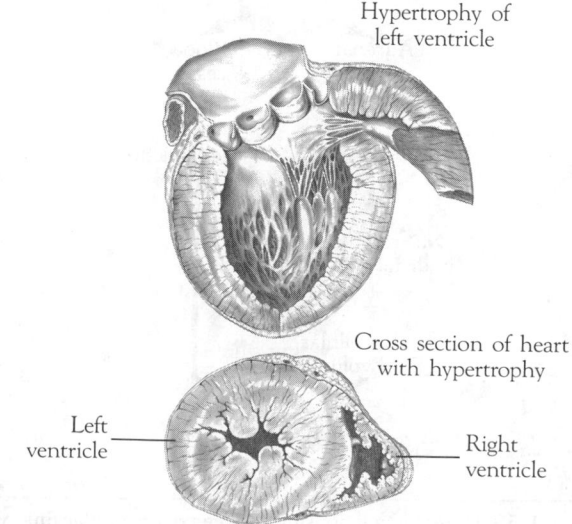

Hypertrophy of left ventricle

Cross section of heart with hypertrophy

Left ventricle

Right ventricle

Figure 1-57 Hypertension. (From Canobbio.[13])

■ TABLE 1-5 Classification of Initial Blood Pressure for Adults Aged 18 Years and Older

Category	Systolic (mm Hg)	Diastolic (mm Hg)
Normal	<130	<85
High normal	130-139	85-89
Hypertension		
Stage 1 (mild)	140-159	90-99
Stage 2 (moderate)	160-179	100-109
Stage 3 (severe)	180-209	110-119
Stage 4 (very severe)	>210	>120

Modified from the 1993 Report of the Joint National Committee on Detection, Evaluation, and Treatment of High Blood Pressure, *Arch Intern Med* 153:154, 1993.

Brain tumor
Neurogenic; psychogenic
Polyneuritis (porphyria)
Coarctation of aorta

The pathogenesis of hypertension is complex because various homeostatic mechanisms contribute to the maintenance of normal arterial pressure.

Cardiac output (stroke volume times heart rate) and peripheral vascular resistance determine arterial pressure. Increases in blood volume (high-output states), heart rate, or arterial vasoconstriction that cause an increase in peripheral resistance can lead to hypertension.

Stimulation and production of high plasma levels of renin (a proteolytic enzyme produced by juxtaglomerular cells) contribute to a complex relationship between extracellular fluid and pressure, leading to sympathetic activation and elevated arterial pressure. Figure 1-58 outlines the conversion of renin to angiotensin I and II.

•••••• Diagnostic Studies and Findings

Urine studies including microscopic examination   Proteinuria, hematuria

Blood chemistry   BUN >20 mg/dl; creatinine >1.5 mg/dl; potassium >5 mEq/L in renal failure; <3.5 mEq/L in primary aldosteronism and with diuretic administration; cholesterol and lipid levels elevated in hyperlipidemia; uric acid level may increase with diuretic therapy; calcium level may increase with diuretic therapy **BP measurements** an average of two or more blood pressure measurements separated by 2-minute intervals; additional measurements are obtained if first two readings differ by more than 5 mm Hg

Electrocardiogram (ECG)   Evaluates presence of left ventricular hypertrophy (increases the segment of electrocardiogram [QRS] voltage) and myocardial ischemia: standard treatment (ST) depression, T wave inversion

Echocardiogram   Evaluates presence of left ventricular hypertrophy

Chest x-ray   Posterior-anterior (PA) view: increased convexity of left heart border; increased cardiothoracic (CT) ratio

•••••• Multidisciplinary Plan

Surgery

None for primary hypertension (see Chapter 11 for surgical interventions for renal disorders)

Medications

Diuretics
    Thiazides (partial listing)
        Chlorothiazide (Diuril) (0.5-1 g/d)
        Chlorthalidone (Hygroton, Thalitone) (12.5-50 mg g/d)
        Hydrochlorothiazide (Esidrix, HydroDIURIL) (50-100 mg/d)
        Bendroflumethiazide (Naturetin) (2.5-10 mg/d)

Loop diuretics
    Furosemide (Lasix) (40-80 mg bid or qid)
    Ethacrynic acid (Edecrin) (initial dose 25-50 mg)
    Bumetanide (Bumex) (0.5-2.0 mg g/d)
Potassium-sparing diuretics
    Spironolactone (Aldactone) (100-400 mg bid or tid)
    Triamterene (Dyrenium) (100-300 mg bid)
    Amiloride (Midamor) (5-20 mg/d or bid)
β-Adrenergic blocking agents
    Propranolol (Inderal) (10-80 mg po bid or qid)
    Metoprolol tartrate (Lopressor) (50-200 mg po qd or bid)
    Pindolol (Visken) (15-60 mg/d)
    Atenolol (Tenormin) (50-100 mg/d)
    Timolol maleate (Blocadren) (20-40 mg/d)
    Nadolol (Corgard) (80-320 mg/d)

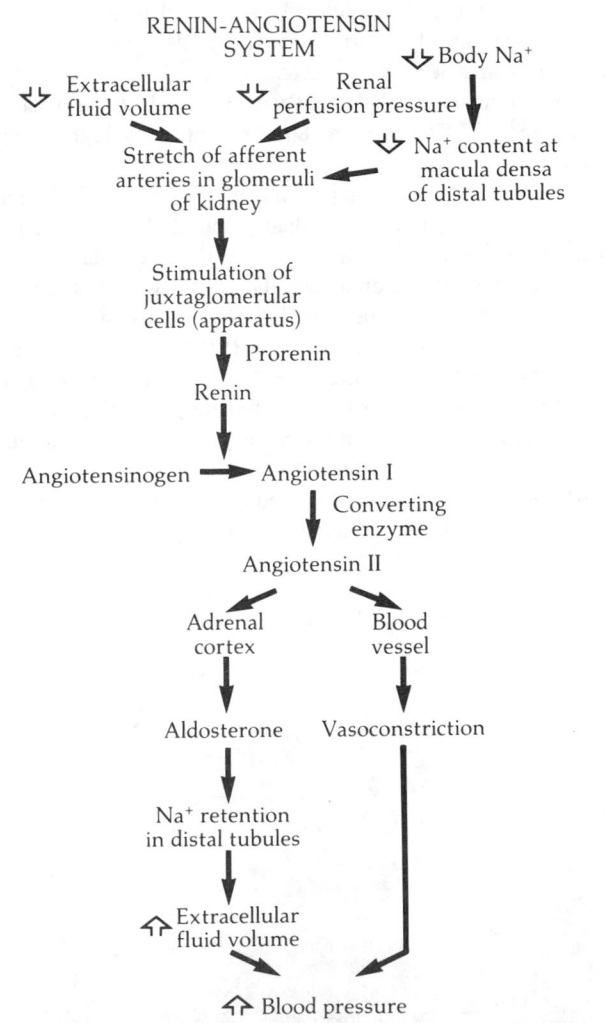

Figure 1-58 Complex relationship between extracellular fluid volume and pressure as mediated by renal hormonal mechanisms. These involve production of renin and angiotensin. Angiotensin is a potent vasoconstrictor that stimulates aldosterone synthesis, resulting in sodium retention and increased volume. (From Kaye.[48])

Antihypertensive agents
   Methyldopa (Aldomet) (up to 2 g/d po bid, tid, or qid)
   Guanethidine (Ismelin) (range 10-200 mg/d po)
ACE inhibitors (partial listing)
   Captopril (Capoten) (24-150 mg tid)
   Enalapril (Vasotec) (2.5-40 mg qd)
   Lisinopril (Zestril) (5.0-40 mg qd)
   Quinapril (Accupril) (5.0-80 mg qd)
   Benazepril (Lotensin) (10-40 mg qd)
Calcium antagonists (partial listing)
   Diltiazem (Cardizem) (90-360 mg)
   Verapamil (Calan, Isoptin) (80-480 mg)
   Nifedipine (Procardia) (30-120 mg)
Central acting α_2-agonists
   Methyldopa
Vasodilators
   Hydralazine (Apresoline) (10-50 mg po qid)
   Sodium nitroprusside (Nipride) (0.5-10 μg/kg/min IV)
   Diazoxide (Hyperstat) (300 mg by rapid IV bolus)
α-Adrenergic blocking agents
   Phentolamine (Regitine) (1-5 mg IV intermittently)
   Prazosin (Minipress) (initial dose 1 mg po, slowly increased to 10-15 mg/d)

General Management

The Stepped care approach (Figure 1-59) in the treatment of high blood pressure (based on recommendations of the 1984 National Joint Committee (JNC)[44] on detection, evaluation and treatment of high blood pressure) is an individualized, systematic approach to treatment
Step 0 nonpharmacologic therapy
   If control is inadequate, drug therapy is initiated

Step 1
   Begins with small doses of a single agent, then increases the dose, adds or substitutes another, or advances the dosages until blood pressure control is achieved; diuretics or β-blockers are suggested as initial treatment
Cardiac monitoring for hypertensive crisis
Arterial pressure monitoring for hypertensive crisis
Dietary management
   Sodium restriction—may range from mild to rigid restriction depending on degree of hypertension; JNC recommended dietary restriction 2-3 g/day

! EMERGENCY ALERT

HYPERTENSIVE CRISIS

Diastolic blood pressure above 130 mm Hg; must determine and treat underlying cause

Assessment

• Rule out renal disease, drug overdose, drug withdrawal, or hyperthyroidism.

Interventions

• Assess end organ function such as urinary output and perfusion.
• Obtain urinalysis, electrolytes, creatinine, uric acid.
• Obtain ECG.
• Obtain chest x-ray.
• Administer high-flow oxygen by mask (10 to 15 L).
• Obtain IV access.
• To lower blood pressures, administer medications that are appropriate for the cause (e.g., sodium nitroprusside, lasix, alpha- and beta-blocking agents).

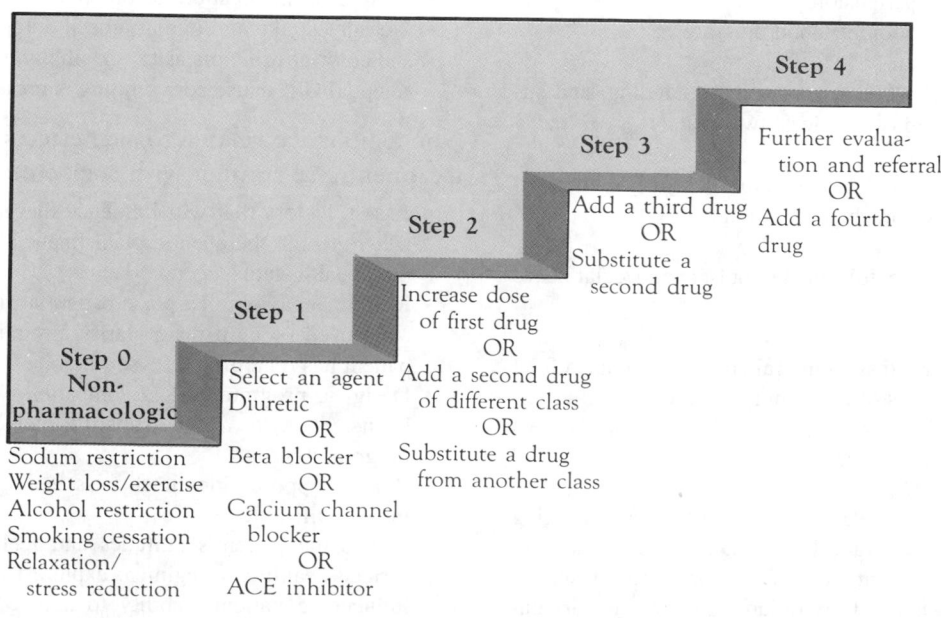

Figure 1-59 Stepped-care approach in treatment of high blood pressure. (From Canobbio.[13])

Alcohol—limit intake to 2 oz 100-proof whiskey, 8 oz wine, 24 oz beer per day

Caffeine—restrict intake

Cholesterol, lipids, saturated fats—reduce intake

Weight control—recommend weight loss of 5% or more in obese patient

Exercise

Regular aerobic exercise appropriate for age and health status

Refer to cardiac rehabilitation for prescribed exercise program

Avoid isometric exercises

Stress reduction and management

Monitor blood pressure on regular basis; frequency determined by blood pressure elevations

NURSING CARE

Nursing Assessment

Symptoms

Mild to moderate hypertension

Asymptomatic

Moderate to severe hypertension

Headaches, dizziness, fatigue, vertigo, palpitations

Severe hypertension

Throbbing suboccipital headache (may be present when patient awakens in morning, disappearing spontaneously after several hours); epistaxis

Physical Examination

Mild to moderate hypertension

Normal with exception of blood pressure

Moderate hypertension

Blood pressure (in both arms; sitting, standing, and supine; determined over at least two visits

Pulse

Tachycardia; bounding; femoral delay as compared with radial or brachial pulsation

Precordium

Displaced but forceful apical impulse; ventricular heave (apical lift)

Auscultation

Bruits over carotid and femoral areas; accentuated S_2 at base; apical systolic murmur; audible S_4; early diastolic blowing murmur (right and left sternal borders and intercostal spaces)

Optic fundi

Retinal changes: grade I—minimal arteriolar narrowing or irregularity; grade II—marked arteriolar narrowing and irregularity with focal tortuosity or spasm; grade III—marked arteriolar narrowing and irregularity with generalized tortuosity, flame-shaped hemorrhages, cotton-wool exudates; grade IV—same as III, plus papilledema

Nursing Dx & Intervention

Pain (headache) related to increased cerebrovascular pressure

- Assess quality of pain and presence of associated symptoms such as nausea, vomiting, and epistaxis.
- Initiate measures *to relieve pain and reduce external stimuli:*
  Maintain a quiet environment with reduced lighting.
  Limit activities.
  Avoid sudden jarring motion.
  Limit visitors.
  Use additional comfort measures such as cold packs and position changes.
- Administer pain relievers and antiemetics as ordered.
- Assist with ambulation *because patient may experience dizziness.*

Altered tissue perfusion (cerebral, renal, vascular) high risk for related to increased peripheral vascular resistance

- Assess and monitor level of consciousness. Check neurologic signs every hour during hypertensive crisis. Notify physician of any sudden changes in mentation, pupillary response, or movement of extremities.
- Maintain seizure precautions as indicated; maintain quiet environment.
- Monitor arterial pressures as indicated; use same arm for blood pressure; use Doppler sensor, if indicated.
- Monitor parenteral fluids with medications as ordered.
- Administer medications as ordered.
- Measure intake and output; check output, noting amount and color of urine; measure specific gravity.
- Keep NPO if nausea or vomiting is present.

Noncompliance related to side effects of prescribed treatment and conflict with sociocultural influences

- Assess factors that will influence the patient's ability to adhere to the therapeutic plan: financial status, age, culture, health status, occupation.
- Review behaviors that place patient at risk for cardiovascular event. Identify and clarify any misconceptions the patient has regarding disease state.
- Design a program that is compatible with the patient's habits, lifestyle, and personality. Include the patient in program design.
- Provide opportunities to discuss feelings toward recommended lifestyle changes.
- Assess the patient's attitudes and feelings toward prescribed health care regimen; explore factors that may be influencing patient's ability to adhere to the treatment plan.

- Explore alternative measures *to increase compliant behaviors,* such as contracting, self-monitoring, behavior modification, shaping behavior, and support groups.

Patient Education/Home Care Planning

1. Instruct the patient and family about high blood pressure, factors that contribute to increasing blood pressure, influencing factors.
2. Instruct patient on home blood pressure monitoring, interpretation of results, and actions to take if significant change occurs. Permit time for practice using home equipment. If patient unable to perform BP monitoring at home, provide information and referrals to have regular BP checks. Refer to home health agency as necessary.
3. Explain diet therapy, including sodium, calorie, and fat restrictions as ordered; include the rationale in explanation. Discuss the importance of restricting alcohol.
4. Explain the role of regular exercise in blood pressure regulation and weight control.
5. Explain the relationship between stress and hypertension, factors that produce stress, and methods to modify stress.
6. Explain antihypertensive therapy, including name, rationale, dosage, and side effects of all prescribed medications.
7. Discuss the importance of not smoking or using tobacco products.

Evaluation

Tissue perfusion is improved   Blood pressure is within acceptable limits. Patient has no complaints of headache or dizziness. Laboratory values are within normal limits.

Patient complies with therapeutic plan   Patient is normotensive, reports taking medication, loses weight, and has no symptoms.

■ PRIMARY PULMONARY HYPERTENSION

Pulmonary hypertension is a vascular abnormality of the pulmonary arterial system.

To be considered primary pulmonary hypertension (PPH), there can be no inciting cause. This diagnosis is uncommon and should be made only after thorough investigation of all possible etiologic factors (thromboembolism, congenital or immunologic abnormalities, collagen-vascular disease, drug ingestion, etc.)

The prevalence and incidence of PPH shows a 3:1 predisposition for females[33] and tends to be diagnosed in the 20s and 30s. There is some evidence of genetic transmission. Despite the overall incidence of PPH being rare, mortality rates of 80% within 5 years of clinical diagnosis make this vascular disease the focus of intense investigation.

••••• Pathophysiology

Many pathologic mechanisms have been postulated to describe the morphologic changes in the pulmonary vascular bed of patients with PPH. The plexogenic pulmonary arteriopathy characteristically seen in PPH may be the result of intense vasoconstriction, secondary to marked vasoreactivity and spasm, with resultant fibrinoid necrosis of the muscular pulmonary arteries. Plexiform or distorted vessels develop subsequently. Eventually these diseased vessels are destroyed and the remaining vessels in this shrinking pulmonary arterial bed suffer a permanent increase in pulmonary vascular resistance.

Signs and symptoms include exertional dyspnea, syncope, chest pain, weakness, fatigue, palpitations, hoarseness (from enlarged pulmonary trunk pressing on recurrent laryngeal nerve), cough, and sometimes hemoptysis. Physical exam: large a wave in the jugular venous pulse (tricuspid valve closure against a hypertensive right ventricle), a left parasternal heave (enlarged right ventricle), a systolic pulsation in the second left interspace, and a loud second heart sound (pulmonary valve closure). In advanced disease, right ventricular function is closely linked to mortality, so careful assessment of tricuspid and pulmonary valve function is important. The systolic murmur of tricuspid regurgitation or the diastolic murmur (Graham-Steele murmur) of hypertensive pulmonary regurgitation must be closely followed.

••••• Diagnostic Studies and Findings

Chest x-ray   Cardiomegaly, prominent central pulmonary arteries, marked tapering of peripheral arteries, RA and RV enlargement.

ECG   RV hypertrophy, RA enlargement, right axis deviation

Two-dimensional echocardiogram   RA and RV enlargement/hypertrophy, RV free wall motion, position and motion of ventricular septum, presence of intraatrial shunt (atrial septal defect or patent foramen ovale), permits estimate of RV systolic pressure and PA pressure.

Cardiac catheterization   Pulmonary artery flotation catheter (Swan-Ganz) can be used to estimate PA pressures and response to vasoactive agents. Pulmonary arteriography can be used to rule out thromboembolic disease but has been associated with some mortality.

Computed tomography (CT) scan   Contrast study of the thorax can define pulmonary artery anatomy and identify thrombus with lower risk than invasive catheterization.

Ventilation/perfusion (V/Q) lung scan   Nuclear contrast study to delineate pulmonary blood flow, identify areas of hypoperfusion possibly secondary to thrombus.

••••• Multidisciplinary Plan

Surgery

No surgical therapy for PPH is available, short of lung or heart-lung transplantation. Currently, donor availability is a major obstacle for most PPH patients awaiting transplant. One-year survival after lung or heart-lung transplant still does not surpass 70% in most institutions, and major complications such as obliterative bronchiolitis significantly affect recipients' quality of life.

Medications

Pulmonary vasodilators—effective only in those patients with PPH who exhibit pulmonary reactivity, rather than fixed pulmonary vascular resistance. Caution must be used to avoid systemic hypotension.

   Hydralazine (Apresoline) (25-50 mg qid orally)
   Nifedipine (Procardia) (10-30 mg qid orally)
   Verapamil (Calan, Isoptin) (80-120 mg tid or qid orally)
   Captopril (Capoten) (6.25-50 mg tid orally)
   Prostacycline (PGl, epusprostenol) (continuous IV infusion through a permanent central venous catheter)
   Oxygen (pulmonary vasodilator at higher concentrations)

Anticoagulation
   Coumadin—may improve prognosis in some patients with PPH, especially if intrapulmonary emboli or thrombus is identified (titrated to INR range of 2-3).

Right heart failure management (as appropriate)
   Digoxin and diuretics

General Management

Medical management is directed at decreasing resistance to pulmonary blood flow and improving circulatory response to right ventricular pressure overload.

Activity restrictions Patients with PPH must avoid all strenuous, heavy isometric exercise, including lifting, pushing, or pulling. No sudden, start-stop exercise, which requires sudden peripheral vasodilation with increased cardiac output is allowed; this can trigger syncope and often death (especially in patients with fixed suprasystemic pulmonary vascular resistance).

Pregnancy/contraception Because many patients diagnosed with PPH are young women, advice must be given to avoid pregnancy because it carries a 50% maternal mortality. Caution must also be taken with use of oral contraceptives (estrogen containing) because these may increase pulmonary vascular resistance, as well as predispose to thrombogenesis.

Altitude/air travel Patients with PPH should be cautioned against traveling or living at high altitudes (>2000 ft) because of decreased concentrations of oxygen secondary to lower atmospheric pressure (predisposing to increased vasoconstriction)

Preventive measures Advise annual flu and pneumonia vaccines

Heart failure management Low-salt diet, daily weighing

Nursing Diagnosis and Intervention

Alteration in oxygenation, decreased, related to ventilation/perfusion mismatch secondary to pulmonary vascular disease

- Optimize pulmonary vasodilator therapy while monitoring for hypotension and increase in symptoms.
- Titrate oxygen therapy as prescribed.
- Increase activity gradually, evaluating tolerance.
- Instruct patient to avoid exposure to community-acquired viruses and to obtain flu vaccine and pneumovax.
- Instruct patient to notify physician at early signs of respiratory infection, new cough, or hemoptysis.

Alteration in cardiac output, decreased, related to fixed pulmonary vascular resistance and systemic vasodilation secondary to isometric activity, vasodilatory medications, dehydration

- Assess BP and vital signs frequently while titrating vasoactive medications; have patient keep home BP diary.
- Instruct patient on activity restrictions for avoidance of syncope.
- Maintain adequate hydration in setting of hot weather, fever, diarrhea.
- Instruct patient on low-salt diet, and obtain daily weights to assess subtle signs of right heart failure.

Anxiety/fear related to poor prognosis, fear of death; syncopal episode secondary to lack of information, lack of perceived control

- Instruct patient on activity guidelines, emphasizing control over adverse symptoms.
- Provide information/explanation regarding procedures, monitoring equipment.
- Provide access for patient to PPH or lung transplant support group.
- Provide supportive/grief counseling in setting of life-threatening condition; provide information regarding advanced directive, chaplain services when appropriate.
- Provide access or timely referral to regional lung transplant program.

Patient Education/Home Care Planning

1. Instruct patient on home BP monitoring when appropriate.
2. Provide access to home IV prostacyclin therapy where available as therapeutic bridge to lung transplant (arrange for home monitoring of IV line).
3. Instruct patient to monitor for fluid accumulation (heart failure) by assessing weights, swelling, and avoiding salts.
4. Monitor anticoagulation where appropriate to maintain INR 2-3.

Evaluation

Patient tolerates therapeutic doses of vasodilator therapy   Patient demonstrates increased exercise tolerance, decreased breathlessness, and absence of syncope.

Patient demonstrates understanding of risky behaviors   Patient understands the risks of isometrics, pregnancy, traveling to high altitudes.

Patient expresses understanding of severity of disease   Patient is able to channel physical reserve to adaptive behaviors such as expression of grief, arrangement for home/family support, and inquiring about potential therapeutic options.

◼ ACUTE ARTERIAL INSUFFICIENCY

Arterial insufficiency is a sudden decrease in the arterial supply to an extremity (Figure 1-60).

Classified as an acute disorder, obstruction of any major artery produces symptoms. The most common causes of acute arterial insufficiency are embolism, thrombosis, and trauma. Cardiac disorders are the main source of thrombi on the left side of the heart.

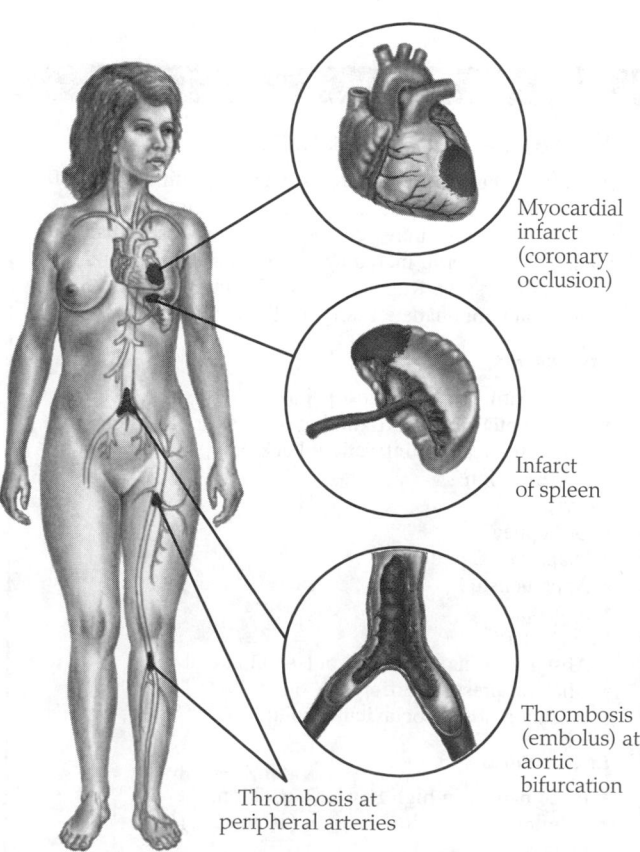

Myocardial infarct (coronary occlusion)

Infarct of spleen

Thrombosis (embolus) at aortic bifurcation

Thrombosis at peripheral arteries

Figure 1-60 Acute arterial insufficiency. (From Canobbio.[13])

The legs are most commonly involved. The femoral artery is most often affected (46%), followed by the popliteal tibial tree (11%) and the iliac arteries (8%).[81]

Acute arterial obstruction may also occur as a result of injury produced by compression, shearing, or laceration of a vessel. Furthermore, severe hypothermia may produce sudden severe vasoconstriction.

•••••• Pathophysiology

Once dislodged, an embolus may travel throughout the systemic circulation, lodging in an arterial branch and stagnating flow in the distal circulation. This leads to the formation of a soft coagulum proximal and distal to the area of stagnant blood flow. The result is the formation of a secondary thrombus, which extends along the arterial wall and progressively compromises collateral circulation. Without adequate collateral circulation, the distal tissues are deprived of oxygenation, a situation that leads to ischemia, pain, and paresthesia in the affected area. With prolonged ischemia, cellular damage occurs, leading to muscle necrosis.

•••••• Diagnostic Studies and Findings

Doppler ultrasonography   Abnormal blood flow pattern proximal to occlusion; "pistal shot" sound characterizes absence of diastolic flow component; ankle/brachial index <0.25 reflects severe ischemia and impending gangrene

Echocardiography   Determines whether heart is source of emboli; transesophageal echo if high suspicion, or question right-to-left shunt, such as patient foramen ovale

Arteriography   Determines location of obstruction and character of arterial circulation proximal and distal to obstruction

•••••• Multidisciplinary Plan

Surgery

Embolectomy—embolus can be removed directly via femoral arteriotomy using soft balloon-tipped catheter known as a Fogarty catheter; catheter is passed distal to occlusion, carefully inflated, and withdrawn

Amputation of limb—for severe advanced ischemia

Medications

Anticoagulants

Heparin sodium (Lipo-Hepin and others)

Indications: Initiated once diagnosis of embolization is made and before operative treatment is performed

Usual dosage: Loading, 5000-10,000 U IV; maintenance dose given to keep partial thromboplastin time to two times normal

Fibrinolytic agents

Streptokinase (Streptase), urokinase (Abbokinase)

Indications: Thrombolytic agents instilled by intraarterial infusion into site of occlusion; method of action is fibrinolysis causing fibrin dissolution

General Management

Percutaneous transluminal angioplasty—nonsurgical procedure involving mechanical dilation of occluded artery performed under local anesthesia with fluoroscopy; lesions considered suitable are stenotic vessels with intraluminal diameter of 2.5 mm and length of not more than 10 cm

NURSING CARE

Nursing Assessment

Peripheral Extremity

Moderate obstruction
  Pain, sudden in onset; numbness; "embolic syndrome" characterized by five Ps: pain, pallor, paresthesia, pulselessness, and paralysis
  Temperature: decreased
  Skin: pale yellow color
  Pulses: absence of distal arterial pulsations of affected extremity
  Poor capillary filling
Severe obstruction
  Leg muscle (gastrocnemius) becomes firm; dorsiflexion of foot produces pain

Nursing Dx & Intervention

Altered tissue perfusion related to interruption of arterial flow

- Assess arterial pulses distal to occlusion every 1 to 2 hours *to determine arterial blood flow patterns.*
- Evaluate signs of further ischemia by checking the color and temperature of the extremity, the presence or absence of sensation, and the level of motor deficit.
- Provide bed rest during acute periods.
- Administer anticoagulants as ordered *to prevent enlargement of thrombus and further embolization.*
- Monitor partial thromboplastin time (PTT), hemoglobin (Hgb), and hematocrit (Hct) daily or as indicated *to maintain therapeutic range and avoid hemorrhagic complications.*
- Keep extremities below level of heart *to maintain optimum gravitational flow.*

Pain related to peripheral ischemia

- Assess quality and degree of pain *to determine if acute or chronic.* Provide for position of most comfort.
- Maintain on bed rest during acute phase.
- Do not raise knee gatch, elevate extremity, or allow hips to be maintained in prolonged flexion *because these procedures can interfere with arterial circulation.*
- Administer analgesics as ordered.
- Protect affected extremity by using a bed cradle, cotton blankets, or sheepskin.

- Provide regular active and passive range of motion exercises unless contraindicated.

Other related nursing diagnosis   High risk for anxiety related to threat or change in health status (possible loss of limb)

Patient Education/Home Care Planning

1. Instruct the patient and family about the disease process, possible causes, and therapeutic modalities.
2. At discharge explain anticoagulant therapy and the need for follow-up monitoring with clotting studies.
3. Explain to the patient and family how to avoid situations that cause blood pooling or interruption of blood flow: crossing legs, smoking, sitting or standing for extended periods of time.

Evaluation

Peripheral perfusion is improved   Pain is relieved. Distal and proximal pulses are present. Extremity has normal color. Normal motor function returns in affected extremity.

   EMERGENCY ALERT

AORTIC ANEURYSM/DISSECTION

An aortic aneurysm/dissection is when the intimal layer of the aorta tears and blood leaks between the intimal and medial layers. This may occlude the major vessels that branch off the aorta, including the myocardial, cerebral, or mesenteric vessels. Rupture of the dissection can cause pericardial tamponade, exsanguination, and shock.

Assessment

- Excruciating/tearing chest pain
- Pain: center of chest, radiating to back or abdomen; may mimic myocardial infarction, back pain, or ulcer
- Hypertension
- Dyspnea
- Orthopnea
- Diaphoresis, pallor
- Apprehension
- Syncope
- Tachycardia
- Absence of major arterial pulse, unilateral
- Bilateral pressure difference
- Pulsation at sternoclavicular joint

Interventions

- Place patient in high Fowler's position.
- Administer high-flow oxygen (10 to 12 L).
- Obtain IV access.
- Anticipate nipride and inderal drips.
- Prepare patient for angiography or surgery.
- Provide support and reassurance.

CHRONIC ARTERIAL INSUFFICIENCY

Chronic arterial insufficiency is inadequate blood flow in arteries. It is caused by occlusive atherosclerotic plaques or emboli, damaged or diseased vessels, aneurysms, hypercoagulability states, or heavy use of tobacco (Figure 1-61).

Atherosclerosis obliterans is the primary cause of chronic arterial insufficiency. Other causes, although rare, may lead to arterial insufficiency of the legs. These include thromboangiitis obliterans (Buerger's disease), cystic degeneration of the popliteal artery, popliteal entrapment, and some connective tissue disorders.

Arteriosclerosis obliterans, a progressive ischemic syndrome, is more common in men, and the incidence rises with age and in women after menopause. It is a diffuse process but is generally confined to short segments of arteries near bifurcations and origins. The aortoiliac and femoropopliteal areas are common sites.

• • • • • Pathophysiology

Progressive narrowing of the arterial tree by atherosclerotic plaques gives rise to collateral vessels that tend to ensure adequate blood supply and prevent peripheral ischemia. However, the effectiveness of these collateral pathways is limited by their small size and high resistance, as well as by the extent of occlusive disease. Progressive occlusion leads to hypoperfusion and ischemia. These are related directly to the number of occlusions and to the adequacy of collateral vessels. The arms and legs are the most vulnerable to ischemia.

• • • • • Diagnostic Studies and Findings

Doppler ultrasonography Quantitates degree of ischemia; ankle/branchial index: arterial pressure less than pressure in brachial artery; normal: ≥0.9, severe: 0.5 or less

Plethysmography Evaluates blood flow and determines degree to which peripheral circulation is decreased

Transcutaneous Po$_2$ (TcPo$_2$) Assess cutaneous oxygen delivery and oxygen demand

• • • • • Multidisciplinary Plan

Surgery

Percutaneous transluminal angioplasty (PTA)—mechanically enlarges diameter of stenotic artery

Arterial revascularization, reconstruction—performed to restore unimpeded pulsatile blood flow, usually beginning with proximal segments (aortoiliac-femoral)

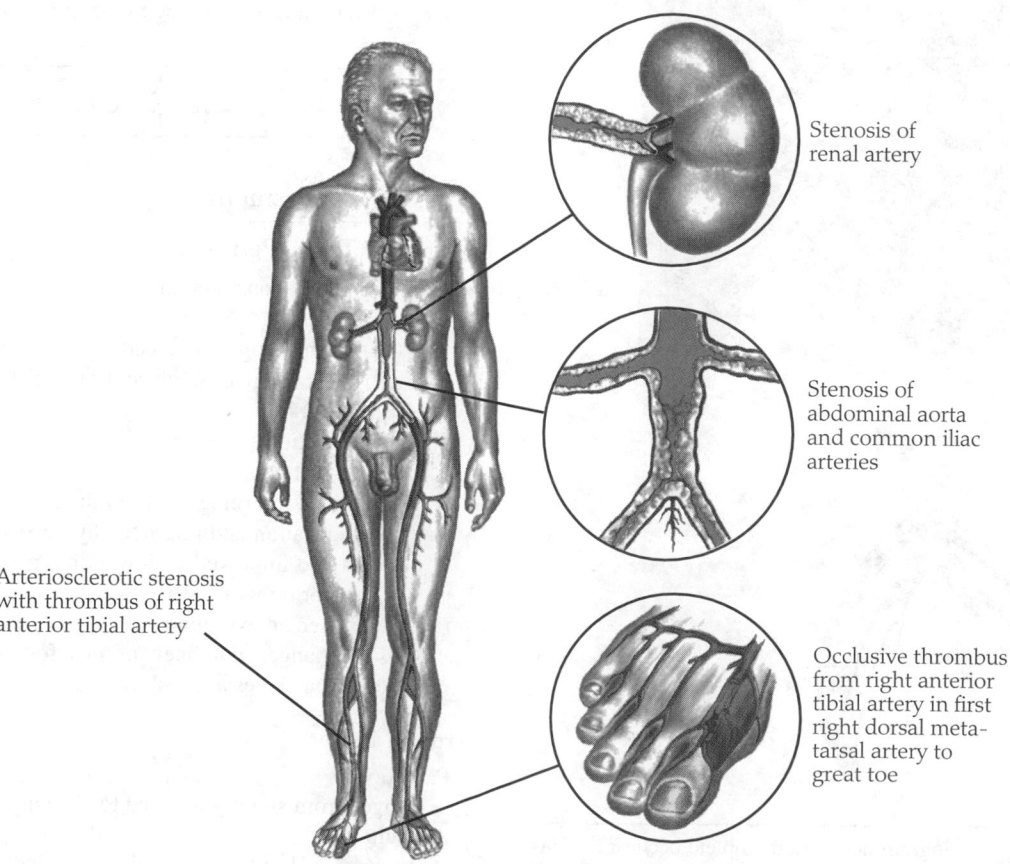

Stenosis of renal artery

Stenosis of abdominal aorta and common iliac arteries

Occlusive thrombus from right anterior tibial artery in first right dorsal metatarsal artery to great toe

Arteriosclerotic stenosis with thrombus of right anterior tibial artery

Figure 1-61 Chronic arterial insufficiency. (From Canobbio.[13])

Endarterectomy—removal of atheromatous intima from artery

Bypass graft surgery—use of Dacron conduit to deliver blood from aorta to femoral vessels, bypassing diseased segments (Figure 1-62)

Femoropopliteal reconstruction
  Femoropopliteal bypass
Profundoplasty—local endarterectomy of proximal profunda femoris artery

Lumbar sympathectomy—removal of second and third lumbar ganglia; performed to improve blood flow to skin

Amputation of limb—for severe, irreversible ischemia (gangrene)

Medications

Anticoagulants, vasodilators, and antiplatelets have been used but tend to be unhelpful or only palliative

Pentoxifylline (Trental) decreases blood viscosity, improves tissue oxygen delivery; used to increase claudication distance

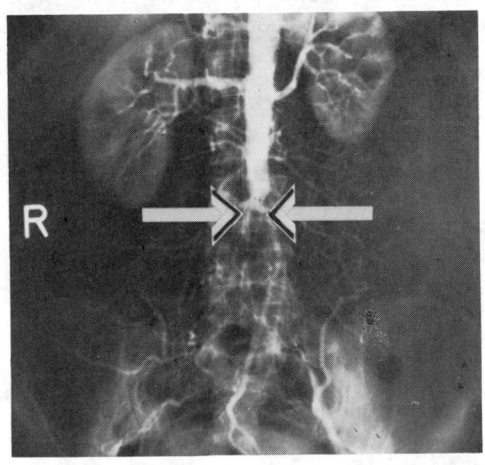

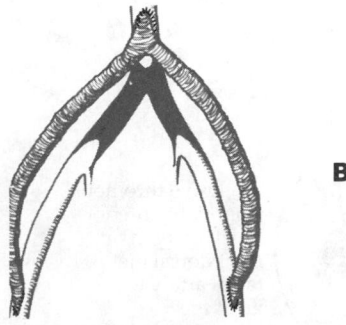

Figure 1-62 **A,** Arteriogram depicting complete occlusion of distal abdominal aorta *(arrows).* **B,** Aortobifemoral bypass graft using synthetic conduit. (From Guzzetta.[40])

General Management

Peripheral angioplasty (PTA)—with inflatable balloon-tipped catheter, atheromatous plaque is mechanically compressed to increase lumen patency; vessels of iliac or femoral arteries are reported to respond best to PTA, but success has been reported for vessels of aorta, popliteal, superior mesenteric, subclavian, and brachial systems, as well as stenoses in peripheral arterial grafts[28]

Laser thermal angioplasty (LTA)—a new, experimental method of obliterating the atheromatous plaque by heat vaporization; with a fiberoptic catheter, energy from laser source is applied to occlusive lesion; often performed in conjunction with PTA

Risk reduction program aimed at weight reduction for the obese patient, smoking cessation, and a low-cholesterol, low–saturated fat diet; evaluation and control of diabetes and hyperlipidemia should be carried out to slow progression of atherosclerotic process

Daily foot care—inspection; cleaning; use of cotton socks; attention to nails, corns, calluses

Regular walking program to point of claudication several times a day may improve patient's walking distance; improvement may be due to development of increased collateral arterial flow, progressive adaptation to discomfort or gait modification, metabolic changes in the muscles, or redistribution of blood flow to the muscles[99]

NURSING CARE

Nursing Assessment

Peripheral Tissue Perfusion

Mild to moderate obstruction
  Intermittent claudication
    Calf pain, fatigue induced by walking and relieved by rest, pain in thigh and buttocks (foot rarely involved)
Severe obstruction
  Ischemic rest pain
    Continuous burning pain confined to toes, aggravated by elevation and improved by dependence; occurs at rest and improved with walking; may occur at night, interfering with sleep
Edema of affected extremity
  Sensory changes: numbness of toes, foot, or lower portion of leg; paresthesia

Arterial Pulses

Palpation
  Ranges from slightly reduced to absent
Auscultation
  Presence of bruits at rest and after exercise; sites are abdominal aorta and iliac and femoral arteries

Skin, Nails, Hair

Ulcerations; glossy, cold, smooth skin; pallor—increasing with elevation of extremity; atrophic nails; hair loss; delayed capillary refill time (>3 sec)

Sexual Function

Impotence in men (reflects decrease in arterial blood flow to branch of internal iliac artery, which may interfere with penile erections)

Nursing Dx & Intervention

Altered peripheral tissue perfusion (chronic) related to interruption of arterial flow

- Assess arterial pulses, determining pulse volume; auscultate for bruits before and after exercise.
- Observe skin color changes (pallor) and venous filling with elevation and dependency procedures *to estimate the degree of ischemia.*
- Avoid procedures or bed positions that *interfere with gravitational blood flow* (arterial flow is downward), such as elevating affected extremity or using knee gatch.
- Protect the affected extremity: place bed cradle over affected areas, avoid use of heating devices on lower extremities.
- Instruct the patient to avoid nicotine *because it causes both small and larger vessels to constrict and damage intimal cells.*

Pain related to peripheral ischemia

- Assess quality and degree of pain; assist the patient to identify activities that precipitate or aggravate pain *to define a baseline for activity intolerance.*
- Provide position of most comfort.
- Frequent, small position changes may be helpful during periods of restlessness brought on by pain.
- Instruct the patient on methods to relieve pain: to stand or dangle at bedside *to obtain relief from ischemic pain.*
- Begin a slow, progressive exercise program.

Impaired skin integrity (actual and high risk for) related to impaired circulation

- Assess skin color, temperature, and integrity *to observe for signs of necrosis.*
- Provide daily skin care *to prevent fissures and infection.*
- Ensure that skin is thoroughly dried.
- Treat ulcerations as they occur.
- Administer soaks, medications, and dressings as ordered.
- Avoid using adhesive tape directly on skin.
- Avoid use of tight constricting socks or hose; use cotton or wool socks that are proper length and size.

Patient Education/Home Care Planning

1. Provide information regarding the disease process and precipitating risk factors (risk factor profile on p. xx).
2. Explain the importance of daily skin care. Tell the patient to wash with mild soap, dry well, and apply lanolin-based lotions.
3. Clean small cuts or abrasions with soap and water; report cuts or skin breaks that do not begin to heal within 2 to 3 days.
4. Nails, corns, and calluses should be managed professionally. Encourage the patient to wear well-fitted, hard-soled shoes.
5. Discuss a daily progressive walking program with the patient: walk until pain increases, stop and stand still to decrease pain, then continue walking.
6. Explain the need to avoid the use of nicotine.
7. Provide weight counseling for obese patients.
8. Explain the need for a low-cholesterol, low-fat diet.
9. Instruct the patient to avoid crossing legs and long periods of sitting or standing.

Evaluation

Peripheral perfusion is improved Patient reports relief of pain (claudication). Pulses are present, equal, and bilateral. Skin color is normal; skin is warm to touch.

Comfort level is achieved Patient verbalizes absence or control of pain. Patient demonstrates use of variety of strategies to reduce pain level.

Skin integrity is maintained Skin shows no signs of ulcerations. Skin color and temperature are normal.

■ RAYNAUD'S DISEASE

Raynaud's disease is a disorder of small cutaneous arteries, most frequently involving the fingers; it is marked by episodic vasospasm.

Raynaud's disease may occur by itself or may follow other disorders. By itself it occurs more commonly in young women, is often triggered by emotional stress and cold, and involves both hands.

•••••• Pathophysiology

Raynaud's disease involves three phases. First, severe constriction of cutaneous vessels results in blanching of the fingers. The vessels then dilate, slowing blood flow. This allows hemoglobin to release more oxygen into the tissues. During this ischemic phase the fingers are first white and then cyanotic, numb, and cold. This phase is followed by a reactive hyperemic phase during which the fingers become red and the patient has throbbing pain. Because attacks are often triggered by stress and cold, the disease may be related to vasoconstriction caused by the release of catecholamines. The attacks may last a few minutes or, in severe cases, several hours.

In severe cases, progressive ischemia with trophic skin changes may lead to recurring infection and gangrene. However, Raynaud's disease is rare and is most often seen in mild form.

•••••• Diagnostic Studies and Findings

Digital plethysmography   Abnormal perfusion pressure and pulsatile contour

Peripheral arteriography   Visualization of distal arteries of hands

•••••• Multidisciplinary Plan

Surgery

Sympathectomy
Lumbar ganglionectomy for relief of symptoms involving feet
Ganglionectomy for relief of symptoms involving hands
Amputation of terminal phalanges (very rare)

Medications

Antihypertensive agents
Reserpine (Serpasil, others)
Indications: Rauwolfia alkaloids that decrease vasoconstriction
Usual dosage: 0.25-0.5 mg/d po
α-Adrenergic blocking agents
Phenoxybenzamine (Dibenzyline)
Dosage is variable
Tolazoline (Priscoline)
Usual dosage: 25-50 mg po tid; 10-50 mg parenterally qid
Vasodilators
Nicotinyl alcohol (Roniacol)
Usual dosage: 50-100 mg po tid or 150 mg bid

General Management

Avoidance of exposure to irritants such as cold, mechanical or chemical injury, and stressful situations

NURSING CARE

Nursing Assessment

Hands and Fingers

Initially blanched and numb after exposure to cold or stress; then fingers become cyanotic; this is followed by change in color to red; trophic changes (ulcerations, chronic paronychia) may occur in long-standing disease

Nursing Dx & Intervention

Pain related to ischemia

- Assess for aggravating factors leading to vasospasm.
- Remove aggravating factors when possible; for example, provide warmth to fingers, have the patient stop smoking.
- Assist the patient to modify stressful periods that may *aggravate vasospasm.*
- Instruct the patient as to cause of pain.

High risk for impaired skin integrity related to progressive ischemia

- Perform daily assessment for color changes and ulcerations.
- Treat ulcerations if they occur.
- Avoid exposure to cold, mechanical and chemical irritants, or other stressful factors.

Patient Education/Home Care Planning

1. Discuss with the patient how to avoid exposure to cold temperatures and the need to wear gloves or mittens when handling cold items or in cold weather.
2. Explain to the patient the need to avoid smoking.
3. Explain the need to avoid stressful situations. Teach ways to deal with stress, such as relaxation techniques.
4. Explain the purpose, side effects, and dosage of medications.

Evaluation

Circulation in hands and fingers is improved   There is no pain. Color is normal and skin is warm. Skin integrity is maintained.

■ VENOUS THROMBOSIS

Venous thrombosis is an abnormal vascular condition; a thrombus develops within a blood vessel (Figure 1-63).

Venous thrombosis is the most common venous disorder. The greatest incidence is in those having surgery (30% to 60%) and in patients receiving intravenous therapy, because of the embolization of a thrombus to the lungs. The incidence of pulmonary embolism in surgical patients has been estimated to be 7.3% to 54%, with the estimated number of deaths 200,000 per year.[13] The following terms are commonly used to describe venous disorders that reflect thrombus formation or inflammation:

phlebitis   Inflammation of vein

phlebothrombosis (venous thrombosis)   Intraluminal thrombus with minimal or no inflammation; have greater tendency to embolize

thromboembolism   Thrombus dislodgement and migration

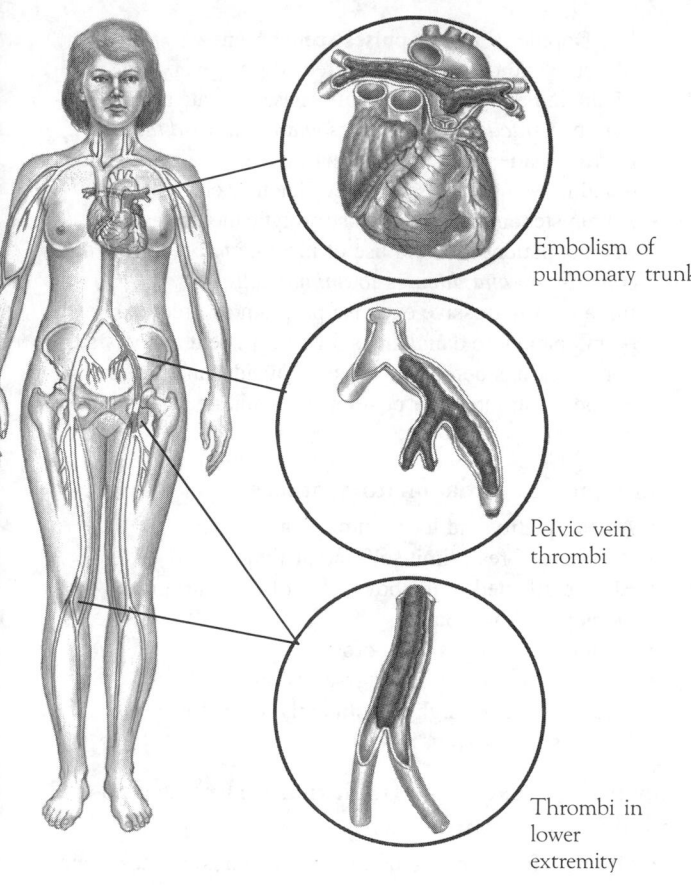

Embolism of
pulmonary trunk

Pelvic vein
thrombi

Thrombi in
lower
extremity

Figure 1-63 Venous thrombosis. (From Canobbio.[13])

thrombophlebitis Acute condition marked by thrombus and inflammation in deep or superficial veins

•••••• Pathophysiology

The triad of stasis, intimal damage, and hypercoagulability is responsible for most venous thrombosis.

Venous stasis occurs in persons who are inactive for a time because of bed rest or immobilization of the lower extremities. Thrombus formation results from a reduction of flow-induced dilution and a decrease in natural circulating anticoagulants (antithrombin III, platelet factor IV, and some prostaglandins).[81] Stasis caused by reduced flow increases the contact between platelets and coagulation factors that enhance platelet aggregation.

Intimal damage may occur as a result of internal or external trauma, usually involving IV therapy. Endothelial damage leads to exposure of the subintimal collagen membrane, which promotes platelet adherence, and activation of intrinsic coagulation factors, which contribute to thrombus formation.

Hypercoagulability reflects an alteration in coagulability. This occurs in some patients with disorders such as polycythemias and anemias, excessive estrogen or steroid use, or malignancies.

Once formed, the thrombus begins an inflammatory process leading to fibrosis. The enlarging thrombus eventually occludes the lumen of the vein or detaches and migrates to the systemic circulation.

Frequent sites for venous thrombus formation are the soleal and gastrocnemius venous sinuses and the larger veins. Thrombosis of these veins is linked to increased risk of clotting. Thrombosis in subcutaneous veins rarely leads to pulmonary embolism.

Diagnostic Studies and Findings

Plethysmography Shows decreased circulation distal to affected area

Doppler ultrasonography Identifies reduced blood flow to specific area; shows obstruction to venous flow

Phlebography Confirms diagnosis; shows filling defects

^{125}I fibrinogen scan Defines location of clot and any emboli that may have dislodged

Multidisciplinary Plan

Surgery

Rarely indicated

Techniques used for deep vein thrombophlebitis necessitating venous interruption—ligation, vein plication, or clipping

Iliofemoral thrombectomy—may be considered for patients with acute iliofemoral thrombosis and compromised arterial perfusion that fail to respond to conventional therapy

Procedures to prevent distal embolization

Extravascular vena cava interruption—application of a partitioning clip around the vein; used prophylactically for patients who are considered at high risk for embolization and are undergoing abdominal surgery for another reason

Intracaval filters (Mobin-Uddin umbrella, Kimray-Greenfield filter)—interruption devices inserted into right internal jugular vein and advanced to vena cava via catheter; once in place, devices permit continuous venous flow while filtering clots, thus preventing further embolization

Medications

Anticoagulants

Heparin sodium

Indications: Initially administered IV to augment fibrinolytic activity and aid in thrombolysis

Usual dosage: 300-500 U/kg followed by infusion of 1000 U/h

Warfarin

Indications: Given later to maintain prothrombin time to twice control level or INR 1.5-2.5; usually for 3 mo

Fibrinolytic agents
  Streptokinase (Streptase)
    Indications: Produces total clot lysis and restores normal venous valve function
    Usual dosage: IV initially 250,000 IU/30 min; maintenance 100,000 IU/h for 24-72 h
Antiplatelet agents (used in prevention of thrombus)
  Dipyridamole (Persantine)
    Usual dosage: 800 mg/d; 400 mg/d if used with anticoagulants

General Management

Bed rest with elevation of affected extremity above level of right atrium
Warm, moist heat
Custom-fitted elastic stockings when ambulatory
Monitoring the partial thromboplastin time or prothrombin time while patient is receiving anticoagulant therapy

NURSING CARE

Nursing Assessment

Lower Extremity (Deep Veins)

Calf pain and tenderness; Homans' sign (calf pain on dorsiflexion of foot); dilated superficial veins; edema of involved extremity (30% to 50% of deep vein thromboses may be clinically silent); pain and tenderness over involved vein (for example, groin); increased size compared with unaffected side

Upper Extremity (Superficial Veins)

Redness, warmth, and tenderness over affected vein; veins visible and palpable

Nursing Dx & Intervention

Impaired skin integrity related to venous stasis and fragility of small blood vessels

- Assess skin integrity daily; observe for signs of redness, breakdown, or ulcerations *reflective of venous stasis.*
- Raise affected extremity above heart *to eliminate venous hypertension.*
- Use elastic compression gradient stockings *to minimize peripheral edema.*
- Administer daily hygiene measures. Use mild soap, rinse well, and dry gently but thoroughly. Avoid vigorous rubbing or massaging that may *lead to dislodgment of clot.*
- If ulceration is present, initiate treatment as indicated: administer warm saline soaks.

Altered tissue perfusion related to interruption of venous flow

- Assess circulation of affected extremity and check pulses in all extremities.

- Use Doppler sensor if pulses seem absent.
- Measure and record size of affected limb every day.
- Maintain bed rest during acute phase; elevate affected extremity *to facilitate venous circulation toward the heart.*
- Instruct patient to avoid positions that restrict venous blood flow such as use of knee Gatch or crossing legs.
- Administer anticoagulant and fibrolytic therapy as ordered.
- Instruct patient to avoid use of nicotine *to prevent further constriction and damage to intimal cells.*
- Initiate a progressive exercise program as ordered. Never permit patient to dangle legs. Instruct patient to apply support stockings before ambulating, avoid standing for long periods, and alternate position by standing on toes, then on heels.

Pain related to inflammatory process

- Assess quality and location of pain.
- Provide bed rest; limit self-care activities.
- Elevate affected limb above level of right atrium.
- Do not use knee Gatch.
- Administer analgesics as ordered.
- Apply warm, moist compresses as ordered.
- Measure calf or thigh or both daily and record.
- Use elastic stockings as ordered.

Impaired gas exchange (high risk for) related to embolization of thrombus

- Observe for signs of pulmonary embolism: chest pain, dyspnea, tachypnea.
- Auscultate lung sounds every 8 hours or as indicated.
- Monitor vital signs every 4 to 8 hours.
- Maintain bed rest during acute period.
- Avoid exercising and massage of affected extremity during acute phase.
- Administer anticoagulant therapy as ordered.
- Use elastic stockings during periods of ambulation.

Other related nursing diagnoses   Impaired physical mobility related to imposed activity restriction secondary to disease process.

Patient Education/Home Care Planning

1. Discuss with the patient and family the nature of the disorder and methods of preventing recurrence.
2. The patient must understand the need to avoid constrictive clothing and crossing legs when sitting.
3. The patient and family must understand the need for skin care.
4. Explain the value of rest periods with legs raised.
5. Explain the need to lose weight if the patient is obese.
6. Discuss with the patient the need to avoid use of nicotine and oral contraceptives.
7. Explain the need for a regular or moderate exercise program.
8. Explain anticoagulant therapy and precautions.

Evaluation

Skin integrity is maintained or improved   Patient exhibits no ulcerations. Skin is free of infections.

Tissue perfusion is improved   Patient has relief of pain, swelling, and redness.

Patient exhibits no signs of respiratory distress   Arterial blood gases (ABGs) are within normal limits. Respirations are at baseline. Lungs are clear. Chest x-ray is normal.

Comfort level is achieved   Patient verbalizes absence or control of pain. Patient demonstrates appropriate strategies to reduce pain.

MEDICAL INTERVENTIONS AND RELATED NURSING CARE

AUTOMATIC IMPLANTABLE CARDIOVERTER-DEFIBRILLATOR

Description and Rationale

The automatic implantable cardioverter-defibrillator (AICD) is a self-contained system capable of identifying and treating life-threatening ventricular dysrhythmias. Originally designed to correct ventricular fibrillation, AICD units now also have the capability to identify and treat ventricular tachycardia.

The surgically implanted device continuously monitors and analyzes the patient's heart rate and waveform configuration. In the presence of rapid ventricular tachycardia and ventricular fibrillation, electrical countershock is delivered directly to the heart via two transcardiac electrodes. One catheter electrode is positioned in the superior vena cava; the second may be a ventricular patch lead made of titanium mesh that is placed on the pericardium or myocardium during surgery.[99]

Patients for whom the AICD device is indicated include those who have survived sudden cardiac death not associated with acute MI and whose dysrhythmias are not controlled with antidysrhythmic therapy, those who have had more than one cardiac arrest but whose dysrhythmia cannot be induced during electrophysiologic testing, and those with sustained ventricular tachycardia not controlled with conventional antidysrhythmic agents.

Contraindications include uncontrollable congestive heart failure, severe physiologic fear of the device, a history of severe chronic obstructive pulmonary disease (COPD), or use of a unipolar pacemaker.

Cautions

Avoidance of strong magnetic fields should be ensured because they can activate or deactivate the AICD device.

Preprocedural Care

1. Initiate preoperative instruction for the patient and family, including information about the AICD device, its benefits and risks, the implantation procedure, and postoperative care. Include discussion regarding surgical approaches that may be used (thoracotomy, median sternotomy, or subxiphoid and subcostal approaches) and routine postoperative procedures and equipment of the intensive care unit where patients receiving implants stay for the first 24 to 48 hours postoperatively.
2. Ensure that written informed consent is obtained.
3. Obtain baseline data as ordered: ECG (baseline rhythm), vital signs, and laboratory work (CBC, blood type and cross-match, electrolytes).
4. Perform skin preparation of chest and abdomen.
5. Permit nothing by mouth (NPO).
6. Deal with preoperative anxiety and fears of discomfort associated with shocks and possible malfunction of the device.

•••••• Multidisciplinary Plan

Surgery

Approach for implantation determined by various clinical circumstances, such as whether the patient has had previous chest surgery or will also undergo corrective cardiac surgery; surgical approaches used for AICD implantation include the following:

Thoracotomy—for patient who previously underwent cardiac surgery and may have scar tissue around the heart

Median sternotomy—used for patients undergoing concomitant cardiac surgery such as antidysrhythmic surgery or coronary artery bypass graft (CABG) surgery

Subxiphoid—incision is made below the xiphoid process entering the pericardial space anteriorly

Subcostal—similar to thoracotomy but requires a smaller incision and shorter recovery time

Medications

Antidysrhythmics—carefully selected to avoid interfering with defibrillation threshold

General Management

Continuous ECG monitoring during and after implantation, observing for inappropriate shocks during sinus rhythm or patient's preestablished rhythm

Hemodynamic monitoring may be required until the patient stabilizes

Diet as ordered

Intravenous therapy as ordered

Activity level determined by clinical status and postprocedural exercise stress test

NURSING CARE

Nursing Assessment

Malfunction of AICD Device

Failure to sense and discharge
Sudden death

ECG Rhythm

Appropriate discharge for ventricular tachycardia (VT)/ventricular fibrillation (VF)

Transient episodes of supraventricular dysrhythmias, nonsustained ventricular tachycardia

False-positive discharges of shocks in the presence of normal sinus rhythm; spurious shocks may be caused by fractured leads or by miscounting of the heart rate because of oversensing

Infection of the Pulse Generator Pocket Site

Redness, swelling, heat, fluid collection or drainage, skin irritation or breakdown

Nursing Dx & Intervention

Fear related to anticipated shock, possible battery failure, and death

- Assess level of understanding, encouraging the patient to verbalize subjective feelings and perceptions.
- Provide information to correct distorted perceptions.
- Assist the patient to identify sources of fear.
- Assist the patient to cope with fears.
- Review strategies to cope with unpredictability of the dysrhythmias and discomfort from the shocks.
- Offer a brief description of the shock, including symptoms that may accompany it.
- Review the signs and symptoms of battery failure or device malfunction and interventions to take if suspected.
- Refer to AICD support group.

Activity intolerance (actual and high risk for) related to functional limitations and prolonged immobility

- Assess the patient's tolerance or intolerance for activities of daily living.
- Determine whether intolerance is related to progressive heart disease or to perceived fear of the AICD device.
- Discuss activity allowances and limitations.
- Encourage the patient to engage in exercise activities as tolerated.
- Participation in a monitored exercise program may give the patient a sense of security when engaging in routine activities.

Other related nursing diagnoses   High risk for decrease in CO related to recurrent ventricular dysrhythmias.

Patient Education/Home Care Planning

1. Explain to the patient and family the purpose and basic function of the AICD device. Describe benefits and limitations.
2. Describe the AICD device, discussing the signs and symptoms of defibrillation discharge.
3. Describe the signs and symptoms of AICD malfunction, such as inappropriate shocks or loss of consciousness, and the need to notify physician if suspected.
4. Explain the need for regular follow-up magnet testing to predict the end of generator life. Describe the use of the transtelephonic system if available.
5. Explain the signs and symptoms of wound or pocket infection, and instruct the patient or family to report any fever or drainage to the physician.
6. Explain to the patient the need to protect the implantation site and to avoid constricting clothing such as belts and girdles.
7. Describe activity allowances and limitations. Explain that most former activities may be resumed, that driving is permitted unless the patient is bothered by neurologic symptoms or continues to have syncope after AICD implantation, and that sexual activity can be resumed without danger to patient or partner.
8. Discuss the need to avoid strong magnetic fields that may activate or deactivate the AICD unit, such as areas around radio or television transmitting towers and use of diathermy motors. Instruct the patient not to touch spark plugs of a running motor, as on a lawn mower or car.
9. Assure the patient that normal household appliances such as microwave ovens and hair dryers will not interfere with the AICD unit.
10. Assure the patient that routine contact with another person will not activate the unit; if the unit discharges during physical contact, the other person may feel a slight muscular contraction but will not be harmed.
11. Explain need to carry AICD identification card and wear Medic Alert bracelet at all times.
12. Direct patient to AICD support group when available, if appropriate.

Evaluation

AICD unit functions properly   Patient demonstrates no further episode of syncope or cardiac arrest. AICD unit shows appropriate discharge response during magnet testing.

Fear level is reduced   Patient is able to verbalize specific fears and concerns regarding AICD unit. Patient verbalizes comfort with AICD unit and asks appropriate questions regarding home maintenance hemodynamic monitoring.

Activity level returns to normal for patient   Patient is able to return to activities of daily living and participates in exercise as allowed. Heart rate ≤120 BPM during exercise (or within 20 BPM of resting heart rate if taking beta blockers); BP within 20 mm Hg of baseline range.

■ CARDIAC SURGERY

(Coronary artery bypass graft, valve surgeries, repair of septal defects, ventricular aneurysm resection, mapping, congenital defect repairs)

Description and Rationale

Surgical intervention for cardiac disorders may be employed as a corrective measure in congenital heart disease or as an alternative treatment modality when a patient's clinical course becomes refractory to medical management.

Cardiac surgery may be broadly classified as an open or a closed procedure. Open-heart techniques were made possible with the development of the cardiopulmonary bypass machine (extracorporeal circulation) in the early 1950s. Since that time advances in myocardial preservation, in preoperative and postoperative support devices, and in pharmacology have contributed to improved mortality and morbidity rates and to a greater number of operative procedures for cardiac disorders.

Procedures for Acquired Disorders

Coronary artery bypass graft (CABG) surgery—myocardial revascularization for coronary artery disease; aimed at relief of unstable angina pectoris; Figures 1-64 and 1-65 show a saphenous vein used as a graft to the coronary artery; because of the need at times for multiple grafts or repeat CABG surgeries, arterial grafts using the internal mammary arteries, the gastric-epiploic artery, and even radial arteries have been used with success

Valve surgery—valvulotomy (commissurotomy), valvuloplasty (repair of valve), replacement with prosthetic valve, Ross procedure (pulmonary autograft implanted in aortic valve location, homograft used to replace pulmonary valve)

Resection of ventricular aneurysm—resection of nonviable myocardium

Septal defects—closure of atrial or ventricular septal defect by direct suturing or placement of Dacron patch across defect

Antidysrhythmia surgery—mapped (directed endocardial resection), and aneurysmectomy

Procedures for Congenital Defects

Closure of patent ductus arteriosus
Closure of atrial or ventricular septal defect
Repair of coarctation of aorta
Repair of tetralogy of Fallot
Fontan or modified Fontan procedure for tricuspid atresia and single ventricle
Mustard procedure or arterial switch for transposition of great vessels
Rastelli (valved-conduit) repair for severe pulmonary stenosis (or pulmonary atresia) and ventricular septal defect

Contraindications

Contraindications to cardiac surgery include bleeding disorders and acute (recent) cerebrovascular accident (stroke).

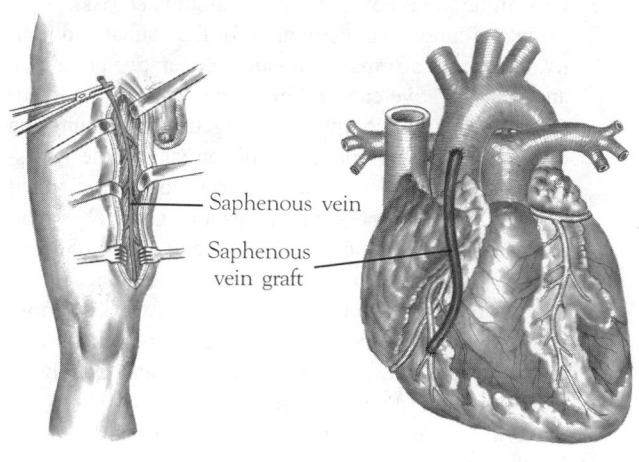

Figure 1-64 Coronary artery bypass graft using saphenous vein. (From Thelan.[85])

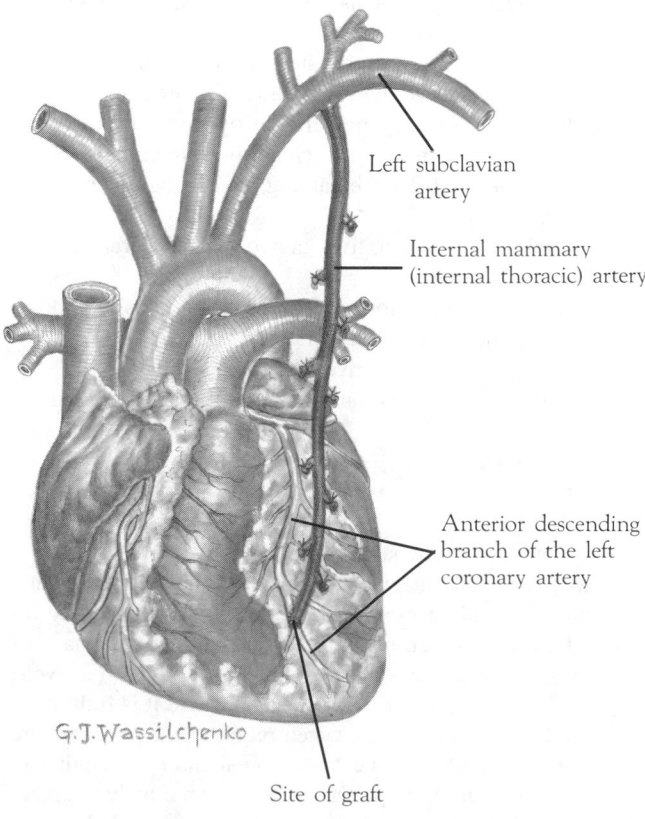

Figure 1-65 Coronary artery bypass graft using internal mammary artery. (From Thelan.[85])

Cautions

Cardiac surgery may be performed with added risk in the presence of pulmonary hypertension, in patients with an active infectious process, or in refractory ventricular failure.

Preprocedural Care

1. Determine the type of lesion and associated risks.
2. Initiate preoperative instruction for the patient and family, including information about the operative procedure and postoperative care: routine procedures of the intensive care unit (suctioning, coughing, turning, monitoring of vital signs); various tubes (endotracheal, chest, gastrointestinal, urinary catheter, intravenous); equipment (respirators, monitors); pain management; level of consciousness and emotional response; and visitor policies.
3. Ensure that written informed consent is obtained.
4. Obtain baseline data: chest x-ray; ECG; laboratory work; complete blood count, blood type, and cross-match, electrolytes, serum chemistries, and urinalysis; weight; height; and vital signs.
5. Perform skin preparation: chest; legs for vein harvesting.
6. Hold or modify preoperative medications:
    Digoxin—discontinued 24 to 36 hours before surgery
    Antiplatelets—instruct patient not to take these up to 1 week before surgery
    Anticoagulants—discontinue warfarin; initiate heparin therapy
    Antidysrhythmics, antihypertensives—in most cases continue until 24 to 48 hours before surgery
7. Initiate pulmonary preparation by instructing the patient to stop smoking, teaching the patient methods for coughing and deep breathing, and using an incentive spirometer.
8. Deal with preoperative anxiety, offering reassurance and support.
9. Assist with insertion of pulmonary artery balloon flotation catheter, if ordered, before surgery.
10. Administer preoperative sedation.
11. Permit nothing by mouth for 12 hours before procedure.

•••••• Multidisciplinary Plan

Surgery

Cardiopulmonary bypass machine (extracorporeal circulation; heart-lung machine)—assumes function of heart and lungs, providing bloodless operative field; procedure involves cannulation of great vessels, allowing drainage of unoxygenated blood that is emptied into venous reservoir; blood is then passed to oxygenator where it is fully saturated; to reduce tissue oxygen requirements, temperature of blood circulating in extracorporeal unit is lowered; cold blood is returned to patient, reducing total body temperature and slowing metabolic processes; myocardial preservation is required while the heart is arrested and includes coronary perfusion, topical cooling (profound hypothermia), and cold cardioplegia arrest

Medications

Preoperative management consists of maintenance of medical management plan to provide inotropic support, dysrhythmia management, hypertension control, and fluid and electrolyte balance

Postoperative management is based on clinical symptoms, complications, and progress of patient
    Parenteral fluids administered based on postoperative hemodynamic parameters
        Volume expanders (Hespan, albumin)
        Blood replacement (packed cells, fresh frozen plasma)
    Inotropic support administered to maintain blood pressure and increase cardiac output
        Dopamine
        Dobutamine
    Vasodilator therapy administered to improve circulation and venous return during high catecholamine surgery immediately postoperatively
        Nipride
        Nitroglycerin

General Management

Intraaortic balloon pump—used when severe ventricular dysfunction occurs as patient is removed from bypass; provides circulatory support to failing myocardium

Hemodynamic monitoring—arterial, left atrial, pulmonary artery, and pulmonary capillary wedge pressures; cardiac output, cardiac index, and SVR measurements may be required

Ventricular assist devices (VAD)—for severe ventricular dysfunction or inability to wean patient from cardiopulmonary bypass support

ECG monitoring—continuous evaluation of heart rate, rhythm

Pacemakers

Immediate postoperative
    Assisted mechanical ventilation
    Suctioning
    Chest tubes

Diet therapy—sodium and fluid restrictions on basis of patient's clinical status

Pulmonary toilet—encourage coughing, deep breathing, and use of incentive spirometry

Physical therapy—range-of-motion exercises and early ambulation

NURSING CARE

Nursing Assessment

Level of Consciousness

Early
    Arousable
Late
    Alert and oriented

Pupils

May be small, but reactive to light

Sensory-Motor Function

As patient awakens, moves all extremities; shivering may occur during rewarming

Respiratory Function

Early

Atelectasis; diminished breath sounds at base

Late

Clear with full aeration; arterial blood gases normal

Cardiovascular System

Postoperative problems

Pleural effusions: diminished breath sounds at the bases, low-grade fever, shallow respiration; positive E to A egophony

Low cardiac output

Narrow pulse pressure; thready, rapid pulse; decreased urine output; labored respiration; disorientation; increased pulmonary capillary wedge pressure (PCWP) and left atrial pressure (LAP)

Dysrhythmias

Atrial fibrillation and flutter; junctional rhythms; heart block; ventricular rhythms: premature ventricular contractions, tachycardia, fibrillation

Cardiac tamponade

Hypotension; narrowed pulse pressure (10 mm Hg); pulsus paradoxus; widened mediastinal shadow on chest x-ray; increased venous pressure

Bleeding

Chest tube drainage at least 250 ml/hour; hypotension; disorientation; prolonged prothrombin time and partial thromboplastin time; decreased platelet levels

Infection

Elevated temperature; purulent drainage from suture sites; chills; diaphoresis; malaise

Pericarditis; postpericardiotomy syndrome

Pericardial friction rub; low-grade fever; chills; diaphoresis; malaise; chest pain

Nursing Dx & Intervention

Decreased cardiac output (high risk for) related to mechanical problems (altered preload, afterload, contractility, heart rate)

- Assess and monitor for signs and symptoms of decreased cardiac output: skin pallor, diaphoresis, hypotension, decreased urine output, tachycardia, diminished peripheral pulse, dyspnea.
- Monitor PAP, PCWP, mixed venous oxygen saturation (Svo_2) and arterial pressures every 15 minutes during the immediate postoperative period, decreasing frequency as the clinical status stabilizes.
- Monitor vital signs every 2 to 4 hours.

- Obtain cardiac output and calculate cardiac index (CI) and systemic vascular resistance (SVR) as indicated.
- Measure urine output every hour; report output of less than 30 ml per hour in an adult patient.
- Monitor and record ECG ratio and rhythm every 4 to 6 hours; initiate pacing as indicated.
- Check peripheral perfusion: pulses, skin temperature, color.
- Auscultate chest for heart sounds to detect gallops, murmurs, or rubs.
- Administer fluids and medications as ordered.

Ineffective breathing pattern related to decreased lung expansion, incision pain, or anxiety

- Assess and monitor respirations, lung sounds, skin color, use of accessory muscles, and arterial blood gases *to determine lung expansion and detect diminished sounds that may be due to increased fluid or atelectasis.*
- Auscultate chest for diminished breath sounds, initially every 1 to 2 hours and later every 4 to 6 hours.
- Observe and maintain patency of chest tubes *to ensure proper drainage and lung expansion.*
- Reposition the patient from one side to the other during the immediate postoperative period *to encourage lung expansion.*
- Assist and encourage the patient to cough and deep breathe, and use incentive spirometry.
- Administer pain medications before coughing procedure; individualize pain management as needed, such as patient-controlled analgesia or epidural anesthesia.
- Obtain serial chest x-rays *to check for progressive or resolving atelectasis and pleural effusions.*

Impaired gas exchange related to hypoventilation, ventilation-perfusion abnormalities

- Assess and monitor respirations, observing rate and quality as the patient is weaned from the respirator.
- Administer oxygen therapy with assisted ventilation; check fraction of inspired oxygen (FIo_2) tidal volume to yield Pao_2 of about 100 mm Hg.
- Observe for signs of progressive atelectasis: diminished breath sounds over affected area, restlessness, rales.
- Obtain and monitor arterial blood gases for signs of respiratory acidosis or alkalosis and Svo_2 for signs of decreased O_2 delivery.
- Auscultate the chest for diminished or adventitious breath sounds every 1 to 2 hours.
- Suction every 1 to 2 hours to maintain a patent airway.
- Oxygenate before suctioning procedure per institutional policy.
- Monitor and record any dysrhythmia experienced during the procedure.

Convalescent care:

- Assist and teach the patient to turn, cough, and deep breathe.
- Encourage use of the incentive spirometer.
- Auscultate lung sounds every 4 to 8 hours.

Fluid volume excess related to postoperative expanded extracellular fluid volume and to postoperative sodium and water retention

- Monitor for signs of fluid volume excess; monitor filling pressures: right atrial pressure (RAP), pulmonary artery diastolic pressure, and left atrial pressure (LAP).
- Inspect for increased JVD and dependent edema.
- During rewarming, check right atrial pressure, left atrial pressure, and PAP every 5 minutes until stable, then every 30 to 60 minutes.
- Titrate parenteral fluids according to hemodynamic parameters per protocol.
- Measure output every hour. Check specific gravity as ordered.
- Limit fluid intake as ordered.
- Monitor electrolyte, hemoglobin, and hematocrit values.
- Weigh daily as indicated by clinical picture.

Risk for infection related to compromised host defense and increased exposure to invasive lines

- Observe for signs of generalized sepsis; elevated temperature, chills, diaphoresis.
- Observe suture sites for local redness, drainage, and swelling; clean incisions and change dressing daily.
- Check temperature every 2 hours for 48 hours, then every 4 hours for 48 hours, then every 8 hours.
- Change IV and pressure lines and dressing as ordered, maintaining aseptic technique *to prevent nosocomial infections and cross-contamination.*
- Obtain blood cultures as ordered *to identify infecting organisms; to guide medical therapy.*
- Obtain complete blood count with differential as ordered.

Risk for hemorrhage related to disruption in platelet function and clotting factors

- Observe for signs of hemorrhage: decreased blood pressure, disorientation, and falling hemoglobin level.
- Observe for signs of coagulopathy: blood oozing from incisions, bloody secretions from endotracheal tube, increased chest tube drainage, and hematuria.
- Observe and measure chest tube drainage every 30 to 60 minutes.
- Report output in excess of 150 ml/h for an adult or 5 ml/kg/h for a child.
- Check hemoglobin, hematocrit, and clotting studies on the patient's arrival in the intensive care unit and every 2 to 4 hours as ordered.
- Administer blood and blood products as ordered.
- Administer drugs as ordered.

Anxiety related to actual or perceived threat to biologic integrity

Preoperative
- Assess anxiety level.
- Provide adequate instruction, answering questions and offering reassurance.

- Explain the method of communication to be used after the operation while the patient is intubated.

Postoperative
- Implement measures that will reduce level of anxiety.
- Orient the patient to time, situation, and location.
- Inform the patient that the surgery is over.
- Assist with communication.
- Anticipate needs if possible.
- Provide pain management as necessary.
- Allow family support and participation.
- Provide reassurance of daily progress.
- Encourage verbalization of fears and questions regarding the operation, recovery, and discharge.
- Begin postoperative instruction.

Patient Education/Home Care Planning

General
1. Review the surgical procedure, emphasizing any precautions or complications that may be associated with it.
2. Clarify what action(s) should be taken if symptoms of infection, bleeding, ventricular failure, or dysrhythmias develop.
3. Review diet and fluid restrictions.
4. Review discharge medication, including purpose, dosages, side effects, and need for specific follow-up laboratory studies as indicated.
5. Discuss activity allowances or limitations. Refer patient to cardiac rehabilitation for progressive ambulation.
6. Discuss the importance of avoiding fatigue and sitting for long periods of time.
7. Discuss care of incisions and symptoms of wound infection to report to the physician.

After valve replacement
1. Discuss the importance of anticoagulation therapy.
2. Discuss the importance of reporting signs of endocarditis (p. 71).
3. Discuss the importance of prophylactic antibiotic therapy before procedures that predispose to bacteremia (p. 61).
4. Provide Medic Alert card for artificial valve/anticoagulation.

Evaluation

Hemodynamic and electromechanical stability is achieved; cardiac output is adequate   Blood pressure, pulmonary artery pressure, and cardiac output are within acceptable range. There is no dysrhythmia. ECG findings are within acceptable limits.

Oxygenation, ventilation, and lung perfusion are adequate Pao_2 and Pco_2 are within normal limits. There is no dyspnea or tachypnea. Lungs are clear on auscultation and radiography.

There is no infection Patient is afebrile.

Hematologic hemostasis is achieved Hematocrit and hemoglobin level are within normal limits. A progressive decline in chest drainage occurs.

Anxiety is reduced There is no pain. Anxiety is absent or decreased. Patient demonstrates appropriate behavior patterns: asking questions and participating in self-care.

Patient has knowledge and understanding of primary cardiac disorder, surgical procedure performed, and discharge instructions Patient is able to describe specific action to take regarding diet, medications, and care of incision(s). Patient is able to describe activity allowances and limitations.

CARDIAC TRANSPLANTATION

Description and Rationale

Cardiac transplantation has evolved rapidly during the past 20 years, yet it was first performed in 1905 when Carrel and Guthrie transplanted the heart of one dog to another. However, it was not until 1967, when Christian Barnard performed the first human cardiac transplantation, that serious interest was stimulated. Because early survival rates were poor, transplantations continued to be performed on a limited basis. Since the introduction of the immunosuppressant agent cyclosporine in 1980, the number of centers performing heart transplantations has grown steadily.

To date there have been nearly 27,000 heart transplants worldwide. In 1993 there were 2290 heart transplants performed in the United States by 164 heart transplant centers.[23,32,64] One-year survival rates are reported to be 88%, and 5-year survival is 78%.

Infection and organ rejection continue to be the most common medical complications and the primary causes of death in long-term follow-up. However, as survival time increases, other medical problems are being identified, and these have contributed to the increased morbidity and mortality of patients over time.

Infection remains a major cause of morbidity and mortality for long-term, immunosuppressed transplant recipients, although the incidence and severity of infections decrease after the first year. The more common sites of infections in this population include the respiratory tract, urinary tract, mediastinum, and retina.

Infection/Rejection

Bacterial infections *(Escherichia coli, Pseudomonas)* make up 66% of all infections in the transplant recipient; 17% are viruses (cytomegalovirus, herpes simplex, herpes zoster); 12% are fungal *(Candida, Aspergillus, Cryptococcus)*; and 5% are protozoal.[92]

Rejection of the transplanted heart remains the primary lifelong threat to the recipient. Cardiac rejection can occur as an acute episode or a chronic condition. The risk of acute rejection is highest in the first days and weeks after transplantation while the immunosuppressant therapy is being adjusted. Although rejection rates decrease with each year of survival, the recipient is always at risk if therapy is interrupted or stopped. Immunosuppression is the only safeguard against acute rejection.

Graft atherosclerosis, or chronic rejection, has been reported to occur in approximately 35% to 40% of patients who survive 5 years after transplantation. The incidence among patients who had coronary artery disease before receiving the transplant is similar to that among patients with pretransplant cardiomyopathy. Furthermore, because the donor heart has been denervated, patients who develop diffuse occlusive CAD do not present clinically with angina pectoris. Thus, if not monitored carefully, they can die suddenly or develop ventricular failure.

Malignancies, particularly lymphomas of the histiocyte type, have been reported.[80] Their occurrence is thought to be associated with immunosuppression therapy, particularly including antithymocyte globulin in addition to cyclosporine. Other reported malignancies include epithelial tumors of the skin and leukemia.

Other late complications associated with lifelong immunosuppression in long-term survivors include osteoporosis (18.2%), spinal disorders (8.8%), and visual problems (14.3%).[23,32]

The quality of life after cardiac transplantation has also been evaluated. It is currently estimated that between 32% and 50% of heart transplant recipients return to work, although nearly 60% report that they are able to do so.[32] Lough and associates[59] reported that an average of 3.7 years after surgery 89% of heart recipients perceived their quality of life as good to excellent, and 82% reported satisfaction with life as good to very satisfactory. Factors associated with negative life change were reported to be financial status, physical appearance, and sexual function. All recipients were bothered by the side effects associated with immunosuppression therapy, but these were found to have little effect on their evaluation of quality of life and life satisfaction.

Immunosuppression Increased understanding of immune suppression and the introduction of various immunosuppressive agents have made organ transplantation a viable treatment modality. Since the late 1960s a variety of nonselective immunosuppressive agents had been used in transplantations, but these were associated with impairment of the immune system, leaving the host vulnerable to any number of infections. With the introduction of cyclosporine A, morbidity and mortality figures have been significantly reduced.

The primary goal of immunosuppressive therapy is to prevent rejection of the foreign graft (heart), yet retain the host's natural immune system, which protects against infections.

The immune system is a complex response mechanism. Its purpose is to destroy any tissue invasion or foreign material to maintain hemostasis. There are two primary types of immune response, humoral and cell-mediated. Both are derived from lymphocytes.

The primary indication for cardiac transplantation is end-stage heart disease that is refractory to medical therapies, surgical interventions, or both. The box on p. 100 shows donor selection criteria.

CARDIAC DONOR SELECTION CRITERIA

GENERAL

Imminent or established brain death (by two medical physicians)
Absence of systemic sepsis
No history of insulin-dependent diabetes
Absence of hepatitis, autoimmune disease
No history of heavy alcohol or intravenous drug use
No strong family history of heart disease

SPECIFIC

Age: males <55 yr; females <40 yr (variable depending on age of recipient)
No history of cardiac disease; no history of severe chest trauma
No history of prolonged cardiac arrest; no prolonged hypoxia
No history of prolonged hypotension; no prolonged use of dopamine
ECG: normal (nonspecific ST, T wave changes may be acceptable)
Laboratory values: normal WBC, creatinine phosphokinase–MB isoenzyme (CPK-MB); within normal limits—arterial blood gases, hemodynamic parameters
Echocardiogram: normal left and right ventricular (LV and RV) function

Contraindications

Absolute contraindications

Pulmonary hypertension (pulmonary vascular resistance [PVR] >6-8 Wood units)
Active infectious process
Kidney failure or liver failure
Severe peripheral vascular disease
Active peptic ulcer disease
Malignant or terminal systemic disease
Emotional or psychologic instability
Insulin-dependent diabetes

Relative contraindications

Age: older than 65 years
Lack of support systems
Non–insulin-dependent diabetes
History of drug or alcohol abuse

•••••• Multidisciplinary Plan

Surgery

Heart transplantation procedures:

Orthotopic   Recipient's heart is excised, leaving the posterior walls of the atria, and is replaced with donor heart

Heterotopic "piggyback"   Donor heart is placed in right chest adjacent to the recipient's heart; anastomosis of the two hearts permit blood to pass through one or both hearts

Medications

A variety of immunosuppressant agents are available. Maintenance immunosuppression protocols for cardiac transplant patients can include the following:

Cyclosporine (Sandimmune)—naturally occurring polypeptide antibiotic produced by fungi; inhibits T cell lymphocyte proliferation and activity, which is responsible for tissue graft rejection

Usual dosage: 2-8 mg/kg/d po; daily dose adjusted to maintain therapeutic levels (NOTE: therapeutic level is dependent on biologic fluid, assay method)
Half-life: 18-40 h (average 27 h)
Excretion: Metabolized by liver; excretion in bile and urine
Side effects: Hirsutism, acne, fragile skin, gingival hyperplasia, free hand tremor
Adverse reaction: Nephrotoxicity, hypertension, hepatotoxicity, infection (viral, bacterial, and fungal), lymphoma

Azathioprine (Imuran)—antimetabolite that produces immunosuppression by inhibiting purine and DNA synthesis

Usual dosage: 1.5-2 mg/kg/d po (NOTE: dosage adjusted to keep WBC above 4500)
Half-life: Approximately 3 h
Excretion: Metabolized by liver; excreted in urine
Side effects: Rash, bruising, nausea, vomiting, stomatitis, muscle wasting, arthralgia, fatigue, decreased libido, impotence
Adverse reaction: Leukopenia, thrombocytopenia, anemia, hepatotoxicity, pancreatitis, jaundice

Antithymocyte globulin (ATG)—reduces T lymphocytes; used to prevent rejection, or as an adjunct to immunosuppression therapy during rejection episodes

Usual dosage: Rabbit ATG-2 mg/kg/d IM, adjusted according to circulating T lymphocytes (WBCs); equine ATG-10 mg/kg/d IV, adjusted according to circulating T lymphocytes (rosette count)
Side effects: Localized pain and inflammation with IM injection; chills, fever, hypotension
Adverse reactions: Anaphylaxis

Orthodone (OKT$_3$, Ortho)—New monoclonal antibody similar to antithyroglobulin (ATG); reduces T cell function; used to prevent graft rejection

Usual dosage: 5 mg IV push daily for 10-14 days; given in less than 1 minute
Side effects: fever, chills, dyspnea, chest pain, vomiting, wheezing, nausea, diarrhea, tremor

Corticosteroids—antiinflammatory agents used to suppress both T and B lymphocyte function and to reverse capillary permeability, vasodilation, and edema; may be used as part of maintenance program to prevent rejection or as adjunct therapy when there is evidence of rejection

Prednisone (Meticorten, Deltasone)—used as part of maintenance therapy

Usual dosage: 0.1-0.2 mg/kg/d po (NOTE: may be increased with rejection)

Methylprednisolone (Medrol, Depo-Medrol, Solu-Medrol)—used when there is evidence of rejection
Usual dosage: 1 g/d for 3 d IV
Half-life: $3\frac{1}{2}$ h
Side effects: Cushingoid appearance, mood changes, GI distress, fragile skin, bruising, delayed wound healing
Adverse reactions: Infection, diabetes, thrombocytopenia, pancreatitis
Antihistamines and acetaminophen—given before therapy to reduce incidence of side effects

Pravastatin (HMG-CoA reduction inhibitor)—used to treat hypercholesterolemia to minimize graft atherosclerosis; found to have immunosuppressant qualities[55]
Usual dosage: 10-40 mg qd
Side effects: rash, nausea, muscle cramps, headache
Adverse reaction: liver dysfunction, rhabdomyolysis

General Management

ECG changes—reflect lack of autonomic innervation of heart that occurs as result of denervation when donor heart is removed
Heart rate—resting heart rate generally higher (90-100 BPM); response to metabolic demands such as fever or exercise in a denervated patient is one in which heart rate changes gradually; as result of these changes, response to drugs whose effect on the heart is mediated by autonomic nervous system is also altered
Rhythm—normal sinus but without respiratory variation
P wave—transplant procedure generally involves retaining posterior portion of recipient's atria, which includes S-A node; therefore second P wave is visible

Endomyocardial biopsy—after first year, endomyocardial biopsies are performed on an interval basis, depending on recipient's clinical status

Diet—low saturated fat and cholesterol; moderate decrease in sodium intake

Laboratory studies—regular monitoring to detect adverse reactions to immunosuppressive therapy: CBC, serum BUN and creatinine, liver function (SGOT, SGPT, LDH), glucose, urinalysis

Serum cholesterol: triglycerides; high-density, low-density lipoproteins (HDL, LDL); magnesium; potassium

Lymphocyte count; T cell studies—while receiving ATG or OKT$_3$

Cyclosporine levels

NURSING CARE

Nursing Assessment

Acute Rejection

Mild or early rejection—generally no symptoms associated; to detect early rejection, diagnosis is done with EMB

Severe rejection
Weakness, fatigue, malaise
Anorexia
Nausea, vomiting
Decreased urine output
Weight gain
Peripheral edema
Distended neck veins
Increased jugular venous pulsations and decreased perfusion: cool pale skin, diminished pulses, diaphoresis, confusion, restlessness
Pulmonary venous congestion: dyspnea on exertion, cough, tachypnea
Development of S$_3$ and S$_4$

Electrocardiogram (ECG)

Using conventional immunosuppression; 20% decrease in QRS voltage; right axis shift; atrial dysrhythmias, e.g., PAC, atrial fibrillation, atrial flutter (with cyclosporine these ECG changes may not be seen)

Chest X-ray

Increased cardiothoracic ratio (cardiomegaly)

Echocardiogram

Thickening of left ventricle; decreased left ventricular function; decreased contractility

Endomyocardial Biopsy (EMB)

Changes in lymphocytes; finding varies according to degree of rejection
Mild—occasional WBCs
Severe—extensive perivascular infiltration of lymphocytes, interstitial edema, and myocyte necrosis
Increased CPK-MB, SGOT, LDH

Infection

Usual signs and symptoms of infection often absent in immunosuppressed patient
Fever—low grade; baseline temperature may be lower than before transplant, so elevation to 37.2° C (99°F) may be significant
Malaise

Nursing Dx & Intervention

Risk for injury: rejection related to noncompliance with prescribed medical regimen

- Assess and evaluate patient for understanding and cognitive appraisal of prescribed lifelong therapy *to identify misconceptions and cues that may indicate potential adherence problems.*
- Encourage discussion regarding changes in lifestyle that have been positive or negative.

- Anticipate and allow questions regarding prescribed therapy.

Risk for infection related to immunosuppressive drug therapy

- Assess and monitor for signs of infection, as discussed previously.
- Take temperature every 4 hours.
- Obtain cultures as indicated: sputum, throat, urine, any suspicious drainage sites in wounds.
- Obtain and assess complete blood count and chest X-ray as indicated. NOTE: Laboratory values may be altered because of steroids.
- Minimize or avoid use of invasive procedures that increase risk of infection: IV, indwelling catheters.
- Change IV tubings, bags, and dressings daily using aseptic technique.
- Avoid placing patient in room with other patient who is at risk for infection *to avoid potential cross-contamination;* initiate reverse isolation for staff and family.
- Minimize number of visitors.
- Restrict visitors who show signs of infections, such as colds, herpes simplex.
- Administer antibiotic therapy as ordered.

Risk for decreased cardiac output related to severe rejection

- Assess and monitor for signs and symptoms of decreased cardiac output and signs of rejection, as discussed on p. 101.
- Auscultate heart sounds, *assessing for changes in rhythm and presence of S_3 and S_4.*
- Auscultate chest for lung sounds, *assessing for signs of increased pulmonary congestion.*
- Weigh daily.
- Prepare patient for EMB.
- Administer immunosuppressive therapy as ordered.

Other related nursing diagnosis Ineffective individual coping related to threat of disease process and inadequate coping resources

---

Patient Education/Home Care Planning

1. Discuss and review signs and symptoms of rejection. Emphasize the importance of keeping scheduled EMB appointments because there are usually *no* signs of early rejection and appearance of symptoms is associated with moderate to severe rejection.
2. Discuss and review the need to take medications lifelong and the need to take them *exactly* as prescribed. Caution the patient *never to stop* taking medication. Notify the physician if a dose was skipped. Review medications, checking dosage, method of administration, and side effects.

---

3. Discuss signs and symptoms of infection to report: elevation of baseline temperature; early signs of sore throat, cold, or flu; and cuts and lesions that do not heal.
4. Discuss the need to reduce the risk of infection by avoiding individuals with infections or contagious diseases, avoiding large crowds, and wearing a face mask when traveling in crowded areas.
5. Discuss the importance of lifelong follow-up: clinic visits, EMB appointments, and periodic stress tests, radionuclide studies, and cardiac catheterization.
6. Discuss activities, allowances, and limitations. Tell the patient to check with the physician before engaging in strenuous or competitive activities or sports.

Evaluation

There is no infection The patient maintains baseline temperature. There is no sign of infection: complete blood count, urinalysis, and cultures are within normal limits.

There are no signs of rejection on biopsy There are no new changes in EMB results. There are no clinical signs of rejection.

Patient complies with therapeutic regimen Serum drug levels are maintained. Patient keeps follow-up appointments and offers questions and concerns appropriately.

HEMODYNAMIC MONITORING

Description and Rationale

Monitoring to assess a patient's circulatory status may be done by indirect (noninvasive) or direct (invasive) methods. Indirect methods include arterial pressure monitoring by sphygmomanometer and stethoscope, heart rate monitoring by chest electrode replacement, and cardiac monitoring. Direct methods are indicated by the term *hemodynamic monitoring.*

Hemodynamic monitoring is a technique that permits close examination of cardiac function in acutely ill patients. Used primarily in critical care units, hemodynamic monitoring permits rapid identification of complications of myocardial infarction, guides the diagnosis and management of patients with low cardiac output, and helps to differentiate pulmonary disease from left ventricular failure.[40]

With use of a balloon-tipped, flow-directed catheter to provide continuous monitoring of the PAP and PCWP, myocardial function can be evaluated in terms of preload, afterload, and contractility. From these parameters the LVEDP can be estimated. Other possible measurements include cardiac output by the thermodilution method and sampling of arteriovenous oxygen differences. Hemodynamic monitoring also provides a direct means of assessing the patient's progress and response to fluid and drug management and permits careful titration of specific therapies.

Pulmonary artery pressure and pulmonary capillary wedge pressure Although the LVEDP is the major determinant of left ventricular function, it cannot be measured at the bedside. However, the LVEDP can be reflected by the pressure in the pulmonary capillaries and by the PAP at the end of diastole. The catheter, which is introduced via the subclavian vein or by cutdown, is passed through the right side of the heart into the pulmonary artery (Figure 1-66). There the balloon is inflated, occluding the artery. With the balloon inflated, the catheter is wedged in a distal branch of the capillaries (Figure 1-67). The pressure recorded reflects left atrial pressure, which corresponds to the LVEDP and is called the pulmonary capillary wedge pressure.

Intraarterial pressure (arterial line) Direct continuous monitoring of systemic arterial pressure is made possible by placement of an indwelling catheter, connected to a transducer and monitor, into a major artery. Central artery pressures, although more accurate, are used less frequently. The radial artery is the most common site for placement. The line also facilitates obtaining blood samples to measure arterial blood gases.

Cardiac output The cardiac output, the volume of blood the heart pumps per minute, can be measured using a calibrated thermistor located near the tip of the pressure catheter. Based on the Fick principle, a thermodilution technique using blood temperature changes is used to produce cardiac output determinations. A known volume of solution is injected at a specific rate into the right atrium via the proximal port of a three- or four-lumen pulmonary pressure catheter. Although the standard practice has been to use an iced solution, studies now show that room temperature injectate produces the same results.[76] The temperature-sensitive thermistor records the temperature of the blood as it passes through the catheter. The difference in temperature between the iced injectate and the blood is calculated, and the cardiac output is then digitally displayed by a special computer.

Contraindications and Cautions

Patients with left bundle-branch block should be observed for development of right bundle-branch block during insertion and while the flotation catheter is in place. Insertion of the flotation catheter in a patient with right-sided endocarditis may cause dislodgment of septic emboli to the lung. Use of the radial artery for monitoring is contraindicated in the presence of inadequate circulation. Relative contraindications include severe bleeding disorders and severe immunosuppression.

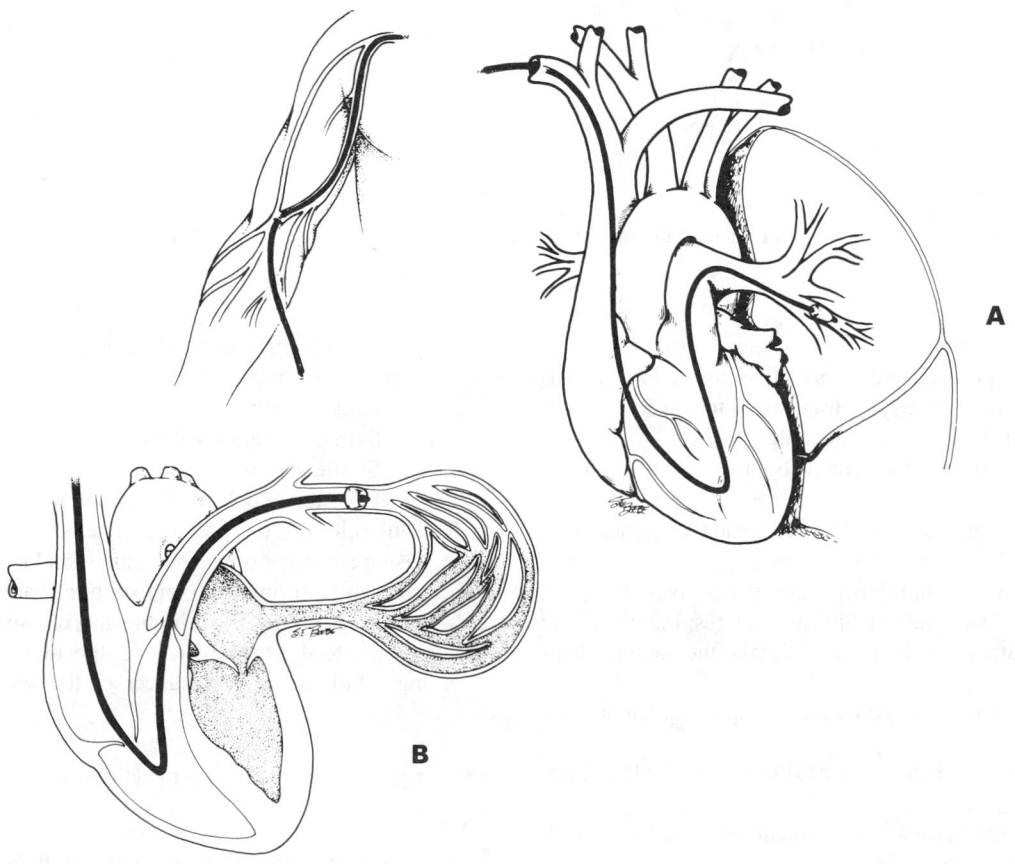

Figure 1-66 Balloon-tipped flow-directed catheter. **A,** Placement of flow-directed catheter via superior vena cava. **B,** Balloon inflated and wedged in pulmonary artery. (From Tucker.[89])

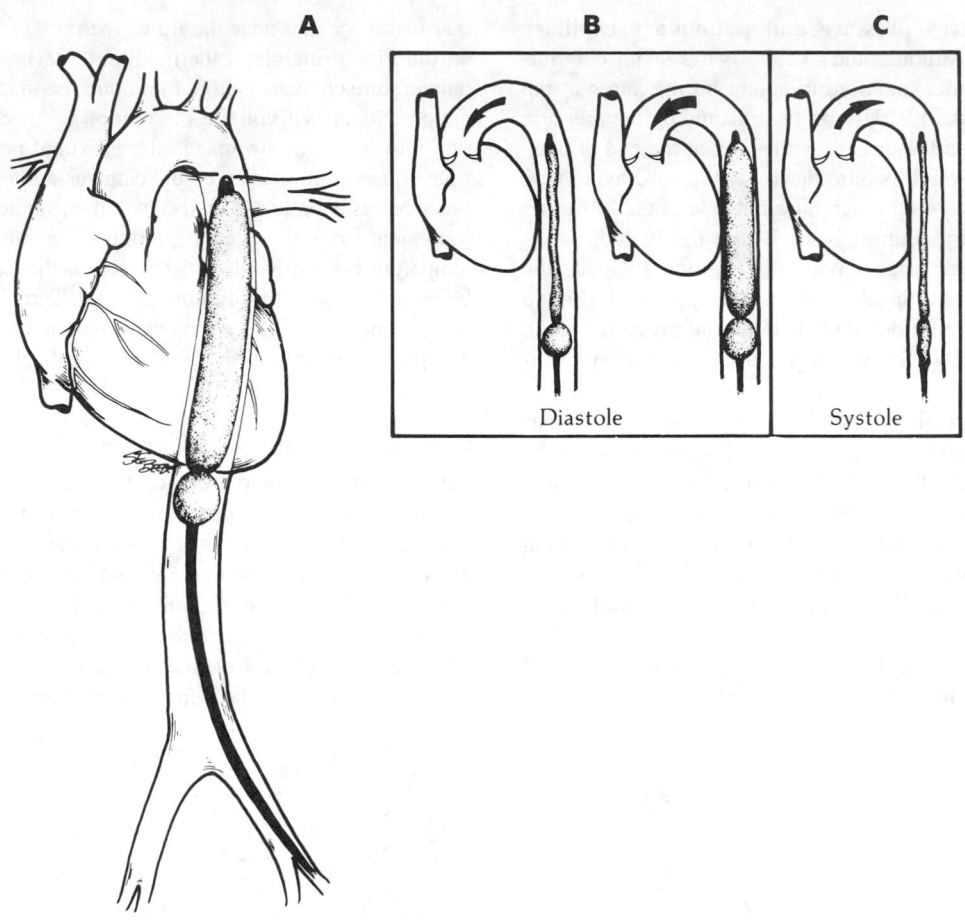

Figure 1-67 Intraaortic balloon. **A,** Position of balloon catheter. **B,** During inflation (diastole). **C,** During deflation (systole). (From Tucker.[89])

Preprocedural Care

1. Pulmonary pressure catheters can be inserted at the bedside, or the patient may be transferred to a special procedure room for insertion under fluoroscopy. Intraarterial lines are inserted at the bedside by means of sterile technique.
2. Explain the purpose, risks involved, and techniques of insertion.
3. Ensure that written, informed consent is obtained.
4. Measure blood pressure, pulse, and respiration. If the cardiac output is to be measured, take the patient's temperature.
5. Connect the patient to a cardiac monitor; obtain a baseline rhythm strip.
6. Place the patient in a supine or slight Trendelenburg's position.
7. Assemble the necessary equipment and supplies according to routine hospital policies:
   Monitoring equipment
      Pressure catheter with flush solution, related closed tubing, stopcocks, and a low-flush pressurized system
      Transducer with oscilloscope
   Insertion equipment
      Local anesthetic
      Skin preparation solution
      Sterile gloves
      Dressing supplies
8. Calibration of the pressure system is recommended to ensure accuracy of measurements, and to avoid spurious readings resulting from temperature changes, or changes in transducer level. Calibrate the pressure monitor according to the manufacturer's directions; for PAP readings calibrate the transducer to the level of the right atrium.

•••••• Multidisciplinary Plan

Surgery

Pulmonary pressure catheter (balloon flotation)—inserted via jugular, subclavian, brachial, or right femoral vein by cutdown or percutaneous puncture under local anesthesia

Arterial catheter—inserted via radial, brachial, or femoral artery by percutaneous method

Medications

Flushing system—continuous microdrip of heparinized solution (5% dextrose), kept in closed system under pressure greater than patient's systolic pressure (usually 300 mm Hg) by pressurized bag

General Management

Continuous ECG monitoring

Monitoring and recording of pressures every 1 to 2 hours or as ordered

Calibration of transducer and monitoring every 4 to 8 hours or as specified by manufacturer

Maintaining patency of catheters with continuous pressurized flushing device

NURSING CARE

Nursing Assessment

Pulmonary Artery Pressure Catheters (Table 1-6)

Pneumothorax and dysrhythmias during insertion; pulmonary air embolism; pulmonary infarction; pulmonary perforation; sepsis or infection; thrombophlebitis at insertion site

Arterial lines

Hemorrhage; clot formation; diminished or absent pulse distal to insertion site; hematoma at insertion site; infection

Nursing Dx & Intervention

Impaired gas exchange (high risk for) related to embolization of thrombus from catheter migration or wedging

- Observe for signs of pneumothorax and pulmonary air embolism: chest pain, dyspnea, hemoptysis, tachypnea.

NORMAL RANGES OF HEMODYNAMIC PARAMETERS

Right atrial pressure	2-6 mm Hg (mean pressure)
Right ventricular pressure	Systolic: 20-30 mm Hg
	Diastolic: 0-5 mm Hg
	End-diastolic: 2-6 mm Hg
Pulmonary artery pressure (PAP)	Systolic: 20-30 mm Hg
	End-diastolic: 8-12 mm Hg
	Mean: 10-20 mm Hg
Pulmonary arterial wedge pressure (PAWP)	4-12 mm Hg (mean pressure)
Arterial pressure (intraarterial)	Peak systolic: 100-140 mm Hg
	End-diastolic: 60-80 mm Hg
	Mean: 70-90 mm Hg
Cardiac output (CO)	4-8 L/min
Cardiac index (CO/body surface area)	2.5-4 L/min
Systemic vascular resistance (SVR)	800-1200 dynes/sec/cm^5
Pulmonary vascular resistance (PVR)	37-250 dynes/sec/cm^5

TABLE 1-6 Problems Observed in Pressure Waveforms

Observation	Etiologic Factors	Interventions
Loss of waveform on oscilloscope	Displacement of catheter	Reposition patient: notify physician
Loss of PAP; PCWP is displayed on monitor	Self-wedging	Instruct patient to cough
		Obtain x-ray examination
Loss of PWP	Displaced into PAP; balloon rupture	Use diastolic of PAP
Decreased amplitude of waveform (damped waveform)	Damping due to:	Flush lines: *Do not force if resistance is met*
	Clot in catheter tip	Check all connections for air leaks: flush air bubbles
	Air bubbles	
	Kinking of catheter	Notify physician
	Occluded catheter	Reposition patient; have patient cough
	Tip against artery wall	
Loss of PCWP; no resistance with inflation	Rupture of balloon	Seal off balloon lumen: *Do not allow any injection of air*
Air bubbles in pressure lines	Air leak in system	Check that all connections are secure
Damping of waveform		
Inaccurate reading		
Artifacts and inadequate pressure readings	Respiratory interference from handling of pressure equipment during readings	Record pressure at end exhalation using printed waveform
	Inaccurate calibration of equipment	Check for possible interference with tubing during readings
	Faulty equipment	Check electrical system for grounding
		Check calibration of and level to RA of transducer
		Check all equipment for proper functioning

From Tucker.[89]

- Observe for and prevent balloon rupture:
  Inflate balloon for few seconds only.
  Ensure balloon is deflated after wedge pressure measurement.
  Observe waveform for signs of self-wedge or damped tracing.
  Secure and label catheter and injection ports to avoid confusion of lines.
- Obtain chest x-ray in first 12 hours or as ordered, and check for catheter placement.
- Auscultate chest sounds every 4 hours *to assess for signs of diminished or adventitious sounds.*
- Monitor arterial blood gases as ordered *to identify fall in arterial Pao2 or increase in Pco2.*
- Administer oxygen therapy as ordered.
- Check patency of lines, tubes, and connections.
- Never use force to flush or irrigate a line that is resistant.

Infection, high risk for related to contamination

- Observe for signs of local inflammation or infection.
- Take measures to prevent infection:
  Maintain aseptic technique during insertion.
  Change flushing solution and tubing to catheter every day.
  Change dressing every day, cleaning insertion site with antiseptic agents.
  Observe for signs of local inflammation or infection.

Anxiety related to perceived threat or change in health status

- Provide continuous explanation of procedure.
- Offer frequent reassurance, encouraging verbalization and questions regarding progress.
- Allow family and significant others to visit when feasible.

Decreased cardiac output (high risk for) related to dysrhythmias

- Observe and monitor ECG rhythm for ventricular dysrhythmias (premature ventricular contractions, ventricular tachycardia) during and after insertion.
- Keep lidocaine available at bedside during insertion.
- Monitor vital signs every 30 to 60 minutes as ordered.

Patient Education/Home Care Planning

1. Explain to the patient and family the purpose of the procedure, as cited in preprocedural care.
2. Explain to the patient not to move the insertion area.

Evaluation

Pressure lines are patent   Waveform is normal.
There is no infection   Patient is afebrile.
Anxiety is reduced   Patient verbalizes absence of anxiety or decrease in anxiety level.

Lung aeration and perfusion are normal   Lung sounds are clear to bases. There is bilateral aeration. Chest x-ray is normal.

INTRAAORTIC BALLOON PUMPING

Description and Rationale

An intraaortic balloon pump (IABP) is a mechanical device that provides circulatory assistance to the failing myocardium. Using the principles of counterpulsation, the balloon inflates with diastole and deflates during systole.

A sausage-shaped balloon is inserted through the common femoral artery and passed upward into the aorta. It lies in the descending aorta just distal to the left subclavian artery (see Figure 1-67). Externally the catheter is connected to a power console that has ECG input. Helium or carbon dioxide gas is used to inflate the balloon.

The IABP is used in the treatment of cardiogenic shock in low–cardiac output states, following cardiopulmonary bypass, in drug-resistant dysrhythmias caused by ischemia, and in unstable angina. The effect of counterpulsation on left ventricular function is produced by diastolic augmentation and afterload reduction.

The first phase of balloon pumping (Figure 1-68), with diastolic augmentations, occurs when the balloon inflates during diastole. This displaces the blood remaining in the aorta after

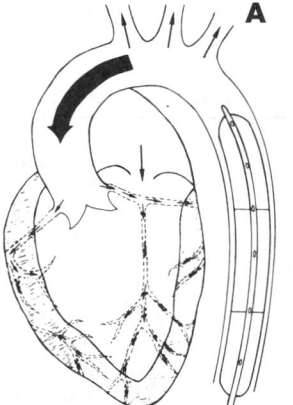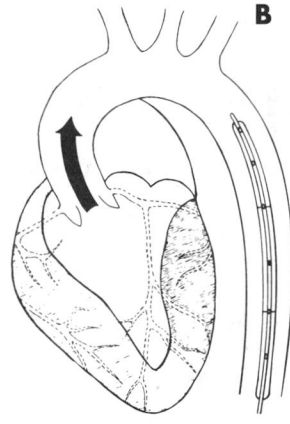

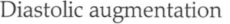

Diastolic augmentation   Systolic unloading

Figure 1-68 Two phases of balloon pumping. **A,** Balloon inflation occurs from closure of aortic valve to end of diastole. Inflation causes retrograde flow of blood in aorta, increasing coronary perfusion pressure without increasing myocardial work or oxygen demand. Inflation also causes antegrade flow, increasing mean arterial pressure, renal flow, and cerebral flow. **B,** Balloon deflation occurs from just before opening of aortic valve to closure of aortic valve. Deflation encourages antegrade flow, decreasing afterload or resistance to left ventricular ejection. Deflation also decreases oxygen required by left ventricle, shortens systolic ejection, and increases stroke volume. (From Michaelson CR, editor: *Congestive heart failure,* St Louis, 1983, Mosby.)

ventricular ejection back into the aortic root. The increased blood in the aortic root results in an elevation of diastolic pressure, increasing coronary blood flow and perfusion.

Afterload reduction, the second phase of balloon pumping, occurs when the balloon deflates during systole. With balloon deflation blood flow is encouraged forward out of the left ventricle. This produces decreased myocardial wall tension during diastole (decreased resistance), decreased myocardial oxygen consumption, and improved left ventricular output.

Contraindications

Contraindications to IABP include severe aortic regurgitation, aortic dissection, abdominal aortic aneurysm, and terminal illness.

Cautions

The cannulated extremity should not be flexed or bent.

Preprocedural Care

1. Explain procedure, insertion technique, equipment to be used, and sensations that may be felt.
2. Ensure that written informed consent from the patient or family is obtained.
3. Prepare the patient:
   a. Assess and record peripheral circulation, checking pulses and noting color and warmth of extremities; vital signs, including heart and breath sounds; hemodynamic status (arterial pressure, PAP, PCWP, cardiac output); and level of awareness (mentation).
   b. Obtain baseline laboratory data (clotting studies, hemoglobin, hematocrit, white blood cell count, and platelets).
   c. Obtain baseline ECG rate and rhythm.
   d. Prepare groin area.

•••••• Multidisciplinary Plan

Medications

Local anesthetic agents
Lidocaine (Xylocaine)

General Management

Continuous monitoring during and after insertion, including ECG, arterial pressure, PAP, cardiac output
Diet as ordered
Intravenous therapy as ordered
Oxygen therapy as indicated
Bed rest; turning every 2 hours with assistance

NURSING CARE

Nursing Assessment

Cannulated Extremity

Normal
   Decreased pulse volume and contour

Complications at insertion site
   Infection
      Fever, local tenderness, swelling, purulent drainage
   Bleeding, hematoma
      Ecchymosis, swelling
   Ischemia
      Diminished or absent pulses, numbness, pallor, pain
   Arterial thrombus formation
      Diminished or absent pulses, numbness, pallor, pain

General Complications

Aortic dissection, perforation
   Sudden, severe, sharp pain in abdomen and back; hypotension; tachycardia; decreased hematocrit value
Thrombocytopenia
   Bleeding; decreased platelet count (fewer than 150,000/ml)
Progressive myocardial failure
   Decreased cardiac output, arterial pressure, and urine output; increased PCWP; rales, rhonchi
Dysrhythmias
   Ventricular ectopy: pulmonary ventricular contractions and ventricular tachycardia; atrial fibrillation

Machine Console and Equipment

Balloon synchronization
   Inflation (augmentation) at dicrotic notch of aortic waveform; deflation at end of diastole
Complications
   Catheter kinking; malposition; balloon rupture

Nursing Dx & Intervention

Altered peripheral tissue perfusion (high risk for) related to interruption of flow, arterial

- Assess skin color, temperature, and pulses, which are indicators of peripheral tissue perfusion.
- Monitor peripheral extremities for decreased perfusion every 1 to 2 hours.
- Provide protection to cannulated extremity with sheepskin, lamb's wool, or foot cradle.
- Perform passive range of motion exercises every 4 hours.
- Avoid bending extremity.
- Check dressings every hour.

Decreased cardiac output (high risk for) related to mechanical factors (preload, afterload, or contractility)

- Monitor arterial pressure, PAP, and PCWP every hour.
- Assess cardiac output as ordered.
- Monitor ECG rhythm every hour.

Altered cerebral, renal, and pulmonary tissue perfusion (high risk for) related to interruption of flow, arterial

- Assess level of consciousness.
- Auscultate breath sounds.

- Monitor arterial blood gases as ordered.
- Maintain oxygen therapy as ordered.
- Measure intake and output every hour.
- Ensure that ordered chest x-ray is obtained.

Impaired skin integrity related to mechanical and internal factors; bed rest, impaired circulation

- Assess for skin breakdown and decubitus formation.
- Turn and position every 2 hours.
- Provide skin care every 2 to 4 hours.

Anxiety related to perceived health status

- Provide continued explanations of procedure and treatments.
- Offer frequent reassurance, encouraging verbalization and questions regarding progress.
- Allow family and significant others to visit patient when feasible.

Evaluation

Perfusion of cannulated extremity is adequate Extremity is warm. Capillary filling time is normal. Pulses are palpable. Color is normal. Mobility of extremity is normal.

Myocardial function is restored Arterial pressure, cardiac output, and PCWP are within normal limits. Urine output is restored to normal. Lungs are clear. S_3 and S_4 are absent.

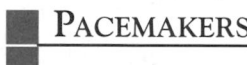

PACEMAKERS

Description and Rationale

Pacemakers are battery-operated generators that initiate and control the heart rate by delivering an electrical impulse via an electrode to the myocardium. Implantation of myocardial electrodes is initiated when a patient has symptomatic atrioventricular block. However, since the development of pacemakers in 1960, their use has expanded to include treatment of symptomatic brachydysrhythmias from other causes and refractory tachydysrhythmias.

Pacemaker implantation may be performed for temporary or long-term pacing. Temporary cardiac pacing is most commonly used for hemodynamic or life support purposes. The therapeutic indications include prophylactic pacing for complete heart block, symptomatic bradydysrhythmias, particularly in the setting of acute myocardial infarction, and as an emergency measure for malfunction of an implanted permanent pacemaker. In addition to control of heart rate, temporary pacing is often used in the electrophysiologic laboratory to evaluate cardiac dysrhythmias and to interrupt refractory tachydysrhythmias (e.g., supraventricular tachydysrhythmias, ventricular tachycardia).

Permanent cardiac pacing is indicated in the presence of symptomatic bradydysrhythmias.

Based on a universal code, pacemakers are described using a three-letter designation for the mode of pacing and the cham-

bers to be sensed and paced. The first letter describes the chamber that will be paced: the atrium (A), ventricle (V), or both (dual) chambers (D). The second letter represents the chamber that will be sensed: atrium (A), ventricle (V), dual (D), or none (O). The third letter reflects the mode that will be used: triggered (T), inhibited (I), or both (D), For example:

VVI
V The pacemaker will pace the ventricle.
V The pacemaker will sense the ventricle.
I   The pacemaker will inhibit pacing when the patient's own impulse is sensed.

There are three types of pacemakers:

Asynchronous or fixed rate, in which rate and rhythm of pacemaker beats are unaffected by spontaneous beats

Demand pacing or standby pacing, which discharges (fires) only when spontaneous beats drop below a preset rate

Synchronous pacemakers, in which a sensing circuit is used to detect atrial and ventricular activity

Contraindications

Pacemaker implantation is contraindicated for patients with active infections. Potential contraindications include the presence of atrial fibrillation or any poorly controlled supraventricular tachycardia.

Cautions

Safety from electrical hazards should be ensured.

Preprocedural Care

1. Initiate preoperative instruction for the patient and family, including purpose and indications for pacemaker implantation, benefits and associated risks, information regarding method of insertion, type and mode of pacemaker to be used, and postoperative care including need for routine 24-hour ECG monitoring and need to restrict activities for 4 to 6 hours.
2. Ensure that written informed consent is obtained.
3. Perform skin preparation.
4. Obtain baseline assessment data: underlying ECG rhythm, heart rate, pulse, respirations, blood pressure, and level of consciousness.
5. Permit nothing by mouth (NPO) 6 to 8 hours before procedure.
6. Initiate intravenous line.
7. Check functioning of external generator (for a temporary unit).

• • • • • • Multidisciplinary Plan

Surgery

Method of implantation depends on whether pacing will be temporary or permanent

Temporary

Transvenous approach—most common technique for temporary pacing; catheter electrode is passed into right ventricle via peripheral vein (brachial, femoral, subcla-

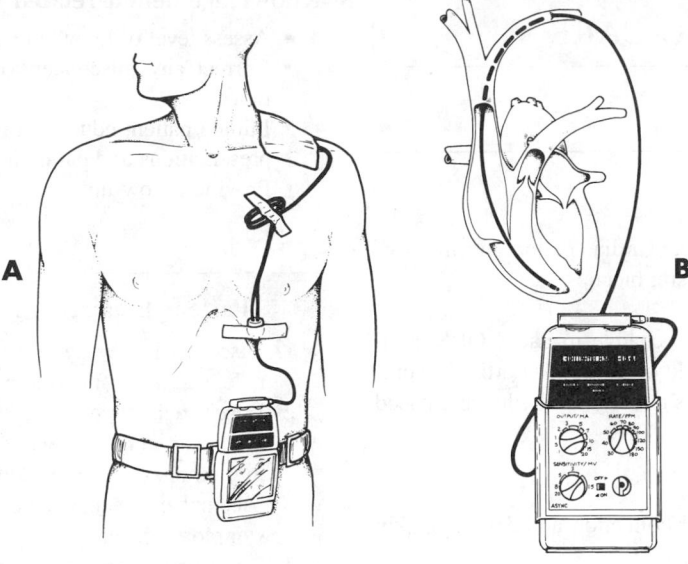

Figure 1-69 A, Temporary external pacemaker. **B,** Temporary pacemaker unit, transvenous approach. (From Tucker.[89])

vian, or internal jugular); electrode is connected to external pulse generator that can be set manually for direct or demand pacing mode (Figure 1-69)

Transthoracic approach—used primarily after open heart surgery; catheter is passed directly into heart through chest wall

Permanent

Transvenous pacing—catheter electrode is passed into right ventricle and attached to small, sealed, battery-operated pulse generator that is planted subcutaneously in shoulder or upper left quadrant (Figure 1-70)

Epicardial pacing—performed less frequently; electrode is sutured to epicardial surface of right ventricle; procedure requires a thoracotomy

Medications

Preoperative

Mild sedation, tranquilizers

Intraoperative

Local anesthesia, used for temporary and long-term transvenous pacing

General anesthesia, used for transthoracic approach

General Management

Cardiac monitoring—ECG pattern observed for rate, pacemaker response, signs of pacemaker failure, and dysrhythmias

Pacemaker unit

Pulse generator—self-contained device consisting of electronic circuit and power source of lithium batteries; device is hermetically sealed for protection from biologic environment; lithium-powered pacemakers can last 8 to 10 years before battery change is required

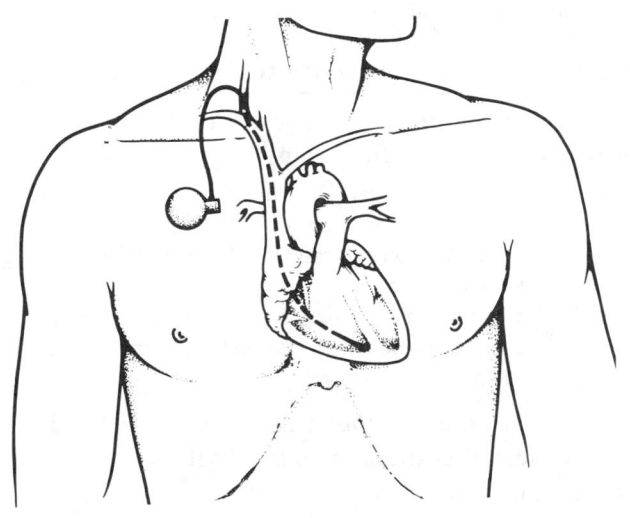

Figure 1-70 Permanent pacemaker. (From Tucker.[89])

Pacing leads—pulse generators use either unipolar or bipolar leads, and most generators are programmable to both; with unipolar leads, electrode (negative terminal) is at distal tip of catheter touching endocardium or myocardium; with bipolar lead two electrodes are located at distal tip of catheter; current flows from pulse generator through distal electrodes into heart, where it stimulates myocardial contraction

Bed rest for 8 hours after implantation, keeping arm below level of shoulder

Range of motion exercises to affected extremity when ordered after third postoperative day

NURSING CARE

Nursing Assessment

Pacemaker Failure

Clinical symptoms
  Syncope, hypotension, bradycardia, pallor, shortness of breath, chest muscle spasm, hiccups
ECG rhythm
  Loss of pacemaker artifact, change in paced QRS complex, decreased amplitude of pacemaker artifact, competition between patient's underlying rhythm and paced beats, dysrhythmias

Infection at Incision Site

Redness, swelling, heat, fluid collection and drainage, skin breakdown, soreness

Dysrhythmias

Premature ventricular beats, ventricular tachycardia, patient complaints of palpitations

Nursing Dx & Intervention

Anxiety related to perceived or actual change in health status, role functioning

- Assess level of anxiety, level of understanding, and fears associated with pacemaker implantation.
- Provide explanation and rationale for pacemaker, gauging the patient's reactions.
- Anticipate and allow the patient's questions regarding changes in lifestyle, cautions, and concerns over pacemaker management.

Decreased cardiac output (high risk for) related to electrical alterations in rate, rhythm, and conduction

- Assess the patient and pacemaker unit for signs of low cardiac output that is *reflective of pacemaker failure:* decreased blood pressure, pulse rate less than 60 beats per minute, light-headedness, decreased amplitude of pulse, cool, pale skin.
- Monitor vital signs every 4 hours after insertion.
- Monitor ECG rhythm strip every 4 hours for 24 hours after insertion.
- Discourage use of nicotine, which causes vasoconstriction and reduces oxygen availability.

Pain related to incision and physical mobility of affected arm

- Assess quality and source of pain.
- Administer pain medication as ordered.
- Encourage range of motion exercises to affected shoulder as ordered.

Knowledge deficit related to lack of information

- Assess level of knowledge.
- Correct any misconceptions regarding pacemaker function.
- Initiate patient education program, providing audiovisual presentations and pamphlets.
- Provide follow-up.

Patient Education/Home Care Planning

1. Discuss with the patient and family the purpose, rationale, and basic function of the permanent pacemaker.
2. Describe the type of pacemaker and the pacemaker's set rate. Instruct the patient on pulse rate and rhythm checking, emphasizing that pulse rate monitoring in lithium pacemakers needs to be done once a week or when symptoms occur.
3. Describe the signs and symptoms of pacemaker failure, including dizziness, weakness, light-headedness, and drop in pacemaker's set rate. Discuss actions to take if pacemaker malfunction is suspected, including calling for a pacemaker check via transtelephonic monitoring and notifying the physician or pacemaker clinic.
4. Describe activity allowances and limitations. Tell the patient to avoid traveling and driving for first 4 weeks after insertion. Encourage the patient to resume normal daily activities and recreational interests, except competitive contact sports, which can increase the risk of lead dislodgment.
5. Discuss the need to avoid and protect against hazards from high-output electrical generators such as diathermy motors, welding equipment, and radar. Most household electrical devices (such as microwave ovens and blow dryers) are considered safe, but review symptoms that may reflect electromagnetic interference and the action to take if symptoms occur.
6. Explain the need for continued medical follow-up and the need for periodic battery replacements; refer the patient to a pacemaker clinic where available.
7. Describe the use of telephone transmitters where available.
8. Explain the signs and symptoms of wound or pocket infection; and instruct the patient or family to report to the physician if fever or drainage develops.
9. Explain to the patient the need to protect the pacemaker site: avoid constricting clothing and direct contact or blows to the site; contact sports are usually contraindicated.
10. Explain the need to carry an identification card.
11. Reassure a female patient in her reproductive years that pregnancy is not contraindicated. Tell her to inform her physician of the desired pregnancy before conception so the pacemaker program can be checked and adapted to rate changes commonly associated with pregnancy.

Evaluation

Pacemaker functions properly Patient is normotensive and without dizziness, syncope, palpitations, chest pain, shortness of breath, or fatigue. Heart rate is acceptable. A temporary pacemaker fires at preset rate, sensing mechanism is visualized, and pacemaker artifact is visualized on ECG. A permanent pacemaker fires at preset rate, and pacemaker artifact is visualized on ECG.

Anxiety level is reduced Patient demonstrates reduced anxiety level and appears relaxed and less tense. Patient verbalizes feeling less fearful and asks appropriate questions. Patient verbalizes understanding of procedures. Misconceptions are corrected.

Cardiac output is maintained Patient remains normotensive. Skin is warm and dry. Patient verbalizes no chest discomfort and rests quietly. Vital signs remain stable.

Patient is free of infection and pain Patient is afebrile. Incisional site is clean with no swelling or redness. Patient verbalizes comfort.

Tissue perfusion is maintained Pulses distal to cannulation site are palpable. Extremities are warm and dry. Coagulation studies are within normal limits.

INTERVENTIONAL TECHNIQUES FOR CORONARY ARTERY REVASCULARIZATION

PERCUTANEOUS TRANSLUMINAL CORONARY ANGIOPLASTY

Description and Rationale

Percutaneous transluminal coronary angioplasty (PTCA) is an invasive, nonsurgical, therapeutic procedure that restores arterial luminal patency, thereby relieving myocardial ischemia by compressing atheromatous plaques. PTCA has evolved over the past 2 decades as an extension of peripheral balloon angioplasty. Intracoronary transluminal dilation, first developed by Andreas Gruntzig in 1977, was at first used only on a highly selected population of patients with stable angina and discrete proximal noncalcified lesions of the coronary arteries. Since then, because of advances and modifications of the percutaneous catheter, the selection criteria of candidates for angioplasty has also widened. Current patient selection criteria focus on accessibility, complexity, and location of the lesion and its compressibility. In 1979 the National Heart, Lung, and Blood Institute issued the following conservative guidelines:

Stable angina with symptoms refractory to medical therapy; single-vessel coronary stenosis

Objective evidence of myocardial ischemia by exercise treadmill, thallium scintigraphy with exercise, or gated blood pool studies

Lesions that are proximal, discrete, concentric, and noncalcified

These guidelines define the ideal situation for angioplasty; however, improvements in equipment and operator experience have gone beyond these early guidelines. Multivessel angioplasty involving complex lesions is now routinely performed.

In fact, much current debate revolves around the treatment of acute myocardial infarction with emergent angioplasty in lieu of thrombolytic therapy. There are distinct advantages to this aggressive interventional approach; however, the limitations surround the emergent availability of the catheterization laboratory. Thus this approach is reserved for larger cardiac specialty centers. The procedure, which is technically similar to a standard cardiac catheterization, involves passing a balloon-tipped catheter into a stenosed coronary artery where the balloon is then inflated and deflated using a handheld syringe or pressure-controlled device (Figure 1-71). Successful dilation is usually accompanied by reduction in the systolic gradient across the stenosis; however, the gradient may not be abolished and the inflation-deflation cycle may have to be repeated several times until the postangioplasty arteriogram demonstrates improved luminal diameter. Successful PTCA is defined as an increase of at least 20% in lumen size. Currently, primary success rates are being achieved in 85% to 90% of patients undergoing PTCA. Symptomatic relief is being achieved in 80%, and long-term follow-up shows continued lumen patency and symptomatic improvement from 6 months to 2 years.[50] The restenosis rate, however, is currently 30%, which is the major driving force behind the development of new interventional devices (described later).[50]

The angioplasty procedure involves using a two-catheter system. First a guiding sheath is introduced percutaneously via the femoral or brachial artery cutdown. After the guiding catheter is at the orifice of the stenosed coronary artery, a second double-lumen dilation catheter is inserted and advanced under fluoroscopy until the balloon straddles the lesion. Pressure is applied at 5 to 10 atmospheres for 30 seconds or longer at a time, depending on patient tolerance or ischemia. After angioplasty, the deflation catheter is removed, leaving the sheath in place.

Arteriograms are performed before and after the procedure, using the guiding catheter in the angiographic catheter. This allows evaluation of the results and decisions regarding the need for further dilation.

Directional coronary atherectomy (DCA) DCA reduces stenosis by removing atheromatous material rather than by compressing the plaque or stretching the arterial wall. DCA is most appropriate for lesions in medium to large coronary arteries, especially in the proximal and middle portion of the vessel. Highly eccentric lesions are appropriate for DCA. The safety is comparable to PTCA, and restenosis rates are modestly better. The device consists of a catheter-mounted cylindrical metallic housing with a central rotating blade.[36] The blade shaves off atherosclerotic plaque and deposits it in the nose cone of the housing so it can be extracted.

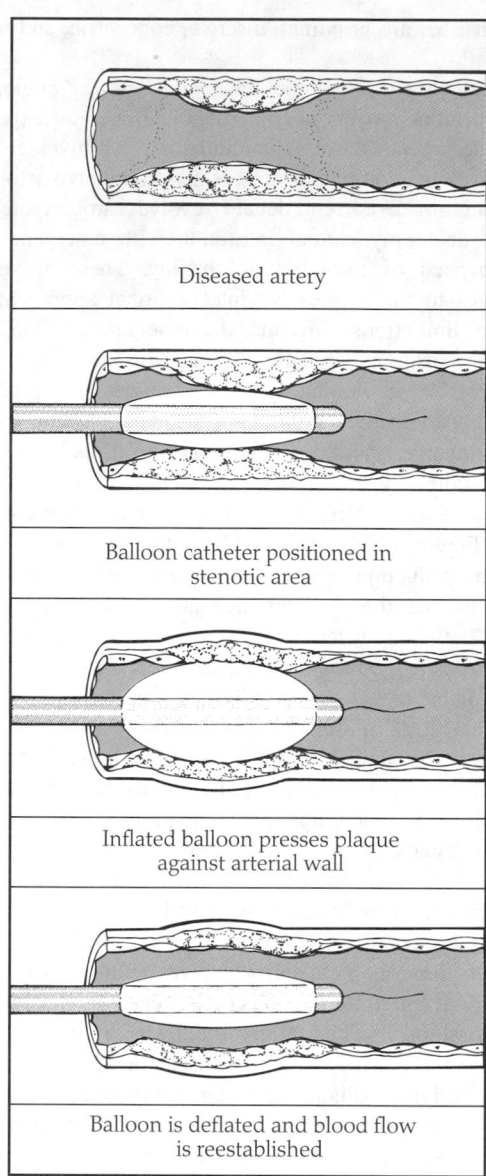

Diseased artery

Balloon catheter positioned in
stenotic area

Inflated balloon presses plaque
against arterial wall

Balloon is deflated and blood flow
is reestablished

Figure 1-71 Coronary angioplasty procedure. (From Canobbio.[13])

Rotational atherectomy (Rotablator) The Rotablator device is an elliptical brass burr coated with diamond chips that is attached to a flexible, high-speed rotating shaft.[36] The plaque is microbraded and the debris is flushed into the distal coronary circulation. Particles should be small enough to pass through the distal vascular bed. This device is best used in small coronary arteries with tortuous anatomy, diffuse disease, or distal stenoses. It is particularly useful with heavily calcified lesions. Acute success rates are good, but size limitations may necessitate adjunctive PTCA for optimal result.

Laser angioplasty Short pulses of laser energy are delivered through a catheter consisting of concentric bundles of optical fibers. Indications for laser angioplasty are long, diffuse, calcified, ostial, and vein graft lesions, as well as totally oc-

cluded vessels. Capable of increasing lumen size, laser ablation is often combined with PTCA to gain access for balloon insertion over a guide wire.

Coronary stents Designed to reduce restenosis and prevent acute occlusion resulting from angioplasty. A stent can maintain dissected vessel patency by compressing the intimal flap against the vessel wall. Several stents are near final approval for clinical use in the United States. Balloon-expandable stents[36] and self-expandable stents are now under clinical evaluation. A major complication of stent placement is acute thrombosis in the first several weeks, before endothelialization of the stent occurs. Aggressive anticoagulation can lead to vascular complications related to bleeding, and thus prolonged hospitalizations. Strategies to minimize potential bleeding while protecting against stent thrombosis are under consideration for this promising technique.

Indications

    Chronic stable angina
    Unstable angina
    Acute myocardial infarction
    Clinical features that make bypass surgery unacceptable

Contraindications

    Left main coronary artery disease
    Coronary artery spasm

Preprocedural Care

1. Initiate preprocedural instruction for patient and family.
2. Ensure that written informed consent for PTCA or interventional revascularization is obtained. Operating room and cardiothoracic team must be on standby throughout procedure for emergency CABG; may be indicated for angioplasty procedures involving large proximal lesion.
3. Obtain baseline data for PTCA and CABG: complete blood count; coagulation studies; electrolyte, BUN, and creatinine levels; blood type and cross-match; ECG; chest x-ray; vital signs.
4. Perform skin preparation of both right and left groin areas.
5. Permit nothing by mouth (NPO) for at least 8 hours before procedure.
6. Establish a patent intravenous line.
7. Administer medications as ordered.
8. Administer preoperative sedatives as ordered.

•••••• Multidisciplinary Plan

Medications

Before procedure
    Antiplatelet agents: aspirin, 325 mg bid; dipyridamole 75 mg tid 48 h before procedure to decrease risk of platelet adhesion, which is thought to be cause of early restenosis after procedure[87]

Diphenhydramine to reduce risk of allergic reaction

Nitrates, calcium channel blockers to reduce risk of coronary artery spasm

Beta-blockers are held

During procedure

Heparin infusion, 10,000 U by continuous drip

Intracoronary nitroglycerin (100-300 mg), sublingual nifedipine (10 mg), or both to prevent coronary artery spasm as catheter is introduced

Thrombolytic agents as necessary (p. 116)

After procedure

Immediate

Heparin infusion (800-1200 U/h); tapered doses for 12-24 h to prevent coronary thrombosis from possible intimal tear

Long-term

Aspirin po for 6 mo; dosage will vary; 60 mg/d (baby aspirin); 325 mg po qid or bid

Nitrates and calcium channel blockers resumed while patient is in hospital and continued for 3-6 mo; dosage varies

Dipyridamole 75 mg po tid for 3 mo, low-dose Coumadin, or both

General Management

Cardiac monitoring—ECG pattern observed for rate, dysrhythmias, signs of ischemia

Intraarterial blood pressure—observed during and after procedure

Intraaortic balloon pump—must be available on standby during procedure

Bed rest for first 6 hours after successful angioplasty, after removal of arterial and venous sheath and until hemostasis has been reestablished

Laboratory studies: careful monitoring of partial thromboplastin time (PTT) and hemoglobin (Hgb), creatinine phosphokinase (CPK), potassium, and sodium levels

Diet—as ordered; force fluids for 24 h

Intake and output—record 4 to 8 h

NURSING CARE

Nursing Assessment

Complications Related to Procedure

Failure to dilate artery

Development of acute thrombosis or occlusion

Myocardial infarction

Coronary artery rupture/dissection

Clinical symptoms

Chest pain, ST depression or elevation, drop in blood pressure, tachycardia, dysrhythmias

Renal hypersensitivity to contrast material, decreased urine output, increased circulating blood volume, increased jugular venous pressure (JVP), dyspnea, crackles

Hemorrhage Related to Prolonged PTT; Drop in Hgb

Cannulated Extremity

Complications at insertion site

Bleeding, hematoma

Ecchymosis, swelling

Ischemia

Diminished or absent pulses, numbness, pallor, pain

Arterial thrombosis formation

Diminished or absent pulses, numbness, pain, swelling, pale skin

Nursing Dx & Intervention

Anxiety (preoperative) related to perceived and actual threat to biologic integrity

- Assess level of anxiety and understanding associated with procedure *to determine source of fears and any misconceptions.*
- Provide explanations and description of procedure, including sensations to be experienced.
- Provide an opportunity for questions.
- Assist the patient to explore fears and discuss feelings.
- Provide the patient with an opportunity to meet the catheterization staff and visit the laboratory and postangioplasty unit.

Decreased cardiac output (high risk for) related to myocardial ischemia or electrical instability (dysrhythmias)

- Assess for signs of diminished cardiac output.
- Monitor blood pressure, heart rate, and respirations every 15 minutes immediately after the procedure, decreasing frequency as clinical status stabilizes.
- Monitor vital signs every 4 hours for 24 hours.
- Monitor ECG, observing for signs of ischemia or dysrhythmias.
- Obtain 12-lead ECG without any episode of chest pain.
- Monitor urine output hourly or for every voiding if the patient is not catheterized.
- Report outputs of less than 30 ml per hour or inability to void within first 4 hours.
- Check peripheral perfusion: pulses, skin temperature, color.
- Auscultate heart sounds, noting diminished or extra sounds *to detect presence of LV failure.*
- Auscultate lung sounds for presence of adventitious sounds or diminished aeration.
- Administer medications as ordered: IV nitroglycerin *to decrease incidence of coronary spasm* and antiplatelet agents *to reduce risk of restenosis.*

Altered peripheral tissue perfusion (high risk for) related to thrombus formation

- Inspect cannulated extremity for ecchymosis, swelling, pain, and warmth *reflective of hematoma formation or bleeding.*

- Assess pulses distal to the site every 15 minutes for 1 hour, noting any decrease in amplitude.
- Decrease frequency as ordered.
- Note skin color and temperature.
- Maintain bed rest in flat position until arterial sheaths are removed.
- Instruct the patient to keep the catheterized extremity immobile and extended *to decrease risk of bleeding.*
- After the catheter sheaths are removed, maintain pressure dressing with 5- to 10-pound sandbags over site.
- Monitor coagulation studies, reporting prolonged partial thromboplastin time or abnormal results to the physician.
- Administer antiplatelet agents as ordered *to reduce risk of restenosis.*

Patient Education/Home Care Planning

Preoperative
1. Explain to the patient and family the purpose and indications for PTCA, its benefits, and associated risks.
2. Describe the procedure, explaining its similarity to cardiac catheterization; it may last 2 to 5 hours. Review sensations to be experienced, such as pressure during insertion of catheter, but explain that there is no discomfort with actual balloon inflation.
3. Explain and review postprocedure routines: that 24-hour monitoring in the coronary care unit is needed, that the affected leg must be kept immobile immediately after the procedure, that patient will remain on bed rest for up to 8 hours, and that discharge home is usually within 24 to 48 hours.
4. Explain the need for consent for CABG surgery. Provide a brief review of differences in patient care after open-heart surgery.

After procedure
1. Reinforce explanation of procedure and postprocedure results.
2. Describe activity allowances and limitations. Explain that, unless contraindicated by postprocedure status, the patient may resume work within a week after discharge.
3. Discuss the importance of avoiding nicotine, which is associated with an increased incidence of restenosis after PTCA.
4. Discuss the need to modify or continue to modify coronary risk factors.
5. Discuss the importance of continued follow-up. Explain that a postexercise ECG treadmill test will be required at 2 weeks and again at 3 months after PTCA.
6. Review medications, discussing dosage, method of administration, and side effects.
7. Discuss the need to modify or continue to modify coronary risk factors.

Evaluation

Anxiety level is reduced Patient appears relaxed. Patient verbalizes less fearfully and asks appropriate questions. Misconceptions are corrected.

Cardiac output is maintained Patient remains normotensive. Skin is warm and dry. Patient verbalizes having no chest pain or discomfort. Vital signs remain stable.

Tissue perfusion is maintained Pulses distal to cannulation site are palpable. Extremities are warm and dry. Coagulation studies are within normal limits.

THROMBOLYTIC THERAPY FOR ACUTE MYOCARDIAL INFARCTION

(Fibrolytic therapy, acute myocardial infarction therapy)

Description and Rationale

It has long been recognized that long-term survival after myocardial infarction depends on maintaining ventricular function. However, only in the past decade have investigators actively sought interventions to retard myocardial necrosis. Thrombolytic therapy has emerged as a successful modality in the treatment of acute myocardial infarction (AMI); its use is based on studies that examined the role of coronary thrombosis as the precipitating factor of myocardial infarctions and on studies that demonstrated how clot lysis and reperfusion of an infarct-related vessel can reduce infarct size and preserve myocardial function.[35] In the acute stage of myocardial infarction (first 6 hours); abrupt coronary occlusion in the setting of an already narrowed coronary artery is caused by intracoronary thrombosis.[35] Total coronary occlusion from intraluminal thrombosis occurs in 80% to 90% of patients with transmural infarctions, and subtotal occlusion occurs in 15% to 20% of patients.[35,41]

Intracoronary infusion of thrombolytic agents, first reported by Rentrop,[73] achieves clot lysis, restores coronary blood flow, and limits myocardial ischemia. However, the extent to which thrombolytic therapy salvages myocardial function is time dependent. Kennedy and co-workers[49] found that the time from onset of clinical symptoms to initiation of intracoronary thrombolysis was the strongest predictor of achieving coronary reperfusion. It is now generally accepted that thrombolytic therapy initiated within the first 4 to 6 hours for patients with an evolving AMI can reduce in-hospital and 1-year mortality rates.

Because early intervention is critical in achieving clot lysis, intravenous administration of thrombolytic agents is more practical unless there is immediate access to an interventional laboratory.[36] Its effectiveness is similar to that of intracoronary administration; each has certain advantages and disadvantages (Table 1-7).

Intracoronary thrombolysis is performed in the cardiac catheterization laboratory with selective angiography, whereas intravenous thrombolysis may be initiated in either the emer-

TABLE 1-7   **Comparison of Intracoronary and Intravenous (Systemic) Thrombolytic Therapy of Acute Myocardial Infarction**

Comparative Features	Intracoronary	Intravenous
Widespread availability	No	Yes
Delay in institution	1-2 h frequent	None
Complexity	Yes	No
Risks of coronary catheterization	Yes	No
Risk of arterial puncture site complications	Yes	No
Risk of systemic bleeding complications	Probably less	Probably more
Cost	High	Low
Success in achieving prompt coronary thrombolysis*	75%-80%	50%-60% (75% with t-PA)
Risk of rethrombosis*	20%	20%
Time required for thrombolysis*	25-35 min	50-60 min
Doses of thrombolytic agent used*	Generally less; therefore early surgery possible	Larger—early surgery risks bleeding complications
Coronary anatomy	Known (initial and residual)	Not known or deferred to later study
Coronary angioplasty	May be first approach or may follow thrombolytic therapy	Not available
Documentation of success or failure	Yes	Not always possible

From Tilkian.[87]
*Applies to conventional agents (streptokinase, urokinase, activase).

gency department or the coronary care unit. In intravenous thrombolytic therapy, administration is via a peripheral vein.

Thrombolytic agents Thrombogenesis, the result of a complex interplay of coagulation factors, begins with platelet aggregation and adhesion. Prothrombin is then converted to thrombin, which contributes to the conversion of fibrinogen to fibrin. Fibrin stabilizes platelet aggregation, forming a hemostatic plug. The development of fibrin-specific thrombolytic agents has been the key to the dissolution of coronary thrombi. Lysis of thrombi results from two actions: invasion of the injury site by leukocytes and activation of the fibrinolytic system. Normally the fibrinolytic system, which involves plasminogen activators, converts plasminogen, a circulating proenzyme, to plasmin. Plasmin, the proteolytic enzyme responsible for clot lysis, degrades fibrin into soluble fragments that are removed in the microcirculation. This system is inadequate to dissolve the fibrin mass of a large thrombus. However, the introduction of exogenous plasminogen activators produces more plasmin, which depletes circulating fibrinogen and generates high titers of fibrinogen degradation products (FDPs), which promote lysis. Exogenous plasminogen activators also destroy coagulation factors V and VIII, causing a systemic lytic state that increases the risk of bleeding.[88a,99]

Streptokinase. Streptokinase (SK, Streptase, Kabikinase), a synthetic protein, is derived from group C-hemolytic streptococci. It forms an activator complex with plasminogen to activate the fibrinolytic process.[88a] In addition, SK depletes fibrinogen levels and other coagulation factors such as V and VIII, predisposing the patient to bleeding. Furthermore, because SK is a bacterial protein with antigenicity, it can lead to a variety of allergic reactions.

Urokinase. Urokinase (Abbokinase), a naturally occurring human proteolytic enzyme, is produced by the parenchy-

mal cells of the kidney. It acts directly on circulating plasminogen to produce the fibrinolytic enzyme plasmin.

Tissue plasminogen activator (Activase) Tissue plasminogen activator (t-PA) is a naturally occurring human enzyme present in endothelium, circulating blood, and human tissue. Unlike SK and urokinase, which activate plasminogen systemically, t-PA is fibrin specific, activating plasminogen only after binding to the plasminogen bound to fibrin contained in the thrombus.[16] Thus t-PA is a clot-specific agent; because it produces relatively little circulating plasmin, it does not deplete other clotting factors, and therefore it reduces the risk of bleeding. Activase has emerged as the thrombolytic agent of choice.[88a]

Indications

Recent (within 30 minutes but not to exceed 4 to 6 hours) onset of chest pain unresponsive to conventional sublingual nitroglycerin therapy

ECG changes documenting acute myocardial injury: ST elevation greater than 0.1 mm with reciprocal changes

Less than 75 years of age

Contraindications
Absolute

Active internal bleeding

History of cerebrovascular event

Previous treatment with SK 6 months to 1 year (does not apply to t-PA)

Intracranial neoplasm, aneurysm

Major Relative

Major surgery (within 10 days)

Recent GI or GU bleeding

Serious trauma

Traumatic CPR

Uncontrolled hypertension (>180 mm Hg systolic or >110 mm Hg diastolic)

Minor Relative

Left-sided heart thrombus

Bacterial endocarditis

Existing bleeding diathesis

Pregnancy

Advanced age (≥75 years)

Diabetic hemorrhagic retinopathy

Cautions

Current anticoagulant therapy

Acute pericarditis

Renal or liver disease

Preprocedural Nursing Care

Initiate preprocedural explanation of procedure to patient and family

Instruct patient and family about purpose and indications for thrombolytic therapy, its benefits, and associated risks

Describe intracoronary procedure, that it is similar to cardiac catheterization and that the procedure may last from 1 to 2 hours; review sensations to be experienced, such as pressure during insertion of catheter but no discomfort with infusion

Explain and review procedures and routines associated with procedure: monitoring in CCU, heart rhythm problems, and bleeding; explain need for bed rest during and after administration and for frequent blood sampling to monitor clotting times

Instruct patient to inform nurse if chest pain develops

Consents are required to perform cardiac catheterization, angioplasty, and CABG surgery

Obtain baseline laboratory data to determine hemostatic status and degree of myocardial injury: CBC with platelets, PT, fibrinogen and fibrin split-product levels, CPK-MB, blood type and cross-match, BUN, creatinine

Obtain diagnostic data such as 12-lead ECG, chest x-ray; obtain vital signs and perform clinical assessment

Administer medication as ordered; give IV lidocaine prophylactically

Prepare for cardiac catheterization if indicated

Establish at least two or three patent IV lines

•••••• Multidisciplinary Plan

Medications

Streptokinase*

Intracoronary—25,000-50,000 U bolus followed by continuous infusion of 2000-4000 U/min for 60 min (total dose 150,000-500,000 U); procedure is carried out in conjunction with angiography; infusions are continued for 30-60 min after antegrade flow has been established

IV—10,000-20,000 U bolus followed by continuous infusion of 10,000-20,000 U administered over 30-60 min (total dose 750,000-1.5 million IU); infusion may be initiated in emergency room or coronary care unit

Precede with diphenhydramine (Benadryl), 50 mg IV, to reduce allergic reaction (does not prevent anaphylactoid reaction)

Half-life: α and β half-life during which serum levels can be detected is 18 min and enzymatic action persists 18 to 80 min; enzymatic action on coagulation system persists up to 24 h

Side effects: Hypotension, which has been reported to occur in 15% of patients, may occur during rapid bolus infusion, allergic reactions, which are reported to occur in 5% of patients, include fever, flushing, rash, periorbital swelling, and bronchospasms; anaphylaxis is rare

Urokinase*

Intracoronary—10,000-30,000 U by bolus followed by continuous infusion of 2000-24,000 U/min; infusion procedure must be performed in conjunction with coronary angiography

IV—10,000-20,000 U by bolus followed by continuous infusion of 10,000-20,000 U/min up to total of 2 or 3 million U

Half-life: 10-20 min; prolonged action on coagulation persists up to 24 h

Side effects: None specified; may be administered rapidly either by bolus or infusion without side effects

Tissue plasminogen activator

Usage dosage: Intravenous

Standard dose—100 mg (concentration 1.0 mg/ml for patients <65 kg; patients >65 kg: 1.25 mg/kg over 3 hours)

Lytic dose, first hour—60% of total dose, 10 mg of which (10%) is administered as an IV bolus

Maintenance dose, second hour—20% of total dose; third hour, 20% of total dose

Half-life: 5 to 7 min

Side effects: bleeding

Heparin

During streptokinase or urokinase infusion, 5000-10,000 U IV bolus followed by continuous infusion to maintain PTT, 1½ to 2 times control value; used to reduce risk of reocclusion immediately and after initial perfusion

After procedure, 600-700 U continuous IV after PTT levels have reached two times control value

General Management

Intraarterial blood pressure—observe for changes in blood pressure during and after infusion; used for drawing of blood sample

---

*Drug dosages are not standardized; bolus and maintenace dosages may have a wide range.

Cardiac monitoring—ECG pattern observed for signs of reperfusion: resolution of preprocedure ECG changes; dysrhythmias

Hemodynamic monitoring—pulmonary artery and pulmonary capillary wedge pressures as indicated

PTCA—may be performed immediately after reperfusion or delayed 1 to 2 days

Coronary arteriograms—postprocedure arteriograms performed before discharge or as indicated by clinical signs

Bed rest—12 hours after intracoronary infusion; intravenous requires no bed rest restrictions

Diet—as ordered

Laboratory studies—careful monitoring during and after thrombolysis: serum fibrinogen levels (will be less 50 mg/dl after infusion of thrombolytic agent, returning to baseline within 24 hours of completion of thrombolytic infusion); partial thromboplastin time (PTT); hemoglobin; creatinine phosphokinase (CPK)

NURSING CARE

Nursing Assessment

Myocardial Ischemia

Preprocedure: 30 minutes of pain; chest discomfort of less than 4 to 6 hours' duration from onset of symptoms; ST elevation of 0.1 mm on ECG; hypotension; dysrhythmias

Reperfusion

Develops within 30 to 60 minutes of administration of thrombolytic therapy; abrupt cessation of chest discomfort; rapid fall in ST elevation; appearance of reperfusion dysrhythmias (may not be accurate indicator of reperfusion): sinus bradycardia and atrioventricular block with hypotension; accelerated idioventricular rhythm; ventricular ectopy; early peaking of CPK-MB levels within 12 hours after onset of symptoms

Bleeding and Hemorrhage

Surface bleeding: intermittent oozing from peripheral venous, arterial punctures

Related to intravascular fibrinogenolysis, which induces lytic state that is associated with bleeding,[99] bleeding at puncture sites; gastrointestinal or intracranial hemorrhage and hemopericardium

Recurrent Ischemia or Infarction

Related to reocclusion, which has been reported to occur in 20% to 40% of patients following successful recanalization[36,41]

Chest pain

ECG: ST-T wave changes

Dysrhythmias

Skin cool, clammy, diaphoretic

Hypotension, tachycardia

Nursing Dx & Intervention

Fluid volume deficit, high risk for related to bleeding or hemorrhage secondary to thrombolysis-induced coagulopathy

- Assess for signs of bleeding: swelling, pain, or discoloration at puncture sites; petechiae; hematoma; flank pain indicating retroperitoneal bleeding; signs of internal bleeding or hemorrhage: tachycardia, tachypnea, hypotension, coolness of skin, pallor, thirst, restlessness, hematuria, occult blood in emesis or stool.
- Monitor blood pressure, heart rate, and respiratory rate every 15 minutes during first hour, decreasing frequency as condition stabilizes.
- Inspect puncture sites every 15 minutes.
- Apply manual pressure when removing catheters and after venipunctures *to control superficial bleeding.*
- Monitor coagulation values until hemostasis has been reestablished.
- Avoid any interruption of vascular integrity after fibrinolytic therapy.
- Avoid use of venous or arterial punctures.
- Use heparin lock for blood sampling and IV access.

Decreased cardiac output (high risk for) related to reperfusion dysrhythmias

- Assess and record changes in ECG tracing during and after thrombolytic therapy *to determine any changes in baseline cardiac rate or appearance of reperfusion dysrhythmias.*
- Monitor vital signs frequently according to protocol and the patient's condition.
- Administer antidysrhythmic medications as ordered.
- Notify the physician promptly of any signs of decreased cardiac output as evidenced by changes in heart rate, blood pressure, and mental status.
- Initiate prompt treatment for life-threatening dysrhythmias per protocol: CPR, drug therapy, and preparation for pacemaker insertion.

Pain: chest (high risk for or actual), related to decreased myocardial oxygen supply; secondary to reocclusion of coronary artery

- Assess and record level of comfort, including patient's verbal and nonverbal expressions.
- Compare with preprocedural chest pain complaints.
- Record any activity that preceded onset of pain to determine etiology.
- Maintain bed rest *to reduce myocardial oxygen demand.*
- Obtain 12-lead ECG *to document recurrent ischemia.*
- Administer drug therapy as ordered to relieve pain; assess and record response.

- Prepare for possible cardiac catheterization, repeat thrombolysis, percutaneous coronary angioplasty (PTCA) or coronary artery bypass graft (CABG).

Altered cerebral, renal, or gastrointestinal tissue perfusion related to thrombolytic drug-induced coagulopathy

- Assess for changes in neurologic status, complaints of headache, or evidence of gastrointestinal bleeding such as occult blood in emesis or stool or hematuria for up to 24 hours after thrombolytic infusion.
- Report any abrupt change from baseline *to determine need for change in or discontinuation of thrombolytic or anticoagulation therapy.*

Patient Education/Home Care Planning

Preoperative

1. Explain to the patient and family about purpose and indications for thrombolytic therapy, its benefits, and associated risks.
2. Describe the procedure: intracoronary—that it is similar to cardiac catheterization and may last 2 to 5 hours. Review sensations to be experienced, such as pressure during insertion of the catheter, but explain that there is no discomfort with infusion.
3. Explain and review procedures and routines associated with the procedure: monitoring in the coronary care unit for heart rhythm problems and bleeding, need for bed rest during and after administration of thrombolytic therapy, and need for frequent blood sampling to monitor clotting times.
4. Inform the patient to notify a nurse if chest pain develops.

After procedure

1. Review the explanation of the procedure and postprocedure results.
2. Discuss with the patient the need to report any signs of bleeding: bruising, bleeding gums, hematuria, or tarry stools.
3. Instruct the patient to report pain relief or new onset of pain.
4. Discuss activity allowances and limitations.
5. Discuss the need to modify or continue to modify coronary risk factors.
6. Discuss the importance of continued follow-up. Explain that coronary angiography may be necessary to evaluate the patency of coronary arteries.
7. Review medications, discussing dosage, method of administration, and side effects.

Evaluation

There is no evidence of bleeding Hemostasis is reestablished. Coagulation studies are within acceptable limits. There are no overt or covert signs of bleeding: no hematomas or petechiae. Vital signs are within normal limits. Patient is alert and oriented.

Cardiac output (CO) is maintained ECG remains stable; dysrhythmias are absent. Vital signs are stable.

Comfort level is achieved Patient verbalizes absence of chest discomfort or pain. Patient is able to resume previous activity level without complaints of pain.

References

1. American Heart Association: Recommendation for prophylaxis of infective endocarditis, *Circulation* 56:139A, 1985.
2. American Heart Association: Standards and guidelines for cardiopulmonary resuscitation and emergency cardiac care, *JAMA* 225:2841, 1986.
3. American Heart Association: *Heart and stroke facts—1995,* Dallas, 1995, National Center.
4. Andreoli K et al: *Comprehensive cardiac care,* ed 2, St Louis, 1987, Mosby.
5. Ball M, Mann J: Lipids and heart disease: a guide for the primary care team, ed 2, Oxford, 1994, Oxford University Press.
6. Belloni FL: The local control of coronary blood flow, *Cardiovasc Res* 13:63, 1979.
7. Blake S: The clinical diagnosis of constrictive pericarditis, *Am Heart J* 106:432, 1983.
8. Braunwald E, editor: *Heart disease: a textbook of cardiovascular medicine,* ed 4, Philadelphia, 1992, Saunders.
9. Brown KK: Surgical therapy of chronic heart failure and severe ventricular function, *Crit Care Nurs Q* 18:45, 1995.
10. Brown WJ: A classification of microorganisms frequently causing sepsis, *Heart Lung* 5:397, 1976.
11. Calafiore AM et al: Coronary revascularization—the radial artery: new interest for an old condition, *J Cardiovasc Surg* 10:140, 1995.
12. Califf RM, Bengtson GR: Cardiogenic shock, *New Engl J Med* 330(24):1724, 1994.
13. Canobbio M: *Cardiovascular disorders,* St Louis, 1990, Mosby.
14. Canobbio M: Eisenmenger syndrome, *Nurs Clin North Am* 19:573, 1984.
15. Cohn LH: Aortic valve prostheses, *Cardiol Rev* 2:219, 1994.
16. Collen D et al: Coronary thrombolysis with recombinant human tissue-type plasminogen activator: a prospective randomized, placebo controlled trial, *Circulation* 70:1012, 1984.
17. Conover MB: *Cardiac arrhythmias: exercises in pattern interpretation,* ed 2, St Louis, 1978, Mosby.
18. Conover MB: *Exercises in diagnosing ECG tracings,* ed 3, St Louis, 1984, Mosby.
19. Conover MB: *Understanding electrocardiology: physiological and interpretative concepts,* ed 3, St Louis, 1980, Mosby.
20. Dajani AS et al: Prevention of endocarditis: recommendations by the American Heart Association, *JAMA* 264:299, 1990.
21. Dalen JE, Alpert JS: Natural history of pulmonary embolism, *Prog Cardiovasc Dis* 17:259, 1975.
22. D'Alonzo GE et al: Survival in patients with primary pulmonary hypertension, *Ann Int Med* 115:343, 1991.
23. De Campli WM et al: Characteristics of patients surviving more than 10 years after cardiac transplantation, *J Thorac Cardiovasc Surg* 109:1103, 1995.
24. Deshpande S et al: Catheter ablation in supraventricular tachyarrhythmias, *J Interven Cardiol* 8:59, 1993.
25. Dole WP, O'Rourke RA: Pathophysiology and management of cardiogenic shock, *Curr Probl Cardiol* 8:1, 1983.
26. Douglas PS, editor: *Cardiovascular Health and diseases in women,* Philadelphia, 1993, Saunders.
27. Doyle B: Nursing challenge: the patients with end-stage renal failure. In Kerr LS, editor: *Cardiac critical care,* Rockville, Md, 1988, Aspen.
28. Doyle JE: Treatment modalities in peripheral vascular disease, *Nurs Clin North Am* 58:139, 1983.
29. Earp JK: The gastroepiploic arteries as alternative coronary artery bypass conduits, *Crit Care Nurs* 14(1):24, 1994.

30. English MA: Dynamic cardiomyoplasty, *Crit Care Nurs Q* 18:56, 1995.
31. Essop R: Transesophageal echocardiography in infective endocarditis: the standard for the 1990's? *Am Heart J* 120:402, 1995.
32. Evans RW: Socioeconomic aspects of heart transplantation, *Curr Opin Cardiol* 10:169, 1995.
33. Fuster V et al: Primary pulmonary hypertension: natural history and importance of thrombosis, *Circulation* 70(4):580, 1984.
34. Gallego-Alvarezz M, Obrien M: Right gastroepiploic artery conduit use in myocardial revascularization, *AORN* 60:763, 1994.
35. GISSI trial: Effectiveness of intravenous thrombolytic treatment in acute myocardial infarction, *Lancet* 1:397, 1986.
36. Gist HC, Messobian HD, Ziskind AA: New interventional techniques for coronary revascularization, *Heart Dis Stroke* 2:198, 1993.
37. Goldberger E: *Textbook of clinical cardiology,* St Louis, 1982, Mosby.
38. Groer MW, Shekleton ME: *Basic pathophysiology: a conceptual approach,* St Louis, 1983, Mosby.
39. Guyton AC: *Textbook of medical physiology,* ed 8, Philadelphia, 1980, Saunders.
40. Guzzetta CE, Dossey BM: *Cardiovascular nursing: bodymind tapestry,* St Louis, 1984, Mosby.
41. Habib GB: Current status of thrombolysis in acute myocardial infarction, part II. Optimal utilization of thrombolysis in clinical subsets, *Chest* 107:528, 1995.
42. Harris L et al: The cardiovascular effects of caffeine on postmyocardial infarction, *Circulation* 72(suppl III):116, 1985.
43. Hirman JA: Nursing assessment/nursing diagnosis in patients with peripheral vascular disease, *Nurs Clin North Am* 21:219, 1986.
44. Joint National Committee: The 1984 report of the national committee on detection, evaluation, and treatment of high blood pressure, *Arch Intern Med* 144:1045, 1984.
45. Joint National Committee: The fifth report of the Joint National Committee on detection, evaluation and treatment of high blood pressure, *Arch Intern Med* 153:154, 1993.
46. Kannel WB, McGee D, Gordon T: A general cardiovascular risk profile: the Framingham study, *Am J Cardiol* 38:46, 1976.
47. Kaushik RR: Surgery for cardiac arrhythmia, *J Interven Cardiol* 8:83, 1995.
48. Kaye D, editor: *Infective endocarditis,* ed 2, New York, 1992, Raven Press.
49. Kennedy JW et al: Acute myocardial infarction treated with intracoronary streptokinase: a report of the society for cardiac angiography, *Am J Cardiol* 55:871, 1985.
50. Kent KM: Transluminal coronary angioplasty. In Rackey CE, editor: Advances in critical care cardiology, *Cardiovasc Clin* 16:53, 1986.
51. Kinney MR et al, editors: *AACN's clinical reference for critical care nurses,* New York, 1981, McGraw-Hill.
52. Kirchhoff KT: An examination of the physiologic basis for "coronary precautions," *Heart Lung* 15:874, 1981.
53. Kistner RL et al: Incidence of pulmonary embolism and thrombophlebitis of lower extremities, *Am J Surg* 124:169, 1972.
54. Kloner RA, Braunwald E: Effects of calcium antagonist on infarcting myocardium, *Am J Cardiol* 30:59(3):84B, 1987.
55. Kobashigawa JA et al: Effect of pravastatin on outcomes after cardiac transplantation, *N Engl J Med* 333(10):621, 1995.
56. Konstam MA, Dracup K: *Heart failure: evaluation and care of patients with left ventricular systolic dysfunction, clinical practice guidelines,* 1994, US Dept Health and Human Services Pub. No. 94-061.
57. Lai WT, Huycke EC, Sung RJ: Supraventricular tachyarrhythmias: mechanism, types, and management, *Postgrad Med J* 83:209, 1988.
58. LeFrock JL et al: Transient bacteremia associated with nasotracheal suctioning, *JAMA* 236:1610, 1977.
59. Lough ME: Quality of life issues following heart transplantation, *Prog Cardiovasc Nurs* 1:17, 1986.
60. Manapat AE et al: Gastroepiploic and inferior epigastic arteries for coronary artery bypass. Early results and evolving applications, *Circulation* 90(II):144, 1994.
61. Maron BJ et al: Management of hypertrophic cardiomyopathy, *Heart Dis Stroke* 2:203, 1993.
62. Moroney DA, Reedy JE: Understanding ventricular assist devices: a self-study guide, *J Cardiovasc Nurs* 8:1, 1994.
63. Mueller HS: Role of intra-aortic counterpulsation in cardiogenic shock and acute myocardial infarction, *Cardiology* 84:168, 1994.
64. Muirhead J: Heart and heart-lung transplantation, *Crit Care Nurs Clin North Am* 4(1):97, 1992.
65. Nagelhout J: Pharmacologic treatment of heart failure, *Nurs Clin North Am* 26:401, 1991.
66. Noel DK et al: Challenging concerns for patients with automatic implantable cardioverter defibrillators, *Focus Crit Care* 13:50, 1986.
67. Otten MW: The effect of known risk factors on excess mortality of black adults in US, *JAMA* 263:845, 1990.
68. Parsonnet V, Furman S, Symth N: A revised code for pacemaker identification: pacemaker study group, *Circulation* 64:60A, 1981.
69. Perez MM, Pintos Diaz G: Arteriosclerosis obliterans of the lower limbs, *Cardiovasc Rev* 4:1357, 1983.
70. Perloff JK: *Clinical recognition of congenital heart disease,* Philadelphia, 1994, Saunders.
71. Perry AG, Potter PA: *Shock: comprehensive nursing management,* St Louis, 1983, Mosby.
72. Rao AK, TIMI Investigators: Thrombolysis in myocardial infarction trial (phase I): effect of intravenous tissue plasminogen activator and streptokinase on plasma fibrinogen and the fibrinolytic system, *Circulation* 72(III):416, 1985.
73. Rentrop KP et al: Effects of intracoronary streptokinase and intracoronary nitroglycerin infusion on coronary angiographic patterns and mortality in patients with acute myocardial infarction, *N Engl J Med* 311:1457, 1984.
74. Rubin LT et al: Treatment of primary pulmonary hypertension with continuous intravenous prostacyclin, *Ann Intern Med* 112:485, 1990.
75. Schneider JR: Effects of caffeine ingestion on heart rate, blood pressure, myocardial oxygen consumption, and cardiac rhythm in acute myocardial infarction patients, *Heart Lung* 16:167, 1987.
76. Shellock FG, Riedinger MS: Reproducibility and accuracy of using room temperature vs. ice temperature for thermodilution cardiac output determination, *Heart Lung* 12:175, 1983.
77. Shinn AE, Joseph D: Concepts of intra-aortic balloon counterpulsation, *J Cardiovasc Nurs* 8:45, 1994.
78. Silva J: Anaerobic infections, *Heart Lung* 5:406, 1976.
79. Skidmore-Roth L: *Mosby's 1996 drug reference,* St Louis, 1996, Mosby.
80. Sklarin NT, Dutcher JP, Wiernik PH: Lymphomas following cardiac transplantation, *Am J Hematol* 37(2):105, 1991.
81. Spittell JA, editor: *Contemporary issues in peripheral vascular disease,* Philadelphia, 1992, Davis.
82. Steinberg JS et al: Radiofrequency catheter ablation of atrial flutter: procedural success and long term outcome, *Am Heart J* 130:85, 1995.
83. Swearingen PL, Sommers MS, Miller K: *Manual of critical care: applying nursing diagnoses to adult critical illness,* St Louis, 1988, Mosby.
84. Tavilian G et al: Complete arterial myocardial revascularization using right gastroepiploic artery and both internal thoracic arteries as pedicled grafts, *J Cardiovasc Surg* 36(3):257, 1995.
85. Thelan L, Urden L, Davie J: *Textbook of critical care: diagnosis and management,* St Louis, 1990, Mosby.
86. Thibodeau GA, Patton KT: *Anatomy and physiology,* ed 3, St Louis, 1996, Mosby.
87. Tilkian AG, Daily EK: *Cardiovascular procedures: diagnostic techniques and therapeutic procedures,* St Louis, 1986, Mosby.
88. TIMI Study Groups: The thrombolysis in myocardial infarction (TIMI) trial: phase I findings, *N Engl J Med* 312:932, 1985.
88a. Topol EJ, editor: *Textbook of interventional cardiology,* ed 2, Philadelphia, 1994, WB Saunders.
89. Tucker SM et al: *Patient care standards: nursing process, diagnosis, and outcome,* ed 6, St Louis, 1996, Mosby.
90. Uber LA, Umber WF: Hypertensive crisis in 1990's, *Crit Care Nurs Q* 16:27, 1993.
91. Urban N: Integrating hemodynamic parameters with clinical decision making, *Crit Care Nurse* 6:48, 1986.

92. Vaska PL: Common infections in heart transplant patients, *Am J Crit Care* 2:145, 1993.
93. Wang WWT: Hypertension update: highlights from 1993 National Report, *Prog Cardiovasc Nurs* 8:13, 1993.
94. Wilkerson JT, Cohn JN, editors: *Cardiovascular medicine,* New York, 1995, Churchill Livingston.
95. Willerson JT, editor: *Treatment of heart diseases,* New York, 1992, Gower.
96. Winslow EH: Cardiovascular consequences of bed rest, *Heart Lung* 14:236, 1985.
97. Wirsing P, Andriopoulous A, Botticher R: Arterial embolectomies in the upper extremity after acute occlusion, *J Cardiovasc Surg* 24:40, 1983.
98. Wit AL, Rosen MR: Pathophysiologic mechanisms of cardiac arrhythmias, *Am Heart J* 106:798, 1983.
99. Wood S et al: *Cardiac nursing,* ed 3, Philadelphia, 1995, Lippincott.

Respiratory System

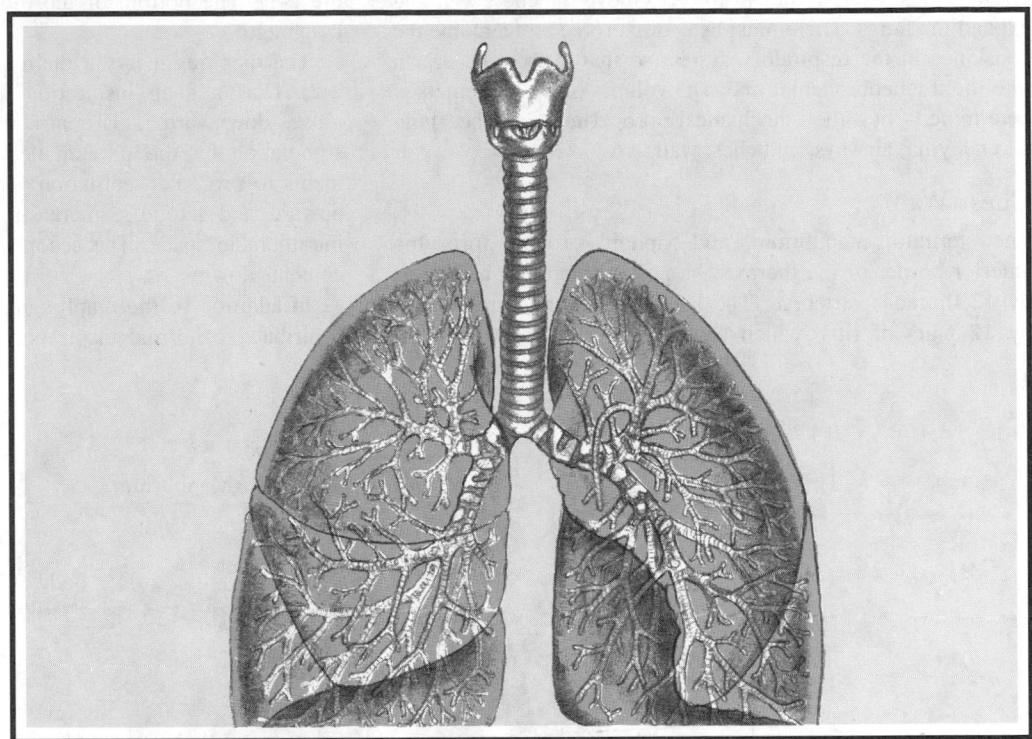

2

OVERVIEW

The major functions of the pulmonary system are ventilation, gas exchange, and lung defense. Ventilation is a major component of the gas exchange function, but is also a measure of the mechanical function of the lung. Gas exchange is the transfer of oxygen and carbon dioxide between the external environment and the blood. Oxygen is then transported throughout the body for use at the cellular level, where it combines with adenosine diphosphate (ADP) and simple sugar (CHO) to produce energy in the form of adenosine triphosphate (ATP). Carbon dioxide and water are metabolic by-products of energy consumption. This cellular use of oxygen and production of carbon dioxide is termed cellular respiration. The third function, lung defense, prevents the entry of noxious substances and microorganisms into the lung and subsequently into the body.

Smoking is the single most common cause of respiratory problems in the adult. It is the major cause of chronic bronchitis, emphysema, and lung cancer in the United States. Environmental factors have become more important over the last several decades as by-products of industrialization and urbanization have polluted the air. Small particles of inhaled air pollutants may cause disease. Major air pollutants include sulfur dioxide and sulfur trioxide, nitrogen dioxide, carbon monoxide, chlorine, ammonia, hydrocarbons, silica, cobalt, asbestos, and coal dust. These chemicals also cause smog and haze, which affect crop growth. Other factors influencing the incidence of respiratory problems include genetic predispositions (asthma, cystic fibrosis) and acute infectious disease.[34]

The following sections discuss the physiologic factors contributing to the major functions of the pulmonary system: ventilation, diffusion, perfusion, lung defense, and control of ventilation. Abnormalities of these factors is discussed in relation to specific disease states.

••••••• Anatomy, Physiology, and Related Pathophysiology

The anatomy of the respiratory system is discussed from a functional perspective within each of the following levels:

1. Ventilation—the movement of air from outside to inside the body and its distribution within the tracheobronchial system to the gas exchange units of the lungs.
2. Diffusion—the movement of oxygen and carbon dioxide across the alveolar-capillary membrane to the blood in the pulmonary capillaries.
3. Perfusion—the movement of blood through the pulmonary and arterial circulation, the distribution and exchange of oxygen and carbon dioxide.
4. Defense mechanism—the regulation of the internal environment involving mechanical barriers, cough, and immune function.
5. Control of breathing—the regulation of ventilation to maintain adequate gas exchange, usually in accord with changing metabolic demands or other special needs.

Ventilation is the process that moves air from outside the body to the gas exchange units of the lungs. The muscles of respiration must exert sufficient force to move the chest wall and expand the lungs. There must be enough force to overcome the resistance in the respiratory system so that air will be drawn into the tracheobronchial tree. The volume of air that enters is determined by the mechanical properties of the lung parenchyma, airways, and chest wall.

Chest Wall

The sternum, manubrium, and xiphoid process form the anterior border of the thorax. The posterior portion is formed by 12 thoracic vertebrae. The lateral boundaries are formed by 12 pairs of ribs, which have a posterior connection di-

rectly to the thoracic vertebrae. The first seven ribs also connect anteriorly to the sternum by the costal cartilages (Figure 2-1). The bottom of the thoracic cage is formed by the diaphragm.

The diaphragm is the main muscle of inspiration (Figure 2-2). During deep inspiration the diaphragm contracts and moves downward. This contraction, which occurs because of stimulation by the phrenic nerve, forces two major movements to promote ventilation. The first raises the lower ribs upward and laterally, increasing the transverse and lateral intrathoracic space. The second action forces the abdominal contents downward.

In addition to the diaphragm, the chest wall muscles that contribute to normal inspiration are the external intercostals

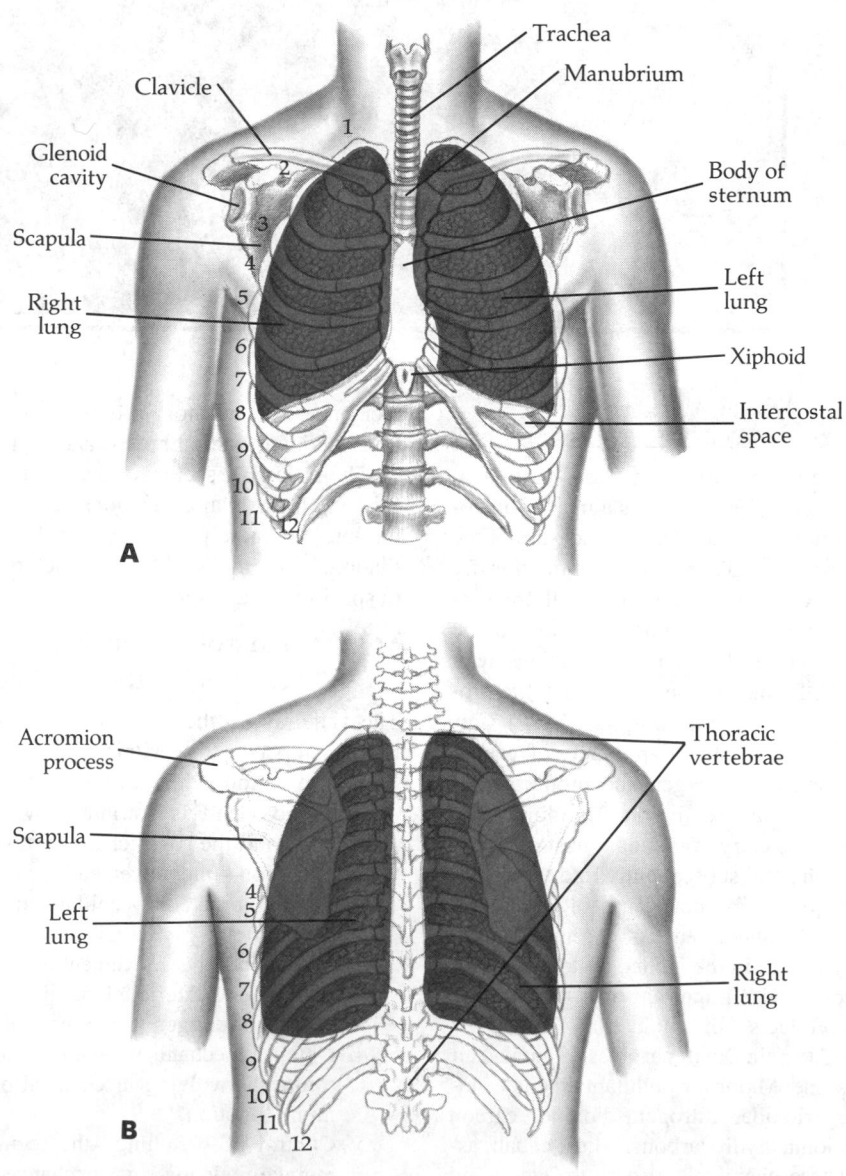

Figure 2-1 Structures of chest wall. **A,** Anterior view. **B,** Posterior view.

and parasternal muscles. With increased inspiratory effort, the accessory muscles raise the first two ribs, stabilize the chest wall, and raise the sternum.

Normal relaxed expiration requires no muscle force. Forced expiration is assisted by contraction of abdominal muscles and internal intercostals.

Thoracic cavity The main structures of the thoracic cavity include the pleura, pleural space, mediastinum, and lungs. Figure 2-3 details this anatomy.

The pleura is a two-layered protective membrane. The first layer is the parietal pleura, which lines the thoracic cavity. The second is the visceral or pulmonary pleura, which covers each lung. Although each is given a separate name, the pleurae are continuous with one another and form one closed sac. Between the two pleurae is a potential space, the pleural space, which contains a serous lubricant film that allows one pleural surface to slip over the other and thus helps the lungs move. The intrapleural space also maintains a subatmospheric pressure.

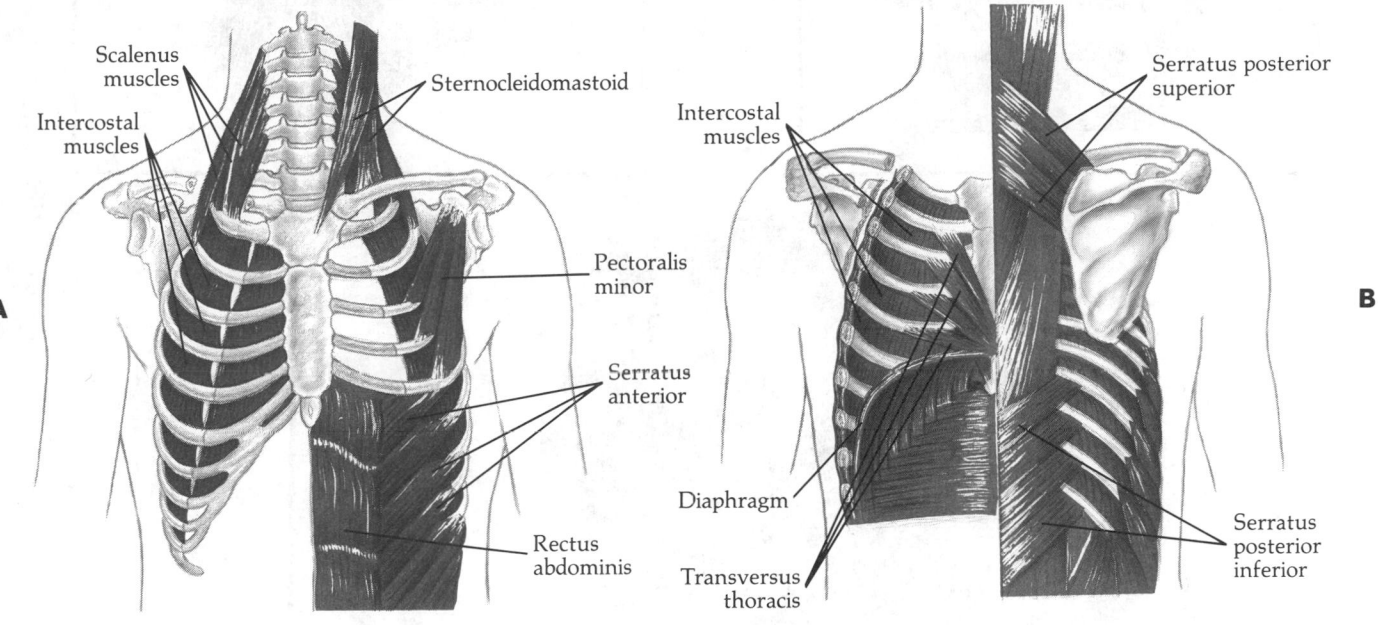

Figure 2-2 Muscles of ventilation. **A,** Anterior view. **B,** Posterior view.

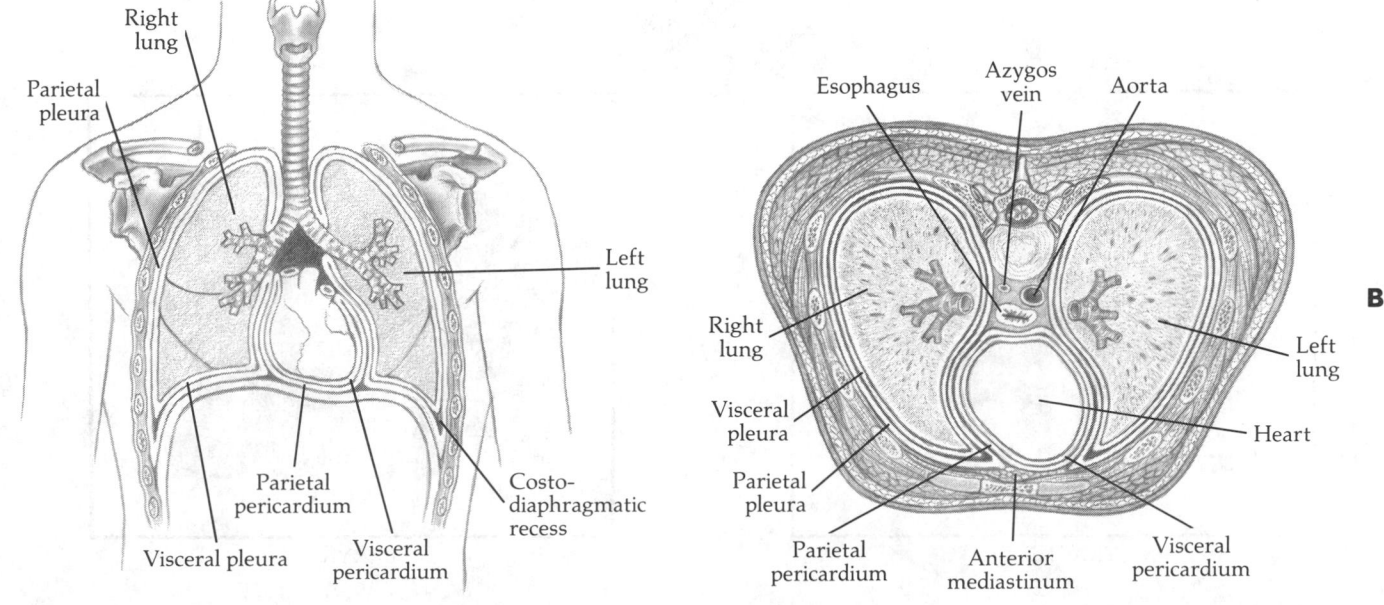

Figure 2-3 Chest cavity-related structures. **A,** Anterior view. **B,** Cross section.

NASAL WALL

PHARYNX

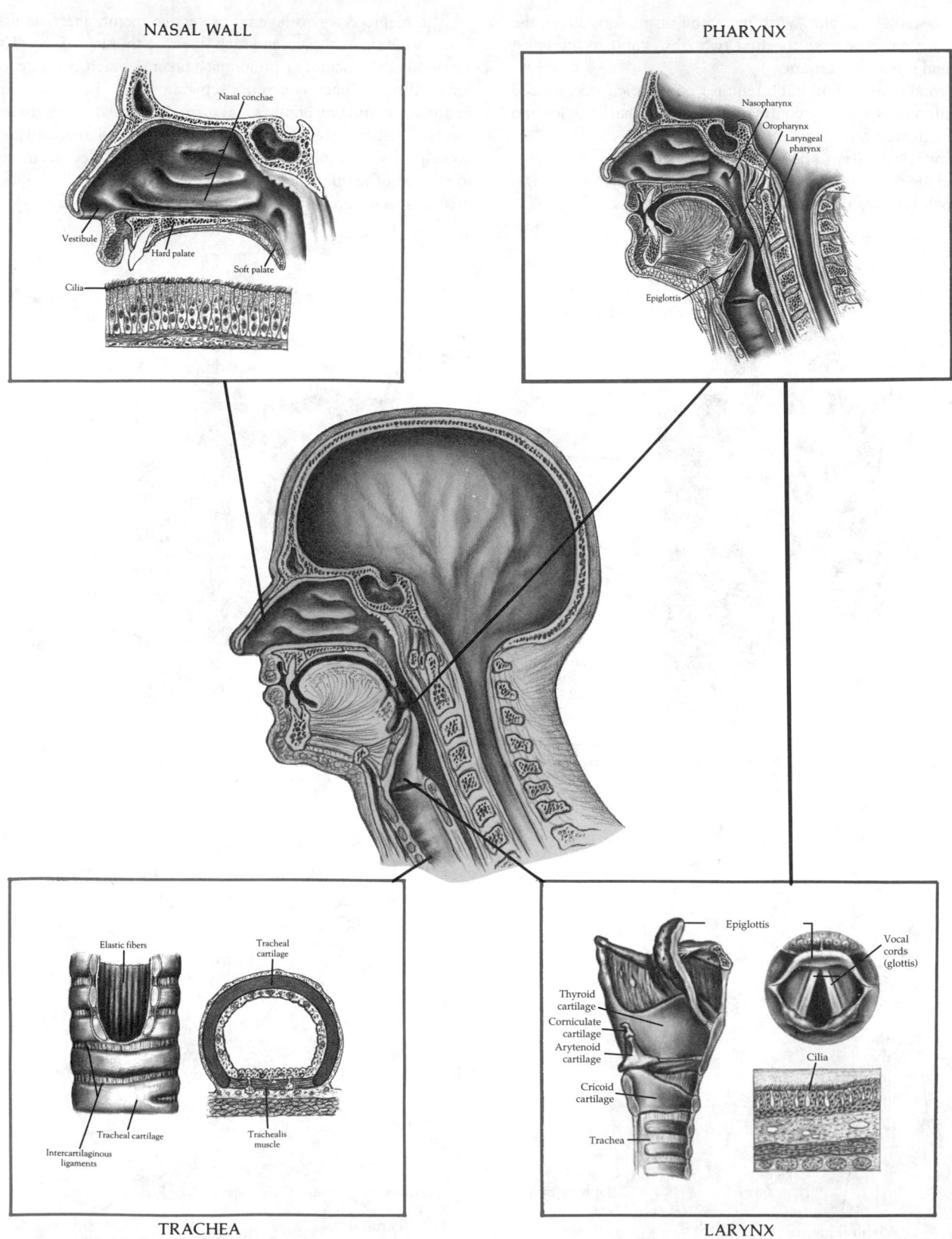

TRACHEA

LARYNX

Figure 2-4 Structures of upper airway.

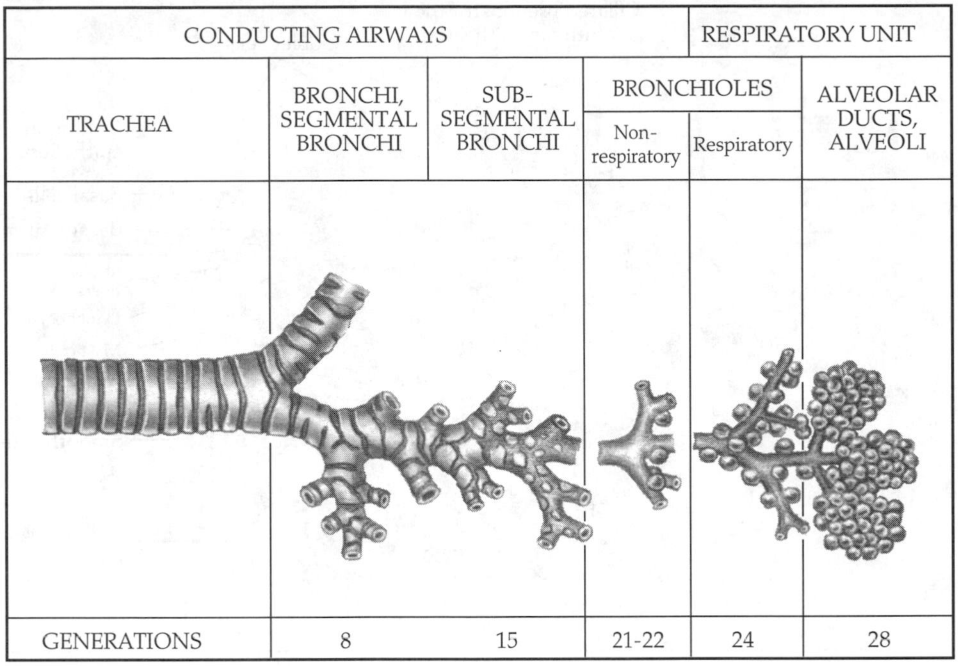

CONDUCTING AIRWAYS					RESPIRATORY UNIT
TRACHEA	BRONCHI, SEGMENTAL BRONCHI	SUB-SEGMENTAL BRONCHI	BRONCHIOLES		ALVEOLAR DUCTS, ALVEOLI
			Non-respiratory	Respiratory	
GENERATIONS	8	15	21-22	24	28

Figure 2-5 Structures of lower airway.

The mediastinum is the region between the right and left parietal pleurae. It is bordered by the sternum on the front and the thoracic vertebrae on the back. The heart, contained in its own pericardial sac, is in the middle of the mediastinum. Also in the mediastinum are the great vessels that enter and leave the heart, the bifurcation of the trachea, the mainstem bronchi, most of the esophagus, the thymus gland, lymph nodes, and various nerves including the phrenic nerve, cardiac and splanchnic branches of the sympathetic system, and recurrent laryngeal and vagus branches of the parasympathetic system.

The hilum is the area where the visceral and parietal pleurae form a sheath around the bronchi. Blood vessels and nerves connect with the lungs through this sheath.

The right lung has three lobes, which are further subdivided into 10 bronchopulmonary segments, and accounts for 55% of total ventilation. The left lung has two lobes and eight bronchopulmonary segments, and accounts for 45% of all ventilation.

Upper airway The upper airway, consisting of the nose, pharynx, larynx, and extrathoracic trachea (Figure 2-4), has three major functions:

1. To conduct air to the lower airway
2. To protect the lower airway from foreign matter
3. To warm, filter, and humidify inspired air

The nose warms, moistens, and filters inspired air. Temperature adjustment and proper humidification begin as soon as air hits the anterior nasal cavity. The structure of the nose, with its two nasal cavities, turbinates, and rich vasculature, provides maximum contact between inspired air and the nasal mucosa. By the time inspired air reaches the bronchi, it is 100% water vapor saturated and has reached body temperature.

Another function of the nose is to clear debris from the inspired air. The nasal cilia, hair, and moisture cluster small airborne particles. Sneezing is a means of clearing the upper airway. When a mechanical or chemical irritation occurs, sensory receptors in the nasal mucosa send impulses to the brain via the trigeminal and olfactory nerves, thus causing a sneeze.

Air passes from the nasal cavity into the three divisions of the pharynx: the nasopharynx, oropharynx, and laryngeal pharynx. The pharynx, covered with ciliated epithelium, continues the process of filtering and humidifying inspired air.

The larynx contains the vocal cords for phonation, prevents aspiration of food into the trachea, and is innervated with irritant receptors. The larynx extends up to the level of the sixth cervical vertebra (C6) and is covered with the same pseudostratified, ciliated, columnar epithelium found in the nose and the pharynx.

The main cartilages of the larynx are the thyroid, cricoid, and arytenoid. Attached to the anterior surface of the thyroid cartilage is the epiglottis. The cricoid cartilage, beneath the thyroid cartilage, forms the narrowest part of the airway for infants and children. The larynx is innervated by two separate branches of the vagus nerve. The recurrent laryngeal nerve innervates the larynx, and the superior laryngeal nerve provides some motor and all sensory innervation. The sensory fibers are responsible for initiating the cough reflex.

Lower airway The lower airway is made up of the trachea, mainstem bronchi, lobar bronchi, segmental bronchi, subsegmental bronchi, terminal bronchioles, and gas exchange units (Figure 2-5).

A range of 23 to 26 levels of branches is found between the trachea and the terminal respiratory units. Down to the level of

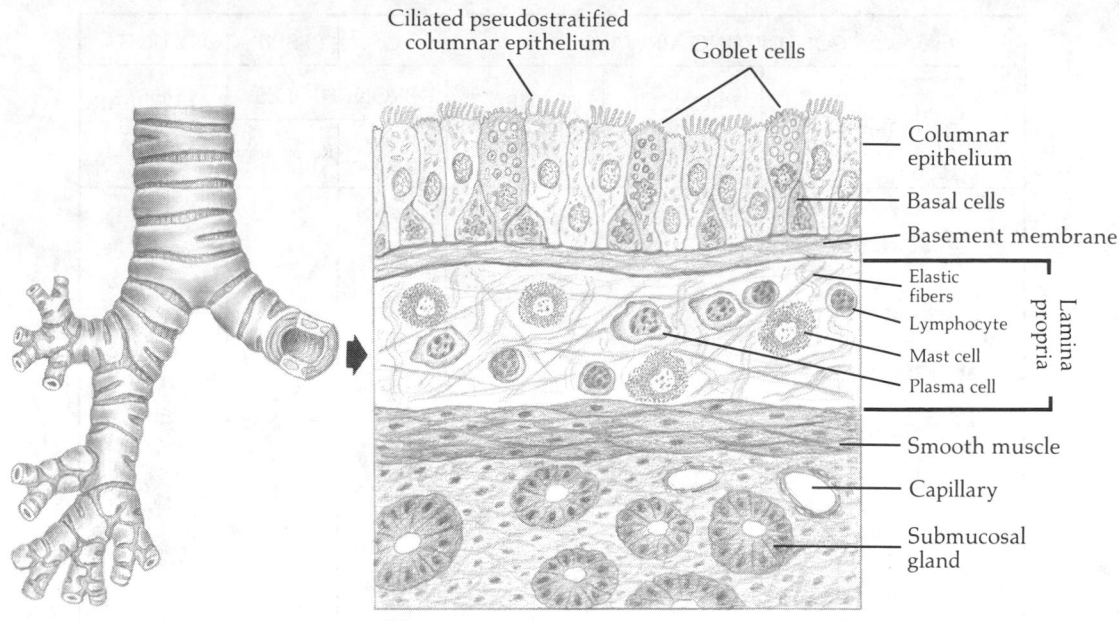

Figure 2-6 Structures of the ventilatory mucosa.

terminal bronchioles, air passages are conducting airways only. At the level of respiratory bronchioles, gas exchange begins.

The trachea, which is 4 to 5 cm wide, and 11 to 12 cm long, is supported by C-shaped rings of cartilage. It extends from the larynx and cricoid cartilage to the division of the right and left mainstem bronchi at the level of the fifth thoracic vertebra (T5) in the chest. The lining of the trachea consists of a pseudostratified, ciliated columnar epithelium mixed with mucus-producing goblet cells (Figure 2-6).

The right and left mainstem bronchi conduct air between the trachea and the lobar bronchi. The right mainstem bronchus, which is about 5 cm shorter than the left bronchus, is fairly vertical. Its position makes it more likely that aspirated material will be drawn into the right lung. The right bronchus then divides into three branches, each of which supplies one of the three lobes of the right lung. The left mainstem bronchus lies more horizontal and divides into two branches, which supply the two lobes of the left lung.

All of the bronchi contain cartilaginous plates and mucous glands. The amount of cartilage decreases toward the periphery. The epithelium is ciliated.

The small airways or bronchioles do not contain cartilage or mucous glands. Cilia and goblet cells are still present. The bronchioles have a complete concentric ring of smooth muscle with two sets of smooth muscle fibers. When the muscle rings constrict, as in asthma, the airways narrow.

The lower part of the bronchioles consists of units, called the *terminal bronchi,* that conduct air from the subsegmental bronchi to the alveolar ducts. The most distal section of the lower respiratory tract consists of the terminal respiratory units (acini), which include the respiratory bronchioles, the alveolar ducts, the alveolar sacs, and the terminal air sacs, called the alveoli. An acinus is the site of gas exchange. Figure 2-7 shows

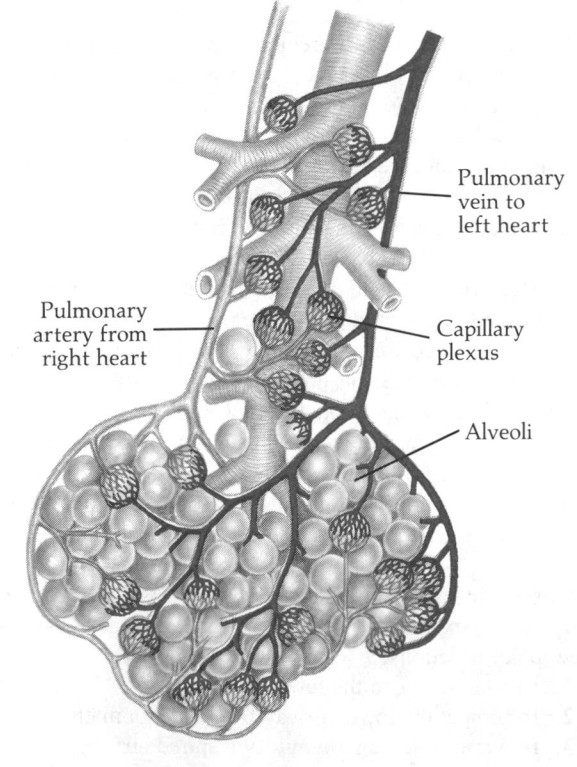

Figure 2-7 Terminal respiratory units.

the cluster arrangement of these units. Note the intertwinement of alveoli and capillary plexus.

The membrane surface of the terminal respiratory units is a flattened, one-cell-thick epithelial surface, the type I cell. The type II cell of the alveolar epithelium secretes the lipoprotein

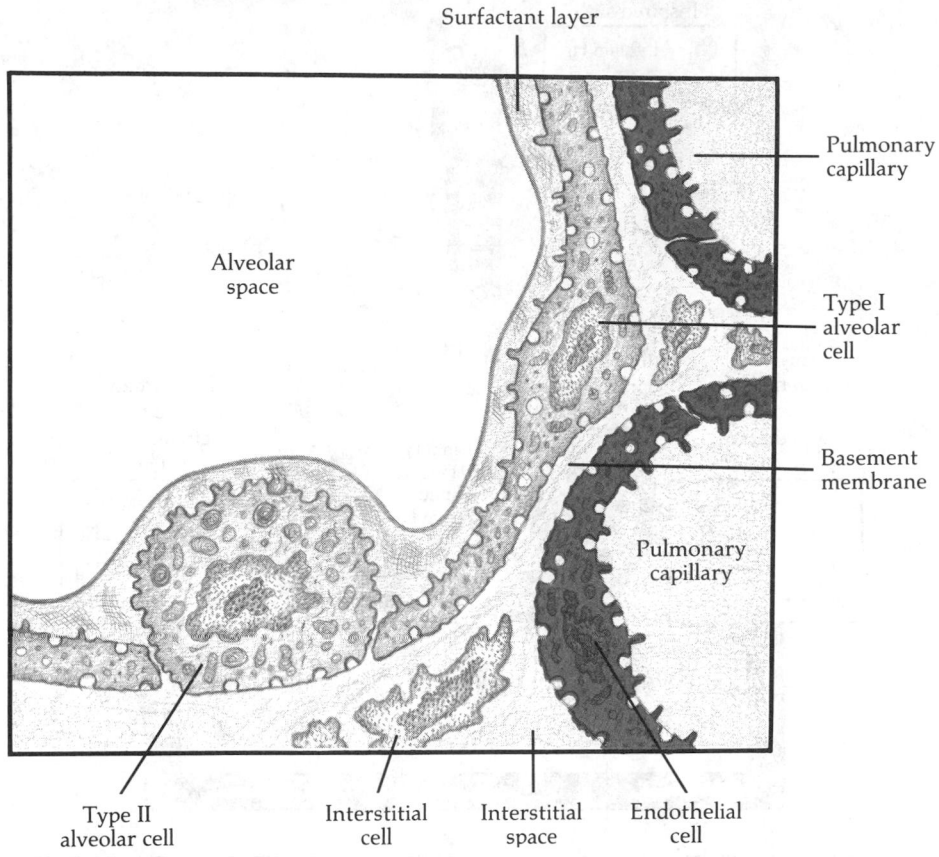

Surfactant layer

Alveolar
space

Pulmonary
capillary

Type I
alveolar
cell

Basement
membrane

Pulmonary
capillary

Type II
alveolar cell

Interstitial
cell

Interstitial
space

Endothelial
cell

Figure 2-8 Alveolar wall and space.

substance called surfactant. Surfactant forms a thin layer between the surface of the alveoli and the air; it decreases the surface tension of the air-liquid interface in the alveoli. Without adequate surfactant, as occurs in hyaline membrane disease or respiratory distress syndrome, it is difficult for the alveoli to inflate with inspiration because of the high pressure gradients needed to overcome the high surface tension.

The alveolar-capillary membrane, shown in Figure 2-8, forms the division between the alveolar space and the pulmonary capillary.

Process of ventilation The term *pulmonary mechanics* refers to the forces and resistances to moving air in and out of the lung. Decreases in the forces or increases in the resistances will impair ventilation.

The forces. The ventilatory forces for inspiration are the inspiratory muscles, the diaphragm, and the chest wall muscle groups. When the inspiratory muscles contract, the thorax is enlarged, and intrapleural and alveolar pressures fall. A pressure gradient between the atmosphere and the alveoli is thus created, and air is "pulled into" the lungs. The force for expiration during normal relaxed breathing is the elastic recoil of the lung. Once the expanding forces are withdrawn, the lung becomes smaller. When a forced expiration (cough for example) or more rapid expiration is required, the abdominal muscles contract,

pushing the abdominal contents against the diaphragm and increasing expiratory force.

The resistances. The basic resistances to ventilation are airways resistance (the caliber of the airway lumen) and the elastic properties of the lung. The airway caliber has a major impact on the rate of air movement into and out of the lung. The airway caliber normally changes with breathing: The airway is larger during inspiration and smaller during expiration. Similarly, the deeper the breath, the larger the airway caliber. Abnormal conditions that affect caliber are excessive mucus, bronchospasm, and edema.

The elastic properties of the lung have a major impact on the volume of lung expansion. The elastic properties are measured and expressed in several ways. One is the *elastic recoil* of the lung. The higher the recoil pressure, that is, the greater the pressure that must be used to inflate the lung, the stiffer the lung. Note that the recoil pressure varies with lung volume. As an analogy, for a single balloon, the larger the volume of the balloon, the greater its tendency to recoil. Another important factor affecting recoil and ability to inflate the lung is surface tension. At a fluid/air interface, surface tension makes it difficult to inflate small "bubbles." In the lung, the inner surface of alveoli is lined with a lipoprotein material called surfactant. This material reduces surface tension, making it easier to

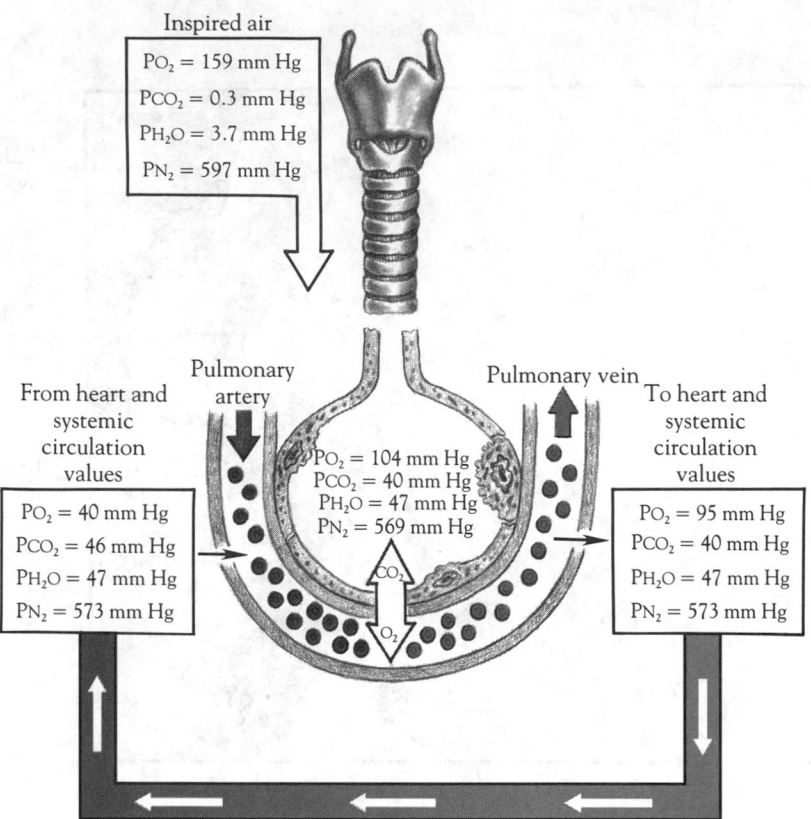

Inspired air

PO_2 = 159 mm Hg
PCO_2 = 0.3 mm Hg
PH_2O = 3.7 mm Hg
PN_2 = 597 mm Hg

Pulmonary artery

Pulmonary vein

From heart and systemic circulation values

PO_2 = 40 mm Hg
PCO_2 = 46 mm Hg
PH_2O = 47 mm Hg
PN_2 = 573 mm Hg

PO_2 = 104 mm Hg
PCO_2 = 40 mm Hg
PH_2O = 47 mm Hg
PN_2 = 569 mm Hg

CO_2

O_2

To heart and systemic circulation values

PO_2 = 95 mm Hg
PCO_2 = 40 mm Hg
PH_2O = 47 mm Hg
PN_2 = 573 mm Hg

Figure 2-9 Partial pressure of respiratory gases in normal respiration.

inflate alveoli. When surfactant is absent or decreased in amount, the lung is much more difficult to inflate and lung recoil increases. *Compliance* is another measure of the elastic properties of the lung. Compliance measures the amount of volume change accomplished per unit of pleural pressure change and is thus a measure of distensibility. When lung recoil is increased, the lung is stiffer and more difficult to inflate, and lung compliance is usually reduced (less volume change per unit of pleural pressure change). Conversely, decreased recoil means that the lung is easier to inflate and compliance is usually increased.

Although the elastic properties of the lung receive the most attention, it must be remembered that the chest wall also exhibits elastic properties. The stiffness of the chest wall will also affect the volume of air drawn into the lung with inspiration.

Diffusion

Once the air reaches the surface of the alveoli, the oxygen must cross the alveolar-capillary membrane and enter the pulmonary capillary system. Likewise the carbon dioxide in the unoxygenated venous blood must cross the alveolar-capillary membrane to be exhaled from the lungs. Diffusion of the gases, oxygen and carbon dioxide, is a constant process, with both gases moving across the membrane simultaneously.

The process of diffusion depends on the thickness of the respiratory membrane, the surface area of the membrane, the diffusion coefficients of the gases, and the partial pressure differences of the gases being diffused.

Any changes in the alveolar membrane or the interstitial spaces between the alveoli and the capillary can affect the rate of gas diffusion. The rate of diffusion is inversely proportional to the thickness of the membrane.

The total alveolar surface for a normal adult is approximately 80 square meters (M^2). Pulmonary capillaries contact 85% to 90% of this surface. Therefore the total surface for gas diffusion is about 70 M^2. Any alteration such as the removal of a lung or emphysema decreases the total surface area available for gas exchange. The pressures that gases exert against a surface are proportional to their concentrations. Carbon dioxide diffuses much more readily than oxygen. Even so, in the normal healthy individual, complete equilibration of the oxygen between the alveolus and capillary occurs in one third of the time available.

The process of gas exchange between the air in the alveoli and the blood in the lung capillaries occurs because of a difference in the partial pressures of the gases. Figure 2-9 shows the partial pressures. Each gas diffuses from an area of high partial pressure to an area of low partial pressure. When the concentration of oxygen is altered, as occurs during

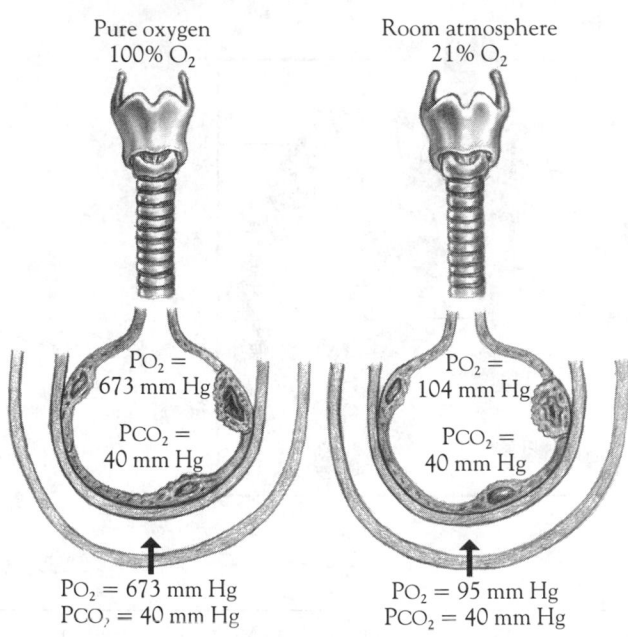

Pure oxygen
100% O_2

$PO_2 =$
673 mm Hg

$PCO_2 =$
40 mm Hg

$PO_2 = 673$ mm Hg
$PCO_2 = 40$ mm Hg

Room atmosphere
21% O_2

$PO_2 =$
104 mm Hg

$PCO_2 =$
40 mm Hg

$PO_2 = 95$ mm Hg
$PCO_2 = 40$ mm Hg

Figure 2-10 Alteration of gas diffusion by varying oxygen concentration.

oxygen therapy, the partial pressures of the gases are also altered (Figure 2-10).

Perfusion

The major purpose of the pulmonary circulation is to deliver blood in a thin film to the alveoli so that oxygen can be taken in and carbon dioxide taken out. The pulmonary vascular system is a high volume-low pressure system. This means that a large amount of blood flows through the lungs and that the capillary resistance to that blood flow is very low.

Blood from the right ventricle of the heart is pumped into the right and left pulmonary arteries, which branch into the alveolar capillaries. At the alveolar-capillary membrane, the blood picks up oxygen and loses carbon dioxide. After being oxygenated, the blood flows into the four pulmonary veins, which return it to the left atrium of the heart.

Under normal resting conditions only a portion of the pulmonary capillaries are actively perfused. As cardiac output increases, the pulmonary arterial pressure remains fairly constant because of two mechanisms:

1. Recruitment of previously unperfused capillaries, which decreases pulmonary vascular resistance and thus permits increased blood flow through the vessels.
2. Capillary dilation, which directly increases the capillary size and decreases the resistance to flow.

Both of these mechanisms can adjust to an increase in cardiac output. A malfunction of these mechanisms could lead to pulmonary hypertension. The pulmonary artery catheter is commonly used to measure the pulmonary arterial pressure in critically ill persons. Pulmonary artery pressures may also be measured during cardiac catheterization.

Common Alterations in Ventilation/Perfusion Matching

Ventilation and perfusion are normally well matched, with an average ventilation perfusion ratio (V/Q) of 0.8 overall. The normal ratio is not a perfect 1.0 match because relatively more blood flows to dependent lung areas. Disease states that alter normal V/Q also alter gas exchange.

1. Alveolar dead space, or high V/Q, occurs when ventilation is normal but the perfusion of a variable number of alveoli is reduced or absent. Either there is not enough blood, or the blood is blocked from reaching the alveoli. Among the many causes of this are gravitational shifts in pulmonary blood flow in a normal subject, impaired blood flow in an ill patient, and pulmonary emboli.
2. Physiologic shunting, also known as low V/Q, occurs when the pulmonary circulation is adequate but the ventilation is inadequate for normal diffusion. Thus part of the blood passing from the right heart to the left heart through the pulmonary system does not become oxygenated.

A normal anatomic shunt is the 2% to 5% of the cardiac output that normally bypasses the pulmonary arterial system. This blood is part of the bronchial, pleural, and coronary circulations. Additional areas of shunt are seen in disease states when alveoli are unventilated or underventilated. Matching of ventilation and perfusion is easily measured by radioisotopes (Figure 2-11).

The arterial blood gases (Table 2-1) indicate the effectiveness of the ventilation, diffusion, and perfusion processes. Blood gases, especially the PaO_2, are influenced by elevation in comparison to sea level. The higher the elevation, the lower the PaO_2. The normal PaO_2 also decreases with age. For example, at an elevation of 3000 ft, a normal PaO_2 would be about 75 mm Hg for a 40-year-old man, but only about 65-70 mm Hg for an 80-year-old man.

Gas Transport

After the diffusion of the gases at the alveolar level, they must be transported to the tissues for use. The following includes the analysis of oxygen and carbon dioxide movement and a discussion of blood gases that can be used to evaluate gas exchange.

Oxygen Oxygen in the blood is carried two ways: dissolved in the liquid part of the blood plasma and in chemical combination with hemoglobin. Most oxygen is transported in the second manner.

The amount of dissolved oxygen carried in the plasma is directly proportional to the partial pressure of oxygen (Henry's law). There is 0.003 ml of oxygen dissolved in each 100 ml of blood for each 1 mm Hg partial pressure of oxygen. Thus at an ideal PaO_2 of 100 mm Hg, only 0.3 ml of oxygen would be carried per 100 ml of plasma.

Most oxygen in the body is transported to the cells in combination with hemoglobin. Oxygen combines loosely and reversibly with the heme portion of hemoglobin. When the PO_2 is low, as in the tissue capillaries, the oxygen is released from the hemoglobin. The average individual has about 15 g of

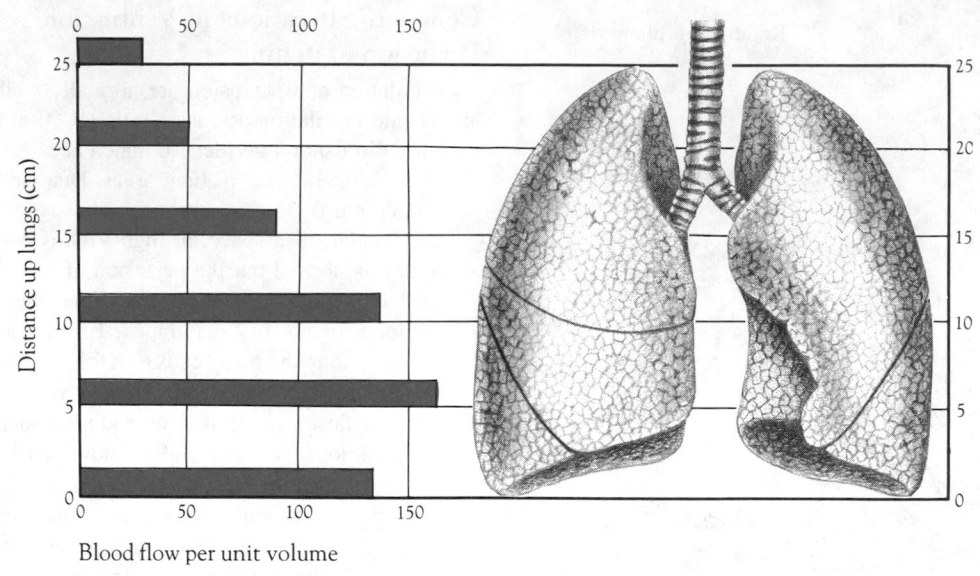

Figure 2-11 Measurements of distribution of blood flow in lungs of individual sitting in an upright position. (Modified from West.[91])

TABLE 2-1 Normal Values for Arterial Blood Gases (at sea level)

Pao$_2$	90 ± 10 mm Hg
O$_2$ saturation	96% ± 1%
Paco$_2$	40 ± 3 mm Hg
pH	7.4 ± 0.03
Bicarbonate	22-26 mEq/L

hemoglobin in each 100 ml of blood. Each gram of hemoglobin has the maximum capability to combine with 1.34 ml of oxygen. Hemoglobin $\times$ 1.34 = O$_2$ capacity. Therefore at 100% saturation, a hemoglobin level of 15 g/100 ml would result in 20.1 ml of oxygen.

Three terms must be differentiated:

1. Oxygen content is the total amount of oxygen carried in both a dissolved and combined state per 100 ml of blood.
2. Oxygen capacity is the maximum amount of oxygen that can be carried.
3. Oxyhemoglobin saturation is the relationship between the amount of oxygen that is carried on the hemoglobin and the amount of oxygen that can be carried. For example, a 90% saturation means that the hemoglobin is carrying 90% of its potential capacity.

The amount of oxygen combined with hemoglobin depends on the partial pressure of oxygen dissolved in the arterial blood (Pao$_2$). The oxyhemoglobin saturation at different partial pressures is shown in the oxyhemoglobin dissociation curve (Figure 2-12). When the blood leaves the lungs, the Pao$_2$ is about 100 mm Hg and the percent saturation is 97.5. In normal mixed venous blood, the P$\bar{v}$o$_2$ is about 40 mm Hg with a 75% saturation. Two important areas along the curve are: (1) at a Po$_2$ of 55 mm Hg the percent saturation is about 88, and (2) at a Po$_2$ of 100 mm Hg the percent saturation is 97.5. On the steep portion of the curve, large changes in saturation occur with relatively small changes in oxygen tension. On the flat portion of the curve, the changes are much smaller. For example, a change in Po$_2$ from 100 mm Hg to 55 mm Hg decreases saturation by only 10%.

Various changes in the blood can also cause changes in the oxyhemoglobin dissociation curve (see Figure 2-12). Shifts to the right are produced by a decrease in pH, a rise in Pco$_2$, and an increase in body temperature. The curve can also be shifted to the right by an increase in 2,3-diphosphoglycerate (DPG) inside the red blood cells, which occurs as a result of prolonged hypoxia. A dissociation curve shift to the right means that the hemoglobin's bond on to oxygen is weakened and that higher gas pressure is needed for binding. Oxygen escapes hemoglobin more easily and is more available to the tissues.

Shifts to the left are produced by an increase in pH, a decrease in PCO$_2$, and a decrease in body temperature. When there is a shift to the left, the affinity of hemoglobin for oxygen is increased. The hemoglobin binds the oxygen more firmly than normal, and although less pressure is needed to bind the two, it is more difficult to separate them at the cellular level. Tissues may be hypoxic because the oxygen remains bound to hemoglobin instead of being released for tissue use.

Carbon dioxide Carbon dioxide transport must be understood clearly because the amount of carbon dioxide in transit

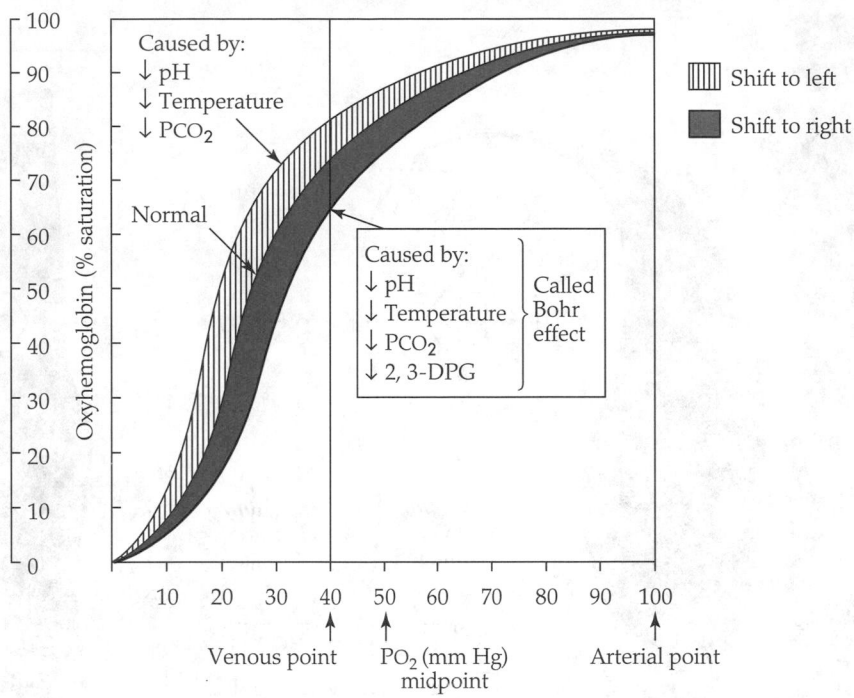

Figure 2-12 Oxyhemoglobin dissociation curve. (Modified from Guenter and Welch.[36])

helps determine the acid-base balance of the body. Carbon dioxide is carried in a variety of forms. The majority (70%) is carried as a bicarbonate (HCO_3), with a lesser amount carried in dissolved forms as carbonic acid (H_2CO_3) and as carbamino compounds. One such carbamino compound is carboxyhemoglobin. Figure 2-13 summarizes the transport of carbon dioxide in the blood.

Acid-Base Balance and Blood Gases

For body cells to function best, body fluids and blood must remain within a specific, narrow acid-base range (pH). Deviations of body pH outside this narrow range interfere with cellular metabolism and can cause cell death. Interactions of substances in the body should produce a hydrogen ion concentration sufficient to maintain a blood pH of 7.35 to 7.45. This normal acid-base balance is maintained by respiratory and kidney function. The acid-base balance is evaluated using the HCO_3/carbonic acid system. The respiratory system determines the carbon dioxide concentration, thereby regulating the hydrogen ion concentration.

$$H_2CO_3 = PCO_2 \times .03$$

The renal system uses buffering mechanisms to regulate bicarbonate concentrations. Following is the Henderson-Hasselbach equation for the calculation of blood pH:

$$pH = 6.1 + \log \frac{HCO_3}{H_2CO_3}$$

Blood pH depends on the ratio of bicarbonate to dissolved carbon dioxide. As long as that ratio is 20:1, the pH is 7.4. If the blood pH falls below that level, alkalemia occurs.

Acid-base imbalances are classified according to whether the person is acidemic or alkalemic, and by the causative mechanism, either respiratory or metabolic. An acid-base imbalance is referred to as acidosis or alkalosis. Acidosis caused by a respiratory disease is marked by an elevated arterial carbon dioxide tension. When acidosis has a metabolic cause, arterial bicarbonate concentration is lowered. Alkalosis is marked by lowered arterial carbon dioxide tension when it is the result of a respiratory disease and by an elevated arterial bicarbonate concentration when it is caused by a metabolic problem.

Disorders of the respiratory system upset the denominator of the acid/base ratio because ventilation disrupts the blood carbon dioxide concentration, and the body attempts to adjust the numerator. Metabolic disorders upset the numerator of the ratio because the bicarbonate is either raised or lowered, and compensation attempts to adjust the denominator.

Acidosis states

Respiratory acidosis ($\downarrow$ pH, $\uparrow$ Paco$_2$) Respiratory acidosis is the result of alveolar hypoventilation. This may occur in response to cardiopulmonary, neuromuscular, skeletal, or airway diseases; to acute infections; or to the actions of drugs such as narcotics or sedatives. The partial pressure of arterial carbon dioxide increases and pH drops.

The body attempts to compensate for the raised Paco$_2$ by removing excess hydrogen ions in the urine in exchange for

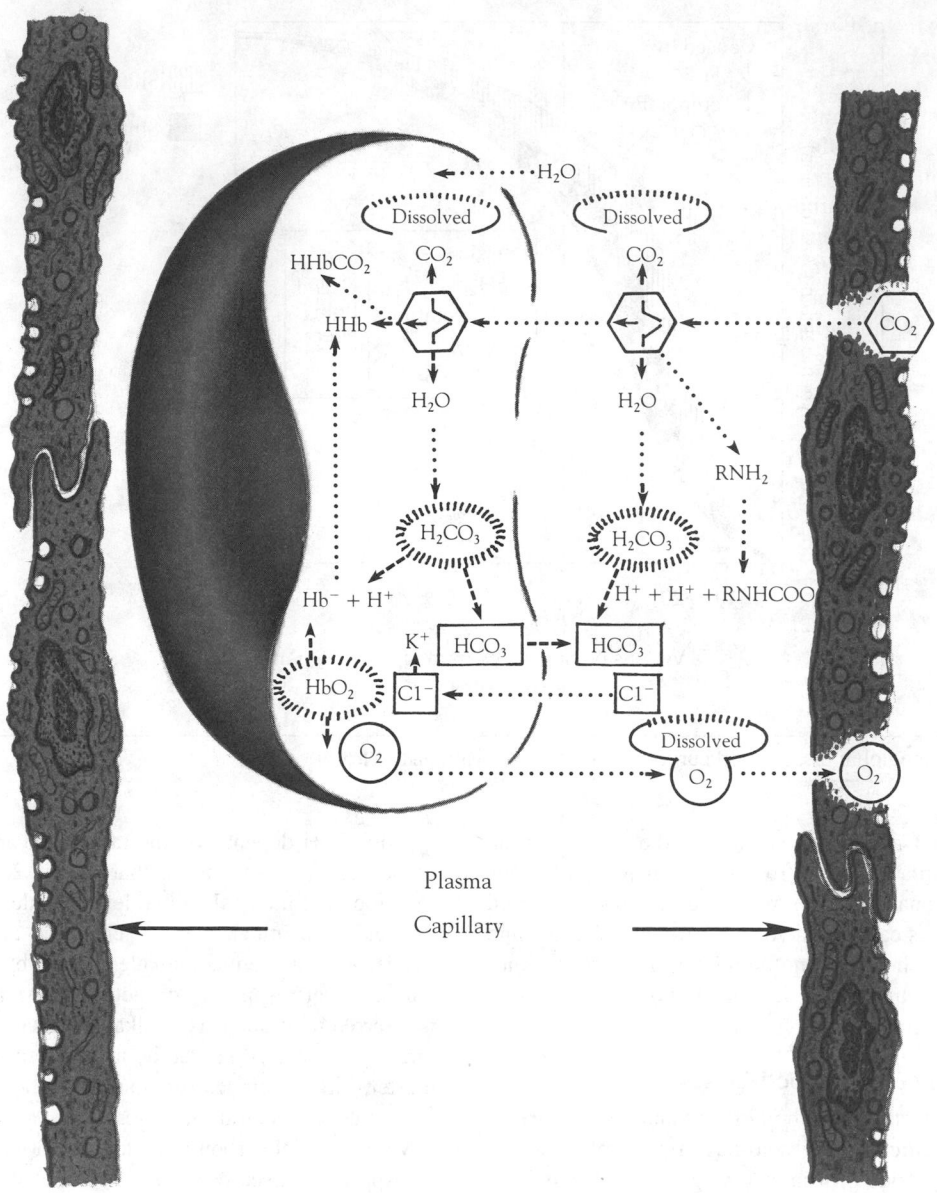

Figure 2-13 Transport of carbon dioxide and other gases in the blood.

bicarbonate ions. The bicarbonate ions are then concentrated in the blood plasma, where they help to restore the acid/base ratio and thus return the pH to normal. Through the process of compensation, the patient may have a high PaCO₂, although the pH returns to normal.

Metabolic acidosis (↓ ph, ↓ HCO₃)   Metabolic acidosis is caused in one of two ways: through the increase of fixed metabolic acids or through the loss of bicarbonate in the body fluids.

Examples of acid increase include salicylate poisoning, renal failure, diabetic ketoacidosis, and circulatory failure that produces a buildup of lactic acid. Persistent diarrhea causes bi-

carbonate loss. In such situations of acidosis, the body responds to the increase in body acids by using bicarbonate ions as sa buffer. As a result the serum bicarbonate levels are low. To compensate, the respiratory system increases ventilation immediately, and the kidneys retain bicarbonate eventually. Table 2-2 summarizes this process.

Alkalosis states

Respiratory alkalosis (↑ pH, ↓ PaCO₂).   Respiratory alkalosis occurs when excess amounts of carbon dioxide are exhaled. Alveolar hyperventilation removes carbon dioxide from the blood, decreasing the PaCO₂ and elevating the pH. Hyperventilation from anxiety is perhaps the best example. Other causes of alkalosis include brain injury or brain tumors, gram-negative sepsis, response to increased ventilatory drive, and hyperventilation with a mechanical ventilator.

The body attempts to compensate by increasing kidney excretion of bicarbonate, retaining chloride, and reducing the formation of ammonia and excretion of acid salts. These mechanisms lower the blood bicarbonate level and thus bring the acid/base ratio back into balance.

Metabolic alkalosis ($\uparrow$ ph, $\uparrow$ HCO_3^-). Metabolic alkalosis is caused by an increase in the body's level of bicarbonate. This occurs when the patient ingests too much base or receives too much bicarbonate during cardiopulmonary resuscitation. Acid loss results from vomiting or gastric suctioning. In all cases the acid/base ratio is altered, and the pH rises. Although in some cases the respiratory system compensates by slowing breathing, this compensation is unusual due to the normal effectiveness of ventilatory drive. The kidneys respond by increasing the removal of bicarbonate ions, thereby conserving hydrogen ions. As a result the pH decreases to normal levels. Table 2-3 summarizes these processes.

Arterial blood gases are usually drawn only intermittently. New arterial catheters have been developed that allow continuous monitoring of arterial blood gases using electrochemical or optical fiber technology.[18,79]

Lung defense mechanisms Lung defenses include both nonspecific and specific mechanisms of protection. Nonspecific mechanisms work to prevent entry of any foreign substance or particle. Nonspecific mechanisms of lung defense include mucociliary clearance, cough, and macrophage clearance.

Mucociliary clearance. Conducting airways are coated by a layer of mucus, which traps inhaled particles. Ciliary movement transports the particles and mucus to the pharynx, where the mucus is swallowed without conscious awareness.

Cough. Chemical or mechanical stimulation of the irritant receptors in the airway initiates a cough reflex. The high velocity created during a cough expels noxious materials and mucus.

Macrophage clearance. Macrophages are specialized leukocytes that defend against particles that reach the alveolar level. Particles are either engulfed or transported out of the area by the macrophages.

TABLE 2-2 Summary of the Acidosis Process

$$CO_2 + H_2O <=> H_2CO_3 <=> H^+ + HCO_3^-$$

	Initial Cause	Buffering	Compensation

Respiratory acidosis	$\uparrow$ P_{CO_2}	Reaction moves to right to handle excess CO_2*
		 $\uparrow$ HCO_3^-
			Lungs
			   Elimination of CO_2
			 Kidneys
			   Elimination of H^+
			   HCO_3^- conserved (the higher the P_{CO_2}, the more HCO_3^- reabsorbed)

Metabolic acidosis	$\downarrow$ Base
	 $\uparrow$ Fixed acids
		Reaction moves to the left to handle excess H^+
		 $\downarrow$ HCO_3^-
			Lungs
			   Elimination of CO_2
			 Kidneys
			   Conserve HCO_3^- (lower the HCO_3^-, the more HCO_3^- conserved)

From Harper.[39]

*Movement to the right refers to moving from the left side of the equation above to the right side, therefore decreasing CO_2 production.

TABLE 2-3 Summary of the Alkalosis Process

$$CO_2 + H_2O = H_2CO_3 = H^+ + HCO_3^-$$

	Initial Cause	Buffering	Compensation

Respiratory alkalosis	$\downarrow$ P_{CO_2}	Movement to left to form more CO_2*
		 $\downarrow$ HCO_3^-
			Kidneys
			   Conservation of H^+
			   HCO_3^- excretion (the lower the P_{CO_2}, the less HCO_3^- reabsorbed)

Metabolic alkalosis	$\uparrow$ Base
	 $\downarrow$ Fixed acids
		Movement to right to form more H^+ to offset increased base HCO_3^- $\uparrow$	Kidneys
			   Conserve H^+ by excreting HCO_3^- (the higher the plasma HCO_3^-, the greater the HCO_3^- excretion)
			 Lungs (in severe alkalosis)
			   $\downarrow$ Ventilation to $\uparrow$ P_{CO_2}

From Harper.[39]

*Movement to the left refers to moving from the right side of the equation above to the left side, therefore increasing CO_2 production.

Specific lung defense mechanisms protect against particular types of noxious substances or initiate an injury response of the lung. Specific mechanisms include immunoglobulins, cellular components, and activation of complement. In the process of normal aging, specific lung defenses become less effective. Elderly persons are therefore increasingly vulnerable to respiratory infections.[62,85]

Control of Breathing

In the past, the control of ventilation was believed to be in a single respiratory center located in the medulla of the brain. However, more recent studies clearly indicate that the control mechanisms of breathing are complex and not entirely understood.

The following discussion represents those factors generally accepted to be the prime determinants of ventilation.[81]

There are at least three respiratory centers: one in the medulla and two in the pons. In addition, a less well-delineated area in the medulla contains chemoreceptors. These are referred to as the central chemoreceptors. Their major stimulus is pH change; they are depressed by hypoxia. The central respiratory centers also receive input from the cerebral cortex and the periphery. Voluntary breath holding is an example of higher cerebral input. Peripheral inputs include mechanical stimulation (irritant receptors in airways, J receptors in lung) and carotid body chemoreceptor response to Pa_{O_2}, Pa_{CO_2}, and pH (Figure 2-14).

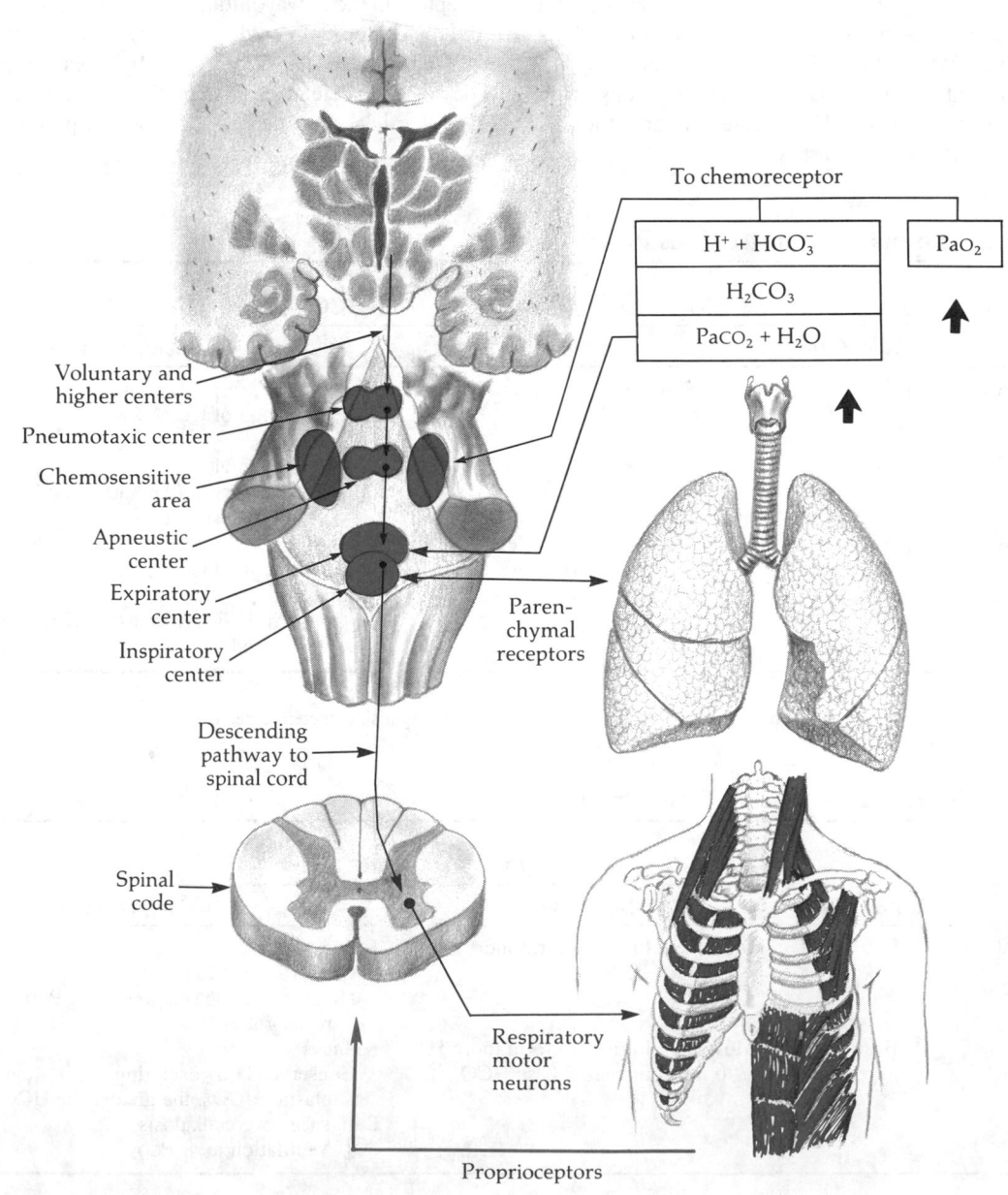

To chemoreceptor

$H^+ + HCO_3^-$

H_2CO_3

$Pa_{CO_2} + H_2O$

Pa_{O_2}

Voluntary and higher centers
Pneumotaxic center
Chemosensitive area
Apneustic center
Expiratory center
Inspiratory center
Descending pathway to spinal cord
Spinal code
Parenchymal receptors
Respiratory motor neurons
Proprioceptors

Figure 2-14 Respiratory control system.

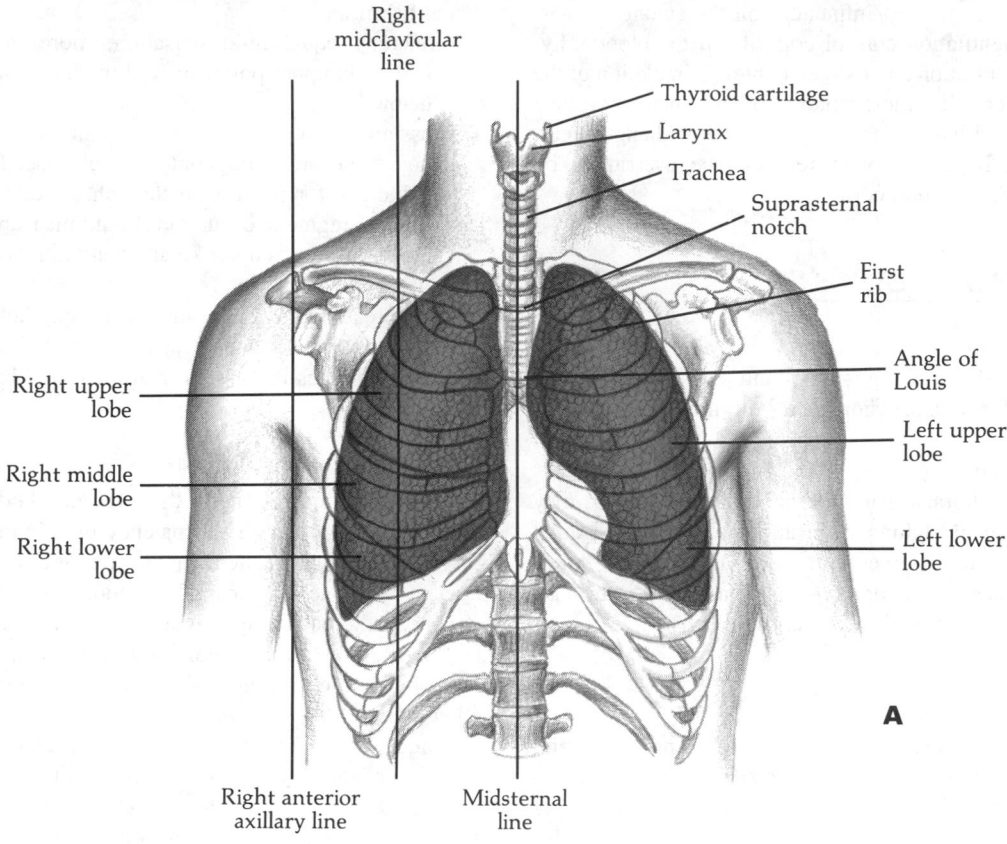

Right
midclavicular
line

Thyroid cartilage

Larynx

Trachea

Suprasternal
notch

First
rib

Angle of
Louis

Right upper
lobe

Left upper
lobe

Right middle
lobe

Right lower
lobe

Left lower
lobe

Right anterior
axillary line

Midsternal
line

A

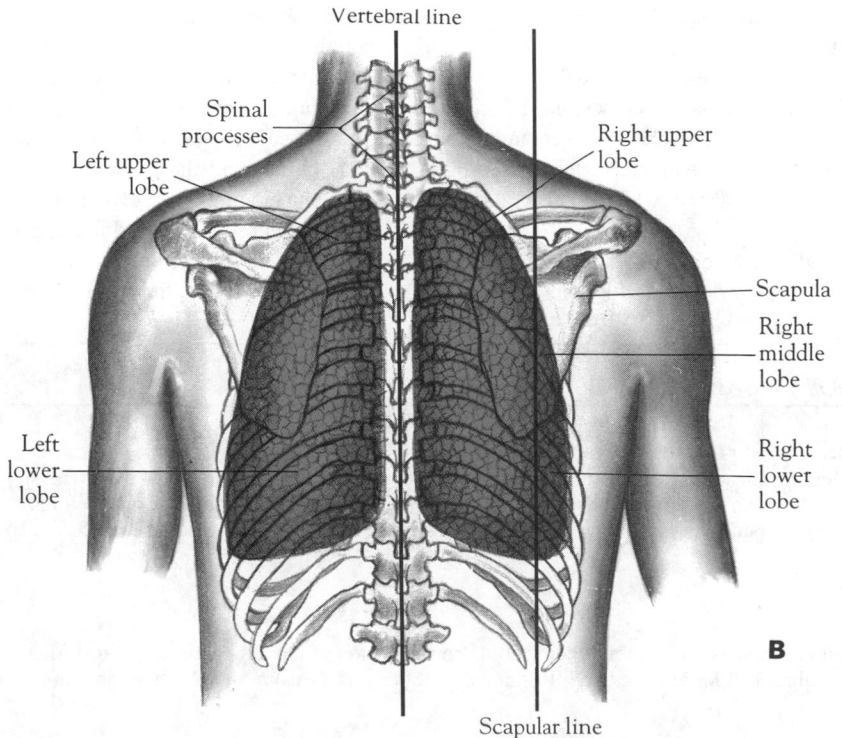

Vertebral line

Spinal
processes

Right upper
lobe

Left upper
lobe

Scapula

Right
middle
lobe

Left
lower
lobe

Right
lower
lobe

Scapular line

B

Figure 2-15 Landmarks and structures of chest wall. **A,** Anterior view. **B,** Posterior view.

In summary, the greatest influences on the autonomic nervous system's ventilation control come from the blood's hydrogen ion concentration and oxygen content stimulation of the medullary center's chemoreceptors. These help correlate breathing with acid-base balance and with gas exchange needs. The whole breathing control system can be overridden by higher areas of the cerebral cortex.

NORMAL FINDINGS

General appearance
Appears relaxed; breathing is quiet and easy without apparent effort; facial expressions and limb movements are relaxed

Breathing pattern
Diaphragmatic-thoracic pattern is smooth and regular; may have occasional sighing respirations; breathing is quiet and passive with symmetric chest expansion; *older adult:* pattern is the same as for adults, but calcification at rib articulation points may decrease chest expansion[24]

Respiratory rate
12-20 resp/min

Skin
Mucous membranes are pink; no cyanosis or pallor present; palpation of skin and chest wall reveals smooth skin and a stable chest wall; there are no crepitations, bulging, or painful areas.

Nail bed, nail configuration
Angulation between base of nail and finger; no thickening of distal finger width (no clubbing)

Chest wall configuration (Figure 2-15)
Symmetric, bilateral muscle development; A-P to transverse ratio is 1:2 to 5:7; straight spinal processes; downward and equal slope of ribs; *older adult:* kyphosis is a common finding in elderly persons; A decrease in intervertebral disk space size may cause a slight increase in A-P/transverse ratio

Tracheal position
Midline and straight; directly above the suprasternal notch; *older adult:* may be slightly deviated if kyphosis is present

Vocal fremitus
Bilaterally equal mild sensation; more intense vibratory feeling in upper posterior wall medial to scapula: see box below

Percussion
Resonance heard throughout lung fields; see Figure 2-16 and Table 2-4 for percussion tone characteristics; percussion of diaphragmatic excursion should measure 4 to 6 cm; inhaled position is approximately at tenth posterior rib level

Auscultation
Quiet breathing heard throughout all lung fields; Figure 2-17 shows normal sounds heard in each lung field, and Table 2-5 describes the normal and abnormal breath and voice sounds

Common Abnormal Findings

Cough Cough is one of the important body reflexes. It is intended to maintain airway patency by eliminating materials accumulated or deposited on the mucosa of the respiratory tract, such as tracheobronchial secretions, blood, aspirated substances, and other foreign bodies. A nonproductive cough may be the result of acute inflammation of the respiratory mucosal membranes, the presence of a tumor, or a reflex initiated in other areas.

Cough of recent onset frequently is caused by an acute infection of the larynx, trachea, bronchi, lung, or pleura.

The intensity of cough has no relationship to the severity or seriousness of underlying bronchopulmonary disease. It is not unusual for a patient with serious pulmonary disease to have minimal or no cough. On the other hand, a mild viral infection involving the trachea or the bronchi may cause a troublesome cough.

Expectoration Expectoration is the act of coughing up and spitting material raised from the lower respiratory tract. Sputum consists of secretions formed continuously by the mucous glands and the goblet cells of the tracheobronchial tree. The cilia along the mucosal lining of the bronchi propel the thin mucous secretions toward the upper airway.

In pathologic conditions, increased tracheobronchial secretions may be due to the stimulation of normal secretory cells or

---

OVERVIEW OF VOCAL FREMITUS

Vocal fremitus is the sensation of sound vibrations produced when the patient speaks.

The examiner may feel for these vibrations by placing the extended hand gently on the chest wall. The spoken voice produces low-frequency vibrations through the vocal cords, the airways, and the pleura. These vibrations are felt and compared bilaterally.

The examiner instructs the patient to say "one-two-three" or "how-now-brown-cow." As these words are spoken, the examiner feels for the vibrations.

ABNORMAL RESPONSES
Increased Fremitus

An increase in the vibratory sensation is felt when there is consolidation of the lung caused by fluid-filled or solid structures, which would transmit the vibrations better than air-filled lungs. This occurs, for example, with pneumonia or a tumor of the lung.

Decreased Fremitus

A decrease in the vibratory sensation is felt when more air than normal is blocked or trapped in the lungs or pleural space; vibrations of the spoken voice are decreased. This occurs, for example, with emphysema or a pneumothorax.

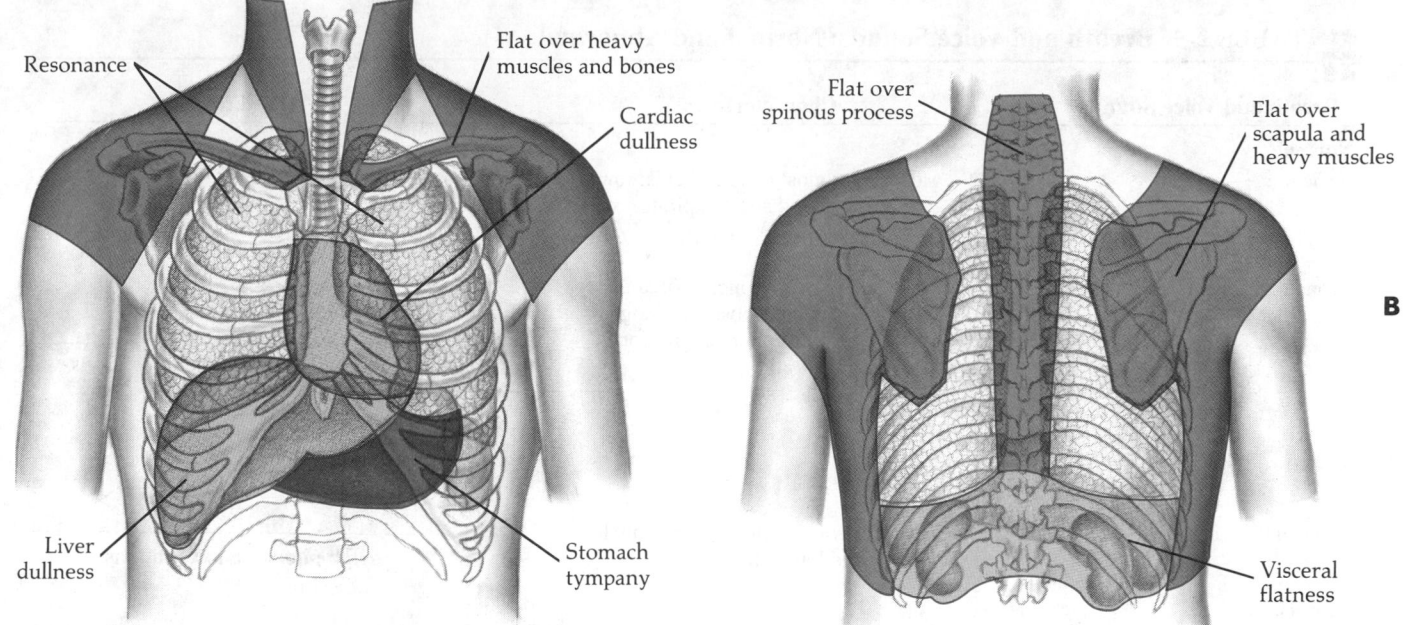

Figure 2-16 Percussion tones. **A,** Anterior view. **B,** Posterior view.

TABLE 2-4 Percussion Tones

Type of Tone	Intensity	Pitch	Duration	Quality
Resonant	Loud	Low	Long	Hollow
Flat	Soft	High	Short	Extremely dull
Dull	Medium	Medium-high	Medium	Thudlike
Tympanic	Loud	High	Medium	Drumlike
Hyperresonant*	Very loud	Very low	Longer	Booming

*Hyperresonance is abnormal sound heard during percussion in adults. It represents air trapping such as occurs in obstructive lung diseases.

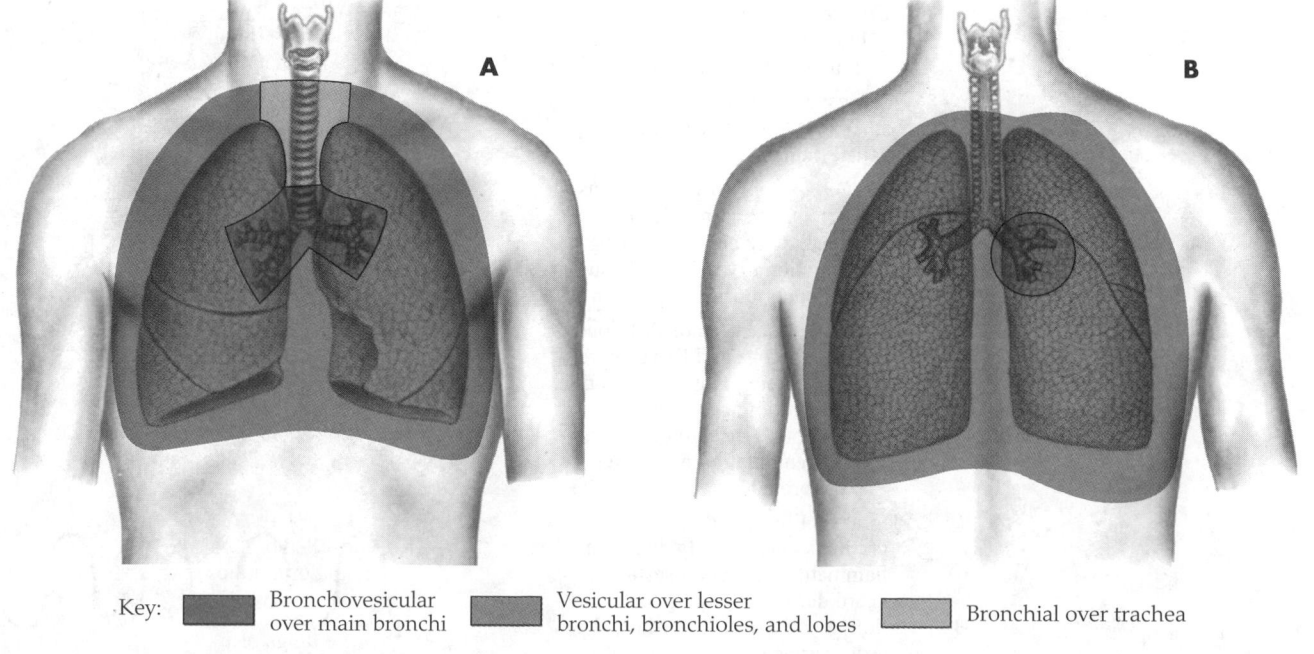

Key: ▮ Bronchovesicular over main bronchi ▮ Vesicular over lesser bronchi, bronchioles, and lobes ▮ Bronchial over trachea

Figure 2-17 Normal auscultatory sounds. **A,** Anterior view. **B,** Posterior view.

TABLE 2-5 Breath and Voice Sounds: Normal and Abnormal

Breath and Voice Sounds	Characteristics	Findings
Normal		
Vesicular	Heard over most of lung fields; low pitch; soft and short expirations (Figure 2-17)	Low pitch, soft expirations
Bronchovesicular	Heard over main bronchus area and over upper right posterior lung field; medium pitch; expiration equals inspiration	Medium pitch, medium expirations
Bronchial	Heard only over trachea; high pitch; loud and long expirations	High pitch, loud expirations
Abnormal		
Bronchial when heard over peripheral lung fields		
Bronchovesicular sounds when heard over peripheral lung fields		
Adventitious	Crackles: discrete, noncontinuous sounds	
	Fine crackles (rales): high-pitched, discrete, noncontinuous crackling sounds heard during end of inspiration (indicates inflammation or congestion)	
	Medium crackles (rales): lower, moister sound heard during midstage of inspiration; not cleared by a cough	
	Coarse crackles (rales): loud, bubbly noise heard during inspiration; not cleared by a cough	
	Wheezes: continuous musical sounds; if low pitched, may be called rhonchi	
	Sibilant or musical wheeze: musical noise sounding like a squeak; may be heard during inspiration or expiration; usually louder during expiration	
	Sonorous wheeze (rhonchi): loud, low, coarse sound like a snore heard at any point of inspiration or expiration; coughing may clear sound (usually means mucus accumulation in trachea or large bronchi)	
	Pleural friction rub: dry, rubbing, or grating sound, usually due to inflammation of pleural surfaces; heard during inspiration or expiration; loudest over lower lateral anterior surface	

■ **TABLE 2-5 Breath and Voice Sounds: Normal and Abnormal—cont'd**

Breath and Voice Sounds	Characteristics	Findings
Adventitious—cont'd	*Stridor:* harsh, high-pitched sound; louder on inspiration than expiration (usually means partial upper airway obstruction)	
Resonance of spoken voice	*Bronchophony:* using diaphragm of stethoscope, listen to posterior chest as patient says "ninety-nine"	Negative response: muffled "nin-nin" sound heard Positive response: clear, loud, "ninety-nine" response heard because lung tissue is consolidated
	Whispered pectoriloquy: listen to posterior chest as patient whispers "one, two, three"	Negative response: muffled sounds heard Positive response: clear "one, two, three" is heard because of lung consolidation
	Egophony: listen to posterior chest as the patient says "e-e-e"	Negative response: muffled "e-e-e" sound heard Positive response: sound of "e" changes to "a-a-a" sound because of consolidation

to an increase in the number of these cells. In acute situations, increased sputum production is the result of transient stimulation of mucous glands and goblet cells.

In addition to mucus, expectorated material may contain other fluids from various sites in the respiratory tract, including the alveoli. It may contain white blood cells accumulated for the purpose of fighting infection, necrotic material, blood, aspirated vomitus, or other foreign material.

The gross appearance of sputum may suggest the underlying condition. Yellow sputum generally indicates the presence of large numbers of white blood cells, which are the major component of pus. Green discoloration signifies the production of an enzyme from stagnant pus. Red or brownish sputum is usually due to the presence of red blood cells.

Dyspnea Dyspnea is a shortness of breath or a difficulty in breathing. The awareness of breathing may range in intensity from mild discomfort to extreme distress. Dyspnea, like pain, is a subjective sign that is likely to be influenced by the patient's reaction, sensitivity, and emotional state. Dyspnea involves both a physiologic and a cognitive component.

Dyspnea as a result of impaired mechanical function occurs under numerous clinical conditions. Some basic causes are increased airway resistance, as in upper airway obstruction, asthma and airway obstructive diseases; reduced pulmonary compliance as a result of pulmonary fibrosis, congestion, edema, and a variety of other parenchymal lung diseases; mechanical interference with the expansion of the lungs because of massive pleural effusion or pneumothorax; and abnormality of chest wall and respiratory muscles resulting in inefficient respiratory efforts.

The circumstance in which the symptom occurs has diagnostic importance. Breathlessness may occur with certain body positions. Orthopnea refers to dyspnea upon lying down. Paroxysmal nocturnal dyspnea is the sudden onset of shortness of breath during the night that occurs in cardiac patients. The cause is thought to be transient pulmonary edema.

 EMERGENCY ALERT

DYSPNEA/RESPIRATORY DISTRESS

Objective finding when the patient is short of breath

Assessment

- PMH/medications.
- Obtain thorough history of this episode.
- Onset gradual or sudden.
- Cigarette smoker.
- Assess respiratory rate and depth noisy respiration.
- Observe for nasal flaring, pallor, decreased level of consciousness.
- Auscultate lung sounds.

Interventions

- Maintain airway, breathing, and circulation.
- Place patient in position of comfort (usual Fowler's).
- Administer high flow oxygen by mask (unless COPD) (10-15 liters).
- Maintain IV access at keep open rate.
- Monitor oxygen saturation.

COPD, chronic obstructive pulmonary disease.

A recent increase in dyspnea in a patient with chronic respiratory disease is indicative of an acute event. This may be due to increased airway resistance as with bronchospasm, secretions, and infection or to reduced pulmonary compliance as with pulmonary congestion or edema.[25]

Hemoptysis Hemoptysis is the expectoration of blood originating from the respiratory tract below the pharynx. Blood-tinged or blood-streaked sputum is not usually called hemoptysis. Hemoptysis is the coughing up of a quantifiable amount of blood pure or mixed with sputum.

The causes of hemoptysis are many. The three major underlying pathologic conditions are infection, neoplasm, and

! EMERGENCY ALERT

CARBON MONOXIDE (CO) POISONING

CO poisoning is often associated with smoke inhalation from fires, engine exhaust, and faulty home heating systems. CO's affinity is 200 times greater than oxygen for hemoglobin. Hypoxia results from the reduced oxygen-carrying capacity of the blood, impaired release of oxygen to the tissues, and impaired cellular respiration.

Assessment

MILD

- Throbbing headache, nausea/vomiting
- Impaired function of complex tasks

MODERATE

- Irritability, weakness, visual changes
- Palpitations
- Loss of dexterity, decreased mentation

SEVERE

- Tachycardia, tachypnea, collapse, syncope

LIFE-THREATENING

- Coma, seizures, Cheyne-Stokes respirations
- Cherry red mucous membranes

Interventions

- Maintain airway, breathing, and circulation.
- Obtain IV access.
- Monitor cardiac status.
- Administer high-flow oxygen (10 to 15 L) by tight fitting mask for 4 hours or $HbCO_2$ <5%.
- Consider hyperbaric oxygen.
- Monitor arterial blood gases.

cardiovascular disease. Common infectious causes of hemoptysis are pneumonia, tuberculosis, bronchiectasis, lung abscess, fungal infection, and parasitic lung diseases. Bronchogenic carcinoma is the neoplastic disease most commonly causing hemoptysis. Hemoptysis is a symptom of certain cardiovascular diseases, such as pulmonary embolism, congestive heart failure, and mitral stenosis.

Chest pain   Chest pain of pulmonary origin can derive from the chest wall, parietal pleura, or visceral pleura. The thoracic wall is the most common source of chest pain; skin, muscles, nerves, and bones may be its cause in association with various clinical conditions. The lung parenchyma is insensitive to painful stimuli, and only the parietal layer of the pleura is very pain sensitive. Its direct or indirect involvement by various pathologic processes commonly causes a dull, constant ache or poorly localized chest pain. Pain with pneumonia and the other inflammatory diseases of the lung is usually due to pleural reaction. In lung cancer, chest pain is frequently indicative of pleural reaction or chest wall invasion.

Pulmonary arterial hypertension sometimes causes chest pain because of increased tension of arterial walls or strain of the right side of the heart muscle. The sudden and transient chest pain of pulmonary embolism results from a pleural reaction.

Pleuritic pain is a well-localized, constant ache or sharp chest pain that is produced or aggravated by deep breathing or other chest wall movement.[25]

CONDITIONS, DISEASES, AND DISORDERS

■ ACUTE RESPIRATORY FAILURE[44,58,81]

Respiratory failure is not a disease, but an acute onset of inadequate gas exchange secondary to another condition or disease process. Respiratory failure is manifested by a PaO_2 of less than 50 mm Hg.

Acute respiratory failure may be present during exacerbation of chronic respiratory conditions, or as a result of an acute situation such as postoperative airway obstruction, severe pneumonia, or trauma. Respiratory failure is generally considered in two categories, hypoxemic respiratory failure and ventilatory respiratory failure.

Hypoxemic Respiratory Failure

Hypoxemic respiratory failure is manifested by a PaO_2 less than 50 mm Hg on room air, with either a normal or low $PaCO_2$. The low PaO_2 stimulates respiratory efforts, resulting in hyperventilation and lowering of the $PaCO_2$ until fatigue sets in. Causes of hypoxemic respiratory failure include V/Q mismatch and intrapulmonary right-to-left shunting. Examples of diseases associated with hypoxemic respiratory failure include the following:

1. Increased pulmonary capillary pressure and edema resulting from such conditions as the following:
   a. Left ventricular heart failure
   b. Fluid overload
2. Lung parenchymal injury
   a. Pneumonia
   b. Tuberculosis
   c. Fungal infections
   d. Near drowning
   e. Chemical or smoke inhalation
   f. Liquid aspiration
3. Increased pulmonary capillary permeability, as in adult respiratory distress syndrome (ARDS)

Hypoxemic respiratory failure is due to areas of low V/Q, including areas of shunt (a complete lack of ventilation with continued blood flow). The more extensive the areas of shunt, the less the response to supplemental oxygen. If severe hypoxemia (PaO_2 <40 mm Hg) cannot be corrected, a metabolic acidosis will result from increased anaerobic metabolism. Cardiac output and alveolar ventilation increase, if possible, to compensate for the hypoxemia.

Diagnostic studies for hypoxemic respiratory failure include evaluating the $Paco_2$ (which is initially low when the body is still trying to compensate but then increases when compensation is no longer possible).

Ventilatory Respiratory Failure

Ventilatory respiratory failure is manifested by a $Paco_2$ acutely elevated over 50 mm Hg, with a low Pao_2 on room air. Ventilation, the actual movement of air between the environment and the alveolar/capillary membrane, is inadequate. Acute alveolar hypoventilation results from either pulmonary disease or central nervous system (CNS)/neuromuscular dysfunction and leads to respiratory acidosis. Examples of diseases and disorders that cause ventilatory respiratory failure include the following:

1. Respiratory center depression caused by a malfunctioning CNS, which can result from the following:
   a. Drug overdoses
   b. CNS lesions or infections
2. Inability of the nervous system to generate respiratory muscle contraction; examples include the following:
   a. Guillain-Barré syndrome
   b. Multiple sclerosis
   c. Spinal cord injury
   d. Myasthenia gravis
   e. Muscular dystrophies
   f. Poliomyelitis
   g. Tetanus
3. Pulmonary disorders
   a. Chronic bronchitis
   b. Emphysema
   c. Massive obesity
   d. Severe kyphoscoliosis
   e. Asthma

The primary problem in ventilatory respiratory failure is the inability to generate enough alveolar ventilation, although right-to-left shunting and V/Q mismatch may also contribute to the hypoxemia with hypercarbia.

The patient may have difficulty performing forced expiratory tests because of shortness of breath. In addition, because of the retention of carbon dioxide, the kidneys tend to retain bicarbonate, so the arterial pH remains above 7.3.

Respiratory failure from CNS depression most commonly follows an overdose of opiates, alcohol, tricyclic antidepressants, barbiturates, or other sedative drugs. After the body takes in large quantities of any of these drugs, stimulation of the respiratory center is depressed and the rate of breathing is lowered, with little change in tidal volume. The respiratory center does not respond to the rising $Paco_2$.

The main difficulty for patients with a neuromuscular disease is the inability to generate enough force for deep-breathing or coughing. Exercise or a need for deep breathing may cause difficulty.

The diagnostic evaluation and nursing care of the patient with respiratory insufficiency and respiratory failure are cause

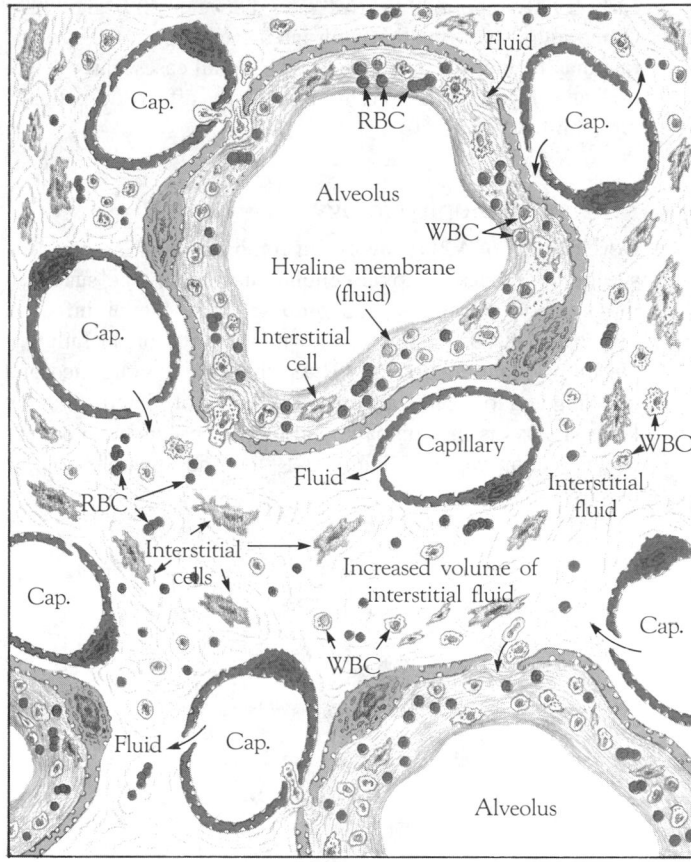

Figure 2-18 Adult respiratory distress syndrome. (From Wilson.[93])

specific. The reader is referred to the specific causes for a detailed discussion.

ADULT RESPIRATORY DISTRESS SYNDROME

In ARDS, capillary permeability is increased, creating a condition in which the lungs are wet and heavy, congested, hemorrhagic, stiff, and unable to exchange oxygen (Figure 2-18).

ARDS is one cause of acute hypoxemia respiratory failure. The following are many of the disorders that may lead to ARDS:

Trauma
Inhaled toxins
Liquid aspiration
Hematologic disorders
Infections
Drug overdose
Toxic metabolic disorders

Because of the variability of its diagnosis, the incidence and survival rates of ARDS are difficult to state. Studies since the early 1970s reported survival rates between 30% and 50%. Other authors suggest that with intensive support, the survival rate may be increased to 60% to 70%. In all cases, early detection and aggressive interventions directly affect the patient's probability of survival.[59]

Pathophysiology

Development of ARDS involves a combination of ischemic tissue injury, release of toxic cellular substances, and sustained inflammatory response. Superimposed nosocomial infection may cause ARDS to progress to multisystem organ failure.[75] On biopsy examination of ARDS, the lung is congested and bleeding and looks like a liver. The amount of secretions in the large airways is insignificant, and there is no visible blockage of the major vessels. Figure 2-19 outlines the physiologic process.

As a result of this process, the following major problems occur:

1. A reduction in the functional residual capacity (FRC)
2. Bronchovascular edema, resulting in a higher interstitial pressure, distal atelectasis, and decreased vital capacity
3. Decreased lung compliance caused by congestion, resulting in a decreased FRC
4. Hypoxemia caused by V/Q mismatch in the lungs, not resolved by oxygen administration alone
5. Increased oxygen consumption, increased airway resistance

Diagnostic Studies and Findings

Pulmonary function   Alveolar-arterial oxygen gradient increased to $P(A-a)O_2$ (also A-a Do_2): 300 to 500 mm Hg; reflects the number of alveolar-capillary units with low V/Q; shunt fraction (Qs/Qt): May be greater than 15% to 20%; measures the degree of intrapulmonary shunting; normal value <6%; compliance (C): below normal; pulmonary capillary wedge pressure (PCWP): low to normal pressure seen in ARDS, less than 15 mm Hg.

Arterial blood gases Pao_2 <55 mm Hg indicates hypoxemia; initially normal to low $Paco_2$ may rise; pH increased in beginning secondary to hyperventilation, as ARDS becomes worse, pH decreases

Lactic acid levels   May be increased in tissue hypoxia; normal values: 0.5-2.2 mEq/L (venous blood)[28]

Chest roentgenograms   There must be a large increase in lung fluid before abnormalities are observed on chest roentgenograms; early diagnostic radiographic changes include thickened or blurred margins of the bronchi or vessels; Figure 2-20 shows diffuse and hazy blurred appearance throughout the lung fields

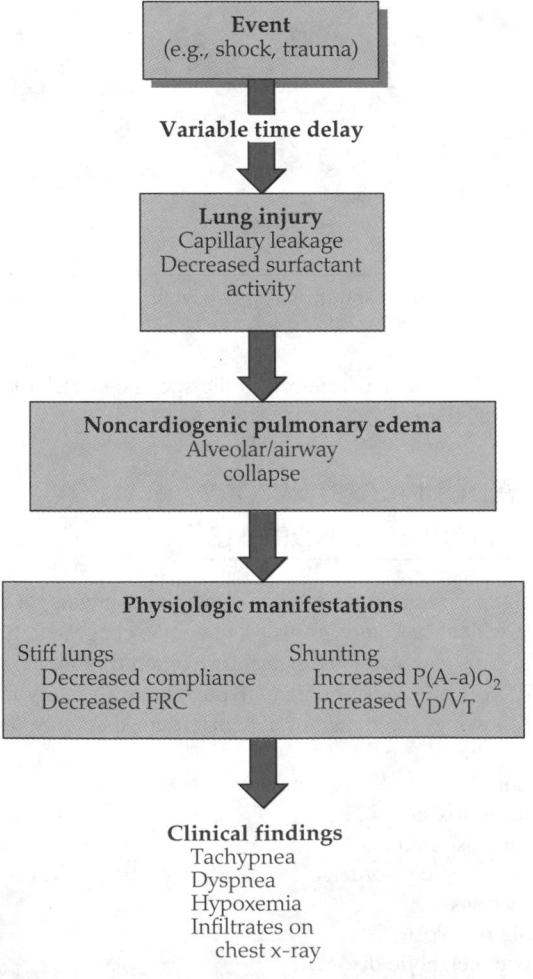

Figure 2-19 Pathogenesis of adult respiratory distress syndrome. (From Wilson.[93])

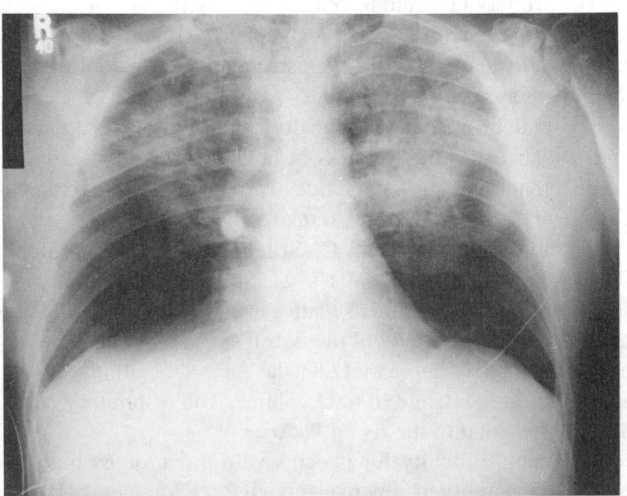

Figure 2-20 Chest roentgenogram of patient with adult respiratory distress syndrome. Heart is normal size; note diffuse infiltrates in upper and middle zones of lungs. (Courtesy R. Keith Wilson, MD, Baylor College of Medicine, Houston, Texas.)

•••••• Multidisciplinary Plan

The major medical plan is focused in three areas:

1. Supportive, to provide adequate oxygenation and mechanical ventilation to reverse the hypoxemia and expand the distal gas exchange units so as to prevent further airway and alveolar collapse
2. Therapeutic, to treat the systemic responses caused by the alterations in pulmonary function
3. Curative, to locate and halt the causal insult (if possible)

Mechanical Ventilation

The purpose of mechanical ventilation for ARDS is to produce a rapid inspiratory flow rate while also exerting a continuous positive end-expiratory pressure (PEEP). PEEP results in decreased shunt and an increase in PaO_2. The effects of PEEP in ARDS are:

1. Pulmonary
   a. Increased mean airway pressure
   b. Increased functional residual capacity
   c. Increased compliance
   d. Decreased shunting
   e. Increased lung volumes
   f. Clearing of lung fields
2. Potential complications
   a. Decreased venous return
   b. Increased pulmonary vascular resistance
   c. Peripheral vasoconstriction
   d. Hypotension
   e. Tachycardia
   f. Oliguria
   g. Increased PCWP (>15 mm Hg), not reflective of left ventricular end-diastolic pressure (LVEDP)
   h. Possible increased incidence of pneumothorax[46]

Guidelines for use of mechanical ventilation with PEEP for ARDS:

1. Tidal volume of 10 to 12 ml/kg body weight. Tidal volumes greater than this may cause alveolar-overinflation, increasing alveolar injury.
2. PEEP should be regulated to maintain oxygenation without undue side effects. The purpose of PEEP is to decrease the intrapulmonary shunting and to improve pulmonary compliance. Therefore PEEP should be considered for use when an inspired oxygen concentration of >50% is required to maintain an adequate PaO_2 level. Optimal use of PEEP is to add it in small increments in an attempt to decrease the intrapulmonary shunt to the 15% to 20% range. PEEP is generally started at 5 cm H_2O if needed, while monitoring for adverse effects of PEEP on cardiac output. Hypotensive patients may require additional fluid volume to compensate for the decreased venous return secondary to PEEP.
3. The goal of mechanical ventilation is to keep the $PaCO_2$ in the range of 35 to 45 mm Hg. A level below this will decrease cardiac output, increase airway resistance, and increase oxygen consumption. A current trend, permis-

EMERGENCY ALERT

SMOKE/TOXIC INHALATION

Occurs when a person has inhaled a noxious gas that was a product of combustion.

Assessment

- Obtain history including duration of exposure, if patient was in a confined area, and the material that was burning
- Burning pain to throat and/or chest
- Upper airway irritation
- Singed facial/nasal hairs, facial burns
- Carbonaceous sputum
- Auscultate for rales, rhonchi, wheezes
- Dyspnea, restlessness, cough, hoarseness
- Signs of pulmonary edema

Interventions

- Maintain airway, breathing, and circulation.
- Administer high-flow, humidifed oxygen by mask (10 to 15 L).
- Obtain IV access.
- Monitor arterial blood gases and/or O_2 saturation.
- Admit and observe.
- Prepare to intubate, emergently as needed.
- Encourage coughing, deep breathing, and raising of sputum.

---

sive hypercapnia, is to allow higher $PaCO_2$ levels to decrease the physical stress of mechanical ventilation on injured pulmonary tissue.[86]

Medications

There are no specific drugs to treat the syndrome. Drugs used are primarily supportive to other therapeutic measures such as mechanical ventilation.

Morphine (3 to 5 mg/hr IV) may be given as sedation for patients on a ventilator who are restless and experiencing tachypnea.

Vecuronium bromide may be used as a neuromuscular blocking agent to completely paralyze the voluntary respirations of the patient and decrease oxygen consumption, while allowing effective mechanical ventilation. Neuromuscular blockers do not have a sedative effect, so must be used in combination with continuous sedation to prevent patient panic during chemical paralysis.[60]

Corticosteroid use is controversial.

Vasoactive medications may be used to optimize hemodynamic responses and fluid volume, based on pulmonary artery catheter readings.

Surfactant replacement therapy is being evaluated for future use. Drug therapy aimed at altering responses to various chemical mediators is under investigation.[75]

General Management

Fluid and electrolyte therapy: Fluids are monitored carefully to optimize cardiac output. Patients with capillary damage from ARDS are especially susceptible to fluid leakage into the alveolar spaces.

Fluid types   There is some controversy with regard to the use of colloids and crystalloids. It is most generally believed that colloidal fluids should be used in hypoalbuminemic patients. All other patients should receive crystalloid fluids.

Quantity of fluids   PCWP is much more reliable than the central venous pressure (CVP) when trying to determine the quantity of fluids to be administered. In most situations, maintenance of the PCWP at 10 to 15 mm Hg provides adequate, but not excessive, intravascular volumes. Certainly clinical parameters such as pulse, urinary output, and peripheral vasoconstriction should also be considered as assessment variables.

Oxygenation   Oxygen support via mask may be used in the very early stages of ARDS but will not be sufficient as the syndrome becomes worse. The goal is to provide the lowest oxygen concentration to maintain the mixed venous oxygen at a level of 40 mm Hg (this may be measured by obtaining a blood sample from the distal lumen of the pulmonary artery catheter or by continuous readings from a mixed venous oxygen pulmonary artery catheter). Continuous pulse oximetry is generally used to monitor oxygen saturation. The $P\bar{v}O_2$ and PaO_2 must both be carefully monitored.

If oxygen concentrations of greater than 50% are required to maintain adequate blood gas oxygen levels, intubation and mechanical ventilation are indicated. See specific mechanical ventilation techniques on p. 205.

Electrocardiogram: Monitor Cardiac Response.

Alimentation   Alimentation should be undertaken from the onset. Enteral alimentation via a small feeding tube is best, but intravenous hyperalimentation should be instituted if enteral alimentation is not possible. The use of H_2 blockers to maintain gastric pH above 4 may be warranted for gastric ulcer prophylaxis.

Tracheobronchial suctioning   To remove mucus secretions and to ensure patient airway.

Monitoring of blood gases and pressure response   The patient's blood gases, PCWP, and alveolar-arterial oxygen gradient ($PA-aO_2$) should be monitored. SpO_2 is monitored continuously via pulse oximeter.

Monitoring of sputum and bronchial secretions   Laboratory analysis of bronchial secretions should be made if secretions are not clear to white, or if other signs of infection are present (elevated white blood cell [WBC], elevated temperature).

Monitoring of chest roentgenograms   Frequent chest roentgenograms: Frequent chest roentgenogram analysis is useful in monitoring the patient's response to the therapeutic treatment.

Alternative Therapies

Patients who are unable to maintain adequate gas exchange on mechanical ventilation may be candidates for extracorporeal membrane oxygenation or carbon dioxide removal. These involve creating a bypass circuit from the patient's vascular system through special membranes.[14]

NURSING CARE

Nursing Assessment

One of the most important assessment rules in the care of the patient with ARDS or potential ARDS is to have good baseline data. If the patient's condition deteriorates, subtle changes can be identified.

Respiratory Status

Respiratory distress: nasal flaring, chest wall retractions, tachypnea, decreased chest wall movement, labored breathing

Breath sounds: crackles, wheeze, decreased, bilaterally unequal

Breathing pattern: labored, irregular

Persistent cough with or without sputum production

Pulmonary function: decreased vital capacity, increased intrapulmonary shunting

Hypercapnia: headache, dizziness, confusion, unconsciousness, twitching, hypertension, sweating, flushed face

Hypoxia: restlessness, confusion, impaired motor function, hypotension, cyanosis, tachycardia

Laboratory Values

Monitor blood gases: $PaCO_2$, PaO_2, $P\bar{v}O_2$, $PA-aO_2$, pH, HCO_3^-, lactic acid levels

Cardiovascular Status

Cardiac output: decreased cardiac output (CO), restlessness, lethargy, tachycardia, hypotension, decreased urinary output

Pulmonary pressures: increased pulmonary wedge pressure (PWP), pulmonary artery pressure (PAP)

Fluid and Electrolytes

Intake and output, potassium, and bicarbonate

Psychosocial

Fear of suffocation, fear of being out of control if on ventilator, fear of unknown, family understanding, support, ability to communicate

Nursing Dx & Intervention[11,37,47,48,83]

Ineffective breathing pattern related to decreased compliance

- Assess ventilation to include evaluation of breathing rate, rhythm, and depth, chest expansion, presence of respiratory distress such as dyspnea, shortness of breath, nasal flaring, cyanosis, and changes in skin color including nail beds and mucous membranes. *Signs of respiratory distress may be present because of stiff lungs and shunting.*

- Assess tidal volume, vital capacity and minute volume, and intrapulmonary shunting.
- Identify contributing factors such as airway clearance or obstruction problem, pain, level of consciousness, or weakness.
- Maintain patient position to facilitate ventilation (i.e., in semi-Fowler's position or tripod position with arms supported), cough, and deep breathing *to maximize breathing potential.*
- Help to protect patient from known sources of secondary infection.
- In collaboration with physician, prepare for and institute mechanical ventilation when patient cannot maintain adequate blood gas levels or demonstrates tiring with breathing efforts.
- When patient is receiving mechanical ventilation, provide care and monitoring consistent with the guidelines presented on pp. 205 to 207.

Impaired gas exchange related to altered ventilation/perfusion relationship

- Monitor arterial blood gases; report increases or decreases of $PaCO_2$ and PaO_2 of more than 10 mm Hg.
- In collaboration with the physician, administer oxygen *to maintain PaO_2 of at least 60 to 65 mm Hg; if blood gas levels cannot be maintained or if the concentration of oxygen exceeds 50%, mechanical ventilation must be considered.*
- *Monitor pulse oximetry. Maintain SpO_2 >90%. If SpO_2 >92%, consider decreasing administered oxygen to decrease potential for oxygen toxicity.*
- Monitor alveolar-arterial oxygen gradient.
- Prevent physiologic factors that promote restlessness or anxiety. Restlessness increases oxygen consumption and CO_2 production.
- Monitor for signs of cor pulmonale: pulmonary hypertension, gradually increasing edema of the legs, increasing CVP and PCWP, jugular venous distention, blood gas abnormalities, and hepatomegaly *related to hypoxemic pulmonary vasoconstriction.*
- Monitor electrocardiogram and cardiac status for arrhythmias *secondary to alteration in blood gases.*
- Monitor and record kidney functioning and urinary output, which may be affected *secondary to chronic tissue hypoxia, alterations in metabolism, and decreased venous return.*
- Carefully monitor body temperature; *this may fluctuate because of alterations in metabolism or secondary infections.* Elevated temperature increases oxygen demand.
- In collaboration with physician, administer respiratory-related medications and assess and document patient's response.

Fatigue related to increased respiratory effort, hypoxia

- Assess factors related to fatigue and strategies for dealing with them.
- Assess support systems and available resources.
- Administer treatments or medications to relieve discomfort.
- Enhance patient's ability to rest between specified activities.
- Assist patient to perform activities of daily living (ADLs) or provide all ADLs as necessary.

Risk for aspiration related to impaired airway

- Avoid triggering gag mechanism when performing caretaking activities, including mouth care.
- Assess and document amount of secretions present, patient's level of consciousness, and patient's ability to swallow secretions effectively.
- Suction when necessary to remove secretions and maintain patent airway.
- For patients with reduced level of consciousness, ensure that head of bed is elevated, unless contraindicated.

Altered nutrition: less than body requirements related to impaired body state

- Assess for adequacy of fluid and caloric intake and ensure intake of required fluids and nutrients.
- Maintain tube feedings or hyperalimentation in collaboration with physician.
- Monitor for signs and symptoms of malnutrition. Calorie requirements are increased by labored breathing.
- Carbohydrate breakdown increases production of carbon dioxide. Enteral or parenteral feeding must be monitored *to avoid excessive carbohydrate or calorie loads.*[19]

Risk for fluid volume deficit related to physiologic stress

- Assess for evidence of gastrointestinal bleeding *secondary to physiologic stress;* monitor serial hemoglobin and hematocrit; check all stools, emesis, and nasogastric aspirate *for presence of blood;* observe changes in vital signs or abdominal girth.
- Initiate prevention measures: for example, minimize activities for uninterrupted periods of time, maintain calm and restful environment, encourage patient to participate in care as tolerated, explain all therapy before administering.
- Provide enteral feedings if tolerated to maintain gut mucosal integrity.

Risk for infection related to equipment and bypass of normal defenses

- Use sterile procedures and sterile equipment.
- Good handwashing before and after patient or equipment contact.
- Tracheobronchial suction only when required by presence of secretions *to avoid traumatizing tissue and introducing bacteria.*

Impaired verbal communication related to intubation or demonstration of significant dyspnea

- Provide alternative method of communication appropriate to the patient's comprehension ability.
- If patient is intubated, assure patient that speech will return as soon as endotracheal tube is removed.
- Observe for signs of frustration or patient withdrawal secondary to the inability to speak.
- Teach family members appropriate methods to communicate with patient.

Patient Education/Home Care Planning

1. Teaching includes the disease process of ARDS as well as the underlying disorder that triggered ARDS.
2. During the critical phase of ARDS, neuromuscular blocking agents and sedatives may be used to allow effective mechanical ventilation. Teach the family appropriate ways to reorient and communicate with the patient.
3. Teach the patient/family the purpose of procedures and equipment used to promote oxygenation and prevent complications of immobility.
4. See the section on mechanical ventilation near the end of this chapter for additional teaching points.

Evaluation

Breathing pattern occurs without tiring patient   Breath sounds are clear in all areas.

Tissue oxygenation is adequate   Blood gases, pulse oximetry within normal limits. Signs of hypoxia or hypercapnia are resolved.

ADLs are completed without fatigue   Behavior is modified to conserve energy.

Aspiration is avoided   Breath sounds are clear. Absence of fever. No evidence of acute aspiration on chest roentgenogram.

Nutritional level is maintained   Weight stabilizes. Serum electrolytes, serum albumin normal.

Fluid volume balance is achieved   Vital signs, PCWP normal. Urine output adequate. Hematocrit within normal limits.

Immune defenses are maintained   Temperature, WBC within normal limits. Sputum clear to white. Absence of infiltrates on chest roentgenogram.

Communication is facilitated   Patient uses alternative methods to express needs and concerns. Patient and family anxiety relieved.

AIRWAYS OBSTRUCTIVE DISEASE

The term airways obstructive disease refers to a group of diseases, all of which are characterized by airway narrowing

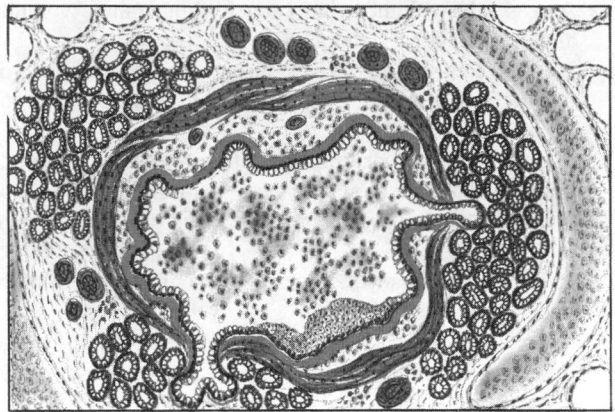

Chronic bronchitis

Figure 2-21   Chronic obstructive pulmonary disease. (From Wilson.[93])

(obstruction) and slowing of forced expiration. The diseases most commonly included are asthma, chronic obstructive bronchitis, and emphysema. The term *chronic obstructive pulmonary disease* (COPD) (Figure 2-21) is a general term for chronic obstructive bronchitis and emphysema, diseases with irreversible airways obstruction. Another less common disease included as one of the airway obstructive diseases is bronchiectasis. Many of these diseases can coexist in the same patient. It is important for the health care professional to identify the sources of obstruction for each individual so that maximal therapeutic benefit can be attained. (See Figure 2-22 for an overview of the relationships between the major airway obstructive diseases.)

COPD: CHRONIC BRONCHITIS AND EMPHYSEMA*

These diseases are a major cause of death and disability in the United States. It is estimated that 14 million people in the United States have COPD. While the mortality rates for other diseases are decreasing, the mortality rate for COPD is increasing, making it the fourth leading cause of death in the United States. Both chronic bronchitis and emphysema are usually associated with a significant smoking history, and patients usually have a component of each.

Chronic bronchitis (chronic obstructive bronchitis) is characterized by excessive mucus secretion and cough. Prolonged exposure to irritants such as cigarette smoke not only increase mucus production and impair clearance, but also result in irreversible narrowing of the small airways. Emphysema refers to abnormal enlargement of the distal air spaces and destruc-

---

*References 27, 35, 49, 53, 57, 72, 74.

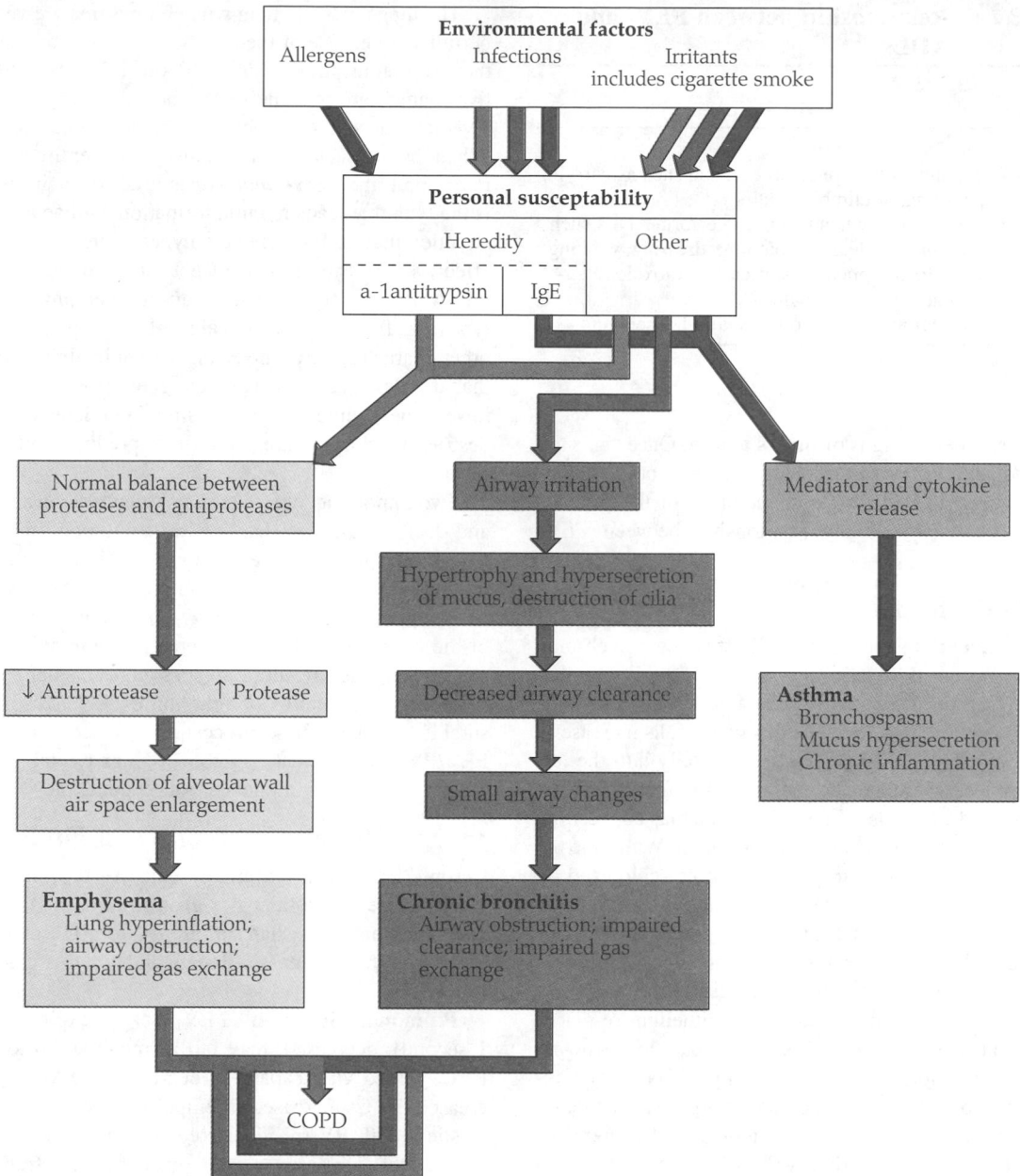

Figure 2-22 Pathogenesis of airways obstructive diseases: The figure demonstrates the interaction between environmental and personal susceptibility factors in the development of airways obstructive disease. The black lines trace the development of emphysema; the blue lines, chronic bronchitis; and the red lines, asthma.

tion of the lung distal to the terminal bronchiole. The result is a loss of lung recoil. The loss of recoil is reflected in increased compliance and the loss of small airway support with subsequent airway narrowing. The destruction of alveolar walls also means that there is a loss of gas exchange surface. In both of these diseases there is persistent, irreversible, progressive airways obstruction.

The development of chronic bronchitis or emphysema is determined by the interrelatedness of the individual's genetic vul-

nerability and environmental factors. The incidence of the diseases has increased dramatically in recent years. The American Lung Association attributes this increase to smoking and airborne irritants and to a better understanding of the physiologic processes and diagnostic criteria. The incidence of chronic bronchitis and emphysema remains greater in men than in women, possibly because of smoking history and choice of occupation.

The course of the diseases before the symptoms develop is unclear. Probably the forced expiratory volume in 1 second

TABLE 2-6 Relationship between FEV$_1$ and ADLs

FEV$_1$ (L)	Activity Response
>3	Normal value for adult
2-1.5	Complaints of dyspnea on exertion such as carrying packages or climbing stairs
about 1	Breathlessness when trying to perform ADLs such as cooking, cleaning, bathing, dressing, walking
	Subject to complications of carbon dioxide retention and cor pulmonale
<0.75	Individual unable to work, usually housebound

Data from Fries.[29]

(FEV$_1$) decreases before signs of illness appear. Once signs are evident, the FEV$_1$ measurement (after bronchodilator administration) may be the best indicator of the prognosis. Table 2-6 summarizes the relationship between FEV$_1$ and ADLs.

•••••• Pathophysiology

Chronic bronchitis   One of the earliest changes in chronic bronchitis appears in the secondary glands. Hypertrophy and hypersecretion occur in the goblet cells and bronchial mucous glands. The goblet cells and the mucous gland cells increase in size and number. The goblet cells extend distally into the terminal bronchioles, where they are not normally found. The net result is increased amounts of sputum, bronchial congestion, and narrowing of bronchioles and small bronchi. With time the normally sterile lower respiratory tract becomes colonized by bacteria, and an increased number of polymorphonuclear neutrophil (PMN) leukocytes is found in the secretions. These leukocytes probably stimulate further bronchial swelling and eventual tissue destruction. As the bronchial wall becomes diseased, granulated and fibrotic squamous epithelium re-places the normal ciliated epithelium. This scarring leads to narrowing and airway obstruction.[31,78] The narrowing results in an increased work of breathing, air trapping, and gas exchange abnormalities related to V/Q mismatching. Measurements demonstrate an increased residual volume, reduced FEV$_1$ and FEV$_1$/forced vital capacity (FVC) ratio, hypoxemia, and, as the disease progresses, CO$_2$ retention.

Emphysema   The main defect underlying emphysema is the derangement of lung elastin by the neutral proteases, the most important of which is elastase. Elastase is made and released by PMN leukocytes and alveolar macrophages. Protease and antiprotease activity is normally in balance to prevent lung destruction. Stimuli such as cigarette smoking appear to increase protease activity and therefore make the person susceptible to lung destruction. One of the antiproteases is alpha-1 antitrypsin. Some individuals have a genetic abnormality and do not produce alpha-1 antitrypsin. These persons often develop severe emphysema in early adulthood. Alpha-1 antitrypsin deficiency is relatively rare and accounts for less than 1% of cases of emphysema.

The lungs of the patient with emphysema are very large, hyperinflated because of the loss of recoil with the destruction of the terminal respiratory units (Figure 2-23). When the destructive changes are concentrated in the respiratory bronchioles and alveolar ducts, the emphysema is described as centriacinar. When the destructive changes involve the entire terminal respiratory unit, the term *panacinar* is used. Panacinar emphysema is the type that leads to bulla formation. Bullae are areas of destruction that become severely hyperinflated due to a ball valve effect; air gets in but cannot get out. (Bullae look like large, thin-walled, empty balloons). Panacinar emphysema is also the type most frequently seen in alpha-1 antitrypsin deficiency. Another characteristic of the changes seen in alpha-1 deficiency is that the destructive changes are seen most commonly in the lower lobes, while in the usual smoking related emphysema the destructive changes are often more predominant in the upper lobes.

Two important consequences of emphysema are air trapping and decreased gas exchange. The air trapping is caused by a loss of elastic recoil. Ventilation is regionally decreased, not only because of the elastic recoil problems, but also because of poor support of terminal airways. This increases collapsibility of the noncartilaginous peripheral bronchioles. The decreased gas exchange is a result of the loss of gas exchange surface and the uneven distribution of ventilation and perfusion. The measurable result of these processes is a decrease in FEV, and FEV/FVC, an increase in the FRC and total lung capacity (TLC), increased compliance, and hypoxemia.

•••••• Diagnostic Studies and Findings

Chronic bronchitis and emphysema are typically "silent" for years before the patient has even minimal symptoms. When symptoms appear, usually at age 50 to 60, diagnostic studies evaluating the shortness of breath and cough are generally performed.

Pulmonary function   FEV$_1$ (forced expiratory volume in 1 second): decreased, may fall as much as 50 to 75 ml/year; FVC (forced vital capacity): decreased; FEV$_1$/FVC ratio: decreased; TLC: increased in emphysema because of decreased elastic recoil; RV (residual volume): increased in emphysema because of decreased elastic recoil and air trapping and in chronic bronchitis because of air trapping; FRC: increased in C (compliance): increased in emphysema; R$_{aw}$ (airway resistance): increased in both chronic bronchitis and emphysema.

Arterial blood gases   Alveolar-arterial (A-a) oxygen gradient: widened; Pao$_2$: decreased; Paco$_2$: increased in late, severe disease (more common in patients with chronic bronchitis than those with emphysema).

Chest roentgenogram   Big lung with flattened diaphragm and increased A-P diameter; in emphysema, vascular markings may be decreased and bullae may be present.

Laboratory values   Hemoglobin and hematocrit may be elevated if patient chronically hypoxemic.

ECG   May show atrial arrhythmias; tall, symmetric P waves in leads II, III, and AVF; vertical QRS axis; and signs of right ventricular hypertrophy late in the disease.

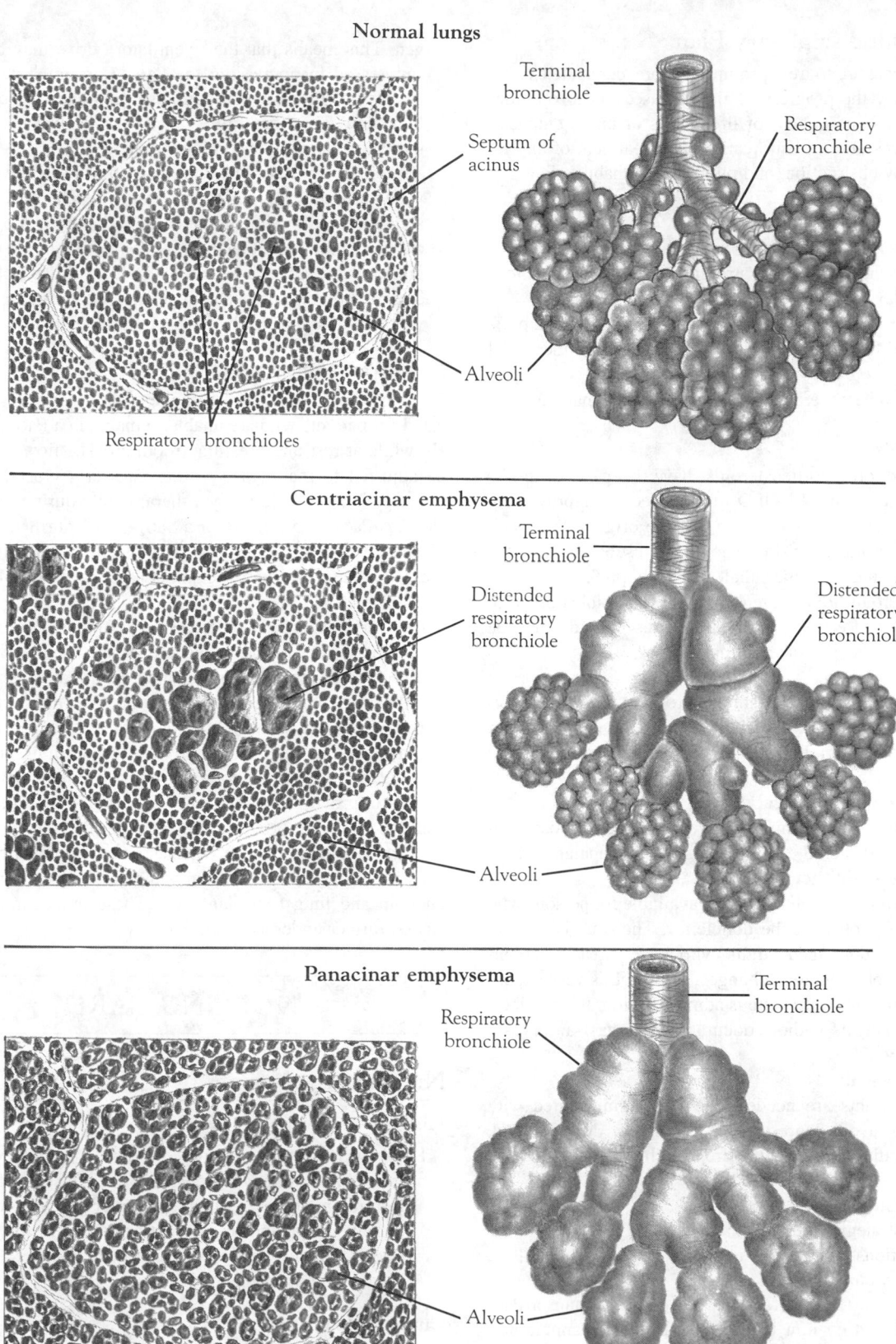

Figure 2-23 Types of emphysema. (From McCance and Huether.[56])

•••••• Multidisciplinary Plan

The goals of care are to treat promptly or prevent acute exacerbations, to slow the progress of the disease, and to optimize functional status and quality of life. Areas of major emphasis are smoking cessation, identification and treatment of any reversible airway obstruction, and pulmonary rehabilitation.

Medications

Bronchodilators

Inhaled anticholinergics (ipratropium): 2 to 3 puffs 3 to 4 times a day

Inhaled beta agonists (albuterol, metaproterenol, etc): 2 puffs as needed for shortness of breath up to 4 to 5 times in 24 hours

Methyl xanthines: therapeutic levels should be maintained at 8 to 15 $\mu g/ml$

Corticosteroids

Inhaled and oral corticosteroids have been used in the chronic treatment of COPD. If no objective improvement is evident after 2 weeks (longer if the original trial is on inhaled steroids), the drug should be discontinued. If the drug is maintained, the inhaled form is preferred. If oral corticosteroids are required, the lowest possible dose with therapeutic effect is used. Intravenous steroids may be used during acute exacerbations

Antibiotics

Broad-spectrum antibiotics are used to treat infectious exacerbations (should be evidence of infection such as fever, leukocytosis, etc.). In chronic management, antibiotics are begun without culture reports

Influenza and pneumococcal vaccines

Influenza vaccine is administered yearly. Pneumococcal vaccine is administered every 6 years in this population[77]

Alpha-1-antitrypsin therapy

Antitrypsin replacement therapy is available for persons who are homozygotes for the deficiency. The drug is used in younger middle-aged adults who have already demonstrated emphysematous changes. The drug is very expensive and requires intravenous administration. It is not indicated in patients without documented alpha-1-antitrypsin deficiency

Psychoactive agents

If antidepressants are needed, they are administered with caution to avoid depression of ventilatory drive; if used, the benzodiazepines are the drug of choice

General Management

Acute exacerbations

Treatment strategies are aimed at the underlying cause of the exacerbations when known (e.g., infection, heart failure, pulmonary emboli)

Oxygen Administered at rates sufficient to maintain a PaO_2 between 55 and 65 mm Hg, usually by nasal cannula at a flow rate of 1 to 3 L/minute. Because patients with chronic bronchitis and emphysema may have chronic hypercapnia, they are considered to be sensitive to increased alveolar oxygen. This means that their ventilatory drive may be further suppressed by increasing the PaO_2. Care must be taken to closely monitor oxygen administration and to increase the flow slowly and carefully. Use of the Venturi mask allows more precise oxygen administration

Mechanical ventilation: Noninvasive mechanical ventilation via a mask may be used to improve gas exchange. Intubation and mechanical ventilation may be necessary if supplemental oxygen cannot maintain the PaO_2 above 40 mm Hg with a pH greater than 7.25. If a patient with severe airways obstructive disease requires surgery with general anesthesia, mechanical ventilation is likely to be required postoperatively

Long-Term Management

Oxygen: Continuous oxygen therapy via nasal prongs is indicated for patients who are unable to maintain a PaO_2 of 55 mm Hg while at rest and breathing room air. The flow rate should be adjusted to maintain a resting PaO_2 close to 60 mm Hg. Some patients require oxygen therapy only during exercise or sleep. A PaO_2 <55 mm Hg or a SaO_2 <88% during activity indicates oxygen need. Oxygen is most often administered to these patients by nasal cannula or transtracheal oxygen catheter.

Chest physiotherapy: Breathing techniques are taught to control dyspnea. Cough techniques are taught to improve airway clearance. Percussion and postural drainage are used only for patients with large amounts of sputum production (p. 200 for techniques).

Physical Training: Although physical training (bicycling, walking, arm exercises) does not improve pulmonary function, it does improve oxygen consumption and work tolerance. In addition, there are often psychosocial benefits to training.

Surgical intervention: In selected cases, surgical treatment is used for emphysema. Procedures include bullectomy, lung reduction, and lung transplantation. These procedures are discussed further under Thoracic Surgery.

NURSING CARE

Nursing Assessment

History

Smoking history and history of known respiratory irritants including duration of exposure to each; history of previous respiratory diseases, infections, allergies, etc.; history of chronic cough and characteristics; family history of respiratory diseases; description of activity tolerance including fatigue and dyspnea precipitation

Current Medications

Careful and complete history of current respiratory-related medications, as well as use of over-the-counter medications and inhalers; observe and evaluate use of inhalers

Use of Oxygen

History of use of oxygen. Include when initiated, delivery device, liter flow, when used, therapeutic response

Use of Home Ventilator

Home (usually night time) ventilation is used only in selected cases. If used, note when it was initiated, ventilator settings, when the modality is used, and therapeutic response

Respiratory Status

Assessment data are derived from a variety of sources. Observed symptoms of impaired status include dyspnea, cough, sputum production, use of accessory muscles, tripod posture, barrel chest. Observe for a paradoxic inward movement of the lower chest with inspiration (usually associated with severe hyperinflation). Auscultory findings in COPD include prolonged expiratory phase, decreased breath sounds, wheeze, hyperresonance. Pulsus paradoxus may be present. Pulmonary function studies should be viewed if available, especially FEV_1 level. Assess for changes in respiratory excursion related to fatigue

Gas Exchange

Note that symptoms are indicators of a gas exchange problem, but arterial blood gases are needed for verification. Not uncommonly, symptoms will appear worse than blood gases and vice versa. Gas exchange problems are not anticipated until the FEV_1 falls below 50% predicted

Symptoms of severe hypoxemia include restlessness, tachycardia, confusion, hypotension, cyanosis, and dysrhythmias. Signs and symptoms of chronic hypoxemia include fatigue, poor memory, problems concentrating, morning headache. If the Pao_2 is less than 55 mm Hg chronically, a secondary erythrocytosis may be seen. Symptoms of an acute rise in $Paco_2$ include asterixis, mental status changes (the changes are variable; some become somnolent, some become combative). More chronic changes may be detected from changes in electrolytes: an increase in CO_2 and a decrease in cardiac index (CI) (other problems may also cause these changes)

Infection

Elevated temperature; purulent sputum; foul mouth odor or taste; pleuritic pain

Nutrition

Malaise and anorexia; weight loss

Major Complications

Cor pulmonale, respiratory failure, severe hypoxemia, pneumothorax, pulmonary emboli

Nursing Dx & Intervention

Ineffective airway clearance related to tenacious secretions, impaired mucociliary clearance, impaired cough effectiveness

- Ensure adequate hydration to replace fluid loss.
- Teach cough techniques to improve cough effectiveness.
- Administer bronchodilators as ordered (may improve mucociliary function; higher flow rates will improve cough effectiveness).
- Administer aerosol therapy and perform postural drainage, if ordered, at least 1 hour after meals.
- Perform airway clearance techniques (e.g., cough) following bronchodilator treatments when airway maximally dilated.
- Note changes in adventitial sounds on chest auscultation, changes in cough, sputum characteristics.

Ineffective breathing pattern related to fatigue, hyperinflation, airway obstruction

- Teach and ensure correct use of bronchodilator inhalers to promote bronchodilation.
- Position patient in tripod position to maximize use of respiratory muscles.
- Instruct and encourage use of controlled breathing pattern and pursed lip exhalation to avoid tachypnea and excessive hyperinflation.
- Avoid use of upper limb activity during episodes of dyspnea (impairs use of accessory muscles).
- Implement airway clearance techniques as indicated above to reduce obstruction.
- Avoid exposure to irritants such as cigarette smoke and perfumes, which might precipitate bronchospasm.
- Plan care to ensure adequate rest periods.
- Should mechanical ventilation become necessary, provide care and monitoring as discussed in that section.

Impaired gas exchange related to hypoventilation and/or altered ventilation/perfusion matching

- Monitor pulse oximetry (continuous or periodic checks).
- Monitor arterial blood gases; report increases in $Paco_2$ and decreases in Pao_2 of more than 10 mm Hg. Any Pao_2 below 50 mm Hg or pH less than 7.3 should be reported.
- Administer oxygen as ordered to maintain Pao_2 of no less than 55 mm Hg (value in 60s is preferred); this usually may be maintained by administration of oxygen by nasal cannula at a flow rate of 1 to 3 L/min; if needed a Venturi mask may be used. Caution must be exercised to avoid overoxygenation and possible depression of ventilation.
- Ensure that oxygen is not discontinued during times of increased need (e.g., walking, going to bathroom, sleep).
- During acute exacerbations avoid unnecessary increases in oxygen consumption by activity, medications, etc.
- Avoid depressing ventilation by excessive sedation, sleeping medications, etc.

- Monitor electrocardiogram and cardiac status for dysrhythmias secondary to alterations in blood gases.
- Monitor for signs of cor pulmonale such as increasing pedal edema, jugular venous distention, weight gain, positive fluid balance, hepatomegaly; other signs include pulmonary hypertension and elevated CVP.
- Monitor serum electrolytes, especially CO_2 and Cl, which may indicate changes in $Paco_2$ and/or acid base status.

Altered nutrition: less than body requirements related to dyspnea and fatigue

- Assess for signs and symptoms of malnutrition.
- Assist patient to choose foods that are easy to chew and swallow; assist by cutting and feeding if patient tires easily. *Medications, sputum, and shortness of breath may cause anorexia, nausea, and vomiting.*
- Avoid gas-producing foods.
- Encourage smaller, more frequent meals.
- If indicated, and in consultation with physician, administer stool softeners *to relieve constipation.*

Risk for infection related to impaired airway clearance and immune function

- Assess for signs and symptoms of infection, fever, dyspnea, and change in sputum color, amount, or odor.
- Obtain sputum for culture and sensitivity.
- Protect patients from known sources of secondary infection.

Knowledge deficit related to disease process

- Explain and reinforce explanation of the disease, medications, and other treatment, including oxygen and exercise.
- Encourage patient and family to ask questions.
- Explain and discuss different medications necessary for treating the disease.

Impaired physical mobility related to deconditioning

- Encourage patient to use adaptive breathing techniques during activity to *decrease the work of breathing.*
- Assist patient to space activities *to provide periods of rest in between* and prolong endurance.
- Encourage gradual increase of activities as tolerated to increase muscle mass.
- Problem solve with patient to determine methods of conserving energy while still performing ADL (e.g., using stool to sit while in the bathroom shaving).
- Assess and document activities that cause patient to tire easily and become short of breath.
- If patient is seriously ill and maintained on bed rest, encourage or provide active or passive range of motion exercises to *maintain adequate muscle mass.*
- Evaluate during activity for possible increased oxygen need during exercise.

Patient Education/Home Care Planning

1. Teach patient adaptive breathing techniques, and work with family to teach postural drainage techniques.
2. Teach airway clearance techniques.
3. Teach importance of avoiding contact with persons who have upper respiratory infections and influenza.
4. Teach facts about and importance of prescribed medications such as bronchodilators and corticosteroids, including use of inhalers and spacers.
5. Provide patient and family with information regarding chronic lung diseases, how to assess individual capabilities and responses, and what to do during an acute episode of difficult breathing.
6. Teach change in health status that must be reported to the patient's health care providers; indicators of change may include change in sputum characteristics or color, decreased activity tolerance, increased use of oxygen, decreased appetite, and fever.
7. Teach importance of adequate fluid intake.
8. Teach importance of not smoking and of avoiding dust-producing articles (feathers, animal dander, cleaning equipment), strong cooking odors and perfumes, which may irritate the respiratory tract.
9. Teach eating and food choice modifications.
10. Provide patient and family with information regarding the care, cleaning, and maintenance of inhalation or oxygen equipment to be used at home.
11. Provide patient and family with respiratory-related health information such as pollution indexes, secondary infection exposure, and community support and exercise groups.
12. Advise patient to avoid using powders and aerosol products, which may cause bronchospasm.

Evaluation

Airway clearance   Sputum and cough are absent or minimal. Sputum, if present, should be clear or white. No rhonchi on auscultation. Chest roentgenogram shows no infiltrates. Patient can demonstrate effective cough techniques.

Breathing pattern   Lung function improved following exacerbation; FEV_1 and FVC are at patient's usual level. Dyspnea reduced; patient able to speak in complete sentences. Patient demonstrates techniques to control dyspnea. Patient and family can discuss energy-conserving strategies.

Gas exchange Pao_2 is greater than 60 mm Hg. $Paco_2$ is normal for patient; pH is in normal range. Patient understands use of home oxygen if indicated.

Nutrition   Patient and family can describe modifications in meal scheduling and food selection to improve nutritional status.

Activity level   Patient and family understand importance of regular exercise program. Patient and family are able to state ways to maintain/increase exercise in the home setting.

Knowledge Patient and family can state medications, their dosage, and schedule. Patient demonstrates correct use of inhalers. Patient and family can state signs and symptoms for which they should contact health care provider.

■ ASTHMA[10,15,57,63,91]

Asthma, although a common problem, does not have a universally accepted definition. Certain characteristics generally accepted to define asthma are hyperresponsive airways, inflammation, and airway obstruction that is reversible either spontaneously or with treatment. The results of these changes include episodic dyspnea with wheeze, mucus hypersecretion, which may progress to mucus plugging, and chronic airway inflammation (Figure 2-24). Status asthmaticus is the term used to describe an asthma exacerbation that does not respond to usual therapy.

Asthma affects more than 10 million people in the United States, and the prevalence is increasing. In those under the age of 20, the prevalence is about 5%; in adults the prevalence rate is about 3.4%. Hospitalization rates and health care costs are also increasing, as are mortality rates. In 1988, more than 4500 persons died from asthma in the United States. Certain risk factors for mortality have been identified. Prevalence and mortality rates are significantly higher in African Americans than in whites. Also, patients with asthma who have had a prior episode of respiratory failure during an asthmatic attack are at greater risk. The most important factor, however, is inadequate treatment.

In recognition of the increasing asthma problem, a National Asthma Education Program (NAEP) was initiated by the National Institutes of Health. Experts from a variety of health care disciplines and care consumers reviewed the current literature and current practice. In 1991, the *Guidelines for the Diagnosis and Management of Asthma* was published. Subsequent publications have included a *Clinicians Guide, Guidelines for the Diagnosis and Management of Asthma during Pregnancy,* and *Diagnosis and Management of Asthma in the Elderly.* The purpose of the NAEP is to educate health care professionals and consumers so as to improve the management of asthma and thus reduce morbidity and mortality.

•••••• Pathophysiology

Bronchial hyperreactivity and airway inflammation are the hallmarks of asthma. The origin of these changes can be related to allergy in the majority of cases. The allergic reaction is one of immediate hypersensitivity mediated by IgE. The reaction of an aeroallergen and IgE causes mast cells to degranulate with the release of mediators. Many of these mediators can directly cause bronchospasm. Others stimulate cytokine production and the influx of inflammatory cells. Many believe that the chronic inflammation contributes to the bronchial hyperreactivity. The mediators and inflammation also contribute to mucus hypersecretion and airway edema. In addition to allergens, other stimuli such as infections, chemical irritants, and physical stim-

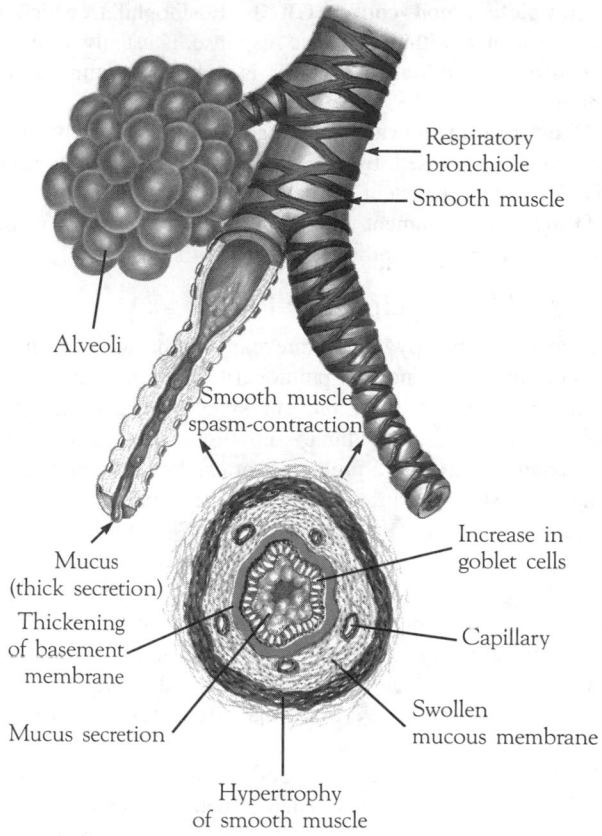

Figure 2-24 In bronchial asthma, the bronchiole is obstructed by muscle spasm, edema of the mucosa, inflammation, and thick secretions. (From Wilson.[93])

ulation can stimulate mediator release. In addition, the irritant receptors are stimulated, resulting in an increase in vagal tone.

All of these factors lead to airways obstruction. Air trapping occurs and the FRC increases. As a result of the overinflation, the patient uses the accessory muscles of respiration. Gas exchange abnormalities occur because of ventilation/perfusion mismatching. There is hypoxemia, but the patient is usually able to hyperventilate. In severe exacerbations, when the FEV_1 falls to 25% of predicted value, hypoventilation may occur.

•••••• Diagnostic Studies and Findings

Pulmonary function Decrease in peak expiratory flow (PEF) and FEV_{-1} with exacerbations. In mild disease these measurements may be near 80% predicted; as the severity of disease worsens, so does the fall in FEV_1 and PEF. Increased variability in flows between AM and PM measures is usually present, and there is at least a 15% increase in FEV_{-1} postbronchodilator administration. The FEV_{-1}/FVC ratio is decreased during attacks and FRC is increased.

Arterial blood gases Pao_2 is decreased; there is usually hyperventilation with a respiratory alkalosis. Hypoventilation with a rise in $Paco_2$ does not occur until the FEV_{-1} falls to approximately 25% of predicted.

Complete blood count (CBC)   Eosinophilia, which is often associated with the allergic response, is usually seen.

Sputum examination   There is usually sputum eosinophilia.

Chest roentgenogram   The radiograph is usually clear. Hyperinflation caused by air trapping may occur in acute episodes and in persistent, chronic cases.

Other   Measurement of IgE antibodies; evaluation of pH if gastric reflux a possibility; evaluation of sinuses.

•••••• Multidisciplinary Plan

The goals of therapy are to prevent asthma attacks, maintain normal or near normal pulmonary function, prevent side effects from medications, prevent symptoms, and maintain normal activity levels. Asthma is now looked on as a chronic illness and is treated as a problem that can be controlled rather than cured. Most important, however, is the goal of preventing symptoms.

Medications

Pharmacologic therapy for asthma includes bronchodilators and antiinflammatories. The use of the drugs is determined by the severity of the disease. The mild and moderate forms are treated at home; severe asthma often requires hospitalization.

Mild disease (infrequent episodes of cough and/or wheeze):
Inhaled beta-agonists (albuterol, metaproterenol, and others): 2 puffs every 3 to 4 hours as needed to treat symptoms (should not need more than 1 to 2 times a week); also used before exposure to known triggers such as exercise
Cromolyn may be used before trigger exposure; usually used in younger adults
Moderate disease (symptoms more than 1 to 2 times a week)
Inhaled beta-agonist as above
May add theophylline, a bronchodilator
May add ipratropium, a bronchodilator, especially in the elderly patient with coexisting bronchitic symptoms
Add inhaled steroids (beclomethasone and others) 4 to 6 puffs twice a day
Severe disease (continuous symptoms; pulmonary function less than 60% baseline)
As above for moderate disease
Increase dose of inhaled steroids
add burst of oral corticosteroids
Exacerbations requiring hospitalization: in addition to above
Inhaled beta-agonist treatments increased to q20-30 min. × 3 and then adjusted according to response (usually initially delivered by small volume nebulizer; eventually by metered dose inhaler [MDI])
If inhaled beta-agonists ineffective may give subcutaneous epinephrine (not usually used in adults >40 years)
Systemic corticosteroids, 80 to 125 mg methylprednisolone intravenously in adults (oral prednisone is also used); may require 60 to 80 mg every 6 to 8 hours
Theophylline, oral or intravenous; maintain serum level of 5 to 15 micrograms/ml

General Management

Oxygenation: humidified oxygen is administered by nasal cannula or mask to maintain PaO_2 in 60 to 70 mm Hg range; oxygen saturation should be ≥93%

Fluid and electrolyte therapy: fluids are given to maintain water balance (insensible loss increased with rapid respiratory rate and intake often decreased due to shortness of breath)

Environment: avoid exposure to triggers; maintain calm environment

Immunotherapy: desensitization is used in patients for whom allergen avoidance is not possible; allergens most likely to be involved are house dust mite, cat dander, alternaria, and grass pollen

Mechanical ventilation: in severe disease that does not respond to pharmacologic therapy, intubation and mechanical ventilation may be required; the goal of therapy is to improve gas exchange without excessive peak inflation pressures; as the patient improves, the $PaCO_2$ will normalize. Patients requiring mechanical ventilation may require sedation. (Sedation is avoided in the nonintubated patient with asthma.)

Follow-up: it is imperative that any patient seen in the emergency room or hospitalized for an asthma exacerbation have a follow-up appointment with a caregiver (Table 2-7)

NURSING CARE

Nursing Assessment

Asthma must be assessed not only in the areas of concern listed but also as to its overall severity on both a short- and long-term basis. Table 2-8 summarizes this assessment.

History

Known family or personal history of allergy, infantile eczema, or previous episodes of asthma
Previous recent severe attack
Prolonged attack (>4 to 36 hours)

TABLE 2-7   Assessment of Asthma Severity in Patients Requiring Urgent Care

Assessment	Action
Good outcome: PEFR or FEV_{-1} ≥70% predicted no wheezes	Discharge home with follow-up
Incomplete response: PEFR or FEV_{-1} 40%-70% predicted; wheezing; shortness of breath	Continue care and assessment
Poor response: PEFR of FEV_{-1} <40% predicted wheezing; pulsus paradoxus >12 mm Hg; accessory muscle use; SpO_2 <90%	Admit to hospital
Respiratory failure: poor response with $PaCO_2$ ≥40 mm Hg	Admit to intensive care

■ TABLE 2-8 Assessment of Severity of Asthma

Mild	Moderate	Severe
PEFR > 80% predicted Variability <20%	PEFR 0-80% predicted Variability 20-30%; 15% response to bronchodilators	PEFR < 60% predicted Variability > 30%
Attacks no more than once or twice a week	Cough and wheeze episodes more than 2 per week	Daily wheezing Frequent severe episodes
Responds to bronchodilators in 12 to 24 hours	Cough and low-grade wheeze between acute episodes	Hospitalization frequently required to break cycle
No signs of asthma between episodes	Exercise tolerance diminished	Poor exercise tolerance
No sleep interruption due to asthma	May be up at night because of cough and wheeze	Much sleep interruption
No hyperventilation	Hyperinflation seen on chest roentgenogram	
Normal chest roentgenogram	Lung volumes may be increased	Airway obstruction may not be completely reversed by bronchodilators
Minimal evidence of airway obstruction	Urgent care or Emergency Department visits <3/year	Lung volumes increased
No to minimal degree of increase in lung volume	Exacerbations take 7 or more days to respond	
Continuous drug therapy not required	Steroids needed during exacerbation	

Modified from Berkow,[5] Ellis.[21]

Previous hospitalization for asthma
Previous history of respiratory failure
Previous requirement for steroids

Current Medications

Careful and complete history of current respiratory-related medications, as well as most recent dose and time before hospital arrival

Respiratory Status

Peak flow measures (see Table 2-8)
Airway clearance: presence of cough/sputum
Respiratory distress: dyspnea, tachypnea, cough, prolonged expiration, use of accessory muscles during breathing, retractions; speaks in short phrases; sits upright
Breath sounds: with increasing obstruction, progress from expiratory wheeze to inspiratory/expiratory wheeze, to decreased wheeze with barely audible breath sounds

Skin

Increased diaphoresis as respiratory distress increases

Hypoxia

Restlessness, tachycardia; confusion, hypotension, cyanosis, premature ventricular contractions, fatigue

Hydration

Intake and output to monitor hydration

Psychosocial

Anxiety
Fear of suffocation

Nursing Dx & Intervention

Ineffective breathing pattern related to airways obstruction, anxiety, fatigue

- Identify contributing factors such as allergens in immediate environment or other irritants that may exacerbate condition.
- Maintain patient positioning *to facilitate ventilation* (i.e., sitting upright and leaning forward on overbed table).
- Instruct patient in pulmonary hygiene routines *that facilitate breathing and minimize pulmonary congestion that could lead to secondary infections.*
- Initiate preventive measures such as uninterrupted periods of quiet time; maintain calm and restful environment; encourage patient to participate in care as tolerated; explain all therapy before administering *to improve breathing pattern.*
- Encourage patient to use adaptive breathing techniques to prolong expiratory time.
- Assist patient to space activities *to provide periods of rest in between.*
- Cover pillows with allergen-proof covers *to eliminate dust and other irritants.*
- Problem solve with patient to determine methods of conserving energy while still performing activities of daily living *to prevent further depression of respiratory status.*
- Assist to protect patient from known sources of secondary infection.
- If mechanical ventilation is required, provide care and monitoring consistent with the guidelines presented on pp. 205 to 207.

Risk for infection related to steroid therapy and ineffective airway clearance

- Assess mouth and oral mucosa for presence of mouth irritation *to prevent possible mouth infection secondary to inhaled corticosteroids.*
- Instruct patient using inhaled corticosteroids to perform thorough mouth washing after each use *to prevent mouth irritation and oral candidiasis.*
- Assess for secondary respiratory infection resulting from congested condition.
- Monitor results of CBC and report abnormal leukocyte level.

Altered health maintenance related to asthma

- Assess with patient or family home and environmental stimulants (allergens) that may exacerbate asthma episode.
- Provide education regarding need to avoid contact with irritant allergens.
- Assist with allergy testing and desensitization if indicated.
- Assess for adverse systemic allergic response during allergy testing or desensitization process.
- Instruct patient in use of peak flow meter and in interpretation of results.
- Listen carefully to collect information regarding significance of asthma and patient's perception of ability to deal with alterations it is causing.

Patient Education/Home Care Planning

1. Teach facts about and importance of prescribed medications such as bronchodilators and corticosteroids, including use of inhalers, spacers, and small-volume nebulizers if indicated.
2. Teach the patient how and when to use the peak flow monitor, and how to report results.
3. Provide the patient and family with information about asthma as a disease, how to assess an asthmatic response, what to do during the process of care, criteria for requesting professional assistance, and acute emergency care.
4. Assist the patient and family to examine secondary factors that may precipitate asthmatic episodes such as emotional stress, fatigue, or environmental changes or specific allergen contacts such as dust, animal dander, feathers, and pollen.
5. Teach the patient adaptive breathing techniques and breathing exercises such as pursed-lip breathing and positioning for use during acute exacerbations.
6. Provide the patient and family with information regarding the care, cleaning, and maintenance of inhalation equipment to be used at home.
7. Provide the patient and family with respiratory-related health information such as pollution indexes, secondary infection exposure, and community support groups.

Evaluation

Air moves optimally in and out of lungs. Lungs are fully aerated as visualized on chest roentgenogram Vital capacity measurements including FEV_1 are optimum for patient's status. WBC is within normal limits. Blood gas values are within normal limits. Airways are clear, breath sounds are clear, and breathing occurs without obstruction.

Physiologic function is stable There are no secondary infections.

Patient preserves pulmonary functioning by maintaining optimum activity level, preventing infection, and following prescribed treatments Patient demonstrates correct use of peak flow meter and interpretation of results.

Patient and family have sufficient information to comply with discharge regimen Patient and family are able at time of discharge to discuss medications (purpose, side effects, route, and schedule), activity regimen, signs of infection or respiratory deterioration, and plan for long-term follow-up maintenance.

Patient and family have sufficient information to assist with preventing further asthma episodes or reduce severity of episodes Patient and family discuss pathophysiology of asthma, precipitating factors, and factor avoidance techniques, as well as treatment interventions should episode occur.

■ BRONCHIECTASIS

Bronchiectasis is the chronic dilation of the medium-sized bronchi with eventual destruction of the bronchial elastic and muscular elements. Usually the result of repeated pulmonary infections or bronchial obstruction, this chronic dilation leads to the eventual malfunctioning of bronchial muscle tone and elasticity (Figure 2-25).

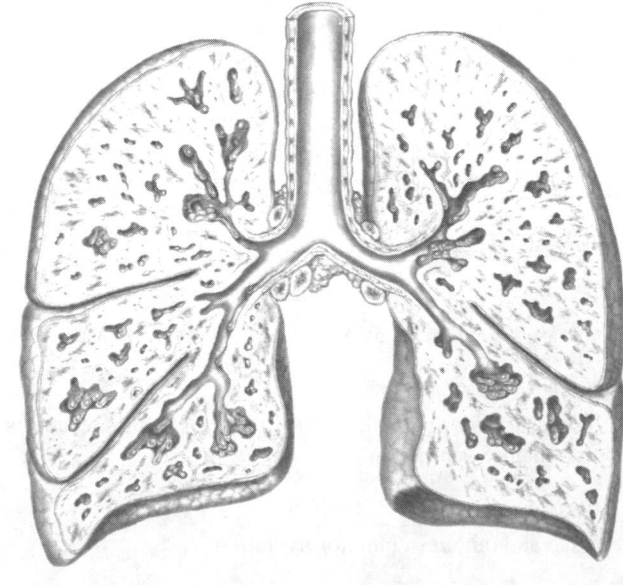

Figure 2-25 Bronchiectasis. (From Wilson.[93])

The incidence of this acquired disorder has decreased greatly since the development of antibiotics and aggressive management of pulmonary infections. Before the use of antibiotics, pulmonary infections sometimes lingered and a sec-ond pulmonary obstruction occurred below the buildup of sputum and bronchial secretions. The chronic obstruction and tissue stretching eventually progress to the destruction of bronchial elasticity and actual malfunctioning of bronchial muscle tone.

Children are at high risk for the development of bronchiectasis. This is because their bronchi are small and soft and easily damaged by prolonged overinflation caused by infection or bronchial foreign body obstruction. The prevalence of childhood bronchiectasis is decreasing because of the use of antibiotics, but it is still seen in children with cystic fibrosis and immune deficiency diseases.

Although disease onset, especially in children, may follow a single episode of pulmonary disease, most adults have a history of numerous pulmonary infections such as pneumonia and a chronic bronchitis type of cough. Delayed resolution of any type of pulmonary disease should raise suspicion of bronchiectasis.

• • • • • • Pathophysiology

Bronchiectasis is almost always caused by a failure of normal lung defenses to infection and a failure to clear bronchial se-cretions. This may be the result of primary or secondary ciliary dysfunction, aspiration of gastric acid or a foreign body, bronchial obstruction by a tumor, or abnormal mucus clearance of cystic fibrosis or allergic aspergillosis. Failure of the immune system may also predispose an individual to infection leading to bronchiectasis. These various factors often occur together and are more likely to cause severe, chronic airway and pulmonary injury in the developing bronchial tree of the child. The most important interrelationships are shown in Figure 2-26.[13]

The development of bronchiectasis usually occurs over a period of time where a recurrence of an inflammatory and infectious process slowly alters the structure of the bronchial walls and their elastic and muscular response. Once the alterations have occurred, they are irreversible.

• • • • • • Diagnostic Studies and Findings

Clinical examination   Severe and chronic, mucopurulent, sputum-producing cough; hemoptysis; moist rales and rhonchi heard over the lower lobes; dyspnea; fatigue; and general signs of pulmonary insufficiency

Bronchography   Definitive diagnostic procedure of bronchiectasis; bronchography outlines walls of bronchi and clearly shows bronchiectatic areas

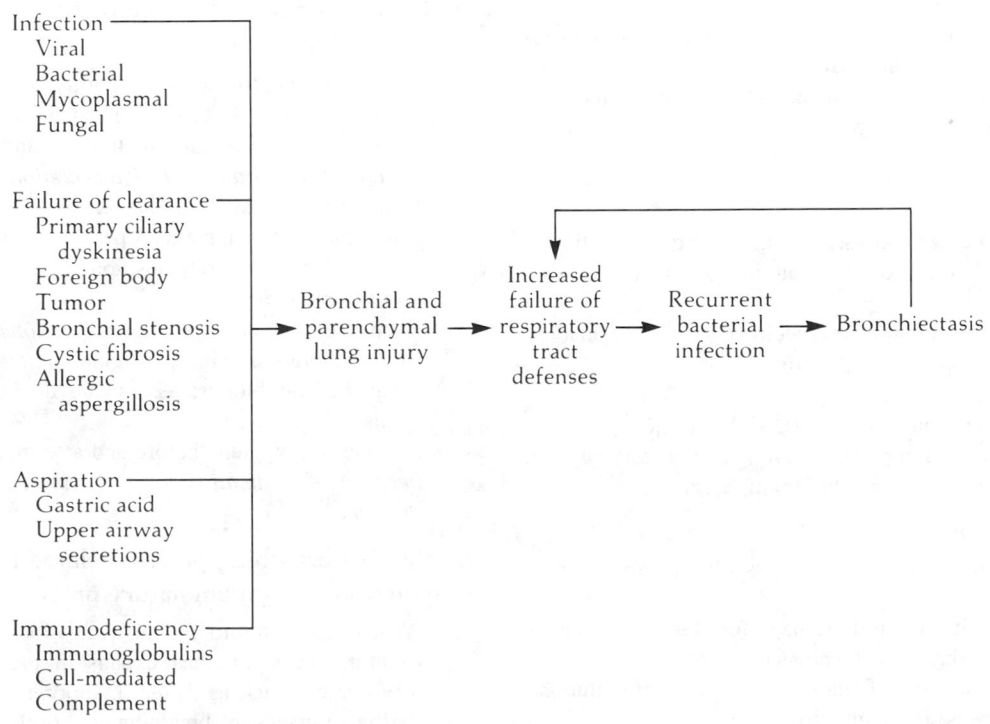

Figure 2-26 Pathogenesis of bronchiectasis. (From Cherniack.[13])

Sputum examination   Gross examination shows that the sputum has three layers (sediment, fluid, and foam); a sputum smear is done to rule out tuberculosis and identify secondary bacterial infections such as those caused by pneumococci, *Pseudomonas,* and *Enterobacter;* large numbers of white blood cells and bacteria that mostly include pharyngeal flora, including anaerobic organisms, are usually seen; the decision on choice of antibiotics in the treatment of the intercurrent infection depends on the result of culture and sensitivity studies of sputum

Complete blood count (CBC)   With severe hypoxia may show polycythemia secondary to pulmonary insufficiency

Pulmonary function   Spirometry may reveal a decreased forced expiratory volume (FEV_1) and a decreased forced vital capacity (FVC); many patients with mild to moderate bronchiectasis will have no abnormality detectable by routine spirometry and arterial blood gas analysis

Chest roentgenogram   Clear but may show patches of inflammation with increased pulmonary markings at the lung bases

•••••• Multidisciplinary Plan

The goals of the medical plan are to maintain maximum ventilation by controlling infections and removing secretions.

Surgery

Bronchial resection—may rarely be performed on patients with isolated areas of bronchiectasis that do not respond to conservative treatment; this disease may be localized enough to permit complete resection without compromising pulmonary function

Chest Roentgenogram

Clear, but may show some areas of inflammation with increased markings at the base

Mediastinal shift may be seen secondary to overinflation of specific lobes of the lung

Medications

Mucolytic agents

Acetylcysteine (Mucomyst), nebulization q2-6h with 20% solution (1-10 ml) or 10% solution (2-20 ml)

Antiinfective agents

Antibiotic therapy should be specific to the organism identified in the sputum evaluation

Bronchodilators

Ipratropium bromide (Atrovent), 40-80 μg q6h

Theophylline used in rare cases, long acting, 200 mg q12h increased in a few days to 300 mg q12h

General Management

Warm or cool mist via vaporizer to assist in liquefying of secretions

Physiotherapy with postural drainage for at least 10 minutes 3 or 4 times a day (p. 200 shows technique)

Warm, dry climate void of smoke, fumes, and air pollution

Patient discouraged from smoking

Fluid increase to liquefy secretions and maintain hydration

Periodic sputum culture to identify presence of secondary infections

---

NURSING CARE

Nursing Assessment

Respiratory Status

Breath sounds: rales and rhonchi over lower lobes

Breathing patterns: may be labored with prolonged expiration; increased dyspnea

Cough: chronic with production of large quantities of purulent sputum (coughing and sputum production may become worse with changes in posture and activity)

Hemoptysis in 50% of cases

Chest wall may have retractions during breathing and decreased expiratory excursion

Respiratory failure will eventually develop

Cardiovascular Response

In advanced cases, cyanosis and clubbing of fingers

Generalized Response

Weight loss, night sweats, fever, gradual emaciation may be indications of disease progression with possible secondary infections

Nursing Dx & Intervention

Ineffective airway clearance related to mucopurulent sputum

• Assess patient to identify inability to move secretions; promote aggressive techniques such as positioning, postural drainage, coughing, suctioning, and fluid promotion *to liquefy and drain excessive secretions.*(See p. 200 for techniques of postural drainage.)

• Assist patient to maintain proper body positioning and frequent alteration of body position *to ensure patient airway and secretion drainage.*

• Suction if necessary *to remove secretions.*

• In collaboration with physician, administer mucolytic drugs and antibiotics; assess and document patient response.

• Provide oral hygiene before and after respiratory therapy *because of medication taste and increased sputum production.*

Ineffective breathing pattern related to bronchial obstruction and inflammatory process

• Assess ventilation to include evaluation of breathing rate, rhythm, and depth, chest expansion, presence of respiratory distress such as dyspnea, shortness of breath, nasal flaring, pursed-lip breathing or prolonged expiratory phase, use of abdominal muscles.

• Periodically assess FEV_1 and FVC *to evaluate pulmonary function.*

- Instruct patient in hygiene routines that facilitate easy and effective breathing.
- Assess patient for tiring in relation to attempts to breathe.

Impaired gas exchange related to compromised airway exchange

- Assess patient to identify signs such as restlessness, confusion, and irritability, which *may indicate the body's response to altered blood gas states.*
- Carefully monitor body temperature, sputum characteristics, and cough characteristics, which *may indicate the presence of secondary infection and which may lead to respiratory insufficiency if not properly treated.*
- Assist patient to avoid environmental irritants such as smoke, fumes, and air pollution; patient should also be instructed not to smoke.
- Monitor and record kidney function and urinary output, which *may be affected secondary to chronic tissue hypoxia and alterations in metabolism.*
- Monitor serum electrolytes, which *may change because of alterations in oxygenation and metabolism.*

Risk for infection related to decreased physiologic state

- Assess for signs and symptoms of infection, fever, dyspnea, and change in sputum color, amount, or odor.
- Obtain sputum for culture and sensitivity.
- Protect patient from known source of secondary infection, which may lead to respiratory insufficiency.

Altered nutrition: less than body requirements related to decompensated physical state

- Assess for signs and symptoms of malnutrition.
- Assist patient to choose foods that are easy to chew and swallow; assist by cutting and feeding if patient tires easily.
- Encourage smaller, more frequent meals.
- Encourage fluid intake of at least 2 L/day to *facilitate liquefying of secretions and promote urinary output.* (If patient has compromised cardiac or renal condition, fluid intake must be determined in collaboration with physician.)

Impaired physical mobility related to decompensated physical state

- Encourage patient to use adaptive breathing techniques *to decrease the work of breathing.*
- Assist patient to space activities *to provide periods of rest in between.*
- Encourage gradual increase of activities as tolerated *to prevent "pulmonary crippling."*
- Problem solve with patient to determine methods of conserving energy while still performing activities of daily living.
- Assess and document activities that cause patient to tire easily and become short of breath.
- If patient is seriously ill and maintained on bed rest, encourage or provide active or passive range of motion exercises *to maintain adequate muscle tone.*

Patient Education/Home Care Planning

1. Teach patient adaptive breathing techniques such as pursed-lip and abdominal breathing.
2. Teach patient to prevent secondary infections by coughing and deep breathing, which will prevent the accumulation of secretion buildup in the lungs.
3. Teach importance of not smoking and avoiding fumes or smoke during active disease state.
4. Teach adaptive exercise and rest techniques.
5. Teach eating and food choice modifications.
6. Teach importance of getting immunizations to prevent illnesses.
7. Teach facts about and importance of prescribed medications.
8. Provide patient and family with respiratory-related health information such as pollution indexes, home humidification techniques, and climate changes.
9. Teach importance of avoidance of contact with other persons who may expose patient to a secondary infection.
10. Teach signs of secondary infection such as change in characteristics of sputum or prolonged fever.

Evaluation

Air moves optimally in and out of lungs   Coughing if present is productive of sputum.

Airway is patent   Airways are clear and breathing occurs without obstruction.

Chest roentgenogram is clear   No evidence of overinflation or infiltration is seen.

Patient is free of secondary respiratory infection   Sputum evaluation shows no evidence of a secondary respiratory infection.

Breathing pattern occurs without tiring patient   Patient demonstrates modified breathing techniques that facilitate ventilatory capacity. Behavior is modified to conserve energy expenditure.

Physiologic function is stable   Nutrition level is maintained.

Patient relates importance of daily pulmonary exercises   Patient demonstrates pulmonary exercises and states rationale and importance of maintaining daily exercise routine.

Patient preserves pulmonary functioning by maintaining optimal activity level, preventing infection, and following prescribed treatment   Patient demonstrates a variety of methods indicating ability to preserve and facilitate optimal respiratory functioning (e.g., breathing exercises, modified activities or exercise, taking medications as prescribed).

Patient and family have sufficient information to comply with discharge regimen   Patient and family are able at time of discharge to discuss medications (purpose, side effects, route, and schedule), activity progression regimen, signs of infection or respiratory deterioration, and plan for follow-up visits.

CYSTIC FIBROSIS[38,42,51,52]

Cystic fibrosis (CF) is an autosomal recessive disorder of the exocrine glands that causes those glands to produce abnormally thick secretions of mucus. The glands most affected are the respiratory, pancreatic, and sweat glands (Figure 2-27).

In the United States, CF is the most common cause of life-threatening pulmonary disease of whites during childhood and adolescence. The disease incidence is 1 in 2500 to 3500 live births. One in 25 persons in the United States carries the CF gene. CF is least prevalent in blacks, American Indians, and persons of Asian ancestry. Boys and girls are equally affected.

CF is the primary cause of pancreatic deficiency and chronic malabsorption in children. It is also responsible for many cases of intestinal obstruction in newborns. Although CF is a widespread multisystem disease, the progressive pulmonary infections are the most important clinical problem and are responsible for most of the morbidity and mortality. Advances in the treatment of the respiratory components of the disease have been important in improving the prognosis, but maximum success cannot be achieved unless gastrointestinal, hepatic, and psychologic components and sweat abnormalities are also managed.

There is no known cure for CF, but much has been done to lengthen the survival of patients. Today the median survival time is 28 years, so that CF is a disease of both children and adults. In 1989, a CF gene was identified. Since then, it has been determined that several genes are involved. Future therapy may involve genetic manipulation to prevent the disease.

Therapy for patients with CF is aimed at improving the nutritional status and minimizing pulmonary involvement. Respiratory and cardiac complications (e.g., hemoptysis, pneumothorax, pulmonary insufficiency, cor pulmonale, and cardiac failure) are additive and tend to become more severe with increasing age. Death is most commonly caused by cardiac and respiratory insufficiency. Lung transplantation is an option that has recently become available in CF.

•••••• Pathophysiology

CF (mucoviscidosis) is a pancreatic enzyme deficiency affecting the exocrine glands throughout the body, both mucus producing and other. The goblet cells of the mucus-producing (exocrine) glands of the body produce abnormal secretions. These secretions, instead of being thin and free flowing, are thick mucoproteins that coagulate to form eosinophilic concentrations in the glands or ducts. The glands and ducts clog and widen, causing pathologic changes and thus symptoms. The pathologic changes are thought to be caused by the obstruction, not the abnormal condition, of the secretions. Abnormalities of the non-mucus-producing glands are seen in saliva and sweat.

CF has a significant and predictable impact throughout the body.

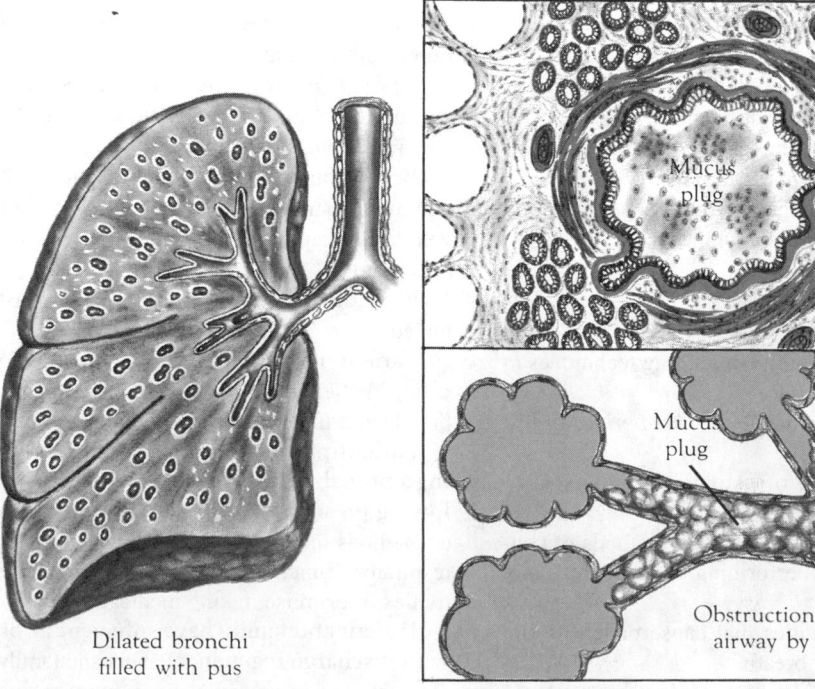

Increased goblet cells in airway epithelium
Increased submucosal size glands

Mucus plug

Mucus plug

Obstruction of small airway by mucus

Dilated bronchi filled with pus

Figure 2-27 Cystic fibrosis. (From Wilson.[93])

Pancreas Thick secretions block the pancreatic ducts, causing cystic widenings of the small lobes of the acini. Degenerative and fibrotic changes in the pancreas result and the essential pancreatic enzymes (trypsin, amylase, and lipase) are unable to participate in food digestion. Thus absorption of fats, proteins, and carbohydrates is disturbed, as evidenced by increased stool fat and protein. Generalized pancreatic dysfunction places patients with CF at higher risk for diabetes mellitus.

Pulmonary system The thick mucus causes bronchial and bronchiolar obstruction. Mucus stasis supports bacterial growth. *Staphylococcus aureus* and *Pseudomonas aeruginosa* are the most common causes of bacterial infection. Antibiotic-resistant *P. aeruginosa* is common as the patient with CF ages.

Tissue damage from the cycle of obstruction, infection, and inflammation results in bronchiectasis. As involvement progresses, hypoxemia, hypercapnia, and acidosis occur. Sequelae are cor pulmonale and heart failure. Major episodes of hemoptysis may occur because of damaged bronchial vessels.

Cardiac system Cardiac changes such as right ventricular hypertrophy occur as a result of hypoxemia and pulmonary hypertension.

Biliary system Foci of biliary blockage and fibrosis are common and become progressively worse, resulting in a type of multilobular biliary cirrhosis. If liver involvement is extensive, portal hypertension and an enlarged spleen may also occur. Jaundice may be evidence of gallbladder obstruction.

Reproductive organs In girls the cervical mucous glands may be dilated. Boys may have abnormal development and function of the epididymis, vas deferens, and seminal vesicles as a result of abnormal secretions during fetal development, rendering 98% of men with CF sterile.

Non-mucus-producing glands Sweat and salivary gland secretions have abnormally high levels of sodium and chloride. There are no histologic abnormalities.

Figure 2-28 summarizes the cystic fibrosis process.

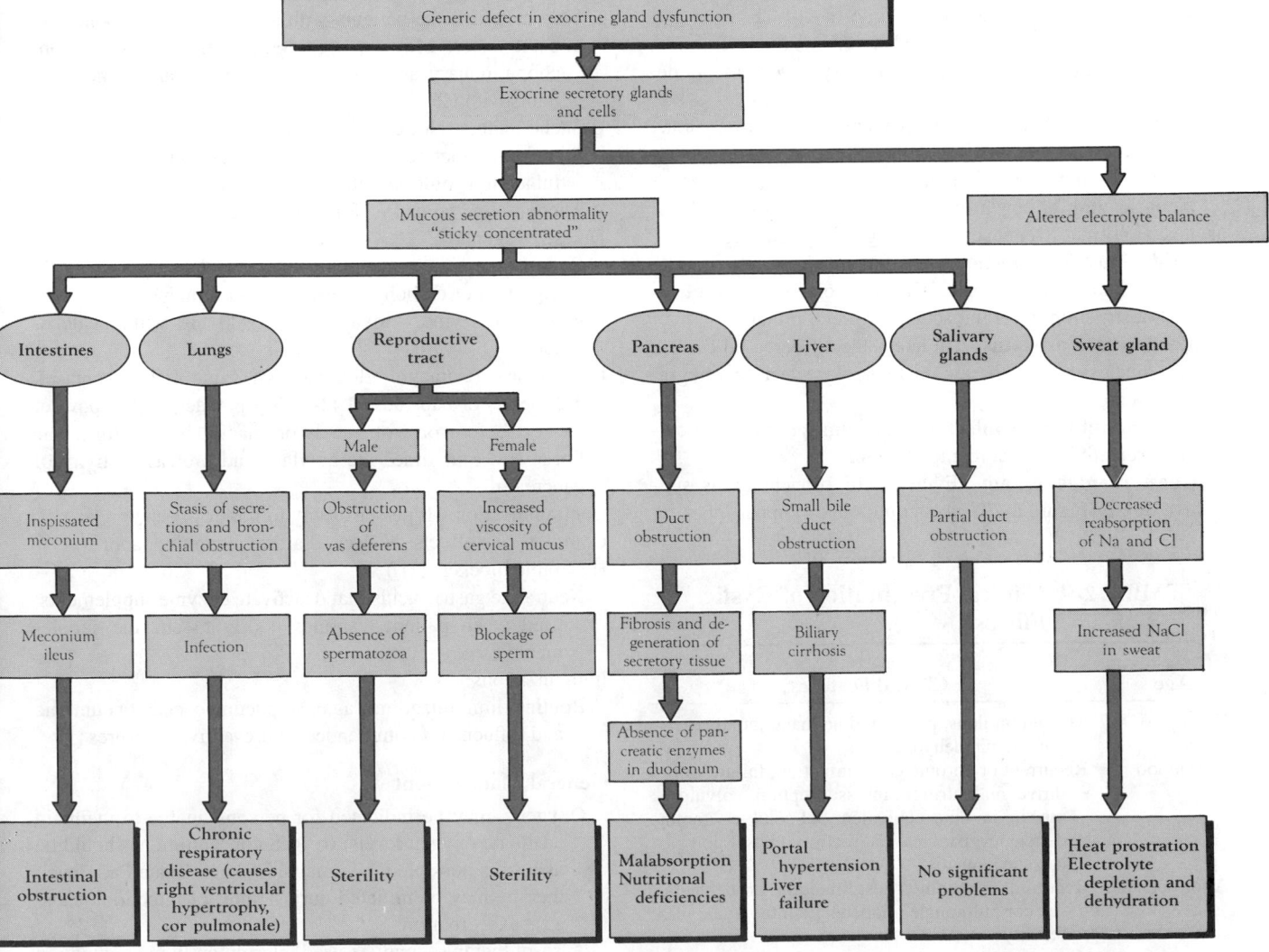

Figure 2-28 Pathogenesis of cystic fibrosis. (From Wilson.[93])

••••• Diagnostic Studies and Findings

Cystic fibrosis may be diagnosed at any age from infancy to adulthood. Diagnosis is based on clinical presentation (Table 2-9) and is confirmed by an elevated sweat chloride level, the most consistent diagnostic test available, although even this has a 2% false-positive and false-negative rate. A sweat chloride concentration greater than 60 mEq/L is considered diagnostic.

History   Frequent pulmonary infections; history of siblings or other family members with CF

Sweat electrolytes   Normal mean value approximately 18 mEq/L (varies with age); sweat chloride 40 to 60 mEq/L suggestive of CF; sweat chloride over 60 mEq/L diagnostic of CF

Pancreatic enzymes   Examination of duodenal secretions or stool for presence of trypsin and chymotrypsin; absence of enzymes suggestive of potential CF

Stool examination for fat   Fat absorption tests conducted for 3 days to calculate ratio of fat in oral intake to fat in stool; impaired fat absorption in intestine, resulting in large volumes excreted in the stool (steatorrhea), suggestive of CF

Laboratory values   Decreased serum sodium, chloride; blood sugar. In late stages of pulmonary involvement, decreased PaO_2, increased $PaCO_2$

Nutritional status   Appetite; percentages of carbohydrate, fat, and protein in diet; salt supplementation; evidence of malnutrition; albumin level, prealbumin

Hepatic and biliary function   Jaundice; enlarged liver; ascites; abnormal liver function findings; enlarged spleen

Gastrointestinal function   Insufficient absorption producing bulky, foul-smelling, pale, watery stools; evidence of intestinal obstruction, fecal impaction, or rectal prolapse

Cardiovascular status   (In late stages) Decreased cardiac output: restlessness; lethargy; tachycardia; electrocardiography; echocardiography

Bronchopulmonary infection   Sputum specimens for culture and sensitivity; chest roentgenogram

Chest roentgenogram   Evidence of bronchiectasis suggestive of CF (Figure 2-29) most commonly in upper lobes

▮ TABLE 2-9   Clinical Presentation of Cystic Fibrosis

Age	Clinical Features
Infancy	Meconium ileus, protracted neonatal jaundice, hyponatremic dehydration
Childhood	Recurrent or chronic chest infection, failure to thrive, malnutrition, intussusception, volvulus, meconium ileus equivalent, fat-soluble vitamin deficiency, pancreatitis, recurrent nasal polyps, chronic sinusitis
Adolescence	Recurrent or chronic chest infection, bronchiectasis, cor pulmonale, diabetes mellitus, male infertility

From Cherniack.[13]

••••• Multidisciplinary Plan

The primary objectives for CF treatment are to slow progression of bronchiectasis and prevent other complications.

Surgery

Bilateral double lung transplantation (usually without heart transplantation) may be an option

Medications

Antiinfective agents

  May be prescribed only at time of illness and infection or prophylactically; if prescribed for infection, antibiotic of choice depends on organism. Antibiotics given orally, IV, or aerosolized. Fluoroquinolones are the only oral antibiotics specific for *P. aeruginosa*

Mucolytics

  Dornase alfa (Pulmozyme). Given daily by aerosol to hydrolyze DNA in sputum, decreasing sputum viscosity and elasticity

Corticosteroids

  May benefit those patients with an asthmatic component in burst doses. May be used long term in allergic bronchopulmonary aspergillosis. Not beneficial for most patients with CF

Bronchodilators (Not used in all patients)

  Salbutamol, metered aerosol 1 to 2 puffs q4 to 6h
    Inhalation solution, inhalation 0.01 to 0.03 mg/kg/day
  Theophylline po or IV 18 to 24 mg/kg/day

Digestive agents

  Rationale: Provide enzymatic activity necessary to assist in digestion of carbohydrates, fats, and proteins

Pancreatin (Elzyme, Viokase), 325-1000 mg with meals or snacks

Pancrelipase (Cotazym, Ilozyme, Ku-Zyme HP, Pancrease), 1-3 tablets or capsules, 0.43-1.29 g powder, or 1-2 powder packets before or with meals or snacks; has 12 times the lipase and four times the amylase and protease activity of pancreatin

Contraindication: Hypersensitivity to pork or beef

Common side effects: Nausea, diarrhea, vomiting, anorexia

Histamine blockers (H_2)

  Neutralize gastric acids that deactivate enzyme supplements; used when patient responds poorly to enzyme supplements

Immunizations

  Routine immunizations against pneumococcal pneumonia and influenza recommended as preventive measures

General Management

  Oxygen—may be indicated for persons unable to maintain adequate oxygen levels; oxygen concentrations should be as low as possible while maintaining adequate PaO_2 level; therapy may be initiated during times of infection or disease exacerbation

  Aerosol therapy—may be used intermittently in conjunction with physiotherapy

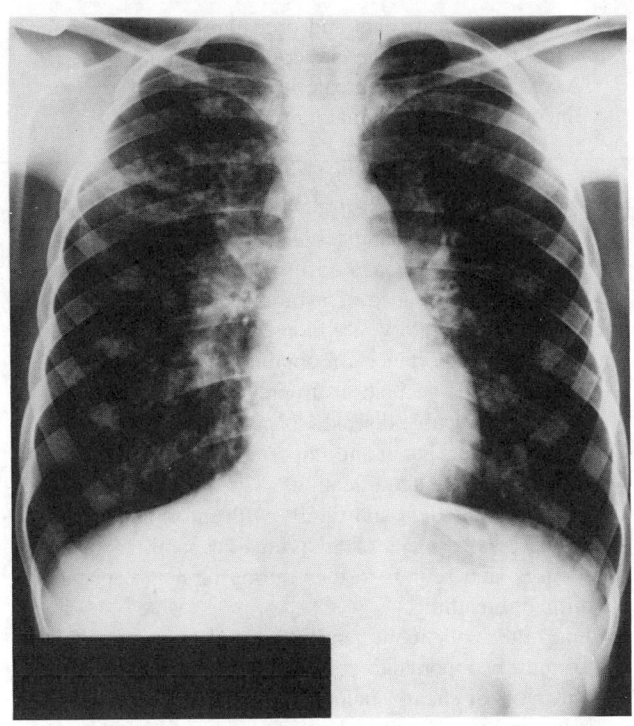

Figure 2-29 Chest roentgenogram of patient with cystic fibrosis. Note bronchial thickening and ill-defined shadows. (Courtesy of Keith Wilson, MD, Baylor College of Medicine, Houston, Texas.)

Diet—sufficient calories; increased work of breathing may increase energy expenditure by 150%; at least 40% of calories should be from fat; supplemental enteral or parenteral feedings may be required during acute illness

Airway clearance—a significant priority of daily health maintenance for the patient with CF; techniques used 1 to 2 times a day in stable disease, increased to 4x or more daily during acute illness; may include postural drainage, percussion, use of flutter valve, percussion vests, forced expiratory technique, and others; see p. 200 for techniques

NURSING CARE

Nursing Assessment

Respiratory Status

Respiratory distress: cough, congestion; tachypnea; retractions; decreased chest wall movement; labored breathing; dyspnea

Examination: barrel chest; dull percussion tone over consolidation or areas of atelectasis; clubbing of fingers and toes

Breath sounds: crackles; decreased or unequal breath sounds

Sputum: productive cough with thick sputum; hemoptysis

Pulmonary function: decreased vital capacity; decreased FEV_1; decreased tidal volume; increased airway resistance

Acute respiratory complications: lobar atelectasis; lung abscess; spontaneous pneumothorax; cor pulmonale; congestive heart failure (rarely)

Hypercapnia

Headache; dizziness; confusion; unconsciousness; twitching; sweating

Hypoxia

Restlessness; confusion; impaired motor function; cyanosis; tachycardia

Psychosocial

Support systems; networking with CF resource groups; ADLs; self-esteem; interaction with peers; sexuality; body image

Nursing Dx & Intervention

Ineffective airway clearance related to tracheobronchial obstruction

- Assess patient's ability to move secretions. If inability is identified, assist with airway clearance techniques.
- Promptly administer mucolytics and expectorants as ordered. Observe for therapeutic response and side effects.
- Assist patient to maintain body position that *ensures maximum airway availability* (semi-Fowler's position or sitting upright).
- Provide hydration *to replace fluids.*
- Administer aerosol and perform airway clearance measures at least 1 hour before meals; provide oral hygiene after treatment.
- Carefully and frequently auscultate chest for quality of breath sounds and adventitious sounds. Note cough and sputum characteristics.

Ineffective breathing pattern related to tracheobronchial obstruction

- Maintain patient positioning *to facilitate use of accessory muscles of ventilation* (tripod position).
- Instruct patient in pulmonary hygiene routines *that will promote easy and effective breathing and facilitate removal of secretions from the tracheobronchial tree.*
- Encourage patient to use adaptive breathing techniques *to decrease work of breathing and to alternate activities with periods of rest.*
- Protect patient from known sources of secondary infection or breathing irritation such as smoking.

Impaired gas exchange related to alveolar-capillary membrane changes

- Assess patient to identify signs, such as restlessness, confusion, and irritability, *that may indicate body's response to altered blood gas states.*

- If patient is very ill, monitor arterial blood gases. Report increases or decreases of more than 10 mm Hg in $Paco_2$ and Pao_2.
- Administer oxygen as ordered and monitor *to maintain Pao_2 between 55 and 65 mm Hg.*
- Venturi mask may be used if needed. If adequate blood gas levels cannot be maintained, noninvasive pressure support ventilation (NIPSV) or continuous positive airway pressure (CPAP) support may be used. See mechanical ventilation on p. 205.
- If patient is very ill, monitor electrocardiogram and cardiac status *for arrhythmias resulting from alterations in blood gases.*
- Monitor and record kidney functioning and urinary output, which may be affected by chronic tissue hypoxia and alterations in metabolism.
- Monitor serum electrolytes, which *may change owing to alterations in oxygenation and metabolism.*
- Carefully monitor body temperature. Elevations in temperature increased tissue demands for oxygen.

Altered nutrition: less than body requirements related to increased caloric needs and impaired nutrient absorption

- Assess nutritional status by daily weighing, monitoring intake and output.
- Provide small, frequent feedings of high-calorie, high-protein, low-fat foods with supplemental vitamins.
- Assist by cutting food and feeding if patient tires easily.
- Administer pancreatic enzyme medications at mealtime.
- If indicated and in consultation with physician, administer stool softeners *to relieve constipation.*
- Monitor for signs and symptoms of malnutrition.

Constipation related to exocrine dysfunction

- Assess stool; note odor, color, amount, frequency, and consistency.
- Observe for signs of intestinal obstruction.
- Administer stool softener as ordered and report results.

Ineffective individual coping related to chronic illness

- Assess patient's perception of present and chronic disease state.
- Assess patient's level of frustration related to feeling of air hunger.
- Determine patient's ability to cooperate with health care providers in interventions such as breathing techniques, exercise progression, and alterations in ADLs.
- Listen carefully to collect information regarding significance of current health care problem and patient's perception of *ability to deal with alterations caused by CF.*
- Assist patient to develop appropriate coping strategies based on personal strengths and past experience.

- Explain all treatments and procedures in manner appropriate for patient's age and comprehension.
- Assist patient to participate in care.
- Encourage patient to maintain usual activities.

Patient Education/Home Care Planning

1. Teach the patient adaptive breathing techniques and work with the family to teach postural drainage techniques.
2. Teach the importance of avoiding contact with persons who have respiratory infections.
3. Teach the importance of obtaining appropriate immunizations and vaccinations to prevent as many childhood and communicable diseases as possible.
4. Teach the facts about and importance of prescribed medications and diet modifications.
5. Provide the patient and family with information regarding CF, assessment of individual capabilities and responses, and actions to take during an acute episode of difficult breathing.
6. Inform the patient and family that a change in health status must be reported to the patient's health care providers. Indicators of change include change in sputum characteristics or color, decreased activity tolerance, nutrition or gastrointestinal changes, weight loss, fever, or stress symptoms indicating an inability to tolerate the disease state.
7. Teach adaptive exercise and rest techniques.
8. Provide the patient and family with information regarding the care, cleaning, and maintenance of inhalation or oxygen equipment used in the hospital or at home, as well as signs of oxygen toxicity.
9. Provide the patient and family with information related to respiratory health, such as pollution indexes, secondary infection exposure, and community support groups.

Evaluation

Airway is patent   Airways are clear.

Breathing occurs without tiring patient. Breath sounds are clear in all areas   Patient demonstrates modified breathing techniques that facilitate ventilatory capacity. Patient's behavior is modified to conserve energy expenditure.

Oxygenation is adequate Pao_2 is maintained at 55 to 65 mm Hg.

Patient understands importance of daily pulmonary exercises   Patient demonstrates pulmonary exercises and states rationale and importance of maintaining daily exercise routine.

Patient preserves pulmonary functioning by maintaining optimum activity level, avoiding infection, and following prescribed treatments   Patient demonstrates variety of methods indicating ability to preserve and facilitate respiratory functioning (breathing exercise, taking medications as prescribed).

Patient and family have sufficient information to comply with discharge regimen   Patient and family at time of discharge are able to discuss medications (purpose, side effects, route, and schedule), dietary therapy regimen, activity progression regimen, signs of infection or respiratory deterioration, and plan for follow-up visits.

Patient and family understand disease process and complications   Patient and family discuss CF as disease: its consequences, outcome, and support strategies.

ATELECTASIS[7,8]

Atelectasis is an acquired condition in which all or part of the normally aerated and expanded lung collapses.

It is a common complication of thoracic or upper abdominal surgery. The problem is caused most often by regional hypoventilation, which commonly leads to a bronchial obstruction with mucus. Atelectasis may also be caused by compression of the lung tissue from hemothorax, pneumothorax, or tumor. (Figure 2-30) High level oxygen therapy may cause absorption atelectasis.

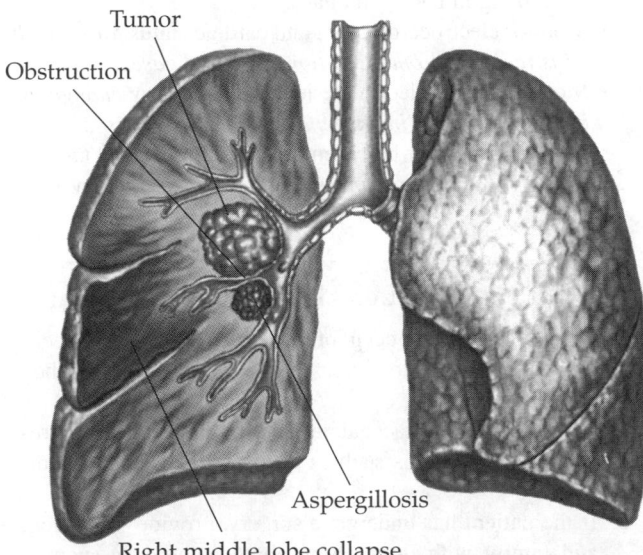

Tumor

Obstruction

Aspergillosis

Right middle lobe collapse

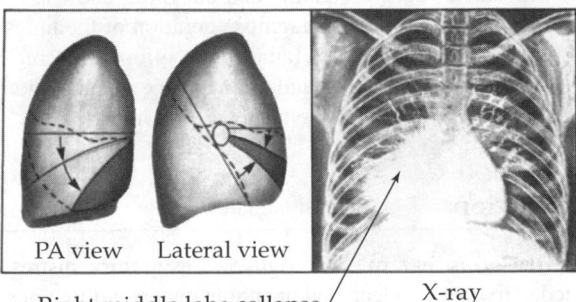

PA view   Lateral view

Right middle lobe collapse   X-ray

Figure 2-30 Atelectasis. (From Wilson.[93])

⋯⋯ Pathophysiology

Atelectasis may occur suddenly and be extensive, or it may occur slowly and cause minor pulmonary problems. Atelectasis may be defined as collapse of the lung from absence of air within the alveoli. The extent of the atelectasis depends on the site and rapidity of the blockage. If the mainstream bronchus to one lung is blocked, the entire lung becomes atelectatic and respiratory compromise is great. If only a small bronchiole becomes slowly blocked because of a buildup of secretions, symptoms may be minor and the respiratory system is able to compensate. In both cases, infection and lung tissue damage are possible.

When airway blockage has occurred, the gas distal to the obstruction is absorbed into the circulation because the oxygen tension in the pulmonary arteries is lower than in the alveoli. The higher the oxygen concentration (FIO_2) of the inspired gas at the time of the blockage, the faster the alveolar collapse. Alveolar collapse results in hypoxemia unless lung compensatory mechanisms transfer blood flow to unaffected areas.

Surfactant levels may be an important factor in atelectasis because decreased surfactant levels are thought to be a cause of the collapse of alveoli. Decreased blood flow after surgery may cause decreased surfactant levels. Another explanation is that the lack of periodic deep breaths or sighs contributes to decreased surfactant activity.

⋯⋯ Diagnostic Studies and Findings

Arterial blood gases Pao_2 less than 80 mm Hg initially, often improving during first 24 hours; $Paco_2$ often normal or low owing to hyperventilation

Serial chest roentgenograms   Airless area visualized; trachea and heart in mediastinum deviated toward atelectatic area; diaphragm elevated on affected side; rib spaces narrowed

Clinical examination   Rapid occlusion with massive collapse: hyperventilation, dyspnea, cyanosis, tachycardia, elevated temperature, diminished breath sounds over affected area, dull or flat percussion tones, restlessness, rales on auscultation; slow occlusion with minor collapse; may be asymptomatic or have minor pulmonary symptoms

Bronchoscopy   May show bronchial obstruction

⋯⋯ Multidisciplinary Plan

The ultimate treatment plan for atelectasis is removal of the underlying cause.

Surgery
Surgical excision of tumor
   Insertion of drainage tube—performed to relieve atelectasis caused by compression component such as hemothorax or pneumothorax
   Bronchoscopy—may be performed to remove retained secretions or possible foreign bodies when atelectasis is not relieved by suction, coughing and deep breathing, or postural drainage

Medications

Bronchodilators

Isoetharine (Bronkosol), 2-4 ml of 0.125%-0.25% solution q4h

Metaproterenol sulfate (Alupent), 2-3 inhalations q3-4h

Anti-infective agents (use is controversial)

Broad-spectrum antibiotic (such as penicillin or ampicillin) given as soon as symptoms are noted; drug may be modified appropriately if specific pathogen is isolated from bronchial secretions

Mucolytic agents such as *N*-acetylcysteine can be given by intermittent positive-pressure breathing (IPPB) or nebulizer

General Management

High tidal volumes and/or PEEP used to maintain open alveoli if patient is intubated

Incentive spirometry

Positioning—patient placed with uninvolved side in dependent position to promote drainage of affected area; patient repositioned at least every hour

Chest physiotherapy with coughing and deep breathing

Ambulation as soon and as often as tolerated

NURSING CARE

Nursing Assessment

Respiratory Status

Tachypnea; retractions; labored breathing; dyspnea; nasal flaring; retractions; rales, bilaterally unequal, diminished over affected area; labored or irregular breathing; hyperventilation; percussion tones dull or flat over affected area

Hypoxia

Restlessness; confusion; hypertension early; hypotension late; cyanosis; tachycardia

Inspired air should be humidified to avoid inspissation of tracheobronchial secretions; supplemental oxygen may be given to maintain arterial $PO_2 \geq 80$ torr (must accept lower value in patients with severe chronic pulmonary diseases)

Bronchopulmonary Infection

Temperature; characteristics of sputum; sputum specimens for culture and sensitivity

Nursing Dx & Intervention

Ineffective airway clearance (high risk for) related to bronchial obstruction

- Teach patient and family deep breathing and cough techniques preoperatively.
- Assess patient's respiratory status frequently after surgery.

- Prevent buildup of respiratory secretions after surgery by encouraging deep breathing and coughing; repositioning patient every hour; ambulating patient as soon as possible; not administering large doses of sedatives, which depress cough reflex and respirations; liquefying secretions by administering aerosol treatments, humidifying inspired air, and maintaining body hydration; and using incentive spirometer *to encourage deep breathing.*
- After surgery, position patient with pillow along incision site *to function as splint.* Administer analgesic medications before initiating deep breathing and coughing exercises.
- Mobilize secretions by use of postural drainage. See later sections for technique.

Impaired gas exchange related to alveolar collapse

- Assess patient to identify signs, such as restlessness, confusion, and irritability, *that may indicate body's response to altered blood gas states.*
- In collaboration with physician's order, monitor arterial blood gases. Report increases or decreases of more than 10 mm Hg in $PaCO_2$ and PaO_2.
- Monitor electrocardiogram and cardiac status *for arrhythmias resulting from alterations in blood gases.*
- Monitor serum electrolyte levels, *which may change owing to alterations in oxygenation and metabolism.*
- Carefully monitor body temperature, *which may fluctuate owing to alterations in metabolism or secondary infections.*

Patient Education/Home Care Planning

1. Teach the patient deep breathing and coughing techniques, as well as to increase activity and to splint when coughing.
2. Teach the patient facts about and the importance of prescribed medications such as bronchodilators and antibiotics.
3. If the patient has undergone surgery, provide the patient and family with information about techniques such as movement, deep breathing, and coughing and use of an incentive spirometer to facilitate aeration of the lungs.
4. Provide the patient and family with information regarding the care, cleaning, and maintenance of inhalation or oxygen equipment in the hospital or at home.

Evaluation

Airway is patent No signs of respiratory distress are noted. Airways are clear, and breathing occurs without obstruction. Breath sounds are clear throughout.

Gas exchange is effective Arterial blood gases are within normal limits: PaO_2 equals 80 to 100 mm Hg. $PaCO_2$ equals 35 to 45 mm Hg; pH equals 7.35 to 7.45.

PLEURAL EFFUSION
(Pleurisy with effusion)

A pleural effusion develops when excess nonpurulent fluid accumulates in the pleural space between the visceral and parietal pleurae (Figure 2-31).

Pleural effusion is rarely a disease by itself. It generally occurs as a secondary problem when the physiologic processes of capillary fluids, lymphatic drainage, membrane hydrostatic pressures, and colloidal osmotic pressures are disturbed.

Pleural effusions may be divided into two categories, transudates and exudates. They are determined by the presence and amount of protein in the aspirated fluid. Following are the common causes of pleural effusions:

Exudates
  Viral infections
  Tuberculosis
  Bacterial infections
  Chest trauma
  Pancreatitis
  Rheumatic fever
  Collagen-vascular diseases
  Metastatic diseases
  Uremia
  Subphrenic abscess
  Pulmonary infarction
Transudates
  Peritoneal dialysis
  Pericarditis
  Cirrhosis
  Congestive heart failure
  Myxedema
  Kidney disease

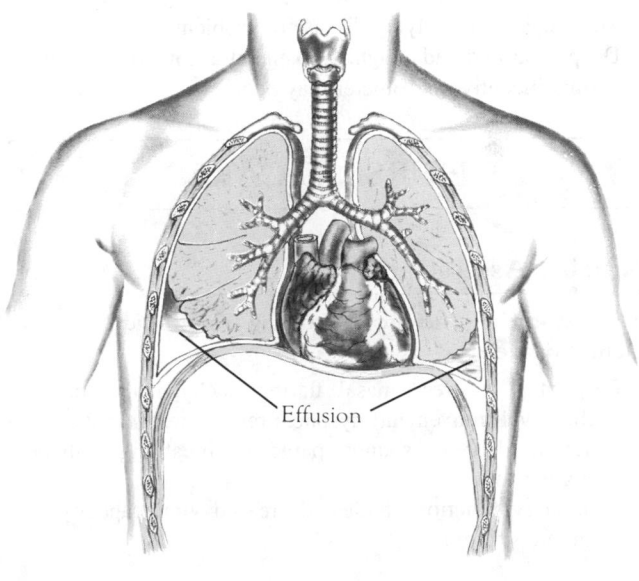
Effusion

Figure 2-31 Pleural effusion. (From Wilson.[93])

Sarcoidosis
Hypoproteinemia

Pathophysiology

The visceral and parietal pleurae form a continuous sac between the lung and the chest wall. Normally only a potential space containing less than 10 ml of fluid separates these surfaces. The fluid is continuously moving in and out of this space because of a balance between hydrostatic pressures, colloidal osmotic pressures, and the surface characteristics of capillaries and the pleurae. Any alteration in pressure gradients or surface characteristics can lead to the formation of an effusion.

The distinction between transudate and exudate is based on protein content. Transudates (hydrothorax) are produced when the flow of protein-free fluid into the pleural space is disturbed. Aspirated fluid is clear or pale yellow, has a specific gravity of 1.015 or less, and has a protein content that is either normal or less than 3 g/dl. Exudates result from a disease of the pleural surface or an obstruction in the lymphatic system that inhibits the drainage of proteins. The fluid is often dark yellow or amber and has a specific gravity greater than 1.016 and a protein content greater than 3 g/dl.

When fluid accumulates as the result of a disturbance in plasma oncotic pressure, it is a transudate. Increased capillary pressure in heart failure and reduced plasma oncotic pressure in certain kidney or liver diseases are the known causes of transudate fluid.

When increased fluid formation is the result of capillary permeability, as in inflammation, it is an exudate. The exudative fluid often has an increased cell count. It may have a large number of white cells, to the point of gross purulent appearance.

Diagnostic Studies and Findings

Clinical examination Dullness to percussion, which shifts with change in position; decreased or absent breath sounds over affected area; egophony above effusion site; dyspnea if effusion has occurred rapidly; if effusion is large, intercostal bulging or decreased chest wall movement during breathing

Chest roentgenogram Effusions typically located at base of pleural space; moderate amount of fluid (250 to 300 ml) must accumulate to be seen on upright posterior-anterior, decubitus, or lateral chest roentgenogram; effusion seen as dense opacity (Figure 2-32); large effusions may obliterate hemothorax, simulating lung collapse; distinction between effusion and collapse based on shift of mediastinum away from effusion but toward lung collapse[61]

Thoracentesis For pleural fluid analysis; submit several hundred milliliters if possible (Table 2-10)

Stain, culture, and sensitivity of pleural fluid Identification of causative agent (bacterial, fungal, or viral)

Cytologic examination of pleural fluid Evaluation of potential neoplastic involvement; bloody effusion without history of chest trauma suggestive of malignancy or pulmonary embolism

Reaccumulation of fluid in pleural space after drainage by thoracentesis Assessment of potential respiratory distress as per discussion

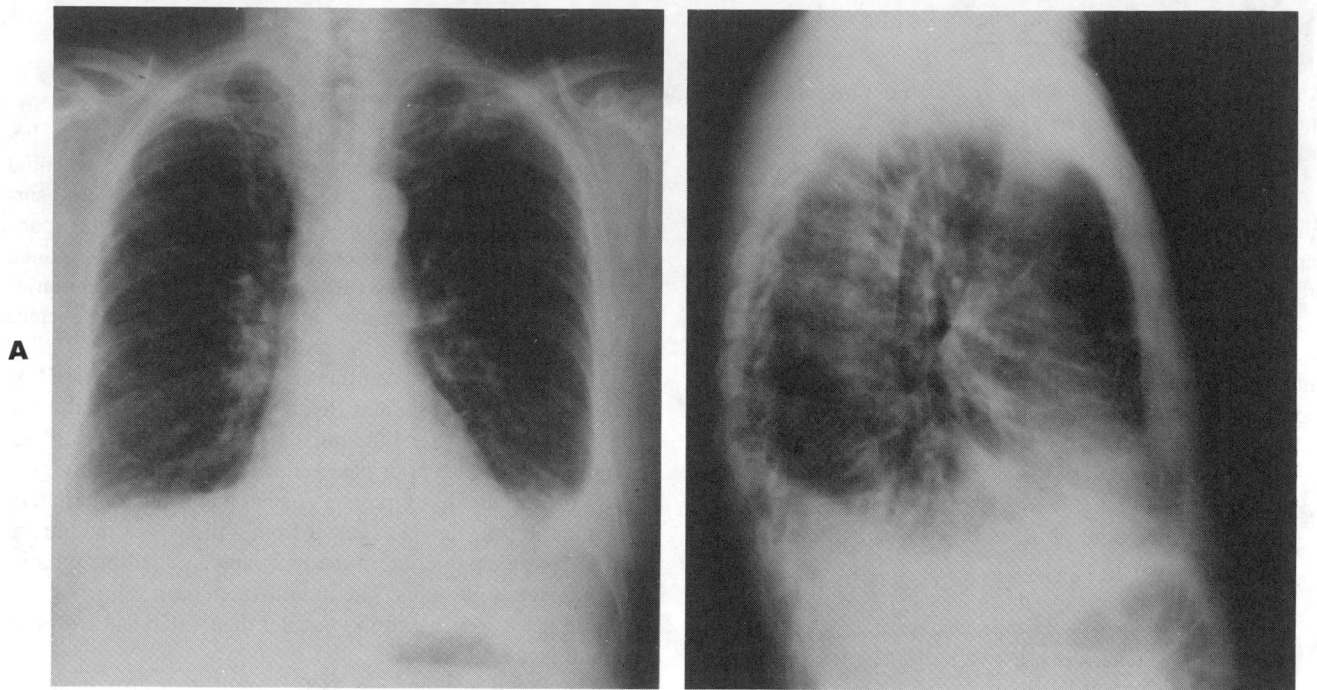

Figure 2-32 Chest roentgenogram of patient with pleural effusion. **A,** PA view: note obliteration of costophrenic angles bilaterally; pulmonary vasculature appears normal. **B,** Lateral view: note lack of costophrenic angles. (Courtesy R. Keith Wilson, MD, Baylor College of Medicine, Houston, Texas.)

Cardiovascular response to removal of large quantity of pleural fluid during thoracentesis Hypotension; tachycardia; cardiac arrhythmias; syncope; clammy skin; paleness

Pleural biopsy with tissue analysis Indicated when fluid analysis fails to establish cause

•••••• Multidisciplinary Plan

Treatment of pleural effusion depends on the etiology and clinical consequences. The following discussion refers to the general treatment of effusion. The reader is referred to the section of the text dealing with the cause of the effusion.

Surgery

Thoracentesis—to drain excess fluid from pleural space and relieve dyspnea or hypoxemia; with rapid removal of large quantities of pleural fluid, the patient may experience dyspnea during lung reexpansion; another complication of thoracentesis is pneumothorax

Insertion of small chest tube

Tube may be connected to underwater seal drainage system and left in place if accumulation of fluids is large and compromising respiratory function

If pleural effusion is caused by malignancy, tube may be inserted to drain fluid and left in place to provide insertion point for medications and therapeutic techniques

Medications

Antibiotics

Antibiotics specific to cause administered if effusion is thought to be caused by infectious process

General Management

Treatment of underlying disease or problem

Deep breathing and coughing to encourage maximal ventilation; incentive spirometer may be used

NURSING CARE

Nursing Assessment

Respiratory Insufficiency Resulting from Fluid in Pleural Space

Respiratory distress: nasal flaring; tachypnea; decreased chest wall movement; dyspnea; restlessness; tachycardia; decreased breath sounds; paradoxic breathing; dull percussion tone

Pulmonary function studies: decreased vital capacity and minute volume

Bronchopulmonary Infection

Temperature; sputum specimen for culture and sensitivity

TABLE 2-10 Pleural Fluid Analysis

Measurement	Transudate	Exudate
Color	Pale yellow	Dark amber, blood or pus
Red blood cells (RBCs)	May increase	>5000 RBCs/mm^3; may increase
Protein	<3 g/dl	>3 g/dl
Specific gravity	<1.016	>1.016
Lactic dehydrogenase (LDH)	<200 U/dl	>200 U/dl
Pleural LDH/serum LDH	<0.6	>0.6
White blood cells (WBCs)		Increase indicates empyema or infected effusion
Amylase		Exceeds serum amylase level
Glucose		Less than serum glucose level
Triglyceride		May be increased
pH	>7.3	Varies

Modified from Miller and Kazemi.[61]

Psychosocial

Fear of dyspnea or not being able to get enough air; potential fear of unknown cause of pleural effusion

Nursing Dx & Intervention

Impaired gas exchange related to alveolar collapse

- Assess for signs of restlessness, confusion, change in respiratory pattern, or irritability *that may indicate altered blood gas levels resulting from compromised breathing.*
- Monitor for atelectasis.
- Turn patient frequently *to prevent pooling of secretions within lungs and pleural space.*
- Assist with thoracentesis procedure and *monitor patient's response after procedure.*
- Assess for signs of secondary infection in pleural area or in lungs themselves.
- If chest tube is in place, assess and provide care as indicated on pp. 203 to 205.

Patient Education/Home Care Planning

1. Teach the patient the importance of positioning to facilitate ventilatory effort.
2. Teach the patient the importance of deep breathing and coughing to keep the lungs aerated and to prevent complications.
3. If pleural effusion is a recurrent problem, ensure that the patient is able to identify signs of accumulating fluid so care can be sought early.
4. Prepare the patient for thoracentesis.

Evaluation

Gas exchange is optimal Blood gases within normal limits.
Minimal fluid remains in pleural space Chest roentgenogram shows no evidence of fluid accumulation. Breath sounds are clear and bilaterally equal; percussion tone is resonant over all lung fields.

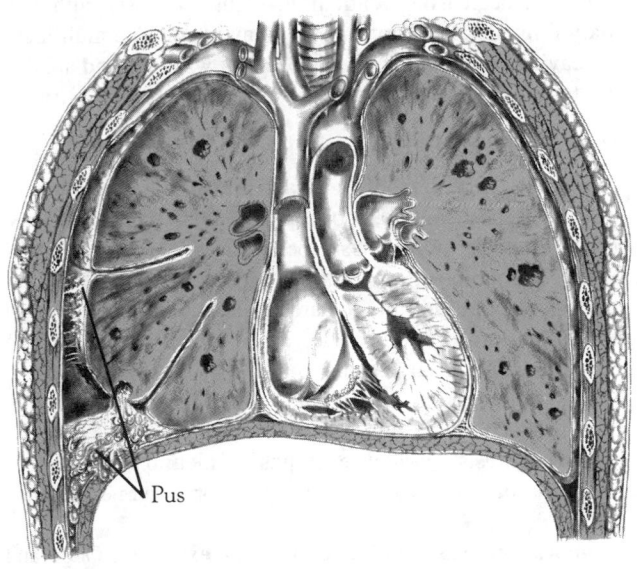

Figure 2-33 Empyema. (From Wilson.[93])

Cause of pleural effusion is identified and treated There is no recurrence of disease.

INFECTIOUS AND INFLAMMATORY DISEASES

EMPYEMA

Empyema is the accumulation of infected fluid or pus in the pleural space (Figure 2-33).

The accumulation of purulent exudate in the pleural cavity may occur in several ways. The most common cause is direct extension from adjacent structures as occurs in pneumonia, tuberculosis, pulmonary abscess, or esophageal rupture. Exudate accumulation may also occur from direct contamination such as that caused by penetrating chest wounds or chest surgery. Empyema is an uncommon but serious disorder that occurs most often in debilitated patients. If identified early and treated promptly with antibiotics, it can usually be controlled.

Pathophysiology

Empyema may affect a small area of pleura or may involve the entire pleural cavity. In the acute stage the affected area appears inflamed and has a thin layer of exudate with a low leukocyte count. If untreated, the exudate thickens and pus may accumulate. The pleura may thicken, and adhesions may occur. The empyema may be loculated, or found in pockets versus freely moving within the pleural space. Chronic empyema develops when there are recurrent infections or when treatment of a previous infection was incomplete. Treatment of chronic empyema is difficult because the pleura often becomes thickened and fibrous, and the lung may stick to the chest wall, decreasing ventilation. Pleural fibrosis with secondary limited ventilatory capacity may result. The multiloculated cavities within the pleural space fill with pus and are difficult to drain.

Diagnostic Studies and Findings

History   Recent thoracic or abdominal surgery; blunt or penetrating chest trauma; esophageal fistula; lung infections; aspiration; recent thoracentesis; persistent fever during administration of antibiotics

Physical examination   Pleural friction rub; localized chest pain; dullness to percussion; decreased breath sounds at lung bases; decreased vocal fremitus

Chest roentgenogram   Pleural fluid, usually unilateral, with associated lung lesion

Thoracentesis   Evidence of pus in pleural exudate (because pus is difficult to aspirate, 18-gauge or larger needle must be used)

Laboratory examination of pleural exudate   Odor and general appearance; specific gravity; cell count; Gram stains; aerobic and anaerobic cultures (NOTE: When materials are sent for culture, all air must be expressed from syringe and sample must be quickly transported to laboratory for anaerobic evaluation)

Multidisciplinary Plan

Surgery

Thoracentesis—may be performed to drain purulent drainage if area is small and localized

Thoracic drainage—closed drainage system; a large diameter tube is usually required and connected to closed system under water-seal drainage

Intrapleural aspiration and instillation of medications—chest tube may be used to aspirate pleural drainage and as vehicle for instillation of antibiotics and fibrinolytic enzymes

Thoracotomy—may be necessary for patients not effectively treated by tube drainage system; area with empyema is resected and thickened membrane is stripped by process called decortication to permit reexpansion of lung

Medications

Antiinfective agents

Antibiotic therapy based initially on results of Gram stain; alterations made if necessary when culture results are available

Fibrinolytic agents

Controversial; recommended by several researchers as method to decrease viscosity of pus and dissolve fibrin clots

General Management

Oxygen support—may be necessary if signs of hypoxia are present

Irrigation of pleural cavity with sterile solution—periodically for patient with thoracotomy tube in place to flush out purulent and necrotic materials

Deep breathing and coughing—to encourage maximum ventilation and decrease congestion resulting from pulmonary problem and bed rest; incentive spirometer may be used

NURSING CARE

Nursing Assessment

Respiratory Insufficiency Resulting from Presence of Pus in Pleural Space

Nasal flaring; tachypnea; decreased chest wall movement; dyspnea; restlessness; tachycardia; decreased breath sounds; paradoxic breathing; dull percussion tone; decreased vital capacity and minute volume; arterial blood gases must be assessed if signs of hypoxia are present

Characteristics and Amount of Purulent Drainage from Pleural Cavity and Physiologic Response to Accumulation

Amount, odor, and color of drainage; specimens sent periodically to laboratory for analysis and culture; response to purulent accumulation, including fever, respiratory distress, and pain

Bronchopulmonary Infection

Temperature; sputum specimen for culture and sensitivity

Nursing Dx & Intervention

Ineffective breathing pattern related to pain and lung compression on inspiration and expiration

- Assess ventilation, including evaluation of breathing rate, rhythm, and depth; chest expansion; and presence of respiratory distress such as dyspnea, shortness of breath, nasal flaring, or prolonged expiratory phase.
- Assess potential of purulent collection to interfere with ventilation and vital capacity.
- Maintain patient in position *that facilitates easy ventilation* (head of bed in semi-Fowler's position).

- Encourage deep breathing, coughing, and use of incentive spirometer.
- Provide analgesics to promote effective cough and deep breathing.

Impaired gas exchange related to inflammation and alveolar collapse

- Assess for signs of restlessness, confusion, and irritability, *which may indicate altered blood gas levels resulting from compromised breathing.*
- Assess blood gases if hypoxia is anticipated.
- Monitor for signs of atelectasis *resulting from decreased ventilation.*
- Encourage deep breathing and coughing *to loosen secretions and facilitate expectoration.* Incentive spirometry may be used.
- Turn patient frequently *to prevent pooling of secretions within lungs and pleural space, and to promote drainage of empyema via chest drainage tube.*

Patient Education/Home Care Planning

1. Teach the patient the importance of positioning to facilitate the ventilatory effort.
2. Teach the patient the importance of deep breathing and coughing to keep the lungs aerated and prevent complications.
3. If empyema is a recurrent problem, teach the patient to identify signs of the problem so care can be sought early.
4. Prepare the patient for thoracentesis or the insertion of chest tubes (see pp. 203 to 205).
5. If the patient is to go home with an open chest tube left in place for drainage, teach care techniques (such as aseptic dressing change).
6. Teach the patient and family about empyema; inform them that the healing process may be slow and that repeated treatments, drainage, irrigation, and chest roentgenograms may be necessary.

Evaluation

Movement of air in and out of lungs is optimum Breath sounds are clear and bilaterally equal; percussion tone is resonant over all lung fields. No purulent material remains in pleural space. Chest roentgenogram shows no evidence of pus accumulation.

Gas exchange is effective Blood gases are within normal limits.

■ ACUTE BRONCHITIS

Acute bronchitis is an inflammation of the bronchi or trachea or both that results from irritation or infection (Figure 2-34).

Acute bronchitis usually heals by itself. It is most common in winter. Acute bronchitis may occur alone and also occurs with many chronic diseases such as bronchiectasis, emphysema, or tuberculosis. It may also be linked to systemic illnesses such as chickenpox, measles, and influenza. Exposure to air pollutants or physical disabilities such as malnutrition or fatigue may make bronchitis worse. If the patient already has a chronic pulmonary or cardiovascular disease, acute bronchitis may become serious. Pneumonia is perhaps the most common complication. If the patient already has impaired cough, lung, or bronchial functioning, acute bronchitis may lead to respiratory failure.

In most cases infective acute bronchitis is viral, but bacterial causes (e.g., *Streptococcus pneumoniae, Haemophilus influenzae*) are also common. Irritative bronchitis may be caused by dust or fumes, such as from strong acids, ammonia, chlorine, bromide, or smoke.

•••••• Pathophysiology

Congestion of the bronchial mucous membranes is the earliest physiologic change. This is followed by desquamation or shedding of the submucosa. The congestion and shedding process causes submucosal edema with leukocyte infiltration. This process interferes with the normal function of the ciliated bronchial epithelium and the phagocytes. The result is a sticky or mucopurulent exudate that stays in the bronchi until coughed out.

Because the normally sterile bronchial system is contaminated, bacteria may move in to cause secondary bacterial infection. At the beginning of the disease process, the sputum of a patient with acute bronchitis is normally mucoid. If the sputum becomes mucopurulent or purulent, a superimposed bacterial infection can be suspected (Table 2-11).

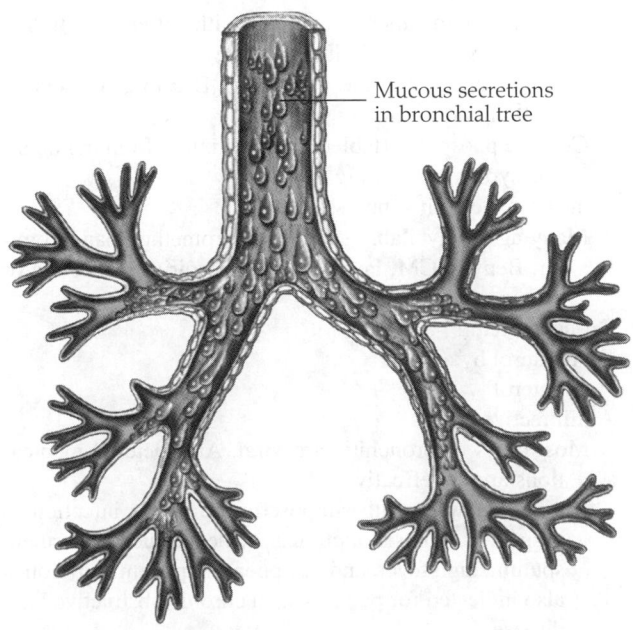

Mucous secretions in bronchial tree

Figure 2-34 Acute bronchitis. (From Wilson.[93])

■ TABLE 2-11 Agents Commonly Causing Acute Bronchitis and Pneumonitis

Product	Industry	Injury
Aldehydes (acrylaldehyde, form-aldehyde, and acetaldehydes)	Plastic, rubber, textiles, resins, disinfectant	Bronchitis, asthma
Ammonia	Fertilizer, explosives, refrigeration	Tracheobronchitis, pulmonary edema
Chlorine and hydrochloric acid	Bleaches, disinfectants, plastics, refining, dye making, organic chemical synthesis	Tracheobronchitis, pulmonary edema
Nitrogen dioxide	Fertilizer, dyes, explosives, farming, rockets, arc welding	Tracheobronchitis, pulmonary edema, bronchiolitis obliterans
Ozone	Arc welding, sewage and water treatment	Tracheobronchitis
Phosgene	Chemical industry, dyes, insecticides	Tracheobronchitis, pulmonary edema
Sulfur dioxide	Bleaching, smelting, paper manufacture, refrigeration	Tracheobronchitis, pulmonary edema (rare)

From Cherniack.[13]

・・・・・ Diagnostic Studies and Findings

Clinical examination Cough initially dry and nonproductive but may produce mucoid sputum within a few days; fever (38.3° to 38.9° C [101° to 102° F]) if cause is bacterial, midsternal chest pain, malaise, sore throat, scattered rales and rhonchi; if patient already has chronic lung disease, sputum may change from clear and thin to thick and tenacious or purulent

Chest roentgenogram Clear; no evidence of lung consolidation

・・・・・ Multidisciplinary Plan

The goals of the treatment plan are to provide supportive therapy during the course of the self-limited disease and to prevent secondary infections.

Medications

Antitussive agents
  Narcotic cough suppressants (use with extreme caution in patients with chronic lung disease)
  Hydrocodone bitartrate (Codone, Dicodid, Hycodan), 5-10 mg tid or qid
  Codeine phosphate (tablets and in mixture form in numerous syrups), 10-20 mg q4-6h
Nonnarcotic cough suppressants
  Many agents available such as dextromethorphan (Romilar, Benylin CM, Pertussin, Congespirin), 10-20 mg or 30 mg q6-8h
Bronchodilators
  Albuterol by aerosol
  Albuterol
Antiinfective agents
  Most cases of bronchitis are viral. Antibacterial medications are not effective.
  Antibiotics when superimposed respiratory infection is suspected on basis of clinical evidence such as purulent sputum, high fever, and ill-appearing patient; antibiotics also indicated for patients with chronic obstructive lung disease
Antipyretic-analgesics
  To reduce fever and relieve malaise

General Management

Increase in fluid intake to maintain hydration
Steam or mist vaporizer to humidify air surrounding patient
Rest to conserve energy
Culture of sputum if sputum becomes purulent or patient's illness becomes progressively worse

NURSING CARE

Nursing Assessment

Because acute bronchitis is generally a self-limited disease, assessment is important to identify complications, superimposed infections, or adverse effects of therapy.

Respiratory Status

Sibilant and sonorous rhonchi; crackles at base; labored or irregular breathing; dyspnea; substernal tightness with breathing; back pain; cough characteristics and duration

Nursing Dx & Intervention

Ineffective airway clearance related to mucopurulent sputum and airway inflammation

• Assess patient to identify inability to move secretions. If inability is identified, assist with appropriate measures (coughing, positioning, suctioning, liquefying secretions, and so on).
• Provide adequate hydration *to avoid viscous secretions.*
• Assist with frequent oral care after sputum expectorated and before meals.

Risk for infection related to debilitated state

• Assess for signs and symptoms of infection, fever, dyspnea, and change in sputum color, amount, or odor.
• Obtain sputum for culture and sensitivity.
• Protect patient from known sources of secondary infection.

Fatigue related and frequent cough

- Assess patterns of fatigue.
- Assess factors related to fatigue and strategies for dealing with them.
- Assess support systems and available resources.
- Administer treatments or medications to relieve discomfort.
- Enhance patient's ability to rest between specified activities.
- Administer antitussive medications to allow rest from cough.

Patient Education/Home Care Planning

1. Teach the patient the importance of consuming large quantities of fluid.
2. Teach the patient the importance of not smoking and of avoiding fumes or smoke when the disease is active.
3. Teach the patient the importance of rest during the course of the disease.
4. Teach the patient facts about and the importance of prescribed medications.
5. Teach the patient how to use antipyretic analgesics to reduce fever and relieve malaise.
6. Teach the patient the importance of avoiding contact with others, who may transmit infection.
7. Teach the patient signs of secondary infection such as a change in sputum characteristics or prolonged fever that may be suggestive of secondary infection.

Evaluation

Airways are patent Breathing occurs without cough or substernal tightness. Breath sounds are clear.

Secondary infection is prevented Temperature and WBC within normal limits. Sputum expectorated effectively, appears clear to white.

Fatigue is minimized Cough is decreased. Sufficient sleep/rest is obtained.

LUNG ABSCESS

Lung abscess is an inflammatory lesion in the lung accompanied by necrosis. The abscess usually has well-defined borders and may be putrid (containing anaerobic bacteria) or nonputrid (containing aerobic bacteria) (Figure 2-35).

The incidence of lung abscess has dropped significantly because of the availability of effective antibiotics and the increased willingness of individuals to seek medical care. Lung abscesses are generally caused by aspiration of infected material, which may occur during unconsciousness, general anesthesia, alcoholism, near-drowning, diabetic coma, or drug sedation.

An abscess can occur as a result of poor oral hygiene, gum disease, infected tonsils, or aspiration of food. Patients with an

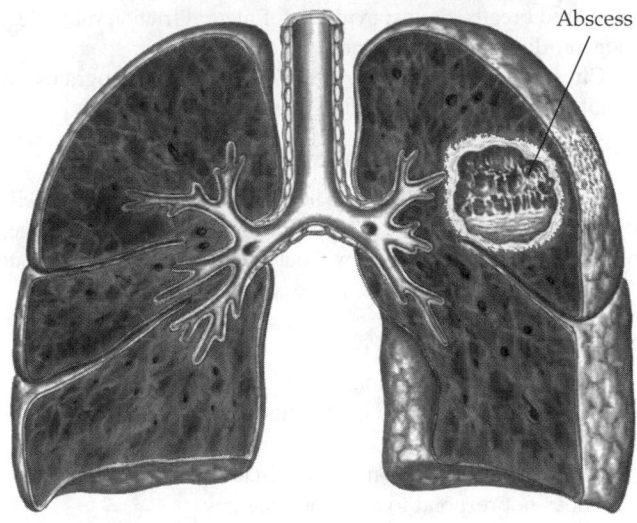

Figure 2-35 Lung abscess. (From Wilson.[93])

obstructing airway lesion (tumor) may develop a postobstructive pneumonia and abscess. In rare instances, infection in other parts of the body will produce septic emboli, which lodge in the lung.

• • • • • • Pathophysiology

The site of the abscess is determined by the body's position at the time of the inhalation. The aspirated material moves to the most dependent position in the lung. Once it has settled, a fibrous granulation tissue forms around it and it embeds itself in the parenchyma.

As the abscess develops, it fills with pus. Pressure develops, and the infected tissue ruptures into the bronchus. Drainage of foul-smelling, pus-filled, or bloody sputum results. The expectoration of purulent sputum may lead to partial healing and cavity formation. However, if the cavity does not drain adequately, small abscesses may form within the lung. Organisms causing lung abscess include bacteria, fungi, and parasites.

• • • • • • Diagnostic Studies and Findings

Clinical examination Initial signs resembling pneumonia; cough producing bloody, purulent, foul-smelling sputum; general malaise; sporadic fever; pleuritic pain; dyspnea if abscess is large; dull percussion tone; rales; if abscess left untreated and becomes chronic may be weight loss, anemia

Chest roentgenogram To follow progress of therapy

Laboratory examination of abscess fluid. Culture and sensitivity When material is sent for culture, all air must be expressed from syringe and sample must be quickly transported to laboratory for anaerobic evaluation

White blood cell count Leukocytosis common

Bronchoscopy Unnecessary if roentgenography shows rapid resolution of abscess but may be needed to verify presence of abscess or determine its severity if patient's condition does not improve

Respiratory insufficiency resulting from presence of abscess in pleural cavity Dyspnea; restlessness; tachycardia;

decreased breath sounds; evidence of pleural friction rub; rales; rhonchi; dull percussion tones

Chest roentgenogram   Serial chest roentgenograms to monitor healing process of lung abscess

•••••• Multidisciplinary Plan

The ability of the lung abscess to heal depends primarily on its ability to drain adequately through the bronchus. With free drainage, resolution occurs; however, without free drainage, and without prompt antibiotic therapy, the abscess may become chronic.

Surgery

Bronchoscopy—occasionally necessary to remove thick, tenacious sputum. Used cautiously to avoid flooding the lung with secretions

Pulmonary resection—necessary in rare cases if lung abscess does not respond to antibiotic therapy

Medications

Antiinfective agents

Antibiotic therapy directed at causative agent; should be monitored and perhaps changed depending on patient's clinical response; should begin as soon as initial sputum specimens have been collected

Intravenous antibiotics usually required for an extended period

Antibiotic therapy continued until all signs of abscess are resolved on serial chest roentgenograms

General Management

Postural drainage—extremely important to drain abscess. Positions may need to be modified for optimal abscess drainage

Percussion—to loosen secretions and enhance their removal

Daily measurement of sputum volume output and assessment of sputum characteristics

NURSING CARE

Nursing Assessment

Respiratory Response

Monitor breath sounds and mucus production
Note which positions promote sputum production

Response to Antibiotic Therapy

Monitoring of response to treatment process; if not improved, assessment for additional underlying cause of abscess such as tumor or foreign body

Psychosocial

Concern that there is infection that must be treated for extended period

Nursing Dx & Intervention

Ineffective airway clearance related to mucopurulent sputum

- Assess patient to identify inability to move secretions. If inability is identified, assist with appropriate measures (such as coughing, positioning, suctioning).
- Assist patient to maintain proper body positioning *to ensure maximum airway availability and to promote drainage position that will facilitate drainage of lobe.*
- Provide hydration to liquefy secretions and replace fluids.
- Perform postural drainage with percussion at least 1 hour before meals; actively encourage coughing after treatment; provide oral hygiene after treatment to eliminate foul taste of drainage.
- Carefully and frequently auscultate chest for quality of breath sounds and adventitious sounds.
- Assess potential of purulent collection to interfere with ventilation.
- Note color, odor, and amount of sputum daily.
- Administer antibiotics as ordered.

Ineffective breathing pattern related to inflammatory process and pleuritic pain

- Identify contributing factors such as airway clearance, obstruction problem, or weakness.
- Assess patient for tiring in relation to attempts to breathe.
- Protect patient from known sources of secondary infection or breathing irritation such as smoking.
- Provide analgesics as needed.

Ineffective individual coping related to fatigue

- Assess patient's ability to cooperate with health care providers regarding intervention strategies, such as frequent postural drainage sessions.
- Balance the need to promote drainage with the need for sleep and rest.
- See p. 1739 for additional strategies.

Patient Education/Home Care Planning

1. Teach the patient the importance of positioning to facilitate abscess drainage.
2. Teach the patient the importance of deep breathing and coughing to keep the lung aerated and to prevent secondary complications.
3. Teach the patient facts about and the importance of prescribed medications such as antibiotics.
4. Provide the patient and family with information regarding lung abscess and the treatment protocol, which may last as long as 6 to 8 weeks.
5. Teach the patient the importance of good oral hygiene, especially as long as there is active lung drainage.

6. Teach the patient methods to reduce the chances of a lung abscess in the future, such as good oral hygiene, avoidance of aspiration, and prompt medical attention for potential bacterial infection of the mouth or respiratory tract.

Evaluation

Movement of air in and out of lung is optimum *Airways are clear* and breathing occurs without obstruction. Breath sounds are clear and bilaterally equal; percussion tone is resonant over all lung fields. No purulent material remains in lungs, and there is no evidence of lung abscess. Serial chest roentgenograms show progressive improvement and healing. Temperature and laboratory values return to normal.

Cause of lung abscess has been identified and treated Disease state does not occur. Discomfort resolves.

Patient describes strategies to cope with fatigue.

Patient and family have sufficient information to comply with discharge regimen Patient and family at time of discharge are able to discuss medications (purpose, side effects, and route) and signs of additional infection or respiratory deterioration.

▌PNEUMONIA AND PNEUMONITIS

Pneumonia is an inflammatory process of the respiratory bronchioles and the alveolar spaces that is caused by infection. Pneumonitis is noninfectious bronchial and alveolar inflammation. Together, these terms are used to refer to inflammatory processes of the parenchyma of the lung (Figure 2-36).

Pneumonia is the most common cause of death from infectious disease in North America. It is also considered to be a major source of disease and death in critically ill patients.[51]

Pneumonia may be caused by bacteria, viruses, *Mycoplasma,* fungi, and parasites. Currently about half of pneumonia cases are caused by bacteria and half by virus. Up to 96% of bacterial pneumonia is caused by three organisms. Since most of the organisms require specific therapy, it is important to identify the agent causing the disease.

Pneumonia occurs most often during the winter and early spring and in persons 60 years or older. Persons most at risk for nosocomial (hospital-acquired) pneumonia are the very young or very old, and those with cardiopulmonary disease, immunosuppression, decreased level of consciousness, or post chest/abdominal surgery.[80]

Bacterial Pneumonia

***Streptococcus pneumoniae* (pneumococcal) pneumonia** *S. pneumoniae* (hemolytic streptococcus type A), a gram-positive diplococcus, is by far the most common and important cause of bacterial pneumonia, accounting for 90% of cases. The infection usually involves extensive consolidation of part

or all of the parenchyma of the lobe. *S. pneumoniae* pneumonia is often seen in infants, the elderly, and patients with sickle cell disease, congestive heart failure, alcoholism, or diabetes mellitus. A vaccine is now available and is 80% to 90% effective against this type of pneumonia in adults.

***Staphylococcus aureus* pneumonia** *S. aureus,* a gram-positive coccus, may cause pneumonia in infants and the elderly and commonly causes pneumonia as a complication of influenza or in hospitalized patients as a secondary infection after surgery, tracheostomy, coma, or immunosuppressive therapy. It accounts for 3% to 5% of bacterial pneumonia.

***Haemophilus influenzae* (type B) pneumonia** *H. influenzae,* a gram-negative bacillus, causes lobar-type pneumonia, bronchopneumonia, or bronchiolitis in adults. It accounts for 1% of bacterial pneumonia.

Nonbacterial Pneumonia

Atypical Pneumonia

***Mycoplasma pneumoniae* pneumonia** Infection with *M. pneumoniae,* which is most common in school-aged children and young adults, spreads among family members. Transmission

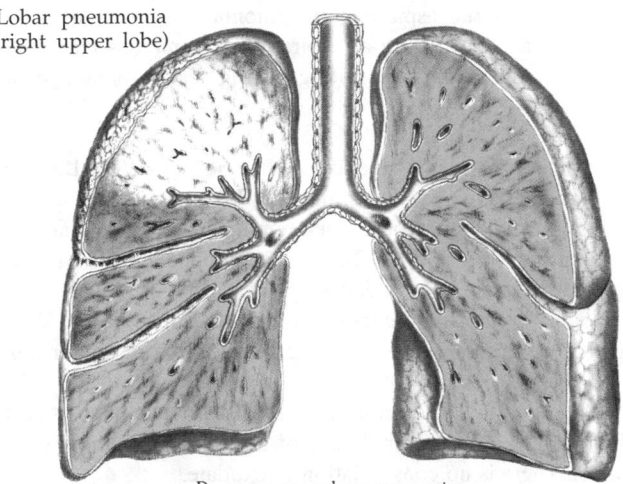
Lobar pneumonia (right upper lobe)

Pneumococcal pneumonia

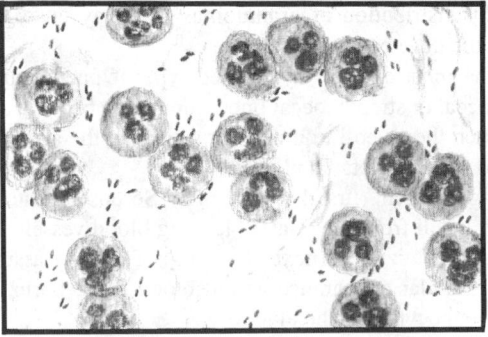
Purulent sputum with pneumococci and polymorphonuclear leukocytes

Figure 2-36 Pneumonia. (From Wilson.[93])

is believed to occur by infected respiratory secretions. *M. pneumoniae* pneumonia is a type of bronchopneumonia.

Legionnaires' disease   *Legionella pneumophila* is a weakly organized gram-negative organism that is identified with a special fluorescent antibody stain. Legionnaires' disease occurs most commonly in older adults and in persons who smoke or have chronic disease such as diabetes, renal disease, cancer, chronic bronchitis, or emphysema. It is three times more common in men than in women.

Pneumocystis carinii pneumonia   *P. carinii* pneumonia, caused by a protozoal organism, is discussed in Chapter 14.

Aspiration Pneumonia Syndrome

Aspiration pneumonia syndrome occurs most commonly as a result of inhalation of substances into the lower airways and alveoli when the patient is in an altered state of consciousness owing to a seizure, drugs, alcohol, anesthesia, acute infection, or shock. It may also occur when the anatomy is altered by esophageal stricture, tracheal fistula, or a nasogastric tube. Aspiration pneumonia may be acquired through foreign body aspiration or aspiration of body substances such as saliva or gastric contents. Nonbacterial aspiration pneumonia may follow aspiration of toxic materials such as toxic fluids and inert substances; bacterial aspiration pneumonia may occur as a secondary problem. Bacterial aspiration pneumonias may cause extensive lung damage resulting in lung abscess or empyema.

•••••• Pathophysiology

The pathophysiology depends on the etiologic agent. Bacterial pneumonia is marked by an intra-alveolar suppurative exudate with consolidation. Lobar pneumonia causes consolidation of the entire lobe (Figure 2-37). Bronchopneumonia causes a patchy distribution of infectious areas around and involving the bronchi. A chest roentgenogram of bronchopneumonia shows patchy segmental or subsegmental infiltration in one or more dependent lobes.

Mycoplasmal and viral pneumonias produce interstitial inflammation with accumulation of an infiltrate in the alveolar walls. There is no consolidation or exudate.

Fungal and mycobacterial pneumonias are marked by patchy distribution of granulomas that may undergo necrosis with the development of cavities.

The most extensively studied type of pneumonia is pneumococcal or streptococcal pneumonia. The bacteria are thought to reach the alveoli in mucus or saliva. In the alveoli, they undergo four predictable phases:[68]

Engorgement (first 4 to 12 hours). Serous exudate pours into alveoli from the dilated, leaking blood vessels.

Red hepatization (next 48 hours). The lung assumes a red granular appearance as red blood cells, fibrin, and PMN leukocytes fill the alveoli.

Gray hepatization (3 to 8 days). The lung assumes a grayish appearance as the leukocytes and fibrin consolidate in the involved alveoli.

Resolution (7 to 11 days). Exudate is lysed and resorbed by macrophages, restoring the tissue to its original structure.

These stages represent the course of untreated pneumococcal pneumonia. With the use of antibiotics the course should run 3 to 5 days.

Viral pneumonia affects the tissues differently. The inflammatory response in the bronchi damages the ciliated epithelium. The lungs are congested and in some cases hemorrhagic. The inflammatory response is composed of mononuclear cells, lymphocytes, and plasma cells in proportions that vary with the type of virus causing the disease. In severe types of viral pneumonia, the alveoli contain hyaline membranes. Characteristic intracellular viral inclusions may be seen in adenovirus, cytomegalovirus, respiratory syncytial virus, or varicella virus infections.

Aspiration pneumonia presents a still different physiologic response, which is based on the pH of the aspirated substance. If the pH is 2.5 or above, little necrosis results. However, if the pH is below 2.5, as is common with gastric acid, atelectasis occurs, followed by pulmonary edema, hemorrhage, and type II cell necrosis. The alveolar-capillary "membrane" may be damaged, leading to exudation and in severe cases ARDS.[61]

•••••• Diagnostic Studies and Findings

Clinical Examination (Depends on Type of Pneumonia)

Bacterial   Sudden onset; chest pain; chills; fever; headache; cough; rales and possibly friction rub; hypoxemia; cyanosis; area of consolidation visible on chest roentgenogram;

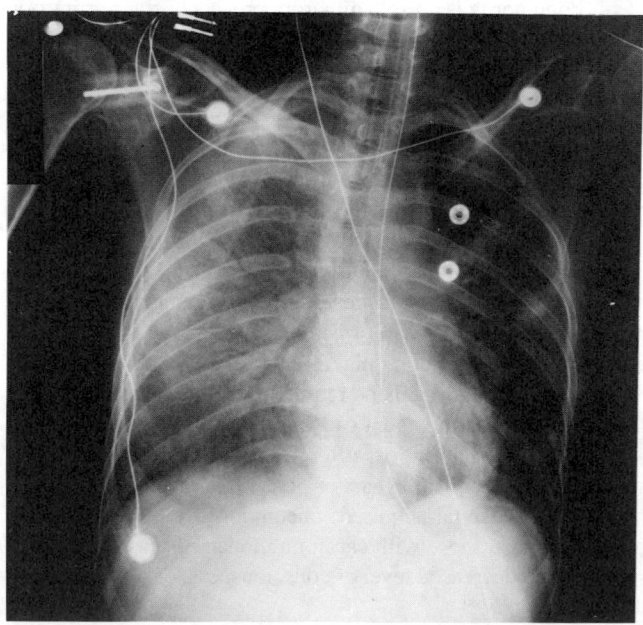

Figure 2-37 Chest roentgenogram of patient with pneumonia. Note infiltrate of right middle and lower zones with air bronchogram seen; right heart border not obliterated. Also note monitor electrodes, gown snaps, endotracheal tube, and ventilator tubing. (Courtesy R. Keith Wilson, MD, Baylor College of Medicine, Houston, Texas.)

sputum culture needed to determine causative agent; egophony; sputum color varies with different organisms

Mycoplasmal Gradual onset; headache; fever; malaise; chills; cough severe and nonproductive; decreased breath sounds and rales; chest roentgenogram clear; white blood cell count normal

Viral Symptoms generally mild; cold symptoms; headache; anorexia; fever; myalgia; irritating cough that produces mucopurulent or bloody sputum; bronchopneumonic type of infiltration on chest roentgenogram; white blood cell count usually normal; rise in antibody titers

Sputum examination Sputum from lower respiratory tract needed for sputum culture. If patient is unable to expectorate sputum, it usually may be obtained by suction or fiberoptic bronchoscopy; macroexamination for odor, consistency, amount, color (see above for anticipated color); microexamination including Gram stain for etiologic agent, neutrophilia, increased epithelial cells, presence of other organisms; sputum culture for organism identification

Blood cultures May be transient bacteremia in pneumococcal pneumonia

Acid-fast stains and cultures To rule out tuberculosis

White blood cell count Leukocytosis (15,000 to 25,000/mm^3) in bacterial infection; normal or low white blood cell count in mycoplasmal or viral infection

Blood gases Hypoxemia ($\downarrow$ Pao$_2$). Usually hyperventilation ($\downarrow$ Paco$_2$) but in the presence of other comorbid conditions, may see hypoventilation ($\uparrow$ Paco$_2$)

Chest roentgenogram Presence of alveolar filling defects (Figure 2-40)

••••• Multidisciplinary Plan

Medications

Antiinfective agents specific to cultured organisms

General Management

Oxygenation—if patient has Pao$_2$ less than 60 mm Hg; Venturi mask or nasal prongs commonly used

Physiotherapy—patient should be encouraged at least to cough and deep breathe to maximize ventilatory capabilities

Hydration—monitoring of intake and output; supplemental fluids to maintain hydration and liquefy secretions

NURSING CARE

Nursing Assessment

Respiratory Status

Tachypnea; retractions; labored breathing; dyspnea; nasal flaring; rales; pleural friction rub; diminished breath sounds over area of consolidation; labored or irregular breathing; breathing tiring for patient; percussion tone dull over area of consolidation

Hypoxia

Restlessness; confusion; tachycardia; cyanosis

Laboratory Values

Evidence of elevated leukocyte count

If patient seriously ill, monitor for decreased pH and Pao$_2$ and increased Paco$_2$

Temperature

Monitored for elevation

Cough and Sputum

Amount and productivity of coughing; color, consistency, odor, and amount of sputum; fatigue related to coughing; periodic laboratory evaluation of sputum needed to evaluate patient's response to treatment; pair with coughing

Hydration State

Intake and output; tissue turgor; liquidity of sputum; electrolytes

Potential Complications

Complications that may occur with pneumonia are pleurisy, atelectasis, empyema, lung abscess, meningitis, and sepsis

Nursing Dx & Intervention

Ineffective airway clearance related to mucopurulent sputum

- Assess patient to identify inability to move secretions. If inability is identified, assist with appropriate measures such as coughing, positioning, suctioning, and liquefying secretions; assist to splint chest wall with coughing if painful.
- Promptly administer bronchodilators, mucolytics, and expectorants per protocol *to dilate bronchioles*. Observe for therapeutic response and side effects.
- Provide hydration *to liquefy secretions and replace fluids*.
- Carefully and frequently auscultate chest for quality of breath sounds and adventitious sounds. Note cough and sputum characteristics.

Ineffective breathing pattern related to inflammatory process, pleuritic pain, and increased ventilatory drive

- Assess ventilation to include evaluation of breathing rate, rhythm, and depth; chest expansion; presence of respiratory distress such as dyspnea, shortness of breath, nasal flaring, pursed-lip breathing, or prolonged expiratory phase; and use of accessory muscles.
- Identify contributing factors such as airway clearance or obstruction problem or weakness.

- Maintain patient in position *that facilitates ventilation* (head of bed in semi-Fowler's position or patient sitting and leaning forward on overbed table).
- Instruct patient in proper pulmonary hygiene routines *that will promote easy and effective breathing, facilitate removal of secretions from tracheobronchial tree, and minimize pulmonary congestion,* which could lead to superinfections.
- Assess patient for tiring in relation to attempts to breathe.

Impaired gas exchange related to altered V/Q relationships

- Assess patient to identify signs, such as restlessness, confusion, and irritability, *that may indicate body's response to altered blood gas states.*
- If necessary and with physician consultation, administer oxygen by nasal cannula or Venturi mask *to maintain* PaO_2 *above 60 mm Hg.*
- Monitor serum electrolytes that may change *because of alterations in oxygenation and metabolism.*
- Carefully monitor body temperature.

Fatigue related to debilitated state, frequent cough

- Assess patterns of fatigue.
- Assess factors related to fatigue and strategies for dealing with them.
- Assess support systems and available resources.
- Encourage patient to use adaptive breathing techniques *to decrease work of breathing.*
- Assist patient to alternate activities with periods of rest.
- Encourage gradual increase of activities as tolerated.
- If patient is seriously ill and maintained on bed rest, encourage or provide active or passive range of motion *to maintain adequate muscle tone.*
- Administer treatments or medications to relieve discomfort.

Altered nutrition: less than body requirements related to debilitated state

- Help patient choose foods that are easy to chew and swallow.
- Assist by cutting and feeding if patient tires easily.
- Consider additional consultation.
- See p. 1546 for additional strategies.

Risk for fluid volume deficit related to fever

- If patient is seriously ill, assess for evidence of dehydration resulting from fever and lack of fluid intake.
- Carefully monitor intake and output.
- Encourage fluid intake if needed.

Family coping: potential for growth

- Assess family's understanding of diagnostic procedures, disease process and prognosis, and therapies used.
- Involve family in care as appropriate.
- Teach family about strict handwashing *to prevent spread of pneumonia.*

Patient Education/Home Care Planning

1. Teach the patient deep breathing and coughing techniques.
2. Teach the family the importance of handwashing when working with the patient to prevent the spread of organisms.
3. Teach the patient and family facts about and the importance of prescribed medications such as antibiotics, including finishing prescribed duration of therapy.
4. Provide the patient and family with information regarding the specific type of pneumonia the patient has, treatment, anticipated response, possible complications, and probable disease duration.
5. Inform the patient and family that a change in health status must be reported to the patient's health care providers. Indicators of change may include a change in sputum characteristics or color, decreased activity tolerance, fever despite the antibiotics, increasing chest pain, or a feeling that things are not getting better.
6. Teach the patient the importance of consuming large quantities of fluid.
7. Teach the patient adaptive exercise and rest techniques.

Evaluation

Airway is patent   There is no cough or pulmonary congestion and no sputum production.

Breath sounds are clear in all areas   There are no areas of decreased breath sounds or consolidation.

Gas exchange is within normal limits PaO_2 equals 80 to 100 mm Hg. Arterial pH equals 7.35 to 7.45.

Activities of daily living are accomplished with minimal fatigue   Patient states importance of gradual activity progression.

Nutrition level is maintained   Patient maintains adequate dietary intake.

Fluid volume status is optimized   Vital signs return to baseline. Urine output is adequate. Serum electrolytes are within normal limits.

Patient and family have sufficient information to comply with discharge regimen   Patient and family at time of discharge are able to discuss medications (purpose, side effects, route, and schedule), dietary therapy regimen, activity progression regimen, and signs of secondary infection.

COR PULMONALE AND PULMONARY HYPERTENSION

Cor pulmonale is a condition of hypertrophy and dilation of the right ventricle of the heart resulting from a disease process that affects the function or structure of the lung or its vasculature. This may occur with or without heart failure (Figure 2-38). Pulmonary hypertension is an increase in the main pulmonary artery pressure at rest or during exercise. This means that the systolic/diastolic pressure in the pulmonary artery exceeds 30/15 mm Hg at rest (Figure 2-39).

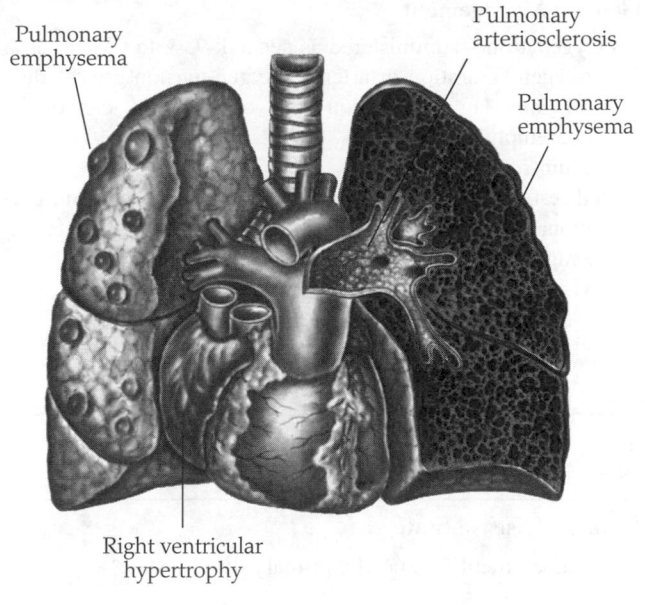

Figure 2-38 Cor pulmonale. (From Wilson.[93])

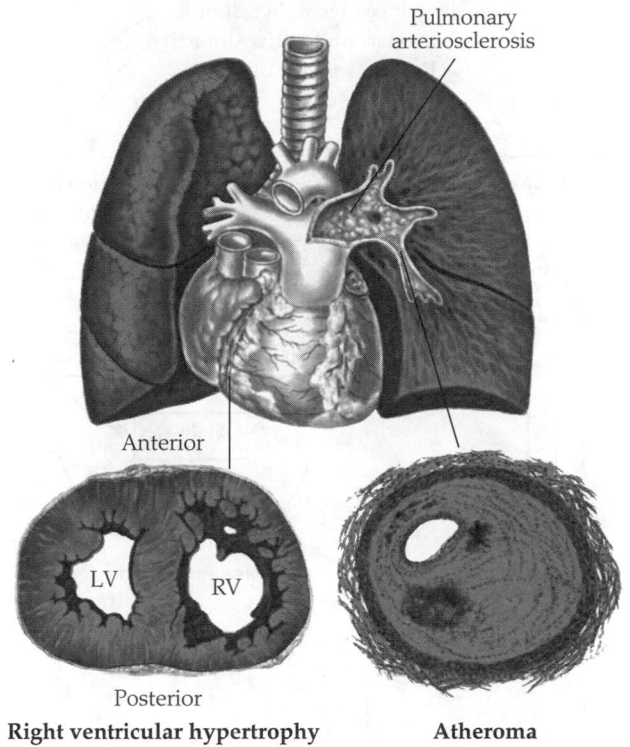

Figure 2-39 Pulmonary hypertension. (From Wilson.[93])

Cor pulmonale occurs as a secondary process following a primary pulmonary disease. The four most common disorders leading to cor pulmonale are obstructive lung diseases, vascular diseases, restrictive lung diseases, and chest wall disorders.

Obstructive lung diseases
  Chronic bronchitis
  Emphysema
  Asthma
  Cystic fibrosis
  Bronchiectasis
Vascular disease—thromboembolism
Restrictive lung diseases
  Atelectasis
  Pneumonia
  Interstitial fibrosis
  Sarcoidosis
Chest wall disorders—kyphoscoliosis
Chronic obstructive pulmonary disease accounts for about 75% of cases of cor pulmonale in the United States.

There are three primary factors in the development of cor pulmonale and right-sided failure: (1) reduction in the size of the pulmonary vascular bed as a result of destruction of pulmonary capillaries or loss of large amounts of lung tissue; (2) increased resistance in the pulmonary vascular bed; and (3) the effect of reduced oxygen in causing pulmonary vasoconstriction and elevation of pressure in the pulmonary artery.

••••• Pathophysiology

The pulmonary circulation is normally a low-pressure, low-resistance system that may increase output, without increasing pulmonary pressure, to increase cardiac output. As pulmonary vascular resistance of the small arterioles and arteries increases in some types of disease, pulmonary hypertension results. Pulmonary hypertension, in turn, increases the workload of the right side of the heart, causing it to hypertrophy and eventually fail.[68]

A second major process causing pulmonary hypertension is an alteration in pulmonary arteriolar vasoconstriction. Chronic vasoconstriction, resulting from hypoxemia, and acidosis may lead to pulmonary hypertension. Figure 2-40 shows the pathogenesis of cor pulmonale.

••••• Diagnostic Studies and Findings

Clinical examination Evidence of other chronic lung diseases; dyspnea; cough; cyanosis; wheezing; distended neck veins; loud pulmonic secondary sound on cardiac auscultation; gallop rhythm and occasional murmur resulting from functional insufficiency of tricuspid and pulmonic valves; dependent edema; liver enlargement

Chest roentgenogram Enlarged pulmonary arteries; right ventricular hypertrophy

Echocardiogram Right ventricular enlargement

Arterial blood gases Decreased Pao_2 in range of 40 to 60 mm Hg; $Paco_2$ varies with underlying disease

Electrocardiogram Arrhythmias resulting from hypoxia; right bundle-branch block; right axis deviation; right ventricular hypertrophy

Complete blood count Elevated hemoglobin level and hematocrit value and polycythemia resulting from chronic hypoxia

Pulmonary arterial pressure Systolic pressure above 30 mm Hg; diastolic pressure above 15 mm Hg

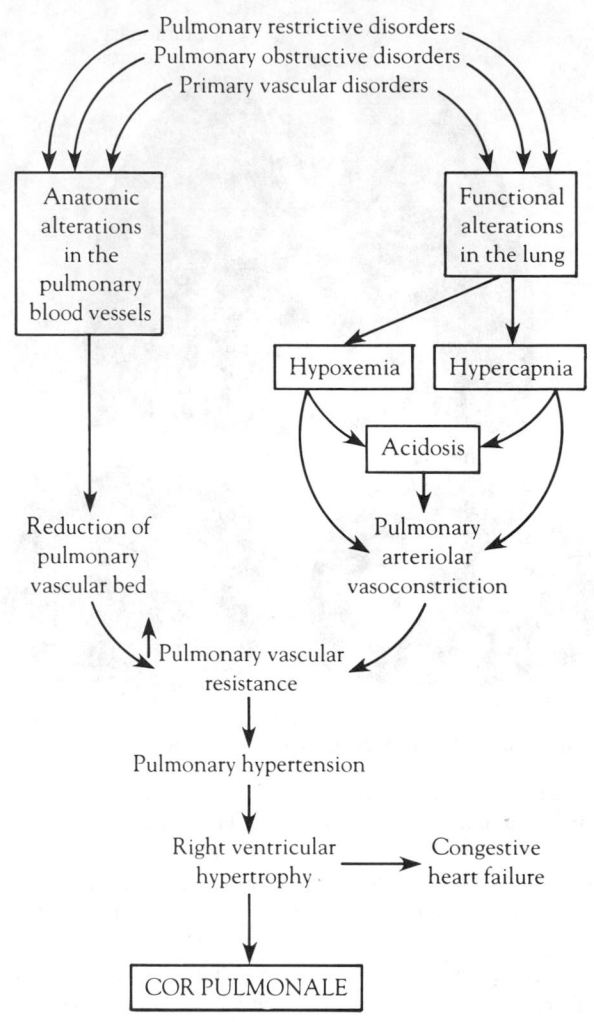

Figure 2-40 Etiology and pathogenesis of cor pulmonale. (From Price and Wilson.[67])

•••••• Multidisciplinary Plan

The underlying pulmonary and cardiac diseases must be treated as well. (See Chapter 1 for cardiac disease guidelines.)

Medications

Diuretics
    Initial diuresis can lower pulmonary artery pressure by decreasing total blood volume; careful monitoring of serum electrolytes needed when administering diuretics
Furosemide (Lasix), 20-80 mg/d to maximum of 600 mg/d
Bronchodilators
    Theophylline recommended to improve airway obstruction and reduce afterload on right side of heart, thereby improving cardiac output
    Theophylline (Theo-Dur, Theolair, Elixophyllin, others), 16 mg/kg divided into 3 or 4 doses

General Management

Oxygenation—administered as needed; 93% to 95% arterial oxygen saturation or arterial oxygen tension greater than 60 mm Hg; ventilation and oxygenation cannot be overemphasized
Sodium-restricted diet
Bed rest during acute episodes to conserve energy and pulmonary effort
Therapeutic phlebotomy—to reduce polycythemia and blood viscosity, used when Hct >58%

NURSING CARE

Nursing Assessment

Primary Disease State

See assessment for specific primary disease state

Fluid Retention

Careful monitoring of intake and output; weight

Presence of Complications

Ankle edema; distended neck veins; abdominal pain; hepatomegaly; cardiac ventricular gallop (S_3); tachycardia; tachypnea

Nursing Dx & Intervention

The primary nursing diagnoses and nursing care should be directed toward the primary disease state. In addition, the following diagnoses and care strategies are specific for cor pulmonale.

Impaired gas exchange related to V/Q mismatch

- Assess patient to identify signs, such as restlessness, confusion, and irritability, that may indicate body's response to altered blood gases.
- In collaboration with physician, order and monitor arterial blood gas studies.
- In collaboration with physician, administer oxygen *to maintain oxygen saturation between 90% and 95%.*
- If patient has chronic hypercapnia, keep oxygen saturation at 88% to 93% to avoid depressing ventilatory drive.
- Monitor electrocardiogram and cardiac status for arrhythmias resulting from alterations in blood gases.
- Monitor for signs of increasing cor pulmonale such as increased pulmonary artery pressure, increased edema in extremities, jugular venous distention, and hepatomegaly.

Fluid volume excess related to right ventricular failure

- Monitor and record weight daily.
- Carefully monitor and record intake and output.
- In collaboration with physician, administer diuretic medications.

- Assist patient to maintain sodium-restricted diet.
- Assist patient to limit fluid intake.
- Monitor serum electrolytes, which may change owing to administration of diuretics or alterations in metabolism.

Patient Education/Home Care Planning

The primary education is directed toward the patient's primary disease state; refer to patient education for specific primary disease.

1. Teach the patient the importance of restricting salt intake and limiting fluid intake.
2. Teach the patient to weigh self daily and report greater than a 2 lb or 1 kg gain per week.
3. Teach the patient facts about and importance of prescribed medications.
4. Provide the patient and family with information regarding the care, cleaning, and maintenance of inhalation or oxygen equipment being used in the hospital or to be used at home, as well as the signs of oxygen toxicity.
5. Emphasize that oxygen ordered continuously must be used at least a total of 22 out of 24 hours for improvement of right heart failure.

Evaluation

Also see the patient outcomes for the underlying disease state.

Optimum gas exchange occurs throughout lungs Blood gas values are within normal limits for patient's condition.

Fluid and electrolyte balance is restored There is no evidence of fluid retention; serum electrolytes are within normal limits.

Patient and family have sufficient information to comply with discharge regimen Patient and family at time of discharge are able to discuss medications, dietary therapy, activity progression, evidence of respiratory infection or compromise, and plan for follow-up visit.

■ PULMONARY EDEMA

Pulmonary edema is the accumulation of serous fluid in the interstitial lung tissue and alveoli. Pulmonary edema may be described as cardiogenic or noncardiogenic. The most common cause of cardiogenic pulmonary edema is increased hydrostatic pressure caused by left ventricular failure. See the section on congestive heart failure (p. 38) for further discussion of cardiogenic pulmonary edema.

Noncardiogenic pulmonary edema results from increased capillary permeability, as occurs with ARDS or from decreased colloid osmotic pressure, as occurs in nephritis or hepatic fail-

! EMERGENCY ALERT

PULMONARY EDEMA

Results from back pressure into lungs and left atria that leads to increased pressures in the pulmonary capillaries that causes fluid to leak into the alveoli. Pulmonary edema is a symptom of an underlying disorder, not a diagnosis.

Assessment

- Sudden onset, S.O.B.
- Chest tightness, anxiety
- Inability to lie down
- Decreased exercise tolerance
- Paroxysmal nocturnal dyspnea and orthopnea
- Cough, rales, rhonchi, wheezes
- Jugular venous distention (JVD), S_3 gallop, decreased heart sounds
- Peripheral edema
- Tachycardia
- Pink, frothy sputum

Interventions

- Place patient in high Fowler's position.
- Administer high-flow oxygen by mask (10 to 15 L).
- Obtain IV access.
- Relieve pain using narcotic such as morphine sulfate.
- Administer diuretics.
- Consider bronchodilators and digitalis.
- Monitor arterial blood gases.
- Provide reassurance.
- Constantly monitor patient.

ure. See the section on ARDS (p. 141) for further description of noncardiogenic pulmonary edema.

When interstitial lung spaces are engorged with fluid, the fluid moves across alveolar capillary membranes into the alveoli. If fluid accumulates faster than it can be cleared, acute pulmonary edema interferes with oxygen diffusion, resulting in acute respiratory failure. See the discussion of acute respiratory failure in this chapter (p. 140).

■ PULMONARY EMBOLISM AND PULMONARY INFARCTION

Pulmonary embolism is the blockage of a pulmonary artery by foreign matter such as a thrombus that usually arises from a peripheral vein, fat, air, or tumor tissue. Subsequent to the blockage is obstruction of blood supply to the lung tissue (Figure 2-41).

Pulmonary infarction is an uncommon complication of pulmonary embolism resulting in a localized area of lung tissue ischemic necrosis distal to the area of embolus.

The formation of a pulmonary embolism usually occurs in patients with well-defined risk factors. Following are the most common predisposing factors:

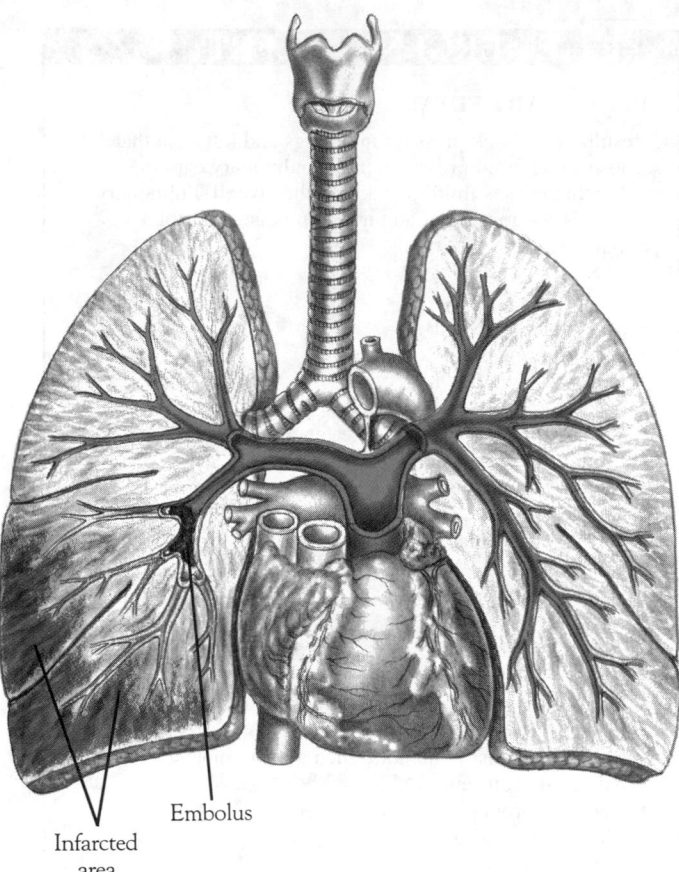

Embolus

Infarcted
area

Figure 2-41 Pulmonary embolism. (From Wilson.[93])

Thrombophlebitis	Elderly
Major surgery	Chronic illness
Use of estrogens	Congestive heart failure
Pregnancy	Obesity
Recent childbirth	Venous insufficiency
Leg trauma	Immobilization from fracture
Myocardial infarction	Polycythemia vera

Pulmonary embolism is the third most common cardiovascular disease in the United States. Overall, predisposing factors are most often surgery/trauma (43%), idiopathic (40%), heart disease (12%), or neoplastic disease (4%).[88]

Death from massive pulmonary embolism usually occurs within the first 24 hours. After that time and with proper treatment, the death rate drops significantly. Resolution of the embolus usually occurs within 7 to 10 days.

•••••• Pathophysiology

Three factors (Virchow's triad) are related to the development of a venous thrombus: venous stasis, injury to the vein wall, and increased blood coagulability.

The most common sites for thrombus formation are the deep veins of the legs, especially iliac, femoral, and popliteal, and the pelvic veins.[32] At some point, the thrombus breaks loose and travels to and lodges in one of the pulmonary arteries.

EMERGENCY ALERT

PULMONARY EMBOLUS

Often confusing and very difficult to diagnose. A pulmonary infarction results from a detached venous thrombus that forms an embolus that then lodges in a branch of the pulmonary artery, tachypnea, causing a partial or total occlusion.

Assessment

- Symptoms often nonspecific
- SOB, trachypnea, tachycardia
- Angina-like chest pain, pallor, or cyanosis
- Anxiety
- Decreased blood pressure
- Wheezes, rales on auscultation
- Abnormal ECG, possible
- Elevated temperature

Interventions

- Obtain arterial blood gases, chest radiograph, ECG.
- Obtain ventilation/perfusion scan (VQ).
- Maintain airway, breathing, and circulation.
- Administer high-flow oxygen by mask (10 to 15 L).
- Obtain IV access.
- Administer analgesia.
- Consider bronchodilators.
- Monitor clotting times and prepare to anticoagulate with heparin.
- Thrombolytic therapy and/or surgical interventions may be considered.

A pulmonary embolism produces an area of the lung that is ventilated but underperfused. This results in an increase in physiologic dead space ventilation. Reflex bronchoconstriction occurs in the affected area and is thought to result from the release of histamine or serotonin from the clot. If the embolism is large and sufficiently reduces the pulmonary perfusion, pulmonary hypertension may result.

If the embolism lodges in a large or medium-sized artery, there may be insufficient collateral bronchial blood circulation. If this occurs, there may be significant tissue hypoperfusion, and pulmonary infarction may result.

•••••• Diagnostic Studies and Findings[54,88]

Clinical examination   Dyspnea, pleuritic pain, apprehension, cough, unexplained hemoptysis, sweats, tachypnea, localized rales, pleural friction rub, tachycardia, cyanosis, low-grade fever, thrombophlebitis

Blood gases PaO_2 less than 60 mm Hg. Hyperventilation leads to $PaCO_2 < 40$ mm Hg; alveolar arterial oxygen tension gradient ($PA-aO_2$) increased

Electrocardiogram   The following classic signs help to differentiate pulmonary embolism from myocardial infarction: ST segment depression, right axis deviation, incomplete or complete right bundle-branch block, tall peaked P waves, S wave in lead I, a Q wave in lead III, T wave inversion in V_1-V_2

Chest roentgenogram   Unilateral diaphragm elevation, enlarged main pulmonary artery associated with decreased vascular markings on one side, unilateral pulmonary effusion, enlargement of heart size

Lung scans   Rapid, relatively safe and easy screening tests for establishing the diagnosis (Figure 2-42); if the patient has a chronic lung disease, asthma, or congestive heart failure, the lung scan is of little diagnostic value; two scans are commonly used sequentially: perfusion lung scan and ventilation lung scan; comparison of scans may be diagnostic of pulmonary embolism: *perfusion lung scan:* this study involves the intravenous injection of serum albumin tagged with tracer amounts of a radioisotope; the radioactive particles pass through the right side of the heart and lodge in the pulmonary capillary bed; significant diagnostic findings reveal an area deficient in radioactivity; *ventilation lung scan:* the patient initially breathes a radioactive gas through a carefully sealed system for several minutes; during this time the lungs are scanned by a gamma camera

Pulmonary angiography   Although it is the most specific diagnostic procedure, pulmonary angiography also has the most risk; the two diagnostic criteria of this technique are intraarterial filling defects and complete obstruction of a pulmonary artery branch

Noninvasive ultrasonography   Evidence of a residual clot in the leg veins is presumptive for a diagnosis of embolus

Potential complications   Cardiac arrhythmias, cor pulmonale, hypotension, severe hypoxemia, pulmonary hypertension, atelectasis

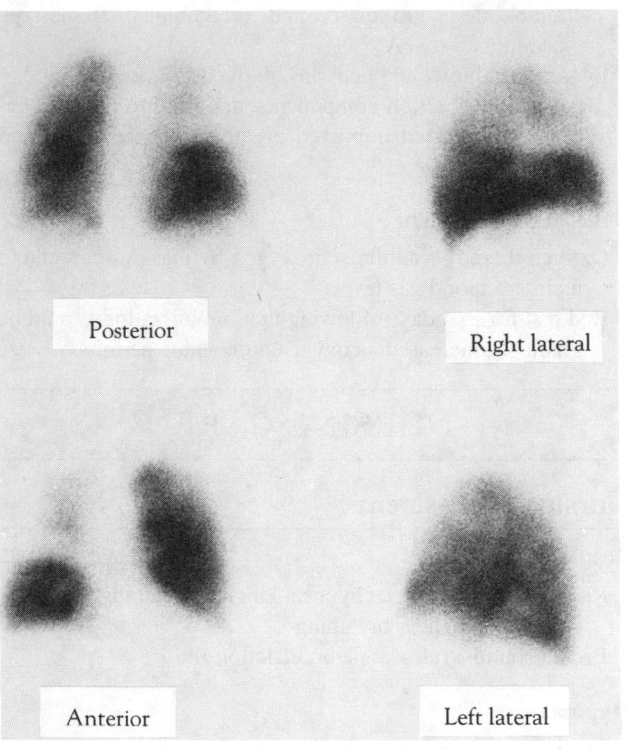

Figure 2-42 Lung scan showing pulmonary embolism. Note decreased perfusion of right upper lobe indicative of pulmonary embolism. (Courtesy R. Keith Wilson, MD, Baylor College of Medicine, Houston, Texas.)

•••••• Multidisciplinary Plan

Surgery

Surgical therapy of pulmonary embolism infrequently indicated; when there are multiple emboli, umbrella filter may be surgically placed in inferior vena cava; other techniques are surgical removal of the embolus, which requires cardiopulmonary bypass, and interruption of blood flow through inferior vena cava via ligation

Medications

Anticoagulants—main purpose of this therapy is supportive

Heparin: does not directly lead to clot lysis; instead, heparin halts clot propagation, enabling endogenous fibrinolytic mechanisms to remove the clot.[63] Heparin may be administered by continuous intravenous infusion or by intermittent intravenous injections

Continuous infusion is associated with fewer hemorrhagic side effects than intermittent bolus doses, and therapeutic levels are attained sooner[1]

Continuous infusion: 18-20 U/kg/hr or 800-1500 U/H to start, adjusted as necessary

The dose of heparin is best monitored and regulated by obtaining serial venous samples for partial thromboplastin time (PTT) coagulation studies. The dose should be adjusted to maintain clotting times in the range of 1.5 to 2.5 times the control values. The drug is generally continued until warfarin (Coumadin) elevates the prothrombin time (PT) therapeutically

Should a severe bleeding event occur secondary to the use of heparin, protamine sulfate may be given intravenously. In such a case, 1 mg of protamine is given for every 100 U of heparin received in the dose before the bleeding episode. The drug should be administered slowly over 3 to 5 minutes in 20 ml saline. The total amount of protamine should not exceed 100 mg

Long-term anticoagulation: necessary when the patient is predisposed to another pulmonary embolus

Warfarin should be started as soon as oral therapy is possible to decrease the length of time heparin is required. Warfarin levels are monitored by PT and also reported as an international normalized ratio (INR). When INR levels reach 2.0 to 3.0 on warfarin, then heparin is discontinued[33]

Oral dose: 5-10 mg daily, titrated to PT level

Warfarin may be used for 6 months up to life in some cases

Fibrinolytic enzymes: fibrinolytic therapy may be used in massive pulmonary embolus associated with hemodynamic instability. Examples of fibrinolytic enzymes are streptokinase, urokinase, and recombinant tissue-type plasminogen (rt-PA)[33]

Low molecular weight heparins, derived from separating heparins into fraction components, are coming into use because of reported improved predictability in dosing and longer half-lives[1]

General Management

Oxygen therapy—administer oxygen by mask or cannula to maintain blood gas levels

Bed rest for first day; following that, mobilization should be gradually increased as oxygenation status permits

NURSING CARE

Nursing Assessment

Respiratory Status

Respiratory distress: tachypnea, labored breathing, dyspnea, coughing, shallow breathing

Breath sounds: rales or pleural friction rub

Hypoxia

Restlessness, confusion, tachycardia, cyanosis

Cough, Sputum

Characteristics of cough and sputum should be monitored daily

Chest Roentgenogram

Should be monitored periodically for changes

Psychosocial

Fear, air hunger, pain, confusion

Potential Risk for Pulmonary Embolism

Identification of persons at risk for development of pulmonary embolism

Nursing Dx & Intervention

Impaired gas exchange related to ventilation/perfusion abnormalities

- Assess patient to identify signs such as restlessness, confusion, and irritability, which may indicate the body's response to altered blood gas states.
- In collaboration with physician order, monitor arterial blood gases; report increases or decreases in $Paco_2$ and Pao_2 of more than 10 mm Hg.
- In collaboration with physician, administer oxygen *to maintain adequate blood gas levels.*
- Monitor electrocardiogram and cardiac status *for arrhythmias secondary to alterations in blood gases.*
- If patient is seriously ill, monitor for signs of cor pulmonale such as pulmonary hypertension, cardiac compromise, jugular venous distention, blood gas abnormalities, and hepatomegaly.
- Monitor and record kidney functioning and urinary output, which may be affected *secondary to tissue hypoxia and alterations in metabolism.*
- As long as patient is in respiratory distress, maintain bed rest; proceed with ambulation as quickly as possible after anticoagulation attained.

Ineffective breathing pattern related to substernal pain

- Assess ventilation to include evaluation of breathing rate, rhythm, and depth, chest expansion, presence of respiratory distress such as dyspnea, shortness of breath, tachypnea, shallow breathing, ineffective breathing, and use of accessory muscles.
- Carefully and frequently auscultate chest for quality of breath sounds and adventitious sounds; *note cough and sputum characteristics.*
- Identify contributing factors such as airway clearance or obstruction problem, or weakness.
- Maintain patient positioning *to facilitate easy ventilation* (i.e., head of bed in semi-Fowler's position).
- Assess patient for tiring in relation to attempts to breathe.
- Encourage patient to space activities *so as to provide periods of rest in between.*
- Administer analgesics as needed to relieve pain and promote effective ventilation.

Patient Education/Home Care Planning

1. Teach the patient about medications (including side effects) that are currently being used to treat the pulmonary embolism. Include information on monitoring for bleeding, as well as information about ongoing laboratory studies needed for medication dosage adjustment. Teach patient to inform all physicians and dentists about anticoagulated status.
2. Teach preventive measures to all high-risk patients preoperatively and initiate interventions postoperatively that will help prevent pulmonary embolism.
3. Teach strategies for persons at high risk to prevent venous pooling, which may lead to thrombophlebitis.
4. Changes in the health status of a patient recovering from pulmonary embolism must be reported immediately to the patient's health care provider. Changes include chest pain, shortness of breath, tachypnea, blood-tinged sputum, and blood in the stool or urine.

Evaluation

Blood gas values are within normal limits for patient Airways are clear, and breathing occurs without obstruction. Chest roentgenogram or lung scan shows no evidence of pulmonary embolism.

Breathing pattern is adequate   There is no shortness of breath, dyspnea, tachypnea, or shallow breathing. Clear breath sounds are heard in all areas. Chest discomfort is relieved.

Patient and family have sufficient information to comply with discharge regimen   Patient and family are able at time of discharge to discuss medications (purpose, side effects, route, and schedule), dietary therapy regimen; activity progression regimen, signs of infection or respiratory deterioration, and plan for follow-up visits.

PNEUMOTHORAX AND HEMOTHORAX[17,30]

The presence of air in the pleural space between the parietal and visceral pleurae is a pneumothorax. The presence of blood in the pleural space is a hemothorax. Many times, especially with trauma, victims have both pneumothorax and hemothorax. In these cases the term *hemopneumothorax* is used (Figure 2-43).

A pneumothorax may be caused by trauma or surgery or may occur spontaneously. A penetrating injury to the chest wall can permit air to enter the pleural space directly. An injury may also cause a broken rib, which tears the lung surface from the inside. Iatrogenic causes of pneumothorax include thoracentesis or subclavian venipuncture, which penetrate the chest wall, as well as application of positive pressure ventilation, which may tear the lung surface internally. In each case, air may gather in the pleural space, resulting in a pneumothorax.

A spontaneous pneumothorax occurs suddenly without injury and may or may not be the result of underlying pulmonary disease. Specifically, there is a rupture of the bronchus or alveolus. Pulmonary diseases such as emphysema, pneumonia, and neoplasms may result in weak tissue where a spontaneous pneumothorax may occur. It may occur in apparently healthy persons, usually tall men between 20 and 40 years of age. For these persons there may be a rupture of a subpleural bleb after a hard cough or sneeze, allowing air to leak from the lungs into the pleural space.

• • • • • Pathophysiology

The pleural space normally maintains a negative pressure, which facilitates lung expansion during ventilation. When there is penetration into the pleural space by an object external to the chest wall (such as a knife or needle) or when there is penetration into the pleural space by an internal mechanism (such as a broken rib or bleb rupture of the lung), air enters the pleural space. The pressure in the pleural space approaches atmospheric pressure. In tension pneumothorax, pleural pressure can exceed atmospheric pressure (becomes positive). Depending on the amount of air that enters initially and the amount that continues to enter, such as with a tension pneumothorax, the lung is no longer able to remain fully inflated.

As the pleural space pressure increases and the lung collapses, there is a mediastinal shift toward the unaffected side. This shift causes pressure on the great vessels returning to the heart and thus a decreased venous return. If pneumothorax is left untreated, cardiac output is compromised.

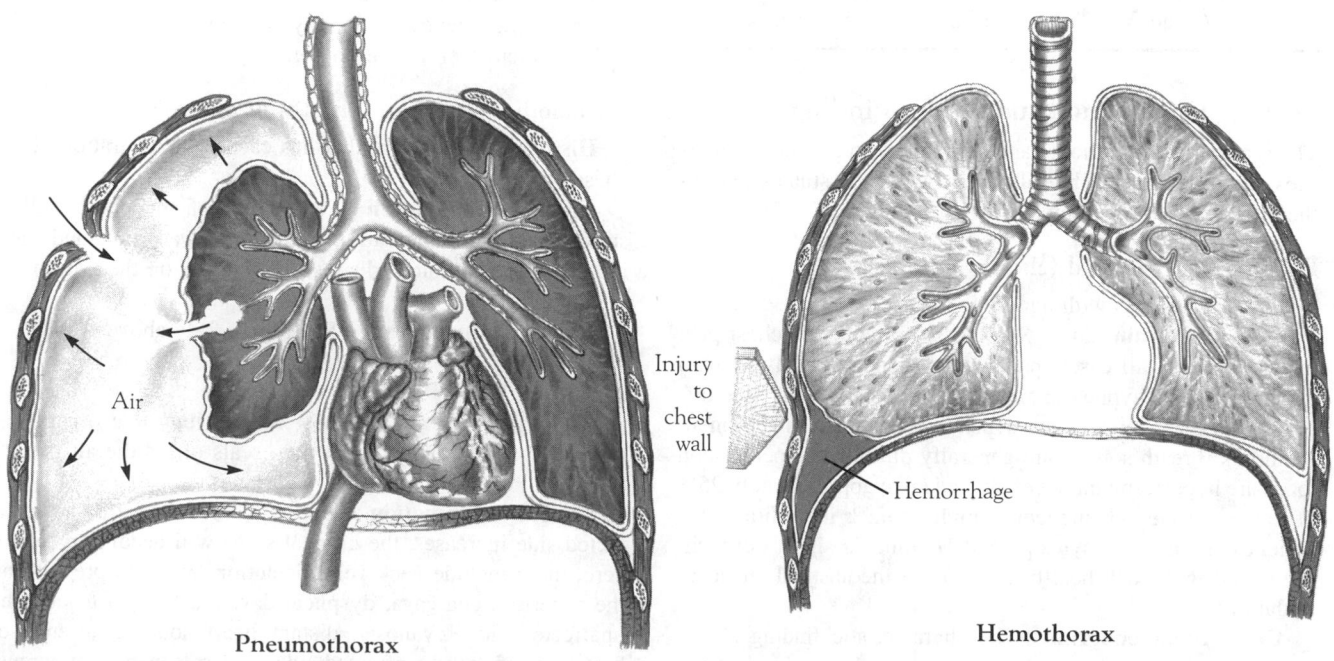

Pneumothorax   Hemothorax

Figure 2-43 Pneumothorax and hemothorax. (From Wilson.[93])

⚠ EMERGENCY ALERT

PNEUMOTHORAX OR HEMOTHORAX

A *pneumothorax* occurs when injury to the lung results in an accumulation of air in the pleural space that leads to loss of pressure and partial or total collapse of the lung. An open wound to the chest wall produces an *open pneumothorax* where air enters through the wound and trachea. A *tension pneumothorax* is a life-threatening situation where the pressure increase is significant and air cannot escape resulting in total collapse of the affected lung leading to mediastinal shift and complete cardiovascular compromise. A *hemothorax* refers to the accumulation of blood in the pleural space.

Assessment

- Dyspnea, tachypnea, tachycardia
- Chest pain
- Decreased or absent breath sound on the affected side
- Hyperresonance (pneumothorax)
- Dullness (hemothorax)
- Open, sucking chest wound (open pneumothorax)
- Hypotension, distended neck veins and tracheal shift plus worsening of vital signs (tension pneumothorax)

Interventions

- Maintain airway, breathing, and circulation.
- Administer high-flow O_2 by mask (10 to 15 L).
- Prepare for chest tube insertion.
- Obtain IV access.
- *If open pneumothorax:* cover wound with sterile, non-porous dressing and tape on three sides.
- *If tension pneumothorax:* perform needle thoracentesis.
- *If hemothorax:* prepare for blood administration, auto-transfusion.
- Prepare patient for corrective surgical intervention.

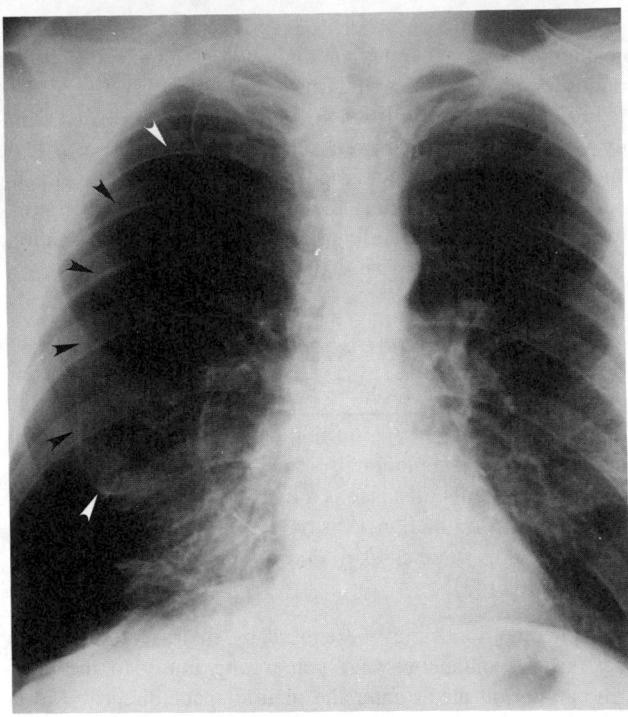

Figure 2-44 Chest roentgenogram of patient with pneumothorax. Note narrowing of pleural edge at arrow point and lack of lung markings beyond pleural line. (Courtesy R. Keith Wilson, MD, Baylor College of Medicine, Houston, Texas.)

•••••• Diagnostic Studies and Findings

The types of pneumothorax and hemothorax have both similarities and differences. The following diagnostic studies discuss the differences where they exist.

Pneumothorax-Closed (chest wall intact)

History   Varies with underlying cause

Clinical examination   Shortness of breath and chest pain in only 50% of all cases; patient may appear acutely ill with cyanosis and tachypnea or may appear to be healthy; the difference in the clinical signs depends on the size of the pneumothorax; breath sounds are generally diminished; percussion tones are hyperresonant over involved area; approximately 25% of patients have subcutaneous emphysema[90]; in addition, the patient demonstrates syncope and Hamman's sign (a crunching sound with each heartbeat owing to mediastinal air accumulation)

Chest roentgenogram   The characteristic finding shows air in the pleural cavity without the lateral markings of the lungs; instead there is a sharp pleural margin seen medially, indicating that the lung has collapsed; if the lung is not entirely collapsed, this margin may not be as obvious; it is therefore desirable to take an expiratory film with the patient sitting upright; because intrapleural air first collects in the apex, partial pneumothorax identification may be made; Figure 2-44 shows a classic picture of a pneumothorax

Pneumothorax—Open (chest wall not intact)

History   Some event that has caused a penetration of the chest wall

Clinical examination   Penetration of the chest wall, a sucking sound on inspiration as the chest wall rises, and varying signs of respiratory distress, depending on the size of the pneumothorax

Chest roentgenogram   See Figure 2-44 above

Tension Pneumothorax

History   Injury to the chest wall or lung that permits air to enter the pleural space but then seals off as the air tries to escape

Clinical examination   As the positive pressure on the affected side increases, the clinical signs will become severe; these include neck vein distention owing to pressure on the superior vena cava, dyspnea, deviated trachea toward the unaffected side, cyanosis, distant heart sounds, absence of breath sounds on the affected side, hyperresonance on percussion of the affected side, and cardiogenic shock; the chest roentgenogram of an individual with a tension pneumothorax shows complete lung collapse, a shift of mediastinal structures toward the unaffected side, and widened intercostal spaces on the affected side.

Hemothorax

History   Chest trauma

Clinical examination   Same as above, with the addition of tachycardia, hypotension, dullness on chest percussion, and signs of hypovolemic shock such as pallor and anxiety; the severity of the hemothorax may be determined by the amount of blood accumulation: less than 300 ml is considered minor and may not cause significant clinical signs; 300 to 1400 ml is moderate; and over 1400 ml is severe, indicating that most clinical signs will also be present

Chest roentgenogram   A minimum of 250 ml of intrapleural fluid is required to show a blunting of the costophrenic angle on an upright chest roentgenogram; it is desirable, therefore, to obtain an upright chest roentgenogram if possible; findings are decreased lung expansion as in Figure 2-44.

Blood gases   Decreased PaO_2

•••••• Multidisciplinary Plan

Surgery

Tube thoracostomy (chest tube): this technique is used to treat most types of pneumothorax or hemothorax. The exception is a small, spontaneous pneumothorax in an otherwise healthy individual

The chest tube should be inserted in the fifth or sixth intercostal space at the midaxillary line. If the tube is positioned posteriorly and toward the apex of the lung, it can effectively remove air and fluid. The lateral placement is preferred not only because it is most efficient but also because it does not produce a cosmetic defect, as does the anterior site of the second intercostal space at the midclavicular line.[90] See pp. 203 to 205 for discussion of chest tubes

Tension pneumothorax requires immediate and specific medical intervention. The building pressure in the pleural space must be reversed. The most effective way to release the pressure is to insert a large-bore needle (16 to 18 gauge) anteriorly at the midclavicular line between the second and third intercostal spaces. Once the needle is inserted, the patient's condition should improve remarkably[46]

Thoracotomy: A hemothorax may require a thoracotomy for correction. Indications for this procedure include an initial thoracostomy tube drainage greater than 1500 ml of blood; a persistent bleeding rate greater than 500 ml/hr; an increasing hemothorax seen on chest roentgenogram; the patient is in an unstable and hypotensive state despite adequate blood replacement

Medications

Hemothorax requires aggressive intravenous therapy to restore the circulating blood volume

Narcotic analgesics: Analgesics may be given for pain if respirations are adequate

Adrenergic agents: Antihypotensives such as dopamine may be indicated, but do not take the place of adequate blood volume

Dopamine (Intropin)

Dilute 1 ampule (200 mg) in 250 ml D5W; use with microdrip administration set; usual dose is 2-5 μg/kg/min initially; then titrate to gain the desired response

General Management

Airway maintenance—done by positioning, a simple airway, or endotracheal intubation, depending on patient's condition

Oxygenation—provide oxygen to maintain adequate blood gas levels

If patient has active and communicating pneumothorax, entrance wound into the chest wall should be immediately covered by petrolatum jelly gauze; three sides of the gauze pad should be taped; the fourth is left open to permit escape of excessive pressure; if gauze is placed on too tightly, tension pneumothorax may result. The respiratory status of the patient is monitored continuously until stabilized

NURSING CARE

Nursing Assessment

Respiratory Status

Respiratory distress to include dyspnea, tachypnea, retractions, labored breathing, nasal flaring

Breath sounds distant, bilaterally unequal, diminished; decreased vocal fremitus on the affected side; hyperresonance to percussion on affected side (pneumothorax); dullness to percussion on affected side (hemothorax)

Breathing pattern may show presence of splinting or hypopnea that may lead to atelectasis

Evaluate chest wall for stability and movement, presence of subcutaneous emphysema

Tracheal deviation noted with palpation

Cough, frequency and characteristics; sputum, amount and characteristics

Hypoxia

Restlessness, confusion, tachycardia, cyanosis; note mucous membranes, nail beds

Cardiovascular Status

Blood pressure, heart rate, auscultation quality, tissue perfusion, urinary output, jugular venous distention with tension pneumothorax

Chest Tube Drainage

Assess intact drainage system and amount and characteristics of drainage

Anxiety

Fear, air hunger, pain, confusion

Secondary Complications

Atelectasis, ARDS, infection, reexpansion pulmonary edema after chest tube insertion[46]

Nursing Dx & Intervention

Ineffective breathing pattern related to decreased lung expansion

- Assess ventilation to include evaluation of breathing rate, rhythm, and depth, chest expansion, presence of respiratory distress such as dyspnea, shortness of breath, nasal flaring, anxiety, retractions, use of accessory muscles.
- Assist to insert chest tubes as indicated.
- Provide chest tube care consistent with the guidelines presented on pp. 203 to 205; carefully maintain *to avoid interruption in the airtight system via dislodgment of the tubing or breaking of the drainage system.*
- Teach patient to splint area of chest tube insertion with a pillow to decrease discomfort when coughing.
- Provide analgesia as needed to promote effective ventilation and coughing.
- Identify contributing factors such as airway clearance or obstruction problem or weakness that may contribute to the patient's respiratory distress.
- Maintain patient positioning *to facilitate easy ventilation* (i.e., head of bed in semi-Fowler's position).
- Reposition patient every 1 to 2 hours to promote drainage of pleural fluids into chest tube.
- Suction if necessary *to remove secretions* from airway.
- Assess patient for tiring in relation to attempts to breathe.
- Encourage patient to breathe deeply but also to use adaptive breathing techniques *to decrease the work of breathing* and to space activities *so as to provide periods of rest in between.*
- Assist to protect patient from known sources of secondary infection.
- Should mechanical ventilation become necessary, provide care and monitoring consistent with the guidelines on pp. 205 to 207.

Impaired gas exchange related to alveolar-capillary membrane changes

- Assess patient to identify signs such as restlessness, confusion, and irritability, *which may indicate the body's response to altered blood gas states.*
- In collaboration with physician, monitor arterial blood gases; report increases or decreases in $PaCO_2$ and PaO_2 of more than 10 to 15 mm Hg.

- Administer oxygen *to maintain the arterial blood gases as ordered.*
- Monitor electrocardiogram and cardiac status *for arrhythmias secondary to alterations in blood gases.*
- Monitor and record kidney functioning and urinary output, which may be affected *by tissue hypoxia and alterations in metabolism.*

Fear related to suffocation and uncertain progress

- Assess patient's level of fear related to the present health state.
- Provide feedback to patient on progress, emphasizing each level of improvement.

Patient Education/Home Care Planning

1. Teach the patient and family about the chest tubes and their purpose and function, and the care that must be taken during their use.
2. Teach the patient adaptive breathing techniques to maximize lung reexpansion and prevent complications.
3. Teach importance of regular medical reevaluations for an extended period following the pneumothorax.

Evaluation

Optimum movement of air in and out of lungs occurs Vital capacity measurements are optimum for patient. Full expansion of lungs is achieved. Chest roentgenograms show full lung expansion with no evidence of pneumothorax or hemothorax.

Blood gas values are within normal limits Clear breath sounds are heard in all areas. Behavior is modified to conserve energy expenditure.

Patient describes a reduction in level of fear Vital signs normalize.

Patient and family have sufficient information to comply with discharge regimen Patient and family are able at time of discharge to discuss medications (purpose, side effects, route, and schedule), dietary therapy regimen, activity progression regimen, signs of infection or respiratory deterioration, and plan for follow-up visits.

IDIOPATHIC PULMONARY FIBROSIS

Idiopathic pulmonary fibrosis (IPF) is one of the interstitial lung diseases. Historically, this aggressive form of idiopathic fibrosis was called Hamman-Rich syndrome. Many of the interstitial lung diseases have a known cause; there is a known insult to the lung and a response. Examples include the pneumoconioses discussed in the next section, granulomatous diseases, venoocclusive disease of the lung, lung radiation, and many others. In IPF, the precipitating event that initiates the lung scarring is unknown. The entire process is thought to be an excessive immune response; the lung is trying to heal itself, but instead overresponds, resulting in extensive scarring.

Idiopathic pulmonary fibrosis is a highly lethal disease; death rates from IPF are comparable to the mortality rates for lung cancer. Newer therapies are aimed at the inflammatory mechanisms, but outcomes remain poor.

····· Pathophysiology

The pathogenesis of IPF has not been well delineated. There is an inflammatory response in the lung with edema and influx of inflammatory cells (e.g., neutrophils). Collapse of alveoli occurs and the inflammation progresses to extensive fibrosis. Over time there is a remodeling of the lung parenchyma. The disease is usually patchy, with areas of normal lung, areas demonstrating inflammation but not fibrosis, and finally areas of extensive fibrosis.[45]

The inflammation and scarring result in a stiff lung; there is increased recoil, decreased compliance. Lung volumes (TLC, RV, VC) are reduced. There is *not* slowing of expiration as the defect is in the lung parenchyma, not the airway. (The FEV_1 will not be reduced but proportionately to the FVC; the FEV_1/FVC ratio is normal.) The dramatic symptom of pulmonary fibrosis is dyspnea. The patient has a relatively rapid respiratory rate; the expiratory time is short.

Gas exchange is also affected. Early in the disease gas exchange is maintained. The patient's arterial oxygenation will be adequate at rest, but the patient often has to hyperventilate (low $PaCO_2$) to maintain the PaO_2. With exercise, the level of oxygenation often falls dramatically. Because the alveoli are filled with debris, these patients are much more difficult to oxygenate than are patients who have diseases such as COPD. At end-stage disease, hypoventilation (CO_2 retention) may occur.

····· Diagnostic Studies and Findings

The diagnosis of IPF is one of exclusion—other reasons for developing fibrosis must be excluded

History   An extensive history is taken to rule out any possibility of immune suppression (e.g., HIV), inhalation exposure (e.g., birds, drugs, workplace), presence of a collagen-vascular disease (e.g., lupus, arthritis); a variety of conditions are capable of producing the roentgenographic picture seen in IPF, and many known diseases can produce inflammation and fibrosis.

Clinical examination   Rapid respiratory rate, short expiratory time. Crackles on auscultation. Chest roentgenogram: Increased interstitial markings (pattern varies with different etiologies of the fibrosis); bilateral patchy infiltrates; lung volumes decreased. Obtaining old films is helpful to determine the time of onset, progression of the changes. A high resolution CT (computed tomography) scan is often required to visualize the presence and/or extent of the changes.

Pulmonary function studies   Decreased lung volumes (TLC, RV, VC). FEV_1/FVC is normal (FEV_1 will be decreased proportionate to decrease in VC). Diffusing capacity of the lung for carbon monoxide (DLco) decreased. Arterial blood gases often demonstrate hyperventilation; PaO_2 is usually maintained. Rest and exercise pulse oximetry (or arterial blood gases) often demonstrates a fall in oxygenation with exercise.

Bronchoscopy   Bronchoscopy with bronchoalveolar lavage (BAL) and/or transbronchial biopsy is performed to obtain a sample of the inflammatory cells in the alveoli (BAL) or an actual piece of lung tissue (biopsy). The presence of an infectious process must be ruled out; cultures from the bronchoscopy will facilitate this process.

Lung biopsy   A thoracoscopy, guided or open lung biopsy, may be done to obtain a sample of lung tissue. The so-called "gold standard," the study to which other results are compared, is the open lung biopsy. The tissue is cultured, the pathologic changes described, and, if indicated, a variety of stains and immunochemical studies can be performed to help identify the cause and extent of the process.[69]

····· Multidisciplinary Plan

If all other causes of the fibrosis are ruled out, the diagnosis of IPF is made. There is no known cure and pharmacologic interventions offer little improvement in the majority of cases (only about 20% respond); there is also the risk that many of the pharmacologic interventions have a high incidence of side effects.

Medications

Corticosteroids—prednisone is given in relatively large doses ($\geq$60 mg/day) initially; if there is a therapeutic response (improved pulmonary function, roentgenographic changes), the dose is tapered to a lower dose to reduce side effects but maintain the therapeutic response. In patients where there is no response, the steroids are discontinued if possible.

Cytotoxic agents such as cyclophosphamide (Cytoxan), azathioprine (Immuran), methotrexate may be used; recently cyclosporin has also been used. Dosages are individualized and monitored by leukocyte count.

Oxygen therapy

Oxygen by cannula; may require flows greater than 6 liters per minute (LPM) with exercise

Surgery

Lung transplantation has been used in idiopathic pulmonary fibrosis; both single and double lung procedures have been done.

NURSING CARE

Nursing Assessment

Respiratory Status

Tachypnea, use of accessory muscles with inspiration, dyspnea, tachycardia; crackles (note crackles are usually present); dry, nonproductive cough

Pulmonary Function Studies reduction in vital capacity and FEV$_1$; changes in oxygenation with exercise (pulmonary function studies will assist nurse to evaluate/set goals for patient's activity, tolerance level)

Hypoxia: tachycardia, tachypnea, restlessness, cyanosis, impaired judgment

White Blood Cell Count

Monitored to follow response and determine dosage of immunosuppressive therapy

Cardiovascular Status

Assess for signs and symptoms of cor pulmonale (see p. 178)

Infection

Assess for signs of infection, lung and elsewhere; note may not demonstrate usual febrile response or high WBC due to immunosuppressive therapy

Anxiety

Fear, air, hunger

Other

Assess for specific drug side effects (see p. 189)

Nursing Dx & Intervention

Ineffective breathing pattern related to decreased compliance, increased ventilatory drive

* Position to improve efficiency of the accessory muscles of inspiration (tripod position); note that position can also be maintained during walking by having patient push a cart, wheelchair, etc.
* Time activities to provide rest periods.
* Ensure that patient is receiving supplemental oxygen to avoid increasing drive related to hypoxemia.

Impaired gas exchange related to alveolar-capillary membrane changes, low V/Q

* Administer oxygen as ordered to maintain Pao$_2$; flow rates usually increased with activity.
* In collaboration with physician, monitor arterial blood gases; report increases or decreases in Pao$_2$ or Paco$_2$ $\geq$10 mm Hg.
* Avoid unnecessary increases in oxygen consumption; plan and pace activities.

Risk for infection due to altered immunologic status

* Ensure that appropriate immunizations (influenza, pneumococcal pneumonia, etc.) received.
* Teach patient/family to avoid exposure to infections.
* Monitor for signs and symptoms of infection—changes in amount, characteristics of sputum, febrile response (will frequently be smaller than usual), WBC response, pain, cuts that do not heal.

Patient Education/Home Care Planning

1. Use of home oxygen—these patients often require complex home systems to provide the high flows required (for example, to attain flows greater than 6 LPM, two home oxygen systems may be needed; some patients use a cannula and mask for oxygen therapy). The patient and family must know how to use and care for the equipment.
2. Discuss with patient and family the need to pace activities to avoid increasing dyspnea, oxygen need, fatigue.
3. Teach the patient and family about the medications being used; include side effects and necessity for monitoring (varies with drug used).
4. At end-stage disease may require referral to home care or hospice for care and support.

Evaluation

Breathing pattern is optimal   For patient's level of pulmonary function; as patient's condition progresses moderate to severe dyspnea may be constantly present.

Gas exchange is adequate   Pao$_2$ is maintained >55 mm Hg at rest and exercise.

Infection is not present.

PNEUMOCONIOSES

(Occupational lung disease)

Industrial and work-related lung diseases are caused by inhaling inorganic dusts or gaseous or particulate matters in the air. They are referred to as pneumoconioses (*pneuma*, lung; *konia*, dust; *osis*, condition). The three major pneumoconioses are silicosis, asbestosis, and coal workers' pneumoconiosis (Figure 2-45). These diseases cause a type of interstitial pulmonary fibrosis.

•••••• Pathophysiology

Particulate matter that is inhaled is deposited in various areas of the respiratory tract. Particles deposited on the mucous surfaces of the nose and upper airways are readily moved toward the pharynx, from which they are swallowed or coughed out. The majority of particles with an aerodynamic diameter >2 to 3 μm are cleared by the normal defense mechanisms of the lower airway. Very small particles and gases are less readily removed from the lung.

The irritating effects of certain particles and gases increase mucus production. With repeated exposures the mucous glands hypertrophy and secrete more mucus in response to a variety of inhaled irritants. This may result in a type of chronic bronchitis.

Bronchioles and alveoli have no mucous glands; therefore particles deposited in their lumen are not as easily removed. Alveolar clearance involves more complex pathways of cellular and fluid transport. Phagocytic cells in the alveoli play the

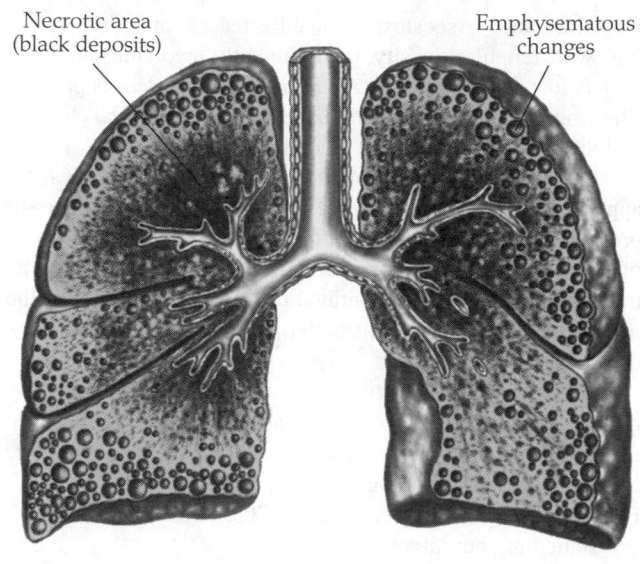
Necrotic area (black deposits)

Emphysematous changes

Figure 2-45 Pneumoconioses. (From Wilson.[93])

major role in disposing of the particles reaching this part of the respiratory tract. In addition, alveolar surfactant and fluid produced from capillary transudation help in moving the particles to the lymph channels. Disposal of particles from the alveoli is a very slow process, and the respiratory membrane remains exposed to their harmful effects until they are removed. Coating of the particles by surfactant and certain chemical reactions, as well as some enzymatic actions, reduce their harmful effects.

Once phagocytized, the particles are processed by the metabolic and enzymatic apparatus of the alveolar macrophages. The phagocytic effectiveness of these cells is influenced by many exogenous and endogenous factors. Sometimes the offending agents impair the function of these cells.

When the primary disposing mechanisms fail to control the agents' harmful effects, the secondary cellular and humoral defense mechanisms are brought into action. These mechanisms result in inflammation, which consists of dilation and increased permeability of capillaries, exudation of fluid, and infiltration of white blood cells. The immunologic system plays a major part in this process. It therefore seems that the pathologic changes are at least partly the result of these secondary defense mechanisms.[25]

Silicosis

Silicosis is the most important of the pneumoconioses. It is a progressive pulmonary disease marked by nodular lesions, which often progress to fibrosis. This disease often shows no symptoms. It is caused by the inhalation and pulmonary deposition of crystalline silicon dioxide dust, mostly from quartz.

Industrial sources of silica in its pure form include the manufacture of ceramics (flint) and building materials (sandstone). It occurs in mixed form in the production of construction materials such as cement. Silica is found in powder form in paints,

porcelain, scouring soaps, and wood fillers. It may also be found in the mining of gold, coal, lead, zinc, and iron. Sources of free silica dust include industries such as mining, quarrying, tunneling, stone cutting, abrasive industry, pottery, and tile manufacturing.

The development of silicosis depends on the size of the silica particle, its concentration in the air, length of exposure, and susceptibility of the individual. Very heavy exposure, as sometimes occurs in sandblasters, may result in a more acute form of silicosis after brief exposure.

Pathophysiology The silica particles deposited in the alveoli are 1 to 3 μm in diameter. These are phagocytized by the macrophages. In the process, part of these cells containing the particles is damaged. Cellular enzymes dispersing in cytoplasm cause death of the macrophages and release of their contents, including the silica particles. More macrophages are attracted to the area and are also killed. The production of fibrosis, the major pathologic finding, has been attributed to the release of certain fibrogenic factors. The pathologic process continues even after the environmental exposure has ceased.

The characteristic pathologic changes are the silicotic nodules, which are fibrotic lesions. In simple silicosis the nodules may measure 2 to 3 mm in diameter and are unevenly scattered throughout the lungs. They are surrounded by distorted lung tissue, which may show emphysematous changes. As the disease state progresses, these changes are characteristic of progressive massive fibrosis (PMF) and indicate complicated silicosis. With progressive massive fibrosis, the upper lobes may show evidence of emphysema, sometimes with large bullous changes.[25]

Asbestosis

Asbestos, the name given to a number of fibrous silicates, is mined principally in Canada, South Africa, and Russia. Raw asbestos is first processed to release asbestos fibers from the parent rock and then transported for use in a variety of industries. In the United States most asbestos is used to fireproof and insulate buildings. Workers in these industries may be exposed to asbestos dust. Symptoms of asbestosis do not usually appear until the individual has been exposed to asbestos dust for at least 10 years.[92]

Pathophysiology Asbestosis is caused by deposition of small asbestos particles on bronchioles or alveolar walls where they are ingested by cells. This swells the alveolar wall by a process that is not fully understood.

Fibrosis in asbestosis, unlike silicosis, is nonnodular, involves mostly the lower lungs, and often has pleural thickening. Pleural thickening, plaque formation, and pleural calcification are common with asbestos exposure. Pleural effusion, sometimes bloody, is a fairly common form of pleural reaction.

Bronchogenic carcinoma often occurs with asbestosis. However, the relationship is mostly because of the combined effect of asbestos and cigarette smoking. Heavy smokers who are also exposed to asbestos have 80 to 90 times the risk of nonsmokers for having bronchogenic carcinoma.[25]

Coal Workers' Pneumoconiosis (Black Lung)

Coal workers' pneumoconiosis (CWP) is a chronic pathologic condition resulting from prolonged exposure to coal dust. Although carbon is not a fibrogenic agent, with massive and prolonged exposure the clearance mechanisms of the lung are overwhelmed, and coal dust accumulates in terminal air spaces, resulting in pulmonary problems.

The incidence of pneumoconiosis in anthracite mining is much higher than in soft (bituminous) coal mining. An estimated 10 to 12 years of mining work is needed for the development of this disease.

Pathophysiology   After the deposition of coal dust in the respiratory bronchioles and alveoli, the first reaction is phagocytosis of the particles by increasing numbers of macrophages, which move to the terminal bronchioles. An excessive dust load overwhelms the pulmonary clearing mechanism. Fibroblasts appear in this area, laying a thin network of reticulin fibers without significant collagen formation. The aggregations of macrophages and dust particles enmeshed in reticulin fibers are called coal macules because they appear as black dots on the lung sections. These spots are often linked with dilation of respiratory bronchioles, called focal centrilobular emphysema. These changes are often seen in simple CWP. The complicated form of the disease is marked by massive fibrosis, involving mostly the upper lobes.[25]

•••••• Diagnostic Studies and Findings

Clinical history   Occupational exposure to silica dust, asbestos, or coal dust

Clinical examination   Patients with all three of these diseases are often asymptomatic; the main symptoms may be tachypnea and dyspnea with or without a dry cough; the cough is worse in the morning; the severity of dyspnea is usually progressive; the dyspnea is more evident in patients who also smoke; patients may have 10 or more years of exposure before clinical symptoms are noticed; as the disease progresses, respiratory failure may develop and clinical evidence of respiratory failure, pulmonary hypertension, or cor pulmonale may appear; relatively few physical findings are apparent until the development of cor pulmonale; rales, clubbing, and other findings associated with chronic lung disease may or may not be present; other clinical signs are decreased chest expansion, diminished breath sounds, and areas of hyporesonance and hyperresonance; patients with CWP have expectorations of black material

Chest Roentgenogram

Silicosis   The initial manifestation of silicosis is the development of small nodules on the chest roentgenogram; at this point in the disease the patient is usually asymptomatic; exposure to silica may have been going on for 10 to 20 years; with the development of massive fibrosis, the upper lobes show evidence of volume loss; the lower lobes show emphysematous changes; in complicated silicosis, massive densities may be seen in the fields; progressive changes from simple nodular form to massive fibrosis may take place within 5 years

Asbestosis   Asbestosis is manifested as interstitial markings with reticular density, predominantly involving the lower lung fields; sometimes a marked honeycomb pattern is present. The lung volume is often diminished; common pleural changes include thickening, plaques, calcification, and effusion

Coal workers' pneumoconiosis   CWP usually does not appear until the worker has been exposed to coal dust for approximately 10 years; the roentgenogram shows the presence of small opacities or nodular densities through the lung fields; these lesions are usually confined to the upper lung fields; the nodular densities are often smaller and less defined than those of silicosis

Pulmonary function tests   These may be normal in early disease; as the disease progresses, abnormalities may be seen; these changes may indicate both obstructive and restrictive lung damage; test findings may include decreases in FVC, FEV_1, reduced diffusing capacity of CO (DL_{CO}), reduced TLC, and static lung compliance

Blood gas studies   These are normal early in the diseases; as the diseases progress, decreased Po_2 and increased Pco_2 may occur; hypoxemia may become severe

Laboratory values   Monitor blood gas values

Secondary infection   Resulting decreased ability to move secretions; increased risk of tuberculosis; monitor temperature, sputum amount, and characteristics

Cor pulmonale and pulmonary hypertension   Monitor for presence

•••••• Multidisciplinary Plan

Surgery

Biopsy—may be necessary for diagnostic evaluation

Medications

None specific; treat complications of disease such as infection, pulmonary hypertension, and cor pulmonale

General Management

Prevention of secondary infections
Chest physical therapy
Steam inhalation
Oxygen by cannula, 1 to 2 L/minute
Increased fluids

NURSING CARE

Nursing Assessment

Respiratory Status

Dyspnea, respiratory distress
Breath sounds: decreased, bilaterally unequal, rales, rhonchi
Persistent cough
Pulmonary function: decreased vital capacity, minute volume, and functional residual capacity; increased intrapulmonary shunting

Hypoxia: restlessness, confusion, impaired motor function, hypotension, tachycardia

Nursing Dx & Intervention

Knowledge deficit related to unfamiliarity with disease process

- Assess patient's and family's level of knowledge about these pneumoconioses.
- Inform patient that prevention is the most important aspect of the management of the disease. The disease may not become apparent until after 20 years of exposure. Protective hoods and clothing should be used during times of exposure.
- Instruct patient to maintain regular follow-up examinations and to report new symptoms or exposure to other respiratory diseases.

Risk for infection related to compromised state

- Instruct patient about increased risk for acquiring tuberculosis and other infectious diseases and about need for frequent medical evaluations.
- Instruct patient to avoid persons with known respiratory infections.
- Assess patient for weight loss, anorexia, and fever, which may be present in the presence of an infection.

Impaired gas exchange related to chronic inhaling of inorganic dusts or particulate matters in the air

- Assess patient to identify signs, such as restlessness, confusion, and irritability, *that may indicate the body's response to altered blood gases.*
- Administer and monitor bronchodilators as ordered.
- Schedule blood gases and pulmonary function testing on a periodic basis.
- Ensure that patient is aware that the disease progresses even if the patient is removed from further dust exposure. The patient should be frequently monitored for condition deterioration.

Patient Education/Home Care Planning

Education should be directed to the predisease state. These diseases are preventable if precautions are taken on a regular basis.

1. Teach the patient that protective head hoods should be used at work when dust production is heavy. Exposure to crystalline silica, asbestos, or coal dust may occur during mining or quarrying for the material. In addition, individuals who work in foundries; who are involved in abrasive blasting, stone cutting, or other masonry work; or who work in areas where glass, pottery, or porcelain is manufactured may be at risk for silicosis.
2. Teach the patient and family to watch for other pulmonary signs that may indicate infection or complications of the disease. Such signs may be dyspnea, cough, worsening expectoration, or hemoptysis.
3. Teach the patient the importance of avoiding environmental pollutants and not smoking.
4. Teach the patient adaptive breathing techniques if dyspnea and shortness of breath are present.

Evaluation

Further lung injury is prevented Patient uses protective headwear so further respiratory damage is prevented.

Patient preserves pulmonary functioning by maintaining optimum activity level, preventing infection, and following prescribed treatments Patient demonstrates a variety of methods indicating ability to preserve and facilitate optimum respiratory functioning (e.g., breathing exercises, modified exercises, modified activities or exercises, taking medications as prescribed).

Patient and family have sufficient information to comply with discharge regimen Patient and family are able to discuss medications, activity progression, signs of infection, breathing exercises, and plan for follow-up visits.

Physiologic function is stable There are no secondary infections.

Blood gases are within normal limits for the patient.

▌ OBSTRUCTIVE SLEEP APNEA[3,6]

Sleep apnea is a diagnosis of disordered breathing. Persons with this syndrome have episodes where they do not breathe during sleep. Although many persons have some brief periods with no breathing during sleep, the occurrence of more than five apneic episodes per hour is abnormal. (To be called apnea, the episode of absence of airflow must last at least 10 seconds.) In addition, many patients have periods of hypopnea (extremely shallow breathing). These periods of apnea and hypopnea are often associated with significant hypoxemia.

Sleep apnea is a relatively commonly occurring problem, with 2% to 9% of the general population having the disorder. The diagnosis is more prevalent among men than among women. The diagnosis is uncommon in premenopausal women. Sleep apnea is also associated with obesity; approximately 50% of persons with obstructive sleep apnea are obese.

Apnea occurring during sleep is categorized as central, obstructive, or mixed. In obstructive apnea, respiratory efforts are made, but there is no airflow because the upper airway is obstructed. Central sleep apnea refers to the loss of ventilatory drive resulting in apneic periods; no respiratory efforts are made. In the mixed type of apnea, a central apnea is followed by obstructive apnea. The majority of the patients have a combination of obstructive and mixed apnea and are diagnosed as having obstructive sleep apnea. Primary central apnea is relatively rare.

Clinical symptoms associated with obstructive sleep apnea include:

- Loud snoring—the bed partner is often forced to sleep in another room due to the noise
- Daytime hypersomnolence—may be so severe that the person will fall asleep while driving a car
- Restless sleep—in addition to general restlessness, may also be excessive arm and leg movement during sleep
- Personality changes
- Diminished cognitive function
- Impotence
- Cardiovascular disease: hypertension, arrhythmias, congestive heart failure

•••••• Pathophysiology

During normal breathing there is enough tone in the muscles of the pharyngeal structures that the opening of the upper airway is maintained during inspiration. (The extrathoracic or upper airway is normally smaller during inspiration and larger during expiration, the opposite of the caliber changes in the lower, intrathoracic airways.) During normal sleep the tone in these muscles is decreased. In patients with sleep apnea, the muscle tone is dramatically decreased. In addition, patients with obstructive sleep apnea often have a smaller than normal pharyngeal opening (for example, anatomic changes such as receding chin, large tongue, large tonsils, excessive fat deposits). When the person inhales, the upper airway is obstructed by the tongue or soft palate, preventing air flow into the lung even though respiratory efforts are made. There are frequently snoring noises, and an abrupt "snort" when the obstruction is broken and the patient inhales. During the apneic periods, the patient's arterial oxygen level can drop dramatically. If untreated, nighttime hypoxemia can lead to pulmonary hypertension and right heart failure.

•••••• Diagnostic Studies and Findings

Clinical history   snoring, observed apnea, daytime hypersomnolence

Physical examination   demonstrates small pharynx, large tongue, receding chin, etc.

Polysomnography (PSG; a sleep study)   the patient is monitored during sleep. Monitoring includes electroencephalogram so that the stages of sleep can be identified, ECG, chest movements, nasal air flow, and pulse oximetry. The sleep study includes monitoring at baseline to identify the problem and then with interventions to ensure that oxygenation is maintained and that the apneic and hypopneic periods are abolished or at least reduced to normal levels

•••••• Multidisciplinary Plan

Surgery   Tracheostomy (the tracheostomy is closed during the day and opened at night to bypass the upper airway obstruction); uvulopalatopharyngoplasty: this procedure widens the posterior pharynx

Medications   Respiratory stimulants may be used in patients with central sleep apnea; examples are medroxyprogesterone, acetazolamide, and theophylline.

Oxygen   Via nasal cannula during sleep or via CPAP apparatus

CPAP (continuous positive airway pressure)   CPAP is applied via a nasal mask or nasal pillows; in some patients, a full face mask may be used. Some patients, especially those who require high pressures (>15 cm H_2O), may not tolerate a continuous pressure. In some situations, BiPAP may be applied.

Appliances   To reposition the mandible (move it anteriorly)

Weight loss   Weight loss has not been a very successful approach to care

NURSING CARE

Nursing Assessment

Clinical History

Question family as well as patient regarding snoring, apnea; if previously diagnosed, ascertain usual home therapy (CPAP, or other device)

Clinical Observation

Observe the patient during sleep for snoring, apnea, excessive limb movements; observe for signs of right sided heart failure (see p. 38)

Oxygenation

Monitor pulse oximetry at night

Nursing Dx & Intervention

Ineffective breathing pattern related to upper airway obstruction

- Apply CPAP as ordered during sleep.
- If tracheotomized, be sure tracheostomy tube is unplugged while patient is sleeping.

Impaired gas exchange related to apneic and hypopneic periods

- Apply oxygen as ordered.

Nutrition

- Obtain dietary consultation.
- Assist patient with dietary selections.
- Encourage patient for weight reduction efforts.

Patient Education/Home Care Planning

1. Teach patient and family about the importance of treating sleep apnea.

2. Instruct patient and family in use of home equipment, CPAP, oxygen.
3. If necessary, instruct patient and family on tracheostomy care (see p. 667).
4. Teach patient and family about dietary changes.

Evaluation

Respiratory pattern during sleep void of apneic, hypopneic episode

Oxygenation maintained at saturation >90% during sleep

Patient demonstrates weight loss; demonstrates change in eating habits, food selection

COLLABORATIVE INTERVENTIONS AND RELATED NURSING CARE

 ### AIRWAY MAINTENANCE

Airway maintenance includes the following:
Suctioning
Oropharyngeal airway
Nasopharyngeal airway
Endotracheal intubation
Tracheostomy (see Chapter 7 for procedures)
Artificial airways are used to assist in the maintenance of a patent airway. In addition, endotracheal tubes and tracheostomy tubes are used as routes for mechanical ventilation.

Preprocedural Care

Clinical Assessment Indicating Airway Obstruction

Restlessness
Wheezing
Noisy respirations
Difficulty breathing
Tachycardia
Rhonchi over large airways
Decreased breath sounds
Retractions: intercostal, suprasternal, supraclavicular, nasal flaring
Stridor
Mouth breathing
Low tidal volume

Preprocedural Teaching

If the patient's situation requiring airway maintenance procedures is an emergency, preprocedural teaching may seem inappropriate. A very simple explanation before the emergency procedure can be supplemented with additional information after the airway is safety secured.

•••••• Procedural Techniques and Associated Care[2,12,44,66,71]

Orotracheal, Nasotracheal, or Endotracheal Suctioning

Indications
Signs of respiratory distress
Noisy, wet breathing
Auscultated rhonchi
Ineffective cough effort

Contraindications
Tight wheeze with bronchospasm or croup

Procedural guidelines
1. If possible, position patient in semi-Fowler's position.
2. Use sterile, gloved technique.
3. Use smallest catheter size possible to remove secretions.
4. Hyperoxygenate patient and hyperinflate before suctioning procedure, or ask the patient to deep breathe.
5. Lubricate catheter tip with sterile saline or water before procedure. Use water-soluble gel lubricant only for nasotracheal approach.
6. Do not apply suction while catheter is being inserted.
7. Insert and advance catheter. If resistance is met, withdraw catheter 0.5 cm.
8. Apply suction for 5- to 10-second interval; rotate and slowly withdraw catheter during suctioning.
9. Administer oxygen and hyperinflate between suctioning periods. Monitor SpO_2.
10. Note and record amount and character of sputum.
11. Note and record patient's response to suctioning procedure.
12. Discard catheter after each treatment.
13. Change vacuum container and tubing every day.

! EMERGENCY ALERT

EMERGENCY AIRWAY MANAGEMENT

An airway obstruction or absence of airway patency can be a life-threatening emergency. Swift action is necessary to resolve this situation.

Assessment
- Tongue, foreign body, bleeding, vomit, or edema obstructing airway
- Inability to vocalize

Interventions
- Maintain cervical spine stabilization if injury is suspected.
- Position the patient supine.
- Open and clear the airway; jaw thrust, chin lift, removal of foreign bodies.
- Suction patient as needed.
- Consider endotracheal intubation.
- Consider needle or surgical cricothyroidotomy.

Alternative method

Closed, in-line suction catheter systems are available for use with endotracheal or tracheostomy tubes. Advantages include the ability to maintain ordered PEEP and hyperoxygenate via a mechanical ventilator during suctioning, as well as elimination of the nurse's exposure to sputum.[71]

Complications

Wheezing or stridor after or during procedure indicating potential bronchospasm or laryngospasm (if noted, administer oxygen and contact physician)

Prolonged spasmodic coughing

Traumatic ulceration of the airways with blood-streaked sputum

Infection

Hypoxemia

Cardiac rhythm and rate disturbance

Oropharyngeal or Nasopharyngeal Airways[16,68]

Indications

Potential or actual upper airway obstruction owing to altered levels of consciousness, resulting in relaxation of the tongue against the hypopharynx

Trauma-induced upper airway obstruction

Procedural guidelines

1. Determine type of airway according to individual patient needs:
   a. Oropharyngeal airway: (poorly tolerated in awake patients, causes gagging) length should be from front teeth to the mandibular angle of jaw.
   b. Nasopharyngeal airway: may be indicated if patient has associated mouth injury; the width should be slightly narrower than the nares diameter.
2. Insertion techniques:
   a. Oropharyngeal airway: approaching from the side of the mouth, insert airway upside down (with distal end pointing up), then rotate the airway over the tongue 180 degrees; the flange of the airway should be securely positioned outside the teeth.
   b. Nasopharyngeal airway: elevating the tip of the nose, the airway should be inserted in anatomic line with the nasal passage. Use water-soluble gel as a lubricant.
3. Position patient on side to facilitate drainage.
4. Remove and clean oral airway at least every 6 to 8 hours; observe for ulcerations of mucous membranes.
5. Remove and clean nasal airway every 12 to 24 hours; rotate to other nares; observe for ulcerations of mucous membranes.
6. Carefully observe position of airway at least every hour; suction if needed via the airway.
7. Provide mouth and nose care at least every 2 hours.
8. Airway removal: observe patient's level of consciousness and presence of gag and swallow reflexes; when patient is awake, instruct him to push oral airway out with tongue; carefully observe patient for adequate airway maintenance after removal.

Complications

Will not prevent aspiration of secretions; suction must be available

May cause patient to gag

May become clogged

May become dislodged if not secured in place

Bleeding secondary to trauma of insertion

Potential infection secondary to airway

Ulceration of nares or pharynx secondary to prolonged insertion

Observe for mucous plugs or other signs of noisy breathing, restlessness, or malpositioning of airway, which indicate blockage of airway or malpositioning

Endotracheal Intubation[12,85]

Indications

Intubation:

Airway obstruction that occurs despite the use of an oral airway

To prevent possible aspiration in an unconscious patient

To remove secretions from the tracheobronchial tree

To provide mechanical ventilation

Extubation:

Should be attempted only in a planned and controlled environment

Procedural guidelines

1. Assemble all equipment before attempting intubation procedure.
2. Check the cuff on endotracheal tube for leakage.
3. Assist to position patient so the neck is flexed and the head is extended; this should bring the mouth, larynx, and trachea in line.
4. Before intubation, explain the procedure and ensure that any false teeth or bridges have been removed.
5. Before intubation, hyperventilate patient using self-inflating bag with supplemental 100% oxygen.
6. If intubation attempt is prolonged, interrupt the procedure and oxygenate the patient. Monitor SpO_2 and electrocardiogram throughout intubation procedure.
7. Once the endotracheal tube is in place, assist to determine proper endotracheal tube placement; this is done by considering the following:
   a. Correct placement: bilateral lung inflation, breath sounds heard equally throughout all lobes.
   b. Incorrect placement:
      Esophagus: absence of breath sounds, respiratory distress and cyanosis; if these are noted, the endotracheal tube should be removed and reinserted.
      Right mainstem bronchus or carina: the endotracheal tube has been inserted too far; clinical signs include unilateral breath sounds, and coughing; if this is noted and confirmed by radiographic examination, the endotracheal tube should be retracted slightly and resecured; reassessment should indicate proper placement.

8. Once the endotracheal tube is in correct position, tape it securely so movement of tube is impossible.
9. If patient is not able to cooperate with maintaining tube placement, consider use of soft wrist restraints to prevent self-extubation with potential laryngeal injury.
10. Monitor tube placement and patency at least every hour; this assessment should include:
   a. Tube position
   b. Tube patency
   c. Lung inflation
   d. Absence of respiratory distress
   e. Generalized respiratory response
11. Provide ongoing care for patients with endotracheal tube in place:
   a. Provide mouth care every 2 hours.
   b. Clean nares and around endotracheal tube at least every 6 to 8 hours.
   c. Reposition and retape endotracheal tube at least daily.
   d. Take precaution not to dislodge tube position.
12. If tube has cuff, use minimal occlusive volume technique to maintain the airway seal; record the amount of air inserted to inflate the cuff; monitor cuff pressures each shift; attempt to maintain pressures <20 mm Hg to avoid tracheal pressure injury.
13. Use bite block or oral airway if the patient bites the endotracheal tube.
14. Patient should receive oxygen while intubated that is at near 100% humidification.
15. If patient is awake, provide writing materials for communication, or agree on use of sign language/communication board. Remind patient that ability to speak returns after tube removal.
16. Extubation:
   a. Assess patient's ability to breathe on own and protect airway before extubation.
   b. Determine that patient is able to maintain spontaneous respiratory rate and tidal volume sufficient to maintain stable blood gas values.
   c. Carefully suction endotracheal tube and pharynx above endotracheal cuff before deflating cuff for extubation.
   d. Immediately after extubation, assess for signs of respiratory distress or laryngeal spasm such as dyspnea, noisy breathing, use of abdominal or accessory muscles, restlessness, irritability, tachycardia, tachypnea, decreased Pao_2, increased $Paco_2$; if these are noted, consult physician immediately and prepare for reinsertion of endotracheal tube.
   e. Teach patient that throat discomfort from the endotracheal tube generally resolves in 24 to 48 hours.

Complications

Delay of oxygenation or ventilation during intubation procedure

Placement of endotracheal tube into right mainstem bronchus, resulting in unilateral aeration with potential for pneumothorax on right side, atelectasis on left side

Ulceration of trachea or tracheoesophageal fistula

Mucous plugs or other blockage of endotracheal tube may lead to hypoxia and respiratory distress

Unplanned extubation by combative patient or secondary to poorly secured tube will require immediate airway and ventilatory assessment by the nurse, as well as potential need for oral airway, patient positioning, and ventilation by Ambu-bag with supplemental oxygen

Aspiration of secretions secondary to poorly inflated cuff, inadequate suctioning before cuff deflation, or too small noncuffed endotracheal tube used

Potential laryngospasm or edema following intubation or extubation

NURSING CARE

Nursing Assessment

Inability to Maintain Patent Airway

Despite the selected technique, patent airway is not obtained; patient continues to have same or different airway obstruction signs as noted during preprocedural assessment (see above)

Carefully assess for patent airway, presence of bilaterally equal breath sounds, and bilateral expansion of chest wall

Carefully observe patent condition of tubing; clean or reposition as necessary to maximize airway potential

For tracheostomy and endotracheal intubation, obtain a chest roentgenogram after insertion to ascertain exact positioning of tube

Bleeding or Trauma Caused by the Airway Maintenance Technique

Observe for blood from mouth, nose, or suctioned mucus. Bleeding is usually self-limited unless the patient is receiving anticoagulants or has a bleeding disorder

Potential Dental Damage Secondary to Insertion

Observe condition of patient's teeth

Ulcerations of Nasal Tissue, Pharynx, or Mouth

Carefully observe tissue around the airway mechanism; when possible, change position of the mechanism or its taped location

Infection Secondary to Airway Maintenance Mechanism

Observe for signs of infection such as increased temperature, change in secretions, foul odor

Nursing Dx & Intervention

Ineffective airway clearance related to tracheobronchial secretions

- Assess patient for signs of hypoxia or airway blockage as indicated in the preprocedural assessment section.

- Position patient *to maximize airway potential.*
- Using sterile technique, suction as needed *to maintain airway.*
- Auscultate chest for presence and quality of bilateral breath sounds and adventitous sounds.
- If patient has oral endotracheal tube in place, teach him or her to avoid biting the tube. If necessary, provide oropharyngeal airway or bite block *to prevent biting on the endotracheal tube.*

Anxiety related to difficulty in breathing and difficulty in communication

- Assess for signs of anxiety secondary to airway blockage or hypoxia.
- Observe for signs of anxiety secondary to the airway maintenance procedure.
- Provide frequent information about procedures in progress.
- Provide emotional support.
- Teach family how to support patient and use the alternative means of communication.

Impaired gas exchange related to tissue hypoxia

- Assess arterial blood gases secondary to airway maintenance procedure; in collaboration with physician, prepare to administer oxygen therapy secondary to airway maintenance procedure.
- Continuously monitor SpO_2.

Risk for aspiration related to excessive oral secretions and presence of tube in airway

- Avoid triggering gag mechanism when performing caretaking activities, including mouth care.
- If swallowing reflex is diminished, elevate head of bed when performing mouth care.
- Assess and document amount of secretions present, patient's level of consciousness, and patient's ability to swallow secretions effectively.
- Administer suction when necessary to remove secretions and maintain patent airway.
- If secretions are thick and inspissated, ensure adequate humidification to help liquefy secretions.
- For patients with reduced level of consciousness, ensure head of bed is elevated, unless contraindicated.
- Position patients laterally to allow drainage of oral secretions out of mouth, unless position is contraindicated.

Evaluation

Airway is patent   Breath sounds are clear and bilaterally equal. There are no adventitious sounds. Breathing occurs easily and seems to be adequate for patient's attempt.

Gas exchange is adequate   Blood gas values are within normal limits.

Anxiety is reduced   Patient verbalizes, writes, or signs feelings of less anxiety. Patient appears more calm and relaxed. Patient is able to communicate.

Aspiration did not occur   Temperature and respiratory rate are within normal limits. Lung fields are clear on chest radiograph.

BREATHING TECHNIQUES

Following are some breathing techiques that may be taught to the patient to facilitate effective ventilation:

Abdominal or diaphragmatic breathing
Cough techniques
Deep breathing and coughing
Incentive spirometry

These are useful and specific measures to increase the volume of air entering the lungs, as well as being expelled from the lungs. These techniques are discussed according to indications and procedural techniques.

Abdominal or Diaphragmatic Breathing

Indications

Patients with chronic and acute obstructive ventilatory disorders may be taught to use a prolonged expiratory time. A longer, slow expiration allows the diaphragm to attain a higher and thus more efficient position. Note: this pattern may be detrimental in patients with severe hyperinflation because of advanced obstructive disease and in patients with restrictive disease.

Procedural Guidelines

1. Assist patient to attain position of comfort, usually sitting or in semi-Fowler's position in bed. Abdominal muscles should be relaxed and knees and hips flexed.
2. Instruct patient to inhale slowly. As patient inhales, the focus should be to pull the diaphragm down and to relax the abdominal wall, allowing the abdomen to bulge outward. If a hand is placed on the patient's abdomen, the hand should rise. In traditional diaphragmatic breathing, upper chest movement should be minimal. Note that in patients who are severely hyperinflated, upper chest movement is usually necessary to maintain ventilation and should not be discouraged.
3. Instruct patient to pause slightly after a deep and even inspiration and then, using a pursed-lip technique, to exhale quietly and naturally.
4. Explain the expiration should last two to three times longer than inspiration.
5. Have patient practice the diaphragmatic breathing technique so that it can be used easily at times of stress, increased respiratory rate, etc.

Pursed-Lip Breathing

Indications

This technique is used to control expiration and to facilitate emptying of the lung. The technique probably decreases the dynamic compression of airways and thus keeps them open longer. Many patients, especially those with emphysema, do pursed lip breathing spontaneously, without instruction.

Procedural Guidelines

1. Assist patient to a position of comfort.
2. Instruct patient to inhale deeply and to pause slightly at end of inspiration.
3. Instruct patient to exhale slowly through pursed lips, a blowing effect occurs.
4. Explain that exhalation should be slow and purposeful.
5. Have patient practice technique for use at times of stress, increased respiratory rate (maintaining adequate expiration will decrease hyperinflation and dyspnea at times of stress).

Cough Techniques

Indications

Cough techniques are taught to improve cough effectiveness and maintain airway clearance. Many types of patients need assistance with cough—those that are postoperative, those with inability to take a deep breath (neuromuscular disease, pain), that are unable to generate rapid expiratory flows (airways obstructive diseases).

Procedural Guidelines

There are several cough techniques that can be used:

1. In the normal cough the individual inhales to a large inspiratory volume and then performs several "coughs," each with less air in the lung. Patients should be instructed to cough in a similar manner. Inhale deeply, hold the breath for several seconds, and then perform several coughs before inhaling again.
2. For the patient with easily collapsible airways, an open glottic technique is used. This type of cough has been called huff coughing and forced expiratory technique (FET) cough. The same maneuver is followed as described for normal cough. The difference is that the repeated expiratory maneuvers are performed without glottic closure/opening; therefore there is no cough noise. Again, several forced expiratory maneuvers should be done on the one deep breath before the patient inhales again. The huff cough may not result in expectoration, but it usually stimulates a natural cough; because secretions have been moved mouthward by the "huffing," the natural cough becomes effective. The huff cough is also effective in postoperative patients.
3. A type of cough used in patients with bronchiectatic types of disease is the end-expiratory cough. The patient inhales deeply, does a short breath hold, and breathes out slowly through pursed lips. Just before the next inhalation, a short cough is done, exhaling the air remaining in the lung. The cough should be performed after most of the air has been exhaled. Several end-expiratory cough maneuvers will often move secretions to a point

in the airway where they can be expectorated using a normal cough maneuver.

4. Another type of cough is the augmented cough. This maneuver has several variations and is used in patients who are unable to produce sufficient expiratory force during a cough maneuver. Patients with chest wall pain/discomfort will often attempt to refrain from coughing or cough with less force. Wrapping a towel around the chest and pulling it snugly during the forced expiratory maneuver will often contribute to expiratory force and reduce pain. The abdominal thrust maneuver is used in patients with neuromuscular disease who are unable to generate sufficient abdominal pressure to produce an effective cough. (Examples are tetraplegics, paraplegics with loss of abdominal muscles, amyotrophic lateral sclerosis, muscular dystrophy). The patient is instructed to take a deep breath (or "stack" several breaths); then as the patient attempts to cough, the caregiver abruptly compresses the abdomen with an in-and-up motion. (The caregiver's hand is placed on the abdominal wall throughout the inspiratory and expiratory maneuver so the action is one of compressing, not hitting.)

Deep Breathing and Coughing

Indications

Patients having upper abdominal or thoracic surgery are at very high risk for the development of postoperative pulmonary complications, especially atelectasis and pneumonia. Patients with pneumonia and those who immobilized are also susceptible to secretion retention and atelectasis. Deep breathing and coughing are used to expand underventilated alveoli and to prevent retention of secretions.

Procedural Guidelines

1. Position patient to faciliate deep inspiration and coughing in a sitting or semi-Fowler's position if possible.
2. Instruct patient to take a slow, deep inspiration. Placing one's hands on the lateral chest and telling the patient to "push my hands out" will help the patient feel the chest motion you are trying to accomplish. The patient should do a breath hold (to a count of 5) at the peak of inspiration. (The term *sustained maximal inspiration* (SMI) describes the slow deep breath and breath hold.) If the patient is postoperative, pain medications may need to be administered 20 to 30 minutes before initiating the procedure.
3. After several deep breaths, the patient is instructed to cough. See above for cough techniques; provide the patient with tissues to collect expelled sputum.
4. Splinting, if required to reduce pain, may be accomplished in several ways. An abdominal incision can be splinted by a pillow and hand pressure over the incision. A sternotomy is splinted by a pillow "hugged" to the chest. A lateral thoracotomy incision is splinted by hand pressure over the incision area or by a towel wrapped around the chest.

Incentive Spirometry

Indications

The incentive spirometer may be used to encourage deep breathing. It provides visual feedback to encourage the patient's efforts; it does not "make" the person deep breathe. Incentive spirometry does not replace other deep breathing and coughing interventions.

Most incentive spirometers are of the volume type, although some are of the flow design. In the volume type, there is a measure of how much air the person inhaled. A marker is placed at the desired volume to provide a goal for the patient.

Procedural Guidelines

1. Position patient in semi-Fowler's position if possible.
2. Instruct patient to seal mouth around mouthpiece and to inhale slowly after a *normal* exhalation. Be sure the patient is inhaling from the mouthpiece and not around it, not through the nose.
3. Instruct the patient to hold the deep breath for a few seconds before exhaling.
4. The incentive spirometry should be used at least every 3 or 4 hours during the postoperative period until the patient is ambulatory and initiates effective deep breathing and coughing without assistance.

Evaluation

All of the breathing techniques have similar evaluation criteria.

Optimum movement of air in and out of lungs occurs Airway is clear, and breathing occurs without obstruction. Patient is able to inhale deeply and exhale effectively. There is no evidence of dyspnea or hypoxia.

Airway is patent There is no evidence of excessive secretions, or condition is optimal for patient; if sputum is present, patient is able to demonstrate productive sputum cough.

Clear breath sounds are heard in all areas Bronchovesicular breath sounds are heard throughout, or optimum breath sounds for patient. No areas of decreased breath sounds or consolidation are heard; rhonchi are absent.

Patient is comfortable during coughing and deep breathing Patient is able to ask for splinting assistance or splints self during deep breathing and coughing exercises.

▌ POSTURAL DRAINAGE, PERCUSSION, AND VIBRATION[20,26]

Postural drainage, percussion, and vibration are effective methods for loosening and moving secretions when patients are unable to maintain airway clearance. The techniques are most helpful in patients who raise copious amounts of sputum (>30 ml/day) and are frequently used in the chronic management of cystic fibrosis and bronchiectasis. These techniques may also be used in other patients where airway clearance is a problem, but the effectiveness needs to be individually evaluated. Postural drainage with percussion and vibration has also been demonstrated to be an effective means of reinflating atelectatic lung.

Contraindications

1. Patients with significant hemoptysis
2. Patients in whom a head-down position is contraindicated (e.g., head injury)
3. Patients with bleeding disorders
4. Patients with rib fractures, or predisposition to pathologic fractures
5. Patients in whom the techniques cause increased dyspnea, wheezing

Procedural Guidelines

Postural drainage consists of positioning the patient in specific positions so that the different segments of the lung are drained by gravity. The postural drainage treatment may be done to drain all areas, or may concentrate on one or two positions (for example, to concentrate on a left lower lobe atelectasis). Each position is maintained for at least 5 minutes. (Postural drainage positions are depicted in Figure 2-46.) After each position the patient should do several deep breaths with prolonged exhalation and end-expiratory cough, followed by a cascade cough.

If positioning and coughing are not effective, percussion and vibration may be added. The percussion and vibrations are done over the areas being drained (see Figure 2-46); these techniques should always be done over ribs, not over the sternum, vertebral bodies, or below the ribs.

To percuss, cup the hands and rhythmically strike the chest wall. The percussion is usually done over one thin layer of clothing. A hollow, deep sound indicates the technique is being performed correctly; there should not be a slapping sound. The area being drained is percussed for 1 to 3 minutes.

Following the percussion, the hand is flattened and applied to the chest wall (same area that was percussed). Have the patient take a deep breath. As the patient does a prolonged exhalation, vibrate and compress the chest wall. Vibration is usually repeated for 2 to 3 breaths. If the vibration does not stimulate a productive cough, have the patient voluntarily cough. If necessary, repeat the percussion and vibration before moving to the next position.

Alternatives to Postural Drainage With Percussion and Vibration

Flutter valve

The flutter valve is a small handheld device. The patient takes a slow deep breath and then exhales through the flutter valve. The flutter creates a vibrating column of air in the airway, much the same sensation as the percussion and vibration. After a few normal exhalations, the patient exhales more forcefully. The maneuver often stimulates a spontaneous cough. Studies have demonstrated that the technique is beneficial in cystic fibrosis, and it has also been used for patients with bronchiectasis. Many

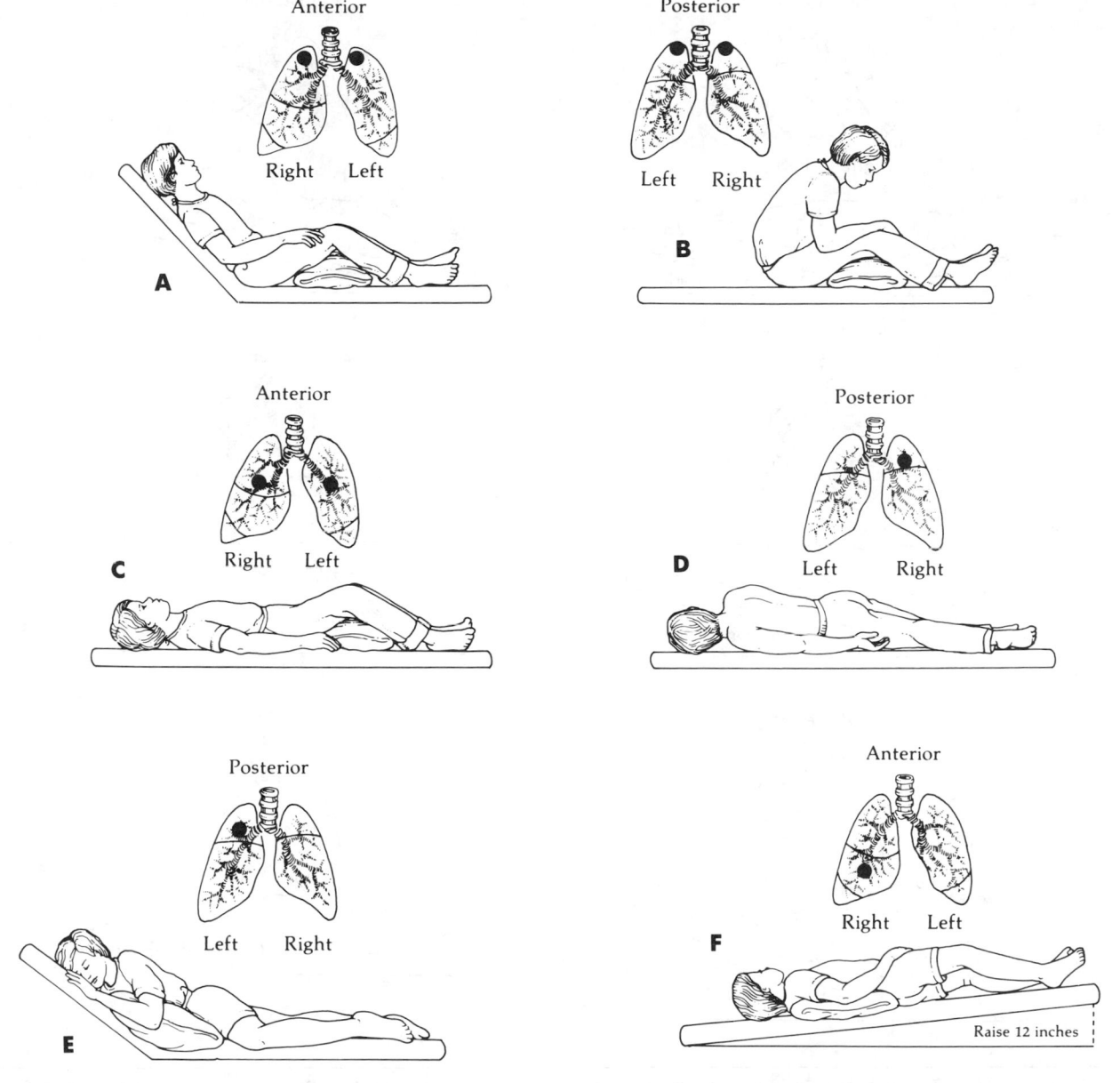

Figure 2-46 Positions for postural drainage. **A,** Anterior apical segment; sitting. **B,** Posterior apical segment; sitting. **C,** Anterior segment; lying flat on back. **D,** Right posterior segment; lying on left side. **E,** Left posterior segment; lying on right side. **F,** Right middle lobe; lying on left side.

patients have been able to replace postural drainage with daily use of the flutter valve. When the technique is effective, patients appreciate the simplicity of treatments, the ability to use the technique while away from home, and the fact that they do not require assistance from others.

High Frequency Chest Oscillation

This technique has been used to replace postural drainage in patients with cystic fibrosis and bronchiectasis. The technique can be used in the hospital or in the home. The procedure is carried out with the patient in a sitting position. A vest is put on

the patient; the vest is attached to a device that creates high frequency vibration of the chest wall. Several different frequencies are used to optimize airway clearance. Treatments require about 15 minutes (less time than full postural drainage). After each change in frequency, the patient is requested to cough.

Patient Education/Home Care Planning

1. Patients may be taught to perform postural drainage at home; a specific routine should be encouraged.

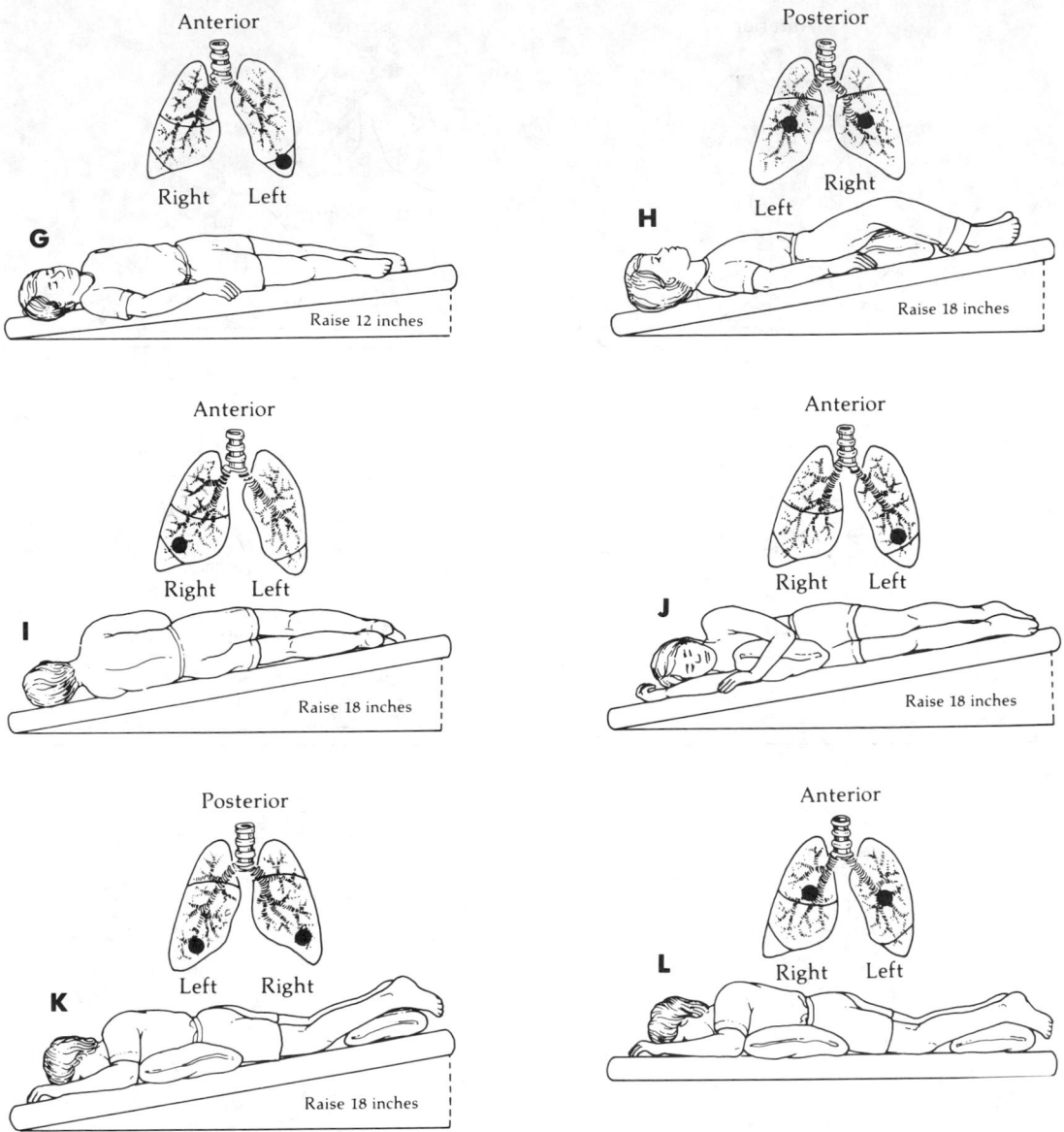

Figure 2-46, cont'd G, Left lingula, lying on right side. **H,** Anterior segments; lying on back. **I,** Right lateral segment; lying on left side. **J,** Left lateral segment; lying on right side. **K,** Posterior segments; lying on stomach. **L,** Superior segments; lying on stomach. (From Hirsch and Hannock.[41])

2. Head-down positioning does not require a complete tilt—only that the shoulders are lower than the hips. Sofa cushions or tilt tables can be used in the home.
3. Adaption of small handheld vibrators will allow patients to do their own postural drainage and percussion without help from another person. The vibrators are also helpful when another family member is doing the percussion/vibration.

Evaluation

Airways are clear   Breath sounds are clear bilaterally following techniques.

Productive sputum specimen is produced   Patient is able to expectorate sputum after each postural drainage position.

Breathing patterns are effective without dyspnea   Respiratory rate and rhythm are adequate; there is an absence of dyspnea.

Gas exchange is adequate   The ABGs are within acceptable range; there is no dyspnea.

CHEST TUBES AND CHEST DRAINAGE SYSTEMS[22,23,66]

Description and Rationale

Chest tubes with attached drainage systems are placed in the pleural cavity to drain fluid, blood, or air from the pleural cavity and to reestablish a negative pressure that will facilitate expansion of the lung. Chest tubes may be inserted postoperatively, as an emergency procedure following chest trauma, or therapeutically as a disease treatment modality. Chest tubes are also used to allow drainage for the mediastinum after cardiac surgery. Following are chest tube insertion sites:

Pneumothorax: usually in second and third intercostal spaces (anterior or lateral)

Hemothorax: usually in seventh, eighth, or ninth intercostal space (posteriolateral)

Thoracotomy: one tube generally inserted in second or third intercostal space (anterior) and another in lower posterior axillary line

Mediastinal: generally two tubes, inserted below xiphoid process

Chest tubes may be terminated when radiographic examination determines that the lung is reexpanded and when the drainage is minimal.

Cautions

Chest tubes are inserted by a physician and sutured into place. Cautions specific to chest tubes and drainage systems include the following:

Sterility must be maintained so as not to introduce infection into pleural cavity.

The system must remain patent: the tubing must not become blocked; if this occurs, a tension pneumothorax may result.

If the drainage tubing becomes dislodged from the patient or a drainage bottle breaks, reestablish drainage with a sterile system as soon as possible.

If the chest tube becomes dislodged from the patient's chest, the patient should exhale forcefully, and the chest wall incision should be quickly covered with a petrolatum jelly gauze.

Preprocedural Nursing Care

Carefully assess patient's preprocedural condition including respiratory rate and quality. Note evidence of dyspnea, labored breathing, tachypnea, tachycardia, quality and distribution of breath sounds, mediastinal shift, subcutaneous emphysema, and crepitus.

Set up drainage equipment appropriately for the type of system being used.

Single-Bottle System (Figure 2-47, A)

1. Unwrap bottles and tubing; maintain sterility.
2. Fill bottle with sterile water until the long glass tubing is submerged 2 cm. This bottle is called the water-seal bottle.
3. The short glass tubing (air vent) should never be covered with water.
4. The long glass tubing is connected to the patient's chest tube, and the short tubing air vent may be open to the air or connected to gravity drainage.

Double-Bottle System (Figure 2-47, B)

1. Prepare first bottle as described for the single-bottle system.

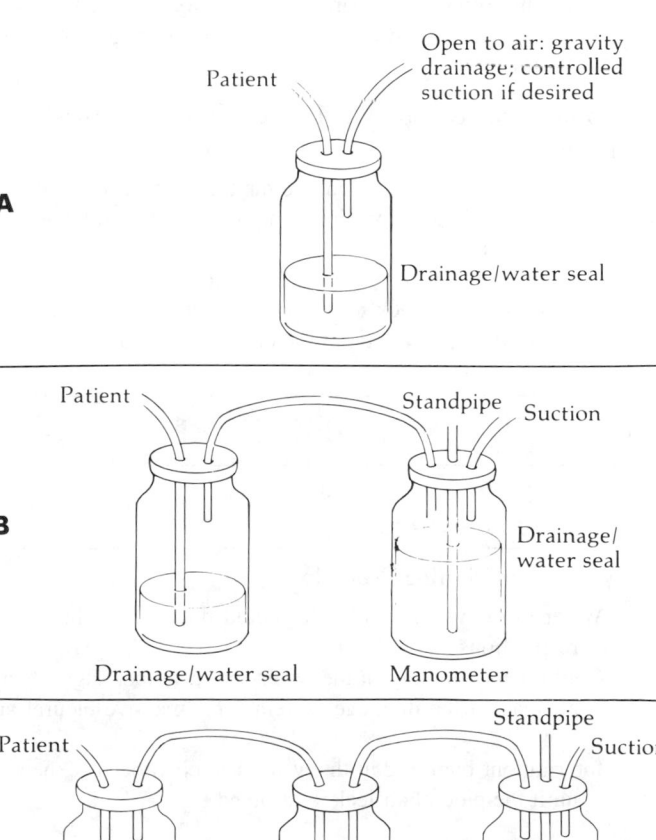

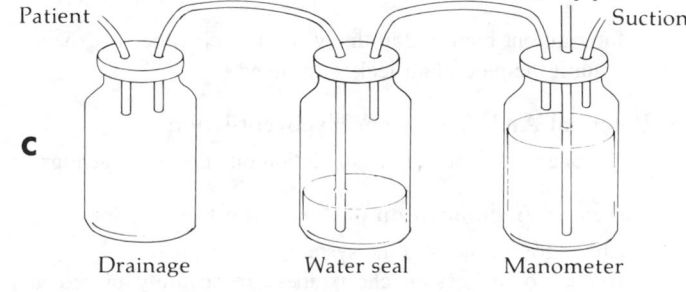

Figure 2-47 Bottle chest drainage system. **A,** Single-bottle system. **B,** Double-bottle system. **C,** Triple-bottle system.

2. Prepare the second bottle (the suction control or manometer bottle) by running a tube from the air vent of the first bottle to an air vent in the second bottle. This is the bottle that regulates the amount of vacuum in the system.
3. Fill the second bottle with sterile water to the designated depth.
4. The second bottle contains a long glass middle tube that acts as the air vent. The length of the large tube submerged under water determines the amount of negative pressure required to drain the chest. A common depth of water is 10 to 20 cm.
5. The suction control or manometer bottle is generally connected to a suction device such as an Emerson or Stedman pump.

Triple-Bottle System (Figure 2-47, C)

1. Prepare first two bottles as previously described.
2. A third bottle is prepared for a position closest to the patient. This bottle acts entirely as a drainage collection bottle.

Commercial Disposable Three-Chamber Units
(Figure 2-48)

1. These systems function like the three-bottle systems.
2. Setup and operation directions are provided with the sterile units.
3. Some systems provide access to collected blood for autotransfusion back to the patient, either with or without additional processing of the collected blood.

NURSING CARE

Nursing Assessment

System Functioning Properly

Water in the water-seal bottle should fluctuate slightly with respirations

Continuous bubbling in the water-seal chamber suggests an air leak in the drainage system (or a massive pleural air leak)

Intermittent bubbling in the water-seal chamber is expected until the pleural air leak is resolved

Potential Atelectasis from Hypoventilation

Dyspnea, evidence of consolidation on chest roentgenogram

Increased Accumulation of Air in the Pleural Space

Check for air leaks in the system

Assess to make sure chest tubes are securely placed and patent

Clinical signs include increased evidence of dyspnea, tachypnea, tachycardia, anxiety, and restlessness, increased subcutaneous emphysema

Infection

Elevated WBC, increased temperature, evidence of purulent drainage

Nursing Dx & Intervention

Ineffective breathing pattern related to pain and decreased lung expansion

- Assess and ensure patency of chest tubes by maintaining a continuous drainage path without kinks or dependent loops.
- Observe for signs of intrapleural fluid accumulation such as decreased breath sounds on affected side, increased dyspnea, and mediastinal shift.
- Always keep chest tube drainage system lower than the patient's chest.
- Observe volume, shade, color, and consistency of drainage from lung and record findings regularly.
- Observe for "tidaling" or fluctuation of fluid in the water-seal bottle; this should rise and fall with breathing; if fluctuation is not seen, carefully evaluate the patency of the tubing.
- Ensure that all tubing connections are securely attached and taped.

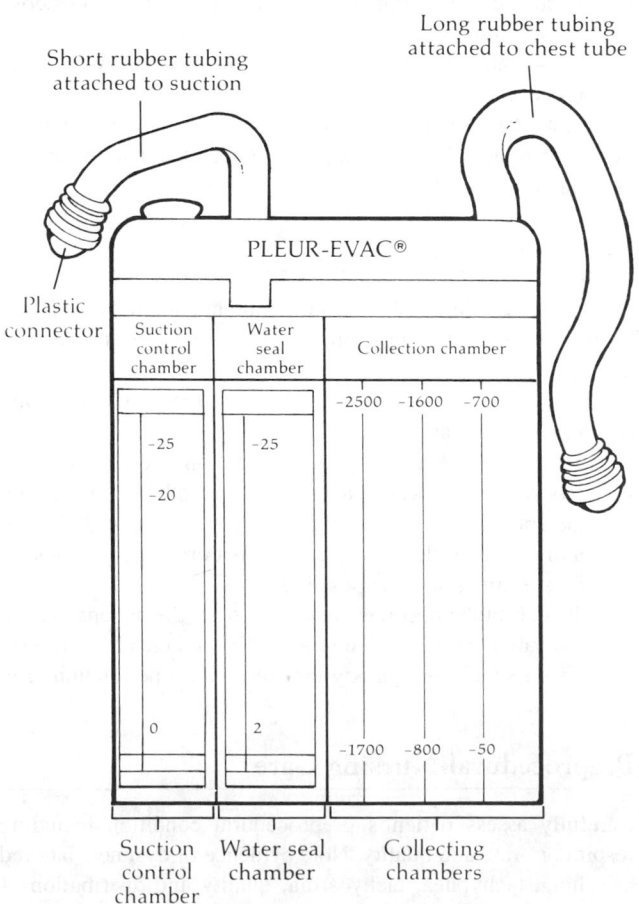

Figure 2-48 Commercial chest drainage system.

- Assist patient to cough, deep breathe, and change position at least every 2 hours.
- Observe special positioning if indicated because of special technique or surgery.
- Auscultate breath sounds at least every 2 to 4 hours.
- Assist patient to splint areas of incision and chest tube insertion.
- Provide analgesia as needed to promote effective ventilation.

Removal of Chest Tubes

Chest tubes may be removed after the lung has been reinflated for 24 hours to several days. Indications for removal are usually confirmed by chest radiographic examination. Removal of either pleural or mediastinal chest tubes are associated with significant discomfort. Analgesics should be administered prior to tube removal.[49] Removal procedures include the following:

1. Place patient in semi-Fowler's position or on side.
2. Physician instructs patient to take a deep breath and hold it.
3. The chest tube suture is clipped and the tube is quickly removed.
4. An occlusive dressing or petrolatum jelly gauze is placed over chest wall wound.
5. Patient is instructed to breathe normally, and the dressing is taped securely.
6. Careful patient assessment should follow on a continuing basis, including rate of respirations, quality of breath sounds, any drainage from chest tube dressing, sudden chest pains, or shortness of breath.

Evaluation

Breathing pattern is adequate   Breath sounds are clear bilaterally. Patient is able to breathe deeply without pain.

Chest tube drainage system is intact and operational System remains intact. Water fluctuates in water-seal container. Drainage accumulates in drainage bottle.

Lungs reexpand   Roentgenograms confirm lung reexpansion. Breath sounds are bilaterally equal and clear. Blood gases are within normal limits for patient. There is no atelectasis, consolidation, or associated infection.

MECHANICAL VENTILATION[2,50,67,81]

Mechanical ventilation is indicated for patients who are unable to maintain adequate ventilation on their own. The ventilator does not cure; it is a temporary support that merely "buys time" for correction of the underlying situation. The following is a brief overview. Refer to specialty texts for more information.

Volume-Cycled Ventilators

Volume-cycled (volume-preset) ventilators terminate inspiration after delivering a preset volume of gas. The desired volume of gas is delivered unless a preset pressure limit is reached. The ventilator continues to deliver a constant tidal volume regardless of the changes in the airway resistance or in compliance of the lungs and thorax.

Inspiratory time is determined by adjusting the flow rate of gas to be delivered (more rapid the flow, shorter the inspiratory time; slower the flow, longer the inspiratory time).

Expiratory time is most commonly determined by setting the respiratory rate. The operator must preset the following:

Tidal volume
Inspiratory pressure limit
Respiratory rate
Peak flow
Degree of sensitivity required by patient to trigger inspiration
Frequency of sighs per hour
Sigh volume—or amount of gas to be delivered during a sigh
Sigh pressure limit during a sigh inspiration
Oxygen percent concentration to be delivered
PEEP

Pressure-Cycled Ventilators

Pressure-cycled (pressure-preset) ventilators terminate inspiration when a preset pressure is achieved. When the pressure is reached, the gas flow stops and the patient passively exhales. The largest patient variable is that varying degrees of resistance interfere with gas flow. Thus the delivered volume may vary as the degree of resistance varies.

External Body Ventilator, Cuirass

External body ventilators function by applying intermittent subatmospheric pressure to the thorax and trunk of the body, thus assisting the patient to breathe. Negative pressure ventilators include tank ventilators, turtle shells, and poncho wraps.

Continuous Positive Airway Pressure (CPAP)

CPAP, delivered to spontaneously breathing patients via exotracheal tube, tracheostomy, or special mask, provides a positive pressure throughout the respiratory cycle. CPAP is helpful in conditions that decrease the FRC.

Noninvasive Pressure Support Ventilation (NIPSV)

Originally used for sleep apnea, NIPSV does not require intubation. It can be provided via nasal pillows and alternates levels of pressure with inspiration and expiration.

NURSING CARE

Nursing Assessment

Preprocedural

$Pa_{CO_2} > 55$ mm Hg
$Pa_{O_2} < 50$ mm Hg on a $FIO_2 > 0.60$ or $Pa_{O_2} > 50$ mm Hg
pH < 7.35

Dead space to tidal volume (V_D/V_T) >0.60
Inspiratory force (IF) <25 cm H_2O
Tidal volume (V_T) <5 ml/kg
Vital capacity (VC) <10 ml/kg

Procedural Problems

PaO_2 >110 mm Hg
    Response to therapy/gas exchange
PaO_2 >20 mm Hg above goal*
    Determine FIO_2; report FIO_2 setting and PaO_2 to physician
    (make sure FIO_2 was not left on 100% oxygen)
PaO_2 or SpO_2 below goal, depending on patient's underlying
    disease*
    Assessment of problem should include:
        Machine or tubing malfunction
        Patient's need for suctioning
        Diminished patient lung function
        Malplaced endotracheal tube
$PaCO_2$ above goal*
    Verify that patient is connected to ventilator and that venti-
    lator tubing is clear of obstruction or water accumulation
    Suction airway if necessary and determine position and
    patency of endotracheal tube
    Evaluate patient for metabolic alkalosis
    Determine whether patient has recently received respira-
    tory depressing sedation, which would affect respira-
    tory status
$PaCO_2$ more than 10 mm Hg below goal level*
    Assess patient's respiratory rate and depth
    Assess for metabolic acidosis

Nursing Dx & Intervention

Ineffective airway clearance related to neuromuscular impairment, inflammatory process, or decreased lung expansion

- Secure endotracheal tube in place (see associated procedure in airway maintenance section).
- Ensure 100% humidification and warming (between 32°
  and 36° C) of inspired gases as ordered.
- Suction as indicated *to maintain airway patency.*
- Monitor airway pressure frequently; one cause of an increased airway pressure is retained secretions. Empty water from ventilator circuit as it accumulates; it may partially obstruct tubing and increase airway pressure.

Ineffective breathing pattern related to neuromuscular impairment, inflammatory process of decreased lung expansion

- Consistently evaluate ventilatory pattern for rate, quality,
  signs of respiratory distress, or inappropriate inspira-
  tory/expiratory ratio (should >1:1).

*Note: Actual goals for individuals on mechanical ventilation may vary; collab-
orate with medical and respiratory professionals to determine goals of therapy.

- Monitor patient for signs of fighting the ventilator, which
  indicate that the patient's respiratory cycle is inconsistent
  with the mechanical cycle; may be due to pain, hypoxemia, secretions, fear, and anxiety; to correct, clear airways as indicated, give emotional support or give sedatives as ordered.
- Ensure that the alarm on the ventilator is ON.
- Carefully check all connections of the ventilator tubing
  regularly to ensure that they are tightly secured.
- PEEP may be used *to prevent alveolar collapse. The
  major goal of PEEP is to improve FRC and oxygen exchange.*
- CPAP functions similar to PEEP but is intended for patients who are breathing spontaneously.

Impaired gas exchange related to alveolar-capillary membrane changes

- Position patient so all lobes of lungs are adequately ventilated and perfused.
- Reposition patient every 30 to 60 minutes; rotate positioning from right and left lateral positions to a semi-
  Fowler's position.
- Carefully monitor ventilator pressure readings and the patient's breath sounds for presence and quality; pneumothorax, pneumomediastinum, and subcutaneous emphysema may be signs of barotrauma secondary to a high
  mechanical ventilator pressure.
- Pneumothorax may be anticipated by seeing an abrupt
  rise in the peak inspiratory pressure for a constant tidal
  volume.
- Carefully monitor all ventilator settings, as well as patient's arterial blood gas response.

Risk for infection related to loss of respiratory defense mechanisms, decreased ciliary action, and stasis of secretions

- Because of warm, moist nature of the ventilator equipment, the patient is prone to nosocomial infections.
- Send sputum specimens to the laboratory for analysis as
  ordered.
- Carefully monitor patient's temperature and characteristics of sputum.

Weaning from the Ventilator[11,81,90]

Physiologic guidelines (before beginning the weaning
process):
1. Vital capacity at least 10 to 15 ml/kg body weight.
2. Maximum inspiratory force greater than 25 cm H_2O.
3. Tidal volume >5 ml/kg.
4. Minute ventilation >10 L/minute.
5. $PaCO_2$ near or below patient's normal.
6. PaO_2 >60 mm Hg on 0.5 FIO_2.

Factors that increase the chance of successful weaning from
mechanical ventilation include adequate nutrition and sleep, relief of pain and anxiety, and development of a trusting relationship between the patient and the care team.

A number of different modes may be used for weaning, including alternating assisted ventilation with periods of spontaneous ventilation, gradual reduction of the rate of synchronized intermittent mandatory ventilation (SIMV), and use of decreasing levels of pressure-support ventilation (PSV).

Risk for dysfunctional ventilatory weaning response

- Involve patient and family in weaning plans. Allow patient to share control of the process.
- Provide patient and family with frequent support and feedback during the process.
- Minimize other activity demands during active weaning *to avoid excessive fatigue.*
- Assess for dysfunctional responses to weaning, indicating a need to slow the pace, provide more support, or possibly resume ventilator support.

Evaluation

Airway patency is maintained Breath sounds are heard in all lobes of lungs. Bilaterally equal lung expansion occurs. Tidal volume is >5 ml/kg. Vital capacity is >10 ml/kg. Inspiratory force is >25 cm H_2O. Dead space to tidal volume ratio is <0.60.

Effectiveness of ventilation or oxygenation is maintained $Paco_2$ is 35 to 45 mm Hg. Pao_2 is >0 mm Hg with FIO_2 0.4 or below. pH is >7.35. There are no clinical signs of dyspnea, restlessness, or cyanosis.

Absence of nosocomial infection Temperature and WBC are normal. Sputum is clear to white.

Weaning from mechanical ventilation is accomplished Patient's spontaneous ventilation is effective and adequate.

OXYGEN THERAPY[43,64,65,67]

Description and Rationale

The goal of oxygen therapy is to provide sufficient amounts of oxygen to the tissues so that normal metabolism can occur. Clinically this means to provide oxygen at the lowest fractional inspired oxygen (FIO_2) to maintain a Pao_2 of at least 60 mm Hg. Therapy is indicated when the patient is unable to maintain an adequate Pao_2 by his own ventilatory efforts.

Spearman, Sheldon, and Egan[85] give the following clinical objectives for oxygen therapy:

To reduce or correct arterial hypoxemia and tissue hypoxia

To reduce or correct the need for physiologic compensatory mechanisms to hypoxemia

Hypoxemia may be caused by a variety of factors. Following are the most common:

Reduced alveolar oxygen: results from either low ambient oxygen or hypoventilation

Ventilation/perfusion ratio imbalance: anatomic shunting that occurs secondary to congenital defects, disease or trauma, or physiologic shunting

Impaired alveolar-capillary diffusion: occurs secondary to pathologic changes such as fibrosis, increased connective tissue, interstitial edema, or tumors

Contraindications and Cautions

Following are risks and precautions regarding the use of therapeutic oxygen:

1. Oxygen-induced hypoventilation: when the arterial carbon dioxide tension is greater than 50 mm Hg, the risk of oxygen-induced hypoventilation increases. It is therefore advised, especially for patients with chronic lung diseases, to maintain oxygen therapy so the arterial oxygen tension remains about 60 to 65 mm Hg.

   To prevent induced hypoventilation, use low concentrations of oxygen if the patient is not mechanically ventilated. It is equally important, however, to adequately oxygenate the patient.

2. Atelectasis: the collapse of alveoli may occur secondary to high concentrations of oxygen in inspired air.

   To prevent this complication, if possible limit the duration of 100% inspired oxygen to no more than 20 minutes.

3. Oxygen toxicity: Although it is not clear exactly what FIO_2 causes oxygen toxicity, it is most probable that an FIO_2 of over 50% administered for longer than 24 hours increases the risk.

Preprocedural Nursing Care: Assessment of Need for Supplemental Oxygen

Hypoxia	Altered blood gas states
Hypotension	Pao_2 <55 mm Hg
Cyanosis	$Paco_2$ >42 mm Hg
Dyspnea	Bradycardia
Disorientation	Cardiac arrhythmias
Anxiety	Tachypnea
Nausea	Drowsiness
Nasal flaring	Headache
Retractions	Poor judgment
Atelectasis	Shortness of breath
Pulmonary edema	Pneumonia
Central nervous system depression	Emphysema
Muscle weakness	Airway obstruction

•••••• Multidisciplinary Plan

Oxygen therapy equipment may be divided into two major types: low-flow and high-flow systems

Low-flow systems do not supply all of the inspired gases that the patient breathes. This means that the patient breathes some room air along with the oxygen. For the system to be effective, the patient must be able to maintain a normal tidal volume, have a regular ventilatory pattern, and be able to cooperate. As the patient's ventilatory pattern changes, so does the concentration of inspired oxygen. Examples of low-flow systems include nasal cannula, simple oxygen mask, partial rebreathing mask with reservoir bag, and nonrebreathing mask with reservoir bag.

High-flow systems supply all gases at a preset FIO_2. These systems are generally not affected by changes in ventilatory pattern. The Venturi mask is the most common example of the high-flow system. Another example is a mechanical ventilator.

Table 2-12 summarizes the major types of oxygen therapy systems, their benefits, problems, and precautions.

NURSING CARE

Nursing Assessment

Respiratory Status

Ventilatory pattern
Tachypnea
Retractions
Work of breathing
Accessory muscle tone
Posturing

Tissue Oxygenation

Restlessness
Irritability
Disorientation
Confusion

Cardiovascular

Hypotension
Sudden hypertension
Tachycardia
Cardiac arrhythmia

Mucosa Hydration

Nasal and mucous membranes

Skin Integrity

Protect bony prominences against pressure

Absorption Atelectasis

This can occur when oxygen washes out nitrogen in the alveoli; without nitrogen the residual volume decreases and the alveoli collapse.
Patients at risk for developing:
    Low tidal volume
    Normal tidal volume without sighing
    Airway trapping such as in chronic lung disease
Problem may be prevented by:
    Limiting 100% oxygen delivery to no more than 20 minutes at a time
    Patent airway
    Mobilizing secretions

Oxygen Toxicity

Clinical signs that may occur after:
    6 hours of 100% oxygen therapy:
        Sharp chest pain
        Dry cough

Guidelines to prevent oxygen toxicity:
1. Limit use of 100% oxygen to brief periods
2. As early as possible reduce FIO_2 to lowest possible level to maintain oxygenation

Equipment

Patency of tubing and bags
Cleanliness
Humidification
Correct size for the patient

Safety

While oxygen is in use, prohibit smoking in the area.

Nursing Dx & Intervention

Ineffective airway clearance related to fatigue, tracheobronchial obstructions, or secretions

- Assess patient to identify inability to move secretions, *which would interfere with oxygenation.*
- Assist patient to maintain proper body positioning *to ensure maximal airway patency.*
- Carefully and frequently auscultate chest for quality of breath sounds and adventitious sounds *that could indicate complications of oxygen therapy.*

Impaired gas exchange related to altered oxygen supply and alveolar-capillary membrane exchange

- Assess patient to identify signs such as restlessness, confusion, and irritability, *which may indicate the body's response to altered blood gas states.*
- In collaboration with physician, monitor arterial blood gases; report increases or decreases of $PaCO_2$ of more than 10 mm Hg.
- In collaboration with physician consultation, administer oxygen *to maintain PaO_2 above 55 mm Hg.*
- Assess patient to determine which oxygen therapy system is best to maintain the required PaO_2 level.
- Monitor electrocardiogram and cardiac status *for arrhythmias secondary to alterations in blood gases.*
- Carefully observe effectiveness of selected oxygen equipment to *maintain determined FIO_2 levels.*
- Clean equipment regularly.

Patient Education/Home Care Planning

1. Assess the patient's knowledge and skills regarding the use of oxygen equipment.
2. Teach the patient the purpose and process of the selected type of oxygen equipment.
3. Teach importance of not smoking (and not permitting others in the area to smoke) during administration of oxygen.
4. Provide the patient and family with information regarding the care, cleaning, and maintenance of oxygen equipment being used in the hospital or to be used at home.

TABLE 2-12 Oxygen Therapy Systems

Type of System	Description	Flow Rate (L/min)*	Approximate Oxygen Concentration Delivered (%)	Benefits	Problems	Nursing Care
Low-Flow Systems						
Nasal cannula		1 2 3 4 5 6	22-24 26-28 28-32 32-36 36-40 40-44 (concentration delivered varies with patient's respiratory rate and volume)	Comfortable, convenient method of delivering concentration of oxygen ranging from 22%-44%. Major advantages of this method are low cost of equipment, allowance for patient mobility, ability to deliver oxygen and still permit patient to eat and talk, and lack of necessity for humidification of inspired gas mixture. Practical system for long-term therapy. Mouth breathing will not affect concentration of delivered oxygen.	Nasal, cheek, and ear irritation. Unable to deliver oxygen concentration over 44%. Assumes a stable breathing pattern. Equipment may not be used if patient has nasal problem or if unable to tolerate nasal prongs. Patient must be able to cooperate to keep prongs in place.	Clean equipment. Evaluate for pressure areas over ears and cheek areas. Liter flow above 6 L/min will *not* increase the FIo₂.
Simple face mask		6 6-7 7-8	40 50 60	If patient's ventilatory needs exceed flow of gas, holes on sides of mask allow for entry of room air. Permits higher oxygen delivery than nasal cannula. System does not tend to dry out mucous membranes of nose or mouth	Mask must be removed prior to patient's eating. Should be operated at flow >5L/min. A tight face mask seal may cause facial irritation. Face mask may increase anxiety in some patients. Not practical for long-term therapy. May feel hot and confining for some patients.	Do not operate at flow less than 5-6 L/min (will not flush out accumulated CO₂). Should not be used for patients with chronic lung diseases. Equipment should be removed and cleaned several times each day.

Continued.

TABLE 2-12 Oxygen Therapy Systems—cont'd

Type of System	Description	Flow Rate (L/min)*	Approximate Oxygen Concentration Delivered (%)	Benefits	Problems	Nursing Care
Partial rebreathing mask with reservoir bag	Masks similar to simple face mask with addition of a reservoir oxygen bag; the purpose of the rebreathing mask is to increase FIO_2 by inhaling from a reservoir; some rebreathing of CO_2 also occurs	8 10-12	40-50 60	The bag makes possible delivery of oxygen concentration between 40% and 60% provided that the reservoir is kept full by a continuous flow of oxygen	Requires tight face seal similar to regular mask. Must be removed for eating and talking. Bag may kink or twist. Impractical for long-term therapy.	Must maintain flow sufficient to keep reservoir bag from completely deflating during inspiration. Check mask for leaks around face; FIO_2 may decrease if mask is not tight fitting. All other functions as with simple mask.
Nonrebreathing mask with reservoir bag	Similar to rebreathing bag, but this mask has one-way expiratory valve that prevents rebreathing of expired gases	6 8 10 12-15	55-60 60-80 80-90 90	Effective as short-term therapy. May deliver oxygen concentration up to 90%.	Requires tight face seal. Impractical for long-term therapy. Must be removed for eating and talking.	Check mask for leaks around face; FIO_2 may decrease if mask is not tight fitting. All other functions as with simple mask.
High-Flow Systems						
Venturi mask	Works on Bernoulli principle of air entrainment: for each liter of oxygen that passes through a fixed orifice, a fixed proportion of room air will be entrained; by varying size of orifice and flow of oxygen, precise FIO_2 is maintained.	Varies with equipment used	24 28 31 35 40 50	Delivers exact concentration. FIO_2 remains constant regardless of the patient's ventilatory pattern. FIO_2 may be measured directly by an oxygen analyzer. FIO_2 dial may be changed and set to deliver a calculated oxygen concentration.	May irritate face skin. Interferes with eating and drinking. If greater than 50% concentration is desired, must switch to different oxygen delivery system.	Check mask for leaks around face; FIO_2 may be altered if system not properly fitting. All other functions as with simple face mask.
Transtracheal oxygen catheter	Small, percutaneous tracheal catheter secured by a neck chain	¼-4 L/min		Avoids nasal drying and facial/ear irritation. May be concealed by clothing. Decreased liter flow of oxygen required compared to nasal cannula.	Requires regular cleaning. May be prone to more frequent lower respiratory infections. May develop mucous balls.	Varies with phase of therapy. Catheter cleaned in place while tract immature. Catheter removed for cleaning after tract mature.

*Normal breathing patterns are assumed.

Evaluation

Airway is patent   Airways are clear, and breathing occurs without obstruction.

Optimum movement of air in and out of lungs occurs   Vital capacity measurements including FEV_1, FVC, TLC, RV, and FRC are optimum for patient's status.

Gas exchange is optimum   Blood gas values, pulse oximetry within normal limits for the patient.

Patient and family have sufficient information to comply with oxygen therapy plan   Therapy plan is maintained.

▌THORACIC SURGERY

Description and Rationale

Thoracotomy   Thoracotomy refers to a surgical incision of the chest wall. An exploratory thoracotomy may be performed to obtain a biopsy specimen or locate a source of bleeding. During the procedure the ribs are spread and the pleura is opened. Closed chest drainage is generally required postoperatively.

Pneumonectomy   Pneumonectomy refers to surgical removal of an entire lung. The surgeon severs and sutures off the main arteries, veins, and the mainstream bronchus at the bifurcation. The major indication for pneumonectomy is lung cancer. Closed chest drainage is generally not done postoperatively. It is desirable for the thoracic cavity on the affected side to fill with serous exudate. The exudate eventually consolidates. The phrenic nerve on the affected side may be severed by the surgeon. This permits the diaphragm to assume an elevated position, which also assists to fill the empty thoracic space.

Lobectomy   Lobectomy refers to removal of a lobe of the lung. Major indications for this procedure include isolated tumors, cysts, tuberculosis, abscess, or localized injury. Closed chest drainage is used following a lobectomy.

Segmental resection   Segmental resection refers to the removal of one or more segments of the lung lobe. Indications for the procedure include tuberculosis, bleb, localized abscess, or bronchiectasis. Closed chest drainage is used following this procedure.

Wedge resection   Wedge resection refers to the removal of a small, wedge-shaped localized area near the lung surface. Indications for the procedure include biopsy and removal of a small area of tuberculosis. The resected area is sutured off before removal. There is generally little disruption of overall lung function. Closed chest drainage is used after the procedure.

Decortication   Decortication refers to the stripping off of a thick fibrous membrane that may develop over the visceral pleura secondary to empyema or the prolonged presence of blood or fluid in the pleural space. Closed chest drainage is required postoperatively.

Lung reduction   This type of surgery is a therapeutic intervention in a highly select group of patients with emphysema. The principles are that a reduction of lung volume will (1) decrease the tension of the respiratory muscles and therefore decrease dyspnea and (2) allow normal lung that was previously compressed to expand and thus improve gas exchange. Two approaches are used. In one, a midline sternotomy is performed and both lungs "trimmed." Strips of bovine pericardium are usually used to help seal the cut surface of the lung and prevent large postoperative air leaks. In the other procedure, a laser beam is used to trim the lung, most usually through multiple thorascopic incisions.

The outcome of the procedure is variable and partly dependent on patient selection. Early studies have demonstrated a reduction in dyspnea and in some patients a reduction in supplemental oxygen requirement. The long-term benefit is unknown.

Lung transplant   Lung transplantation originally required a heart lung transplantation. Today, lung transplantation (without transplanting the heart) is possible. Depending on the recipients underlying pulmonary pathology a heart lung, single lung, or double lung transplantation can be done.

Heart lung transplantations are done for patients with primary pulmonary hypertension and for cardiac defects associated with pulmonary hypertension (Eisenmenger's syndrome). Heart lung transplantations are done via a midline sternotomy incision.

Double single lung transplantation (in other words, a right and left lung are transplanted; the trachea is native to the recipient) is the procedure done in patients with cystic fibrosis. Because of the risk of infection if one native lung were left, single lung transplantation is avoided. The double lung transplantation is usually the procedure of choice in younger candidates. The double lung transplantation is usually done via a clam shell incision (anteriorly from side to side at the lower thoracic border). Some surgeons also prefer the double lung transplantation for patients with emphysema.

The single lung transplantation is done for patients with interstitial fibrosis. Some surgeons also use this approach for patients with emphysema. This procedure allows more persons to receive a transplant; a consideration when donors are not always available. A lateral thoracotomy incision is usually used. In single lung transplantation, one must always remember that the native lung with its disease is still present. The aim is for the native lung to essentially shut down, with blood flow and ventilation going to the new lung.

Whenever a lung is transplanted, consideration is given not only to blood type but also to the size of the donor and recipient. (If the lung is too small, it may not fill the thorax; if the transplanted lung is too large, it may be difficult to fully inflate it.) Lung transplantation patients receive immunosuppression, as do other transplantation patients. Another specific consideration in lung transplantation is the problems with airway clearance. The donor lung has no cough reflex (the lung is denervated), and the bronchial arteries are not attached to the recipient's systemic circulation. Mucus tends to be more tenacious and mucociliary clearance is often impaired; coupling this finding with loss of the cough reflex means that nursing care and patient care regarding airway clearance are of prime importance. Patients are taught to voluntarily cough several times a day, and most are taught to do postural drainage at least once or twice a day.

Both acute and chronic rejection are more difficult to diagnose than in heart transplantations. It is often difficult to differentiate a pulmonary infection (high risk for infection because of immunosuppression) from rejection. Also lung function can be impaired and the patient may be unaware of the change. Thus, patients do daily monitoring of spirometry (FEV$_1$ and FVC); a fall in FEV$_1$ or FVC is a signal to contact their caregivers. Bronchoscopy may be done to assist in diagnosing the cause of the fall in function, but patients are often treated for both infection (antibiotics) and rejection (corticosteroids). Chronic rejection in lung transplantation results in bronchiolitis obliterans with severe airways obstruction.

Contraindications and Cautions

The following are potential complications of thoracic surgery:
    Respiratory insufficiency
    Tension pneumothorax
    Atelectasis
    Bronchopleural fistula
    Pulmonary edema
    Subcutaneous emphysema
    Infection

Preprocedural Nursing Care

Carefully determine preoperative status of patient including the following:
    Baseline pulmonary function studies
    Electrocardiogram
    Arterial blood gases
    Electrolytes
    Other existing health problems
    Current respiratory status: amount and extent of dyspnea, cough, and respiratory distress
    General nutrition and hydration state
Provide preoperative teaching to include the following:
    Need to stop smoking preoperatively
    Coughing and deep breathing techniques
    Overview of equipment and procedures that will most likely occur postoperatively
    Listen preoperatively to patient and family questions and concerns; provide information and clarification when indicated
    Assure patient that pain medication will be available postoperatively to assist with discomfort
    Teach patient the need for postoperative range of motion and leg exercises, early ambulation

NURSING CARE

Nursing Assessment

Blood Gases

pH, Pao$_2$, Paco$_2$, HCO$_3^-$, O$_2$ saturation to monitor ventilator assistance or patient's ability to ventilate self

Chest Tube Drainage

Amount of drainage, characteristics of drainage, patency of closed drainage system, presence of air leak

Incision Status

Suture line characteristics

Respiratory Status

Lung expansion status, signs of atelectasis, consolidation, infection, pulmonary embolus, mediastinal shift, paradoxical motion
Dyspnea, tachypnea, shallow respirations, crackles, rhonchi, decreased tidal volume, cough

Cardiovascular Status

Electrocardiogram changes, hypovolemia, pulmonary edema, venous stasis, cardiac arrhythmias, central venous pressure within normal limits for patient

Pain

Pain with activities of turning, coughing, deep breathing, and range of motion

Fluid and Electrolyte Balance

Adequate urinary output
Electrolytes

Infection

Increased WBC, fever, purulent drainage, redness around incision area

Nutrition

Food intake

Nursing Dx & Intervention

Ineffective airway clearance related to tracheobronchial secretions

- Maintain patent airway by suctioning and adequate position; if patient has endotracheal tube, see p. 1614 for additional strategies.
- Assess for signs of airway obstruction including restlessness, inadequate chest expansion, stridor, noisy respirations, cyanosis, or dyspnea (atelectasis may be preventable with proper nursing care).
- Evaluate for signs of atelectasis that may result secondary to airway obstruction; signs include increased respiratory rate, rapid pulse, increased temperature, cyanosis, and diaphoresis.

Ineffective breathing pattern related to pain and fatigue

- Carefully monitor status of closed chest drainage system; note fluctuation or tidaling in the water-seal chamber and the drainage tubing near the patient; see closed-chest drainage system for additional strategies.

- If patient is on mechanical ventilator, see p. 1616 for specific nursing strategies.
- When patient is ventilating independently, carefully assess respiratory rate, depth, and quality; note signs of dyspnea and respiratory distress, hemoptysis.
- Administer intermittent positive-pressure breathing (IPPB) as ordered; evaluate and record response.
- Encourage coughing and deep breathing on a regular basis until patient is able to maintain procedure by self; observe and record response.
- Facilitate patient rest between activities.

Impaired physical mobility related to incisional pain and chest tubes

- Initiate passive and encourage active range of motion throughout the postoperative period.
- The patient is at risk for developing stiffness and ankylosis of the shoulder on the side with the chest tubes; encourage range of motion for that shoulder on a regular schedule.
- Encourage passive and active range of motion of the legs *to decrease the potential for thrombosis.*
- Ambulate patient as soon as possible and in accord with patient's ability to tolerate ambulation.
- Make sure a call button is conveniently placed for patient's use.

Patient Education/Home Care Planning

1. Explain the need to continue coughing and deep breathing.
2. Explain the need to move and ambulate frequently, increasing the amount of exercises gradually.
3. Explain that numbness, heaviness, or pain in the operative site is normal.
4. Explain the need to report the following symptoms to physicians:
   Persistent dyspnea
   Cough
   Elevated temperature
   Upper respiratory infection
   Redness, swelling, pain, or drainage from incision

Evaluation

Evaluation criteria are based on the individual procedure performed and the underlying disease state.

Airways are patent   Breath sounds are clear.

Breathing pattern is effective without pain or fatigue Arterial blood gases are within acceptable range.

Patient is able to move around without pain.

References

1. Agnelli G: Anticoagulation in the prevention and treatment of pulmonary embolism, *Chest* 107(1):39S-57S, 1995.
2. Ahrens TS, Nelson G: *Pulmonary anatomy and physiology.* In Kinney MR, Packa DR, Dunbar SB, editors: *AACN's clinical reference for critical-care nursing,* St Louis, 1993, Mosby.
3. American Thoracic Society: Indications and standards for use of nasal continuous positive airway pressure (CPAP) in sleep apnea syndromes, *Am J Respir Crit Care Med* 150:1738-1745, 1994.
4. American Thoracic Society: Standards for the diagnosis and care of patients with chronic obstructive pulmonary disease, *Am J Respir Crit Care Med* 152:S77-S120, 1995.
5. Berkow R: *Merck manual of diagnosis and therapy,* ed 14, Rahway, NJ, 1982, Merck.
6. Bootzin RR, Quan SF, Bamford CR, Wyatt JK: Sleep disorders, *Compr Ther* 21:401-406, 1995.
7. Brooks-Brunn J: Postoperative atelectasis and pneumonia, *Heart Lung* 24:94-115, 1995.
8. Brooks-Brunn J: Postoperative atelectasis and pneumonia: risk factors, *Am J Crit Care* 4:340-349, 1995.
9. Burrows B: An overview of obstructive lung diseases, *Med Clin North Am* 65:455, 1981.
10. Busse WW, et al: Stress and asthma, *Am J Respir Crit Care Med* 151:249-252, 1995.
11. Carpenito LJ: *Nursing diagnosis application to clinical practice,* ed 5, Philadelphia, 1993, JB Lippincott.
12. Chang VM: Protocol for prevention of complications of endotracheal intubation, *Crit Care Nurse* 15(5):19-27, 1995.
13. Cherniack RM: *Current therapy of respiratory disease,* ed 2, Philadelphia, 1986, BC Decker.
14. Chillcott S, Sheridan PS: ECCO2R: an experimental approach to treating ARDS, *Crit Care Nurse* 15:50-56, 1995.
15. Corbridge TC, Hall JB: The assessment and management of adults with status asthmaticus, *Am J Respir Crit Care Med* 151:1296-1316, 1995.
16. Cummins RO: *Textbook of advanced cardiac life support,* Dallas, 1994, American Heart Association.
17. Despars JA, Sassoon CSH, Light RW: Significance of iatrogenic pneumothoraces, *Chest* 105(4):1147-1150, 1994.
18. Dirks JL: Innovations in technology: continuous intra-arterial blood gas monitoring, *Crit Care Nurse* 15:19-27, 1995.
19. Donahoe M, Rogers RM: In Tierney D, editor: Nutritional aspects of lung disease, *Current Pulmonary* 17:275-302, 1995.
20. Eid N, Buchheit J, Neuling M, Phelps H: Chest physiotherapy in review, *Respir Care* 36:270-282, 1991.
21. Ellis EF: Asthma in childhood, *J Allergy Clin Immunol* 72:526, 1983.
22. Erickson RS: Mastering the ins and outs of chest drainage. Part I, *Nursing 89* 19:37, 1989.
23. Erickson RS: Mastering the ins and outs of chest drainage. Part 2, *Nursing 89* 19:46, 1989.
24. Evers BM, Townsend CM, Thompson JC: Organ physiology of aging, *Surgical Clin North Am* 74:23-39, 1994.
25. Farzan S: *A concise handbook of respiratory diseases,* ed 3, Norwalk, CT, 1992, Appleton & Lange.
26. Fedorovich C, Littleton MT: Chest physiotherapy: evaluating the effectiveness, *Dimens Crit Care Nurs* 9:68-74, 1990.
27. Ferguson GT, Cherniack RM: Management of chronic obstructive pulmonary disease, *N Engl J Med* 328:1017-1022, 1993.
28. Fishbach FT: *A manual of laboratory & diagnostic tests,* ed 4, Philadelphia, 1992, JB Lippincott.
29. Fries JF, Ehrlich GE: *Prognosis: contemporary outcomes of disease,* Bowie, MD, 1981, Charles Press.
30. Gammon RB, Shin MS, Buchalter SE: Pulmonary barotrauma in mechanical ventilation, *Chest* 102:568-572, 1992.
31. George RB, Light RW, Matthay RA: *Chest physiology,* New York, 1983, Churchill Livingstone.
32. Giuntini C, et al: Epidemiology, *Chest* 107:3S-9S, 1995.
33. Goldhaber SZ: Contemporary pulmonary embolism thrombolysis. *Chest* 107:45S-57S, 1995.
34. Gong H, Linn WS: Health effects of criteria air pollutants, *Current Pulmonary* 15:341-397, 1994.
35. Gosselink RAA et al: Diaphragmatic breathing reduces efficiency of breathing in patients with chronic obstructive pulmonary disease, *Am J Respir Crit Care Med* 151:1136-1142, 1995.

36. Guenter CA, Welch MH: *Pulmonary medicine,* Philadelphia, 1977, JB Lippincott.
37. Hammer J: Challenging diagnosis: adult respiratory distress syndrome, *Crit Care Nurse* 15:46-51, 1995.
38. Hansen LG, Warwick WJ, Hansen KL: Mucus transport mechanisms in relation to the effect of high frequency chest compression (HFCC) on mucus clearance, *Pediatric Pulmona* 1994; 17(2):113-118.
39. Harper RW: *A guide to respiratory care: physiology and clinical approaches,* Philadelphia, 1981, JB Lippincott.
40. Hill D: Transtracheal oxygen—setting up a home care program, *Caring Magazine* 5:44-47, 1995.
41. Hirsch J, Hannock L: *Mosby's manual of clinical nursing practice,* St. Louis, 1981, Mosby.
42. Hodson ME: Aerosolized dornase alfa (rhDNase) for therapy of cystic fibrosis, *Am J Respir Crit Care Med* 151:S70-S74, 1995.
43. Hoffman LA: Novel strategies for delivering oxygen: reservoir cannula, demand flow, and transtracheal oxygen administration, *Respir Care* 39:363-377, 1994.
44. Hudak CM, Gallo BM, Benz JJ: *Critical care nursing: a holistic approach,* ed 6, Philadelphia, 1994, JB Lippincott.
45. Hunninghake GW, Kalica AR: Approaches to the treatment of pulmonary fibrosis, *Am J Respir Crit Care Med* 151:915-918, 1995.
46. Jantz MA, Pierson DJ: Pneumothorax and barotrauma, *Clin Chest Med* 15:75-91, 1994.
47. Kim MJ: Ineffective airway clearance and ineffective breathing patterns: theoretical and research base for nursing diagnosis, *Nurs Clin North Am* 22:125, 1987.
48. Kim MJ, McFarland GK, McLane AM: *Pocket guide to nursing diagnoses,* ed 6, St Louis, 1995, Mosby.
49. Kinney MR, Kirchhoff KT, Puntillo KA: Chest tube removal practices in critical care units in the United States, *Am J Crit Care* 4:419-424, 1995.
50. Knebel A, Strider VC, Wood C: The art and science of caring for ventilator-assisted patients, *Crit Care Nurs Clin North Am* 6:819-829, 1994.
51. Konstan MW, Stern RC, Doershuk CF: Efficacy of the flutter device for airway mucus clearance in patients with cystic fibrosis, *J Pediatr* 124:689-693, 1994.
52. Korst RJ et al: Gene therapy for the respiratory manifestations of cystic fibrosis, *Am J Respir Crit Care Med* 151:S75-S87, 1995.
53. Larson JL: Ineffective breathing patterns related to respiratory muscle fatigue, *Nurs Clin North Am* 22:207, 1987.
54. Manganelli D, Palla A, Donnamaria V, Giuntini C: Clinical features of pulmonary embolism, *Chest* 107:25S-38S, 1995.
55. Martin L: *Pulmonary physiology in clinical practice: the essentials for patient care and evaluation,* St Louis, 1987, Mosby.
56. McCance KL, Huether SE: *Pathophysiology: the biologic basis for disease in adults and children,* ed 2, St Louis, 1994, Mosby.
57. McFadden ER: Improper patient techniques with metered dose inhalers: clinical consequences and solutions to misuse, *J Allergy Clin Immunol* 96:278-283, 1995.
58. Melot C: Ventilation-perfusion relationships in acute respiratory failure, *Thorax* 49:1251-1258, 1994.
59. Milberg JA, Davis DR, Steinberg KP, Hudson LD: Improved survival of patients with acute respiratory distress syndrome (ARDS): 1983-1993, *JAMA* 273:306-309, 1995.
60. Miller JN: Comprehensive review: neuromuscular blocking agents in critical care, *Crit Care Nurs Q* 18:60-73, 1995.
61. Miller LG, Kazemi H: *Manual of clinic pulmonary medicine,* New York, 1983, McGraw-Hill.
62. Morris JF: Physiological changes due to age, *Drugs Aging* 4:207-220, 1994.
63. Nunn JF: *Nunn's applied respiratory physiology,* ed 4, Oxford, 1993, Butterworth Heinemann.
64. Pfister S: Management of a transtracheal oxygen catheter in a mechanically ventilated patient, *Crit Care Nurse* 13:52-58, 1993.
65. Phipps WJ, Cassmeyer VI, Sands JK, Lehman MK: *Medical-surgical nursing,* ed 5, St Louis, 1995, Mosby.
66. Pierce LN: *Guide to mechanical ventilation and intensive respiratory care,* Philadelphia, 1995, WB Saunders.
67. Price SA, Wilson LM: *Pathophysiology: clinical concepts of disease processes,* ed 5, St Louis, 1996, Mosby.
68. Raghu G: Interstitial lung disease: a diagnostic approach, *Am J Respir Crit Care Med* 151:909-914, 1995.
69. Rakel RE: *Conn's current therapy,* Philadelphia, 1987, WB Saunders.
70. Redick EL: Closed-system, in-line endotracheal suctioning, *Crit Care Nurse* 13:47-51, 1993.
71. Renston JP, DiMarco AF, Supinski GS. Respiratory muscle rest using nasal BiPAP ventilation in patients with stable severe COPD, *Chest* 105:1053-1060, 1994.
72. Rhodes M: Update on chest trauma, *Crit Care Q* 6:59, 1983.
73. Ries AL: In Tierney D, editor: Pulmonary rehabilitation, *Current Pulmonary* 15:441-467, 1994.
74. Rinaldo JE: In Tierney D, editor: The adult respiratory distress syndrome, *Current Pulmonary* 15:137-156, 1994.
75. Seidel HM et al: *Mosby's guide to physical examination,* St Louis, 1991, Mosby.
76. Shapiro ED et al: The protective efficacy of polyvalent pneumococcal pollysaccharide vaccine, *N Engl J Med* 325:1435-1460, 1991.
77. Smith L, Thier S: *Pathophysiology: the biological principles of disease,* Philadelphia, 1981, WB Saunders.
78. Szaflarski NL: Emerging technology in critical care: continuous intraarterial blood gas monitoring, *Am J Crit Care* 5:55-65, 1996.
79. Tablan OC, et al: Guideline for prevention of nosocomial pneumonia. Part I. Issues on prevention of nosocomial pneumonia—1994, *Am J Infect Control* 22:247-292, 1994.
80. Thelan LA, Davie JK, Urden LD, Lough ME: *Critical care nursing: diagnosis and management,* ed 2, St Louis, 1994, Mosby.
81. Tisi GM: *Pulmonary physiology in clinical medicine,* Baltimore, 1980, Williams & Wilkins.
82. Traver GA: Ineffective airway clearance: physiology and clinical application, *Dimens Crit Care Nurs* 4:198-208, 1985.
83. Traver GA, Cline MG, Burrows B: Asthma in the elderly, *J Asthma* 30:81-91, 1993.
84. Traver GA, Mitchell JT, Flodquist-Priestley G: *Respiratory care: a clinical approach,* Gaithersburg, MD, 1991, Aspen.
85. Tuxen DV: Permissive hypercapnic ventilation, *Am J Respir Crit Care Med* 150:870-874, 1994.
86. U.S. Department of Health and Human Services: *Guidelines for the diagnosis and management of asthma,* Bethesda, MD, 1991, National Institutes of Health.
87. Vincent JE: Medical problems in the patient on a ventilator, *Crit Care Q* 6:33, 1983.
88. Wagenvoort CA: Pathology of pulmonary thromboembolism, *Chest* 107:10S-24S, 1995.
89. Weilitz PB: Weaning a patient from mechanical ventilation, *Crit Care Nurse* 13:33-41, 1993.
90. Weiss EB: Bronchial asthma, *Clin Symp* 27:39, 1975.
91. West J: *Respiratory physiology: the essentials,* Baltimore, 1979, Williams & Wilkins.
92. West JB: *Respiratory physiology—the essentials,* ed 5, Baltimore, 1995, Williams & Wilkins.
93. Wilson SF, Thompson JM: *Mosby's clinical nursing series: respiratory disorders,* St Louis, 1990, Mosby.
94. Young T et al: The occurrence of sleep-disoriented breathing among middle-aged adults, *N Engl J Med* 328:1230-1235, 1993.

Neurologic System

3

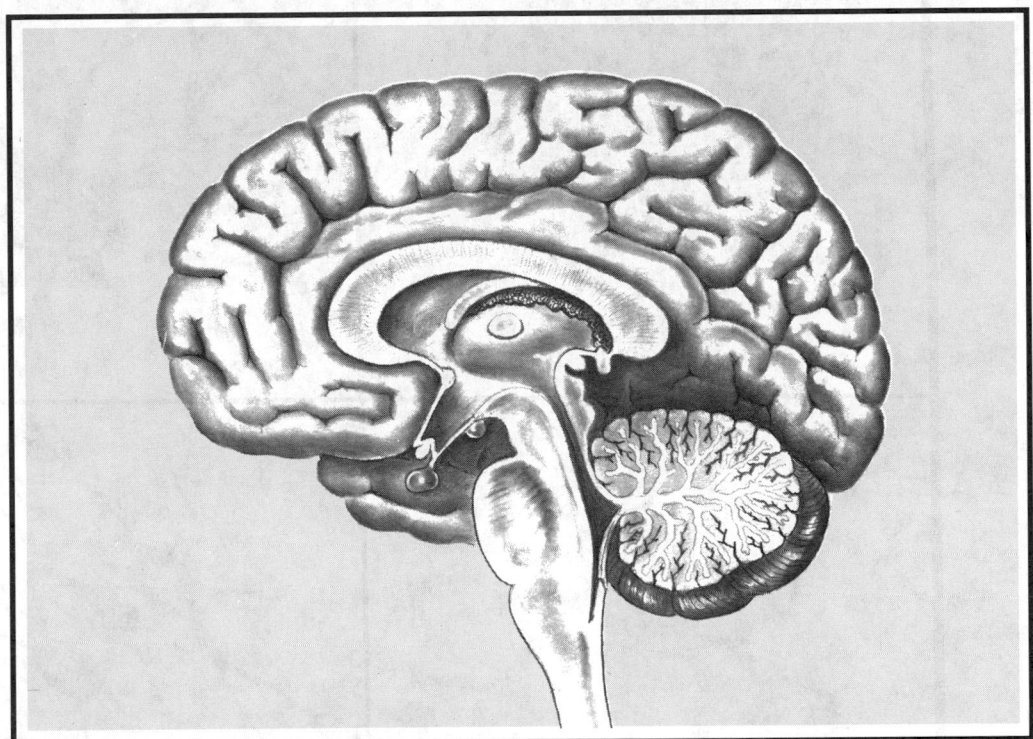

(Figure 3-1)

OVERVIEW

The human nervous system consists of complex structures and processes that provide an intricate circuit board through which the various functions of the body are integrated. Because these functions are integrative, the physiologic and psychologic ramifications of a neurologic dysfunction can be devastating for both patients and their families.

•••••• Anatomy, Physiology, and Related Pathophysiology

The nervous system is divided into two fairly distinct structural categories: the central nervous system (CNS), which consists of the brain and spinal cord, and the peripheral nervous system (PNS), which is made up of 12 pairs of cranial nerves, 31 pairs of spinal nerves, and the sympathetic and parasympathetic subdivisions of the autonomic nervous system. Functionally, the central and peripheral nervous systems are interdependent in that each is made of millions of shared neurons and neuroglia cells. The neuron is the basic unit of the nervous system. The neuroglia cells support the neuron.

Neuroglia Cells

About 40% of the structures of the brain and spinal cord are neuroglia cells. These cells protect, support, and nourish the cell bodies and processes of the neurons. There are four distinct types of neuroglia cells: astrocyte, ependyma, microglia, and oligodendroglia (Figure 3-1). All of these cells, except the microglia, come from the embryonic ectoderm. Unlike neurons, neuroglia cells can divide and multiply by mitosis and are a main source for nervous system tumors.

Astrocyte cells (astroglia) look like stars because of the many processes extending from their cell bodies. Their functions include helping to conduct impulses, helping to supply nutrition, storing information, supporting the neuron's structures, and helping to maintain the blood-brain barrier. Astrocytes are further divided into fibrillary astrocytes, which are found in white matter, and protoplasmic astrocytes, which are found in gray matter.

Ependymal cells are found within the epithelial lining of the cerebral ventricles, the choroid plexuses, and the spinal cord's central canal. Their main function is to help produce cerebrospinal fluid.

Microglia are stationary cells scattered throughout the central nervous system, mainly in white matter. These cells come from the embryonic mesoderm. The function of microglia is phagocytosis, during which the microglia become mobile and ingest and digest tissue debris.

Oligodendroglia cells synthesize a lipid-protein complex that forms myelin sheaths around the axonal projections of neurons in the central nervous system. Functions of the myelin sheath include holding nerve fibers together, providing insulation, promoting ionic flow, and transmitting nerve impulses (saltatory conduction). Oligodendroglia begin forming at about

Ependymal cell　　　　　　　　　　　　　　Astrocyte

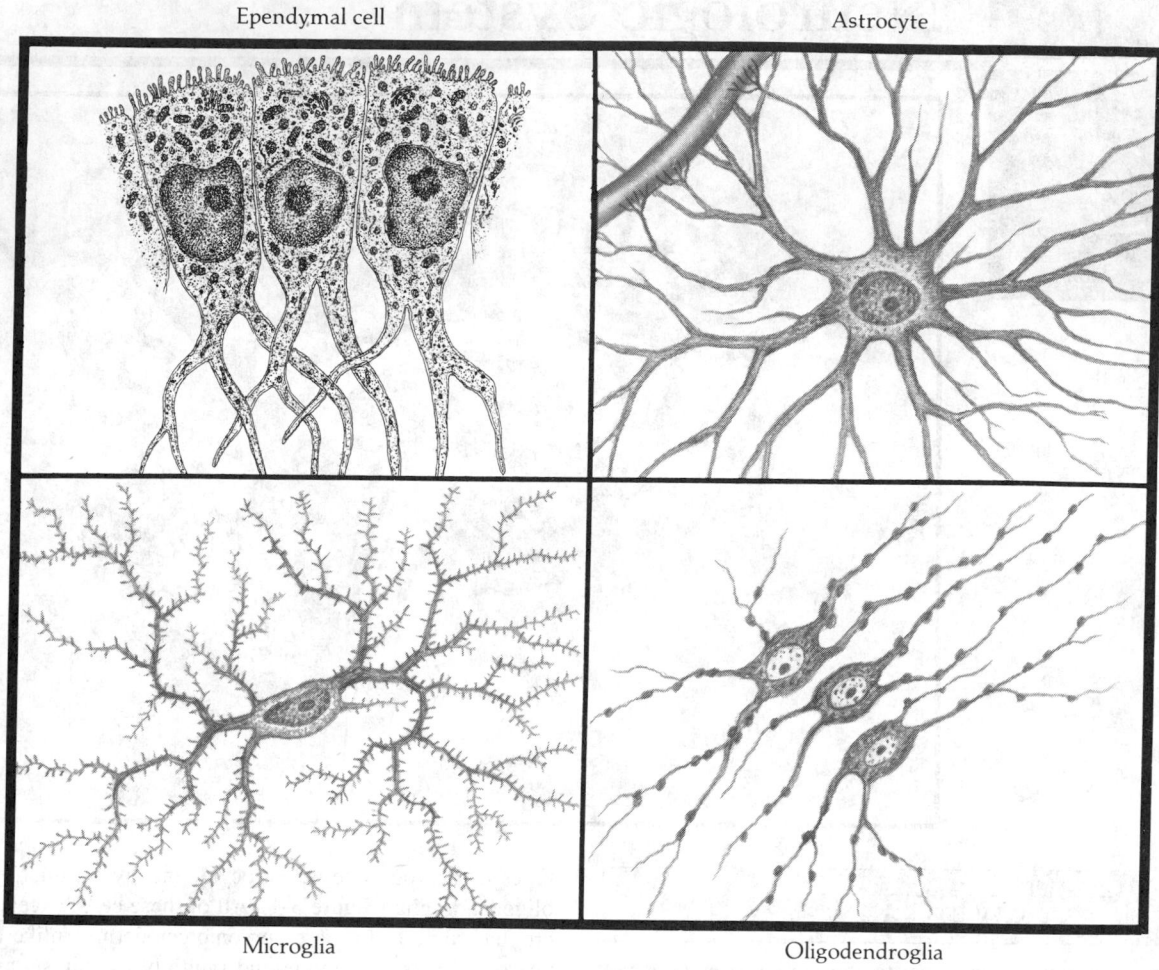

Microglia　　　　　　　　　　　　　　Oligodendroglia

Figure 3-1 Types of neuroglia cells.

the fourth fetal month and continue until about 20 years of age. Unlike Schwann cells, the oligodendroglia cannot regenerate. Instead, damaged neuronal structures are replaced with astrocytes, forming a gliotic scar that can disrupt the neuronal tissue.

Neurons

Neurons (Figure 3-2) come in many sizes and shapes, and each transmits specific nervous stimuli. The neurons have properties of excitation and electrical-chemical conductivity. In the central nervous system, groups of neurons are called nuclei; in the peripheral nervous system they are called ganglia.

Cytologic features　The neuron is made of a *cell body,* or perikaryon; *prosections,* called dendrites; and an axon. The nerve cell body is the gray matter of the nervous system.

Each neuron contains only one centrally located *nucleus.* The nucleus is a large, double-membraned structure containing deoxyribonucleic acid (DNA). Inside the nucleus is a single nucleolus containing ribonucleic acid (RNA). Surrounding the nucleus is granular *cytoplasm* containing many organelles, including Nissl bodies, mitochondria, the Golgi complex, neuro-

filaments, and microtubules. Nissl bodies help to synthesize protein. *Mitochondria* are rod-shaped organelles that regulate the cell's respiratory metabolism. Metabolic energy is stored as adenosine triphosphate (ATP). The *Golgi complex,* located in the cytoplasm, condenses and stores substances needed to transmit impulses. Dense neurofilaments are found throughout the cytoplasm and in the axonal and dendritic processes. Neurofilaments are made of structures called neurotubules or microtubules. Together, they form the neurofibril, which is involved in axoplasmic transport with cells.

Processes　Extending from the cell body is a long, smooth projection called the *axon,* or *axis cylinder* (Figure 3-2). The axon originates from the neuron's cell body at a point called the axon hillock. The myelin around the axon protects and insulates it. Axons, which carry efferent impulses away from cell bodies, form the white matter of the central nervous system. Terminal branches of the axon are called terminal filaments, or boutons (axon telodendria).

Extending from the cell body to the immediate surrounding areas are short receptive processes, or *dendrites.* The branch-

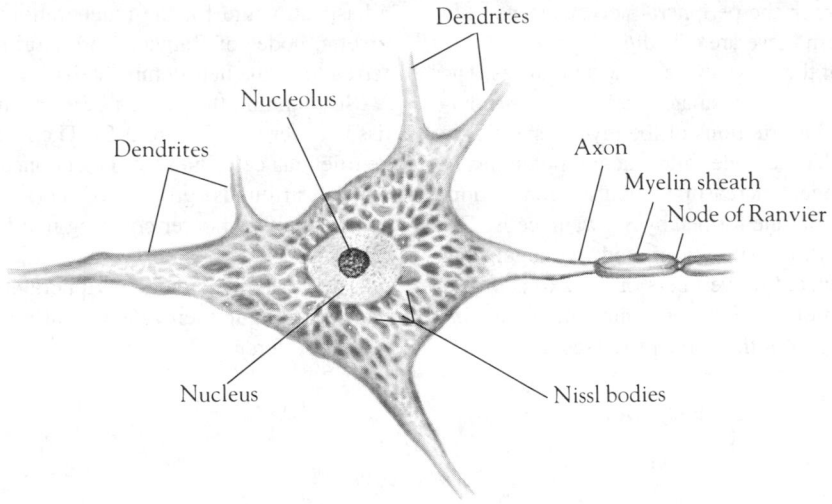

Figure 3-2 Diagram of neuron with composite parts. (From Rudy.[55])

like dendrites have no myelin sheath and lie with the cell body in the gray matter. The dendritic branches increase the surface area from which neuronal impulses can be picked up. Dendrites transmit afferent impulses toward the cell body. Rootlike terminal endings of the dendrite, or dendritic spines, help to transmit synapses.

Classification Structurally, neurons can be subdivided according to the number of processes and the axon lengths (Figure 3-3).

Unipolar neurons have only one process or pole, which divides close to the cell body. One branch of this division, called the peripheral process, carries afferent impulses toward the cell body. The other branch, the central process, conducts efferent impulses away from the body. *Bipolar* neurons have two processes: one axon and one dendrite. Bipolar neurons are found in the spinal ganglia, the nasal mucous membrane, and the rod and cone cells of the retina. *Multipolar* neurons make up most of the central nervous system, including all association (internuncial) and motor neurons. Multipolar neurons consist of a cell body, one long projection, and one or more shorter branches.

Neurons can also be classified by the axon length. Subdivisions within this classification are Golgi type I and Golgi type II (see Figure 3-3). *Golgi type I* neurons are large and have long axons. They are found in the long fiber tracts located in the cerebral cortex, cerebellum, and spinal cord. *Golgi type II* neurons are small cells that are found between larger neurons and that establish complex circuits in the nervous system. These neurons are found throughout the brain and spinal cord. Golgi type II neurons have short axons that branch repeatedly and end near the cell body.

Functionally, the neurons are classified as afferent, internuncial (association), or efferent (see Figure 3-3). *Afferent* (sensory) neurons conduct impulses to the central nervous system. *Internuncial* (association) neurons are in the central ner-

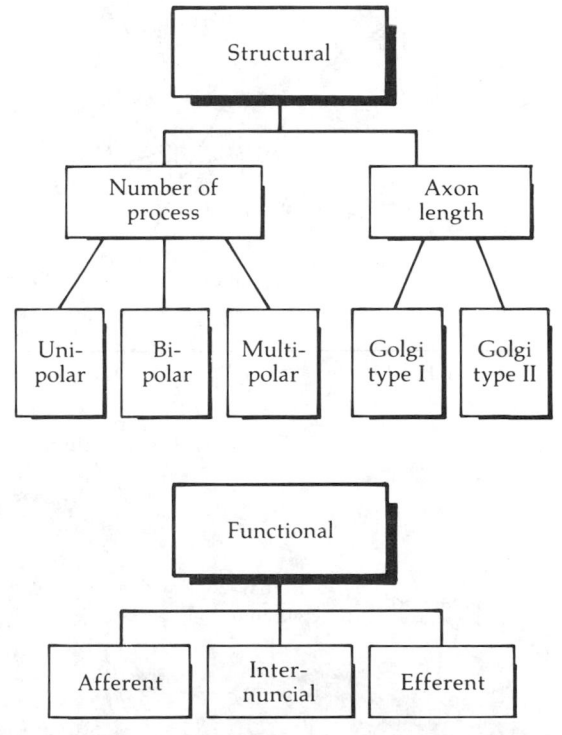

Figure 3-3 Structural and functional neuron classification.

vous system and conduct afferent and efferent impulses. *Efferent* (motor) neurons transmit impulses to effector organs and tissue.

Nerves

In the peripheral nervous system the neuron carries impulses to and from the central nervous system via the chainlike grouping of neuron cell fibers into *nerves* (Figure 3-4). (The term *nerve* applies only to cell fibers in the peripheral nervous system. In the central nervous system these are called *fiber tracts.*)

The axon is the part of the nerve that conducts impulses. The myelin sheath around the axon insulates, protects, and nourishes the axon. Periodic interruptions of the myelin sheath are called *nodes of Ranvier.* These nodes allow action potentials to skip from node to node, increasing impulse conduction. *Neurilemma* is a thin membrane formed by Schwann cells. The neurilemma membrane wraps spirally around the segmented myelin sheaths of myelinated nerve fibers or the axons of unmyelinated nerves. Functions of the neurilemma membrane include protection and support of the nerve processes. It provides

a basic structure for the regeneration of nerve processes. The myelin, nodes of Ranvier, and neurilemma are sometimes referred to as the neurilemma cells.

Surrounding the nerve fibers are three layers of connective tissue coverings (Figure 3-5). The *endoneurium* surrounds the neurilemma cells. Next to the endoneurium is the *perineurium,* which surrounds groups of nerve fibers (fascicles). The *epineurium* is an outer covering that binds the groups of fascicles together.

The nerve fibers in the peripheral nervous system are classified according to their function: afferent, internuncial (association), or efferent.

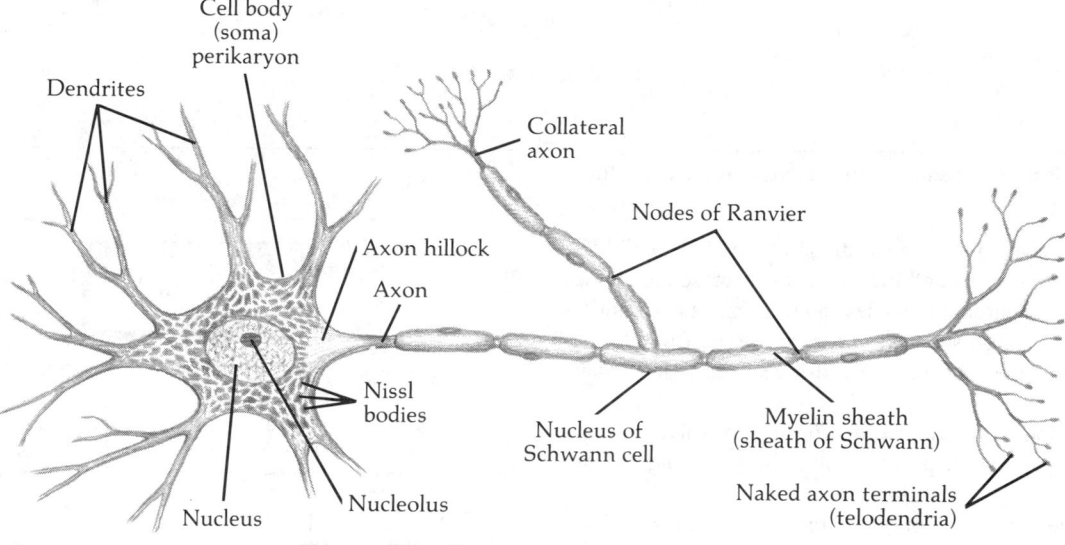

Figure 3-4 Peripheral nerve.

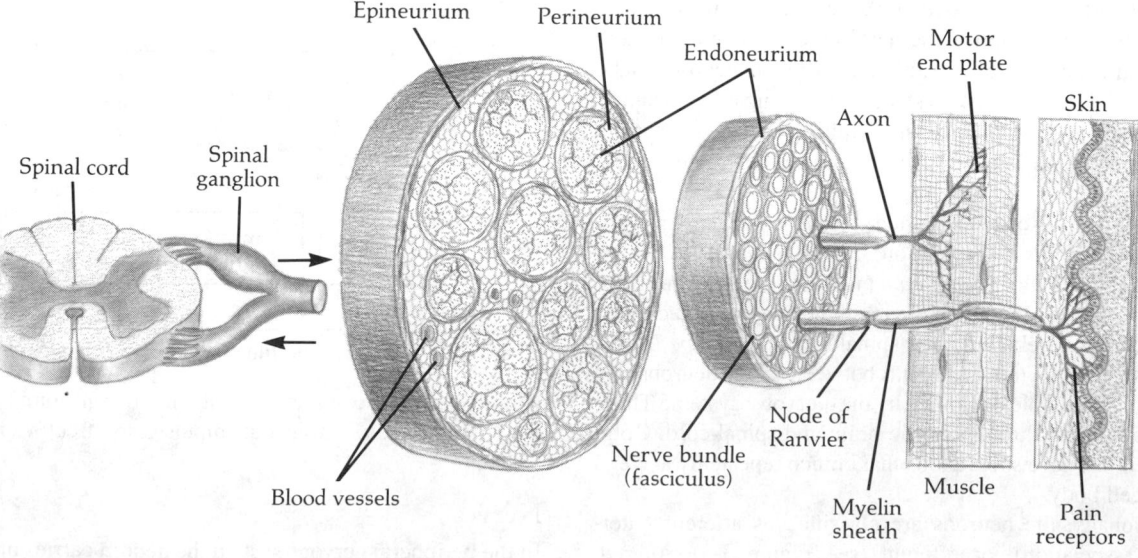

Figure 3-5 Peripheral nerve trunk and coverings.

Nerve impulse. Nerve fibers are charged (polarized) in their resting state. In this state the cells have a resting membrane potential of -70 mV, which means the inside of the cell membrane has a negative charge in relation to the outside. There is a high concentration of sodium (Na^+) outside the cell and a high concentration of potassium (K^+) in the cell. This results in unequal electrical charges across the cell membrane. This difference is the result of the relative impermeability of the cell to sodium and the sodium-potassium pump mechanism, whereby sodium is pumped continuously out of the cell and potassium is pumped in.

When a strong enough stimulus (referred to as the threshold intensity) begins, there is a rapid, marked change in the cell membrane permeability. This change results in a gain of sodium and a loss of potassium in the cell. With the gain of sodium the cell becomes positive relative to the interstitial space, and an action potential or depolarization results. The depolarization stimulus excites one area, which then excites other parts of the cell membrane (conduction), until the entire membrane is stimulated at the same intensity. Thus the wave of depolarization moves cyclically along the entire length of the nerve process. Following depolarization, the ionic flow reverses. Sodium is pumped out as potassium is pumped back into the cell. This is the repolarization process, whereby the membrane is returned to its resting potential. During depolarization and one third of the repolarization process, the neuron cell cannot be restimulated with another action potential. This time interval (or *absolute refractory period*) prevents repeated excitation of the neuron. Figure 3-6 illustrates this process.

The speed of impulse conduction depends on whether the nerve has a myelin sheath. In the unmyelinated nerve the action potential must travel the entire length of the nerve fiber. In myelinated nerves the axon is exposed only at the nodes of Ranvier; therefore the action potential is not transmitted along the entire axon membrane. Instead, the action potential "skips," discontinuously, from one node of Ranvier to the next. With this node-to-node conduction, termed *saltatory transmission,* the action potential travels faster. This increases the speed of the impulses and decreases the demand for energy.

Synapse. Because neurons occur in chainlike pathways, impulses must travel from one cell to another via functional junctions called *synapses*. Actual synaptic transmission is a chemical process that occurs because of the release of neurotransmitters. In addition, synapses are polarized so the impulse flows in one direction only (e.g., from the axon of one neuron to the axon, dendrites, or cell body of another neuron in a pathway).

The anatomic structures of the synapse consist of presynaptic terminals, the synaptic cleft, and the postsynaptic membrane (Figure 3-7). The presynaptic terminals (also called presynaptic knobs) contain hundreds of very small circular vesicles that store excitatory or inhibitory neurotransmitters.

There are three types of interneuronal synapses: *axosomatic,* in which the axon of one neuron contacts the cell body of another neuron; *axodendritic,* in which the axon of one neuron contacts the dendrites of another nerve cell; and *axoaxonic,* in which one axon contacts with another axon.

Neurotransmitters

At least 30 different neurotransmitters can affect chemical transmission of an impulse at the synapse. When an impulse stimulates the presynaptic terminals, they secrete neurotransmitters into the synaptic cleft. This changes the permeability of the postsynaptic membrane. Neurotransmitters either excite or inhibit activity in the postsynaptic cell.

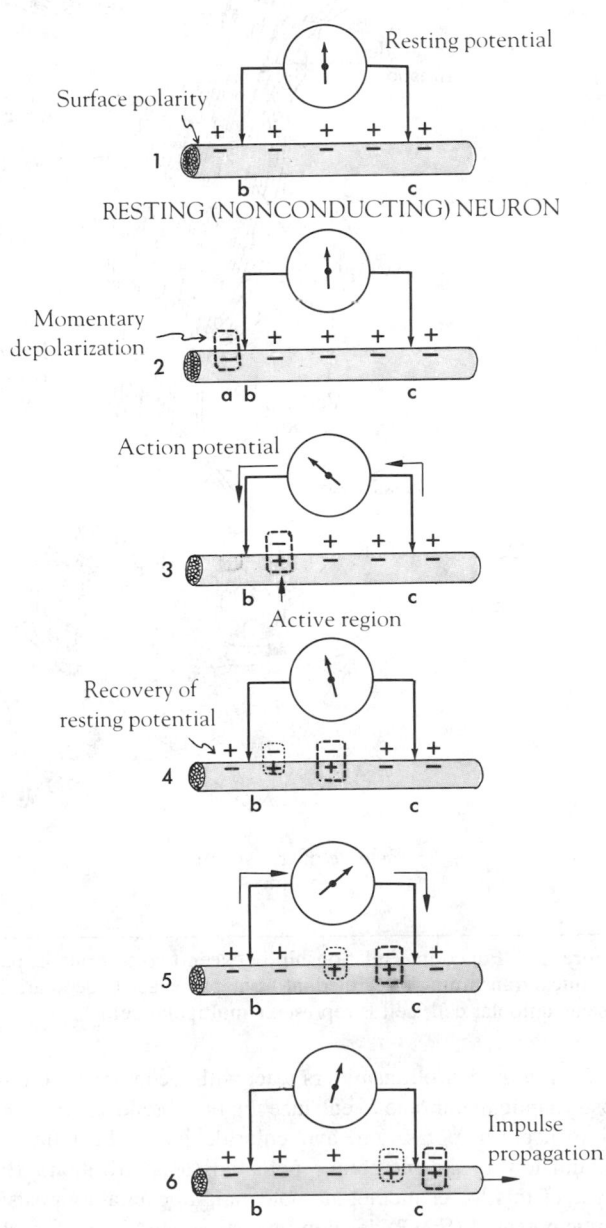

Figure 3-6 Stages in impulse propagation. (From Schottelius and Schottelius.[57])

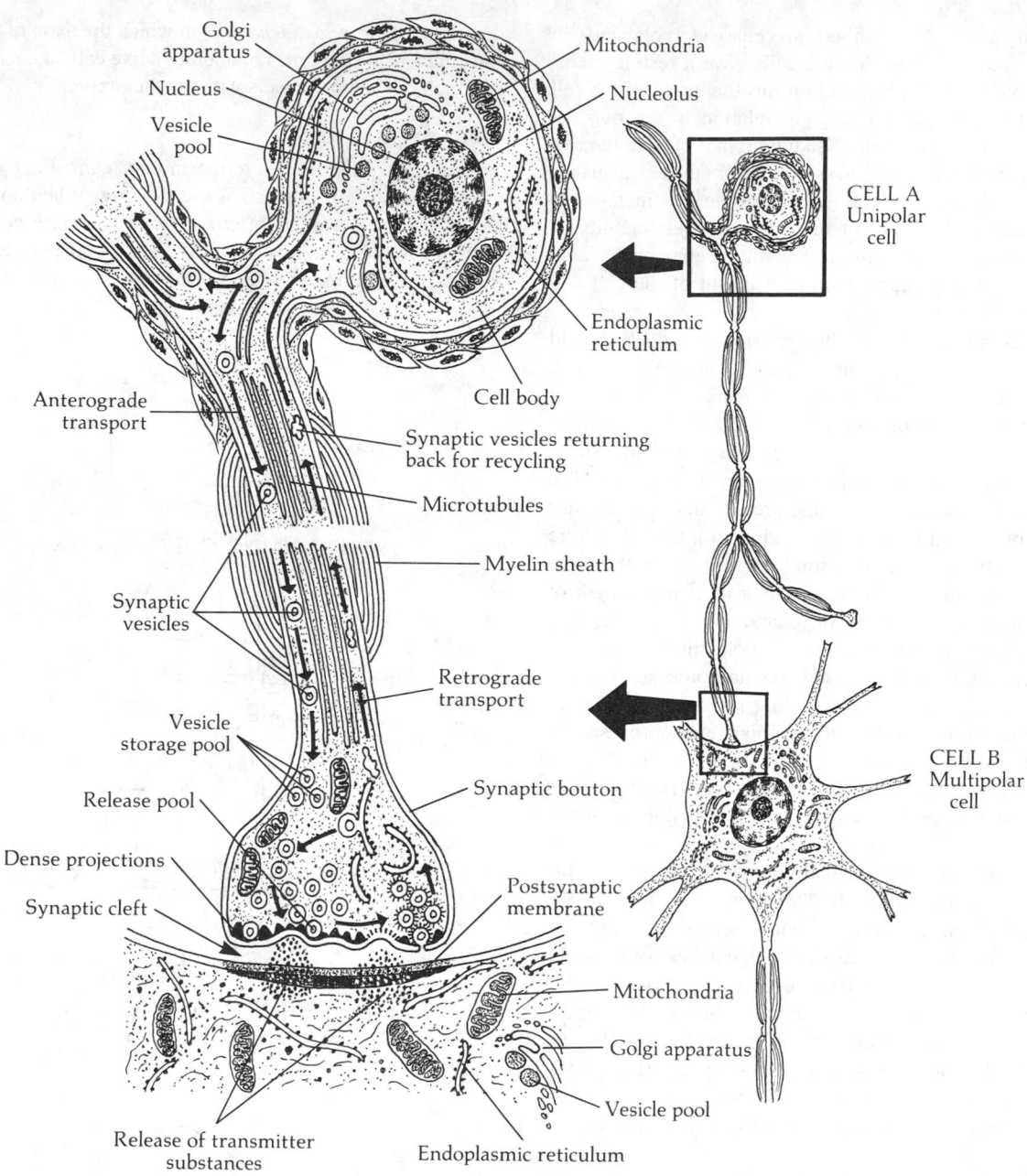

Figure 3-7 Functional relationship between two neurons in pathway. Electrical impulse travels along axon of first neuron to synapse. Chemical transmitter is secreted into synaptic space to depolarize membrane (dendrite or cell body) of next neuron in pathway. Cell A represents unipolar cell; cell B represents multipolar cell.

Excitatory neurotransmitters react with receptor sites on the postsynaptic membrane to enhance the membrane's permeability to sodium, potassium, and chloride ions. The influx of sodium lowers the membrane potential (depolarization). Because of this lower membrane potential, an excitatory postsynaptic potential (EPSP) develops and stimulates the postsynaptic neuron toward an action potential. Acetylcholine is the principal excitatory neurotransmitter of the voluntary nervous system and the parasympathetic division of the autonomic ner-

vous system. Other central excitatory neurotransmitters are norepinephrine, dopamine, serotonin, L-aspartate, and glutamic acid. Norepinephrine is the major postsynaptic excitatory neurotransmitter in the sympathetic division of the autonomic nervous system.[17]

Inhibitory neurotransmitters decrease the permeability of the postsynaptic membrane to sodium but increase its permeability to potassium and chloride ions. The potassium ion flows out and chloride flows in, hyperpolarizing (the opposite of

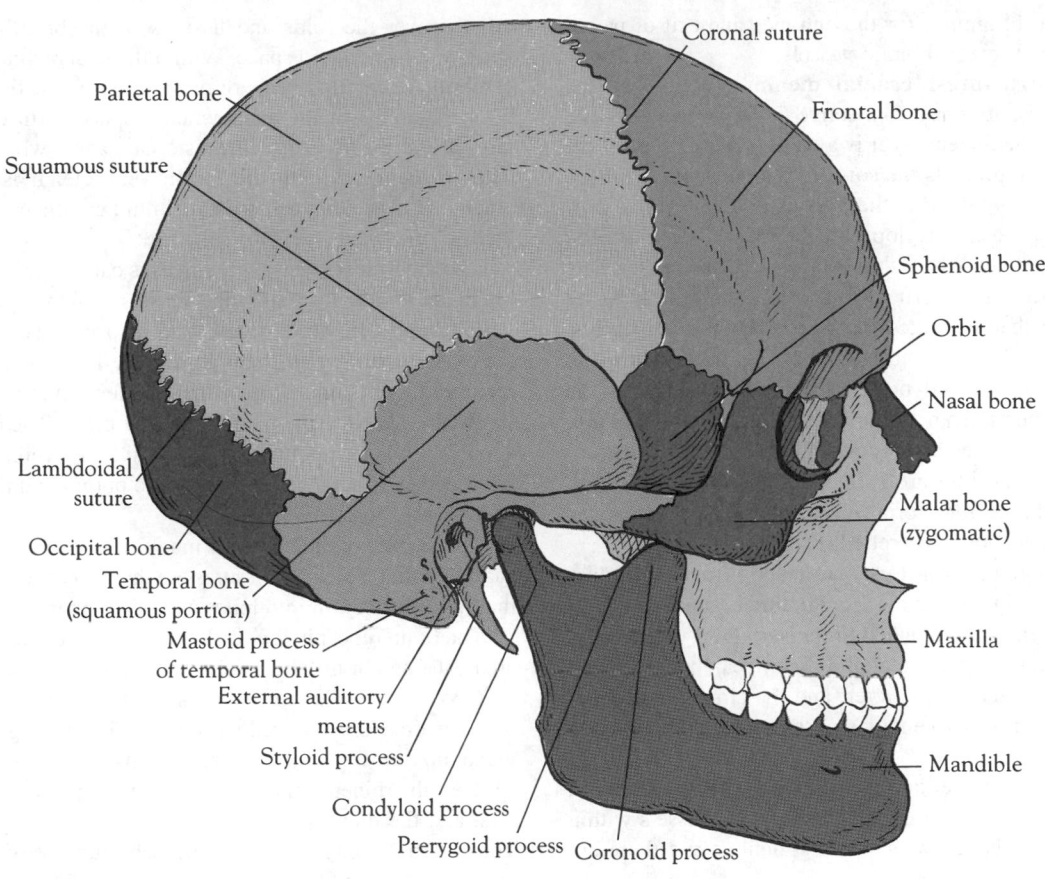

Figure 3-8 Lateral view of skull. (From Anthony and Kolthoff[3].)

depolarizing) the postsynaptic cell membrane and forming an inhibitory postsynaptic potential (IPSP). The formation of the IPSP is called direct inhibition. Another type of inhibitory action is presynaptic inhibition, which occurs when the excitatory presynaptic terminals are stimulated by an inhibitory neuron. In presynaptic inhibition there is partial depolarization of the excitatory presynaptic terminals so that less excitatory neurotransmitters are released from these endings. This decreases the amplitude of the action potential as it arrives at the presynaptic terminals and decreases end-excitation of the neuron. Inhibitory neurotransmitters include γ-aminobutyric acid (GABA) (presynaptic) and glycine (postsynaptic).

The number of neurotransmitters depends on the rate and number of impulses that stimulate the presynaptic terminals. Therefore, to form an action potential on the postsynaptic membranes, one presynaptic terminal may have to depolarize repeatedly (referred to as temporal summation) or many presynaptic terminals may have to depolarize and release neurotransmitters (spatial summation).

To prevent overstimulation of the postsynaptic membrane, the neurotransmitter is inactivated chemically after synaptic transmission. The neurotransmitter is inactivated by enzyme degradation (i.e., acetylcholine is inactivated by acetylcholin-

esterase), retaken up by presynaptic terminals (i.e., dopamine, serotonin, and GABA), or diffused from the postsynaptic membrane.

Central Nervous System

Protective structure: skull The brain is protected by the bony structure of the skull (Figure 3-8). The skull is divided into two primary sections, the cranium and the skeleton of the face. The cranial portion of the skull is made up of eight relatively flat and irregular bones joined together by a series of fixed joints called sutures. These bones are composed of three layers: the solid *outer table,* the spongy middle *diploë,* and the solid *inner table.* The inner table of the skull forms a cavity filled with ridges and convolutions that are custom designed for holding the brain. This internal cavity has three major regions: the anterior fossa, the middle fossa, and the posterior fossa. The anterior fossa contains the frontal lobes; the middle fossa contains the temporal, parietal, and occipital lobes; and the posterior fossa contains the brainstem and cerebellum.[17]

At the base of the skull in the inferior anterior portion of the occipital bone is a large oval opening called the foramen magnum. It is at the foramen magnum that the brain and spinal cord become continuous. Also at the base of the skull is a series of openings (called foramina) for the entrance and exit of paired cranial nerves and cerebral blood vessels.

Protective structures: cranial meninges   Between the skull and the brain are three connective tissue layers called the meninges. Each meningeal layer is a continuous separate sheet that, like the skull, protects the soft brain tissue (Figure 3-9).

The outermost meninge is the fibrous double-layered *dura mater*. The dura mater envelops the brain and separates the skull into compartments by its various folds or processes. The falx cerebri process is a vertical fold of the dura mater at the midsagittal line that separates the two cerebral hemispheres. The tentorium cerebelli is a horizontal double fold of dura that supports the temporal and occipital lobes and separates the cerebral hemispheres from the brainstem and the cerebellum. (The tentorium provides an important line of division. Structures above the tentorium are called supratentorial, and those below it are called infratentorial.) The falx cerebelli separates the two hemispheres of the cerebellum.

The cranial dura mater differs significantly from spinal dura mater in the following ways: the cranial dura is attached firmly, but the spinal dura is not attached to the vertebrae; cranial dura is made of two layers, periosteal and meningeal, but the spinal dura has only one meningeal layer; and the cranial dura separates in places and forms venous sinuses, which the one-layer spinal dura does not.[13]

Between the dura mater and the middle meningeal layer is a narrow serous cavity called the subdural space. Vessels within the subdural space have few support structures and therefore are easily injured.

The middle layer of the meninges is called the arachnoid. It is made of a two-layered, fibrous, elastic membrane that crosses over the folds and fissures of the brain, creating the spongy subarachnoid space. Within the subarachnoid space are cerebral arteries and veins of different sizes. At the base of the brain, dilations in the subarachnoid space form cisterns. The largest of these cisterns is the cisterna magna, which communicates or connects with the fourth ventricle. It is in the subarachnoid space that cerebrospinal fluid circulates over the surfaces of the brain.

The innermost layer of meninges is called the pia mater. The pia mater is rich in small blood vessels, which supply the brain with a large volume of blood. It is also in direct contact with the external surface of the brain tissue. The arachnoid and pia membranes are collectively called the leptomeninges.

Brain   Next to the pia mater is the brain. The brain is only about 2% (about 3 pounds) of the total body weight of an adult but receives about 20% of the cardiac output and requires 20% of the body's oxygen use.[51]

The surface of the brain has many convolutions separated by shallow folds. Sulci and fissures are the deeper folds or grooves that divide the brain into lobes and hemispheres.

The brain (encephalon) is divided into three major anatomic areas: the cerebrum, the cerebellum, and the brainstem.

Cerebrum.   The cerebrum is the largest anatomic portion of the brain and is covered with several layers of gray cells that make up the cerebral cortex. It consists of cerebral hemispheres, the rhinencephalon, the internal capsule and basal ganglia, and the diencephalon (i.e., thalamus and hypothalamus). The internal white matter of the cerebrum consists of many myelinated nerve fibers and neuroglia cells. The cerebrum is divided lengthwise into symmetric right and left sides by the longitudinal fissure. Each half is called a lateral cerebral hemi-

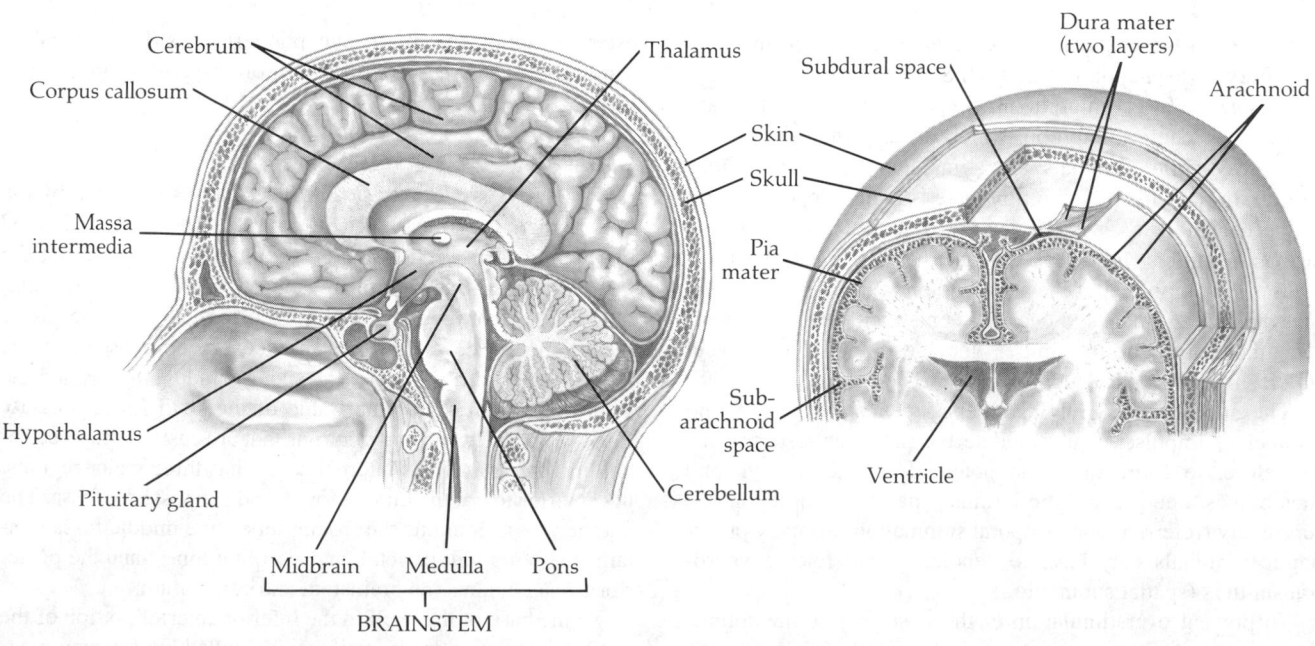

Figure 3-9 Meninges of brain.

sphere. The hemispheres are joined lengthwise by a large tract of white commissural fibers, the corpus callosum, that serves as the communication link between the hemispheres. The major folds of the cortex divide each lateral hemisphere into four lobes, or cerebral hemispheres, which are named for the overlying cranial bones: frontal, parietal, occipital, and temporal (Figure 3-10).

Certain areas of the cerebral cortex are responsible for specific functions of the cerebrum. Probably the best-known classification of these areas is *Brodmann's map.* On the basis of histologic studies, Brodmann developed a map of 47 different areas of the cerebral cortex (Figure 3-11) and classified them as primary function areas or association areas.

Primary function areas are those in which movement or the perception of movement occurs. *Association areas* surround the primary function areas. They provide higher levels of integration (i.e., memory, learning) for sensory experiences.

The *frontal lobe* is located in the anterior fossa and extends from the anterior portion of each hemisphere to the central sulcus (fissure of Rolando) posteriorly. The inferior border is the lateral cerebral fissure (fissure of Sylvius). The frontal lobe controls psychic and higher intellectual functions. It also contains higher-level centers for autonomic functioning, such as cardiovascular responses and gastrointestinal activity. Broca's area, which assists in the formation of words, is also located in the frontal lobe.

The *parietal lobe* is located in the middle fossa in the area between the central sulcus (fissure of Rolando) and the parieto-occipital fissure. The major functions of the parietal lobe are position sense, touch, and motor movement.

The *occipital lobe* is a pyramidal structure in the middle fossa, behind the parieto-occipital fissure and just above the cerebellum. The occipital lobe contains the primary vision centers (primary vision cortex).

The *temporal lobe* also is located in the middle fossa. It lies inferior to the lateral cerebral fissure (fissure of Sylvius) and extends posteriorly to the parieto-occipital fissure. Primary functions of the temporal lobe are memory storage and hearing. Wernicke's area, the auditory association area, is found in the temporal lobe.

The *rhinencephalon* (limbic lobe) is anatomically part of the temporal lobe but has different functions. It consists of cortical and subcortical structures that form the border of the lateral ventricles of each cerebral hemisphere. The functions of the rhinencephalon involve self-preservation, visceral activities, instincts, feeling states, and moods.

The *basal ganglia* are gray nuclei located deep within the white matter of each cerebral hemisphere. They consist of the paired anatomic structures of the lenticular nucleus, caudate nucleus, amygdaloid body, and claustrum. The lenticular and caudate nuclei together are called the corpus striatum. Functions include motor control of fine body movements, particularly in the hands and lower extremities.

The internal capsule, located in the thalamic-hypothalamic area, is a massive bundle of white matter. It consists of afferent

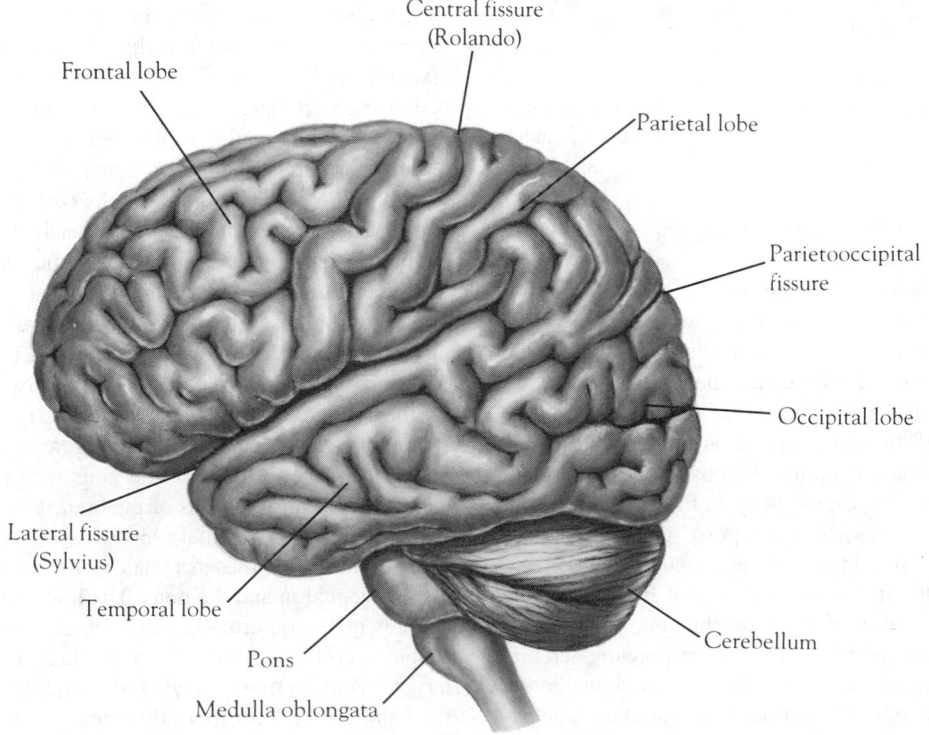

Figure 3-10 Lateral view of cerebral hemisphere (showing lobes and principal fissures), cerebellum, pons, and medulla oblongata. (From Rudy.[55])

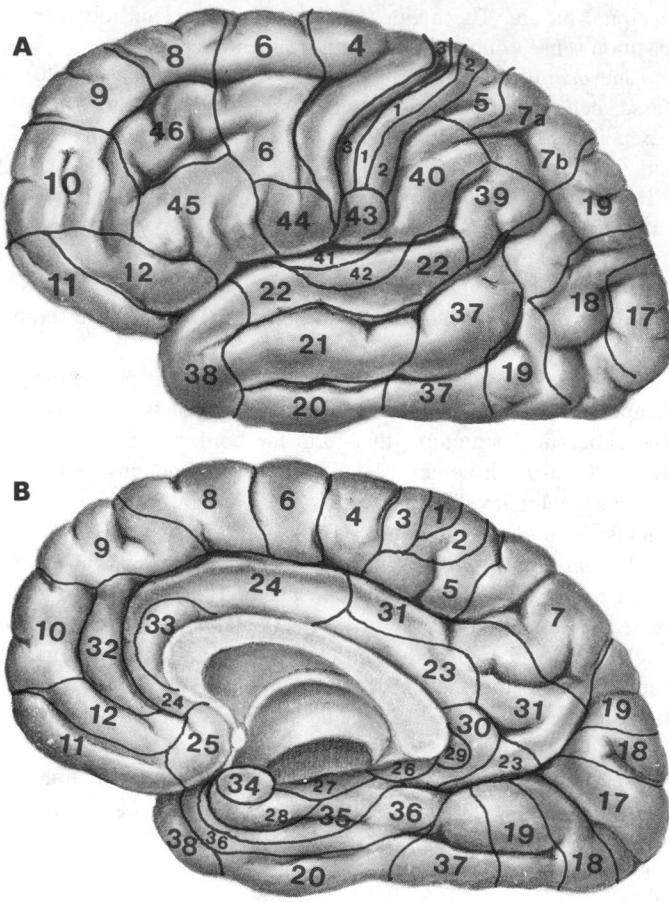

Figure 3-11 Cytoarchitectural map of the lateral and medial surface of the human cortex according to Brodmann's map. **A,** Lateral surface. **B,** Medial surface. (From Rudy.[55])

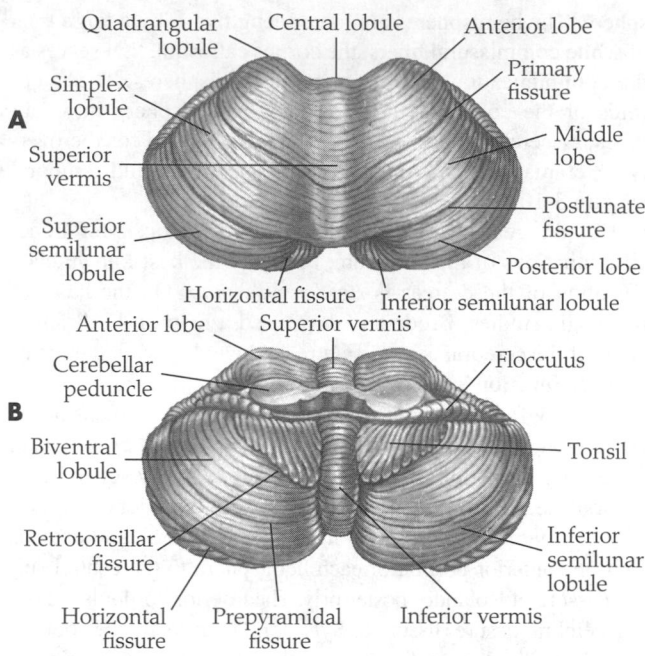

Figure 3-12 Cerebellum. **A,** Superior surface. **B,** Inferior surface.

and efferent fiber tracts that transmit impulses from the cerebrum to the brainstem and spinal cord.

The oval *diencephalon* forms the rostral (toward the head) end of the brainstem and consists of gray matter.[36] The diencephalon contains pathways for visceral, sensory, somatic, and motor impulses and consists of the epithalamus, thalamus, hypothalamus, and subthalamus. The epithalamus, located in the most dorsal aspect of the diencephalon, is made of the pineal body, habenula, habenular commissure, posterior commissure, and striae medullares. The pineal body is the most important structure of the epithalamus and is composed primarily of neuroglia cells. It plays a role in growth and sexual development. The thalamus consists of two connected oval masses of gray matter in the dorsal portion of the diencephalon. Each half of the thalamus is located deep within the corresponding cerebral hemisphere.[34] The thalamus functions as a relay and integration station for cerebral, cerebellar, and brainstem activity. The hypothalamus lies inferior to the thalamus, forming the floor and portions of the walls of the third ventricle. Functions of the hypothalamus are indicated in Table 3-1. The subthalamus is situated between the tegmentum of the midbrain and the dorsal

aspect of the thalamus. Its functions are part of the extrapyramidal system of the autonomic nervous system.

Cerebellum. The cerebellum (Figure 3-12) is approximately one-fifth the size of the cerebrum and consists of two lateral hemispheres and a medial portion, the *vermis*. It is separated from the cerebrum by the tentorium cerebelli. The cerebellum has an outer cortex of gray matter and an internal medulla of white matter. Embedded deep within the white matter are four pairs of nuclei: dentate, emboliform, globose, and fastigial. The midbrain connects the cerebellum to the cerebral cortex. The cerebellum attaches on each side of the brainstem by three large bundles of nerve fibers, the *cerebellar peduncles.* The cerebellum also connects with the semicircular canals, or organs of balance. It is involved primarily in coordinating movement, equilibrium, muscle tone, and position sense. Each of the cerebellar hemispheres con-trols movement coordination for the same side of the body (ipsilateral).

Brainstem. The brainstem (Figure 3-13) consists of the midbrain (mesencephalon), the pons, and the medulla oblongata. The overall functions of the brainstem are to maintain involuntary reflexes for vital functioning of the body.

The *midbrain* (mesencephalon) forms a junction between the diencephalon and the pons. The lower surface contains two bundles of fibers, crura cerebri, which are made of the corticospinal, corticopontine, and corticobulbar tracts of the voluntary nervous system carrying descending motor fiber tracts from the cerebral cortex to the pons. The upper surface of the midbrain consists of four rounded elevations called the corpora quadrigemina. The rostral pair of elevations is the superior colliculi (eye tracking), and the caudal pair is the inferior colliculi (auditory reflexes). The major function of the midbrain is to

TABLE 3-1 Principal Thalamic Nuclei

Neuroanatomic Classification	Functional Classification	Principal Connections		General Functions
		Afferent Fibers	Efferent Fibers	
Anterior nuclei				
Anteromedial	Nonspecific projection	From hypothalamus via mammillothalamic tract (of Vicq d' Azyr); higher-order of olfactory neurons	To cingulate gyrus of cerebral cortex	Part of circuit involved in limbic system, convey olfactory impulses
Anterodorsal	Nonspecific projection			
Anteroventral	Nonspecific projection			
Midline nuclei				
Cell groups beneath lining of wall, third ventricle	Nonspecific projection	From spinothalamic, trigeminothalamic tracts, medial lemniscus, reticular formation, other thalamic nuclei, hypothalamus	To hypothalamus and cortex (few to anterior rhinecephalon); basal ganglia; other thalamic nuclei	Center for integrating crude visceral and somatic sensations
Massa intermedia	Nonspecific projection			
Medial nuclei				
Scattered cells in internal medullary lamina (intralaminar nuclei)	Nonspecific projection	From prefrontal cortex, septal areas, basal ganglia, and other thalamic nuclei	To prefrontal cortex	Integrate somatic and visceral sensory impulses before projecting information to cortex; association center for synthesis of crude somatic sensations
	Nonspecific projection	From thalamic nuclei, prefrontal cortex, basal ganglia	To prefrontal cortex	
Dorsomedial	Nonspecific projection	From putamen, caudate nucleus, other thalamic nuclei	To basal ganglia, other thalamic nuclei	Intrathalamic integrating center
Centromedial	Nonspecific projection			
Lateral nuclei				
Anterior ventral	Nonspecific projection	From globus pallidus via thalamic fasciculus	To corpus striatum; cortex (frontal lobe)	Part of circuit involved in voluntary motor functions
Lateral ventral	Specific projection	From cerebellum via superior cerebellar peduncle; globus pallidus via thalamic fasciculus	To cerebral cortex (premotor areas) via posterior limb of internal capsule	Relays sensory impulses from trunk and limbs*
Posterolateral ventral	Specific projection	Termination of spinothalamic tracts, medial lemniscus	To sensory areas of cortex (postcentral gyrus) via posterior limb of internal capsule	Relays sensory impulses from face†
Posteromedial ventral	Specific projection	Termination of secondary trigeminal and taste fibers		Primary sensory relay nuclei
Dorsal lateral	Specific projection	From other thalamic nuclei; parietal lobe of cerebral cortex	To cerebral cortex (parietal lobe)	Functions controversial
Posterior lateral	Specific projection			
Reticular	Nonspecific projection	From entire cerebral cortex, other thalamic nuclei, reticular formation of brainstem	To other thalamic nuclei, tegmentum of midbrain	
Posterior nuclei				
Pulvinar	Specific projection	From other thalamic nuclei, cerebral cortex (parietal, temporal, occipital lobes)	To cerebral cortex (parietal, temporal, occipital lobes)	Integrates auditory, visual, somatic impulses
Medial geniculate†	Specific projection	From brachium of inferior colliculus	To auditory cortex via sublenticular portion of internal capsule (bilateral projection)	Audition
Lateral geniculate†	Specific projection	From optic tract (cranial nerve II)	To ipsilateral striate cortex via retrolenticular portion of internal capsule	Vision

From Jensen.[37]

*The posterolateral and posteromedial ventral nuclei of the thalamus are important because they are the principal thalamic relay system for somesthetic afferent fibers.

†The medial and lateral geniculate bodies sometimes are classed together as the *metathalamus*.

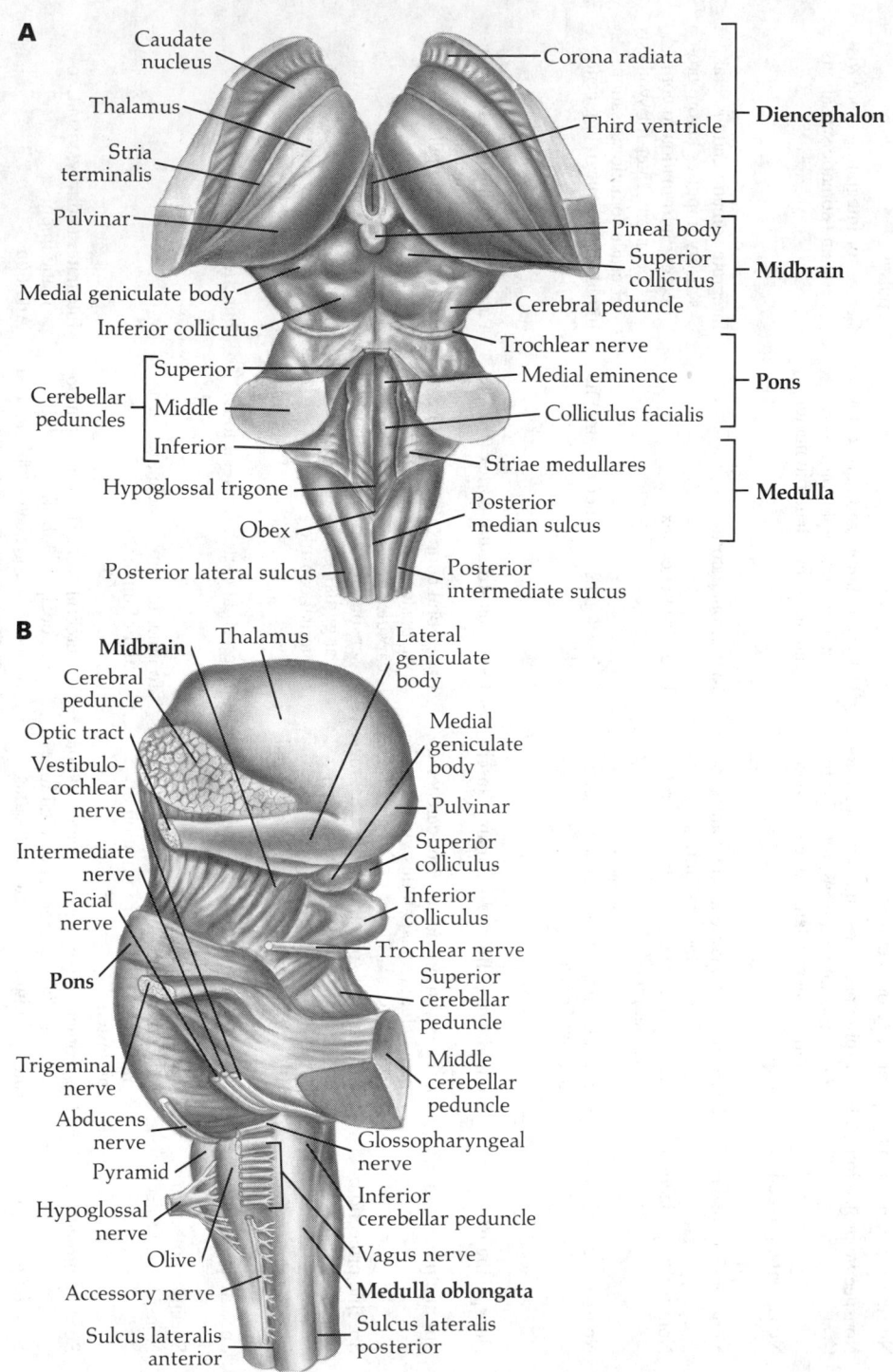

A

Caudate nucleus

Thalamus

Stria terminalis

Pulvinar

Medial geniculate body

Inferior colliculus

Cerebellar peduncles
- Superior
- Middle
- Inferior

Hypoglossal trigone

Obex

Posterior lateral sulcus

Corona radiata

Third ventricle — **Diencephalon**

Pineal body

Superior colliculus — **Midbrain**

Cerebral peduncle

Trochlear nerve

Medial eminence — **Pons**

Colliculus facialis

Striae medullares — **Medulla**

Posterior median sulcus

Posterior intermediate sulcus

B

Midbrain

Thalamus

Lateral geniculate body

Cerebral peduncle

Optic tract

Vestibulo-cochlear nerve

Medial geniculate body

Pulvinar

Intermediate nerve

Facial nerve

Superior colliculus

Inferior colliculus

Trochlear nerve

Superior cerebellar peduncle

Pons

Trigeminal nerve

Middle cerebellar peduncle

Abducens nerve

Pyramid

Glossopharyngeal nerve

Hypoglossal nerve

Inferior cerebellar peduncle

Olive

Vagus nerve

Accessory nerve

Medulla oblongata

Sulcus lateralis anterior

Sulcus lateralis posterior

Figure 3-13 Brainstem. **A,** Posterior view. **B,** Lateral view.

relay stimuli dealing with muscle movement, visual reflexes, and auditory reflexes from the spinal cord, medulla oblongata, and cerebellum and to the cerebrum.

The *pons* (metencephalon; Figure 3-13) connects the midbrain to the medulla oblongata and relays impulses to the brain centers and to the lower spinal centers of the nervous system.

Sensory and motor nuclei of the trigeminal (cranial V), abducens (cranial VI), facial (cranial VII), and acoustic (cranial VIII) nerves originate in the pons. The corticobulbar and corticospinal tracts make up the white matter of the pons.

The *medulla oblongata* (myelencephalon; Figure 3-13) contains the reflex centers for controlling involuntary functions such as breathing, sneezing, swallowing, coughing, salivation, vomiting, and vasoconstriction. The medulla also provides points of origin for the glossopharyngeal (cranial IX), vagus (cranial X), spinal accessory (cranial XI), and hypoglossal (cranial XII) nerves.

Reticular formation. The reticular formation is a scattered, interconnected complex of sensory nerve fibers extending from the upper spinal cord through the midventral portion of the medulla, pons, midbrain, and diencephalon. Located in the reticular formation are centers that regulate respiration, blood pressure, heart rate (medulla), and vegetative functions (Figure 3-14).

Reticular activating system. The reticular activating system (RAS) is a polysynaptic, nonspecific sensory pathway considered to be an integral regulatory center of the central nervous system. It extends from the superior level of the brainstem to the cerebral cortex. Most of the RAS is excitatory and is involved in maintaining attention, the sleep-awake cycle, regulation of visceral functions such as respiration and vasomotor tone, consciousness, perception of sensory input, regulation of temperature, emotional states, learning, conditioned reflexes, and regulation of skeletal muscle tone and activity.[36]

Spinal vertebrae The vertebral column (Figure 3-15, *A*) is made up of 33 vertebrae divided into five anatomic and functional regions: cervical, thoracic, lumbar, sacral, and coccygeal. Vertebrae are joined together by numerous ligaments and intervertebral discs that provide strength and flexibility.

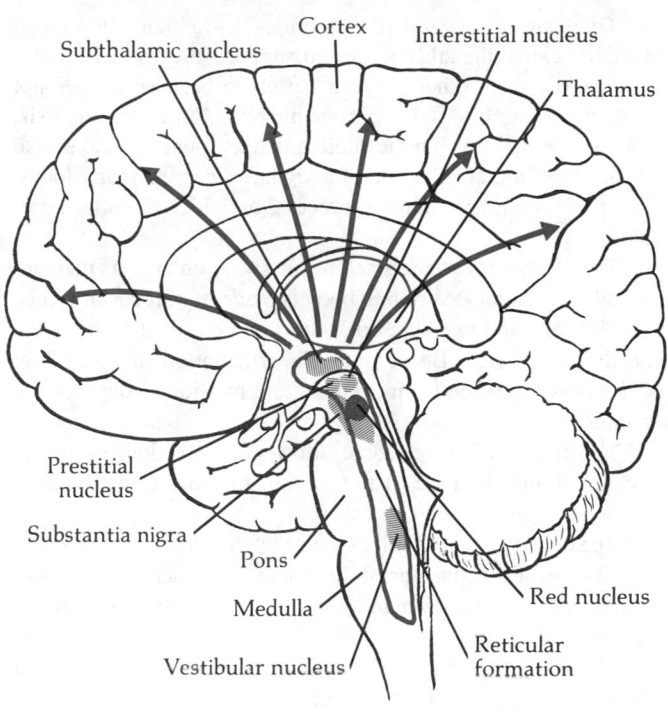

Figure 3-14 Reticular activating system.

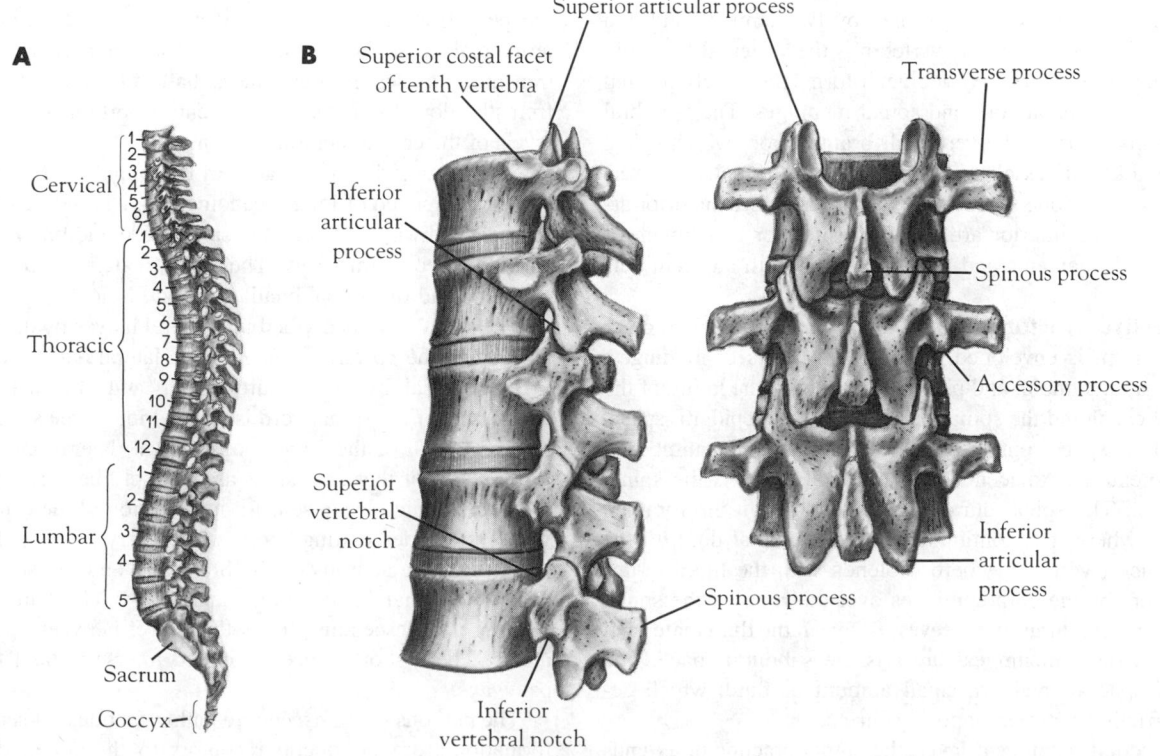

Figure 3-15 A, Vertebral column. **B,** Anatomic structure of vertebrae. (From Rudy.[55])

There are seven *cervical* vertebrae. C1 is a highly developed vertebra called the atlas because it supports the head. The atlas is different from other cervical vertebrae because it does not have a vertebral body or spinous process. C2, called the axis, forms a pivot on which the skull and atlas rotate. The axis also is different in that its vertebral body has a perpendicular tooth-like projection, the odontoid process, on which the atlas articulates.

The 12 *thoracic* vertebrae progressively enlarge as they descend. The thoracic vertebral body is made of four costal facets, two inferior and two superior, that provide articulation for the heads of the ribs. Because of rib articulation, the vertebral column is least free for movement and rotation in the thoracic region.

The five *lumbar* vertebrae allow great freedom of movement. L5 and the base of the sacrum together form the lumbosacral angle.

The *sacrum* in the adult is a wedge-shaped bone formed by the fusion of the five sacral vertebrae. The sacral canal, containing the cauda equina and filum terminale, originates in this region.

The *coccyx* in the adult is also a fused bone consisting of three to five coccygeal vertebrae.

The typical vertebra (Figure 3-15, *B*) found in the cervical, thoracic, lumbar, or sacral regions has several important anatomic characteristics. The vertebral body is the cylindric weight-bearing ventral portion. It is separated from the vertebral bodies above and below it by cartilage and fibrous tissue called intervertebral discs. The dorsal portion of the vertebra is the vertebral arch, which is formed by two laminae and two pedicles. In the center of the vertebra is the vertebral foramen. In conjunction with other vertebrae, it forms the vertebral canal containing the spinal cord and spinal meninges. The vertebral notch forms a part of the vertebral foramen from which spinal nerves and blood vessels exit the spinal cord. Finally, the vertebral processes (one spinous, two transverse, two superior articular, and two inferior articular) are sites for attachment of muscles and ligaments and for articulation with adjacent vertebrae.

Protective structures: spinal meninges   The spinal cord, like the brain, is enveloped by the three layers of meninges: dura mater, arachnoid, and pia mater. Between the lining of the vertebral canal and the spinal dura mater is the epidural space. The epidural space contains areolar tissue, fat, and a number of venous plexuses. Adjacent to the epidural space is the spinal dura mater. The spinal dura mater extends from the foramen magnum, where it is continuous with the cranial dura, to the second sacral vertebra, where it blends with the filum terminale. Laterally, the dura continues over the roots of the spinal nerves, forming dural root sleeves. Between the dura mater and the intermediate meningeal layer is the subdural space. The subdural space contains a small amount of fluid, which decreases friction between opposing surfaces.

The second meningeal layer, the spinal arachnoid, extends superiorly from the foramen magnum, to the inferior surfaces of the cauda equina and filum terminale. Laterally, the spinal arachnoid encloses the spinal nerve roots to the point of exit from the vertebral canal. The space between the arachnoid and the pia mater is the subarachnoid space, which contains cerebrospinal fluid.

The innermost layer, the spinal pia mater, extends downward to the filum terminale, where it is connected by the denticulate ligaments to the spinal dura mater between the ventral and dorsal spinal nerve roots.

Spinal cord   The spinal cord (Figure 3-16) originates at the foramen magnum and ends at the superior border of L2. It is a continuation from the medulla oblongata. The cord tapers in the lower thoracic area into a cone-shaped structure called the *conus medullaris*. Extending inferiorly from the conus medullaris is a thin prolongation, the *filum terminale,* that anchors the spinal cord to the coccyx. The spinal cord consists of 31 segments, each giving rise to a pair of spinal nerves.

Microscopically, the spinal cord consists of gray (unmyelinated) and white (myelinated) matter. The *gray matter* integrates the cord reflexes and is concentrated into an internal core. When this internal core is viewed in cross section, it resembles a butterfly (Figure 3-17). The paired gray matter projections forming the front "wings" of the butterfly are the anterior, or ventral, horns. The pair of projections forming the back "wings" is called the posterior, or dorsal, horns. The ventral horn consists of multipolar neuron structures (e.g., cell bodies, dendrites) that together form the motor efferent neurons of the ventral roots and spinal nerves. The dorsal horn contains cell bodies and dendrites of sensory (afferent) neurons and sensory receptors from the periphery. The gray matter also contains internuncial (association) neurons. The internuncial neurons transmit impulses from one lateral half of the cord to the other, from the dorsal portions to the ventral portions, and to other levels of the central nervous system.

Surrounding the gray matter of the spinal cord is the *white matter,* comprised of long ascending and descending tracts that serve as pathways between the spinal cord and brain for afferent and efferent impulses. The white matter is grouped into anatomic and functional bundles called fasciculi.

The spinal cord is divided into lateral halves by the *anterior fissure* and the *posterior sulcus.* Each lateral half is connected to the other half by commissures of gray and white matter. Each lateral half of the spinal cord is divided into three sections that run the length of the spinal cord: dorsal, lateral, and ventral. Within each of these divisions are distinct fiber tracts: ascending fibers, which bring sensory information to the central nervous system; descending fibers, which carry impulses from the brain to motor neurons of the brainstem and the spinal cord; and internuncial (association) neurons, which form short ascending and descending tracts that travel between spinal segments. These short tracts are called intersegmental tracts or pathways.

The neurons in the *ascending* pathways transmit sensory information from peripheral receptors to the spinal cord and brain. The sensory chain consists of a three-neuron pathway.

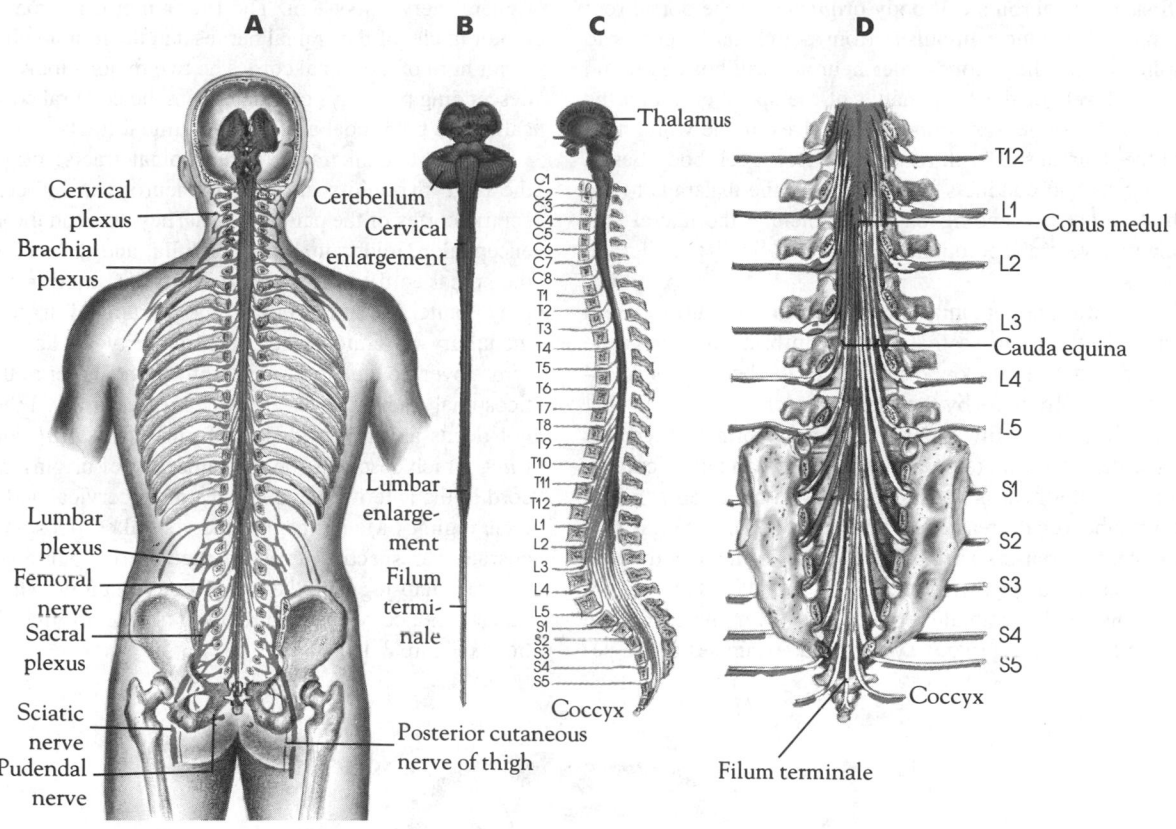

A
Cervical plexus
Brachial plexus
Lumbar plexus
Femoral nerve
Sacral plexus
Sciatic nerve
Pudendal nerve

B
Cerebellum
Cervical enlargement
Lumbar enlargement
Filum terminale
Posterior cutaneous nerve of thigh

C
Thalamus
C1
C2
C3
C4
C5
C6
C7
C8
T1
T2
T3
T4
T5
T6
T7
T8
T9
T10
T11
T12
L1
L2
L3
L4
L5
S1
S2
S3
S4
S5
Coccyx

D
T12
L1 — Conus medul
L2
L3
Cauda equina
L4
L5
S1
S2
S3
S4
S5
Coccyx
Filum terminale

Figure 3-16 Spinal cord within vertebral canal and exiting spinal nerves. **A,** Posterior view of brainstem and spinal cord in situ with spinal nerves and plexuses. **B,** Anterior view of brainstem and spinal cord. **C,** Lateral view showing relationship of spinal cord to vertebrae. **D,** Enlargement of caudal area showing termination of spinal cord (conus medullaris) and group of nerve fibers constituting the cauda equina. (From Rudy.[55])

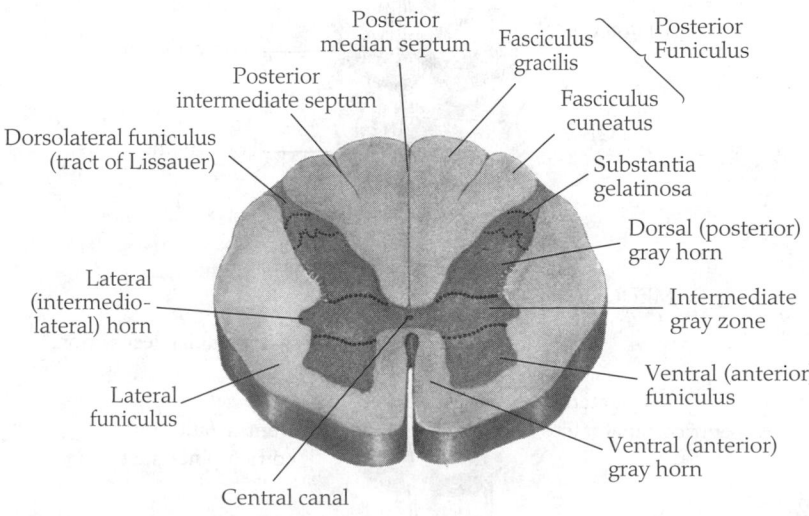

Posterior median septum
Fasciculus gracilis
Posterior Funiculus
Posterior intermediate septum
Fasciculus cuneatus
Dorsolateral funiculus (tract of Lissauer)
Substantia gelatinosa
Dorsal (posterior) gray horn
Lateral (intermediolateral) horn
Intermediate gray zone
Ventral (anterior) funiculus
Lateral funiculus
Ventral (anterior) gray horn
Central canal

Figure 3-17 Cross section of spinal cord illustrating subdivisions of white and gray matter. (From Rudy.[55])

The first-order neuron's cell body originates in the dorsal root ganglion and conducts impulses from peripheral receptors to the spinal cord. The second-order neuron's cell body is found at various levels of the gray matter of the spinal cord and the brainstem. These neurons conduct impulses, in the white matter, to the thalamus. The third-order neuron's cell body lies in the thalamus and conducts impulses from the thalamus to the cerebral cortex. Ascending pathways include the lateral spinothalamic, ventral spinothalamic, and fasciculi gracilis and cuneatus.

The pathways are organized according to body surface areas and cross in the brain so that sensory information enters the cerebral cortex from the opposite side of the body. This crossing over is usually done by the second-order neuron.

The *descending* pathways are made of two principal types of neurons, the upper motor neurons and lower motor neurons. The upper motor neuron has its cell body in the cerebral motor areas or subcortical areas (i.e., brainstem) of the central nervous system. It transmits impulses from the brain to motor neurons in the anterior (ventral) horn of the spinal cord and to motor neurons in the cranial nerves. The lower motor neuron begins in the central nervous system and terminates in the pe-

ripheral nervous system. The lower motor neurons consist of motor nuclei of the cranial nerves and the motor cells in the anterior horn of the spinal cord. The two major subdivisions of the descending pathways originate from the cerebral cortex and are called the pyramidal and extrapyramidal tracts.

The pyramidal tracts (corticospinal tracts) originate from the large pyramid-shaped motor neurons in the cerebral precentral cortex of the parietal lobe. They descend through the diencephalon, midbrain, pons, medulla, and the white matter of the spinal cord to the motor cells in the anterior horns of the gray matter. In the medulla the pyramidal tracts form the medullary pyramids where the majority of fibers decussate (cross over) to the other side and form the larger of the two corticospinal tracts, the *lateral corticospinal tract*. Fibers that do not decussate at the medulla form the *ventral corticospinal tract,* which descends (on the same side of origin) in the spinal cord in the anterior white matter to the cervical and upper thoracic regions. Many fibers of the ventral corticospinal tract decussate at respective levels of the anterior white commissure before synapsing with the lower motor neurons. The pyramidal tracts conduct voluntary impulses and reflex muscle contractions (Figure 3-18).

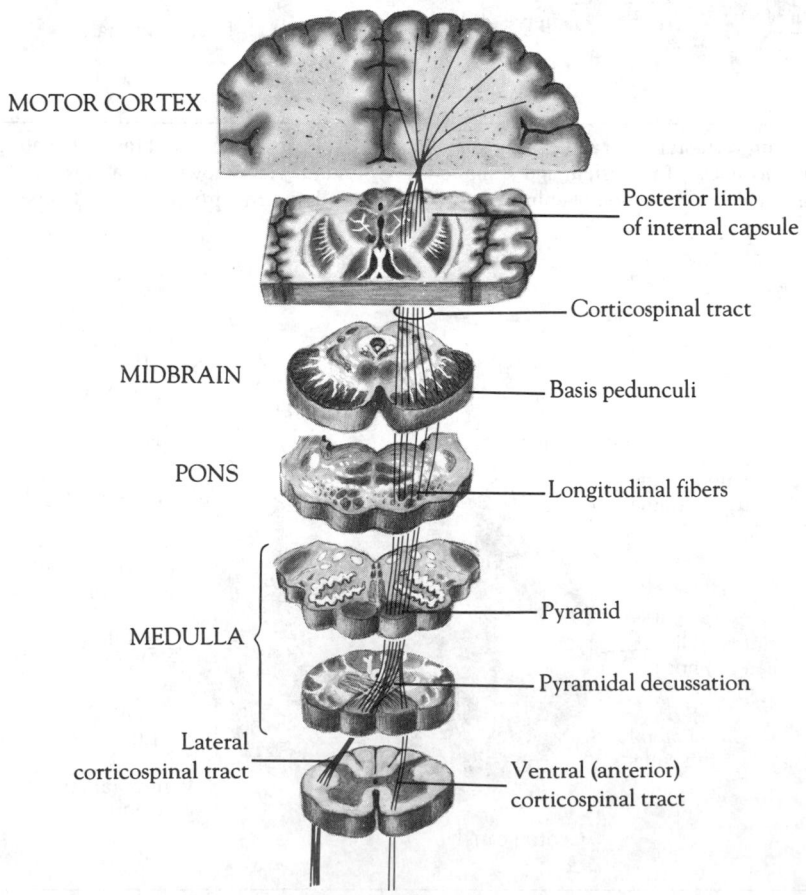

MOTOR CORTEX

Posterior limb of internal capsule

Corticospinal tract

MIDBRAIN

Basis pedunculi

PONS

Longitudinal fibers

MEDULLA

Pyramid

Pyramidal decussation

Lateral corticospinal tract

Ventral (anterior) corticospinal tract

Figure 3-18 Schematic drawing to show decussation of pyramids at level of medulla. (From Rudy.[55])

The extrapyramidal tracts (Figure 3-19) originate in the brainstem, basal ganglia, and cerebellum. These pathways are motor systems that coordinate muscular activity. The *medial reticulospinal* tract originates in the reticular formation of the brainstem and descends uncrossed. It stimulates flexor responses and inhibits extensor responses. The *lateral reticulospinal* tract also originates from the brainstem and is primarily uncrossed. The lateral tract stimulates extensor responses and inhibits flexor responses to maintain posture. Table 3-2 summarizes the principal ascending and descending tracts of the spinal cord and their respective functions.

The *extrapyramidal system* is a functional unit, not an anatomic one, and depends on an intact pyramidal system. This system consists of extrapyramidal areas of the cerebral cortex, the corpus striatum, thalamic nuclei connected to the corpus striatum, the subthalamus, and the rubral and reticular systems. The extrapyramidal system coordinates associated movements and changes in posture and integrates functions of the autonomic nervous system.[36] The system has fibers that originate from the cerebral cortex and project to the basal ganglia. The basal ganglia of the extrapyramidal system act to coordinate movement.

Reflexes

The reflex arc (Figure 3-20) is the basic functional unit that maintains body integrity by automatically conducting impulses from sensory receptors (afferent) to efferent neurons. In the reflex arc or loop, a sensory nerve ending is stimulated and then conveys the impulse via sensory (afferent) neurons to gray matter nuclei in the spinal cord. In the gray matter the afferent neuron may synapse directly with lower motor neurons, or it may synapse with one or more internuncial (association) neurons, which transfer the impulse to the lower motor neuron. The lower motor neurons (efferent) carry the impulse via the ventral roots of the spinal cord to the neuroeffector junction. The effector organ then responds to stimulation (e.g., by muscle contraction or glandular secretion). An example of a simple reflex involving only two neurons and one synapse is the knee-jerk (patellar) reflex. When the knee is tapped, afferent receptors are stimulated and send the impulse to the spinal cord. In the spinal cord the impulse is directly relayed to the lower motor neuron. As a result, the quadriceps muscles contract and jerk the leg.

Unlike the knee-jerk reflex, which is the only monosynaptic reflex in the body, most reflex pathways involve numerous synaptic connections (polysynaptic). Reflex response time increases proportionately with the number of synapses. Some reflexes involve only one half of the body (e.g., flexor reflex) and are called ipsilateral reflexes. Other reflexes cross over, eliciting responses on the opposite side of the body (e.g., crossed extensor reflex). These are called contralateral reflexes. For example, when someone steps on a tack, there is a reflex flexion in one leg to move away from the tack, while in the opposite leg there is extension to maintain body balance.

Finally, both the brain and the spinal cord contain reflex centers that provide important data about level of functioning. Pupillary response, cardioregulatory mechanisms, and the medullary vasomotor mechanisms are all brain reflexes. Reflexes controlled predominantly by the spinal cord include emptying of the bowel and bladder, withdrawal from painful stimuli (known as a nociceptive reflex), increased blood flow to the skin, and stretch reflexes that maintain normal posture and position. Specific reflexes and responses elicited are discussed in the section on normal findings of the neurologic system.

Peripheral Nervous System

Cranial nerves The 12 pairs of cranial nerves (Table 3-3) form the peripheral nerves of the brain. Some have only motor fibers (five pairs), some have only sensory fibers (three pairs),

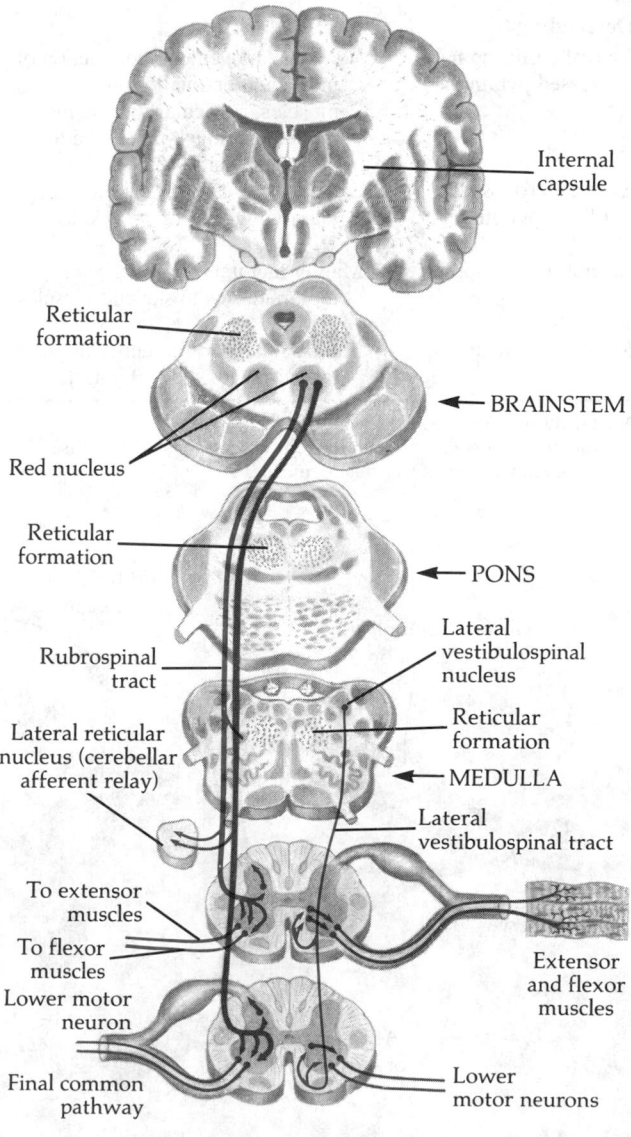

Figure 3-19 Extrapyramidal descending tracts. Upper motor neurons originate below level of cortex and converge on lower motor neurons (final common pathway) along with upper motor neurons of pyramidal tracts. Rubrospinal tract originates in red area.

■ TABLE 3-2 Major Ascending and Descending Spinal Cord Tracts

Name	Function	Location	Origin*	Termination†
Ascending				
Lateral spinothalamic	Pain, temperature, and crude touch opposite side	Lateral white columns	Posterior gray column opposite side	Thalamus
Ventral spinothalamic	Crude touch, pain, and temperature	Anterior white columns	Posterior gray column opposite side	Thalamus
Fasciculi gracilis and cuneatus	Discriminating touch and pressure sensations, including vibration, stereognosis, and two-point discrimination; also conscious kinesthesia	Posterior white columns	Spinal ganglia same side	Medulla
Spinocerebellar	Unconscious kinesthesia	Lateral white columns	Posterior gray column	Cerebellum
Descending				
Lateral corticospinal (or crossed pyramidal)	Voluntary movement, contraction of individual or small groups of muscles, particularly those moving hands, fingers, feet, and toes of opposite side	Lateral white columns	Motor areas of cerebral cortex (mainly areas 4 and 6) opposite side from tract location in cord	Intermediate or anterior gray columns
Ventral corticospinal (direct pyramidal)	Same as lateral corticospinal except mainly muscles of same side	Lateral white columns	Motor cortex but on same side as tract location in cord	Intermediate or anterior gray columns
Lateral reticulospinal	Mainly facilitatory influence on motorneurons to skeletal muscles	Lateral white columns	Reticular formation, midbrain, pons, and medulla	Intermediate or anterior gray columns
Medial reticulospinal	Mainly inhibitory influence on motorneurons to skeletal muscles	Anterior white columns	Reticular formation, medulla mainly	Intermediate or anterior gray columns

Modified from Thibodeau.[64]
*Location of cell bodies of neurons from which axons of tract arise.
†Structure in which axons of tract terminate.

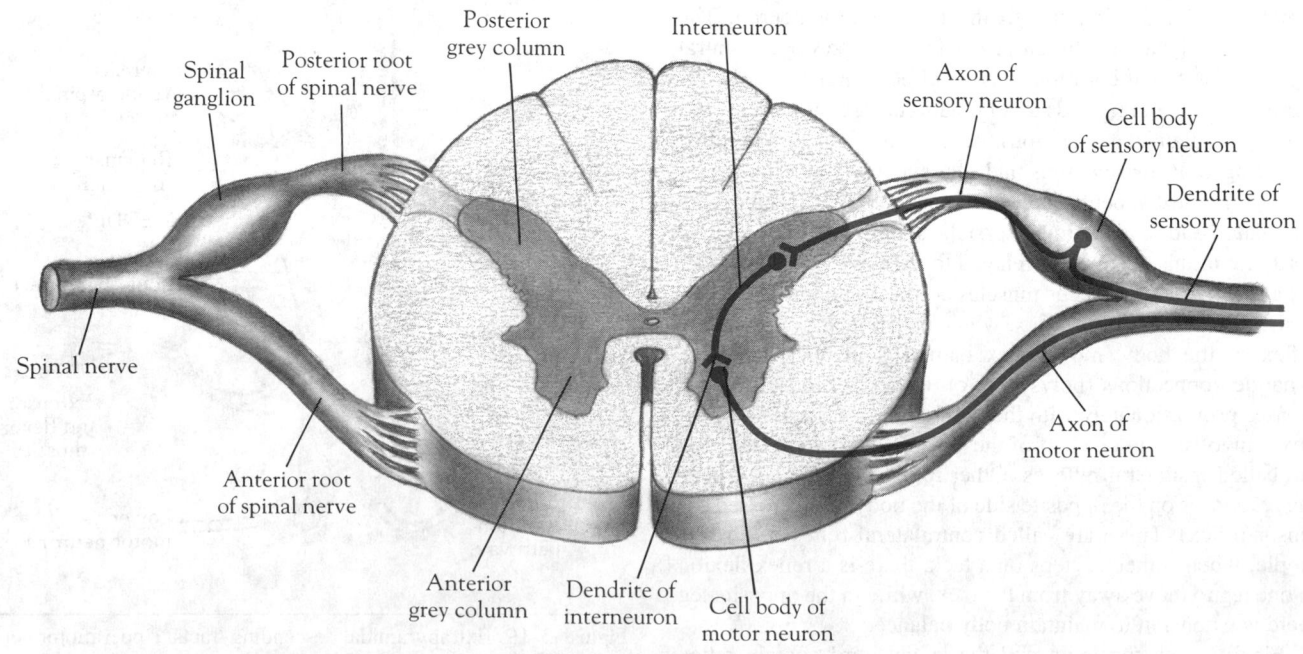

Figure 3-20 Three-neuron reflex arc.

TABLE 3-3 Cranial Nerves

Nerve*	Sensory Fibers†			Motor Fibers†		Functions‡
	Receptors	Cell Bodies	Termination	Cell Bodies	Termination	
I Olfactory	*Nasal mucosa*	*Nasal mucosa*	*Olfactory bulbs (new relay of neurons of olfactory cortex)*			*Sense of smell*
II Optic	*Retina*	*Retina*	*Nucleus in thalamus (lateral geniculate body): some fibers terminate in superior colliculus of midbrain*			*Vision*
III Oculomotor	*External eye muscles except superior oblique and lateral rectus*			**Midbrain (oculomotor nucleus and Edinger-Westphal nucleus)**	**External eye muscles except superior oblique and lateral rectus; fibers from Edinger-Westphal nucleus terminate in ciliary ganglion and then to ciliary and iris muscles**	**Eye movements, regulation of size of pupil, accommodation,** *proprioception (muscle sense)*
IV Trochlear	*Superior oblique*			**Midbrain**	**Superior oblique muscle of eye**	**Eye movements,** *proprioception*
V Trigeminal	*Skin and mucosa of head, teeth*	*Gasserian ganglion*	*Pons (sensory nucleus)*	**Pons (motor nucleus)**	**Muscles of mastication**	*Sensations of head and face,* **chewing movements,** *muscle sense*
VI Abducens	*Lateral rectus*			**Pons**	**Lateral rectus muscle of eye**	**Abduction of eye,** *proprioception*
VII Facial	*Taste buds of anterior two thirds of tongue*	*Geniculate ganglion*	*Medulla (nucleus solitarius)*	**Pons**	**Superficial muscles of face and scalp**	**Facial expressions, secretion of saliva,** *taste*
VIII Acoustic						
1 Vestibular branch	*Semicircular canals and vestibule (utricle and saccule)*	*Vestibular ganglion*	*Pons and medulla (vestibular nuclei)*			*Balance or equilibrium sense*
2 Cochlear or auditory branch	*Organ of Corti in cochlear duct*	*Spiral ganglion*	*Pons and medulla (cochlear nuclei)*			*Hearing*

Continued.

From Thibodeau.[64]

*The first letters of the words in the following sentence are the first letters of the names of the cranial nerves. Many generations of anatomy students have used this sentence as an aid to memorizing these names. It is "On Old Olympus' Tiny Tops, A Finn And German Viewed Some Hops." (There are several slightly differing versions of this mnemonic.)

†Italics indicate sensory fibers and functions. Boldface type indicates motor fibers and functions.

‡An aid for remembering the general function of each cranial nerve is the following 12-word saying: "Some say marry money but my brothers say bad business marry money." Words beginning with "S" indicate sensory function. Words beginning with "M" indicate motor function. Words beginning with "B" indicate both sensory and motor functions. For example, the first, second, and eighth words in the saying start with "S," which indicates that the first, second, and eighth cranial nerves perform sensory functions.

TABLE 3-3 Cranial Nerves—cont'd

Nerve*	Sensory Fibers†			Motor Fibers†		Functions‡
	Receptors	Cell Bodies	Termination	Cell Bodies	Termination	
IX Glossopharyngeal	*Pharynx; taste buds and other receptors of posterior one third of tongue*	*Jugular and petrous ganglia*	*Medulla (nucleus solitarius)*	**Medulla (nucleus ambiguus)**	**Muscles of pharynx**	*Taste and other sensations of tongue, swallowing movements, secretion of saliva, aid in reflex control of blood pressure and respiration*
	Carotid sinus and carotid body	*Jugular and petrous ganglia*	*Medulla (respiratory and vasomotor centers)*	**Medulla at junction of pons (nucleus salivatorius)**	**Otic ganglion and then to parotid gland**	
X Vagus	*Pharynx, larynx, carotid body, and thoracic and abdominal viscera*	*Jugular and nodose ganglia*	*Medulla (nucleus solitarius), pons (nucleus of fifth cranial nerve)*	**Medulla (dorsal motor nucleus)**	**Ganglia of vagal plexus and then to muscles of pharynx, larynx, and thoracic and abdominal viscera**	*Sensations and movements of organs supplied; for example, slows heart, increases peristalsis, and contracts muscles for voice production*
XI Spinal accessory				**Medulla (dorsal motor nucleus of vagus and nucleus ambiguus)**	**Muscles of thoracic and abdominal viscera and pharynx and larynx**	**Shoulder movements, turning movements of head, movements of viscera,** *voice productions, proprioception?*
				Anterior gray column of first five or six cervical segments of spinal cord	**Trapezius and sternocleidomastoid muscle**	
XII Hypoglossal				**Medulla (hypoglossal nucleus)**	**Muscles of tongue**	**Tongue movements,** *proprioception?*

■ TABLE 3-4 Spinal Nerves and Peripheral Branches

Spinal Nerves	Plexuses Formed from Anterior Rami	Spinal Nerve Branches from Plexuses	Parts Supplied
Cervical 1 2 3 4	Cervical plexus	Lesser occipital Great auricular Cutaneous nerve of neck Anterior supraclavicular Middle supraclavicular Posterior supraclavicular Branches to numerous neck muscles	Sensory to back of head, front of neck, and upper part of shoulder, motor to numerous neck muscles
		Phrenic (branches from cervical nerves before formation of plexus; most of its fibers from fourth cervical nerve)	Diaphragm
		Suprascapular and dorsoscapular	Superficial muscles* of scapula
		Thoracic nerves, medial and lateral branches	Pectoralis major and minor
		Long thoracic nerve	Serratus anterior
Cervical 5 6	Brachial plexus	Thoracodorsal	Latissimus dorsi
		Subscapular	Subscapular and teres major muscles
		Axillary (circumflex)	Deltoid and teres minor muscles and skin over deltoid
7 8		Musculocutaneous	Muscles of front of arm (biceps brachii, coracobrachialis, and brachialis) and skin on outer side of forearm
Thoracic (or dorsal) 1 2		Ulnar	Flexor carpi ulnaris and part of flexor digitorum profundus; some of muscles of hand; sensory to medial side of hand, little finger, and medial half of fourth finger
3 4 5		Median	Rest of muscles of front of forearm and hand; sensory to skin of palmar surface of thumb, index, and middle fingers
6 7 8	No plexus formed; branches run directly to intercostal muscles and skin of thorax	Radial	Triceps muscle and muscles of back of forearm; sensory to skin of back of forearm and hand
		Medial cutaneous	Sensory to inner surface of arm and forearm
9		Iliohypogastric ⎱ Sometimes fused	Sensory to anterior abdominal wall
10 11		Ilioinguinal ⎰	Sensory to anterior abdominal wall and external genitalia; motor to muscles of abdominal wall
12		Genitofemoral	Sensory to skin of external genitalia and inguinal region
		Lateral cutaneous of thigh	Sensory to outer side of thigh
Lumbar 1 2 3		Femoral	Motor to quadriceps, sartorius, and iliacus muscles; sensory to front of thigh and medial side of lower leg (saphenous nerve)
4 5		Obturator	Motor to adductor muscles of thigh
Sacral 1	Lumbosacral plexus	Tibial† (medial popliteal)	Motor to muscles of calf of leg; sensory to skin of calf of leg and sole of foot
2 3		Common peroneal (lateral popliteal)	Motor to evertors and dorsiflexors of foot; sensory to lateral surface of leg and dorsal surface of foot
4 5		Nerves to hamstring muscles	Motor to muscles of back of thigh
		Gluteal nerves, superior and inferior	Motor to buttock muscles and tensor fasciae latae
Coccygeal 1		Posterior cutaneous nerve	Sensory to skin of buttocks, posterior surface of thigh, and leg
		Pudendal nerve	Motor to perineal muscles; sensory to skin of perineum

From Thibodeau.[64]

*Although nerves to muscles are considered motor, they do contain some sensory fibers that transmit proprioceptive impulses.

†Sensory fibers from the tibial and peroneal nerves unite to form the *medial cutaneous* (or sural) *nerve* that supplies the calf of the leg and the lateral surface of the foot. In the thigh the tibial and common peroneal nerves are usually enclosed in a single sheath to form the *sciatic nerve*, the largest nerve in the body with its width of approximately ¾ inch. About two thirds of the way down the posterior part of the thigh, it divides into its component parts. Branches of the sciatic nerve extend into the hamstring muscles.

and the rest (four pairs) have both sensory and motor fibers. The cranial nerves "correspond to the spinal nerves serving common sensation, voluntary control of muscles, and autonomic functions in the head; in addition, they include the mechanism for the special senses of vision, hearing, smell, and taste."[32]

Table 3-3 summarizes origin, functional class, and primary functions of the cranial nerves. Assessment of their functions is in the section on neurologic assessment.

Spinal nerves The 31 pairs of spinal nerves arise from different segments of the spinal cord. Each pair of spinal nerves is formed by the union of anterior and posterior roots attached to the spinal cord. Each pair of spinal nerves and its corresponding part of the spinal cord constitute a *spinal segment*. Individual spinal segments in turn innervate specific body segments.

Some spinal nerves join at the anterior rami to form a complex network of nerve fibers called a plexus. The *cervical* and *brachial plexuses* provide peripheral nerves for innervation to the upper extremities. The lower extremities are innervated by peripheral nerves from the *lumbar* and *sacral plexuses*. Unlike the cervical and thoracic spinal nerves, the lumbar and sacral nerves do not exit from the intervertebral foramen at right angles. Instead, these nerves extend obliquely and inferiorly and form a large bundle of nerve fibers called the *cauda equina*.

Table 3-4 summarizes the spinal nerves, corresponding plexuses, and peripheral innervation (see also Table 3-5).

Dermatomes Each spinal nerve root innervates a specific area, or dermatome, of the body surface for superficial or cutaneous sensation. Although there is a great deal of overlap in the spinal nerves, knowledge of the distribution of dermatomes is useful for assessment and evaluation purposes (Figure 3-21).

Autonomic Nervous System

The autonomic nervous system is considered part of the peripheral nervous system. It regulates the body's internal environment in close conjunction with the endocrine system. It is responsible for the unconscious moment-to-moment functioning of all internal systems, including visceral organs (e.g., digestive, urogenital), involuntary muscle fibers (e.g., smooth muscle), and glandular functions (e.g., adrenal medulla, islets of Langerhans in the pancreas). The autonomic nervous system is activated by centers in the hypothalamus, brainstem, and spinal cord. It is characterized by a two-neuron chain consisting of a preganglionic neuron and a postganglionic neuron.

Preganglionic neurons have cell bodies in the central nervous system and efferent fibers that terminate in the autonomic ganglia. *Postganglionic* neurons have cell bodies outside the central nervous system in the autonomic ganglia and innervate the target, or effector, organ (e.g., cardiac muscle). The purpose of the postganglionic neuron is to relay impulses beyond the ganglia.

The autonomic nervous system has two major subdivisions (sympathetic and parasympathetic), and both consist of autonomic ganglia and nerves. Generally each effector organ has both sympathetic and parasympathetic innervation. The subdivisions differ in the type of neurotransmitters released, distribution of nerve fibers, and effects on organs innervated, in that the subdivisions produce antagonistic physiologic responses.

The *sympathetic* (thoracolumbar) subdivision is activated during internal and external stress situations (the flight-fight phenomenon). During those stressful situations, sympathetic responses include increases in blood pressure and heart rate and vasoconstriction of peripheral blood vessels. The sympathetic division is also called *adrenergic* because the transmitter substance norepinephrine (noradrenalin) is secreted by its postganglionic nerve terminals.

The preganglionic fibers of the sympathetic system are located in the intermediolateral columns of the thoracic and first two lumbar segments in the spinal cord (i.e., T1 to T2); thus this system is sometimes called the thoracolumbar system. After leaving the spinal nerves, the small, myelinated, preganglionic, sympathetic fibers enter the sympathetic trunk via the white ramus. The sympathetic trunk is a chain of ganglions extending from the base of the skull to the coccyx on either side of the spinal cord.

Most axons of sympathetic neurons synapse in the sympathetic trunk or travel up and down the trunk before synapsing. Some axons do not synapse within the sympathetic trunk; instead they exit to synapse in collateral ganglia nearer to the organ of innervation. Acetylcholine is the neurotransmitter at all preganglionic nerve terminals of the sympathetic division. Norepinephrine is the neurotransmitter at all postganglionic nerve terminals of the sympathetic system. Because of the sympathetic chain ganglia, the nerve fibers of the sympathetic system generally have short and long postganglionic fibers. Fibers terminate on two receptor sites (α or β), which determine the effects of the neurotransmitters. β receptors are divided into β_1 and β_2 receptors because some drugs affect some, but not all, β receptors.

The adrenal medulla is a functional extension of the sympathetic nervous system. Its postganglionic neurons are specialized secretory cells. Epinephrine and norepinephrine are secreted by the adrenal medulla at the same time the sympathetic nerves are stimulating afferent organs and have almost the same effect as direct sympathetic stimulation. As a result, body tissues are stimulated simultaneously, directly by the sympathetic nerves and indirectly by the hormones of the adrenal medulla. After their release, the hormones are rapidly metabolized, primarily by the liver. Approximately one half of the catecholamines are excreted in the urine as free or conjugated normetanephrine and metanephrine. Daily normal urinary output of the catecholamines equals approximately 6 mg of epinephrine and 30 mg of norepinephrine.[30,36] Chapter 11 gives further detail on the adrenal medulla and the catecholamines.

The *parasympathetic* (craniosacral) subdivision of the autonomic nervous system consists of preganglionic fibers arising from cell bodies in cranial nerves III, VII, IX, and X, as well as sacral spinal nerves II through VII. This division is activated when an individual is at rest or relaxed, protecting and restoring the body's resources. It works slower than the sympathetic division, has a more discrete effect, and dominates control over

TABLE 3-5 Cranial Nerves Contrasted with Spinal Nerves

	Cranial Nerves	Spinal Nerves
Origin	Base of brain	Spinal cord
Distribution	Mainly to head and neck	Skin, skeletal muscles, joints, blood vessels, sweat glands, and mucosa except of head and neck
Structure	Some composed of sensory fibers only; some of both motor axons and sensory dendrites; some motor fibers belong to somatic nervous system, some to autonomic	All of them composed of both sensory dendrites and motor axons; some of latter somatic, some autonomic
Function	Vision, hearing, sense of smell, sense of taste, eye movements	Sensations, movements, and sweat secretion

From Anthony and Kolthoff.[3]

the sympathetic subdivision during nonstressful conditions. Parasympathetic fibers in the cranial and sacral nerves form synaptic connections only with terminal ganglia located near the organs innervated. Therefore in the parasympathetic division, preganglionic fibers are long and postganglionic fibers are short. Both preganglionic and postganglionic fibers secrete the neurotransmitter *acetylcholine;* therefore the parasympathetic subdivision is called *cholinergic.*

The organs innervated and effects of stimulation by sympathetic and parasympathetic subdivisions are summarized in Tables 3-4 and 3-5.

Vascular Supply to Brain and Spinal Cord

Maintaining adequate blood supply to the brain and spinal cord is vital for proper functioning of the nervous system. The blood removes metabolic waste products and supplies the cells with nutrients.

Brain The blood supply to the brain comes principally from two pairs of arteries, the internal carotid and the vertebral arteries. The *internal carotid* arteries arise from the common carotid artery at the level of the thyroid cartilage. They supply approximately 80% of the blood to the brain. The internal carotid arteries then give rise to the anterior and middle cerebral arteries at about the level of the optic chiasm. The *anterior cerebral artery* supplies portions of the medial surfaces of the frontal and parietal lobes, nuclei of the basal ganglia, caudate putamen, and portions of the internal capsule and corpus callosum. The *middle cerebral artery* supplies lateral surfaces of the parietal, frontal, and temporal lobes. It is the major source of blood supply to the precentral (motor) and postcentral (sensory) gyri. The vertebral arteries arise from the right and left *subclavian arteries* and provide the remaining 20% of cerebral blood supply. The vertebral arteries join at the base of the brain and form the basilar artery. The *basilar artery* enters the skull at the foramen magnum and ascends to the midbrain. Branches of the vertebral and basilar arteries supply the brainstem and cerebellum. In the midbrain the basilar artery splits into the pair of *posterior cerebral arteries.* The posterior cerebral arteries supply portions of the temporal and occipital lobes of each hemisphere, the vestibular organs, and the cochlear apparatus. Figure 3-22 illustrates the vessels supplying the brain tissue.

At the base of the brain the cerebral arteries are connected, by their communicating branches, into an arterial circle called the *circle of Willis* (Figure 3-23). More specifically, the poste-

rior cerebral artery is connected to the middle cerebral artery by the posterior communicating branches. The anterior cerebral arteries are connected by the anterior communicating branches. The purpose of the circle of Willis is to ensure circulation if one of the four main blood vessels is interrupted.

Branches of cerebral arteries extend throughout the brain. These branches are called end arteries because they have few branching connections. This lack of branching results in decreased potential for collateral circulation.

Dense networks of capillaries are found in the gray matter of the brain. These capillaries are surrounded by a protective membrane formed by the end-feet of *astrocyte cells.* The capillary blood enters the deep veins, which then empty into the superficial venous plexuses and dural sinuses (principally the superior longitudinal sinus). The venous blood is drained from these sinuses by the internal jugular veins, which return the blood to the general circulation (a small volume of blood drains via the *pterygoid* and ophthalmic venous sinuses).

The anterior, middle, and posterior meningeal arteries provide an abundant blood supply to the cranial meninges.

Spinal cord The arterial blood supply to the spinal cord comes from three main vessels: the one spinal artery and the two radicular arteries. The *spinal artery* arises from branches of the vertebral arteries at the level of the foramen magnum. It then divides into one anterior and two posterior branches. These branches then enter the vertebral canal with the dorsal and ventral nerve roots. The *radicular* artery arises from the thoracic and abdominal aorta and divides into anterior and posterior branches that enter the spinal cord at the intervertebral foramina. At the spinal segments the radicular arteries connect with the spinal arteries to form an extensive vascular plexus around the entire spinal cord.

The spinal venous system is extensive, with many intradural veins exiting from the ventral median fissure. In addition numerous extradural veins form a dense venous plexus in the pia mater. Venous blood is drained from the plexus by veins accompanying roots of the spinal nerves.

Brain barriers The neuronal tissues of the brain are extremely sensitive to any changes in the ionic concentration of their environment. Therefore the composition of the brain's internal environment must be delicately balanced to ensure normal functioning. The *blood-brain barrier* is a physiologic mechanism that helps maintain and protect this homeostatic balance by way of selective capillary permeability. Since

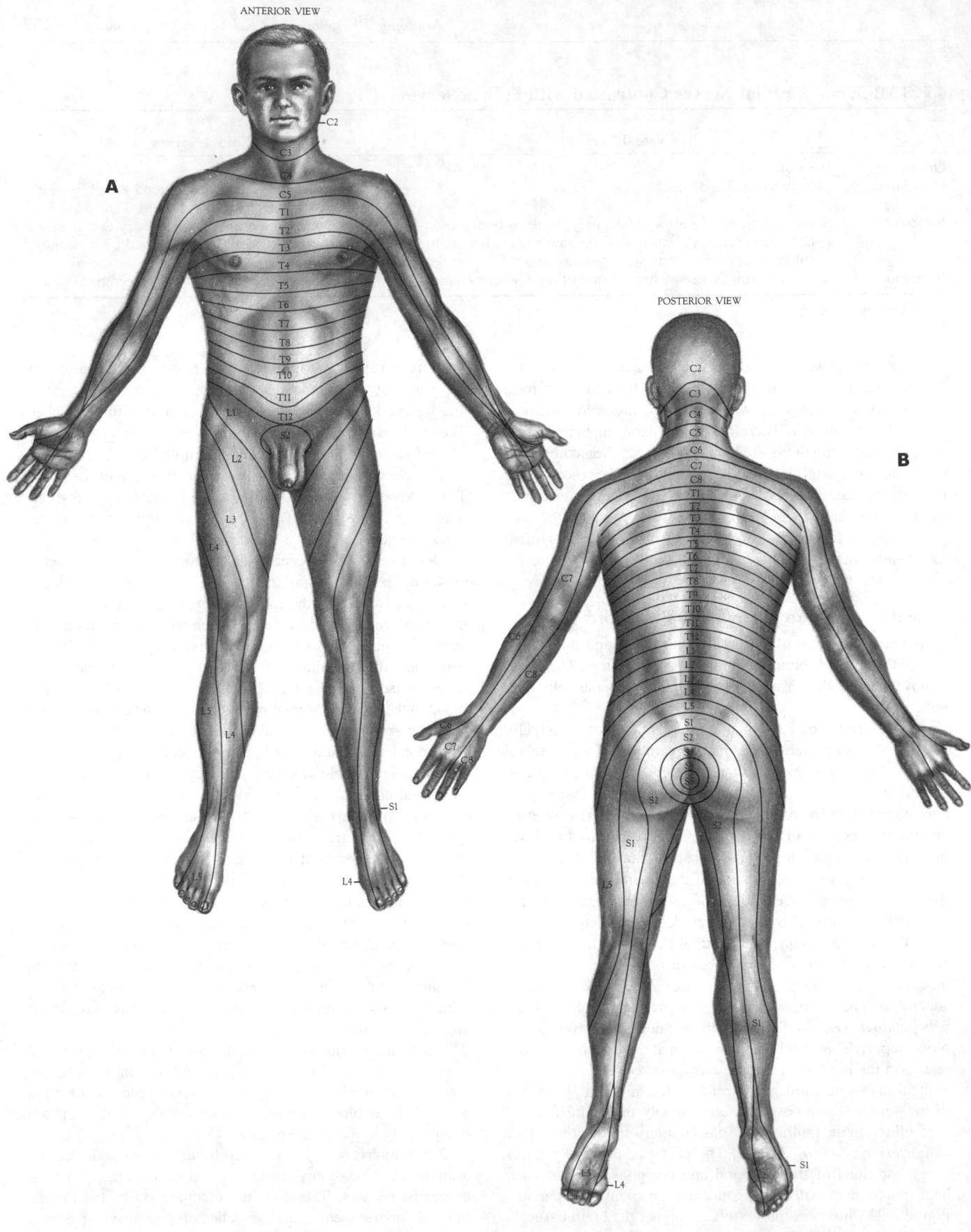

Figure 3-21 Dermatomes of the body: the area of body surface innervated by particular spinal nerves. It appears that there is a distinct separation of surface area controlled by each of the dermatomes; however, there is almost always overlap between spinal nerves. **A,** Anterior view. **B,** Posterior view. (From Rudy.[55])

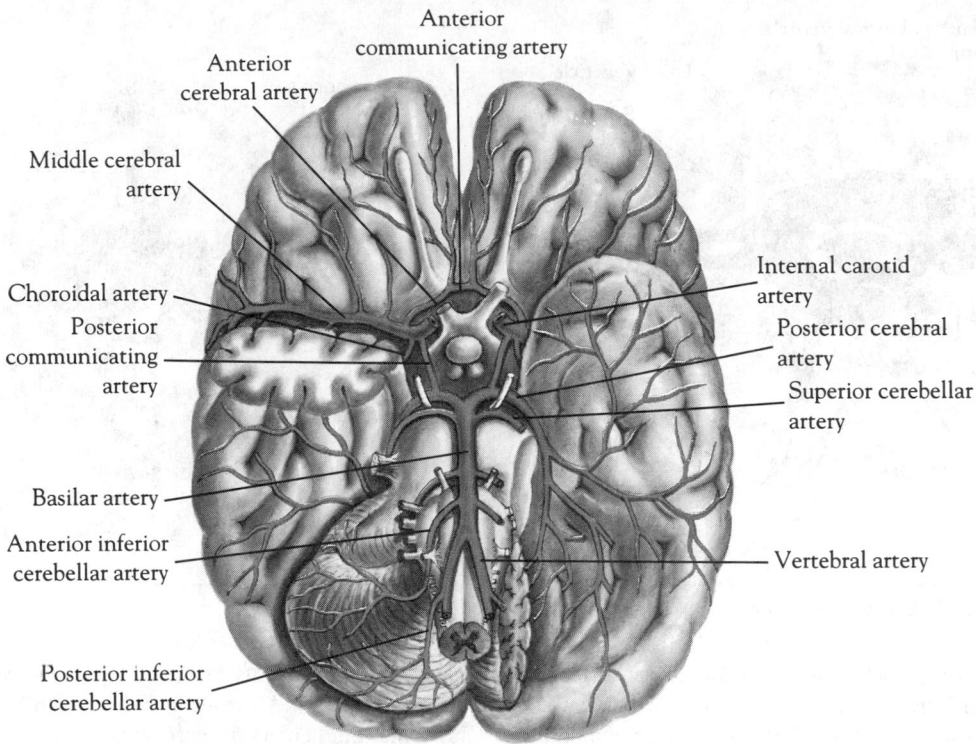

Figure 3-22 Blood supply of the brain. (From Rudy.[55])

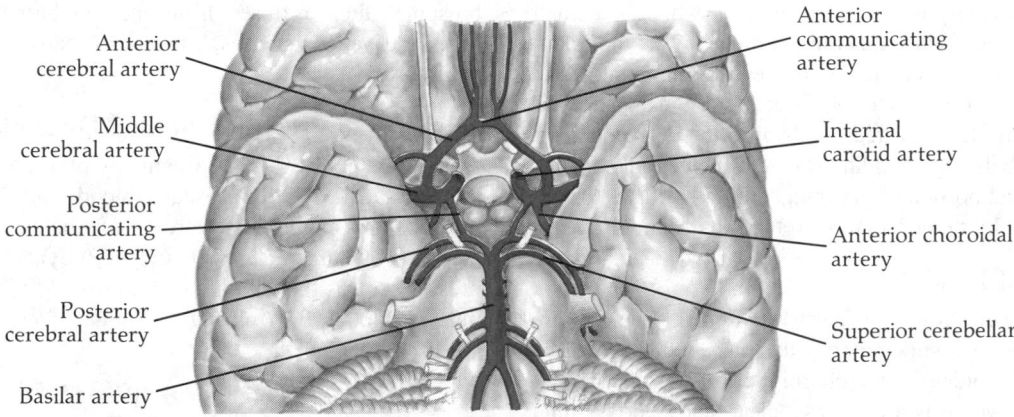

Figure 3-23 Anatomic diagram of circle of Willis.

substances from the blood enter the brain either through capillaries into the cerebrospinal fluid or through capillaries into the extracellular fluid, there are actually two barrier mechanisms. The blood-brain and blood-cerebrospinal barriers function together to protect the neuronal brain tissue. The complex of intermembranes that form these barriers is found in most regions of brain parenchyma, the choroid plexus, and the vasculature of the brain. Unlike most capillaries in the body, these capillaries are surrounded by astrocyte end-feet that form tight junctions of the endothelial cells. It is thought the tight junctions and glial end-feet affect capillary permeability. Both the blood-brain and blood-cerebrospinal barriers are permeable to oxygen, carbon dioxide, and water. They are slightly permeable to electrolytes (e.g., Na^+, K^+, Cl^-) but are impermeable to fixed acids and bases and many drugs. These barriers develop in the postnatal period; thus the cerebral capillaries of the newborn are far more permeable than those of the adult.

Cerebral Ventricular System

The cerebral ventricular system is a series of four ependymal-lined cavities (Figure 3-24). The ventricles are interconnecting structures that originate from the single cavity of the embryonic

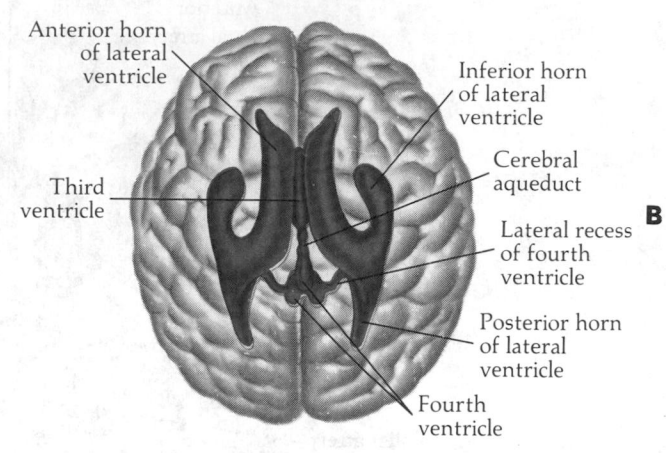

Figure 3-24 Cerebral ventricles. **A,** Lateral view. **B,** Superior view.

neural tube. The two largest cavities, the lateral ventricles, are located within each cerebral hemisphere. Each lateral ventricle consists of a body and anterior (frontal), inferior (temporal), and posterior (occipital) horns. The lateral ventricles in each hemisphere are separated from each other by a thin layer called the septum pellucidum. Each of these ventricles communicates, via the interventricular foramen of Monro, with a central cavity. This central cavity is the third ventricle, which is a small cleft space between the thalamic structures of the diencephalon. In the midbrain the third ventricle communicates with the fourth ventricle via the aqueduct of Sylvius. The rhomboid fourth ventricle is located posterior to the pons and anterior to the cerebellum, extending down to the central canal of the upper cervical portion of the spinal cord. The fourth ventricle is connected by three foramina to the subarachnoid space.

Cerebrospinal Fluid

Parts of the lateral, third, and fourth ventricular structures are lined with dense networks of capillaries called the *choroid plexus* (tela choroidea). The choroid plexus secretes cerebrospinal fluid, which is a colorless, clear, and odorless fluid that contains glucose, electrolytes, oxygen, water, carbon dioxide, small amounts of protein, and a few leukocytes. The cerebrospinal fluid removes metabolic wastes, provides nutrition, performs some mechanical function (i.e., shock absorber), and participates in maintaining normal intracranial pressure. In 24 hours the choroid plexuses secrete approximately 500 to 750 ml of cerebrospinal fluid; however, only about 125 to 150 ml is present in the system at any one time.

From the choroid plexuses in the lateral ventricles, the cerebrospinal fluid passes through the foramen of Monro to the third ventricle. From there, it slowly flows through the aqueduct of Sylvius to the fourth ventricle. The fluid then leaves the fourth ventricle through the single medial foramen of Magendie (located in the roof of the fourth ventricle) and the

paired foramina of Luschka (located in the lateral portion of the fourth ventricle). After leaving the fourth ventricle, the cerebrospinal fluid enters the subarachnoid space, where it fills the spinal cisterns and slowly diffuses upward over the convexities of the brain. The fluid is slowly absorbed from the subarachnoid space by the arachnoid villi, which are clusterlike protrusions extending into the superior sagittal sinus. The cerebrospinal fluid diffuses from the arachnoid villi into the intradural venous sinuses, where it is reabsorbed into the venous system.

Intracranial Pressure: Normal Dynamics

Approximately 88% of the contents of the cranial cavity is brain tissue, 2% is intravascular blood, and the final 10% is cerebrospinal fluid. These three components are the essential elements of intracranial pressure (ICP) dynamics. Intracranial pressure equals the volume of brain tissue (BTV) plus the volume of blood (BV) plus the volume of cerebrospinal fluid (CSFV).

$$ICP = BTV + BV + CSFV$$

The normal intracranial pressure in the recumbent position is about 0 to 15 mm Hg (110 to 140 mm H_2O). Standing decreases intracranial pressure, whereas such activities as sitting, sneezing, coughing, isometric exercises, sexual intercourse, and the Valsalva maneuver cause a transient rise in intracranial pressure. Because the skull limits brain expansion, these activities are normally compensated for by a redistribution of cerebrospinal fluid to the spinal subarachnoid space or by partial collapse of the cisterns and cerebral ventricles. (The skull of a young child is not rigid, so expansion is not so severely limited.)

Another important determinant in the dynamics of intracranial pressure is the autoregulation of cerebral blood flow. This blood flow is generally expressed as cerebral perfusion pressure

(CPP) and is maintained by the regulation of resistance vessel diameters. The cerebral perfusion pressure equals the mean arterial blood pressure (MABP) minus the mean intracranial pressure (MICP).

$$CPP = MABP - MICP$$

The normal range of cerebral perfusion pressure is 80 to 100 mm Hg. Cerebral perfusion pressure must be at least 50 mm Hg for the brain to receive an adequate blood supply. To maintain normal cerebral perfusion, the blood vessels constrict or dilate, thereby directly affecting intracranial pressure.

The last component in intracranial pressure is the actual brain tissue. The compensatory mechanism of brain tissue displacement or shifting is not usually considered a part of normal dynamics.

Any activity or condition that causes a sustained increase in one of the essential elements listed above must be compensated for by a decrease in one or both of the other two essential elements. This principle is known as the Monro-Kellie doctrine and must be understood in relation to normal dynamics of intracranial pressure as well as pathologic states that lead to increased intracranial pressure.

Variations in Older Adult

Like other systems in the body, the neural structures undergo significant changes as a person ages. Understanding these anatomic and physiologic changes assists the practitioner to establish realistic normative behaviors for the elderly population.

Brain The neuronal cells of the central nervous system (brain and spinal cord) of all adults are postmitotic and therefore do not regenerate once destroyed. Studies indicate that the aging process causes a loss of brain cells, and that cells not destroyed may undergo significant structural changes. Brain cells decrease in number at a rate of about 1% a year after 50 years of age. However, this rate of loss is not consistent throughout the brain, so that certain areas may lose cells at a faster (e.g., cortex) or slower (e.g., brainstem) rate than others. Other cells, such as the neurons of the prefrontal neocortex, undergo structural changes that result in a progressive decline in dendritic interconnections. In addition, neuronal cells of the elderly contain the age pigment *lipofuscin* in the storage granules, as well as senile plaques and neurofibrillary tangles.

Cerebral blood flow studies indicate there is a change with age in cerebral blood flow and oxygen utilization. Cerebral blood flow showed a decline from 79.3 ml/min/100 g of brain tissue at the mean age of 17 to 46 ml/min/100 g at the mean age of 80, a net loss of 33.3 ml/min/100 g of brain. The rate of cerebral oxygen consumption declined from 3.6 ml/min/100 g of brain tissue at the mean age of 17 to 2.7 ml/min/100 g at the mean age of 80.[13]

Nerve conduction velocity of the individual over 50 years also differs from that of younger adults. By 80 to 90 years of age, conduction velocity equals about 50 m/sec, whereas a young adult has a conduction velocity of approximately 60 m/sec. This loss of conduction velocity appears to be slightly greater in aging women. Nerve conduction velocity in the elderly is also affected by an increased synaptic delay and a change in neurotransmitters. Recent studies indicate that in the human brain, monoamine oxidase (MAO) and serotonin increase with age while norepinephrine decreases. This reciprocal increase may explain the depression and apathy often associated with aging.[13]

Vertebrae The vertebral column may show advancing kyphosis in the thoracic region of the elderly patient. This degenerative change is the result of osteoporosis, vertebral collapse, or changes in vertebral cartilage. As the vertebral cartilage calcifies, there is decreased mobility of the vertebral column.

Spinal cord The basic reflex arc does not change with the aging process. However, the spinal cord may show changes in sensory conduction because of decreased vascularity of the white matter in the cord. Therefore diminished reflexes in the distal portion of the lower extremities (i.e., ankle) are not uncommon. Degenerative changes in the peripheral nerves are responsible for the loss of vibratory sense at the ankles. Reflexes of the upper extremities should be intact in the healthy elderly individual.

■ NORMAL FINDINGS

"Normal" behaviors must be evaluated in terms of the patient's baseline pattern, as well as significant variables (i.e., anxiety) affecting the assessment process. One way to establish the patient's baseline is through a careful and thorough health history. Whenever the health history or the physical examination provides data indicating a deviation from normal, that symptom or complex of symptoms requires a comprehensive symptom analysis.

Normative behaviors of the geriatric patient may vary from source to source. Therefore it is recommended that the examiner cross reference the assessment findings with the patient's previous patterns of behavior. The examiner also must carefully consider the effect on behavior of such variables as physical illness, displacement, examiner approach, change in self-image, and physiologic changes (i.e., diminished sense of hearing or vision).

General Cerebral Functions

Appearance and behavior Age, height, weight; body proportionate in size in terms of body parts; clean; groomed; dressed appropriate to age, sex, peers, and background; *older adult:* Length of trunk decreased in relation to extremities

Posture Shoulders back and relaxed; arms rest at sides; feet rest on floor (if applicable); stands with narrow base; *older adult:* may assume posture with slight semiflexion at principal joints; stands with narrow to medium base; may exhibit kyphosis in thoracic spine region with accompanying backward tilt of head

Gestures Smooth; coordinated; deliberate

Movements Coordinated; smooth; deliberate; able to change positions with smooth, even movements; *older adult:* changes position with slow, even movements

Facial expression   Facial features symmetric; establishes eye contact; acknowledges examiner presence; uses eye contact throughout interview

Attention   Able to complete thought processes (i.e., able to repeat series of numbers forward and backward); has continuity of ideas

Level of consciousness   Responds appropriately to visual, auditory, tactile, and painful stimuli; oriented to person, place, time; able to carry out simple and complex commands; opens eyes spontaneously; extraocular eye movement present; *older adult:* may respond more slowly but still appropriately to visual, auditory stimuli; may demonstrate diminished response to tactile and painful stimuli; able to carry out simple and complex commands, with slower response time

A reliable guide to the quick determination of the level of neurologic status in an individual who may or may not be able to participate in more advanced testing is the Glasgow coma scale (GCS) (Table 3-6). This scale measures three faculties: eye opening, best motor response, and best verbal response. Numbers are assigned to each of the responses in the three categories. The lowest possible score is 3; 15 is the highest. A GCS of less than 7 indicates a coma state. Serial scores have value in trending patient status. To score, the patient's best response is elicited in each category and the points added

Intellectual functions   Memory: immediate; able to repeat a series of numbers (e.g., 12, 9, 5, 1, 6); recent: able to repeat correct series of numbers after 5 min; remote: able to state correct birthplace; able to correctly state personal and vocational history; abstract reasoning: able to describe meaning of simple proverbs such as "A stitch in time saves nine," or "Rome wasn't built in a day"; insight: demonstrates consistent awareness of reality and perception of self; *older adult:* may demonstrate increased resistance to "new" ideas

---

 EMERGENCY ALERT

ALTERED LEVEL OF CONSCIOUSNESS

Changes in a person's level of consciousness (LOC) can be serious, must be assessed further, and are a symptom not a diagnosis. LOC is an important vital sign because it reflects cerebral perfusion and function.

Assessment

• Determine patient's baseline status.
• Assess ability to verbalize.
• Assess ability to follow commands.
• Assess orientation to person, time, place, and situation.
• Assess response to pain, light pressure.
• Assess pupillary response.
• Use the Glasgow Coma Scale to score.

Interventions

• Maintain airway, breathing, and circulation.
• Ensure patient safety.
• Interventions are directed as underlying cause is discovered.

Specific Cerebral Functions

Sensory interpretation   Visual: recognizes objects; differentiates between size and shape; auditory: able to identify sound made by ringing bell; tactile: able to recognize familiar objects through use of touch (stereognosis); *older adult:* longer response time

Cortical   Motor integration: able to carry out a skilled act such as protruding tongue, using a comb; comprehension: able to answer questions correctly throughout history, interview, and examination; judgment: able to discuss plans for future

Language and speech   Smooth, flowing; easily able to formulate words; varied inflections; pace, clarity, tone, volume, and vocabulary appropriate to age and educational level; demonstrates ability to read appropriate to educational level; able to write letters and numbers to dictation; *older adult:* flow may be slightly decreased

Emotional status   Affect: appropriate to verbalization; body behaviors indicative of mild to moderate anxiety; mood: consistent with conversation; cooperates with examiner

Thought processes   Content: spontaneous, natural, logical, and free flowing; *older adult:* thought patterns become more concrete; thought patterns increase in orderliness

Cranial Nerves

Olfactory (I)   Able to identify aromatic, volatile, nonirritating substances (e.g., lemon, peppermint) with each nostril;

TABLE 3-6 Glascow Coma Scale

Category	Response	Score (points)
Eye opening	Eyes open spontaneously	4
	Eyes open in response to voice	3
	Eyes open in response to pain	2
	No eye opening response	1
Best verbal	Oriented (e.g., to person, place, time)	5
	Confused, speaks but is disoriented	4
	Inappropriate, but comprehensible words	3
	Incomprehensible sounds but no words are spoken	2
	None	1
Best motor	Obeys command to move	6
	Localizes painful stimulus	5
	Withdraws from painful stimulus	4
	Flexion, abnormal decorticate posturing	3
	Extension, abnormal decerebrate posturing	2
	No movement or posturing	1
TOTAL POINTS POSSIBLE		**3-15**

older adult: may demonstrate diminished sense of smell; able to identify changes in aromatic substances with each nostril

Optic (II) See Chapter 6

Oculomotor, trochlear, abducens (III, IV, VI) Eyelids symmetric and not drooping; pupils equal in size, regular in outline, with prompt and equal reaction (direct and consensual) to light stimulus; conjugate gaze; smooth conjugate eye movements intact through six cardinal positions of gaze; prompt accommodation to distant and near objects; bilaterally, equal corneal light reflex; *older adults:* eyelids appear less elastic; eye movements intact with some limitation of upward gaze; eyes may be unable to converge

Trigeminal (V) Sensory: bilateral blink when limbus of cornea touched with cotton wisp; symmetric tickling sensation when cotton wisp touched to anterior scalp, paranasal sinuses, and jaws; symmetric pressure and pain sensation when alternating blunt and sharp ends of a safety pin are touched to anterior scalp, paranasal sinuses, and jaws; symmetric warm and cold sensation felt when patient is tested for temperature over anterior scalp, paranasal sinuses, and jaws; motor: patient experiences bilaterally strong contractions of temporal and masseter muscles

Facial (VII) Sensory: able to correctly identify sweet, sour, salty, and bitter substances placed on anterior tongue; motor: symmetry of facial movements such as smiling, frowning, closing eyes, raising eyebrows, showing teeth, and puffing out cheeks

Acoustic (VIII)
Cochlear division: bilateral ability to hear whispered voice (from distance of 1-2 ft); able to hear watch ticking (from distance of 1-2 in); Weber test: sound heard equally in both ears; Rinne test: Sound heard twice as long by air conduction as by bone conduction

Vestibular division (tested only with history of vertigo)
Bárány test: demonstrates a feeling of nausea, slow horizontal nystagmus toward side irrigated, with past pointing and falling; Bárány chair rotation: nystagmus, past pointing, and postural deviation in direction of chair movement; vertigo and sensation of continued movement in opposite direction of chair movement; electronystagmography: No displacement of corneal-retinal potential bilaterally

Glossopharyngeal and vagus (IX, X) Immediate contraction of pharyngeal muscles, with or without gagging, with lateral, upper, lower, and posterior stimulation; speech smooth, without hoarseness; able to identify tastes of sweet, salty, sour, and bitter on posterior third of tongue

Spinal accessory (XI) Able to turn head against resistance: sternocleidomastoid muscle bilaterally equal in strength and symmetry; able to shrug shoulders against resistance with bilaterally equal strength of upward movement

Hypoglossal (XII) Able to protrude tongue in midline; able to move tongue in and out of mouth rapidly; able to wiggle tongue from side to side (Table 3-7)

Proprioception; Cerebellar and Motor Function

Gait Maintains upright posture of trunk; walks unaided with narrow base, weight shifts from one extremity to another, pelvis approximately at right angle to weight-bearing extremity; maintains balance; opposing arm swing; *older adult:* maintains upright posture of trunk (if no kyphosis); walks with narrow to medium base

Romberg test Slight swaying, but upright posture and narrow foot stance maintained

Tandem walk Able to walk heel to toe in straight line

One-foot balance Able to maintain position for at least 5 sec; bilaterally equal response with eyes open and eyes closed

Hop in place Able to maintain balance, hop on one foot, and stay in place: bilaterally equal response

Knee bends Able to perform knee bends while maintaining balance

Upper extremity testing Able to rapidly pronate and supinate hands with bilaterally equal timing, purposeful movement; able to touch nose repeatedly with alternate index finger in rhythmic fashion (eyes open and eyes closed); able to rapidly and purposefully touch each finger to thumb; able to move index finger from nose to examiner's finger in coordinated fashion (each hand tested)

Lower extremity testing Able to purposefully run heel down contralateral shin with bilaterally equal coordination

Muscle strength and tone See Chapter 4

Sensory Functions

Primary Light touch: able to perceive light or tickling sensation; able to identify location touched correctly; pain: able to perceive pain sensation as sharp or dull; able to identify area touched correctly; temperature: able to perceive sensation as hot or cold; vibration: able to perceive sensation of vibration

Discriminating sensation Stereognosis: able to identify common object (e.g., key, pencil) by handling it; two-point discrimination: able to distinguish whether touched by one or two objects; palms, 8-12 mm; dorsum of hands, 20-30 mm; fingertips 2.8-5 mm; dorsa of fingers, 4-6 mm; chest

TABLE 3-7 Mnemonic for Learning Cranial Nerves

#	Nerve	First Initial
I	Olfactory	On
II	Optic	Old
III	Oculomotor	Olympus
IV	Trochlear	Towering
V	Trigeminal	Top
VI	Abducens	A
VII	Facial	Finn
VIII	Acoustic	And
IX	Glossopharyngeal	German
X	Vagus	Viewed
XI	Spinal Accessory	Some
XII	Hypoglossal	Hops

and forearm, 40 mm; back, 40-70 mm; upper arms and thighs, 75 mm; shins, 30-40 mm; *older adult:* may evidence diminishment from normal adult findings; graphesthesia: can recognize traced letter or number on hand, back; double simultaneous sensation: able to distinguish if touched on one or two sides of body (at same level); *older adult:* may not be able to distinguish; kinesthetic: able to identify change in position of fingers as up or down

Reflexes

Superficial   Upper abdominal (T8, T9, T10): upward movement of umbilicus toward area of stimulus; *older adult:* may be diminished or absent; lower abdominal (T10, T11, T12): downward movement of umbilicus toward area of stimulation; *older adult:* may be diminished or absent; cremasteric (T12, L1): elevation of ipsilateral testicle as cremaster muscle contracts (males only); gluteal (L4 to S3): Contraction of anal sphincter

Deep tendon   Biceps (C5, C6): flexion of arm at elbow; triceps (C6, C7, C8): extension of arm at elbow and contraction of triceps muscles; finger flexion (C7 to T1): fingers flexed; brachioradialis (C5, C6): flexion at elbow and pronation of forearm; patellar (L2, L3, L4): extension of leg at knee and contraction of quadriceps; *older adult:* may be diminished; achilles (S1, S2): plantar flexion of foot at ankle; *older adult:* may be absent; see box for grading and recording of deep tendon reflexes

Pathologic   Plantar (Babinski) (L4, L5, S1, S2): dorsal flexion of great toe with fanning of other toes; chaddock (L4, L5, S1, S2): dorsal flexion of great toe with fanning of other toes; clonus: no movement of foot

CONDITIONS, DISEASES, AND DISORDERS

▌BRAIN ABSCESS

A brain abscess is a suppurative infection consisting of a collection of pus within the parenchyma of the brain.

The incidence of brain abscesses is site specific, depending on such factors as the size of the area and the amount of cerebral blood flow. As a result, 80% of the abscesses are found in the cerebrum, and 20% are found in the cerebellum. Statistics indicate that 5% to 20% of brain abscesses occur in more than one site. The individual with a brain abscess presents a difficult clinical situation, since a 30% to 60% mortality rate is associated with the disorder. Surgical intervention may reduce the mortality, but this depends on accessibility of the abscess and the general condition of the patient. Morbidity following a brain abscess presents continued difficulties. Individuals surviving brain abscesses may experience different types of neurologic deficits including paralysis and seizures.

▌GRADING AND RECORDING OF DEEP TENDON REFLEXES

Deep tendon reflexes (DTR) are graded according to the following scale:

0	absent
1+	present, but diminished
2+	normal
3+	increased, slightly hyperactive
4+	brisk, hyperactice; clonus may also be present

Patient's reflex scores are recorded by entering the correct scores at the correct location on a stick figure.

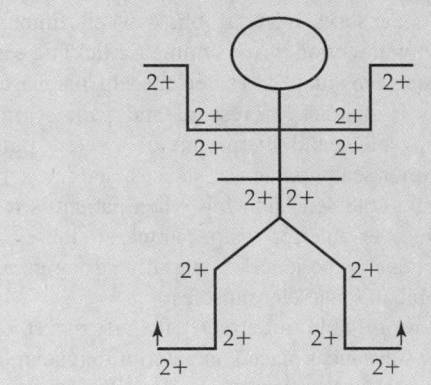

•••••• Pathophysiology

The majority of brain abscesses result from extension of chronic middle ear, sinus, or mastoid infections. The bacteria of these infections can invade the cranial vault directly through the bone, through spinal dura mater, across the subdural and subarachnoid spaces, or along venous channels as in the extension of a septic thrombophlebitis. Suppuration from the ear accounts for one third to one half of all brain abscesses and produces disease either in the ipsilateral cerebellar hemisphere or in the temporal lobe. Extended infections from the frontal sinuses primarily affect the anteroinferior parts of the frontal lobes. Sphenoidal sinusitis may extend to the frontal or temporal lobes, and ethmoid sinusitis may extend to the frontal lobes.

Penetrating head injuries, compound skull fractures, and osteomyelitis of the skull also may lead to the formation of a brain abscess. Patients with right-to-left cardiac shunts are susceptible to the formation of brain abscesses because of polycythemia, which causes cerebral ischemia and necrosis. Most abscesses disseminated through the bloodstream are multiple and found in the white matter, particularly in areas distal to those perfused by the middle cerebral artery.

Organisms commonly isolated as the cause of brain abscesses include streptococci, aerobic Enterobacteriaceae, and the staphylococci. Anaerobic bacteria (i.e., *Bacteroides fragilis*) and aerobic Enterobacteriaceae (i.e., *Escherichia coli, Klebsiella*) are found in suppurative ear infections. Anaerobic and microaerophilic streptococci, *Bacteroides, Fusobacterium,* and *Veillonella* species are found in suppurative lung infections. Staphylococci frequently are associated with penetrating head injuries and endocarditis. In patients with impaired host resistance, disseminated fungal infections (e.g., candidiasis) may also result in brain abscesses. In the patient with AIDS, brain abscess may be caused by the protozoal organisms, *Toxoplasma gondii.*

Following the initial implantation of bacteria there is a localized inflammatory reaction (i.e., cerebritis or encephalitis), which is characterized by local edema, hyperemia, leukocyte infiltration, and parenchymal softening. Several days to weeks after bacterial invasion of the brain tissue, there is central liquefaction and necrosis of brain tissue that produce a cystic mass of pus. The cystic mass is encapsulated by a wall of granulated tissue from migration of fibroblasts. Continued fibroblastic activity and gliosis result in replacement of granulation tissue of the abscess wall by collagenous connective tissues. The encapsulation process usually is completed within about 3 weeks. The abscess wall generally is thinnest on the ventricular side, predisposing this side to rupture. Infiltration of the leptomeninges (subarachnoid and pia mater) may lead to low-grade cerebrospinal fluid pleocytosis (greater than normal number of cells in cerebrospinal fluid). When the infection extends toward the cortex, meningitis results; when it extends toward the ventricles, ventriculitis results.

•••••• Diagnostic Studies and Findings

Lumbar puncture *Contraindication: may precipitate brain herniation if intracranial pressure is elevated severely;* rebound increases in intracranial pressure may occur during or after lumbar puncture

Roentgenograms: skull, sinuses, mastoid processes, chest Helpful in locating associated suppurative processes

CT scan Locates well-formed and encapsulated abscesses; visualizes ventricle size and midline displacement

Brain scan Locates abscesses over 1 cm in size; sensitive in early cerebritis when local alteration in permeability of blood-brain barrier can be visualized

CSF studies (if done) Slight increase in pressure; increase in WBC; increased protein; normal glucose levels; CSF cultures nonspecific unless abscess has ruptured

Carotid arteriography Locates temporal lobe abscesses; posterior circulatory arteriography used to locate cerebellar abscesses

Magnetic resonance imaging (MRI) Same as CT scan without radiation

Electroencephalogram (EEG) Marked slowing at sites of abscess

Brain biopsy Isolates pathogen

•••••• Multidisciplinary Plan

Surgery

Aspiration or complete excision and evacuation of abscess (method depends on site and accessibility of lesion)

Stereotaxic biopsy (for lesions deep in the brain)

Craniotomy (done only when abscess is encapsulated)

Medications

Anti-infective agents; course of therapy may be 6 wk
  Penicillin G, 20 million units IV qd
  Chloramphenicol (Chloromycetin), 50 mg/kg/d in divided doses q6h IV
  Nafcillin (Unipen), 500 mg IV q4h
    Semisynthetic, resistant penicillin used *if Staphylococcus aureus* isolated
  Metronidazole (Flagyl)
  Loading: 15 mg/kg IV over 1 h
  Maintenance: 7.5 mg/kg IV over 1 h q6h
  Used if anaerobic bacteria such as *Bacteroides fragilis* are isolated
Dexamethasone (Decadron), 6-12 mg IV q6h
Pyrimethamine (Daraprine, Fansidar for T. gondii)
Sulfadiazine for T. gondii

Anticonvulsants-Phenytoin (Dilantin)

General Management

Serial-order CT scans or brain scans to monitor progression
Support of vital functions (e.g., ventilator) if indicated
Physical therapy
Nutritional services: high caloric intake
Treatment of elevated intracranial pressure
Social services
Occupational therapy

NURSING CARE

Nursing Assessment

Pain Related to Increased Cerebral Pressure

Headache (70% of patients) that becomes increasingly severe
Activation phase
  Increased pulse
  Increased blood pressure
  Increased respiratory rate
  Dilated pupils
  Pallor
  Increased muscle tension
  Cold perspiration
  Raised hairs on some parts of body
Rebound phase
  Blood pressure lower than before pain experience
  Pulse rate slower than before pain experience
Adaptation phase
  Pain occurring frequently or for long duration: pulse rate and blood pressure not increased as much as in activation phase

Stress reaction
  Pain persisting for many days
  Increased production of 17-ketosteroids
  Increased production of eosinophils
  Increased susceptibility to other infections
Vocalizations
  Grunt
  Whimper
  Groan
  Sob
  Cry
  Gasp
Facial expressions
  Clenched teeth
  Eyes open wide or tightly shut lids
  Wrinkled forehead
  Biting lower lip
Other
  May withdraw socially
  May not initiate conversation

Airway Clearance

Patient's ability to handle secretions
Airway patency

Breathing Patterns

Arterial blood gases as per protocol
  a. Report changes in arterial oxygen pressure (PO_2) of 10-15 mm Hg
  b. Report changes in P_{CO_2} of 10-15 mm Hg

Level of Consciousness

Note level of consciousness, orientation, and ability to understand
Lethargy
Irritability
Confusion or coma

Increased Intracranial Pressure

Arterial blood gases, blood chemistry, and serum electrolytes are appraised
Changing level of consciousness (see p. 242 for additional signs and symptoms of increased intracranial pressure)
Papilledema (late sign)
Changes in respiratory patterns

Meningeal Irritability

Nuchal rigidity (25% of patients)

Seizure Activity

Generalized or focal (30% of patients)
Preconvulsive (preictal) stage
  Aura: flash of light; sense of loss, fear; weakness; dizziness; peculiar taste, smell, and sounds

  Cry or scream
  Fall to floor
  Loss of consciousness
  Tachypnea
Convulsive stage
  Tonic: rigid body; flexed jaws; clenched fists; extended legs; cyanosis; holding breath
  Clonic: urinary and/or fecal incontinence; jerking of facial muscles and extremities; biting tongue; frothing at mouth
Postconvulsive (postictal) stage
  Altered level of consciousness
  Headache
  Nausea and/or vomiting
  Malaise
  Muscle soreness
  Aspiration
  Breathing difficulty, choking, cyanosis, decreased breath sounds, tachycardia, tachypnea

Other

Selective aphasia (if temporal lobe involved)
Weakness of lower facial muscles
Ataxia, nystagmus, incorrdination of extremities, and occasionally intention tremors (cerebellar abscess)
Impaired two-point discrimination, altered position sense, astereognosis, visual inattention, and impaired opticokinetic nystagmus (parietal lobe abscess)

Fluid Balance

Intake and output

Anxiety

Appearance
  Increased perspiration, clammy skin
  Fatigue
  Increased muscle tension (rigidity)
  Skin blanches; pale
  Increased small motor activity (i.e., tremors, restlessness)
Behavior
  Decreased attention span
  Increased immobility
  Decreased ability to follow directions
Other
  Increased rate or depth of respirations
  Increased heart rate
  Rapid shifts in body temperature, blood pressure
  Urinary urgency
  Diarrhea
  Dry mouth
  Decreased appetite
  Pupillary dilation

Skin Integrity

Assess skin turgor and pressure for areas of breakdown

Assessment Findings Related to Specific Location of Brain Abscess

Temporal Lobe

Dysphasia (sensory)
Cranial nerves III and VI palsies
Disturbances in visual fields
Contralateral facial paresis

Frontal Lobe

Localized frontal headache
High fever
Seizures
Scalp tenderness
Lethargy, disorientation
Contralateral paralysis/hemiparesis
Dysphagia (motor)

Cerebellum

Nuchal rigidity (stiff neck)
Ipsilateral ataxia
Dystonia
Suboccipital headache
Nystagmus
Dysfunction of III, IV, V, and VI cranial nerves

Nursing Dx & Intervention

Ineffective airway clearance related to altered cerebrovascular status

- Maintain patent airway; avoid flexion of neck if patient is comatose.
- Suction as needed *to prevent obstruction.*
- Assist ventilation as per protocol.
- Monitor vital signs and neurologic status every 1 to 2 hours and PRN.
- Keep emergency drugs and ventilator at bedside.
- Maintain nothing-by-mouth status *to prevent risk of choking and aspiration.*

Ineffective breathing pattern related to altered cerebrovascular status

- Maintain patent airway; intubation and assisted ventilation may be indicated *to maintain adequate respiratory status.*
- Note respiratory rate, depth, and level of consciousness every 15 to 30 minutes and as needed.
- Check blood pressure, temperature, and pulse rate every 1 to 2 hours and as needed *to monitor cardiovascular status.*
- Administer medications as per protocol.
- Limit fluid intake as ordered; may include titrating fluids according to pulmonary artery pressure, central venous pressure, or pulmonary capillary wedge pressure.

Altered cerebrospinal tissue perfusion related to high risk for intracranial hypertension

- Take and record ECG rhythm strips every 2 to 4 hours and as needed, noting rate and rhythm.
- Measure intake and output. Report hourly output less than 30 ml *to identify potential hypotension or fluid overload.*
- Monitor hemodynamics (central venous pressure, arterial pressure, pulmonary artery pressure, pulmonary capillary wedge pressure) as per protocol.
- Monitor intracranial pressure (if monitoring device is used) every 30 minutes to 1 hour *to monitor neurologic status. **Continuous flushing devices must not be used for measuring ICP.***
- Monitor vital signs every 1 to 2 hours and as needed.
- Maintain head of bed at 20- to 30-degree elevation *to facilitate cerebral venous drainage.*
- Maintain body alignment.

Pain related to increased cerebral pressure

- Assess and document patient's degree of pain.
- See general intervention strategies listed on p. 1637.

Risk for impaired skin integrity related to prolonged immobility

- Administer skin care every 2 to 4 hours *to stimulate circulation.*
- Turn patient every 2 hours *to minimize pressure points on the skin.*
- Use air mattress or egg-crate mattress *to prevent skin breakdown.*
- Use sandbags or footboard *to prevent footdrop.*
- Keep skin dry.

Sensory/perceptual alterations related to altered cerebrovascular status

- Keep side rails up at all times when patient is alone. Maintain patient safety at all times *to prevent injury.*
- Maintain quiet environment, reducing external stimuli to a minimum *to reduce sensory overload.*
- Reorient patient frequently to time, place, and person. Introduce yourself each time you reorient patient.
- Repeat explanations frequently and simply *to facilitate understanding.*
- Have family bring in familiar objects *to provide sense of security.*
- Maintain planned rest periods *to allow sufficient time for REM sleep.*
- Use day and night lighting appropriately *to facilitate normal sleep-wake patterns.*
- Stimulate senses of touch, taste, and position.

Personal identity disturbance related to altered sensory and perceptual states

- See general intervention strategies listed on p. 1688.

Risk for injury related to seizure activity

Preconvulsive

- Have oral airway at bedside *to prevent airway obstruction.*
- Have suction equipment available at bedside.
- Pad side rails, if indicated, *to prevent injury if patient is restless.*
- Administer oxygen per protocol.
- Identify auras if possible.

Convulsive

- Maintain patent airway.
- Support and protect head; turn to side if possible *to protect airway.*
- Prevent injury.
- Ease to floor if patient is in chair.
- Place pillows along side rails if patient is in bed *to prevent injury.*
- Remove surrounding furniture.
- Loosen clothing *to prevent constriction.*
- Provide privacy as necessary.
- Stay with patient; remain calm *to provide reassurance.*
- Note frequency, time, involved body parts, and length of seizure *to establish the type of seizure activity.*

Postconvulsive

- Maintain patent airway.
- Suction as indicated.
- Check vital signs and neurologic status every 15 minutes.
- Administer oxygen per protocol.
- Reorient patient to environment *to minimize sensory-perceptual alteration.*
- Provide emotional support *to minimize fear and anxiety.*
- Place patient in position of comfort; turn head to side.
- Administer oral hygiene as necessary for secretions and bleeding.
- Prepare for diagnostic tests if ordered: CT scan, skull series, arteriogram, EEG.

Potential for infection related to hematogenous dissemination of pathogen

- Monitor temperature q 4 hours and WBC daily to monitor effectiveness of drug therapy.
- Maintain strict use of universal precautions to prevent secondary infections.
- Monitor heart rate, respiratory rate, and BP q 4 hours and PRN.
- Administer selected anti-infective therapy as prescribed.
- Monitor for signs of meningitis: nuchal rigidity, headache, chills, and diaphoresis.

Patient Education/Home Care Planning

1. Ensure the patient and family know and understand the following:
   a. Nature of a brain abscess, treatments, and procedures; explain as they occur
   b. Need to ambulate as tolerated
   c. Importance of maintaining planned rest periods
   d. Names of medications, dosages, frequency of administration, purposes, and toxic or side effects
   e. Need to avoid taking over-the-counter medications without consulting physician
   f. Possible residual effects such as headaches, sensory or motor deficits, seizures
2. Discuss with the patient and the family ways to recognize seizure activity and appropriate course of action:
   a. Sit or lie down.
   b. Avoid trying to stop seizure or restraining patient.
   c. Protect patient from injury.
   d. Observe and record body parts involved and duration of seizure activity.
3. Ensure that the patient and family understand importance of ongoing outpatient care (i.e., physician's visits and physical therapy).
4. Explain to the patient and family the importance of maintaining a well-balanced diet.

Evaluation

Patient demonstrates effective airway clearance Breath sounds are normal. Chest excursion is symmetric. Rate and depth of respirations are normal. Cough is effective. There are no subjective or objective findings of shortness of breath, air hunger, or dyspnea on exertion.

Patient demonstrates an effective breathing pattern Patent airway is maintained. Chest excursion is symmetric. Breath sounds are normal, or there is no increase in adventitious sounds. Arterial blood gas values are within normal ranges or consistent with patient's baseline. Vital signs are within normal ranges or consistent with patient's baseline. Hemoglobin levels are 14 to 18 g/dl (male) and 12 to 16 g/dl (female). Intake and output are stable. There are no signs of respiratory distress. Resonance of all lobes is evident on percussion. Skin color is without cyanosis.

Patient maintains adequate cerebral and spinal tissue perfusion There is no change in level of consciousness. There is no evidence of neurologic deficits. Pattern of electrolytes is stable. There is no seizure activity.

Patient demonstrates intact skin integrity Skin is intact. Nutritional status is adequate. Electrolyte balance is maintained. Patient is free of pressure sores from contractures.

Patient experiences minimal alterations in comfort Patient openly verbalizes feelings of discomfort when they occur. Patient is able to use measures to decrease discomfort. Patient verbalizes a decrease in subjective feelings of discomfort. There is a decrease in objective findings of pain.

Patient demonstrates minimal complications of sensory-perceptual alterations Patient maintains optimal level of mobility. Patient remains free of injury. Skin integrity is maintained. Nutritional status is adequate. Patient demonstrates minimal self-care deficits. Patient demonstrates social participation appropriate to physiologic status.

Patient demonstrates intact self-concepts Patient openly verbalizes feelings of grief, loss, etc. Patient verbalizes positive feelings about self. Patient acknowledges actual changes in self-image. Patient focuses on present and future appearance and function. Patient verbalizes feelings of hopefulness and helpfulness.

Patient remains free of traumatic injury Safety measures appropriate to level of physiologic status are used. Skin integrity is maintained. Skin is free of bruises, burns, abrasions, redness, etc. Environment is safe. Patient is free of nosocomial infections.

Patient is free of signs and symptoms of infection Patient is afebrile and WBC is 5000 to 10,000/mm³. Patient's vital signs are stable.

HYDROCEPHALUS

Hydrocephalus is characterized by an abnormal accumulation of cerebrospinal fluid within the cranial vault with subsequent dilation of the cerebral ventricles.[48]

Hydrocephalus has an incidence of 4 per 1000 births through the age of 3 months, but can occur at any age. In infants it is considered a primary disease, whereas in later life it occurs as a complication of other diseases.

Hydrocephalus has several known causes, which can be categorized as congenital or acquired. Congenital abnormalities obstruct the flow of cerebrospinal fluid; 70% of these obstructions result from stenosis of the aqueduct of Sylvius. Other anomalies causing or associated with hydrocephalus are the Arnold-Chiari malformation, Dandy-Walker syndrome, and spina bifida cystica.[47] Flow and absorption of cerebrospinal fluid also can be affected by fibrosis of meninges and obstruction of the aqueduct and basal cisterns caused by inflammatory lesions.

Causative mechanisms of hydrocephalus are (1) excessive secretion of cerebrospinal fluid as a result of a choroid plexus papilloma, (2) obstruction of cerebrospinal fluid flow in the ventricles or subarachnoid space, (3) obstruction by pacchionian granulations, and (4) hemodynamic production. Common sites for obstruction of cerebrospinal fluid are the third ventricle, the fourth ventricle, the foramina of Monro, and the aqueduct of Sylvius. Each site may be obstructed by a mass within or outside the lumen. Pacchionian granulations caused by inflammatory processes and fibrosis can occlude the arachnoid villi, preventing the escape of cerebrospinal fluid from the subarachnoid space and resulting in hydrocephalus.

Although most causes of hydrocephalus are associated with intraventricular hypertension, there are two types in which intraventricular pressure is not elevated. *Hydrocephalus ex vacuo* results in ventricular dilation to fill spaces caused by a decreasing neural mass (e.g., Alzheimer's disease and stroke). *Normal pressure hydrocephalus* is characterized by dilated ventricles, normal neural tissue mass, and normal intracranial pressure.

The etiology and pathology of normal pressure hydrocephalus remain to be elucidated.

Communicating vs. Noncommunicating Hydrocephalus

A *communicating* or extraventricular hydrocephalus occurs when the obstruction is outside the ventricular system; therefore flow between the ventricles is not blocked. Excessive cerebrospinal fluid accumulates in the ventricles because the fluid is not adequately absorbed from the cerebral subarachnoid space. The *noncommunicating,* or intraventricular, hydrocephalus results in an accumulation of cerebrospinal fluid from a block of the normal flow at some point in the ventricular system. The cerebral ventricles proximal to the block then dilate.

•••••• Pathophysiology

When there is an obstruction in the ventricular system or in the subarachnoid space, the cerebral ventricles dilate, causing the ventricular surface to stretch, disrupting its ependymal lining. The underlying white matter atrophies and may be reduced to a thin ribbon. There is selective preservation of the gray matter, even when the ventricles have attained enormous size. The dilation process may be an insidious or acute process and may be selective, depending on the site of blockage. The acute process may cause a medical emergency. In the infant and young child the cranial sutures split and widen to accommodate the increasing cranial mass. If the anterior fontanel is not closed, it bulges and feels tense to palpation. Aqueductal stenosis, a sex-linked familial disease, causes a marked dilation of the lateral and third ventricles. This dilation gives the head a characteristic dominant frontal brow appearance. The Dandy-Walker syndrome occurs when there is an obstruction of the exit foramina of the fourth ventricle. Consequently the fourth ventricle dilates, with the posterior fossae becoming prominent and bossing below the tentorium. This type of hydrocephalus gives the patient generalized symmetric enlargement of the cerebrum, and the face appears disproportionately small.

In the older individual the cranial sutures have closed; therefore the space is fixed and limits expansion of the brain mass. As a result the older person usually exhibits the signs and symptoms of increased intracranial pressure before the cerebral ventricles become greatly enlarged.

Defects of cerebrospinal fluid absorption and circulation in hydrocephalus are not complete. Formation of cerebrospinal fluid exceeds the capacity of the normal ventricular system every 6 to 8 hours, and a total lack of reabsorption is incompatible with life. Ventricular dilation causes a disruption of the normal ependymal lining of the walls of the cavities, permitting increased absorption. If the collateral route is adequate to prevent progressive ventricular dilation, a state of compensation may exist.[12]

•••••• Diagnostic Studies and Findings

Angiography Detection of vessel abnormalities caused by stretching; vascular lesions

CT scan/MRI   Detection of variations in tissue density; presence of cysts or masses; visualization of the ventricular system

Lumbar puncture   Diagnosis of communicating hydrocephalus; *contraindication:* elevated intracranial pressure; *performing lumbar puncture on patient with increased ICP may result in brain herniation.*

Subdural/ventricular puncture   As for lumbar puncture

Ventriculography   Visualization of ventricular system configuration; shows ventricular dilation with hydrocephalus

•••••• Multidisciplinary Plan

Surgery*

Correction of CSF obstruction such as resection of cyst, neoplasm, or hematoma

Ventricular bypass into normal intracranial channel (i.e., Torkildsen procedure where CSF is shunted from lateral to cisterna magna) in noncommunicating hydrocephalus

Ventricular bypass into extracranial compartment (i.e., ventriculoperitoneal or ventriculoatrial shunt)

Reduction of CSF production as in third or fourth ventriculostomy or endoscopic choroid plexus extirpation (plexectomy or electric coagulation)

Medications

Acetazolamide (Diamox), 8-30 mg/kg in divided doses, IV

Mannitol (Osmitrol), in initial management of severe increased intracranial pressure

Dexamethasone (Decadron), 6-20 mg q6h IV

General Management

Intracranial pressure monitoring
Cardiac monitoring
Respiratory monitoring
Physical therapy
Speech/Occupational therapy
Dietary consultation

NURSING CARE

Nursing Assessment

Head Circumference (Pediatrics)

Severely enlarged head
Bulging fontanels after pulsation
Fixed downward gaze of eyes with visible sclera above (sunset gaze)
Visible, distended scalp veins
Radiation of light throughout accumulated cerebrospinal fluid with translumination

*Therapy of choice.

Vomiting

More frequent in older patient
Likely to occur in morning (frequency may increase with increased intracranial pressure)

Seizures

Focal or general tonic-clonic seizures
May assume opisthotonic position

Behavioral Changes

Feeds poorly (pediatrics)
Lethargy
Irritability when stimulated
Apathy, inattentiveness

Increased Intracranial Pressure

Change in level of consciousness, restlessness, lethargy
Decreased pulse
Increased systolic blood pressure
Widened pulse pressure
Irregular and decreased respirations
Pupillary changes—papilledema (late)
Seizures
Worsening of focal neurologic signs

Muscle Tone

Alteration of muscle tone in extremities

Later Assessment Findings

Physical and/or mental development lag
Prominence of forehead
Scalp shiny, with scalp veins prominent
Optic atrophy, strabismus, nystagmus, exposed sclera

Nursing Dx & Intervention

Ineffective breathing pattern related to impaired respiratory mechanics

- Assess arterial blood gases as ordered:
    Report decrease of Po_2 of 10 to 15 mm Hg.
    Report increase of Pco_2 greater than 10 to 15 mm Hg.
- Maintain patent airway.
- Have intubation and assisted ventilation equipment at bedside.
- Suction as needed.
- Auscultate breath sounds before and after suctioning *to determine effectiveness of secretion removal.*
- Position for maximum lung expansion; elevate head of bed slightly (10 to 20 degrees).
- Note respiratory rate and depth and level of consciousness every 15 to 30 minutes and as needed.
- Check pulse rate, temperature, and blood pressure every 1 to 2 hours and as needed.
- Administer medications as per protocol.
- Limit fluid intake as per protocol; include titrating according to intracranial pressure.

- Measure and record intake and output; report hourly output less than 30 ml *to detect hypervolemia.*
- Administer tube feedings per protocol *to ensure adequate nutrition.*

Altered cerebral tissue perfusion related to enlarged ventricular system

- Assess values and waveforms of intracranial pressure line, if appropriate **(Continuous flushing devices are not used for ICP measurement):**
  - Maintain patency and sterility of system.
  - Monitor effects of treatments on intracranial pressure.
  - Correlate neurologic status with intracranial pressure values, and notify physician if inconsistent.
- Assist with drainage of cerebrospinal fluid from system, if indicated, *to prevent or control intracranial hypertension.*
- Intervene *to prevent increased intracranial pressure:*
  - Administer medications, treatments, and intravenous fluids per protocol.
  - Maintain elevation of head of bed per protocol *to maximize cerebral venous drainage.*
  - Accurately record intake and output.
  - Monitor serum electrolytes, blood count, and arterial blood gases for abnormalities.
- Intervene to monitor or prevent seizures:
  - Assess seizure history of patient.
  - Institute seizure precautions *to minimize potential for injury to the patient:*
    - Airway at bedside
    - Bed height at lowest level *to prevent falls*
    - Side rails up at all times and padded, if needed, *to prevent patient injury*
    - Oxygen and suction equipment at bedside
    - Emergency medications at bedside
  - Administer anticonvulsants as per protocol:
    - Monitor effects and side effects.
    - Monitor serum for therapeutic levels of anticonvulsant.
- Provide preoperative nursing care for patient who will have shunt implantation:
  - Monitor vital signs and neurologic status every 15 minutes to 1 hour and as needed.
  - Suction or aspirate mucus as needed *to prevent airway obstruction.*
  - Observe for signs and symptoms of shock.
  - Administer medications (i.e., antibiotics and anticonvulsants).
  - Turn every 2 hours and provide skin care every 2 hours *to protect skin integrity.*
  - Insert nasogastric tube to decompress abdomen.
  - Avoid hyperthermia and hypothermia.
- Provide postoperative nursing care after shunt implantation:
  - Position patient and pump shunt per protocol *to maintain maximum effectiveness.*

Compress valve specified number of times at regular intervals.
Accurately measure intake and output and record on flow sheet.
Administer parenteral fluids per protocol.
Administer feedings per protocol *to provide adequate nutrition.*
Monitor for signs of complications, such as dehydration, infection, or fluid overload.
Monitor serum antibiotic levels.

Sensory/perceptual alterations related to altered sensory integration

- Assess and record patient's level of orientation.
- Have side rails up at all times when patient is alone *to prevent injury or fall.*
- Maintain patient safety at all times.
- Judiciously use soft restraints; monitor patient's response.
- Involve family in aspects of care as appropriate *to minimize feelings of powerlessness.*
- Frequently reorient patient to time, person, and place.
- Reintroduce yourself each time you reorient patient.
- Have family bring in familiar objects *to promote sense of security.*
- Allow family to stay with patient.
- Maintain planned rest periods *to allow sufficient time for REM sleep.*
- Use day and night lighting appropriately *to promote normal sleep-wake cycle.*
- Stimulate patient's sense of touch, taste, and position.

Impaired skin integrity related to physical immobilization

- Assess patient's skin condition for redness when turning or providing skin care.
- See general intervention strategies listed on p. 1559.
- Prevent pressure sores and contractures:
  - Keep scalp dry and clean.
  - Reposition every 2 hours, and turn head frequently.
  - (Maintain neck in neutral alignment *to facilitate cerebral venous drainage and prevent increased intracranial pressure*).
- Rotate head and body together *to prevent strain on neck.*
  - Provide passive ROM exercises, especially to lower extremities, every 4 hours and as needed *to prevent contractures.*

Patient Education/Home Care Planning

1. Make certain the patient and family know and understand the following:
   a. Nature of hydrocephalus, treatments, and procedures; explain as they occur
   b. Care of shunt devices if indicated
   c. Need to ambulate as tolerated

d. Importance of maintaining planned rest periods
e. Names of medications, dosages, frequency of administration, purposes, and toxic or side effects
f. Need to avoid taking over-the-counter medications without consulting physician
g. Possible residual effects such as headaches, sensory or motor deficits, seizures
2. Discuss with the patient and the family ways to recognize seizure activity and the appropriate course of action:
   a. Assist patient to sit or lie down.
   b. Avoid trying to stop seizure or restraining patient.
   c. Protect patient from injury.
   d. Observe and record body parts involved and duration of seizure activity.
3. Ensure that the patient and family understand the importance of ongoing outpatient care (i.e., physician's visits and physical therapy).
4. Explain to the patient and family the importance of maintaining a well-balanced diet.

Evaluation

Patient demonstrates an effective breathing pattern Patent airway is maintained. Chest excursion is symmetric. Breath sounds are normal or there is no increase in adventitious sounds. Arterial blood gas values are within normal ranges or consistent with patient's baseline. Vital signs are within normal ranges or consistent with patient's baseline. Hemoglobin levels are 14 to 18 g/dl (male) and 12 to 16 g/dl (female). Intake and output are stable. There are no signs of respiratory distress. Resonance of all lobes is evident on percussion. Skin color is without cyanosis.

Patient maintains adequate cerebral tissue perfusion There is no change in level of consciousness. There is no evidence of neurologic deficits. Pattern of electrolytes is stable. There is no seizure activity.

Patient demonstrates minimum complications of sensory-perceptual alterations Optimum level of orientation is maintained. The patient remains free of injury. Skin integrity is maintained. Nutritional status is adequate. Self-care deficits are minimal. Social participation is appropriate to physiologic status.

Patient demonstrates skin integrity Skin is intact. Nutritional status is adequate. Electrolyte balance is maintained. Patient remains free of pressure sores and contractures.

CRANIAL AND PERIPHERAL NERVE DISORDERS

BELL'S PALSY

Bell's palsy (facial paralysis) is the paralysis of the facial nerve (cranial nerve VII), resulting in a sudden loss of ability to move the muscles of expression of the face (Figure 3-25).

Any or all of the three branches of the facial nerve may be affected. The disorder can be unilateral or bilateral, transient or permanent. Generally the disorder appears static for about

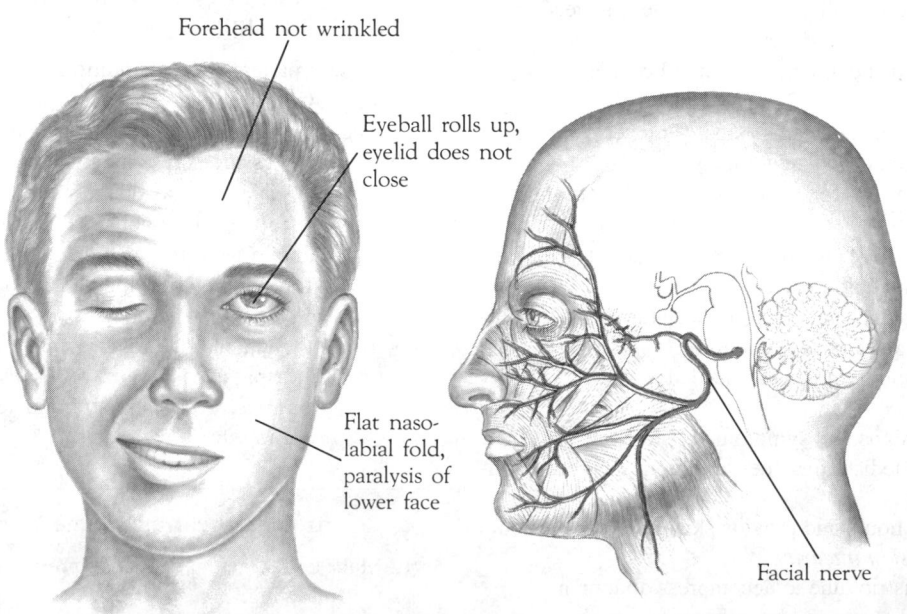

Forehead not wrinkled

Eyeball rolls up, eyelid does not close

Flat naso-labial fold, paralysis of lower face

Facial nerve

Figure 3-25 Bell's palsy. (From Chipps et al.[16])

10 days to 2 weeks, at which time muscle tone begins to reappear. Voluntary movement of the muscles may appear within 3 or 4 weeks. However, some individuals manifest no recovery for almost 6 months, and maximum recovery (which may not be complete) may occur in approximately a year. More than 80% of the patients with Bell's palsy recover without residual neurologic deficits.[17]

•••••• Pathophysiology

The pathogenesis and pathophysiology of Bell's palsy are unclear. One hypothesis is that a viral infection of the geniculate ganglion is responsible for the disorder. Other possible mechanisms include local ischemia and edema or emotional trauma and the resulting vasoconstriction.[24]

The disorder can occur at any age but most frequently occurs in individuals between 20 and 60 years. Men and women are affected about equally. The diagnosis of Bell's palsy is made by clinical features and a characteristic history.

•••••• Multidisciplinary Plan

Medications

Corticosteroids
   Prednisone (Deltasone), 20-60 mg/d po; dosage is gradually reduced
Analgesics as required

General Management

Electrical stimulation of nerve
Warm, moist heat
Massage
Facial sling to prevent muscle stretching and to facilitate eating (by improving lip alignment)
Facial exercises (i.e., wrinkling brow, forcing eyes closed, puffing out cheeks) for 5 minutes three or four times daily, as muscle tone returns
Swallowing precautions
Nutritional consultation

NURSING CARE

Nursing Assessment

Pain

Usually begins behind the ear
May or may not be accompanied by herpetic vesicles in the external ear

Paralysis

Drawing sensation on affected side, followed by complete paralysis of affected side of face: all muscles powerless and flaccid (i.e., cannot smile, wrinkle forehead, or close eye; drooling of saliva; constant eye tearing)

Taste

Loss of taste sensation over anterior two thirds of tongue on affected side

Eating and Drinking Difficulties

May see anorexia and weight loss
Impaired ability to chew and swallow increases the potential for choking and aspiration

Nursing Dx & Intervention

Pain related to cranial nerve VII irritation

* Establish baseline and ongoing assessment of patient's perception of discomfort.
* Provide gentle massage as needed *to relieve pain and promote relaxation.*
* Provide warm moist heat per protocol.
* Provide for electrical stimulation per protocol *to relieve severe pain.*
* Apply facial sling as needed *to prevent muscle stretching and facilitate eating.*
* Administer pain medications per protocol.
* Provide eye care every 1 to 2 hours and as needed *to prevent corneas from drying and injury.*
* Apply moist eye pads as indicated *to prevent injury and to minimize eye strain.*
* Teach patient to perform facial exercises three or four times daily for 5 minutes *to promote muscle tone:*
   Wrinkling brow
   Grimacing
   Whistling
   Puffing out cheeks
   Forcing eyes closed
* Provide patient with sunglasses as needed *to prevent eye strain.*

Altered nutrition: less than body requirements related to inability to ingest foods

* Assess patient's ability to chew and swallow.
* Offer patient frequent, small feedings *to maintain adequate caloric intake.*
* Maintain soft diet as indicated *to minimize choking.*
* Avoid hot fluids and foods *to prevent burns to insensitive areas.*
* Provide patient with privacy at mealtimes *to minimize anxiety and embarrassment.*
* Provide patient with adequate time for eating meals.
* Teach patient to take foods on unaffected side *to minimize discomfort.*
* Apply facial sling *to improve lip alignment.*
* Teach patient to chew food on unaffected side.
* Provide meticulous mouth care before and after meals.
* Provide dietary supplements as indicated *to maintain adequate caloric intake.*

Impaired verbal communication related to pain

• See general intervention strategies listed on p. 1715.

Anxiety related to threat to self-concept

• See general intervention strategies listed on p. 1669.
• Assist patient to deal with anxiety about the disorder, discomfort, changes in self-image, and fear of recurrence; explain possible causes and treatments for the disorder:
  State explanations simply and monitor reactions.
  Repeat explanations as indicated.

Impaired social interaction related to self-concept disturbance

• See general intervention strategies listed on p. 1702.

Patient Education/Home Care Planning

1. Discuss with the patient the possible causes, involvement, symptoms, treatments, and usual course of Bell's palsy (explain procedures as they occur).
2. Discuss signs of complications and progression of the disorder.
3. Explain special techniques such as the use of facial slings, massage, dietary adjustments, and exercise program to minimize discomfort.
4. Stress importance of continued eye care.
5. Explain safety measures for minimizing trauma to insensitive areas.
6. Explain names of medications, dosage, frequency of administration, purpose, and toxic or side effects of the medication.
7. Stress importance of ongoing outpatient care: physician's visits, physical therapy and exercise program, and support groups.

Evaluation

Patient and family demonstrate adequate knowledge of Bell's palsy Patient is able to explain possible causes of Bell's palsy. Patient is able to explain treatment modalities for the disorder. Patient is able to explain the usual course of the disorder.

Patient demonstrates minimal discomfort Patient is able to use measures such as facial sling and warm massage as needed. Patient openly expresses feelings of discomfort when they occur. Patient is able to perform facial exercises as indicated.

Patient demonstrates adequate nutritional status Weight pattern is stable: normal for height, age, sex, and previous baseline. Intake and output are balanced and stable. Diet is appropriate to age. Skin turgor is good. There is fluid and electrolyte balance. Dietary supplements are used as appropriate.

Patient does not demonstrate the complications of impaired communication

Patient demonstrates a low level of anxiety Patient openly verbalizes concerns and feelings of grief, loss, and dis-

comfort. Open verbalization of feelings is supported by the health care professionals and family.

Patient demonstrates an intact, realistic body image Patient openly verbalizes feelings of grief and loss. Patient verbalizes positive feelings about self. Patient acknowledges actual changes in self-image. Patient focuses on present appearance and function. Patient verbalizes feelings of hopefulness, helpfulness, and powerfulness.

Patient demonstrates social participation Patient can state the importance of interpersonal relationships. Patient can relate to self and others. Patient participates in unit or group activities. Patient participates in family activities as appropriate to his condition.

■ GUILLAIN-BARRÉ SYNDROME

Guillain-Barré syndrome is an acute syndrome characterized by widespread inflammation or demyelination of ascending or descending nerves in the peripheral nervous system that results in impaired nerve impulse conduction between the nodes of Ranvier (Figure 3-26).

Guillain-Barré syndrome has an incidence of 1.7 per 100,000 persons. Eighty-five percent of individuals affected by the Guillain-Barré syndrome have complete functional recovery. The recovery period usually extends over several weeks, but it may last months or even years. The remaining 15% of affected individuals experience some degree of permanent neurologic deficit.

Guillain-Barré syndrome is also known as acute idiopathic polyneuritis, acute polyradiculoneuropathy, postinfectious polyneuritis, Landry-Guillain-Barré-Strohl syndrome, infectious neuronitis, infectious polyneuritis, acute polyradiculitis, acute idiopathic polyradiculoneuritis, and acute inflammatory polyradiculoneuropathy.

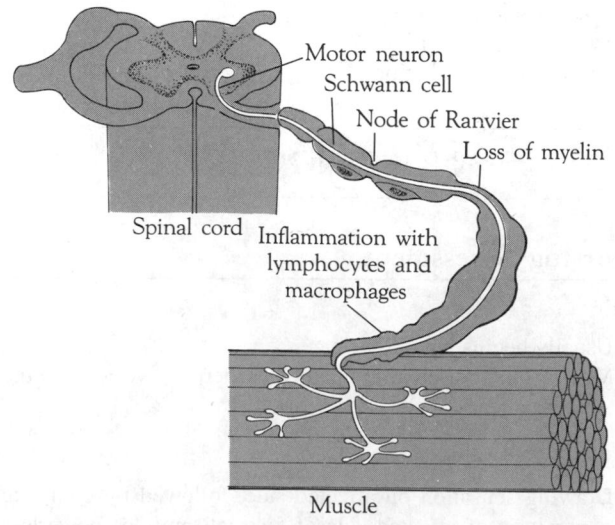

Figure 3-26 Demyelination of nerve segments in Guillain-Barré syndrome. (From Chipps et al.[16])

······ Pathophysiology

The pathogenesis of Guillain-Barré syndrome is thought to be related to the sensitization of peripheral nerve myelin and is characterized by infiltration of mononuclear cells at all levels of the peripheral nervous system. Over half of the individuals affected have had a mild, nonspecific infection 10 to 14 days before the onset of Guillain-Barré symptoms, suggesting that sensitized lymphocytes may produce demyelination. A significant number of persons have developed symptoms characteristic of Guillain-Barré syndrome after being inoculated for the swine flu. The syndrome occurs in both sexes and can affect persons of any age.

Morphologic alterations that characterize Guillain-Barré syndrome include (1) widespread monocytic inflammatory infiltrate around blood vessels throughout the cranial and spinal nerves, including nerve roots, ganglia, and distal nerves; (2) segmental demyelination of peripheral nerves; and (3) in severe cases, axon destruction with resultant axonal reaction and wallerian degeneration. Anterior horn cells and neurons in dorsal root ganglia occasionally show central chromatolysis. If the axon loss is severe, denervation group atrophy can be seen in distal muscles. Electron microscopic studies have shown a breakthrough of the basement membrane of the Schwann cell by phagocytic cells that insinuate themselves beneath the myelin layers and are then stripped away.[53]

Complications from Guillain-Barré syndrome, although rare, may occur in the acute phase. These complications may include respiratory failure, cardiovascular collapse, bradycardia, hypertension, infection/sepsis, and syndrome of inappropriate secretions of antidiuretic hormone (SIADH).

Diagnostic Studies and Findings

CSF sampling Albuminocytologic dissociation: decreased protein initially (15 to 45 mg); then increases as high as 600 mg; followed by return to normal; lymphocyte count normal

Electromyography (EMG) Reduced nerve conduction velocity when tested near peak of illness (usually 4 to 8 weeks after onset); low voltage potentials; fibrillations and positive sharp waves (more common in late stages). *Pulmonary function tests (PFT)* below normal for patient's height and weight

······ Multidisciplinary Plan

Surgery

Tracheotomy (see Chapter 2) indicated if respiratory failure occurs

Medications

Pituitary hormones
  Corticosporin (ACTH), 25-40 U IM or subcutaneously tid (possibly valuable if given early in course of the disorder; dosage and frequency individually determined)
Corticosteroids
  Prednisone (Deltasone), 5-80 mg/d in divided doses

Anti-infective agents
  Prophylactic antibiotics
Anticoagulants (Heparin)

General Management

Cardiac monitoring
Hemodynamic monitoring
Mechanical ventilation/respiratory support
Intubation or tracheostomy
Plasmapheresis (plasma exchange)
Chest physiotherapy
Arterial blood gas monitoring
Nutritional maintenance (e.g., IV or nasogastric feedings)
Nutritional consultation
Special eye care
Bowel/bladder management
Physical therapy
Psychosocial counseling

NURSING CARE

Nursing Assessment

Autonomic Function

Hypertension
Sinus tachycardia or bradycardia
Postural hypotension
Chest and abdominal tightness
Profuse diaphoresis
Urinary incontinence, constipation
Paroxysmal facial flushing
Heart block

Cranial Nerve Function

Cranial nerve VII most commonly involved; abnormal testing response elicited
Dysphagia
Dysarthria

Motor Function

Patient's ability to provide self-care varies
Weakness following paresthesia
Most common type of weakness is ascending (i.e., lower to upper limbs to trunk)
Equal involvement of proximal and distal muscles
Atrophy possible

Reflex Status

Deep tendon reflexes absent or diminished

Sensory Function

Usually less severe than motor involvement
Superficial or deep sensory involvement: usually stocking-glove distribution

Level of Consciousness

Not usually affected
Patient's anxiety level is a factor

Respiratory Function

Airway patency
Assess breath sounds, arterial blood gases as per protocol
Respiratory muscle paralysis

Nursing Dx & Intervention

Ineffective breathing pattern related to neuromuscular impairment

- Auscultate breath sounds every 1 to 2 hours; assess quality and any increase in adventitious sounds.
- Maintain patent airway. Intubation, tracheostomy, and mechanical ventilation may be indicated.

Risk for aspiration related to depressed gag reflex

- Suction as needed *to prevent airway obstruction and aspiration.* Hyperoxygenate lungs with 100% oxygen for 1 minute before and 1 minute after suction, unless contraindicated. Maintain aseptic technique.
- Monitor mechanical ventilation, if used:
    Ensure that tidal volume, rate, mode, and oxygen concentration are set as ordered.
    Ensure that ventilator alarms are on and functional.
- Monitor arterial blood gases per protocol *to check for signs of respiratory failure:*
    Report decrease in Po_2 of 10 to 15 mm Hg.
    Report increase in Pco_2 greater than 10 to 15 mm Hg.
- Note respiratory rate, depth, and level of consciousness every 15 to 30 minutes and as needed.
- Check blood pressure, temperature, and pulse rate every 1 to 2 hours and as needed based on patient's condition *to monitor for signs of autonomic dysfunction.*
- Assist and teach patient to cough and deep breathe every 2 hours *to improve respiratory functioning.*
- Administer medications per protocol.
- Limit fluid intake per protocol: may include titrating fluids according to pulmonary artery, pulmonary capillary wedge, or central venous pressure.
- Measure and record intake and output; report hourly output less than 30 ml.
- Monitor hemodynamics (central venous pressure, arterial pressure, pulmonary artery pressure, pulmonary capillary wedge pressure) per protocol.

Impaired physical mobility related to neuromuscular impairment

- See general intervention strategies listed on p. 1597.

Feeding, bathing/hygiene, dressing/grooming, and toileting self-care deficit related to impaired mobility status

- Avoid giving oral feedings *to minimize risk of aspiration;* administer IV or nasogastric feedings per protocol.

- Administer oral hygiene every 2 hours and as needed.
- Provide daily hygiene care *to promote cleanliness and self-esteem.*
- Provide eye care every 2 hours *to prevent injury:*
    Cleanse eyes and remove crust.
    Apply eye shields or tape eyes closed *to protect cornea.*
    Administer artificial tears or eye drops per protocol *to provide lubrication.*
- Maintain bowel function with regular evacuation *to prevent constipation.*

Anxiety related to altered sensory and motor functions

- Deal realistically and honestly with patient's anxiety about the disorder, the discomfort, and the change in self-image.
- Explain potential treatments for the disorder:
    State simply and monitor patient's reactions.
    Repeat explanations, as indicated.
- Teach basic relaxation techniques. Reinforce teaching, as indicated.
- Teach the essential aspects of care, as indicated by the patient's condition.
- Assist the patient to participate in making decisions about care, as indicated by patient's condition.
- Alert staff to possible emotional changes; expect mood swings.

Body image, personal identity, and self-esteem disturbances related to altered sensory and motor functions

- See general intervention strategies listed on pp. 1680, 1685, and 1688.

Ineffective individual coping related to sudden illness and physiologic crisis

- Assess coping mechanisms and behavior patterns *to determine baseline information.*
- Provide patient with opportunity to express fears and concerns *to help reduce tension.*
- Encourage participation in care as tolerated *to reduce feelings of powerlessness.*
- Encourage family participation in care and emotional support *to reinforce importance of emotional care.*
- Obtain psychologic consult if indicated.

Patient Education/Home Care Planning

1. Encourage open verbalization regarding fears of permanent disability, loss of function, and dying, as well as changes in body image.
2. Stress importance of avoiding individuals who have upper respiratory infections.
3. Emphasize importance of maintaining planned rest periods.

4. Stress need for independence and socialization:
   a. Encourage self-care.
   b. Encourage patient to eat meals with family.
5. Explain each medication, dosage, frequency of administration, purpose, and toxic or side effects.
6. Stress need to check with physician before taking any over-the-counter medication.
7. Emphasize need to exercise to tolerance level and avoid fatigue.
8. Stress need for high-caloric, high-protein diet; progress from soft to solid as tolerated.
9. Emphasize need to arrange utensils and food so they are easily managed by the patient.
10. Discuss need to maintain fluid intake at 2000 ml daily, unless contraindicated.
11. Stress need to avoid constipation:
    a. Drink fluids.
    b. Use stool softeners (as approved by physician).
    c. Eat foods and fruits high in roughage.
12. Emphasize need for diversional activities (e.g., watching television, reading, listening to radio).
13. Stress importance of ongoing outpatient care: physician's visits, physical therapy, and occupational therapy.
14. Ensure the patient or family demonstrates the following: speech exercises, active and/or passive ROM exercises with massage to all extremities, and exercises that increase strength and mobility of fingers (e.g., squeeze toys, balls, clay).
15. Discuss importance of warm baths to alleviate pain and stiffness.

Evaluation

Patient demonstrates an effective breathing pattern Airway remains patent. Chest excursion is symmetric. Vesicular, bronchial, and bronchovesicular breath sounds are normal with no adventitious sounds. Arterial blood gas values are within normal ranges or consistent with patient's baseline. Vital signs are within normal limits or consistent with patient's baseline. Hemoglobin levels are 14 to 18 g/dl (male) and 12 to 16 g/dl (female). Intake and output are stable. There are no signs of respiratory distress (i.e., nasal flaring, increased pulse rate, air hunger). All lobes are resonant on percussion. Skin color is not cyanotic.

Patient remains free of aspiration Airway is patent. Vital signs are stable. Patient reports no sensation of choking. Breath sounds are normal.

Patient demonstrates minimum complications of impaired physical mobility Skin integrity is maintained. Contractures and deformities do not form. Level of mobility is appropriate to physiologic status. Intake and output pattern is stable. Nutritional status is adequate. There are no signs or symptoms of thrombophlebitis. There are no signs or symptoms of local infection.

Patient demonstrates minimum self-care deficits Outcome criteria stated for impaired physical mobility are met.

Level of self-care is appropriate to physiologic status. Diet is high in calories and protein. Physical and occupational therapy is given as indicated.

Patient demonstrates a low level of anxiety Patient openly verbalizes concerns and feelings of grief, loss, and discomfort. Patient openly verbalizes feelings, supported by health care professionals and significant others. Patient verbalizes essential aspects of care. Patient is able to demonstrate relaxation techniques when feelings of anxiety begin.

Patient demonstrates intact self-concept Patient openly verbalizes feelings of grief and loss. Patient verbalizes positive feelings about self. Patient acknowledges actual change in self-image. Patient focuses on present and future appearance and function. Patient verbalizes feelings of hopefulness, helpfulness, and powerfulness.

Patient demonstrates adequate individual coping Effective coping mechanisms are used, and patient shows no irritability, insomnia, or tension.

TRIGEMINAL NEURALGIA
(Tic douloureux)

Trigeminal neuralgia, or tic douloureux, is a neurologic condition that affects the sensory distribution of the trigeminal facial nerve (cranial nerve V) and is characterized by flashing, stab-like paroxysms of pain radiating along the course of a branch of cranial nerve V from the angle of the jaw (Figure 3-27).[67]

Terminal neuralgia is caused by degeneration of or pressure on the nerve. Any of the three branches of the nerve may be

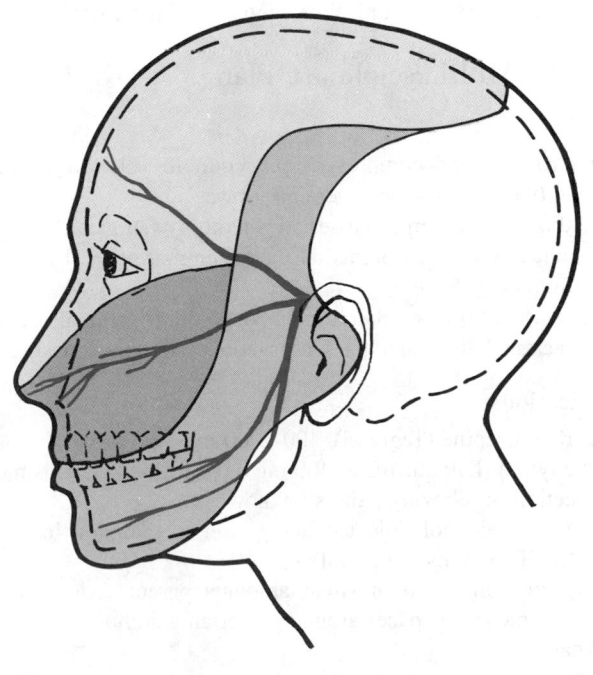

Figure 3-27 Pathway of trigeminal nerve and facial areas innervated by each of the three main divisions of this nerve. (From Phipps et al.[49])

affected. Attacks of lancinating pain, caused by trigeminal neuralgia, often cause the person to wince with facial contractions, thus the term "tic douloureux."

• • • • • • Pathophysiology

The etiology of trigeminal neuralgia is unknown. The term "neuralgia" is used because there is no demonstrable structural lesion along the course of the nerve. A similar syndrome can occur in cases of multiple sclerosis, gasserian ganglion tumor, cerebellopontine tumor, or brainstem infarction.[37] The idiopathic form of trigeminal neuralgia affects 15,000 individuals in middle adult to late adulthood each year. There is slightly higher incidence in women.

Although any of the trigeminal nerve's three branches can be affected, the second (maxillary) and third (mandibular) divisions are most commonly involved. Neuralgia of the first division (ophthalmic) results in pain over the forehead and around the eyes. Neuralgia of the second division results in pain in the nose, cheek, and upper lip, and when it occurs in the third division it causes pain in the lower lip and on the side of the tongue. Episodes of the pain recur over weeks or months, although there may be spontaneous remissions. Tender areas (trigger zones) and any mechanical activity such as smiling, talking, or touching the face can set off an attack.[35] These trigger points are the parts of mucous mem-brane or skin that are close to the involved nerve. Common trigger points are:

First division: supraorbital notch
Second division: infraorbital foramen close to the junction of the cheek and nose
Third division: side of the tongue or the mental foramen

The diagnosis of trigeminal neuralgia is based on the characteristic history and clinical presentation of the disorder.

• • • • • • Multidisciplinary Plan

Surgery

Microvascular decompression procedure for selective cutting of fibers within the trigeminal nerve
Radio frequency retrogasserian rhizotomy (surgical lesions, made at selected points on the trigeminal nerve, by radio frequency current)
Avulsion of the peripheral branches of the trigeminal nerve
Intracranial division of the sensory root of the trigeminal nerve

Medications

Carbamazepine (Tegretol), 400-1000 mg/d po or IV
Phenytoin (Dilantin), 200-400 mg/d po or IV (mechanism of action in relieving pain is unknown)
Absolute alcohol: injected into gasserian ganglion in very small amounts (i.e., 1 ml)
Glycerol: injection of small amounts percutaneously into subarachnoid spaces around gasserian ganglion
Analgesics

General Management

Semisolid, fluid diet; nutritional consult
Psychosocial counseling

Social services
Home health consult

NURSING CARE

Nursing Assessment

Pain

Severe, shooting pain, starting at a particular point with a repetitive tic and increasing in severity to where it shoots violently and with explosive force through the face on the affected side
Discover what precipitates pain

Apprehension

Protects face from any stimulation

Personal Identity

Actual change in function of facial nerve
Protection of face from any form of stimulation
Change in social involvement
Verbalization of:
    Negative feelings about self
    Preoccupation with change or loss
    Focus on past appearance and function
    Feelings of powerlessness, helplessness, hopelessness
Change in life-style
Fear of rejection by others

Altered Nutrition

Food must be proper temperature and consistency

Social Isolation

Preoccupation with own thoughts and meaningless, repetitive activities
Dull, sad affect
Hostility projected in voice and behavior
Seeks to be alone
Withdrawn, uncommunicative, no eye contact
Activities and interests inappropriate for developmental stage and age
Verbalizes feelings of rejection
Verbalizes interests inappropriate for developmental stage and age
Insecurity in public
Expresses feeling different from others
Inability to meet others' expectations
Absence of, or insecurity in, significant purpose in life

Nursing Dx & Intervention

Anxiety related to threat to self-concept

• See general strategies on p. 1669.

Pain related to pressure on trigeminal nerve

• Promote rest and relaxation *to increase coping skills.*
• Modify anxiety associated with the pain experience.

- Provide other sensory input *to serve as diversional therapy.*
- Administer medications per protocol.
- Remain with the patient *to minimize anxiety.*
- Improve effectiveness of pain relief measures by using them before the pain becomes intense.
- Administer anticonvulsant therapy.

Altered nutrition: less than body requirements related to inability to ingest food because of pain

- Offer small, frequent feedings *to encourage adequate intake.*
- Complete nursing care before feeding times.
- Allow ample time for feeding.
- Encourage a high-protein diet; semisolid food.
- Accurately measure and record intake on a flowsheet *to establish if intake is adequate.*
- Administer parenteral fluids per protocol.
- Administer tube feedings per protocol.

Body image disturbance related to threat to self-concept

- See general intervention strategies listed on p. 1685.
- Assist patient to become involved in self-care.
- Assist patient to become involved in unit activities.

Social isolation related to altered physical appearance

- Allow the patient to express perceptions regarding the illness. Offer support and clarification.
- Foster a sense of relatedness to self.
- Foster a sense of relatedness to family:
  Provide for physical closeness of family member.
  Include family in care as appropriate.
  Have patient teach family about the disorder.
- Encourage patient to personalize the environment. Allow personal items to be brought from home.
- Use touch as therapeutic intervention *to minimize depersonalization.*
- Encourage patient to verbalize needs met through interpersonal relationships.
- Encourage group activities *to enhance social skills.*
- Encourage patient to maintain good grooming habits *to promote self-esteem.*

Patient Education/Home Care Planning

1. Ensure patient's understanding of involvement, symptoms, treatments, and usual course of trigeminal neuralgia (explain procedures as they occur).
2. Discuss signs of complications and progression of the disorder.
3. Discuss measures for minimizing stimulation of affected areas and trigger zones.
4. Discuss name of medications, dosage, frequency of administration, purpose, and toxic or side effects of the medication.
5. Stress the importance of ongoing outpatient care and physician's visits.
6. Refer patient to support groups.
7. Ensure family members' understanding of possible dietary alterations.

Evaluation

Patient and family demonstrate adequate knowledge of trigeminal neuralgia Patient is able to explain treatment modalities for the disorder. Patient is able to explain the usual course of the disorder.

Patient demonstrates a low level of anxiety Patient openly verbalizes concerns and feelings of grief, loss, and discomfort. Patient openly verbalizes feelings, supported by health care professionals and family. Patient verbalizes essential aspects of care.

Patient demonstrates minimum discomfort from the disorder Patient openly expresses feelings of discomfort when they occur. Patient is able to use measures to decrease discomfort such as decreasing stimuli to affected areas and judicious use of analgesics.

Patient demonstrates adequate nutritional status Weight pattern is stable. Intake and output pattern is stable. Skin turgor is good. There is fluid and electrolyte balance. Dietary supplements are taken as appropriate.

Patient demonstrates an intact, realistic body image Patient openly verbalizes feelings of grief and loss. Patient verbalizes positive feelings about self. Patient scknowledges actual changes in self-image. Patient focuses on present appearance and function. Patient verbalizes feelings of hopefulness, helpfulness, and powerfulness.

Patient demonstrates social participation Patient states the importance of interpersonal relationships. Patient experiences a sense of relatedness to self and to others. Patient participates in unit or group activities. Patient participates in family activities, as appropriate to patient's condition.

DEGENERATIVE DISORDERS

ALZHEIMER'S DISEASE

Alzheimer's disease is a chronic neurologic disorder that is characterized by progressive and selective degeneration of neurons in the cerebral cortex and certain subcortical structures.

Alzheimer's disease was originally described in 1907 by a German neuropsychiatrist named Alois Alzheimer. At that time Alzheimer published a brief report that depicted the pathologic and clinical manifestations of a 55-year-old institutionalized woman who experienced unexplained "premature aging." Although the woman's motor function, gait, muscle strength, coordination, and reflexes remained fairly normal, she experienced severe and progressive deterioration in mental functions. At autopsy Alzheimer found that the woman's brain had widened sulci and small gyri and was smaller than those of other 50-year-old women.[6]

Alzheimer's disease is the fourth leading cause of death among alderly persons in the United States.[50] An estimated 4.4% of individuals over 65 years of age demonstrate the manifestations of moderate to severe dementia syndromes, and two thirds of this group are believed to have Alzheimer's disease.[23] Both men and women may be affected, but the incidence is higher in women. Current research efforts indicate that Alzheimer's disease is age related; it is uncommon in young persons and rare in middle age. However, as age increases, so does the incidence of the disorder such that its prevalence in individuals over the age of 80 is estimated at greater than 20%.[7]

To date, only genetics and female gender have been identified as risk factors for Alzheimer's disease. The genetic factor is believed to be inherited in the form of an autosomal dominant trait.[72] The risk associated with female gender has been attributed to two factors. First, Alzheimer's disease is age related and women live longer than men. Second, it is believed that development of Alzheimer's disease is sometimes related to a gene on the X chromosome.[6]

The onset of Alzheimer's disease is usually subtle and insidious. The duration and rate of progression vary, but for the well-cared-for patient, the average survival rate from onset is approximately 8 to 9 years.[6]

•••••• Pathophysiology

Grossly, the primary pathologic feature of Alzheimer's disease is the degeneration and loss of selective neuronal cells in the cerebral cortex that utlimately results in symmetric and extensive convolutional atrophy, particularly in the frontal and medial temporal regions. This cerebral atrophy is accompanied by an enlargement of the cerebral ventricles, which is not severe unless concomitant hydrocephalus exists.[7]

Characteristic microscopic lesions in the brain tissue of persons with Alzheimer's disease include neuritic plaques, neurofibrillary tangles, granulovacuolar degeneration, and Hirano bodies. Neuritic plaques consist of degenerated intracortical foci of clustered and thickened neurites (axons and dendrites) that surround a spherical deposit of amyloid (starchlike protein) fibrils.[7] These plaques usually are found most prominently in the frontal cortex and hippocampus. Neurofibrillary tangles (neurofibrils) consist of masses of twisted and tangled intracellular protein that are deposited primarily in the cytoplasm of neuronal cell bodies. These neurofibrils are found primarily in the hippocampus and adjacent areas of the temporal lobe and are most abundant in areas of severe neuronal loss. Granulovacuolar degeneration consists of membrane-bound vacuoles containing finely granular material that is found most prominently in the pyramidal neurons of the hippocampus. Hirano bodies are found in the neuropil and consist of intracytoplasmic eosinophilic rods.[6] Cell loss in the hippocampus is believed to correlate with the memory loss of Alzheimer's disease.

Characteristic cell loss found in the brain of an individual with Alzheimer's disease includes both cortical and subcortical structures. Cell loss in the cortex includes the larger cells of the association cortex and cholinergic cells at the rostal portion of the reticular activating system (RAS). The loss of cholinergic cells results in reduced levels of the neurotransmitter acetylcholine. Recent studies have suggested that deficiencies in cholinergic transmission may lead to a breakdown of neuronal structures and play a role in the clinical expression of Alzheimer's disease.[72] Cell loss in subcortical structures includes noradrenalin cells in the locus ceruleus and dopamine-secreting cells of the pars compacta of the substantia nigra.[6]

The basic pathophysiology processes of brain damage occurring with Alzheimer's disease are not known. One proposed etiology is related to chronic aluminum toxicity. However, recent studies indicate that while aluminum apparently does accumulate in tangle-bearing neurons, it does not appear that such an accumulation is a necessary condition for Alzheimer changes in the cell. Further, epidemiologic data does not indicate a higher incidence of Alzheimer's disease in individuals who chronically ingest aluminum (i.e., antacids).[6]

One possible reason that brain cells degenerate and die may be the reduced rate in overall cerebral metabolism in Alzheimer's disease. This cerebral metabolic reduction is approximately 25% compared to age- and sex-matched cognitively intact controls.[6] Another possibility regarding the pathophysiology of Alzheimer's is that it may be linked to some type of generalized membrane abnormalities or abnormal cellular calcium metabolism.[6]

As previously stated, the pathophysiology of Alzheimer's is not known. However, many current research efforts are targeted at unraveling the mystery of this devastating disease.

•••••• Diagnostic Studies and Findings

CT scan (serial)   Cerebral ventricular and subarachnoid space enlargement because of diffuse brain atrophy (later stages)

Magnetic resonance imaging (MRI)   Same as CT scan

Electroencephalogram   Diffuse slowing of brain waves and diminished voltage (advanced stages)

Comprehensive history   Identification of symptoms listed in the assessment section for this disorder; family history of similar disorders; careful attention to medication history

Psychometric and behavioral rating scales   Mini Mental State (MMS); Mental Status Questionnaire (MSQ); Haycox behavior scale; Hamilton depression scale

•••••• Multidisciplinary Plan

Medications

Psychotropic agents
   Haloperidol (Haldol), 2-4 mg/d po (NOTE: Haloperidol has reported risk of inducing dyskinesia tarda[6])
Sedative/Hypnotic
   Chloral hydrate, 0.5-1 g po

Antianxiety agents
  Lorazepam (Ativan), 2-6 mg/d po in divided doses
  Diazepam (Valium), 2-20 mg/d po in divided doses
  Alprazolam (Xanax), 0.75-1.5 mg/d po in divided doses
Tricyclic agents (NOTE: Agents have anticholinergic side effects that may impair cognitive function)
  Nortriptyline (Aventyl), 75-100 mg/d po
  Amitriptyline (Elavil), 25-100 mg/d po
Laxatives/stool softeners
  Ducosate sodium (Colace)

General Management

Cardiac monitoring
Support of vital functions (i.e., ventilator) if indicated
Nutritional support: soft or liquid diet
Social services consultation
Physical therapy
Psychologic counseling and support
Community referrals
Occupational therapy
Home nursing services
Extended care facility referrals

NURSING CARE

Nursing Assessment

The literature has described three stages of Alzheimer's disease.[71]

Initial Stage (2 to 4 Years)

Level of consciousness is a factor to document

Absentmindedness

Lack of spontaneity
Time and spatial disorientation
Loss of memory and emotional control
Changes in affect
Depression
Diminished ability to concentrate
Perceptual alterations
Neglectfulness in appearance
Careless actions
Judgment mistakes
Delusions (transitory) of persecution
Muscle twitching
Epileptiform seizures
Ability to provide self-care is a factor
Patient has potential for injury
Patient's level of mobility is a factor

Middle Stage (2 to 12 Years)

Assess and document level of consciousness
Nocturnal restlessness

Apraxia (impaired ability to perform purposeful activity)
Alexia (inability to comprehend written words)
Asterognosia (inability to identify objects by touch)
Auditory agnosia (total or partial inability to recognize familiar objects by the sense of sound)
Agraphia (inability to write)
Hypertonia
Increased aphasia
Hyperorality
Complete disorientation
Unsteady gait
Progressive memory loss
Increase in socially unacceptable behaviors
Decreased ability to comprehend
Preservation phenomenon (i.e., repetitive actions such as chewing, tapping)
Ability to provide self-care is a factor
Patient's skin condition may become red when cleaned
Patient's potential for injury is a factor
Patient's level of mobility is a factor

Terminal Stage (Up to 1 Year)

Level of consciousness is documented
Seizures (rare)
Marked weight loss; emaciation
Decreased appetite
Bulimia
Apraxia
Visual agnosia
Incontinence (bowels and/or bladder)
Hyperorality
Paraphasia
Hypermetamorphosis
Increased irritability
Feelings of helplessness
Bedridden
Unresponsive or comatose

Anxiety

Appearance
  Increased perspiration, clammy skin
  Fatigue
  Increased muscle tension (rigidity)
  Skin blanches: pale
  Increased small motor activity (i.e., tremors, restlessness)
Behavior
  Decreased attention span
  Increased immobility
  Decreased ability to follow directions
Other
  Increased rate or depth of respirations
  Increased heart rate
  Rapid shifts in body temperature, blood pressure
  Urinary urgency
  Diarrhea
  Dry mouth

Decreased appetite

Pupillary dilation

Seizure Activity

Generalized or focal

Preconvulsive (preictal) stage

Aura: flash of light; sense of loss, fear; weakness; dizziness; peculiar taste, smell, and sounds

Cry or scream

Fall to floor

Loss of consciousness

Tachypnea

Convulsive stage

Tonic: rigid body; flexed jaws; clenched fists; extended legs; cyanosis; holding breath

Clonic: urinary and/or fecal incontinence; jerking of facial muscles and extremities; biting tongue; frothing at mouth

Postconvulsive (postical) stage

Altered level of consciousness

Headache

Nausea and/or vomiting

Malaise

Muscle soreness

Aspiration

Breathing difficulty, choking, cyanosis, decreased breath sounds, tachycardia, tachypnea

Altered elimination

Patients demonstrate varying voiding patterns

Urine is checked for sediment, concentration, and color

Altered sleep patterns

Current sleep patterns can be compared with normal sleep patterns

Various factors may cause sleep pattern to be interrupted

Patient's daytime habits and activities should be noted

Nursing Dx & Intervention

Sensory/perceptual alterations related to neurologic disease

- Keep side rails up at all times when patient is alone *to minimize risk for falls and injury.*
- Maintain patient safety at all times.
- Maintain quiet environment, reducing external stimuli to a minimum.
- Reorient patient frequently to time, place, and person.
- Introduce yourself each time you reorient patient.
- Repeat explanations frequently and simply *to facilitate understanding;* speak slowly in a calm voice.
- Have family bring in familiar objects *to provide memory aids.*
- Maintain planned rest periods *to allow sufficient time for REM sleep.*
- Use day and night lighting appropriately *to promote normal sleep-wake cycle.*
- Stimulate senses of touch, taste, position.
- Have visitors or staff wear name tags.

- Document observation of patient's memory skills.
- Call patient by preferred name *to aid in self-recognition.*
- Maintain consistent caregivers.
- Maintain a simple and consistent schedule of care activities.
- Post large calendar *to aid in time and date orientation.*

Feeding, bathing/hygiene, dressing/grooming, and toileting self-care deficit related to progressive neuromuscular impairment

- Assist with feeding, as indicated; use IV or nasogastric feedings per protocol.
- Administer oral hygiene every 2 hours and as needed *to remove secretions and promote comfort.*
- Assist with daily hygiene care as indicated.
- Administer eye care every 2 to 4 hours if indicated *to prevent dryness and injury.*
- Perform intermittent urinary catheterization per protocol.
- Maintain bowel function with regular evacuation *to prevent constipation.*

Risk for impaired skin integrity related to altered mobility and sensation

- Prevent pressure sores and contractures:
  Keep skin dry and clean.
  Reposition every 2 hours; massage pressure areas after turning *to stimulate circulation.*
  Provide passive ROM exercises every 4 hours and as needed *to prevent contractures.*
    Perform ROM exercises gently, slowly, and rhythmically.
    Repeat each ROM exercise three times, every 4 hours.
  Use footboard or Spence boots *to prevent footdrop.*
- Maintain high-protein, low-calcium diet *to prevent muscle wasting.*

Risk for injury related to seizures

- Institute safety measures.
- Maintain bed in low position at all times unless side rails are up or when nurse is with the patient.
- Provide the patient with a call light within easy reach.
- Maintain side rails in up position at bedtime, after sedation, when patient is confused, and as needed.
- Maintain wheelchairs and stretchers in locked position when transferring patient.
- Pad side rails if patient is overactive.

Preconvulsive

- Have oral airway at bedside *to prevent obstruction.*
- Support and protect head; turn to side if possible *to prevent aspiration.*
- Prevent injury:
  Ease to floor if in chair.
  Place pillows along side rails if in bed.
  Remove surrounding furniture.
  Loosen constrictive clothing.
- Provide privacy as necessary *to protect patient's dignity.*
  Stay with patient; remain calm.

- Note frequency, time, involved body parts, and length of seizure *to determine type of seizure.*
  Postconvulsive
- Maintain patent airway.
- Suction as indicated.
- Check vital signs and neurologic status.
- Administer oxygen per protocol *to minimize cerebral hypoxia.*
- Reorient patient to environment *to minimize perceptual alteration.*
- Place patient in position of comfort; turn head to side *to prevent aspiration.*
- Administer oral hygiene as necessary for secretions and bleeding.

Impaired physical mobility related to perceptual-cognitive impairment

- Assess and document patient's level of mobility.
  - Change position slowly *to prevent orthostatic hypotension.*
  - Position in proper body alignment.
- Use firm mattress or bed board *to support back and spine.*
- Apply antiembolus stockings to lower extremities *to promote venous return.*
- Administer anticoagulation therapy per protocol *to prevent embolus formation.*
- Observe for signs of thrombophlebitis
- Provide passive range of motion exercises *to maintain joint mobility.*

Altered patterns of urinary elimination related to sensory and neuromuscular impairment

- Perform intermittent catheterization per protocol.
- Monitor intake and output. Maintain fluid intake at 2000 ml/day unless contraindicated.
- Assess urine for sediment, concentration, color, and odor.
- Acidify urine with foods such as orange juice and cranberry juice *to minimize potential for infection.*
- Administer urinary tract germicides (e.g., methenamine mandalate [Mandelamine]) as ordered.

Altered nutrition: less than body requirements related to sensory and neuromuscular impairment

- Offer small, frequent feedings *to encourage adequate intake.*
- Complete nursing care before feeding times.
- Allow ample time for feeding.
- Encourage a high-protein, low-calcium diet.
- Accurately measure and record intake on a flowsheet *to establish adequate intake.*
- Administer parenteral fluids per protocol.
- Administer tube feedings per protocol.
- Elevate head *to prevent aspiration.*

Anxiety related to altered self-concept

- See general intervention strategies listed on p. 1669.

- Support the family:
  Provide for ongoing contact.
  Give appropriate referrals to support groups.
- Assist patient to deal realistically and honestly with anxiety about inability to predict course of the disorder and change in self-image and self-esteem.

Powerlessness related to sensory and neuromuscular impairment

- Assist patient to reestablish as much physiologic control as condition allows:
  Share information about physiologic functioning with the patient.
  Focus on functions that remain intact.
- Assist patient to reestablish some means of psychologic control:
  Encourage patient to express feelings as long as possible.
  Encourage patient to participate in care as long as able to do so.
  Encourage patient to become an active decision maker about care and immediate environment as able.

Social isolation related to altered mental status

- See general intervention strategies listed on p. 1700.

Impaired adjustment related to impaired cognition

- Encourage patient to express feelings and fears regarding disease and disabilities.
- Recognize possibility of emotional responses such as anxiety, depression, withdrawal, anger, helplessness, powerlessness, and crying.
- Assist patient to examine own responses to the threatening situation.
- Avoid judgment, criticism, or belittling of feelings and ideas.
- Encourage focus on remaining strengths and intact roles.
- Support patient's spiritual beliefs.
- Encourage a sense of control:
  Include patient in specific aspects of care as appropriate.
  Share observations with patient regarding physical status and progress.
- Teach patient to understand and manage feelings of anger and helplessness.
- Assist patient to develop problem-solving skills regarding disappointments and dissatisfactions.
- Assist patient to develop a stress management plan with simple relaxation exercises, self-monitoring activities, and use of imagery.

Altered family processes related to situational transition and/or crisis

- Assist family to identify and understand what is occurring as specifically as possible *to focus on the situational factors.*
- Assist family to redefine situation in favorable terms.

- Support family in efforts to clarify family interactions.
- Assist family to express ideas assertively *to resolve the problem or situation.*
- Assist family in exploring alternatives for problem solution.
- Provide family with information about family dynamics *that enhance family's problem-solving skills.*
- Assist family in identification of consequences of proposed options for resolutions of the problem.
- Support family members in efforts to implement problem resolution.
- Assist family in evaluating effectiveness of problem solving.

Anticipatory grieving related to potential for loss of loved one

- Encourage patient and family to identify and describe their perceptions of potential loss.
- Encourage patient and family to verbalize fears and concerns *to determine need for appropriate information.*
- Recognize the following factors as influencing coping behaviors: previous experiences with life-threatening situations, socioeconomic background, spiritual beliefs, cultural beliefs, educational background.
- Identify current sources of social support to the patient and family, as well as disruptions in present life-style related to anticipated loss such as finances or living arrangements.
- Identify grieving stage the patient and family are experiencing. Recognize patient and family may differ in stages of grieving.
- During stage of shock and disbelief, provide quiet environment *to minimize noxious environmental stimuli.*
- Allow for use of denial and other defense mechanisms. *To avoid false hope,* do not reinforce denial.
- Do not confront patient or family members who have distorted perceptions.
- Facilitate expression of emotions.
- Provide assurance that intense feelings and reactions are normal.
- Enlist support from other sources of support to patient and family *to encourage appropriate use of support resources.*
- During stage of developing awareness:
  Provide family with ongoing information regarding patient's progress, care, and prognosis.
  Encourage family to express need for information and desires in caring for the patient.
  Facilitate family participation in patient's care as appropriate *to decrease feelings of isolation and loss.*
  Arrange flexible visiting hours *to promote family interactions.*
  Assist patient and family to share feelings, concerns, and fears with each other.
  Assist family members to maintain own self-care needs *to promote and maintain physical health.*

Evaluate need for referral to resources such as the social services department.
- During period of mourning before patient's death:
  Promote expression of what family expects when death occurs.
  Discuss indicators of impending death as appropriate.
  Provide comfort measures for the patient.
  Encourage family to maintain verbal communication and touch with patient even though patient may not respond.
  Provide privacy *to protect patient and family dignity.*

Sleep pattern disturbance related to sensory alterations

- Assess for factors that interfere with sleep *to determine potential causes for inadequate sleep.*
- Encourage patient to express concerns when unable to sleep.
- Assess patient's daytime habits and activities:
  Assist in planning of daytime activities.
  Discourage daytime napping if it negatively affects nighttime sleep patterns.
- Provide comfortable environment *to promote rest or sleep.*
- Teach patient simple relaxation techniques *to promote rest or sleep.*
- Decrease fluid intake before bedtime.
- Discourage intake of food or caffeine at bedtime.
- Discourage strenuous mental or physical activity before bedtime.
- Assist patient to maintain a normal day-night pattern *to facilitate sleeping at night.*
- Provide sedation per protocol if necessary. Evaluate effectiveness and side effects of sedatives.

Ineffective individual coping related to sudden illness and physiologic crisis

- Assess coping mechanisms and behavior patterns *to determine baseline information.*
- Provide patient with opportunity to express fears and concerns *to help reduce tension.*
- Encourage participation in care as tolerated *to reduce feelings of powerlessness.*
- Encourage family participation in care and emotional support *to reinforce importance of emotional care.*
- Obtain psychologic consult if indicated.

Aspiration, risk for related to enteric feeding via nasoenteric tube

- Confirm feeding tube placement after insertion, q 4 H and PRN.
  Confirm tube placement before and after each intermittent tube feeding.
  Confirm initial enteral tube placement by physician examination of chest x-ray.
- Tape nasogastric tube securely per protocol.
- Aspirate stomach contents *to determine gastric pH.*

- Assess bowel sounds q 4 H and PRN.
- Assess patient for abdominal distention, nausea/vomiting, and diarrhea/constipation.
    Hold tube feedings if bowel sounds are absent and if diarrhea/constipation or nausea/vomiting is present.
- Maintain proper patient positioning.
    Elevate head-of-bed 30 to 40 degrees.
    Turn patient to right side *to facilitate stomach drainage through pylorus.*
- Discontinue continuous feedings 30 to 40 minutes before activity/procedure that require lowering the patient's head.
- Check vital signs q 2 H and PRN.
- Check pulmonary-tracheal secretions q 4 H and PRN *to detect presence of enteral feeding.*
- Monitor for signs of aspiration including cough, wheezing, dyspnea, hyperthermia, and tachycardia.
- Auscultate breath sounds q 4 H and PRN.

Confusion, chronic related to organic or cognitive impairment

- Assess baseline physical, functional, and psychosocial status.
- Evaluate previous interests.
- Ensure optimal sensory input (i.e., eyeglasses, hearing aid) is available.
- Evaluate stimulation threshold *to prevent overstimulation.*
- Provide for structured repetitive group activities.
- Provide rest periods between activities *to minimize fatigue.*
- Monitor for changes in physical, functional, and psychologic status.
- Maintain calm, reassuring demeanor when interacting with patient *to promote sense of trust.*
- Encourage patient to participate in care as tolerated *to minimize feelings of powerlessness.*
- Provide positive feedback for tasks/activities that are mastered.

Caregiver role strain, related to severity of patient's illness

- Obtain assistance with meeting of caregiver role.
    Assist caregiver to identify/utilize caregiving resources such as family members, friends, community agencies, etc.
- Assist caregiver to develop plan of care with paced, direct care activities.
- Assist caregiver to develop support systems with alternate caregivers/friends.
- Assist caregiver to identify and address personal health care needs.

Patient Education/Home Care Planning

1. Discuss each medication's dosage, time of administration, purpose, and side effects.
2. Reinforce physician's explanation of medical management.

3. Emphasize need to avoid taking over-the-counter medications without notifying the physician.
4. Emphasize need for adequate nutritional status:
    a. Give diet as tolerated.
    b. Offer small, frequent feedings.
    c. Instruct to chew thoroughly and eat slowly and in small pieces.
5. Emphasize need for activity and exercise to tolerance:
    a. Plan activities of daily living.
    b. Maintain rest periods as planned.
    c. Do active and passive ROM exercises.
    d. Get at least 8 hours of sleep at night, if possible.
6. Encourage independent activities, as possible:
    a. Alert patient to limitations.
    b. Avoid overprotection.
    c. Stress need for supportive devices, as indicated.
7. Emphasize importance of ongoing outpatient care.
8. Give outpatient, home nursing care or extended care facility referral, as appropriate.
9. Emphasize safety measures: side rails, ramps, shower chairs, walkers, and canes.

Evaluation

Patient demonstrates minimal complications of sensory/perceptual alterations Level of orientation is optimum. Patient is free of injury. Patient demonstrates skin integrity. Self-care deficits are minimum. Social participation is appropriate to physiologic status.

Patient demonstrates minimal self-care deficits Outcome criteria listed for impaired physical mobility are met. Level of self-care activities is appropriate to physiologic status. Patient participates in physical and occupational therapy.

Patient demonstrates skin integrity Skin is intact. Nutritional status is adequate. Electrolyte balance is maintained. Patient is free of pressure sores and contractures.

Patient remains free of traumatic injury Safety measures are appropriate to physiologic status. Skin integrity is maintained. Skin is free of bruises, burns, abrasions, and redness. Environment is safe. Patient is free of nosocomial infections.

Patient demonstrates an optimum level of mobility Skin integrity is maintained. Patient remains free of contractures and deformities. Level of mobility is appropriate to physiologic status. Intake and output pattern is stable. Nutritional status is adequate. Patient is free of thrombophlebitis. Patient is free of local infection. Patient participates in an ongoing physical therapy program.

Patient demonstrates minimum complications from alterations in urinary elimination patterns Intake and output pattern is stable. Urine is clear, yellow to amber in color, and without sediment. Skin in perineal area is clean and dry. Urine is acidic (pH 6.0). Patient is free of urinary tract infections. Patient is free of bladder distention. Patient or family can describe symptoms of urinary tract infections that require medical intervention.

Patient demonstrates adequate nutritional status Weight pattern is stable. Intake and output pattern is stable. Diet is appropriate to physiologic status. Skin turgor is good. Fluid and electrolyte balance is maintained. Patient takes dietary supplements, as appropriate.

Patient demonstrates a low level of anxiety Patient openly verbalizes concerns and feelings of grief, loss, and discomfort. Patient openly verbalizes feelings, supported by health care professionals and family. Patient verbalizes essential aspects of care. Patient identifies methods to effectively deal with anxious feelings.

Patient demonstrates minimal feelings of powerlessness Optimum level of physiologic control, as possible for current health status, is maintained. Optimum level of psychologic control, as possible, is maintained. Patient participates, as possible, in decision making about care. Patient participates, as possible, in self-care.

Patient demonstrates intact self-concepts Patient openly verbalizes feelings of grief and loss. Patient acknowledges actual change in self-image. Patient verbalizes positive feelings about self. Patient focuses on present and future appearance and function. Patient verbalizes feelings of hopefulness, helpfulness, and powerfulness.

Patient demonstrates social participation Patient states importance of interpersonal relationships. Patient relates to self and others. Patient participates, as possible, in unit and group activities. Patient participates, as possible, in family activities.

Patient demonstrates optimum level of adjustment Patient actively involves self in future goal setting that is consistent with changed health status. Patient seeks and cooperates with assistance provided by competent caregivers. Patient demonstrates active self-care practices as appropriate to health status. Patient uses strengths and potentials to engage in maximally independent and constructive lifestyle.

Patient's family demonstrates intact family processes Family demonstrates role congruence. Family demonstrates clear communication. Family demonstrates constructive interactions. Family achieves resolution to the problem situation. Family learns and utilizes new approaches to problem solving.

Patient demonstrates minimum sleep-pattern disturbances Actual and potential causes of disturbances for inadequate sleep are identified. Management plan to correct or minimize causes of inadequate sleep is developed. Patient verbalizes feelings of being rested or refreshed.

Patient and family demonstrate constructive anticipatory grief work Patient and family demonstrate ability to discuss thoughts and feelings about impending loss. Patient and family verbalize needs for information. Patient and family demonstrate appropriate use of available resources. Patient's family demonstrates ability to meet ongoing self-care needs. Patient (as appropriate) and family participate in mutual decision making regarding anticipated loss. Patient and family demonstrate constructive interactional patterns.

Patient demonstrates effective coping mechanisms Patient is able to express fears and concerns. Patient participates in care as able.

Patient demonstrates minimal confusion Available sensory aids (i.e., eyeglasses, hearing aid) are used appropriately. Patient is able to participate in structured repetitive group activities. Rest periods between activities are maintained. Patient is able to participate in care to tolerance.

Caregiver demonstrates minimal role strain Caregiver appropriately utilizes available resources. Caregiver develops adequate support systems. Caregiver addresses personal needs.

Patient remains free of aspiration Airway is patent. Vital signs are stable. Patient reports/demonstrates no signs of choking. Breath sounds are normal. Nasoenteric tube placement is verified.

AMYOTROPHIC LATERAL SCLEROSIS
(Lou Gehrig's disease)

Amyotrophic lateral sclerosis (ALS) is a rapidly progressive degenerative disease of the motor neurons of the cortex, brainstem, and spinal cord. It is characterized by atrophy of the muscles of the hands, forearms, and legs that eventually spreads to involve most of the body.[67]

Amyotrophic lateral sclerosis, also called Lou Gehrig's disease, is the most common variant of motor neuron disease. The cause and the cure of amyotrophic lateral sclerosis remain unknown.

Amyotrophic lateral sclerosis usually occurs between the ages of 40 and 70 years, but it also may occur in the very aged. The disorder has an incidence of 2 to 7 cases per 100,000 persons in the United States. In the United States, 95% of the cases are sporadic, and 5% are familial. Approximately two to three men are affected with amyotrophic lateral sclerosis to each woman, and the disease is more common among whites than blacks. The disorder usually is fatal within 2 to 3 years after diagnosis, but one fifth of the patients may survive for between 5 and 20 years. A clustering of cases occurs in the western Pacific regions of Guam and Mariana Islands, where a form of amyotrophic lateral sclerosis is perhaps 50 to 100 times more common than in other regions.

The cause of amyotrophic lateral sclerosis is unknown. Virologic studies have not revealed any disease-specific abnormality, and most ultrastructural studies for virus material have been inconclusive or negative. Immunologic factors have been suggested by the finding of immune complex deposition in the glomeruli of some patients with the disease and the cytotoxicity of amyotrophic lateral sclerosis serum to anterior horn cells in tissue culture.[37] Epidemiologic studies in Guam support a genetic or external agent as a possible causative agent. Other proposed causes include metabolic disturbances (i.e., metal imbalances), inappropriate nutrition, and systemic stimuli responses (i.e., infection, trauma).

•••••• Pathophysiology

Amyotrophic lateral sclerosis is characterized by the deterioration of the anterior horn cells. Atrophy of the cortex, particularly of the precentral gyrus, may be grossly apparent in the cerebrum. Other pathologic changes include reduced numbers and size of the Betz cells of the motor cortex. In the brainstem there is loss of the motor neurons except for those serving the extraocular muscles. In the spinal cord there is a loss of large motor neurons and degeneration of the corticospinal tract.[37] The surviving motor neurons are atrophic and show pyknotic nuclei. The loss of the anterior horn cells results in denervation of the muscle fibers.

•••••• Diagnostic Studies and Findings

Serum   Creatinine phosphokinase may be twice normal value

CSF sampling   Mild elevation of total protein with a normal IgG concentration and normal cell count

Myelography   Normal or shrunken spinal cord

CT scan (brain)   Normal; shows cerebral atrophy

Muscle biopsy   Abnormalities and changes of denervation

Electromyography   Remarkable fibrillations indicating muscle wasting and denervation; useful in confirming diffuse process in monoparetic or unilateral forms of the disease

•••••• Multidisciplinary Plan

No specific treatment for amyotrophic lateral sclerosis has been established. Present modalities are aimed at treating symptoms when they occur.

Surgery

Cricopharyngeal myotomy to alleviate dysphagia

Cervical esophagostomy

Transtympanic neurectomy to control neural supply to parotid glands

Tracheostomy

Medications

Antianxiety agents (used for muscle relaxant effect)

    Diazepam (Valium), 5 mg po bid to tid

    Ativan, 1 mg po bid

Muscle relaxants

    Baclofen (Lioresal), 5 mg po tid; up to 15-25 mg po tid (therapy initiated at low dosage and increased gradually until optimum results are achieved)

General Management

Cardiac monitoring

Mechanical ventilation (respiratory support)

Prosthesis to support weakened muscles

Physical therapy to maintain muscle strength

Psychosocial counseling and support

Nutritional support: soft or liquid diet

Occupational therapy to assist with performance of activities of daily living

Community referrals

Social service referral

NURSING CARE

Nursing Assessment

Symptoms of amyotrophic lateral sclerosis vary, depending on which motor neuron cells are affected.

Muscle Functioning

Respiratory muscle paralysis

Loss of swallow and choking reflex

Assess ability to handle secretions and swallow

Fasciculation of muscles; may be accompanied by weakness

Upper extremity (usually unilateral) atrophy evident in palms and both sides of thumbs

Loss of dexterity for fine hand movements

Lower extremities

    Spasticity and progressive weakness until flaccidity and atrophy occur

Sensory Function

Not affected

Bulbar Palsy

Fasciculations and atrophy of the tongue

Dysphagia

Dysphonia

Dysarthria

Excessive drooling

Patient is at increased risk for choking and aspiration due to dysphagia

Reflexes

Progressive decrease

Increase in pathologic reflexes

Mental Faculties

Not affected

Altered Communication

Patient's ability to communicate may be altered

Fear

Subjective statements of feeling fearful about health status and future life-style

Altered Nutrition

Nutritional needs are altered

Nursing Dx & Intervention

Ineffective airway clearance related to high risk for obstruction

- Maintain patent airway; avoid flexion of the neck if patient is comatose.

- Auscultate for breath sounds every 1 to 2 hours; report any changes.
- Suction as needed *to prevent obstruction and manage secretions;* maintain equipment at bedside.
- Assist ventilation per protocol.
- Monitor vital signs every 1 to 2 hours; monitor neurologic status every 1 to 2 hours.
- Keep emergency drugs at the bedside.
- Maintain nothing-by-mouth status *to prevent risk of choking or aspiration.*
- Maintain quiet, nonstressful environment whenever possible *to minimize anxiety and fear.*
- Remain with patient during meals.
- Administer crushed pills in gelatin or custard.
- Elevate head of bed before eating *to minimize risk of choking.*

Ineffective breathing pattern related to neuromuscular impairment

- See general intervention strategies on p. 1616.

Altered nutrition: less than body requirements related to impaired ability to ingest food

- Offer patient frequent, small feedings *to promote adequate nutrition and fluid intake.*
- Maintain soft or liquid diet as indicated *to prevent aspiration.*
- Have suction equipment at bedside at all times *to prevent aspiration.*
- Have patient eat and drink in an upright position with neck flexed.
- Apply soft cervical collar if patient is unable to hold head upright.
- Avoid mucus-producing foods such as milk *to control secretion production.*
- Institute IV, nasogastric, or gastric feedings per protocol *to minimize risk of aspiration.*
- Administer anticholinergic drugs *to reduce oral secretions.*
- Provide frequent mouth care.

Impaired physical mobility related to progressive muscle weakness

- Use braces (hand splint; ankle-foot braces) *to maintain function.*
- Teach family turning, positioning, and transfer techniques.
- Turn and reposition patient every 2 hours and as needed *to reduce potential for spasticity* that occurs as a result of spinal cord involvement.
- Schedule activities and nursing care *to allow rest periods.*
- Provide relaxation techniques.
- Encourage participation in care *to promote self-esteem.*
- Perform passive ROM exercises *to maintain muscle strength.*
- Assist patient in use of mobility aids.
- Administer skeletal muscle relaxants *to reduce spasticity.*

Feeding, bathing/hygiene, dressing/grooming, toileting self-care deficit related to neuromuscular impairment

- See general intervention strategies on p. 1600.

Impaired verbal communication related to neuromuscular impairment

- Develop a means of communication with patient:
  When patient is restricted to eye or eyelid movement, develop a code with the patient.
  Reinforce the techniques established.
- Assist patient and family to identify other outlets for communication.
- Continue to use sense of touch and nonverbal forms of communication.

Body image disturbance related to biophysical changes

- See general intervention strategies on p. 1685.

Social isolation related to altered state of wellness

- See general intervention strategies on p. 1700.

Aspiration, risk for related to enteric feeding via nasoenteric tube

- Confirm feeding tube placement after insertion, q 4 H and PRN.
  Confirm tube placement before and after each intermittent tube feeding.
  Confirm initial enteral tube placement by physician examination of CXR.
- Tape nasogastic tube securely per protocol.
- Aspirate stomach contents *to determine gastric pH.*
- Assess bowel sounds q 4 H and PRN.
- Assess patient for abdominal distention, nausea/vomiting, and diarrhea/constipation.
  Hold tube feedings if bowel sounds are absent and if diarrhea/constipation or nausea/vomiting are present.
- Maintain proper patient positioning.
  Elevate head-of-bed 30 to 40 degrees.
  Turn patient to right side *to facilitate stomach drainage through pylorus.*
- Discontinue continuous feedings 30 to 40 minutes before activity/procedure that require lowering the patient's head.
- Check vital signs q 2 H and PRN.
- Check pulmonary-tracheal secretions q 4 H and PRN *to detect presence of enteral feeding.*
- Monitor for signs of aspiration including cough, wheezing, dyspnea, hyperthermia, and tachycardia.
- Auscultate breath sounds q 4 H and PRN.

Ineffective individual coping related to sudden illness and physiologic crisis

- Assess coping mechanisms and behavior patterns *to determine baseline information.*
- Provide patient with opportunity to express fears and concerns *to help reduce tension.*

- Encourage participation in care as tolerated *to reduce feelings of powerlessness.*
- Encourage family participation in care and emotional support *to reinforce importance of emotional care.*
- Obtain psychologic consult if indicated.

Caregiver role strain, related to severity of patient's illness

- Obtain assistance with meeting of caregiver role.

    Assist caregiver to identify/utilize caregiving resources such as family members, friends, community agencies, etc.
- Assist caregiver to develop plan of care with paced, direct care activities.
- Assist caregiver to develop support systems with alternate caregivers/friends.
- Assist caregiver to identify and address personal health care needs.

Patient Education/Home Care Planning

1. Encourage open verbalization of feelings and fears about loss of function, changes in body image, and dying.
2. Emphasize importance of maintaining planned rest periods.
3. Stress need for independence and socialization:
   a. Encourage self-care to tolerance.
   b. Encourage family to eat meals together for as long as possible.
4. Emphasize need to exercise to tolerance levels.
   a. Tell the patient to avoid fatigue.
   b. Teach the patient and family active exercises and ROM exercises.
5. Discuss name of each medication, dosage, frequency of administration, purpose, and toxic and side effects.
6. Stress need to check with physician before taking any over-the-counter medications.
7. Emphasize need to maintain fluid intake at 2000 ml daily, unless contraindicated.
8. Discuss proper techniques for turning, positioning, and transfer.
9. Stress importance of ongoing outpatient care:
   a. Physician's visits
   b. Physical therapy
   c. Occupational therapy
   d. Home nursing care, if indicated
   e. ALS Foundation referral
10. Ensure that the patient and family can demonstrate application of hand splints and ankle-foot braces.

Evaluation

Patient demonstrates adequate airway clearance   Airway remains patent. Breath sounds can be auscultated in all lobes. Chest excursion is symmetric during respiratory cycle. There are no signs of respiratory distress.

Patient demonstrates an effective breathing pattern   Airway remains patent. Chest excursion is symmetric. Vesicular, bronchial, and bronchovesicular breath sounds are normal. Arterial blood gas values are within normal limits or consistent with patient's baseline. Vital signs are within normal limits or consistent with patient's baseline. Hemoglobin levels are 14 to 18 g/dl (male) or 12 to 16 g/dl (female). Intake and output are stable. There are no signs of respiratory distress. Skin tone is appropriate to racial background. All lobes are resonant on palpation.

Patient demonstrates adequate nutritional status   Weight pattern is stable. Intake and output pattern is stable. Diet is appropriate to physiologic status. Skin turgor is good. There is fluid and electrolyte balance. Dietary supplements are taken, as appropriate.

Patient experiences a minimum level of impaired physical mobility   Skin integrity is maintained. Patient remains free of contractures or deformities. Patient demonstrates a level of mobility appropriate to physiologic status. Intake and output are stable. Nutritional status is adequate. There are no signs or symptoms of local infection.

Patient demonstrates minimum self-care deficits   Outcome criteria listed for impaired physical mobility are met. Level of self-care is appropriate to physiologic status. Patient participates in physical and occupational therapy.

Patient demonstrates minimum impaired verbal communication   Patient verbalizes feelings as long as physically able to do so. Patient develops alternative methods of communication.

Patient demonstrates intact self-concepts   Patient verbalizes, as possible, positive feelings about self. Patient acknowledges actual change in self-image. Patient verbalizes, as possible, feelings of grief, loss of functioning, and dying.

Patient remains free of aspiration   Airway is patent. Vital signs are stable. Patient reports/demonstrates no signs of choking. Breath sounds are normal. Nasoenteric tube placement is verified.

Patient demonstrates effective coping mechanisms   Patient is able to express fears and concerns. Patient participates in care as able.

Caregiver demonstrates minimal role strain   Caregiver appropriately utilizes available resources. Caregiver develops adequate support systems. Caregiver addresses personal needs.

■ MULTIPLE SCLEROSIS

■ Multiple sclerosis (MS), or disseminated sclerosis, is a chronic progressive neurologic disease that is characterized by disseminating demyelination of nerve fibers of the brain and spinal cord.[67]

Multiple sclerosis is the most prevalent of the human demyelinating diseases, with an incidence of 40 to 60 per 10,000 persons in the United States and Canada. Women are affected with the disorder slightly less often than men. The onset of symptoms occurs between 20 and 40 years of age in 75% of the cases. Incidence of the disease is rare in childhood, and the onset of symptoms rapidly decreases in old age. The severity, duration, and prognosis of multiple sclerosis vary. The survival rate of individuals with multiple sclerosis is approximately 85% of that for the general population. The diagnosis of this disorder is made on the presence of multiple lesions in the central nervous system and dissemination over time.

Studies show an association between the prevalence of multiple sclerosis and distance from the equator. Multiple sclerosis is most prevalent in western Europe, southern Canada, southern Australia, and New Zealand.[37] Within the United States, the prevalence of multiple sclerosis is higher in the Great Lakes region, the northern Atlantic states, and the Pacific Northwest.

Studies have shown that persons who move from areas of higher prevalence to areas of lower prevalence after 15 years of age retain the risk of multiple sclerosis at the level of their previous environment. Individuals below 15 years of age acquire the risk prevalence of the new environment.[37]

The cause of multiple sclerosis is unknown. Etiologic hypotheses include genetic, virologic, epidemiologic, and immunologic features.

Studies indicate that first-degree relatives of a family member with multiple sclerosis have a 15 times greater incidence of multiple sclerosis than the general population. A person who has an identical twin affected with multiple sclerosis has a 20% risk of the disease, 300 times greater than in the general population.

Individuals with multiple sclerosis have elevated (i.e., up to twofold) serum and cerebrospinal fluid titers of antibodies to many viruses including herpes simplex type I, parainfluenza, rubella, mumps, measles, and Epstein-Barr virus.

Approximately 90% of individuals affected with multiple sclerosis have abnormalities of the cerebrospinal fluid, particularly increased IgG and oligoclonal bands. Suppressor lymphocyte function is altered, and acute deteriorations are accompanied or perhaps preceded by defective immunoregulation, allowing unimpeded damage to the myelin membrane and oligodendrocytes. Remission is accompanied by a rebound elevation in suppressor function.[37]

•••••• Pathophysiology

The neuropathologic changes in multiple sclerosis include multifocal plaques of demyelination distributed randomly within the white matter of the brainstem, spinal cord, optic nerve, and cerebrum. In the acute stages, perivenular cuffs of inflammatory cells have been noted. The active changes include three essentially concurrent processes: breakdown of myelin structure, lysis of oligodendrocytes, and activation of astroglial processes.[37] Within the cerebrum there is a predilection of plaques in the periventricular areas, particularly around the third and fourth ventricles. A mild lymphocytic meningitis mainly in deep sulcal recesses may accompany the parenchymal changes. The external surface of the brain appears normal. Brain weight may be diminished, and the ventricles may be enlarged. The most characteristic feature of the chronic lesions is a proliferation of astrocytic processes, which transform the lesion into a glial scar. As lesions age, the lipid products of myelin breakdown are phagocytosed.[24]

During the demyelination process (termed primary demyelination), the myelin sheath and the myelin sheath cells are destroyed. The demyelination process leads to four significant central disturbances: a decrease in nerve conduction velocity, nerve conduction block (frequency related), differential rate of transmission of impulses, and complete failure of impulse transmission. These disturbances account for the variety of clinical signs and symptoms. Symptom remission occurs when demyelinated areas are healed by sclerotic tissue. However, when the nerve fiber degenerates, symptoms become permanent.[33]

•••••• Diagnostic Studies and Findings

CSF sampling Elevated CSF γ-globulin; normal or low CSF protein; negative VDRL; increased WBC count; abnormal colloidal gold curve (in absence of neurosyphilis); presence of myelin basic pattern

CT scan May show ventricular enlargement and cerebral atrophy (with long-term disease); areas of low attenuation around cerebral ventricles

Positron emission tomography (PET) May show altered locations and patterns of cerebral glucose metabolism

•••••• Multidisciplinary Plan

Surgery

Contralateral thalamotomy
Rhizotomy

Medications

Corticosteroids
  Prednisone, 40-60 mg/d po for 8 d (dosage is reduced gradually)
  Dexamethasone (Decadron), initial dose of 0.75-9 mg/d; maintenance dose individually adjusted to maintain an adequate clinical response
Pituitary hormones
  Corticotropin (ACTH, Athcar), 40-50 U bid for 7-10 d
Muscle relaxants
  Dantrolene sodium (Dantrium), initial dose of 25 mg po qid; maintenance dose up to 400 mg/d po
Psychotherapeutic agents
  Chlorpromazine (Thorazine), 10 mg po tid
Muscle relaxants
  Baclofen (Lioresal), 15-25 mg po tid
β-Adrenergic blocking agents
  Propranolol (Inderal), 40-240 mg/d po
Potassium supplements if ACTH is administered

General Management

Braces
Splints
Wheelchair, walker, cane

Nutritional consultation
Physiotherapy
Occupational therapy
Home nursing services
Extended care facility referrals
Hydrotherapy
Speech therapy
Social services
Home health consultation

NURSING CARE

Nursing Assessment

Sensory Symptoms

Numbness and tingling of involved extremity or face
Loss of joint sensation and proprioception (generally accompanies extremity edema)
Loss of sense of position, shape, texture, and vibration (50% of patients)

Ocular Symptoms

Optic neuritis (pain with eye movement, visual clouding, decrease in visual field)
Nystagmus (70% of patients)
Diplopia
Marcus-Gunn phenomenon (dilation of affected pupil when light is shone into eye)
Swinging-flashlight sign (dilation of affected pupil when light is moved from intact eye to eye with defect)

Motor Symptoms

Weakness in lower extremities (initially)
Decline in motor function after hot bath or shower (Uhthoff's phenomenon)
Incoordination
Intentional tremors of upper extremities and ataxia of lower extremities
Motor weakness and ability to carry out ADL varies
Staggering gait and spastic weakness of speech muscles
Facial palsy

Vestibular/Auditory Functions

Vertigo

Mental/Behavioral Symptoms

Patient's anxiety level is a factor
Irritability
Inattentiveness
Emotional lability
Mild depression
Poor judgment
Later: memory deficits; depression; confusion; disorientation; impaired communication patterns; dementia

Other

Hyperactive reflexes
Positive Babinski's sign
Ankle clonus (50%)
Impotence
Loss or impairment of sphincter control
Loss of abdominal reflexes (80%)
Lhermitte's phenomenon
Charcot triad (intentional tremors, nystagmus, and staccato speech) with brainstem involvement
Urine and fecal incontinence
Respiratory insufficiency or respiratory failure
Loss of swallow and gag reflex
Nutritional status changes

Nursing Dx & Intervention

Ineffective airway clearance related to decreased energy and fatigue

- Auscultate for breath sounds every 1 to 2 hours and as needed; report changes in breath sounds.
- Maintain patent airway, and avoid flexion of the neck if patient is immobile.
- Suction as needed *to prevent obstruction.*
- Assist ventilation as indicated.
- Monitor vital signs every 1 to 2 hours; monitor neurologic status every 1 to 2 hours.
- Keep emergency drugs at bedside.
- Maintain nothing-by-mouth status *to prevent risk of choking or aspiration.*

Ineffective breathing pattern related to musculoskeletal impairment

- See general intervention strategies on p. 1616.

Anxiety related to change in health status

- Assist patient to deal realistically with anxiety about inability to predict course of the disorder, discomfort from spasticity, and change in self-image and self-esteem.
- Explain potential treatments for the symptoms of the disorder:
    State in basic terms and monitor patient's response.
    Repeat explanations as needed.
- Alert other health care professionals and family to potential emotional changes.

Bathing/hygiene, dressing/grooming, feeding, and toileting self-care deficit related to neuromuscular weakness

- Assist with feeding, as indicated:
    Use of hand braces
    Use of IV or nasogastric feedings, as ordered
- Administer oral hygiene every 2 hours and as needed.
- Assist with daily hygiene care, as indicated.
- Administer eye care every 2 to 4 hours.

- Perform intermittent catheterization as per protocol *to maintain adequate bladder elimination and prevent infection.*
- Maintain bowel function with regular evacuation.

Altered nutrition: less than body requirements related to decreased strength and ability to ingest food

- See general intervention strategies on p. 1546.

Altered patterns of urinary elimination related to neuromuscular impairment

- See general intervention strategies on p. 1576.

Impaired verbal communication related to decreased musculoskeletal strength

- Develop means of communication with the patient: pad and pencil, Magic Slate.
- Teach patient to speak in a slow, unhurried manner.
- Obtain referral for speech therapy. Reinforce techniques established.
- Assist patient and family to identify other outlets for communication.
- Continue to use sense of touch and other nonverbal forms of communication.

Aspiration, risk for related to enteric feeding via nasoenteric tube

- Confirm feeding tube placement after insertion, q 4 H and PRN.
    - Confirm tube placement before and after each intermittent tube feeding.
    - Confirm initial enteral tube placement by physician examination of CXR.
- Tape nasogastric tube securely per protocol.
- Aspirate stomach contents *to determine gastric pH.*
- Assess bowel sounds q 4 H and PRN.
- Assess patient for abdominal distention, nausea/vomiting, and diarrhea/constipation.
    - Hold tube feedings if bowel sounds are absent and if diarrhea/constipation or nausea/vomiting are present.
- Maintain proper patient positioning.
    - Elevate head-of-bed 30 to 40 degrees.
    - Turn patient to right side *to facilitate stomach drainage through pylorus.*
- Discontinue continuous feedings 30 to 40 minutes before activity/procedure that require lowering the patient's head.
- Check vital signs q 2 H and PRN.
- Check pulmonary-tracheal secretions q 4 H and PRN *to detect presence of enteral feeding.*
- Monitor for signs of aspiration including cough, wheezing, dyspnea, hyperthermia, and tachycardia.
- Auscultate breath sounds q 4 H and PRN.

Ineffective individual coping related to sudden illness and physiologic crisis

- Assess coping mechanisms and behavior patterns *to determine baseline information.*

- Provide patient with opportunity to express fears and concerns *to help reduce tension.*
- Encourage participation in care as tolerated *to reduce feelings of powerlessness.*
- Encourage family participation in care and emotional support *to reinforce importance of emotional care.*
- Obtain psychologic consult if indicated.

Caregiver role strain, related to severity of patient's illness

- Obtain assistance with meeting of caregiver role.
    - Assist caregiver to identify/utilize caregiving resources such as family members, friends, community agencies, etc.
- Assist caregiver to develop plan of care with paced direct care activities.
- Assist caregiver to develop support systems with alternate caregivers/friends.
- Assist caregiver to identify and address personal health care needs.

Patient Education/Home Care Planning

1. Discuss nature of multiple sclerosis and treatment modalities (explain procedures as they occur).
2. Stress importance of routines for activities of daily living.
3. Emphasize importance of avoiding fatigue, overwork, and emotional stress.
4. Stress importance of regular exercise and planned rest periods.
5. Emphasize importance of diversional activities.
6. Stress importance of speech therapy, physical therapy, and occupational therapy.
7. Encourage verbalization about feelings.
8. Emphasize need for socialization with significant others.
9. Stress need for independence and self-care to level of tolerance:
    a. Support the patient when ambulating.
    b. Help the patient to walk with a wide base.
10. Discuss symptoms of disease progression and flu or cold to report to the physician.
11. Emphasize need to avoid persons with upper respiratory infections.
12. Stress need to avoid extremes of hot and cold.
13. Discuss the name of medication, dosage, frequency of administration, purpose, and toxic or side effects.
14. Emphasize importance of avoiding over-the-counter medications.
15. Stress importance of ongoing outpatient care:
    a. Physician's visits
    b. Physical therapy
    c. Speech therapy
    d. Occupational therapy

e. Home nursing services

f. MS Society referral

16. Ensure that the patient and family demonstrate the following:

a. Active and/or passive ROM exercises

b. Proper techniques of ambulation

c. Proper techniques for turning, positioning, and transfer

d. Application of hand splints and braces

e. Methods for maintaining patient safety

17. Ensure the patient understands factors that exacerbate symptoms of multiple sclerosis

a. Overexertion

b. Hot baths

c. Fever

d. Emotional stress

e. Cold

f. High humidity

g. Pregnancy

Evaluation

Patient demonstrates a patent airway Breath sounds are normal. Chest excursion is bilateral and symmetric. Rate and depth of respiration are normal. Cough is effective. There are no subjective or objective findings of shortness of breath, air hunger, or dyspnea on exertion.

Patient demonstrates an effective breathing pattern Airway is patent. Chest excursion is symmetric. Breath sounds are normal, or there is no increase in adventitious sounds. Arterial blood gas values are within normal ranges or consistent with patient's baseline. Hemoglobin levels are 14 to 18 g/dl (male) or 12 to 16 g/dl (female). Intake and output are stable. There are no signs of respiratory distress. All lobes are resonant on percussion. Skin color is not cyanotic.

Patient demonstrates a low level of anxiety Patient openly verbalizes concerns and feelings of grief, loss, and discomfort. Patient openly verbalizes feelings, supported by health care professionals and family. Patient verbalizes essential aspects of care. Patient identifies methods to deal effectively with anxious feelings.

Patient demonstrates minimum self-care deficits Level of orientation is optimum. Patient remains free of injury. Skin integrity is maintained. Nutritional status is adequate. Self-care deficits are minimal. Social participation is appropriate to physiologic status.

Patient demonstrates adequate nutrition Weight pattern is stable. Intake/output pattern is stable. Diet appropriate. Good skin turgor. Fluid and electrolyte balance.

Patient demonstrates minimum complications from alterations in urinary elimination patterns Intake and output patterns are stable. Urine is clear, yellow to amber in color, and without sediment. Skin in perineal area is clean and dry. Urine is acidic (pH 6.0). Patient remains free of urinary tract infections. Patient remains free of bladder distention. Pa-

tient can describe symptoms of urinary tract infections that require medical intervention.

Patient demonstrates minimum impaired verbal communication Patient verbalizes feelings for as long as physically able to do so. Patient develops alternative methods of communication.

Patient and family demonstrate adequate knowledge of multiple sclerosis Patient and family state that the disorder is not hereditary. Patient and family state the nature of the disease in basic terms. Patient and family can identify possible treatment modalities. Patient and family can identify symptoms of progression.

Caregiver demonstrates minimal role strain Caregiver appropriately utilizes available resources. Caregiver develops adequate support systems. Caregiver addresses personal needs.

Patient remains free of aspiration Airway is patent. Vital signs are stable. Patient reports/demonstrates no signs of choking. Breath sounds are normal. Nasoenteric tube placement is verified.

Patient demonstrates effective coping mechanisms Patient is able to express fears and concerns. Patient participates in care as able.

PARKINSON'S DISEASE

(Paralysis agitans)

Parkinson's disease is a chronic, slowly progressive degeneration of the brain's dopamine neuronal systems. It is characterized by the clinical symptoms of masklike facies, trunk-forward flexion, muscle weakness and rigidity, shuffling gait, resting tremors, finger pill-rolling, and bradykinesia (Figure 3-28).

The progressive, degenerative course of Parkinson's disease varies from individual to individual. Approximately 30% of persons with Parkinson's disease experience dementia.

The cause of Parkinson's disease includes known genetic, viral, vascular, and toxic factors and many unknown factors. Parkinson's disease occurs throughout the world in all racial and ethnic groups. Surveys indicate an incidence of about 130 per 100,000 standard population. The disorder is uncommon in individuals under 40 years of age, with the mean age of onset at 60 years. The prevalence of Parkinson's disease increases with age, and statistics indicate that 1% of the population over 60 years of age are afflicted with the disorder. Family studies indicate that approximately 2% of the adult siblings of individuals with Parkinson's disease also have the disorder.

•••••• Pathophysiology

Parkinson's disease can be divided into three major types in terms of pathophysiologic mechanisms: parkinsonism-dementia complex, Lewy body Parkinson's disease, and neurofibrillary tangle Parkinson's disease. Parkinsonism-dementia complex is unique to certain Pacific islands and is often associated with amyotrophic lateral sclerosis. The pathologic characteristics of this complex include neurofibrillary tangles found throughout the neuraxis, atrophy of the thalamus and temporal

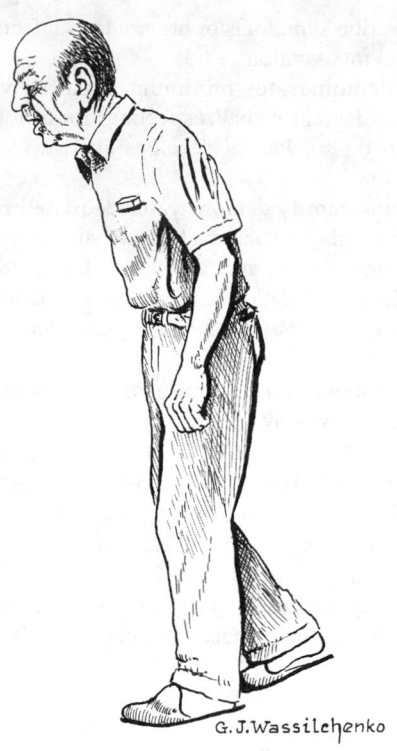

G.J.Wassilchenko

Figure 3-28 Posture and shuffling gait associated with Parkinson's disease. (From Rudy.[55])

and frontal lobes, and granulovascular degeneration in structures such as the hippocampus.

Lewy body Parkinson's disease involves the degeneration of the pigmented neurons of the substantia nigra and locus ceruleus. Other melanin-bearing neurons of the brainstem and spinal cord also degenerate, such as the dorsal motor nucleus of the vagal nerve, and paravertebral ganglia. The surviving melanin-bearing cells contain structures known as Lewy bodies, which are cytoplasmic inclusions consisting of a central core of filamentous proteins. Radiating from the central core is a less dense array of tubules that may represent excess axoplasmic transport material or degenerated storage granules.[41]

Neurofibrillary tangle parkinsonism demonstrates the following pathologic changes: atrophy of the cerebral cortex with an increased subarachnoid space and narrow gyri, depigmentation (usually) of the substantia nigra, and the presence of neurofibrillary tangles in the surviving neuronal cells of the substantia nigra. These neurofibrillary tangles consist of helically twisted pairs of filaments and result from proliferation of the neurofilaments. Studies suggest a possible relationship between this form of Parkinson's disease and viral encephalitis.

Iatrogenic parkinsonism, which closely resembles Parkinson's disease, may be induced by different drugs, such as the major tranquilizers or, rarely, methyldopa, α-methyl-

paratyrosine, and reserpine. These agents interfere with the synthesis or the storage of dopamine or block the striatal dopamine receptors.[37] The effects of chemical-induced parkinsonism are reversible within 1 to 2 weeks after discontinuation of the offending agent.

Progression of Parkinson's disease and resultant disabilities may be evaluated by the use of the following classification system:

Stage I: Unilateral involvement
Stage II: Bilateral involvement
Stage III: Mild to moderate impairment; impaired postural reflexes
Stage IV: Marked impairment; fully developed, severe disease
Stage V: Confined to bed or wheelchair

•••••• Diagnostic Studies and Findings

Serum examination   Mild microcytic anemia
Chest roentgenograms   Slight scoliosis
CT scan, skull films   Normal results (CT scan may show cerebral atrophy, with history of chronic dementia)
Electroencephalogram (EEG)   Normal results or shows minimum slowing and/or disorganization; with marked dementia and bradykinesia, may show moderate to marked slowing and diffuse disorganization
Swallowing studies   (see Part Two) Abnormal pattern: delayed relaxation of cricopharyngeal muscles
Gastrointestinal studies   (see Part Two) Hypomotility; delayed emptying of stomach; varying degrees of large bowel distention (frank megacolon in patients with severe constipation)

•••••• Multidisciplinary Plan

Surgery

Stereotactic thalamotomy: produces small lesion in ventrolateral nucleus of thalamus to alleviate contralateral tremor and rigidity

Medications

Antiparkinsonism agents
  Carbidopa (Sinemet), 10-25 mg po tid or qid
  Trihexyphenidyl (Artane), 2-5 mg po tid or qid
  Benztropine mesylate (Cogentin), 0.5-6.0 mg/d po
  Amantadine (Symmetrel), 100 mg/d po for 5-7 d
  Ethopropazine (Parsidol), 20-600 mg/d po
  Bromocriptine mesylate (Parlodel), 2.5 mg po bid or tid
  L-Dihydroxyphenylalanine (levodopa), 100-250 mg po tid or qid
  Orphenadrine (Disipal), 50 mg po tid
Antidepressant agents
  Amitriptyline (Elavil), 75-150 mg/d po
Antihistamine
  Diphenhydramine (Benadryl), 10-50 mg po q6h prn

General Management

Heat massage
Walkers, canes, wheelchairs

Physiotherapy
Bowel and bladder program
Nutritional program
Social services
Occupational therapy
Extended care facility referral
Speech therapy
Resources available (National Parkinson Foundation)

NURSING CARE

Nursing Assessment

Initial Symptoms

Weakness, tendency to tremble (usually in one hand)
Slowness or awkwardness of affected limb
Some loss of facial expression
Deliberate quality of speech
Tendency to maintain arm flexed at elbow
May progress to other side of the body after 1 to 2 years

Autonomic Dysfunction

Increased secretion of sebum resulting in scaly erythematous
    eruptions of skin (particularly by ears and eyebrows and in
    scalp and nasolabial folds)
Intermittent, profuse diaphoresis
Gastric retention
Urgency or hesitancy in micturition
Urinary retention
Orthostatic hypotension
Dysphagia

Equilibrium

Festination (leaning of the trunk farther and farther with
    each step):
    Propulsion (forward stepping with leaning of trunk)
    Retropulsion (backward stepping with leaning of trunk)
    Lateropulsion (sidewise stepping with leaning of trunk)

Face

Masklike facies
Decreased eye blinking

Gradual Dementia

Initial
    Forgetfulness
    Minor confusional episodes
    Depression
Later
    Irritability
    Paranoia and visual hallucinations
    Frank delirium
    Social isolation

Hands

Fingers extended, with metacarpophalangeal joints flexed
    approximately 30 degrees

Handwriting

Letters becoming progressively smaller (micrographia)
Tremulous writing

Nutrition

Impaired deglutition
Drooling
Weight loss
Failure of cricopharyngeal muscles to relax—choking
Bowel dysfunction—constipation

Posture and Rigidity

Shuffling gait without arm swing (Figure 3-28)
Akinesia (most evident in spinal musculature)
Hypertonicity
Stooped body posture
Impaired mobility
    Patient's level of mobility is a factor
    Self-care deficits

Speech

Involuntary repetition of sentences
Decreased amplitude
Soft, rapid monotone

Toes

Toe flexion with dorsiflexion of proximal phalanges
Great toe may assume continuous dorsiflexion position

Tremors

Lips, jaws, tongue, facial muscles, axial muscles, and limb
    muscles
Usually resting tremors (most apparent when affected area is
    at rest): paralysis agitans

Nursing Dx & Intervention

Risk for aspiration related to impaired swallowing

- Maintain patent airway, and avoid flexion of the neck if
  patient is immobile.
- Suction as needed *to prevent obstruction.*
- Assist ventilation as indicated.
- Monitor vital signs every 1 to 2 hours; monitor neurologic
  status every 1 to 2 hours.
- Keep emergency drugs and ventilator at bedside.
- Help patient select foods that are easy to swallow.
- Provide frequent mouth care.
- Remain with patient during meals.
- Give oral medications (crushed) in gelatin or custard.
- Teach family members Heimlech maneuver.
- Maintain choking precautions.

Constipation related to neuromuscular impairment

- Assess and document presence of bowel sounds.
- Provide high-residue diet *to promote gastrointestinal motility.*
- Maintain activity level to tolerance.
- Maintain regular bowel evacuation with stool softeners, rectal suppositories, mild cathartics, and natural laxatives such as prune juice.

Sensory/perceptual alterations related to impaired neuromuscular function

- See general intervention strategies on p. 1643.

Impaired physical mobility related to decreased neuromuscular functioning

- Institute gait-retraining program if indicated *to maintain balance and to improve walking.*
- Apply splints and braces as indicated.
- Continue with physiotherapy program.
- Encourage outdoor ambulation (avoid extremes of hot and cold).
- Encourage patient to dress daily *to promote self-esteem.*
  - Avoid shoes with laces or snaps.
  - Avoid clothes with buttons; use zippers.
  - Place head of bed or chair on blocks *to facilitate getting up.*
  - Provide raised toilet seat and side rails *to facilitate sitting and standing.*
- Administer medications in a timely fashion *to avoid symptom aggravation.*

Bathing/hygiene, dressing/grooming, toileting self-care deficit related to impaired neuromuscular function

- Perform range-of-motion exercises to prevent stiffness, muscle wasting, and contractures.
- Assist with feeding, as indicated:
  - Use of hand braces
  - Use of IV or nasogastric feedings, as ordered
- Administer oral hygiene every 2 hours and as needed *to control drooling.*
- Assist with daily hygiene care, as indicated.
- Administer skin care every 2 to 4 hours and as needed *to remove skin oil and perspiration.*
- Administer eye care every 2 to 4 hours *to remove crustations.*
- Perform intermittent urinary catheterization per protocol *to maintain adequate bladder elimination and to prevent infection.*

Anxiety related to change in health status

- See general intervention strategies on p. 1669.
- Support the family:
  - Provide for ongoing contact.
  - Give appropriate referrals to support groups.

- Assist patient to deal realistically and honestly with anxiety about inability to predict course of the disorder, discomfort from spasticity, and change in self-image and self-esteem.
- Explain potential treatments for the symptoms of the disorder:
  - State in basic terms and monitor patient's response.
  - Repeat explanations as needed.
- Alert other health care professionals and family to potential emotional changes.
- Instruct family that patient is intellectually normal, despite physical disability.

Impaired verbal communication related to neuromuscular status

- Assess patient's ability to communicate and develop means of communication with the patient, such as pad and pencil, Magic Slate, call light.
- Teach patient to speak in a slow, unhurried manner. Provide electronic amplifiers as needed *to augment decreased amplitude of speech.*
- Obtain referral for speech therapy. Reinforce established techniques.
- Assist patient and family to identify other outlets for communication.
- Continue to use sense of touch and other nonverbal forms of communication.

Altered nutrition: less than body requirements related to impaired neuromuscular function

- Assess patient's nutritional status and ability to chew and swallow.
- Offer small, frequent feedings *to minimize risks of dysphagia and aspiration.*
- Complete nursing care before mealtimes.
- Apply braces to minimize tremors.
- Encourage a high-bulk, high-roughage diet. Provide supplements as needed. Control protein intake *to minimize blocking of effects of L-dopa.*
- Allow ample time for eating and keep food warm.
  - Place utensils within easy reach.
  - Cut foods for patient.
  - Use blender for thick foods.
- Use bib or straw as indicated.

Body image disturbance related to biophysical and cognitive perceptual changes

- Provide an ongoing assessment of the patient's interpersonal strengths. Focus on strengths and potential.
- Reorient to time, person, and place as appropriate.
- Carefully explain what you are doing and why you are doing it.
- Answer questions simply and honestly.
- Correct misinformation.

- Protect the patient's privacy.
- Provide gentle physical care in a caring environment.
- Assist patient to become involved in self-care.
- Assist patient to become involved in unit activities.

Social isolation related to alterations in mental status

- See general intervention strategies on p. 1700.

Altered patterns of urinary elimination related to neuromuscular impairment

- Assess characteristics of patient's voiding pattern (frequency, amount).
- Perform intermittent catheterization per protocol.
- Monitor intake and output. Maintain fluid intake at 2000 ml/day unless contraindicated.
- Assess urine for sediment, concentration, color, and odor.
- Acidify urine with foods such as orange juice and cranberry juice *to minimize potential for infection.*
- Administer urinary tract germicides (e.g., methenamine mandalate [Mandelamine]) as ordered.

Confusion, chronic related to organic or cognitive impairment

- Assess baseline physical, functional, and psychosocial status.
- Evaluate previous interests.
- Ensure optimal sensory input (i.e., eyeglasses, hearing aid) is available.
- Evaluate stimulation threshold to prevent overstimulation.
- Provide for structured repetitive group activities.
- Provide rest periods between activities to minimize fatigue.
- Monitor for changes in physical, functional, and psychologic status.
- Maintain calm, reassuring demeanor when interacting with patient to promote sense of trust.
- Encourage patient to participate in care as tolerated to minimize feelings of powerlessness.
- Provide positive feedback for tasks/activities that are mastered.

Caregiver role strain, related to severity of patient's illness

- Obtain assistance with meeting of caregiver role.
  Assist caregiver to identify/utilize caregiving resources such as family members, friends, community agencies, etc.
- Assist caregiver to develop plan of care with paced direct-care activities.
- Assist caregiver to develop support systems with alternate caregivers/friends.
- Assist caregiver to identify and address personal health care needs.

Patient Education/Home Care Planning

1. Discuss causes, symptoms, and treatments modalities for Parkinson's disease (explain procedures as they occur).
2. Stress importance of verbalization about loss of self-esteem, sexuality, and body functions.
3. Emphasize importance of verbalization about feelings.
4. Encourage social participation.
5. Emphasize capabilities.
6. Encourage independence and self-care; avoid overprotection.
7. Stress need for daily exercise program.
8. Emphasize need for high-calorie, soft diet; instruct the patient to eat slowly and take small bites.
9. Stress need for diversional activities.
10. Discuss safety measures to prevent injury.
11. Emphasize need for speech therapy.
12. Stress need for frequent skin care and oral hygiene.
13. Emphasize need for bowel and bladder programs.
14. Discuss name of medication, dosage, frequency of administration, purpose, and toxic or side effects.
15. Ensure that the patient understands he or she must take medications with food to reduce gastric irritation and nausea.
16. Stress importance of ongoing outpatient care:
    a. Physician's visits
    b. Physical therapy
    c. Home nursing care
    d. Parkinson's Disease Information Center; Parkinson's Foundation

Evaluation

Patient and family demonstrate adequate knowledge of Parkinson's disease Patient and family state the nature of the disease in basic terms. Patient and family can identify possible treatment modalities. Patient and family can identify symptoms of progression.

Patient demonstrates a patent airway Breath sounds are normal. Chest excursion is bilateral and symmetric. Rate and depth of respiration are normal. Cough is effective. There are no subjective or objective findings of shortness of breath, air hunger, or dyspnea on exertion.

Patient demonstrates minimum complications of constipation Dietary intake is adequate. Fluid intake is adequate (2000 ml/day unless contraindicated). Intake and output patterns are stable. Patient remains free of fecal impaction. Patient demonstrates a regular bowel evacuation pattern.

Patient demonstrates minimum complications of sensory/perceptual alterations Optimum level of orientation is maintained. Patient remains free of injury. Skin integrity is maintained. Nutritional status ia adequate. Self-care deficits are minimum. Social participation is appropriate to physiologic status.

Patient demonstrates optimum level of mobility Skin integrity is maintained. There are no contractures and deformities. Patient's level of mobility is appropriate to physiologic status. Intake and output pattern is stable. Nutritional status is adequate. There is no thrombophlebitis. There is no local infection. Patient participates in an ongoing physical therapy program.

Patient demonstrates minimum self-care deficits Outcome criteria listed for impaired physical mobility are met. Level of self-care activities is appropriate to physiologic status. Patient participates in physical and occupational therapy.

Patient demonstrates a low level of anxiety Patient openly verbalizes concerns and feelings of grief, loss, and discomfort. Patient openly verbalizes feelings, supported by health care professionals and family. Patient verbalizes essential aspects of care. Patient can identify methods to effectively deal with anxious feelings.

Patient demonstrates minimum impaired verbal communication Patient verbalizes feelings for as long as physically able to do so. Patient develops alternative methods of communication.

Patient demonstrates adequate nutritional status Weight pattern is stable. Intake and output pattern is stable. Diet is appropriate to physiologic status. Skin turgor is good. Fluid and electrolyte balance is maintained. Patient takes dietary supplements, as appropriate.

Patient demonstrates intact self-concepts Patient openly verbalizes feelings of grief and loss. Patient verbalizes positive feelings about self. Patient acknowledges actual change in self-image. Patient focuses on present and future appearance and function. Patient verbalizes feelings of hopefulness, helpfulness, and powerfulness.

Patient demonstrates social participation Patient states importance of interpersonal relationships. Patient relates to self and others. Patient participates, as possible, in unit and group activities. Patient participates, as possible, in family activities.

Patient demonstrates minimum complications from alterations in urinary elimination patterns Intake and output pattern is stable. Urine is clear, yellow to amber in color, and without sediment. Skin in perineal area is clean and dry. Urine is acidic (pH 6.0). Patient is free of urinary tract infections. Patient is free of bladder distention. Patient can describe symptoms of urinary tract infections that require medical intervention.

Caregiver demonstrates minimal role strain Caregiver appropriately utilizes available resources. Caregiver develops adequate support systems. Caregiver addresses personal needs.

Patient demonstrates minimal confusion Available sensory aids (i.e., eyeglasses, hearing aid) are used appropriately. Patient is able to participate in structured repetitive group activities. Rest periods between activities are maintained. Patient is able to participate in care to tolerance.

■ MYASTHENIA GRAVIS

Myasthenia gravis is a neuromuscular disease involving lower motor neurons and muscle fibers that is characterized by abnormal fatigue and motor weakness of skeletal muscles that increases with effort and improves with rest. Voluntary muscles most commonly affected in myasthenia gravis include the oculomotor, facial, laryngeal, pharyngeal, and respiratory muscles.

The cause of myasthenia gravis is unknown, although considerable data suggest that it is a systemic autoimmune disease. Myasthenia gravis is not a hereditary condition, but 15% of infants born to myasthenic mothers manifest transitory symptoms lasting from 7 to 14 days after birth. The incidence of myasthenia gravis is 3 to 6 per 100,000 individuals. There are two characteristic ages of onset: between the ages of 20 and 30 years and in late middle age. When the disorder begins in the second or third decade, women are more commonly affected than men. When the disorder begins in late middle age, men are affected more often than women. Epidemiologic studies have not produced any specific socioeconomic or racial factors. Clinical studies have indicated that 80% of the patients with myasthenia gravis have thymic abnormalities (10% have a thymoma, and 70% have thymic hyperplasia). The role of the thymus in the pathogenesis is unclear. Mortality for individuals with myasthenia gravis is 15 times greater than for the general population.

••••• Pathophysiology

Regardless of the cause of myasthenia gravis, the basic physiologic defect is that nerve impulses do not pass onto the skeletal muscle at the myoneuronal junction. This defect appears to result from either a deficiency in release of acetylcholine from the presynaptic terminals or a deficiency (i.e., blockage or reduced numbers) in the postsynaptic membrane receptor sites. Biopsy studies of myasthenic patients have shown that small end-plate potentials are normal in frequency but have markedly decreased amplitudes. Postsynaptic potentials are slightly smaller than normal but contain the normal number of acetylcholine quanta.[24]

Research pursuing the prospect that myasthenia gravis is produced by an autoimmune mechanism has shown that a major feature in the pathogenesis is an attack on end-plate acetylcholine receptors by circulating antibodies.[23] The reason that these antibodies to acetylcholine receptors develop remains to be elucidated.

There is no evidence in myasthenia gravis of central or peripheral nervous system disease. Involved skeletal muscles usually do not atrophy, and there is no loss of sensation. The primary signs are extreme fatigability and weakness of voluntary muscles.

••••• Diagnostic Studies and Findings

Chest roentgenogram, CT scan of chest May indicate presence of thymoma

Edrophonium chloride (Tensilon) test Intramuscular injection of 2 mg of edrophonium chloride (Tensilon); if no symptoms occur, an additional 8 mg is injected and the patient is observed for improvement in muscle tone; in 30 seconds to 1 minute, patients with myasthenia gravis demonstrate marked improvement in muscle tone that lasts 4 to 5 minutes

Electromyogram (EMG) Muscle fiber contraction with progressive decremental response

Curare test Myasthenia gravis patient will be curarized with $\frac{1}{32}$ of the normal curare dose; done by a neurologist with anesthesia at the bedside, ready to intubate; done only if all the other findings are normal or questionable; frequently seen as the ultimate diagnostic technique for myasthenia gravis; serum Anti-AChR antibody titer may be elevated

Four-test panel
1. ACh-R-binding antibody test
2. ACh-R-modulating antibody test
3. ACh-R-blocking antibody test
4. Striational antibody test

Cerebrospinal fluid (CSF) analysis
CSF protein levels elevate as disease progresses

•••••• Multidisciplinary Plan

Surgery

Tracheotomy (see Chapter 7)
Thymectomy
    Suprasternal approach
    Transsternal approach

Medications

Cholinergic agents
    Neostigmine (Prostigmin), 7.5-45 mg q2-6h
    Pyridostigmine (Mestinon), individualized size and frequency of dosage (range 15-90 mg/d po)
    Ambenonium chloride (Mytelase), 10-25 mg po tid or qid
Corticosteroids
    Prednisone, 100 mg po qod (dose gradually reduced)

Immunosuppressants

(Immunosuppressive drug therapy may produce false-negative of four-test panel results)
    Azathioprine (Imuran)
    Cyclophosphamide (Cytoxan)
Diphenoxylate hydrochloride (Lomotil), prn
Pituitary hormones
    ACTH, 100-160 U/d for 10 d (rarely used)

General Management

Mechanical ventilation, if indicated
Plasma exchange (plasmapheresis)
Bronchoscopy (see Part Two for additional information)
Physical therapy
Occupational therapy
Social Services
Swallow Precautions

NURSING CARE

Nursing Assessment

Eye Muscles (Usually Affected First)

Ocular palsy
Ptosis (unilateral or bilateral)
Diplopia

Facial Muscles

Masklike expression and mobility (weakness) of face
Weak voice that may fade to a whisper
Dysphagia
Choking
Aspiration, impaired swallowing
Drooling
Nasal speech

Neck Muscles

Head bobbing up and down

Respiratory Muscles

Breathlessness
Respiratory weakness
Respiratory failure, reduced tidal volume, and vital capacity

Other Muscles

Stress incontinence
Anal sphincter weakness

Other

Altered nutrition—ability to chew and swallow is a factor

Reflexes

Normal or brisk

Myasthenia Gravis Crisis

Respiratory distress
Tachycardia
Tachypnea
Generalized muscular weakness
Extreme fatigue
Anxiety
Restlessness
Irritability
Facial weakness
Dysphagia
Inability to chew
Elevated temperature
Ptosis
Speech impairment
Hypertension

Cholinergic Crisis

Respiratory distress
Vertigo
Blurred vision
Sweating
Lacrimation
Salivation
Anorexia
Dysarthria
Dysphagia
Abdominal cramps; diarrhea
Nausea and vomiting
Muscular spasms or cramps
Generalized muscle weakness
Dyspnea and wheezing
Bradycardia
Hypotension

Nursing Dx & Intervention

Risk for aspiration related to impaired swallowing

- Auscultate for breath sounds every 1 to 2 hours, and report any changes to the physician.
- Maintain patent airway, and avoid flexion of the neck if patient is comatose.
- Suction as needed *to prevent obstruction.*
- Assist ventilation as indicated.
- Monitor vital signs every 1 to 2 hours; monitor neurologic status every 1 to 2 hours.
- Keep emergency drugs and suction equipment at the bedside.
- Provide a quiet, supervised nondistracting environment.
- Assess for presence of gag reflex.
- Teach family members Heimlich maneuver.

Ineffective breathing pattern related to impaired neuromuscular function

- See general intervention strategies listed on p. 1616.
- If patient has a thymectomy, assess for signs of pneumothorax: restlessness, tachycardia, respiratory distress, cyanosis, diaphoresis.
- Maintain patency of chest tubes.
- Provide chest physiotherapy *to mobilize secretions.*
- Monitor tidal volume and vital capacity every hour in acute stage.

Impaired physical mobility related to neuromuscular impairment

- See general intervention strategies on p. 1597.

Feeding, bathing/hygiene, dressing/grooming, and toileting self-care deficit related to neuromuscular impairment

- See general intervention strategies on p. 1600.

Altered nutrition: less than body requirements related to impaired swallowing

- Offer small, frequent feedings.
- Encourage a high-protein, high-bulk, high-roughage diet.
- Administer medications 30 minutes before eating *to maximize muscle strength needed for chewing and swallowing of food.*
- Allow ample time for eating. Stay with patient.
- Accurately measure and record intake on a flowsheet.
- Administer parenteral fluids per protocol *to ensure adequate fluid intake.*
- Monitor the patient's weight pattern, and report any significant changes.
- Obtain nutritional services consultation.
- Administer enteral feedings as ordered.
- Maintain swallow precautions.

Impaired verbal communication related to neuromuscular impairment

- Assess patient's ability to communicate.
- Develop means of communication with patient: pad and pencil, Magic Slate, call light.
- Teach patient to speak in a slow, unhurried manner *to avoid voice strain.*
- Obtain referral for speech therapy. Reinforce technique established.
- Assist patient and family to identify other outlets for communication.
- Continue to use sense of touch and other nonverbal forms of communication.

Powerlessness related to illness-related regimen

- See general intervention strategies on p. 1677.

Ineffective individual coping related to sudden illness and physiologic crisis

- Assess coping mechanisms and behavior patterns *to determine baseline information.*
- Provide patient with opportunity to express fears and concerns *to help reduce tension.*
- Encourage participation in care as tolerated *to reduce feelings of powerlessness.*
- Encourage family participation in care and emotional support *to reinforce importance of emotional care.*
- Obtain psychologic consultation if indicated.

Aspiration, risk for related to enteric feeding via nasoenteric tube

- Confirm feeding tube placement after insertion, q 4 H and PRN.
  Confirm tube placement before and after each intermittent tube feeding.
  Confirm initial enteral tube placement by physician examination of CXR.
- Tape nasogastic tube securely per protocol.

- Aspirate stomach contents *to determine gastric pH.*
- Assess bowel sounds q 4 H and PRN.
- Assess patient for abdominal distention, nausea/vomiting, and diarrhea/constipation.

  Hold tube feedings if bowel sounds are absent and if diarrhea/constipation or nausea/vomiting are present.
- Maintain proper patient positioning.

  Elevate head-of-bed 30 to 40 degrees.

  Turn patient to right side *to facilitate stomach drainage through pylorus.*
- Discontinue continuous feedings 30 to 40 minutes before activity/procedure that requires lowering the patient's head.
- Check vital signs q 2 H and PRN.
- Check pulmonary-tracheal secretions q 4 H and PRN *to detect presence of enteral feeding.*
- Monitor for signs of aspiration including cough, wheezing, dyspnea, hyperthermia, and tachycardia.
- Auscultate breath sounds q 4 H and PRN.

Patient Education/Home Care Planning

1. Discuss names of medications, dosage, time of administration, purpose, and side effects. For anticholinesterase medications:
   a. Stress importance of dosage.
   b. Instruct patient to take at scheduled times.
   c. Instruct patient not to skip doses.
   d. Instruct patient to avoid taking with fruit, tomato juice, coffee, or other medications.
   e. Instruct patient to take medications with food to minimize gastric irritation and nausea.
   f. Inform patient of toxic side effects (i.e., diarrhea, abdominal cramping, muscular weakness).
2. Stress need to avoid taking over-the-counter medications without notifying the physician.
3. Discuss symptoms of progression or recurrence to report to physician.
4. Emphasize need to wear medical alert tag.
5. Stress importance of avoiding individuals with upper respiratory infection.
6. Discuss symptoms of upper respiratory infection to report to physician (i.e., chills, cough, low-grade temperature).
7. Stress need to avoid alcohol, tobacco, and prolonged exposure to heat or cold.
8. Emphasize need for adequate nutritional status:
   a. Give diet as tolerated.
   b. Arrange food and utensils so they can be managed by patient.
   c. Instruct to chew thoroughly, and eat slowly and in small pieces.
9. Stress need for activity and exercise to tolerance:
   a. Plan activities of daily living.
   b. Maintain rest periods as planned.
   c. Do active and passive ROM exercises.
   d. Get at least 8 hours of sleep at night.
10. Emphasize need for diversional activities.
11. Stress importance of avoiding physical and emotional stress.
12. Emphasize need for speech therapy.
13. Stress importance of avoiding constipation.
14. Emphasize importance of ongoing outpatient care.
15. Give available agencies for reference (e.g., Myasthenia Gravis Foundation).
16. Give outpatient or home nursing care referrals.

Evaluation

Patient and family demonstrate adequate knowledge of myasthenia gravis Patient states the nature of the disorder in basic terms. Patient can identify treatment modalities. Patient can state treatment regimen. Patient can identify symptoms of progression.

Patient demonstrates a patent airway Breath sounds are normal. Chest excursion is bilateral and symmetric. Rate and depth of respirations are normal. Cough is effective. There are no subjective or objective findings of shortness of breath, air hunger, or dyspnea on exertion.

Patient demonstrates an effective breathing pattern Airway is patent. Chest excursion is symmetric. Breath sounds are normal, or there is no increase in adventitious sounds. Arterial blood gas values are within normal ranges or consistent with patient's baseline. Vital signs are within normal ranges or consistent with patient's baseline. Hemoglobin levels are 14 to 18 g/dl (male) or 12 to 16 g/dl (female). Intake and output are stable. There are no signs of respiratory distress. All lobes are resonant on percussion. Skin is not cyanotic.

Patient demonstrates an optimum level of mobility Skin integrity is maintained. Patient is free of contractures and deformities. Level of mobility is appropriate to physiologic status. Intake and output pattern is stable. Nutritional status is adequate. Patient remains free of thrombophlebitis. Patient remains free of local infection.

Patient demonstrates minimum self-care deficits Outcome criteria stated for impaired physical mobility are met. Level of self-care is appropriate to physiologic status. Diet is high in calories and protein. Patient participates in physical and occupational therapy as indicated.

Patient demonstrates minimum impaired verbal communication Patient verbalizes feelings for as long as physically able to do so. Patient develops alternative methods of communication.

Patient demonstrates minimum feelings of powerlessness Optimum level of physiologic control, as possible for current health status, is maintained. Optimum level of psychologic control, as possible, is maintained. Patient participates, as possible, in decision making about care. Patient participates, as possible, in self-care.

Patient demonstrates minimum complications of bowel incontinence Skin in perineal area is clean and dry. Dietary intake is adequate. Fluid intake is adequate (2000 ml daily, unless contraindicated). Intake and output pattern is stable. Patient remains free of fecal impaction. Patient demonstrates a regular bowel evacuation pattern.

Patient demonstrates effective coping mechanisms Patient is able to express fears and concerns. Patient participates in care as able.

Patient remains free of aspiration Airway is patent. Vital signs are stable. Patient reports/demonstrates no signs of choking. Breath sounds are normal. Nasoenteric tube placement is verified.

TUMORS

INTRACRANIAL TUMORS
(Brain tumors)

Intracranial tumors include both benign space-occupying (primary) and malignant (metastatic) lesions. The incidence of intracranial tumors in the United States is about 10,000 per year. Intracranial tumors can occur in any structural area of the brain and in all age groups. Growth rates range from the rapid growth of glioblastomas to the almost imperceptible changes of some meningiomas (Figure 3-29).[37]

Brain tumors are named according to the tissues from which they arise. Primary brain tumors include oligodendrogliomas, ependymomas, astrocytomas and glioblastomas, medulloblastomas, and meningiomas. Secondary or metastatic tumors include metastatic carcinoma or sarcoma. (See Chapter 16 for a discussion of malignant brain tumors.)

Gliomas

Oligodendrogliomas form in the oligodendroglia cells that are responsible for the formation of the central nervous system myelin sheaths. These tumors evolve slowly and may be detected on a routine skull roentgenogram because of intracranial calcification. The most common sites for oligodendrogliomas are the frontal and temporal lobes; but they are also found in the brainstem, cerebellum, and spinal cord. This type of tumor makes up only 5% of all intracranial tumors. There is a high incidence of this tumor among young adults who have a childhood history of temporal lobe epilepsy.[41]

Ependymomas are fairly rare in the general adult population and make up only 5% of all intracranial tumors. They are more commonly found in young children and adolescents and account for 20% of brain tumors in this age group. Ependymomas form in the ependymal cells and astrocytes that line the walls of the cerebral ventricular system and most commonly affect the fourth ventricle.

Astrocytomas form in astrocyte cells at any level of the central nervous system. In the adult they are usually lateral and supratentorial, whereas astrocytes in children are in or near the midline.[39] Cerebellar astrocytomas, which constitute 30% of all pediatric brain tumors, are usually located just lateral to the midline in the cerebellar hemisphere. Simple surgical excision provides a long survival rate. Brainstem astrocytomas primarily affect school-aged children, who have a high mortality rate because of destruction of the local cranial nerve nuclei and the long tracts.

Cerebral astrocytomas are classified by grade (Table 3-8). Cerebral astrocytomas are common between 30 and 50 years of age, making up 30% of the brain tumors for this age group. These tumors have a growth rate proportional to their grade. For example, grades I and II grow slowly, whereas grades III and IV grow rapidly.[41]

Neuronal Cell Tumor

Medulloblastomas constitute 20% of brain tumors in children and occur most frequently in children under 10 years of age.

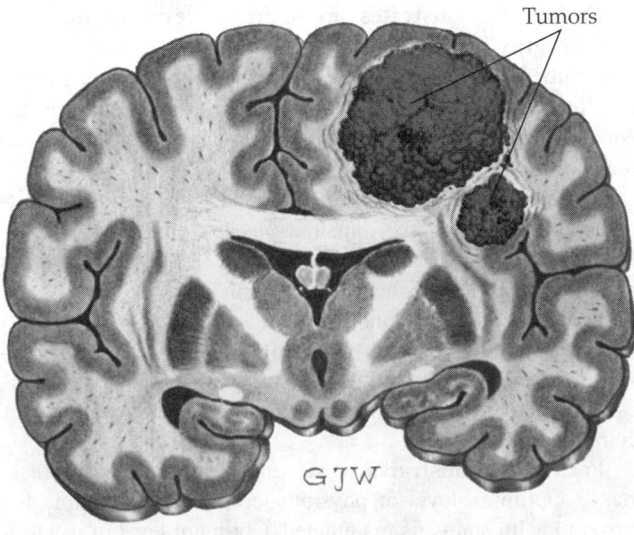

Figure 3-29 Intracranial tumor. (From Chipps et al.[16])

TABLE 3-8 **Grades of Astrocytoma**

Grade	Growth Rate	Prognosis
Astrocytoma		
Grade I	Slow	Good; 15-20 yr after surgery
Grade II	Slow	Good; 10-15 yr after surgery
Glioblastoma		
Grade III	Rapid, invasive	Poor; less than 2 yr without therapy
Grade IV (glioblastoma multiforme)	Rapid, invasive	Very poor; 6-9 mo without surgery

Medulloblastomas are found in the posterior cerebellar vermis and roof of the fourth ventricle. The tumor eventually obstructs the flow of cerebrospinal fluid from the aqueduct, resulting in hydrocephalus and cerebellar signs. Without irradiation, the tumor is fatal; with irradiation there is a 30% survival rate.

Meningiomas are adult tumors arising from the cells of vessels, pia-arachnoid, and surrounding fibroblasts. Meningiomas make up 15% of all adult tumors of the central nervous system and its coverings. These tumors are found in the parasagittal falx of the frontal lobe, sylvian fissure region, olfactory groove wing of the sphenoid bone, superior surface of the cerebellum and cerebellopontine angle. They occur more frequently in women and are found in approximately 40% to 50% of patients with von Recklinghausen's disease (neurofibromatosis). The symptoms of a meningioma are manifested as the tumor indents a local area of the brain and raises the intracranial pressure.

• • • • • • Pathophysiology

An *oligodendroglioma* can be seen microscopically as small round cells with spheric nuclei. Many of these tumors have an astrocytic component; therefore recurrence of the tumor may have astrocytic characteristics.

An *ependymoma* has several variants. The *myxopapillary ependymoma* is a special variant occurring in adolescents. It develops in the fifth ventricle (ventriculus terminalis), formed by the caudal opening of the central canal of the spinal cord.[41] Generally symptoms of increased intracranial pressure are manifested when the ependymoma fills the fourth ventricle, blocking the flow of cerebrospinal fluid.

An *astrocytoma* of low grade (I or II) is gelatinous and frequently indistinguishable from cerebral gliosis. This type of tumor is slow growing and infiltrative. Astrocytomas commonly arise in the white matter. Their cellularity is almost normal.[41] Astrocytomas of grades III and IV are rapid-growing tumors characterized by a high degree of macroscopic necrosis. An as-

trocytoma of this grade is not confined to white matter and may grow into areas of the subarachnoid space and the brainstem. These tumors are very cellular, pleomorphic, and necrotic and demonstrate marked endothelial proliferation.[41]

A *medulloblastoma* arises in the caudal cerebellar vermis and is markedly cellular. The cells in the tumor have little cytoplasm and are undifferentiated. When medulloblastomas occur beyond the first decade of life, they arise more rostrally and laterally in the cerebellar hemispheres.[41]

A *meningioma* may have one of several cell types, each with a different prognosis depending on the cellular variety. The tumor cells are commonly uniform and may form characteristic whorls.[37] Frequent locations for these tumors include the ethmoid regions, parasagittal region, sphenoid ridge, and the dorsal roots of the spinal cord.

Regardless of the pathologic type of intracranial tumor, signs and symptoms reflect progressive neurologic deficits caused by focal disturbances and increased intracranial pressure. Focal disturbances are caused by increasing compression of brain tissue and the infiltration or direct invasion of brain parenchyma resulting in destruction of neural tissue.[51] Cerebral blood supply may also be altered by the tumor's compression of blood vessels, resulting in necrotic cerebral tissue or seizures. Approximately 30% of adults with intracranial tumors develop focal or generalized seizure activity. Increased intracranial pressure may result from regional edema, alterations in cerebrospinal fluid circulation, and an increase in tissue within the skull. Hydrocephalus results from disruption in the circulation of cerebrospinal fluid from the cerebral ventricles to the subarachnoid spaces (Figure 3-30).

The size and location of the specific tumor can cause shifts of brain tissue with associated brain herniation syndromes. If left untreated, herniation can lead to infarction and hemorrhage in the upper pons and the midbrain, resulting in pontomedullary decompensation.[24]

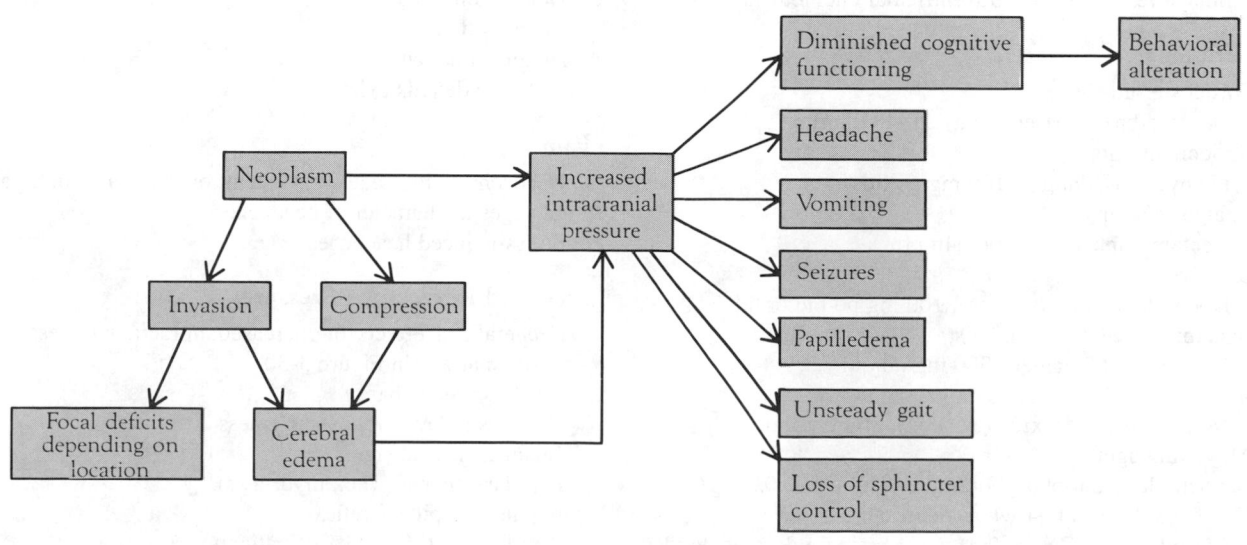

Figure 3-30 Origin of clinical manifestations associated with an intracranial neoplasm. (From McCance and Huether.[43])

•••••• Diagnostic Studies and Findings

Skull roentgenograms Erosion of posterior clinoid process or presence of intracranial calcifications

Chest roentgenograms Detection of primary lung tumor or metastatic disease

CT scan Identification of vascular tumors; shifts in midline structures; changes in cerebral ventricular sizes

Electroencephalogram (EEG) Marked focal slowing (with rapidly developing tumors); rhythmic, periodic, and high-voltage slowing (with increased intracranial pressure)

Dural sinus venography May indicate narrowed sinuses and interference with cranial damage

Echoencephalogram Shifts in midline structures

Ophthalmoscopic examination Papilledema (late sign of increased intracranial pressure)

Brain scan Increased uptake of isotope in the tumor

Pneumoencephalogram Tumor localization; contraindicated if increased intracranial pressure is suspected

Cerebral angiography Cerebral vascularity; blood vessel deviations

Magnetic resonance imaging (MRI) Same as CT scan, without radiation

Positron emission tomography (PET) Same as CT scan, but also details sites of glucose metabolism in the brain under various conditions

Stereotaxic biopsy Identifies histologic cell type

•••••• Multidisciplinary Plan

Surgery

Intracranial pressure monitoring

Tumor excision; craniotomy (supratentorial; infratentorial)

Shunting procedure to treat secondary complications of hydrocephalus

Laser therapy

Ommaya reservoir for intraventricular chemotherapy

Medications

Corticosteroids
  Dexamethasone (Decadron), 20-40 mg/d po
Anticonvulsants
  Phenytoin (Dilantin), 100 mg po tid
Analgesic/antipyretics
  Acetaminophen, gr X po q4h prn
Laxatives
  Docusate sodium (Colace), 100 mg po bid or tid
Histamine receptor antagonist
  Cimetidine (Tagamet), 300 mg po qid
Antacids
  Magnesium hydroxide (Maalox), 30 ml po qid
Alkylating agents
  Triethylene thiophosphoramide (Thiotepa), 0.2 mg/kg IV for 5 d; repeat q4 wk as necessary
  Carmustine (BCNU), 200 mg/m^2 (single dose or divided doses of 100 mg/m^2) IV q6 wk

Antimetabolites
  Floxuridine (FUDR), 0.1-0.6 mg/kg/d intra-arterial infusion or 0.4-0.6 mg/kg/d via hepatic artery
  Fluorouracil (5-FU), 12.5 mg/kg/d IV for 3-5 d; repeat q4 wk as necessary
Other
  Procarbazine (Matulane), 100-150 mg/m^2 po for 10 d
  Vincristine (Oncovin), 1-2 mg/m^2 IV q wk

General Management

Radiation therapy
Mechanical ventilation, if indicated
Cardiac monitoring
Nutritional consultation
Physical therapy
Speech therapy
Occupational therapy
Social services

NURSING CARE

Nursing Assessment

Focal Neurologic Disturbance

Gradually increasing weakness
Subtle sensory loss
Adult-onset seizures not always relieved by medications

Mentation

Patient's level of consciousness must be noted (See Table 3-6)
Personality changes (i.e., loss of emotional restraints)
Insidious decrease in mentation
Depression
Memory deficits
Judgment deficits
Self-care deficits exist

Pain

Headaches with steady, persistent, or intractable dull pain
Changes in character of headaches
Stress-induced headaches

Increased Intracranial Pressure

(Generalized effects of increased intracranial pressure are summarized in Figure 3-30)
Restlessness, lethargy
Changes in level of consciousness
Changes in vital signs
Pupillary changes (i.e., mydriasis)
Impaired pupillary reflex
Papilledema (70%-75% of patients)
Vomiting (may be projectile)

Fluctuations in temperature—temperature must be taken every 20 minutes and prn
Seizures
Worsening of focal neurologic signs
Changes in respiratory patterns

Seizure Activity

Seizure history
Potential for injury
Initial symptom in 15% of patients
Preconvulsive (preictal stage)
Aura: flash of light; sense of loss; fear; weakness; dizziness; peculiar taste, smell, and sounds
Cry or scream
Fall to floor
Loss of consciousness
Tachypnea
Convulsive stage
Tonic: rigid body; fixed jaws; clenched fists; extended legs; cyanosis; holding breath
Clonic: urinary and/or fecal incontinence; jerking of facial muscles and extremities; biting tongue; frothing at mouth
Postconvulsive (postictal stage)
Altered level of consciousness
Headache
Nausea or vomiting
Malaise
Muscle soreness
Aspiration: breathing difficulty, choking, cyanosis, decreased breath sounds, tachycardia, tachypnea

Pituitary Dysfunction

Cushing's syndrome
Acromegaly
Giantism
Hypopituitarism

Nursing Dx & Intervention

Ineffective airway clearance related to high risk for tracheobronchial obstruction

- See general intervention strategies listed on p. 1614.

Ineffective breathing pattern related to potential ineffective airway clearance

- See general intervention strategies listed on p. 1616.

Altered cerebral tissue perfusion related to high risk for interruption of flow and exchange problems

- Establish baseline and ongoing neurologic assessment every 1 to 2 hours and as needed as indicated by the patient's condition, level of consciousness, motor or sensory deficits, cranial nerve functioning, auditory functioning, nausea and vomiting, reflex status, pupillary size, reaction, behavior and personality changes, abnormal posturing spontaneously, or to stimulus response.
- Intervene *to monitor and prevent increased intracranial pressure:*
  Administer medications, treatments, and IV lines per protocol.
  Maintain elevation of head of bed per protocol *to facilitate venous drainage.*
  Accurately record intake and output *to monitor for imbalance.*
  Monitor serum electrolytes, blood count, and arterial blood gases for abnormalities.
- Monitor values and wave forms of intracranial pressure line, if appropriate *(Continuous flushing systems must not be used for ICP measurement).*
- Maintain patency and sterility of the system.
- Monitor effects of treatments of intracranial pressure.
- Correlate neurologic status with intracranial pressure values; notify physician if inconsistent.
- Assist with drainage of cerebrospinal fluid from the system *to lower intracranial hypertension.*
- Plan nursing care *to minimize elevation in ICP.*
- Avoid flexion of hip, isometric exercises, Valsalva maneuver, hypoxemia, and hypercapnia.
- Maintain normothermia.
- Provide adequate ventilation and oxygenation.
- Elevate head of bed 30 to 45 degrees *to facilitate cerebral venous drainage.*
- Monitor for signs of brain herniation.
  Change in LOC
  Change in response to painful stimuli
  Change in pupil size or shape
  Widening pulse pressure
  Change in respiratory pattern
  Bradycardia
- Intervene *to monitor and prevent seizures.*
  Institute seizure precautions: padded tongue blade and airway at bedside, bed height at lowest level, side rails up at all times and padded, oxygen and suction equipment at bedside, emergency medications at bedside.
  Administer anticonvulsants as per protocol:
  Monitor effects and side effects.
  Monitor serum for therapeutic levels of the anticonvulsant.
  Administer corticosteroids *to control cerebral edema.*

Ineffective thermoregulation related to cerebral edema or increased intracranial pressure

- Administer steroids per protocol *to reduce cerebral edema.*
- Administer antipyretic agents per protocol.
- Administer IV fluids at room temperature *to promote adequate fluid intake and prevent chilling.*

- Monitor vital signs q2h and prn.
- Adjust environmental temperature as indicated.
- Adjust patient temperature as indicated, using cooling blanket, heat mattress, or warm blankets.

Sensory/perceptual alterations related to neurologic impairment

- Maintain quiet environment *to reduce external stimuli to a minimum.*
- Reorient patient frequently to time, place, and person. Introduce yourself each time you reorient patient.
- Repeat explanations frequently and simply.
- Assist patient in judgments, perceptions, and reorientation as needed.
- Have family bring in familiar objects.
- Maintain planned rest periods *to allow sufficient time for REM sleep.*
- Use day and night lighting appropriately *to promote nocturnal wake-sleep pattern.*
- Stimulate senses of touch, taste, and position.
- Address patient by preferred name *to promote self-recognition.*

Risk for injury related to seizure activity

- Maintain bed in low position at all times unless side rails are up or when nurse is with the patient.
- Provide the patient with a call light within easy reach.
- Maintain side rails in up position.
- Pad side rails if patient is overactive.
- Monitor for occult bleeding (gastric, stools, urine).

Preconvulsive

- Have oral airway at bedside.
- Support and protect head; turn to side if possible.
- Prevent injury:
    Ease patient to floor if in chair.
    Place pillows along side rails if in bed.
    Remove surrounding furniture.
    Loosen constrictive clothing.
- Provide privacy as necessary.
- Stay with patient; remain calm.
- Note frequency, time, involved body parts, and length of seizure.

Postconvulsive

- Maintain patent airway.
- Suction as indicated *to prevent airway obstruction.*
- Check vital signs and neurologic status.
- Administer oxygen per protocol *to minimize cerebral hypoxia.*
- Reorient patient to environment.
- Place patient in position of comfort; turn head to side.
- Administer oral hygiene as necessary *to remove or control secretions and blood.*

Impaired physical mobility related to perceptual cognitive impairment

- See general intervention strategies listed on p. 1597.

Bathing/hygiene, dressing/grooming, feeding self-care deficit related to perceptual cognitive impairment

- Assist with feeding as indicated. Use IV or nasogastric feedings per protocol.
- Assist with daily hygiene care as indicated.
- Administer eye care every 2 to 4 hours if indicated *to prevent crustation and infection.*
- Maintain bowel function with regular evacuation.

Risk for impaired skin integrity related to impaired physical mobility

- See general intervention strategies listed on p. 1557.
- Provide frequent skin care.
- Monitor for signs of phlebitis.
- Protect skin from tape application, sunlight, and friction.

Powerlessness related to perceptual cognitive impairment

- See general intervention strategies listed on p. 1677.

Constipation related to neuromuscular impairment

- See general intervention strategies listed on p. 1571.

Diarrhea related to neuromuscular impairment

- See general intervention strategies listed on p. 1573.

Altered patterns of urinary elimination related to neuromuscular impairment

- See general intervention strategies listed on p. 1576.

Adaptive capacity, decreased

Intracranial

- Perform neurologic assessment q 2 H and PRN *to detect signs of increased ICP.*
- Monitor vital signs q 1 H and PRN *to detect changes in blood pressure with widening pulse pressure and bradycardia.*
- Assess for changing levels of consciousness.
- Assess for pupillary changes.
- Assess patient's motor and sensory functions *to detect potential changes in ICP.*
- Assess for headache, vomiting, and seizure activity.
- Monitor cardiac status.
- Measure and record ICP per protocol.
- Maintain neutral body alignment with head of bed elevated at 30 degrees, unless contraindicated *to facilitate cerebral venous drainage.*
- Avoid procedures that result in increased thoracic and abdominal pressure such as hip flexion, coughing, isometric exercises, and Valsalva maneuver.
- Log roll patient *to minimize increases in BP and ICP.*
- Minimize patient activity.
- Administer supplemental oxygen *to prevent hypoxia and hypercapnia.*

- Hyperoxygenate with 100% oxygen before suctioning and limit ETS to <15 seconds *to minimize cerebral ischemia.*
- Monitor ABGs and regulate mechanical ventilation *to maintain $PaCO_2$ 25 to 30 mm Hg to reduce cerebral vasodilation.*
- Administer diuretics, hyperosmotics, and corticosteroids as directed.
- Limit fluid intake *to maintain slight state of dehydration.*
- Maintain normothermia *to minimize cerebral metabolic demands.*

Confusion, chronic related to organic or cognitive impairment

- Assess baseline physical, functional, and psychosocial status.
- Evaluate previous interests.
- Ensure optimal sensory input (i.e., eyeglasses, hearing aid) is available.
- Evaluate stimulation threshold *to prevent overstimulation.*
- Provide for structured repetitive group activities.
- Provide rest periods between activities *to minimize fatigue.*
- Monitor for changes in physical, functional, and psychologic status.
- Maintain calm, reassuring demeanor when interacting with patient *to promote sense of trust.*
- Encourage patient to participate in care as tolerated *to minimize feelings of powerlessness.*
- Provide positive feedback for tasks/activities that are mastered.

Aspiration, risk for related to enteric feeding via nasoenteric tube.

- Confirm feeding tube placement after insertion, q 4 H and PRN.
    - Confirm tube placement before and after each intermittent tube feeding.
    - Confirm initial enteral tube placement by physician examination of chest x-ray.
- Tape nasogastric tube securely per protocol.
- Aspirate stomach contents *to determine gastric pH.*
- Assess bowel sounds q 4 H and PRN.
- Assess patient for abdominal distention, nausea/vomiting, and diarrhea/constipation.
    - Hold tube feedings if bowel sounds are absent and if diarrhea/constipation or nausea/vomiting are present.
- Maintain proper patient positioning.
    - Elevate head-of-bed 30 to 40 degrees.
    - Turn patient to right side *to facilitate stomach drainage through pylorus.*
- Discontinue continuous feedings 30 to 40 minutes before activity/procedure that requires lowering the patient's head.
- Check vital signs q 2 H and PRN.
- Check pulmonary-tracheal secretions q 4 H and PRN *to detect presence of enteral feeding.*

- Monitor for signs of aspiration including cough, wheezing, dyspnea, hyperthermia, and tachycardia.
- Auscultate breath sounds q 4 H and PRN.

Patient Education/Home Care Planning

1. Involve the family in care, as possible; teach essential aspects of care.
2. Reinforce the physician's explanation of medical management.
3. Stress importance of ongoing outpatient care and follow-up visits.
4. Encourage independent activities, as possible:
    a. Alert the patient to limitations.
    b. Avoid overprotection.
    c. Stress need for supportive devices as indicated.
5. Stress need for a regular exercise program. Teach ROM exercises to family.
6. Stress importance of diet as ordered:
    a. Offer supplemental feedings.
    b. Offer small portions, and instruct the patient to chew slowly.
7. Stress importance of safety measures: side rails, ramps, shower chairs, and walkers and canes.
8. Discuss each name of medication, dosage, time of administration, and toxic or side effects.
9. Ensure the patient understands the need to avoid over-the-counter medications without first consulting physician.
10. Encourage socialization with friends and family.
11. Stress importance of verbalization of feelings about anxiety, fear, and body image changes.
12. Discuss with the patient and family about seizures: safety measures and whom to contact.

Evaluation

Patient demonstrates a patent airway Breath sounds are normal. Chest excursion is bilateral and symmetric. Rate and depth of respirations are normal. Cough is effective. There are no subjective or objective findings of shortness of breath, air hunger, or dyspnea on exertion.

Patient demonstrates an effective breathing pattern Airway is patent. Chest excursion is symmetric. Breath sounds are normal, or there is no increase in adventitious sounds. Arterial blood gas values are within normal ranges or consistent with patient's baseline. Vital signs are within normal ranges or consistent with patient's baseline. Hemoglobin levels are 14 to 18 g/dl (male) or 12 to 16 g/dl (female). Intake and output are stable. There are no signs of respiratory distress. All lobes are resonant on percussion. Skin color is not cyanotic.

Patient maintains adequate cerebral tissue perfusion Level of consciousness is unchanged. There is no evidence of neurologic deficits. Pattern of electrolytes is stable. There is no seizure activity.

Patient demonstrates adequate body temperature regulation   Vital signs are within normal range for patient. Serum electrolytes and fluid balance are within normal limits. Patient's body temperature is maintained between 35.8° and 37.3° C (96.4° and 99.2° F). Patient remains free of symptoms of hypothermia or hyperthermia including flushing or cyanosis, irritability, and seizures.

Patient demonstrates minimal complications of sensory/perceptual alterations   Level of orientation is optimum. Patient is free of injury. Patient demonstrates skin integrity. Self-care deficits are minimum. Social participation is appropriate to physiologic status.

Patient remains free of traumatic injury   Safety measures are appropriate to physiologic status. Skin integrity is maintained. Skin is free of bruises, burns, abrasions, and redness. Environment is safe. Patient is free of nosocomial infections.

Patient demonstrates an optimum level of mobility   Skin integrity is maintained. Patient remains free of contractures and deformities. Level of mobility is appropriate to physiologic status. Intake and output pattern is stable. Nutritional status is adequate. Patient is free of thrombophlebitis. Patient is free of local infection. Patient participates in an ongoing physical therapy program.

Patient demonstrates minimum self-care deficits   Outcome criteria listed for impaired physical mobility are met. Level of self-care activities is appropriate to physiologic status. Patient participates in physical and occupational therapy.

Patient demonstrates minimum feelings of powerlessness   Optimum level of physiologic control, as possible for current health status, is maintained. Optimum level of psychologic control, as possible, is maintained. Patient participates, as possible, in decision making about care. Patient participates, as possible, in self-care.

Patient demonstrates minimum complications of bowel alteration   Skin in perineal area is clean and dry. Dietary intake is adequate. Fluid intake is adequate (2000 ml/day unless contraindicated). Intake and output patterns are stable. There is no fecal impaction. Bowel evacuation pattern is regular. Diarrhea is controlled or absent.

Patient demonstrates minimum complications from alterations in urinary elimination patterns   Intake and output patterns are stable. Urine is clear, yellow to amber in color, and without sediment. Skin in perineal area is clean and dry. Urine is acidic (pH 6.0). Patient remains free of urinary tract infections. Patient remains free of bladder distention. Patient can describe symptoms of urinary tract infections that require medical intervention.

Patient demonstrates minimal confusion   Available sensory aids (i.e., eyeglasses, hearing aid) are used appropriately. Patient is able to participate in structured repetitive group activities. Rest periods between activities are maintained. Patient is able to participate in care to tolerance.

Patient remains free of aspiration   Airway is patent. Vital signs are stable. Patient reports/demonstrates no signs of choking. Breath sounds are normal. Nasoenteric tube placement is verified.

Patient demonstrates maximal intracranial adaptive capacity   Vital signs are stable. No signs of increased intracranial pressure are present. Patient is normothermic. Arterial blood gas values are within normal limits or consistent with patient's baseline. Intake and output are stable. Skin color is not cyanotic.

SPINAL TUMORS

Spinal tumors, although less common than intracranial tumors, are similar in pathologic types. They can arise from spinal nerve roots, the meninges, parenchyma of the cord, vertebral column, or the spinal vascular network (Figure 3-31).

Spinal tumors frequently affect young and middle-aged adults, and usually involve the thoracic (50%), cervical (30%), and lumbosacral (20%) areas. The tumors are rare in children and elderly persons. Spinal tumors are classified according to their location; those occurring within the spinal cord tissue are called *intramedullary,* and those outside the spinal cord are called *extramedullary.* Extramedullary tumors are categorized further as intradural, extradural, or extravertebral. Spinal lesions constitute approximately 1% of all tumors in the general population. Men and women are affected about equally, except that meningiomas affect women more frequently. Approximately 85% of intraspinal tumors are benign.

•••••• Pathophysiology

Intramedullary tumors within the tissue of the spinal cord arise primarily from astrocyte or ependymal cells. Expanding intramedullary lesions may compress the spinal cord and nerve roots and destroy the parenchyma. Extramedullary tumors can be inside or outside the dural sac and produce spinal cord and spinal nerve root compression. Lesions outside the dural sac are called *extradural* and include herniated vertebral discs, acute and chronic infectious processes, metastatic lesions, meningiomas (5% to 10%), schwannomas (25% to 30%), and epidural hemorrhages. Tumors located within the dural sac but outside the spinal cord and nerve roots are called *extramedullary intradural* and include several types of glial tumors (e.g., ependymoma), most meningiomas and schwannomas, hemorrhages, and embryonic or congenital lesions. *Extramedullary extravertebral* tumors are commonly associated with bony destruction of vertebrae.[32]

Schwannomas are the spinal tumors most commonly arising from the nerve sheath and can be found in all portions of the spinal cord. These tumors appear as a firm, encapsulated, rounded mass that contains many small cysts. Schwannomas consist of interlacing bands of cells with parallel intracellular fibrils and elongated nuclei that are usually arranged in parallel rows. There are also a number of star-shaped cells resembling astrocytes loosely arranged in the microscopic structure. Small foci of degeneration with cysts are common. First, the schwannoma compresses as the spinal nerve root in the foramen of the

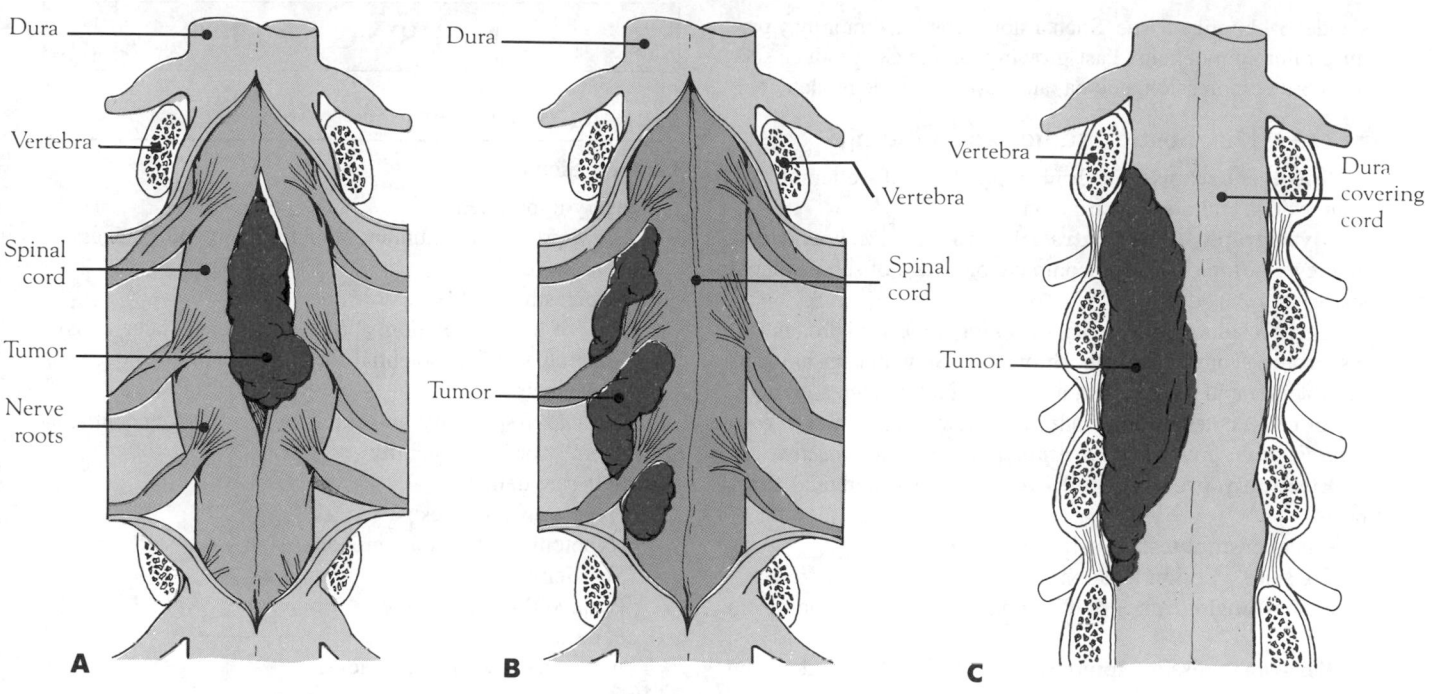

Figure 3-31 Spinal cord tumors. **A,** Intramedullary tumor. **B,** Intradural-extramedullary tumor. **C,** Extradural-extramedullary tumor.

canal, producing localized nerve root symptoms. As the lesion progresses, it further compresses other nerve roots and the spinal cord, producing neurologic findings of cord compression. Symptoms are usually asymmetric. Extradural schwannomas are often hourglass or dumbbell in shape with a portion in the spinal canal attached by a narrow band of tumor through the foramen to a part outside the spinal canal. This type of tumor can compress cervical, mediastinal, or abdominal tissue.[4]

Meningiomas constitute approximately 22% of all primary spinal tumors. Most meningiomas are extramedullary. Eighty percent of meningiomas affect women, usually in the fourth, fifth, or sixth decade of life. These tumors can appear anywhere in the spinal canal but are most common in the region of the nerve roots, particularly in the thoracic region (two thirds of meningiomas occur in this region). They appear as small, rounded, nodular masses that frequently attach to the insertion of the denticulate ligament and extend dorsally or ventrally. Meningiomas consist of groups of elongated cells with round or oval nuclei. There is a tendency toward the formation of whorls, and calcification frequently is present in the center of the whorls. Symptoms are initially produced by traction or irritation of the nerve roots (i.e., radicular pain) and progress to long motor tract signs (i.e., spasticity) as a result of compression. Meningiomas can undergo malignant changes.[4]

Ependymomas make up approximately 13% of all spinal cord tumors. They arise from the lining of the internal spaces of the central nervous system and are usually intramedullary. Ependymomas are found throughout the spinal cord but commonly are located caudally in the conus medullaris and the filum terminale (cauda equina ependymoma). They are more common in men, generally appearing in the fourth or fifth decade of life. These tumors occur as loculated masses in the spinal canal, frequently with fusiform swelling. Microscopically, an ependymoma appears as a crowded mass of polygonal-type cells. In the filum it appears as a central core of connective tissue and blood vessels that is surrounded by a single layer of ependymal cells. Ependymomas may extend to 10 vertebral spaces in length and produce symptoms resulting from cord compression.[4]

Astrocytomas and oligodendrogliomas are similar clinically. The oligodendroglioma is a rare type of spinal cord tumor. Astrocytomas are less common than ependymomas, generally intramedullary, and more common in men. Astrocytomas appear as elongated, fusiform swellings of the spinal cord. (See Table 3-6 for grading of astrocytomas.) Symptoms result from compression of the long tracts of the spinal cord.

The pathologic processes occurring with any spinal tumors can result from spinal cord destruction and infiltration, spinal cord displacement and compression, spinal nerve root irritation and compression, disruption in spinal blood supply, or disruption of cerebrospinal fluid circulation.[32]

Most benign lesions produce neurologic symptoms by compression and displacement of the spinal cord and by irritation and compression of the spinal nerve roots rather than by invasion and destruction of the spinal cord. The severity of neurologic symptoms depends on the degree of compression and how rapidly it develops. With slower-growing tumors, the spinal cord can accommodate the mass by compressing itself into a slender, ribbonlike tissue. Such a slow-growing tumor may produce minimum deficits. Fast-growing tumors can produce sudden cord compression, edema, and severe neurologic deficits.[29]

•••••• Diagnostic Studies and Findings

Roentgenograms   Determine presence of vertebral column lesions and bony destruction

Myelography (with contrast)   Identifies size, boundaries, and level of tumor (with incomplete blockage of subarachnoid space)

Cerebrospinal fluid (CSF) sampling   Elevated protein levels; Froin's syndrome (xanthochromatic CSF with large amounts of protein, rapid coagulation, and absence of an increased number of cells) noted if CSF collected below level of tumor; *contraindication: if elevated intraspinal pressure is suspected*

Electromyogram (EMG)   Assistive in differential diagnosis

Queckenstedt test   Positive

CT scan   Lesion location identified

Spinal angiograms   Differentiates vascular lesions from tumors

Positron emission tomography (PET)   Lesion location identified

•••••• Multidisciplinary Plan

Surgery

Tumor excision
Laminectomy
Tracheotomy, if indicated
Spinal fusion
Lumbar puncture

Medications

Corticosteroids (to control cord edema)
    Dexamethasone (Decadron), 10-40 mg IV qid
Antacids
    Maalox, 15-30 ml po or nasogastric q4h
Histamine antagonist
    Cimetidine (Tagamet), 300 mg po or IV
Analgesic/antipyretics
    Acetaminophen, gr X po q4h prn
Systemic chemotherapy

General Management

Radiation therapy
Mechanical ventilation, if indicated
CT scans
Soft cervical collar, if indicated, to alleviate discomfort
Spinal prostheses
Physiotherapy
Nutritional consultation
Psychosocial counseling and support
Extended care facility referral, if appropriate
Social services

NURSING CARE

Nursing Assessment

General Signs

Sensory impairment
    Slow, progressive numbness or tingling, and coldness in an extremity
    Hyperesthesia at level of lesion
    Loss of touch, vibration, and position sense (later signs)
    Skin integrity has potential for breakdown
Motor impairment
    Weakness, spasticity, and clumsiness: spreading contralaterally or homolaterally
    Self-care deficit
    Hyperactive reflexes
    Hypotonia and ataxia (cerebellar signs)
    Spasticity
    Positive Babinski's reflex
    Paresis
    Assess patient's mobility level
Pain
    Intermittent nerve root (radicular) pain, aggravated by straining, movement, and coughing
    Persistent back pain
Sphincter disturbances
    Urinary urgency
    Difficulty in initiating urination
    Retention and overflow incontinence
    Decreased sphincter control (later sign)
Other
    Brown-Séquard syndrome
    Contralateral loss of temperature and pain
    Ipsilateral motor loss
    Ipsilateral loss of vibration, touch, and position sense
    Potential for injury exists

Cervical Tumors

C4 and above
    Sensory
        Vertigo
    Motor
        Quadriparesis
        Atrophy of sternocleidomastoid muscles
        Dysphagia
        Dysarthria
        Tongue deviation
        Respiratory insufficiency
        Respiratory failure
    Other
        Occipital headaches
        Nuchal rigidity
        Down-beat nystagmus
        Papilledema

C4 and below
  Sensory
    Paresthesia
    Horner's syndrome (ipsilateral pupillary constriction, ptosis, and anhidrosis)
  Motor
    Weakness
    Muscle fasciculations
    Muscle atrophy
  Other
    Shoulder and arm pain

Thoracic Tumors

Sensory
  Hyperesthesia band immediately above level of lesion
Motor
  Spastic paresis of lower extremities
  Positive Babinski's sign
  Lower motor neuron deficits
Other
  Sphincter impairment

Lumbar Tumors

Sensory
  Localized loss in legs and saddle area
Motor
  Footdrop
  Diminished or absent patellar and Achilles reflexes
Other
  Severe low back pain with radiation down legs
  Perineal and bladder discomfort
  Decreased libido
  Impotence
  Bladder disturbances

Nursing Dx & Intervention

Ineffective breathing pattern related to impaired respiratory muscle function

- Auscultate for breath sounds every 1 to 2 hours. Assess quality and any increase in adventitious sounds *to prevent pulmonary complications:*
    Suction as needed *to prevent airway obstruction and secretion stasis.*
    Hyperoxygenate lungs with 100% oxygen for 1 minute before and 1 minute after suctioning, unless contraindicated, *to minimize hypoxia during suctioning.*
- Monitor mechanical ventilation, if used:
    Ensure that tidal volume, rate, mode, and oxygen concentration are set as ordered.
    Ensure that ventilator alarms are on and functional.
- Monitor arterial blood gases per protocol *to minimize risks of respiratory insufficiency and failure:*
    Report decrease in Po_2 of 10 to 15 mm Hg *to prevent hypoxemia.*

Report increase in Pco_2 greater than 10 to 15 mm Hg *to prevent hypercapnia.*
- Check blood pressure, temperature, and pulse rate every 1 to 2 hours and as needed.

Altered cerebral or spinal tissue perfusion related to altered cerebrovascular dynamics

- Establish baseline and ongoing neurologic assessment every 1 to 2 hours and as needed.
- Intervene *to monitor or prevent increased intracranial pressure:*
    Administer medications, treatments, and IV lines per protocol.
    Maintain elevation of head of bed per protocol *to facilitate cerebral venous drainage.*
    Accurately record intake and output *to monitor for imbalance.*
    Monitor serum electrolytes, blood count, and arterial blood gases for abnormalities.
    Monitor values and waveforms of intracranial pressure line *to minimize risks of increased intracranial pressure.*
    Continuous flushing systems must not be used for measuring ICP.
    Maintain patency and sterility of the system.
    Monitor effects of treatments on intracranial pressure.
    Correlate neurologic status with intracranial pressure values; notify physician if inconsistent.
    Assist with drainage of cerebrospinal fluid from the system *to decrease intracranial hypertension.*
- Intervene *to monitor or prevent seizures.* Institute seizure precautions:
    Padded tongue blade and airway at bedside
    Bed height at lowest level to prevent falls
    Side rails up at all times and padded
    Oxygen and suction equipment at bedside
    Emergency medications at bedside
- Administer anticonvulsants per protocol:
    Monitor effects and side effects.
    Monitor serum for therapeutic levels of the anticonvulsant.
- Maintain balance between hyperthermia and hypothermia.

Sensory/perceptual alterations (kinesthetic, tactile) related to motor/sensory changes

- See general intervention strategies on p. 1643.

Risk for trauma related to seizures

- Maintain bed in low position at all times unless side rails are up or nurse is with patient *to prevent patient falls.*
- Provide patient with a call light within easy reach.
- Maintain side rails in up position at bedtime, after sedation, when patient is confused, and as needed.

- Maintain wheelchairs and stretchers in locked position when transferring patient *to minimize risks for falling.*
- Pad side rails if patient is overactive.

Preconvulsive
- Have oral airway at bedside.
- Support and protect head; turn to side if possible.
- Prevent injury:
    Ease patient to floor if in chair.
    Place pillows along side rails if patient is in bed.
    Remove surrounding furniture.
    Loosen constrictive clothing.
- Provide privacy as necessary. Stay with patient; remain calm.
- Note frequency, time, involved body parts, and length of seizure *to determine type of seizure.*

Postconvulsive
- Maintain patent airway.
- Suction as needed, as indicated.
- Check vital signs and neurologic signs.
- Administer oxygen per protocol *to minimize cerebral hypoxia.*
- Reorient patient to environment.
- Place patient in position of comfort; turn head to side *to prevent aspiration.*
- Administer oral hygiene as necessary for secretions and bleeding.

Risk for impaired skin integrity related to musculoskeletal impairment

- Administer skin care every 2 hours *to prevent breakdown and decubitus ulcers.*
    Turn patient every 2 hours and as needed, unless contraindicated:
    Change position slowly.
    Position in proper body alignment.
    Massage pressure points every 2 hours *to stimulate circulation;* give gentle back rubs every shift and as needed.
    Keep skin dry and clean.
    Provide passive ROM exercises every 4 hours and as needed *to maintain joint mobility.*
    Perform ROM exercises gently, slowly, and rhythmically.
    Repeat each ROM exercise three times, every 4 hours.
- Maintain high-protein, low-calcium diet.

Impaired physical mobility related to neuromuscular impairment

- Assess patient's mobility level and document the following interventions:
    Use firm mattress or bed board *to support back and spine.*
    Use footboard or Spence boots *to prevent footdrop.*
    Apply antiembolus stockings to lower extremities *to promote venous return.*
    Administer anticoagulation therapy per protocol.

Encourage self-care activities to tolerance.
Plan all activities and maintain planned rest periods *to avoid fatigue.*
Obtain physical therapy referral.

Feeding, bathing/hygiene, dressing/grooming, and toileting are self-care deficits related to altered motor/sensory changes

- Assist with feeding, as indicated; use IV or nasogastric feedings per protocol.
- Administer oral hygiene every 2 hours and as needed.
- Assist with daily hygiene care as indicated.
- Administer eye care every 2 to 4 hours if indicated.
- Perform intermittent urinary catheterization per protocol.
- Maintain bowel function with regular evacuation *to prevent constipation.*

Pain related to spinal cord compression

- Modify anxiety associated with the pain experience.
- Provide other sensory input *to minimize focus on painful stimuli.*
- For patients receiving radiation or chemotherapy:
    Explain procedure or medication before implementing.
    Administer antiemetic and antidiarrheal medications as needed *to prevent nausea and control diarrhea.*
    Provide frequent skin care.
    Monitor for signs of phlebitis.

Body image disturbance related to physical, cognitive, and perceptual alterations

- Assess degree of orientation and ability to communicate.
- Provide for a safe, comfortable, secure environment.
- Reorient to time, person, and place, as appropriate *to maintain sense of personal identity.*
- Carefully explain what you are doing and why you are doing it.
- Answer questions simply and honestly.
- Correct misinformation.
- Protect the patient's privacy.
- Provide gentle physical care in a caring environment.

Patient Education/Home Care Planning

1. Involve family in care, as possible; teach essential aspects of care.
2. Reinforce physician's explanation of medical management.
3. Stress importance of ongoing outpatient care and follow-up visits.
4. Encourage independent activities, as possible:
    a. Be alert to limitations.
    b. Avoid overprotection.
    c. Stress need for supportive devices as indicated.
5. Stress need for regular exercise program: teach ROM exercises to family.

6. Stress importance of diet as ordered:
   a. Offer supplemental feedings.
   b. Give small portions, and instruct patient to chew slowly.
7. Stress importance of safety measures:
   a. Side rails
   b. Ramps
   c. Shower chairs
   d. Removal of scatter rugs
   e. Walker, canes
8. Discuss name of medication, dosage, time of administration, and toxic or side effects.
9. Stress need to avoid over-the-counter medications without first consulting physician.
10. Encourage socialization with friends and family.
11. Stress importance of verbalization of feelings about anxiety, fear, and body image changes.
12. Ensure patient and family understand about seizures (i.e., safety measures and whom to contact).

Evaluation

Patient demonstrates an effective breathing pattern Airway is patent. Chest excursion is symmetric. Breath sounds are normal, or there is no increase in adventitious sounds. Arterial blood gas values are within normal ranges or consistent with patient's baseline. Vital signs are within normal ranges or consistent with patient's baseline. Hemoglobin levels are 14 to 18 g/dl (male) and 12 to 16 g/dl (female). Intake and output are stable. There are no signs of respiratory distress. All lobes are resonant on percussion. Skin color is not cyanotic.

Patient maintains adequate cerebral and spinal tissue perfusion Level of consciousness is unchanged. There is no evidence of neurologic deficits. Electrolyte pattern is stable. There is no seizure activity.

Patient demonstrates minimal complications of sensory/perceptual alterations Level of orientation is optimum. Patient remains free of injury. Patient demonstrates skin integrity. Nutritional status is adequate. Self-care deficits are minimum. Social participation is appropriate to physiologic status.

Patient remains free of traumatic injury Safety measures are appropriate to level of physiologic status. Skin integrity is maintained. Skin is free of bruises, burns, abrasions, and redness. Environment is safe. Patient is free of nosocomial infections.

Patient demonstrates skin integrity Skin is intact. Nutritional status is adequate. Electrolyte balance is maintained. Patient is free of pressure sores and contractures.

Patient demonstrates an optimum level of mobility Patient exhibits skin integrity. Patient is free of contractures and deformities. Level of mobility is appropriate to physiologic status. Nutritional status is adequate. Intake and output pattern is

stable. Patient is free of thrombophlebitis. Patient is free of local infection. Patient participates in an ongoing physical therapy program.

Patient demonstrates minimum self-care deficits Outcome criteria listed for impaired physical mobility are met. Level of self-care activities is appropriate to physiologic status. Patient participates in physical and occupational therapy.

Patient experiences minimum alterations in comfort Patient openly verbalizes feelings of discomfort when they occur. Patient can use measures to decrease discomfort. Patient verbally validates a decrease in subjective feelings of discomfort. Patient verbally validates a decrease in objective findings of pain.

Patient demonstrates intact self-concepts Patient openly verbalizes feelings of grief and loss. Patient acknowledges actual change in self-image. Patient verbalizes positive feelings about self. Patient focuses on present and future appearance and function. Patient verbalizes feelings of hopefulness, helpfulness, and powerfulness.

VASCULAR DISORDERS

■ ANEURYSM
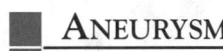
(Cerebral aneurysm)

An intracranial aneurysm is a localized dilation that develops secondary to a weakness of the arterial wall.

Cerebral aneurysm is the fourth most frequent cerebrovascular disorder, with an incidence of 9.6 cases per 100,000 in the general population. The peak incidence is in the 35- to 60-year-old age group, and women are affected slightly more often than men. Cerebral aneurysms rarely occur in children and adolescents. Saccular aneurysms are associated with an increased incidence of congenital polycystic disease of the kidney and coarctation of the aorta.[48] Hypertension is found more frequently in persons who have aneurysms than in the average population; however, aneurysms also occur in normotensive individuals.

Ruptured cerebral aneurysm is the most common cause of nontraumatic subarachnoid hemorrhage. At least 28% of individuals with ruptured cerebral aneurysm die immediately. Of individuals who survive the initial hemorrhage but are not treated, approximately 50% experience rebleeding within a year. Approximately one third of individuals who survive ruptured cerebral aneurysms demonstrate some residual paralysis, headaches and mental changes, or epilepsy. Aneurysmal rupture often is associated with physical exertion (e.g., sports or coitus), severe emotional excitement, and a sudden rise in blood pressure, but it can also occur during sleep.

•••••• Pathophysiology

No single mechanism has been identified in the pathogenesis of intracranial aneurysm. Possible causes are congenital structural defects in the media and elastica of the vessel wall, incomplete involution of embryonic vessels, and secondary factors such as arterial hypertension, atherosclerotic changes, hemodynamic disturbances, and polycystic disease. Intracranial aneurysms also may result from the shearing forces produced during craniocerebral trauma. These shearing forces may weaken the arterial wall, which expands or dilates with each arterial pulsation until bleeding or symptoms occur.

Aneurysms are generally classified according to their predominant characteristics into (1) saccular, or berry; (2) fusiform, or atherosclerotic; and (3) mycotic (Figure 3-32). *Saccular* aneurysms constitute 95% of all ruptured aneurysms. They appear as small, thin-walled "berries" protruding from arteries primarily at points of bifurcations and branchings. Because of the local weakness in the vessel, the intima bulges outward and the sac slowly enlarges until finally wall dissolution and rupture occur.[24]

Fusiform (giant) aneurysms are spindle-shaped dilations of the entire circumference of an artery for several centimeters. They are characterized by degenerative changes in the elastic fibers and deposits of cholesterol in the intima and by fibrous replacement of smooth muscle.[3] These aneurysms most commonly occur along the trunk of the basilar artery. They infrequently rupture and generally produce symptoms by compression of adjacent cerebral tissue or cranial nerves. When rupture does occur, the atherosclerotic or fusiform aneurysm is often fatal.

Mycotic aneurysms are rare and can result when a septic embolus from acute or subacute bacterial endocarditis or other infectious process causes arterial necrosis that may lead to thrombosis or aneurysm formation. Mycotic aneurysms usually arise in a characteristic location along the distal branches of the middle and anterior cerebral arteries.[72] They tend to be multiple.

The majority of ruptured aneurysms are saccular, or berry, aneurysms. Saccular aneurysms characteristically occur at specific locations in the intracranial circulation. Approximately 85% of berry aneurysms are found in the anterior portion of the circle of Willis, and 15% are situated in the vertebral or basilar arteries. Within the anterior portion, there are three main sites of rupture: termination of the internal carotid artery (25%), the

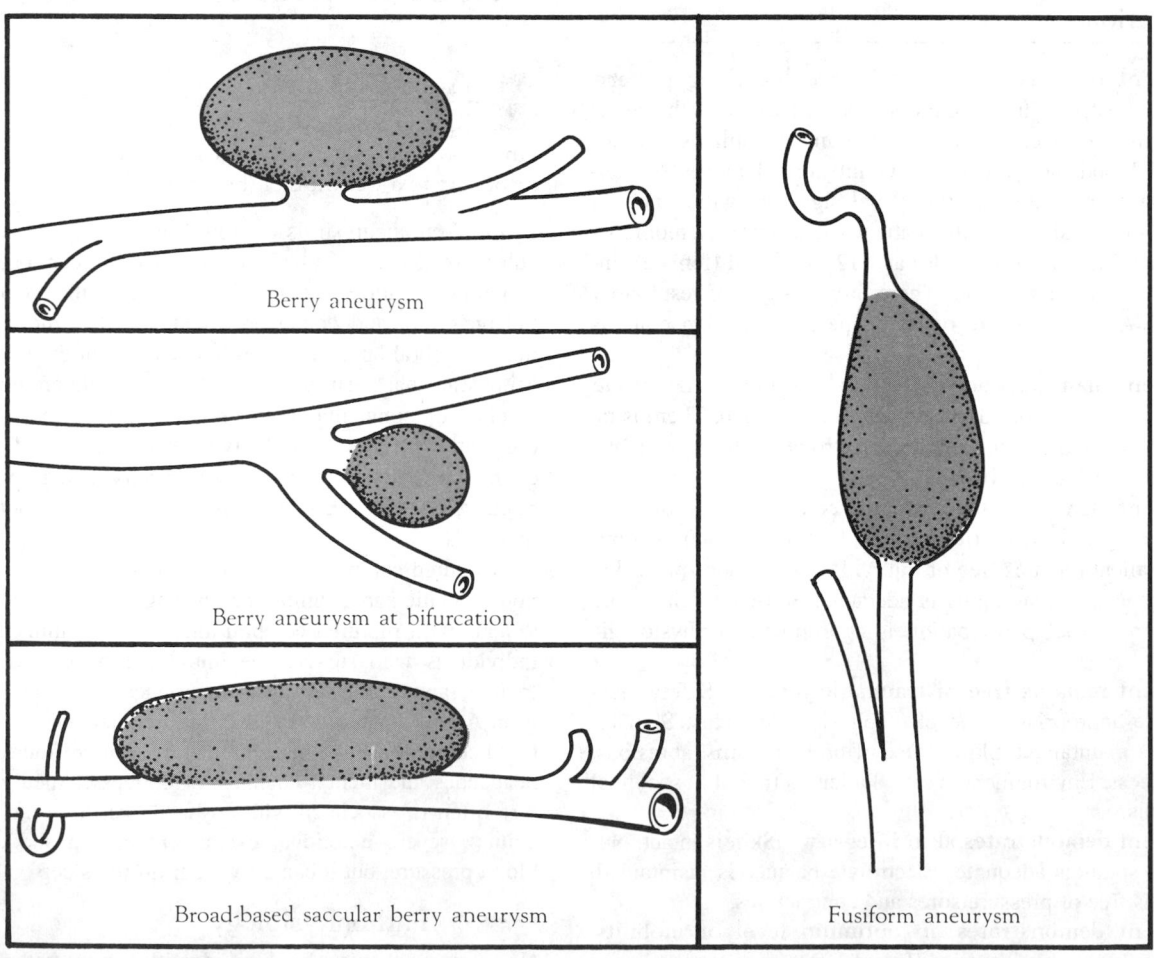

Berry aneurysm

Berry aneurysm at bifurcation

Broad-based saccular berry aneurysm

Fusiform aneurysm

Figure 3-32 Types of aneurysms. (From McCance and Huether.[43])

anterior communicating artery (23%), and the middle cerebral artery bifurcation (16%).[53] Aneurysms of the internal carotid are frequently large and may be situated either in the angle formed by the internal carotid and the posterior communicating artery or at the site of bifurcation of the internal carotid into the anterior and middle cerebral arteries. Aneurysms of the middle cerebral artery usually are located approximately 2 to 3 cm from the vessel's origin, at the site of origin of the first main branches.[28] Multiple aneurysms, often bilateral and symmetric, may be found in 15% to 20% of cases.

Most saccular cerebral aneurysms have a definable neck, and many are multilobular. Thickening, thrombosis, and wall calcification frequently are seen.[18] The aneurysms may vary from 2 mm to 5 cm in diameter. Most aneurysms are at least 10 mm in diameter at the time of rupture. Larger aneurysms may result in erosion of the bones of the skull and compression of cerebral tissue and adjacent cranial nerves.[18] Histopathologic examination shows thinning of the arterial wall with fragmentation of internal elastica and degeneration or absence of its smooth muscle wall.

Aneurysmal rupture occurs when the pulse pressure tears a very small hole in the fundus of the aneurysm, which results in direct hemorrhage into the leptomeningeal compartment (subarachnoid hemorrhage) under arterial pressure. Such a hemorrhage spreads rapidly, producing localized changes in the underlying cortex and focal irritation of the cranial nerves and arteries.[25] The bleeding commonly is stopped by the formation of a fibrin-platelet plug at the point of rupture and by tissue compression. Within approximately 3 weeks the hemorrhage undergoes *resorption.* Resorption occurs by the arachnoidal villi after the leukocytes and macrophages have begun their scavenging.[25] There is a serious risk of recurrent rupture 7 to 10 days after the original hemorrhage.

Massive hemorrhage (i.e., 30 to 50 ml) may produce rapid filling of the ventricular system and vasal cisterns or produce a hematoma that locally distorts the subarachnoid space and brain tissue. Aneurysms of the anterior communicating artery lying next to the medial surfaces of the frontal lobes and aneurysms of the middle cerebral artery within the sylvian fissure next to the frontal and temporal lobes are particularly prone to rupture into the parenchyma of the brain. Aneurysms of the anterior communicating artery may rupture into the frontal lobes. Aneurysms of the basilar artery may rupture into the midbrain or diencephalon. Secondary rupture into the cerebral ventricles can occur because these intracerebral hemorrhages commonly extend through the brain tissue.[18] Aneurysmal rupture may include bleeding in nearby cranial nerves. The most commonly affected cranial nerve is the oculomotor, or cranial nerve III, because of rupture of an aneurysm at the origin of the posterior communicating artery from the internal carotid artery. The optic nerve frequently is involved with ophthalmic artery aneurysms. Carotid aneurysms in the cavernous sinus involve cranial nerves III, IV, and VI, which act on the muscles and the first division of the trigeminal nerve. Increased intracranial pressure results in distortions that can produce unilateral or bilateral sixth nerve palsies. Most of the cranial nerve palsies that develop result from hemorrhage in the nerve and not from compression of the nerve by the aneurysm.[18]

Increased intracranial pressure is frequently a sequela of acute subarachnoid hemorrhage and occurs because of several mechanisms. First, an expanding hematoma acts as a rapidly enlarging space-occupying lesion that compresses or displaces adjacent brain tissue. Second, blood in the basal cistern may impede or interrupt the flow of cerebrospinal fluid. Last, if the pacchionian granulations become distended with blood, the spinal fluid resorption is impeded.[24] The increased intracranial pressure may retard subsequent hemorrhage.

Cerebral vasospasms are a frequent complication of subarachnoidal hemorrhage and occur in 35% to 40% of individuals with ruptured intracranial aneurysms. The pathophysiology of vasospasms is not clearly understood, but it is believed that certain substances, such as prostaglandins, serotonin, catecholamines, and methemoglobin, are released by the blood into the subarachnoid space. These vasoactive substances are thought to precipitate the vasospasms.[24] Edema, media necrosis, and proliferation of the intima have been described as sequelae to the initial vasospasms. Cerebral vasospasms usually appear 4 to 10 days after the hemorrhage and are characterized by measurable constriction or reactive narrowing of the cerebral arteries. The vasospasms are most evident in arteries adjacent to the site of hemorrhage and tend to be lessened when bleeding is minimal. Vasospasms can produce focal neurologic deterioration, cerebral ischemia, and infarction. Angiography shows severely constricted cerebral vessels and confirms the diagnosis.

Subarachnoid hemorrhages are graded according to their severity and clinical status. In one method for grading hemorrhages, individuals in grades I and II are managed medically for an average of 10 days and then treated surgically to prevent recurrent bleeding. Individuals in grades III and IV are managed medically for 3 to 4 weeks to stabilize them for surgery. Individuals in grade V are not surgical candidates unless they have life-threatening complications. The complete cerebral aneurysm classification system is listed in Table 3-9.

TABLE 3-9 Cerebral Aneurysm Rupture Classification System

Grade	Criteria
I (minimal bleed)	Asymptomatic: alert, minimal headache and minimum nuchal rigidity; no neurologic deficits
II (mild bleed)	Mild to severe headache; alert; nuchal rigidity; minimum neurologic deficits
III (moderate bleed)	Lethargic or confused; severe headache; nuchal rigidity; mild focal neurologic deficits
IV (moderate to severe bleed)	Stuporous, nuchal rigidity; mild to severe hemiparesis; may exhibit decerebrate posturing
V (severe bleed)	Comatose; decerebrate posturing

•••••• Diagnostic Studies and Findings

Lumbar puncture   NOTE: *Should be done with caution in presence of suspected increased intracranial pressure;* elevated protein content (80 to 130 gm/dl); increased WBC count; slightly decreased glucose; bloody cerebrospinal fluid with xanthochromia (hemolyzed RBCs)

CT scan (serial)   Demonstration of blood in the subarachnoid space; displaced cerebral midline structures; localized blood clots

Magnetic resonance imaging (MRI)   Same as CT scan

Cerebral angiogram   Identification of local or general vasospasm; outlining of cerebral vasculature

Skull roentgenograms   May reveal calcified wall of aneurysm and areas of bone erosion

Echoencephalogram   Shifts in midline structure

Brain scan   May indicate the presence of local diminution of flow

Serum tests   Electrolyte imbalances; changes in bleeding parameters (i.e., prothrombin time, partial thromboplastin time, and platelet count)

Regional cerebral blood flow (rCBF)   Mean flow values for both hemispheres and determination of status of cerebral vasospasm

•••••• Multidisciplinary Plan

Surgery

Tracheostomy or endotracheal intubation
Intracranial pressure monitoring
Cerebral ventriculostomy to treat increased intracranial pressure and hydrocephalus
Ventriculoatrial shunting (hydrocephalus)
Clipping of aneurysm
Ligation of aneurysm
Wrapping of aneurysmal sac
Trapping of aneurysm with bypass grafting
Embolization of aneurysm
Evacuation of intracerebral clot

Medications

Anticonvulsants
  Phenytoin (Dilantin), 100 mg po or IV tid or qid (do not exceed 50 mg/min IV to prevent hypotension and cardiac arrhythmias)
  Phenobarbital, 50-100 mg po in 2 or 3 divided doses
Antihypertensive agents
  Hydralazine (Apresoline) as ordered
  Methyldopa (Aldomet), 250-500 mg IV q6h
Antifibrinolytic agents
  Aminocaproic acid (Amicar), 24-36 g/d IV for 3 wk (not given with coagulopathies) (Use is controversial)
Corticosteroids
  Dexamethasone (Decadron), 6-10 mg IV q6h
Analgesic/antipyretics
  Acetaminophen (Tylenol), gr X po or rectal suppository q4h prn

Pituitary hormone
  Vasopressin injection (Pitressin), 5-10 U IM or subcutaneously tid or qid (treatment of diabetes insipidus)
Narcotic analgesics
  Acetaminophen with codeine, 30 mg po or IV q4-6h prn
Stool softeners
  Docusate sodium (Colace), 100 mg po or nasogastric bid
Agents to control vasospasms
  Antihistamine (antiserotonin effect)
    Methysergide maleate (Sansert), 4-8 mg/d po
    Phenoxybenzamine (Dibenzyline), 10-40 mg po bid or tid
  Reserpine (Serpasil), 0.1 mg subcutaneously qid
  Kanamycin sulfate (Kantrex), 1 g po tid
  Calcium-blocking agents
    Nifedipine (Procardia), 10-20 mg po tid (dosage tirated)

General Management

Ventilatory support
Hypothermia blanket
ECG; cardiac monitoring
Arterial blood pressure monitoring
Elevation of head of bed
Serial arterial blood gases
Subarachnoid precautions
Strict intake and output
Intermittent catheterization
Seizure precautions
Antiembolus stockings
Hemodynamic monitoring
Complete bed rest
Soft, high fiber diet
Social services consult
Home health referral
Nutritional consultation

NURSING CARE

Nursing Assessment

Assessment findings depend on the location of the hemorrhage.

Level of Consciousness

Varies from brief loss of consciousness to persistent coma
Level of consciousness checked every 15 to 30 minutes

Meningeal Irritation

Nuchal rigidity
Positive Kernig's sign
Positive Brudzinski's sign
Fever
Irritability
Restlessness
Later stages: seizures and blurred vision

Visual Disturbances

Blurred vision
Double vision
Visual field defects: unilateral blindness

Cranial Nerve Involvement

Ptosis and dilation of pupil
Inability to move eye upward or inward
Papilledema
Photophobia

Autonomic Function

Diaphoresis
Chills
Heart rate changes
Changes in blood pressure
Slight temperature elevation (37.8° to 38.9° C; 100° to 102° F)
Altered respiratory rhythm

Motor Function

Onset and worsening of hemiparesis
Aphasia
Dysphagia
Hemiplegia
Unilateral or bilateral transient paresis of lower extremities
Ability to communicate varies

Increased Intracranial Pressure

Restlessness and lethargy
Changes in level of consciousness
Changes in vital signs (i.e., Cushing response with increased systolic blood pressure, wide pulse pressure, and decreased pulse rate)
Pupillary changes (i.e., mydriasis)
Impaired pupillary reflex
Papilledema (late symptom)
Vomiting
Fluctuations in temperature
Seizures
Worsening of focal neurologic signs
Changes in respiratory patterns

Seizure Activity

Preconvulsive (preictal stage)
Aura: flash of light; sense of loss; fear; weakness; dizziness; peculiar taste, smell, and sounds
Cry or scream
Fall to floor
Loss of consciousness
Tachypnea
Convulsive state
Tonic: rigid body; fixed jaws; clenched fists; extended legs; cyanosis; holding breath
Clonic: urinary and/or fecal incontinence; jerking of facial muscles and extremities; biting tongue; frothing at the mouth

Postconvulsive (postictal) stage
Altered level of consciousness
Headache
Nausea or vomiting
Malaise
Muscle soreness
Aspiration: breathing difficulty, choking, cyanosis, decreased breath sounds, tachycardia, tachypnea
Pneumonia

Pain

Sudden onset of a violent headache usually beginning as localized frontally or temporally and then generalizing to involve entire head

Vasospasms

Drowsiness followed by hemiplegia or hemiparesis
Aphasia
Focal neurologic deficits
Seizures

ECG Abnormalities

Q waves
Elevated ST segments
ST and T wave changes

Other

Dizziness, nausea, and vomiting frequent
Cranial bruits may sometimes be auscultated on affected side
Babinski's sign

Nursing Dx & Intervention

Ineffective airway clearance related to impaired cough reflex

- See general intervention strategies on p. 1614.

Ineffective breathing pattern related to neuromuscular dysfunction

- See general intervention strategies on p. 1616.

Altered cerebral tissue perfusion related to increased intracranial pressure secondary to subarachnoid hemorrhage

- Report any changes to physician.
- Monitor closely for signs of increased intracranial pressure (greater than 15 mm Hg for 5 minutes or longer).
- Maintain patency and sterility of intracranial pressure monitoring device, if used:
    Use surgical asepsis for all dressing changes.
    Monitor intracranial pressure responses to care and treatments.
    Continuous flushing devices must not be used for measuring ICP.

- Administer medications per protocol: anticonvulsants, steroids, antibiotics, antifibrinolytics (monitor prothrombin time, partial thromboplastin time, and platelet count), and analgesics.
- Elevate head of bed 30 to 40 degrees, unless contraindicated, *to facilitate venous return.*
- Maintain strict intake and output (1500 to 1800 ml/24 hours) *to maintain fluid balance.*
- Observe for signs of dehydration or overhydration.
- Maintain normothermia per protocol *to minimize cerebral metabolic demands.*
- Institute subarachnoid precautions, if appropriate:
    Provide private room with controlled lighting (i.e., dim artificial lighting).
    Maintain complete bed rest *to keep physical activity and exertion to a minimum.*
    Provide *all* nursing care for the patient.
    Limit visitors to immediate family members *to prevent overstimulation.*
    Have patient wear elastic stockings or sequential compression devices *to prevent venous stasis.*
    Maintain dietary restrictions (no stimulants such as coffee, tea, or soda).
    Administer stool softeners *to prevent straining during bowel movement.*
    Instruct patient on need to avoid coughing and sneezing *to prevent sudden increases in intracranial pressure.*
    Instruct patient not to watch television, listen to radio, or read.
- Avoid hip flexion.
- Maintain head and neck in neutral position *to facilitate venous drainage.*
- Administer calcium (CA) and channel blocking agents as per protocol *to treat cerebral vasospasms.*
- Provide adequate ventilation (Pao_2 >80 mm Hg; $Paco_2$ <40 mm Hg).
- Monitor for signs of brain herniation.
    Change in LOC.
    Change in response to painful stimuli.
    Change in pupil size or shape.
    Widening pulse pressure.
    Change in respiratory pattern.
    Bradycardia.

Sensory/perceptual alterations (kinesthetic, tactile) related to altered sensory perception

- See general intervention strategies on p. 1643.

Risk for injury related to seizures

- Maintain bed in low position at all times unless side rails are up or nurse is with patient.
- Provide patient with a call light within easy reach.
- Maintain side rails in up position at bedtime, after sedation, when patient is confused, and as needed *to prevent falls.*
- Maintain stretches in locked position when transferring patient *to prevent falls.*

Preconvulsive
- Maintain seizure precautions.
- Have oral airway at bedside *to maintain patent airway.*
- Have suction equipment available at bedside *to prevent aspiration.*
- Pad side rails, if indicated.
- Administer oxygen per protocol *to prevent cerebral hypoxia.*
- Establish means of communication.
- Identify auras if possible.

Convulsive
- Maintain patent airway.
- Support and protect head; turn to side if possible *to maintain airway.*
- Prevent injury:
    Ease patient to floor if in chair.
    Place pillows along side rails if patient is in bed.
    Loosen constrictive clothing.
- Provide privacy as necessary; stay with patient.
- Note frequency, time, involved body parts, and length of seizure *to provide accurate description of seizure activity.*

Postconvulsive
- Maintain patent airway.
- Suction as indicated *to maintain open airway.*
- Check vital signs and neurologic status per protocol.
- Administer oxygen per protocol *to prevent hypoxia.*
- Reorient patient to environment *to minimize sensory-perceptual alteration.*
- Place patient in position of comfort, and turn head to side.
- Administer oral hygiene as necessary *to remove secretions and bleeding.*

Impaired physical mobility related to prolonged bed rest

- See general intervention strategies listed on p. 1597.
- Encourage mobility to tolerance, unless contraindicated by subarachnoid hemorrhage precautions.
- Encourage self-care activities to tolerance unless contraindicated by subarachnoid hemorrhage precautions.
- Plan all activities to avoid fatigue; maintain planned rest periods.
- Obtain physical therapy referral.

Risk for impaired skin integrity related to sensory and perceptual alterations

- See general intervention strategies listed on p. 1557.

Anxiety related to altered self-concept

- See general intervention strategies listed on p. 1669.

Impaired verbal communication related to altered sensory and neuromuscular function

- Develop a means of communication with the patient: pencil, Magic Slate, or call light within easy reach. Reinforce the techniques established.

- Assist patient and family to identify other outlets for communication.
- Continue to use sense of touch and nonverbal forms of communication.

Adaptive capacity, decreased

Intracranial

- Perform neurologic assessment q 2 H and PRN *to detect signs of increased ICP.*
- Monitor vital signs q 1 H and PRN *to detect changes in blood pressure with widening pulse pressure and bradycardia.*
- Assess for changing levels of consciousness.
- Assess for pupillary changes.
- Assess patient's motor and sensory functions *to detect potential changes in ICP.*
- Assess for headache, vomiting, and seizure activity.
- Monitor cardiac status.
- Measure and record ICP per protocol.
- Maintain neutral body alignment with head of bed elevated at 30 degrees, unless contraindicated *to facilitate cerebral venous drainage.*
- Avoid procedures that result in increased thoracic and abdominal pressure such as hip flexion, coughing, isometric exercises, and Valsalva maneuver.
- Log roll patient *to minimize increases in BP and ICP.*
- Minimize patient activity.
- Administer supplemental oxygen *to prevent hypoxia and hypercapnia.*
- Hyperoxygenate with 100% oxygen before suctioning and limit ETS to <15 seconds *to minimize cerebral ischemia.*
- Monitor ABGs and regulate mechanical ventilation to maintain $PaCO_2$ 25 to 30 mm Hg *to reduce cerebral vasodilation.*
- Administer diuretics, hyperosmotics, and corticosteroids as directed.
- Limit fluid intake *to maintain slight state of dehydration.*
- Maintain normothermia *to minimize cerebral metabolic demands.*

Patient Education/Home Care Planning[66]

1. Involve family in patient care, as possible; teach essential aspects of care.
2. Reinforce physician's explanation of medical management.
3. Stress importance of ongoing outpatient care and follow-up visits.
4. Stress need for regular exercise program:
   a. Teach ROM exercises to family.
   b. Instruct patient or family to perform ROM exercises to all body joints every 2 to 4 hours.
5. Encourage independent activities, as possible:
   a. Be alert to limitations.
   b. Avoid overprotection.
   c. Instruct regarding need for supportive devices as indicated (wheelchair, braces, walker, canes, overhead trapeze).
6. Stress importance of diet as ordered:
   a. Offer supplemental feedings.
   b. Offer small portions, and instruct patient to chew slowly.
   c. Arrange food and utensils within easy reach.
   d. Avoid foods such as soft breads, mashed potatoes, semicooked vegetables, and large pieces of meat that can cause choking.
7. Stress importance of safety measures:
   a. Side rails
   b. Ramps
   c. Shower chains
   d. Removal of scatter rugs
   e. Walker, canes, flat shoes
8. Discuss each name of medication, dosage, time of administration, and toxic or side effects.
9. Ensure that patient understands need to avoid over-the-counter medications without first consulting physician.
10. Encourage socialization with friends and family.
11. Stress importance of communication:
    a. Speak slowly and distinctly.
    b. Use one-word commands and short sentences. Repeat as needed.
    c. Use gestures and touch when giving directions. Maintain eye contact.
    d. Implement speech exercises twice a day.
12. Stress importance of verbalization of feelings about anxiety, fear, and body image changes.
13. Discuss with patient and family about seizures (i.e., safety measures and whom to contact).

Evaluation

Patient demonstrates a patent airway Breath sounds are normal or no increase in adventitious sounds. Chest excursion is bilateral and symmetric. Rate and depth of respirations are normal. Cough is effective. There are no subjective or objective findings of shortness of breath, air hunger, or dyspnea on exertion.

Patient demonstrates an effective breathing pattern Airway is patent. Chest excursion is symmetric. Breath sounds are normal, or there is no increase in adventitious sounds. Arterial blood gas values are within normal ranges or consistent with patient's baseline. Vital signs are within normal ranges or consistent with patient's baseline. Hemoglobin levels are 14 to 18 g/dl (male) and 12 to 16 g/dl (female). Intake and output are stable. There are no subjective or objective signs of respiratory distress. All lobes are resonant on percussion. Skin color is not cyanotic.

Patient maintains adequate cerebral tissue perfusion Level of consciousness is unchanged. There is no evidence of neurologic deficits. Pattern of electrolytes is stable. There is no seizure activity.

Patient demonstrates minimum complications of sensory/perceptual alterations   Level of orientation is optimum. Patient remains free of injury. Skin integrity is maintained. Nutritional status is adequate. Self-care deficits are minimum. Social participation is appropriate to physiologic status.

Patient remains free of injury   Safety measures are appropriate to level of physiologic status. Skin integrity is maintained. Skin is free of bruises, burns, abrasions, and redness. Environment is safe. Patient is free of nosocomial infections.

Patient demonstrates optimum level of mobility   Skin integrity is maintained. Patient remains free of contractures and deformities. Level of mobility is appropriate to physiologic status. Nutritional status is adequate. Intake and output pattern is stable. Patient remains free of thrombophlebitis. Patient remains free of local infection. Patient participates in an ongoing physical therapy program.

Patient demonstrates skin integrity   Skin is intact. Nutritional status is adequate. Electrolyte balance is maintained. Patient remains free of pressure sores and contractures.

Patient demonstrates a low level of anxiety   Patient openly verbalizes concerns and feelings of grief, loss, and discomfort. Patient openly verbalizes feelings, supported by health care professionals and family. Patient verbalizes essential aspects of care. Patient can identify methods to effectively deal with anxious feelings.

Patient demonstrates minimum impaired verbal communication   Patient verbalizes feelings for as long as physically able to do so. Patient develops alternative methods of communication.

Patient demonstrates maximal intracranial adaptive capacity   Vital signs are stable. No signs of increased intracranial pressure are present. Patient is normothermic. Arterial blood gas values are within normal limits or consistent with patient's baseline. Intake and output are stable. Skin color is not cyanotic.

STROKE

(Cerebrovascular accident)

In stroke, or cerebrovascular accident (CVA), the cerebral vessels are occluded by an embolus or cerebrovascular hemorrhage, resulting in ischemia of the area of the brain normally perfused by the damaged vessels.[63]

The sequelae of a stroke depend on the extent and the location of the ischemia (Figure 3-33). Stroke is the third leading cause of death in the United States and accounts for approximately 200,000 deaths annually. Furthermore, stroke is the second leading cause of chronic disability and illness, with approximately 200,000 individuals experiencing some degree of disability from the residual effects. Statistics from 1980 indicate that stroke has an incidence of 196 per 100,000 general population. Persons 25 to 64 years of age are affected, but incidence increases rapidly from age 35 upward. The greatest increase in frequency occurs between 75 and 85 years of age.[33] Epidemiologic studies indicate variations in incidence in different geographic areas in the United States and in other parts of the world.

Certain risk factors may predispose an individual to a stroke; hypertension is the major risk factor. Risk factors showing some familial tendencies include diabetes mellitus, hyper-

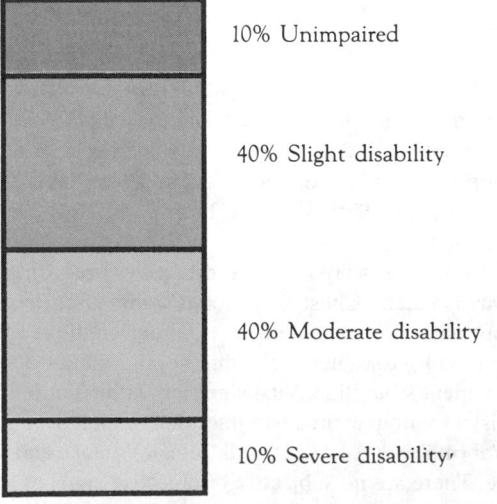

Figure 3-33 Degree of disability in survivors of stroke. (From Chipps et al.[16])

  EMERGENCY ALERT

CEREBROVASCULAR ACCIDENT

Cerebrovascular accident (CVA) is a cerebral infarct that results from a decrease in cerebral blood flow, cerebral embolus, and commonly cerebral thrombosis. Patients at risk are those with hypertension, diabetes, cardiac disease, hyperlipidemia, polycythemia, family history, smoking, and use of oral contraceptives.

Assessment

- HA, progressive or sudden neurologic deficits
- Decreased carotid pulse or carotid bruit
- Hypertension
- Signs of cerebral ischemia: hypotension, shock, arrest

Interventions

Maintain airway, breathing, circulation.
- Closely monitor vital signs.
- Administer anticoagulant therapy if indicated.
- Obtain IV access.
- *If patient is hypertensive,* reduce blood pressure slowly to minimize risk of hemorrhage or extension of the infarct.
- Administer diuretics and/or corticosteroids as ordered to reduce cerebral edema.

tension, cardiac disease, subclavian steal syndrome, and high serum cholesterol level. Obesity, sedentary life-style, cigarette smoking, stress, and high serum levels of cholesterol, lipoprotein, and triglycerides make the individual a high-risk candidate for stroke. In women the use of oral contraceptives and cigarette smoking increase the risk of stroke. Combinations of risk factors put the individual at a greater risk.[17]

••••• Pathophysiology

The pathologic mechanisms of stroke are commonly listed as hemorrhagic, thrombotic, and embolic in the most recent vascular literature. Hemorrhage may be subarachnoid from rupture of the subarachnoid artery or intraparenchymal from rupture of an intraparenchymal artery. Embolic occlusion stems from tumors, valvular cardiac diseases, and, most commonly, plaques released from cerebral vessels that produce infarction. Thrombotic arterial occlusion produces various ischemic or hypoxic insults.[41]

Cerebral Hemorrhage

The pathogenesis of hypertensive cerebral hemorrhage is not completely understood. However, several facts are known: the hemorrhage usually occurs in relation to some mild exertion, and it occurs in individuals who have experienced significant increases in systolic-diastolic pressures for several years. Some researchers theorize that microaneurysms, known as *Charcot-Bouchard aneurysms,* in small arteries or arteriolar necrosis may precipitate the bleeding. The major sites of bleeding in hypertensive cerebral hemorrhage include the putamen (55%), cortex and subcortex (15%), thalamus (10%), pons (10%), and cerebellar hemisphere (10%).[53]

Hypertensive vascular disorders primarily affect the smaller arteries and arterioles, causing thickening of vessel walls, increase in cellularity of some vessels, and hyalinization, possibly with necrosis.[53]

Resolution of the hemorrhage occurs via resorption and begins when macrophages and reactive fibrillary astrocytes appear. After the tissue has been cleared of blood by the macrophages, there is a cavity surrounded by dense, fibrillary gliosis and hemosiderin-laden macrophages.[53]

Cerebral Infarction

Cerebral infarction occurs when a local area of brain tissue is deprived of blood supply because of vascular occlusion. Several hypotheses regarding the pathogenesis of cerebral infarcts include: abrupt vessel occlusion (e.g., embolus) that results in tissue infarction in the distribution supply of the occluded vessel; gradual vessel occlusion (e.g., atheroma), which may not result in an infarction if collateral blood supply is sufficient; and vessels that are stenosed but not completely occluded. This may precipitate an infarction if the collateral blood supply to the hypoxic area becomes compromised.[53]

Common causes of vascular occlusions are cerebral thrombi and cerebral emboli. Thrombi usually occur in larger vessels (e.g., internal carotid arteries) and are associated with localized damage to the vessel wall at the point of occlusion. Atherosclerosis and hypotension are important underlying processes, but other types of vascular injury (e.g., arteritis) can initiate thrombosis. Emboli usually affect smaller vessels and are commonly found at points of narrowed vessel lumen and bifurcation. The sources of cerebral emboli vary, but the most common is a mural thrombus is the left atrium or ventricle. Septic emboli may originate from bacterial endocarditis. Cerebral infarcts from embolic occlusions frequently are hemorrhagic, whereas thrombotic infarcts are bland or ischemic. Emboli occur most frequently in the middle cerebral artery.

A cerebral infarction may be ischemic or hemorrhagic. *Ischemic* infarctions usually are not demonstrable on gross examination for 6 to 12 hours. The initial change of the affected area is a slight discoloration and softening, with the gray matter taking on a muddy color and the white matter losing its normal fine-grained appearance.[53] After 48 to 72 hours, infarction, necrosis, circumlesional swelling, and mushy disintegration of the affected area are evident. Eventually there is liquefaction and formation of a cyst surrounded by a firm glial tissue.

Histologic changes after an infarction include cell body changes, interruption and disintegration of the myelin sheath and axis cylinder, and loss of oligodendroglia and astrocytes. Polymorphonuclear leukocytes begin to appear 48 hours after infarct. At 78 to 96 hours, macrophages appear about blood vessels.

Hemorrhagic infarctions usually occur in the cerebral cortex and result from a reflow of blood into the infarcted area. This reperfusion is caused by a fragmentation or lysis of the embolus or a reduction of vascular compression and reestablishment of blood flow.[53] Hemorrhagic infarcts therefore are ischemic in origin.

••••• Diagnostic Studies and Findings

CT scan Infarct: appears initially (24 hours) as area of decreased density surrounded by area of intermediate density; shifts in midline structures and ventricular system; older infarct: area of low density extending toward cortex or shift in ventricular system toward lesion

Magnetic resonance imaging (MRI) Same as CT scan; hemorrhage: rounded shape and uniformly high density

Lumbar puncture *NOTE: Perform with caution in presence of intracranial hypertension;* increased pressure; bloody spinal fluid

Electroencephalography May show focal slowing around area of lesion

Brain scan Diminished perfusion; detection of infarction, encapsulated hemorrhage, hematoma, and arteriovenous malformations

Cerebral angiography Shows occlusion or narrowing of large vessels, particularly carotid artery occlusions

B mode ultrasound Outlines with ultrasound the flow of blood through large neck vessels

Skull roentgenogram Pineal body position; intracranial calcifications

Echoencephalography Shifts in midline structures; displaced ventricles

Doppler ultrasonography Direction and velocity of blood flow through vessels

•••••• Multidisciplinary Plan

Surgery

Carotid endarterectomy

Anastomosis of superior temporal artery and middle cerebral artery (STA-MCA anastomosis)

Intracranial pressure monitoring

Endotracheal intubation or tracheostomy

Evacuation of intracerebral clot or hematoma

Medications

Anticoagulants

Warfarin sodium (Coumadin), loading doses: 40-60 mg (adult), 20-30 mg (elderly); maintenance dose: 5-10 mg

Antihypertensives

Diazoxide (Hyperstat), 5 mg/kg IV

Diuretic

Furosemide (Lasix), 40-80 mg IV, 30-60 min before each dose of diazoxide

Corticosteroids

Dexamethasone (Decadron), 10 mg initially, then 4 mg q4-6h IV or IM

Anticonvulsants

Phenytoin (Dilantin), 100-600 mg/d orally or IV

Narcotic analgesic

Codeine, 30-60 mg q3-4h

Analgesic/antipyretics

Acetaminophen, gr X q4h po or rectal suppository

Antacids

General Management

Mechanical ventilation

Hypothermia blanket

ECG and cardiac monitoring

Subarachnoid precautions

Strict intake and output

Bed rest

Elevation of head of bed

Nasogastric tube

Foley or indwelling catheter

Elastic stockings

Serial arterial blood gases

Seizure precautions

Hemodynamic monitoring

Nutritional consultation

Social services

Home health referral

NURSING CARE

Nursing Assessment

The following table summarizes assessment findings and diagnostic studies in seven types of strokes.

	Intracerebral Hemorrhage	Subarachnoid Hemorrhage	Subdural Hemorrhage
Onset	Rapid; minutes to 1-2 h	Sudden; varied progression	Insidious; occasionally acute
Duration	Permanent if lesion is large; small lesions are potentially reversible	Variable; complete clearing may occur in days or weeks	Hours to months
Relation to activity	Usually occurs during activity	Most commonly related to head trauma	Usually related to head trauma
Contributing or associated factors	Hypertensive cardiovascular disease; coagulation defects	Intracerebral arterial aneurysm; trauma; vascular malformations	Chronic alcoholism
Sensorium	Coma common	Coma common	Generally clouded
Nuchal (neck) ridigity	Frequently present	Present	Rare
Location of cerebral deficit	Focal; arterial syndrome not common	Diffuse aneurysm may give focal sign before and after	Frontal lobe signs; ipsilateral pupil may dilate
Convulsions	Common	Common	Infrequent
Cerebrospinal fluid	Bloody unless hemorrhage entirely intracerebral	Grossly bloody; increased pressure	Normal to slightly elevated protein
Skull roentgenograms	Pineal shift, edema, hemorrhage, or hematoma	Normal or calcified aneurysm	Frequent contralateral shift of pineal gland

Nursing Dx & Intervention

Altered cerebral tissue perfusion related to hemorrhage and/or increased intracranial pressure

- Monitor closely for signs of increased intracranial pressure.
- Maintain patency and sterility of intracranial pressure monitoring device, if used:
  Use surgical asepsis for all dressing changes.
  Monitor intracranial pressure responses to care and treatments.
  Continuous flushing devices must not be used for measuring ICP.
- Administer medications per protocol: anticonvulsants, steroids, antibiotics, antifibrinolytics (monitor prothrombin time, partial thromboplastin time, and platelets), analgesics, and agents for control of vasospasms.
- If steroids are being administered:
  Check stools *to detect occult blood.*
  Test urine for glucose and acetone *to detect glycosuria.*
  Administer phytonadine, MSD (Aquamephyton) intramuscularly daily or every other day *to control tendency for bleeding.*

Administer antacids per protocol *to decrease or prevent gastric irritation.*
- Elevate head of bed 30 to 40 degrees, unless contraindicated, *to facilitate cerebral venous drainage.*
- Maintain strict intake and output (1500 to 1800 ml/24 hours).
- Observe for signs of dehydration and overhydration.
- Maintain normothermia per protocol.
- Institute subarachnoid precautions, if appropriate:
  Provide private room with controlled lighting (i.e., dim artificial lighting).
  Maintain complete bed rest *to keep physical activity and exertion to a minimum.*
  Provide *all* nursing care for the patient.
  Limit visitors to immediate family members only *to prevent overstimulation.*
  Have patient wear elastic stockings at all times *to prevent venous stasis.*
  Maintain dietary restrictions (no stimulants).
  Administer stool softeners *to prevent straining during bowel movement.*
  Instruct patient on need to avoid coughing and sneezing *to prevent sudden increases in intracranial pressure.*
  Instruct patient not to watch television, listen to radio, or read.

Extradural Hemorrhage	Focal Cerebral Ischemia	Cerebral Thrombosis	Cerebral Embolism
Rapid; minutes to hours	Rapid; seconds to minutes	Minutes to hours	Sudden
Initially fluctuating; then steadily progressive	Seconds to minutes	Permanent if lesion is large; potentially reversible if lesion is small	Rapid improvement may occur depending on collateral flow
Almost always related to head trauma	Occurs during activity if related to decreased cardiac output	Usually occurs at rest	Unrelated to activity
Any condition that predisposes to trauma	Peripheral and coronary atherosclerosis; hypertension	Peripheral and coronary atherosclerosis; hypertension	Atrial fibrillation; aortic and mitral valve disease; myocardial infarct; atherosclerotic plaque
Rapidly advancing coma	Usually conscious	Usually conscious	Usually conscious
Rare	Absent	Absent	Absent
Temporal lobe signs; ipsilateral pupil may dilate; high intracranial pressure	Focal; or arterial syndrome	Focal; or arterial syndrome	Focal; or arterial syndrome
Common	Rare	Rare	Rare
Increased pressure; color and cells usually normal	Usually normal	Usually normal	Usually normal
Frequently fracture across middle meningeal artery groove	May show calcification of intracranial arteries	Possible arterial calcification and pineal shift from edema	Usually normal

Sensory/perceptual alterations (visual, auditory, kinesthetic, gustatory, tactile, olfactory) related to cerebral hemorrhage and/or increased intracranial pressure

- See general intervention strategies on p. 1643.

Risk for injury related to seizures

- Maintain bed in low position at all times unless side rails are up or nurse is with patient.
- Provide patient with a call light within easy reach.
- Maintain side rails in up position at bedtime, after sedation, when patient is confused, and as needed.
- Maintain wheelchairs and stretchers in locked position when transferring patient *to prevent falls.*

Preconvulsive

- Maintain seizure precautions:

    Have oral airway at bedside *to provide for adequate oxygenation.*

    Have suction equipment available at bedside *to prevent aspiration.*

    Pad side rails if indicated.

    Administer oxygen per protocol *to prevent cerebral hypoxia.*

    Establish means of communication; identify auras if possible.

Convulsive

- Maintain patent airway.
- Support and protect head; turn to side if possible *to prevent aspiration.*
- Prevent injury:

    Ease patient to floor if in chair.

    Place pillows along side rails if patient is in bed.

    Loosen constrictive clothing.

- Provide privacy as necessary. Stay with patient.
- Note frequency, time, involved body parts, and length of seizure.

Postconvulsive

- Maintain patent airway.
- Suction as needed.
- Check vital signs and neurologic status.
- Administer oxygen per protocol.
- Reorient patient to environment *to minimize sensory-perceptual alteration.*
- Place patient in position of comfort, and turn head to side.
- Administer oral hygiene as necessary *to remove secretions and bleeding.*

Impaired physical mobility related to altered sensory and neuromuscular status

- Administer skin care every 2 hours *to prevent skin breakdown.*

    Turn patient every 2 hours and as needed, unless contraindicated, *to prevent skin breakdown and to prevent respiratory complications.*

    Change position slowly *to prevent potential orthostatic hypotension.*

    Position in proper body alignment.

    Keep skin dry; administer perineal care as needed.

    Massage pressure points every 2 hours *to stimulate circulation;* give gentle back rubs every shift and as needed.

    Use air mattress *to prevent pressure points.*

    Use firm mattress *to provide support for the patient's back.*

    Perform active or passive ROM exercises every 2 to 4 hours *to prevent contractures.*

- Perform dorsiflexion of quadriceps muscles and ankles every 2 to 4 hours unless contraindicated.
- Assist patient out of bed to chair two or three times daily unless contraindicated *to promote mobility.*
- Use footboard or Spence boots *to prevent footdrop.*
- Apply elastic stockings *to prevent thrombus and embolus formation.*
- Administer anticoagulation therapy per protocol:

    Monitor serum coagulation studies.

    Check stool for occult bleeding.

    Check urine for occult bleeding.

    Monitor for signs of thrombophlebitis and deep vein thrombosis including redness, tenderness, localized swelling, warmth, and upward red streaking on an extremity.

- Monitor nutritional status.
- Encourage mobility to tolerance unless contraindicated by subarachnoid hemorrhage precautions.
- Encourage self-care activities to tolerance unless contraindicated by subarachnoid hemorrhage precautions.
- Plan all activities and maintain planned rest periods *to avoid fatigue.*
- Obtain physical therapy referral.
- Encourage diversional activities if appropriate.

 SIGNS AND SYMPTOMS FOR STROKE

Restlessness and lethargy

Changes in level of consciousness

Changes in vital signs (increased systolic BP; widened pulse pressure, decreased pulse rate)

Pupillary changes (i.e., mydriasis)

Improved pupillary reflexes

Papilledema (late sign)

Nausea and vomiting (may be projectile)

Other

Feelings of powerlessness

Improved mobility—skin condition and pressure points should be checked every 20 minutes, as well as phonation, respiration, and articulation-resonance (PRA)

Impaired communication—assess ability to communicate

Feeding, bathing/hygiene, dressing/grooming, and toileting self-care deficit related to neurologic impairment

- Assess degree of self-care deficit and institute the following:
  - Assist with feeding, if indicated; use IV or nasogastric feedings, as ordered.
  - Administer oral hygiene every 2 hours and as needed *to keep mucous membranes moist.*
  - Assist with daily hygiene care as indicated *to promote self-esteem.*
  - Administer eye care every 2 to 4 hours if indicated.
  - Insert indwelling urinary catheter or perform intermittent urinary catheterizations per protocol.
  - Maintain bowel function with regular evacuation.

Risk for impaired skin integrity related to prolonged immobility

- See general intervention strategies on p. 1557.

Powerlessness related to neurologic impairment

- Reestablish as much physiologic control as possible.
- Share knowledge of physiologic functioning with patient and family.
- Assist patient to reestablish some means of psychologic control:
  - Encourage patient to express feelings.
  - Encourage patient and family to participate in care.
  - Encourage patient to become an active decision maker about care and immediate environment.

Impaired verbal communication related to altered cerebrovascular status

- Develop a means of communication with patient: pencil, Magic Slate, or call light within easy reach. Reinforce the techniques established.
- Assist patient and family to identify other outlets for communication *to minimize frustration.*
- Continue to use sense of touch and nonverbal forms of communication.

Adaptive capacity, decreased

Intracranial
- Perform neurologic assessment q 2 H and PRN *to detect signs of increased ICP.*
- Monitor vital signs q 1 H and PRN *to detect changes in blood pressure with widening pulse pressure and bradycardia.*
- Assess for changing levels of consciousness.
- Assess for pupillary changes.
- Assess patient's motor and sensory functions *to detect potential changes in ICP.*
- Assess for headache, vomiting, and seizure activity.
- Monitor cardiac status.
- Measure and record ICP per protocol.

- Maintain neutral body alignment with head of bed elevated at 30 degrees, unless contraindicated *to facilitate cerebral venous drainage.*
- Avoid procedures that result in increased thoracic and abdominal pressure such as hip flexion, coughing, isometric exercises, and Valsalva maneuver.
- Log roll patient *to minimize increases in BP and ICP.*
- Minimize patient activity.
- Administer supplemental oxygen *to prevent hypoxia and hypercapnia.*
- Hyperoxygenate with 100% oxygen before suctioning and limit ETS to <15 seconds *to minimize cerebral ischemia.*
- Monitor ABGs and regulate mechanical ventilation *to maintain $PaCO_2$ 25 to 30 mm Hg to reduce cerebral vasodilation.*
- Administer diuretics, hyperosmotics, and corticosteroids as directed.
- Limit fluid intake *to maintain slight state of dehydration.*
- Maintain normothermia *to minimize cerebral metabolic demands.*

Confusion, chronic related to organic or cognitive impairment

- Assess baseline physical, functional, and psychosocial status.
- Evaluate previous interests.
- Ensure optimal sensory input (i.e., eyeglasses, hearing aid) is available.
- Evaluate stimulation threshold *to prevent overstimulation.*
- Provide for structured repetitive group activities.
- Provide rest periods between activities *to minimize fatigue.*
- Monitor for changes in physical, functional, and psychological status.
- Maintain calm, reassuring demeanor when interacting with patient *to promote sense of trust.*
- Encourage patient to participate in care as tolerated *to minimize feelings of powerlessness.*
- Provide positive feedback for tasks/activities that are mastered.

Caregiver role strain, related to severity of patient's illness

- Obtain assistance with meeting of caregiver role.
  - Assist caregiver to identify/utilize caregiving resources such as family members, friends, community agencies, etc.
- Assist caregiver to develop plan of care with paced direct care activities.
- Assist caregiver to develop support systems with alternate caregivers/friends.
- Assist caregiver to identify and address personal health care needs.

Ineffective individual coping related to sudden illness and physiologic crisis

- Assess coping mechanisms and behavior patterns *to determine baseline information.*
- Provide patient with opportunity to express fears and concerns *to help reduce tension.*
- Encourage participation in care as tolerated *to reduce feelings of powerlessness.*
- Encourage family participation in care and emotional support *to reinforce importance of emotional care.*
- Obtain psychologic consult if indicated.

Aspiration, risk for related to enteric feeding via nasoenteric tube

- Confirm feeding tube placement after insertion, q 4 H and PRN.
    - Confirm tube placement before and after each intermittent tube feeding.
    - Confirm initial enteral tube placement by physician examination of CXR.
- Tape nasogastic tube securely per protocol.
- Aspirate stomach contents *to determine gastric pH.*
- Assess bowel sounds q 4 H and PRN.
- Assess patient for abdominal distention, nausea/vomiting, and diarrhea/constipation.
    - Hold tube feedings if bowel sounds are absent and if diarrhea/constipation or nausea/vomiting are present.
- Maintain proper patient positioning.
    - Elevate head-of-bed 30 to 40 degrees.
    - Turn patient to right side *to facilitate stomach drainage through pylorus.*
- Discontinue continuous feedings 30 to 40 minutes before activity/procedure that requires lowering the patient's head.
- Check vital signs q 2 H and PRN.
- Check pulmonary-tracheal secretions q 4 H and PRN *to detect presence of enteral feeding.*
- Monitor for signs of aspiration including cough, wheezing, dyspnea, hyperthermia, and tachycardia.
- Auscultate breath sounds q 4 H and PRN.

Patient Education/Home Care Planning

1. Involve the family in care, as possible. Teach essential aspects of care.
2. Reinforce the physician's explanation of medical management.
3. Stress importance of ongoing outpatient care and follow-up visits.
4. Stress need for regular exercise program:
    a. Teach ROM exercises to family.
    b. Perform ROM exercises to all body joints every 2 to 4 hours.
5. Encourage independent activities, as possible:
    a. Be alert to limitations.
    b. Avoid overprotection.
    c. Emphasize need for supportive devices as indicated (wheelchair, braces, walker, canes, overhead trapeze).
6. Stress importance of diet as ordered:
    a. Offer supplemental findings.
    b. Offer small portions, and instruct patient to chew slowly.
    c. Arrange food and utensils within easy reach.
    d. Avoid foods such as soft breads, mashed potatoes, semicooked vegetables, and large pieces of meat that can cause choking.
7. Stress importance of safety measures: side rails; ramps; shower chains; removal of scatter rugs; and walker, canes, and flat shoes.
8. Discuss name of each medication, dosage, time of administration, and toxic or side effects.
9. Stress need to avoid over-the-counter medications without first consulting physician.
10. Encourage socialization with friends and family.
11. Stress importance of communication:
    a. Speak slowly and distinctly.
    b. Use one-word commands and short sentences. Repeat as needed.
    c. Use gestures and touch when giving directions. Maintain eye contact.
    d. Implement speech exercises twice a day.
12. Stress importance of verbalization of feelings about anxiety, fear, and body image changes.
13. Ensure the patient and family understand about seizures (i.e., safety measures and whom to contact).

Evaluation

Patient maintains adequate cerebral tissue perfusion Level of consciousness is maintained or improved. There is no evidence of neurologic deficits. Electrolyte pattern is stable. There is no seizure activity.

Patient demonstrates minimal complications of sensory/perceptual alterations Optimum level of orientation is maintained. Patient remains free of injury. Patient demonstrates skin integrity. Nutritional status is adequate. Self-care deficits are minimum. Social participation is appropriate to physiologic status.

Patient remains free of injury Safety measures are appropriate to physiologic status. Skin integrity is maintained. Skin is free of bruises, burns, abrasions, and redness. Environment is safe. Patient is free of nosocomial infections.

Patient demonstrates an optimum level of mobility Skin integrity is maintained. Patient remains free of contractures and deformities. Level of mobility is appropriate to physiologic status. Intake and output pattern is stable. Nutritional status is adequate. Patient remains free of thrombophlebitis. Patient remains free of local infections. Patient participates in an ongoing physical therapy program. Patient demonstrates minimum self-care deficits. Outcome criteria listed for impaired physical mobility are met. Level of self-care activities is appropriate to physiologic status. Patient participates in physical and occupational therapy.

Patient demonstrates optimal self-care activities Level of self-care is appropriate to physiologic status. Patient participates in self-care to optimal level.

Patient demonstrates skin integrity Skin is intact. Nutritional status is adequate. Electrolyte balance is maintained. Patient remains free of pressure sores and contractures.

Patient demonstrates minimum feelings of powerlessness Optimum level of physiologic control, as possible for current health status, is maintained. Optimum level of psychologic control, as possible, is maintained. Patient participates, as possible, in decision making about care. Patient participates, as possible, in self-care.

Patient demonstrates minimum impaired verbal communication Patient verbalizes feelings for as long as physically able to do so. Patient develops alternative methods of communication.

Patient demonstrates effective coping mechanisms Patient is able to express fears and concerns. Patient participates in care as able.

Patient demonstrates minimal confusion Available sensory aids (i.e., eyeglasses, hearing aid) are used appropriately. Patient is able to participate in structured repetitive group activities. Rest periods between activities are maintained. Patient is able to participate in care to tolerance.

Patient remains free of aspiration Airway is patent. Vital signs are stable. Patient reports/demonstrates no signs of choking. Breath sounds are normal. Nasoenteric tube placement is verified.

Patient demonstrates maximal intracranial adaptive capacity Vital signs are stable. No signs of increased intracranial pressure are present. Patient is normothermic. Arterial blood gas values are within normal limits or consistent with patient's baseline. Intake and output are stable. Skin color is not cyanotic.

Patient demonstrates effective coping mechanisms Patient is able to express fears and concerns. Patient participates in care as able.

TRAUMA

▮ CRANIOCEREBRAL TRAUMA

▮ Craniocerebral trauma is severe physical injury to the brain or structures within the cranium.

Trauma is the leading cause of death for individuals between 1 and 35 years of age. Craniocerebral trauma is a major factor in half the deaths resulting from physical injuries and is the second most common cause of neurologic deficits. In addition to the 77,000 individuals who die each year in the United States from traumatic brain injury, 50,000 to 60,000 individuals survive head injuries with varying levels of permanent deficit. Injury to the brain is the most serious complication of head trauma.

General effects of moderate to severe head injuries include cerebral edema, sensorimotor deficits, and increased intracranial pressure. After the initial brain injury, secondary damage can result from brain herniation, cerebral ischemia, and hypoxemia. Leading causes of craniocerebral trauma include falls, industrial accidents, vehicular accidents (70% of victims sustain head injuries), assaults, sport accidents (e.g., football, boxing, diving), and intrauterine and birth injuries.

•••••• Pathophysiology

Craniocerebral injuries can result from primary or secondary trauma to the head. Primary trauma occurs when traumatic forces directly impact the head, setting into action the mechanisms of injury. The mechanisms of primary trauma that produce actual brain deformation include acceleration-deceleration with cavitation, as well as rotation of the skull and its cranial contents. These forces can occur simultaneously or in succession and damage the brain by compression, shearing, or tension. Acceleration injuries result when the head is struck by a moving object and set in motion. The slower-moving brain tissue is damaged by sudden contact with the edges of the dural membrane or the bony prominences of the skull. As a result of acceleration forces, there may be bruising or contusion of the undersurfaces of the occipital lobes, the brainstem, the superior surface of the cerebellum at the edge of the tentorium, or the tips of the frontal and temporal lobes. Another factor in the acceleration mechanism is the effect of positive and negative pressure waves traversing the skull. A high-pressure wave (positive) occurs at the point of impact, whereas a low-pressure wave (negative) occurs opposite the site of impact. If the negative pressure reaches vapor pressure, theoretically it may produce cavitation and a contrecoup injury (injury in area opposite the site of impact).

Deceleration occurs when the moving head strikes a solid, immovable object (as when the head hits a windshield). There is rapid deceleration of the skull, but the brain decelerates more slowly (20 msec), and the brain tissue may travel 2 to 3 cm in that time period.

Acceleration-deceleration movements from lateral flexion, hyperflexion, hyperextension, and turning movements during the injury cause the cerebrum to rotate about the brainstem and produce shearing, straining, and distortion of neural tissue. Microscopically, the stretching or tension causes fracture of axons in the longitudinal bundles of the cerebrum and the long axons in the brainstem. This rotational mechanism is a major cause of contrecoup lesions and may account for most of the contusions to the brain tissue. Areas most frequently injured during rotation are the frontal and temporal lobes.

Primary trauma to the head may be followed by secondary injury that increases the morbidity and mortality of head-injured patients. Secondary trauma to the head may result when tension strains and shearing forces are transmitted to the cranium by extreme torsion and stretching of the neck, as in a hard fall on the buttocks. Other factors such as sustained intracranial hypertension, sustained cerebral edema, hypercapnia, hypoxemia, systemic hypotension, infections, and respiratory trauma and its complications may contribute to secondary injury to the brain.

Head injuries can be classified as open or closed. *Open* head injuries result from skull fractures or penetrating wounds (Figure 3-34). The velocity, mass, shape, and direction of impact are the major determinants of brain injury. With an open head injury there is some type of skull fracture, such as linear, comminuted, depressed, or perforated.

A linear fracture is a simple break in bone continuity that produces an inbending of the bone at the point of impact and an outbending of the skull in the surrounding area. A comminuted skull fracture occurs when two or more communicating breaks divide the bone into two or more fragments. Depressed fractures result when the bone is forced below the line of normal contour from impact with a moving object. Compound fractures may be linear, comminuted, or depressed.

Another and serious type of skull fracture is the basal fracture, which can be linear, comminuted, or depressed. Structures most commonly damaged with this type of fracture include the internal carotid artery and cranial nerves I, II, VII, and VIII. Basal skull fractures usually traverse the paranasal sinuses (frontal, maxillary, or ethmoid). The fragility of the bones and the close adherence of the dura account for the frequency of this type of fracture and the subsequent leakage of cerebrospinal fluid through the dural tear.[32]

With open head injuries there can be high- or low-velocity impacts. The higher the velocity of impact, the greater the explosive effect within the cranium. For example, in high-velocity impacts, such as with gunshot wounds, there is lacera-

tion at the entry site, cerebral edema, hemorrhage into the destroyed area, and remote contusions (secondary to tissue displacement).[59] Lower-velocity impacts usually result in distortion and linear fractures of the skull.

A *closed,* blunt head injury can produce the pathologic signs of cerebral concussion, contusion, or laceration. A concussion is a transient neurologic dysfunction of paralysis and is the least serious type of brain injury. With a concussion there may be immediate and transitory disturbances in equilibrium, consciousness, and vision. *Contusions* result in bruising of brain tissue, usually accompanied by hemorrhages of surface vessels. *Lacerations* are the actual tearing of the cortical surface. Contusions and lacerations result in microscopic hemorrhages around blood vessels with destruction of surrounding brain tissue.

A contusion or laceration directly beneath the site of impact is a *coup* lesion; those occurring opposite the site of impact are *contrecoup* lesions (Figure 3-35). The two major factors that determine the distribution of coup and contrecoup lesions are the ability of cerebrospinal fluid to act as a shock absorber and shifts of the intracranial contents. With a coup lesion the impact causes greater displacement of the skull than the brain. At the site of impact the cerebrospinal fluid is squeezed out from between the brain and skull, and the skull hits the brain at the point of impact.[41] Contrecoup lesions occur because of dissipation of the cerebrospinal fluid between the trailing edge of the brain and the trailing surface of the skull and because of a compensatory increase in the volume of cerebrospinal fluid between the leading edge of the brain and the leading surface of the skull.[41] The coup or contrecoup lesion may be accompanied by cavitation, which is the release of dissolved gases from cerebrospinal fluid, blood, or brain tissue. The release of these gases produces microscopic bubbles that extensively disrupt neural tissue, primarily in cerebrospinal pathways and near blood vessels.

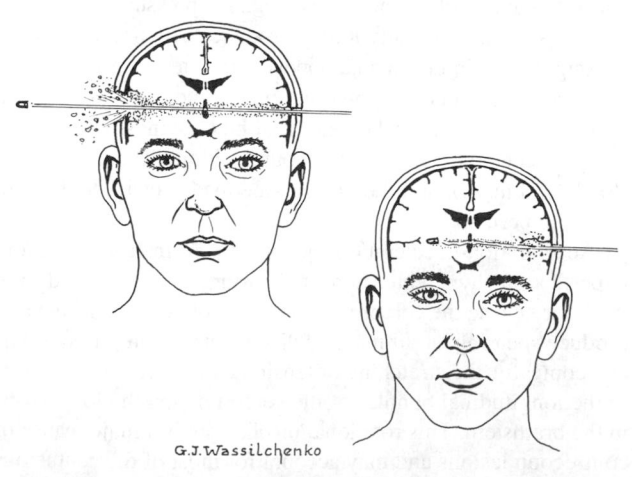

G.J. Wassilchenko

Figure 3-34 Penetrating bullet wound of the head. Bullet wound or other penetrating missile will cause an open (compound) skull fracture and damage to brain tissue. Shock wave effects are transmitted throughout the brain. (From Thelan et al.[62])

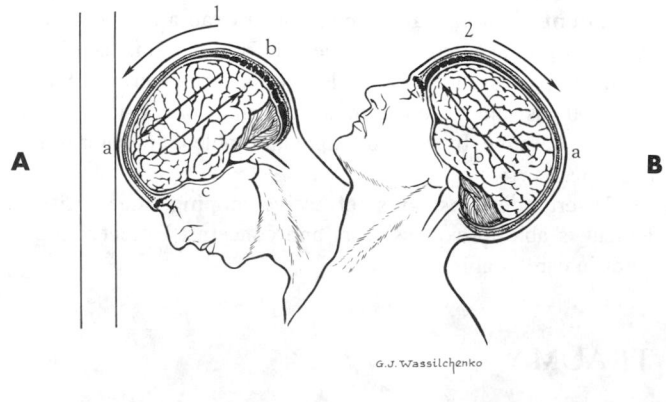

G.J. Wassilchenko

Figure 3-35 Coup and contrecoup head injury following blunt trauma. **A,** Coup injury: impact against object: a, site of impact and direct trauma to brain; b, shearing of subdural veins; c, trauma to base of brain. **B,** Contrecoup injury: impact within skull: a, site of impact from brain hitting opposite side of skull; b, shearing forces through brain. These injuries occur in one continuous motion—the head strikes the wall (coup), then rebounds (contrecoup). (From Rudy.[55])

Secondary responses to craniocerebral trauma may include the formation of an epidural, subdural, or intracerebral hematoma, a subarachnoid hemorrhage, cerebral edema, and brain herniation (Figure 3-36). An *epidural* hematoma usually occurs when there is a linear fracture of one of the skull's membranous bones, such as the temporal area near the meningeal artery and vein. After rupture the arterial blood forms a convex mass that indents the brain. If the hemorrhage continues, the hematoma may break periosteal attachments and the dural collagen.

A *subdural* hematoma may result from cerebral hemorrhage in the temporal, frontal, or midline region or in any region where there is a laceration of brain tissue or its parenchymal vessels. Because the subdural hematoma is venous, symptoms appear much later than with the arterial epidural hematoma and therefore can be classified as acute, subacute, or chronic. *Acute* subdural hematomas usually manifest symptoms within 24 to 48 hours after severe trauma. Symptoms of *subacute* subdural hematoma may develop anywhere from 48 hours to 2 weeks after severe head injury. *Chronic* subdural hematomas develop weeks, months, and possibly years after an apparently minor head injury. The chronic type of subdural hematoma is most common for those individuals in the 60- to 70-year age group because atrophy of the brain permits more room for expansion.

An *intracerebral hematoma* is a collection of blood within the actual brain tissue that usually occurs in the temporal or frontal region. Extensive removal of the hematoma and surrounding necrotic brain tissue generally is necessary to prevent further brain injury.

Subarachnoid hemorrhage is a frequent complication of head trauma. The pathologic processes of subarachnoid hemorrhage are presented in the discussion of vascular lesions.

Cerebral edema after craniocerebral trauma can occur locally around the injury and throughout the brain. Cerebral edema that develops after a traumatic head injury is not a single clinical or pathologic entity but exists in three forms: vasogenic, cytotoxic, and ischemic.[39] Vasogenic edema results from an increase in capillary permeability, which then permits transudation of plasma out of the cerebral vessels and into the compliant brain tissue. Cytotoxic edema occurs with impairment or failure of the cation pump, allowing infiltration of water and sodium into the intracellular space. Ischemic edema encompasses both previous types. Mechanisms of ischemic cerebral edema are initiated by the infiltration of water and sodium into the intracellular space (cytotoxic edema). This intracellular edema then affects the tight junction of the endothelial cell, with resultant infiltration of plasma across the damaged capillaries into the extracellular space (vasogenic edema).[41]

The mechanisms of traumatic cerebral edema are significant factors affecting both an individual's physiologic responses and survival after a severe head injury. If untreated or uncontrolled, cerebral edema produces a cycle of intracranial hypertension, reduced cerebral perfusion, and increased cerebral hypoxia. These mechanisms then produce more cerebral edema, and results are often fatal.[24]

The peak of cerebral edema is usually around 72 hours after the traumatic injury. Responses to the cerebral edema include increased intracranial pressure and the cerebral herniation syndromes.

Brain herniation is a secondary complication that can develop as a result of a primary head injury. The main types of brain herniation syndromes are uncal, transtentorial, and cerebellar. *Uncal* (lateral transtentorial) herniation involves displacement of the medial portion of the temporal lobe across the tentorium into the posterior fossa, compressing the midbrain and brainstem. *Transtentorial* (central) herniation involves downward displacement of the cerebral ventricles through the diencephalon against the midbrain. *Cerebellar* herniation results when the cerebellar tonsils move downward through the foramen magnum and compress the medulla.

•••••• Diagnostic Studies and Findings

Skull roentgenograms Detection of calvaria fractures (simple, compound, depressed, or comminuted); visualization of bone fragments

Cervical roentgenogram To confirm or rule out cervical spinal injury (assume neck injury until proven negative)

Chest roentgenogram Indicates presence of aspiration, chest injuries, and atelectasis; indicates placement of endotracheal tube

CT scan May indicate subdural hematoma, intracerebral hematoma, or shift and distortion of cerebral ventricles

Magnetic resonance imaging (MRI) Same as CT scan

CSF sampling *May be contraindicated with increased intracranial pressure;* Normal in cerebral edema and brain concussion; increased pressure and blood with laceration and contusion

Cerebral angiography May indicate intracerebral or subdural hematoma by showing avascular areas with displacement of surrounding vessels

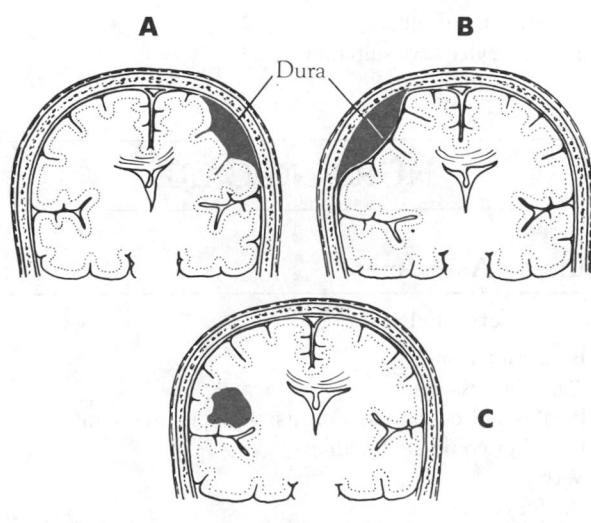

Figure 3-36 Different types of hematomas. **A,** Subdural. **B,** Epidural. **C,** Intracerebral. (From Thelan et al.[62])

Pneumoencephalogram Demonstration of cerebral ventricular shift, distortion, or dilation

Electroencephalogram (EEG) (done serially) Appearance or development of pathologic waves; determination of brain death

Cisternogram Identification of dural tear site with basal skull fracture

Echoencephalogram Detects shifts in midline structures

Serum osmolarity Hyperosmolar state (i.e., diabetes insipidus and syndrome of inappropriate secretion of antidiuretic hormone [SIADH]); hypo-osmolar state

Serum electrolytes Natriuresis; hypernatremia and hyponatremia; elevated plasma cortisol; increased serum lactic dehydrogenase

Urine osmolarity Dilute urine or concentrated urine

Arterial blood gases Hypoxemia; hypercapnia

•••••• Multidisciplinary Plan

Surgery

Suturing of head and scalp lacerations
Debridement of wounds
Ventricular catheter, subarachnoid bolt, and epidural sensor
Ventriculostomy
Cranioplasty
Shunting procedures for hydrocephalus
Craniectomy
Craniotomy
Tracheostomy
Skull trephine (burr holes)

Medications

Diuretics
  Mannitol 20% (osmotic diuretic), 0.25 mg/kg IV q4-6h (Used with caution)
  Furosemide (Lasix) (Loop diuretic), 20-40 mg IV q6-8h
Anticonvulsants
  Phenytoin sodium (Dilantin), 18 mg/kg; then maintenance dose of 5 mg/kg/d
  Phenobarbital sodium, 30-120 mg/d in 2 or 3 individual doses
  Carbamazepine (Tegretol), 200 mg bid initially; gradually increased up to 800-1200 mg/d in divided doses
Corticosteroids (to control cerebral edema)
  Dexamethasone (Decadron), 4-10 mg IV q6h
Histamine antagonist
  Cimetidine (Tagamet), 300 mg IV q6h
Analgesic/antipyretics
  NOTE: Avoid morphine sulfate because of medullary depressant effects
  Acetaminophen, 325-650 mg po or rectal suppository q4h prn
Antacids
  Maalox, 30 ml po or nasogastric q2h
Artificial tears, prn

Stool softeners
  Colace, 100 mg po tid
Muscle relaxants and paralyzers
  Pancuronium (Pavulon), 1-4 mg IV q4h
  Pentobarbital (Nembutal) for barbiturate coma; loading dose 3-5 mg/kg IV by slow push; maintenance dose 1-3 mg/kg IV by continuous infusion
Thiopental, 1-5 mg/kg; slow IV push and maintenance dose of 1-3 mg/kg/hr
Antibiotics
  Broad-spectrum agents used to prevent or control infection

General Management

Controlled mechanical ventilation
Hyperventilation to control intracranial hypertension
Cervical collars
Central venous pressure line
Arterial pressure line
Intracranial pressure monitoring
Hypothermia-hyperthermia balance
Incentive spirometry
Cardiac monitoring
Salem sump, nasogastric tube
Swan-Ganz catheterization
Glasgow Coma Scale
Endotracheal intubation
Nutritional support (i.e., enteral feedings, intravenous hyperalimentation)
Physical therapy program
Warm or cold compresses for periorbital edema and ecchymosis
Indwelling urinary catheter
Speech therapy, if indicated
Psychosocial counseling
Seizure precautions
Nutritional consultation
Social services consultation
Home health referral

NURSING CARE

Nursing Assessment

Cranial Nerve Palsies

Bilateral anosmia
Agnosia (less common)
Paralysis of ocular movements: diplopia, nystagmus
Partial or complete blindness
Vertigo
Deafness
Numbness, paresthesias, or neuralgia of areas supplied by trigeminal nerve
Strabismus

Level of Consciousness

Mental changes
  Irritability
  Anxiety
  Restlessness
  Confusion
  Delirium
  Stupor
  Coma
Posttraumatic amnesia (loss of day-to-day memory after the injury)
Retrograde amnesia (loss of memory regarding events immediately preceding the injury)

Pain

Headache

Motor Function

Concussion
  Transitory extensor spasms
Contusion
  Weakness
  Paresis
  Paralysis
  Decorticate (flexor) posturing: upper extremity flexion, lower extremity extension
  Decerebrate (extension) posturing: extension and internal rotation of upper extremities, extension of lower extremities
  Areflexia

Meningeal Irritability

Nuchal rigidity
Positive Kernig's sign
Positive Brudzinski's sign

Skull Fracture

Linear
  No bone displacement
  Possible epidural hematoma
Depressed
  Focal neurologic deficits
  Cranial nerve injuries
Basilar
  Conjunctival hemorrhage
  CSF rhinorrhea (drainage from nose)
  Bilateral periorbital ecchymosis (raccoon eyes)
  CSF otorrhea (drainage from ear)
  Mastoid bone ecchymosis (Battle's sign)
  Hearing impairments
  Positive halo sign (drainage of blood encircled by CSF)

Cerebral Edema/Increased Intracranial Pressure

Changes in level of consciousness
Inability to clear secretions
Slow, labored respirations
Changes in arterial blood pressure and pulse pressure (later sign)
Bradycardia
Anorexia
Pupillary dysfunction
Papilledema (late sign)
Changes in motor function (i.e., posturing)
Nausea and vomiting (may be projectile)
Positive Babinski's sign (usually contralateral to lesion)
Visual abnormalities (i.e., diplopia, visual blurring, decreased visual acuity)
Monoparesis or hemiparesis (usually contralateral)
Seizures

Brain Herniation

Uncal
  Decreased level of consciousness with almost simultaneous rapid motor function changes (decerebrate or decorticate posturing) and rapid changes in pupillary equality
  Respiratory acidosis or alkalosis
  Loss of oculocephalic reflex
Transtentorial
  Decreased level of consciousness
  Nuchal rigidity
  Headache
  Unilateral or bilateral pupil dilation
  Elevated blood pressure
  Bradycardia
  Cheyne-Stokes respiration
  Cardiac arrhythmias
  Decerebrate or decorticate posturing
Cerebellar
  Pupils constricted and nonreactive
  Decreased level of consciousness
  Apnea or ataxic respiration

Hemorrhage

Epidural hematoma
  Transient loss of consciousness
  Increasing intracranial pressure (rapid development)
  Ipsilateral dilated pupil
Subdural hematoma
  Increasing lethargy
  Headache
  Increasing intracranial pressure
  Seizures
  Minimal dilation of unilateral pupil
Intracerebral hematoma
  Increasing intracranial pressure
  Sensory and motor deficits

Reflexes

Pupils dilated
Loss of cutaneous and tendon reflexes (concussion)
Babinski's reflex positive (with increased intracranial pressure)

Vital Signs

Decreased blood pressure

Pulse slow (associated with intracranial hypertension) or rapid and feeble (associated with hemorrhage)

Respirations shallow or temporary cessation (concussion)

Hyperventilation

Cheyne-Stokes, apneustic, ataxic, or cluster respirations (dependent on level of function)

Hyperthermia associated with hypothalamic injury

Widening pulse pressure with hypertension and bradycardia (Cushing's syndrome) associated with intracranial hypertension and cerebral ischemia

Other

Punch-drunk encephalopathy: memory impairment, dysarthria, ataxias, tremors, parkinsonian manifestations

Postconcussion syndrome: headache, insomnia, nervousness, fatigability, giddiness

Dehydration

Polyuria

Shock

Extracranial Complications

Cervical fracture not diagnosed

Chest injuries

Fat emboli

Gastrointestinal hemorrhage

Hypoxia

Hypercapnia

Anemia

Hypotension

Nursing Dx & Intervention

Ineffective airway clearance related to impaired cough reflex

- Maintain patent airway; avoid flexion of the neck until cervical films rule out neck injury.
- Auscultate for breath sounds every 1 to 2 hours and as needed. Suction as needed *to remove secretions and blood.*
- Monitor vital signs every 1 to 2 hours; monitor neurologic status every 15 to 30 minutes until stable, then every 1 to 2 hours.
- Keep emergency drugs and ventilator at bedside.
- Maintain nothing-by-mouth status, if indicated, *to prevent risk of choking or aspiration.*
- Maintain neck in neutral position to promote optimal cerebral venous drainage.

Ineffective breathing pattern related to neuromuscular impairment and/or increased intracranial pressure

- Auscultate breath sounds every 1 to 2 hours; note quality and any increase in adventitious sounds; suction as needed; hyperoxygenate lungs with 100% oxygen for 1 minute before and 1 minute after suctioning, unless contraindicated; limit suctioning to less than 15 seconds *to prevent suction-induced hypoxemia.*
- Maintain patent airway; intubation/tracheostomy and mechanical ventilation may be indicated.
- Monitor mechanical ventilator, if used:
  Ensure that tidal volume, rate, mode, and oxygen concentration are set as ordered.
  Ensure that ventilator alarms are on and functional.
- Monitor arterial blood gases per protocol:
  Report decrease in Po_2 of 10 to 15 mm Hg *to prevent hypoxemia.*
  Report increase in Pco_2 greater than 10 to 15 mm Hg *to prevent hypercapnia.*
- Check blood pressure, respirations, and pulse rate every 1 to 2 hours and as needed based on patient's condition.
- Administer muscle relaxants per protocol.

Altered cerebral tissue perfusion related to primary injury or increased intracranial pressure

- Establish baseline and ongoing neurologic assessment every 15 to 30 minutes and as needed as indicated by patient's condition.
- Intervene *to monitor or prevent increased intracranial pressure:*
  Administer medications, treatments, and IV lines as per protocol.
- If steroids are being administered:
  Check stools *to detect occult blood.*
  Test urine for sugar and acetone *to detect glycosuria.*
  Administer phytonadine, MSD (Aquamephyton) intramuscularly daily or every other day *to control tendency for bleeding.*
  Administer antacids per protocol *to decrease or prevent gastric irritation.*
- Maintain elevation of head of bed as per protocol *to facilitate cerebral venous drainage.*
- Accurately record intake and output; monitor for imbalance.
- Test urine pH every two hours *to detect onset of diabetes insipidus.*
- Post fluid restriction chart that clearly indicates amount of fluid permitted for a 24-hour period and how restriction is allocated for each work shift.
- Monitor serum electrolytes, blood count, and arterial blood gases for abnormalities.
- Monitor values and waveforms of intracranial pressure line if appropriate:
  Maintain patency and sterility of the system.
  Monitor effects of treatments on intracranial pressure.
  Correlate neurologic status with intracranial pressure values; notify physician if inconsistent.
  Assist with drainage of cerebrospinal fluid from the system *to control intracranial hypertension.*
  Prevent initiation of Valsalva maneuver *to prevent increase in intrathoracic pressure.*
  Continuous flushing systems must not be used for measuring ICP.

- Intervene to monitor or prevent seizures:
  Monitor serum levels of anticonvulsant agents.
  Administer anticonvulsant agents per protocol. Monitor effects and side effects.
  Maintain seizure precautions.

Sensory/perceptual alterations (visual, auditory, gustatory, kinesthetic, tactile, olfactory) related to altered cerebrovascular status

- Keep side rails up at all times when patient is alone *to prevent falls.*
- Maintain patient safety at all times.
- Avoid sedative agents, if possible.
- Maintain quiet environment, reducing external stimuli to a minimum.
- Reorient patient frequently to time, place, and person. Introduce yourself each time you reorient the patient.
- Repeat explanations frequently and simply.
- Have family bring in familiar objects *to minimize depersonalization.*
- Maintain planned rest periods, allowing sufficient time for REM sleep.
- Use day and night lighting appropriately *to promote natural sleep-wake cycle.*
- Stimulate senses of touch, taste, and position.
- Support family members to understand what is happening as a result of perceptual alterations.
- Address patient by preferred name.

Risk for injury related to seizures

- Maintain bed in low position at all times unless side rails are up or nurse is with patient.
- Provide patient with a call light within easy reach.
- Maintain side rails in up position at bedtime, after sedation, when patient is confused, and as needed.
- Maintain wheelchairs and stretchers in locked position when transferring patient.

Preconvulsive

- Maintain seizure precautions:
  Have oral airway at bedside *to provide for adequate oxygenation.*
  Have suction equipment available at bedside *to prevent aspiration.*
  Pad side rails if indicated *to prevent injury.*
  Administer oxygen per protocol *to prevent cerebral hypoxia.*
  Establish means of communication; identify auras if possible.

Convulsive

- Maintain patent airway.
- Support and protect head; turn to side if possible.
- Prevent injury:
  Ease patient to floor if in chair.
  Place pillows along side rails if patient is in bed.
  Remove surrounding furniture.
  Loosen constrictive clothing.
- Provide privacy as necessary; stay with patient.

- Note frequency, time, involved body parts, and length of seizure.

Postconvulsive

- Maintain patent airway.
- Suction as needed, as indicated.
- Check vital signs and neurologic status.
- Administer oxygen as per protocol *to prevent hypoxia.*
- Reorient the patient to environment.
- Provide emotional support.
- Place patient in position of comfort; turn head to side.
- Administer oral hygiene as necessary for secretions and bleeding.

Impaired physical mobility related to neuromuscular or musculoskeletal impairment

- Assess skin condition and pressure points when administering skin care.
- Administer skin care every 1 to 2 hours:
  Turn patient every 2 hours and as needed, unless contraindicated.
  Change position slowly *to prevent orthostatic hypotension.*
  Position in proper body alignment; may need to use log-roll technique when turning.
  Massage pressure points every 2 hours *to stimulate circulation;* give gentle back rubs every shift and as needed.
- Use firm mattress or bed board *to support back and spine.*
- Use footboard or Spence boots *to prevent footdrop.*
  Instruct patient not to push against footboard *to prevent Valsalva maneuver.*
- Apply antiembolus stockings or sequential compression devices to lower extremities *to promote venous return.*
- Administer anticoagulation therapy per protocol *to prevent thrombus or embolus formation:*
  Monitor serum coagulation studies.
  Check stool *to detect occult bleeding.*
  Check urine *to detect occult bleeding.*
  Monitor for signs of thrombophlebitis and deep vein thrombosis including redness, tenderness, localized swelling, warmth, and upward red streaking on an extremity.
- Monitor nutritional status.
- Encourage mobility to tolerance or per protocol.
- Avoid isometric exercises.
- Encourage self-care activities to tolerance.
- Plan all activities to avoid fatigue; maintain planned rest periods.
- Obtain physical therapy referral.

Feeding, bathing/hygiene, dressing/grooming, and toileting self-care deficit related to neurologic disorder

- Assess degree of deficit and institute necessary interventions.
- Assist with feeding as indicated.
- Use IV or nasogastric feedings per protocol.

- Administer oral hygiene every 2 hours and as needed.
- Assist with daily hygiene care as indicated.
- Administer eye care every 2 to 4 hours if indicated *to prevent drying of corneas.*
- Maintain bowel function with regular evacuation.

Risk for impaired skin integrity related to prolonged immobility

- See general intervention strategies on p. 1557.

Body image, self-esteem, and personal identity disturbances related to cognitive changes

- Assess and document patient's degree of concern and confusion.
- Provide for a safe, comfortable, secure environment.
- Reorient the patient to time, person, and place, as appropriate.
- Carefully explain what you are doing and why you are doing it.
- Answer questions simply and honestly.
- Correct misinformation.
- Protect patient's privacy.

Anxiety related to threat of self-concept and change in health status

- See general intervention strategies listed on p. 1669.
- Assist patient to reestablish as much physiologic control as condition allows.
- Share knowledge of physiologic functioning with the patient and family.
- Assist patient to reestablish some means of psychologic control.
- Encourage patient to express feelings.
- Encourage patient and family to participate in care.
- Encourage patient to become an active decision maker about care and immediate environment.

Impaired verbal communication related to neurologic impairment

- Assess patient's ability to communicate.
- Develop a means of communication with the patient: pencil, Magic Slate, or call light within easy reach.
- Reinforce the techniques established.
- Assist patient and family to identify other outlets for communication.
- Continue to use sense of touch and nonverbal forms of communication.

Adaptive capacity, decreased

Intracranial

- Perform neurologic assessment q 2 H and PRN *to detect signs of increased ICP.*
- Monitor vital signs q 1 H and PRN to detect changes in blood pressure with widening pulse pressure and bradycardia.
- Assess for changing levels of consciousness.

- Assess for pupillary changes.
- Assess patient's motor and sensory functions *to detect potential changes in ICP.*
- Assess for headache, vomiting, and seizure activity.
- Monitor cardiac status.
- Measure and record ICP per protocol.
- Maintain neutral body alignment with head of bed elevated at 30 degrees, unless contraindicated to facilitate cerebral venous drainage.
- Avoid procedures that result in increased thoracic and abdominal pressure such as hip flexion, coughing, isometric exercises, and Valsalva maneuver.
- Log roll patient *to minimize increases in BP and ICP.*
- Minimize patient activity.
- Administer supplemental oxygen *to prevent hypoxia and hypercapnia.*
- Hyperoxygenate with 100% oxygen before suctioning and limit ETS to <15 seconds *to minimize cerebral ischemia.*
- Monitor ABGs and regulate mechanical ventilation to maintain $Paco_2$ 25 to 30 mm Hg to *reduce cerebral vasodilation.*
- Administer diuretics, hyperosmotics, and corticosteroids as directed.
- Limit fluid intake *to maintain slight state of dehydration.*
- Maintain normothermia *to minimize cerebral metabolic demands.*

Caregiver role strain, related to severity of patient's illness

- Obtain assistance with meeting of caregiver role.
    Assist caregiver to identify/utilize caregiving resources such as family members, friends, community agencies, etc.
- Assist caregiver to develop plan of care with paced direct care activities.
- Assist caregiver to develop support systems with alternate caregivers/friends.
- Assist caregiver to identify and address personal health care needs.

Aspiration, risk for related to enteric feeding via nasoenteric tube

- Confirm feeding tube placement after insertion, q 4 H and PRN.
    Confirm tube placement before and after each intermittent tube feeding.
    Confirm initial enteral tube placement by physician examination of chest x-ray.
- Tape nasogastic tube securely per protocol.
- Aspirate stomach contents *to determine gastric pH.*
- Assess bowel sounds q 4 H and PRN.
- Assess patient for abdominal distention, nausea/vomiting, and diarrhea/constipation.
    Hold tube feedings if bowel sounds are absent and if diarrhea/constipation or nausea/vomiting are present.

- Maintain proper patient positioning.
  Elevate head-of-bed 30 to 40 degrees.
  Turn patient to right side *to facilitate stomach drainage through pylorus.*
- Discontinue continuous feedings 30 to 40 minutes before activity/procedure that require lowering the patient's head.
- Check vital signs q 2 H and PRN.
- Check pulmonary-tracheal secretions q 4 H and PRN *to detect presence of enteral feeding.*
- Monitor for signs of aspiration including cough, wheezing, dyspnea, hyperthermia, and tachycardia.
- Auscultate breath sounds q 4 H and PRN.

Ineffective individual coping related to sudden illness and physiologic crisis.

- Assess coping mechanisms and behavior patterns *to determine baseline information.*
- Provide patient with opportunity to express fears and concerns *to help reduce tension.*
- Encourage participation in care as tolerated *to reduce feelings of powerlessness.*
- Encourage family participation in care and emotional support *to reinforce importance of emotional care.*
- Obtain psychologic consult if indicated.

Confusion, chronic related to organic or cognitive impairment

- Assess baseline physical, functional, and psychosocial status.
- Evaluate previous interests.
- Ensure optimal sensory input (i.e., eyeglasses, hearing aid) is available.
- Evaluate stimulation threshold *to prevent overstimulation.*
- Provide for structured repetitive group activities.
- Provide rest periods between activities *to minimize fatigue.*
- Monitor for changes in physical, functional, and psychologic status.
- Maintain calm, reassuring demeanor when interacting with patient *to promote sense of trust.*
- Encourage patient to participate in care as tolerated *to minimize feelings of powerlessness.*
- Provide positive feedback for tasks/activities that are mastered.

Patient Education/Home Care Planning

1. Involve family in care, as possible; teach essential aspects of care.
2. Reinforce physician's explanation of medical management.
3. Stress importance of ongoing outpatient care and follow-up visits.

4. Encourage independent activities, as possible:
   a. Alert to limitations
   b. Avoid overprotection.
   c. Stress need for supportive devices as indicated.
5. Emphasize need for regular exercise program. Teach ROM exercises to family.
6. Stress importance of diet as ordered:
   a. Offer supplemental feedings.
   b. Offer small portions; instruct patient to chew slowly.
7. Stress importance of safety measures: side rails; ramps; shower chairs; walker, canes.
8. Instruct patient regarding name of medication, dosage, time of administration, and toxic or side effects.
9. Stress need to avoid over-the-counter medications without first consulting physician.
10. Encourage socialization with friends and family.
11. Emphasize importance of verbalization of feelings about anxiety, fear, and body image changes.
12. Ensure that patient and family understand about seizures (i.e., safety measures and whom to contact).

Evaluation

Patient demonstrates a patent airway Breath sounds are normal. Chest excursion is bilateral and symmetric. Rate and depth of respirations are normal. Cough is effective. There are no subjective or objective findings of shortness of breath, air hunger, or dyspnea on exertion.

Patient demonstrates an effective breathing pattern Airway is patent. Chest excursion is symmetric. Breath sounds are normal, or there is no increase in adventitious sounds. Arterial blood gas values are within normal ranges or consistent with patient's baseline. Vital signs are within normal ranges or consistent with patient's baseline. Hemoglobin levels are 14 to 18 g/dl (male) or 12 to 16 g/dl (female). Intake and output are stable. There are no signs of respiratory distress. All lobes are resonant on percussion. Skin color is not cyanotic.

Patient maintains adequate cerebral tissue perfusion Level of consciousness is unchanged. There is no evidence of neurologic deficits. Electrolyte pattern is stable. There is no seizure activity.

Patient demonstrates minimum complications of sensory/perceptual alterations Optimum level of orientation is maintained. Patient remains free of injury. Patient demonstrates skin integrity. Nutritional status is adequate. Self-care deficits are minimum. Social participation is appropriate to physiologic status.

Patient remains free of traumatic injury Safety measures are appropriate to level of physiologic status. Skin integrity is maintained. Skin is free of bruises, burns, abrasions, and redness. Environment is safe. Patient is free of nosocomial infections.

Patient demonstrates minimum self-care deficits Outcome criteria listed for impaired physical mobility are met.

Level of self-care activities is appropriate to physiologic status. Patient participates in physical and occupational therapy.

Patient demonstrates skin integrity Skin is intact. Nutritional status is adequate. Electrolyte balance is maintained. Patient remains free of pressure sores and contractures.

Patient demonstrates on optimum level of mobility Patient exhibits skin integrity. Patient remains free of contractures and deformities. Level of mobility is appropriate to physiologic status. Intake and output pattern is stable. Nutritional status is adequate. Patient remains free of thrombophlebitis. Patient remains free of local infection. Patient participates in an ongoing physical therapy program.

Patient demonstrates intact self-concepts Patient openly verbalizes feelings of grief and loss. Patient verbalizes positive feelings about self. Patient acknowledges actual change in self-image. Patient focuses on present and future appearance and function. Patient verbalizes feelings of hopefulness, helpfulness, and powerfulness.

Patient demonstrates a low level of anxiety Patient openly verbalizes concerns and feelings of grief, loss, and discomfort. Patient openly verbalizes feelings supported by health care professionals and family. Patient verbalizes essential aspects of care. Patient identifies methods to effectively deal with anxious feelings.

Patient demonstrates minimum impaired verbal communication Patient verbalizes feelings for as long as physically able to do so. Patient develops alternate methods of communication.

Patient demonstrates maximal intracranial adaptive capacity Vital signs are stable. No signs of increased intracranial pressure are present. Patient is normothermic. Arterial blood gas values are within normal limits or consistent with patient's baseline. Intake and output are stable. Skin color is not cyanotic.

Caregiver demonstrates minimal role strain Caregiver appropriately utilizes available resources. Caregiver develops adequate support systems. Caregiver addresses personal needs.

Patient remains free of aspiration Airway is patent. Vital signs are stable. Patient reports/demonstrates no signs of choking. Breath sounds are normal. Nasoenteric tube placement is verified.

Patient demonstrates effective coping mechanisms Patient is able to express fears and concerns. Patient participates in care as able.

Patient demonstrates minimal confusion Available sensory aids (i.e., eyeglasses, hearing aid) are used appropriately. Patient is able to participate in structured repetitive group activities. Rest periods between activities are maintained. Patient is able to participate in care to tolerance.

SPINAL CORD TRAUMA

Spinal cord trauma is physical injury to the spinal cord caused by violent or disruptive action.

Injuries to the spinal cord constitute approximately 10% of traumatic injuries to the nervous system. Approximately 10,000 spinal cord injuries occur each year in the United States, and spinal cord trauma from vehicular accidents accounts for one half to two thirds of the total incidence. Approximately one third of the individuals with spinal cord injuries die before reaching an acute care facility. About 80% of individuals sustaining a spinal cord injury are between the ages of 18 and 25 years, and most are male. Causes of spinal cord trauma include assaults (e.g., bullet wounds), falls, sport injuries (e.g., diving accidents), industrial accidents, birth injuries, degenerative changes (e.g., vertebral disk deterioration), and vehicular accidents. At present more than 100,000 individuals in the United States are paralyzed as a result of spinal cord trauma.

The most common sites of injury are the lower cervical region (C4-7 and T1) and the thoracolumbar junction (T12, L1, and L2). Trauma to the spinal cord causes concussion, contusion, laceration, hemorrhage, transection (partial or complete), or impairment in the spinal vascular supply.

•••••• Pathophysiology

As with craniocerebral trauma, the spine (and spinal cord) can be injured by direct or indirect forces. Direct injuries such as falls on the head or buttocks can cause spinal cord lesions from fractured vertebrae or direct compression of the cord by depressed bone fragments. Indirect injuries (the major type of spinal cord injuries) can occur when excessive forces accelerate the cranium in relation to the trunk (i.e., whiplash injury) or when the trunk is suddenly decelerated in regard to the lumbar spine. Whether the forces are direct or indirect, the subsequent fractures of vertebrae seriously injure the neural elements of the spinal cord.

 EMERGENCY ALERT

NEUROGENIC (SPINAL) SHOCK

Neurogenic shock is a form of vasogenic or distributive shock that results when the vascular system dilates. In neurogenic shock this generally occurs when there is disruption of the spinal cord leading to loss of sympathetic tone and resultant dilation of the arterioles and venules.

Assessment

- Decreased blood pressure
- Rapid, shallow respirations
- Slowed pulse rate
- Paraplegia, quadriplegia, or priapism
- Diaphoresis above the level of the cord injury
- Loss of vasomotor tone and ability to control heat
- Warm and dry skin

Interventions

- Maintain airway, breathing, and circulation.
- Protect cervical spine from displacement or injury.
- Obtain IV access and administer fluids (avoid overload).
- Administer vasoconstricting medications as ordered.
- Monitor vital signs.
- Monitor urinary output.

Vertebral Injuries

The primary mechanisms of vertebral injury, occurring alone or in combination, include hyperextension, hyperflexion, vertical compression trauma, and rotation.[32]

Hyperextension injuries (Figure 3-37) (commonly termed *whiplash*) are common in the cervical region, and damage results from the forces of acceleration-deceleration and the sudden reduction in the anteroposterior diameter of the spinal canal. Since the spinal canal is full of neural tissue in the cervical area, injury can produce profound disability. With a hyperextension injury the cord can be compressed between the body of one vertebra and the leading edge of the laminal arch of adjacent vertebrae, causing complete or partial transection. In addition, the ligamentum flavum may be torn or bulge inward, and intervertebral discs may tear. Severe hyperextension injuries can produce complete transverse fracture of the vertebral body. With the compression and shearing forces of a hyperextension injury, gray matter of the cord is destroyed and microcirculation at and around the level of the injury is disrupted.

Hyperflexion injury (Figure 3-38) results in an overstretching, compression, and deformation of the spinal cord from a sudden and excessive force that propels the neck forward or an exaggerated lateral movement of the neck to one side or another. Hyperflexion injuries can occur with wedge or compression fractures of the vertebral body with or without dislocation, fracture of the pedicle with or without dislocation of intraspinal ligaments, or fracture of the vertebral body and rupture of the intervertebral discs.

Vertical compression (Figure 3-39) trauma primarily occurs around the area of the thoracolumbar junction (T12 to L2) and results from a force applied along an axis from the top of the cranium through the vertebral bodies. With compression injuries the vertebral body bursts, compressing the spinal cord and damaging nerve roots with bony fragments.

Rotation (Figure 3-40) can involve all portions of the vertebral body including pedicles, ligaments, and the articulation. Fracture of the pedicles or locked facets of the vertebrae can rupture ligaments and shear spinal cord tissue.

Vertebral injuries can be classified as simple fractures, compressed or wedged fractures, comminuted fractures, and vertebral dislocation.[32] A *simple* fracture is a single break usually affecting transverse or spinous processes. Vertebral alignment usually remains intact, and compression of the spinal cord is not usually present.

Compressed, or *wedged,* vertebral fractures occur when the vertebral body is compressed anteriorly. Spinal cord compression may or may not be present with a wedged fracture.

Comminuted, or *burst,* fractures can cause serious injury to the spinal cord. The vertebral body shatters into multiple fragments, and these fragments may penetrate the spinal cord. Burst fractures occur at the cervical, thoracic, and lumbar regions.

Dislocation of a vertebra may rupture the ligamentum flavum, resulting in dislocation of the vertebral facets, which can be unilateral or bilateral. This dislocation disrupts alignment of the vertebral column, and injury to the spinal cord may or may not be present. Partial dislocation of the spinal cord is called *subluxation.*

Spinal Cord Injuries

The neural elements of the spinal cord and spinal nerve roots are injured by compression from bone, disc herniation, hematoma, and ligaments; edema following compression or concussion; overstretching or disruption of neural tissue; and disturbances in spinal circulation.[24]

The sequence of pathologic processes following impact injury to the spinal cord are localized hemorrhaging, which advances from the gray to the white matter; reduced vascular

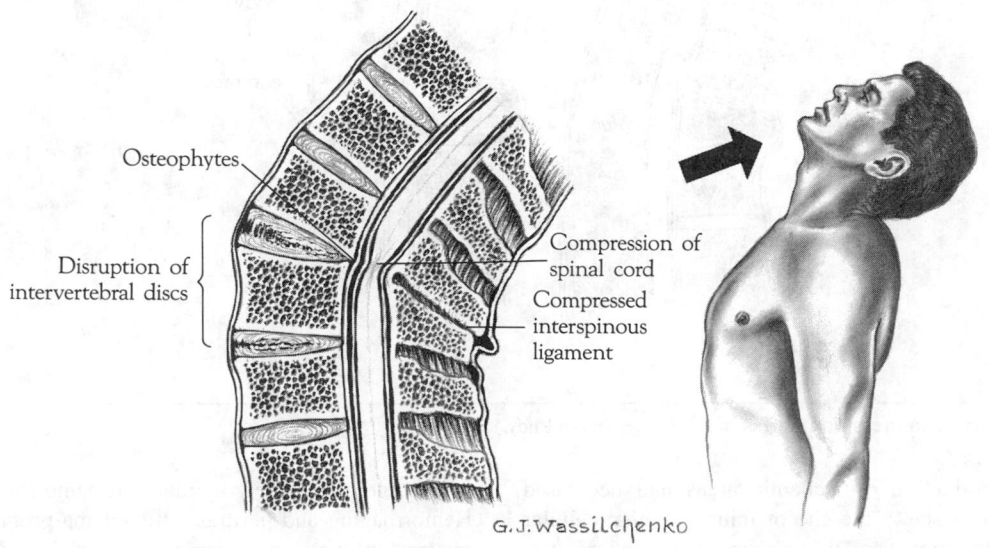

Figure 3-37 Hyperextension injuries of the spine. (From Rudy.[55])

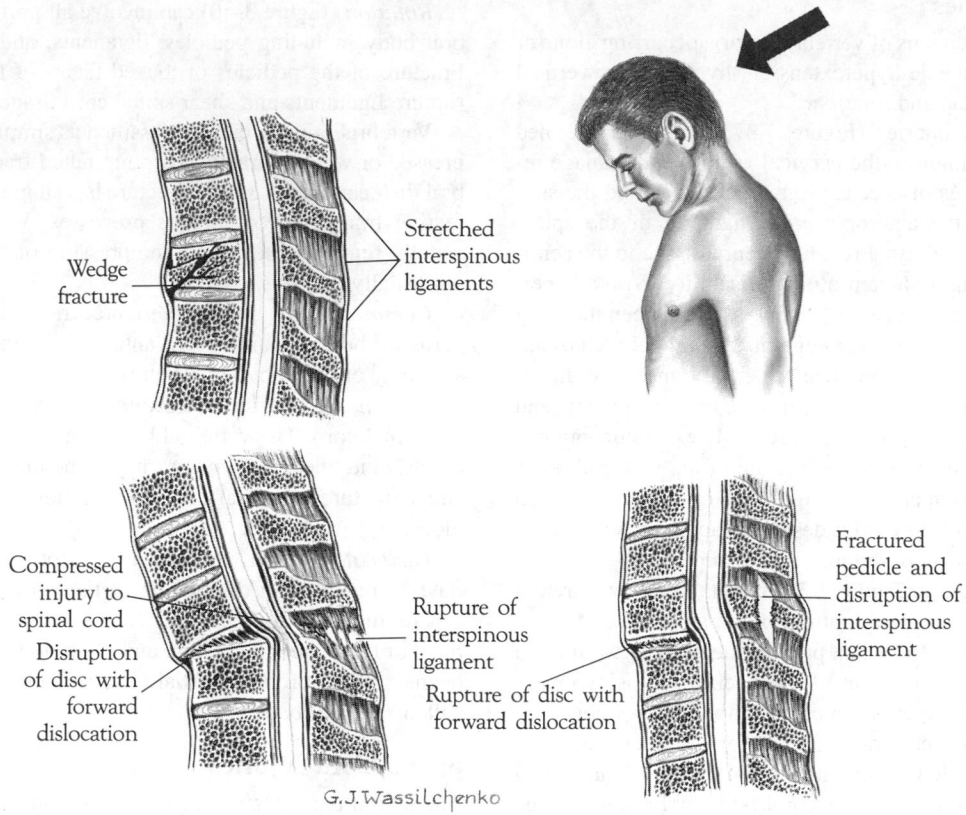

Figure 3-38 Hyperflexion injury of the spine. (From Rudy.[55])

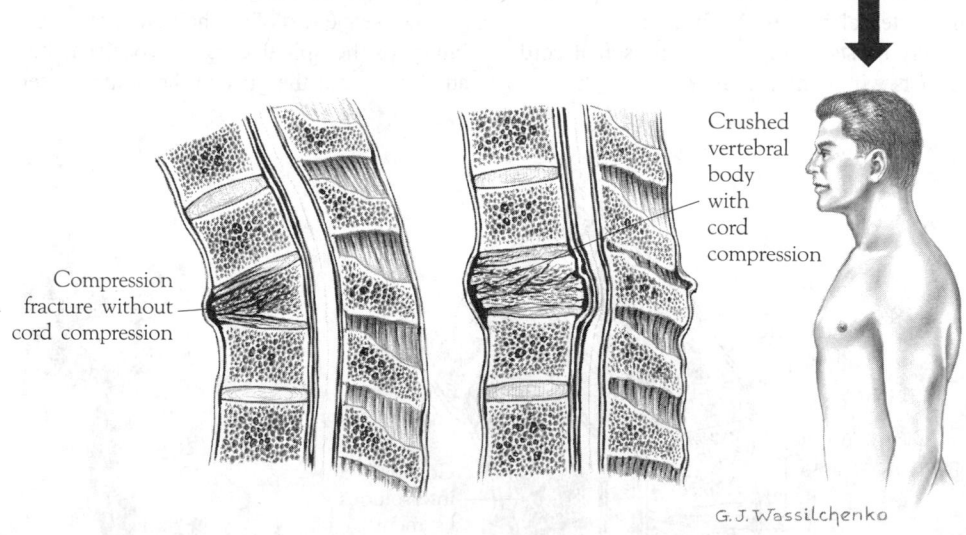

Figure 3-39 Vertical compression injuries of the spine. (From Rudy.[55])

perfusion and production of ischemic areas and decreased oxygen tension in tissue at the site of injury; edema; cellular and subcellular alterations; and tissue necrosis. Several minutes after the traumatic injury, microscopic hemorrhages appear in the central gray matter and in the pia-arachnoid. They increase in size until the entire gray matter is hemorrhagic and necrotic. Hemorrhaging and peritraumatic edema progress to the white matter, forming vacuolation and wedge-shaped foci that impair the microcirculation to the spinal cord. This impairment produces ischemia or vascular stasis.

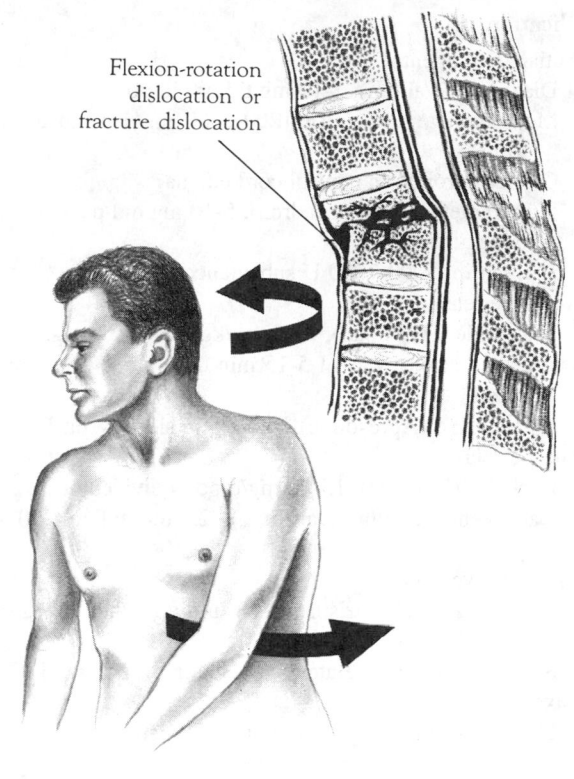

Flexion-rotation
dislocation or
fracture dislocation

Figure 3-40 Flexion-rotation injuries of the spine. (From Rudy.[55])

Circulation in the white matter returns to normal within approximately 24 hours, but circulation in the gray matter remains altered.

Changes in the chemistry and metabolism of the traumatized regions include a transitory increase in tissue lactate, a rapid decrease in tissue oxygen tension within 30 minutes of the injury, and increased norepinephrine concentration. Increased concentrations of norepinephrine released to the cord tissue may produce ischemia, vascular rupture, or necrosis of neuronal tissue.[4]

Localized ischemia of neural tissue may result from compression on the vasculature of the cord or nerve roots by bony fragments or herniated discs. If the flow of blood from the vertebral artery to the anterior spinal artery or to the branches of the radicular arteries is impaired, severe cord ischemia results. Hemorrhage, other than with contusion and edema, usually does not produce significant neural impairment. Epidural and subdural hematomas rarely are large enough to cause serious compression. Although subarachnoid bleeding is usual, it is of little clinical significance. Larger intramedullary hematomas, on the other hand, may produce a tubular hematomyelia that can cause partial or complete interruption in spinal cord functioning.[24]

After the necrosis that occurs immediately after the injury, a phase of resorption and organization begins. This state is characterized by the appearance of phagocytes within 36 to 48 hours after injury, proliferation of microglial and mesenchymal cells, and changes in astroglias. Blood gradually is re-moved from the tissue by disintegration of red cells and resorption of hemorrhages. Macrophages engulf degenerating axons in the first 10 days after injury.[4]

The traumatized section of the cord is removed in the third to fourth week after the injury and gradually replaced with connective scar tissue or glial fibers. Injured segments of the spinal cord are replaced with connective scar tissue or glial fibers. Injured segments of the spinal cord are replaced with acellular collagenous tissue, which connects the meninges to the cord and central canal. Scarring in the injured area consists mainly of thickened meninges and connective tissue.

Spinal Shock

Spinal shock at the area of transection occurs after complete or incomplete severing of the spinal cord. It causes a complete loss of sensory, motor, autonomic, and reflex functioning below the level of the lesion. Spinal shock results from the loss of inhibition from descending tracts, continued inhibition of supraspinal impulses, and axonal degeneration of the interneurons.

Autonomic Hyperreflexia

Autonomic hyperreflexia may occur after spinal shock has been resolved and reflex activity has returned. The syndrome is associated with a massive uncompensated cardiovascular response to stimulation of the sympathetic division of the autonomic nervous system.[17] Individuals most likely to be affected with autonomic hyperreflexia have lesions at the level of T6 or above. If symptoms of autonomic hyperreflexia are not treated, serious damage and possibly even death can result.

Cord Syndromes

Trauma to the spinal cord results in several syndromes that develop from the specific area of cord damaged and vary in severity depending on the amount of cord compression or transection.

The *anterior* cord syndrome occurs after an acute flexion injury to the cervical area and is the most common syndrome. Damage to the anterior spinal artery, the ventral portion of the spinal cord, or both accounts for the loss of upper and lower motor function.

The *posterior* cord syndrome, although rare, is associated with cervical hyperextension trauma.

Central cord syndrome may result from hyperextension injuries or flexion injuries. The central cord syndrome is characterized by central edema of the spinal cord and compression on the anterior horn cells. Neurologic deficits include mixed upper and lower motor neuron loss (disproportionately more impairment in upper extremities) and spasticity below the level of injury.

The *Brown-Séquard* syndrome results from rotation-flexion injuries where subluxation or dislocation of the fracture occurs by unilateral pedicle-laminar injuries.[17] Neurologic deficits include ipsilateral paresis, loss of proprioception, and contralateral loss of pain and temperature sensations.

The *herniated disc* syndrome is one of the most common spinal cord syndromes. Degenerative changes with the fraying and tears of the anulus fibrosus predispose the intervertebral discs to posterior displacement through a laceration of the anulus fibrosus and the posterior longitudinal ligament. The extrusion of fibrocartilaginous material may occur spontaneously or in response to activity (e.g., lifting) or slight injury. The severity of symptoms depends on quantity of herniated disc tissue, number of involved discs and amount of nerve root compression, and amount of spinal canal narrowing.[32] Herniated discs most frequently (90%) affect the lower lumbar and lumbosacral regions.

Motor Neurons

Motor neurons are the nerve cell responsible for transmitting impulses from the brain or spinal cord to muscular or glandular tissue. Spinal cord trauma can cause varying degrees of motor neuron impairment, so it is important to understand the difference between the upper and lower motor neurons. *Upper* motor neuron lesions result from damage in the corticobulbar or corticospinal tract. *Lower* motor neuron lesions result in the loss of reflex and voluntary responses of muscles because of destruction of anterior horn cells, peripheral nerves, or ventral nerve roots or motor fibers.[32]

•••••• Diagnostic Studies and Findings

Roentgenograms (anterior-posterior and lateral) Vertebral fractures

Serum chemistry Hypoglycemia or hyperglycemia; electrolyte imbalance; possibly decreased hemoglobin and hematocrit

CT scan Spinal cord edema

Magnetic resonance imaging (MRI) Spinal cord edema and compression

Spinal puncture Establishes presence or absence of spinal block

Myelography Establishes presence of spinal block

•••••• Multidisciplinary Plan

Surgery

Laminectomy
Tracheostomy or endotracheal intubation (nasal)
Spinal fusion for stabilization
Wound debridement; suturing of lacerations
Cervical tongs (i.e., Cone, Vinke, Crutchfield, Gardner-Wells)
Halo traction
Halo with femoral traction
Body casts
Spinal cord cooling
Myotomies, tenotomies, neurectomies, rhizotomies, and muscle transplants (treatment for spasticity)
Harrington rod insertion for stabilization of thoracic deformities

Medications

Antianxiety agents
    Diazepam (Valium), 2-10 mg tid or qid po
    Meprobamate (Equanil), 1200-1600 mg/d po in divided doses
    Corticosteroids (to control cord edema)
        Dexamethasone (Decadron), 5-10 mg qid po
    Anticoagulants
        Heparin, 5000-7000 U subcutaneously q12h
Antihypertensive agents
    Diazoxide (Hyperstat),* 1-3 mg/kg, up to 150 mg, IV, repeated at intervals of 5-15 min until blood pressure reduced
    Hydralazine (Apresoline),* 20 mg in slow IV push
Muscle relaxants
    Baclofen (Lioresal), 15-80 mg/d po in divided doses
    Dantrolene sodium (Dantrium), 25 mg tid to 200 mg qid
Antiinfective agents
    Sulfisoxazole (Gantrisin), 2-4 g initially, then 4-8 g/d in divided doses
    Methenamine mendelate (Mandelamine), 1-2 g qid
Laxatives
    Glycerin or bisacodyl (Dulcolax), as rectal suppository

Antacids

Magnesium hydroxide and aluminum hydroxide (Maalox T.C.), 20 ml po q4h

General Management

Mechanical ventilation
Stryker or Foster frame bed
Skeletal traction
Vital capacity and tidal volume measurements
Splints and braces
Phrenic nerve stimulator
Bed board and firm mattress
Cardiac monitoring
Intermittent urinary catheterization
Intake and output recording
Dietary consultation
Sex counseling
Psychosocial counseling for individual and family
Cervical collar (soft or hard)
Immobilization of part with sandbags
Serial measurement of arterial blood gases
Urine sugar and acetone; guaiac
Antiembolus stockings or sequential compression devices
Nasogastric tube
Physical therapy
Occupational therapy
Social services

*Treatment for autonomic hyperreflexia.

NURSING CARE

Nursing Assessment

Spinal Shock

Complete neurologic assessment every 15 to 30 minutes until stable

Complete transection

Flaccid paralysis below level of lesion

Loss of proprioception, pain, temperature, touch, and pressure below level of lesion

Loss of all spinal reflexes below level of lesion

Loss of vasomotor tone

Loss of visceral and somatic sensations below level of lesion

Loss of ability to perspire below level of lesion

Dysfunction of bowel and bladder

Possible priapism[32]

Partial transection

Asymmetric flaccid paralysis below level of lesion

Asymmetric loss of reflexes below level of lesion

Some senses of proprioception, pain, temperature, touch, and pressure intact below level of injury

Some visceral and somatic sensations intact below level of lesion

Less vasomotor instability

Less bowel and bladder dysfunction

Possible priapism

Autonomic Hyperreflexia

Complete neurologic assessment every 15 to 30 minutes until stable

Paroxysmal hypertension

Pounding headache

Diaphoresis above level of lesion

Flushing above level of lesion

Cutis anserina below level of lesion

Nasal stuffiness

Nausea

Bradycardia

Other

Altered body image—determine the degree of concern or confusion

Herniated Disc Syndrome

Lumbar

Pain in lower back with radiation down back of one leg

Restricted spinal mobility

Walking painful

Back appears straight with loss of lumbar curve

Spastic paravertebral muscles

Impaired sensation of affected leg and foot

	MUSCLE FUNCTION ACCORDING TO LEVEL OF SPINAL CORD INJURY
C4 and above	Loss of all muscle function including respiratory (usually fatal)
C5	Quadriplegia with poor respiratory functioning
C6-C8	Quadriplegia with sparing of some arm and hand muscles
T1-T3	Quadriplegia with loss of muscle function below nipple line
T4-T10	Paraplegia with some chest and trunk muscles intact
T11-L2	Paraplegia with muscles intact through upper thigh
L3-S1	Paraplegia with muscles of chest, trunk, thigh, and most of leg intact; loss of voluntary bowel and bladder control
S2-S4	Loss of voluntary bowel and bladder control

Less active ipsilateral ankle jerk may be present

Pain aggravated by jugular compression

Cervical

Stiffness of neck

Pain radiating down arm to fingers

Pain

Hyperesthesia immediately above level of lesion

Intense tingling and burning pain below level of lesion (in paraplegia)

Spasticity

Partial or complete loss of voluntary control

Exaggerated deep tendon reflexes

Sexual Function Irregularities

Varies from normal function to complete impotence

Menstrual irregularities for short time after injury

Trophic Skin Changes

Trophic ulcers

Skin and nail changes

Skin condition may show signs of breakdown when skin care is administered

Nursing Dx & Intervention

Ineffective airway clearance related to impaired cough reflex

- Auscultate for breath sounds every 1 to 2 hours as needed.
- Maintain patient airway, and avoid flexion of the neck.
- Suction as needed *to remove secretions and prevent aspiration.*
- Assist ventilation as indicated. Keep Ambu bag at bedside.
- Monitor vital signs every 1 to 2 hours; monitor neurologic status every 15 to 30 minutes.

- Maintain nothing-by-mouth status if indicated *to prevent risk of choking or aspiration.*

Ineffective breathing pattern related to neuromuscular impairment

- Auscultate for breath sounds every 1 to 2 hours; note quality and increase in adventitious sounds; suction as needed; hyperoxygenate lungs with 100% oxygen for 1 minute before and 1 minute after suctioning, unless contraindicated, *to prevent hypoxemia.*
- Maintain patent airway. Intubation/tracheostomy and mechanical ventilation may be indicated.
- Monitor mechanical ventilator, if used:
  Ensure tidal volume, rate, mode, and oxygen concentration are set as ordered.
  Ensure ventilator alarms are on and function *to prevent accidental disconnection.*
- Monitor arterial blood gases, as ordered:
  Report decrease in Po_2 of 10 to 15 mm Hg.
  Report increase in Pco_2 greater than 10 to 15 mm Hg.
- Check blood pressure, temperature, and pulse rate every 1 to 2 hours and as needed based on patient's condition.

Altered cerebral and spinal tissue perfusion related to increased intracranial pressure and/or respiratory exchange impairment

- Ensure immobilization of vertebral column:
  Maintain skeletal traction.
  Maintain cervical skeletal traction:
  Crutchfield tongs:
    Check traction and orthopedic frame every 4 hours.
    Make sure tongs are secure.
    Ensure weights hang freely.
    Assess tong sites every 4 hours and as needed.
    Provide tong site skin care: clean with hydrogen peroxide, and then apply povidine-iodine solution *to prevent sepsis.* Cover with sterile dressing.
  Halo traction:
    Assess traction pins *to ensure they are tight and secure.*
    Assess fiberglass cast jacket for proper fit (should be able to insert index finger between cast and skin).
    Assess cast edges for roughness and crumbling; petal rough edges:
      Provide routine cast care.
      Provide pin site skin care: clean site with hydrogen peroxide, and then apply povidone-iodine solution *to prevent infection.*
      Cover with sterile dressing.
  Stryker frame:
    Inspect pressure points (face, chin, scapula, coccyx, and heels) every 2 to 4 hours *to prevent skin breakdown.*
    Administer skin care every 2 to 4 hours *to prevent breakdown.*
    Secure all bolts before turning patient.
    Assess pulse and respirations before and after turning.
    Check position of canvas under patient after turning.
    Use arm rests *to maintain alignment.*
    Establish method of elimination.
  Maintain *strict* body alignment; keep body straight and head flat:
    Do not move head or spinal column.
    Use sandbags, if needed, *to maintain alignment.*
  Administer medications as ordered:
    Give steroids *to control cord edema.*
    When steroids are being administered:
      Check stools *to detect occult blood.*
      Test urine for sugar and acetone *to detect glycosuria.*
      Administer phytonadione, MSD (AquaMEPHYTON), intramuscularly daily or every other day *to control tendency for bleeding.*
      Administer antacids per protocol *to decrease or prevent gastric irritation.*
  Avoid injection below the level of the lesion.
  Maintain parenteral fluids per protocol.
  Measure intake and output every hour. Immediately report urine output of less than 30 ml/hour.

Sensory/perceptual alterations (visual, auditory, kinesthetic, gustatory, tactile, olfactory) related to neuromuscular dysfunction

- See general intervention strategies listed on p. 1643.

Risk for injury related to tissue hypoxia and/or integrative dysfunction

- Assess and document potential for injury and strategies for prevention.
- Maintain bed in low position at all times unless side rails are up or nurse is with patient.
- Provide patient with a call light within easy reach.
- Maintain side rails in up position at bedtime, after sedation, and as needed.
- Maintain stretchers in locked position when transferring patient.
- Pad side rails if patient is overactive.

Impaired physical mobility related to neuromuscular and musculoskeletal impairment

- Assess skin condition for signs of breakdown when administering skin care.
- Administer skin care every 2 hours:
  Turn patient every 2 hours and as needed, unless contraindicated, *to prevent respiratory complications.*
  Change position slowly *to prevent orthostatic hypotension.*
  Position in straight body alignment; use log-roll technique when turning.
- Keep skin dry; give perineal care as needed.
- Massage pressure points every 2 hours *to stimulate circulation;* give gentle back rubs every shift and as needed.
- Use heel and elbow guards as needed *to prevent skin irritation and breakdown.*
- Use firm mattress.

- Perform active or passive ROM exercises every 2 to 4 hours *to promote circulation and improve muscle tone.*
- Use footboard or Spence boots *to prevent footdrop.*
- Apply antiembolus stockings or sequential compression devices to lower extremities.
- Administer anticoagulation therapy per protocol:
  Monitor serum coagulation studies.
  Check stool *to detect occult bleeding.*
  Check urine *to detect occult bleeding.*
  Monitor for signs of thrombophlebitis and deep vein thrombosis including redness, tenderness, localized swelling, warmth, and upward red streaking on an extremity.
- Encourage mobility to tolerance or per protocol.
- Encourage self-care activities to tolerance.
- Plan all activities to avoid fatigue.
- Maintain planned rest periods.
- Obtain physical therapy referral.

Feeding, bathing/hygiene, dressing/grooming, and toileting self-care deficit related to neuromuscular impairment

- See general intervention strategies listed on p. 1600.

Bowel incontinence related to neuromuscular impairment

- Maintain fluid intake of 2000 ml/day, unless contraindicated.
- Monitor intake and output.
- Provide patient with diet that is high in roughage, protein, and bulk.
- Keep patient's skin clean and dry.
- Check patient for impaction every 1 to 2 days.
- Institute a regular bowel evacuation program:
  Begin bowel retraining program *to prevent constipation.*
  Instruct patient to take 8 to 10 ounces of prune juice 12 hours before time set for defecating; insert glycerin suppository high in rectum 15 to 20 minutes before set time; then place patient on bedpan, toilet, or commode.
  Insert lubricated glycerin suppository 2 hours before set time, and position patient in sitting position or transfer to bedpan or commode at set time.
  Instruct patient to drink 4 to 8 ounces prune juice each night.
  Instruct patient to drink a warm drink (water, coffee, milk) 30 minutes before set time.
  Insert laxative suppository for 2 to 4 days, then glycerin suppository for 2 to 4 days; note length of time between insertion and defecation; place patient on bedside commode at appropriate time; if no bowel movement, give small tap water enema.[62]

Altered patterns of urinary elimination related to neuromuscular and/or sensory motor impairment

- Observe for bladder distention every 2 to 4 hours.

- Perform intermittent catheterization per protocol.
- Perform catheter care every shift:
  Maintain closed system.
  Tape catheter to thigh *to prevent pulling and tension* (female).
  Tape catheter to lower abdomen *to prevent pulling and tension* (male).
- Monitor intake and output. Maintain fluid intake of 2000 ml daily unless contraindicated.
- Acidify urine with foods such as cranberry juice.
- Administer urinary tract germicides (e.g., Mandelamine) as ordered.
- Begin bladder retraining program:
  Upper motor neuron bladder:
  Administer fluids between 7 AM and 7 PM.
  Remove urinary catheter at 7 AM.
  Force fluids (i.e., 240 ml) every hour.
  After approximately 3 or 4 hours, trigger area (i.e., digital stimulation of rectum) until stimulated and attempt to void is made; if patient is able to void, residual urine is immediately checked:
  Residual urine of less than 100 ml is needed to continue with training.
  Residual urine of greater than 100 ml requires catheter reinsertion. Bladder retraining is then resumed another day.
  Lower motor neuron bladder:
  Administer fluids between 7 AM and 7 PM.
  Remove urinary catheter at 7 AM.
  Force fluids (i.e., 240 ml) every hour.
  After approximately 3 to 4 hours, patient attempts to void by Valsalva maneuver, Credé maneuver of bladder, or contraction of abdominal muscles.
  If patient is able to void, residual urine is immediately checked:
  Residual urine of less than 50 to 75 ml is needed to continue with training.
  Residual urine of greater than 75 ml requires catheter reinsertion. Retraining is then resumed on another day.

Risk for impaired skin integrity related to prolonged immobility

- See general intervention strategies listed on p. 1557.

Body image disturbance related to change in body functioning

- Provide a safe, comfortable, secure environment.
- Carefully explain what you are doing and why you are doing it.
- Listen to the feelings the patient expresses (i.e., feelings of grief and loss).
- Answer questions simply and honestly.
- Correct misinformation.
- Protect the patient's privacy.
- Provide gentle physical care in a caring environment.

- Provide an ongoing assessment of the patient's interpersonal strengths. Focus on strengths and potential.
- Assist the patient to become involved in self-care.
- Assist the patient to become involved in unit activities.

Anxiety related to threat to self-concept

- See general intervention strategies on p. 1669.

Powerlessness related to lack of control over self-care

- See general intervention strategies listed on p. 1677.

Caregiver role strain, related to severity of patient's illness

- Obtain assistance with meeting of caregiver role.
    Assist caregiver to identify/utilize caregiving resources such as family members, friends, community agencies, etc.
- Assist caregiver to develop plan of care with paced, direct care activities.
- Assist caregiver to develop support systems with alternate caregivers/friends.
- Assist caregiver to identify and address personal health care needs.

Patient Education/Home Care Planning

1. Discuss name of each medication, dosage, time of administration, purpose, and side effects.
2. Avoid over-the-counter medications without first checking with physician.
3. Discuss muscle-building exercises: rubber balls, clay, trapezes, pulleys, squeeze toys, and sit-ups.
4. Stress importance of bladder retraining:
   a. Avoid food low in calcium.
   b. Force fluids to 2000 ml/day unless contraindicated.
   c. Maintain an acidic urine by drinking cranberry juice and taking ascorbic acid if ordered.
   d. Avoid alcoholic beverages, coffee, and tea.
   e. Maintain mobility as tolerated.
   f. Stress that rehabilitation may be a long process.
   g. Instruct regarding signs of full bladder.
   h. Avoid use of penile clamp to control incontinence.
   i. Avoid persons with infections, especially upper respiratory infections.
   j. Instruct regarding care of indwelling catheter.
   k. List symptoms to report to physician: urinary tract infection, kidney stone, upper respiratory infection, or skin lesions.
5. Ensure that the patient or family demonstrates:
   a. Bladder exercises every 2 to 4 hours:
      (1) Tighten rectum or vaginal vault.
      (2) Hold contraction for 5 seconds; then relax.
      (3) Continue tightening and relaxing for 5-min period.
   b. Credé maneuver for manual bladder stimulation:
      (1) Apply manual pressure over suprapubic region.
      (2) Contract abdominal muscles.
   c. Palpation of bladder distention
   d. Intake and output measurement
   e. Recording of time and amount of fluid intake
   f. Recording of time and amount of urine voided
   g. Testing of urine for pH
   h. Application of condom catheter if necessary
   i. Self-catheterization
6. Discuss importance of bowel retraining program:
   a. Encourage patient participation in developing program.
   b. Evaluate previous bowel habits.
   c. Establish regular bowel habits: (1) time of day that will be convenient for patient once discharged (e.g., after breakfast) and (2) development of program to have bowel evacuation at same time of day or every 3 days.
   d. Discuss exercises that will help to develop abdominal muscles and tone: pushing up, bearing down, and contracting abdominal muscles.
   e. Ensure privacy.
   f. Provide bedside commode rather than bedpan when possible: encourage sitting position rather than lying position.
   g. Keep equipment easily available at bedside.
   h. Ensure that the patient recognizes signals that may indicate full bowel: goose pimples, perspiration, rising of hair on arms or legs, and sense of fullness.
   i. Assist the patient to develop exercise or signals that may help to stimulate urge to defecate: (1) pressure on inner thigh, (2) stroking anus, (3) digital rectal stimulation, (4) drinking coffee, and (5) massaging abdomen downward or side to side.
   j. Discuss ways to respond to signals of defecation promptly.
   k. Discuss importance of establishing well-balanced diet that includes bulk and roughage.
   l. Discuss foods to avoid: bananas, beans, and cabbage.
   m. Assist the patient to recognize impaction: (1) no formed stool for 3 days, (2) semiliquid stools, and (3) restlessness and increased feeling of discomfort.
   n. Discuss treatment for impaction: (1) laxative suppository, (2) tap water or oil retention enema, or (3) manual clearing of bowel followed by enema.
   o. Stress importance of reporting symptoms of autonomic hyperreflexia to physician immediately.
   p. Discuss possibility of accidental incontinence once program has been established.
   q. Instruct the patient to relate incontinence to change in diet or daily routine.
7. Stress importance of ongoing outpatient care such as physician's visits and physical therapy.
8. Refer to Spinal Cord Injury Foundation.

Evaluation

Patient demonstrates a patent airway Breath sounds are normal. Chest excursion is bilateral and symmetric. Rate and depth of respirations are normal. Cough is effective. There are no subjective or objective findings of shortness of breath, air hunger, or dyspnea on exertion.

Patient demonstrates an effective breathing pattern Airway is patent. Chest excursion is symmetric. Breath sounds are normal, or there is no increase in adventitious sounds. Arterial blood gas values are within normal ranges or consistent with patient's baseline. Vital signs are within normal ranges or consistent with patient's baseline. Hemoglobin levels are 14 to 18 g/dl (male) or 12 to 16 g/dl (female). Intake and output are stable. There are no signs of respiratory distress. Skin color is not cyanotic.

Patient demonstrates adequate cerebral and spinal tissue perfusion Neurologic and vital signs are stable. Spinal column is immobilized via appropriate method. Straight body alignment is maintained. Intake and output are adequate.

Patient demonstrates minimum complications of sensory/perceptual alterations Level of orientation is optimum. Patient remains free of injury. Nutritional status is adequate. Skin integrity is maintained. Self-care deficits are minimum. Social participation is appropriate to physiologic status.

Patient remains free of traumatic injury Safety measures are appropriate to level of physiologic status. Skin integrity is maintained. Skin is free of bruises, burns, abrasions, and redness. Environment is safe. Patient is free of nosocomial infections.

Patient demonstrates an optimum level of mobility Skin integrity is maintained. Patient remains free of contractures and deformities. Level of mobility is appropriate to physiologic status. Intake and output pattern is stable. Nutritional status is adequate. Patient remains free of thrombophlebitis. Patient remains free of local infection. Patient participates in an ongoing physical therapy program.

Patient demonstrates minimum self-care deficits Outcome criteria listed for impaired physical mobility are met. Level of self-care activities is appropriate to physiologic status. Patient participates in physical and occupational therapy.

Patient demonstrates minimum complications of bowel incontinence Skin in perineal area is clean and dry. Dietary intake is adequate. Fluid intake is adequate (2000 ml/day unless contraindicated). Intake and output pattern is stable. Patient remains free of fecal impaction. Patient demonstrates a regular bowel evacuation pattern.

Patient demonstrates skin integrity Skin is intact. Nutritional status is adequate. Electrolyte balance is maintained. Patient remains free of pressure sores and contractures.

Patient demonstrates intact self-concepts Patient openly verbalizes feelings of grief and loss. Patient verbalizes positive feelings about self. Patient acknowledges actual change in self-image. Patient focuses on present and future appearance and function. Patient verbalizes feelings of hopefulness, helpfulness, and powerfulness.

Patient demonstrates a low level of anxiety Patient openly verbalizes concerns and feelings of grief, loss, and discomfort. Patient openly verbalizes feelings supported by health care professionals and family. Patient verbalizes essential aspects of care. Patient identifies methods to effectively deal with anxious feelings.

Patient demonstrates minimum feelings of powerlessness Patient maintains optimum level of physiologic control, as possible for current health status. Patient maintains optimum level of psychologic control, as possible. Patient participates, as possible, in decision making about care. Patient participates, as possible, in self-care.

Caregiver demonstrates minimal role strain Caregiver appropriately utilizes available resources. Caregiver develops adequate support systems. Caregiver addresses personal needs.

HEADACHE
(Vascular, tension, traction-inflammatory)

Headache, or cephalalgia, is any ache or pain in the head that results from the stimulation of pain-sensitive structures in the cranium or the extracranial tissues in the head and neck.

Approximately 30 million individuals in the United States seek health care for recent or recurring headaches. Headaches range in severity from a benign and transient discomfort to a

> **! EMERGENCY ALERT**
>
> **HEADACHE**
>
> Headache is an extremely common complaint. Causes may include acidosis, hypoglycemia, dehydration, *glycemia,* toxicologic factors, infections both local and systemic, trauma, and toothaches. Each is treated accordingly.
>
> *Assessment*
> - Nausea, vomiting, family history
> - Use PQRST assessment
> - Pain: mild, throbbing, stabbing, unilateral, localized, photophobia, buzzing sounds, euphoria, intense yawning, depression
> - Weight gain, generalized edema
> - Visual field changes
> - Miscellaneous paraesthesia
>
> *Interventions*
> - Assess stability of vital signs.
> - Rule out injury and try to determine underlying cause of headache.
> - Place patient in darkened room (decreased light may relieve visual disturbances).
> - Administer medications and obtain laboratory work as indicated.

severe, incapacitating pain. They may be the symptom of some potentially destructive pathologic process such as cerebral hypoxia, head trauma, inflamed meninges, cerebral hemorrhage, or expanding cranial mass. Therefore headaches, and particularly *recurring* headaches, require thorough investigation, including a complete history and neurologic examination.

Headaches may be classified as vascular, muscle contraction, and traction-inflammatory. Vascular headaches include migraine, cluster, and hypertensive headaches, as well as headaches from secondary responses (e.g., to infectious process). Muscle contraction headaches may occur from psychogenic problems, such as response to trauma or as a result of medical disorders such as cervical arthritis. Traction-inflammatory headaches may result from infection, intracranial or extracranial lesions, occlusive vascular disorders, diseases of facial structures, and medical disorders such as arteritis.[17]

•••••• Pathophysiology

Afferent pain fibers carry sensory stimuli to the tissue of the central nervous system by the three divisions of the trigeminal nerve, the first three cervical nerves, and cranial nerves IX (glossopharyngeal) and X (vagus). Intracranially, the trigeminal nerve supplies structures in the anterior and middle fossae of the skull above the tentorium. Trigeminal innervation extracranially includes all or most of the nervous supply to the facial skin; the subcutaneous tissues, and especially the blood vessels in this region; the eyes, nose, sinuses, and teeth; and most of the ear and external auditory canal.[4] The first three cervical nerves serve structures in the posterior fossae and the infradural region. Cranial nerves IX and X also supply portions of the posterior fossae and refer pain to the throat and ear.

Head pain can be caused by distention, dilation, or traction of intracranial or extracranial arteries; traction, compression, or disease states affecting sensory cranial or spinal nerves; meningeal irritation and increased intracranial pressure; displacement or traction of large intracranial veins or their dural envelopes; and voluntary or involuntary spasms and possible interstitial inflammation or traction of cervical and cranial muscles.

Extracranial causes of headaches include emotional tension, disorders of extracranial arteries, sinusitis, and inflammatory lesions of the bone and its coverings. Pain results from chronic sustained contractions of skeletal muscles, changes in intracranial pressure, vessel dilation and stretching of surrounding tissue, or a combination of the preceding factors.

·Intracranial causes of headaches, such as mass lesions, produce pain from the compression, inflammation, distortion, or traction of the pain-sensitive blood vessels and meninges at the base of the brain.

Headaches of diffuse meningeal irritation are most likely caused by the chemical irritation of nerve endings and the stretching of pain-sensitive structures by dilation and congestion of inflamed meningeal vessels. This type of headache typically is throbbing because of the transmission of arterial pulsation to cerebral tissues already under increased tension.[58]

Vascular Headaches

Migraine headaches   Migraine headache generally begins in childhood, adolescence, or early adult life and is found in approximately 5% of the general population. It is frequently familial. Young women appear most susceptible, particularly just before or during the menstrual period. Migraine is characterized by a paroxysmal, throbbing, unilateral head pain that frequently is accompanied by autonomic symptoms such as nausea and vomiting. Attacks generally decrease in frequency and intensity with advancing age.

The exact pathogenesis of migraine is unknown. The initial physiologic change is that of vasospasm in the intracranial and extracranial arteries and their branches on one side of the head. Ten to 30 minutes later, dilation of the same vessels occurs. The constriction of the arteries is responsible for the symptoms of the aura, while vessel dilation produces the headache part of the syndrome. In headache-free intervals the cranial vessels of the migraine patient are hypersensitive to inhalation of carbon dioxide and intravenously administered histamine.[48]

Recent studies indicate that serotonin levels rise during the prodromal phase and drop during the headache phase. Also, the urinary excretion of 5-hydroxyindoleacetic acid (5-HIAA), a metabolite of serotonin, is increased during the migraine episodes. Platelet aggregability, which increases just before a migraine attack, is thought to be responsible for the release of serotonin.[37]

Agents and circumstances thought to precipitate migraine attacks include emotional stress and tension, menstruation, too much or too little sleep, and dietary agents such as tyramine, nitrate, and glutamate. However, none of these affect all individuals or consistently produce attacks in the same individual.[16] There is no evidence to support allergy or autonomic disorders as responsible for migraine attacks.

Cluster headaches   Cluster headaches (Horton's syndrome, histamine headache, migrainous neuralgia, or paroxysmal nocturnal cephalalgia) are intense repetitive vascular events. Cluster headaches are four times more common in men and generally occur in the third and fourth decades of life.[37] They are characterized by a distinct episode of excruciating pain, usually unilateral, which lasts from ½ to 1 hour, and is accompanied by ipsilateral lacrimation, nasal stuffiness, and drainage.[16] Usually, the same side of the head is involved in the cluster of attacks. There is no prodrome and usually only slight nausea. The attack may occur at any time (generally they are nocturnal), and multiple attacks are common.

Headaches may occur in a episodic or chronic pattern. The episodic pattern of cluster headaches is characterized by recurring headaches for several weeks to months, followed by months to years during which no headaches occur.

Chronic cluster headaches are either primary or secondary in type. The primary chronic pattern is characterized by persistent, repetitive attacks for years at a time. The secondary chronic type occurs when the episodic attacks evolve into chronic, unremitting attacks.[16]

The exact mechanism of cluster headaches is unknown. Increased histamine with resultant vasodilation has been implicated.

Tension Headaches

Muscle contraction headaches Muscle contraction headaches are the most common type of head pain. Research studies indicate a preponderance of muscle contraction headaches in women and a higher incidence in adults from 20 to 40 years of age. This headache is usually bilateral and may be diffuse or confined to the frontal, temporal, parietal, or occipital area. The onset of an attack is more gradual than with a migraine, and duration is highly variable, but it may last for several days up to several months or years.

Muscle contraction headaches are frequently accompanied by contraction of skeletal muscles of the face, jaw, and neck. Concurrent arterial vasodilation may contribute further to the discomfort. There are no structural changes in the involved muscle groups.

Traumatic headaches The posttraumatic, or postconcussion, headache, which consists of a dull, generalized pain, may develop after head injury and may be coupled with other symptoms such as lack of concentration, giddiness, or dizziness. Symptoms are much the same whether the head injury is mild or severe. Traumatic headaches usually are nonfocal, appearing for at least part of every day and persisting over days, weeks, or months. The headache is made worse by coughing and straining, which raises the pressure in both intracranial and extracranial venous systems.

Posttraumatic headaches are thought to be caused by vascular dilation, muscle contraction, or direct injury to the scalp.

Traction-Inflammatory Headaches

Traction headaches Traction headaches may result from increased intracranial pressure, cerebral hemorrhage, decreased intracranial pressure (e.g., lumbar puncture), and inflammatory processes (e.g., encephalitis, meningitis). The discomfort produced with traction headaches occurs because of referred pain when the pain-sensitive structures (cranial nerves, arteries, etc.) are stretched or displaced by a mass lesion.

Temporal arteritis Temporal arteritis, also called cranial arteritis or giant cell arteritis, generally affects individuals over 60 years of age. This headache usually is located in the temporal area and may be accompanied by visual loss, which is caused by ophthalmic artery involvement.[37]

Temporal arteritis is thought to result from an autoimmune mechanism and is included in the group of collagen-vascular diseases. The temporal arteries may be palpated as firm, tender cords or may be seen as tortuous, enlarged vessels.

• • •

Other clinical types of headaches include those from angioma and aneurysm, chronic subdural hematoma, brain tumor, and medical disorders such as hypothyroidism, Cushing's disease, fevers of any cause, chronic lung disease with hypercapnia, hypertension, acute anemia, chronic nitrate or ergot exposure, corticosteroid withdrawal, carbon monoxide exposure, adrenal tumors producing aldosterone, and sometimes Addison's disease.

• • • • • • Diagnostic Studies and Findings

Cervical and skull roentgenograms Detection of abnormalities at base of brain

Funduscopic eye examination Possible irritation of iris and ciliary body

Serum Increased sedimentation rate; anemia (lithium serum level *not* to exceed 1 mEq/L)

CT scan Possible intracranial lesions

Magnetic resonance imaging (MRI) Same as CT scan

Cerebral angiography Detection of vascular abnormalities

Neurologic history and examination Identification of precipitating influences; effects on activities of daily living; neurologic deficits

• • • • • • Multidisciplinary Plan

Medications

Analgesic/anti-inflammatory agents
    Ergot preparations (Table 3-10)
Adrenergic agents
    Isometheptene mucate (Midrin, Octinum), 1-2 capsules at onset of headache; followed by 1-2 capsules 1 h later; maximum dosage: 5 capsules/12 h
Psychotherapeutic agents
    Chlorpromazine (Thorazine), 25 mg IM, po, or rectal suppository
    Promethazine (Phenergan), 25 mg IM or rectally; 50 mg po
    Hydroxyzine (Vistaril), 75 mg IM or 50-100 mg po
    Lithium carbonate (Lithane; others), initial dose of 300 mg po bid to qid; *must* be monitored by serum levels
Analgesic/antipyretics
    Acetaminophen (Tylenol), 600 mg po q4h prn
Narcotic analgesics
    Meperidine (Demerol), 50-75 mg IM q4-6h prn
Corticosteroids
    Dexamethasone (Decadron), 8-12 mg IM
β-Adrenergic blocking agent
    Propranolol (Inderal), initial dose 20 mg po bid or tid; titrated gradually up to 80-200 mg/d in divided doses
    Methysergide maleate (Sansert), 2 mg tid or qid; for up to 5-6 mo; followed by mandatory discontinuance for at least 1 mo
    Cyproheptadine (Periactin), 4 mg po bid-qid
Antidepressants
    Phenelzine (Nardil), 10-15 mg po bid-qid
Antihypertensive agents
    Clonidine hydrochloride (Catapres), 0.2 mg po bid-tid

Antianginal agents
  Dipyridamole (Persantine), 25-50 mg po tid or qid
Nonsteroidal anti-inflammatory agents
  Sulfinpyrazone (Anturane), 200 mg po bid-qid
Antidepressants
  Amitriptyline (Elavil), 25-100 mg po qid
  Amitriptyline (Elavil), 10-100 mg at bedtime of (HS)
  Imipramine (Tofranil), 10-75 mg HS in divided doses
  Desipramine (Norpramin), 25-75 mg HS in divided doses

General Management

Application of heat or cold to affected areas
Dietary counseling to eliminate food items that may provoke headaches: vinegar, chocolate, pork, onions, excessive caffeine, citrus fruits, bananas, yogurt, sour cream, alcohol, canned figs, ripened cheeses, herring, doughnuts, cured sandwich meats, chicken livers, broad bean pods, fermented or marinated foods, avocados, and MSG
Psychologic counseling for behavioral modification, stress management, and biofeedback

TABLE 3-10 Drugs Used in the Treatment of Vascular Migraine Headaches

Drug	Use	Dose	Action	Side Effects
Methysergide maleate (Sansert)	For prophylactic treatment of vascular headaches such as migraine, cluster, and others which have been difficult to control; not effective for an acute attack; a serotonin antagonist. *Alert:* Patient must be under medical supervision because this drug has such serious side effects	2 mg orally tid with meals; after taking drug for 5 mo, it should be discontinued for 3-4 wk to reduce the incidence of serious side effects; dosage should be reduced gradually to prevent rebound headache	The action is not clear, but it decreases the frequency of headache in patients that are difficult to control with other drugs	Fibrotic changes in the retroperitoneal and pleuropulmonary tissue and in the mitral and aortic valves are the most serious complications; any of the following symptoms should be reported at once: urinary tract obstruction, dysuria, back pain, peripheral vascular insufficiency, cold, numb, or painful extremities and diminished pulse, dyspnea, and chest pain. *Contraindications:* Cardiac conditions, severe hypertension, pregnancy, peripheral vascular disease, and atherosclerosis
Ergotamine tartrate (Gynergen)	Treatment of vascular migraine headaches. A single dose of ergotamine (1 or 3 mg by injection at bedtime) is effective for *cluster headaches*	2 mg orally; 2 mg sublingually, initially to be followed by 2 mg every 30 min until the headache subsides, or until 6 mg have been taken (Some texts suggest that up to a total of 9 mg may be taken.); 0.25-0.5 mg *subcutaneously* or *IM* at onset; dose may be repeated hourly up to 1.0 mg in 24 h; 0.25 mg intravenously at onset; no more than 0.5 mg/24 h; rarely given IV; 2-4 mg by *rectal suppository* at onset; 2 mg may be repeated hourly, up to 6-8 mg	Ergot alkaloids result in cerebral vasoconstriction, which decreases the amplitude of the pulsations of the cranial arteries; in addition to its powerful vasoconstrictive property, it constricts the smooth muscles of the uterus; however, the major use of ergot alkaloids is for the treatment of migraine headaches	Has a *cumulative action,* so it must be taken sparingly and as ordered or ergotism will develop (*Ergotism:* numbness and tingling of fingers and toes, muscle pain and weakness, gangrene, and blindness). *Contraindications:* Diabetes mellitus, sepsis, hepatorenal disease, peripheral and coronary disease, hypertension, and pregnancy

From Hickey.[34]

■ TABLE 3-10 Drugs Used in the Treatment of Vascular Migraine Headaches—cont'd

Drug	Use	Dose	Action	Side Effects
Ergotamine with caffeine (Cafergot)	Same as ergotamine	Each tablet contains 1 mg of ergotamine tartrate and 100 mg of caffeine; usual dose is 1-2 tablets at onset and another tablet in 30 min, not to exceed 6 tablets per attack (also available in suppositories if vomiting occurs)	The caffeine increases the effectiveness of the ergotamine by its vasoconstrictive action	Same as ergotamine
Dihydroergotamine (DHE 45)	Treatment of migraine headaches which tend to be severe	1 mg IM or IV at onset; repeat in 1 h	Action is not clear, but a majority of patients receive relief in 15 min to 2 h after administration	Less toxic and fewer side effects than ergotamine; less likely to cause vomiting than ergotamine
Ergotamine tartrate, 0.3 mg Phenobarbital, 20 mg Belladonna alkaloid, 0.1 mg (Bellergal)	Reduces the number of attacks in patients who have one or more weekly	Give 2 or 3 times daily for a few weeks	Vasoconstriction, sedation, and reduction of spasm	Same as ergotamine, along with dryness of mucous membrane and drowsiness *Contraindications:* In addition to those of ergotamine, do not give to patients with glaucoma

Others
  Analgesics
    Codeine sulfate, 30 mg
        or
    Meperidine (Demerol), 50 mg
    Aspirin, 0.6 g   Either drug may be given for severe pain once the headache has become full-blown; narcotics are avoided unless the pain is very severe, and precautions should be taken to avoid addiction

    Butalbital (Fiorinal), 2 tablets   These drugs may be tried for less severe pain
  Diuretics
    Hydrochlorothiazide (Esidrix) or acetazolamide (Diamox)   These drugs are given 1 wk before menstruation if premenstrual tension predisposes the individual to headaches; in addition, mild tranquilizers and analgesics such as aspirin may be given
  Antihistamines
    Diphenhydramine (Benadryl) and others   May be helpful in cluster headaches

NURSING CARE

Nursing Assessment

Classic migraine	Throbbing, high-intensity; unilateral discomfort in temporal area, upper cranium, or lower hemicranium (rare)	Usually unilateral in temporal area, but may occur in any area of the head	Hours	Hours to days	Prodrome/aura: Visual disturbances Sensory symptoms Mild paresis Nausea, vomiting, or anxiety
Common migraine	Throbbing, intense pain; progresses to generalized nonthrobbing head pain	Usually frontal or temporal region	Gradual	Hours to days	Prodrome; photophobia; nausea; irritability; vomiting; anxiety
Cluster	Sudden, intense, and unilateral pain	Orbitotemporal area; may begin in area of nostril and spread to adjacent eye and sometimes forehead	Sudden	Hours; occurs in clusters	No prodrome; anxiety; lacrimation; rhinorrhea; nasal congestion; flushing of face; Horner's sign with ptosis and pupillary constriction
Muscle contraction	Aching, tightness, or pressure	Suboccipital, occipital, frontal areas	Gradual	Hours to days	Muscle tension; anxiety

Continued.

Posttraumatic headaches	Dull, generalized pain	Varies	Gradual	Varies	Intensified by physical exertion; anxiety; personality changes; insomnia; lack of concentration; nausea, vomiting; dizziness; fatigue; unsteadiness
Traction headaches	Deep, dull, steady ache usually worse in morning and aggravated by coughing or straining	Varies	Varies	Varies	Varies
Temporal arteritis	Variable intensity; unilateral or bilateral tenderness of painful area	Temporal, occipital, fronto-occipital regions; may be accompanied by tenderness of painful areas	Gradual	Weeks	Visual loss

From Hickey.[32]

Nursing Dx & Intervention

Anxiety related to change in health status

- See general intervention strategies listed on p. 1669.

Pain related to severe headache

- Assess and document degree of pain and effect of medication administered.
- Promote rest and relaxation.
- Decrease noxious stimuli.
- Modify anxiety associated with the pain experience.
- Provide other sensory input *to reduce focus on noxious stimuli.*
- Administer medication per protocol. Dosages of ergot drugs greater than 10 mg/week can lead to ergotism and cumulative effects.
- Remain with patient *to reduce anxiety.*
- Use whatever measures the patient believes will alleviate the pain.
- Teach patient about his discomfort.
- Use other professionals, as appropriate.
- Improve effectiveness of pain relief measures by using them before the pain becomes intense. Lie in quiet, dark room after taking the medication.
- Apply cold compresses or dry heat to head and neck to increase circulation and to decrease muscle tension.

Patient Education/Home Care Planning

1. Reinforce physician's explanation of medical management.
2. Instruct regarding name of medication, dosage, time of administration, and toxic or side effects.
3. Instruct regarding proper use of ergot drugs:
   a. Take medication at earliest symptom of a headache.
4. Stress need to avoid over-the-counter medications without first consulting physician.
5. Emphasize need for regular exercise program.
6. Instruct regarding possible food causes of headaches.

Evaluation

Patient demonstrates a low level of anxiety Patient openly verbalizes concerns and feelings of grief, loss, and discomfort. Patient openly verbalizes feelings, supported by health care professionals and family. Patient verbalizes essential aspects of care. Patient identifies methods to deal effectively with anxious feelings.

Patient experiences minimal alterations in comfort Patient openly verbalizes feelings of discomfort when they occur. Patient can use measures to decrease discomfort. Patient verbally validates a decrease in subjective feelings of discomfort. Objective findings of pain are decreased.

 SEIZURE DISORDER

(Convulsions, epilepsy)

Seizures, or convulsions, are paroxysmal episodes in which there are sudden and violent involuntary contractions of a group of skeletal muscles and disturbances in consciousness, behavior, sensation, and autonomic functioning.

Seizures may be tonic or clonic, focal, and unilateral or bilateral. The term *epilepsy* denotes a group of neurologic disorders characterized by the repeated occurrence of any of the various forms of seizures. Approximately 2 to 4 million Americans are affected with epilepsy, many are children. There are many social consequences of a seizure disorder including possible loss of driving or educational privileges. Of all persons with epilepsy, 25% have recurrent seizures while receiving medication, 10% are institutionalized, and 5% are home-bound invalids.[41]

• • • • • • Pathophysiology

Seizure disorders can be classified as resulting from pathologic processes, endogenous or exogenous poisons, metabolic disturbances, fever, and idiopathic. *Pathologic processes* include formation abnormalities (e.g., vascular anomalies), space-occupying lesions (e.g., brain abscess, tumors, hematomas), craniocerebral trauma, acute cerebral edema (e.g., secondary to

! EMERGENCY ALERT

SEIZURE

Seizures are classified as partial, generalized, and unclassified and are a symptom rather than a diagnosis. Seizures are characterized as an abnormal period of electrical activity in the brain.

Assessment

- Patient may report an aura.
- Can be localized and then progress (partial).
- Sudden loss of consciousness with contractions of large muscle groups, apnea, dilated/unresponsive pupils, bite the tongue, incontinence of bladder/bowel, hyperventilation, sweating, rapid pulse, excessive salivation.
- Frequently a postictal phase follows a seizure where muscles relax, loss of consciousness is depressed, and respirations are deep; confusion, disorientation, and headache may follow; the patient may be fatigued and sleep for several hours.

Interventions

- Ensure patent airway.
- Position patient on side if possible.
- Protect the patient's body from injury.
- Treat underlying cause.
- Administer high-flow oxygen by mask (10 L), if possible.
- Obtain IV access; administer medications to suppress seizures if required.

---

acute renal failure), infection (e.g., encephalitis), degenerative changes (e.g., leukodystrophies), vascular lesions (e.g., embolus, cerebrovascular accidents, and hemorrhages), and neuronal injury (e.g., anoxia from deficient oxygen).

Toxic endogenous substances (e.g., uremia) or *exogenous* substances such as certain medications (e.g., phenothiazines), lead ingestion, and alcohol intoxication or sudden withdrawal may precipitate seizure activity.

Metabolic disturbances (i.e., electrolyte imbalances) that cause an interference with crucial substances such as oxygen, glucose, or calcium being delivered to cerebral tissues can result in seizures.

Individuals with decreased neuronal thresholds may experience a seizure secondary to a *febrile* state.

Finally, *idiopathic* seizures may occur without any identifiable cause. The basis of idiopathic seizure disorders may be a biochemical imbalance.

These causative agents are either genetic factors or acquired factors. *Genetically,* epilepsy is rarely a predictable, inherited entity. The only well-defined inherited seizure pattern is that of the classic 2.5 to 3/s spike-and-wave pattern on the electroencephalogram (EEG).[37] Therefore, although inheritance may be a risk in developing seizures, environmental risk factors (e.g., trauma) play a significant role. *Acquired* factors include pathologic processes (e.g., infection), trauma that produces epileptogenic lesions, toxic substances, metabolic disturbances, and febrile states.

Traditionally, seizures have been classified as grand mal, petit mal, psychomotor (temporal lobe), and focal motor (jacksonian). With advanced technology it became evident that many neurologic manifestations of seizures did not fit into these categories. In 1969 the International League Against Epilepsy formulated a revised classification that incorporated pathophysiologic principles of all types of seizure activity.

Partial seizures start with a localized activation of neurons and generally do not involve the whole brain or significantly impair consciousness or memory. Partial seizures with simple symptoms produce symptoms of which the individual is aware, including autonomic, sensory, or focal motor symptoms. Simple partial seizures start with focal motor symptoms (jacksonian seizures), generally in the contralateral precentral gyrus. Symptoms first occur in the part of the body controlled by that brain area and then can spread to involve the entire limb and frequently the entire half of the body. The seizure ends with a gradual reduction of clonic, jerking movements. Seizure activity that occurs usually in the hand or face and is continuous, clonic, and localized is called *epilepsia partialis continua.* Simple sensory seizures are uncommon, but when present, they originate from hyperexcitable neurons in the postcentral gyrus. Symptoms of a partial sensory seizure include various degrees of numbness and paresthesias. Autonomic seizures result from hyperexcitable neurons of the frontal, temporal, mesial, orbital, or insular cortices. These seizures may begin with disturbances in gastric motility, which may progress to nausea and vomiting, tenesmus, or sudden bowel evacuation.[24] Partial seizures with only autonomic symptoms are rare.

Partial seizures with complex symptoms generally produce some type of spisodic loss of consciousness. This type of seizure may include cognitive, affective, psychosensory, or psychomotor symptoms. Events that trigger the seizure occur within the structures of the temporal lobe. Complex partial seizures begin with various types of auras such as sensory illusions, déjà vu, or unusual smells. The individual may recognize these auras, or memory of them may be lost in postictal amnesia. In complex partial seizures, EEG abnormalities are localized in temporal or frontotemporal areas, including rhinencephalic structures. Complex partial seizures are characterized by purposeful behavior that is inappropriate for the time and place.[4] Automatisms such as lip smacking, walking aimlessly, or picking at one's clothing are common. The individual with this type of seizure usually cannot remember the seizure, but consciousness is not lost totally.

Psychomotor seizures in children can be confused with absence attacks because of the relative paucity of memory patterns in the temporal lobe of the young child. Complex partial attacks in children can be distinguished from absence attacks by the fact that the psychomotor attacks occur much less frequently and are of longer duration.

Generalized seizures begin locally but almost immediately result in bilateral involvement of the corticoreticular and reticulocortical systems of the diencephalon. Generalized seizures are usually petit mal (absence seizures) or grand mal (tonic-clonic) in nature. Petit mal seizures usually affect children after the age of 4 years and before puberty,[32] and although rare, they can occur in adults up to 70 years of age. Petit mal seizures consist of a sudden cessation of conscious activity without convulsive motor activity or loss of postural control.[48] These absence attacks usually last for seconds or minutes. The brief lapses of consciousness may be accompanied by minor motor manifestations (e.g., eyelid flickering and isolated myoclonic jerks). After a petit mal seizure, the individual quickly regains consciousness or awareness and usually experiences no postictal confusion.

Grand mal seizures are one of the most common epileptic paroxysms and may be generalized seizures or the result of secondary generalization of partial seizures. Grand mal seizures usually occur without warning and follow a common pattern: (1) *tonic* phase; forceful contraction of axial and appendicular muscles, loss of postural control, epileptic cry, cyanosis; usually lasts 2 or 3 minutes; (2) *clonic* phase, characterized by gradual transition from tonic contractions to intermittent bilateral brisk clonic movements; this phase represents recurring inhibition phases interrupting the initial tonic phase; (3) *postictal* phase: amnesia of seizure and possibly even retrograde amnesia.

Generalized seizures also can result from secondary generalization of focal cortical discharges and are identical to primary generalized seizures. These facts make it difficult to distinguish secondary generalized seizures from primarily generalized tonic-clonic seizures. With secondary generalized seizures, however, there are usually diffuse cerebral pathologic findings.[4]

Generalized seizures such as myoclonic seizures, tonic seizures, infantile spasms, and atonic seizures usually occur during childhood and generally are associated with some type of genetic, perinatal, or metabolic brain disease. *Myoclonic* seizures may occur alone or coexist with other types of seizures. Individuals with severe and generalized myoclonus demonstrate evidence of disturbances in function of the reticular substance in relevant areas of the sensory cortex.

Tonic seizures are a less common type of primary generalized seizure marked by sudden rigid posturing of trunk and extremities, frequently with deviation to one side of the head and eyes. Tonic seizures are frequently of a shorter duration than tonic-clonic seizures and are not followed by a clonic phase. These seizures usually indicate a lesion in the area of the midbrain and are sometimes seen in individuals with severe cerebral palsy.

Infantile spasms (hypsarrhythmia) are generalized seizures occurring between birth and approximately 12 months of age. They consist of brief synchronous contractions of the neck, torso, and arms.[48] Infantile spasms rarely occur in an apparently normal infant; rather, they usually occur in children with an underlying neurologic disorder (e.g., anoxic encephalopathy). Approximately 90% of children with infantile spasms develop mental retardation.

Atonic seizures consist of brief loss of consciousness and postural tone; these symptoms are not associated with tonic muscular contractions.[48] This type of seizure frequently is accompanied by other forms of seizure activity.

Unilateral seizure is a type of seizure in which clinical signs usually occur on one side of the body and the EEG discharges are recorded over the contralateral cerebral hemisphere.[4] Unilateral seizures may shift from one side to another but generally do not become symmetric.

The microscopic changes leading to pathologic processes occurring during the different types of seizure activities are essentially the same. The major alteration in the physiologic state is a hypersynchronous discharge in a localized area of the brain.[48] This localized area of hypersynchronized discharge is called the *epileptogenic focus,* producing a large, sharp EEG waveform known as the spike discharge.

Metabolic changes occurring within the cerebrum during the epileptic discharges include release of unusually large amounts of neuropeptides and neurotransmitters during the seizure, increased cerebral blood flow to primary involved areas, increased extracellular concentrations of potassium and decreased extracellular concentrations of calcium, changes in oxidative metabolism and local pH, and increased utilization of glucose.

Termination of seizure activity appears to be related to the large and lasting hyperpolarization of the neuronal cell membrane. This hyperpolarization is possibly generated by an electrogenic sodium pump. As the hyperpolarization is sustained, the neuronal cells cease firing, and the surface potentials of the brain are suppressed.[24]

•••••• Diagnostic Studies and Findings

CT scan   Structural changes

Magnetic resonance imaging (MRI)   Structural changes

Skull roentgenogram   Evidence of fractures; shift of calcified pineal gland; bony erosion; separated sutures

Echoencephalogram   Possible midline shifts of brain structures

Cerebral angiography   Possible vascular abnormalities; evaluation of a subdural hematoma

Electroencephalogram (EEG)   Grand mal: high, fast voltage spiked in all leads; petit mal: 3/s, rounded spike wave complexes in all leads; psychomotor (temporal lobe): square-topped 4-6/s spike wave complexes over involved lobe; delta waves: usually associated with destroyed brain tissue; theta waves: not always abnormal

Urine screening   Indicates presence and levels of certain medications

Serum chemistry   Hypoglycemia; electrolyte imbalance; increased blood urea nitrogen; blood alcohol levels

History and neurologic examination   Pattern of onset and characteristics of seizure activity; precipitating factors

•••••• Multidisciplinary Plan

Surgery

Excision of epileptogenic focus
Stereotactic lesions

Medications

Anticonvulsants

  Grand mal, simple partial, and complex partial

    Phenytoin (Dilantin), 100 mg po or IV tid or qid

    Phenobarbital, 2-5 mg/kg/day

    Primidone (Mysoline)

      Day 1-3: 100-125 mg po hs

      Day 4-6: 100-125 mg po bid

      Day 7-9: 100-125 mg po tid

      Day 10 and maintenance: 250 mg po tid

    Carbamazepine (Tegretol), initially 200 mg po bid; increase dosage gradually until desired response is obtained (should not exceed 120 mg/d)

  Petit mal

    Ethosuximide (Zarontin), initially at 3-6 yr of age, 250 mg/d po; 6 yr and older, 500 mg po qd; maintenance dose, individually determined according to patient's response

General Management

Emergency equipment at bedside

Serum chemistry monitoring (complete blood count, platelet count)

Routine urinalysis

Dietary therapy (i.e., ketogenic diet)

Serum drug levels (e.g., Dilantin, phenobarbital)

Seizure precautions

NURSING CARE

Nursing Assessment

Simple Partial Seizures

Motor signs

  Involuntary recurrent contractions of muscles (e.g., face, hand, arm, finger) of one body part; may be confined to one body area or spread to contiguous ipsilateral body parts (spread of activity such as left thumb to left hand to left arm to left side of face is known as jacksonian march)

Behavioral manifestations

  Sensory: auditory or visual hallucinations; paresthesias; vertigo

  Autonomic and psychic: sensation of déjà vu; complex hallucinations; illusions; unwarranted feelings of anger or fear; pupillary dilation; sweating

Level of consciousness

  No loss of consciousness

Complex Partial Seizures

Onset

  May consist of variety of auras (e.g., sensory hallucinations, déjà vu, unusual smells)

Motor activity

  Compulsive patting or rubbing of body parts, lip smacking, walking aimlessly, swallowing, picking at clothing (termed automatisms)

  Unconscious performance of highly skilled acts

Level of consciousness

  Episodic loss of conscious contact with environment

Postictal amnesia

  Amnestic for seizure events

  May be amnestic of auras

Generalized Seizures

Petit mal

  Transient loss of consciousness for few seconds to minutes

  May be accompanied by flickering eyelids or intermittent jerking movements of hands

Grand mal

  See findings listed on p. 332

Myoclonic

  Sudden brief contraction of muscle groups producing rapid jerky movements in one or more extremities or entire body

  May be accompanied by violent fall without loss of consciousness

Tonic

  Sudden assumption of an abnormal dystonic posture for a few seconds to minutes

  Consciousness usually retained

  Head and eyes may deviate toward one side

Infantile spasms

  Brief synchronous contractions (usually flexion) of both arms, neck, and trunk

  Mental retardation

Atomic "drop attacks"

  Brief loss of consciousness and postural tone without associated tonic muscular contractions

Unilateral Seizures

Clonic, tonic, or tonic-clonic seizures affecting only or affecting predominantly one side of body

May be with or without impairment in level of consciousness

Seizures may shift from one side to another (usually not symmetric)

Unclassified Seizures

Any atypical seizure activity

Nursing Dx & Intervention

Ineffective airway clearance related to perceptual impairment

- See general intervention strategies listed on p. 1614.

Ineffective breathing pattern related to neuromuscular impairment

- See general intervention strategies listed on p. 1616.

Sensory/perceptual alterations (visual, auditory, kinesthetic, gustatory, tactile, olfactory) related to change in level of consciousness

- See general intervention strategies listed on p. 1643.

Risk for injury related to seizures

- Maintain bed in low position at all times unless side rails are up or nurse is with patient.
- Provide the patient with a call light within easy reach.
- Maintain side rails in up position at bedtime, after sedation, when patient is confused, and as needed *to prevent accidental falls.*
- Maintain wheelchairs and stretchers in locked position when transferring patient.

Preconvulsive

- Maintain seizure precautions:

    Have oral airway at bedside.

    Have suction equipment available at bedside *to prevent aspiration.*

    Pad side rails, if indicated.

    Administer oxygen per protocol *to prevent cerebral hypoxia.*

    Establish means of communication. Identify auras if possible.

Convulsive

- Maintain patient airway.
- Support and protect head; turn to side if possible *to maintain airway.*
- Prevent injury:

    Ease patient to floor if in chair.

    Place pillows along side rails if patient is in bed.

    Loosen constrictive clothing.

- Provide privacy as necessary; stay with patient.
- Note frequency, time, involved body parts, and length of seizure *to provide accurate description of seizure activity.*

Postconvulsive

- Maintain patent airway.
- Suction as indicated.
- Check vital signs and neurologic status.
- Administer oxygen per protocol *to prevent hypoxia.*
- Reorient patient to environment *to minimize sensory-perceptual alterations.*
- Place patient in position of comfort, and turn head to side.
- Administer oral hygiene as necessary *to remove secretions and bleeding.*

Anxiety related to change in health status

- See general intervention strategies listed on p. 1669.

Social isolation related to alteration in physical appearance during seizure activity

- See general intervention strategies listed on p. 1700.

Patient Education/Home Care Planning

1. Discuss with patient the nature of the seizure disorder and need to adopt positive attitude.
2. Stress importance of verbalizing feelings of shame, humiliation, anxiety, and fears regarding seizure disorder. Assist in clarifying common fears and myths about epilepsy (i.e., not a form of insanity).
3. Emphasize need to avoid overprotection.
4. Stress need to continue with normal work and recreation routines. Assure patient that activity may inhibit seizure activity.
5. Emphasize need to avoid excessive stress or emotional excitement.
6. Discuss importance of wearing a medical alert band or carrying a medical alert card at all times.
7. Stress importance of well-balanced diet and avoidance of excessive use of stimulants such as alcohol.
8. Emphasize importance of identifying aura and course of action to take.
9. Discuss name of medication, action, side effects, dosage, and frequency of administration.
10. Stress need to avoid taking over-the-counter medications without first consulting physician.
11. Emphasize importance of ongoing outpatient care.

Evaluation

Patient demonstrates a patent airway Breath sounds are normal. Chest excursion is bilateral and symmetric. Rate and depth of respirations are normal. Cough is effective. There are no subjective or objective findings of shortness of breath, air hunger, or dyspnea on exertion.

Patient demonstrates an effective breathing pattern Airway is patent. Chest excursion is symmetric. Breath sounds are normal, or there is no increase in adventitious sounds. Arterial blood gas values are within normal ranges or consistent with patient's baseline. Vital signs are within normal ranges or consistent with patient's baseline. Hemoglobin levels are 14 to 18 g/dl (male) or 12 to 16 g/dl (female). Intake and output are stable. There are no signs of respiratory distress. All lobes are resonant on percussion.

Patient remains free of traumatic injury Safety measures are appropriate to physiologic status. Skin integrity is maintained. Skin is free of bruises, burns, abrasions, and redness. Environment is safe. Patient is free of nosocomial infections.

Patient demonstrates a low level of anxiety Patient openly verbalizes concerns and feelings of grief, loss, and discomfort. Patient openly verbalizes feelings, supported by health care professionals and family. Patient verbalizes essential aspects of care. Patient can identify methods to effectively deal with anxious feelings.

Patient demonstrates social participation Patient can state importance of interpersonal relationships. Patient relates to self and others. Patient participates, as possible, in unit and group activities. Patient participates, as possible, in family activities.

MEDICAL INTERVENTIONS AND RELATED NURSING CARE

CHORDOTOMY

Description and Rationale

A chordotomy is a surgical procedure in which the lateral spinothalamic tract of the spinal cord is divided to relieve pain. The lesion is created on the contralateral side, approximately two to three spinal segments above the desired level of anesthesia, which then severs the pain pathways. If the pain is midline, the lesions must be made bilaterally. The preferred surgical technique is the *percutaneous chordotomy.*

The procedure consists of stereotactic insertion of a spinal lumbar puncture needle laterally between C1 and C2 (at the cervical level). A wire electrode then is inserted into the anterior quadrant, and a lesion is made by use of a radio frequency generator at a designated site to destroy ascending pain fibers. The percutaneous chordotomy may be repeated if pain recurs or the level of anesthesia falls. The other method for performing a chordotomy consists of a *surgical thoracic resection approach.* Following exposure of the spinal cord, the dendate ligament is divided at the level selected for the chordotomy.

Following a chordotomy, the patient may experience an interruption in respiratory reflex pathways causing periods of apnea or respiratory arrest, temporary paralysis, permanent loss of temperature sensation, and loss of bowel and bladder control.

•••••• Multidisciplinary Plan

Surgery

Tracheotomy, if indicated
Swan-Ganz catheterization

Medications

Local anesthesia (percutaneous chordotomy)
General anesthesia
Regional anesthetic blocks (preoperatively)

General Management

Radio-frequency generator (percutaneous chordotomy)
Mechanical ventilator, if indicated (i.e., high cervical chordotomy)

Pulmonary function testing (preoperatively and postoperatively)
Cardiac monitoring
Counseling and support regarding coping effectively with diffuse pain
Occupational therapy
Physical therapy

NURSING CARE

Nursing Assessment

Pain

Discomfort at puncture or incision site

Complications

Paralysis
  Leg weakness
  Temporary paralysis
Bowel/bladder control
  Temporary (i.e., several weeks) urine retention
  Incontinence
Respiratory function
  Periods of apnea
  Respiratory arrest (with cervical chordotomy)
Sensation
  Permanent loss of temperature sensation below level of interruption
  Paresthesias
  Decreased position sense

Other

Postural hypotension
Potential for skin breakdown related to impaired physical mobility

Nursing Dx & Intervention

Ineffective breathing pattern related to interrupted respiratory reflex pathway

- Maintain patent airway; intubation/tracheostomy and mechanical ventilation may be indicated:
    Suction as needed. Hyperoxygenate lungs with 100% oxygen for 1 minute before and 1 minute after suctioning, unless contraindicated, *to prevent hypoxemia.*
- Maintain aseptic technique during suctioning *to prevent infection.*
- Monitor mechanical ventilator, if used:
    Ensure that tidal volume, rate, mode, and oxygen concentration are set as ordered.
    Ensure that ventilator alarms are on and functional.

- Monitor arterial blood gases as ordered:
    Report decrease in Po_2 of 10 to 15 mm Hg.
    Report increase in Pco_2 greater than 10 to 15 mm Hg.
- Note respiratory rate, depth, and level of consciousness every 15 to 30 minutes and as needed.
- Stay with patient in acute distress *to monitor and minimize feelings of anxiety.*

Altered spinal tissue perfusion related to high risk for spinal cord edema

- Perform neurologic assessment every 1 to 2 hours and as needed:
    Check level of consciousness.
    Assess pupillary size, reaction, and equality.
    Check for extraocular eye movements.
    Note motor and sensory deficits (i.e., color and strength of extremities). Report any increase in deficits immediately to the physician.
- Administer medications as ordered (e.g., steroids *to control cord edema.*)
- If steroids are being administered:
    Check stools *to detect occult blood.*
    Test urine for sugar and acetone *to detect glycosuria.*
    Administer phytonadine, MSD (Aquamephyton), intramuscularly daily or every other day *to control tendency for bleeding.*
    Administer antacids per protocol *to decrease or prevent gastric irritation.*
- Maintain parenteral fluids as ordered.
- Measure intake and output every hour. Immediately report urine output of less than 30 ml/hour.

Sensory/perceptual alterations related to potential loss of neuromuscular function

- See general intervention strategies on p. 1643.

Impaired physical mobility related to surgical procedure

- Administer skin care every 2 hours:
    Turn patient every 2 hours and as needed unless contraindicated:
    Change position slowly.
    Position in straight body alignment.
    Use log-roll technique when turning.
    Keep skin dry; give perineal care as needed.
    Massage pressure points every 2 hours *to stimulate circulation;* give gentle back rubs every shift and as needed.
- Use heel and elbow guards as needed.
- Use firm mattress or bed board.
- Perform active or passive ROM exercises every 2 to 4 hours.
- Apply antiembolus stocking to lower extremities *to prevent thrombus and embolus.*
- Administer anticoagulation therapy as ordered:
    Monitor serum coagulation studies.
    Check stool *to detect occult bleeding.*

- Check urine *to detect occult bleeding.*
- Monitor for signs of thrombophlebitis and deep vein thrombosis including redness, tenderness, localized swelling, warmth, and upward red streaking on an extremity.
- Monitor nutritional status.
- Encourage mobility to tolerance or as ordered.
- Encourage self-care activities to tolerance.
- Plan all activities to avoid fatigue.
- Maintain planned rest periods.
- Obtain physical therapy referral.

Patient Education/Home Care Planning

1. Stress need to continue with physical and occupational therapy as ordered.
2. Discuss methods of avoiding injury (e.g., burns) to lower trunk and legs.
3. Discuss methods and routine for inspecting lower portion of the body and feet for infection and breaks in the skin.
4. Discuss care of surgical incision (with thoracic approach chordotomy).
5. Emphasize importance of ongoing outpatient care by physician.

Evaluation

Patient demonstrates an effective breathing pattern Airway is patent. Chest excursion is symmetric. Breath sounds are normal or there is no increase in adventitious sounds. Arterial blood gas values are within normal ranges or consistent with patient's baseline. Vital signs are within normal ranges or consistent with patient's baseline. Hemoglobin levels are 14 to 18 g/dl (male) or 12 to 16 g/dl (female). Intake and output are stable. There are no signs of respiratory distress. All lobes are resonant on percussion. Skin color is not cyanotic.

Patient demonstrates adequate cerebral tissue perfusion Level of consciousness is unchanged. There is no evidence of further neurologic deficits. Pattern of electrolytes is stable. There is no seizure activity. Vital signs are stable.

Patient demonstrates minimum complications of sensory/perceptual alterations Level of orientation is optimum. The patient remains free of injury. Skin integrity is maintained. Nutritional status is adequate. Self-care deficits are minimum. Social participation is appropriate to physiologic status.

Patient demonstrates an optimum level of mobility Skin integrity is maintained. Patient remains free of contractures and deformities. Level of mobility is appropriate to physiologic status. Intake and output pattern is stable. Nutritional status is adequate. Patient remains free of thrombophlebitis. Patient remains free of local infection. Patient participates in an ongoing physical therapy program.

Patient demonstrates skin integrity Skin is intact. Nutritional status is adequate. Electrolyte balance is maintained. Patient remains free of pressure sores and contractures.

Patient experiences minimum alterations in comfort
Patient openly verbalizes feelings of discomfort when they occur. Patient uses measures to decrease discomfort. Patient verbally validates a decrease in subjective feelings of discomfort. There is a decrease in objective findings of pain.

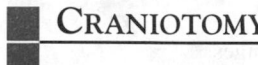

CRANIOTOMY

Description and Rationale

A craniotomy is a surgical procedure in which an opening is made into the cranium for removal of a tumor, control of bleeding, or relief of intracranial pressure. A flap is created by leaving the bone attached to the muscle so that the tissue can be turned down.[17] Next the dura is incised in the opposite direction so its base is near the midline. After the surgery's purpose is accomplished, closure is done in layers (i.e., dura, muscles, fascial, galea, and scalp).[5] Craniotomies can be classified into two major categories: supratentorial and subtentorial.

Supratentorial craniotomy refers to a surgical procedure performed on the brain structures located above the tentorium for removal of space-occupying lesions in the frontal, temporal, parietal, and occipital lobes. The incision usually is made behind the hairline. *Subtentorial* craniotomy is performed to relieve the discomfort of trigeminal neuralgia and for tumor removal from the cerebellum or cerebellar-pontine angle.[32] The incision usually is made slightly above the nape of the neck.

Complications following a craniotomy can include any or all of the following: increased intracranial pressure, seizures, meningitis, respiratory distress, cardiac arrhythmias, wound infection, diabetes insipidus, thrombophlebitis, visual disturbances, personality changes, bowel or bladder dysfunction, periocular edema, motor and sensory disturbances, headache, and postoperative hydrocephalus.

If part of the cranium is removed without replacement (i.e., to provide decompression from cerebral edema), the procedure is termed a *craniectomy*. *Cranioplasty* is the surgical repair of a cranial defect to reestablish the integrity and normal contour of the skull. The area of cranial defect is repaired through the use of substitute bone materials (i.e., tantalum, vitallium, or plastic).

•••••• Multidisciplinary Plan

Surgery

Intracranial pressure monitoring

Medications

Corticosteroids
　　Dexamethasone (Decadron), 20-40 mg/d po (dosage gradually tapered)
Anticonvulsants
　　Phenytoin (Dilantin), 100 mg po tid
Stool softener
　　Docusate sodium (Colace), 100 mg po bid or tid

Histamine-blocking agents
　　Cimetidine (Tagamet), 300 mg po qid
Antacids
　　Magnesium hydroxide (Maalox), 30 ml po or NG qid
Anti-infective agents
　　Organism specific

General Management

Mechanical ventilation, if indicated
Cardiac monitoring
Nutritional consultation
Physical therapy

NURSING CARE

Nursing Assessment

Focal Neurologic Disturbance

Gradually increasing weakness
Subtle sensory loss
Adult-onset seizures not always relieved by medications

Mentation

Personality changes
Insidious decrease in mentation
Depression
Memory deficits
Judgment deficits

Pain

Headaches with steady, persistent, or intractable dull pain
Changes in character of headaches
Stress-induced headaches

Increased Intracranial Pressure

Restlessness, lethargy
Changes in level of consciousness
Changes in vital signs (i.e., Cushing response with increased systolic blood pressure, wide pulse pressure, and decreased pulse rate)
Pupillary changes (i.e., mydriasis)
Impaired pupillary reflex
Papilledema (late sign)
Vomiting
Fluctuations in temperature
Seizures
Worsening of focal neurologic signs
Changes in respiratory patterns
Impaired swallow/gag reflex

Seizure Activity

Preconvulsive (preictal) stage
　　Aura: flash of light; sense of loss; fear; weakness; dizziness; peculiar taste, smell, and sounds

Cry or scream

Fall to floor

Loss of consciousness

Tachypnea

Convulsive stage

Tonic: rigid body; fixed jaws; clenched fists; extended legs; cyanosis; holding breath

Clonic: urinary or fecal incontinence; jerking of facial muscles and extremities; biting tongue; frothing at mouth

Postconvulsive (postictal) stage

Altered level of consciousness

Headache

Nausea and/or vomiting

Malaise

Muscle soreness

Aspiration

  Breathing difficulty

  Choking

  Cyanosis

  Decreased breath sounds

  Tachycardia

  Tachypnea

  Pneumonia

Diabetes Insipidus

Marked polyuria

Marked polydipsia

Anorexia

Weight loss

Dehydration

Dry skin

Poor turgor

Headache

General weakness

Irritability

Apathy

Laboratory studies

  Urinary specific gravity of 1.001 to 1.005

  Electrolyte imbalance

  Increased plasma osmolality

Other

Periocular edema

Thrombophlebitis

Nursing Dx & Intervention

Ineffective airway clearance related to impaired cough reflex

- See general intervention strategies on p. 1614.

Ineffective breathing pattern related to high risk for increased intracranial pressure

- See general intervention strategies on p. 1616.

Altered cerebral tissue perfusion related to increased intracranial pressure

- Monitor

  Cranial nerve functioning

  Auditory functioning

  Nausea and vomiting

  Reflex status

  Pupillary size and reaction

  Behavior and personality changes

  Posturing spontaneously or stimuli response

- Intervene to monitor and prevent increased intracranial pressure:

  Administer medications, treatment, and IV lines as ordered.

- If steroids are being administered:

  Check stools *to detect occult blood.*

  Test urine for glucose and acetone *to detect glycosuria.*

  Administer phytonadione, MSD (AquaMEPHYTON) intramuscularly daily or every other day *to control tendency to bleeding.*

  Administer antacids per protocol *to decrease or prevent gastric irritation.*

- Maintain elevation of head of bed as ordered *to facilitate venous return.*

- Accurately record intake and output; monitor for imbalance.

- Monitor serum and urine osmolarity *to detect onset of diabetes insipidus.*

- Monitor urine specific gravity.

- Administer replacement fluids per protocol.

- Monitor serum electrolytes, blood count, and arterial blood gases for abnormalities.

- Monitor values and waveforms of intracranial pressure line if appropriate:

  Maintain patency and sterility of system.

  Monitor effects of temperature on intracranial pressures.

  Correlate neurologic status with intracranial pressure values; notify physician if inconsistent.

  Assist with drainage of cerebrospinal fluid from the system.

- Intervene to monitor and prevent seizures:

  Obtain patient's seizure history.

  Institute seizure precautions:

    Padded tongue blade and airway at bedside

    Bed height at lowest level

    Side rails up at all times and padded *to prevent injury*

    Oxygen and suction equipment at bedside *to prevent hypoxia and aspiration*

    Emergency medications at bedside

  Administer anticonvulsants as ordered:

    Monitor effects and side effects.

    Monitor serum for therapeutic levels of the anticonvulsant.

Impaired skin integrity related to impaired physical mobility

- Maintain head elevation at 30 to 45 degrees if supratentorial approach used *to promote cerebral venous return.*
- Keep head of bed flat with infratentorial approach *to prevent pressure on brainstem;* avoid neck flexion *to prevent stress on suture line.*
- Check head dressing every hour and as needed. Report any new or increased drainage. Measure and mark all drainage.
- Change head dressing as needed *to prevent infection.*
- Maintain patency of ventricular drainage system if used.
- Provide wound care every shift and as needed when head dressing is removed.
- Monitor laboratory results for elevated white blood cell count.

Sensory/perceptual alterations related to altered neurologic status

- Keep side rails up at all times when patient is alone.
- Maintain patient safety at all times.
- Maintain quiet environment, reducing external stimuli to a minimum.
- Reorient patient frequently to time, place, and person.
- Introduce yourself each time you reorient the patient.
- Repeat explanations frequently and simply.
- Set realistic goals.
- Assist patient in judgments, perceptions, and reorientation as needed.
- Have family bring in familiar objects.
- Maintain planned rest periods, allowing sufficient time for REM sleep.
- Use day and night lighting appropriately.
- Stimulate senses of touch, taste, and position.
- Support family members to understand what is happening as a result of perceptual alterations.

Risk for trauma related to seizures

- Maintain bed in low position at all times unless side rails are up or when nurse is with patient.
- Provide patient with a call light within easy reach.
- Use restraints judiciously.
- Maintain side rails in up position at bedtime, after sedation, when patient is confused, and as needed.
- Maintain wheelchairs and stretchers in locked position when transferring patient.
- Pad side rails if patient is overactive.

Preconvulsive
- Maintain seizure precautions:
    Have oral airway at bedside *to provide for adequate oxygenation.*
    Have suction equipment available at bedside *to prevent aspiration.*
    Pad side rails if indicated.

Administer oxygen per protocol *to prevent cerebral hypoxia.*
Establish means of communication; identify auras if possible.

Convulsive
- Maintain patent airway.
- Support and protect head; turn to side if possible.
- Prevent injury:
    Ease patient to floor if in chair.
    Place pillows along side rails if patient is in bed.
    Remove surrounding furniture.
    Loosen constrictive clothing.
- Provide privacy as necessary *to protect patient's dignity.*
- Note frequency, time, involved body parts, and length of seizure.

Postconvulsive
- Maintain patent airway.
- Suction as needed *to prevent aspiration.*
- Check vital signs and neurologic status. Administer oxygen as ordered *to prevent hypoxia.*
- Reorient patient to environment *to minimize sensory-perceptual alteration.*
- Place patient in position of comfort; turn head to side.
- Administer oral hygiene as necessary *for secretions and bleeding.*

Impaired physical mobility related to postoperative recovery

- See general intervention strategies listed on p. 1597.

Self-care deficit related to neurologic change

- Assist with feeding as indicated; use IV or nasogastric feedings as ordered.
- Administer oral hygiene every 2 hours and as needed.
- Assist with daily hygiene care as indicated *to promote self-esteem.*
- Administer eye care every 2 to 4 hours if indicated.
- Perform intermittent urinary catheterization as ordered.

Pain related to craniotomy incision

- Promote rest and relaxation.
- Modify anxiety associated with the pain experience.
- Provide other sensory input.
- Remain with patient.
- Improve effectiveness of pain relief measures by using them before the pain becomes intense.
- For patients receiving radiation or chemotherapy:
    Explain procedure or medication before implementing.
    Administer antiemetics and antidiarrheal medications as needed.
    Provide frequent skin care.
    Provide frequent mouth care *to promote comfort.*
    Monitor patient's laboratory values for depressed red blood cells, white blood cells, or platelets. Report to physician.

Maintain planned rest periods.

Offer frequent, small feedings *to combat anorexia and discomfort of nausea.*

Body image, personal identity, and self-esteem disturbances related to neurologic changes/deficits

- See general intervention strategies listed on pp. 1665, 1680, and 1688.

Adaptive capacity, decreased

Intracranial

- Perform neurologic assessment q 2 H and PRN *to detect signs of increased ICP.*
- Monitor vital signs q 1 H and PRN *to detect changes in blood pressure with widening pulse pressure and bradycardia.*
- Assess for changing levels of consciousness.
- Assess for pupillary changes.
- Assess patient's motor and sensory functions *to detect potential changes in ICP.*
- Assess for headache, vomiting, and seizure activity.
- Monitor cardiac status.
- Measure and record ICP per protocol.
- Maintain neutral body alignment with head of bed elevated at 30 degrees, unless contraindicated *to facilitate cerebral venous drainage.*
- Avoid procedures that result in increased thoracic and abdominal pressure such as hip flexion, coughing, isometric exercises, and Valsalva maneuver.
- Log roll patient *to minimize increases in BP and ICP.*
- Minimize patient activity.
- Administer supplemental oxygen *to prevent hypoxia and hypercapnia.*
- Hyperoxygenate with 100% oxygen before suctioning and limit ETS to <15 seconds *to minimize cerebral ischemia.*
- Monitor ABGs and regulate mechanical ventilation to maintain $PaCO_2$ 25 to 30 mm Hg *to reduce cerebral vasodilation.*
- Administer diuretics, hyperosmotics, and corticosteroids as directed.
- Limit fluid intake *to maintain slight state of dehydration.*
- Maintain normothermia *to minimize cerebral metabolic demands.*

Confusion, chronic related to organic or cognitive impairment

- Assess baseline physical, functional, and psychosocial status.
- Evaluate previous interests.
- Ensure optimal sensory input (i.e., eyeglasses, hearing aid) is available.
- Evaluate stimulation threshold *to prevent overstimulation.*
- Provide for structured repetitive group activities.
- Provide rest periods between activities *to minimize fatigue.*

- Monitor for changes in physical, functional, and psychologic status.
- Maintain calm, reassuring demeanor when interacting with patient *to promote sense of trust.*
- Encourage patient to participate in care as tolerated *to minimize feelings of powerlessness.*
- Provide positive feedback for tasks/activities that are mastered.

Aspiration, risk for related to enteric feeding via nasoenteric tube

- Confirm feeding tube placement after insertion, q 4 H and PRN.

Confirm tube placement before and after each intermittent tube feeding.

Confirm initial enteral tube placement by physician examination of CXR.

- Tape nasogastic tube securely per protocol.
- Aspirate stomach contents *to determine gastric pH.*
- Assess bowel sounds q 4 H and PRN.
- Assess patient for abdominal distention, nausea/vomiting, and diarrhea/constipation.

Hold tube feedings if bowel sounds are absent and if diarrhea/constipation or nausea/vomiting are present.

- Maintain proper patient positioning.

Elevate head-of-bed 30 to 40 degrees.

Turn patient to right side *to facilitate stomach drainage through pylorus.*

- Discontinue continuous feedings 30 to 40 minutes before activity/procedure that require lowering the patient's head.
- Check vital signs q 2 H and PRN.
- Check pulmonary-tracheal secretions q 4 H and PRN *to detect presence of enteral feeding.*
- Monitor for signs of aspiration including cough, wheezing, dyspnea, hyperthermia, and tachycardia.
- Auscultate breath sounds q 4 H and PRN.

Patient Education/Home Care Planning

1. Involve family in care, as possible; teach essential aspects of care.
2. Reinforce physician's explanation of medical management.
3. Emphasize the importance of ongoing outpatient care and follow-up visits.
4. Encourage independent activities, as possible:
   a. Alert the patient to limitations.
   b. Avoid overprotection.
   c. Stress need for supportive devices as indicated.
5. Explain the need for regular exercise program and need for ROM exercises to family.
6. Discuss the importance of diet as ordered:
   a. Offer supplemental feedings.
   b. Offer small portions; instruct the patient to chew slowly.

7. Discuss the importance of safety measures: side rails, ramps, shower chairs, removal of scatter rugs, walker, and canes.
8. Explain name of medication, dosage, time of administration, and toxic or side effects.
9. Explain need to avoid over-the-counter medications without first consulting physician.
10. Encourage socialization with friends and family.
11. Explain the importance of verbalization of feelings about anxiety, fear, and body image changes.
12. Instruct the patient and family about seizures (i.e., safety measures and whom to contact).

Evaluation

Patient's airway is patent Breath sounds are normal. Chest excursion is bilateral and symmetric. Rate and depth of respirations are normal. Cough is effective. There are no subjective or objective findings of shortness of breath, air hunger, or dyspnea on exertion.

Patient's breathing pattern is effective Airway remains patent. Chest excursion is symmetric. Breath sounds are normal, or there is no increase in adventitious sounds. Arterial blood gas values are within normal ranges or consistent with patient's baseline. Vital signs are within normal ranges or consistent with patient's baseline. Hemoglobin levels are 14 to 18 g/dl (male) or 12 to 16 g/dl (female). Intake and output are stable. There are no signs of respiratory distress. All lobes are resonant on percussion. Skin color is not cyanotic.

Cerebral tissue perfusion is adequate Level of consciousness is unchanged. There is no evidence of neurologic deficits. Pattern of electrolytes is stable. There is no seizure activity.

Patient experiences minimum complications of sensory/perceptual alterations Patient maintains an optimum level of orientation. Patient remains free of injury. Skin integrity is maintained. Nutritional status is adequate. Self-care deficits are minimal. Social participation is appropriate to physiologic status.

Patient remains free of traumatic injury Safety measures are appropriate to level of physiologic status. Skin integrity is maintained. Skin is free of bruises, burns, abrasions, and redness. Environment is safe. Patient is free of nosocomial infections.

Patient's level of mobility is optimum Skin integrity is maintained. Patient remains free of contractures and deformities. Level of mobility is appropriate to physiologic status. Intake and output pattern is stable. Nutritional status is adequate. Patient remains free of thrombophlebitis. Patient remains free of local infection. Patient participates in an ongoing physical therapy program.

Self-care deficits are minimized Criteria listed for impaired physical mobility are met. Level of self-care activities is appropriate to physiologic status. Patient participates in physical and occupational therapy.

Alterations in comfort are minimized Patient openly verbalizes feelings of discomfort when they occur. Patient can use measures to decrease discomfort. Patient verbally validates a decrease in subjective feelings of discomfort. There is a decrease in objective findings of pain.

Patient maintains intact self-concepts Patient openly verbalizes feelings of grief and loss. Patient verbalizes positive feelings about self. Patient acknowledges actual change in self-image. Patient focuses on present and future appearance and function. Patient verbalizes feelings of hopefulness, helpfulness, and powerfulness.

Patient demonstrates maximal intracranial adaptive capacity Vital signs are stable. No signs of increased intracranial pressure are present. Patient is normothermic. Arterial blood gas values are within normal limits or consistent with patient's baseline. Intake and output are stable. Skin color is not cyanotic.

Patient remains free of aspiration Airway is patent. Vital signs are stable. Patient reports/demonstrates no signs of choking. Breath sounds are normal. Nasoenteric tube placement is verified.

Patient demonstrates minimal confusion Available sensory aids (i.e., eyeglasses, hearing aid) are used appropriately. Patient is able to participate in structured repetitive group activities. Rest periods between activities are maintained. Patient is able to participate in care to tolerance.

INTRACRANIAL PRESSURE MONITORING

Description and Rationale

Intracranial pressure (ICP) monitoring devices now make it possible to reliably measure the parameters of intracranial dynamics such as volume-pressure relationships, pressure waves, and cerebral perfusion pressures. Indications for intracranial pressure monitoring include any of the following: head trauma; cerebral hemorrhage; massive brain lesions; encephalitis; congenital hydrocephalus; hydrocephalus resulting in an alteration of cerebrospinal fluid production or absorption; and symptoms of increased intracranial pressure such as change in level of consciousness, headache, vomiting, or deterioration in respiratory status and motor function.[31] Intracranial pressure can be measured continuously via three basic monitoring systems: the ventricular catheter, the subarachnoid bolt, and the epidural sensor (Figure 3-41).

The *ventricular* catheter consists of a cannula that is implanted, via burr holes, into the anterior horn of the lateral ventricle of the nondominant cerebral hemisphere. The catheter then is connected by pressure-resistant, fluid-filled tubing to a transducer and recording instrument.[17] (NOTE: Continuous flushing devices are not used for intracranial pressure measurement.) The transducer is positioned so the dome is at the level of the foramen of Monro. The external anatomic landmarks for this position are the tragus of the ear or the edge of the brow.

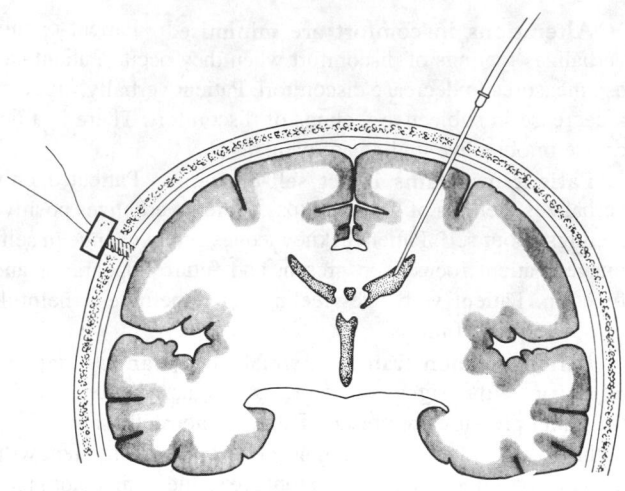

Figure 3-41 Subarachnoid screw monitoring *(left)* and intraventricular *(right)* devices for measuring intracranial pressure. Both require attachment to transducer using a stopcock or pressure tubing. (From Budassi and Barbar.[9])

An error of approximately 2 torr exists for each inch of discrepancy between the level of the transducer and the pressure source.

Advantages of the ventricular catheter include accurate measurement of intracranial pressure; instillation of a contrast medium; evaluation of pressure/volume responses; and ability to drain large amounts of cerebrospinal fluid, if needed.

Disadvantages of the ventricular catheter are that catheter placement may be difficult if the lateral ventricle is displaced, swollen, or collapsed; the catheter is the most invasive type of monitoring and can provide another route for infection; excessive cerebrospinal fluid drainage can occur if stopcock is not positioned properly; brain tissue or blood may occlude the catheter; false pressure readings may occur if the ventricle collapses and compresses the catheter; and frequent recalibration of the transducer and monitor is necessary for accurate readings.

The *subarachnoid bolt* method of intracranial pressure measurement began in the early 1970s. The device consists of a metal screw with a sensor tip that is inserted through a twist drill hole into the subdural or subarachnoid space. Although the cerebrum is not penetrated, the intracranial pressure is measured directly from the cerebrospinal fluid. The bolt is connected to a transducer and recording device via pressure-resistant, fluid-filled tubing. Here, as with the intraventricular catheter, continuous flushing devices are contraindicated. Indications for use of the subarachnoid bolt are to provide a means to measure and monitor intracranial pressure and to provide access for sampling of the cerebrospinal fluid.

Advantages of the bolt are that intracranial pressure is measured directly and accurately from cerebrospinal fluid; it provides access for cerebrospinal fluid sampling and drainage; it provides access for volume-pressure responses; and it can be placed quickly without penetrating the cerebrum.

 EMERGENCY ALERT

INCREASED INTRACRANIAL PRESSURE

Increased intracranial pressure (ICP) reflects three volumes in the cranial vault: brain, cerebrospinal fluid, and blood. Normal ICP is 10 to 15 mm Hg. ICP is controlled by autoregulatory mechanisms that may fail after injury. This failure leads to cerebral vasodilatation, increased blood volume, and cerebral engorgement as well as edema.

Assessment

- Cerebral ischemia, evidence of hypoxia
- Headache, nausea, vomiting
- Amnesia, altered level of consciousness
- Altered speech, drowsiness, agitation
- Dilated, nonreactive pupil
- Unresponsive to verbal, painful stimuli
- Abnormal posturing
- Increased blood pressure and decreased pulse
- Altered respiratory pattern
- Herniation of the brain may occur

Interventions

- Maintain airway, breathing, circulation.
- Administer high-flow oxygen by mask (10-15 L).
- Obtain IV assess.
- Position patient's head to decrease ICP (usually low Fowler's); local guidelines may vary.
- Hyperventilate patient to maintain $Paco_2$ (26 to 30 mm Hg); local guidelines may vary.
- Administer mannitol, anticonvulsant, antipyretic as ordered.
- Do not occlude CSF leak from nose, ears, etc.
- Obtain CT scan, MRI.
- If patient has been injured and if there is drainage from nose or ears, test drainage with dextrose stick to determine whether fluid is cerebral spinal fluid.

Disadvantages of the bolt are that it may become occluded with tissue or blood; the infection rate is comparable to that of the ventricular catheter; it requires a closed skull; and frequent recalibration of the transducer and monitor is necessary for accurate readings.

The *epidural sensor* consists of placement of a fiber-optic sensor, radio transmitter, or tiny balloon with radioisotopes in the epidural space through a burr hole in the skull. The sensor cable then plugs directly into the monitor.

Advantages of the sensor are that it is less invasive; it can be easily placed; and it cannot become occluded.

The major disadvantage of the sensor is its questionable reliability. Other disadvantages are that the system cannot be recalibrated if the sensor is affected by pressure or heat; cerebrospinal fluid sampling and drainage are not possible; and volume/pressure responses cannot be evaluated.

The fiberoptic transducer-tipped catheter is a relatively new device for monitoring ICP. This catheter can be placed intraventricularly, intraparenchymally, in the subarachnoid space, or in the subdural space. Advantages of the fiberoptic

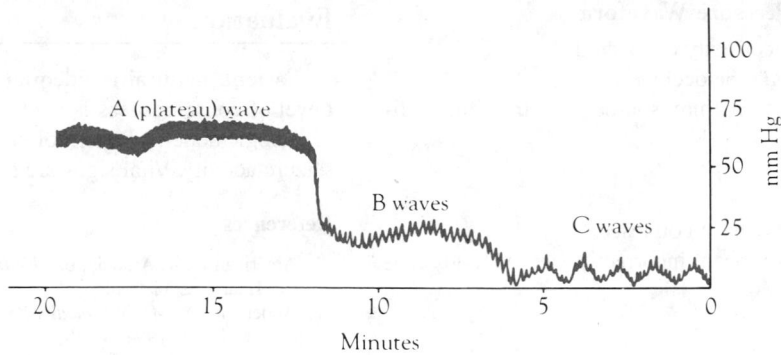

Figure 3-42 Intracranial pressure waves. Composite drawing of A (plateau) waves, B waves, and C waves. (From Holloway.[35])

transducer-tipped catheter are that it may be placed in three different areas of the cerebrum, is capable of monitoring intraparenchymal pressure, provides for CSF drainage with a ventricular system, and requires no adjustment of the transducer with head movement. Disadvantages of the fiberoptic catheter are that it is relatively fragile, cannot be recalibrated or reset to zero after placement, and requires a separate monitoring system.

Pressure waves Intracranial pressure's dynamic state is reflected by the pressure waves produced. These waveforms are most commonly known as A-waves, B-waves, and C-waves (Figure 3-42).

A-waves (or plateau waves), which occur at variable intervals, are spontaneous, rapid increases in pressure between 50 to 200 torr. Plateau waves usually occur in patients with moderate intracranial pressure elevations and last 5 to 20 minutes, falling spontaneously. Factors that can trigger plateau waves include REM sleep, emotional stimuli, isometric muscle contractions, the rebound phase of the Valsalva maneuver, hypercapnia, hypoxemia, sustained coughing and sneezing, arousal from sleep, and certain positions such as neck flexion or extreme hip flexion. A-waves are known to cause cerebral ischemia and brain damage and can produce paroxysmal or transient symptoms of change in level of consciousness, headache, nausea and vomiting, altered motor function, abnormal pupillary reactions, changes in vital signs (i.e., increased blood pressure, widened pulse pressure, and decreased pulse rate), and respiratory patterns (i.e., ataxic breathing and central neurogenic hyperventilation).[17] Because of the ischemia and previously stated symptoms, A-waves are the most clinically significant intracranial pressure waveforms and require immediate intervention to prevent further brain injury.

B-waves appear as sharp, rhythmic, sawtooth waves that occur every ½ to 2 minutes and have pressures up to 50 torr. B-waves correlate to changes in respiration, such as Cheyne-Stokes respirations. B-waves can also occur in patients with normal intracranial pressure.

C-waves are small, rapid, rhythmic waves that occur at a rate of approximately 4 to 8 per minute and increase pressures up to 20 torr. C-waves are also called Traube-Herring-Mayer

waves. These waveforms correspond to normal changes in the systemic arterial pressure and are not clinically significant.

•••••• Multidisciplinary Plan

Surgery

Intracranial pressure monitoring
Tumor excision
Shunting procedure

Medications

Corticosteroid agents
    Dexamethasone (Decadron), 20-40 mg/d po
Anticonvulsant agents
    Phenytoin (Dilantin), 100 mg po tid
Laxative agents
    Docusate sodium (Colace), 100 mg po bid or tid
Antiemetic agents
    Cimetidine (Tagamet), 300 mg po tid
Antacids
    Magnesium hydroxide (Maalox), 30 ml po qid
Anti-infective agents
    Organism specific

General Management

Radiation therapy
Mechanical ventilation, if indicated
Cardiac monitoring
Arterial blood pressure monitoring
Nutritional consultation
Physical therapy

NURSING CARE

Nursing Assessment

The reader is referred to the appropriate disorder for specific physical assessment findings.

Loss of Intracranial Pressure Waveform

Transducer may be incorrectly connected
Monitoring device could be occluded
Air may be between pressure source and transducer diaphragm

Low Intracranial Pressure

Cerebral ventricles may have collapsed
Transducer may have been incorrectly zeroed and calibrated

High Intracranial Pressure

Excessive activity
Body posture with neck or extreme hip flexion
Use of positive end-expiratory pressure (PEEP)
Hyperthermia
Respiratory distress
Fluid and electrolyte imbalances
Infection
Blood pressure changes

False High Intracranial Pressure

Transducer too low or incorrectly balanced
System incorrectly calibrated
Air in system

False Low Intracranial Pressure

Transducer too high
Air in system

Nursing Dx & Intervention

Altered cerebral tissue perfusion related to altered cerebrovascular dynamics

- Maintain sterility of the intracranial pressure monitoring equipment:
   Maintain strict sterile technique *to prevent infection.*
   Change equipment (i.e., tubing) daily or as ordered.
- Maintain patency of intracranial pressure monitoring device:
   Keep all stopcock ports capped *to keep system closed to air.*
   Never flush the system.
   Observe for cerebrospinal fluid leaks and blood in the tubing.
- Obtain accurate pressure measurements:
   Place patient in baseline position.
   Obtain measurements when patient is at rest—not when moving, coughing, sneezing, etc.
   Level the transducer.
   Recalibrate the transducer according to the manufacturer's instructions.
   Obtain measurements and record.
   Report significant changes in intracranial pressure to physician immediately.

Evaluation

Patient maintains adequate cerebral tissue perfusion
Level of consciousness is unchanged. There is no evidence of neurologic deficits. Pattern of electrolytes is stable. There is no seizure activity. Vital signs are stable.

References

1. American Heart Association: *1990 Stroke facts,* Dallas, 1991, American Heart Association.
2. Anderson KN: *Mosby's medical, nursing, and allied health dictionary,* ed 4, St Louis, 1994, Mosby.
3. Anthony CP, Kolthoff NJ: *Textbook of anatomy and physiology,* ed 9, St Louis, 1975, Mosby.
4. Baker AB, editor: *Clinical neurology,* ed 2, New York, 1983, Harper & Row.
5. Barkauskus VH, Stoltenberg-Allen K, Baumann LC, Darling-Fischer C: *Health & physical assessment,* St Louis, 1994, Mosby.
6. Bates B: *A guide to physical assessment,* ed 3, Philadelphia, 1983, JB Lippincott.
7. Blass J: Alzheimer's disease, *Diabet Med* 31:4, 1985.
8. Braunwald E et al, editors: *Harrison's principles of internal medicine,* ed 11, New York, 1983, McGraw-Hill.
9. Budassi SA, Barbar JM: *Emergency nursing: principles and practice,* St Louis, 1981, Mosby.
10. Sheehy SB: *Emergency nursing: principles and practice,* ed 3, St Louis, 1992, Mosby.
11. Burns KR, Johnson PJ: *Health assessment in clinical practice,* Englewood Cliffs, NJ, 1980, Prentice-Hall.
12. Cahill M: *Diagnostics,* ed 2, Springhouse, Penn, 1986, Springhouse.
13. Caird FI, Judge TG: *Assessment of the elderly patient,* ed 3, California, 1977, Pitman Medical.
14. Carnevali DL, Patrick M: *Nursing management for the elderly,* Philadelphia, 1979, JB Lippincott.
15. Carotenuto R, Bullock J: *Physical assessment of the gerontologic client,* Philadelphia, 1980, FA Davis.
16. Chipps E, Clanin N, Campbell V: *Neurologic disorders,* St Louis, 1992, Mosby.
17. Conn HG, Conn RB Jr: *Current diagnosis,* Philadelphia, 1980, WB Saunders.
18. Crowell RM, Zervas NT: Management of intracranial aneurysm, *Med Clin North Am* 63:695, 1979.
19. Davis GT, Hill PM: Cerebral palsy, *Nurs Clin North Am* 15:35, 1980.
20. Davis JE, Mason CB: *Neurologic critical care,* New York, 1979, Van Nostrand Reinhold.
21. Demyer W: *Technique of the neurologic examination: a programmed text,* ed 3, New York, 1980, McGraw-Hill.
22. De Young S: *The neurologic patient: a nursing perspective,* Englewood Cliffs, NJ, 1983, Prentice-Hall.
23. Dietsche L, Pollman J: Alzheimer's disease: advances in clinical nursing, *J Gerontol Nurs* 8:2, 1982.
24. Eliasson SG et al, editors: *Neurological pathophysiology,* ed 2, New York, 1978, Oxford University Press.
25. Escourolle R, Poirier J: *Manual of basic neuropathology,* ed 2, Philadelphia, 1978, WB Saunders.
26. Geffner ES, editor: *Compendium of drug therapy,* New York, 1983, Biomedical Information.
27. Go KG et al: Interpretation of nuclear magnetic resonance tomograms of the brain, *J Neurosurg* 59:574, 1983.
28. Groer MW, Shekleton ME: *Basic pathophysiology: a holistic approach,* ed 3, St Louis, 1989, Mosby.
29. Grundy JH: *Assessment of the child in primary health care,* New York, 1981, McGraw-Hill.
30. Guyton A: *Textbook of medica physiology,* ed 5, Philadelphia, 1976, WB Saunders.
31. Ham RJ, Sloane PD: *Primary care geriatrics: a case-based approach,* ed 2, St Louis, 1992, Mosby.
32. Hazinski MF: *Nursing care of the critically ill child,* ed 2, St Louis, 1992, Mosby.

33. Hickey J: *The clinical practice of neurological and neurosurgical nursing,* Philadelphia, 1981, JB Lippincott.

34. Hickey J: *The clinical practice of neurological and neurosurgical nursing,* ed 2, Philadelphia, 1995, JB Lippincott.

35. Holloway NM: *Nursing the critically ill adult,* Reading, Mass, 1979, Addison-Wesley.

36. Hudak CM et al: *Critical care nursing,* ed 3, Philadelphia, 1982, JB Lippincott.

37. Jensen D: *The principles of physiology,* ed 2, New York, 1982, Appleton-Century-Crofts.

38. Kaye D, Rose LF: *Internal medicine for dentistry,* ed 2, St Louis, 1990, Mosby.

39. Kim MJ, McFarland GK, McLane AM, editors: *Pocket guide of nursing diagnoses,* ed 6, St Louis, 1995, Mosby.

40. Kinney MR, editor: *AACN's clinical reference for critical-care nursing,* New York, 1981, McGraw-Hill.

41. Kintzel K, editor: *Advanced concepts in clinical nursing,* ed 2, Philadelphia, 1977, JB Lippincott.

42. Leech RW, Shuman RM: *Neuropathology: a summary for students,* New York, 1982, Harper & Row.

43. McCance KL, Huether SE: *Pathophysiology: the biologic basis for disease in adults and children,* ed 2, St Louis, 1994, Mosby.

44. McElroy DB: Hydrocephalus in children, *Nurs Clin North Am* 15:23, 1980.

45. Merrit HH: *A textbook of neurology,* ed 6, Philadelphia, 1979, Lea & Febiger.

46. Nikas DL, editor: *The critically ill neurosurgical patient: contemporary issues in critical care nursing,* vol 3, New York, 1982, Churchill Livingstone.

47. Passo S: Malformations of the neural tube, *Nurs Clin North Am* 15:%, 1980.

48. Petersdorf RG, editor: *Harrison's principles of internal medicine,* ed 10, New York, 1983, McGraw-Hill.

49. Phipps WJ, Sands J, Lehman MK, Cassmeyer V: *Medical-surgical nursing: concepts and clinical practice,* ed 5, St Louis, 1995, Mosby.

50. Pluckhan M: Alzheimer's disease: helping the patient's family, *Nursing 86,* Nov 1986.

51. Price SA, Wilson LM: *Pathophysiology: clinical concepts of disease processes,* ed 5, St Louis, 1997, Mosby.

52. Ramirez B: When you're faced with neuro patients, *RN* 42:67, 1979.

53. Robbins SL, Cotran RS: *Pathologic basis of disease,* ed 2, Philadelphia, 1977, WB Saunders.

54. Robinson J, editor: *Coping with neurologic problems proficiently, Nursing Skillbook Series,* Springhouse, Pa, 1982, Intermed Communications.

55. Rudy EB: *Advanced neurological and neurosurgical nursing,* St Louis, 1984, Mosby.

56. Selzer P: Understanding NMR imaging with the aid of a simple mechanical model, *Med Times* 114:1, 1986.

57. Schottelius BA, Schottellius DD: *Textbook of physiology,* ed 18, St Louis, 1978, Mosby.

58. Smith LH, Thier SO: *Pathophysiology: the biological principles of disease,* Philadelphia, 1981, WB Saunders.

59. Stub RL, Black FW: *The mental status examination in neurology,* Philadelphia, 1997, FA Davis.

60. Swaiman KF: *Pediatric neurology: principles and practice,* ed 2, St Louis, 1994, Mosby.

61. Taylor JW, Ballinger S: *Neurological dysfunctions and nursing interventions,* New York, 1980, McGraw-Hill.

62. Thelan LA, Davie JK, Urden LD, Lough ME: *Critical care nursing: diagnosis and management,* ed 2, St Louis, 1994, Mosby.

63. Thibodeau GA, Patton KT: *Anatomy and physiology,* ed 3, St Louis, 1995, Mosby.

64. Thibodeau GM: *Structure and function of the body,* ed 9, St Louis, 1995, Mosby.

65. Thompson JM, Wilson SF: *Health assessment for nursing practice,* St Louis, 1996, Mosby.

66. Tucker SM et al: *Patient care standards: collaborative practice planning guides,* ed 6, St Louis, 1996, Mosby.

67. Urosevich PR: *Coping with neurologic disorders, Nursing Photobook Series,* Springhouse, Pa, 1981, Intermed Communications.

68. Walleck C: Head trauma in children, *Nurs Clin North Am* 15:115, 1980.

69. Wong DL: *Whaley and Wong's nursing care of infants and children,* ed 5, St Louis, 1995, Mosby.

70. Williams L: Alzeheimer's: the need for caring, *J Gerontol Nurs* 12:2, 1986.

71. Wyngaarden JB, Smith LH, editors: *Cecil's textbook of medicine,* Philadelphia, 1985, WB Saunders.

Musculoskeletal System

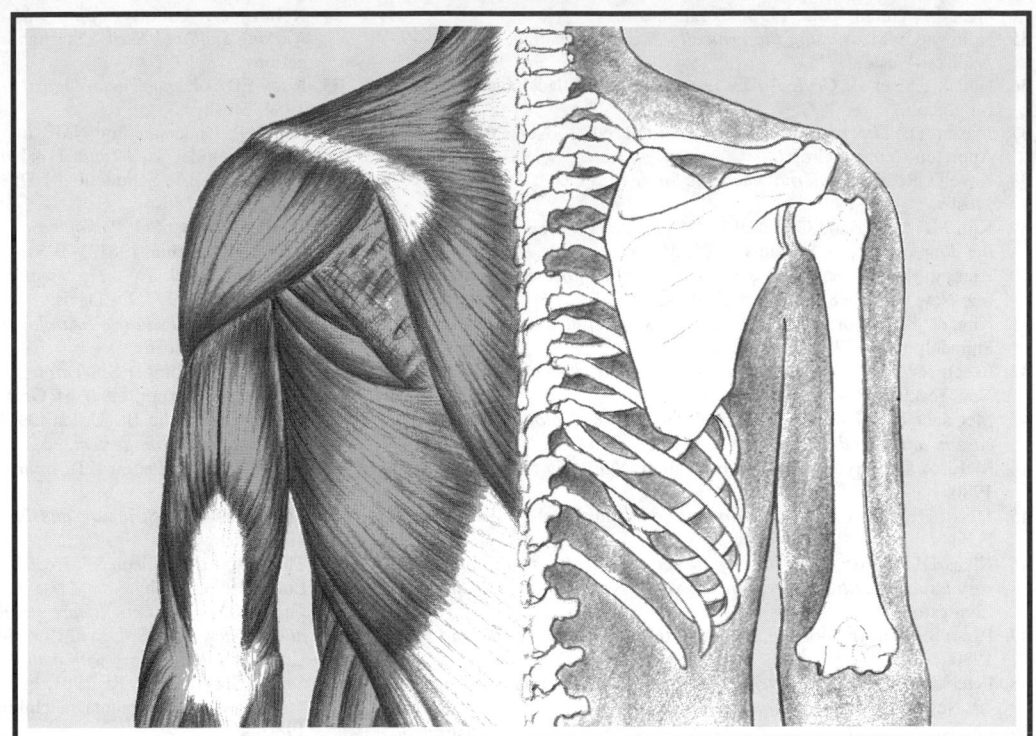

4

OVERVIEW

The tissues of the musculoskeletal system are the framework for the rest of the body and provide the means for easy, comfortable movement. Because of their many important structures and functions, they greatly affect the body's general health when they are inflamed, injured, or anomalous. Musculoskeletal anomalies and birth injuries affect newborns and lead to disability in growth, development, and productivity throughout life. Injuries from sports or physical fitness activities are major factors in the health of young to middle-aged adults. Trauma, primarily from automobile accidents, is the number-one cause of death among people aged 16 to 24 years. Inflammatory, rheumatic, and degenerative diseases of the musculoskeletal tissues are significant causes of death among young adults and account for a large portion of the illness and disability of middle-aged and elderly adults. Billions of dollars are spent yearly for care and treatment of people of all ages with musculoskeletal conditions. The economic cost is a major health care problem.

•••••• Anatomy, Physiology, and Related Pathophysiology

Skeleton

According to Wolff's law, which states that bones are shaped according to their function, the 206 bones of the skeleton are shaped according to their specific functions. Thus they may be long (arm or leg), short (wrist or ankle), flat (sternum or scapula), irregular (vertebrae), or rounded (patella). The skull, face and auditory ossicles, vertebrae, ribs, sternum, and hyoid bone make up the axial skeleton; the appendicular skeleton consists of the bones in the upper and lower extremities, shoulders, and pelvis (Figure 4-1).

Bones support the body, enabling it to stand erect; protect internal organs and other soft tissues; assist movement by leverage and in coordination with muscles; make blood cells within the red bone marrow; and provide for storage of minerals, particularly calcium and phosphorus.

Structure of bone tissue Long bones of the extremities and thorax consist of a long shaft, the diaphysis, and two ends, the epiphyses. The epiphyses are covered with cartilage and are separated from the shaft by the growth plate and nutrient arteries of the metaphysis (Figure 4-2). The outer surface (cortex) of a bone is hard, dense tissue called compact bone. The ends of long bones, the flat bones, and the ridges or crests of the ilium and tibia contain cancellous bone, which is soft and spongy and has cavities containing the red bone marrow for hematopoiesis. Red bone marrow depletions are replaced by fat cells of the yellow bone marrow, which is found in the shafts of long bones.

The periosteum is the tough outer membrane that covers each bone and provides protection and nutrition. Blood vessels in the inner layer of the periosteum bring nutrients and remove wastes. The periosteal blood vessels communicate with vessels in the central canal of the haversian system, which is the microscopic unit of compact bone.

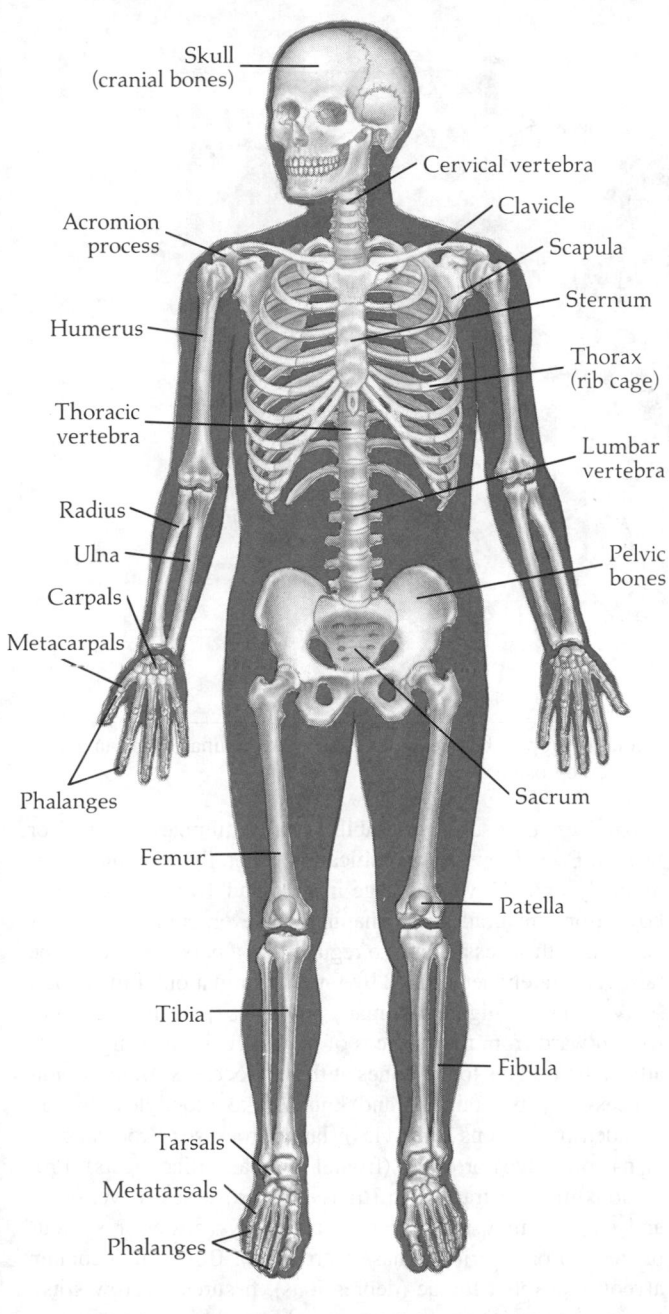

Figure 4-1 Bones that make up axial and appendicular skeletons (see text for content).

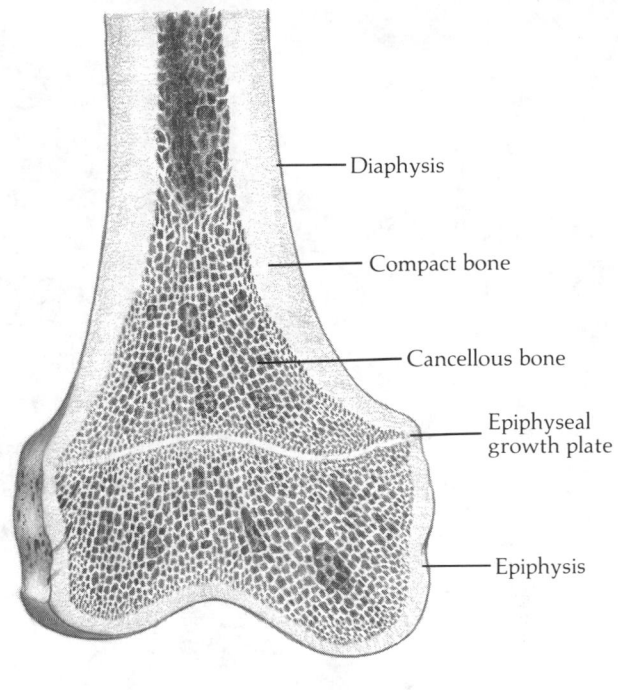

Figure 4-2 Bone showing relationships of compact and cancellous bone, epiphysis, epiphyseal plate, and diaphysis.

The haversian system contains layers or plates of compact bone cells called lamellae. These lamellae surround the haversian canal, which contains two blood vessels and a nerve. The lamellae are aligned parallel to the shaft of the bone and encompass the lacunae, which are small cavities filled with bone cells and tissue fluids. The lacunae are connected to the blood vessels in the haversian canal by smaller canals, the canaliculi (Figure 4-3). The haversian canal provides nutrients to osteocytes for bone building and removes wastes and debris from

bone growth and resorption. Osteocytes, the major bone-forming cells, develop from osteoblasts, which are spindle-shaped cells found beneath the periosteum and in the inner region of bones, the endosteum. Osteoblasts remain dormant until needed for bone growth, when they mature into osteocytes. A third type of cell, the osteoclast, also is needed for shaping and remodeling bone. It is used for resorption of unneeded or necrotic bone cells. The skeleton replaces itself every 3 months.[31]

Bones are in a constant process of resorption counterbalanced by new bone formation. This process prevents bones from becoming excessively thick or heavy from new bone formation or from becoming thinner or weakened from resorption. The formation and resorption process is related to calcium and phosphate levels and metabolism in the body.

Approximately 99% of the calcium in the body is contained in bones; the remaining 1% circulates in the blood plasma and interstitial fluid. Extracellular calcium and phosphate concentrations are regulated by secretions of parathyroid hormone from the parathyroid glands, by absorption in the intestinal tract, and by retention or excretion by the kidneys so that relatively stable concentrations are maintained. Low calcium levels stimulate parathyroid hormone production, which stimulates osteoclasts to break down bone structure. The breakdown of bone frees calcium phosphate crystals to be available to increase serum calcium concentrations. The gastrointestinal ion transport system absorbs calcium and moves the ion from the gut lumen to the blood. Resorption of calcium increases in the renal tubules to raise serum calcium levels, which concurrently

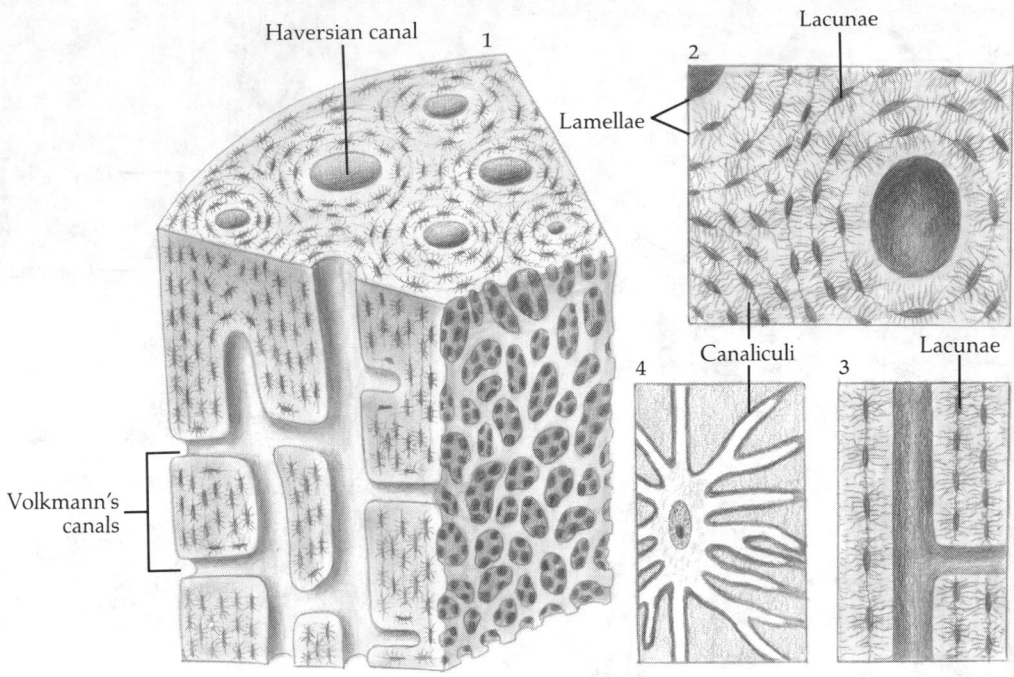

Figure 4-3 *1,*Three-dimensional view of compact bone; *2,* transverse section of compact bone depicting lamellae, lacunae, and canaliculi; *3,* longitudinal section of bone with lacunae and canaliculi; *4,* lacunae occupied by osteocyte.

reduces the resorption of phosphate. Through these processes, calcium levels remain relatively constant in healthy people, and bone remains strong with relatively stable calcium concentration through formation and resorption.

Bone strength, formation, and resorption are affected by the amount and metabolism of vitamin D, which facilitates the absorption of calcium and phosphorus from the intestine. A deficiency of either vitamin D or sunshine (needed to activate sterol precursors to vitamin D in the skin) will cause changes in bones, known as rickets in children and osteomalacia in adults.

The skeleton begins to develop from mesenchymal cells in the first prenatal month and is completely formed by the third month. Bones form through intramembranous and endochondral formation. In both processes, the first stage involves formation of cancellous or spongy bone tissue, which later becomes compact bone through deposition of bone matrix. The bone matrix then becomes calcified. The bones of the skull and other flat bones are formed through intramembranous pathways, and all long bones are formed from endochondral tissues within a preformed cartilage framework. After birth, secondary centers for ossification develop in the epiphyseal regions of the bones. The cartilage that remains in this region becomes the epiphyseal plate. The growth or proliferation of the cartilage cells in this region results in the increased length of bones as the body grows. When the bone has reached its final size, these growth zones are resorbed and replaced by bone. As the bone grows longer, its outer diameter increases slightly. The volume in the bone marrow cavity also increases. New bone is continuously deposited on the outer surfaces with resorption from the inner surfaces, until the final bone shape is achieved. The shape of each bone

maximizes its load-bearing ability and minimizes its mass or weight. Bone growth and ossification generally continue longitudinally until 15 years of age in girls and 16 years of age in boys. Bone maturation and shaping, however, continue until 21 years in both sexes and are so regular that a person's age can be fairly accurately determined by x-ray examination of the bones.

As shown in Figure 4-4, many processes (prominences) project outward from the surfaces of bones. Tendons or ligaments attach themselves to the bones at these processes. Bony prominences may be rounded and knucklelike (condyles); small, rounded projections (tubercles); large processes (trochanters); or narrow ridges or crests (frontal bone and iliac crests). Projections may be transverse (transverse processes of vertebrae and ear), or they may project posteriorly (posterior spinous processes) or anteriorly (nasal cartilages). Bones also contain alveoli (sockets), fossae (depressions), fissures (narrow slits), foramina (openings for nerves, muscles, and blood vessels), sinuses (cavities), and sulci (grooves).

Muscles

Structure of skeletal muscles   Skeletal muscles make up 40% to 45% of the body's weight (Figure 4-5). Through their contractions, they move the whole body or just parts of it. They cover the skeletal bones and help produce the contours of the body. Muscles are attached at each end to a bone, ligament, tendon, or fascia. One end of the muscle, the more fixed end, is referred to as the origin; the more movable end is the muscle insertion. Muscles of the skeletal system are voluntary muscles controlled by the will; in contrast, visceral muscles move involuntarily.

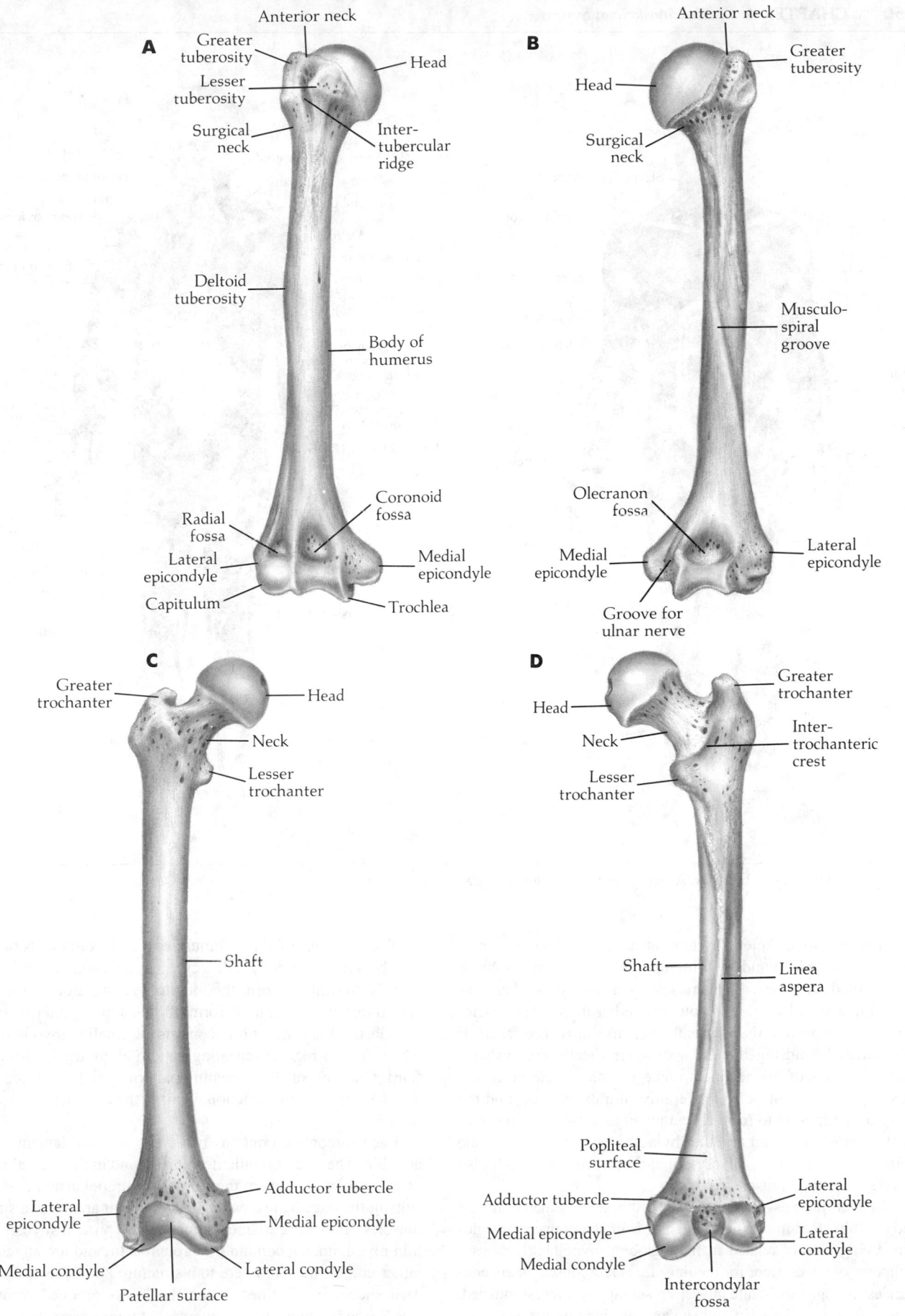

Figure 4-4 A, Anterior and **B,** posterior views of right humerus. **C,** Anterior and **D,** posterior views of right femur.

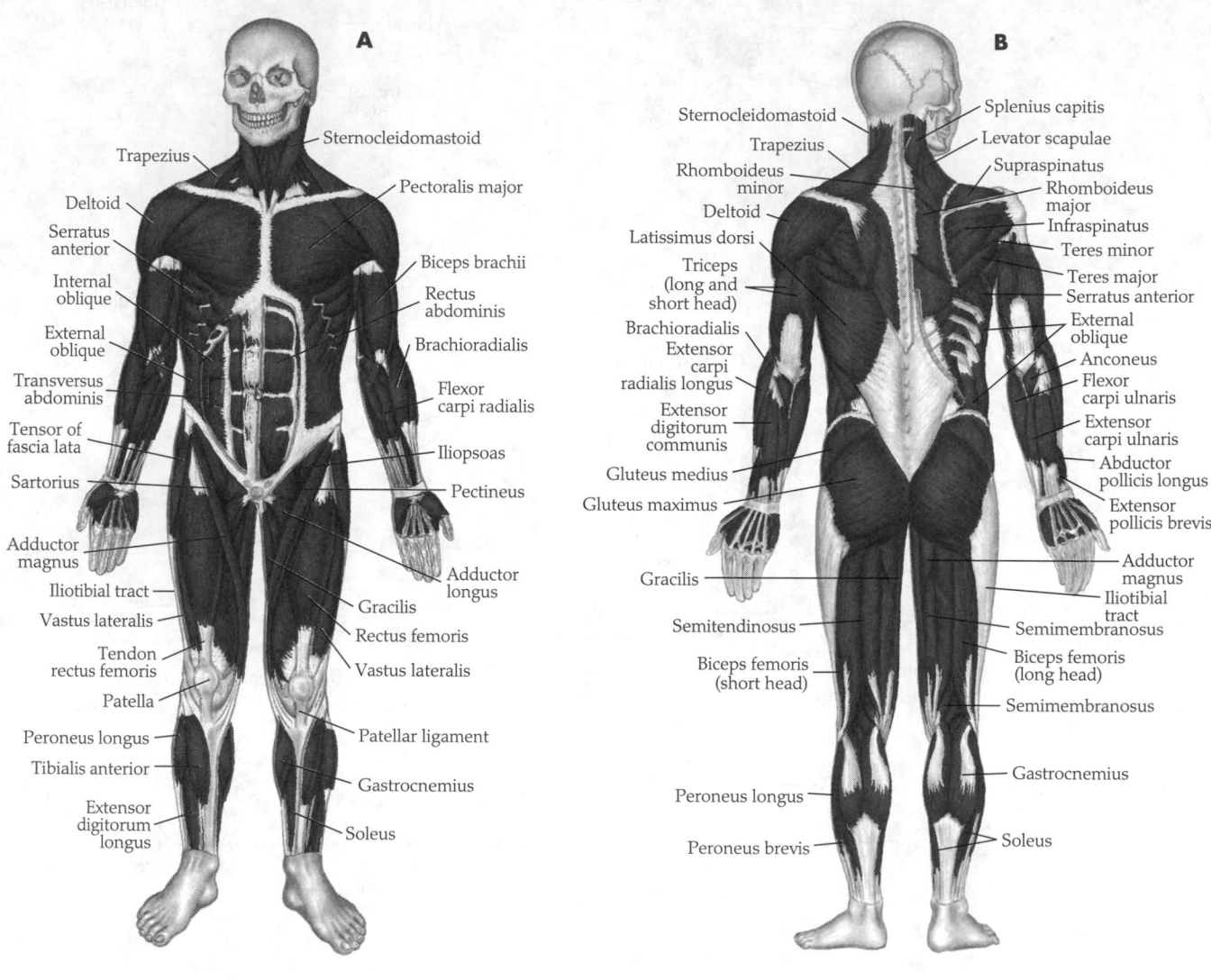

Figure 4-5 Muscles of body. **A,** Anterior view. **B,** Posterior view.

Muscles of the skeletal system (striated muscles) are generally long, slender bundles containing dark cross-markings or lines called striations. Each muscle is made up of fibers enclosed in a sarcolemma and bound together in bundles (fasciculi) by a connective tissue sheath (perimysium). The fasciculi are further bound together by a stronger sheath (epimysium). These bundles of bound fibers make up the muscle belly, the fleshy part of the muscle. The epimysium extends beyond the belly of the muscle to form a tendon (Figure 4-6). The muscles of the limbs are bound together by a layer of connective tissue called fascia, a tough, silvery-appearing covering, which also covers individual muscle groups.

Skeletal muscles vary in length, width, and diameter and are red or white. Red muscle gets its color from the pigment myoglobin. Being closely related to hemoglobin, myoglobin acts as a temporary oxygen store for the muscle. White muscle fibers contain less myoglobin. White muscles react rapidly when stimulated, whereas red muscles carry out slower, sustained movements.

The striations of skeletal muscles result from bands of muscle fibers made up of cylindric cytoplasmic elements called myofibrils. Myofibrils form the longitudinal striation of the muscle; transverse striations form the banding patterns in the myofibrils. Each myofibril consists of smaller myofilaments, which form a regular repeating pattern along the length of the fibril. One unit of this repeating pattern is called a sarcomere. The sarcomere is the functional unit of the contractile system in muscles.

Each sarcomere contains two types of myofilaments: thick and thin. The thick myofilaments are found in the central region of the sarcomere, where their orderly, parallel arrangement results in the dark bands, called A bands, that are seen in striated muscles. The thick filaments contain the protein myosin. The thin myofilaments contain the protein actin and are attached at either end of the sarcomere to a structure known as the Z line. Two successive Z lines define the limits of one sarcomere. The Z lines contain short elements that interconnect the thin fil-

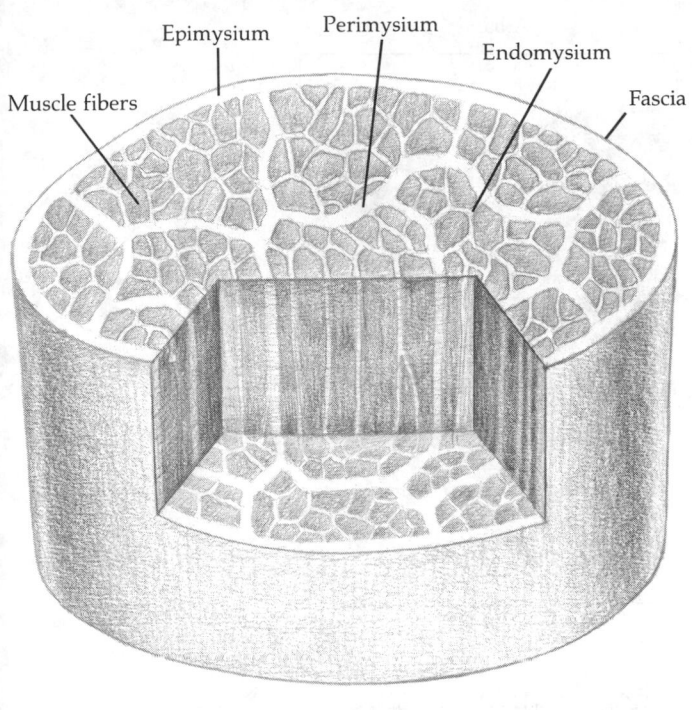

Epimysium Perimysium
Endomysium
Muscle fibers   Fascia

Figure 4-6 Structure of muscle fibers and their coverings.

aments from two adjoining sarcomeres to provide an anchoring point for the thin filaments. The thin elements extend from the Z lines toward the center of the sarcomere, where they overlap with the thick filaments (Figure 4-7).

Two other bands, the I band and the H zone, change during contraction in relation to the positions of the thick and thin filaments in the sarcomere. The I band is between the ends of the A bands in two adjoining sarcomeres. Because it contains only thin filaments, it usually appears as a light band separating the dark A bands. The H zone is a thin, lighter band in the center of the A band that corresponds to the space between the ends of the thin filaments. Only thick filaments are found in the H zone.

Muscle contraction Muscles move the body through tightening and shortening of their fibers (contraction) brought about through the motor unit. Each motor unit has 100 to 200 muscle fibers innervated by a single motor nerve axon that stimulates the motor unit and sends the contraction through the muscle body. The muscle responds either entirely or not at all to the stimulus. The strength of the muscle contraction is determined by the number of motor units contracting and by the number of times per second each motor unit is stimulated.

During contraction the thick and thin filaments slide past each other, but the lengths of the individual thick and thin filaments do not change. As the thin filaments move past the thick filaments, the width of the H zone between the ends of the thin filaments becomes smaller and shorter. These changes in the banding pattern during contraction led to the sliding-filament theory of muscle contraction, that is, that muscle shortening re-

sults from the relative movement of the thick and thin filaments past each other.

Sliding of the filaments is produced by the myosin cross-bridges, which swivel in an arc around their fixed positions on the surface of the thick filament. The cross-bridges undergo many repeated cycles of movement during a contraction. The myosin bridges detach themselves from actin, rebind to new actin sites, and repeat these cycles of movements, brought about by the binding of a molecule to adenosine triphosphate (ATP) to myosin. The process of binding ATP appears to break the linkage between actin and myosin. The reaction returns the bridge to its initial state so it can repeat the cycle of bridge movement.

Muscle contraction results from a series of interactions at the myoneural junction in the muscle tissue. The stimulus travels along the motor nerve to the motor end plate (myoneural junction) of the muscle fiber. Acetylcholine is produced at this synapse (junction) and released. It causes the muscle to contract by depolarizing the sarcolemma. Depolarization permits interstitial calcium ions to enter the muscle membrane to aid the contraction. The wave of depolarization travels through the muscle fiber until it is deactivated by the enzyme acetylcholinesterase (Figure 4-8). The fiber is then ready for reactivation. The positive calcium ions catalyze an energy-releasing reaction to cause the actin to slide along the myosin, which results in contraction and shortening of the muscle.

The energy for muscle contraction comes from the hydrolysis of ATP into ADP + phosphate + energy. Additional energy sources are phosphocreatine, a protein-energy source found only in muscle tissues, and oxygen, which aids contraction by oxidizing the lactic acid that results from the anaerobic hydrolysis of the high-energy ATP bonds.

Muscle spasm is an involuntary contraction of one muscle or a group of muscles caused by repetitive activation of entire motor units from the repetitive firing of a motor nerve. Tetanus is a sustained contraction caused by a repetitive series of stimuli conducted along the sarcolemmal membrane.

Muscles also have the ability to relax. A relaxing factor called relaxin acts by rendering ATP inactive until the next stimulus reaches a particular fiber, thereby keeping the muscle relaxed.

Muscle twitch A muscle twitch occurs when a minimal stimulus is attained. All muscle fibers associated with the stimulated nerve contract and then relax.

An isotonic twitch causes the muscle to change length when constant tension is applied throughout its contraction. An isometric twitch is one in which the muscle remains or retains a constant length even with a sudden increase in muscle tension.

Muscle tone Tone in muscles provides resistance to passive elongation or stretch and ensures a rapid reaction to an external stimulus. It results from a continuous flow of stimuli from the spinal cord to each motor unit. Muscle tone can be increased or decreased depending on the activity within the nervous system. Tone is increased in anxiety states and decreased during restful periods.

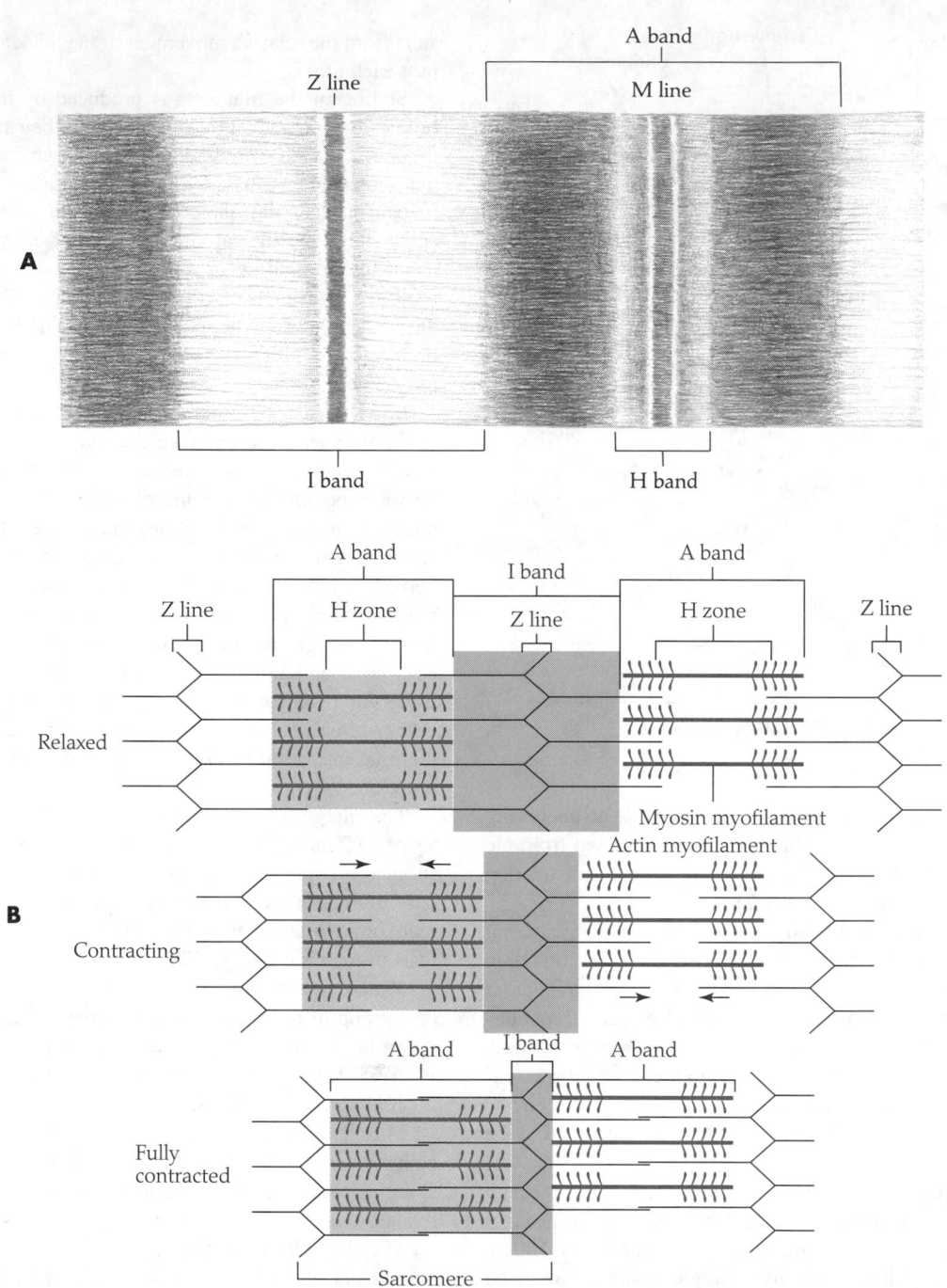

Figure 4-7 A, Lines and bands in striated muscle. **B,** Sarcomere shortening in response to cross bridge formation. During contraction, the I bands shorten, but the A bands do not. The H zone narrows or even disappears as the actin myofilaments meet at the center of the sarcomere. (**B** from Seely.[134])

Ligaments

Ligaments hold bones to bones. They may encircle a joint to add strength and stability, as they do around the hip joint (Figure 4-9), or they may hold obliquely or parallel to the ends of bones across the joint, as they do in and around the knee joint (Figure 4-10). Ligaments are relatively long bands. They are made up of tough bands of collagen fibers arranged in parallel bundles of fibers to add strength. Type I collagen produces these large, densely packed fibers (see p. 355 for discussion of collagen structure and types). Type I collagen gives ligaments great tensile strength with limited extensibility. When ligaments are taut, they provide the greatest stability to the specific joint. Ligaments allow movement in some directions while restricting movement in other directions. Ligaments differ from tendons by their lower percentage of collagen and higher percentage of ground substance.[169]

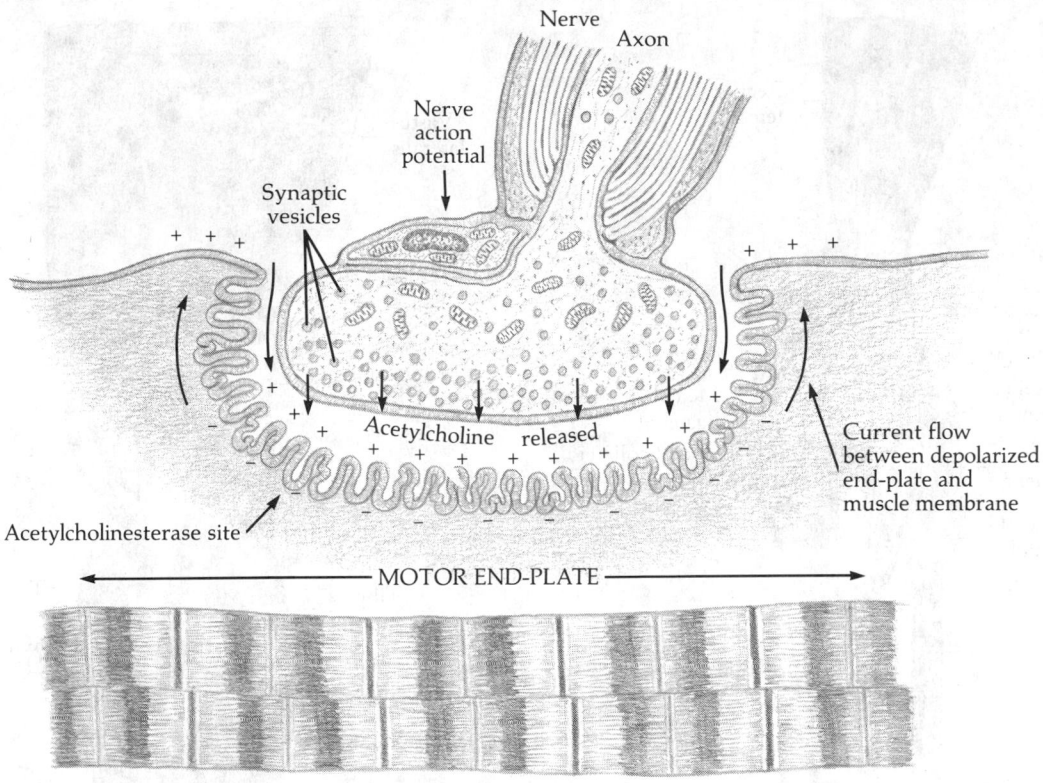

Figure 4-8 Motor end plate and myoneural junction involved in muscle contraction (see text for content).

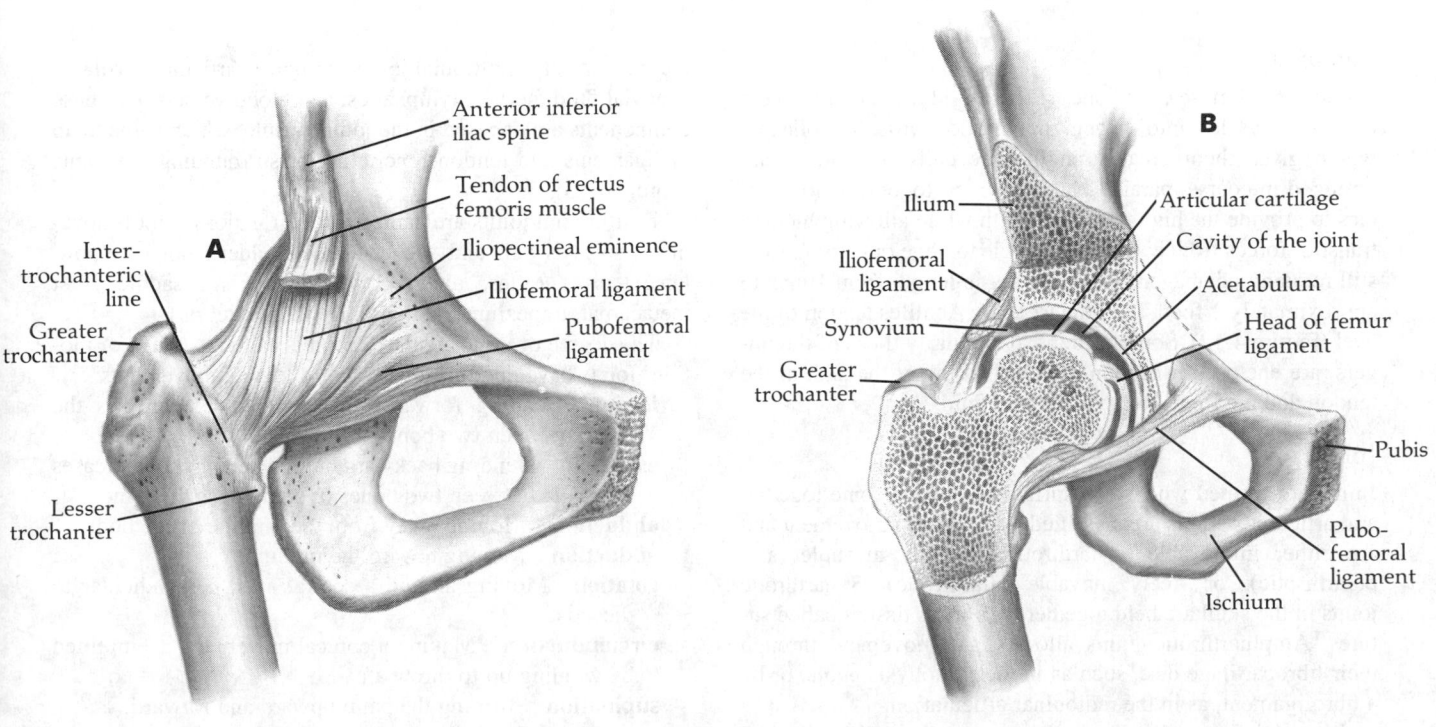

Figure 4-9 A, Ligaments surrounding hip joint. **B,** Ligaments holding structures in hip joint.

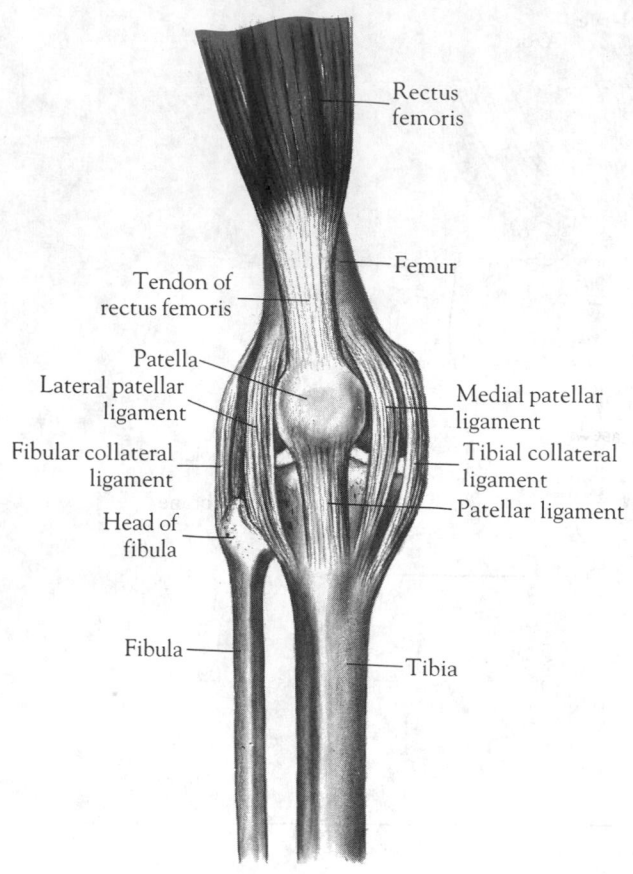

Figure 4-10 Ligaments of knee joint.

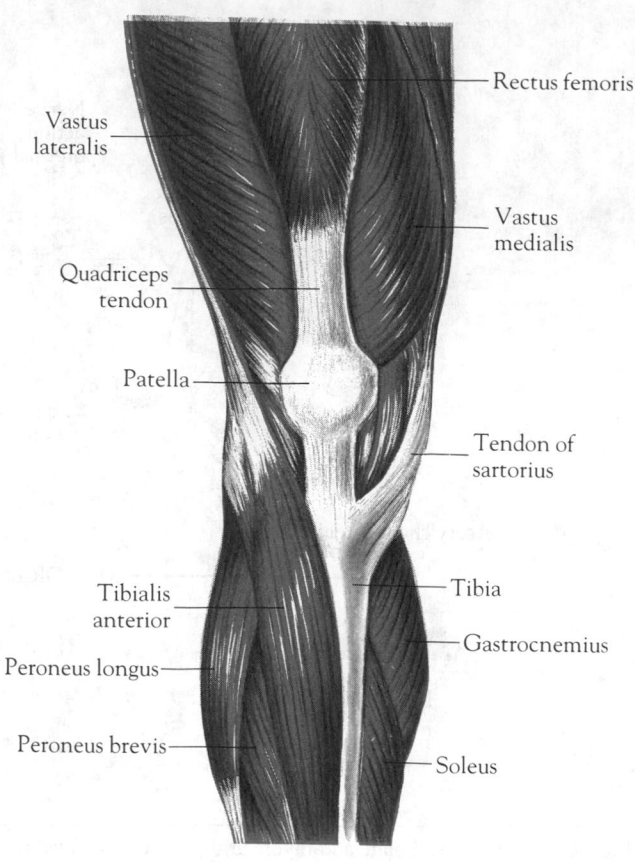

Figure 4-11 Tendons and muscles around knee joint (anterior view).

Tendons

Tendons hold muscles to bones (Figure 4-11). They form at the ends of muscles into strong, nonelastic cords of collagen, which gives them great strength. The cells of tendons are arranged in coarse, parallel bundles bound together into fascicles to provide the high tensile strength while allowing them to transmit forces from contractile muscle to bone or cartilage and still remain undamaged. Tendons vary in length from 1 inch to approximately 1 foot. The longest is the Achilles tendon of the heel (Figure 4-12). Some tendons, particularly those of the fingers, are enclosed in tendon sheaths that direct the path of the tendon and are lubricated by synovial fluid.

Joints

Joints are formed where two surfaces of bones come together and articulate. Joints are classified by degree of movement and are either immovable (synarthrotic), slightly movable (amphiarthrotic), or freely movable (diarthrotic). Synarthrotic joints in the skull are held together by fibrous tissues called sutures. Amphiarthrotic joints allow slight movement through their fibrocartilage disc, such as in the symphysis pubis, or by a fibroligament, as in the radioulnar articulation.

Most joints are diarthrotic. They are also called synovial joints because they are lined with synovial membranes. Other components of diarthrodial joints are bones, articular cartilage, synovial fluid, nerves, lymphatics, and blood vessels. All these components are encased in the joint capsule, which is made up of ligaments and tendons encircling or surrounding the joints (Figure 4-13).

Diarthrodial joints are named for their major form of movement, such as ball and socket (hip, shoulder), hinge (elbow, knee), pivot (atlas, axis), condyloid (wrist), saddle (first metacarpal, trapezium), and gliding (intervertebral).

The degree of movement of a joint is called its range of motion. Joints have one or more of the following movements:

flexion   Bending forward; shortening that decreases the angle between two bones.

extension   Bending backward or lengthening that increases the angle between two bones or straightens the joint.

abduction   Moving away from the midline of the body.

adduction   Moving toward the midline.

rotation   Moving around a central axis, perpendicular to the axis.

circumduction   Making a conical movement, exemplified by winding up to throw a ball.

supination   Turning the palm upward and forward.

pronation   Turning the palm downward and backward.

eversion   Turning the sole of the foot outward.

Gastrocnemius muscle
(Lateral head)
(Medial head)
Soleus muscle
Achilles tendon
Calcaneus

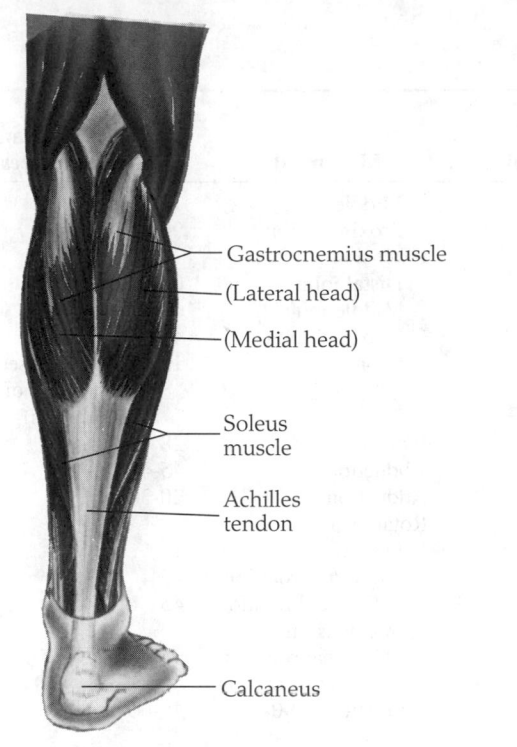

Figure 4-12 Achilles tendon in leg.

inversion Turning the sole of the foot inward.

dorsiflexion Pulling the foot and toes upward and forward.

plantar flexion Pushing the foot and toes downward and backward.

elevation Lifting upward.

depression Lowering.

protraction Moving a part forward.

retraction Moving a part backward.

apposition Moving the thumb toward the little finger to touch together.

When joints cannot or do not maintain their usual ranges of movement, they affect all musculoskeletal tissues and other body tissues. Table 4-1 gives ranges of motion of major joints.

Synovium

The synovium is a membrane that completely lines the inner surfaces of the joint (see Figure 4-13). It forms from cells within the inner layer of the joint capsule. The membrane has villous folds that contain the blood vessels and lymphatics. The membrane is made up of cells derived primarily from type I collagen molecules, although the blood vessels are derived from type III collagen (see p. 356).

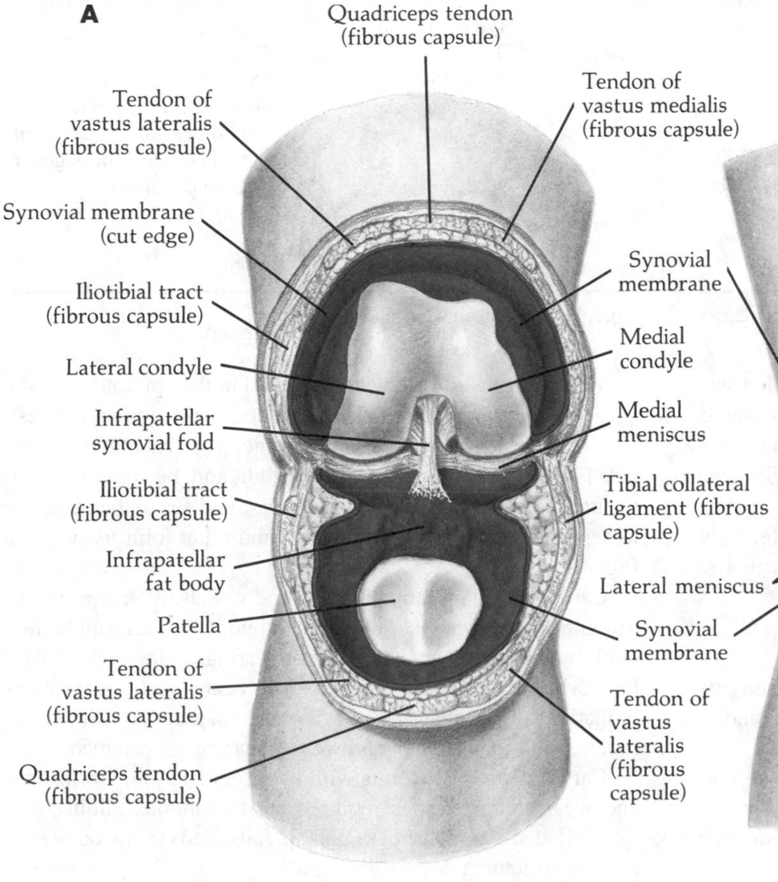

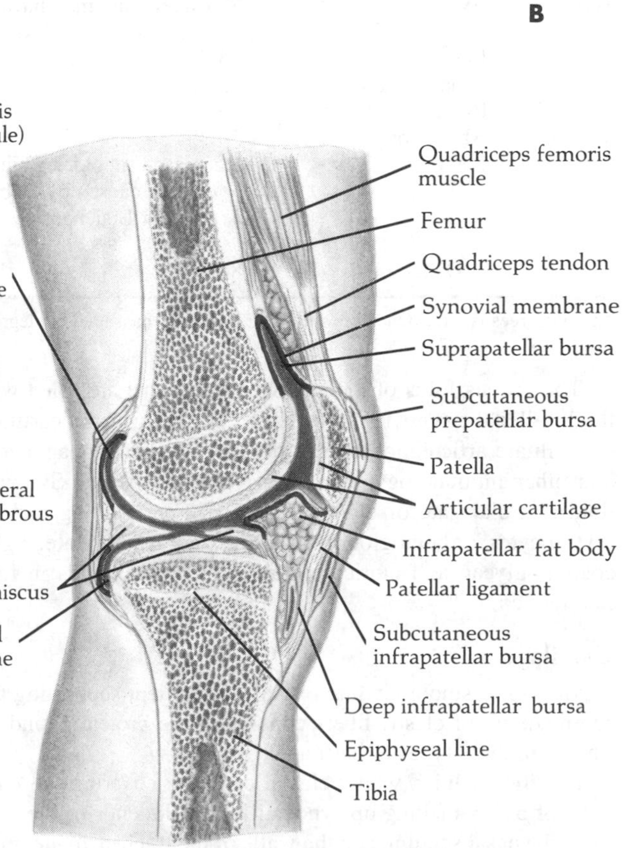

A
Quadriceps tendon (fibrous capsule)
Tendon of vastus lateralis (fibrous capsule)
Tendon of vastus medialis (fibrous capsule)
Synovial membrane (cut edge)
Iliotibial tract (fibrous capsule)
Synovial membrane
Lateral condyle
Medial condyle
Infrapatellar synovial fold
Medial meniscus
Iliotibial tract (fibrous capsule)
Tibial collateral ligament (fibrous capsule)
Infrapatellar fat body
Lateral meniscus
Patella
Synovial membrane
Tendon of vastus lateralis (fibrous capsule)
Tendon of vastus lateralis (fibrous capsule)
Quadriceps tendon (fibrous capsule)

B
Quadriceps femoris muscle
Femur
Quadriceps tendon
Synovial membrane
Suprapatellar bursa
Subcutaneous prepatellar bursa
Patella
Articular cartilage
Infrapatellar fat body
Patellar ligament
Subcutaneous infrapatellar bursa
Deep infrapatellar bursa
Epiphyseal line
Tibia

Figure 4-13 Knee joint (synovial joint). **A,** Frontal view. **B,** Lateral view.

TABLE 4-1 Range of Motion of Major Joints

Joint	Movements	Average Ranges (in Degrees)*	Joints	Movements	Average Ranges (in Degrees)*
Cervical spine	Flexion	35-45 (older adult 35)		Middle joint	100
	Extension	35 (older adult may have pain and some stiffness)		Proximal joint	90
				Extension	
	Lateral bending	45		Distal joint	0
	Rotation	45		Middle joint	0
	Hyperextension	45		Proximal joint	45
Thoracic and lumbar spine	Flexion	80-90	Hip	Flexion	120-135 (decreased in older adult because of degenerative changes)
	Extension	30			
	Lateral bending	28-35			
	Rotation	35-38 (older adult 30)		Extension	28
	Hyperextension	30		Abduction	45-48
Shoulder	Flexion	90 (some stiffness in older adult)		Adduction	20-30
				Rotation	
	Backward extension	44-55		In flexion	
	Abduction	90		Internal rotation	45
	Adduction	45-50		External rotation	45
	Circumduction	360 (older adult may have crepitation)		In extension	
				Internal rotation	35
Elbow	Flexion	145-160 (older adult may only be able to flex 135 degrees)		External rotation	48
				Abduction in 90-degree flexion	45-60
	Hyperextension	0	Knee	Flexion	120-130 (same or decreased in older adult but with soreness and stiffness; may have crepitation)
Forearm	Pronation	70-90			
	Supination	85-90			
Wrist	Extension	70 (older adult may have soreness or stiffness)		Hyperextension	10
	Flexion	73-90	Ankle	Flexion	48-50
	Ulnar deviation	33-55		Extension	18-20
	Radial deviation	19	Forefoot	Inversion	30-33 (same or decreased in older adult because of hallux valgus or degenerative changes)
Thumb	Abduction	58			
Fingers	Flexion	Decreased (in older adult may be caused by Heberden's or Bouchard's nodes)			
				Eversion	18-20
				Dorsiflexion	20
	Distal joint	80		Plantar flexion	45-50

*Zero degrees is the extended position; movement is measured by degrees in the specific directions in which the joint moves.

The villous folds of the synovial membrane are filled with fluid, called the synovial fluid, that bathes the articular cartilage to facilitate articulation and to provide nutrients, phagocytes, and other immunologic functions within the joints. Synovial fluid is a dialysate of blood plasma, without clotting factors, erythrocytes, or hemoglobin, but containing hyaluronate, a glycoaminoglycan and lubricating glycoprotein that aids in friction reduction.[104]

Cartilage

Cartilage is a smooth, white or yellow, resilient supporting tissue made up of elastic fibers containing the protein chondrin. There are three types of cartilage:

hyaline Bluish white, elastic cartilage covering the ends of bones making up synovial joints, the ends of the ribs, the nasal septum, and the walls of the trachea; made up of type II collagen molecules with some type I cells.

fibrous White fibers that are particularly resistant to tension and are found in the symphysis pubis and the knee; made up of type I collagen molecules.

yellow Elastic yellow fibers found in the epiglottis and the pinna (outer ear); made up of type I collagen molecules.

Cartilage serves as a smooth surface for articulating bones (see Figure 4-13). It also absorbs weight and, because it is elastic and moldable, absorbs shock, stress, and strain to prevent or lessen injury to bones within joints and other joint tissues (see Figure 4-13).

Cartilage contains no intrinsic blood vessels. It receives its nutrition from the synovial fluids forced into its porous cellular network by the movements and weight bearing of the joints. Therefore, when a particular joint ceases to bear weight or develops limitations of its usual range of movements, articular cartilage atrophies until joint motion and weight bearing are resumed.

Cartilage provides joints with excellent friction, lubrication, and wear characteristics required for continuous gliding motion.[92] It also absorbs shocks and spreads loads to the bony supporting structures.

Water is the most abundant component of normal articular cartilage, making up 65% to 80% of the wet weight of the cartilage.[92]

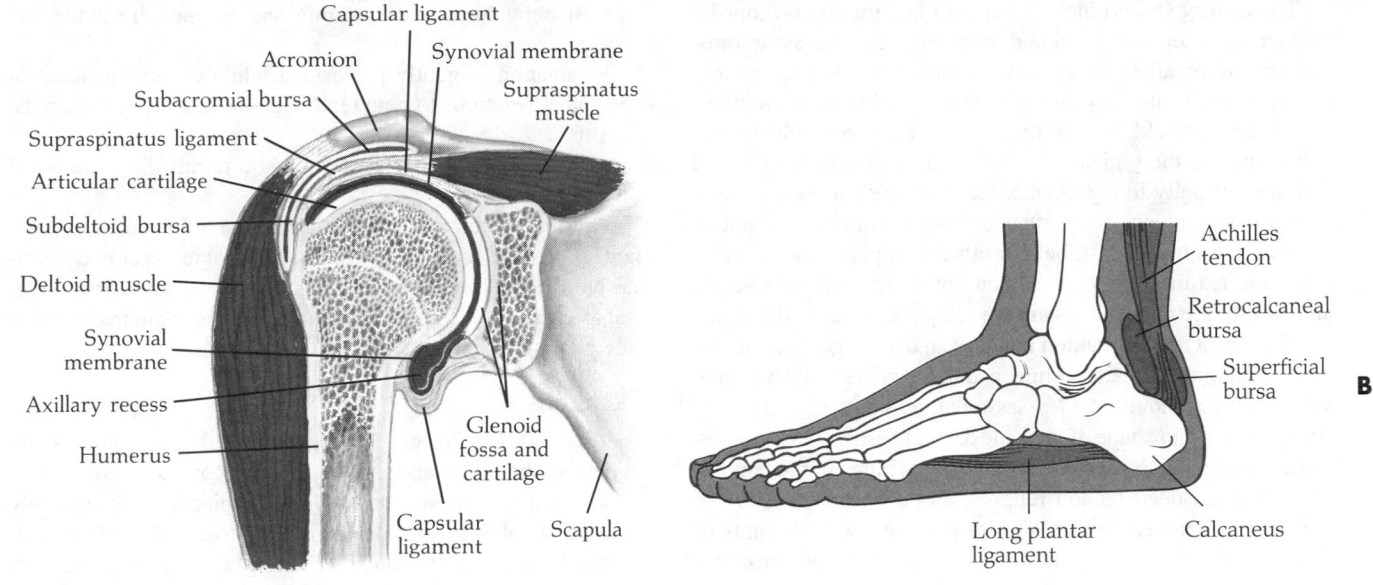

Figure 4-14 A, Bursae of shoulder joint. **B,** Bursae of the heel.

Bursa

A bursa is a small sac or cavity in the tissues (usually the tendons) surrounding or near a joint (Figure 4-14). The bursa is lined with synovial membrane and contains synovial fluid. Normally the bursa is a part of the musculoskeletal tissues, but a bursa can also form as a result of pressure or friction over a prominent part. Just such a bursa forms over a bunion in hallux valgus deformity.

The bursa reduces friction between tendons and bones or between tendons and ligaments by lubrication with synovial fluid from the bursal sac. New bursae can develop as a result of increased pressure or friction. Their formation may increase the pressure and cause pain.

Collagen

The protein collagen is the principal supporting element in connective tissues. It makes up approximately half the total body protein in fully developed adults. Collagen also plays an active role in developmental processes, cell attachment, chemotaxis, and the binding of antigen-antibody complexes. Thus collagen is more than an inert structural protein.

The collagen molecule is an asymmetric, rigid, rodlike structure made up of three individual polypeptide strands that are aligned colinearly throughout the molecule. The three individual strands of collagen are tightly coiled together in the form of a left-handed helix (the minor helix). They are then coiled around a common central axis to form a right-handed helix (the major helix). This coiled-coil configuration is stabilized by interchain hydrogen bonds.

Collagen molecules are referred to as type I, II, or III, and so on; there are presently 15 known types of collagen.[92] Types I, II, and III make up the most extensively occurring molecules. They are also called interstitial collagens because fibers from these types are found predominantly in spaces between the cellular elements of a tissue or organ.

Fibers from type I collagen molecules are found in all major connective tissues and in the stroma of several organs. Tissues such as bone, tendon, and dentin and fibrocartilage appear to be formed exclusively of type I collagen molecules. Type I molecules play a major role as supporting elements in tissues that normally exhibit very little distensibility under mechanical stress. It also appears that type I collagen molecules can be synthesized by the connective tissue cells in which they are found.

Type I collagen molecules are made up of two identical α-1 strands and a different but homologous α-2 chain. Type II is made of three α-1 chains, found primarily in hyaline cartilage, where they lend their special tensile properties to the mechanical strengths of the cartilage. Type III collagen molecules, which are also made up of three identical α-1 chains, are found in tissues that are the most distensible, such as the skin, blood vessel walls, and the uterine walls, and in several organs. Type III fibers coexist as fine reticular networks with type I molecules with larger fibers in the same tissues.

Differences in the three chains can be seen by electron microscopy. Each chain yields a unique set of peptides when examined, and each type of collagen develops from or under the control of separate and distinct structural genes. Thus the specific chain type and arrangement gives the particular collagen the strength and distensibility most suited to its specific tissue and distribution within the connective tissues of the body.

■ NORMAL FINDINGS

■ The orthopedic examination should take into account both the history and the physical examination.

The history should include any past and present orthopedic problems, patterns of local and systemic signs and symptoms, and review of all body systems; social, marital, employment (occupational), and psychologic state; and habits or hobbies. Assessment should include the effects of any musculoskeletal conditions on the patient's lifestyle, employment, family, and activities of daily living (ADL). The patient's age, sex, general appearance, and any deformities or assistive devices are noted. Presence of a brace, cast, belt, or other wrapping is noted. Skin color and texture are observed and noted. The patient's height and weight are checked, as are the temperature and vital signs.

The physical examination includes an overall general inspection; observance of gait, posture, and movements while walking, sitting, and standing; and assessment of bilateral symmetry, strength, size and shape of musculoskeletal tissues, muscular development, generalized or localized edema, range of movements of each joint, deep tendon reflexes, and condition of skin, of body, and of fingers and toes (with presence or complaints of Raynaud phenomenon). Note lesions, rash (color and site), pain at rest or with movement in one or more joints, temperature of skin over and around joints, texture of skin and nails, nodules in or around joints, hair growth and distribution, and evidence of bruises, hemorrhage, bone or joint deformity, congenital defects or deformities, condition of blood vessels, peripheral pulses, color of tissues, lymph nodes, leg length equality, and "point" tenderness (patient can point to area of greatest tenderness).

The following equipment is needed: goniometer to measure range of movements, percussion hammer, paper clip, cotton, sphygmomanometer, thermometer, tourniquet, tape measure, and stethoscope.

The following principles should be kept in mind in performing an orthopedic examination:

- Normal tissues are examined before injured, inflamed, or otherwise involved ones.
- Local signs and symptoms are assessed along with systemic findings.

NEUROVASCULAR ASSESSMENT OF EXTREMITIES*

The five *P*'s can help the nurse recall quickly the parameters to assess when evaluating the neurovascular status of an extremity:

Pain
Paresthesia
Pulses (peripheral or distal to the injury)
Pallor (color)
Paralysis
Plus:
Presence of edema
Temperature of injured tissues
Capillary refill in 2 to 4 seconds
Compare injured limb or part with tissues of opposite side

---

*Neurovascular assessment consists of all nine parameters listed.

- Bilateral local and systemic observations are made and compared.
- Palpation is gently performed while observing facial or other reactions to note tenderness or sensitivity within the tissues.
- Movements are assessed within norms for ranges of movements.

Physical examination is one part of the orthopedic examination, along with the history and the radiologic, serologic, surgical biopsy or exploratory, and consultative examinations. Special assessment techniques may also be done to aid in diagnosis (see p. 359).

Skeleton

Posture   Stands upright; head perpendicular to shoulders and pelvis; shoulders and pelvis aligned; convex curve to thoracic spine; concave curve to lumbar spine; arms hang freely from shoulders; feet aligned with toes pointing straight ahead; *older adult:* stance less upright, with head and neck more forward; thoracic curvature more pronounced; lumbar curvature less pronounced; shoulders may be hunched or rolled forward; angle of head of femur into acetabulum changes, leading to varus planting or placement of thighs, legs, and feet; height is decreased; may have kyphotic thoracic curve; may have less lordotic curve; *elderly adult**: frail; functional disabilities in walking, maintaining balance, and pain-free mobility caused by osteoporosis and decreased muscle mass

Gait   Smooth, coordinated, easy, rhythmic with push off and swing through; arms move freely at sides; easy acceleration and deceleration; can stand still without swaying or tilt; *older adult:* gait slow to initiate and stop; gait may be shuffling at times, with less knee and ankle lifts; more stiffness of hips, knees, and back; steps may be shorter and more rapid but cover less overall distance, may limp; *elderly adult:* slow gait, may need to hold onto furniture or another person to maintain balance; shuffles when stepping; less bending at knees; may have varus planting of feet if female

Muscles

Shape and contour   "Full-bellied"; firm and supple; muscle mass in overall conformity with body build; tapered at either end of muscle mass; *older adult:* shape and contour decrease, with less belly and mass common

Strength   Peak of muscle strength is 25 to 30 years; able to perform work of movements on demand and to maintain work activity over time; smooth and firm when contracted; loose when relaxed; strong grip, push, and pull strength; *older adult:* initial work energy strong, but strength lessens over time (gradual 10% loss in muscle strength between 30 and 60 years); movements may be somewhat uncoordinated and jerky; grip, push, and pull strength weaker than young adults; *elderly adult:* poor muscle mass or strength; weak grip, push,

---

*Elderly adult is a person aged 85 and above.[56]

and pull strength; uncoordinated movements; fears going to unfamiliar places because of possibility of falling

Range of movements Able to move bones and joints through movements required or permitted by the bone and joint structures; movements are smooth and sustained if necessary; muscle action begins smoothly without jerking; usual length is regained when muscle is relaxed; paired opposing actions are smooth; there should be no limitation of movement (see Table 4-1); *older adult:* all muscles can be put through passive range of movement slowly; active range of movement may be slower or limited in one or more joints, either symmetrically or asymmetrically; slight to moderate tenderness or pain may accompany movement; *elderly adult:* may have moderate loss of full range of motion; may have flexion contractures of elbows, which can be straightened carefully with assistance; movements may be uncoordinated and jerky; may have tenderness of spinal areas and joints of wrists, hips, knees, and ankles

Joints

Shape and contour Depends on specific type and position in body; bones of joint should articulate without deformity on one another in alignment; joint is firm and strong; *older adult:* joints appear larger than surrounding tissues; contour may be irregular in one or more joints; bones may glide over one another with slightly audible click or sound; joint is stiffer than younger adult; *elderly adult:* joints are misshapen and irregular; are large; do not glide easily; may have pain on weight bearing in back and hips or knees; may have limp

Temperature Warmth around joint should be same as surrounding tissues; may have some redness (erythema)

Swelling/edema None; *older adult:* may have slight edema of fingers, feet, or lower legs; *elderly adult:* may have edema under lower eyelids and edema of fingers, feet, and legs

Ligaments, Cartilage, and Tendons

Shape and contour Taut, elastic, and firm; permit weight bearing; *older and elderly adults:* taut but may be tighter and less elastic; may limit bone and joint contour

Movements Easily moves through range of motion and holds joints and muscles according to place or function; movements of joints can be sustained without deformity or curvature; weight bearing is pain free; *older adult:* less ease and range of movements; joints are stiffer; may have some joint laxity and weakness; weight bearing may cause some soreness or pain; *elderly adult:* jerky, uncoordinated movements; movements are slower and with some soreness and pain; joints are stiff, weaker, and with some to moderate laxity

■ Special Assessment Techniques*

Examination or Test	Site	Normal Findings	Abnormal Findings
Joint range of movements	Any or all joints	Specific range of motion (ROM) as per Table 4-1; no soreness or pain; no edema or elevated temperature in or around joints	Limitation of range of movements in one or more spheres; pain, soreness, muscle weakness, edema, elevated temperature in or around joint or joints
Straight leg raising (Lasègue)	Legs (one at a time)	No pain or soreness in back, buttocks when leg is raised while fully extended at knee; patient lies on back	Pain, soreness, or radiation of pain from low back to buttocks; may spread down leg to toes
McMurray	Knee	No excessive or palpable pop or click in knee noted when ankle is grasped to turn knee medially and laterally, and while moving knee backward and forward from full flexion to extension	Click or pop felt or heard; pain or local tenderness is positive for meniscal damage or tears
Fabere-Patrick	Knee and hip	Knee can be flexed and brought to almost horizontal position to body with heel resting on opposite knee	Knee cannot be brought to horizontal position; limitation may be in hip, knee, or back (usually hip disease prevents knee rotation to horizontal position)
Drawer: anterior and posterior	Knee	Knee has slight forward or backward movement while flexed on tibia and fibula	Knee has more movement forward or backward (direction indicates tear of either anterior or posterior cruciate ligaments)
Trendelenburg	Pelvis and gluteus muscles	With weight on one leg, pelvis on opposite side will be slightly elevated (observed posteriorly)	With weight on one leg, pelvis will drop (due to weakness or pain in hip joint or its muscles) on opposite side
Thomas	Hip, knee, and lumbar spine	With patient on back, hip and knee are flexed to abdomen without flexion simultaneously occurring in lumbar spine	When patient flexes knee and hip to abdomen, lumbar spine will flex if there is a pathologic condition of the hip, and opposite leg will rise from table

*These tests are examples of those most commonly done. The reader is referred to Seidel et al: *Mosby's guide to physical examination,* ed 3, 1995, Mosby, or to Thompson J, Wilson SF: *Health assessment for nursing practice,* 1996, Mosby, for additional special assessments.

Continued.

■ Special Assessment Techniques*—cont'd

Examination or Test	Site	Normal Findings	Abnormal Findings
Phalen	Wrists	No tingling of fingers with wrists maximally flexed against each other and held for 1 minute	Tingling felt in the thumb, the index finger and the middle and lateral half of the ring finger
Tinel	Carpal tunnel of wrist	No tingling into thumb, index, and middle fingers when median nerve is tapped at the wrist	Tingling felt as above for Phalen test
Burdzinski	Back and neck	With patient lying on back, no pain is felt in neck or back when head is passively flexed to chest	Pain in back and neck felt with passive flexion of head; knees and hips involuntarily flex to relieve pain (sign of meningeal irritation)
Kernig	Back and leg	No back or leg pain felt when leg is extended (patient lies on back with hip and knee flexed)	Pain is felt in lower back, neck, or head when leg is extended from flexed position (sign of meningeal irritation)

CONDITIONS, DISEASES, AND DISORDERS

INFLAMMATORY CONDITIONS

Inflammatory conditions are those that result in local or systemic responses to noxious stimuli (temperature extremes, chemicals, microorganisms, and others). These conditions can affect cells locally, resulting in cellular and tissue alterations while attempting to initiate, maintain, and resolve the inflammatory reaction. Initial reactions are referred to as acute, which are rapid and short lived; reactions that are longer lasting or prolonged are referred to as chronic inflammatory conditions. Inflammatory conditions of musculoskeletal tissues involve both acute and chronic conditions.

Inflammatory conditions can affect one or more muscles, tendons, ligaments, bones, and structures in and around the joints. Because of the interaction of the structures, diagnosis and treatment of specific tissue inflammations may be difficult. Overlapping therapy may be needed to ensure relief of the condition. Treatment methods for many specific musculoskeletal inflammatory conditions are identical. Also, inflammatory or degenerative effects in one musculoskeletal tissue may have long-term effects on contiguous tissues. Therefore inflammatory conditions must be considered serious alterations even if only one small area of localized inflammation is noted.

■ ANKYLOSING SPONDYLITIS

Ankylosing spondylitis is a localized chronic inflammatory condition that begins with low back (lumbar) pain and progresses throughout the spinal column, eventually resulting in hardening and fusing (ankylosing) and severe deformity of the vertebral column and adjacent tissues.

Ankylosing spondylitis (formerly Marie-Strümpell disease) progressively inhibits mobility. This disease occurs more commonly in men than women; it occurs between 20 and 40 years of age and rarely occurs after 50 years of age. A marked hereditary factor, histocompatibility antigen HLA-B27, is associated with ankylosing spondylitis. It is inherited as a mendelian-dominant trait.[58]

•••••• Pathophysiology

The exact pathologic condition in ankylosing spondylitis is unknown; the disease appears to begin insidiously in the enthesis, which is the site of insertion of ligaments and joint capsules in the sacroiliac bones and joints. The intervertebral discs become inflamed and are infiltrated by vascular connective tissue that then ossifies. The peripheral portions of the anulus fibrosus are the major areas initially affected, but as the disease progresses, the entire anulus, intervertebral ligaments, and the vertebrae themselves undergo similar inflammatory and ossifying changes. The disease gradually moves up the entire spinal column. The vertebral calcifications are called bamboo spines because the x-ray signs look like bamboo canes. The disease may also involve the hips, knees, and shoulders, but the primary sites are the spine and sacroiliac joints.

•••••• Diagnostic Studies and Findings

Physical examination of back and all musculoskeletal tissues   Local or systemic limitations and pain; Reiter's syndrome of conjunctivitis with uveitis, urethritis, and arthritis may be the complaint of patients with ankylosing spondylitis, along with morning stiffness and backache; there may be progressive kyphosis of the cervical, thoracic, and lumbar spine with the patient eventually being unable to look forward; hip abnormalities may result in severe disability

Roentgenograms   Inflammatory or degenerative changes referred to as bamboo spine

Serologic examination   Positive test for histocompatibility antigen HLA-B27, present in more than 90% of patients with ankylosing spondylitis but in less than 10% of general population; HLA-B27 is found in only 50% of African-Americans with ankylosing spondylitis[58]; rheumatoid factor is negative in most patients

Erythrocyte sedimentation rate Elevated during the disease activity (normal elevations [male, 0 to 9 mm/h; female, 0 to 20 mm/h] increase to 10 to 15 mm/h and 20 to 25 mm/h, respectively)

•••••• Multidisciplinary Plan

Surgery

Total hip replacement to correct postinflammatory fixed flexion of hip joints

Osteotomy of the midlumbar vertebrae, only if patient cannot see straight ahead because of kyphosis

Cervical spinal fusion to aid in maintaining upright position of neck

Osteotomy of thoracic vertebrae if marked thoracic deformity is present

Medications

Analgesic-antipyretic agents
  Salicylate analgesics (aspirin), 600 mg q4h (with buffering)
Nonsteroidal antiinflammatory agents
  Ibuprofen, 400-600 mg tid or qid
  Naprosyn, 250-500 mg bid or tid
  Clinoril, 150-200 mg bid
  Indomethacin (Indocin), 25-50 mg tid; may be increased to a maximum of 200 mg/d

General Management

If smoker, patient should stop smoking

Occupational therapy for identification and learning of modifications in ADL, employment, and changes in lifestyle necessary because of rigidity and curvature of spinal column

Consultations with social service and community nursing personnel to plan for long-term care and follow-up

Exercises to maintain mobility, including swimming and walking (rest is not beneficial in ankylosing spondylitis)

Physical therapy for exercises of the entire back, specific joint and muscle exercises, and deep-breathing exercises or other respiratory exercises

A firm mattress and bed with only a small pillow

Occasionally, use of a back brace or other orthosis

Occasionally, use of cervical or pelvic belt traction

Education related to avoidance of trauma to prevent vertebral fracture

NURSING CARE

Nursing Assessment

Lumbar Area of Back

Pain (may alternate side to side and is usually worse on getting up or when rising in the morning)
Stiffness
Limitation of motion
Radiation to buttocks or down one or both legs

Cervical or Thoracic Areas

Loss of normal curves; kyphosis; fixed flexion of cervical vertebrae—patient unable to look forward

Systemic Responses

Polyarthritis (asymmetric and affecting the large joints of the lower limbs)
Malaise, fatigue, weight loss, vague chest pains
Reiter's syndrome possible (Table 4-2)
Limitation of respiratory functions

Spread

Throughout spinal column as disease progresses and to sacroiliac, hips, knees, neck, and shoulder joints
Cannot hold head upright

Psychosocial Concerns

Self-concept and body image concerns from limitation of social interactions and loss of mobility and independence

Nursing Dx & Intervention

Impaired physical mobility (actual and high risk for) related to spinal inflammatory condition

- Assess for extent of impaired joint movements; assess posture and gait.

■ TABLE 4-2 Syndromes Associated with Arthritic Diseases

Syndrome	Patterns	Associated Diseases
Reiter	Triad of conjunctivitis, urethritis, and arthritis; oral, genital, and mucocutaneous lesions (stomatitis, ulcerations, papules)	Ankylosing spondylitis; rheumatoid arthritis
Behçet	Triad of iritis, oral lesions, and genital lesions; cutaneous lesions; phlebitis; colitis; polyarthritis	Polyarthritis of unknown etiology
Sjögren	"Sicca" patterns of dryness (sicca) of conjunctiva and salivary glands; arthritis; swelling of parotid gland; Raynaud's phenomenon in some patients	Connective tissue diseases such as systemic lupus erythematosus (SLE), progressive systemic sclerosis (PSS), polymyositis
Stevens-Johnson (variant of erythema multiforme)	Stomatitis with ulcerations of oral mucosa; high fever; genital ulcerations; erythematous skin eruptions; arthritis	Erythema multiforme; erythema nodosum; rheumatic fever; rheumatoid arthritis and juvenile rheumatoid arthritis; ulcerative colitis

- Observe movements for signs of relief or progressive impairment *to note patient's condition.*
- Assist with range of motion (ROM) exercises *to maintain joint mobility.*
- Encourage performance of prescribed exercises (swimming and walking) *to maintain mobility.*
- Massage back as needed *to relieve tense or tired muscles.*
- Assist patient to positions of comfort; keep bed flat *to maintain extension of the spine.*
- Assist with immersion in Hubbard tank or spa *to lessen muscle spasms and strengthen extensor muscles.*
- Teach deep-breathing exercises *to maintain respiratory functions and to aid peripheral oxygenation.*

Pain related to muscle/joint limitation of movements

- Assess patient for the presence, amount, and severity of pain.
- Administer analgesic and antiinflammatory medications as prescribed *to relieve pain and inflammation.*
- Observe patient's movements for increasing ease and frequency *to note effects of medications.*
- Listen for patient's verbalization of pain relief or continuing pain *to determine if changes are needed.*
- Observe all involved points *to note abatement or continuation of inflammation.*
- Encourage proper use of pillow and mattress *to prevent additional trauma and pain.*
- Observe for side effects of medications (e.g., gastric irritation or burning; changes in complete blood count [CBC] and erythrocyte sedimentation rate [ESR]; diarrhea or constipation) *to note reactions to medications.*

Body image disturbance and altered role performance related to severe kyphosis and rigidity of spine

- Assess for implicit and expressed concerns.
- Encourage socialization with family and friends *to help maintain usual roles.*
- Encourage team recreational activities and games, such as team swimming and walking with others, *to maintain patient's inclusion in activities.*
- Encourage compliance with treatment regimen *to prevent severe deformity.*
- Encourage patient to continue seeing physician for continuity of care and for current or recent developments in treatment of ankylosing spondylitis *to aid in maintaining long-term healthy status.*

Injury, risk for, related to potential vertebral fracture

- Assess for complaint of increased pain and soreness in neck or back.
- Teach patient about avoidance of trauma *to prevent possible fracture of vertebra resulting from osteoporosis or spinal rigidity.*
- Encourage patient to seek medical care for increased pain in back *to differentiate cause of pain increase.*

- Discuss ways to lessen development of osteoporosis, including activity, exercises, and weight bearing, *to lessen possibility of fracture.*
- Observe patient for weakness or loss of motor functions *to note possible signs of paraplegia.*

Patient Education/Home Care Planning

1. Reiterate explanations of inflammatory processes and rationale for medical care to ensure that patient and family understand.
2. Discuss rationale for exercise as opposed to rest of affected tissues: rest is harmful in ankylosing spondylitis.
3. Explain actions and side effects of salicylates and other antiinflammatory medications. The patient should understand and be alert to the many side effects of ordered medications. List common side effects for patient safety.
4. Demonstrate deep-breathing, ROM, and joint mobility exercises to encourage patient to comply.
5. Include family members in evaluation, practice, and performance of ADL as necessary for home care continuity.
6. Explain benefits of aquatherapy (especially swimming and water aerobics) to maintain mobility.

Evaluation

Patient retains adequate vertebral mobility and satisfactory curvature　Patient's inflammation abates without ankylosis or severe curvature.

Patient experiences pain relief with medications　Patient continues own ADLs and usual employment activities, interactions, and recreation.

Patient maintains independence, social interactions, and self-care activities　Patient states pain is tolerable with analgesic medication and other treatments. Patient does not experience vertebral fracture. Patient appears to accept change in appearance.

BURSITIS

Bursitis is the inflammation of a bursa.

Because the bursa is an enclosed sac situated between muscles or tendons and bony prominences, the inflammation may spread to certain structures or may simply be an inflammation of the bursal fluid and sac.

One or more bursae can become inflamed, but the most common sites are the subdeltoid and subacromial bursae of the shoulder (see Figure 4-14), the olecranon (elbow) bursa, the greater trochanteric bursa lateral to the hip, and the anserine bursa in the medial aspect of the upper tibia. One common but often overlooked site of bursitis is the obturator internus bursa.[155]

Bursitis is more common in athletes and persons who do repetitive motions. It can cause significant morbidity. It may also be associated with low back pain.

•••••• Pathophysiology

Bursitis usually results from constant friction between the skin and musculoskeletal tissues around the affected joint. Bursitis from friction would be sterile or aseptic without pathogenic organisms. Rarely, bursitis results from a foreign body or microorganism invasion. The area around the bursa becomes exquisitely tender. Motion is either partially or greatly limited by the swollen, enlarged sac, which causes pressure and pain when the tissues are moved. The area may be reddened, hot, and edematous with only point tenderness (the patient can point to the spot or area of greatest tenderness) or with soreness radiating to the tendons at the site. Tendinitis may also occur, further limiting motion and prolonging recovery. Calcium may be deposited in the bursal sacs in long-standing or recurring bursitis.

•••••• Diagnostic Studies and Findings

History   Repetitive motions for throwing; running long distances; overuse; low back pain

Physical examination   Localized inflammation in bursal area; point tenderness; limitation of motion of one or more bursae and involved joints

Roentgenograms   May or may not show calcified deposits

•••••• Multidisciplinary Plan

Surgery

Open removal of the calcified deposits
Aspiration of fluid within the sac (infrequently) for persistent edema and pressure
Removal of the bursal sac (rarely needed)

Medications

Analgesic-antipyretic agents
  Salicylates (aspirin), 600-1000 mg q4h
Nonsteroidal antiinflammatory agents
  Ibuprofen, 400-600 mg qid or tid
  Indomethacin (Indocin), 25 mg bid, tid, or qid
If the bursa is infected, antibiotics specific for the offending organism following culture
Injections of steroids into the sac to relieve the inflammation; dosage is individualized

General Management

Avoidance of activities (such as kneeling) that cause pressure
Avoidance of constant friction movements (such as throwing or hitting a ball) that cause the inflammatory reaction
Avoidance of repetitive motions that affect bursa and joint
Moist heat applications every 4 hours to the inflamed area
ROM exercises to help regain or maintain motion
Wrapping with elastic bandages, if bursa is accessible, to reduce edema

NURSING CARE

Nursing Assessment

Inflammatory Process

Area around joint
Heat
Redness
Swelling
Tenderness and pain with use; aching around joint
Limitation of motion

Systemic Response

Similar responses in one or more joints or bursae
Fever and malaise if pathogen is involved

Psychosocial Concerns

Limitation of use of muscles and joint, possibly curtailing income or livelihood

Nursing Dx & Intervention

Impaired physical mobility (limitation of motion) related to inflammation of bursa

- Assess degree of limitation of movement of involved joint.
- Encourage stretching exercises to maintain ROM as prescribed *to maintain functions.*
- Caution against continuing activities that may cause recurrence *to lessen chance of chronicity.*
- Observe for edema, pain, and redness related to limiting or increasing motion *to note progression.*
- Apply warm compresses every 4 hours as ordered *to aid resolution or easing of inflammation.*
- Remove bandages, observe site, and rewrap bandages (if used) *to prevent disarrangement or tightening of bandages.*

Pain related to inflammation of bursa

- Assess amount, severity, and duration of pain.
- Administer medications as prescribed *to relieve pain and inflammation.*
- Note continuation or relief of pain, tenderness, or inflammation *to note efficacy of medications.*
- Observe for side effects of medications *to note presence or need for other medications.*
- Handle inflamed tissues gently *to prevent additional trauma.*
- Discourage activities that increase pain or discomfort.

Patient Education/Home Care Planning

1. Discuss ROM exercises to lessen possibility of bursal inflammation.

2. Give the patient a list of side effects of medications and instruct the patient to report to physician as needed.
3. Alert the patient to the possibility that pain may increase temporarily after injection of steroids (1 to 24 hours), to be followed by noticeable pain relief and increasing ROM.
4. Caution the patient to avoid activities that could cause exacerbation until inflammation is resolved (4 to 6 weeks).

Evaluation

Patient regains ROM of affected joint   Patient can engage in usual activities with affected joint and contiguous tissues.

Patient no longer needs medication to relieve pain   Patient feels no pain with ROM actions or when using joint for usual activities.

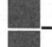

EPICONDYLITIS AND TENDINITIS
(Tenosynovitis)

Epicondylitis is an inflammation of the tendons of the medial or lateral epicondyles of the radius, ulna, or other bones. Tendinitis (tenosynovitis) is an inflammation of the tendons and their sheaths.

Epicondylitis and tendinitis may occur together and, with some variations, the local sites of inflammation are next to one another, which makes proper diagnosis more challenging.

Lateral epicondylitis, commonly called tennis elbow, is caused by repetitive twisting and swinging movements of the elbow that accompany, among other activities, swinging a tennis racket or using a hammer or other tools. Inflammation affects the tendons that originate in the medial or lateral epicondyles of the radius or ulna. The tendons and their sheaths may both become inflamed (tendinitis and tenosynovitis, respectively). Medial epicondylitis is called golfer's elbow and is primarily related to repetitive swings of the elbow, such as those made by the golfer.

Tenosynovitis affects joints other than the elbow, with the shoulder and knee joints frequently affected in baseball pitchers, football players, soccer players, and other athletes. Tenosynovitis also frequently affects tendons of the fingers of one or both hands.

Tenosynovitis is a common condition. It may be caused by infection, diabetes, or gout and can accompany pregnancy.

•••••• Pathophysiology

Repetitive trauma damages and tears the fibers of the common extensor tendon of the involved joint. Extravasation of tissue fluids sets up inflammatory reactions, and healing produces scar tissue and adhesions that limit the range of motion of the joint. The joint can then become inflamed by repetitive trauma to the scarred, inelastic fibers. The inflammation can spread to the tendon sheath, with fibrosis binding the sheath to the tendon and thus further limiting joint movements. Classic symptoms of epi-

condylitis include tenderness (frequently point tenderness), pain, and edema. Pronation or supination of the hand when the elbow is in 45 degrees of flexion causes severe medial and epicondylar pain if the inflamed joint is the elbow. In the hand, pain is increased on passive extension of the affected digit or digits.

•••••• Diagnostic Studies and Findings

History   Flexion, rotation, and repetitive ROM actions from occupational or sports activities resulting in localized joint pain, tenderness, and limitation of motion in involved joint, such as elbow, shoulder, or knee

Physical examination   Point of tenderness and increased pain with supination and pronation of hand or arm; edema and tenderness radiating along the tendon and its sheath; weak grasp or loss of strength of affected joint; decreased ROM of affected joint

•••••• Multidisciplinary Plan

Surgery

Removal of calcium deposits from the inflammatory processes occasionally required

Removal of a degenerated (scarred and bound-down) tendon sheath for chronic, persistent synovitis of a shoulder, elbow, or heel because of calcium deposits from repeated trauma

Incision of infected tissues, if indicated by severity of condition

Medications

Corticosteroids orally in individualized doses

Injection of steroids into the inflamed area to relieve pain; may need to be repeated at intervals for complete pain relief; dosage and type individualized

Analgesic-antipyretic/antiinflammatory medications
  Ibuprofen, 400-800 mg tid or bid
  Salicylates (aspirin), 600 mg q4h for mild conditions
Antibiotics
  Specific to organism; may be Ancef or other broad-spectrum antibiotic, given intravenously (IV)

General Management

Cold or moist heat applications to area q4h

Rest to the part or parts for varying periods of time

Occasionally, splint or other orthosis applied to the forearm and elbow, sling for shoulder; knee immobilizer (rarely used)

ROM exercises per physical therapist

NURSING CARE

Nursing Assessment

Inflammatory Process

Localized pain in shoulder, elbow, wrist, hand, or knee, and pain radiating to forearm or leg

Tenderness with movement or use
Edema in shoulder, elbow, or knee
Edema in one or more fingers

Range of Motion

Pain increased with supination and pronation of hand or flexion and extension of fingers; pain with throwing motions of shoulder; pain with lateral movements of knee

Systemic

Elevated temperature if infection present

Psychosocial Concerns

Concern for ability to earn a living if in an occupation requiring full elbow, hand, shoulder, or knee ROM or other joint movements

Nursing Dx & Intervention

Impaired physical mobility related to limitation of joint functions and pain

- Assess degree and amount of joint movements.
- Encourage exercises *to maintain ROM if prescribed.*
- Caution against continuing activities that may cause recurrence.
- Observe for edema, pain, and redness related to limiting or increasing motion *to note progression of symptoms.*
- Apply prescribed cold or warm compresses every 4 hours as ordered *to relieve inflammation* (whirlpool may be used).

Pain related to inflammation of tendons

- Assess amount, severity, sites, and type of pain.
- Administer medications as prescribed *to relieve pain.*
- Note continuation or relief of pain, tenderness, or inflammation *to assess effect of medications.*
- Observe for side effects of medications *to note problem that may need treatment.*
- Handle inflamed tissues gently *to avoid additional pain.*
- Apply splint, sling, or joint immobilizer as ordered, if used.
- Administer prescribed antibiotic *to resolve infection, if present.*

Altered role performance related to presence and severity of condition

- Assess for evidence of concerns.
- Encourage expression of concerns; seek guidance to resolve concerns about employment or recurrence of condition.
- Encourage patient to comply with treatment regimen and to continue medical care *to note recovery.*
- Discuss preventive techniques, therapies, or other strategies *to ease concerns.*

Patient Education/Home Care Planning

1. Explain inflammatory processes and effects of repetitive trauma to lessen painful episodes and inflammation.
2. Give a list of the side effects of medications to the patient. Clarify to ensure understanding.
3. Alert the patient to the possibility that pain may increase temporarily after injection of steroids (1 to 24 hours), to be followed by noticeable pain relief and increasing ROM.
4. Caution the patient to avoid activities that could cause exacerbation until inflammation is resolved (4 to 6 weeks).
5. Discuss the effects of application of heat or cold with patient and family.

Evaluation

Patient regains joint mobility without limitation Patient can put joint through normal ROM without limitation, hesitation, or loss of strength.

Patient experiences relief of pain Patient has no pain on usual ROM activities and has stopped use of oral steroids and analgesics.

Patient returns to employment as before No restrictions are necessary on employment activities.

■ RHEUMATOID ARTHRITIS

Rheumatoid arthritis is a chronic systemic disease characterized by inflammation of the connective tissues throughout the body.

Rheumatoid arthritis affects 7 million persons in the United States, occurring 3:1 in females over males. It affects about 1% of the population worldwide and affects about 5% of population aged 70 years and above.[145]

This severely disabling chronic disease is one of the major rheumatic diseases. Although the disease is a systemic disorder, this discussion concerns the local effects on the tissues in and around the joints. The disease appears to be decreasing in its incidence and severity.[141]

Rheumatoid arthritis is thought to be an autoimmune phenomenon, although there is evidence of a genetic predisposition, especially related to HLA-DR4, HLA-DR, HLA-DP, and HLA-DQ.[145]

Most patients develop rheumatoid arthritis between 25 and 55 years of age, although the disease also occurs in children between 8 and 15 years old, when it is referred to as juvenile rheumatoid arthritis or Still's disease. Over 200,000 new cases are diagnosed each year. Asians and Hispanics have low incidence of this disease.

•••••• Pathophysiology

The disease begins in the synovial membrane within the joint, usually in one of the smaller joints of the wrist, fingers, or hand.

However, bilateral symmetric joint involvement is a characteristic finding. The synovial membrane becomes inflamed from the autoimmune antigen-antibody effects, and the membrane becomes swollen, irritated, and painful. There is an abundance of activated T-cells in joints affected by rheumatoid arthritis, whereas virtually no T-cells are present in normal joints. These T-cells are antigen specific,[141] although their relevance has yet to be determined. There are also abundant macrophages and monocytes present in affected joints, which produce cytokines that affect immune responses and inflammatory reactions. These cytokines include interleukins 1 through 8, tissue necrosis factor, transforming growth factor alpha and beta, granulocyte-macrophage colony–stimulating factors, and platelet-derived growth factors alpha and beta.[141] Some of these cytokines cause cartilage destruction and amplify the inflammatory focus.

Fibrotic changes and hypertrophy of the synovial membrane occur. These changes are called pannus formation. The inflammatory reaction spreads to other joint tissues, including the cartilage, and eventually to the bones. Ligaments and tendons also are involved; they are scarred and shortened, which eventually contributes to deformities, subluxations (partial dislocations), and contractures. Cartilage degeneration results in pain and grating with weight bearing and movements. As the cartilage erodes and degeneration continues, the bone ends are exposed and also develop erosions, bone cysts, or fissures. Eventually bone spurs and osteophytes (outgrowths of bone) develop, further limiting joint mobility and use. The entire joint and its structures remain inflamed, edematous, and painful. Also, collections of fibroblasts in collagen tissues near joints enlarge into rheumatoid nodules, a classic feature of rheumatoid arthritis.

Characteristically, rheumatoid arthritis affects smaller joints symmetrically before involving the larger weight-bearing joints. Bouchard's nodes are the classic enlargements of the proximal phalangeal and metacarpophalangeal joints.

Eventually the local disease in the joints involves major organ systems in the remainder of the body, including the heart, kidneys, lungs, skin, eyes, and hematologic tissues.

•••••• Diagnostic Studies and Findings

History Monoarticular or polyarticular inflammation

Physical examination Criteria for the diagnosis of rheumatoid arthritis have been established by the American Rheumatism Association (ARA); presence of five or more of the following confirms the diagnosis: morning stiffness on arising; pain and tenderness in at least one joint; swelling in at least one and possibly two joints; symmetric joint swelling bilaterally; fatigue, malaise, and weight loss; paresthesias of hands or feet; Raynaud's phenomenon of fingers and toes; development of subcutaneous nodules; involvement of major organs such as heart and kidney; pericarditis; valvular lesions; vasculitis; pneumonitis; fibrosis; tenosynovitis; ankylosis of joints; joint contractures; presence of Bouchard's nodes; Felty's syndrome (splenomegaly and leukopenia); deformities of joints; ulnar drift of wrists; sicca syndrome and scleritis of eyes

Serologic examination Rheumatoid factor (a large immune globulin): Positive in 80% of patients with rheumatoid arthritis[165]

Erythrocyte sedimentation rate (ESR): elevated (moderate to severe elevation [to 15 mm/h in males and 25 mm/h in females]); normal: 0-9 mm/h in males and 0-20 mm/h in females

C-reactive protein: present during acute phases

Red cell count: anemia, primarily hypochromic (normocytic is common)

White cell count: elevated over all cell types

Serum complement decreased

Antinuclear antibody may be positive

MULTIPLE TREATMENTS* IN MANAGEMENT OF RHEUMATOID ARTHRITIS

Education for patient and family
Heat/cold applications
Therapeutic exercises
Rest
Salicylates at therapeutic doses
Occupational and physical therapies
Orthotic devices
Gold salts, antimalarial drugs, D-penicillamine
Nonsteroidal antiinflammatory drugs and analgesic drugs
Glucocorticoids in low or high doses
Intraarticular glucocorticoids
Reconstructive surgery
Immunosuppressive drugs, such as azathioprine
Cytotoxic drugs, such as methotrexate

*Treatments generally include each of the above modalities during the course of the disease process.

NEW APPROACHES IN THE TREATMENT OF RHEUMATOID ARTHRITIS

Total lymphoid irradiation
Antibodies
    Immunoglobulin preparations
    Monoclonal antibodies
Cytokines and cytokine inhibitors
    Interleukin-1 and its inhibitors
    Interleukin-2 and its inhibitors
    Interferon gamma
Peptides
Collagen II
Immunotoxins
Photopheresis
T-cell vaccination

Data from Smolen.[141]

Synovial fluid aspiration and analysis   May reveal immune complexes and elevated white cell counts

Synovial membrane biopsy   Positive for pannus formation and inflammatory changes

Roentgenograms   Rarefaction of bones, plus erosions of involved bone, as disease progresses; subluxation (partial dislocation) of bones from joints

NOTE: Laboratory studies are not "diagnostic" of rheumatoid arthritis but are used in conjunction with careful evaluation of the history, physical findings, laboratory tests, and radiographs.[165]

• • • • • • Multidisciplinary Plan

Surgery

Synovectomy of inflamed synovial membranes to relieve pain and maintain muscle and joint balance

Repair of ruptured or fibrotic tendon sheaths to prevent deformity and subluxations

Total joint replacement to increase mobility

Arthrodesis (fusion of a joint): may be done to decrease deformity and joint instability; spinal fusion may be required to treat subluxation

Osteotomy to change weight-bearing surfaces and relieve pain

Arthroplasty to correct deformities

Medications

Analgesic-antipyretic agents
  Aspirin, divided doses up to 5 g/d
Nonsteroidal antiinflammatory agents
  Ibuprofen (Motrin), 1200-3200 mg/d
  Fenoprofen (Nalfon), 1200-3200 mg/d
  Tolmetin (Tolectin), initially 400 mg tid to reach optimum daily dose of 600-1800 mg/d
  Naproxen (Naprosyn), 750-1500 mg/d
  Diclofenac (Voltaren), 75-150 mg/d
  Piroxicam (Feldene), 20 mg/d
Antirheumatic agents
  Gold thiomaleate (Myochrysine), 20-50 mg/wk IM, or auranofin (Ridaura), 6 mg/d po, to decrease inflammation
  Penicillamine (Cuprimine, Depen), 125-250 mg/d increased to 500-750 mg/d; may be used as a substitute for patients sensitive to gold
Immunosuppressive agents
  Azathioprine (Imuran), 305 mg/kg/d initially; then 1-2 mg/kg/d maintenance dose
Antimalarial agents
  Hydroxychloroquine, 40 mg/d po
Antineoplastic agents
  Methotrexate (Rheumatrix), 2.5-15 mg po or IM weekly
  Cyclophosphamide; dosage is individualized
Corticosteroids
  Primarily prednisone (Deltasone, others) or prednisolone (Delta-Cortef, others) in titrated doses of 2-10 mg/d, used after other medications for antiinflammatory effects

Hydrocortisone (Cortef, others), 100 mg, injected into the joint to reduce inflammation

General Management (see box)

Immersion in paraffin "glove" (rarely used currently)

Immersion in whirlpool or spa; aquatherapy for joint exercises

Application of splints to inflamed joints to maintain proper position

Moist, warm applications to joints

Applications of cold alternating with heat

ROM exercises to maintain motion

Prescribed rest periods in morning and afternoon

Well-balanced diet; avoidance of obesity because of increased joint stress

Providing instruction and practice in home maintenance technique

Providing knowledge about the disease to ease patient's fears and increase compliance with treatment regimen

NURSING CARE

Nursing Assessment

Local Inflammatory Processes in Joint

Edema; boggy joint
Pain
Heat
Redness
Limitation of motion
Deformity; numbness of fingers or toes
Flexion contractures

Systemic Processes

Malaise
Pale color of skin; anemia
Marked fatigue; weakness
Fever
Multiple joint involvement
Subcutaneous rheumatoid nodules
Weight loss
Color of fingers or toes (redness, whiteness, blueness) changes at times

Psychosocial Concerns

Lack of thorough understanding of rheumatoid arthritis
Concerns with self-concept, body image disturbances, loss of mobility because of chronicity, and deformity
Multiple treatments without cure in near future
Interference with roles

Economic Concerns

Major costs for treatments over extended periods of time
Possible loss of employment because of nature of disease and joint involvement

Nursing Dx & Intervention

Anxiety related to newness of diagnosis and present lack of curative therapies

- Assess patient's level of anxiety *to determine optional nursing measures.*
- Clarify physician's explanations, if needed, because anxiety may preclude patient's and family's clear understanding of proposed regimen.
- Review specifics of patient's regimen, as needed, *to aid understanding and patient's participation.*
- Review characteristics of patient's "stage" of rheumatoid arthritis; correlate patient's symptoms with relief to be achieved by treatment regimen *to lessen anxiety.*
- Discuss patient's daily roles and responsibilities to determine optimal times for specific care (e.g., time of day for aquatherapy if employed during day or evening hours) *to facilitate achieving treatment goals.*
- Remind patient and family of nurse's and physician's availability *to clarify regimen if needed.*
- Answer questions as honestly as possible *to establish trust and ease concerns.*

Activity intolerance related to anemia and disease state

- Assess levels of energy, tiredness, and fatigue.
- Provide rest periods in morning and afternoon *to maintain strength.*
- Provide 8 to 10 hours for uninterrupted nighttime sleep *to help maintain strength.*
- Alternate activities with rest periods *to prevent fatigue.*
- Provide trapeze, assistive devices, and side rails as needed to help conserve energy and muscle and joint functions.
- Provide a diet high in iron-containing foods *to aid relief of anemia.*
- Seek consultation with physical therapists for exercises *to maintain strength.*
- Monitor laboratory data such as hematocrit and hemoglobin *to note current anemia* (levels of hematocrit <30% and hemoglobin <12 g are indicative of anemia).

Pain related to inflammatory process

- Assess presence, amount, site, and severity of pain.
- Administer medications as prescribed *to relieve pain and inflammation.*
- Have patient sleep and rest on a firm mattress with a small head pillow *to prevent deformities.*
- Massage back *to ease tightness and pressure of muscles and joints.*
- Encourage patient to be active during periods of pain relief *to maintain usual roles.*
- Encourage patient to express thoughts and feelings about pain, disease, and loss of independence *to ease concerns.*

- Encourage diversionary activities *to decrease focus on pain.*
- Encourage patient to participate actively and positively in each type of treatment *to increase comfort and sense of control.*
- Provide list of common side effects of medications *for safety and to relieve concern.*

Impaired home maintenance management related to joint and muscle weakness

- Assess ability and strength to carry out homemaking activities.
- Use occupational therapists to teach modifications in home environment *to lessen joint and systemic stress.*
- Use community health nurses *for home evaluation and continuity of care.*
- Have patient practice with and use implements and utensils *to gain skill and independence.*
- Encourage self-care, modify utensils, and provide learning experience *to gain skills.*
- Explain safety measures for home maintenance *to lessen possibility of injury.*

Impaired physical mobility related to joint and systemic involvement

- Assess degree and amount of joint movements or limitations.
- Assist with treatment regimen (such as heat, cold, paraffin) *to maintain joint mobility.*
- Provide ROM exercises as able *to prevent stiffening of joints.*
- Provide splints and walking aids such as cane or crutch *to lessen joint stress.*
- Turn and position the patient every 2 to 4 hours *to prevent joint deformity.*
- Provide joint rest during acute exacerbation *to prevent further joint damage.*
- Maintain joints in functional (extended) positions *to prevent joint contractures.*

Sleep pattern disturbance related to pain and joint or muscle disease

- Assess sleep patterns over time.
- Prepare patient for rest with massage and straightening of bed linens *to aid relaxation.*
- Position with small pillows under head and lower back *to prevent flexion contractures.*
- Administer medications *to relieve pain and inflammation.*
- Give warm milk or snack *to induce sleep.*
- Maintain a quiet environment *to promote and maintain sleep periods.*
- Avoid caffeine-containing foods *to promote restful sleep.*
- Monitor, and possibly change, hours of administration of medications, such as diuretics and steroids, that could interfere with sleep *to promote sleep.*

Body image disturbance and altered role performance related to deformities and chronic disease

- Assess concerns about condition and role performance.
- Encourage active participation in usual roles as able *to maintain self-concept.*
- Allow patient to ventilate feelings about deformities and limitation of movements to determine needs.
- Offer support and encouragement *to help maintain a positive attitude about the disease and its treatment.*
- Encourge family members to maintain open communication with the patient *to help maintain usual roles.*
- Employ team concept (occupational therapy, physical therapy, medicine, nursing, and others) to discuss plan of care *to provide continuity of care and to build trust relationships with patient and family.*

Injury, potential for, related to medications, their side effects, and treatments with hot and cold applications

- Assess knowledge and understanding of purposes for specific medications and use of hot and cold applications *to determine patient's current education needs.*
- Provide a written list of common side effects of patient's medications, along with expected action of the medications *to increase patient's comfort and knowledge.*
- Discuss measures to lessen side effects of medications, such as enteric coatings, taking with food or sufficient fluids, or use of antacids.
- Discuss responsibility of patient to report occurrence of side effects to physician or nurses *for safe care.*
- Discuss expected actions and purposes of hot and cold applications; provide written list of actions *to increase patient's understanding and compliance.*
- Clarify specific methods for prescribed applications *to increase knowledge and compliance.*
- Discuss safety factors related to use of heat and cold because of patient's skin or joint conditions *to increase safe care for patient.*
- Remind patient to report untoward responses, such as increased pain, blistering, or stiffness, *to prevent injury to susceptible tissues.*

Coping, ineffective, individual, related to depression of chronic illness of R.A.

- Assess for signs of mild, moderate, or severe depression; *mild:* sadness; dejected appearance; needs extra effort to concentrate or do usual activities; *moderate:* inability to experience joy; feelings of powerlessness, lack of energy; pessimistic; sleep disturbances; slowed speech and thought processes; *severe:* despair, hopelessness, emptiness; limited ability to respond to teaching, stimuli, or do life-sustaining activities; anorexia; constipation; decreased libido.
- Ascertain from patient if the patient has suicidal ideations *to provide safe care.*

- Ascertain patient's ability to do self-care: grooming, hygiene, nutrition, and elimination *to determine present status of depression.*
- Observe patient's interactions with health professionals, family members, friends: does patient initiate or wait to be addressed?
- Discuss patient's perceptions of rheumatoid arthritis as a chronic condition and outlook on treatments *to find areas of concern to patient.*
- Encourage patient to express expectations of self, family members, health care professionals *to determine feelings of being wanted, appreciated, or tolerated, anger, or other feelings.*
- Ascertain patient's ability or desire to participate in goal setting *to determine patient's self-esteem or sense of passiveness.*
- Monitor patient's energy level and sleep patterns *to determine depth of depression or need for protective measures.*
- Assist with self-care activities and make decisions for patient until energy levels and self-esteem increase *to aid patient's recovery efforts.*
- Provide care for physical symptoms, such as anorexia, constipation, or insomnia, *to demonstrate acceptance of patient's concerns.*
- Prepare patient for any diagnostic tests to determine personality traits or as part of patient interview or history *to provide data for physician's evaluation.* (Tests include symptom checklist 90R, Center for Epidemiologic Studies—Depression Scale, Beck Depression Inventory, and Arthritis Impact Measurement Scale.[84])
- Assist patient to identify people to turn to for assistance *to help patient feel more hopeful and positive.*
- If prescribed, administer antidepressant medication *to aid efforts to overcome depression.*
- When energy level rises, have patient do simple to complex care as condition permits *to strengthen patient's self-esteem and sense of accomplishment.*
- Assist patient to set goals for self and others *to help patient develop realistic expectations for self and others.*
- Seek guidance from health care professionals to help deal with patient's depression *for safe and effective care and environment.*

Altered nutrition: less than body requirements, related to inadequate intake of iron, anorexia, and depression

- Assess mealtime intake for types and amounts of foods; appetite; and presence of nausea, vomiting, or lack of interest in eating.
- Discuss food likes and dislikes *to determine if changes are needed.*
- Weigh daily before breakfast *to note weight losses or gains.*
- Provide oral hygiene before meals *to enhance taste for foods.*

- Encourage eating of 4 to 6 smaller meals daily instead of 3 large ones *to conserve energy because eating smaller meals is less fatiguing.*
- Discuss, and assist patient to select from menu, iron-containing foods *to increase iron intake to lessen anemia.*
- Clarify that iron absorption is increased by intake of orange juice, and provide when taking medication *to lessen anemia.*
- Provide food or milk when administering nonsteroidal antiinflammatory medications *to reduce or prevent gastric irritation.*
- Provide snack at bedtime *to aid intake and lessen effects of gastric secretions on empty stomach.*
- Utilize health care professionals for guidance to deal with patient's depression to provide safe and effective care and environment.

Knowledge deficit related to disease and progression

- Assess knowledge and understanding of disease.
- Explain inflammatory process *to increase understanding.*
- Explain the different treatments and their purposes *to increase compliance.*
- Provide a quiet environment *to aid teaching/learning process.*

Patient Education/Home Care Planning

1. Reiterate explanations of chronicity and controllability of rheumatoid arthritis and its symptoms to aid understanding.
2. Reiterate necessity for patient compliance with treatment regimen for maximum benefits.
3. Discuss with patient and family members each medication and common side effects to be noted or reported to the physician.
4. Encourage patient to participate actively and fully in each aspect of the disease, its treatments, and alternatives for long-term care.
5. Explain the necessity for cooperative family relationships in the patient's care and treatments to maintain self-worth and role relationships.
6. Teach foods needed for a balanced diet.
7. Explain community resources to deal with future depressive episodes, if they occur.

Evaluation

Patient experiences only mild anxiety   Patient's anxiety is relieved by repeated explanations and physician visits over time.

Patient has a satisfactory tolerance of daily activities   Patient can maintain ADL with mild restrictions of lifting because of limited strength and slight joint deformities.

Patient has adequate pain relief   Patient has long, pain-free periods when complying with analgesic regimen.

Patient can maintain activities at home   Patient has learned to use modified utensils to maximize muscle strengths. Patient can use home appliance by self.

Patient has satisfactory physical mobility   Patient can walk several miles daily with assistive aid. Patient can walk up and down stairs, using the railing for support. Patient uses aquatherapy daily.

Patient has long periods of sleep   Patient has 6 to 7 hours of restful sleep at night. Patient can return to sleep after changing position.

Patient has manageable side effects from medications   Patient experiences no injury from hot/cold applications.

Patient regains positive outlook   Depression is treated with appropriate medications. The patient sets realistic goals.

Patient has intake of iron-containing foods and proteins to overcome anemia   Patient has normal hematocrit (over 33%) and hemoglobin (over 12 g). Patient has increased appetite and eats 4 to 6 small meals per day. Patient has not lost weight and is maintaining satisfactory weight for size, age, and sex.

Patient has a positive body image and has returned to usual roles   Patient verbalizes acceptance of rheumatoid arthritis and its possible progression over time. Patient has slowly regained roles in family hierarchy and usual behaviors.

Patient maintains physical mobility over time   Patient moves slowly and deliberately with use of cane or other assistive device. Patient can walk recreationally for 1 to 2 miles several times a week. Demonstrates proper use of assistive devices. Medications and massage ease backache.

OSTEOMYELITIS

Osteomyelitis is an infection of the bone and its marrow.

Osteomyelitis concerns those who have a fractured bone and an open wound. It may start by direct invasion into bone tissues from the open wound or fractured bone (exogenous spread), or it may spread from an infected throat or from bacterial pneumonia to a distant site in the host bone (hematogenous spread). Long-standing or inadequately treated osteomyelitis can be destructive and life threatening.

Some of the major organisms causing osteomyelitis are *Staphylococcus aureus, Streptococcus pneumoniae, Escherichia coli, Pseudomonas aeruginosa,* and *Haemophilus influenzae.* Children usually develop osteomyelitis from hematogenous spread from a sore throat. Adolescents and adults develop it from direct invasion after trauma and surgical procedures. Sickle cell disease also predisposes the person to osteomyelitis after a "sickling" episode in which ischemia may lead to necrosis of bone.[97] Some persons with pulmonary tuberculosis also develop osteomyelitis of joints or vertebra. Persons with pressure sores may develop osteomyelitis in underlying bones.[40]

• • • • • Pathophysiology

The invading organisms travel to the site within the metaphysis (the part of the bone between the shaft and the epiphyseal area). The longer and larger the bone, the more susceptible it is to osteomyelitis. The metaphysis provides a secluded, warm, well-nourished area in which the organisms can grow and multiply. The pathogens produce pus, which at first remains localized and confined. As more purulent matter is produced, the enlarging mass blocks blood flow in the bone, causing an area of infarction and causing the bone to become necrotic. An inflammatory response to the mass and necrotic tissue brings polymorphonuclear macrophages to the site to combat the pathogens. Purulent matter continues to be produced, and the enlarging mass spreads out of the confined area, through the cortex of the bone, into contiguous tissues, and into the bone marrow. Pain ensues as the mass presses against the rigid walls of the infected bone. The exudate matter flows through the least resistant pathways to the skin surface through a sinus tract. The infected bone attempts to keep the infection localized by forming new bone trabeculae called involucrum (the necrotic or dead bone tissues are called sequestrum). The infection spreads into the bone marrow, along fascial planes in the affected area, and to the skin through the sinus tract. The weakened, infected bone may fracture, and the patient may be hesitant to move, may have pain or soreness, and may experience edema or increased warmth in the area as the osteoclasts attempt to destroy or resorb small, dead, sequestered bone. Large sequestra must be surgically removed because they are a source for continued infection (Figure 4-15). Osteomyelitis may spread to a joint, leading to septic arthritis, or to the vertebra, especially if the osteomyelitis is due to tuberculosis.[129]

Occasionally, a Brodie's abscess may develop in an area of osteomyelitis if the pathogenic organisms are insufficient in number or virulence to lead to a full-scale infection. The macrophages enclose the area, and a cold abscess forms, surrounded by fibrous (scar) tissue and a ring of dense bone. The pathogens inside the abscess may remain alive and virulent. If so, they may flare up and cause a reinfection, or they may die. The resultant cavity will eventually fill with serum or blood.

Osteomyelitis may become subacute or chronic related to incomplete resolution of the initial infection, which occurs in 15% to 30% of patients.[129] Children and adolescents may also develop chronic recurrent multifocal osteomyelitis with multiple sites of bone involvement.[147]

• • • • • Diagnostic Studies and Findings

History   Antecedent infection or open trauma in the previous 3 to 4 weeks; history of pulmonary tuberculosis; sickle cell disease

Physical examination   Area of tenderness, edema, warmth, redness, and possibly mass or drainage near the ends of long bones; increased pain with movement or weight; spiking fevers in 39° to 40° C (103° to 104° F) range intermittently noted, chills, and diaphoresis; headache and nausea; fracture of involved bone; presence of open pressure sore or puncture wound of foot

Aspiration of mass   May aspirate purulent material

Culture of mass or drainage   Infecting pathogenic organisms: bacteria or fungi; an increasing number of joint-replacement patients have fungal infections[119]

White blood cell count   Elevated with increased levels of polymorphonuclear neutrophils (PMNs) indicative of bacterial infection

Erythrocyte sedimentation rate   Increased

X-rays   Initially may not reveal the destructive processes but will later show rarefaction of the involved bone with evidence of formation of sequestrum and involucrum; chest x-ray may reveal lesions of tuberculosis

CT scan   May show spread along fascial planes into surrounding tissues

Serum cultures   Pathogenic organism, most commonly *S. aureus*—55% of cases[129]

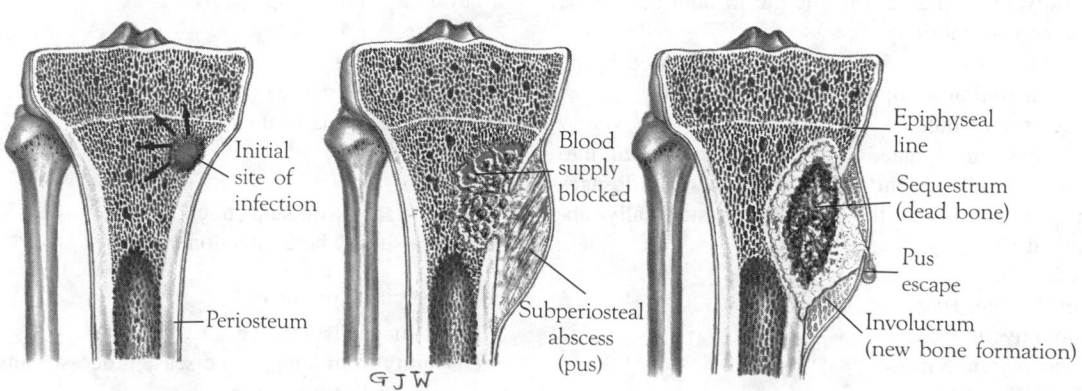

Figure 4-15 Development of osteomyelitis infection with involucrum sequestrum. Infection begins in metaphyseal area of bone. (From Mourad.[104])

Magnetic resonance imaging May show soft tissue mass or sinus tract, bone marrow changes, or vertebral osteomyelitis

Bone scan May show "hot" area of inflammation or "cold" area if the bone is avascular at the time of the scan[43]

•••••• Multidisciplinary Plan

Surgery

Aspiration of abscess for culture purposes only

After "sterilization" of abscess, sequestrum is removed and replaced by bone grafts

Saucerization is performed: involved bone is scraped to remove all necrotic cells, after which bone regenerates; if the defect is pronounced, bone grafts may be applied or metallic fixation may be applied (never used in infected areas or if uncertainty exists about the possibility of lingering pathogens remaining)

External fixation devices such as Hoffman or Ilizarov apparatus (pp. 436 to 439) may be used to hold bones weakened from the initial infection, from saucerization during treatments, or from fracture

Amputation of limb (done less frequently now because of improved treatment modalities)

Removal of implants until infection is cleared

Reaming of intramedullary canal for long-term chronic osteomyelitis[111]

Oxygen Therapy

Hyperbaric oxygen therapy: 100% oxygen at 2 atmospheres pressure for 2 hours 6 times a week, given in hyperbaric chamber

Medications

Antibiotics/Antibacterials
  Children
    Oxacillin 150 mg/kg/d for staphylococcal organisms
    Cefazolin 100 mg/kg/d if child allergic to penicillins
    Clindamycin 25 mg/kg/d
    Vancomycin 40 mg/kg/d if allergic to both penicillins and cephalosporins[43]
    Antibiotics given for 5 to 10 days IV, followed by po administration for up to 6 wk
  Adolescents and adults
    Antibiotics impregnated in bone and cemented into beads for placement at site of infection (dosages are large because they are not systemically absorbed[119])
    Cefazolin or moxalactam, 6 g
    Cefotaxime, 10 g
    Tobramycin, 9.6 g
    Vancomycin, 5 g
    Ticarcillin, 12 g
    Ciprofloxacin, po or IV for 4 to 6 weeks, individualized dose (IV 2 wk, 4 wk po or longer)

For fungal osteomyelitis
  Fluconazole or itraconazole, individualized dose
Analgesics/antipyretics
  Acetaminophen, 325-500 mg q4h prn
  Aspirin, 500-650 mg, 1-2 tabs q4h prn (Only for adolescents 18 or over to avoid Reye's syndrome)
  Oxycodone (Percodan), 15 to 60 mg q4h prn
  Morphine, 10-15 mg q4h po or IM for severe pain

General Management

Splints to decrease joint pain

Bed rest to conserve energy

Sling for the arm, if site of infection is in arm

Cast to prevent a fracture of weakened bones; should have "windows" for dressing changes, if needed

Frequent dressing changes of draining area

Frequent checks of external fixation apparatus, if in use

Ambulation to maintain muscle and joint strength after initial bed rest

Ilizarov fixator to prevent pathologic fracture of weakened bone

As condition permits, child may be taken to playroom

NURSING CARE

Nursing Assessment

Inflammatory Processes

Redness

Increased warmth at site

Edema

Tenderness on use or palpation of involved bone

Mild to severe pain or sharp pain with bone fracture

Affected part may not be used or have decreased ROM

May have palpable mass or sinus tract

Systemic Processes

Fever and chills; diaphoresis

Malaise

Weakness

Headache and nausea

Concurrent or past infection

Spread

Local tissues with sinus tract

Distant sites, where infection continues

Psychosocial Concerns

Body image disturbance

Disability from long-term disease processes and compliance with medication regimen

Concern about possible amputation

Economic cost

Nursing Dx & Intervention

Impaired physical mobility related to bone involvement

- Assess effects on mobility and joint use.
- Encourage ROM to unaffected joints *to decrease tiredness and prevent weakening.*
- Encourage self-care *to maintain muscle strength.*
- Encourage hobby and diversionary activities *to maintain motion and strength in all uninvolved joints.*
- Use wheelchair or crutches *to aid ambulation if necessary and to increase socialization.*

Body temperature, altered, actual and risk for elevations of, related to infection in bone and soft tissue

- Assess body temperature and other vital signs q4h as prescribed; assess presence and amount of wound drainage.
- Administer prescribed antipyretic medication *to reduce hyperpyrexia if present.* Antipyretics will mask fevers.
- Monitor for diaphoresis and patient's response to drop in fever; change clothing and bed linens as needed *to maintain skin integrity.*
- Monitor for additional signs of pyrexia: flushed skin, headache, malaise, sleepiness, or restlessness *to determine patient's reaction to fever and infection.*
- Maintain room temperature; keep consistently in normal temperature (70° to 74° F [21° to 23.3° C]) *to aid patient's comfort.*
- Provide light bed covers only *to lessen possible elevation of temperature* from excess covers.
- Provide adequate fluid replacement *to prevent dehydration.*
- Record and report temperature elevations as necessary.

Pain related to presence of abscess in bone and soft tissue

- Assess for amount, site, severity, and duration of pain.
- Maintain bed rest or limited activity *to lessen stress on involved tissues* (initially).
- Administer analgesics as prescribed *to relieve pain.*
- Handle affected limb gently *to lessen pressure and pain.*
- Use sling when appropriate for arm infections.
- Administer intravenous antibiotics in collaboration with physician *to clear infection and thereby lessen pain.* Monitor patient's response.
- Use care when initiating intravenous therapy per physician prescription and during therapy *to preserve venous integrity for long-term need* (therapy may be via a central venous catheter).
- Use care to maintain asepsis of all equipment *to prevent nosocomial infection.*
- Encourage activities to divert attention from condition (e.g., with children, take to playroom, outside).

Infection, risk for spread related to pathogens and site of osteomyelitis

- Assess site of infection: observe for local changes (sinus tract with purulent drainage; palpate contiguous tissues and joints for signs of inflammation or infection.
- Listen to patient's complaints of pain in back or joints distant to initial site of osteomyelitis *to determine if infection has spread,* especially if infection is due to tubercle bacilli.
- Monitor patient's body temperature *to determine if infection is systemic.*
- Monitor initial infection site for increase in drainage and patient's hesitancy to use part *to determine if infection is abating or increasing.*
- Monitor serum hematologic study or culture results *to determine if patient's defenses are responding to the infectious process;* check complete blood count, including hematocrit and hemoglobin, blood or wound culture results, and antibiotic sensitivity data.
- Use universal precautions *to prevent spread of infection to others or patient.*
- Wash hands after patient contacts *to prevent nosocomial infection.*

Altered peripheral tissue perfusion related to surgery or oxygen therapy

- Perform postoperative neurovascular checks (see p. 358) *to determine tissue perfusion in affected areas.*
- Note skin color and condition of wound after each treatment in hyperbaric chamber.
- Monitor patient's response to being in enclosed chamber for hyperbaric therapy (may become claustrophobic) *for greatest patient benefits.*
- Remove jewelry, watch, synthetic clothing, and perfume before hyperbaric therapy *for patient safety and to prevent possible combustion.*

Impaired skin integrity related to incision and surgery

- Assess skin surfaces *for wound closure and condition.*
- Remove splint *for care and to check skin condition.*
- Change dressings as needed *to remove drainage and to lessen odor and skin maceration.*
- Reposition patient every 2 hours *to maintain healthy skin tissues.*
- Massage skin areas *to increase tissue perfusion.*

Body image disturbance related to pathology

- Assess concerns related to condition or treatments.
- Explain rationale for long-term therapy *to clear disease.*
- Assess equipment (splint, Hoffman or Ilizarov apparatus, etc.) for proper functioning, as well as patient's responses, *to monitor effects of treatments.*
- If amputation is required, do preoperative preparation, allowing patient to talk about concern over loss of

body part. After amputation, do necessary care to promote wound healing and prevent complications (see p. 410).

- Encourage patient and family interaction *to maintain relationships and usual roles.*

Anxiety related to economic costs of prolonged treatments

- Assess patient's and family's verbalized concern about cost of treatments, hospitalization, lack of insurance, or extent of insurance imbursement.
- Assess for signs of anxiety, such as sighing, crying, wringing hands, restlessness, apprehension, irritability, ability to listen, and ability to understand explanations.
- Provide privacy to discuss concerns *to learn extent of problems.*
- Maintain a safe and quiet atmosphere.
- If a child patient, take child to playroom for supervision while discussing concerns with parents *to lessen child's anxiety.*
- Teach or explain to patient and family self-care activities *to help ease anxiety.*
- Seek consultation with social worker for explanation of financial or home care needs *to lessen anxiety or seek solutions.*
- Discuss option of home care with patient and family *to provide a sense of control of future care or needs.*
- Discuss home care needs with community health nurse *to determine feasibility of home treatment plan or regimen.*
- Secure home care equipment, if needed, and teach patient and family how to use and maintain *for safe care.*
- Discuss community resources available for family's use such as Meals on Wheels, Home I.V. Therapy Team, and others *to ease anxiety about home care.*

Patient Education/Home Care Planning

1. Reiterate the need for prompt medical attention to local or systemic infections to prevent the recurrence or the spread of infection; discuss how osteomyelitis occurs.
2. Discuss the rationale, purposes, and expected outcomes for long-term antibiotic therapy to increase the patient's understanding and compliance.
3. Discuss home care for long-term IV antibiotic treatments and other home care needs as necessary.
4. List the side effects of long-term antibiotic therapy, and clarify with patients and family.
5. Discuss purposes for continuing ROM exercises to maintain strength and mobility.
6. Use pictures to clarify characteristics of the hyperbaric oxygen chamber and the external fixator.
7. Discuss community resources available for care or financial aid.

Evaluation

Patient's temperatures are within normal ranges Wound drainage has ceased.

Patient has experienced relief of pain   Patient takes no analgesic for pain. Patient states that no longer has pain in wound site at any time.

Patient has satisfactory mobility   Patient walks about easily without aid. Patient has no muscle or joint soreness.

Patient has satisfactory tissue integrity   Patient has well-healed, 3-inch scar on right lateral surface of thigh. Patient has no tenderness, numbness, or unusual skin color at site. Patient's neurovascular checks are all in normal limits.

Patient has no evidence of continuing infection   Patient has no wound drainage and wound is healing well. Vital signs and laboratory data are within normal ranges.

Patient has regained skin integrity (see Nursing Dx & Intervention for impaired skin integrity)   Patient's scar edges are approximated with scar, remaining slightly pink. Patient has no skin lesions or pressure areas.

Patient has a positive body image   Patient is outward looking, in high spirits, eager for new experiences, and seems to have no fear of recurrent disease.

Patient's and family's anxiety has markedly lessened Restlessness no longer; no crying noted; responses to questions are pertinent to discussion. Family's financial concerns have been addressed by appropriate personnel. Patient and family are looking forward to discharge and home treatments.

DEGENERATIVE CONDITIONS

As people age, they experience some musculoskeletal conditions resulting from degeneration. Even though such conditions may begin in a specific tissue, such as the cartilage or bone, they affect not only that tissue but also other musculoskeletal tissues because of their anatomic and physiologic interrelationships. Therefore these conditions have local and systemic effects, as do the conditions previously discussed.

Age-related changes in the feet are listed in Table 4-3.

HALLUX VALGUS

Hallux valgus is deviation of the great toe toward the other toes.

In hallux (great toe) valgus, the great toe deviates toward the other toes either from congenital abnormality or from tendon and ligament degeneration caused by increasing weight and weight-bearing activities. The forefoot becomes splayed (spread out), allowing the first metatarsal bone to deviate into a more varus position (Figure 4-16).

Usually hallux valgus is bilateral, with one side more prominent and symptomatic than the other. It is most commonly

TABLE 4-3 Age-Related Changes in Feet

Tissue	Common Changes
Skin	Dryness; atrophy; hyperkeratosis (marked thickening, especially skin of heels and balls of feet); cracking, scaling; corns, calluses; ulcerations
Bones	Osteoporosis with diffuse osteopenia
Toenails	Onychauxis (thickened and discolored nails) Onychocryptosis (ingrown nails) Onychomycosis (fungal infections of nails) Corns on top of or between toes
Ligaments and tendons	Tendinitis; rupture of tendon (Achilles); claw or hammer toes; overlapping toes; weakened ligaments; bursitis retrocalcaneal (above heel); tendinitis of tibialis posterior tendon; flattening of arch; splaying of toes and metatarsal bones, mid-foot pronation
Joints	Hallux valgus; hallux rigidus; joint instability
Nerves and circulation	Acrocyanosis (blue color) of feet; cold feet; ulcerations; hair loss; smooth skin; inelastic skin; edema; nail dystrophy; limb or foot ischemia leading to gangrene; paresthesia; numbness

noted in women during the sixth decade, with a strong familial tendency. Adolescents also may have hallux valgus (hallux refers to the great toe and valgus refers to lateral deviation away from the midline).

The etiology of hallux valgus remains controversial related to its basis in wearing constrictive footwear or having a genetic basis. Its genetic role was first addressed in 1925,[33] but studies have continued to yield conflicting information about genetic influence. It is possible that juvenile hallux valgus is transmitted as an autosomal dominant trait, but it is also possible that it may be passed as an X-linked dominant trait or as a polygenic trait, and studies are presently ongoing to determine whether constrictive footwear merely aggravates hallux valgus or if a significant hereditary predisposition is the major causative factor in its development.[33]

•••••• Pathophysiology

Hallux valgus is most obvious from the increasing prominence and deformity of the first metatarsal bone, with this bone's shaft deviated medially away from the second metatarsal. The head of the first metatarsal bone develops a protective bursa (bunion) wherever it rubs against a shoe. As the valgus deformity of the proximal phalanx of the great toe increases, the second toe is crowded and may also become deformed.

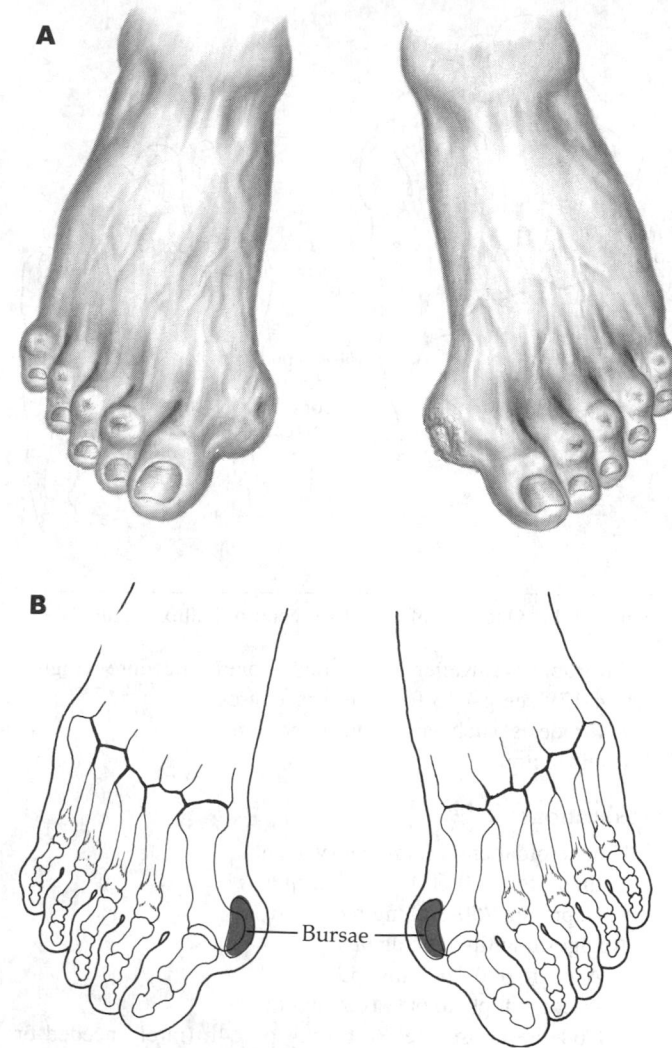

Figure 4-16 Hallux valgus with bunion. **A**, External view. **B**, Anatomic view. (From Mourad.[104])

•••••• Diagnostic Studies and Findings

Physical examination   Valgus deformity of great toe, with or without bursa development (bunion), hammer toe, corns, calluses, and often bilateral; great toe and second toe may be over or under each other; forefront splaying bilaterally; arch of foot weakened (may show "flat" foot); tailor's bunion may be present at the outer base of the small toe

X-ray   Deformities described above

History   Familial occurrence, primarily in mother, rarer in father

•••••• Multidisciplinary Plan

Surgery

   Osteotomy to realign bones, such as Mitchell osteotomy or other osteotomy

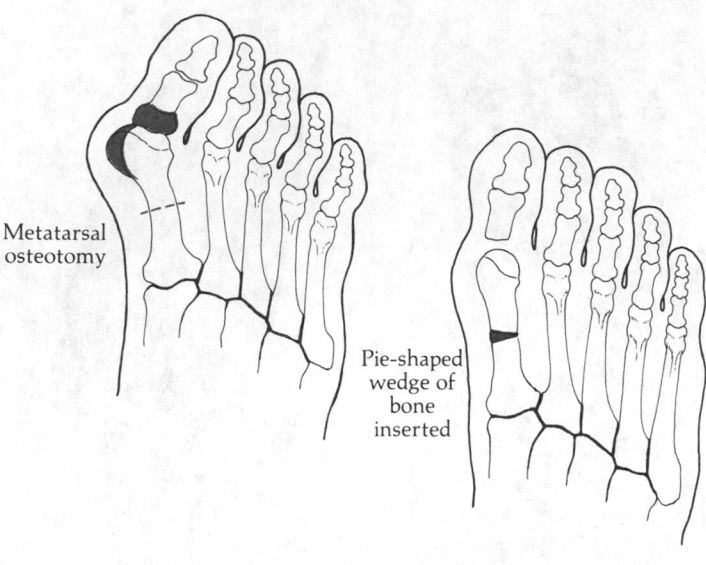

Metatarsal
osteotomy

Pie-shaped
wedge of
bone
inserted

Figure 4-17 One type of operative repair of hallux valgus.

Arthroplasty: Keller operation; Stone procedure (Figure 4-17); see p. 415 for other procedures
Arthrodesis, such as Lapidus operation
Bunionectomy

Medications

Nonsteroidal antiinflammatory agents
  Ibuprofen 400-600 mg tid or qid
  Naproxen 250-500 mg bid or tid
Analgesic-antipyretic agents
  Aspirin, 600-1000 mg qid
  Acetaminophen, 600-1000 mg qid
  Codeine phosphate, 30-60 mg po q4h (rarely needed or used because of side effects)

General Management

Taping pad under metatarsal heads to change weight-bearing pressure
Changing shoe style to wider, open-toed shoe with soft upper portions, cushioned sole
Foot exercises to lessen splayfoot
Application of ice bag to site of bunion
Form-fitting insole in shoe to cushion foot
Use of toe pad over corn or bunion
Custom-molded shoes occasionally necessary

NURSING CARE

Nursing Assessment

Signs of Degeneration

Valgus (away from midline) deformity of great toe and varus deformity of first metatarsal bone; splaying of metatarsal bones

Presence of bunion on great toe
Corn development from pressure on other toes; may have corns between toes
Deformity or crowding of second toe
Hammer toe possible in other toes
Callus possible under metatarsal heads of other toes
Possible presence of tailor's bunion at base of small toe
Toenails: thickened, discolored; may have ingrown toenails; fungal infections

Other Accompanying Signs

Presence of inflamed bursa, producing tenderness and often exquisite pain in and around joint (metatarsophalangeal joint of great toe)
Condition usually bilateral
Hallux rigidus: painful hallux valgus with marked movement limitations
Skin appearance: may be dry, itching, loss of patches of skin, if vigorous scratching; hyperkeratosis of heel with marked thickening; cracks in heel areas

Psychosocial Concerns

Concern with body image from deformity and pain
Concern with need to change shoe styles and sizes

Nursing Dx & Intervention

Impaired physical mobility related to pain and deformity

- Assess effects of condition on mobility and body image.
- Encourage use of padding in shoes *to change weight-bearing sites.*
- Encourage usual activities when pain is relieved *to increase mobility.*
- Encourage consulting with physician to remove bursa if necessary *to relieve condition and increase mobility.*
- Encourage consultation with physician or podiatrist for need to change shoe styles or sizes *to decrease progression of foot abnormalities.*

Pain related to bunion, inflammation, and deformity

- Assess amount, duration, site, and severity of pain.
- Administer ordered medication *to ease discomfort.*
- Teach side effects of medications.
- Apply ice bag to inflamed bursa *to lessen edema and pain.*
- Encourage temporary cessation of weight bearing when pain is acute *to increase comfort.*
- Encourage wearing of shoes with wider box and soft tops *to increase comfort and lessen pressure on tender areas.*

Body image disturbance related to deformities

- Assess concerns about presence of hallux valgus.
- Encourage wearing of well-fitted footwear *to lessen progression.*

- Encourage consulting with physician for possible surgical removal *to aid in positive feeling.*
- Encourage exercises *to lessen progressive deformity.*
- Consult physician for placement or use of orthoses in shoes *to lessen effects of deformities.*

Patient Education/Home Care Planning

1. Clarify bunion as accompanying hallux valgus.
2. Instruct about preventive measures with proper footwear, use of orthoses, and exercises.
3. Explain surgical options previously discussed with physician, if necessary, for clarity.
4. Provide list of medication side effects and instruct to notify physician if any occur.
5. Teach care of the feet to prevent infection or deal with age-related changes.

Evaluation

Patient walks without deformity of toe joint Patient uses orthotic devices as ordered, wears well-fitted shoes, applies ice during acute inflammation, and rests the joint. Patient undergoes surgical correction if necessary to relieve deformity and regain painless mobility.

Patient's pain and inflammation are relieved Surgical procedure removes bunion and corrects toe alignment, thereby relieving pain. Orthoses ease discomfort of splay foot. Side effects of medications are few and manageable.

Patient has positive body image Better-looking feet have a positive effect on patient's body image.

Patient states principles and practices for proper foot care Keep skin of feet clean and dry; dry between toes after cleansing; apply moisturizing lotion to prevent drying or cracking. Check feet daily to note early signs of inflammation or pressure. Wear properly fitted shoes with low heels. Alternate shoes to permit shoes to dry between uses.

■ OSTEOARTHRITIS

Osteoarthritis (OA) is a condition characterized by degenerative changes initially in the cartilage covering the ends of bones, primarily in the major weight-bearing joints: hip and knee.

The development of OA involves a process of changes taking place initially in the joint cartilage. The exact cause or causes for these changes have not been determined; however, in 1990 several researchers reported locating the gene that might be associated with OA cartilage degradation. This gene may not allow cartilage to repair itself after injury, causing the cartilage to wear down (erode) more easily. The exact role of the gene has not been determined.

Osteoarthritis is a disease of older persons. More than 50 million Americans are affected. It is the most prevalent clinical entity within the domain of the orthopedist.[92] More women than men are affected, and the incidence increases after women experience menopause and after aging progresses. Nearly 100% of persons 75 and older have OA. It occurs in all countries and climates. Obesity is thought to play some part in the degenerative changes, although its exact role has not been determined.

Osteoarthritis is either primary (idiopathic) or secondary to joint effects from trauma, metabolic conditions, and endocrine conditions.

•••••• Pathophysiology

Osteoarthritis is characterized by successive destruction of the musculoskeletal tissues of the affected joint. Early changes in the normal, whitish, smooth hyaline cartilage include an increase in its water content and a decrease in the amount of proteoglycan (complex protein-carbohydrate molecules). The cartilage looks irregular and pitted and is softer. It undergoes fibrillation, and cartilage flakes (detritus) are shed into the joint. This shedding rubs away the cartilage, primarily from sites where the maximum load is greatest. Repeated wear and erosion thin the cartilage.

Although the cartilage is not rubbed away or thinned in nonstress areas, it is unhealthy from undernourishment. Cartilage is nourished during compression by synovial fluid and transudates from subchondral vessels. This pumping action does not occur in nonstress areas, so there is undernourishment. The subchondral vessels hypertrophy and invade the cartilage, which calcifies and later ossifies, forming osteophytes. The hyperemia spreads into the bone beneath the stress area, but pressure in this area prevents the vessels from penetrating into the cartilage. The cartilage continues to be rubbed away, exposing the underlying bone. Stress (fatigue) fractures occur in the subchondral trabeculae, and cysts and osteophytes develop where pressure is greatest. Bone ends become reshaped or remodeled as OA develops.

During cartilage erosion, detritus is deposited on the synovial lining, which then hypertrophies. Flakes of cartilage also penetrate into the subsynovial layer, where they induce fibrosis that extends into the capsule. The ligaments and tendons of the capsule become thickened, inelastic, and stiff. The fibrous tissue shrinks as it matures, thereby limiting joint movement and causing deformity (Figure 4-18). Thus all the joint tissues—cartilage, bone, synovium, ligaments, tendons, muscles, and skin—are involved in OA.

Restriction of movement resulting from fibrosis is the main feature of osteoarthritis. Symptoms appear early in joints such as the hip, where full extensions and stability are required for walking. Because the hip joint capsule is well supplied with pain fibers, slight restriction is noted by pain with attempts at full extension. Thus major weight-bearing joints show earlier symptoms. Weight bearing continues as an aggravation in osteoarthritis.

Besides the hip and knee, the carpometacarpal joint at the base of the thumb, the vertebrae and sacroiliac joints, and the distal joints of the fingers are also affected by osteoarthritis.

Limitation of movements and pain are the major symptoms. Pain frequently occurs during and after a night's rest. Usually there are no systemic signs, just the local signs confined to the joints and their contiguous tissues.

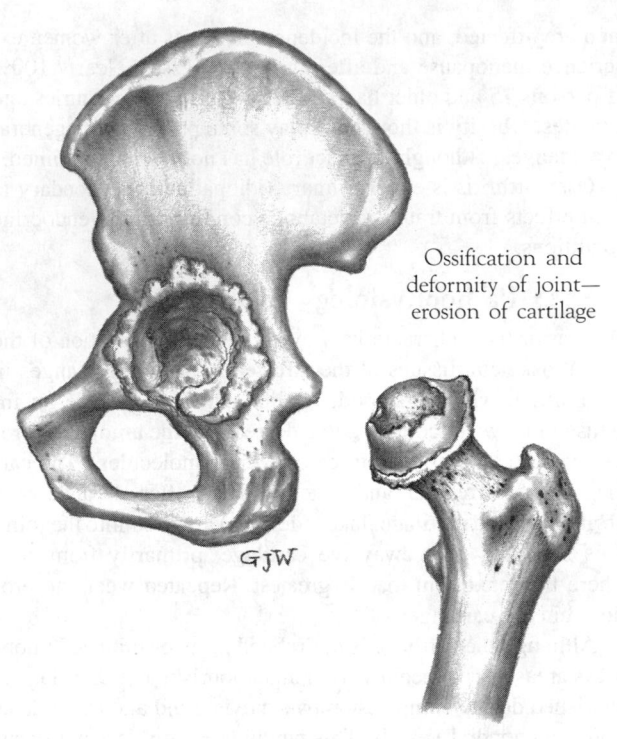

Ossification and deformity of joint— erosion of cartilage

Figure 4-18 Osteoarthritis of hip joint. Note erosion of cartilage from head of femur and osteophytes around acetabulum. (From Mourad.[104])

•••••• Diagnostic Studies and Findings

Physical examination Enlarged edematous joint with some stiffness and deformity; usually only one joint has most pronounced signs, although more than one can be involved; if hip is involved, patient may hold it flexed, adducted, and externally rotated; joint may be tender but rarely feels hot; movements of joint limited; crepitus common; Heberden's nodes may be present in distal interphalangeal joints of fingers, and Bouchard's nodes occur in the proximal interphalangeal joints; gait analysis is done to determine weight-bearing patterns and stability

Erythrocyte sedimentation rate Usually normal; may be elevated in generalized polyarticular OA[4]

X-ray Decreased or diminished joint space; necrotic or sclerotic bone; osteophytes and lipping in some joints; subchondral bone cysts

•••••• Multidisciplinary Plan

Surgery

Arthroscopic debridement of joint
Arthroplasty to repair the joint
Total joint replacement to replace diseased tissues
Osteotomy to change weight-bearing surfaces
Arthrodesis to limit joint movements (done to abolish pain)
Spinal fusion to maintain posture and eliminate pain
Muscle release

Medications

Analgesic-antipyretic agents
  Aspirin (enteric-coated), 600-1000 mg 3-4 times daily
Nonsteroidal antiinflammatory agents
  Ibuprofen (Motrin), 300-400 mg 3-4 times daily
  Naproxen (Naprosyn), 250-375 mg bid
  Tolmetin (Tolectin), 200-400 mg 3-4 times daily
  Indomethacin (Indocin), 25-50 mg 3-4 times daily
  Sulindac (Clinoril), 150-200 mg bid
  Piroxicam (Feldene), 20 mg/d
  Diclofenac (Voltaren), 25-75 mg bid
  Oxaprozin (Daypro), 600-1200 mg/d
  Choline magnesium trisalicylate (Trilisate), 500-1000 mg
    tid or 1500 mg bid

Intraarticular Agents[86]

Betamethasone, 3 mg/ml, 0.25-2.0 ml, based on joint size—
  small, medium, or large
Dexamethasone, 8 mg/ml, 0.5-2.0 ml
Hydrocortisone acetate, 25-50 mg/ml, 0.2-2.0 ml
Prednisolone tebutate, 20 mg/ml, 0.4-2.0 ml
Triamcinolone acetonide, 10-40 mg/ml, 0.25-1.0 ml

General Management

Moist heat applications with diathermy, ultrasound, and radiant heat
Aerobic exercises in water to loosen stiff joints and ease soreness
Rest and modified weight-bearing activities beneficial
Canes, crutches, or walkers to aid walking, decrease joint stress, and increase stability
Soft collar and cervical traction to lessen pain in neck areas
Back brace or support to lessen pain and maintain posture
Elastic bandage to wrist or knee for support; orthosis for knee (brace)
Massage around painful joints
Wearing sturdy, low-heeled shoes
Weight reduction, if overweight

NURSING CARE

Nursing Assessment

Local (Joint) Signs of Degeneration

Limitation of full extension, pain on arising and on weight bearing in joint; gait may be antalgic (pain avoiding)
Pain disturbing sleep as disease progresses
Joint stiffness and deformity from fibrosis, shrinkage, and muscle imbalance
Limp
Joint feels unstable and may give way
Pain radiating to soft tissues around joint
Heberden's nodes on distal phalangeal joints and Bouchard's nodes on proximal phalangeal joints

Systemic Signs

None

Psychosocial Concerns

Body image changes
Pain
Limitation of movement or weight bearing
Loss of socialization/isolation

Nursing Dx & Intervention

Impaired physical mobility related to joint pathology

- Assess ROM, mobility limitations, and gait.
- Encourage and assist with ambulation as needed *to maintain joint functions and mobility.*
- Assist with ADL as needed *to aid in completing activities.*
- Use ambulatory aid as prescribed *to facilitate walking with less discomfort and more stability.*
- Assist with ambulation after pain is relieved with heat or medication *to increase distances and muscle strength.*
- Encourage aerobic exercises in water to increase joint movement without increasing joint stress (immersion in water removes most of effects of gravity on joints).

Pain related to joint pathology and pressure on contiguous tissues

- Assess amount and severity of pain.
- Administer prescribed analgesic or antiinflammatory medications *to lessen pain and aid relaxation.*
- Assess effects of medications for pain relief *to note efficacy.*
- Use heat and diathermy as prescribed *to relieve pain.*
- Discuss other strategies to relieve pain such as imagery, relaxation techniques, and diversion *to increase patient's sense of control over pain episodes.*
- Stress proper posture when walking, standing, or sitting *to aid in proper muscle use.*
- Encourage weight loss, if overweight, *to decrease joint stress.*
- Apply traction or collar if necessary and prescribed *to lessen muscle pain; use knee brace as prescribed.*
- Encourage use of assistive devices *to aid homemaking activities.*

Body image disturbance and altered role performance related to progressive degenerative condition

- Assess effects of condition on ADL.
- Encourage patient to perform usual activities and ADL *for self-esteem and to maintain fitness and strength.*
- Encourage patient to comply with plan of medical care *to lessen joint deformity and decrease pain.*
- Encourage planned rest *to maintain strength.*
- If surgery is contemplated, review and clarify options previously discussed by physician with patient *to lessen anxiety.*
NOTE: Nursing care after surgical treatments for OA begins on p. 417.

NOTE: Nursing care after surgical treatments for OA begins on p. 417.

Patient Education/Home Care Planning

1. Clarify understanding of degenerative nature of this disease and effects on mobility.
2. List side effects of medications; clarify with patient.
3. Caution about effects of heat on less sensitive tissues.
4. Discuss benefits of aerobic exercises in water.
5. Discuss weight loss if overweight.

Evaluation

Patient walks with minimum limitation of motion Patient maintains self-care, ADL, and employment for as long as desired without experiencing uncontrollable pain or joint movement limitations or deformity.

Patient has relief of severe pain Patient takes medications as prescribed without nausea, vomiting, gastrointestinal burning, bleeding, pain, or hematologic changes. Pain is relieved with medications, and joint mobility is enhanced. Patient uses imagery and relaxation techniques periodically.

Patient returns to social interactions, with positive body image Patient returns to usual family, social, and employment roles. Patient engages in aerobic exercises in water alone and in groups.

MUSCULAR DYSTROPHY

The muscular dystrophies consist of a group of x-linked recessively inherited diseases of childhood characterized by progressive weakness and atrophy of symmetric groups of skeletal muscles. The prototype of all muscular dystrophies is Duchenne's muscular dystrophy.

The study of muscle pathology began in 1849 with a paper presented to the French Academy of Science on the subject of progressive muscular atrophy with fatty transformation by a physician named Guillaume-Benjamin-Amaut Duchenne.[50] However, the most rapid strides toward understanding the bases of many muscle pathologic conditions have been made since 1978 with the emergence of molecular genetics[50] and the discovery of the structure of the gene, with the analysis of the human genome, which is still ongoing. Since 1978 the protein product of the muscular dystrophy gene, dystrophin, has been localized to the sarcolemma membrane of muscles. Much research has since been done attempting to devise new treatments for a great many hereditary human diseases.

One group of muscular diseases are the muscular dystrophy diseases listed in Table 4-4, with their sexual and genetic transmission, rates of occurrence of children affected, symptoms, diagnostic studies, and usual treatments. The muscular dystrophy diseases cause degeneration of skeletal muscle fibers by progressive, symmetric weakness and wasting of these muscle groups leading to increasing disability and deformity.

TABLE 4-4 Classifications of Muscular Dystrophy

Type	Sex Affected	Prevalence (Rate of Occurrence)	Symptoms	Diagnostic Studies	Usual Treatments
Duchenne's muscular dystrophy (major)	Males only, X-linked, recessive	1:3500 births	Progressive muscle wasting and weakness leading to difficulty running, stair climbing, rising from the floor without use of the upper extremities for "climbing up the legs" support (positive Gower's sign); may have hypertrophy of calf muscles from fatty degeneration; loss of ability to walk; may develop scoliosis and joint contractures; many have cardiac sinus tachycardia and right ventricular hypertrophy; eventually develop dysrhythmias and heart failure; may have poor gastric motility; moderate mental retardation may be noted; pulmonary failure; waddling gait	Creatine phosphokinase elevated (often up to 100 times normal [normal:cord blood, 70-380 U/L; 5-8 h, 214-1175 U/L; 24-33 h, 130-1200 U/L; 72-100 h, 87-725 U/L]; electrocardiogram may show units of decreased amplitude and short duration; muscle biopsy shows dystrophic degeneration and fibrosis, with some regeneration but no dystrophin; dystrophin immunotesting; DNA mutation analysis by polymerase chain reaction and Southern blot analysis—help determine correct diagnosis; dystrophin RNA testing can detect some DNA mutations; electromyogram shows lack of contractility	Physical therapies; education of patient/family related to use of orthotic devices, braces, wheelchair, exercises, and use of parallel bars; myoblast cell therapy (recent development) with myoblasts injected into muscles of boys with Duchenne's—unknown yet if muscle functions will be restored; prednisone therapy has some short-term benefit to slow progression of muscle weakness; pulmonary breathing exercises; spinal fusion with metallic implants, such as Harrington, Luque, or Cotrel-Dubousset (CD) rods (less use of CD rods)
Becker's muscular dystrophy (milder form of Duchenne's)	Males; X-linked; female carriers	1:30,000 live births	Develops later in childhood than Duchenne's; has longer course and less severe involvement; can usually walk fast and longer in teen years; less muscle degeneration and fewer respiratory problems	Same as for Duchenne's; DNA analysis differentiates Duchenne's from Becker's	Release of contracted muscles of hips, knees, ankles, and feet and tenotomy of tendons; electromyogram shows lack of contractility (same as for Duchenne's but later in course of disease)
Variant of Becker's muscular dystrophy: myalgia without weakness	Males only; female carriers	None noted yet	Milder symptoms than Becker's; less skeletal muscle weakness	Same as above	Individualized according to patient's symptoms; physical therapy, education as above
Emery-Dreifuss muscular dystrophy	Males only, X-linked recessive; female carriers		Muscle weakness in first few years of life; awkward gait; tendency to toe-walk; by the middle of the second decade may see fixed equinus ankle deformities, flexion contracture of the elbows, extension contracture of the neck, tightness of the lumbar paravertebral muscles, and cardiac abnormalities (bradycardia; later complete heart block); patient is able to walk up to ages 50 to 60	Electromyogram shows muscle myopathy; muscle biopsy shows muscle myopathy; creatine phosphokinase: only mild to moderate elevations	Heel-cord lengthening for equinus contracture; transfer of posterior tibial tendon; release of elbow contractures; medications for cardiac involvement and use of a pacemaker if indicated

Type	Inheritance	Clinical Features	Diagnosis	Treatment
Facioscapulohumeral muscular dystrophy	X-linked, autosomal dominant	Slowly progressive weakness of face, shoulder girdle, and shoulder muscle; begins in late childhood or early adulthood; limited abduction of arms; weakness in dorsiflexion of foot; foot drop; weakness of muscles of forearms, thighs, and pelvis; scoliosis is rarer than in other muscular dystrophies; affected person can usually live a full life	Similar to above	Operative stabilization of shoulders to eliminate winging of scapulae; arthrodesis of scapula to ribs with metallic plate and screws; other treatments for individual patient needs
Infantile facioscapulohumeral muscular dystrophy (variant of adult form)	Autosomal recessive	More severe than adult form; infant develops facial diplegia in early months of life; sensorineural hearing loss, often by 5 years of age; scapular winging; lumbar lordosis; foot drop; loss of ability to walk by second decade of life; severe weakness of gluteus maximus muscles		Use of ankle-foot orthosis; heel-cord lengthening; use of spinal orthosis; scapulopexy; use of hearing aid; use of wheelchair; spinal arthrodesis
Limb-girdle muscular dystrophy	Autosomal recessive; autosomal dominant in some families	Shoulder and hip weakness; weak distal muscles of the limbs	Creatine phosphokinase levels may be 10 times higher than normal; electromyogram (EMG) shows myopathy; muscle biopsy shows myopathy	Similar to that for Becker's
Congenital muscular dystrophy (Fukuyama type congenital muscular dystrophy is prevalent in Japanese infants)	Males and females; autosomal recessive	Affected babies are weak at birth; have severe joint stiffness; variable course—some have rapid degeneration and do not survive beyond first year, whereas others live full life expectancy; muscle/joint contractures; Japanese infants have central nervous system involvement	Creatine phosphokinase levels elevated; dystrophin gene or protein have no abnormalities; EMG abnormal; muscle biopsy shows perimysial and endomysial fibrosis	Passive ROM exercises; use of splints; osteotomy rarely done; use of various orthoses
Myotonic dystrophy	Males and females; autosomal dominant	Delayed muscle relaxation (delayed release of hand grip); frontal baldness in affected males; glaucoma in both sexes; normal muscle motor strength	Serum creatine phosphokinase levels normal; EMG shows "dive bomber pattern"—diagnostic of this condition	Treatments are individualized
Congenital myotonic dystrophy		Severe hypotonia; facial diplegia; long, narrow face; problems feeding; respiratory problems; club foot common; many have moderate to severe mental retardation; walking onset delayed	Radiologic studies of feet and lungs, prenatal gene study may show presence of this condition	Use of serial manipulation of feet; cast immobilization; ankle-foot orthosis; possible use of Lofstrand crutches for foot problems; use of foot-leg brace; spinal fusion for scoliosis if develops in adolescence

Data from Shapiro and Specht.[135]

Presently, the majority of children with the major muscular dystrophies rarely live beyond 20 to 25 years of age.

Not only are the skeletal muscles affected in the muscular dystrophies, but also other organs, joints, and bones. Cardiac involvement, smooth muscles, and at times moderate mental retardation may affect some children. Many variations or mutations are now being diagnosed because of DNA and genetic research and studies of the human genome.

•••••• Pathophysiology

The muscular dystrophies listed in Table 4-4 appear to be X-linked recessive genetic diseases. They are associated with progressive muscle degeneration of predominantly male children. Duchenne's muscular dystrophy is the most severe form of muscular dystrophy; it affects 1:3500 boys in early childhood.[163] Mutations of the gene lead to a premature termination of dystrophin, a protein vital to normal muscle function, which is localized to the sarcolemmal membrane covering muscle fibers. Dystrophin is a large protein consisting of domains referred to as A through D. The A and C domains have homology (similarity) with α-actinin, the B domain has homology to spectrin, and the D domain has recently been shown to be homologous to a chromosome 6–encoded dystrophin-like protein.[163] The D domain is essential in the association of dystrophin with the sarcolemma. No dystrophin has been detected in muscle biopsies of patients with Duchenne's muscular dystrophy, whereas in a milder form (Becker's muscular dystrophy) the dystrophin is of abnormal size or quantity. During fetal development, COOH-truncated dystrophin is initially present in the myotubes of fetuses with Duchenne's muscular dystrophy, with the same location as in a normal fetus. It is thought that the COOH-terminal domain of dystrophin is involved in the integration in the plasma membrane and that this domain is missing in the dystrophin of fetuses with Duchenne's muscular dystrophy mutations; it is a plausible proposal that dystrophin is degraded when no integration in the sarcolemma of the muscle cell can take place.[163] Without dystrophin, muscles suffer complete loss of function, resulting in progressive muscle wasting and leading to early death. Dystrophin deficiency probably leads to instability of the plasma membrane of skeletal muscle fibers, with two immediate consequences: leakage of cellular contents out of the cell and influx of extracellular material into the cell.[68] The extremely high muscle creatine kinase (CK) found in dystrophin-deficit species from birth is evidence of the efflux of cytoplasm from muscle fibers. However, the unregulated influx of extracellular material into the myofiber, especially calcium ions, usually leads to cell death. Biochemical and physiologic differences between specific muscle fibers and muscle groups may explain the different degrees of muscle cell death noted.

•••••• Diagnostic Studies and Findings

Physical examination   Marked wasting and muscle weakness progressing to increasing disability, deformity, and eventually death; loss of strength; atrophy of muscle mass; delayed motor development; difficulty in running, climbing, and riding tricycle; abnormal gait; enlarged calves (hypertrophy of muscle with fatty infiltration); positive Gowers' sign: process of rising from sitting or squatting position by using hands to "walk up" thighs until upright (Figure 4-19); mild mental retardation; decreased deep tendon reflexes

X-ray   Contractures of hips, knees, and ankles; lordosis of lumbar spine; scoliosis

Muscle biopsy   Reveals lack of dystrophin, degeneration of muscle fibers; fatty infiltration

Blood serum studies   Greatly elevated CK; serum glutamic-oxaloacetic transaminase (SGOT) levels are sharply elevated

Electromyogram (EMG) studies   Reveal decreased amplitude and duration of motor unit potentials[167]

•••••• Multidisciplinary Plan

Surgery

Release of contractures

General Management

Gentle ROM exercises to maintain functions
Assistance with ADL
Use of brace to affected joints to prevent contractures
Consultation with Muscular Dystrophy Association for guidance and support as needed
Use of wheelchair for movement from place to place
Home teaching for educational progress
Specialized nursing assistants as muscular weakness progresses for home care
Nutritional guidance as needed
Genetic counseling

NURSING CARE

Nursing Assessment

Whole Body Assessment

Muscle strength, grip, pull and push strength
Deep tendon reflexes charted
Presence of contractures
Muscle atrophy
Age-related motor development
Gait
Posture: lordosis, scoliosis
Enlarged calves
Age-related mental development

Systemic Processes

Pulmonary functions
Breath sounds
Cardiac size and heart sounds
Systemic infections
Obesity

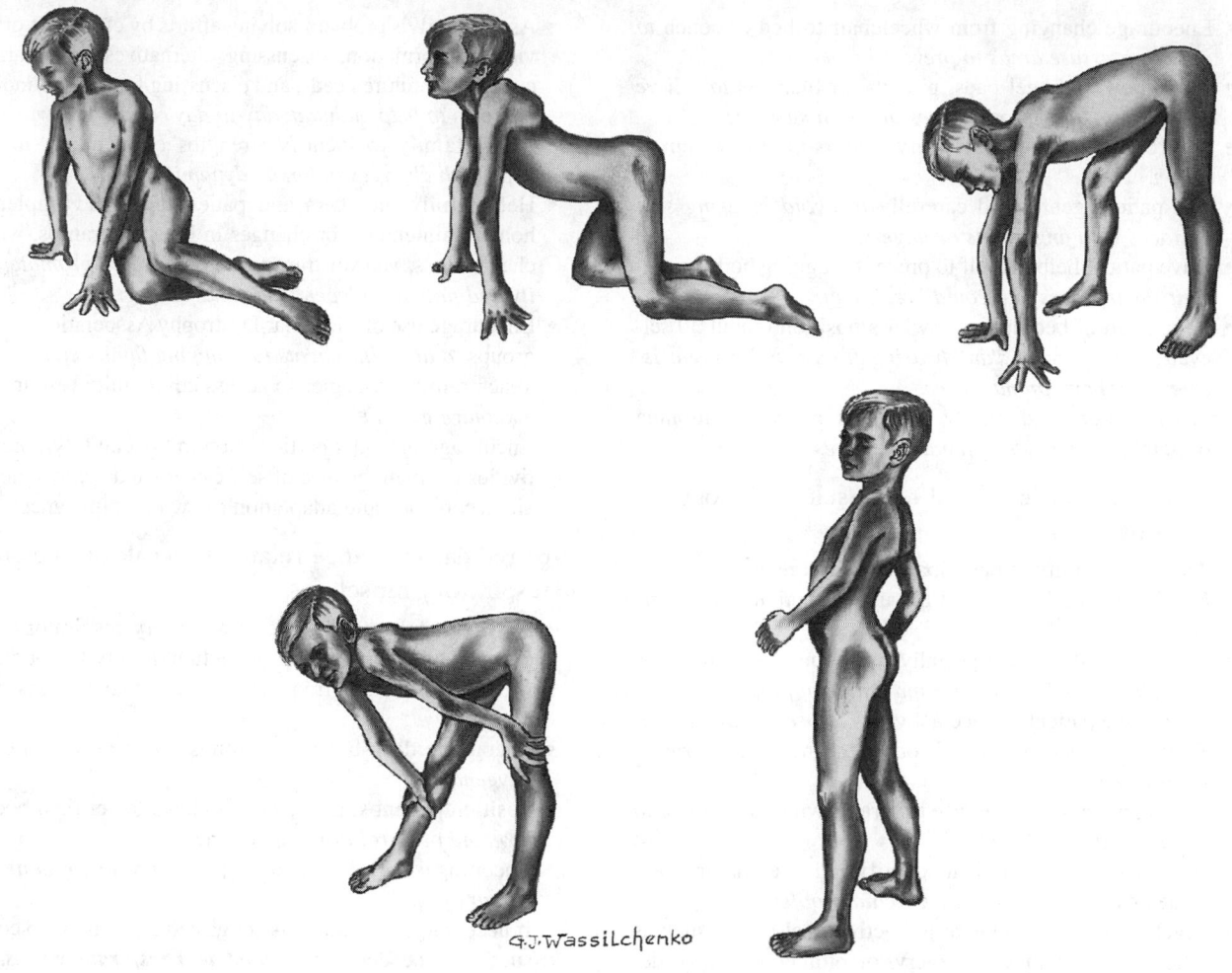

Figure 4-19 Child with Duchenne's muscular dystrophy attains standing posture by assuming a kneeling position, then gradually pushing his torso upright (with knees straight) by "walking" his hands up his legs (Gowers' sign). Note marked lordosis in upright position. (From Wong.[167])

Psychosocial Concerns

Parental guilt related to transmittal of disease
Self-concept and independence
Eventual fatal nature of muscular dystrophy
Progressive weakness and muscle atrophy
Loss of social contacts and socialization

Nursing Dx & Intervention

Impaired physical mobility/high risk for disuse syndrome related to progressive muscle wasting and atrophy

- Assess muscle strength or weakness (as listed above).
- Assist with ROM exercises *to maintain functions as able.*
- Assist with ambulation, if needed, *to maintain muscle strength.*
- Provide wheelchair, if muscle weakness is severe, *to conserve energy and assist with mobilization.*
- Encourage child to do ADL as able *to maintain independence and self-esteem.*

- Seek assistance or guidance from Muscular Dystrophy Association *for optimal supportive care to patient and family.*
- Encourage camping activities with other disabled children *to aid in self-identity and socialization.*

Risk for impaired skin integrity related to pressure on bony prominences from wheelchair or brace use

- Assess all skin surfaces and bony prominences carefully.
- Assist to bathe and carefully dry all skin surfaces *to prevent skin abrasion or maceration.*
- Teach patient and family to do "minishifts" *to relieve pressure on bony prominences and skin surfaces.*
- Apply lotion to skin tissues *to help keep skin surfaces supple* and moisturized.
- Encourage fluid intake *to maintain skin hydration.*
- Monitor patient for bowel or bladder incontinence, diarrhea, and excess perspiration *to prevent skin maceration or breakdown.*

- Encourage changing from wheelchair to bed or couch *to change pressure areas to prevent breakdown.*
- Use elbow and heel pads, pillows, or blankets *to relieve pressure on bony prominences and skin surfaces.*
- Turn or reposition patient every 2 hours *to promote circulation.*
- Lift patient gently and carefully *to avoid breaking skin surfaces with fingernails or fingers.*
- Have patient help lift self to prevent dragging body *to prevent shear forces that could break skin.*
- Keep head of bed in low Fowler's position (about 30° elevation) *to prevent skin shearing forces and prevent ischemia of bony prominences.*
- Teach patient and family members proper positioning principles *to provide optimal safe care.*

Activity intolerance related to muscle pathology and weakness

- Assess for ability to participate in self-care activities.
- Monitor strength of patient throughout activities *to determine ability to function.*
- Monitor vital signs, especially pulse and respirations, *to note changes with activities indicative of fatigue.*
- Encourage patient to pace activities *to prevent overtiring.*
- Provide planned rest periods or quiet times *to conserve or restore energy.*
- Assist patient to do exercise programs when well rested *to achieve maximal benefits.*
- Assist patient and family to identify activities that increase or decrease activity tolerance *to aid problem solving.*
- Teach patient strategies to aid activity tolerance, such as relaxation techniques, imagery, or biofeedback (age dependent), *to increase activity tolerance.*
- Encourage family members to promote self-care and independence while monitoring patient's responses *to aid coping behaviors of patient and family.*
- Collaborate with patient and family to develop a daily plan of activities, rest, and quiet times *for optimal patient benefits.*
- Teach family to help patient pace self *to conserve energy.*
- Encourage patient's and family's use of community resources *for maximal care and benefits.*

Altered family processes and coping: potential for growth related to ultimate death of child with muscular dystrophy

- Assist patient and family to identify changes in family situation and dynamics because of illness and its eventual outcome *to determine effects and possible options for change.*
- Assist patient and family to adapt to muscular dystrophy and to continue living rather than dealing with dying *to foster adjustment to muscular dystrophy.*
- Offer support and guidance to help family deal with the stress of an ill child on individual members and the family as a whole *to determine requirements for resources if needed.*

- Assist family's problem-solving efforts by clarifying or providing information, discussing alternatives, summarizing current and future needs, and discussing family and individual roles *to help maintain day-to-day coping behaviors.*
- Assist family to identify strengths of members *to help cope with changes in family dynamics.*
- Help family members and patient plan and implement home maintenance or changes in lifestyle (ramps, wheelchair access, van for transportation, etc.) *to promote family and patient independence and comfort.*
- Encourage use of Muscular Dystrophy Association support groups *to aid adjustments to changing family situation.*
- Teach family strategies to access community resources *to maximize growth.*
- Encourage patient's participation in Special Olympics activities for maintenance of self-esteem and achievement to aid acceptance and adaptation to own circumstances.[57]

Impaired gas exchange related to weak pulmonary or respiratory muscles

- Assess breath sounds, use of accessory respiratory muscles, dyspnea, production of sputum, ability to cough.
- Monitor vital signs frequently *to detect early signs of infection.*
- Encourage deep-breathing exercises *to promote maximal oxygenation.*
- Position patient side to side with head lower than body *to promote postural drainage* if able.
- Encourage use of incentive spirometry *to promote pulmonary functions.*
- If necessary, and patient is congested and unable to cough, suction as needed *to maintain clear respiratory passages.*
- Use aseptic technique for suctioning *to prevent introducing infective organisms.*
- Teach patient and family members positioning, postural drainage, and suctioning, if necessary, *to lessen their anxiety and increase comfort.*

Decreased cardiac output related to cardiac muscle decompensation

- Assess vital signs, heart sounds, pulse for rate or dysrhythmias.
- Monitor vital sign changes with activity *to determine severity of condition.*
- Administer prescribed medications, if any, *to strengthen cardiac functions.*
- Observe for edema throughout body *to determine peripheral circulatory status or decompensation.*
- Monitor patient's color and mental alertness *to determine peripheral circulation and oxygenation.*
- Monitor ECG, if on monitoring, for changes in rhythms *to determine need for additional medications or physician visit.*
- If on IV therapy, monitor type of solution and medication infusion, rate, and effects on patient *to determine if changes are needed.*

- Monitor laboratory data, such as complete blood count (CBC), electrolyte levels, and CK, *to determine patient's response to therapy.*
- Administer oxygen therapy, if prescribed, *to promote oxygenation and avoid hypoxia.*

DEFICIENCY DISEASES

■ OSTEOMALACIA

Osteomalacia is a disease of adults characterized by increasing softening, brittleness, flexibility, and deformity of bones.

Osteomalacia is the adult equivalent of rickets in children; both may result from a vitamin D deficiency, which leads to reduced absorption of calcium and phosphorus. The vitamin D deficiency may be from inadequate dietary intake, insufficient sunshine, malabsorption in the intestines, or defective metabolism of vitamin D. Other causes include chronic phosphate depletion, anticonvulsant therapy, administration of etidronate over time, renal tubular diseases, and gluten entropathy.[82]

Osteomalacia is a rare disease of adults with musculoskeletal disease. It is slightly more common in women.

•••••• Pathophysiology

Without vitamin D, the amount of calcium and phosphorus available for bone calcification is inadequate to maintain strong bones. Defective growth and replacement of rigid bones are noted first in immature skeletal bones at sites of growth and in mature bones at points of stress, where turnover is most rapid. The physiologic balance of bone growth and resorption is disrupted. Defective replacement at the sites mentioned is noticed first because of the increased demand for new bone formation. Failure of mineralization and the bones' resultant inability to resist stress because of lack of rigidity are evident through the patient's symptoms and by x-ray examination.

•••••• Diagnostic Studies and Findings

History Decreased intake or absorption of vitamin D, from unfortified milk, after gastrectomy, or other cause

Physical examination Bone pain, muscle weakness, and general malaise; pelvic deformities; waddling gait

Serum calcium levels Lower than normal (4.5 to 5.5 mEq/L); serum parathyroid hormone (PTH) levels are elevated if hypocalcemia is present

Serum alkaline phosphatase Elevated above 13 King-Armstrong units

Vitamin D level Below normal

Erythrocyte sedimentation rate May be slightly elevated

X-ray General decalcification of bones; pseudofractures (Looser's zones): incomplete fractures in various stages of healing; distal shaft of bones may show widening, fraying, and cupping[82]

Biopsy of iliac crest Excessive uncalcified bones

Renal osteodystrophy (chronic renal failure) From lack of completion of vitamin D metabolism

•••••• Multidisciplinary Plan

Medications

Nutritional supplements: vitamin D, 400-600 USP units, po or IV, daily, until deficiency is corrected

Calcium supplements when serum phosphate level is normal

General Management

Supplying well-balanced diet with fortified milk and sources of vitamin D (egg yolks, tuna, cod-liver oil, and salmon)

Avoiding use of antacids containing aluminum (aluminum prevents absorption of phosphate in intestines)[82]

Having sufficient exposure to sunlight to aid utilization of vitamin D

NURSING CARE

Nursing Assessment

Skeleton: Bone Growth, Maturation

Bone pain present and severe (most common manifestation of osteomalacia)

Strength of bone impaired; fractures common

May have backache and muscle weakness

Deformation of bones that are not able to bear normal weights

Systemic Processes

General weakness throughout body; may have malaise and fatigue

Psychosocial Concerns

Body image disturbances

Possibility of fractures

Nursing Dx & Intervention

Impaired physical mobility related to weakened, deformed bones

- Assess musculoskeletal tissues *to note deformities.*
- Position to support affected tissues; use pillows appropriately *to aid in maintaining positions.*
- Assist with ambulation if no fracture is present *to increase mobility.*
- Prevent additional injury through maintenance of a safe environment: side rails, nonskid surfaces, and clean, dry areas *for safety.*

Altered nutrition: less than body requirements related to inadequate or inappropriate intake

- Assess intake of milk and other foods containing calcium and vitamin D.

- Administer medications (vitamin D) per physician's prescription *to correct deficiency.*
- Explain how therapy will improve patient's condition *to increase compliance.*
- Supply well-balanced diet high in vitamin D and calcium-containing foods; explain how this will affect condition *to aid compliance and relieve condition.*

Patient Education/Home Care Planning

1. Discuss sources of vitamin D and calcium and need for adequate intake.
2. Discuss exposure to sunlight to aid absorption of vitamin D.
3. Discuss avoiding use of aluminum-containing antacids; may consider use of ranitidine or cimetidine.

Evaluation

Patient improves mobility as bones become stronger Patient moves freely without aid. Patient states that bones do not feel as if they will break or give way.

Patient regains and maintains adequate vitamin D levels Patient has normal serum levels of vitamin D and serum calcium levels. Bones regain proper calcification, and x-rays show increased density with minimum or no deformity. Patient avoids use of aluminum-containing antacids.

OSTEOPOROSIS

Osteoporosis is a systemic condition of overall reduction in bone mass or density in which bone resorption has outstripped bone formation, thereby upsetting the normal balance.

Osteoporosis is classified as type I—primary, consisting of juvenile and postmenopausal osteoporosis; and type II—secondary, consisting of cases caused by endocrine abnormalities; estrogen and testosterone deficiency; medications such as corticosteroids, heparin, anticonvulsants and methotrexate; and chronic diseases of the lungs or kidneys.

The disease is most common in postmenopausal women, probably because of endocrine involution and inactivity. Younger people may develop osteoporosis after severe injuries, with paralysis and long periods of immobility that can lead to osteoporosis. People with rheumatoid arthritis, endocrine abnormalities, and chronic pulmonary or renal disease may also develop osteoporosis. Men can develop osteoporosis but do so less frequently than women (ratio is 1:4). It has been estimated that 33% of postmenopausal women have osteoporosis, and risk of an osteoporotic fracture is 1 in 3.[81]

Annual expenditure on short-term care after an osteoporotic hip fracture exceeds $8 million. There are approximately 275,000 new osteoporotic hip fractures each year in the United States.[81]

······ Pathophysiology

Patients with osteoporosis have normal bones but less overall bone quantity. The remaining bone becomes weakened from the demands of weight bearing. Pathologic fractures can occur with little force, especially in the lower radius, femoral neck, and vertebrae. The vertebral column's overall mass is diminished, leading to increasing kyphosis (dowager's hump) and loss of height. Backache is common and can radiate down the legs. Dull, constant pain is common in the back and chest. Women at greater risk for osteoporosis with fracture are those who have had oophorectomies with loss of estrogen, have used steroids over a prolonged period of time, are Caucasian, have excessive alcohol intake, smoke cigarettes, and are inactive.[81]

······ Diagnostic Studies and Findings

History Prolonged immobility; menopause; decreased activity; oophorectomy; chronic disease; smoker; excessive alcohol intake; bed rest; lack of weight bearing

Physical examination Increased kyphosis; backache or neck ache with radiation to legs and arms; fractures; small frame; few other symptoms

X-ray Soft vertebral bodies that are indented by the discs and become biconcave; vertebrae possibly wedged from fractures; thoracic vertebral curvature increased; absorptiometry studies: single-photon, dual-photon, dual-energy x-ray, and quantitative computed tomography; each will show specific peripheral bone or cortical bone mass according to its purpose

Blood serum study Low levels of alkaline phosphatase (alkaline phosphatase increases bone formation); high levels of serum total hydroxyproline (increases bone resorption); high levels of serum osteocalcin may indicate a high rate of bone loss[39]

······ Multidisciplinary Plan

Medications

Etidronate (Didronel), 400 mg daily for 2 wk only every 3 mo with 1500 mg calcium daily during etidronate-free periods

Alendronate (recently approved by the Food and Drug Administration [FDA]) for women unable to take estrogen, in individualized dose

Estrogens for postmenopausal women who have undergone hysterectomy; because of increased risk of endometrial cancer and cardiovascular complications, use of estrogens for osteoporosis is controversial; however, estrogen-progesterone combinations are now advocated as estrogen 0.625 mg/d; progesterone may be added to the estrogen (estrogen taken for 25 d/mo, combined with progesterone for days 16-25, then both stopped for rest of month) or 50-100 µg/d of transdermal estradiol; addition of progesterone may not protect against breast cancer *risk,* although there is no increase in breast cancer noted related to these medications[146]

Nutritional Supplements

Calcitonin, subcutaneously, individual dosage
Calcium carbonate (Os-Cal or Os-Cal-Fluor), 1 g/d
Vitamin D, 50,000 IU once or twice per week
High-protein diet

General Management

Application of back corset or neck support to prevent stress
  fractures
Ambulation and maintaining active weight-bearing exercises
  to hold calcium in bones
Passive exercises if unable to do active exercises

NURSING CARE

Nursing Assessment

Skeletal Tissues

Degree of strength in muscles and joints
Presence of increased kyphosis
Loss of height
Fracture of hip, compression fractures of vertebrae, or frac-
  ture of radius

Other Tissues

Backache
Neck pain
Pain radiating to legs and arms

Psychosocial Concerns

Self-concept: disturbances in self-esteem and body image
Alteration in physical mobility; possibility of fractures
Pain
Fear of falling

Nursing Dx & Intervention

Impaired physical mobility related to decreased bone mass and pain

- Assess pain as it affects mobility.
- Administer medications as prescribed; monitor response *to modify condition.*
- Perform ROM exercises actively and passively if neces-sary *to maintain muscle and joint strength.*
- Use sling or ambulatory aid (cane or crutch) if needed *to lessen stress on bones.*
- Apply back corset or neck collar *to lessen pain and in-crease mobility* (use is controversial because such aids limit muscle movements).
- Encourage aerobic exercise in water *to maintain ROM of joints.*
- Do weight-bearing exercises *to stimulate bone mineral-ization.*

Self-esteem disturbance and altered role performance related to kyphosis and pain

- Assess ability to carry out self-care, ADL, and usual roles.
- Explain or clarify the processes accompanying meno-pause as normal and natural *to ease concerns.*
- Encourage usual ADL and other activities *to maintain bone mass.*
- Encourage fashion consultation for clothing to lessen evi-dence of increased kyphosis *to increase self-esteem.*
- Administer prescribed medications *to help retain bone mass and lessen pain.*

Impaired gas exchange related to kyphosis

- Assess respiratory rates, depth, and breath sounds *to eval-uate effects of kyphosis.*
- Encourage attempts to maintain upright posture *to aid ventilation.*
- Check vital capacity to determine if level is satisfactory.
- Encourage deep-breathing exercises *to aid gas exchanges.*
- Encourage shoulder-strengthening exercises *to enhance breathing.*

Injury, risk for, related to fall or fracture of radius, hip, or vertebra

- Assess ability to move easily and freely or limitations on movements.
- Assess gait and placement of feet when walking, espe-cially in postmenopausal women, *to determine risk of a hip fracture.* (With aging the normal 150° angle of fit of the femur into the acetabulum shortens to 135°, resulting in a more varus placing of each foot when walking. Varus placement puts a strain on the neck of the femur, which in the case of a minor twist in the presence of osteoporosis can easily lead to a fractured femoral neck.)
- Caution patient to walk carefully and to observe surfaces ahead to lessen possibility of a slip, ankle twist, or fall *to prevent possible fracture.*
- Encourage gentle extension hip exercises in pool (with wa-ter above waist level to negate effects of gravity) *to increase hip ROM to help maintain 150° angle of hip and femur.*
- Instruct patient to remove loose rugs or carpeting and long cords from walking areas *to lessen danger of tripping or falling.*
- Clarify effects of shadows or wearing bifocal glasses as influencing depth perception when walking on uneven surfaces *to lessen risk of falling.*
- Encourage wearing of well-repaired shoes and, in rain and in icy conditions, wearing proper footwear *to prevent slip-ping or falling.*

Patient Education/Home Care Planning

1. Discuss perception of osteoporosis as "thin" bones; bone mass is decreased, but bones are not thinner, there is just less bone mass.

2. List advantages of exercise and activity to maintain bone mass and calcium in bones.
3. Clarify effects of increased calcium intake and reiterate need for serial examinations of serum calcium levels.
4. Encourage a program of active exercises to maintain strength of muscles and bones.
5. Encourage patient to read current research data and treatment modalities and discuss with physician.
6. Encourage compliance with taking prescribed medications to increase bone mass.

Evaluation

Patient maintains pain-free ambulation and joint mobility   Patient's disease is controlled by medication, calcium intake, or activity. Patient has no continued major loss of bone density on x-ray.

Patient has positive self-esteem and has maintained roles   Patient is outward looking. Patient participates in usual roles and responsibilities. Patient wears clothing to disguise kyphosis.

Patient has satisfactory gas exchange   Patient has normal color, respiratory rates, and depth; vital capacity is in low normal range.

Patient does not experience a fractured radius, vertebra, or hip   Patient exercises in water several times weekly.

TRAUMA

Musculoskeletal injury or trauma occurs in all age groups. One in five emergency department visits is associated with musculoskeletal trauma, and one in four patient visits to physicians correlates with musculoskeletal conditions. Among older people, musculoskeletal conditions and trauma rank second only to respiratory conditions as reasons for hospital admission. Because of our fast-paced lifestyles, the injured person may suffer injuries not only to the musculoskeletal tissues but to other tissues as well. Even when these injuries are not fatal or life threatening, they may require periods of hospitalization and recovery. Also, there is no assurance that there will be no future disability or pain, and periods of decreased mobility are likely.

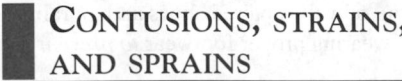

CONTUSIONS, STRAINS, AND SPRAINS

A contusion is a bruise without an external break in the skin.

A strain is a "pull" in a muscle, ligament, or tendon caused by excessive stretch.

A sprain is a tear in a muscle, ligament, or tendon; it may be mild to severe.

Trauma to the musculoskeletal tissues may involve one specific tissue, such as one ligament, one tendon, or a single muscle mass, although injury to single tissues is rare. Injury to several tissues is more common, such as multiple fractures of bones, with many fracture fragments associated with skin, nerve, and blood vessel trauma. Such injuries frequently are life threatening.

Less serious injuries comprise bruises or contusions of the skin; strain (stretch) of tendon or ligament fibers; and sprains (tearing) of some, many, or all tendons, ligaments, or even bones in and around a joint. These three conditions (contusion, strain, or sprain) have similar initial signs, require similar assessments, and have similar treatments.

•••••• Pathophysiology

Contusions are bruises from sudden external pressure that tears the subcutaneous circulatory veins and capillaries. Bleeding occurs in the injured subcutaneous tissues and is noted by bluish discoloration of the injured tissues, with edema or swelling accompanying the vessel or tissue injury. Depending on the extent or severity of the contusion, the edema and discoloration begin to abate in 48 to 72 hours. A charleyhorse is a contusion of a muscle.

A *strain* is caused by an undue force applied to muscles, ligaments, or tendons. It stretches the fibers, causing a temporary weakness, numbness, and some bleeding if the veins or capillaries within the injured tissues are excessively stretched. The weakness may last 24 to 72 hours, but the numbness usually disappears within hours. Bleeding may continue for 30 minutes or longer unless pressure or cold is applied to stop it. A strained muscle, ligament, or tendon can regain its full function after conservative treatments, which are discussed later. Muscles that are frequently strained are the hamstring and pectineus (hamstring and groin pull, respectively).

A *sprain* is a partial or full tearing off or away (avulsion) of one or more ligaments or tendons or portions of the bone in and around a joint. Sprains are caused by undue force, twisting, or pull exerted during sports or work activities. Most sprains occur in the ankles, wrists, fingers, and toes. Other joints can be sprained if undue force, pressure, or pull is applied without relief.

Sprains are classified as first degree (some tearing of fibers with some bleeding); second degree (moderate tearing and more extensive bleeding or hemorrhage); and third degree (full tearing or avulsion of the tendon or ligament from its bony attachment, with or without some bone attached, accompanied by marked hemorrhage, pain, edema, and loss of function).

•••••• Diagnostic Studies and Findings

History   Pressure applied to area, usually unanticipated; undue force; pull without relief (if strain or sprain); pain with use; mechanism of injury; surface where injury occurred

Physical examination   Skin, circulatory, and musculoskeletal signs as described on pp. 356 to 359

•••••• Multidisciplinary Plan

	Contusion	Strain	Sprain
Surgery			
Open reduction and repair of torn or avulsed tissues	None	None	May be needed for full joint function; ligament or tendon may be reattached or may need to be removed if severely damaged; avulsed fragment may require screw for reattachment
Medications			
Analgesics	None	Aspirin, 300-600 mg qid prn; acetaminophen, 300-600 mg qid prn	Aspirin, 300-1000 mg q4h to relieve pain and inflammation; nonsteroidal antiinflammatory medications in individualized doses
Narcotics	None	None	Codeine, 30-60 mg po q4-6h for severe pain
General Management*			
Cold application	Ice application for 24 h	Ice application for 24 h	Ice application for 24 h or longer
External wrap	None	Elastic wrap or sling	Elastic wrap or cast; sling for upper extremity
Elevation	None	Elevate if extremity	Elevate if extremity
Exercises (ROM)	Gentle exercises after 48 h	Gentle exercises and use as able after 48 h	No exercises while severe edema and bleeding present; gentle exercises may be begun after 3-5 d, depending on tissue injured and severity of sprain
Weight bearing	Full use	As able; full use	Cessation of weight bearing with crutch use for 7 d or longer, depending on tissues involved

*Part of treatment of musculoskeletal injuries referred to as RICE.

R = Rest for injured part. May be temporary nonuse or more prolonged non–weight bearing, depending on injury.

I = Ice. Applications of ice lessen bleeding and edema. Ice is needed for 24 to 72 hours or longer, depending on the injury.

C = Compression. Elastic bandages or at times a circular cast may be used for compression. Compression is to be of the *venous* vessels; therefore the wrapping should be applied only snugly enough that it does not compromise the *arterial* flow. Application of the bandages or cast should be from distal to proximal on the limb to aid venous constriction and venous return.

E = Elevation. The injured part is elevated to heart level to aid venous return and thereby lessen edema. Elevation of the part too high (or above the patient's central venous pressure) should be avoided because too high elevation could impede arterial flow and increase rather than decrease edema. Normal central venous pressure (CVP) ranges from 6 to 13 cm H_2O pressure. Elevation should not exceed 5 inches above the heart level (2.5 cm = 1 inch; 5 inches = 12.5 cm), assuming the patient has the highest CVP. Accurate elevation can be achieved if the patient has a CVP line in place. If not, elevation to heart level is safest.

NURSING CARE

Nursing Assessment

	Contusion	Strain	Sprain
Specific tissue or tissues	Skin and subcutaneous tissue	Tendon, ligament, bone, and entire joint	Same as with strain
Local processes	Bluish discoloration and edema; skin openings; pain; soreness	Weakness, numbness, bleeding noted by discoloration; assess for skin opening; joint mobility, stability, or laxness; pain; edema; ability to bear weight or use joint normally	Same as with strain only more pronounced: more edema, bleeding, and discoloration; inability to use joint, muscles, or tendons normally; cannot bear weight; pain more severe and constant
Systemic processes	Other bruises or contusions possibly present	Distant joints possibly sore from initial injury; generalized muscle soreness	Same as with strain
Psychosocial concerns	Minor discomfort; no major concerns	Temporary (24-72 h) impairment of mobility	Mobility impaired for varying periods (10 days to 3 or more weeks); may develop posttraumatic arthritis later

Nursing Dx & Intervention

Impaired physical mobility related to specific injury

- Assess injured area *to determine condition.*
- Handle injured tissues gently *to avoid further trauma.*
- Provide support under affected joints *to prevent lever actions of muscles.*
- Apply ice or bag of frozen peas to site *to decrease edema and bleeding.*
- Cover ice bag or frozen pea bag with dry cloth *to prevent tissue damage.*
- Elevate injured part or parts to heart level *to decrease edema and increase venous return.*
- Assist with ROM exercises when allowed; perform as able *to increase mobility.*
- Use sling for upper extremity injury *to lessen pain and increase comfort.*
- Perform neurovascular checks (see p. 358) as prescribed *to determine condition and to note possible complications.*
- Assist with crutch walking, as needed; assess crutches for proper length *to provide for safety.*
- Caution patient not to rest axillae on crutches *to prevent nerve damage.*
- Administer analgesics and nonsteroidal antiinflammatory medications *to lessen pain and aid in relief of inflammation.*
- Assist with personal hygiene as needed *to maintain healthy tissues.*
- Assess concerns with immobility *to lessen anxiety.*

Altered role performance related to injury

- Assure patient that full function should be regained after treatment *to ease concerns.*
- Encourage resumption of ADL and usual activities as able *to enhance self-concept.*
- Caution about possibility of reinjury if self-care and preventive measures are not learned.
- Discuss concerns related to employment or future sports activities *to elicit thoughts or fears,* if present.

Patient Education/Home Care Planning

1. Be sure the patient knows the nature and extent of injury.
2. Demonstrate to the patient the use of crutches, if necessary.
3. Discuss the effects of cold applications if the patient has future trauma.
4. Consult physicians or trainers to teach the patient preventive measures in sports or exercise activities.
5. Clarify with the patient or family the use of medications, dressing changes, and need for limited mobility, if necessary.
6. List for the patient or family the signs and symptoms that require physician's attention.

Evaluation

Patient recovers ROM of affected joints and tissues without limitations   Patient experiences no pain, tenderness, limitation of motion, edema, or loss of function of tissues. Patient needs no analgesic medication.

Patient regains social interactions and usual role   Patient returns to usual family, social, and employment roles.

▌ DISLOCATION

A dislocation is a displacement of a part, usually a bone, from its normal anatomic position within a joint.

Dislocations may be complete or partial (called subluxations). They usually result from a blow, force, or pull strong enough to cause the bone to be forced or pulled from the joint. For some people, repeated dislocations are common because of repetitive or chronic trauma to a joint, which weakens ligaments, tendons, or muscles. Some joints, such as the shoulder, elbow, fingers, and knee, are more commonly dislocated than others.

Subluxations are partial dislocations and are more common in people with long-standing rheumatoid arthritis because fibrosis shortens the tendons, forcing the bones to sublux; this is referred to as a swan-neck boutonniére deformity, common in some arthritic conditions.

•••••• Pathophysiology

The major signs of dislocation are deformity and inability to use the part or joint normally. Tendons or ligaments can become interposed, making reduction and replacement of the dislocated part into the joint difficult or impossible without open surgical reduction. Reduction and replacement within the joint space without surgery is more commonly impossible in cases of subluxations associated with rheumatoid arthritis because of the shortening of the tendon from inflammatory changes. Trapping of nerves or blood vessels between dislocated bones is a surgical emergency.

•••••• Diagnostic Studies and Findings

History   Repetitive trauma, such as throwing or hitting a ball; presence of rheumatoid arthritis; acute injury during work or recreational activity

Physical examination   Head or other part of bone out of the normal anatomic position; tendon shortening; deformity; inability to use joint normally; tenderness; possible edema

X-ray   Dislocated parts noted; position of parts not in normal anatomic sites

•••••• Multidisciplinary Plan

Surgery

Open reduction of the dislocated bone or bones, if not able to reduce dislocation manually

Tendon debridement or transplant for swan neck and bou-tonniére deformities to prevent recurrence

General Management

Manual closed reduction of the dislocated bone into the joint

Application of a sling for the upper extremity to lessen stress on shoulder joint

Elastic wrap of lower extremity joint

Ice applications for 24 hours, then warm applications to joint

Active exercises under physical therapist's direction as pre-scribed by physician

Application of skin traction, especially Buck extension, for a short period of time if hip dislocated with acetabular damage

NURSING CARE

Nursing Assessment

Joint and Bones of Joint

Palpation of dislocated part out of usual position

Deformity

Inability to use joint normally

Tenderness, soreness, or pain

Psychosocial Concerns

Self-concept

Disturbances of role expectations

Impaired mobility and ROM

Nursing Dx & Intervention

Impaired physical mobility related to dislocation

- Assess effects of dislocation on patient's mobility and ROM.
- Apply sling or elastic wrap *to maintain reduction.*
- Perform ROM to all unaffected joints *to maintain strength.*
- Assist with ambulation four or more times daily *to main-tain strength,* depending on which joint is involved.

Role performance disturbance related to injury or condition

- Assess patient's statements of limitations.
- Assure that full ROM should be regained after reduction and healing *to lessen concerns.*
- Assist with hygiene and ADL as needed *to lessen patient stress.*
- Provide postoperative care as needed *to aid recovery.*

Injury, risk for, related to shortening, laxity, or weakness of joint ligaments, tendons, or muscles

- Assess previously dislocated joints for stability, laxness, or weakness of joint tissues.

- Discuss current activities related to affected joints regard-ing possible recurrence (Is person doing same activities as previously? Is person using a protective device to prevent recurrence? Is person doing strengthening exercises?) *to determine risk of recurrence.*
- Consult with physical therapist for exercises to strengthen joint tissues *to lessen risk of recurrence.*
- Encourage patient to comply with prescribed medical plan *to lessen risk of recurrence.*

Patient Education/Home Care Planning

1. Clarify how repetitive trauma weakens joint supports and predisposes to repeated dislocations.
2. Explain that prompt treatment lessens long-term effects of repetitive dislocations.
3. Encourage continued compliance to prescribed therapy to lessen risk of recurrence.

Evaluation

Patient has normal ROM of affected joint and no lim-itation of mobility Patient performs ROM exercises without pain, limitation, or recurrence of dislocation.

Patient returns to usual roles and activities Patient does own ADL unassisted. Patient has returned to employment or sports activities as before dislocation. Patient has no dis-comfort with use. Patient has experienced no recurrence of dis-location.

▮ FRACTURES

A fracture is a discontinuity or break in a bone.

Fractured bones cause major trauma to musculoskeletal tis-sues. Not only is the most vital part (bone) unable to perform its normal functions, but all the surrounding tissues also are un-able to function normally. The cumulative effects may or may not be in direct relationship to the severity of the injury because of the interrelationship of these tissues.

The type of fracture is usually related to the source or force of the blow (see box on pp. 392 to 394). Only minor force may be needed for a greenstick fracture of one bone cortex, whereas more powerful forces cause comminuted fractures with associ-ated soft tissue trauma. Anyone is susceptible to fractures; however, younger children and elderly people may suffer frac-tures from minor forces. Young and middle-aged adults have stronger musculoskeletal tissues; therefore greater force is re-quired to fracture a bone, and there is more associated soft tis-sue trauma.

Each year, more than 150,000 persons die from trauma and fractures with an additional 4 million or more persons treated

TYPES AND CAUSES OF FRACTURES

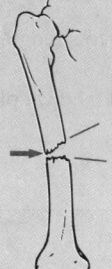

Angulated: Fracture with fragments at angles to each other   *Cause:* Direct or lateral force, causing break and loss of anatomic positions

Angulated

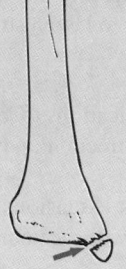

Avulsed: Fracture that pulls bone and other tissues from usual attachments   *Cause:* Direct energy or force, with resisted extension of bone and joint

Avulsed

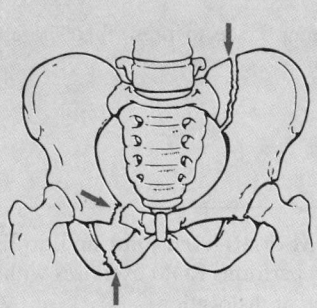

Bucket-handle: Double vertical fractures of pelvis on same side, resulting in pelvic dislocation   *Cause:* Direct blow or anterior compression force, with or without sacral torsion

Bucket-handle

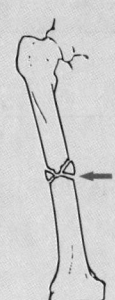

Butterfly: Butterfly-shaped piece of fractured bone, usually accompanying comminuted fracture   *Cause:* Direct, indirect, or rotational force to bone

Butterfly

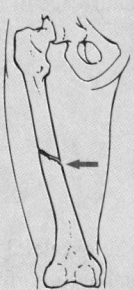

Closed: Skin intact over fracture *Cause:* Minor force or energy

Closed

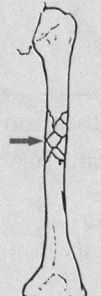

Comminuted: Fracture with more than two pieces; may have significant associated soft tissue trauma   *Cause:* Direct crushing injury or force to tissues and bone

Comminuted

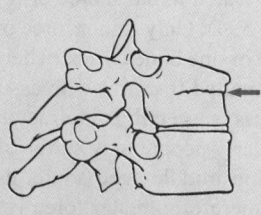

Compression: Fracture is squeezed or wedged together at one side   *Cause:* Compressive, axial energy or force applied directly from above fracture site

Compression

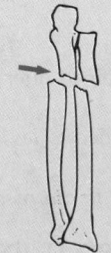

Displaced: Fracture with one, both, or all fragments out of normal alignment   *Cause:* direct energy or force to site

Displaced

From Mourad.[104]

TYPES AND CAUSES OF FRACTURES—cont'd

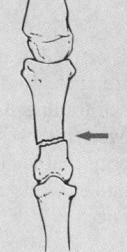

Extraarticular: Fracture near but outside a joint *Cause:* Direct energy above or below a joint

Extraarticular

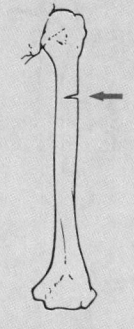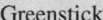

Greenstick: Break in only one cortex of bone *Cause:* Minor direct or indirect energy

Greenstick

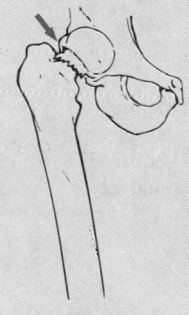

Impacted: Fracture with one end wedged into opposite end or inside fractured fragment *Cause:* Compressive axial energy or force directly to distal fragment

Impacted

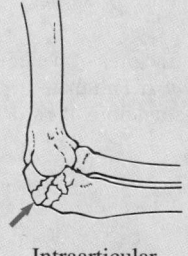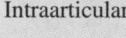

Intraarticular: Fracture involving bones inside a joint *Cause:* Direct or indirect energy or force to joint

Intraarticular

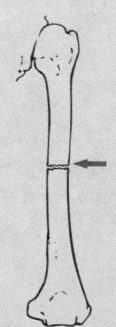

Linear: As a line, so can be transverse or oblique *Cause:* Minor or moderate energy or force directly to bone

Linear

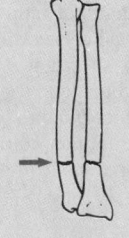

Nightstick: Fracture of ulna caused by blow to forearm elevated in defensive position *Cause:* Direct force or blow to forearm

Nightstick

Nonangulated: Fracture with fragments in anatomic relationship to each other *Cause:* Minor force or energy

Nonangulated

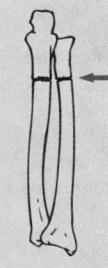

Nondisplaced: Fracture fragments in close approximation and anatomic position to each other *Cause:* Minor to moderate force or energy

Nondisplaced

Continued.

TYPES AND CAUSES OF FRACTURES—cont'd

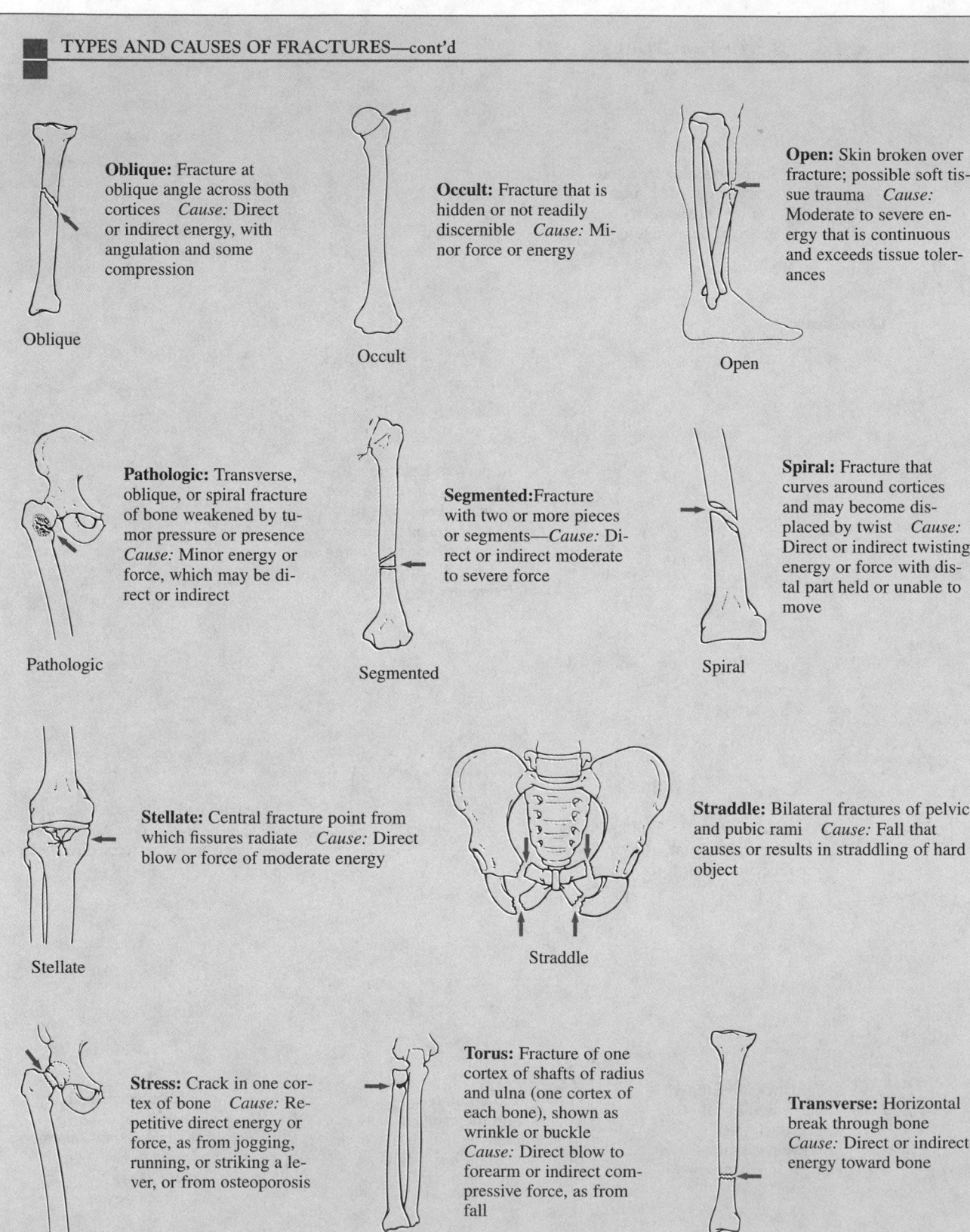

Oblique: Fracture at oblique angle across both cortices *Cause:* Direct or indirect energy, with angulation and some compression

Oblique

Occult: Fracture that is hidden or not readily discernible *Cause:* Minor force or energy

Occult

Open: Skin broken over fracture; possible soft tissue trauma *Cause:* Moderate to severe energy that is continuous and exceeds tissue tolerances

Open

Pathologic: Transverse, oblique, or spiral fracture of bone weakened by tumor pressure or presence *Cause:* Minor energy or force, which may be direct or indirect

Pathologic

Segmented: Fracture with two or more pieces or segments—*Cause:* Direct or indirect moderate to severe force

Segmented

Spiral: Fracture that curves around cortices and may become displaced by twist *Cause:* Direct or indirect twisting energy or force with distal part held or unable to move

Spiral

Stellate: Central fracture point from which fissures radiate *Cause:* Direct blow or force of moderate energy

Stellate

Straddle: Bilateral fractures of pelvic and pubic rami *Cause:* Fall that causes or results in straddling of hard object

Straddle

Stress: Crack in one cortex of bone *Cause:* Repetitive direct energy or force, as from jogging, running, or striking a lever, or from osteoporosis

Stress

Torus: Fracture of one cortex of shafts of radius and ulna (one cortex of each bone), shown as wrinkle or buckle *Cause:* Direct blow to forearm or indirect compressive force, as from fall

Torus

Transverse: Horizontal break through bone *Cause:* Direct or indirect energy toward bone

Transverse

at hospitals. Trauma costs Americans over $200 billion annually.

• • • • • Pathophysiology

Bones are held relatively firmly in their normal anatomic positions by their shape, bony projections and processes, and the strong ligaments and tendons that hold them in their joints. Muscles surrounding the bones along their shafts also provide protection. However, either direct or indirect forces against the bone that are superior to the strength of the bone, muscles, tendons, or ligaments cause the tissues to "give in." Bones break when they cannot continue to resist the strength, duration, or repetitive nature of the applied forces.

Aging also affects bones, making them more subject to a fracture. Cortical bone in the human femur, for example, becomes less stiff, less strong, and more brittle with aging.[74] Age-related fractures are an enormous problem in the United States, especially related to the vertebrae, proximal femur, and distal radius, which are frequent sites of fractures. Aging causes trabecular loss, less bone mass, and changes in the "architecture" of the bones. Bone mineral density is decreased, more so in females than males, leading to fracture risk. Osteoporotic changes in bones, especially in the lumbar spine, have shown a decrease in trabecular bone density of approximately 50% from ages 20 to 80 years.[74]

A fractured bone can no longer maintain its normal length unless the two fragments impact into each other at the time of the fracture. Usually there will be shortening of the tissues around the fractured bone because of muscle contraction and spasms as the muscles respond to the stimulus of trauma. As the muscles contract and shorten, they move the distal fragment upward (cephalad). The distal fragment is less stable and more movable than the proximal fragment, which is held more firmly from the muscles' originations (the origins of muscles are less movable than their insertions). The shortening of the muscles and the displacement of the distal fragment result in deformity, overriding, and displacement, characteristic signs of a fracture. The deformity can generally be noted on physical examination as a deviation from the normal appearance of the tissues. Displacement of the distal fragment is a significant sign because the distal fragment must be replaced in continuity with the proximal fragment for healing and bone union. The amount of displacement and the angulation and rotation of the distal fragment are caused by the loss of the bone's continuity and the severity or strength of the muscle spasms and contraction. Force must be applied to the distal fragment and to the muscles to overcome the muscle contraction so that the two or more fracture fragments can again become aligned. Terms used to describe the position of the distal fragment include varus or valgus displacement, rotation, and medial, lateral, anterior, or posterior displacement.

When a bone is fractured, many or all of the following processes occur. These processes begin immediately with the injury and continue for weeks, months, and in some situations even years before they are completed and bone union has been achieved:

Hematoma formation. Blood and blood cells move into the injured tissues from vessels broken or bruised at the time of injury and from the inflammatory response to release of histamine, bradykinins, and serotonin into the injury site. White blood cells, especially monocytes, phagocytize debris to keep the area of injury localized and prevent spread to contiguous tissues. Bleeding into the tissues causes a hematoma to form. Blood cells, especially thrombocytes, begin to work with fibroblasts to form a fibrin (clot) meshwork within the hematoma. Usually the hematoma is well formed in 24 to 48 hours, and frank or continued bleeding slows or ceases completely. There appears to be an optimum-size hematoma to facilitate bone union. Healing is delayed or prevented by hematomas that are too small or too large, although the exact favorable size is still undetermined. Along with fibroblasts, platelets also make platelet-derived growth factor, macrophages, T-lymphocytes, and hematopoietic growth factors such as transforming growth factor-β.

Consolidation, angiogenesis, and cartilage formation. During this period of fracture healing, a fascinating phenomenon occurs because osteoblasts (bone-forming cells) move into the fibrin meshwork to make new *bone,* not scar tissue. No other tissue except the liver regenerates itself as itself. The osteoblasts help in firming the fracture site, intertwining it with collagen connective tissue fibers to form strong cartilage and then with new bone to bridge the gap between the fractured ends. Capillary buds develop into new blood vessels (angiogenesis), which bring more nutrients and calcium molecules into the area to form soft bone callus. A tissue oxygen gradient is necessary for the maintenance of angiogenesis in the injury area. This bone-forming period lasts 3 to 6 weeks or longer.

Callus formation. This is probably the most vital period for bone healing for two reasons: (1) Enough nutrients must be present to provide a continuous supply to support bone formation to its completion. Oxygen is a major nutrient, as is alkaline phosphatase, along with sufficient amounts of vitamins A, B, C, and D, carbohydrates, proteins, minerals, and water. Alkaline phosphatase may be a key enzyme that governs much of the mineralization process. Insulin, a potent growth factor, must be present in proper amounts for healing at this stage. This may be one reason that diabetics have impaired fracture healing; not only do they have circulatory disturbances, but their fracture callus cells may respond ineffectively to other signals because of inadequate insulin. (2) Callus formation must be enhanced by the "right" amount of compression of the fractured fragments. Too little compression may result in pseudobone (false bone), and too much compression may decrease oxygen supply and tension, resulting in bone-end absorption and creating too large a gap for the collagen fibers to bridge. This decreases or prevents formation of strong callus.

! EMERGENCY ALERT

DISLOCATIONS AND FRACTURES

Fractures and dislocations occur frequently. Attention to circulatory and neurovascular status is essential to minimize further damage. One classification of fractures is closed or simple and open or compound. Dislocations occur when a joint exceeds its range of motion and joint tissues are disrupted (usually a bone).

Assessment

- Assess vital signs; rule out life-threatening injury.
- Assess for swelling, discoloration, abrasions, contusions, or obvious deformity.
- Assess neurovascular status (the five *P*'s and others; see box on p. 358), and reassess frequently.

Interventions

- Immobilize limb; note and observe for swelling.
- Elevate and apply cold pack as possible (protect skin from direct contact with ice).
- Assist with traction application if neurovascular status is compromised.
- If open wound is present, apply a dry sterile dressing.
- Apply a pressure dressing if profuse bleeding is present.
- Manage pain.

Osteoclast activity is greater when compressive forces are too great, because osteoclasts act to absorb or resorb bone cells, whereas osteoblasts aid bone formation. The balance is disrupted between the two cells, and callus or new bone formation is decreased. This period lasts 3 to 6 months or longer, depending on the type of fracture and the above conditions.

Remodeling. If present, excess bone is resorbed during this period. The collagen fibers and fibrous tissues are aligned to form trabeculae along the lines of stress according to Wolff's law, which states that bone will respond to stress by becoming thicker and stronger and that the structure of a bone depends on its function. Osteoclasts resorb the excess callus or poorly aligned trabeculae until they are firm and strong. Remodeling may continue for up to 2 years after injury.

Bone healing, then, depends on several *local* factors, including the severity of the injury, nutrient supply, amount of bone bridge or gap, degree of immobilization, infection or necrosis of bone cells, and type of bone fractured. Cancellous bone fractures heal more quickly than fractures of compact bone because of the presence of blood and blood cells in greater quantities than in compact bone. *Systemic* factors influencing bone healing include the patient's age (children heal more quickly), concomitant diseases such as diabetes, hormonal balances (growth hormones aid healing and excess corticosteroids delay healing), and stress, immobility, or mobility at the fracture site. Application of electric current aids bone healing and has become a valuable adjunct in recent years.

Fractures of bones may not heal well or form bone union in the usual amount of time, or they may not even unite. There may be *delayed* union, in which bone union does not occur for 9 months or longer after a fracture; there may be *malunion,* in which the bones unite in a less than optimal position; and there may be *nonunion,* in which no fracture healing has occurred. Open fractures (fractures in which the skin has been torn or disrupted) must be carefully cleaned, definitively treated, and closed as soon as feasible to prevent possible infection and to promote proper healing.

••••• Diagnostic Studies and Findings

History   Sudden, unexpected trauma; chronic, repetitive forces rather than sudden force usually cause stress fractures

Physical examination   Local deformity; edema or a mass; distal tissues held at abnormal angles or positions; limitation of use of part; crepitation; pain or tenderness at or around the site; subjective signs of numbness, tingling, weakness, or inability to use part normally; distal tissues cooler than proximal; peripheral pulses should be palpable; skin over injury site open or intact

X-ray   Complete break in bone continuity or in one cortex; rarely, may fail to reveal fracture initially; repeat in 10 days for certainty because bone resorption at fracture site makes diagnosis easier

••••• Multidisciplinary Plan

Emergency Care

Application of splint to hold fractured bones to prevent additional injury

Nonuse or non–weight bearing

Application of cryotherapy

Transport to medical facility

Surgery

Open reduction of the fracture with interal fixation (ORIF) of the fracture fragments with pins, nails, screws, staples, plates, intramedullary nails, or wire

Arthroplasty with replacement with prosthesis

Total joint replacement for crush injuries

Amputation for severe crush injuries

Microvascular surgery (see box on p. 412)

Application of external apparatus such as the Hoffman, Ilizarov, Ace-Fischer, or other device

Medical Care

Closed reduction with cast

Application of skin or skeletal traction (depends on type of bone or fracture severity; traction less used now because of extended hospitalization and costs)

Experimental use of bone "glue" to aid fracture "setting" and healing

Medications

Narcotic analgesics

Meperidine (Demerol), 50-100 mg q3h IM for acute pain

Morphine, 5-20 mg q4h subcutaneously, or hydromorphone (Dilaudid), 2-4 mg q4h subcutaneously, for acute pain (may use patient-controlled analgesic pump intravenously)

Analgesic-antipyretic agents

Aspirin, 600-1000 mg q4h between narcotic administration times; aspirin also has anticoagulant effects to prevent deep vein thrombosis

Acetaminophen (Tylenol), 600-1000 mg q4h between narcotic administration times

Anticoagulants

Heparin in individualized doses IV (after bleeding ceased), then Lovenox (enoxaparin), 30 mg subcutaneously bid, then Coumadin (warfarin), individualized doses po

Tranquilizers

Hydroxyzine (Vistaril), 25-50 mg IM, with narcotic as a narcotic potentiator

Muscle relaxants

Flexeril (cyclobenzaprine), 10-20 mg po tid

Robaxin (methocarbamol), 500-750 mg po q4-6 h; Skelaxin (metaxalone), 400-800 mg tid or qid

Antiinfective agents specific to the invading organisms (noted by culture) if the skin is open; after surgery, antibiotics

Cefoxitan (mefoxin), 1 g q8h IV for 3 days

Cefobid (cefoperazone), 2-4 g q12h IV for 48-72 h (or longer)

Vancomycin (Vancocin), 1 g q12h or 400 mg q6h IV

Antiinflammatories

Ibuprofen, 400-800 mg tid or bid

Toradol (Ketorolac), 15-30 mg IM or IV q4h

General Management

Placing on bed rest, if necessary, because of severity of injuries

Ensuring patient does not bear weight on affected bone and joints; having patient use cane, crutches, or walker to avoid bearing weight on injured extremity initially

Well-balanced diet high in vitamins, proteins, carbohydrates, and minerals

Forcing fluids

Concurrent treatment of systemic diseases if present

Beginning physical therapy exercises early in postoperative period

Use of cryotherapy to decrease bleeding and edema for 48 to 72 hours postoperatively

NURSING CARE

Nursing Assessment

Fracture Site and Surrounding Tissues

Edema

Color changes in fracture site and distal to site

Deformity

Paresthesia with numbness and tingling

Pain, acute and unremitting

Limitation of movement or inability to use part

Skin closed or open

Crepitation (movement of parts normally not movable, causing noise, crackling, or rubbing together of fractured ends)

Bruising; blisters on skin at fracture site

Bleeding or hematoma (noted by mass)

Presence or absence of pulses distal to injury

Systemic Concerns

Pallor

Confusion

Dyspnea

Shock

Changes in blood pressure

Sweating or perspiring

Fear and anxiety

Concomitant diseases or other injuries to distant organs

Psychosocial Concerns

Self-concept

Disturbances in body image and impairment of physical mobility

Alteration in comfort, severe pain

Inability to carry out usual roles and responsibilities

Nursing Dx & Intervention

Impaired physical mobility related to fractured bone and soft tissue trauma

- Assess area around fractured bone.
- Gently handle injured tissues by supporting joint above and below site *to prevent additional injury and lessen pain.*
- Apply ice pack to site *to lessen edema formation and bleeding.*
- Elevate extremity as prescribed; support with pillows *to aid venous return.*
- Put patient on bed rest, if prescribed, *to put body and part at rest.*
- Explain purposes for rest and not bearing weight on injured extremity *to ease patient's concerns.*
- Perform neurovascular checks *to note condition of affected tissues.*
- Assess integrity of cast or function of traction or wrapping every 1 to 2 hours initially, then every 4 hours *to note condition or functions.*
- Explain position required for maximum healing *to aid compliance.*
- Assist to proper position; change position every 2 hours or help patient position self correctly *to ease tired muscles.*
- Teach patient the "post position" for lifting self (patient plants [posts] unaffected foot flat on bed with knee bent at right angle; lifts body using trapeze while pushing down

with foot and leg). Help by lifting patient's buttocks if needed *to encourage independence and self-care.*

- Teach exercises to maintain strength and facilitate resolution of inflammation; quadriceps, buttocks, and triceps setting exercises done every 4 hours when allowed *to maintain muscle strength.*

Pain related to pressure on nerve endings

- Assess amount, type, severity, and duration of pain.
- Help patient assume a position of comfort if possible *to lessen pain or discomfort.*
- Monitor patient's use of narcotic in patient-controlled analgesia or administer prescribed narcotic analgesics: every 3 hours for meperidine (action is lost after 3 hours) or every 4 hours for opiate narcotics. Administer narcotics around the clock for 3 to 5 days or longer as prescribed *to maintain adequate blood levels to relieve pain.* Periods between narcotics may be increased with use of muscle relaxants for acute muscle spasms *to lessen dependence on narcotics and to decrease muscle spasms.*
- Administer nonnarcotic analgesics or nonsteroidal antiinflammatory medications as prescribed every 4 hours between narcotic administrations to enhance pain relief. Antiinflammatory medications *aid resolution of inflammation.*
- Change position every 2 hours *to lessen muscle fatigue.*
- Massage back and buttocks *to decrease pressure and fatigue and to increase circulation in those areas.*
- Administer muscle relaxant or sedatives as prescribed *to aid reduction of muscle spasms and lessen pain.*

Body image disturbance and altered role performance related to temporary loss of independence

- Assess self-concept and dependency concerns.
- Maintain privacy while helping patient perform ADL and hygienic care *to aid personal cleanliness and self-esteem.*
- Offer oral hygiene and back care frequently *to maintain healthy tissues.*
- Explain that proper positioning and non–weight bearing are required *to facilitate bone healing.*
- Encourage patient to express feelings about enforced immobility and displacement from familiar surroundings *to foster comfort.*
- Arrange for physical therapy and occupational therapy consultations *to maintain muscle strength and self-esteem and to prepare for self-care after discharge.*
- Encourage family members to interact with patient *to maintain customary roles and esteem.*
- Help patient comply with high-nutrient diet *to lessen weight loss (a patient in skeletal traction may lose weight quickly) and to maintain positive body image.*

Knowledge deficit related to shock (from severity of injury) and to unfamiliar terms or treatments

- Assess patient's understanding of condition, if feasible; if in shock or unconscious, do assessment when patient's condition has improved.

- Clarify needed misconceptions or lack of understanding; may use pictures or patient's x-rays *to provide needed explanations.*
- Show videotape, if available, of similar-aged or same-sex patient with same type of injury or treatment *to clarify a specific regimen or action.*
- Ask patient if understands by having patient draw picture *to ascertain level or degree of understanding.*
- Continue teaching patient as needed at present time or later period *if patient appears tired or uncomfortable.*
- Provide a quiet, calm atmosphere *for optional learning to proceed.*
- Seek questions from patient and family *to determine if additional teaching is needed.*

Altered tissue perfusion related to impaired circulation from trauma

- Assess condition of affected tissues.
- Perform all parts of neurovascular checks every hour initially. Check color; temperature; peripheral pulses; edema; presence, amount, and type of pain; motor functions (patient should be able to move parts proximal to injury; sensory functions (complaints of numbness, tingling, or pins and needles indicate sensory compromise); and capillary refill (compress nail of middle finger or toe, release; nail should pink up in 2 to 4 seconds for normal capillary refill; 4 to 6 seconds is abnormal and should be reported); compare the injured area with the same tissues on the opposite side of the body. Another critical finding, along with prolonged capillary refill, is increased pain on passive movement of the fingers or toes or pain not relieved by narcotic administration, which could signify that the patient may be developing compartment syndrome. Increased anoxia caused by the stretching of the muscle with the passive movement causes the increased pain (see Figure 4-29). Report abnormal findings to physician.
- Elevate limb to heart level to increase venous return, thereby lessening edema.
- Loosen circumferential dressings, if present, or bivalve cast *to increase arterial circulation to tissues.*

Risk for impaired skin integrity related to immobility, presence of a cast, or traction equipment

- Assess skin surfaces for signs of pressure, such as redness, blistering, soreness, or open lesion.
- Reposition patient every 2 hours *to relieve pressure.*
- Turn to side if permitted *to distribute pressure to other areas and to relieve tired or sore muscles.*
- Massage around bony prominences *to increase circulation.*
- Use foam or lamb's wool bed pads *to distribute pressure.*
- Encourage patient to eat adequately from a high-protein, high-carbohydrate, high-vitamin diet *to maintain healthy cellular tissues and to aid fracture healing.*
- Be sure patient gets at least 3000 ml of fluid daily *to maintain skin turgor and renal functions.*
- Teach patient how to move self in bed *to lessen friction and shearing forces and maintain healthy skin surfaces.*

- Use turning sheet, if allowed, to turn side to side *to relieve pressure on skin and bony prominences.*

Patient Education/Home Care Planning

1. Reiterate reasons for rest and not bearing weight on injured limb (anxiety may prevent the patient from hearing or understanding initial explanations).
2. Explain reasons for weight loss and how the patient can lessen it through exercise and diet.
3. Explain measures for dealing with acute pain and changes in using medications as pain decreases.
4. Show pictures of bone healing processes to elicit the patient's cooperation and understanding.
5. Explain turning and moving techniques to prevent skin breakdown.
6. List purposes and techniques for neurovascular checks.
7. Encourage patient to notify physician if concerned about healing processes or prolonged pain.
8. Discuss signs and symptoms to report to physician and signs and symptoms that require medical atttention.
9. Coordinate teaching with physical or occupational therapists for self-care at home.
10. Provide needed aids (walker, crutches) or equipment (bed pad, abduction pillow) before discharge for self-care at home.

Evaluation

Patient resumes walking and bearing full weight on limb without limitation or discomfort in usual time frame after healing—may be 6 weeks to 2 months or longer Patient feels no discomfort or pain when walking or bearing weight on limb or using part normally.

Pain is relieved as bone union occurs in anatomic position Patient can use part without pain. No deformity is present. Patient is using no analgesics for pain after 2 to 3 months.

Patient resumes social interactions and roles Patient returns to family, social, and employment roles after 3 months or later, according to bone fractured and treatment.

Patient has normal tissue perfusion Patient has normal color, temperature, capillary refill, motor and sensory functions, and no edema of healed tissues after 6 to 9 months.

Patient has healthy skin turgor without developing pressure areas Patient has pink, well-nourished skin with good turgor. Is regaining lost weight over 3 months or longer.

Patient able to explain type of injury, purposes, and results of treatments

CURVATURES OF THE SPINAL COLUMN

The spine develops its characteristic curves during fetal growth (Figure 4-20). Both prenatally and postnatally the curves may become abnormal because of defective bone, muscle, nerve, or

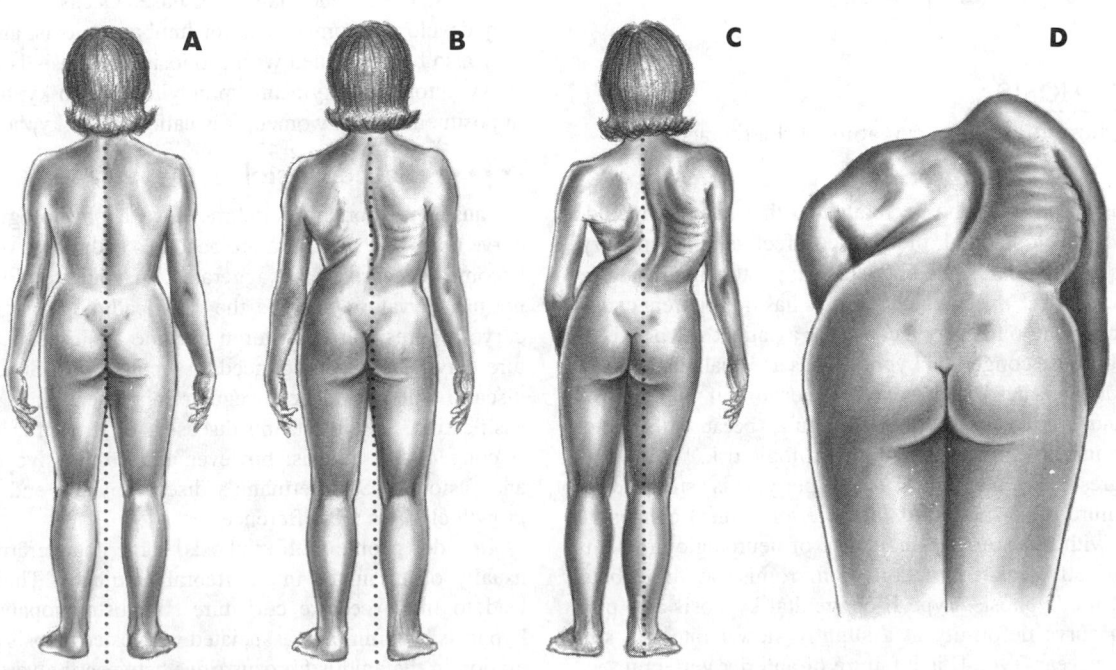

Figure 4-20 Normal spinal alignment and abnormal spinal curvatures associated with scoliosis. **A,** Normal. **B,** Mild. **C,** Severe. **D,** Rotation and curvature of scoliosis.

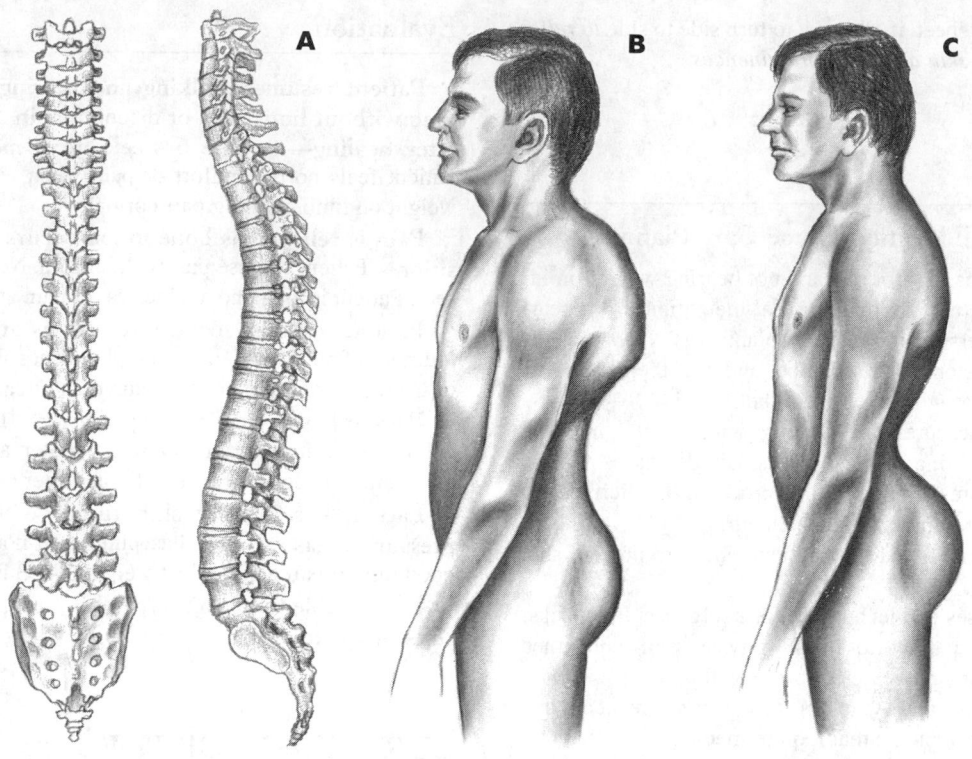

Figure 4-21 A, Normal spinal alignment and curvatures. **B,** Kyphosis. **C,** Lordosis.

other growth factors. The abnormal curves are called kyphosis (excessive curvature of thoracic spine), scoliosis (lateral or rotary curvature of thoracic spine), and lordosis (excessive curvature of lumbar spine) (Figure 4-21).

KYPHOSIS

Kyphosis is excessive curvature of the thoracic vertebrae.

Various types of kyphosis, related to their causes, include congenital, developmental, metabolic, infective, inflammatory, neuromuscular, tumor, skeletal dysplasia, posttraumatic and iatrogenic kyphosis.[61] Idiopathic kyphosis has no apparent cause.

It is important to identify a cause for a patient's kyphosis, if possible, because congenital kyphosis has a virtual guarantee of progression. It is also important to determine if the curve is smooth and gradual or sharp and angular because the latter curves are usually associated with neurologic risk.[61]

A progression of curve of 5° to 10° per year is estimated for type I (failure of formation of the anterior bodies) congenital kyphosis, with an estimated incidence of neurologic problems of 25% to 30% related to cord compromise at the gibbus (hump) of the kyphosis. Type II congenital kyphosis also progresses in curve deformity at a slightly slower rate, but still about 5° per year. Type II is a failure of anterior vertebral segmentation. Type III is a condition of mixed anomalies and has no specific curve progression rates.[61]

Kyphosis occurs in various age groups. When it occurs in young children, it is usually congenital. It may become apparent in the adolescent years, when it is referred to as juvenile kyphosis, or Scheuermann's disease. Occasionally kyphosis may develop to compensate for lumbar lordosis, and kyphosis may also be associated with scoliosis. Kyphosis is also a classic symptom of ankylosing spondylitis. When kyphosis occurs in postmenopausal women, it is called senile kyphosis.

•••••• **Pathophysiology**

Because the thoracic vertebrae have a physiologic posterior curve normally, the curvature becomes pathologic only when it becomes excessive or exaggerated. In young children the abnormal curvature may be the only pathologic sign until the curve progresses. As children become adolescents, the curvature may become pronounced, especially with Scheuermann's disease, which produces irregular epiphyseal plate growth and ossification. Scheuermann's disease is often confused with type II congenital kyphosis; however, the progressive ossification and fusion of Scheuermann's disease by the end of skeletal growth clarifies the difference.

In older people with kyphosis, some degenerative changes usually occur in the intervertebral cartilages. These changes lead to the excessive curvature. In postmenopausal women kyphosis is commonly associated with osteoporosis and degeneration in the anulus fibrosus rings between the vertebrae.

Kyphotic curves may occur mainly in the thoracic vertebra or lower in the thoracolumbar vertebrae, primarily in congenital kyphosis, where the progressive curve growth compromises the spinal cord leading to motor and sensory changes in the lower body and extremities if the curve progression is left untreated.

Diagnostic Studies and Findings

Physical examination Excessive thoracic spinal curvature, rounded shoulders; occasional low back pain (40% of adolescents with Scheuermann's disease have back pain, as do many children with congenital kyphosis); easy fatigability; exaggerated lumbar lordosis to compensate for the kyphosis; respiratory deficit

X-ray Marked curvature of thoracic spine; *geriatric patients:* possible osteoporosis with vertebral wedging; wedging and narrowing of anterior portions of thoracic vertebral bodies (T6 to T10); lateral tomograms may show spinal deformities not clear on plain x-ray; MRI or myelograms may show sites of neurologic pressures

Histocompatibility testing Serum HLA-B27 antigen present in young adults with ankylosing spondylitis

Multidisciplinary Plan

Surgery

Halo traction; osteotomy
Spinal fusion for severe kyphosis, especially if signs of neurologic deficit begin
Spinal instrumentation (see p. 448)

Medications

Older adults may have hormonal treatment or mineral administration
Young adults with ankylosing spondylitis receive several drugs (pp. 360 to 361) for treatment of their disease processes

General Management

Milwaukee brace for adolescents
Back corset for older adults
Orthotic devices (plastic or canvas/metal splint) for adolescents
Teaching patient to stand up as straight as possible
Exercise program to strengthen muscles and ligaments
Deep-breathing exercises for any respiratory compromise

NURSING CARE

Nursing Assessment

Thoracic Spine

Adolescent
Rounded shoulders
Backache
Excessive curvature of thoracic spine
Lumbar lordosis increased

Young adult
Stiff, sore back when rising on awakening
Low back pain not relieved with rest
Increasing curvature of thoracic spine
Older adult
Female
Postmenopausal
Loss of height
Excessive curvature of thoracic spine

Systemic Processes

Young adult
Positive HLA-B27 histocompatibility antigen
Reiter's syndrome (conjunctivitis, uveitis, genital lesions, low back pain)
Pulmonary compromise
Neurologic compromise

Psychosocial Concerns

Self-concept
Disturbances in self-esteem, body image, and role expectations
Neurologic: possible paralysis; need to use ambulatory aid (crutches, wheelchair)

Nursing Dx & Intervention

Self-esteem and body image disturbances and altered role performance related to spinal deformity

- Assess back and spine for excessive thoracic curvature by having patient bend over, turn side to side, face front and back.
- Discuss principles of proper posture *to aid in maintaining upright posture.*
- Explain that condition is not life threatening *to ease concern.*
- Assist with application of brace or orthosis, if used, until patient can do it alone *to aid compliance.* Patient should wear cotton T-shirt under orthosis or brace *to protect skin surfaces.*
- Discuss clothing to make brace less obvious *to increase self-confidence.*
- Discuss exercises to strengthen back muscles.
- Discuss patient's life goals and review need for possible alteration (patient should set goals so as to be able to do what he or she desires without many limitations; see p. 361 for limitations with ankylosing spondylitis).

Impaired physical mobility related to back pain and deformity

- Nursing care is discussed under ankylosing spondylitis, p. 361.

Impaired gas exchange related to pulmonary compromise

- Nursing interventions are discussed under care of a person in a cast, p. 432.

Impaired peripheral tissue perfusion

- Neurologic effects are discussed under spinal fusion, p. 451.

Patient Education/Home Care Planning

1. Reiterate that patient can help self through exercises, posture changes, and using a brace, orthosis, or splint, in most instances.
2. Reiterate that patient should be able to achieve life's goals even with kyphosis.
3. Explain clothing types to lessen curvature noticeability.
4. Teach preoperative and postoperative care if patient is to have surgical treatment.

Evaluation

Patient returns to social interactions and roles   Patient has improved self-concept and body image, is better able to regain family and social roles, and is positive about self and the future.

Patient's posture has improved and curvature is lessened after treatment and mobility is increased   Patient stands straighter with less curvature or rotation, hips and shoulders are more normally aligned, and mobility is improved.

Patient has adequate gas exchange   Patient has normal breath sounds in all lobes; has respiratory excursions of normal rates and depth. Color is normal.

Patient is regaining muscle strength and normal sensory functions after surgical repair

SCOLIOSIS

Scoliosis is lateral curvature of the vertebral column.

Scoliosis has been noted in infants (infantile scoliosis), young children (juvenile), teenagers (adolescent), and adults. For most patients the cause of the scoliosis is unknown; thus it is called idiopathic scoliosis (70% of patients with scoliosis)[168] and constituting 1% to 4% of all children.[142] A familial genetic factor, hormonal and metabolic factors, and skeletal growth factors may also play parts in causing some cases of scoliosis. Most cases of scoliosis become more prominent and noticeable in the early teenage years because of uneven shoulders and hip levels and more pronounced laterality and rotatory curvatures. Curvatures may vary from 20° (considered the lowest limit of clinically important scoliosis) to curves of 60° or more. Girls are affected more than boys. Approximately 1.5 per 1000 population have scoliosis. Scoliosis associated with Rett syndrome occurs only in females as a dominant gene on the chromosome[70] and is its most common orthopedic problem.

•••••• Pathophysiology

The curvatures of scoliosis have more than one dimension because they occur in the vertically stacked vertebrae. Three curve planes are involved: concave curvature on the anterior vertebral bodies, convex posterior curves, and lateral rotation of the thoracic spine on bending or flexing forward. Lordosis is present in the thoracic vertebral curve. As the person with scoliosis bends forward, the thoracic lordosis causes lateral flexion of the affected thoracic vertebrae. The lateral curvature is thus secondary to the thoracic lordosis. Also, the larger the lordosis, the greater the rotation and lateral curvature on flexion. The risk of curve progression is greatest for children with larger curves who are in the adolescent growth spurt.[143]

Curves can also stop growing and restart during adult years. Muscles, ligaments, and other soft tissues become shortened on the concave side of the curve and can influence the "growth" of the curve, or compression of one side of the vertebral bodies. Usually curves greater than 20° require treatment. Curves of 60° affect pulmonary functions.

Scoliotic curves are referred to as thoracic (the most common thoracolumbar) and lumbar. Curves may be double, with a right thoracic curve and left lumbar curve, left thoracic curve and right lumbar curve, or variations of these. Interestingly, true wry neck (torticollis) is scoliosis of the cervical spine.

•••••• Diagnostic Studies and Findings

History   Asymmetry of shoulders or hips; uneven hemlines, pant length, or waistline; forward bending in school screening indicates lateral curvature

Physical examination   Lateral deviation with or without rotation or vertebrae; curvature may become more pronounced when patient bends forward; rotation may also be more noticeable when patient bends forward; when hands of examiner are placed on patient's hips, one hand is higher than other when patient is standing upright; examination of leg length reveals one leg is shorter, and when patient sits, the curvature disappears, rib angles may protrude, and one hip may stick out; asymmetric shoulder levels; prominence of one shoulder, parents may be unaware of curvature until it is significant; muscle wasting; decreasing mobility and gait ataxia (with Rett syndrome); deep tendon reflexes may be abnormal; absent abdominal reflexes

X-ray   Curvature and angle of curvature, plus rotation; special x-ray studies can detect lordosis, concave curves, and convex curves; in Rett syndrome, a long, C-shaped thoracolumbar curvature is most common

Risser's sign   X-rays show skeletal maturity by evaluating ossification of the iliac apophysis (anterior iliac spine), classified as Risser 1 through 4—ranges from 25% to 100% ossification; Risser 5—fusion of the apophysis, cessation of skeletal growth[142]

Bone scan   Bone scans, MRI, CT, tomogram, or myelogram may be done if patient has back pain or abnormal neurologic findings on physical exam

Pulmonary consultation   Arterial blood gases

•••••• Multidisciplinary Plan

Surgery

Straightening of curve with Harrington or Luque rods, Wisconsin segmental system, Texas Scottish Rite Hospital system, Isola spine implant system, the Moduloc posterior spinal system,[89] or Cotrel-Dubousset instrumentation (CDI) for internal fixation with bone grafts to fuse spine; may be anterior, posterior, or both

Dwyer procedure: staples and screws fixed to the vertebral bodies; a cable is inserted through the screw heads; tightening the cable closes the vertebral areas and straightens the curve

Anterior discectomy with interbody fusion

Pedicle screw fixation is investigational under FDA regulations

General Management

Use of Milwaukee, Boston, or similar brace or orthotic device

Application of Cotrel's traction or halo-femoral traction

Regimen of exercises to strengthen back muscles

Electrical stimulation to paraspinous muscles—no longer used because does not alter the natural history of curve progression[143]

NURSING CARE

Nursing Assessment

Entire Spinal Column

Spinal column will curve away from the midline in thoracic and lumbar areas.

One shoulder or hip will be a different height than the other; legs of unequal length

Spine will rotate laterally when patient bends over; use of scoliometer to measure angle of trunk rotation

May have upper and lower (sacral) curves

Arm-to-body space will be different on one side

Systemic Concerns

Patient may have muscle weakness through body

Cardiac or respiratory signs such as pulse rate or rhythm changes, dyspnea, or shortness of breath may be noted in more severe scoliosis of thoracic area; vital capacity may be decreased

Psychosocial Concerns

Self-concept

Alteration on body image and role expectations

Impaired physical mobility

Impaired gas exchange

Nursing Dx & Intervention

Body image disturbance and altered role performance related to spinal deformity

- Assess degree or severity of curvature.
- Discuss patient's feelings of inadequacy because of deformity *to aid in ventilation of feelings.*
- Discuss clothing to make brace less noticeable *to ease concerns.*

- Discuss need to continue wearing brace *to prevent increase in rotation or lateralization.* Orthosis or brace is worn for 23 hours per day in most instances.
- Discuss adjustments to clothing hemlines *to negate effects of scoliosis.*
- Encourage usual peer relationships and activities *to aid psychosocial development.*

Risk for impaired skin integrity related to presence and use of brace or other orthotic device

- Assess all skin tissues for condition, presence of skin irritation, color changes, or open areas.
- Clarify necessity to wear proper clothing such as cotton T-shirt under brace or orthosis *to maintain skin integrity.*
- Encourage proper skin cleansing and use of lotions *to maintain intact and healthy skin tissues.*
- Monitor fit of brace or orthosis *to detect early signs of improper fit or pressure areas.*
- Encourage child or parents to check with orthotist if signs of skin pressure develop *to prevent progression of skin irritation.*

Impaired physical mobility related to deformity or treatment

- Assess effects of condition on mobility.
- Discuss purposes of bed rest and Cotrel's or halo-femoral traction before surgical correction.
- Change patient's position every 2 to 3 hours *to maintain tissue integrity.*
- Discuss need to limit activities to maintain traction or brace use *to increase compliance.*
- If surgery is performed, discuss need to bed rest *to permit healing.* (See p. 451 for nursing care for spinal fusion.)
- Encourage patient to maintain peer visits and interactions while movement is restricted *to foster personal growth and esteem.*
- Arrange for tutoring *to help patient keep up with schoolwork,* if needed.
- Arrange for occupational therapy and physical therapy consultations *to maintain muscle strength and keep spirits up.*
- Provide well-balanced diet *to promote healing after surgery and to lessen risk of infection.*

Impaired gas exchange related to pulmonary compromise

- Nursing care is discussed under fracture/cast care, p. 432.

Patient Education/Home Care Planning

1. Clarify usual progression of lateralization without treatment.
2. Encourage continuity of medical care to monitor status of scoliosis and postoperative progress and healing.
3. Reiterate need to wear brace as prescribed to prevent progression of scoliosis before surgical correction.

4. After surgery, explain bone healing processes and cautions to permit healing to proceed.
5. Teach pulmonary and breathing exercises to improve pulmonary functions postoperatively.
6. Encourage communication and use of National Scoliosis Foundation or Scoliosis Association materials and services.
7. Encourage continuance of school-age children's screening for early detection of spinal abnormalities.

Evaluation

Patient returns to social interactions and roles Patient has improved self-concept and body image, is better able to regain family and social roles, and is positive about self and future.

Posture and mobility have improved and curvature is lessened after treatment Patient stands straighter with less curvature and rotation, hips and shoulders are more normally aligned, and mobility is improved.

Patient has satisfactory gas exchange Patient has clear breath sounds and normal respiratory rates. No cough is noted. Patient's color is normal. Vital capacity has decreased minimally.

Patient uses brace or orthosis as prescribed Skin tissues develop no redness or chafing. Patient wears proper underclothing under device.

LORDOSIS

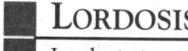

Lordosis is a normal curvature of the lumbar spine.

Lordosis may become exaggerated during pregnancy or in cases of large abdominal tumors or obesity, when overcorrection may be necessary to maintain balance when upright. Structural changes do not occur, and the condition is relieved with delivery, removal of the tumor, or weight loss.

Hyperlordosis, or "swayback," is fairly common in young children, especially girls, before puberty. The cause is thought to be rapid skeletal growth without appropriate stretching of the posterior soft tissues, such as the lumbar fascia and paraspinal muscles.

Permanent hyperlordosis, although very rare, can occur from degenerative conditions (e.g., osteoporosis) of the lumbosacral discs or vertebral bodies. Treatments for hyperlordosis include use of a brace or lumbar belt, spinal fusion, or osteotomy.

PERIPHERAL NERVE INJURIES

During a difficult delivery the baby may be injured around the neck and shoulder because of the force required for delivery through a tight pelvis and vagina. The injuries may be traction injuries to the nerves of the brachial plexus, but the results of such injuries are musculoskeletal from weakness and atrophy. Table 4-5 presents several injuries that can occur at birth or develop later in life from trauma. Nerve damage at any time of life causes significant musculoskeletal defects.

Without stimuli, muscles become weakened and flaccid and eventually shrink and atrophy. As muscles atrophy, they pull the tendons, ligaments, bones, and skin with them. Because the flexor muscles are generally stronger than the extensors, flexion contractures usually result. Adduction is frequently more noted than abduction, although either may be present. Rotation and pronation of the muscles and joints are also common. Changes may also accompany the motor losses.

CARPAL TUNNEL SYNDROME

Carpal tunnel syndrome is a cluster of symptoms affecting the functions of the wrist, hand, and fingers. It is caused by compression of the median nerve.

Carpal tunnel syndrome results from compression of the median nerve in the tendon sheath under the transverse ligament on the ventral surface of the wrist (Figure 4-22). Because the tissues in this part of the wrist normally fit closely together, any swelling will usually bring on the compressive symptoms. The syndrome usually develops after trauma with subsequent fibrosis and scarring of the tendon sheath. However, no previous trauma may be noted.

Certain repetitive movements involving wrist twisting, turning, or pounding, such as those experienced when using a computer for many hours daily or a jackhammer, may cause the syndrome. Carpal tunnel syndrome has become one of the three most common industrial or work-related conditions and is related to the increased computer usage in all industries and departments in industries and government.

Curiously, pregnant women may develop carpal tunnel syndrome during their last trimester. The reasons for this have not yet been determined, although fluid retention and edema may be contributing factors. Recently, chronic hypoxia from decreased circulation has been suggested as a potential precipitating event.[173]

More women than men develop carpal tunnel syndrome. Menopausal women and people with rheumatoid arthritis also show a higher incidence of the condition. It is seen bilaterally in nearly half of those affected.[173]

•••••• Pathophysiology

Carpal tunnel syndrome develops secondary to repetitive motions of the wrist area, secondary to trauma, ganglion or neuroma, or tenosynovitis.

Pain is one of the first symptoms of carpal tunnel syndrome. It often occurs at night, waking the patient with burning, tingling, and numbness. The fingers feel swollen, and the hand feels heavy. The patient must usually hang the arm over the bed or get up and walk around to relieve the pain. The fingers may have paresthesias, including the thumb and the second, third, and radial side of the fourth fingers.

TABLE 4-5 Musculoskeletal Effects of Nerve Injuries

Nerve	Site of Injury	Cause of Injury	Effects of Injury
Brachial plexus	Cervical roots of C5-7	Traction to arm or shoulder during delivery; gunshot wound; avulsion of nerves from excess traction accidentally applied; injury to cervical vertebrae	Erb's palsy: affected arm, forearm, and hand internally rotated and pronated. Injury may cause temporary weakness and palsy; if severe, it will cause permanent paralysis with contracture of lower forearm, wrist, and fingers; sensory loss to outer arm
Brachial, axillary, and musculocutaneous	Cervical roots of C8 and T1	Breech delivery with arm above head; gunshot wound	Klumpke's palsy: intrinsic muscles of hand and flexor muscles of fingers are paralyzed; some sensory loss may be present in ulnar forearm and hand; permanent effects: a claw hand develops in a flaccid, weak limb
Radial	Shoulder or elbow	Leaning on crutches in axillae; elbow: fracture; other: cutting of nerve, pressure of cast at wrist	Radial weakness from leaning on crutches with axillary pressure is fully reversible; elbow lesions; may have paralysis of wrist extensor and supinator muscles; eventually may need tendon transplants to wrist and fingers
Ulnar	Shoulder to elbow and to forearm	Open wounds (cut); fracture of medial epicondyle or lateral condyle; osteoarthritic or rheumatoid arthritis changes	Ring and little fingers may be temporarily or permanently held in hyperextended positions while rest of the hand is clawed; sensation is lost over ring and little fingers; there is muscle wasting of intrinsic muscles of hand
Median	Wrist under transverse carpal ligament	Trauma; pregnancy; rheumatoid arthritis; postmenopausal state; overuse (carpal tunnel syndrome)	Wasting of palmar thenar prominence (base of thumb); edema of hand; heavy, "clumsy" hand; sensory loss over radial $3^1/_2$ fingers; if median nerve is several without repair, paralysis of middle finger or index finger causes it to point ahead while other fingers are held in flexion; muscle wasting of hand (see below for carpal tunnel syndrome)
Peroneal	Neck of fibula	Pressure of splint; traction with leg in external rotation	Patient cannot dorsiflex or evert foot and toes; outer side of leg is wasted; footdrop is present; sensation is lost over front and outer half of leg and dorsum of foot and toes; posterior tibial nerve injuries may cause tarsal tunnel syndrome (p. 406)

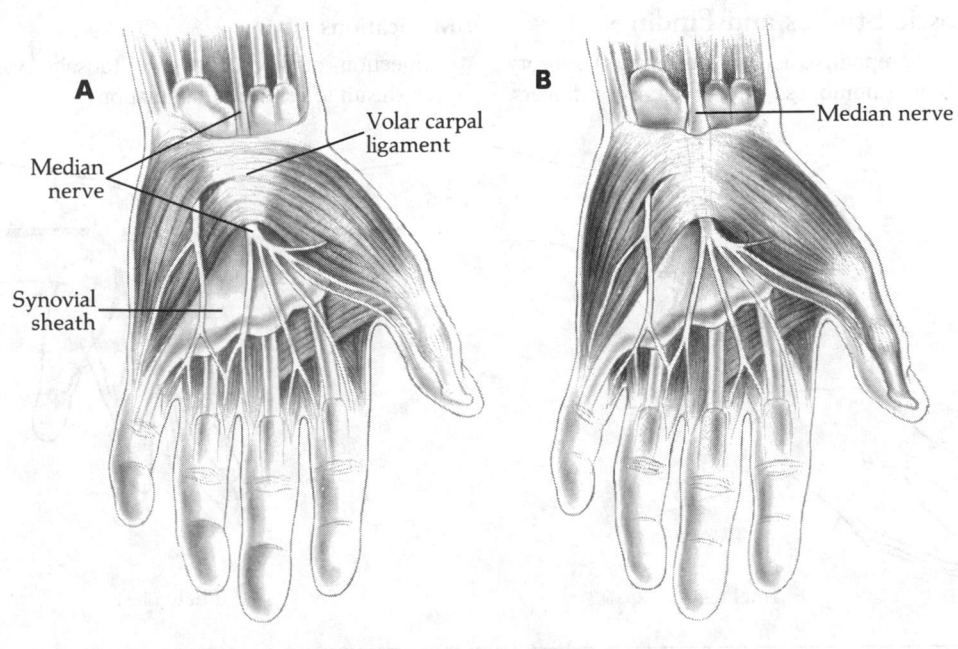

Figure 4-22 **A,** Wrist structures affected in carpal tunnel syndrome. **B,** Decompression of median nerve.

During the day the patient has few symptoms except when doing things that require turning the wrist, such as word processing and construction work. The hand is weaker and feels clumsy, and sometimes pain may radiate up the arm. The thenar muscles develop atrophic changes with noticeable loss of muscle mass. Either one hand or both hands may be involved.

Five factors have been found to correlate with carpal tunnel syndrome caused by repetitive motion[46]:

- Age 50 years or older
- Symptoms that have occurred for more than 10 months
- Constant tingling and burning sensation
- Trigger finger (one finger locks, indicating that a broader area of inflammation is present)
- Positive Phalen's test (see below)

A condition similar to carpal tunnel syndrome can occur in one or more other peripheral nerves, including the radial and ulnar tunnels in the upper extremity. Tarsal tunnel syndrome, which is similar to carpal tunnel syndrome, may occur in the lower extremity. Radial nerve weakness can temporarily occur from improper use of crutches. This clears when the person stops resting on the axillary supports of the crutches. Ulnar nerve injuries frequently accompany elbow trauma. When severe, such upper extremity nerve injuries can cause clawing of and loss of sensation in the ring and little fingers.

Trauma to the posterior tibial nerve or entrapment in the transvere tunnel over the Achilles tendon can cause tarsal tunnel syndrome. The symptom patterns are the same as those of carpal tunnel syndrome, but the symptoms appear in the foot and ankle instead of the hand and wrist. Treatments for tarsal tunnel syndrome are the same as for other entrapment syndromes and are specific to the particular nerve, ligament, and tendon sheath involved.

•••••• Diagnostic Studies and Findings

History   History of repetitive activities of wrist(s); sensory changes; paresthesia and numbness of thumbs, index fingers, and ring fingers; pain waking patient at night; motor changes, with clumsiness, heaviness of hand, and edema; thenar muscle atrophy; pain, possibly radiating up arm; correlation with pregnancy, rheumatoid arthritis, postmenopausal state, diabetes, thyroid dysfunction; similar symptoms in lower extremity with tarsal tunnel syndrome

Physical examination   Deficits in sensory mapping along median nerve innervation pathways; positive Tinel's sign (Figure 4-23): increased tingling with gentle tap over tendon sheath on ventral surface of central wrist; edema of fingers noted; thenar surfaces of palm thinner than normal (wasting); holding wrists against each other in forced palmar flexion for 1 minute can elicit sensory changes of numbness and tingling, which is a positive Phalen's test (Figure 4-23), one indication of carpal tunnel syndrome

Electromyogram   Weakened muscle response to stimulation

Magnetic resonance imaging   Shows compression and flattening of the median nerve; increased signal intensity within the median nerve, abrupt changes in diameter of the median nerve[173]

Handheld electroneurometer   Used if EMG services not available; predicts motor latency of median nerve diagnostic of carpal tunnel syndrome[10]

•••••• Multidisciplinary Plan

Surgery

Release of carpal ligament and tendon to relieve compression (see Figure 4-22); surgery may be done endoscopically

Medications

Injection of hydrocortisone (dosage varies) into tendon sheath to relieve inflammation

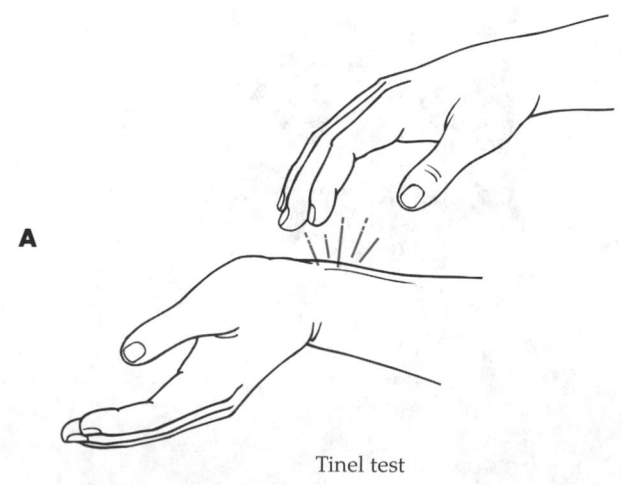

Tinel test

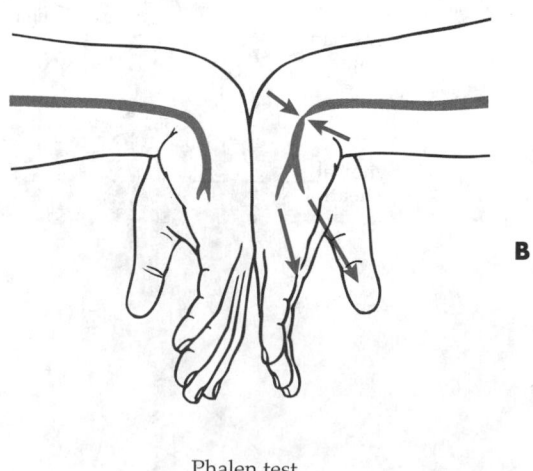

Phalen test

Figure 4-23 **A,** Tinel sign. **B,** Phalen test.

Antiinflammatory medication
Ibuprofen 400-600 mg bid

General Management

Use of a cock-up splint to relieve pressure and to lessen wrist flexion

Elevation to relieve edema

ROM exercises to lessen sense of clumsiness

Restriction of twisting and turning activities of wrist

Continuation of usual medical care for systemic illness (rheumatoid arthritis) if present

NURSING CARE

Nursing Assessment

Wrist, Hand, and Fingers (Both Extremities)

Inability to use hands and fingers through normal ranges of motion

Movements limited

Presence or absence of edema, numbness, tingling, pain

Assessment of time when pain is present, severity, and activities that increase or decrease pain

Assessment of palmar thenar (base of thumb) surfaces for atrophy

Assessment of distribution of paresthesia (if present) into fingers or up arm

Systemic Concerns

Rheumatoid arthritis
Postmenopausal state
Pregnancy in last trimester
Diabetes
Thyroid dysfunction

Psychosocial Concerns

Self-concept, disturbance in: body-image, role performance
Impaired physical mobility

Nursing Dx & Intervention

Altered peripheral tissue perfusion related to compression and edema of nerve

- Assess circulatory status of limb by neurovascular checks (p. 358).
- Apply ice bag to wrist area *to decrease edema.*
- Report increasing numbness to physician *for patient safety.*
- Apply splint *to prevent flexion of wrist;* flexion increases numbness and tingling in presence of syndrome.
- Compare both wrists and hands *to note if symptoms are bilateral.*

Impaired physical mobility related to pain, edema, and motor changes

- Assess effects of condition on wrist and hand ROM.
- Explain inflammatory processes to correlate need to limit activities of wrist and hand *to ease concerns or anxiety.*
- Assist with and teach proper splint application and need to wear at night *to prevent flexion of wrist;* assist with hygienic care if necessary *to increase independence and compliance.*
- Elevate hand and wrist if edema present *to aid venous return.*
- Assist with ROM exercises if ordered *to maintain functions.*
- Continue care for concomitant illnesses *to relieve symptoms.*
- Observe and assess site for relief of symptoms after injection of hydrocortisone, if used, or after surgical release *to note effects of treatment.*
- Encourage continuing follow-up medical care until recovery is complete *to aid resolution of condition.*

Pain related to edema and compression of nerve

- Assess amount, type, and severity of pain.
- Administer pain medication as prescribed; monitor and report patient's response *to note efficacy.*
- Apply ice bags *to decrease edema and pain.*
- Do preoperative preparation and teaching *to ease anxiety and promote safe care.*
- Monitor relief of numbness, tingling, and pain after surgical procedure *to determine effect of ligament release.*

Patient Education/Home Care Planning

1. Reiterate explanations of inflammatory processes as bases for symptoms.
2. Discuss activities to lessen stress on inflamed tissues.
3. Reassure about relief of symptoms after surgical release or injection of steroids that follows reduction of edema and healing of involved tissues.
4. If patient is pregnant, discuss probable relief of symptoms after delivery.
5. If condition employment-related, discuss possible need for changing to alternate job activities or seek changes in equipment to prevent recurrence.

Evaluation

Patient regains adequate tissue perfusion   Patient has no numbness, tingling, or edema after treatments.

Patient regains joint ROM and muscle strength over time   Patient performs self-care and regains strength after incision heals; thenar pad gradually regains muscle mass

Patient experiences pain-free wrist and hand functions Patient has no pain, edema, numbness, or tingling when using wrist and hand.

SCIATIC NERVE INJURY

Sciatic nerve injury is a pathologic condition usually caused by external trauma to the nerve.

Injury to the sciatic nerve may be primary, from a gunshot wound, stabbing, fall, or other cause, or it may result from pressure from rupture of an intervertebral nucleus pulposus. The pathologic nucleus pulposus exerts pressure on the spinal nerves as they exit the spinal cord and traverse the sciatic nerve. The intervertebral discs that most often rupture (95%) are at L5-S1 and L4-L5 interspaces. Cervical intervertebral discs rupture less frequently, although they can become painful from degenerative changes and may lead to spinal stenosis from osteophyte formation.

The following discussion focuses on pathologic findings in the sciatic nerve resulting from herniation (rupture) of one or more lumbar intervertebral nuclei pulposi.

Low back pain, with or without sciatica, is a symptom complex reported in nearly 60% to 80% of persons in the general population with a cost of $24 billion per year. The medical treatment of low back pain is the leading compensable cost of injury in the workplace.[53] The primary role of the orthopedist is to help patients with their primary treatment and to minimize the chance of patients subsequently having chronic low back pain with all its attendant psychologic, social, and economic costs.[133]

‧‧‧‧‧‧ Pathophysiology

The nucleus pulposus is a semigelatinous mass inside the cartilaginous anulus (disc) between the bodies of each vertebra. It plays a key role in the structural stability of the spine by providing load absorption and distribution while anchoring the vertebral bodies to one another through a wide range of motions.[8] When the cartilage of the anulus cracks or degenerates, it allows the nucleus pulposus to rupture through the cracks. A ruptured disc is a twofold process of degeneration of the anulus with herniation of the nucleus pulposus material. It appears that the intervertebral disc undergoes the most dramatic age-related changes of all connective tissues.[8]

Rupture of the anulus is generally caused by degenerative changes in the cartilaginous structures of the anulus. As the disc (anulus) ages, it loses elasticity, partly from changes and increases in proteoglycans in its collagen fibers and partly from decreases in its fluid content. These changes weaken the disc, making it unable to tolerate even usual body weight. The disc flattens or bulges, and additional pressure from lifting, straining, increased weight, or a sudden twist, turn, or sharp bending of the back may cause the anulus to bulge backward or tear. The nucleus pulposus can then extrude through the crack. The mass can extrude anteriorly toward the cord, laterally toward the lamina and facets, or posteriorly toward the posterior spinous processes (Figure 4-24). The extruded mass presses on the dura mater or nerve roots or both, causing pain in the back that radiates to the sciatic nerve. The presence of the extruded mass plus the pressure cause edema to develop, which also increases pain. At times, if the entire nucleus mass has not extruded, it may move back inside the disc when the edema subsides. If the mass stays extruded, it can adhere to the nerve roots or their dural sheaths, adding to the scarring and pain. Eventually the prolapsed material can also disturb the functioning of the facets of the vertebrae, leading to further degeneration of these joints.

The incident that causes the acute rupture can be as trivial as a sneeze or cough while the person is bent forward. Usually it is caused by lifting something while the body is not in optimum lift position, an unexpectedly heavy load, or a load that shifts suddenly. Excessive pressure is referred from tensed abdominal and back muscles to the anulus and then to the nucleus, which

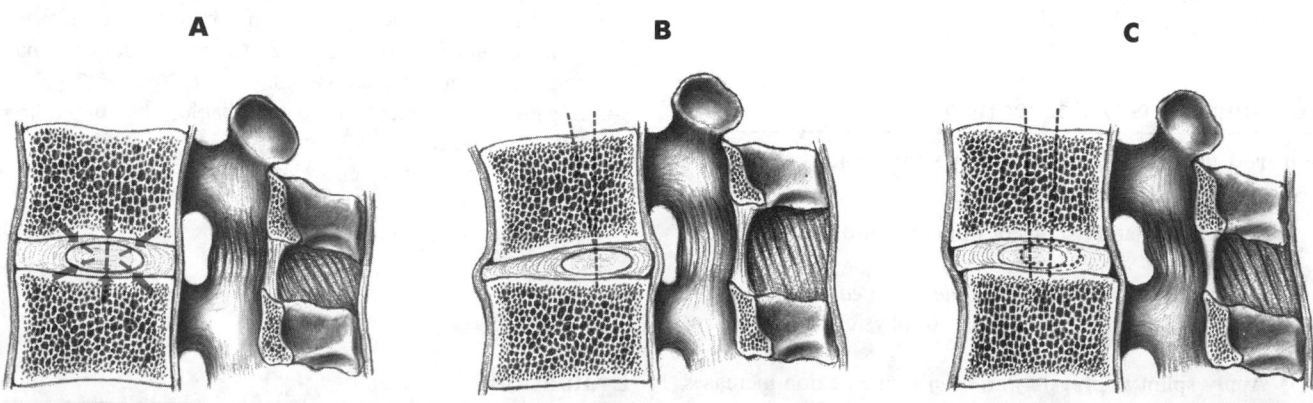

A   **B**   **C**

Figure 4-24 Mechanisms that can cause degeneration of the anulus leading to herniation of the nucleus pulposus. **A,** Axial pressure. **B,** Lateral pressure. **C,** Posterior pressure.

ruptures through the weakened, cracked anulus. Signs of sciatic nerve pressure follow the rupture. Approximately one third or more patients who have a first episode of back pain are still having significant problems 2 years later.[133]

• • • • • Diagnostic Studies and Findings

History   Sudden acute pain in low back, with or without radiation to hips or down one or both legs.

Physical examination   Loss of normal lordotic curve; "list" or tilt to side; tense, tight back muscles; tenderness in low back that may radiate to buttocks; ROM movements limited in forward flexion, in lateral flexion, and sometimes in extension; pain radiating down (usually) one leg to foot and toes; straight leg raising limited by pain; pain increased with foot dorsiflexion; sensations impaired on outer thigh, calf, and foot; paresthesia with numbness and tingling; knee and ankle reflexes possibly diminished or absent (knee reflex rarely lost)

X-rays of back   Tilt; diminished disc space (not necessarily diagnostic)

Myelogram   Location of rupture revealed by impaired dye flow (see p. 1479 for myelography)

CT scan   Ruptured disc or spinal stenosis

MRI   Ruptured disc shows clearly and shows where pressure is on nerves or other tissues; also identifies changes in facet joints

Discogram   Should differentiate between disc infection or rupture

• • • • • Multidisciplinary Plan

Surgery

Arthroscopic discectomy
Percutaneous discectomy
Microdiscectomy
Nuclear discectomy
Hemilaminectomy with removal of extruded nucleus and degenerated anulus
Spinal fusion, if more than one disc is involved and patient does heavy lifting
Fenestration to open nerve root exit sites

Chemonucleolysis

Done less frequently now and tends to be concentrated in a few centers

Medications

Analgesic-antipyretic agents
   Aspirin (ASA), 600-1000 mg q4h
   Acetaminophen (Tylenol), 600-1000 mg q4h
Antianxiety agents
   Diazepam (Valium), 2-10 mg po q4-6h
Narcotic analgesics
   Oxycodone (Percodan), 30-60 mg q4h for severe pain uncontrolled by aspirin
   Meperidine (Demerol), 50-150 mg IM q3h

Muscle relaxants
   Cyclobenzaprine (Flexeril), 10-20 mg po tid
   Methocarbamol (Robaxin), 500-750 mg po q4-6h
   Metaxalone (Skelaxin), 400-800 mg tid or qid
Nonsteroidal antiinflammatory drugs
   Naproxen (Naprosyn), 250-500 mg bid
   Diclofenac (Voltaren), 25-75 mg bid
   Choline magnesium trisilicate (Trilisate), 750-1000 mg q4h
   Ibuprofen (Motrin), 400-60 mg bid or tid
   Toradol, 10 mg q4-6h

General Management

Application of skin traction (pelvic belt) (no study indicates any influence on low back pain with traction[29])
Williams' position in bed (head of bed and knee gatch each elevated 45° to relax lumbosacral muscles
Diathermy to low back three or four times daily; ice massage; hydrotherapy
Application of canvas back support or metal back brace
Physical therapy with specific exercises to strengthen back and abdominal muscles
Bed rest on firm mattress during acute rupture for 1 to 3 days only because there is a 3% loss of muscle strength per day during bed rest[29]
Cessation of lifting and stooping
Back massage after diathermy
Use of transcutaneous electrical nerve stimulation (TENS)
Avoidance or cessation of smoking (nicotine decreases discal circulation[29])
Maintenance of normal weight (some patients overeat and gain weight with chronic low back pain[123])

NURSING CARE

Nursing Assessment

Vertebral Column, Lumbar Back, and Sciatic Nerve Dermatomes (Areas on the Skin Surface Ennervated by Spinal Nerve Roots)

Degree of lumbar lordotic curve
Range of movements of back (forward, backward, lateral to each side) are slightly less than normal
   "List" or tilt to either side
   Tenderness or painful areas
Pain in back or buttocks, radiating down posterior thighs and legs to feet and toes; may be only unilateral
Assessment of muscles for spasm, tenseness, tightness, or weakness
Leg-raising assessments—may be diminished or less than 90°
Sensory functions around thigh, leg, and foot (bilaterally)
Strength or absence of knee and ankle reflexes
Bowel or bladder function changes; may have constipation and bladder retention

Systemic Concerns

Concomitant systemic diseases
  Rheumatoid arthritis
  Ankylosing spondylitis
  Osteoarthritis
  Osteoporosis

Psychosocial Concerns

Body image disturbance and altered role performance
Impaired physical mobility
Acute pain in lower back with radiation
Failure of conservative care necessitating surgery

Nursing Dx & Intervention

Impaired physical mobility related to back and leg pain and muscle spasms

- Assess ability to move and limitations of movements.
- Explain purposes of hospitalization, temporary bed rest, and traction *to increase compliance.*
- Explain use of firm mattress and bed position (Williams' position) *to relax spasm of back muscles.*
- Prepare patient for physical therapy, diathermy, and massage; assist with hygienic care to have patient ready and to lessen strain on back *to aid compliance and lessen anxiety.*
- Help apply back support, brace, or belt; teach self-application *to increase independence.*
- Place in skin traction belt; observe responses; remove traction while sleeping *to lessen muscle spasms and muscle strain.*
- Monitor relief of pain or numbness *to determine efficacy of treatments.*

Body image disturbance and altered role performance related to condition

- Assess condition's effects on usual roles and self-concept.
- Encourage to discuss usual roles and temporary adjustments needed with family members *to ease patient's concerns.*
- Seek assistance from social services *for continuity of care after discharge.*
- Encourage to ventilate stresses or other concerns *to aid relaxation.*

Pain in back and legs related to condition

- Assess amount, sites, and severity of pain.
- Keep patient on bed rest *to relieve inflammation with acute low back pain,* if prescribed— usually not longer than 48 to 72 hours because it decreases muscle strength.
- Administer analgesics around the clock as prescribed *to maintain an adequate blood level for first 2 or 3 days.*
- Administer nonsteroidal antiinflammatory medications as prescribed *to block effects of prostaglandins to relieve pain.*[24]
- Administer muscle relaxants as ordered *to relieve spasms.*
- Assess effect of Williams' position *in relieving spasms and pain.*

- Offer back massage *to relax muscles and relieve inflammation.*
- Assess relief of pressure signs on sciatic nerve by determining relief of paresthesia, numbness, and so forth *to note resolution of symptoms.*
- Perform "laminectomy checks" *to note progression or regression of symptoms:* assess sites and amount of numbness, tingling, motor functions, leg strength, temperature of extremities, sites and amount of pain, sites of radiation of pain, color, and warmth of affected tissues.
- Report continued presence of pain, paresthesia, and muscle spasms to physician.
- Teach muscle relaxation techniques *to aid relaxation of tense muscles.*
- Use dietary measures, high fluid intake, and medication *to prevent constipation (straining increases pain).*
- Encourage weight loss through diet, if overweight, *to lessen strain on weak muscles of back and abdomen.*

Patient Education/Home Care Planning

1. Discuss purposes of bed positions to relieve pain and inflammation.
2. Demonstrate proper lifting postures, when feasible.
3. Demonstrate exercises to strengthen muscles.
4. Encourage maintenance of normal weight for size, sex, and age.
5. Provide pamphlet and explain use of proper body mechanics.
6. Encourage to seek medical care if symptoms recur.
7. Stress cessation of smoking.

Evaluation

Patient regains physical mobility with treatments   Patient resumes walking with less back pain. Patient returns to work while continuing treatments. Back muscle spasms are no longer present.

Patient resumes social interactions and roles   Patient returns to family, social, and employment roles and activities. Patient takes rest periods periodically.

Patient's back pain and muscle spasms are relieved   Patient uses back for ADL without pain, numbness, radiation to legs, or muscle spasms. Patient has no limitations in ROM. Patient needs only nonnarcotic analgesics for discomfort.

MEDICAL INTERVENTIONS AND RELATED NURSING CARE

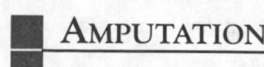 **AMPUTATION**

Description and Rationale

An amputation is the removal of all or part of a specific tissue or organ. Musculoskeletal tissues are frequently amputated because of crush injuries, severe sepsis, malignant tumors, or gangrene resulting from loss of arterial or venous circulatory integrity. Less frequently a limb may be amputated because of intractable pain from paralysis or because of multiple recurrent flare-ups of osteomyelitis that threaten not only the limb but also the individual's life.

The following terms refer to amputations involving the extremities:

forequarter Removal of entire arm, forearm, and hand; extremity disarticulated at shoulder joint.

arm Amputation above elbow or along forearm.

hemipelvectomy Removal of thigh at hip joint, leg, and foot; also referred to as hindquarter amputation or hip disarticulation.

thigh Amputation above the knee (above-knee amputation, AKA).

lower leg Amputation below the knee (below-knee amputation, BKA).

foot Amputation of toes and foot at metatarsal joints (Syme's amputation).

finger or toe Amputation of part or all of one or more fingers or toes.

The three types of amputations are *provisional,* which is done when primary healing is unlikely; *definitive end bearing,* which is done when weight will be borne through the end of the stump; and *definitive non–end bearing,* which is done when weight will not be borne at the end of the stump. When weight will be borne through the end of the stump, the incision is not made at the end but is cut through or near a joint; if weight will not be borne at the end of the stump, the incision can be terminal (at the end of the stump). Also, the incision may be cut perpendicularly to the bone through all the tissues, called a guillotine incision, with little or no incisional closure and only loosely applied dressings. The guillotine incision is used in grossly infected tissues. The more frequently used incision is closed and snugly dressed after the tissues are amputated; it is commonly done in noninfected tissues.

During the surgical procedure, bleeding is controlled through application of a tourniquet unless there is arterial insufficiency. Skin flaps are made, usually of equal length for

MICROVASCULAR REPAIR AND REPLANTATION

Although not thoroughly discussed here, major advances in the care of patients with severe musculoskeletal trauma have been made with the development of microvascular surgical techniques. These include replantation of completely amputated body parts and revascularization of crush, avulsion, and other soft tissue injuries.

Before replantation or microsurgical repair, data are gathered and evaluated to determine whether functional return is possible, particularly if the injuries involve an upper extremity. Functional return is more likely when the injury is to a finger or fingers or low on the forearm because of the shorter distances for nerve regeneration. Repair or replantation should be performed as soon as possible after the injury because ischemic tissues must be reperfused within 12 hours for function to be regained. Necrosis of tissues may preclude functional return if tissues are ischemic longer than 24 hours.

Surgical repair or replantation is done under a microscope and usually follows a pattern of stabilization of fractured bones followed by repair of arteries for restoration of blood flow. With circulation restored, nerves, veins, tendons, and ligaments are repaired, and skin closure, which may necessitate placement of a skin graft, is done. Nerves may not be repaired during the initial surgery but may be repaired 2 to 3 weeks later because the injuries or scarring from inflammatory processes and healing may delay or preclude nerve regeneration.

Postoperatively, nursing observations and care are critical for the success of the repair or replantation. Tissue pressure monitoring may be required in crush injuries to detect rising interstitial pressures, which may signal the development of compartment syndrome (see Figure 4-27). The digits are monitored closely for evidence of capillary refill and arterial flow through the use of Doppler detectors, arteriography, and plethysmography. Tissue temperatures are checked with thermometers, and edema, skin color, and turgor are closely assessed. Bleeding is carefully monitored, especially if anticoagulants are being administered. The external fixator or splint is checked for proper position and function. Dressings are changed as required to aid healing, and antibiotics are administered to prevent infection.

Leeches *(Hirudo medicinalis)* may be used in the early postoperative period to decrease venous congestion and edema by promoting bleeding. At times each leech will ingest 5 to 10 times its own weight in secretions and fluid. Leeches are used carefully and are closely monitored. They loosen their hold after 10 to 30 minutes of feeding. Each leech is placed individually in a congested area. The leech is placed on a bleeding puncture wound made by a sterile needle. The leech quickly attaches to the site. Its bite is painless because the leech secretes a natural anesthetic to lessen pain. Once the leech has become attached to the site, it is covered and confined with a sterile clear specimen cup taped over the area. The leech will loosen its hold or attachment when it is full (some leeches can ingest up to 50 ml). As the leech loosens its hold, it is removed and put in alcohol or saline to destroy it. Leeches may be needed for 3 to 5 days or until the congestion is markedly lessened.

A complication of the use of leeches is a bacterial infection that responds to cephalosporin or aminoglycoside therapy.

The patient, relatives, visitors, and all health care personnel in contact with the patient are not permitted to smoke because the nicotine in the tobacco could lead to vasospasm, vasoconstriction, and ischemia, which could threaten the tissue perfusion and healing processes.

Initial outcomes after repair or replantation vary with the extent of trauma, the adequacy of tissue repairs, the degree of inflammatory responses, scarring, and absence of complications of arterial and venous occlusion and infection. Long-term success depends greatly on physical therapies and psychosocial rehabilitation.

EMERGENCY ALERT

UNINTENTIONAL TRAUMATIC AMPUTATION

Unintentional traumatic amputation occurs when a limb or digit is partially or totally severed from the body.

Assessment and Interventions

- Maintain airway, breathing, and circulation.
- Control bleeding, support limb in functional position.
- Administer high-flow oxygen by mask (10 to 15 L).
- Obtain IV access.
- Locate amputated part; wrap part in gauze saturated with normal saline or lactated Ringer's solution.
- Maintain amputated part at 40° C; *do not* place directly on ice.
- Keep limb in anatomically correct position.
- Transport to medical facility.

---

upper limb or above-knee amputations and with a longer posterior flap for below-knee amputations. The muscles are divided distal to the intended site of bone resection, and later opposing muscle groups are sutured over the bone end to each other and to the periosteum to provide better muscle control and circulation. Nerves are divided proximal to the bone end. After the bone is cut, all vessels and bleeders are ligated carefully and the skin flaps are sutured closed (unless tissues are infected), drains are inserted, and the stump is firmly dressed.

Contraindications and Cautions

1. If the amputation is to be done to remove a malignant tumor, metastasis to distant sites is usually a contraindication.
2. Lack of arterial circulation requires that the amputation be proximal to the gangrenous or necrotic tissues.
3. Enough tissues must be left on and over the stump for fitting of a prosthesis when possible.

Preprocedural Nursing Care

1. Meticulous skin cleansing with antiseptic solutions removes transient and some resident bacteria.
2. Determine presence of peripheral pulses as distally as possible; for crush injuries, may need Doppler for most accurate assessment.
3. Compare edema, color, temperature, skin condition, and pain (when present) with tissues on the opposite side of the body. Edema may be pronounced in venous obstruction.
4. Observe the skin for open or draining areas.
5. Check vital signs for evidence of systemic infection and to monitor the patient's general condition.
6. With crush injuries, observe the patient for hemorrhage, possible shock, and renal functions.
7. If the patient is a child or older adult, determine factors related to age and developmental or educational level that could affect recovery and self-care after the amputation.

8. A rehabilitated person with a similar amputation may visit the patient preoperatively when possible or when requested by the patient.
9. Monitor control of chronic diseases, such as diabetes or peripheral vascular diseases, related to preoperative and postoperative care.
10. Begin discussion of phantom limb pain before surgery to enhance positive patient outcomes and to reduce anxiety and fear.[128]

•••••• Multidisciplinary Plan

Surgery

Wound suction continuously postoperatively
Change of dressings as needed

Medications

Antiinfective agents
    Cephalothin sodium (Keflin), 500-1000 mg IV q4-6h for 48-72 h (or longer, if prescribed)
    Cefazolin (Ancef), 250-1000 mg q4-6h IV for 5-7 d
    Vaucomycin (Vancocin), 500-1000 mg q6-8h for 24 h
Narcotic analgesic agent
    Meperidine (Demerol), 50-100 mg IM q3h for pain (may use patient-controlled analgesia intravenously)
Intravenous fluid replacement with 5% dextrose in 0.45 normal saline, 2000-3000 ml for 24 h

General Management

Stump elevated for 24 hours, then kept flat and extended (elevation depends on presence or amount of edema in stump)
Adduction exercises of amputated extremity, 10 times per hour after 24 hours
For lower extremity amputation, turning to prone position four times daily to extend hip and knee
Thigh (hamstring) tightening exercises in prone position begun after 24 hours (10 times every 4 hours)
Up with crutches three times daily on first postoperative day
Physical therapy consultation for exercise regimen, to assist with ambulation, and for shoulder or elbow exercises, if upper extremity amputation
Occupational therapy consultation for rehabilitation care
Regular diet as desired
Stump wrapping after sutures are removed
Orthotic technician (prosthetist) to measure for prosthesis
Stump check every hour for first 24 hours to note color, drainage, edema, bleeding, sutures (wound), and pulses proximal to incision site; measure amount of drainage in suction system, if used
Tourniquet always present at bedside
Up in chair after recovery from anesthesia
Pulmonary deep breathing and coughing every 4 hours
Analysis of gait problems and progress by gait laboratory personnel
NOTE: Some patients may return from surgery with a prosthesis already in place, held to the stump with plaster (an im-

mediate postsurgical fitting). It is usually left in place up to 10 days, after which it is removed, the sutures are removed, and a new cast is applied. This fitting lessens edema and pain, although the rigidity of the plaster delays the shaping of the stump into a conical shape. However, the immediate postsurgical prosthesis does permit earlier ambulation and discharge, particularly in younger patients.

NURSING CARE

Nursing Assessment

Site of Amputation (Stump)

Drainage or bleeding scant and serosanguineous
Edema slight
Dressing intact without constriction
Pain may be sharp and acute in incisional area
If rubber drain is present, drainage may be scant to moderate, although still serosanguineous; drainage in a suction setup, such as a Hemovac or Jackson-Pratt, may be moderate and serosanguineous
Tourniquet should be at bedside

Entire Extremity

Extremity should remain extended to prevent contraction
Range of motion of muscles and joints may be slightly limited by pain, stiffness, or edema
Only incisional area edema or erythema unless infection develops

Psychosocial Concerns

Concern with alteration in body image and appearance
Presence of phantom pain—feeling as if fingers or hand, toes and foot, or arm or leg are still present, are pinched, or are painful; may have burning or crushing sensations or cramping or spasmodic sensation[128]
Alteration in mobility and ability to maintain livelihood and income

Complications

Hemorrhage, wound infection, or dehiscence
Development of contractures
Persistence of phantom pain
Development of neuromas
Excessive scar formation
Inability to use prosthesis for ADL and mobility
Development of limp

Nursing Dx & Intervention

Body image disturbance related to loss of limb

- Assess effects of amputation on body image.
- Allow and encourage patient to express feelings of mutilation, grief, anger, and loss, as well as avoidance of looking at stump, *to aid adaptation processes.*

- Encourage patient to help with dressing changes and wrapping of stump as able. Teach family member wrapping techniques if necessary *to increase competence and independence.*
- Encourage family members to walk with patient *to maintain strength and social contacts.*
- Encourage grooming and wearing of personal clothing *to maintain individuality and personality.*
- Encourage activities for self-care and ambulation *to maintain positive outlook and maximum strength.*
- Arrange for consultation with gait laboratory *for assistance with gait management to increase self-esteem in use of prosthesis.*
- Encourage or arrange for social services consultation *for economic and employment aid.*
- Arrange for follow-up care referral *to aid rehabilitation.*

Impaired physical mobility related to loss of limb

- Assess ability to use remaining limbs.
- Turn and position on side, back, and abdomen (after 24 hours) *to maintain muscle and joint ROM.*
- Teach adduction and extension exercises and help patient perform them every 4 hours *to prevent abduction and flexion contractures.*
- Assist with sitting in chair and ambulation with aid as able *to maintain muscle strength.*
- Prepare patient for physical therapy, transportation for exercises, and stump wrapping if appropriate.
- Encourage family members to learn wrapping (Figure 4-25).
- Encourage family members to walk with patient during initial ambulation periods, accompanied by health professionals, *to increase independence.*
- Teach purposes of prone and extension positions *to prevent contractures.*
- Assist prosthetist with prosthesis measurements and fitting as needed *to aid rehabilitation.*
- Contact personnel in gait laboratory, per physician's prescription, for gait analysis *to increase patient's mobility and confidence.* Gait analysis determines the optimal type of prosthetic foot for amputee.[155]

Pain (nerve trauma after surgery) related to surgical transection

- Assess type, amount, and severity of pain.
- Administer narcotics as ordered every 3 hours for first 24 to 48 hours until surgical trauma is lessened; then administer as needed *to aid pain relief* (may have patient-controlled analgesia).
- Explain causes for phantom pain sensations and techniques to overcome them *to ease concerns.* Phantom limb pain can be triggered by urination, defecation, ejaculation, barometric pressure changes, angina pectoris, and herpes zoster.[127]
- Teach patient other pain-relieving techniques, including use of diversionary measures such as listening to music, listening to radio, watching television or videotapes, using

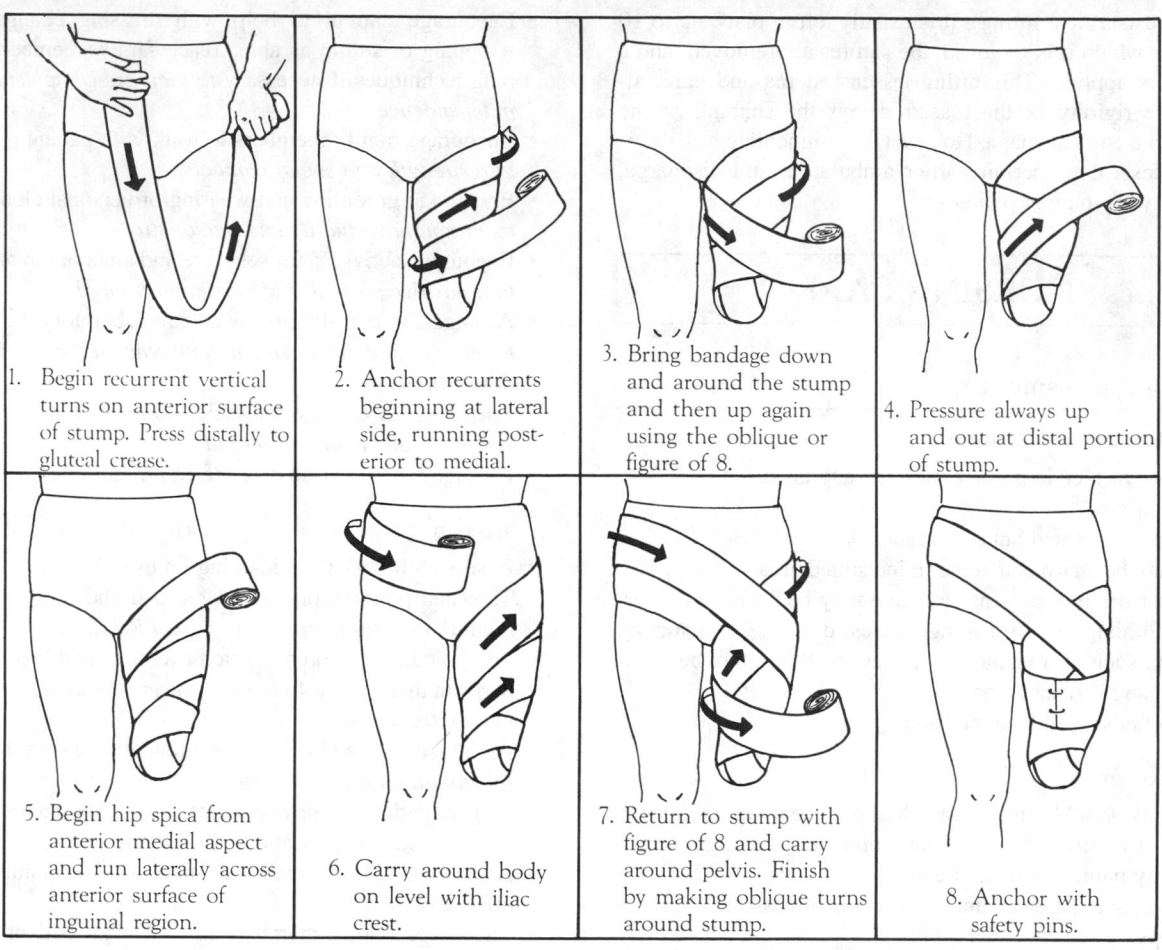

1. Begin recurrent vertical turns on anterior surface of stump. Press distally to gluteal crease.

2. Anchor recurrents beginning at lateral side, running posterior to medial.

3. Bring bandage down and around the stump and then up again using the oblique or figure of 8.

4. Pressure always up and out at distal portion of stump.

5. Begin hip spica from anterior medial aspect and run laterally across anterior surface of inguinal region.

6. Carry around body on level with iliac crest.

7. Return to stump with figure of 8 and carry around pelvis. Finish by making oblique turns around stump.

8. Anchor with safety pins.

Figure 4-25 Method of wrapping to help shape stump after above-knee amputation. (From Mourad.[104])

relaxation techniques, and guided imagery, *to lessen need for narcotic usage and divert attention.*

- Massage back and other bony prominences *to ease soreness or pain.*
- Administer antibiotics as ordered to prevent infection, thereby *lessening pain and scarring.*

Impaired skin integrity related to healing wound on stump

- Assess wound for signs of healing: amount of redness: edema; condition of sutures or skin clips, if present; a proximation of wound edges, pain, functions, sensory deficits.
- Reinforce or change wound dressings using strict aseptic technique *to hasten wound healing and to prevent wound infection.*
- Monitor cast, if present, for tightness or loosening, edema above edges, and other signs of integrity of the cast *to determine the viability of the cast and need for changes.*
- Monitor the pressure in the Jobst air splint, if in use. Pressure is usually inflated to 20 mm Hg for 22 hours per day *to control edema and aid shaping the stump.*

- Wrap stump when prescribed with proper techniques (see Figure 4-25) *to aid molding and shaping of stump and control edema.*
- Demonstrate proper wrapping techniques to patient and family members *to increase self-reliance and self-care.*
- Teach patient and family that elastic wraps must be removed and reapplied *to maintain their snugness and effectiveness.*
- Assist with removal of (or remove, if unit policy) sutures or skin clips, as prescribed, *to permit wound maturation and reduce inflammation.*
- Teach stump skin care; clean incisional area with prescribed solution or soap and water *to decrease resident bacteria to reduce possibility of infection.*
- Assist with measuring and fitting of prosthesis, if necessary, *to facilitate regaining physical mobility.*
- Continue extension and adduction exercises *to maintain proper limb muscle functions for prosthesis use.*

Impaired skin integrity related to pressure of prosthesis

- Assess stump daily for skin integrity: healing of incisional area, presence or amount of edema, redness, hot areas, conical shape, abrasions, or irritated areas.
- Teach patient to wear stump sock, if required with specific prosthesis, over stump, and to change daily, or more often if damp, *to prevent skin breakdown.*
- Teach patient to wash stump every evening with warm water, dry the stump carefully and gently, and apply a coating of cornstarch or powder *to help maintain skin integrity.*
- Teach patient to wash and dry prosthesis and stump sock each evening *to keep them clean and dry to maintain their integrity.* The sock should be laid flat after washing on a smooth surface, not dried in a dryer, which could cause shrinkage.
- Teach patient to do careful daily checks of stump, sock, and prosthesis for any signs of pressure, wear, or breakdown *to prevent any wound or skin breakdown.* Skin damage can take months to heal.

Patient Education/Home Care Planning

1. Show the patient and family proper positions, exercises, and ambulation techniques.
2. Demonstrate stump-wrapping techniques to the patient and family.
3. Explain to the patient and family that prolonged phantom pain experiences are unusual and should receive medical attention, if persistent.
4. Discuss skin care with the patient and family to prevent stump irritation or breakdown.
5. List signs of a wound infection, and discuss these with the patient and family.
6. Provide information about gait analysis to patient and family.
7. Explain community resources available for financial, rehabilitative, or home care as needed.
8. Discuss daily care principles of stump, sock, and prosthesis.

Evaluation

Alteration in body image and self-concept is achieved Patient has positive outlook about condition and can take up personal and employment roles after convalescence.

Patient has regained mobility after wound healing Patient's scar has healed well on stump. Stump fits into prosthesis well. Patient walks with slight limp only. Patient uses upper extremity prosthesis satisfactorily and continues care with occupational and physical therapists. Patient uses gait analysis personnel and techniques to increase ambulation skills.

Patient experiences pain relief over time Patient needs no analgesics. Patient has no phantom pain.

ARTHROPLASTY

Arthroplasty refers to repair or refashioning of one or both sides of upper or lower extremities, parts, or specific tissues within a joint. Parts of a joint repaired during an arthroplasty include bones, cartilage, synovium, ligaments, and tendons. Bursae are outside a joint, but they may be removed during an arthroplastic procedure.

Arthroplasties are described as *interpositional arthroplasty,* in which a metal barrier is interposed between the bones after reshaping one or both bone ends (e.g., cup arthroplasty, currently done to preserve as much bone as possible, particularly the head of the femur), *gap arthroplasty,* in which one of the bones in the joint is excised (e.g., Girdlestone arthroplasty, now performed mainly to remove infected bones), *partial joint replacement arthroplasty,* or *hemiarthroplasty,* in which one joint bone end is replaced with a prosthesis (e.g., prosthesis replacing head and neck of femur), and *total joint replacement arthroplasty,* in which both bone ends are replaced (e.g., total hip or knee replacement). Synovectomy is an example of an excisional arthroplasty, as is a meniscectomy with removal of the meniscus within the knee joint.

Refashioning or repairing a joint usually follows trauma, degeneration, or inflammation of one or more tissues within the joint. The surgery may be performed within hours of a traumatic injury, such as a hip fracture or meniscus tear, or it may be done after years of inflammation in a joint, such as occurs with rheumatoid arthritis or after degenerative erosions accompanying osteoarthritis.

An arthroplasty, therefore, is usually performed to relieve restrictive movements of a joint, to relieve pain, to remove loose or torn tissues (ligaments, cartilage, or calcium deposits), to reshape one or both bone ends to make a joint perform more smoothly, or to remove overgrown, hypertrophied tissue (synovium) or atrophic, avascular tissue (avascular head of femur).

Contraindications and Cautions

The age of a specific patient may be a contraindication to a particular arthroplasty. Arthroplasties are performed infrequently in children because they may damage the growth epiphyses and the immature cartilage and bones. Surgical repair of childhood conditions such as Legg-Perthes disease is undertaken only after more conservative medical treatments fail to resolve the condition. Adolescents with large, unsightly bunions may have an arthroplasty to correct them, but often surgical correction is required again in later years. Older adults with rheumatoid arthritis or degenerative osteoarthritis may have their surgical procedures delayed to correct a concurrent endocrine, cardiac, or respiratory condition, as also will those patients having arthroplastic surgery after trauma.

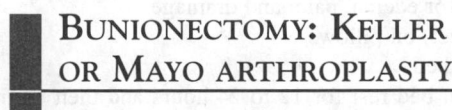

BUNIONECTOMY: KELLER OR MAYO ARTHROPLASTY

Description and Rationale

Keller arthroplasty is one of the most commonly performed corrective procedures for hallux valgus and bunions. It involves excision of the proximal part of the proximal phalanx plus trimming of the prominent portion of the metatarsal head. Mayo procedure involves excision of the first metarsal head and trimming of the prominent portion of the proximal phalanx. Both procedures are examples of gap arthroplasty; the gap is usually filled with a Silastic implant. The bunion (enlarged bursa and knob of bone) is also removed during the arthroplasty. A plaster toe cap or splint is then applied to some patients.

Contraindications and Cautions

1. Hallux valgus in an adolescent is primarily unsightly and deforming; surgical correction may be delayed until the patient is older because osteotomy is a radical procedure at this age.
2. Surgery may be delayed or avoided in some patients through careful attention to wearing properly fitted footwear. Padding may protect the bunion to lessen pain. Exercise and use of a metatarsal arch support may lessen splayfoot.
3. Surgery may not be entirely successful or satisfactory. Bunions can recur, and surgery may weaken the foot slightly.

•••••• Multidisciplinary Plan

Surgery

Arthroplasty or osteotomy
Bunionectomy

Medications

Narcotic analgesics
    Meperidine (Demerol), 75-100 mg IM q3h for 24-48 h for severe pain (may have patient-controlled analgesia pump with smaller doses)
    Codeine (codeine sulfate or phosphate), 30-60 mg
    Oxycodone (Percodan), 5-10 mg po
Analgesic-antipyretic agent
    Aspirin, 600-1000 mg po q4h for minor pain
Nonsteroidal antiinflammatory medications
    Ibuprofen, 400-600 mg q4-6h
    Toradol, 10 mg po q4-6h

General Management

Up with crutches when edema lessens, usually in 1 day (depends on whether surgery is bilateral)
Check cast or splint for tightness, intactness, and drainage
Wear wooden shoe in place of splint
Assess wound for edema, pain, and drainage
Elevate foot (feet) on pillows
Elevate foot of bed
Keep patient on bed rest for 12 to 24 hours and then up in chair without weight bearing, if prescribed
Apply ice bags to operative site continuously
Assess motor and sensory functions in toes and feet postoperatively

NURSING CARE

Nursing Assessment

Preoperative

Area of great toe (bilateral)
    Presence of deformity
    Swelling over first metatarsal head (bursa)
    Pain and throbbing in bunion area
    Limitation of movement of joint with or without pain
    Presence of hallux valgus deviation
    Hammer toe
    Crowding of second toe
    Splayfoot
    Calluses or corns
Foot
    Varus or valgus deviation of one or both feet usually noted
Shoes
    Condition
    Type
    Evidence of wear; sites of wear
    Softness
    Data indicative of footwear contributing to hallux condition
Systemic
    Evidence of gout
        Tophi
        Elevated serum uric acid levels
        Pattern of acute pain in great toe joint and other joints

Postoperative

Great toe or toes and incisional site
    Assessment of plaster cast, splint, or wooden shoe for intactness
    Visible portions of toes
        Color
        Edema
        Pain
        Pulses proximal or distal to incision (if able to locate in toe)
        Drainage
        Bleeding
    Dressing
        Tightness
        Drainage
    Amount of sensation and motion in operative area (splint, shoe, or dressing may limit movement)
Psychosocial concerns
    Alteration in body image, comfort, and mobility
    Possibility of recurrence or lack of wound healing
Other complications
    Excessive scarring or recurrence of bursa
    Weakening of foot joint or joints of or near one or more toes

Nursing Dx & Intervention

Pain related to corrective procedures

- Assess amount, type, and severity of pain.
- Put bed cradles on bed to cover feet without pressure of linens *to aid comfort.*
- Keep foot of bed and feet elevated *to lessen edema.*
- Administer narcotics as prescribed *for acute pain relief.*
- Administer analgesics or antiinflammatory medications after acute pain is relieved *to continue pain relief.*
- Apply ice bags *to lessen bleeding and edema.*
- Assist with position changes and skin care; do back massage as needed *to relieve tired muscles.*
- Instruct patient about analgesic and antiinflammatory effects of medications and ice *to increase compliance and use.*

Impaired physical mobility related to foot surgery

- Assess limitations on mobility.
- Help patient up in chair when prescribed *to increase mobility.*
- Assist with use of crutches when up *to aid mobility efforts.*
- Encourage activities as strength and cast, splint, or wooden shoe permit *to maintain mobility.*
- Encourage return to social activities in spite of cast, splint, or crutches *to lessen isolation.*
- Help with fitting of soft shoes if or when cast is removed (to lessen pressure or rubbing on tender tissues) *to prevent additional injury.* Often, open, laced shoes are used after bunion surgery.

Altered peripheral tissue perfusion related to surgery or cast

- Assess neurovascular functions.
- Remainder of nursing care is discussed on p. 433.

Patient Education/Home Care Planning

1. Explain wound healing and signs of wound dehiscence to report to physician.
2. Discuss principles and examples of proper footwear.
3. Explain that friction and pressure of snug footwear can precipitate recurrence.
4. Discuss bone and wound healing for long-term follow-up.
5. Provide list of signs or symptoms of infection.

Evaluation

Patient is relieved of acute pain Patient can walk easily without pain. Deformity has been removed. ROM in normal scar formation is not excessive. Pain in and around joint is gone.

Patient has satisfactory physical mobility Patient returns to usual activities with unassisted, pain-free mobility. Footwear is comfortable. Patient feels better about body image.

Patient has normal peripheral perfusion Neurovascular checks are within normal limits with minimal edema of toes; operative wound is well approximated with minimal edema of suture line; no drainage is present.

TOTAL JOINT REPLACEMENT ARTHROPLASTY

Description and Rationale

Work done since the late 1950s and early 1960s has made it possible to repair and replace bone surfaces on both sides of

---

■ TOTAL HIP REPLACEMENT

Sir John Charnley of England first reported his experiences with low friction arthroplasty in the hip joint in 1961. Since that time, total hip replacement has become one of the most frequently performed orthopedic surgical procedures. Over 275,000 total hip replacements are done yearly in the United States, and over 1 million are done worldwide. Also, 75,000 total hip replacement revisions are done yearly. Revisions are often required 8 to 10 years after placement because of the loosening of one or both prostheses in the joint. Approximately three fourths of the revisions are done because of loosening; others are done because of deep infection (about 5%), implant fracture (5%), or because of other individual reasons, such as marked pain or discomfort or the need to replace a particular prosthesis (some last longer than others).

Currently, prostheses are being developed with new instruments and techniques for inserting them (Figure 4-26). Prostheses now have matching parts that fit snugly into each other, allowing only one part (not two, three, or more) to be replaced as needed; they also have a porous coating to be press fit into the bone shaft or socket. The porous coating blends with the bone through bioingrowth of bone cells. Another substance, hydroxyapatite, now is being applied to prostheses, bonding the replacement directly to bone without intervening fibrous tissue. This substance may strengthen the bone-prosthesis bonding. At present, methylmethacrylate polymer (a substance that helps glue the prostheses in place) is used in about 40% to 50% of total hip replacements because it was found to contribute to loosening, as well as joint infection.

Ball-and-socket joints (hip and shoulder joints) succeed better when replaced than do joints that are more complex and have more functions, such as the knee, wrist, elbow, or ankle (Figure 4-27).

Total joint replacement requires special operative tables and instruments, and careful extensive physician-patient contact with consultation before and after surgery. When successful, as are the great majority of joint replacements, this surgery provides the patient with relief from pain, increased mobility, and a freedom not available with more conservative procedures.

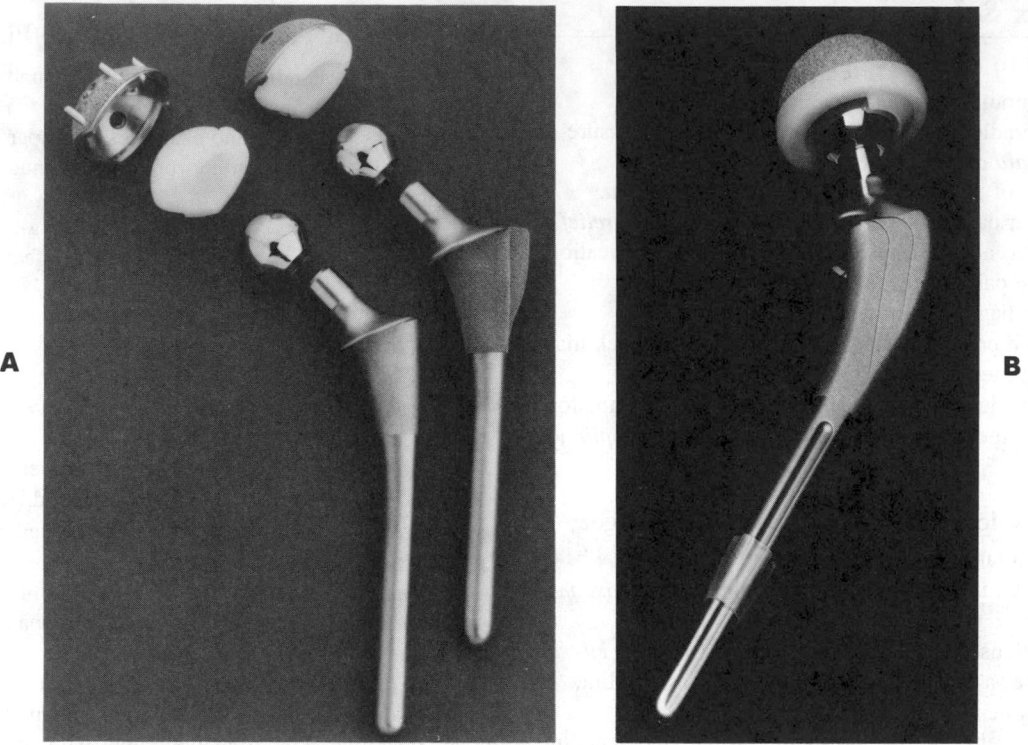

Figure 4-26 Several types of total hip replacement prostheses. **A,** Courtesy Zimmer, Warsaw, Indiana. **B,** Courtesy Biomet, Warsaw, Indiana. (From Mourad.[104])

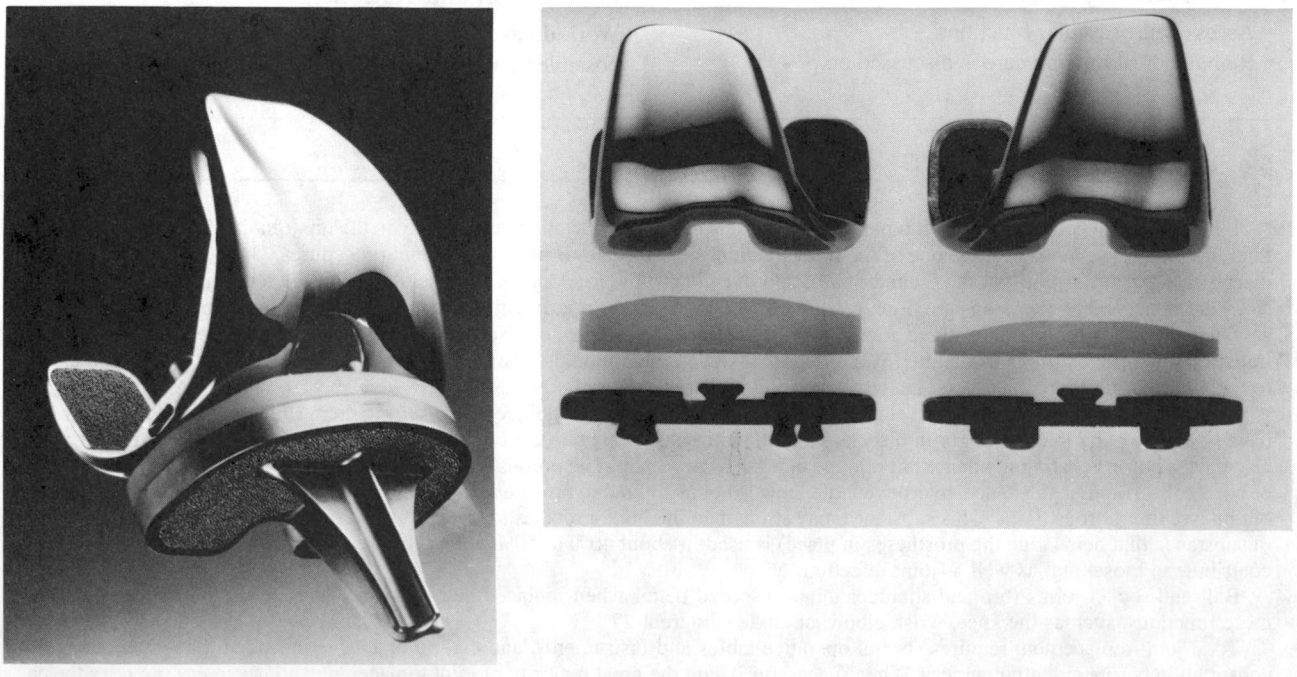

Figure 4-27 Several types of total knee replacement prostheses. Courtesy Zimmer, Warsaw, Indiana. (From Mourad.[104])

many joints. Work with total replacement of hip joints has led to the ability to totally replace many joints, including ankles, knees, shoulders, elbows, wrists, and joints of the fingers and toes. Not all prosthetic materials or arthroplastic procedures work entirely satisfactorily in the joints with more and varied movements, such as the elbow, wrist, knee, and ankle. To date more successful replacements have been achieved in the ball-and-socket joints, the hip and shoulder. Research and design changes continue to perfect the prostheses and the techniques for all total arthroplastic procedures.

Replacement of both joint surfaces is required primarily in inflammatory or degenerative conditions within the joint, such as those accompanying rheumatoid arthritis or osteoarthritis from deterioration of the synovium or cartilage. As one or more of the normal joint tissues deteriorate or degenerate, the bone ends are exposed, causing pain and limitation of joint movements. Joint stiffness and muscle atrophy follow, further increasing pain and limiting movement and mobility, both locally in the involved joint and systemically as other joints become involved. Exposed bone surfaces will lead to bone growth that may eventually adhere to the opposing bone ends, causing bony ankylosis and loss of joint movements. Therefore replacement of the deteriorated or degenerated tissues and bones restores movement and relieves pain.

Total joint replacements involve removal of some or all of the synovium, cartilage, and bone on both sides of the joint. One of the joint bone surfaces is then replaced with a metallic prosthesis while the other surface is replaced with a ceramic or plastic, silicone-lined prosthesis. This metallic-plastic approximation is necessary to prevent metal-to-metal wear, friction, and possible electrolytic reactions from the interactions and intermingling of joint fluids. Individual physicians prefer specific combinations of prostheses for particular joints according to the patient's condition. Also, the timing for total joint replacement varies with physician and patient because this procedure is usually elective except in situations of trauma.

Currently each prosthetic replacement on both sides of the joint may be secured with or without methyl methacrylate, a pliable polymer that hardens to hold the prostheses more firmly. Through research and development, ceramic and metallic components have been designed that are self-adhering and immovable and do not require methacrylate adherence. These self-adhering replacements currently are being used in many centers. They have become more widespread as the technique for their insertion and the differences in postoperative recovery and rehabilitation were accepted. Patients take longer to start walking

---

■ TOTAL SHOULDER ARTHROPLASTY

Total shoulder arthroplasty (TSA) dates to 1973 preceded by more than 20 years of shoulder surgical approaches and development of improved prostheses.

Total shoulder arthroplasty is performed as treatment to relieve intractable pain associated with arthritic conditions, osteonecrosis of the humeral head, fracture of the humeral head or neck, rotator cuff arthropathy, and neoplasms and for chronic shoulder pain and instability problems. Because it is similar to a ball-and-socket joint, the TSA arthroplasty has achieved promising successful outcomes. However, because the shoulder lacks a true bony socket it relies heavily on the support and integrity of its soft tissue for stability through its extensive range of motion (the shoulder is capable of a wider range of motion than any other joint in the body).[71] It has flexion/extension, abduction/adduction, and internal rotation/external rotation. (See Table 4-1 for shoulder ROM compared with other joints.)

Total shoulder arthroplasty is a technically challenging surgery because of all the structures articulating with the humerus and glenoid cavity, including the tendons and muscles of the rotator cuff, the deltoid muscle, the subacromial and subscapular bursae, the acromion process of the scapula, and the multiple nerve plexes around the joint.

The designs of the humeral prosthesis and the glenoid component are vital to the successful outcome of TSA. The humeral prosthesis is now a two-piece modular unit that permits the best fitting of the distal humeral shaft portion, coupled with the best fit of available proximal stem portion, thus producing a custom-fit prosthesis. The glenoid component is vital for the ultimate success of TSA because the weight of the extremity when in 90° abduction causes a force against the glenoid that may represent 10 times the weight of the extremity,[71] which can lead to loosening of the glenoid component. This component may be all plastic, metal-backed plastic, all metal, smooth-fit cemented, porous-coated cementless with screw fixation, or pegged,[71] there being no consensus as to the best glenoid component among the varieties.

Total shoulder arthroplasty involves removal of the head of the humerus, preparing the humeral shaft for the distal and proximal humeral components, and smoothing the glenoid for placement of the glenoid component, which may be cemented or held in place with screws.

Complications include infection, dislocation or subluxation, intraoperative fracture, nerve weakness, loosening, impingement, pulmonary embolus, and pneumonia.

The ultimate success of TSA involves a planned rehabilitative coordinated recovery protocol involving exercises to restore ROM and strengthen muscles. The patient must actively participate in the program for the time required. For the relief of preoperative pain, patients usually are highly motivated and compliant.

Preoperative preparations and postoperative care are similar to those for other joint arthroplasties discussed on p. 417. Specific nursing diagnoses and interventions include impaired physical mobility; pain, intractable; high risk for injury related to infection, dislocation, nerve palsy, pulmonary embolus, and pneumonia; impaired peripheral neurovascular integrity; and impaired skin integrity (see the box on total hip replacement on p. 417 for care).

■ TOTAL ELBOW REPLACEMENT

Total elbow replacement (TER) is done primarily to relieve the severe pain and repair the destruction of the elbow joint secondary to rheumatoid arthritis.

Total elbow replacement involves resurfacing and use of either nonconstrained or semiconstrained implants. The resurfacing components provide resurfacing areas for the bones making up the joint. The semiconstrained implants are either hinged or of snap-fit designs. The most successful replacements are those that have the fewest constraints and most closely resemble the anatomic elbow.[37] Additionally, there must be sufficient metaphyseal bone stock and intact collateral ligaments for stability.[37]

Total elbow replacement consists of removal of the diseased trochlea of the intraarticular humerus and ulna with replacement by the capitellocondylar nonconstrained resurfacing implant made of metal with a long humeral stem, and the diseased ulnar surfaces with a metal-stemmed polyethylene ulnar "tray." Each prosthetic component is cemented in place with the use of methyl methacrylate. After the incision is closed and a drain inserted, the operative arm is placed in a protective posterior plaster splint secured with elastic bandages. The elbow and splint are placed in approximately 90° flexion.

Postoperative physical therapy, occupational therapy, administration of IV antibiotics, neurovascular checks, pain management, and wound care are all vital to the successful outcome of TER.

Vital nursing diagnoses include self-care deficit: ADL; impaired peripheral neurovascular and tissue integrity; high risk for injury: delayed wound healing; high risk for infection; impaired skin integrity; and risk for injury: displacement of prostheses or loosening.

Complications of TER are similar to other total joint arthroplasties, including wound or joint infection, dislocation of prostheses, deep vein thrombosis or pulmonary embolism, joint instability, and loosening of prostheses. Nursing interventions are given in the box on total hip replacement on p. 417.

---

and use crutches or other aids for a longer time with the self-adhering replacements because the bone particles used as the natural interfacing material must granulate and ossify for solid adherence to the prosthetic replacements. Obviously, using the patient's own bone for the interface with the prosthesis is desirable because methyl methacrylate sets up an inflammatory response that may eventually lead to loosening or instability within the joint (see the box on specific joint replacements).

The most important goal in replacement of the hip or knee, after pain relief, is restoration of function so the patient can walk effectively and carry out the activities desired.[1]

Contraindications and Cautions

1. Joint infection with or without an associated systemic infection is the major deterrent to total replacement. Infection loosens components, prevents healing, and may eventually lead to osteomyelitis.
2. Active flare-up of a chronic rheumatic or other inflammatory disease is another deterrent. Flare-ups of such disorders as rheumatoid arthritis, ulcerative colitis, or systemic lupus preclude surgery until the condition is controlled or becomes quiescent.
3. Respiratory diseases and limitations from chronic conditions may preclude surgery. Methyl methacrylate is excreted through the lungs; this may set up a pneumonitis that could severely limit respiratory reserves.
4. Chronic renal conditions or mild failure may also preclude replacement because prolonged hypotension could lead to acute renal shutdown.
5. Bleeding or clotting disorders would usually preclude surgery unless special care is taken to prevent hemorrhage, such as use of fresh frozen plasma for hemophiliacs.
6. Insertion of the femoral component into the femoral shaft during total hip replacement causes pressure changes in

the venous system, which can lead to thrombophlebitis and pulmonary or fat embolization.[54]
7. Limb length inequality can occur from inadequate muscle strength or improper operative fit. If limbs are unequal in length preoperatively, the inequality can possibly be corrected with the surgical procedure.
8. Porous-coated prostheses used for noncemented total joint replacements must be "press fit" for bioingrowth to occur.

PREPROCEDURAL NURSING CARE

1. Preadmission patient data are gathered (usually by phone).
2. Blood serum studies and chest x-ray, ECG, and x-rays of operative joints are done, either in family physician's or orthopedic surgeon's office. Leg length measurements are also done, and a thorough physical examination is done.
3. Begin respiratory care preoperatively, including deep-breathing and coughing exercises and use of respiratory aids such as Triflow or Respirex apparatus for incentive spirometry.
4. Begin antibiotics intravenously 30 minutes preoperatively to establish a therapeutic blood level.
5. Design physical therapy teaching 2 to 10 days before surgery.
6. Patient is made NPO at midnight the day of surgery.
7. Patient is admitted to hospital on morning of surgery, and all preparations are completed expeditiously.
8. Patient or family may have donated blood for use during surgery as needed.

• • • • • Multidisciplinary Plan

Medications

Antiinfective agents

Cefamandole (Mandol), 1000 mg q8h IM or IV

Cefazolin (Ancef), 1000 mg q6-8h for 24 h

Ciprofloxacin (Cipro), 500 mg q12h

Cephalexin (Keflex), 250-500 mg q6h po when IV antibiotics are discontinued

Narcotic analgesic agents (may be administered per patient-controlled analgesia)

Morphine, 1.5-2 mg q10min with 20-30 mg lockout

Nonsteroidal antiinflammatory agents

Ibuprofen, 400-800 mg tid or qid

Toradol, 10-20 mg tid or qid

Antianxiety agents

Hydroxyzine (Vistaril), 25-50 mg IM q6h

Anticoagulants

Low-molecular-weight heparin, 30 mg q12h subcutaneously

Warfarin (Coumadin), 5 mg/d beginning after heparin has been discontinued

Sedative-hypnotics

Flurazepam (Dalmane), 15-30 mg at bedtime

Cathartic or laxative agents

Bisacodyl (Dulcolax), 1-2 tablets or rectal suppository prn

Analgesic-antipyretic agents

Acetaminophen (Tylenol), 600 mg q4h prn for elevated temperature

If rheumatic or inflammatory disease is present, antirheumatic or antiinflammatory medications are begun postoperatively as soon as patient can tolerate oral intake

General Management

Empty and record suction drainage every 4 hours, if prescribed; otherwise, empty as needed (some physicians have discontinued use of drainage systems)[78]

Give oxygen at 2 to 3 L per nasal cannula for 12 to 24 hours, then as needed

Perform respiratory therapy with IPPB every 4 hours, or instruct patient in use of incentive spirometer every 2 to 4 hours

Help patient do deep breathing and coughing every 2 hours

Record intake and output every 8 hours

Maintain bed rest for 8 to 16 hours (varies with specific joint replaced, the security of the replacement prostheses, and physician's choice)

Change dressing after 24 to 48 hours; may reinforce dressing as necessary

Give nothing by mouth for 12-24 hours; then clear liquids and advance to regular diet as tolerated

Perform neurovascular checks every hour for 24 hours, then every 2 hours for 24 hours, and then every 4 hours (see p. 358)

Check vital signs every 8 hours initially, then every 2 to 4 hours

Maintain position of operative area with sling, splint, abduction pillow, immobilizer, brace, or elastic wrappings (varies with specific joint replaced); after a total knee replacement, a continuous passive motion (CPM) machine may be present and in use

Patient should be up but bearing no weight on operative limb after bed rest order expires (may be after 12 or 24 hours, depending on joint replaced and whether cemented or noncemented replacement was done); some phyicians may permit touch-down weight bearing

Begin physical therapy exercises on first or second postoperative day; exercises and schedule vary with joint replaced; exercises are either active or passive to all joints, excluding the operated joint, and include quadriceps setting, straight leg raising, flexion and extension, or other individually prescribed exercises for the particular joint replaced

Patient should be up with walker or crutches four times daily; ambulation should increase as patient is able with up to 25 pounds weight to operative limb, gradually increasing to full weight bearing with crutches (time frame varies with type of prostheses used, cemented or uncemented replacement, and physician's choice)

Patient should sit in chair for 10 to 15 minutes only (after hip replacement), two or three times daily for first week; then may sit in chair 20 or 30 minutes four times daily

Patient should wear antiembolism hose or have an athrombic (pneumatic compression) pump system in use for operative extremity

Encourage fluid intake and high-fiber foods (if tolerated) to prevent constipation; administer rectal suppository if needed to empty rectum; indwelling bladder catheter is in place for 12 to 24 hours, then removed

Patient should use toilet riser for toilet (prevents hyperflexion of hip after total replacement—may lead to dislocation of prosthesis)

Patient should wear a sling and swathe after total shoulder replacement for 7 to 10 days

Monitor suction-reinfusion drainage system for possible reinfusion or for homologous transfusion of blood (some postoperative suction-reinfusion drainage systems are neither physiologically beneficial nor cost effective,[11] but the blood obtained by postoperative salvage is better than banked blood because platelets and clotting factors remain intact[49]

NURSING CARE

Nursing Assessment

Joint and Incisional Area

Presence, amount, and type of drainage

Edema

Color of tissues and capillary refill of fingers or toes

Presence, type, and tightness of dressing or bandages

Presence of peripheral pulses

Pain in incision or distal to operative site

Presence of immobilizing device, splint, or pillow to maintain proper position of prosthesis within joint

Leg in abducted position after total hip replacement

Systemic Concerns

Respiratory functions

Excursion

Dyspnea

Orthopnea

Pain in chest or lung areas

Cough; sputum expectoration

Decreased lung sounds

Urinary

Presence of indwelling catheter in urinary bladder

Intake and output

Vascular and cardiac

Hypertension, peripheral vascular disease, cardiac irregularities

Psychosocial Concerns

Concern with body image

Acute pain

Regaining mobility and weight bearing

Risk of death with surgery

Other Complications

Pneumonitis

Pneumonia

Wound infection (superficial or deep)

Limb inequality or limp

Urinary tract infection after catheter use

Dislocation of prostheses

Thrombophlebitis or deep vein thrombosis (it is estimated that deep vein thrombosis occurs after total hip replacement in over 50% of patients; it occurs in 65% of patients after total knee replacement [TKR])[116]

Pulmonary embolism—fatal in 2% to 3% after total hip replacement and 1% to 3% after knee arthroplasty[116]

Fat embolism—occurs in 0.5% to 0.8% after total joint replacement[106a]

Nursing Dx & Intervention

Impaired physical mobility related to surgical and soft tissue trauma

- Assess ROM of unaffected joints.
- Maintain bed rest as prescribed *to promote recovery.*
- Begin ambulation with ambulatory aid and weight-bearing restrictions as prescribed *to aid early rehabilitation and to prevent complications.* Start slowly with rest periods; increase gradually.

- Encourage performance of active and passive ROM exercises, isometric exercises, and other specific exercises *to aid muscle strength and decrease complications of immobility.*
- Encourage use of trapeze to assist with lifting, turning, and positioning *to increase independence.*
- Assist to be up in chair twice daily with increases to four times daily.
- Secure physical therapist's assistance with being up and ambulating.
- Encourage participation in activities such as swimming, stationary bike riding, and calisthenics *to increase physical and cardiovascular fitness.*

Impaired skin integrity related to incision through to joint structures

- Assess condition of all skin surfaces.
- Reinforce and then change dressing with strict aseptic technique: note wound edge approximation, redness, edema, hematoma, or unusual tenderness of wound *as signs of possible wound infection.* Infection after total hip arthroplasty varies from 0.1% to 1%; after total knee arthroplasty (TKA) infection varies from 1% to 4%.[172]
- Measure and empty drainage (may reinfuse) in suction setup as prescribed.

Altered peripheral tissue perfusion related to surgery and immobility

- Assess circulatory condition of operative limb; compare with unoperative limb.
- Apply ice to operative site for 24 hours *to lessen edema and bleeding.*
- Do circulation checks and record findings; note presence or absence of pain, swelling, redness, or heat in calf and positive Homans' sign *as signs of thrombophlebitis.*
- Check drainage in suction apparatus and record. Report unusual amounts *as signs of hemorrhage.*
- Remove antiembolism hose twice daily; check color, presence of pulses, and skin condition; replace hose after 15 to 30 minutes off *to aid circulation.*
- Check vital signs; note presence of hypotension and elevated pulse or temperature; record and report *as signs of infection or sepsis.*
- Maintain prescribed flexion, extension, or abduction of operative tissues according to specific joint replaced *to aid recovery and increase mobility.*
- Maintain IV therapy as prescribed *to aid tissue perfusion and means for antibiotic administration.*
- Administer low-molecular-weight heparin or coumadin as prescribed *to prevent thrombophlebitis.*
- Check antithrombotic hose and external compressive system functioning for normal or abnormal status; correct as needed *to maintain a safe environment.*

Pain related to tissue trauma

- Assess amount, type, and severity of pain.
- Monitor narcotics use via patient-controlled analgesia to determine if change is needed *to increase comfort.*
- Turn, raise, or adjust position *to prevent pressure and lessen fatigue.*
- Administer medications for concomitant disease as prescribed *to relieve symptoms and pain.*
- Administer sedative at bedtime as prescribed *to provide for restful sleep.*
- Assess bowel and bladder output; may need laxative, suppository, or enema *to aid elimination.*
- Convalescent care: encourage self-care and return to ADL as able *to aid recovery.*
- Stress alternatives to medication for restful sleep (activity to become tired, reading, warm milk, snack or massage) *to lessen dependence on medications.*

Impaired physical mobility related to bed rest and bone surgery

- Assess ROM of unaffected tissues.
- Encourage walking as able *to aid recovery.*
- Assist with ROM, gluteal, and quadriceps setting exercises *to maintain muscle strength.*
- Monitor use of crutches or walker *to ascertain proper amount of weight bearing.*
- Complete care referral for home care follow-up *to foster continuity of care.*
- Stress compliance with prescribed rehabilitation program after discharge *for full recovery.*
- Encourage continued contact with physician for follow-up care *for safety and patient comfort.*

Injury, risk for, related to dislocation of prosthesis

- Assess postoperative position for required position *to maintain prostheses inside joint* (abduction of operative limb after hip replacement).
- Reiterate preoperative instructions *to prevent dislocation:* avoid adduction of legs and not to cross ankles; keep head of bed below 90° *to prevent unsafe hip flexion;* keep operative leg abducted by using abduction pillow or 2 to 3 pillows placed between legs; use the knee immobilizer, if prescribed, *to prevent knee flexion, which could cause hip flexion;* keep leg abducted when turned to side.
- Teach the "post" position *to prevent dislocation:* patient bends knee of unoperative leg and firmly plants (posts) foot on mattress, then grasps trapeze, stiffens back and pelvis and lifts body from bed by pushing on posted foot and leg while pulling up. Assist with lifting as needed.
- Maintain patient on bed rest for 1 to 2 days, then help patient up in a chair, cautioning to avoid adduction of the operative limb and to avoid 90° flexion of the hip.

- Listen to patient's complaints of increased pain in operative area and observe position of the limb—if it is held in external or internal rotation, could indicate dislocation of hip prostheses.
- Use toilet riser to elevate seat *to prevent hyperflexion of hip, which could dislocate prosthesis.*

Injury, risk for, related to development of deep vein thrombosis

- Elevate legs as prescribed *to increase venous return and lessen stasis.*
- Keep patient well hydrated *to decrease blood viscosity to lessen stasis.*
- Encourage deep breathing *to promote venous return through vena cava.*
- Maintain antiembolism hose or pneumatic compression device *to promote venous return.*
- Administer low-molecular weight heparin, 30 mg every 12 hours, *to lessen possibility of deep vein thrombosis.* Orthopedic surgery patients are at high risk of developing deep venous thrombosis and pulmonary embolism.[110]
- Monitor bleeding and clotting times while patient is receiving heparin (therapeutic range of partial thromboplastin time is up to 1.5 times normal—normal is 30 seconds). Prothrombin times are done with warfarin administration; therapeutic ranges are 1.3 to 1.5 times the patient's control.[48]
- Monitor stools, urine, and emesis for blood and skin areas for bruising or ecchymosis while patient is receiving heparin or warfarin.
- Use external pneumatic compression devices as prescribed *to lessen possibility of deep vein thrombosis.*
- Continue anticoagulation with warfarin (Coumadin) as prescribed after heparin discontinued *to continue to prevent deep vein thrombosis.*
- Advise patient and family of agents that interact with warfarin anticoagulation such as cefamandole, cimetidine, phenytoin, and trimethoprim.[48]

Risk for infection related to wound or joint infection

- Assess wounds for signs of infection.
- Perform wound care aseptically *to prevent introduction or transfer of organisms.*
- Observe wound for redness, edema, abscess, or purulent drainage *as signs of infection.*
- Monitor patient's vital signs and note elevations *as signs of possible infection.*
- Listen to patient's complaints of deep, dull, aching pain in hip operative area *as signs of possible joint infection;* report findings to physician.
- Maintain blood levels of IV antibiotics as prescribed *to lessen possibility of infection.*

TOTAL KNEE ARTHROPLASTY

Total knee arthroplasty (TKA) is a more difficult procedure than total hip arthroplasty because of the multiple functions of the knee, including flexion, extension, and rotation, in the course of weight bearing. No single prosthetic design type for the femoral, patellar, or tibial components has been entirely satisfactory because of the knee joint's complexity, and the prostheses have undergone revisions and are continuing to be redesigned. When a primary knee implant is well aligned, balanced, and firmly fixed, it can withstand 20 years or more of wear in some patients, and 90% to 95% of all primary knee replacements still perform well up to 15 years postoperatively.[148] However, revisions of TKA are being done in up to 20% of patients.[14]

Total knee arthroplasty is done to relieve the constant pain associated with osteoarthritis, rheumatoid arthritis, traumatic arthritis, or chondromalacia. Lingering pain may not entirely disappear, occasionally remaining up to 1 year after TKA.[14] Such lingering pain may be associated with reflex sympathetic dystrophy[26] or to the components in the TKA themselves.[13]

Total knee arthroplasty involves preparing the femoral condyles for the femoral prosthesis; preparing the tibial surface for the prosthesis while attempting to preserve as much bone stock as possible and creating a level surface in the bone; and preparing the patella for the patellar component. Diligence must be taken to carefully align the femur and tibia in as anatomically correct a position as possible to prevent undue wear or loosening of either prosthesis. It is also vital to prevent shearing of the patellar component by recessing it to help maintain joint stability.

Prostheses presently being used include a cobalt-chrome femoral prosthesis, usually noncemented, with a cemented or noncemented polyethylene tibial prosthesis, with additional fixation with screws, stems, or pegs. The patellar component is usually a metal-backed polyethylene prosthesis. Bioingrowth occurs on the porous-coated prostheses over about 30% of the surface, 30% of the time, in 30% of cases.[14]

Meticulous preoperative preparation and postoperative care must be done to prevent complications after TKA, which include superficial wound and deep, periprosthetic infections; deep vein thromboses; pulmonary emboli; acute compartment syndrome; osteolysis, especially in the tibial plateau; aseptic loosening; patellar maltracking; patellar fracture; reflex sympathetic dystrophy; and hemorrhage or blood loss, which can be up to 1500 ml, not always reinfused.[4,30]

Rehabilitative exercises must be performed by the patient to restore stability and improve motion, under the guidance of physical therapists, over a long (6 months to 1 year) period of time.

Nursing diagnoses include impaired physical mobility; high risk for injury: infection; impaired skin integrity; pain; high risk for peripheral neurovascular compromise; risk for skin necrosis; and altered role performance. Nursing interventions for these diagnoses are discussed under total hip arthroplasty.

TOTAL ANKLE REPLACEMENT

Total ankle replacement (TAR) has been available to orthopedic surgeons since the early 1970s. It is indicated as treatment for the severe pain and disability of older patients with rheumatoid arthritis and less frequently for older patients with posttraumatic arthritis of the ankle. Total ankle replacement is indicated after there have been less than satisfactory results with nonoperative management, including use of antiinflammatory medications, analgesics, and supportive devices. Younger patients may have an ankle arthrodesis, considered the "gold standard" for younger patients with posttraumatic arthritis who place a high physical demand on their ankle joints.[85]

Total ankle replacement involves preparation of the patient as for other surgical procedures, meticulous skin cleansing, and administration of an intravenous prophylactic antibiotic after the induction of anesthesia. Anesthesia may be given as general anesthesia or regional anesthesia via a spinal-subarchnoid block.[85] Total ankle replacement is done in an operating room with vertical laminar air flow and operating personnel wearing body exhaust suits.

Preparation of the dome of the talus is done for the prosthesis, along with subperiosteal dissection of the distal tibia. Osteophytes are removed, as is some synovial tissue. The medial malleolus is resected, and trial spacers are inserted to assess the sufficiency of the preparations. The tibial prosthesis is placed, after removal of the trial components, and held with the use of polymethyl methacrylate cement. The talar component is inserted and held in place with a small amount of cement. The ankle joint is reduced and held in dorsiflexion compression until the cement is fully polymerized. The types of prostheses used include two types of porous-coated prostheses, not currently used without cement.[85] Tibial components may be multiaxial, allowing unrestricted movement about any of the three major axes, or a single-axis joint prosthesis that allows flexion or extension only, with various degrees of constraint to internal-external rotation and abduction-adduction.[85] After the components are inserted, the tourniquet is released, and hemostasis is done. Sutures are placed, and a small drain may be inserted. The wound is covered with a bulky, soft compressive dressing, and a plaster splint is placed. The operative leg and ankle are kept elevated for up to 3 days. A short-leg walking cast is applied and worn for 2 to 3 weeks to permit soft tissue healing. After cast removal, ROM exercises are done by the patient, and ambulation progresses as tolerated.

Complications include infection (2.9%), incomplete pain relief (up to 6%), reoperation to remove excess (impinging) bone (up to 6%), and loosening of one or both components (4.9%). Results varied from 61% to 88% satisfactory in rheumatoid arthritis patients to 63% satisfactory results in posttraumatic arthritis patients.[85] Previous same ankle surgery also led to a high rate of failure.[80]

Nursing diagnoses include high risk for infection; impaired physical mobility; acute or chronic pain; high risk for injury: loosening of components; and alteration in body image or self-esteem.

Patient Education/Home Care Planning

1. Stress that rehabilitation of muscles and joint tissues, locally and systemically, will require daily practice over time.
2. Discuss compliance with medication regimen for chronic disease, if present.
3. Discuss that joint ROM and mobility should be regained after recovery and rehabilitation are accomplished.
4. Stress use of antiembolism hose as prescribed to prevent deep vein thrombosis.
5. Caution patient to notify physician if chest pain or calf pain develop after discharge.
6. Avoid sources of infection (e.g., use prophylactic antibiotics before dental or genitourinary procedures).
7. Teach signs of dislocation of prosthesis and to notify physician if one or more occur.
8. Provide list of medications that interact with warfarin.

Evaluation

Patient has regained physical mobility Patient walks with ambulatory aid as required until healing occurs. Patient walks daily without pain or soreness of operative joint.

Patient has regained skin integrity Patient's incision heals well without excess scarring or keloid. Scar is maturing normally (beginning to contract).

Patient has regained peripheral tissue integrity Patient does not develop any neurological deficit. Patient performs ROM and ankle exercises as required. Patient's color and temperature of extremities are within normal ranges.

Patient has minimal pain Patient no longer needs narcotic or nonnarcotic analgesics, but continues to take nonsteroidal antiinflammatory medication two or three times daily for muscle and joint soreness. States is doing well with pain control.

Patient has experienced no displacement of prostheses X-rays show excellent position of prostheses. Patient has no joint deformity.

Patient developed no thrombophlebitis Patient has no vein problems during postoperative period. Patient is taking coumadin 3 months postoperatively.

Patient developed no wound or joint infection Patient's incision heals well with no drainage. There are no fluctuant masses, no temperature elevations, and no joint pain or soreness.

ARTHROSCOPY

Description and Rationale

With the advent and development of the arthroscope, startling changes have occurred in operative examination and treatment of pathologic joint conditions. Although the knee joint is still a major focus, nearly all joints can be examined with the arthroscope. The multiple benefits of early arthroscopic treatment with specialized techniques and instruments in the hands of a skilled practitioner include lessened inflammation, degeneration, and posttraumatic arthritis. With the advent of same-day surgical settings, patients experience decreased hospital stays and can usually return to their daily activities sooner with full use of the involved joint after arthroscopic examination and repair.

Arthroscopy is most frequently done for diagnosis and treatment of knee injuries, primarily torn or damaged menisci. The menisci, C-shaped rings of cartilage covering the ends of the tibia within the knee joint, are subject to degeneration, tears, and wear (Figure 4-28). Cartilage has no intrinsic blood supply, and if torn, worn, or degenerated, it rarely heals without developing unsatisfactory fibrocartilage. Trauma to the meniscus is

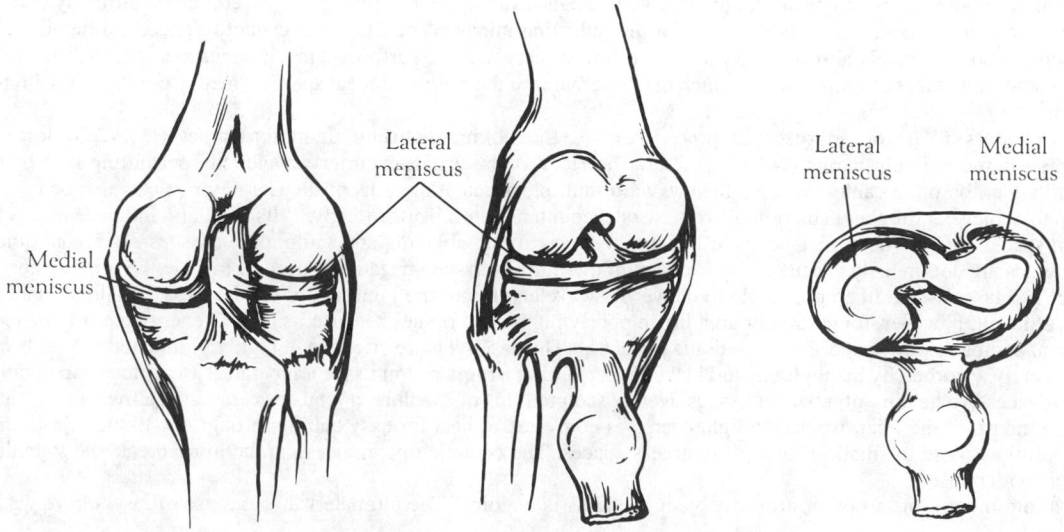

Figure 4-28 Medial and lateral menisci of knee. (From Mourad.[104])

greatest among athletes who suffer tears from external forces, such as a tackle, or from internal forces when a load exceeds the compressibility and resiliency of the cartilage; this may occur in a single incident or over time from repeated stressors. The meniscal tear may cause slight, partial, or complete avulsion from adjoining bone tissues.

The discussion that follows focuses on the knee because it is the joint most commonly examined and treated arthroscopically, although it is commonly done in the shoulder, ankle, elbow, and hip. In the hip, arthroscopy is the most useful procedure for diagnosing and treating loose bodies, torn labra, foreign bodies, and synovial pathology of the hip joint.[76]

Loose or torn pieces of menisci 1 inch or slightly larger in size can be removed arthroscopically. One or more small incisions may be required for full visualization of the joint. Incisions or "ports" for arthroscopic procedures are on the mediolateral or posterolateral surfaces of the knee joint superior to the patella. The exact incidence of knee arthroscopic procedures is difficult to determine; however, it is a common procedure.

Contraindications and Cautions

1. Arthoscopy requires skilled practitioners, as well as more specialized techniques and equipment than extensive arthrotomy procedures.
2. Using more than one port for visualization of the joint may lead to infection.
3. Small pieces of torn or loose cartilage may be missed if hidden under other joint tissues.

4. Hemorrhage must be prevented to lessen posttraumatic arthritis.
5. Scar formation may predispose to future tears in ligaments or cartilage.
6. Postoperative physical therapy and individualized exercise programs must be prescribed and performed to maintain or regain the muscles' and joints' mobility, stability, and strength.
7. Many arthroscopic procedures are same-day surgeries; the patient must be stable for discharge.

•••••• Multidisciplinary Plan

Medications

Finish IV fluids, as prescribed, then discontinue
Narcotic/analgesics
   Toradol, 30 mg IV or IM q4h while hospitalized
   Oxycodone (Percodan), 30-60 mg q4h prn
Antiinfective agent
   Ancef, 1000 mg IV preoperatively and q8h × 3 doses postoperatively
Antiinflammatory agent
   Ibuprofen, 600-800 mg q4h

General Management

Bed rest until patient is fully alert; then can be up with crutches four times daily, depending on operative findings, and joint examined or treated

---

■ LASER ARTHROSCOPY

Use of the laser for arthroscopy is now being done by laser-use specialists. A CO_2 laser is used where precision cutting and ablation of tissues are desired.[137] The energy of the CO_2 laser heats the water in cells and surrounding tissue to over 100° C, almost immediately causing it to vaporize, leaving a precise defect in the exposed tissues. Also, when the laser is focused through a lens in the handpiece, the focused photon beam makes a narrow path through the tissues; if the photon beam is wider and defocused, it causes clotting in small vessels and denaturation of protein.[137] Disadvantages of using the CO_2 laser include difficulty delivering the laser beam without cumbersome articulating arms for the reflecting mirrors. The CO_2 laser cannot be used in a liquid medium because its energy is so completely absorbed by water; therefore surgery must be performed in a gaseous medium to distend the joints, resulting in some subcutaneous emphysema, which may migrate into the retroperitoneal space or mediastinum even with the use of the tourniquet.[137]

Two other lasers used for arthroscopic procedures are the holmium:yttrium-aluminum-garnet (Ho:YAG) laser and the neodymium:yttrium-aluminum-garnet (Nd:YAG) laser. The Ho:YAG laser has a shorter wavelength, permitting it to be delivered into the joint via a fiberoptic cable, avoiding the awkward multiple articulating arms of the CO_2 laser. It can also be used in a liquid medium to achieve cutting and ablation of the tissues encountered during arthroscopy.[137] Its smaller handpiece makes access to narrow joint spaces easier. The higher-powered lasers make the cutting, ablation, and sculpting of tissues easier and quicker. The vaporized tissues are continously evacuated by a saline inflow-outflow system negating a need to irrigate the joint postoperatively.

The Nd:YAG laser uses a fiberoptic cable to deliver its wavelength into the joint, and it can be used in a liquid medium. This laser is less efficient, however, for cutting or ablating in poorly pigmented tissues because its beam's energy tends to be lost by forward dispersal and backward scatter from the tissue surface.[137] This laser is more effective in highly pigmented tissues because it is almost completely absorbed by hemoglobin and melanin, permitting a rapid rise in tissue temperature to achieve vaporization of the cells without excessive heating of adjacent tissues. Newly sculpted tips of sapphire crystals or ceramic coatings aid in transmitting the energy to the tip of the fiber, where the light energy is converted to heat for easy cutting through the tissues. Also, this laser's small size permits its use in small or difficult to access spaces. The ceramic tips, rather than the more breakable sapphire-crystal tips, are most widely used.

Research into the use of lasers for arthroscopic procedures is ongoing. The ultimate value and use of lasers have yet to be determined.

Check of vital signs every 2 hours for 6 hours; then every 4 hours as needed

Neurovascular checks every hour for 24 hours

Ice bags to knee continuously; keep leg elevated, if knee joint operated

Change dressing as needed

Advancement to regular diet as tolerated

Physical therapy consultation for knee exercises

Knee immobilizer to operative knee as prescribed

Perform discharge preparation and teaching if to be discharged same day

Continuous passive motion machine, degrees of motion, and times prescribed for postoperative treatment after ligament repairs

NURSING CARE

Nursing Assessment

Neurovascular Status of Knee Joint and Lower Extremity

Color: may be slightly paler, but capillary refill and perfusion should be within 2 to 4 seconds

Temperature: slightly cooler than opposite knee and leg

Peripheral pulses: should be present and full

Movement: should be normal in ankle; knee should be able to be flexed with moderate discomfort, if no ligament repair done

Sensations: should be normal

Pain: varies with severity of injuries and patient's pain threshold

Psychosocial Concerns

Concern with regaining knee mobility and strength to return to usual ADL and activities without impairment

Complications

Hemorrhage

Thrombus formation (deep vein thrombosis)

Posttraumatic degeneration and arthritis

Infection

Weak ligaments with possibility of tear or retear

Compartment syndrome

Nursing Dx & Intervention

Altered peripheral tissue perfusion related to use of tourniquet during arthroscopy

- Assess neurovascular status as prescribed *to determine current status;* report abnormal data to physician.
- Apply ice bags to knee continuously *to lessen bleeding and edema.*
- Encourage patient to report severity of pain *to help determine if amount is normal or if a complication (arterial occlusion) is developing.*

- Determine amount of active and passive movement (increased pain on passive movement is one indication of compartment syndrome).

Impaired physical mobility related to knee arthroscopy

- Assess effects of surgery on mobility.
- Assist to positions of comfort; assist to ambulate as needed *to maintain strength.*
- Assess drainage and change dressing as needed (drainage should be scant, serosanguineous) *to note condition of wound and healing.*
- Assist with physical therapy exercises as needed *to regain joint functions.*
- Teach walking up and down stairs *to regain joint motion.*
- Assist with straight leg raising exercises as needed *to increase muscle strength.*

Pain related to removal of part of meniscus or to ligament repair and arthroscopy

- Assess site, amount, and severity of pain.
- Administer medications as prescribed for pain *to aid comfort.*
- Help male patient to stand to void (easier while standing if male).
- Assist with and prepare tray for meals *to aid intake of food and fluids.*
- Elevate leg as prescribed *to aid venous return and to decrease edema.*
- Apply ice bags *to lessen edema and thereby decrease pain.*
- Apply knee immobilizer *to prevent flexion;* may have long layered dressing on operative leg.
- Monitor use of continuous passive motion machine, if and when in use.

Patient Education/Home Care Planning

1. Discuss physical therapy exercises needed to gradually increase strength and mobility.
2. List for the patient the signs or symptoms that would require return to see physician, such as increased pain, redness around arthroscopy portals, drainage from portals, swelling of knee, pain in calf, redness and heat in calf, or elevated body temperature.
3. Discuss with the patient appropriate use of pain medications and adequate diet to promote healing.

Evaluation

Patient regains normal peripheral perfusion Patient has pink color to skin. Patient has capillary refill in 2 to 4 seconds. Color is the same in both legs. Patient has no numbness or swelling.

Patient regains joint motion   Patient has full ROM without pain or limitation, has returned to usual activities, and does not have degenerative changes at this time.

Patient has relief of pain   Patient needs only an occasional analgesic for pain.

 # MENISCECTOMY/MENISCAL REPAIR

Description and Rationale

Traditional meniscectomy for removal of larger portions of damaged or degenerated cartilage from the knee joint is still required at times, although the incidence of this more extensive procedure continues to lessen as arthroscopic techniques and skilled practitioners have become more available. The techniques and equipment have been in use in the United States only since 1974, but the knowledge and understanding gained in the past 15 years are revolutionizing the thinking and surgical treatment of meniscal lesions. Open meniscectomy is still required for some patients, however, and some nursing care differs from that of closed arthroscopy (see Figure 4-28 and p. 425 for content).

Meniscal repair is now the major treatment for meniscal injuries because the importance of meniscal preservation has been recognized, primarily influenced and aided by the use of arthroscopy.[42]

Meniscal tears suitable for repair include those that are located no more than 3 mm from the meniscosynovial junction; those in which there is minimal damage to the body of the meniscus; and those in which the length of the tear is such that it subluxes into the joint and is obviously unstable.[42]

A meniscal tear should be suspected in a patient with a history of intermittent locking, joint effusions, pain, a positive McMurray's test (see p. 359), and an unstable knee. Meniscal repairs involve a short hospital stay but extensive postoperative rehabilitation.

Diagnostic studies needed to determine the repairability of a torn meniscus include a double contrast arthrogram and an MRI. The patient's age must be considered because vascular penetration has been shown to be greater in skeletally immature individuals.[42] Acute tears also yield slightly improved results compared with the repair of chronic tears. The repairable meniscus is finally determined through arthroscopy.

Tears not suitable for arthroscopic repair include those that are greater than 5 mm from the meniscosynovial junction and tears in which the displaceable portion of the meniscus is grossly deformed or torn.[42]

Meniscal repair is preferred to partial meniscectomy because it offers the chance to restore the normal anatomy and function of the knee.[114]

Contraindications and Cautions

1. Small pieces of torn or loose cartilage may be missed if hidden under other joint tissues during arthroscopy; however, newer positioning techniques help locate the torn meniscal pieces.

2. Hemorrhage must be prevented to lessen posttraumatic arthritis.
3. Scar formation may predispose to future tears of ligament or cartilage (menisci).
4. Postoperative physical therapy and individualized programs of exercises must be prescribed and performed to maintain or regain the joint's mobility, stability, and strength.
5. The long-term effects of loss of cartilage are not yet fully understood, although degenerative arthritis is common.[113]
6. Newer arthroscopic equipment permits better visualization and operative repairs of menisci and ligaments.

•••••• Multidisciplinary Plan

Medications

Narcotic analgesic agents
   Meperidine (Demerol), 75-100 mg IM q3h for severe pain or use of PCA protocol according to age
Analgesic-antipretic agents/antiinflammatory agents
   Aspirin, 600-1000 mg po q4h prn
   Ibuprofen, 400-800 mg q4h
   Acetaminophen, 650 mg q4h
Antiinfective agents
   Cefazolin sodium (Ancef) or cephalothin sodium (Keflin) (or other cephalosporin), 500-1000 mg q6-8h for 3 doses
   Cephalexin (Keflex), 250-500 mg q6h po, after IV antibiotic is discontinued, if necessary to prevent infection

General Management

Crutch walking with minimal weight bearing; varies with specific procedure but may begin as early as 6 to 8 hours postoperatively, continued for 6 weeks
Knee immobilizer splint applied between exercise periods, prescribed for 4 to 6 weeks after meniscal repair
Use of hinged knee brace for 2 weeks postoperatively, locked in extension; followed by ROM from 20° to 80°, then free motion is permitted after 4 weeks
Maintain postoperative dressing and immobilization as prescribed (varies with specific procedure; for meniscectomy, 24 hours and then up with crutches four times as tolerated)
Check peripheral pulses every 2 hours with neurovascular checks
Elevate operative leg and foot of bed
Apply ice or cryocuff to incisional area
On first postoperative day, begin straight leg raising exercises if prescribed; may not begin until second to third postoperative day with anterior cruciate ligament repair
Begin active and passive ROM knee exercises in physical therapy on first postoperative day (varies with procedure and patient need, but specific program will be prescribed)
Do quadriceps setting exercises, 10 repetitions per set, every hour (see box on muscle setting exercises)

TECHNIQUES FOR MUSCLE SETTING EXERCISES

MUSCLE	TECHNIQUE
Quadriceps setting	Ask patient to straighten leg and thigh; then ask patient to lower knee joint to bed while contracting quadriceps muscle. Have patient hold contraction for 4 to 6 seconds, then relax muscle and knee joint. Repeat exercise 10 to 15 times every 3 to 4 hours. Knee joint should move proximally when quadriceps contracts.
Gluteal setting	Have patient either flat in bed or in low Fowler's position; ask patient to tighten (squeeze) buttocks (gluteal muscles) and hold for 5 seconds; relax buttocks muscles, and repeat tightening (setting) 10 to 15 times every 3 to 4 hours.
Triceps setting (in preparation for crutch walking)	Have patient extend forearm and hold elbow straight, with fingers spread apart on bed; then have patient press hands into mattress while trying to lift shoulders (tenses triceps muscles). Head of bed can be in low Fowler's to aid in doing this exercise. Repeat exercise 10 to 15 times every 3 to 4 hours.

! EMERGENCY ALERT

COMPARTMENT SYNDROME

Compartment syndrome occurs after soft tissue or musculoskeletal injury or surgery in which the amount of swelling, accumulation of fluid, or hematoma constricts circulation, perfusion, and oxygenation to the area. Each compartment contains at least one muscle, nerve, artery, and vein.

Assessment

- Assess capillary refill (normal refill is 2 to 4 seconds).
- Assess for pulses above and below the site of trauma.
- Assess neurovascular status (the five *P*'s).
- Assess for presence of infection, condition of affected tissues.
- Increased pain is common.

Interventions

- Elevate limb and reposition frequently.
- Apply cold packs to area (protect skin from direct contact with ice).
- Perform frequent neurovascular assessments (once every hour).
- Monitor interstitial pressures as prescribed.
- Manage pain.
- Obtain IV access.
- Prepare for surgical incision and fasciotomy, if indicated.

NURSING CARE

Nursing Assessment

Knee Joint and Incisional Area

Presence, amount, and type of drainage (usually is scant, serosanguineous)

Skin color (paler than unoperative knee)

Edema and pain (increasing edema and pain are untoward signs of excessive bleeding)

Ability or inability to move leg with knee extended

Complaint of increasing amounts of pain; may signify compartment syndrome (see box)

Psychosocial Concerns

Alteration in or concerns with body image and ability to return to usual activities and sports (if an athlete)

Limitation of mobility over time

Development of arthritis

Other Complications

Development of hematoma or thrombus in or distal to knee or calf

Instability of knee joint; knee stiffness

Recurrence of pain with or without degeneration or reinjury of tissues of knee joint (patellofemoral pain)

Reflex sympathetic dystrophy

Compartment syndrome also possible (ischemia of muscles leading to necrosis of tissues)

Reinjury of same or injury of opposite knee

Nursing Dx & Intervention

Impaired physical mobility related to surgery and meniscal repair

- Assess ROM of unaffected joints.
- Maintain bed rest as prescribed *to aid recovery.*
- Begin straight leg raising exercises as prescribed *to regain strength.*
- Encourage performing quadriceps setting exercises every 2 hours when prescribed *to maintain strength.*
- Encourage setting of gluteus muscles every 2 hours when prescribed *to maintain functions.*
- Help patient up in a chair with minimal weight bearing initially; then progress to helping patient walk with crutches as needed. Monitor patient's response *to note progress.*
- Emphasize necessity to continue exercise program at home and in rehabilitation setting *to aid recovery.*

- Apply continuous passive motion machine (used when meniscal repair is combined with anterior cruciate ligament reconstruction).[96] The machine is kept at full extension and 30° of flexion of knee.[136]
- Teach patient how to put on knee immobilizer, splint, or brace if required *to aid independence and self-care.*
- Assist with ADL as required *to increase independence.*
- Encourage weight lifting of operative leg as prescribed *to regain full function* (usually done in rehabilitation center).

Altered peripheral tissue perfusion related to surgery and use of tourniquet

- Assess color and temperature of operative limb.
- Perform neurovascular checks every 2 hours, including check of color, edema, temperature, pain, sensory or motor changes, ability to use or lift leg, peripheral pulses, extension of inflammation to contiguous tissues above or below knee, and comparison of operative leg

characteristics with unoperative leg *to note current status.*
- Report changes in findings; may require removal of constricting dressings or additional surgery if pulses are absent *to aid perfusion and relieve pressure.*
- Elevate leg and foot of bed *to increase venous return.*
- Note patient's complaint of increased pain on passive movement *as one sign of compartment syndrome* (see box).
- Apply ice to site *to decrease edema.*
- Continue checks every 4 to 6 hours *to note changes early.*

Impaired skin integrity related to surgical incision

- Assess condition of wound or incision.
- Change dressings of wound as needed *to aid healing.*
- Observe drainage characteristics and amount; report findings to physician if drainage cloudy or odorous—may be sign of infection.
- Obtain culture of cloudy or odorous drainage *to determine type or presence of infective organisms.*

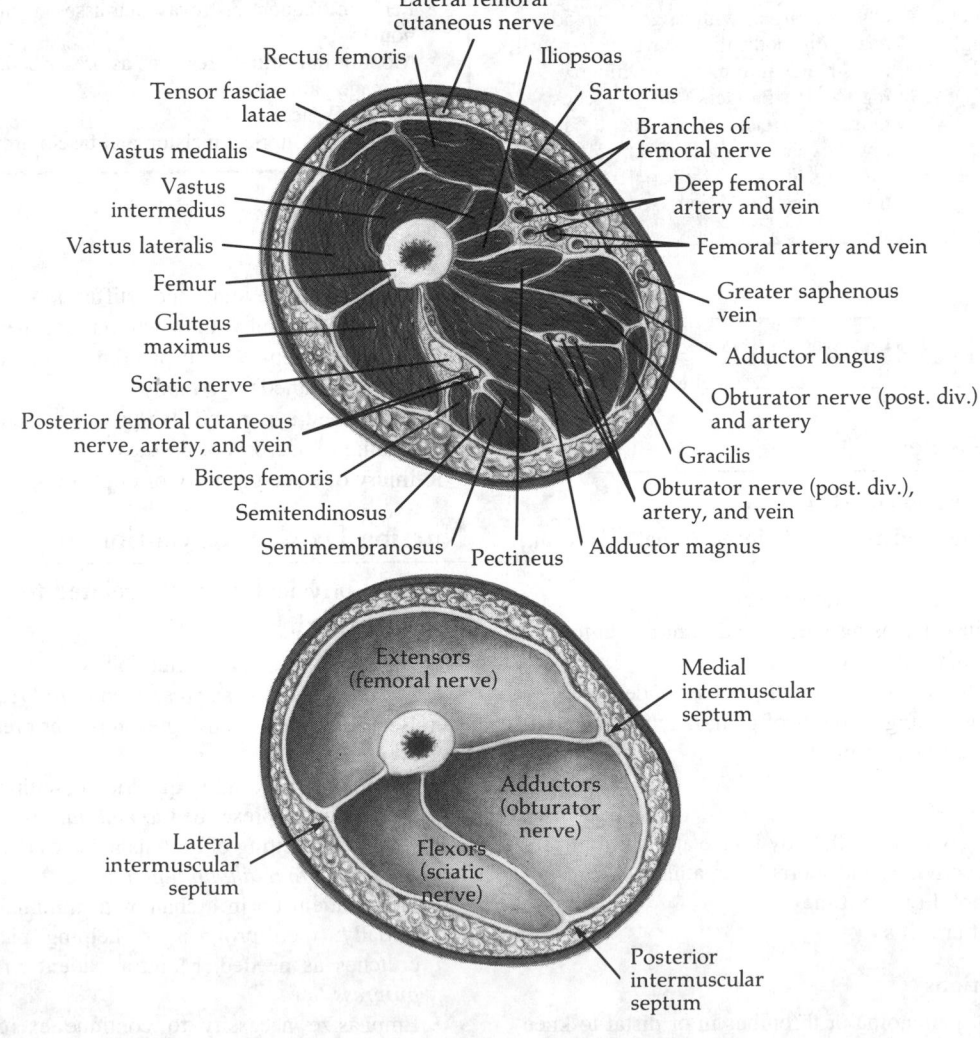

Figure 4-29 Compartments and cross section of the thigh. Each compartment contains at least one muscle, nerve, artery, and vein.

Pain related to surgical procedure

- Assess presence, amount, type, and severity of pain.
- Administer narcotics per order every 3 hours, or encourage patient's use of PCA medication. Increase time between administration of narcotics or analgesics as acute pain abates *to lessen need.*
- Administer aspirin or ibuprofen between narcotics (enhances pain relief and relief of inflammation). Encourage use of aspirin as antiinflammatory drug if prescribed (patients are usually discharged with either aspirin or acetaminophen "prescription" to buy over the counter) *to substitute for narcotics.*
- Encourage position changes *to lessen pressure and fatigue.*
- Report continuing severe pain, change in peripheral pulses, or increasing edema as signs *indicative of ischemia, thrombus formation, or developing compartment syndrome** (Figure 4-29).

Patient Education/Home Care Planning

1. Clarify recovery program and exercises to aid recovery.
2. Clarify rationale for each part of neurovascular check to gather thorough information about tissues.
3. Reiterate the need for continuing the exercise and walking programs prescribed for long-term recovery.
4. Encourage return to social contacts to regain mobility and comfort even though having only partial weight bearing initially.
5. Stress need to refrain from sports activities that could retraumatize unhealed tissues until physician permits resumption.
6. Encourage compliance with low-impact, in-line sports activities such as swimming, rowing machine, or level surface jogging *to aid full recovery.*

Evaluation

ROM of knee joint is regained Patient has 90° to 125° flexion and full extension of knee with minimal pain over time.

Patient has normal peripheral tissue integrity Patient returns to sports activities or usual ADL with protective knee covering, if required. Patient has normal color, normal temperature of legs, and no swelling.

---

*A compartment contains one or more muscles, along with at least one artery, vein, and nerve held enclosed in a covering of inflexible fascia. The interstitial pressure rises with edema and bleeding into injured muscles. The pressure rises because the fascia does not allow the muscle to swell with the edema and bleeding. Unless the fascia is opened, the muscle will die in 6 to 12 hours from ischemia as the elevated venous and interstitial pressure or slow arterial inflow of blood delay removal of wastes.

Patient has relief of pain Patient takes no nonnarcotic analgesics and has no lingering pain. Patient has no compartment syndrome.

ARTHROSCOPIC LIGAMENT REPAIR

Ligaments in and around joints, particularly of the knee, shoulders, fingers, and ankles, are often injured or torn in athletic activities or are torn from repetitive stresses causing, initially, microscopic tears and eventually complete tears of one or more ligaments in a joint. The most frequently torn ligament is the anterior cruciate ligament in the knee (see Figure 4-10). The tear can be partial or complete. It usually occurs from hyperextension or abnormal rotation of the knee.[131] A complete tear creates laxity in the knee and must be repaired to restore joint stability. Tears in ligaments are also called sprains (see p. 388), referred to as first-, second-, or third-degree sprains. Posterior cruciate ligaments can also be torn inside the knee.

The medial and lateral collateral ligaments surrounding the knee joint are also torn frequently in sports activities. Swelling, tenderness, and at times mild to moderate pain along the ligament pathways are indications of these tears. The person is unable to continue to play after the injury and is more comfortable keeping the affected knee partially flexed. Often, a tear of the medial collateral ligament of the knee is accompanied by a medial meniscal injury.[131] One half of anterior cruciate ligament tears are accompanied by meniscal injury.[154]

Cruciate ligament tears, both anterior and posterior, must be repaired carefully for the knee to be fully rehabilitated. With the development of the arthroscope, these injuries decrease the overall rehabilitative process, but the athlete faces a long, intense process of exercises to restore strength and stability to the knee. Often rehabilitation takes 1 year or longer.

Contraindications and Cautions

1. Arthroscopic repairs are done by skilled physicians, frequently by sports medicine physicians or orthopedic surgeons.
2. Multiple ports for arthroscopic surgery may predispose to infection.
3. Younger patients or children whose growth plates are still open may be treated more conservatively with braces and rehabilitative exercises.
4. If the young child or athlete's knee remains unstable, surgery may be considered despite the risk of growth arrest.[131]
5. Surgery may be done within a day or two after injury to the athlete or may be delayed until some of the bleeding and edema have subsided.
6. The injured athlete will be placed on crutches to preclude additional injury related to the knee instability.
7. The knee and anterior cruciate ligament have a direct relationship to the foot and hip for walking during which a stable knee is required.[60]

•••••• Multidisciplinary Plan

Medications

Antiinflammatory agents
    Ibuprofen, 400-800 mg tid or qid
    Toradol, 30 mg IV or po q4h
Antiinfective agent
    Ancef, 1000 mg IV before surgery, and q8h × 3 IV post-
        operatively
Narcotic analgesic
    Oxycodone (Percodan), 30-60 mg po q4h prn
Muscle relaxant
    Metaxalone (Skelaxin), 10-20 mg q4-6h

General Management

Ambulation with crutches
Elevation of affected leg and knee
Ice to knee
Neurovascular checks every 1 to 2 hours as prescribed
Dressing changes as needed
Elastic bandages or bulky dressing postoperatively
Regular diet as tolerated
Up without weight bearing or as prescribed on crutches
Continuous passive motion machine, degrees of motion and
    times prescribed
Physical therapy rehabilitative exercises as prescribed

NURSING CARE

Nursing Assessment

Neurovascular Status of Knee Joint and Lower Extremity

Color and capillary refill: refill in 2 to 4 seconds is
    normal
Temperature: slightly cooler than opposite leg
Discoloration or contusions around knee joint
Peripheral pulses: should all be present and full
Movement: knee may be slightly flexed, but can be moved;
    extension will cause pain
Sensation: should be within normal limits
Edema: may have marked edema around knee
Pain: varies with number and site of ligament tear or
    sprain

Psychosocial Concerns

Severity of injury
Limitation after injury and surgical repair
Prolonged rehabilitation needed
Possible end of career or sports activities
Reinjury possible

Complications

Hemorrhage or hematoma
Thrombus formation or deep vein thrombosis
Infection
Posttraumatic degeneration and arthritis
Possible retear
Compartment syndrome
Loss of livelihood, financial problems

Nursing Dx & Intervention

See pp. 429 to 430.

FIXATION FOR IMMOBILIZATION OF BONES (EXTERNAL)

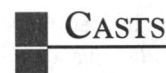

CASTS

Description and Rationale

Casts are hard structures of plaster, fiberglass, or plastic materials used to immobilize musculoskeletal tissues after injuries. Although plaster (gypsum) is still the most frequently used material for casts, newer fiberglass, soft plastic, and cast-tape casts are being used more often. Each of the particular materials requires specific application techniques and has advantages and disadvantages, such as being heavy, cumbersome, or expensive or requiring special drying procedures and care to prevent skin breakdown. The use of a particular material is determined by the patient's injury, length of time needed for immobilization, and the physician's preference (Figures 4-30 and 4-31).

Preparation for encasement in a cast varies from simply explaining its application and purpose to complete physical preparation, including an enema, bath, and skin cleansing with antiseptic solutions. Explanations and care should be geared to the patient's level of comprehension and need to prevent undue fear or anxiety. Handling the patient gently, especially the parts to be encased in a cast, alleviates tension and facilitates application without additional trauma.

Depending on the type of cast and the materials used, all supplies should be assembled and assistance for positioning and holding arranged in advance. Privacy is required when the skin is exposed, and breast and genital areas should be covered for the patient's ease of mind. Padding may be used over bony prominences before the cast is applied.

Once a cast is applied, drying times vary with the material used, the amount of plaster used, the areas of the body put into the cast, and the weather conditions. Plaster casts dry more slowly in damp, high-humidity conditions and can take 2 or 3 days to dry thoroughly. While drying, the areas in a cast must remain uncovered for drying to proceed from inside out. Drying is also facilitated by using fans (except with open wounds) and lamps with low-wattage bulbs.

During the drying periods, care must be taken to avoid making finger indentations in the cast, which would be reflected inward and cause a pressure area on the skin under the indented area. Pressure is also eased by turning the patient every 2 hours while the cast is drying to prevent molding and deformation. Propping or elevating with pillows helps maintain proper positioning. The

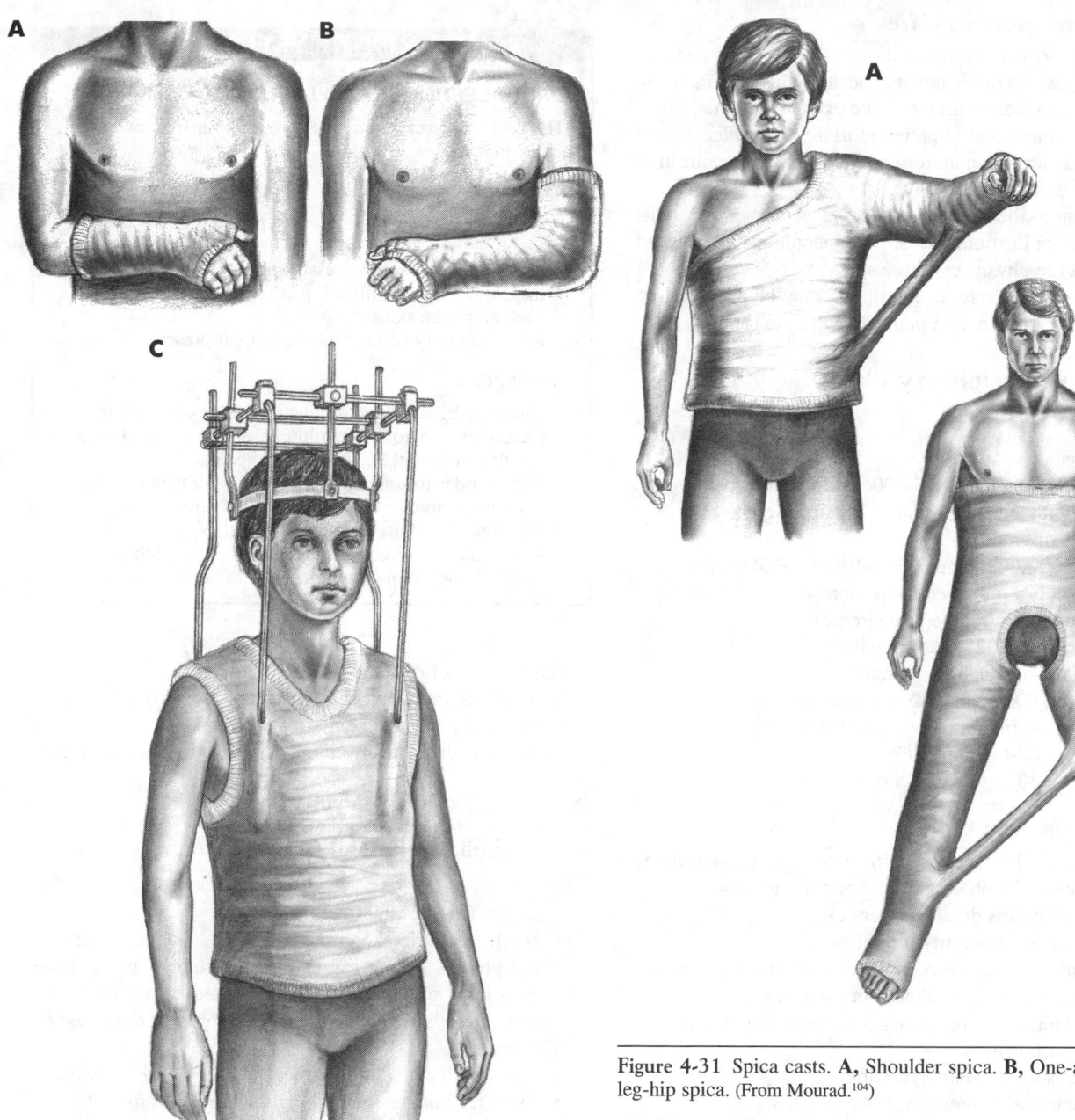

Figure 4-31 Spica casts. **A,** Shoulder spica. **B,** One-and-one-half leg-hip spica. (From Mourad.[104])

Figure 4-30 Examples of casts for upper extremity injuries. **A,** Short arm cast. **B,** Long arm cast. **C,** Body jacket with halo apparatus attached; it may be used with brace, not cast. (From Mourad.[104])

pillows used should not have a plastic or rubber covering because the heat given off by the cast material will be trapped by the rubber or plastic and reflected back to the tissues in the cast, causing injury to the skin. Plastic and rubber also delay drying of plaster.

Contraindications and Cautions

1. Open fractures may not be treated with casts initially because of the need to observe the injury site over an ex-

tended period. If in a cast, a window may be cut for dressing changes.
2. Plaster casts must be kept dry to prevent disintegration and weakening of the cast.
3. Fiberglass, plastic, and cast-tape casts can become wet without weakening; however, the skin under the cast must be dried if it becomes very wet to prevent maceration under the cast.
4. Abdominal distention should be treated before placing a patient in a spica cast because the distention may increase, causing respiratory or circulatory compromise. A circular abdominal window may be cut out of the cast to lessen pressure over tissues.

Preprocedural Nursing Care

1. The skin areas to be encased must be clean, dry, and free of open lesions or blisters that occur with some fractures.
2. X-rays are taken to ascertain the extent of trauma.
3. All equipment and supplies must be assembled before the procedure is begun for ease and safety of application without unnecessary delay.
4. Sufficient skilled personnel should be present to assist with the application; two or three people may be needed to assist the physician with a spica or body cast.
5. A sedative, narcotic, or anesthetic may be given before cast application to ease pain and calm the patient.

•••••• Multidisciplinary Plan

Medications

Narcotic analgesic agent
  Meperidine (Demerol), 25-100 mg IM q3h (exact dosage varies with age and trauma), if pain severe
Analgesic-antipyretic agents
  Aspirin, 300-600 mg po or rectally (if NPO) for moderate pain q4h prn (not used for persons under 18 because of association with Reye's syndrome)
  Acetaminophen, 325-600 mg q4h
Sedative-hypnotics, nonbarbiturate
  Flurazepam (Dalmane), 30 mg po at hs, prn
Nonsteroidal antiinflammatory medications
  Ibuprofen, 400-600 mg q46h
  Toradol, 15-30 mg IV or IM q4h

General Management

Ice bags prescribed to a specific site—place carefully to avoid causing indentation of a damp plaster cast
Bed rest until cast is dry, if plaster cast
Elevation of cast (extremity) on pillows
Neurovascular checks every hour for 24 hours, then every 2 hours for 24 hours, and then every 4 hours
For open reduction, recording and reporting amount of drainage or bleeding
Forcing fluids to maintain hydration
Begin regular diet as prescribed
Seek consultation with physical therapist for exercises to maintain muscle strength, use of crutches, if needed, and for assistance with ambulation
Apply sling for cast to upper arm for comfort and safety

NURSING CARE

Nursing Assessment

Cast and Contiguous Tissues

Extent of cast and type of materials used
Neurovascular condition of tissues around cast
Position of tissues in cast (e.g., in flexed or extended position) or functional position of fingers in forearm cast
Condition of cast (damp or dry)

EMERGENCY ALERT

TROUBLESHOOTING SPLINTS AND CASTS

The goal is to prevent circulatory compromise or extension of the injury.

Assessment

- Assess neurovascular status (see p. 358 for 9 checks areas).
- Assess for new injury, pressure sores.
- Inspect for signs of infection at suture lines, surgical sites, and open skin.
- Assess stability of surgical hardware if present.

Interventions

- Obtain order to loosen or bivalve cast or splint while maintaining anatomic position; assess for restored color, circulation sensation, and lessened pain.
- Obtain order for radiographs to assess for new injury or to ensure corrective measures were effective.
- Pad pressure points and areas adequately.
- Reposition limb frequently (every 2 hours, minimum).
- Maintain elevation of affected area to lessen edema.

Temperature of cast and tissues around cast
Ice bags: ice melted or still frozen and properly placed
Reaction of patient to being in a cast
Compare with tissues from opposite side to detect changes

Nursing Dx & Intervention

Impaired physical mobility related to presence of the cast

- Assess ROM of unaffected muscles.
- Teach isometric exercises as feasible, such as quadriceps and gluteus setting exercises. If fracture is below knee, quadriceps setting exercises of affected leg are vital *to retain muscle strength and prevent atrophy of thigh and leg muscles.*
- Assist with ambulation as needed *to increase mobility.*
- Teach techniques for walking with crutches *for safety.*
- Apply sling to upper extremity *to hold cast snugly and lessen edema formation.*
- Teach patient to allow cast to lie in sling with shoulder loose *to prevent shoulder pain or "freeze" of muscles of joint, for upper extremity cast.*
- Assist physical therapist with rehabilitation program.

Pain related to cast or trauma

- Assess presence, site, and degree of pain.
- Stress that return of pain after pain-free period should be reported to physician (may indicate loss of reduction or other complication).
- Administer narcotic or analgesic as necessary and prescribed *to relieve pain.*
- Note increase in pain, numbness, or tingling and decrease or absence of pulses as indicative of compart-

ment syndrome or that cast may be too tight; report promptly to physician because cast may need to be cut (bivalved).
- Stress need to elevate extremity if edema recurs after discharge *to relieve edema by increasing venous return.*
- With body cast note signs of increasing anxiety, dyspnea, nausea or vomiting, or eructation or complaints of abdominal distention; may be caused by "cast syndrome" from excessive aerophagia (air swallowing) or from kinking of the superior mesenteric artery, leading to gastric or intestinal distention and ileus; cast may need to be bivalved, and a nasogastric tube may be inserted *to relieve ileus and vascular compromise.* If no abdominal window is present, one may be cut in cast.
- Consult occupational therapist and physical therapist for activities *to relieve boredom and maintain muscle strength.*

Risk for peripheral neurovascular dysfunction related to fracture and soft tissue trauma and cast

- Assess status of injured leg or arm and compare with opposite extremity: skin color, edema, temperature, presence of contusions or other lesions; cast, type and dryness.
- Perform neurovascular checks as prescribed: check color, temperature, edema, peripheral pulses and capillary refill, motor and sensory functions, and pain (type, amount, and site) *to determine current neurovascular status.*
- Elevate casted tissues *to increase venous return, thereby decreasing edema.*
- Change patient's position every 2 hours *to lessen pressure on sensitive tissues and relieve muscle tension.*
- Monitor patient's complaint of increasing severity of pain and increasing pain on passive movement *as one sign of developing compartment syndrome.* Report to physician, if present.
- Monitor interstitial tissue (compartment) pressures as prescribed *to detect rising venous pressures as a sign of developing compartment syndrome.*
- Perform capillary refill of toes or fingers to detect prolonged refill as a sign of decreased arterial inflow and developing ischemia *as a sign of compartment syndrome.*
- Release constricting dressings or bivalve cast to relieve compressive forces *to reduce interstitial pressures.*
- Prepare patient for surgical fasciotomy, if physician determines its necessity, from unrelieved increased interstitial pressures.

Impaired physical mobility after cast removal related to edema and muscle weakness after cast removal

- Assess for presence of edema and amount of muscle function after cast is removed.
- Explain that affected tissues may develop edema and tenderness with reuse *to ease concern.*
- Explain to patient that he or she must elevate extremity for 24 hours and when sitting thereafter *to lessen edema.*

- Caution patient to resume usual activities slowly *to lessen edema and soreness.*
- Explain that soreness and pain are common after cast removal *to ease concern;* explain that patient should take nonnarcotic analgesic to ease soreness for 24 to 48 hours.
- Explain that patient should continue ROM exercises as usual *to regain or maintain strength.*
- Explain that muscle atrophy and an accumulation of dead skin cells is common after cast removal *to prepare patient for appearance of tissues.*

Patient Education/Home Care Planning

1. Explain techniques to keep cast clean and dry.
2. Explain not to put anything inside cast.
3. Explain use of hair dryer on cool setting to ease itching under cast.
4. Explain need for well-balanced meals and adequate fluids.
5. Explain proper crutch and walking techniques, including not to lean on axillae supports and to bear weight on hand grips.
6. Explain skin care after cast removal: gently cleanse skin with cold-water wash containing enzymes; allow to soak into skin for 20 to 30 minutes, then flush with clear water; dry carefully and apply a lubricating lotion to prevent cracking or drying of the skin. Caution not to scrub skin tissues because this could cause skin openings and sores.
7. Explain that the patient should report persistent pain, weakness, and edema to the physician (usually all symptoms are relieved in 3 or 4 days after cast removal, although muscle weakness may persist longer); at times special exercises may be prescribed.
8. Teach signs and symptoms of compartment syndrome (see p. 429).

Evaluation

Patient regains mobility and ROM Patient uses muscles and joints normally, without limitation or edema, and has minimum initial postremoval pain and discomfort.

Patient is relieved of pain Patient needs only occasional analgesic for muscle soreness. Acute pain is gone. Patient has only occasional sore joint pain. X-rays show fracture union.

Patient regains usual peripheral vascular perfusion Patient has no numbness or edema of extremity or digits. Color returns to normal 1 to 2 days after cast removal. Patient has not developed compartment syndrome.

▪ EXTERNAL FIXATION DEVICES

Description and Rationale

Several types of externally applied fixation devices are currently used for immobilization of bones, including the Roger Anderson, Ilizarov, Monticelli-Spinelli, Hoffman, and Ace-Fischer apparatuses. The Hoffman apparatus consists of pins placed at right angles to the long axis of a bone and held by the clamps and screws of the device. The Ilizarov or Ace-Fischer devices have pins, rods, and rings placed in oblique and vertical angles to the long axis of the bone and then attached to the retaining devices. The use of one or the other device depends on the patient's condition and physician choice, as with any medical treatment (Figure 4-32).

Externally applied fixation is use in many sites and for many conditions. Sites where such fixation may be applied include bones of the face, jaw, upper and lower arm or leg, pelvis, ribs, and fingers or toes. Pins used vary in number, length, and thickness according to the bones or area to be treated. The major reasons for use of these devices are that they allow increased use of contiguous joints while maintain-ing local immobility, permit the patient's discharge to home, hold unstable fractures or reductions and weakened muscles while allowing ambulation, and hold bones with tissue or bone infection (pins are above and below the infected areas). They are also currently used for nonunions and for leg-lengthening procedures. They are also used for traumatic injuries that have a lot of soft tissue damage that precludes use of a cast and for bone transport for limb salvage. A portion of bone is moved to a new site to fill a void, and new bone forms behind the transported segment through distraction osteogenesis.[63]

Contraindications and Cautions

1. Severely comminuted bone fractures may be a contraindication because the multiple pins needed may cause more fractures or weakening. Comminution with good alignment may be an indication for use, as it is for the Ilizarov or Monticelli-Spinelli fixators.
2. Severe or *spreading* osteomyelitis may be another contraindication because the multiple sites can be sources for progressive infection; localized osteomyelitis may al-

low use of an external fixator to help hold the weakened bones to prevent fracture.
3. Overuse or excessive muscular movements may cause loosening or pin movements.
4. The multiple pin entrance and exit sites can be sources of skin and bone infection.
5. After removal of the pins, bones can be refractured because of the multiple tracts through the bones; patients must be cautioned to increase activities slowly to prevent reinjury.
6. Self-care techniques must be learned by the patient and family.
7. Limb-length discrepancy of less than 2 cm requires no specific treatment.[108]

•••••• Multidisciplinary Plan

Surgery

Pin care according to institution policy—some physicians do not prescribe pin care
Turning of nuts as required every 6 hours for some fixators

Medications

Narcotic analgesic agent
    Meperidine (Demerol), 50-100 mg IM q3h (dosage varies with age and trauma); may use patient-controlled analgesia with age-appropriate dosage
Antiinfective agents
    Cefamandole (Mandol) or cefazolin (Ancef), 250-1000 mg IV q6h for 7 d
    Cephalexin (Keflex), 500 mg q6h po after IV antibiotic is discontinued
Analgesic-antipyretic agents
    Aspirin, 600 mg po q4h for moderate pain or temperature

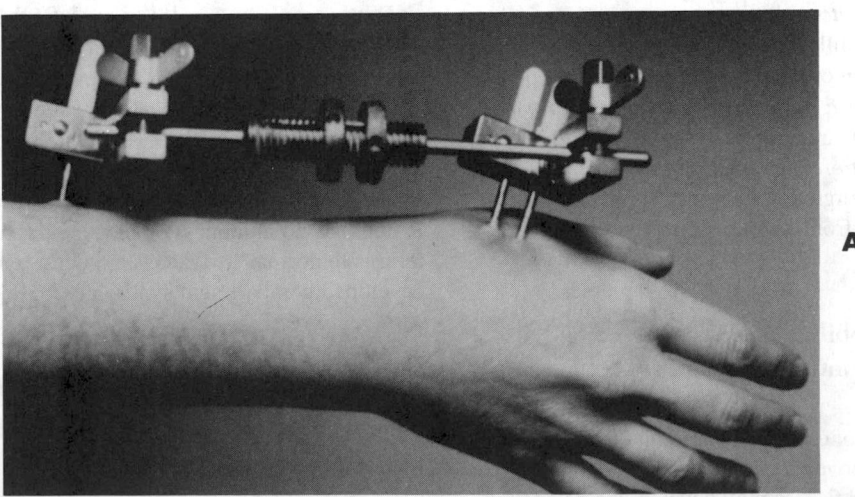

Figure 4-32 External fixation apparatuses. **A,** Hoffman. (From Mourad.[104])

above 38.3° C (101° F) (aspirin should not be given to persons younger than 18 years of age because of its association with Reye's syndrome.)

Acetaminophen 325-650 mg po q4h prn for moderate pain or temperature above 38.3° C (101° F)

General Management

Neurovascular checks every hour for 24 hours, then every 2 hours for 24 hours, and then every 4 hours

Ice bags to site continuously

Elevation of extremity on pillows

Up with sling (if upper extremity) or with crutches and no weight bearing (if lower extremity; after recovery from anesthetic); may also use wheelchair.

ROM to unaffected joints and muscles

Turning (tightening) nuts as ordered every 6 hours for limb lengthening only

Begin regular diet as prescribed

Inspect pin sites every shift for signs of inflammation or infection; do pin site care per institution policy or physician's prescription

NURSING CARE

Nursing Assessment

Site of Injury and External Apparatus

Assessment of each pin entrance and exit site

Color—marked redness and purulent drainage may signify infection, and the pin may need to be removed[108]

Temperature and edema of tissues

Drainage

Peripheral pulses

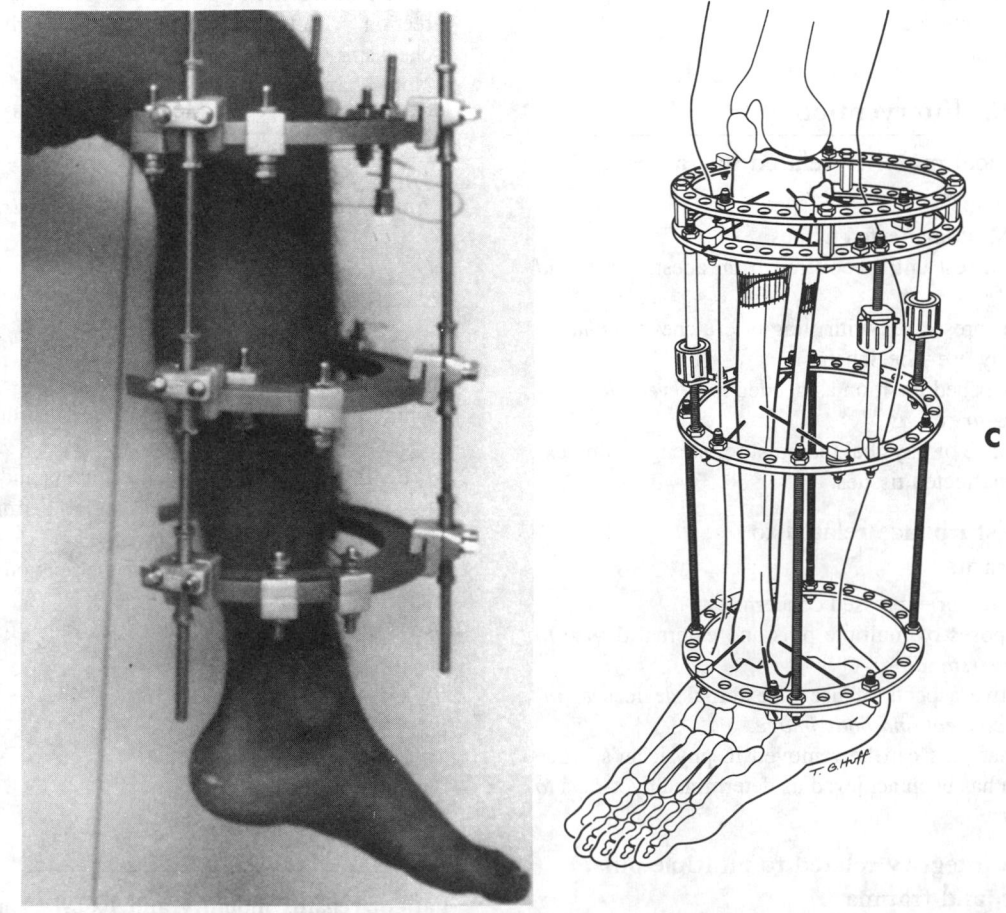

Figure 4-32, cont'd. External fixation apparatuses. **B,** Monticelli-Spinelli Circular Fixator. **C,** Ilizarov apparatus with corticotomies for lengthening lower leg. (From Mourad.[104])

Ability to move contiguous muscles and joints (unless to be held immobilized)
Pain, numbness, or tingling
Position of fixator
Intactness of fixator parts

Systemic Concerns

Temperature and other vital signs
Nausea
Headache or other pain

Psychosocial Concerns

Concern with body image
Degree of mobility or immobility
Acute pain
Possibility of infection

Other Complications

Nonunion or malunion
Infection, including osteomyelitis and rarely toxic shock syndrome
Muscle or nerve damage or injury
Compartment syndrome
Fat embolism syndrome
Deep vein thrombosis

Nursing Dx & Intervention

Impaired physical mobility related to trauma and fixation device

- Assess ROM of unaffected tissues.
- Maintain bed rest until recovered from anesthesia *to aid recovery.*
- Ambulate as prescribed with sling or crutches *to enhance mobility;* may use wheelchair.
- Turn and alter bed position as needed *to prevent development of pressure areas.*
- Seek assistance of physical therapist for strengthening exercises to unaffected tissues.

Body image disturbance related to external apparatus

- Assess implicit or expressed concerns.
- Clarify purposes of multiple pins and external device *to increase understanding.*
- Stress positive aspects of use of external devices *to increase self-concept and body image.*
- Reiterate that pins can be removed in physician's office when union has been achieved as determined by x-rays *to ease concern.*

Impaired skin integrity related to multiple pins, skin openings, and trauma

- Assess skin areas for signs of pressure or inflammation.
- Wound care as needed. Pin care: clean each site with hy-

drogen peroxide–soaked swabs; remove drainage with normal saline; then dry. Topical antibiotic ointment may or may not then be lightly applied, depending on physician or institutional policy. (Pin care may not be done or is stopped if sites are clean, dry, and without drainage and may vary according to institutional policy or physician prescription.[72])
- Clean all sutures if present with antiseptic and redress if drainage is present. Sutures may be left open to air if unit policy.

Pain related to trauma or fixation apparatus

- Assess site and amount of pain (may initially be acute, sharp pain at pin insertion sites on skin) *to determine current status.*
- Administer narcotics and analgesics as needed and prescribed *to relieve pain or discomfort.*
- Stress that recurrence of pain at site is a sign to be reported to physician—may indicate a developing problem.
- Stress that acute pain episodes will lessen in 24 to 48 hours and that most pain will be relieved in approximately 7 to 10 days *to ease concern.*
- Note localization of pain to one site (may be sign of infection or inflammation); continue hourly neurovascular checks *to note early changes.*
- Note change in sensation or numbness and tingling as signs of neurovascular pressure; report increases in either sign because these may signify beginning compartment syndrome.
- Apply ice bags as prescribed *to lessen edema and pain.*

Patient Education/Home Care Planning

1. Explain to the patient and family pin care techniques to continue at home as needed; provide instructions in writing to avoid confusion.
2. Stress the need to increase movements and weight bearing slowly to lessen tenderness and to permit the muscles to regain strength.
3. Discuss and list side effects of medications and what to report to physician.
4. Reiterate treatment goals and stress need for compliance with regimen.
5. Stress 24-hour availability of health care personnel to ease concerns.

Evaluation

Patient regains mobility and ROM   Patient uses muscles and joints normally, without limitation or edema, and with minimum initial postremoval pain and discomfort.

Patient has a positive body image Patient has equal leg lengths. Patient has become more outgoing and sociable.

Wound sites remain free of infection No drainage, redness or erythema is noted at pin sites. No fracture has occurred. Skin openings are closing without signs of infection.

Patient is relieved of pain Patient has only occasional pain or muscle soreness.

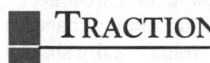

TRACTION

Description and Rationale

Traction is the application of force to the skin, muscles, and bones to aid in reduction of fractures, hold the reduced bones in alignment for healing, relieve muscle spasms and pain, and ex-

ert sufficient pull on muscles and bones to relieve pressure on peripheral spinal nerves. Traction can be applied to the skin and thus indirectly to the bones and muscles, or it can be applied directly to the bones through skeletal pins inserted through the skin and bones with the pins then being attached to ropes, pulleys, and weights. The particular type of skin or skeletal traction applied is determined by the physician with regard to the patient's injury or condition, the purpose of the traction, the age of the patient, the weight of the patient, the condition of the skin tissues to be placed in traction, and the length of time the patient will need to be kept in traction. Table 4-6 summarizes the various types of skin and skeletal traction and the specific points pertinent to each type of traction (Figures 4-33 and 4-34).

Because time is required to overcome muscle spasms, bone overriding, angulation, and shortening, patients may be in

■ TABLE 4-6 Traction

Type	Patient's Age	Amount of Weight	Purposes and Principles	Considerations for Care
Buck's extension (one or both legs) (Figure 4-33, *A*)	Any age; most commonly used in adults	5-8 lb/leg	Applied preoperatively for hip fractures; for "pulling" contracted muscles; for relieving muscle spasms of legs or back; patient usually lies in recumbent position; may be turned to either side if no fracture is present; if there is a fracture, patient is turned to unaffected side; pillows to back and between legs	Skin of older patients is more "friable" and subject to loosening because of less subcutaneous fat; patient's complaints of burning under tape, moleskin, or traction boot should be assessed; traction may be removed for skin care even in presence of fracture; check heels for pressure areas
Russell's (one or both legs) (Figure 4-33, *B*)	Children 5 years or older to older adults	2-5 lb/leg	Applied for "pulling" contracted muscles; preoperatively for hip fractures; uses principle that "for every force in one direction, there is an equal force in the opposite direction" for the pulley placement and amount of weight used, because weight pull is doubled	Patient is positioned on back for most effective pull; knee sling can be loosened for skin care and checking pulses in popliteal area
Pelvic belt or girdle (abdomen and pelvis are enclosed) (Figure 4-33, *C*)	Adults or older adolescents	20-35 lb	Relieve muscle spasms and pain associated with "disc" conditions; pull is from iliac crests to relieve spasm	Patient may be positioned in Williams' position, which permits 45° of flexion of the knees and hips to relax the lumbosacral muscles; orders usually state to be "in traction 2 hours, out 2 hours" and out of traction at night; traction straps should not put pressure over sciatic nerves
Pelvic sling (under pelvis and buttocks like a hammock)	Adults	20-35 lb	For holding fractured pelvic bones; buttocks must be slightly off bed	Patients are comfortable in the sling even with extensive pelvic bruising; they may become dependent on being in the sling, and gradual "weaning" may be required; the sling should be kept clean and dry, and the patient can be removed from the sling for care and toileting, if institutional policies permit

Continued.

◼ TABLE 4-6 Traction—cont'd

Type	Patient's Age	Amount of Weight	Purposes and Principles	Considerations for Care
Cervical head halter (under chin, around face, head, and back of head)	Adults	5-15 lb	For relieving muscle spasms caused by degenerative or arthritic conditions in or of the cervical vertebrae; halter should be applied so pull comes from occipital area, not through chin portion	Patients may be in low or high Fowler's position depending on the purpose of the traction; halter is usually incorrectly positioned if the patient complains of pain of chin, teeth, or temporomandibular joint; the side straps usually should be adjusted to relieve these conplaints; patients should be removed from the traction for sleeping; patients may also use this type of traction at home for cervical arthritic conditions
Cotrel's (cervical head halter and pelvic belt to pelvis)	Adolescents	5-7 lb to head halter and 10-20 lb to pelvic belt	For stretching muscles preoperatively for scoliosis; principle is to pull muscles and joints apart	Patient is put in this traction to relax muscles and curvature; should be in traction except for sleeping; rarely, patient may be placed in Cotrel's postoperatively, too, although less frequently because of newer operative techniques such as Harrington or Luque rod or Cotrel-Dubousset instrumentation
Dunlop's (lower humerus and forearm)	Children to adults	5-7 lb to humerus; 3-5 lb to forearm	For realigning fractures of the humerus; body is used for counteraction by slightly elevating side of bed of arm in traction; forearm is merely held at right angles to the humerus for comfort, by using Buck's extension to the forearm	Dunlop's can be totally skin traction by Buck's extension to the humerus or can be skeletal with a Steinmann pin inserted through the distal humerus; use of either depends on the patient's injury; traction to the *forearm* should be removed daily for skin care, pulse checks, and ROM exercises because the forearm traction is merely a means to keep the forearm vertically at a right angle to the humerus; patients must have assistance during ADL because they are held flat on their backs; they can turn enough for back care only
Cervical via skull tongs (skull bones bilaterally)	Any age (most commonly young adults)	20-30 lb (depends on weight of patient)	To realign fractures of cervical vertebrae and to relieve pressure on cervical nerves; patient must be on a special bed or frame such as a Circ-Olectric bed or Stryker frame to facilitate care; traction weights must never be "lifted"; traction must be continuous	Patients with this traction may be severely injured, having either upper or lower spinal cord injury or complete transection, making them develop quadriplegia or paraplegia; neurovascular checks are required hourly to assess progression or relief of symptoms; patients also may develop paralytic ileus (therefore are given nothing by mouth), may have a nasogastric tube inserted to suction, and have an indwelling urinary catheter; pin care is done according to institutional policies and physician's preference
Balanced suspension to femur (Steinmann pin or Kirschner wire inserted through upper tibia; thigh and leg are suspended in a splint and leg attachment) (see Figure 4-34)	Any age from 3 yr	20-35 lb	For realignment of fractures of the femur; to overcome muscle spasms associated with fractures of the femur; suspension of the thigh and leg is "balanced" by countertraction attached to the top of the thigh splint with weights equal to those of suspension (usually 7-8 lb)	Patients in this traction should be recumbent for best effects; they can turn approximately 30° to either side briefly for back care or can lift themselves using the trapeze and by using the uninjured leg and foot; neurovascular checks are vital to assess circulatory status and to prevent compartment syndrome (see p. 429)

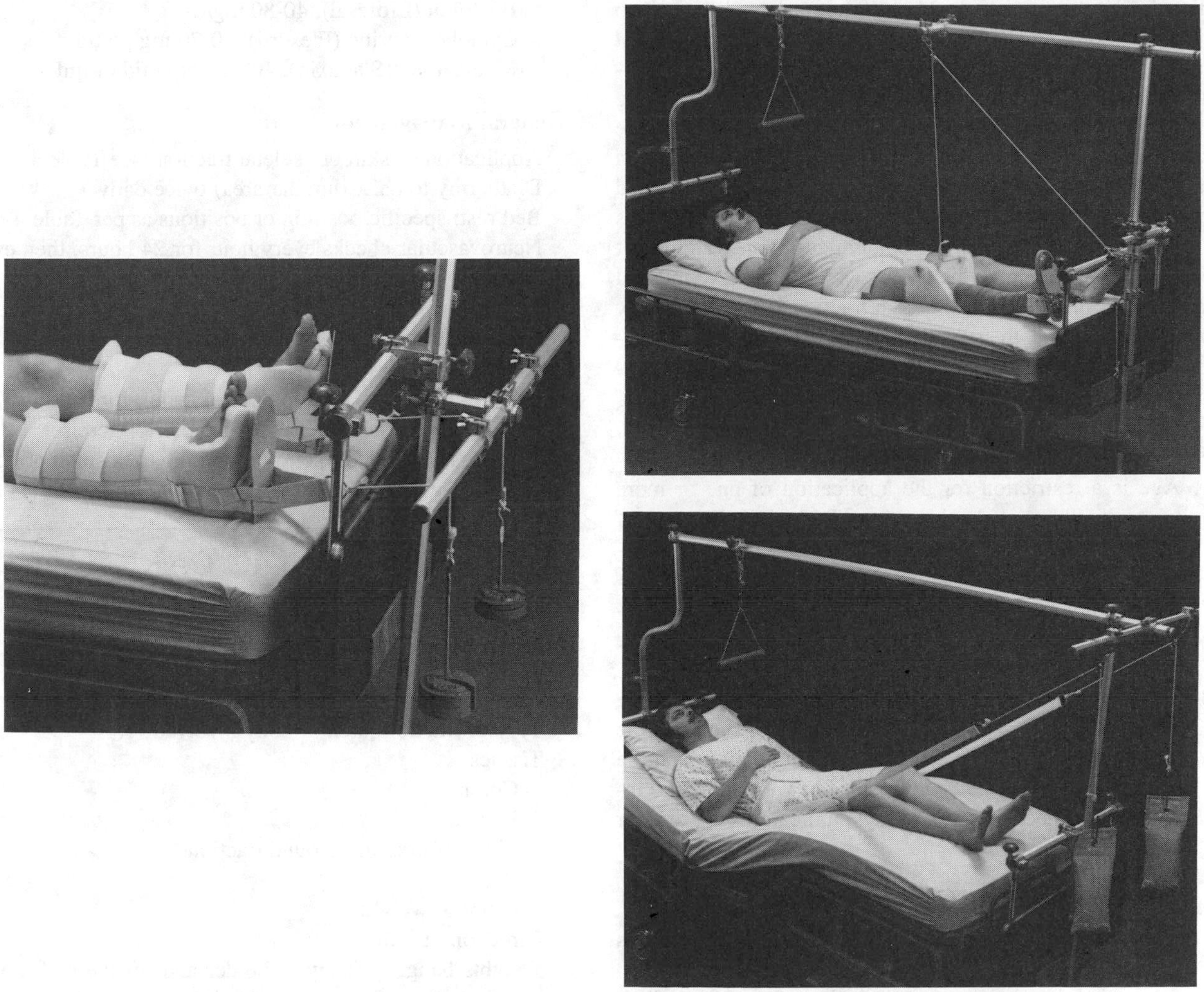

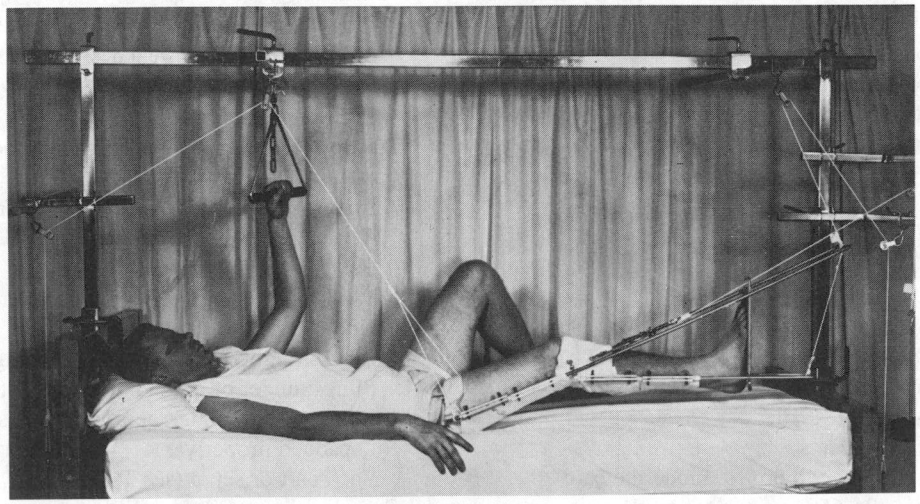

Figure 4-33 Types of skin traction. **A,** Buck extension. **B,** Russell. **C,** Pelvic belt.

Figure 4-34 Balanced suspension skeletal traction to the femur. (From Brashear.[120])

traction for as short a time as 24 to 48 hours or as long as 4 to 6 weeks or more. Generally, patients in skeletal traction must remain hospitalized for the entire time because of the specialized care and equipment required (except for patients being treated with home cervical traction with a head halter, or in rare instances in other types of traction). Because hospitalization in traction is extensive and also expensive, patients may be placed in traction for periods only to achieve relief of muscle spasms and to correct fracture overriding or angulation; once alignment is regained, the patient may be taken to surgery to have internal metallic fixation. Therefore although traction is still frequently required for specific treatment of an individual patient's injuries, the traction may be removed sooner than in the past because metallic implants may be used to maintain the reduction.

Contraindications and Cautions

1. Age is a restriction for the application of one or more types of skin or skeletal traction (Table 4-6). Because of lack of muscle mass or strength, a newborn baby or an elderly adult may not benefit from traction.
2. Open draining wounds or lesions are also contraindications to the use of either skin or skeletal traction because such wounds predispose to infection.
3. The amount of weight applied must be determined by the physician, who will consider the amount of muscle spasm, the degree of overriding and angulation, and the specific purposes of the treatment. The weight may be increased or decreased as x-rays indicate the need for weight changes.

Preprocedural Nursing Care

1. Reiterate or clarify upcoming events for patient's traction.
2. Assess local and systemic physical condition for indications or contraindications to placement in traction (such as open lesions or blisters, drainage, or deep calf pain).
3. Assist with hygienic self-care for clean, dry skin surfaces.
4. Assist with positioning for x-rays.
5. Administer preprocedural medication if prescribed.
6. Assemble all equipment for application of specific traction.
7. Assist with application of specific traction.

•••••• Multidisciplinary Plan

Medications

Narcotic analgesic agents
    Meperidine (Demerol), 50-100 mg IM q3h for 72 h (may use patient-controlled analgesia with age-specific dosages)
    Morphine, 10-15 mg IM q4h
Analgesic-antipyretic agents
    Aspirin, 600-1000 mg q4h prn for moderate pain
    Acetaminophen, 325-650 mg q4h for moderate pain
Tranquilizers
    Diazepam (Valium), 2-10 mg po q4-6h
Muscle relaxants
    Baclofen (Lioresal), 40-80 mg/d
    Cyclobenzaprine (Flexeril), 10-20 mg po tid
    Metaxalone (Skelaxin), 400-800 mg tid or qid

General Management

Application of skin or skeletal traction (see Table 4-6)
Diathermy to back (lumbar area) twice daily
Bed rest: specific position or positions as per Table 4-6
Neurovascular checks every hour for 24 hours, then every 2 hours, and then every 4 hours
Monitoring of tissue pressure if prescribed
Ice bags to affected tissues (site always indicated for application)
Diet: high protein, high vitamin, low fat; force fluids
Physical therapy for ROM and isometric exercises
Pin care for skeletal traction according to hospital policies or physician's preference

NURSING CARE

Nursing Assessment

Area of Body in Traction*

Type of traction; area of body involved
Tissues
    Color
    Edema
    Signs of pressure around traction
    Pain
Amount of weight
Direction of pull
Weights hanging freely in holder and off the bed, not over patient[149]

Systemic Concerns

Patient
    Pressure areas over bony prominences
    Muscle strength or weakness
    Weight loss
    Position in bed
Traction (entire traction setup) and principles of maintaining traction
    Ropes: riding freely in pulleys, no frayed ends; knots intact; *never reuse rope*[149]
    Pulleys: moving freely
    Weights: Hanging freely in holder; correct prescribed amount
    Knots: intact; no rope fraying
    Pins: straight, unbending; not moving in tissues
    Slings: under or around appropriate tissues
    Belts: intact; under appropriate tissues; clean and dry; padded properly
    Each part of setup (see Table 4-6)
Complications of immobility
    Weight loss

*See Table 4-6 for specific tissues.

Development of osteoporosis
Possible pulmonary infections
Pressure areas or sores

Psychosocial Concerns

Concern with changes in body image
Immobility and loss of livelihood
Acute pain
Bone healing over time

Other Complications

Nonunion
Malunion
Embolic phenomena
Pin necrosis
Skin lesions or pressure areas

Nursing Dx & Intervention

Pain related to trauma and traction

- Assess pain experiences to determine extent, etiology, and patient's reactions.
- Help patient alter position within traction limitations *to relieve muscle and joint stiffness or soreness.*
- Administer narcotic analgesics as prescribed *to relieve acute pain* and nonnarcotic analgesic (aspirin or acetaminophen) *to relieve inflammation.*
- Assess patient's entire pain experiences: *local* pain at site of injury and *systemic* spread (e.g., chest pain, dyspnea, calf pain, headache, confusion); *may be indications of pulmonary, circulatory, neurologic, or other complications.*
- Assess for evidence of fat embolism with symptoms of mental confusion, dyspnea, chest pain, and vital sign changes. A petechial rash may also develop over upper chest and neck with fat emboli, which are more common with long-bone fractures.
- Assess and perform Homans' procedure to determine possible cause of calf pain; could indicate thrombophlebitis if positive Homans' sign; may also have redness, swelling, increased warmth in calf.
- Assess degree of muscle spasms in injury site; clarify causes of and measures *to relieve spasms through traction and muscle-relaxant medications.*
- Compare both legs *for similarities or differences.*
- Monitor entire traction setup for proper functioning *to decrease friction, which decreases effectiveness of traction.*[149]
- Observe all bony prominences for signs of pressure or irritation on skin and nerves.
- Clarify use of ice bags and apply ice bags *to help relieve muscle spasms, bleeding, and edema.*
- Assist with ROM exercises *to maintain strength in unaffected muscles.*
- Assess affects of diathermy *in relieving pain and muscle spasms* if pertinent to injury.
- Perform pin care if needed *to remove secretions and to lessen possibility of infection.* Follow institutional policies or physician's preference for pin care.

Body image disturbance related to weight loss and weakness

- Assess effects of injury on body image and self-concept.
- Explain purposes of traction repeatedly because patient's anxiety and pain may preclude hearing or full understanding.
- Explain reasons for bed rest, weakness, and anorexia. Encourage patient to eat more as appetite returns *to help regain weight and to aid in tissue and bone healing.* Patients can lose from 10 to 20 pounds in skeletal traction because of decreased muscle activity over time.
- Explain purposes of position changes: *to maintain healthy tissues.*
- Assess appetite and intake and output *to note current status and to encourage intake.*
- Maintain 3000 ml fluid intake *to maintain hydration and to perfuse kidneys properly to prevent renal complications.*

Impaired physical mobility related to traction, hospitalization, and loss of livelihood

- Assess effects of injury and traction on mobility.
- Clarify use of traction as one part of treatment regimen for patient's specific injury *to increase understanding and compliance.*
- Encourage patient and family communications with physician for "timetable" of plans for overall treatment *to aid compliance.*
- Seek consultations (per physician's order) for occupational therapy and physical therapy *to assist patient's recovery and adjustment to treatment regimen and hospitalization.*
- Seek consultation with social service personnel to help patient and family plan and prepare for possible economic needs *to regain livelihood* (may lose employment while hospitalized).
- Encourage patient's self-care activities *to maintain mobility within traction limits.*
- If surgical repair follows traction use, assist to ambulate *to regain mobility.*

Patient Education/Home Care Planning

1. Ensure that patient and family can apply traction correctly if it is to be used in the home.
2. Explain to patient and family the use of muscle relaxants and pain medications if prescribed for home use.
3. Ensure that patient and family recognize when to contact physician if symptoms recur.
4. Explain that patient should maintain intake of well-balanced diet to regain weight and strength.

Evaluation

Patient has minimal pain experiences   Patient has moderate soreness of operative site after surgical repair, relieved with narcotic, analgesic, and muscle relaxant occasionally. No other pains are noted.

Patient has a positive body image   Patient has positive outlook toward full recovery in 3 to 6 months. Patient regains some weight (5 lb), some muscle strength, and feels positive and sure of full recovery.

Patient regains more physical mobility and ROM   Patient tolerates traction well and undergoes insertion of intramedullary rod to fractured femur. Patient walks with crutches and cane for next 10 days or longer. Performs ROM for unaffected muscles.

FIXATION FOR IMMOBILIZATION OF BONES (INTERNAL)

Surgical implantation of metallic pins, nails, screws, plates, and other devices for immobilizing or repairing traumatized or damaged bones and joints is major orthopedic treatment. With the development in the early 1930s of nonreactive metal alloys, surgical repair has provided greatly decreased hospitalization periods, a more rapid return to home and social and employment opportunities, and a more rapid regaining of mobility. Surgical repair requires the concurrent administration of antibiotics to prevent infection, the major hazard and deterrent to use of more orthopedic surgical and metallic implants for a wider range of injuries. However, in most instances the advantages of internal metallic fixation far exceed the disadvantages.

Fractures of bones may be surgically immobilized by screws attached to a compression plate; nails or pins, as in a hip nailing; a rod or nail placed within the intramedullary canal (intramedullary rod) or parallel to the bones (Harrington rod, Cotrel-Dubousset instrumentation, or Luque rod); screws or staples to hold fracture fragments together; or natural bone grafts to fill in gaps in bones or to fuse two bone surfaces together, as in a spinal fusion.

This section will focus on several procedures representative of internal fixation procedures: hip nailing or pinning, spinal fusion by Harrington or Luque rods or Cotrel-Dubousset instrumentation, spinal fusion by natural bone grafts, and internal fixation with compression plate and screws.

INTERNAL FIXATION WITH HIP NAILS OR PINS

Description and Rationale

The patient's specific injury, general physical and mental condition, and the physician's choice from the many available metallic nails and pins determine which type will be used for the particular patient. The injury may be a fairly stable fracture that requires only a single nail, such as a compression nail or screw or a sliding compression nail. Unstable fractures may require multiple pins, such as Knowles pins, or use of a nail with a side plate.

The type of internal fixation used is also determined by the particular fracture type and site. Hip fractures are referred to as intracapsular or extracapsular. Intracapsular fractures are those of the femoral head or neck that are contained within the hip capsule (Figure 4-35). Intracapsular fractures may disrupt the blood supply of the head of the femur, with subsequent development of avascular necrosis of the head of the femur. Therefore fractures of the head or proximal femoral neck may be treated with insertion of a femoral prosthesis (hemiarthroplasty). Subcapital or distal neck fractures may heal without avascular necrosis; thus these latter fractures may be nailed or pinned (Figure 4-36).

Extracapsular fractures are those around or through the trochanters and are referred to as intertrochanteric or subtrochanteric fractures. These fractures heal well with the use of compression screws or nails because the blood supply to the fracture site comes from the surrounding vessels outside the capsule. Side plates attached to the nails help maintain a stable reduction while healing progresses (Figure 4-36, *A*).

Finally, the patient's physical and mental condition may also help determine which type of internal fixation is performed. The weak or confused patient would benefit from a compression interlocking nail, which can withstand some weight bearing; a single nail with or without a side plate would be appropriate for a stable fracture in a mentally clear patient who could be cautioned and expected to walk with only minimum or touchdown weight bearing.

Thus the specific internal fixation and repair require careful evaluation and assessment by the surgeon and other health professionals for the patient's greatest benefit.

There is a level of morbidity and mortality associated with hip fractures and hip surgery in older patients. Many patients never regain ambulatory status after surgery and require long-term care. The mortality rate of postoperative hip surgery patients who experience pulmonary embolism approaches 200,000, secondary to thromboembolic disease. Without anticoagulation, as many as 75% of patients will show deep vein thrombosis with a mortality rate of 2%.[48]

Preprocedural Nursing Care

1. The patient may be placed in traction, usually Buck's extension or Russell's, while preparations for surgery are completed.
2. Chest and injury site x-rays are evaluated.
3. An enema is given, if needed, and an indwelling catheter may be inserted.
4. An electrocardiogram is done to determine cardiovascular status.
5. Complete consultation for medical clearance is done before surgery, if patient is older or elderly.

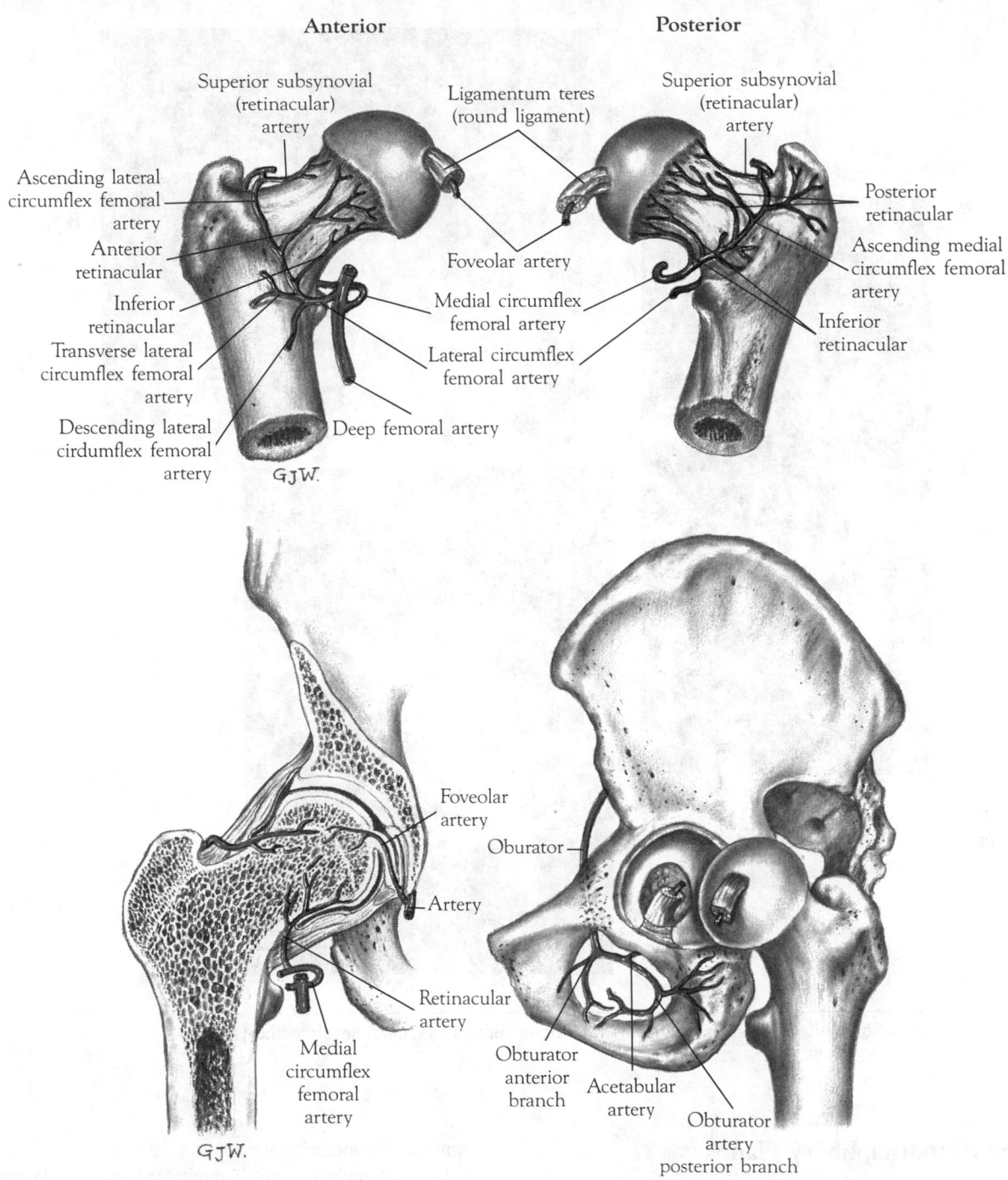

Anterior   **Posterior**

Superior subsynovial (retinacular) artery

Ligamentum teres (round ligament)

Superior subsynovial (retinacular) artery

Ascending lateral circumflex femoral artery

Anterior retinacular

Inferior retinacular

Transverse lateral circumflex femoral artery

Descending lateral cirdumflex femoral artery

Foveolar artery

Medial circumflex femoral artery

Lateral circumflex femoral artery

Deep femoral artery

Posterior retinacular

Ascending medial circumflex femoral artery

Inferior retinacular

GJW.

Foveolar artery

Oburator

Artery

Retinacular artery

Medial circumflex femoral artery

Obturator anterior branch

Acetabular artery

Obturator artery posterior branch

GJW.

Figure 4-35 Blood supply to hip joint. (From Mourad.[104])

6. Serologic studies are done for chemistry analysis; urinalysis is done.
7. Preoperative medication is administered.
8. Intravenous therapy is initiated for fluid intake.

9. Skin cleansing is done to decrease organisms in the operative site in the prep room.
10. Type and cross-match for packed red blood cell replacement is done.

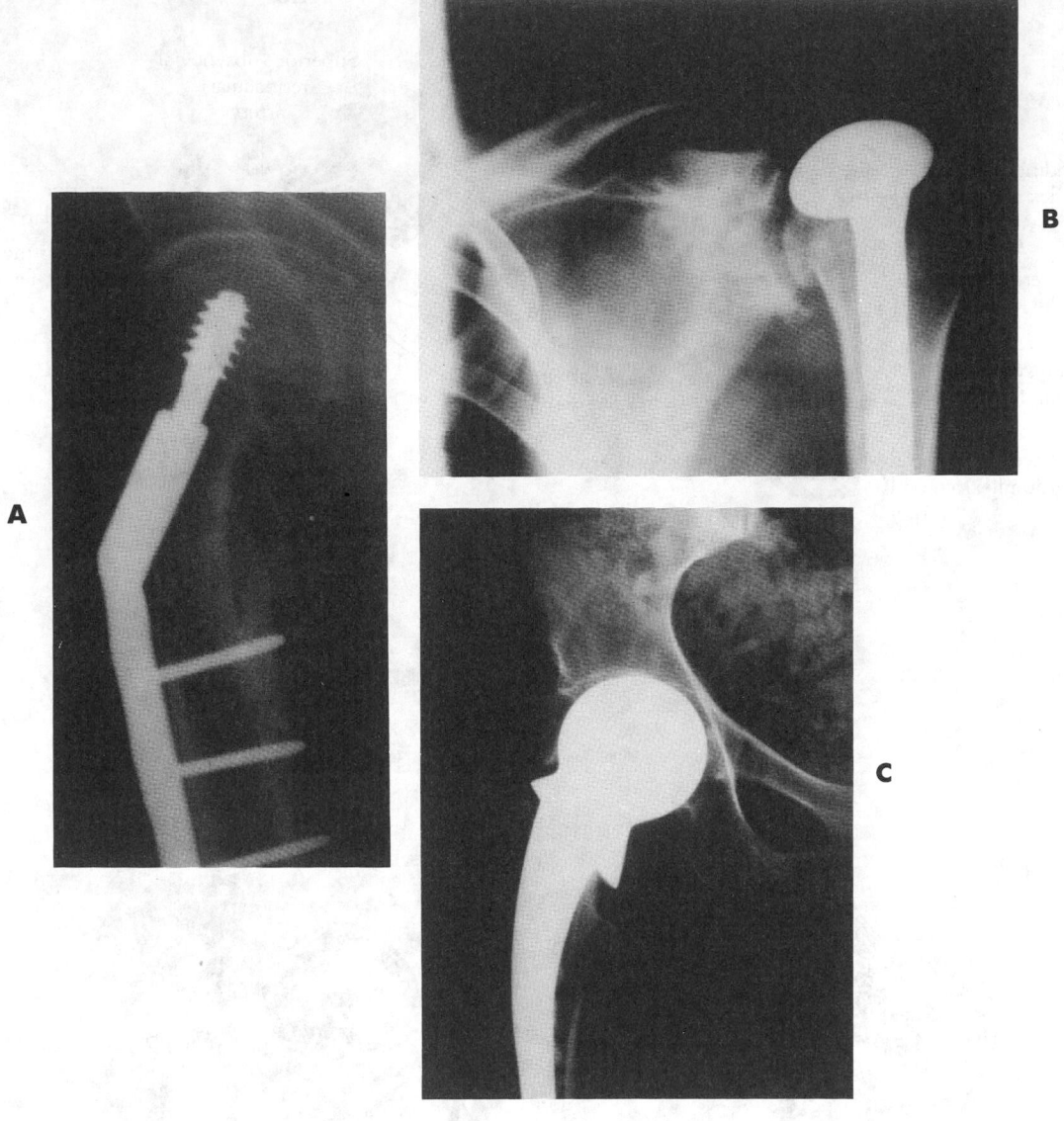

Figure 4-36 A, Type of hip nail. **B,** Prosthesis replacing head of humerus. **C,** Femoral head prosthesis.

Multidisciplinary Plan

Medications

Antiinfective agents
  Cefazolin (Ancef), 250-1000 mg IV q6h
Narcotic analgesic agents
  Meperidine (Demerol), 50-100 mg q3h for 24 h, then q3h
    prn (may have PCA administration in smaller dosages)
Analgesic-antipyretic agents
  Aspirin, 600 mg q4h for temperature elevation above
    38.3° C (101° F) and for moderate pain
Nonsteroidal antiinflammatory medications
  Ibuprofen, 400-600 mg q4-6h
  Toradol, 10 mg po q4h or 15-30 mg IM or IV q4h

Antiembolic medications
  Low-molecular-weight heparin (enoxaparin [Lovenox],
    30 mg subcutaneously bid, followed by warfarin
    (Coumadin) 5-10 mg po to keep International Normal-
    ized Ratio (INR) (2.0-3.0)[115]
Intravenous 1000 ml 5% D/.2N/S at 125 ml/h; add 20 mEq
  KCl to each liter

General Management

Oxygen therapy, 1-4 L for 8-24 h postoperatively
Deep breathing and coughing every 2 hours
Respirex (or Triflow) 10 times every hour for incentive
  spirometry
Pulmonary IPPB every 4 hours

Bed rest with operative leg in neutral position

Turning to unoperative side and back every 2 hours

Change of dressing as needed; reinforce as needed

Record input and output; record wound drainage separately

Vital signs every 15 minutes for four times, every 30 minutes for four times, every hour for four times, then every 4 hours

Up in chair three times on first postoperative day with no or touch-down weight bearing on operative leg

Up with walker on second postoperative day; weight bearing on operated leg must be specifically prescribed

Clear liquids after nausea has subsided; advance to regular diet as tolerated

CBC, electrolytes, and CO_2 measurements in morning and daily for 4 days

Physical therapy to help with walking and ROM exercises

Perform neurovascular checks as prescribed

Apply antithrombotic hose, pneumatic compression hose, or plexipulse to prevent deep vein thrombosis

NURSING CARE

Nursing Assessment

Hip and Upper Thigh Incisional and Wound Area

Assessment
  Dressing—type
  Drainage—type, amount
  Wound suction equipment, if present—may not be used
  Drainage in container or on dressing
Presence of edema at wound site
Position of thigh and leg
Complaints of pain in operative area or calf
Color of tissues
Antiembolism hose presence

Systemic Concerns

Respiratory and circulatory status
Vital signs: temperature elevation
Mental state and recovery from anesthesia
Muscle strength or weakness
Urinary output, catheter-drainage setup, and voiding after catheter removal
Intravenous fluid type, amount, and rate

Psychosocial Concerns

Concern with body image
Immobility
Confusion
Acute pain
Postoperative lack of ambulation
Fear of falling

Complications

Loss of reduction or dislocation
Thrombophlebitis
Pneumonia

Cardiac arrhythmias
Wound infection
Compartment syndrome

Nursing Dx & Intervention

Body image disturbance related to trauma

- Assess concerns.
- Maintain bed rest; clarify need for bed rest *to aid compliance.*
- Massage back *to aid comfort and circulation.*
- Help walk with walker and weight bearing as prescribed (may continue partial weight bearing for up to 1 month, gradually increasing to full weight by 2 to 3 months) *to prevent undo stress on prosthesis or tissues.*
- Discuss how to prevent recurrence of trauma *to ease fears or concerns.*

Impaired physical mobility related to modification in weight bearing

- Assess ability to understand instructions and limitations.
- Assist to dangle at bedside on first postoperative day, then to pivot to chair with no weight on operative leg, or touch-down weight if prescribed.
- Stress that operative foot should be placed on floor but weight should be borne on unoperative leg (refer to limb as either left or right leg so patient has a clear understanding) *to maintain safety in care.*
- Turn every 2 hours; prop with pillows between legs or back *to maintain position.*
- Assist with ROM quadriceps and gluteal sitting exercises *to maintain muscle strength.*
- Help physical therapist walk patient with walker and limited weight to operative limb (if assistance is needed) *for comfort and safety.*
- Encourage patient and family members to walk together *for patient's safety.* Instruct family about weight-bearing techniques *for clarity and safety.*

Pain related to trauma and surgery

- Assess wound for evidence of resolution of surgical trauma and inflammation.
- Assess patient's complaints of pain; clarify site, type, and amount of pain.
- Administer analgesics judiciously because of patient's age.
- Dosage should be sufficient to relieve pain without causing confusion (may need to vary dosage within ordered ranges) *for safety in care.*
- Turn or reposition patient and massage back *to increase comfort.*
- Perform Homans' test to determine development of thrombophlebitis, which could lead to pulmonary embolism and a mortality rate of 2%.[48] Observe for chest pain, dyspnea, and changes in vital signs, *which could indicate pulmonary embolism, atelectasis, or pneumonia.*
- Observe autologous blood transfusion equipment for amount and type of reinfusion, if needed and prescribed.

- Assist with meal and food selections *to aid in healing, resolution of inflammation, and enhancement of bone calcification.*
- Force fluids *to aid digestion and bowel and bladder elimination.*

Patient Education/Home Care Planning

1. Clarify need for weight-bearing restrictions for bone union.
2. Clarify signs to report to the physician: increased soreness or pain at operative site, fever, decreased urine output or burning with urination.
3. Reiterate techniques for use of walker or crutches.
4. Teach patient and family necessity to continue eating a well-balanced diet and drinking plenty of fluids for healing, circulation, and elimination.

Evaluation

Patient has positive body image Patient has positive outward-looking demeanor. Patient appreciates ability to get around.

Patient regains mobility Patient walks with progressive weight bearing as healing occurs, with minimum discomfort and satisfactory ROM.

Patient is free of pain Patient has no pain in fracture site. Muscle and joint strength is regained. Has lessened fear of falling.

INTERNAL FIXATION WITH HARRINGTON OR OTHER RODS TO VERTEBRAL COLUMN

Description and Rationale

Harrington rods are long metallic implants attached posteriorly to the vertebral column after corrective repair and fusion as treatment for scoliosis or vertebral burst fractures. The rod or rods (they may be bilaterally used) hold the vertebrae in the corrected alignment to permit the bone grafts to heal and fuse the vertebrae solidly. The rods may remain in the site for extended periods or may be removed (rarely done) after x-rays indicate there is sound, solid fusion. In the early postoperative period some patients may wear a fitted brace to help the rods maintain spinal immobility if the curvature was marked preoperatively and multiple grafts were implanted during surgery. The brace is worn during waking hours and is removed for sleep.

Luque rods are another kind of metallic implant used for corrective spinal surgery. Luque rods are used on both sides of the spinal column with multiple attachments to each spinal segment to add corrective forces throughout the deformity. Addi-

tionally, Luque rods are contoured to aid in correcting the deformation. Luque rods can also be combined with an L-shaped segment in a new technique for spiral instrumentation referred to as STIF spinopelvic transiliac fixation (STIF), providing a more stable construct.[157]

Cotrel-Dubousset rods are a third type of internal fixation rod that are used to straighten and fuse the vertebrae. The patient's specific condition and the physician's preference determine which rods will be used (Figure 4-37).

Contraindications and Cautions

1. Harrington and other rods are foreign bodies, as are all metallic implants; thus they may cause a severe inflammatory reaction and infection, which may necessitate their removal.
2. Open surgery may predispose to local wound infection or may lead to meningeal infections.

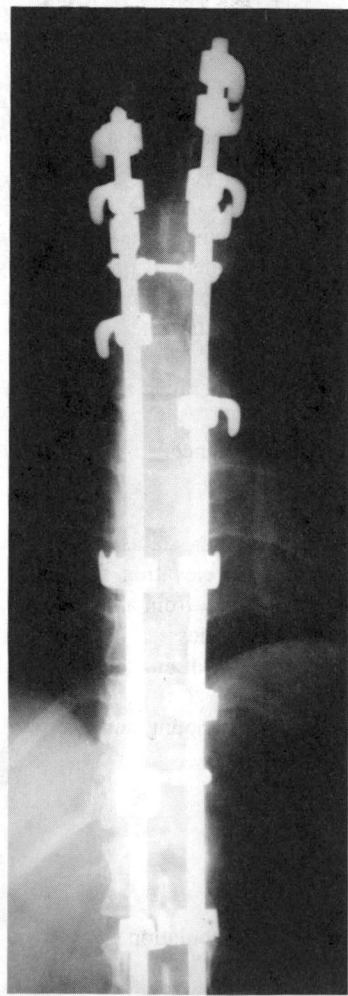

Figure 4-37 Cotrel-Dubousset rods used to treat scoliosis. (From Mourad.[104])

3. One or more bone grafts may be needed to maintain the correction of the curvature or fracture; parts of or whole grafts may not unite firmly, which may necessitate prolonged wearing of a brace, encasement in a plaster cast, or even reoperation.

4. The spinal attachments holding the rods may loosen, allowing the rods to move. Major movement of either end of the attachments would necessitate reoperation.

5. Complete medical evaluation is done to determine current status of chronic conditions, if present.

Preprocedural Nursing Care

1. The patient may be placed in Cotrel's or halo-femoral traction (see Table 4-6) before surgery to stretch muscles contracted from scoliosis.

2. Meticulous skin cleansing is done to remove organisms to prevent infections.

3. X-rays determine respiratory and spinal conditions; respiratory therapy with IPPB and a respiratory apparatus, such as Respirex or Triflow, is done every 4 hours.

4. Serologic and urologic studies are done.

5. An enema is administered to clear the lower bowel.

6. An indwelling catheter is inserted into the urinary bladder.

7. A full-length bed pad or alternating pressure mattress is placed on mattress.

8. Autologous blood donations may be made every 7 to 14 days and stored frozen before use.[52]

•••••• Multidisciplinary Plan

Medications

Narcotic analgesic agents
   Meperidine (Demerol), 50-100 mg IM q3h
   Morphine, 10-15 mg IM q4h or PCA with 1 to 2 mg (depending on patient's age) q10min with 20 mg lockout
Analgesic-antipyretic agents
   Aspirin, 600 mg rectal suppository for moderate pain q4h prn or for temperature over 38.3° C (101° F) (aspirin should not be given to persons under age 18 yr because of its association with Reye's syndrome)
   Acetaminophen, 325-650 mg q4h prn
Antiinfective agents
   Cefazolin (Ancef) or cefamandole (Mandol), 250-500 mg q6h IV
Intravenous 1000 ml 5% D/.45N/S at 75 ml/h with 10 mEq KCl in every other liter
Muscle relaxants
   Cyclobenzaprine (Flexeril), 10-20 mg tid
   Diazepam, 10-15 mg q4-6h
Nonsteroidal antiinflammatory agent
   Ibuprofen, 400-800 mg tid or qid

General Management

IPPB every 4 hours
Maintain patient flat in bed
Logroll patient every 2 hours
Help patient deep breathe and cough every 2 hours; use respiratory aid 10 times every hour
Do not change dressing; reinforce if needed
Do neurovascular checks every hour
Give clear liquids after patient has had nothing by mouth for 24 hours; advance to regular diet as tolerated
Force fluids after intravenous line is discontinued
Do ROM exercises to arms and legs every 4 hours
Keep cast uncovered until dry or keep brace on at all times (if prescribed and in place)
Consult physical therapist for ROM and isometric exercises
Begin ambulation with assistance as prescribed

NURSING CARE

Nursing Assessment

Vertebral Column, Incisional Wound Site

Check alignment and position of back and entire patient
Check wound
   Drainage (may have suction drainage)
   Edema
   Dressing
   Presence of brace or plaster cast with open window in back portion
Skin condition of formerly contracted tissues
Respiratory excursions; depth, rate, and character of respirations
Site and amount of pain

Systemic Concerns

Assessment of motor and sensory functions by neurovascular checks
Catheter drainage
Intravenous fluid infusion site, solution, and rate
Presence of nausea or vomiting
Abdominal distention or ileus

Psychosocial Concerns

Self-concept and body image
Immobility
Acute pain
Length of convalescence

Other Complications

Shock
Hemorrhage
Wound infection
Nonunion
Loss of reduction
Pneumonia
Urinary tract infection
Meningitis

Nursing Dx & Intervention

Body image disturbance related to deformity and dependence because of bed rest and surgery

- Assess patient's concerns with self-concept and image.
- Stress patient's improved appearance after fusion *to aid positive self-concept.*
- Encourage self-care as able; help with placement and removal of supplies *to maintain an esthetic atmosphere*
- Assist with bath or shower *to provide security and encourage self-care.*

Impaired physical mobility related to prolonged convalescence and muscle weakness and spasms

- Assess ROM of unaffected tissues.
- Turn, with assistance of another health professional, by logrolling every 2 hours. (Teach family logrolling technique if possible, and use their assistance.) Do not let patient turn self; logrolling cannot be accomplished safely this way because patient would twist. Twisting could disrupt fibrin meshwork (see pp. 391 to 395 for bone healing), thereby delaying or preventing bone union and fusion. Brace will hold back sufficiently rigid after discharge so patient can safely turn or get up unassisted.
- Encourage deep breathing and leg exercises *to increase self-activities and independence and promote healing and circulation.*
- Perform neurovascular checks every hour; that is, observe and compare in all four extremities: color, temperature, edema; ROM; grip, push, and pull strength; sharp and dull discrimination; and presence and type of pain, radiation, numbness, and tingling *to note signs of pressure.*
- Massage exposed areas of shoulders, neck, back, and buttocks *to relieve tiredness and muscle spasms.*
- Assist with stretching exercises if needed *to relieve skin restrictions from preoperative curvature limitations.*
- Caution patient to avoid bending, twisting, stooping, or lifting more than 10 lb.[52]

Risk for altered neurologic function related to insertion of metallic implants and bone grafts

- Assess muscle strength or weakness in muscle groups to detect early signs of pressure or palsy.
- Monitor urinary and bowel output *to detect early signs of paralysis or weakness.*
- Perform neurovascular checks to all extremities as prescribed *to determine current status;* compare with previous data *to note any deterioration;* report untoward changes to physician.
- Consult with physical therapist for exercises *to increase or maintain muscle functions.*

Impaired gas exchange related to operative procedure and anesthesia

- Assess rate, quality, and depth of respirations, cough, or sputum production and color of sputum and skin tissues.
- Encourage deep breathing and coughing *to enhance and clear respiratory efforts and excursions.*
- Have patient use respirex or triflow *to increase respiratory excursions and strengthen respiratory muscles.*
- If chest tube is present, splint the chest or incision area while assisting patient to cough *to enhance respiratory excursions and lessen pain during procedure.*
- Monitor breath sounds in all lobes *to detect signs of respiratory complications.*
- Encourage family members to assist patient with pulmonary exercises *to encourage their participation in care as able.*

Pain related to surgical trauma and muscle stretching

- Assess patient's complaints of pain; clarify site, type, and amount of pain.
- Administer medication (dosage adjusted to age, if younger child or adolescent, and severity of pain) as ordered *to maintain therapeutic levels,* or monitor use of PCA medications. Carefully monitor children to determine amount of pain and pain medication dosage and administration *to help maintain pain relief.*
- Assess wound as pain source; note signs of resolution of inflammation and surgical trauma. Report continued edema, redness, and increased drainage *as untoward signs.*
- Help patient increase amount and time of walking (when allowed up) *to help resolve muscle soreness and weakness and to lessen soreness and pain in operative site.*
- Change dressings over incision (after initial dressing change by physician) as needed; note lessening of soreness and acute pain as healing proceeds *to note resolution of inflammation.*
- Check bowel sounds, abdominal distention, passage of flatus (ileus may be source of pain).
- Administer prescribed muscle relaxant medication *to relieve muscle spasms.*

Patient Education/Home Care Planning

1. Demonstrate to the patient and family how to put on brace.
2. Clarify that muscle stiffness, weakness, and soreness may increase with increase in activities but will last for brief periods only.
3. Reiterate stages of bone healing for strong union; stress need for caution against sudden position changes and need to continue wearing the brace.
4. Stress that the patient must eat a well-balanced diet to regain muscle strength, promote healthy bone growth, and promote wound healing.
5. Explain that sudden or gradually increasing pain should be reported to physician.
6. Stress walking program to increase strength and endurance.

7. Stress need to refrain from sexual activity until incisions are healed and patient has few aches or pains; should wear thoracolumbosacral orthosis during sexual activity.[52]

Evaluation

Self-concept is positive Patient resumes social contacts after convalescent period. Patient wears brace without difficulty or embarrassment. Patient enjoys new "straightened" appearance.

Patient regains independence, mobility, and spinal motion with limited flexion Patient moves freely without muscle weakness, discomfort, or pain and has learned to use muscles of lower extremities and hips to assist lumbar muscles (must kneel or bend from hips rather than from lumbar area).

Patient is relatively pain free Patient takes only occasional nonnarcotic analgesic for muscle and bone pain.

SPINAL FUSION WITH BONE GRAFTS

Spinal fusion with natural autogenous bone grafts is done as treatment of a herniated nucleus pulposus. Nursing care of patients after spinal fusion for treatment of a ruptured disc is similar to that discussed previously, with the addition of assessing relief of sensory pressure signs, numbness, and tingling as surgical wound healing progresses. Autogenous bone grafts usually provide solid union without the problems associated with metallic implants, such as foreign body reactions, loosening, or infections.

Nursing care for spinal fusion is the same as for internal fixation with Harrington rods.

HEMILAMINECTOMY (LAMINECTOMY)

Description and Rationale

Hemilaminectomy is the partial removal of the lamina to gain access to the intervertebral space to remove a ruptured disc. It may also be called a laminectomy. From 200,000 to 500,000 laminectomies are done yearly in the United States.[17] The pathophysiology leading to disc degeneration and rupture is discussed on p. 408 (Figures 4-38 and 4-39).

Automated percutaneous discectomy (APD) was developed in 1984 as an alternative to the use of chymopapain for percutaneous removal of a herniated disc. By 1991 more than 80,000 APDs had been performed worldwide.

Automated percutaneous discectomy requires a thorough physical examination and history, plain x-rays, either a CT scan or MRI, and discography to determine the exact pathology of the disc. As one criterion for APD, the herniated disc fragments must be contained within paraspinal ligaments to achieve removal of the herniated particles by the pituitary rongeur or the Nucleotome instrument. Another criterion for APD is that the patient's pain is greater in the leg than in the back because it has been found that the higher the percentage of leg pain, the more suitable the decompression, and the lower the percentage of leg pain, the poorer the results from decompression. Additionally, APD indications are that MRI, CT, or discographic evidence indicates only one single herniation within the anulus of the disk and failure to be benefited with a well-managed course of conservative treatment to relieve the pain and symptoms.[59]

Automated percutaneous discectomy is done with the patient in the lateral decubitus position. The skin is anesthetized locally, and the 18-gauge diamond-tipped trocar is inserted, directed to the posterolateral corner of the affected disc. Correct site is confirmed fluoroscopically, after which the cannula is inserted against the anulus, and the anulotomy is done. An aspiration probe is inserted into the disc space, its position also confirmed by fluoroscopy. The aspiration probe, containing an 8-inch long, 2 mm–diameter needle with a sharpened blade, can be turned 180° in a reciprocal cutting action of up to 180 cycles per minute.[59] Suction is applied through the inner cannula, aspirating the nucleus pulposus, which is then collected in a collection bottle with saline. The equipment is removed and the stab wound is covered with a small adhesive dressing. Leg pain should be relieved as the herniated fragments are removed, stated by the patient, who is awake.[17]

The success rate is approximately 75%, varying from 49% to 85% in various groups studied.[59] The patient is discharged the next day.

Complications include hematoma and disc-space infection, nerve root injury, and occasional cauda equina injury.

Contraindications and Cautions

1. Determination of the cause and location of one or more degenerated or ruptured discs requires physiologic and psychologic diagnostic profiles before surgery.
2. Removal of a degenerated or ruptured disc may not relieve the patient's complaints of pain.
3. Patients for lumbar spine surgery are admitted the morning of surgery after extensive preadmission testing has been done.
4. Postoperative rehabilitation requires the patient's cooperation and performance of daily exercises to strengthen the spinal and abdominal muscles.
5. The specific operative procedure varies with the site of disc rupture and the patient's and physician's preference. Percutaneous discectomy and microdiscectomy are now more frequently being done because these are less invasive procedures for a single herniated disc.
6. The patient should stop smoking, if a smoker, because of the vascular effects of nicotine on the disc.[51]

•••••• Multidisciplinary Plan

Medications

Narcotic analgesic agents
  Meperidine (Demerol), 50-100 mg q3-4h for pain before surgery

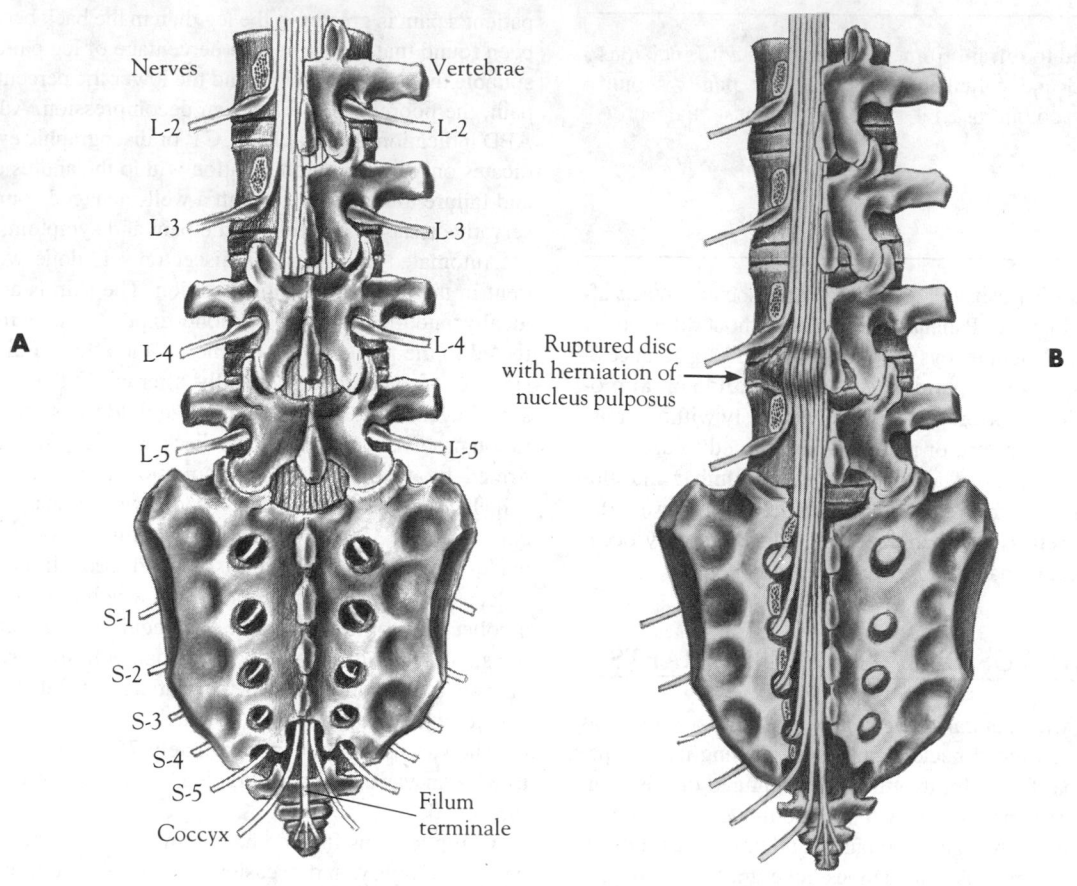

Figure 4-38 A, Spinal nerves exiting from cord. **B,** Herniated nucleus pulposus; note pressure on nerve.

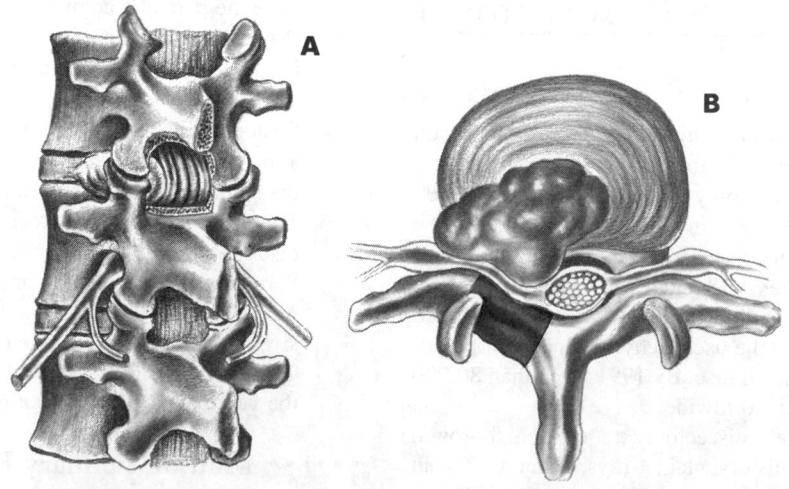

Figure 4-39 Laminectomy for herniation of nucleus pulposus. **A,** Area of lamina removed during a hemilaminectomy. **B,** Herniated nucleus pulposus.

Antiinfective agents
    Cefazolin (Ancef) or cefamandole (Mandol), 250-500 mg
      q6h IV
Intravenous, 1000 ml 5% D/.45N/S at 75-100 ml/h
Postoperative PCA analgesia may be used, if needed (rarely
    used because pain is relieved by the surgical procedure)

General Management

Nothing by mouth until morning; then clear liquids and ad-
    vance to regular diet
Bed rest until evening of surgery
Turn side to side every 2 hours
Patient up at bedside evening of surgery and up as tolerated
    thereafter
Neurovascular checks every hour for 4 hours, then every 2
    hours for four times, and then every 4 hours
Male patient may stand to void if necessary
Reinforce dressing if needed; change dressing after 24 hours
Check vital signs every hour for 4 hours, then every 2 hours
    for four times, and then every 4 hours
Have patient deep breathe and cough every 2 hours; use
    Respirex 10 times every hour
Physical therapy consultation for exercise regimen and pro-
    gram
Ambulate as prescribed
Discharge as physician prescribes

NURSING CARE

Nursing Assessment

Incisional Area of Lumbar Back or Cervical Area

Assessment of motor strengths and sensory condition of feet
    and legs or arms and hands bilaterally (usually are within
    normal limits for push, pull strength; may have some re-
    maining sensory changes such as lingering numbness or
    decreased sensitivity to sharp pinpricks) (Figure 4-40)
All peripheral pulses palpable
Skin temperature of feet, legs, arms, and hands: may be
    slightly cool and pale
Drainage on dressing scant to moderate amount and sero-
    sanguineous
Pain mild to moderate in operative area with some radiation
    to shoulders and occipital area (if cervical) and to hips and
    buttocks (if lumbar)
If cervical ruptured disc, may have soft surgical collar in
    place

Systemic Concerns

Headache
Nausea
Abdominal distention
Urinary retention (may need to stand to void)

Psychosocial Concerns

Acute pain
Lingering chronic pain
Limitation of neck or back muscle and joint mobility and
    strength

Other Complications

Hemorrhage, hematoma
Motor and sensory weakness
Continued pain
Wound infection
Disc infection

Nursing Dx & Intervention

Pain related to pressure on the nerve and surgical trauma

• Assess degree, site, type, and amount of pain; medicate as
  necessary.

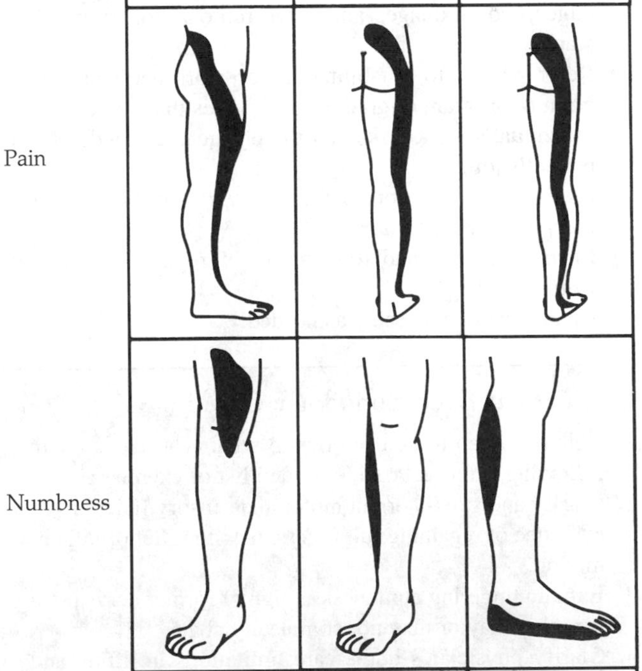

Nerve root	L4	L5	S1
Pain			
Numbness			
Motor weakness	Extension of quadriceps.	Dorsiflexion of great toe and foot.	Plantar flexion of great toe and foot.
Screening exam	Squat & rise.	Heel walking.	Walking on toes.
Reflexes	Knee jerk diminished.	None reliable.	Ankle jerk diminished.

Figure 4-40 Testing for lumbar nerve root compromise. (From Bigos.[14a])

- Turn or adjust position *to relieve fatigue and discomfort.*
- Get patient up to change position and ease pain. Instruct on proper techniques to turn, sit up, and walk *to maintain safe care.*
- Increase up time as able *to increase activity.*
- Perform neurovascular checks. Report any decreases in motor or sensory functions.

Impaired physical mobility related to surgery

- Assess ROM of unaffected tissues.
- Encourage physical therapy as ordered and prescribed *to increase muscle strength.*
- Note and assess muscle spasms or limitation of movements when moving and doing wound care or hygienic care *to note current conditions or continuation of pain or soreness.*
- Teach patient how to logroll, if required or prescribed.

Impaired skin integrity, risk for, related to wound infection

- Assess incisional area for relief of inflammation and evidence of wound healing (approximation of wound edges, no drainage, and later removal of sutures or staples).
- Refer patient to rehabilitation for work-hardening program (a program of graduated activities that stimulate the individual's work tasks and the physical demands of the patient's job).[19]
- Assess vital signs for fluctuations *that could indicate inflammation or infection.*
- Encourage fluid and food intake of regular diet *to aid wound healing.*
- Change wound dressing as needed.

Patient Education/Home Care Planning

1. Reiterate need to do exercises to regain muscle strength following surgery. Provide written list of exercises.
2. Clarify and stress normal motor and sensory functions as evidence of regaining full functions with relief of inflammation.
3. Explain lingering numbness as sign of former nerve pressure that may or may not completely abate.
4. Clarify physician's home care limitations in lifting and driving for 1 to 3 weeks or longer (individualized, based on specific condition). Stress follow-up visit to physician to determine recovery status.
5. Explain signs of fever, continued pain, and wound drainage as reportable to physician.

Evaluation

Neck or back pain is relieved Patient has some residual motor or sensory impairment with less pain, locally or systemically.

Patient has satisfactory ROM without muscle spasms Patient can move about more comfortably and easily, can do prescribed exercises satisfactorily, and returns to family, social, and, later, employment activities.

Patient has no wound or disc infection Patient's wound and incision heals well. There is no drainage. Scar is contracting normally.

References

1. deAndrade JR: Activities after replacement of the hip and knee, *Orthop Spec Ed* 2(6):7, 1993.
2. Agency for Health Care Policy and Research: Acute low back pain guideline, *Orthop Today* 15(1):19, 1995.
3. Althizer L: Total hip arthroplasty, *Orthop Nurs* 14(4):7, 1995.
4. Altman RD: Laboratory findings in osteoarthritis. In Moskewitz RW et al, editors: *Osteoarthritis: diagnosis and medical/surgical management,* ed 2, Philadelphia, 1992, Saunders.
5. Altman GT, Rogers VP: Is salvage reinfusion necessary in primary total knee replacement? *Contemp Orthop* 30(1):15, 1995.
6. Angelini C, Danieli GA, Fontanari D: *Muscular dystrophy research: from molecular diagnosis toward therapy,* New York, 1991, Excerpta Medica.
7. Baker CL, Todd JL: Intervening in acute ankle sprain and chronic instability, *J Musculoskeletal Med* 12(7):51, 1995.
8. Ballard WT, Weinstein JN: Biochemical aspects of aging and degeneration in the intervertebral disc, *Contemp Orthop* 24(4):453, 1992.
9. Barnes CL: Duplex scanning in orthopaedic patients, *Contemp Orthop* 22:283, 1991.
10. Beckenbaugh RD, Simonian PT: Clinical efficacy of electroneurometer screening in carpal tunnel syndrome, *Orthopedics* 18(6):549, 1995.
11. Berg EE: Postoperative blood salvage systems, *Orthop Nurs* 12(3):8, 1993.
12. Berkowitz SD: Treatment of established deep vein thrombosis: a review of the therapeutic armamentarium, *Orthopedics* 18(suppl):18, 1995.
13. Berman AT et al: Symposium: the painful total knee replacement and the influence of component design, *Contemp Orthop* 28(6):523, 1994.
14. Bert JM et al: Symposium: total knee replacement, *Contemp Orthop* 28(3):267, 1994.
14a. Bigos S, Bowyer O, Braen G, et al: Acute low back problems in adults. Clinical practice guideline, quick reference guide, number 14. Rockville, MD: US Department of Health and Human Services, Public Health Service, Agency for Health Care Policy and Research, AHCPR Public no. 95-0643, Dec 1994.
15. Birrer RB, Poole B: Athletic taping, part 3: the knee, *J Musculoskeletal Med* 12(7):43, 1995.
16. Bobyn JD: PE (polyethylene) quality is researcher's concern in prosthesis success, *Orthop Today* 15(7):10, 1995.
17. Bonati AO: Arthroscopic nuclectomy, *Am J Arthroscopy* 1(1):16, 1991.
18. Booth RE Jr: Critical care pathways in thromboembolic disease, *Orthopedics* 18(suppl E):6, 1995.
19. Brewer CC, Storms BS: The final phase of rehabilitation: work hardening, *Orthop Nurs* 12(6):9, 1993.
20. Brashear RH Jr, Raney RB Sr: *Shand's handbook of orthopaedic surgery,* ed 10, St Louis, 1986, Mosby.
21. Brillhart AT: Arthroscopic laser surgery, *Am J Arthroscopy* 1(2):5, 1991.
22. Brillhart AT: Arthroscopic laser surgery: the CO$_2$ laser and its use, *Am J Arthroscopy* 1(2):7, 1991.
23. Brillhart AT: Arthroscopic laser surgery: the holmium:YAG laser and its use, *Am J Arthroscopy* 1(3):7, 1991.
24. Buck M, Paice JA: Pharmacologic management of acute pain in the orthopaedic patient, *Orthop Nurs* 13(6):14, 1994.
25. Buckwalter JA, Lohmander S: Operative treatment of osteoarthrosis, *J Bone Joint Surg* 76-A(9):1405, 1994.

26. Cameron HU, Park YS, Krestow M: Reflex sympathetic dystrophy following total knee replacement, *Contemp Orthop* 29(4):279, 1994.

27. Castello PH, Enzenaur RJ, Jones DEC: Multifocal avascular necrosis in scleroderma, *Contemp Orthop* 31(2):97, 1995.

28. Charness AL: Matching skills with services, *Biomechanics* 2(7):85, 1995.

29. Chase J: Outpatient management of low back pain, *Orthop Nurs* 11(1):11, 1992.

30. Cherf JM et al: Roundtable: complications of total knee arthroplasty, *Orthop Spec Ed* 3(2):14, 1994.

31. Chopra D: Body, mind and soul, Columbus, Ohio, August 20, 1995, WOSU-TV (television broadcast).

32. Colwell CW: Consortium data: comparative efficacy of low molecular weight heparin and warfarin following total hip replacement, *Orthopedics* 18(suppl):21, 1995.

33. Coughlin MJ: Hallux valgus: heredity or bad shoes? *Biomechanics* 2(8):31, 1995.

34. Crosbie J, McConnel J, editors: *Key issues in musculoskeletal physiotherapy*, London, 1993, Butterworth Heinemann.

35. Cummings SR et al: Risk factors for hip fracture in white women, *N Engl J Med* 332(12):767, 1995.

36. Cunningham ME: Bursitis and tendinitis, *Orthop Nurs* 13(5):13, 1994.

37. Dale KG, Orr PM, Harrell PB: Total elbow replacement, *Orthop Nurs* 11(5):23, 1992.

38. Damiano DL, Abel MF, Vaughan CL: Muscle strengthening in normal and pathological gait, *Biomechanics* 2(7):81, 1995.

39. Delmas PD: Markers of bone formation and resorption. In Favus MJ, editor: *Primer on the metabolic bone diseases and disorders of mineral metabolism*, ed 2, New York, 1993, Raven Press.

40. Deloach ED, Check WE, Long R: Diagnosing osteomyelitis underlying pressure sores, *Contemp Orthop* 27(3):240, 1993.

41. Dempster DW, Lindsay R: Pathogenesis of osteoporosis, *Lancet* 341:797, 1993.

42. Diment MT, DeHaven KE, Sebatianelli WJ: Current concepts in meniscal repair, *Orthopedics* 16(9):973, 1993.

43. Dirschl DR: Acute pyogenic osteomyelitis in children, *Orthop Rev* 23(4):305, 1994.

44. Drucker DA et al: Total hip arthroplasty using a hydroxypatite-coated acetabular and femoral component, *Orthop Rev* 20(2):179, 1991.

45. Dubin S: The physiologic changes of aging, *Orthop Nurs* 11(3):45, 1992.

46. Eaton RG: Carpal tunnel syndrome treatment options revealed by applying five-factor test, *Orthop Spec Ed* 2(1):8, 1993.

47. Eckhouse-Ekeberg DR: Promoting a positive attitude in pediatric patients undergoing limb lengthening, *Orthop Nurs* 13(1):41, 1994.

48. Einhorn TA et al: Conditions affecting orthopaedic surgical practice. In Simon SR, editor: *Orthopaedic basic science*, Chicago, 1994, American Academy of Orthopedic Surgeons.

49. Evans RL, Rubash HE, Albrecht SA: The efficacy of postoperative autotransfusion on total joint arthroplasty, *Orthop Nurs* 12(3):11, 1993.

50. Fardeau M: A new era for muscular dystrophy research. In Angeline C, Danieli GA, Fontanari D, editors: *Muscular dystrophy research*, New York, 1991, Excerpta Medica.

51. Feingold DJ et al: Complications of lumbar spine surgery, *Orthop Nurs* 10(4):39, 1991.

52. Ficner HB: Revision surgery in adult scoliosis patients, *Orthop Nurs* 12(2):23, 1994.

53. Fischgrund JS, Montgomery DM: Diagnosis and treatment of discogenic low back pain, *Orthop Rev* 22(3):311, 1993.

54. Fitzgerald RH Jr: Preventing DVT following total knee replacement: a review of recent clinical trials, *Orthopedics* 18(suppl):10, 1995.

55. Fitzgerald RH et al: Symposium: The National Hip Registry: a new resource for measuring and improving the quality of health care, *Contemp Orthop* 31(2):127, 1995.

56. Fried LP, Williamson JD, Kasper J: The epidemic of frailty: scope of the problem. In Perry HM III, Morley JE, Coe RM, editors: *Aging and musculoskeletal disorders*, New York, 1993, Springer.

57. Gagliardi BA: The impact of Duchenne muscular dystrophy on families, *Orthop Nurs* 10(5):41, 1991.

58. Gerscovich EO, Greenspan A, Montesana RX: Treatment of kyphotic deformity in ankylosing spondylitis, *Orthopedics* 17(4):335, 1994.

59. Gill K: Percutaneous lumbar diskectomy, *J Am Acad Orthop Surg* 1(1):33, 1993.

59a. Gill K, Blumenthal SL: Clinical experience with automated percutaneous discectomy: The Nucleotome system, *Orthopedics* 14(7):757, 1991.

60. Gray GW: Treating the ACL, *Biomechanics* 2(4):63, 1995.

61. Guille JT, Forlin E, Bowen JR: Congenital kyphosis, *Orthop Rev* 22(2):235, 1993.

62. Hanna LG: When the shoe doesn't fit, *Biomechanics* 2(8):41, 1995.

63. Hart K: Using the Ilizarov external fixator in bone transport, *Orthop Nurs* 13(1):35, 1994.

64. Heinrich JT, McBeath AA: The gluteus minimus muscle pedicle graft in the treatment of femoral head avascular necrosis, *Am J Orthop* 24(8):615, 1995.

65. Hernandez MA III, Corley FG: Finger joint injury: intervene early to minimize dysfunction, *J Musculoskeletal Med* 12(8):66, 1995.

66. Higgins KR: Growth factors in the treatment of problem diabetic foot wounds, *Biomechanics* 2(8):83, 1995.

67. Higgins RM: Replantation of digits, *Orthop Nurs* 10(3):11, 1991.

68. Hoffman EP: Current knowledge on dystrophin structure and function. In Angelini C, Danieli GA, Fontanari D, editors: *Muscular dystrophy research*, New York, 1991, Excerpta Medica.

69. Hockberg MC et al: The association of body weight, body fatness and body fat distribution with osteoarthritis of the knee: data from the Baltimore Longitudinal Study of Aging, *J Rheumatol* 22(3):488, 1995.

70. Huang TJ, Lubicky JP, Hammerberg KW: Scoliosis in Rett syndrome, *Orthop Rev* 23(7):931, 1994.

71. Johnson RL: Total shoulder arthroplasty, *Orthop Nurs* 12(1):14, 1993.

72. Jones-Watson P: Clinical standards in skeletal traction pin site care, *Orthop Nurs* 10(1):12, 1991.

73. Joyce ME, Jingushi S, Bolander ME: Transforming growth factor-beta in the regulation of fracture repair, *Orthop Clin North Am* 21(1):199, 1990.

74. Kaplan FS et al: Form and function in bone. In Simon SR, editor: *Orthopaedic basic science*, Chicago, 1994, American Academy of Orthopaedic Surgeons.

75. Kaye R: Ankylosing spondylitis: a common and treatable condition, *J Musculoskeletal Med* 9(1):3, 1992.

76. Kearns L: Arthroscopy found useful for treating hip conditions, *Orthop Today* 14(7):1, 1994.

77. Khan MA et al: Recognizing and managing fractures in ankylosing spondylitis, *J Musculoskeletal Med* 10(1):45, 1993.

78. Kim MJ, McFarland GK, McLane AM: *Pocket guide to nursing diagnoses*, St Louis, 1995, Mosby.

79. Kim Y-H, Franks DJ: Cementless revision of cemented stem failures associated with massive femoral bone loss, *Orthop Rev* 21(3):375, 1992.

80. Kitaoka HB et al: Survivorship analysis of the Mayo total ankle arthroplasty, *J Bone Joint Surg* 76-A(7):974, 1994.

81. Kleerekoper M, Avioli LV: Evaluation and treatment of postmenopausal osteoporosis. In Favus MJ, editor: *Primer on the metabolic bone diseases and disorders of mineral metabolism*, ed 2, New York, 1993, Raven Press.

82. Klein GL: Nutritional rickets and osteomalacia. In Favus MJ, editor: *Primer on the metabolic bone diseases and disorders of mineral metabolism*, ed 2, New York, 1993, Raven Press.

83. Koval KJ, Zuckerman JD: Functional recovery after fracture of the hip, *J Bone Joint Surg* 76-A(5):751, 1994.

84. Krug HE, Woods SR, Mahowald ML: Tests that detect depression in RA, *J Musculoskeletal Med* 12(8):27, 1995.

85. Lachiewicz PF: Total ankle arthroplasty, *Orthop Rev* 23(4):315, 1994.

86. Lee SH, Abramson S: Stepped-care guide to osteoarthritis therapy, *Orthop Spec Ed* 1(1):45, 1995.

87. Liang MH, Logigian MK: *Rehabilitation of early rheumatoid arthritis,* Boston, 1992, Little, Brown.
88. Liscum B: Osteoporosis: the silent disease, *Orthop Nurs* 11(4):21, 1992.
89. Logue E, Sarwark JF: Idiopathic scoliosis: new instrumentation for surgical management, *J Am Acad Orthop Surg* 2(1):67, 1994.
90. Lonner BS, Harwin SF: Treatment of sepsis of the hip following total hip arthroplasty, *Contemp Orthop* 31(1):23, 1995.
91. Malmivaara A et al: The treatment of acute low back pain—bed rest, exercises, or ordinary activity? *N Engl J Med* 332(6):351, 1995.
92. Mankin HJ, Mow VC, Buckwalter JA, et al: Form and function of articular cartilage. In Simon SR, editor: *Orthopaedic basic science,* Chicago, 1994, American Academy of Orthopaedic Surgeons.
93. Marcus RE, Goodfellow DB, Pfister ME: The difficult diagnosis of tibialis tendon rupture in sports injuries, *Orthopedics* 18(8):715, 1995.
94. Margulies JY et al: Cotrel Dubousset and Wisconsin segmental spine instrumentation: comparison of results in adolescents with idiopathic scoliosis King type II, *Contemp Orthop* 30(4):311, 1995.
95. McCarthy JC, Busconi B: The role of hip arthroscopy in the diagnosis and treatment of hip disease, *Orthopedics* 18(8):753, 1995.
96. McLaughlin J et al: Rehabilitation after meniscus repair, *Orthopedics* 17(5):463, 1994.
97. Meier DE et al: Hematogenous osteomyelitis in the developing world: a practical approach to classification and treatment with limited resources, *Contemp Orthop* 26(5):495, 1993.
98. Metcalf EM: The orthopaedic critical path, *Orthop Nurs* 10(6):25, 1991.
99. Michael JW: The biomechanics of prosthetic knee mechanisms, *Biomechanics* 2(8):45, 1995.
100. Minter JE, Dorr LD: Indications for bilateral total knee replacement, *Contemp Orthop* 31(2):108, 1995.
101. Moehring HD, Voigtlander JP: Compartment pressure monitoring during intramedullary fixation of tibial fractures, *Orthopedics* 18(7):631, 1995.
102. Mosher CM: The Papineau bone graft: a limb salvage technique, *Orthop Nurs* 10(1):27, 1991.
103. Moskowitz RW et al: *Osteoarthritis: diagnosis medical/surgical management,* ed 2, Philadelphia, 1992, Saunders.
104. Mourad L: *Mosby's clinical nursing series: orthopedic disorders,* St Louis, 1991, Mosby.
105. Mow AC, Flatow EL, Foster RJ: Biomechanics. In Simon SR, editor: *Orthopaedic basic science,* Chicago, 1994, American Academy of Orthopaedic Surgeons.
106. Mueller TJ: Healing the heel, *Biomechanics* 2(7):61, 1995.
106a. Müller C, Rahn BA, Pfister U, Meinig RP: The incidence, pathogenesis, diagnosis, and treatment of fat embolism, *Orthop Rev* 23(2):107-117, 1994.
107. Murphy CD: The small pin circular fixator for proximal tibial fractures with soft tissue compromise, *Orthopedics* 14(2):273, 1991.
108. Nance DK, Mardjetko SM: Technical aspects and nursing considerations of limb lengthening, *Orthop Nurs* 13(1):21, 1994.
109. Nelson CL: Blood conservation techniques in orthopaedic surgery—one expert's protocol, *Peer to Peer* 7(4):3, 1995.
110. NIH Consensus Conference: Total hip replacement, *J Am Med Assoc* 273(24):1950, 1995.
111. Ochsner RE, Brunazzi MG: Intramedullary reaming and soft tissue procedures in treatment of chronic osteomyelitis of long bones, *Orthopedics* 17(5):433, 1994.
112. Oldaker SM: Live and learn: patient education for the elderly orthopaedic client, *Orthop Nurs* 11(3):51, 1992.
113. Olson B, Ustanko L, Warner S: The patient in a halo brace: striving for normalcy in body image and self-concept, *Orthop Nurs* 10(1):44, 1991.
114. O'Meara PM: Surgical techniques for arthroscopic meniscal repair, *Orthop Rev* 22(7):781, 1993.
115. Paiement GD: Prophylaxis is in—be it warfarin, LMW heparin, aspirin, or mechanical device, *Peer to Peer* 7(4):7, 14, 1995.
116. Paiement GD: Thromboembolic complications following trauma surgery: incidence and outcomes, *Orthopedics* 18(suppl):12, 1995.
117. Pappagallo M: Putting a cap on pain, *Biomechanics* 2(7):25, 1995.
118. Parr JE et al: Symposium: polyethylene wear and osteolysis, *Contemp Orthop* 31(1):51, 1995.
119: Patzakis MJ et al: Symposium: current concepts in the management of osteomyelitis, *Contemp Orthop* 28(2):157, 1994.
120. Paulos LE: Autograft is ACL "tissue of choice," *Orthop Today* 14(9):1, 1994.
121. Perry HM III, Morley JE, Coe RM, editors: *Aging and musculoskeletal disorders,* New York, 1993, Springer.
122. Pons F et al: Purification of dystrophin and visualization by rotary-shadowing in electron microscopy, and deletion detection using domain-specific antibodies. In Angelini C, Danieli GA, Fontanari D, editors: *Muscular dystrophy research: from molecular diagnosis toward therapy,* New York, 1991, Excerpta Medica.
123. Popkess-Vawter S, Patzel B: Compounded problem: chronic low back pain and overweight in adult females, *Orthop Nurs* 11(6):31, 1992.
124. Ranawalt CS et al: Symposium: cemented versus bony ingrowth prostheses, *Contemp Orthop* 25(5):511, 1992.
125. Reid IR et al: Long term effects of calcium supplementation on bone loss and fractures in post-menopausal women: a randomized controlled trial, *Am J Med* 98(4):331, 1995.
126. Renstrom PAFH, editor: *Clinical practice of sports injury prevention and care,* Oxford, 1994, Blackwell Scientific.
127. Rougraff BT et al: Limb salvage compared with amputation for osteosarcoma of the distal end of the femur, *J Bone Joint Surg* 76-A(5):649, 1994.
128. Rounseville C: Phantom limb pain: the ghost that haunts the amputee, *Orthop Nurs* 11(2):67, 1992.
129. Salisbury JR, Woods CG, Byers PD, editor: *Disease of bones and joints,* New York, 1994, Chapman & Hall Medical.
130. Schaefer S: Fundamentals of hyperbaric oxygen therapy, *Orthop Nurs* 11(6):9, 1992.
131. Schenck RC Jr, Heckman JD: Injuries of the knee, *Clin Symp* 45(1):17, 1993.
132. Schmalzreid TP et al: The relationship between the design, position, and articular wear of acetabular components inserted without cement and the development of pelvic osteolysis, *J Bone Joint Surg* 76-A(5):677, 1994.
133. Schofferman J: Low back pain guideline released, *Orthop Today* 15(1):1, 1995.
134. Seeley RR, Stephens TD, Tate P: *Anatomy and physiology,* St Louis, 1995, Mosby.
135. Shapiro F, Specht L: The diagnosis and orthopaedic treatment of inherited muscular diseases of childhood, *J Bone Joint Surg* 75-A(3):439, 1993.
136. Shelbourne KD, Wilckens JH: Current concepts in anterior cruciate ligament rehabilitation, *Orthop Rev* 20(12, suppl):35, 1991.
137. Sherk HH, Lane GJ, Black JD: Laser arthroscopy, *Orthop Rev* 21(9):1077, 1992.
138. Simon SR, editor: *Orthopaedic basic science,* Chicago, 1994, American Association of Orthopaedic Surgeons.
139. Sipos D: MP implants for rheumatoid arthritis in the hand, *Orthop Nurs* 12(5):7, 1993.
140. Sipos DA: Carpal tunnel syndrome, *Orthop Nurs* 14(1):17, 1995.
141. Smolen JS, Kalden JB, Maini RN, editors: *Rheumatoid arthritis,* New York, 1992, Springer-Verlag.
142. Song K, Herring JA: Early recognition and assessment of idiopathic scoliosis, *J Musculoskeletal Med* 10(4):63, 1993.
143. Song K, Herring JA: Management options for idiopathic scoliosis, *J Musculoskeletal Med* 10(11):40, 1993.
144. Spence RK: Vascular surgeon details approach to surgical anemia, *Peer to Peer* 7(4):5, 1995.
145. Springfield DS, Friedlander GE, Lane N: Molecular and cellular biology of inflammation and neoplasia. In Simon SR, editor: *Orthopaedic basic science,* Chicago, 1994, American Academy of Orthopaedic Surgeons.
146. Stanford JL et al: Combined estrogen and progestin hormone replacement therapy in relation to risk of breast cancer in middle-aged women, *J Am Med Assoc* 274(2):137, 1995.
147. Stanton RP, Lopez-Sosa FH, Doidge R: Chronic recurrent multifocal osteomyelitis, *Orthop Rev* 22(2):229, 1993.

148. Stiehl JB et al: Symposium: revision total knee replacement, *Contemp Orthop* 30(3):249, 1995.

149. Styrcula L: Traction basics part I, *Orthop Nurs* 12(2):71, 1994.

150. Styrcula L: Traction basics part II, *Orthop Nurs* 13(3):55, 1994.

151. Styrcula L: Traction basics part III, *Orthop Nurs* 13(4):34, 1994.

152. Sullivan PM et al: Total hip arthroplasty with cement in patients who are less than fifty years old, *J Bone Joint Surg* 76-A(5):863, 1994.

153. Swedlar WI, et al: Rheumatic changes in diabetes: shoulder, arm and hand, *J Musculoskeletal Med* 12(8):45, 1995.

154. Swenson EJ Jr: Diagnosing and managing meniscal injuries in athletes, *J Musculoskeletal Med* 12(5):35, 1995.

155. Swezey RL: Obturator internus bursitis: a common factor in low back pain, *Orthopedics* 16(7):783, 1993.

156. Thomas SS, Barnett J: Walking through gait analysis, *Orthop Nurs* 13(6):7, 1994.

157. Thomas KA et al: Enhanced spino-pelvic fixation for segmental spinal instrumentation: a preliminary biomechanical evaluation, *Orthopedics* 17(6):527, 1994.

158. Tibone JE, Shaffer B: A functional approach to managing shoulder impingement, *J Musculoskeletal Med* 12(7):37, 1995.

159. Timmons ME, Bower FL: The effect of structure preoperative teaching on patients' use of patient-controlled analgesia (PCA) and their management of pain, *Orthop Nurs* 12(1):23, 1993.

160. Tomaino MM: Lower limb salvage: microvascular reconstruction of post-traumatic soft tissue and skeletal defects, *Orthopedics* 18(7):665, 1995.

161. Touchet RII: Floating through pregnancy, *Biomechanics* 2(8):87, 1995.

162. Turpie AGG: Deep vein thrombosis prophylaxis in the outpatient setting: preventing complications following hospital discharge, *Orthopedics* 18(suppl):15, 1995.

163. vanOmmen GJB et al: Duchenne and Becker muscular dystrophy mutations studied at the gene and protein level. In Angelini C, Danieli GA, Fontanari D, editors: *Muscular dystrophy research,* New York, 1991, Excerpta Medica.

164. Watson TW, Stanitski CL, Stanitski DF: External fixation costs less than traction in children, *Orthop Today* 15(7):12, 1995.

165. Weinstein SL, Buckwalter JA, editors: *Turek's orthopaedics,* ed 5, Philadelphia, 1994, Lippincott.

166. Weisman MH, Weinblatt ME: *Treatment of the rheumatic diseases,* Philadelphia, 1995, Saunders.

167. Williamson VC: Amputation of the lower extremity: an overview, *Orthop Nurs* 11(2):55, 1992.

168. Wong DL: *Whaley and Wong's nursing care of infants and children,* ed 5, St Louis, 1995, Mosby.

169. Woo L-Y, An K-N, Arnoczky SP, et al: Anatomy, biology, and biomechanics of tendon, ligament, and meniscus. In Simon SR, editor: *Orthopaedic basic science,* Chicago, 1994, American Academy of Orthopaedic Surgeons.

170. Woo SL-Y et al: Biomechanical considerations. In Moskowitz RW et al, editors: *Osteoarthritis: diagnosis and medical/surgical management,* Philadelphia, 1992, Saunders.

171. Yagi T: Considering drains and tourniquets, *Peer to Peer* 7(4):11, 1995.

172. Yandrich TJ: Preventing infection in total joint replacement surgery, *Orthop Nurs* 14(2):15, 1995.

173. Yu JS: Magnetic resonance imaging of the wrist, *Orthopedics* 17(11):1041, 1995.

Integumentary System

5

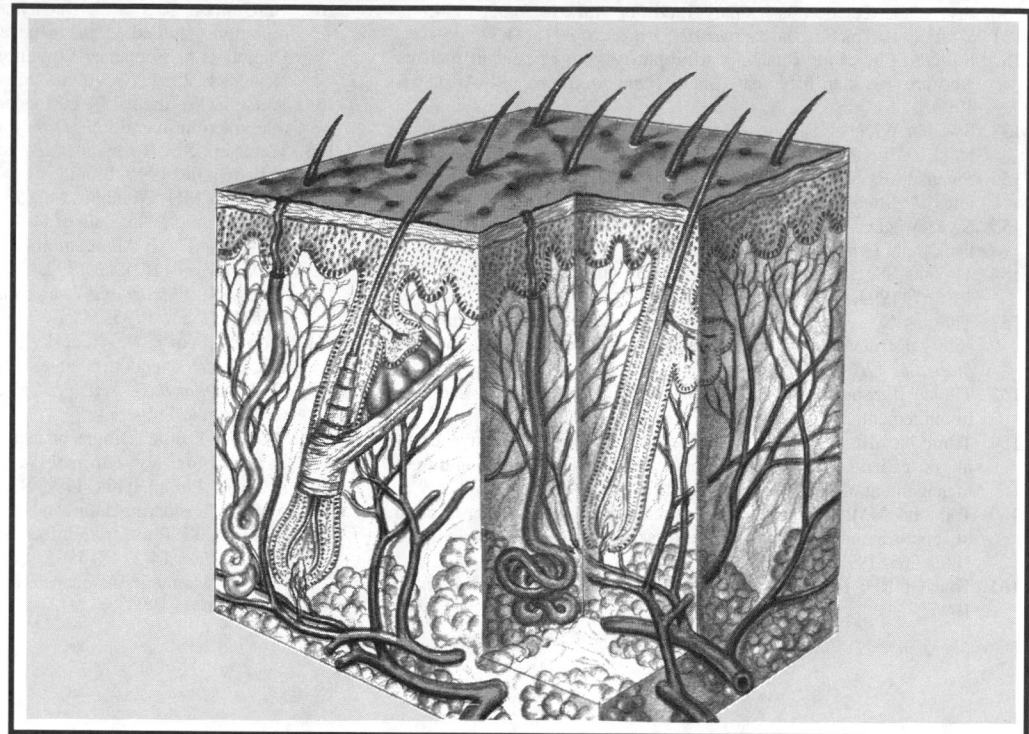

OVERVIEW

The integument, or skin, is the largest organ of the body. It is a protective barrier between the internal structures of the body and the external environment. It is tough, resilient, and virtually impermeable, but it is also affected by changes within the body. The condition of the skin can indicate a great deal about a person's health and how the environment affects that person.

Skin disorders and diseases are common; approximately 3% of all annual office vists are made to dermatologists. An estimated 2% of the U.S. population experiences an acute skin condition, but the true extent of skin disorders is difficult to determine because many persons with skin problems treat themselves rather than seek medical care. The economic cost of skin diseases is substantial.[57,58]

•••••• Anatomy, Physiology, and Related Pathophysiology

Structure

The skin comprises two principal layers: an outler layer, called the epidermis, and an underlying connective tissue layer, called the dermis. Beneath the dermis is the hypodermis (subcutaneous tissue), which technically is not part of the skin. The hypodermis is composed of loose connective tissue and fat cells that provide a layer of insulation. Specialized structures of the epidermis include glands, hair, and nails.

The anatomy of the skin varies from one part of the body to another, so the diagram of the skin in Figure 5-1 shows only the main parts and their approximate relationships. The pathologic conditions that arise in skin disorders occur in one or more of the various layers. The variation in anatomy often accounts for the distribution of skin diseases.

Epidermis The epidermis is composed of stratified squamous epithelium. Two cell types, keratinocytes and melanocytes, make up most of the epidermal cells. The epidermis is composed of two major sublayers: the stratum corneum, which protects the body against harmful environmental substances and restricts water loss; and the cellular stratum, where keratin cells are synthesized. The basement membrane lies beneath the cellular stratum and connects the epidermis to the dermis. The epidermis has no blood or lymph channels and depends on the underlying dermis for its nutrition.

The *stratum corneum* is the outer horny layer of closely packed dead squamous cells that contain the waterproofing protein keratin and form the protective barrier of the skin. The variation in skin thickness (0.5 mm in the eyelids to 4 mm in the palms and soles) is due mostly to differences in the thickness of the stratum corneum.

The *cellular stratum* is composed of three or four layers; from the most superficial to the deepest they can be identified as follows:

Stratum lucidum. This is a thin translucent layer of protein-filled cells found only in the thicker skin of the palms and

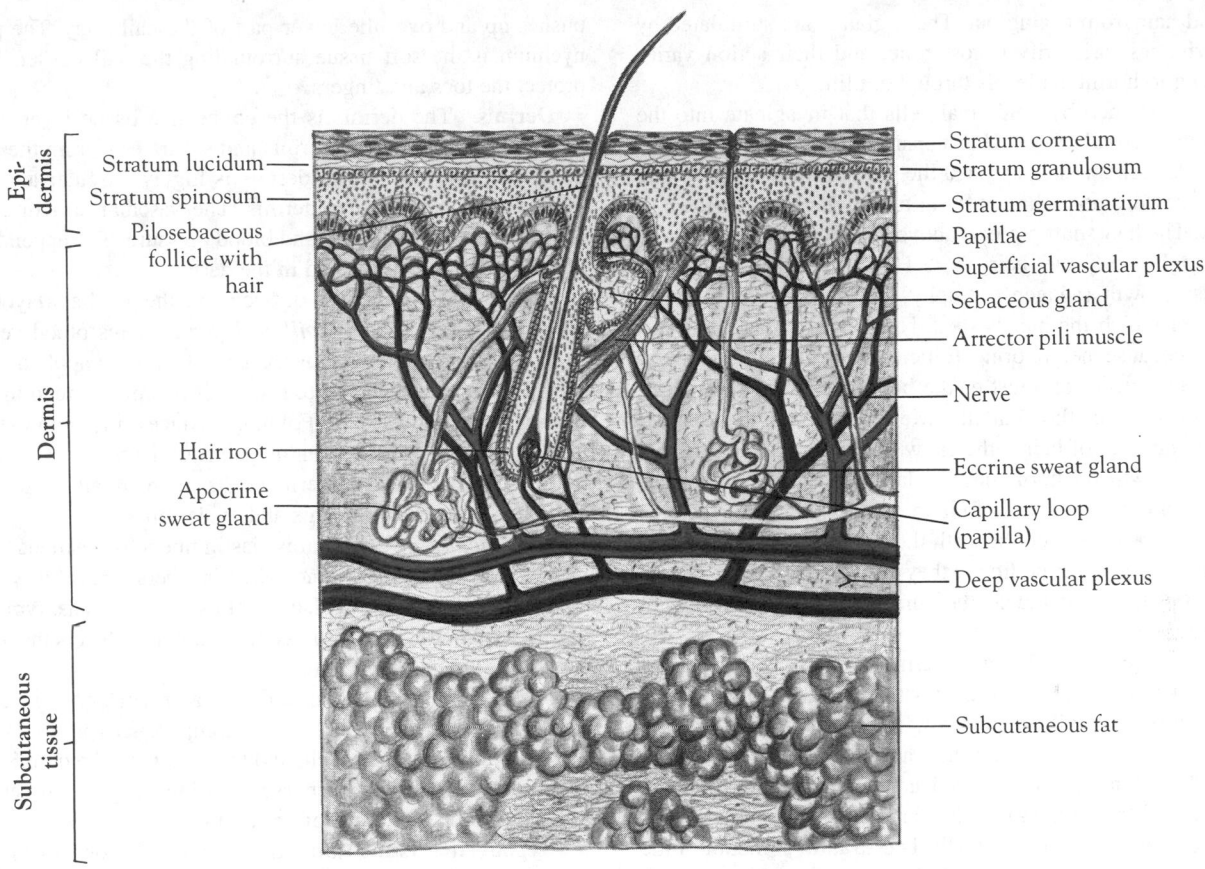

Figure 5-1 Structures of skin.

in the soles. The cells of this layer are filled with a transparent substance that appears to be a precursor of keratin.

Stratum granulosum. This granular layer is composed of cells containing granules of keratohyalin, an intermediate in keratin formation.

Stratum spinosum. This is the prickle cell layer, where cells begin to flatten and precursors of keratin appear.

Stratum germinativum. This is the basal cell layer, where mitotic activity occurs to replace the cells in the upper epidermal layer. The basal layer also contains the melanocytes, which synthesize the melanin that gives the skin its color.

The keratinocytes in the basal layer evolve into cells of the stratum corneum as they mature (keratinize) and make their way to the surface, where they are eventually desquamated. The transit time of basal layer cells to the final stage of desquamation is approximately 28 days.

Appendages The epidermis invaginates into the dermis and forms eccrine sweat glands, apocrine sweat glands, sebaceous glands, hair, and nails.

The *eccrine sweat glands* are small, convoluted secretory coils that extend from the dermis and open directly on the surface of the skin. Only humans have eccrine glands. They are distributed throughout the body except for the lip margins,

eardrums, nail beds, inner surface of the prepuce, and glans penis. The main function of the sweat glands is regulation of body temperature through water secretion. The eccrine sweat glands are innervated by sympathetic cholinergic nerve fibers, and heat is the primary stimulus for their secretion. Muscle exertion and emotional stress also stimulate secretion of water, chlorides and other electrolytes, and waste products such as lactate and urea.

The *apocrine sweat glands* are special structures found only in the axilla, nipple and areola, anogenital area, eyelids, and external ear. They do not develop fully until puberty. These glands are much larger and located deeper than the eccrine glands. The secretory duct of an apocrine sweat gland enters the hair follicle above the entrances of the sebaceous duct. The apocrine glands are adrenergic, and they secrete a white fluid containing water, salt, protein, carbohydrate, and other substances in response to emotional stimulation. Secretions from these glands are initially odorless, but bacteria on the skin decompose the organic components of sweat and cause distinctive body odors.

The *sebaceous glands* occur everywhere on the body except the palms and soles. They are continuous with and secrete into a pilosebaceous follicle, which may or may not contain a hair. They occasionally open directly onto the skin. Sebaceous glands secrete sebum, a lipid-rich substance that helps keep the skin and hair from drying out. These glands are stimulated by sex hormones, primarily testosterone, and their action varies according to hormonal levels throughout life.

Hair is formed by epidermal cells that invaginate into the underlying dermal layers. Hair consists of keratin that is synthesized by cells in the papilla at the base of the hair shaft. The papilla provides nourishment for mitosis, which causes the hair to grow. The hair shaft projects above the skin surface and at an acute angle with the hair root. Hair goes through cyclic changes: growth (anagen), atrophy (catagen), and rest (telogen), after which the hair is shed. Normal hair loss is not noticeable because neighboring follicles have differently timed cycles. Hair grows on most of the body except for the palms, soles, and parts of the genitalia. Men and women have about the same number of hair follicles, which are stimulated to differential growth by hormones. Melanocytes in the hair shaft give the hair its color. Hair follicle muscles, called arrectores pilorum, are immediately beneath the sebaceous glands. When innervated by adrenergic fibers, they elevate the hair to a more vertical position and indent the surrounding skin, producing "goose bumps."

The *nails* (Figure 5-2) are epidermal cells converted to hard plates of keratin. The nail root lies beneath the skin; the nail body (plate) is the visible part lying on the nail bed. The nail bed is highly vascular, giving the transparent nail body a pink color. The white crescent-shaped area extending beyond the proximal nail fold (lunula) marks the end of the matrix. This is the site of mitosis and nail growth. The stratum corneum of the skin covering the nail root is the cuticle, or eponychium, which

pushes up and over the lower part of the nail body. The paronychium is the soft tissue surrounding the nail border. Nails protect the toes and fingers.

Dermis   The dermis is the connective tissue layer of the skin that supports the epidermis and separates it from the cutaneous adipose tissue. The dermis is highly vascular and provides nutrition for the epidermis. The vascular structure also controls body temperature and blood pressure. The appendages of the epidermis are located in the dermis.

The dermis is composed of two parts, the papillary layer and the reticular layer. The *papillary layer* contains blood vessels and some nerve elements that respond to stimuli applied to the skin. This layer is folded into ridges, or papillae, extending into the upper epidermal layer. Folding produces ridges on the surface of the skin—notably on the palms of the hands. The papillae also nourish living epidermal cells and maintain a strong attachment between the dermis and epidermis.

The *reticular layer* contains elastin fibers for resilience, collagen fibers for strength, and reticulin fibers for stability. This connective tissue portion also contains blood vessels, lymphatics, nerves, matrix, and various cells. Collagen forms the greatest part of the dermis.

The skin is actually the body's major sensory organ. The sensory fibers in the dermis form a complex network to provide the sensations of pain, touch, and temperature. The dermis also contains autonomic motor nerves that innervate blood vessels, glands, and the arrectores pilorum muscles.

Hypodermis (subcutaneous tissue)   The dermis is connected to underlying organs by a layer of subcutaneous tissue

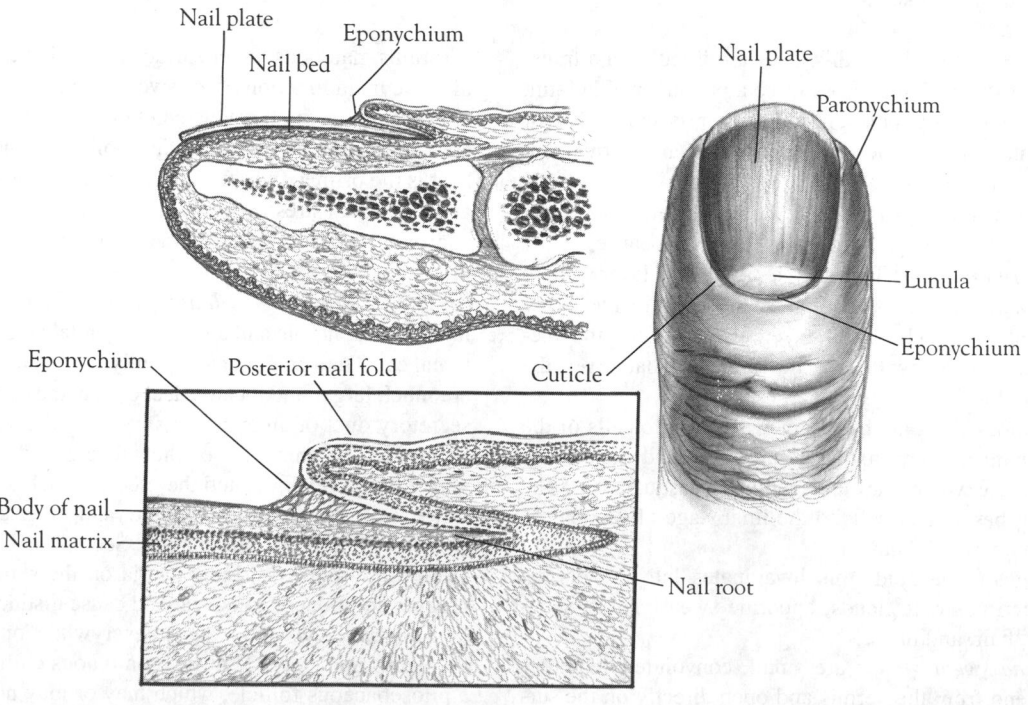

Figure 5-2 Structures of nail.

that is composed of loose connective tissue filled with fatty cells. This layer of adipose tissue provides heat, insulation, shock absorption, and a reserve of calories. Sensory and autonomic motor nerve fibers are located in the subcutaneous tissue.

Function

The skin provides several functions that are integral to the functioning of the entire body.

Protection   An intact stratum corneum creates a physical barrier against invasion by bacteria and foreign substances and minor physical trauma. Glandular secretions wash microorganisms from the pores, and colonies of nonpathogenic bacteria on the skin retard the growth of pathogens. Hairs in the nose, ears, anogenital areas, eyebrows, and eyelids act as barriers against the entry of foreign materials. Sebaceous gland secretions, along with the skin, prevent absorption of water during immersion. The skin reduces potential damage to deoxyribonucleic acid (DNA) from ultraviolet radiation through thickening of the stratum corneum that disperses radiation and through melanin production that forms a protective cap over the nucleus of the cell.

Retardation of body fluid loss   The skin acts as a barrier to minimize loss of internal contents and to prevent the internal fluid environment from leaking out.

Excretion   The skin acts a a minor organ of excretion. Some urea and lactic acid are lost through the skin, along with sweat and sodium chloride.

Regulation of body temperature   The skin controls body temperature by four processes: *radiation* of heat energy from the body surface; *conduction* of heat from the skin to other objects or the air; *convection* or removal of heat by air currents; and *evaporation* of perspiration stimulated by the sympathetic nervous system when the body is overheated.

Blood vessels of the skin help control body temperature by dilating in warm environments to promote heat loss through radiation and by constricting in cold environments to help conserve heat. If the skin is directly exposed to temperatures below 15° C (59° F), blood vessels begin to constrict to prevent the tissues from freezing.

Blood pressure regulation   During strenuous exercise, anxiety, or hemorrhage, constriction of skin blood vessels through sympathetic stimulation reduces blood flow to the skin, promotes increased venous return, increases cardiac output, and thereby increases blood pressure.

Tissue repair   The skin maintains itself and repairs its own wounds through exaggeration of the normal process of replacement of desquamated stratum corneum and formation of scar tissue.

Vitamin D production   The skin provides an area for irradiation of vitamin D precursors. Through catalytic action, ultraviolet light converts the precursor found in the skin to vitamin D_3, which is reabsorbed into blood vessels. Vitamin D is necessary in the metabolism of calcium and phosphorus.

Sensory perception   Free nerve endings and special receptors in the skin function alone or together to detect environmental stimuli, including pain, touch, heat, cold, pressure, vibration, tickle, itch, wetness, oiliness, and stickiness.

Expression   Feelings such as anxiety, fear, and anger may be visible on the skin through sweating, pallor, or flushing. Because of its visibility, skin is also closely connected with an individual's body image.

NORMAL FINDINGS

Skin

Tone   Deep to light brown in blacks; whitish pink to ruddy with olive or yellow overtones in whites; *older adult:* skin of whites tends to look paler and more opaque

Uniformity   Sun-darkened areas; areas of lighter pigmentation in dark-skinned people (palms, lips, nail beds); labile pigmented areas associated with use of hormones or pregnancy; callused areas appear yellow; crinkled skin areas darker (knees and elbows); dark-skinned (Mediterranean origin) people may have lips with bluish hue; vascular flush areas (cheeks, neck, upper chest, or genital area) may appear red, especially with excitement or anxiety; skin color masked through use of cosmetics or tanning agents; *older adult:* more freckles; uneven tanning; pigment deposits; hypopigmented patches

Moisture   Minimum perspiration or oiliness felt; dampness in skin folds; increased perspiration associated with warm environment or activity; wet palms, scalp, forehead, and axilla associated with anxiety; *older adult:* increased dryness, especially of extremities; decreased perspiration

Surface temperature   Cool to warm

Texture   Smooth, even, soft; some roughness on exposed areas (elbows and soles of feet); *older adult:* flaking and scaling associated with dry skin, especially on lower extremities

Thickness   Wide body variation; increased thickness in areas of pressure or rubbing (hands and feet); *older adult:* thinner skin, especially over dorsal surface of hands and feet, forearms, lower legs, and bony prominences

Turgor   Skin moves easily when lifted and returns to place immediately when released; *older adult:* general loss of elasticity; skin moves easily when lifted but does not return to place immediately when released; skin appears lax; increased wrinkle pattern more marked in sun-exposed areas, in fair skin, and in expressive areas of face; pendulous parts sag or droop (under chin, earlobes, breasts, and scrotum)

Hygiene   Clean, free of odor

Alterations   Striae (stretch marks) usually silver or pinkish; freckles (prominent in sun-exposed areas); some birthmarks; *older adult:* nevi often become lighter or disappear; seborrheic keratose (pigmented, raised, warty, slightly greasy lesions most often found on trunk or face); senile (actinic) keratose on exposed surfaces, first seen as small reddened areas and then as raised, rough, yellow to brown lesions; senile sebaceous adenomas (yellowish flattened papules with central depressions); cherry adenomas (tiny, bright, ruby red, round; may become brown with age)

Nails

Configuration   Nail edges smooth and rounded; nail base angle 160 degrees; nail surface flat or slightly curved; *older adult:* toenails may be thickened and distorted.

Consistency   Smooth, hard surface; uniform thickness; *older adult:* fingernails may be more brittle or peel

Color   Variations of pink; pigment deposits in nail beds of dark-skinned individuals; *older adult:* toenails may lose translucence and luster and become yellow

Adherence to nail bed   Nail base feels firm when palpated

Hair

Surface characteristics   Scalp smooth; hair shiny; vellus hair short, fine, inconspicuous, and unpigmented; terminal hair coarser, thicker, more conspicuous, and usually pigmented; *older adult:* sebaceous hyperplasia may extend into scalp

Distribution and configuration   "Normal" varies with individual; hair present on scalp, lower face, nares, ears, axillae, anterior chest around nipples, arms, legs, back, buttocks; female pubic configuration forms inverted triangle; hairline may extend up linea alba; male pubic configuration is upright triangle with hair extending up linea alba to umbilicus; *older adult;* increased facial hair (especially in women), bristly quality; men may have coarse hair in ears, nose, and eyebrows; decreased scalp hair; symmetric balding in men (most often frontal or occipital); decreased pubic and axillary hair

Texture   Scalp hair may be fine or coarse; fine vellus hair over body; coarse terminal hair in pubic and axillary areas; *older adult:* facial hair coarse; body hair fine

Color   Wide variation from pale to black; color may be masked or changed with rinses or dyes; *older adult;* graying; whitening; hairs that do not lose pigment often become darker

Quantity   "Normal" varies with individuals; gradual symmetric balding of scalp hair in some men; *older adult;* general decrease of body and scalp hair

•••••• Descriptions and Characteristics of Skin Lesions

Primary Skin Lesions

Primary skin lesions occur as initial spontaneous manifestations of an underlying pathologic process.

Lesion

Macule—flat; nonpalpable; circumscribed; less than 1 cm in diameter; brown, red, purple, white, or tan in color
Examples: Freckles; flat moles; rubella; rubeola; drug eruptions

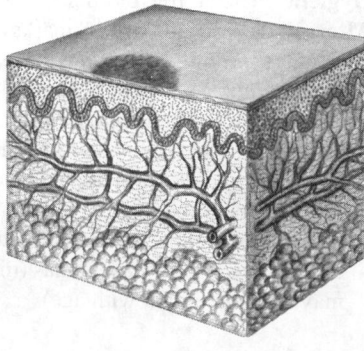

Patch—flat; nonpalpable; irregular in shape; macule greater than 1 cm in diameter
Examples: Vitiligo; port-wine marks

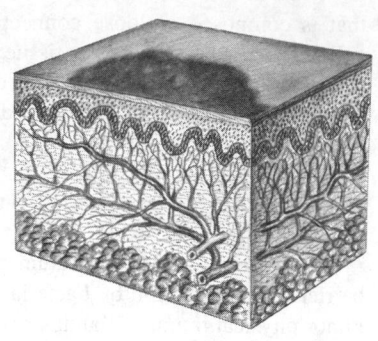

Papule—elevated; palpable firm; circumscribed; less than 1 cm in diameter; brown, red, pink, tan, or bluish red in color
Examples: Warts; drug-related eruptions; pigmented nevi

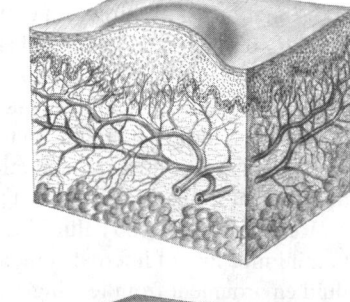

Plaque—elevated; flat topped; firm; rough; superficial papule greater than 1 cm in diameter, may be coalesced papules
Examples: Psoriasis; seborrheic and actinic keratoses; eczema

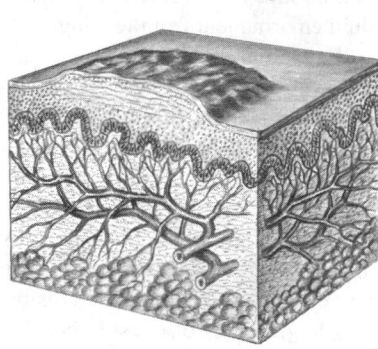

Wheal—elevated, irregular-shaped area of cutaneous edema; solid, transient, changing; variable diameter; pale pink in color
Examples: Urticaria; insect bites

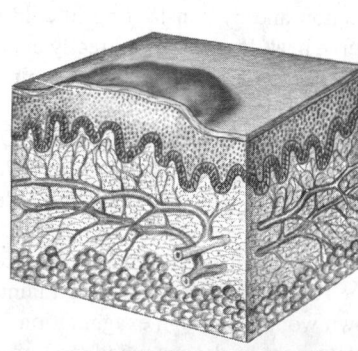

Nodule—elevated; firm; circumscribed; palpable; deeper in dermis than papule; 1 to 2 cm in diameter
Examples: Erythema nodosum; lipomas

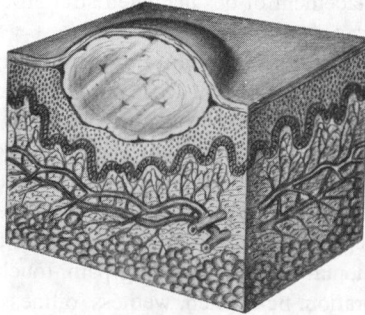

Tumor—elevated; solid; may or may not be clearly demarcated; greater than 2 cm in diameter; may or may not vary from skin color
  Examples: neoplasms

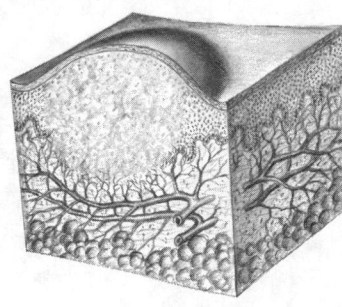

Vesicle—elevated; circumscribed; superficial; filled with serous fluid; less than 1 cm in diameter
  Examples: Blister; varicella

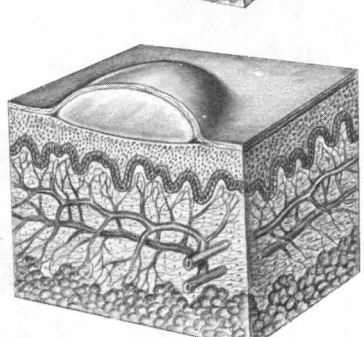

Bulla—vesicle greater than 1 cm in diameter
  Examples: Blister; pemphigus vulgaris

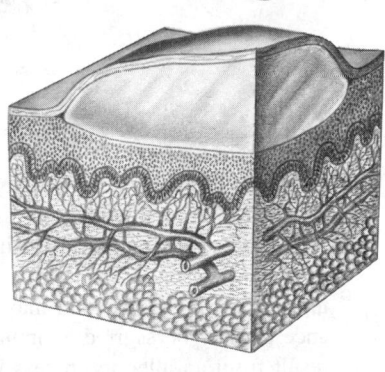

Pustule—elevated; superficial; similar to vesicle but filled with purulent fluid
  Examples: Impetigo; acne; variola; herpes zoster

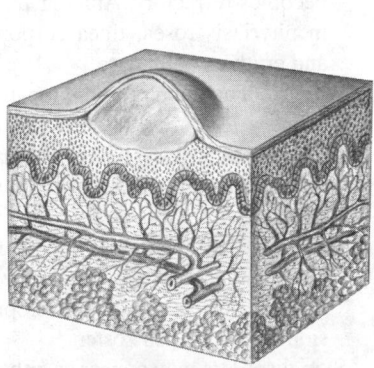

Cyst—elevated; circumscribed; palpable; encapsulated; filled with liquid or semisolid material
  Example: Sebaceous cyst

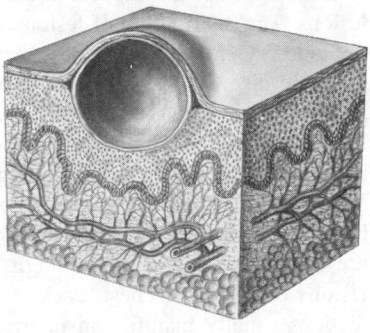

Telangiectasia—fine, irregular red line produced by dilation of capillary
  Example: Telangiectasia in rosacea

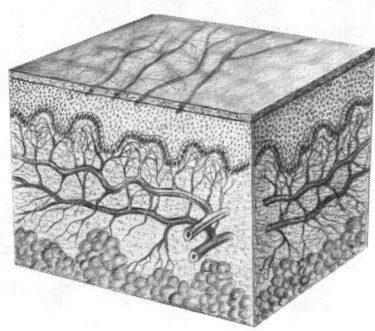

Secondary Skin Lesions

Secondary lesions are a result of later evolution of a primary lesion or are induced by external trauma to the primary lesion.

Lesion

Scale—heaped-up keratinized cells; flaky exfoliation; irregular; thick or thin; dry or oily; varied size; silver, white, or tan in color
  Examples: Psoriasis; exfoliative dermatitis

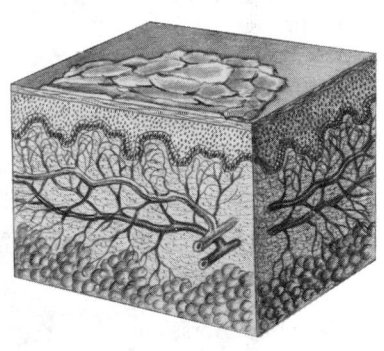

Crust—dried serum, blood, or purulent exudate; size varies; brown, red, black, tan or straw in color
  Examples: Scab on abrasion; eczema; impetigo

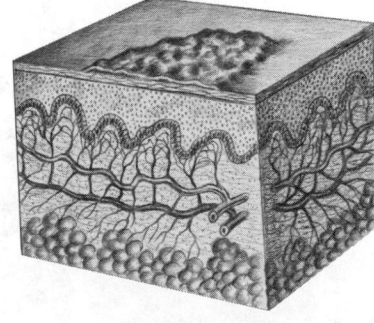

Lichenification—rough, thickened epidermis; accentuated skin markings due to rubbing or irritation; often involves flexor aspect of extremity
  Example: Chronic dermatitis

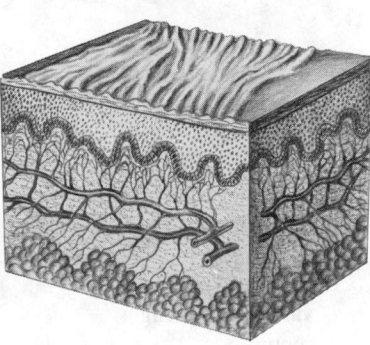

Scar—thin to thick fibrous tissue replacing injured dermis; irregular; pink, red, or white in color; may be atrophic or hypertrophic
Examples: Healed wound or surgical incision

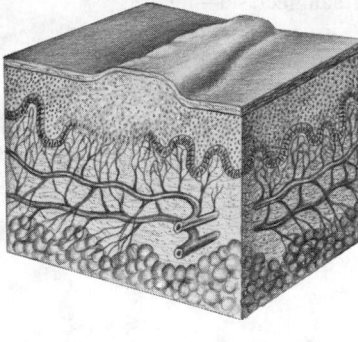

Keloid—irregularly shaped, elevated, progressively enlarging scar; grows beyond boundaries of wound; due to excessive collagen formation during healing
Examples: Keloid from ear piercing or burn scar

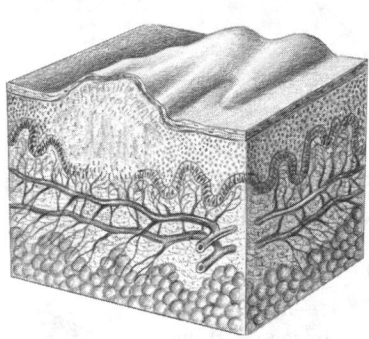

Excoriation—loss of epidermis; linear or hollowed-out crusted area; dermis exposed
Examples: Abrasion; scratch

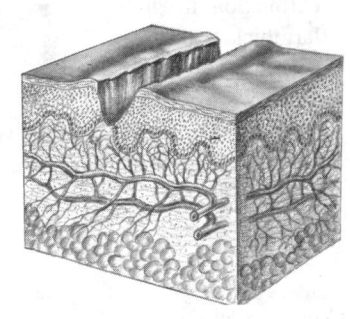

Fissure—linear crack or break from epidermis to dermis; small; deep; red
Examples: Athlete's foot; cheilosis

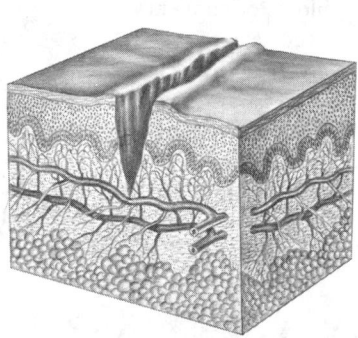

Erosion—loss of all or part of epidermis; depressed; moist; glistening; follows rupture of vesicle or bulla; larger than fissure
Examples: Varicella; variola following rupture

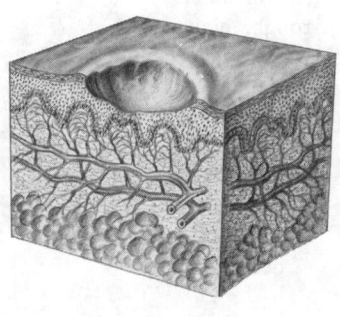

Ulcer—loss of epidermis and dermis; concave; varies in size; exudative; red or reddish blue
Examples: Decubiti; stasis ulcers

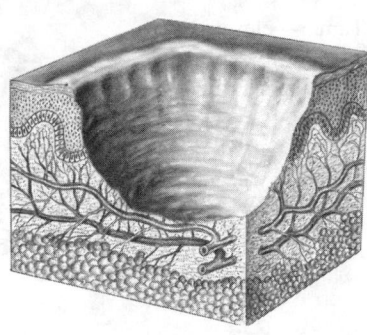

Atrophy—thinning of skin surface and loss of skin markings; skin translucent and paperlike
Examples: Striae; aged skin

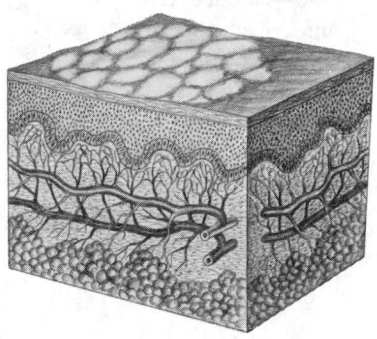

Attributes of Lesions

The configuration of skin lesions often has diagnostic value. These patterns can sometimes be explained by their pathogenesis. There are three common patterns of arrangement:

Annular. The formation of rings indicates extension of the lesion from the initial location to the periphery with clearing in the center. The skin may revert to normal appearance or may be scarred. Annular configuration can also result from an allergic process in which the central area becomes refractory. Annular patterns are commonly seen in pityriasis rosea, tinea corporis, tinea cruris, urticaria, and erythema annulare.

Grouped. This pattern is the localization of numerous small primary lesions in one area. It may be from mechanical factors (as in insect bites) or from a predisposition of a particular body area to a specific lesion, as in herpes simplex.

Linear. This arrangement may be caused by external factors such as trauma or may occur in contact dermatitis. It may also be determined by developmental origins of the lesions, as in herpes zoster.

Skin disorders may appear as either generalized or localized lesions. The distribution of lesions may also provide diagnostic clues. Generalized lesions may indicate an underlying systemic disorder, as in erythema multiforme; an allergic response, as with drug reactions; or a genetic disorder, as with lamellar ichthyosis. Localized lesions occur frequently as the result of a primary irritant or allergic eczematous dermatitis. Many disorders produce lesions in specific regions of the body. For example, erythema nodosum produces nodules that are limited to the legs and thighs. Acne vulgaris produces lesions on the face, chest, back, and shoulders. Candidal infections usually manifest in interriginous areas. Tinea cruris produces lesions in the perineal region. Pityriasis rosea may be distinguished from tinea corporis by the absence of lesions on the face and scalp. Pediculosis corporis is characterized by lesions along clothing lines, while scabies lesions are found in interdigital webs along the fingers and on the wrist and penis. In contrast, lesions from flea bites are limited to the ankles and lower legs.

In assessing skin lesions, the following characteristics should be considered and described:

Characteristics of the lesion
    Size
    Shape or configuration
    Color
    Consistency
    Elevation or depression
Pattern of arrangement
    Annular
    Grouped
    Linear
Location and distribution
    Generalized or localized
    Region of the body
    Discrete or confluent

CONDITIONS, DISEASES, AND DISORDERS

BACTERIAL CONDITIONS

■ FURUNCLES AND CARBUNCLES

A furuncle is an acute localized staphylococcal infection that is initially limited to a hair follicle but spreads rapidly to the surrounding dermis and subcutaneous tissue. A carbuncle is a group of furuncles combind as one larger lesion and involving adjoining hair follicles.

Furuncles and carbuncles usually occur in areas exposed to friction, pressure, or plugging, such as sweat glands in the axilla. These skin lesions tend to develp in people who are debilitated, malnourished, fatigued, or obese. They also develop in people who have altered immune mechanisms, diabetes mellitus, severe acne, or seborrheic dermatitis. Poor personal hygiene is another predisposing factor.

Furuncles occur most frequently on the neck, breasts, face, and buttocks. The condition may be recurrent and troublesome (furunculosis) and often occurs in healthy young adults.

Carbuncles develop more slowly than single furuncles. They occur most frequently on the nape of the neck in men.

•••••• Pathophysiology

A furuncle develops as a small perifollicular abscess that ordinarily destroys the hair and follicle during its early stages. A carbuncle involves more than one pilosebaceous unit and may involve many.

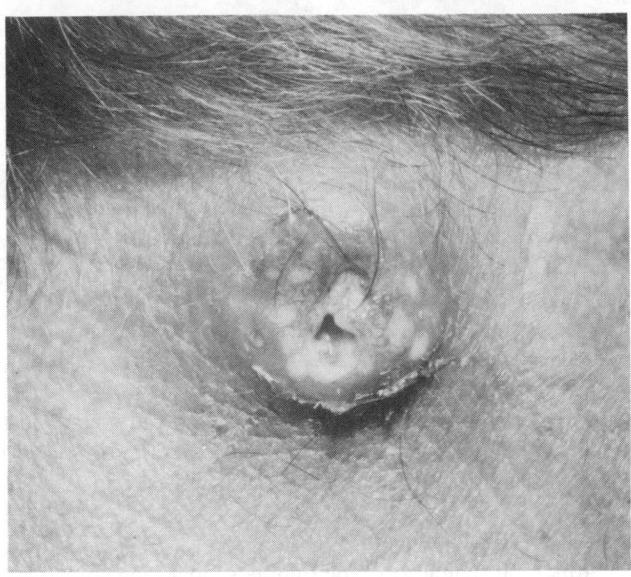

Figure 5-3 Furuncle. (Courtesy of Jaime A. Tschen, M.D., Department of Dermatology, Baylor College of Medicine, Houston.)

The invading organism is usually *Staphylococcus aureus,* which is found anywhere on the body. It usually gains entry after trauma causes a break in the skin. The organism produces an acute inflammatory process around the hair follicle. The initial nodule becomes a pustule that is 5 to 20 mm in diameter at the base of the hair follicle. The surrounding skin becomes red, hot, and tender. Local edema occurs in 3 to 5 days. The center of the lesion fills with yellow pus and forms a core that may rupture spontaneously or require surgical incision (Figure 5-3). The initial drainage is purulent and progresses to a serosanguineous discharge. Healing occurs gradually, usually with residual scarring.

The infection is usually walled off by local defense mechanisms. However, if the inflammatory process spreads to the deeper structures of the dermis and subcutaneous tissue (cellulitis), the bacteria may reach the dermal vascular plexus and cause septicemia. This complication is more likely to occur in people with altered immune status and in infants, whose defense mechanisms are less efficient.

•••••• Diagnostic Studies and Findings

Physical examination   Characteristic lesion
Culture of lesion discharge   Presence of infecting organism *(Staphylococcus aureus)*

•••••• Multidiscplinary Plan

Surgery
    Incision to promote drainage after lesion has become localized and filled with pus

Medications
    Antiinfective agents
        Systemic antibiotics

Teicoplanin 200 mg intramuscular (IM) or IV qd
Pencillinase-resistant penicillin for 4-6 wk to prevent subsequent development of new lesions
Cloxacillin (Cloxapen, Tegopen), 250-500 mg q8h
Dicloxacillin (Dycill, Dynapen, Pathocil, Veracillin), 250-500 mg po q6h
Nafcillin (Nafcil, Unipen), 250-1000 mg po q4 6h
Cefazolin (Kefzol) for patients allergic to penicillin, 250-500 mg po q6h
Rifamycin (Rifampin), 600 mg po qd for recurrent furunculosis
Mupirocin (Bactroban) 2% topical, applied intranasally tid to eliminate nasal carriage of *S. aureus*
Topical antibiotics once the lesions begin to drain, bacitracin or Neosporin applied locally tid or qid
Analgesics if lesions are extensive or pain is severe

General Management

Warm, moist compresses to promote suppuration
Nutritional therapy for underlying malnourishment, obesity, or debilitation
Appropriate therapies for underlying disease

NURSING CARE

Nursing Assessment

Inflammatory Process

Tenderness; pain; swelling; redness around infected follicle

Systemic Response to Infection

Malaise; fever; regional lymphadenopathy; increased white blood count; increased eosinophils; decreased neutrophils; increased lymphocytes; increased erythrocyte sedimentation rate

Spread of Infection

Personal hygiene; family hygiene

Psychosocial Concerns

Concern with body image

Nursing Dx & Intervention

Impaired skin integrity related to inflammatory process

- Assess for inflammation, drainage, and signs of systemic infection.
- Use meticulous hand washing *to prevent spread of infection.*
- Apply hot, moist compresses *to promote suppuration.*
- Change sterile dressing frequently after spontaneous drainage or surgical incision; properly dispose of contaminated articles *to prevent spread of infection.*

- Teach importance of not picking or squeezing lesions *to decrease the spread of infection and the risk of scarring.*
- Instruct patient in correct use of antibiotic therapies.

Risk for impaired skin integrity related to exudates

- When drainage begins, eliminate compresses *to prevent skin maceration and infection.*
- Teach meticulous hand washing and proper hygiene practices *to prevent autoinoculation.*

Risk for infection related to inadequate primary or secondary defenses

- Instruct patient to bathe daily with bacteriostatic soap and to avoid using oily preparations *to reduce the risk of recurrence.*
- Address predisposing factors such as altered nutritional status and obesity; patient should modify intake of fats and sugars.

Body image disturbance related to cognitive-perceptual factors

- Assess for presence of defining characteristics.
- Recognize importance of body image in growth and development.
- Teach importance of not picking or squeezing lesions *to decrease the risk of scarring.*
See p. 1685 for additional strategies.

Pain related to injuring agents: biologic factors

- Assess for discomfort.
- Apply warm, moist compresses.
- Instruct patient in use of analgesics.

Patient Education/Home Care Planning

1. Discuss with the patient or family members to make sure that
   a. The patient bathes daily with a bacteriostatic soap
   b. The patient uses towels, linens, and clothing separate from the rest of the family
   c. The patient's clothing, linen, and towels are changed and washed daily
   d. A clean washcloth is used each time lesions are cleaned or soaked; lesions should be washed gently, not scrubbed
2. Ensure that the patient and family know how to apply warm compresses and to change dressings using aseptic technique.
3. Ensure that the patient and family understand the need to maintain the correct regimen of antibiotic therapy.

Evaluation

Therapeutic effect is achieved Existing lesions heal. Skin is intact and free of infection. Scarring is minimal. Pain is alleviated.

Hygiene measures to prevent spread or recurrence are instituted Lesions do not recur. Infection does not spread to family members.

Patient evaluates appearance in a realistic manner Patient engages in usual activities and relationships.

◼ FOLLICULITIS

Folliculitis is a superficial or deep bacterial infection and irritation of the hair follicle usually caused by *Staphylococcus aureus*.

The bacterial infection can be limited to the hair follicle, resulting in its destruction, or the process can extend deeper to involve all of the hair follicle and the surrounding dermis.

Newborns have multiple lesions of the forehead, face, and neck. In adults the lesions are found in hairy areas such as the thigh, face, scalp, groin, or axilla.

Folliculitis may become chronic where the hair follicles are deep in the skin, as in the bearded area. Stiff hairs in the bearded area may emerge from the follicle, curve, and reenter the skin, producing a chronic low-grade irritation without significant infection (pseudofolliculitis). Pseudofolliculitis occurs most often in black men.

•••••• Pathophysiology

Folliculitis is a variable condition, with lesions ranging from minute, white-topped pustules in newborns to large, yellow, tender, pus-containing lesions in adults.

The primary lesion is a small pustule 1 to 2 mm in diameter located over the pilosebaceous orifice. It is sometimes perforated by a hair. The pustule may be surrounded by inflammation or nodular lesions. A crust develops after the pustule ruptures.

Predisposing factors include superficial damage to the skin, exposure to certain chemicals, solvents, and greases, and the presence of staphylococci. Other bacteria can also cause folliculitis, especially after antibiotic therapy. Gram-negative folliculitis occurs in patients who receive long-term tetracycline or erythromycin therapy for acne.

•••••• Diagnostic Studies and Findings

Physical examination Characteristic lesions

Culture of lesions Presence of infecting organism: gram-positive *Staphylococcus aureus* or gram-negative organisms

•••••• Multidisciplinary Plan

Medications

Antiinfective agents
 Systemic antibiotics
  Erythromycin (Delta-E, E-Mycin, Ery-Tab, Eryc, others), 250 mg po q6h for 10 d
  Penicillin V (Pen-Vee-K, V-Cillin K), 125-500 mg po q6h for 10 d
  Penicillinase-resistant penicillins
   Cloxacillin (Cloxapen, Tegopen), 250-500 mg po q6h

   Dicloxacillin (Dycill, Dynapen, Pathocil, Veracillin), 125-250 mg po q6h
  Cephalexin (Keflex), 250-500 mg po q6h
  Rifampin (Rifadin, Rimactane) 600 mg/d po for recalcitrant condition
  Clindamycin hydrochloride (Cleocin) 150 mg/d for prophylaxis[18,37]
 Topical antibiotics
  Bacitracin or Neosporin, applied locally tid or qid

NURSING CARE

Nursing Assessment

Inflammatory Process

Tenderness; pain; swelling, redness around infected follicle

Spread of Infection

Personal hygiene; presence of precipitating factors such as exposure to oils, greases, and solvents

Nursing Dx & Intervention

Impaired skin integrity related to inflammatory process

- Assess for inflammation.
- Use meticulous hand washing *to avoid spread of infection.*
- Apply hot, moist compresses *to promote suppuration.*
- Prevent maceration of skin *to avoid delay in healing.*
- Instruct patient to use antibacterial soap.
- Instruct patient in correct use of antibiotic therapies.
- Assess predisposing factors.

Risk for impaired skin integrity related to exudates, chemical substance, or mechanical factors

- Teach meticulous hand washing and proper hygiene practices *to avoid autoinoculation.*
- Help patient identify and eliminate precipitating factors such as skin maceration and exposure to oils, greases, and solvents *to prevent occurrence of new lesions.*
- Encourage men with chronic folliculitis or pseudofolliculitis in bearded area to grow a beard *to prevent occurrence of new lesions.*

Body image disturbance related to cognitive perceptual factors

- Assess for presence of defining characteristics.
- Recognize importance of body image in growth and development.
- Help patient express feelings about body and body appearance *to begin process of realistic assessment.*
- See p. 1685 for additional strategies.

Patient Education/Home Care Planning

1. Discuss with the patient or family members to make sure that
   a. The patient bathes daily with a bacteriostatic soap
   b. The patient uses towels, linens, and clothing separate from the rest of the family
   c. The patient's clothing, linen, and towels are changed and washed daily

---

Evaluation

Lesions heal   Skin is intact and free of infection.

Hygienic measures to prevent spread of recurrence are instituted   Lesions do not spread; no new lesions develop. Lesions do not spread to family members.

Precipitating factors are avoided   No new lesions develop.

Patient evaluates appearance in a realistic manner   Patient engages in usual activities and relationships.

▌ IMPETIGO AND ECTHYMA

▌   Impetigo (impetigo contagiosa) is a superficial vesiculopustular infection. Echthyma is an ulcerative form of impetigo.

Impetigo and echthyma occur primarily in infants, children, and the elderly. They are highly contagious among newborns in nurseries and young children and less contagious in older people.

The arms, legs, and face are more susceptible to impetigo and ecthyma than unexposed areas, although lesions may occur anywhere. Impetigo occurs most commonly on the face. It usually appears first around the nose and mouth. Ecthyma occurs most often on the legs, the posterior aspect of the thighs, and the buttocks.

Impetigo occurs most frequently during the late summer and early fall. Biting insects, mosquitoes, and flies appear to be the most frequent transmitters. Predisposing factors include poor hygiene, anemia, and malnutrition. The infection spreads easily among family members and from one child to another in a classroom or playgroup.

•••••• Pathophysiology

Impetigo is produced by coagulase-positive staphylococci and β-hemolytic streptococci. The bacteria may be found alone or in combination. Staphylococci are usually seen in very early lesions, but streptococci predominate in chronic lesions.

The infectious process is located beneath the corneum. The initial lesion is a small erythematous macule that changes into a vesicle or bulla with a thin roof. In streptococcal impetigo the vesicle becomes pustular in a matter of hours. A characteristic thick, honey-colored crust forms when the vesicle ruptures. In staphylococcal impetigo the thin-walled bulla breaks and a thin clear crust forms from the exudate. Both forms usually produce pruritus, burning, and regional lymphadenopathy. Autoinoculation from scratching may cause satellite lesions to form. Because the process is superficial, healing can occur spontaneously in the center of the lesion. This results in the formation of annular or circinate patterns.

A serious complication that develops in 2% to 5% of patients is acute glomerulonephritis from a nephritogenic strain of β-hemolytic streptococci. Impetigo in adults may have a more serious prognosis than impetigo occurring during childhood.

Ecthyma is a deeper infection than impetigo. It often develops in neglected superficial abrasions or from the scratching of insect bites. The inflammatory process is deeper and involves both the dermis and epidermis, so scarring results.

Ecthyma is characterized by localized thick, adherent crusted plaques with underlying ulceration and purulent exudate. The early lesions may appear as a vesicle or pustule surrounded by an area of erythema. Itching is common, an autoinoculation from scratching can transmit ecthyma to other parts of the body.

•••••• Diagnostic Studies and Findings

Physical examination   Characteristic lesion

Gram stain   Identification of infecting organism (gram positive or gram negative)

Culture   Identification of infecting organism (coagulase-positive staphylococci; β-hemolytic streptococci)

•••••• Multidiscplinary Plan

Medications

Antiinfective agents
  Systemic antibiotics
    Penicillin V (Pen-Vee-K, V-Cillin K), 125-500 mg po q6-8h for 10-14 d
    Penicillin G benzathine (Bicillin, Permapen), 1.2 million U IM as single injection
    Erythromycin (Delta-E, E-Mycin, Ery-Tab, Eryc, others), 250-500 mg po q6h for 10-14 d
    Dicloxacillin (Dynapen) if initial treatment fails, 250-500 mg po q6h
    Cephalexin (Keflex) if initial treatment fails, 250-500 mg po q6h
  Topical antibiotics
    Mupirocin 2%, Bacitracin, or Neosporin applied locally tid or qid
  Antihistamines for itching

General Management

Crust removal through soap and water washing and cool, moist compresses
Nutritional therapy for underlying malnourishment or debilitation
Appropriate therapies for underlying disease

NURSING CARE

Nursing Assessment

Lesion

Vesicle, bulla, exudate, or ulceration; satellite lesions; itching

Spread of Infection

Personal hygiene, particularly fingernails; family hygiene; contact with others; presence of lesions in other family members

Psychosocial Concerns

Concern that others may react to highly contagious disease; concern with body image

Nursing Dx & Intervention

Impaired skin integrity related to infectious process

- Assess lesions for characteristics.
- Use meticulous hand washing *to prevent spread of infection.*
- Remove crusts: clean lesion with bactericidal soap and water; apply compresses of Burow's solution and cool water *to soften crust;* gently scrub crust; dispose of contaminated articles *to prevent spread of infection.*
- Apply topical antibiotics to area of lesion for 2 days after lesion disappears.
- Cut patient's fingernails short *to minimize damage to lesion and to prevent autoinoculation from scratching.*
- Assess for symptoms of glomerulonephritis.

Risk for impaired skin integrity related to exudates and mechanical factors

- Cut patient's fingernails short *to prevent autoinoculation and new skin breaks.*
- Teach patient and family meticulous hand washing *to prevent autoinoculation and spread to family members.*
- Have patient and family bathe daily with bactericidal soap *to reduce recurrences and prevent spread to family members.*

Risk for infection related to inadequate primary defenses and environmental exposure

- Check family members for lesions *for early detection and treatment.*
- Address predisposing factors such as insect control and nutrition.

Body image disturbance related to cognitive-perceptual factors

- Assess for presence of defining characteristics.
- Recognize importance of body image in growth and development.

- Encourage patient to express feelings about body appearance and fear of reaction or rejection by others *to begin process of realistic self-evaluation.*
- See p. 1685 for additional strategies.

Patient Education/Home Care Planning

1. Ensure that the patient or family members understand that
   a. The patient and all family members must bathe daily with bacteriostatic soap
   b. The patient or any family member with lesions must use towels, linens, and clothing separate from the rest of the family
   c. The patient's clothing, linen, and towels must be changed and washed daily
   d. A clean washcloth must be used each time lesions are cleaned or soaked
2. Ensure that the patient and family know how to remove the crust from the lesions: apply cool compresses of water and Burow's solution to soften the crust, and then scrub the crust gently.
3. Instruct parents to check other family members, particularly other children, for lesions, and have infected family members treated.
4. Ensure that the patient and family understand the need to maintain the correct regimen of antibiotic therapy even though the skin lesions have healed.

Evaluation

Lesions resolve Skin is intact and free of infection.

Hygienic measures are instituted Lesions do not spread to other areas of the body; lesions do not recur.

Measures to prevent spread of infection are instituted Infected family members are treated. Infection does not spread to noninfected family members.

Patient evaluates self-concept in realistic manner Engages in usual activities and relationships.

■ CELLULITIS AND ERYSIPELAS

■ Cellulitis is a diffuse, acute streptococcal or staphylococcal infection of the skin and subcutaneous tissue. Erysipelas is a rarer form of streptococcal cellulitis.

Cellulitis occurs most frequently in the lower extremities, usually from bacterial invasion through a wound in the skin or an open lesion. The infection may also spread through the lymphatic system from an existing infection site, but often there is no predisposing condition or site of entry.

Erysipelas occurs on the face (bilaterally), ears, arms, and legs. Recurrences in the same area are not uncommon.

•••••• Pathophysiology

Cellulitis is most commonly caused by group A β-hemolytic *Streptococcus* or *Staphylococcus aureus.* Diffuse spread of the infection occurs because enzymes produced by the organism break down cellular components that would otherwise localize the inflammatory process. Areas of skin trauma, ulceration, or lymphedema are especially susceptible to developing cellulitis.

The area of infection is diffuse and involves all layers of the skin and subcutaneous tissue, with ill-defined borders. The skin is red, hot, indurated, and tender. Sometimes pitting is evident with pressure. Irregular lymphangitic streaks (seen as red streaks) may extend from the periphery, and regional lymphadenopathy may be present. The skin frequently has an infiltrated surface resembling the skin of an orange (peau d'orange). Breakdown of the infected area can occur with purulent discharge. Local abscesses form occasionally and require surgical incision.

Erysipelas occurs at the dermal level of the skin. It is caused specifically by group A β-hemolytic streptococci. The inflammatory process is acute with sudden onset. The area of infection is characterized by an erythematous, hot, and tender raised plaque with well-defined, sharply demarcated margins. Burning and pain, which may be severe, are common at the lesion site. Vesicles and bullae may develop and rupture, occasionally with necrosis of the involved skin. There is a great deal of exfoliation of the overlying skin as erysipelas heals.

Both cellulitis and erysipelas may be accompanied by systemic symptoms.

•••••• Diagnostic Studies and Findings

Physical examination   Characteristic lesion

Culture of lesion   For infecting organisms (group A β-hemolytic *Streptococcus* or *Staphylococcus aureus);* organism difficult to isolate unless drainage is present

Blood culture   For infecting organism: only occasionally positive

•••••• Multidisciplinary Plan

Surgery

  Incision and drainage of localized abscesses
  Debridement of devitalized structures

Medications

  Antiinfective agents
    Systemic antibiotics
      Should be continued for 1 wk after infection has cleared; may need to be prolonged for several weeks for erysipelas
      Oxacillin (Bactocill) 2.0 g IV q4h
      Cefazolin (Kefzol) 1.0 g IV q8h
      Nafcillin (Unipen) 250-500 mg po q6h
      Dicloxacillin (Dynapen) 500 mg po q6h
      Erythromycin (Delta-E, E-Mycin, Ery-Tab, Eryc, others), 250-500 mg po q6h for 10-14 d

! EMERGENCY ALERT

CELLULITIS

Cellulitis is an infectious process in which devitalized tissue or a dirty wound becomes infected with growth of often anaerobic bacteria.

Assessment

• There is an erythemous area and an open wound.
• Exudate and foul smell may be present.
• Pain is usually minimal.
• Patient appears healthy otherwise.

Interventions

• Obtain IV access.
• Administer antibiotics as ordered.
• Physician may consider incision and drainage or fasciotomy.
• Physician may consider hyperbaric oxygen treatments if gas formation is present.

      For severe infections requiring hospitalization; penicillin G aqueous, 400,000-1.2 million U IV q6h followed by oral therapy after 36-48 h
  Analgesics
    Aspirin (ASA) or acetaminophen (Tylenol), alone or combined with codeine

General Management

  Immobilization and elevation of affected limb to reduce edema
  Hospitalization for patients with severe infections or systemic symptoms
  Cool compresses for discomfort alternated with warm compresses or soaks to increase circulation
  Appropriate therapies for underlying disease

NURSING CARE

Nursing Assessment

Inflammatory Process

  Cellulitis: tenderness, pain; redness; heat; swelling; lymphangitic streaks; peau d'orange skin; purulent discharge; abscesses
  Erysipelas: tenderness, pain; redness; heat; swelling; raised plaque; vesicles; bullae; purulent exudate

Systemic Response to Infection

  Regional lymphadenopathy; fever; chills; tachycardia; headache; hypotension; malaise; increased white blood count; decreased neutrophils; increased eosinophils; increased lymphocytes; increased erythrocyte sedimentation rate

Nursing Dx & Intervention

Impaired skin integrity related to the inflammatory process

- Assess for inflammatory process.
- Elevate and immobilize affected area for 2 to 3 days *to decrease edema and increase circulation for healing.*
- Use meticulous hand washing *to prevent spread of infection.*
- Use sterile dressing changes for ulcers and open or draining lesions *to prevent spread of infection.*
- Observe for signs of systemic infection (see under Nursing Assessment).
- Instruct patient in correct use of antibiotic therapies *to obtain maximum benefit.*

Pain related to injuring agents: biologic

- Assess for discomfort.
- Elevate and immobilize affected area *to promote lymphatic drainage.*
- Apply cool wet compresses alternated with warm compresses or soaks.
- Instruct patient in use of analgesics.

Impaired physical mobility related to pain and discomfort

- Elevate affected area *to decrease edema and pain.*
- Explain need to maintain elevation and immobility for at least 2 to 3 days.
- Discuss with patient options to maximize elevation and immobility depending on patient's situation and severity of infection: bed rest, sling, crutches, or leg propped above heart level.

Patient Education/Home Care Planning

1. Explain the need to elevate and immobilize the affected area for at least 2 to 3 days or until redness and edema decrease.
2. Demonstrate how to wash an open or draining wound gently with clean washcloth and soap and water and to change dressings using aseptic technique.
3. Demonstrate how to apply a cool compress for discomfort, alternating with a warm compress or warm soak to increase circulation.

Evaluation

Infection resolves   Lesions heal. Skin is intact and free of infection.

Pain is relieved   Symptoms of pain, burning, and discomfort are alleviated.

Mobility is regained   Patient engages in usual activities.

Systemic infection does not occur or is quickly resolved   Laboratory values are normal; temperature is normal.

ACNE VULGARIS

Acne vulgaris is an inflammatory disease of the pilosebaceous follicles characterized by comedones, pustules, papules, or nodular lesions.

Acne occurs during puberty, although lesions may occur as early as 8 years of age and continue through the twenties and thirties. The peak incidence appears to be around 14 years of age for girls and 16 years for boys. Acne occurs more frequently in boys but tends to be more severe and prolonged in girls. Almost all adolescents experience some degree of acne, and about 80% have substantial lesions that range from superficial noninflammatory comedones to cysts and scars. Only a small percentage of these people seek medical attention; most treat themselves with over-the-counter preparations that may be ineffective.

Acne lesions occur most frequently on the face, neck, upper back, and chest. The precise cause of acne is unknown. Research now centers on overproduction of sebum, follicular keratinization, bacterial proliferation, and the development of inflammation as the primary pathogenic factors.[6] The course and severity of the disease seem to be genetically determined. Dietary factors have little or no influence on the development of the disease, although certain foods may aggravate the condition in some patients. Predisposing factors include the use of cosmetics, steroids, oral contraceptives, and certain drugs (iodides, bromides, phenytoin, phenobarbital, trimethadione, isoniazid, ethionamide, rifampin, and lithium); exposure to heavy oils, greases, and tars; friction or occlusion from clothing such as sweatbands, shoulder straps, and football shoulder pads; emotional stress; hyperalimentation; or an unfavorable climate. Acne seems to improve during the summer and worsen in the fall and winter. This is probably because exposure to sunlight lessens the severity of acne during the summer months. However, a hot, humid climate can produce severe acne in some people.

The clinical presentation of acne can range from a mild noninflammatory form to severe inflammatory cystic acne. In the mildest forms only comedones may be present. Moderate involvement also produces some papules or pustules. The most severe forms manifest inflammatory papules, pustules, cysts, abscesses, and scarring.

•••••• Pathophysiology

The sebaceous gland increases in size and produces more sebum because of androgenic activity. This is accompanied by abnormal keratinization of the middle third of the hair follicle, which results in obstruction of the pilosebaceous unit. This blockage prevents the normal flow of sebum to the skin surface, causing retention of cells, lipids, fatty acids, hair, and focal masses of *Corynebacterium acnes (Propionibacterium acnes).* Comedones then form either as open comedones (blackheads) or closed comedones (whiteheads). Open comedones have a raised opening that allows the contents to escape to the skin surface. The black appearance is caused by melanin granules or oxidation of the keratinous material. Closed comedones have a skin covering that prevents extrusion of the contents and promotes further retention of keratin and sebum. The open or closed comedones can remain free of inflammation, despite the presence of bacteria. As the contents of the structure continue to accumulate, the enlarging comedone becomes visible. This process may take weeks, months, or a year. If the wall of the upper third of the hair follicle becomes disrupted, its contents are discharged onto the epidermis and a pustule develops.

An enlarged follicle can eventually rupture and discharge its contents into the surrounding dermis. The result is the development of the inflammatory papule, nodule, or cyst. There is usually a combination of acute inflammation and foreign body reaction induced by keratin and hair in the dermis. Rupture of the follicle can occur spontaneously because of the inflammatory effects of the bacteria or can be caused by trauma such as squeezing the comedone. The deeper the lesions, the more severe the potential for and degree of scarring.

The regeneration of the ruptured follicular wall is accomplished by proliferating keratinizing epidermis, but cystic structures with surrounding fibrosis can form in the process. These can develop into deep cystic processes with interconnecting channels, gross inflammation, and abscess formation. Chronic, recurring lesions produce distinctive acne scars.

••••• Diagnostic Studies and Findings

Physical examination   Characteristic lesions and scarring

••••• Multidisciplinary Plan

Management usually includes a combination of modalities that depends on the severity and type of lesions.

Surgery

Surgical removal of fibrotic cysts that have not responded to intralesional injections or liquid nitrogen therapy; excision should not be performed on actively inflamed acne cysts

Intralesional injections of corticosteroids (triamcinolone [Aristocort, Kenalog]) into cysts, 2.5-5 mg/ml of injectable steroid in saline or lidocaine, 0.1-0.3 ml in each cyst

Medications

Vitamins
  Oral retinoids
    Isotretinoin (Accutane), 0.521 mg/kg/d po in 2 divided doses for 20 wk; initial dose individualized for patient's weight and severity of disease, with dosage adjusted after 2 wk according to response of disease; second course may be initiated for persistent acne after 2 mo without therapy
  Topical
    Vitamin A acid (retinoic acid) (Retin-A) gel or cream, 0.01%-0.1% applied nightly 30 min after washing face and 1 h before bedtime

Antiinfective agents
  Systemic antibiotics (for severe acne)
    Tetracycline, 250-500 mg po qid for 4 wk, then decreased to lowest maintenance dose that gives good response; ibuprofen (Motrin) 2.4 g/d will enhance the effect of 1 g of tetracycline daily
    Minocycline (Minocin), 100 mg/d po in divided doses when no response to tetracycline
    Erythromycin (Delta-E, E-Mycin, Ery-Tab, Eryc, others), 250-500 mg po qid; same regimen as with tetracycline, if response to tetracycline is poor
    Doxycycline (Vibramycin, Monodox) 100 mg po qd
  Topical antibiotics
    Clindamycin 1%, apply tid or qid to lesions
    Erythromycin 2%, apply tid or qid to lesions
    Tetracycline, apply tid or qid to lesions
Keratolytic agents
    Salicyclic acid gel, apply nightly to affected areas
    Benzoyl peroxide 2.5%-10%, 3-4 h/d for 4 d, then overnight if tolerated; patient establishes own level of tolerance for strength and time
Hormones
    Mestranol, 0.075-0.1 mg or equivalent po in cyclic monthly routine
    Ethinyl estradiol, 0.035-0.05 mg po in cyclic monthly routine
    Spironolactone (Aldactone), 50-200 mg po in divided doses with meals; for antiandrogenic effect
    Prednisone, 5.0-7.5 mg po qd, PM administration

General Management

Cryotherapy—liquid nitrogen applied with cotton-tipped applicator or fine spray onto cysts

Expression of comedones by means of Schamberg or other extractor

Ultraviolet light in increasing doses at least once a week

Well-balanced diet to eliminate foods known to aggravate condition; foods will be specific to each individual

NURSING CARE

Nursing Assessment

Lesion

Presence of comedones (open or closed), pustules, papules, nodules, cysts, pitting scars on face, neck, shoulders, upper back, or chest; seasonal or monthly pattern and history of past inflammatory lesions; evidence of picking or squeezing lesions

Inflammatory Process

Tenderness; pain; swelling; redness and infected follicle

Psychosocial Concerns

Concern with body image and social relationships

Nursing Dx & Intervention

Impaired skin integrity to inflammatory process; high risk for infection related to mechanical factors and internal factors

- Assess for inflammatory process.
- Encourage patient to seek medical attention when acne develops.
- Stress importance of adhering to therapeutic regimen; assist in setting up overall schedule for managing regimen on daily basis.
- Plan schedule for facial hygiene; clean skin with acne soap or mild soap once or twice a day, keep skin clean and dry, and avoid abrasive soaps.
- Give written instructions for use of peeling agents such as benzoyl peroxide or retinoic acid. Alternating the creams can give better results. Never apply the two together.
- Discourage squeezing, picking, and rubbing of lesions *to prevent infection.*
- Teach patient how to use comedone extractor. Set up criteria for which comedones can be removed. Establish limited schedule for removal *to prevent further tissue damage.*
- Apply hot packs to cystic lesions *to promote circulation and suppuration.*
- Encourage frequent shampooing and hairstyle that keeps hair off face.
- Analyze diet and help patient identify foods that cause flare-ups.
- Help patient deal with stress; help patient label feelings, identify alternative courses of action, and set reachable goals.
- Identify and eliminate predisposing factors.
- Dispel myths that sexual activity or abstinence causes or affects acne.
- Instruct patient in correct use of antibiotic therapies.

Situational low self-esteem; body image disturbance related to cognitive perceptual factors

- Recognize importance of body image in growth and development.
- Assess patient's perception of his or her appearance.
- Teach importance of not picking or squeezing lesions, *to decrease risk of scarring.*
- Encourage patient to express feelings about body, body appearance, or fear of reaction or rejection by others *to begin process of realistic self-evaluation.*
- Encourage patient to develop interests and other attributes *to support positive self-image, feelings of self-worth, and self-confidence.*
- Help patient evaluate facial scarring in realistic perspective *so it does not become focal point of existence.*
- Advise patient of availability of tinted acne lotions that can mask lesions and scars.
- Arrange for individual or group therapy *if patient is unable to adjust to appearance.*

Patient Education/Home Care Planning

1. Discuss and provide written instructions regarding the following:
   a. Side effects of systemic antibiotics and oral retinoids (isotretinoin should not be given to women of childbearing potential because fetal abnormalities have been reported with use of this drug)
   b. Need for and schedule of follow-up laboratory work for long-term antibiotic therapy or with oral retinoids
   c. Untoward effects of topical preparations:
      (1) For increased redness and peeling, reduce time and strength of preparation until symptoms subside, then increase slowly
      (2) Photosensitizing properties of retinoic acid: use only at bedtime; do not go out into sunlight with it on; use sunscreen with SPF of 15
   d. Safe use of ultraviolet lamp: eyes covered, timed exposure with backup timer, and measured distance
2. Discuss good hygiene practices to prevent secondary infection.
3. Discuss with the patient how to maintain a well-balanced diet and get adequate rest.
4. Encourage the patient to go out into the sunlight unless contraindicated.
5. Discuss with the patient and family that successful therapy requires the patient's full cooperation and patience and that therapy is long-term and results may not be immediate.
6. Discuss with the patient the importance of continuing local lesion care even after the lesions have resolved.

Evaluation

Disease condition improves   Patient has fewer comedones, pustules, papules, nodules, or cysts.

Acne lesions improve   Lesions heal with as little scarring as possible. There is no secondary infection.

Inflammatory process recedes   There is no pain, tenderness, swelling, or redness around affected follicle.

Side effects or untoward effects of medications are recognized and treated quickly   Patient seeks medical attention for untoward or side effects.

Patient has realistic self-concept   Acne disorder is not used as excuse for unsuccessful interpersonal relationships. Patient has realistic perception of his or her appearance.

ROSACEA

Rosacea is a chronic inflammatory disorder involving the central area of the face, which is characterized by erythema, telangiectasia, papules, and pustules.

Rosacea tends to occur in people who blush easily and sunburn easily. It appears most often in white women in their forties and fifties. When it occurs in men, it is usually more severe and is often associated with rhinophyma. Rhinophyma is characterized by thickened red skin on the nose that can be disfiguring.

The cause of rosacea is unknown, although alcohol, coffee, spicy foods, stress, and sun exposure may precipitate or exacerbate it in some people. Physical activity, infection, endocrine abnormalities, use of tobacco, and extreme heat or cold—anything that produces flushing—can also aggravate rosacea. The use of fluorinated steroid creams can also cause rosacea.

• • • • • • Pathophysiology

The main pathologic processes of rosacea are instability of the superficial blood vessels, which results in persistent erythema and telangiectasia; overgrowth of normal bacteria, which results in pustules; and a granulomatous inflammation, which results in papular localization.

Rosacea develops gradually, beginning with periodic flushing across the forehead, nose, chin, and cheeks. The redness is intermittent at first but later becomes permanent. Telangiectasia develops along with pustules and papules. The inflammatory process causing the papules is granulomatous, differentiating it from the papules of acne. The pustules of rosacea appear similar to those of acne but do not have the characteristic comedones of acne. Rhinophyma is seen in advanced cases, where there is marked hyperplasia of the sebaceous glands of the nose. Rhinophyma develops on the lower half of the nose and produces red, thickened, bulbous skin with dilated follicles.

Rosacea is sometimes associated with ocular symptoms of keratitis, corneal vascularization and blepharitis, and uveitis.

Rosacea usually spreads slowly and does not subside without treatment.

• • • • • • Diagnostic Studies and Findings

Physical examination Characteristic vascular flushing and acneform lesions without comedones of acne vulgaris; rhinophyma

• • • • • • Multidiscplinary Plan

See Chapter 6 for treatment of eye symptoms.

Surgery

Excision of excess tissue in rhinophyma

Medications

Antiinfective agents
   Systemic antibiotics
      Tetracycline, 250-500 mg po qid initially for 1- to 2-wk periods to prevent pustules; decrease doses as symptoms subside
      Metronidazol (Flagyl), 200 mg po bid
      Erythromycin, 250 mg po q6h
   Topical erythromycin 2% or clindamycin 2% alternated with hydrocortisone cream
   Topical metronidazole gel 0.75% or cream 1%
Corticosteroids (topical preparations)
   Sulfur 20% in hydrocortisone cream 1% applied bid
   Hydrocortisone cream 1% applied bid

Isotretinoin (Accutane), 0.5 mg/kg/d for 20 wk
Spironolactone, 50 mg/d for 4 wk for antiandrogenic effect

General Management

Electrolysis for large dilated blood vessels
Cryotherapy for rhinophyma
Carbon dioxide laser therapy for rhinophyma[27,28]
Avoidance of hot food, drinks, and activities that precipitate or aggravate condition

NURSING CARE

Nursing Assessment

Inflammatory Process

Erythema, telangiectasia, papules, and pustules across forehead, nose, chin, and cheeks; rhinophyma

Extension of Inflammation

Ocular symptoms of keratitis, conjunctivitis, uveitis, and vascular dilation

Precipitating Factors

Erythema in response to sunlight, hot beverages, spicy foods, vegetables, vinegar, alcohol, physical activity, and stress

Psychosocial Concerns

Concern with body image

Nursing Dx & Intervention

Impaired skin integrity related to inflammatory process

- Assess for inflammatory process.
- Instruct patient not to squeeze or pick pustules *to prevent infection.*
- Instruct patient to keep skin clean and oil free but to avoid excessive dryness and irritation *to prevent aggravation of condition.*
- Instruct patient to shampoo hair often *to avoid oiliness.*
- Instruct patient in correct use of antibiotic and medication therapies *to maximize therapeutic benefit.*

Risk for impaired skin integrity related to environmental or internal factors

- Help patient identify factors that cause exacerbations, and work with patient to eliminate them.

Body image disturbance related to cognitive-perceptual factors: situational low self-esteem

- Assess patient's perception of his or her appearance.
- Encourage patient to express feelings about body, body appearance, and fear of reaction or rejection by others *to begin process of realistic self-evaluation.*
- Help patient evaluate his or her appearance in a realistic manner.

Impaired tissue integrity related to the
inflammatory process

- Assess for ocular symptoms of keratitis, conjunctivitis, uveitis, vascular dilation.
- See Chapter 6 for nursing interventions.

Evaluation

Pustular lesions resolve   Skin is intact with no papules or pustules.

Exacerbations are not triggered by avoidable factors Patients avoids factors leading to facial hyperemia.

Side effects or untoward reactions from long-term antibiotic therapy are recognized and treated   Patient seeks medical attention for untoward or side effects.

Patient evaluates appearance in a realistic manner Patient engages in usual activities and relationships.

BENIGN SKIN CHANGES

CORNS AND CALLUSES

A corn (clavus) is a painful circumscribed area of hyperkeratosis caused by external pressure. A callus is a superficial area of hyperkeratosis that forms at the site of repeated pressure or friction.

A corn is a flat or slightly elevated circumscribed lesion with a smooth hard surface. "Soft" corns are caused by the pressure of a bony prominence. They appear as whitish thickenings usually between the fourth and fifth toes. "Hard" corns have a sharply defined conical appearance. They appear most frequently over bony prominences, such as the interphalangeal joints of the toes at the site of pressure from footwear. Hard corns are usually painful. The pain may be dull and constant or sharp when pressure is applied, similar to the sensation of stepping on a pebble.

Calluses are not well demarcated and may be large. They are elevated, with a normal pattern of skin ridges running over the surface. Calluses usually occur on the weight-bearing areas of the feet, overlying bony prominences. Calluses may form over plantar warts and must be differentiated from them. They are also common on the palmar surface of the hands, particularly in people who work with their hands. Calluses are usually not tender, but pressure may produce dull pain.

Pathophysiology

A corn contains a localized pinpoint accumulation of keratin that forms an elongated hard plug in the horny layer of the epidermis with thinning of the underlying epidermis. The plug presses downward on the dermal structures.

In callus formation the epidermis reacts to repeated friction with an increased mitotic rate that results in hyperkeratosis and thickening of the stratum corneum.

The severity of a corn or callus depends on the degree and duration of the trauma that caused it to form.

Diagnostic Studies and Findings

Physical examination Characteristic lesion consistent with history of chronic pressure or friction

Multidisciplinary Plan

Surgery

Excision of superficial cornified layer of corn

Medications

Keratolytics
40% salicyclic acid plaster or ointment
Corticosteroids
Injection of triamcinolone (Kenalog, Aristocort), 10 mg/ml at base of corn to relieve pain

General Management

Orthopedic correction of weight-bearing mechanics through use of bars and support devices
Corn pads to redistribute weight and relieve pressure

NURSING CARE

Nursing Assessment

Lesion

Thickened skin; may be tender to touch

Pain

Location, duration, and intensity

Nursing Dx & Intervention

Impaired skin integrity related to mechanical factors

- Assess lesion for characteristics.
- Teach patient how to apply keratolytic substance and to avoid normal skin *to prevent tissue damage.*
- Demonstrate proper application of corn pads.

Pain related to physical factors

- Assess for pain and tolerance.
- Teach patient use of corn pads to relieve pressure.

Knowledge deficit related to cause and prevention

- Teach patient that most corns and calluses on feet are caused by tight, ill-fitting shoes and that new lesions can be avoided by wearing shoes that fit properly.
- Show patient potential areas of pressure and how shoes should fit.

Patient Education/Home Care Planning

1. Explain the importance of not paring away existing corns and calluses.
2. Discuss with the patient the use of keratolytic plaster: apply sticky side to skin, making sure plaster is large enough to cover affected area; cover the plaster with adhesive tape and leave in place for designated period of time (overnight to 7 days); after the plaster is removed, soak the area in warm water and rub the soft macerated skin with a rough towel or pumice stone; reapply the plaster and repeat the process until all hyperkeratotic skin is removed.

Evaluation

Source of pressure is relieved Shoes fit properly. Orthopedic correction is used. Corn pads redistribute weight. New lesions do not form.

Existing lesions resolve Symptoms of pain are alleviated. Thickened areas disappear.

SEBACEOUS, EPIDERMAL, AND DERMOID CYSTS

Sebaceous, epidermal, and dermoid cysts are slow-growing, benign, cystic, intradermal, or subcutaneous tumors.

Cysts are classified into three basic types depending on their histopathology: epidermal cysts, pilar or trichilemmal cysts (sebaceous cysts), and dermoid cysts.

Epidermal cysts are usually found on the face, scalp, neck, and back. Epidermal cysts include milia, acne cysts, and traumatic inclusion cysts. Only a few lesions are usually present unless the patient has had severe acne, in which case multiple lesions may be present.

Pilar or trichilemmal cysts (wens) occur most frequently on the scalp but may also occur elsewhere. These cysts are usually referred to as sebaceous cysts. However, this is a misnomer. True sebaceous cysts are seen only in steatocystoma multiplex, a relatively rare inherited condition.

Dermoid cysts are usually found at birth. They are located deep in the subcutaneous tissue and may adhere to the periosteum.

Cystic lesions vary in size from 1 mm to several centimeters. Most cysts are less than 3 cm in diameter but can enlarge to the size of an orange. On palpation the mass is firm, movable, round, globular, and nontender unless infected.

•••••• Pathophysiology

The wall of the epidermal cyst is composed of keratinizing epidermis. The cyst contains keratin in laminated layers. The wall of the pilar cyst is made up of epidermal cells from the central part of the hair follicle. The contents of the pilar cyst are homogeneous rather than in laminated layers. The walls of the dermoid cyst are composed of keratinizing epidermis containing hair follicles, sebaceous glands, and sweat glands.

Cyst formation may occur after inflammation, trauma, or rupture of closed comedones. A person may also have a genetic predisposition to cyst formation. The contents of the cyst are the result of the obstructed hair follicle, and the exact nature depends on the level of the obstruction. The contents are soft and yellow-white and have a rancid odor.

•••••• Diagnostic Studies and Findings

Physical examination Characteristic lesion

•••••• Multidisciplinary Plan

Surgery

Excision of cyst, including wall, to prevent recurrence incision and drainage of infected cysts

Medications

Corticosteroids
Triamcinolone (Aristocort, Kenalog) by intralesional injection

---

NURSING CARE

Nursing Assessment

Lesion

Size; location; number; presence of tenderness, inflammation, or infection; on palpation, firm, movable, round, globular, and nontender

Pyschosocial Concerns

Concern about body image

Nursing Dx & Intervention

Risk for impaired skin integrity related to mechanical factors

- Assess for number, size, location, and characteristics of lesions.
- Teach importance of not picking or squeezing lesions *because this may lead to infection of cyst.*

Body image disturbance related to cognitive-perceptual factors

- Assess for presence of defining characteristics.
- Recognize importance of body image in growth and development.
- Teach importance of not picking or squeezing lesions, *which may lead to infection and result in scarring.*
- Encourage patient to express feelings about body, body appearance, and fear of reaction or rejection by others, *to assist in process of realistic self-evaluation.*

Patient Education/Home Care Planning

1. Demonstrate and discuss with the patient dressing changes and suture care after excision of the cyst.

Evaluation

Nonexcised lesions do not become infected   There is no redness, swelling, tenderness, pus, or fever; scarring is minimal.

Excised lesions heal   Skin is intact and smooth.

Patient evaluates appearance realistically   Patient engages in usual activities and relationships.

CUTANEOUS TAG

(Acrochordon)

Cutaneous tags are common, small, flesh-colored or pigmented pedunculated lesions.

Acrochordons are found most often in middle-aged and elderly people. The number increases with pregnancy and menopause. The lesions occur most frequently around the neck, upper chest, axilla and groin and with seborrheic keratoses. They may occur singularly or in the hundreds. Although the lesion is benign, it may cause concern because of cosmetic embarrassment or because of irritation by clothing.

•••••• Pathophysiology

The cutaneous tag consists of an outpouched core of loose connective tissue and dilated capillaries covered by normal epidermis. The papilloma is pedunculated and varies in size from 1 to 2 mm in diameter to considerably larger, soft, baglike, fibrous lesions.

•••••• Diagnostic Studies and Findings

Physical examination   Characteristic lesion

•••••• Multidisciplinary Plan

Surgery

Removal with scalpel or scissors, with electrocoagulation of central vessel if needed

General Management

Removal through electrodesiccation or cryotherapy

NURSING CARE

Nursing Assessment

Lesion

Location; number; size; presence of irritation, tenderness, and inflammation

Psychosocial Concerns

Concern about body image

Nursing Dx & Intervention

Risk for impaired skin integrity related to mechanical factors

- Assess for location, number, and size of lesions and presence of irritation, tenderness, or inflammation.
- Evaluate with patient the potential for irritation of tags through friction from clothing or rubbing against other body parts.

Body image disturbance related to cognitive-perceptual factors

- Assess for presence of defining characteristics.
- Encourage patient to express feeling about body, body appearance, or fear of reaction by others *to assist in process of realistic self-evaluation.*

Patient Education/Home Care Planning

1. Discuss with the patient the benign nature of the lesions.
2. Explain to the patient that lesions can be removed relatively easily for cosmetic purposes or if tags become irritated.

Evaluation

Patient evaluates lesions in realistic manner   Patient seeks treatment for lesions that are irritated or inflamed. Lesions are removed if they become irritated or if patient is embarrassed.

KELOID

A keloid is an overgrowth of fibroelastic tissue that occurs spontaneously or at the site of dermal trauma.

The factors that trigger keloid formation are unknown. There appears to be a genetic predisposition and a regional susceptibility because keloids commonly occur on the sternum, chest, upper back, and earlobes and where an injury crosses normal flexion creases. Keloids occur predominantly in children or young adults, particularly in dark-skinned persons (Figure 5-4).

•••••• Pathophysiology

In susceptible people keloids form after any skin trauma, or they may arise spontaneously. Keloids are an abnormal progressive deposition of collagen that exceeds the requirements for wound repair. This may be the result of immune activity. The lesions are soft and pink in the early stages and then become firm and white. Keloids are raised, smooth, or ridged, extend beyond the edges of the initial wound, and

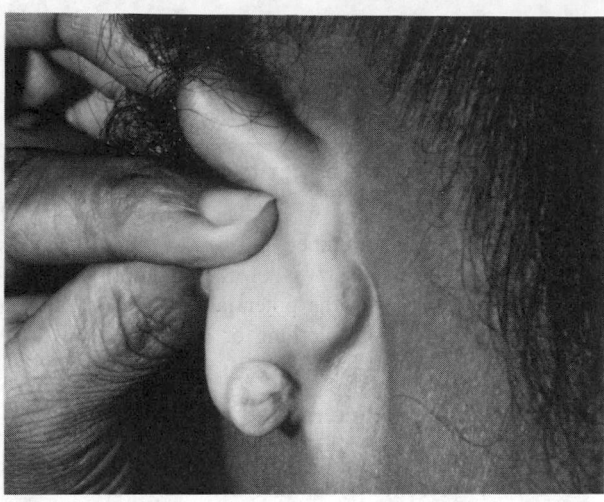

Figure 5-4 Keloid. (Courtesy of Stephen B. Tucker, M.D., Department of Dermatology, University of Texas Health Science Center at Houston.)

may continue to grow for many months or years to form large irregular lesions. Keloid scars are frequently tender and pruritic.

•••••• Diagnostic Studies and Findings

Physical examination   Characteristic lesion; clinical differentiation from hypertrophic scar not possible in first 3 months of lesion, but thereafter any continued increase in size and sensitivity of firm, indurated scar is indicative of keloid formation

•••••• Multidisciplinary Plan

Keloids may become worse as the result of treatment; therefore the need for intervention must first be carefully assessed. Small keloids are often best left untreated. Many keloids gradually soften and flatten out over a period of years, even without treatment

Surgery

Surgical or carbon dioxide laser excision combined with radiation therapy or intralesional injection of steroids for large keloids—surgical excision alone will result in the formation of new and larger keloids

Medications

Corticosteroids

Triamcinolone (Aristocort, Kenalog), 20-40 mg/ml by intralesional injection; may require repeated injections at monthly intervals until keloid remains flattened and asymptomatic

Topical retinoic acid, 0.05% applied bid for 3 mo

General Management

Solid carbon dioxide or liquid nitrogen applied topically at 2-week intervals

NURSING CARE

Nursing Assessment

Lesion

Size; location; color; tenderness; pruritus

Psychosocial Concerns

Concern about body image

Nursing Dx & Intervention

Impaired skin integrity related to mechanical factors

- Assess lesion for size, location, color, tenderness, pruritus.
- Discuss nature of keloid formation and help patient find skilled practitioners for therapeutic intervention.
- Inform patient that optimum time for treatment is within first few months of scar formation, while lesions are still vascular and growing, and that older keloids may be resistant to treatment.
- Instruct patient not to scratch keloid that itches *to avoid skin trauma that could cause further keloid formation.*

Risk for impaired skin integrity related to mechanical factors

- Discuss safety habits *to avoid injury that leads to keloid formation:* protective clothing, proper equipment, and so on.

Body image disturbance related to cognitive-perceptual factors; situational low self-esteem

- Assess patient's perception of his or her appearance.
- Help patient express feelings about body, body appearance, and fear of reaction or rejection by others *to assist in process of realistic self-evaluation.*

Patient Education/Home Care Planning

1. Discuss with the patient the nature of keloid behavior and the need to evaluate therapeutic intervention carefully with practitioners familiar with and skilled in treating keloids.
2. Explain to the patient that many keloids gradually soften and flatten out over a period of years, even without treatment.

Evaluation

Patient is knowledgeable about keloid therapies and risks   Patient seeks intervention early and from practitioners familiar with and skilled in keloid treatment. Patient avoids surgical excision of keloids.

Patient takes measures to prevent injury that would result in keloid formation   Patient uses safety measures, such as protective clothing and use of proper equipment, to avoid injury. Patient refrains from scratching or irritating scar tissue.

Patient evaluates appearance in a realistic manner Patient engages in usual activities and relationships.

■ SEBORRHEIC KERATOSES

■ Seborrheic keratoses are common, benign, superficial, epithelial, pigmented tumors.

The cause of seborrheic keratoses is unknown. They occur most frequently after 40 years of age. They most commonly occur on the back, central chest, face, and scalp. In blacks the lesions tend to be more numerous and smaller and to occur earlier. The lesions are inherited as a dominant trait.

Seborrheic keratoses vary in color from yellow to brownish black. They are elevated plaques with sharply circumscribed borders and appear to be stuck on the skin. The size of the lesion varies from a few millimeters to several centimeters. They almost always occur in multiples rather than singly. These lesions do not become malignant, but a sudden increase in the number and degree of itching of the lesions can occur in association with an internal malignancy.

•••••• Pathophysiology

Immature keratinocytes accumulate, causing formation of seborrheic keratoses. Keratinization eventually occurs, causing the lesions to become warty, dry, and fissured. The surface of the lesions often appears greasy, with pits filled with keratotic material. These represent invaginations of the epidermis. There is also a papular variant of the lesion that has a smooth surface. Epidermal thickening is associated with an increase of dermal papillae and the formation of the verrucous surface. The lesions grow slowly and are round or oval.

Seborrheic keratoses are usually asymptomatic unless they become irritated. They may itch occasionally. Irritation of the lesions by physical or chemical trauma results in tenderness, itching, erythema, and an increase in the size of the lesion.

•••••• Diagnostic Studies and Findings

Physical examination   Characteristic lesion
Biopsy   Done if squamous cell carcinoma is suspected

•••••• Multidisciplinary Plan

In most instances small, asymptomatic seborrheic keratoses require no treatment. Treatment is instituted for lesions that itch, are irritated, or are cosmetically embarrassing.

Surgery

Shave ablation or curettage using local anesthesia

General Management

Liquid nitrogen cryotherapy at 2- to 3-week intervals
Carbon dioxide pencil applied with light to moderate pressure for 12 to 20 seconds

NURSING CARE

Nursing Assessment

Lesion

Location; size; number; appearance; color; surface characteristics; borders; pruritus; changes in characteristics

Irritation of Lesion

Erythema; tenderness; increased pruritus

Psychosocial Concerns

Concern with body image

Nursing Dx & Intervention

Risk for impaired skin integrity related to mechanical factors

- Assess lesions for characteristics.
- Reassure patient that this lesion has no potential for malignancy.
- Have patient identify lesions that itch, are irritated, or are cosmetically embarrassing *for potential treatment.*
- Evaluate with patient lesions that are likely to become irritated from clothing or rubbing against other body parts *to identify for potential treatment.*

Body image disturbance; situational low self-esteem related to cognitive-perceptual factors

- Assess patient's perception of his or her appearance.
- Encourage patient to express feelings about body, body appearance, or fear of reaction or rejection by others *to assist in process of realistic self-evaluation.*
- Inform patient that bothersome lesions can be removed, usually with minimal or no scarring.

Patient Education/Home Care Planning

1. Explain to the patient that the lesion has no potential for malignancy.
2. Discuss with the patient the availability of medical therapy for lesions that become irritated or bothersome or that are cosmetically embarrassing.

Evaluation

Treated lesions heal   Skin is intact with minimum scarring and is free of infection.

Patient evaluates lesions realistically   Patient seeks treatment for lesions that itch, are irritated, or are cosmetically embarrassing.

Patient evaluates appearance realistically Patient engages in usual activities and relationships.

ERYTHEMA MULTIFORME

Erythema multiforme is an acute inflammatory eruption characterized by symmetric erythematous, edematous, or bullous lesions precipitated by numerous factors.

The cause and pathogenesis of erythema multiforme are unknown. The mechanism of response seems to be an allergic hypersensitivity.

The disease is associated with herpes simplex, bacterial and other infections, endocrine changes, and internal malignancies. Almost any drug can cause erythema multiforme; penicillin, sulfonamides, salicylates, and barbiturates are the most commonly implicated drugs. Bacterial and viral infections are often implicated in children and young adults, but association with drugs and malignancy is more common in adults. Attacks sometimes last for 2 to 4 weeks and recur in the fall.

•••••• Pathophysiology

In mild cases of erythema multiforme, eruption occurs only in cutaneous lesions of erythematous macules, papules, and plaques located predominantly in the distal portion of the extremities and face and symmetrically distributed. The classic lesion (target or iris lesion) is a dark, urticarial plaque with elevated circular borders and a depressed inner ring (Figure 5-5). After a few days the central area of erythema develops a dusky purplish discoloration that can become bullous.

In more severe cases fever, coryza, malaise, and athralgia may also occur. In these cases the lesions are predominantly vesiculobullous and involve mucous membranes as well as skin. In children and young adults a severe and sometimes fatal form of erythema multiforme known as Stevens-Johnson syndrome can develop. In this syndrome mucous membrane lesions are present and may or may not be accompanied by cutaneous lesions. Vesicles and ulcerations develop in the mucous membrane of the lips, mouth, nasal passages, eyes, and genitalia. Conjunctival and corneal lesions are present in 90% of the cases.

Genitourinary lesions in erythema multiforme can compromise bladder function, and the inflammatory process can involve the kidneys with consequent hematuria and renal tubular necrosis. Mucous membrane ulceration can extend into the pharynx, esophagus, larynx, trachea, and bronchi.

The variety of histologic changes in erythema multiforme depends on the site of involvement and the degree of the inflammatory process. The blood vessels are dilated and are surrounded by lymphohistiocytic infiltrate with substantial edema of the papillary dermis. Edema of the upper dermis leads to the formation of bullae that are subepidermal without acantholysis. Epidermal necrosis occurs primarily in the center of the lesion, the site of the dusky iris (target) lesion.

•••••• Diagnostic Studies and Findings

Physical examination Characteristic lesion, particularly iris or target lesion; lesions fixed and do not fade or change location; absence of itching

Complete blood count Increased white blood count, increased erythrocyte sedimentation rate

Urinalysis Red blood cells and albumin in urine if genitourinary lesions are present

Antistreptolysin titer Elevated if disease occurs after streptococcal infection

•••••• Multidisciplinary Plan

Mild erythema multiforme clears spontaneously and may require no treatment other than elimination of the precipitating factor. For treatment of eye symptoms see Chapter 6.

Medications

Antiinfective agents
    Systemic antibiotics for underlying infection or control secondary infection; specific drug and dosage depend on infection and its severity and age of patient
Corticosteroids
    Systemic glucocorticoids
        Prednisone, 60-80 mg po qd in divided doses, then decreased; controversial[1]
Clobetasol propionate (Temovate) 0.025% ointment in adhesive paste to yield a 0.25% concentration for oral lesions; under investigation[48]
Local anesthetic agents
    Viscous lidocaine (Xylocaine) swish for mouth lesions
Analgesics
    Aspirin (ASA), 600 mg po q4-6h

General Management

Wet dressings to debride crusted lesions
Bed rest; hospitalization for severe cases
Bland diet for mouth lesions
Intravenous fluids for hydration in severe cases

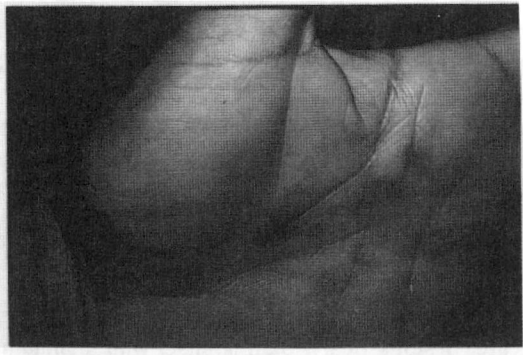

Figure 5-5 Erythema multiforme (target lesion). (Courtesy of Stephen B, Tucker, M.D., Department of Dermatology, University of Texas Health Science Center at Houston.)

NURSING CARE

Nursing Assessment

Lesion

Erythematous macules, papules, vesicles, or bullae at distal aspect of extremities and face; target or iris lesion; vesicles or ulcerations of mucous membranes

Systemic Involvement

Fever; coryza; arthralgia; malaise; chest pain; vomiting; diarrhea; hematuria; albuminuria; increased erythrocyte sedimentation rate; increased white blood count; radiologic changes in lungs

Nutrition

Inability to eat because of mouth ulcerations

Psychosocial Concerns

Concern about body image

Nursing Dx & Intervention

Impaired skin integrity related to mechanical factors

- Assess lesions for characteristics.
- In collaboration with physician, apply wet dressings *to debride lesions* (see p. 527).
- Scrub crusted lesions gently with antibacterial soap *to promote healing and prevent infection.*
- Teach meticulous hand washing and good hygiene *to prevent secondary infection.*

Altered oral mucous membrane related to pathologic condition

- Assess for presence of lesions.
- Provide soft, bland diet *to prevent tissue damage.*
- Avoid astringent or acidic liquids *to promote comfort.*
- Provide mouth care with alkaline or saline mouthwash *to promote comfort and prevent infection.*
- Instruct patient in use of viscous lidocaine mouth swish *to promote comfort.*

Pain related to physical factors

- Assess for discomfort.
- Apply cool compresses or soaks.
- Encourage bed rest.
- Instruct patient in use of analgesics.

Altered nutrition: less than body requirements related to inability to ingest food

- Assess nutritional status.
- Provide soft, bland diet *to promote comfort while eating.*
- In collaboration with physician, offer viscous lidocaine mouth swish 15 minutes before eating *to promote comfort.*

Body image disturbance related to cognitive-perceptual factors

- Assess for defining characteristics.
- Help patient express feelings about body, body appearance, or fear of reaction or rejection by others *to assist in process of realistic self-evaluation.*

Patient Education/Home Care Planning

1. Demonstrate to the patient and family the application of cool compresses or soaks using aseptic technique.
2. Discuss with the patient and family the need for follow-up urinalysis to detect the presence of renal tubular necrosis.
3. Discuss with the patient and family signs and symptoms of secondary infection and to seek medical attention if they occur.
4. Help the patient identify potential precipitating factors and to eliminate those factors when possible.

Evaluation

Existing lesions heal   Lesions resolve. Ulcerations and erosions reepithelialize. Skin and mucous membrane heal. Discomfort is alleviated.

Secondary infection is avoided   There is no swelling, redness, or pus in healing lesions.

Nutritional status is adequate   Weight is maintained. Lesions heal.

Systemic involvement resolves   There are no red blood cells or protein in urine. White blood count is 5000 to 10,000/mm^3. Erythrocyte sedimentation rate is normal (depends on method).

Complications are recognized early   Patient has follow-up urinalysis. Patient seeks medical attention for vision changes.

Patient evaluates appearance in a realistic manner   Patient engages in usual activities and relationships.

ERYTHEMA NODOSUM

Erythema nodosum is an acute inflammatory nodular eruption that involves primarily the lower extremities and is precipitated by various factors.

Erythema nodosum is found equally in boys and girls but is more common in adults, particularly young women. It occurs more commonly from January to June.

There are many precipitating factors, including various infections, drugs, diseases, and pregnancy. Erythema nodosum frequently follows an infection of the upper respiratory tract, especially from streptococci. In adults streptococcal infections and sarcoidosis are the most common causes. An underlying systemic cause is identifiable in more than 50% of cases. The remainder of the cases occur in apparently healthy young adults.

The prodromal symptoms may be fever, chills, malaise, and arthralgia, which occur a few days or several weeks before the onset of the eruption. Some of the prodromal symptoms may be from the underlying condition.

•••••• Pathophysiology

Erythema nodosum is a vascular reaction pattern, most likely a hypersensitivity response involving both cellular and humoral mechanisms (see Chapter 14).

The eruption is sudden with discrete, erythematous, hot, and very tender nodules on the shins, knees, ankles, thighs, buttocks, and sometimes lower arms. The nodules are bright red initially but change to a purplish color and finally become a flat brown pigmentation that slowly fades completely. The total evolution of lesions takes 3 to 4 weeks.

The nodules vary in size from 6 to 8 mm and are usually bilaterally symmetric. There may be only a few lesions or many appearing in crops. New crops may occur periodically. Edema of the ankles and general aching of the legs are common and are aggravated by ambulation.

Cellular changes are probably due to the immunologic processes. Deep dermal inflammation extends down into subcutaneous tissue. Small blood vessels experience mild vasculitis and inflammatory infiltrate with partial obstruction of blood flow.

•••••• Diagnostic Studies and Findings

Physical examination   Characteristic lesion; history consistent with possible precipitating factors

Complete blood count   Increased erythrocyte sedimentation rate; platelet estimate

Biopsy   Deep excision biopsy including subcutaneous tissue; shows histologic changes described previously

Diagnostic studies to isolate underlying disorders   Antistreptolysin titer; throat culture; tuberculosis test; rheumatoid factor; antinuclear factor

•••••• Multidisciplinary Plan

Management of the disease is aimed at identifying and treating the precipitating factor or underlying disorder.

Medications

Analgesics
   Aspirin (ASA), 600 mg po q4-6h
Antiinfective agents
   Systemic antibiotics for underlying infection; may require long-term therapy; specific antibiotic depends on the underlying infection
Corticosteroids
   Intralesional injection of triamcinolone (Aristocort, Kenalog), 5 mg/ml
Potassium iodide, 360-900 mg po qd for 3-4 wk

General Management

Bed rest with legs elevated to reduce pain and swelling
Cool compresses applied to nodules
Support stockings or elastic bandages

NURSING CARE

Nursing Assessment

Lesions

Red, hot, tender nodules (initially) on anterior aspect of lower extremities

Systemic Involvement

Fever; chills; malaise; arthralgia; ankle edema; aching legs

Underlying Disorder

Complete blood count; urinalysis; antistreptolysin titer; tuberculosis test; rheumatoid factor; throat culture; antinuclear factor

Psychosocial Concerns

Concern about body image

Nursing Dx & Intervention

Pain related to biologic factors

* Assess for discomfort.
* Encourage bed rest and elevation of legs *to alleviate aching.*
* Have patient use support hose and elastic bandages *to prevent venous pooling.*
* Apply cool compresses.

Body image disturbance related to cognitive-perceptual factors

* Assess for defining characteristics.
* Encourage patient to express feelings about body, body appearance, or fear of reaction or rejection by others *to begin process of realistic self-evaluation.*
* Assure patient that lesions heal without scarring.

Patient Education/Home Care Planning

1. Help the patient identify potential precipitating factors and eliminate them when possible (such as with drugs).
2. Explain the effects of long-term antibiotic therapy if indicated.
3. Discuss with the patient the management of symptoms: elevation of legs, rest, use of support hose or elastic bandages, and application of cool compresses.

Evaluation

Discomfort is alleviated   Nodules resolve. Skin integrity is restored.

Underlying condition is identified and treated   Symptoms of underlying disorder improve and resolve.

Precipitating factors are eliminated when possible Condition does not recur.

Patient evaluates appearance in realistic manner Patient engages in usual activities when possible and in usual relationships.

INFESTATIONS AND PARASITIC DISORDERS

◼ PEDICULOSIS

Pediculosis is an infestation by lice of the head (pediculosis capitis), the body (pediculosis corporis), or the genital area (pediculosis pubis).

Pediculosis is a highly pruritic and often secondarily infected disorder that results from two species of lice: *Pediculus humanus,* which affects the head and body, and *Pthirus pubis,* which infects the pubic area, the lower abdomen, and sometimes the eyebrows, eyelashes, and scalp.

Pediculosis capitis occurs most frequently in schoolchildren and is easily transmitted by personal contact and by objects such as combs and hats. Itching and excoriation are present. The posterior aspect of the scalp commonly shows the most involvement. The posterior occipital nodes may be enlarged and tender.

Pediculosis corporis is characterized by pruritus and parallel linear excoriations that are frequently secondarily infected. The infesting lice live in the seams of clothing and move onto the skin to feed frequently. Lesions are most common on the shoulders, buttocks, and abdomen. Infestation is associated with unhygienic living conditions ("vagabond's disease").

Pediculosis pubis is transmitted by close personal contact, usually through sexual contact. Infestation is usually in the pubic hair but may occur in the chest or axillary hair, eyebrows, or eyelashes. A sign of infestation is the presence of reddish-brown specks on undergarments as a result of the excreta of lice.

• • • • • Pathophysiology

In pediculosis capitis, injection of saliva from the lice during feeding produces severe pruritus. Scratching causes excoriation, and secondary infection is common. Each day the female louse lays 7 to 10 eggs that hatch in 8 days. The eggs (nits) are cemented to the hair shaft and cannot be dislodged.

In pediculosis corporis the primary lesion is an urticarial papule, which is often obscured by secondary excoriation and infection. With prolonged infestation the skin becomes dry, scaly, and hyperpigmented.

Pediculosis pubis is manifested primarily by itching. The lice ova are commonly attached to the skin at the base of the hair follicle. Discrete, small, 1 to 3 cm, gray-blue macules can be seen on the trunk, thighs, and axillae. These lesions are due to a reaction of the lice's saliva with bilirubin, converting it to biliverdin. Excoriation and secondary infection are uncommon.

• • • • • Diagnostic Studies and Findings

Physical examination Presence of lice or eggs; presence of nonspecific lesion with characteristic distribution

Wood's light Fluorescence of adult louse

Microscopic examination Examination of hair shaft for eggs

• • • • • Multidisciplinary Plan

Medications

Antiinfective agents

Lindane (Kwell) shampoo, cream, or lotion, applied qd for 2 d; application repeated in 10 d; used with caution with young children because of neurotoxicity

Synthetic pyrethrin (RID) liquid applied to dry hair, scalp, and any other infested area; left on 10 minutes then rinsed with warm water, soap, and shampoo; dead lice and eggs removed with nit comb; treatment repeated in 7-10 d; must not exceed two consecutive applications within 24 h

Permethrine (NIX) 1% creme rinse for head lice; applied to towel-dried hair; left on 10 minutes and rinsed out

Ophthalmic preparation of yellow mercury oxide qd for infested eyelashes

Cholinergic agents

Physostigmine (Eserine) 0.25% ophthalmic ointment qd for infested eyelashes

General Management

Rinsing with white vinegar diluted with equal amounts of water followed by washing to remove residual nits from hair

Lice removed from eyelashes with forceps

Body lice eliminated from clothing and bedding by thorough hot washing, hot ironing, boiling, and steaming

Personal articles sealed in a plastic bag for 10 days

NURSING CARE

Nursing Assessment

Local Response to Infestation

Pruritus; excoriation; secondary infection

Infestation

Location and distribution of lesions or local responses

Psychosocial Concerns

Concern that others may react to transmissible infestation

Nursing Dx & Intervention

Impaired skin integrity related to mechanical factors

- Assess for presence of lice, eggs, and lesions.
- Isolate patient until treatment is complete *to prevent transmission.*

- Instruct patient in use of lindane *to kill parasite.*
- Instruct patient to comb hair with fine-toothed comb *to remove eggs after preparation is used.*
- Instruct patient to remove lice from eyelashes with cotton-tipped applicator.
- Instruct patient in good hygiene, meticulous hand washing, and need for short fingernails *to avoid secondary infection.*

Risk for impaired skin integrity related to mechanical factors

- Teach patient how to decontaminate sources of infestation.
- Treat all family members and sexual partners.
- Advise patient that recurrence is common.
- Teach patient importance of not borrowing personal items such as combs.

Situational low self-esteem related to negative self-appraisal

- Assess for defining characteristics (see p. 1680).
- Encourage patient to express feelings about the infestation, embarrassment, or fear of rejection by others *to begin the process of realistic self-evaluation.*
- Assure patient and family that infestation can be treated successfully.

Patient Education/Home Care Planning

1. See under Nursing Dx & Intervention.
2. Explain to the patient that prolonged use of lindane may result in dermatitis.
3. Advise that all household members and sex partners be treated.[6]

Evaluation

Infestation is cleared in patient and affected family members and partners   Pruritus subsides. No new areas of itching or excoriation develop. There are no lice or eggs on examination.

Lesions heal   Excoriations resolve. Skin is intact.

Secondary infection is resolved or avoided   Lesions heal without redness, swelling, or pus.

Infestation does not spread to unaffected family members or intimate contacts   Associates of patient do not develop symptoms. Hair and skin are free of lice or eggs. All family members and sexual partners receive treatment.

Patient evaluates self realistically   Patient verbalizes positive feelings about self.

■ SCABIES

Scabies is a transmissible parasitic infestation chracterized by burrows, pruritus, and excoriations with secondary infection.

Scabies is caused by the *Sarcoptes scabiei* mite. The infestation and lesions occur most commonly on the finger webs, the flexor surfaces of the wrist, and the elbows and axillary folds, along the belt line, and on the lower buttocks. The areolae in women and the genitals in men are particularly susceptible. Lesions do not extend to the face in adults but may do so in infants.

Scabies is transmitted readily by personal contact. It characteristically spreads to other family members, to intimate contacts, and between schoolchildren. It is not transmitted by clothing, bedding, or inanimate objects. Infestation can occur from cats, dogs, and other small animals, but the animal scabies mite does not burrow, only feeds.

••••• Pathophysiology

The impregnated female mite burrows into the stratum corneum and forms a small tunnel that is seen as a fine, wavy, dark line. The burrow is a few millimeters to 1 cm long with a minute papule at the open end. The mite extends the burrow daily and deposits eggs and feces in it (Figure 5-6).

The lesions are at first asymptomatic. After several weeks, the person becomes sensitized to the mite and itching becomes noticeable. The itching is intense and more severe at night. The itching intensifies over a period of several weeks. The burrows and papules are often obscured by secondary excoriation, bacterial infection, crusting, and lichenification. A fine rash is present that consists of papules of various sizes.

••••• Diagnostic Studies and Findings

Physical examination   Burrows; nonspecific excoriations; papules with characteristic distribution; intense itching that worsens at night; burrow ink test (BIT): blue or black felt-tipped pen is applied to suspected lesions and partially removed with alcohol pad: ink is retained in the burrows

Scrapings   Taken from burrow and placed in oil; presence of mite on microscopic examination

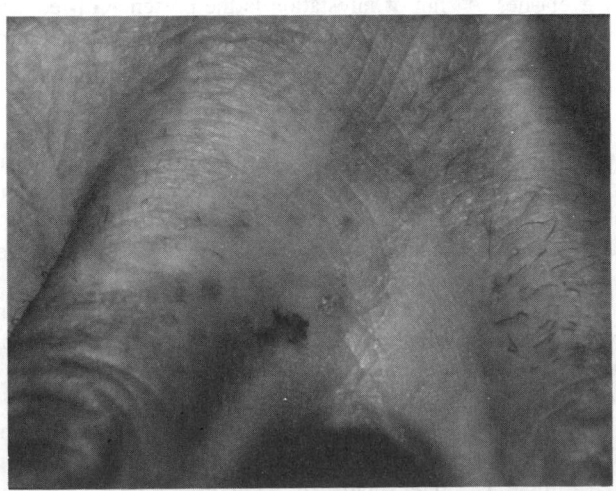

Figure 5-6 Scabies burrow. (Courtesy of Stephen B, Tucker, M.D., Department of Dermatology, University of Texas Health Science Center at Houston.)

•••••• Multidisciplinary Plan

Medications

Antiinfective agents

Permethrine cream 5% (Elimite) applied to entire body and left on 18-24 h and then washed off; lacks systemic toxicity

Benzyl benzoate topical emulsion 20%-25%; applied to entire cutaneous surface from neck down; left on 12-24 h and then washed off; procedure repeated after 2 d; third treatment may be necessary in 2 wk

Lindane (Kwell) 1% cream or lotion applied according to above instructions; not used for young children because of neurotoxicity; not recommended during pregnancy

Sulfur ointment 5%-10% applied nightly for 3 nights, with previous applications washed off before new application; washed off thoroughly 24 h after final application; used for infants

Crotamiton (Eurax) applied with benzyl benzoate; less irritating than benzyl benzoate

Corticosteroids

Fluorinated corticosteroid ointment 1% applied topically bid, tid, or qid for persistent itching

General Management

Clothing and linens washed and dried on hot cycles

Personal articles sealed in a plastic bag for 10 days

NURSING CARE

Nursing Assessment

Lesion

Linear gray-brown burrows a few millimeters in length; excoriation; secondary infection; crusting; papules; vesicles; lichenification

Local Response to Infestation

Intense itching out of proportion to visible signs; itching worse at night

Psychosocial Concerns

Concern that others may react to transmissible infestation

Nursing Dx & Intervention

Impaired skin integrity related to mechanical factors

- Assess lesions for characteristics.
- Isolate patient until treatment is completed *to prevent transmission.*
- Instruct patient in meticulous hand washing and good hygiene *to avoid secondary infection.*
- Have patient's fingernails cut short *to avoid excoriation from scratching.*
- Instruct patient in use of treatment lotion; all skin surfaces except face must be covered.

Risk for impaired skin integrity related to mechanical factors

- Have all family members and sexual partners treated.
- Have patient notify sexual contacts.
- Instruct patient and family in modes of infestation and transmission.

Situational low self-esteem related to negative self-appraisal

- Assess for defining characteristics.
- Prepare patient and family for potential reaction of others to transmissible infestation.
- Encourage patient to express feelings about the infestation, embarrassment, or fear of rejection by others *to begin the process of realistic self-evaluation.*
- Assure patient and family that infestation can be treated successfully.

Patient Education/Home Care Planning

1. Explain to the patient and family that treatment irritates the skin and does not quickly reduce the pruritus; discomfort may persist for a few weeks.
2. Demonstrate the use of cool soaks and compresses to reduce itching after treatment is complete.
3. Stress the importance of the correct use of treatment lotion to avoid neurotoxicity and undue irritation.
4. Advise that all family members and sex partners be treated.

Evaluation

Infestation is cleared in patient and affected family members and partners No new papules, burrows, or areas of itching develop.

Lesions heal Excoriations resolve. Skin is intact.

Secondary infection is resolved or avoided Lesions heal without redness, swelling, crusts, or pus.

Infestation does not spread to seemingly unaffected family members or sexual partners These people do not develop symptoms of infestation, or they seek treatment if symptoms develop.

Patient evaluates self realistically Patient verbalizes positive feelings about self.

▌ ARACHNID AND HYMENOPTERA BITES

▌ Arachnids are ticks, spiders, and scorpions; Hymenoptera are bees, wasps, yellow jackets, and ants. Their bites cause toxic and allergic reactions as a result of the injection of a venom or toxin.

Tick bites Tick bites are common in woods and fields throughout the United States. The tick attaches itself to a passing animal or person and after biting remains attached to the skin for several days or longer. Ticks transmit Rocky Mountain spotted fever, Q fever, relapsing fever, and Lyme disease. (See Chapter 13.) The tick bite is initially painless but begins to itch after several days. Infiltration and erythema develop around the bite with formation of firm, discrete, intensely pruritic nodules that may be present for several months or longer.

Systemic symptoms attributed to a toxin include fever, malaise, headache, and abdominal pain. Several species of ticks inject a salivary neurotoxin that causes paralysis. Paresthesia and pain in the lower extremities, weakness, and incoordination develop. The condition may progress to respiratory failure and death from bulbar involvement. Symptoms clear dramatically once the tick is removed.

Spider bites   The most important spider bites are caused by the black widow and brown recluse spiders. The black widow is common throughout the United States and southern Canada. It lives in old lumber, unused sheds, and outdoor toilets and may be found in attics, drawers, and closets. Only the female bites and only in self-defense. The female is recognized by her coal black coloring with an hourglass-shaped red or orange marking on the underside of the abdomen.

The black widow bite results from the injection of a neurotoxic venom through a clawlike appendage. The bite, which may go unnoticed, is felt as a pinprick followed by a dull numbing pain. Local necrosis may cause a small ulcer at the site. Within 10 to 60 minutes muscle spasms occur locally and then spread to include all extremities and the trunk. Excruciating pain is felt in waves. The attack subsides after several hours.

Systemic symptoms may include restlessness, vertigo, sweating, chills, pallor, hyperactive reflexes, hypertension, tachycardia, thready pulse, nausea and vomiting, headache, eyelid edema, urticaria, pruritus, and fever. Ascending paralysis, severe hypotension, circulatory collapse, convulsions, and death may result. Mortality is less than 1%.

The brown recluse spider is common in the south-central United States and is usually found in dark areas such as drawers and closets. It commonly bites people when they are asleep. The spider is small and light to dark brown, with a light violin-shaped mark on its head. The female is more dangerous than the male. Most bites occur between April and October.

Brown recluse venom is coagulotoxic. Pain and local symptoms develop 2 to 8 hours after the bite. Localized vasoconstriction causes ischemic necrosis at the site. The area is red with blisters and blebs surrounded by ischemia. After several days the center becomes dark and hard. After 2 weeks it becomes depressed, demarcated, and necrotic, and a large open ulcer forms. The ulcer may take several weeks to heal and may require grafting.

Systemic symptoms include fever, chills, malaise, weakness, arthralgia, nausea, vomiting, petechiae, hemolysis, and thrombocytopenia.

Scorpion bites   Scorpions are found throughout the United States but are most common in the southern United States and Mexico. The two deadly species are found in the southwest United States.

Scorpions are nocturnal and photophobic. They sting by means of a hooked caudal stinger that discharges venom. Most stings occur during the warmer months. Nonlethal bites cause local swelling, tenderness, pain, a sharp burning sensation, skin discoloration, paresthesia, regional lymphadenopathy, and rarely, anaphylaxis. Lethal bites are neurotoxic and result in pain, hyperesthesia followed by hypoesthesia, drowsiness, itching of the nose, mouth, and throat, slurred speech, incontinence, vomiting, and convulsions. Symptoms last 24 to 48 hours. Death may follow cardiovascular or respiratory failure. Mortality is less than 1%.

Bee, wasp, hornet, yellow jacket, and ant stings   All female Hymenoptera have an egg-laying organ (stinger) that can be used for defense or offense. The venom of bees, hornets, wasps, and yellow jackets contains four to six distinct chemical compounds, each of which can produce an allergic reaction. The venoms of all stinging Hymenoptera are closely related and therefore cross-sensitizing.

Local reactions include swelling, pain, erythema, urticaria, and pruritus. Generalized allergic reactions include nausea, vomiting, diarrhea, urticaria, pruritus, and anaphylaxis, with shortness of breath, tightness in the chest, difficulty swallowing, anxiety, convulsions, or unconsciousness. Delayed reaction (serum sickness) occurs 1 to 4 weeks after the sting and is characterized by fever, malaise, lymphadenopathy, rash, urticaria, and arthralgia.

•••••• Pathophysiology

The local or systemic response to injection of a venom occurs as a result of direct action of the venom on susceptible cells, IgE-mediated humoral immune response (type I), and immune complex humoral response (type III).

The arthropod or Hymenoptera venom is toxic to all humans. The biologically active venom works directly on susceptible cells (such as nerve cells and blood cells). The protein component of the venom may contain enzymes that cause cell lysis, histamine release, anticoagulation, or interference with neuromuscular transmission.

The IgE-mediated immune response occurs in people who are sensitive to the protein component of the venom, which acts as an antigen. These people have come in contact with the allergen in the past and have become sensitized rather than immunized. Sensitization triggers the synthesis of specific antiallergenic IgE antibodies. On subsequent contact with the allergen, the person responds with a type I immune reaction.

IgE immunoglobulins are bound to mast cells and basophils. Mast cells are found in all body tissues, close to blood vessels, and in abundance in the skin. Basophils circulate as leukocytes in the blood. Both mast cells and basophils contain potent pharmacologically active substances such as histamine, bradykinin, serotonin, and other vasoactive amines. The venom (antigen) becomes bound to the IgE on the surface of the cell, creating degranulation of the cell that releases the active agents. These mediators cause increased vascular permeability and smooth muscle contraction. Histamine seems to be the most important agent. Its release causes peripheral vasodilation, increased permeability of capillaries with subsequent loss of plasma from the circulation, smooth muscle constriction (as in the bronchi), and increased mucous gland secretion. If the agents remain confined to the area of the bite, the tissue reaction remains localized (local anaphylaxis) with tissue swelling, wheal formation, and itching. If the mediators are released systemically, systemic anaphylaxis (anaphylactic shock) may result. The widespread response to histamine release causes profound bronchoconstriction and vasodilation with subsequent circulatory collapse. The severity of the reaction depends on the amount of the sensitizing dose, the amount and distribution of the IgE antibodies, and the dose of toxin that causes the reaction.

A type III (immune complex) reaction, or serum sickness, can develop 1 to 3 weeks after the antigen is injected. The antigen initiates an immune response, and antibodies are formed. The response is mediated by IgG or IgM and complement. The immune complexes are deposited in joints, blood vessels, kidneys, and the heart. Platelet aggregation is caused by the collection of immune complexes and complement along blood vessel walls. Anaphylatoxins are released during activation of the complement system, causing a severe inflammatory response.

•••••• Diagnostic Studies and Findings

Physical examination Puncture wound with characteristic symptoms

Complete blood count Eosiniphilia in type I reaction

Direct immunofluorescence Presence of antigen, immunoglobulin, or complement in type III reaction

•••••• Multidisciplinary Plan

Surgery

Skin grafting—split-thickness graft to close brown recluse spider bite

Medications

For anaphylaxis

Bronchodilators

Epinephrine (Adrenalin), 1:1000 for allergic reactions, 0.3-0.5 ml subcutaneously or IM for mild or severe reactions repeated q5-20min as needed; 0.1-0.2 ml subcutaneously injected into site to decrease absorption of antigen; 0.25-0.5 ml IV in 10 ml saline repeated in 5-10 min for severe anaphylaxis with cardiovascular involvement

Epinephrine 1:200 aqueous suspension, 0.3 ml subcutaneously; long-acting for severe reactions without cardiovascular involvement after edema has subsided

Aminophylline (Aminodur, Lixaminol, Phyllacontin, Somopyllin) for bronchospasm, 6 mg/kg IV over 10-20 min followed by 0.5 mg/kg/h IV

Antihistamines

Diphenhydramine (Benadryl), 50-100 mg IV

Adrenergic agents

Isoproterenol (Isuprel, Proterenol), 1 mg diluted in 500 ml D_5W infused at rate of 0.5-1 ml/min for myocardial insufficiency

Vasoconstrictors for prolonged hypotension

Norepinephrine (Levophed, Levarterenol), 8-12 µg/min IV of 4 µg/ml dilution, titrated

Metaraminol (Aramine), 15-100 mg/500 ml D_5W IV, titrated, for adults; 0.4 mg/kg IV for children

Corticosteroids

Hydrocortisone, 100 mg IV for prolonged symptoms

Oral antihistamines

Diphenhydramine (Benadryl), 25-50 mg po qid for mild reaction

For toxins

Antivenin, 1 ampule IV in 10-50 ml saline for black widow and scorpion bites

Anticonvulsant muscle relaxants

Calcium gluconate 10% 10 ml IV slowly q4h

Methocarbamol (Delaxin, Forbaxin, Metho-500, Robaxin, others), 300 mg/min IV to total of 3 g/d

Orphenadrine (Flexon, Flexoject, Norflex, others), 60 mg IV q12h

For convulsions from scorpion bites

Phenobarbital, 30-60 mg/min IV up to 600 mg

Corticosteroids

Dexamethasone (Decadron, Hexadrol), 4 mg IM q6h for brown recluse spider bites during acute phase, then in decremental doses

Antihistamines

Diphenhydramine (Benadryl), 25-50 mg po qid

Antiinfective agents

Bacitracin or Neosporin applied tid or qid as topical antibiotic for brown recluse spider bite

Immunologic agents

Tetanus prophylaxis as indicated with tetanus toxoid, 0.5 ml IM

Intravenous infusion with D_5W or lactated Ringer's solution

General Management

Scraping to remove stinger if present; do not squeeze or pinch because retained venom sacs discharge residual venom

Application of meat tenderizer paste (containing proteolytic enzyme) to sting site

Hospitalization for observation or ventilator support

Prevention (see under Patient Education)

NURSING CARE

Nursing Assessment

Local Response

Presence or absence of stinger; pain, itching; edema; blister; ulcerations; tissue necrosis

Systemic Response

Anxiety; feeling of doom; fever; malaise

Respiratory

Respiratory distress; tightness in chest; shortness of breath; wheezing; dyspnea

Cardiovascular

Tachycardia; bradycardia; hypotension; imperceptible pulse; pallor

Musculoskeletal

Cramping; pain; rigidity; weakness

Gastrointestinal

Nausea; vomiting; diarrhea; cramping; constipation

Skin

Flushing; diffuse erythema; urticaria; pruritus

Delayed Response

One to 4 weeks after sting; fever; malaise; lymphadenopathy; arthralgia; rash; urticaria

Psychosocial Concerns

Concern about body image as a result of disfigurement, depending on severity of tissue damage; fear of insects, spiders, bees, and scorpions

Nursing Dx & Intervention

Ineffective breathing pattern related to tracheobronchial obstruction

- Assess for shortness of breath, wheezing, dyspnea.
- Maintain airway.
- In collaboration with physician, perform oropharyngeal suctioning as needed *to clear secretions.*
- Provide oxygen by cannula or mask.
- Position *for ease of respiration.*
- Administer drugs as indicated *for control of symptoms.*

Decreased cardiac output related to mechanical factors; fluid volume deficit related to failure of regulatory mechanisms

- Monitor vital signs *to detect circulatory compromise.*
- Initiate intravenous line in collaboration with physician *to provide vascular access for fluids and medications.*
- Administer drugs as indicated *to control symptoms.*

Impaired skin integrity related to chemical substance

- Apply meat tenderizer paste *to neutralize venom.*
- Apply ice packs *to decrease pain and swelling and to limit venom absorption.*
- Keep patient quiet *to limit venom circulation.*

- Remove stinger by scraping *to prevent further discharge of retained venom by squeezing.*
- Remove tick; do not pull because head and mouth may remain embedded; apply heat to body and tick will back out, or cover with oil, which blocks its breathing and causes it to withdraw.
- Clean bite with antiseptic *to prevent infection.*
- Clean brown recluse bite with 1:20 Burow's solution *to prevent infection.*

Pain related to biologic factors

- Assess for discomfort.
- Apply ice packs to area *to reduce swelling.*
- Apply meat tenderizer *to neutralize venom.*

Fear (of arachnids and Hymenoptera) related to environmental stimuli

- Assess for defining characteristics.
- Encourage patient to express fears.
- Help patient develop preventive measures (see under Patient Education).

Body image disturbance related to cognitive-perceptual factors

- Assess for presence of defining characteristics.
- Encourage patient to express feelings about body, body appearance, or fear of reaction or rejection by others *to begin process of realistic self-evaluation.*
- Reassure patient with disfiguring ulcer that skin grafting can improve appearance.

Patient Education/Home Care Planning

1. Explain to patients who are sensitive to stings the need to carry an emergency kit that has an antihistamine and epinephrine. Teach the patient or a family member or friend how to inject epinephrine.
2. Explain to patients who are sensitive to stings to wear or carry medical alert information and identification.
3. Refer the patient to an allergist for desensitization.
4. Explain to the patient how to remove ticks and stingers.
5. Discuss with the patient and family preventive measures such as wearing protective clothing when outdoors, spraying areas of spider infestation with creosote every 2 months, inspecting clothing before putting it on in infested areas, not wearing bright colors or scents that attract bees when outdoors, and inspecting pets and people for ticks after a visit to a tick-infested area.
6. Encourage the patient and family to keep the site of the bite clean by washing two or three times daily with warm soapy water or water with hydrogen peroxide; apply antibiotic ointment as needed.
7. Demonstrate how to change the dressing if needed.

Evaluation

Local toxic reaction is minimized   Stinger or tick is removed correctly, and treatment is initiated immediately. Areas of ulceration and necrosis are limited. Pain is alleviated.

Systemic response is avoided or resolved   Cardiovascular, neurologic, musculoskeletal, or gastrointestinal symptoms are avoided or resolved. Respirations are regular and easy. Pulse rate is 60 to 100 and regular. Blood pressure is within patient's usual limits. Reflexes, sensation, and motion are intact. Patient has urinary continence and bowel function. There is no malaise, fever, lymphadenopathy, arthralgia, rash, or urticaria after delayed response.

Lesions heal   Areas of necrosis, ulceration, and blistering reepithelialize. Skin is intact and free of infection.

Sensitized patients institute precautionary measures   Patient carries medical alert information and identification. Patient carries emergency kit. Patient, family member, or friend demonstrates injection of epinephrine. Patient arranges to see allergist for desensitization.

Psychosocial concerns are addressed   Patient expresses feelings about body appearance. Patient with disfiguring ulcer has opportunity to seek surgical interventions. Patient expresses fears about arachnids and hymenoptera. Patient discusses preventive measures.

LESIONS CAUSED BY BEETLES AND CATERPILLARS

Toxic reactions to beetles and caterpillars occur from contact with the toxin on the skin.

Blister beetles produce local irritation and blistering if they are crushed while on the skin surface. Damage to the beetle causes release of a toxic substance in the insect's body fluids.

More than 50 species of caterpillars possess spines that contain a venom capable of producing dermatitis on human skin. These caterpillars are widely distributed throughout the United States and Canada. Contact with the venom occurs from direct contact with the insect or its nest or from windblown hairs. Papular lesions or urticaria may develop at the site or elsewhere on the body. The venom produces a stinging sensation followed by swelling and erythema. Symptoms can occur systemically, depending on the species and the amount of venom the person receives. Painful and persistent nodules are formed if the toxin comes in contact with the conjunctiva.

• • • • • • Pathophysiology

The venom produces a direct toxic response to human tissue. The caterpillar's venom is biologically active and causes histamine release, anticoagulation, fibrinolysis, and plasminogen activity. The toxins are capable of producing impaired cellular activity or cellular destruction.

• • • • • • Diagnostic Studies and Findings

Physical examination   Lesion consistent with history of beetle or caterpillar contact

• • • • • • Multidisciplinary Plan

Medications

Corticosteroids
   Topical corticosteroid for skin inflammation; hydrocortisone, 1% applied tid
   Ophthalmic corticosteroid and analgesic for eye injury; cortisporin ophthalmic solution, 1-2 drops qid

NURSING CARE

Nursing Assessment

Local Reaction

   Pain; swelling; blister; papule; urticaria; necrosis

Systemic Reaction

   Widespread papular lesions; urticaria

Nursing Dx & Intervention

Impaired skin integrity related to chemical factors

- Assess for lesions.
- Flush skin with copious amounts of water and scrub gently with soap and water *to remove toxin.*
- Irrigate eye with copious amounts of normal saline *to remove toxin.*

Patient Education/Home Care Planning

1. Instruct the patient to avoid crushing beetles.
2. Teach the patient how to flush the skin and eye.
3. Teach the patient to keep the site clean by washing two or three times a day with soap and water.
4. Show the patient how to use eye drops.

Evaluation

Lesions heal   Urticaria, blisters, or papules resolve. Necrotic areas reepithelialize. Pain is alleviated. Skin is intact and free of infection. Eye symptoms or visual disturbances resolve.

LESIONS CAUSED BY FLEAS, FLIES, AND MOSQUITOES

Toxic reactions to fleas, flies, and mosquitoes occur as a result of saliva that is injected during feeding.

Fleas   Any of the human or domestic animal fleas will attack humans. Adult fleas are attracted to moving objects and leap to attack them. Thus flea bites are often found on the ankles or lower legs. The bites are characteristically found in groups of three on the ankles, legs, or waist. The flea penetrates the skin, feeds, and then crawls to a higher location until stopped by constrictive clothing.

A flea bite usually results in a small wheal with a hemorrhagic puncture at the center. In susceptible persons the flea bite produces larger wheals, urticaria, intensely pruritic papules, bullae, and small necrotic ulcers. Flea bites are usually harmless but can produce a severe reaction in sensitive persons.

Flies   There are innumerable biting flies in the United States. Most common are the blackflies, houseflies, deer flies, gadflies, and dog or stable flies. Most flies feed during the day or at dusk and attack in swarms on exposed parts of the body such as the face, neck, and arms. Fly-transmitted tularemia occurs in the central and western United States.

Fly bites are painful and pruritic for several days. Urticaria may occur as a result of a protein in the fly's saliva.

Mosquitoes   Mosquitoes are important because they transmit viral encephalitis, dengue fever, yellow fever, malaria, and filariasis. Lesions are produced on the skin when the mosquito feeds and deposits droplets of saliva. These lesions commonly occur on exposed areas of the hands, arms, face, and legs.

Mosquitoes are attracted by lights, dark clothing, and the presence of arm-blooded creatures. In most species the female mosquito is the bloodsucking biter.

The usual mosquito bite produces transient local irritation and pruritic erythematous papules. Large numbers of bites can produce intense pruritus. Urticaria and serum sickness can develop in sensitive people.

•••••• Pathophysiology

For an explanation of toxic reactions and antigen-antibody reactions see p. 486.

•••••• Diagnostic Studies and Findings

Physical examination   Puncture wound with characteristic symptoms

•••••• Multidisciplinary Plan

For treatment of systemic reactions see p. 487.

Medications

Corticosteroids
   Glucocorticoid ointment (e.g., hydrocortisone 1%) with 0.5% menthol and 0.5% phenol applied topically to lesions ql-2h
Antiinfective agents
Topical antibiotics
   Bacitracin or Neosporin applied qd or bid

General Management

Prevention (see under Patient Education)

NURSING CARE

Nursing Assessment

Local Response

Puncture wound with any of the following: pain, pruritus, wheal, urticaria, erythematous papule, bullae, or small necrotic ulcer; secondary infection; pain, swelling, tenderness, exudate

Systemic Response

See p. 488.

Serum Sickness

Fever; malaise; lymphadenopathy; arthralgia; rash; urticaria

Nursing Dx & Intervention

Impaired skin integrity related to chemical and mechanical factors

- Assess for lesion, pain, and pruritus.
- Apply ice to puncture wound *to decrease pain and swelling.*
- Instruct patient to trim fingernails *to decrease damage and prevent secondary infection from scratching.*
- Instruct patient in good hygiene and hand washing *to prevent secondary infection.*

Risk for impaired skin integrity related to chemical and mechanical factors

- Instruct patient in personal and prophylactic environmental control; see under Patient Education.

Patient Education/Home Care Planning

1. Discuss with the patient how to keep the lesion clean by washing two or three times a day with soap and water.
2. Teach the patient how to change the dressing for infected lesions.
3. Explain to the patient the correct use of appropriate insect repellents:
   a. For flies: repellent should contain at least 20% *N,N*-diethyl-*m*-toluamide, reapply every 1 to 2 hours or after swimming.
   b. For mosquitoes: repellent should contain at least 20% *N,N*-diethyl-*m*-toluamide, indalone, or dimethyl pthalate; reapply every 1 to 2 hours or after swimming.
4. Explain to the patient the control of fleas in the environment and on animals.
   a. Environment: apply dimpylate 1%, lindane 1%, malathion 3%, methoxychlor 5%, ronnel 1%, or trichlorfon 1% in kerosene; use according to instructions on container.

b. Animals and furniture: dust with malathion 4% powder, rotenone 1% powder, or methoxychlor 10%; use according to instructions on container. Repeat procedure at 2-week intervals to eliminate newly hatching fleas.

Evaluation

Lesions heal   Puncture wound resolves. Pain disappears. Skin is intact and free of infection.

Systemic responses resolve   There is no fever, malaise, lymphadenopathy, arthralgia, rash, or urticaria. Cardiovascular, neurologic, gastrointestinal, and musculoskeletal symptoms are also resolved.

Patient takes precautionary measures and uses environmental control   No new lesions occur.

DERMATITIS

ECZEMATOUS DERMATITIS (ECZEMA)

Eczematous dermatitis is a superficial inflammation of the skin that is characterized by vesicles, redness, edema, oozing, crusting, scaling, and itching.

Eczematous dermatitis is a reaction pattern of the skin. Several forms of dermatitis occur, including primary contact dermatitis, allergic contact dermatitis, atopic dermatitis, diaper dermatitis, and seborrheic dermatitis. The common feature of the various forms is the breakdown of the epidermis, usually as a result of intracellular vesiculation. Eczematous dermatitis is the model for understanding the other forms of dermatitis. The treatments are similar, and the nursing care is virtually the same. Individual differences are identified in the following discussion when appropriate.

•••••• Pathophysiology

Eczematous dermatitis can be classified as acute, subacute, or chronic. The skin responds to a wide variety of noxious stimuli with a limited number of changes, including vasodilation, edema of the upper dermis, inflammatory cell infiltration of the upper dermis and epidermis, and breakdown of epidermal cells. Vesicles or bullae form when fluid accumulates between epidermal cells (spongiosis) or when there are changes within the cell itself.

The result of this inflammatory process is a skin surface that is erythematous (from vasodilation), edematous, exudative, or eroded (from vesicle formation), and crusted or scabbed (from infection or an accumulation of serous exudate). Thickening and scaling occur from attempted or exaggerated repair efforts (hyperkeratosis or parakeratosis).

Table 5-1 summarizes the clinical features and changes occurring in eczematous dermatitis. Acute dermatitis becomes subacute as it heals, as a result of either treatment or natural repair processes. Subacute eczematous dermatitis can resolve or become chronic if exposure to noxious stimuli persists. Acute, subacute, and chronic eczematous dermatitis may occur simultaneously.

•••••• Diagnostic Studies and Findings

See discussions of contact dermatitis, atopic dermatitis, and seborrheic dermatitis.

Physical examination   Characteristic eruption; history congruent with specific forms of eczematous dermatitis

•••••• Multidisciplinary Plan

Table 5-2 summarizes the specific treatment measures for the different classes of eczematous dermatitis.

■ TABLE 5-1 Clinical Features and Changes in Eczematous Dermatitis

	Acute	Subacute	Chronic
Clinical features	Erythema; exudate; weeping vesicles; crusts; pruritus	Less erythema; involuting vesicles; excoriation; some scaling; pruritus	Dryness; scaling; lichenification; pruritus
Microscopic changes	Vasodilation; edema; inflammatory infiltrates; spongiotic vesicles	Less vasodilation, inflammatory infiltrates, and vesiculation; parakeratosis; hyperkeratosis; acanthosis	Hyperkeratosis; no frank vesicles; acanthosis

■ TABLE 5-2 Summary of Treatments for Eczematous Dermatitis

	Acute	Subacute	Chronic
Chemotherapeutic	Antihistamines; systemic corticosteroids; topical corticosteroids (water miscible); topical antibacterials; topical antifungals	Topical corticosteroids in emollient base	Keratolytic agents; tars; topical corticosteroids
Supportive	Wet dressings (Burow's, saline, or tap water)	Oil-in-water compresses; emollient creams	Oil soaks or compresses; occlusive dressings; hydration

Medications

Antipruritic agents

Antihistamines

Cyproheptadine (Cyprohepadine, Periactin), 12-16 mg/d po in divided doses

Trimeprazine (Temaril), 2.5 mg po qid

Hydroxyzine (Atarax, Vistaril), 25-100 mg po tid or qid

Corticosteroids

Systemic

Prednisone, 40-80 mg po in divided doses; dosage depends on severity of condition

Topical

Hydrocortisone (Cort-Dome, others), 1% tid or qid

Betamethasone valerate (Valisone), 0.1% tid or qid

Antiinfective agents

Systemic—for secondary infection; specific drug and dosage depend on infecting organism and severity of condition

Topical antibacterials

Bacitracin or Neosporin applied tid or qid

Topical antifungals

Nystatin (Mycostatin, Nilstat, others), miconazole (Monistat-Derm), or clotrimazole (Lotrimin, Mycelex), applied bid

Keratolytics

Salicylic acid, 3%-5% added to topical corticosteroid

Urea, 10%-20% added to topical corticosteroids

General Management (see pp. 526 to 528)

Wet Burow's dressings, saline, and plain water dressings

Occlusive dressings

Oil-in-water compresses

Hydration

NURSING CARE

Nursing Assessment

Eruption

Clinical features as described in Table 5-1

Secondary Infection

Purulent drainage; fever; tenderness; regional lymphadenopathy

Psychosocial Concerns

Concern with body image; inability to sleep because of pruritus

Nursing Dx & Intervention

Impaired skin integrity related to mechanical factors

- Assess for characteristics of lesions (Table 5-1).
- Instruct patient in hand washing and good hygiene *to prevent secondary infection.*
- Instruct patient to cut fingernails short *to decrease trauma and secondary infection.*
- Apply dressings; wet, oil, or occlusive, as indicated (see p. 527).
- Scrub crusted lesions gently with antibacterial soap *to debride.*
- Establish realistic therapeutic regimen with patient *to alleviate patient's frustration.*
- Instruct patient in use of medications.

Patient problem: pruritus related to inflammatory process

- Assess for discomfort.
- Apply cool compresses for wet skin or oil compresses for dry skin *to soothe itching and discomfort.*
- Instruct patient in use of antipruritics *to relieve itching.*

Body image disturbance related to cognitive-perceptual factors

- Assess patient's perception of personal appearance.
- Encourage patient to express feelings about body, body appearance, or fear of reaction or rejection by others *to begin process of realistic self-evaluation.*
- Encourage development of other interests *so skin condition does not become focal point of patient's existence.*

Patient Education/Home Care Planning

1. Demonstrate the application of compresses, soaks, and scrubs using aseptic technique.
2. Discuss with the patient the use and side effects of medications.
3. Explain to the patient and family that successful therapy requires patience, that therapy may be long term, and that results may not be immediate.
4. Discuss with the patient the signs and symptoms of secondary infection and the necessity of seeking medical treatment if they occur.

Evaluation

Eruption improves Erythema, exudate, crusts, dryness, scaling, and pruritus are decreased. Excoriated areas reepithelialize.

Pruritus is alleviated There are fewer areas of excoriation. Patient is able to sleep.

Secondary infection is avoided Lesions heal without purulent exudate. Temperature is normal.

Patient evaluates his or her appearance in a realistic manner Patient engages in usual activities and relationships.

■ CONTACT DERMATITIS

Contact dermatitis is an acute or chronic inflammation of the skin caused by external factors (primary irritant dermatitis) or specific sensitizers (allergic contact dermatitis).

Contact dermatitis is a form of eczematous dermatitis (see p. 491). Primary irritant dermatitis is caused by irritation from various chemical and biologic substances, including acids, alkalies, solvents, detergents, oils, salts, secretions, and excretions. Chronic hand dermatitis ("housewife's eczema") and industrial dermatoses are common primary irritant dermatoses. The degree of irritation depends on the physical and chemical characteristics of the substance and the degree and time of exposure. The amount of inflammation varies from person to person and depends on factors such as race, degree and pH of perspiration, type of skin, preexisting disease, and family history. People with little skin pigmentation are more susceptible to the effects of irritants.

Allergic contact dermatitis is a manifestation of delayed hypersensitivity. The allergen is an environmental substance to which the person has become sensitized. Genetically predisposed people and those who have had a previous episode of allergic contact dermatitis are more likely to experience episodes of the disorder. The most common causes of allergic contact dermatitis are chemicals that have a high sensitizing index, including certain plants (tulips and chrysanthemums), plant oils (poison ivy, oak, and sumac), nickel, chrome, rubber, and paraphenylenediamine (an ingredient in many dyes).

The severity of the reaction depends on how long and frequent the contact is. Because allergic contact dermatitis is enhanced by friction and pressure, the addition of these factors to simple exposure produces a more severe reaction.

•••••• Pathophysiology

The irritating substances of primary irritant dermatitis cause damage to the stratum corneum, alters its elasticity, and change the physical features of the skin's lipid film. This impairs the barrier function of the skin and allows absorption of the irritating substance and the subsequent changes of eczematous dermatitis. The basic features of primary irritant dermatitis are the same as those of eczematous dermatitis (see pp. 491 to 492). The condition can be acute, subacute, or chronic. Primary irritant dermatitis is frequently complicated by secondary bacterial infection.

Allergic contact dermatitis is a cell-mediated, type IV immune response (see Chapter 14). The sensitizing chemical (hapten) enters the epidermis through the stratum corneum and combines with epidermal proteins to form a new molecule (hapten-protein or hapten-carrier complex) that has antigenic potential. This molecule enters the local cutaneous lymphoid tissue, where specific committed lymphocytes are developed and selectively directed against the antigen. Subsequent exposure to the hapten results in release of the committed lymphocytes around the capillary endothelial cells with the development of inflammation and eczematous dermatitis.

•••••• Diagnostic Studies and Findings

Physical examination   Characteristic history of contact with irritating or sensitizing substance; detailed history essential

Patch test (see Part Three)   Usually positive to allergen in allergic contact dermatitis; should not be performed if patient has active acute dermatitis

•••••• Multidisciplinary Plan

Management is directed toward identification and elimination of the precipitating factor.

General Management

Tepid tub baths with Aveeno, 1 cup to ½ tub, bid-tid for acute, severe conditions with marked edema and bullae

NURSING CARE

Nursing Assessment

Eruption

Erythema; exudate, vesicles; crusts; scaling; dryness; lichenification; pruritus; location and distribution of eruption; history of eruption; site of initial eruption; history of contact with irritating or sensitizing substances; pattern of flare-ups

Secondary Infection

Purulent drainage; fever; tenderness; regional lymphadenopathy

Psychosocial Concerns

Concern with body image; inability to sleep

Nursing Dx & Intervention

See p. 492.

Patient Education/Home Care Planning

1. Discuss with the patient how to eliminate or avoid the precipitating factors.

Evaluation

Precipitating factor is identified and avoided   There are no recurrent episodes of dermatitis.

▪ ATOPIC DERMATITIS

Atopic dermatitis is a chronic, superficial, pruritic, inflammatory response of the skin that is often associated with other atopic diseases (asthma, hay fever, and allergic rhinitis).

Atopy refers to a type I immunologic response that is hereditary (see Chapter 14). Patients with atopic dermatitis usually have high serum levels of IgE. Patients with atopic dermatitis experience vasomotor changes, great susceptibility to environmental irritants, and susceptibility to bacterial and viral infections. Atopic dermatitis is associated with ichthyosis and xerosis and with numerous abnormalities of humoral and cell-mediated immunity.

Patients with atopic dermatitis have dry, highly sensitive skin with a lowered threshold to pruritus, so that a minor stimulus causes exaggerated itching. Scratching leads to epidermal breakdown and damage to nerve endings, which in turn increase the itch sensation. This itch-scratch cycle is characteristic of atopic dermatitis.

Atopic dermatitis can begin at any time. There are usually three phases: an infantile phase (3 or 4 months to 2 years of age), the childhood phase (4 to 10 or 12 years), and the adolescent and young adult phase. The condition gradually improves.

This section addresses only the adolescent and young adult phase.

•••••• Pathophysiology

The disease is the result of a type I immunologic response. The findings are the same as those of eczematous dermatitis and may be acute, subacute, or chronic (see discussion of eczematous dermatitis).

There is a great tendency toward vasoconstriction of superficial blood vessels, decreased response to cooling and warmth, increased sweat production in flexor areas, and a blanch phenomenon on stroking (white dermographism). Cold and low humidity are poorly tolerated. Heat and high humidity are also poorly tolerated; vasodilation increases the inflammatory response, thereby aggravating the dermatitis and causing increased itching. Psychologic and emotional factors do not play a causative role but do modify symptoms. Food allergies may exacerbate the skin disease in some patients, and a good history is extremely important.

•••••• Diagnostic Studies and Findings

Physical examination Characteristic eruption with typical distribution; personal or family history of allergies

Immunofluorescence Serum IgE may be elevated

•••••• Multidisciplinary Plan

Atopic dermatitis presents the whole range of eczematous process from acute to chronic, and treatment must be directed accordingly. The focus of therapy is to interrupt the itch-scratch cycle.

Medications

Corticosteroids
  Topical steroids with menthol or camphor 0.25%-0.5% applied bid or tid
  Systemic
    Prednisone (Deltasone, Orasone, others), 60-80 mg/d as single morning dose for 1-2 wk only
Keratolytics
  Coal tar 2% (Alphosyl, Tar-Doak) applied topically at bedtime

Antihistamines
  Hydroxyzine (Atarax, Vistaril), 25-100 mg po tid or qid
  Diphenhydramine (Benadryl) 25-50 mg po tid or qid
  Tripelennamine (Pyribenzamine, PBZ), 10 mg po bid or tid
  Third-generation multifunction antihistamines (ketotifen, cetrizine, azelastine)
Antiineffective agents
  Systemic antibiotics for secondary infection; drug and dosage dependent on causative organism and severity of infection

General Management

Burow's dressings and saline compresses (see pp. 526 to 528)
Oatmeal and oil baths (see pp. 526 to 528)
Occlusive dressings (see pp. 526 to 528)
Allergy diet (controversial)
House humidified
Light, cotton clothing

NURSING CARE

Nursing Assessment

Eruption

Lichenification; excoriation; subacute papular eruptions; generalized erythema; pruritus

Location

Face; neck; upper chest; flexor surfaces; wrists, feet; upper back; generalized

Special Disease Manifestations

Chronic hand eczema; nummular eczema (coin-shaped eczematous plaques)

Secondary Infection

Purulent drainage; fever; tenderness; regional lymphadenopathy

Psychosocial Concerns

Concern with body image; inability to sleep because of pruritus; exacerbations caused by stress

Nursing Dx & Intervention

See p. 492.

Patient Education/Home Care Planning

1. Discuss with the patient and family that the patient should avoid the following:
   a. Heat, high humidity, and rapid changes of temperature

b. Sweating
c. Excessive bathing
d. Strong soaps and detergents that can irritate skin
e. Emotional stress
f. Wools, coarse synthetic fabrics, and tight-fitting clothing
g. Primary irritants
2. Discuss with the patient and family that the patient should
   a. Keep skin well lubricated
   b. Wear light, loose, cotton clothing that "breathes"
   c. Bathe in lukewarm, not hot, water
3. Discuss with the patient and family the signs and symptoms of secondary infection and the need to seek medical attention if they occur.
4. Explain to the patient and family that therapy requires patience and results may not be immediate.
5. Teach the adolescent or young adult to manage the skin condition as soon as possible.

Evaluation

Known causative agents are avoided   Eruption subsides. Exacerbations are limited.

Pruritus is relieved   Scratching decreases. Excoriations heal. Patient is able to sleep.

Secondary infection is avoided   Eruption is free from tenderness and purulent exudate. There is no fever or lymphadenopathy.

Patient assesses appearance in realistic manner   Patient engages in usual relationships and activities when possible.

■ SEBORRHEIC DERMATITIS

Seborrheic dermatitis is a chronic, recurrent, erythematous scaling eruption that is localized in areas where sebaceous glands are concentrated.

In infants, seborrheic dermatitis may develop on the scalp, back, and intertriginous and diaper areas. The scalp lesions are scaling, adherent, thick, yellow, and crusted. Lesions elsewhere are erythematous, scaling, and fissured.

After puberty lesions tend to occur in the scalp, eyebrows, eyelids, nasolabial areas, postauricular areas, and presternal and intertriginous areas (Figure 5-7). Lesions may be mild or severe and vary from dry, greasy scales to erythema, excoriation, and crusting. Secondary bacterial or fungal infection may occur. Genetic factors seem to affect the incidence and severity of the disease. The disorder is worse during the winter months.

•••••• Pathophysiology

The cause of seborrheic dermatitis is unknown. Histologic changes include vasodilation and discharge of inflammatory cells into the epidermis from the capillary loops. Epidermal in-

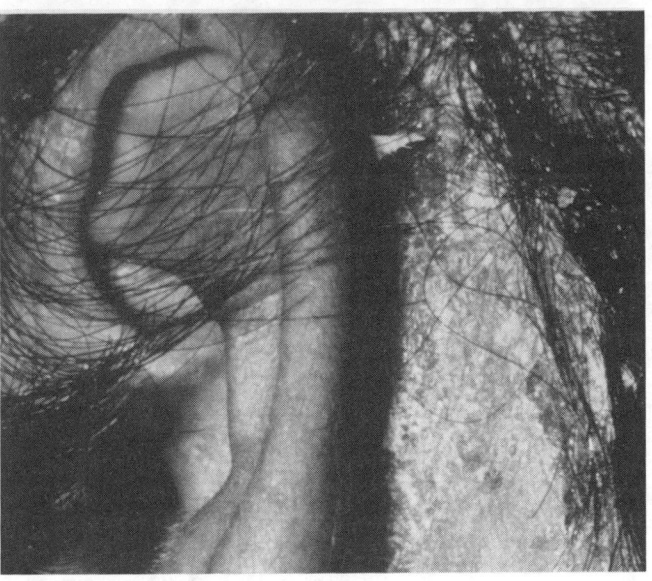

Figure 5-7 Seborrheic dermatitis. (Courtesy of Stephen B, Tucker, M.D., Department of Dermatology, University of Texas Health Science Center at Houston.)

flammation and eczema may be present. Scales are produced as a result of an increased mitotic rate and an accumulation of corneocytes. Despite the name, the composition, production, and flow of sebum are normal.

•••••• Diagnostic Studies and Findings

Physical examination   Characteristic lesions and distribution

•••••• Multidisciplinary Plan

Medications

Corticosteroids
   Topical
      Fluccinolone (Synalar), 0.01% bid
      Flucinonide (Lidex), 0.05% bid
      Hydrocortisone (Hytone), 2.5% bid
      Betamethasone (Valisone), 0.05% bid in hairy areas
Antiseborrheic shampoos
   Coal tar (Denorex, 9%; DHS tar 0.5%; others), 2-3 times wk in the first week, then once weekly as needed; leave on for 5 min before rinsing
   Selenium sulfide (Selsun Blue 1%; others), 2-3 times wk; leave on 2-3 min before rinsing
   Pyrithone zinc (Danex 1%; DHS zinc 2%; others), 2 times/wk
   Combinations (Sebulex, 2% sulfur, 6% salicylic acid; others) 2 times/wk
Antiinfective agents
   Topical antibiotics for secondary infection
      Neomycin 0.1% bid or tid
      Chloramphenicol (Chloromycetin cream) 0.1% bid or tid

Keratolytics
  Salicylic acid 1%-3% topically bid
  Precipitated sulfur 1%-5% topically bid
  Tar cream 4% topically bid

General Management

Oils—castor, mineral, and olive, rubbed into scalp lesions and left overnight
Frequent shampooing
Burow's solution for weeping lesions

NURSING CARE

Nursing Assessment

Eruption

Erythema; scaling; fissures; inflammation; pruritus

Secondary Infection

Purulent discharge; fever; tenderness; increased inflammation; regional lymphadenopathy

Psychosocial Concerns

Concern about body image

Nursing Dx & Intervention

Impaired skin integrity related to pathologic process and mechanical factors

- Assess for characteristics and distribution of lesions.
- Instruct patient in use of medications and topical preparations.
- Instruct patient to shampoo daily *to alleviate scaling and crusting.*
- Instruct patient not to scratch or rub lesions *because that will prolong course of disease.*

Body image disturbance related to cognitive-perceptual factors

- Assess for defining characteristics.
- Encourage patient to express feelings about body, body appearance, or fear of reaction or rejection by others *to begin process of realistic self-evaluation.*
- Assure patient that treatment can be successful.

Patient Education/Home Care Planning

1. Explain to the patient the use of medications and preparations.
2. Explain the care regimen to the patient.
3. Discuss with the patient the signs and symptoms of secondary infection and how to seek medical care if these occur.
4. Explain to the patient to avoid external irritants, excessive heat, and excessive perspiration.

Evaluation

Eruption resolves Erythema and inflammation disappear. Scaling decreases. Fissures heal. Pruritus is relieved. Skin is intact.

Secondary infection is resolved or prevented There is no purulent discharge, fever, or lymphadenopathy.

Patient evaluates his or her appearance in a realistic manner Patient engages in usual activities and relationships.

HERPES ZOSTER

Herpes zoster is an acute cutaneous vesicular eruption caused by the varicella-zoster virus.

Herpes zoster, also known as shingles, occurs as a result of reactivation of a dormant varicella virus. Reactivation can occur at any time. Older adults and HIV-positive individuals are more likely to develop the condition because of their diminishing immunologic functioning.

The eruption is generally limited to the skin of a single dermatome, although one or two adjacent dermatomes may be involved. Pain, itching, and burning along the dermatome precede the eruption by 4 to 5 days. The pain is often mistaken for pleurisy, myocardial infarction, or appendicitis, and diagnosis may be difficult until the characteristic eruption occurs. The eruption begins with erythematous plaques of various size that involve all or part of a dermatome. Purulent, fluid-filled vesicles arise in clusters from the erythematous base. Successive crops continue to appear for 7 days. The vesicles either involute or rupture and then heal in 10 to 14 days, frequently with residual scarring.

Postherpetic neuralgia, the most common complication, is a dermatomal pain syndrome that persists beyond the time of complete cutaneous healing. Pain can persist in a dermatome for months or years after the lesions have disappeared. Most cases resolve in a few months. The pain is often severe, intractable, and exhausting. The incidence of postherpetic neuralgia increases with the age of the patient.

•••••• Pathophysiology

Herpes zoster occurs as a result of reactivation of the varicella virus that entered the cutaneous nerves during an earlier episode of acute infection with the virus. The virus remains dormant in the sensory root ganglia of the lifetime of the patient and can be reactivated at any time. Reactivation can be triggered by local trauma, acute illness, a compromised immunologic state, fatigue, emotional upsets, or chronic debilitation. Once reactivated the virus travels down the sensory nerve and infects the skin of the affected ganglion.

•••••• Diagnostic Studies and Findings

Physical examination Characteristic lesion: clusters of painful, itching vesicles along a single dermatome.

Cytologic smear Direct identification of multinucleated cells

Culture Vesicular fluid to determine presence of virus

•••••• Multidisciplinary Plan

Medications

Analgesic agents

ASA (Aspirin), 300 mg po q4h for mild pain

Acetaminophen (Tylenol, Datril), 250 mg po q4h for mild pain

Codeine po in dosages sufficient for more severe pain relief during eruptive phase or for postherpetic neuralgia

Tranquilizers

Chlorpromazine (Thorazine), 25 mg po qid for severe postherpetic neuralgia

Antiviral agents

Acyclovir (Zovirax), 800 mg po q4h for 7-10 d during eruptive phase

Acyclovir sodium (Zorivax), 10 mg/kg IV q8h; for immunocompromised patients

Famciclovir (Famvir), 500 mg po tid for 7 d

Systemic steroids

During eruptive phase for prevention of postherpetic neuralgia; use is controversial[1,24]

Prednisone, 20 mg po tid for 7 d, followed by 20 mg po bid for 7 d, followed by 20 mg each morning for 7 d

For postherpetic neuralgia

Capsaicin cream (Zostrix), 0.075% applied topically

Amitryptyline (Elavil), 75-100 mg po qd, with perphenazine (Trilafon), 4 mg po tid-qid, or fluphenazine hydrochloride (Permitil), 1 mg po tid-qid, or thioridazine (Mellaril), 25 mg po qid; may be necessary to continue medication for months

Chlorprothixene (Taractan), 25-50 mg po q6h for 4-10 d

Carbamazepine (Tegretol), 600-800 mg p qd, with nortriptyline (Pamelor), 50-100 mg po qd

Intralesional injection of triamcinolone (Aristocort, Kenalog), 0.2 mg/ml daily

General Management

Cryosurgery (for postherpetic neuralgia)

Affected area sprayed with refrigent (freon, Frigiderm) until blanching occurs, repeated every 2 weeks for three to six treatments; if relief occurs, it is rapid and limited to specific area treated; produces relief in about 50% of affected patients

Transcutaneous electric nerve stimulation (TENS) treatments (for postherpetic neuralgia)

NURSING CARE

Nursing Assessment

Lesions (Eruptive Phase)

Location and characteristics; crusting; scarring with healing

Secondary Infection (Eruptive Phase)

Erythema, swelling, purulent drainage from lesions

Discomfort (Eruptive Phase)

Pain, burning, itching of lesions; intensity

Discomfort (Postherpetic Phase)

Intensity and location; interference with activity

Nursing Dx & Intervention

Impaired skin integrity related to pathologic process and mechanical factors

- Assess for lesion characteristics and location.
- Apply wet compresses with Burow's solution for 20 minutes three times a day *to macerate vesicles, remove serum and crust, and suppress bacterial growth.*
- Assess for secondary infection from scratching.
- Trim fingernails short *to prevent secondary infection.*

Pain related to biologic agents

- Assess for pain, itching, and burning during eruptive phase.
- Assess for pain during postherpetic phase.
- As physician directs, provide analgesic medications.
- Provide empathy, understanding, and emotional support for patient with persistent pain.
- Investigate alternate means of pain management with patient and physician, e.g., biofeedback, transcutaneous nerve stimulation.

Patient Education/Home Care Planning

1. Discuss with the patient the course of the disease process.
2. Discuss the correct use of analgesics.
3. Demonstrate the application of wet compresses with Burow's solution (p. 527).

Evaluation

Eruption improves   Lesions resolve; secondary infection does not occur.

Pruritus is alleviated   Areas of excoriation resolve or do not occur.

Pain is relieved   Patient is able to resume usual activities without fear of triggering paroxysms of pain.

Patient successfully manages intractable pain   Patient engages in usual activities and maintains interpersonal relationships; patient is not withdrawn or suicidal.

▌ ICHTHYOSIS

Ichthyosis is a common inherited keratinization disorder that is characterized by varying degrees of dryness, scaling, and exfoliation. Several genetic keratinization abnormalities result in dry, scaly skin. The most common condition is ichthyosis vulgaris, an autosomal dominant inherited disease that occurs in 1 in 1000 people. The other forms of ichthyosis are rarer.

••••• Pathophysiology

In ichthyosis vulgaris the mitotic rate is decreased and the stratum corneum fails to desquamate normally. The granular layer is reduced or absent, and sweat and sebaceous glands may be reduced. The follicular orifices are hyperkeratotic and are often plugged with keratin. The ability of the stratum corneum to retain water is decreased. Aggravation during the winter months and improvement during the summer are common. The other forms of ichthyosis show similar pathologic changes.

Table 5-3 summarizes the clinical, pathologic, and genetic features of the four patterns of inherited ichthyosis (Figure 5-8).

••••• Diagnostic Studies and Findings

Physical examination Characteristic lesion

••••• Multidisciplinary Plan

Medications

Emollients (apply to moist skin bid after bathing)
   Propylene glycol 40%-50%
   Propylene glycol 60%, ethanol 2%, and salicylic acid 6% in gel base under occlusive dressing for 1-4 d and then every third night
   Hydrophilic petrolatum
   Water-miscible bath oil
Keratolytics (apply after bathing to moist skin or 3-7 times/wk)
   Salicylic acid 5% in emollient base
   Urea 10% in water-miscible base
   Sodium chloride 10% and salicylic acid 5%

Vitamins
   Tretinoin (Retin-A) 0.1% (vitamin A, retinoic acid), applied topically for lamellar ichthyosis
Oral synthetic retinoids
   Etretinate (Tegison), 0.3-0.5 mg/kg/d; up to 0.75 mg/kg/d as tolerated for lamellar ichthyosis

NURSING CARE

Nursing Assessment

Lesions

Type of scale and distribution as in Table 5-3; severity

Secondary Infection

Redness; tenderness; swelling; exudate; odor

Comfort and Mobility

Discomfort from dry, cracked skin; limitation on mobility

Psychosocial Concerns

Concern about body image

Nursing Dx & Intervention

Impaired skin integrity related to biologic and mechanical factors

- Assess for distribution and severity of lesions.
- Instruct patient and parent in use of topical preparations.

■ **TABLE 5-3 Summary of Ichthyosis Disorders**

Disorder	Inheritance Pattern	Age of Onset	Prognosis	Histopathology	Type Scale	Distribution
Vulgaris	Dominant	Childhood (1 to 4 years)	Improves during adult years	Increased mitotic rate; retained stratum corneum; decreased granular layer; plugged follicular orifices	Fine, small, thin, light	Back and extensor surfaces; flexures spared; increased markings on palms and soles
Male, sex linked	Recessive X linked	Birth	Persistent	As above; increased plugging	Large, brown	Neck and trunk; total extremities; flexures spared; normal markings
Lamellar nonbullous	Recessive	Birth	Persistent	Increased mitotic rate; granular layer present; acanthosis; hyperkeratosis; plugged follicular orifices	Large, coarse, yellow, raised corners	Generalized; thick palms and soles
Bullous epidermolytic hyperkeratoses	Dominant	Birth	Persistent; severe forms may cause death in early infancy from secondary infection	As above; vacuolation of epidermal cells	Thick, gray-brown, coarse, warty, vesicular, and bullous lesions	Patchy or generalized; flexures affected

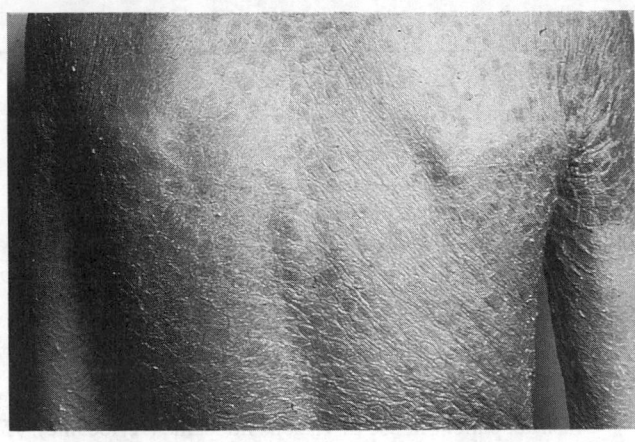

Figure 5-8 Lamellar ichthyosis. (Courtesy of Stephen B, Tucker, M.D., Department of Dermatology, University of Texas Health Science Center at Houston.)

- Stress importance of good hygiene *to prevent secondary infection.*

Chronic pain related to physical factors; impaired physical mobility related to pain and discomfort

- Instruct patient in use of emollients *to decrease dryness.*
- Instruct patient not to use soap or to use it sparingly while bathing *to prevent drying and cracking of skin.*
- Instruct patient to maintain humidity in living environment *to prevent drying and cracking of skin.*

Body image disturbance related to cognitive-perceptual factors

- Assess patient's or parent's perception of patient's appearance.
- Encourage patient to express feelings about body, body appearance, and fear of reaction or rejection by others *to begin process of realistic self-evaluation.*
- Encourage patient to develop interests and other attributes *to support positive self-image, feelings of self-worth, and self-confidence.*
- Help patient evaluate appearance in a realistic manner *so it does not become focal point of existence.*
- Inform parents that condition may improve as child matures.

Patient Education/Home Care Planning

1. Instruct the patient and family in the use of emollients and keratolytics.
2. Instruct the patient in the signs and symptoms of secondary infection and to seek medical care if they occur.
3. Inform the patient and family that successful therapy requires the patient's full cooperation and patience, that therapy is long term, and that results may not be immediate.

Evaluation

Secondary infection is avoided There is no redness, tenderness, swelling, or purulent exudate.

Discomfort is relieved Dryness decreases. Cracks and fissures improve. Limitations on mobility lessen.

Patient makes successful adaptations in self-concept Patient develops interests and participates in activities compatible with degree of mobility. Patient engages in satisfying relationships. Patient does not use disorder as excuse for unsuccessful relationships.

▌LICHEN PLANUS

Lichen planus is a chronic pruritic inflammatory eruption of the skin and mucous membrane. It is characterized by small angular papules that may combine to form larger plaques.

Lichen planus occurs most frequently in adults. The onset may be gradual or abrupt. The average duration of the disease is 15 to 24 months, but it may persist or recur for years. Healing is followed by residual pigmentation that eventually fades.

• • • • • • Pathophysiology

The cause of lichen planus is unknown. However, certain drugs and chemicals used in developing color photographs can cause an eruption.

Inflammation occurs primarily at the dermal level with lymphocytic infiltrate. There are hyperkeratosis and prominence of the granular layer. Vacuolation, degeneration, and inflammatory changes occur in the basal layer. Fibrin and IgM are deposited in the papillary dermis.

Cutaneous lesions are pruritic, flat-topped, reddish-violet, angular papules that are 0.5 to 5 mm in diameter. The papules have a sheen on cross-lighting. Whitish-gray lines (Wickham's striae) are seen on the skin. The individual papules can combine to form larger plaques, becoming more scaly and verrucous. The lesions are usually symmetrically distributed and occur most commonly on the flexor surfaces of the wrist, forearm, and ankles and on the abdomen and sacrum. The face, palms, and soles are rarely affected. Eruption can occur at the site of minor trauma (Köbner's phenomenon).

Lesions of the buccal mucosa are present in 50% to 60% of the cases. These gray lacy lesions may ulcerate and be painful. Malignant degeneration occurs in about 1 in 100 cases.

Clinical variants of lichen planus include annular, bullous, hypertrophic, and atrophic lesions. Nails can be involved, with pitting, thinning, and increase in longitudinal ridging. In severe cases the nail may be shed completely.

• • • • • • Diagnostic Studies and Findings

Physical examination Characteristic lesion
Biopsy Characteristic histologic findings
Immunofluorescence IgG deposits in papillary dermis

•••••• Multidisciplinary Plan

Medications

Corticosteroids

Topical

Hydrocortisone (Cort-Dome, others), 0.1% or triamcinolone (Aristocort, Kenalog, others) 0.1% in occlusive dressing at bedtime; must be maintained until all signs of lesions disappear

Triamcinolone, 0.1% in dental paste (Kenalog in Orabase), applied q3-5h for mouth lesions

Intralesional injection

Triamcinolone (Aristocort, Kenalog), 5 mg/ml (see p. 529)

Systemic corticosteroids for very severe or generalized lesions

Prednisone, 40-60 mg/d po, then decreasing doses

Clobetasol propionate (Temovate), 0.025% ointment in adhesive paste to yield a 0.25% concentration for oral lesions; under investigation[48]

Vitamins

Tretinoin (Retin-A), 0.1% applied with cotton-tipped applicator at night followed by triamcinolone 0.1% tid

Local anesthetics

Viscous lidocaine (Xylocaine), mouth swish before meals

Antipruritics

Antianxiety agents

Hydroxyzine (Atarax, Orgatrax, Vistaril), 25-100 mg po tid or qid

Antihistamines

Cyproheptadine (Cyproheptadine, Periactin), 4 mg po tid

Terfenadine (Seldane), 60 mg po bid

General Management

Withdrawal of all current medications and replacement with substitutes

NURSING CARE

Nursing Assessment

Lesion

Angular papules; bullous, hypertrophic, and atrophic lesions; coalesced plaques; mucosal plaques, or ulceration; distribution of lesions

Discomfort

Pruritus; pain from buccal ulceration

Nutrition

Inability to eat because of buccal ulceration

Psychosocial Concerns

Concern with body image

Nursing Dx & Intervention

Impaired skin integrity related to inflammatory process

- Assess for location and characteristics of lesions.
- Instruct patient in good hygiene and need for short fingernails *to prevent secondary infection.*
- Apply cool compresses *to relieve itching.*
- Instruct patient in use of occlusive dressing (see p. 527) *to promote healing.*

Altered oral mucous membrane related to pathologic condition

- Instruct patient in use of viscous lidocaine (Xylocaine): 15 minutes before eating, swish in mouth *to promote comfort.*
- Instruct patient to avoid astringent and acidic fluids *to avoid tissue trauma.*
- Provide mouth care with alkaline or saline mouthwash *to promote comfort and prevent infection.*

Pain related to physical factors

- Assess for discomfort.
- Provide soft diet *to prevent mechanical irritation.*
- Provide bland foods *to prevent mechanical irritation.*

Body image disturbance related to cognitive-perceptual factors

- Assess patient's perception of his or her appearance.
- Encourage patient to express feelings about body, body appearance, or fear of reaction or rejection by others *to begin process of realistic self-evaluation.*

Patient Education/Home Care Planning

1. Discuss with the patient the treatment regimen, medications, and dressings.
2. Discuss with the patient the side effects of medications.
3. Teach the patient the signs and symptoms of secondary infection and to seek medical treatment if they occur.
4. Discuss the long-term nature of the disorder and the fact that treatment requires persistence and patience.
5. Discuss with the patient the avoidance of precipitating drugs and chemicals.

Evaluation

Eruption improves Papules, bullae, and plaques resolve. Ulcerations reepithelialize. Pruritus resolves. Secondary infection does not occur.

Discomfort from buccal lesions is alleviated Patient is able to eat and does not lose weight.

Pruritus is alleviated Areas of excoriation resolve or do not recur.

Patient evaluates appearance in realistic manner Patient engages in usual activities and relationships.

PIGMENTED DISORDERS

PIGMENTED NEVI, BLUE NEVI, AND MONGOLIAN SPOTS

Pigmented nevi, blue nevi, and mongolian spots are benign skin lesions that are caused by accumulation of pigment in the dermis.

Pigmented nevi occur in various forms that vary in size and degree of pigmentation. Nevi are present on most persons and may occur anywhere on the body. They may be flat, slightly raised, dome shaped, smooth, rough, or hairy. Their color ranges from tan, gray, and shades of brown to black.

The blue nevus usually occurs as a single nodular lesion on the dorsal surface of the hands, face, or buttocks. The nevus is present at birth and remains unchanged through life.

Mongolian spots have a dusky blue color and blend into the surrounding normal skin. The spots occur primarily in Asian and dark-skinned infants, usually in the lumbosacral area. The spots vary in diameter from 1 cm to several centimeters. They cause no symptoms and usually disappear during childhood.

•••••• Pathophysiology

The lesions occur as the result of nevus cells that migrate to the dermis during embryonic development. The nevus cells have the same origin as melanocytes and are closely associated with them. The nevus cells contain melanin pigment, which give the lesions their color. The blue color of the blue nevus and the mongolian spots is caused by the concentration of melanin and its depth below the epidermis.

Table 5-4 summarizes the features of the various types of pigmented nevi.

•••••• Diagnostic Studies and Findings

Physical examination   Characteristic lesion
Biopsy   Shows histologic configuration

•••••• Multidisciplinary Plan

Most nevi do not require any treatment. Surgical removal may be indicated for cosmetic purposes or if changes occur in the nevus (see box below). Mongolian spots require no treatment.

Surgery

Shave ablation with electrodessication of base for intradermal nevus
Excisional or punch biopsy removal of junction nevus
Excision of hairy nevus with full-thickness skin grafting (see p. 530)

Laser Therapy

Argon laser treatment for some pigmented lesions[3,27,28]
Pulsed tunable dye laser for some pigmented lesions[10]
Q-switch ruby Candela laser for some pigmented lesions[46]

 MALIGNANT CHANGES IN NEVI

Some changes in preexisting nevi may indicate malignancy. Moles that exhibit any of the following changes or irregularities should receive medical evaluation:

A—Asymmetry of one half compared to the other
B—Borders irregular
C—Color blue-black or variegated, with red, white, blue, pink, gray
D—Diameter >6 mm
E—Elevation from change in thickness
F—Fading of the borders, with notches or streams of pigmentation
G—Growing
H—Halo formation (depigmented area) around the nevus

TABLE 5-4 Features and Occurrence of Various Types of Pigmented Nevi

Type	Features	Occurrence	Comments
Halo nevus	Sharp, oval, or circular; depigmented halo around mole; may undergo many morphologic changes; usually disappears and halo repigments (may take years)	Usually on back in young adult	Usually benign; biopsy indicated because same process can occur around melanoma
Intradermal nevus	Dome shaped; raised; flesh to black color; may be pedunculated or hair bearing	Cells limited to dermis	No indication for removal other than cosmetic
Junction nevus	Flat or slightly elevated; dark brown	Nevus cells lining dermoepidermal junction	Should be removed if exposed to repeated trauma
Compound nevus	Slightly elevated brownish papule; indistinct border	Nevus cells in dermis and lining dermoepidermal junction	Should be removed if exposed to repeated trauma
Hairy nevus	May be present at birth; may cover large area; hair growth occurring after several years		Should be removed if changes occur

NURSING CARE

Nursing Assessment

Lesion

Location; size; color; shape

Lesion Changes

Enlargement; darkening; crusting; bleeding; inflammation; ulceration; appearance of satellite lesions

Psychosocial Concerns

Concern about body image

Nursing Dx & Intervention

Body image disturbance related to cognitive-perceptual factors

- Assess for presence of defining characteristics.
- Encourage patient to express feelings about body, body image, or fear of reaction or rejection by others *to begin process of realistic self-evaluation.*

Patient Education/Home Care Planning

1. Discuss with the patient the benign nature of the lesions.
2. Explain to the patient about changes that might indicate malignancy, and encourage the patient to seek medical attention if they occur.

Evaluation

Patient seeks treatment for changes in lesions   Patient seeks medical attention if color or size of nevus changes, if it bleeds, or if it is exposed to repeated trauma.

Patient evaluates appearance in realistic manner   Patient seeks removal if lesion is cosmetically embarrassing.

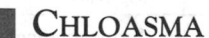

CHLOASMA

Chloasma is a diffuse, mottled brown pigmentation that appears over areas of the face and forehead.

•••••• Pathophysiology

Chloasma is a blotchy brown pigmentation that involves the forehead, malar prominences, and preauricular areas. The distribution is usually symmetric. Chloasma occurs primarily in women during and after childbearing years. Increased activity of melanocytes and the increase in melanin deposits in the basal cells of the epidermis can occur with pregnancy or from the use of anovulatory hormones. Exposure to sunlight exaggerates the pigmentation. It fades somewhat after childbirth or after the hormones are discontinued. Rarely, chloasma occurs idiopathically in dark-skinned men.

•••••• Diagnostic Studies and Findings

Physical examination   Characteristic pigmentation and distribution; in women, history congruent with pregnancy or anovulatory hormones

•••••• Multidisciplinary Plan

Medications

Topical depigmenting agents

Hydroquinone (Eldopaque, Eldoquin), 2%-4% applied sparingly bid

Compound of retinoic acid 0.1% hydroquinone 5%, and dexamethasone 0.1% applied sparingly bid

Sunscreen—para-aminobenzoic acid (PABA) 5% (Pabanol, Sunbrella) in ethyl alcohol 95%, applied twice a day and after swimming and bathing

Laser Therapy

Argon laser treatment[27,28]

Q-switch ruby laser treatments[46]

General Management

Discontinuation of anovulatory hormones

NURSING CARE

Nursing Assessment

Pigmentation

Severity and extent of pigmentation; questioning to determine if woman is pregnant or taking anovulatory hormones

Psychosocial Concerns

Concern about body image

Nursing Dx & Intervention

Body image disturbance related to cognitive-perceptual factors

- Assess patient's self-perception.
- Encourage patient to express feelings about body, body image, or fear of reaction or rejection by others *to begin process of realistic self-evaluation.*
- Inform patient that pigmentation fades in time.
- Instruct patient in use of medications.

Patient Education/Home Care Planning

1. Discuss with the patient the need to avoid sun exposure, which will worsen the condition.
2. Explain to the patient the need to use sunscreens.
3. Discuss with the patient the side effects of depigmenting agents.

Evaluation

Existing pigmentation fades   Blotchy brown areas become less noticeable.

Patient avoids sunlight and use of anovulatory hormones   New areas of pigmentation do not occur.

Patient evaluates appearance in realistic manner   Patient seeks treatment for areas that are cosmetically embarrassing. Patient engages in usual activities and relationships.

DEPIGMENTATION: ALBINISM AND VITILIGO

Albinism and vitiligo are depigmentation that results from a congenital or acquired decrease in melanin production.

Albinism is a rare inherited disease that may be complete or partial. Partial albinism is autosomal dominant. The affected areas are usually linear and unilateral. The same area may be affected in more than one family member. A small area on the scalp with a streak of white hair is frequently seen.

Complete or universal albinism is autosomal recessive or irregularly dominant. There is no pigmentation in the skin, hair, and eyes. (Some pigmentation may occur with increasing age.) The skin is pale, the hair white, and the iris pink or red. Nystagmus and errors of refraction are common. Skin cancer and premature actinic keratosis are common.

Vitiligo is localized areas of depigmentation that are caused by the disappearance of previously active melanocytes. Vitiligo is fairly common, occurring in 1% of the world's population. It is a familial trait and can occur at any age. It has been associated with autoimmune and endocrine disorders. The depigmentation can also result from exposure to phenols, thiols, and quinones. Initial lesions frequently develop in areas exposed to the sun. The process may remain stable for years and involve only small areas, or it may progress to affect more extensive areas or the entire skin surface and hair. The eyes do not lose their pigment.

The lesions are completely depigmented and have well-demarcated borders that may be hyperpigmented. Vitiligo usually develops symmetrically and may follow trauma to the area. The hands, axillae, perineum, and periorbital areas are usually involved. The surface of the depigmented skin is normal except for the absence of pigmentation. There is no scaling. Some spontaneous repigmentation occurs in about 10% of patients, but complete repigmentation is rare.

Vitiligo is associated with thyroid dysfunction, diabetes mellitus, Addison's disease, and pernicious anemia.

•••••• Pathophysiology

In partial albinism melanocytes are not present in the depigmented area because they failed to migrate to the skin during embryonic development. In complete albinism melanocytes are present in the dermis, but they are unable to synthesize pigment because of a block in the formation of melanin from its precursor.

The cause of vitiligo is unknown. It is considered an autoimmune process that causes destruction of preexisting melanocytes. The melanocytes are abnormal and in various stages of cell death at the periphery of the lesions. Repigmentation is thought to result from the migration of melanocytes from residual areas of melanocytic activity within hair follicles.

•••••• Diagnostic Studies and Findings

Physical examination   Distinctive lesions with characteristic configuration and distribution

•••••• Multidisciplinary Plan

There is no treatment for albinism other than protection from sun exposure and actinic damage. The treatment for vitiligo is protracted and has mixed results.

Medications

Photosensitizers
  Psoralen therapy with 8-methoxypsoralen or methoxsalen (Oxsoralen, Trisoralen) to repigment
    Psoralen, 40-50 mg po 2 h before sun exposure; sun exposure time initially 20 min then gradually increased
    Psoralen, 40-50 mg po with long-wave ultraviolet light (PUVA), exposure time gradually increased (see p. 532)
Sunscreens
  PABA 5% (Pabanol, Sunbrella) as protection against sunburn, applied topically q3h and after swimming
Skin dyes containing dihydroxyacetone (Vitadye) to stain stratum corneum; applied topically several times a week
Corticosteroids
  Oral glucocorticoids or topical glucocorticoids used in occlusive dressings to repigment
Depigmenting agents
  For surrounding area in extensive vitiligo 20% monobenzyl ether or hydroquinone

NURSING CARE

Nursing Assessment

Lesions
  Location and distribution; extent of involvement

Psychosocial Concerns
  Concern about body image

Nursing Dx & Intervention

Risk for impaired skin integrity related to radiation

- Instruct patient *to protect skin exposure* to sun through use of protective clothing and hats.
- Instruct patient to use PABA as sunscreen *to protect skin from actinic damage.*

Body image disturbance related to cognitive-perceptual factors; situational low self-esteem

- Assess patient's perception of his or her appearance.
- Encourage patient to express feelings about body, body image, or fear of reaction or rejection by others *to begin process of realistic self-evaluation.*
- Encourage development of interests and other attributes *to support positive self-image and feelings of worth and self-confidence.*
- Help patient evaluate appearance in realistic way *so it does not become focal point of patient's existence.*
- Advise patient of cosmetic products (Covermark) available for use on small areas.
- Facilitate initiation of counseling if patient is unable to adjust to appearance.

Patient Education/Home Care Planning

1. Discuss with the patient the need to protect against exposure to the sun to prevent premature actinic damage.
2. Discuss with the patient the use and side effects of medications and preparations.
3. Explain to the patient that treatment for vitiligo is protracted and results vary.

Evaluation

Actinic damage is avoided   Epidermis is not dry or fissured. There are no actinic keratoses. Skin remains smooth and elastic.

Patient evaluates appearance in realistic manner   Disorder is not used as excuse for unsuccessful interpersonal relationships. Patient develops interests and relationships so appearance is not focal point of existence.

PITYRIASIS ROSEA

Pityriasis rosea is a self-limiting inflammation of unknown etiology.

The disease peaks in spring and fall. It is less likely to occur on tanned skin, and sunlight apparently hastens the course. Onset is sudden, with occurrence of a herald patch followed 1 to 3 weeks later by a generalized eruption. New lesions continue to appear for about a week after onset of the generalized eruption. A gradual involution follows. Total duration is 4 to 12 weeks with rare recurrence. The disease is not infectious or contagious.

•••••• Pathophysiology

The cause of pityriasis rosea is unknown. Pathogenesis may be related to a cell-mediated immunity. The primary (herald) patch is a single oval or round plaque with fine superficial scaling. The remainder of the lesions are smaller but similar in configuration to the primary lesions. The lesions develop in the trunk and extremities. The palms and soles are not involved, and facial involvement is rare. The lesions are characteristically distributed in parallel alignment following the direction of the ribs

in a Christmas tree-like pattern. An inverse pattern can occur, with concentration of the lesions on the extremities and few lesions on the trunk. The lesions are usually pale, erythematous, and macular with the fine scaling, but they may be papular or vesicular. Pruritus may be present.

Microscopic examination reveals nonspecific inflammation of the dermis, perivascular infiltrates, and localized epidermal changes with spongiosis and focal parakeratosis.

•••••• Diagnostic Studies and Findings

Physical examination   Characteristic lesion with distinct distribution and congruent history

VDRL or rapid plasma reagin (RPR) test   Done to rule out secondary syphilis

•••••• Multidisciplinary Plan

Treatment is usually unnecessary

Medications

Antipruritic effects
  Antipruritic agents
    Menthol 0.25% in cream base applied topically bid or tid
  Antihistamines
    Cyproheptadine (Cyproheptadine, Periactin), 4 mg po tid
  Antianxiety agents
    Hydroxyzine (Atarax, Orgatrax, Vistaril), 25-100 mg po tid or qid
Corticosteroids
  Prednisone, 10 mg po qid for severe pruritus until itching subsides, then in decremental doses over 14 d

General Management

Exposure to short wave ultraviolet light (UVB)—five consecutive daily doses to level of erythema to decrease pruritus and extent of eruption

---

NURSING CARE

Nursing Assessment

Lesion

Pale, erythematous macules with fine scaling or papules and vesicles; herald patch larger than new lesions; characteristic distribution

Psychosocial Concerns

Concern with body image

Nursing Dx & Intervention

Impaired skin integrity related to inflammatory process and mechanical factors

- Assess for lesions and pruritus.
- Lubricate skin with emollient and water-miscible bath oil *to alleviate dryness and scaling.*

- Stress importance of good hygiene *to avoid secondary infection.*
- Have patient cut fingernails short *to avoid tissue trauma from scratching.*

Body image disturbance related to cognitive-perceptual factors

- Reassure patient that lesions will clear in 4 to 12 weeks.
- Encourage patient to express feelings about body, body appearance, or fear of reaction or rejection by others *to begin process of realistic self-evaluation.*

Patient Education/Home Care Planning

1. Explain to the patient that the disease is self-limiting and will resolve.
2. Explain to the patient that exposure to sunlight may hasten the course of the disease.
3. Teach the patient the signs and symptoms of secondary infection and to seek medical attention if they occur.
4. Discuss with the patient the use and side effects of medications.

Evaluation

Lesions resolve Macules, papules, vesicles, and scaling disappear. Pruritus is relieved. Skin is intact.

Secondary infection is resolved or avoided There is no tenderness, swelling, purulent discharge, or fever.

Patient evaluates appearance in realistic manner Patient engages in usual activities and relationships.

PSORIASIS

Psoriasis is a chronic and recurrent disease of keratin synthesis that is characterized by dry, well-circumscribed, silvery, scaling papules and plaques.

Psoriasis occurs in 3% to 5% of the population. Onset is usually between the ages of 10 and 40 years. A family history of psoriasis is common.

The onset of the disease is slow, and the course is characterized by periods of inactivity and exacerbation. Emotional stress may cause exacerbations. Spontaneous remission may occur.

Psoriasis characteristically involves the back, buttocks, and extensor surfaces of the extremities, particularly the knees and elbows, and the scalp. The nails, axillae, umbilicus, eyebrows, and anogenital areas may be affected. Generalized eruptions can occur. Approximately 5% of people with psoriasis have associated arthritis. Lesions may develop at sites of recent epidermal injury.

The characteristic lesions of psoriasis are raised, erythematous, sharply demarcated papules covered with overlapping, silvery or shiny scales. The papules may combine as large plaques. When the scales are removed, a deep red base, covered with a thin membrane that bleeds, is revealed.

•••••• Pathophysiology

The basic defect in psoriasis is in the control of the growth of epidermal cells. This defect may be genetic, biochemical, or immunologic. The three main components of the psoriatic process are increased mitotic rate that results in rapid cellular turnover and shortened transit time of the epidermal cell from the basal layer to the epidermis (4 to 7 days versus the normal 28 days), faulty keratinization of the horny layer, which desquamates readily and affords little protection to the underlying skin, and dilation of upper dermal vessels and intermittent discharge of polymorphonuclear leukocytes into the dermis.

The three processes occur in different degrees that result in varying forms of psoriasis with differing clinical features. If the increased mitotic rate predominates, the result is a thick silvery scale because of the separation of corneocytes and the presence of air between them. If vasodilation predominates, the result is diffusely red, hot, slightly scaling skin.

The forms of psoriasis and their clinical features are summarized in Table 5-5.

•••••• Diagnostic Studies and Findings

Physical examination Characteristic lesions

•••••• Multidisciplinary Plan

Medications

Corticosteroids
  Topical nonfluorinated corticosteroids for lesions on face and intertriginous areas
    Hydrocortisone (Cort-Dome, others), 2%-3% applied sparingly bid

---

TABLE 5-5 Clinical Features and Distribution of the Various Forms of Psoriasis

Clinical Pattern	Clinical Features	Distribution
Localized plaques	Erythematous plaques with silver scales; nails pitted, thickened, discolored, and crumbling beneath free edge	Extensor aspect of extremities; elbows; knees; scalp; nails
Generalized plaques	As discussed above	Disseminated
Guttate	Tiny plaques (0.5-2 cm); sudden onset usually after streptococcal infection; may progress to other types; may itch	Disseminated
Pustular	Pustular lesions covered by thin scale	Palms and soles only or generalized
Erythrodermic exfoliative	More inflammatory; skin red and hot; deep erythema with massive shedding of scales; usually follows overly aggressive therapy; can cause temperature and fluid imbalances	Generalized

Topical corticosteroids for lesions on scalp, body, and extremities

Fluocinolone (Fluonid, Synalar), 0.025%-0.01% applied sparingly bid, tid, or qid

Betamethasone (Valisone), 0.05%-0.1% applied sparingly bid, tid, or qid

Triamcinolone (Aristocort, Kenalog), 0.05%-0.1% applied sparingly bid, tid, or qid

Mometasone furoate (Elocon), 0.1% applied once daily

High-potency topical steroid[61]

Clobetasol propionate (Temovate), 0.05% applied sparingly bid or tid

Betamethasone dipropionate (Diprolene), 0.05% applied sparingly bid or tid

Topical corticosteroids in conjunction with tar preparations or in occlusive therapy (see p. 527)

Intralesional injections of corticosteroids

Triamcinolone (Kenalog), 10 mg/ml

Systemic corticosteroids—individualized treatment regimen; use is controversial[1]

Topical Vitamin D_3 preparations[44,49]

Keratolytics

Coal tar preparations (Alphosyl, Psorigel, Balnetar), added to bath oil or shampoo or applied sparingly to lesions

Dianthrol compounds

Anthralin (Anthra-Derm), 0.1%-2% applied sparingly at bedtime or bid; very irritating and stains clothing permanently; cannot be used simultaneously with corticosteroids

Phenol-saline mixture (P & S liquid), massaged into scalp and left for 3-4 h for scalp lesions, followed by tar shampoo

Photosensitizing agents

Psoralen (Trisoralen, Oxsoralen), 0.6 mg/kg 2-4 h before exposure to ultraviolet light; used as photoactivator in combination with long-wave ultraviolet light therapy (see p. 532)

Oral retinoids

Etretinate (Tegison), 1 mg/kg/d po up to maximum of 75 mg/d; for severe recalcitrant forms; used especially in combination therapy

Acetritin (Etretin); investigational[47] for severe recalcitrant forms; used especially in combination therapy

Antineoplastic agents (used for antimetabolite effect)

Methotrexate 5-7.5 mg in a single weekly po, IM, or IV dose, increased by a 2.5-5 mg increment q wk up to 30 mg/wk, then tapered after clearing; or 2.5 mg q12h in 3 doses in a 24 h period, increased by 2.5 mg each wk up to 30 mg/wk, then tapered after clearing; for severe recalcitrant disease[2]

Cyclosporin 3 mg/kg/d as initial dose, altered according to clinical state; dose not to exceed 5 mg/kg/d; for severe disease[53]

Antiinfective agents

Penicillin (Pen Vee-K, V-Cillin, others), 250 mg po qid for 10 d for underlying streptococcal infection in guttate psoriasis

General Management

See p. 531

Exposure to short-wave ultraviolet light (UVB)—one to three times weekly with increasing UVB exposure; kept below level that would cause erythema

Goeckerman therapy—UVB therapy in combination with coal tar applications that are photosensitizing; coal tar ointment applied and left on for several hours and then washed off; UVB therapy then administered in doses to account for photosensitization; tar finally reapplied

Long-wave ultraviolet light (UVA) in combination with psoralen as a photosensitizer (PUVA therapy)—psoralen administered in initial dose of 0.6 mg/kg; UVA irradiation delivered 2 to 4 hours after psoralen administration; dosage and exposure determined by individual response; special equipment and careful monitoring required, so therapy is usually provided in special treatment centers; treatment usually reserved for chronic, severe, refractory psoriasis[31,32]

Combination therapies

PUVA-UVB—PUVA plus UVB

Methotrexate-PUVA—methotrexate plus PUVA

Methotrexate-UVB—methotrexate plus UVB

RePUVA—etretinate plus PUVA

Acitretin-UVB—etretin plus UVB

Topical, soak or both PUVA—topical oxsolaren plus PUVA

X-ray therapy and Grenz-ray therapy—used to provide temporary clearing of stubborn plaques; of limited value as therapeutic tools in psoriasis therapy

Occlusive dressings with topical corticosteroids or tar preparations or both (see p. 527)

Day care treatment centers for psoriasis—patients with severe psoriasis can undergo treatment regimens that are intensive or that require special equipment and supervision

NURSING CARE

Nursing Assessment

Lesions

Characteristics and distribution as in Table 5-5

Psoriatic Arthritis

Pain; tenderness; stiffness in small distal joints (early); larger joints involved later

Environment

Presence of mechanical injury that can exacerbate lesions; stress factors

Nursing Dx & Intervention

Impaired skin integrity related to the pathologic process and mechanical factors

- Assess for lesion characteristics, distribution, and severity.
- Explain disease process regarding exacerbations and remissions.

- Stress importance of adhering to therapeutic regimen; help patient set up overall schedule for managing regimen on daily basis *to maximize therapeutic value.*
- Give written instructions for use of topical preparations, tar baths, and shampoos.
- Instruct patient in application of occlusive dressings.
- Instruct patient to scrub scales gently during daily bath with soft brush and to apply medications after removing scales *to maximize absorption and therapeutic value.*
- Instruct patient not to apply keratolytics and tar to unaffected areas *because they may precipitate new lesions.*
- Explore stress factors affecting patient and alternatives for dealing with stress *to help prevent exacerbations.*

Body image disturbance related to cognitive-perceptual factors

- Recognize importance of body image in growth and development.
- Assess patient's perception of his or her appearance.
- Encourage patient to express feelings about body, body appearance, or fear of reaction or rejection by others *to begin process of realistic self-evaluation.*
- *Encourage patient to develop interests and other attributes* to support positive self-image, feelings of worth, and self-confidence.
- *Facilitate initiation of individual or group therapy* if patient is unable to adjust to appearance.

Social isolation related to alterations in physical appearance

- Involve family members in treatment regimen.
- Stress that psoriasis is not communicable.
- Refer patient for counseling *if patient is socially disabled by disease.*

Powerlessness related to illness-related regimen

- Assess for presence of defining characteristics.
- Observe for signs of depression and apathy.
- Involve patient in decision making *to increase sense of power and control.*
- Encourage patient to express dissatisfaction and frustration.

Patient Education/Home Care Planning

1. Discuss with the patient the treatment regimen and the use of medications.
2. Discuss with the patient the side effects of medications.
3. Explain to the patient that anthralin (Dithranol) stains skin, sheets, and clothing. Skin discoloration resolves in a few weeks as the stratum corneum is shed.
4. Evaluate the patient's ability to carry out home care and reteach procedures as necessary.
5. Discuss with the patient the need for good hygiene to avoid secondary infection.

Evaluation

Lesions improve Scaling, pustules, erythema, and size of plaques decrease.

Exacerbating factors are avoided Patient takes precautions against skin trauma. Patient avoids or tries alternative strategies for reducing stress factors.

Untoward effects from therapies are minimized Patient seeks medical attention for untoward or side effects from medications or therapies.

Patient copes with disorder in an effective manner Patient engages in satisfying relationships. Patient seeks counseling when feeling overwhelmed by disease. Patient does not use disorder as excuse for failures in life or in relationships. Patient participates actively in treatment regimen.

■ PRURITUS

Pruritus is a localized or generalized itching sensation that elicits the desire to scratch.

Pruritus may occur as a primary disorder or may be a symptom of a systemic disorder. Pruritus may result from inflammations caused by various factors, including irritation, infection, infestations, and allergic reactions. It may be the result of systemic disease, malignancy, and altered physiologic states.

Three areas of the body are most frequently affected by pruritus: the anus (pruritus ani), vulva (pruritus vulvae), and ear (otitis externa). These are body orifices that have an abundance of sensory nerve endings.

Pruritus ani occurs primarily in men. It is caused by many factors and is associated with various diseases. Perianal erythema and scratches or gross excoriation are evident. Lichenification or fissures occur in long-term cases. The entire gluteal fold may be involved. Aggravating factors include contact dermatitis, anatomic abnormalities, infection, and systemic disorders. Common irritating factors include feces, irritation from toilet tissue, tight clothing, sweating, and long periods of sitting. The itching is often associated with tension, irritability, and depression.

Pruritus vulvae is caused by many factors and is associated with various diseases. Pruritus vulvae begins with intermittent episodes that can develop into unremitting pruritus. Erythema develops in the labia majora, with lichenification in longstanding disease. The perianal region may also be affected. Tight clothing, heat, perspiration, motion, sitting, and lying down aggravate the condition.

Otitis externa occurs in the external ear usually as a result of trauma, moisture in the ear, and bacterial colonization. The distal third of the external canal and the meatal skin develop a scaling erythema that becomes moist and oozing as the condition worsens. Itching is the main complaint. Otitis externa is aggravated by heat, humidity, moisture, and overzealous cleansing (see Chapter 7).

Generalized pruritus can signify a systemic disorder. Diabetes mellitus, thyroid disorders, HIV infection, drug reactions, biliary obstruction, renal disease, malignancy, and pregnancy are common causes of generalized pruritus.

•••••• Pathophysiology

The exact mechanism of pruritus is undetermined. The itch sensation seems to arise from nerve endings just below the epidermis and in the dermis. Itching may be a result of repetitive, low-frequency stimulation of C fibers that are similar to but distinct from those that transmit pain.

Persistent scratching may produce erythema, urticarial papules, excoriation, and fissures. Prolonged scratching and rubbing may produce lichenification and pigmentation. Many factors, including personality, determine whether itching will be ignored, rubbed, or scratched and excoriated.

•••••• Diagnostic Studies and Findings

Physical examination and history To determine underlying cause or systemic disorder

Laboratory studies with generalized pruritus To determine possible systemic cause: complete blood count, blood urea nitrogen, serum bilirubin, serum iron, blood glucose, sulfobromophthalein retention, stool for occult blood, and parasites.

Biopsy To determine histopathologic changes

•••••• Multidisciplinary Plan

Treatment is aimed at the specific underlying cause (see specific diseases for treatments) and at eliminating aggravating factors (see under Patient Education/Home Care Planning).

Medications

Topical preparation: combination of menthol 0.5%, phenol 0.5%, and betamethasone 0.1% applied sparingly tid
Antiinfective agents
  Topical antibiotics if pruritus has bacterial etiology; gentamicin (Garamycin) or polymycin, applied tid
Antianxiety agents (used for antipruritic effect)
  Hydroxyzine (Atarax, Orgatrax, Vistaril), 25 mg po at bedtime or q6h for localized itching
Antihistamines (used for antipruritic effect)
  Trimeprazine (Temaril), 5 mg po at bedtime or q6h for localized itching
  Terfenadine (Seldane), 60 mg po in the morning, with diphenhydramine (Benadryl), 50-100 mg po at bedtime
Psychotherapeutic agents (used for antipruritic effect)
  Chlorpromazine (Thorazine), 10-25 mg po q6-8h for severe generalized itching

General Management

Sitz baths
Burow's compresses
Emollients for dry skin
UVB phototherapy in suberythemogenic doses

NURSING CARE

Nursing Assessment

Pruritus

Severity; localization; diurnal or seasonal patterns; distribution

Lesion

Erythema; scaling; excoriation; fissures

Environment

Aggravating factors; stress, tension; depression; irritability

Nursing Dx & Intervention

Impaired skin integrity related to mechanical factors

- Instruct patient in good hygiene *to prevent secondary infection.*
- Instruct patient to cut fingernails short *to avoid tissue damage from scratching.*

Pain related to biologic and physical factors

- Help patient identify and eliminate potentially aggravating factors (see under Patient Education/Home Care Planning).
- Help patient identify stress factors and alternative approaches to dealing with stress *to avoid aggravating the condition.*
- Apply cool compresses and Burow's compresses *to alleviate itching.*
- Offer sitz baths *to alleviate itching.*
- Apply emollients *to prevent dry skin.*
- Instruct patient in use of medications.

Patient Education/Home Care Planning

1. Explain to the patient the need to avoid aggravating factors:
   a. Heat and humidity
   b. Rubbing and friction from clothing
   c. Tight clothing
   d. Wool and rough fabrics
   e. Fabrics that do not allow ventilation
   f. Excessive perspiration
   g. External irritants (such as soap)
   h. Dry skin
   i. Temperature changes
2. Discuss with the patient the use and side effects of medications.
3. Discuss with the patient the use of compresses (see p. 527).
4. Discuss with the patient the signs and symptoms of secondary infection.

Evaluation

Aggravating factors are avoided Pruritus decreases. Exacerbations do not occur.

Underlying disease is identified and treated Erythema, scaling, excoriation, and fissures resolve. Pruritus is alleviated.

Secondary infection is resolved or avoided There is no tenderness, swelling, or purulent exudate in resolving lesions.

Discomfort is alleviated   Scratching and excoriations decrease. Patient is able to sleep.

TINEA (DERMATOPHYTOSIS)

Tinea is a group of superficial fungal infections.

Dermatophytes (ringworm fungi) cause various superficial fungal infections through invasion of the stratum corneum, nails, or hair. The disorders are usually classified according to the anatomic location because treatment of most superficial fungal disorders is the same and the clinical appearance of the eruption is not always related to the species of fungus. The disorder varies from mild inflammation to acute vesicular infection. Remissions and exacerbations may occur. Itching is usually present. The condition is transmissible from other persons or from animals.

•••••• Pathophysiology

The local response to fungal invasion is inflammation, scaling, erythema, and pruritus. A cell-mediated immunologic response may develop, with the production of further erythema, spongiosis, vesicles, and oozing. Table 5-6 summarizes the features of tinea.

•••••• Diagnostic Studies and Findings

Physical examination   Characteristic lesion and distribution

KOH (potassium hydroxide) scraping   Presence of branching mycelia or spores

Fungal culture   Infecting organism

Wood's light   Affected hairs fluoresce

•••••• Multidisciplinary Plan

Medications

Antiinfective agents

Griseofulvin (Fulvicin, Grifulvin, Grisactin, Gris Owen, Gris-Peg) for tinea capitis and severe cases of other tineas, 1 g po in divided doses with meals; may require more than 4 mo therapy; continue therapy for 2 wk after last sign of clinical activity

Ketaconazole (Nizoral), 200-400 mg/d po for up to 3 mo

Itraconazole (Sporonax) 100 mg/d po for 15 d for tinea corporis and tinea cruris; 100 d po for 30 d for tinea pedis; 100 mg/d po for 6 mo for onychomycosis

Terbinafine, 250 mg po bid for 6 weeks; under investigation[1,30]

Topical antifungals rubbed in bid for 3 wk

Tolnaftate 1% (Aftate, Tinactin)

Miconazole 2% (Monistat-Derm)

Clotrimazole 1% (Lotrimin, Mycelex)

Econazole 1% (Spectazole)

Cyclopiroxolamine 1% (Loprox)

Ketaconazole cream 2% (Nizoral), qd

Naftifine cream 1% qd, qel 1% bid (Naftin)

Terbinafine cream 1% (Lamisil)

Keratolytic agents (for noninflammatory scaling)

Salicylic acid 3% and benzene acid 6% in ointment or alcohol

TABLE 5-6 Summary of Tinea

Type	Distribution	Occurrence	Clinical Features
Tinea corporis	Nonhairy parts of body; face; neck; extremities	More common in hot and humid climates; more common in rural than in urban settings; occurs in both adults and children	Pruritus; papulosquamous annular lesions with raised borders; lesions expand peripherally with central clearing
Tinea cruris	Groin; inner thigh; scrotum or labia not involved	More common in adult men; tends to recur; flare-ups common in summer; aggravated by tight clothes, perspiration, and physical activity	Pruritus; hypopigmented; well-demarcated lesions; dryness and scaling; pustules present at margins; central clearing sometimes present; secondary bacterial or candidal infection and maceration common
Tinea capitis	Scalp	More common in children; contagious	Lesions vary: small gray scaly patches with short broken hairs; mild erythematous papules; raised, boggy, inflamed nodules dotted with perifollicular abscesses; thick, yellow, suppurative lesions; lesions may be small, coalesced, or cover entire scalp; hairless patches
Tinea pedis	Feet; begins in third and fourth interdigital spaces and spreads to involve plantar surface; may involve nails	Rare in children; not transmitted by simple exposure	Lesions vary: maceration, scaling, fissuring of interdigital space; vesicular scaling, erythema of plantar surface; chronic, noninflamed, diffuse scaling; nails brittle, discolored; pruritus
Tinea unguium	Toenails and (less commonly) fingernails	—	Nails thickened, lusterless, and discolored; subungual debris; nail plate crumbling or absent

General Management

Preventative measures (see under Patient Education)

NURSING CARE

Nursing Assessment

Lesion

For description and distribution see Table 5-6

Secondary Infection (Bacterial or Candidal)

Itching; exudate; inflammation; odor; tenderness; maceration

Environment

Aggravating factors; hygiene; contacts

Nursing Dx & Intervention

Impaired skin integrity related to infectious process and mechanical factors

- Assess for lesion characteristics and distribution.
- Decrease moisture in affected areas.
- Stress importance of good hygiene and hand washing *to prevent secondary infection.*
- Have patient's fingernails cut short *to avoid tissue trauma from scratching.*
- For tinea capitis, remove scales with shampoo and gently scrub before medication is applied *to maximize absorption of medication.*
- Instruct patient in use of medications and preparations *to avoid recurrence.*

Risk for infection related to transmissibility

- Inform patient that contacts should be screened and referred for treatment if symptoms appear *to avoid reinfection.*
- Instruct patient that pets should be checked and treated for fungal infection *to avoid reinfection.*
- Instruct patient and family to protect themselves and others by not sharing towels or personal articles and by wearing protective footwear in public showers.

Pain related to biologic and physical factors

- Assess for discomfort and itching.
- Instruct patient to avoid tight clothing *to avoid aggravating the condition.*
- Instruct patient to wear cotton next to skin *to avoid aggravating the condition.*
- Instruct patient to stay in areas of decreased humidity *to avoid aggravating the condition.*
- Instruct patient in use of medications and preparations as prescribed.

Patient Education/Home Care Planning

1. Teach the patient and family about the transmission, recurrence, and reinfection of the disease.
2. Discuss with the patient the necessity of avoiding aggravating factors: tight clothing, moist skin, and excessive humidity.
3. Teach the patient to thoroughly dry intertriginous and interdigital areas after bathing; to wear nonocclusive footwear; to wear cotton socks; and to change clothes and towels frequently and to launder them in hot water.
4. Stress the importance of following the therapeutic regimen to avoid recurrence of reinfection.
5. Discuss with the patient and family the side effects of medications.
6. Discuss with the patient and family the signs and symptoms of secondary infection and the necessity of seeking medical attention if they occur.

Evaluation

Eruption clears up   Papules, scaling, pustules, erythema, vesicles, and pruritus resolve. Nails resume smooth texture.

Secondary infection is avoided or resolved   There is no tenderness, swelling, or purulent exudate.

Spread of infection is contained   Contacts are notified and treated if symptoms appear. Personal articles and items are not shared.

Aggravating environmental factors are avoided   Eruption clears. Exacerbations do not recur.

Discomfort is alleviated   Patient stops scratching

■ URTICARIA

Urticaria is a reaction pattern characterized by hives or wheals.

Urticaria is a common disorder tha can occur at any age. It can be acute, chronic, or physical. Most cases are acute, lasting from hours to a few weeks. This condition is self-limited, and most people do not seek medical treatment. Patients who have a history of hives lasting 6 weeks or longer are considered to have chronic urticaria. The course of chronic urticaria is unpredictable and may last for months or years, followed by spontaneous resolution. The physical urticarias include dermographism, pressure urticaria, and cholinergic urticaria. Hives are elicited by physical stimuli to the skin; the attacks are brief and transient.

Drugs, foods, and environmental antigens are common causes of acute and chronic urticaria. Emotional stress should also be considered in the evaluation of chronic urticaria.

•••••• Pathophysiology

A hive or a wheal is a nonpitting edematous plaque that results from localized capillary vasodilation followed by transudation of protein-rich fluid into the surrounding tissue. The hive may be erythematous or white with irregular borders that extend or recede during the evolution of the hive. The hive resolves when the fluid is reabsorbed.

Histamine is the primary chemical mediator of urticaria. Histamine induces vascular changes resulting in vasodilation and pruritus. It also causes endothelial cell contraction, which allows vascular fluid to leak between the cells through the vessel wall. A variety of immunologic, nonimmunologic, physical, and chemical stimuli may cause release of histamine from the mast cells. Other factors that contribute to vascular dilation include alcohol ingestion, emotional stress, endocrine factors, exercise, fever, and heat.

•••••• Diagnostic Studies and Findings

Physical examination   Characteristic lesion, location, pattern, and history; inducement of hive by physical stimuli to determine physical urticaria

Sinus and dental radiographic examination   For chronic urticaria; a percentage of these patients exhibit sinusitis

Change of environment   For chronic urticaria; separation from the home and work environment for a 1- to 2-week trial period

Food challenge   For chronic urticaria, foods containing salicylate, azo dyes, and benzoic acid preservative; to elicit hive development

Biopsy   For chronic urticaria; to rule out urticarial vasculitis

Laboratory tests   For specific suspected causes in internal diseases such as hyperthyroidism, systemic lupus erythematosis, and carcinomas; there are no routine laboratory studies for acute urticaria

•••••• Multidisciplinary Plan

Treatment is aimed at identifying and eliminating known causes or aggravating factors.

Medications

For symptom control
  Epinephrine 1:1000, 0.2-1 ml subcutaneously or IM for severe urticaria and laryngeal edema
Antihistamines
  Hydroxyzine (Atarax, Vistaril), 10 mg q4h, then increase dosage as required to 25-100 mg q4h
  Cyproheptadine (Periactin), 4 mg qid
  Terfenadine (Seldane), 60 mg/po/bid
  Astemizole (Hismanal), 10 mg/po/qid
  Lorataine (Claritin), 10 mg/po/tid
  Cromolyn sodium (Intal) oral nebulizer, 20 mg tid for refractory chronic urticaria

NURSING CARE

Nursing Assessment

Lesion

Edematous plaques of 1-3 mm; erythematous or white, either uniformly or varied; approximately round or oval with borders that extend and recede; new hives appear as old ones resolve; duration varies from hours to weeks; generalized distribution with inhalants, ingestions, and internal disease; localized distribution with contact urticaria

Pruritus

Intensity and interference with activities

Secondary Infection

Erythema, excoriation, purulent exudate from scratching

Nursing Dx & Intervention

Impaired skin integrity related to mechanical factors

- Assess for lesion characteristics and distribution.

Pain related to physical factors

- Assess for excoriation and secondary infection from scratching.
- Trim fingernails short *to prevent secondary infection.*
- Apply cool compresses to localized lesions or use cool baths for generalized eruption *to soothe pruritus.*

Patient Education/Home Care Planning

1. Discuss with the patient the possible causes of condition and help identify and eliminate precipitating or aggravating factors: foods, drugs, emotional stress, exercise, heat, pressure or physical stimuli, other vasodilating factors.
2. Discuss with the patient a diet free of salicylates, azo dyes, and benzoic acid preservatives if indicated.
3. Discuss with the patient the use of antihistamines.
4. Discuss with the patient the chronic nature of urticaria, that evaluation may be lengthy and unrewarding, and that in most cases the disorder resolves spontaneously.

Evaluation

Eruption improves   Hives resolve and do not recur.

Pruritus is alleviated   Areas of excoriation resolve or do not occur. Patient stops scratching.

VASCULAR DISORDERS OF CUTANEOUS BLOOD VESSELS

■ HEMANGIOMAS

Hemangiomas are congenital vascular lesions of the skin and subcutaneous tissue.

•••••• Pathophysiology

The three common types of hemangiomas are nevus flammeus, capillary hemangiomas, and cavernous hemangioma.

Nevus flammeus (port-wine stain) is a flat purple-red lesion that is present at birth and is caused by a mass of mature, dilated, congested capillaries in the dermis. The color depends on whether the superficial, middle, or deep dermal vessels are involved. The lesion does not disappear or fade over time, does not enlarge, and may develop a thickened nodular surface.

The occipital area of the scalp is the most common site of occurrence. The lesion may occur elsewhere and is frequently seen on the face. The lesion are usually unilateral and tend to follow the course of a cutaneous nerve.

Capillary hemangioma (strawberry mark) is a common, raised, bright red lesion that usually appears in the third to fifth week of life. It consists of a proliferation of endothelial cells arranged in strawberry-like lobules. It may occur anywhere on the body. It may enlarge for the first several months but rarely enlarges after the first year. It involutes spontaneously and is usually completely regressed by 3 to 5 years of age. Involution begins with an area of fibrosis in the center. The lesion may leave a brownish pigmentation or scarring and wrinkling of the skin as it involutes. No treatment is required unless the lesion is massively disfiguring or is near the eye or a body orifice where it might interfere with body functioning.

Cavernous hemangioma is a large vascular pool lined with mature epithelial cells that are located in the subcutaneous tissue of the dermis. It is deeper than the other types of hemangiomas and may contain many arteriovenous shunts and vascular formations.

The lesion, which is present at birth, is reddish blue and round and may be elevated and compressible. It can occur on any part of the body. Most lesions eventually involute at least partially.

•••••• Diagnostic Studies and Findings

Physical examination   Characteristic lesion and congruent history

•••••• Multidisciplinary Plan

Laser Therapy*

Nevus flammeus: argon laser, pulsed-dye laser, candela laser, CW dye laser, copper vapor laser
Capillary hemangioma: argon laser, pulsed-dye laser
Cavernous hemangioma: argon laser, Nd-YAG laser

Surgery

Used for capillary or cavernous hemangiomas only if lesion does not involute; may leave more scarring than spontaneous resolution
Excision with grafting
Cryosurgery (see p. 528)

Medications

Capillary or cavernous hemangiomas
Corticosteroids; efficacy questionable[1]
Prednisone, 10 mg po bid or tid with decremental doses until lesion resolves
Intralesional injection of triamcinolone (Kenalog, Aristocort); may cause scar formation

---

*References 3, 4, 10, 14, 27, 28, 39, 46.

NURSING CARE

Nursing Assessment

Lesion History

Present or absent at birth; rate of growth or involution

Lesion

Size; color; texture; elevation; location; secondary trauma or bleeding

Nursing Dx & Intervention

Risk for impaired skin integrity related to mechanical factors

- Assess lesion for characteristics.
- Instruct patient in ways to protect lesions from scratching (cut nails short) and trauma *to avoid tissue damage and bleeding and secondary infection.*
- Stress importance of good hygiene *to avoid secondary infection.*
- Advise patient that it is better to wait for involution of capillary and cavernous hemangiomas *to avoid complications and scarring through early treatment.*

Body image disturbance related to cognitive-perceptual factors

- Assess for defining characteristics.
- Advise patient of excellent prognosis for involution of capillary and cavernous hemangiomas, but warn that lesion may grow before it involutes.
- Use accurate measurements or photographs *to show progress of involution.*
- Assess patient's self-perception or parents' perception of child's appearance.
- Encourage patient to express feelings about body, body image, and fear of reaction or rejection by others *to begin process of realistic self-evaluation.*
- Help patient or parent evaluate appearance in realistic manner *so lesion does not become focal point of existence.*

Patient Education/Home Care Planning

1. Discuss with the patient and family the likelihood of involution.
2. Discuss with the patient and family the hazards of unnecessary treatment.

Evaluation

Secondary trauma and infection are minimized   Lesion remains intact and free of bleeding, crusting, excoriation, and purulent exudate.

Unnecessary scarring is avoided Family waits for spontaneous involution in capillary and cavernous hemangiomas before seeking treatment.

Patient and parents evaluate appearance in realistic manner Patient develops interest and attributes and engages in activities so hemangioma is not focal point of existence. Lesion is not used as excuse for unsuccessful interpersonal relationships.

TELANGIECTASIA AND HEREDITARY HEMORRHAGIC TELANGIECTASIA

Telangiectasia is a network of dilated superficial dermal capillaries and venules.

•••••• Pathophysiology

Essential telangiectasia is a disorder that is characterized by a network of small dilated veins on the thighs and calves of adult women. The condition is localized and often symmetric. The vessels involved are the superficial venous plexuses. The condition affects the appearance only, not the health, of the person.

Telangiectasia is also a component of certain systemic diseases, such as lupus erythematosus and scleroderma, and certain hereditary disorders. Hereditary hemorrhagic telangiectasia (Rendu-Osler-Weber disease) is a rare, autosomal dominant, inherited disorder. Telangiectatic lesions of the skin, mucous membranes, and internal organs are present in this disease. Lesions occur most commonly after puberty and increase throughout adult life. The small, red to violet lesions consist of thin, dilated vessels that blanch with pressure and tend to bleed spontaneously or with minor trauma. Bleeding may also occur from lesions in the mouth, pharynx, and gastrointestinal and genitourinary tracts. Anemia may result from continued oozing. Bleeding tends to become more severe with age. Systemic problems may arise from associated pulmonary arteriovenous fistulas and cerebrovascular malformations.

•••••• Diagnostic Studies and Findings

Physical examination Characteristic lesions
Complete blood count Iron deficiency anemia

•••••• Multidisciplinary Plan

For treatment of anemia see Chapter 15. For treatment of underlying systemic disorders see the specific diseases.

Medications

For Rendu-Osler-Weber disease
   Estrogens
      Cyclic therapy to decrease bleeding tendency
   Corticosteroids
      Nasal spray to control bleeding
   Hematinic agents
      Iron po for iron loss through repeated bleeding

General Management

For localized lesions
   Electrolysis—free hydrogen via electric current to obliterate vessels
Blood transfusion for acute hemorrhage

Laser Therapy

Argon or pulsed dye laser[4,27,28]

NURSING CARE

Nursing Assessment

Lesion

Number, location and bleeding tendency; symptoms of anemia (see Chapter 15)

Nursing Dx & Intervention

Impaired skin integrity related to pathologic process and mechanical factors

- Assess lesions for characteristics.
- Instruct patient *to avoid trauma to lesions;* wear protective clothing and cut fingernails short.

Altered oral mucous membrane related to pathologic condition and trauma

- Instruct patient to eat soft foods *to avoid mechanical trauma.*
- Instruct patient to use soft toothbrush *to avoid mechanical trauma.*

Body image disturbance related to cognitive-perceptual factors

- Assess for defining characteristics.
- Encourage patient to express feelings about body, body image, or fear of reaction or rejection by others *to begin process of realistic self-evaluation.*
- Advise patient of availability of covering makeup (Covermark).

Patient Education/Home Care Planning

1. Discuss with the patient protective measures to avoid trauma that may cause bleeding (see under Nursing Dx and Intervention).
2. Discuss with the patient the use and side effects of medications.
3. Discuss with the patient the advisability of seeking medical attention if unable to stop a bleeding episode.

Evaluation

Trauma is minimized Bleeding episodes are less frequent.

Patient assesses self-concept in realistic manner   Patient engages in activities compatible with limitations of disorder. Patient engages in interpersonal relationships. Patient employs protective measures and seeks medical attention as needed.

▍VASCULITIS

▍Vasculitis is a range of cutaneous lesions associated with inflammation of the wall of blood vessels of the skin and subcutaneous tissue.

Vasculitis is a general term for a large number of disorders that cause skin lesions as a result of inflammation of the walls of cutaneous blood vessels. The diseases range in severity from mild to fatal. The cutaneous lesions appear as erythematous papules and plaques, nodules, urticaria, purpuric or hemorrhagic papules and vesicles, and pustular and necrotic lesions.

Lesions, which tend to develop in crops, occur most commonly on the legs, thighs, and buttocks. Some lesions begin as erythematous papules or plaques and progress to ulcerations that heal slowly. In severe ulcerative forms, lesions are progressive and involve other body organs. There is currently no universal or satisfactory classification system for the vasculitis disorders.

•••••• Pathophysiology

Vasculitis involves intravascular and extravascular changes. The sequence of events occurs as a result of damage to the vessel that is precipitated by numerous factors and modified by the body's response to noxious stimuli.

The inflammatory process of the vessel includes increased permeability; epithelial shedding; increased deposition of fibrin, platelets, and leukocytes; changes in endothelial cells during repair; and thrombosis. The cutaneous changes that occur as a result of the inflammation processes depend on the degree of inflammation and the size of the involved vessel.

The pathogenesis of vasculitis can be summarized as follows:
Intravascular component
   Deposition of circulating antigen-antibody complexes with chemotaxis of leukocytes and release of mediators of inflammation
   Direct toxic effect of circulating chemicals, drugs, and bacterial antigens
   Bacterial emboli and reaction to products of bacterial breakdown
Vascular wall component
   Endothelial proliferation in reparative attempt
   Infiltration by lymphocytes and polymorphonuclear leukocytes
   Fibrinoid necrosis and scarring from fibrin deposits
   Granulomatous infiltrates
Extravascular component
   Leakage of red blood cells and fibrin into surrounding tissue

Deposition of inflammatory infiltrates
Thrombosis of small vessels with secondary tissue; ischemia
Increased fibrosis
Venous stasis

•••••• Diagnostic Studies and Findings

Physical examination   Lesions and history as described under Nursing Assessment
Biopsy of blood vessel   Immunofluorescence shows cellular changes as described above; will determine type and severity of vasculitis
Further studies to determine systemic involvement and underlying conditions   Complete blood count; antinuclear factor, serum protein, and rheumatoid factor; serum fibrinolytic activity; VDRL test or rapid plasma reagin test; culture and antistreptolysin titer; urinalysis for red blood cells and casts; serum complement and cryoglobulin; x-rays of chest, sinuses, and teeth; of gastrointestinal tract if symptoms indicate

•••••• Multidisciplinary Plan

Specific treatment is aimed at the particular clinical condition or underlying disease process.

Medications
   Antihypertensive agents
      If needed to minimize small vessel damage
   Antiinfective agents
      Agent-specific to clear infection
   Corticosteroids
      Systemic glucocorticoids for deep tender nodular lesions
   Nonsteroidal antiinflammatory agents
      Aspirin, potassium iodide, indomethacin (Indocin), ibuprofen (Motrin), phenylbutazone (Butazolidin, Azolid)

NURSING CARE

Nursing Assessment

Lesion
   Erythematous papules, plaques, or nodules; persistent urticaria; purpuric papules and vesicles; pustules; necrotic lesions

Surrounding Tissue
   Abnormal vascular patterns; abnormal reactions to cold

History
   Precipitating factors; infection; food and drug allergies or sensitivity

General Medical Problems
   Diabetes mellitus; arthritis; cardiovascular diseases; respiratory diseases; connective tissue diseases

Nursing Dx & Intervention

Nursing interventions other than those listed depend on the symptoms produced by the particular clinical condition and disorder.

Impaired skin integrity related to inflammatory process

- Assess lesions for characteristics.
- Instruct patient in good hygiene and hand washing *to prevent secondary infection.*
- Apply dressings on open or draining lesions.

Risk for impaired skin integrity related to altered circulation

- Encourage elevation of affected part *to promote lymphatic drainage.*
- Initiate range-of-motion exercises *to maintain blood flow.*
- Protect affected area from cold *to prevent vasoconstriction.*

Pain related to physical factors

- Assess for defining characteristics.
- Encourage patient to rest affected area.
- Apply cool compresses to hot, nodular lesions.

Patient Education/Home Care Planning

1. Teach the patient how to change dressings, if indicated, using aseptic technique.
2. Teach the patient how to use cool compresses as needed.
3. Discuss with the patient the use of medications and their side effects.
4. Discuss with the patient the signs and symptoms of secondary infection and the need to seek medical attention if they occur.

Evaluation

Clinical disorder is identified and treated Inflammatory response is not exacerbated or does not recur.

Cutaneous lesions improve Erythema and lesions resolve. Necrotic areas reepithelialize. Discomfort is alleviated. Skin is intact.

Secondary infection is resolved or avoided There is no swelling, purulent exudate, fever, or lymphadenopathy.

BURNS (THERMAL, CHEMICAL, AND ELECTRICAL)

Thermal burns are caused by exposure to flames, hot liquids, and radiation. Chemical burns are caused by contact, ingestion, inhalation, or injection of acids, alkalies, or vesicants. True electrical burns occur when electrical current passes through the body to the ground. Electrical current can also cause secondary flash or flame burns.

More than 2 million people in the United States are burned each year. Although most of these burn injuries are minor, approximately 3% to 5% are life threatening. Burn injury is the second-leading cause of death among young children and is the fourth overall cause of accidental death for people of all ages.

•••••• Pathophysiology

Thermal and chemical injury disrupts the normal protective barrier function of the skin, causing a wide range of sequelae. In electrical injury heat is generated as the electricity passes through tissues. The thermal energy released is the cause of the injury.

The extent and depth of the burn injury determine the extent and severity of burn sequalae. Injury to the stratum corneum results in evaporative heat and water loss as a result of the loss or disruption of the lipid-water barrier of that layer. Injury to the stratum germinativum results in delayed or absent reepithelization and healing. Injury to the deeper structures results in scarring and tissue damage that may require skin grafting.

Vascular changes are caused by direct cellular damage or inflammatory processes. During the first few hours after the burn, vasoactive substances are released from the injured cells and vasoconstriction occurs. Vasodilation then occurs as a result of kinin release. During this period histamine causes increased capillary permeability, which allows plasma to leak into the burn area.

There are three zones of associated tissue damage:

Zone of coagulation. This is the area of greatest destruction, where coagulation and irreversible cellular death occur. The area remains white because all viable tissue has been destroyed. Leukocytosis is inhibited or totally blocked. The zone can extend deeply into the tissue structures, causing full-thickness skin destruction.

Zones of stasis. This area surrounds the zone of coagulation and involves the vasculative dermis. Shortly after the burn, leukocytes and platelets aggregate in underlying capillaries, causing thrombosis. This, combined with the vasoconstriction, causes decreased circulation and transient ischemia to the area. With appropriate protection and treatment, circulation to the area can be restored and the tissue saved. However, the tissue in this area is very fragile, and any further trauma because of rough handling or infection can convert this zone to one resembling the zone of coagulation.

Zone of hyperemia. This area, which is the least affected, forms the border of the burn wound. Vascular integrity is maintained with no cellular death. The area is bright red and blanches with pressure. The inflammatory processes are present.

In electrical injury, vessel wall changes occur that are characterized by cellular disintegration of the media of the arteries and arterioles and by severe arterial spasm.

Vascular changes and tissue loss cause fluid shifts. The first of these shifts, the hypovolemic stage, occurs during the first 24 to 48 hours. It is characterized by a rapid shift of fluid and protein from the vascular compartment into the interstitial spaces, causing blisters, edema, and fluid escape. Deep in the wound, sodium is translocated into skeletal muscle and other tissues and pulls water with it, which results in hyponatremia and hyperkalemia. This fluid shift, along with evaporative fluid loss from the surface of the wound, causes an abrupt decrease in the circulating blood volume resulting in hypovolemic shock. In turn hypovolemic shock causes decreased cardiac stroke volume, decreased blood pressure, increased peripheral resistance, decreased tissue perfusion, and circulatory collapse. Anuria, renal failure, and death result if treatment is delayed or inadequate.

Uninjured cells may become dehydrated as a result of this fluid shift. Hypoproteinemia develops from continued loss of protein as a result of increased capillary permeability. Nitrogen is lost through renal catabolism, and a negative nitrogen balance develops. Metabolic acidosis can occur as a result of decreased tissue perfusion, anaerobic metabolism, and retained acid end products.

Within 18 hours after the burn injury, the sodium and water shunting reverse. Within 48 to 72 hours of the burn, a second fluid shift occurs in the opposite direction that causes fluid to return to the vascular compartment. In this phase the rapidly increasing blood volume causes diuresis and hemodilution that may result in dehydration, hyponatremia, and hypokalemia. Metabolic acidosis may occur because of bicarbonate loss in the urine and the catabolic state. Protein continues to be lost through the burn wound. Hypovitaminosis and weight loss also occur.

The evaporative fluid loss that occurs after the burn may be 5 to 19 times the normal loss. Associated with this fluid loss are tremendous heat loss and hypermetabolism that cause enormous caloric expenditure and hypothermia.

Erythrocyte hemolysis and a decrease in red cell mass occur as a result of direct damage and a decreased half-life of damaged red cells. Platelet function and half-life are also diminished. Hemoconcentration occurs as a result of fluid loss from the vascular system, which causes hematocrit values to rise.

Patients who have been injured in a fire may also have carbon monoxide poisoning from inhaling the gas that results from incomplete burning of some materials. Poisoning occurs because carbon monoxide has 200 times the affinity of oxygen to combine with hemoglobin.

•••••• Diagnostic Studies and Findings

Physical examination   Determination of extent of injury using rule of nines (Figure 5-9); Lund and Browder charts (Figure 5-10); determination of degree of injury (Tables 5-7 and 5-8)

Determination of mechanism of injury   Thermal, chemical, or electrical

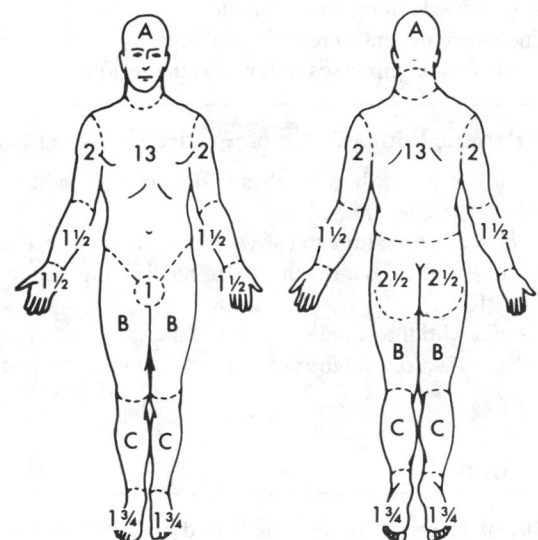

Relative percentages of areas affected by growth (age in years)

	0	1	5	10	15	Adult
A: half of head	9½	8½	6½	5½	4½	3½
B: half of thigh	2¾	3¼	4	4¼	4½	4¾
C: half of leg	2½	2½	2¾	3	3¼	3½

Second degree _____ and
Third degree _____ =
Total percent burned____

Figure 5-10 Estimation of burn injury: Lund and Browder chart. Areas designated by letters (**A, B,** and **C**) represent percentages of body surface area that vary according to age. The accompanying table indicates the relative percentages of these areas at various stages in life. (From Sabiston.[64])

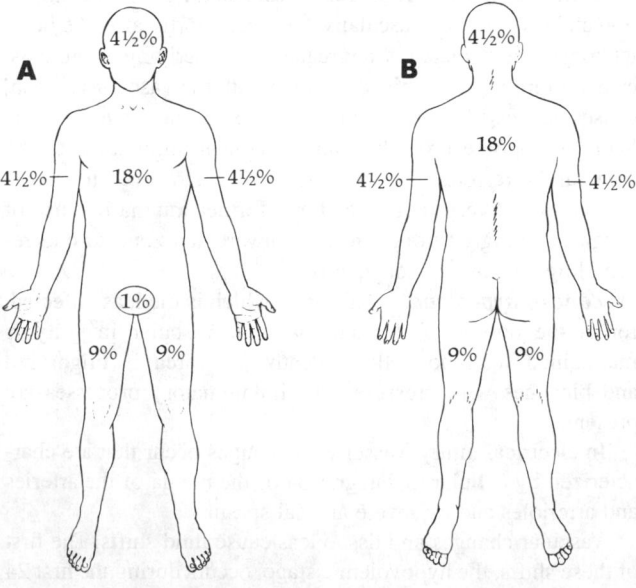

Figure 5-9 Estimation of adult burn injury: rule of nines. **A,** Anterior view. **B,** Posterior view.

TABLE 5-7 Assessment of Burn Injury

Degree	Depth	Characteristics
Superficial (first degree)	Epidermis only; devitalization of epidermis and dilation of intradermal vessels	Pain; erythema; blanching with pressure; normal texture
Partial-thickness (second degree)	Destruction of epidermis and part of dermis	Erythema; blisters; pain; blanching with pressure; firm texture
Full-thickness (third and fourth degree)	Destruction of all layers of skin extending into subcutaneous tissue, muscle, nerves, and bone	Dryness; pale, white, brown, or red color; charring; no capillary refill; no pain; firm and leathery texture

TABLE 5-8 American Burn Association Classification of Burn Injury

Class	Description
Major	Full-thickness burns over 10% or more of body surface area (BSA)
	Partial-thickness burns over 25% of BSA
	All burns on face, hands, eyes, ears, feet, or perineum
	All inhalation and electrical burns
	All burns complicated by trauma
	All burns in poor-risk patients
Moderate	Full-thickness burns over 2%-10% of BSA
	Partial-thickness burns over 15%-25% of BSA
Minor	Full-thickness burns over less than 2% of BSA
	Partial-thickness burns over less than 15% of BSA

Baseline laboratory studies Complete blood count; serum electrolytes; glucose; blood urea nitrogen; creatinine; arterial carboxyhemoglobin; arterial blood gases; bilirubin; phosphorus; alkaline phosphatase; clotting studies; urine for myoglobin and hemoglobin levels

Fiberoptic bronchoscopy Inspection of major and proximal airways to determine upper airway injury

Xenon lung scan Determination of small airway and parenchymal burns; bolus of xenon is injected; as xenon gas is expired from lungs, injured areas trap gas and show high-density levels.

●●●●●● Multidisciplinary Plan

Short-Term Care of Major Burns

Surgery

Escharotomy—may be needed for circumferentially burned extremities or chest

Fasciotomy—may be needed for electrical injuries

Medications

Narcotic analgesics
  Meperidine (Demerol) for pain, 20-25 mg IV
Immunologic agents
  Tetanus immunization
Diptheria tetanus (DT)
  0.5 ml IM for immunized patients
  0.5 ml IM plus 250 U tetanus immune globulin (Hypertet) for nonimmunized patients

! EMERGENCY ALERT

THERMAL INJURY: BURNS

Burn injury occurs from human contact with flame, hot liquids and objects, chemicals, electricity, and radiation. The surface burn is a low priority during initial contact with the patient; maintaining airway, breathing, and circulation is the top priority.

Assessment

- Assess airway and respiratory status for burns and inhalation injury; prepare for emergency intubation.
- Obtain history of events, time of incident, duration, and nature of chemicals if known.
- Assess physical area of injuries and burns.
- Assess circulatory status of affected extremities.

Interventions

- Maintain airway, breathing, and circulation.
- Stop burn process by removing clothing.
- Administer high-flow humidified oxygen (10 to 15 L) by mask.
- Obtain IV access and administer fluids.
- Maintain temperature by covering burns with *dry* sterile dressings and ensuring warm room temperature.
- Elevate affected extremities.
- Manage pain.
- Physician may consider escharotomies for compromised circulation.
- Prevent infection by using aseptic technique.
- If chemical burn: thoroughly rinse off chemical.
- If electrical burn: be alert that as electricity passes through the body muscle damage, including to the heart, may have occurred.
- If tar burn: cool tar, remove with oil-based product such as antibiotic ointment or De-Solv-It solvent.

General Management

Airway maintenance; intubation if needed

Humidification with 10% oxygen for inhalation injuries

Emergency treatment of musculoskeletal injuries or hemorrhage

Fluid replacement

  Parkland (Baxter formula)—2-4 ml lactated Ringer's solution/kg/% of BS burned/24 hr; give one half of total amount in first 8 hours and one half during next 16 hours

Brooke formula (after first 24 hours)—colloids (plasma, plasmanate, or dextran) 0.5 ml/kg/% of BSA burned plus 2000 ml of dextrose in water

Electrical and inhalation injuries require more fluids

Urethral catheterization

Nasogastric tube insertion

Wound cleansing with povidone-iodine (Betadine), saline, or hydrogen peroxide

Central venous line insertion

Swan-Ganz catheter to monitor pulmonary arterial and capillary wedge pressures

Long-Term Care of Major Burns

Surgery

Skin grafts (see p. 530)

Split-thickness—autograft from unburned area; postage stamp or strip application

Mesh graft—split-thickness graft meshed with special instrument to cover large areas; held in place by dressing or sutures

Homograft—skin from deceased person; used as temporary cover for about 10 days; may survive 4 to 5 weeks

Heterograft—pigskin or synthetic substitute; acts as biologic dressing

Autologous cultured human epithelium—epidermal cells from unburned area cultured into sheets in flask; cultured sheets then attached to petrolatum gauze squares and sutured in place in wound; petrolatum gauze removed 7 to 10 days later

Amputation of limb severely injured from electrical injury

Medications

Antiinfective agents

Topical (Table 5-9)

Mafenide acetate 10% (Sulfamylon); sterile application of amounts sufficient to just cover wound; wound left open to air; reapplied bid after washing off previous application and debriding wound

Silver sulfadiazine 1% (Silvadene) cream applied tid or qid; left open or covered with mesh gauze dressing;

washed off before application, but no wound debridement done

Silver nitrate solution 0.5%; saturated thick gauze pads replaced q12-24h

Parenteral

Aq. Penicillin G for prophylaxis against gram-positive organisms; 1.2-2 million U IV in divided doses

Narcotic analgesics

Codeine, meperidine (Demerol), methadone (Dolophine); dosage determined on individual basis

General Management

Wound debridement (see p. 528)

Hydrotherapy (see p. 527) once or twice daily for 20 to 30 minutes for dressing removal and debridement

Dressings, wet or dry (see p. 527 for wet dressings)

Dry dressing—single layer of nonadherent fine mesh gauze held in place by coarse gauze wrap

Nutrition

2 to 4 protein/kg/d

3500 to 5000 calories daily

Vitamin and iron replacement

Total parenteral nutrition (hyperalimentation) if needed

Physiotherapy

Care of Minor Burns

Medications

Immunologic agents

Tetanus immunization, 0.5 ml IM for immunized patients

Diphtheria tetanus

0.5 ml IM plus 250 U tetanus immune globulin (Hypertet) for nonimmunized patients

Antiinfective agents

Topical (applied with sterile tongue blade to completely cover wound with 1/8-inch thickness)

Mafenide acetate (Sulfamylon) 5%

Silver sulfadiazine (Silvadene) 1%

Povidone-iodine (Betadine)

Polymyxin B, Bacitracin, Neosporin

Nystatin combined with Silvadene

■ **TABLE 5-9   Comparison of Topical Burn Agents**

Agent	Advantages	Disadvantages
Mafenide acetate (Sulfamylon)	Penetrates rapidly; not inactivated by pus or body fluids; softens wound, allowing better mobility; more effective in established infection	Painful; sulfa sensitivities; acidosis with renal or pulmonary impairment; antibacterial activity lasts 4-6 h
Silver sulfadiazine (Silvadene)	Penetrates slowly; not inactivated by pus or body fluids; minimum systemic absorption; painless; antibacterial activity lasts up to 48 hours	Sulfa sensitivities; not as effective in established infection
Silver nitrate	Wet dressings retain heat, moisture, and reduce evaporation; no sensitivities	Painful; staining

Narcotic analgesics
Codeine, 30-60 mg po or subcutaneously q4-6h
Morphine, 8-10 mg subcutaneously
Meperidine (Demerol), 50-100 mg po q4-6h
Analgesic-antipyretics
Aspirin, 650 mg po q4-6h

General Management

Wound cleansed with one-half-strength Betadine solution
Wound debridement (see p. 528)
Dressing—innermost layer of nonadherent, porous, fine mesh gauze (fine enough to prevent epithelialization into gauze); second layer of bulky, fluffed coarse mesh gauze to absorb exudate; outer layer of semielastic coarse mesh to apply even pressure and hold dressing in place; change once or twice daily
Polyurethane dressing (Epi-Lock), left on for one week
Hydrocolloid dressings (Duoderm), left on for several days
Dimac with silver sulfadiazine (Sildimac), dressing left on for several days

NURSING CARE

Nursing Assessment

Wound

Degree and extent of injury; see Tables 5-7 and 5-8; mechanism of injury (thermal, chemical, or mechanical)

First Fluid Shift and Hypovolemic Shock

Vital signs: decreased blood pressure, increased pulse; urinary output (desirable:50 ml/h); monitoring of central venous pressure; potassium levels increased

Second Fluid Shift

Hyperpnea; blood pH less than 7.35; CO_2 combining power less than 21 mEq/L; $PaCO_2$ less than 40 mm Hg

Airway

Pulmonary edema (see Chapter 2); singed nasal hair; soot in mouth or nose; darkened septum; rales, cough, or cyanosis; dyspnea or stridor

Carbon Monoxide Poisoning

Vomiting; chest pain; tachycardia; confusion; agitation; decreased coordination

Neurologic

Changes in level of consciousness

Cardiovascular

Vital signs; dysrhythmias; fluid shifts; cyanosis; capillary refill; pulses

Musculoskeletal

Fractures; decreased mobility; deformities; exposed bone or muscle

Hypermetabolism and Heat Loss

Body temperature; weight loss

Hemopoietic

Increased hematocrit; hemoglobinuria

Gastrointestinal

Mouth injuries; nausea and vomiting; blood in gastric contents; bowel sounds; paralytic ileus; stress ulcer

Renal

Renal failure resulting from hypovolemic shock; oliguria; anuria; desirable output 50 ml/h for adults, 1 ml/kg/h for children; myoglobinuria; hemoglobinuria; diuresis (second phase)

Pain

Presence or absence; location; intensity; severity

Psychosocial

Body image

Infection

Inflammation; exudate; odor

Nursing Dx & Intervention

Impaired skin integrity related to hyperthermia

- Assess for degree and extent of injury.
- Handle wounds gently *to avoid converting zone of stasis to zone of coagulation.*
- Provide hydrotherapy *to debride burn.*
- Provide wound care to graft donor site *to promote healing.*
- Use bed cradles *to prevent pressure to injured tissue.*
- Assess for signs and symptoms of first and second fluid shifts.

Infection, risk for, related to impaired skin integrity

- Implement isolation precautions *to prevent infection.*
- Use sterile technique in wound care: debridement, topical preparations, and dressing changes *to prevent infection.*
- Use sterile linen *to prevent infection.*

Fluid volume deficit related to active loss

- Observe patency of urinary catheter.
- Monitor input and output.
- Replace fluids to achieve output of 50 ml/h.
- Monitor vital signs.
- Monitor urine specific gravity.
- Monitor central venous pressure.

Altered renal, cardiopulmonary, gastrointestinal, and peripheral tissue perfusion related to hypovolemia

- Maintain adequate fluid replacement *to maintain circulating volume.*
- Maintain optimum mobility *to promote circulation.*
- Provide adequate nutrition *to promote tissue healing.*

Impaired physical mobility related to musculoskeletal impairments; high risk for disuse syndrome related to immobilization

- Provide active and passive range-of-motion exercises *to prevent muscle wasting and contractures.*
- Use CircOlectric bed per physician order.
- Refer patient for physiotherapy *to establish therapeutic regimen of motion and exercise.*
- Apply splints *to prevent contractures.*
- Have patient participate in water exercises *to maintain limb mobility.*
- See p. 1597.

Altered nutrition: less than body requirements related to hypermetabolism

- Assess for nutritional status and weight loss.
- Monitor protein intake: 2 to 4 g/kg/d.
- Monitor caloric intake: 3500 to 5000 calories daily *to meet necessary requirements and promote healing.*
- Monitor vitamin replacement.
- In collaboration with physician, institute total parenteral nutrition *to replace or supplement oral intake.*
- Provide high-protein powdered milk preparations.
- Encourage self-feeding.
- Offer favorite foods *to stimulate appetite.*
- Avoid performing painful procedures near mealtime.
- Offer snacks.

Constipation related to immobilization, altered tissue perfusion, medications

- Assess for defining characteristics.
- Give nothing by mouth until bowel sounds return.
- Provide bulk foods *to promote peristalsis.*
- Provide fruit juices *to promote peristalsis.*
- Administer stool softeners *to aid elimination.*

Hypothermia related to fluid loss

- Keep patient warm through control of environmental temperature *to prevent heat loss.*
- Maintain adequate caloric intake (see under Nutrition) *to provide energy and heat replacement.*

Pain related to chemical or physical agents

- Assess for pain.
- Administer analgesics as ordered.
- Position patient for comfort.
- Provide or refer patient for hydrotherapy.
- Instruct in relaxation techniques.
- Refer patient for biofeedback training.

Body image disturbance related to cognitive-perceptual factors; situational low self-esteem

- Assess for defining characteristics.
- Encourage patient to express feelings about body, body appearance, or fear of reaction or rejection by others *to begin process of realistic self-evaluation.*
- Spend time with patient *to reassure patient that appearance is not repulsive.*
- Prepare visitors for patient's appearance *to reduce overt negative reactions.*
- Encourage self-esteem by continued interest in patient and attentiveness to patient's needs.

Anticipatory grieving related to potential loss of physiosocial and psychosocial well-being

- Assess for defining characteristics.
- Encourage patient to express distress, anger, sorrow, guilt, and fear *to assist patient in movement through stages of grieving.*

Powerlessness related to illness-related regimen

- Observe for signs of depression or apathy.
- Involve patient in decision making *to increase sense of control.*
- Encourage patient to express dissatisfaction and frustration.
- Accept patient's feelings of anger.

Patient Education/Home Care Planning

1. Demonstrate to the patient the care of minor burns:
   a. Cleanse wound with one-half-strength Betadine using sterile gauze; rub gently to remove existing topical agent.
   b. Apply topical agent thickly enough to cover wound with $1/8$ inch of agent to provide healing and prevent bandage from adhering.
   c. Apply nonadherent fine mesh gauze (fine enough not to be epithelialized), then fluffed bulky coarse gauze to trap exudate; hold in place with semielastic net to exert even pressure.
2. Discuss with the patient the care of healed burns:
   a. Wash skin gently, rinse well, dry thoroughly, and apply cream.
   b. Avoid exposure to sunlight, harsh detergents, fabric softeners, and irritation by rubbing of clothing.
3. Discuss with the patient the importance of watching for signs of infection and the need to seek early treatment to avoid further complications.
4. Explain to the patient that increased calories and protein may be required until healing is complete.
5. Advise the patient of available support groups and community resources to assist in the resumption of usual activities and relationships.

Evaluation

State of homeostasis exists Normal blood values include the following: pH of 7.35-7.45; $PaCO_2$ of 40-43; CO_2 combining power of 21-28 mEq/L; sodium 136-145 mEq/L; potassium 3.5-5 mEq/L; chloride 100-106 mEq/L. Nitrogen is in balance. Fluids are in balance. Patient has usual elimination pattern.

Burn area heals Reepithelialization occurs. Skin is intact and free of infection.

Nutrition is adequate Patient eats diet high in protein, calories, minerals, and vitamins. Patient does not lose weight. Wounds heal.

Patient is free of contractures Patient has full extremity flexion and extension.

Patient resocializes and evaluates appearance in realistic manner Patient returns or plans to return to former activities if possible. Patient develops interests and activities compatible with degree of limitation. Patient engages in satisfactory interpersonal relationships.

Home care is satisfactory Healing remains uninterrupted. New tissue is free of irritation or infection. Scar tissue remains soft and pliable.

Complications are recognized and treatment is sought Patient seeks medical attention for infection, weight loss, contracture, or changes in scar tissue.

■ COLD INJURY (FROSTBITE)

Frostbite is a localized cold injury caused by exposure to freezing temperatures.

Several predisposing factors are associated with the occurrence of frostbite. People who are not acclimated to the cold and those from warmer climates have more vasospasm and less heat production in their extremities when exposed to cold temperatures; thus their risk of cold injury is increased. A racial predisposition of blacks to cold injury has been noted. Fatigue, hunger, young or old age, circulatory disorders, fear, use of alcohol, and hypoxia increase the risk of cold injury. Factors that promote heat loss such as contact with metal, wet skin, and high wind velocity contribute to the occurrence and severity of frostbite injuries.

•••••• Pathophysiology

Cellular injury in frostbite is caused by direct freezing of cells at the time of injury or by inadequate tissue perfusion resulting from vascular spasm and occlusion of small vessels in the injured area.

With direct freezing of cells (crystallization), ice crystals form in extracellular fluids and osmotically draw intracellular fluid, thereby causing cel dehydration. Vascular changes include vasoconstriction, decreased capillary perfusion, and increased viscosity of the blood with sludging and thrombus formation.

After thawing, vascular stasis occurs in the injured area as a result of obstruction in the vascular bed. Edema occurs in the injured area and peaks 2 to 3 days after thawing. Thrombi, interstitial hemorrhaging, and leukocyte infiltration are present. Tissue necrosis occurs and becomes more prominent as the edema resolves. It may take 60 to 90 days before the necrotic tissue becomes fully evident.

The extent of the injury is determined by the amount and rate of heat loss from the skin. Frostbite is classified as superficial or deep. Superficial injury involves the skin and subcutaneous tissue. The injured area is white, waxy, soft, and anesthetic. Capillary refill is absent. On thawing the area becomes flushed, edematous, and painful and then may turn mottled or purplish. Large blisters may develop within 24 hours and resolve in about 10 days, leaving a hard dark eschar. After 3 to 4 weeks the eschar separates, leaving sensitive new epithelium. Throbbing and burning pain lasts for several weeks. The area is sensitive to heat and cold for months, and the frostbitten part may perspire excessively.

Deep frostbite injures the skin, subcutaneous tissue, muscle, tendon, and neurovascular structures. The injured part is hard and solid and remains cold, mottled, and blue or gray after thawing. Blisters may be absent or may form after several weeks at the point where viable and nonviable tissue meet. Edema occurs in the entire limb and may take months to resolve. When the blisters dry, blacken, and slough off, a line of demarcation remains where the viable tissue separates and retracts from the dead tissue.

•••••• Diagnostic Studies and Findings

Physical examination Characteristic findings with congruent history

•••••• Multidisciplinary Plan

Surgery

Escharotomy

Sympathectomy for severe vasospasm and pain

Debridement after retraction of viable tissue (13 weeks to 4 months after injury)

Amputation of nonviable extremity after retraction of viable tissue and medical intervention; may be several months after injury

Medications

Immunologic agents

Tetanus immunization, 0.5 ml IM for immunized patients

Diphtheria tetanus

0.5 ml IM plus 250 U tetanus immune globulin (Hypertet) for nonimmunized patients

Plasma expanders

Low-molecular-weight dextran 40, 20 ml/kg IV q24h to decrease sludging; this therapy is controversial[62]

Antiinfective agents

Tetracycline or ampicillin (Amcill, Omnipen, others) for prophylaxis, 250 mg po q6h

Narcotic analgesics

Morphine, up to 15 mg IM q3h

EMERGENCY ALERT

THERMAL INJURY: COLD

Frostbite is irreversible, however, minimizing the damage is of top priority. Frostbite occurs when ice crystals form in the intracellular space, they then enlarge and compress cells. This results in rupture that ultimately leads to microvascular occlusion. *Hypothermia* may also be present. Frostbite is classified as superficial and deep.

Assessment

Superficial:
- Assess for tingling, numbness, burning sensation, and whitish color, usually on tips of toes.
- Assess circumstances, duration of exposure, temperature, wind chill, and other risk factors (e.g., homeless, peripheral vascular disease).

Deep:
- White to waxy appearance
- Burning pain followed by warmth, then numbness
- Edema, blistering 1 to 7 days after injury
- Black or gray mottling

Interventions

Superficial:
- Handle skin extremely gently; do *not* rub.
- Apply warm soaks and elevate injured area.
- Avoid friction and weight on affected parts.
- Manage pain.

Deep:
- Handle skin extremely gently; DO NOT RUB.
- Obtain IV access.
- Manage pain (thawing tissue is extremely painful).
- Prevent body heat loss by keeping patient covered and ensuring warm room temperature.
- Assess neurovascular status frequently.
- Once at health care facility, immerse injured part in warm water: 38° to 41° C (100° to 106° F).

Analgesic-antipyretics
    Aspirin, 650 po q3h
Fibrinolytic agents, antiprostaglandins, thromboxane inhibitors, calmodulin antagonists: experimental therapies[62]

General Management

Rapid rewarming by immersion for 20 minutes in water at 38° to 41° C (100° to 106° F)
Protective isolation of patient or extremity
Whirlpool baths three times a day at 32° to 37° C (90° to 98° F)

NURSING CARE

Nursing Assessment

Injured Area

Color of skin; resilience of tissue; extent of limb involvement; duration of contact with cold; superficial injury: white, waxy, soft, no capillary refill; deep injury: hard, solid, mottled, blue or gray

Healing Process

Pain; edema; color; blister formation; eschar formation; line of demarcation between viable and nonviable tissue

Infection

Pus; odor; redness; heat; fever

Complications

Vasospasm; pain; hyperesthesia; increased perspiration

Nursing Dx & Intervention

Altered tissue perfusion related to interruption of arterial or venous flow

- Assess injured area for characteristics.
- In collaboration with physician, initiate rapid rewarming in water at 38° to 41° (100 ° to 106° F) until the skin becomes soft and pliable and develops color.
- Completely immerse affected area in water, avoiding contact of skin with container.
- Instruct patient not to smoke *to avoid vasoconstriction.*

Impaired skin integrity related to hypothermia

- Use sterile sheets *to prevent infection.*
- Isolate patient or extremity if necessary *to prevent infection.*
- Use bed cradle *to prevent mechanical trauma to injured tissue.*
- Keep blisters intact *to avoid introducing pathogens.*
- Keep extremity exposed to air *to prevent maceration.*
- Avoid debridement *to prevent further tissue injury.*

Impaired physical mobility related to pain and tissue damage

- Assess for impaired mobility.
- Elevate extremities periodically *to promote venous return and prevent stasis.*
- Initiate range of motion exercises *to promote circulation and prevent contractures.*

Pain related to physical factors

- Assess for pain.
- Keep sheets off extremity *to avoid pressure.*
- Administer analgesics as ordered.
- Instruct patient in relaxation techniques.
- Refer patient for biofeedback training.

Body image disturbance related to cognitive-perceptual factors

- Assess for defining characteristics.
- Encourage patient to express feelings about body, body appearance, or fear of reaction or rejection by others *to begin process of realistic self-evaluation.*

Anticipatory grieving related to high risk for loss of physiosocial or psychosocial well-being

- Encourage patient to express distress, anger, sorrow, guilt, and fear about potential loss of extremity part or function *to assist in movement through stages of grieving.*

Powerlessness related to illness-related regimen

- Observe for signs of depression and apathy.
- Inform patient that healing process is long-term, slow, and uncertain; provide accurate information about healing.
- Encourage patient to express dissatisfaction and frustration.
- Involve patient in decision making *to increase sense of control.*
- Accept patient's feelings of anger.

Patient Education/Home Care Planning

1. Discuss with the patient the need to protect the extremity from temperature extremes and rapid changes in temperature because the tissue is sensitive to temperature changes and refreezing will cause tissue loss.
2. Discuss with the patient the need to avoid tight, constrictive clothing or pressure to an area that might decrease circulation.
3. Demonstrate to the patient the application of dry, sterile dressing to small, open areas.
4. Explain to the patient the need to avoid smoking to reduce vasoconstriction.
5. Discuss with the patient preventive measures to avoid future episodes of reinjury of the frostbitten part: protective, multilayered, warm, nonconstrictive clothing; avoidance of fatigue, hunger, and use of alcohol when exposed to the cold.

Evaluation

Maximum tissue is preserved Initial rapid thawing with no refreezing of tissue occurs. Tissue is free of infection. Healing is allowed to occur without premature surgical intervention.

Pain is alleviated Patient verbalizes relief of pain.

Joints are functional Patient has full extension and flexion of joints.

Patient evaluates self in realistic manner Patient resumes former activities if possible. Patient develops interests and activities compatible with degree of limitation. Patient engages in satisfactory interpersonal relationships.

Patient prevents further injury to area Patient avoids tight, constrictive clothing or pressure to area. Patient does not smoke.

Patient prevents further episodes of cold injury Patient wears protective clothing and avoids hunger, fatigue, and use of alcohol when exposed to cold.

DISEASES OF THE NAILS

▮ FUNGAL INFECTIONS

See "Tinea."

▮ PARONYCHIA

Paronychia is an acute or chronic inflammation of the proximal nail fold.

Erythema, induration, and swelling of the nail folds and consequent pain and tenderness are the primary features of paronychia. Staphylococci, streptococci, and sometimes *Candida* are the organisms usually responsible for the infection. One or more fingers or toes may be involved. Paronychia may be acute or chronic. Acute paronychia usually results from minor trauma or a hangnail. Chronic paronychia occurs in people whose hands are exposed to chronic irritation and moisture.

•••••• Pathophysiology

In acute paronychia organisms enter through a break in the epidermis. The infection may follow the nail margin or extend beneath the nail and suppurate. Purulent exudate may drain from beneath the nail fold. The eponychium remains attached to the nail plate. This separation creates a space in which foreign material and inflammatory exudate accumulate. Such an environment is conducive to bacterial and yeast growth. Chronic paronychia usually leads to nail ridging, distortion, and discoloration.

•••••• Diagnostic Studies and Findings

Physical examination Characteristic lesion
Culture Growth of infecting organism

•••••• Multidisciplinary Plan

Surgery

Incision and drainage of purulent pocket

Medications

Antiinfective agents
Systemic antibiotics; depending on infecting organism
Anticandidal solutions or lotions applied topically tid, clotrimazole (Lotrimin, Mycelex), miconazole (Monistat-Derm)
Naftifine (Naftin), terbinafine (Lamasil), cicloprox (Loprox)
Thymol 4% in chloroform solution, 1 drip tid to affected area

---

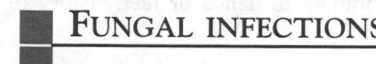

NURSING CARE

Nursing Assessment

Inflammatory and Infectious Processes

Erythema; swelling; heat; tenderness; pain; purulent exudate; nails ridged, distorted, and discolored

Environmental Factors

Constant moisture and trauma to hands or feet; history of previous infections

Nursing Dx & Intervention

Impaired skin integrity related to inflammatory and infectious processes

- Assess nail folds for inflammation and infection.
- Apply hot soaks *to promote suppuration and drainage.*
- Instruct patient in proper hand washing *to reduce existing pathogens.*
- Instruct patient to scrupulously dry hands and feet, especially around nails, and to use hot air drying rather than towel when possible *to prevent a wet environment that predisposes to infection.*

Risk for impaired skin integrity related to mechanical factors

- Instruct patient to protect hands and feet from moisture by wearing cotton socks and rubber gloves with cotton liners when hands are in water.
- Discuss with patient role of environmental factors such as moisture and trauma, and explore ways to eliminate them.

Pain related to physical factors

- Offer hot soaks *to decrease swelling.*
- Elevate affected limb *to prevent throbbing.*

Patient Education/Home Care Planning

1. Discuss with the patient prevention strategies regarding handwashing, drying, protection from moisture, and trauma (see under Nursing Dx & Intervention).
2. Discuss with the patient the use of medications and their side effects.
3. Demonstrate to the patient aseptic dressing changes if needed for draining lesions or after incision and drainage.

Evaluation

Inflammation subsides, and infection resolves   There is no erythema, swelling, heat, tenderness, pain, or purulent exudate   Chronic moisture and trauma are avoided   Paronychia does not recur.

DISEASES OF THE HAIR

ALOPECIA

Alopecia is a partial or complete loss of hair.

Alopecia may occur as a result of genetic factors, the aging process, or local or systemic disease. Alopecia can be scarring or nonscarring and localized, patterned, or diffuse. The biologic dysfunctions of hair have little clinical importance, but the psychologic and social importance is substantial (Figure 5-11).

•••••• Pathophysiology

Table 5-10 summarizes the clinical features and pathophysiology of the various types of hair loss.

•••••• Diagnostic Studies and Findings

Physical examination   Hair loss distribution, characteristics, and history
Biopsy   Reveals hair phase and structural damage
Damage   Infecting bacteria or fungus

•••••• Multidisciplinary Plan

Surgery

Hair transplant for androgenetic hair loss

Medications

Topical minoxidil 2%-3% for androgenetic alopecia[12]
Topical minoxidil 2% plus Retin-A for androgenetic alopecia; under investigation[12]
Topical minoxidil 5% plus 0.5% anthralin for alopecia areata
Topical sensitizers
   Dinitrochlorobenzene (DNCB); for many months
Corticosteroids
   Intralesional injection of 1-2 ml of triamcinolone (Kenalog), 10 mg/ml
   Topical glucocorticoids under occlusive dressing (see pp. 527 to 528)
     Betamethasone (Valisone), 0.1%
     Fluocinolone (Fluonid, Synalar, Fluosyn, Synemol), 0.025%
Chemotherapeutic agents
   Cyclosporine, 6 mg/kg/d po

General Management

Prolonged phototherapy (PUVA)

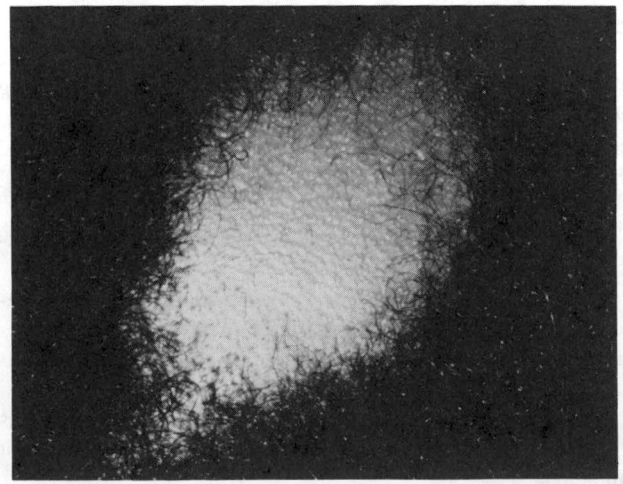

Figure 5-11 Alopecia areata. (Courtesy of Stephen B, Tucker, M.D., Department of Dermatology, University of Texas Health Science Center at Houston.)

▪ TABLE 5-10 Clinical Features and Pathology of Various Forms of Alopecia

Disease	Type	Features	Pathology
Areata	Nonscarring; localized or general	Occurs on any part of body; associated with family incidence; skin soft, smooth, not inflamed; one or several patches of loss; loss sudden; regrowth may occur with fine, light hair; hair pigments eventually	Inflammatory infiltrate around hair bulb; retraction in anagen hair; abnormal keratinization; loss of melanin and melanocytes; increased number of hair follicles in telogen phase
Androgenetic	Nonscarring; patterned	Occurs on scalp; in men frontal and temporal loss; thinning over vertex in women; mild, severe, or complete loss; familial trait	Androgens cause hair follicles to become smaller in size; terminal hair no longer formed; most hair follicles eventually disappear
Mechanical and chemical	Nonscarring; localized	Acute or chronic; attributable to hairdressing procedures or habitual hair pulling; skin may show trauma from tight braids or curlers	Trauma to hair shaft; localized breakage of hair
Telogen effluvium	Nonscarring; diffuse	Occurs 6 to 16 weeks after precipitating episode; hair loss seen on shampooing or brushing; occurs as diffuse thinning; common precipitating factors are pregnancy, hormone therapy, stress, surgery, fever, and illness	Increased percentage of hairs in resting phase and subsequently in normal process of shedding
Drug related	Nonscarring; diffuse	Caused by antimitotic drugs (anagen hair loss) or by oral contraceptives, anticoagulants, propanolol (telogen hair loss); usually temporary	Antimitotic drugs cause decreased mitosis and decreased number of anagen hairs; hair shaft constricted; cause increase in percentage of hairs in telogen phase and subsequently in normal process of shedding
Scarring	Scarring	Due to systemic diseases such as lupus erythematosus, scleroderma, lichen planus, folliculitis decalvans; regrowth does not occur	Follicle destroyed by infection or scarring

NURSING CARE

Nursing Assessment

Lesion

As described in Table 5-10; location; distribution; scarring

Precipitating Factors

Trauma; drugs; family history; systemic diseases

Psychosocial Concerns

Concern about body image

Nursing Dx & Intervention

Body image disturbance related to cognitive-perceptual factors: situational low self-esteem

- Assess patient's self-perception.
- Encourage patient to express feelings about body, body appearance, or fear of reaction or rejection by others *to begin process of realistic self-evaluation.*
- Advise patient that regrowth will occur in certain temporary conditions.
- Discuss use of wigs and hairpieces.

Patient Education/Home Care Planning

1. Advise the patient that commercial preparations will not restore hair or encourage hair growth.
2. Discuss with the patient the cause and course of the disease.
3. Discuss with the patient the use of glucocorticoids under an occlusive dressing when indicated (see pp. 527 to 528).

Evaluation

Underlying cause of hair loss is diagnosed and treated There is no new hair loss. Hair regrowth occurs in some conditions.

Patient evaluates appearance in realistic manner Patient does not use commercial hair restorative preparation. Patient uses wigs or hairpieces. Patient engages in satisfactory interpersonal relationships.

▪ HYPERTRICHOSIS AND HIRSUTISM

Hypertrichosis refers to nonspecific hair growth of all types. Hirsutism is excessive hair growth induced by androgens in women.

▪▪▪▪▪▪ Pathophysiology

Hypertrichosis occurs as a result of increased activity of the hair follicle with the production of a coarse terminal hair. Localized hypertrichosis can be the result of persistent trauma that causes chronic hyperemia and inflammation of the dermis.

Hypertrichosis can also be caused by systemic disorders, including severe infection, gross malnutrition, and gluten enteropathy.

Hirsutism occurs as a result of increased androgen activity and simulates the male pattern of hair distribution, with increased coarse terminal hair on the face, areolae, midline of the abdomen, and extremities. Hirsutism may be familial. Onset usually occurs slowly with no other symptoms of virilization. It may occur after menarche. Sudden onset of hirsutism may be from increased androgen production from adrenal, ovarian, or pituitary sources or by certain drugs such as systemic steroids, androgens, testosterone, progesterone, norethindrone, and phenytoin.

•••••• Diagnostic Studies and Findings

Physical examination   Distribution of hair with congruent history

Screening for adrenal, ovarian, and pituitary disorders

•••••• Multidisciplinary Plan

For treatment of adrenal, ovarian, or pituitary disorders, see the specific diseases. Generally, tumors are removed surgically; glucocorticoids are used for adrenal hyperplasia.

General Management

Electrolysis—hair follicle destroyed by passage of galvanic electric current

Diathermy—tissue destroyed through electrocoagulation; not recommended because it may cause scarring

Depilatories (wax or chemical)—chemicals can be irritating

Shaving

Bleaching with hydrogen peroxide and ammonia to depigment hair

NURSING CARE

Nursing Assessment

History

Onset; menstrual history; family history of hirsutism

Hair Characteristics

Description of hair; type; distribution and pattern

Systemic Features

Signs of virilization; size of ovaries and clitoris; uterine development

Psychosocial Concerns

Concern about body image

Nursing Dx & Intervention

Body image disturbance related to cognitive-perceptual factors: situational low self-esteem

- Assess patient's self-perception.
- Encourage patient to express feelings about body, body image, and fear of reaction or rejection by others *to begin process of realistic self-evaluation.*
- Advise patient of treatments available for hair removal or bleaching.

Patient Education/Home Care Planning

1. Discuss with the patient the advantages and disadvantages of the methods to remove or bleach the hair.
2. Discuss with the patient the cause and course of the disorder.

Evaluation

Underlying or systemic disorders are diagnosed and treated   Hair growth diminishes or ceases.

Patient chooses acceptable method for removing or bleaching hair   Patient is satisfied with method and appearance.

Patient evaluates appearance in realistic manner   Patient engages in usual activities and relationships.

MEDICAL INTERVENTIONS AND RELATED NURSING CARE

Common Therapeutic Interventions and Topical Preparations and Medications

Common Therapeutic Interventions	Therapeutic Effect	Nursing Care/Patient Education
Balneotherapy	Treat large areas of body or widely disseminated lesions	Fill tub full (20 to 25 gallons) at room temperature. Keep water from cooling. Bathe for 20 to 30 minutes. Use safety mat because medications make tub slippery. Keep room warm. Remove loose skin and crusts after bath. Apply medications while skin is still moist. Blot dry. Have patient dress in light, loose clothing.
Tap water	Antipruritic cooling; antiinflammatory	
Colloid, oatmeal, 1 cup	Antipruritic; nondrying	
Colloid, cornstarch, 2 cups	Antipruritic; drying	
Tar, commercial preparations, 2 teaspoons	Antipruritic; nondrying	
Carbonis detergens liquor, 1 ounce	Antipruritic; nondrying	
Oil (Alpha-Keri, Domol, Lubath, Jeri-Bath, etc.)	Lubrication	

Common Therapeutic Interventions and Topical Preparations and Medication—cont'd

Common Therapeutic Interventions	Therapeutic Effect	Nursing Care/Patient Education
Burn hydrotherapy May add prescribed amounts sodium chloride, potassium chloride, calcium hypochlorite, or detergent	Facilitate dressing change and debridement	Immerse in water at temperature of 100° F (37.8° C) for 20 to 30 minutes. Stay with patient. Administer pain medications. Plug catheter. Shave and debride as needed. Use aseptic technique.
Occlusive dressings	Increased absorption and penetration of topical preparations; produces moisture retention, skin maceration, and decreased evaporation to increase effect of topical preparations	Apply airtight plastic film over medicated skin. Remove for 12 of 24 hours to prevent complications. Watch for complications: bacterial and candidal infections, sweat retention, folliculitis, and side effects of medications.
Shampoos Selenium sulfide Betadine Zinc pyrithione 2% Carbonis detergens liquor, 5% Triethanolamine sulfate 40%	 Antiseborrheic Antibacterial Antiseborrheic Antiseborrheic Antipruritic Bland (can add medications)	Lather sufficiently. Gently work into scalp. Avoid contact with eyes.
Wet dressings and compresses Tap water or normal saline Aluminum acetate (Burow's) Potassium permanganate 1:10,000 solution; 5 grains/ 3 quarts water	Cool and dry acute inflammation through evaporation Antipruritic; antiinflammatory used in acute oozing dermatoses As above; also antibacterial As above; also antifungal and antibacterial	Soak compress to point of dripping. Keep at room temperature. Remoisten every few minutes. Apply for 15 to 30 minutes every 2 to 3 hours. Do not rub or blot. Do not treat more than one third of the body at one time. Keep patient warm and covered. Advise patient that potassium permanganate stains skin, clothing, and tub. Instruct patient to use soft towels or cotton sheeting for home care to avoid irritating skin. Instruct patient to use clean towel or sheet each time compress is used, to keep them separate from rest of family linens, and to launder between each use.
Dry burn dressing Nonadherent, porous, fine mesh gauze Bulky, fluffed, coarse, mesh gauze Semielastic coarse mesh	 First layer; nonadherent; fine enough to prevent epithelialization into gauze Second layer; absorbs exudate Outer layer; applies even pressure; holds dressing in place	Cleanse wound with one-half strength Betadine using sterile gauze; rub gently to remove existing topical agent. Apply topical agent thick enough to cover wound with $\frac{1}{8}$ inch of agent to provide healing and prevent bandage from adhering. Apply layers of dressing: fine gauze, bulky coarse gauze; semielastic mesh. Change dressing one or two times daily.
Topical Preparations		
Creams and ointments Petrolatum, mineral oil, lanolin, Eurin, Qualatum, Unibase, Dermabase	Lubrication; protection; vehicle for medications; decrease water loss; ointments greasy with oil base; creams lighter and water washable	Rub into skin by hand. Cover ointments with light dressing to protect clothing. Apply frequently. Wash off before reapplication.
Gels Contain propylene glycol and carboxymethylene	Like creams and ointments; clear and nongreasy; may be used on hairy areas	Apply with fingers. Avoid rubbing because gels are thixotropic agents (become thinner with rubbing). Apply frequently.
Lotions With 0.5% menthol and 0.25% phenol	Liquid vehicles for medications; lubrication; cooling through evaporation Antipruritic; drying	Apply with cotton gauze. Lotions are usually not washed off between applications.
Pastes	Stiff vehicle of powder and ointment; porous and less occlusive than ointments; protective	Apply with tongue depressor. Wash off between applications. Scrub gently if paste is difficult to remove.
Powders Talc, zinc, oxide, cornstarch	Absorbent; hygroscopic (take up water); reduce friction	Apply with shaker. Avoid accumulation in intertriginous areas.
Topical Medications		
Antiseptic agents Chlorhexidine, povidone iodine, hexachlorophene	Treat carriers of pathogens; reduce overall skin bacterial count	Observe for sensitivities. Do not use hexachlorophene for infants and children.

Continued.

Common Therapeutic Interventions and Topical Preparations and Medications—cont'd

Topical Medications	Therapeutic Effect	Nursing Care/Patient Education
Antibacterial agents	Like antiseptic agents	Observe for sensitivities. Cover with light dressing to protect clothing. Apply two to four times a day. Wash off before reapplication. With sulfamylon, debride wound before reapplication.
Neomycin	For gram-negative and gram-positive organisms	
Bacitracin	For gram-negative organisms and *Pseudomonas*	
Silver sulfadiazine (Silvadene)	For burns; for gram-negative and gram-positive organisms and yeast	
Sulfamylon	For burns; bacteriostatic only; for gram-negative and gram-positive organisms	
Precipitated sulfur 3%	Antiseborrheic	Observe for irritation.
Salicylic acid 3%-5%; urea 10%-20%	Keratolytic; increases absorption of other medications	Observe for irritation.
Corticosteroids	Decrease inflammation through vasoconstriction and direct action on leukocytes; decrease prostaglandin synthesis; decrease mitotic rate of epidermal cells	Apply sparingly to skin or apply in occlusive dressing. When used for prolonged periods, especially under occlusive dressings, watch for thinning of skin, striae formation, telangiectasia, and follicular hyperkeratosis.
Hydrocortisone 1%; fluocinolone 0.01%; triamcinolone 0.025%-0.1%; betamethasone		

CRYOSURGERY

In cryosurgery tissue is frozen to remove hyperkerolytic growths (such as warts) or to cause involution of cysts.

Contraindications and Cautions

1. Overfreezing can cause scarring and hyperpigmentation.
2. Application of liquid nitrogen can be painful and is not well tolerated by children.

Procedure

1. Liquid nitrogen is applied with a cotton-tipped applicator and is held in place for 10 to 20 seconds.
2. Carbon dioxide is applied via CO_2 pencil, which is held in place with moderate pressure for 20 to 30 seconds.

Nursing Interventions

1. Inform patient before treatment of possibility of scarring or hyperpigmentation, and help patient evaluate the benefit/risk trade-off.
2. Instruct patient in the procedure.
3. Observe for blister formation immediately with CO_2 or in 5 to 10 hours with liquid nitrogen.
4. Instruct patient to prevent infection by keeping area clean and dry, not puncturing blister, and not picking at scab.
5. Instruct patient to observe for signs of infection and to seek medical attention if they occur.

DEBRIDEMENT

In debridement dead tissue or eschar is removed to facilitate healing or in preparation for skin grafting.

Procedure

Surgery

Surgical excision—large areas removed down to fascia
Tangential excision—layers of eschar removed with dermatome or scalpel to point of capillary bleeding; edge of tissue picked up with forceps and necrotic tissue cut with scissors; margin of 0.5 cm left to avoid cutting viable tissue; debridement limited to area of 10 cm; bleeding controlled by direct pressure; topical agent applied

Medications

Proteolytic enzymes applied with saline to erode and consume eschar

Mechanical

Removal through mechanical action in dressing changes, hydrotherapy, and showers

Nursing Interventions

1. Describe procedure to patient.
2. Administer analgesics 20 minutes before debridement.
3. After procedure, assess area for exudate, color, sensation, bleeding, and size of area debrided.
4. Assess patient's response; pain, stress, or fear.

DISSECTION, BLUNT

This technique is an office surgical procedure for removal of epidermal tumors, using a blunt dissector. Normal tissue is not disturbed, and scarring does not usually occur.

Procedure

1. Before procedure, the patient is given systemic analgesics if lesions are such that postoperative pain is anticipated, such as with large plantar or periungual warts.
2. Local anesthesia with lidocaine is provided via needle injection or jet injector.
3. The plane of dissection is established by inserting the tip of blunt-tipped scissors between the lesion and the normal skin and cutting the skin circumferentially.
4. The blunt dissector is then inserted into the opened plane, which is separated from the normal underlying tissue with short firm strokes.
5. After the lesion is removed, the dissector is drawn back and forth over the exposed surface of the bed to remove tissue fragments.

Nursing Interventions

1. Instruct patient in the procedure.
2. After procedure cover wound with Band-Aid. Advise patient to change it daily for 3 to 4 days and thereafter to leave wound exposed to air.
3. Advise patient that moderate to intense pain may occur for 30 minutes to 2 hours after blunt dissection of periungual and plantar warts.

ELECTRODESICCATION AND CURETTAGE

In electrodesiccation an electric current is used to remove superficial lesions. In curettage a dermal curette with round or oval sharp surfaces is used to remove superficial lesions. The procedures may be used together or separately.

Contraindications and cautions

1. High-frequency current can deactivate a pacemaker. Special precautions are required in patients with indwelling cardiac pacemakers.
2. Electrodes should be changed after each use or sterile disposable needle electrodes used to prevent the transmission of viral-associated infections.

Procedure

Fulguration

1. The surface to be treated is cleaned so it is dry and free of blood.
2. The pointed electrode is held slightly away from the tissue surface, and the unit is activated.
3. A sparking occurs, resulting in tissue dehydration and charring of immediate surrounding area.

Desiccation

1. The pointed electrode is placed in contact with the skin surface or inserted slightly in the tissue, and the unit is activated.
2. The resulting tissue char is produced by fulguration.

Electrocoagulation

1. The bipolar setting is used.
2. The active electrode is placed in contact with the tissue, and the unit is activated.
3. Tissue necrosis is more extensive than with fulguration or desiccation.

Curettage

1. The area is anesthetized with lidocaine via needle injection or jet injector.
2. The skin around the lesion is supported with the fingers of the hand not holding the instrument.
3. With several smooth strokes, the curette is drawn through the tissue.

Nursing Interventions

1. Instruct patient in the procedure.
2. Clean surrounding skin with antibacterial agent.
3. If oozing occurs after procedure, cover with sterile gauze.
4. Leave area exposed to air or covered with light dressing.
5. Encourage daily washing with soap and water.

INTRALESIONAL INJECTIONS

Intralesional injections are injections of a corticosteroid into a lesion. The antiinflammatory action helps clear lesions and reduce the size of cysts.

Contraindications and Cautions

1. Injection into subcutaneous tissue can result in transient or permanent atrophy and local tissue depression.

Procedure

1. Aqueous suspension (usually triamcinolone, 5-10 mg/2 ml) is injected intracutaneously into the lesion or cyst with a fine-gauge needle. The more superficial the injection, the better the result.

Nursing Interventions

1. Inform patient before treatment of the possibility of atrophy, and help the patient evaluate the benefit/risk trade-off.
2. Instruct patient to observe for side effects of treatment: bleeding, hemorrhaging, pigmentation, and atrophy; adrenal suppression may occur with multiple injections.
3. Instruct patient to observe for desired effects: cyst decreases in size and lesion clears.
4. Instruct the patient to keep the area clean to avoid secondary infection.

LASER THERAPY

Laser (light amplification by stimulated emission of radiation) therapy is used to treat certain vascular, pigmented, and other lesions of the skin. The most commonly used laser systems are the pulsed-dye laser, argon laser, and carbon dioxide laser.

Procedure

Pulsed-dye Laser

1. Anesthesia is seldom required. Topical or local anesthesia is sometimes used, especially in children.
2. Most patients feel the laser pulse as a snapping sensation against their skin.
3. A gray-blue bruise is produced that resolves in 7 to 14 days, or the bruise may take up to 3 months to resolve in darker-skinned patients.
4. Wound care is usually not necessary.

Argon Laser

1. Local or general anesthesia is usually administered.
2. The potential for scarring is higher than with the pulsed-dye laser.
3. Testing is usually performed with both the argon and pulsed-dye laser to select the most effective treatment.
4. A superficial burn wound is created that requires dressing changes for 1 week or for several weeks.

Carbon Dioxide Laser

1. The laser beam can be focused to bloodlessly excise lesions, or it can be defocused to vaporize tissue.
2. Local anesthesia is usually used.
3. Evaporation of tissue during excision and vaporization produces steam that requires removal by smoke evacuation equipment.
4. Postoperative pain is minimal.
5. Excision produces an incision that may require closure with sutures, staples, or other wound-closure materials. Wound healing may be delayed; therefore sutures or staples are commonly left in place longer than with a comparable scalpel wound.
6. Vaporization produces minimal thermal damage to surrounding tissue that will turn it brown; it will remain brown until it is healed.

Nursing Interventions

1. Assist in discussing all treatment options with the patient. Discuss with the patient that patch testing may be used to assist in determination of efficacy, or it may be used to select the most effective system of treatment. Such testing may delay actual therapy.
2. Assist in discussing potential adverse outcomes with the patient: hypertrophic scarring, hypopigmentation, hyperpigmentation, incomplete removal of the lesion, and infection.

3. Prepare the patient for any draping or safety equipment that may be used during the procedure, such as patient eye protectors and wet draping, depending on the laser and on the area being treated.
4. Assist in ensuring appropriate safety precautions:
   a. Limited access to the surgical area
   b. Internally controlled door locks
   c. Proper testing of equipment before each use
   d. Eye protection designed for the specific laser being used
   e. Removal of reflective jewelery and surgical instruments
   f. Wet draping if required
5. Cleanse the area to be treated. Remove all makeup or skin lotions, and dry the area.
6. Provide assistance and support to the patient to remain stationary during the procedure.
7. Discuss postprocedure care with the patient, depending on the laser system used. Discuss with the patient the need to
   a. Avoid trauma to the area
   b. Pat dry the skin after bathing, rather than rubbing it
   c. Avoid sunlight to the area, and use a sunscreen with an SPF of 15 or higher; this precaution may need to be observed for several months

SKIN GRAFT

In a skin graft a section of skin tissue that is separated from its blood supply is transferred to a recipient site to provide tissue for epithelization.

split-thickness graft Composed of epidermis and superficial layers of dermis.

full-thickness graft Composed of epidermis and all layers of dermis.

homograft (allograft) Skin from a deceased person that is used as temporary cover for about 10 days, and may survive for 4 to 5 weeks.

heterograft (xenograft) Pigskin or synthetic substitute that acts as biologic dressing.

autograft Skin from another part of the patient's own body.

mesh graft Split-thickness graft meshed with a special instrument to cover large areas and held in place by a dressing or sutures.

autologous cultured human epithelium Unburned epidermal cells cultured into sheets in a flask. The cultured sheets are then attached to petrolatum gauze squares and sutured in place in the wound. The petrolatum gauze is removed 7 to 10 days later.

Procedure

1. The donor site is prepared by surgical scrub. The recipient site is debrided and cleansed.
2. A split- or full-thickness graft is taken from the donor site with a dermatome. The graft is cut as "postage stamps" or strips or is meshed and is placed on recipient sites.

3. The graft is held in place by a presure dressing or sutures.
4. The donor site is covered with nonadherent gauze held in place by a gauze dressing.

Nursing Interventions

Donor Site

1. Remove the outer dressing in 24 hours.
2. Inspect the site daily.
3. Assess for bleeding, pain, and infection.
4. Leave nonadherent gauze in place until it separates spontaneously.
5. If infection occurs, treat it with medicated wet dressing.

Recipient (Graft) Site

1. Inspect the site daily.
2. Assess for edema, hematoma formation, fluid collection, infection, and viability of graft tissue.
3. Immobilize the affected part to avoid disrupting the graft.
4. Elevate the grafted extremity for 7 to 10 days.
5. Protect the graft from scratching by the patient.
6. If infection occurs, treat it with a medicated wet dressing.
7. The heterograft acts as a biologic dressing; expect it to slough off in 10 days to 5 weeks.

Healing Phase

1. Inform the patient about the changing hues of graft scar tissue; pale, then pink, then red, then fading to resemble surrounding skin; a full-thickness graft may remain deeply red for several months.
2. Anticipate skin scaling with a full-thickness graft.
3. Lubricate the donor site with lanolin or cocoa butter to keep the tissue soft and pliable.
4. Apply mineral oil or lanolin to the graft site after the second or third week to remove superficial crusts, moisten the graft, and stimulate circulation.
5. Instruct the patient who will be at home to avoid overexposure of the graft site to the sun because the site is sensitive to the sun and can burn easily.
6. Encourage the patient to express feelings about body, body appearance, or fear of reaction or rejection by others.

■ SYSTEMIC STEROID THERAPY

In systemic steroid therapy parenteral or oral glucocorticoids are used for their antiinflammatory action.

Contraindications and Cautions

1. Hypertension and diabetes mellitus can be exacerbated.
2. Concurrent infections can be masked.
3. Therapy is used with caution in patients who are predisposed to peptic ulceration, thrombophlebitis, adrenal suppression, and mood swings.

Procedure

The dose and duration of treatment depend on the severity of the disease and the patient's response. The patient should receive a dose sufficient to produce a therapeutic response and then be maintained with a minimum effective dose; the dose should be tapered slowly after the lesions have cleared.

Approximate equivalent doses of various steroids are as follows:

Betamethasone, 0.5 mg	Methylprednisolone, 4 mg
Dexamethasone, 0.75 mg	Prednisolone, 5 mg
Fludrocortisone, 2 mg	Prednisone, 5mg
Hydrocortisone, 20 mg	Triamcinolone, 4 mg

Nursing Interventions

1. Inform the patient about the side effects to watch for and to seek medical attention if they occur: euphoria, gastrointestinal pain or bleeding, bruising, thrombophlebitis, hypertension, moon face, cushingoid features, acne, hirsutism, osteoporosis, and mood swings.
2. Instruct the patient to take medication with milk or antacids to decrease gastric irritation.
3. Instruct the patient to increase protein intake to combat osteoporosis.

■ TOPICAL STEROID THERAPY

Topical steroids are used therapeutically for their antiinflammatory, immunosuppressant, and antimitotic effects on the skin.

Contraindications and Cautions

For use of superpotent topical steroids:

1. All of the local side effects from less potent topical steroids may be accentuated with superpotent steroids.
2. Systemic side effects may include the suppression of the hypothalamic-pituitary-adrenal axis or the development of Cushing's syndrome.
3. Superpotent topical steroids should not be used in children because of their increased ratio of skin surface to body weight.
4. Superpotent topical steroids should not be used in occlusive dressings because enhanced absorption could lead to atrophy and bacterial infection.
5. Superpotent topical steroids should not be used for longer than 2 weeks in flexor areas because these areas are sites of natural occlusion.
6. Prolonged usages of superpotent topical steroids should be avoided in the elderly because they have thinner skin and the drug clears more slowly.
7. Superpotent topical steroids should not be used on the face, eyelids, scrotum, or mucous membranes because of the enhanced degree of penetration in these areas.

Procedure

Topical steroids in general are used alone, or often they are used under occlusive dressings. Topical steroids can be classified in terms of their relative potency. The superpotent (i.e., betamethasone dipropylene, clobetasol propionate, and difloasone diacetate) produce a highly effective and enhanced therapeutic effect; however, they require special guidelines for use.

1. The proper potency is selected. The lowest-potency preparations are used for dermatoses that are mild and chronic and involve the face, intertriginous regions, and genitalia. Medium- and high-potency preparations are used for dermatoses that are more severe and recalcitrant to treatment.
2. The proper vehicle is selected. Ointments are occlusive and are best used for chronic inflammation characterized by dryness, scaling, and lichenification. Lotions, creams, and gels are nonocclusive and are used for acute and subacute inflammations that are oozing or vesiculated. Lotions and gels are best used on hairy areas such as the scalp.
3. Frequency of application is determined. The stratum corneum acts as a reservoir and continues to release topical steroid into the skin after the initial application. Application one to two times is usually sufficient. Some chronic dermatoses become less responsive after prolonged or more frequent use of topical steroids.

Nursing Interventions

1. Instruct the patient in the proper application of the preparation. Application right after bathing improves penetration of the preparation into the skin. The product should be spread as thinly as possible until it disappears. It is not necessary to leave a visible layer.
2. Inform the patient of potential topical side effects: atrophy and striae formation, acne, enhanced fungal infection, retarded wound healing, and contact dermatitis. Glaucoma or cataracts can occur with application to the eyelids.
3. Inform the patient of the potential risk of systemic absorption and side effects with extensive and chronic use of potent topical steroids.

■ ULTRAVIOLET LIGHT THERAPY

Short-wave ultraviolet light (UVB) is used for the treatment of psoriasis and acne. In Goeckerman therapy ultraviolet light therapy is used in combination with coal tar applications that are photosensitizing; it is used for the treatment of psoriasis. In PUVA therapy long-wave ultraviolet light (UVA) is used in combination with psoralen, which is a photosensitizer (P + UVA = PUVA); it is used for treating psoriasis.

Procedure
Short-Wave Ultraviolet Light

1. The patient is exposed one to three times per week.
2. The exposure time is increased to keep skin just below erythema level.

Goeckerman Therapy

1. Coal tar ointment is applied, left on for several hours, and then washed off.
2. UVB therapy is given in doses to account for photosensitization.
3. The skin is kept just below erythema level.
4. Coal tar ointment is reapplied after UVB exposure.

PUVA Therapy

1. Psoralen is administered in an initial dose of 0.6 mg/kg.
2. UVA irradiation is delivered 2 to 4 hours after psoralen administration.
3. Dosage and exposure are determined by individual response.
4. Therapy is usually provided in specific treatment centers because specialized equipment, careful calibration, and close monitoring are required.

Contraindications and Cautions
PUVA Therapy

1. Long-term effects of PUVA therapy remain controversial, and treatment is usually reserved for chronic, severe, refractory psoriasis.

Nursing Interventions

1. Instruct the patient in the procedure.
2. Assist the patient in setting up a schedule to maintain the therapeutic regimen.
3. Instruct a patient who is using short-wave ultraviolet light therapy at home to
   a. Use a lamp with an automatic timer to shut off.
   b. Use a backup timer.
   c. Measure the distance from the lamp carefully and maintain the correct distance.
   d. Increase exposure time slowly and keep the skin below erythema level.
   e. Wear an occlusive protective eye covering.
4. Advise a patient who is using concomitant photosensitizing agents to avoid lengthy exposure to sunlight.
5. Advise a patient who is receiving PUVA therapy of the undetermined long-term effects, and assist the patient in evaluating the risk/benefit trade-off.

References

1. Arndt K: *Manual of dermatologic therapeutics,* ed 5, Boston, 1995, Little, Brown.
2. Auerbach R: Psoriasis symposium: methotrexate, *Semin Dermatol* 11(4) (suppl 1):23, 1992.
3. Bailin P, Ratz J, Wheeler R: Laser therapy of the skin, *Otolaryngol Clin North Am* 23(1):123, 1990.

4. Bandoh Y, Yanai A, Tsuzuki K: Dye laser treatment of portwine stains, *Aesthetic Plast Surg* 14:287, 1990.

5. Berger B: Lyme disease, *Semin Dermatol* 12(4):357, 1993.

6. Berson D, Shalita A: The treatment of acne: the role of combination therapies, *J Am Acad Dermatol* 32(5):s31, 1995.

7. Billstein S, Mattaliano V: The "nuisance" sexually transmitted diseases: molluscum contagiosum, scabies, and crablice, *Med Clin North Am* 74(6):1487, 1990.

8. Blondell R: Parasites of the skin and hair, *Prim Care,* 18(1):167, 1991.

9. Bowers A, Thompson J: *Clinical manual of health assessment,* ed 4, St Louis, 1992, Mosby.

10. Cotterill J: New lasers for old diseases. In Marks R, Cunliffe W, editors: *Skin therapy,* United Kingdom, 1994, Martin Dunitz.

11. Cunliffe W: Treatment of the difficult acne patient. In Marks R, Cunliffe W, editors: *Skin therapy,* United Kingdom, 1994, Martin Dunitz.

12. DeVillez R: The therapeutic use of minoxidil, *Dermatol Clin* 8(2):367, 1990.

13. Devlin J, David J, Stanton R: Elemental diet for refractory atopic eczema, *Arch Dis Child* 66:93, 1991.

14. Diwan R: Laser therapy in the treatment of congenital vascular abnormalities, *Md Med J* 39(4):343, 1990.

15. Ellison M, Crabtree D: Antibiotic therapy for common infections, *Prim Care* 17(3):521, 1990.

16. Farr P: New lamps for psoralen photochemotherapy of psoriasis. In Marks R, Cunliffe W, editors: *Skin therapy,* United Kingdom, 1994, Martin Dunitz.

17. Feingold D: Staphylococcal and streptococcal pyodermas, *Semin Dermatol* 12(4):331, 1993.

18. Ferrante J: Infectious skin diseases, *Prim Care* 17(4):867, 1990.

19. Fiedler V et al: Treatment-resistant alopecia areata, *Arch Dermatol* 126:756, 1990.

20. Finlay A: Treatment of onychomycosis. In Marks R, Cunliffe W, editors: *Skin therapy,* United Kingdom, 1994, Martin Dunitz.

21. Fischbach FT: *A manual of laboratory diagnostic tests,* ed 4, Philadelphia, 1992, Lippincott.

22. Fry L: Cyclosporin in the treatment of psoriasis. In Marks R, Cunliffe W, editors: *Skin therapy,* United Kingdom, 1994, Martin Dunitz.

23. Goldstein S: Advances in the treatment of superficial candidal infections, *Semin Dermatol* 12(4):315, 1993.

24. Goodpasture H: Antiviral drug therapy, *AFP* 43(1):197, 1991.

25. Habif T: *Clinical dermatology: a color guide to diagnosis and therapy,* ed 3, St Louis, 1995, Mosby.

26. Hanifin J: The role of antihistamines in atopic dermatitis, *J Allergy Clin Immunol* 86(4)(pt 2):666, 1990.

27. Hanke CW: Lasers in dermatology, *Indiana Med,* June, 394, 1990.

28. Hartwig P: Lasers in dermatology, *Nurs Clin North Am* 25(3):657, 1990.

29. Hay R et al: A comparative study of terbinafine versus griseofulvin in "dry-type" dermatophyte infections, *J Am Acad Dermatol* 24(2)(pt 1):243, 1991.

30. Hay R et al: Itraconazole in the management of chronic dermatophytosis, *J Am Acad Dermatol* 23(3)(pt 2):561, 1990.

31. Helm T et al: PUVA therapy, *AFP* 43(3):908, 1991.

32. Honigsmann H: Phototherapy and photochemotherapy. *Semin Dermatol* 9(1):84, 1990.

33. Jacobson M et al: Acyclovir-resistant varicella zoster virus infection after chronic oral acyclovir therapy in patients with the acquired immunodeficiency syndrome (AIDS), *Ann Intern Med*112(3):187, 1990.

34. Janniger C, Schwartz R: Seborrheic dermatitis, *Am Fam Physician* 52(1):149, 1995, Mosby.

35. Kim MJ, McFarland G, McLane A: *Pocket guide to nursing diagnoses,* ed 6, St Louis, 1995.

36. Koo J: Psoriasis symposium: phototherapy, *Semin Dermatol* 11(4)(suppl 1):11, 1992.

37. Kremer M et al: Long-term antimicrobial therapy in the prevention of recurrent soft-tissue infections, *J Infect* 22:37, 1991.

38. Lanigan S: Intoxicated by port wine stains—the treatment of port wine stains with a pulsed tunable dye laser. In Marks R, Cunliffe W, editors: *Skin therapy,* United Kingdom, 1994, Martin Dunitz.

39. Lanigan S, Cotterill J: The treatment of port-wine stains with the carbon dioxide laser, *Br J Dermatol* 123:229, 1990.

40. Lawrence C: The cutting edge. In Marks R, Cunliffe W, editors: *Skin therapy,* United Kingdom, 1994, Martin Dunitz.

41. Lazarus G: Psoriasis symposium: new aspects of pathogenesis of psoriasis, *Semin Dermatol* 11(4)(suppl 1):2, 1992.

42. Levine G: Sexually transmitted parasitic diseases, *Prim Care* 18(1):101, 1991.

43. Leyden J, Aly R: Tinea pedis, *Semin Dermatol* 12(4):280, 1993.

44. Lookingbill D, Marks J Jr: *Principles of dermatology* ed 2, Philadelphia, 1993, Saunders.

45. Lowe N et al: Advances in photochemotherapy. In Marks R, Cunliffe W, editors: *Skin therapy,* United Kingdom, 1994, Martin Dunitz.

46. Lowe N: Laser therapy of vascular benign pigmented lesions. In Marks R, Cunliffe W, editors: *Skin therapy,* United Kingdom, 1994, Martin Dunitz.

47. Lowe N: Psoriasis symposium: retinoids, *Semin Dermatol* 11(4)(suppl 1):17, 1992.

48. Lozada-Nur F, Min ZH, Guang Z: Open preliminary clinical trial of clobetasol propionate ointment in adhesive paste for treatment of chronic vesiculoerosive diseases, *Oral Surg Oral Med Oral Pathol* 71(3):283, 1991.

49. Lynch P: *Dermatology,* ed 3, Baltimore, 1994, Williams & Wilkens.

50. Mandy S: Dermabrasion. In Marks R, Cunliffe W, editors: *Skin therapy,* United Kingdom, 1994, Martin Dunitz.

51. Marks R, Cunliffe W, editors: *Skin therapy,* United Kingdom, 1994, Martin Dunitz.

52. Marks R: New indications for topical retinoids. In Marks R, Cunliffe W, editors: *Skin therapy,* United Kingdom, 1994, Martin Dunitz.

53. Menter A: Psoriasis symposium: cyclosporin, *Semin Dermatol* 11(4)(suppl 1):30, 1992.

54. Menter A: Psoriasis symposium: topical therapy, *Semin Dermatol* 11(4)(suppl 1):5, 1992.

55. Miller L et al: Sildimac: a new delivery system for silver sulfadiazine in the treatment of full-thickness burn injuries, *J Burn Care Rehabil* 11(1):35, 1990.

56. Motley R: Electrosurgery and electrocautery in dermatology. In Marks R, Cunliffe W, editors: *Skin therapy,* United Kingdom, 1994, Martin Dunitz.

57. National Center for Health Statistics: *Advance data from vital and health statistics,* Series 16, No. 4, Public Health Service, Washington, DC, 1990, US Government Printing Office.

58. National Center for Health Statistics: *Current estimates from the National Health Interview Survey, 1992,* Series 10, No. 189, Public Health Service, Washington, DC, 1994, US Government Printing Office.

59. Orkin M, Maibach H: Scabies therapy 1993, *Semin Dermatol* 12(4):22, 1993.

60. Perrone C et al: Varicella in patients infected with the human immunodeficiency virus, *Arch Dermatol* 126:1033, 1990.

61. Prawer S, Katz I: Guidelines for using superpotent topical steroids, *AFP* 41(5):1531, 1990.

62. Rosen P, Barkin R, editors: *Emergency medicine concepts and clinical practice,* ed 3, St Louis, 1992, Mosby.

63. Ruzicka T: Efficiency of acitretin in combination with UV-B in the treatment of severe psoriasis, *Arch Dermatol* 126:482, 1990.

64. Sabiston DC Jr, editor: *Textbook of surgery: the biological basis of modern surgical practice,* ed 11, Philadelphia, 1977, Saunders.

65. Saul A, Bonifaz A: Itraconazole in common dermatophyte infections of the skin: fixed treatment schedules, *J Am Acad Dermatol* 23(3)(pt 2):554, 1990.

66. Seidel H et al: *Mosby's guide to physical examination,* ed 3, St Louis, 1995, Mosby.

67. Tung J, Maibach H: The practical use of methotrexate in psoriasis, *Drugs* 40(5):697, 1990.

68. Van der Steen P et al: Treatment of alopecia areata with diphenylcyclopropenone, *J Am Acad Dermatol* 24(2)(pt 1), 1991.

69. Williams R: Antihistamines—useful in atopic eczema? *Practitioner* 234:624, 1990.

70. Wyatt D, McGowan D, Najarian M: Comparison of a hydrocolloid dressing and silver sulfadiazine cream in the outpatient management of second-degree burns, *J Trauma* 2097:857, 1990.

71. Young E, Newcomer V, Kligman A: *Geriatric dermatology,* Philadelphia, 1993, Lea & Febiger.

The Eye

6

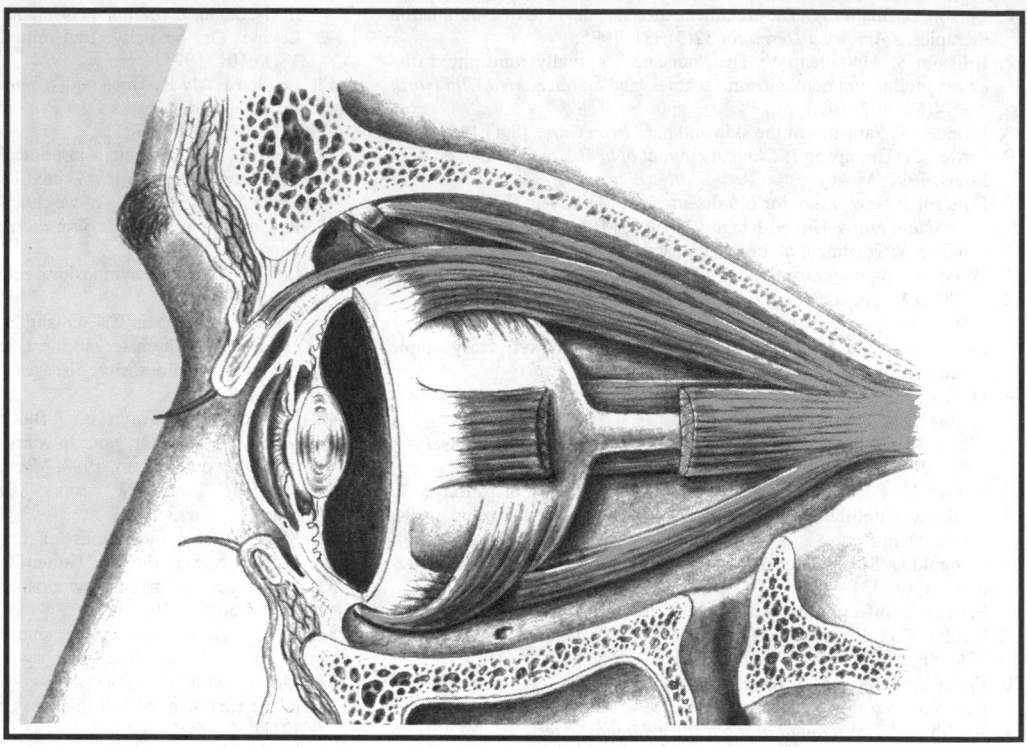

OVERVIEW

Preserving vision and preventing blindness are important to everyone. A recent poll found that Americans fear blindness more than any other disorder except cancer.[6] The American Academy of Ophthalmology's Committee on Eye Care for the American People reports that "approximately 1,000,000 Americans are legally blind, more than 11.4 million are visually impaired because of chronic or permanent defects, 80 million have a disease in one or both eyes, and additional millions need eyeglasses or contact lenses to see clearly."[6] Eye care has become the focus of more attention in recent years because expanding knowledge and technology have increased the opportunity for early diagnosis and successful treatment of eye disorders. Technologic advances include microsurgical techniques, laser surgery, contact lens refinement, development of intraocular lenses, and corneal replacement. Screening programs offered by schools and community agencies have enhanced public awareness of eye disorders and preventive eye care. This greater awareness of the need for periodic eye examinations, of specific measures for preventing eye injuries, and of the early signs or symptoms of eye disorders has contributed to the prevention of visual impairment. Major eye disorders include cataract, corneal impairments and injuries, glaucoma, retinal diseases, strabismus, and amblyopia. All these impairments can cause blindness, but most of them are partially or fully treatable if diagnosed early. Nurses can contribute signif-

icantly to the prevention of visual impairment by becoming knowledgeable about the cause and prevention of eye disorders and by urging patients to follow through with self-care and health promotion measures. For example, the American Academy of Ophthalmology's Committee on Eye Care for the American People has made the recommendations in the box on p. 535.

•••••• Anatomy, Physiology, and Related Pathophysiology

External Structures

Orbit and its contents   The human eye is approximately 24 mm in diameter. It rests within a fatty cushion in a bony orbit of the skull. The orbit comprises six bones forming a cavity that converges into two major posterior openings, the optic foramen and the superior orbital fissure (Figure 6-1). Through these openings run blood vessels and nerves that connect the eyeball to the brain and the body's blood supply. The ophthalmic artery, the optic nerve, and sympathetic nerves from the carotid plexus enter the orbit through the optic foramen. The oculomotor nerve (CN III), trochlear nerve (CN IV), abducent nerve (CN VI), and ophthalmic branch of the trigeminal nerve (CN V) pass through the superior orbital fissure.[34]

The orbit contains the eyeball, which is cradled in the anterior portion; six oculomotor muscles, which surround and insert into the eyeball; a muscle for elevating the eyelid; and fat, ligaments, and connective tissue in the posterior section that

GUIDELINES FOR EYE EXAMINATIONS FOR ADULTS AND THE ELDERLY

All adults with decrease in visual acuity for distant or near objects should have an ophthalmologic eye examination or refractive eye examination.

All adults should have an eye examination by a family physician, internist, or other health care professional as a component of regular health care.

Adults with risk factors such as a family history of glaucoma, cataract, retinal detachment, or significant degenerative eye disease should have an ophthalmologic eye examination early in adult life and at medically appropriate intervals thereafter.

Adults with diabetes mellitus should have an ophthalmologic eye examination at the time of diagnosis and at medically appropriate intervals thereafter.

Adults with systemic disease and/or medical treatment known to be associated with increased risk of eye disease should have an ophthalmologic eye examination at time of diagnosis and/or treatment onset.

All adults 65 or more years of age should have an ophthalmologic eye examination at least every 2 years.

Adults should participate in vision screening programs conducted by eye care and health care professionals, industry representatives, or volunteer organizations annually or every 2 years.

From Comprehensive Adult Eye Examination.[6]

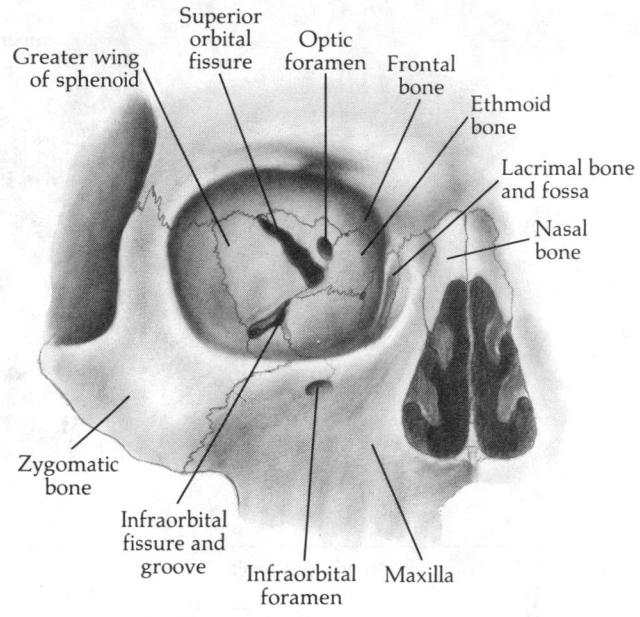

Figure 6-1 Right bony orbit.

cushion and support the eyeball and the extrinsic muscles. The anterior orbital walls are relatively thick and provide good protection for the eye. The medial wall which separates the orbit from the ethmoid sinus, is extremely thin and vulnerable to ethmoid sinus infection.[34] The medial wall also contains a fossa for the lacrimal sac, which extends downward through the nasal lacrimal duct into the nose. The lateral posterior wall is also very thin and separates the orbit from the temporal lobe.

The anterior roof of the orbit contains the fossa for the lacrimal gland. The floor of the orbit is supported primarily by the orbital plate of the maxilla, which contains the infraorbital fissure. The maxillary branch of the trigeminal nerve (CN V) passes through this infraorbital fissure. The posterior wall of the orbit contains a fibrous sheet that encircles the optic foramen and is the origin for the extrinsic muscles, which stretch forward to encircle and insert into the anterior and medial aspects of the eyeball (Figure 6-2). The orbital contents are supported and separated from the bone by a periosteal lining and fascial tissue that form the eye socket in which the eyeball rests.

Eyelid   The exposed part of the eye is protected by a lid that serves as a shield from external injury and exposure to excessive light. As the upper lid blinks, it distributes tears over the surface of the eye to keep it moist. When the lids are open, they form the palpebral fissure (the elliptic opening). As a result, the upper lid covers part of the iris (Figure 6-3). The lids meet at the medial (inner) canthus and fold over a small elevation, called the lacrimal caruncle. This caruncle contains large sebaceous

glands. The inner canthus is sometimes obscured by a vertical skin fold (epicanthus) in Asian people and young children. The central portion of the upper and lower lid is thickened with a firm connective tissue (tarsal plate) that protects the eye and maintains the shape of the lid. The eyelids are lined with a thin, transparent mucous membrane (palpebral conjunctiva) that continues as an outer cover for the sclera of the eyeball (bulbar conjunctiva) (see Figure 6-2). The conjunctiva contains blood vessels, nerves, hair follicles, and sebaceous glands (meibomian glands). The meibomian glands are found along the margin of the lids. Their secretions prevent rapid evaporation and overflow of tears and create an airtight seal when the eyelids are closed.

Lid movement is supplied from the superior division of the oculomotor nerve (CN III), which activates the superior palpebral levator muscle for upper lid elevation and the retractor muscle for lower lid retraction. The facial nerve (CN VII) activates the orbicularis oculi muscle, an oval sheet of fibers that surrounds the palpebral fissure, for lid closure. Superior and inferior palpebral smooth muscles and a central portion of the orbicularis oculi muscle respond to sympathetic innervation for involuntary blinking. The upper lid receives its sensory innervation from the ophthalmic division of the trigeminal nerve (CN V), and the lower lid is innervated by the maxillary branch of the trigeminal nerve.

The eyelids are the only portion of the eye that has a lymphatic system. The medial portions of the upper and lower lids drain into the submaxillary nodes, and the lateral aspects drain into the preauricular nodes.[34]

Lacrimal apparatus   The lacrimal system secretes and drains a fluid that moistens and lubricates the anterior surface of the eye. Tears are produced in the lacrimal gland, which is located in the anterior lateral fossa of the orbit. Smaller

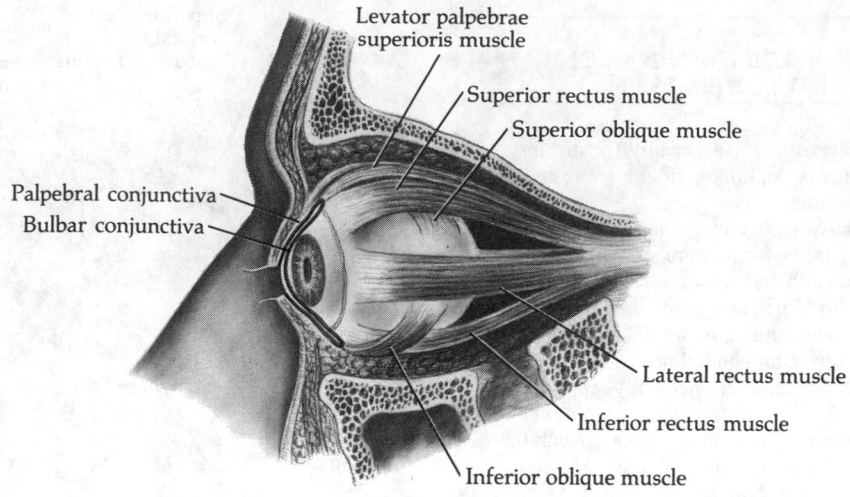

Figure 6-2 Diagrammatic section of orbit.

accessory glands scattered throughout the palpebral conjunctiva also secrete fluid. Lacrimal fluid is normally clear and does not overflow unless reflex or mental-emotional stimuli produce excessive tearing or unless there is a blockage in the normal drainage channels. Sebaceous gland secretion and a thin mucin layer combine with the aqueous portion of tears to maintain a constant film over the cornea. Lacrimal fluid contains immunoglobulins, lymphocytes, phagocytes, and lysozyme as protective substances.[34]

Lid blinking helps distribute tears over the eye and draws the tears inward to the puncta, which are small openings in the margins of the upper and lower lids at the inner canthus (Figure 6-3). The puncta empty into the lacrimal canaliculi, which join to form the common canaliculus. Tears empty next into the lacrimal sac (see Figure 6-3). The adjacent lacrimal duct empties into the nasal cavity in the inferior nasal meatus.

Eyeball

Layers of the Eye

Outer layer: cornea and sclera The eyeball is surrounded by the sclera, the "white" of the eye. It is a tough fibrous layer that covers the posterior five sixths of the eye.

The cornea covers the anterior one sixth of the eye. It is transparent, avascular, and richly innervated with sensory nerves (trigeminal [CN V]). The anterior surface of the cornea is convex, and irregularities of the curvature cause astigmatism. Because the cornea is avascular, it depends on the atmosphere, tears, and aqueous humor for oxygenation and nourishment. The cornea has five layers: the superficial epithelial layer, which is continuous with the bulbar conjunctiva; Bowman's membrane; stroma, which constitutes 90% of corneal thickness; Descemet's membrane; and an endothelial layer.[44]

The epithelial layer is a regenerative multilayered barrier. If its cells are injured, uninjured cells migrate to the traumatized area and form a new barrier one cell thick within an hour of the injury.[34] Total repair of the corneal epithelium takes approxi-

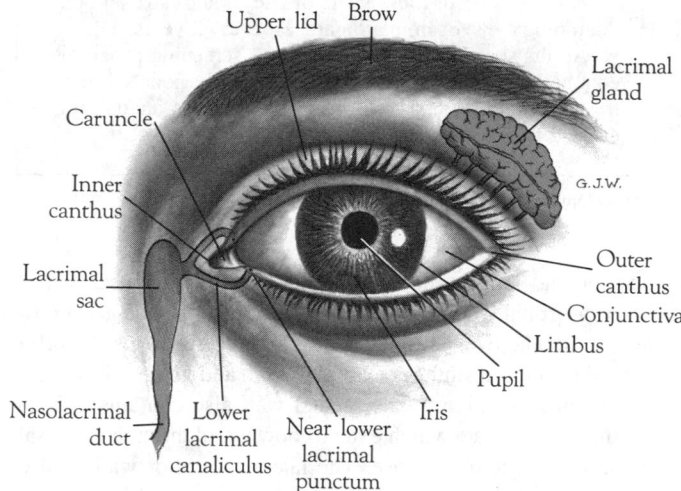

Figure 6-3 Visible surface of eye.

mately 48 to 72 hours in a normal, healthy person. Because of its dependence on exposure to tears, corneal epithelium is subject to edema if deprived of oxygen. (The implications for contact lenses are discussed later.) The stroma is faced anteriorly with a collagenous membrane (Bowman's membrane) that resists infection and trauma. If Bowman's membrane is destroyed, it re-forms with scarring and irregular cell formation that contribute to astigmatism. The endothelial layer pumps fluid from the other corneal layers into the aqueous humor. A relatively diminished fluid volume is necessary for corneal transparency. If the endothelium is destroyed, it does not regenerate, and the remaining corneal layers become edematous.

The sclera and cornea merge at a junction called the limbus (see Figure 6-3). The corneoscleral limbus has a rich vascular supply that encircles and nourishes the outer edges of the cornea. At the limbus, corneal cells are mixed with conjunctival and scleral layers. Bowman's membrane ends abruptly at this junction. The posterior inner surface of the limbus adjoins the trabecular meshwork and the canal of Schlemm, which drain aqueous fluid from the anterior chamber.[44]

The sclera is the outer layer that surrounds most of the eye. It is adjacent to the second layer, the uveal tract, which includes the choroid layer, the ciliary body, and the iris (Figure 6-4). The sclera has three layers. The outermost is the episclera, which merges with fascial tissue at the limbus; it is vascular and dense, and the minute vessels can be seen through the conjunctiva. The middle layer, the scleral stroma, is composed of tough collagenous fibers that create the white appearance of the sclera. The innermost layer, the lamina fusca, contains melanocytes that may contribute to a yellow-brown scleral hue in dark-skinned people. The lamina fusca contains collagenous fibers that filter into the choroid layer for adherence. The oculomotor muscles attach to the sclera at various points near the midsection of the eyeball (see Figure 6-2). The sclera also has numerous openings through which nerves and blood vessels pass. The two major openings are the posterior foramen, which admits the optic nerve into the eye, and the anterior foramen, where the ciliary muscle adjoins at the limbus in the anterior chamber.

Middle layer: choroid, ciliary body, and iris   The middle layer of the eyeball (the uveal tract) comprises the choroid, a vascular layer; the ciliary body; which contains smooth muscles attached to the lens and an epithelial portion for secreting aqueous humor; and the iris, which surrounds the pupil (see Figure 6-4).

The choroid adheres to the sclera at the entrance point of the optic nerve and extends anteriorly to the ciliary body. It has five layers. The outer layer, the suprachoroid, contains melanocytes, smooth muscle fibers, and ciliary arteries that nourish a portion of the choroid. The three middle layers contain veins and arte-

rioles that feed into the ciliary body, the iris, and the outer portion of the retina. The inner layer of the choroid is called Bruch's membrane. It is multilayered and collagenous and contains cells from the adjacent retinal and choroid layers.

The ciliary body has both a muscular and a secretory function. The ciliary muscles expand from the choroid and extend anteriorly and medially toward the lens (Figure 6-5). The body

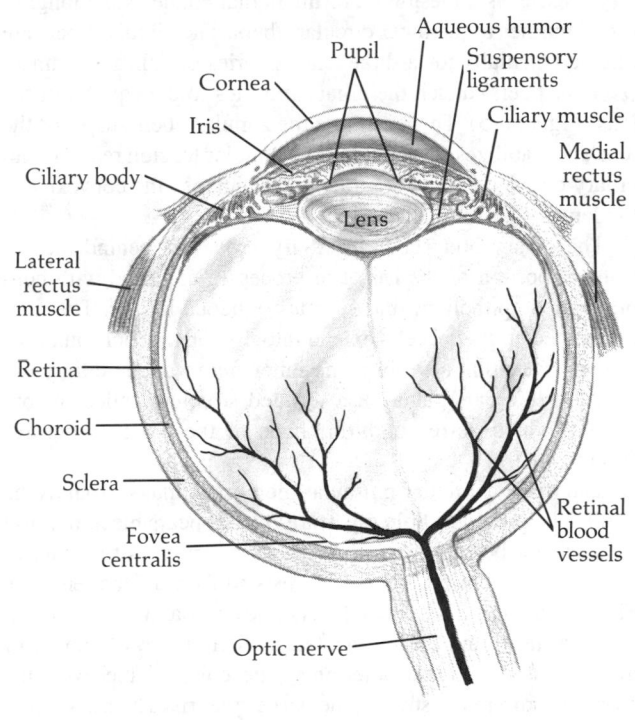

Figure 6-4 Cross section of eye.

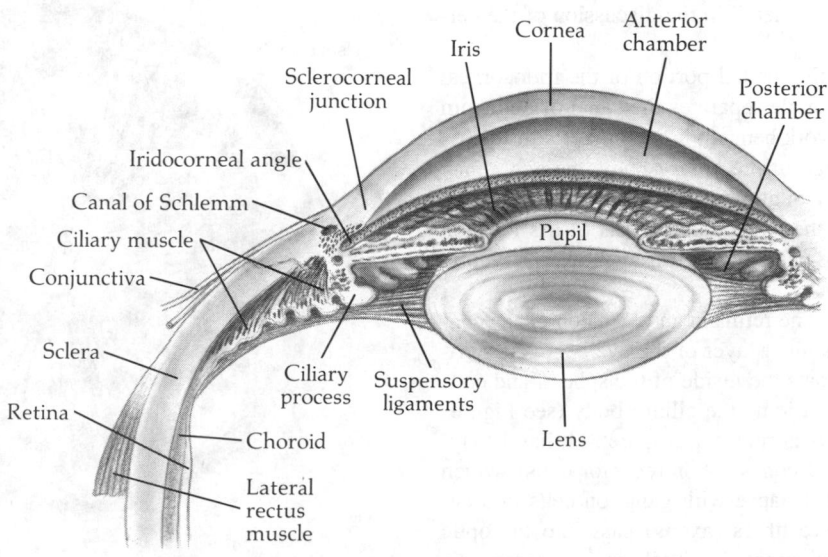

Figure 6-5 Close-up view of ciliary body, zonules, lens, and anterior and posterior chambers.

forms a ring of smooth ciliary muscle that surrounds the lens and parallels the overlying sclera. There are three groups of ciliary muscles. Muscles in the outer division are longitudinal and parallel and adjacent to the sclera. Contraction of these fibers opens the canal of Schlemm, a thin-walled vessel that encircles the eye and drains aqueous fluid from the anterior chamber. The canal of Schlemm is located at the inner aspect of the sclerocorneal junction (limbus) (Figure 6-5). The middle layer of ciliary muscles is a meshwork of fibers that connects the longitudinal muscles to the inner circular fibers. The circular fibers are directed medially toward the lens. A series of delicate ligament (zonular fibers) attach the ciliary muscles to the equator of the lens (Figure 6-5). The tension of the zonular fibers suspends the lens and stabilizes its position. The zonular tension relaxes with ciliary circular muscle contraction to increase the convexity of the lens for accommodation.[34]

The ciliary body ends in ciliary processes behind the peripheral portion of the iris. The processes are lined with nonpigmented epithelium that secretes aqueous humor. The nonpigmented epithelial cells extend into the sensory portion of the retina. The retina also joins the inner lining of the ciliary epithelium (the pars plana) at a serrated structure called the ora serrata, which corresponds in shape to the ciliary processes (Figure 6-6).

The iris is a circular muscular membrane that surrounds the pupil. The pupil is a hole (aperture) that appears black because light cannot be seen behind it. The iris separates the anterior and posterior eye chambers and rests in front of the lens (see Figure 6-5). The iris has two layers: the stroma, which is the anterior surface, and the pigmented epithelium. The amount of melanin in the stroma determines the color of the eyes; the more melanin in the stroma, the darker the iris. The iris sphincter surrounds the pupil, and its contraction decreases pupil size. The pigmented epithelial layer contains the dilator pupillae muscle, which dilates the pupil when contracted. Pupillary response is described in more detail in the discussion of the nervous system of the eye.

The iris is located at the medial portion of the iridocorneal angle (Figure 6-5). This angle separates the canal of Schlemm and the trabecular meshwork beneath it from the iris. If the iris inserts at the anterior edge of the ciliary body, the angle may become narrow. Pupillary dilation also thickens the iris which may affect the width of the angle. The effects of iris location and shape on the iridocorneal angle are discussed in the section on glaucoma.

Inner layer: retina   The retina is an extension of the central nervous system. This inner layer of the eye begins posteriorly at the optic nerve, coats the inside of the sphere, and ends at the ora serrata, where it joins the ciliary body (see Figures 6-4 and 6-6). The retina is normally transparent. It has 10 layers and contains rods and cones (photoreceptor cells), which are connecting cells that synapse with ganglion cells in a peripheral layer. Optic nerve fibers (axons) pass into the optic nerve (Figure 6-7). The pigmented epithelium (adjacent to the choroid surface) contains enzymes and protein binding sites for vitamin A. These protein sites are necessary for the photochemical visual process. The rods and cones are elongated cells that respond to light and convert it into electrical energy. They pass through the next four layers. Both types of cells contain light-sensitive pigments that undergo chemical changes necessary for neural transmission of light. Rods are light sensitive in low levels of light (scotopic vision). Cones perceive images and color in higher levels of light (photopic vision). Rods and cones are so named because of their microscopic appearance; rods are more cylindric and generally more elongated. Rods and cones connect with each other in the plexiform layer and synapse with a variety of cells that ultimately reach the ganglion cells. The ganglion cells transmit electrical discharges through their axons to the midbrain.

Rods and cones are scattered throughout the retinal surface. If the retina were laid out on a flat surface, its center would be the fovea centralis. The fovea is a small depression that contains no rods but is densely packed with cones. Each cone synapses with more than one foveal photoreceptor and ganglion cell but with fewer of these cells than elsewhere in the retina. Visual acuity is sharpest in this area if enough light is available for photopic vision. The fovea is surrounded by the macula lutea, a pigmented area about 4.5 mm in diameter. Rods are densely packed in the periphery of this region (approximately 150,000 rods/mm^2) and become less dense as they extend toward the periphery. Cones average about 4500/mm^2 and also become sparse in the periphery.[34] The optic disc (the head of the optic nerve) perforates the retina about 3 mm toward the nose from the fovea. The disc is approximately 1.5 mm in diameter and contains no rods or cones. This results in a small blind spot for each eye located about 15 degrees laterally from the center of vision. The viewer is not aware of this because the

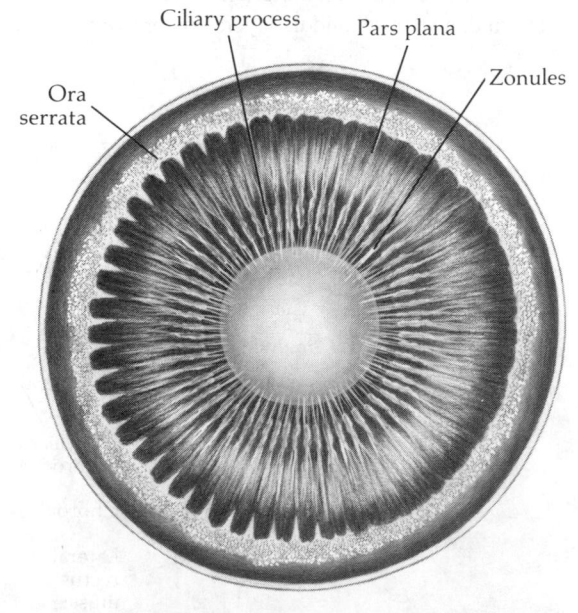

Figure 6-6 Posterior view of ciliary body and surrounding structures. (Retina and ciliary body join at ora serrata.)

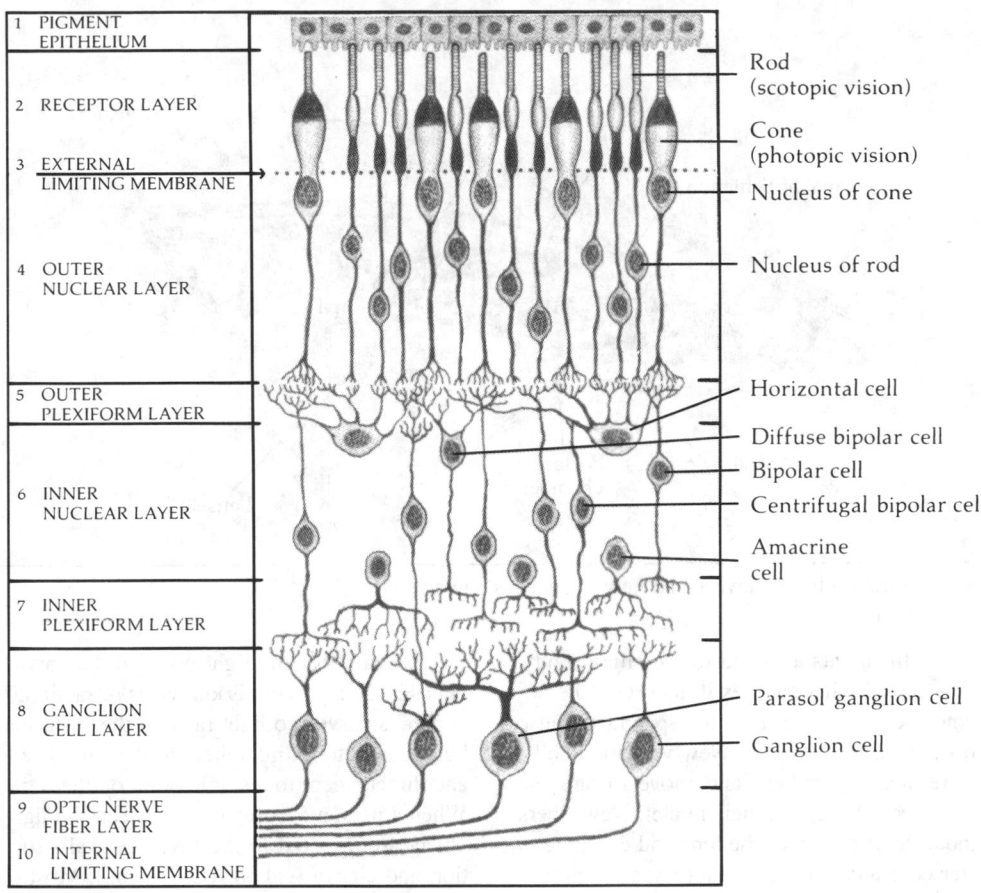

Figure 6-7 Layers of retina.

other eye compensates for the loss. The periphery of the retina contains primarily rods. When viewed through the ophthalmoscope, the fovea appears as a small pinpoint of light surrounded by a yellow-brown pigmented area (the macula). The head of the optic nerve appears as a pink or cream-colored circle with a white depression in the center. This depression is where the central retinal artery and central vein bifurcate, emerge, and feed into smaller branches throughout the retinal surface.

Chambers, Fluids, and Inner Structures of the Eye

Aqueous fluid and intraocular pressure   The eye contains three chambers: the anterior, the posterior, and the vitreous body. The anterior chamber rests between the cornea (in front) and the iris (behind). It maintains a depth of approximately 3 mm between the center of the cornea and the pupil. It is filled with approximately 0.2 ml of aqueous humor, which flows from the posterior chamber and empties at the canal of Schlemm (see Figure 6-5). The canal of Schlemm is a highly permeable oval channel that surrounds the anterior chamber. It is adjacent to the trabecular meshwork, which filters the fluid before it enters the canal (Figure 6-8). The meshwork also encircles the anterior chamber and lies at the apex of the iridocorneal angle.

The posterior chamber is a narrow passage behind the iris and in front of the lens and the ciliary body. Aqueous humor flows into the anterior chamber through the pupil (see Figure 6-8).

Aqueous humor is secreted by the ciliary processes. It maintains intraocular pressure (normally within a range of 10 to 22 mm Hg), contributes to metabolism of the lens, and nourishes the cornea. Intraocular pressure is maintained by the rate of fluid secretion and the resistance to outflow by the trabecular meshwork. Eyeball pressure must exceed atmospheric pressure to maintain the shape of the sphere. Intraocular pressure fluctuates 1 to 2 mm Hg with each heartbeat. Pressure fluctuations are based on the pressure within the episcleral veins, which connect to the canal of Schlemm, and the osmotic pressure of the blood. Normal pressure changes (up to 5 mm Hg) are usually quickly compensated for by trabecular meshwork distention, which lowers outflow resistance.[34] Valsalva's maneuver (bearing down to complete a bowel movement) increases venous pressure and so greatly increases intraocular pressure, which quickly returns to normal when the maneuver ends. Drinking large quantities of water or receiving saline intravenous fluids causes a slight increase in intraocular pressure.

Lens   The lens separates the posterior chamber from the vitreous body. It is biconvex and transparent and is held in

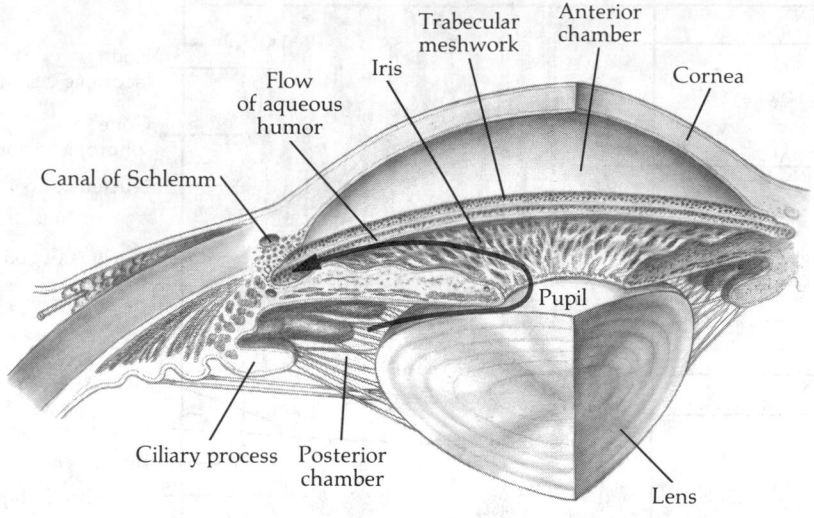

Figure 6-8 Close view of trabecular meshwork and flow of aqueous humor.

position by suspensory ligaments attached to the ciliary body. The lens comprises a capsule that encases it, a cortex (the peripheral portion), and a central core. It is transparent because most of its cells do not have a nucleus. Newly formed cells, with nuclei, originate at the periphery and move toward the center, where mature fibers have lost their nuclei. New fibers are formed throughout the life span of the lens and continue to migrate to the center core and become compressed. Therefore an older lens is larger, denser, less elastic, and less able to contract to accommodate for near vision. The lens also maintains transparency by avoiding excessive hydration. The lens is surrounded by media that are high in sodium. The lens membrane is relatively impermeable to sodium, and lens metabolism pumps out sodium, which decreases osmotic activity. The lens becomes yellow in middle age, which diminishes the intensity of blue-toned light on the retina.[44]

Vitreous body The vitreous cavity contains approximately 4.5 ml of vitreous humor, which is a gelatinous substance that adheres firmly to the retina, the ciliary epithelium (at the base of the lens), and the margin of the optic nerve. If the vitreous humor diminishes in volume or degenerates, retinal tears may occur because of traction on the retina.

Image Formation

Light reception and refraction The receptors of the eye are sensitive to only a small portion of the light spectrum. Light in wavelengths less than 400 nm or greater than 700 nm is not absorbed by rods and cones and therefore is not seen.

To reach the retina, light must pass through the clear media of the cornea, aqueous fluid, the lens, and the vitreous body. Light rays are emitted in all directions from any source. These light rays pass through the optic system, which focuses them at a specific point to achieve image accuracy.

A ray of light that passes from one clear medium into another is affected by the density of the medium. The density of the cornea slows the light ray, and the curvature of the cornea bends it. This process is known as refraction. The surface of the cornea is curved so light rays hit the surface at different angles but are bent to redirect them to the lens. The lens further bends and directs them to a single point on the retina (Figure 6-9, *A*). When a person focuses on an object, the light waves from that object are directed to the fovea centralis for image identification and clarity (called focal vision). Most objects have more than one point of focus. As different points of focus from an object reach the retina, they form an image that is upside down and reversed (Figure 6-9, *B*). Light waves also enter the eye from a wide visual field (approximately 170° arc for each eye) that surrounds the object of focus. These peripheral sources focus on the outer areas of the retina (ambient vision) and help with spatial sense.[34]

The anterior surface of the cornea is the primary refractive area of the eye. The more a surface bends light rays, the greater the refractive power. The shift in the direction of light when it moves through the corneal surface is greater than the second shift at the lens surface.

Accommodation Accommodation is the process by which the lens alters its shape for visual clarity when the eye is viewing an object at close range. In other words, the lens surface increases its refractive power by becoming thicker and more convex to accommodate near objects. Normally the lens is somewhat flattened and held tight by the ligaments that attach to the circular ciliary muscle. When the muscles contract, the ligaments relax and release their tension on the lens. The lens contracts and becomes more spheric. The lens is constantly adjusting to stimuli at different distances. Ciliary branches of the oculomotor nerve respond to brain signals for this automatic response.

Binocular vision and vergence Normal eyes are aligned in their orbits so that they can direct light rays to the fovea centralis of each eye. The visual axis is an imaginary line drawn

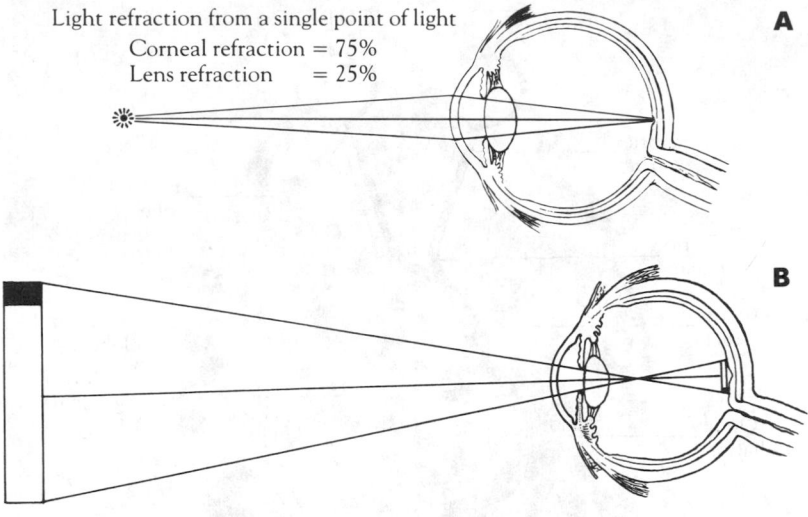

Light refraction from a single point of light
Corneal refraction = 75%
Lens refraction = 25%

Figure 6-9 **A,** Light refraction from single point of light. **B,** Light refraction from object with more than one point of light.

from each fovea centralis to a fixation point. When a three-dimensional object is focused on the back of both eyes, there is a slight difference in the horizontal placement of the two images. This slight difference sets up two images in the brain, which permits the binocular viewer (using both eyes) to experience the visual sensation of depth (stereopsis).

Vergence is a visual reflex of simultaneous eye movements. When distant objects are viewed, the visual axes of the eyes become more parallel and the eyes are rotated outward (divergence). As the object draws nearer, the medius rectus muscles contract and pull the eyes inward (convergence).[44] This reflex is necessary to prevent diplopia (double vision). If a person holds a finger about 10 inches in front of his nose and focuses on the finger, he sees one finger. If he suddenly shifts his focus to a distant object, he sees two fingers because the parallel visual axes do not meet at the finger.

Image Interpretation

Visual pathway　We are able to see because refracted light rays stimulate retinal photoreceptors and are changed into electrical energy. This energy is transmitted to different cerebral cortical areas for interpretation. Light rays constantly stimulate photoreceptors. Rods and cones contain specific pigments (opsins) that combine with a form of vitamin A to absorb light and convert it to an electrical potential. These photoreceptors synapse with second- and third-order neurons within the retina, which converge into fibers that enter the optic nerve. The optic nerve forms the optic disc and exits the eyeball at the posterior region. The choroid and all the retinal layers except the nerve fiber layer end at the edge of the disc.

The optic nerve contains more than 1 million fibers (axons of ganglion cells) that control vision, eye movement, and pupillary reflexes. As the optic nerve exits the sphere, it is encased in dura mater, an arachnoid sheath, and pia mater. It forms an S-shaped curve that allows it to stretch when the eye is moved.

The orbital portion of the nerve is about 30 mm long. The optic nerve also contains the central retinal artery and vein, which bifurcate and branch into the eyeball near the head of the nerve (the disc). The central artery and vein exit the optic nerve about 12 mm behind the eyeball.[34]

The optic nerves from each eye pass through the optic foramen and meet at the optic chiasm, which lies above and in front of the pituitary gland. Optic tracts emerge from the chiasm and encircle the hypothalamus. They terminate in the lateral geniculate bodies in the temporal lobes (Figure 6-10). Cells in the lateral geniculate bodies send fibers (optic radiation) to the occipital lobe of each cerebral hemisphere. The visual cortex in the posterior aspect of the occipital lobe receives most of the visual fibers representing central vision (stimuli from the fovea centralis and surrounding macula). Adjacent occipital lobe areas receive fibers representing the more peripheral portions of the retina. Reversed images are righted when perceived in the cortex.

Objects in the visual field stimulate the opposite side of the retina. When nerve fibers pass into the optic nerve, the nasal (closest to the nose) and temporal (closest to the side of the face) fibers are separate within the sheath. Temporal fibers pass on the temporal side of the nerve, nasal fibers are on the nasal side, and central (foveal) fibers are in the center of the nerve. When the nerves merge at the chiasm, nasal fibers cross (decussate) to the opposite optic tract. Temporal fibers do not cross but continue in the optic tract on the same side as the nerve that conveys them to the chiasm (Figure 6-11). Therefore the pathway of vision for an object seen on a person's right side would be through nasal receptors in the right eye and then through the nasal side of the optic nerve to the chiasm, where it would cross to the left optic tract and proceed to the left cerebral occipital lobe. Visual field defects can often be traced to disorders in specific anatomic locations because of the arrangement of nerve fibers. A left or right optic nerve lesion would cause a

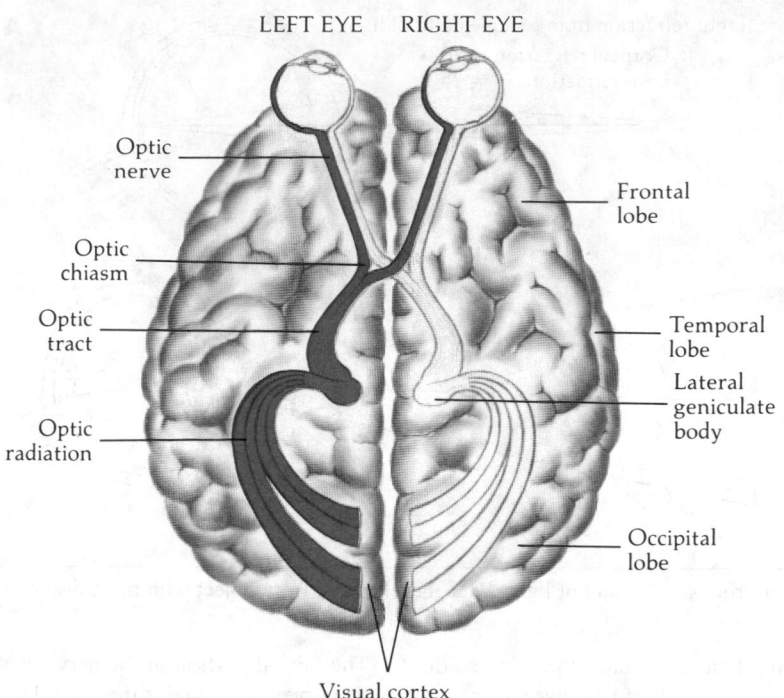

LEFT EYE RIGHT EYE

Optic nerve

Optic chiasm

Optic tract

Optic radiation

Frontal lobe

Temporal lobe

Lateral geniculate body

Occipital lobe

Visual cortex

Figure 6-10 Visual pathway.

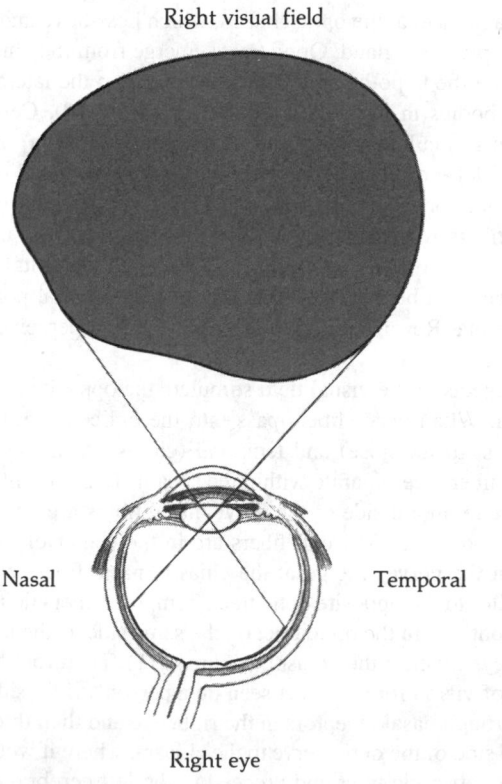

Right visual field

Nasal

Temporal

Right eye

Figure 6-11 Image placement on retina.

corresponding defect in the left or right eye. Chiasm lesions can cause a variety of defects depending on the location of the lesion. A common defect is bitemporal hemianopia, which results from a pituitary tumor. A left optic tract lesion would result in a bilateral right visual field deficit. These defects are depicted in Figure 6-12.

Light and dark adaptation The concentration of pigment in the photoreceptor cells of the retina determines the sensitivity of these cells to light. Photoreceptive pigments are constantly being used and replaced through chemical changes in the retina. When the eyes are exposed to bright light, the pigments become bleached and the sensitivity of the photoreceptors diminishes. Bright light causes discomfort for several minutes until breakdown of the photopigments produces a gradual rise of the visual threshold. Together with pupillary constriction, decreased rod and cone sensitivity to light protects the retinal cells in bright light. This is called light adaptation.[44]

Exposure to darkness tends to increase photopigment regeneration to increase sensitivity to light. Rhodopsin, the photopigment in rods, is particularly sensitive to dim light and enables a person to visualize dim forms and shapes in near darkness. Rhodopsin does not absorb color wavelengths, so color is not perceived in dim light.

Color perception Light waves do not contain color. Color is perceived according to the wavelength (frequency) of a light ray. Colors are determined by hue (the standard recognition of a particular shade) and saturation (the intensity of a color). A less intense color contains larger amounts of white and appears

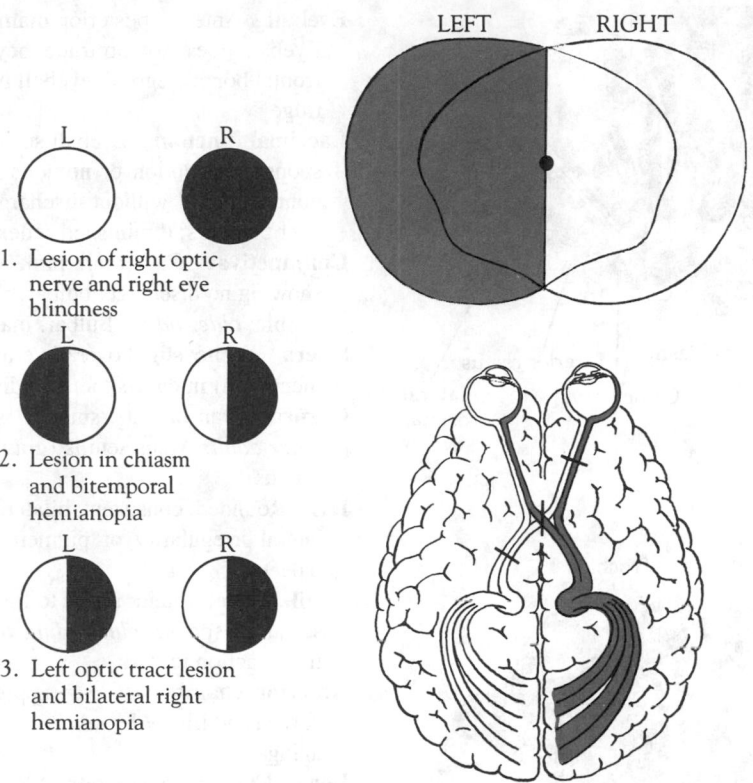

LEFT   RIGHT

L   R

1. Lesion of right optic
nerve and right eye
blindness

L   R

2. Lesion in chiasm
and bitemporal
hemianopia

L   R

3. Left optic tract lesion
and bilateral right
hemianopia

Figure 6-12 Visual pathway defects.

relatively pale. Any object that reflects all visible light rays evokes a sensation of white. The absence of light rays is perceived as black.

The retina contains three types of cones, and each has a different photopigment that absorbs light waves of different frequencies. Each type of cone responds to a primary color: red, green, or blue. If all of the cones are equally stimulated, white is perceived. Rods do not perceive color.

Eye Movement

The movement of each eye is controlled by six muscles. Four of these (the recti) originate behind the eyeball, move forward around the sphere, and insert into the sclera about 7 mm behind the limbus (Figure 6-13, *A*). The superior oblique muscle begins at the posterior orbit, passes forward to the anterior orbital rim, loops through the trochlea (a fibrocartilaginous structure) to return to the eyeball, and inserts into the sclera under the belly of the superior rectus muscle (Figure 6-13, *B*). The sixth muscle, the interior oblique, originates at the nasal side of the orbit and passes under the eyeball to attach at its lateral surface (Figure 6-13, *B*). The oculomotor nerve (CN III) supplies the medial, inferior, and superior rectus muscles and the inferior oblique muscle. The trochlear nerve (CN IV) supplies the superior oblique muscle, and the abducent nerve (CN VI) supplies the lateral rectus muscle (Figure 6-14).

Contraction of an eye muscle turns the eye toward that muscle. All six muscles are constantly coordinating stretch and contraction functions to permit full and continuous eye movement.

Both eyes must move together to maintain a clear focus. When a person looks to the right, the right lateral rectus muscle and the left medial rectus muscle contract. The innervation stimulus to both muscles is equal, so the speed and destination of the two eyeball movements are equal. Muscles that produce equal movement of each eye in the same direction are called yoke muscles. Eye movements that are simultaneous, equal, and coordinated are called conjugate eye movements.

The fibers within the extraocular muscles are highly differentiated. Eye muscles are capable of slow graded contractions and very rapid contractions. Rapid eye movements may be voluntary or involuntary. One type of rapid reflex movement is called saccade. Saccadic movements are small rapid jerks that alternate with steady fixation (particularly when the eye is focusing on a near object). Saccadic movements bring peripheral retinal images to the fovea centralis for clarity. These movements also sweep images over retinal receptors to prevent light adaptation. If a person continued to focus an image in one retinal area, color and detail would fade in a few seconds. Saccade also occurs during sleep as rapid eye movement (REM).

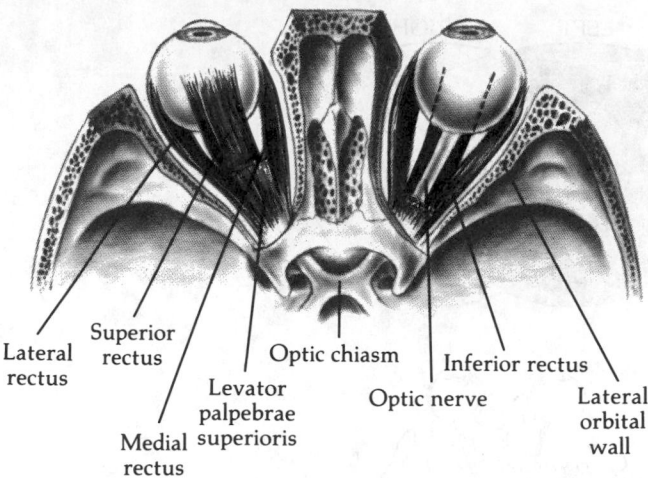

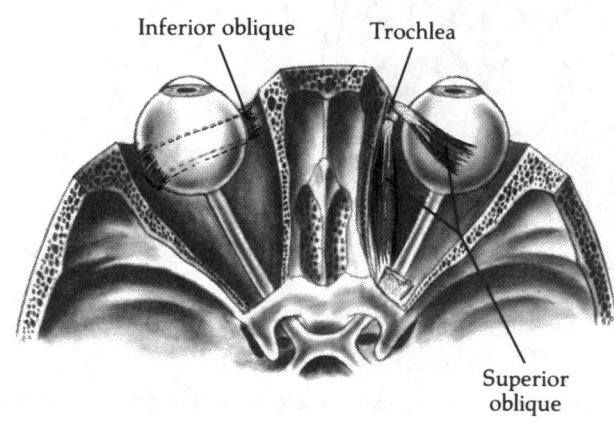

Figure 6-13 Extraocular muscles.

Certain reflexes also allow the eyes to maintain a steady gaze of fixation despite head movements. If the head turns to the right, the eyes can shift an equal rotation to the left. Upward head movement causes downward rotation of the eyes.

In summary, eye movements can be classified as tracking (slow, smooth, coordinated rotations for maintaining the image of an object on the fovea centralis); vergence (slow, smooth movements that rotate the eyes inward or outward to track an object as being near or far); saccadic movements (rapid reflexes that alternate with fixation to keep the image clear and steady); and compensatory movements (reflexes that coordinate head movement with object fixation and steady gaze). Table 6-1 summarizes the major nervous system mechanisms of the eye.

▪ NORMAL FINDINGS

Eyelids Blink response to light or corneal touch; frequent involuntary bilateral blinks (average 15 to 20 per minute); lid margins rest over inferior and superior borders of cornea

Eyeball Anterior-posterior diameter 22-27 mm; Caucasian: Eyeball does not protrude beyond supraorbital bridge of frontal bone; Negroid: eyeball may protrude slightly beyond ridge

Lacrimal function Eyeball surface moist; excess tears in response to emotion or noxious atmospheric stimuli; puncta nontender and without discharge on palpation; *older adult:* over 50 years; diminished reflex response for excess tearing

Conjunctivae Palpebral: pink with uniform small vessels showing no discharge; bulbar; clear, tiny, red vessels may be visible; *older adult:* Bulbar: may lack luster of young adult.

Sclera White; slight overall yellowish cast or black dots (pigmentation) in dark-skinned individuals

Cornea Transparent, smooth surface; convex curvature; *older adult:* Arcus senilis (gray ring of lipid deposit around limbus)

Iris Rounded; consistent, bilateral coloration; *older adult:* bilateral irregularity of pigment density (color may appear paler)

Pupil Equal; round; reacts to light and accommodation; consensual response; *older adult:* often miotic with slower dilation reaction to dark

Anterior chamber Clear; approximately 3.3 mm between cornea and iris; *older adult:* becomes slightly shallower with aging

Lens Clear, biconvex refractile body, enclosed in a capsule. Becomes yellowish with age. When opaque deposits are numerous enough to cause vision deficit that interferes with normal activities of daily living (ADL), a significant cataract exists and may ethically be surgically removed

Internal eye Full, round, bilateral red reflex

Retina Uniform pink and granular texture (Negroid surface uniformly more pigmented); choroid layer may be visible showing linear light orange vessels; *older adult:* may appear slightly paler

Vessels Central vein and artery emerge on nasal side of physiologic cup within disc, and each immediately breaks into two branches; arteries light red and 25% narrower than dark red veins; narrow band of light may appear at center of arteries; vessel caliber regular and uniformly decreases as vessel branches toward periphery; venous pulsations more prominent in young adults; *older adult:* arteries slightly narrower; arterial light reflex may be widened; arterial caliber may be slightly irregular

Disc, cup Whitish, cream, or pink; vertically oval or round with distinct border (nasal side may be slightly less demarcated and temporal border may appear as grayish crescent); approximately 1.5 mm diameter (magnified 15 times through ophthalmoscope); cup is small, white or pale depression in center of disc and occupies approximately half of disc diameter; *older adult:* disc may appear slightly smaller and more opaque

Macula, fovea Macula is darker area two disc diameters temporally from disc; fovea is pinpoint bright light in center of macula

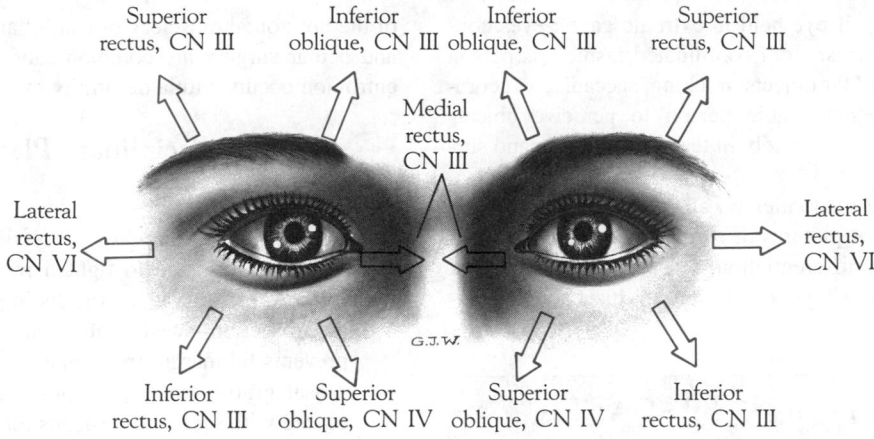

Figure 6-14 Innervation of movement of extraocular muscles.

TABLE 6-1 Summary of Major Nervous System Mechanisms of the Eye

Function	Mechanism
Lid movement	
Oculomotor (CN III)	Innervates levator palpebrae superioris and inferior rectus
Facial (CN VII)	Innervates orbicularis oculi
Sensation (trigeminal [CN V])	Ophthalmic division for upper lid; maxillary division for lower lid
Reflex response	Sympathetic fibers from superior cervical ganglion innervate palpebral muscles
Tears	Normal moisture maintained by secretory function of palpebral accessory glands; excess tears mediated through stimulation of facial nerve (CN VII) and trigeminal nerve (CN V)
Corneal sensation	Trigeminal nerve (CN V)
Pupil	
Constriction	Light stimulates retina and afferent fibers that pass through optic nerve (CN II) and chiasm and then deviate from tract to area of midbrain (superior colliculus); axons leave this area and connect to nucleus of oculomotor nerve (CN III), which sends efferent fibers to ciliary ganglion (between optic chiasm and posterior orbit); parasympathetic fibers leave ciliary ganglion and enter eye to stimulate iris sphincter
Consensual response	Both pupils constrict when only one is stimulated; oculomotor nucleus responds to afferent fibers from one eye and sends signals through its fibers and parasympathetic fibers to both iris muscles
Dilation	Reduction of parasympathetic tonic flow to iris sphincters in dim light; sympathetic stimulation of fibers from carotid plexus occurs with startle or pleasure responses
Lens accommodation	Oculomotor nerve (CN III) mediates parasympathetic stimulation for ciliary muscle contraction and resultant lens convexity
Vision	Light focuses on retinal receptors; axons pass into optic nerve (CN II), chiasm, optic tracts, lateral geniculate bodies, and optic radiation to occipital lobe and visual cortex
Eye movement	Conjugate movements occur because nuclei of CN III, IV, and VI connect in fiber tract in midbrain
Oculomotor nerve (CN III)	Innervates superior rectus, medial rectus, inferior rectus, and inferior oblique muscles
Trochlear nerve (CN IV)	Innervates superior oblique muscle
Abducent nerve (CN VI)	Innervates lateral rectus muscle

Data from Newell[34] and Vaughan.[44]

Visual acuity

Distant vision   20/20 (able to read designated size letter on standardized chart at 20 feet distance); *older adult:* 20/20 to 20/30

Near vision   Able to read newsprint at 14 inches; *older adult:* presbyopic owing to loss of lens refractive power (average person over 60 years cannot focus more closely than 3 feet without corrective lenses)

Peripheral vision   Temporal vision 90° from central visual axis; upward: 50°; nasalward: 60°; downward: 70°; *older adult:* may be slightly diminished but usually not measurable with confrontation testing

Eye movement, coordination, and interpretation   Both eyes demonstrate coordinated, parallel movements in six cardinal fields of gaze; physiologic nystagmus (mild rhythmic twitching if eye held in extreme gaze); eyes converge and diverge in smooth coordinated fashion as person focuses on near and far objects; tracking, saccadic, and compensatory movements enable person to perceive objects clearly in depth and accurately in terms of distance and surrounding space

Color perception Able to identify all colors accurately when tested with series of pictures or cards that present multicolored field for color differentiation; *older adult:* brightness of colors may be dimmed; yellow overcast to hues owing to aging lens

CONDITIONS, DISEASES, AND DISORDERS

DISORDERS OF THE EYELID

Lid disorders are extremely common and varied. Because the lids are responsible for tear maintenance and dispersion, structure and position defects can result in excess tears or drying of the eyeball surface. Deformities and movement abnormalities interfere with the lid's vital protective function and with vision. Structure and movement malfunctions alter facial expression and appearance and create cosmetic concerns. Many pain receptors are near the lid margin, and stretching and inflammation of the tissue result in acute discomfort. Because the palpebral conjunctiva is adjacent to the lid margin, disorders in this area can produce acute and diffuse redness of the eye.

Two types of lid disorders will be discussed: those involving position, structure, and movement and those involving inflammatory disorders. Most disorders of lid structure and function require surgical intervention if localized nerve or muscle malfunction is diagnosed as the causative factor. Inflammatory disorders can affect the glands in the eyelids, the eyelid margins, and the meibomian glands. The skin of the eyelids may also be involved in a variety of inflammations because of the skin's looseness, its exposed position, and the secondary involvement of the eye. Contact dermatitis is common in the eye area because of use of cosmetics and frequent rubbing of the eyes.[34]

▪ ENTROPION

Entropion is an abnormal inward turning of the margin of the eyelid.

•••••• Pathophysiology

The lower lid is most commonly involved. Involution of the lid can be caused by atrophy of the lower lid retractor muscle (atonia), spasms of the orbicularis oculi muscle, or scarring and deformity of the tarsal plate resulting from trauma or chemical or inflammatory assaults. Atonia is relatively common in the elderly and can occur in varying degrees of severity. If the lashes are turned inward, corneal and conjunctival inflammation may occur. Spastic entropion results from chronic or acute irritation

of the horizontal muscle. Corneal inflammation, conjunctivitis, and ocular surgery are common causes of spasm. Congenital entropion occurs with a deformity of the tarsal plate.[34]

•••••• Multidisciplinary Plan

Surgery

Orbicularis procedure—small section of orbicularis oculi muscle is resected to tighten remaining muscle farthest from lid margin, which results in peripheral lid eversion

Tarsal resection—wedge of tarsal plate is removed, which prevents lid margin from rotating inward

Mucosal graft—scarred, atrophied conjunctiva may be replaced with section of mucous membrane from mouth[34]

General Management

For entropion (spasm from irritation), remove irritation (such as eye dressing) to reduce or relieve spasms; stabilize lower lid with pressure patch or tape lower lid to cheek for temporary relief

NURSING CARE

Nursing Assessment

Eyelid and Lashes

Lashes turned inward; possible tear spillage

Cornea and Conjunctiva

Possible conjunctivitis; secondary corneal infection
Possible corneal abrasion or erosion from eyelashes rubbing on cornea

Pain

Impaired vision and depth perception

Psychosocial

Anxiety

Nursing Dx & Intervention[22]

Risk for injury: cornea and conjunctiva, related to entropion spasms or inverted eyelashes

- Assess conjunctiva and cornea for inflammatory signs or signs of abrasion.
- Remove irritation if possible (e.g., by removing eye dressing) *to reduce spasms.*
- Splint or stabilize everted lid by taping to cheek *to maintain normal lid position.*
- Place pressure patch over eye *to stabilize lower lid.*

Anxiety related to fears about vision or surgery

- Assess patient's level of anxiety.
- Listen to patient's concerns *to allay fears about vision or surgery.*

- Provide supportive counseling and explanations about disorder and upcoming surgical procedure.

Sensory/perceptual alterations (visual) related to use of unilateral eye patch

Before surgery
- Warn patient that depth perception will be lost and that 50% of peripheral vision will be lost on affected side.

After surgery
- Help patient with ADL.
- Caution patient to bring hand forward slowly to touch objects (especially containers of hot liquid and containers receiving poured liquids) *to ensure safety.*
- Explain that patient should turn head fully toward affected side to view objects or obstacles.
- Teach patient to use up and down head movements to judge stair dimensions and oncoming objects when walking and to proceed slowly *to avoid injury.*

Sensory/perceptual alterations (visual) related to use of bilateral eye patches

Before surgery
- Warn patient that eyes will be patched *to promote healing.*
- Orient patient to bedside equipment and room arrangement.
- Arrange for placement of personal belongings in advance and review plan with patient.
- Warn patient that side rails will be raised for safety.

After surgery
- Raise side rails *to ensure safety.*
- Address patient by name from doorway and identify yourself *to reduce anxiety.*
- Complement voice stimulation with touch *to notify patient of your proximity.*
- Reorient patient to equipment (such as call light) and personal belongings at bedside by directing patient's hand.
- Encourage patient to perform self-care with personal hygiene *to maximize independence.*
- Ensure patient's privacy, and assure patient that privacy is provided.
- Provide patient with television set or radio *to encourage mental and memory stimulation.*
- Engage patient in discussions about news or other items heard.
- Provide patient with clock that can be felt and remind patient of date *to promote orientation.*
- Discourage napping, which patient may want to do as he or she loses track of time.
- Help patient with meals *to ensure needed caloric intake:*
    Read menu selections.
    Guide hand to utensils and food on tray.
    Describe food on tray in clock terms (e.g, coffee is at 2 o'clock, knife and spoon are at 3 o'clock).
    Help with cutting meats, removing lids from containers, buttering bread, and so on.

- Help with walking *to ensure patient's safety:*
    Walk slowly and slightly ahead of patient; patient's hand should rest on your arm at elbow.
    If possible, allow patient to trace progress by running the dorsal aspect of his or her free hand along a wall.
    Describe surroundings as you proceed.
    Warn of steps, turns, and narrow passageways in advance.
    Allow patient to feel chair, toilet, or bed before turning to sit.

Pain (postoperative) related to eyelid surgery
- Assess patient's level of discomfort.
- Give pain medication as ordered *to keep patient as comfortable as possible.*

Risk for injury to surgically repaired lid related to nausea or vomiting
- Assess patient's feelings of nausea.
- Request order for antiemetic and administer if needed *to prevent vomiting that puts strain on surgically repaired lid.*

Risk for infection related to surgical alteration in skin integrity
- After removal of patch(es), administer antibiotic ointment as ordered *to prevent infection.*

Patient Education/Home Care Planning

1. Ensure that the patient understands the need to avoid rubbing or picking at the eyes.
2. Demonstrate to the patient the application of prescribed ointment to eyes, and watch the patient perform a demonstration.

Evaluation

Cornea and conjunctiva are healthy Cornea is transparent, smooth, glossy, and moist. Palpebral conjunctiva is homogeneous pink color, and bulbar conjunctiva is clear. There is no burning, itching, or evidence of infection.

Patient experiences decreased anxiety Patient is able to discuss the disorder and the treatment and is able to cope with concerns about vision.

Visual alteration is improved Patient is able to perform ADL and return to preoperative level of function.

Surgically repaired eyelid maintains proper position and movement Lid margins are flush against eyeball surface. Eyelids close completely. Lid margins rest over inferior and superior borders of cornea. There is no tear spillage.

Patient is able to care for abnormally positioned lid that is not surgically repaired Patient administers prescribed medications successfully. Patient is able to monitor condition of eye and report conjunctival or corneal irritation in early stage.

Postoperative pain is minimized   Patient experiences no pain in the affected eye.

ECTROPION

Ectropion is an abnormal outward turning of the margin of the eyelid.

•••••• Pathophysiology

Ectropion occurs in two main forms, atonic and cicatricial. Only the lower eyelid is involved in the atonic type, which is the more common. Older adults are frequently subject to the atonic type from the bulbar conjunctiva owing to relaxation of the orbicularis oculi muscle. This condition can occur in all degrees of severity and may cause corneal drying, irritation and conjunctivitis. Paralysis of the orbicularis oculi muscle (CN VII) also results in atonic ectropion. Cicatricial ectropion can affect either the upper or lower eyelid and follows burns, lacerations, and infections of the eyelid skin.

•••••• Multidisciplinary Plan

Surgery

Ectropion repair—wedge of skin, muscle, and tarsal plate removed to tighten lower lid(s)[11]

Skin grafting—replacement of scar tissue that relieves constriction of inferior part of lower lid

General Management

Monitoring of exposed conjunctiva for infection and drying

Lubricating ointment as needed

NURSING CARE

Nursing Assessment

Eyelid

Possible tear spillage

Cornea and Conjunctiva

Corneal drying; conjunctivitis; pain or irritation

Psychosocial

Anxiety

Talk of knowledge about disorder

Embarassment about eyelid deformity

Nursing Dx & Intervention[22]

Risk for injury: cornea and conjunctiva, related to inadequate tear drainage and eyelid malposition

- Assess conjunctiva and cornea for symptoms of dryness.
- Administer artificial tears or lubricating ointment as ordered.
- Be certain that lid is closed when applying dressing.

Body image disturbance related to eyelid deformities

- Assess patient's concerns.
- Encourage family members to be supportive.
- See pp. 1685 to 1687.

Knowledge deficit related to disorder and eye care

- Educate patient about disorder.
- Discuss alternative care plans, rationale, and consequences.

Anxiety related to fears about vision or surgery

- Assess patient's level of anxiety.
- Listen to patient's concerns *to allay fears about vision or surgery.*
- Provide supportive counseling and explanations about disorder and upcoming surgical procedure.

Sensory/perceptual alterations (visual) related to use of unilateral eye patch

Before surgery

- Warn patient that depth perception will be lost and that 50% of peripheral vision will be lost on affected side.

After surgery

- Help patient with ADL.
- Caution patient to bring hand forward slowly to touch objects (especially containers of hot liquid and containers receiving poured liquids) *to ensure safety.*
- Explain that patient should turn head fully toward affected side to view objects or obstacles.
- Teach patient to use up and down head movements to judge stair dimensions and oncoming objects when walking and to proceed slowly *to avoid injury.*

Sensory/perceptual alterations (visual) related to use of bilateral eye patches

Before surgery

- Warn patient that eyes will be patched.
- Orient patient to bedside equipment and room arrangement.
- Arrange for placement of personal belongings in advance and review plan with patient.
- Warn patient that side rails will be raised for safety.

After surgery

- Raise side rails *to ensure safety.*
- Address patient by name from doorway and identify yourself *to reduce anxiety.*
- Complement voice stimulation with touch *to notify patient of your proximity.*
- Reorient patient to equipment (such as call light) and personal belongings at bedside by directing patient's hand.
- Encourage patient to perform self-care with personal hygiene *to maximize independence.*
- Ensure patient's privacy, and assure patient that privacy is provided.

- Provide patient with television set or radio *to encourage mental and memory stimulation and to prevent withdrawal.*
- Engage patient in discussions about news or other items heard.
- Provide patient with clock that can be felt, and remind patient of date.
- Discourage napping, which patient may want to do as he or she loses track of time.
- Help patient with meals *to ensure needed caloric intake:*
  Read menu selections.
  Guide hand to utensils and food on tray.
  Describe food on tray in clock terms (e.g., coffee is at 2 o'clock, knife and spoon are at 3 o'clock).
  Help with cutting meats, removing lids from containers, buttering bread, and so on.
- Help with walking *to ensure patient's safety:*
  Walk slowly and slightly ahead of patient; patient's hand should rest on your arm at elbow.
  If possible, allow patient to trace progress by running the dorsal aspect of his or her free hand along a wall.
  Describe surroundings as you proceed.
  Warn of steps, turns, and narrow passageways in advance.
  Allow patient to feel chair, toilet, or bed before turning to sit.

Pain (postoperative) related to eyelid surgery

- Assess patient's level of discomfort.
- Give pain medication as ordered *to keep patient as comfortable as possible.*

Risk for injury to surgically repaired lid related to nausea or vomiting

- Assess patient's feelings of nausea.
- Request order for antiemetic and administer if needed *to prevent vomiting, which puts a strain on the surgically repaired lid.*

Risk for infection related to surgical alteration in skin integrity

- After removal of patch(es), administer antibiotic ointment as ordered to prevent infection.

Patient Education/Home Care Planning

1. Ensure that the patient understands the need to avoid rubbing or picking at the eyes.
2. Demonstrate to the patient the application of prescribed ointment to the eye(s), and watch a demonstration.

Evaluation

Cornea and conjunctiva are healthy Cornea is transparent, smooth, glossy, and moist. Palpebral conjunctiva is homogeneous pink color, and bulbar conjunctiva is clear. There is no burning or itching or evidence of infection.

Patient experiences decreased anxiety Patient is able to discuss disorder and treatment and is able to cope with concerns about eyelid deformity.

Postoperative pain is minimized Patient experiences decreased pain and irritation in the affected eye.

Surgically repaired eyelid maintains proper position and movement Lid margins are flush against eyeball surface. Eyelids close completely. Lid margins rest over inferior and superior borders of cornea. There is no tear spillage.

Patient is able to care for abnormally positioned lid that is not surgically repaired Patient administers prescribed medications successfully. Patient is able to monitor condition of eye and report conjunctival or corneal irritation in early stage.[11]

Visual alteration is improved Patient is able to perform ADL and returns to preoperative level of function.

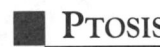

PTOSIS

Ptosis is a drooping of the upper eyelid.

•••••• Pathophysiology

Ptosis can be bilateral or unilateral, constant or intermittent, and congenital or acquired. Congenital deformity usually involves malfunction of the levator muscle and is often accompanied by limited eye movement associated with superior rectus muscle failure. Acquired ptosis is mechanical, neurogenic, or myogenic in origin. Mechanical factors usually stem from abnormal weight of the eyelid imposed by such conditions as chronic edema, tumor, or excess tissue. Malfunction of the oculomotor (CN III) interferes with lid elevation, eye movement, and pupillary constriction. Carotid aneurysms and diabetic neuropathy are common causes of CN III degeneration. Interruption of the sympathetic innervation of the smooth muscle that maintains lid tone and dilates the pupil causes ptosis. Horner's syndrome (a miotic pupil and drooping lid) occurs with sympathetic pathway lesions such as goiter, cervical lymph node enlargement, or apical bronchogenic carcinoma.[34] Unilateral ptosis is frequently the first sign of myasthenia gravis, which is characterized by fatigability of striated muscles. Bilateral involvement with progressive diminished eye movement may ensue. Aging eyes lose muscle tone of the lid elevator and the smooth muscle within the lid, and a general mild lid sag may occur.[34]

•••••• Multidisciplinary Plan

Surgery

Resection of levator palpebrae superioris muscle—if functioning, muscle is reattached to tarsus at shorter length to increase muscle strength and lid-raising capacity

Upper eyelid suspension—when levator muscle is not functioning, supportive band of material is threaded within lid and attached to frontalis muscle to provide sling effect; lid movement is not affected, but cosmetic effect is improved[34]

General Management

Glasses with "crutch" can be worn to suspend inoperable lid
Treatment of systemic disorders (such as treatment of myasthenia gravis or removal of sympathetic pathway lesion) may relieve lid drooping[34]

NURSING CARE

Nursing Assessment

If both lids are involved, head may be thrown back and forehead constantly furrowed as frontalis muscle is flexed to suspend eyelids upward.

Nursing Dx & Intervention[22]

Body image disturbance related to eyelid deformities

- Assess patient's concerns.
- Encourage family members to be supportive.
- See pp. 1685 to 1687.

Pain (postoperative) related to eyelid surgery

- Assess patient's level of discomfort.
- Give pain medication as ordered *to promote comfort.*
- Apply ice compresses as ordered *to decrease swelling.*

Risk for infection related to surgical alteration in skin integrity

- Administer antibiotic ointment *to prevent infection.*

Patient Education/Home Care Planning

1. Explain to the patient about disorder.
2. Discuss alternative care plans, rationale, and consequences with patient and family.
3. Ensure that patient or family can administer antibiotic ointment if ordered and can verbalize signs and symptoms of infection.

Evaluation

Cornea and conjunctiva are healthy Cornea is transparent, smooth, glossy, and moist. Palpebral conjunctiva is homogeneous pink color, and bulbar conjunctiva is clear. There is no burning or itching or evidence of infection.
Body image is intact Patient experiences decreased concern about eyelid deformities.
Pain is minimized Patient experiences no pain.
Surgically repaired eyelid maintains proper position and movement Lid margins are flush against eyeball surface. Eyelids close completely. Lid margins rest over inferior and superior borders of cornea. There is no tear spillage.

Patient is able to care for abnormally positioned lid that is not surgically repaired Patient administers prescribed medications successfully. Patient is able to monitor condition of eye and report conjunctival or corneal irritation in early stage.[42]

LAGOPHTHALMOS

Lagophthalmos is inadequate closure of the eyelids.

Lagophthalmos may result from facial nerve (CN VII) weakness or enlargement or protrusion of the eyeball.[34]

•••••• Multidisciplinary Plan

Surgery

Immediate surgical closure of lids may be necessary to prevent corneal drying and trauma; upper and lower eyelid adhesions can be temporarily or permanently created

General Management

When only small portion of central cornea is exposed:
Lubricating ointment instilled at bedtime for protection during sleep
Soft contact lens worn or artificial tears administered several times a day
Sustained-release tear insert in each eye once a day[34]

NURSING CARE

Nursing Assessment

Cornea

Corneal drying; secondary keratitis; pain or irritation

Psychosocial

Anxiety
Body image concerns

Nursing Dx & Intervention[22]

Risk for injury: cornea and conjunctiva, related to inadequate tear dispersion

- Assess eye for symptoms of dryness.
- Administer artificial tears, sustained-release tear insert, or lubricating ointment as ordered.
- Be certain lid is closed when applying dressing *to prevent injury to cornea and conjunctiva.*

Body image disturbance related to eyelid deformities

- Assess patient's concerns.
- Encourage family members to be supportive.
- See pp. 1685 to 1687.

Knowledge deficit related to disorder and eye care

- Educate patient about disorder.
- Discuss alternative care plans, rationale, and consequences.

Anxiety related to fears about vision and surgery

- Assess patient's level of anxiety.
- Listen to patient's concerns *to allay fears about vision or surgery.*
- Provide supportive counseling and explanation about disorder and upcoming surgical procedure.

Sensory/perceptual alterations (visual) related to use of unilateral eye patch

Before surgery

- Warn patient that depth perception will be lost and 50% of peripheral vision will be lost on affected side.

After surgery

- Help patient with ADL.
- Caution patient to bring hand forward slowly to touch objects (especially containers of hot liquid and containers receiving poured liquids) *to ensure safety.*
- Teach patient to turn head fully toward affected side to view objects or obstacles.
- Tell patient to use up and down head movements to judge stair dimensions and oncoming objects when walking and to proceed slowly *to avoid injury.*

Sensory/perceptual alterations (visual) related to use of bilateral eye patches

Before surgery

- Warn patient that eyes will be patched.
- Orient patient to bedside equipment and room arrangement.
- Arrange for placement of personal belongings in advance and review plan with patient.
- Warn patient that side rails will be raised for safety.

After surgery

- Raise side rails.
- Address patient by name from doorway and identify yourself *to reduce anxiety.*
- Complement voice stimulation with touch *to notify patient of your proximity.*
- Reorient patient to equipment (such as call light) and personal belongings at bedside by directing patient's hand.
- Encourage patient to perform self-care with personal hygiene *to maximize independence.*
- Ensure patient's privacy, and assure patient that privacy is provided.
- Provide patient with television set or radio *to encourage mental and memory stimulation and to prevent withdrawal.*
- Engage patient in discussions about new or other items heard.
- Provide patient with clock that can be felt and remind patient of date *to promote orientation.*
- Discourage napping, which patient may want to do as he or she loses track of time.
- Help patient with meals *to ensure needed caloric intake:*
  Read menu selections.
  Guide hand to utensils and food on tray.
  Describe food on tray in clock terms (e.g., coffee is at 2 o'clock, knife and spoon are at 3 o'clock).
  Help with cutting meats, removing lids from containers, buttering bread, and so on.
- Help with walking *to ensure patient's safety:*
  Walk slowly and slightly ahead of patient; patient's hand should rest on your arm at elbow.
  If possible, allow patient to trace progress by running the dorsal aspect of his or her free hand along a wall.
  Describe surroundings as you proceed.
  Warn of steps, turns, and narrow passageways in advance.
  Allow patient to feel chair, toilet, or bed before turning to sit.

Pain (postoperative) related to eyelid surgery

- Assess level of discomfort.
- Give pain medication as ordered *to keep patient as comfortable as possible.*

Risk for injury to surgically repaired lid related to nausea or vomiting

- Assess patient's feelings of nausea.
- Request order for antiemetic and administer if needed *to prevent vomiting that puts strain on surgically repaired lid.*

Risk for infection related to surgical alteration in skin integrity

- After removal of patch(es), administer antibiotic ointment as ordered *to prevent infection.*

Patient Education/Home Care Planning

1. Ensure that the patient can administer eye drops, lubricant, or tear insert if ordered; discuss with the patient the need to wash hands before and after the procedure.
2. Caution the patient to avoid rubbing or picking at the eyes.
3. Encourage the patient to avoid noxious odors or fumes such as cigarette smoke.
4. Suggest that the patient use a humidifier in the home if the atmosphere is dry.
5. Show the patient how to monitor the eye for signs and symptoms of dryness or irritation.

Evaluation

Cornea and conjunctiva are healthy Cornea is transparent, smooth, glossy, and moist. Palpebral conjunctiva is homogeneous pink color, and bulbar conjunctiva is clear. There is no burning, itching, or evidence of infection.

Patient experiences decreased anxiety Patient is able to discuss the disorder and the treatment and is able to cope with concerns about eyelid deformity.

Surgically repaired eyelid maintains proper position and movement Lid margins are flush against eyeball surface. Eyelids close completely. Lid margins rest over inferior and superior borders of cornea. There is no tear spillage.

Patient is able to care for abnormally positioned lid that is not surgically repaired Patient administers prescribed medications successfully. Patient is able to monitor condition of eye and report conjunctival or corneal irritation in early stage.

Postoperative pain is minimized Patient experiences decreased pain and irritation in the affected eye.

Visual alteration is improved Patient can perform ADL and returns to preoperative level of functioning.

■ BLINKING DISORDERS

Blinking disorders may occur as excessive blinking or a diminished rate of blinking.

······ Pathophysiology

Blinking is both a voluntary and an involuntary action. The rate of involuntary blinking varies among individuals, but blinking occurs frequently enough to spread tears over the surface of the eye. Reflex blinking increases in response to conjunctival or corneal irritation or pain in the eye. Chronic irritation may result in a continuous clonic response that is sustained until the stimulus is removed. Rapid blinking also accompanies anxiety and may become a prolonged pattern with chronic stress. Spasms of the orbicularis oculi muscle (blepharospasm) sometimes occur in elderly people. These spasms are involuntary, tonic, spasmodic, usually bilateral contractions. They range from an annoying tic to a dangerous level during which the person cannot see. They are also unattractive. Causes include irritation of the eyes, facial nerve lesions, fatigue, and anxiety. Absence or diminution of blinking may accompany parkinsonism or hyperthyroidism.

······ Multidisciplinary Plan

Blinking disorders may be relieved when the cause (systemic origin, anxiety, or local irritation) is treated or removed. When a systemic origin cannot be determined, rapid bilateral blinking is labeled as essential blepharospasm. In many cases, botulinum toxin is injected, in minute doses, every few months, to paralyze the obicularis oculi muscle and decrease the frequency and intensity of the spasms.[11,35]

NURSING CARE

Nursing Assessment

Blinking Disorder

Rapid bilateral blinking
    Multiple anxiety behaviors
Tics
    Anxiety; statements of stress

Cornea and Conjunctiva

Diminished blinking
    Conjunctival drying and irritation or corneal drying; keratitis

Psychosocial

Anxiety

Nursing Dx & Intervention[22]

Risk for injury: cornea and conjunctiva, related to inadequate tear dispersion

- Assess eye for symptoms of dryness.
- Administer artificial tears, sustained-release tear insert, or lubricating ointment as ordered *to improve lubrication.*
- Be certain lid is closed when applying dressing *to prevent injury to cornea.*

Knowledge deficit related to disorder and eye care

- Educate patient about disorder.
- Discuss alternative care plans, rationale, and consequences.

Anxiety related to fear about disorder

- Assess patient's level of anxiety and stressors.
- Listen to patient's concerns.
- Provide supportive counseling.

Patient Education/Home Care Planning

1. Ensure that the patient can administer eye drops, lubricant, or tear insert if ordered; discuss with the patient the need to wash hands before and after the procedure.
2. Caution the patient not to rub or pick at the eyes.
3. Encourage the patient to avoid noxious odors or fumes such as cigarette smoke.
4. Suggest that the patient use a humidifier in the home if the atmosphere is dry.
5. Show the patient how to monitor the eye for signs and symptoms of dryness or irritation.

Evaluation

Cornea and conjunctiva are healthy   Cornea is transparent, smooth, glossy, and moist. Palpebral conjunctiva is homogeneous pink color, and bulbar conjunctiva is clear. There is no burning, itching, or evidence of infection.

Lid movement is normal   Open and closure movement of lid is not excessive. Vision is not obscured. Source of nervous mannerisms or local irritant has been removed.

Anxiety is decreased   Patient is able to discuss and cope with the disorder.

BLEPHARITIS

Blepharitis is an inflammation of the eyelid margins.

•••••• Pathophysiology

Blepharitis is a chronic condition that can be caused by organisms (chiefly *Staphylococcus*), associated with seborrheic dermatitis, or aggravated by allergies. Often the causative factors are inseparable. Other conditions commonly associated with chronic blepharitis are diabetes, gout, anemia, and rosacea.[34] Infections of the nose and mouth can be transferred to the eyes and lids by frequent eye rubbing. Staphylococcal lesions usually ulcerate and often involve the conjunctiva and meibomian glands. Chalazions and hordeola (styes) may develop and recur. Seborrheic blepharitis is frequently accompanied by dermatitis of the scalp, eyebrows, and external ears. Some people first have this chronic condition in childhood and continue to have intermittent exacerbations throughout life.

•••••• Multidisciplinary Plan

Medications[28,34,44]

Antiinfective agents
  Ointment applied locally qd or bid, usually at bedtime if infection is present
    Sulfacetamide sodium (Sulamyd, others), 10%-30% solution or 10% ointment
    Bacitracin (Baciguent), 500 U/1 g ointment
    Neomycin sulfate (Myciguent), 0.5% ointment
  Systemic medication
    Tetracycline (Achromycin), 250 mg bid
  Selenium sulfide shampoo and soak for brows, eyelids[11]

General Management

Eyelid hygiene
  Drape warm washcloth over both eyes for 10 minutes; warm the cloth every 2 minutes
  Wash the face with warm soap and water
  Mix one part "no-tears" baby shampoo with two parts water in a clean container
  Wrap your finger in a washcloth
  Rub the eyelids (along the lashes) with a wet, warm washcloth dipped in the baby shampoo and water mixture
  Rinse face with warm water and dry
  Do above 3 to 4 times a day for 4 to 6 weeks; thereafter only once daily

NURSING CARE

Nursing Assessment

Eyelids and Lashes

Red lid margins; flaking and scaling around lashes; localized discomfort; loss of lashes; ingrown lashes; thickening and eversion of lid margins; tear spillage; in ulcerative staphylococcal blepharitis, pus, multiple lesions and crusting at lid margins, development of ulcers, lids glued shut by dried drainage

Cornea and Conjunctiva

Light sensitivity; possible chronic conjunctivitis; possible corneal inflammation[34]

Nursing Dx & Intervention[22]

Impaired skin integrity; high risk for impaired skin integrity related to lesions or ulcerations

- Assess lids and conjunctivae for crusting or inflammation.
- Perform eyelid hygiene as appropriate *to minimize skin injury.*

Risk for infection related to organism transfer from nose or mouth

- Assess patient's self-care and hygiene habits (e.g., hand washing, avoidance of rubbing eyes).
- Instruct patient in self-care *to prevent reinfection.*
- Demonstrate and instruct patient in self-administration of ointment *to prevent injury and contamination.*

Patient Education/Home Care Planning

1. Ensure that the patient can perform eyelid hygiene regimen, and apply antibiotic ointment if ordered.
2. Discuss with the patient hygiene practices related to self-care of the eye, such as washing hands before and after self-care and avoiding fumes and smoke.
3. If the patient uses eye makeup, encourage the patient to avoid use during the acute phase of lid infection because makeup is a common allergen and also may become contaminated with the causative organisms.

Evaluation

Eyelids are normal   Lid margins are smooth and without scaling.

Conjunctiva is normal   Palpebral conjunctiva is homogeneous pink color, and bulbar conjunctiva is clear. There is no excessive tearing or evidence of infection.

CHALAZION

Chalazion is a granulomatous inflammation of a meibomian gland.

Pathophysiology

A chalazion forms on the conjunctival aspect of the upper or lower eyelid as glands in both are affected. It begins as a nontender swelling and may take several weeks to develop. It does not appear inflamed unless a secondary infection occurs. If large enough, the nodule can compress the eyeball and cause an astigmatism, resulting in blurred vision. A large nodule also produces discomfort as the upper lid closes, causing pressure on the cornea. Some chalazia disappear in a few months without ever causing symptoms. Chronic chalazia tend to subside partially and reactivate periodically.[34,44]

Multidisciplinary Plan

Medical Treatment

Hot-packing chalazia several times daily often causes them to open and drain; however, unless antibiotic eyedrops are prescribed to destroy the bacteria, they recur chronically

Surgery

Localized excision of chronic chalazion with patient under local anesthesia; antibiotic eye drops administered three or four times a day before and after surgery

Medications

Antiinfective agents
Ointment applied locally 4 times/d postoperatively
Sulfacetamide sodium (Sulamyd, others), 10%-30% solution or 10% ointment
Bacitracin (Baciguent), 500 U/1 g ointment
Neomycin sulfate (Myciguent), 0.5% ointment

NURSING CARE

Nursing Assessment

Eyelids

Small, nontender, noninflamed lump on outer lid; lid eversion reveals nodule that points toward conjunctiva; secondary infection produces redness, pain, and suppuration; sensitivity to light

Nursing Dx & Intervention

Risk for infection related to surgical alteration in skin integrity or secondary contamination

- Assess entire lid for inflammatory signs *to evaluate for presence of infection.*
- Apply warm compresses with clean cloth for 10 to 20 minutes two to three times a day after excision of chalazion *to expedite healing.*

Patient Education/Home Care Planning

1. Discuss with the patient hygiene practices related to self-care of the eye, such as washing hands before and after self-care and avoiding fumes and smoke.
2. If the patient uses eye makeup, encourage the patient to avoid use during the acute phase of lid infection because makeup is a common allergen and also may become contaminated with the causative organism.
3. Demonstrate to the patient how to administer ointment.
4. Demonstrate to the patient how to apply warm compresses to eyes.

Evaluation

Eyelids are normal   Lid margins are smooth, without lesions. There is no evidence of infection.

Conjunctiva is normal   Palpebral conjunctiva is homogeneous pink color, and bulbar conjunctiva is clear. There is no excessive tearing.

HORDEOLUM

A hordeolum (sty) is an acute infection of an eyelash follicle or the glands of Moll or Zeis (sebaceous glands).

Pathophysiology

The offending organism is usually *Staphylococcus.* The lesion becomes a pustule that eventually points and may rupture. Multiple pustules may occur along adjacent lash follicles because of reinfection.[34,44]

Multidisciplinary Plan

Medications

Antiinfective agents (ointment applied locally 2-4 times/d)
Sulfacetamide sodium (Sulamyd, others), 10%-30% solution or 10% ointment
Bacitracin (Baciguent), 500 U/1 g ointment
Neomycin sulfate (Myciguent), 0.5% ointment

General Management

Warm compresses with clean cloth for 10 to 20 minutes two or three times a day
Local incision of pustule if rupture is not spontaneous

NURSING CARE

Nursing Assessment

Eyelids

Initial tenderness with localized redness and swelling that forms pustule at lid margin; may be multiple pustules; generalized lid edema; pain that increases as pustule enlarges and ceases with rupture

Nursing Dx & Intervention

Risk for infection related to secondary contamination

- Assess patient's hygiene practices (e.g., handwashing before touching the eye) *to prevent spread of infection.*
- Assess the patient for *Staphylococcus* infections or lesions elsewhere on the body *to monitor potential for or presence of systemic staphylococcal infection.*

Impaired skin integrity; high risk for impaired skin integrity related to presence of pustule

- Apply warm compresses with clean cloth for 10 to 20 minutes two or three times a day *to expedite healing.*

Patient Education/Home Care Planning

1. Demonstrate to the patient the application of warm compresses and antibiotic ointment if ordered.
2. Discuss with the patient hygiene practices related to self-care of the eye, such as washing hands before and after self-care and avoiding fumes and smoke.
3. If the patient uses eye makeup, encourage the patient to avoid use during the acute phase of lid infection because makeup is a common allergen and also may become contaminated with the causative organism.

Evaluation

Eyelids are normal Lid margins are smooth, without lesions. There is no evidence of infection.

Conjunctiva is normal Palpebral conjunctiva is homogeneous pink color, and bulbar conjunctiva is clear. There is no excessive tearing.

LACRIMAL APPARATUS DISORDERS

Patients with lacrimal disorders usually complain of "dry eyes," excessive tearing, or pain and swelling of the lacrimal duct. Inadequate tearing can result in drying and severe damage to the cornea. Excessive tearing can be caused by overproduction of tears by the lacrimal gland or a faulty drainage system that results in tear spillage. Tear accumulation can interfere with vision and irritate the eyeball. Inflammation of the lacrimal sac and adjacent canaliculi can be associated with conjunctivitis, nasal disease, or drainage obstruction.

■ DRY EYE SYNDROME

Dry eye syndrome is a condition in which tear production is inadequate. The signs and symptoms may occur in any age group; however, they are most common in women 50 to 60 years old.

•••••• Pathophysiology[34,44]

Dry eye syndrome occurs for three primary reasons: lacrimal gland malfunction, mucin deficiency, and mechanical abnormalities that interfere with the spread or maintenance of tears over the eyeball surface. Lacrimal gland malfunctions can be congenital or acquired. The most common congenital disorders are lacrimal gland aplasia, ectodermal dysplasia, and trigeminal nerve (CN V) malfunction, which disrupts sensory stimulation to the upper lid. Acquired disorders that affect lacrimal gland function can be systemic, infectious, or related to trauma. Common systemic disorders that may be associated with diminished tear production are rheumatoid arthritis (Sjögren's syndrome), leukemia, lymphoma, sarcoidosis, and systemic sclerosis. Facial nerve (CN VII) palsy inhibits tearing. Mumps and some forms of conjunctivitis may obstruct tear flow. Chemical burns and irradiation may reduce lacrimal gland function. Some medications such as antihistamines, atropine, and β-adrenergic blockers decrease tear production. Even if the lacrimal gland is not functioning, accessory glands in the palpebral conjunctiva may secrete sufficient tears to prevent severe corneal damage.

A layer of mucin, produced by goblet cells in the lid, maintains a homogeneous tear spread over the eyeball surface. The absence of mucin causes the tear film to break up, leaving "dry holes" over the cornea. Mucin deficiency is commonly associated with some forms of chronic conjunctivitis, vitamin A deficiency, and medications such as antihistamines and β-adrenergic blockers.

Mechanical defects that contribute to dry eyes include abnormalities of eyelid structure and function, protrusion of the eyeball (proptosis), and use or misuse of contact lenses.[34,44]

The symptom most commonly associated with inadequate tearing is keratoconjunctivitis sicca (KCS). The person experiences burning, itching, and a foreign body sensation in the eyes. The cornea and conjunctiva may show inflammation, erosion, or keratinization. Untreated or severe KCS can result in blindness.

•••••• Diagnostic Studies and Findings[34,44]

Rose Bengal staining Drop of 1% or 2% solution placed in conjunctival sac; 2% solution demonstrates loss of corneal and conjunctiva epithelium in keratoconjunctivitis sicca; 1% solution valuable in demonstrating conjunctival and corneal epithelial cell loss and degeneration; patients with deficiency of aqueous portion of tears have punctate staining of lower two thirds of cornea and bright red staining of bulbar conjunctiva in area corresponding to palpable aperture.

Schirmer's test Strip of filter paper, 3.5×0.05 cm, placed in temporal aspect of conjunctival cul-de-sac of lower lid for 5 minutes; 10 to 15 mm length of paper wetted with tears considered normal; more than 25 mm moistened paper indicates excessive tearing.

Basic secretion test Topical anesthetic administered to eyeball before filter paper inserted; anesthesia reduces lacrimal output to allow measurement of tear production of accessory glands in eyelid

•••••• Multidisciplinary Plan[11,34]

A correlation does not always exist between the failure of tear production and inflammatory or degenerative changes on the surface of the eye. The mechanisms that connect tear and mucin production to ocular surface maintenance are not fully understood. Depending on the cause and severity of the condition, the examiner may select from or combine the following therapeutic approaches.

Restoration or stimulation of tears
  Estrogen replacement therapy has been associated with relief of dry eye symptoms in some postmenopausal women[9,44]
  Elimination of systemic medications that have created the problem
  Treatment and resolution of eyelid or conjunctival inflammation
  Alteration in contact lens prescription or patient's self-care methods
Preservation of existing tears
  Surgically induced punctal occlusion
  Eyelid repair (ectropion) or lid closure repair
  Wearing of airtight goggles to prevent tear evaporation
Tear replacement
Maintenance and treatment of ocular surface
  Antibiotic ointments
  Lubricating ointments
  Some studies have reported success with the use of topical vitamin A preparations in the maintenance of healthy conjunctival tissue[11]

Surgery

Occlusion of puncta to conserve tears
Surgical repair of lid position or movement abnormalities

Medications

Antiinfective agents
  Ointment applied locally for existing inflammation
  Polysporin Ophth. Oint. (Polymixin, 10,000 U; Bacitracin, 500 U), 2-4 times/d
Tear substitute
  Adsorbobase hydroxylethyl Cellulose Thimeros 1 0.002% edetate disodium 0.05% (Tears Naturale), 1-2 drops tid prn
  Duasab Polymeric system with Dextran, benzalkonium chloride 0.01% edetate disodium 0.05% (Tears Naturale), 1-2 drops prn
Ointment to lubricate and protect the eyes
  White petroleum and mineral oil (Duolube, Akwa Tears), instill in conjunctival sac prn

General Management

Humidifier in environment
Airtight goggles or eye shield

NURSING CARE

Nursing Assessment

Dry Eyes

Burning; itching; foreign body sensation; sensitivity to light; blurred vision; lack of tears; loss of glossy appearance of cornea; tear film interspersed with mucus strands

Nursing Dx & Intervention[11,22,34]

Risk for injury: cornea and conjunctiva, related to lack of tears

- Assess eye for signs and symptoms of irritation (itching, burning, and loss of glossy appearance of eyeball surface).
- Administer artificial tears, sustained-release tear insert, or lubricating ointments as ordered *to prevent tissue damage to ocular surface.*

Sensory/perceptual alterations (visual) related to decreased vision or to lid closure

- Raise side rails.
- Address patient by name from doorway and identify yourself.
- Complement voice stimulation with touch *to notify patient of your proximity.*
- Orient patient to bedside equipment (such as call light, bed control, and side rails) and personal belongings at bedside by directing patient's hand over objects.
- Encourage patient to perform self-care with personal hygiene *to maximize independence.*
- Provide support and supervision with ADL.
- Provide patient privacy, and assure patient that privacy is provided.
- Help with meals. (Patients may become so frustrated at mealtime that they may not eat without this assistance.)
  Read menu selections.
  Guide hand to utensils and food on tray.
  Describe food on tray in clock terms.
  Teach patient to "trail," that is, to use dorsal aspect of index and middle fingers to find objects on food tray.
  Fill glasses only half full because patient may spill easily.
  Help patient with cutting meat, removing lids from cartons, buttering bread, and so on.
- Help with walking *to ensure patient safety.*
  Walk slowly and slightly ahead of patient.
  Patient's hand should rest on your arm at your elbow.
  If possible, allow patient to trace progress by running the dorsal aspect of his or her free hand along a wall.

Describe surroundings as you proceed.

Allow patient to feel chair, toilet, or bed before turning to sit.

Pain related to localized inflammation

- Assess patient's degree of discomfort.
- Provide analgesics as ordered *to promote patient's comfort.*

Patient Education/Home Care Planning

1. Demonstrate to the patient how to administer eye drops, lubricant, or a tear insert; stress the importance of washing hands before and after the procedure.
2. Ensure that the patient knows to avoid rubbing or picking at the eyes.
3. Encourage the patient to avoid noxious odors or fumes and to use a humidifier in the home if the atmosphere is dry.
4. Demonstrate to the patient how to monitor the eye for signs and symptoms of dryness or irritation.

Evaluation

Cornea and conjunctiva are healthy Cornea is transparent, smooth, glossy, and moist. Palpebral conjunctiva is homogeneous pink color, and bulbar conjunctiva is clear. There is no burning, itching, or evidence of infection.

Visual alteration is improved Patient experiences no sensitivity to light; blurred vision improves.

■ EXCESSIVE TEARS

Excessive tears can occur from overproduction or inadequate drainage of tears.

•••••• Pathophysiology[34,44]

Tear spillage most commonly occurs because the drainage system is faulty (epiphora). The puncta can be occluded because of congenital absence of an opening or because of infection in the lacrimal sac. Lid abnormalities, such as ectropion, cause abnormal alignment of the lacrimal tear pool and the puncta. An accumulation of tears in the inner canthus is an irritant that stimulates more tear production. Obstructions may also occur in the lacrimal duct or the meatus in the nasal cavity.

Lacrimation (excessive tear production) occurs most commonly with reflex stimulation of the lacrimal gland. Corneal injury, eye pain, noxious odors, eyestrain, bright light, and allergies are examples of sensory stimuli affecting the trigeminal nerve (CN V). Glaucoma often stimulates tear production because of trigeminal irritation. Facial nerve (CN VII) irritation during vomiting or laughter also stimulates tear production. Abnormal regeneration of the facial nerve following Bell's palsy causes "crocodile tears," a phenomenon of excess tearing that occurs during eating. Parasympathetic stimulants (cholinergic drugs) and some endocrine disorders (such as hyperthyroidism) can also increase tearing.

•••••• Diagnostic Studies and Findings

Dye disappearance Cul-de-sac of lower lid flooded with 2% fluorescein solution; fluorescein normally disappears from cul-de-sac in 1 minute

Computed tomography Computed tomography (CT), with or without contrast, shows normal vs. abnormal lacrimal passages

•••••• Multidisciplinary Plan

Surgery

Repair of lid structure abnormalities to enhance punctal access to tear pool

Probing of obstructed punctum

Construction of tube connecting conjunctival cul-de-sac to nasal cavity

Dacryocystorhinostomy (DCR): creation of a new pathway for tear drainage, bypassing the nasolacrimal duct by making an opening in the nasal bone

General Management

Related to removal of cause of lacrimation

NURSING CARE

Nursing Assessment

Eyes

Tear spillage; blurred vision; puncta red and swollen; puncta may exude purulent material on mild compression over lacrimal sac; conjunctivitis (reddened conjunctiva)

Nursing Dx & Intervention

Risk for infection related to secondary contamination

- Assess eye for amount of lacrimation or increased symptoms of irritation or infection.
- Encourage patient to maintain hygiene *to prevent infection.*

Patient Education/Home Care Planning

1. Discuss with the patient hygiene practices related to self-care of the eyes, such as washing hands before and after self-care and keeping hands away from the eyes.

Evaluation

Lacrimal drainage system is patent   There is no excess tearing. Inner canthus of eye is homogeneous pink color. When eye is compressed at medial infraorbital rim, punctum does not exude any material.

Underlying endocrine cause, if any, is corrected   Amount of tears produced is not excessive.

■ DACRYOCYSTITIS

■ Dacryocystitis is an inflammation of the lacrimal sac.

•••••• Pathophysiology

Dacryocystitis can be acute or chronic and is caused by block-age of tear drainage from the punctum or lacrimal sac.

Normal newborns often do not have patent nasolacrimal ducts. The duct usually opens about the third week of life. If the duct fails to open, tearing occurs and eventually puru-lent material exudes from the punctum. The condition often corrects itself by 3 to 6 months of age. Lacrimal probing may be performed if spontaneous patency does not occur. Surgical construction of a duct is rarely needed, but if nec-essary it is performed when the child reaches 3 or 4 years of age.[44]

Chronic dacryocystitis most often occurs in middle-aged adults. Spontaneous punctum obstruction is followed by bacte-rial infection with a mucopurulent discharge. The nasolacrimal duct can also be obstructed by injury or nasal lesions, causing an inflammatory response.

Acute dacryocystitis has a rapid onset, with marked swelling and tenderness of surrounding tissue.[44]

•••••• Multidisciplinary Plan[34,44]

Surgery

Incision and drainage of abscess
Dacryocystorhinostomy for construction of passage between lacrimal sac and nasal cavity

Medications

Antiinfective agents
Systemic antibiotics for acute, severe infection
Instillation of antibiotic or sulfonamide eye drops 4-5 times/d until infection subsides

General Management

Daily massage of lacrimal sac to rid it of purulent material (often assists spontaneous opening of the nasolacrimal duct system in newborns)
Warm compresses over affected eye during acute phase
Lacrimal probing with graduated sizes of probe while patient is under local anesthesia

Nursing Assessment

Lacrimal Inflammation

Tear spillage; purulent material exuding from punctum on compression; punctum swollen, and surrounding tissue may be reddened; localized pain

Nursing Dx & Intervention

Risk for infection related to obstruction of tear drainage

- Assess punctum and surrounding tissue for inflammation.
- Apply warm compresses over affected eye for 10 or 20 minutes three or four times a day.
- Lightly massage lacrimal sac at medial infraorbital rim *to rid sac of accumulated purulent material.*
- Administer antibiotic or sulfonamide eye drops or oint-ment as ordered.
- Wash hands thoroughly before and after care of affected eye *to prevent spread of infection.*

Patient Education/Home Care Planning

1. Discuss with the patient hygiene practices related to self-care of the eyes, such as washing hands before and after self-care and keeping hands away from the eyes.

Evaluation

Cornea and conjunctiva are healthy   Cornea is trans-parent, smooth, glossy, and moist. Palpebral conjunctiva is ho-mogeneous pink color. Bulbar conjunctiva is clear. There is no burning, itching, or evidence of infection.

Lacrimal drainage system is patent   There is no excess tearing. Inner canthus of eye is homogeneous pink color. Punc-tum does not exude any material when eye is compressed at medial infraorbital rim.

CONJUNCTIVAL DISORDERS

The bulbar conjunctiva is a protective coating for the scleral portion of the eyeball. It can be affected by many injuries or in-fections from the environment. It adjoins the palpebral con-junctiva in the lid cul-de-sac and is susceptible to infection be-cause it is close to the eyelid. The conjunctiva also responds to internal infections or diseases such as measles, diabetes melli-tus, or riboflavin deficiency. This outer layer contains blood vessels that dilate rapidly and pain receptors that register mild to moderate discomfort in response to inflammation. The conjunctiva is adjacent to the cornea and can be an avenue for spreading infection to this vital area.

■ CONJUNCTIVITIS

■ Conjunctivitis is an inflammation or infection of the conjunctiva.

Conjunctival tissue can become inflamed by dust, smog, tobacco smoke, noxious fumes, wind, sun, and airborne allergens. Conjunctivitis is common and easily spread, particularly in crowded environments such as schools and nursing homes.

•••••• Pathophysiology[34,44]

Conjunctivitis varies in severity. Vascular dilation and engorgement can be a response to external irritants such as smog, hair sprays, or noxious fumes. The person may experience lacrimation and a foreign body sensation, but no discharge or progressive infectious process appears. Generalized hyperemia and burning are initial responses to insufficient tearing, and a secondary infection can follow rapidly. Allergic responses may be seasonal and include vascular injection, moderate tearing, and severe itching.

Viral conjunctivitis is characterized by generalized hyperemia, profuse tearing, and little exudate. Preauricular nodes are commonly associated with viral infections. Some adenoviruses invade the upper respiratory or gastrointestinal systems, causing fever and acute systemic signs along with the conjunctivitis. Viral infections may be mild and self-limited or may quickly invade the cornea and surrounding tissue and cause severe ocular surface and periorbital pain. Type 1 herpes simplex conjunctivitis has been diagnosed more often in recent years with fluorescent antibody staining of corneal scrapings. Herpes conjunctivitis often invades the cornea with inflammation, erosion, and ulceration. Usually only one eye is involved initially, but both may be affected eventually. Recurrent eye lesions that may cause scarring and diminished vision can be brought on by stress, immunosuppression, menstruation, fever, or exposure to ultraviolet light.

Bacterial conjunctivitis, the most common type, is frequently called pinkeye. Almost any bacterium can be involved, but *Pneumococcus, Staphylococcus,* and *Streptococcus* organisms are common. The infection usually begins in one eye and is transferred to the other eye through contamination. The onset is acute, with a mucopurulent exudate, tearing, generalized hyperemia, and moderate discomfort. This form of conjunctivitis is highly contagious.

Some organisms rapidly invade the cornea and the conjunctiva and lead to corneal ulceration and perforation. Two of the most virulent organisms are *Neisseria gonorrhoeae* and *Chlamydia trachomatis*. Ophthalmia neonatorum, a conjunctivitis that occurs in newborns, is commonly transmitted from the mother with acute gonorrheal urethritis during birth. Ophthalmia neonatorum occurs within the first 10 days of life and is characterized by a rapid progression of signs from mild inflammation to marked redness, swelling, and purulent exudate. Corneal involvement is common and severe. *Chlamydia trachomatis* organisms can also be transmitted during a newborn's passage through the vagina. The early symptoms are similar to those of gonococcal conjunctivitis, but the incubation period is slightly longer (5 to 14 days). *Chlamydia* organisms do not respond to silver nitrate, which has been traditionally administered prophylactically to newborns. Since 1980, erythromycin has been more commonly used because it is effective against both *N. gonorrhoeae* and *Chlamydia*. Both gonococcal and chlamydial organisms (which are transmitted venereally) can invade adult conjunctivae and cause severe, acute, purulent infection.

The conjunctival infections that have been described are generally acute and can be successfully treated. Some persons have a chronic recurrent conjunctivitis characterized by periodic eye discomfort, redness, and discharge. Repeated inflammatory episodes can cause thickening of the conjunctiva and lid margins. The causes are numerous, but the most common are contact allergens (such as cosmetics or chlorine), airborne allergens, excessive meibomian gland secretions, and chronic blepharitis. Trachoma (a chronic *Chlamydia trachomatis* conjunctivitis) has been described as the leading cause of blindness in the world. It is prevalent in warm climates where living conditions are crowded and hygienic practices are poor. Insects may transmit the disease. In some cases the disease heals spontaneously, but in other cases it leads to conjunctival or corneal scarring and loss of vision if left untreated.

•••••• Diagnostic Studies and Findings[34,44]

Microscopic examination of stained conjunctival scrapings Numerous polymorphonuclear neutrophils in bacterial infections; monocytes in viral infections or trachoma; eosinophils and basophils in allergies

Culture of exudate or conjunctival scrapings Organism identification

•••••• Multidisciplinary Plan[11,34,44]

Medications

Antiallergic agents (decongestants, antihistamines)
    Naphzoline HCl (Naphcon, Opcon, Vasocon Reg)
    Phenylephrine HCl (Velva-Kleen, Preferin, Eye Cool)
    Tetrahydrozoline HCl (Collyrium, Murine Plus)
Nonsteroidal antiinflammatory drugs
    Ketorolac tromethamine (Acular)
Antiinfective agents (medication varies with causative organism)
    Sulfacetamide sodium (Sulamyd, Bleph 10), 10%-30% solution or 10% ointment for 3-7 d
    Erythromycin (Ilotycin), topical 0.5% ointment for 3-7 d
    Gentamicin sulfate (Garamycin, Genoptic), topical 3 mg/ml solution or 3 mg/g ointment for 3-7 d

Antiviral agents
Idoxuridine (IDU, Dendrite Herplex), 0.1% solution, 1 drop q1h during day and q2h at night
Adenine arabinoside (Ara-A, Vira-A), 3% ointment instilled 5 times/d
Trifluridine (TFT, Viroptic), 1% solution, 1 drop q2h during waking hours during epithelial healing, then 1 drop q4h for 7 d
For gonococcal or chlamydial conjunctivitis or severe purulent conjunctivitis
Tetracycline (Achromycin, Terramycin), 250-500 mg po qid for 21 d
Erythromycin (E-Mycin, others), 250 mg qid for 21 d
Prophylactic dose within first hour of life for newborns
Erythromycin ophthalmic ointment, 0.5%, in each eye
Tetracycline ophthalmic ointment, 1% in each eye

General Management

Saline irrigation for purulent discharge
Warm compresses for discomfort and inflammation, 10 to 15 minutes two to three times a day
Cold compresses for allergic itching, 10 to 15 minutes two or three times a day
Eyelid hygiene regimen for softening, loosening, and removing crusts on eyelids[34]

NURSING CARE

Nursing Assessment

Allergic and General Irritant Responses

Lacrimation; generalized hyperemia; gritty, sandy sensation; severe itching (with allergies)

Viral Inflammation

Lacrimation, minimum mucopurulent discharge; generalized hyperemia; possible preauricular nodes; some lid swelling; moderate discomfort; possible photophobia

Bacterial Inflammation

Purulent discharge; lid swelling; generalized hyperemia; moderate discomfort; possible photophobia; complaints of blurred vision (owing to excess exudate over eye surface); blurring may disappear with blinking

Severe (Corneal) Involvement

Moderate discomfort that becomes severe

Nursing Dx & Intervention[22]

Risk for infection related to organism contamination

- Assess patient's eyes for presence of mucopurulent discharge *to confirm presence of bacterial, possible gonococcal, or chlamydial infection.*

- Isolate patient from others (in institutional setting) and use precautions *to prevent spread of infection.*
- Administer prescribed topical ointments or systemic antibiotics.

Risk for injury related to excessive irritation

- Administer saline irrigations for excessive discharge *to prevent crusting and expedite healing.*
- Cleanse lids and lashes with mild shampoo and water mixture and clean, wet washcloth *to remove crusts.*

Pain related to localized inflammation

- Apply warm compresses to eyes *to increase comfort.*
- Administer analgesics as ordered.

Patient Education/Home Care Planning

1. Demonstrate to the patient how to perform saline irrigation of the eye.
2. Demonstrate to the patient how to apply warm compresses with a clean cloth or cold compresses (ice should not be applied directly to eyelids).
3. Instruct the patient to wash hands thoroughly before and after treating each eye.
4. Encourage the patient to keep the hands away from the face.
5. Encourage the patient to avoid crowded environments when possible.
6. Discuss with family members the need to avoid touching their faces and to wash hands thoroughly when contact has occurred.
7. Encourage the patient to avoid noxious fumes and smoke.
8. Discuss with the patient the importance of not wearing contact lenses during the suppuration period.

Evaluation

Conjunctiva and cornea are healthy Palpebral conjunctiva is homogeneous pink color. Bulbar conjunctiva is clear and glossy. Cornea is clear and glossy. There is no eye discomfort, lacrimation, or discharge.

■ SUBCONJUNCTIVAL HEMORRHAGE

Subconjunctival hemorrhage is a common phenomenon caused by the rupture of a blood vessel. It appears suddenly as a well-defined bright red area on the surface of the eyeball and gradually disappears in 2 to 3 weeks. A large hemorrhage may be darker in color and expand for the first few days. The patient feels no discomfort but is usually alarmed. The ruptured vessel is usually the result of localized increased pressure (following severe coughing, vomiting, or sneezing) or minor trauma. Often a cause cannot be found, and no treatment exists. In rare instances blood dyscrasias, hypertension, or viral conjunctivitis is associated with this hemorrhage.[34,44]

CONJUNCTIVAL DISCOLORATION AND GROWTHS

The conjunctiva is subject to a large variety of growths, tumors, and discoloration. Bilirubin is absorbed in the conjunctiva with jaundice and gives the underlying sclera a yellow coloring. This discoloration is different from the normal yellowish pigmentation that occurs with increased melanin deposits in dark-skinned people.

Two of the most common benign growths are pterygium and pinguecula. A pterygium is a triangular growth of connective tissue that usually advances from the nasal side of the conjunctiva and encroaches on the cornea. It occurs more commonly among people who are frequently exposed to the sun and wind. It is not surgically removed unless it creates a cosmetic concern or threatens to involve the central cornea. A pinguecula is common in older adults and appears as a yellow nodule on either side of the cornea at the limbus. It usually involves both eyes. It may be periodically inflamed but does not invade the cornea and is usually not treated unless the patient is concerned about its appearance.

DISORDERS OF THE CORNEA AND SCLERA

The cornea is the main exterior protector of vision. Visual clarity depends on uniformity, smoothness, and transparency throughout the corneal layers. The avascular central cornea depends on its periphery (the limbus) for nourishment and on its epithelial (outer layer) and endothelial (inner layer) activity for hydration stability. Because the cornea is exposed to the external environment, it is more vulnerable to trauma and infection. Injury to the outer epithelial layer exposes Bowman's membrane and the substantia propria (stromal layer) to infection. If untreated infection perforates the cornea, the eye may be lost. The epithelial layer regenerates rapidly without scarring, but the deeper layers form opacities that may cause astigmatism or mild to severe visual loss.

Recently developed surgical techniques for corneal transplantation involving new microscopic and illuminating systems have greatly improved the prognosis for patients needing new corneas.[38] Corneal transplant and implications for nursing are covered in the last section of this chapter (p. 603).

The sclera surrounds the eyeball and is adjacent to the uveal tract (including the choroid layer). It opens posteriorly to admit the optic nerve and other nerves and vessels into the eye. Scleral inflammation and disease are often associated with systemic connective tissue disorders.

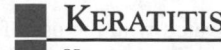

KERATITIS

Keratitis is an inflammation of the cornea.

• • • • • • Pathophysiology[34,44]

The cornea can be injured by exposure (drying), ischemia, nutritional deficiency, microbe invasion, anesthesia (sensory interruption), and trauma. Keratitis (corneal inflammation) may be superficial (epithelial), invade the stroma (subepithelial) or eventually break through the inner layer (Descemet's membrane) to the endothelium. Most organisms require a break in the epithelium before they can enter the cornea. The epithelium can be damaged by hypersensitivity to conjunctival inflammation, corneal drying, mechanical injury, or chemical irritants. Because the epithelium is richly innervated, superficial inflammation causes moderate to severe pain. Epithelial erosions may appear in the form of tiny pits or small or coarse lesions scattered over the surface. Central ulcers (or craters) may invade deeply into the underlying layers. Some of the medical treatments prescribed for therapy or relief of discomfort may facilitate bacterial invasion. People whose immune systems have been suppressed are more vulnerable to infection; the misuse of local corticosteroid therapy increases the tissue destruction activity of collagenase, which is produced when epithelial cells are injured. Immunosuppression also makes a person more vulnerable to invasion by fungi which easily penetrate Descemet's membrane. Fluorescein solution, which is used to stain and detect epithelial damage, is easily contaminated and can inoculate the epithelium with organisms. A patient who is given local anesthetics (particularly for use at home) can further abrade the cornea without knowing it. Besides inhibiting the protective corneal reflex, anesthesia of the eye interrupts epithelial regeneration.

Almost any bacterium can invade the cornea. *Pneumococcus, Staphylococcus, Streptococcus,* and *Pseudomonas* organisms are the most common. Fungal infections have become much more common since the introduction of topical corticosteroids and antibiotics. Chronic debilitating disease increases vulnerability to fungal infections. Viral infections, most commonly caused by herpes simplex, are also prevalent.

Herpes zoster can also invade the eye through inflammatory lesions of areas served by the trigeminal nerve. The lesions, in the form of scattered erosions or plaques, may be superficial or embedded in the deeper corneal layers. Residual corneal stromal infiltrates and scarring may ensue. The acute phase of herpes zoster keratitis resolves in 4 to 6 days. Treatment is primarily aimed at relieving the symptoms. Topical and systemic steroids and some newly approved antiviral topical medications speed recovery.

Pneumococcus and *Pseudomonas* organisms tend to spread rapidly and form ulcers that penetrate deep into the stroma. Herpes keratitis can be recurrent; it is triggered by stress, exposure to ultraviolet light (sunlight), or by other illness. It is relatively asymptomatic because it attacks the trigeminal nerve (CN V) and diminishes pain. Corneal ulceration and optic atrophy develop rapidly in neonates contaminated with herpes virus at birth. Adults with recurrent herpes keratitis may heal with or without scarring. Herpesvirus is also activated with the use of topical steroids. Some virus forms are highly contagious and cause outbreaks, especially in schools, institutions, and eye clinics. Chronic disabling illness increases an individual's vulnerability to corneal damage, as do certain diseases, such as diabetes mellitus, leukemia, chronic alcoholism, severe vitamin A deficiency, and autoimmune diseases.

Recent reports have created concern about the increasing incidence of *Acanthamoeba* keratitis. *Acanthamoeba* is commonly found in fresh water, soil, and airborne dust. The organisms have been recovered from the nose and throat of seemingly healthy individuals, suggesting that they can be inhaled as well as acquired through contaminated water. The amoebae are resistant to freezing, to most antimicrobial agents, and to levels of chlorine used to disinfect swimming pools, public drinking water, and hot tubs. Most people who have this infestation are contact lens wearers who use distilled or tap water to clean or rinse their lenses. The organism is devastating because it is resistant to most antimicrobials, it is often misdiagnosed as herpes simplex keratitis and treated without success, and it tends to cause recurrent epithelial breakdown. A large percentage of patients with this disorder have had to undergo a corneal transplant to regain useful vision.[11]

The severity of corneal destruction depends on the virulence of the organism, the degree of corneal destruction, the accuracy and promptness of therapy, and the immunocompetence of the host.

•••••• Diagnostic Studies and Findings[34,44]

Fluorescein stain (2%)   Sterile paper strips most commonly used; breaks in epithelium are stained green.

Ulcer scrapings for microscopic viewing (Gram or Giemsa stain)   Organism identification

Ulcer scrapings for culture   Organism identification

•••••• Multidisciplinary Plan[34]

Surgery

Corneal transplantation
Enucleation (or evisceration)

Medications

Mode, frequency, and duration of therapy depend on identified organism and degree of corneal penetration[11,34,44]
Antiinfective agents
  Topical
    Erythromycin, 5 mg/g
    Gentamicin, 3-8 mg/ml
    Penicillin G, 10,000-20,000 U/ml
    Bacitracin, 10,000 U/ml
    Sulfacetamide sodium, 10% solution
    Amphotericin B, 1.5-3 mg/ml
    Idoxuridine, 0.1% solution or 0.5% ointment
  Subconjunctival injections of antibiotics for acute, severe central ulcerations

Systemic antibiotics (IV or po) for acute severe central ulcerations, if sclera is involved, or if perforation threatens
Antiviral agents
  Idoxuridine (IDU, Dendrite, Herplex), 0.1% solution, 1 drop q1h during day and q2h at night
  Adenine arabinoside (Ara-A, Vira-A), 3% ointment, instill 5 times/d
  Trifluridine (TFT, Viroptic), 1% solution, 1 drop q2h during waking hours during epithelial healing, then 1 drop q4h for 7 d
Mydriatic-cycloplegic agents
  Atropine, 1% solution bid or tid for painful inflammation of iris and inflammatory constriction of pupil
Mucolytics
  Acetylcysteine, 10%-20% solution for inhibiting collagenase
Analgesics (for severe pain)
  Acetaminophen (Tylenol), 650 mg po q4h prn
  Acetaminophen (Tylenol 650 mg) with codeine (30 mg), 1-2 tablets po q4h prn
  Codeine, 30-60 po q4h prn
Antiamoeba agents
  Brolene
  Polyhexamethylene biguanide (PHMB), 0.02%
  Chlorhexidine, 0.02%
  Clotrimazole, 1% gtts
  Ketoconazole, 200 mg bid po
  Itraconazole, 200 mg bid po

General Management

Supportive therapy according to severity of condition
Hospitalization for extensive central ulcer (over 2-3 mm diameter or penetrating deep into stroma)
Pressure dressings (often over both eyes) for discomfort
Loose epithelium mechanically removed with applicator and local anesthetics for viral keratitis.
Ice compresses for 10 to 15 minutes two or three times a day for discomfort and inflammation
Therapeutic soft contact lenses for recurrent corneal erosion or other chronic keratopathy

NURSING CARE

Nursing Assessment

Corneal Epithelium

Moderate to severe pain; blurred vision; haloes seen around lights; lacrimation; generalized hyperemia; fluorescein stains green on corneal surface; possible photophobia; possible purulent exudate, especially with accompanying conjunctivitis

Scarring

Opacity or irregular light reflection may be visible on corneal surface; diminished vision if opacity in visual axis

Edema

Cornea appears dull and uneven; visual loss (blurring)

Ulceration

Ulcers vary in appearance and size; whitish gray opacity with overhanging margins; fungous ulcer may be white, fluffy, and elevated; severe pain with epithelial damage or iritis; lacrimation and possible purulent discharge; generalized hyperemia

Nursing Dx & Intervention

Risk for infection related to epithelial erosion

- Assess for purulent exudate. If purulent exudate is present, isolate patient (in institutional setting) and practice precautions *to prevent spread of infection.*
- Administer topical and systemic medications as ordered for infection.

Risk for injury related to epithelial erosion

- Assess cornea for epithelial disruption with inspection and with fluorescein stain.
- Instill mydriatic-cycloplegic topical solutions as ordered *to prevent inflammatory constriction of pupil and iritis.*

Pain related to localized inflammation

- Administer topical anesthetic if ordered.
- Apply pressure bandage to eye; be certain eye is closed before covering (one or both eyes may be covered) *to prevent further damage to ocular surface.*
- Apply warm compresses for 10 to 15 minutes two or three times a day *to relieve discomfort.*
- Provide systemic analgesic as ordered *to promote comfort.*

Sensory/perceptual alterations (visual) related to use of bilateral eye patches or decreased vision

- Raise side rails *to ensure safety.*
- Address patient by name from doorway and identify yourself.
- Complement voice stimulation with touch *to notify patient of your proximity.*
- Orient patient to bedside equipment (such as call light, bed control, and side rails) and personal belongings at bedside by directing his or her hand over objects.
- Encourage patient to perform self-care with personal hygiene *to promote independence.*
- Provide patient's privacy, and assure patient that privacy is provided.
- Help with meals *to promote needed caloric intake:*
  Read menu selections.
  Guide hand to utensils and food on tray.
  Describe food on tray in clock terms.
  Help with cutting meat, removing lids from cartons, buttering bread, and so on.

- Help with walking *to avoid injury:*
  Walk slowly and slightly ahead of patient; patient's hand should rest on your arm at the elbow.
  If possible, allow patient to trace progress by running the dorsal aspect of his or her free hand along a wall. Describe surroundings as you proceed.
  Allow patient to feel chair, toilet, or bed before turning to sit.

Patient Education/Home Care Planning

1. Explain to the patient the self-care of corneal abrasion.
2. Demonstrate to the patient how to instill eye drops or ointments as ordered.
3. Demonstrate to the patient the application of warm or cold compresses.
4. Discuss with the patient the need to wear dark glasses if a cycloplegic drug is ordered.
5. Discuss with the patient the need to wash hands before and after treating each eye.
6. Encourage the patient to keep hands away from the face and eyes except when treating condition.
7. Explain to the patient not to use a soiled handkerchief or tissue on the eyes.
8. Encourage the patient to avoid noxious fumes and smoke.
9. Discuss with the patient how to monitor the eye for increased pain or change in discharge.
10. Explain visual changes (increased blurring) or visual blockage.

Evaluation

Cornea is healthy Cornea is clear and glossy. There is no eye discomfort, lacrimation, or discharge.

Visual alteration is improved Patient is able to perform ADL and return to precondition level of functioning.

CORNEAL INJURIES

Corneal injuries are injuries to the surface epithelium or deeper layers of the eye in the form of contusions, abrasions, perforations, lacerations, burns, or damage from chemical irritants.

•••••• Pathophysiology[34,44]

Contusions result from blows that do not penetrate the corneal surface. Frequently the protective lid suffers the most damage, with edema and bruising. A subconjunctival hemorrhage may result, which looks alarming but usually heals spontaneously over 2 to 3 weeks without residual effects. The anterior chamber should be examined for repository blood, which gravitates to the lower segment and is absorbed within a few days, leaving no aftereffects. If the entire chamber is filled with blood, normal intraocular pressure is threatened and surgical evacuation through an incision at the corneal margin may be required. Severe blows may dislocate the lens, which causes visual distortion and possible ciliary spasms that are extremely painful. Surgical intervention with lens removal may be necessary. Retinal hemorrhages may occur; they are usually self-limited and without complications unless the macula is the site of bleeding. A large retinal hemorrhage might invade the vitreous, permanently obscuring vision, and increase the risk of a retinal tear.

Corneal abrasion is the disruption of cells and the loss of the superficial epithelium. This outer surface is easily separated from the underlying layers and can be injured or destroyed by exposure (lack of moisture), chemical irritants that dissolve in the protective tear film, and scrapes from foreign bodies. Drying of the surface occurs with structural or functional alterations of the eyelids, which normally blink and spread tears to maintain moisture. Some studies have shown that eye surface irritation is a risk with individuals who work with computer visual display terminals (VDTs) for prolonged periods. There is some evidence that the rate of blinking is reduced during the intense staring at the VDTs, and heated or air-conditioned offices with low humidity contribute to drying and irritation of the eye surface. Contact lenses, eyelashes, dust and dirt particles, fingernails, and crusted matter from purulent eye drainage are among the most common offenders for scraping the corneal surface. The industrial disaster in Bhopal, India, in 1984 is an example of an irritant, methyl isocyanate (MIC), causing edema and permanent destruction of the exposed epithelial surface of the eyes of thousands of victims.

The epithelium heals quickly (within 24 to 48 hours) and leaves no scarring or residual damage. However, severe pain occurs with even minor abrasions because of the numerous pain receptors in the epithelium. Lacrimation and photophobia accompany the pain. Short-acting anesthetic drops may be administered to provide immediate relief and ease the eye examination, but the drops are not given after the examination because the anesthetic slows epithelial repair. The extent of the abrasion can be viewed with fluorescein dye. Foreign bodies are often spotted during examination of the surface. If no foreign bodies are found, the upper eyelid may need to be everted and examined. Even with removal of the foreign body and rapid healing, the eye surface must be monitored (and is often treated) for possible secondary infection because epithelial breaks invite a variety of bacteria that cannot normally invade an intact epithelium.

Lacerations and perforations are serious emergencies because of invasion and disruption of the underlying stroma, endothelium, lens, and vitreous. The eye should be patched or shielded (if a foreign body is protruding) until surgery is performed. The iris may fall forward to close a corneal wound and may need to be partially excised before the wound is closed. Lens perforations usually result in cataract formation, which may result in a need to remove the lens. After surgical repair the eye is treated for potential massive infection and monitored for uveitis (see p. 567), vitreous clouding, scarring, and changes in vision. Mydriatic-cycloplegic agents may be given to maintain pupil dilation and thus prevent adhesions from forming on the underlying lens.

Many perforations occur in industrial settings, where flying metal flakes or particles are produced by high-speed drilling, riveting, and grinding. Workers are encouraged to wear protective goggles to prevent such injuries. The Occupational Safety and Health Administration (OSHA) mandates the use of protective eyewear or goggles whenever there is even minimal risk. Foreign bodies with iron or rusted particles may leave a deposit in the form of a rust ring. This deposit can be surgically removed after the epithelium has healed if it is superficially deposited. Deeply dispersed iron particles may interfere with an individual's vision in the future. Some foreign bodies, such as glass, are inert and can remain embedded in the eye tissue for years without harmful effects.

Chemical irritants, depending on the substance, can burn and destroy the underlying corneal layers. Regardless of the substance, the eye should be irrigated with copious amounts of water or sterile saline. Alkaline substances (such as ammonia, lime and cement dust, and sodium hydroxide) penetrate the tissues rapidly and continue to burn into the cornea unless they are removed. Acids coagulate the protein and often result in relatively superficial reversible damage. Local anesthetic drops may be used initially to provide comfort and ease irrigation and examination, but they are not used more than twice because they obstruct the healing process of the epithelium.

Ultraviolet burns (or irritation) can occur with sun exposure and are a risk for welders who are not protected from welding flashes. Epithelial irritation, swelling, and possible desquamation may occur. Desquamation is usually repaired without visual loss or changes.

 EMERGENCY ALERT

TRAUMA TO THE EYE

Reasons vary greatly, but over half of eye injuries are occupational incidents.

Assessment

- Obtain through history; sensation of foreign body.
- Assess area; obtain visual acuity if possible.
- Assess for tearing.
- Look for hemorrhage, hyphema, foreign body, impaled object, and eviscerated eye tissue or vitreous humor.
- Assess for facial fractures, head injury.

Interventions

- Do not install anesthetic drops before eye is examined or without an order from the physician.
- If patient is in severe pain, patch both eyes.
- Check to see if patient is wearing contact lenses.
- Prevent drying by instilling ointment or artificial tears.
- Lightly apply ice pack for ecchymosis or abrasions.
- Decrease intraocular pressure by keeping patient's head still and head of bed elevated.
- Prepare for an ophthalmology consultation.
- If an impaled object is in the eye, stabilize the object and patch both eyes. Do not attempt to remove the object.

EMERGENCY ALERT

CHEMICAL BURNS TO THE EYE

Chemical burns are caused by acids, alkaline substances, or irritants such as Mace. Acid burns are usually superficial whereas alkaline burns are progressive and represent an extreme emergency.

Assessment

- Determine the chemical.
- If burn is from an alkaline source there may be tissue destruction, which may be seen as white spots on the eye.
- The damage from an alkaline burn may not be evident until 3 to 4 days after the injury.

Intervention

- Regardless of the chemical, irrigate the eye immediately with copious amounts of normal saline or tap water. Continue to irrigate until the pH of the eye returns to 7.0, which is normal. The irrigation may take as long as 30 minutes. Do not be afraid to irrigate too much.

ACID

- Irrigate as directed above.
- Apply topical applications of antibiotics and cycloplegic agents as ordered.

ALKALINE

- Irrigate as directed above.
- Apply topical applications of antibiotics, steroids, and cycloplegic agents as ordered.

•••••• Diagnostic Studies and Findings

Fluorescein stain (2%)   To identify corneal surface disruption

Slitlamp examination   To view the eye surface, anterior chamber, deeper layers of the cornea, and anterior eye.

Indirect ophthalmoscopy   To view vitreous and retina

•••••• Multidisciplinary Plan

Surgery

Removal of foreign objects
Removal of damaged or prolapsed eye tissue
Repair of wounds

Medications[11]

Mode, frequency, and duration of therapy depend on degree of corneal penetration and potential for secondary infection.

Topical anesthetics (administered once or twice for pain relief during examination or removal of foreign body)
Proparacaine (Alcaine, Ophthetic), 0.5% solution, 1-2 drops in injured eye; onset within 2 min; duration, 20 min
Tetracaine (Pontocaine), 0.5% solution or ointment, 1-2 drops in injured eye; onset within 1 min; duration, 20 min

 EMERGENCY ALERT

CORNEAL ABRASION

Corneal abrasion is common; it usually occurs when a foreign body scratches the corneal epithelium.

Assessment

- Tearing and eyelid spasms
- Pain
- Diagnosed by using fluorescein staining and observing the abrasion with a blue light

Intervention

- Test visual acuity.
- Apply topical anesthesia if indicated and in collaboration with a physician.
- Patch eye for 24 hours after examination.
- Instruct patient to avoid blinking eyelid as much as possible.
- Instruct patient to avoid driving while patch is in place.

Antiinfective agents (type and duration of medication depend on extent of injury)
Topical
Erythromycin (Ilotycin), 1% ointment applied qd or bid in conjunctival cul-de-sac
Combination of Bacitracin 400 U, Polymixin B 5000 U, and Neomycin 0.25% (Neosporin) ointment, applied tid or qid in conjunctival sac
Tetracycline (Achromycin), 1% suspension or ointment, 1-2 drops bid or qid
Mydriatic-cycloplegic agents (may be given to prevent inflammatory pupillary constriction, uveitis)
Scopolamine hydrobromide (Isopto Hyoscine), 0.25% solution, 1-2 drops in injured eye; duration, 48-72 h
Systemic antibiotics may be prescribed for severe invasive trauma
Systemic analgesics may be prescribed for severe invasive trauma

General Management

Protective eye patch or shield applied until patient is examined
Eye irrigation—normal saline is commonly used
Bilateral pressure dressing often prescribed for 24-72 h to promote rest, reduce discomfort, and aid corneal reepithelialization
Tinted glasses to reduce discomfort of photophobia

NURSING CARE

Nursing Assessment

Corneal Epithelium

Moderate to severe pain; blurred vision; lacrimation; photophobia; generalized redness; fluorescein stains green on disrupted corneal surface; presence of foreign body

Surrounding Conjunctivae

Generalized redness, bleeding, excoriation, presence of foreign body; evert upper lid to inspect for foreign body if discomfort persists and foreign body is not present on eye surface

Anterior Chamber

May be partially or completely filled with blood

Surrounding Eye Tissue

A portion of the iris may prolapse through open corneal wound

Nursing Dx & Intervention

Pain related to corneal injury

- Assess patient's level of discomfort. If discomfort is severe, delay visual testing or other assessment until topical or systemic anesthetic or analgesic has been ordered and has taken effect.
- Administer medications as ordered immediately *to relieve discomfort.*
- After treatment, apply pressure bandage to eye *to relieve discomfort* (be certain eye is closed before applying bandage).
- Apply a warm compress for 10 to 15 minutes as ordered *to relieve discomfort and inflammation.*
- Administer cycloplegic medication as ordered *to prevent pain from inflammatory pupil constriction and iritis.*
- Ensure the safety and comfort of hospitalized patient.

Risk for injury related to corneal surface disruption

- Assess surface of eye for foreign body. If foreign body is not visible on surface, evert upper eyelid and assess conjunctival surface for foreign body.
- Assess eye for surface injury.
- Assess eye for corneal epithelial breaks with fluorescein stain.
- Apply bandage or shield to eye until patient can be examined.
- Warn patient not to touch eye for duration of topical anesthetic *to avoid self-injury.*

Risk for infection related to corneal surface disruption

- Administer topical and systemic medications as ordered *to prevent infection.*

Fear related to discomfort and uncertainty about present and future visual loss

- Relieve discomfort as quickly as possible.
- Assess patient for signs of fear.
- Provide comfort and realistic reassurance.
- Keep patient informed about all procedures as they occur *to alleviate as much uncertainty as possible.*

Sensory/perceptual alterations (visual) related to use of eye patch or decreased vision

- Warn patient that depth perception will be lost and 50% of peripheral vision will be lost on affected side.
- Caution patient to bring hand forward slowly to touch objects (especially containers of hot liquid and containers receiving poured liquids) *to ensure safety.*
- Explain that patient should turn head fully to affected side to view objects or obstacles.
- Teach patient to use up and down head movements to judge stair dimensions and oncoming objects *to promote safety.*
- Teach patient to proceed slowly with all movement *to prevent injury.*

Sensory/perceptual alterations (visual) related to use of bilateral eye patches or bilateral vision loss

- Assess patient for level of fear or disorientation related to sudden loss of vision.
- Review events since injury and present situation with patient *to reorient patient and to maximize patient's capacity to deal with present circumstances.*
- Raise side rails *to ensure safety.*
- Address patient by name and identify yourself *to reduce anxiety.*
- Complement voice stimulation with touch *to notify patient of your proximity.*
- Orient patient to equipment (such as call light) and personal belongings at bedside by directing patient's hand.
- Encourage patient to perform self-care with personal hygiene *to maximize independence.*
- Ensure patient's privacy, and assure patient that privacy is provided.
- Provide patient with television set or radio *to encourage mental and memory stimulation.*
- Provide patient with a clock that can be felt, and remind patient of date.
- Continue to assess patient for evidence of sensory deprivation signs (e.g., withdrawal, anxiety, depression).
- Balance privacy and quiet with stimulation events.
- Help patient with meals *to promote the needed caloric intake.*
  Read menu selections.
  Guide hand to utensils and food on tray.
  Describe food on tray in clock terms.
  Help with cutting meals, removing lids from containers, buttering bread, and so on.
- Help with walking *to promote safety.*
  Walk slowly and slightly ahead of patient; patient's hand should rest on your arm at elbow *to maximize patient's capacity to maintain balance and assurance of attending support.*
  If possible, allow patient to trace progress by running the dorsal aspect of his or her free hand along a wall.
  Warn of steps, turns, and narrow passageways in advance.
  Allow patient to feel chair, toilet, or bed before turning to sit.

1. Demonstrate to the patient how to apply eye drops or ointment as ordered.
2. Demonstrate to the patient how to apply warm or cold compresses as ordered.
3. Tell the patient to wash hands well before treating eye(s).
4. Discuss with the patient the need to wear dark glasses if a cycloplegic drug is ordered.
5. Encourage the patient to keep the hands away from face and eyes except when treating condition.
6. Instruct the patient not to use a soiled handkerchief or tissue on the eyes.
7. Encourage the patient to avoid noxious fumes and smoke.
8. Discuss with the patient how to monitor the eye for increased pain and for blood or discharge from the eye or on the dressing.
9. Intepret any temporary or permanent visual alterations the patient might experience (e.g., blurring with corneal healing, swelling, blurring with ointment over eye surface, blurring and photophobia with pupil dilation).
10. Review with the patient the need for eye protection at work (e.g., protective goggles) or at other times (e.g., care of contact lenses—see p. 598.)

Evaluation

Cornea is healthy   Cornea is clear and glossy. There is no discomfort, visual loss, distortion, or evidence of infection.

Visual alteration is improved   Patient is able to perform ADL and has returned to preinjury level of function. Fear has disappeared.

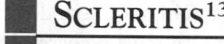 SCLERITIS[13]

Scleritis is an inflammation of the sclera.

Scleral inflammations are uncommon. The sclera has a poor blood supply and a low metabolism that does not encourage infection. Deep-seated aching and tenderness to touch without loss of vision are early indicators of the disease. An ocular muscle may contract and turn the eye if the inflammation is near its insertion. Because of the proximity of the sclera to the uveal tract, secondary choroiditis or retinal detachment may occur.

The episclera (located anteriorly) is more vascular than the rest of the sclera, and infections in this area may be worse. Infection is usually unilateral, has a sudden onset, and is accompanied by marked generalized hyperemia and pain. The cause is not always apparent, and the inflammation often subsides spontaneously.

Chronic or recurrent scleritis may result in scleral thinning with a localized outward bulging of the choroid layer. Perforation may occur.

DISORDERS OF THE UVEAL TRACT AND PUPIL

The uveal tract comprises the iris, ciliary body, and choroid layer. The iris surrounds the pupil and controls its size; and ciliary body secretes aqueous humor and controls accommodation; and the vascular choroid nourishes the anterior uveal tract and part of the retina. The location and extent of uveal lesions determine the variety and severity of signs, symptoms, and visual alterations. Deep corneal inflammation often spreads to the iris and results in a painful contraction of the iris and ciliary body. Iris abnormalities or inflammation can alter the shape of the pupil, disrupt the pupillary light reflex, or form adhesions to the cornea or lens to cause glaucoma. Ciliary body lesions can interfere with accommodation or cause anterior chamber or vitreous clouding with exudates, which diminishes visual acuity. Choroidal inflammation can spread to the sensory retinal layer and destroy central or peripheral vision. Retinal detachment may occur because of vitreous pull on the retina.

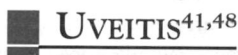 UVEITIS[41,48]

Uveitis is an inflammation or infection of the uveal tract.

Uveitis is the most common uveal condition. Organisms can be identified if the inflammation is peripheral enough to give the examiner access to infected tissue for staining or culture. Often the cause is unknown, and the inflammation is treated on the basis of the presumed cause. Some inflammatory processes are associated with endogenous causes or chronic conditions that can be diagnosed and treated systemically. Acute inflammations vary in severity and may subside without residual alterations. The uveal tract is also subject to congenital or developmental lesions that may or may not affect vision.

•••••• **Pathophysiology[34,44]**

Inflammation of the uveal tract can be acute or chronic, can be mild or severe, and can involve primarily the anterior tract (iris, ciliary body, and anterior choroid), the posterior choroid, or the entire eye. The most common form of uveitis is acute anterior inflammation. The onset is sudden, and the symptoms of pain and visual loss appear abruptly and are sometimes severe. The arteries of the anterior ciliary body become engorged and dilated, creating a purplish discoloration around the limbus (circumcorneal flush). The iris and the ciliary body release an exudate that increases protein and inflammatory cells in the anterior chamber. The protein causes clouding of the chamber (aqueous flare), and the cells form in clumps that adhere to the posterior cornea (keratic precipitates). Keratic precipitates, a diagnostic determinant, can be viewed with a slitlamp and occasionally with the ophthalmoscope if the deposits are large enough. A massive production of cells forms pus in the anterior chamber (hypopyon). The ciliary body also releases exudate into the vitreous to cause clouding and cell production. The iris is usually constricted (miotic pupil) and does not respond to light. The constriction is painful, and pain intensity increases with light stimulation. If the pain is severe, it is difficult to open the lid for examination. If the iris remains constricted, it quickly forms adhesions to the underlying lens (posterior synechiae) that may obstruct aqueous flow and cause a pupillary block glaucoma. With anterior inflammation the iris, ciliary body, and anterior choroid are usually all involved because of a common blood supply.

Posterior uveitis is usually confined to the posterior choroid and quickly spreads to the sensory retina. The vitreous becomes clouded with cells and exudate that can be viewed with an ophthalmoscope. Chorioretinal lesions can also be seen as irregular gray-white areas on the retinal surface. Vision impairment is the chief symptom of posterior choroiditis. Often there is no pain, redness, or photophobia. The degree of visual impairment depends on the extent of vitreous clouding and the location of retinal sensory layer inflammation. If the macula is involved, central vision is severely impaired. Retinal inflammations often leave scars that permanently impair the patient's vision.

Acute uveitis results from external infection, trauma (laceration, puncture, or contusion) or chemical burns. Herpes simplex, herpes zoster, and fungal infections are common causes of iritis. There are many endogenous sources. Rubella, rubeola, or mumps may cause a mild, transient uveitis. A hypermature cataract may release exudate into the anterior chamber and cause severe inflammation. Systemic diseases such as rheumatoid arthritis, regional enteritis, ankylosing spondylitis, and collagen disorders may contribute to uveitis. Many uveitis exacerbations are idiopathic and treated symptomatically. Acute uveitis can recur, particularly if the cause is endogenous and chronic.

Chronic uveitis is usually a continuous and progressive inflammation that involves cell production in the anterior and posterior chambers, frequent posterior synechia formation, retinal involvement, minimum exterior inflammatory signs or pain, and residual scarring of inflammatory sites. Some organisms invade and remain in the uveal tract. Tuberculosis, herpes zoster, and some forms of fungi are common causes of chronic inflammation. Systemic diseases such as sarcoidosis, rheumatoid arthritis (Still's disease), and histoplasmosis may be implicated. Some of the chronic syndromes are caused by local eye degenerative reactions. Chronic infections resulting from the degenerative changes in blind eyes may force a decision to perform enucleation for relief. Pars planitis is a chronic inflammation of the posterior choroid that involves vitreous opacites with a chief complaint of "floaters," retinal inflammation, and scarring. The cause is unknown, and the disease extends over 5 to 10 years.

In severe infections the entire inner eyeball may become inflamed (panophthalmitis). Pyogenic bacteria may penetrate to the uvea with trauma, through rupture of a corneal ulcer, or through endogeneous sources such as septicemia, meningitis, or bacterial endocarditis. *Staphylococcus aureus, Pseudomonas,* and *Proteus* are commonly involved organisms. Suppurative panophthalmitis is acute and severe. Severe pain, visual loss, and necrosis of the sclera may be followed by rupture of the globe. Sometimes the infection does not invade the sclera but remains confined to the inner eyeball (endophthalmitis). In this case the onset and course are less severe and the infection is more responsive to treatment.

Diagnostic Studies and Findings[34,44]

Staining and culture of scraping Performed if uveitis is associated with peripheral inflammation or ulceration; organism is identified through culture and Gram stain

Slitlamp (binocular microscope) examination Focuses on thin sections of cornea, anterior chamber, lens, or anterior vitreous; presence and extent of inflammatory cells or pus in anterior chamber and anterior vitreous can be viewed.

Gonioscopy Corneal contact lens (goniolens) is placed over anesthetized cornea to permit viewing of anterior chamber angles with microscopic lens; cellular debris and adhesions are seen in anterior chamber; angles can be viewed

Ophthalmoscopy Vitreous opacities and chorioretinal lesions can be viewed

Diagnostic studies to rule out or identify systemic disease

Multidisciplinary Plan[34,44]

Acute uveitis is often treated symptomatically because the cause cannot be identified.

Surgery

Enucleation for ruptured globe or marked eye degeneration[20]
Lens extraction for lens-induced uveitis

Medications

Mydriatic-cycloplegic agents (duration of administration depends on severity of infection)
  Atropine sulfate (Atroprisol, Isopto Atropine), 1% solution bid or tid to maintain full pupillary dilation
Corticosteroids—topical (often the choice with anterior uveitis)
  Instilled as frequently as q1-2h initially for severe inflammation, or bid or tid; to reduce inflammation and prevent iritic adhesions; patient response must be carefully supervised because herpes simplex and fungal organisms increase in activity and growth with steroid therapy; immunosuppression may increase host susceptibility to secondary infection; because open-angle glaucoma is a common complication of topical steroid treatment, ocular tension must be carefully monitored.
  Dexamethasone alcoholic suspension (Maxidex), 0.1% suspension, 1-2 drops 4-6 times/d
  Fluorometholone suspension (FML Liquifilm), 0.1%, 1-2 drops 4-6 times/d
Corticosteroids—subconjunctival injections (sometimes administered along with topical medication; administration and dosage determined by physician)
  Dexamethasone sodium phosphate (Decadron phosphate, Hexadrol), 4 mg/ml
  Hydrocortisone acetate (Hydrocortone Acetate, Cortef Acetate), 25 mg/ml or 50 mg/ml

Topical antiinfective agents (type and duration of medication depend on severity of infection)

Erythromycin (Ilotycin), 1% ointment applied qd or bid in conjunctival sac

Combination of Bacitracin 400 U, Polymixin B 5000 U, and Neomycin 0.25% (Neosporin) ointment, applied tid or qid in conjunctival sac

Tetracycline (Achromycin), 1% suspension or ointment, 1-2 drops bid or qid

Systemic medications

Analgesics

Acetaminophen (Tylenol), 650 mg po q4h prn

Acetaminophen (Tylenol), 650 mg with codeine (30 mg), po q4h prn

Corticosteroids

For posterior uveitis and inflammations that do not respond to local treatment

NURSING CARE

Nursing Assessment

Anterior Uveitis

Moderate pain; severe pain if associated with keratitis; intense photophobia; no visual change; possible blurred vision if eye chambers clouded with exudate, or possible blurred distant vision with ciliary spasm; circumcorneal flush (purplish coloration); pupillary constriction

Posterior Uveitis

Minimum or no pain; blurred vision from vitreous opacities or sensory retina inflammation (may be central [macular] or peripheral, depending on extent and location of inflammation); ophthalmoscopy may reveal vitreous opacities as black dots

Nursing Dx & Intervention

Pain related to acute anterior iridocyclitis

- Assess patient for degree of discomfort.
- Administer cycloplegics as ordered *to reduce painful pupillary constriction.*
- Apply warm and cold compresses for 10 to 15 minutes two or three times a day as ordered.
- Administer systemic analgesics as ordered *to promote comfort.*
- Instruct patient to wear dark glasses or avoid light *to reduce photophobic discomfort.*

Risk for injury: adhesions and increased intraocular pressure, related to iridocyclitis

- Administer cycloplegics as ordered *to prevent adhesions from iris to lens.*
- Assess patient for signs of increased intraocular pressure, increased haziness of vision (corneal edema), extreme pain, nausea, vomiting, or onset of conjunctival injection.

Risk for infection related to penetration of bacteria to the uvea

- Administer topical and systemic medications (steroids, antiinfective agents) as ordered *to prevent infection.*

Patient Education/Home Care Planning

1. Demonstrate to the patient how to apply eye drops and ointments.
2. Demonstrate to the patient how to apply warm and cold compresses.
3. Encourage the patient to wear dark glasses.
4. Discuss with the patient how to monitor the eye for increased pain, visual changes (increased blurring), and inflammatory signs.
5. Review with the patient that vision will be blurred because the pupil will be dilated.

Evaluation

Uveal tissue is healthy Cornea is clear and glossy. There is no photophobia, eye discomfort, inflammation (corneal, circumcorneal, or conjunctival), or discharge.

Vision is restored There is no blurring at close or distant range.

UVEAL TRACT DEFORMITIES[36,41,43]

Uveal tract deformities range from minor defects to severe impediments to visual functioning.

A coloboma is a localized absence of uveal tissue. An absence of a portion of the iris may cause a pupil shape defect (see p. 571) with no visual defects. If the choroidal coloboma is large, the overlying retina is deprived of blood supply in that area, which affects sensory vision. Aniridia is absence or diminishment of the iris. The pupil appears greatly enlarged, and no iris is showing. Photophobia and severe reduction of visual acuity follow. Aniridia may be inherited or associated with other chromosomal disorders such as mental retardation, Wilms' tumor, and urogenital abnormalities. The iris can atrophy over a period of years, leaving a misshapen pupil or holes (looking like additional pupils) over the visible surface of the iris. The presence of holes can cause diplopia. Atrophy can follow severe eye inflammation or trauma or occur as a primary disease. Choroid atrophy can be a benign disorder or result in marked retinal degeneration. Some forms of choroid atrophy cause progressive night blindness and diminished visual acuity.

The size of the pupil is controlled by dilator and constrictor muscles in the iris. There are no disorders of the pupil, but its size, response to light (accommodation), uniformity of shape, and symmetric responses with the corresponding eye are indicators of iris, eye, or systemic disorders.[34,43] Table 6-2 gives a summary of pupil abnormalities.

TABLE 6-2 Pupil Abnormalities

Abnormality	Contributing Factors	Appearance
Bilateral		
Miosis (pupillary constriction; usually less than 2 mm in diameter)	Iridocyclitis; miotic eye drops (such as pilocarpine given for glaucoma)	
Mydriasis (pupillary dilation; usually more than 6 mm in diameter)	Iridocyclitis; mydriatic or cycloplegic drops (such as atropine); midbrain (reflex arc) lesions or hypoxia; oculomotor (CN III) damage; acute-angle glaucoma (slight dilation)	
Failure to respond (constrict) with increased light stimulus	Iridocyclitis; corneal or lens opacity (light does not reach retina); retinal degeneration; optic nerve (CN II) destruction; midbrain synapses involving afferent pupillary fibers or oculomotor nerve (CN III) (consensual response is also lost); impairment of efferent fibers (parasympathetic) that innervate sphincter pupillae muscle	
Argyll Robertson pupil	Bilateral, miotic, irregular-shaped pupils that fail to constrict with light but retain constriction with convergence; pupils may or may not be equal in size; commonly caused by neurosyphilis or lesions in midbrain where afferent pupillary fibers synapse	
Oval pupil	Sometimes occurs with head injury or intracranial hemorrhage; transitional stage between normal pupil and dilated, fixed pupil with increased intracranial pressure (ICP); in most instances returns to normal when ICP is returned to normal	
Unilateral		
Anisocoria (unequal size of pupils)	Congenital (approximately 20% of normal people have minor or noticeable differences in pupil size, but reflexes are normal) or caused by local eye medications (constrictors or dilators), amblyopia, or unilateral sympathetic or parasympathetic pupillary pathway destruction (NOTE: Examiner should test whether pupils react equally to light; if response is unequal, examiner should note whether larger or smaller pupil reacts more slowly [or not at all] because either pupil could be abnormal size)	
Iritis constrictive response	Acute uveitis is frequently unilateral; constriction of pupil accompanied by pain and circumcorneal flush (redness)	Normal eye Affected eye
Oculomotor nerve (CN III) damage	Pupil dilated and fixed; eye deviated laterally and downward; ptosis	Normal eye Affected eye

TABLE 6-2 Pupil Abnormalities—cont'd

Abnormality	Contributing Factors	Appearance
Horner's syndrome	Miotic pupil; ptosis; interruption of sympathetic nerve supply to dilator pupillae muscle; may be caused by goiter, cervical lymph enlargement, apical bronchogenic carcinoma, or surgical injury to neck	Normal eye Affected eye
Adie's pupil (tonic pupil)	Affected pupil dilated and reacts slowly or fails to react to light; response to convergence normal; caused by impairment of postganglionic parasympathetic innervation to sphincter pupillae muscle or ciliary malfunction; often accompanied by diminished tendon reflexes (as with diabetic neuropathy or alcoholism)	Normal eye Affected eye

Other Irregularities

Iridectomy	Sector iridectomy	
	Peripheral iridectomy Surgical excision of portion of iris usually done in superior area so upper lid will cover additional exposure	
Coloboma (localized absence of portion of iris)	Congenital absence of area of iris; remaining iris shows normal light response	
Iridodialysis (circumferential tearing of iris from scleral spur)	Blunt trauma; more than one "pupil" in eye can cause diplopia	

GLAUCOMA

Glaucoma incorporates a variety of diseases that exhibit all or at least one of the following abnormalities: increase in intraocular pressure, degeneration of the optic nerve (disc), and visual field losses that may lead to total loss of vision.

The prevalence of glaucoma is difficult to determine because of the different screening methods and criteria for diagnosis among physicians and regions of the world. An estimated 1.5% of persons over 40 years of age have glaucoma, and approximately 100,000 persons in the United States are blind as a result of this disease.[8]

Glaucoma is detected in a variety of ways. Simple tonometry testing reveals intraocular pressure (IOP) that exceeds the normal range of 10 to 22 mm Hg. Only 5% to 10% of persons with IOP over 21 mm Hg have visual defects or optic nerve changes. A variety of variables (discussed later) determine whether an unaffected person with a high IOP will only be monitored or will be treated for glaucoma. When screening methods include ophthalmoscopy or perimetry testing for visual field defects, some patients with a normal IOP exhibit optic nerve degeneration or visual field losses. Approximately one third of the visual defect population have a normal IOP when first examined.[15] Tonometry alone is not an adequate screening method for detecting glaucoma, and higher incidences are reported when persons are more thoroughly examined.

Glaucoma occurs because aqueous fluid cannot be drained adequately from the anterior chamber to maintain a normal IOP. Excessive pressure results in optic nerve degeneration.

Primary glaucomas (from an unknown cause) include open-angle, closed-angle, and glaucoma "suspect" disorders. Open-angle glaucoma is the more common and generally affects adults over 40 years of age. The onset is insidious and asymptomatic, and the disease progresses slowly. Many elderly persons with glaucoma are successfully treated with medications and retain vision. Closed-angle glaucoma occurs because of eye structure defects or changes and results in a mechanically blocked drainage system. The onset is usually acute and dramatic. The category of glaucoma "suspect" disorders includes individuals with an elevated IOP (above 24 mm Hg) who exhibit no ocular changes and persons with normal IOP levels (low tension) who show abnormal optic disc and peripheral field changes. Secondary glaucomas can be caused by inflammation, trauma, corticosteroid administration, systemic disorders, or local eye changes. In addition, a number of congenital syndromes include glaucoma.

Glaucoma can be classified as follows[34]:

Primary
  Chronic open-angle
  Glaucoma "suspect"
    Low-tension/normal tension
    Ocular hypertension
  Closed-angle
    Pupillary block
    Plateau iris
      Ciliary body block
Secondary open-angle
  Pretrabecular
  Foreign cells within trabecular meshwork
  Trabecular meshwork abnormality
  Increased venous pressure
Secondary closed-angle
  Membrane contracture
  Pupillary block
  Angle shift
Developmental glaucoma
  Primary
  Secondary

•••••• Pathophysiology[15,21,29,34,44]

Open-Angle Glaucoma

Approximately 90% of cases of primary glaucoma are of the open-angle type. The incidence of this disease increases with age. Population studies have shown that less than 1% of persons under 65 years of age have glaucoma and that approximately 3% of the population over 75 years of age have this disorder. Other risk factors for open-angle glaucoma have been identified. Nonwhites have a much higher incidence and frequently exhibit an earlier onset and a more rapid eye degeneration. Hypertension has been linked to glaucoma, as have the hypotensive episodes associated with treatment for hypertension. Approximately 20% to 25% of patients with elevated IOP have a family history of this disease. Persons with myopia and diabetes are reported to have a higher incidence of glaucoma.

Increased IOP occurs because of degenerative changes of unknown cause in the trabecular meshwork and the canal of Schlemm. Excess fluid cannot be emptied from the anterior chamber.

Intraocular pressure is not static but normally varies 2 to 5 mm Hg with increased heart rate, activity, or excitement. One high reading does not constitute a basis for diagnosis. Some persons exhibit visual field defects and optic nerve changes with normal or near-normal IOP, whereas others are able to tolerate elevated IOP without eye damage. Elevated IOP without ocular damage is called ocular hypertension. Some physicians believe that this elevation is a precursor of glaucoma, but others think that a mildly elevated IOP (20 to 24 mm Hg) is a normal state. The risk for eye damage increases with age, a family history of glaucoma, diabetes, and systemic vascular disorders.

Early open-angle glaucoma may be difficult to diagnose because it is asymptomatic. Even persons with visual field defects do not usually perceive them until they become extensive. There is no pain or blurred vision, and the outer eye does not appear inflamed or abnormal to the examiner. Tonometry usually shows an elevated IOP. The Schiötz tonometer is less accurate in higher pressure ranges and consistently shows lower pressures than applanation or noncontact tonometers. Direct ophthalmoscopy may reveal the earliest finding if the examiner is sufficiently skilled. The physiologic cup (a depression in the center of the disc) may be larger in one eye than the other. As the disease progresses, the cup widens and extends toward the disc temporal margin. The temporal vessels appear to drop (or bend) abruptly into the cup. The large vessels become displaced and crowded toward the nasal side of the disc. The temporal disc border atrophies and loses its pink coloration to appear a flat white. The cup widens and deepens (excavation) as the surrounding optic nerve margin diminishes and atrophies.

Visual field testing often shows the most tangible alterations. Visual field testing by confrontation does not measure early or limited defects. The Goldmann perimeter measures both central and peripheral losses. Characteristic defects (blind areas or scotomas) appear and enlarge as the disease progresses. Nerve fiber bundles originating from the optic nerve cease to function as the nerve head atrophies. The nasal visual field is often first affected, and eventually the periphery is diminished. The person may retain only a small portion of central vision with acuity of the unaffected area.

Many older adults are treated successfully with medication. Parasympathomimetic agents (miotic eye drops) increase the outflow of fluid by enlarging the area around the trabecular meshwork. β-Adrenergic blocking agents (eye drops) and orally administered carbonic anhydrase inhibitors decrease aqueous production. These drugs are given in various combinations. Miotic drops disturb vision because of pupillary constriction and may cause ciliary spasms. β-Blockers must be administered cautiously to asthmatic patients. Epinephrine drops are sometimes prescribed to increase outflow, but their use should be evaluated carefully because of potential systemic effects (tachycardia) and occasional local effects (macular edema). Diuretics deplete potassium and may cause thirst and drinking of large amounts of fluids, which could increase pressure. Patients receiving medication need careful and continuous supervision.

If IOP cannot be controlled through medication, laser trabeculoplasty (creating openings in the trabecular meshwork with laser beams), laser iridotomy, or surgery may be performed. Surgery usually involves the creation of an opening between the anterior chamber and the subconjunctival space. Many physicians prefer laser therapy because it is less damaging to the eye (see p. 605). Success rates for laser and surgical therapies are variable. The openings or filter systems may not remain patent. Invasive therapy for open-angle glaucoma is a last resort for eyes that do not respond to chemotherapeutic regimens.

Normal Tension Glaucoma
Closed-Angle Glaucoma[5]

Closed-angle glaucoma occurs because mechanical blockage of the anterior chamber angle results in accumulation of aqueous fluid and increased IOP. Most persons with closed-angle glaucoma have shallow anterior chambers (less than 3 mm depth between the iris and the posterior corneal surface), which is often a familial trait. These persons do not exhibit IOP elevations unless the angle is closed and obscures the trabecular meshwork, which ordinarily drains fluid from the anterior chamber. The shallow chamber is often accompanied by narrowed anterior angles (Figure 6-15). Narrow angles are more vulnerable to other physiologic events that cause further crowding of the angles.

Angle closure occurs because of pupillary dilation or forward displacement of the iris. In some instances pupillary dilation (physiologic or induced) causes the iris to crowd into the anterior angle, resulting in obstruction. Forward displacement of the iris occurs with enlargement of the lens, which normally thickens with aging. The iris can also be pushed forward with physiologic pupillary block. In a shallow anterior chamber the iris may press against the lens and obstruct aqueous flow from the posterior chamber to the anterior chamber. As fluid accumulates posteriorly, it bulges forward against the iris. A bulging iris can be viewed by an examiner with a penlight aimed obliquely at the cornea. The bulge casts a shadow on the opposite side of the light source (Figure 6-16).

Angle closure can occur in a subacute, acute, or chronic form. Subacute episodes often precede an acute attack. These episodes may involve transient angle obstruction with symptoms of blurred vision, mild to severe pain, and halos seen around lights. Persons with subacute angle closure may not exhibit increased IOP during an examination, but provocative testing with rapid drinking of water, sitting in a dark room to cause pupil dilation, or induced mydriasis may elicit an increased IOP.

Acute angle closure causes a dramatic response. A sudden onset of blurred vision, severe ocular pain, and halos seen around lights is followed by a progression of symptoms as the pressure increases. Ciliary injection (a purplish red coloration around the limbus), profuse lacrimation, a mildly

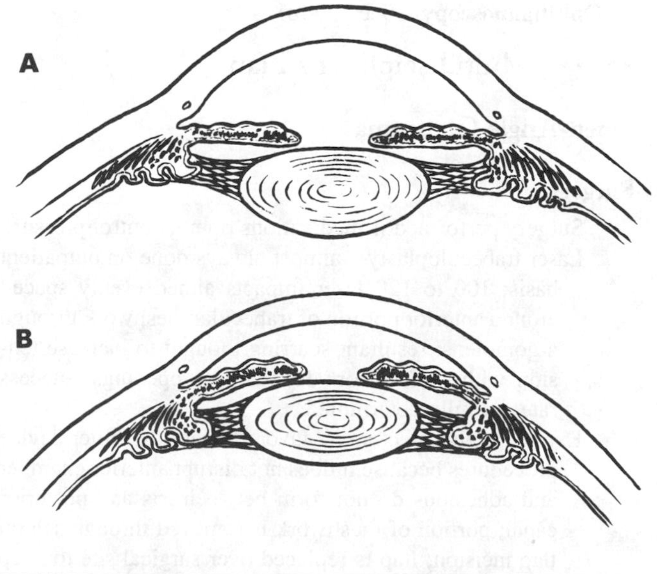

Figure 6-15 A, Normal anterior chamber. **B,** Shallow anterior chamber. Shallow chamber shows forward displacement of iris and narrow anterior angle.

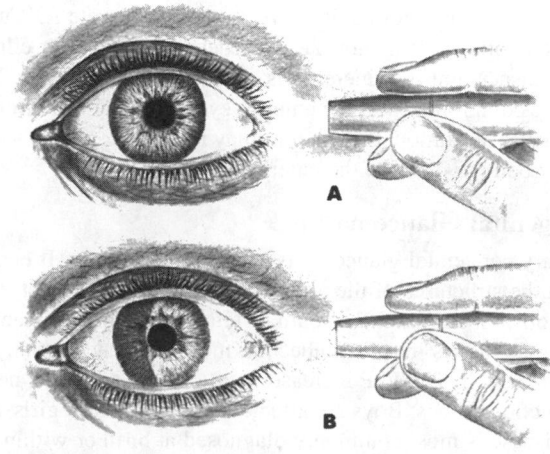

Figure 6-16 A, Normal anterior chamber: iris is flat. **B,** Shallow anterior chamber: iris is bulging, and crescent shadow appears on far side. (From Seidel.[37])

dilated, nonreactive pupil (5 to 6 mm in diameter), and nausea and vomiting may occur. Corneal edema causes the cornea to appear hazy. An acute episode constitutes a medical emergency. If the pressure is not relieved within several hours, eye damage occurs. Adhesions (anterior synechiae) begin to form between the iris and the cornea, which eventually closes the angle. Within a few days the iris and ciliary body begin to atrophy, the cornea shows permanent changes because of chronic edema, and optic atrophy and deterioration of nerve fibers occur. Total loss of vision is the result.

Emergency medical treatment consists of oral or intravenous administration of carbonic anhydrase inhibitors to suppress aqueous humor secretion, miotic eye drops to pull the iris away from the inner angle, osmotic agents to reduce pressure, and systemic analgesics to reduce pain. Surgical treatment (usually laser iridotomy) follows as soon as ocular pressure is stabilized.[2] Although usually only one eye is affected at a time, surgery is eventually performed on the other eye as a preventive measure.

Chronic episodes of increased IOP can occur when anterior angles are sufficiently narrowed to partially obstruct outflow. The patient may have minimal symptoms (hazy vision, mild pain) or none, and the IOP is usually elevated when measured. Subacute and chronic forms of angle closure are often treated medically or surgically to prevent insidious eye damage, such as slow formation of anterior adhesions.

Secondary Glaucomas

Trabecular meshwork obstruction or closed-angle glaucoma can occur because of eye deformities, inflammation, or trauma (surgical or accidental). Corticosteroid therapy increases IOP; this may be transient or may cause permanent eye damage.

A displaced, enlarged, hypermature, or ruptured lens can result in a crowding of the angle, an associated trabecular meshwork obstruction, or uveitis. Uveitis may cause a pupillary block with ciliary spasms or posterior synechiae (adhesions of the iris to the lens), which ultimately obstructs angle drainage. Trabeculitis with resultant scarring and damage may follow iridocyclitis when inflammatory cells and fibrous material are deposited in the anterior angles. Eye contusions elevate IOP, usually temporarily. If hemorrhage or edema of the iris or ciliary body ensues, the IOP increase is sustained and the angle flow may be compromised. If the anterior eye is traumatized through surgery or laceration, the iris root may re-form or adhere to the ciliary body to obstruct the anterior angle.

Congenital Glaucoma[47]

Primary congenital glaucoma is a hereditary disease. It occurs when the structures of the anterior chamber angle do not fully develop at about the fifth month of fetal life. A thin remnant of iris tissue inserts into the trabecular meshwork and partially or fully covers it. The IOP increases, and corneal and optic nerve destruction ensues. Boys are affected more often than girls, and the disease is most commonly diagnosed at birth or within the first 2 years of life. The disease is most often bilateral. The earlier the symptoms, the less favorable the prognosis because earlier onset indicates a greater anatomic abnormality. Other systemic congenital defects may accompany primary congenital glaucoma. Early symptoms are excessive tearing and photophobia. A hazy cornea eventually becomes opaque because of edema and stretching with breaks in Descemet's membrane, which allows fluid into the cornea. The eye enlarges because the tissue is elastic, and the diameter of the cornea increases. Optic nerve deterioration occurs rapidly, resulting in total loss of vision. If the symptoms are diagnosed early, goniotomy (cutting away the tissue covering the meshwork) is performed. In some instances the goniotomy must be repeated a number of times to ensure adequate drainage. Approximately 80% of these surgeries are successful.

Secondary congenital glaucomas are associated with a variety of systemic and eye disorders. Aniridia, the absence of an iris, may be associated with other anterior eye deformities to cause glaucoma. A dystrophic cornea or a congenital cataract may be associated with glaucoma. Neurofibromatosis and Sturge-Weber syndrome (hemangioma of the face) are two of the more common systemic disorders that accompany congenital glaucoma. Usually filtering or trabeculoplasty procedures are performed with varying success, depending on the severity of the anatomic abnormality.

•••••• Diagnostic Studies and Findings

Tonometry (Schiötz, applanation, or contact methods) Normal range 10 to 22 mm Hg

Visual field studies Central field tangent screen: blind spots are outlined by using 1 to 3 mm white target placed on board; normal blind spot is 13 to 18 degrees temporal from central fixation; abnormal isolated spots (scotomas) or confluent areas can be identified; nasal areas are usually lost first; automated perimetry: various automated machines (such as Goldmann perimeter) measure both central and peripheral fields

Gonioscopy Cellular debris and adhesions in anterior chamber angles can be viewed

Ophthalmoscopy See p. 1461

•••••• Multidisciplinary Plan

Open-Angle Glaucoma[39]

Surgery

Surgery performed if medications do not control pressure

Laser trabeculoplasty—almost always done on outpatient basis; 100 to 120 laser impacts aimed evenly spaced around anterior portion of trabecular meshwork through a goniolens; resultant scarring thought to increase tension within meshwork to maintain openings; success rate not fully determined

External trabeculectomy—favored over other filter device procedures because it does not disrupt anterior chamber and adhesions do not form between iris and posterior canal; portion of meshwork is removed through scleral flap incision; flap is replaced over surgical site to keep anterior chamber intact; procedure performed in hospital with patient under general anesthesia

EMERGENCY ALERT

SUDDEN VISUAL CHANGES

Sudden changes in vision may be suggestive of an acute eye emergency, which may lead to blindness.

Central Retinal Artery Occlusion

ASSESSMENT

- Produces sudden blindness; prognosis is poor.

INTERVENTIONS

- Interventions are directed at returning the blood supply to the retina and dilation of the artery.
- Possible interventions include amyl nitrate inhalation, sublingual nitroglycerin, and alternating administration of carbon dioxide and oxygen.

Retinal Detachment

ASSESSMENT

- Once detached, the retina is unable to perceive light because the blood and oxygen supply to the retina is compromised.
- Patient may report flashes of light, veil in visual field, or dark spots or particles in the visual field.

INTERVENTIONS

- Immediate bed rest.
- Patch both eyes.
- Obtain ophthalmology consultation as soon as possible; surgery may be indicated.

Glaucoma

Glaucoma causes 1 of every 10 cases of blindness in the United States. Acute angle closure glaucoma occurs when the aqueous humor is trapped in the anterior chamber of the eye leading to increased intraocular pressure. *Acute glaucoma is an emergency and may lead to blindness in hours.*

ASSESSMENT

Patient complains of severe eye pain, foggy cornea, severe headache, halos around lights, fixed and slightly dilated pupil, visual changes, and sometimes nausea and vomiting.

INTERVENTIONS

- In consultation with physician, administer miotic drops every 15 minutes to decrease the pupil size to allow for drainage of aqueous humor.
- In consultation with physician, administer pain medications and medications that will lower intraocular pressure (Diamox is generally used).
- Surgical intervention may be necessary.

Medications

β-Adrenergic–blocking agents

Timolol maleate (Timoptic), 0.25%-0.5% solution, 1 drop in each eye, usually bid; reduces aqueous production; serious side effects include bradycardia, palpitation, bronchial asthma, hypotension, and congestive heart failure; these necessitate discontinuation in 5%-10% of patients

Betaxolol (Betopic), 0.5% solution, 1 drop in each eye qd; reduces aqueous production; side effects are similar to Timolol, but air flow obstruction responses may be less common

Miotics

Pilocarpine (Isopto carpine, Pilocar), 0.25%-8% solution, 1-2 drops 2-6 times/d

Pilocarpine continuous-release insert device (Ocusert)—device is placed in conjunctival sac and releases medication over 7-day period; reduction in IOP is same as with drops; some patients have difficulty removing and inserting

Anticholinesterase drops (long-acting, strong miotics) for aphakic glaucoma; these agents should not be used for narrow-angle glaucoma because pupillary block may occur

Echothiophate iodide (Phospholine, Echodide), 0.03%-0.25% solution, 1 drop qd or bid

Adrenergic agents (to increase aqueous outflow)

Epinephrine drops (Epifrin, Glaucon), 0.25%-2% solution bid (possible side effect of tachycardia and extrasystole may occur)

Dipivefrin (Propine), 0.1% solution, 1 drop bid in each eye

Carbonic anhydrase inhibitors (CAIs)

Suppress aqueous production; contraindicated if allergic to sulfa

Oral

Acetazolamide (Diamox) 125-250 mg po 1-4 × daily or Diamox time-released sequellae 500 mg 1-2 × daily

Dichlorphenamide (Daranide) 50 mg 1-4 × daily

Methazolamide (Neptazane) 25-50 mg 1-4 × daily

Topical

Dorzolamide HCl ophthalmic solution 2% (Trusopt) 1 gtt tid

Closed-Angle Glaucoma

Surgery

Laser iridotomy—lens placed over anesthetized cornea; argon laser aimed at iris for approximately 50 deliveries to penetrate iris and create openings for aqueous flow; laser sessions repeated several times if necessary; ultimately both eyes usually treated

Peripheral iridectomy—3 to 4 mm incision made at limbus or parallel to limbus over cornea; iris prolapses through limbus, or forceps is inserted into anterior chamber to pull portion of iris outward so small wedge or piece of iris can be excised; remaining iris is massaged back into chamber, and pupil is constricted to assure surgeon that it is intact and round surrounding excised wedge; incision is then closed; pupil is dilated postoperatively, and steroid eye medication is given for few days so inflamed iris will not form adhesions; iridectomy opens channel between anterior and posterior chambers and creates opening in anterior angle for aqueous flow

Medications

In acute attacks, medications given to lower and control IOP so surgery can be performed

Hyperosmotic agents

Glycerin (Glycerol, Osmoglyn), 50% solution, 1.5 g/kg body weight po; duration, 4-6h

Mannitol (Osmitrol), 20% solution, 2 g/kg body weight, IV

Carbonic anhydrase inhibitors

Acetazolamide (Diamox), 250 mg po bid or qid, or 500 mg followed by 250 mg IV q4h; should be given immediately to abort acute attack

Narcotic analgesics

Meperidine (Demerol), 100 mg IM q4-6h prn

Miotics

Pilocarpine hydrochloride (Isopto carpine, Pilocar) 0.25%-8% solution, 1-2 drops q4-6h

Congenital Glaucoma

Surgery

Goniotomy—knife inserted near limbus to penetrate anterior chamber and reach area of trabecular meshwork in anterior angle; special goniolens used to scrutinize angle while knife tears away tissue covering meshwork; procedure may be repeated a number of times to ensure patency of drainage system

Medications

Medications not usually given; surgery necessary for alleviation; miotics sometimes given in preparation for surgery

NURSING CARE

Nursing Assessment

Open-Angle Glaucoma

Asymptomatic (no blurring, pain, or inflammatory signs, early visual defects not perceived by patient); outer eye appears normal

Tonometry

IOP usually elevated (more than 24 mm Hg) but may be within normal limits (under 22 mm Hg)

Visual fields (perimetry)

Typical central blind spots (scotomas) identifiable; superior/nasal vision usually lost before peripheral vision

Closed-Angle Glaucoma

Excessive lacrimation; acute, severe ocular pain (usually bilateral); blurred vision; halos seen around lights; pupil in mild dilation (5 to 6 mm diameter); corneoscleral flush (purplish red coloration at limbus); cornea may appear hazy; possible nausea and vomiting

Tonometry

IOP usually sharply elevated (may be over 50 mm Hg)

Congenital Glaucoma

Excessive lacrimation; photophobia; hazy opaque cornea; affected eye enlarged (both eyes may be affected); affected cornea enlarged in diameter

Tonometry

IOP usually elevated but elastic eye tissue may stretch and give false low reading

Nursing Dx & Intervention[29,42,45]

Open-Angle Glaucoma

Noncompliance related to side effects of eye medications

- Assess patient's needs and response to medications *to see if negative responses are occurring* (physician may be able to change medication if side effects are severe).
- Assess patient's knowledge about disease and its insidious progress unless treated *to anticipate noncompliance.*
- Be certain patient can read medication labels.
- Explain that number of medications and number of administrations can be confusing, inconvenient, and easy to forget. Enlist patient's assistance and understanding in devising medication schedule that patient can meet *to reduce noncompliance.*
- Discuss with patient that medications do not relieve any symptoms and may cause unpleasant side effects.
- Ensure that patient is aware of possible side effects:
    Miotics—blurred vision for 1 to 2 hours after administration, diarrhea
    Timolol—fatigue, weakness, depression
    Diamox—numbness, tingling of extremities and lips, decreased appetite or nausea, impotence

Risk for injury related to side effects of medications

- Instruct patient with new prescription that frequent checkups by physician are needed *to detect side effects and other symptoms such as increased IOP, sudden blurred vision, and inflammation of eyes.*
- Teach patient about possible side effects:
    Miotics—pupillary block, myopia from excessive accommodation
    Timolol—keratitis, asthma, bradycardia
    Epinephrine—eye irritation, periorbital edema, tachycardia
    Diamox—hypokalemia, confusion, urinary calculi
- Inform patient that examination (tonometry, health history, ophthalmoscopy, gonioscopy, and perimetry) will be needed every 2 to 3 months until physician determines that IOP is stable and there is no further optic nerve damage or visual field loss. Examination should be performed annually thereafter.

- Demonstrate correct method for administration and storage of eye drops. Have patient repeat demonstration *to ensure proper technique.*

Sensory/perceptual alterations (visual) related to symptoms of disease or side effects of medication

- Assess and review patient's family and support system for assistance in dealing with visual loss.
- Assess patient's feelings about visual loss or changes.
- Review patient's lifestyle and suggest adjustments to blurred vision associated with miotics.
- Offer support for feelings of loss and helplessness.

Risk for injury related to diminished peripheral vision

- Inform patient that diminished peripheral vision is a great safety hazard and that peripheral vision may be markedly reduced with advanced glaucoma.
- Explain that patient must learn to turn head to visualize either side *to ensure safety.*
- Ask patient to reduce clutter in home (such as electrical cords, loose rugs, and items on floor) *to prevent falls.*
- Inform patient that home should be well lighted (especially stairways) and that night light in bathroom is helpful.
- Warn patient that seeing at night, at dusk, or in dim lighting will be difficult *because miotic pupils do not dilate to admit more light to retina in subdued lighting or darkness.*

Laser Trabeculoplasty

Knowledge deficit related to lack of information about the procedure

- Describe procedure carefully to patient and family members, including discussion of equipment, length of procedure, nature of procedure, and postoperative events.
- Educate patient about administering eye medications and necessity for maintaining prescribed therapy because iris may become inflamed postoperatively and IOP may be increased:

  Glaucoma medications—resumed until inflammatory process subsides and then discontinued or adjusted

  Topical steroid drops—often prescribed for approximately 1 week after surgery; reduce inflammation but may raise IOP
- Inform patient that IOP may rise postoperatively and must be carefully monitored.
- Educate patient about necessity for keeping appointments for monitoring IOP.
- Educate patient about self-monitoring for symptoms (especially sudden onset):

  Excessive lacrimation

  Photophobia

  Severe ocular pain
- Advise patient that vision will be blurred for first day or two after procedure.

Anxiety related to uncertainty about discomfort and outcome of laser procedure

- Assess patient's level of anxiety.
- Offer support, comfort, and information *to ease anxiety.*
- Administer anesthetic eye drops immediately before procedure as ordered.
- Inform patient that headache and blurred vision may occur for first 24 hours after procedure.

Pain related to surgical procedure

- Administer systemic analgesics as ordered for headache that may occur a day or two after procedure.
- Apply eye patch or wear sunglasses for a few hours postoperatively *to avoid discomfort associated with light exposure.*

Peripheral Trabeculectomy

Knowledge deficit related to lack of information about the procedure

- Describe procedure carefully to patient and family members, including discussion of equipment used, length of procedure, nature of procedure, and postoperative events.

Anxiety related to uncertainty about discomfort and outcome of procedure

- Assess patient's level of anxiety.
- Offer support and comfort.
- Orient patient to surroundings and inform patient that affected eye will be patched postoperatively.
- Explain to patient that damaged vision cannot be restored, but further damage probably will be prevented.

Risk for injury related to postoperative complications

- Assess patient's vital signs until stable.
- Observe eye dressing for excessive bleeding (small amount of serosanguineous drainage may be present).
- Inform patient that periodic tonometry measurements are usually performed *because IOP may temporarily increase postoperatively.*
- Administer antiemetics as ordered for nausea *to avoid elevated IOP associated with emesis.*
- Administer mydriatics as ordered; pupil of affected eye is dilated immediately or within 2 or 3 days postoperatively *to prevent formation of iris adhesion.*
- Administer glaucoma medications for unoperated eye.

Sensory/perceptual alterations (visual) related to unilateral eye patch

Before surgery
- Warn patient that depth perception will be lost and 50% of peripheral vision will be lost on affected side.

After surgery
- Help patient with activities of daily living.

- Caution patient to bring hand forward slowly to touch objects (especially containers of hot liquid and containers receiving poured liquids).
- Teach patient to turn head fully toward affected side to view objects or obstacles.
- Tell patient to use up and down head movements to judge stairs and oncoming objects and to go slowly *to avoid injury.*

Pain related to surgical procedure

- Assess patient for postoperative discomfort and give systemic analgesics as ordered *to promote comfort.*

Closed-Angle Glaucoma

Pain related to increased IOP

- Assess patient's level of discomfort.
- Give medications as ordered *to reduce discomfort* (meperidine may not be ordered for some patients because it tends to cause nausea and vomiting).
- Administer osmotics or carbonic anhydrase inhibitors as ordered *to reduce aqueous production.*

Anxiety related to fear of vision loss

- Assess patient's level of anxiety.
- Offer comfort and support.
- Give realistic assurance about maintenance of vision if IOP is brought under control quickly.
- Keep patient informed of progress and planned medical and surgical interventions.
- Describe impending surgical procedures, including equipment, length of procedure, nature of procedure, and postoperative events.

Laser Iridotomy

Pain related to procedure

- During procedure, help patient to hold still (head is stabilized on chin rest).
- Offer reassurance and support.
- Administer topical anesthetic as ordered.
- Administer systemic analgesics as ordered if headache and mild eye pain continue for day or two.
- Eye patch or sunglasses usually applied for a few hours postoperatively *to avoid discomfort associated with light exposure.*

Knowledge deficit related to lack of information about procedure

- Educate patient about necessity of maintaining prescribed therapy.
- Educate patient about necessity of keeping appointments for monitoring IOP. (This procedure may be done on outpatient basis, and patient compliance is a vital factor.)

- Educate patient about self-monitoring for symptoms (especially sudden onset):
  Excessive lacrimation
  Photophobia
  Severe ocular pain
- Advise patient that vision will be blurred for first day or two after procedure.
- Advise patient that procedure may have to be repeated several times to ensure patency of angle.

Risk for injury related to postoperative complications

- Assess patient's vital signs until stable.
- Observe eye dressing for excessive bleeding.
- Observe patient for sudden onset of severe pain in operated eye and administer medications as ordered *to avoid eye injury related to elevated IOP.*
- Inform patient that tonometry measurements will probably be performed periodically.
- Administer antiemetics as ordered for nausea *to avoid elevated IOP.*
- Administer mydriatics and steroid drops for operated eye as ordered *to avoid inflammation and adhesions.* (Unoperated eye may need to be maintained with glaucoma medications if patient has previously received them.)

Sensory/perceptual alterations (visual) related to unilateral eye patch

Before surgery
- Warn patient that depth perception will be lost and 50% of peripheral vision will be lost on affected side.

After surgery
- Help patient with activities of daily living.
- Caution patient to bring hand forward slowly to touch objects (especially containers of hot liquid and containers receiving poured liquids).
- Teach patient to turn head fully toward affected side to view objects or obstacles.[22]
- Tell patient to use up and down head movements to judge stairs and oncoming objects and to go slowly.

Pain related to procedure

- Assess patient for postoperative discomfort and give systemic analgesics as ordered.

Patient Education/Home Care Planning

Specific knowledge needs are described under Nursing Dx & Intervention because glaucoma is commonly managed on an outpatient basis.
1. Review with the patient that glaucoma is not curable but can be controlled.
2. Explain to the patient that medications *must* be taken regularly and at the prescribed intervals.

3. Encourage the patient to visit the physician regularly as prescribed.
4. Ensure that the patient understands the need to monitor himself or herself for side effects[29] and report any to the physician because therapy may be changed according to the patient's response to medications (either undesirable side effects or ineffective therapy).
5. Explain to the patient to watch for sudden changes, including severe eye pain, inflamed eye, excessive lacrimation, marked photophobia, and visual field losses (inability to use peripheral vision), which may be noted because of bumping into obstacles from the side or at the patient's feet.
6. Remind the patient of any existing limited vision and related safety concerns.
7. Review with the patient factors that may increase IOP, such as constrictive clothing around the neck or torso, constipation (straining), heavy exertion or lifting, and sneezing or coughing (upper respiratory infection).
8. Explain that family members should be examined regularly because glaucoma and shallow anterior chambers are often familial.

Evaluation

IOP is under control Tonometry shows IOP of less than 24 mm Hg.

Eye damage is not present or not increasing There are no visual field defects, or existing field defects are not increasing. Eye examination shows normal findings. Eyeball surface is moist without excessive tearing. Conjunctiva is clear without injection. Cornea is clear, and no redness appears at limbus. Pupil may be constricted because of medication. Red reflex is full and round. Retinal surface is pink, granular, and uniform in color and consistency. Optic disc is pinkish white and translucent with physiologic cup that occupies no more than half of disc diameter. Both optic cups are same size. Central vessels emerge evenly from optic disc and are not crowded toward nasal side.

Pain is diminished Patient experiences no eye pain or headache.

Visual alteration is improved Patient can perform ADL and returns to usual level of function.

DISORDERS OF THE LENS[16,34,44]

The lens is a 4 mm (sagittal diameter) by 9 mm (equatorial diameter) transparent structure between the anterior chamber and the vitreous body. Its transparency and biconvex shape enable it to focus light rays on the retina through refraction. The lens is suspended by fibers (zonule) that attach to the ciliary muscles, and it is stabilized behind the iris. The elasticity of the lens enables it to increase its spheric shape in response to ciliary contraction for near vision (accommodation). Loss of elasticity with aging results in diminished refractive power for near vision (presbyopia).

Diseases of the lens result in either opacity or dislocation of the lens. Because the lens contains no pain fibers or blood vessels, usually the only symptom is blurred vision without discomfort.

■ LENS DISLOCATION[34,44]

The lens can be dislocated by trauma (a blow to the eye), systemic congenital disorders, or deformities of the lens itself.

In most instances the lens loses the full support of the zonular fibers and is either partially dislocated or fully detached and floating in the vitreous. Iritis and glaucoma are common complications of a lens in the vitreous. The detached lens may be surgically removed to prevent further eye damage, although complications may ensue because of disruption and loss of vitreous. Partially dislocated lenses are often successfully treated with glasses to correct blurred vision.

■ CATARACT[18,19,26,34]

Cataract is an opacity of the lens.

The prevalence of the disease is difficult to determine because in some studies cataracts are defined as lens changes, whereas in others the disease is reported when vision is altered or the lens must be surgically removed. A summary of available data states that visible lens changes occur in 42% of the 52- to 64-year-old population and that 5% of these people demonstrate some visual impairment. Between 60% and 91% of the 65- to 85-year-old group show senile lens opacities, and approximately 25% to 46% of these people demonstrate visual impairment. Cataracts are the third-leading cause of blindness.

No one has perfectly transparent lenses. Minor imperfections do not impair vision and are not apparent with gross examination. Gradual opacification of the lens is a physiologic process; if all people lived long enough, they would develop cataracts. The diagnosis of cataract is usually confirmed when a patient reports visual impairment. Considerable opacification may occur before the patient notices visual changes.

Congenital cataracts are relatively rare and occur in all degrees of severity. Newborns can exhibit total or minimal opacification. Surgery may be performed in infancy or the eyes may be observed and surgically treated at a later time. In many instances opacification does not impair vision sufficiently to warrant surgical removal.

The only therapy for lens opacities that impair vision is surgical removal of the lens. Surgical procedures for the eye have changed dramatically in the last 20 years. Fine suture materials, the operating microscope, microsurgical instruments, improved general anesthetic procedures, and ultrasonic probes for lens emulsification and lens suction have all contributed to an improved prognosis and rapid recovery from surgery. In the past, patients had to wait for the cataract to become "ripe" (develop marked edema and liquefaction) before surgery was possible. Newer techniques permit the decision to be made jointly by the patient and physician on the basis of visual impairment and the patient's need for visual clarity. Extended-wear soft contact lenses and surgically implanted lenses allow monophakic persons (those with one lens removed) to enjoy binocular vision. Over 95% of surgically treated cataract patients can now look forward to restored useful vision.

Pathophysiology

Acquired cataracts can occur because of trauma, heat, toxins, intraocular inflammation, systemic disease, or aging. Aging is considered the primary risk factor for cataract formation. Senile cataracts occur because of protein alterations, accumulation of water, increasing edema, and migration and disruption of normal fibers within the lens. The exact cause for these changes is unknown. Cataracts are usually bilateral but progress more rapidly in one eye than the other.

Opacities occur in different formations and in different areas of the lens (Figure 6-17). The central part of the lens (nucleus) is harder and denser than the periphery (cortex) because newly formed fibers continuously migrate toward and pack together in the central nucleus. The lens is surrounded by the capsule, a semipermeable membrane. The most common type of senile cataract occurs in the posterior subcapsular area. These opacities tend to obscure central vision relatively early. Cortical (or peripheral) cataracts, called soft cataracts, may cause marked opacification without interfering with vision. Eventually the opacities encroach on the visual axis and decrease visual acuity. Nuclear (or hard) cataracts occur in the central area of the lens. As the central lens changes, it enlarges and increases its spheric shape, which permits some persons to enjoy "second sight," an increase in near vision. This diminished presbyopia is a temporary improvement and is followed by increased opacities that ultimately reduce vision. Opacities may develop very slowly and form different configurations. An early symptom may be glare (especially at night) because the opacities reflect light rays inefficiently. In some instances central opacities split light rays and cause a monocular diplopia. This symptom disappears as the opacity increases. Vision may improve in dim light (or with pupil dilation) because the person has more pupil available to see around the opacity. Some patients are able to "see" the dark spots, which remain fixed in the visual field, unlike floaters (debris in the vitreous) that move around.

If the cataract is not removed, it may eventually cause the entire lens to be opaque. This can be seen with gross observation as a whitish discoloration of the entire pupil. Less advanced opacities may be seen through the ophthalmoscope as dark spots, patches, or networks of lines that disrupt the red reflex.

Decision for removal of the lens is usually based on the patient's need to see. Vision is evaluated by examining both eyes. If one eye enables the patient to maintain adequate vision, the failing eye may not be surgically treated. In some instances the lens swells and encroaches on the anterior chamber angle to cause glaucoma. Hypermature cataracts may release toxic products that cause a secondary uveitis or glaucoma or both. Surgical intervention is sometimes undertaken to prevent eye damage regardless of visual acuity.

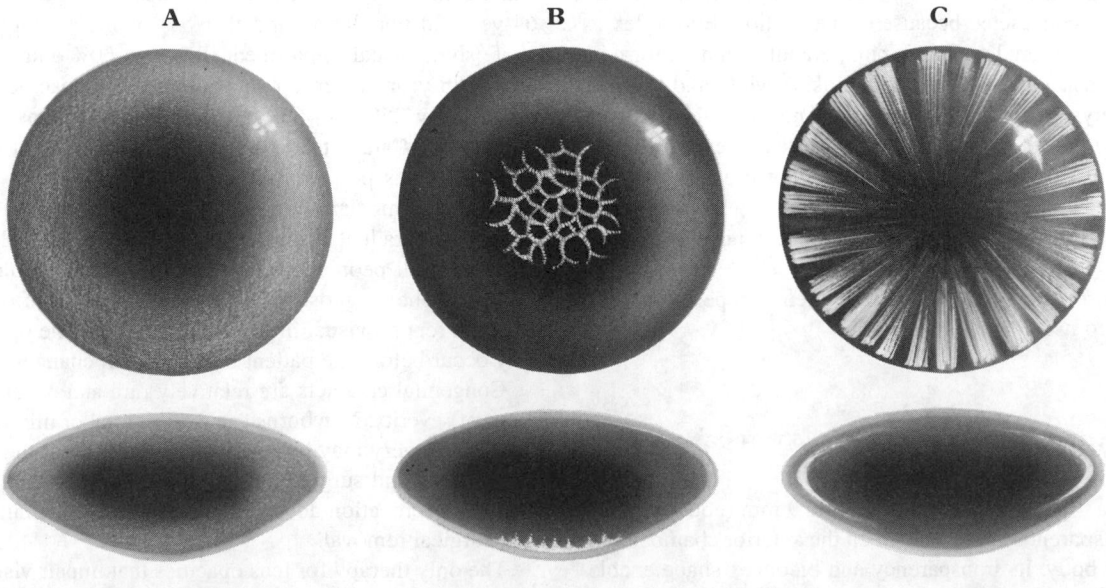

Figure 6-17 Appearance of various types of aging cataracts. **A,** Nuclear sclerosis. **B,** Nuclear sclerosis and posterior subcapsular cataract. **C,** Nuclear sclerosis and anterior and posterior cortical cataracts. (From Newell.[34])

Risk factors other than age have been identified as possible sources for cataract formation. Women over 65 years of age are reported to have a higher rate of cataract formation than men. Some studies have shown that people living in warm, sunny climates have a significantly higher incidence of cataracts. The correlation between cataract formation and ultraviolet light exposure is under further investigation. The lens is susceptible to heat because its avascular tissue does not transfer heat efficiently.

High-dose radiation has been proved to cause cataracts. Survivors of atomic bomb explosions have exhibited a high prevalence of this disease. Study findings of the effects of exposure to low doses of radiation over a prolonged period are not conclusive. Some concern has been raised about computed tomography scans of the skull as a direct source of radiation to the eyes.

Some drugs are reported to be associated with early cataract formation. Corticosteroids, phenothiazines, and some cancer chemotherapy agents are commonly used medications cited in clinical and animal studies.

Diabetes is associated with an earlier onset of cataracts. Young adults with poorly controlled diabetes may rarely exhibit fulminating bilateral cataracts. Sorbitol, a by-product of excessive glucose, is known to accumulate in and damage the lens. Hypertensive patients also have a higher incidence of cataracts.

Blunt trauma (contusion) to the eye may result in opacification of the lens that occurs several months after the injury. If the trauma is invasive, localized opacification occurs as a response to rupture of the lens capsule.

Congenital cataracts may be associated with multiple systemic disorders or other eye deformities, or they may occur in the absence of other signs or symptoms. Maternal rubella in the first trimester often results in infant cataracts that may be accompanied with other signs of deformity. Down syndrome is commonly associated with cataracts, which usually do not progress sufficiently to impair vision. Infants with identifiable cataracts should be examined and monitored for other physical abnormalities, developmental delay, impaired hearing, and mental retardation.[50]

Most infants and children with cataracts do not exhibit enough opacification to interfere with normal vision. If a newborn has dense opacities, surgery is often performed shortly after birth to prevent permanent sensory loss from disuse of the eye. Foveal stimulation must occur in both eyes in the first 4 months of life to allow normal visual development. Long-wearing contact lenses may be prescribed for monophakic infants if the parents are able to manage the care involved. Children with slowly progressive cataracts have a better prognosis for normal binocular vision if surgery can be delayed until 10 to 12 years of age.

Congenital cataracts can be detected at birth if severe opacification is present. Marked density can be seen with gross observation. The newborn normally manifests a full round red reflex when examined with an ophthalmoscope. Lens opacities interrupt the red reflex and require further examination with a gonioscope. In some instances the parent may notice that the infant is not responding visually at home. The family of the affected child should be examined for cataracts.

•••••• Diagnostic Studies and Findings

Cataracts are identified through ophthalmoscopy or slitlamp examination. Visual acuity is measured periodically to assess visual function in both the impaired eye and the less impaired eye.

•••••• Multidisciplinary Plan[31,33,34,44]

Surgery

Surgical removal of the lens   Indications for surgical intervention include diminished visual acuity (by definition of the patient's lifestyle needs), hypermature cataracts that threaten to cause eye damage (glaucoma, uveitis), and the necessity to treat or view the structure behind the lens.

Two procedures are used for extraction: intracapsular and extracapsular. Intracapsular extraction is removal of the entire lens, including its surrounding capsule. An 18 to 20 mm incision is made at the superior limbus arc, and the entire lens is extracted through the incision. A peripheral iridectomy may be performed at the same time. The lens is extracted by forceps or a cryoprobe (which has a low-temperature tip that freezes and adheres to the lens surface so that it can be easily extracted). Chymotrypsin, a protolytic enzyme, is sometimes briefly instilled in the anterior chamber to dissolve resistant zonular fibers in younger patients. Total lens extraction has traditionally been performed on elderly patients. This procedure is no longer common in the Western Hemisphere.

Extracapsular extraction is removal of the anterior portion of the capsule and the lens, leaving the posterior capsule intact. This is the standard in the United States and most of the Western Hemisphere. A 2 to 3 mm incision at the limbus provides access to the anterior capsule, which is mechanically disrupted so the lens nucleus can be removed. The remaining lens cortex is irrigated and suctioned out, leaving the posterior capsule in place. Leaving the capsule in place avoids disruption and loss of vitreous. This method is favored by some surgeons to accommodate placement of a lens implant. The posterior capsule often becomes opaque and has to be opened with the use of a laser. This creates a clear pathway for light to reach the retina, and visual acuity returns to its previous level.[3]

With younger adults, ultrasonic fragmentation (phacoemulsification) is used to disintegrate the lens so it can be aspirated. A rapidly vibrating needle powered by ultrasonic energy breaks up the lens tissue. This method is not used with older adults because the lens nucleus is hardened and resistant to emulsification. The incision for this procedure is only 3 mm. The patient is usually able to leave the hospital the same day, often within hours of the surgical procedure.

The lens can be removed with either general or local anesthesia. General anesthesia is used only when local anesthesia is not possible.[7]

Postoperative care is usually uncomplicated. The patient is ambulatory within an hour. An eye patch may be applied to the operative eye for a brief period or longer if the physician prefers. A metal eye shield is applied to the eye at night for several weeks to prevent accidental rubbing or injury. The postoperative phase requires patient precautions to avoid increased intraocular pressure.

Lens implantation   Lens implantation offers many advantages over the use of eyeglasses and is particularly useful for patients with good vision in the unoperated eye. Binocular vision is rapidly restored, with improved depth perception and good distant visual acuity. The lens implant provides accurate distant vision, and glasses are prescribed to correct near vision difficulties.

Polymethylmethacrylate (Plexiglas), the lens material originally discovered to be nonirritating to the eyes, is still used today. A wide variety of sizes, shapes, and lens placements have been devised and are selected according to the surgeon's preference, the overall condition of the patient's eye, and the cataract extraction method used. The implant is usually placed at the time of the cataract removal, and the limbus incision may have to be enlarged to allow implantation. The two common types of implant lenses are the anterior chamber lens, which rests over the pupillary opening and lodges in the anterior angle and the posterior chamber lens, which is held in position either in the capsule of the lens or sutured to the iris (Figure 6-18).

However, many patients are not good candidates for implantation because of potential postoperative complications. Patients with severe myopia, a history of chronic iritis, retinal detachment, diabetic retinopathy and glaucoma, congenital cataracts, or complications during surgery would not be advised to receive an implant. The rate of surgical complications is reported to be 2% to 5% of implantations performed, and complications include corneal edema, secondary glaucoma, iritis, hemorrhage, retinal detachment, and lens displacement.

Some surgeons believe that implants should be used only if the patient cannot tolerate contact lenses. The long-range dura-

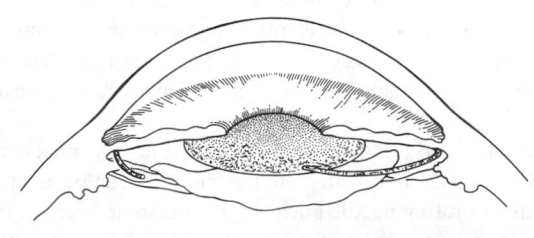

Figure 6-18 A posterior chamber lens located between the iris and the posterior lens capsule. The haptics, the delicate supporting structures, rest either in the remnants of the capsule of the crystalline lens that is still connected by the lens zonule to the ciliary body or in the recess between the posterior iris and the ciliary body. (From Newell.[34])

bility of the lenses is uncertain, and in most instances they are used only for patients over 65 years of age. Some surgeons believe that extended-wear lenses will eventually replace lens implants as methods for the manufacture and use of contact lenses improve.

Medications[34,44]

A wide variety of preoperative and postoperative medications are ordered according to the surgeon's preference, the patient's condition, and the nature of the procedure.

Preoperative

Topical antiinfective agents (usually prescribed 1 wk before surgery)

Gentamicin sulfate (Genoptic, Garamycin), 3 mg/ml, 1-2 drops q4h

Mydriatic-cycloplegic agents (usually prescribed 2h before surgery)

Atropine sulfate (Atroprisol, Isopto Atropine), 1% solution 1 drop

Cyclopentolate (Cyclogyl), 1 drop of 1% solution or 2 drops of 0.5% solution q5min for 15 min.

Hyperosmotic agents

Glycerin (Glycerol, Osmoglyn), 50% solution, 1.5 g/kg body weight, po

Mannitol, IV 500 mg by slow drip

Sedative-hypnotics

Secobarbitol (Seconal), 100 mg po

Antiemetics

Promethazine (Phenergan), 25 mg IM

Narcotic analgesics

Meperidine (Demerol), 50-100 mg IM

Postoperative

Mydriatic-cycloplegic agents (not used with lens implant)

Atropine sulfate 1%, 1 drop bid for 2-6 wk after surgery

Corticosteroids

Prednisolone suspension (Metimyd, others), 1 drop of 0.2%-0.5% suspension qid

Hydrocortisone acetate (Cortef, others), 1 drop of 0.5%-2.5% suspension qid

Analgesics

Acetylsalicylic acid with codeine (Empirin #3), po q4h prn

Acetaminophen (Tylenol), 650 mg po q4h prn

General Management

Corrective lenses should be prescribed for aphakic patients.

The removal of the lens causes a severe hyperopia because of loss of accommodative powers and a marked magnification of visual objects. Adults must receive some type of corrective lens to maintain visual function. Based on the patient's overall condition, the physician performs lens implantation or prescribes contacts. Spectacle correction is reserved as a last resort. Aphakic infants must have corrective lenses to permit development of vision in the first 6 months of life.

Eyeglasses are still prescribed for patients who cannot tolerate contact or implanted lenses. Adjusting to eyeglasses is difficult because image magnification of approximately 30% is still present and peripheral vision and depth perception are obscured. Binocular vision is not possible with a unilateral cataract removal unless contact lenses are prescribed. Corrective lenses are usually bifocal, and the prescription may have to be changed several times over a period of months until the most effective visual correction is attained.

Contact lenses are usually the prescription of choice for adults and infants if the wearer can tolerate them. Increased depth perception, less image magnification (approximately 7%), and binocular vision are attained. Many elderly patients who cannot remove and insert lenses visit a physician weekly and later monthly or quarterly for removal and cleansing of extended-wear lenses and examination of the eyes. Parents of infants receiving contact lenses must be capable of removing, inserting, and cleansing the lenses and monitoring the eyes for complications. For further discussion of contact lens care and precautions see p. 598. A permanent corrective lens can usually be prescribed within 4 to 6 weeks after surgery.

A protective patch is worn postoperatively for 24 to 72 hours. Dark glasses are worn to relieve photophobic discomfort, if the patient's pupil(s) are dilated, and a protective eye shield is worn at night to prevent injury to the eye during sleep.

NURSING CARE

Nursing Assessment

Cataract

Glare at night and in bright light; blurred vision; peripheral vision may diminish before central vision; near vision may improve temporarily (with nuclear cataract); monocular diplopia if central opacity splits visual axis

Advanced Cataract

Pupil cloudy and white on gross examination; total blindness

Aphakia with Eyeglass Correction

Thick lenses; 30% magnification of images; clear vision perceived only when looking through center of lens; diminished and distorted peripheral vision; good near vision; monocular aphakic patient unable to use binocular vision (diminished depth perception)

Aphakia with Contact Lens Correction

7% to 10% magnification of images; peripheral vision intact; monocular aphakic patient able to experience binocular vision (improved depth perception); improved near and far visual acuity; reading glasses may be needed

Aphakia with Implanted Lens Correction

Most often treatment performed today; full binocular vision restored; minimum magnification; peripheral vision intact; improved near and far visual acuity; reading glasses are needed because unlike the human lens, the lens implant can only focus vision at either distance or near (reading); most patients receive implants designed for distant viewing; occasionally, a lens is implanted that corrects to near viewing (e.g., if the patient's occupation is performed with mostly near vision, such as accounting)

Psychosocial

Fears regarding blindness, pain, and surgical procedure

Nursing Dx & Intervention

Sensory/perceptual alterations (visual) related to cataract formation

- Review patient's lifestyle needs and suggest possible alterations *for adjustment to blurred vision or reduced peripheral vision.*
- Assess patient's family and support system *to provide assistance in dealing with visual loss.*
- Review with patient and family safety measures in home and community and necessary lifestyle changes and resultant feelings *to clarify decisions about surgery to remove cataract(s).*

Fear related to anticipation of eye surgery

- Discuss with patient concerns about cataract surgery and correct any misconceptions, such as that the remaining eye will deteriorate faster after surgery or that total immobilization is necessary postoperatively for a prolonged period.
- Assess patient for visual acuity, other physical problems, frailty, knowledge about condition, and available support system.
- Offer support and comfort.
- Orient patient to room and surroundings (if admitted to hospital).
- Describe procedure carefully to patient and family members, including equipment, length of procedure, nature of procedure, and postoperative events, *to reduce fear.*

Risk for trauma related to lack of preoperative measures

- Tell patient to refrain from squeezing eyelids shut or touching eyes postoperatively.
- Encourage older patient to wear glasses during day as reminder not to rub eye.
- Teach patient to avoid heavy lifting, straining, or bending over at the waist *because this might cause dizziness and precipitate a fall.*
- Administer preoperative medications as ordered (antibiotic drops or ointments, mydriatic or cycloplegic drops, ocular hypotensive agents, and preanesthetic medications).

Risk for injury: postoperative complications related to cataract surgery

- Position head of bed at 30° elevation.
- Observe dressing for excessive drainage or bleeding.
- Assess patient for marked temperature elevation or sudden onset of severe pain.
- Report temperature elevation or pain increase to physician *to avoid eye injury from inflammation or increased ocular pressure.*
- Help patient avoid nausea, vomiting, sneezing, coughing, straining with elimination, and touching operated eye *to avoid increased ocular pressure.*
- Help patient to turn to unoperated side.
- Approach patient from unoperated side *to aid in recognition.*
- Help patient walk the night of surgery *to prevent injury.*
- Maintain eye patch in place (usually for first or second day).
- Apply eye shield at night *to prevent injury during sleep.*
- Give postoperative medications as ordered (mydriatic drops, miotic medication [lens implant], antibiotic or steroid drops *to prevent infection,* laxative as needed, and antiemetic as needed).

Sensory/perceptual alterations (visual) related to unilateral eye patch

Before surgery
- Help in measuring visual acuity of unoperated eye preoperatively.
- Have patient's glasses available for immediate use postoperatively.
- Warn patient that depth perception will be lost and 50% of peripheral vision will be lost on affected side.

After surgery
- Help patient with activities of daily living.
- Caution patient to bring hand forward slowly to touch objects (especially containers of hot liquids and containers receiving poured liquids).
- Teach patient to turn head fully toward affected side to view objects or obstacles *to avoid falls.*
- Tell patient to use up and down head movements to judge stairs and oncoming objects and to go slowly.

Pain related to surgery

- Assess patient for postoperative discomfort (which is usually mild) and itching and administer analgesics as ordered *to prevent patient from inadvertently rubbing eye.*

Patient Education/Home Care Planning

1. Discuss with the patient the need to avoid heavy lifting, straining with elimination, and strenuous exercise for 6 weeks because increased intraocular pressure should be avoided until the eye is healed.
2. Alert the patient to wear an eye shield at night for 2 to 6 weeks to avoid injury to the eye.

3. Inform the patient that dark glasses may be worn during the day to avoid pupil constriction and glare associated with mydriatic medication. The eye is sensitive to light after surgery, and tearing or squinting may occur in bright natural or artificial light.
4. Review with the patient the correct procedures for instilling eye drops and ointments and applying an eye shield (without touching or applying pressure on the eyeball) to avoid self-inflicted injury.
5. Discuss with the patient and family that patient's lifestyle must be altered to deal with continued diminished vision in one or both eyes because final prescription eyeglasses or contact lenses take 4 to 8 weeks to attain.
6. Explain to a patient receiving eyeglasses that images will be magnified 30%, peripheral vision will be obscured and distorted, and the lenses will probably be bifocal or trifocal. Therefore lifestyle changes and safety concerns will need to be assessed; for example, the patient must learn to judge distances when descending stairs or viewing oncoming objects and must turn the head from side to side to see the peripheral environment. Several recent studies have shown an association between loss of peripheral vision and driving performance. A few states require some form of visual field testing before awarding or renewing a driver's license, but most do not. The visual acuity testing that is ordinarily performed does not usually pick up peripheral loss. Patients with peripheral loss will need to be evaluated and counseled about their driving potential. Losing the ability to drive is a huge alteration for most people. Follow-up in the form of support is necessary to ensure compliance with the driving ban, continued access to the community, and maintenance of the patient's well-being in the face of this loss of independence.
7. Explain to a patient receiving contact lenses that images will be magnified 7% to 10%, peripheral vision will be intact, and reading glasses may also be prescribed. Therefore the patient must learn to care for, insert, and remove lenses (see p. 598) or arrange to visit a physician routinely for removal, cleansing, and reinsertion of extended-wear lenses (see p. 598).
8. Review with the patient that it will be necessary to adjust to mild magnification when performing daily activities.
9. Alert the patient and family to signs and symptoms of complications to watch for and report; sudden onset of eye pain, redness and watering of eyes; photophobia, and sudden onset of visual changes.

Evaluation

Patient with cataracts has adjusted to visual changes. Lifestyle needs are not hampered by diminished vision. Patient is able to participate in activities requiring near and far vision. Patient understands cause of visual changes and recognizes that further changes will ensue. Patient expresses feeling of self-control in terms of participating in future decisions about cataract surgery. Patient is not endangering himself or herself with activities requiring more vision than patient has, such as driving, venturing into the community without assistance, home maintenance, self-care activities (self administering medication), or working at a job.

Patient with cataract removal has adjusted to visual correction with contact lenses Patient can demonstrate insertion, removal, and cleansing of lens or schedules regular visits to practitioner for lens care. Peripheral vision is intact. Binocular vision is intact. There is no eye pain, further marked visual change, eye redness, lacrimation, or photophobia.

Patient with cataract removal has adjusted to visual correction with lens implant Peripheral vision is intact. Binocular vision is intact. There is no eye pain, marked visual change, eye redness, lacrimation, or photophobia.

DISORDERS OF THE RETINA[34,44]

The retina, the inner lining of the eyeball, is a multilayered extension of the central nervous system that receives images and transmits them to the brain. Lesions or disorders affecting this surface result in altered vision without pain because sensory fibers do not exist in this area. The degree and type of diminished vision depend on the extent and location of the lesions. Central retinal lesions encroach on the macula and the fovea centralis, severely reducing central vision, near vision, and color differentiation. Peripheral (rod) lesions affect peripheral vision, causing isolated blind spots, night blindness, or gradual peripheral loss until the person is reduced to tunnel (or tubular) vision. Retinal diseases can be congenital or acquired through inflammation, trauma, vascular insufficiency, or aging. The diseases vary in severity from total blindness at birth or a slowly deteriorating condition to minor defects that are unnoticed by the person. The cause and cure for many of these diseases are unknown. Photocoagulation can sometimes arrest the pathologic process, but treatment is difficult if the lesion is in the macular area because photocoagulation causes scarring and further vision reduction. Alterations in the configuration of the retina can cause traction, hole formation, and tearing that are surgically treatable.

■ RETINAL VASCULAR OCCLUSION

Occlusion of the retinal artery or vein can cause loss of vision.

•••••• Pathophysiology

Retinal arterial occlusion causes a sudden, unilateral, painless loss of vision. The severity of vision diminishment ranges from total loss with an occluded central artery to a visual field defect that corresponds to blockage of a branch. Emboli associated with atherosclerosis, valvular heart dis-ease, and blood hyperviscosity are among the most common causes. Emboli sometimes form in elderly patients with carotid plaques. Retinal arterial spasms cause transient vision losses that often progress to a permanent loss. Treatment for occlusion must be swift (within 2 hours) to restore vision. Massage of the eyeball (intermittent moderate pressure on the globe) may dislodge an embolus and send it to a more peripheral branch. Evaluation and treatment of the systemic disorder that led to the retinal artery occlusion follow emergency treatment.

Retinal vein occlusion results in a more gradual loss of vision, occurring over several hours in contrast to the abrupt loss with arterial blockage. Venous blockage usually occurs in only one eye, and the degree of vision interruption depends on whether the central vein or one of its branches is occluded. Vein occlusion is associated with systemic vascular disease, venous stasis, arterial hypertension, and blood hyperviscosity. Branch occlusion is more common than central blockage and is sometimes successfully treated with photocoagulation. Photocoagulation does not cure the vascular or systemic disease but deters localized hemorrhage and neovascularization (formation of new vessels). When retinal veins are obstructed, they become engorged and tortuous, and neovascularization occurs in the retina and iris and may extend into the vitreous. The new vessels leak protein and blood. Hemorrhage from dilated veins, retinal edema, and neovascularization may result in anterior synechia formation (adhesions at the anterior angle) and acute glaucoma. Some patients recover from venous stasis retinopathy without treatment. Others respond to photocoagulation. Some patients are left with irreversible visual defects.

•••••• Diagnostic Studies and Findings[34,44]

Direct ophthalmoscopy Venous dilation and tortuosity; arterial narrowing or obliteration; opacities; hemorrhage; microaneurysms; neovascularization; retinal pallor, detachment, breaks, and folds.

Fluorescein angiography Abnormal placement of vessels (crowding, shunts, obliteration); vessel leakage; microaneurysms; neovascularization

•••••• Multidisciplinary Plan[11,14,34,44]

Retinal Artery Occlusion

Surgery

Anterior chamber paracentesis—with patient under local anesthesia, needle is inserted through limbus into anterior chamber; 1 or 2 drops of aqueous fluid is removed to cause sudden lowering of intraocular pressure, which might dislodge embolus

Medications

Anticoagulant agents (may be prescribed in early phases of occlusion)

Heparin, IV loading dose of 5000-10,000 U followed by 5000-10,000 U q4-6h for adult

General Management

Intermittent massage of eyeball—physician applies moderate pressure to globe for 5 seconds, releases pressure for another 5 seconds, and then repeats maneuver in attempt to dislodge embolus to more peripheral branch

Oxygenation—95% oxygen for 10 minutes each hour over period of hours

Evaluation and treatment of systemic cardiovascular dysfunction

Retinal Vein Occlusion

Recovery may be spontaneous, and no curative therapy exists. Therapy is given to prevent further retinopathy in the affected eye and occlusive responses to the other eye.

Surgery

Photocoagulation (see pp. 605 to 606) to burn small or new vessels

Medications

Anticoagulant agents

Heparin, for adult, IV loading dose of 5000-10,000 U followed by 5000-10,000 U q4-6h, followed by bishydroxycoumarin (Dicumarol), 25-150 mg/d as maintenance dose

Acetylsalicylic acid (aspirin), for adult, 200 mg every third day; may be given for antithrombotic effect as preventive measure for remaining eye

Corticosteroids

Prednisone (Deltasone, others), 30 mg qd in divided doses for retinal edema

General Management

Monitoring of eye for increased intraocular pressure

NURSING CARE

Nursing Assessment

Central Retinal Artery Occlusion

Monocular event; sudden (within seconds), painless loss of vision; fovea cherry red in contrast to surrounding whiteness; no pupil constriction response; consensual response present

Central Retinal Vein Occlusion

Usually monocular event; gradual (within hours), painless loss of vision; retinal veins dilated and tortuous; neovascularization; cotton wool patches; visible hemorrhages

Psychosocial

Anxiety

Nursing Dx & Intervention

Sensory/perceptual alterations (visual) related to sudden unilateral loss

- Assess extent of visual impairment.
- Offer support and comfort.
- Keep patient informed of status, progress, and events during emergency care *to decrease anxiety.*

Anxiety related to threat of further visual loss

- Assess patient's level of anxiety.
- Inform patient of related systemic disease and its effect on present and future visual dysfunction *to reduce anxiety.*
- Be realistic in describing health status assessment and prognosis to patient.
- Offer continuing support and comfort to patient and family.

Patient problem: bleeding related to anticoagulant therapy

- Assess patient for spontaneous bleeding, such as hematuria, tarry stools, bleeding gums, or bruising *to determine response to anticoagulant therapy.*
- Observe patient for allergic responses (pruritus, rash, or wheals).
- If medication is continued at home, educate patient concerning dosage, frequency, signs of bleeding, necessity for keeping appointments with physician, drug interactions, and necessity for keeping laboratory appointments for prothrombin time monitoring.

Patient Education/Home Care Planning

1. Review with the patient the systemic disease that contributes to the vascular problem.
2. Explain the degree of visual loss (usually unilateral) and its effect on the patient's lifestyle.

Evaluation

Outcomes vary from a fully restored healthy retina with fully functional vision to total loss of central vision, peripheral vision, or both, with marked retinal destruction.

Vision returns   Vision returns to or approaches previous acuity.

Condition of retina is normal for patient   Appearance of retina returns to normal or shows improvement.

Patient has adjusted to partial or complete loss of vision   Patient is fully informed about present visual status and prognosis. Patient is able to draw on effective support system to supplement self-care. Patient is aware of safety measures to use at home or in the community related to visual changes or loss.

Patient experiences no bleeding   There are no hematuria, bruising, tarry stools, or bleeding gums from anticoagulant therapy.

■ DIABETIC RETINOPATHY[4,25,30,34,40]

■ Diabetic retinopathy is a vascular disorder that occurs in patients with diabetes.

Diabetic retinopathy is one of the leading causes of blindness in the Western world. The prevalence of retinal pathology is directly related to the length of time that diabetes has been present. Newell[34] states that 7% of diabetics who have had the disease less than 10 years have retinopathy, as do 26% of those with diabetes of 10 to 14 years' duration and 63% of those with diabetes for 15 years or more. These figures are estimates because the onset of non–insulin-dependent diabetes is not easily determined. The incidence of retinopathy is increasing as diabetics receive better treatment and live longer. Retinopathy is also related to the degree of control of diabetes in early years of the disease.

•••••• Pathophysiology[34,44]

Diabetic retinopathy exists in all degrees of severity, and the loss of visual acuity depends on the location of the lesion rather than its extent. An early lesion in the central retina (macular area) can obliterate central vision. Multiple scattered lesions throughout the periphery may not affect visual acuity. Clinicians divide retinopathy into background retinopathy and proliferative retinopathy on the basis of severity. Both conditions involve the same lesions of deterioration, but proliferation is marked by the onset of neovascularization and greater tissue destruction.

Initially the venous capillaries lose vascular tone, dilate, and develop permeable microaneurysms that contribute to ischemia and edema of the surrounding retinal tissue. Hard yellow exudates (lipid deposits) form in the edematous tissue as the fluid is being reabsorbed. The remaining retinal veins become dilated, tortuous, and irregular in caliber. Soft deposits (cotton wool patches) also form in response to vascular insufficiency. These small, white, fluffy patches indicate microinfarction in the nerve fiber area of the retina. Hemorrhages within the layers of the retina appear as small red dots that eventually are reabsorbed and disappear. Larger hemorrhages also occur between the vitreous and the retina. Opacities and hemorrhages obscure vision to the extent that they occur in the visual axis. A preretinal hemorrhage might suddenly obliterate vision as it spills into the vitreous.

The formation of new vessels (neovascularization) marks the onset of proliferative retinopathy. A network of fine, permeable vessels, venous in origin, leaks protein and blood into the surrounding tissue, which becomes edematous and opaque in appearance. More hard and soft deposits form in the retina in response to edema and vascular insufficiency. The tiny vessels spread out over the inner surface of the retina and contribute to further hemorrhage and vitreous detachment from the retina. Eventually the vessels and surrounding tissue become fibrous and the vitreous contracts and fully detaches.

The course of retinopathy varies greatly. The pathologic changes may take many years to develop, and the patient may or may not lose functional vision.

Photocoagulation of the vascular abnormalities frequently slows the progress of microaneurysm formation and neovascularization. However, photocoagulation cannot be used in the macular area. Control of diabetes after retinopathy has begun is less effective in reducing retinal damage than careful control at the onset of diabetes.

•••••• Diagnostic Studies and Findings

Indirect ophthalmoscopy   Venous dilation and tortuosity; arterial narrowing or obliteration; opacities, hemorrhage; microaneurysms; neovascularization.

Slitlamp examination (biomicroscopy)   Magnification of lesions

Fluorescein angiography   Vessel leakage; microaneurysms; neovascularization

•••••• Multidisciplinary Plan

Surgery

Photocoagulation (see pp. 605 to 606) to destroy neovascularization sites, prevent retinal edema, and seal small leaking vessels

Vitrectomy—if portion of vitreous is clouded with blood or fibrous membrane, opacities can be removed with fine probe passed through anterior scleral incision; fiberoptic light attached to probe permits direct viewing of vitreous and retina with microscope and special contact lens; cannulated probe cuts and removes vitreous fragments; removed vitreous is replaced with a basic salt solution; simultaneous infusion and aspiration maintain intraocular pressure during surgery; after surgery, gas (sulfur hexafluoride or perfluorocarbon) mixed with air may be introduced into the eye to support the retinal layer in proper position until adequate scar formation creates permanent adhesion of the detached area; silicone oil may also be used as a vitreous replacement; air-gas mixtures are absorbed and replaced by aqueous humor; silicone oil remains in the eye permanently

Medications

For vitrectomy

Cycloplegic agents (prescribed before and for 4-6 wk after surgery)

Atropine sulfate (Atroprisol, Isopto Atropine), 1% solution bid or tid

Topical antiinfective/steroid agent (to prevent inflammation and secondary infection)

Combination of dexamethasone, alcohol 0.1%, neomycin 3.5 mg, polymixin B, 6000 U (Maxitrol), suspension or ointment, 1-2 drops qid for 4 wk

Systemic analgesics

Acetaminophen (Tylenol), 650 mg po q4h prn

Acetaminophen (Tylenol) with codeine (30 mg) po q4h prn

General Management

Vitrectomy

Pressure patch to operative eye immediately after surgery

Ice packs to operative eye as ordered to reduce inflammation and discomfort

For 4 to 5 days, patient must spend most of the time on abdomen or sitting forward with unoperative side of the head resting on a table (to permit air in eye to float against retina); this positioning is not necessary if oil is injected into the eye

Dark glasses worn postoperatively to reduce discomfort from photophobia

Assessment and careful control of diabetes; some think this is more effective in preventing or delaying retinopathy during first 5 years of disease, although this is controversial

The Diabetes Complications Control Trial (DCCT), a national, multi-center randomized clinical trial, proved that tight glucose control reduces the incidence and severity of diabetic retinopathy, heart and kidney disease by 50%[8,23]

NURSING CARE

Nursing Assessment

Background Retinopathy

General Factors

Visual loss may be total, partial, or absent; may not correspond to number or severity of lesions seen; possible complaints of glare; absence of pain; visible retinal changes

Hard Yellow Exudates

Yellow, waxy, confluent deposits that surround microaneurysm area

Cotton Wool Patches

Fluffy, white, soft deposits scattered over retinal surface

Subretinal Hemorrhages

Small, round, red spots, less circumscribed and usually larger than microaneurysms

Preretinal Hemorrhages

Larger, blotchy, red spots

Dilated Retinal Veins

Enlarged and tortuous; may appear "beaded" (irregular in caliber)

Proliferative Retinopathy

Neovascularization

Minute network of fine vessels (often at arteriovenous crossing)

Retinal Opacification

Increased clouding or whitening of area surrounding neovascularization

Vitreous Hemorrhage

Large, red blotches (may obscure much of retina); patient may "see" vitreous hemorrhage as red shower over eyes or multiple floaters, or vision may suddenly be obscured; lesions described in background retinopathy may also be present

Nursing Dx & Intervention[22,44]

Sensory/perceptual alterations (visual) related to bilateral gradual loss of vision

- Assess visual acuity and review ADL that are affected or diminished because of loss of vision.
- Be alert for patient's feelings of guilt about lack of self-care. (Patient may express misconceptions and blame himself or herself for present condition.)
- Devise strategies for carrying out ADL with patient *to maximize patient independence.*
- Assess patient's support system at home, and encourage full use of it.
- Give realistic encouragement for maintenance of independent functioning.

Knowledge deficit related to self-care and monitoring of diabetes mellitus

- Assess patient's knowledge of disease status and self-care practices.

Risk for injury related to self-care and safety threatened by diminished vision

- Help patient to adapt self-care practices to visual handicaps.
- Review activities that require close vision and color differentiation (such as urine testing, reading medication labels [use large print], and administering insulin injections).
- Review patient's support system and encourage full use of it.
- Help patient identify resources available in community for other assistance as needed.

Anxiety related to hospitalization and uncertainty about outcome of vitrectomy

- Assess patient's level of anxiety, which may be increased because of poor vision.
- Assess patient for present visual acuity, other physical problems, frailty, knowledge about condition, and available support system.
- Offer support and comfort.
- Orient patient to room and surroundings.
- Ensure that small personal items are within easy reach.
- Describe procedure and warn patient that one or both eyes may be patched after surgery and that operative eye will be swollen and bruised for a period of time.

- Explain that patient will not be totally immobilized for a long period. Bathroom privileges are usually permitted by second day.
- Inform patient that outcome for functional vision depends on condition of retina.
- Patient should be able to learn his or her visual status from physician (to the extent that physician can offer prognosis).
- Inform patient that decision for using general or local anesthetic will be made by physician.

Risk for injury (postoperative) related to vitrectomy

Before surgery
- Administer antibiotic, cycloplegic eye drops as ordered.

After surgery
- Assess patient's vital signs until stable.
- Be alert for fever.
- Help patient assume and maintain position on abdomen or sitting forward with unoperated side of head resting on table if ordered *to permit air injected in eye to float against retina.*
- If position of head is not stipulated, semi-Fowler's position or side-lying position with operated eye upward is favored.
- Check dressing for excessive bleeding (swelling and serous drainage will exist for first 24 to 48 hours).
- Give postoperative eye drops as ordered (cycloplegic, antibiotic, and antiinflammatory).
- Assess patient for nausea, coughing, excessive restlessness, and disorientation.
- Give narcotics and antiemetics as ordered *to prevent excessive restlessness, bumping head, sneezing, coughing, and vomiting to avoid increased intraocular pressure.*
- Report any signs of upper respiratory infection to physician.
- Encourage patient to do periodic deep breathing *to avoid respiratory infection associated with bed rest.*

Pain related to postoperative status and restricted positioning

- Monitor patient's ocular-orbital-muscle discomfort, and administer analgesic-muscle relaxant as ordered.
- Offer frequent (every 2 to 4 hours) neck and back rubs *to relieve discomfort and muscle tension occurring from prolonged positioning restriction.*
- Provide skin care for knees and elbows; consider sheepskin if at risk for skin breakdown.
- Limit time in elbow-flexed position and with head resting on forearms *to prevent ulnar and radial nerve compression, respectively.*

Sensory/perceptual alterations (visual) related to monocular vision with postoperative eye patch

Before surgery
- Be sure patient's glasses are available for immediate use postoperatively.

- Warn patient that depth perception will be lost and 50% of peripheral vision will be lost on affected side.
- Notify patient that no reading will be permitted while operative eye is patched *to prevent eye movement;* however, watching television may be permitted.

After surgery
- Help patient with activities of daily living.
- Caution patient to bring hand forward slowly to touch objects (especially containers of hot liquids and containers receiving poured liquids).
- Teach patient to turn head fully toward affected side *to view objects or obstacles.*
- Tell patient to use up and down head movements to judge stairs and oncoming objects and to go slowly.

Sensory/perceptual alterations (visual) related to binocular patches

- Assess patient for restlessness, anxiety, depression, or disorientation.
- Keep side rails up at all times *to ensure safety.*
- Identify yourself when entering room; touch patient as you approach and identify yourself and what you are doing *to maintain patient orientation.*
- Put note at door instructing all who enter to identify themselves and explain reason for being there (e.g., cleaning staff).
- Help with feeding and hygienic measures as needed. (Patient may have entered hospital with severely diminished vision and may have some self-care skills).
- Place call bell and all personal articles within reach; have patient locate them with hand.
- Maintain patient's independence as much as possible.
- Describe events and nursing activities as they occur.
- Visit patient frequently and offer back rubs, deep breathing, range of motion exercises, and conversation *to provide stimulation.*

Patient Education/Home Care Planning

1. Maintain the patient's awareness of the diabetic state and self-care needs.
2. Reinforce with the patient the need for regular visual examinations.
3. Ensure that the patient knows to monitor visual responses and changes at home and to report any sudden changes to the physician:
   a. Sudden loss of vision (usually unilateral; loss may be within seconds or persist over a day or two)
   b. Increase in floaters or persistent floaters
   c. Flashes of light
   d. Sharp pain in or around eyes
4. Ensure that the patient is aware of any changes in visual status, especially changes in peripheral vision (as evidenced by running into large objects, "blind" spots on either side of central vision, or changes in ability to differentiate colors).

5. Review with the patient that visual changes may be very gradual (over many years). Give the patient realistic reassurance to help him or her continue an independent lifestyle to the fullest extent and develop ways to adapt to diminishing vision.

6. If the patient has had a vitrectomy:
   a. Cycloplegic, antibiotic, and antiinflammatory eye drops will be continued at home. Review the procedure for administering eye drops, and emphasize the importance of maintaining the prescribed dosage. Tell the patient to wash hands before administering drops.
   b. Tell the patient to avoid constipation (straining), sneezing, coughing, heavy lifting (more than 5 pounds), rapid or jarring head movements, and heavy exercise the first week or two at home.
   c. Watching television or reading is acceptable.
   d. Have the patient make an appointment with the physician for a week after discharge.
   e. Visual function should be restored to the extent that the retina is intact. Tell the patient to review visual prognosis with the physician.

7. If gas or air bubble was injected intraoperatively, caution the patient to secure advice from the ophthalmologist regarding air travel while the bubble is present.

Evaluation

Outcomes vary from a healthy retina with fully functional vision to total loss of central vision, peripheral vision, or both, with marked retinal destruction.

Condition of retina is optimal for patient Changes in retinal appearance are slowed or stopped.

Pain has decreased or been eliminated Patient experiences no pain or discomfort in eye area or in other areas because of restricted positioning.

Patient has adjusted to partial or complete loss of vision Patient is fully informed about present visual status and prognosis. Patient is able to draw on effective support system to supplement self-care. Patient is aware of safety measures to use in home or in community related to visual changes or loss.

■ RETINAL DEGENERATION[34,44]

Degenerative changes in the retina cause a partial or complete loss of vision.

•••••• Pathophysiology

Retinal degeneration may occur because of genetic defects, inflammation, vascular insufficiency, or aging. In many instances the cause of the disorder is unknown; the defect is often familial. Some defects occur at birth, with total blindness, whereas others develop insidiously and lead to severe visual loss. Some degenerative changes only minimally affect vision or are considered harmless. The extent, spread, and location of the deterioration and ensuing lesions determine the effect on visual acuity. Lesions that encroach on the macula often diminish vision dramatically.

Age-related macular degeneration (ARMD) occurs because layers of the choroid thicken and the capillaries of the choroid are sclerosed and deprive the fovea centralis of nourishment. It is divided into two forms: dry (atrophic) and exudative (wet). The onset of dry form is slow, involving both eyes, but deterioration may progress faster in one eye than the other. Near and central vision diminishes over a period of years, but some of the peripheral vision remains intact.[1]

The wet form of ARMD comes on acutely, over a period of days or weeks. It involves serous detachment of the pigment epithelium, followed by neovascularization, hemorrhaging, and eventually scarring of the overlying retina. Photocoagulation destroys the neovascular network and may prevent further visual loss if the macula is not destroyed in the process. Elderly adults (9 out of 10) with macular degeneration experience the dry form with gradual (bilateral) loss of central vision and are eventually classified as legally blind.[12] One out of ten develops the wet form.

•••••• Diagnostic Studies and Findings

Indirect ophthalmoscopy Opacities; hemorrhage; microaneurysms; neovascularization; retinal pallor, detachment, breaks, and folds.

Slitlamp examination (biomicroscopy) Magnification of lesions

Fluorescein angiography Retinal vessel irregularities, neovascularization, vessel leakage, and detached pigment epithelium

•••••• Multidisciplinary Plan

Surgery

Photocoagulation (see pp. 605 to 606) used when degenerative site is not over macula to destroy neovascularization sites, prevent retinal edema, and seal small leaking vessels

NURSING CARE

Nursing Assessment

Age-related Macular Degeneration

Bilateral event (pathologic progress usually not the same in both eyes); gradual diminishment of vision over months or years

Psychosocial

Ability to carry out ADL with level of independent functioning

Nursing Dx & Intervention[22,27]

Sensory/perceptual alterations (visual) related to gradual bilateral loss

- Assess visual acuity and review ADLs that are affected or diminished because of loss.
- Devise strategies for carrying out activities of daily living.
- Refer patients with 20/70 or worse vision to a low vision center to access specialized magnifying devices and other daily living aids for the visually impaired. (For a national listing contact the Light House, New York City.)
- Assess patient's support system at home and encourage full use of it.
- Give realistic encouragement for maintenance of independent functioning.
- See pp. 1643 to 1646.

Patient Education/Home Care Planning

Education depends on the extent of visual changes (usually bilateral) and whether the prognosis indicates that further changes will occur.
1. Inform the patient or family that the patient should have regular visual examinations.
2. Provide full information to the patient or family about visual status and prognosis (realistic reassurance about a gradual loss may help the patient maintain an independent lifestyle).

Evaluation

Outcomes vary from mild to severe loss of vision.

Patient has adjusted to loss of vision   Patient is fully informed about present visual status and prognosis. Patient is able to draw on effective support system to supplement self-care. Patient is aware of safety measures to use in the home or community.

RETINAL HOLES, TEARS, AND DETACHMENT

Retinal holes and tears are breaks in the continuity of the retina. Detachment is a separation of the sensory layers of the retina from the pigmented epithelium.

•••••• Pathophysiology[24,34,44]

The retina is a smooth, unbroken, multilayered surface that attaches to the hyaloid membrane of the vitreous on its inner aspect. The posterior retinal lining (pigmented epithelium) attaches to Bruch's membrane of the choroid layer on its outer aspect. Breaks in the continuity of the retina can occur in the form of small holes caused by degeneration or tearing (tears are ∪ shaped, with flaps over the holes).

Degenerative holes usually occur in the retinal periphery and are the result of retinal thinning that often parallels the ora serrata. Multiple holes form a row of latticework that is fluid filled and covered by vitreous that adheres to either side of the series of holes. Latticework degeneration occurs in about 8% of the population in all age groups, and contributes to about 30% of hole-formation retinal separations. The holes are often missed during general ophthalmoscopic inspection and can be seen only with scleral depression and an indirect ophthalmoscope. Many of these patients are asymptomatic, and retinal detachment does not occur. They are carefully monitored for further degeneration or tearing throughout their lifetimes.

Retinal tears occur most often because of vitreous traction. The vitreous degenerates with age and falls forward, resulting in fluid-filled cavities and collagenous areas that tug on the inner lining of the retina. The vitreous also contracts with fibrous band formations associated with retinal degeneration or diabetic retinopathy. Aphakic and myopic persons are at a higher risk for separation because the posterior chamber space is enlarged, which increases vitreous pull. A tear may be small or large, and underlying tissue bulges through it. Holes and tears may lead to detachment, a pulling away of the sensory retinal layers from the pigmented epithelium. The inner layers buckle or fold into the vitreous.

Holes and tears in the retina do not cause pain. Visual diminishment may go unnoticed unless the retinal break is in the macular area or the tear enlarges over time. Vitreous pull often stimulates a sensation of lightning flashes or bright streaks of light that are momentary and unilateral. The light sensation may be a harmless phenomenon or may signal potential retinal damage. If the retina breaks or tears with vitreous pull, the patient may experience a shower of floaters (black spots or dots) because minute papillary hemorrhages send particles floating through the vitreous within the visual axis.

Retinal detachment occurs because of traction holes or breaks in the retina (rhegmatogenous) or because fluid, blood, or a mass separates the sensory portion from the pigmented epithelium (exudative) (Figure 6-19). Inflammation, hemorrhage, and tumors are common contributors to retinal separation.

Detachment often begins in the periphery and continues to spread posteriorly. The circumferential spread may occur over a few hours or may continue for several years. A relatively rapid separation gives the sensation that a curtain is being pulled over the eyes. A slow separation may offer no symptoms until the macular area is invaded or the person closes the unaffected eye and notes decreased vision in the affected eye.

Examination with an indirect ophthalmoscope shows the detached portion of the retina as a gray bulge, ripple, or fold in contrast to the pink attached retina. If holes or tears are within the examiner's visual range, the choroid layer shows through as a contrasting cherry red spot.

•••••• Diagnostic Studies and Findings[34,44]

Indirect ophthalmoscopy   Retinal pallor, detachment, breaks, and folds

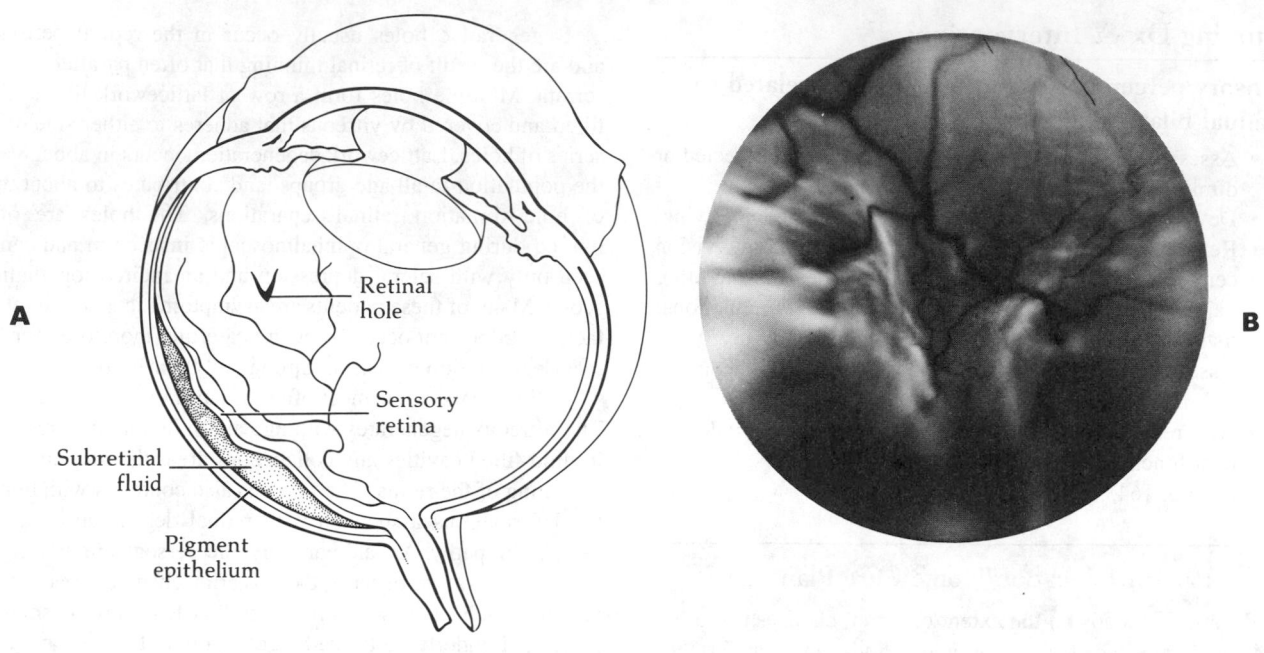

Figure 6-19 A, Retinal detachment with horseshoe-shaped hole in superior temporal quadrant. **B,** Ophthalmoscopic appearance of a retinal detachment. (From Newell.[34])

Slitlamp examination (bimicroscopy)   Magnification of lesions

Three-mirror gonioscopy   Magnified view of retinal lesions

•••••• Multidisciplinary Plan

The use and type of surgical therapy depend on the extent and location of the retinal detachment.

Surgery

Photocoagulation (see pp. 605 to 606)—used to burn and eventually seal localized tears or breaks in posterior portion of eyeball[3]

Cryothermy—frozen-tipped probe placed on sclera directly over area of retinal hole; borders of hole are "frozen," inflammatory response ensues, and eventual scarring seals hole

Diathermy—heat applied by means of ultrasonic probe to scleral surface directly over site of retinal break; resultant burn causes inflammatory response with eventual scarring and sealing

Scleral buckle—sclera indented by means of local implant or encircling strap so it is flattened against retinal tissue that has fallen away from inner surface; conjunctiva pulled back to expose scleral surface; indirect ophthalmoscopy and diathermy probe used to identify areas of detachment; partial thickness of sclera is incised and pulled back to form flaps that eventually hold implant in place; rectus muscles tied with sutures so eyeball can be rotated to expose equator; detached area may be treated with diathermy before implant is put in place; encircling rod or strap often used if multiple retinal holes exist; implant sutured in place, and subretinal fluid drained from site of detachment; air, other gases such as sulfur hexafluoride, or liquids such as silicone oil may be injected into vitreous to flatten detached retina against choroid surface; air or liquid is absorbed and eventually replaced with vitreous fluid

Medications

Adrenergic-mydriatic agents

Phenylephrine (Neo-Synephrine) 2.5%-10%, 1-2 drops instilled for preoperative pupil dilation

Mydriatic-cycloplegic agents

Cyclopentolate (Cyclogyl), 1 drop of 1% solution or 2 drops of 0.5% solution preoperatively and postoperatively; frequency and duration of postoperative dosage vary with degree of inflammation

Antiinfective agents (postoperative eye drops to prevent uveitis complications)

Gentamicin sulfate (Garamycin), 3 mg/ml topical solution, 1-2 drops qid

Neomycin sulfate and prednisolone sodium phosphate, neomycin 3.5 mg/ml and prednisolone 5 mg/ml; frequency and duration of prescription vary according to physician's order, usually 1 drop tid or qid for 4-6 wk

General Management

Postoperative monocular or binocular eye patches (according to physician's preference) to rest eyes for day or two (usually bilateral patches because operated eye may move when unoperated eye moves)

If air is injected into vitreous cavity, head positioned so air bubble will rise and remain flush against detached retinal segment; physician specifies optimum head position and duration for positioning (usually 4 to 8 days); usual position is face down or angled to unoperated side; pillows or rubber or plastic ring used to support head; pillows under abdomen for support

Dark glasses to reduce discomfort from photophobia

NURSING CARE

Nursing Assessment

Visual Symptoms Reported by Patient

Flashing lights (unilateral, may be repeated over a period of days, months, or years); shower of floaters (black dots within visual field); sensation of curtain folding over eyes

Appearance of Retina

Vessels over detached portion dark red in color; holes or breaks within detached area cherry red, in contrast to the grayish area

Nursing Dx & Intervention

Anxiety related to sudden loss of unilateral vision

- Assess patient's level of anxiety.
- Offer comfort, support, and realistic reassurance (about 90% of retinal detachment repairs are successful).
- Inform patient that both eyes may be patched postoperatively *to promote healing.*

Risk for injury related to preoperative status: detached retina

- Supervise limited activities or bed rest as ordered.
- Maintain bilateral eye patches if ordered.
- Keep room dark.
- Keep patient supine.
- Keep side rails up if patient is bedfast.
- Assist with walking and avoid jarring, bumps, or fall *to prevent further detachment.*
- Administer cycloplegic drops as ordered.

Sensory/perceptual alterations (visual) related to preoperative or postoperative binocular-patching

- Assess patient for disorientation and agitation.
- Identify yourself when entering room; touch patient as you approach and identify yourself *to notify patient of your proximity.*
- Instruct others to identify themselves and state purpose of entering room.
- Help with feeding, hygienic measures, and walking as needed.

- Provide frequent sensory stimulation with visits and conversation postoperatively.

Risk for injury related to postoperative status

- Assess patient's vital signs until stable.
- Position patient as ordered. (If gas or air has been injected into vitreous, head position may need to be maintained for 4 to 8 days.)
- Supervise bed rest or limited activities as ordered (bathroom privileges are usually ordered on second day.)
- Keep patient's head parallel to floor when patient is out of bed for brief periods.
- Check dressing for excessive bleeding.
- Report sudden severe pain.
- Assess and document marked swelling and serous drainage, which is present for first 42 to 48 hours.
- Initiate deep-breathing exercises four times a day, if indicated, *to prevent respiratory infection.*
- Administer cycloplegic, mydriatic, antibiotic, and antiinflammatory eye drops as ordered.
- Assess patient for nausea, coughing, excessive restlessness, and disorientation.
- Administer antiemetics as ordered *to prevent elevated intraocular pressure.*
- Avoid excessive restlessness, jarring or bumping head, sneezing, coughing, or vomiting.

Pain related to postoperative status

- Monitor patient's pain (which is usually moderate), and administer narcotics according to physician's orders.

Patient Education/Home Care Planning

1. Inform the patient that cycloplegic and antibiotic eye drops will be continued at home. Review the procedure for administering eye drops, and emphasize the importance of maintaining the prescribed dosage and washing the hands thoroughly before administration.
2. Tell the patient to avoid constipation (straining), sneezing, jarring head movements, and heavy exercise for the first 4 to 6 weeks at home.
3. Inform the patient that television watching is permitted but reading should generally be avoided for the first week (physician will specify).
4. If the patient's occupation is sedentary, work may be resumed after the second week at home (physician will specify).
5. Discuss with the patient the need to be aware of visual changes or sensation and to report sudden loss of vision, severe pain in the eyeball, a heavy shower of floaters, or flashing lights to the physician. (Usually some floaters are seen for a period of weeks postoperatively, but they should be reported.)
6. Have the patient schedule an appointment with the physician a week after hospital discharge.

7. With the patient and physician, review and ensure that the patient understands visual status, including the possibility of recurrence of detachment in the affected eye, ultimate visual acuity and macular damage, and potential for retinal detachment or holes in the other eye.

Evaluation

Outcomes vary from a fully restored healthy retina with fully functional vision to total loss of central vision, peripheral vision, or both, with marked retinal destruction.

Vision returns   Vision returns to or approaches previous acuity.

Condition of retina is optimal for patient   Appearance of retina returns to normal or shows improvement.

Patient adjusts to partial or complete loss of vision   Patient is fully informed about present visual status and prognosis. Patient is able to draw on effective support system to supplement self-care. Patient is aware of safety measures to use in home or community.

Pain is diminished   Patient experiences no pain that is unrelieved by acetaminophen or similar analgesia after discharge from the hospital.

◼ VISUAL IMPAIRMENT (BLINDNESS)

Visual impairment is a state of diminished visual acuity that ranges from low vision (partial vision) to total blindness.

Legal blindness was defined in the United States in the 1920s and 1930s as a means to identify people who could not function in society without official assistance. The legally blind category, still used today, includes individuals with a maximum acuity of 20/200 (with optimum correction) or a visual field that is reduced to a range of 20 degrees (rather than the normal range of 180 degrees). This definition is unique to the United States and does not reflect the universal visual status and complementary needs for visual assistance that people present to the health professions.

The World Health Organization and a variety of experts have attempted to define and standardize categories of visual impairment to serve as guidelines for research and reporting. Table 6-3 is adapted from the International Classification of Diseases, published by the World Health Organization in 1977.

•••••• Pathophysiology[9,10,32,37]

The categories of impairment are helpful to health professionals but still do not incorporate the vast array of visual alterations that must be assessed, managed, or prevented. Regardless of the specific disorder or the degree of impairment, most visual alterations are frightening, immobilizing, and handicapping to an individual. Uncorrected myopia can seriously hamper a person's performance in school. A lack of near vision can

cause the loss of a job. Visual field loss can contribute to an automobile accident or a disastrous fall at home. Even a minor transient incident such as a mild corneal abrasion arouses fear of further visual loss and temporarily incapacitates the individual. Nurses are called on to provide comfort, education, and skilled care whether a patient has a symptom, a specific disease, a concern, or simply healthy vision that can be maintained with knowledgeable health promotion practices. The purpose of this section is to present some of the major causes of blindness or visual impairment throughout the world and to identify the major disorders that are treatable, correctable, and preventable.

More than 79.5 million Americans have a disorder of one or both eyes, not including the millions who have refractive errors. The chief causes of blindness in the United States are retinal degeneration, glaucoma, cataract, and amblyopia. With the exception of amblyopia, most of these diseases are associated with aging and are increasing in incidence as the American population grows older. Laser therapy has helped slow or stop visual deterioration associated with retinal degeneration in recent years. Macular degeneration is still often untreatable, as are some forms of congenital retinal disorders. The DCCT proved the efficacy of tight glucose control in reducing the incidence of diabetic retinopathy by 50%. However, as more diabetic individuals survive early and middle adulthood because of better care, the number of visually handicapped people is likely to increase. At present, about 413,000 people in this country have visual impairments, and 192,500 are legally blind because of retinal diseases. Further research is in progress in the areas of diabetic care, laser therapy, and other forms of retinal therapy. Genetic counseling and research are expected to reduce the incidence of some disorders. Early detection and careful monitoring of a number of systemic diseases, especially diabetes and cardiovascular disorders, will eliminate or slow visual complications. In addition, rehabilitative services for the visually handicapped continue to improve the quality of life for these individuals.

◼ TABLE 6-3 Categories of Visual Impairment

Category	Visual Acuity (with Optimum Correction)	Visual Field Radius
Low Vision Status		
1	20/70	Not defined
2	20/70 to 20/200	Not defined
Blindness Status		
3	Able to count fingers at 3 m; 20/200 to 20/400	Radius reduced to 5-10° regardless of visual acuity status
4	Able to count fingers at 1 m; 20/400 to 20/1200 (5/300)	Radius reduced to 5-10° regardless of visual acuity status
5	No light perception	—

Cataract, another disease associated with aging, is usually treatable with surgery (removal of the lens), and vision is usually restored so the individual can function at least as well as before the surgery. The surgical procedure has become more available and simpler because patients no longer have to wait for surgery until they are severely handicapped and they do not have to endure long recovery periods. The incidence of cataract is increasing because Americans are living longer. One study reported that 18% of the group between the ages of 65 and 74 years showed a decrease in vision to 20/30 or less, and 46% of those between 75 and 85 years of age showed the same effect; in both sets the effect was related to cataract. Yet even with improved and simplified treatment, about 71,500 people in this country are legally blind because of cataract.

Glaucoma is still a leading cause of blindness in this country, but it is becoming less so because detection and early care have enabled people to control intraocular pressure and prevent optic nerve deterioration. Vision screening, compliance with prescribed care, and familial screening and counseling are major issues with this disorder.

Blindness from ambylopia can be prevented with comprehensive eye examination of infants and acuity screening and follow-up with preschool children.[10,32]

The World Health Organization[10] estimates that 10 million people throughout the world are totally blind and that millions more have incapacitating impairments. The leading worldwide causes of blindness are trachoma, leprosy, onchocerciasis, and xerophthalmia. Trachoma, a form of chronic keratoconjunctivitis caused by *Chlamydia trachomatis,* currently affects about 400 million people. It exists primarily in rural areas of the Middle East, Africa, and Asia, where poverty, crowding, flies, lack of sanitation, and malnutrition dominate. It can be cured with sulfonamides and tetracyclines, but if it is not treated, recurrent scarring leads to total blindness. In the United States, the disease exists among Indians in the Southwest and in some rural areas. Leprosy (Hansen's disease) affects about 15 million people throughout the world. Chronic eyelid inflammation, keratoconjunctivitis, and iritis result in granuloma formation and eventual blindness. The disease is treated systemically, and topical rifampin is used with severe corneal involvement. Because international reporting systems are vague, the estimates of the percentage of eye involvement from the systemic disease range from 6% to 90%. The disease is uncommon in the United States. Onchocerciasis (river blindness) is transmitted by black fly bites. Infected larvae are deposited in clear running streams in Central Africa, Mexico, and Central and South America. Microfilariae from the adult female enter the eyes and cause corneal opacification, inflammation and atrophy of the iris, and eventual destruction of the eyes. Treatment is not very effective, and attempts are being made to rid areas of the fly with insecticides. It is estimated that this disease affects about 40 million people. Xerophthalmia (dry eye) is caused by protein, calorie, and vitamin A deficiency. If the cornea is not protected with moisture, it softens, becomes vulnerable to fungal and bacterial invasion, or becomes necrotic. Eventually retinal deterioration and destruction of the optic nerve result in blindness. In countries where malnutrition is common (India, Somalia), infants with this disorder frequently die of infection or pneumonia before reaching adulthood. Supplemental vitamin A (along with antiinfective agents) can reverse early eye complications and prevent blindness.

Besides the most common causes of blindness, other disorders contribute greatly to visual impairment. Corneal diseases and infestations are not the major contributors to blindness that they are in other parts of the world because Americans have better access to a higher quality of care. However, herpes simplex virus is being reported and treated increasingly in the United States. The treatments are partially successful, and new antiviral agents are being explored, but the disease tends to recur or reactivate and threatens the corneal structure. Some corneal problems have occurred because of use or misuse of contact lenses (see p. 598). The cornea is also vulnerable to damage from exposure to toxic agents (in vapor, spray, dust, or liquid form) such as ammonia, butanol, lime and cement dust, some forms of detergents and pesticides, and other concentrated liquid alkalies or acids. People must be educated and counseled about early symptoms of eye irritation or inflammation and measures to protect the eyes.

Safety regulations need to be explored and put into practice to assist the public with eye protection. Protective goggles should be worn in some work settings and while traveling in vehicles in the open air. Some sports activities require eye protection. The scrutiny of children's toys and the laws that some states have passed regulating the sale of BB guns have helped reduce eye injuries.

Many other varieties of eye diseases threaten visual functioning. Most are treatable if detected early and followed by skilled therapy. The American Academy of Ophthalmology's Committee on Eye Care states, "Despite the fact that an increasing number of people seek out and utilize eye care services, approximately a third of all new blindness is potentially avoidable if only Americans had access to or could take full advantage of existing and available technology."[6]

NURSING CARE

Nursing Assessment

Signs and Symptoms for Further Evaluation or Referral

Blurred vision (uncorrectable with lenses; uncorrectable by wiping film from eyes); double vision; sudden loss of vision; alternating dimming and clearing of vision; red eye; traumatized eye; eye pain; loss of side vision; halos (colored rays or circles around lights); crossed, turned, or wandering eye; twitching or shaking eye; flashes or streaks of light; floaters (dots, streaks, or strands, especially in showers or large numbers, or a floater that does not go away); a sense of pressure or "pulling" within the eye; discharge, crusting, or excessive tearing; swelling of any part of the eye; bulging of one or both eyes; difference in size of eyes or pupils

Emotional Reactions

Fear; immobilization (physical and emotional); anxiety; disorientation; altered self-esteem; and altered body image

Chronic Visual Impairment

Possible unsafe living conditions; possible isolation; possible nutritional deficit (related to self-care); possible general ineffective coping (with activities of daily living; earning income; maintaining support system; intellectual stimulation; or recreational activities)

Nursing Dx & Intervention

Risk for injury related to sudden onset of alteration in eye or vision

- Assess eye surface and lid for signs listed above.
- Assess patient for visual symptoms listed above.
- Apply pressure patch or shield (with trauma) *to protect from further injury.*
- Refer patient to physician *to secure medical diagnosis, care, and prognosis.*
- Provide wheelchair, put up side rails, or assist with walking by offering arm for patient's hand *to ensure safety while transporting patient.*

Fear related to sudden onset of alteration in eye or vision

- Assess patient's level of fear.
- Orient patient to surroundings, people in the vicinity, and procedures taking place *to alleviate as much uncertainty as possible.*
- Constantly reassure patient that he or she is being cared for: speak in a soothing voice and use touch as a comfort.
- Avoid lengthy and complicated explanations *to avoid sensory overload.*
- Maintain a quiet atmosphere.

Pain related to traumatic eye injury

- Administer topical analgesic as soon as ordered.
- Apply eye patch after treatment as ordered *to alleviate discomfort from photophobia.*
- Administered cycloplegics as ordered *to reduce painful pupillary constriction.*
- Administer systemic analgesics as ordered.

Risk for infection related to alteration in eye integrity

- Administer topical and systemic antiinfectives as ordered.

Sensory/perceptual alterations (visual) related to use of unilateral eye patch

Before surgery or treatment

- Warn patient that depth perception will be lost and 50% of peripheral vision will be lost on affected side.

After surgery

- Help patient with activities of daily living.
- Caution patient to bring hand forward slowly to touch objects (especially containers of hot liquids and containers receiving poured liquids) *to ensure safety.*
- Explain that patient should turn head fully toward affected side *to view objects or obstacles.*
- Teach patient to use up and down head movements to judge stairs and to proceed slowly *to compensate for loss of three-dimensional vision.*

Sensory/perceptual alterations (visual) related to use of bilateral eye patches

Before surgery or treatment

- Warn patient that eyes will be patched.
- If possible, orient patient to bedside equipment and room arrangement *to avoid or reduce disorientation.*
- Arrange for placement of personal belongings in advance, and review plan with patient.
- Warn patient that side rails will be raised *for safety.*

After surgery (most patients are admitted after surgery)

- Assess patient's level of anxiety and disorientation.
- Reorient patient to equipment (such as call light) and personal belongings at bedside by directing patient's hand.
- If necessary, review immediate past events and procedures with patient *to assist in reorientation.*
- Raise side rails *to ensure safety.*
- Address patient from doorway and identify yourself.
- Complement voice stimulation with touch *to notify patient of your proximity.*
- Help family members and other staff to use vocal and touch approach *to reduce patient's anxiety.*
- Encourage patient to perform self-care with personal hygiene.
- Ensure patient's privacy, and assure patient that privacy is being provided.
- Provide patient with television set or radio *to encourage mental and memory stimulation.*
- Provide patient with clock that can be felt and remind patient of date.
- Help patient with meals. Read menu selections *to encourage patient to eat.*
   Guide hands to utensils and food on tray.
   Describe food on tray in clock terms.
   Help with cutting meats, removing lids from containers, buttering bread, and so on.
- Assist with walking *to prevent injury.*
   Walk slowly and slightly ahead of patient; patient's hand should rest on your arm at elbow.
   If possible, allow patient to trace progress by running the dorsal aspect of his or her free hand along the wall.
   Describe surroundings as you proceed.
   Warn of steps, turns, and narrow passageways in advance.
   Allow patient to feel chair, toilet, or bed before turning to sit.

Decisional conflict related to knowledge deficit of cause of visual loss and ways to prevent further loss or maintain present vision

- Assess patient's knowledge about events and localized or systemic causes for visual alteration.
- Assess patient's level of knowledge about the treatment prescribed.
- Assess patient's capacity and motivation for further learning *to avoid patient education that is not usable* (because of anxiety, inability to take in too much or too complicated information at one time, or because patient cannot read directions or labels).
- Plan to extend elaborate teaching beyond hospital stay *to avoid sensory overload.*

Impaired adjustment related to irreversible loss of vision

- Assess patient's personal reactions to present level of visual functioning.
- Assess patient's reactions to anticipated discharge from hospital and functioning at home.
- Help patient identify specific fears in terms of self-care.
- Provide specific information about visual capacity and changes that will have to be made at home.

Risk for trauma related to self-care at home with impaired vision

- Assess patient's visual functioning in relation to self-care potential (e.g., ability to drive an automobile, maneuver in home, maneuver in community, support system available to assist, access to community).
- Help patient and family identify specific changes that must be made to ensure safety (e.g., driving prohibited, placing furniture in home in familiar locations) *to prevent falls and increase independence.*
- Plan for assessment and counseling beyond hospital stay *to monitor safety and deal with problems as they arise at home.*

Self-esteem disturbance related to irreversibly impaired vision

- Assess patient's feelings about himself or herself in the context of living and functioning with visual loss.
- Assess family's perception of patient's ability to function with impaired vision.
- Identify specific self-care capabilities in the hospital and encourage patient to exercise self-care *to help patient achieve a sense of independence.*
- Encourage patient to make as many decisions as possible about daily routines *to enhance competence.*

Family coping: potential for growth related to acceptance of patient's altered visual status

- Assess family's reaction to patient's altered visual status.
- Discuss family's changed perceptions with family members *to make them more aware of altered behavior toward patient.*

- Encourage family to help patient toward independent living as quickly as possible.
- Recognize that family dynamics will change over a long period of time and that continued counseling should be available.

Patient Education/Home Care Planning

1. Describe the anatomy and function of the normal eye.
2. Describe the alterations in visual function that have occurred.
3. Clarify the prognosis so that the patient understands the time frame and degree of recovery or the degree of irreversible visual impairment.
4. While the patient is in the hospital or clinic teach and help him or her practice self-assistance skills to maximize independence:
   a. Exploring and mapping out furniture, steps, and doorways in the room through guidance and touch
   b. Using another's arm to serve as a guide when walking
   c. Tracing the wall (or rail) with free hand to orient to perimeters of the room while walking
   d. Using a lightweight walking stick when walking alone to identify obstacles
   e. Exploring food, containers, liquids, and utensils with touch before eating
   f. Feeling chairs or toilet before turning to sit
   g. Obtaining assistance for selection of clothing before dressing and approval and support of appearance afterward
   h. Placing articles for grooming and hygiene near bed and arranging them so they can be retrieved whenever patient wishes
5. On discharge, review specific hazards in the home with patient and family:
   a. The patient's room arrangement and living quarters should not be altered once the patient is familiar with the placement of furniture and furnishings.
   b. The patient should proceed slowly and with assistance in exploring living arrangements.
   c. The family must evaluate and maintain living quarters for a clutter-free environment (e.g, loose throw rugs, loose articles on floor or stairways, electric cords).
   d. Exploration of the outdoors must proceed carefully and with assistance (uneven ground, steps, loose gravel, and icy sidewalks are some of the additional hazards of the outdoors).
   e. Exploration of the community must proceed slowly and with assistance.
6. Discuss with the patient and family that progress will be slow; they must allow for frustration and should seek additional support from community or health agencies.

7. Encourage the family to explore the future for increased independence when the patient has made initial adjustments to impaired vision. The state agency for the blind should be contacted immediately upon discharge; this agency can give early assistance and provide support for future concerns (e.g. computer-assisted reading, talking books, time and temperature devices, rehabilitation for future employment, acquisition of new skills).

8. In collaboration with the physician, demonstrate to the patient how to care for eye(s) at home:
   a. Administering drops or ointment as prescribed
   b. Keeping eye(s) free of infection by washing hands, not contaminating dropper, using clean tissues or cloth to wipe eyes, and gently wiping from inner to outer canthus
   c. Monitoring eye(s) for signs and symptoms of infection (pain, itching, redness, swelling, discharge)
   d. Monitoring eye(s) for signs and symptoms of the specific disorder

Evaluation

No injury occurs after alteration in vision   No signs of injury are present during acute phase of visual impairment.

Patient adjusts to visual impairment   Patient reports no signs or symptoms of infection or disease. Patient reports no accidents in the home or community. Patient reports satisfaction with self-care abilities. Patient reports progress with (or mastery of) selected visual handicap aids. Patient reports ability to earn income or is seeking or getting employment training. Patient reports interpersonal relationships are satisfactory. Patient reports resumption of old recreational or diversional skills or acquisition of new ones. Patient exhibits confidence in caring for himself or herself and in relating to others.

Pain is absent   Patient experiences no pain or discomfort from photophobia or pupillary constriction.

Infection is absent   No signs or symptoms of infection exist.

MEDICAL INTERVENTIONS AND RELATED NURSING CARE

CONTACT LENSES

Description and Rationale

Contact lenses are rounded plastic discs that are curved and shaped to fit over the cornea and beneath the eyelid. As methods for producing them improve, they are being used increasingly as a substitute for eyeglasses to correct refractive errors.

Contact lenses, introduced in the 1940s, are available in many forms and serve a multitude of purposes. Hard lenses were originally used to correct refractive errors and high astigmatism associated with corneal irregularities.[44] The introduction of soft lenses in 1971, extended wear lenses in 1981, and disposable lenses in 1990 has expanded the benefits of contact lenses and the indications for their use. Some of the major indications for contact lenses are cosmetic preference over eyeglasses, monocular aphakia, bullous keratopathy, keratoconus, marked difference in refractive error between eyes (anisometropia), active occupation or sports participation, and severe corneal irregularities.

A major concern with all types of lenses is to maintain an adequate oxygen supply to the corneal surface. The cornea receives most of its oxygen from precorneal tears. Contact lenses float on the precorneal tear film and act as foreign bodies that interrupt normal tear flow.

Hard or rigid lenses often cover only the corneal surface (7 to 9 mm in diameter).[34] Blinking action pumps tear fluid under the lens to keep the corneal surface moist. The corneal lens is small enough to shift during blinking so tears can be pumped under the lens and debris can be carried away from the cornea. Hard lens materials have been improved technologically, and most allow permeation of oxygen through the lens. These lenses, called gas permeable rigid (hard) lenses, vary in their percentage of permeability. Hard lenses are still prescribed for correction of marked corneal irregularities because their shape does not conform to the corneal surface as readily as soft lenses and they provide better peripheral vision. Hard lenses can be worn only for a limited time (10 to 14 hours) and are not worn during sleep. They eventually change the shape of the corneal surface and therefore cannot be worn alternately with eyeglasses.

Soft lenses are made of hydrophilic plastics that increase access of fluid to the cornea. They are usually larger in diameter and more easily tolerated than hard lenses and can be worn longer. They are regarded as a medical device and are regulated by the Food and Drug Administration. Soft lenses absorb medications, cleaning solutions, and chlorinated water from swimming pools and gradually release them into the tear film.[34] This can cause local irritation and systemic side effects. Soft lenses are removed every day for cleansing and are not worn during sleeping hours to allow the cornea to recover.

Extended-wear lenses are designed to provide continuous oxygen to the cornea. One type of lens is ultrathin and permits absorption of oxygen through it. The other type is thicker but has a higher concentration of water (70% to 80%), which continuously bathes the corneal surface. Extended-wear lenses can be worn for periods ranging from a few days to several months, depending on patient tolerance, self-care habits, and the patient's eye condition. The effects of extended wear and the development of new materials are the subjects of considerable research. In late 1993 the introduction of daily wear disposable lenses began a movement to change the way people think about contact lenses. New materials enabled the creation of an ultrathin, highly oxygen permeable lens, which can be used for 24 hours and then disposed of for about the same cost as a standard set of contact lenses and the cleaning solutions needed to maintain them for 1 year.

Contact lenses are successfully worn by many people but are definitely contraindicated in some instances. Corneal infection and damage can occur if lenses are not handled appropriately. People who wear lenses must have a clear understanding of how to insert, remove, and care for them. Misuse can result in severe eye damage and loss of vision.

Contraindications

Chaotic or disorganized lifestyle

Lack of motivation to monitor eye responses and care for lenses

Manual dexterity problems or any condition that interferes with daily removal and insertion and lens care (daily-wear lenses can sometimes be replaced with extended-wear lenses that are monitored, removed, and cleaned by a professional)

Poor blinking or lid function

Diminished corneal sensation

Chronic blepharitis or conjunctivitis

Occupation or lifestyle that involves heavy fumes or dust in the environment

High astigmatism (contraindicated for soft and extended-wear lenses)

······ Multidisciplinary Plan[44]

The patient is evaluated for indications and contraindications for lens wearing and the appropriate type of lens. After the lenses are prescribed and fitted, the patient is closely followed for signs of complications. The major complications are corneal abrasion, corneal edema, infection, ulceration, tight lens syndrome, and giant papillary syndrome.

Corneal Abrasions

Corneal abrasions occur when hard lenses are left in too long (overwear syndrome) and drying of the corneal surface results in minute epithelial breaks. Abrasions also form if foreign bodies lie between the lens and the cornea or if the corneal surface is scraped during insertion or removal. A fluorescein stain can be used to identify epithelial breaks. The patient experiences severe pain and usually seeks care immediately. Epithelial abrasions can heal in 24 to 48 hours.

Medications

Antiinfective agents

Sulfacetamide sodium (Sulamyd, Bacitracin, Ilotysin, Neomycin) 10% ointment applied to affected eye before 24-h patching

Anesthetics

Proparacaine (Ophthaine) 0.5% solution, 1-2 drops in each eye, gives relief for 10-15 min (used to facilitate exam; never sent with patient)

Cycloplegic agents

Cyclogyl 0.5%-1% solution, 1-2 drops bid or tid for 24 h

General Management

Binocular tight patches for 24 hours (if patient has someone to care for him or her) or monocular patch on more painful

eye and cycloplegic drops in open eye to reduce ciliary spasm and pain (see above for dosage); reexamination of patient in 24 hours

Corneal Edema

Corneal edema most commonly occurs with soft or extended-wear lenses because of a more gradual oxygen deprivation to the cornea. The epithelium becomes edematous, and vision becomes blurred. There is usually no pain, but slight redness of the eye may be evident.

General Management

Removal of contact lens reverses condition; lens prescription may have to be changed.

Corneal Ulceration and Infection

Corneal ulceration and infection occur if corneal abrasions or edema are not successfully treated. A secondary uveitis may ensue and require intensive emergency care to prevent loss of vision (see pp. 567 to 569 for pathophysiology and interventions). Infection also occurs if insertion, removal, and lens care are not managed hygienically by the patient.

Medications

Antiinfective agents

Sulfacetamide sodium (Sulamyd) 10% or 30% solution, 1-2 drops several times/d for 3-7 d (varies with severity of infection)

Fortified Bacitracin, fortified gentamycin, or other antiinfective appropriate to the invading organism is prescribed

General Management

Cool compresses for discomfort and inflammation for 10 to 15 minutes two or three times a day

Culture and sensitivities laboratory test of corneal and conjunctival mucous and drainage

Tight Lens Syndrome

Tight lens syndrome occurs in soft lens wearers. The lens tends to change shape and become more curved and less mobile over the cornea. The change may take place within hours after the fitting or within several days (with extended-wear lenses). The wearer experiences decreased visual acuity and conjunctival congestion.

General Management

Removal of lens reverses process; wearer may have to be refitted with new prescription

Giant Papillary Syndrome

Giant papillary syndrome occurs after several months or years of lens wearing and manifests itself as a cobblestone-appearing inflammation of the inner lining of the upper lid. Redness, tearing, and discharge accompany the tissue inflammation. The cause is unknown, and the treatment is removal of the lens.[44]

NURSING CARE

Nursing Assessment[34,44]

Corneal Abrasion (Epithelial)

Moderate to severe pain; blurred vision; halo seen around lights; generalized hyperemia; lacrimation; fluorescein stains (green) on corneal surface; patient unable to open eyes (because of pain)

Corneal Edema

Blurred vision; absence of pain; dull appearance of cornea; slightly reddened conjunctiva

Corneal Ulceration

Ulcers varying in appearance and size; severe pain associated with epithelial damage; iritis; lacrimation and possible purulent discharge; generalized hyperemia

Localized Infection

Purulent discharge; generalized hyperemia; moderate discomfort; possible photophobia; crusting around lids; eyes may be "stuck together" in morning (or on awakening); complaints of blurred vision (because of excessive exudate over eye surface), which disappears with blinking

Tight Lens Syndrome

Eye discomfort; decreased visual acuity (onset may be sudden [within hours] or more gradual); patient unable to remove lens; conjunctival congestion with some redness

Giant Papillary Syndrome

Slow onset over months or years; lacrimation; conjunctival redness; discharge may be present

Nursing Dx & Intervention

Knowledge deficit related to care of contact lenses

- See under Patient Education for specific instructions.
- Deficit exists with new prescription or if medical problems arise after lenses are fitted.

Risk for injury related to epithelial damage to cornea with potential for stroma injury

- Assist with identification of epithelial breaks with fluorescein stain as ordered.
- Instill medications as ordered, such as topical antibiotics and cycloplegic drops.

Pain related to corneal epithelial damage

- Apply pressure bandage to eye(s) as ordered, being certain that covered eye is closed *to reduce blinking and eye movement.*
- Apply topical anesthetic as ordered *to reduce pain.*
- Apply cool compress as ordered for 10 to 15 minutes *to reduce inflammation or discomfort.*
- Administer systemic analgesic as ordered and document response.
- Discourage patient from reading *to reduce eye movement.*

Sensory/perceptual alterations (visual) related to total loss of vision with binocular patches

- Raise side rails *to ensure safety.*
- Address patient by name from doorway, and identify yourself and reason for presence.
- Complement voice stimulation with a touch *to notify patient of your proximity.*
- Orient patient to bedside equipment (such as call light, bed control, and side rails) and personal belongings at bedside by directing his or her hand over objects.
- Encourage patient to perform self-care with personal hygiene *to maximize independence.* Provide support and supervision.
- Provide privacy, and assure patient that privacy is provided.
- Help with meals *to ensure adequate intake.*
  Read menu selections.
  Guide hand to utensils and food on tray.
  Describe food on tray in clock terms.
  Assist with cutting meat, removing lids from cartons, and so on.
- Help with walking *to prevent injury.*
  Walk slowly and slightly ahead of patient with patient's hand resting on your arm at your elbow or on your shoulders.
  If possible, allow patient to trace progress by running the dorsal aspect of his or her free hand along the wall.
  Describe surroundings as you proceed.
  Allow patient to feel chair, toilet, or bed before turning to sit.
- Visit frequently to be certain patient is sufficiently stimulated *to avoid withdrawal.*
- Be certain that someone wil be at home to supervise patient's activity after discharge.
- Review above safety and comfort measures with caretaker.

Sensory/perceptual alterations (visual) related to blurred vision with corneal edema or tight lens

- Assure patient that condition is temporary.
- Review activities of daily living (such as driving, preparing food, housekeeping, personal hygiene, toileting, and maneuvering around house) and responsibilities at work *to be certain that they can be performed safely by patient or with assistance from someone else.*

Patient Education/Home Care Planning[34,44]

1. Caution the patient to wash hands and dry well before inserting and removing lenses.
2. Explain to the patient that eyelashes and face should be thoroughly cleansed before lenses are inserted.
3. Inform the patient that instructions for care and follow-up should be carried out meticulously.
4. Explain the care of hard contact lenses.
   a. Encourage the patient to monitor himself or herself for sudden onset of pain, excessive eye redness, sudden decrease in vision, mucus discharge, or foreign body sensation. Tell the patient to remove the lenses and report to the physician.
   b. Inform the patient that adjustment to new lenses may take 2 to 3 weeks and that mild photophobia, tearing, and lid edema may occur.
   c. Inform the patient that hard lenses are not recommended for wearing alternately with glasses or on a part-time basis after initial adjustment and that wearing time will increase to 10 to 14 hours after the adjustment period.
   d. Inform the patient that hard lenses should not be worn when engaging in contact sports.
   e. Tell the patient that lenses must be removed at night or before sleeping.
   f. Explain that lenses must be cleaned after each removal according to the manufacturer's directions and stored in their case.
   g. Explain that the lens is wetted with an approved wetting solution before being placed over the cornea.
   h. Review the insertion and removal procedure with the patient and have the patient demonstrate it to ensure competence.
   i. Inform the patient of the importance of consistently applying one lens before the other to avoid mixing the lenses. If vision is blurred immediately after application, the lenses may be reversed.
   j. Tell the patient to check the lenses daily for scratches, tears, loose debris, or clouding. Tell the patient to report to the physician if unable to wash the lenses clear.
   k. Emphasize the need to keep appointments with the physician. Eyes may change shape, or refractory error may cause changes. Lenses should be replaced regularly (usually every 1 to 2 years).
5. Explain the care of soft and extended-wear lenses.
   a. Encourage the patient to monitor himself or herself for sudden onset of pain, excessive eye redness, sudden decrease in vision, mucus discharge, or foreign body sensation. Tell the patient to remove the lenses and report to the physician.
   b. Inform the patient that the adjustment time for soft lenses is usually shorter and involves less eye irritation than with hard lenses.
   c. Inform the patient that soft lenses are less likely to pop out.
   d. Tell the patient that soft lenses can be alternated with glasses.
   e. Caution the patient not to wear soft lenses while swimming, applying eye medications, or using hair or body sprays because soft lenses absorb chemicals easily.
   f. Explain that soft lenses are usually removed at night and that the wearing time will increase to 12 to 14 hours after adjustment time.
   g. Tell the patient that lenses must be cleaned after each removal according to the manufacturer's instructions and stored in a specified solution. Soft lenses should not be permitted to dry out.
   h. Explain that the storage solution must be changed as directed.
   i. Inform the patient that soft lenses are fragile and can be damaged by exposure to makeup, creams, or mascara or nicked by fingernails.
   j. Tell the patient that lenses should be checked daily for scratches, tears, loose debris, or clouding. Tell the patient to report to the physician if unable to wash the lenses clear.
   k. Explain that the lens must be wetted with an approved wetting solution before being placed in the eye.
   l. Review the insertion and removal procedure with the patient, and have the patient demonstrate it to ensure competence.
   m. Inform the patient of the importance of consistently applying one lens before the other to avoid mixing the lenses. If vision is blurred immediately after application, the lenses may be reversed.
   n. Stress the need to keep appointment with the physician because the eyes and lenses should be checked regularly.

Evaluation

Cornea is healthy Cornea is clear and glossy without eye discomfort, redness, or discharge.

Contact lenses are successfully worn Visual acuity is 20/20 OD, OS, and OU. Near vision is clear at 14 inches.

Patient is aware of high risk for injury with lenses Patient can verbalize the need to care for lenses properly; no signs or symptoms of infection, corneal damage, or lack of proper fit are present.

ENUCLEATION

Description and Rationale

Enucleation, or surgical removal of the eyeball, is performed when other treatment of the eyeball is insufficient to prevent pain, disfigurement, or spread of malignant disease. Indications include severe infections, malignancies such as melanoma and retinoblastoma, large and infiltrating tumors, extensive trauma to the eye, blindness when severe eye pain is also present, and end-stage glaucoma, when the patient is blind with no light perception and has increased intraocular pressure. Enucleation may also be performed as a prophylactic measure when sympathetic ophthalmia is likely to occur. Sympathetic ophthalmia is a rare granulomatous inflammation that usually develops within 3 months of an injury to one eye and involves the entire area. The injured eye is called the exciting eye, and the other eye (the sympathizing eye) can also become inflamed with uveitis unless the exciting eye is enucleated before the inflammation spreads.

Enucleation can be performed with the patient under local or general anesthetic. During surgery a 360-degree peritomy is performed at the limbus, opening the conjunctiva and allowing Tenon's fascia to be separated between the rectus muscles. The rectus muscles are separated, hooked, and cut with scissors near their insertion into the sclera. The inferior oblique muscle and superior oblique tendons are hooked and cut, the medius rectus muscle is clamped, and enucleation scissors are placed between the sclera and Tenon's capsule. The optic nerve is then cut as far behind the globe as possible, and the eye is removed. After adequate hemostasis is obtained at the socket, the muscles may be sutured to each other around a plastic or the muscles may be sutured to each other around a plastic or Teflon sphere to build up the eye and provide a more acceptable cosmetic appearance.

After the enucleation a "conformer" is placed in the socket until postoperative edema subsides and an artificial eye can be placed, usually 10 to 14 days after enucleation.

Two relevant surgical procedures are evisceration and exenteration. In evisceration the entire contents of the eyeball and sometimes the cornea are removed but the sclera remains. This procedure may be used when panophthalmitis, an inflammation of the entire inner eye including the sclera, is present. Exenteration is a more radical procedure in which the eyelids, eyeball, and orbital contents are removed, usually in cases of malignancies of the lacrimal gland, extension of eyelid malignancies in the orbit, malignant melanoma of the conjunctiva, or melanoma or retinoblastoma that has invaded the orbit.

Contraindications and Cautions

Panophthalmitis is a contraindication to enucleation because the risk of postoperative meningitis is increased after removal of an actively infected eyeball.

•••••• Multidisciplinary Plan

Surgery

Removal of the eyeball as described previously

Medications

Narcotic-analgesic agents
Meperidine (Demerol), 50-75 mg IM q4-6h prn for severe pain

Acetaminophen with codeine (Tylenol with Codeine), 30-60 mg po q4-6h prn for less severe pain

General Management

Firm pressure dressing applied to operative site for 24 to 48 hours
Activity progression without restrictions as tolerated
Progressive diet as tolerated

NURSING CARE

Nursing Assessment

Eye Socket

Pain at enucleation site; headache on side of enucleation; no fever or bleeding

Nursing Dx & Intervention

Pain related to surgical intervention

- Administer pain medications as ordered by physician and document response.
- Notify physician if pain or headache persists *because this may indicate infection.*
- Notify physician if temperature is elevated *because this may indicate infection.*

Risk for injury related to postoperative bleeding

- Assess dressing at operative site frequently for signs of oozing or frank bleeding.
- Document absence of blood or amount if present.
- Maintain firm pressure dressing at operative site until removal is ordered by physician.
- Monitor and document patient's vital signs according to protocol, and report any change in pulse and blood pressure.

Sensory/perceptual alterations (visual) related to enucleation procedure

- Help patient walk as tolerated *to avoid injury.*
- Ensure that patient's call light and personal belongings are close by on unaffected side.
- Help patient with meals as needed *to ensure adequate caloric intake.*

Body image disturbance related to loss of eye

- Assess patient for depression and anxiety.
- Assure patient that appearance will be normal when patient is fitted with artificial eye and that satisfactory visual adjustment usually occurs.
- Listen to patient's fears and concerns in comforting, supportive manner.
- Assure patient that period of depression is normal after procedure such as removal of eye.

Evaluation

There is no infection or pain Patient and family demonstrate ability to care for eye socket and artificial eye after discharge from hospital. Patient verbalizes signs and symptoms of possible infection: pain, headache, drainage, and elevated temperature.

Body image is adequate Patient is fitted with and wears artificial eye, if appropriate, after discharge from hospital, to improve appearance. Patient verbalizes understanding of need for eye removal and expresses concerns and frustrations regarding disease process and body image.

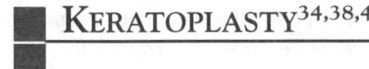

KERATOPLASTY[34,38,44]

Description and Rationale

Keratoplasty, or corneal transplant, is the excision of corneal tissue and its replacement by a cornea from a human donor.[34] This procedure may be performed to replace a corneal opacity, which is a lack of corneal transparency resulting from injury or inflammation, or to correct a variety of corneal abnormalities called corneal dystrophies. Certain bilateral hereditary disorders may be present at birth but usually develop during adolescence and progress through adulthood. Some do not affect vision, but many do. The success of corneal transplantation as a treatment for these dystrophies depends on the type and extent of the corneal abnormality. The dystrophy may possibly recur in the donor graft. One of the dystrophies for which keratoplasty is particularly successful is keratoconus, a condition in which the symmetric curvature of the cornea is distorted by an abnormal thinning and forward bulging of the central portion of the cornea. A penetrating corneal transplant restores useful vision with a 95% success rate.[34] Corneal perforation, which is usually a complication of a corneal ulcer, is a serious condition that may destroy vision if not treated rapidly. Keratoplasty may be performed if there is imminent danger of perforation of a corneal ulcer.

There are two types of keratoplasty: lamellar and penetrating. Lamellar or nonpenetrating keratoplasty is a partial-thickness graft in which the surgeon removes and replaces a superficial layer of cornea without entering the anterior chamber. In a penetrating keratoplasty the entire thickness of cornea is removed and replaced by donor corneal tissue. This is the traditional type of keratoplasty and can be either complete or partial, depending on whether the entire cornea is excised.

Donor eyes are obtained from cadavers of noninfected people who have died as a result of injury or acute disease or from patients whose eyes have been surgically removed for some reason but whose corneas are normal. Ideally the donor is between 25 and 35 years of age. Corneas should not be used from patients who were ill for a long time before death or who had such diseases as leukemia, sepsis, hepatitis, HIV positivity, or certain tumors of the eye.

If it is known when a patient dies that the eyes are to be donated, the lids should be closed and covered with small ice bags. Nothing should touch the corneas themselves. The donor eyes should be enucleated within an hour after death, but up to 5 hours is acceptable if ice bags have been placed on the eyes at death. Ideally corneas are transplanted into the recipient immediately after removal, but many eye banks can now safely store corneas for longer periods. Whole eyes can be stored from 24 to 48 hours if refrigerated; corneal tissue can be kept longer if removed with a 3 mm rim of scleral tissue attached. Corneas must not be folded during storage, because this damages the endothelium. They must be stored at a temperature of 4° C (39° F) in a modified tissue culture medium.[34]

Transplantation is usually performed with the patient under topical and retrobulbar anesthesia. The surgeon removes the cornea from the donor's eye with a trephine and then removes the impaired areas from the recipient eye using another trephine the same size or slightly larger. The donor cornea, called the donor button, is sutured into place with continuous or interrupted sutures to align and graft and ensure a watertight wound (Figure 6-20).

Contraindications and Cautions

Light perception and projection must be normal before surgery will be considered.

There is the possibility that some corneal dystrophy will occur in the transplanted cornea.

Corneal graft rejection may occur. This starts 3 weeks or more after keratoplasty and is limited to the donor cornea, since there are no blood vessels or lymphatics to sensitize the recipient. The inflammatory process begins at the graft margin and spreads to involve the entire graft.

•••••• Multidisciplinary Plan

Surgery

Lamellar or penetrating keratoplasty as described previously

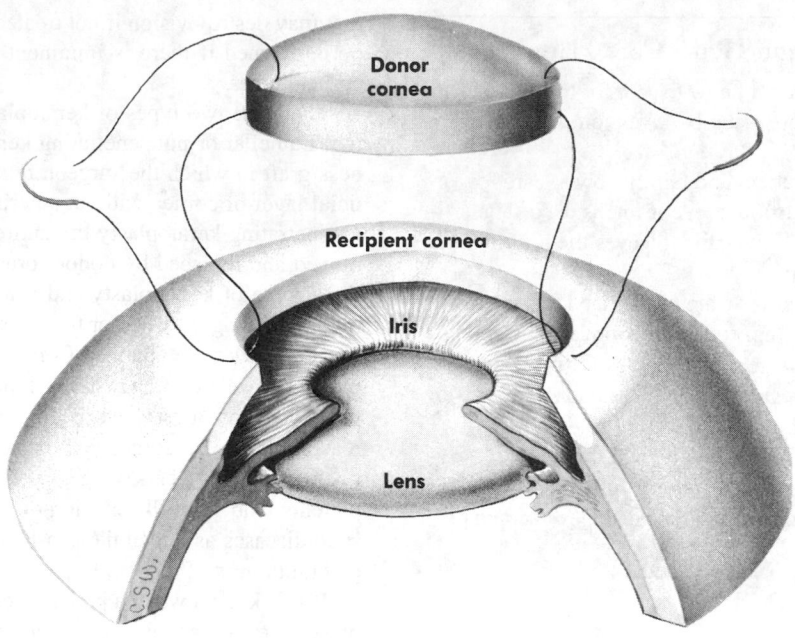

Figure 6-20 The excised portion of the cornea is being replaced with a clear donor cornea in a partial penetrating keratoplasty. (From Newell.[34])

Medications

Narcotic analgesic agents
    Meperidine (Demerol), 50-100 mg IM q4h for pain
Antiemetic agents
    Prochlorperazine (Compazine), 25 mg by rectum bid or 5-10 mg IM q4-6h for nausea
Corticosteroids
    Pred-Forte eye drops, 1 drop qid
Laxatives
    Docusate sodium (Colace), 240 mg to prevent straining during bowel movement

General Management

Unilateral eye patch for 24 hours
Activity and diet progress as tolerated

NURSING CARE

Nursing Assessment

Cornea

Wound edema; inflammation; photophobia; decreased vision; clouding caused by vascularization as result of graft rejection

Nursing Dx & Intervention

Sensory/perceptual alterations (visual) related to unilateral eye patch

- Ensure that eye patch remains securely in place for at least 24 hours.
- Help patient with walking postoperatively because patient may be unsteady and must be prevented from falling and injuring eye.
- If the patient stays in the hospital overnight, ensure that call light is in place, side rails are up, and items at bedside are in familiar place for patient *to ensure safety.*
- Administer eye drops, as ordered by physician.

Pain related to surgical intervention

- Administer pain medication as ordered, particularly on first postoperative night if the patient remains in the hospital, *to decrease discomfort and promote rest and healing of eye.*

Risk for injury related to potential increase in IOP causing displacement of graft

- Institute measures designed to prevent increases in intraocular pressure that might push healing graft forward.
- Administer antiemetics as ordered *to prevent vomiting.*
- Encourage patient not to cough but to breathe deeply often *to increase lung expansion.*

- Avoid using any material that may cause sneezing: talcum powder, perfumes, room sprays, or pepper on meal trays.
- Instruct patient not to lean over, lift, or push heavy objects and to avoid straining when having a bowel movement *to avoid increased intraocular pressure.*

Patient Education/Home Care Planning

1. Review with the patient the need to prevent increases in intraocular pressure because eye tissue requires more time to heal than other tissue. Warn the patient to avoid extreme exertion or emotion, sudden jerky movements, lifting or pushing heavy objects, or straining at stool.
2. Discuss with the patient that the sutures will remain in the eye for as long as a year to ensure adequate healing.
3. Discuss with the patient that the photophobia experienced after surgery will gradually decrease, that vision will slowly improve, that dark glasses may be worn, if needed, and that further correction with eyeglasses may be necessary.
4. If the patient is discharged with eye drops, ensure that the patient or family can demonstrate the appropriate technique of instillation.
5. Review with the patient and family the signs and symptoms of graft rejection (inflammation, clouding, drainage, and pain at graft site), and tell them to notify the physician immediately so treatment can begin promptly.

Evaluation

Corneal graft heals adequately   Wound edema and inflammation dissipate. Photophobia decreases. Vision improves slowly. No evidence of graft rejection occurs. No injury is caused to the graft from increase in intraocular pressure.

Pain is absent   No pain is experienced after graft heals.

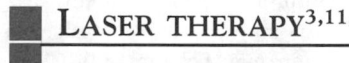

LASER THERAPY[3,11,44]

Description and Rationale

The word "laser" is an acronym for *l*ight *a*mplification by *s*timulated *e*mission of *r*adiation. Experimentation with the effect of light on the retina began in the 1800s after the invention of the ophthalmoscope, when ophthalmologists began noticing solar burns in patients' eyes after solar eclipses. Early investigators used the effects of the sun or the carbon arc to produce a lesion in the retina. Since that time, research with laser therapy has refined and broadended its use, and lasers are now the treatment of choice for a wide variety of ophthalmic disorders.

Ophthalmic lasers differ by the type of energy they create and the color(s) they are able to emit. Interestingly, over time and with research, we have come to use specific colors in the light spectrum to treat specific ophthalmic disease and conditions. For example, an early study compared the effects of blue/green light to green light in the treatment of diabetic retinopathy. Green light created by argon gas is now the color of choice for most laser treatments for diabetic retinopathy.

Lasers in ophthalmology create energy by photocoagulation, photoradiation, photodisruption, or photovaporization. Laser treatment is not selective; it is unable to discriminate healthy tissue from diseased tissue. Also, it destroys the treated tissue and creates a small but permanent scar. Therefore most ophthalmic laser treatments are aimed at stabilizing vision and preventing further vision loss.

Photocoagulation occurs when light is absorbed by pigment and converted into heat energy. This can be likened to a sunburn of the skin. When the sun's rays are absorbed by the melanin in skin, they are converted into heat energy. If the heat created is strong enough or long lasting, a burn of the skin results. The iris, retina, and choroidal layers of the eye are heavily pigmented and usually photocoagulate easily.

Photoradiation laser therapy uses a photosensitizing drug in conjunction with a laser. The photosensitizing drug is injected intravenously 24 to 48 hours before the patient is exposed to laser light. The dye is absorbed by abnormal cells like those in ocular malignant melanomas or in basal cell carcinomas of the ocular and head area. The tumor areas are exposed to laser light that excites the dye in the abnormal cells, resulting in destruction and necrosis of the abnormal tumor tissues.

Photodisruption is the term used to describe the effect of the neodymium:yttrium-aluminum-garnet (Nd:YAG) laser. This white laser light is aimed at the target tissue extremely precisely. When the light impacts the tissue, small explosions occur on the surface that eventually disrupt the tissue and create a hole or opening. This technique is most commonly performed on patients who have had cataract surgery. At the time of primary extracapsular cataract surgery the posterior lens capsule is left intact. This provides support for the vitreous jelly and retina and is proven to lower the incidence of retinal detachments in postcataract patients. However, approximately 6 months to 2 years after surgery this capsule, which is clear at the time of surgery, becomes cloudy or opaque to light, and patients note a loss in visual acuity. The Nd:YAG laser is used to "blast" an opening in the center of this capsule, re-creating a clear pathway for light. This usually results in a sudden and dramatic improvement in visual acuity. It is one example where laser treatment does result in visual improvement rather than a stabilization of vision and prevention of further loss.

Photovaporization therapy is the use of carbon dioxide laser radiation to vaporize malignant intraocular and extraocular tumors in a precise manner. When repeated surface impacts are made with the carbon dioxide laser, carbon dioxide radiation is highly absorbed by ocular tissue, with almost complete absorption and conversion to heat within a tissue depth of 100 μm.[3]

Laser therapy provides a nonsurgical approach to many ophthalmic disorders and can usually be performed on an outpatient basis. The goal of most ophthalmic laser therapy is to stabilize vision and to prevent further visual loss. It offers hope to patients with diabetic retinopathy and glaucoma.

Two types of laser treatments are performed for the treatment of diabetic retinopathy. Panretinal photocoagulation (PRP) treatment is the application of several thousand laser spots or burns to the peripheral areas of retina. The laser burns create scars, destroying the retinal tissue where it is applied. The macular area is spared to maintain central vision. Theoretically, abnormal blood vessels, which occur in diabetic retinopathy and threaten vision by hemorrhaging or causing traction retinal detachments, regress after laser therapy because they are perceived by the body as no longer needed. The goal of the treatment is to sacrifice some areas of retinal tissue to spare and protect central vision.

Focal laser treatment is performed for diabetic persons whose blood vessels are leaking fliud and plasma into the retina, creating edema and blurring central vision. A localized application of laser spots is aimed directly at the leaky blood vessels to seal them closed, preventing additional leakage. In approximately 2 months the remaining fluid is absorbed and the macular area dries out. Vision usually does not improve after focal laser therapy; however, if diabetic-related edema is identified early, when vision is minimally affected, good stabilization is usually accomplished, as well as no further vision loss.

Photocoagulation has also become useful in the treatment of glaucoma to control intraocular pressure. A procedure called laser trabeculoplasty can control pressure successfully in about 85% of cases, especially in eyes with wide angles and slight pigmentation of the trabecular meshwork.

Laser therapy is also useful in treating chronic primary closed-angle glaucoma. The aim of therapy is to prevent the pressure in the posterior chamber from exceeding that of the anterior chamber by creating an opening that eliminates the accumulation of aqueous humor in the posterior chamber. The surgeon performs a laser iridotomy in which a localized area of the midperipheral iris is caused to bulge forward by means of mild laser burns. The central portion of this area is then perforated by laser burns of much higher energy. Many applications of the beam may be necessary.[3]

Contraindications and Cautions

Before photocoagulation therapy each segment of the eye must be closely examined for factors that would diminish the effectiveness of therapy.

NURSING CARE

Nursing Assessment

Vision

Constriction of peripheral fields; temporary decrease in central vision; slight decrease in night vision; headache from bright laser light; pain unrelieved by acetaminophen

Nursing Dx & Intervention

Decisional conflict related to lack of information about laser procedure

- Explain purpose of laser therapy.
- Assure patient that procedure causes little pain and that topical anesthetic (eye drops) wil be administered *to alleviate anxiety related to fear of pain.*
- Describe the procedure to the patient and the family. Explain that patient will be awake and sitting up in a chair and may have special contact lens placed on eye.
- Describe bright lights caused by laser beam that patient will see during procedure.
- Explain that procedure may take 15 to 40 minutes.
- Tell patient that family member or friend should accompany patient and drive home *because patient's eyes will be dilated and vision may be temporarily blurred.*

Pain related to laser treatment

- Explain to patient that headache may develop after treatment because of bright laser light. Suggest acetaminophen *to relieve discomfort.* Warn patient not to use aspirin for 24 hours after the procedure *because of its anticoagulant effect.*

Patient Education/Home Care Planning

1. Emphasize the importance of not increasing the venous pressure in the head, neck, and eyes, particularly with Valsalva's maneuver. Instruct the patient to keep the head up and to move slowly and not to bend over or make sudden movements.
2. Caution the patient not to lift anything heavier than 5 pounds and not to strain for any reason, as when having a bowel movement, for 24 hours after the procedure. Encourage the patient to take a stool softener to avoid constipation.
3. Explain that spots may be seen before the eyes for 24 to 48 hours after treatment. Inform the patient that the eye may be bloodshot, the vision may be somewhat blurred temporarily, and night vision may be temporarily decreased.
4. Advise the patient to avoid coughing and sneezing and not to blow the nose vigorously. (However, sneezes should not be stifled because this raises the pressure in the eyes.)
5. Teach the patient not to rub the eyes.
6. Instruct the patient to avoid medications that contain epinephrine, such as nose drops or sprays, because these may raise the blood pressure.
7. Instruct the patient to use nonaspirin pain relievers for 24 hours after laser surgery to avoid bleeding and to reduce the antiinflammatory response. (Laser creates scarring by heat and inflammation.)

Evaluation

Vision is restored or improved   Blurred vision decreases after about 3 weeks, and normal vision returns.

◼ RADIAL KERATOTOMY

Radial keratotomy is the most accepted procedure designed to correct or modify mild myopia (nearsightedness). Radial incisions, like the spokes of a bicycle wheel, are made around the periphery of the cornea, ultimately resulting in a flattening of the cornea (Figure 6-21). The flattened cornea redirects the light rays to a more appropriate level on the surface of the retina to reduce the myopia. A calibrated diamond knife is used to make anywhere from four to eight equally spaced incisions in the corneal surface. The central portion of the cornea (3 to 4 mm diameter) is left untouched so resultant scarring does not cause glare or interfere with central vision.

Candidates for this procedure are mildly or moderately myopic patients who usually attain 20/40 vision without further correction after the surgery. However, some patients may still need eyeglasses to attain maximum correction.

The procedure is controversial because a variety of unknowns can cause problems after surgery. For example, the cornea heals and reshapes differently in each patient, and the visual acuity is not fully predictable in any indvidual. Although the procedure does not threaten vision, the outcome may be increased astigmatism for some patients and less-than-expected reduction in myopia for others. The danger of perforating the cornea and cutting into the anterior chamber is always present during the procedure. Slight perforations heal quickly with no complications; deeper perforations cause loss of the pressure stability in the chamber and may delay the completion of surgery for a month or so. Fluctuating chamber pressures cause visual impairment until healing is complete. In some patients the corneal scars may become pigmented and visible in 6 to 12 months. Long-term follow-up research is still being done.

The procedure has been approved for outpatient therapy and is accomplished with the use of a topical anesthetic. The eye is pressure patched for 24 hours after the procedure, and the patient may experience foreign body sensations for the first 12 to 24 hours.

In February 1995, the FDA approved the excimer laser to be used by ophthalmologists for performing photorefractive keratectomy (PRK), an alternative therapy to reduce myopia for astigmatism. Through computerized technology, the excimer laser is provided data used to calculate the depth and pattern of the corneal tissue to be removed.

Unlike radial keratotomy, in which partial-thickness incisions that completely avoid the optical center (the pupil) are made in the cornea, PRK laser pulses are aimed directly at the center of the optical zone.

A third procedure used to reduce myopia is automated lamellar keratectomy (ALK). Still under investigation, ALK utilizes a diamond blade attached to a mechanized plane. After precise calculations are made the plane is rolled over the corneal center, slicing away exact amounts of corneal tissue to reduce myopia.

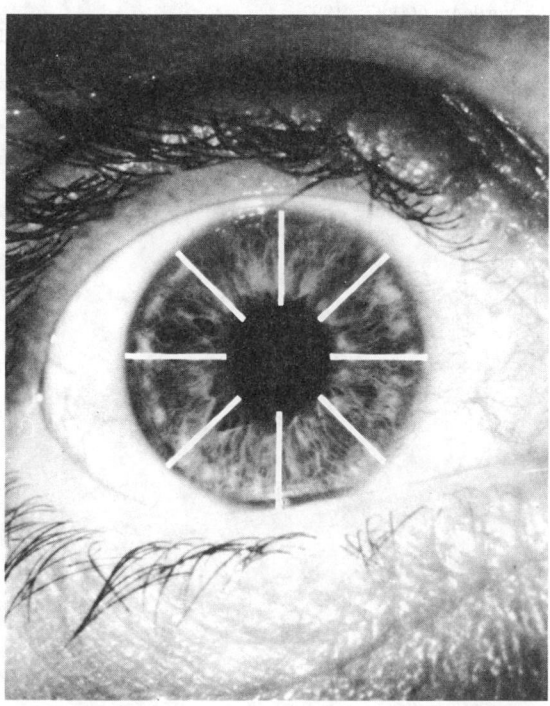

Figure 6-21 Location of incisions in radial keratotomy. Central 3 to 4 mm optical zone of cornea is not incised, and incisions do not extend beyond corneoscleral limbus. Four, eight, or sixteen radial incisions are made. (From Newell.[34])

References

1. Alexander LJ: Age-related macular degeneration: the current understanding of the status of clinicopathology, diagnosis and management, *J Am Optom Assoc* 64(12):822, 1993.
2. Anonymous: Laser peripheral iridotomy for pupillar-block glaucoma, *Ophthalmology* 101(10):1749, 1994.
3. Benson WE, Coscas G, Katz LJ, editors: *Current techniques in ophthalmic laser surgery,* Philadelphia, 1995, Current Medicine.
4. Bienkowski J: An overview of the progression of diabetic retinopathy with treatment recommendations, *Nurse Pract* 19(7):50, 1994.
5. Chi TS, Netland PA: Angle recession glaucoma, *Int Ophthalmol Clin* 35(1):117, 1995.
6. Comprehensive adult eye examination: preferred practice pattern, *Am Acad Ophthalmol,* 1995.
7. Davis DB 2nd, Mandel MR: Anesthesia for cataract surgery, *Int Ophthalmol Clin* 34(2):13, 1994.
8. DCCT Research Group: the diabetes complications and control trial (DCCT): update, *Diabetes Care* 13:427, 1990.
9. Ferri FF, Fretwell MD: *Practical guide to the geriatric patient,* St Louis, 1992, Mosby.
10. Flynn JT: 17th Annual Frank Costenbader lecture, amblyopia revisited, *J Pediatr Ophthalmol Strabismus* 28(4):183, 1991.
11. Fraunfelder FT, Roy FN, editors: *Current ocular therapy,* Philadelphia, 1995, Saunders.

12. Freund KB, Yannuzzi LA, Sorenson JA: Age-related macular degeneration and choroidal neovascularization, *Am J Ophthalmol* 115(6):786, 1993.

13. Friedlander MH: The eye in immunologic disease, *J Fl Med Assoc* 81(4):252, 1994.

14. Groer MW, Shekleton ME: *Basic pathophysiology: a holistic approach,* ed 3, St Louis, 1989, Mosby.

15. Grosskreutz C, Netland PA: Low tension glaucoma, *Int Ophthalmol Clin* 34(3):173, 1994.

16. Hart W Jr, editor: *Adler's physiology of the eye,* ed 9, St Louis, 1992, Mosby.

17. Helveston EM: *Surgical management of strabismus: an atlas of strabismus surgery,* ed 4, St Louis, 1993, Mosby.

18. Hockwin O: Cataract classification, *Doc Ophthalmol* 88(3-4):264, 1994-1995.

19. Hurst MA, Douthwaite WA: Assessing vision behind cataract: a review of methods, *Optom Vis Sci* 70(11):903, 1993.

20. Jaffe NS: *Atlas of ophthalmic surgery,* ed 2, St Louis, 1995, Mosby.

21. Jay JL: Primary open angle glaucoma, *Practitioner* 236(1511):199, 1992.

22. Kim MJ, McFarland GK, McLane AM: *Pocket guide to nursing diagnoses,* ed 6, St Louis, 1995, Mosby.

23. Kohner EM: The effect of diabetic control on diabetic retinopathy, *Eye* 7(pt 2):309, 1993.

24. Lewis H, Ryan SJ, editor: *Medical and surgical retina: advances, controversies, and management,* St Louis, 1994, Mosby.

25. MacCuish AC: Early detection and screening for diabetic retinopathy, *Eye* 7(pt 2):254, 1993.

26. MacInnis B: Update in cataract and refractive surgery, *Can J Ophthalmol* 30(1):1, 1995.

27. Mattingly WB: Advanced low vision optics, *Ophthalmic Nurs Technol* 13(4):161, 1994.

28. Mauger TF, Craig EL: *Mosby's ocular drug handbook,* St Louis, 1995, Mosby.

29. Migdal C: What is the appropriate treatment for patients with primary open-angle glaucoma: medicine, laser or primary surgery, *Ophthalmic Surg* 26(2):108, 1995.

30. Murphy RP: Management of diabetic retinopathy, *Am Fam Physician* 51(4):785, 1995.

31. Murray S: Cataract surgery: new techniques, better results, *Practitioner* 239(1549):272, 1995.

32. Navon SE, McKeown CA: Amblyopia, *Int Ophthalmol Clin* 32(1):35, 1992.

33. Nelson LB, Wagner RS: Pediatric cataract surgery, *Int Ophthalmol Clin* 34(2):165, 1994.

34. Newell FW: *Ophthalmology: principles and concepts,* ed 7, St Louis, 1992, Mosby.

35. Osako M, Keltner JL: Botulinum A toxin (oculinum) in ophthalmology, *J Am Optom Assoc* 65(9):621, 1994.

36. Salasche SJ et al: The retinoblastoma gene and its significance, *Ann Med* 26(3):177, 1994.

37. Seidel HM et al: *Mosby's guide to physical examination,* ed 3, St Louis, 1995, Mosby.

38. Serdarevic ON: Refractive corneal transplantation: control of astigmatism and ametropia during penetrating keratoplasty, *Int Ophthalmol Clin* 34(4):13, 1994.

39. Serle JB: Pharmacologic advances in the treatment of glaucoma, *Drugs Aging* 5(3):156, 1994.

40. Smith SC: Diabetic retinopathy, *Nurs Clin North Am* 27(3):745, 1992.

41. Swanson MW: Ocular metastatic disease, *Optom Clin* 3(3):79, 1993.

42. Thompson JM, Wilson SF: *Health assessment for nursing practice,* St Louis, 1996, Mosby.

43. Tusa RJ, Newman SA, editors: *Neuroophthalmological disorders: diagnostic work-up and management,* New York, 1995, Marcel Dekker.

44. Vaughn D, Abury T, Riordan-Eva P: *General ophthalmology,* ed 14, Norwalk, Conn, 1995, Appleton & Lange.

45. Vernon S: How to screen for glaucoma, *Practitioner* 239(1549):257-260, 1995.

46. vonNoorden GK: *Binocular vision and ocular motility: theory and management of strabismus,* ed 5, St Louis, 1996, Mosby.

47. Wagner RS: Glaucoma in children, *Pediatr Clin North Am* 40(4):855, 1993.

48. Weiter JJ, Roh S: Viral infections of the choroid and retina, *Infect Dis Clin North Am* 6(4):875, 1992.

49. Wright KW: *Pediatric ophthalmology and strabismus,* St Louis, 1995, Mosby.

50. Wong DL: *Whaley and Wong's nursing care of infants and children,* ed 5, St Louis, 1995, Mosby.

Ear, Nose, and Throat

7

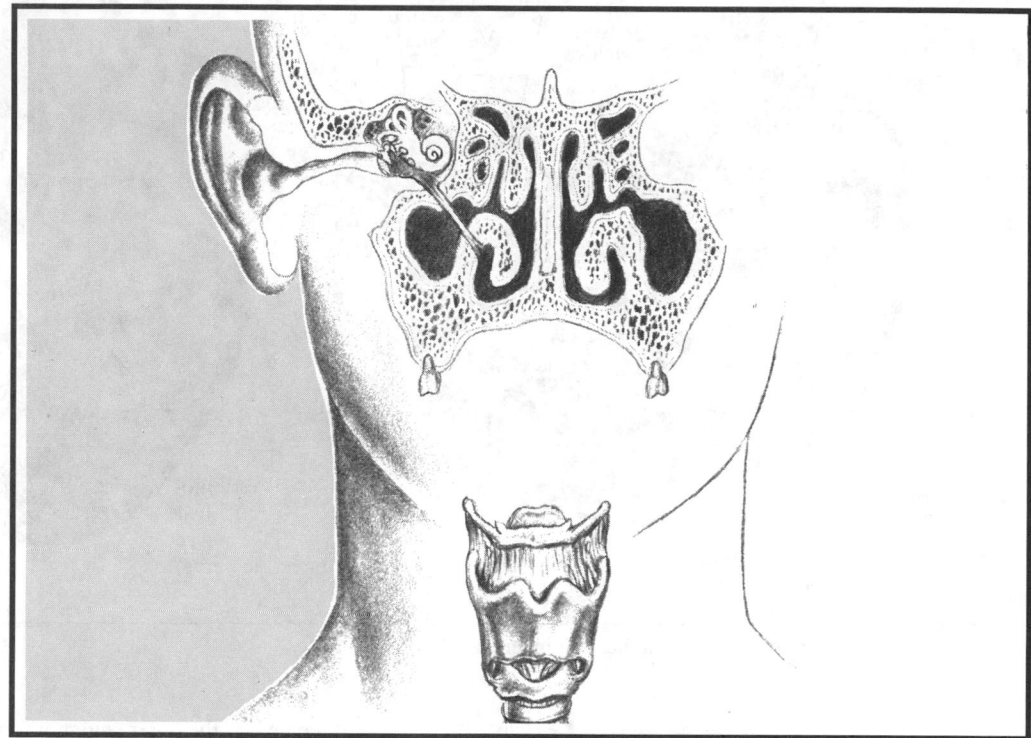

OVERVIEW

The ears, nose, and throat (ENT) are responsible for many of the body's senses, such as sound, smell, and taste, and for balance and speaking. Health professionals who care for patients with disorders affecting these areas must be highly sensitive and skilled in assessing the symptoms of disorders that may have a great impact on a patient's life or self-perception.

Ear, nose, and throat disorders can cause painful, incapacitating illnesses and major disruptions in communication, appearance, eating, swallowing, and breathing. Neoplastic disorders of the ear, nose, and throat may be fatal.

Because many ENT disorders are treated on an outpatient basis, patient and family education is a focus of this chapter.

The development of antibiotics and new surgical techniques has greatly reduced the impact of many ENT diseases. Hearing loss was once a common occurrence after severe or repeated ear infections, but now infection-related hearing loss has been nearly eliminated in the United States. Other diseases that once were life threatening are now considered minor if treated early. Surgical techniques such as microsurgery, stapedectomy, cochlear implant, and tympanoplasty have greatly improved the management of the patient with a hearing loss.

•••••• Anatomy, Physiology, and Related Pathophysiology

Ear

The ears are responsible for both hearing and equilibrium. The ear is divided into three anatomic sections: the external ear, the middle ear, and the inner ear (Figure 7-1).

External ear The function of the external ear is to receive sound waves and direct them to the tympanic membrane. The external ear includes the outer projection (known as the auricle or pinna) and the ear canal called the external auditory meatus, or the external auditory canal. The auricle is attached to the head by muscles innervated by the facial nerve. It is composed of cartilage and covered by skin, except for the ear lobe, which contains fat but no cartilage (Figure 7-2). The auricle is highly susceptible to frostbite because it has little subcutaneous fat to protect it and only one layer of blood vessels. The sensory nerve supply of the auricle is provided by the greater auricular nerve, the lesser occipital nerve, the auricular branch of the vagus nerve, the auriculotemporal nerve, and the fifth, seventh, and tenth cranial nerves.

The external auditory meatus or ear canal has a slight downward curve; it ends at the tympanic membrane. The outer half is cartilaginous, and the inner half is bony except in infants, in whom ossification has yet not occurred. The skin that lines the cartilaginous portion of the canal is thick and contains fine

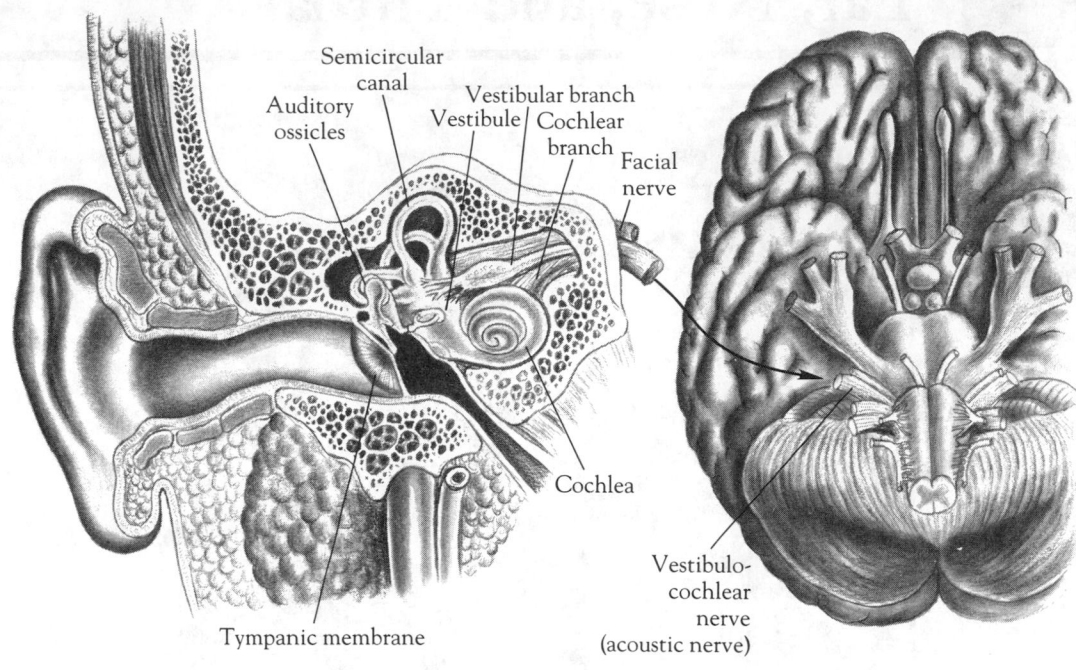

Figure 7-1 Relationship of external, middle, and inner ear.

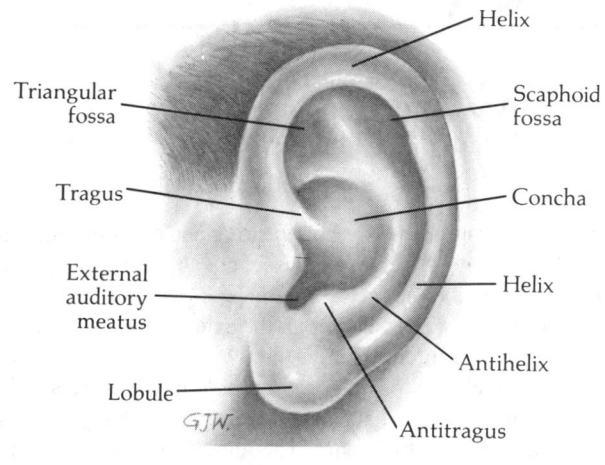

Figure 7-2 Anatomic structures of the external ear. (From Seidel.[44])

hairs, large sebaceous glands, and ceruminous glands. Cerumen (earwax), the combined secretion of the sebaceous and ceruminous glands, may accumulate so much that it obstructs sound transmission. The epithelium that lines the bony half of the external canal is very thin and does not contain hair or glands. In adults the external canal is approximately 24 mm long, and the bony portion is slightly longer than the cartilaginous portion (Figure 7-3).

The temporomandibular joint is anterior to the ear canal. Diseases of this joint can cause referred pain to the ear.

Tympanic membrane The tympanic membrane, which separates the external ear from the middle ear, is composed of three layers: the outer squamous layer, the inner cuboidal layer, and a middle layer of fibrous collagen tissue. New cells of the tympanic membrane are produced in the periphery and migrate toward the center of the drum. The drum is somewhat conical and slightly inclined; the concavity of the drumhead (umbo) and its position in relation to the ear canal vary and may be greatly altered during disease.

The fibers of the tympanic membrane condense into an incomplete, dense, fibrous ring called the anulus, which fits into the tympanic sulcus. The anulus contains a superior break, the notch of Rivinus, between the anterior and posterior malleolar ligaments. The portion of the tympanic membrane closing this area is the pars flaccida, so named because it does not contain a fibrous collagen layer.

The tympanic membrane is described as a translucent window through which the middle ear may be viewed. The color is usually a translucent pearl gray, although this may vary slightly in normal membranes (Figure 7-4).

Middle ear The middle ear, or tympanic cavity, is covered by the tightly stretched tympanic membrane. It is a small, roughly oblong, flattened space that is lined with nonciliated, single-layered mucous membrane and contains bony walls. During an infection the mucous membrane becomes ciliated and multilayered. This area holds air and three small bones, or ossicles: the malleus, the incus, and the stapes (Figure 7-5).

The ossicles connect the tympanic membrane with the oval window and represent the normal pathway of sound transmission across the middle ear space. The first bone is the malleus (hammer); it has a head, neck, handle, and short process. The manubrium (handle) and the short process attach to the

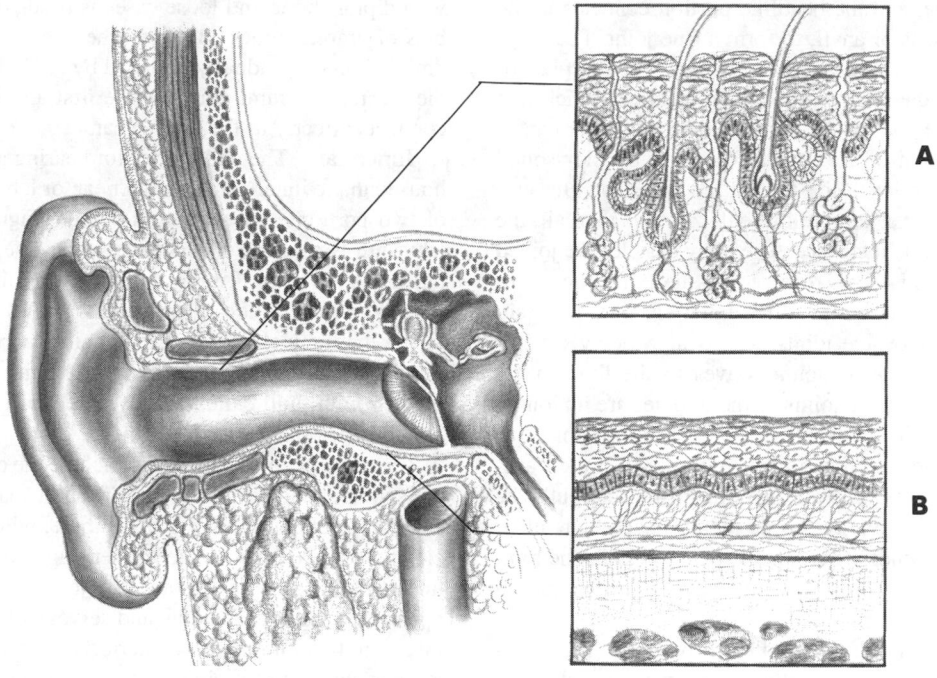

Figure 7-3 External auditory canal. **A,** Cartilaginous ear canal showing hair follicles, sebaceous glands, and cercuminous glands, **B,** Bony ear canal with thin epithelial lining, containing no hair or glands.

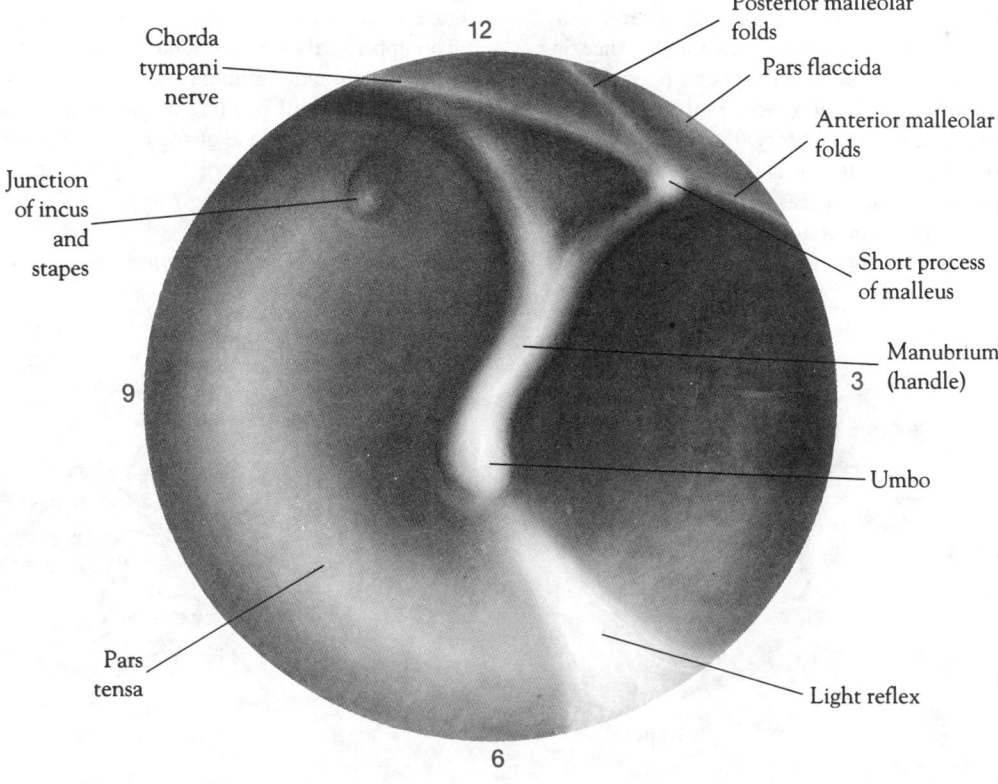

Figure 7-4 Normal tympanic membrane. (From Wong.[54])

tympanic membrane, and the headlike portion connects to the second bone, the incus or anvil, to form a true joint. The incus connects to the third bone, the stapes (stirrup). The footplate of the stapes fits into the oval or vestibular window, which is a small opening in the wall between the middle and inner ear.

The major function of the middle ear is to transfer sound waves from the outer ear to the fluid-filled inner ear. Because the fluid in the inner ear is more difficult to move than air, the pressure waves must be increased. The bony ossicles are joined so they amplify sound waves received by the tympanic membrane and transmit these waves to the inner ear by a lever action of their freely movable joints. The oval window's membrane vibrates and conducts sound waves to the fluid in the inner ear. In otosclerosis the joints of the ossicles are no longer freely movable, resulting in decreased sound transmission. Two small skeletal muscles attached to the ossicles affect the transmission of sound waves. The tensor tympani muscle pulls the malleus inward to tense the tympanic membrane, which attenuates high-pitched sounds. The stapedius muscle pulls the footplate of the stapes outward, possibly making low-frequency sounds more audible.

The middle ear communicates directly with the nasopharynx by means of the eustachian tube. This tube, which leads downward and medially to the nasopharynx, carries air into the middle ear to equalize pressure on both sides of the tympanic membrane. The mucosal lining of the middle ear is continuous with that of the nasopharynx by way of the eustachian tube. Normally the eustachian tube is passively closed; it opens by action of the tensor and levator muscles of the palate, usually, although not always, during swallowing, yawning, or sneezing to equalize middle ear pressure with atmospheric pressure. The eustachian tube can serve as a direct route for infection to reach the middle ear from the upper respiratory tract.

A third structure of the middle ear is the collection of mastoid air cells. These are air-filled spaces in a portion of the temporal bone in the skull. They communicate posteriorly with the middle ear. They are present at birth but are small and filled with diploic bone and loose osseous tissue between the two tables of cranial bones. Between the ages of 2 and 6 years the diploic bone is gradually replaced by air cells that bud off from the mastoid antrum, which is the first and largest air cell and connects directly to the middle ear.

Inner ear   The end organs for hearing and equilibrium are housed in the inner ear. The inner ear, or labyrinth, is composed of two portions, one inside the other (Figure 7-6). The bony labyrinth is a series of channels within the petrous portion of the temporal bone. Lining the bony labyrinth is the membranous labyrinth, which is the same shape as the bony channels. Inside the bony channels is fluid called perilymph, which surrounds the membranous labyrinth. The membranous labyrinth is filled with fluid called endolymph. There is no communication between the fluid-filled spaces.[11]

Components of the inner ear include the cochlea for hearing, the semicircular canals for equilibrium, that is, rotational and angular acceleration, and the vestibule, which houses the utricle and saccule responsible for sensing changes in gravity and linear and angular acceleration. The vestibule is a space that opens onto the oval window and serves as the entrance into the inner ear. It communicates anteriorly with the cochlea and posteriorly with the semicircular canals and utricle.

Cochlea.   The cochlea is a snail-shaped bony tube that contains the organ of Corti, which is the neural end organ for hearing. The cochlea is about 3.5 cm long with about $2\frac{1}{2}$ spiral turns. Throughout its length, the basilar and Reissner membranes separate it into three tubes or chambers called scalae (Figure 7-7).[2]

The upper scala vestibuli and the lower scala tympani contain perilymph and communicate with each other through the helicotrema, a small opening at the apex of the cochlea. The scala vestibuli at the base of the cochlea ends at the oval window, where the footplate of the stapes is attached. The scala

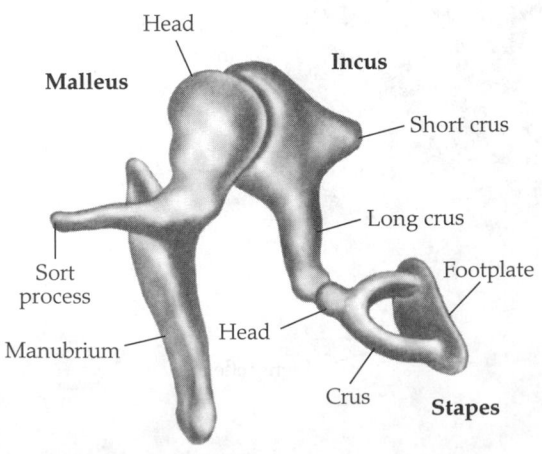

Figure 7-5 Ossicles of right middle ear.

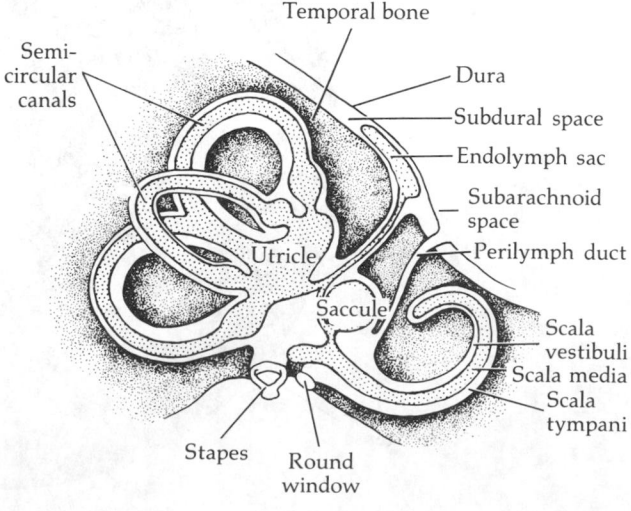

Figure 7-6 Bony labyrinth and membranous inner labyrinth. (From Ganong.[11])

tympani ends at the base of the cochlea into or at the round window, which is an opening enclosed by a secondary tympanic membrane. The round window bulges outward to dissipate the pressure waves that are set up in the inner ear fluid during sound transmission. The scala media, or the middle cochlear chamber, contains endolymph and does not communicate with the other two scalae (Figures 7-8 and 7-9).[2]

The organ of Corti is located on the basilar membrane and contains the receptors of hearing (Figure 7-10, *A)*. It extends from the base of the cochlea to the apex and has a spiral shape. The receptors for hearing are hair cells arranged in two rows. There are approximately 3500 inner and 20,000 outer hair cells, and their tips are embedded in the tectorial membrane (Figure 7-10, *B*). When these hair cells are bent or distorted by pressure waves, sound is changed (transduced) into electromechanical impulses. These impulses are carried by the afferent neuron to the spiral ganglion in the bony core of the cochlea. The axons of these nerves form the auditory division of the eighth cranial nerve (vestibulocochlear nerve) and terminate in the dorsal and ventral cochlear nuclei of the medulla oblongata. From the cochlear nuclei, axons carry auditory information to the inferior canaliculi for reflexes associated with hearing, such as turning the head to locate a sound. The fibers then pass to the medial geniculate body in the thalamus and to the primary auditory cortex, Brodmann areas 41 and 42, which are located in the superior portion of the temporal lobe.[35]

Semicircular canals.   The semicircular canals are perpendicular to each other on each side of the head. Three canals are on each side: a superior, posterior, and horizontal canal; they are so oriented to sense changes in the three planes of space. Inside the bony canals are the membranous canals suspended in the perilymph. Near the end of each canal is an enlargement called the ampulla, which houses the crista ampullaris, or the vestibular receptors. The hair cells of the crista ampullaris are stimulated with rotation. The pattern of stimulation varies with the direction and plane of rotation. Nerve fiber tracts compose the vestibular portion of the vestibulocochlear nerve, or cranial nerve VIII, to the vestibular nuclei and terminate in the four vestibular nuclei at the level of the pons and medulla in the brainstem. Tracts that descend from the vestibular nuclei into the spinal cord are responsible for head-righting reflexes and changes with muscle tone associated with rotation. Ascending fibers from the vestibular nuclei are concerned with eye movements, that is, nystagmus associated with rotation.

Utricle and saccule.   Housed within the vestibule are the utricle and saccule, which are responsible for sensing changes in gravity and forward and backward movement. Hair cells in the macula of the utricle and saccule are stimulated by head tilting and by jumping or falling, respectively. Both macular structures are sensitive to forward and backward movement. Fibers from the utricle and saccule compose portions of the vestibular division of cranial nerve VIII, which is the vestibulocochlear nerve. The vestibular division is important for the control of posture and the maintenance of balance. The cochlear division is responsible for hearing.

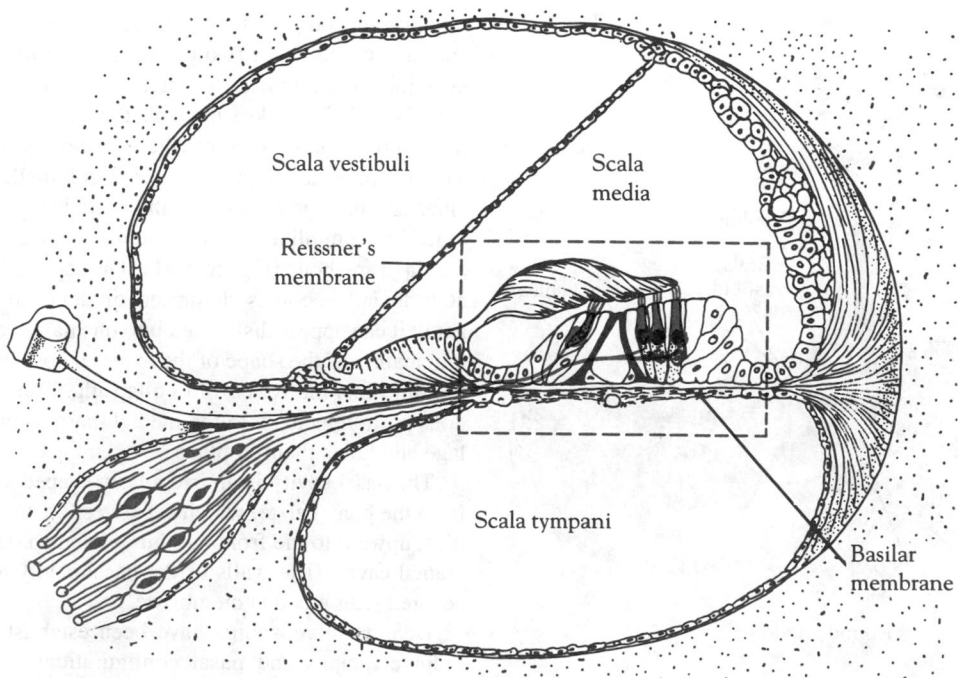

Figure 7-7 Scalae of the cochlea, separated by Reissner's membrane and basilar membrane. *X* and *Y* indicate orientation via-a-vis drawing on right in Figure 7-9. (From Berne & Levy.[2])

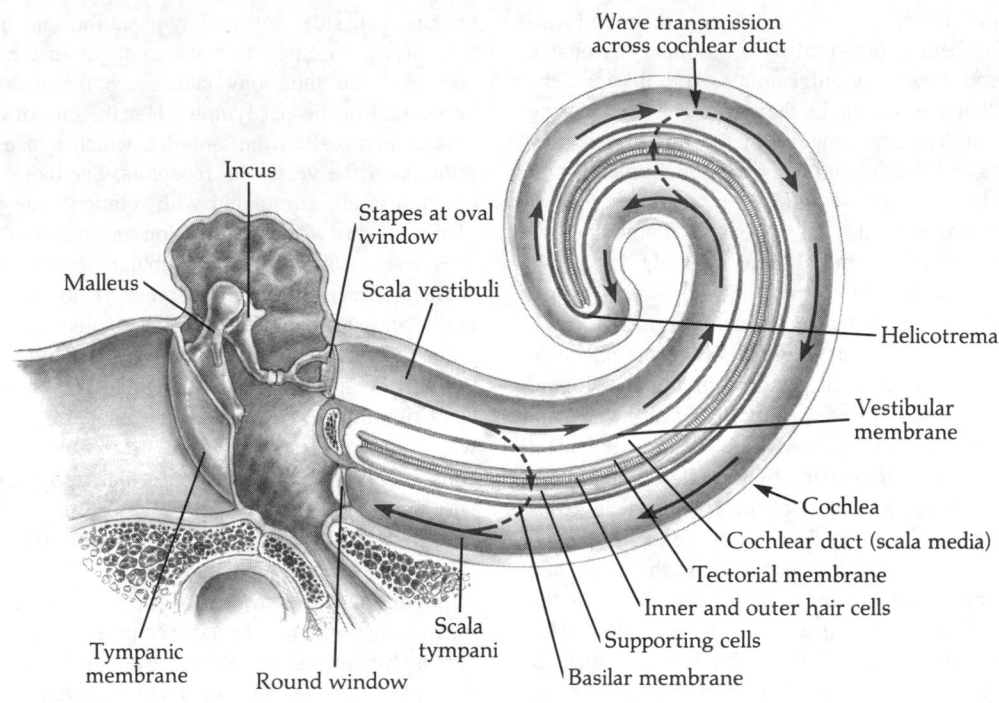

Figure 7-8 Middle ear, showing relationship of ossicles and cochlea. Communication between scala vestibuli and scala tympania is shown. Arrows indicate displacement of liquid inside bony cochlea and round window from movement of stapedial footplate and displacement of oval window.

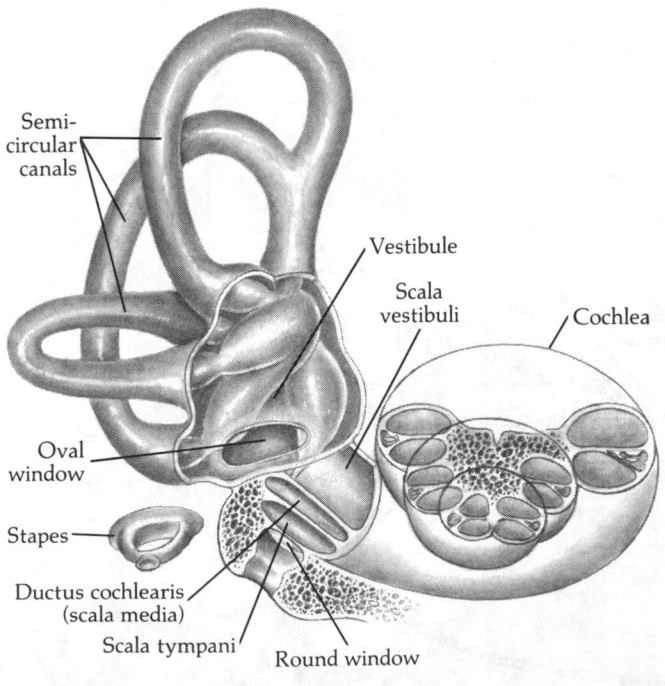

Figure 7-9 Coiled structure of cochlea showing relationships of oval window, scala vestibuli, scala media, and scala tympani. Arrows indicate path of continuous flow from scala vestibuli through helicotrema to scala tympani.

Nose

The nose is composed of bone in the upper third segment and cartilage in the lower two thirds. The midline point where the nose joins the forehead is called the nasion. The bridge of the nose is called the dorsum, and the base, which includes the nares (nostrils), is the point where the nose joins the upper lip.[27] The two nares are separated by the columella and allow air to enter and pass posteriorly to the nasopharynx. The nose is divided in the midline by the septum, which is composed of both cartilage and bone (Figure 7-11). The septum is usually straight at birth but becomes deformed or deviated in almost every adult; it can appear dislocated into one nasal vestibule. The septum maintains the shape of the external nose by acting as a strut that prevents the roof from collapsing. The anterior cartilaginous portion melds into the medial margins of the lateral cartilage and holds them in place.[27]

The nasal cavity is an irregularly shaped space that extends from the bony palate, which separates the nose and mouth cavities, upward to the frontal, ethmoid and sphenoid bones of the cranial cavity. The walls of the nasal cavity are made of bone covered with mucous membrane.

Definite relationships have been established between geographic regions and nasal configurations. In warm climates with high absolute humidity, noses tend to be flat; in areas with low absolute humidity, noses are narrow and protrude farther from the face. This latter configuration probably improves the air-conditioning efficiency of the nose.[3]

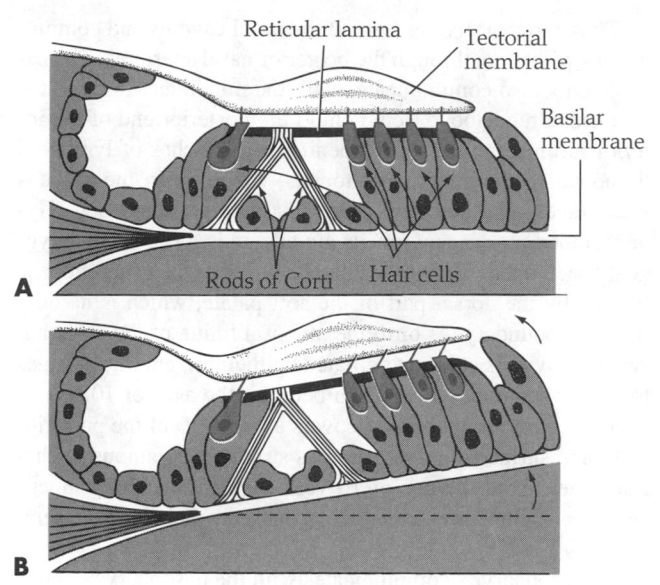

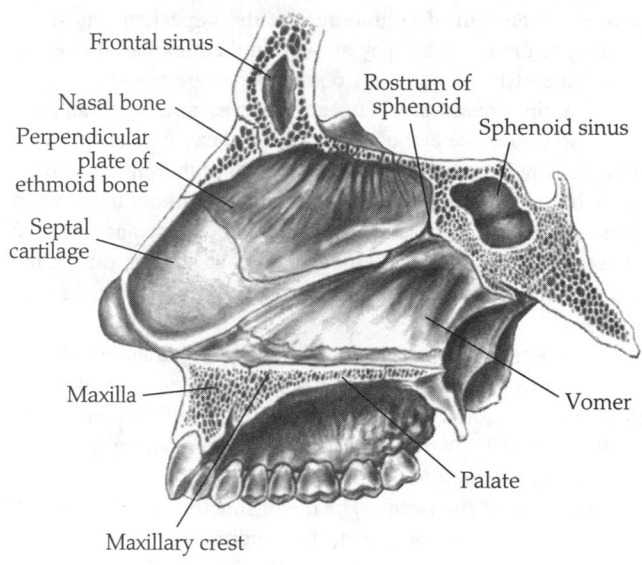

Figure 7-10 A, Organ of Corti on basilar membrane. **B,** Hair cells embedded in tectorial membrane. (From Berne & Levy.²)

Figure 7-11 Nasal septum.

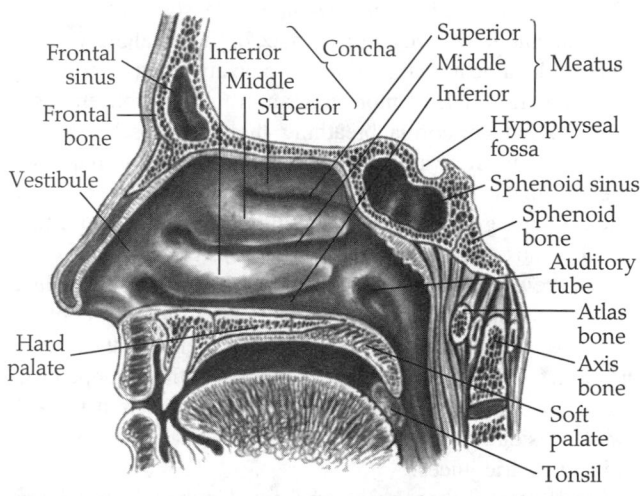

Figure 7-12 Lateral wall of nose.

The vestibule of the nostril is lined with skin containing vibrissae, or nasal hairs, and some sebaceous and sweat glands. The nose is lined with respiratory mucosa, except for the skin in the vestibule and the olfactory epithelium. Mucus secreted by the mucosa is carried back to the nasopharynx by the cilia of the mucosa. The nasal mucosa is extremely vascular, which makes it appear redder than the oral mucosa.

The lateral wall of the nose has three and occasionally four nasal turbinates or conchae: the inferior, middle, superior and supreme (Figure 7-12). The supreme turbinate, if present, is quite small and cannot be seen during examination. The inferior turbinate is a separate bone, but the other three are part of the ethmoid bone. The turbinates greatly increase the surface area of the mucous membrane over which air travels as it passes through the nasal passages and into the nasopharynx. The nasolacrimal duct communicates indirectly with the lacrimal gland and opens onto the lateral surface of the inferior meatus of the nose. Tears drain continuously into the nose. If any part of the system becomes blocked or if tears are formed at an unusual rate, the fluid runs out onto the face.

The blood supply to the nose comes from the external and internal carotid arteries. The external carotid artery supplies blood primarily through one of its terminal divisions, the internal maxillary artery. This artery and its terminal branch, the sphenopalatine artery, supply blood to most of the posterior nasal septum and the lateral wall of the nose. The second largest vessel that supplies blood to the internal nose is the anterior ethmoidal artery, which derives its blood from the internal carotid system. The ethmoidal artery supplies blood to the anterosuperior part of the septum and the lateral wall of the nose. The external nose receives blood mostly from the same arteries as the internal nose; but venous drainage is partly through the angular vein, which leads into the inferior oph-

thalmic vein and the cavernous sinus. Most venous drainage is downward through the anterior facial vein.

The muscles of the external nose receive their nerve supply from the seventh cranial nerve. The external skin is innervated by the first and second divisions of the fifth cranial nerve. The nerve supply to the internal nose is from the olfactory nerve and the first and second divisions of the fifth cranial nerve.

The paranasal sinuses, which lighten the weight of the skull and give resonance and timbre to the voice, are air-filled, mucous membrane–lined cavities in the facial and cranial bones surrounding the nasal cavities. They drain into the nasal cavities through the ostia of the middle meatus (openings between the inferior and middle turbinates). The sinuses are in the frontal, sphenoid, ethmoid, and maxillary bones. The maxillary sinuses (or antrum of Highmore) are the largest and most accessible of the sinuses. They are within the maxillary bones on either side of the nose. The frontal sinuses are above the eyes, the ethmoid sinuses are between the eyes and nose, and the sphenoid sinuses lie at the rear of the nasal cavity. The sphenoid sinuses, which are the most deeply placed of the sinuses, are directly below the sella turcica, from which pituitary tumors can erode downward to fill them. Only the maxillary and ethmoid sinuses are present at birth; the frontal sinuses form during the second year of life, and the sphenoid sinuses form during the third year.

The normal physiologic functions of the paranasal sinuses are unknown.[27] It has been proposed that they did not develop for any specific biologic reason but were formed incidentally to the forward and downward growth of the face during transition from infancy to adulthood.[27,36]

Functions of the nose   The major functions of the nose are air conditioning and olfaction; air conditioning refers to temperature and humidity control and to filtering of particles and bacteria in inspired air before it reaches the trachea, bronchi, and lungs. Inspired air reaches the nasopharynx in about ¼ second; during this short period, the temperature of the air reaches 97° to 98° F and the humidity becomes a constant 75% to 80%.

Serum and mucus cover the surface of the nasal mucosa and can provide large amounts of water to be absorbed by cold, dry air. As much as 1 L of moisture can evaporate from the nose during 24 hours of normal breathing; the submucosal glands replenish this moisture as the water evaporates. The turbinates are covered with erectile tissue that can rapidly fill with blood, which allows greater control of temperature and humidification. The nose, sinuses, pharynx, trachea, bronchi, and bronchioles are covered by a continuous mucous blanket to which airborne particles cling on contact. The blanket contains lysozyme, an enzyme that causes most bacteria to disintegrate on contact. Cilia carry the mucous blanket with its trapped particulate matter back toward the nasopharynx where it is swallowed. Residual bacteria are then destroyed by hydrochloric acid and gastric juices.

The olfactory sense organs are located in the olfactory membrane that covers the roof of the nose and is reflected medially downward over the superior turbinate. The olfactory receptors are hair cells or chemoreceptors that are stimulated when air is inspired through the nose.

Pharynx

The pharynx, from the Greek word for throat, is the muscular tube that is behind the oral cavity and extends downward from the base of the skull to the larynx. The pharynx is a somewhat conical chamber. It conducts air between the nasal cavities and larynx and conducts food from the mouth to the esophagus.

The pharynx is divided into three sections: nasopharynx, oropharynx, and laryngopharynx. The nasopharynx is above the margin of the soft palate posterior to the nose; the oropharynx is the area behind the mouth that is visible when the tongue is depressed with a tongue blade; and the laryngopharynx is dorsal to the larynx (Figure 7-13).

The nasopharynx lies behind the nasal cavities and communicates with them through the posterior nasal apertures. The nasopharynx also communicates with the middle ear through the eustachian tube about 1 cm behind the posterior end of the inferior turbinate. Near these openings are patches of lymphoid tissue called the pharyngeal tonsils, which lie in the mucous membrane at the junction of the posterior wall and roof. (Hypertrophied pharyngeal tonsils are adenoids.) The nasopharyngeal space opens inferiorly into the oropharynx so the floor is formed by the dorsal part of the soft palate, which is its only movable boundary. At birth the mucosal lining of the nasopharyngeal cavity is columnar ciliated epithelium, but this changes to patchy squamous epithelium between the ages of 10 and 80 years. Squamous epithelium covers about 80% of the posterior wall, and surface mucosa becomes stratified squamous epithelium after about the age of 10 years. Glands secreting mucus and serous fluid are scattered throughout the mucous membrane.

The oropharynx communicates with the nasopharynx above and the laryngopharynx below to the level of the epiglottis. The oropharynx contains the palatine tonsils, which with the pharyngeal and lingual tonsils (on the dorsum of the tongue) comprise Waldeyer's ring. This ring is a protective barrier of lymphoid tissue between the mouth and throat and the respiratory and digestive tracts. This lymphoid tissue is considered important in the development of immune bodies. If stimulated by bacterial infection, immune bodies promote the production of additional immune factors that provide future protection from bacterial infection.[8]

The laryngopharynx boundaries are the superior constrictor muscle and vertebrae posteriorly, the larynx and pyriform fossa below, and the hyoid bone, base of the tongue, and constrictor muscle above. The upper end of the epiglottis projects into the laryngopharynx.

The oropharynx and laryngopharynx are spaces surrounded by muscles that provide support to the surrounding tissue and a passageway through which air, food, and fluids can be ingested. Swallowing is accomplished by the action of the constrictor muscles in the pharynx and by the suprahyoid and infrahyoid muscles. Action of these muscles and their nerves is also responsible for the gag reflex, which protects the air and food passages from the entrance of any unwanted material. Two cranial nerves are responsible for the gag reflex: the glossopharyngeal nerve (cranial nerve IX) and the vagus nerve (cranial nerve X). The glossopharyngeal nerve has sensory and motor divisions. The sensory division supplies sensation to the pharynx, and the motor division innervates the posterior wall of the pharynx. The vagus nerve innervates all of the thoracic and abdominal viscera and conveys impulses from the walls of the intestines, the heart, and the lungs.[35]

Tonsils   The tonsils are small masses of primarily lymphoid tissue. They are covered by mucous membrane and contain small openings that deliver phagocytes to the mouth and pharynx.

In the past, removal of the tonsils and adenoids was commonplace, but it is now known that the lymphoid tissue of the

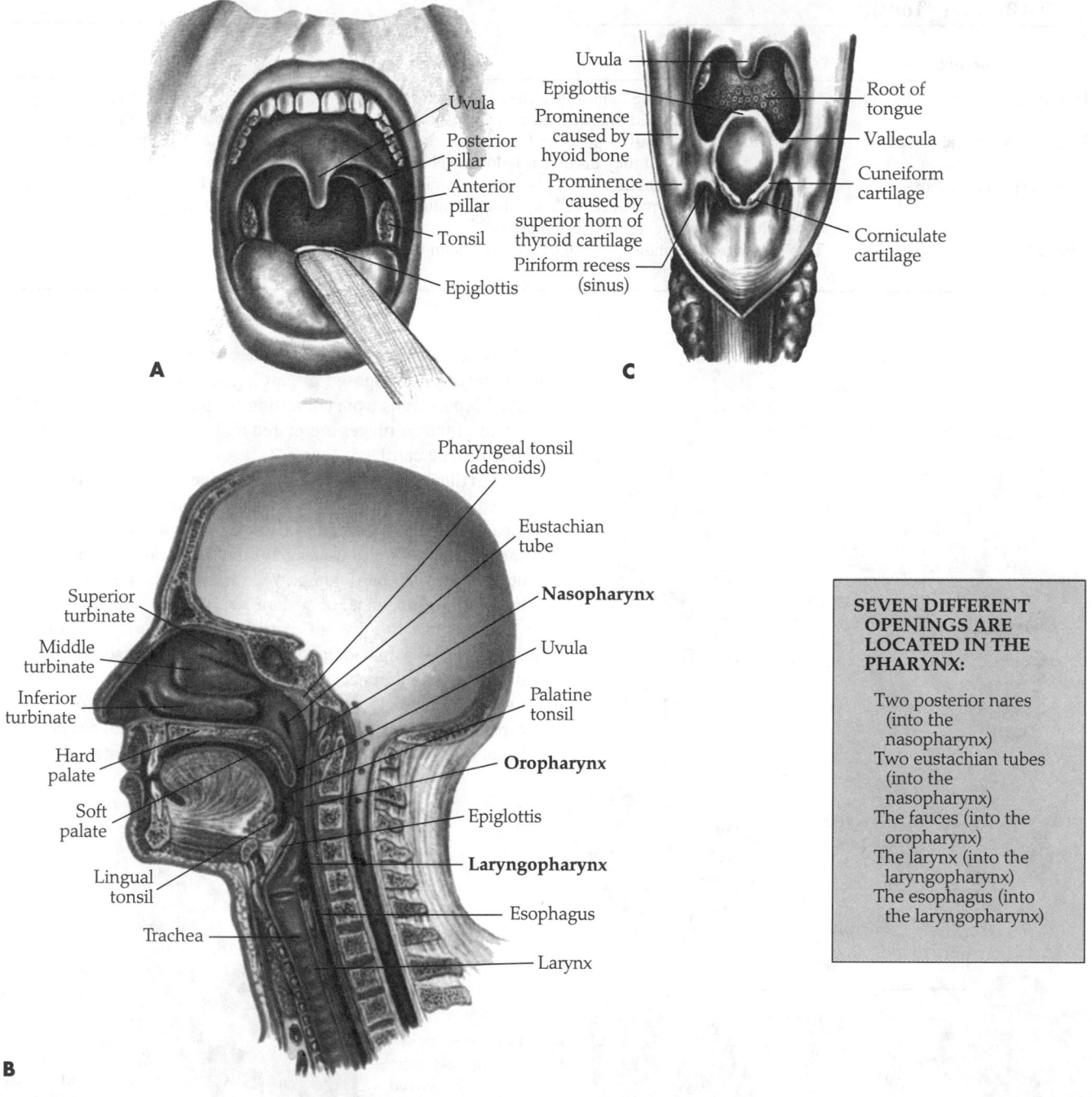

Figure 7-13 A, Structures of pharynx: uvula, epiglottis, and tonsils. **B,** Structures of upper respiratory tract. **C,** Hypopharynx (posterior view).

pharynx plays an important role in the immune system of the body, and they are not removed as frequently (Table 7-1).

The lymphoid tissues of Waldeyer's ring drain into the lymph nodes of the neck. The adenoids in the nasopharynx drain into the posterior cervical lymph glands, and the palatine and lingual tonsils drain into the anterior cervical lymph nodes.

Larynx

The larynx has several functions: (1) it is the air passageway between the pharynx and the lungs; (2) it prevents food and fluid from entering the lungs; and (3) it is involved in sound production or phonation.

The larynx is a roughly tubular structure with an irregular shape. It is somewhat wider at the top where it is attached to the

■ TABLE 7-1 Tonsils

Structure	Description
Pharyngeal tonsil or adenoid	Mass of lymphoid tissue in nasopharynx; extends from its roof almost to free end of soft palate; present in all infants and children; starts to regress just before puberty; normally absent in adults
Lateral pharyngeal bands	Extend down lateral wall of pharynx from adenoids; located behind posterior tonsillar pillar; gradually become thinner until they disappear below level of faucial tonsil
Faucial (palatine) tonsil	Located laterally at junction of oropharynx and oral cavity; composed of large lymphoid follicles; contains numerous crypts lined with squamous epithelium; supplied by tonsillar and palatine arteries, which come from external carotid artery
Lingual tonsils	Two masses of lymphoid tissue located on dorsum of tongue; extend from circumvallate papillae of tongue to epiglottis

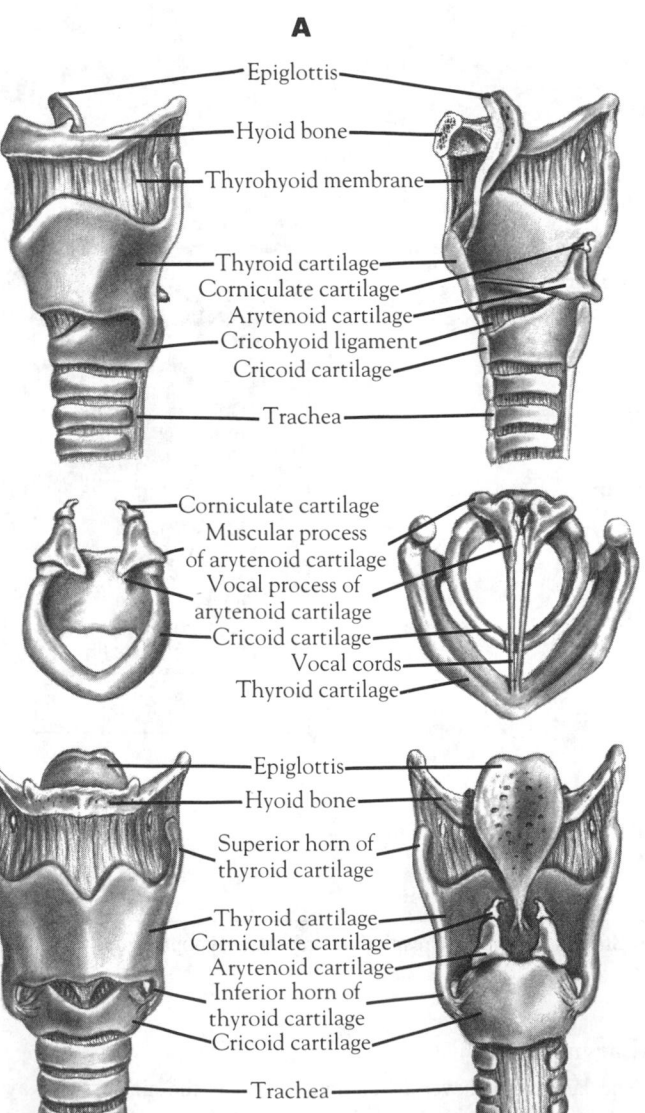

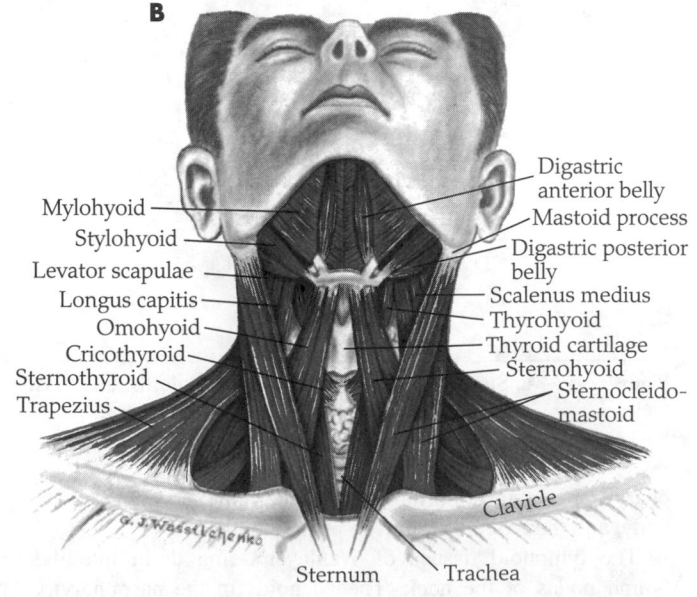

pharynx and narrower below where it attaches to the trachea. The larynx is composed of cartilages, ligaments, and muscles that keep its walls from collapsing on inspiration (Figure 7-14). Three of the cartilages are paired and three are unpaired, for a total of nine cartilages (Table 7-2).

Cartilages and muscles of the larynx   The larynx is protected on its front and sides by the thyroid cartilage (thyroid means shieldlike) and from behind by vertebrae. The thyroid cartilage is the largest cartilage of the larynx. Its midline prominence forms the hard bump in the front of the neck called the laryngeal prominence, or "Adam's apple."

Just below the thyroid cartilage lies the cricoid cartilage, which can be palpated in normal necks and can usually be seen in people with thin necks. The cricoid (ring-shaped) cartilage is the only complete ring of cartilage in the respiratory tract. Structurally it resembles a signet ring, with the signet portion located posteriorly. The cricoid cartilage articulates with the

Figure 7-14 Larynx. **A,** Cartilages and ligaments. **B,** Neck muscles.

TABLE 7-2 Cartilages and Muscles of the Larynx

Structure	Description
Unpaired Cartilages	
Thyroid	Largest cartilage of larynx; forms anterior midline shield called laryngeal prominence or Adam's apple
Cricoid	Only complete cartilaginous ring in respiratory tract; located just below thyroid cartilage
Epiglottis	Leaf shaped; projects upward at base of tongue and guards opening of larynx
Paired Cartilages	
Arytenoid, corniculate, and cuneiform	Serve as attachment for vocal ligaments; movement of cartilages controls tension of vocal ligaments
Instrinsic Muscles	
Thyroarytenoideus	Tilts arytenoid cartilages toward thyroid; results in shortening and relaxation of vocal cords
Arytenoideus	Approximates arytenoid cartilages and closes glottis
Cricothyroideus	Lifts anterior section of cricoid cartilage; results in increased tension on vocal cords
Posterior	
Cricoarytenoideus	Produces lateral rotation of arytenoid cartilages; results in separation of vocal cords and opening of glottis
Lateral	
Cricoarytenoideus	Produces medial rotation of arytenoid cartilages; results in approximation of vocal cords and closing of glottis

thyroid and arytenoid cartilages. The cricoid and thyroid cartilages are attached by the cricothyroid membrane.

The arytenoid, corniculate, and cuneiform cartilages are the paired cartilages of the larynx and serve as attachments for the vocal ligaments. The arytenoid cartilages swing in and out. This action opens or closes the space between the vocal cords because the posterior end of each vocal cord is attached to an arytenoid cartilage and thus must move with it.

The epiglottis is a leaf-shaped cartilaginous structure that is attached to the thyroid cartilage by ligaments and projects upward and posterior to the base of the tongue to guard the opening of the larynx.

The larynx contains extrinsic and intrinsic striated muscles. The extrinsic muscles connect the larynx to adjacent structures of the neck (the hyoid and sternum) and assist in swallowing. The five intrinsic muscles (Table 7-2) connect the laryngeal cartilages and alter the shape of the laryngeal cavity by contracting. The intrinsic muscles act as constrictors, dilators, and

tensors, so they are important in sound production or phonation. A branch of the vagus nerve, the recurrent laryngeal nerve, supplies the intrinsic muscles except for the cricothyroid muscle, which is supplied by the superior laryngeal nerve. This innervation becomes particularly significant during endotracheal intubation; mechanical manipulation of the vocal cords and musculature may result in bradycardia from vagal stimulation.

Internal structures of the larynx The internal structures are protected by the thyroid cartilage in front and include the vestibule, the false vocal cords, the true vocal cords, the laryngeal ventricle, and the glottis.

The inlet to the larynx lies in the anterior wall of the pharynx and is bordered by the epiglottis and arytenoid cartilages. From the inlet the larynx expands into a wide vestibule that ends at the level of the true vocal folds.

Inside the larynx are two pairs of shelflike folds that project inward from the lateral walls of the larynx. The superior folds, or false vocal cords, are attached to the cartilage anteriorly and the arytenoid cartilage posteriorly. They do not produce sound. Just under the false vocal cords are the true vocal cords. The true vocal cords are joined anteriorly where they attach to the inner surface of the thyroid cartilage. This is a fixed point at which the cords are held immobile, but they attach posteriorly to the movable arytenoid cartilages, which allow them to adduct and abduct.

The laryngeal ventricle, a fold of mucous membrane between the true and false cords, extends up under the thyroid cartilage. Glands in the upper portion of the ventricle secrete mucus that lubricates the vocal cords.

The narrowest portion of the larynx is the glottis; this is the space between the vocal cords. The glottis is somewhat larger in men than in women. It is very small in infants, thereby causing much greater danger when the airway becomes edematous as with laryngitis.

Additional structures of the larynx The larynx is lined with mucous membrane that is continuous with the pharynx above and the trachea below. The mucosa folds over the false cords beneath the epiglottis, invaginates into the laryngeal ventricle, and comes out again to cover the true vocal cords before descending into the trachea.

Most of the blood supply to the larynx is provided by the superior and inferior thyroid arteries through their branches, the superior and inferior laryngeal arteries.

Lymphatic drainage is provided by lymph nodes in the middle and upper cervical chains along the internal jugular vein. All parts of the extrinsic larynx and the arytenoid area contain a somewhat rich lymphatic network, but the true vocal cords have a sparse supply of lymphatic vessels.

Functions of the larynx The most important function of the larynx is to form an airway between the pharynx and the trachea. The larynx is not merely a tube, as is the trachea. It is an organ with sphincter functions that help prevent aspiration and assist in coughing. During swallowing the aryepiglottic folds, the arytenoids, and the tubercle of the epiglottis fold inward, close the larynx, and prevent food from entering the trachea. Other actions close the glottis when a foreign body enters the throat and assist in expelling it by increasing intrathoracic pressure when coughing. The cough reflex is an important protective mechanism and is set off whenever the highly sensitive laryngeal mucosa is touched by a foreign body.

Phonation, or the formation of speech sounds, is also an important function of the larynx. Although phonation is not its chief purpose, the larynx is sometimes called the "voice box." During phonation, tracheal air pressure increases and decreases; as the edges of the cords firm and relax, the larynx moves up and down so the air columns above and below are lengthened and shortened. The larynx creates sounds (humming or buzzing) as a result of vocal cord vibration. Words are formed when the vibrating column of air comes up from the larynx to the tongue, lips, palate, and teeth (Figure 7-15). Movements of the mouth (articulation) actually form the words.

 ## Normal Findings

Ear

External ear   Height and size equal; skin clean; no evidence of injury or trauma; *older adult:* earlobes may appear pendulous

Auricle   Moves freely without causing pain; *older adult:* may be more prominent

Tympanic membrane   Drumhead slightly conical, quite shiny, and pearl gray in color; oblique position when viewed with otoscope; cerumen color varying from black to brown to creamy pink; cerumen waxy or flaky; depending on translucency, should be possible to visualize following in normal drumhead: malleus, anterior and posterior malleolar folds, anulus (whiter and denser than rest of drumhead), long process of incus (frequently seen posterior to manubrium of malleus), occasionally chorda tympani nerve seen crossing transversely behind drumhead at about level of short process of malleus;

older adult: some landmarks may appear more pronounced because of atrophied or sclerotic tympanic changes; cerumen may appear very dry as fewer sebaceous glands are active

Eustachian tube   Eardrum moves with Valsalva maneuver if tube is patent

Vestibulocochlear nerve (cranial nerve VIII)   Patient able to hear whisper from distance of 2 feet; tuning fork placed in middle of head heard equally well in both ears; *older adult:* presbycusis (hearing loss from senile degenerative changes) may be present

Nose

Nares   Oval and symmetric

Mucosa   Nose mostly lined with respiratory mucosa that is deep pink and glistening; *older adult:* may be somewhat drier

Septum   Septum usually not straight but deviates from midline; posterior two thirds bony, anterior one third cartilaginous; *older adult:* usually deviates

Turbinates   Turbinates deep pink and similar in color to rest of nasal mucosa; firm consistency

Sinuses   No tenderness, swelling, or purulent secretions from sinus ostia

Olfactory nerve (cranial nerve I)   Patient able to identify odor of substances such as lemon or coffee; *older adult:* sense of smell may be somewhat depressed

Pharynx

Oropharynx   Soft palate pink, showing fine vessels under mucosa; hard palate white, more irregular, showing rugae running transversely; ducts of mucous glands may be seen in back of hard palate; uvula may vary greatly in size and may be bifid or "split"; tonsils same color as rest of oral mucosa, with crypts of whitish epithelium showing; small irregular red or pink spots of lymphoid tissue commonly seen in mucosa of posterior pharyngeal wall; gag reflex induced by touching posterior wall of pharynx

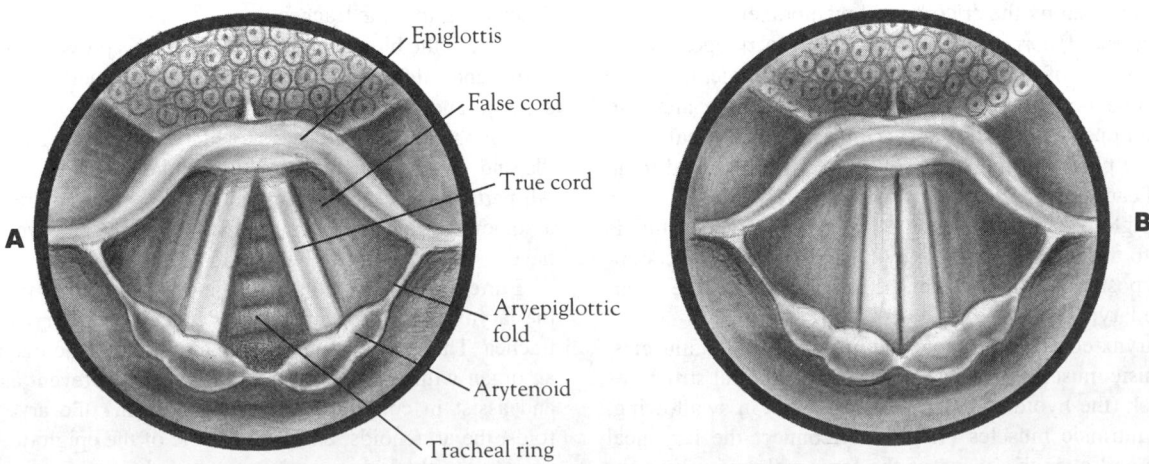

Figure 7-15 Larynx. **A,** In quiet respiration. **B,** In phonation.

Nasopharynx Superior, middle, and inferior turbinates can be seen and may vary in size and appearance; orifice of eustachian tube seen, usually pale, yellowish, and small; orifice normally closed but opens during yawning and swallowing; adenoids seen growing from roof and posterior wall if not surgically removed, usually small after puberty

Hypopharynx Circumvallate papillae in inverted V found on posterior tongue, may vary greatly in size; lingual tonsils on either side of tongue, may vary in size; small white spots that are debris in tonsillar crypts frequently seen; valleculae seen as cup-shaped spaces between tongue and epiglottis, may have large veins; epiglottis varies in size, shape, and color, free edge thin and slightly curved

Larynx

External (by visual examination) Thyroid cartilage (Adam's apple) protrudes, more obvious in men; laryngeal crepitation should occur when thyroid cartilage is grasped between thumb and forefinger and is moved from side to side; cricoid cartilage can be seen in thin persons with head extended and can be easily palpated; hyoid bone palpable above thyroid cartilage; cricoid cartilage drawn upward when patient says high-pitched E-E-E as normal cricothyroid muscle contracts; *older adult:* thyroid cartilage may be very noticeable

Internal (by indirect laryngoscopy) Cords move only slightly during normal respiration; phonation causes adduction of cords, which should approximate perfectly; true vocal cords appear white and sharp edged, although they are actually pink with rounded edges; a few tracheal rings sometimes seen all the way to carina; false vocal cords appear dull pink and thicker than true vocal cords; arytenoids dull red, mobile, and swing in and out with phonation; they appear as small mounds at posterior end of glottis; *older adult:* musculature control decreases, producing characteristic hoarseness and quavering voice; atrophy of muscles and mucosa in trachea; fatty infiltration of trachea

Normal variations in pregnancy Increased vascularity of upper respiratory tract from elevated estrogen levels; nasal stuffiness, epistaxis, fullness in ears, and impaired hearing may result from engorgement of capillaries of nose, pharynx, and eustachian tubes[45]

CONDITIONS, DISEASES, AND DISORDERS

EAR DISORDERS

◼ BENIGN TUMORS

Benign tumors affecting the ear are nonmalignant growths such as keloids, nodules, sebaceous cysts, polyps, and exostoses.

Nonmalignant tumors may develop on the external ear or anywhere in the ear canal. They rarely become malignant, but they may occlude the ear canal and cause retention of cerumen and a conductive hearing loss. The prognosis is excellent with proper diagnosis and treatment.

•••••• Pathophysiology

Keloids are large overgrowths of hypertrophied scar tissue that result from surgery or trauma. They are much more common in blacks than in whites. In the ear keloids commonly form as a result of ear piercing; however, other trauma to the auricle can also cause them. Keloids may also appear with no history of trauma. The treatment is excision, followed by repeated injections of a long-lasting steroid. Recently, carbon dioxide laser resection of the keloid has been performed, allowing the wound bed to heal by secondary intention with good results.

Nodules may form along the superior rim of the auricle and become indurated or painful. The cause is unknown. Treatment is excision or injection of a long-lasting steroid such as methylprednisolone or triamcinolone (Kenalog).

Sebaceous cysts are sebaceous glands that become obstructed with sebum, a soft, cheesy material. These cysts may occur in the meatus of the canal or just behind the earlobe. They are normally painless, but can enlarge quickly and become painful if infected. Acute sebaceous cysts are incised and drained, and hot, moist compresses are applied.

Exostoses are small, hard, bony lumps covered with normal epithelium. They arise from the osseous ear canal near the tympanic membrane and are attached to the posterior wall. The bases of these exostoses are close to the facial nerve. Exostoses are usually bilateral and frequently occur in multiples. They rarely occur during childhood and are more common in men than in women. They are usually asymptomatic and seldom cause an obstruction of the canal. It is believed that exostoses form from an irritation of the periosteum as a result of swimming in cold water. Treatment is usually unnecessary, although removal may be indicated if they grow too large.

◼ HEARING IMPAIRMENT
(Deafness)

Hearing impairment is a state of diminished auditory acuity that ranges from partial to complete loss of hearing.

Hearing loss can be partial or total and can occur in low, medium, or high frequencies or in combination. Hearing is measured in decibels (dB), which is a ratio that compares the relationship between two sound intensities.

The American Medical Association's formula for hearing loss is that hearing is impaired 1.5% for every decibel that the pure tone average exceeds 25 dB. A hearing loss of 40 dB in both ears, or a 22.5% hearing impairment, usually impairs a person's ability to function normally in social situations and requires the use of a hearing aid unless it can be medically or surgically treated. True deafness, however, is defined as 85 to 90 dB below normal. Hearing losses can occur in one or both ears, depending on the etiology and may imply only a partial loss of function, depending on the severity.

Many individuals in industrialized societies are exposed to high levels of noise. Noise exposure is the major cause of acquiring hearing loss in the United States; it is ranked as one of the country's major health problems by the National Institute of Occupational Safety and Health. Permanent threshold shifts can also result from exposure to a number of ototoxic agents—ototoxic compounds, such as aspirin, are the most commonly used drugs in industrialized societies. Current debate discusses whether a combination of salicylates and noise produces more hearing loss or hair cell loss than noise exposure alone.[48]

•••••• Pathophysiology

The six types of hearing loss are sensorineural, conductive, mixed, congenital, simulated, and central.

Sensorineural hearing loss   Sensorineural hearing loss is the result of disease within the cochlea, the cochlear nerve, or the brain. It usually results from trauma, an infectious process, a degenerative process such as presbycusis, a senile degenerative change in the hair cells in the organ of Corti (see box), a congenital abnormality, or exposure to ototoxic substances such as certain drugs.[47]

Exposure to high level noise appears to damage the cochlea in a temporary and in a permanent manner. Extremely high-level exposures, such as impulse noise, may cause direct mechanical damage of the hair cells and supporting cells in the organ of Corti and the lateral wall of the cochlea.

Ototoxic drugs (aminoglycoside antibiotics and cisplatin) clearly increase damage caused by concurrent exposure to noise; ototoxic drugs also cause permanent damage when administered alone. The initial site of damage appears to be the hair cells.[48]

 HEARING AND BALANCE DISORDERS IN THE ELDERLY

Presbycusis is hearing loss in the aged patient. Changes in the inner ear result in a predominantly high-frequency sensorineural hearing loss. The hearing loss may be associated with tinnitus (ringing in the ears). Although presbycusis cannot be cured, some patients may benefit from the use of a hearing aid. Consultation with an audiologist will allow the patient to experiment with various techniques to enhance hearing and communication.

Presbyvertigo (presbyastasis) is the vestibular disorder associated with aging. When a balance disorder occurs in this group of patients, it is usually associated with a decrease in visual acuity and altered proprioception. The three systems are necessary to maintain balance, therefore the elderly may have more difficulty ambulating, resulting in falls and injury. As with presbycusis, presbyvertigo cannot be cured but the symptoms can be controlled. Consultation with a physical therapist can provide the patient with vestibular (balance) exercises to help accommodate to the vertigo. In addition, the use of a cane or walker can be attempted to compensate for the loss of stability.

This may also be called perceptive or nerve-type hearing loss. Patients with sensorineural hearing losses are often unable to use hearing aids satisfactorily.

Conductive hearing loss   Conductive hearing loss is also called transmission hearing loss. It occurs in disorders of the external or middle ear such as otitis media, otosclerosis, or a perforated eardrum. These patients have a normal inner ear, but sound waves are prevented from reaching the inner ear normally. If sound is amplified, these patients may be able to hear very well, and therefore a hearing aid can be beneficial. With the exception of otosclerosis in which the drumhead usually appears normal, disorders that cause conductive hearing loss also cause changes in the normal appearance of the drumhead, such as thickening or retraction.

Mixed hearing loss   Some patients have both conductive and sensorineural hearing losses.

Congenital hearing loss   Congenital hearing loss is present from birth or early infancy. "Neonatal" causes may be anoxia, trauma during delivery, or Rh incompatibility. Other causes may be maternal exposure to syphilis or rubella during pregnancy or the use of ototoxic drugs during pregnancy. Infants with serum bilirubin levels greater than 20 mg/dl may also incur hearing losses from the toxic effect of high bilirubin levels on the brain.

Simulated hearing loss   Simulated hearing loss is also called functional, psychogenic, or nonorganic hearing loss. It means that an apparent hearing loss is not the result of an organic cause and may represent malingering or a functional disorder.

Central hearing loss   Central loss is caused by damage to the brain's auditory pathways, as in a cerebrovascular accident.

•••••• Diagnostic Studies and Findings

Weber test   The tip of the handle of a vibrating tuning fork is placed on the patient's forehead or front teeth. The patient is asked if the sound is heard in the head, right ear, or left ear. Sound is heard in the head or equally in both ears if the patient has normal hearing. Lateralization of sound to the deaf ear occurs in conductive hearing loss; lateralization of sound to the better ear occurs in sensorineural hearing loss.

Rinne test   A vibrating tuning fork is alternately placed against the mastoid bone (to determine bone conduction) or in front of the ear (for air conduction). Bone conduction is heard longer than or equal to air conduction in conductive hearing loss; air conduction is heard longer but not twice as long as bone conduction in sensorineural hearing loss.

Schwaback test   The Schwaback test compares the hearing of the examiner with the patient. The vibrating tuning fork is placed on the mastoid bone of both the examiner and patient. The patient hears longer than the examiner in conductive hearing loss; the examiner hears longer than the patient in sensorineural hearing loss.

Audiometric tests   Speech and impedance audiometry, tympanometry, and electrocochleography are used to differentiate between types of hearing loss and to identify degree of hearing impairment.[47]

•••••• Multidisciplinary Plan

Surgery

Depending on the type of hearing impairment, a variety of surgical interventions may be appropriate

Stapedectomy—see p. 665

Cochlear implant—provides auditory sensation to patients with severe bilateral hearing loss who have not had any successful hearing with a hearing aid; complex procedure in which inferior aspect of the basal scala tympani is exposed; bone is removed from inferior margins of scala tympani for distance of approximately 4 to 5 mm from round window; surgeon then negotiates the tip of the silastic-sheathed multielectrode around the first turn of the basal cochlea in the bony groove in the posterior canal wall, which is then covered with cortical bone and temporalis fascia[47]; device electrically stimulates remaining, intact, and excitable auditory neurons in profoundly deaf individuals; electronic "heart" of device is small processor that can be carried on belt and can receive sound through microphone and electronically break signal into four channels; a tiny transmitter, which is mounted behind ear, sends signal to receiver implanted under skin; from internal receiver, fine wire leads to electrode, which is implanted against auditory nerves in cochlea.

Environmental and speech sounds are picked up by a microphone and sent to a sound processing unit that filters the stimuli. The auditory stimuli are changed into an electrical pattern that goes to the external transmitter. An internal receiver is under the external transmitter. The electrical stimuli are transmitted to the cochlea by an electrode that stimulates cochlear nerve fibers.

The patient, physician, nurse, and audiologist form the cochlear implant team. Extensive testing, counseling and rehabilitation is required for the patient before, during, and after a cochlear implant.

Cochlear nucleus implant—clinical studies are underway on cochlear nucleus implants; they are made up of an externally placed microphone and transmitting device; the surgically implanted external receiver is connected to a stimulating patch electrode that is placed on the surface of the brainstem overlying the cochlear nucleus; the implant may be useful for patients with bilateral acoustic neuromas and for persons whose deafness is a result of congenital, traumatic, ototoxic, or inflammatory causes—those who are not candidates for cochlear implant because they lack excitable auditory nerve fibers.[9]

General Management

Hearing aids—amplifier- or transducer-type hearing aids prescribed, depending on nature of hearing impairment

Bone conduction hearing aids—these aids may be implanted under the scalp in patients with unilateral sensorineural hearing loss after acoustic neuroma surgery; the aids may be effective in some cases; however, they are not yet routinely recommended

---

NURSING CARE

Nursing Assessment

Stares blankly or has strained facial expression; speaks loudly; asks to have things repeated; gives irrelevant answers to questions; may not participate in conversations; withdraws; may hear much better when watching speaker's face; inattentive; daydreams; scholastic performance below apparent ability (if school age); delayed speech and language development (if small child); may complain of sound distortion; intolerant of loud noise

Nursing Dx & Intervention

Sensory/perceptual alterations (auditory) related to hearing impairment

- Assess patient's degree of hearing impairment and concomitant ability to communicate with others.
- Ensure that other health-care providers are aware of patient's hearing impairment—place a note on Kardex, on door, and at intercom at nursing station.
- When conversing, speak slowly and distinctly and face patient directly *so patient can see your face.* Do not shout or overexaggerate words.
- Ensure that patient has heard and understood everything said.
- Ascertain whether patient hears better from one ear than from the other and speak toward that ear when talking with patient.
- Obtain speaker phone or pocket talker and a pillow speaker for television set *so patient can use telephone and television comfortably.*
- Discuss with family members any strategies used at home to assist patient with hearing.
- If patient is hospitalized for problem unrelated to hearing impairment, ascertain whether patient has been evaluated for hearing problem and discuss with physician, patient, and family the possibility of audiology consultation and follow-up, if appropriate.
- If patient is completely deaf, provide Magic Slate or notepad *so patient can communicate in writing.*
- If patient wears a hearing aid at home, encourage patient to wear it in the hospital also. Check hearing aid for power level, battery, and proper functioning.
- If patient is being fitted for a hearing aid, encourage and assist patient to wear it for progressively longer periods of time and assure patient that any discomfort is temporary.
- If patient is hospitalized for ear surgery to improve or stabilize hearing, provide patient with appropriate preoperative and postoperative care and assess and record any improvements in hearing after operation.

Patient Education/Home Care Planning

1. Demonstrate for the patient the proper use and maintenance of hearing aid, if prescribed. (See "Care of a Hearing Aid" and "What to Do If a Hearing Aid Fails to Work" below.)
2. Ensure that the patient and family are aware of any post-operative instructions, if appropriate.
3. Encourage the patient to ask people to speak more slowly or clearly or to repeat statements so the patient does not feel left out of conversations.
4. Encourage referral for aural rehabilitation, if indicated.

Patient Education/Home Care Planning

Care of a hearing aid
1. Turn the hearing aid off when not in use.
2. Open the battery compartment at night to avoid accidental drainage of the battery.
3. Keep an extra battery available at all times.
4. Wash the earmold frequently (daily if necessary) with mild soap and warm water, using a pipe cleaner to cleanse the cannula.
5. Dry the earmold completely before reconnecting it to the receiver.
6. Do not wear the hearing aid if an ear infection is present.

Patient Education/Home Care Planning

What to do if hearing aid fails to work
1. Check the on-off switch.
2. Inspect the earmold for cleanliness.
3. Examine the battery for correct insertion.
4. Examine the cord plug for correct insertion.
5. Examine the cord for breaks.
6. Replace the battery, cord, or both, if necessary. The life of batteries varies according to the amount of use and the power requirements of the aid. Batteries last from 2 to 14 days.
7. Check the position of the earmold in the ear. If the hearing aid "whistles," the earmold is probably not inserted properly into the ear canal, or the person needs to have a new earmold made.

Evaluation

Patient recovers uneventfully (if surgery performed) Hearing level is improved to normal. Patient verbalizes ear regimen and any symptoms to be reported to physician.

Patient copes well with hearing impairment   Patient verbalizes and demonstrates use and maintenance of hearing aid (if used). Hearing level is improved with use of hearing aid. Patient has learned to use strategies, such as lip reading or sign language.

EXTERNAL OTITIS

External otitis is a general term used to describe inflammatory diseases of the auricle and the external auditory canal.

External otitis may be acute or chronic and may be localized, as with furunculosis, or diffuse, involving the entire canal. The disorder may be caused by either infections or dermatosis or by a combination of the two. It is more common in summer and is sometimes called swimmer's ear. External otitis varies in severity; occasionally no infection is present, and it may result from either contact or seborrheic dermatitis. Either bacteria or fungi may produce infectious external otitis. Bacterial causes are usually attributed to *Pseudomonas, Proteus, Streptococcus,* or *Staphylococcus.* Fungi, which are most common in the tropics, are usually *Aspergillus* and *Candida.* Predisposing factors include allergies that may increase the likelihood oi external otitis; irritants such as hair sprays, hair dyes, or dust that causes the person to scratch the ear canal, resulting in excoriation; cleaning or scratching the ear canal with a foreign object, such as a cotton swab, bobby pin, or finger, which causes irritation and possible introduction of infectious organisms; continual use of earphones, earplugs, hearing aid, or earmuffs, which trap moisture in the ear, thereby creating a medium for infection; and swimming in contaminated water, which is absorbed by the wax in the ear, macerates the skin of the canal, and allows the introduction of organisms.

•••••• Pathophysiology

Acute external otitis is frequently caused by *Pseudomonas,* which can be cultured from the auditory canal. The infection begins in the external auditory canal, usually after minor trauma. It may spread from the canal through Santorini's fissures in the conchal cartilage, after involving the perichondrium. It then invades the periauricular tissue, including the parotid gland, temporomandibular joint, and soft tissues at the base of the skull. The infection can progress along the base of the skull, causing paralysis of the seventh cranial nerve at the stylomastoid foramen, the ninth, tenth, and eleventh cranial nerves at the jugular foramen, and the hypoglossal nerve and the hypoglossal canal. The jugular vein may become thrombosed, progressing to a lateral sinus thrombosis. The infection could also progress from the external auditory canal, through the tympanic membrane, and into the middle ear, and through the mastoid air cells and into the petrous apex and brainstem. Mortality is 67% among patients with facial nerve paralysis and 20% for those with other cranial nerve involvement.

Acute external otitis can range from mild to severe. In the mild stage, pain is moderate to severe and is aggravated by traction on the auricle or pressure on the tragus. The patient may have a low-grade fever and a sticky, yellow discharge from the ear canal. There may be a partial loss of hearing or the feeling of a blocked ear if the ear canal is swollen or obstructed with debris.

Pain is more intense during the severe stage of external otitis. Often the entire side of the head aches, and the patient cannot tolerate examination of the auricle. A sticky, yellow discharge from the ear canal is usually present; hearing may be diminished, and the ear feels blocked. The patient's temperature may be as high as 40° C (104° F). The external auditory canal is swollen or entirely closed, and the tragus and external meatus are also swollen. The epithelium of the canal is usually soggy and pale. Desquamated epithelium and wax are often present in the canal. However, the canal may be reddened rather than pale, or the epithelium may be dry instead of wet. Patients may also have lymphadenopathy anterior to the tragus, behind the ear, or in the upper neck. If the auricle is involved, the skin is crusted and oozing. Pustules may be present and the ear may be swollen and tender. If the infection did not originate on the face or scalp, it may spread to these areas. The eardrum frequently cannot be seen well in acute external otitis because the ear canal is so swollen. An infected canal usually causes much more pain than if the auricle alone is affected because the epithelium of the ear canal cannot stretch much without causing pain.

With chronic external otitis, itching rather than pain is the usual complaint. There is no pain even with manipulation of the auricle or tragus. The epithelium is thickened and red, and the canal and drumhead are insensitive to pressure from cotton applicators. A discharge is usually present.

A rare, lethal type of external otitis, which is called malignant external otitis, is caused by *Pseudomonas* and occasionally by *Staphylococcus epidermidis;* it is a fulminant bone-destroying infection. It occurs most commonly in elderly diabetic patients. It quickly involves all contiguous structures and has a mortality of 50% to 75% unless recognized early and treated with potent parenteral antibiotics.

In fungal external otitis, a characteristic mass (black or grayish with *Aspergillus niger*) forms in the ear canal. Its removal reveals a hyperemic, edematous epithelium that may be denuded. Fungal infections may be asymptomatic because frequently the growth is found only on wax or other debris in the ear and has not invaded the tissue.

Furunculosis is a localized type of external otitis in the outer half of the ear canal. Glands and hair follicles in this area may become infected and form boils or furuncles. The onset of a furuncle may be acute; the patient may notice a feeling of fullness in the ear, loss of hearing, adenopathy, and swelling behind the ear. The area is reddened. It may be very swollen and may obstruct the entire canal. Pain is intense; even a small furuncle causes severe pain until it is surgically drained or breaks spontaneously. Movement of the auricle and tragus causes pain, as does chewing if the furuncle is on the canal floor or anterior wall.

•••••• Diagnostic Studies and Findings

Culture of drainage   Identification of causative organisms; usual organisms are *Pseudomonas, Proteus, Streptococcus, Staphylococcus, Aspergillus,* and *Candida*

•••••• Multidisciplinary Plan

Surgery

Surgery not performed unless furuncle needs incision and drainage

Medications

Narcotic analgesics such as codeine, 30 mg po q4h
Corticosteroids
  A wick is inserted into the ear canal; hydrocortisone and acetic acid otic solution may be used to reduce swelling and to allow penetration of antibiotics
Antiinfective agents
  Antibiotic or antifungal ear drops may be prescribed, which usually contain 0.5% neomycin or 10,000 U/ml of polymyxin; if ear canal is swollen, a wick may be inserted to allow drops to reach ear canal
Systemic antibiotics may be prescribed if infection is severe; specific drug depends on causative organism

General Management

Careful cleaning of ear canal to remove debris and impacted cerumen
Heat therapy to external ear for pain relief
For malignant external otitis: hyperbaric O_2 therapy may be used to reverse tissue hypoxia and augment the action of aminoglycoside antibiotics (for advanced or recurrent cases)[7]

NURSING CARE

Nursing Assessment

Infection of External Ear

Acute
  Moderate to severe pain in the ear, which is exacerbated by chewing and manipulation of the auricle or tragus; headache; fever; feeling of fullness or blockage in ear; foul-smelling, yellow, sticky discharge from ear (black if from fungal infection); hearing normal or decreased; tinnitus; localized swelling; erythema; lymphadenopathy behind ear and in upper neck
Chronic
  Chief complaint itching rather than pain; discharge usually present

Nursing Dx & Intervention

Pain related to ear infection

- Assess need for pain medication and in collaboration with physician, provide medication as required *for pain relief;* evaluate and document effectiveness.
- Monitor vital signs, especially temperature.
- If chewing is painful, arrange for soft or full-liquid diet.

Impaired skin integrity related to involvement of skin by infectious process

- Assess ear canal and auricle for swelling, crusting, scabs, pustules, and discharge.

- Keep ear canal clean: Cleanse gently with cotton swab soaked with Burow's solution (as ordered) and also apply directly to auricle. Dry gently and completely.
- Administer antibiotics as ordered.
- Instill medicated ear drops as ordered.
- Observe and record amount of aural drainage.

Sensory/perceptual alterations (auditory) related to obstruction of ear canal from edema or debris

- Assess degree of hearing impairment.
- If patient's hearing is diminished, be sure that adequate method of communication is used.
- Speak slowly and clearly and stand directly in front of patient when speaking.
- Instruct patient and family about factors contributing to development of external otitis and encourage patient to keep foreign objects such as bobby pins out of ears.
- Encourage patient to use earplugs when swimming and to minimize amount of water that gets into ears when showering and shampooing.

Patient Education/Home Care Planning

1. Discuss with the patient and family the necessity of completing the prescribed course of medication, whether antibiotics or ear drops, to avoid inadequate treatment or possible recurrence.
2. Demonstrate to the patient and family the proper way to instill ear drops. (See "Instructions for Using Ear Wash and Drops" below.)
3. If Burow's soaks are done, give instructions in the proper method.

Patient Education/Home Care Planning

Instructions for using ear wash and drops

The patient will need a 2- or 3-ounce ear syringe and a prescription for ear wash and drops. The patient should have a family member or another care giver perform the ear washing according to the following instructions:

1. Wash hands before and after the earwashing procedure.
2. Fill the ear syringe with the solution.
3. The solution must be at body temperature. If the solution is too warm or too cool, the patient will feel dizzy. Warm the solution by placing the syringe in a pan of hot water. Do *not* warm the solution on the stove or in the microwave.
4. Have the patient lie down with the ear to be washed facing up. Pull up and out on the external ear. Place the tip of the ear syringe into the ear canal. Do not be afraid to push it down into the ear. However, a return flow of solution should be noted. If not, the syringe is in too far. Pull the syringe out slightly.

5. Pump the warmed solution from the syringe back and forth into the ear by squeezing and releasing the bulb of the syringe. Do this very vigorously and repeatedly. The ear wash must be forced back and forth, in and out of the ear canal.
6. Have the patient lean over the side of the sink or basin and let the solution run out of the ear.
7. Pull the ear up, back, and out to straighten the ear canal.
8. Put 3 to 5 warmed drops into the ear.
9. If the solution burns too much at first, it may need to be diluted. Mix 2 ounces of water with 2 ounces of the solution. Later, decrease the amount of water used with each irrigation.
10. Use the solution and drops twice a day for 2 weeks and then until the ear stops running or becomes dry. If it is uncertain whether the ear is dry, check it by putting a cotton swab down into the ear canal. If the cotton swab comes out dry, stop using the solution and drops. If the cotton swab is wet or there is an odor from the ear, continue using the solution and drops for 4 days.
11. Do not use the solution and drops as long as the ear remains dry and is not running, and as long as there is no odor. Should the ear start to run after being dry for a period of time, start using the ear solution and drops until the ear is once again dry.

Instruct the patient to prevent any water from getting into the ear. Instruct the patient to refrain from swimming. Whenever there is a chance that water may get into the ear, such as when the patient showers or washes his hair, the patient should put cotton in the ear. First, place a dry piece of cotton in the ear, then a second piece of cotton that has been saturated with petroleum jelly.

Instruct the patient to call the physician if there are questions.

Evaluation

Inflammation of external ear and canal is cleared   No pain is present in the ear. Patient's temperature is within normal limits. There is no discharge from ear canal. Hearing is within normal limits for patient. There is no cervical lymphadenopathy.

Patient and family verbalize increased knowledge of disease and its treatment   Patient and family verbalize understanding of cause of, contributing factors to, and ways to prevent recurrence of disease. Patient and family verbalize understanding of necessity of completing prescribed course of antibiotics.

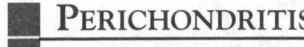

PERICHONDRITIS

Perichondritis is an inflammation of the auricular cartilage.

Perichondritis may follow a skin infection or trauma, which causes exposure of the cartilage to bacteria.

••••• Pathophysiology

Perichondritis may be initiated by trauma, insect bites, or incision of superficial infections of the pinna, which causes pus to accumulate between the cartilage and the perichondrium. The causative organism is usually a gram-negative rod, frequently *Pseudomonas*. Perichondritis can cause a loss of blood supply to the cartilage, resulting in breakdown and necrosis of the cartilage. The pinna appears enlarged, inflamed, and shiny. Pain is usually severe, and localized fluctuant areas may be present on the auricle. Perichondritis must be treated early and aggressively to prevent a lengthy, destructive course.

••••• Diagnostic Studies and Findings

Culture of purulent material Identification of causative organism

••••• Multidisciplinary Plan

Surgery

Incision and drainage of any purulent material; removal of any necrotic cartilage

Medications

Antiinfective agents
  Systemic parenteral antibiotic therapy, depending on cultured organisms; local irrigations with antibiotic solutions (usually polymyxin B [10,000 U/ml], bacitracin, neomycin 0.5%, or a combination)
Narcotic analgesics or analgesic/antipyretic agents
  Analgesia for pain relief; aspirin or acetaminophen (Tylenol) 650 mg, with codeine, 30 mg po q4h

General Management

Small polyethylene tube inserted into area beneath nonpressure dressing to facilitate irrigation
Local heat applications for relief

NURSING CARE

Nursing Assessment

Auricular Cartilage

Inflammation, erythema, and swelling of the cartilage, usually with pus; fluctuant areas on auricle; severe pain; may have fever or lymphadenopathy; history of trauma, insect bite, or incision of superficial infection on pinna

Nursing Dx & Intervention

Pain related to inflammation of auricular cartilage

- Assess need for pain medication and provide analgesic medications for pain relief as ordered. Evaluate and document effectiveness.

Sensory/perceptual alterations (auditory) related to obstruction of ear canal or use of ototoxic drugs

- Assess patient's hearing ability before and during treatment with ototoxic drugs.
- Administer antibiotics as ordered.
- Perform irrigations as ordered with room-temperature antibiotic solution.
- Be aware that irrigating solution contains potentially ototoxic drugs.
- Monitor vital signs, especially temperature.

Impaired skin integrity related to inflammation of and altered circulation to auricular cartilage

- Assess auricular cartilage for inflammation, swelling, and presence of pus.
- Perform wound care of affected area if incision and drainage have been done.
- Apply local heat for comfort as ordered.

Patient Education/Home Care Planning

1. Discuss with the patient and family the necessity of completing the prescribed course of antibiotics to avoid recurrence or complications.
2. If wound care is being done, be sure that the patient and family know the procedures to change the dressing and aseptic techniques to avoid wound contamination.

Evaluation

Patient is free of pain Patient can tolerate pain or is comfortable with analgesia prescribed.

No hearing impairment exists Patient's hearing remains at pretreatment level.

Inflammation of auricular cartilage is absent There is no drainage from affected ear. Temperature is within normal limits for patient. There are no fluctuant areas on auricle. Patient and family demonstrate ability to change dressing properly using aseptic technique.

Patient and family verbalize and demonstrate knowledge of treatment Patient and family verbalize understanding of necessity of completing prescribed course of antibiotics to prevent recurrence of infection.

INFECTIOUS MYRINGITIS

Infectious or bullous myringitis is an inflammation of the tympanic membrane.

Vesicles in the tympanic membrane and at the end of the external auditory canal appear hemorrhagic and rupture spontaneously, which is revealed by serosanguineous fluid in the external ear. The cause is either viral or bacterial, and the disorder sometimes occurs after infections of the ear canal or acute otitis media. It is common in children.

The patient experiences severe ear pain and some tenderness over the mastoid area. Occasionally fever and mild hearing loss are present. Untreated infection can result in perforation of the tympanic membrane. Treatment consists of pain management with aspirin or other analgesics, local heat for comfort, and either local or systemic antibiotic therapy to prevent secondary infection. Infectious myringitis usually resolves spontaneously within 3 days to 2 weeks.

OTITIS MEDIA

Otitis media is an inflammation of the middle ear and can be classified as acute and suppurative or subacute (otitis media with effusion).

Acute Otitis Media

Acute otitis media is very common in young children and is usually the result of a bacterial or viral infection of the upper respiratory tract. Organisms travel from the nasopharynx to the middle ear by way of the eustachian tube. Infants and children have shorter, straighter eustachian tubes than do adults; this easier access to the middle ear is probably the reason otitis media is common in children. Another contributing factor is that children have not developed immunities to the organisms that cause the infection. Children also have a large mass of adenoid tissue that usually disappears during adolescence. If this lymphoid tissue is swollen, it can obstruct the opening of the eustachian tube and contribute to the development of otitis media by preventing equalization of the atmospheric pressure in the ear, thereby causing a vacuum and effusion of the middle ear.

Most episodes of recurrent acute otitis media occur between 6 and 36 months of age and in the winter and early spring. Prophylactic antibiotics, prescribed and used appropriately, may be helpful in protecting children during this period.[19]

Although the prognosis for acute otitis media is good, successful treatment requires patients to follow medical regimens and to keep scheduled appointments with caregivers for proper follow-up.

Epidemiologic studies have shown that up to 80% of all children who have not yet attained school age have episodes of eustachian tube dysfunction and secretory otitis media of varying duration. In addition to causing reduced hearing and various eardrum changes, secretory otitis media predisposes to acute middle ear infection and perhaps even chronic otitis media and cholesteatoma later in life.[49]

Otitis Media With Effusion (Subacute)

Otitis media with effusion results from incomplete resolution or inadequate treatment of acute otitis media. The most recent evidence indicates that in a large number of cases, bacteria or bacterial products are trapped in the middle ear as a result of poor tubal muscular function. This situation causes a high negative pressure in the middle ear and produces transudation of fluid from the blood vessels in the membranes of the middle ear. Ciliostasis may be another factor; it causes stagnation of the collected effusion. Yet another factor may be failure to clear the bacteria and bacterial products by dysfunctional phagocytes or inadequate host-immune response to eradicate bacteria. These trapped bacteria in the middle ear initiate a host response that causes tissue injury leading to otitis media with effusion.[31] Otitis media with effusion can also be caused by allergies that produce edema in the lumen of the eustachian tube or by barotrauma that results from external pressure markedly exceeding lowered pressure of the middle ear, as during diving or the descent of an airplane. It is common in children.

Patients feel a fullness in their ears but have no pain or fever. A conductive hearing loss may occur, especially in chronic otitis media with effusion. Otoscopic examination reveals mild retraction of the tympanic membrane with a clear transudate from the blood vessels. The tympanic membrane is immobile and amber colored, and a fluid level or air bubbles may be seen through the tympanic membrane. The meniscus of the fluid may appear as a thin black hair or line across the tympanic membrane. If blood is present, as with barotrauma, the fluid may appear blue-black.

Treatment consists of inflation of the eustachian tube, a Valsalva maneuver (in which the patient inspires, holds the breath, and bears down as though having a bowel movement) several times a day, myringotomy to drain fluid from the middle ear, or antihistamine or decongestant therapy to improve eustachian tube function. A small plastic tube may be inserted following myringotomy and left in place for several weeks to promote drainage and equalize air pressure; this is most commonly done in children but also occasionally in adults.

Chronic otitis media with effusion that results from inadequate treatment of acute otitis media or from overgrowth of the lymphoid tissue in the nasopharynx caused by sino-nasal infections or allergies poses a serious threat to the patient's hearing. There are few symptoms; a fluctuating hearing loss or a feeling of heaviness on one side of the head is most common. Treatment is directed at the underlying cause and the removal of fluid by myringotomy. A small tube is frequently inserted during myringotomy to equalize pressure on both sides of the eardrum and is left in place for 8 to 9 months, when it usually falls out by itself. These tubes may need to be replaced. Patients should be instructed not to swim while a tube is in place.

Not to be overlooked as a cause of chronic otitis media with effusion in adults is carcinoma of the nasopharynx; if the effusion is unilateral, a thorough workup must be done to rule out carcinoma.[8]

Chronic otitis media caused by repeated attacks of acute otitis media, and acute mastoiditis may result in a permanent perforation of the tympanic membrane. Chronic changes such as thickening and scarring of the mucosa eventually occur in the middle ear, and the ossicles may be destroyed. These permanent tympanic perforations result in a slight conductive hearing loss. If the ossicles are involved, the hearing loss may be greater.

There are two types of perforations, central and marginal. In central perforations, the margin of the eardrum is not involved; in marginal perforations, the anulus or margin of the drum is destroyed. Central perforations are more benign than marginal ones and less likely to result in cholesteatomas. Cholesteatomas occur when the marginal perforation of the eardrum allows squamous epithelium of the external auditory canal to grow into the middle ear, which then becomes lined with squamous epithelium. As the epithelium grows, it desquamates and the debris collects inside the middle ear. Cholesteatomas enlarge slowly, expand into the mastoid antrum, and destroy adjacent structures.

The most common symptom of chronic otitis media is a constant, painless, serous discharge from the ear, which varies from foul smelling to nearly odorless. The discharge becomes much worse when the patient has an infection of the upper respiratory tract, and it occasionally causes slight discomfort in the ear.

Treatment consists of thoroughly cleaning the ear and instilling a solution of 0.5% acetic acid with 1.0% hydrocortisone three times a day for 5 to 7 days. Severe cases require systemic antibiotic therapy. Tympanoplasty can also be performed to restore and reconstruct the mechanisms of the middle ear (see p. 671).

•••••• Pathophysiology

The usual pathogens of acute otitis media are gram-positive cocci; *Streptococcus* is cultured from approximately 30% of effusions, but *Haemophilus influenzae* is also frequently found (20% of cases).[19] The inflammation usually results from an infection that ascends through the eustachian tube and involves the lining of the whole middle ear. This has several effects. Exudate and edema interfere with ciliary action in the eustachian tube so its efficiency as a barrier to infection is lost. The opening of the tube is also abnormal because edema has decreased the size of the lumen and inflammation has caused hyperemia of the mucosal lining of the middle ear, which results in increased oxygen absorption. This leads to decreased aeration, development of a partial vacuum, retraction of the tympanic membrane, and serous exudation. This stage is common in viral infections of the upper respiratory tract, but the infection does not progress if the middle ear is reaerated. However, if bacterial superinfection is present, the exudate becomes purulent and causes bulging of the tympanic membrane as the pus collects behind it. This is called purulent otitis media.

•••••• Diagnostic Studies and Findings

Culture of purulent drainage Identification of causative organisms

•••••• Multidisciplinary Plan

Surgery

Myringotomy—to drain pus and fluid from middle ear (see p. 664)

Medications

Antiinfective agents
Amoxicillin (Amoxil, Larotid), 500 mg po tid for 10 d
Sulfamethoxazole (Septra or Bactrim), 1 tab po bid or qid (if allergic to penicillin)

Penicillin G or V, 250-500 mg po q6h for 10 d for patients older than 8 yr
Ampicillin (Amcil, others), 50-100 mg/kg/d for 10 d for children under 8 yr because of frequency of *H. influenzae* infections in this age group
Efixime 4 mg/kg bid po
If patient is allergic to penicillin, erythromycin (E-Mycin, others), 250 mg po q6h for adults and older children; combination of erythromycin and sulfisoxazole for children younger than 8 yr
Analgesic/antipyretic or narcotic analgesics
Codeine, 30 mg po q4h (for severe pain); sedatives sometimes given to small children
Antihistamines
Chlorpheniramine (Chlor-Trimeton), 4 mg po q4-6h for 7-10 d for adults; 0.35 mg/kg qid for children
Decongestants
Pseudoephedrine (Sudafed), 30 mg po q4-6h for adults

General Management

A new therapy involves teaching children a method of autoinflation using a special tube designed to improve middle ear ventilation and thereby reduce the need for inserting ventilation tubes

NURSING CARE

Nursing Assessment

Tympanic Membrane

Severe, deep, throbbing pain behind tympanic membrane; pain may disappear if eardrum ruptures; feeling of fullness in ears; partial loss of hearing

Infectious Process

Fever that may be as high as 40° C (104° F); chills; malaise, weakness and dizziness; nausea and vomiting; tympanic membrane appears red, inflamed, and bulging; if it is perforated, pulsating purulent material can be seen coming through drum after ear is cleaned of pus and debris

Nursing Dx & Intervention

Pain related to buildup of pus behind tympanic membrane

- Assess need for pain medication and provide analgesia as ordered; evaluate and document effectiveness.
- Administer sedatives, if ordered, to young children as needed, *to assist with relaxation and sleep.*
- Instruct parents in appropriate dosages of medication to give child at home.
- Encourage bed rest if patient is weak, complains of malaise, or has nausea and vomiting.

Impaired skin integrity related to skin contamination by purulent material

- Assess patient's outer ear for purulent drainage.
- If patient has had myringotomy, keep ear clean and dry.
- Place sterile cotton in outer ear *to absorb drainage and prevent possible contamination of outer ear, which leads to development of external otitis media.*
- Monitor vital signs, especially temperature, and report any changes.
- Instruct patient/family to avoid introduction of water in ear canals, which can produce an environment for bacterial growth.

Sensory/perceptual alterations (auditory) related to fluid in middle ear

- Assess patient for symptoms of hearing deficit.
- If patient is child, ask parents if they have noticed any signs of hearing loss: inattentiveness, blank stares, lack of response to questions, or pulling at affected ear. (Ear pain is frequently so severe that hearing loss is not noticed.)
- Administer antibiotics as ordered and instruct patients and family about appropriate dosages.
- Instruct patient or family to monitor level of hearing (it should return to normal with appropriate antibiotic therapy).

Patient Education/Home Care Planning

1. Discuss with the patient and family the necessity for completing the entire course of antibiotics to prevent a recurrence or complications.
2. Explain to the parents the need to feed children in an upright position and not lying down to prevent reflux of nasopharyngeal flora through the eustachian tube into the middle ear.
3. Explain to the patient the need to avoid blowing the nose forcefully, which can force contaminated material into the eustachian tube.
4. If the patient has had a myringotomy, demonstrate to the patient and family how to change the cotton in the outer ear at least twice a day.
5. Instruct patient/parents to avoid the introduction of water in ear by using earplugs or inserting a cotton ball coated with petroleum jelly into ear canal when showering or shampooing hair.

Evaluation

Patient's comfort level is increased   Pain is decreased. Patient can sleep through the night and experiences no nausea or vomiting. Patient is afebrile. Activity level is normal.

Skin integrity is maintained   There is no purulent drainage from tympanic membrane. Tympanic membrane appears normal with no bulging, redness, retraction, or inflammation.

Hearing is intact   Patient's hearing is at preinfection level, or the family knows to monitor carefully for return of hearing.

Patient and family have increased knowledge of treatment   Patient and family verbalize understanding of necessity for completing prescribed course of antibiotics and the need to seek medical intervention if symptoms persist or recur.

MASTOIDITIS

Mastoiditis is an inflammation of the air cells of the mastoid cavity.

Usually of bacterial origin, mastoiditis is the result of the extension of a middle ear infection. It was quite common before the discovery of antibiotics but is now found only in patients whose otitis media was untreated or inadequately treated.

•••••• Pathophysiology

Mastoiditis occurs when pus is left in the middle ear from otitis media, and infection progresses into the bony portion of the mastoid antrum and cells. This can cause bony necrosis of the mastoid process and breakdown of its bony structure. If untreated, the infection can lead to formation of subperiosteal abscesses and other complications, including meningitis, facial paralysis, brain abscesses, and sigmoid sinus thrombosis.

With mastoiditis, large amounts of thick purulent material usually fill the external auditory canal, which indicates perforation of the tympanic membrane. The soft tissue that is next to the eardrum may be ruptured and sagging. X-ray examinations of the mastoid are needed to determine the extent of involvement. Findings vary from clouding of the air cells and some decalcification of the bony walls to complete coalescence of the air cells. If early decalcification is present, intense antibiotic therapy and myringotomy can usually cure mastoiditis; if it has progressed to further destruction, simple mastoidectomy is necessary.[8] Chronic infection can also lead to the development of a cholesteatoma.

•••••• Diagnostic Studies and Findings

Mastoid x-ray examinations   May show cloudy air cells and decalcification of cell walls; cholesteatoma

Audiometric testing   to show and document amount of hearing loss and middle ear impedance

•••••• Multidisciplinary Plan

Surgery

Mastoidectomy if necessary; involves removing involved bone and cleansing area; can be performed through postaural or endaural incision

Myringotomy to drain fluid and pus from middle ear (see p. 664)

Medications

Antiinfective agents

Penicillin G procaine suspension (Wycillin, Duracillin), 600,000-1,200,000 U IM

Penicillin G aqueous, 1.5 million U q4-6h for severe infections

Other agents specific to organism

Analgesics

Acetaminophen 650 mg with/without codeine 30 mg q4h prn

NURSING CARE

Nursing Assessment

Ear

Thick purulent discharge from ear; dull aching behind ear; low-grade fever; auricle may be pushed out from head by edema; erythema; hearing loss; presence of cholesteatoma

Nursing Dx & Intervention

Pain related to perforation of tympanum and necrosis of mastoid process

- Assess need for pain medication, and administer analgesics as ordered. Evaluate and record effectiveness of pain relief.
- Administer antibiotics as ordered.

Impaired skin integrity related to bony necrosis of mastoid process

- Assess dressings and reinforce as necessary after mastoidectomy.
- Place gauze between ear and head *to avoid pressure of ear against head and to promote adequate circulation.*
- Record amount and color of wound drainage and patient's temperature.
- Assess incision for separation, abscess, erythema, tenderness after mastoidectomy.
- Avoid introduction of water into ear canal.

Sensory/perceptual alterations (auditory) related to rupture of tympanic membrane or ear surgery

- Assess patient's hearing before and after mastoidectomy and myringotomy.
- If patient experiences hearing loss, speak slowly and clearly when talking with patient.
- Ensure that family and other staff members are aware of hearing loss and use appropriate methods of communication.
- Assist patient with standing and ambulation initially *because patient may experience some vertigo.* Administer antivertiginous medications, as ordered.

Patient Education/Home Care Planning

1. Discuss with the patient and family the necessity of completing the prescribed course of antibiotics to prevent recurrence or complication.
2. Demonstrate dressing change technique to patient and family, if necessary.
3. Discuss possible hearing loss with the patient and family and refer to medical or community resources as appropriate.
4. Reassure patient that cracking and popping noises are normal if mastoid surgery performed.
5. Inform the patient that ear discomfort is normal. Increased ear pain should be reported to the physician.
6. Instruct the patient to avoid the introduction of water into the ear. Demonstrate the procedure of inserting a cotton ball coated with petroleum jelly into the ear canal when showering or shampooing the hair.
7. Advise the patient to consult with physician regarding specific instructions on flying.

Evaluation

Patient's comfort is increased   There is no pain in ear. Patient's temperature is within normal limits. Activity level is normal for patient.

Skin integrity is intact   There is no drainage in external canal. If mastoidectomy was performed, wound is well healed.

Hearing is maintained   Patient's hearing is assessed and, if diminished, the patient is referred to appropriate medical and community resources.

Patient and family verbalize knowledge of treatment of mastoiditis   Patient and family verbalize understanding of necessity for completing the prescribed course of medication.

LABYRINTHITIS

Labyrinthitis is an inflammation of the labyrinth of the inner ear.

Labyrinthitis is quite rare, and it is usually classified into four types: paralabyrinthitis, serous, purulent, and viral. Because the membranous labyrinth is protected by bone, it is difficult for microorganisms to enter the area unless the bony labyrinth is eroded, as it is with cholesteatoma formation in chronic otitis media. However, organisms can gain entry through the oval and round windows during acute otitis media or through the cochlear aqueduct or internal auditory canal during meningitis. Symptoms are usually severe vertigo and nystagmus followed by total sensorineural hearing loss on the affected side.

Paralabyrinthitis causes the least serious symptoms of the four types of labyrinthitis. A fistula between the bony and membranous labyrinths is caused by erosion of the bone from granulation or cholesteatoma formation, but no inflammation or infection exists. There is no spontaneous nystagmus, and vertigo may be present only because the membranous labyrinth is exposed when exogenous stimulation occurs. A diagnosis is usually made when alternating positive and negative pressures are applied to the external meatus: applying positive pressure may induce nystagmus toward the affected ear, and negative pressure has the opposite effect. Nystagmus is not always produced, however, and the presence of vertigo usually assists in making the diagnosis. Treatment consists of surgically exteriorizing the fistula.

In *serous labyrinthitis* the membranous labyrinth is inflamed and direct labyrinthine stimulation occurs, probably by a direct effect on the nerve endings. This stimulation produces nystagmus on the affected side. Nystagmus may also result from the caloric effect caused by the hyperemia. The patient experiences severe vertigo and nausea and vomiting, characteristically lies quietly with the affected side down, and looks up in an attempt to decrease the nystagmus. The patient may experience some deafness. Any type of movement may worsen the vertigo, and an attempt to stand results in a fall. Heavy sedation, bed rest, and systemic antibiotics in high doses are indicated. If the patient's hearing returns, the labyrinthitis was serous rather than purulent.

Purulent labyrinthitis causes destruction of the labyrinth and cochlea, resulting in permanent deafness in the affected ear. Symptoms and treatment are the same as for serous labyrinthitis; massive doses of antibiotics are administered to prevent the spread of infection and pus and resultant meningitis. Drugs such as ampicillin are usually prescribed because pencillin does not easily cross into the labyrinth. Patients may require intravenous hydration and administration of antivertigo drugs such as meclizine.

Viral labyrinthitis is a common condition that can affect both hearing and balance. It may occur after an infection of the upper respiratory tract; as a sequelae of mumps, measles, rubella, or encephalitis; or following herpes infections of cranial nerves VII or VIII.

Nursing care is aimed at preventing falls. Bed rails are kept up, and the patient is instructed to lie quietly and not to get out of bed without assistance. Antiemetic and antivertigo medications are administered for patient comfort. Antibiotics are given if ordered. The patient's intake and output are monitored for symptoms of dehydration, and IV fluids are given if ordered.

If not hospitalized, the patient should stay in bed at home and request assistance from a family member before getting up during acute episodes. Vestibular suppressants (buclazine, meclizine) may be prescribed to decrease severity of vertigo. Labyrinthine (vestibular) exercises may also be suggested to assist the patient in compensating for the dizziness.[47] See box for exercises to strengthen your balance system.

If the symptoms persist for a prolonged period, vestibular nerve resection or labyrinthectomy may be performed.

Patient Education/Home Care Planning

Exercises to strengthen your balance system

Balance exercises can decrease dizziness. Although the exercises are accomplished by turning the head and neck, the exercises are performed to help the brain compensate for the injury to the balance system.

The balance exercises are done while the patient is sitting with feet on the floor for stability. The balance exercises may make the patient dizzy. If dizziness occurs, have the patient wait for the dizziness to subside, but then continue with the exercises.

The head is turned quickly in 6 different directions. A "sequence" consists of quickly jerking the head right; left; up; down; tilt right; and tilt left. The distance that the head is turned is unimportant. An inch in each direction is sufficient as long as the head is stopped suddenly. After each position, the head should be returned to the midline before beginning the next position. The entire sequence should be repeated 10 times, twice per day. The diagrams illustrate how these balance system exercises should be done. Over a period of months, these will help the balance system to compensate.

Any physical activity or movement that causes dizziness should be repeated several times. For example, if turning quickly to the right or looking up causes dizziness, these maneuvers should be repeated often. Instead of avoiding certain situations or positions that cause dizziness, repeat them. These repetitions will hasten the recovery process. Although avoiding dizziness is more comfortable for most patients, the only way for the patient to regain complete balance function is to use the balance system. The goal of these exercises is to improve compensation over a period of several months.

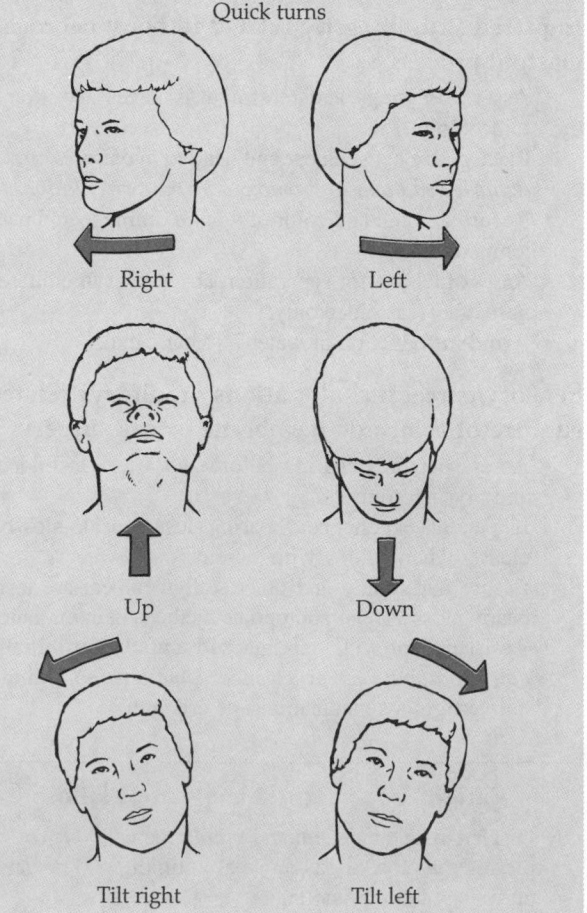

Quick turns

Right   Left

Up   Down

Tilt right   Tilt left

OBSTRUCTION

Obstruction of the ear canal is usually caused by excessive secretion or impaction of cerumen or by foreign bodies, including insects.

Young children put various objects, such as beads, pebbles, beans, and small toys, into their ears. An obstruction of the ear canal can lead to infection and to conductive hearing loss if auditory function is disrupted.

•••••• Pathophysiology

Cerumen is normally produced in small amounts and dries in the ear, where it is forced out bit by bit during chewing and talking. Some people, however, have overactive glands that produce excessive amounts of cerumen that can completely occlude the ear canal. Others have narrow or tortuous ear canals that can become impacted with cerumen.

Insects occasionally fly into the ear, which causes an unpleasant sensation as they beat their wings.

Foreign objects, which children frequently put into their ears, may not cause symptoms or may cause intense pain if deep in the canal. Physicians occasionally find foreign objects in children's ears during a routine examination.

•••••• Diagnostic Studies and Findings

Otoscopic examination   Visualization of obstructing object

•••••• Multidisciplinary Plan

Surgery

Surgical removal of foreign object under anesthesia may be necessary if patient, who is often a child, is unable to remain still during removal

Medications

Carbamide peroxide 6.5% (Debrox drops), 5-10 gtt in ear canal to soften cerumen

General Management

Removal of cerumen by irrigation or with cerumen spoon
If insect is cause of obstruction, it is smothered with drops of oily substance and removed with forceps
Other foreign objects removed with forceps if possible (see Emergency Alert box)

NURSING CARE

Nursing Assessment

Auditory Function

Ear feels occluded; some tinnitus or "buzzing" may be present; pain in ear; slight hearing loss; canal may be completely occluded by cerumen; may be insect or foreign body in canal

---

! EMERGENCY ALERT

FOREIGN BODY REMOVAL: EAR, NOSE

Assessment

- Patient complains of a foreign body (FB) in the ear or nose.

EAR

- There may be evidence of purulent drainage or odor from the ear. This is most commonly seen in children.
- Examine the ear canal with an otoscope to determine presence of foreign body.
- Carefully assess if there is perforation of the eardrum before irrigation of the ear canal.

NOSE

- There may be evidence of purulent drainage or odor from one nostril. This is most commonly seen in children.

Intervention

EAR

- Remove the foreign body by suction, water irrigation, or forceps. (If object is a food product, do not use water to irrigate. This may make the food substance swell.)
- If the object is a living insect: drop mineral oil into the ear, shine a light into the ear canal and the insect will crawl toward the light.
- If necessary, restrain patient and manage pain to prevent further injury.

NOSE

- Administer nasal decongestants and topical anesthetic drops.
- Place patient in a head-down Trendelenberg position.
- Remove the foreign body with alligator or ring forceps.
- If necessary, restrain patient and manage pain to prevent further injury.

Nursing Dx & Intervention

Sensory/perceptual alterations (auditory) related to obstruction of ear canal

- Assess degree of hearing impairment or tinnitus.
- Instill ear drops or perform irrigation if ordered. Use solution at room temperature *to avoid stimulating a caloric response.*
- Warn patient and family not to put foreign objects in ears.

Pain related to obstruction deep in ear canal

- Assess need for pain medication and provide instruction about safe analgesic medications.

Patient Education/Home Care Planning

1. For patients who produce excessive cerumen, suggest a method for preventing impaction or obstruction: once a week put 1 or 2 drops of an oily substance in the ears at night. In the morning put 1 or 2 drops of hydrogen peroxide in the ears and clean gently with a soft cotton wick.

Evaluation

Sensory/perceptual integrity is restored Obstruction, if present, is removed. There is no feeling of occlusion or tinnitus in the ear. Hearing is normal for the patient.

Pain is absent Patient experiences no pain in the ear.

■ OTOSCLEROSIS

■ Otosclerosis is a disease of the bone in the bony labyrinth (cochlear otospongiosis) or the otic capsule, in which normal bone is replaced by the formation of highly vascular, "spongy" otosclerotic bone.

Otosclerosis most commonly (85%) occurs at the oval window and eventually causes a conductive hearing loss. Most patients have the disease in both ears, although not to the same degree. It is unilateral in about 10% to 15% of patients.[23]

Otosclerosis is present to some degree in about 10% of whites. It is not found as frequently in Asians and blacks but is reported as common in southern India. About half of patients with otosclerosis have a family history of the disease. Women are apparently affected more often than men, and although the etiology is unclear, pregnancy frequently triggers a rapid onset of this condition. It is usually noticed first in the late teens or early twenties.[8]

•••••• Pathophysiology

The precise pathophysiologic process that causes otospongiotic and otosclerotic disease is still unclear. It is not thought to have any relationship to previous ear infections. During the process, however, normal bone in the otic capsule is gradually replaced by otosclerotic bone that is highly vascular and described as spongy. Although it is controversial, one theory postulates that the destructive process causes the release of proteolytic enzymes, which destroy the capsular bone, freeing other destructive enzymes. As these enzymes enter the labyrinthine fluid, they may affect the neural elements of the inner ear, causing vestibular and cochlear functional impairment. The second stage of this process is the body's natural reaction to heal the involved area by calcification. The calcification causes local expansion of the bone and leads to progressive fixation of the stapes with physical intrusion into labyrinthine spaces and virtual immobilization of the footplate in the oval window.[23] This produces a conductive hearing loss because sound pressure vibrations can no longer be transmitted to the fluid media. Patients may also experience a sensorineural hearing loss if the cochlea is involved. This is referred to as a mixed hearing loss.

In otosclerosis the eardrum usually appears normal, although a pink blush called Schwartz's sign can occasionally be seen through the eardrum. This indicates a high degree of vascularity in active otosclerotic bone.

•••••• Diagnostic Studies and Findings

Rinne test Bone conduction lasts longer than air conduction in affected ear (negative Rinne)

Weber test Tone lateralizes to poorer ear

Audiometric tests Hearing loss ranges from 60 dB in early stages to total loss in later stages; sound lateralizes more to affected ear; on examination with otoscope tympanic membrane appears normal

•••••• Multidisciplinary Plan

Surgery

Stapedectomy (see p. 665)

Stapedotomy—minimal (0.4 mm) opening of oval window; ribbon-shaped, platinum Teflon prosthesis is crimped to long process of the incus through opening into footplate before rather than after disrupting the incudostapedial joint and breaking off the stapes arch; this causes less trauma to inner ear, prevents migration of prosthesis, and produces better hearing results[47]

Medications

Antiinfective agents

Tetracycline (Achromycin), 250 mg po q6h for 10 d (after surgery)

Amoxicillin, 250 mg po tid for 10 d (after surgery)

Vestibular suppressants may be ordered to control postoperative vertigo

General Management

Air conduction hearing aid if stapedectomy is not indicated

NURSING CARE

Nursing Assessment

Auditory Function

Slowly progressive conductive hearing loss; low- to medium-pitched tinnitus

Nursing Dx & Intervention

Risk for activity intolerance related to bed rest and vertigo after stapedectomy

- Assess patient for pain, nausea, or dizziness.
- Encourage activity level within physician's protocol. (Some patients can be up the day of surgery, others require bed rest for at least a day.)
- Instruct the patient to lie flat with head turned to side and operated ear facing upward *to maintain position of inserted prosthesis.*
- Point out to the patient that vertigo, pain, nausea, and vomiting may occur.
- Administer analgesic, vestibular suppressant, or antiemetic medication as needed.
- Keep side rails up *to prevent fall from bed.*
- *Convalescent care:* Assist patient to begin ambulation gradually *to minimize vertigo.*

Patient Education/Home Care Planning

1. Encourage the patient not to cough, sneeze, or blow the nose for at least 1 week to prevent increased pressure by way of the Eustachian tube, which may dislodge the prosthesis and graft over the oval window. Instruct the patient to cough or sneeze with the mouth open, if coughing or sneezing cannot be avoided. Nose should be blown *gently* if necessary.

2. Discuss with the patient to avoid loud noises, although no evidence exists that any damage is caused.

3. Explain to the patient that a decrease in hearing may occur after surgery because of increased fluid in the middle ear.

4. Encourage the patient to discuss with the physician when flying will be permitted because pressure changes may cause injury to the prosthesis and graft. This varies greatly from physician to physician and can range from 2 to 3 days after surgery to 1 to 2 months after surgery.

5. Caution the patient to avoid the introduction of water in the ear. Demonstrate technique of placing cotton ball coated with petroleum jelly into ear canal when showering or shampooing hair.

Evaluation

Patient activity level returns to normal Patient experiences no vertigo. Patient experiences no pain. Hearing is improved to normal (remember that patient may experience decrease in hearing after surgery until packing is removed and blood in middle ear is reabsorbed).

Patient and family verbalize understanding of treatment Patient verbalizes understanding of importance of completing antibiotic regimen and knowledge of convalescent care.

■ ACOUSTIC NEUROMA

Neuromas are benign lesions that arise from the neurilemma or Schwann cell sheath in the covering of the axon of a neuron.

Acoustic neuromas actually arise from the vestibular portion rather than from the cochlear portion of the eighth cranial nerve; the origin is only occasionally found to be the acoustic nerve. Thus these tumors are also called vestibular schwannomas, tumors of the eighth cranial nerve, or cerebellopontine angle tumors. Because most of these neuromas arise within the internal auditory meatus, early effects may be from pressure on the meatus, the cochlear division of the eighth cranial nerve, and the vestibular nerve. Initially patients usually have tinnitus, unilateral hearing loss, and nystagmus.[31] Although these tumors can affect people at any age, most patients are 40 to 50 years of age, with women affected slightly more frequently (60%) than

men. Acoustic neuromas comprise approximately 8% to 10% of all intracranial tumors.[5]

During the past 20 years, advances in diagnosis and techniques for removal of these tumors, such as the use of lasers and microsurgery, have greatly reduced morbidity and mortality.

•••••• Pathophysiology

The neuroma is a well-defined, fleshy, lobulated mass that is soft and cystic in some areas. It has a variegated appearance that may be caused by areas of old hemorrhage, although the tumor itself is quite avascular. Small, white, patchy areas of calcification may also be present.

The tumor usually arises in the internal auditory meatus. It is called an intracanalicular tumor if it lies entirely within the auditory canal and is considered an ear tumor. Small tumors measure between 2 and 5 cm, and large tumors have a minimum diameter of 5 cm.[51] As the tumor increases in size, it grows into the cerebellopontine angle and may begin to erode the wall of the internal meatus above and below. After the tumor grows out of the bony canal, it can expand medially, anterosuperiorly, and posteroinferiorly. As it grows medially, the tumor encroaches on the brainstem in the region of the pons. By this time the neuroma is usually about 2.5 cm in diameter and may be in contact with the anterior inferior cerebellar artery, which is responsible for the blood supply to the side of the pons and medulla. Continued enlargement medially compresses and distorts the pons and aqueduct, producing brainstem signs and causing an obstructing hydrocephalus.

As the tumor expands anterosuperiorly, it displaces the facial nerve and stretches it over the surface of the tumor. Although it may adhere to the facial nerve, the tumor can usually be separated from the nerve at surgery because the tumor does not normally wrap itself around the nerve. As the tumor extends farther, it usually involves the trigeminal nerve, lifting it up from below, causing facial numbness, pain, and decreased corneal sensation.

If the tumor extends inferiorly and posteriorly, it may compress the middle cerebellar peduncle and the cerebellum. It also stretches the ninth, tenth, and eleventh cranial nerves as it approaches the foramen magnum.

Most acoustic neuromas grow within the subarachnoid space. They are usually considered slow growing, although this can vary from patient to patient. Tumors seem to grow fairly rapidly in young adults and more slowly in the elderly.

Substantial cochlear and labyrinthine changes occur with these space-occupying lesions of the internal meatus (Figure 7-16), causing abnormalities of the cochlear and eighth cranial nerves. There may be chemical alterations, such as high concentrations of protein in the perilymph, and the sense organs themselves may be destroyed, although the hair cells of the organ of Corti often remain quite normal.

Von Recklinghausen's disease, or neurofibromatosis, can also cause acoustic neuromas that are usually bilateral and expand within the nerve rather than against the nerve, such as in isolated neuromas.[54]

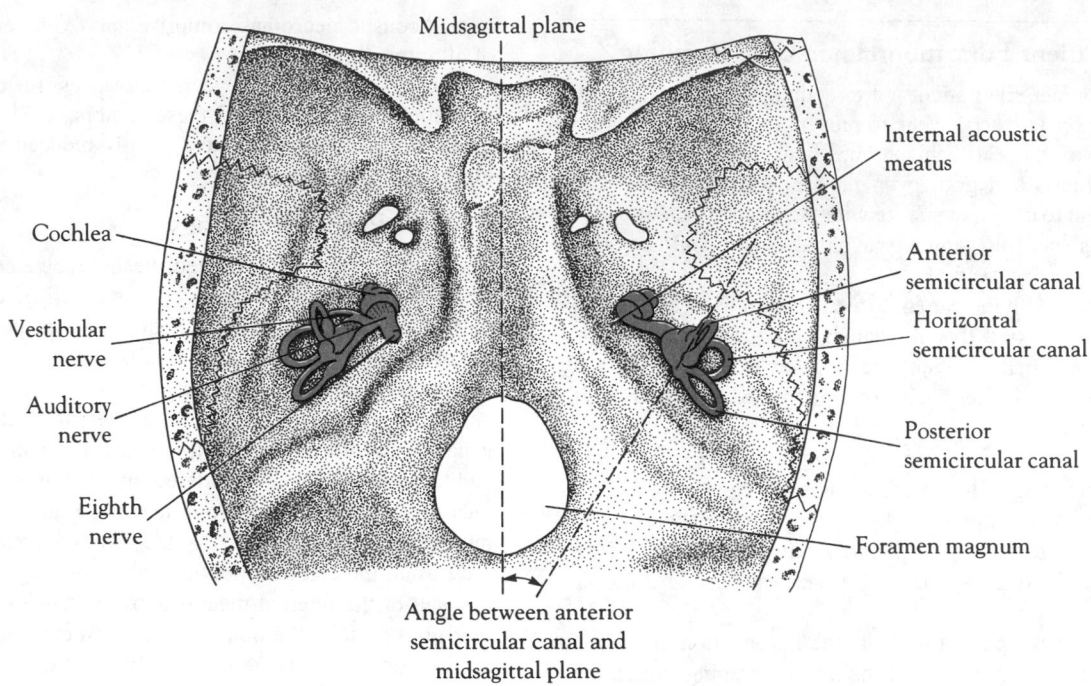

Midsagittal plane

Cochlea

Vestibular nerve

Auditory nerve

Eighth nerve

Internal acoustic meatus

Anterior semicircular canal

Horizontal semicircular canal

Posterior semicircular canal

Foramen magnum

Angle between anterior semicircular canal and midsagittal plane

Figure 7-16 Inner ear viewed from above, showing relative location of internal meatus and vestibular, auditory, and eighth nerves. (From Berne & Levy.[2])

•••••• Diagnostic Studies and Findings

Audiology, electrocochleography, and brainstem response to audiometry   Performed to evaluate degree of hearing loss and to differentiate between conductive and sensorineural hearing losses

Cerebral arteriography   Used less frequently in recent years but may be performed to diagnose aneurysms, to outline size and location of tumors, and to determine location and deviation of major vessels (see p. 1491, for description)

Computed tomography (CT) and magnetic resonance imaging (MRI) scan   Can indicate presence of tumor, pinpoint location, and show evidence of enlarged ventricles (see p. 1489, for description)

Lumbar puncture   Cerebrospinal fluid examined for increased protein; should not be performed if increased intracranial pressure is suspected to prevent herniation of cerebellar tonsils through foramen magnum or uncal herniation through tentorial notch[23,54] (see p. 1509, for description)

•••••• Multidisciplinary Plan

Surgery

Surgery is the treatment of choice because these tumors do not respond well to chemotherapy or radiation; the objective is to remove the tumor completely while saving the facial nerve and acoustic nerve; surgery can last from 9 to 14 hours; suboccipital or transpetrosal approach can be used for tumor of any size; for suboccipital approach, small portion of hair at base of neck is shaved; some surgeons prefer translabyrinthine approach, which is most appropriate for the patient with a tumor 1.5-4 cm in size and no usable hearing; one instatition reports that all acoustic neuromas, regardless of size, can be removed with this approach, although there may be technical problems with very large tumors; translabyrinthine approach associated with lower mortality, better facial nerve function, less postoperative ataxia, and much less postoperative hydrocephalus than with suboccipital approach but greater loss of hearing[31]; advantage is avoidance of pressure on cerebellum[31]

If tumor is large and adheres to facial nerve, total removal of tumor may necessitate sacrifice of facial nerve; if possible, end-to-end anastomosis of nerve stumps is done at time of surgery and should result in return of nerve function[54]

Ventriculostomy—sometimes performed during surgery so intracranial pressure can be monitored after surgery

Medications

Corticosteroids
   Dexamethasone (Decadron), 4-6 mg IV q4h to decrease cerebral edema
Antihypertensives
   Propranolol (Inderal), 160 mg po over 24 h before operation for prophylaxis, then nitroprusside (Nipride) during operation and after operation as needed
Osmotic diuretics to decrease cerebral edema

General Management

Cardiac, hemodynamic, and intracranial pressure monitoring; intubation with mechanical ventilation during and immediately after surgery; oxygen administered by face mask after extubation

Nothing by mouth and intravenous feedings until patient is able to eat; tube feedings necessary in some patients until gag reflex or ability to chew returns

Physical therapy and possibly speech therapy after surgery

NURSING CARE

Nursing Assessment

Symptoms Depend on Size and Location of Tumor

Auditory Function

Sensorineural hearing loss, usually unilateral and slowly progressive; tinnitus; dizziness and transient unsteadiness; true vertigo (sense of rotation, nausea, or vomiting) in some patients; otalgia (ache within ear or mastoid); tension or neck pain on same side as otalgia; occasional facial numbness; occasional tic douloureux

Visual Function

Decreased tear production; eyes feel dry and gritty; nystagmus, with eye movement slower and coarser toward side of tumor[14]; with large tumors, diplopia, ataxia, headaches, loss of vision

Gustatory Function

Diminished sense of taste on anterior two thirds of tongue; difficulty chewing and/or swallowing

Motor Function

Poor coordination and gait disturbances; patient leans toward affected side; impairment of fine movements[14]

Nursing Dx & Intervention

Altered cerebral tissue perfusion related to surgical procedures

- Establish neurologic baseline and assess neurologic status and vital signs every 15 minutes until stable, then every 1 hour, then every 4 hours. Notify physician of any changes.
- Monitor and record amount of and describe ventricular drainage, if used.
- Assess for signs of increasing intracranial pressure: widening pulse pressures, decreased level of consciousness, papilledema, seizures, hyperactive deep tendon reflexes, complaints of headache, vomiting.
- Avoid or limit any activity that may increase intracranial pressure.

- Administer osmotic diuretics or dexamethasone as ordered *to decrease cerebral edema.*
- Observe for symptoms of hydrocephalus from edema or bleeding into ventricles, which is possible after surgery.
- Assess for presence of cerebrospinal fluid leak.
- Observe cardiac monitor *to detect any dysrhythmias* resulting from cerebral edema or vagal stimulation during surgery.
- Keep head of bed elevated 45 degrees *to promote venous drainage and limit cerebral edema.*
- Assess for seizure activity.

Altered peripheral tissue perfusion related to rebound hypertension

- Assess patient's blood pressure frequently; be alert for hypertension, which could be significant after surgery.
- Monitor Nipride drip per protocol.

Ineffective breathing pattern related to decreased gag reflex, mechanical ventilation

- Assess patient's arterial blood gases and chest expansion for adequate ventilation.
- Maintain ventilator settings and suction airway as needed (patient may be mechanically ventilated for 1 or 2 days after surgery).
- Observe patient after extubation for return of gag reflex and ability to cough effectively.
- Provide oxygen by face mask as ordered after extubation.
- Continue suctioning or physical therapy of the chest as needed.

Risk for fluid volume deficit related to dehydration necessary to decrease congestion in vasculature and to minimize effects of postoperative swelling[47]

- Assess skin turgor, mucous membranes, and lung sounds *to monitor fluid status.*
- Maintain and record intravenous infusions at ordered rate. *Titrate to maintain serum osmolarity between 300 and 310 mOsm/L.*
- Permit nothing by mouth initially.
- Maintain strict intake and output records.
- Monitor electrolyte levels *because patients are given diuretics to decrease brain bulk during surgery.*
- Perform care of Foley catheter *to prevent urinary tract infection;* patient will have catheter until able to void normally.
- Provide frequent mouth care; patient may suck on lollipops.

Pain related to surgical procedure

- Assess for pain and give medication as needed *to minimize pain, nausea, and vomiting.* Evaluate and document effectiveness.

Altered nutrition: less than body requirements related to NPO status; decreased gag reflex; discomfort from surgery

- Administer antacids *to decrease increased gastric acidity and prevent stress ulcers.*
- Begin offering patient soft or pureed foods when gag reflex has returned, feeding on unaffected side if patient experiences difficulty or facial weakness or numbness.
- Evaluate need for dietary consultation.

Sensory/perceptual alterations (auditory, visual, gustatory) related to surgical procedure

1. Visual
   - Assess cornea for excessive dryness.
   - Provide artificial tears/lubricants to patient's eyes as needed (every few hours) to maintain lubrication because of loss of corneal reflex and decreased ability to close eye.
   - Place moisture chamber (clear plastic occlusive eye patch) over affected eye to collect moisture and protect the cornea.
   - Tape eye closed and apply patch, if indicated. Check frequently to ensure eyelid closure under patch.
   - Adapt patient's environment to accommodate for visual changes.
2. Auditory
   - Assess for hearing loss.
   - Indicate **patient with hearing loss** on chart, room intercommunication system.
   - Speak slowly and distinctly with adequate lighting on your face. Face the patient directly and do not shout or overexaggerate words.
   - Place telephone, call light, etc. on unaffected side.
3. Gustatory (swallowing)
   - Maintain nothing by mouth until gag reflex returns.
   - Assess for gag reflex; symmetry and movement of tongue, soft palate, and pharynx; patient's ability to swallow without evidence of aspiration or collection of food in mouth.
   - Provide tube feedings, as ordered, until patient is able to swallow.
   - Inspect oral cavity and provide oral care after meals.
   - Consult with dietitian and/or swallowing therapist to determine food consistencies best tolerated and techniques to improve swallowing.

Impaired skin integrity related to surgical incision

- Assess dressing for drainage and bleeding and reinforce or change as needed.
- Remove dressing 3 to 5 days after surgery. Observe for redness, inflammation, drainage, or edema near operative site. Edema may be from accumulation of subgaleal fluid because dura was entered; fluid should be reabsorbed in few days. Position patient comfortably and change position frequently until patient is mobile *to prevent skin breakdown.*

- Provide adequate support to head and back when positioning *because neck muscles may be weak.*

Body image disturbance related to facial weakness/paralysis

- Encourage patient to discuss feelings and concerns.
- Discuss patient's perception of body.
- Assess coping mechanisms used in the past.
- Encourage participation in self-care activities.
- Facilitate social interactions with family, other patients, staff.
- Assist patient to identify realistic goals and ways to achieve these goals.
- Provide information on support groups.

The Acoustic Neuroma Association, PO Box 12402, Atlanta, GA 30355; 404-237-8023.

Patient Education/Home Care Planning

1. Explain to the patient and family signs and symptoms of wound infection.
2. Discuss with the patient and family signs and symptoms of hydrocephalus or increased intracranial pressure, which in rare cases occurs several weeks after surgery (onset of new motor weakness, stiff neck, fever, visual disturbance, seizures, drainage from incision or ear).
3. Ensure that the patient and family understand the need for continued physical therapy rehabilitation and possible speech therapy.
4. Explain to the patient and family the need for maintenance of nutrition, especially if a chewing or swallowing deficit remains. If the patient is discharged but will continue tube feedings, be sure that the patient or a family member can perform the procedure safely.
5. Ensure that the patient and family understand that deficits may take several months to resolve or may not resolve at all; assess family's coping mechanisms and the possible need for assistance in dealing with these deficits.
6. Instruct patient to avoid crowds, persons with upper respiratory infections.
7. Provide instruction on eye care/protection, if facial weakness present.
8. Provide written information on support group (The Acoustic Neuroma Association).

Evaluation

Adequate cerebral tissue perfusion is maintained Neurologic signs are stable. Ventricular drainage is minimal to absent. Intracranial pressure remains normal; patient experiences no seizures, vomiting, decreased level of consciousness, or cerebrospinal fluid (CSF) leak. Cardiac status is stable.

Peripheral tissue perfusion remains normal Patient's blood pressure is normal.

Breathing pattern improves   Arterial blood gases (ABGs) are normal; patient is weaned from ventilator soon after surgery. Gag reflex returns to normal. Patient experiences no need for suctioning.

Patient's fluid volume status is normal   Patient experiences no dehydration. Electrolyte levels remain within normal limits for patient. Patient voids with no problems when Foley catheter is removed.

Comfort level is maintained   Patient experiences minimal pain at operative site. Nausea and vomiting are absent. Headaches are absent. Hearing, dizziness, and tinnitus have improved or are stable.

Nutritional status is maintained   Patient receives adequate nutrition while NPO; when gag reflex returns, patient is able to maintain normal caloric intake by mouth. Dietary consult is provided if appropriate.

Patient can swallow normally   Gag reflex returns to normal soon after extubation.

Skin integrity is maintained   Operative site heals normally, with no inflammation or drainage. Patient experiences no skin breakdown caused by bed rest or decreased activity. Preoperative gait and coordination difficulties have improved.

Corneal tissue is maintained   Corneal lubrication is protected and maintained, and patient experiences no dryness or loss of corneal reflex.

Body image change is accepted   Discusses feelings. Uses appropriate coping strategies. Interacts with family and friends. Sets realistic goals.

■ MÉNIÈRE'S DISEASE

Ménière's disease, also called endolymphatic hydrops, is a labyrinthine dysfunction associated with dilation of the membranous labyrinth with a resultant abnormal fluid balance of the inner ear.

Ménière's disease has three typical symptoms: severe vertigo, tinnitus, and a sensorineural hearing loss, which is usually fluctuating, progressive, and initially of low tones. Although never fatal, Ménière's disease is nonetheless quite incapacitating during attacks, which occur periodically between intervals of remission. As hearing decreases, the attacks become less frequent, and they may stop altogether when the patient's hearing loss is almost total. The acute attacks usually last for several hours, but between attacks the patient may have no symptoms except for tinnitus and a gradually progressive hearing loss. In severe or untreated cases, however, the patient may have daily attacks, although with periods of complete relief from vertigo between attacks.

Adults between the ages of 30 and 60 years are usually affected. Although it can occur at any age, Ménière's disease is rare in children (it has been seen in a 6-year-old). It is distributed equally by sex; the condition is more often unilateral than bilateral, although the likelihood of bilaterality increases as patients grow older. Half of those who had the disease develop in the second ear did so within 2 years of onset in the first ear, and another 27% developed it after 5 years or longer.[31]

A likely cause has been found in approximately 25% of those affected, and a positive family history noted for 10% to 20%, so that genetic Ménière's disease remains a possibility.[31]

Some researchers believe that the incidence of Ménière's disease may have increased since World War II, possibly because of a correlation between the disease, current living habits, and environmental conditions, such as increased stress and increased salt intake.

A subgroup of female patients with Ménière's disease experiences symptoms that are correlated with the luteal phase of the menstrual cycle. Many hormonal effects occur during the premenstrual period; compartmental fluid redistribution within the body may be the most pertinent.

•••••• Pathophysiology

The most widely accepted theories regarding the cause of Ménière's disease are (1) an overproduction of endolymph from some disturbance in the formation of fluid in the inner ear and (2) a decreased absorption of endolymph from a disturbance in the sac, which leads to an accumulation of endolymph.

Many other theories have been postulated, but few have been widely accepted. Endolymphatic hydrops, however, is thought to cause degeneration of the neural end organ of the labyrinth and cochlea. Some researchers believe that fluid disturbances are caused by sodium retention, allergies, or vascular spasm. Small vesicles may form in the walls of the endolymphatic system, and the sudden rupture of these vesicles may cause acute attacks of vertigo. The cause of the formation of these vesicles is unclear.

The principal cause appears to be failure of the resorption mechanisms of the endolymphatic sac, resulting in slow accumulation of endolymph with distention and rupture of the membranous labyrinth. Potassium-rich neurotoxic endolymph may then enter the perilymphatic space, causing temporary paralysis of sensory and neural structures. As the disease progresses, there are permanent morphologic changes in sensory and neural structures and persistent losses in auditory and vestibular function.[31,33]

These patients have hypocellular mastoid processes and deficiencies of the vestibular aqueduct. Trautmann's triangle is often small or distorted, primarily because of the anatomy of the lateral sinus, which is displaced anteriorly and more medially in most patients.

A fundamental problem seems to be malabsorption in the duct or sac. All forms of Ménière's disease develop after some inciting cause that may have occurred years earlier. Known or inciting factors include infection, trauma, otosclerosis, and syphilis, although the disease may be idiopathic. The syndrome is probably related to developmental abnormalities of the endolymphatic duct or sac, hypodevelopment of Trautmann's triangle, anterior displacement of the lateral sinus, and sometimes vascular anomalies, especially in venous drainage. Thus the quality of the endolymph is affected.[31,33]

Characteristically, in advanced Ménière's disease, endolymphatic hydrops is seen in the scala media and saccule. It fills the vestibule and scala vestibuli in many cases. Because of the displacement of perilymph in advanced disease, the radial fluid flow decreases and longitudinal blood flow becomes dominant. Less often, the utricle or cochlear duct extends to occupy the vestibule. Stagnation of outflow can occur, and such distention can interfere with traveling waves and alter cochlear function.[31,33]

•••••• Diagnostic Studies and Findings

Audiology   Tuning fork test shows sensorineural deficit; Rinne test may be false positive if severe unilateral hearing loss is present; pure tone test shows sensorineural hearing loss involving low tones

Electrocochleography   Used frequently to aid in differential diagnosis of auditory diseases

Electronystagmography   (ENG)   Measurement and graphic recording of electrical potentials of eye movements during spontaneous, positional, and caloric evoked nystagmus. Normal to decreased vestibular response on affected side

Caloric tests   5 ml ice water instilled into each ear with patient's head elevated 30 degrees to cause acute attack with nausea, vomiting, vertigo, and nystagmus; response is occasionally hypoactive in involved ear and sometimes in both ears

X-ray examinations of petrous bones   Internal auditory meatus examined carefully; patients with Ménière's disease usually have shorter, straighter vestibular aqueducts than do patients without Ménière's disease

•••••• Multidisciplinary Plan

Goals are preservation of hearing and control of vertigo.

Surgery

Recent increased interest in surgical therapies because medical therapy has failed to halt hearing losses; if medical therapy has failed, two surgical procedures may be performed

Decompression of endolymphatic sac—done by inserting Teflon endolymphatic subarachnoid shunt or by incision in sac kept patent by muscle flap or Teflon sheet; has some benefit in about two thirds of patients

Destruction of end organ and neural connections by labyrinthectomy or vestibular neurectomy; labyrinthectomy performed only as last resort when vertigo is persistent and little or no hearing is left because cochlear function is destroyed; vertigo disappears in almost every case, but tinnitus may remain; vestibular neurectomy may be regarded as operation of choice; middle cranial fossa approach is used; 90% of patients have relief from vertigo, some with improvement in hearing[23]

Medications

Vasodilators

Histamine (Diphosphate), 2.75 mg given in 200-500 ml of 5% glucose; drip over 1 h (in remission); based on theory that labyrinthine ischemia is cause of disease; most have not been found to be effective, but β-histamine may improve vertigo, hearing, and tinnitus

Papaverine hydrochloride (Pavabid) 150 mg po bid

Nicotinic acid (Niacin) 50-200 mg/d po

Vestibular suppressants

Acetyl-D-leucine, 500 mg po q12h

Prochlorperazine (Compazine), 10 mg po q6h

Droperidol (Inapsine), 25-50 mg/d IV

Haloperidol (Haldol), 5 mg IV q8h

Diazepam (Valium), 2.5-5 mg po q6h

Lorazepam (Ativan), 0.5-1 mg po q4-6h prn

Diuretics (used as vestibular compressant)

Hydrochlorothiazide (Hydrodiuril), 25-200 mg/d

Cholinergic blocking agents

Atropine, 0.01 mg/kg to maximum of 0.04 mg/kg subcutaneously or IM

Scopolamine (transderm Scop) 0.5 mg patch q3d

Adrenergic agents

Epinephrine, 0.2-0.5 mg IV may be administered to stop an attack; sedatives and antiemetics such as meclizine (Antivert), 25 mg po qid, and prochlorperazine (Compazine), 10 mg po q6h, may be used

General Management

Bed rest maintained during acute attack

Low sodium diet (2 gm) may be used to control symptoms

Restriction of salt and water intake

Avoidance of tobacco, alcohol, caffeine, and high triglycerides

NURSING CARE

Nursing Assesssment

During Acute Attack

Balance

Sudden onset of acute vertigo (sensation of movement)

Auditory function

Tinnitus described by patient as a persistent background hum; decreased hearing

Visual function

Nystagmus

General

Nausea and vomiting; sweating; abdominal pain; diarrhea; and bradycardia

Between Attacks

Auditory function

Gradually progressive sensorineural hearing loss; tinnitus; loudness intolerance; some patients describe a fullness, pressure, or dull ache in ear; normal tympanic membranes

Nursing Dx & Intervention

Risk for trauma related to fall during vertigo attacks

- Assess patient for vertigo, nystagmus, nausea, and vomiting.
- Keep side rails of bed up *to prevent a fall.*
- Encourage patient to lie quietly and *not* to get up without assistance during attack.
- Instruct patient to avoid sudden head movements or position changes, since *attacks may begin without warning.*
- Administer antiemetics, antivertiginous medications, and/or vestibular sedatives *to help prevent vomiting and promote rest.*

Sensory/perceptual alterations (auditory) related to degeneration of neural end organs of hearing

- See Part IV.

Patient Education/Home Care Planning

1. Discuss with the patient theories about the etiology of the disease and acute attacks.
2. Ensure that the patient is aware that hearing loss may be progressive unless treatment is successful.
3. Explain to the patient ways to minimize tinnitus if the patient is bothered by it.
4. Explain to the patient that the attacks will last a few hours and will stop on their own, but that treatment is available to diminish or stop them if necessary.
5. Ensure that the patient understands the danger of trying to walk unassisted during an attack because of vertigo.
6. Assist patient and family to identify hazards in home environment. Recommend adaptations.
7. Discuss with the patient and family dietary or medical regimen, if used, or about surgical interventions, if used.
8. Reinforce vestibular/balance exercise, if ordered.

Evaluation

Patient safety is maintained Patient verbalizes understanding that attacks will eventually stop of their own accord. Patient verbalizes understanding that sudden movements and hazardous tasks should be avoided because of sudden onset of vertigo. Patient expresses knowledge of side effects of medical regimen if ordered or of surgical intervention if used.

Auditory function is monitored Patient understands possibility of hearing loss.

▮ TINNITUS

Tinnitus is the perception of sound in the absence of an acoustic stimulus.

Tinnitus is usually described as a ringing in the ears, although it may also be perceived by the patient as roaring, sizzling, whistling, or humming. Although usually a subjective experience, tinnitus occasionally can be heard as a blowing sound or bruit by the examiner.

The intensity of tinnitus varies greatly from patient to patient. It is often slight and is noticed by the patient only at night when other sounds are minimal. At other times it can be loud and continuous to the point that some patients may even consider suicide. It can be intermittent or continuous and may be accompanied by a hearing loss. It may also be unilateral or bilateral.

Although the mechanism that produces tinnitus is not thoroughly understood, it can be a symptom of nearly all ear disorders. In many cases it is the first or only symptom of disease, and any patient complaining of tinnitus must have a thorough examination to determine the cause. It is widely estimated that 30 million Americans have tinnitus.

•••••• Pathophysiology

The exact mechanism that causes tinnitus is unknown. However, it is known that tinnitus can be caused by a disturbance anywhere in the ear, as well as in the acoustic nerve, brainstem, or cortex (Figure 7-17). Two disorders with tinnitus as a major symptom, Ménière's disease and acoustic neuroma, are discussed separately in this section.

External ear causes include obstruction of the canal by foreign bodies or cerumen; patients usually describe the sound as low pitched, muffled, and intermittent. These patients may perceive their own voices as having a hollow sound.

Most middle ear disorders can also cause tinnitus. Otosclerosis is usually accompanied by tinnitus, which is described by patients as a ringing or whistling. It is constant, and some patients experience more than one sound. Infectious or inflammatory processes usually produce tinnitus, which is described as pulsating. This type of tinnitus usually ends when the infection is cleared.

Acoustic trauma caused by very loud noises frequently produces high-pitched tinnitus and may be associated with a temporary hearing loss. These symptoms should warn the patient that the ears should be protected before exposure to loud noises or a permanent hearing loss may result. The pitch of tinnitus in these patients is usually near the frequency where their hearing loss is the greatest.

Tinnitus is commonly caused by certain drugs. Quinine, salicylates, some diuretics, aminoglycoside antibiotics, and cisplatin frequently cause tinnitus and can also cause a hearing loss. These drugs damage the cochlea and the eighth cranial nerve; the tinnitus is usually high pitched and may or may not continue after the drug is stopped.

Other causes of tinnitus include anemia and hypotension. This tinnitus usually resolves when the underlying condition is corrected. Cardiovascular diseases, such as arteriosclerosis and hypertension, may also produce a tinnitus that may fluctuate with the patient's blood pressure.

Audible or objective tinnitus can be heard by another person. It is better understood, and the cause usually is easily diagnosed. If a patient complains of a blowing sound that

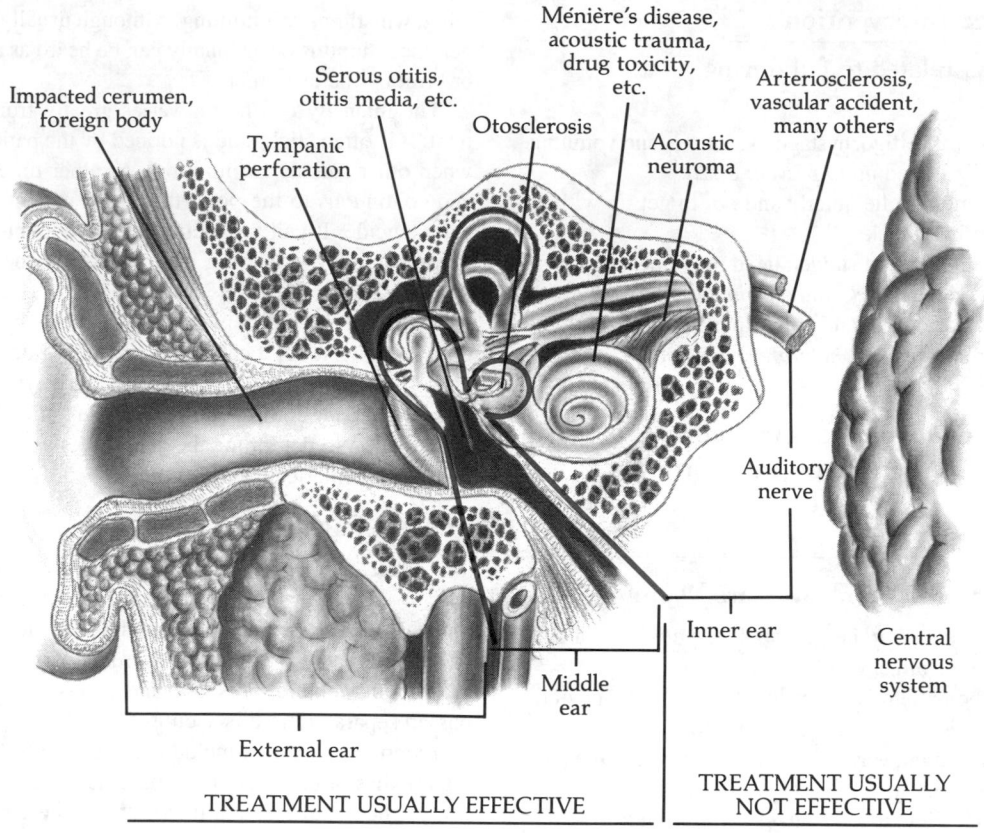

Impacted cerumen, foreign body

Serous otitis, otitis media, etc.

Tympanic perforation

Ménière's disease, acoustic trauma, drug toxicity, etc.

Otosclerosis

Acoustic neuroma

Arteriosclerosis, vascular accident, many others

Auditory nerve

Inner ear

Central nervous system

Middle ear

External ear

TREATMENT USUALLY EFFECTIVE

TREATMENT USUALLY NOT EFFECTIVE

Figure 7-17 Areas where tinnitus may occur.

coincides with respirations or complains of clicking sounds, the physician should suspect audible tinnitus and may be able to hear it by placing an ear or a stethoscope over the patient's ear. An abnormally patent eustachian tube is usually the cause of blowing tinnitus, and this is quite annoying to patients. Luckily it may be of short duration, and patients can improve the condition somewhat by performing repeated Valsalva maneuvers to increase the negative pressure in the nasopharynx or equalize the pressure in the middle ear with the atmosphere. The clicking noises are fairly rare, are usually intermittent, and are produced by tetanic contractions of the muscles of the soft palate. The cause of this condition is unknown, but it is a reflex action, and the palate can be seen to contract, sometimes 175 to 200 times a minute. This is usually treated with injections of lidocaine on the involved side to stop the contraction of the palate.

Diagnostic Studies and Findings

Audiology   Presence or absence of concurrent hearing loss; any diagnostic study may be performed to rule out the presence of systemic or ear diseases known to produce tinnitus; pitch—the patient manipulates the frequency of tone until the pitch is equal to the most prominent pitch of the tinnitus; loudness—can be evaluated by adjusting the level of pure tone until it has the same loudness as tinnitus; if a profound hearing loss is present, the measurement may be only a few decibels

sensation level, whereas in regions of normal hearing, the measurement may be 40 dB sensation level; pure tone masking—measures the minimum level of a pure tone required to mask the tinnitus as a function of the masker frequency.

Multidisciplinary Plan

Surgery

None, unless surgery is indicated for particular disorder that is found to be cause of tinnitus

Medications

Vasodilators
   Nicotinic acid (Niacin), 50-200 mg/d po to vasodilate blood vessels that supply inner ear; its efficacy is questionable
Antianxiety agents (used for sedative effect)
   Diazepam (Valium), 5 mg po q4-6h
Anticonvulsants (used for sedative effect)
   Carbamazepine (Tegretol), 200 mg po bid for 1 d, then maintenance dose of 800 mg-1.2 g qd
   Phenytoin (Dilantin), 100 mg po tid
   Primidone (Mysoline), 100-125 mg/d at bedtime for 3 d, then 250 mg tid or qid, and carbamazepine in combination; have helped in some cases, but exact mechanism is unknown

General Management

Hypnosis, biofeedback helpful in some cases; radios or masking units to drown out tinnitus or to make it less noticeable to the patient

NURSING CARE

Nursing Assessment

Auditory Function

Patient describes sound in one or both ears as ringing, sizzling, whistling, roaring, humming, or hissing; may be intermittent or continuous; may be high pitched; history of acoustic trauma, that is, exposure to loud noise; history of ototoxic drugs; hearing may be normal to decreased; may be associated with vertigo

Nursing Dx & Intervention

Sensory/perceptual alterations (auditory) related to tinnitus; hearing impairment

- Assess patient for hearing impairment or degree of tinnitus.
- Encourage use of background noise, that is, radios or masking units *to present a more pleasant noise.*
- Ensure that the use of any ototoxic substances is discontinued, if possible.
- Assist with any procedures necessary for diagnosis or treatment.

Anxiety related to constant tinnitus

- Assess successful coping mechanisms used in past.
- Provide information about tinnitus, its causes, and treatment.
- Encourage patient to verbalize concerns.

Patient Education/Home Care Planning

1. Explain to the patient that tinnitus is usually a symptom of a systemic or ear disease and that a thorough examination should be performed.
2. Encourage the patient to avoid exposure to loud noises that may cause acoustic trauma.
3. Discuss with the patient the ototoxic effects of some drugs. If the patient must take an ototoxic drug, be sure that periodic audiologic testing is performed to detect any hearing loss.
4. Refer to counseling or support group, if necessary.

Evaluation

Auditory symptoms are improved or managed Patient verbalizes understanding of cause of tinnitus if known. Patient verbalizes understanding that tinnitus can be a side effect of certain drugs. Patient understands that loud noises may be damaging and cause tinnitus and hearing loss. Patient verbalizes knowledge of various ways to diminish or minimize the tinnitus, that is, radios or masking units.

NOSE DISORDERS

▌ EPISTAXIS

Epistaxis is bleeding from the nose caused by irritation, trauma, coagulation disorders, hypertension, chronic infection, or tumor.

Epistaxis is thought to have occurred at least once in over 10% of the normal population. It is either a primary disorder or secondary to another condition such as hemophilia or leukemia and many cases are idiopathic.

In children, who are twice as likely to have epistaxis as adults, the bleeding is usually mild and tends to originate from the anterior nasal septum. In older adults bleeding is more likely to originate from the posterior septum so that the bleeding point is more difficult to locate and the bleeding may be profuse.[35,47] Epistaxis is equally common in men and in women and occurs more frequently in winter, probably because of the dryness of the air.

Although epistaxis is a frightening experience for the patient, it generally looks and feels worse than it actually is. The blood is usually bright red and the patient may swallow some of it, which is an unpleasant sensation. Although adults can lose up to 1 L per hour during severe bleeding, the mortality is extremely low. When the patient bleeds enough to show signs of shock, the nosebleed usually stops because of low blood pressure. Some deaths are thought to have been caused by coronary ischemia from blood loss.[27]

•••••• Pathophysiology

The most common cause of epistaxis is trauma to the nasal mucosa from damage by a foreign object, picking crusts from the nasal septum, or dryness of the nasal mucosa. Nosebleeds are fairly common in patients with coagulation defects such as hemophilia, leukemia, and purpura. Infection, tumors, and some drugs and toxins may cause nosebleeds; in many instances, however, the cause is simply not identified or is considered idiopathic.

There may be some relationship between menstruation and epistaxis. It may be that in some women with premenstrual syndrome the nasal mucosa becomes congested at the time of menstruation, setting the stage for epistaxis.[23,27]

The incidence of epistaxis is no higher in hypertensive patients than in normotensive patients. However, hypertensive patients may bleed more profusely, partly because of the direct effect of the increased pressure and also because the small nasal arteries and arterioles of hypertensive patients tend to have much of their muscular walls replaced by fibrous tissue and are incapable of contracting adequately to attain hemostasis.[23,27]

Children experience frequent nosebleeds from the anteroinferior part of the septum known as Little's area or Kiesselbach's plexus (Figure 7-18). The etiology is not clear, but the area is richly vascular, and children have hyperemic and congested upper respiratory tracts. Children also pick and rub their noses in the area where the mucosa is stretched over cartilage and bone.

Intractable nose picking is another cause of anterior nosebleeds. Some patients cannot stop picking their noses, either because of a nervous habit or because crusts are present from an earlier ulceration or perforation. Constant nose picking can cause septal ulceration or even a perforation, which leads to epistaxis.

A hereditary disease that is an unusual cause of epistaxis is Rendu-Osler-Weber disease or hemorrhagic hereditary telangiectasia. This disease is gene dominant and may be passed from either parent to a child of either sex. Epistaxis is usually the initial symptom, but telangiectasis is commonly found in other mucous membranes or anywhere on the external surface of the body. Bleeding usually occurs from the nose and gastrointestinal tract because mucosa in those areas is very fragile, whereas other areas have protective layers of squamous epithelium.

Most nosebleeds in the anterior part of the nose originate from Kisselbach's plexus, the highly vascular network in the anterior nasal septum. It is also anatomically closer to the rapid inspiratory air flow, which may dry the normal mucus flow, especially in cold, dry weather.[47] Because the vessels are fairly small and easily accessible, these nosebleeds are the easiest to treat. If bleeding is from the posterior part of the nose, the exact source of bleeding is more difficult to locate because it is sometimes impossible to see and bleeding is more profuse. (See Emergency Alert box.) Usually just one source on one side of the nose bleeds, although bleeding frequently originates from both sides in patients with blood dyscrasias.

•••••• Diagnostic Studies and Findings

Hematocrit, hemoglobin, platelets, prothrombin time, partial thromboplastin time, reticulocyte count, and differential   Done to rule out coagulation defect; results usually

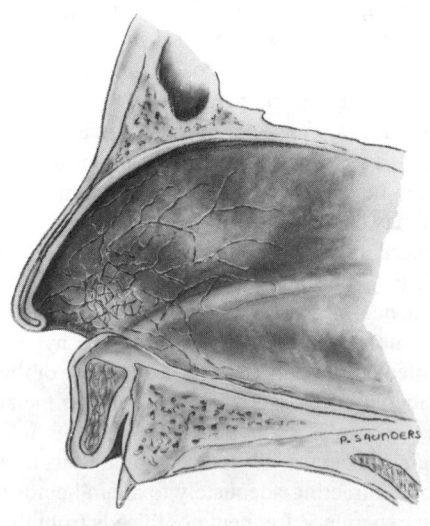

Figure 7-18 Kisselbach's plexus. (From DeWeese & Saunders.[8])

normal; bleeding from other parts of body likely in patients with hematologic disorders.

Rhinoscopy and nasopharyngoscopy   To detect and localize site of bleeding

•••••• Multidisciplinary Plan

Surgery

Arterial ligation of ethmoid, maxillary, or carotid artery if proper packing fails to control nosebleed

Endoscopic cautery—chemical or electrical cauterization of bleeding vessels using nasal endoscope to visualize bleeding

Septal dermoplasty for Rendu-Osler-Weber disease—skin graft is placed in nose to cover anterior parts of septum

---

 EMERGENCY ALERT

EPISTAXIS

Epistaxis is common. It may be minor or major and may actually become so severe that it is life threatening. Patients at risk for bleeding and those taking anticoagulants are more prone to nosebleeds. Epistaxis is most commonly seen in children and individuals 50 years of age and older.

Assessment/Intervention

ANTERIOR BLEEDING

The most common spot for bleeding is from the anterior and posterior septum.

- Assess the location of the bleeding.
- Pinch the nose firmly and hold for at least 10 minutes. It is best if you pinch the patient's nose instead of asking the patient to do so. This way, you can ensure steady and firm pinching.
- If bleeding continues beyond the pinching 10-minute period, prepare the patient for additional treatment.
- With the patient in a high Fowler position, slightly hyperflex the head and suction the clots in the nasal passage.
- Observe the canal for continued bleeding. If present, and in conjunction with physician, apply vasoconstricting agent such as 10% cocaine solution.
- If bleeding continues, the nose may need to be cauterized with silver nitrate or anterior nasal packing inserted.

POSTERIOR EPISTAXIS

Posterior bleeding is more difficult to manage. It usually results from a chronic condition such as hypertension, atherosclerotic heart disease, or blood dyscrasia. The bleeding usually originates from the sphenopalatine artery, anterior ethmoid artery, or the nasopalatine artery.

- Assess that the bleeding is posterior.
- Place the patient in a high Fowler position.
- In conjunction with a physician, anesthetize the posterior nasal passage with 10% cocaine solution.
- Pack the bleeding site with packing materials such as an epistaxis catheter, Foley catheter tip, and/or tampon.
- Monitor vital signs and estimate blood loss. If necessary, provide fluid volume replacement.
- Instruct patient to (1) tilt head forward if bleeding occurs; (2) not to blow nose; and (3) to apply steady pressure to nose for at least 5 minutes if bleeding recurs.

and floor and walls of nose anteriorly to provide protective covering over fragile mucosa; combined with laser therapy gains control of epistaxis for several years

Medications

Fibrinolytics

Vitamin K (Aquamephyton), 10 mg/po or IM; useful in some cases of epistaxis, but packing remains therapy of choice

Antiinfective agents

Penicillin, 1.5 million U IV q6h recommended for prophylaxis because packing obstructs drainage of paranasal sinuses and may precipitate a sinus infection

General Management

Nosebleed from anterior part of nose

Easiest to treat; source of bleeding located, and clots and fresh blood aspirated with suction; cotton ball saturated with 1:1000 epinephrine inserted into bleeding nostril, and strong pressure applied to compress cotton ball against septum for several minutes; after cotton ball is removed, cauterization performed by means of silver nitrate or electric cautery; packing unnecessary if bleeding is controlled with cauterization; pressure alone may control bleeding. If bleeding is not controlled, the nose may be packed with gauze strips saturated with antibiotic ointment

Epistaxis from posterior part of nose

Postnasal packing: with patient sitting to prevent aspiration of blood, bleeding site located by advancing strong suction tip until nose fills with blood when suction tip has passed; large postnasal pack introduced through mouth by attaching it to catheter that is inserted into nostril and out mouth (Figure 7-19); catheter pulled through nose, lodging pack in posterior part of nose and providing compression to bleeding site; packing remains in place for 5 days; if both choanae occluded because of large size of pack, patient must be checked daily for ear or eustachian tube symptoms; patient will have some difficulty swallowing

Posterior nasal pack: a silicone balloon is used to occlude the posterior choana; this configuration provides a good fit, using several ml of fluid without placing painful pressure on the soft palate that is often associated with Foley catheters; a suction channel is opened when the stylette, which allows accurate placement along the floor of the nose or around a septal deviation, is removed; to control epistaxis, an anterior pack may be placed easily because the parallel suction and inflation channels have a narrow diameter; discomfort is minimal and patient may often be treated in an outpatient setting

NURSING CARE

Nursing Assessment

Nasal Bleeding

Bright red blood comes from the nares; patient may also swallow or expectorate blood; history of trauma, nose picking, hypertension, or other known cause

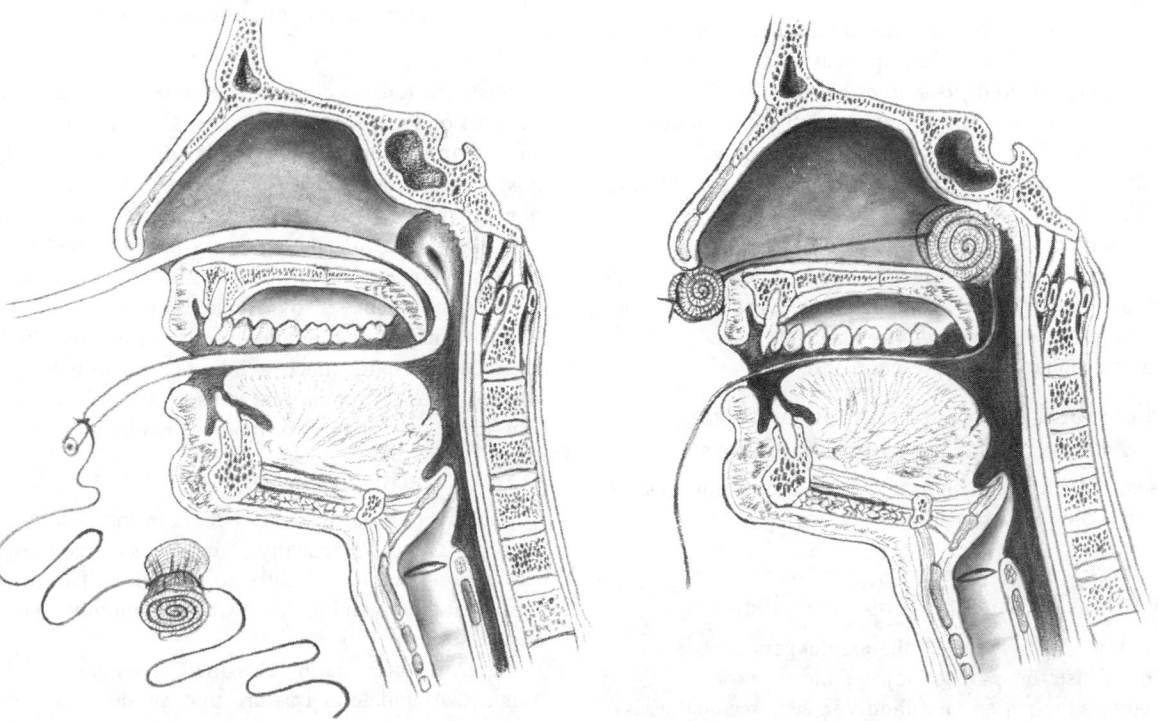

Figure 7-19 Postnasal packing for epistaxis.

General Examination

Examination of patient's body for bruises or petechiae that may indicate underlying hematologic disorder

Nursing Dx & Intervention

Risk for fluid volume deficit related to nasal bleeding

- Practice universal precautions.
- Maintain patient in sitting position to prevent aspiration of blood.
- Obtain history.
- Initiate first aid measures such as pinching anterior nasal ala(e) for 10-15 minutes; apply ice compresses to promote vasoconstriction.
- Encourage patient to minimize activity.
- Monitor fluid, electrolyte, and hemodynamic values.
- Assess blood pressure, pulse, and level of consciousness.

Fear related to loss of blood

- Prepare patient for all procedures.
- Assess patient's emotional state.
- Reassure patient that amount of blood lost looks worse than it probably is.
- Encourage patient not to swallow blood *to prevent nausea and vomiting.*
- Have patient breathe through mouth.
- Have basin nearby for patient *to expectorate blood.*

Risk for aspiration related to inability to clear secretions; gagging

- Assess patient's ability to expectorate and clear secretions.
- Elevate head of bed or have patient sit with head tipped forward *to prevent aspiration of blood.*
- Pinch patient's nostrils together for 5 to 10 minutes *to compress soft portion of nostril against septum.*
- Apply ice or cold compress to nose *to help stop bleeding.*
- Notify patient's physician.
- Assist with packing if necessary.
- If nasal packing is in place, encourage fluids, and provide frequent oral hygiene *to decrease mucosal dryness because patient will be breathing through mouth.*
- Inspect oropharynx for presence of blood.

Altered cerebral and cardiopulmonary tissue perfusion related to large-volume blood loss

- Assess patient's vital signs and level of consciousness.
- Record color and amount of blood loss.

Patient Education/Home Care Planning

1. Explain to the patient the inherent dangers in nose picking or of inserting foreign objects into the nose.
2. Encourage the patient and family to seek medical assistance immediately if nasal infection or epistaxis occurs.

3. If epistaxis is from dryness of mucous membranes, discuss with the patient possible benefits of using a humidifier or vaporizer to provide additional humidity in the home especially during the winter months.
4. Encourage patient to sneeze with mouth open and avoid vigorous nose blowing.
5. Instruct patient in first aid measures if nasal bleeding recurs.
   - Pinch nostrils tightly for 10 to 15 minutes.
   - Apply ice compresses.
   - Instill nasal decongestant spray to provide vasoconstriction, per physician's order.

Evaluation

Epistaxis is well controlled and patient's fear is minimized Bleeding is absent. Patient's hematocrit value and hemoglobin level are normal. Mucous membranes are healed if bleeding is from picking or ulceration. Patient verbalizes understanding of cause of epistaxis, if known, and ways to prevent bleeding in the future.

Breathing pattern is normal Patient experiences no aspiration of blood during epistaxis and is able to clear secretions.

Tissue perfusion remains adequate Patient experiences no loss of consciousness, and vital signs remain stable.

NASAL FRACTURES

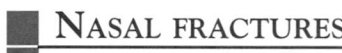

A nasal fracture is a traumatic injury to the nasal bones.

Nasal fractures occur quite commonly and more often than fractures of the other facial bones. Common causes are accidents, sports injuries, and assaults. In children, falls are the most common cause of nasal fractures. They occur more commonly in men.[3,27] However, when nasal fractures are diagnosed, it is essential to rule out fractures of associated facial bones such as zygomatic or mandibular fractures because facial injuries or trauma may also damage these bones.

Even a nasal fracture that appears simple usually has associated damage to the mucosal lining of the nose. If a patient has suffered a facial trauma that causes epistaxis, damage to the bone-cartilage structures of the nose is likely.

• • • • • • Pathophysiology

A nasal fracture occasionally occurs in the birth canal during delivery. These are usually "greenstick" fractures, and the baby's nose inclines slightly to one side. The nose can be grasped at the tip and pulled toward the midline to realign it in these cases.

Nasal fractures can be classified as unilateral, bilateral, or complex. A unilateral fracture may produce little or no displacement and may appear on an x-ray examination as a simple crack. Bilateral fractures, which are the most common, may be caused by a swinging punch or blow that pushes both nasal bones to one side or by a frontal blow that depresses the nasal bones and gives a flattened look to the nose. The entire nose may be deviated, and the nose may have a C or S deformity.

Complex fractures are usually caused by powerful frontal blows. Such blows may shatter the nasal pyramid and frequently the frontal bones as well, causing a marked depression of the nasal and facial bones.

The usual findings are epistaxis, a noticeable facial deformity, and a history of trauma. Edema occurs quickly at the injury site and depending on the severity may include periorbital swelling. Ecchymosis is common, the nose is exquisitely tender, and nasal obstruction occurs. Complex fractures of the nose and face may result in diplopia or subscleral hemorrhage.

•••••• Diagnostic Studies and Findings

X-ray examination of face and nose Show fractures and depressed areas of facial and nasal bones; done to complement clinical, visual evaluation

Ophthalmoscopy Performed to rule out eye injury such as corneal abrasion or laceration, also to check lacrimal apparatus and orbit

•••••• Multidisciplinary Plan

Surgery

Reduction and fixation of the fractures as quickly as possible after injury (within first hour or two before swelling begins, or after 3 or 4 days when swelling has decreased) because fragments tend to stabilize quickly; bilateral nasal packing or nasal splints usually inserted during surgery to maintain stability and position of nasal structure; wiring or splinting may be required for complex fractures

Medications

Narcotic analgesics or analgesic/antipyretics
Acetaminophen (Tylenol), 325-650 mg q4-6h with/without codeine, po q4-6h prn

General Management

Simple thumb pressure on convex side of the nose occasionally enough to push bones back together

NURSING CARE

Nursing Assessment

Facial Swelling

Deformity; ecchymosis; epistaxis; nose very tender; history of trauma to face and nose; possible accompanying lacerations; possible bony crepitus; if leak of cerebrospinal fluid is present, clear fluid dripping from nose and/or ears

Respiratory Status

Difficulty in breathing through the nose; mouth breathing

Nursing Dx & Intervention

Pain related to facial trauma

- Assess need for pain medication and provide adequate analgesia for pain relief; evaluate and document effectiveness.

Ineffective breathing pattern related to nasal obstruction and swelling

- Assess for shortness of breath, dyspnea from nasal obstruction, or difficulty in swallowing.
- Apply ice to face and nose *to minimize swelling and bleeding without pressure to nose.*
- Monitor amount and color of epistaxis and record.
- Keep head of bed elevated, even when sleeping, *to prevent aspiration of blood or secretions and minimize edema.*
- Prevent patient from swallowing blood or aspirating; encourage patient to breathe through mouth.
- Have basin nearby for patient *to expectorate blood.*
- Provide frequent oral hygiene and encourage intake of oral fluids.
- Monitor vital signs and level of consciousness.

Sensory/perceptual alterations (visual) related to periorbital edema

- Assess for eye swelling; apply ice *to minimize edema.*
- Observe for scleral hemorrhage and periorbital edema.
- If eyes are not completely closed, assess patient's ability to see.

Patient Education/Home Care Planning

1. Ensure that the patient knows to keep head elevated, even while sleeping.
2. Explain to the patient the timing of pain medication for maximum effectiveness.
3. Encourage the patient to seek medical assistance immediately if there is a decrease in vision, level of consciousness, or ability to breathe.

Evaluation

Comfort is maintained Pain is minimized or managed effectively with oral pain medications.

Breathing pattern There is no facial deformity. There is no nasal obstruction; patient can breathe normally through nose.

Vision remains normal for patient Sclera is clear without redness or swelling.

■ NASAL POLYPS

Polyps are benign growths that appear as soft, pale gray, nontender masses and gradually form from recurrent localized swelling of the sinuses or nasal mucosa (Figure 7-20).

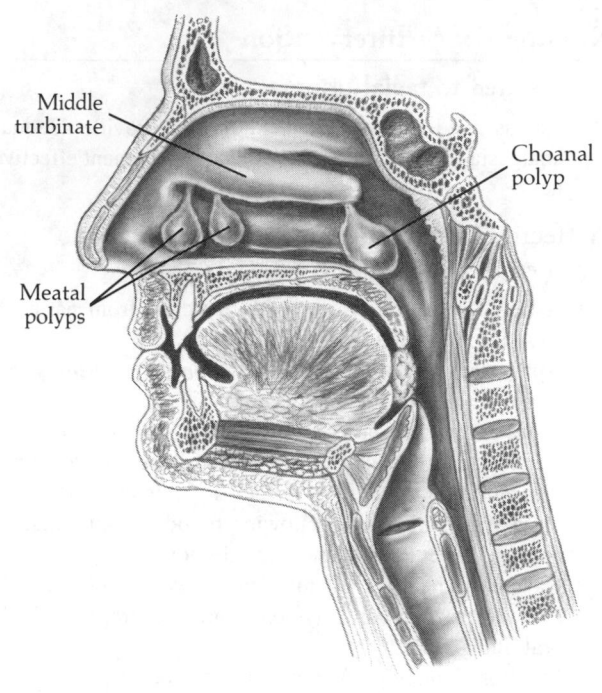

Figure 7-20 Nasal polyps.

Polyps are seen in about 90% of patients with chronic maxillary sinusitis. Polyps may become quite large. They are usually bilateral, occur in multiples, and may cause actual distention and enlargement of the bony structures of the nose. Even after surgical removal, some nasal polyps recur. Although rare in children, polyps are occasionally found in children with cystic fibrosis and allergies and in those with Peutz-Jeghers syndrome. The symptoms of this syndrome include pigmented spots on the skin, especially around the mouth, and polyposis of the gastrointestinal tract.

Many patient with polyps have anosmia or hyposmia.[44,47]

Pathophysiology

The etiology of nasal polyps is not clear. They are often pedunculated and suspended in the nasal cavity by stalks of varying lengths. The polyps and stalks usually originate in the paranasal sinuses, particularly the ethmoid sinuses, and pass into the middle meatus of the nose through the ostia connecting them to the nasal cavities. They are often called pseudotumors. Their pathogenesis is thought to be the result of focal mucosal edema that causes a polypoid swelling. Because of the polyp's weight, the swelling tends to enlarge and eventually becomes suspended on a stalk.[3]

Polyps are usually found in the middle meatus near the openings of the sinuses and occasionally in the roof of the nose. They are never found on the septum or in the lower meatus; the reason for this is not known.[3,23]

Nasal polyps are often found in patients with allergy, cystic fibrosis, asthma, disorders of ciliary motility, chronic rhinitis, and chronic sinusitis. The exact relationship is unknown but may be related to an inflammatory response causing hypertrophy of the mucosa, edema, and thinning of the mucous membranes.

An interesting phenomenon that occurs in some patients with asthma and nasal polyposis is an intolerance to aspirin, in-domethacin, and some coal tar dyes. This intolerance is severe and can cause respiratory arrest if these substances are ingested. This is thought to be related to the inhibitory action of these substances on prostaglandin synthesis.[24]

Diagnostic Studies and Findings

X-ray examinations of sinuses Shadows over affected areas; ethmoid sinuses and sometimes maxillary sinuses appear opaque

Immunologic assessment Performed if allergy is considered a causative factor

Multidisciplinary Plan

Surgery

Polypectomy—each polyp avulsed with wire snare
Caldwell-Luc procedure—may be performed if polyps originate in maxillary sinus
Functional endoscopic sinus surgery—removal of polyps using nasal endoscope

Medications

Corticosteroids
Deltasone (prednisone) high dose for 5 days
Methylprednisolone (Medrol dosepack) decreasing doses may be used for severe nasal obstruction to decrease size of polyps
Steroids are not recommended for long-term use; local steroid sprays, such as beclomethazone diproprionate (Beconase, Vancenase), dexamethasone sodium phosphate (Decadron turbinaire), triamcinolone acetonide (Nasacort) can be used for long-term control of the size of polyps and to prevent recurrence by reducing the inflammatory response[25]
Antihistamines
Terfenadine (Seldane), 60 mg po bid
Aztemizole (Hismanal), 10 mg po qd
Loratadine (Claritin), 10 mg po qd
Decongestants
Pseudoephedrine hydrochloride (Sudafed), 30 mg po q 4-6 h
Phenylpropanoline hydrochloride (Entex, Ornade), 1 po bid
Pseudoephedrine hydrochloride with guaifenesin (Deconsal II, Guaifed), 1 po bid
Aniinfective agents
Organism-specific antibiotics to treat infection

NURSING CARE

Nursing Assessment

Nasal Obstruction

Feeling of fullness in face or nose; nasal obstruction; difficulty breathing through nose; nasal discharge; anosmia; symptoms of allergic rhinitis, such as sneezing, watery eyes, eczema, and asthma

Nursing Dx & Intervention

Ineffective airway clearance related to swelling of the nasal mucosa and nasal obstruction.

- Assess patient's ability to clear secretions.
- Assess amount of swelling.
- Increase humidification.
- After polypectomy, elevate head of bed, and apply ice compresses to nose *to minimize swelling and bleeding.*
- Change nasal drip pad as indicated and record amount and consistency of drainage.
- Encourage patient not to swallow blood or secretions but to expectorate into basin *to prevent nausea.*
- Monitor patient's vital signs.
- Instruct patient not to blow nose *to prevent tissue trauma and promote healing.*
- Convalescent care: *Observe for bleeding.*
- *If bleeding occurs, instruct patient to notify physician, elevate head of bed, check vital signs, compress outside of nose against septum, and apply ice compresses to nose.*
- *If bleeding persists, packing may be necessary.*

Sensory/perceptual alterations (olfactory) related to anosmia, presence of nasal edema

- Assess patient's ability to smell.
- Assure patient that sense of smell should return postoperatively after swelling has decreased.
- Instruct patient to make appropriate adaptations to environment.

Patient Education/Home Care Planning

1. Ensure that the patient knows how to reach the physician immediately if bleeding begins after surgical removal of polyps.
2. Encourage the patient with allergies to avoid known allergens if possible and to take antihistamines early to minimize allergic reactions. May be referred for immunologic evaluation if local treatment ineffective.
3. Explain to the patient the need to use decongestant nose drops and sprays cautiously because of the rebound effect on the mucous membranes.
4. Instruct patient to make appropriate changes in environment.
   - Install smoke detectors.
   - Check appearance of food for spoilage.
   - Check gas lines for leaks.

Evaluation

Normal airway clearance is maintained Bleeding, nasal obstruction, shortness of breath, or nausea are not present after surgery.

Olfactory sense is maintained Patient verbalizes understanding that sense of smell will return after swelling decreases.

Patient's knowledge of polyps is increased Patient verbalizes understanding of possible causes and ways to prevent recurrence of nasal polyps. Patient seeks early treatment for sinusitis or minimizes severity of allergies by taking antihistamines, receiving immunologic evaluation and treatment.

SEPTAL DEVIATION AND PERFORATION

A deviated septum is a shift of the septum from the midline, which is common in many adults. It is either S or C shaped.

Although the septum is usually straight at birth, it may shift from one side to another as a result of trauma or injury.

A septal perforation is a hole in the nasal septum between the nostrils, which is usually in the anterior or cartilaginous septum but may occasionally occur in the bony septum. A small perforation, which can be caused by infections, nasal crusting, or nose picking, is often asymptomatic, although a slight whistle may be heard as the patient breathes. Larger perforations may produce rhinitis, nasal crusting, or epistaxis.

•••••• Pathophysiology

The nasal septum is usually straight. The septum is occasionally bent during birth, and the infant may have a twisted-appearing nose. This can usually be corrected when first noticed by placing light pressure on the convex side of the nose. There is no need for packing or a splint. Minor degrees of deviation go unrecognized in the newborn period[27]

With aging, the septum has a tendency to become deviated or to form a hump. There is frequently no history of injury to account for the deviation. As a result, few adults have a totally straight septum. Trauma during childhood may also contribute to septal deviation in the adult.

Although frequently no symptoms are associated with a deviated septum, some patients have moderate to severe degrees of nasal obstruction. Other, less well-defined symptoms include headaches, which occur in some patients who have a septal spur impinging on the inferior turbinate; epistaxis; and symptoms of sinusitis, which are rare but may be influenced by a deviated septum that obstructs a sinus opening.

Septal perforations may be small or large. They may be asymptomatic or may cause annoying symptoms, such as crusting, a watery discharge, or a whistling noise as the patient breathes. Small perforations are usually caused by repeated irritation of the nose such as picking it; they may also be caused by septal surgery. Less frequent causes are repeated cauterizations because of epistaxis, abuse of intranasal cocaine, and chronic nasal infections. Once quite common, perforations resulting from syphilis and tuberculosis are now rare. Approximately 25% to 30% of perforations are of unknown etiology.[27] Ninety percent of perforations are in the anterior cartilaginous portions of the nose, less than 10% are in posterior or superior bony portions. The margins of many are lined by smooth, shiny, flat mucosa; others have elevated edges of granulation tissue and crusted edges. These latter types should be fully evaluated for the presence of serious underlying disease.[27]

•••••• Diagnostic Studies and Findings

Facial x-ray examination; examination with nasal speculum or endoscope Show a shift of the septum or septal perforation

•••••• Multidisciplinary Plan

Surgery

For deviation

Submucous resection—may be performed to reposition septum and relieve nasal obstruction

Rhinoplasty—may be done to correct nasal structure deformity

Septoplasty to replace septum in midline—may be done to relieve nasal obstruction and to enhance external appearance of nose

For perforation

Surgical closure—possible but not always successful; a Silastic "button" prosthesis may be inserted to close perforation[27]

Medications

Analgesic/antipyretics

Acetaminophen (Tylenol), 650 mg po q4-6h to relieve headache if present (for deviation)

Antihistamines

Terfenadine (Seldane), 60 mg po bid

Aztemizole (Hismanal), 10 mg po qd

Loratadine (Claritin), 10 mg po qd

Decongestants

Pseudoephedrine hydrochloride (Sudafed), 30 mg po q4-6h

Phenylpropanolamine hydrochloride (Entex, Ornade), 1 po bid

Pseudoephedrine hydrochloride with guaifenesin (Deconsal II, Guaifed), 1 po bid

Antiinfective agents

Antibiotic ointment topically applied to prevent infection; bacitracin (Baciquent), 500 U/g in petrolatum base

General Management

Local application of lanolin or petrolatum twice a day to prevent crusting (for perforation)

Irrigate nose with normal saline or a dilute solution of sodium bicarbonate two or three times a day to keep the nasal mucosa hydrated (for perforation) (See bottom, right for instructions for "Nasal Irrigations")

Packing to control bleeding if present (for deviation)

NURSING CARE

Nursing Assessment

Nasal Obstruction

Irregularities or deformity of external nose; obstruction to nasal breathing; feeling of facial fullness, headaches, epis-

taxis; crusting of nasal mucosa; whistle sound when breathing (perforation); or sinusitis

Nursing Dx & Intervention

Ineffective breathing pattern related to septal deformity causing obstruction

- Assess and record respiratory status.
- Postoperative care includes explanation to patient that facial and periorbital edema may be present and that nasal packing or nasal splints may be used.
- Instruct patient to breathe through mouth during this time.

Impaired skin integrity related to surgery on septum

- Keep head of bed slightly elevated *to prevent edema and promote drainage.*
- Use ice compresses on face *to decrease edema, pain, and bleeding.*
- Use cool mist vaporizer *to assist in liquefying secretions.*
- Point out that patient may experience difficulty swallowing if nasal packing used.
- Change drip pad as necessary, recording color, consistency, and amount of drainage.
- Provide meticulous mouth care *because the patient is breathing through mouth.*

Risk for injury related to bleeding or tissue trauma

- Assess and report presence of excessive bleeding, swallowing, or purulent drainage.
- Caution patient against attempting to blow nose, *which may cause bruising, edema, and bleeding.*
- Caution patient not to smoke for at least 2 days and to limit physical activity for several days *to prevent irritation or trauma to tissues, which may cause bleeding.*

Patient Education/Home Care Planning

1. To prevent tissue trauma, encourage the patient not to smoke or blow the nose.
2. Encourage the patient to avoid strenuous activity and exercise for several days.
3. Instruct patient in techniques for supplemental humidification.
   - Vaporizer or humidifier
   - Normal saline nasal spray
   - Normal saline irrigations (see box)
   - Apply ointment to nose

Patient Education/Home Care Planning

Nasal irrigations
Using a syringe
1. Purchase an "ear syringe" (small rubber bulb syringe) from the drugstore.

2. Mix solution of normal saline: 1 teaspoon salt per 1 quart water (boiled). Store solution in a clean bottle.
3. Squeeze bulb of syringe to withdraw solution from storage container.
4. Leaning over a sink, insert tip of syringe about 1½ to 2 inches into nostril.
5. Gently squeeze bulb to irrigate nose.
6. Blow nose gently after first irrigation.
7. Repeat the irrigation with second syringeful.

Note: The normal saline solution also can be placed in a nasal spray bottle for moisturizing the nasal mucosa.

Using a water pik
1. Mix solution as above.
2. Set irrigator to lowest pressure setting.
3. Insert irrigator tip into nose or oral cavity.
4. Leaning over a sink, irrigate nose or sinus through oral cavity defect. Keep your mouth open as some solution will come out through the mouth.
5. Repeat the irrigation.

Evaluation

Nasal obstruction is lessened The patient breathes comfortably. No epistaxis or headache is present.

Skin integrity is maintained Septum heals well, with no evidence of infection.

Injury does not occur to nasal tissue Patient verbalizes understanding of the need not to blow the nose, smoke, or participate in excess physical activity for several days.

■ SINUSITIS

Sinusitis is an inflammatory process caused by bacterial, viral, fungal, or allergic conditions that change the mucosa of a sinus.

Sinusitis is frequently blamed for such symptoms as headaches or nasal problems and accounted for 25 million visits to a health care facility in 1993-94.[20] Sinusitis can be acute or chronic.

The changes in the sinus mucosa caused by sinusitis produce definite signs and symptoms, most of which can be assessed during a physical examination or on an x-ray examination.

An attack of sinusitis may follow a common cold (0.5% of the time) because nasal edema results in blockage of the sinus ostia, resulting in retained secretions in the sinuses; excessive or forceful nose blowing may also force infected material into the sinuses. Because the sinuses normally drain secretions through their normal routes into the meatus, any condition that obstructs these openings and forces the secretions to remain in the sinuses may cause sinus infection. These conditions may in-

clude the presence of nasal polyps, a deviated nasal septum, or nasal edema resulting from an allergic disorder.[3]

The maxillary sinus (antrum) is the one most frequently affected with acute sinusitis, although the entire group of sinuses may be involved. These are maxillary, frontal, ethmoid and sphenoid sinuses, all of which drain into the middle meatus of the nose.

The prognosis for sinusitis is usually good with identification and adequate treatment, but some complications may result from sinusitis if the infection spreads. These complications include septicemia, periorbital abscesses, brain abscesses, and osteomyelitis.

Regardless of the type of sinusitis, patients should avoid cold, damp conditions and maintain a constant room temperature and humidity. Air conditioning may aggravate sinusitis, as does smoking because smoke irritates the mucous membranes and inhibits the normal self-cleansing ciliary action.

•••••• Pathophysiology

Acute suppurative sinusitis may follow a common cold, or during swimming or diving when infected water may be forced into the nose resulting in a bacterial infection, or following dental manipulation.

Bacteria that are commonly responsible include gram-positive cocci, such as *Streptococcus, Staphylococcus moraxella catarrhalis,* and *H. influenzae.* Other organisms are less commonly responsible.

Swimming and diving may cause an acute onset of sinusitis; otherwise the symptoms occur gradually as the involved sinus becomes more inflamed. The nasal mucosa appears red and swollen, and purulent discharge is obvious in the middle meatus. The discharge increases, may be blood tinged in the first 24 to 48 hours, and may cause an inflamed, sore throat from the postnasal discharge. As fluid fills the sinuses, they become opaque to transillumination and an actual fluid level may be seen on x-ray examinations of the sinus.

Pain varies from low-grade to intense as the oxygen in the sinus is absorbed into the blood vessels. This creates negative pressure in the sinus and allows it to be filled with exudate, which produces a painful positive pressure. Tenderness is also present over the involved sinus.

Most cases of acute sinusitis are cured with conservative treatment, including antibiotics, decongestants, and mucoevacuants. Purulent secretions may be present for 3 to 4 days and then slowly resolve over the next 10 days to 2 weeks. In a few cases, however, a purulent nasal discharge persists, and the patient may continue to complain of nasal congestion and vague discomfort over the sinuses or face. This is classified as subacute sinusitis. These patients may have persistent pus in the nose for more than 3 weeks after the acute infection. Because antibiotic therapy will be needed, a culture of the exudate should be obtained and x-ray examinations may be taken to determine if more than one sinus is involved.

Frontal sinusitis can cause severe intracranial complications because these sinuses are in close physical relationship with the orbits and are separated from them by thin bony walls. Infection spreads easily from these sinuses to the orbits either through dehiscences in the bones or through infected thrombophlebitic veins. Spread of the infection is made easier by the rich plexus of valveless veins passing between the frontal and ethmoid sinuses and the orbits.[3,20,23] Fungal sinusitis may occur both in healthy persons and in persons who are compromised by immunosuppression, debilitation, diabetes, or malignancies being treated with cytotoxic drugs. Depending on the particular fungus and the health of the affected person, fungal sinusitis may be fatal. It is being increasingly recognized in otherwise healthy individuals and should be suspected as well in immunocompetent individuals who have nasal polyposis and sinusitis refractory to standard medical management.[56]

The most common infecting fungal agent is *Aspergillus.* Patients usually have a unilateral infection of the maxillary sinus after a long-standing sinus infection. Similar infections may be caused by *Alternaria, Petriellidum,* or *Paecilomyces,* all commonly found soil organisms.[19]

Patients with persistent subacute sinus infections may have an allergy; recognition of this obviously aids in treatment.

If sinus infections are neglected or a patient has repeated attacks, the mucosal lining of the sinus may become permanently damaged. This is known as chronic suppurative sinusitis. Often the only symptom is continued purulent nasal discharge. If the patient seems unable to overcome the infection, the physician must look for systemic conditions that may lower resistance to infection, such as anemia, malnutrition, or hypometabolism.

Allergic sinusitis occurs only in conjunction with allergic rhinitis. The symptoms are the same, and the sinus mucosa undergoes the same changes as the nasal mucosa. Patients with allergic rhinitis probably also have allergic sinusitis; polyps, which are common with allergic rhinitis, also occur with regularity in the mucosal lining of the sinuses.

Purulent sinusitis superimposed on allergic rhinitis and sinusitis is called hyperplastic sinusitis. The lining of the mucosa and submucosa becomes chronically thickened, and nasal polyps tend to form and recur even after surgical removal. These polyps may block the natural openings to the meatus and obstruct drainage of purulent material. Tissue swelling remains severe, and the nasal tissue does not respond to the usual decongestant solutions. The nose feels plugged most of the time, and a frontal headache is common.

•••••• Diagnostic Studies and Findings

Transillumination   Examiner shines bright light in patient's mouth with lips closed around bulb; involved sinus appears dark, whereas normal sinus transilluminates; has limited use but is a good screening tool.

Sinus x-ray examinations   Involved sinuses appear clouded or actual fluid level may be seen (Figure 7-21); screening sinus CT—best diagnostic method to evaluate significant sinonasal inflammatory disorder

Culture of sinus discharge   To identify causative organism

Sinus endoscopy   To evaluate drainage, edema, obstruction of sinus ostia

•••••• Multidisciplinary Plan

Surgery

Most now can be performed through sinus endoscopy (functional endoscopic sinus surgery)—to open sinus ostia and drain sinuses

For acute maxillary sinusitis
  Creation of nasal window—to open sinus and allow pus and secretion to drain through nose

For chronic maxillary sinusitis
  Caldwell-Luc procedure (radical antrum operation) through incision under lip to remove diseased mucosa and periosteum

For chronic ethmoid sinusitis
  Ethmoidectomy—to remove infected tissue through incision into ethmoid sinus

For chronic frontal sinusitis
  Creation of osteoplastic flap—involves incision across skull and behind hairline to drain sinuses
  Frontoethmoidectomy—allows removal of infected frontal sinus tissue through external ethmoidectomy

For sphenoid sinusitis
  External sphenoethmoidectomy—performed through incision that begins under eyebrow and extends along side of nose, allowing removal of infected sinus tissue

For fungal sinusitis
  Aggressive comprehensive surgical debridement of diseased tissue

Medications

Antiinfective agents
  Penicillin G or V, 250 mg po q6h for 10 d
  Erythromycin (E-Mycin), 250 mg po q6h for 10 d
  Clarithromycin (Biaxin), 500 mg po bid for 10-14 d

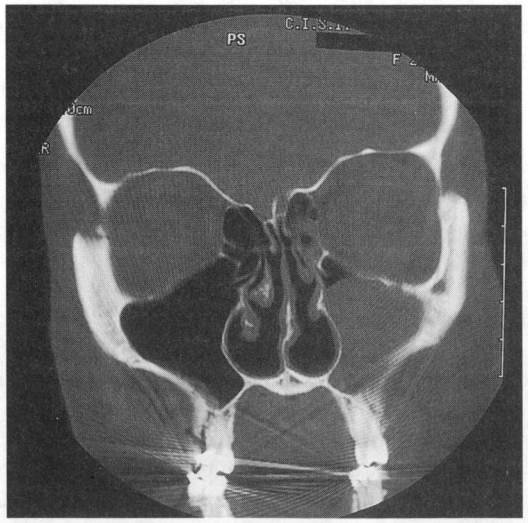

Figure 7-21 CT scan showing ethmoid and maxillary sinusitis. (From Sigler & Schuring.[46])

Amoxicillin (Amoxil, Larotid), 500 mg po tid for 10 d

Amoxicillin—Clavulanate (Augmentin), 500 mg po q6h for 10-14 d

Sulfamethoxazole (Bactrim, Septra), 1 tab po bid or qid

Cefaclor (Ceclor) 250 mg po tid

Cephalexin (Keflex), 500 mg po qid

Ampicillin, 500 mg po q6h (for chronic sinusitis)

Loracarbef (Lorabid), 400 mg po bid for 10-14 d

Amphotericin (Fungizone), 1 mg in 250 D5W over 2-4 h, or 0.25 mg/kg daily by slow infusion over 6 h; increase gradually as patient's tolerance develops, to a maximum of 1 mg/kg/d; dosage must not exceed 1.5/mg/kg/d; premedicate patient with acetaminophen (Tylenol) and diphenhydramine (Benadryl) as a prophylactic measure to avoid some of the unpleasant side effects

Narcotic analgesics (used to relieve headache from acute sinusitis)

Codeine, 30-60 mg po q4-6h

Meperidine (Demerol), 50 mg po q4-6h

Antihistamines (used to decrease secretions and congestion in patients with allergic component)

Iodinated glycerol, 2 tablets qid, with liquid

Azatadine (Optimine), 1 or 2 mg po q12h

Decongestants

Pseudoephedrine (Sudafed), 30 mg po q4-6h prn

Phenylpropanolamine Hcl (Entex) po bid for 10-14 d

Vasoconstrictors

Nose drops or nasal spray containing vasoconstrictor to keep the nose open; Afrin or Neo Synephrine (1 spray in each nostril q12h) is commonly prescribed for 3-5 days only

General Management

Drainage of involved sinus if usual therapy fails

Antral puncture (puncture of medial wall of maxillary sinus) to provide means of irrigation (may also be done to collect specimen for diagnosis)

Steam inhalation to encourage drainage and promote vasoconstriction

Hot, wet packs applied locally for relief of pain and congestion at least four times a day

NURSING CARE

Nursing Assessment

Acute Sinusitis

Malaise; anorexia; nasal congestion; purulent nasal discharge; cough; sore throat; fever, usually low grade; pain over sinus areas that worsens as patient lowers head; pressure over involved areas and upper teeth; orbital or facial edema; constant, severe headaches; loss of vocal resonance, hyposmia; halitosis

Subacute Sinusitis

Stuffy nose; vague intermittent discomfort in involved areas; fatigue; pus in nose more than 3 weeks after acute infection; nonproductive cough

Chronic Sinusitis

Persistent purulent nasal discharge; occasional slight headache (from nasal edema or allergic rhinitis, and not necessarily from sinuses) that is worse in the morning and relieved slightly during the day; postnasal drip; halitosis

Allergic Sinusitis

Nasal stuffiness; symptoms of allergic rhinitis; watery eyes, eczema, and asthma; itching and burning of nose and eyes; sneezing; frontal headache; thin nasal discharge

Nursing Dx & Intervention

Pain related to edema of nasal tissue

- Assess and document level of comfort.
- Encourage bed rest with head of bed slightly elevated *to promote drainage of secretions.*
- In collaboration with physician, give analgesics, decongestants, and antihistamines as needed for relief. Assess and document effectiveness.
- Administer antibiotics as ordered.
- Encourage steam inhalation *to liquefy secretions and promote drainage.*
- Apply warm, moist compresses locally at least four times a day *for pain relief and promotion of drainage.*
- Monitor vital signs, especially temperature.
- Watch for and report increase in headaches, blurred vision, periorbital edema, chills, or vomiting.

Sensory/perceptual alterations (olfactory) related to nasal congestion

- Assess patient's ability to smell.
- Administer antihistamines, decongestants, and nose drops or spray in collaboration with physician *to relieve nasal congestion.*
- Reassure patient that condition is temporary.

Sleep pattern disturbances related to headache and nasal stuffiness

- Assess patient's comfort and relaxation level at bedtime.
- Give analgesic medications per physician's orders before patient goes to bed *to minimize headaches.* Administer antihistamines, decongestants, or nose drops at bedtime *to clear nasal passages.*
- Make sure that patient understands importance of using nose drops as prescribed *to prevent rebound effect on mucous membranes if drops are used for a long time.*

Risk for ineffective breathing pattern related to the presence of nasal packing

- Assess and document patient's respiratory status frequently.

- Inform patient before surgery that nasal packing may be in place, that breathing through the mouth will be necessary, and that nose blowing cannot be performed postoperatively *to prevent tissue trauma and bleeding.*

Risk for bleeding after surgery related to postoperative hemorrhage

- Assess patient for bleeding after surgery.
- Monitor vital signs and watch for frequent swallowing, which may indicate hemorrhaging and swallowing of blood.

Impaired skin integrity related to surgical intervention

- Assess surgical site every 1 to 2 hours.
- Place patient in semi-Fowler's position *to minimize edema and promote drainage.*
- Use iced compresses *to minimize swelling and bleeding for first 24 hours.*
- Apply cool or warm vapor inhalations as ordered.
- Provide meticulous mouth care *because patient will be breathing through mouth and may have copious bloody secretions.*
- Change dressing or nasal drip pad and record amount and color of drainage. (There will normally be small amounts of bright red blood with some clots.)
- Inform patient that some numbness of upper lip and teeth may be present after Caldwell-Luc procedure and that black eye and some swelling of operative area are not uncommon for about a week after sinus surgery.
- Instruct patient not to brush teeth in the surgical area during this time *to prevent tissue trauma.*

Patient Education/Home Care Planning

1. Encourage the patient not to smoke after surgery to minimize irritation of the mucous membranes.
2. Discuss with the patient the need to watch for bleeding after surgery and to notify the physician immediately if it occurs.
3. Explain to the patient the early signs and symptoms of sinusitis so prompt treatment can be sought.
4. Caution patient about overuse of nasal decongestant sprays (longer than 3-5 days), which can cause rebound edema.

Evaluation

Pain and sensory alterations are improved   There is no headache, nasal congestion, or purulent discharge. Patient's ability to smell remains normal.

Patient is able to sleep comfortably   Patient verbalizes an understanding of ways to enhance relaxation and the ability to sleep by using relaxation techniques, analgesics, decongestants, and antihistamines.

Normal breathing pattern is maintained   Patient verbalizes an understanding of the need for postoperative mouth breathing, being unable to blow the nose. Patient's breathing returns to normal when edema subsides.

There is no blood loss after surgery   Patient's vital signs remain stable; no hemorrhage occurs.

Tissue integrity is maintained   There is no excessive bleeding or postoperative infection; the wound is completely healed. Patient returns to preoperative level of activity.

Patient's knowledge of sinusitis is increased   Patient verbalizes an understanding of the causative factors of sinusitis, signs and symptoms of infection, and when to seek medical assistance.

THROAT DISORDERS

ABSCESSES

Throat abscesses are infections in the fascial spaces.

The most common throat abscesses are peritonsillar (quinsy), retropharyngeal, and pharyngomaxillary. These abscesses may form after tonsillitis or an infection of the upper respiratory tract. A peritonsillar abscess forms in the space between the tonsil and the fascia that covers the superior constrictor muscle; a retropharyngeal abscess forms between the posterior pharyngeal wall and the prevertebral fascia; and a pharyngomaxillary abscess forms in the deep space between the fascia of the parotid gland, the internal pterygoid muscle, and the superior constrictor muscle (Figure 7-22).

•••••• Pathophysiology

A peritonsillar abscess usually forms after a patient has had tonsillitis for a few days and appears to improve. Peritonsillar abscesses are usually caused by group A β-hemolytic streptococci, *Staphylococcus aureus*, or occasionally anaerobic organisms. They are rare in children but fairly common in young adults.

Retropharyngeal abscesses historically were found almost exclusively in infants and children less than 6 years old because the lymph nodes in the retropharyngeal space have usually disappeared by young adulthood. Adult cases have been reported with increasing frequency in the medical literature, possibly because of underlying systemic pathologic conditions, or anaerobes and multiple organisms involved with deep neck infections.[19,45] These are usually found as complications of infections that have spread from the pharynx, sinuses, adenoids, or ears to the retropharyngeal lymph nodes.

Pott's disease, or tuberculosis of the cervical spine, can also cause a "cold" retropharyngeal abscess that may appear at any age.

Pharyngomaxillary abscesses are less common than peritonsillar abscesses but more common than retropharyngeal abscesses. Pharyngomaxillary abscesses usually occur as a result of direct contamination with a needle or by the spread of an adjacent infection.

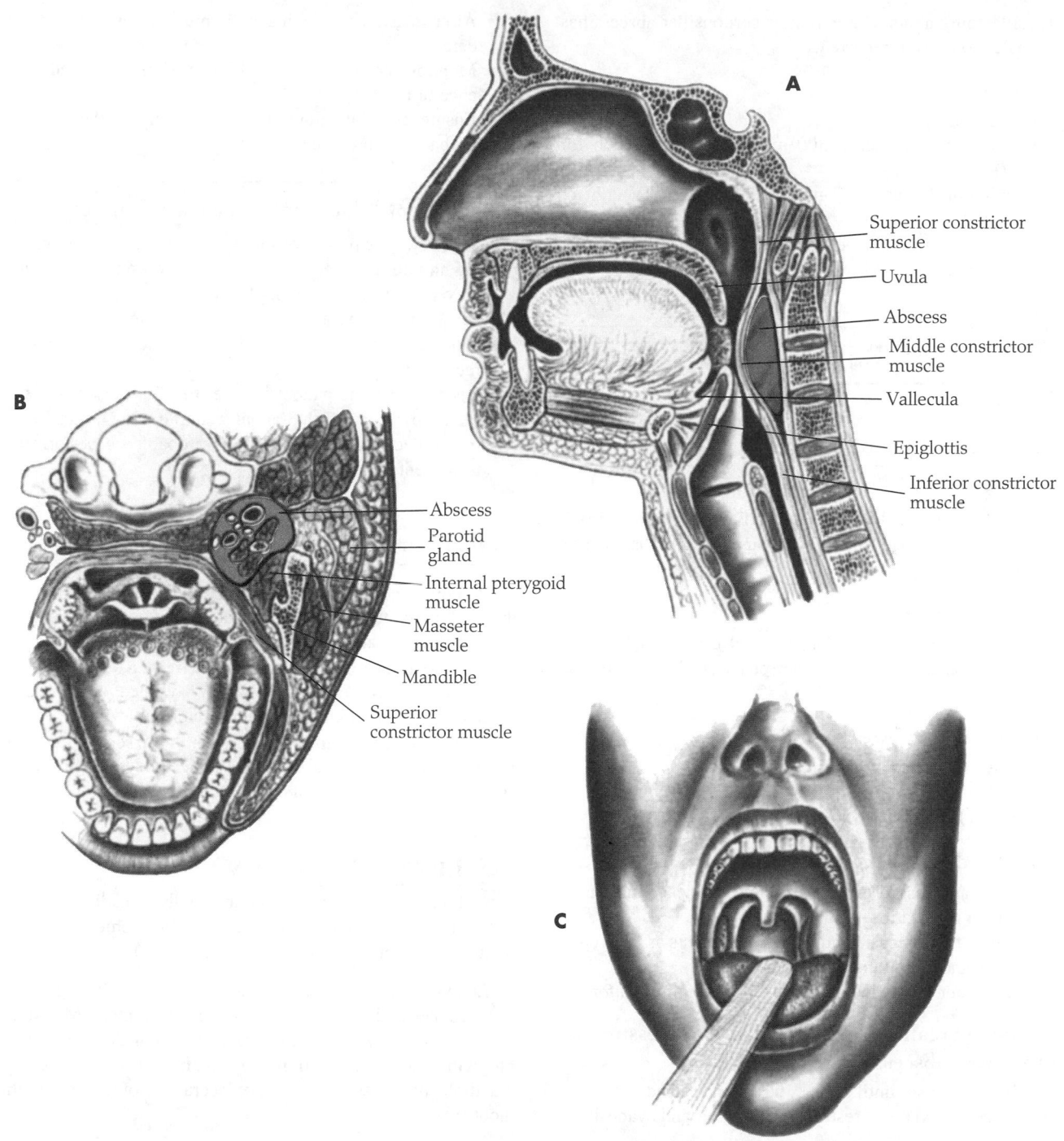

Figure 7-22 A, Retropharyngeal abscess. **B,** Pharyngomaxillary space infection. **C,** Peritonsillar abscess.

•••••• Diagnostic Studies and Findings

CT or MRI scan   Larynx appears pushed forward; mass shows in posterior pharynx with retropharyngeal abscesses

Culture of abscess   To identify causative organism

Visual examination   Tonsil appears pushed toward midline forward and downward; uvula may rest against tonsil or palate

•••••• Multidisciplinary Plan

Surgery

Guided needle aspiration with CT

Incision and drainage of abscess with or without local anesthetic, if needed

Tonsillectomy about 1 month after peritonsillar abscess has healed to prevent recurrence

Medications

Antiinfective agents

Clindamycin (Cleocin), 300 mg IV, IM, or po q6h for 10-14d

Ampicillin-Sulbactam (Unasyn), 1.5-3 g IM, IV q6h for 7-10 d

Amoxicillin-Clavulanate (Augmentin), 500 mg po q8h for 10-14 days

NURSING CARE

Nursing Assessment

Peritonsillar Area

Severe sore throat; difficulty in swallowing; trismus; drooling; muffled voice; thick secretions; fever, chills, nausea, and malaise

Retropharyngeal Area

Stridor and nasal obstruction; muffled cry; child lies with head extended; fever; posterior pharyngeal wall soft, red, and bulging

Pharyngomaxillary Area

Fullness behind jaw; trismus

Nursing Dx & Intervention

Pain related to swelling from abscess

- Assess and record amount of pain experienced and need for pain medication.
- Administer analgesic and antipyretic agents as ordered.
- Assess and document effectiveness.
- Administer hot saline gargles or irrigation *for comfort.*

Ineffective breathing pattern related to pressure on airway from abscess

- Observe airway until abscess has been drained.
- Assess for dyspnea, restlessness, stridor, and cyanosis.

Risk for aspiration related to spontaneous rupture of abscess

- Before abscess is drained, assess patient closely for signs of spontaneous rupture of abscess and possible asphyxiation from pus. (When abscesses are drained, it is not unusual for pus to pour out.)
- Avoid use of oral thermometer and gargles, which could precipitate spontaneous rupture of abscess.
- Keep patient upright with oral suction available *to prevent aspiration of pus that would result in suffocation.*

- After incision and drainage, administer antibiotics as ordered.
- Monitor and document vital signs, skin color, and presence of bleeding.
- Ensure adequate fluid intake; intravenous therapy will probably be ordered.

Patient Education/Home Care Planning

1. Explain to the patient or family the necessity of continuing antibiotic therapy for the entire prescribed course to prevent recurrence or complications.
2. Review signs of abscess with patient and family. Encourage patient to seek medical attention if symptoms recur.
3. Discuss with the patient that peritonsillar abscesses are likely to recur and that about a month after the abscess has healed, a tonsillectomy will probably be performed to prevent recurrence.

Evaluation

Patient's comfort is improved   There is no pain in throat. Temperature is within normal limits for patient. Trismus and drooling are absent. Incised area is healing well.

Normal breathing pattern is maintained   Patient's airway is maintained. There is no stridor, dyspnea, or aspiration. Vital signs and fluid intake remains at normal levels.

The patient and family understand course of treatment for abscess   Patient and family verbalize understanding about completing prescribed course of antibiotic therapy.

█ LUDWIG'S ANGINA

Ludwig's angina is a virulent, rapidly spreading cellulitis of the floor of the mouth that occurs in the submental, sublingual, and submaxillary spaces (Figure 7-23).

Ludwig's angina is actually not an abscess, although it resembles one, and there is no lymphatic involvement. More than 80% of cases develop in patients with dental disease such as gingivitis, tooth extraction, or trauma (fractures of the mandible, peritonsillar abscess, or lacerations of the floor of the mouth).[8]

•••••• Pathophysiology

These patient's lower molars oddly have the roots closer to the inner than to the outer side of the jaw, and the tips of the roots may extend below the mylohyoid line. The infection usually begins around a tooth root that drains into the submandibular space rather than into the sublingual space because of root placement. The usual causative organisms are *Streptococcus viridans* and *Escherichia coli.*

The infection spreads rapidly to the sublingual space, which causes the floor of the mouth to become very swollen. It may

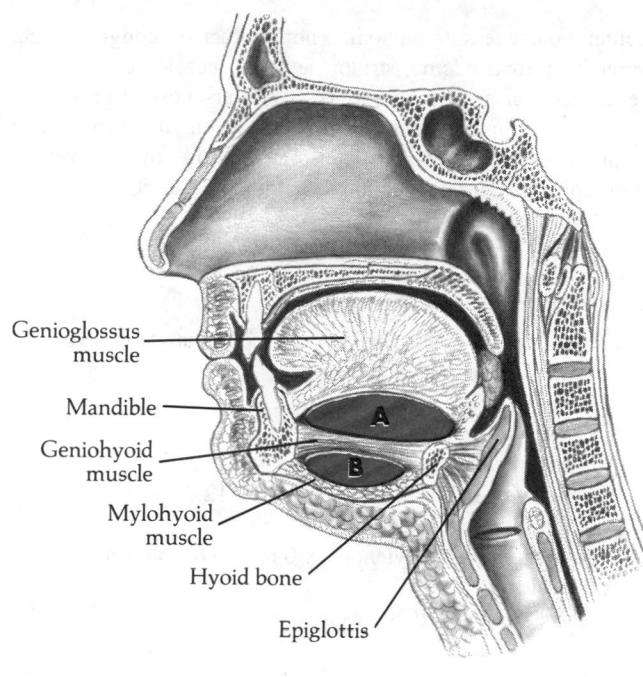

Genioglossus muscle

Mandible

Geniohyoid muscle

Mylohyoid muscle

Hyoid bone

Epiglottis

Figure 7-23 Ludwig's angina. **A** and **B** indicate spaces in which infection may start.

involve all the tissues under the mandible and usually one or both submandibular spaces. The swelling may extend all the way down to the clavicle. Because the tongue is elevated in the back of the mouth, airway obstruction is a danger. The patient has a fever and systemic signs of illness.

Pus is seldom found if an incision and drainage are performed, although they must occasionally be done to drain fluid and relieve the pressure on the swollen tissues.

Tracheotomy must often be performed because the patient's airway is greatly compromised from both swelling and excessive secretions.

•••••• Diagnostic Studies and Findings

Identification of causative organism   Culture of exudate; visual examination

CT scan   Indicates presence of and pinpoints location of abscess

•••••• Multidisciplinary Plan

Surgery

Incision and drainage—to relieve pressure
Tracheotomy if airway is impaired

Medications

Antiinfective agents
Penicillin G aqueous, 1-2 million U q4h IV
Cefotaxime (Claforan), 1-2 g q6-8h IM or IV (given if patient is allergic to penicillin)

NURSING CARE

Nursing Assessment

Infectious Process in Mouth

Severe pain in involved tooth area; trismus (difficulty opening mouth); dysphonia; patient unable to eat; excessive secretions and drooling; tongue elevation from swelling of the floor of the mouth

Respiratory Function

Dyspnea and stridor from laryngeal edema

Nursing Dx & Intervention

Ineffective airway clearance related to swelling, airway obstruction

- Assess patient for signs of airway obstruction.
- Perform usual tracheostomy care and frequent suctioning; assist patient in suctioning secretions.
- Encourage patient to expectorate secretions, if possible.
- Observe vital signs and symptoms of dyspnea and stridor.
- Elevate head of bed.

Pain related to swelling in the floor of the mouth

- Assess level of pain experienced and need for pain medication.
- Provide adequate analgesia for pain relief; assess and document effectiveness.
- Perform wound care gently but thoroughly if incision and drainage were performed.

Fear related to inability to open mouth, pain, and airway obstruction

- Assure patient that he or she is closely monitored
- Explain all procedures, progress, and areas of concern.
- Explain tracheostomy procedure and suctioning, and assure patient it will assist with breathing.

Altered nutrition: less than body requirements, related to trismus, pain, and swelling in the floor of the mouth

- Assess and document patient's fluid and nutrition status.
- Ensure adequate fluid intake *to prevent dehydration.*
- Monitor intravenous line closely.
- As soon as patient can take food and fluids orally, have nutritionist visit patient to plan diet *to provide needed caloric intake.*

Patient Education/Home Care Planning

1. Stress the importance of good dental hygiene to prevent recurrence of Ludwig's angina or other oral or dental problems.

2. Ensure that patient and family can perform wound care if tracheotomy is performed.
3. Discuss with patient and family the nutritional needs after discharge.
4. Discuss the need for the patient to complete course of antibiotics.

Evaluation

Airway clearance is adequate   Airway is patent without respiratory difficulty. Tracheostomy stoma is healing well. There is no swelling in the floor of the mouth. Tongue is not elevated.

Comfort is increased   Pain is diminished to absent. Temperature is within normal limits. Wound is healing normally if incision and drainage is performed. Fear is resolved.

Patient's nutritional status is adequate   Patient eats with no difficulty and understands the need to maintain adequate caloric and fluid intake.

Patient's knowledge base is increased   Patient verbalizes understanding of importance of prophylactic dental care and early treatment of any oral inflammation.

▇ LARYNGITIS

Laryngitis, or inflammation of the larynx, is a common disorder that may be either acute or chronic.

Acute laryngitis may be found as part of a viral or bacterial infection of the upper respiratory tract, or it may be an isolated infection limited to the vocal cords. Trauma such as voice abuse or gastroesophageal reflux may also cause acute laryngitis.[22]

Chronic laryngitis implies inflammatory changes in the laryngeal mucosa. It can be progressive and may lead to a serious voice disability.

•••••• Pathophysiology

Acute laryngitis is often found in combination with viral or bacterial infections of the upper respiratory tract. Viral infections are the most common, but organisms such as β-hemolytic streptococci and *Streptococcus pneumoniae* are also causative agents. Laryngitis may occur with colds, bronchitis, pneumonia, or influenza.

Noninfectious causes include excessive use of the voice, such as public speakers or singers; chronic reflux of gastric acid; inhalation of toxic or irritating fumes; or aspiration of caustic chemicals.

Chronic laryngitis can be caused by frequent attacks of acute laryngitis, chronic abuse of the voice, and smoking. Chronic tonsillitis and adenoiditis, allergies, or hypermetabolic states may occasionally cause chronic laryngitis.

•••••• Diagnostic Studies and Findings

Laryngoscopy, direct or indirect   Shows abnormalities in true cords, reddened mucosa, and secretions on vocal cords;

acute: hoarseness to aphonia; nonproductive cough; rough, scratchy throat; edema, stridor, and dyspnea in severe cases; fever or malaise; chronic: progressive hoarseness, if present, is worse in morning because of dried secretions in larynx; voice improves during day and deteriorates again toward evening with voice use; usually no throat pain; nonproductive cough

•••••• Multidisciplinary Plan

Surgery

None unless tracheotomy is required because of severe laryngeal edema

Medications

Antiinfective agents
   Penicillin G, 250 mg po q6h for 10-12 d
Analgesic/antipyretics
   Acetaminophen (Tylenol), 650 mg po q4-6h prn
Analgesics
   Throat lozenges (Chloraseptic or Cepacol) if necessary for throat pain
Antitussive agents
   Guaifenesin (Robitussin), 100-400 mg q4h to relieve cough

General Management

Voice rest
Steam inhalation
Speech therapy for chronic laryngitis

NURSING CARE

Nursing Assessment

General

Hoarseness; rough, scratchy throat; fever, malaise; cough

Nursing Dx & Intervention

Pain related to sore throat, laryngeal edema

- Assess level of pain experienced.
- Administer analgesics, throat lozenges, or antitussives *for comfort.*
- Administer antibiotics as ordered.
- Provide for inhalation of warm steam *for symptomatic relief.*
- Enforce that patient does not smoke.

Impaired verbal communication related to poor voice quality, hoarseness

- Assess patient's understanding of need for voice rest.
- Encourage complete voice rest or minimal use of voice. Encourage patient not to whisper as more force is needed to approximate vocal cords.

- Provide Magic Slate or paper and pencil *to facilitate communication.* Provide communication board, if patient is illiterate.
- Anticipate patient's needs as much as possible *to eliminate need for patient to talk.*
- Encourage family and friends to assist patient by asking questions patient can answer by nodding.
- If patient is hospitalized, mark on intercom that patient cannot respond and notify patient that someone will come to room when light is turned on.

Patient Education/Home Care Planning

1. Ensure that the patient understands possible sequelae of constant voice abuse and smoking and encourage improvement of these habits.

Evaluation

Comfort is improved There is no hoarseness and voice is normal for patient. Raw, tickling feeling in throat is gone. Cough and throat pain are absent. Temperature is within normal limits for patient. There is no inflammation or swelling in laryngeal mucosa or vocal cords.

Patient's understanding of laryngitis is increased Patient verbalizes understanding of causes of laryngitis and preventive measures: no smoking, no voice abuse, early treatment of colds, and recognition of symptoms of bronchitis.

■ PHARYNGITIS

Pharyngitis is an acute or chronic inflammation of the pharynx, including the pharyngeal walls, tonsils, uvula, and palate.

•••••• Pathophysiology

Pharyngitis is the most common of the throat disorders. It frequently precedes or accompanies the common cold and is characterized by a mild sore throat, difficulty and pain in swallowing, and a low-grade fever. In more than 50% of cases pharyngitis is viral in origin.[19] The bacterial cause is usually *Streptococcus,* especially in children. Unless complicated by other bacteria, pharyngitis usually resolves in 4 to 6 days. It is communicable for 2 to 3 days after the initial symptoms appear. Fungal pharyngitis is usually seen in immunocompromised patients and may result from prolonged use of antibiotics.

If follicular pharyngitis develops, usually from infection by β-hemolytic streptococci, the mucous membrane becomes severely inflamed and studded with white or yellow follicles. If these follicles are present, most are on the tonsils; if the tonsils have been removed, the follicles appear on the lymphoid areas in the posterior pharynx and also on the lingual tonsil and in the nasopharynx.

In approximately 10% of cases, pharyngitis is a result of infection with adenovirus. Primary infections occur during childhood; summer epidemics may result from waterborne vectors. In winter the mode of transmission is mainly respiratory. This can cause a severe and rapidly infectious, diffuse respiratory infection known as acute febrile respiratory disease, often accompanied by primary atypical pneumonia.[19] Infectious mononucleosis, caused by the Epstein-Barr virus, may also cause pharyngitis.

•••••• Diagnostic Studies and Findings

Throat culture Taken to determine causative organism
Heterophil agglutination antibody (monospot) To rule out mononucleosis
WBC

•••••• Multidisciplinary Plan

Medications

Antiinfective agents
  Penicillin G or V, 250 mg po q6h for 10 d (if pharyngitis has bacterial cause)
  Fluconazole (Diflucan), 100-200 mg po qd for 1-5 d
  Nystatin (Mycostatin), 100,000 U/ml 400,000-600,000 U po (swish and swallow) qid for 10-14 d
  Clotrimazole (Mycelex Troche), 10 mg (dissolve in mouth) qid for 14 d
Analgesic/antipyretics
  Acetylsalicylic acid (aspirin), 300-600 mg po q4-6h

General Management

Bed rest
Humidification
Warm saline throat irrigations
Adequate fluid intake; if throat is so painful and swollen that adequate fluids cannot be taken orally, the patient is often hospitalized for intravenous fluid intake for 24 to 72 hours or until inflammation subsides

---

NURSING CARE

Nursing Assessment

Infectious Process in Throat

Sore throat, with slight difficulty swallowing, including saliva; mild fever; headaches, malaise, and joint pain; cervical lymphadenopathy; pharynx reddened and inflamed; blisters or follicles on tonsils or lymphoid areas
Patients with mononucleosis may have enlargement of the spleen in addition to local symptoms

Nursing Dx & Intervention

Pain related to infectious process in throat

- Assess level of pain experienced.
- Administer antiinfective agents and analgesics as ordered.

- Assess and document effectiveness.
- Provide warm saline throat irrigations *for comfort*.
- Encourage bed rest.

Risk for fluid volume deficit related to pain and an inability to drink fluids normally

- Assess patient's fluid intake, skin turgor, and urine output.
- Encourage a fluid intake of at least 2500 ml/day.
- Monitor intake and output, observe for signs of dehydration (dry skin, cracked lips, and decreased urine output).
- If intravenous fluid is ordered, maintain adequate flow rate.
- Assist patient with frequent oral hygiene; patient may be mouth breathing, which adds to discomfort.
- Monitor patient's temperature and report abnormalities.

Patient Education/Home Care Planning

1. Instruct the patient and family about the necessity of completing the prescribed course of antiinfective agents to prevent complications or recurrence of infection.
2. Inform the patient and family of possible irritants (smoking and lack of humidity) and ways to prevent inflammation.

Evaluation

Pharyngitis is resolved   Sore throat is gone. Patient is afebrile. Activity level is normal for patient. There is no swelling or infection in throat. Cervical lymphadenopathy is absent.

Patient verbalizes knowledge of treatment   Patient verbalizes understanding of necessity of completing prescribed course of antiinfective agents.

Patient maintains adequate hydration   Fluid and nutritional status are adequate for patient's needs. Skin turgor is normal.

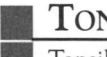 TONSILLITIS

Tonsillitis is an inflammation of the palatine tonsil(s).

Tonsillitis may be acute or chronic. It usually remains localized in the tonsillar tissue and is considered mildly contagious. It is characterized by a sore throat, but the patient may experience referred pain to the ears.

Tonsillitis is usually an airborne bacterial infection. It can occur at any age but is most frequently found in children between the ages of 5 and 10 years. If uncomplicated, it usually resolves after 5 to 7 days. Treatment makes the patient more comfortable and may prevent serious complications such as arthritis, glomerulonephritis, or chronic tonsillitis. A less common cause of tonsillitis is viral infection.

Several years ago the role of the tonsils and adenoids in the immune system was not as well known as it is today, and sur-

gical removal of the tonsils and adenoids was common. However, these procedures are performed less today because the importance of this lymphoid tissue to the body's immune system has been established.

•••••• Pathophysiology

Tonsillitis begins as a sore throat accompanied by fever, chills, headache, myalgia, joint pain, and anorexia. The patient may also have enlarged and tender anterior cervical lymph nodes. The tonsils appear enlarged, reddened, and inflamed with pus or exudate projecting from between the pillars of the fauces or in the crypts. Some of the exudate can be pulled away from the tonsil, which causes bleeding. The white blood cell count is frequently increased.

A throat culture should be obtained to identify the infecting organism. *Streptococcus* (β-hemolytic streptococci group A) is the most common organism. If this is the cause, the tonsils appear studded with yellow follicles. Other causative agents are *Pneumococcus* and gram-negative organisms (*Proteus, Pseudomonas,* or coliforms) and viruses.

•••••• Diagnostic Studies and Findings

Throat culture   Identification of causative organism

•••••• Multidisciplinary Plan

Surgery

Tonsillectomy, if indicated, after acute infection has subsided (see p. 666)

Medications

Analgesic/antipyretics
  Acetaminophen (Tylenol), 650 mg po q4-6h for adults
Antiinfective agents
  Penicillin V (PenVee), 125 -250 mg po q6h
  Penicillin G (Bicillin), 600,000-1,200,000 U IM

NURSING CARE

Nursing Assessment

Infectious Process in Throat

Moderate to severe sore throat; pain referred to ears; anterior cervical lymphadenopathy; fever and chills; headache; muscle and joint pain; anorexia; increased secretions from throat; enlarged, reddened, inflamed tonsils; pus or exudate on tonsils; halitosis; edematous or inflamed uvula; elevated white blood count

Nursing Dx & Intervention

Pain related to severe sore throat

- Assess level of pain experienced and need for pain medication.

- Provide adequate analgesia *for relief of throat pain;* assess and document effectiveness.
- Administer antibiotics as ordered.
- Perform throat irrigations; provide hot saline gargles or ice collar as comfort measures.
- Maintain bed rest during acute phase and emphasize importance of rest while convalescing.

Risk for fluid volume deficit related to difficulty in swallowing fluids

- Assess skin turgor, intake and urine output, and ability to swallow fluids.
- Encourage increased fluid intake, keeping in mind that children can become dehydrated very quickly. Note that the child may like ice cream, sherbet, or flavored drinks; avoid citrus juices *because they may irritate throat.*
- If patient is hospitalized, monitor intravenous intake *to ensure adequate intake of fluid.*

Altered nutrition: less than body requirements related to difficulty in swallowing food

- Assess patient's nutritional status and ability to eat.
- Ensure that patient has adequate intake of soft, nourishing foods.
- Encourage patient to eat foods that are minimally irritating to throat and provide adequate caloric intake, that is, soups and milkshakes.

Patient Education/Home Care Planning

1. Stress to the patient and family the importance of completing the prescribed course of antibiotics to prevent complications or recurrence.
2. Ensure that patient and family understand which foods and fluids maintain adequate nutrition and hydration without irritating sore throat.

Evaluation

Comfort is improved   Patient is afebrile. Tonsils are normal in size and free of pus and exudate. There is no pain in throat. Lymph nodes are not enlarged, although this might persist after other symptoms have disappeared. White blood count is within normal limits. Patient and family verbalize understanding of necessity of completing the required course of medication.

Nutrition and hydration are adequately maintained   Patient is able to eat and drink to maintain nutritional and hydration status within normal limits.

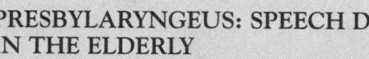 VOCAL CORD PARALYSIS

Vocal cord paralysis is the loss of nerve and motor supply to the vocal cords resulting in fixation and abnormal position of one or both cords.

Paralysis of the vocal cords is the result of either disease or injury to the superior laryngeal nerve or the recurrent laryngeal nerve, which is the branch of the vagus nerve that provides the entire motor supply to the larynx.

Vocal cord paralysis may be unilateral or bilateral. The quality of the voice depends on whether one or both cords are affected, as well as the position and tenseness of the affected cords. Paralysis of the vocal cords may also be described as complete versus incomplete or abductor versus adductor. Lesions of the central nervous system, such as multiple sclerosis, syringomyelia, brain tumors, and vascular accidents can produce paralysis of the vocal cords.

•••••• Pathophysiology

The left recurrent laryngeal nerve, which follows a longer path, is paralyzed in more than 70% of cases, in contrast to about 15% for the right recurrent laryngeal nerve. Men are affected about 10 times more commonly than women, and the most common age is during the seventies. The most common cause is thyroid surgery, with other causes following surgery such as anterior cervical fusions or carotid endarterectomy.[6] Other vocal cord paralyses are caused by malignant disease, possibly because of an increased incidence of smoking, leading to cancer of the lung and larynx.

One study shows a relationship between the degree of vocal cord dysfunction and the patient's age and sex. The normal aging process (see box below) may make compensation of vocal fold paralysis more difficult in the older population. Similarly, weight loss or presence of cancer may result in vocal fold atrophy and loss of pulmonary support, thereby leading to a more severe disability than might be expected from vocal cord paralysis alone. Some patients can compensate well after injury; others cannot. This requires more research.[37]

Peripheral causes are also common. These include stretching of the nerve, as occurs with aortic aneurysms and mitral stenosis. Stretching causes enlargement of the left auricle and also stretches the left recurrent laryngeal nerve. The nerve can be infiltrated or stretched by lung or bronchial tumors. Thyroid carcinomas may cause paralysis, and tumors of the vocal cords eventually cause fixation of one or both cords as the tumor invades the muscle or nerve.

Probably 10% of the cases of vocal cord paralysis are unexplained and are called idiopathic. These cases may be from viral infections that remain undiagnosed. In many of these cases

---

■ PRESBYLARYNGEUS: SPEECH DISORDER IN THE ELDERLY

Presbylaryngeus is dysphonia of the elderly. The patient's vocal cords undergo a loss of muscle tone resulting in bowing of the vocal cords. This bowing prevents the normal approximation of the cords causing a breathy, weak voice. Consultation with a speech therapist may provide the patient with strengthening exercises to improve the voice.

the function of the vocal cord recovers spontaneously; this is probably true in 80% of the patients with vocal cord paralysis if recovery has begun before 6 months has passed. The high incidence of infections of the upper respiratory tract suggests a viral cause in many cases.

The most common form of paralysis is unilateral; one cord is paralyzed and the other remains normal. If the affected cord is paralyzed in the midline, the normal cord can usually approximate it and the patient may have a normal voice. However, if the paralyzed cord is abducted, the normal cord cannot meet it and the patient has a husky, "breathy" voice and may be at risk for aspiration.

Dyspnea is not associated with unilateral cord paralysis because the laryngeal airway is adequate; the good cord abducts enough for the airway. However, bilateral cord paralysis affects the airway more seriously. The cords are usually paralyzed in the adducted position. The cords may be within 2 to 3 mm of the midline, and the patient suffers both stridor and dyspnea on exertion. Anything causing even minimal vocal cord edema may precipitate respiratory distress.

•••••• Diagnostic Studies and Findings

Laryngoscopy Shows paralyzed condition of cords
Bronchoscopy and esophagoscopy Done as part of malignancy workup
Videostroboscopy Records vocal cord movement
Electromyography Determines vocal cord innervation
Skull x-ray examinations, CT scan to visualize the course of the recurrent laryngeal nerve from the skull base to the chest, thyroid scan, upper gastrointestinal series, and complete neurologic examination Performed to rule out other causes

•••••• Multidisciplinary Plan

Surgery

For unilateral paralysis

Injection of measured amounts of Teflon into paralyzed cord under direct laryngoscopy; enlarges or swells cord and brings it closer to midline so normal cord can better approximate it; strengthens voice and prevents aspiration

Thyroplasty—involves an external incision in the neck with insertion of a stent to move the paralyzed cord toward the midline[18]

For bilateral paralysis

Tracheotomy may be needed because of inadequate airway

Alternative therapy is arytenoidectomy in which one arytenoid cartilage is removed and glottis is opened posteriorly

King procedure is another alternative in which suture is passed around arytenoid cartilage and through adjacent cricoid cartilage; arytenoid is rotated and fixed laterally; improves airway patency but may adversely affect quality of voice; many patients decide to conserve their voices and keep tracheotomy tube

Medialization laryngoplasty—generally performed under local anesthesia with little discomfort to the patient; involves creation of a window into the larynx, centered over the thyroid alar; a Silastic implant (1×0.5 cm) is placed after the cartilage is pushed inward[18,23,37]

NURSING CARE

Nursing Assessment

Voice

Vocal weakness; hoarse, breathy quality

Respiratory Function

Stridor and dyspnea on exertion if paralysis is bilateral

Nursing Dx & Intervention

Impaired verbal communication related to poor voice quality and to surgical procedure

- Assess and document quality of patient's voice before and after operation.
- Ensure that patient understands surgical procedure.
- Indicate to patient that voice will be improved but may not be completely normal.

Ineffective breathing pattern related to excessive secretions

- Assess patient closely for excessive secretions and need for suctioning.
- Increase humidification.
- Elevate head of bed.
- Minimize patient's activity.
- Encourage patient to avoid upper respiratory infection.
- Provide usual postoperative care after tracheotomy is performed.
- After assessing patient's readiness, teach patient to care for tracheotomy tube: suctioning, cleaning, and changing tube.

Patient Education/Home Care Planning

1. Instruct patient to avoid smoking, smoke-filled environment.
2. Encourage follow-up with rehabilitation team members (speech therapist, gastroenterologist).
3. Encourage patient to avoid crowds, upper respiratory infections, strenuous exercise.
4. If a tracheotomy has been performed:
   - Remind the patient that speaking can be accomplishd normally by using a tracheotomy plug or by occluding the lumen of the tracheotomy with a finger.
   - Advise the patient to wear a Medic-Alert bracelet indicating that a tracheotomy is present.

- Ensure that the patient and family can care safely for the tracheotomy tube at home; evaluate the need for community resource assistance to provide care.

Evaluation

Communication has improved　Voice maintains good quality. Secretions have diminished and patient requires minimal suctioning.

Breathing pattern improves　Patient demonstrates ability to suction, clean and humidify tracheotomy tube.

VOCAL CORD POLYPS AND NODULES

Polyps usually develop on the vocal cords from chronic abuse of the voice, allergies, or chronic inhalation of irritants, which frequently starts during an acute infection of the upper respiratory tract. Polyps are edematous masses of mucous membrane that attach to the vocal cords by either broad or narrow bases. Most have a broad base so there is permanent interference with voice production; however, some polyps are pedunculated, hang under the vocal cord, and cause only intermittent symptoms. Polyps are usually unilateral and may appear anywhere on the cord. They are common in adults who smoke, have allergies, or live in very dry climates. Polyps are far more common in men and rarely found in children. Because the cords are inhibited from approximation, painless hoarseness is the only symptom.

Polyps are gelatinous and telangiectatic, but mainly transitional types of polyps can be seen. Examination may show a change in the permeability of blood vessels, allowing extravasation of fluid, fibrin, or erythrocytes. After this, reactive processes develop and labryinthine vascular spaces form. This process is similar to the formation of a thrombus. The polyps develop at the site of maximum muscular and aerodynamic forces exerted during phonation and are considered a sequela of phonotrauma.

Vocal cord nodules, also called singer's, teacher's, or screamer's nodules, are caused by chronic voice abuse, such as singing, screaming, or constantly speaking outside the natural voice range. Nodules occur at any age and usually in girls and women, although they are sometimes found in young boys who scream and shout excessively.

The nodules are benign growths that first appear red and raised above the vocal cord surface. They later change into small white lumps that touch when the cords approximate. Because they are raised, the cords are kept apart and produce a characteristic hoarse, breathy voice (Figure 7-24).

Conservative treatment of nodules and complete voice rest often cause even large nodules to disappear. After voice rest, speech therapy may be indicated to prevent recurrence of the nodules and restore a normal voice. In contrast, polyps usually require surgical removal; they do not disappear with voice rest. Direct laryngoscopy is performed, and the polyps are excised.

If a patient has bilateral polyps, the excision should be done in two stages because doing both sides at the same time may cause a laryngeal web to form between the two raw surfaces.

Nursing Dx & Intervention

Impaired verbal communication related to prescribed voice rest

- Assess patient's understanding of need for voice rest.
- Ensure that patient does not speak during period of voice rest; provide patient with Magic Slate or paper and pencil *to encourage nonverbal written communication.*
- Remind visitors and staff members that patient is not to speak; attempt to anticipate patient's needs so patient will not have to speak.
- Use humidifier in room *to provide adequate moisture in air and decrease throat irritation.*
- Encourage patient to avoid smoking to minimize exposure to irritants.

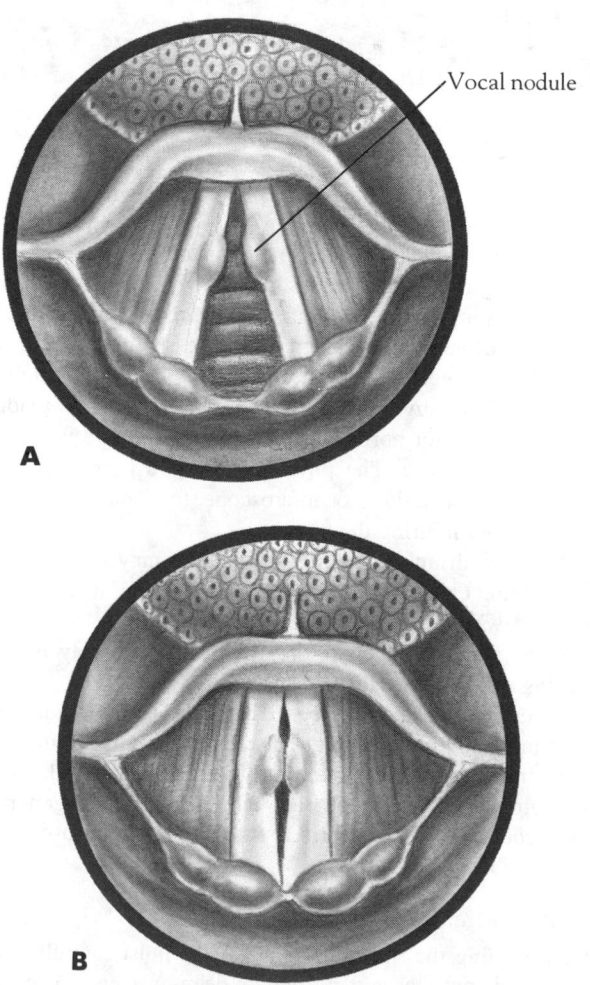

Vocal nodule

A

B

Figure 7-24 Vocal cord nodules. **A,** During respiration. **B,** During phonation.

Evaluation

Patient's communication has improved There are no nodules or polyps on vocal cords. Patient is able to speak in a normal voice. Patient verbalizes understanding of stresses on voice and how to minimize these: no smoking, avoidance of allergens, and no excessive shouting or screaming.

MEDICAL INTERVENTIONS AND RELATED NURSING CARE

■ Myringotomy
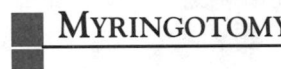

Description and Rationale

Myringotomy is an incision of the tympanic membrane, usually to drain pus or fluid from the middle ear. Myringotomy was once performed routinely for ear infections such as otitis media, but the advent of antibiotics has greatly decreased the need for it.

A local or general anesthestic may be used, although the procedure is relatively painless. A curved incision is made in the posteroinferior portion of the drumhead with a very sharp myringotomy knife. The physician wears a head mirror and uses an aural speculum, or microscope, to visualize the drumhead to avoid injuring the ossicles.

After the drumhead is incised, suction may be used to remove fluid. Cotton is then placed in the ear to absorb the drainage, which may continue for several days.

A myringotomy incision heals quickly with only minimal scarring and does not disrupt hearing.

A ventilating tube may be inserted after a myringotomy to assist in equalizing pressure. The ventilating tube normally remains in place for 6 to 9 months. The tube usually falls out of the tympanic membrane as the membrane regenerates. Myringotomy can be performed with or without the use of ventilating tubes.

Contraindications and Cautions

When making the incision the physician must carefully avoid injuring the ossicles and cutting too deep. A deep incision may cut the mucous membrane covering the promontory, causing bleeding and pain. If it is cut, however, the injury is not serious. The drumhead can be easily visualized posteriorly and inferi-

orly, which is where the incision should be made to avoid injury to the medial wall of the middle ear and the ossicles.

There are no apparent contraindications to myrinogotomy if the disease process requires its performance. Most third-party payers require precertification and evidence of alternative therapy before approving a myringotomy.

•••••• Multidisciplinary Plan

Surgery

Incision of eardrum with sharp myringotomy knife for evacuation of pus and fluid; possible insertion of ventilating tubes.

Medications

Antiinfective agents
Tetracycline (Achromycin), 250 mg po q6h
Gentamicin otic drops indicated only if patient has mucoid effusions because risk is significantly higher for developing postoperative otorrhea
Analgesics
Acetaminophen (Tylenol), 650 mg with codeine 30 mg q4-6h prn

General Management

Cotton in ear to absorb drainage

NURSING CARE

Nursing Assessment

Tympanic Membrane

Drainage from eardrum; bleeding and pain at incision site; no impairment of hearing

Nursing Dx & Intervention

Pain related to surgical incision

- Assess degree of discomfort.
- Provide analgesia as needed *for pain relief;* assess and document effectiveness.
- Administer antibiotics and ear drops as ordered.
- If patient is child, instruct parents in treatment regimen and proper instillation technique for ear drops.

Impaired tissue integrity related to surgical incision

- Assess amount of drainage from ear.
- Change cotton as needed.
- Teach technique to patient or to parent.
- Because drainage is usually infected, wash hands well after handling drainage and teach patient or parents to do same *to prevent contamination.*
- Keep external ear dry and clean.
- Assess for and report symptoms such as headache, nausea, fever, or increased ear pain.

Patient Education/Home Care Planning

1. Explain to the patient and family the necessity for completing the prescribed course of antibiotics to prevent recurrence or complications.
2. Discuss with the patient or family the need to monitor for hearing loss or increased ear pain. Myringotomies occasionally need to be performed again for reaccumulation of fluid.
3. Ensure that the patient and family understand how to assess the amount of drainage and how to change cotton in the ear.
4. Explain to the patient and family that no water should enter the ear. Ear plugs or cotton balls coated with petroleum jelly may be used.

Evaluation

Comfort is improved Patient experiences no pain at myringotomy site. Patient is afebrile.

Tissue integrity is maintained Myringotomy incision is healed well with no evidence of pus or fluid behind eardrum. There is no drainage from eardrum. Patient does not experience hearing loss.

STAPEDECTOMY

Description and Rationale

Attempts to reverse hearing losses that result from otosclerosis have been made for almost 100 years. Stapedectomy is the result of refinement of these various attempts and is now the operation of choice in many patients with hearing losses from otosclerosis. During stapedectomy the surgeon partially or completely removes the footplate and the stapes and replaces them with a prosthesis that allows the reestablishment of normal sound pathways. The prostheses are made of various materials, depending on the physician's preference.

If patients are appropriately selected for the procedure and the surgeon has the necessary skills, 90% of patients experience an improvement in the level of hearing and in many instances hearing is almost normal.

Patients who may benefit from stapedectomy include those with a negative Rinne test of at least 572 Hz with a vibrating tuning fork and an air-bone gap of at least 20 dB for speech frequencies. Patients with otosclerosis and accompanying tinnitus may experience relief from tinnitus after stapedectomy.

Because the "worst" ear is the one operated on, patients selected for this surgery must have one ear functioning at a fairly adequate level. The operative ear must have a mobile malleus and a normally situated tympanic membrane.

Contraindications and Cautions

Active external otitis or otitis media must be well healed before stapedectomy will be considered

Severe vertigo from Ménière's disease

Occupation that requires frequent or large changes in barometric pressure, that is, divers, pilots, and those who work at heights

"Dead" or nonfunctioning ear on one side, unless patient has reached stage at which hearing aid can no longer be satisfactorily used

Patients younger than 25 years of age because otosclerosis may still be in an active stage

Older patients assessed carefully for general health status and adequate sensorineural reserve and for evidence of vestibular damage; caution exercised in patients with any vestibular damage and poor sensorineural reserve because results may not be satisfactory

Perforation of tympanic membrane

•••••• Multidisciplinary Plan

Surgery

With patient under local anesthetic and sedation surgeon turns eardrum back on itself like omelette; microscope used to magnify bones of middle ear; stapes and footplate removed by means of various picks and sometimes electric drill; when footplate is removed, open oval window sealed with fascial graft from temporal muscle, and prosthesis connected to incus to restore normal sound conduction; several types of prostheses used; one end attached to the incus and other to graft or plug in oval window; external ear canal packed to ensure healing of tympanum; packing left in place 5 or 6 days

Medications

Analgesics
  Meperidine (Demerol), 50-100 mg IM q4h prn
  Toradol, 30-45 mg IM q6h prn
Antiemetic agents
  Prochlorperazine (Compazine), 10 mg IM q6h prn
  Meclizine (Antivert) for vertigo effect, 25 mg po 1/2 h ac and hs
Sedative agents
  Sedation, such as pentobarbital (Nembutal), 60-100 mg po before surgery
  Phenobarbital, 60-100 mg po or Versed, 2.5-5 mg IM before surgery
Antiinfective agents
  Tetracycline (Achromycin), 250 mg po q6h for 10 d
  Amoxicillin, 250 mg po tid for 10 d

General Management

Bed rest for 24 hours (may vary with physician) with operative side facing upward to maintain position of prosthesis and graft

---

NURSING CARE

Nursing Assessment

Infectious Process

Fever or other symptoms of infection; pain in operated ear

Auditory Function

Hearing ability: vertigo

Gustatory Function

Ability to taste with anterior tongue

Reparative Granuloma

Occurs in about 1% of stapedectomies; cause is unknown, but it may be related to contamination of the implant or trauma to the tissue; can be recognized if the flap and tympanic membrane still appear reddened and inflamed and there has been no hearing improvement 1 week after surgery; granulomas can fill much of middle ear and must be completely removed along with prosthesis; different type of prosthesis must then be inserted

Nursing Dx & Intervention

Impaired physical mobility related to the need for bed rest; vertigo

- Assess patient's understanding of need for bed rest and immobility.
- Enforce bed rest as ordered; patient should lie flat with operative side up *to maintain position of prosthesis and graft.*
- Do not turn patient.
- Keep side rails up *to prevent falls.*
- When patient is allowed to be up, assist patient because *vertigo may be present.*
- Begin movement and ambulation gradually and provide medication for pain or dizziness as needed.

Sensory/perceptual alterations (auditory) related to ear packing postoperatively

- Assess patient's hearing levels before and after operation.
- Improvement in hearing may not be noticeable immediately because of packing in ear and bleeding. Make sure that patient is aware of this fact *to avoid disappointment immediately after surgery.*
- Speak distinctly, facing patient.

Risk for impaired skin integrity related to surgical intervention, draining, and possible bleeding

- While patient is hospitalized, assess for excessive bleeding, drainage, fever, and ear pain and report any symptoms immediately.

- Inform patient that after packing is removed, a piece of cotton may be placed in ear for few days *to provide protection.*
- Instruct patient in appropriate technique of changing cotton and tell patient to do it once or twice a day.

Pain related to surgical procedure

- Assess patient's degree of pain and report excessive ear pain immediately.
- Administer pain medication and antiemetics as needed; assess and document effectiveness.
- Encourage patient to move gradually, avoiding sudden movement *to minimize pain at operative site and vertigo.*

Patient Education/Home Care Planning

1. Encourage the patient to avoid sneezing or nose blowing for at least 1 week to prevent dislodgment of the prosthesis and graft.
2. Ensure that the patient is aware of the necessity for careful ear care both immediately before surgery and on an ongoing basis.
3. Explain to the patient that the ear must not become wet (as by shampooing) while deep external packing remains in place. Instruct patient to insert cotton coated with petroleum jelly into ear canal.
4. Explain to the patient that smoking is contraindicated after stapedectomy.
5. Instruct patient to confer with surgeon about instructions for flying and exercise.

Evaluation

Patient mobility is normal   Activity level is normal for patient; no weakness or vertigo is present.

Hearing improves after surgery   Hearing is improved to normal.

Tissue integrity is maintained   There is no pain or excessive drainage from operated ear. Patient verbalizes understanding of ear care regimen and symptoms to report to physician.

Comfort is improved   Patient experiences no pain and is afebrile.

TONSILLECTOMY

Description and Rationale

Tonsillectomy is the surgical removal of the tonsils and usually the adenoids (adenoidectomy). The rationale for this procedure is usually the removal of chronically infected tissue. A general anesthetic is used; the most common method for removal of the tonsils is dissection and snare because it can be used for all sizes of tonsils whether they are in shallow or deep fossae. Although it has disadvantages, the guillotine method is chosen by some physicians. Injury to the tonsillar pillar is more common with this method, and it is not suitable for deeply recessed tonsils. It may also not reach the base of the tonsils and will leave a tonsil tag. Adenoids are removed with an adenotome; a curette may also be used to remove adenoid tissue.

Contraindications and Cautions

Presence of any acute infection, especially tonsillitis

Active tuberculosis

Presence of hematologic disorders, such as hemophilia, leukemia, or aplastic anemia

•••••• Multidisciplinary Plan

Surgery

Tonsil and adenoidal tissue removed

Medications

Narcotic analgesics

Acetaminophen (Tylenol), 650 mg with codeine, po q4-6h prn (avoid aspirin because of possibility of bleeding)

Antibiotics

May be prescribed by some physicians

General Management

Intravenous fluids until nausea has subsided and patient is drinking well

Soft or liquid diet

Minimize activity

NURSING CARE

Nursing Assessment

Postoperative Status

Vital signs stable; no fever; pulse and blood pressure normal for patient; skin warm and dry; level of consciousness appropriate for recovery from anesthesia; no bleeding at operative site; if adenoidectomy is done, there may be some serosanguineous nasopharyngeal drainage trickling down back of throat

Complications

Bleeding from failure to secure bleeding points during surgery; airway obstruction from blood or secretions; aspiration of blood or secretions

Nursing Dx & Intervention

Pain related to surgical intervention

- Assess patient's degree of pain.
- Provide adequate pain relief; assess and document effectiveness.

- Ensure adequate fluid intake.
- Monitor intravenous intake at prescribed rate until discontinued and then provide soothing fluids *to prevent dehydration.*
- Instruct patient to avoid citrus juice, *which would cause irritation in the throat.*
- Offer ice chips or popsicles *to encourage fluids and provide comfort.*
- Monitor vital signs, level of consciousness, and presence of bleeding and report any change immediately.
- Provide ice collar for comfort, if ordered.

Risk for aspiration related to postoperative bleeding

- Maintain patent airway; keep patient on bed rest lying on side as much as possible *to prevent aspiration.*
- Observe for vomiting of dark brown fluid because of "swallowed" blood during surgery.
- Watch for frequent swallowing, which may indicate bleeding; check frequently with flashlight *to see if blood is trickling down back of throat.*

Patient Education/Home Care Planning

1. Explain to the patient the need to avoid clearing the throat, to watch for bleeding, and to call the physician immediately if any symptoms occur. They may occur about 5 to 10 days after surgery when the scab sloughs from the operative area.
2. Because tonsillectomy is routinely performed as outpatient surgery, give the patient a preprinted list of instructions for postoperative care at home (see box on p. 668).

Evaluation

Comfort is improved There is no bleeding from operative site. Patient is afebrile and takes fluids and food well. Activity level is normal for patient. Patient verbalizes understanding of necessity of watching for late postoperative bleeding and calling physician immediately. Patient verbalizes knowledge of when to return to physician for postoperative visit.

Airway remains patent Patient experiences no bleeding; no aspiration occurs.

■ TRACHEOTOMY

Description and Rationale

A tracheotomy is an incision into the trachea to form a temporary or permanent opening, which is called a tracheostomy. The incision is made through the second, third, or fourth tracheal ring, and a tube is inserted through the opening to allow passage of air and the removal of tracheobronchial secretions.

POSTOPERATIVE INSTRUCTIONS OF TONSILLECTOMY AND ADENOIDECTOMY

1. For the first 7 to 10 days after surgery there may be pain and soreness in the throat and ears.
2. Small amounts of bleeding occur during this period. If bleeding persists, call the physician immediately.
3. If signs and symptoms of infection occur, such as purulent exudate or increase in pain or fever, call the physician immediately.
4. Keep the fluid intake high for the first few days after surgery, which will help keep the temperature down.
5. The diet should consist of soft bland foods, gelatin, cooked cereals, ice cream, soft-boiled eggs, custard, broth, mashed potatoes, and noncitrus juices for about 1 week. Apple and grape juice are the best liquids. Carbonated beverages may be taken if the patient tolerates them. Well-ground meat should be added as soon as tolerated.
6. Activity should not cause overexertion for the next 7 to 10 days. If tolerated, the patient may go outside after the second day. Persons with acute infections should be kept away. Bathing may be carried out in the usual manner.
7. Acetaminophen (Tylenol) (if patient is not allergic) may be taken by mouth, 650 mg every 4 hours for pain, especially ½ hour before meals. If the patient is given medications to take home from the hospital, they may be substituted for Tylenol.
8. The patient should not gargle but only gently rinse mouth.
9. Avoid throat clearing.
10. Do not smoke.
11. If you have any questions or concerns, call your physician to discuss these areas.

Courtesy Ruth Weddle, RN, and Eden Rivera, RN, University of California, San Francisco.

EMERGENCY ALERT

FOREIGN BODY IN THROAT

Foreign bodies in the throat may penetrate or obstruct the airway or the object may be aspirated into the lungs. Fish and chicken bones are commonly found foreign bodies.

Assessment

- History of foreign body.
- The patient may appear fearful and anxious.
- Assess for difficult breathing, noisy respirations, coughing and/or choking.
- The patient may complain of pain or sharpness in the throat.

Intervention

- If the patient is coughing, do not perform the Heimlich maneuver. This may actually suck the foreign body deeper into the airway.
- If the patient is not able to cough and evidence of complete airway obstruction exists, attempt to clear the airway with a finger sweep.
- Proceed with the Heimlich maneuver. Four abdominal thrusts, and repeat if necessary.
- Attempt to clear airway with suction, and prepare for an emergency tracheotomy.

Except in the cases of head, neck, and face trauma, a tracheotomy is rarely performed as an emergency procedure. If immediate airway control is needed and the patient is hospitalized, endotracheal intubation is usually performed; a tracheotomy is performed as an elective procedure if an artificial airway is necessary longer than an endotracheal tube should be left in place.

Aside from tracheotomy performed to reduce anatomic dead space (by approximately 150 cc) in patients with chronic pulmonary disease or to aid in mechanical ventilation of an unconscious patient, most tracheotomies are performed on patients in two categories. Patients in the first group have an obstruction at or above (see Emergency Alert box) the level of the larynx, such as foreign body obstruction, carcinoma of the head and neck, severe infection (such as Ludwig's angina), trauma to the tongue or mandible, or stenosis from prolonged intubation. Patients in the second group have no actual obstruction but are unable to raise their own secretions and are in danger of anoxia if secretions accumulate and are not removed from the chest. These patients include those with paralysis of the chest muscles and diaphragm (as in Guillain-Barré syndrome), patients who are unconscious or semiconscious with head injuries, and patients with fractured ribs or other chest injuries causing severe pain that inhibits them from coughing. Tracheotomy is an excellent way to provide access to the trachea when a patient needs frequent suctioning. Other indications include patients with smoke inhalation or severe burns around the head and neck and patients who are at risk of edema from surgery in the head and neck.

Contraindications and Cautions

Caution exercised in infants because of extremely small size of their tracheas and small size of tube that must be used.[8]

Caution exercised if surgical incision in neck would increase risk of infection

•••••• Multidisciplinary Plan

Surgery

Vertical incision in midline of neck from lower border of thyroid cartilage to slightly above suprasternal notch; soft tissue and muscle layers divided and isthmus of thyroid exposed and divided between clamps or retracted upward, which exposes rings of trachea; vertical incision made, usually between third and fourth rings, secretions thoroughly suctioned, and tracheostomy tube of correct size for patient inserted; first tracheal ring should not be cut (Figure 7-25); complete hemostasis ensured after procedure; if procedure is elective, endotracheal tube left in place and tracheotomy performed over tube; endotracheal tube can be removed after airway is secured; traction sutures may be inserted above and below the opening (stoma) for reopening the stoma in case of accidental decannulation

Medications

Drugs prescribed depending on reason for tracheotomy, that is, infection or laryngeal edema

General Management

Tracheobronchial suctioning
Humidification of inspired air

NURSING CARE

Nursing Assessment

Respiratory Function

Respiratory rate; amount and color of tracheal secretions; need for and frequency of suctioning; anxiety level; arterial blood gases; presence of bleeding at tracheostomy site (should be absent); no excessive coughing after suctioning; adequate humidification provided to tracheostomy (mucus is thin and without thick plugs); breath sounds audible in all lobes after suctioning; tracheostomy ties securely fastened

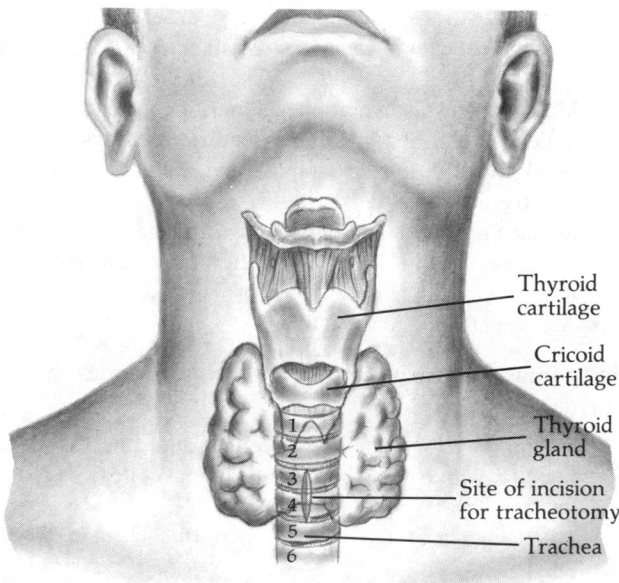

Figure 7-25 Correct area of trachea for incision and insertion of tracheotomy tube.

Pneumomediastinum

No dyspnea, crepitus, or edema of face and neck

Pneumothorax

No cough, anxiety, sharp chest pain, or tachycardia

Cardiac Tamponade

No increase in central venous pressure, narrowed pulse pressure, paradoxic pulse, decreased pressure, dyspnea, or decreased level of consciousness

Nursing Dx & Intervention

Ineffective airway clearance; high risk for aspiration; impaired gas exchange related to obstruction or excessive secretions

- Assess for and report any symptoms suggesting pneumomediastinum, pneumothorax, cardiac tamponade, hemorrhage, or subcutaneous emphysema.
- Assess rate, rhythm, depth of respirations; auscultate lung fields; monitor ABG's and pulse oximetry.
- Encourage coughing and deep breathing.
- Elevate head of bed.
- Suction airway as often as necessary *to maintain patent airway and remove secretions.* This can be done as frequently as every 5 to 10 minutes immediately after surgery to every 3 to 4 hours after tracheostomy has been in place awhile. Use catheter that is no greater than half diameter of tracheostomy tube. Preoxygenate and hyperinflate patient using Ambu bag before suctioning. Give patient five sigh breaths. Do not suction for more than 5 to 10 seconds *because suctioning decreases alveolar oxygen pressure by 30 mm Hg.* Keep bypass port open on catheter while inserting it *to minimize oxygen removal.* Gentle twisting motion of catheter should be used when removing catheter.
- Stop suctioning immediately if any signs of respiratory distress occur *because mucus blockage may be present and patient may quickly become hypoxic.* Postoxygenate patient after suctioning by giving five sigh breaths with Ambu bag to reopen small airways. Maintain adequate humidification *to keep secretions loose and minimize difficulty in secretion removal.* (Sputum is 95% water and mucous membranes dry out easily without proper hydration.) If necessary, 3 to 5 ml of sterile saline can be instilled into tracheostomy tube before suctioning *to facilitate removal of secretions.*[17]
- Clean inner cannula (if present) of tracheostomy tube every 4 hours as necessary or discard disposable inner cannula.
- If appropriate, ensure that patient receives chest physiotherapy, depending on condition and reason for tracheostomy.
- Document suctioning, patient response, result of chest assessment, and all treatments.
- If patient is receiving ventilation assistance or intermittent positive pressure breathing treatments, a cuffed

tracheostomy tube will be used. The cuff pressure should be maintained at level that just occludes trachea. Pressure should be less than 20 mm Hg.

- *Convalescent care:* Observe for any frank bleeding from tracheostomy or pulsation of cannula. (*Innominate artery is in close proximity, and tracheostomy tube may erode through the artery wall.*)
- Ensure that tracheostomy ties are secured at all times *to prevent tube from falling out or becoming dislocated.*
- When tracheotomy has just been performed, change ties with assistance *so tracheostomy tube is held in place while ties are replaced.* Institutional policy may vary regarding whether nurses may change tracheostomy ties within first 48 hours after surgery. Two nurses should be present during tracheostomy tie changes.
- Avoid using aerosol sprays, talcum powder, or tissue or gauze containing cotton *to prevent patient from inhaling foreign particles.*
- Use precut tracheostomy gauze or unlined gauze opened full length and folded into U shape under neck plate of outer cannula. Replace when soiled.

Anxiety related to presence of tracheostomy, the inability to speak, and concern about breathing pattern

- Assess patient's level of anxiety and carefully explain suctioning procedure to patient.
- Provide assurance that patient will be closely observed for respiratory distress or need for suctioning and that call light will be answered promptly.

Impaired verbal communication related to the inability to talk

- Assess patient's understanding of inability to communicate verbally.
- Evaluate patient's ability to read and write.
- Provide patient with Magic Slate or pen and paper *to facilitate communication.*
- Use word cards with commonly used phrases or flash cards/picture communication board, if patient is illiterate.
- *Convalescent care:* Instruct patient to occlude tracheostomy opening with finger or plug *to allow verbal communication,* only if tube is uncuffed.
- Consult with physician and speech therapist to use alternative speech devices (electrolarynx, speech valve, fenestrated tracheostomy tube).
- Observe patient for nonverbal cues.

Impaired skin integrity related to stoma incision, to decreased activity, or to immobility

- Assess stoma during every shift and note any bleeding, purulent drainage, and condition of surrounding tissue.
- Check skin under tracheostomy dressing and note areas of breakdown.
- Wear gloves to change dressing when soiled or at least every shift.

- Clean wound thoroughly with hydrogen peroxide and water or normal saline when changing dressing.
- Clean inner cannula of tracheostomy tube during every shift or as necessary.
- Ensure that sterile technique is maintained while suctioning.
- Make sure that patient is turned at least hourly if condition warrants and that areas of breakdown are noted and treatment begun promptly.
- Change tracheostomy ties, as needed.

Altered nutrition: less than body requirements related to the inability to eat or drink normally, to discomfort, and to anorexia

- Assess closely for signs of dehydration and malnutrition and report immediately.
- Monitor intravenous or tube feedings as necessary and document appropriately.
- Weigh patient daily.
- *Convalescent care:* Assess patient's ability to swallow.
- If patient is eating, has a cuffed tracheostomy tube, and is prone to aspiration, inflate cuff while patient eats and deflate after meals.
- Instruct patient to assume sitting position for meals and for 1 hour afterward.
- Consult nutritionist and swallowing therapist to determine food consistency and adequate calories.
- Provide high-calorie snacks and supplements if needed.
- Provide attractive, clean environment at meals and meticulous mouth care before meals *because patient may experience loss of taste because of decreased sense of smell.*
- Weigh patient daily and maintain accurate record of intake and output.
- If patient is receiving tube feedings, ensure that they are of sufficient caloric value *to maintain weight and promote wound healing.*
- Monitor patient's hydration and nutritional status.
- Follow established guidelines for tube feedings; that is, check for placement in stomach and residual before next tube feeding.
- Replace residual, and hold feeding if greater than 100 ml.
- Feed patient with head of bed elevated *to prevent aspiration.*
- Assess patient's bowel activity.

Body image disturbances related to presence of tracheostomy

- Encourage patient to discuss feelings and concerns.
- Identify, with patient, successful coping strategies used in the past.
- Assess patient's readiness to perform self-care procedures.
- Remain with patient during self-care to provide needed support.
- Demonstrate techniques/coverings to camouflage tracheostomy.

- Provide privacy for patient and significant other to discuss possible societal reactions, sexual concerns.
- Encourage participation in support/self-help organizations.

Impaired home maintenance management related to the need for continued tracheostomy care and the possible invalid status of patient

Convalescent care

- If patient will be discharged with tracheostomy, ensure that patient and family have been instructed in and understand management of tracheostomy at home, including suctioning, cleaning, wound care, humidification, changing tracheostomy ties, and tube feeding if necessary. Discuss changes in activities of daily living, such as, no water in stoma; tracheostomy tube protection; sexual activity.
- Ensure that family and patient know where to purchase supplies and when to return to see physician.
- Arrange for home health services and equipment, as ordered.
- Provide patient and caregivers with resources and emergency instructions (cardiopulmonary resuscitation, Medic-Alert).

To prepare patient for tracheostomy tube removal

- Assess patient's ability to breathe and cough effectively, gag reflex, and swallowing reflexes.
- Report any symptoms of distress to physician immediately.
- "Plug" tracheostomy tube intermittently and increase length of time for occlusion as patient tolerates.
- Remove tracheostomy tube or assist physician with removal of tube when patient tolerates occlusion well.
- Apply Steri-Strips or tape *to approximate wound edges.*
- Apply occlusive dressing over Steri-Strips.
- Stress need for patient to splint stoma site with finger when coughing or speaking.
- Check and cleanse wound site daily.
- Observe for signs of infection; opening should heal within few days.
- Make referral to visiting nurse or public health nurse.

Patient Education/Home Care Planning

(See "Impaired home maintenance management" on p. 1606.)
1. Inform the patient that there will be frequent suctioning, a loss of speech, and decreased ability to smell and that he will not be breathing through the nose or mouth while the tracheostomy is present.
2. Refer the patient to a speech therapist, if appropriate, to learn esophageal or alternative method of speech.
3. Reinforce need for supplemental humidification (normal saline instillation, humidifier, moist bib).

Evaluation

If short-term tracheostomy is used, respiratory status is within normal limits Patient has no excess secretions,

and tracheostomy stoma is healed without signs of infection. Patient does not experience dyspnea or shortness of breath.

Patient and family anxiety is decreased Patient and family demonstrate an understanding of and are at ease in caring for the tracheostomy tube and in the suctioning procedure.

Verbal communication is improved Patient can enhance speech by occluding tracheostomy tube with finger or plug, uses alternative devices as indicated.

Skin integrity is maintained Stoma is healed. No drainage or bleeding is present.

Nutritional status is maintained Weight and caloric intake are normal for patient. Patient eats regularly; patient and family demonstrate the ability to administer tube feedings as necessary.

If long-term tracheostomy is needed, patient and family demonstrate ability to care for all aspects of tracheostomy at home Patient and family demonstrate suctioning and cleaning techniques, wound care, changing ties, and methods for humidification. Visiting or public health nurse assists patient and family if necessary.

Patient/family adjusts to changes in body image Patient and significant other able to provide care, able to socialize with others.

TYMPANOPLASTY

Description and Rationale

Tympanoplasty is a reconstructive or reparative procedure of the middle ear that is usually performed to correct conductive hearing loss caused by chronic suppurative otitis media. The procedure involves rebuilding the structures of the middle ear or replacing them with prostheses. Tympanoplasty may also be occasionally performed to close a perforation of the tympanic membrane (myringoplasty or type I tympanoplasty) or to assist with clearing infections in patients with chronic suppurative otitis media and a sensorineural (rather than conductive) hearing loss. There is no chance of correcting the hearing loss in these patients. Tympanoplasty may also be indicated in patients with ossicular problems such as dislocation of the incus from trauma, congenital middle ear problems, or tympanosclerosis, in which the malleus is fused to the incus. In these cases metal or plastic prostheses, autogenous material, or cadaveric ossicles are commonly used. Because these patients have no concomitant infection, the results are often good.[8,13]

The principal rationale for tympanoplasty is to improve hearing in patients with conductive hearing loss but intact nerve function or cochlear reserve. The greatest improvement is seen in patients with bilateral disease and a large difference between air and bone measurements. In chronic otitis media the tympanic membrane, malleus, and incus are frequently damaged or destroyed. If this occurs, sound waves can enter the oval and round window with equal intensity and cancel each other, because the tympanic membrane is not there to protect the round window from sound pressure. Chronic otitis media also disrupts the tympanic membrane to stapes footplate ratio or the tympanic membrane–footplate ratio, thereby negating the transformer action of the middle ear.

Tympanoplasty, of which there are five types described below, improves hearing by reestablishing two important middle ear functions: restoring the tympanic membrane to stapes footplate ratio and creating sound protection for the round window.

Contraindications and Cautions

Presence of infection; procedure to clear infection must be performed before tympanoplasty

Patients with poor nerve function as determined by bone conduction tests

Hearing loss from otosclerosis or serous otitis media rather than chronic suppurative otitis media

• • • • • Multidisciplinary Plan

Surgery (Figure 7-26)

Postaural or endaural approach; with operating microscope at high magnification, surgeon performs one of five types of tympanoplasty, using either temporal fascia or tissue from nearby vein as graft; tympanic membranes from human cadavers sometimes used as graft, although this technique is still being evaluated. Teflon or stainless steel wires also used occasionally

Type I (myringoplasty)—performed for closure of perforation; epithelium removed from edge of perforation and graft of autogenous tissue, usually fascia or vein placed under tympanic membrane; TM footplate ratio and round window sound protection restored

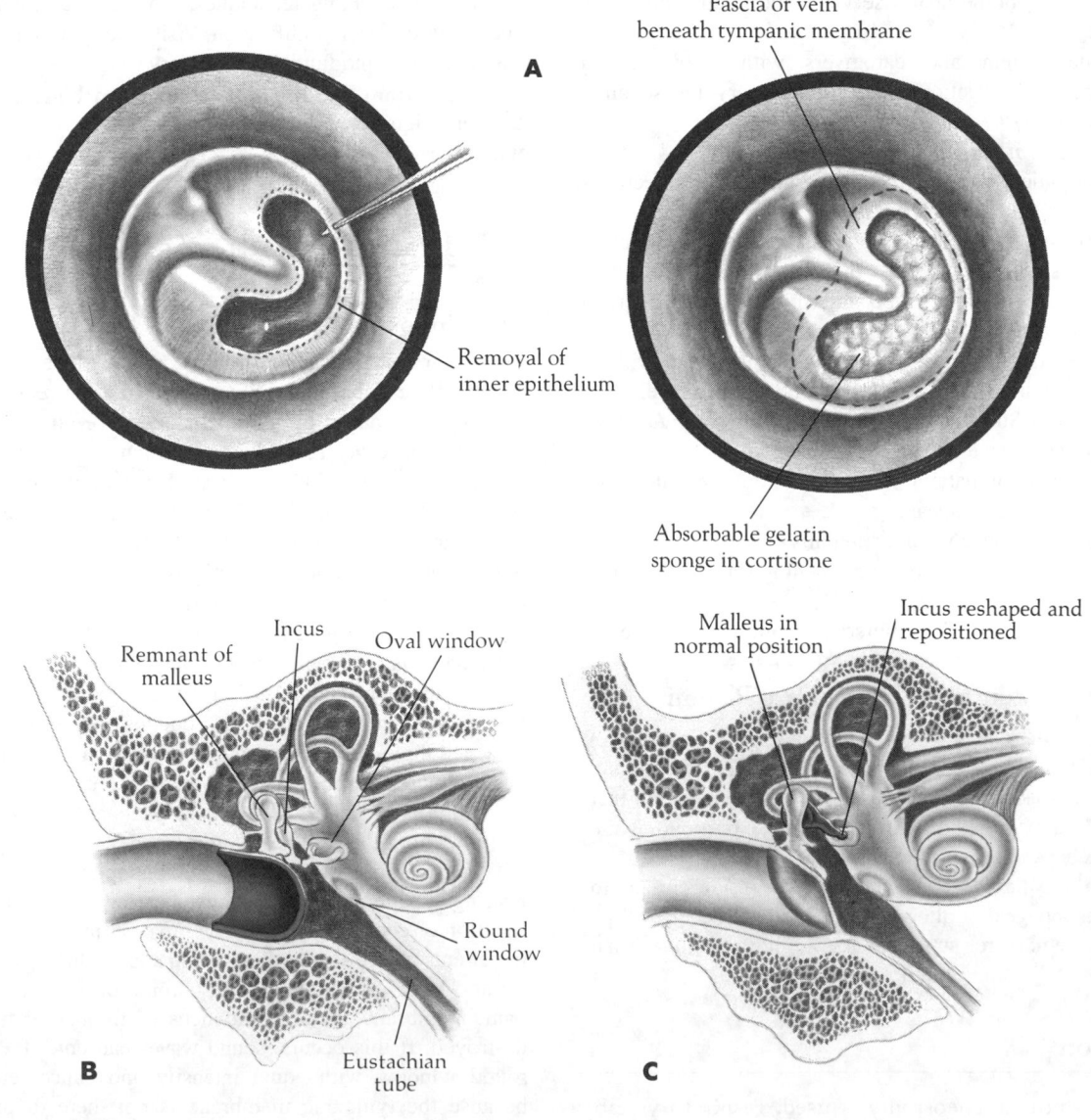

Figure 7-26 Various types of tympanoplasty. **A,** Type 1 (myringoplasty). **B,** Type 2. **C,** Variation of type 2.

Type II—performed when malleus is eroded; perforation closed with graft against incus or what remains of malleus; enough ossicular chain must remain to create new TM footplate ratio

Type III—also restores both areal ratio and sound protection of round window by means of autogenous graft; performed when tympanic membrane and ossicular chain are destroyed but normal stapes remains; graft is placed in contact with stapes

Type IV—TM footplate ratio cannot be restored, but round window sound protection is provided; only footplate remains intact, and air pocket is placed between round window and graft to provide sound protection

Type V—only round window sound protection provided; footplate is fixed and fenestration into inner ear must be performed; replaced by stapes surgery

Medications

Narcotic analgesics
  Meperidine (Demerol), 50 mg IM q4h prn
  Acetaminophen (Tylenol), 650 mg with codeine q4-6h prn

Antiinfective agents
  Tetracycline (Achromycin), 250 mg po q6h, or penicillin G, 250-500 mg po q6h
Antiemetics (for antivertigo effect)
  Meclizine (Antivert), 250 mg po 1/2 h ac and hs

General Management

Bed rest until next morning with head of bed elevated 40 degrees and operative side facing upward

NURSING CARE

Nursing Assessment

Middle Ear Function

Bleeding; amount, color, and consistency of drainage; temperature elevation; dizziness when getting out of bed or with sudden movement; nausea; vertigo

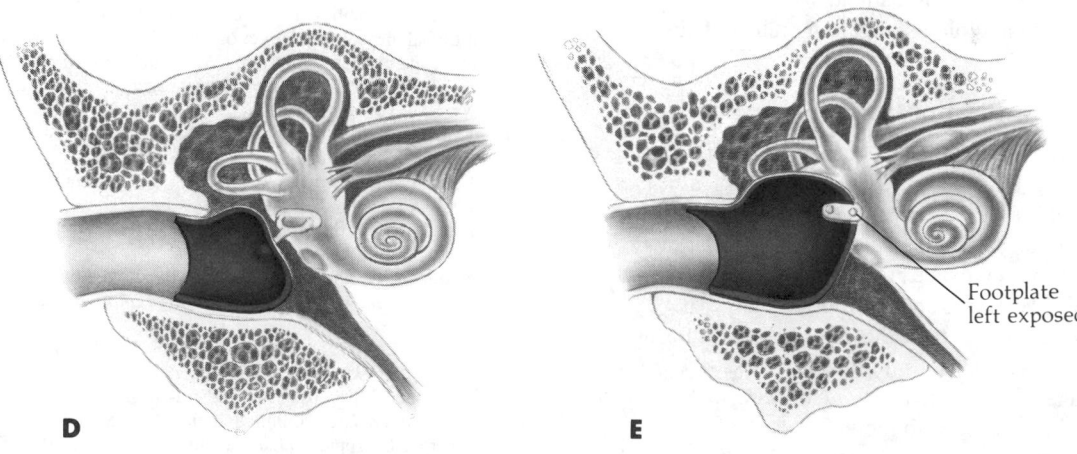

D   **E**

Footplate left exposed

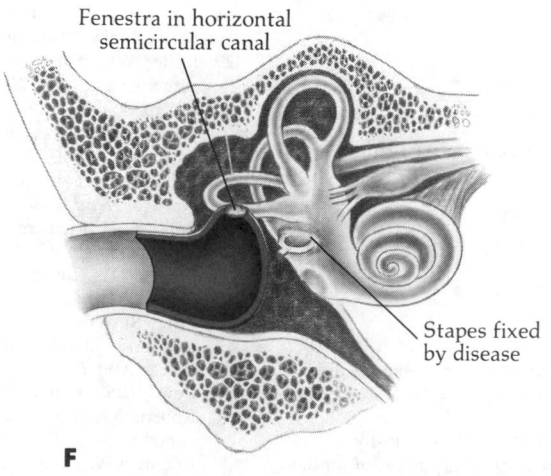

Fenestra in horizontal semicircular canal

F

Stapes fixed by disease

Figure 7-26, cont'd. Various types of tympanoplasty. **D,** Type 3. **E,** Type 4. **F,** Type 5.

Nursing Dx & Intervention

Risk for injury related to a fall or a disruption of graft

- Assess, record, and report unusual bleeding or drainage from operative site.
- Encourage patient to maintain bed rest until first morning after surgery.
- Keep patient from lying on operative side *to prevent pressure on graft.*
- Elevate head of bed 40 degrees.
- Assist with ambulation when patient is allowed to get up.
- Administer antivertiginous medications, as ordered.

Sensory/perceptual alterations (auditory) related to postoperative edema

- Assess patient's hearing ability before and after operation.
- Reassure patient that hearing improvement, if expected, will not be noticed until edema and drainage at operative site have decreased.
- Speak distinctly, facing patient.
- Consult with audiologist regarding rehabilitation.

Patient Education/Home Care Planning

1. Explain to the patient the need to avoid showering or shampooing until permitted by the physician to prevent contamination of the ear canal.
2. Explain to the patient the need to notify the physician immediately if evidence of fever, bleeding, increased drainage, or dizziness exists after discharge.
3. Discuss with the patient the use of Antivert for about 1 month after surgery to minimize dizziness.
4. Encourage the patient to avoid blowing the nose with force and to sneeze with mouth open.
5. Inform the patient to avoid strenuous activity until approved by physician.
6. Encourage patient to discuss restrictions for flying with physician.

Evaluation

Graft heals well   There is no fever, excessive drainage, or dizziness.

Hearing is improved if this was reason for procedure Increased hearing is verified by audiometric testing.

References

1. Andrews J et al: The exacerbation of symptoms in Ménière's disease during the premenstrual period, *Arch Otolaryngol Head Neck Surg* 118(1):74, 1992.
2. Berne RM, Levy M: *Physiology,* ed 3, St Louis, 1992, Mosby.
3. Blitzer A, Lawson W, Friedman WH: *Surgery of the paranasal sinuses,* ed 2, Philadelphia, 1991, Saunders.
4. Britton BH: *Common problems in otology,* St Louis, 1991, Mosby.
5. Clayton H et al: Acoustic neuroma standard of care, *ORL-Head Neck Nursing* 13(1):15, 1995.
6. Cummings CW et al: *Otolaryngology head and neck surg, Update II,* St Louis, 1990, Mosby.
7. Davis J et al: Adjuvant hyperbaric O_2 in malignant external otitis, *Arch Otolaryngol Head Neck Surg* 118(1):89, 1992.
8. DeWeese DD, Saunders WH: *Textbook of otolaryngology,* ed 8, St Louis, 1994, Mosby.
9. El-Kashlan HK et al: Direct electrical stimulation of the cochlear nucleus: surface vs penetrating stimulation, *Otolaryngol Head Neck Surg* 105:4, 1991.
10. Fairbanks DNF: *Antimicrobial therapy in otolaryngology-head and neck surgery,* ed 6, Alexandria, VA, 1991, American Academy of Otolaryngology-Head and Neck Surgery.
11. Ganong WF: *Review of medical physiology,* ed 12, Los Altos, Calif, 1985, Lange Medical Books.
12. Gianoli GJ et al: Retropharyngeal space infection: changing trends, *Otolaryngol Head Neck Surg* 105(1):92, 1991.
13. Glasscock ME, Stambaugh GE: *Surgery of the ear,* ed 4, Philadelphia, 1990, Saunders.
14. Gruppi LA: Acoustic neuromas: nursing management during the acute postoperative period, *Crit Care Nurs* 7(5):16, 1987.
15. Hamid MA: Vestibular rehabilitation, *Adv Otolaryngol Head Neck Surg,* 6:27, 1992.
16. Hirsch JE, Hannock LA, editors: *Mosby's manual of clinical nursing procedures,* St Louis, 1981, Mosby.
17. Hudak M, Domb A: Postoperative head and neck cancer patients with artificial airways: the effect of saline lavage on tracheal mucus evacuation and oxygen saturation, *ORL-Head Neck Nursing* 14(1):17, 1996.
18. Isshiki N: Laryngeal framework surgery, *Adv Otolaryngology-Head Neck Surg* 5:37, 1991.
19. Johnson JT, editor: *Antibiotic therapy in head and neck surgery,* New York, 1987, Marcel Dekker.
20. Kennedy DW: *Sinus disease: guide to first-line management,* Darien, CT, 1995, Health Communications Inc.
21. Kim MJ, McFarland GK, McLane AM: *Pocket guide to nursing diagnosis,* ed 6, St Louis, 1995, Mosby.
22. Koufman JA: The otolaryngologic manifestations of gastroesophageal reflux disease (GERD), *Adv Otolaryngology-Head Neck Surg* 7:115, 1993.
23. Lee KJ: *Essential otolaryngology-head and neck surgery,* ed 6, Norwalk, CT, 1995, Appleton & Lange.
24. Luckmann J, Sorensen K: *Medical-surgical nursing: a psychophysiologic approach,* ed 3, Philadelphia, 1987, Saunders.
25. Mabry RL: Topical pharmacology for allergic rhinitis: new agents, *South Med J* 85(2):149-154, 1992.
26. Malasanos L et al: *Health assessment,* ed 4, St Louis, 1990, Mosby.
27. McCall M: It killed George or managing the peritonsillar abscess patient effectively, *ORL-Head Neck Nursing* 11(1):10, 1993.
28. Meyerhoff WL, Rice DH: *Otolaryngology-head and neck surgery,* Philadelphia, 1992, Saunders.
29. Miller WE: The role of the outpatient nurse in endoscopic sinus surgery, *ORL-Head Neck Nursing* 10(3):20, 1992.
30. Myers E, editor:*New dimensions in otorhinolaryngology, head and neck surgery,* Proceedings of the XIII World Congress, vols 1 and 2, Amsterdam, 1985, Excerpta Medica.
31. Pallanch JF et al: Prosthetic closure of nasal septal perforations, *Otolaryngol Head Neck Surg,* 90:448, 1982.
32. Pollock KJ: Ménière's disease: a review of the problem, *ORL-Head Neck Nursing* 13(2):10, 1995.
33. Preston DY: Chronic suppurative otitis media without cholesteatoma management, *ORL-Head Neck Nursing* 13(4):17, 1995.
34. Price S, Wilson L: *Pathophysiology: clinical concepts of disease processes,* ed 5, St Louis, 1997, Mosby.
35. Proetz AW: *Essays on the applied physiology of the nose,* ed 2, St Louis, 1953, Annals of Otolaryngology.
36. Roberts NK: The selective approach to successful stoma management at home, *ORL-Head Neck Nursing* 13(4):12, 1995.
37. Rothman W: Laryngoplasty of the treatment of vocal cord paralysis in an amateur singer, *Arch Otolaryngol Head Neck Surg* 118(1):209, 1992.

38. Saxton DF et al: *The Addison-Wesley manual of nursing practice,* Menlo Park, Calif, 1983, Addison-Wesley.
39. Schindler RA, Merzenich MM, editors: *Cochlear implants,* New York, 1985, Raven Press.
40. Schlossberg D, editor: *Infections of the head and neck,* New York, 1987, Springer-Verlag.
41. Schuring LT: *Assessment of the ear.* In Phipps WJ et al: *Medical-surgical nursing: concepts and clinical practice,* ed 4, St Louis, 1991, Mosby.
42. Schuring LT: *Management of persons with problems of the ear.* In Phipps WJ et al: *Medical-surgical nursing: concepts and clinical practice,* ed 4, St Louis, 1991, Mosby.
43. Schuring LT et al: *Guidelines for otorhinolaryngology-head and neck nursing practice,* New Smyrna Beach, Fl, 1996, The Society of Otorhinolaryngology and Head-Neck Nurses.
44. Seidel HM et al: *Mosby's guide to physical examination,* ed 3, St Louis, 1995, Mosby.
45. Sigler BA: *Nursing care of clients with disorders of the nose and throat.* In Luckmann & Sorensen's *Medical-surgical nursing: a psychophysiologic approach,* ed 4, Philadelphia, 1993, Saunders.
46. Sigler BA, Schuring LT: *Ear, nose and throat disorders,* St Louis, 1993, Mosby.
47. Spongr VP et al: Effects of noise and salicylates on hair cell loss in the chinchilla cochlea, *Arch Otolaryngol Head Neck Surg* 118(2):157-164, 1992.
48. Stangerup SE et al: Autoinflation as a treatment of secretory otitis media, *Arch Otolaryngol Head Neck Surg* 118(2):149, 1992.
49. Thompson JM, Wilson SF: *Health assessment for nursing practice,* St Louis, 1996, Mosby.
50. Tucker SM et al: *Patient care standards collaborative practice planning guides,* ed 6, St Louis, 1996, Mosby.
51. Ward P, Berci G: Observations on so-called idiopathic vocal cord paralysis, *Ann Otol Rhinol Laryngol* 91:558, 1982.
52. Wehrmaker SL, Wintermute JR: *Case studies in neurological nursing,* Boston, 1978, Little, Brown.
53. Wilson SF, Thompson JM: *Respiratory disorders,* St Louis, 1990, Mosby.
54. Wong DL: *Nursing care of infants and children,* ed 5, St Louis, 1995, Mosby.
55. Yellon RF: Infections of the fascial spaces of the head and neck in the pediatric population, *Adv Otolaryngology-Head Neck Surgery* 9:317, 1994.
56. Zieskela LA: Dematiaceous fungal sinusitis, *Otolaryngol Head Neck Surg* 105:4, 1991.

Gastrointestinal System

8

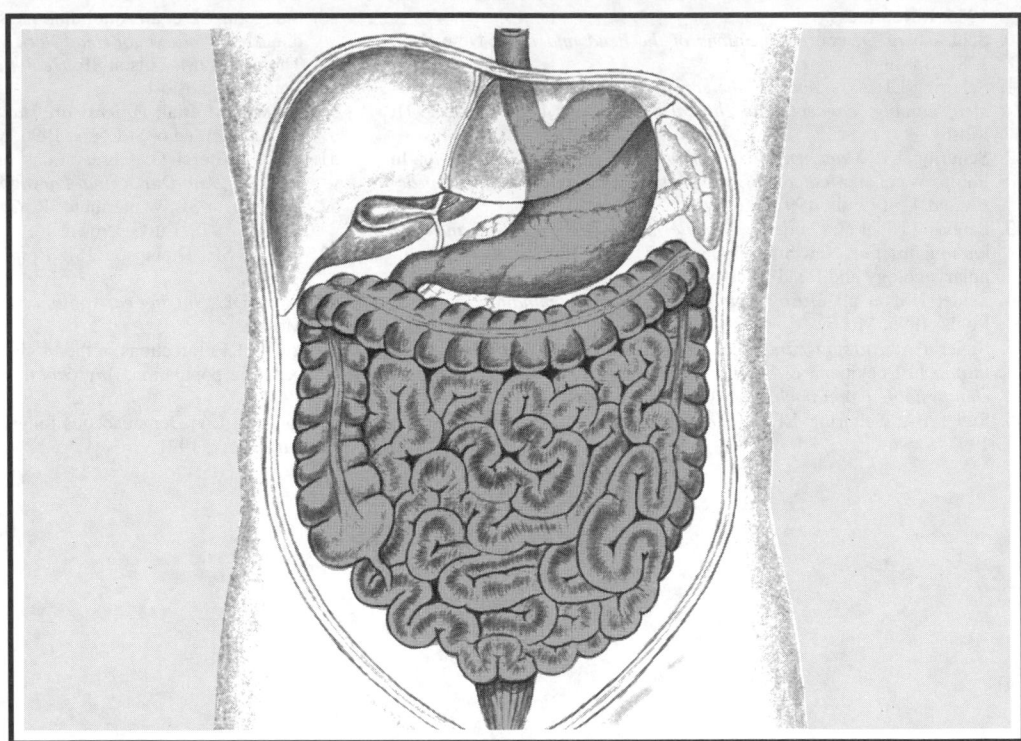

OVERVIEW

Disorders or inflammation of any organs in the gastrointestinal system are commonly called digestive diseases. Examples of digestive diseases are reflux esophagitis, peptic ulcer disease, ulcerative colitis, pancreatitis, and cancer. The diagnosis, treatment, and management vary with each digestive disease.

More Americans are hospitalized with disorders of the digestive system than any other group of disorders. The National Institute of Diabetes and Digestive and Kidney Diseases reports that more than 40 million people are chronically ill with digestive diseases. This results in 158 million restricted activity days and 22 million work-loss days. In 1985, the direct health care costs associated with digestive diseases were more than $40 billion, or at least 10% of all U.S. health care costs. Approximately 191,000 people die each year from digestive diseases.[20] Thus this group of diseases may have devastating long-term personal, social, and economic effects. There are more than 25 lay organizations and 18 professional associations involved in digestive disease programs and education. This reflects the national concern with the management of digestive diseases.

The importance of digestive diseases and their implications for health care have often been minimized. The group of diseases involving the gastrointestinal tract may vary from mild to severe. The chronicity of the diseases and the symptoms can affect the person's ability to maintain a desired lifestyle. Psychosocial stressors often intensify the symptoms.

The National Digestive Disease Advisory Report[50] showed that research involving the gastrointestinal tract is also relevant to the study of acquired immunodeficiency syndrome (AIDS). The immune dysfunction damages the gastrointestinal tract, and this damage contributes to the malnutrition and wasting syndrome observed in AIDS. The latest research on neuropeptides found in the intestine indicates that these substances may modulate immune function. This finding may have significance for future research.[50]

•••••• Anatomy, Physiology, and Related Pathophysiology

The gastrointestinal tract is a series of connected organs and accessory organs whose overall purpose is to break down food products that can be used by the body as a source of energy. Three key processes are associated with the gastrointestinal tract: digestion, absorption, and metabolism. Digestion is the mechanical and chemical breakdown of food into amino acids, glucose, and fatty acids that can be used by the body for cellular functions. Absorption is the passage of the digested food products (essential nutrients) from the lumen of the gastrointestinal tract into the blood and lymphatic system. Metabolism is the use of the basic food product by the cell. Digestion and absorption can be affected by age-associated physiologic changes, infections, inflammatory diseases, surgery, or other alterations of the gastrointestinal tract. To adequately assess the effects of digestive diseases, the nurse must have a basic understanding of the alimentary, or gastrointestinal, system.

The gastrointestinal system consists of the mouth, pharynx, esophagus, stomach, and small and large intestines. Accessory organs include liver, gallbladder, and pancreas. The accessory organs in the mouth are the teeth and salivary glands (Figure 8-1).

The gastrointestinal system produces both exocrine and endocrine secretions. Exocrine secretions prepare food for absorption by diluting it to the osmolality of plasma (isotonic), altering the pH for hydrolysis, and hydrolyzing complex foods. The exocrine secretions also protect the mucosa from physical and chemical irritants. Endocrine secretions are important in the control and coordination of secretory and motor activities involved in the digestion and absorption of food. The types and functions of the secretions are discussed as they appear in the gastrointestinal tract.

Indigenous bacteria, or microflora, are present throughout the gastrointestinal tract. The flora's most important function is to protect the host from pathogens; however, in certain pathologic conditions, otherwise normal flora may have unfavorable effects on the host. Normal flora of the intestinal organs are discussed as they appear in the gastrointestinal tract.

Mouth

The mouth, also called the buccal cavity or oral cavity, is the beginning of the gastrointestinal tract. Mechanical and chemical digestion begins in the mouth. The teeth and tongue aid in mechanical breakdown, and the secretions of the salivary glands begin basic starch digestion and lubricate food to aid in swallowing.

The vestibule is the region between the lips, cheeks, teeth, and gums. The region posterior to the teeth and gums is the mouth cavity proper. Saliva from the salivary glands is received by the mouth cavity proper and aids in digestion.

The lips keep food and saliva in the mouth during chewing (mastication). The lips are sharply demarcated from the surrounding facial skin by the vermilion-cutaneous line. The lips are covered externally by skin and internally by mucous membrane. The bulk of the lips is composed of orbicularis oris, a sphincterlike muscle.

The internal cheeks are composed of muscle, fat, areolar tissue, nerves, vessels, and buccal glands covered by an inner mucous membrane. The gums, or gingivae, are dense fibrous tissue covered by a smooth mucous membrane.

The roof of the mouth is formed by the hard and soft palates. The hard palate is formed by two palatine bones and parts of the superior maxillary bone. The midline of the hard palate is called the linear raphe. The mucous membrane of the hard palate is thick, pale, and corrugated anterior to and to either side of the linear raphe. The posterior mucous membrane is thin, smooth, and a deeper pink. Attached to the posterior portion of the hard palate is the soft palate. The soft palate forms the partition between the mouth and the nasopharynx. In a relaxed position the anterior surface of the soft palate is concave and continuous with the roof of the mouth whereas the posterior surface is convex and continuous with the nasal cavities. The uvula is the conical fingerlike projection of the posterior

border of the soft palate. During swallowing the soft palate moves upward, closing off the nasopharynx and preventing foods and fluids from entering the pharynx.

The tongue is a muscular organ anchored to the hyoid bone and the mandible and covered with a mucous membrane. The frenum, or frenulum, is a fold of mucous membrane under the tongue that attaches the tongue to the floor of the mouth. Mucous membrane also attaches the tongue to the epiglottis, soft palate, and pharynx. The tip of the tongue is the apex.

The tongue contains mucous and serous glands. The mucous glands are behind the apex and secrete mucin. The serous glands, also called Ebner's glands, are found in the back of the tongue. Ebner's glands assist in the distribution of substances to be tasted over the tongue.

The muscles of the tongue are divided into lateral halves by a median fibrous septum. The two groups of muscles can be identified by their role in the tongue's functions. The muscles that assist the tongue in protrusion, retraction, elevation, and

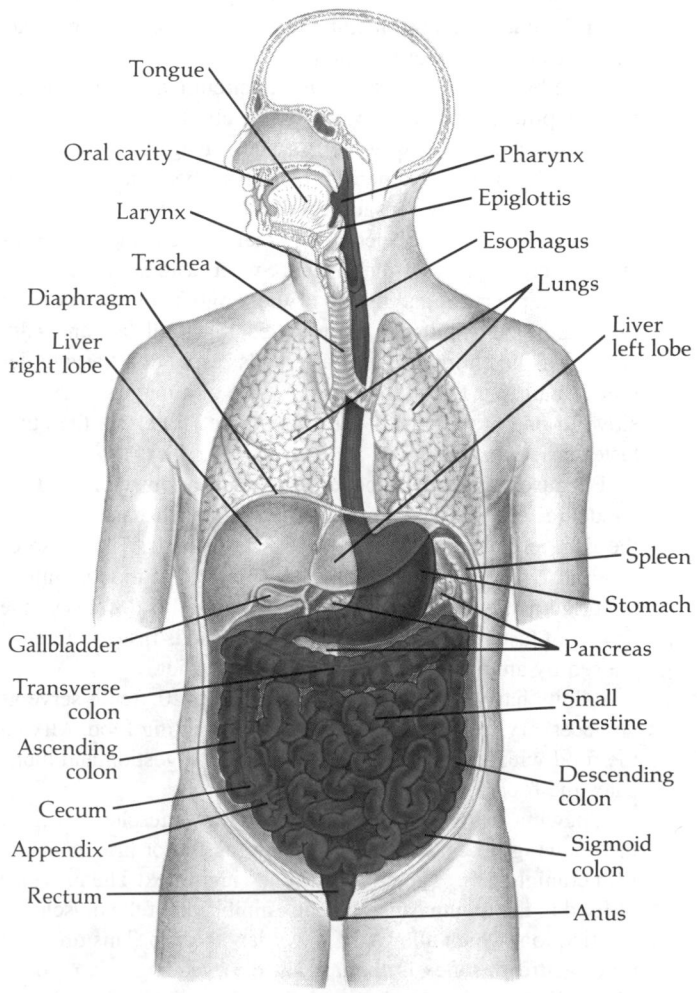

Figure 8-1 Anatomy of gastrointestinal system.

depression during mastication are the genioglossus, hyoglossus, chondroglossus, styloglossus, and palatoglossus. The muscles that are responsible for altering the shape of the tongue (shortened, curved, narrowed) include the longitudinalis superior, longitudinalis inferior, transversus, and verticalis. These movements are important in the enunciation of different letters and words.

The four types of papillae that contain taste buds are located on the anterior two thirds of the dorsum of the tongue. They are papillae vallatae, papillae fungiformes, papillae filiformes, and papillae simplices. Papillae vallatae, or circumvallate papillae, form an inverted V on the posterior dorsal surface of the tongue. These are the largest papillae and are round and flattened. The taste buds are found on their lateral surfaces.

Papillae filiformes are numerous and arranged in tight parallel rows. They contain thick, dense epithelium and appear white on the tongue's surface. The filiform papillae also contain elastic fibers.

The papillae fungiformes are found mainly at the apex and sides of the tongue. They are large and deep red.

The papillae simplices are similar to papillae of the skin and cover the entire mucous membrane of the tongue. The papillae simplices play a minor role in taste sensation.

Taste buds are concentrated in the circumvallate and fungiform papillae. Adults have approximately 10,000 taste buds, and children have a few more.[30] As a person ages, the taste buds begin to degenerate and perception of taste becomes less acute.

The four primary sensations of taste are sweet, sour, salty, and bitter. Taste buds detecting a primary taste tend to be localized in certain areas of the tongue. Sweet taste is primarily on the anterior surface and the tip of the tongue; sour taste on the two lateral sides; bitter taste on the papillae vallatae; and salty taste over the entire tongue. Taste buds respond in varying degrees to all four taste sensations. A taste bud may be very sensitive to one or two tastes but respond moderately to the other taste sensations.

Because taste buds respond to taste sensations with a different degree of sensitivity, the brain determines the taste based on the degree of stimulation of various taste buds. The sense of smell also affects the sense of taste. Odors from food stimulate the olfactory system. When the sense of smell is decreased, the degree of taste is often reported as diminished. Taste preference is used by animals and humans to regulate diet.

Adults have 32 teeth, and children have 20. Teeth serve as an accessory to digestion by cutting and mixing food. Mixing the food with saliva begins some chemical digestion and lubricates the food for swallowing.

Chewing involves the stimulation of jaw muscles. Much of the chewing process is innervated by the motor branch of the fifth cranial nerve. There is also a chewing reflex. The presence of food in the mouth causes a reflex inhibition of the muscles of mastication, which allows the lower jaw to drop. This drop initiates a stretch reflex in the jaw muscles, leading to a rebound contraction: raising the jaw and closing the teeth. The closure of the teeth on the bolus of food inhibits the jaw muscles, allowing the jaw to drop and rebound. This is then repeated.

Because digestive enzymes work only on the surface of food particles, chewing increases the surface area exposed to the enzymes. Chewing food also increases the ease with which food is swallowed and affects the ease of emptying of food from the stomach into the small intestine.

The composition of bacteria varies from place to place in the mouth but adheres most efficiently to the tooth surfaces, the buccal mucosa, and the surfaces of the tongue and pharynx. Normal oral flora is similar to that found in the distal colon. Good dental hygiene removes most detrimental oral flora, although poor dental hygiene contributes greatly to the development of oral disease. Oral bacteria is killed as it enters the stomach and therefore has little significance for the remainder of the gastrointestinal tract.

Salivary Glands

The salivary glands are the parotid, submaxillary, and sublingual glands. Some small salivary glands are found in the lips, buccal mucosa, and palate. These are exocrine glands that secrete a mixture of serous and mucous fluid into the oral cavity.

The parotid gland is anterior to the external ear and wraps around the mandible. The parotid glands are the largest of the salivary glands; each weighs approximately 14 to 30 g. The parotid (Stensen's) duct enters the mouth at its papillae opposite the second maxillary molar tooth. The parotid gland produces ptyalin (salivary amylase), which begins the chemical breakdown of starches. The action of ptyalin in the mouth breaks down only 5% to 10% of ingested starches. The action of the enzyme continues in the stomach for 30 minutes to several hours, until the pH falls, rendering the enzyme inactive.

The submaxillary gland is smaller, weighing 7 to 10 g. It is located in the submandibular fossa. The submaxillary (Wharton's) duct opens on the floor of the mouth adjacent to the base of the frenulum of the tongue. The secretory motor fibers originate in the chorda tympani nerve. The submaxillary gland produces a mixture of mucous and serous secretions.

The sublingual glands are located beneath the floor of the mouth and weigh approximately 3 g. The sublingual glands consist of predominantly mucous acini with a few serous acini, thus producing primarily mucous secretions. The primary purpose of the sublingual gland secretions is lubrication.

Approximately 1000 to 1500 ml of saliva is produced by the salivary glands in 24 hours. The parotid and submaxillary glands account for almost 90% of the total production of saliva. The pH of the saliva is maintained between 6.0 and 7.0 by a complex autonomic mechanism that controls salivary secretion of sodium, potassium, chloride, and bicarbonate ions. The superior and inferior salivatory nuclei are located in the brainstem and may be stimulated by taste and tactile sensations from the tongue and mouth. Pleasant taste stimuli result in more salivation than unpleasant tastes, and smooth-textured foods stimulate more saliva production than rough-textured foods. Less salivation may result in less lubrication of food and more difficulty in swallowing. More saliva is produced when a person is eating a food he or she likes than when eating a disliked food.

Thus salivation may be divided into three phases: psychic, gustatory, and gastrointestinal. The psychic phase occurs when the mouth is preparing itself to receive food. It is stimulated by thoughts or smells of pleasant foods. The gustatory phase occurs while one is chewing or swallowing food. The saliva is stimulated to aid in mastication and lubricate the food for swallowing. The gastrointestinal phase occurs when one has eaten irritating foods. The salivation is a response to reflexes originating in the stomach or upper intestines. The swallowed saliva dilutes or neutralizes the irritant.

Oropharynx

The oropharynx is the midpoint of the upper respiratory tract and digestive tract and is responsible for separating food and air as they pass through this area. The superior boundary is at a horizontal line that would connect the soft palate with the second cervical vertebra. The inferior line would connect horizontally the tip of the epiglottis and the base of the tongue. The nasopharynx lies between the oropharynx and the hypopharynx (see Chapter 7).

The oropharynx is lined by a mucous membrane of stratified squamous epithelium that is continuous with the lining of the mouth, nasal cavities, and larynx. The contents of the oropharynx include the soft palate, the uvula, the tonsils and their pillars, and the base of the tongue.

Esophagus

The esophagus is a hollow muscular tube approximately 25 cm (10 inches) long. It is closed at both ends by the upper esophageal sphincter and the lower esophageal sphincter. The esophagus begins in the neck at the lower border of the fifth cervical vertebra and connects the hypopharynx to the cardia of the stomach. On each side of the esophagus are the thyroid lobes and parathyroid glands. The recurrent laryngeal nerves run directly in front of the esophagus. In the thorax the esophagus is found to the left of the midline with the pericardium and left atrium in front. The arch of the aorta crosses the lateral aspect of the esophagus at the level of the fourth thoracic vertebra. The descending aorta runs laterally and slightly posterior to the esophagus. At the level of the tenth thoracic vertebra the esophagus passes through the diaphragm into the abdominal cavity.

The esophagus narrows slightly at three points: near its origin in the region of the cricoid cartilage, at the arch of the aorta, and as it passes through the diaphragm. The esophagus is more vulnerable to perforation and trauma in these areas.

The arterial blood supply of the esophagus comes from the inferior thyroid artery in the neck, from branches of the descending aorta, and from the left gastric artery. The esophageal veins join the vena azygos, which joins the superior vena cava and the systemic circulation. The veins at the lower end of the esophagus communicate freely with the tributaries of the left gastric vein that join the portal vein. The upper part of the esophageal blood supply drains into the superior vena cava; the middle part drains into the azygos system; and the bottom third drains into the portal system through gastric veins. When there is increased pressure in the portal system, there is increased pressure in the esophageal veins, leading to the development of esophageal varices.

The wall of the esophagus has all the characteristics of the gastrointestinal tract except for the serosa. Absence of serosa becomes important when esophageal surgery (i.e., anastomosis) has been performed because an increased chance for leakage may be present postoperatively. The esophageal lumen is lined with stratified squamous mucosa that is continuous with the oral cavity and pharynx. At the lower end of the esophagus the luminal lining changes to a simple columnar (transitional) epithelium that merges with the gastric mucosa in the cardiac portion of the stomach. The esophageal mucosa functions as a barrier to noxious luminal contents. The mucosa is repeatedly exposed to potentially damaging intraluminal materials, including oral intake and hypertonic gastric contents associated with gastroesophageal reflux. However, esophageal injury does not occur in most individuals. The esophageal mucosa maintains its protective function even when normal protective mechanisms, such as the lower esophageal sphincter, esophageal peristalsis, and salivary bicarbonate, fail.[28]

The submucosa layer underlying the squamous epithelium contains the blood vessels, nerves, mucous cells, and connective tissues. The mucous cells secrete mucus to further lubricate the food and protect the wall of the esophagus. The secretions are amphoteric, neutralizing both acid and base.

The muscle layer is composed of an internal circular and outer longitudinal layer. It differs from the remainder of the alimentary tract in several ways. First, the longitudinal layer is thicker than the inner circular layer. Second, the upper third of the esophagus is striated muscle. This portion of the esophagus receives its innervation from lower motor neurons and is dependent on cholinergic mechanisms. If these nerves are cut, flaccid paralysis of the upper esophagus will occur.[63] The middle third of the esophagus is mixed muscle tissue, and the lower third is primarily smooth muscle. The innervation of the smooth muscle found in the lower two thirds of the esophagus is preganglionic fibers of the autonomic nervous system. No flaccid paralysis develops if these nerves are cut.

Swallowing

Deglutition (swallowing) can be divided into several phases. In the voluntary phase the tongue moves upward and backward, forcing a bolus of food into the pharynx. During the voluntary stage of swallowing, the bolus of food stimulates swallowing receptors around the pharynx. A series of involuntary events follow.

When the swallowing receptors around the pharynx are stimulated, the impulses pass to the brainstem, resulting in a series of autonomic pharyngeal muscular contractions. First, the soft palate rises to meet the posterior pharyngeal wall, closing the nasopharynx. Second, contraction of the suprahyoid muscles elevates the larynx and trachea, which increases the diameter of the pharynx. Third, the epiglottis bends backward and the vocal cords come together, further blocking the respiratory tract.

As the bolus enters the pharynx, the cricopharyngeal muscle relaxes, permitting the bolus to enter the esophagus. This stimulates rapid peristaltic waves. These actions increase the size of the pharynx, pull the pharynx up to receive the food, and close the larynx to prevent aspiration. The nerve impulses of the pharynx, which are stimulated by the bolus of food, travel the trigeminal nerve to the medulla oblongata, where the swallowing center is located. Nerve impulses then travel back along the glossopharyngeal and vagus nerves to move the bolus into the esophagus.

The esophageal phase of swallowing moves the bolus from the pharynx to the stomach by peristalsis. There are three types of esophageal peristalsis: primary, secondary, and tertiary. Primary peristalsis is a continuation of the movement begun in the pharynx. If a person is upright, downward gravity also affects the travel time through the esophagus. If primary peristalsis fails to move all the food that has entered the esophagus into the stomach, secondary peristalsis is stimulated from the distention of the esophagus by the retained bolus. The only difference is that primary peristalsis is initiated in the pharynx and secondary peristalsis is initiated in the esophagus at the level of the aortic arch.

Tertiary contractions may occur in some individuals, particularly after middle age. These are nonperistaltic contractions and do not assist in transport of food through the esophagus. The autonomic mechanisms of swallowing are usually preserved as an individual ages.[33]

Approximately 1 to 3 cm above the junction of the esophagus and stomach lies the lower esophageal sphincter. It has a higher resting pressure than the body of the esophagus or the stomach. Under normal circumstances this area relaxes with primary or secondary peristalsis. The purpose of this high-pressure area is to prevent reflux of acid gastric contents into the esophagus. Certain factors* increase or decrease this high-pressure zone:

Increase high-pressure zone
  Gastrin
  Cholinergic agents
    Methacholine (Mecholyl)
    Bethanechol (Urecholine)
  Metoclopramide
  Prostaglandin F_2
  Gastric alkalinization (antacids)
  α-Adrenergic agonists
  Protein meal
  Nonfat milk
  Ethanol (low dose)
  Bombesin
Decrease high-pressure zone
  Secretin
  Cholecystokinin
  Glucagon

Anticholinergics
Gastric inhibitory polypeptide
Vasoactive intestine peptide
Verapamil
Prostaglandins E, E_2, A_2
Gastric acidification
α-Adrenergic antagonists
Fat meal
Whole milk
Ethanol (high dose)

Peritoneal Cavity

The abdomen is the largest cavity in the human body. It contains the stomach, small intestine, kidneys, adrenal glands, uterus in women, liver, colon, gallbladder, pancreas, and major vessels. The abdomen is bordered anteriorly by the abdominal muscles and iliacus, posteriorly by vertebral column and lumbar muscles, inferiorly by the plane of the superior aperture of the lesser pelvis, and superiorly by the diaphragm.

The structures in the cavity are protected and covered by peritoneum, which is made up of serous membrane composed of mesothelium and a thin layer of irregular connective tissue. The parietal peritoneum is the tissue that lines the abdominal wall. The mesentery is a double fold of parietal peritoneum that is fan shaped and encircles the jejunum and ileum (segments of the small intestines) attaching them to the posterior abdominal wall. The blood vessels and nerves of the small intestine pass through the mesentery. The greater omentum is an apron-shaped double fold of peritoneum that hangs loosely over the intestines. The greater omentum is attached to the upper border of the duodenum, the lower edge of the stomach, and the transverse colon.

A small amount of serous fluid separates the space between the parietal and visceral peritoneum. The fluid provides lubrication between the organs and the abdominal wall.

Stomach

The function of the stomach is to alter the consistency and the composition of ingested foods. The ingested foods are liquefied, increasing the surface area of food particles to facilitate the digestive process. The food particles mixed with gastric secretions create a solution called chyme. The chyme is then released in a regulated manner into the duodenum for further digestion and absorption.

The stomach connects to the esophagus 3 cm below the diaphragm. The stomach lies obliquely beneath the cardiac sphincter of the esophagus, above the pyloric sphincter next to the small intestine, and under the left lobe of the liver and diaphragm. The size, shape, and position of the stomach vary depending on body size, posture, degree of gastric retention, degree of gastric muscle development, and effects of pressures from adjacent organs. Its normal capacity is 1 to 2 L. The stomach functions as a reservoir where mechanical and chemical breakdown of food continues.

The stomach is divided into the cardia, fundus, body, antrum, and pylorus (Figure 8-2). The cardia is the proximal

---

*Adapted from Bolt RJ et al: *The digestive system*, New York, John Wiley & Sons.

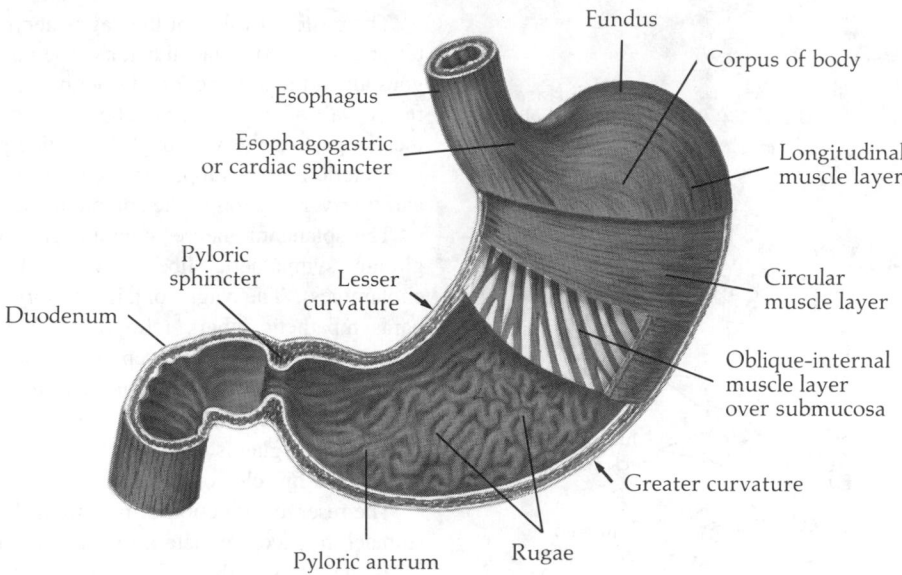

Figure 8-2 Gross anatomy of stomach.

portion of the stomach. The lesser curvature of the stomach extends from the cardiac orifice to the pyloric opening in a downward curve. Attached to this border is the lesser omentum, or gastrohepatic ligament. The greater curvature is almost four times longer than the lesser curvature, and the greater omentum is attached to it.

The fundus is the uppermost portion of the stomach. Although the fundus is distal to the cardia, it is superior to the cardia anatomically. The body of the stomach extends distally from the fundus to the level at which the gastric lumen assumes a transverse direction. The antrum is the peristaltic portion of the stomach and is distal to the body. The pylorus is the portion just before the duodenum.

The wall of the stomach is composed of four layers: (from the innermost lining layer out) the mucosa, the submucosa, the muscle layer, and the serosa. The mucosa layer is separated from the submucosa by the muscularis mucosa and is composed of gastric epithelium. The mucosa is arranged in longitudinal folds called rugae found most predominantly in the fundus and body regions of the stomach. The rugae are invaginated with gastric pits, or openings to gastric glands, which are responsible for gastric acid secretion (Figure 8-3). The rugae are low and flat in the lesser curvature and are sometimes absent in the antrum.

There are three distinct areas of cells within the stomach: the cardia, the oxyntic, and the antral, or pyloric. The mucosa of the cardia is columnar epithelium that secretes mucus. This zone or area has also been referred to as the transitional or junctional mucosa.

The glands of the fundus and body are straight, closely packed, and tubular. These glands contain neck cells, parietal (oxyntic) cells, chief (zymogen) cells, and argentaffin cells. Mucous neck cells are most numerous and play a role in mucosal

cell renewal. Parietal cells are located at the upper portion of the gland. Parietal cells produce hydrochloric acid (HCl) and intrinsic factor. Chief cells are most abundant in the deeper portion of the gland and secrete pepsinogen (type I). Argentaffin cells are in the deeper portion of the gland and produce serotonin.

The fundus and body are often referred to as the acid-pepsin secreting area. The pepsinogen is activated in a pH less than 5.0. The optimum level of pH is 1.8 to 3.5. The hydrochloric acid provides the acidity necessary for the pepsinogen to convert to its active form, pepsin.

The antrum mucosa is thinner than the oxyntic, and the gastric pits are deeper. The glands are tubular and coiled. Gastrin-producing G cells are located in the mucosa adjacent to the tubular glands. The tubular glands secrete mucus and pepsinogen II.

The submucosa is composed of loose areolar and elastic tissue. It contains vascular and lymphatic channels and an intrinsic nerve plexus, Meissner's plexus. The muscle layer is thick and is composed of three separate strata of smooth muscle. The outer, longitudinal layer extends downward from the esophagus along the greater and lesser curvatures to the pyloric sphincter. The middle circular muscle forms a uniform layer over the entire stomach. There is a second nerve plexus found between the two muscle layers, Auerbach's plexus. The inner oblique muscle is continuous with the circular muscle of the esophagus and is thickest in the fundus region. It extends to the pyloric sphincter. The outermost layer is the serosa and is an extension of the peritoneum.

The blood supply to the stomach is from large branches of the celiac artery. There may be variation in the branching pattern of the celiac axis. In approximately one fourth of all people, the left hepatic artery arises in part or totally from the left gastric artery. Gastrectomy in this group of patients may lead to necrosis of the

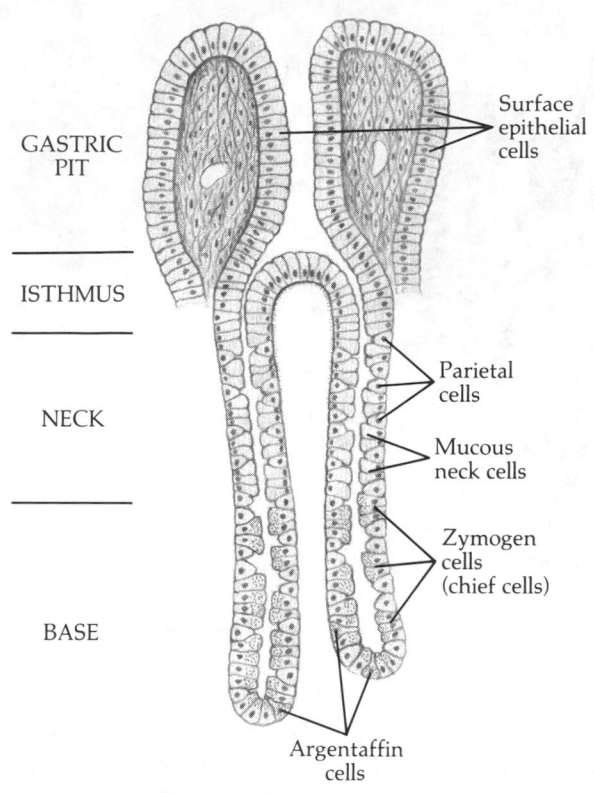

GASTRIC PIT

Surface epithelial cells

ISTHMUS

NECK

Parietal cells

Mucous neck cells

Zymogen cells (chief cells)

BASE

Argentaffin cells

Figure 8-3 Human gastric mucosa. Diagram of tubular gland from fundic area of stomach.

left lobe of the liver unless the surgeon first assesses the pattern of arterial blood flow.[6] Arterial branches passing through the muscle layer form an extensive plexus of blood vessels in the submucosa. These vessels then enter the mucosa and subdivide to form a capillary network in the lamina propria surrounding the gastric glands and pits. Blood can be shunted from one area of the stomach to another or from one layer of the stomach to another by submucosa anastomoses and numerous submucosa arteriovenous communications. Mucosal ischemia can be caused by a redistribution of blood flow from vasoconstrictor activity of the sympathetic nervous system and by vasoconstrictor drugs. Bolt and co-workers[6] state that it is not clearly understood whether the vagus nerve is capable of directly mediating vasodilation of the gastric vascular supply. Venous blood from the right and left gastric veins of the stomach empties directly into the portal vein.

The vagus and splanchnic nerves innervate the stomach. Branches of the left and right vagus nerves join to form the anterior esophageal plexus, and branches of the right vagus form the posterior esophageal plexus. At the distal esophagus they join to form the anterior and posterior vagal trunk. The anterior trunk provides the anterior gastric and hepatic divisions. The anterior gastric division goes along the lesser curvature to the pyloric sphincter with branches to the anterosuperior wall of the stomach. The hepatic division supplies the gallbladder, biliary tree, and proximal duodenum.

The posterior trunk of the vagus nerve divides into the posterior gastric and celiac divisions. The posterior gastric division goes along the lesser curvature with branches to the posteroinferior wall of the stomach. The celiac division descends with the left gastric artery through the celiac plexus to the superior mesenteric plexus, supplying the small intestine and ascending and transverse colon to the splenic flexure.

The splanchnic nerves contain sensory fibers and postganglionic sympathetic fibers (whose transmitters are catecholamines). The vagi contain sensory fibers, preganglionic parasympathetic fibers (cholinergic), and purinergic fibers (adenosine triphosphate receptors).[6] These fibers synapse with the ganglion cells of the myenteric (Auerbach's) plexus and the submucosal (Meissner's) plexus. The postganglionic fibers end in the gastric glands and muscle fibers stimulating gastric secretion and muscle contraction.

The reservoir function of the stomach is the capacity of the stomach to accommodate a meal. A vagal-mediated reflex relaxes the body of the stomach so that it accepts the ingested meal with minimal increase in intragastric pressure. Once swallowing is completed, the gastric wall tension increases and intragastric pressure is proportional to the volume ingested. This also helps to modulate gastric emptying. If the normal vagal reflex activity is inhibited or if the capacity of the stomach is reduced, the reservoir function is altered. People with significantly compromised reservoir functions need to eat frequent, smaller meals to avoid or minimize symptoms such as early satiety, postprandial epigastric pain, and nausea and vomiting.

Gastric secretions include mucus, pepsinogen, hydrochloric acid, intrinsic factor, and the hormone gastrin. Gastric mucus is composed of proteins, glycoproteins, mucopolysaccharides, and blood group substances. The principal component is glycoprotein. Gastric mucus is a thin layer of mucus adherent to the cell surface. The role of gastric mucus in the mucosal barrier is not well defined. The gastric mucosal barrier helps separate acid in the lumen from bicarbonate on the epithelial cell surface. The mucosal barrier prevents diffusion of hydrogen ions from lumen to mucosa and diffusion of sodium ions from mucosa to lumen.

The surface mucous cells are stimulated by vagus nerve and acetylcholine in response to chemicals (i.e., ethanol) and physical contact and friction from roughage in the diet. They protect the mucosa with an alkaline layer of lubricant.

Pepsinogen is secreted by the chief cells of glands in the body and fundus with a small amount secreted by neck cells and by Brunner's glands in the duodenum. Pepsinogen is converted to active pepsin at a pH less than 6.0. The optimum pH of pepsin is 1.8 to 3.5 with no activity greater than a pH of 5.0. Pepsinogen is stimulated by both vagal stimulation and a local reflex activity. Pepsinogen secretion is increased by the presence of gastrin, calcium, histamine, and secretin. Pepsin is responsible for initiating protein digestion, particularly collagen, a major protein component of meat.

Hydrochloric acid is secreted by the parietal cells. Endogenous stimuli for hydrochloric acid production is acetylcholine, gastrin, and histamine. The basal secretion of hydrochloric acid

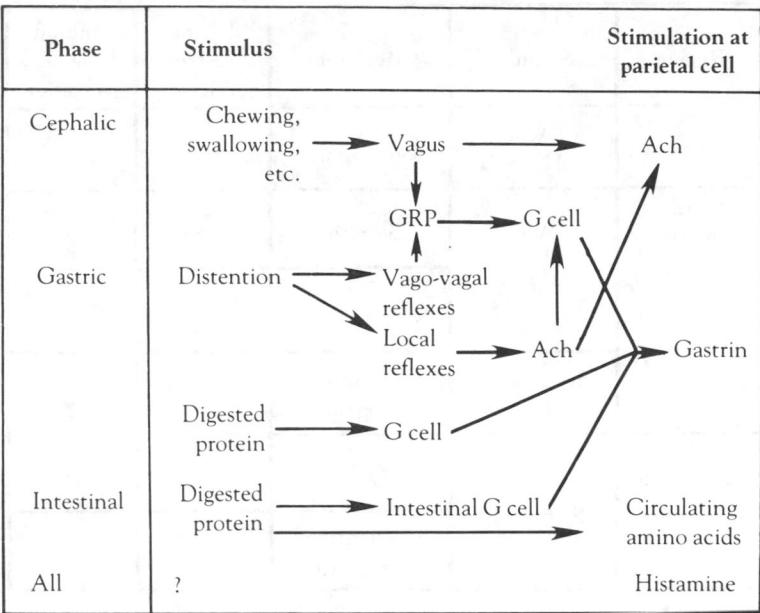

Phase	Stimulus	Stimulation at parietal cell

Figure 8-4 Mechanisms for stimulation of acid secretion. (From Johnson.[37])

is lowest between 5 and 11 AM and highest between 2 PM and 1 AM.[37] Histamine, secreted by mast cells in the stomach, plays a critical role in regulating gastric acid secretion through the activation of the parietal H_2 receptor.

The production of intrinsic factor by the parietal cells is a critical function of the stomach. Intrinsic factor is a mucoprotein that binds with vitamin B_{12}. This bond is essential for the absorption of vitamin B_{12} at specific receptor cells in the terminal ileum. The stimuli that increase secretion of intrinsic factor are the same as those stimulating hydrochloric acid production. The failure to secrete intrinsic factor is associated with achlorhydria and the absence of parietal cells. The condition results in vitamin B_{12} deficiency and subsequent pernicious anemia.

The hormone gastrin is secreted by the antral G cells and is the primary mediator of gastric acid secretion. Gastrin is also secreted by cells in the duodenum, pancreatic islets, and jejunum. Vagal stimulation, gastric distention, and the presence of amino acids, peptides, and calcium ions stimulate the secretion of antral gastrin. Antral gastrin then circulates in the blood system with the parietal cells as the target organ. When the gastric pH is less than 1.5, gastrin release is inhibited. Duodenal gastrin is secreted in response to distention and protein.

Gastric secretion has been divided into three phases (cephalic, gastric, and intestinal) that occur almost simultaneously. The cephalic phase includes the sight, smell, taste, thought, and chewing of food, as well as conditional reflexes and intracellular hypoglycemia. The vagus nerve releases acetylcholine by postganglionic fibers in the gastric mucosa, causing the secretion of hydrochloric acid, intrinsic factor, and pepsinogen. The gastric phase constitutes the major physiologic stimulus for gastric secretion and is activated by the presence of food in the stomach. The intestinal phase serves mainly to inhibit gastric secretions. Duodenal gastrin that is released in response to protein digestion products and distention functions in the same way as antral gastrin (Figure 8-4).

Inhibition of gastric secretions in the intestinal phase is related to the actions of cholecystokinin (CCK), secretin, gastric inhibitory polypeptide (GIP), vasoactive intestinal peptide (VIP), glucagon, and prostaglandins (Figure 8-5). CCK is stimulated by L-amino acids and fatty acids in the duodenum. When CCK and gastrin are both present, a competitive inhibition of gastrin occurs because both have the same active terminal tetrapeptide. Thus the secretory function of gastrin is inhibited. Hydrogen ions in the duodenum stimulate the release of secretin. Secretin inhibits acid output and blocks the secretory effects of gastrin and histamine. Secretin stimulates pepsinogen output. Both CCK and secretin stimulate pancreatic secretion of bicarbonate.

Gastric inhibitory polypeptide (GIP) is composed of 43 amino acids and is found throughout the intestinal tract, although it is concentrated in the duodenum. GIP has a wide range of functions, including inhibition of food-stimulated release of gastrin, gastric acid secretion, and pepsinogen secretions. VIP and glucagon inhibit gastric secretion and stimulate intestinal electrolyte secretion.

Prostaglandins are a group of cyclic fatty acid compounds with 20 carbon acids. Prostaglandins act to inhibit parietal cells, effecting a prostaglandin-mediated negative feedback loop that regulates gastric acid secretion.

Enterogastrone is a general term often used to designate hormones released from duodenal mucosa in response to acid,

Region	Stimulus	Mediator	Inhibit gastrin release	Inhibit acid secretion
Antrum	Acid (pH < 3.0)	Somatostatin	+	
Duodenum	Acid	Secretin	+	+
		Nervous reflex		+
	Hyperosmotic solutions	Unidentified enterogastrone		+
Duodenum and jejunum	Fatty acids	GIP	+	+
		Unidentified enterogastrone		+

Figure 8-5 Mechanisms for inhibition of acid secretion. (From Johnson.[37])

fatty acids, and hyperosmotic solutions that inhibit gastric acid secretions.[63] There are still unanswered questions regarding gastric inhibition. Future research should answer many of the uncertainties in the understanding of hormonal inhibition of gastric secretion.

Gastric motility can be divided into tonic, mixing, and peristaltic contractions. Gastric tone controls luminal volume and maintains a relatively constant pressure despite changes in volume. The fundus and body serve as a receptacle and the antrum as a pump. Circular muscle contractions in the body of the stomach mix the food with the gastric secretions. Contractions in the antrum are stronger and produce considerable mixing motions and propulsion of gastric contents into the duodenum in a controlled fashion.

Antral peristaltic contractions force the chyme into the pyloric canal and then into the duodenum. The pyloric sphincter is a high-pressure zone that relaxes with antral peristalsis and contracts in response to acids, fats, amino acids, and nonisotonic solutions in the duodenum. Gastric distention stimulates stretch receptors, which results in increased gastric peristalsis and increased gastric emptying. The stimulus for rapid gastric emptying is gastric distention.

There are three receptors in the duodenum that release substances inhibiting gastric emptying: osmoreceptors, acid-sensitive receptors, and fat-sensitive receptors. Hormones released in the duodenum (gastrin, CCK, secretin, pancreatic polypeptide, gut glucagon, GIP, VIP, calcitonin, prostaglandins, and bulbogastrone) inhibit gastric emptying. The complete physiologic role of the hormones is not well understood.[6,37]

Gastric emptying can be impaired by drugs, diseases, and surgery. Incomplete emptying may result in early satiety, postprandial epigastric pain, and vomiting. Rapid gastric emptying may occur with duodenal ulcers and after surgery for peptic ulcers. Prokinetic oral medications may be effective in increasing gastric emptying time.

The microflora of the stomach are comparatively sparse. Only relatively acid-resistant organisms survive any length of time. *Lactobacillus, Candida, Streptococcus, Neisseria, Staphylococcus,* and *Peptostreptococcus* are the genera best represented. *Helicobacter pylori* may colonize the stomach; it is not clear whether this organism should be considered part of the indigenous flora or a pathogen.

Small Intestine

In the small intestine, ingested food is mixed, digested, and absorbed. The small intestine is divided into three segments: duodenum, jejunum, and ileum. The first portion is the duodenum; at 20 to 30 cm (8 to 12 inches) long, it is the shortest segment. The ligament of Treitz is the dividing point between the duodenum and jejunum, although histologic changes cannot be demonstrated. The jejunum is 2.5 m (8 feet) long, and the ileum is 3.5 m (11⅓ feet) long. The jejunum and ileum have no specific anatomic division (Figure 8-6).

The wall of the small intestine is divided into four layers: mucosa (innermost layer), submucosa, muscularis externa, and serosa (outer layer). As in other segments of the gastrointestinal tract, the mucosa is separated from the submucosa by the muscularis mucosae. The submucosa contains the connective tissue, lymphatics, blood vessels, and nerves. Meissner's plexus is in the submucosa. The muscularis externa consists of an inner circular layer and an outer longitudinal layer. Auerbach's (myenteric) plexus lies between the two muscle layers.

The duodenum is C shaped. The first portion of the duodenum lies behind and below the right and caudate lobes of the liver and

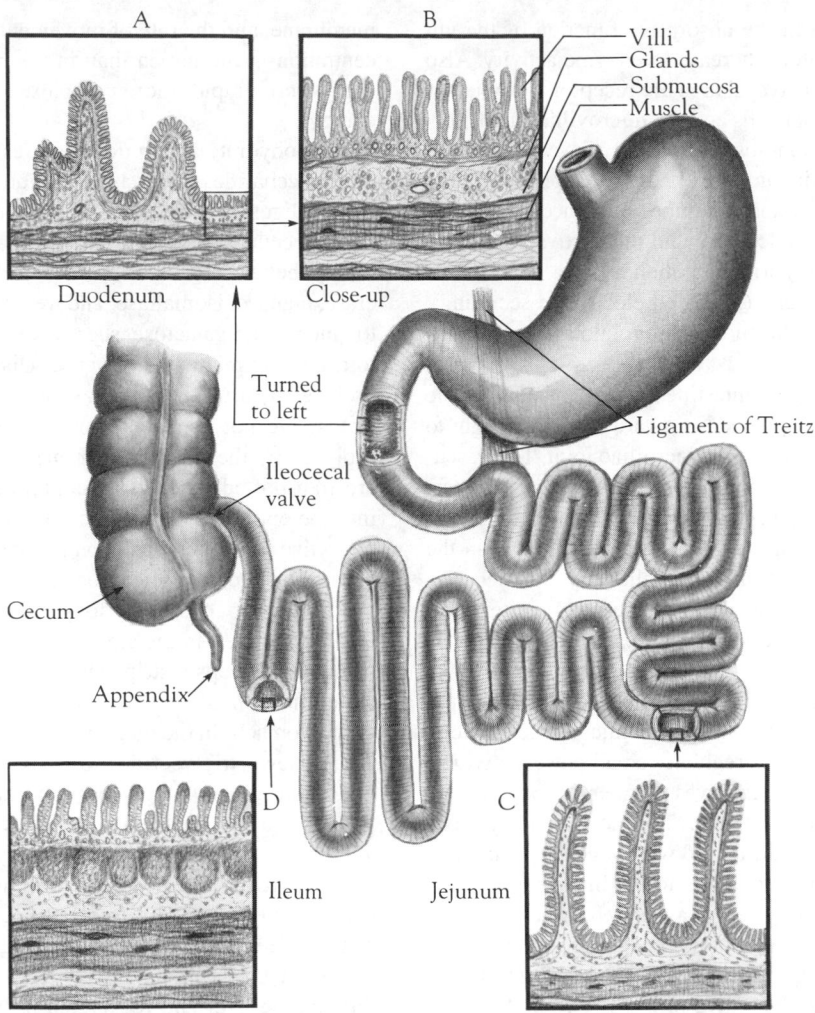

Figure 8-6 Clinical anatomy of small intestine

gallbladder and in front of the common bile duct and portal vein. This portion is suspended from the lesser omentum. The remaining duodenum is located retroperitoneally. The second portion of the duodenum descends vertically to the level of the fourth lumbar vertebra and lies in front of the vena cava, right ureter, and psoas muscle. Ventrally, the second portion is relative to the right lobe of the liver, transverse colon, and small intestine. The common bile duct and main pancreatic duct empty into the duodenum at the ampulla of Vater, 7 to 10 cm distal to the pyloric sphincter.

The third portion, or horizontal segment, crosses the third and fourth lumbar vertebrae, vena cava, and aorta. The superior mesenteric vessel crosses this segment anteriorly. The fourth segment ascends along the left side of the aorta, turns sharply anteriorly, and then descends caudally as the jejunum. The ligament of Treitz, a suspensory ligament of the duodenum, is a band of fibers and muscle tissue originating in the right crus of the diaphragm. The portion of the duodenum proximal to the ampulla of Vater receives its blood supply from the celiac axis. The remainder is supplied by the superior mesenteric artery.

The duodenum contains Brunner's glands in the submucosa, which secrete an alkaline fluid containing pepsinogen. The hormones secreted in the duodenum include gastrin, CCK, secretin, GIP, VIP, and enterogastrone.

The jejunum and ileum have a greatly increased mucosa and submucosa surface area for absorption. Three characteristic features of this portion of the small intestine are a large series of circular folds of mucosa and submucosa; minute, fingerlike projections of the mucosa called villi; and microvilli, or brush border. Mucosal crypts at the base of the villi extend into the wall of the small intestine to the muscularis mucosae. Epithelial cells migrate from the crypts to extrude from the tip of the villi. As an epithelial cell migrates to the tip of the villus, its absorptive capacity increases. The brush border (microvilli) is covered with a glycocalyx (mucopolysaccharide) cover that contains many of the digestive enzymes of the small intestine. Hosoda and associates describe a possible age-related increase in brush border membrane enzymes. This may indicate higher turnover of small intestinal cells with senescence or may reveal an age-related reduction in the absorptive function of the gut that leads to a compensatory increase in enzyme activity. Also found in the microvillus-calyceal area are receptors for vitamin B_{12}.[63] The surface epithelial cells and the microvillus brush border constitute the digestion-absorption unit. Several enzymes are found in this unit, including alkaline phosphatase, folic acid, folic acid conjugase, and a number of disaccharides and peptidases, as well as adenylcyclase and the "active pump" for sodium.[6,63] In addition to surface epithelial cells, goblet cells (mucin secreting), crypt cells (fluid and electrolyte secreting), and enteroendocrine cells (hormonal) are found in the small intestine.

The mesentery of the small intestine is fixed to the left of the second lumbar vertebra and goes downward and to the right to approximately the level of the right sacroiliac joint. The vascular supply of the entire jejunum and ileum (except for the terminal portion of the ileum) arises from the left border of the superior mesenteric artery. The vessels are contained within the mesentery. The terminal ileum is supplied by the ileocolic artery from the right side of the superior mesenteric artery. Venous drainage is through the superior mesenteric vein to the portal vein.

The small intestine has both sympathetic and parasympathetic stimulation. In addition to the autonomic nervous system, the enteric nervous system also regulates small bowel activities. The enteric nervous system involves purinergic, peptidergic, and serotonergic neurotransmitters. The autonomic nervous system stimulation can be interrupted with vagotomy and sympathectomy without significant alteration in intestinal motility. An intact enteric nervous system may therefore be more important for peristalsis than autonomic innervation.

The primary function of the motility of the small intestine is to facilitate the digestive-absorptive process. Two motions are found in the small intestine: mixing, or segmental, and propulsive, or peristaltic. The mixing movements bring the chyme in contact with pancreatic and biliary secretions. The musculature constricts at the rate of 11 to 12 contractions per minute, resulting in segmentation resembling links. Segmentation also increases the contact of the chyme with the intestinal villi and microvilli, enhancing absorption. Peristalsis propels chyme forward at a rate of 2 to 20 cm per minute. This appears as a progressive moving ring. The myenteric plexus supplies the sympathetic and parasympathetic stimulation for segmentation and peristalsis.

The terms "digestion" and "absorption" emphasize two phases of a single continuing process. The digestion of dietary lipids, carbohydrates, and proteins is initiated in the lumen of the duodenum and proximal jejunum and is completed at the glycocalyx and microvilli plasma membrane of enterocytes (jejunal absorptive cells). Most absorption occurs in the jejunum. Vitamin B_{12} is absorbed in the terminal ileum, and bile salts are reabsorbed by active transport in the terminal ileum. Otherwise, minimum absorption occurs in the ileum unless the jejunum is nonfunctioning or diseased. The processes of absorption in the small intestine are passive absorption and active transport. Passive absorption resembles diffusion of a substance through a

membrane, and the rate of movement depends on a higher concentration in the lumen than in the bloodstream. Active transport is more rapid, more complex, more efficient and requires energy.

Carbohydrate absorption requires conversion of starches to monosaccharides. Starch digestion by pancreatic amylase yields oligosaccharides and disaccharides. Active absorption of sugars occurs primarily in the brush border and at the apex of the epithelial cell. Brush border enzymes include lactase, sucrase, maltase, isomaltase, and trehalase. Lactose is hydrolyzed to glucose and galactose, sucrose to fructose, and dextrins, maltotriose, and maltose to glucose. Disaccharides are further hydrolyzed by brush border enzymes. Disaccharides, sucrose, and lactose are not dependent on pancreatic amylase but are hydrolyzed by the brush border enzymes. Glucose and galactose are transported through a sodium-dependent ATPase process into the epithelial cells. Fructose appears to be absorbed by a nonactive facilitated diffusion transport process.[6] Carbohydrate absorption occurs in the duodenum and jejunum.

Dietary fat consists of long-chain triglycerides that are insoluble in water. In the stomach, fat is shaken into a fine emulsion. Gastric pepsin strips fat of its protein wrapper. Lipase secreted from mouth and tongue remains active in digesting fats in the stomach. In the duodenum and jejunum, pancreatic lipase breaks down triglycerides to diglycerides, then to monoglycerides, and finally to glycerol and fatty acids. Glycerol is absorbed into the epithelial cell and capillaries directly. Monoglycerides, fatty acids, and conjugated bile salts form the micelle. At the brush border the micelle breaks up, allowing the monoglyceride and free fatty acid to enter the cells. The bile salts return to the intestinal lumen, where they are reabsorbed in the terminal ileum. Resorbed bile salts are cycled through the liver and reexcreted in bile. Bicarbonate from the pancreas is also important because efficient lipolysis occurs in an alkaline pH.

The absorbed fatty acids and β-monoglycerides are resynthesized to triglycerides, are enclosed in a protein covering, forming chylomicrons, are transported through the lymphatics and thoracic duct, and finally reach the blood. Some medium-chain triglycerides do not depend on micelle formation and after hydrolysis can be absorbed by the epithelial cell as fatty acids and transported directly into the portal venous system.

Although gastric pepsin begins protein digestion, it is not essential for protein digestion. Pancreatic proteases include trypsinogen, chymotrypsinogen, procarboxypeptidases A and B, leucine aminopeptidase, and nucleases. The hormone cholecystokinin (CCK) is the primary stimulator of the pancreatic acinar cells. CCK is released in the duodenum and jejunum in the presence of amino acids and fatty acids. The presence of hydrogen ions, or a low pH, stimulates the release of the hormone secretin. Secretin stimulates the bicarbonate and fluid responses of the pancreas. The activation of the pancreatic enzyme trypsinogen depends on the intestinal secretion of the enzyme enterokinase. Thus pancreatic functioning depends on the presence and functioning of a normal proximal small bowel.

The intraluminal protein digestion by-products are peptides of two to six amino acids. The brush border and intracellular enzymes further break down these products to free amino acids, dipeptides, and some tripeptides that can enter the epithelial cell. The enterocyte has at least three carrier-mediated transport systems, including one for neutral amino acids, one for basic amino acids, and one for peptide-linked amino acids. In the cell the small peptides are hydrolyzed into free amino acids, which are absorbed into the capillary, where further protein breakdown occurs.

Vitamin B_{12} binds with intrinsic factor (gastric secretion) to protect it from gastric digestion and bacterial digestion in the small bowel. The intrinsic factor also is essential for attachment of vitamin B_{12} to receptors of the glycocalyx membrane of the ileal absorptive cell. Calcium, magnesium, and pH greater than 5.6 are also necessary for the attachment of vitamin B_{12} and the transport through the cell. The vitamin B_{12} is then transported in the portal blood bound to a carrier (transcobalamin). Pancreatic insufficiency may be associated with a vitamin B_{12} deficiency because R binders found in saliva, gastric secretions, bile, and intestinal secretions can bind with vitamin B_{12} instead of intrinsic factor. Pancreatic proteases degrade the R binders, making it possible for vitamin B_{12} to bind with the intrinsic factor. Intestinal microflora are capable of synthesizing vitamin B_{12}. When oral vitamin B_{12} is reduced, the use of antibiotics may alter intraluminal flora, resulting in vitamin B_{12} deficiency. The body stores of vitamin B_{12} may be adequate for years. Thus clinical signs of vitamin B_{12} deficiency are unusual.

Calcium absorption is highest in the upper small intestine where the pH is lowest. Its absorption and transport are enhanced by vitamin D. Calcium is transported against a concentration gradient. Passive absorption occurs when intraluminal concentrations are greater than 6 mmol/L. Calcium absorption is decreased by phosphate ingestion, anticonvulsant drugs, alcohol, and steroids.

Dietary folate is composed of multiple glutamyl units, and the linkage is broken by the jejunal brush border enzymes to monoglutamate. Absorption occurs primarily in the proximal small bowel by a saturable, carrier-mediated process that is maximal at a luminal pH between 5.5 and 6.0. Folate enters the portal circulation and functions as a cofactor in many enzyme systems.

Iron absorption depends on the physiologic demands of the body. When iron stores are low or when red blood cells are being rapidly formed, iron absorption is increased. Iron absorption occurs primarily in the duodenum and proximal jejunum against a concentration gradient. Iron is absorbed in the ferrous form, bound to globulin (transferrin), then released into the portal circulation or stored within cells as apoferritin.

One of the major functions of the small intestine is fluid and electrolyte shifts from gastrointestinal lumen to blood and from blood to lumen. In a 24-hour period, approximately 9 L of fluid enters the lumen of the small intestine. Approximately 7.5 to 8.2 L is endogenous secretions (saliva, gastric, intestinal, pancreatic, and bile). Another 1 to 1.5 L is exogenous. Most of the fluid is reabsorbed, and only 500 to 1000 ml passes through the ileocecal valve into the colon. The duodenum and jejunum are primarily responsible for the large amounts of absorption of fluids, electrolytes, and nutrients because of large pores that allow rapid flow of solutes and water in both directions. Isosmolarity in the lumen is rapidly attained and maintained throughout the small intestine. Several factors help prevent osmotic disequilibrium, including the relative impermeability of gastric mucosa, the regulation of gastric emptying, the fact that nutrients are largely macromolecules with low osmotic activity, and rapid absorption of products of macromolecule digestion or breakdown. Fat is high in most diets, but because its osmotic potential is low, it does not impede osmotic equilibrium. Maintaining osmolarity requires rapid flow of salt and water through the intestinal membrane. The direction of the flow is determined by hydrostatic and osmotic forces.

Sodium absorption is a major function of the small intestine, with approximately 1145 mEq being reabsorbed every 24 hours. Sodium absorption plays a part in regulating cellular absorption of electrolytes and water. The brush border contains a carrier that binds sodium and glucose. When intraluminal glucose is present, sodium is actively reabsorbed by the shared carrier. Sodium is also absorbed from the lumen by a sodium-hydrogen exchange mechanism. A sodium pump at the basolateral border of epithelial absorbing cells transports sodium from intracellular to intercellular spaces by means of sodium-potassium ATPase activity. The decrease of intracellular sodium concentration enhances the sodium-glucose carrier mechanism.

In the ileum a chloride-bicarbonate exchange mechanism is present. The bicarbonate concentration in the ileum is much higher than in the jejunum. Potassium is absorbed based on sodium-potassium ATPase and hydrostatic and osmotic forces.

Water transport is passive and depends on osmotic and hydrostatic pressures. Increased solute concentration in the intercellular space (e.g., from sodium pump activity) provides osmotic forces for water absorption. As water flows through the pores, it brings small solutes with it. This is referred to as solvent drag. Hydrostatic forces from the serosa layer will restrict passive water and solute absorption. Water from the interstitial fluid will enter the lumen when solutes accumulate in the lumen. The flow continues until osmotic equilibrium is reached.

The secretory function of the intestinal epithelium appears to be the result of electrogenic activity. If the secretory function is greater than the absorption function, significant fluid and electrolyte loss can occur. This is frequently seen in diseases of abnormal states (malabsorption syndromes).

Immunologic function of the small bowel is regulated through Peyer's patches, lymphoid cells, and nonorganized cells in the lamina propria. Peyer's patches are found in the submucosa and contain small lymphocytes from the mesenteric nodes. Lymphoid cells differing from Peyer's patches are found in the lamina propria. IgA is the prominent immunoglobulin found in the small bowel, but IgM, IgG, IgD, and IgE are also present. The IgA found in the small bowel differs from serum IgA. An infant is born without secretory or serum IgA. The secretory IgA appears first and reaches adult levels sooner. The secretory IgA has antiviral and antibacterial activities. The

TABLE 8-1   Gastrointestinal Hormones and Their Actions

Hormone	Location	Primary Action	Secondary Action
Gastrin	Antrum, duodenum, proximal jejunum	Stimulates gastric acid secretion	Trophic effect on gastrointestinal mucosa
Cholecystokinin	Throughout small intestine, but primarily found in jejunum	Stimulates contraction of gallbladder Stimulates secretion of pancreatic enzymes	Motility of stomach and small intestine
Secretin	Throughout gastrointestinal tract, except colon; primary sites are duodenum and jejunum	Stimulates pancreatic bicarbonate secretions	Numerous interactions with other gastrointestinal hormones
Gastric inhibitory peptide	Small intestine, primarily jejunum	Increases release of insulin from pancreas	Decreases gastric acid secretion Increases intestinal secretion
Enteroglucagon	Primarily lower ileum and colon	Inhibits motility	May be trophic for mucosa
Vasoactive intestinal peptide	Esophagus to rectum	Increases intestinal and pancreatic secretions	Decreases gastric acid secretion Increases insulin secretion Causes peripheral vasodilation

immune system of the small bowel is complex. Clinically important immune responses to invasive intracellular organisms and to tumors include responses of T cells, B cells, M cells, plasma cells, phagocytic cells, and mast cells present in the submucosa, lymphoid, and lamina propria tissues.

Hormonal function of the small intestine is of great interest. The small intestine may be the body's largest and most diffuse endocrine organ. Bolt and associates[6] provide the following criteria for a gut hormone:

Production of a biologic response in another organ

Production of a response with no innervation between the gut and another organ

Similar response in the organ when an extract of the gut tissue is given

Occurrence of biologic response when pure or synthetic exogenous hormone is given

Four hormones meet these criteria: secretin, gastrin, cholecystokinin (CCK), and gastric inhibitory polypeptide (GIP). Hormone candidates include substances that do not necessarily meet all four criteria. Some of the hormone candidates have known structures, whereas the structures of the others have yet to be identified:

Known structure
  Vasoactive intestinal peptide
  Motilin
  Pancreatic polypeptide
  Somatostatin
  Neurotensin
  Substance P
  Urogastrone
  Enkephalins
Unknown structure
  Chymodenin
  Bombesin-like peptides
  Gut glucagon–like immunoreactants
  Gastrozymin
  Anticholecystokinin peptide

Incretin
Villikinin
Enterooxyntin
Bulbogastrone
Pancreatone

The actions of the hormones are complex, and many have more than one action. The activity may be as a paracrine agent, a neuroendocrine or neurotransmitter substance, or an exocrine agent. Based on amino acid sequence and pharmacologic and physiologic action, two categories of hormones in the small intestine can be identified. Family 1 includes gastrin and CCK. The terminal amino acids in the last four positions are the same in gastrin and CCK. Family 2 includes secretin, enteroglucagon, vasoactive intestinal peptide (VIP), and GIP. Numerous amino acids in similar positions can be found in each of the family 2 hormones.

Table 8-1 summarizes small intestinal hormones and their activities.

The numbers and types of bacteria found in the small intestine depend on the flow rate of the intestinal contents and is highest when stasis occurs, such as in a bowel obstruction. Streptococci, lactobacilli, yeasts, staphylococci, clostridia, bacteroides, and coliforms may be present, particularly in the distal ileum.

Large Intestine (Colon) and Rectum

The colon is approximately 150 cm ($4\frac{1}{2}$ to 5 feet) long. The terminal ileum joins the colon at the ileocecal valve. The appendix arises from the cecum medially, about 2 cm below the junction of the ileum and cecum. The cecum is continuous with the ascending colon, which goes from the cecum to the undersurface of the right lobe of the liver. The colon bends to the left, forming the hepatic flexure. The colon then extends to the left, becoming the transverse colon. The transverse colon has a mesentery and therefore a wide range of movement. The cecum, ascending colon, and proximal half of the transverse colon are derived from the midgut. The innervation and vascular supply are shared with the small intestine.

The transverse colon continues to the left and slightly upward, forming the splenic flexure. The splenic flexure is slightly higher than the hepatic flexure and is in front of and above the left kidney. As the colon turns downward, it becomes the descending colon. The sigmoid colon begins at the point where the descending colon crosses the iliac artery at the rim of the pelvis. The mesentery of the sigmoid colon attaches it to the posterior (retroperitoneal) wall of the pelvis. Near the mid-sacrum, the sigmoid colon becomes the rectum. The rectum descends in front of the sacrum and coccyx. The rectum becomes the anal canal approximately 2 cm anterior to the tip of the coccyx. The upper portion of the rectum is in the peritoneal cavity, but the distal 12 to 15 cm has no peritoneal covering. This area lies behind the bladder in the male with the seminal vesicles on either side. In the female the distal 12 to 15 cm is posterior to the uterus. The rectal ampulla is the lowest part of the rectum and is anterior to the posterior aspect of the prostate in the male. In the female the rectal ampulla is attached to the posterior wall of the vagina.

The distal half of the transverse colon, splenic flexure, descending sigmoid, and rectum are derived from the hindgut. The inferior mesenteric artery supplies this portion of the large intestine and rectum. The nervous innervation is from the sacral parasympathetic fibers.

The wall of the colon is divided into the same four layers as the small intestine: mucosa, submucosa, muscularis externa, and serosa. There are no villi in the large intestine. The simple columnar epithelial surface is flat and is broken into polygonal units by clefts. Goblet cell openings occur on the epithelial surface. In the center of polygonal units are crypts of Lieberkühn. These crypts are lined with goblet cells and extend into the muscularis mucosae. At the bottom of the crypts are proliferating undifferentiated epithelial cells and occasionally argentaffin cells. Cell renewal begins in the crypts. The cells then migrate upward to the surface and extrude into the lumen. The renewal time is approximately $3\frac{1}{2}$ to 4 days.

The mucosa, submucosa, and circular muscular layer form semilunar folds (plicae semilunares) dividing the haustra (sacculations). The semilunar folds are crescent shaped and extend one third of the way around the wall of the intestine. The longitudinal muscle layer is incomplete in the large colon. It is called teniae coli and is the noticeable band in the colon wall. Fatty tags (appendices epiploicae) project from the serosa coat of the colon; this is another difference between the large and small intestines.

The musculature of the rectum is a continuation of the colonic muscular layers. The outer longitudinal layer spreads from the teniae of the sigmoid colon to form a continuous even coat. The superficial fibers insert into the perianal body and merge with the levator ani muscles of the pelvic floor. The deep fibers insert into the perianal skin. The circular muscle forms the internal sphincter surrounding the anal canal. The pectinate line marks the boundary between the anal canal and rectum. At this anorectal junction, the lining layer changes from columnar to squamous epithelial cells. The external sphincter is striated muscle and lies outside the internal sphincter. The external sphincter encircles the terminal portion of the anal canal.

The mesenteric attachments of the colon permit considerable mobility of the ileocecal junction and sigmoid colon. Two potential problems are a volvulus, or twisting of the bowel on itself, and intussusception. The hepatic and splenic flexures, descending colon, and rectum are relatively fixed.

The major blood vessels of the large colon and rectum are the superior and inferior mesenteric arteries as previously stated. The superior rectal artery is a branch of the inferior mesenteric and branches as low as the proximal anal canal. The middle and inferior rectal arteries are branches of the internal iliac artery and supply the anal canal and subcutaneous perianal area. The superior hemorrhoidal vein empties into the inferior mesenteric vein, which drains into the portal system. The inferior hemorrhoidal veins drain into pudendal veins and the systemic venous system. Because of the venous relationship with the portal system, portal hypertension can lead to congestion and enlargement of the hemorrhoidal system and hemorrhoids.

The lymph nodes of the colon include epicolic nodes, found on the surface; paracolic nodes, found on the mesenteric border; and intermediate nodes, associated with superior and inferior mesenteric arteries. The lymphatics from the intermediate nodes join the lymph nodes adjacent to the abdominal aorta (Figure 8-7).

Nervous innervation includes external sympathetic and parasympathetic fibers and submucosal and myenteric nerve plexuses. Sympathetic innervation is from segments T2 to L2. These form the mesenteric hypogastric nerves. The parasympathetic fibers to the right colon are through the vagus nerve. The left colon parasympathetic fibers are from the second to fourth sacral segments by way of the pelvic nerves.

The integrated functions of the colon, rectum, and internal and external sphincters require both sensory and motor innervation. The sensory pathways for the anal canal and perianal skin go through the somatic nerves to S2, S3, and S4. Proprioceptive spindles are found in the striated muscle of the external sphincter. Autonomic sensory innervation for the rectum passes through the same segments (S2, S3, and S4), but through parasympathetic pathways. The pudendal nerve and coccygeal plexus originating in S2 to S5 form the motor fibers for the external sphincter. The hypogastric nerve provides excitatory motor stimuli of the parasympathetic fibers. The rectal sympathetic fibers are from L2 through L4 and the parasympathetic fibers are from S2 through S4.

The normal functions of the colon include controlling transit of waste, absorption, and limited secretion. Defecation is the mechanism for eliminating metabolic waste and dietary residue. Colonic motor activity includes segmentation (mixing) and peristaltic movement. Segmentation occurs by alternate formation and relaxation of haustral folds. Peristalsis is a forward movement over longer segments of bowel. Colonic activities increase after a meal. There is an increase in ileal activity resulting in a slow filling of the cecum and ascending colon. The fluid contents of the right colon are moved back and forth (segmentation) over the absorptive epithelium. The proximal colon retains the contents longer than the distal colon.

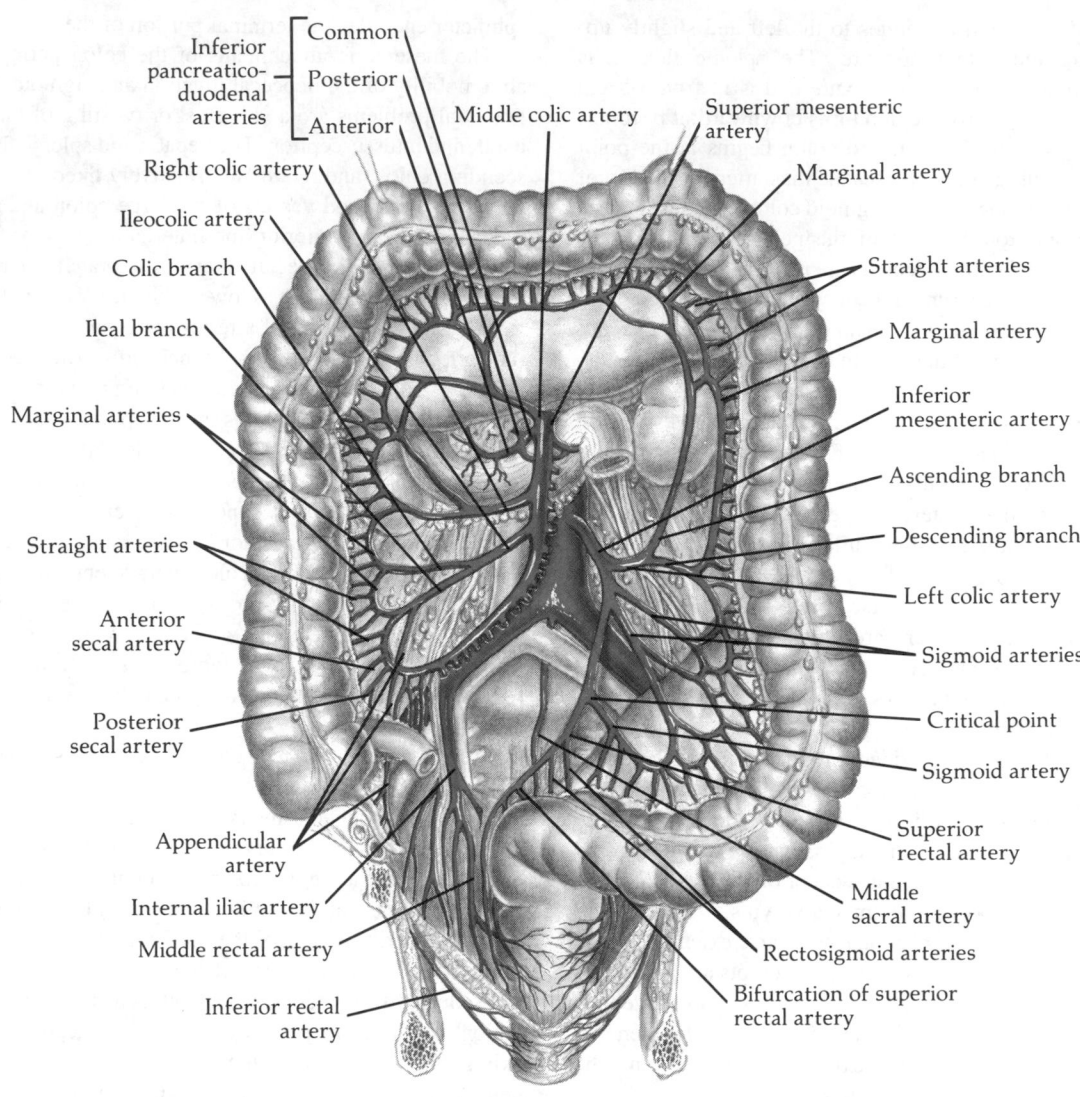

Figure 8-7 Arterial and venous blood supply to primary and accessory organs of alimentary canal.

Gradually the sigmoid colon fills, and the stool periodically passes into the rectum. Distention of the rectum causes an urge to defecate. Defecation can be a simple emptying of the rectal area, or it may stimulate mass propulsion and empty the distal half of the colon. Defecation in a continent person includes voluntary relaxation of external sphincters, relaxation of internal sphincters, increase in intraabdominal pressure, tensing of the pelvic floor, and colon contraction.

Most absorption of fluid and electrolytes occurs in the right colon. The mechanism for water absorption is passive flow in response to an osmotic gradient. The osmotic gradient is produced by active absorption of sodium. The colon is sensitive to aldosterone and other mineralocorticoids, and the response of the colon is to increase sodium absorption and potassium secretion. Potassium is secreted into the colon lumen. The mucus secreted by the goblet cells can contain high quantities of

potassium. If the luminal potassium concentration goes above 15 mEq/L, a shift occurs and potassium is absorbed. Chloride ion is absorbed as a pair with sodium bicarbonate secreted by the colon. As chloride is absorbed, bicarbonate is secreted.

The colon has a minimum digestive or synthetic function. Ingested cellulose is not digested and passes into the colon largely unaltered. In constipated people, when feces remain in the lumen for prolonged periods, the colon can digest and absorb the cellulose. The bacteria in the colon can synthesize folic acid, riboflavin, biotin, vitamin K, and nicotinic acid. The importance of this ability is unknown.

Enterohepatic circulation involving the colon has been identified. The urea-ammonia enterohepatic circulation is related to the hydrolysis of circulating blood urea in the colonic epithelial wall by bacterial ureases. This produces ammonia, which is absorbed into the blood. Any remaining ammonium ion that en-

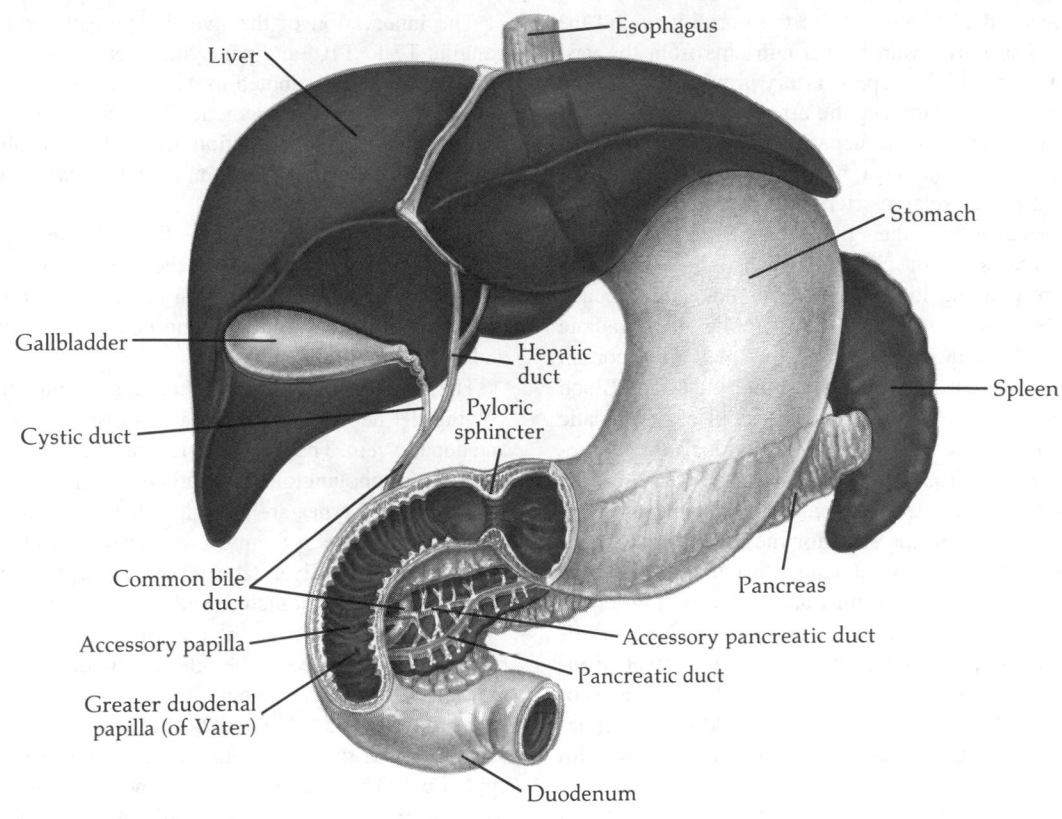

Figure 8-8 Liver, gallbladder, and pancreas.

ters the lumen is converted to free ammonium as a result of the alkaline pH of the lumen. Free ammonium readily penetrates the mucosa and returns to the liver.

A wide variety of drugs can be administered by enema or suppository. The rectum has a poor absorptive capacity, so absorption depends on the level at which the preparation is in the colon and retention time in the colon.

The average amount of gas in the gastrointestinal tract is 100 ml. Gas in the gastrointestinal tract is made up of swallowed air, gas diffusing across the mucosa, and gas produced by bacteria. The major components of flatus are oxygen, nitrogen, carbon dioxide, methane, and hydrogen. Hydrogen and methane are produced by bacteria. The bacteria use substrate found within the lumen, related to diet. Carbon dioxide may be formed as a result of neutralization of acid by bicarbonate, or it may be swallowed. Bacterial use of oxygen may result in low concentrations of oxygen. Flatus passes through the colon more rapidly than liquid or semisolid feces because resistance to flatus flow by haustration is less effective.

Most of the intestinal flora present in the colon is anaerobic, with little invasive potential under normal circumstances. The colon is heavily populated with *Escherichia, Bacteroides,* and *Eubacterium* genera. Potential pathogens such as *Staphylococcus aureus* and *Clostridium difficile* are normally present in low numbers.

Liver

The liver is the largest organ in the body, weighing 1.4 to 1.8 kg (3 to 4 lb). It is a complex organ with many functions, including bile production, protein metabolism, carbohydrate metabolism, fat metabolism, drug metabolism, coagulation, detoxification, and storage of certain minerals and vitamins.

The liver is located under the diaphragm in the upper right portion of the abdominal cavity (Figure 8-8). The superior surface of the liver is under the right and left halves of the diaphragm. The inferior surface is above (from right to left) the hepatic flexure of the colon, the upper pole of the right kidney, the first portion of the duodenum, the inferior vena cava, and the stomach. The liver normally extends from the fifth intercostal space to just below the right costal margin. The right lobe is normally palpable on inspiration 1 to 2 cm below the right costal margin. The left lobe is rarely palpable in the epigastric region of a healthy person.

The liver is divided into two lobes, with the right six times larger than the left in an adult and three times larger in infants. The falciform ligament separates the lobes. The right lobe is further subdivided into quadrate and caudate lobes. Riedel's lobe is a common accessory lobe on the right that is lateral to the gallbladder. This is a functional and anatomic division of the liver created by the falciform ligament. The division is determined largely by the liver's vascular supply.

The liver has a dual blood supply: the portal vein and the hepatic artery. The portal vein brings nutrients from the gastrointestinal system, and the hepatic artery provides the arterial circulation. The origin of the hepatic artery varies. In approximately 55% of individuals the hepatic artery originates from the celiac artery. The remainder have hepatic arteries arising from the left gastric or splenic artery. Off the hepatic artery is the gastroduodenal artery; then the hepatic artery enters the porta hepatis, divides into the right and left hepatic arteries, and enters the corresponding lobes of the liver. A middle hepatic artery originates from one branch and supplies the quadrate lobe. The possible variations in blood flow play an important role in surgical interventions in the gastrointestinal tract. Blood flow to the liver can be disturbed if the origin of the hepatic artery is not carefully noted. In 25% of individuals the left hepatic artery originates from the left gastric artery and this may be the only left hepatic artery present. Occasionally the right hepatic artery arises from the superior mesenteric artery. Another deviation is for the entire hepatic artery to arise from the superior mesenteric artery. In reading arteriograms, it is helpful to know of possible alternative patterns of blood flow. Arteriography can be useful before surgery. Also, for effective intraarterial chemotherapy, a knowledge of possible anomalies of the hepatic arteries is necessary. The right, middle, and left hepatic arteries supply different areas and do not anastomose with each other to any significant degree.

Within the liver, branches of the hepatic artery, the portal vein, and bile ducts in the portal tract, described as the portal triad, accompany each other and empty into sinusoids. The portal vein is formed by the superior mesenteric vein at its junction with the splenic vein. The inferior mesenteric vein also empties into this system. The portal vein has several tributaries, of which the left gastric or coronary vein is the most important. The left gastric vein anastomoses with the esophageal veins, which empty into the vena cava.

The branches of the hepatic artery and portal vein are next to each other within the substance of the liver, with the portal vein emptying into the sinusoids. Approximately 1500 ml of blood passes through the liver every minute. Seventy percent of the blood flow is from the portal vein, which is derived primarily from the inferior and superior mesenteric veins, with one third or less coming from the splenic vein. The remaining 30% of the blood flow is from the hepatic artery.

Sinusoidal outflow is into central veins that flow into the hepatic veins. The three hepatic veins (right, middle, and left) enter the inferior vena cava separately. Normal portal pressure is 8 to 10 mm Hg. Arteriolar resistance, pressure in the aorta, and pressure in the inferior vena cava are important determinants of hepatic blood flow. Exercise, standing, or assuming an erect position reduces hepatic blood flow.

In the liver a superficial subcapsular lymphatic network communicates with the gallbladder and a deep lymphatic network that runs in portal triads with branches of the portal vein, hepatic artery, and bile ducts. The lymphatic drainage is primarily to the nodes at the hilum of the liver and eventually into the thoracic ducts.

The innervation of the liver is sympathetic (paravertebral ganglia, T7 to T10) and parasympathetic (vagus). The sympathetic fibers are distributed to the hepatic arterial branches and bile ducts. The parasympathetic fibers innervate the biliary tree. Although neuronal stimulation affects hepatic blood flow and biliary tree pressures, there are no known direct effects on parenchymal cell function.

The stroma is the connective tissue of the liver. It includes Glisson's capsule, which covers the liver and the connective tissue around the vascular and biliary branches. A reticular framework extends into the lobules and lies between the liver plates and sinusoidal lining cells.

The liver is composed of a complex circulatory system involving the hepatic artery, portal vein, sinusoids, central vein, and hepatic vein. The biliary system includes the bile canaliculi, ductules (or cholangioles), hepatic duct, and common duct.

Several cell types are present in the liver. The parenchymal cell, or hepatocyte, is the most important. The chemical actions that occur in the liver take place in the parenchymal cells. Kupffer (reticuloendothelial) cells line the sinusoids.

The flow of bile is in the opposite direction of the flow of blood through the liver. The bile canaliculi carry the bile from the central vein area to the portal triads. The bile canaliculi are small, intercellular channels between parenchymal cells. The canaliculi join the bile ductules, which are lined by columnar epithelium. The ductules join together to form the bile ducts, which form part of the portal triad with the hepatic artery and portal vein. The bile ducts go toward the hilum of the liver and join, forming the right and left hepatic ducts. The common hepatic duct joins the cystic duct from the gallbladder to form the common bile duct.

The common bile duct is joined by the pancreatic duct, and the two combined ducts form the ampulla of Vater on the duodenal mucosa. Oddi's sphincter at the opening regulates the one-way flow of bile and pancreatic secretions into the duodenum.

Heme, a source of bile pigments, is an end product of the breakdown of hemoglobin and accounts for 80% to 90% of the bilirubin produced daily in adults.[6] Hemoglobin is broken down into globin, iron, and protoporphyrin heme. The metabolic process for the conversion of protoporphyrin heme to bilirubin is poorly understood. It has been suggested that heme is converted to bilirubin by microsomal heme oxygenase found in reticuloendothelial cells of the spleen and liver. This is a multistep process that begins with the oxidation of heme to carbon monoxide and verdoheme. Verdoheme loses its iron to yield biliverdin, which is then reduced to bilirubin. The bilirubin is taken up by the parenchymal cells (hepatocytes) by active transport. This is unconjugated bilirubin, a lipid-soluble pigment that cannot be excreted by the liver unless it is conjugated, increasing its water solubility. Within the parenchymal cell the bilirubin is conjugated. The enzyme located on the endoplasmic reticulum, glucuronyl transferase, stimulates this process.

Conjugated bilirubin is not absorbed from the intestine or gallbladder. In the colon, bacteria hydrolyze conjugated bilirubin to urobilinogen. Urobilinogen is found in feces, bile, and urine. It is partially absorbed and reexcreted by the liver and kidneys. Most urobilinogen is found in the feces.

In the kidneys, urobilinogen is secreted by the proximal tubules and partially reabsorbed. The amount of reabsorption is increased in acid urine. Urine urobilinogen is influenced by the amount of hemolysis of red cells: an increase in hemolysis increases urine urobilinogen. In the presence of decreased bowel motility and stagnation of the small bowel contents, small bowel bacterial colonization and hence bacterial activity are increased. This increases the formation of urobilinogen from bilirubin. Absorption in the small bowel is more efficient, and the absorbed urobilinogen is excreted by the kidney, increasing urine urobilinogen. Hepatocellular disease or transhepatic shunting of portal blood increases the amount of urobilinogen in the systemic circulation, increasing excretion by the renal system. In the presence of biliary tract obstruction, less bilirubin enters the intestines, decreasing both fecal and urine urobilinogen.

The formation of bile is a major function of the liver. Hepatic bile has a specific gravity of 1.009 and an alkaline pH. It contains approximately 97% water, cholesterol, bile salts, phospholipids, mucin, conjugated bilirubin, electrolytes (sodium, potassium, chloride, and bicarbonate), calcium, and many enzymes. The liver secretes approximately 700 ml of bile per day. Although bile is secreted continuously, a meal augments the rate of secretion. The volume of bile produced by the liver is determined by the amount of bile salts synthesized. Conjugated bile salts are secreted by the hepatocytes, and this provides an osmotic pressure for the movement of water into bile. The volume of bile increases as it flows through the biliary tree because of active secretion of an electrolyte solution high in bicarbonate by the biliary epithelium.

Secretion of bile is increased by vagal stimulation and by the action of secretin, cholecystokinin-pancreozymin, vasoactive intestinal peptide, gastrin, and glucagon. Vagal stimulation and cholecystokinin-pancreozymin cause relaxation of the sphincter of Oddi. Exogenous agents that increase hepatic bile secretion and contraction of the gallbladder include bile salts, acetylsalicylic acid, pilocarpine, acetylcholine, choline, histamine, and insulin.

Bile is composed of bile acid, phospholipids, cholesterol, and bile pigments. Bile salts are necessary for micellular solubilization of dietary lipids and to maintain biliary cholesterol in solution. Two primary bile salts are cholic (trihydroxy) and chenodeoxycholic (dihydroxy). They are synthesized in the liver from cholesterol, are conjugated with glycine and taurine, and then form salts with sodium and potassium. Most bile salts are reabsorbed in the terminal ileum by an active transport process. Bile salts entering the colon are deconjugated and dehydroxylated by bacterial enzymes to form secondary bile acids. Cholic acid is broken down to deoxycholic (dihydroxy) acid, which is absorbed, conjugated by the liver, and secreted into bile. Chenodeoxycholic acid gives rise to lithocholic (monohydroxy) acid, which is poorly absorbed. Bile salts are formed when potassium and sodium combine with conjugated bile acids, of which 80% are cholic and chenodeoxycholic acids, with the largest percentage of the remaining bile salts being deoxycholic.

There is approximately 5 g of bile salts with a half-life of 3 to 5 days; these salts are recirculated six to 10 times a day. New bile acids account for 10% of the total amount each day, replacing the amount lost in the feces.

The formation of bile is only one function of the liver. Protein, carbohydrate, and lipid metabolism are additional functions. The liver is the source of albumin, which is 50% to 60% of the total plasma protein. For protein synthesis the liver uses dietary amino acids, amino acids formed by endogenous protein catabolism, and amino acids formed during carbohydrate and fat metabolism. Deamination of amino acids in the liver releases nitrogen, which is converted to urea. The liver also converts ammonia formed in other parts of the body to urea. Other functions related to protein metabolism include uric acid formation from nucleoprotein, creatine formation from glycine, and synthesis of methionine and arginine. Other proteins, of importance to coagulation, include haptoglobin, C-reactive protein, several glycoproteins, transferrin, serum enzymes, and ceruloplasmin.

Albumin has two major functions. First, it helps maintain the plasma colloid osmotic pressure because of its small molecular size and high charge. About one third of the body's albumin (4.5 to 5 g/kg) is intravascular, and the rest is extravascular. Second, albumin plays a role in active transport.

Carbohydrate metabolism involves the liver's ability to store glycogen within the hepatocyte. The liver converts glucose, fructose, and galactose to glycogen. If a diet is low in carbohydrates, or in the presence of prolonged fasting, the liver can convert protein and fat to glycogen. This is referred to as gluconeogenesis. Glucose not stored as glycogen or aminated to amino acids is converted to fatty acids, carbon dioxide, and water.

A normal blood glucose level depends on the liver's ability to remove glucose from the blood, store glucose as glycogen, break glycogen into glucose, and release glucose into the blood. Glycogenolysis (breaking glycogen to glucose) is increased by a decreased blood glucose, exercise, glucagon, and epinephrine. In a fasting state, glucose stores can be significantly depleted in approximately 12 hours. In hepatocellular disease, glycogen stores may be reduced, resulting in hypoglycemia. This may also occur during stress and exercise.

Dietary lipid enters the liver in the form of chylomicrons. Triglycerides are hydrolyzed to glycerol and fatty acids. The liver also takes up fatty acids mobilized from fat depots and synthesizes fatty acids from carbohydrates and amino acids. The fatty acids are used in oxidation for energy production, resynthesis of triglycerides, formation of cholesterol esters, and conversion to phospholipids. Hepatic triglyceride accumulation, or fatty liver, may be the result of an excess of fatty acids, reduced lipid oxidation, or decreased lipoprotein formation.

Cholesterol is synthesized in the liver from acetate. Other sources of cholesterol are kidneys, adrenal glands, and small bowel mucosa. The liver removes cholesterol from the blood and excretes cholesterol into bile, forming a bile acid. Cholesterol may also combine with fatty acids to form cholesterol esters. Serum cholesterol is kept in solution by phospholipids.

The liver plays a major role in coagulation in that it is the site of production of coagulation factors I, II, VI, VII, VIII, IX, and X. Vitamin K is required for the synthesis of factors II, VII, IX, and X. Natural vitamin K is lipid soluble. There are synthetic forms of vitamin K that are water soluble. Vitamin K is stored in the liver. Oral anticoagulants such as coumarin interfere with the action of vitamin K within the parenchymal cell. The liver also removes active clotting factors from the circulation, contributing to coagulation homeostasis.

Plasminogen (profibrinolysin), the inactive form of plasmin (fibrinolysin), is believed to be synthesized by the liver. Plasmin is a proteolytic enzyme that dissolves fibrin, the plasma protein responsible for the semisolid character of a blood clot. Plasminogen levels may be decreased in hepatocellular disease. Antiplasmin, a proteinase inhibitor found in plasma and serum, is also formed in the liver.

Clotting abnormalities may accompany almost any type of liver disease. The severity of acquired clotting problems associated with hepatic disease depends on the extent of hepatocellular damage. Vitamin K deficiency is uncommon because vitamin K is found in food and is synthesized by colonic bacteria. Vitamin K deficiency may be seen in chronically ill people with limited oral intake who are taking broad-spectrum antibiotics. Chronic alcohol abusers may be vitamin K depleted because of their diets and liver disease. Also, patients on long-term total parenteral nutrition have clotting abnormalities develop if their diet is not supplemented with vitamin K. Malabsorption of vitamin K may result from problems that cause a decrease in lipid absorption, for example, biliary obstruction. Coagulation problems seen in hepatocellular damage are usually caused by increased use of clotting factors, decreased production of clotting factors, production of abnormal clotting factors, or platelet abnormalities.

The liver also plays a role in detoxification of many materials, particularly drugs. Most drugs undergo significant metabolism during their first pass through the liver, resulting in a significant drop in their systemic availability. Basically, the liver process involves making the substance water soluble for excretion in bile or urine. Enzymes from the smooth endoplasmic reticulum oxidize, reduce, hydrolyze, and conjugate foreign compounds. The enzymes have a low substrate specificity and readily detoxify substances. The processes that determine whether a compound is excreted in the urine or the bile are multiple and not always understood. Substances that are highly polar and those with molecular weights greater than 200 are excreted in the bile. Substances with smaller molecular weights are excreted in the urine.

The effectiveness of lipid-soluble drugs may be altered by their conversion in the liver to a water-soluble state. Some drugs, such as phenylbutazone, become more potent after conversion in the liver to oxyphenylbutazone. However, oxidation of barbiturates decreases their effect and may produce a toxic by-product. Some drugs require metabolic transformation in the liver for production of a therapeutic action. In a patient with liver disease it is important to know the effects of a drug. Certain medications should be avoided, and others should be given in reduced dosages.

Gallbladder

The gallbladder (see Figure 8-8) is a pear-shaped sac 6 to 8 cm (3 to 4 inches) long and attached to the inferior surface of the liver. It is joined to the biliary tree by the cystic duct at the point where the hepatic duct becomes the common bile duct.

The mucosa of the gallbladder is columnar epithelium overlying a lamina propria. The mucosa is in multiple, irregular folds that increase its absorptive area. The fibromuscular layer forms the framework of the sac. It is a mixture of longitudinal smooth muscle fibers and dense fibrous tissue. The fibromuscular layer is covered by a subserous adventitia. The serous layer is continuous with the serosa of the liver.

The gallbladder is supplied by the superior and inferior cystic artery, which branches off the hepatic artery. The venous system consists of capillary plexuses that drain into superficial veins on the gallbladder surface. These superficial veins empty directly into the liver. The gallbladder also has an extensive lymphatic system that connects with the lymphatic channels draining the liver. This system then combines with the lymphatic vessels of the cystic duct and proximal sections of the extrahepatic ductal system and drains into the nodes at the porta hepatis.

Innervation of the gallbladder and biliary tree is from the sympathetic and parasympathetic systems. Parasympathetic stimulation causes contraction of the gallbladder. Sympathetic stimulation is inhibitory. Preganglionic sympathetic fibers are from the seventh or tenth thoracic segment, and postganglionic fibers from the celiac ganglia.

The hepatic division of the vagal nerve supplies parasympathetic preganglionic fibers that synapse with postganglionic fibers in the gallbladder wall. Afferent fibers travel with the splanchnic nerves and the right phrenic nerve. Right referred shoulder pain in gallbladder disease is related to this shared course with the right phrenic nerve.

The function of the gallbladder is to concentrate and store bile. The organ stores 30 to 50 ml of bile. In the presence of cholecystokinin (CCK) the gallbladder contracts, forcing bile through the cystic duct into the common bile duct and hence the duodenum (see discussion of bile under "Liver").

Pancreas

The pancreas (see Figure 8-8) is an important accessory organ of digestion. It is located transversely across the posterior wall of the abdomen. It is about 20 cm (10 inches) long and weighs 60 to 160 g. The pancreas can be divided into the head, the body, and the tail. The head of the pancreas is situated in the concavity of the duodenal loop on the right side of the vertebral column at the level of the first lumbar vertebra. It lies in front of the inferior vena cava and the superior mesenteric vessels. The common bile duct passes through the head of the pancreas. The body of the pancreas extends leftward and superiorly to the hilum of the spleen. The terminal portion of the pancreas is the pancreatic tail.

The pancreas resembles the salivary glands histologically. The difference between the two is the presence of islets of

Langerhans within the pancreas. The pancreas has both exocrine and endocrine functions. Acinar cells secrete the exocrine products, bicarbonate and pancreatic enzymes, and the endocrine secretions of insulin, glucagon, and gastrin are from the alpha, beta, and delta cells of islets of Langerhans.

The blood supply of the pancreas is from the superior and inferior pancreaticoduodenal arteries and from branches of the splenic artery. The venous flow from the body and tail of the pancreas is through the splenic vein, and the head empties directly into the portal vein. The lymphatic system drains through the pancreaticoduodenal nodes to the celiac nodes.

The innervation of the pancreas is sympathetic and parasympathetic. The sympathetic fibers follow the arterial blood vessels and play a part in regulating blood flow to the pancreas. The parasympathetic fibers terminate at the acinar cells, the islet cells, and the smooth muscle cells and regulate pancreatic secretion.

The pancreas is divided into lobules; each lobule empties into a branch of the main pancreatic duct that joins the common bile duct at the ampulla of Vater before entering the duodenum. Each individual lobule is a group of acini formed from acinar cells and drained by a ductule that forms intralobular ducts that empty into the pancreatic duct. Dark zymogen granules that are the precursors of pancreatic enzymes form the acinar cells. With the enzymes stored and secreted in an inactive form, and with the presence of inhibitors of proteolytic enzymes in the pancreatic juice, the pancreas protects itself from autodigestion.

The exocrine secretion of the pancreas is approximately 1 to 2 L per day. The secretions are aqueous and clear, rich in bicarbonate, digestive enzymes, and electrolytes. The enzymes formed in the acinar cells are secreted into the ducts. Water and electrolytes are secreted by the ductular epithelium. The major pancreatic exocrine function is digestion and absorption in the small intestines. The bicarbonate, calcium, and magnesium in the pancreatic secretions are necessary for creating an optimum environment for enzyme activity. Interference with the exocrine function may lead to severe malabsorption of the dietary fats, fat-soluble vitamins, protein, and carbohydrates in starch form.

The four major enzyme groups secreted by the pancreas are amylolytic, lipolytic, proteolytic, and nucleolytic. Of these, the proteolytic enzymes (trypsinogen, chymotrypsinogen, procarboxypeptidase, and proaminopeptidase) account for most enzymes in the juice.

The hormones involved in the regulation of pancreatic exocrine secretions are gastrin, secretin, and cholecystokinin (CCK). Gastrin is released by the antral mucosa in response to the presence of food in the stomach, distention, a decrease in hydrogen ion concentration, and vagal stimulation. In the duodenum, gastrin release is stimulated by distention and the presence of protein. Cholecystokinin is secreted by the duodenal and proximal jejunal mucosa by the presence of L-amino acids, long-chain fatty acids, and hydrogen ions. The response of the pancreas to gastrin and cholecystokinin is the secretion of enzyme-rich fluid. There is a minimum increase in volume in bicarbonate output, and chloride concentration decreases slightly.

Calcium and magnesium secretions parallel enzyme output. Secretin is released from duodenal and proximal jejunal mucosa in response to hydrogen ion. Secretin stimulates large volumes of pancreatic secretions, which are high in bicarbonate, with little increase in enzyme output. The concentration of cations (sodium and potassium) remains relatively constant. Anion concentration varies with the flow rate. As bicarbonate concentration increases, chloride concentration decreases. Secretin does interact with gastrin and cholecystokinin to augment the secretory response.

Vagal stimulation augments the hormonal stimulation of the exocrine secretions. The sight, smell, and taste of food stimulate the vagus. Also, gastric distention stimulates the vagus nerve. Vagal stimulation of the pancreas results in the secretion of pancreatic enzymes with a minimum increase in bicarbonate concentration or volume.

Any disease process that obstructs the duct system or destroys the acinar cells reduces the secretion of enzymes and bicarbonate and progresses to malabsorption and damage of the duodenal mucosa from unneutralized hydrochloric acid. In the presence of pancreatic disease, secretory functions can be decreased by limiting or eliminating food ingestion, minimizing vagal stimulation with anticholinergics, and reducing acids by nasogastric suctioning and use of H_2 blockers or antacids. A pancreas that is not secreting properly may be partially compensated for by an increase in fat and protein in the diet, use of medium-chain triglycerides, or administration of pancreatic enzyme extracts.

The islets are spheric cells that are outgrowths from the walls of the pancreatic duct during embryonic life. The hormones released from the islets directly enter the circulation.

The endocrine functions are the secretion of glucagon (alpha cells), insulin (beta cells), and gastrin (delta cells). Glucagon causes glycogenolysis in the liver. A blood glucose level less than 60 to 80 mg/dl stimulates the alpha cells to release glucagon, causing the breakdown of glycogen to glucose in the liver. A normal blood glucose level "turns off" the alpha cells.

The beta cells of the islets of Langerhans secrete insulin, which increases glucose use. It carries glucose by active transport through the cellular membrane. An increased blood glucose level, usually after a meal, stimulates the beta cells to release insulin. The insulin carries the glucose across the cell membrane, reducing the blood level to normal.

NORMAL FINDINGS*

Mouth

Temporomandibular joint   Mobility: smooth jaw excursion; 3.5 to 4.5 cm; tenderness: absent on palpitation; crepitus: absent; referred pain: absent on closing jaw

---

*Adapted from Thompson JM, Wilson SF: *Health assessment for nursing practice*, St Louis, 1996, Mosby.

Occlusion Top back teeth rest directly on lower teeth; upper incisors slightly override lowers; *older adult:* may change because of missing teeth; marked overclosure may be associated with edentulous patient; individuals who stoop and thrust head forward tend to habitually protrude lower jaw

Lips Color: pink; symmetry: vertical and lateral symmetry at rest and on movement; moisture: smooth and moist; surface characteristics: slight vertical linear markings; *older adult:* decreased saliva production may contribute to drier lips and difficulty swallowing foods; vertical markings increased; "purse-string" appearance associated with edentulism or overclosure of jaws

Inner lips and buccal membrane Color: pale coral, pink; increased pigmentation, general or localized, in dark-skinned individuals; landmarks; parotid duct; pinpoint red marking; may be slightly elevated; surface characteristics: where teeth meet, occlusion line may appear on adjacent mucosa; clear saliva over surface; *older adult:* surface characteristics: mucosa becomes thinner and less vascular; may appear shinier than in younger adults; Fordyce's granules common

Gums Color: pink, coral; surface characteristics: slightly stippled, clearly defined, tight margin at tooth; patchy brown pigmentation in dark-skinned individuals; hypertrophy may appear during puberty or pregnancy; if inflammation (gingivitis) appears, refer to dentist; *older adult:* color: may be slightly paler; surface characteristics: stippling may be decreased

Teeth Number: 32 (adult); upper and lower third molars may be absent; color: white, yellowish, or grayish hues; form: smooth edges; surface characteristics: smooth; dental restorations; movement: none or slight movement; *older adult:* color: may appear more yellowish or slightly darker; form and surface characteristics: teeth may appear elongated as more root surface or neck of tooth is exposed with resorption of supporting bone

Tongue Symmetry and movement: forward thrust smooth and symmetric; tongue appears symmetric; color: pink; surface characteristics: dorsal and lateral is moist and glistening, with papillae; elongated vallate papillae; fissures; smooth, even tissue; ventral surface: pink and smooth with large veins; *older adult:* papillae may appear slightly smoother and shinier; epithelium is thin and loosely attached; veins may be varicosed

Floor of mouth Frenulum is centered; submaxillary duct opening can be found; color: pale, coral pink

Hard and soft palate Color: hard palate: pale; soft palate: pink; surface characteristics: hard palate: immovable, irregular transverse rugae, midline exostosis (torus palatinus) may be present; soft palate: movable, symmetric elevation, smooth

Mouth odor Absent or sweet

Oropharynx

Landmarks Anterior and posterior pillars symmetric; uvula midline; tonsils; color: posterior wall pink; surface characteristics: smooth; tonsils may be cryptic; slight vascularity on posterior wall

Abdomen

Inspection On inspection the following are normal findings; skin color: may be pale in comparison to body parts that are more exposed; surface characteristics: smooth, soft, silver-white striae; scars: configuration, location, and length; venous network: faint, fine network; umbilicus: centrally located; usually shrunken, but may protrude slightly; should be smooth and noninflamed; contour: flat, rounded, or concave (scaphoid); symmetry: evenly rounded with maximum height of convexity at umbilicus; surface motion: peristalsis usually not visible but may be visible in thin people; pulsations in upper midline may be visible in thin people; movement with respirations: smooth and even; female primarily exhibits costal movements while males evidence primarily abdominal movements; contour remains smooth and symmetric when patient takes a deep breath and holds it; rectus abdominis muscles are prominent; on tightening muscle, midline bulge may appear; *older adult:* contour: geriatric patients may have an increase in fat deposits over abdominal area even though subcutaneous fat over extremities is decreased

Auscultation Bowel sounds: usually 5 to 34 per minute; irregular; gurgles, clicks, and quality vary greatly; all four quadrants; absence of vascular sounds; absence of friction rub

Percussion

- Four abdominal quadrants Tone: general distribution of tympany depending on amount of air and solid material in bowel; suprapubic dullness over distended bladder
- Liver percussion Lower border: usually at costal margin or slightly below; upper border: begins in fifth to seventh intercostal space; midclavicular liver span: 6 to 12 cm (2½ to 4½ inches); liver span usually greater in men than women; liver span greater in taller individuals; right midaxillary liver: liver dullness; may be heard in fifth to seventh intercostal space; midsternal liver span: 4 to 8 cm (1½ to 3 inches); liver descent with deep inspiration: lower border should move inferiorly to 2 to 3 cm (¾ to 1 inch); *older adult:* lower border: in elderly patient with distended lungs, liver border is 1 to 2 cm (½ to ¾ inch) into abdominal cavity; upper border: with distended lung may descend 1 to 2 cm (½ to ¾ inch); deep inspiration may be difficult for elderly individual
- Spleen percussion* Left posterior midaxillary line: small area of splenic dullness at sixth to tenth rib, or tone may be tympanic (colonic); left intercostal space in anterior axillary line: tympanic; left lower rib cage: gastric "bubble"; tympanic; varies in size

Palpation

- Four abdominal quadrants
  Light and moderate palpation Tenderness: none; muscle tone: abdomen relaxed; muscular resistance may be seen in anxious patients; surface characteristics: smooth, consistent tension opposed to localized area of rigidity (increased tension); masses: none; *older adult:* muscle tone: often more lax

---

*If an enlarged spleen is suspected, it may be advisable to perform palpation before percussion.

Deep palpation Tenderness: often present in midline near xiphoid process over cecum, over sigmoid colon; masses: aorta often palpable at epigastrium and pulsates in forward direction; can palpate borders of rectus abdominis muscles; feces may be palpated in ascending or descending colon; sacral promontory may be palpable; umbilicus: check for bulges, nodes, and umbilicus ring; normal findings include umbilicus ring with no irregularities or bulges; umbilicus may be inverted or slightly everted; *older adult:* muscle tone: often more lax

Liver Liver border and contour: liver often not palpable; liver may "bump" against fingers on inspiration, especially in thin people; liver border surface: smooth; tenderness: none; *older adult:* liver commonly palpated 1 to 2 cm ($\frac{1}{2}$ to $\frac{3}{4}$ inch) below costal margin in patients with distended lungs, emphysema, and lowered diaphragm

Spleen Spleen not normally palpable

Kidney Occasionally lower pole of kidney may be palpable in thin individuals; right kidney most often palpable; contour: smooth, firm; tenderness: none

Inguinal nodes Note presence of nodes: small, mobile; none tender; nodes often present; contour: smooth or nonpalpable; consistency: soft or nonpalpable

Assessment for abdominal fluid None should be found; techniques for assessment include flank bulging and fluid shift

Rectal-Anal Region

Perianal area Skin and surface characteristics: Smooth, clear; no tenderness in coccygeal area; anus: surface characteristics include increased pigmentation, coarse skin

Rectal examination Sphincter muscle: tightens evenly around finger with minimal discomfort for patient; anal muscular ring: smooth, even pressure on finger; rectal wall: continuous, smooth surface (examination should cause minimal discomfort for patient); stool: brown, soft

CONDITIONS, DISEASES, AND DISORDERS

ORAL CAVITY DISORDERS

Oral cavity disorders may result in localized inflammation or infection, pain, and difficulty eating. The diagnostic studies, multidisciplinary plan and nursing care will therefore be related to all oral cavity disorders at the end of this section.

◼ GLOSSITIS

Glossitis is a chronic or acute inflammation of the tongue.

Glossitis is manifested as a reddened, inflamed, smooth, and sore tongue, and it usually has one of several causes:

1. Ulcerations, from stomatitis, lichen planus, or carcinomas of the tongue, can cause glossitis.

2. Anemia (usually iron deficiency or pernicious anemia) is one of the most common causes of glossitis. Other vitamin B group deficiencies can also produce glossitis (vitamin B_6, vitamin B_{12}, folate).

3. Sometimes a patient's tongue appears normal, but the patient complains of soreness. In these cases anemia must be ruled out, but depression and other psychogenic causes or factors have been known to cause a painful tongue.

4. Chemical irritants, drug reactions, amyloidosis, microbial infections (candidiasis), vesiculoerosive diseases, and systemic infections may cause glossitis. Median rhomboid glossitis, believed to stem from erythematous candidiasis on the dorsum of the tongue, is a common oral manifestation of patients infected with HIV.[44]

5. Geographic tongue, the cause of which is unknown, is manifest as irregular, smooth, red areas with sharply defined borders that heal and then reappear in a few days. Examination reveals thinning of the epithelium in the middle of the lesion with mild hyperplasia and hyperkeratosis around the edges. Some chronic inflammatory cells can be found in the underlying tissue. Most patients are asymptomatic, but some complain of soreness and hypersensitivity to certain foods.

A variation in geographic tongue is hairy tongue, in which the filiform papillae become elongated and resemble hair. The papillae can vary in length and color; the cause is unknown, but usually only adults are affected. Some drugs, for example, clindamycin, can also cause these papillae.

Treatment for glossitis consists of correcting the underlying cause, if known. Pain relief (both analgesics and viscous lidocaine), meticulous mouth care, and, if necessary, a bland diet may aid patient comfort.

◼ LEUKOPLAKIA

Leukoplakia is persistent white patches in the oral mucosa that cannot be removed by simply rubbing the surface. The term "leukoplakia" is a clinical description and not a pathologic diagnosis. Diagnosis must be made by exclusion.[13]

Increased keratin production is known to cause the whitish appearance, but its development can be the result of many factors. A small percentage of nondysplastic leukoplakias (about 5%) undergo malignant change and become squamous cell carcinomas. Biopsies should be done on all leukoplakias to determine the probable cause.

•••••• Pathophysiology

The causes of leukoplakia vary. Friction from cheek biting or prolonged denture wearing can cause lesions that are initially pale and translucent and later become white and thick with a rough surface. Smoking, usually pipe smoking, may cause a lesion that is probably formed from both chemical components of the smoke and irritation from the heat.

Tertiary syphilis (which is rare today) produces a characteristic leukoplakia on the dorsum of the tongue.

Another uncommon cause is white sponge nevus, a familial disorder characterized by large, soft thickening of the superficial epithelial layers. The entire inner surface of the mouth can be affected by the thick, white plaque. Although untreatable, this is a benign condition.

Patients who have chronic candidal infections in their mouths have plaque formed from epithelial overgrowth. This is another uncommon cause and is treated with local or systemic antifungal agents.

A type of leukoplakia called hairy leukoplakia (so-called for its characteristic hairy or corrugated appearance) has a high association with HIV infection. Eighty percent of people with hairy leukoplakia will develop full-blown AIDS within 2 years. Hairy leukoplakia usually occurs on the side of the tongue and is caused by the Epstein-Barr virus.[36]

Most commonly, leukoplakias are of unknown etiology. In these patients the degree of hyperkeratosis ranges from simple to severe. Treatment of choice may be local excision of the leukoplakia. However, recurrence is common, so many physicians simply choose to see the patient frequently to observe for any changes in the appearance of the leukoplakia; if changes do occur, they perform periodic biopsies to assess for malignancy.

There are three types of leukoplakia: simplex, verrucous, and erosive, depending on its degree and likelihood of malignant transformation. Leukoplakia simplex, which is the smooth and nonindurated type, rarely results in malignant change, whereas verrucous and erosive leukoplakia more commonly become malignant.

◼ PERIODONTAL DISEASE

The term "periodontal disease" refers to diseases of the supporting tissues of the teeth that are usually inflammatory.

The characteristic feature of chronic periodontitis is the destruction of these supporting tissues; almost every case begins with gingivitis, which, if not treated properly, progresses to irreversible chronic periodontitis and loosening, and loss of teeth.

Acute Gingivitis

Acute ulceromembranous gingivitis is usually seen in young adults who have neglected oral hygiene.

Although the exact cause is unclear, plaque bacteria are thought to be implicated in this infection that may also require lowered host resistance. The inflammation starts at the tips of the interdental papillae and progresses quickly to involve the gingival membranes and periodontal tissues. Crater-shaped ulcers with erythematous, edematous edges are characteristic, with a thick yellowish or grayish material over the surface of the ulcer. Bleeding occurs if this material is removed.

The infection remains localized; although the mouth is very sore and the gums bleed, the patient experiences no fever, malaise, or lymphadenopathy.

Acute gingivitis also is seen frequently in patients who are HIV positive, and infection can be progressive and aggressive.

Treatment is with antibiotics for the specific organism and oral hygiene measures to reduce the acute oral infection. The patient and family must be given explicit instructions in the performance of meticulous oral hygiene. Excellent life-long plaque control will decrease or eliminate gingival inflammation in most patients.[35]

Plaque control may be achieved by mechanical or chemical methods. Mechanical plaque removal may be aided by new manual and electric toothbrushes and interproximal cleaning tools. Chemical plaque control with safe and effective agents such as chlorhexidine are available. Chlorhexidine agents, although widely available, may cause tooth staining and altered taste sensation; research is ongoing into improved chemical antiplaque agents.

Chronic Gingivitis

Almost everyone has a degree of chronic gingivitis. It is probably caused by the accumulation of plaque around the neck of the tooth, which if not removed adequately by oral care, involves the epithelium and progresses to the periodontal tissues. Gingivitis can develop in 2 days if plaque is allowed to accumulate, and there is a correlation between the amount of plaque and the severity of the gingivitis.

Although the exact relationship between gingivitis and the destruction of the supporting tissues is not clearly understood, it is probable that the bacteria present in the plaque begin an inflammatory response that is assisted by interactions between antibodies, complement, neutrophils, lymphocytes, and macrophages. Immunologic responses have also been implicated.

As plaque begins to collect at the neck of the teeth, inflammatory changes occur in the gingiva. The epithelium becomes hyperplastic, blood vessels dilate, and some extend almost to the surface, causing the gums to appear darker than normal, even purplish, as a result of congestion. These inflammatory cells spread so that the gingiva appears edematous, soft, and slightly glazed. The gums bleed easily, and there is usually a collection of calculus, or calcified plaque, above the gingival margins.

Chronic gingivitis, if it has not progressed further than the gingiva, will subside if meticulous oral hygiene is begun and followed strictly. Part of the treatment must be aimed at teaching the patient and family about oral hygiene and the progression of the disease if these instructions are not followed.

Periodontitis

Acute periodontitis is quite uncommon and usually does not last long. It can be caused by trauma, most often from biting on a hard object, which may produce some minor damage that heals quickly; a periodontal abscess, which is a complication of periodontal disease; or progression from ulceromembranous gingivitis if untreated.

Premature, progressive periodontitis is common in HIV-infected patients and is thought to be caused by an overgrowth of microorganisms.

Chronic periodontitis is very common and is the main reason for loss of teeth in adults. Up to 70% of adults have at least mild periodontitis, whereas less than 15% are affected by severe disease and tooth attachment loss.[35] Untreated infection of the gingiva leads to progressive inflammation and destruction of the supporting structures of the teeth.

The four main features of chronic periodontitis are destruction of periodontal membrane fibers, resorption of alveolar bone, migration of the epithelial attachment along the root toward the apex, and formation of pockets around the teeth.[35]

The pocket formation is characteristic of periodontitis; these pockets form a closed space where bacteria (and possibly anaerobic bacteria) grow. The infected material cannot drain, and these bacteria irritate the tissues.

Clinical symptoms include bleeding from the gums, a bad taste in the mouth, and foul-smelling breath; later there is gum recession and loosening of the teeth. The gingiva appears purplish and swollen, and plaque and calculus are evident.

The best treatment is prevention; regular and thorough toothbrushing and removal of plaque would make any further treatment or surgery unnecessary. However, surgery is necessary when the disease has been neglected, pockets have formed, and the gingiva cannot be restored to normal without surgical intervention.

Patients who are considered for surgery must realize that they will have to expend some effort to maintain their teeth during the postoperative period. The rationale for surgery includes debridement and removal of plaque and calculus and restoring soft tissue and bone to its normal contour and state of health.

Several surgical procedures may be carried out, depending on the severity of the periodontal disease. A local anesthetic is used in most cases, and patients rarely require hospitalization. Patient education remains a vital part of the overall treatment because, if a patient is unaware of or fails to comply with meticulous oral hygiene measures, the disease will undoubtedly recur or progress. When the disease has reached the point where surgery would not be useful, the teeth must be extracted and the patient will have to wear dentures.

 EMERGENCY ALERT

DENTAL AVULSION

Avulsion of the teeth usually occurs as a result of injury. It may be possible to replant the tooth if medical attention is obtained immediately after the injury.

INTERVENTION

- Ensure that the patient's airway is patent and is not obstructed with teeth/tooth.
- Place the tooth/teeth immediately into a normal saline solution.
- Control bleeding at the site with pressure using a gauze sponge.
- Obtain dental consultation as soon as possible. Time is important for the successful replantation of the tooth/teeth.

SALIVARY GLAND DISORDERS

Disorders or inflammation can occur in the parotid, sublingual, or submaxillary glands.

Salivary gland disorders can be classified into several categories: inflammation, as in mumps and acute and chronic sialadenitis; obstruction, as in calculi; and degenerative diseases and neoplasms, which are not discussed here. Dry mouth (xerostomia), which may be caused by damaged salivary glands, is an unpleasant problem and can be the result of local or systemic causes and chronic anxiety states.

•••••• Pathophysiology

Inflammation of the salivary glands is most commonly caused by mumps. Mumps is discussed further in Chapter 13. Of the salivary glands, the parotid gland is most commonly affected by an inflammatory process.

Less common infections are acute ascending parotitis and chronic sialadenitis. Acute parotitis is most frequently seen in postoperative patients who have poor oral hygiene and who are dehydrated. Usually, the patients have prolonged nasogastric intubation and are elderly, debilitated, and malnourished. Infection is caused by ascending bacteria from the oral cavity (staphylococcal or gram-negative) and can lead to abscesses. If not treated the infection may occlude the trachea, causing acute respiratory failure. Parotitis begins with pain or tenderness in the angle of the jaw.

This disorder can be prevented by proper hydration, good oral hygiene, and care taken during surgery to avoid trauma to the duct orifices. Treatment of acute parotitis includes rehydration, the discontinuation of all medications that may decrease salivary flow, parotid massage, broad-spectrum antibiotic therapy, oral hygiene, and hard candies to suck to stimulate salivary flow. Response to therapy should be observed within 48 to 72 hours after initiating treatment. Despite antibiotic therapy, the mortality rate of acute suppurative parotitis approaches 25%.[54]

Chronic sialadenitis is usually caused by chronic duct obstruction, which may be due to mucus plugs or other causes. It is usually unilateral, and the patient experiences painful swelling of the gland accompanied by an inflamed duct and purulent discharge from the orifice. Treatment is usually conservative, but occasionally removal of the obstruction or excision of the gland is necessary.

Obstructions of the salivary glands are usually caused by calculi, although mucoceles and cysts may also form, and these must be excised. Calculi formation is quite common, and most (80%) of them form in the parotid gland or Stensen's duct; the rest are in the sublingual and minor salivary glands. Although salivary calculi occur at any age, they are uncommon in children. Men are affected twice as often as women. Diagnosis is based on recurrent, painful enlargement of the gland and is confirmed by physical examination, palpation, and imaging techniques.

Calculi are composed mainly of calcium and phosphate and tend to form more frequently in the submandibular gland because its saliva has a high pH and is viscous because of a high mucin content. This gland also may be irritated by the teeth during chewing, and it is larger in diameter and longer than the parotid duct.

Pain and swelling may occur suddenly during eating and subside within a short time. Symptoms may not occur with every meal, and sometimes the patient is asymptomatic until the stone enlarges, moves along the duct, and can be felt in the mouth. Usually no inflammation is present, but occasionally a gland or duct becomes infected, indicated by increased swelling and tenderness over the gland and purulent discharge from the orifice. Pain and fever accompany this infection. Treatment is the same as for acute parotitis.

Xerostomia, or dry mouth, can result from a variety of transient and chronic causes. Fear and acute anxiety are the most common causes of transient dry mouth. Chronic conditions can be caused by mouth breathing; heavy smoking; some drugs such as antihistamines, antidepressants, and sympathomimetics; chronic anxiety states; and treatment with radiation to the head and neck, which causes irreversible damage to the salivary glands. With xerostomia, the lubrication, mastication, and digestion of food may become difficult. This may lead to depression, poor nutrition, and weight loss. The rate of opportunistic infection increases with xerostomia; the most common of these infections is candidiasis.

STOMATITIS

Stomatitis is ulceration in the mouth that may be on the gums or the oral mucosa.

Stomatitis may be a single lesion, as from a local injury, or widespread, caused by systemic factors. Stomatitis is mainly inflammatory, and there are several types: viral, bacterial, noninfective, and drug related. It may result from excessive smoking, spicy foods, poor nutrition, poor oral hygiene, or allergic responses. All types of stomatitis are usually quite painful and therefore may inhibit food ingestion; this can be a major problem in an already debilitated patient.

•••••• Pathophysiology

Herpetic stomatitis is the most common form of viral stomatitis; after an initial infection, usually in infancy or childhood, it begins with vesicle formation. After the rupture of the vesicles and the shedding of the cells, an ulcer is visible. These ulcers are usually scattered over the mucous membranes and are circular and about 3 to 4 mm in diameter. The gingivae are swollen and inflamed, and the local lymph nodes are usually swollen. The patient may have an elevated temperature, increased salivation, and severe mouth pain. These lesions usually clear in 7 to 10 days.

After the primary infection, many people are subject to recurrent infections. These are not usually within the mouth but affect the skin around the lips at the mucocutaneous junctions. These infections, known as herpes labialis, are caused by the herpes simplex virus and are discussed further in Chapter 13.

Angular stomatitis, which is the result of iron deficiency anemia, causes inflammatory changes at the angles of the mouth that vary from reddening to ulcerated, crusting fissures. More common in elderly patients with full dentures, it can cause deep folds at the corners of the mouth, where infection can spread if not treated, making the condition much more extensive. Lack of vitamins such as niacin and riboflavin can cause cellular weakening because cell growth, oxidation, and metabolism are impaired.

Denture stomatitis is caused by occlusion of the mucous membranes by a tight-fitting denture for a long time. This creates a closed environment in which organisms can grow. Although the patient may be asymptomatic, there is normally a reddened, erythematous area corresponding to the area covered by the denture. These patients should leave their dentures out, at least at night, to allow the mucous membranes to heal.

Aphthous stomatitis (canker sores) is one of the more common diseases affecting the mucous membranes. The underlying cause of these small, yellowish, very painful ulcers is unclear, although several factors have been implicated (virus, allergy, gastrointestinal disease, psychosomatic causes). Women are affected slightly more often than men. The disease is most troublesome in adolescence or early adult life and often clears up by early middle age. The first sign of aphthous stomatitis is usually a pricking feeling in the mucous membrane, followed soon after by eruption of painful ulcers that may appear alone or in groups. They resemble craters with red, raised margins, and they usually heal in a week or so without scarring. These lesions do not vesiculate like herpetic lesions.

Thrush, or oral candidiasis, is one of the most common types of stomatitis. This mycotic stomatitis is characterized by white plaques on the oral mucous membrane, gums, and tongue. It is frequently seen in patients who are malnourished, diabetic, immunosuppressed, or taking antibiotics that destroy the normal oral flora.

Although *Candida* is part of the normal mouth flora, some weakening of the body's resistance can permit an increase in its growth (usually *C. albicans* or *C. tropicalis*). Fungal spores lodge between the epithelial cells and cause a gradual separation of the layers, spreading the infection to the surface of the mucous membrane and the rest of the mouth. White patchy growths appear in several areas of the mucous membrane and spread so a continuous membrane forms. Oral candidiasis occurs in more than 79% of patients with HIV infection and AIDS.[26]

One of the more distressing types of stomatitis appears as a result of drug treatment. It is frequently seen in patients who have been taking systemic antibiotics for long periods and who have bacterial overgrowth in the mucous membranes or in patients receiving chemotherapy for cancer treatment, and it may be quite debilitating because the patient may already have a lowered resistance to infection. In a severely leukopenic patient, necrotizing ulceration of the mucous membranes, gums, and throat may occur, which can in turn cause septicemia. Usually, these ulcers appear on the mucous membranes in any number and are very painful. They may cause increased salivation and prevent the patient from eating normally.

• • • • • Diagnostic Studies and Findings

X-ray examination of lateral and oblique views of jaw and upper neck   May demonstrate large stones

X-ray examination using dental film to project through floor of mouth from below   May demonstrate small stones

Sialography   May demonstrate partial or complete filling defects in the ductal system with retention of dye on evacuation films; not advisable in acute stage of inflammation

Ultrasonography   May demonstrate suppuration within the gland or presence of sialoliths

Laboratory studies   Serum B_{12}, folate levels decreased with anemia; WBC normal or slightly elevated in presence of acute inflammation or infection

Microbiologic studies   Culture and sensitivity of oral ulcerations, plaque bacteria, or purulent matter expressed from periodontal pockets/abscesses

• • • • • Multidisciplinary Plan

Surgery

Surgical removal of sialoliths if stone cannot be removed by manual manipulation

Medications

Anesthetic agents
  Topical anesthetics (viscous lidocaine [Xylocaine]) as needed
Vitamins
  Vitamin replacement if condition caused by underlying deficiency
Glucocorticoid ointment
  Kenalog in Orabase (aphthous ulcers)
Antiinfective agents
  Topical
    Nystatin (Mycostatin) oral suspension or lozenges for *Candida* q6h po
    Clotrimazole vaginal tablets for *Candida* q6h po
  Systemic
    Oral or intravenous antibiotics as indicated by culture, sensitivity
Narcotic analgesics
  Acetominophen (Tylenol) with codeine, 30 to 60 mg po q4-6h as needed
  Meperidine (Demerol) 50 to 75 mg IM q4-6h as needed for acute pain relief

General Management

Many sialoliths can be removed by manipulation of duct
Mild mouthwashes for comfort
Synethetic saliva for comfort

Meticulous oral hygiene to include plaque removal
Photodynamic therapy using light-sensitive drugs to selectively identify and destroy diseased cells may be promising modality for treatment of precancerous and cancerous lesions of the pharynx, including recurrent leukoplakia[5]

Dietary

Well-balanced diet; bland if necessary; high in protein, calories, and needed vitamins
Nutritional consultation if necessary

NURSING CARE

Nursing Assessment

General

- Anorexia, weight loss
- Dehydration
- Fever, malaise
- Lymphadenopathy with parotitis, primary herpetic stomatitis
- Recent or recurrent chemotherapeutic or antibiotic regimen

Oral Examination

- Reddened, inflamed, smooth tongue
- Dry oral membranes
- Localized swelling
- Purulent discharge from orifice of duct
- Palpation of stone in gland or duct
- Increased or decreased salivation
- Halitosis
- Painful, ulcerated areas on oral mucous membranes that may appear yellowish with reddened, raised areas
- White coating on the tongue

Nutritional Status

- Sensitivity to spicy foods and discomfort when eating
- History of poor dietary habits
- Debilitated physical appearance
- Presence of dentures in angular and denture stomatitis

Nursing Dx & Intervention

Pain related to inflammation, ulcerations

- Assess patient *for discomfort* related to eating.
- Provide analgesics *for pain relief* as prescribed, especially before meals, and assess and document effectiveness.
- Topical anesthetic agents such as viscous lidocaine (Xylocaine) may be helpful in relieving the discomfort.
- Apply warm, moist packs to affected area *to decrease swelling and discomfort.*
- Advise frequent gargles, mouth irrigation, and synthetic saliva (with xerostomia) *to improve comfort.*

Risk for infection related to presence of plaque bacteria

- Monitor oral temperature bid.
- Examine duct orifices for evidence of purulent discharge. Assess for signs of infection in opened or excised duct, if stone has been surgically removed.
- Administer oral or intravenous antibiotics as ordered *to prevent or treat infection.*

Altered oral mucous membrane related to infection, ulcerations, or inflammation

- Assess oral mucous membranes for evidence of ulcerations.
- Provide mouthwashes, avoiding those with alcohol *because they may be irritating.*
- Assist with and instruct patient about thorough but gentle mouth care.
- Keep lips lubricated *to prevent drying and further irritation.*
- Administer topical antiinfective agents as ordered. Freezing nystatin may make it more tolerable for patient.
- Offer ice chips *for a numbing effect.*
- Provide hard, sour candies for patient to suck *to stimulate salivary flow.*
- Ensure adequate hydration.

Altered nutrition: less than body requirements related to oral pain when eating

- Assess patient's nutritional status.
- Assess patient's oral intake and make note of any decrease in intake associated with discomfort when eating.
- Change the texture of food to soft or pureed if necessary.
- Avoid extremes of temperature in food.
- Provide dietary consultation *to offer a palatable, nourishing diet that is high in protein, calories, and vitamins.*
- Instruct patient to avoid spicy foods, alcohol, and citrus juices if they are irritating. A bland diet may be more tolerable.
- Maintain needed level of hydration; intravenously, if prescribed.

Patient Education/Home Care Planning

1. Explain to the patient the importance of continued meticulous mouth care. Instruct the patient in effective plaque removal techniques.
2. Discuss with the patient and family the need for maintenance of a proper diet.
3. If stomatitis is herpetic, inform the patient of its infective nature and instruct in isolation and handwashing techniques.
4. Ensure the patient's understanding of prescribed medications, including application, dosage, and side effects.
5. Ensure that the patient knows ways to prevent or minimize dry mouth.

Evaluation

Oral pain is manageable   Patient is able to eat with relative comfort. There is no localized pain.

Inflammation/infection is resolved   Patient is afebrile. There is no localized swelling. Patient verbalizes understanding of oral hygiene measures to prevent recurrence.

Oral mucous membrane is healing   Oral ulcers and inflammation decreased or resolved. Absence of halitosis.

Adequate nutrition is maintained   Patient's weight and hydration are maintained at normal levels.

ESOPHAGEAL DISORDERS

ACHALASIA

Achalasia is a neuromuscular disorder of esophageal motility that is characterized by failure of the lower esophageal sphincter to relax, by dilation of the esophagus, and by loss of esophageal peristalsis. Most patients with achalasia have progressive dysphagia, first with solid then with liquid foods. Other classic symptoms include chest pain, hiccups, regurgitation, and weight loss.[2]

Achalasia is more common in adults, but it may also be seen in children and infants. The incidence of achalasia is 1 in 100,000 population per year.[25] In a geriatric patient, achalasia may be related to cancer of the lower end of the esophagus. Also, an increased risk (2% to 7%) of esophageal cancer exists for patients with long-standing achalasia that was never treated or was minimally treated.[67]

The cause is unknown. Although there are reports of several cases of achalasia in one family, the disorder has not been classified as hereditary. Emotional factors may exaggerate or trigger a latent defect. Treatment is palliative, not curative.[26]

•••••• Pathophysiology

There are three pathophysiologic changes in achalasia: elevated resting lower esophageal sphincter pressure, residual pressure after swallowing because of poor relaxation of the lower esophageal sphincter, and loss of peristalsis in the body of the esophagus.

The esophageal sphincter pressure is elevated to approximately 50 mm Hg (twice normal level). This high pressure does not relax with swallowing. In a normal situation the lower esophageal sphincter pressure drops to the level of the stomach pressure. In achalasia the pressure drops but not enough to permit unrestricted passage of food into the stomach.

The changes associated with achalasia are the result of denervation of the smooth muscle segment of the esophageal body and of the lower sphincteric region. Studies have demonstrated that muscle strips from the lower esophageal sphincter (LES) of patients with achalasia do not contract in response to ganglionic stimulation. The muscle strips only contract with direct stimulation from acetylcholine. Studies with cholecystokinin octapeptide demonstrate an unexpected increase in the LES pressure, possibly related to a loss of inhibitory neurons in this region. These and other studies suggest that loss of ganglion cells in the region of the lower sphincter has caused a functional impairment of the esophagus.[61]

Motility disturbances in the body of the esophagus mean that the peristalsis is weak and ineffectual in pushing a bolus of food through the closed sphincter. Aperistalsis may be located throughout the length of the esophagus. The esophagus may empty only when the hydrostatic pressure of its contents is great enough to overcome the pressure resistance in the lower esophageal sphincter. Because esophageal emptying depends on gravity in this case, emptying is improved if the person is sitting rather than lying down.

In the early stages the body of the esophagus is dilated symmetrically. In later stages the esophagus dilates considerably, lengthens, and curves. The body of the esophagus may bend and rest on the diaphragm. A dilated esophagus in achalasia may hold 1 to 2 L of fluid.

•••••• Diagnostic Studies and Findings

Splash-down time   Length of time between swallowing and reaching the stomach (normally 8 to 10 seconds): takes longer or not heard at all

Radiography studies

Chest x-ray (screening): absence of gastric air bubble; air-fluid level in esophagus; possible aspiration pneumonia, pulmonary fibrosis (complications from aspiration); presence of food in esophagus; esophageal dilation and distortion may be observed as mediastinal mass

Barium swallow with fluoroscopy: absent peristalsis in esophageal body; dilated esophagus; conically narrowed LES ("beaklike" tapering); retained food in the esophagus

Manometry

   Pressure readings: elevated resting lower esophageal sphincter pressure (50 mm Hg or greater) and residual pressure after swallowing; intraesophageal resting pressure greater than intragastric pressures; absence of primary peristalsis in esophageal body

Video or line esophagram (cineRadiography-Scintigraphy): barium is swallowed and followed on video tape demonstrating absent peristalsis

Radionuclide scans for esophageal emptying: decreased or delayed esophageal emptying

Endoscopy (to rule out cancer and other conditions that mimic achalasia): dilation, atony of esophageal body; puckered and closed lower sphincter that does not open during the procedure

•••••• Multidisciplinary Plan

NOTE: Therapy chosen depends on availability of local experts in either medical or surgical area.

Forceful pneumatic dilation of esophagus is primary treatment and is done to decrease ability of sphincter to react to stretch

May be required when dilation cannot be done or is unsuccessful; surgical treatment is a distal esophagomyotomy (Heller procedure) in which the muscle fibers enclosing the esophagus are divided, allowing mucosa to pouch out through divisions in muscle layers; when this surgery includes the cardiac end of the stomach, it is referred to as a cardiomyotomy; the most common complication after the Heller procedure is gastroesophageal reflux; an antireflux operation (loose fundoplication) is frequently performed at the same time as myotomy

Medications

All have a direct relaxant effect on the smooth muscle fibers of LES. Not proven to be of substantial value in changing the clinical symptomatology of patients with achalasia; however, may be used in patients with significant concomitant disease where dilation or surgery is considered too risky

Nitrates   Sublingual isosorbide dinitrate (Isordil), 5 to 10 mg before meals

   Oral isosorbide dinitrate (Isordil), 10 mg

Calcium channel blockers   Verapamil (Isoptin) or nifedipine (Procardia capsules or SL); dosage varies in clinical studies; give close to meal times for optimal effect

General Management

Carcinoma after treatment remains a possibility, and diagnosis may be more difficult because of lack of early symptoms; a tumor in the dilated esophagus may be large before obstructive symptoms develop; pain and dysphagia associated with carcinomas may be assumed to be part of the primary diagnosis of achalasia

Pulmonary problems may still develop after dilation from reflux at night, and patient instruction should include refraining from oral intake 1 to 2 hours before bedtime

Nutritional Consultation

To help patient select and plan diet that is easily swallowed

Gradual symptoms and adaptation techniques of patients include fullness after meals; swallowing water or bicarbonate of soda after a meal; and using a modified Valsalva maneuver after a meal

Regurgitation of retained material can be recognized as food eaten hours earlier; nocturnal regurgitation may be severe

Dysphagia becomes continuous and annoying, with difficulty first with solids and later with liquids

Nutritional Status

Gradual weight loss

Vomiting (overflow from esophagus): does not have "sour" characteristics of emesis from stomach (usually undigested or stale food)

Pulmonary

History of hoarseness, night cough, chronic laryngitis, and bronchitis from aspiration of retained food and fluids; chest discomfort and spasms; nocturnal coughing spells

Coping

Impact on work, social activities, relationships; how long patient has had condition; any previous treatment

Nursing Dx & Intervention

Altered nutrition: less than body requirements

- Assess patient to determine which foods patient can and cannot swallow. A soft diet encourages more rapid esophageal emptying.
- Provide diet that avoids alcohol, spicy foods, or foods at temperature extremes *because these items may be irritating to the esophagus.*
- Instruct patient to eat slowly, chew food thoroughly, and arch the back while swallowing *to facilitate swallowing.*
- Instruct patient to eat sitting upright and to remain sitting after completion of the meal *because emptying of the esophagus is improved if patient is sitting.*
- Request nutritional consultation.
- Administer medications as ordered *to relieve discomfort, thus promoting appetite.*

Risk for aspiration related to esophageal regurgitation with food accumulation

- Elevate head of bed while patient sleeps *to avoid regurgitation or aspiration.*
- Assess patient closely for signs of pulmonary problems, especially in the morning after patient awakens.
- Instruct patient to eat evening meal in early evening *to allow food time to pass into stomach before going to sleep.*

Risk for ineffective individual coping related to chronicity of disease and impact on eating

- Allow patient to express concerns and frustration regarding disruption of mealtimes and inability to participate in social functions involving food.
- Assess support systems and provide additional resources.

Patient Education/Home Care Planning

1. Explain to the patient the importance of not eating for at least 2 hours before bedtime to decrease symptoms and to prevent aspiration.
2. Discuss with the patient the need to try using more than one pillow to elevate the head and shoulders slightly or to raise the head of the bed.
3. Instruct the patient to prepare liquid foods to maintain nutritional status, if solid foods cause dysphagia.
4. Discuss with the patient the signs and symptoms of pneumonia or other pulmonary problems related to aspiration of food.
5. Discuss with the patient the relationship between achalasia and a slightly higher incidence of esophageal cancer. If the patient's symptoms change, he or she should be encouraged to see a physician.
6. Explain to the patient the procedure for care before and after dilation, with an explanation of surgical treatment, if necessary.

Evaluation

Nutritional status is adequate Patient maintains stable weight.

There are no pulmonary problems Airway is clear. There is no evidence of aspiration or other pulmonary problem.

Patient is coping with disease Patient understands alternate methods of management and uses support systems. Patient is able to communicate effectively with medical staff.

ESOPHAGEAL DIVERTICULUM

An esophageal diverticulum is a hollow outpouching of one or more layers of the esophageal wall.

The symptoms associated with esophageal diverticulum depend on where the diverticulum is located. Esophageal diverticuli occur in three main areas. The most common, Zenker's diverticulum, develops through the space at the junction of the hypopharynx and the esophagus. A Zenker's diverticulum is three times more common in men than in women, and usually occurs in patients who are 60 years of age or older. It is rare in patients younger than 30.[4]

A second type of diverticulum, traction diverticulum, occurs at the midpoint of the esophagus and is caused by the esophageal wall reaction to local inflammation—usually from inflamed lymph nodes. Fungal or tuberculous inflammation is particularly contributory. Traction diverticula are the least common and the least clinically significant of the three types.

The third type, epiphrenic diverticulum, occurs immediately above the lower esophageal sphincter and is usually acquired.[61] The incidence is greatest in men 50 to 60 years old.

•••••• Pathophysiology

The only diverticula of clinical consequence are those that retain food or fluid. Zenker's diverticulum is related to a developmental weakness of the muscular coat of the posterior portion of the pharynx. A small hernia of the esophageal wall is pushed out with swallowing and forms a diverticulum. Zenker's diverticulum can enlarge and obstruct the esophagus.

Bronchitis and bronchiectasis can result from nocturnal regurgitation and aspiration associated with both Zenker's and epiphrenic diverticulum.

•••••• Diagnostic Studies and Findings

Barium swallow Herniation of esophageal wall

Manometry Epiphrenic diverticulum demonstrates simultaneous repetitive contractions, as well as abnormal lower esophageal sphincter function

•••••• Multidisciplinary Plan

Surgery

Epiphrenic diverticulum (only for severe symptoms): thoracotomy, diverticulectomy, myotomy, and possibly antireflex operation

Zenker's diverticulum: excision of the diverticulum and cricopharyngeal myotomy of the lower esophageal sphincter

General Management

Careful assessment of patient so that other esophageal diseases are not overlooked in managing esophageal diverticulum

---

NURSING CARE

Nursing Assessment

Gastrointestinal

Zenker's diverticulum
  Regurgitation of undigested food eaten hours earlier
  Dysphagia, late symptom, indicates obstruction of esophagus
  Bad taste in mouth (sour metallic)
  Halitosis
  Sloshing fluid in the diverticulum heard as gurgling noises
Esophageal diverticulum
  Regurgitation of food eaten hours before
  Dysphagia with sensation of pressure in lower esophagus after eating
  Intermittent vomiting

Pulmonary

Zenker's diverticulum
  Aspiration at night may lead to chronic pulmonary disease
Epiphrenic diverticulum
  Aspiration with pulmonary symptoms

Nutritional status

Weight loss
Food intolerances and associated nutritional deficiencies

Nursing Dx & Intervention

Risk for aspiration related to inadequate swallowing of food and fluids

- Assess patient closely for signs of pulmonary problems (i.e., choking or aspirating).
- Keep head of bed elevated.
- Encourage patient to sleep with head and shoulders elevated on at least two pillows *to prevent aspiration.*

Altered nutrition: less than body requirements related to difficulty in eating

- Assess nutritional status.
- Consult with nutritionist.

- Weigh patient daily.
- Monitor and record intake and output accurately.
- Ensure that patient's knowledge of food preparation is adequate *to facilitate swallowing and emptying of diverticulum.*

Patient Education/Home Care Planning

1. Ensure that the patient understands the relationship between potential pulmonary problems (aspiration) and lying down after eating.
2. Nutritionist will review with the patient which foods to avoid, will demonstrate menu planning, and will discuss follow-up procedures.

Evaluation

Aspiration is prevented   Breath sounds of the patient are heard over all the lung fields. No evidence of aspiration or other pulmonary problem exists.

Nutrition is adequate   Patient maintains stable weight.

■ HIATAL HERNIA

Hiatal hernia refers to the presence in the chest, above the diaphragm, of part of the stomach that has passed through the normal esophageal hiatus.

Hiatal hernia is very common, occurring in approximately 20% to 50% of the population.[27] It is more common in women and much more common in elderly individuals. A hiatal hernia is clinically significant when it is accompanied by a reflux of acid.

•••••• Pathophysiology

Muscle weakness is a primary factor in a hiatal hernia developing. Loss of muscle tone in middle age or after a long illness weakens the muscles around the diaphragmatic opening, predisposing the person to hiatal hernia. Increased intraabdominal pressure helps to push the upper portion of the stomach through the large opening of the diaphragm.

Intraabdominal pressure may be increased by the effort needed to evacuate firm stools associated with low-residue diets or constipation. Hiatal hernia is uncommon in countries where the diet is high in fiber. Obesity, pregnancy, and ascites are associated with hiatal hernia, as are the use of girdles and tight-fitting belts and clothes. Esophagitis may lead to secondary shortening of the esophagus and spasm, which may pull part of the stomach upward, creating a small hiatal hernia. Esophageal carcinomas may also pull upward on the stomach. This may cause confusion in diagnosing the primary cause. Hiatal hernia is also seen with kyphoscoliosis.

Hiatal hernia may develop after surgical treatment for achalasia. After partial gastrectomy, hiatal hernia may be found because of the straightening and opening of the gastroesophageal junction angle and the elimination of the sphincter.

Paraesophageal and sliding hiatal hernia are two types of hiatal hernia. Paraesophageal hernias involve the herniation of the cardia of the stomach up into the chest, with the gastroesophageal junction remaining below the diaphragm. Acid reflux is not present in this type. Less than 10% of all hiatal hernias are paraesophageal. Complications associated with paraesophageal hernias are incarceration, hemorrhage, obstruction, and strangulation. These disorders are treated operatively.[67]

The sliding hiatal hernia is the most common type of esophageal hernia. In these patients the cardioesophageal junction and a portion of the fundus of the stomach are above the diaphragm. This condition creates a weakened lower esophageal sphincter (LES), allowing reflux of acid into the esophagus. Eighty percent of patients with clinically significant gastroesophageal reflux have a sliding hiatal hernia.[67]

Hiatal hernias interfere with normal protective mechanisms of the lower esophageal sphincter, allowing reflux of acid into the esophagus. Also, if a portion of the stomach is fixed above the diaphragm, congestion of the gastric mucosa may lead to gastritis and ulcerations in the herniated portion of the stomach. The size of the hiatal hernia does not affect the development of esophagitis or the severity of the symptoms.

Diagnostic Studies and Findings

Esophagography (barium swallow) Outpouching, depending on patient's position when the test is performed

Esophagoscopy with biopsy Assessment of degree of esophagitis and rule out carcinoma

Motility studies Demonstration of reflux and low pressure in lower esophageal sphincter

pH monitoring of lower esophagus over a 24-hour period Increase in acidity

Laboratory studies Stool for occult blood; serum for diagnosing anemia

Bernstein test (acid perfusion test) Used to differentiate between cardiac chest pain and pain resulting from esophageal origin (patient has esophageal pain or heartburn if the test is positive)

Radioisotope scintiscan Diagnosis of nocturnal aspiration

Multidisciplinary Plan

Surgery

Conservative medical management usually successful; surgery is indicated in the following situations:

Persistent or recurrent symptoms not responding to medical treatment

Complete mechanical incompetence of the sphincter (<6 mm Hg)

Strictures

Strangulation or incarceration (paraesophageal hiatal hernia)

Types of Procedures

Nissen fundoplication: the fundus of the stomach is wrapped around the lower 3 to 4 cm of esophagus, creating an area of higher pressure; procedure may be done laparoscopically

Belsey fundoplication: the fundus is wrapped around 270 degrees of the lower esophagus and the operation is performed through a left thoracotomy

Medications

Antacids, 1 ounce taken 1 and 3 h after eating and at bedtime

Histamine H_2 receptor blockers—ranitidine (Zantac), 300 mg at dinnertime or bid

Gastrointestinal stimulants—metoclopramide (Reglan), 10 to 20 mg/d; will increase the rate of gastric and esophageal emptying by stimulating the smooth muscles of the intestine; monitor for signs of acute agitation with metoclopramide

Cisapride (Propulsid), 10 to 20 mg qid before meals and at bedtime; improves esophageal peristalsis, increases LES tone, and promotes gastric emptying

General Management

Instruct patient to use 4- to 10-inch bed blocks to raise the head of the bed so that he or she lies on an incline; pillows are not effective

Avoid eating foods that are irritating

Avoid increasing intraabdominal pressure by wearing tight belt, corset, or girdle

Avoid eating 1 to 2 hours before bedtime; avoid lying down after eating

Walk around after eating

Weight reduction

Take medications with an ample amount of water; always take medications in an upright position

NURSING CARE

Nursing Assessment

Pain

Reflux esophagitis: symptoms include heartburn or pain; the condition is worsened by lying down or stooping over; pain is relieved by sitting up or by antacids

Epigastric pain

Pattern of discomfort in relation to food ingestion

Nutrition

History of foods that irritate or worsen symptoms

Dysphagia

Gastrointestinal

Gaseous eructations, water brash (mouth filling with fluid from esophagus), regurgitation

Sudden onset of vomiting, pain, and complete dysphagia indicates incarceration of paraesophageal hiatal hernia

Pulmonary Status

Chronic lung disease after nocturnal regurgitation and aspiration; may include hoarseness, chronic laryngitis, bronchospasm

Nursing Dx & Intervention

Altered nutrition: less than body requirements related to postprandial pain and dysphagia

- Assess patient's nutritional status.
- Provide small meals; avoid gastric distention.
- Provide a bland diet, avoiding foods that are irritating. Chocolate is associated with relaxation of the esophageal sphincter and is contraindicated.
- Have patient avoid eating 1 to 2 hours before bedtime *to reduce the heartburn of reflux esophagitis.*
- Have patient sip a half glass of water after a meal *to cleanse the esophagus.*
- Consult with the nutritionist for meal planning, as well as weight reduction for those who are obese.

Pain related to gastroesophageal reflux

- Assess patient for symptoms of reflux esophagitis: heartburn or pain that increases when lying down, water brash (mouth filling with fluid refluxing from the esophagus), and dysphagia.
- Provide 4-inch blocks to elevate the head of the bed (and help patient find out where they can be brought for home use); *this will maintain the patient in an inclined plane, reducing the abdominal pressure.*
- Provide antacids at the bedside for frequent use during the acute phase. Administer antacids to patients with poor memory or who are confused.
- Explain the relationship between food and the pain the patient is experiencing; that is, that the pain is related to reflux of gastric contents.
- Administer H_2 blockers and gastrointestinal stimulants as ordered.

Patient Education/Home Care Planning

1. Discuss with the patient the relationship between hiatal hernia, reflux esophagitis, and the treatment plan.
2. Provide instructions on use of prescribed medications. If the patient has other medical problems and is taking other medications, check with the pharmacist before choosing the antacid to be used.
3. Provide information on the use of 4- to 10-inch blocks under the head of the bed; the patient may also need help to prevent sliding out of the bed.
4. Other substances that reduce pressure in the lower esophageal sphincter and should be avoided include chocolate, peppermint, nicotine, anticholinergics, calcium channel blockers, nitrates, diazepam, β-adrenergic agonists (Isuprel; Alupent), dietary fat, caffeine, and alcohol.

Evaluation

Nutrition is maximized   Patient takes in small, frequent, low-fat, high-protein meals, avoiding irritating substances. Patient's weight remains stable.

Pain is minimized   Patient understands the medication regimen and the importance of raising the head of the bed; patient reports a decrease in pain associated with eating and sleeping.

ESOPHAGEAL VARICES

Esophageal varices are dilated blood vessels in the esophagus caused by portal hypertension.

Portal hypertension results in the enlargement of collateral blood vessels and the predisposition to ascites. Normally blood flows from the higher pressures of the portal system through the liver sinusoids and then through the hepatic vein to the lower pressure of the vena cava and the systemic venous system. As long as this normal flow is uninterrupted, the potential collateral circulation between the portal and systemic circulations remains closed. Potential collateral circulation exists at the cardioesophageal junction, in the lower rectum, and around the umbilicus. When the normal hemodynamics are disturbed by portal hypertension, the flow of blood that normally goes from the coronary veins into the splenic vein is reversed.[81] This forces open the collaterals between the esophagus and the gastric veins, leading to esophageal varices. Internal hemorrhoids and dilated veins around the umbilicus also occur.

Portal hypertension is the result of blockage or increased resistance to the inflow of blood into the liver or decreased outflow of blood from the portal system into the vena cava. Causes of portal hypertension include congenital obstruction of portal vein, thrombosis of splenic vein from acute pancreatitis, liver parenchymal disease, occlusion of the hepatic vein, and cirrhosis.

Forty percent of all patients who have cirrhosis eventually develop variceal hemorrhage. Acute mortality of variceal bleeding approaches 50%, and approximately 60% of patients with variceal bleeding will die within 1 year after their first episode of bleeding.[51]

•••••• Pathophysiology

The veins from the small segment of the abdominal esophagus and the fundus and cardia of the stomach drain into the left coronary vein. These two venous systems are connected by small veins that lie in the esophageal submucosal plexus and normally remain closed. When these veins become dilated, they quickly become tortuous and variceal because of poor support in the esophageal submucosa. In portal hypertension the pressure of the portal system is transmitted through these collateral vessels, which dilate and then produce large esophageal varices. The focus of care is on the management of massive gastrointestinal hemorrhages that occur in these patients. Priorities of treatment include correction of hypovolemia, achievement of hemostasis at the bleeding site, and prevention of pulmonary aspiration. The long-term goal is to prevent recurrent hemorrhage.

•••••• Diagnostic Studies and Findings

Endoscopy   Tortuous protrusions into lower end of esophagus; may show large amount of blood and possibly source of bleeding

Mesenteric angiography   Demonstrates collateral circulation; may demonstrate bleeding site
Barium swallow   Outlines varices

•••••• Multidisciplinary Plan

Surgery

Surgery is recommended if patient has bled once because 60% to 90% run a risk of further bleeding
  Surgical ligation during acute bleeding episode; does not correct underlying pathologic condition
Shunt procedures: high morbidity caused by anatomic variations created from shunting procedure; hepatic encephalopathy common
  Portacaval shunt: portal vein or one of its tributaries is connected to the inferior vena cava, and portal vein blood flow bypasses diseased liver; complication: hepatic encephalopathy
  Splenorenal shunt: diverts portion of blood flow away from liver to reduce pressure; lower incidence of hepatic encephalopathy
  Mesocaval shunt: unites high-pressure superior mesenteric vein of patient with portal hypertension to low-pressure inferior vena cava, directly or with a synthetic graft
  Distal splenorenal shunt: uses spleen to conduct blood from high pressure of esophageal and gastric varices to low-pressure renal vein
  Transjugular intrahepatic portosystemic shunt (TIPS): catheter-directed percutaneous shunt using stainless steel balloon expandable wire mesh stent to connect portal vein to hepatic vein to decompress portal system; minimizes hepatic encephalopathy; no general anesthesia required
Liver transplantation for intractable esophageal bleeding

Medications

Focus is on management of the massive gastrointestinal hemorrhages that occur
Pituitary hormone
  Vasopressin (Pitressin), to reduce portal and mesenteric blood flow, given intravenously or during endoscopy or angiography; side effects include abdominal cramps, diarrhea, hyponatremia, peripheral vasoconstriction, hypertension, decreased cardiac output, angina, dysrhythmias, and infarction of bowel
Vasodilators
  Nitroglycerin; initial bolus 20 U over 20 minutes, continuous infusion 0.2 to 0.8 U/minute, concurrent administration with vasopressin may help to minimize the undesirable side effects of vasopressin
Histamine receptor antagonist
  Cimetidine (Tagamet), 300 mg qid, or ranitidine (Zantac), 100 mg qid, at meals and bedtime
Antacids
  Maalox, to protect gastric mucosa

Coagulants
  Vitamin K, IM
  Fresh frozen plasma; platelets
Propranolol (β-blocker), 20-80 mg bid
  Lowers portal pressure

General Management

NPO
Sclerotherapy of varices may be done by a transhepatic approach or through an endoscope; involves injecting varices with agents that irritate them, causing thrombosis; complications include perforation of esophagus, aspiration pneumonia, pleural effusions, increased ascites, and ulceration of esophagus; repeated sclerotherapy results in the development of supportive scar tissue around the vessel
Esophageal tamponade to control bleeding
  Minnesota (quadruple lumen) tube: improvement over Sengstaken-Blakemore tube; additional lumen for esophageal aspiration
  Sengstaken-Blakemore tube (triple lumen): gastric aspiration with two balloons (esophageal and gastric); need additional nasogastric tube to empty esophagus if patient is not alert
Complications of esophageal tamponade include rupture or erosion of esophagus, occlusion of airway by balloon, and aspiration of secretions
Blood transfusions: volume replacement; keep Hct about 30% (overtransfusion can contribute to portal hypertension and potentiate variceal rupture)
Removal of ascitic fluid (paracentesis)

NURSING CARE

Nursing Assessment

(See also Cirrhosis)

Gastrointestinal

History of liver disease
Massive hematemesis
Melena
Assess amount of blood lost

Mental Status

(See nursing assessment under Hepatic Coma on pp. 771 to 772)

Nursing Dx & Intervention

Altered cerebral, cardiopulmonary, gastrointestinal, and peripheral tissue perfusion related to variceal hemorrhage

• Assess patient for signs and symptoms of hypovolemic shock related to GI bleeding:
    Postural changes in pulse and blood pressure
    Cool, clammy skin

Increase in respiratory rate

Change in mental status

Decreased urine output

Hemoglobin and hematocrit unchanged immediately but decreased within 24 hours

- Start IV line with large-bore catheter and administer IV fluids as ordered by physicians *to begin fluid replacements and to facilitate possible blood transfusions.*
- Assist with the insertion of Swan-Ganz or CVP catheter and perform ongoing hemodynamic monitoring.
- Assess patient for possible blood transfusion reaction per protocol.
- Perform gastric lavage with room temperature saline or water as ordered by physician. If patient vomiting or at high risk for aspiration, notify physician. Endotracheal intubation may offer best airway protection from aspiration of blood or gastric contents.
- Assist with esophageal tamponade *to control bleeding* if ordered, and monitor patient closely after insertion of the tube.
- Assess for signs of complications associated with esophageal tamponade; rupture or erosion of the esophagus, occlusion of the airway by the balloon, and aspiration of secretions. Monitor esophageal balloon pressure: prevent pressure from exceeding 45 mm Hg. Limit inflation time to 24-36h.
- If patient has diarrhea, assist with gentle cleansing and application of moisture barrier ointment to soothe and protect perianal skin.

Altered thought processes related to biochemical abnormalities associated with shunting of portal blood into systemic circulation

- Assess patient closely for symptoms of hepatic encephalopathy: apathy, euphoria, asterixis (flapping), personality changes, confusion, disorientation, and stupor progressing to coma; document and report to physician immediately if any of these occur.
- If confusion or disorientation occurs, frequently reorient patient to time, date, and place.
- If patient is disoriented or combative, ensure patient's safety by placing side rails up or restraining patient if necessary.
- Stay with patient or enlist assistance from family members *to keep patient from harming himself or herself.*
- Continue to administer lactulose or neomycin as ordered by physician. These agents help eliminate blood from patient's gut; if untreated, hepatic encephalopathy could occur from by-products of protein metabolism produced by bacterial action in gut.
- Provide usual care necessary for comatose patient if hepatic coma should occur.

Other related nursing diagnoses Diarrhea and impaired skin integrity; see Hepatic Coma on pp. 770 to 771.

Patient Education/Home Care Planning

1. Prepare the patient for all diagnostic procedures, treatments, or surgery so the patient will understand what will happen and what to expect.
2. Review with the patient the effects of high-protein diets and alcohol consumption in preventing future complications. Include the nutritionist.
3. Discuss with the patient the relationship of the esophageal varices to the primary diagnosis that resulted in portal hypertension.
4. Instruct the patient to avoid alcohol, salicylates, and other medications that may irritate the gastric or esophageal mucosa.
5. Instruct the patient to avoid activities that increase intraabdominal pressure, including heavy lifting, straining to stool, vomiting, ingestion of large meals.
6. Instruct the patient in early detection of bleeding, including weakness, dizziness, dark stool, "coffee ground" emesis.
7. Assist patient with location of community resources that offer rehabilitation from alcohol abuse, if applicable.

Evaluation

There is no gastrointestinal bleeding Hematocrit and hemoglobin are normal for patient. Vomiting and diarrhea are not present. Vital signs are stable. Skin turgor is normal for patient.

Mental status is normal for patient Patient is alert and oriented to time, date, and place.

STOMACH DISORDERS

GASTRITIS

Gastritis is inflammation of the mucosa of the stomach.

Gastritis has been classified in several different ways, including acute or chronic and erosive or nonerosive. For the purposes of this chapter gastritis will be discussed as two separate but related entities: acute and chronic gastritis. The similarities are histologic; the clinical manifestations and morbidity are discussed separately.

According to Yamada, infections of *Helicobacter pylori* are responsible for most cases of histologic gastritis. Multiple other factors also contribute to the development of or are directly responsible for clinical gastritis; definitive diagnosis must be verified by endoscopic gastric biopsy.[71]

Acute gastritis is predominantly an erosive process. It is responsible for 10% to 30% of upper gastrointestinal bleeding.[67] Predisposing factors include excessive alcohol intake. Alcoholics are five times more susceptible to gastritis than nonalcoholics. Other causes include excessive aspirin intake (2.5 g/d for several days) nonsteroidal antiinflammatory agents (NSAIDs), *Helicobacter pylori* infection, and severe physical stress (burns, sepsis, severe trauma, extensive surgery, shock, and respiratory, hepatic, or renal failure). The mortality rate is less than 5% when the cause of bleeding is aspirin or an alcoholic binge; it is greater than 30% in association with alcoholic cirrhosis and portal hypertension.[71]

Chronic gastritis, also classified as erosive and nonerosive, implies a duration of at least 6 months. Chronic erosive gastritis is rare, and the symptoms, if present, are anorexia, nausea, and a vague upper abdominal discomfort.

The more common, chronic nonerosive gastritis, increases in frequency with age and is seen more often in women than men. The incidence increases given chronic alcoholism and postgastrectomy. By 50 or 60 years of age, 50% or more of the population can be shown to have *Helicobacter pylori* gastritis.[71] Other possible causes include gastric stasis, duodenal regurgitation, repeated mucosal injury, immunologic factors, endocrine disturbances, radiation treatment, ulcerative colitis, genetics, diet, environment, and debility.[26] Gastric ulcer, gastric cancer, and pernicious anemia are associated.

•••••• Pathophysiology

Acute gastritis is a brief inflammatory process affecting the stomach mucosa. It involves erosion of the mucosa. The mucosa is spotted with submucosal hemorrhages that resemble ecchymoses and may be round or linear. There may also be shallow erosions that appear as brown spots or red petechiae or small breaks in the mucosa. The hemorrhagic erosions usually involve only the glandular layer, are extremely shallow, and are found anywhere in the stomach. Acute gastritis is more common in gastric ulcer than duodenal ulcer. The difference between gastritis erosion and gastric ulcer is that in erosion the muscularis mucosa is uninvolved and healing leaves no scar.

Erosion and hemorrhage are caused by a back-diffusion of hydrogen ions and mucosal ischemia. The disruption of the gastric mucosal barrier allows the back-diffusion of the hydrogen ion, which stimulates the release of vasoactive substances, increased capillary permeability, and inflammation (Figure 8-9).

Steroids appear to potentiate the action of other factors in acute gastritis. Nonsteroidal antiinflammatory agents probably affect gastric mucosa because they work by inhibiting prostaglandin synthesis. Prostaglandins have a cytoprotective function on the gastric mucosa. Apparently, patients taking both nonsteroidal antiinflammatory agents and aspirin are at a greater risk for bleeding from acute erosive gastritis. In these cases, the patient must be observed, medications adjusted, and the patient treated for erosion as indicated.

If the irritating agent or stimulus is removed, a spontaneous remission often results.

Chronic gastritis is often referred to as a nonerosive, nonspecific gastritis that is further differentiated by the histologic appearance of the gastric mucosa into superficial gastritis, atrophic gastritis, or gastric atrophy.

Superficial gastritis is characterized by an inflammatory infiltration of the lamina propria. Lymphocytes, plasma cells,

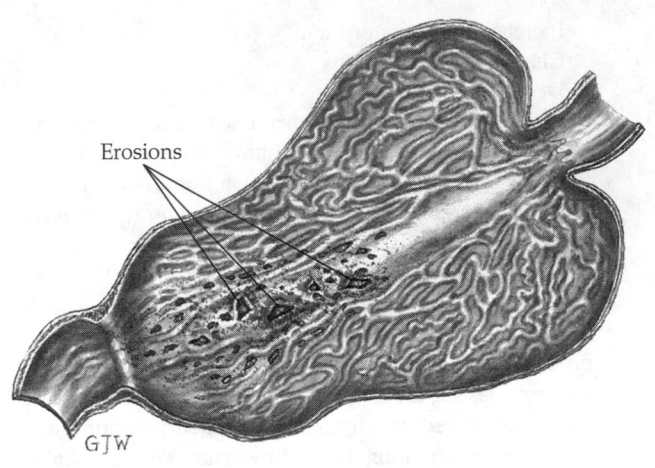

Figure 8-9 Erosive gastritis (disruption of "tight cellular junctions" with back diffusion of H⁺). (From Doughty.[17])

and eosinophils are found in the outer one third of the mucosa. The gastric cells are not involved.

Atrophic gastritis shows a loss of fundic glands, parietal cells, and chief cells. The muscularis mucosa is split and thickened, and marked inflammation is present.

Gastric atrophy refers to marked or total gland loss with minimum inflammation. The mucosa is thinned.

Two additional features, intestinal metaplasia and pseudopyloric metaplasia, may be seen in the three types of chronic gastritis. Intestinal metaplasia is the replacement of normal gastric cells by cells identical to those of the normal small intestine. Intestinal metaplasia is greater in more severe degrees of gastric atrophy. The surface of the normal stomach is columnar, whereas the small intestine has a prominent brush border and may contain goblet and Paneth's cells. When intestinal metaplasia occurs, the stomach acquires the appearance and absorptive capacity of the small intestine. Cancer is much more likely to develop in intestinalized gastric mucosa in comparison to the rare instances of carcinoma of the intestinal epithelium in the small intestine.

In pseudopyloric metaplasia the normal fundic glands are replaced by clear-staining mucous glands that cannot be distinguished from mucous glands in the antral gland or cardial gland mucosa. The replacement may be partial or total. Diagnosis of pseudopyloric metaplasia is made by biopsy. It is imperative that the location of the biopsy be carefully stated on pathology slips so the pathologist does not mistake normal antral gland mucosa for pseudopyloric metaplasia or vice versa.

Chronic gastritis has also been divided into type A and type B. Type A gastritis involves the fundus. There are circulating parietal cell antibodies and high serum gastrin levels. The destruction of parietal cells by the inflammatory process results in a marked reduction in acid secretion and impaired intrinsic factor production or binding. There is decreased binding of intrinsic factor with dietary vitamin B₁₂ in the stomach, impairing vitamin B₁₂ absorption and eventually resulting in pernicious anemia. Pernicious anemia evolves almost exclusively from type A gastritis.[63,71] The relationship of the parietal cell antibodies and intrinsic factor lends support for the hypothesis that type A gastritis has an autoimmune background.

Type B gastritis involves the fundus and the antrum. Type B gastritis increases with age and is probably caused by *Helicobacter pylori* infection. This infection can be eradicated with antibiotic therapy, including metronidazole and bismuth. Type B has less reduction of acid secretions, normal gastrin levels, and only rare impairment of vitamin B_{12} absorption. As the mucosa of the stomach changes with atrophy, the acid secretion is reduced, resulting in achlorhydria or hypochlorhydria.

Atrophic gastritis and gastric atrophy are associated with an increase in gastric malignancies. There is a high rate of cell death and increased cell turnover in atrophic gastritis. Mucosal nuclear activity is increased during the premalignant state. The highest mitotic rates are found in areas of intestinal metaplasia.

Diagnostic Studies and Findings

Acute Gastritis

Nasogastric aspiration   Frank blood or heme-positive aspirate

Stool for guaiac   Positive

Endoscopy   Erosions, superficial ulcerations, and diffuse oozing of blood when procedure is done during acute phase; best performed within 24 hours of admission or lesions will begin to heal

Angiographic visualization   If bleeding has not stopped, used to detect and treat lesions with infusion of vasopressin

Double-contrast barium study   Superficial gastric erosions; cannot be used to detect bleeding lesions

Enzyme-linked immunosorbent assays (ELISA)   For detection of serum antibodies to *Helicobacter pylori*

Urease test   Endoscopic biopsy specimen placed in solution of urea and phenol red; presence of *Helicobacter pylori* turns solution pink; 90% sensitivity to *Helicobacter pylori* after 3 h; biopsy specimens should be sent for histologic examination only if urease test negative after 3 h

Chronic Gastritis

Serum gastrin   Elevated in type A

Serum parietal cell antibodies   Presence in type A, high association with pernicious anemia

Intrinsic factor antibodies   Presence in type A

Antibodies to gastrin-producing cells   Presence in type B

Gastric secretory testing (Pentagastrin)   Requires intubation; superficial gastritis: normal or slightly decreased acid secretion; atrophic gastritis: hypochlorhydric; gastric atrophy: achlorhydric

Serum pepsinogen I levels   Elevated in superficial gastritis; low level in atrophic gastritis reflects absence of chief cells

Schilling test   Assessment of vitamin B_{12} absorption by measuring urinary excretion of an oral dose of radiolabeled vitamin B_{12}

Barium swallow with double contrast   Appearance of a "bald fundus" and thinning of gastric rugae

Endoscopy with biopsy and cytology   Biopsy necessary to obtain a definitive diagnosis; cytologic examination of multiple biopsy sites through the stomach is used to rule out gastric carcinomas

Enzyme-linked immunosorbent assays (ELISA)   For detection of serum antibodies to *Helicobacter pylori*

Urease test   Endoscopic biopsy specimen placed in solution of urea and phenol red; presence of *Helicobacter pylori* turns solution pink; 90% sensitivity to *Helicobacter pylori* after 3 h; biopsy specimens should be sent for histologic examination only if urease test negative after 3 h

Multidisciplinary Plan

Acute Gastritis

Surgery

   Partial gastrectomy, pyloroplasty, or vagotomy (truncal, selective, or highly selective) may be indicated for managing patients with major bleeding from erosive gastritis

Medications

   Histamine receptor antagonists
      Ranitidine (Zantac), 100 mg po qid
      Cimetidine (Tagamet), 300 mg po qid
   Antacids
      Antacids recommended to help maintain alkaline pH
      Antacids (30 ml q2h) have been shown to be 80% to 90% effective in keeping pH above 4.0
   Fluid volume replacement
      Intravenous fluid replacement during a bleeding episode to maintain volume
      Blood replacement may be required when gastrointestinal hemorrhage is associated with acute gastritis
   Pituitary hormone
      Vasopressin (Pitressin) per angiography or IV, 20 U in 100 cc D_5W over 10 min, may be used in severe cases and may be repeated q3-4h if bleeding recurs; may lose efficacy after repeated doses

General Management

   Room temperature water or saline lavage used in patient with gastrointestinal bleeding
   Laser therapy with direct coagulation of bleeding spots through an endoscopic approach may be used
   Removal of causative agents (alcohol, aspirin, nonsteroidal antiinflammatory agents)
   Withholding of food and fluids until vomiting and inflammation subside; then bland diet of medium temperature in acute gastritis without bleeding will assist healing process

Nutritional Consultation

   To help patients identify foods that exacerbate symptoms and select diet that minimizes symptoms

Chronic Gastritis

Symptomatic treatment only

Medications

Antacids to reduce or alleviate symptoms

Vitamins

Vitamin C (ascorbic acid) to facilitate iron absorption in the patient with achlorhydria

Vitamin B_{12} injections (cyanocobalamin), 1 mg/ml (1000 µg) if pernicious anemia diagnosed

Antibacterial agents[22] to eradicate *Helicobacter pylori*

Bismuth subsalicylate,* 2 tabs qid × 2 wk

Metronidazole, 250 mg tid × 2 wk

Tetracycline or Amoxacillin, 500 mg qid × 2 wk

General Management

Endoscopy with any change in symptoms to assess formation of gastric polyps and gastric carcinomas in patients diagnosed with atrophic gastritis and gastric atrophy

Routine Schilling tests or serum vitamin B_{12} levels to evaluate intrinsic factor deficiency

Nutritional Consultation

To help patients identify foods that exacerbate symptoms and select diet that minimizes symptoms

NURSING CARE

Nursing Assessment

Acute Gastritis

General

Malaise

Pain

Asymptomatic; or vague complaints of postprandial distress after a large meal; or vague dyspepsia, particularly relieved by food

Epigastric discomfort or fullness, cramping

Pattern of discomfort in relation to food or drug ingestion

History of ethyl alcohol (ETOH) or aspirin (ASA) intake

Gastrointestinal

Nausea, vomiting, eructation

Hematemesis, melena

Hemorrhage

Abdominal Examination

Abdominal tenderness

---

*Colloidal bismuth subcitrate is the preferred bismuth compound for treatment of *Helicobacter pylori* but is not yet FDA-approved in the United States; bismuth subsalicylate (Pepto-Bismol) is being studied and is currently part of the recommended triple regimen.

Nutritional Status

Anorexia, early satiety

Weight loss

Chronic Gastritis

Often asymptomatic

Gastrointestinal

Dyspepsia, epigastric fullness after eating, diarrhea, flatulence, steatorrhea, bleeding

Pain

No relief with antacids

Nutritional Status

Intolerance of fatty or spicy foods

Anorexia, weight loss

Oral Examination

Cheilosis, glossitis, stomatitis (associated with pernicious anemia)

Extremities

Numbness and tingling

Nursing Dx & Intervention

Fluid volume deficit related to active upper gastrointestinal bleeding

- Observe patient for early signs of gastrointestinal bleeding: hematemesis, melena, blood in nasogastric aspirate or stool.
- Assess for signs of hypovolemic shock and initiate replacement of fluid volume.
- Permit nothing by mouth; keep patient quiet if hemorrhage is considered a possibility.
- Maintain intravenous fluids and blood as ordered and observe for transfusion reactions.
- Prepare patients for endoscopy as a diagnostic or treatment procedure.

Altered nutrition: less than body requirements related to postprandial distress

- Assess patient's nutritional status, since dietary intake may be altered *because of symptoms related to eating*.
- Identify foods or fluids that irritate or exacerbate, and avoid these.
- Monitor intake and output.
- Record nausea and vomiting.
- Administer antiemetics as ordered.
- Provide frequent (approximately six) small feedings a day if acute gastritis *to relieve postprandial distress associated with large meals*.
- Nutritional consultation to help patient identify irritating foods and select diet that minimizes symptoms.

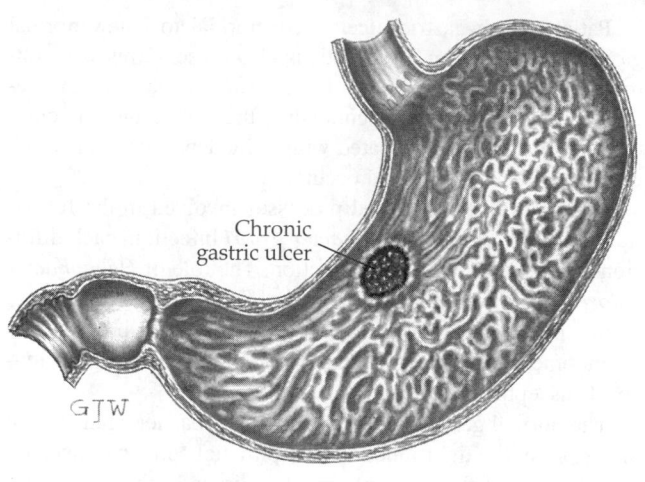

Figure 8-10 Gastric peptic ulcer. (From Doughty.[17])

Evaluation

Volume status is within normal limits Bleeding has stopped (hematemesis and melena are absent). Blood pressure and pulse are within normal limits for patient. Patient is taking oral fluids.

Nutrition is adequate Patient will have an appetite, and weight will be stable. Serum vitamin B_{12} level is within normal limits. Schilling test is normal (8% to 40% of original oral dose of radioactive vitamin B_{12} appears in a 24-hour urine specimen).

GASTRIC ULCERS

A gastric ulcer is a well-defined break in the gastric mucosa that penetrates the muscularis mucosae.

A gastric ulcer (Figure 8-10) must be differentiated from a duodenal ulcer and from gastric erosion. Often gastric ulcers are included with duodenal ulcers and discussed under the classification of peptic ulcer disease. However, the incidence and pathophysiology of gastric and duodenal ulcers are not the same. Duodenal ulcers are three to four times more common than gastric ulcers.[63] *Helicobacter pylori* is the etiologic factor in most patients with gastric and duodenal ulcers, although acid is also implicated.

Gastric ulcers affect males and females equally with a peak incidence at age 55 to 65. Approximately 3000 people die each year from gastric ulcers. The recurrence rate in the first 2 years after healing by medical therapy is approximately 40%, with 70% recurring within the first year. Gastric ulcers account for about 20% of all peptic ulcers. Three percent to 5% of all gastric ulcers are carcinomas, occurring more commonly in the larger ulcers (those that are greater than 2 cm in diameter). Gastric ulcers are strongly correlated with aspirin and alcohol abuse.* Other causative drugs or agents are those that damage the gastric mucosal barrier (nonsteroidal antiinflammatory drugs [NSAIDs], Tylenol, ASA, and salt). Gastric ulcers form scar tissue when they heal. Complications of gastric ulcers include bleeding, obstruction, and perforation.

Nonsteroidal antiinflammatory drugs (NSAIDs) are believed to increase the rate of ulcer complications by fourfold in the elderly. Because of their widespread therapeutic usage, major research investigations are currently focused on the development of new NSAIDs that are devoid of or have reduced gastroduodenal toxicity. The most promising of these are nitric oxide–releasing NSAIDs.[32] Research has also concentrated on coprescribed cytoprotective drugs such as misoprostol (Cytotec) and omeprazole (Prilosec).

Gastric ulcers are more common in people with type A blood (type O is more common in people with duodenal ulcers). Gastric ulcers also occur within family groups. Smokers develop gastric ulcers more frequently than nonsmokers and have slower healing of existing ulcers.[47]

•••••• Pathophysiology

Gastric ulcers are generally found at the junction of the fundic with the pyloric mucosa. Ulcers in the antrum are usually smaller than those in the proximal part of the stomach. Gastritis is more common in patients with gastric ulcers and is often seen around the ulceration. The relationship of gastritis and gastric ulcer can be stated as follows: it appears that a gastric ulcer is more than a localized lesion and that gastritis contributes to the hyposecretion of gastric acid and to the susceptibility of the mucosa to ulcerate.

---

*Aspirin abuse is considered to be the ingestion of 15 or more aspirins per week.[63]

Patients with gastric ulcers have normal to below normal gastric acid secretion. If gastritis is also present, this will contribute to the hyposecretion of acid. An exception to the decreased acid production occurs when the gastric ulcer is close to the pylorus or is associated with a duodenal ulcer, in which case hypersecretion of acid occurs.

There are three proposed processes involved in the formation of gastric ulcers: *Helicobacter pylori* infection, back diffusion of acid, and pyloric dysfunction. The role of *Helicobacter pylori* in gastric ulcer formation is not fully established, but evidence indicates that infection and inflammation promote the development of metaplasia and a consequent increase in mucosal susceptibility to ulceration.[15]

The normal gastric mucosa maintains a barrier against back diffusion by the tight junctions of epithelial cells that mechanically prevent reflux. The plasma membrane of the surface epithelial cells is made up of layers of lipids and contributes to the mucosa barrier.

Agents that are barrier breakers (e.g., aspirin, alcohol, and NSAIDs) disrupt the tight junctions, and acid flows back into the mucosa. Detergents, such as bile salts, and toxic agents can destroy the lipid plasma membrane. When the mucosal barrier is damaged, acid diffuses back from the stomach into the mucosa. Histamine is released, stimulating more acid production, vasodilation, and increased capillary permeability. Bleeding may develop. Protein loss may occur, and an increased sodium content may be found in the stomach.

Bile is generally prevented from contact with the gastric mucosa by a competent pyloric sphincter. In gastric ulcer disease the pyloric sphincter does not respond normally to secretin or cholecystokinin, thus bile is allowed to reflux into the stomach.

Antral motility is also decreased in a patient with a gastric ulcer. The delay in gastric emptying may be observed during barium studies. The effect on antral motility appears to be more common in patients with gastric ulcers near the pylorus. The motility returns to normal when healing occurs.

The four layers of a peptic ulcer include the superficial layer, which lines the ulcer with a white fibrinous coat composed of leukocytes and erythrocytes; a second layer of fibrinoid necrosis; a third layer of inflammatory granulation tissue containing blood vessels; and the fourth layer, a dense scar of fibrous tissue lacking elastic tissue. The dense scar forms the base of the ulcer and extends beyond the margins of the mucosal defect. In a rapidly developing ulceration, massive bleeding may develop in asymptomatic patients when the vessel wall erodes. When the ulceration develops at a slower rate, inflammatory responses, thrombosis, and endarteritis occur and inhibit massive bleeding, and the patient experiences symptoms of peptic ulcer disease.

Ulcers heal slowly because of the scarred avascular tissue. The scarred mucosa over a healed ulcer contains patches of atrophic epithelium and scattered glands. The more scar tissue present, the thinner the mucosal layer. Endarteritis is frequent, and the muscularis mucosae is interrupted and may be partially obliterated. The mucosa and glands that develop are often a simple pyloric type with areas of intestinalization, rather than gastric glands of the fundic type.

••••• Diagnostic Studies and Findings

Endoscopy and biopsy (esophagogastroduodenoscopy) May be used as an initial procedure in actively bleeding patients; may identify gastric ulcers too shallow to detect with barium studies; biopsy to rule out gastric cancer; endoscopy repeated in 4 to 6 weeks for evaluation of treatment

Double-contrast barium study (upper GI) Detection of a gastric ulcer; when present, radiologist must determine whether lesion is a gastric ulcer or a gastric carcinoma

Gastric analysis (pentagastrin stimulation) Average gastric acid output is normal to low

Gastric cytologic findings Abnormal findings would indicate gastric carcinoma

Laboratory studies Hypochromic anemia; gastrin levels normal or slightly elevated; stool for guaiac often positive

Enzyme-linked immunosorbent assays (ELISA) For detection of serum antibodies to *Helicobacter pylori*

Urease test Endoscopic biopsy specimen placed in solution of urea and phenol red; presence of *Helicobacter pylori* turns solution pink; 90% sensitivity to *Helicobacter pylori* after 3 h; biopsy specimens should be sent for histologic examination only if urease test negative after 3 h

••••• Multidisciplinary Plan

Surgery

Medical management usually successful; surgery is indicated in the following situations:
  Recurrent gastric ulcer, persistent bleeding or hemorrhage, perforation, penetration, obstruction, intractability
Types of procedures
  Partial gastrectomy; parietal cell vagotomy and excision of ulcer; vagotomy and pyloroplasty; parietal cell vagotomy

Medications

Histamine receptor antagonists
  Cimetidine (Tagamet), 300 mg po qid, 400 mg po bid, 800 mg po at bedtime
  Ranitidine (Zantac), 150 mg po bid, 300 mg po after dinner
  Famotidine (Pepcid), 40 mg po after dinner
  Nizatidine (Axid), 300 mg po qd, 150 po bid
Proton pump inhibitor
  Omeprazole (Prilosec), 20–40 mg/d (not yet approved by the FDA for treatment of acute gastric ulcers)
Helicobacter pylori
  Bismuth subsalicylate,* 2 tabs qid × 2 wk
  Metronidazole, 250 mg tid × 2 wk
  Tetracycline or Amoxacillin, 500 mg qid × 2 wk

---

*Colloidal bismuth subcitrate is the preferred bismuth compound for treatment of *Helicobacter pylori* but is not yet FDA-approved in the United States; bismuth subsalicylate (Pepto-Bismol) is being studied and is currently part of the recommended triple regimen.

Buffers
  Antacids 500-1000 mmol/d, 1 and 3 h after eating and at bedtime
Cytoprotective
  Sucralfate, 1 g qid on an empty stomach (not yet FDA-approved for this indication)

General Management

Esophagogastroduodenoscopy (EGD) to manage bleeding
Room temperature water or saline lavage if massive hemorrhage
Arteriography with intraarterial vasopressin if intractable bleeding
Avoid spicy foods, coffee (both decaffeinated and caffeinated), tea, 80 proof alcohol, smoking, known ulcerogenic substances (aspirin [ASA], steroids, nonsteroidal antiinflammatory drugs [NSAIDs]); discontinue NSAIDs if possible
Rest

Nutritional Consultation

To help patient identify foods that irritate gastric mucosa and develop dietary plan that minimizes symptoms

NURSING CARE

Nursing Assessment

General

Fatigue

Pain (No Symptoms to Vague Symptoms and Atypical Symptoms)

Heartburn, dyspepsia
Relation of pain to ingestion of food (pain in gastric ulcer usually occurs closer to ingestion of food than in duodenal ulcer)
Location of pain in left midepigastric area or pain radiating to the back (ulcer on posterior wall)
Relief of pain with antacids
Epigastric distress on an empty stomach described as gnawing, burning, hunger pangs
Use of ulcerogenic substances (ASA, NSAIDs, alcohol)

Gastrointestinal

Anorexia
Vomiting, fullness, distention

Nutrition

Weight loss common

Abdominal Examination

Epigastric tenderness, voluntary muscle guarding

Complications

Hemorrhage, perforation, obstruction (see signs and symptoms in "Duodenal Ulcer," p. 718)

Nursing Dx & Intervention

Altered renal, cerebral, cardiopulmonary, gastrointestinal, and peripheral tissue perfusion related to blood loss

- Assess patient for gastrointestinal bleeding: monitor vital signs, central venous pressure, Swan-Ganz catheter pressure, laboratory values, urinary output, early signs of hypovolemic shock.
- Maintain intravenous fluids and blood replacements as ordered to replace fluid volume loss.
- Prepare patient for endoscopic procedures: permit nothing by mouth, explain procedure, and administer preprocedural medications as ordered.
- Institute room temperature lavage if ordered for gastrointestinal bleeding not controlled by endoscopy.

Altered nutrition: less than body requirements related to abdominal pain after eating

- Assess nutritional history, note any weight loss (associated with abdominal pain, distention after eating, and patient's limitation of intake) or gain. *(Some patients may eat more in an attempt to decrease the pain.)*
- Monitor intake and output.
- Record complaints of fullness, nausea, and vomiting *because these symptoms may indicate delayed gastric emptying.*
- Consult with nutritionist.

Pain related to presence of gastric ulcer

- Assess patient for location of pain, relief of pain with antacids, or sudden onset of severe, diffuse abdominal pain *to plan appropriate management and to determine whether perforation occurs.*
- Provide antacids as needed *because pain is often relieved by small amounts of antacids.*

Patient Education/Home Care Planning

1. Discuss with the patient the relationship of causative agents to the development of gastric ulcers, recurrence rate (approximately 40%), and repeat of endoscopy.
2. Provide written information on medication regimen, and ensure that the patient can identify the drugs and when each is to be taken, which require empty stomach or should be taken after a meal, and so forth.
3. Discuss with the patient diet management during the acute phase: avoid spices, avoid alcohol, avoid any type of coffee or tea, avoid citrus acid juices, avoid binges and overdistention.
4. Ensure that the patient understands that milk ingestion is not encouraged because of increased gastric acid secretion.
5. Give the patient a list of over-the-counter remedies that contain salicylates.
6. Discuss the importance of continued treatment, even in the absence of overt symptoms.

Evaluation

Volume status is normal   Bleeding has stopped (hematemesis and melena are absent). Blood pressure and pulse are within normal limits for the patient. Patient is taking oral fluids.

Nutrition is adequate   Patient tolerates recommended diet. Patient has an appetite. Patient's protein and calorie intake is adequate.

Pain is relieved   Patient is able to identify irritating substances in diet and to avoid them. Patient understands medication regimen and how medications are used to alleviate symptoms.

INTESTINAL DISORDERS

■ DUODENAL ULCERS

A duodenal ulcer is a chronic circumscribed break in the duodenal mucosa extending through the muscularis mucosae that leaves a residual scar with healing. The duodenal ulcer is the most common form of peptic ulcer disease.

The incidence of duodenal ulcers has been decreasing since the 1950s. Currently, there are about 200,000 to 400,000 new cases a year.[26] Men are 1.5 to 3 times more likely than women to develop a duodenal ulcer.[26] The incidence increases with age until approximately the age of 60. Risk factors include *Helicobacter pylori* infection, NSAIDs, cigarette smoking,[47] and coffee. Genetic and environmental factors have also been implicated in the development of duodenal ulcer disease.

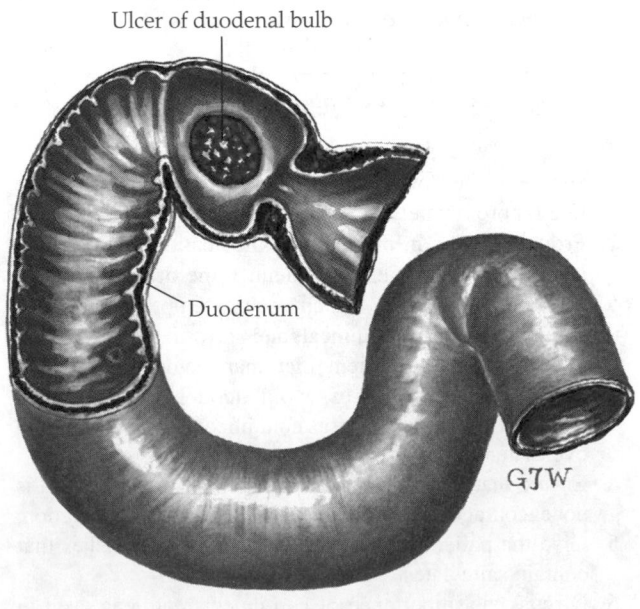

Ulcer of duodenal bulb

Duodenum

GJW

Figure 8-11 Duodenal peptic ulcer. (From Doughty.[17])

More efficient diagnostic techniques and treatment may also have a role in the decline of duodenal ulcers. The duodenal ulcer (Figure 8-11) can be differentiated from dyspepsia, duodenitis, and gastric ulcer. Medical treatment with H_2 receptor antagonists has been successfully used, and patients often undergo diagnostic techniques and treatment as outpatients. Surgery is used only to manage complications of duodenal ulcers such as perforation.

There are also regional differences in duodenal ulcers. For example, prevalence is higher in Scotland and northern England than southern England. In India, duodenal ulcers are more common in the south. Occupational factors have also been associated with duodenal ulcers. The common myth that duodenal ulcers occur in high-pressured professionals and executives is not true.[50,61] Duodenal ulcers are more common in unskilled laborers and lower-income families, and more common in Caucasians than in other races.

Recently the organism *Helicobacter pylori* has been strongly implicated in the possible pathogenesis of duodenal ulcers. The organism has an affinity with gastric-type epithelium (a circumstance that is common in the duodenum of patients with duodenal ulcers). Duodenal hyperacidity causes gastric metaplasia,[51] which may increase mucosal susceptibility to ulceration.

•••••• Pathophysiology

The duodenal ulcer usually is less than 1 cm in diameter and is located 0.5 to 2 cm from the pylorus. Duodenal ulcers occur on both the anterior and posterior walls. The ulcers on the anterior wall appear to have a greater incidence of perforation. Posterior wall ulcers tend to be larger. The four layers of a peptic ulcer are as follows:[63]

1. Superficial layer lining the ulcer with a white fibrinous coat composed of leukocytes and erythrocytes
2. Zone of fibrinoid necrosis
3. Inflammatory granulation tissue
4. Layer of dense fibrotic tissue without elastic tissue (scar), forming the base of the ulcer and extending beyond the margins

Patients with duodenal ulcers secrete more gastric acid than normal in basal states and in response to stimuli. The increased acid production may be the result of an increased capacity to secrete hydrochloric acid because of increased parietal cell mass, or heightened vagal activity increasing the response to stimuli to overproduce acid, or a decreased ability to stop or "turn off" gastric secretions.

The nervous system phase of gastric secretions includes impulses from the cortex (limbic system and hypothalamus) to the vagal nerve. Vagal stimulation acts directly on the parietal cells and indirectly on the antral G cells to release gastrin. Pepsin and hydrochloric acid secretions are stimulated. The stimuli to the nervous system may include food in the mouth (tactile), thoughts and anticipation of food, or the sight of food.

Gastric activity also affects the regulation of secretions. The person with a duodenal ulcer secretes larger amounts of gastric juices and may be unable to stop the release of gastrin in response to normal hormonal stimuli. The concentration of acid in the duodenum is higher than normal. Hypersecretion of acid, in and of itself, does not result in a duodenal ulcer, but has been shown to be a factor in its development.

The emotional aspects of the duodenal ulcer patient must also be considered. Ulcer patients as a group tend to repress external expressions of emotions and feelings. It may be that psychosocial stressors and increased susceptibility to stressful life events plus familial or environmental factors may be related to duodenal ulcers.

The more rapid the development of the ulcer, the more likely that blood vessels in the ulcer will show inflammatory changes, medial hypertrophy, or endarteritis. Blood vessels adjacent to the ulcer will have arteriosclerotic changes. The blood vessels 5 cm away from the ulcer will appear normal. In rapidly developing ulcers, bleeding is more common and may be massive because the blood vessel wall may erode in an asymptomatic patient. In instances where the duodenal ulcer develops slowly, thrombosis, endarteritis, and inflammatory changes result in an avascular, scarred area that heals slowly.

In addition to upper gastrointestinal bleeding, other complications of duodenal ulcer disease include gastric outlet obstruction, perforation, and intractable pain. Obstruction of the gastric outlet may be caused by spasms, edema, or scarring. Protracted vomiting may indicate outlet obstruction.

Perforation is a life-threatening event. Perforation occurs in 2% to 5% of all duodenal ulcers. The overall incidence has been decreasing.

Intractability may develop from other complications of duodenal ulcers, stresses in patients' lives, and other disorders. Primarily, the patient no longer responds to medical management, or recurrences interfere with activities of daily living. Posterior penetration of the ulcer through the duodenal wall and into the pancreas will alter the pain. An increase in pain, loss of antacid relief, and radiation of pain to the back are the primary symptoms. Acute pancreatitis is rare but may occur.

•••••• Diagnostic Studies and Findings

Endoscopy and biopsy (esophagogastroduodenoscopy) May be used as initial procedure in actively bleeding patients; presence of an ulcer; degree of healing

Double-contrast barium studies (Upper GI) Presence of a crater, scar, or deformity in duodenum; delayed gastric emptying of barium (gastric outlet obstruction)

Gastric analysis (pentagastrin stimulation) Hypersecretion of gastric acid (also used to evaluate effectiveness of vagotomy in reducing acidity)

Laboratory studies Creatinine, calcium; hypochromic anemia; stool for guaiac often positive in chronic ulcer; pepsinogen level—high level; serum amylase—increased with posterior penetration (complication)

Enzyme-linked immunosorbent assays (ELISA) For detection of serum antibodies to *Helicobacter pylori*

Urease test Endoscopic biopsy specimen placed in solution of urea and phenol red; presence of *Helicobacter pylori* turns solution pink; 90% sensitivity to *Helicobacter pylori* after 3 h; biopsy specimens should be sent for histologic examination only if urease test negative after 3 h

•••••• Multidisciplinary Plan

Surgery

Medical management usually successful; surgery is indicated usually for complications:
Perforation, penetration, obstruction, and intractability
Types of procedures
Removal of a portion of gastrin-producing portion of stomach (antrectomy or partial gastrectomy) with attachment of duodenum to stomach (Billroth I) or attachment of stomach to jejunum (Billroth II) and vagotomy
Complications of surgical procedures
Alkaline reflux gastritis; afferent loop syndrome; bezoar formation; malnutrition

Medications

Histamine receptor antagonists (do not take within 2 h of antacids)
Cimetidine (Tagamet), 300 mg qid po, 400 mg bid po, 800 mg po at bedtime
Ranitidine (Zantac), 300 mg po after dinner
Famotidine (Pepcid), 20 mg po after dinner
Nizatidine (Axid), 300 mg po after dinner
Antacids
Antacids (aluminum-magnesium regimen), po: provide 144 mEq buffering capacity 1 and 3 h after a meal and at bedtime (amount required varies based on commercial antacid used; Table 8-2)

TABLE 8-2   Relative Potency of Liquid Antacids

Antacid	Potency*
Concentrated aluminum and magnesium hydroxides	
Delcid	100
Maalox Therapeutic Concentrates	75
Mylanta II	75
Gelusil II	60
Regular aluminum and magnesium hydroxides	
Maalox	45
Mylanta	40
Gelusil	40
Riopan	40
Aluminum hydroxide	
Alternagel	40
Amphojel	20

Modified from Sleisenger.[61]
*Millimoles of neutralizing capacity per 15 ml.

Proton pump inhibitor
   Omeprazole (Prilosec), 20 mg/d for 4-8 wk
Helicobacter pylori
   Bismuth subsalicylate,* 2 tabs qid × 2 wk
   Metronidazole, 250 mg tid × 2 wk
   Tetracycline or Amoxicillin, 500 mg qid × 2 wk
Cytoprotective
   Sucralfate (Carafate), 1 g qid on empty stomach for 4-8
   wk; avoid other medications 30 min before and after
   dose
Prostaglandin E Analog
   Misoprostol (Cytotec), 200-400 μg bid to qid; take before
   eating and at bedtime to decrease adverse effects; used
   prophylactically to prevent duodenal ulcer in patients
   taking NSAIDs

General Management

Esophagogastroduodenoscopy (EGD) to manage bleeding
Room temperature water or saline lavage, if massive hemorrhage
Arteriography with intraarterial vasopressin for intractable bleeding
Avoid spicy foods, coffee (both decaffeinated and caffeinated), tea, alcohol, smoking, known ulcerogenic substances (aspirin [ASA], steroids, nonsteroidal antiinflammatory drugs [NSAIDs]) when possible
Rest

Nutritional Consultation

To assist patient in identification of foods and eating patterns that contribute to increased gastric acid secretion and subsequent mucosal irritation, and to develop diet that minimizes gastric acid secretion and ulcer symptoms

NURSING CARE

Nursing Assessment

Pain (No Symptoms to Vague and Atypical Symptoms)

Heartburn, dyspepsia
Relation of pain to ingestion of food (pain in duodenal ulcer) usually occurs 45 to 60 minutes after eating, and there is pain at night
Chronic or periodic symptoms
Relief of pain with antacids
Well-localized epigastric pain occurring when stomach is empty, relieved by food, vomiting, or antacids
Use of ulcerogenic substances (ASA, NSAIDs, alcohol)

---

*Colloidal bismuth subcitrate is the preferred bismuth compound for treatment of *Helibacter pylori* but is not yet FDA-approved in the United States; bismuth subsalicylate (Pepto-Bismol) is being studied and is currently part of the recommended triple regimen.

Gastrointestinal

Constipation (may be related to diet and drugs)
Diarrhea (may be present from antacid therapy)

Nutrition

Weight gain (patient may eat more frequently in attempt to alleviate symptoms)

Abdominal Examination

Epigastric tenderness, voluntary muscle guarding

Complications

Upper Gastrointestinal Bleeding

Hematemesis
Melena
Dizziness or syncope
Decreased blood pressure and increased pulse
Decreased hematocrit

Perforation of Duodenum

Sudden, severe, diffuse upper abdominal pain
Referred pain to shoulder
Rigid, boardlike abdomen
Rebound tenderness
Rapid, shallow respirations

Pyloric Outlet Obstruction

Protracted vomiting

Posterior Penetration

Increased pain
Pain radiating to neck
Loss of antacid relief

Nursing Dx & Intervention

Altered renal, cerebral, cardiopulmonary, gastrointestinal, and peripheral tissue perfusion related to blood loss

- Assess patient for gastrointestinal bleeding: monitor vital signs, central venous pressure, Swan-Ganz catheter pressure, laboratory values, urinary output, and early signs of hypovolemic shock.
- Maintain intravenous fluids and blood replacements as ordered *to replace fluid volume loss.*
- Prepare patient for endoscopic procedures: permit nothing by mouth, explain procedure, administer preprocedural medications as ordered.
- Institute room temperature lavage if ordered for gastrointestinal bleeding not controlled by endoscopy.

Pain related to presence of duodenal ulcer

- Observe patient for changes in nature, location, and relief of pain that would denote impending complications.
- Provide antacids at the bedside *to relieve well-localized epigastric pain.*

Patient Education/Home Care Planning

1. Provide instructions (verbal and written) on medication regimen; ensure that the patient can identify drugs and understand when each is to be taken, which medicines require an empty stomach or should be taken after a meal, and so forth.

2. Provide information on relationship of duodenal ulcers and smoking, alcohol, coffee, aspirin-containing compounds, milk, and various antacids.

3. Discuss with the patient diet management during acute phase: avoid spices, avoid 80 proof alcohol, avoid any type of coffee or tea, avoid citrus acid juices, avoid binges and overdistention.

4. Ensure that the patient understands that milk ingestion is not encouraged as a result of increased gastric acid secretion.

5. Give patient a list of over-the-counter remedies that contain salicylates.

6. Discuss the importance of continuing treatment, even in the absence of overt symptoms.

7. Ingestion of alcohol and H_2 blockers (except famotidine) may result in increased absorption of oral alcohol, higher blood levels, and greater susceptibility to alcohol toxicity.

Evaluation

Bleeding has stopped   Hematemesis and melena are absent. Blood pressure and pulse are within normal limits for patient. Patient is taking oral fluids.

Pain is relieved   Patient is able to identify irritating substances in the diet and avoids them. Patient will tolerate recommended diet.

■ APPENDICITIS

Appendicitis is the inflammation of the vermiform appendix; it may be classified as simple, gangrenous, or perforated. Simple appendicitis involves an inflamed and intact appendix, whereas in gangrenous appendicitis the appendix may have focal or extensive necrosis with microscopic perforations. Gross disruption of the appendix wall occurs in perforated appendicitis.

Acute appendicitis is the most common cause of acute abdomen in the United States and is one of the most common indications for emergency abdominal surgery. The rate of appendicitis is 1 in 15, and the disorder is more common in adolescents and young adults. The diagnosis is difficult to determine in very young and elderly individuals. A very young child is often unable to describe the symptoms that are key clues to the diagnosis. In an elderly person the symptoms are vague and may cause the person to delay seeking medical assistance, and then the physician may not consider appendicitis as a possibility. The abdominal tenderness in the elderly may be mild,

making diagnosis more difficult. Acute appendicitis is more common in some families than others. Statistics show acute appendicitis to be slightly more common in males than females.

·····Pathophysiology

Appendicitis can be compared to a closed loop obstruction in which obstruction occurs first and inflammation and infection second. In acute appendicitis (Figure 8-12) the long narrow tube of the appendix is obstructed, hypoxia develops, the mucosa ulcerates, and bacteria invade the wall. The lumen of the appendix may be obstructed by a kinking of the appendix (this is uncommon), edema of the lymphoid tissue, or a fecalith. The lymphoid hyperplasia or edema may develop in response to a viral or bacterial infection. A fecalith is a formed, hard mass of feces. Fecaliths are associated with diets deficient in fiber. After the lumen becomes obstructed, the mucosa continues to secrete fluid until the intraluminal pressure exceeds the venous pressure. Hypoxia develops because blood flow is impeded. The mucosal wall ulcerates, and bacterial invasion occurs. The infection results in more edema, which further impedes blood flow. Gangrene and perforation occur in 24 to 36 hours. Perforation of the appendix creates serious complications, including periappendiceal abscess, pelvic abscess, or peritonitis.

Atypical appendicitis refers to situations in which the symptoms do not follow the classic presentation of appendicitis. The position of the appendix (retrocecal, pelvic, retroileal, preileal, subcecal), the age of the patient, and pregnancy may affect the symptoms of appendicitis, making diagnosis more difficult.

·····Diagnostic Studies and Findings

White blood cells   Elevated, with shift to the left; 10,000 to 16,000/mm³; 75% neutrophils; 10% have normal differential cell counts

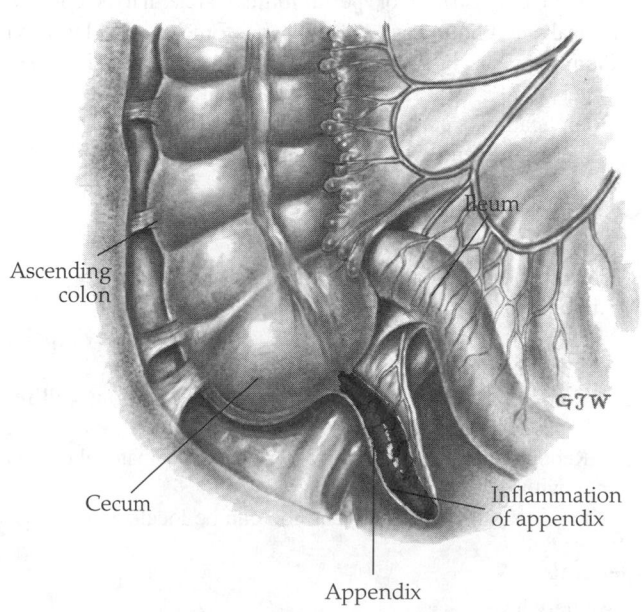

Figure 8-12 Appendicitis (acute). (From Doughty.[17])

Urinalysis   Small number of erythrocytes and leukocytes

Plain films of the abdomen (KUB)   Localized air fluid levels, localized right lower quadrant ileus, increased soft tissue density in the right lower quadrant; altered right psoas shadow, abnormal right flank stripe

Pelvic examination (in females)   To rule out pelvic infection

Ultrasound   May be helpful in patients in whom the clinical features of appendicitis are ambiguous; dilated appendiceal lumen and a thickened wall

CT scan (indicated if mass)   Identifies abscesses and appendicoliths

Intravenous pyelogram (IVP)   To differentiate appendicitis from suspected urinary tract disease

•••••• Multidisciplinary Plan

Surgery

Appendectomy

Medications

Antiinfective agents
   Metronidazole (Flagyl) or cefamandole (Mandol) as a single prophylactic dose before surgery or for a period postoperatively (to prevent wound infection or pelvic abscess)

NURSING CARE

Nursing Assessment

Abdominal Pain (Typical)

Pain in epigastrium or periumbilical area that is colicky, peaks in 4 hours, and subsides (see Emergency Alert box)

Pain reappears in right lower quadrant, is progressively severe, and is exacerbated by movement

Complications: perforation—more severe pain; peritonitis; increasing tenderness and rigidity

Gastrointestinal Functioning

May vomit once or twice; anorexia present

Constipation and failure to pass flatus

Abdominal examination
   Patient can point to localized pain at McBurney's point (midway between iliac crest and umbilicus)
   Coughing or moving abdominal wall up and out will reproduce or exacerbate pain
   Rebound tenderness; muscle rigidity (palpate abdomen with *one* finger)
   Pain on palpation or percussion can be localized to a spot

General

Anxiety level

Low-grade fever, does not usually exceed 39° C (102° F)

Atypical Appendicitis

Retrocecal or retroileal
   Pain less intense (no discomfort with walking or coughing) and poorly localized
   Urinary frequency (irritation of ureter)
Pelvic
   Very severe, constant pain
   Localized pain on left
   Urge to urinate and defecate
   Tenderness on rectal examination
   Absence of muscle rigidity and abdominal tenderness

! EMERGENCY ALERT

ACUTE ABDOMINAL PAIN

Acute onset of abdominal pain needs immediate evaluation

ASSESSMENT

- Determine *PQRST*
   P = Precipitating factors
   Q = Quality
   R = Radiation
   S = Severity
   T = Time of onset
- Assess associated symptoms such as nausea, vomiting, diarrhea, constipation, fever, chills, urinary tract symptoms (frequency, burning, pain), gynecologic symptoms (pain, discharge, missed menses) gastrointestinal upset.
- Conduct a thorough physical assessment of the abdomen, including inspection, auscultation, palpation, and percussion.
- Determine laboratory tests to be obtained specific to symptoms.
- Determine radiologic studies to be obtained specific to symptoms.

INTERVENTIONS

- If indicated, maintain ABC's.
- Obtain IV access as indicated by vital signs and hydration.
- Obtain results of relevant laboratory and radiologic studies.
- If indicated, keep client NPO until possible surgical evaluation is completed.
- Surgical intervention may be indicated for the following problems:
   appendicitis
   bowel obstruction
   cholecystitis
   diverticulitis
   massive GI bleeding
   pancreatitis
   peritonitis
   perforation of viscus
   ruptured ectopic pregnancy
   urethral stone
   ruptured intraabdominal aneurysm

In elderly persons
 Symptoms vague; pain minimal
 Pain
In pregnancy
 Late in gestation, diagnosis more difficult because of displacement of cecum by uterus

Nursing Dx & Intervention

Pain related to appendiceal inflammation

- Assess patient's description of the pain type, duration, changes in, and location because these data are important to the diagnosis.
- Help patient reduce pain by having him or her lie still and avoid sudden movements, such as coughing.
- Administer analgesics as ordered after the diagnosis has been established.

Anxiety related to fear of the unknown and to the impending surgery

- Assess patient and family for increased tension, apprehension, and other characteristics associated with fear.
- Provide emotional support for patient and family because the pain is acute and frightening and surgery is imminent.
- Reassure patient during physical examination of the abdomen because the procedure is extremely painful; limit the number of abdominal examinations performed.

Patient Education/Home Care Planning

1. Wound or incisional care instructions should be provided.
2. A pattern of increasing activities (i.e., walking, driving) should be provided as recommended by the physician.

Evaluation

Comfort level is achieved Reduction or absence of guarding, protective behavior. Uses pain control strategies appropriately. Verbalizes increased control over pain.

Anxiety is reduced Absence or reduction of defining characteristics indicating the presence of anxiety.

DIVERTICULAR DISEASE

Diverticulosis is the presence of diverticula, pouchlike herniations through the muscular wall of the intestine. They may occur anywhere throughout the gut but are most common in the sigmoid colon. Diverticulitis is the most frequent complication of diverticular disease and the result of inflammation or perforation of one or more diverticula.

Diverticular disease is more common in developed Westernized countries. It is probably secondary to a diet that is low in fiber. African, Asian, and Third World countries have low rates of diverticular disease; however, when a Western diet is adopted by blacks in Africa, diverticular disease develops.[63]

It is uncommon to find diverticular disease in persons younger than 40. The incidence of diverticular disease increases with age. One third to one half of all autopsies on persons age 60 and over show that they have diverticular disease.[61] Ninety-five percent of diverticula are in the sigmoid colon.[67] Ten percent to 20% of patients with diverticulosis will have diverticulitis develop (Figure 8-13), or they will hemorrhage over time. Bleeding from diverticular disease is one of the most common causes of lower gastrointestinal hemorrhage.[61]

• • • • • • Pathophysiology

The development of diverticula is related to the pressures generated in the bowel lumen. Normal intraluminal pressure is less than 10 mm Hg in the sigmoid colon. The normal pressure can be increased significantly when the bowel is divided into segments by the muscular contraction rings. The muscular activities in the localized segments can exert enough pressure to increase intracolonic pressure to 90 mm Hg, and this high pressure may push out diverticula through "weak spots" where blood vessels enter the colon wall.[71]

Symptoms of diverticular disease that are considered complications are caused by the associated motility disorder and not to the presence of the diverticula. Intraluminal pressures in diverticular disease are excessive in response to food ingestion, morphine, and parasympathomimetic agents. These pressures are virtually identical to intraluminal pressures recorded in patients with irritable bowel syndrome.

Constipation has been associated with diverticular disease. More pressure is required to move hard, dry fecal material

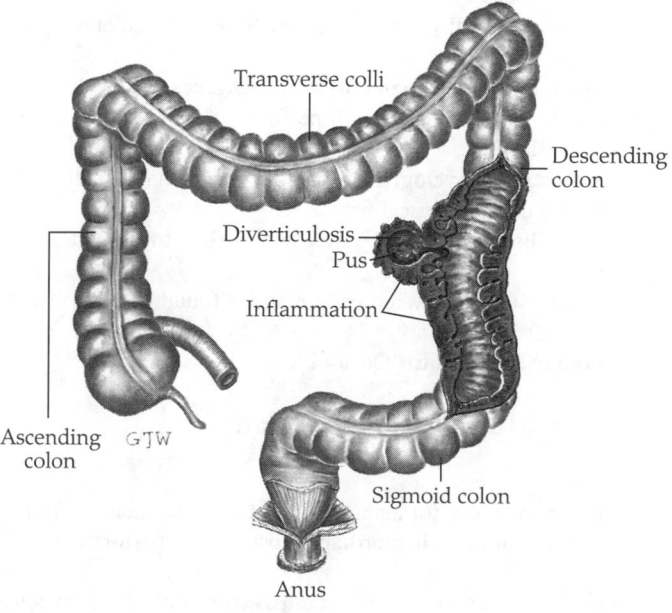

Figure 8-13 Diverticulosis (diverticulitis). (From Doughty.[17])

through the lumen. Moist, soft stools and multiple bowel movements each day are associated with high-fiber diets. The decrease in segmentation and intracolonic pressures with high-fiber diets may lessen the symptoms of diverticulosis and impede progression of the disease.

The blood flow to the large colon runs from the mesentery around the bowel and divides into branches that go subserosally. These vessels enter the circular muscle obliquely from the mesenteric side of the bowel between the mesenteric and lateral teniae. There is a rich submucosa plexus around the circumference of the colon. The diverticulum that pushes out under the muscular coat has a prominent vasculature over the dome of the diverticulum and at the antemesenteric border of the orifice of the diverticulum. Major bleeding in diverticular disease is associated with the large vessel over the dome. Localized inflammation at the base of the diverticulum with vascular granulation tissue may be the source of minor bleeding from diverticula.

Complications include bleeding, intraabdominal abscesses, fistulas (to distant bowel, bladder, vagina, or abdominal wall), bowel obstructions, and generalized peritonitis.

•••••• Diagnostic Studies and Findings

Barium enema (not used in acute diverticulitis) Demonstrates diverticulum, segmental spasms, narrowed lumen, thickened interhaustral folds (sawtooth appearance)

Water-soluble contrast enema (used in acute diverticulitis) Demonstrates abscess cavities, sinus tracts, fistula, intramural abscesses, extrinsic compression.

Plain abdominal films Free abdominal air (perforation); ileus (localized inflammation); small bowel obstruction; normal in uncomplicated diverticular disease

CT scan (with IV and oral contrast) Effacement of pericolic fat, abscess, fistulas (diverticulitis)

Ultrasonography May demonstrate extracolonic fluid collections

Sigmoidoscopy or colonoscopy Orifices of the diverticula may be visible (high risk of perforation if instrument enters a diverticulum)

Intravenous pyelogram To rule out a mass on the left ureter or a colonic vesical fistula

White blood cells Elevated with a shift to the left in diverticulitis

Urinalysis A few red cells may be found in urine if left ureter is affected

Stool examination Occult blood

•••••• Multidisciplinary Plan

Surgery

Surgery reserved for management of complications or for recurrent attacks; hemorrhage, obstruction, perforation, and fistula

Primary resection with anastomosis (if bowel not edematous or if there is not gross infection present)

Primary resection with temporary colostomy (two-stage procedure) if bowel is edematous or in presence of gross infection

Medications

Diverticulosis

Bran, 10 to 25 g/d in divided doses (must slowly increase to develop tolerance; will help relieve abdominal pain; lowers intraluminal pressure)

Laxatives

Hydrophilic colloid laxatives (rather than bran in acute phases may be better tolerated; slowly decrease amount as bran and fiber in diet increase)

Diverticulitis

Intravenous fluid therapy

Narcotic analgesic

Meperidine (Demerol) for analgesia (dose calculated for patient)

Ampicillin (Amcill), 2 g, *or*

Cephalexin (Keflex), 1-4 g/d parenterally in divided doses (mild diverticulitis)

Gentamicin (Garamycin) or tobramycin (Nebcin), 5 mg/kg/d, and clindamycin (Cleocin), 1.6-2.4 g/d parenterally in divided doses (severe diverticulitis or perforation)

Chloramphenicol (Chloromycetin), 4 g/d tapering to 2 g/d (severe diverticulitis)

Cefoxitin (Mefoxin), 4-6 g/d parenterally in divided doses

All antiinfective agents continued for 7-10 d; not all listed would be used; agents chosen should cover the major colon pathogens: anaerobes, gram-negative bacilli, and gram-positive coliforms

General Management

Nasogastric tube inserted if nausea, vomiting, and abdominal distention are severe

Radiographic studies and ultrasonography used to evaluate the response to therapy (i.e., resolution of abscess)

Carcinoma: difficult to detect in bowel with narrowed areas and partial obstruction; use colonoscopy procedures to distinguish between acute diverticular disease and carcinoma after an acute episode

Bleeding: angiographic injection of vasopressin, 0.5 to 1 ml/min

High-fiber diet for managing diverticulosis

Give nothing to eat initially in acute diverticulitis; slowly resume diet; when inflammation has resolved and bowel functioning returns to normal, resume high-fiber diet

For acute diverticulitis, bed rest

Nutritional Consultation

To advise patient in choices for selecting a high-fiber diet

NURSING CARE

Nursing Assessment

Pain

Diverticulosis
Ranges from no pain to intermittent cramping, left lower abdominal pain
Diverticulitis
Pain more intense; may be severe pain; in the elderly it is often difficult to assess pain

Abdominal Examination

Diverticulosis
Tenderness in left lower colon, palpable colon, distention; sometimes there are no symptoms
Diverticulitis
Palpable colon, tenderness in the left lower quadrant, distended and tympanic abdomen, decreased bowel sounds; may hear increased bowel sounds with abdominal distention if obstruction is present

Gastrointestinal

Constipation or alternating constipation and diarrhea
Blood in stools

Urinary

Dysuria; frequency (associated with bladder involvement)
Passage of gas or stool through urethra (colovesicular fistula)

Nursing Dx & Intervention

Altered renal, cerebral, cardiopulmonary, gastrointestinal, and peripheral tissue perfusion related to sepsis and bleeding

- Assess patient for lower gastrointestinal bleeding, a complication of diverticular disease.
- Assess patient for signs and symptoms of sepsis, a complication of diverticulitis.
- Maintain intravenous fluids, monitor vital signs, intake, and output if complications occur *to prevent intravascular fluid imbalance.*

Pain related to colonic inflammation

- In acute phase, provide low-fiber diet *to allow bowel inflammation to resolve.* (Patients with acute and chronic disease should avoid nuts and popcorn.)
- In diverticulosis, provide bran or other good fiber source with instructions on slowly increasing the amount *to promote soft, moist stools.*
- Discuss with patient efficacy of increasing fiber, fluids, and activity *to prevent constipation.*
- Provide analgesic as ordered.

Constipation related to low-fiber diet, inactivity

- Provide bran or hydrophilic colloid laxative, increase oral fluid intake, and increase patient's activity level *to reduce constipation (dry stool).*
- Initiate dietary consultation or provide information on high-fiber diets.
- See pp. 785 to 788 for management of temporary colostomy and interventions related to care and adaptation.

Patient Education/Home Care Planning

1. Dietary instructions on high-fiber diet should be provided. Teach the patient ways to make bran more palatable (e.g., muffins, use on cereals).
2. Discharge instructions should include relationships of diet to diverticular disease, assessment of bowel movements to evaluate dietary intake of bran and fluids, and signs of complications of acute diverticular disease.
3. Instruct the patient in bowel training, that is, to set aside a time daily without anxiety or interruption to have a bowel movement.
4. See pp. 785 to 788 for colostomy care instructions.

Evaluation

There is no gastrointestinal bleeding Hematocrit and hemoglobin are normal for patient. Patient's vital signs are stable. Stool for occult blood negative.

Comfort level is achieved Patient shows a reduction in or absence of guarding or protective behavior. Patient uses pain control strategies appropriately. Patient verbalizes increased control over pain.

Patient experiences regular bowel movements Patient reports that stools are soft, brown, and regular in caliber.

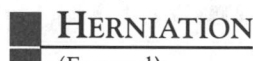 HERNIATION
(External)

A hernia is a protrusion of an organ (usually bowel) through an abnormal opening in the muscle wall. Hernias may be congenital (failure of certain structures to close after birth) or acquired when muscle weakens (associated with obesity, surgery, or illness or from increased abdominal pressure as a result of straining or ascites).

Hernias can occur in any age group. Lifting heavy objects is commonly associated with hernia formation. Approximately 75% of hernias occur in the groin (indirect inguinal, direct inguinal, or femoral). Kinds of hernias include reducible, irreducible, incarcerated, and strangulated. Reducible hernias may be returned to their proper position. They return spontaneously, or they are returned manually. An irreducible hernia (incarcerated) cannot be returned to the abdomen. It is trapped by the narrow neck of the opening or defect. An incarcerated hernia that becomes gangrenous because the contents are constricted is called a strangulated hernia.

•••••• Pathophysiology

External hernias include inguinal, femoral, umbilical, and incisional hernias. The inguinal hernia is the most common. It is a weakness in the abdominal wall where the spermatic cord (men) or the round ligament (women) emerges. In an indirect inguinal hernia the herniation protrudes through the inguinal ring and follows the round ligament or spermatic cord. A direct inguinal hernia goes through the posterior inguinal wall. Inguinal hernias are more common in men.

A femoral hernia, or protrusion through the femoral ring into the femoral canal, is seen as a bulge below the inguinal ligament. It occurs more frequently in women. Femoral hernias strangulate easily.

The umbilical hernia is caused by a gradual yielding of the scar tissue closing the umbilical ring. Predisposing factors include (1) multiple pregnancies with prolonged labor, (2) ascites, (3) obesity, and (4) large intraabdominal tumors.[67] Ventral and incisional hernias are associated with muscle weakness from abdominal incisions. Hernias after surgery are more common in obese persons, the elderly, those with wound infections, and those with general debility.

•••••• Multidisciplinary Plan

Surgery

Herniorrhaphy (surgical repair of hernia) or hernioplasty (reinforcement of weakened area with wire, fascia, or mesh)
Temporary colostomy (for complications of intestinal obstruction or strangulation of hernia)

General Management

Binder or truss (to reduce hernia and to prevent protrusion; danger: strangulation if not reduced properly)

NURSING CARE

Nursing Assessment

Abdominal Examination

Examine patient supine and sitting
Can often see hernia "bulge" or protrude as person changes position or coughs (many patients have a history of being able to reduce their own hernias before seeking repair)
Palpate weakened muscle area
Pain of increasing severity, fever, tachycardia, and abdominal rigidity are signs of strangulations

Nursing Dx & Interventions

High risk for injury related to hernia repair

- Prevent or manage any increased abdominal pressure (coughing, straining at stool, hiccups) that could impair healing at the hernia site.
- Optimize nutrition for adequate wound healing.
- Apply scrotal support for inguinal hernia repairs.

Patient Education/Home Care Planning

1. Inform the patient of the need to lose weight if the patient is obese.
2. The patient should avoid heavy lifting for 6 to 8 weeks, unless otherwise specified by the physician. Give the patient a limit of weight not to carry or lift.
3. If the patient will use a binder at home, provide correct instructions for application. Teach the patient to observe for skin irritation.
4. Teach the patient to splint incision with hands or pillow to provide incisional support if it is necessary to cough or sneeze.
5. Instruct the patient to increase fiber and fluids postoperatively to prevent constipation. If the patient is discharged home on codeine, he or she may need a bulk laxative.
6. See pp. 785 to 788 for management of temporary colostomy and interventions related to care and adaptation.

Evaluation

No injury is present   Patient verbalizes understanding of preventing increased abdominal pressure. Patient is having regular bowel movements. Incision is healing without signs of infection.

■ INTESTINAL OBSTRUCTION

An intestinal obstruction occurs when the contents of the intestines fail to propel forward through the lumen. Intestinal obstructions may be mechanical or functional.

Mechanical obstructions are caused by a blockage of the bowel lumen by adhesion, hernia, volvulus, tumor, inflammation (as in Crohn's disease), impacted feces, or intussusception. Functional obstructions, also referred to as ileus, occur when there is a loss of propulsive peristalsis associated with abdominal surgery, hypokalemia, intestinal distention, peritonitis, severe traumas, spinal fractures, ureteral distention, or the effects of some narcotic drugs and diphenoxylate (Lomotil).

Intestinal obstructions are more common in persons who have undergone abdominal surgery or who have had congenital abnormalities of the bowel. An intestinal obstruction, if untreated, can progress to a life-threatening disorder. The severity and types of symptoms vary according to the cause and location of the intestinal obstruction. Ninety percent of intestinal obstructions are the result of adhesions or incarcerated hernias.

Mechanical obstructions can be caused by factors that block the lumen of the bowel wall, in which case they are referred to as obturation obstructions. This category includes intussusception, large gallstones, feces, bezoars, and ingested foreign objects. Intrinsic factors that may progress to mechanical obstructions include stenosis, strictures associated with chronic inflammation or neoplasms, iatrogenic strictures after intestinal surgery or radiation therapy, and mesenteric vascular occlusion.

Extrinsic factors that may lead to mechanical obstructions of the intestine are the most common cause of intestinal obstructions and include adhesions, hernias, neoplasms, abscesses, and volvulus.

A volvulus is a twisting of the bowel on itself. The two most common sites for the development of a volvulus are the cecum and the sigmoid colon. A cecal volvulus may occur any time from adolescence but is most common in the fifth decade of life. Sigmoid volvulus is more common in the elderly and has been associated with chronic constipation. A volvulus usually develops in an area where an underlying abnormality exists.

Mechanical obstructions may be simple obstructions in the small bowel or colon or strangulation obstructions. The location of a mechanical obstruction is important in determining the sequelae. Simple mechanical obstructions may resolve medically, whereas strangulation obstructions require surgical intervention.

The paralytic ileus or functional obstruction is a state of inhibited motility in the gastrointestinal tract that is temporary and reversible.

•••••• Pathophysiology

An accumulation of fluid and gas proximal to an obstruction occurs in a simple mechanical obstruction of the small bowel. Initially, the pooled fluids include ingested foods and digestive enzymes. Intestinal gas, in obstruction, is primarily made up of swallowed air that has high concentrations of nitrogen and is not absorbed by the intestinal mucosa. The distention of the bowel by the trapped fluids and gases causes the small bowel to secrete water and electrolytes into the obstructed lumen.

The distention impedes venous return and inhibits the absorptive quality of the mucosa. The bowel wall becomes edematous. The bowel continues to secrete water, sodium, and potassium into the obstructed segment. As the obstruction continues, the intestinal distention is self-perpetuating. Distention increases the intestinal secretions of water and electrolytes into the lumen. As fluid and gas pour into the intestine, motility is further compromised and the distention enlarges proximally. Successive loops of proximal bowel distend, fill with fluid, and stop absorbing. Transudation of water through the wall of the obstructed segment may develop, leading to the development of peritoneal fluid. Distention may lead to pressure necrosis of the bowel wall.

Bacteria are not usually found in the small intestine, but during intestinal obstruction an abnormal bacterial flora that rapidly proliferates is found in the intestinal lumen. The bacteria produce hydrogen or methane gases that contribute to the gaseous distention. Also, the small bowel contents become feculent during obstructions as a result of the bacterial proliferation.

The site and duration of intestinal obstruction affect the symptoms and potential metabolic effects. Obstructions in the upper jejunal area usually result in vomiting and little abdominal distention. Dehydration and electrolyte depletion occur.

In distal small bowel obstruction or ileal obstructions, constipation is an early symptom. Vomiting, which is not a promi-

nent symptom, is less effective in reducing intestinal decompression. Reflex vomiting may result from intestinal distention. In distal small bowel obstruction, large quantities of fluid and electrolytes may become trapped in the intestinal lumen, resulting in nausea and passage of gas. As much as 8 L of fluids may be found in the lumen with untreated, prolonged obstructions.[63] The patient has classic signs and symptoms of circulatory shock (severe hypovolemia). Before the development of shock, dehydration and metabolic acidosis accompanied by oliguria, azotemia, and hemoconcentration occur. Early circulatory changes may be detected by tachycardia, low central venous pressure, and hypotension. Hypovolemic shock develops if the obstruction is not treated.

The intestinal distention can impair breathing because abdominal distention causes elevation of the diaphragm. The increased intraabdominal pressure caused by the intestinal distention may impede venous return from the legs.

Death of the bowel wall (bowel necrosis) complicates intestinal obstructions. Shock can quickly develop when long loops of bowel are affected. Short-segment involvement progresses quickly to perforation and peritonitis.

Impaired circulation to the bowel wall during obstructions is referred to as a strangulation obstruction. The circulation may be impeded by a closed-loop obstruction that causes occlusion of the lumen at two points along the length of the bowel segment. Volvulus is an example of a closed-loop obstruction. The closed-loop obstruction progresses to strangulation more rapidly than a simple mechanical blockage of the lumen. The circulation to the bowel may also be impaired by a sustained increase in intraluminal pressure, as with intestinal distention.

When the circulation is impaired, the venous outflow is impaired and the mural veins become engorged. The bowel wall becomes ischemic. An arterial spasm follows, and the bowel responds to anoxia with increased peristalsis. Within 15 minutes, blood escapes from the engorged veins and infiltrates the submucosa and mucosa, resulting in a hemorrhagic infarction of the tissues. Venous thrombosis occurs, further compromising circulation. The necrosis develops from the mucosa outward. Small intravascular thrombi extend the area of necrosis. The lymph channels dilate and may carry bacteria from the lumen into the serosa. Initially, the fluid accumulating resembles plasma, and it gradually becomes bloody and contains bacteria and toxins.

Strangulation results in loss of blood and plasma from the affected segment. Shock occurs quickly if the patient has been dehydrated before strangulation developed. Gangrene may develop and progress to peritonitis. Perforation of the strangulated segment may occur, releasing a toxin that may be absorbed from the peritoneal cavity, producing systemic effects. Bacterial infection and toxemia are generally thought to be responsible for the shock that can quickly develop in strangulation obstructions.

In colonic obstructions the colon may become massively distended by gas. Fluid and electrolyte losses are not as significant as in small bowel obstructions and occur when the obstruction is prolonged. When the ileocecal valve is competent, there is little if any small bowel distention. However, a competent ileocecal valve may resist backward decompression enough to produce a closed-loop obstruction. If this develops, cecal distention may be significant and may progress to perforation of the cecum.

The most common cause of colon obstruction is cancer, and perforation during obstructive episodes is adjacent to the tumor. As in small bowel obstructions, the patient must be carefully observed for signs and symptoms of strangulation obstruction.

•••••• Diagnostic Studies and Findings

Serial abdominal x-rays—plain films   Abnormally large amounts of gas in the bowel; films taken with patient standing or sitting, supine, and on left side; gas- and fluid-filled loops of bowel; gas does not progress downward in serial examinations; cecal volvulus: marked distention of cecum; sigmoid volvulus: large dilated loop, from right to left side of abdomen; two fluid levels can be visualized

Barium enema*   Barium will clear entire colon or stop at site of obstruction; cecal volvulus: conical narrowing at the twist; sigmoid volvulus: narrowing at the twist

Serum electrolytes   Demonstrates electrolyte losses

White blood cell count   Sudden rise greater than 10,000/mm³ indicates strangulation

Serum amylase   Normal value rules out acute pancreatitis; concentration as a result of fluid losses

Arterial blood gas   Acid-base deficits

•••••• Multidisciplinary Plan

Surgery

Used when cause of obstruction is thought to be adhesions, necrosis, tumor, or unresolved inflammatory lesions (e.g., strictures found in Crohn's disease)

Surgical resection of mechanical obstruction after patient's fluid and electrolytes are stabilized; strangulation obstructions are a surgical emergency; in colonic obstructions, surgery is almost always required

Cecal volvulus: untwisting bowel; if viable, the cecum and ascending colon are anchored in place; if gangrene is present, bowel resection of involved parts

Sigmoid volvulus: elective resection of twisted segment; if later viability is questioned, operate without decompression

Obstructing lesions of the right colon

Either a one-stage ileotransverse colostomy or two-stage procedure, with diverting ileostomy in a fragile patient

Obstructing lesions of the left colon

Temporary end colostomy, with resection and later colostomy take-down

Intraoperative colonic lavage, with primary anastomosis

Primary intestinal anastomosis using resection, with intraluminal bypass tube

Cecostomy—in patients with high surgical risk

Transverse colostomy—requires three operations; the first is a decompressing colostomy; the second surgical procedure is resection and anastomosis; the third surgical stage is closure of colostomy

General Management

Nasogastric (for upper or jejunal obstruction) or intestinal suctioning (for distal obstructions); Cantor or Miller-Abbott tubes (used rarely) when obstruction is caused by infection or inflammation and can resolve with medical therapy (intravenous fluids and electrolytes, administration of blood or plasma)

Colonoscopy may assist with reduction of volvulus by releasing trapped gas and fluid (surgery may still be advised after reduction of volvulus if mucosal viability is in doubt)

Medications

Antibiotics if strangulation is present

Prophylactic perioperative antibiotics (for anaerobes and gram-negative organisms) in unprepared bowel; surgery to prevent wound infection and sepsis

NURSING CARE

Nursing Assessment

General

Loss of skin turgor and dry mucous membranes: dehydration

Fever (high fever with strangulation of small bowel; peritonitis)

Anxiety level

Tachycardia and hypotension (may indicate dehydration or peritonitis)

Pain

Crampy abdominal pain; onset clearly recalled

Severe continuous ache (strangulation)

Gastrointestinal

Vomiting

Proximal jejunal obstructions: profuse vomiting unassociated with abdominal distention

Distal small bowel obstruction: feculent odor (secondary to bacterial proliferation in obstructions)

Colonic obstructions: vomiting after prolonged obstructions; usually secondary to pain; may contain fecal material

Obstipation

Obstipation and failure to pass gas are signs of a complete obstruction after the bowel distal to the obstruction has been evacuated

Constipation

---

*Meglucamine diatrizoate (Gastrografin) used if perforation is suspected.

Blood in stools (may indicate strangulation, cancer, intussusception, or infarction of obstructing lesions)

History of previous surgeries, inflammatory bowel disease, diverticulitis, or symptoms of malignancy

Abdominal Examination

Observe and palpate carefully for presence of hernias

Note amount of abdominal distention; girth measurements may be beneficial in observing the progress of an obstruction

Mechanical obstruction: peristalsis is high-pitched, tinkling sound with rushes

Visible peristalsis: seen moving toward obstruction and reversing

Paralytic ileus: absence of bowel sounds or low infrequent sounds

Auscultate abdomen for full 5 minutes before palpating

Localized tenderness, constant pain, guarding, and rebound tenderness are signs of strangulation obstructions

Sigmoid loop volvulus may be palpable

Nursing Dx & Intervention

Fluid volume deficit related to vomiting, third spacing of fluids

- Assess patient carefully for signs and symptoms of severe fluid and electrolyte loss, metabolic acidosis, and hypovolemic shock as a result of accumulation of gas and fluids and distention of intestine and sepsis (if perforation occurs).
- Administer intravenous fluids and electrolytes, blood, and plasma *to replace and maintain fluid volume.*
- Monitor vital signs, central venous pressure, blood pressure, urinary output, and nasogastric aspirations every hour.
- Measure abdominal girth every 4 to 8 hours *to assess distention.*
- Notify physician of changes in patient's status because they generally indicate a decline in patient's stabilization for surgical intervention.

Pain related to intestinal distention, ischemia or obstruction

- Assess abdominal area for signs of perforation and peritonitis: increased severity and diffuseness of pain, rebound tenderness, guarding.
- Help patient assume a comfortable position (one that places minimum stress on the abdominal muscles); limit sudden movement and abdominal examination.
- Provide analgesics as prescribed.

Anxiety related to fear of the unknown and impending surgery

- Assess patient and family for increased tension, apprehension, and other characteristics associated with fear.
- Provide emotional support for patient and family *because the pain is acute and frightening and surgery is often imminent.*
- Reassure patient and explain to patient and family all the tests and procedures. Provide preoperative teaching.

Patient Education/Home Care Planning

1. Do primary postoperative teaching if resection and anastomosis of small bowel obstruction were performed. This includes showering, activity progression, driving, and returning to work.
2. Colonic obstructions are often treated with a temporary diverting colostomy, and the patient requires instruction in colostomy care and plans for continued surgical intervention, and education about the primary cause of the obstruction (see pp. 785 to 788).

Evaluation

Fluid balance is maintained Patient returns to normal hydration levels as assessed by skin turgor, color, and mucous membrane, blood pressure and pulse, and urinary output.

Comfort level is achieved Patient shows reduction or absence of guarding or protective behavior. Patient uses pain control strategies appropriately. Patient verbalizes increased control over pain.

Anxiety is reduced Patient shows absence or reduction of defining characteristics indicating the presence of anxiety.

■ INTESTINAL ISCHEMIA

Intestinal ischemia may develop when the mesenteric vascular supply is insufficient. Acute and chronic occlusion of blood flow to the splanchnic bed, thrombosis or embolus of the superior mesenteric artery, strangulation obstructions, chronic vascular insufficiency, anoxia, hypotension, or other low-flow states may lead to intestinal ischemia.

Intestinal ischemia has in the past been difficult to diagnose. The symptoms initially do not correspond with physical examination and laboratory findings. As the ischemia progresses, the severity of the patient's condition becomes apparent, and perforation and peritonitis may have already occurred. Advances in angiography have assisted the physician in diagnosing intestinal ischemias. Awareness of intestinal ischemias is increasing and angiography is being used to rule out acute occlusion of vessels when patients are seen with sudden onset of severe abdominal pain. Poor perfusion of the intestine is known to result in ischemia, and the syndromes of poor perfusion are gaining more attention. The frequency of thrombosis or embolus as the cause of mesenteric ischemia has been reported to be as high as 75%. Diagnosis of poor perfusion syndromes as the pathologic cause of the ischemic episode has decreased the incidence of occlusions of the large vessels to 25%.[63]

Advances in vascular surgery and advances in nutritional and fluid replacement after intestinal resections have allowed a more aggressive approach in the treatment of intestinal ischemias. Although vascular disorders of the intestines are more common in older persons with arteriosclerosis, cases have been reported in children and pregnant women.[41]

•••••• Pathophysiology

The blood flow to the intestines may be affected by a variety of factors.[41] The following factors increase splanchnic blood flow:

Presence of food

Digestive hormones: gastrin, secretin, and cholecystokinin

Metabolite-produced muscle activity

β-stimulating sympathomimetic amines

The following factors decrease splanchnic blood flow:

Physical activities

Abdominal distention (marked intraluminal pressure)

α-Stimulating sympathomimetic amines

Cardiac glycosides (digitalis)

The response to the alteration in blood flow depends on the degree of obstruction of blood flow, the rapidity of onset, the duration of the process, and the efficiency of the collateral circulation. Disease processes may affect both large and small vessels. This section reviews the normal pattern of blood flow to the intestines; the cause of alteration of blood flow, including a variety of diseases that affect blood distribution to the bowel; and the pathophysiology of events.

The intestine receives its blood supply from the celiac, the superior mesenteric, and the inferior mesenteric arteries. These three major vessels arise from the abdominal aorta and subdivide into a complex collateral circulation. The celiac artery divides into the splenic, left gastric, and hepatic arteries to supply the stomach, proximal duodenum, liver, pancreas, and spleen. The hepatic artery divides into the gastroduodenal artery, which divides to form the superior pancreaticoduodenal and right gastroepiploic arteries. The celiac axis is interconnected with the superior mesenteric artery through pancreaticoduodenal arcades. Ischemic necrosis of the stomach is uncommon because of this rich collateral network.

The superior mesenteric artery divides into the ileocolic, middle colic, and right colic arteries. The terminal ileum, cecum, and proximal ascending colon are supplied by the ileocolic artery. The ascending colon and hepatic flexure are supplied by the right colic artery. The middle colic vessel supplies the proximal portion of the transverse colon.

In addition to the above branches, the superior mesenteric artery divides into smaller arteries that supply the jejunum and ileum. The superior mesenteric artery connects with the celiac axis through the pancreaticoduodenal artery. In this way the small intestine receives its blood flow.

The vessels originating from the superior mesenteric artery ultimately enter the wall of the intestine as end arteries. Few anastomotic connections are found in the bowel wall. Vasculitis may result in the selective occlusion of the distal vessels and may lead to segmental infarction and small bowel ischemia and necrosis.

The superior mesenteric artery is susceptible to atherosclerotic changes and is a common site for thrombosis and embolus. The inverted Y shape of the superior mesenteric artery as it leaves the aorta provides a channel for emboli. Thromboses and emboli tend to occlude the superior mesenteric artery within 2 cm of its origin off the aorta.

The inferior mesenteric artery supplies blood to the distal transverse colon, the descending and sigmoid colon, and proximal portions of the rectum. The distal transverse colon and the splenic flexure appear to be more vulnerable to ischemia. A "watershed" area refers to branches of the inferior mesenteric artery anastomosing with the superior artery branches in the rectosigmoid area. The branches involved are the inferior mesenteric and the hypogastric.

Acute vascular occlusion may be the result of thrombosis or embolus to the superior mesenteric artery. The development of emboli is associated with atrial fibrillation in patients with subacute bacterial endocarditis and cardiac valve disease, mural thrombosis of myocardial infarct, and postintracardiac surgery. Thrombosis of mesenteric vessels is associated with polycythemia, sickle cell trait, intraabdominal sepsis, pancreatic disorders, and blood dyscrasias. It may also occur after bowel surgery, other major surgery, or abdominal trauma, when there may be a decrease in blood flow to the mesentery. Infarction of the bowel results in a sudden onset of severe abdominal pain, distention, fluid loss, and shock.

Chronic intestinal angina is an obstructive vascular disease involving atherosclerotic changes in two of the three major vessels. An increase in mesenteric blood flow is required to supply oxygen for the metabolic processes of digestion, absorption, and increased peristalsis. Abdominal pain occurs when the superior mesenteric artery supply is less than the demand of the smooth muscle activity in the intestine. The patient may fear eating and begin losing weight. Between meals, the patient is free of pain. Diagnosis may be delayed because many physicians first test the patient for cancer because weight loss and pain in older persons are associated with malignancies. Intestinal ischemia may progress to frank infarction of the intestine.

Nonocclusive intestinal ischemia accounts for up to 50% of the cases.[71] Patients with recent myocardial infarctions, severe congestive cardiac failure, shock, anoxia, or hypotension may have a nonocclusive intestinal ischemia develop. An episode of inadequate cardiac output and poor tissue perfusion results in shunting of blood away from the gut to vital organs. The use of α-adrenergic vasoconstrictors in patients in shock adds to the effect of the increased secretions of endogenous catecholamines, further reducing mesenteric blood flow. Other drugs that may negatively influence intestinal circulation include vasopressin, propranolol, estrogens, and ergot derivatives.

The mucosa layer is the most sensitive to oxygen deprivation because it has the highest energy requirement as a result of its high metabolic activity and rapid cell turnover. The mucosa undergoes hemorrhagic necrosis. As the anoxia continues, the necrosis becomes transmural (involving all layers of the bowel wall).

The patient who has nonocclusive intestinal ischemia develop may have evidence of some degree of occlusive or atherosclerotic changes in smaller splanchnic vessels.

Digitalis has been associated with the development of poor perfusion syndromes. Digoxin constricts splanchnic vessels. In patients with early intestinal infarction, considerations should be made regarding discontinuation of digoxin therapy.[60]

Celiac axis compression by the median arcuate ligament of the diaphragm or by neurofibrous tissue of the celiac ganglion is associated with recurrent epigastric pain and an epigastric bruit (which does not radiate to the lower abdomen). Celiac axis compression is more common in young women and is relieved by surgical division of the ligament or bands. The medical profession has challenged the validity of celiac axis compression as a disorder or a syndrome.[61,63] The cause of the pain and the absence of symptoms in many patients with stenosis of the celiac axis have raised unanswered questions.

Vasculitis has been associated with mesenteric infarction in approximately 3% of reported cases. However, the vasculitis associated with systemic disorders may be seen as intestinal angina or frank infarction. The systemic disorders include polyarteritis nodosa, lupus erythematosus, dermatomyositis, rheumatoid vasculitis, scleroderma, anaphylactoid purpura, and Degos' disease. Table 8-3 examines the bowel involvement that occurs as a result of systemic vasculitis.

Certain surgical procedures such as coarctation of the aorta, excision of abdominal aneurysms, and iliac or femoral grafts are associated with mesenteric vascular insufficiency.

The oxygenation of the bowel depends on patency of the major arterial vessels, arteriolar resistance, adequacy of perfusion pressure, arterial oxygen saturation, and oxygen need. Acute or chronic changes of any or all of the above affect the blood flow to the bowel.

The events of intestinal ischemia include structural changes in the cells within 5 minutes of the occlusion of the superior mesenteric artery. The epithelium becomes detached from the basement membrane at the villus tips, and subepithelial blebs form. Within 30 to 60 minutes, the villi are denuded of epithelium. The mucosa undergoes necrosis and ulceration with an inflammatory cell infiltration. A secondary bacterial invasion occurs. In acute ischemic necrosis, massive submucosa edema and bleeding into the mucous membrane develop because of an increase in capillary permeability followed by loss of capillary integrity.

TABLE 8-3 Systemic Disorders Affecting Splanchnic Perfusion

Disorder	Definition	Gastrointestinal Implications
Periarteritis nodosa	A progressive, polymorphic disease of connective tissue characterized by numerous large, palpable or visible nodules in clusters along segments of medium-sized arteries	Segmental ischemia with ulceration, hemorrhage, or perforation to massive infarction of bowel; may also have hepatic artery thrombosis; nodules obstruct lumen of vessels
Lupus erythematosus	A chronic inflammatory collagen disease affecting many systems; includes severe vasculitis, renal involvement, and lesions of skin and nervous system.	Segmental lesions of ischemia progressing to necrosis and perforation; involvement of submucosa and muscularis leads to protein-losing enteropathy; abdominal pain may be caused by serositis or acute pancreatitis; ulcerative colitis and Crohn's disease have been associated with lupus erythematosus; diagnosis of gastrointestinal involvement difficult to evaluate
Dermatomyositis	A disease of the connective tissue characterized by pruritic or eczematous inflammation of skin and tenderness and weakness of muscles	Vasculitis associated with ischemia of bowel; increased incidence of gastrointestinal cancers with this disorder
Rheumatoid arthritis	A collagen disease that affects the connective tissue by inflammation and fibrinoid degeneration	Vasculitis associated with intestinal ischemia; occurs with abdominal pain
Scleroderma	A relatively rare autoimmune disease affecting blood vessels and connective tissue; most common in middle-aged women	Bowel symptoms arise from fibrosis of the intestinal wall and loss of muscle; focal areas of vasculitis may lead to ischemia
Anaphylactoid purpura (Henoch-Schönlein syndrome)	A self-limited hypersensitive vasculitis that occurs primarily in young children; palpable purpuric skin lesions appear on lower abdomen, buttocks, and legs; arthritis and abdominal pain are also seen; occasionally seen in adults, whose prognosis is not as favorable as children	Colicky abdominal pain; surgery demonstrates submucosal and subserosal hemorrhages; may have upper or lower gastrointestinal bleeding; segmental ischemic bowel episodes may occur but do not generally progress to gross infarction or perforation
Degos' disease (malignant atrophic papulosis)	A rare syndrome of progressive occlusive vascular disease affecting small and medium-sized arteries; primarily involves the skin (malignant atrophic papulosis) and intestine; skin lesions usually precede gastrointestinal symptoms; primarily affects young men	Lesions (identical to skin lesion) are found in mucosa and serosa of bowel; weight loss and diarrhea develop; progresses to intestinal infarction and perforation

The submucosal edema and hemorrhage are seen as the "thumbprint" pattern in radiographic studies. The exudation of protein-rich fluid, and later blood, found in the intestinal lumen is the result of the loss of epithelial and vascular integrity. Fluid loss and hypovolemia further compromise blood flow to the intestine.

The development of peritonitis indicates the involvement of the muscle and serosa layer and that the perforation is imminent or has occurred. If the ischemic episode is self-limited and does not progress to perforation and resection, the acute inflammatory response resolves spontaneously with stricture formation.

In chronic or gradual reduction of blood flow, the anoxia damages the mucosa initially. The necrosis may be limited to the mucosa, in which event the mucosa will slough with regeneration occurring in 4 to 5 days. The villi may recover but their shape and functioning abilities are affected and a temporary malabsorption develops that is seen clinically as enterocolitis. As the anoxia continues, the necrosis progresses. A microscopic examination of the bowel may reveal a coagulative necrosis of the inner two thirds of the wall with muscle and serosa uninvolved. A scar may form.

The bowel totally deprived of its blood supply ultimately becomes black and necrotic. The bowel perforates, with leakage of intestinal contents. Bacterial invasion of the necrotic bowel produces gas cysts, massive sepsis, and shock. Repair cannot take place when this degree of injury has occurred, and bowel death usually results. If surgery is performed, it is usually a massive bowel resection resulting often in short bowel syndrome.

• • • • • Diagnostic Studies and Findings

Plain films of the abdomen (KUB)   Dilated loops of bowel with air-fluid levels; complete absence of small bowel air; generalized distention (later sign); thickening of bowel wall with edema and fluid (ischemic colitis); string or ring of gas outside lumen of bowel (marked necrosis); gas in portal vein (evidence of leak of bacteria from infarcted bowel); blunt plicae

Angiography   Abnormal vascular tree (intestinal angina); demonstrates site of arterial blockage or spasm; absence or severe flow impairment of two of the three vessels supplying the bowel (chronic mesenteric ischemia); angiographic studies generally indicated only in patients with disorders predisposing to embolization but may be used when other tests are negative and patient is symptomatic; also used preoperatively to map vessels that are narrowed or occluded

Barium studies   Early stages find appearance of spasm and irritability with narrowing of bowel lumen and thumbprinting; disordered motility (slow or rapid)

Colonoscopy   Swollen folds and mucosa, dusky color, presence of ulcerations similar to those found in Crohn's disease; not diagnostic

Computerized tomography scan (CT)   Small bowel distended with fluid and air; wall thickened; may show immediate cause of ischemia or infarction

Hematocrit   In presence of necrosis, hemocentration (decreased fluid volume)

White blood cell count   Leukocytosis (20,000 and higher)

Amylase and lipase   Elevated (from leakage into peritoneum or from back-pressure resulting from development of intestinal obstruction)

• • • • • Multidisciplinary Plan

Surgery

Chronic
Balloon angioplasty (intestinal angina) to improve blood flow
Bypass graft, embolectomy, endarterectomy, and reimplantation procedures have been used effectively

Acute
Resection of infarcted bowel, temporary colostomy or ileostomy, and subsequent reanastomosis (colonic ischemia)

Medications

Acute
Antiinfective agents
    Agent-specific antibiotics given to reduce bacterial flora of bowel and treat sepsis
Adrenergic agents
    Dopamine in low dosages may be used as a vasopressor if fluid replacement does not correct shock (α-stimulating sympathomimetic amines [e.g., norepinephrine] should be avoided)
Vasodilators
    Intraarterial infusion of vasodilators (papaverine, Urotensin II), for up to 5 d
    Stop digitalis unless absolutely necessary
Anticoagulation with heparin followed by bishydroxycoumarin (dicumarol)(used in patients with mesenteric venous occlusion that tends to recur); dosages adjusted based on patient's coagulation time

General Management

Patients with abdominal pain but no evidence of peritonitis or systemic toxicity should be treated conservatively

Acute
Electromyography
Injection of radioactive microspheres
Intraoperative fluorescein angiography (may be used during surgery to determine viability of bowel and evaluate mesenteric vessels)
Intravenous fluid replacements, volume expanders
Nasogastric or intestinal suctioning preoperatively for treatment of ileus
Hyperalimentation postoperatively

NURSING CARE

Nursing Assessment

This section is divided into assessments of chronic ischemia of the bowel (i.e., intestinal angina) and acute episodes of ischemia. The acute episodes are similar in progression of symptoms, and therefore not all causes are outlined. Acute occlusive ischemia is used as the example. Exceptions are noted. The assessment of abdominal pain is an example of an area where differences do exist in the acute episodes.

Pain (Abdominal)

Intestinal angina: severe crampy or colicky pain around umbilicus; radiates to back; lasts 2 to 4 hours; no pain between meals

Acute occlusive ischemia; severe colicky pain in the periumbilical area; as ischemia progresses, pain becomes more severe and poorly localized

Ischemic colitis; lower abdominal pain of abrupt onset

Mesenteric venous thrombosis: gradual progression of abdominal pain until it resembles acute occlusive ischemia

Gastrointestinal Symptoms (In Response to Ischemia or Necrosis)

History: recurring pain after meals

Sudden onset in patient with atrial fibrillation, prosthetic heart valves, bacterial endocarditis

Intestinal angina: nausea and vomiting; abdominal bloating; malabsorption with steatorrhea and diarrhea

Acute occlusive ischemia; copious vomiting and hematemesis indicate necrosis adjacent to ligament of Treitz; gross rectal bleeding

Enterocolitis symptoms: malabsorption; diarrhea, may be hemorrhagic (seen regardless of cause of ischemia, results from sloughing of mucosa and bacteremia)

Abdominal Examination

Absence of significant abdominal findings initially; hyperperistalsis, with no tenderness or resistance

After necrosis occurs: classic signs of peritonitis with rebound tenderness, rigidity, abdominal distention, and ileus

General

Fever

Nutritional Assessment

Intestinal angina: weight loss; fear of eating because of chronic malabsorption syndrome; malnutrition

Cardiovascular

Shock; hypotension; anoxia; severe congestive heart failure; recent myocardial infarction or some cause that results in shunting of blood away from the gut to "vital" organs; tachycardia

Nursing Dx & Intervention

Fluid volume deficit related to acute ischemic event

- Assess patient carefully for signs and symptoms of severe fluid and electrolyte loss, metabolic acidosis, and hypovolemic shock *resulting from accumulation of gas and fluids and distention of intestine and sepsis* (if perforation occurs).

- Replace intravenous fluids and electrolytes, blood, and plasma as ordered.
- Monitor vital signs, central venous pressure, blood pressure, urinary output, diarrhea, and nasogastric aspirations every hour.
- Measure abdominal girth every 8 hours *to assess distention.*
- Notify physician of changes in patient's status, because they generally indicate a decline in patient's stabilization for surgical intervention.

Pain related to acute ischemia

- Assess abdominal area for signs of perforation and peritonitis: increased severity and diffuseness of abdominal pain, rebound tenderness, guarding, rigidity.
- Help patient assume a comfortable position; limit sudden movement and abdominal examination.
- Provide analgesics as prescribed.

Diarrhea related to colitis caused by ischemia

- Assess patient for signs of steatorrhea and diarrhea (intestinal angina); gross rectal bleeding (acute occlusive ischemia); and hemorrhagic diarrhea (enterocolitis), which are diagnostic assessments of ischemia of the intestine.
- Assist patient with cleansing of perianal area. Apply moisture barrier ointment after cleansing to protect perianal skin.
- Nutritional consult to suggest dietary regimen/selections that may help decrease bowel transit time.

Altered nutrition: less than body requirements; related to chronic intestinal pain after eating or after resection for acute ischemia

- Assess through careful history a "fear of eating" versus other causes of weight loss.
- Provide enteral nutrition as tolerated.
- Initiate and monitor hyperalimentation as ordered after operation for significant small bowel resections.
- Nutritionist to see patient for both ongoing assessment and recommendations.

Patient Education/Home Care Planning

Chronic ischemia
1. Help the patient understand the relationship of eating and pain in intestinal angina.
2. After surgery for venous thrombosis, the patient may need instruction regarding anticoagulant therapy.

Acute ischemia
1. In colonic ischemia a temporary colostomy may be performed. If so, the patient requires colostomy teaching and plans for surgical closure at a later date.

2. The patient who has had a massive bowel resection may be on home total parenteral nutrition. In these cases the patient and family require extensive discharge preparation (i.e., central line care; management of total parenteral nutrition).
3. Help the patient deal with an increase in diarrhea, especially for the first 6 months postoperatively, caused by rapid transit time or varying degrees of malabsorption.

Evaluation

Fluid balance is maintained   Patient returns to normal hydration levels as assessed by skin turgor, color, moist mucous membranes, blood pressure, pulse, and urinary output. Serum electrolytes, hematocrit, and WBC are within normal limits.

Comfort level is achieved   Reduction in or absence of guarding or protective behavior. Patient uses pain control strategies appropriately. Patient verbalizes increased control over pain.

Diarrhea is manageable   Patient's perianal skin is intact. Patient understands the use of diet to decrease bowel transit time.

Nutritional status is normal   Patient maintains normal body weight. Nutritional status is maintained through home hyperalimentation (major resection of small bowel).

IRRITABLE BOWEL SYNDROME

Irritable bowel syndrome (IBS), or functional bowel syndrome, is a disorder of the large bowel that results in altered bowel habits, abdominal pain, and absence of detectable disease.

The patient may have diarrhea or constipation or both. Abdominal pain and distention are common.

It is important to recognize the mislabeling of IBS in the past. Nervous colon, spastic colon, and mucous colitis are incorrect terms. Nervous colon recognizes only one aspect of the possible cause of IBS. Spasticity is one sign or response of the colon to the altered motor activity. Inflammation is not present, making "colitis" a misnomer. IBS does not progress or predispose individuals to inflammatory bowel disease or cancer.

The incidence of IBS is considered high, but accurate data on the prevalence are not available. IBS does not lead to death and therefore does not appear on death certificates. Rarely does IBS require hospitalization. IBS is a leading cause of absenteeism from work. Up to 50% of referrals to gastroenterologists are for irritable bowel syndrome.[19] Many people with IBS do not seek medical attention because they have mild symptoms, making it more difficult to estimate the prevalence.

The incidence of IBS is higher in females than males with a 2.3:1 ratio. There is a higher incidence in whites than nonwhites and in Jews than non-Jews. Symptoms generally begin before the age of 35, and in many patients isolated instances of IBS during adolescence can be identified by the patients. A third of the patients can trace IBS to childhood.[19]

●●●●● Pathophysiology

IBS is a functional disorder of gastrointestinal motility. The abdominal pain and altered bowel pattern are caused by altered motility of the small and large intestines. Motility may be affected by emotions, food, neurohumoral agents, gastrointestinal hormones, toxins, prostaglandins, and colon distention.

Two patterns of IBS are identified: painful IBS with diarrhea, constipation, or both and IBS with painless diarrhea. The two types of IBS may be differentiated on observations of motility recordings.

Segmental contractions are the predominant form of normal motor activity in the colon, consisting of 90% of recorded motor activity. Segmental contractions slow the forward progress of stool, promoting mixing, absorption, and dehydration. Segmental contractions appear as haustral markings on barium studies. Increasing segmental contractions produce constipation, whereas decreasing segmentation results in diarrhea.

Although motility studies demonstrate abnormalities throughout the alimentary tract in patients with IBS, no one abnormality clearly separates IBS from organic gastrointestinal disease or even from normal bowel function.[71] Some of the more common (but not pathognomonic) abnormalities are described below. In general, a diagnosis of IBS is based on recognition of characteristic symptom patterns, probability, and exclusion of organic gastrointestinal disease.

A pattern of hypermotility with high-amplitude pressure waves is common in patients with painful IBS. Motility in the pain-free diarrheal-predominant IBS is normal or lower than normal.

Motility of the bowel may be affected by a variety of factors. For example, sleep lowers the motor activity in the colon. This may account for the infrequency of nocturnal symptoms. The presence of nocturnal symptoms usually indicates an organic etiology rather than the functional cause of IBS.

Anxiety, depression, fear, and hostility have been identified in IBS, as well as other gastrointestinal disorders. Stress and emotions alone do not cause IBS but are related to the clinical course. Stress can be related to the onset of symptoms. Diarrhea can readily be associated with stressful situations such as test taking or job interviews. Constipation is not apparent for several days, and it may be more difficult to pinpoint the source of anxiety or generalized depression.

Meals, or the ingestion of food and caffeine, will stimulate colonic hypermotility in irritable bowel syndrome. The postprandial symptoms are related to this effect. Normally, a meal will lengthen segmental contractions, allowing for additional mixing and absorption, and the effect of the meal slows after approximately 50 minutes. In IBS the meal stimulation of segmental contractions may be blunted and the effect continues postprandially, gradually becoming stronger.

The gastroileocolic response to food ingestion moves intestinal contents forward, emptying material in the distal colon and creating distention. Colon distention may induce exaggerated spastic contractions in IBS. Patients with alternating diarrhea and constipation or diarrhea-predominant IBS often have a bowel movement after every meal. For some this may be the only symptom of IBS.

Neurohumoral agents, such as cholinergic, anticholinergic, adrenergic, and adrenergic-blocking substances, produce hyperactivity of the colon in both normal bowels and in irritable bowel syndrome. In IBS, response to neurohumoral agents is more pronounced and occurs during both symptomatic and asymptomatic periods.

Anticholinergic agents affect colonic activity induced by meals. Anticholinergics suppress an early neurogenic myoelectric and motor reflex component of the gastrocolic reflex in normal subjects. In IBS the myoelectric and motor reflex is not suppressed, but anticholinergics inhibit the second, delayed component of gastrocolic reflex, which is hormonally mediated.

The gastrointestinal hormones that affect motility include cholecystokinin, gastrin, glucagon, and vasoactive intestinal peptide. Cholecystokinin is associated with abdominal pain and colonic hypermotility when given through infusion. Because cholecystokinin is released after a meal, this may account for the postprandial pain in IBS. Also, the delayed hormonally mediated phase of the gastrocolic reflex depends on the fatty content of the meal. This indicates a relationship with cholecystokinin that produces colonic contractions.

•••••• Diagnostic Studies and Findings

No specific radiographic, endoscopic, or biochemical abnormalities are associated with the diagnosis of IBS. Diagnosis is made by the exclusion of organic diseases with similar symptoms, as follows:

Sigmoidoscopy Spastic contractions may prevent passage of the instrument beyond 10 to 12 cm; reproduction of symptoms with air insufflation; mucosa free of ulcers, bleeding, friability, and masses; do not use enemas or cathartics before sigmoidoscopy (may produce edema, obscuring the normal colon appearance); to rule out colon cancer, polyps, colitis, diverticulosis, and hemorrhoids

Manometric studies May be used to evaluate electric response to colon; balloons are placed in rectosigmoidal colon (cephalad balloon) and rectum (caudad balloon), and 20 mm of air is instilled into the cephalad balloon every 20 minutes; balloon mimics presence of stool in the area; a graph recording is made of the bowel response to the stimulus; response in a normal bowel is a brief contraction in rectosigmoid and rectum, with a rapid return to the prestimulus state; in patient with IBS, the distention may produce a diffuse spastic contraction in rectosigmoid and rectum

Biopsy To rule out other disorders; not helpful in diagnosing IBS

Stool test for guaiac To rule out inflammatory bowel diseases and malignancy

Stool stains To rule out motile amebic trophozoites, leukocytes, and mucus

Stool cultures To rule out ova and parasites, specifically *Giardia*

Complete blood count To rule out anemia and inflammation

Differential blood cell count (Eosinophilia) To rule out parasitosis, cytosis (suggests tuberculosis), and vacuolated cells (suggest inflammation)

Three-day trial on lactose-free diet, lactose tolerance test, or breath hydrogen test To rule out lactose insufficiency in patients with distention and bloating or diarrhea

Double-contrast barium enema Exaggerated haustral contractions or absence of haustrations; narrow lumen with pellet stones; lumen easily dilated; rule out colon cancer, polyps, diverticulosis

Cholecystogram or ultrasonography of gallbladder To rule out gallbladder disease in presence of dyspepsia

Small bowel series To rule out obstruction of bowel, if diarrhea and symptoms suggest obstruction

Colonoscopy To rule out inflammatory bowel disease, polyps, diverticulosis, or colon cancer when clinically justified as in change in symptoms in patient with long-standing IBS; uncontrollable exacerbation of IBS

Thyroid function To rule out hyperthyroidism or hypothyroidism if constipation predominates

•••••• Multidisciplinary Plan

Surgery

Rare

Medications

Bulk-forming laxatives
  Psyllium preparations (Metamucil, Konsyl, L.A. Formula, Mitrolan) taken at meal times; in obese patients before meals and in thin patients after meals (hydrophilic properties bind water, preventing excessive dehydration of stool and excess liquidity); may improve symptoms
Antidiarrheal agents
  Diphenoxylate (Lomotil), 2.5 to 5 mg mg q4-6h
  Loperamide (Imodium), 2 mg q6-8h
  Dependency on antidiarrheals can develop; slow withdrawal of medicines as coping abilities are developed is recommended; may improve symptoms
Antispasmodic agents
  Anticholinergics
    Dicyclomine (Bentyl), 20 mg 30-45 min before meals
    Propantheline (Pro-Banthine), 15 mg 30-45 min before meals
    Hyoscyamine (Levsin), 1-2 tablets q4 as needed, *not* before meals
  Calcium channel blockers
    Currently under investigation for treatment of IBS based on smooth muscle relaxant properties and inhibitory effects on gastrocolonic response

General Management

Patient should be placed on high-fiber (12 to 16 g/d as 2 tablespoons of bran qid; gradually reduced), low-lactose, no caffeine diet before trying drug therapy
Low-fat diet (to reduce stimulation of cholecystokinin)

Avoid irritating foods (idiosyncratic)

Relaxation techniques

Nutritional Consultation

To assist patient with food history/diary that may help identify irritating or troublesome foods, because diet may affect motility in IBS

NURSING CARE

Nursing Assessment

General

Tense, anxious patient who may be unaware of features of tenseness

No evidence of weight loss

Pain

Lower abdominal pain

Often patient locates pain by using the palm to describe a circular motion (rather than finger pointing to one discrete spot)

Pain often precipitated by meals

Pain often relieved by defecation

Gastrointestinal

Alternating diarrhea and constipation, diarrhea, or constipation

Constipation

Episodic initially, becomes continuous, increasingly intractable to laxatives and later to enemas

Stools: hard and narrow

Objectively defined as passage of fewer than three stools per week; sometimes patient will have diarrhea following a week of constipation

Subjectively defined as difficult or painful evacuation

Diarrhea

Defined as loose, mushy, or watery stools

Urgency and tenseness in the morning or after meals, followed by evacuation

Initial movement may be of normal consistency and is rapidly followed by a softer, unformed stool and then by increasingly loose stools

Abdominal pain is relieved by bowel movement

Postprandial diarrhea correlating with quantity rather than type of food

Patients with diarrhea only–type IBS more likely to have explosive, watery stools; classically these patients experience no weight loss

Abdominal Examination

Palpable, tender sigmoid colon

Nursing Dx & Intervention

Constipation related to gastrointestinal motility disorder and stress

- Assess history of bowel movements; in IBS patients often experience constipation followed by diarrhea—constipation may be defined as fewer than three stools per week; defecations described as painful or difficult.
- Administer bulk laxatives as ordered.
- Help patient identify irritating or troublesome foods because diet may affect motility in IBS.

Diarrhea related to gastrointestinal motility disorder and stress

- Assess history of bowel movements; in IBS diarrhea is defined as loose, mushy, or watery stools; urgency after meals is common; abdominal pain is relieved by defecation.
- Administer antidiarrheal agents as ordered.
- Help patient identify irritating or troublesome foods because diet may affect motility in IBS.

Ineffective individual coping related to stress

- Assess for related factors that would increase stress, tension, or an emotional state.
- Help patient recognize the role of emotions, stress, and diet in the symptoms of IBS.
- Help patient and family understand that the symptoms are based on functional motility problems and that psychosocial stress accentuates rather than causes the symptoms.
- Help patient identify sources of stress and counterbalancing relaxation techniques.
- Encourage patient to keep a diary of events and symptoms.
- Psychotherapy may be helpful for patients who do not show improvement on medications.

Patient Education/Home Care Planning

1. Provide information on irritable bowel syndrome. Patient education material is available through the National Digestive Disease Education Information Clearinghouse, NIH, 1555 Wilson Blvd., Suite 600, Rosslyn, VA 22209-2461.
2. Instruct the patient in necessary diet alterations. Inform patient that often it is possible to manage with diet and stress reduction without using any medications.
3. Provide written instructions for medications prescribed for the management of IBS by the physician. Ensure that the patient knows the names, amounts, and rationales for the treatment plan.

Evaluation

Bowel functioning is normal   Diarrhea and constipation are relieved, and recurrences are managed through medical regimen and stress reduction.

Psychosocial stress is reduced Patient can identify sources of stress and uses effective coping mechanisms. Combination of counseling, relaxation techniques, modification of diet (avoiding irritating foods), and medications is effective in relieving symptoms. Symptoms are managed so that lifestyle does not center around bowel elimination.

LACTOSE INTOLERANCE

Lactose intolerance results from a deficiency of the enzyme lactase. Lactase (found in the brush border of the intestinal villi) is necessary for the digestion or breakdown of the disaccharide lactose (found in milk and milk products). Lactose intolerance is a common cause of diarrhea, crampy abdominal pain, gas, and bloating.

Lactase deficiency may have a genetic basis, and certainly is expressed more in some population groups than in others. Spiro[63] states that 10% to 20% of the white population of northern European ancestry has a lactase insufficiency and that three fourths of the blacks in Africa, as well as some Chinese, Indians, and Mediterranean inhabitants, have lactase insufficiency.

Primary disaccharidase deficiency is a congenital, hereditary absence of the lactase enzyme. The symptoms may be present from birth or may become apparent in middle life. By the age of 10 to 20 years, most persons with genetic tendencies for lactase deficiency have the same low level of lactase as adults. Primary lactase insufficiency is associated with a normal bowel mucosa and epithelial cells.

Secondary disaccharidase deficiency occurs when injury or disease damages the brush border of the intestinal mucosa. The secondary lactase deficiency may be temporary or permanent. Diseases or disorders associated with secondary lactase insufficiency include gastroenteritis, ulcerative colitis, Crohn's disease, operative procedures (partial gastrectomy, small bowel resection), and cholera.

•••••• Pathophysiology

The basis of the symptoms found in lactose intolerance is an excessive amount of sugar in the bowel lumen. Disaccharides form a large part of the dietary carbohydrate, and the three predominant forms are maltose (glucose and glucose), lactose (glucose and galactose), and sucrose (glucose and fructose). The disaccharides are not digested by enzymes in the lumen of the bowel but are taken into the brush border of the intestinal mucosal cell. The disaccharide is split by enzymes in the brush border into the simple sugars (glucose, galactose, and fructose), which can be further absorbed and metabolized. The enzymes of the brush border are lactase, sucrase, and a series of four enzymes that are called maltase.

The lactose absorption begins in the duodenum, and lactase activity is highest in the jejunum and nearly absent in the ileum. The process of lactose digestion is slower, normally, than sucrose and maltose. The blood sugar level after a meal of lactose will show little increase.

Lactase is present in the microvillus membrane of the columnar epithelial cells. Many intestinal bacteria also contain lactases. The two forms of lactase differ in their actions. Gut lactase splits the disaccharide, lactose, into glucose and galactose. Bacterial lactase results in the formation of hydrogen gas, carbon dioxide, and short-chain organic acids.

The diarrhea associated with lactose intolerance is caused by the osmotic effect of the lactose in the small bowel. The osmotic load of the lactose increases fluid secretion into the small bowel. The organic acids and fermentation products of the bacterial lactase in the colon impede colonic absorption. The pH of the stools in children may drop to 5.5 in response to the presence of organic acids.

The bloating and gaseous symptoms are the end products of bacterial lactase breaking down lactose.

•••••• Diagnostic Studies and Findings

Dietary trial: 3 weeks on a lactose-free diet Absence of gastrointestinal symptoms

Lactose tolerance test Positive for lactose intolerance: blood sugar rise less than or equal to 20 mg/dl after lactose load of 50 g/m^2 in children or 50 g in adults; accompanied by characteristic symptoms

Hydrogen breath test A rise of more than 20 parts per million after administration of oral lactose is consistent with lactose intolerance (NOTE: Oral antibiotics can suppress bacteria that produce hydrogen; smoking increases breath hydrogen concentrations; small percentage of individuals do not normally produce hydrogen gas)

Stool pH Drop from the normal pH of 7.0 or 8.0 to 5.5 (more common in children)

•••••• Multidisciplinary Plan

Medications

Commercial lactase enzyme preparation can be used in milk for patients with limited tolerance to milk
Lactose-free diet

General Management

Low-lactose diet (is tolerated well by most individuals; lactose added until symptoms appear and then decreased until asymptomatic)
Calcium supplements (particularly in postmenopausal women)

NURSING CARE

Nursing Assessment

Gastrointestinal

Excessive gas and flatus
Abdominal gurgling and pain

Persistent to profuse diarrhea
May vary from mild to extreme

Nutritional Status

History as to dietary sources of calcium

Nursing Dx & Intervention

Diarrhea related to osmotic effect of unhydrolyzed sugars in the colon

- Assess for history of milk tolerance or intolerance *to determine onset.*
- Assess for familial tendency for lactose intolerance.
- Assess for relationship between foods and onset of abdominal symptoms.
- Record amount, frequency, and consistency of bowel movements.

Altered nutrition: less than body requirements related to inability to eat calcium-rich (Ca^{++}) foods; related to undiagnosed lactose intolerance with weight loss

- Assess patient for bone disease involvement caused by low intake of calcium and provide calcium supplements.
- Refer mothers of infants with diarrhea and failure to thrive to physician *for evaluation of lactase deficiency versus other malabsorption syndromes.*

Patient Education/Home Care Planning

1. Provide oral and written instructions on lactose-free or low-lactose diets.
2. Patients should be taught to read all labels to avoid packaged foods containing milk, milk products, milk solids, whey, lactose, milk sugar, curd, casein, galactose, and skim milk powder. Restricted foods include milk, yogurt, ice cream (also sherbets), cheese, desserts (made from milk and milk chocolate), sauces or stuffings (made with milk, cream, or cheese), and cream soups.

Evaluation

Bowel elimination is normal   There are no symptoms with low-lactose or lactose-free diet.

Nutritional status is good   Calcium level is normal; there are no signs of bone disease.

◼ CELIAC SPRUE

Celiac sprue is a malabsorption disease that can occur at any age. The mucosa of the small intestine is damaged by gluten-containing grains (wheat, barley, rye, and oats).

Celiac sprue (Figure 8-14) may cause severe malabsorption from the small bowel, resulting in marked malnutrition, debili-

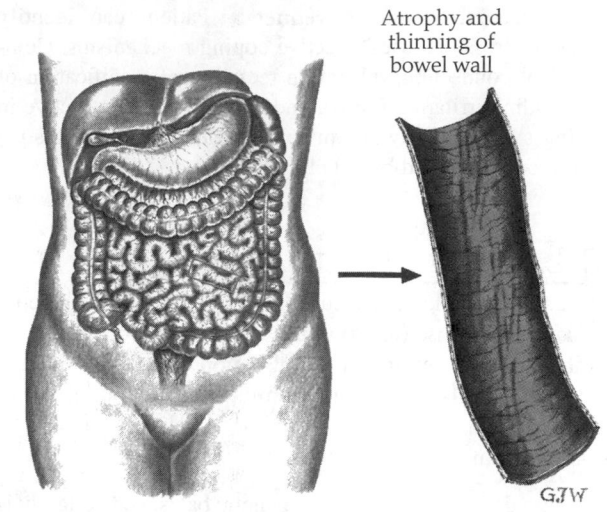

Atrophy and thinning of bowel wall

GJW

Figure 8-14   Celiac sprue (primary malabsorption). (From Doughty.[17])

tation, dehydration, and complications of nutrient and vitamin deficiencies. Other associated disorders include depression, thyroid disease, peptic ulcer disease, and diabetes mellitus.

Celiac sprue was first described in the literature in 1932. In 1950 a landmark study recognized the relationship of certain dietary grains to celiac sprue.[61] The incidence of celiac sprue is estimated at 0.03% of the general population. It appears that the estimate may be low, however, because asymptomatic celiac sprue patients have been identified during studies of familial and genetic tendencies of the disease.[71] The highest incidence of celiac sprue is in western Ireland, but there are cases of celiac sprue worldwide.[61] Celiac sprue is rare among blacks, Jews, and persons of Mediterranean descent. Women are affected more often than men. Celiac sprue is also more common in people with blood type O and less common in people with blood type A.

Only 50% of patients have gastrointestinal symptoms when initially examined. Other complaints include dermatitis herpetiformis, anemia, tetany, osteomalacia, muscle symptoms, allergic complaints, fatigue, and weight loss.[26]

The onset of celiac sprue symptoms occurs at two peak periods. The first peak occurs when the infant's diet is changed to include cereals. There is a period during late childhood when the disease becomes asymptomatic; however, in the fourth and fifth decades the second onset of symptoms occurs. Unequivocal evidence of celiac sprue in childhood indicates a need to remain on a gluten-free diet indefinitely to avoid recurrent disease during adult life.

•••••• Pathophysiology

In celiac sprue the interaction of the water-soluble protein moiety (gluten) with the mucosa of the small bowel changes the absorptive surface structures of the mucosa. Ingestion of gluten-containing foods subsequently causes bloating, malaise, abdominal cramps, and diarrhea within a few hours. The fecal fat excretion increases. The intestinal absorptive cells are damaged. The dying absorptive cells are sloughed from the mucosal surface more rapidly than normal. The number of proliferating cells increases, and the crypts become hyperplastic to compensate for the excessive loss of absorptive cells. Th mucosal layer of the small bowel appears flat, the villi are absent, and the intestinal crypts are markedly elongated and open onto a flat, absorptive surface. These structural changes decrease the amount of epithelial surface available for digestion and absorption. Many of the mucosal enzymes necessary for digestion and absorption are altered in the damaged mucosal cells. Thus the absorptive cells are reduced in number and functionally compromised. The crypt cells are increased in number, which accounts for the elongation of the crypts.

Celiac sprue may involve varying lengths of small intestine. The amount of involved bowel does correlate with the severity of the clinical symptoms. The proximal bowel is always involved and is usually more severely involved than the distal bowel. In mild cases of celiac sprue, some villous structure will remain even in the proximal bowel.

Treatment with a gluten-free diet results in significant improvements in the intestinal mucosa. The absorptive cells improve in days. The mucosa of the distal small intestine improves more rapidly than the proximal bowel, which was more severely involved. It may take months or years to reach its full recovery. Complete reversion to normal is uncommon. This may be in part related to inadvertent gluten ingestion.

The cause of gluten damage to the intestinal mucosa is not known. Four possible mechanisms are an immune response to dietary gluten, a genetic disorder, a metabolic disorder, and a viral disorder. Circulating antibodies to gluten fractions have been found in patients with celiac sprue. However, there does not appear to be a correlation between the presence of the circulating antibodies and the severity of the disease. Researchers have also found that immunoglobulins synthesized by celiac sprue mucosa have antigluten specificity. Other data link celiac disease to a rare virus, human adenovirus 12. This virus may be responsible for initiating the immune system's reaction to gluten, thus causing the disease. Although evidence implicates the immune response theory, it is inconclusive at this time.

Genetic factors do play a role in celiac sprue. The incidence of disease in relatives is higher than in control populations. Approximately 85% to 95%[29] of celiac sprue patients carry the histocompatibility antigen HLA-B8. HLA-DW3 antigen, which is associated with HLA-B8, is also found in more than 80% of patients with celiac sprue. However, not all patients with HLA-B8 or HLA-DW3 have celiac sprue, nor do all patients with celiac sprue have these two antigens.[61]

In addition, antigens have been detected on the surface of B lymphocytes that are identified from antisera of celiac sprue patients. These antigens are present in most patients with celiac sprue and in all the parents of celiac sprue patients. This suggests a recessive inheritance.[53] It may be that the cause is a combined genetic and immune response.

Levels of some specific peptidases have been found to be reduced in the mucosa in untreated celiac sprue. These peptidases are important in the digestion of gliadin (a complex mixture of pro-

teins obtained by alcohol extraction of wheat gluten). In the treatment of celiac sprue, the peptidase levels return to normal. If the lack of the peptidases caused celiac sprue, the deficiency would be apparent in treated and untreated celiac sprue. This does not support the theory of a metabolic disorder as a cause of celiac sprue.

Several factors contribute to the diarrhea in celiac sprue. The stool volume and osmotic load entering the colon are increased by the malabsorption in the small bowel. Water and electrolytes are secreted into the upper small bowel lumen rather than being absorbed. Cholecystokinin and secretin release is impaired in celiac sprue, decreasing pancreatic and biliary secretions and compromising digestion. Thus the digestion and absorption of nutrients, fluids, and electrolytes is impaired in the small bowel, resulting in higher stool volume and the osmotic load. The diarrhea is aggravated by the presence of dietary fats and bile salts. The excessive dietary fat is broken down by the colon bacteria into hydroxy fatty acids, which are potent, irritating cathartics. If the terminal ileum is involved, conjugated bile salts are absorbed and enter the colon. Bile salts have a direct cathartic action in the colon.

Esophageal cancer and intestinal lymphomas have been associated with celiac sprue. The incidence of carcinomas in celiac sprue patients is approximately 10%.[61] Patients who have been responding well to a gluten-free diet and who suddenly have gastrointestinal systems develop (weight loss, malabsorption, abdominal pain, bleeding) should undergo diagnostic studies to rule out carcinoma. Before the diagnostic workup, it is necessary to ask the patient about adherence to the gluten-free diet. Any amount of gluten can damage the mucosa and create symptoms.

Refractory sprue is another complication. In refractory sprue, patients intially respond to a strict gluten-free diet and then relapse despite maintaining the diet. Some of these patients respond to corticosteroids. If patients do not respond, malabsorption becomes progressive and may lead to death. Since the advent of home total parenteral nutrition, however, death is less common.

Mucosal ulceration and intestinal strictures can develop in celiac sprue. The ulcers may perforate, with ensuing peritonitis. Intestinal strictures may lead to intestinal obstructions.

•••••• Diagnostic Studies and Findings

Jejunal biopsy (serial sections) Most valuable diagnostic procedure; flat mucosal surface; shortened or absent villi; elongated intestinal crypts; villous atrophy with crypt hyperplasia.

Quantitative stool for fat, 72- to 96-hour collection Normal results: 2 to 7 g of fat per 24 hours while ingesting 100 g/d

Hemoglobin, hematocrit, folic acid, and vitamin B_{12} levels Anemia common in celiac sprue; anemia may be related to folic acid or vitamin B_{12} deficiencies

Prothrombin time Prolonged if vitamin K deficiency present

Xylose tolerance test Excretion in urine is decreased in severe, untreated celiac disease

Hydrogen breath test for lactose intolerance Secondary lactase deficiency

Serum electrolytes Decreased; metabolic acidosis present

Serum calcium, magnesium, phosphorus, zinc, albumin, globulins, cholesterol, and carotene Decreased

Alkaline phosphatase Increased in patients with osteomalacia

Barium contrast studies: barium swallow Dilation of small intestine; marked coarsening of mucosal pattern or complete obliteration of mucosal folds; fragmentation of barium; delayed transit time of barium

Gluten challenge After response to gluten-free diet, rechallenge bowel to establish diagnosis unequivocally

•••••• Multidisciplinary Plan

The only treatment is a permanent gluten-free diet.

Medications

Used to manage effects of malnutrition and malabsorption
Hematinic agent
   Anemia: iron
Vitamins
   Anemia: folic acid, vitamin B$_{12}$
   Multivitamins daily to replace vitamins A, C, and E; thiamine; riboflavin; niacin; and pyridoxine
Electrolyte and nutritional replacements
Dehydration: intravenous fluid with potassium chloride added
Calcium: tetany, 1 to 2 g IV calcium gluconate
Magnesium: tetany, 0.5 g magnesium sulfate in dilute solution IV, *or*
   100 mEq magnesium chloride po
Osteomalacia: calcium gluconate or calcium lactate, 6 to 8 g/d and oral vitamin D

Nutritional Consultation

To instruct patient regarding gluten-free diet

NURSING CARE

Nursing Assessment

Gastrointestinal

Diarrhea: watery, bulky, semiformed, light tan or grayish, greasy-appearing, rancid odor
Constipation: large quantities of "puttylike" stool

Abdominal Examination

Excessive amounts of malodorous flatus
Protuberant and tympanic
"Doughy" consistency
Ascites (hypoproteinemia)

General

Weakness, fatigue, lassitude, fever
Weight loss (some patients lose little weight because of a tremendous intake of calories and enormous appetite until disease becomes severe)

Orthopedic

Bone pain (low back, rib cage, pelvis)
Pathologic fractures (uncommon)
Signs and symptoms of osteomalacia and osteoporosis
Signs and symptoms of calcium and magnesium depletion

Integument

Purpura
Clubbing of nails
Dry skin
Poor skin turgor
Edema (hypoproteinemia)
Skin pigmentation
Ecchymoses (hypoprothrombinemia)
Hyperkeratosis follicularis (vitamin A deficiency)
Pallor
Dermatitis herpetiformis
Increased skin and mucous membrane pigmentation

Mouth

Cheilosis and glossitis
Decreased papillation of tongue

Extremities

Loss of light touch, vibration, and position (peripheral neuropathy)

Psychosocial

Coping with diagnosis
Compliance with diet
Relationship support

Nursing Dx & Intervention

Altered nutrition: less than body requirements related to malabsorption

- Do thorough nutritional assessment with a physical assessment.
- Consult with nutritionist.
- Weigh patient daily.
- Provide dietary supplements as ordered; in severe malabsorption, hyperalimentation may be used during initial stabilization period.
- Check dietary trays for foods containing gluten.
- Support patient and family as they learn the implications of a gluten-free diet.
- Evaluate patient's comprehension of dietary patient education.
- Evaluate, in outpatient setting, patient's dietary intake and nutritional status (weight gain and stabilization); a diary may be helpful.

Diarrhea related to gluten sensitivity

- Assess frequency, volume, and consistency of bowel movements.
- Assess history or pattern of diarrhea (i.e., onset and duration, symptoms as an infant or child, severity).

- Replace intravenous fluids and electrolytes, vitamins, and minerals as ordered.

Anxiety related to strict nutritional restrictions and increased chances of cancer

- Discuss with the patient the implications of diet restrictions on social functioning, allowing them to verbalize their concerns.
- Enlist the help of family members or significant others in assisting the patient to follow the recommended diet.
- Provide the patient with specific information regarding the increased risk of cancer.

Patient Education/Home Care Planning

1. Provide written and oral instructions on a gluten-free diet (no wheat or wheat products).
2. Encourage the patient to buy a cookbook on gluten-free cooking.
3. Instruct the patient to read labels carefully. Wheat flour is often used as an extender in processed foods and is in many brands of ice cream, salad dressings, canned foods, instant coffee, catsup, mustard, and candy bars.
4. Provide consultation with a nutritionist to teach the patient about the presence of gluten in many foods.
5. Ensure that the patient understands the increased risk of cancer and understands the importance of reporting any changes in symptoms to the provider.

Evaluation

Nutrition is adequate   Patient tolerates recommended diet. Patient has an appetite. Patient is able to plan menus around dietary restrictions. Patient achieves and maintains usual weight.

Gastrointestinal function is normal   Bowel elimination is normal with no steatorrhea.

Anxiety is reduced or decreased   Absence or reduction of defining characteristics indicating presence of anxiety.

SHORT BOWEL SYNDROME

Short bowel syndrome refers to the severe diarrhea and significant malabsorption symptoms that develop after small bowel resections. The severity of short bowel syndrome is influenced by the amount of bowel resected and the portion of small bowel resected. Symptoms are related to the diarrhea (fluid and electrolyte losses) and malnutrition (mineral, vitamin, fat, carbohydrate, and protein deficiencies).

Catastrophic malabsorption may develop from massive resections of the small bowel. The total length of resected bowel and the bowel lost must be considered in establishing the prognosis and treatment. Forty percent of the small bowel may be resected and tolerated well, *if* the duodenum, proximal je-

junum, distal half of ileum, and ileocecal sphincter are spared. In contrast, resection of 25% of the small bowel can result in severe diarrhea and malabsorption if the distal two thirds of the ileum and ilocecal valve are removed.[60] The advent of hyperalimentation has improved the survival rate of people who have lost significant amounts of small bowel.

Short bowel syndrome may develop after major resection of the small intestine for mesenteric thrombosis, volvulus of the small intestine, and strangulated internal or external hernias. Less common causes include Crohn's disease, trauma, and radiation enteropathy. Jejunal bypass procedures for obesity are no longer recommended because of the severe malabsorption associated with the surgery.

•••••• Pathophysiology

The loss of small bowel affects the body's ability to absorb nutrients and vitamins. The pathophysiologic response to resections of small bowel varies, depending on the length and the segments involved. If 3 m or less of the small intestine remain, serious nutritional abnormalities develop. If less than 1 m of normal small bowel remains, many patients will require total parenteral nutrition to sustain life.[67]

The pathophysiologic response to resections of small bowel varies depending on length and segments involved. The ileocecal valve plays an important role in reducing contamination of residual small bowel by colonic flora. The valve also controls transit time of the contents. When short bowel syndrome occurs, absorption of water, electrolytes, fat, protein, carbohydrates, vitamins, and trace elements is reduced. Fluid loss is greatest in the first few days after surgery. Fluid loss is also higher when all or part of the colon has also been resected.

The small bowel absorbs nutrients and vitamins in different segments. Resections of small portions of the midintestine do not generally create clinical problems. However, smaller resections involving proximal or distal segments result in more significant clinical symptoms. The duodenum is responsible for iron, folate, and calcium absorption. Resection or bypass of the duodenum may result in anemia. The distal or terminal ileum is responsible for bile salt and vitamin B_{12} absorption. Reduction or absence of the active absorptive sites for bile salts will disrupt the enterohepatic circulation of bile salts.

Two forms of diarrhea may develop: cholerheic or steatorrheic. Cholerheic diarrhea is a watery diarrhea that is common if less than 100 cm of distal ileum is resected.[71] In cholerheic diarrhea the hepatic synthesis of bile salts partially compensates for the bile salts not being absorbed in the ileum. Fat digestion remains normal. The bile salts in the colon impair fluid and electrolyte absorption and stimulate further secretions of fluid into the colon. Steatorrheic diarrhea occurs when more than 100 cm of distal ileum is removed. Bile salt loss cannot be compensated by hepatic synthesis and fat digestion is impaired (this can be resolved by using an agent such as cholestyramine). Undigested fat in the colon also impairs fluid and electrolyte absorption and stimulates colonic secretions. Steatorrheic diarrhea contains water, electrolytes, bile salts, and undigested fats. After ileal resections, gallstones have been reported to be two to three times higher than in the general population. This has been related to the depletion of the bile salt pool.[71]

Interestingly, the small bowel undergoes an adaptive process after bowel resections. The remaining villi enlarge and lengthen, increasing the absorptive surface area. The epithelial hyperplasia is associated with accelerated cell renewal and migration. It appears that exposure to nutrients (oral feedings), exposure to bile and pancreatic enzymes, and response to trophic gut peptides influence the adaptative process. Cholecystokinin and secretin support the adaptative process. The presence of oral feedings is necessary for adaptation to occur, but the oral intake should be gradually started and advanced. Clinically, the patient tends to improve in absorptive ability with time.

Gastric hypersecretion occurs in approximately half of the patients who have massive small bowel resections and the mucosa distal to the stomach can be injured by high gastric ouput.[18] This can impair intestinal absorption by damaging the mucosa. This is often a temporary effect and decreases to normal levels.

•••••• Diagnostic Studies and Findings

Double-contrast barium films   Estimation of amount of small bowel remaining; increase in caliber of remaining segment several weeks surgery (adaptation)

Laboratory studies: folate, iron, vitamin B$_{12}$, vitamin A, calcium, magnesium, potassium, MCV, MCHC, MCH, sodium, carotene, cholesterol, zinc   Reduced

Prothrombin time   Lengthened

Quantitative stool test for fat   Steatorrhea normal: 2 to 7 g of fat per day on diet of 100 g of fat per day

Lactose intolerance   Lactase deficiency (jejunal loss)

Xylose tolerance   Excretion in urine decreased

Culture of intestinal fluid   Bacterial overgrowth

D-Lactate levels (serum)   Elevated

Bone biopsy   Osteomalacia

•••••• Multidisciplinary Plan

Medications

Parenteral replacement of fluid loss

Antidiarrheal agents (liquid form may be absorbed better than tablets or capsules)

Diphenoxylate (Lomotil), 2.5-5 mg q4h po

Loperamide (Imodium), 2 mg q6h po

Paregoric may be used; dosage varies with degree of resection and diarrhea

Tincture of opium 10 gtt

Codeine, 60 mg IM or po

Somatostatin 50 μg subcutaneously q6h bid to tid (may be added to parenteral nutrition fluids)

Antiinfective agents

Broad-spectrum antibiotic therapy if bacterial overgrowth suspected

Histamine receptor antagonist

Cimetidine (Tagamet), 300 mg IV q6h then qid with meals and at bedtime (for gastric hypersection)

Omeprazole (Prilosec), 60 mg qd

Bile salt binders

Ileal resections with cholerheic diarrhea: cholestyramine, 8 to 12 mg/d

Vitamins

Cyanocobalamin (vitamin B$_{12}$), 1000 μg IM monthly (if extensive ileal resection)

Folate, 1 mg po daily

General Management

Intravenous fluids and replacement of K$^+$, Mg^{++}, Ca^{++}

Hyperalimentation for nutrition, especially immediately postoperatively

Gradual oral feedings: elemental diets initially; followed by polymeric supplements; add milk carefully (a low-lactose diet may be preferred)

High caloric intake; six meals per day

Home total parenteral nutrition

Protection of perianal skin from diarrhea

Nutritional Consultation

To advise on preparation of hyperalimentation; to advise on progression to enteral feedings; to instruct patient regarding dietary selections/avoidance at home (if applicable)

NURSING CARE

Nursing Assessment

General

Purpura

Generalized bleeding

Poor skin turgor

Severe weight loss

Fatigue

Lassitude

Weakness

Nutritional Status

Weight

Diarrhea (cholerheic or steatorrheic)

Monitor for signs and symptoms of nutritional deficiencies

Nursing Dx & Intervention

Altered nutrition: less than body requirements; related to decreased intestinal absorptive area

• Consult with nutritionist for input on diet strategies and monitoring.

- Assess patient for signs of malabsorption: severe weight loss, fatigue, dehydration, osteoporosis, hypokalemia, hyponatremia.
- Help patient design a nutritional plan to meet lifestyle and caloric needs.
- Provide nutritional replacements as ordered *to prevent complications of malabsorption.*
- Provide total parenteral nutrition as ordered.
- Observe catheter site (Broviac, Hickman, central line).
- Change dressing per protocol.
- Observe for signs of infection (fever or redness at insertion site).
- Monitor vital signs, intake and output, urine for sugar and acetone, and daily weights while receiving parenteral nutrition.
- Record description of stools, including frequency, characteristics, and odor.

Fluid volume deficit related to increased fluid losses from diarrhea

- Assess patient carefully for signs of fluid loss and shock: skin turgor, daily weights, intake and output, and blood pressure (sitting and lying).
- Provide fluid replacement as ordered.
- Measure and record stool volume and urinary output.

Diarrhea related to decreased intestinal absorptive area

- Assess stools for signs of cholerheic vs. steatorrheic diarrhea.
- Provide antidiarrheal agents as ordered.
- Record accurate description of stools and frequency.
- Provide fluid replacements as ordered.
- Assist patient with cleansing of perianal area and apply moisture barrier ointment as needed *to prevent skin breakdown.*

Risk for ineffective individual coping related to need for lifestyle change

- Provide opportunities for patient to verbalize concerns and feelings regarding the possibility of home total parenteral nutrition (TPN) for an undetermined time after major bowel resection.
- Consider having the patient meet other home TPN patients *for support and inspiration.*
- Discuss with the family and significant others their fears and concerns related to the new diagnosis and assist them in providing support for the patient.

Patient Education/Home Care Planning

1. Provide information, oral and written, on dietary restrictions, dietary supplements, and medications regarding nutritional effects of malabsorption.
2. Discuss with the patient the possibility of home total parenteral nutrition if necessary. Provide a home care referral to evaluate and assist the patient and family.

3. Provide the patient with information about the signs and symptoms of key electrolyte, fluid, and nutritional losses and complications from increased acidity and oxalate stones.
4. Instruct the patient to notify the physician immediately if gastroenteritis develops because the patient can become seriously dehydrated quickly.

Evaluation

Nutritional status is normal   Patient gains weight. Degree of diarrhea is minimized. Dietary plans provide adequate nutrition for absorptive capacity of the bowel. Nutritionist remains involved with dietary planning.

Fluid status is adequate   Patient has moist mucous membranes. Patient has balanced intake and output. Patient's blood pressure and pulse rate are within normal limits. Patient's urine specific gravity and osmolality are within normal limits.

Diarrhea is controlled   Patient's fluid status and electrolytes are within normal limits.

Patient is coping with the situation or recognizes resources   Patient performs the activities of daily living. Patient appropriately uses others for support. Patient has clear, realistic goals regarding the situation.

▌ PERITONITIS

Peritonitis is the inflammation of the peritoneum. The inflammatory response may be localized or generalized.

The cause of peritonitis is contamination of the peritoneal cavity by bacteria or chemicals. Peritonitis is also classified as primary and secondary. Primary peritonitis is an acute (Figure 8-15) or subacute bacterial infection of the peritoneum not associated with any underlying bowel disorder. It is often seen in children with underlying nephrotic syndromes and urinary tract infections. Cirrhosis with ascites is most commonly associated with primary peritonitis. Secondary peritonitis is the result of contamination of the peritoneum from perforation of the gastrointestinal tract (peptic ulcer, diverticulum, or appendix), gangrene of the bowel, salpingitis, traumatic injuries, and surgical contaminants. Peritonitis is a common complication of many diseases and can progress to perforation or rupture of the organs of digestion. In secondary peritonitis the inflammation is a result of bacterial and chemical irritation.

Secondary (generalized) peritonitis is a serious complication of an acutely ill patient. The overall mortality of generalized peritonitis is 40% with the use of antibiotics and intensive support systems.[67] Three factors that negatively affect the prognosis are age, type of contamination, and tissue perfusion. An older patient is at a higher risk for a poor prognosis or poor response to treatment. Fecal contamination is the most serious. Poor tissue perfusion indicates a poor prognosis. Poor tissue perfusion is associated with hypotension, acidosis,

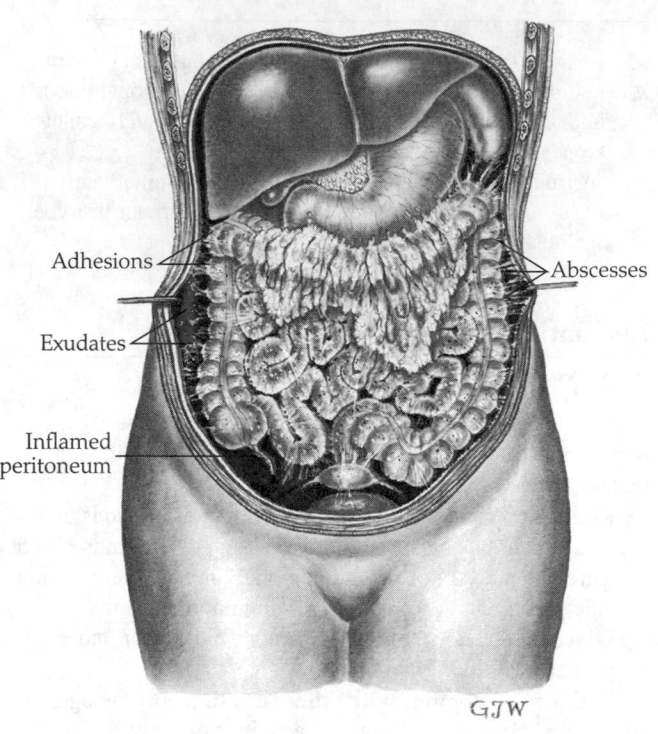

Adhesions

Abscesses

Exudates

Inflamed
peritoneum

GJW

Figure 8-15 Peritonitis (acute). (From Doughty.[17])

hypokalemia, or respiratory difficulties. Perforated peptic ulcer, ruptured appendix, trauma, ischemic bowel disease, intestinal obstruction, pancreatitis, and perforated colon are common causes of a generalized peritonitis.

Primary peritonitis accounts for approximately 1% of the incidence of infectious peritonitis.[41] Primary peritonitis may be divided into idiopathic (or spontaneous) and tuberculous peritonitis. Spontaneous bacterial peritonitis is associated with 2% of all abdominal emergencies and 13% of diffuse peritoneal sepsis in children.[61]

Tuberculous peritonitis is caused by a reactivation of latent tuberculosis in the peritoneum. The patient may not have active pulmonary, intestinal, or genital tuberculosis. Peritonitis from fungi and parasites is uncommon. *Candida albicans* may cause severe peritonitis, but it requires a contamination of the peritoneum, usually from an occult gastrointestinal perforation. *Coccidioides immitis* may result in granulomatous peritonitis in 1% to 2% of patients with coccidioidomycosis. Parasitic infections rarely lead to clinical symptoms of peritonitis but may closely resemble peritoneal carcinomatosis or tuberculosis during laparotomy.

Complications of peritonitis include abscess formation in the pelvis, the subphrenic space, and the abdomen.

•••••• Pathophysiology

The peritoneum is a semipermeable membrane enclosing the abdominal viscera and mesentery. It forms a closed, saclike structure that is opened in the female at the fallopian tubes. The peritoneum is divided into visceral and parietal peritoneum.

The visceral peritoneum covers the intraperitoneal organs and forms the mesenteries of these organs. The parietal peritoneum lines the abdominal wall, the undersurface of the diaphragm, the pelvic floor, and the retroperitoneal viscera (duodenum, ascending and descending colon, portions of the pancreas, kidney, and adrenals). The omentum is formed by a double layer of fused peritoneum and enclosed lymphatic vessels and blood vessels. The omentum plays a primary role in the peritoneal defense mechanism against impending perforations and small perforations.

The nervous innervation of the parietal peritoneum is from the same nerves that supply the abdominal wall. The irritation of the parietal peritoneum stimulates afferent nerves, which are transmitted through the intercostal nerves. The pain is perceived as somatic pain. No pain receptors are identified in the visceral peritoneum, and afferent stimulation is conducted through the visceral sympathetic nervous system. The different responses or symptoms of irritation are related to the nerve pathways. The symptoms of parietal peritonitis include a sharp, localized pain, whereas the pain in visceral peritonitis is poorly characterized and poorly localized.

The diaphragmatic peritoneum is innervated in the central portion from phrenic nerves and in the peripheral portion by branches of the intercostal nerves. Symptoms vary depending on the location of the pathologic process. Phrenic nerve stimulation would result in referred pain to either shoulder. Intercostal nerve stimulation may cause pain in the thoracic or the abdominal wall, as occurs in cholecystitis.

The peritoneal defense mechanism is the body's attempt to localize or wall off any contamination of the peritonal cavity and prevent diffuse peritonitis. The first response is vascular dilation and increased capillary permeability. Large numbers of polymorphonuclear leukocytes pour into the area and through phagocytosis remove bacteria and foreign matter. Fibroblastic exudate is deposited and plasters the adjacent bowel, mesentery, and omentum to the inflamed area, forming a watertight seal. Thus the inflammation is enclosed as an abscess. Peritoneal injuries heal without fibrous adhesions unless infection, ischemia, or foreign bodies are associated with the peritonitis.

The body's response to secondary (acute bacterial) peritonitis includes removal of the bacteria through diaphragmatic lymphatics; phagocytosis and destruction of bacteria by opsonins, polymorphonuclear leukocytes, and macrophages; and localization by the omentum and fibroblastic exudate. Vascular dilation, hyperemia, and a fluid shift occur. The vascular dilation and hyperemia lead to an increase in polymorphonuclear leukocytes and macrophages. The absorption capacity of the peritoneum increases, facilitating the absorption of bacteria and toxins. A fluid shift occurs from the extracellular fluid compartment into the free peritoneal space, into the loose connective tissue (as edema), and into the lumen of the atonic gastrointestinal tract. The translocation of water, electrolytes, and protein into this third-space compartment depletes the circulating fluid volume. The rate of fluid shift is proportional to the degree of peritoneal involvement and the success of the body's peritoneal defense mechanism.

Early diagnosis and treatment are necessary to prevent severe shock from the loss of fluid into the peritoneal space. The principal complications of untreated peritonitis are septicemia, shock, ileus, and major organ failure including respiratory, renal, hepatic, and cardiac systems. The patient has symptoms of an acute condition in the abdomen, and it is necessary to rule out other causes of the symptoms.

•••••• Diagnostic Studies and Findings

Laboratory studies WBC: increased leukocytes; RBC: hemoconcentration; metabolic acidosis; respiratory alkalosis; electrolytes: vary

Plain films of the abdomen (KUB) Intestinal distention (small and large); gas and fluid collections in both the large and small bowel; free air (perforations); bowel walls may appear thickened

Peritoneal aspiration Identification of organisms (primary peritonitis); appearance of aspirate (cloudy, blood-tinged, etc.); amylase, protein measurement, cytologic examination

•••••• Multidisciplinary Plan

Surgery

Operative procedure determined by primary cause

Objectives of surgery are to close perforation, to prevent septicemia, and to prevent abscess formation (or to drain abscess)

Medications

Aggressive volumes of electrolytes and colloid solutions to correct hypovolemia

Analgesics to control pain

Antibiotic therapy to cover multiple bacterial flora contaminating the peritoneal cavity; usually includes aminoglycoside (aerobic gram negative), clindamycin or metronidazole (anaerobes), ampicillin (enterococci), and cephalosporins (broad spectrum). β-lactam antibiotics (carbapenems), a new class of broad-spectrum antibiotics, are being evaluated in the treatment of bacterial peritonitis

General Management

NPO

Nasogastric suctioning

Hourly vital signs, urinary output measurement, CVP

Monitoring: CBC, electrolytes, creatinine, arterial pH, PO_2, PCO_2, blood clotting profiles, liver and renal function tests

CVP or Swan-Ganz catheter for pulmonary capillary wedge and pulmonary artery pressure determinations

Oxygen (increased metabolic demand and respirations decreased because of pain and abdominal distention)

Respiratory assist devices or endotracheal intubation

Cultures: blood, urine, sputum, peritoneal fluid

Nutritional supplements: total parenteral nutrition (TPN), providing 3000 to 4000 calories per day (to avoid major catabolic losses)

NURSING CARE

Nursing Assessment

Abdominal Examination

Abdominal pain; diffuse tenderness and rigidity; often rebound

Diminished or absent bowel sounds

Abdominal distention

Pulmonary Examination

Shallow and rapid; limited intercostal respirations

Pain associated with deep respirations and coughing

Cardiovascular

Rapid, weak, thready pulse

Decreased blood pressure

Kidney

Decreased urinary output

General

Fever

Lying quietly in bed with knees flexed

Guards abdomen against sudden movements or physical examination

Appears "ill"

Gastrointestinal

Vomiting

Nausea

Anorexia

Nursing Dx & Intervention

Pain related to irritation of parietal peritoneum

- Assess abdominal area for signs of perforation and peritonitis: increased severity and diffuseness of abdominal pain, rebound tenderness, guarding.
- Help patient assume a comfortable position (one that places minimum stress on the abdominal muscles); limit sudden movement and abdominal examination.
- Provide analgesics as prescribed. (Some surgeons will not order analgesics because they may mask signs and symptoms.)

Fluid volume deficit related to fluid shifts associated with inflamed peritoneum

- Assess patient carefully for signs and symptoms of severe fluid and electrolyte loss, metabolic acidosis, and hypovolemic shock *resulting from accumulation of gas and fluids, distention of intestine, and sepsis.*
- Replace intravenous fluids and electrolytes, blood, and plasma as ordered.

- Monitor vital signs; central venous pressure, urinary output, and nasogastric aspirations every hour.
- Notify physician of changes in patient's status because they generally indicate a decline in patient's stabilization for surgical intervention.

Anxiety related to pain, fear of death, and fear of the unknown

- Reassure patient and family, providing a calming influence.
- Explain all tests, procedures, and upcoming surgery.
- Use comfort measures.
- Encourage patient to ventilate feelings.

Patient Education/Home Care Planning

1. The patient manages any wounds, abscesses, or incisions that have not closed or continue to drain before and after discharge from the hospital.
2. The patient identifies purpose of discharge medications and appropriate method of administration, including times, route, and length of course of medications.

Evaluation

Body functions normally Pain, fever, and abdominal signs are absent. Urinary output is adequate, and normal bowel pattern is restored. Incision heals. Blood pressure and pulse are normal.

Laboratory studies are within normal limits WBC, hemoglobin, hematocrit, Po_2, PCo_2, and pH are within normal limits.

Pain is tolerable Patient understands that staff is doing all they can for the pain. Pain resolves with resolution of peritonitis.

Adquate fluid volume is maintained Patient has moist mucous membranes. Patient has a balanced intake and output. Patient's urine output and specific gravity are within normal limits. Vital signs are stable.

Anxiety has decreased Patient and family verbalize concerns and understanding of tests and procedures.

■ POLYPS

The term "polyp" refers to a discrete tissue mass that is elevated above the mucosal surface. A polyp may be described according to histologic examination, presence or absence of a stalk, and whether it is one of multiple similar protrusions in the gastrointestinal tract.

The histology of a polyp determines the tissue from which the polyp developed and the descriptive name. For example, adenoma develops from epithelium, myoma from smooth muscle, and hemangioma from blood vessels. The most common type of colonic polyp is an adenoma. Pedunculated polyps are attached to the mucosa by a stalk, whereas sessile polyps rest on a broad base of mucosa. Although polyps may occur throughout the gastrointestinal tract, the predominant site is in the distal 25 cm of the colon. Colonic polyps may be classified as neoplastic or nonneoplastic. Neoplastic polyps include adenomas and carcinomas. Categories of nonneoplastic polyps include mucosal polyps, hyperplastic polyps, pseudopolyps of inflammatory bowel disease, and juvenile polyps. Syndromes that involve multiple gastrointestinal polyps include familial polyposis, Gardner's syndrome, Turcot syndrome, Peutz-Jeghers syndrome, and juvenile polyps.

The frequency of colonic adenomas, although varying widely among populations, tends to be highest in North America and Europe. Autopsy surveys in the United States indicate that 50% of the population have at least one adenomatous colonic polyp. When age is considered as a variable, it is noted that two thirds of those 65 years of age and older have colonic adenomas. Adenomas in the colon and rectum are more likely to become malignant. The diagnosis and removal of polyps play an important role in preventing colon and rectal cancers.

Familial polyposis, an inherited autosomal dominant trait, is characterized by progressive development of hundreds of polyps (adenomas) throughout the colon. Familial polyposis is a precancerous condition. The development of colon cancer in familial polyposis is inevitable without surgical intervention. The polyps begin to develop after puberty, and the patient may remain asymptomatic for several years. The presence of multiple cancers at the time of diagnosis is high. Family assessments and genetic counseling are important in reducing the rates of early death from colon cancer by identifying family members who have the gene for familial polyposis.

Gardner's syndrome is a variant of familial polyposis and consists of gastrointestinal polyposis, osteomas of the skull, mandible, and long bones, and soft-tissue tumors. Gardner's syndrome is inherited as an autosomal dominant trait. The gastrointestinal polyps appear in the small and large intestine and are precancerous.

Turcot syndrome describes the combination of familial polyposis and malignant central nervous system (CNS) tumors. The CNS tumors include glioblastomas and medulloblastomas.

Putz-Jeghers syndrome involves mucocutaneous pigmentation of the mouth, lips, hands, and feet and multiple polyps in the small and large intestines. The polyps are hamartomas; that is, they develop from glandular epithelium supported by smooth muscle. The pigmentation generally fades after puberty with the exception of those found in the mouth.

Juvenile polyps are distinctive hamartomas found in the rectum of children. The polyps do not tend to be precancerous lesions but are removed because of the associated problems of bleeding, obstructions, and intussusception.

•••••• Pathophysiology

Colonic polyps or adenomas are composed of immature epithelial cells that continue to proliferate. Normally, the lower third of the colonic crypt is the site of cell division. As the cells move upward toward the lumen of the colon, they differentiate into colonic epithelium that secretes mucus. When the normal processes of cell proliferation and differentiation are altered, cells migrate to the surface, where they continue to synthesize DNA and divide. The surface epithelium of undifferentiated cells accumulates and leads to the formation of a polyp. The same steps are found in familial polyposis, where normal-appearing mucosa is found to be mature and differentiated epithelium and polyps are composed of proliferative cells.

Adenomatous polyps may develop as tubular adenomas, villous adenomas, or tubulovillous adenomas. Tubular adenoma is used to describe polyps that consist of densely packed colonic cells with loss of goblet cell mucin, branching of glands, and varying degrees of nuclear atypia. Tubular adenomas are more common and usually smaller. Villous adenomas contain a proliferation of villi. Villous adenomas are larger than tubular adenomas. The polyps that contain villi and tubular epithelium are referred to as tubulovillous adenomas. The involvement of the villi is associated with a higher incidence of cancer.

The relationship between polyps and cancer has been developed through longitudinal observations. Dysplasia, in varying degrees, is found during histologic examination of polyps after biopsy. Evidence supporting the relationship between polyps and colon carcinomas is based on three major findings: location of clusters of cancers within adenomatous polyps, findings in patients with multiple polyposis, and epidemiologic studies. Although small, isolated colon carcinomas are rare, small groups of cancers are found within adenomatous polyps. The development of carcinomas in patients with colonic polyps is usually 10 to 15 years after the appearance of benign adenomas. Data supporting the time span are based on patients with familial polyposis. However, residual adenomatous tissue may be found surrounding malignant tissue in patients with early colon cancer lesions at diagnosis and surgery. The same population groups tend to have high rates of colon cancer and colonic adenomas, further supporting the relationship.

When a polyp is removed, cytologic and histologic studies are performed to carefully assess the patient for further medical or surgical intervention. Polyps may be associated with mild to severe degrees of dysplasia. When the polyp contains foci in which the nuclei are large and irregular, cells are crowded, polarity is lost, and cribiform glands are present, the cytologic appearance is malignant. The interpretation of the finding is then made by examining the entire polyp. If the foci do not extend into the muscularis mucosae, the polyp contains carcinoma in situ. If there is extension into the muscularis mucosae and submucosa (and thus lymphatic and blood supply), the polyp is considered invasive carcinoma.

The development of polyps in familial polyposis is through the alteration of the normal cell proliferation and differentiation as previously described. In familial polyposis, young people develop hundreds to thousands of colonic polyps. Cancer, in one or more polyps, generally develops before 40 years of age.

Studies of skin fibroblasts of patients with familial polyposis and Gardner's syndrome have demonstrated abnormal growth characteristics in culture. The cells have normal contact inhibition; they grow in multilayered, crisscrossed patterns and have decreased serum requirements for growth. The study of skin fibroblasts in patients to detect the familial polyposis trait may be a diagnostic tool for the future.[61]

In Gardner's syndrome precancerous polyps may be found throughout the gastrointestinal tract. Duodenal polyps are more common than jejunal or ileal. Multiple polyps may also be found in the stomach. Extracolonic manifestations include osteomas of the mandible, skull, and long bones (e.g. epidermoid cysts, fibromas, lipomas, and desmoid tumors), dental abnormalities (e.g., impacted teeth, mandibular cysts), and soft tissue tumors (e.g., carcinoma of the thyroid and adrenal glands).

••••• Diagnostic Studies and Findings

Stool for occult blood   Positive for blood

Proctosigmoidoscopy   Visualization of bowel lumen demonstrates presence of polyps (flexible fiberoptic sigmoidoscopy is better tolerated, but only 30 cm in length)

Colonoscopy   Visualization and polypectomy; biopsy (total excision of polyp is the accepted method of providing an accurate histologic diagnosis)

Radiography studies   Osteomas found in Gardner's syndrome

Air-contrast barium enema   Used to identify polyps above the rectosigmoid area

••••• Multidisciplinary Plan

Surgery

Colonic adenomas: require colon resection with wide margins for invasive carcinoma, sessile polyps, cancer in stalk, cancer at margin of resection by polypectomy, and undifferentiated cancer in any polyp

Inherited multiple polyposis syndromes: require prophylactic proctocolectomy with end ileostomy, continent ileostomy, or ileoanal reservoir

General Management

Colonic adenomas: colonic polypectomy by colonoscopy for benign polyp, pedunculated polyp, and carcinoma in situ when confined to head of polyp

Juvenile polyps: colonoscopy with polypectomy

Routine or periodic proctosigmoidoscopy or colonoscopy in patients at risk for developing familial polyposis or Gardner's syndrome; screening should begin after 12 years of age if symptoms have not already led to a diagnosis[34]

Genetic counseling

NURSING CARE

Nursing Assessment

Gastrointestinal

Hematochezia (blood per rectum); occult and overt

Abdominal pain

Crampy, lower abdominal pain (caused by intermittent intussusception in Peutz-Jeghers syndrome)

Diarrhea in villous adenoma

Constipation or a change in the caliber of stools

Family history of deaths from colon cancer or known relatives with familial disease

Skin and Mucous Membranes

Macular lesions (brown to greenish black) around the mouth, nose, lips, buccal mucosa, hands, feet, and occasionally in the perianal and genital regions (Peutz-Jeghers syndrome)

Psychosocial

Assess individual's ability to cope in relation to the presence of familial disease that may require surgery

Nursing Dx & Intervention

Risk for altered bowel elimination related to bowel disease workup

- Assess carefully patient's history regarding bowel patterns, changes in pattern, rectal bleeding, and abdominal pain.
- Prepare patient through preprocedural teaching for colonoscopy examination, barium enemas, and proctosigmoidoscopy.

Risk for ineffective individual coping related to treatment of silent disease

- Provide opportunities for patient to verbalize concerns and feelings regarding the possibility of surgery.
- Consider having the patient meet other patients of the same age and with the same disease for support.
- Discuss with the family and significant others their fears and concerns related to the new diagnosis; assist them in providing support for the patient.
- Assess patient who is to undergo surgery for familial polyposis regarding verbal responses to the actual change in the structure of his or her body function; physical changes anticipated with surgery; and age, sex, and developmental level.
- Assist patient by providing information on rationale of total colectomy for familial polyposis and available surgical procedures including conventional ileostomy, continent ileostomy, and anal sphincter–saving surgeries.
- Refer patient to ET nurse and ostomy organization for support.

Patient Education/Home Care Planning

1. Close follow-up should be planned because of recurrence rates. Evaluation will require barium enema, proctosigmoidoscopy, or colonoscopy. The pattern should be as follows:

   Benign colonic adenoma; every 2 to 3 years

   Carcinoma confined to polyp: in 6 months, then yearly

   Multiple polyps and family history of cancer: yearly

   Asymptomatic familial polyposis: every 6 months

   Familial polyposis, following surgery when rectal segment is left: every 6 months

   See pp. 786 to 787 for instructions on ostomy care or care of the patient with an ileoanal reservoir, if appropriate.

Evaluation

Gastrointestinal function is managed Patient has no diarrhea, constipation, rectal bleeding, or abdominal pain.

Patient is coping with situation or recognizes resources Patient performs activities of daily living. Patient appropriately uses others for support. Patient has clear, realistic goals regarding the situation.

▉ PSEUDOMEMBRANOUS COLITIS

(Antibiotic-associated colitis)

Pseudomembranous enterocolitis is an inflammation and necrosis of the bowel that primarily affects the mucosa and occasionally the submucosa. Pseudomembranous exudative plaques are found attached to the mucosal surface of the small bowel (enteritis), colon (colitis), or both (enterocolitis).

Clostridium difficile has been identified as the enteric pathogen responsible for pseudomembranous colitis after antibiotic therapy. Although many antimicrobial agents have been implicated in pseudomembranous colitis, the most common agents include clindamycin, lincomycin, cephalosporins, ampicillin, penicillin, metronidazole, and amoxicillin. Antibiotic-associated pseudomembranous colitis is by far the most common risk factor, although there are others, including surgery of the colon, stomach, or pelvis region complicated by shock during or after the surgery; spinal fractures; intestinal obstructions; Crohn's disease; uremia, leukemia, colonic carcinoma, and heavy metal poisoning.

If untreated, pseudomembranous colitis leads to severe dehydration, electrolyte imbalance, toxic megacolon, and colonic perforation.

• • • • • • Pathophysiology

Antibiotic-induced pseudomembranous colitis develops when the normal bowel flora is altered by antibiotic therapy. The *C. difficile* organisms multiply, producing two toxins. The toxins damage the membranes of the epithelial cells, leading to cell necrosis. Poor vascular perfusion to the mucosa may also progress to necrosis of the mucosal layer of the gut. Antibiotic-induced pseudomembranous enterocolitis tends to be primarily a disease of the colon, whereas studies of pseudomembranous enterocolitis not associated with antibiotics demonstrated lesions in the small bowel as well.

The pseudomembrane is composed of fibrin, mucin, sloughed epithelial cells, and leukocytes. The mildest form of pseudomembranous enterocolitis consists of focal necrosis. A characteristic "summit" lesion develops from a collection of fibrin and polymorphonuclear cells. As the disease progresses, the appearance changes to a "volcanic" lesion that includes glandular cell disruption and the typical pseudomembrane of elevated yellow-white plaques. As the necrosis worsens, there is an extensive involvement of the lamina propria and a thick overlaying of the pseudomembrane. If the pseudomembranes slough, the bowel is left with large denuded areas.

Pseudomembranous colitis can progress to a life-threatening illness. The symptoms may not develop for 4 to 7 weeks after the antibiotic therapy has been discontinued. Patients generally have severe diarrhea, abdominal tenderness, fever, and leukocytosis. As the bowel wall necrosis continues, the patient begins to lose fluids, electrolytes, and albumin. Toxic megacolon may develop. The colon may perforate, leading to the sequelae of peritonitis and sepsis.

Early diagnosis is important in initiating oral treatment and preventing the disorder from becoming fulminant or intractable to medical management. The medical management consists of antimicrobials that are effective against *C. difficile.* In patients with a less severe disease, an anion exchange resin (cholestyramine) has been used to bind the toxins produced by *C. difficile.* Cholestyramine should not be used in combination with antimicrobials because the resin will bind the antimicrobial and reduce the drug levels in the colon.

•••••• Diagnostic Studies and Findings

Plain films of abdomen (KUB)   Markedly edematous colon; distorted haustral markings; colon distention; air fluid levels in toxic megacolon; ileus

Barium air-contrast studies   Rounded filling defects outlining plaques

Colonoscopy and sigmoidoscopy   Yellowish white plaques; erythema; friable mucosa; ulcerations; hemorrhage

Computerized tomography scan (CT)   Thickened colon

Stool analysis   *C. difficile* toxin assay

Laboratory   Leukocytosis (10,000 to 20,000/mm^3 or higher)

•••••• Multidisciplinary Plan

Surgery (For perforation or toxic dilation)

Severely ill patients with fulminant or intractable symptoms may require colectomy or diverting ileostomy (rare)

Medications

Metronidazole, 1.2-2.0 g/d q7-15 d po
Vancomycin, 500 mg to 2 g daily q7-14 d po
Cholestyramine, 4 g q6h for 5 d po
Bacitracin, 2 g/d q7-10 d po

General Management

Intravenous fluids; total parenteral nutrition
Bowel rest
Discontinue inciting antibiotic
No antidiarrheal drugs

NURSING CARE

Nursing Assessment

General

Fever
History—recent exposure to antibiotic agent

Gastrointestinal

Diarrhea consisting of watery stools containing mucus; severity varies up to 30 loose stools per day; may begin during antibiotic therapy or after drug is discontinued; stool may occasionally be bloody
Abdominal cramps
Vomiting

Integumentary

Assess perianal area for irritation from diarrhea

Abdominal Examination

Abdominal pain and tenderness on palpation
Decreased bowel sounds

Cardiovascular

Signs of acute dehydration

Nursing Dx & Intervention

Diarrhea related to effect of C. *difficile* toxin on bowel mucosa

- Assess all patients receiving antibiotics for diarrhea, particularly those receiving clindamycin, ampicillin, and cephalosporins.
- Report to physician patients experiencing loose, watery, frequent diarrheal stools.
- Observe patient for signs and symptoms of fluid loss, electrolyte imbalance, abdominal pain or tenderness, and fever.
- Document number, description, amount, and frequency of bowel movements.
- Follow standard body substance isolation—*C. difficile* toxin is often spread among patients and among patients and staff. Spores can also be found on inanimate objects.
- Replace fluid losses as ordered with isotonic solution.
- Assess for an accurate I and O.

Altered renal, cerebral, cardiopulmonary, gastrointestinal, and peripheral tissue perfusion related to massive fluid shifts and losses

- Assess patient for signs of toxic megacolon, colonic perforation, and intestinal ischemia.
- Assess patient's blood pressure, pulse, temperature, and respirations, reporting any signs of shock.

- Assess for presence of maroon stools and abdominal distention.
- Maintain patient's intravenous fluids as ordered.

Risk for impaired skin integrity related to massive diarrhea

- Assess for skin breakdown and the need for pressure-relieving devices for patients who are not ambulatory.
- Cleanse skin carefully after each bowel movement; warm sitz baths will help cleanse the skin and soothe irritated perianal skin.
- Apply barrier ointments to perianal area as long as the patient has diarrhea.

Patient Education/Home Care Planning

1. Patients will be given oral medications, and it is important that the patient understand the rationale for the agent and the importance of compliance with the prescribed protocol.
2. If surgery is required for fulminating disease, the patient and family will require instructions in management of the diverting or permanent ileostomy. The surgery is rarely necessary.
3. Ensure that the patient understands he or she must notify his or her health provider if diarrhea recurs. Symptoms of a relapse (diarrhea; with or without fever; cramps) occur 3 to 10 days after treatment is discontinued.

Evaluation

Body functions normally   Patient has no diarrhea, nor does diarrhea recur after discontinuation of treatment.

Fluid balance is maintained   Patient returns to normal hydration levels as assessed by skin turgor, mucous membranes, color, blood pressure, and pulse. Serum electrolytes, hematocrit, and WBC are within normal limits.

■ CROHN'S DISEASE

Crohn's disease, a chronic inflammatory disorder of the gastrointestinal tract, may occur in any part of the gastrointestinal tract from the mouth to the anus, but the most common sites are the terminal ileum and colon.

Crohn's disease, granulomatous colitis, regional enteritis, transmural colitis, and transmural ileitis all refer to the same disease process. Crohn's disease is segmental in nature, and normal mucosa will be found between diseased segments (skip lesions). Crohn's disease and ulcerative colitis are often called inflammatory bowel diseases (IBD), and differential diagnosis between the two diseases is important in planning treatment. A chronic disorder, Crohn's disease frequently recurs after surgical resection of diseased segments.

The overall incidence of Crohn's disease has increased by a factor of 1.4 to 4 over the past 20 years, with a prevalence range of 10 to 70 cases per 100,000 population.[61] The disease has also been increasing in the young.[63] It is hard to determine if the increase is in actual numbers of cases or whether it is related to an increased awareness of Crohn's disease and improved diagnostic techniques. Crohn's disease is more common among Jews than non-Jews and among whites than nonwhites. The age at onset of the disease is the early teens and early twenties, with a range of 15 to 30 years of age.[10,61] A positive family history for inflammatory bowel disease may be found in up to 40% of the patients.[10] The frequency among siblings is higher than with more distant relatives, yet no genetic markers have been found to support a genetic basis.

Crohn's disease is described by the anatomic location of the disease. Crohn's disease may be limited to the small bowel, involve both small bowel and colon (ileocolitis), be limited to the colon, or be present in the stomach or duodenum. A small group of patients may have Crohn's disease that is limited to the anorectal region. Most patients have Crohn's disease involving both the small bowel and colon.

The cause of Crohn's disease is unknown. Research funded through the Crohn's and Colitis Foundation of America (CCFA; previously the National Foundation of Ileitis and Colitis) and other digestive disease groups is directed toward discovery of the cause and cure for this chronic illness.

•••••• Pathophysiology

Although the cause of Crohn's disease is unknown, it has been hypothesized that an exogenous agent penetrates the intestinal epithelium, creating a cytopathic immune response in a susceptible individual. Factors that have been examined as possible causes include infectious agents (bacteria and viruses), altered host susceptibility, immune-mediated intestinal damage, psychologic factors, and dietary and environmental factors.

Psychologic factors that cause Crohn's disease[10,61,63] have not been documented; yet stress has been associated with clinical exacerbations.

The role of infectious agents has been studied to identify a specific myobacteria or virus responsible for Crohn's disease. Recent studies have explored the possibility of cell wall–defective variants of enteric bacteria, whereas other research suggests a viruslike agent. Granulomatous lesions have been produced on the footpads of mice by injecting extracts from Crohn's lesions. The same results were discovered when injections were made from intestinal extracts from normal specimens. So far, studies have failed to document a specific cause in Crohn's disease.

Altered host susceptibility has been considered in the cause of Crohn's disease. Although a specific infectious agent has not been identified, some researchers suggest that an impaired immune or inflammatory response to an infectious agent might progress to Crohn's disease. Impairment of various manifestations of cell-mediated immunity has been found in a substantial portion of patients with Crohn's disease, but this may be due to drug therapy or to malnutrition. Genetic transmission of specific histocompatibility antigens has also been explored, without conclusive findings.

Immune mechanisms have been implicated in the cause of Crohn's disease because of the recurrent inflammatory process, presence of granulomatous lesions, systemic manifestations, and the positive response to corticosteroids and other imunosuppressives. Studies have examined the following as possible immune causes: hypersensitivity reaction in the intestines, "autoimmune" antibody–mediated damage to intestinal epithelium, tissue deposition of antigen-antibody complexes, lymphocyte-mediated cytotoxicity, and impairment of cellular immune mechanisms.[10,71]

Sleisenger and Fordtran[61] identify three weaknesses in the immunity basis for inflammatory bowel disease. First, the cytotoxicity of lymphocytes disappears after surgical removal of the diseased bowel. Second, the antibody-dependent, cell-mediated damage to the intestinal mucosa has not been demonstrated in the intact host. Third, it is not confirmed that the K cell–mediated cytotoxicity induced by lymphocytes is specific to inflammatory bowel disease.

Dietary and environmental factors have also been questioned in the cause of Crohn's disease. Chemical food additives, such as carragccnin, reduced dietary fibers, smoking, oral contraceptives, and increased refined sugars have been studied. No evidence firmly links dietary or environmental factors to Crohn's disease at this time.

In Crohn's disease the inflammatory process extends through the layers of the bowel wall, hence the term "transmural." Microscopically the following are found in the intestines: transmural inflammation, submucosal infiltration, submucosal thickening and fibrosis, ulceration through the mucosa, fissures, and focal granulomas. As the disease progresses, the bowel wall thickens and the lumen narrows. Stenosis is common. The mucosa shows skip lesions, with normal bowel between diseased segments. The mesentery thickens and may extend over the serosal surface toward the antimesenteric border of the bowel. The intestinal segment may become fixed as the mesentery becomes fibrotic and contracts. The mesenteric nodes are enlarged and firm and may come together to form an irregular mass. The lymphatic vessels dilate and may be visible in the involved mesentery and serosal layer of the bowel.

The mucosal layer in advanced Crohn's disease consists of deep mucosal ulcerations and nodular submucosal thickening, producing a cobblestone appearance to the surface layer. The ulcers usually extend into the submucosa, and two or more ulcers may coalesce to form deep longitudinal ulcers traversing long segments. These ulcers are often referred to as *rake* ulcers. As the disease progresses, the mucosa becomes denuded.

The inflammation of the serosa and mesentery leads to a characteristic tendency in Crohn's disease for involved loops of bowel to adhere to one another. Fissures extend through the entire wall of the bowel and erode into adjacent loops of bowel or bladder, forming a fistula. It is not unusual for a fistula tract to develop to the skin (enterocutaneous), the umbilicus, or the perineum. When the rectum is diseased, ulcers arising in the rectal crypts may end in the perirectal fat and form abscesses. Rectal abscesses may erode into the anal sphincter and the supporting muscles. Abscesses can occur anywhere in the peritoneum, retroperitoneal area, or pelvis.

The severity of the malabsorption depends on the severity of the Crohn's disease, the amount of gut involved, and the treatment regimen. Crohn's disease in the jejunum and ileum decreases the capacity of the small bowel mucosa to absorb multiple nutrients, including carbohydrates, amino acids, folate, water-soluble vitamins, fats, and fat-soluble vitamins. Disease in the terminal ileum may lead to vitamin B_{12} (cobalamin) malabsorption and bile salt reabsorption, resulting in increased diarrhea because of increased osmolality of bile salt in the colon and decreased fat absorption. Lactase deficiency may develop with small bowel disease. The presence of ulcerations in extensive disease may result in protein loss. Iron deficiency anemia may develop from a chronic, slow blood loss and decrease in iron absorption. Bleeding in Crohn's disease is often mild, and the stool color may not change. The characteristic changes of the lymphatic system in Crohn's disease contribute to an impaired fat absorption.

The strictures and internal fistulas common in Crohn's disease may lead to stasis of intestinal contents in the bypassed segment, which results in bacterial overgrowth in the lumen; bacterial overgrowth impairs absorption of carbohydrates, fats, and vitamin B_{12} and alters bile salt metabolism, affecting fat absorption.

Therapy may also affect nutrition. Some patients impose dietary restrictions on themselves or limit their oral food intake. Patients should be tested for lactose intolerance before a lactose-free diet is imposed. Surgical resection of diseased segments of small bowel and colon may also affect nutrition. Resection or bypass of an intestinal segment may decrease the absorptive surface area. Resection of the terminal ileum may lead to vitamin B_{12} and bile salt malabsorption. The distal ileum is the site for reabsorption of conjugated bile salts, and the loss of ileum results in loss of bile salts through the colon, thereby decreasing the total bile salt pool and decreasing biliary secretion of bile salts, resulting in fat malabsorption. Unabsorbed bile salts stimulate the colon mucosal secretion and reduce the net absorption of water and electrolytes in the colon, and the patient experiences increased diarrhea.

Surgeries that result in enteroenterostomies (bowel anastomosis to bowel), surgical blind loops, and loss of ileocecal valve create conditions in which bacterial overgrowth frequently occurs. The effect of overgrowth of enteric microorganisms was discussed previously.

Folate deficiency is common in patients with Crohn's disease. Decreased dietary intake and decreased absorption affect folate levels. In addition, sulfasalazine (which is frequently used in treating Crohn's disease) impairs the absorption of folate. Patients with Crohn's disease may also have an increased requirement for folate because of increased catabolism and chronic blood loss.

Patients with Crohn's disease frequently have increased caloric and protein requirements because of the catabolic effects of the chronic inflammation and superimposed infection. This further depletes the patient's nutritional status. The consequences of the impaired absorption and nutritional deficiencies are more serious in children than adults. Growth retardation and delayed sexual maturation occur in 20% to 30% of young patients. The use of corticosteroids over a prolonged period also contributes to growth retardation.

Complications of Crohn's disease are either intestinal (e.g., small bowel obstructions, abscesses, cancer, perforation, or fistula formation) or systemic. Obstructions are usually the result of inflammation and edema in a strictured or narrowed segment of bowel. The typical obstruction tends to progress slowly to a complete obstruction. Sudden complete obstruction may occur if the bowel becomes kinked by adhesions.

Fistula formation is very common in Crohn's disease and is a characteristic that often distinguishes Crohn's disease from ulcerative colitis. Perianal and perirectal fistulas and fissures can be extremely severe and may cause more problems for the patient than other clinical symptoms. Enterocutaneous fistulas can also cause severe management problems for the patient. A fistula between the bowel and bladder is infrequent, but when it occurs, it leads to chronic urinary infections and if untreated may progress to irreversible renal damage. Free perforation is rare in Crohn's disease because of the more frequent fistula and abscess formation.

Systemic manifestations include arthritis, iritis, erythema nodosum, ankylosing spondylitis, pyoderma gangrenosum, aphthous mouth ulcers, and occasionally liver disease. Arthritis is the most common systemic manifestation. Arthritic symptoms may be present several years before bowel symptoms appear. Children with arthritic symptoms should have tests done to rule out inflammatory bowel disease. The arthritis may be migratory arthritis involving large joints, sacroiliitis, or ankylosing spondylitis. In Crohn's disease the arthritis does not seem to reflect the degree of intestinal disease. (However, in ulcerative colitis, arthritis tends to be more severe, and the patient experiences exacerbations or remissions depending on the intestinal state.)

Erythema nodosum and pyoderma gangrenosum are inflammatory disorders of the skin that may occur with Crohn's disease. Pyoderma gangrenosum is the more severe disorder and may be found during a recurrence of active Crohn's disease in a patient after a surgical resection. The lesion may develop before the bowel symptoms.

Although liver disease is unusual in patients with Crohn's disease, mild abnormalities of liver function may be observed in hospitalized patients. Sclerosing cholangitis occurs more frequently in patients with Crohn's disease than in the general population. Renal disorders may also be a complication of Crohn's disease. The infections related to enterovesical fistulas may lead to urinary tract infections. The ureters may also be affected by the bowel and mesenteric inflammation, leading to obstruction and hydronephrosis. Oxalate stones and hyperoxaluria have been associated with steatorrhea in patients with Crohn's disease.

Cancer of the colon occurs three times more often in patients with Crohn's disease than in the general population. This is less frequently than colon cancer is found in patients with ulcerative colitis. Crohn's disease may vary from a mild to severely debilitating disease. An individual may experience one

acute episode and be asymptomatic for years. Medical management is the primary form of therapy; however, most patients will require surgery at some time to manage intestinal complications of the long-term effects of the disease. The recurrence of Crohn's disease after surgical resection ranges from 75% to 90% in 15 years.[61]

••••• Diagnostic Studies and Findings

Stool cultures   Negative (used to rule out infections)

Stool guaiac   Positive (shows blood loss)

Laboratory studies   Serum albumin: low (protein loss through lesions and increase in protein catabolism); liver function: abnormal (pericholangitis or fatty liver); serum cobalamin: low (ileal disease); serum folic acid: low (malabsorption); hemoglobin, hematocrit: anemia; leukocytes (marked elevation may suggest presence of abscess or other suppurative condition)

Platelets $>300,000/ml^3$ (may occur with active disease)

Lactose tolerance test   To rule out lactase deficiency

Sigmoidoscopy   Rectum: rectal mucosa may be free of disease; perianal or perirectal fissures, fistulas, or abscesses may be found; distal colon: aphthous ulcers or erosions; deep longitudinal fissures with intervening edematous mucosa

Colonoscopy   Skip lesions; cobblestone mucosa

Biopsy   Presence of granulomas; also aids in differentiation of pseudopolyposis, ulcerative colitis, adenomatous polyp, and cancer

Barium studies   Upper small bowel, barium enemas; asymmetric disease, skip lesions, pseudodiverticula, linear ulcerations, transverse fissures, cobblestone mucosa, strictures, fistulas (NOTE: routine preparation of colon should be omitted because it may initiate an exacerbation of the disease; prepare patient with a clear liquid diet for 2 to 3 days)

••••• Multidisciplinary Plan

Surgery

Strictureplasty–a conservative approach for high-risk patients with chronic bowel obstruction

Surgical resection of diseased segments of bowel (operative therapy reserved for complications of Crohn's disease or unequivocal failure to respond to medical management)

Total colectomy with ileostomy (when disease is limited to the colon and is not responsive to medical management or cancer is found)

Subtotal colectomy with temporary ileostomy or with ileorectal anastomosis (when the rectum is not involved)

Medications

5-ASA formulations (may inhibit inflammatory or immune-mediated injuries)

Sulfasalazine (Azulfidine): acute phase: 3 to 4 g/d in divided doses tid; maintenance: 1 to 2.5 g/d tid

Mesalamine

    Asacol: 800 mg tid po

    Pentasa: 1 g qid po

Prednisone: acute phase: 50 to 80 mg/d (intravenously in severely ill patient); maintenance: 5 to 15 mg/d po

Antibiotics

Metronidazole (Flagyl): 15 mg/kg/d in divided doses

Immunomodulatory agents

"Third-line" drugs—these have significant side effects, and their use is somewhat controversial

6-Mercaptopurine (6-MP): acute phase: 1.5 mg/kg/d po (has a steroid-sparing effect and may be more useful in patients with fistulas and perianal disease)

Azathioprine: 50 mg/day initial dose; may be gradually increased if tolerated

In clinical trials only: cyclosporine A and methotrexate

Diarrhea: loperamide, diphenoxylate, codeine; if diarrhea related to bile salt malabsorption: cholestyramine, aluminum hydroxide; metamucil may be used for watery stools in the chronic phase

Vitamin B_{12} supplementation (q month) if terminal ileum disease is present

Calcium supplement

General Management

Acute phase: intravenous fluids, nothing by mouth, bed rest or limited activity

Complication of small bowel obstruction: nasogastric suctioning

Stenosis or narrowing of lumen: avoid high-fiber foods containing cellulose or those foods that are not readily digested

Nutritional support: vitamin replacement, folic acid, iron, total parenteral nutrition (TPN), enteral alimentation; lactose restrictions (if indicated); some institutions use peripheral amino acids, fat for 1 to 5 days, with bowel rest and then start food or TPN

Nutritional Consultation

To assist patient in identification of foods that exacerbate symptoms; to assist in planning for enteral/parenteral supplementation

NURSING CARE

Nursing Assessment

Gastrointestinal

Initially, diarrhea, abdominal cramping, and fever; as disease progresses, must observe patient for signs of complications

Diarrhea: when disease confined to ileum, five or six loose bowel movements per day; when colon involved, urgency and incontinence frequent

Abdominal cramping: mild to severe, lower quadrant, intermittent periumbilical colic experienced during bowel movements

Gastrointestinal complications

Fistulas

Stool in urine

Passing gas via vagina

Fecal drainage through skin (enterocutaneous)

Small bowel obstructions

Toxic megacolon

Cancer

Free perforations (rare)

Hemorrhage (infrequent)

Nutritional Status

Anorexia, nausea, dietary intolerance, weight loss

Perianal Examination

Presence of fissures, fistulas, or abscesses

Extracolonic Manifestations

Arthritis

Inflammation of eye, skin, or mucous membrane in form of iritis, pyoderma gangrenosum, erythema nodosum, or aphthous ulcers of mouth and tongue

General

Low-grade fever

Low energy level

Coping

Emotional status

Interactions with significant others

Interactions with health care providers

Impact on social activities and work

Involvement with local support organizations; seeks psychiatric help

Impact on sexuality and sexual activity

Knowledge Level

Disease process, complications, manifestations, usual tests and procedures, local support organizations

Musculoskeletal

Joint pains, back pain

Nursing Dx & Intervention

Diarrhea related to intestinal inflammatory process

- Assess the frequency of bowel movements and the appearance of stools for the presence of blood or evidence of steatorrhea.
- Protect the perianal skin with barrier ointments.
- Provide for privacy and odor control.
- Check stools for occult blood.
- Provide antidiarrheal medications as ordered.
- Replace losses as needed (fluids, electrolytes, and blood products).

Altered nutrition: less than body requirements related to decreased intake, nausea, abdominal pain and cramping, food intolerance, and diarrhea

- Monitor weight, serum albumin (or prealbumin if available), folate, hemoglobin, magnesium, iron, and vitamin B_{12}.
- Nutritional consultation.
- Provide nutritional supplements, enteral or parenteral formulas as ordered.
- Assist the patient to identify irritating foods if the disease is new to him or her.

Risk for ineffective family coping related to the nature of the disease symptoms and the chronicity of the disease and the effect on sexuality

- See pp. 1754 to 1755.
- Provide sensitive, caring approach to patient and his or her family.
- Assess the patient and family regarding knowledge of Crohn's disease, problems with medical treatment regimen, myths regarding the disease, coping patterns, and the use of support groups or psychiatric services.
- Help the patient and family support one another as they manage the effects of chronic illness in their lives; refer as needed for support.
- Provide opportunities for the patient and family to express their feelings regarding the illness and to identify their perceptions for a successful outcome (including changes in sexuality patterns).

Pain related to intestinal inflammation

- Monitor changes in intensity of pain, effectiveness of narcotics, the relation of pain to stress, passage of bowel movements, and eating.
- Provide for adjunctive treatments that help manage the pain (relaxation, music, massage, diversion).
- Provide analgesics as ordered.

Risk for impaired skin integrity related to diarrhea, incontinence, and perianal disease

- Assess perianal region for irritation from diarrhea or fistula drainage.
- Protect perianal skin in patients with frequent bowel movements:
    1. Use gentle cleansing solutions, such as Periwash or Tucks.
    2. Do not use toilet paper; have patient use squirt bottle to rinse perineum after bowel movements instead of wiping.
    3. Apply barrier cream to protect skin.
    4. If area is denuded, use Sitz baths or cleanse with cotton balls soaked in mineral oil.
    5. Use Anusol suppositories or Nupercainal Ointment.
- Provide interventions or treatment for perianal fissures as ordered; treatment includes Sitz baths and keeping the perianal area cleansed after bowel movements.

Patient Education/Home Care Planning

1. Discuss with the patient the usual treatments, procedures, and natural history of the disease.
2. Teach the patient the importance of optimal nutrition in cooperation with the nutritionist.
3. Explain to the patient the schedules of medications. Ensure that the patient understands how prednisone affects the adrenal glands and how he or she must not abruptly stop taking the medication.
4. Provide the patient with information on drug toxicities. For example, sulfasalazine is associated with rashes, and patients may be desensitized with small doses.
5. Inform the patient of the Crohn's and Colitis Foundation of America as a source of support and information.
6. Provide specific instructions for procedures and allow return demonstrations: TPN or central line care.

Evaluation

Number and consistency of stools are within normal limits Patient has a decrease in episodes of fecal incontinence. Patient has fewer episodes of diarrhea and incontinence. Patient's perianal skin is intact. Patient knows which foods to avoid.

Nutrition is adequate Patient's weight is in positive nitrogen balance. Patient has an appetite. Patient's protein and calorie intake is adequate.

Patient and family are able to cope with chronic illness or an acute exacerbation Patient and family are able to verbalize factors that create anxiety and stress. Patient and family are aware of resources available to them for further supportive care. Patient and family are able to verbalize mechanisms that help them deal with stressors.

Comfort level is achieved Patient is able to perform ADLs. Patient has stopped using all injectable narcotics by discharge. Patient is able to use alternate methods for relief of pain.

ULCERATIVE COLITIS

Ulcerative colitis is a chronic mucosal inflammatory disease limited to the colon and rectum.

The disease generally starts in the rectum and progresses uninterrupted through the colon. The mucosa and submucosa layers of the colon and rectum are affected by ulcerative colitis. It is often difficult to differentiate the symptoms of ulcerative colitis from Crohn's disease of the large colon. The distinction between the two diseases is important in planning treatment and long-term prognosis. Ulcerative colitis is cured by total proctocolectomy. The incidence of cancer associated with long-standing ulcerative colitis is four times greater than in Crohn's disease. Ulcerative colitis is characterized by bloody, frequent, watery diarrhea. Patients report as many as 20 to 30 diarrheal stools per day. Remissions and exacerbations of the disease are common.

The annual incidence of ulcerative colitis in the United States has been relatively stable, with six to eight cases per 100,000 persons per year.[10,61] The incidence of ulcerative colitis is more common among Jewish than non-Jewish populations and among whites than nonwhites. Interestingly, the incidence of ulcerative colitis is more common among European and American Jews than Jews living in Tel-Aviv.[68] The disease is seen with highest frequency between the age of 15 and 25 years.

There is a higher frequency of additional cases of ulcerative colitis in families than in control populations. It is not uncommon to have family members with ulcerative colitis and Crohn's disease. A small percentage of patients may demonstrate features of both ulcerative colitis and Crohn's disease.

As with Crohn's disease, research continues to focus on discovery of the cause. Surgery is no longer considered a "last resort," and newer surgical techniques have improved the outlook for patients. Continent ileostomies and ileoanal reservoir procedures have eliminated the need for conventional ileostomies in selected patient populations.

•••••• Pathophysiology

The cause of ulcerative colitis is unknown. Proposed causes include infectious agents, genetic factors, immunologic mechanisms, environmental, and psychosomatic determinants. No specific bacterium or virus has been found to be the exogenous agent producing the inflammatory reaction seen in ulcerative colitis. The genetic hypothesis is suggested because of the familial tendency for the disease, the higher incidence in Jews, and the low incidence among nonwhites.

An immunologic origin has been suggested for ulcerative colitis because of the presence of extraintestinal manifestations and the presence of antibodies to colonic epithelial cells and of cytotoxic T cells; also, a clinical and histologic response from immunosuppressive agents may be present.[68] A defect in the immunoregulatory activity of the intestinal epithelium may exist. The association of ulcerative colitis with other autoimmune diseases, such as lupus erythematosus, hemolytic anemia, and vasculitis, strengthen the view that ulcerative colitis is an immunologic reaction.

Environmental factors may have a role in the pathogenesis of ulcerative colitis because of the increased incidence of the disorder in industrialized nations. Also, an increased incidence of ulcerative colitis occurs in nonsmokers or in heavy smokers who quit. "Environmental factors (infectious, noninfectious antigens, or toxins) may trigger a sequence of events in which altered immunologic responses become critical in the pathogenesis of inflammatory bowel disease."[89]

Patients with ulcerative colitis have been labeled in the past with a "colitis personality." Research has documented that psychosomatic factors are not the cause of ulcerative colitis. Social and occupational backgrounds of patients with inflammatory bowel disease do not differ from the general population. It is time to eliminate any reference to personality or psychosomatic mechanisms as the cause. The effects of chronic illness on a person's life should be explored. Twenty to 30 bowel movements per day with urgency and occasional incontinence may interfere with work, social and sexual activities. A patient may need help in learning how to cope with the illness and symptoms. Stress and tension may influence the symptoms of ulcerative colitis and have been known to cause exacerbations.

Ulcerative colitis is an inflammatory disease confined primarily to the mucosa and to a lesser degree to the adjacent submucosa. The primary lesion appears to be crypt abscess formation in the crypts of Lieberkuhn. Polymorphonuclear cells accumulate near the tip of the crypt, and degenerative changes occur in the crypt epithelial cells. As the crypt abscess progresses, frank necrosis of the crypt epithelium occurs and the polymorphonuclear infiltrate extends through the colonic epithelium. A more chronic inflammatory infiltrate composed of mast cells, lymphocytes, plasma cells, and eosinophils develops. Vascular engorgement appears in the submucosa. The microabscesses in the crypts are not visible to an unaided eye. However, as the microabscesses coalesce by lateral enlargement, they produce shallow ulcerations of the mucosa extending down to the lamina propria. In some areas the extensions of the abscesses undermine the mucosa on three sides, producing an area of ulceration adjacent to a hanging fragment of mucosa, which is referred to as a pseudopolyp during radiographic or endoscopic procedures.

The body attempts to heal itself even as the destruction of the mucosa is occurring. Highly vascular granulation tissue may develop in ulcerated, denuded areas. Collagen is deposited in the lamina propria. Fibrosis is minimal. In long-standing disease the muscularis mucosae may hypertrophy. The hypertrophy and spasms of the muscularis mucosae may result in shortening and narrowing of the colon, loss of haustral markings, and apparent stricture formation. All of these are reversible in ulcerative colitis because they are not caused by fibrosis.

The two most prominent symptoms of ulcerative colitis are hematochezia and diarrhea. (See Emergency Alert box on p. 754). The bleeding is the result of the mucosal changes; ulceration, vascular engorgement, and highly vascular, friable granulation tissue. As the mucosa is destroyed or damaged, it loss its ability to absorb sodium and water, resulting in watery diarrha. The absence of involvement of the muscularis and serosa layers accounts for the lack of localized abdominal pain, fistula formation, and well-defined peritoneal signs observed frequently in Crohn's disease.

Complications of ulcerative colitis include perforation, toxic megacolon, adenocarcinoma of the colon, massive hemorrhage, and extracolonic manifestations. Perforation of the colon may develop if the disease process extends through the muscle and serosa layers of the colon. Toxic megacolon is a severe and serious complication of ulcerative colitis. Toxic megacolon is associated with fulminant disease, in which the circular and longitudinal muscles have been destroyed. Damage to the

---

! EMERGENCY ALERT

GASTROINTESTINAL BLEEDING

The upper and lower gastrointestinal (GI) tract may experience hemorrhage and may produce significant pain. Upper GI bleeding is most commonly caused by peptic ulcers that erode through a vessel. Ruptured esophageal varices produce upper GI bleeding and are often associated with chronic hepatic disease; one third of these individuals die. Lower GI bleeding from the large bowel and rectum is typically caused by ulcerative colitis, cancers, ulcers, hemorrhoids, diverticulitis, or polyps.

ASSESSMENT

- History: determine history, including alcohol use, previous bleeding or ulcers, history of pain or gastric upset.
- Assess hemodynamic stability, including vital signs, skin color and moisture, and other signs that may indicate hypovolemia or shock.
- Presence of hematemesis (vomiting of blood), black tarry stools, or bright red stools.
- Presence of epigastic tenderness, jaundice, enlarged spleen, or enlarged liver.

INTERVENTIONS

- If indicated, maintain ABCs.
- Keep client NPO until source of bleeding is determined.
- Obtain IV access and maintain fluid hydration as indicated by signs of hypovolemia.
- Obtain laboratory specimens as indicated, including hemoglobin, hematocrit, and possible specimens for type and cross-matching of blood.
- Prepare for possible endoscopy to determine source of bleeding.

---

myenteric ganglia in the wall of the colon produces a loss of contractibility, and peristalsis ceases with marked dilatation of the colon developing. The transmural inflammation may lead to necrosis and perforation. Narcotics, anticholinergics, and hypokalemia may precipitate toxic megacolon because they produce atony of the smooth muscles of the colon.

Cancer of the colon and rectum occurs at a much higher rate in patients with ulcerative colitis than in the general population. Two factors appear to be related to the incidence of adenocarcinoma of the colon and rectum. First, the duration of the disease process has been related to the cancers. Ulcerative colitis of 10 years' duration increases the risk, and the risk continues to increase thereafter. Second, the extent of colonic involvement influences the risk of colorectal cancers. The more universal (affecting the entire colon and rectum) ulcerative colitis is, the higher the incidence of cancer. Patients with the disease limited to the rectum have no greater risk of colon cancer than persons of the same age and sex without ulcerative colitis. The cancerous lesions tend to be flat and infiltrative in nature and are multicentric. Early diagnosis is important. In patients with

ulcerative colitis of 10 years or longer, frequent colonoscopy with biopsy is recommended (at least yearly). Even with close follow-up, colon cancer may be detected too late for curative therapy.

The question often arises of prophylactic colectomy after a duration of 10 years. Colectomy does cure ulcerative colitis and also prevents colon cancer. Of course, the person will have some type of diversional procedure (conventional ileostomy, continent ileostomy, ileorectal pouch). One question of length of duration is the actual beginning of the disease. Patients may have the ulcerative colitis for a year or two before diagnosis. The decision to have surgery is a serious one with which patients are faced. By the time a patient with long-standing disease is admitted for surgery, he or she has dealt with a variety of emotions and may be "ready" for surgery. Other patients prefer to wait until it is essential that surgery be done. Although it is impossible to generalize and recommend surgical interventions for all patients, the nurse does play an important role in educating patients to the risk of cancer, the long-term effects of the disease, its treatments, and the need for consistent follow-up, even when the patient is asymptomatic.

A medical emergency for a person with ulcerative colitis is a massive hemorrhage, which occurs in approximately 4% of patients.[61] Patients with ulcerative colitis are often severely ill, with high temperatures, tachycardia, and fluid depletion. Massive fluid replacements are required to replace the circulating volume and maintain blood pressure. The hemorrhage usually subsides spontaneously. Surgical intervention (total proctocolectomy) is rarely necessary.

The mortality of an acute initial episode of ulcerative colitis is approximately 5%. The prognosis is negatively affected by total colonic involvement, age at onset older than 60 years, and presence of toxic megacolon.

Extracolonic manifestations can also be serious complications of ulcerative colitis. Arthritis, uveitis, and skin disorders reflect the disease process and will have remissions and exacerbation with the disease. The arthritis of ulcerative colitis involves the larger joints and is migratory. The joint is frequently swollen, erythematous, and tender. Steroids also cause osteonecrosis, and patients should have bone scans or magnetic resonance imaging (MRI) if they complain of bone pain while receiving long-term steroids.

Uveitis (iritis) is the most common eye lesion seen accompanying ulcerative colitis. The patient may experience blurred vision, eye pain, and photophobia. An acute attack of iritis may be followed by atrophy of the iris, anterior and posterior synechiae, and old pigment deposits on the lens.

The extracolonic skin disorders consist of erythema nodosum and pyoderma gangrenosum. Erythema nodosum consists of raised, tender, erythematous swellings of 2 to 3 cm on the arms and legs. The condition often develops during an exacerbation of the colitis and is frequently found when arthritis is associated with the exacerbation of the primary disease. Occasionally arthritis and erythema nodosum appear just before the first overt bowel symptoms of ulcerative colitis. Pyoderma gangrenosum is less frequent than erythema nodosum and is usually associated with severe ulcerative colitis. Pyoderma gangrenosum first appears as a pinpoint lesion, a boil, or an infected hair follicle. The lesion collects purulent drainage that contains few polymorphonuclear cells and no bacteria. The lesion may drain spontaneously. There is a characteristic purple border around the lesion. As the lesion becomes gangrenous, progressive necrosis of the dermis occurs and the area is deeply ulcerated. Healing of the lesions requires control of the ulcerative colitis through corticosteroids or surgical removal of the colon and rectum.

Liver diseases have also been associated with ulcerative colitis. The pathogenesis is not understood, and the incidence of liver disease is approximately 7%. Liver disease may range from minor abnormalities in one or more liver function tests to more serious changes in liver structure and function. Diseases of the liver associated with ulcerative colitis include fatty infiltrations, pericholangitis, chronic active hepatitis, postnecrotic cirrhosis, amyloidosis, and sclerosing cholangitis. The question remains as to the degree of improvement in liver diseases after colectomy.

Renal stone formation is associated with ulcerative colitis and is probably related to dehydration, inactivity of the patient, and changes in the composition of the urine.

Ulcerative colitis may range from mild to severe. The degree of involvement of the colon influences the severity. For many patients, ulcerative colitis will remain in remission for years after an acute phase of the illness. The treatment and the nursing interventions will be influenced by the degree of involvement and the severity of the colitis.

•••••• Diagnostic Studies and Findings

Stool cultures   Negative

Laboratory studies   Hemoglobin, hematocrit: anemia
Liver function: abnormal; serum albumin: low; erythrocyte sedimentation rate (ESR): elevated; white blood cells (acute episode): elevated

Sigmoidoscopy   Submucosal inflammation and edema; subepithelial infiltration and edema; microscopic mucosal erosions; crypt abscesses; granular appearance; friable (bleeds easily)

Rectal biopsy   Inflammatory changes in the mucosa; helps to differentiate between ulcerative colitis and Crohn's colitis

Colonoscopy   Superficial mucosal changes in early disease: hyperemia, mucosal friability, fine granular pattern, shallow ulcerations; late disease: coarse, granular appearance; deep mucosal ulcerations; pseudopolyps; shortening of colon; loss of haustrations; NOTE: colonoscopy should be avoided in acute situations because of danger of perforation

X-ray examination   Plain film of abdomen: shortening of colon; loss of haustrations; irregular mucosa caused by pseudopolyps, ulcerations, and mucosa tags; midtransverse colon dilated with air in toxic megacolon; thickened bowel wall

Double-contrast barium enemas   Evaluates disease above the sigmoidoscopy level (preferred over colonoscopy); early disease: study may appear normal, or there may be a reticulated pattern denoting the denudation of the mucosa; late disease: ulceration of mucosa; shortening of the bowel; pseudopolyps; NOTE: under no circumstances should a patient with

ulcerative colitis be prepared with irritant cathartics; such treatment may worsen the disease; barium enemas should be avoided in acute situations because of danger of perforation

•••••• Multidisciplinary Plan

Surgery

Emergency operations (fulminant disease, hemorrhage, perforation, toxic megacolon)
Total abdominal colectomy (subtotal colectomy) with end ileostomy and distal mucous fistula or Hartmann's pouch
Elective operations (intractability, dysplasia, or cancer)
Mucosal proctectomy with ileoanal anastomosis performed in one or two stages; if the operation is done in one stage, there is no diverting ileostomy; stage I: Subtotal colectomy, rectal mucosal stripping, creation of ileal reservoir, anastomosis of reservoir to upper anal canal after pulling it down through the rectal muscle tube, formation of diverting ilesotomy; stage II: Takedown of the diverting ileostomy and reestablishing bowel continuity
Continent ileostomy: Total proctocolectomy with the creation of an ileal reservoir with an intussuscepted ileal segment or nipple valve formation creating continence
Total proctocolectomy with permanent ileostomy

Medications

Choice depends on location and severity of disease; if the disease is confined to the rectum or left colon, suppositories or enemas may be all that are needed
Corticosteroids
In mild disease (ulcerative proctitis), acute phase: hydrocortisone retention enemas, 100 mg in 60 ml nightly, should retain for 20 min
In mild disease, remission: hydrocortisone retention enemas several times per week slowly tapering down and discontinuing
In moderate disease, acute phase: prednisone, 40 to 60 mg/d po
In moderate disease, remission: taper off prednisone slowly
In severe disease, acute phase: prednisolone, 100 mg IV over 24 h (need intravenous potassium to prevent steroid-induced hypokalemia) q10-14d followed by prednisolone, 60 to 100 mg/d po (If patient does not respond, surgery may be indicated)
5-ASA derivatives (need weeks to months for response)
Rectal preparations
Rowasa enema 4 g/60 ml buffered suspension suppository 0.5 g/kg
Oral preparations
Sulfasalazine (Azulfidine): acute phase, 3 to 4 g tid po; maintenance, 2 g po qid
Pentasa, 250 mg-4 g/d
Asacol, 400 mg
Claversol or Salofalk, 250,000 mg
Dipentum, 500 mg bid

Topical corticoids (decreased systemic effects, decreased systemic absorption—clinical trials only)

Budesonide, 2 mg/dl enema (100 times more potent than topical hydrocortisone)

Tixocortol pivalate, 250 mg nightly enema

Immunosuppressives

6-Mercaptopurine (6-MP), 50 mg/d to 1.5 mg/kg/d

Azathioprine, 50 mg/d initially; dosage may be increased if well tolerated

Cyclosporine (clinical trials only)

Methotrexate (clinical trials only)

For diarrhea:

Loperamide (Imodium) 4 mg/d and 2 mg after each unformed stool up to a maximum of 16 mg

Diphenoxylate hydrochloride (Lomotil), 5 mg qid (codeine and Lomotil used with caution because opiates and atropine in Lomotil can precipitate toxic megacolon)

Metamucil, 1 tsp qid (used to add bulk to watery stools; avoid in the very ill patient)

Folate supplementation

General Management

Acute phase: intravenous fluids, limited activity or bed rest, total parenteral nutrition (TPN) (for severe dehydration and cachexia); blood replacement usually required; nasogastric tube if dilated colon; no opiates or anticholinergics if risk of toxic megacolon

Nutrition: no general restrictions; patients should avoid foods that they identify as irritating; usually a low-fiber diet advanced as tolerated with one food added at a time; milk can be a problem for some patients; need extra calories and protein

NURSING CARE

Nursing Assessment

General

Low energy level, fever

Pain

Location and nature of pain

Use pain scale for rating both intensity of pain and ability to tolerate pain

Nutritional Status

Anorexia, nausea, dietary intolerances, weight loss

Abdominal Examination

Localized areas of tenderness, bowel sounds

Gastrointestinal

Diarrhea—amount and frequency; presence of blood or mucus; relation to eating, stress, activity; tenesmus; incontinence

Hemorrhoids

Skin

Pyoderma gangrenosum, erythema nodosum

Perianal skin for fissures, fistulas, abscesses, irritation

Coping

Emotional status

Interactions with significant others

Interactions with health care providers

Impact on social activities and work

Involvement with local support organizations or psychiatric help

Impact on sexuality and sexual activity

Knowledge Level

Disease process, complications, manifestations, usual tests and procedures, local support organizations

Musculoskeletal

Joint pains; back pain

Complications

Toxic megacolon

Severe abdominal distention

Increasing abdominal pain

Fever

Tachycardia

Sharp decrease in number of stools and in gas

Rectal bleeding

Hypoactive or absent bowel sounds

Nursing Dx & Intervention

Diarrhea related to intestinal inflammatory process

- Assess the frequency of patient's bowel movements and the appearance of stools (presence of blood; evidence of steatorrhea).
- Protect patient's perianal skin with barrier ointments.
- Provide privacy and odor control for patient.
- Check patient's stools for occult blood.
- Provide patient with antidiarrheal medications as ordered.
- Replace patient's losses as needed (fluids, electrolytes, and blood products).

Altered nutrition: less than body requirements related to decreased intake, nausea, abdominal pain and cramping, food intolerance, and diarrhea

- Monitor patient's weight, serum albumin (or prealbumin, if available), folate, hemoglobin, magnesium, iron, and vitamin B_{12}.
- Request a consultation with the nutritionist for the patient.
- Provide the patient with nutritional supplements, enteral, or parenteral formulas as ordered.
- Assist the patient to identify irritating foods if the disease is new to him or her.

Risk for ineffective family coping related to nature of disease symptoms and the chronicity of the disease, and the effect on sexuality

- See pp. 1754 to 1756.
- Provide sensitive, caring approach for patient and his or her family.
- Assess patient and family regarding their knowledge of ulcerative colitis, current medical treatment regimen, myths regarding the disease, coping patterns, and use of support groups or psychiatric services.
- Help patient and family support each other as they manage the effects of chronic illness in their lives. Refer patient for support as needed.
- Provide opportunities for patient and family to express their feelings regarding the illness and to identify their perceptions for a successful outcome (including changes in sexuality patterns).

Pain related to intestinal inflammation

- Monitor changes in patient for the intensity of pain, the effectiveness of narcotics, the relation of pain to stress, the passage of bowel movements, and eating.
- Provide for adjunctive treatments for patient that help manage the pain (relaxation, music, massage, diversion).
- Provide analgesics as ordered.

Risk for impaired skin integrity related to diarrhea, incontinence, and perianal disease

- Assess patient's perianal region for irritation from diarrhea.
- Protect perianal skin in patients with frequent bowel movements:
    1. Use gentle cleansing solutions (Periwash, Tucks) on patient.
    2. Do not use toilet paper; have patient use squirt bottle to cleanse perineal area after bowel movements instead of wiping.
    3. Apply barrier cream to protect patient's skin.
    4. If area is denuded, have patient use Sitz baths or cleanse with cotton balls soaked in mineral oil.
    5. Have patient use Anusol suppositories or Nupercainal ointment.
- Provide interventions or treatment for patient's perianal fissures as ordered: Sitz baths; keep area cleansed after bowel movements.

Patient Education/Home Care Planning

1. Discuss with the patient the usual treatments, procedures, and natural history of the disease.
2. Teach the patient the importance of optimal nutrition, using the nutritionist.
3. Explain schedules of medications. Ensure that the patient understands how prednisone affects the adrenal glands and explain that the patient must not abruptly stop taking the medication.

4. Provide the patient with information about drug toxicities. For example, sulfasalazine is associated with rashes, and patients may be desensitized by taking small doses.
5. Inform the patient of the Crohn's and Colitis Foundation of America as a source of support and information.
6. Provide the patient with specific instructions for procedures and allow return demonstrations: TPN, central line care.

Evaluation

Number and consistency of stools are within normal limits Patient has a decrease in episodes of fecal incontinence and in the number of stools. Patient has fewer episodes of diarrhea and incontinence. Patient's perianal skin is intact. Patient knows which foods to avoid.

Nutrition is adequate Patient is in positive nitrogen balance. Patient has an appetite. Patient's protein and caloric intake is adequate.

Patient and family are able to cope with chronic illness or an acute exacerbation Patient and family are able to verbalize factors that create anxiety and stress. Patient and family are aware of resources available to them for further supportive care. Patient and family are able to verbalize mechanisms that help them deal with stressors.

Comfort level is achieved Patient is able to perform ADLs. Patient has stopped using all injectable narcotics by discharge. Patient is able to use alternate methods for relief of pain.

BENIGN TUMORS

The term "tumor" is used to refer to neoplasm, a new growth of tissue characterized by uncontrolled proliferation of cells. A tumor may be malignant or benign.

The benign tumors of the small and large intestines include colonic adenomas (polyps), villous or papillary adenomas, lipomas, leiomyomas, and lymphoid hyperplasia. Polyps have been discussed on p. 744. A villous adenoma is a rare tumor found most often in the rectosigmoid area; it may be benign or contain foci of carcinoma. Lipomas are smooth, round tumors found in the submucosal layer of the colon. Leiomyomas are found in the small intestine and are submucosal or subserosal growths that protrude intraluminally, extraluminally, or in both directions. Malignant tumors of the colorectal area are covered in Chapter 16.

Benign tumors in the intestines occur equally in men and women. The benign tumors are most often discovered between the ages of 50 and 80. Symptomatic benign tumors are commonly diagnosed between the ages of 30 and 60. Most benign tumors in the small and large intestines are asymptomatic and may be discovered during routine examinations or surgery. Symptoms, when present, are generally related to the size of the tumor. A benign tumor may block the lumen, resulting in obstruction or intussusception. If the mucosa covering a tumor is irritated and becomes ulcerated, the patient may have signs of intestinal bleeding.

The cause of isolated benign tumors of the small intestine is unknown. Benign tumors in the small bowel include adenomas, leiomyomas, lipomas, hamartomas (associated with Peutz-Jeghers syndrome), and neurogenic tumors. Pseudotumors may also be found in the small intestine, and surgical excision is required for histologic studies and differential diagnosis.

The most common benign tumor of the colon is the polyp (or colonic adenoma). Neurofibromas, leiomyomas, and lipomas are found, but the incidence is low. Histologic examination of the tissue is required to determine the type of tumor. Villous adenomas are polyps found in the rectosigmoid area, and they are associated with more symptoms than other tumors. Both colonic polyps and villous adenomas are associated with malignancies.

•••••• Pathophysiology

Adenomas in the intestines may be tubular, villous, or tubulovillous. Adenomas in the small intestine are generally found near the ileum. Villous adenomas are rare in the small intestine and when they occur are found in the duodenum. The villous adenoma is most often found in the rectosigmoid areas. The rectosigmoid villous adenoma appears as a "frondlike, velvety surface."[63] It tends to recur, to secrete large amounts of mucus, and to act as a site for development of cancer.

The primary symptoms of villous adenomas in the rectosigmoid area include increased colonic motility, diarrhea, and electrolyte loss. A villous adenoma higher in the gastrointestinal tract does not seem to precipitate the electrolyte loss, probably because of the reabsorption capacity of the colon distal to the adenoma. Villous adenomas consist of branching papillary fronds lined with goblet cells. The villous adenoma secretes large amounts of mucus. If the villous adenoma is large, the amount of fluid lost through mucous secretions can be significant. Sodium and potassium are lost in the mucous diarrhea. The fluid and electrolyte imbalance may divert attention away from the presence of a villous adenoma as other conditions and causes are considered during diagnosis.

Lipomas may occur anywhere in the small and large intestines, but they are more common in the colon. Lipomas tend to be single lesions averaging 4 cm in diameter. Most lipomas are found incidentally during surgery. Symptoms are associated with intussusception, obstruction, or bleeding. Lipomas in the colon may be detected during water enemas when the returns contain fat. An enlargement of the ileocecal valve may be caused by lipomatosis or by a tumor in the cecum. Lipomatosis is more common, and differential diagnosis can be made by colonoscopy.

Leiomyomas in the small intestine are found in the jejunum and tend to produce more symptoms than other benign tumors of the small intestine. Ulceration of the mucosa is common, and patients' initial complaint is bleeding. Obstruction and intussusception are rare.

Lymphoid hyperplasia of the colon is found more often in children than in adults. An enlarged lymphoid follicle may occur in the rectum. No intervention is required. When lymphoid hyperplasia appears in multiple numbers throughout the rectum and colon, it can be confused with familial polyposis. Differential diagnosis is important because treatment is not indicated in lymphoid hyperplasia and total colectomy is used to treat familial polyposis.

•••••• Diagnostic Studies and Findings

Small bowel   Barium studies; prograde enteroclysis or retrograde infusion through ileocecal valve: small isolated tumors, multiple small tumors; exploratory laparotomy: biopsy and removal of tumor for histologic studies

Colon   Sigmoidoscopy, colonoscopy: visualization, biopsy, and removal of tumor; double-contrast barium enema: villous adenoma; reticulated appearance; presence of tumors in colon and rectum

•••••• Multidisciplinary Plan

Surgery

Laparotomy may be used for diagnosis and removal of tumors in small bowel when patient is symptomatic

Villous adenoma

Above peritoneal reflection: resection of bowel containing villous adenoma

Below peritoneal reflection: local excision

With evidence of frank invasive carcinoma: abdominoperineal resection

NURSING CARE

Nursing Assessment

Abdominal Examination

Signs of intestinal obstruction: abdominal pain, distention, nausea and vomiting, absence of peristalsis, absence of bowel movements

Large bowel or distal small bowel obstructions: fecal odor to emesis

Gastrointestinal

Occult, blood-tinged, or black tarry stools

Nursing Dx & Intervention

Constipation related to partial obstruction of bowel lumen

• Assess patient for signs and symptoms of intestinal obstructions: abdominal pain, abdominal distention, decreased peristalsis, nausea, vomiting.

• Determine whether patient has regular bowel habits and whether bowel pattern has changed.

- Observe stool for shape, consistency, color, quantity, and odor.
- Note and report any signs of blood-tinged stools.
- Check stool for occult blood, an early sign of a bowel tumor.

Patient Education/Home Care Planning

1. Provide patient with information about the type of tumor and any impact regarding long-term care (e.g., after removal of villous adenoma, regular follow-up required if a focus of carcinoma is present).
2. Provide routine postoperative information on activity, diet, driving, and returning to work associated with any abdominal surgery.

Evaluation

Body functions normally   Bowel elimination is adequate.

ANAL AND RECTAL DISORDERS

◼ ANORECTAL ABSCESS

An anorectal abscess is a localized infection with pus found in the tissue spaces adjacent to and in the anorectal area.

Anorectal abscesses are classified according to location (Figure 8-16)

Perianal: beneath perianal skin
Ischiorectal: ischiorectal fossa
Intersphincteric: between internal and external sphincters
Pelvirectal or supralevator: above the levators ani and below the pelvic peritoneum

Anorectal abscesses are more common in men. Certain diseases and conditions increase the likelihood of anorectal abscesses developing. Anorectal abscesses are common in patients with Crohn's disease and in homosexual men who engage in traumatic anal intercourse. Hematologic and immune-deficient conditions have also been associated with anorectal abscesses.

•••••• Pathophysiology

Anorectal abscesses develop from infections beginning in an anal crypt and moving along anal ducts through the internal sphincter before spreading in different directions. An infection may also develop in anal fissures, prolapsed internal hemorrhoids, traumatic injuries, and superficial skin lesions that progress to form anorectal abscesses. Extension of the abscess formation is the most common complication. An abscess may eventually progress to an anorectal fistula.

•••••• Diagnostic Studies and Findings

Anoscopy (proctoscopy)   Visualization of lesions above the pectinate line

•••••• Medical Plan

Surgery

Prompt surgical drainage of abscess, with or without excision of fistula tracts associated with anorectal abscesses

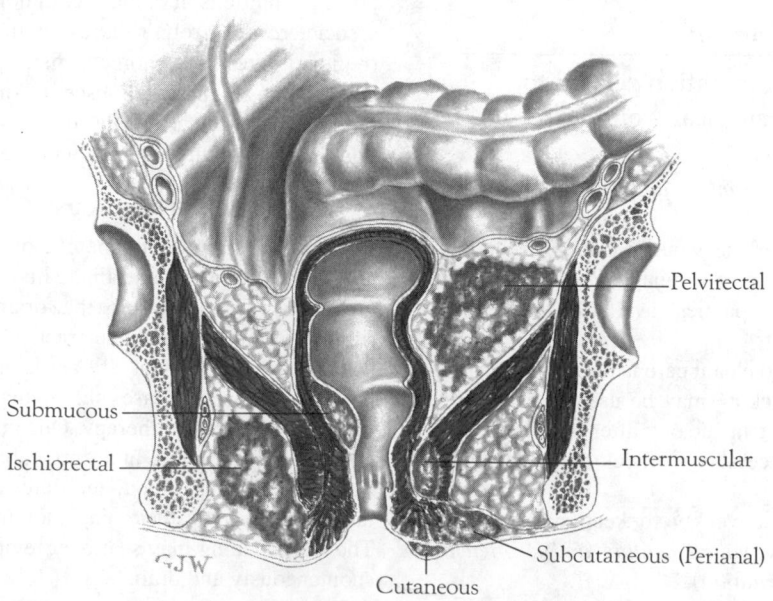

Figure 8-16 Anorectal abscesses. (From Doughty.[17])

Medications

Antibiotic therapy based on causative organisms

Stool softeners: docusate (Colace), 50 to 200 mg/d; dose based on individual's response

General Management

Sitz baths

NURSING CARE

Nursing Assessment

General

Fever, malaise

Pain

Throbbing, constant pain exacerbated by sitting or walking (superficial abscess); pain decreases if abscess drains spontaneously; pain with defecation

Gastrointestinal

Change in bowel habits (purulent discharge, increased odor); last bowel movement; use of laxatives or stool softeners, anal intercourse, anal dilators (e.g., vibrators or other instruments)

Perianal Examination

Assess for signs of a tender, erythematous and indurated area that displaces the anus (superficial abscess), erythema, purulent drainage

Nursing Dx & Intervention

Risk for altered bowel elimination related to presence of infection or surgical wound

- Keep the perianal area clean.
- Provide Sitz baths, *for comfort and for cleansing purposes.*
- Apply the dressing over the wound; change frequently, noting color and amount of drainage; dressing may be held in place with mesh "panties" available for use in incontinence management.
- Keep the surgical wound clean; care is needed after urination and defecation; packing may be used to ensure that the wound heals from the inside out; after bowel and bladder elimination, it is necessary to check the dressing and replace if soiled.
- Shave the perianal area weekly to keep hair from the wound *(hair will delay wound healing and is often the cause of infection or irritation).*
- Irrigate the wound before packing with normal saline or irrigation solution as ordered.

Pain related to infection or inflammation in sensitive area

- Provide analgesics as ordered.
- Provide a thick pillow, cushion, or flotation pad for sitting (avoid air rings and rubber donuts *because they tend to spread the buttocks apart).*

Patient Education/Home Care Planning

1. Demonstrate to the patient how to irrigate the wound (Water Pik or shower massager may be used) and to reinsert dressing. Family member may need to assist the patient. The patient should comprehend the necessity of keeping the wound clean and free of fecal soiling.

Evaluation

Gastrointestinal function is normal Patient has no constipation or hard, formed stools.

Comfort level is achieved Patient verbalizes increased comfort and is able to have pain-free bowel movements.

■ ANORECTAL FISTULA

An anorectal fistula is a hollow, fibrous tunnel or tract with two openings lined by granulation tissue.

The internal opening of an anorectal fistula is inside the anal canal or rectum and leads to the secondary, or external, opening (Figure 8-17). The external opening is in the perianal skin. Fistulas from the colon, small bowel, or urethra may exit through the perineum and be mistaken for anorectal fistulas.

Although an anorectal fistula may occur without predisposing conditions, it is more common to find anorectal fistulas associated with Crohn's disease in the large or the small bowel (regional enteritis). Anorectal fistulas are associated with the presence of an anorectal abscess. An anorectal abscess that is drained may reduce the discomfort and pain, but a fistulous tract may remain through which the abscess continues to drain.

•••••• Pathophysiology

The primary, or internal, opening of an anorectal fistula is usually at a crypt near the pectinate line. Infection in the crypt progresses to form an abscess that drains (spontaneously or with surgical drainage), and the tract is preserved as the abscess heals. Anorectal fistulas are associated with traumatic injury, fissures, Crohn's disease, chlamydial infections, tuberculosis, cancer, and radiation therapy. Once the tract is fibrosed, it will not close on its own and surgical intervention is indicated. Stool, pus, mucus, blood, and flatus may drain through the fistula. Patients may have single or multiple anorectal fistulas. The skin opening may seal over temporarily, but it will reopen spontaneously and drain.

After treatment, recurrent fistulas in the anorectal area are associated with inadequate exposure of the tract, with primary

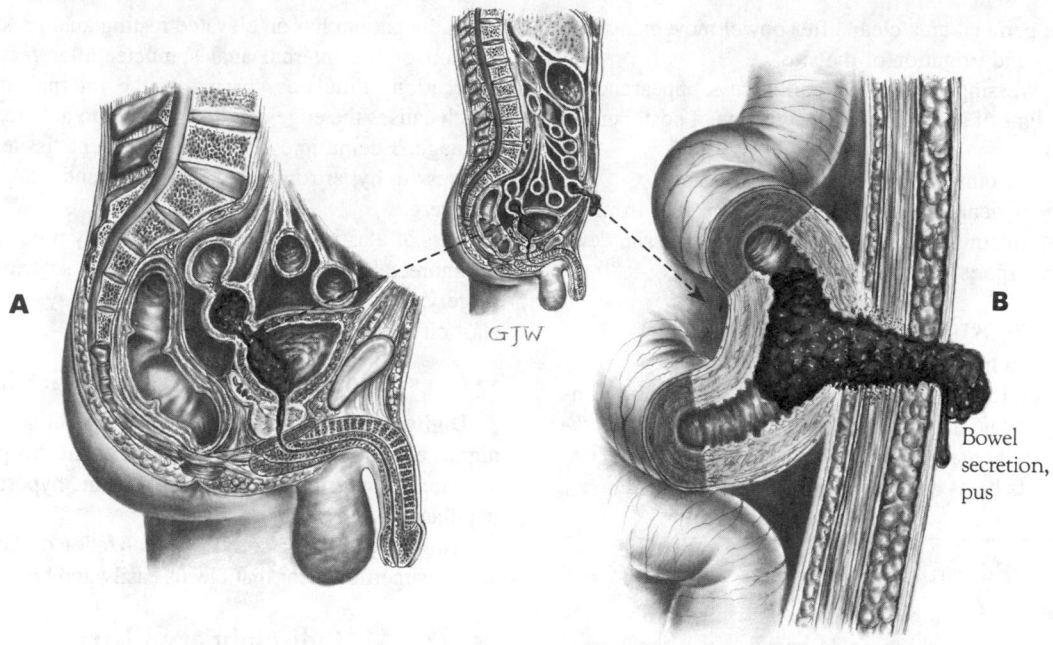

Figure 8-17 Fistulas. **A,** Internal fistula with escape of bowel into the bladder and urethra. **B,** Enterocutaneous fistula into the abdominal wall. (From Doughty.[17])

openings not being identified, and with failure of the tract to heal from the inside out. When a patient has Crohn's disease, recurrent anorectal fistulas are associated with exacerbation of the inflammatory bowel disease.

•••••• Diagnostic Studies and Findings

Digital rectal examination Palpate tract direction internally

Anoscopy (proctoscopy) May reveal the primary opening in a crypt

Sigmoidoscopy Used to rule out other sources of fistula formation

Fistulography Used if the tract is of questionable origin; rules out colonic, small bowel, and urethral fistulas

•••••• Multidisciplinary Plan

Surgery

Fistulotomy or fistulectomy may be indicated depending on location and depth of the fistula tract

Medications

Antibiotics per sensitive organism

Stool softener: docusate (Colace), 50 to 200 mg/d; dose based on individual's response

Metronidazole (Flagyl), 20 mg/kg/d in divided doses (for perianal disease associated with inflammatory bowel disease)

General Management

Sitz baths as needed and after defecation

NURSING CARE

Nursing Assessment

Perianal Examination

Raised, red papules

Drainage of pus, blood, mucus, or stool through the open skin lesions

Pruritus

Inundated, "cordlike" pattern may be palpated from cutaneous opening toward anus

Pain

Complaints of pain and discomfort; complaints are greater when lesions are sealed and not draining

Gastrointestinal

Change in bowel habits (purulent discharge, increased odor); last bowel movement; use of laxatives or stool softeners; anal intercourse; anal dilators (e.g., vibrators or other instruments); history of anorectal abscesses or inflammatory bowel disease

Nursing Dx & Intervention

Risk for altered bowel elimination related to presence of infection or surgical incision

• Estimate amount of drainage; note color, odor, and consistency of drainage.

- Keep the perianal area clean after bowel movements with Sitz baths and irrigation of the site.
- Replace dressings as soiled and assess appearance of wound, signs of healings, and early signs of postoperative infection.
- Irrigate the wound before packing or dressing.
- Shave the perianal area regularly to prevent hair from irritating or infecting the wound as granulation tissue develops after surgery.

Pain related to perianal inflammation

- Provide pain medication as needed.
- Provide a thick foam cushion or pillow for patient to use in sitting (avoid air rings and rubber donuts *because they tend to spread the buttocks apart*).
- Provide Sitz baths or warm compresses as needed.

Patient Education/Home Care Planning

1. Instruct the patient how to irrigate the wound with a Water Pik or shower massager, to shave the perianal area, and to redress the wound.
2. Show the patient how to use a mirror to inspect the area and look for redness or firm reddened areas of increased itching and tenderness.
3. Mesh panties can be used to hold dressings in place, or sanitary pads or belts may be used in the underwear. Jockey shorts will be more effective than boxer shorts for managing dressings.
4. A family member's help may be needed.
5. Sitz baths can be used for cleansing and for comfort. (The Sitz bath does not replace the irrigation procedure.)

Evaluation

Gastrointestinal function is normal   Patient has no constipation or hard, formed stools.

Comfort level is achieved   Patient verbalizes increased comfort and is able to have pain-free bowel movements.

■ ANAL FISSURE

An anal fissure is a small tear in the lining of the anus. The tear resembles a slitlike crack and may extend from the anal verge to the pectinate line.

Fissures are most common in young and middle-aged adults. The posterior midline is the most common site, but occasional anal fissures will be found in the anterior wall. Fissures in other positions on the anal wall are usually associated with Crohn's disease or ulcerative colitis.

• • • • • • Pathophysiology

Anal fissures are usually caused by trauma from passing large, hard stools. Acute fissures are tears that may become chronic

when the patient has an elevated resting anal pressure and contraction of the internal anal sphincter after rectal distention. Defecation stimulates spasms of the internal anal sphincter, which causes the edges of the sphincter to adhere, trapping any drainage. Edema and fibrosis of adjacent tissue develop and progress to hypertrophied anal papillae and a tag of skin at the anal verge.

Loss of elasticity of the anal canal may predispose a person to anorectal fissures. Laxative abuse, scarring from anal surgery, and chronic diarrheal diseases may lead to a loss of elasticity, as will frequent anal intercourse.

• • • • • • Diagnostic Studies and Findings

Digital rectal examination   Use topical anesthesia before digital examination to decrease pain from the procedure; induration; tenderness; sphincter spasm; hypertrophied anal papillae

Anoscopy (proctoscopy)   Visualization of the anorectal fissure: a superficial tear that bleeds easily and has a reddish base

• • • • • • Multidisciplinary Plan

Surgery

Lateral subcutaneous sphincterotomy (internal sphincter is divided up to the pectinate line, hypertrophied papillae and anal tag are excised, and fissure is left to heal)

Medications

Bulk agents
    Psyllium (Metamucil or Effersyllium), 1 tsp (7 g) 1-3 times per day
Emollient suppositories
Analgesic ointments
    Dibucaine (Nupercaine) prn topically
Tucks or witch hazel pads to cleanse

General Management

Topical application of silver nitrate solution or cautery with silver nitrate sticks
Sitz bath
Warm compresses

NURSING CARE

Nursing Assessment

Pain

Complaints of pain and discomfort during evacuation; described as tearing or burning; associated with slight bleeding; evacuation stimulates spasms that result in prolonged, gnawing discomfort for extended periods

Gastrointestinal

Change in bowel habits (constipation, bright red blood after bowel movements); pruritus; last bowel movement; history or use of laxatives or stool softeners, anal intercourse, anal dilators (e.g., vibrators or other instruments), enema abuse, or inflammatory bowel disease; obtain dietary history

Perianal Examination

Rectal tag of skin, rectal discharge

Nursing Dx & Intervention

Constipation related to painful defecation

- After surgery, record consistency of stool and effectiveness of stool softeners.
- Keep the postoperative site clean and free of stool by using Sitz baths and careful cleansing after surgery.
- Administer bulk laxatives as ordered.

Pain related to inflammation of anal area

- Provide warm compresses, Sitz baths, and analgesic ointments for pain and discomfort.
- Patients often postpone or delay having bowel movements because of the pain.
- Premedicate before bowel movement and/or have Sitz bath ready.

Patient Education/Home Care Planning

1. Provide the patient with information on natural methods of relieving or preventing constipation (i.e., diet high in bulk and fiber, increased fluid intake, avoidance of harsh laxatives and constipating medications such as codeine).

Evaluation

Gastrointestinal function is normal Patient has no constipation or hard, formed stools.

Comfort level is achieved Patient verbalizes increased comfort and has no pain with evacuation or delayed pain.

■ HEMORRHOIDS

Hemorrhoids are masses of vascular tissue found in the anal canal.[61]

Internal hemorrhoids are found above the pectinate line, arise from the superior hemorrhoidal venous plexus, and are covered with mucosa. External hemorrhoids are found below the pectinate line, arise from the inferior hemorrhoidal venous plexus, and are covered by anoderm and perianal skin. Patients may have a combination of internal and external hemorrhoids.

Internal hemorrhoids may also be classified according to the degree of involvement:

First-degree: project slightly into the anal canal

Second-degree: prolapse with defecation and reduce spontaneously

Third-degree: prolapse with defecation and reduce manually

Fourth-degree: irreducible

The usual location of internal hemorrhoids is around the anal circumference, including right anterior, right posterior, and left lateral areas.[61]

The commonly accepted cause is that hemorrhoids are varicose veins. This cause has been recently questioned because of weaknesses in the original theory. The basis of the varicose vein theory of hemorrhoids is that increased pressure in the veins results in congestion. Certain occupations, the erect positions of humans, structural absence of valves in the veins, and increased abdominal pressure from straining at defecation, constipation, and pregnancy have been associated with the development of hemorrhoids. The varicose vein and increased pressure cause has been questioned because internal hemorrhoids may appear in early pregnancy before the uterus is large enough to create increased abdominal pressure and because the blood associated with hemorrhoidal bleeding is bright red, not dark as expected with the venous system.

A hypothesis is that the hemorrhoidal plexus is a rich vascular network with direct arteriovenous shunts. The vascular tissue slides easily and may be displaced downward with the evacuation of stool.[61,65,71] High resting anal pressures and failure of the internal sphincter to relax may contribute to the development of hemorrhoids in some people. In older patients, low resting anal pressures and sliding of tissues during bowel movements have been associated with hemorrhoids.

•••••• Pathophysiology

Based on Thompson's description[65] of the hemorrhoidal plexus as a vascular mound on a cushion, an internal hemorrhoid is a prolapse of normal vascular mounds or a prolapse of normal anal canal lining. The prolapse may be caused by spasms of the internal sphincter that require straining or increased pressure to push the stool through the internal sphincter and at the same time push out the hemorrhoid.

The complications associated with internal hemorrhoids include bleeding, prolapse, and thrombosis. Because the hemorrhoid is composed of spongy vascular tissue, bleeding tends to be an oozing of bright red blood. The blood may appear as a bright spot on toilet paper or on the surface of the stool. Blood may drip from the anus for a few minutes after the stool has been expelled. Iron deficiency anemia may develop if blood loss continues over a period of time.

Prolapse of hemorrhoids is first perceived as a mass of tissue that protrudes from the anus after a bowel movement. Initially, it slips back into the anal canal spontaneously. As the condition continues, the hemorrhoid will later need to be manually replaced and may become irreducible. A mucous discharge is associated with irreducible hemorrhoids because of the mucosal covering of the internal hemorrhoid. Protection of undergarments will be required. Pain is associated with prolapsed and inflamed hemorrhoids but is not a general symptom of internal hemorrhoids. Patients whose initial complaint is pain should be assessed for other anorectal conditions (fissure, abscess) and colorectal diseases.

Thrombosis of prolapsed hemorrhoids can create severe pain. This is also referred to as strangulated hemorrhoids. Ulceration and secondary infections can develop. One or all hemorrhoids may be affected.

A thrombosis of an external hemorrhoid is a blood clot within a hemorrhoidal vein. The pectinate line is visible and separate from the mass or lump that forms. Thrombosis of external hemorrhoids has been associated with heavy lifting, straining at defecation, and childbirth. The patient has a painful lump that appears suddenly at the anus. Pain may be constant and is increased with sitting and defecation. It usually disappears in a week. The thrombosed external hemorrhoid should not be confused with prolapsed, thrombosed internal hemorrhoids. If the skin covering the clot becomes ulcerated, bleeding may be noted.

•••••• Diagnostic Studies and Findings

Complete blood count (CBC) and iron studies   To determine presence of anemia and if it is caused by iron deficiency

Digital rectal examination   Tone of internal sphincter; usually increased in young men with hemorrhoids; may be low in older patients and women with hemorrhoids; Palpation of third-degree internal hemorrhoids

Anoscopy   Visualization of hemorrhoids as instrument is removed

Sigmoidoscopy and barium enema   To rule out carcinoma and inflammatory disease; particularly important in patients 40 years old and older

•••••• Multidisciplinary Plan

Surgery

Injection of sclerosing solutions (5% sodium morrhuate or phenol in vegetable oil) submucosally around hemorrhoid; complications: sloughing of overlying mucosa, prostatic or rectal infection, reaction to injected material

Rubber band ligation (placement of rubber band over base of hemorrhoid causes necrosis and sloughing of hemorrhoid in 7 days); complications: rarely, rectal infection

Cryosurgery (application of metal probe cooled by liquid nitrogen or carbon dioxide freezes hemorrhoid); may not heal for several weeks

Lateral internal sphincterotomy (partial division of internal sphincter lowers anal pressure); seldom used unless an anorectal fissure is also present

Hemorrhoidectomy (surgical excision of the hemorrhoidal masses); complication: anal stenosis

Excision under local anesthesia of thrombosed external hemorrhoid if seen in a day or two of onset

Photocoagulation (application of infrared light or lasers to coagulate hemorrhoids)

Medications

Anesthetic ointments and suppositories
   Nupercaine (Dibucaine) prn
Stool softeners
Analgesics

General Management

Manual dilation of anus (anus is dilated 4 cm regularly by patient with a special dilator); complication: incontinence
High-fiber diet, adequate hydration, and exercise to minimize constipation and straining
Warm Sitz baths; compresses

Nutritional Consultation

To educate patient regarding high-fiber dietary selections

NURSING CARE

Nursing Assessment

Perianal Skin Examination

External hemorrhoids visible in subcutaneous skin at anus; if hemorrhoids are thrombosed, tender, bluish spheric mass at anal verge
Prolapsed internal hemorrhoids: moist, red mucosa covering upper portion; presence of mucoid discharge or staining of undergarments

Pain

Size and type of hemorrhoid determine amount of pain: internal hemorrhoids may have no symptoms; thrombosis of prolapsed hemorrhoids causes severe pain

Gastrointestinal

Change in bowel habits (constipation, bright red blood after bowel movements); pruritus; last bowel movement; history or use of laxatives or stool softeners, straining at the toilet, enema abuse; obtain dietary history

Nursing Dx & Intervention

Pain related to inflammation and increased pressure

- Assess amount, character, and threshold of pain or discomfort; relate to bowel pattern.
- Use thick foam pillows or pads under buttock; avoid air or rubber donuts *because they spread the buttocks apart.*
- Promote the use of Sitz baths *for comfort and for cleansing* after bowel movements.
- Assess patient during Sitz bath for hypotension resulting from vasodilation of pelvic blood vessels.
- Provide oral and topical analgesics as ordered.
- Use ice packs as ordered *to reduce congestion and edema.*
- Use warm compresses *to promote circulation* (also soothing).

Constipation related to poor dietary habits and fear of defecation

- Instruct patient to defecate promptly with the urge, to avoid sitting on the toilet for prolonged periods, and to avoid straining.

- Provide adequate fluids *to maintain hydration.*
- Encourage patient to exercise (mild at first).
- Give patient medication before first bowel movement.
- Encourage patient to have a bowel movement after surgery even though patient may be afraid of increased pain *(prevents formation of strictures and preserves lumen size of the anus).*
- Assess patient during the first bowel movement for signs of weakness or dizziness.
- Administer laxatives as ordered.
- Educate patient regarding a high-fiber diet.

Patient Education/Home Care Planning

1. Management and prevention of constipation with diet, fluids, and physical activities should be discussed with the patient.
2. The patient needs to respond to urge to defecate, to avoid straining, and to keep the stool soft and moist.

Evaluation

Gastrointestinal function is normal Patient has no constipation or hard, formed stools. Patient eats a high-fiber diet with good hydration.

Comfort level is achieved Patient verbalizes increased comfort and has no pain with evacuation. Patient has no delayed pain.

PILONIDAL DISEASE

Pilonidal disease occurs in the midline of the upper portion of the gluteal fold. A sinus channel develops that is lined with epithelium and hair.

The sinus channel may appear as a hairy dimple that is asymptomatic unless it becomes infected or inflamed. A cyst or abscess may develop. Pilonidal disease affects men more than women, probably because of the increased amount of hair.

• • • • • Pathophysiology

The trapping of hair beneath the skin and the enlargement of hair follicles probably causes infection and irritation.

• • • • • Diagnostic Studies and Findings

Refer to diagnostic studies on anorectal fistulas.

• • • • • Multidisciplinary Plan

Surgery

Incision and drainage under local anesthesia; removal of hair and granulation tissue; wound may be closed or left open and packed

Medications

Antibiotic therapy to treat the infection per organism

NURSING CARE

Nursing Assessment

Pain Tenderness, erythema, and induration in sacral region

Examination Hairy dimple in gluteal fold; open draining lesion in sacral regon with hair protruding from sinus opening

Nursing Dx & Intervention

Pain related to surgical drainage of cyst or abscess

- Assess perianal area for presence of inflammation of a sinus channel.
- Apply hot moist compresses when an abscess is present.
- Assist patient with Sitz bath.
- Assess patient during Sitz bath for hypotension (related to vasodilation).
- Position patient on abdomen or side.

Patient Education/Home Care Planning

1. Prepare the patient or family member to change dressing as needed, to keep wound free of fecal and urinary contamination, and to cleanse wound as needed.
2. Avoid direct trauma.
3. Shave skin regularly or apply a depilatory regularly to prevent hair growth.

Evaluation

Comfort level is achieved Patient uses pain control strategies appropriately. Patient verbalizes increased control over pain.

LIVER DISORDERS

CIRRHOSIS

Cirrhosis is a chronic degenerative disease of the liver in which diffuse destruction and regeneration of hepatic parenchymal cells have occurred.

In cirrhosis the lobes are covered with fibrotic tissue, and the lobules are infiltrated with fat (Figure 8-18). The diffuse increase in connective tissue results in disorganization of the lobular and vascular structure of the liver, affecting the many functions of the liver and its blood flow. Cirrhosis is characterized by nodular regeneration, which is an attempt by the liver to heal itself by fibrosis or scar tissue. Cirrhosis is the end result of pathologic changes associated with liver disease.

A variety of conditions may progress or lead to cirrhosis of the liver and range from genetic disorders to alcohol abuse. The

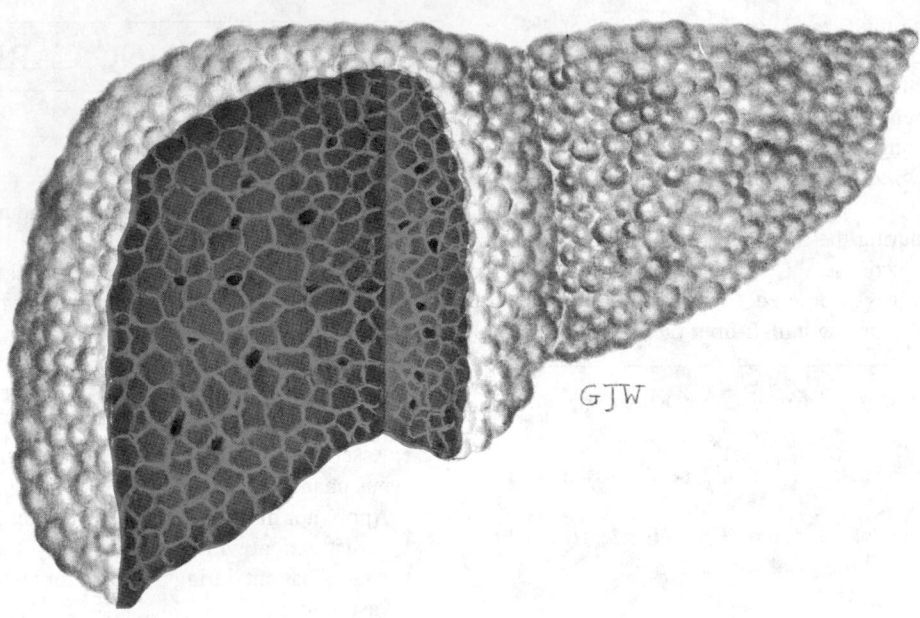

Figure 8-18 Cirrhosis of the liver (septal cirrhosis). (From Doughty.[17])

genetic disorders include galactosemia, α-1-antitrypsin deficiency, and Wilson's disease. Biliary atresia, a congenital malformation of bile ducts, may progress to cirrhosis. Chemical agents that may be toxic to the liver include acetaminophen, thorazine, ether, amitriptyline (Elavil), and various household cleansers (carbon tetrachloride). Infectious causes, such as viral hepatitis, syphilis, and schistosomiasis, may progress to cirrhosis. Alcoholic cirrhosis is the most common and accounts for approximately 80% of the liver disease in urban areas.

Cirrhosis develops in approximately 10% to 20% of alcoholics. Of interest to clinicians and researchers is why all individuals who abuse alcohol do not develop cirrhosis. One theory is that certain individuals have an increased ability to oxidize alcohol that may be familial or heredity based.[63] Thus alcohol ingestion in a susceptible host in the presence of an unknown factor may lead to cirrhosis of the liver.

•••••• Pathophysiology

The pathophysiology of cirrhosis will vary according to the initial cause (viral hepatitis, biliary obstruction, alcohol abuse). The symptoms and results of cirrhosis are the same. For this reason and because of the high incidence of alcohol abuse–related cirrhosis, the pathophysiology of the alcohol-induced cirrhotic changes will be described. Alcoholic cirrhosis is also referred to as portal cirrhosis, Laënnec's cirrhosis, and micronodular cirrhosis.

Several steps occur before the liver becomes cirrhotic. Initially, subcellular changes develop and may progress to a fatty liver. (Fatty livers are not limited to alcoholic cirrhosis.) The fatty liver is a reversible stage if alcohol intake is eliminated. The fatty liver can be recognized by its increased size and the marked degree of fatty infiltration seen microscopically. The fatty liver in the presence of continued alcohol ingestion may

progress to alcoholic hepatitis. It is the continuing use of alcohol that causes development of cirrhosis versus the progression from fatty liver to hepatitis to cirrhosis. These may not be related. The patient could have cirrhosis and acute hepatitis could develop because of a drinking bout if the patient has cirrhotic changes. In alcoholic hepatitis the fatty infiltration is combined with liver cell necrosis, leukocytic inflammation, and fibrosis. As the disease progresses, the inflammatory changes decrease and fibrotic changes increase. Continued alcohol ingestion leads to chronic changes (i.e., alcoholic cirrhosis).

The microscopic changes in cirrhosis consist of degeneration and death of hepatocytes, proliferation of connective tissue, and regeneration of hepatocytes. The connective tissue spreads from the portal tracts and from the central veins throughout the liver, changing the normal lobular architecture. The extension of fibrous cords throughout the liver alters the relationship between the hepatic veins and the portal veins. Scar tissue and nodular regeneration of hepatocytes may compress small branches of the portal vein. The compression of the vessels leads to an increased alteration in the vascular system. The veins become engorged and dilated, and portal hypertension develops. The nodular regeneration of the hepatic cells produces postsinusoidal obstruction, which causes the portal system to become congested and contributes to portal hypertension.

The overall effects of the structural and vascular changes are seen in the resulting dysfunction of the liver and the changes in the portal circulation. The liver is a very complex organ and plays a major role in metabolism, detoxification, blood-forming functions, storage of iron, copper, and various vitamins, and formation of bile. As the liver functions are altered, various clinical manifestations develop, including bleeding disorders (decreased clotting factors), muscle wasting (decreased protein metabolism), hepatic coma (detoxification of ammonia), jaundice (inability to conjugate bilirubin), and peripheral edema (low serum albumin and an increase in hydrostatic pressure). The changes in the portal circulation result in portal hypertension, one of whose clinical manifestations is esophageal varices. Ascites and mesenteric congestion are other clinical manifestations.

Ascites in chronic liver disease has been associated with portal hypertension, low serum albumin, and abnormalities in the lymphatic system. The transudation of fluid between capillaries and tissue spaces is determined by the equilibrium of hydrostatic and osmotic forces in the two compartments. In the normal situation the hydrostatic pressure is higher at the arterial end of the capillary and promotes the passsage of protein-free fluid into the pericapillary space. The hydrostatic pressure is lower than the osmotic pressure and the extravascular tissue pressure at the venous end of the capillary, and reabsorption of the fluid occurs.[58] The patient with advanced cirrhosis and portal hypertension has an increased intravascular hydrostatic pressure (portal hypertension) and decreased vascular osmotic pressure (low serum albumin). The combination of the changes in hydrostatic pressure and osmotic pressure leads to the loss of fluid into the peritoneal cavity, an extravascular space.[58] Abnormalities in the lymphatic system contribute to ascites formation. In cirrhosis with portal hypertension, the thoracic duct is enlarged and lymph flow is significantly increased. The high lymph flow may decompress the hepatic or splanchnic vessels. Lymph from the liver is generally high in protein. When the lymph flow is greater than the thoracic duct can manage, a hepatic venous outflow obstruction develops, with resultant ascites. The ascitic fluid in a venous outflow obstruction is high in protein. When the obstruction is an extrahepatic venous obstruction, the protein concentration is low in the fluid.[63]

The communication between the thoracic duct and the subclavian vein helps to determine the occurrence and severity of ascites. Thoracic duct drainage can decrease ascitic volume and portal pressure. Fluid exudes from the surface of the liver into the peritoneal cavity when the lymph system is unable to manage it.

The formation of ascites is not a simple reaction to increased hepatic venous outflow obstruction. Interrelated factors include aldosterone, antidiuretic hormone (ADH), and prostaglandins. The development of ascites results in a decreased blood volume, which stimulates aldosterone secretion. Reexpansion of blood volume stimulates ascites formation, reducing blood volume, restimulating aldosterone, and creating a cycle. This traditional hypothesis of the relationship between ascites and aldosterone has been challenged. It has been proposed that sodium retention occurs first followed by fluid retention and then ascites.

ADH has been found to be elevated in the serum and urine of patients with ascites from cirrhosis. The increase in ADH may be the result of a decrease in effective plasma volume. Effective plasma volume has been defined as the portion of the total plasma volume that effectively stimulates volume receptors.[58] ADH in patients with ascites may contribute to the retention of water, resulting in hyponatremia.

Prostaglandins have also been suggested in the complexity of the ascites formation in cirrhosis because of sodium retention. Prostaglandins may play a role in determining renal plasma flow and sodium retention in decompensated cirrhosis, Indomethacin, a potent inhibitor of prostaglandins, decreases renal flow and creatinine clearance in cirrhotic patients with sodium retention. Indomethacin also decreases plasma renin activity and aldosterone levels.[58]

There are three types of jaundice: obstructive, hemolytic, and hepatocellular. Obstructive jaundice develops in association with obstruction of the biliary ductal system. There is marked elevation of alkaline phosphatase, mild elevation of serum glutamic-oxaloacetic transaminase (SGOT) and lactate dehydrogenase (LDH), and significant bile in the urine. Hemolytic jaundice is associated with an increased load of bilirubin from hemolysis that a diseased liver is unable to manage. Large amounts of urobilinogen may be found in the urine. Anemia is generally associated with hemolytic jaundice. Hepatocellular jaundice develops because of a failure of the liver cells to metabolize bilirubin. In acute hepatocellular failure, the LDH and SGOT are markedly increased and urine contains both bile and urobilinogen. In chronic cirrhosis or hepatocellular failure, there may be no elevation of enzymes and the jaundice may not correlate with the severity of the liver disease. Its presence usually indicates acute disease, and in the patient with chronic cirrhosis the presence of jaundice indicates a poor prognosis. Severe hepatic parenchymal necrosis may develop in the absence of jaundice.[58] Hemolysis is common in cirrhosis and may contribute to jaundice. Biliary obstruction may also occur in cirrhosis.

Hepatic encephalopathy encompasses several stages of mental deterioration culminating in coma. The pathophysiology and treatment are presented on pp. 771 to 772. Bleeding esophageal varices are a major complication associated with portal hypertension and are discussed on p. 707.

The healthy liver plays a role in the metabolism of estrogens. In cirrhosis, hyperestrogenism develops, which includes an increase in sex hormone–binding globulin and other hormone-binding proteins and an increase in the secretion of prolactin.[58] Clinically, the patient shows signs of feminization, including gynecomastia, spider angiomas, palmar erythema, and testicular atrophy. The distribution of body hair changes, with less chest hair and axillary hair being noted. In women testosterone may accumulate with some masculinization.

Hematologic disorders associated with cirrhosis include impaired coagulation and anemia. The liver is responsible for the synthesis of proteins needed for coagulation: fibrinogen, prothrombin, and various other clotting factors. The liver uses vitamin K to produce prothrombin. Vitamin K absorption depends on bile. Treatment of cirrhosis by wiping out intestinal bacteria will decrease the production of vitamin K.

Anemia in cirrhosis may be microcytic, hypochromic anemia resulting from gastrointestinal blood loss and iron deficiency; macrocytic anemia from folic acid deficiency, leukopenia, or thrombocytopenia; or hemolytic anemia. Hemolysis may be indicated by reticulocytosis, hyperbilirubinemia, or increased levels of serum LDH. Splenomegaly may be associated with leukopenia, thrombocytopenia, and hemolytic anemia.

A major complication of cirrhosis is hepatorenal syndrome. Hepatorenal syndrome occurs when a patient with decompensated cirrhosis has acquired, functional renal failure develop. The usual causes of renal insufficiency are present in hepatorenal syndrome, but the kidneys are normal. The patient has oliguria, azotemia, and a urine of high osmolality and low sodium content. Oliguria and azotemia will persist in hepatorenal syndrome even if blood volume and cardiac output are normal. Hepatorenal syndrome carries a very high mortality rate and does not respond well to medical management.

Hypotension in liver failure is common and may lead to oliguria, azotemia, hyponatremia, and changes in potassium levels. Clinically, the patient may have a high cardiac output and a low total peripheral resistance. Changes in the liver circulatory system may be responsible for this development, and treatment focuses on improving liver function. In addition, oliguria may be associated with a depletion of circulatory blood volume (decreased cardiac output) and decreased renal perfusion. Treatment requires volume expanders.

The patient with cirrhosis has a complex, interrelated group of clinical manifestations. The symptoms observed in cirrhosis can be correlated with a particular dysfunction in the liver or its vascular system. The nurse must be able to identify potential life-threatening complications of advanced liver failure.

•••••• Diagnostic Studies and Findings

Serum bilirubin   Elevated in jaundice

SGOT, SGPT, LDH   Elevated (SGOT may be higher if alcoholic cirrhosis)

Serum albumin   Decreased (tissue edema)

Prothrombin time   Prolonged

Complete blood count   Anemia, leukopenia, thrombocytopenia

Blood glucose   Hypoglycemia (from impaired gluconeogenesis)

Serum ammonia   Elevated (sign of impending hepatic coma)

Urinalysis   Sodium and potassium levels; urine dark, bile colored; presence of urobilinogen

Endoscopic retrograde cholangiopancreatography (ERCP)   May show common bile duct obstruction

Esophagoscopy   Presence of esophageal varices

Percutaneous liver biopsy   Histologic changes found in cirrhosis of liver: fatty infiltration; degeneration and regeneration of hepatocytes; increase in connective tissue

Ultrasonography   Evaluate patency of splenic and portal veins; differentiates biliary obstruction from nonobstructive, parenchymal jaundice; presence of occult ascites; assess liver size

Liver scans   Decreased uptake in liver (caused by intrahepatic shunts that bypass liver cells); cold spots of cirrhosis can be differentiated from hepatocellular carcinoma by gallium scans

Barium contrast esophagography   Documents esophageal varices

Angiography   Detects sites of upper gastrointestinal bleeding

Percutaneous transhepatic portography (angiographic study)   Visualization of portal venous system

Paracentesis   Clear, straw-colored fluid; decreased total protein

•••••• Multidisciplinary Plan

Surgery

Refer to discussions of esophageal varices and hepatic coma

Ascites: peritoneovenous shunt (LeVeen valve, ascites drainage system implanted in abdominal wall and connected to peritoneal cavity and to venous system)

Medications

Diuretics (used to promote fluid loss; recommended weight loss 1-1 1/2 pounds/d)

   Spironolactone (Aldactone, potassium-sparing diuretic), 100 mg/d (higher dosage may be used initially or given in combination with other diuretics)

   Hydrochlorothiazide (Esidrix) or furosemide (Lasix); dosage varies; given with spironolactone

Digestants

   Pancreatin (Panteric), 1 or 2 tablets po with meals; each tablet contains 2400 mg; use in presence of steatorrhea; promotes fat digestion

Vitamins

   Menadiol sodium diphosphate (Synkayvite; vitamin K), 5-15 mg IM, subcutaneously, or IV; repeat dosage in 12 h if no improvement or give 10 mg for 3 d

   Vitamin C (decreased vitamin C associated with gastrointestinal bleeding)

   Folic acid, 1 mg/d po (for anemia)

Cathartics and laxatives

   Stool softeners (to reduce straining and thereby reduce chance of bleeding from hemorrhoids); docusate (Colace), 50-200 mg/d

   Lactulose (Cephulac), 30 ml 3-4 times/d po, 300 ml in 700 ml NS or sorbitol per rectum as retention enema for 30-60 minutes (to decrease serum ammonia levels)

General Management

Paracentesis: indicated for diagnostic purposes, relief of abdominal pain, relief of dyspnea or orthopnea, reduction of intraabdominal pressure; complications: perforation of abdominal viscera, hemorrhage, infection, shock, hyponatremia syndromes

Ascites reinfusion (as an albumin substitute for expanding plasma volume)

Oxygen and incentive spirometer if respiratory complications develop

Intravenous fluids

Fresh whole blood during acute bleeding episodes

Abstinence from alcohol

Adequate rest

Albumin replacement

Vitamin supplements, including thiamine, iron, and vitamins K and C

Fresh frozen plasma or platelets

Diet: high in protein (70 to 90 g), high in carbohydrates, approximately 3000 calories

Diet: with impending liver failure, restrict protein and fluids

Nutritional Consultation

To counsel patients regarding sodium restrictions, salt substitutes, high or low protein dietary selections, fluid restrictions

Psychological Consultation

May be advised to counsel patient, family members regarding alcoholism; refer patient and family members to Alcoholics Anonymous and affiliated family organizations

NURSING CARE

Nursing Assessment

General

Fatigability; fever; weakness

Gastrointestinal

History of hepatitis or previous liver disease; drug use; toxic substance ingestion; alcohol use

Nausea, vomiting, hematemesis

Change in bowel habits; hemorrhoids

Glossitis; cheilosis

Psychosocial Concerns

Ability to give up alcohol ingestion (if alcoholic cirrhosis)

Assess coping level and support

Mental Status

Changes in thinking and mental function resulting from increased serum ammonia levels; may progress to hepatic coma (serum ammonia levels do not always correlate with mental functions; that is, some patients with very high levels have minimum mental function alteration, whereas others with low levels may progress to coma)

Nutrition

Recent changes in weight (loss or gain)

Anorexia

Integumentary

Jaundice, spider angiomas, spider telangiectasis, palmar erythema, purpuric lesions, loss of chest hair

Urinary

Changes in urine output, oliguria

Color of urine: dark yellow, amber, mahogany

Pulmonary

Shortness of breath, decreased lung expansion

Extremities

Nail changes (transverse pale bands)

Signs of tissue wasting (legs)

Asterixis, tremors

Sexuality

Impotence, loss of libido, sterility, amenorrhea

Abdominal Examination

Ascites; abdominal pain

Splenomegaly; hepatomegaly

Caput medusae (dilated veins around the umbilicus secondary to portal hypertension)

Nursing Dx & Intervention

(See also hepatic coma, esophageal varices)

Risk for injury related to altered clotting factors

- Help patient minimize trauma (e.g., forceful nose blowing, harsh toothbrush, safety razors).
- Assess for signs of bleeding.
- Provide stool softener and remind patient not to strain during bowel movements.
- Use small-gauge needles for injections and apply pressure after injections.
- Record any indications of small bleeding sites.
- Monitor platelet count and prothrombin time.

Fluid volume deficit related to use of diuretics and third spacing of fluids (ascites and edema)

- Assess for clinical signs of electrolyte imbalance, particularly sodium, potassium, and magnesium.
- Maintain accurate intake and output records, reporting abnormalities.
- Record daily weights.
- Measure abdominal girth daily *to monitor ascites.*
- Monitor serum and urine electrolytes.
- Provide diuretics as ordered.
- Restrict fluid intake if ordered.
- Perform frequent mouth care.
- Administer IV fluids and colloids as ordered.

Altered nutrition: less than body requirements related to poor nutritional intake and anorexia

- Assess nutritional status.
- Provide small frequent feedings high in calories, carbohydrates, and fats, low in proteins, and low in sodium.

- Provide salt substitutes if ordered.
- Nutritionist to assist in finding palatable low-salt foods.
- Nutritionist to follow patient and assist in making healthy choices.

Ineffective breathing pattern related to ascites

- Assess lung fields for signs of congestion or infection.
- Place patient in semi-Fowler's or high Fowler's position *to increase lung expansion compromised by ascites.*
- Turn frequently from side to side.
- Monitor blood gases.
- Monitor vital signs.
- Assist patient with ADLs if patient is short of breath.

Altered thought processes related to increased serum ammonia levels

- Observe for early signs of mental changes: lethargy, confusion, drowsiness, and irritability.
- Avoid use of sedatives or tranquilizers.
- Refer to section on hepatic coma.

Risk for ineffective family coping related to chronic irreversible illness, progressive debility, and changes in sexuality

- See ineffective family coping.
- Provide sensitive, caring approach to the patient and family.
- Assess the patient's and family's coping patterns and use of support groups or psychiatric services.
- Provide opportunities for patient and family to express fears and concerns regarding the illness.

Patient Education/Home Care Planning

1. Stress the importance of avoiding alcohol and provide information on alcoholic cirrhosis.
2. Help the patient identify community resources available for alcohol rehabilitation.
3. Provide the patient with information on altered drug effects with cirrhosis and caution to use only physician-prescribed or -approved medications.
4. Have the nutritionist ensure that patient and family understand written dietary instructions. Stress the role of nutrition in recovery. Include any restrictions required, specifically sodium or protein.
5. Instructions should include the need for rest and diversional activities to prevent boredom.
6. Provide and ensure that patient understands written instructions of signs and symptoms that warrant seeing a physician: increased abdominal girth, rapid weight gain or loss, edema, fever, blood in urine or stool, bleeding that does not cease with pressure in a short time (nosebleeds, cuts, gums), gross upper gastrointestinal bleeding, or tarry stools.
7. Instruct the family in all of the above plus signs of mental changes: confusion, untidiness, night wandering, personality changes, irritability, and sleeplessness.

Evaluation

Patient's risk of bleeding diminishes Platelet count, bleeding times are normal. Patient verbalizes common signs of abnormal bleeding times and how to minimize trauma during these times.

Fluid volume is maintained Serum electrolytes (sodium, potassium, and magnesium) are normal. Fluid weight loss is 1 to 1 and one-half pounds per day. Abdominal girth decreases. Peripheral edema is reduced. Vital signs are stable. Urinary output is adequate.

Nutrition is adequate Patient does not experience anorexia, nausea and vomiting, indigestion, or muscle wasting. Calorie and protein intake is sufficient for healing. Patient does not drink alcohol.

Breathing pattern is normal Patient does not experience atelectasis or pneumonia. Ascites decreases or disappears; therefore lung expansion improves.

Thought processes are normal Thought processes are not altered. Serum ammonia levels are controlled.

Patient and family are able to cope with chronic illness or an acute exacerbation Patient and family are able to verbalize factors that create anxiety and stress. Patient and family are aware of resources available to them for further supportive care. Patient and family are able to verbalize mechanisms that help them deal with stressors.

■ HEPATIC COMA

In acute and chronic liver diseases, a series of neuropsychiatric manifestations may develop that range from hepatic encephalopathy to precoma to hepatic coma. Hepatic coma is the end stage of the neuropsychiatric manifestations.

The pathophysiology of hepatic coma has become better understood and has been related to the presence of two factors: the shunting of blood around the liver so that substances toxic to the brain are no longer completely metabolized or cleared by the liver, and hepatic insufficiency. The syndrome is currently referred to as portal-systemic encephalopathy (PSE). PSE is characterized by recurrent changes in consciousness, impaired intellectual function, neuromuscular abnormalities, metabolic slowing of electroencephalogram, and elevated serum ammonia levels.[58]

Most patients who have hepatic coma or PSE develop cirrhosis. However, PSE may develop in fulminant liver failure, deficiency of urea cycle enzyme, and Reye's syndrome. PSE occurs in patients with cirrhosis who have portal hypertension or portal-systemic shunting. Hepatic coma also develops in half of those patients who have portacaval shunts.

Several clinical situations have been associated with the initiation of PSE and include azotemia; medications such as sedatives, tranquilizers, and analgesics; gastrointestinal bleeding; high dietary protein; sepsis; hypokalemia; hypovolemia; paracentesis; and hypokalemic alkalosis. An iatrogenic cause occurs in approximately half of the cases of hepatic coma.

• • • • • Pathophysiology

Most episodes of PSE are caused by ammonia intoxication. Ammonia is a by-product of nitrogen metabolism. Nitrogen is a by-product of amino acid digestion. The bacteria in the colon break down nitrogen to ammonia. The ammonia is absorbed and carried through the portal veins to the liver, where it is converted to glutamine, a nontoxic form. Glutamine is later synthesized by the liver into urea, which is excreted.

The colon, when in a fasting state, is a continuous source of ammonia. The colon bacteria responsible for ammonia formation may also be found in the small bowel of patients with cirrhosis.[63] When the portal vein flow bypasses the liver, such as with a portal-systemic anastomosis, the systemic blood ammonia levels increase to toxic levels.

The following equation refers to the ammonia and ammonia hydroxide balance:

$$NH_4OH \rightleftharpoons NH_4^+ + OH^-$$

Only ammonia hydroxide can cross the cell membrane and thus create toxic effects. The pH of the extracellular and intracellular compartments affects this equation. Abnormalities of acid-base balance, primarily alkalosis associated with hypokalemia, result in an increase in ammonia hydroxide and passage of the substance into the cells. Hypokalemia in alcoholic cirrhosis may be related to vomiting, diarrhea, diuretics, and secondary aldosteronism.

Ammonia is also released during muscle activities from the muscles of the extremities. Under normal resting conditions, a small quantity of ammonia uptake occurs. This uptake may increase when arterial levels of ammonia are increased.[58]

PSE may be initiated by conditions that increase nitrogen levels. Endogenous factors include azotemia, blood in the gastrointestinal tract, and constipation. Azotemia affects the kidney's ability to excrete nitrogen. Blood is a source of more ammonia than dietary protein, and the ammonia is liberated from the blood in the colon. Constipation may exaggerate other factors. In constipation the waste products remain in the colon for longer periods, providing more opportunity for colonic bacteria to convert nitrogenous products to ammonia.

Exogenous factors that contribute to the nitrogenous cause of PSE include dietary protein, ammonia salts, urea, cation exchange resins, amino acids, and diuretics. In addition to these factors potassium depletion is associated with nitrogenous PSE.

Several noncirrhotic clinical conditions in which ammonia levels are associated with PSE include hereditary deficiencies of urea cycle enzymes and Reye's syndrome.

The blood ammonia levels do not always correlate well with the clinical manifestations of PSE. Venous blood levels do not reflect what is delivered to the tissues. Arterial ammonia blood levels are recommended, and because individuals respond differently to various levels of ammonia, serial studies of ammonia levels would provide a better indication of the relationship of increasing symptoms to blood levels. Blood ammonia levels are also affected by potassium levels and food ingestion. Hypokalemia results in more tissue uptake of ammonia with a resultant low serum ammonia level. Serum levels of ammonia increase after meals and vary according to the amount of protein

consumed. Fasting and serial arterial ammonia levels are more likely to correlate with the clinical symptoms of PSE.

• • • • • Diagnostic Studies and Findings

Ammonia blood levels (fasting)   Elevated
Serum electrolytes   Hypokalemia; alkalosis
Blood glucose   Hyperglycemia: iatrogenic hyperglycemia may cause coma; in cirrhosis there is little glycogen stored, so patients are usually hypoglycemic
Electroencephalogram (EEG)   Paroxysms of bilateral, synchronous, symmetric slow waves at a rate of 1 $\frac{1}{2}$ to 3/sec. Four grades of EEG: grade 0: normal; grade 1: mild impairment; grade 2: moderate impairment; grade 3: severe impairment; grade 4: coma; rule out other causes of coma such as subdural hematomas and nonnitrogenous causes of PSE

• • • • • Multidisciplinary Plan

Medications

Antiinfective agents (nonabsorbable)
  To decrease bacterial action in colon
  Neomycin sulfate, 0.5-1 g po q6h for 7 d
Broad-spectrum antibiotics
  Ampicillin
Ammonia detoxicants
  Lactulose (Cephulac), 300 ml syrup diluted with 700 ml normal saline (NS) or sorbital by enema (retain 20 to 30 min), or 30 to 45 ml tid or qid po

General Management

Removal of blood from gastrointestinal tract: cathartics
Gastric lavage with room temperature saline or water
Cleansing enemas with dilute acetic acid or neomycin
Discontinuation of any precipitating substance: dietary proteins, sedatives, diuretic therapy, analgesics
Intravenous glucose (minimizes protein breakdown)
Oxygen (respiratory or metabolic alkalosis)
Correction of any electrolyte imbalances
Parenteral or enteral nutrition

NURSING CARE

Nursing Assessment

(See also Cirrhosis)

Mental Status

Appearance and behavior
  Level of consciousness
    Drowsiness, hypersomnia, insomnia, or inversion of sleep pattern; slow responses; lethargy; minimum disorientation, somnolence, confusion, semistupor, stupor, coma
  Posture and motor behavior
    Metabolic tremor
    Muscular incoordination

    Impaired handwriting
    Asterixis (liver flap)
    Hypoactive or hyperactive reflexes
    Ataxia
    Slowed movements of depression
    Nystagmus
Speech and language
    Slurred speech
Mood
    Unusual mood, thoughts of hopelessness
    Exaggeration of normal behavior
    Euphoria or depression
    Garrulousness
    Irritability
    Decreased inhibitions
    Overt changes in personality
    Anxiety or apathy
    Inappropriate behavior
    Bizarre behavior
    Paranoia or anger to rage
Thought processes, thought content, and perceptions
    Shortened attention span, amnesia for past events
Cognitive functions
    Loss of orientation to time, place, and person
    Grossly impaired computations to inability to compute

Integumentary

    Perianal erythema or erosions (diarrhea)

Nursing Dx & Intervention

See also cirrhosis and esophageal varices

Altered thought processes related to impaired liver clearance

- Assess for early signs of changes in consciousness, intellect, personality, behaviors, and neuromuscular activities.
- Record indications of changes.
- Have patient do simple arithmetic computations or use NCT.
- Have patient do serial handwriting to compare differences.
- Monitor arterial ammonia and potassium levels.
- Assess for clinical signs of hypokalemia and alkalosis.
- Provide sedatives, tranquilizers, and analgesics as ordered, note any delayed or prolonged reactions, and report immediately; avoid use of above if possible.
- Protect the patient from injury as personality behaviors become more overt and inappropriate and as neuromuscular activities alter.
- Identify personality and behavior changes and relate them to the progression of the disease and help family and staff understand and learn about the disease progression.
- Document treatment ordered by physician as implemented (e.g., retention or cleansing enemas, gastric lavage, medications).

Risk for injury related to changes in mentation

- Reorient patient frequently.
- Ensure side rails up on bed at all times.
- Ensure that call-light device is within patient's reach or attached to patient's bedclothes.
- Assist patient with ambulation.
- Toilet patient frequently.

Risk for impaired skin integrity related to incontinent diarrhea

- Begin protective perianal skin care before beginning lactulose or neomycin orally or rectally. Diarrhea stools will be more acidic. Cleanse the skin with gentle, nondetergent solutions, such as commercial perineal cleansers.
- Pat the skin dry or use a hair dryer on cool or warm; avoid hot settings.
- Use a barrier ointment, skin sealant, or fecal collector.
- Use ointment on top of protective film. Repeat with each bowel movement.

Impaired skin integrity related to incontinent diarrhea

- Keep in mind that skin impairment is harder to treat than to prevent.
- Cleanse perianal skin with Domeboro (aluminum acetate) solution and cotton balls; dry with hair dryer.
- Evaluate patient for the use of fecal collector.
- Dust eroded areas with stoma powder, and cover with a barrier ointment. Cleanse and remove the barrier with commercial cleanser.
- Assess the skin for fungal infection (itchy red rash with papules, pustules, or white curdy exudate).
- Repeat the procedure with each bowel movement.

Patient Education/Home Care Planning

1. Provide the family with and ensure understanding of written signs of changes in mental functions that are related to early PSE: confusion, untidiness, night wandering, and personality changes. They should notify the physician if symptoms occur.
2. Have the nutritionist ensure that the patient and family understand dietary instructions for reduced protein intake.

Evaluation

Thought processes are not impaired Thought processes, personality, behavior, consciousness, and neuromuscular activities are not altered. Blood ammonia levels are normal. Patient remains injury-free.

Skin integrity is maintained There are no signs of irritation or erosion.

GALLBLADDER DISORDERS

CHOLECYSTITIS WITH CHOLELITHIASIS

(Gallstones)

Cholecystitis refers to the acute or chronic inflammation of the gallbladder.

Acute cholecystitis is associated with gallstones (cholelithiasis) in 95% of cases (Figure 8-19).[67] Less than 5% of cases of acute cholecystitis are acalculous or unrelated to stone formation. Chronic cholecystitis refers to repeated attacks of acute cholecystitis and an abnormal-looking gallbladder. Pain often follows a meal in chronic cholecystitis. Chronic cholecystitis predisposes to acute cholecystitis (Figure 8-20), common duct stones, and adenocarcinoma of the gallbladder.

Acute cholecystitis is common and accounts for one fourth of all gallbladder surgeries. Although it may occur in all ages, it is more common in middle age.

The overall death rate is about 5%, occurring almost entirely in patients over 60 years or in those with diabetes.

Recent research has found that crystals of cholesterol, a major component of gallstones, form in 6 hours. The process can be visualized by video-enhanced, time-lapse photography. Physicians may be able to use this knowledge in the future to "test" bile samples of people at high risk for gallstones and initiate preventive measures.[50]

•••••• Pathophysiology

Acute cholecystitis consists of acute inflammation of the wall of the gallbladder. In calculous cholecystitis an obstruction of the cystic duct by a stone or from edema resulting from the passage of a stone is the underlying problem. The cystic duct is obstructed. The gallbladder distends, and the wall becomes edematous, compressing the capillaries and lymphatics and

resulting in ischemia and inflammation. The inflamed mucosa allows bile salt to be reabsorbed, further damaging the mucosa. If the inflammation continues, the wall will become friable and necrosis may develop. Perforation of the gallbladder may occur. The perforation may be small and localized, forming an abscess, or there may be free perforation, causing generalized peritonitis. In severe acute cholecystitis, inflammation spreads to the serosal layer of the gallbladder and may progress to form inflammatory adhesions to adjacent structures. Bacteria may be found in the bile and is associated with secondary infections.

The gallbladder heals after the acute attack with scarring and decreased absorptive capacity. The mucosa of the gallbladder in a patient with chronic cholecystitis is also ulcerated and scarred. Chronic cholecystitis may develop from repeated intermittent episodes of cystic duct obstruction resulting in chronic inflammation. The gallbladder is contracted, white in color, and thick walled. The bile is turbid and filled with debris.

Acute cholecystitis in the absence of stones has been associated with sudden starvation and immobility. These are changes that affect the regular filling and emptying of the gallbladder. A patient hospitalized for cardiovascular disease, burns, traumas, or biliary surgery may have acalculous acute cholecystitis develop. The patient on TPN may also have cholecystitis develop as a result of gallbladder distention and biliary stasis.

The primary symptom associated with acute cholecystitis is pain. The pain of acute cholecystitis has been described as colicky. However, this is not a true colic pain that waxes and wanes.

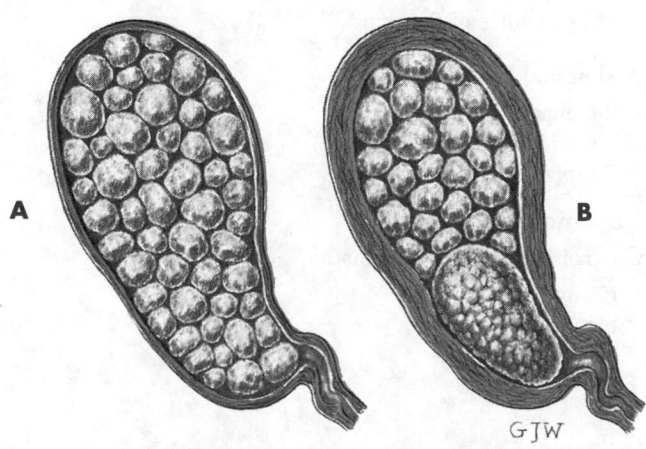

Figure 8-19 Cholelithiasis. **A,** Multiple faced stones. **B,** Large and numerous small stones in chronic cholecystitis. (From Doughty.[17])

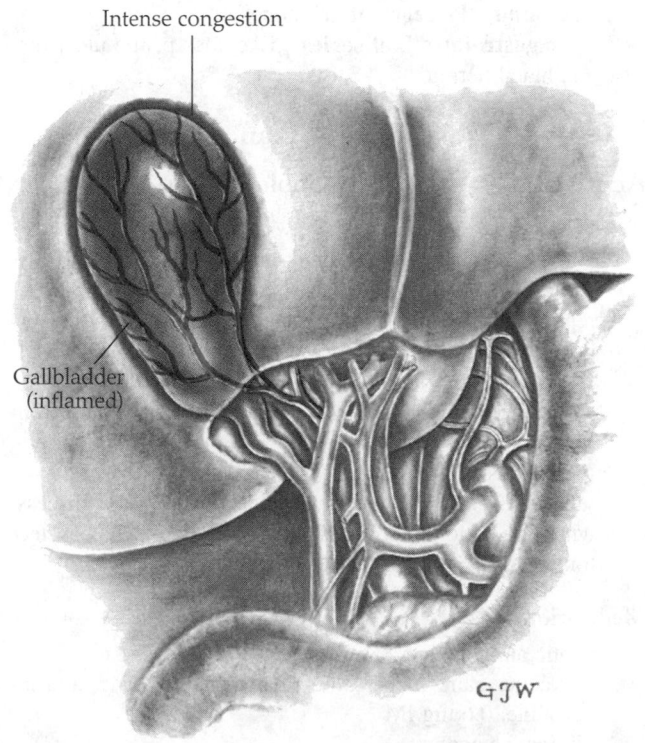

Figure 8-20 Cholecystitis (acute). (From Doughty.[17])

The pain of acute cholecystitis is abrupt in onset, reaches a peak intensity quickly, and remains at that level for 2 to 4 hours. Initially the pain may be poorly localized, but as it becomes more severe it localizes in the right upper quadrant epigastric region. The pain radiates around the midtorso to the right scapular area. Guarding and rigidity represent peritoneal involvement. Tenderness may be elicited at the tip of the ninth costal margin during inspiration (Murphy's sign). Jaundice may be found in acute cholecystitis. The jaundice may be related to edema of the ducts or to direct involvement of the liver by inflammation because stones are not always found in patients with jaundice.

•••••• Diagnostic Studies and Findings

Acute Cholecystitis

Plain films of abdomen   Gallstones visualized

Ultrasound   Gallstones; thickening of wall

Biliary scintigraphy   Scans 15 to 30 minutes after IV injection of radionuclide show the ducts but not the obstructed gallbladder; recommend repeat scan 4 hours after injection to rule out late filling of gallbladder

Serum amylase   Elevated may indicate concomitant acute pancreatitis; usually indicates common duct stone

White blood count   Leukocyte count of 12,000 to 15,000/mm^3

Chronic Cholecystitis

Double-dose oral cholecystogram   Nonfunctioning gallbladder

Ultrasound   Presence of gallstones

Upper gastrointestinal series   Excludes peptic ulcer disease and hiatal hernia

•••••• Multidisciplinary Plan

Acute Cholecystitis with Cholelithiasis
Surgery

Laparoscopic cholecystectomy—the gallbladder and the stones can be removed laparoscopically; this will probably replace most open cholecystectomy because more surgeons are learning the laparoscopic technique, and hospital stays are shorter

Cholecystectomy with operative cholangiography and exploration of common bile duct

Percutaneous cholecystotomy (in critically ill patients—a tube is inserted into the gallbladder to drain the abscess; when the patient recovers from acute attack, cholecystectomy can be performed)

Medications

Narcotic analgesics
> For acute pain, meperidine (Demerol), 100 mg, and atropine, 0.6 mg IM

Antiinfective agents
> Average severity
>> Ampicillin, 4 g/d IV
>> Cefazolin, 2-4 g/d IV

Severe disease
> Penicillin, 20 mU/d IV
> Clindamycin and aminoglycosides

General Management

Intravenous fluids to correct dehydration
Nasogastric tube; nothing by mouth

Chronic Cholecystitis

Surgery

Cholecystectomy with exploration of common bile duct

Medical Management

Stone dissolution—ursodiol
> For stones <5 mm and devoid of calcium

Extracorporeal shock wave lithotripsy used in conjunction with dissolution for stones that are initially larger than 5 mm

General Management

Avoidance of offending foods

NURSING CARE

Nursing Assessment

Acute Cholecystitis with Cholelithiasis
Pain

> Severe right upper quadrant pain with referral to right scapula
> Sudden, generalized abdominal pain indicates free perforation

General

> Fever 37° to 39° C (99° to 102° F)

Gastrointestinal

> Anorexia, nausea, vomiting
> Mild jaundice of the skin

Abdominal Examination

> Rebound tenderness; rigidity
> Positive Murphy's sign
> Gallbladder may be palpable

Chronic Cholecystitis
Gastrointestinal Symptoms

> Fat intolerance
> Flatulence
> Nausea, vomiting
> Anorexia

Pain

> Nonspecific abdominal pain and tenderness in right hypochondrium
> Episodic abdominal pain
> Dyspepsia

Biliary colic—steady pain that begins abruptly and subsides gradually; pain lasts from a few minutes to several hours

Nursing Dx & Intervention

Pain related to biliary colic (obstruction of cystic duct)

- Assess and document characteristics, location, and severity of pain.
- Provide pain medication as ordered and record patient's response.
- Allow patient to assume position that is least painful.
- Allow patient to express feelings and fears.

Risk for fluid volume deficit related to emesis and nothing by mouth (NPO) status

- Assess patient for signs of dehydration: dry mouth and mucous membranes, dry skin, blood pressure, and pulse.
- Maintain careful intake and output records, including emesis and nasogastric aspiration.
- Monitor serum electrolytes.
- Provide intravenous fluids as ordered.
- Maintain frequent oral hygiene.

Patient Education/Home Care Planning

1. During the acute phase, the patient will need explanation of all procedures and may require pain medication before moving. The patient should be made aware that the nurse recognizes the severity of the pain during acute cholecystitis.
2. After or during the resolution of the acute phase, the patient will need information about cholecystectomy to make an informed decision regarding surgery.

---

3. Patients electing medical management will need information on chronic cholecystitis; signs and symptoms of recurrence; signs of potential complications (recurrent attacks, jaundice, obstruction of common bile duct, cholangitis, pancreatitis, internal biliary fistula, carcinoma); and low-fat diets.

Evaluation

Comfort level is achieved Patient verbalizes increased control over pain. Patient uses pain control strategies appropriately.

Adequate hydration is maintained Intake and output equal; vital signs stable; mucous membranes moist; serum electrolytes within normal limits.

PANCREATIC DISORDERS

■ PANCREATITIS

Pancreatitis is an inflammation of the pancreas that may be acute or chronic

Acute pancreatitis (Figure 8-21) involves a diffuse inflammation caused by premature activation of pancreatic enzymes into active, potent proteolytic enzymes. Acute pancreatitis is a process of autodigestion. The two types of acute pancreatitis are interstitial or edematous pancreatitis and hemorrhagic or necrotizing pancreatitis. The two forms may be a continuum of the same process. Interstitial pancreatitis is milder and characterized by interstitial edema, with exudation into the surrounding retroperitoneal structures. As the disease progresses, frank

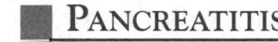

Advanced hemorrhagic
pancreatitis

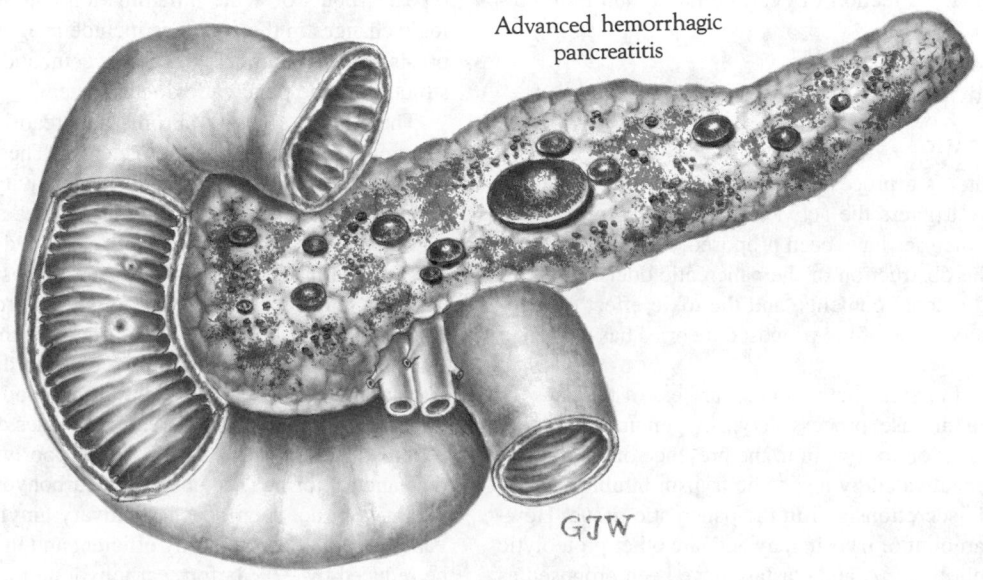

GJW

Figure 8-21 Pancreatitis (acute). (From Doughty.[17])

necrosis develops with disruption and thrombotic occlusion of blood vessels. Bleeding, ischemic necrosis, and fat necrosis are found throughout the pancreas.

Most cases of acute pancreatitis are caused by biliary tract disease or heavy alcohol intake; yet many other causes of acute pancreatitis exist, including postoperative states (pancreas, stomach, biliary tract), infections (mumps, hepatitis, coxsackie B), drugs (thiazides, steroids, azathioprine, pentamidine), and vasculitis. More conditions are being recognized all the time. The incidence varies with location and is higher in urban populations. Local or systemic complications occur in 20% of attacks.[69] Complications include abscess, pseudocyst formation, hemorrhage, ascites, and local effects on contiguous organs (portal vein thrombosis, bowel necrosis, intraperitoneal bleeding, and obstruction of the common duct). Systemic effects include pleural effusions, atelectasis, acute renal failure, gastritis, disseminated intravascular coagulation (DIC), hypotension, hypoglycemia, and hyperglycemia. Mortality of acute necrotizing pancreatitis ranges from 10% to 50%.[21]

Chronic pancreatitis is characterized by progressive functional damage to the pancreas even if the initiating cause is removed. The primary causative factor is chronic excessive alcohol ingestion. Clinical features include pain, malabsorption, diabetes mellitus, and intraductal calcifications. Complications consist of loss of exocrine and endocrine function, pseudocysts, biliary and duodenal obstruction, malnutrition, and drug addiction.

A pseudocyst occurs when an accumulation of tissue debris, blood, fat droplets, and pancreatic juice develops within confluent areas of necrosis. A pseudocyst may arise within or adjacent to the pancreas. Pancreatic ascites develops when the accumulation of active pancreatic enzymes and leukocytes irritates the peritoneal surfaces and fluid accumulates in the peritoneal cavity. The same process of irritation through the diaphragmatic lymphatics leads to pleural effusion. Abscesses result from secondary infection of necrotic tissue and fluid collection.

•••••• Pathophysiology

Acute Pancreatitis

Acute pancreatitis is a process of autodigestion, but the agent that prematurely triggers the activation of the enzymes is unknown. Several theories have been proposed, including the theory involving the obstruction of the pancreatic ducts, reflux of bile, reflux of duodenal contents, and the toxic effect of alcohol. Unfortunately, none of the proposed theories has proven to be the cause.

The process of enzyme activation regardless of the cause is the basis of the disease process. Trypsinogen may undergo spontaneous activation to trypsin in the presence of an alkaline pH. Trypsin is inactivated by a specific trypsin inhibitor found in the pancreatic secretions and in the pancreatic tissue. However, the small amount of trypsin may activate other proteolytic enzymes. Phospholipase A and elastase have been proposed as the primary enzymes responsible for autodigestion. Phospholipase A, in the presence of bile, results in severe pancreatic parenchymal and adipose tissue necrosis. Elastase dissolves the elastic fibers of blood vessels and is implicated in the hemorrhage associated with necrotizing pancreatitis.

Many substances released from the injured pancreas will have systemic effects. Two low–molecular weight vasoactive peptides (kinins) are released and result in vasodilation and increase in vascular permeability, resulting in circulatory shock. Severe pulmonary edema and pain are also associated with the vasoactive peptides.

Hypocalcemia develops when a decreased binding of calcium to serum protein occurs as a result of a drop of albumin levels. In addition, a decrease in ionized serum calcium occurs in acute pancreatitis. Damage to the islet cells results in mild, transient hyperglycemia from release of glucagon and decreased release of insulin. The glucose levels are too high for the insulin production to control.

Patients with acute pancreatitis are at risk for developing adult respiratory distress syndrome (ARDS). Arterial hypoxia occurs when intrapulmonary right-to-left shunting develops. Pulmonary edema from disruption of the alveolar-capillary membrane is a serious complication. In addition, renal function may be altered during acute pancreatitis. Hypovolemia and shock are not always the causative factors in altered renal function. The blood flow may be reduced and the vascular resistance increased in the kidney in the absence of hypovolemia.

Another major potential complication of acute pancreatitis is disseminated intravascular coagulation (DIC), which involves the development of microthrombi and consumption of clotting factors. Mild DIC may play a role in the development of early hypoxia and renal impairment.

Chronic Pancreatitis

Chronic pancreatitis generally develops from an insidious sclerosing process in the pancreas; however, it may develop from repeated bouts of acute inflammation and necrosis. The histologic changes in the pancreas include irregularly distributed fibrosis, reduced number and size of acini and islet cells, and obstruction of the pancreatic ductal system.

The clinical signs of chronic pancreatitis include pain and functional impairment of the pancreas. The pain may be intermittent or chronic and affects the productivity of the patient and his or her activities of daily living. Nausea and vomiting often accompany the pain. The pain is described as steady, boring, dull, or sharp and radiates from the epigastrium to the back. The pain may be lessened by leaning forward from a sitting position. Eating or lying down may increase the pain.

Malabsorption and weight loss develop during the course of the chronic illness. Patients may limit food intake because of the pain. Secretions of pancreatic enzymes decrease in chronic pancreatitis, and fat and protein are poorly digested. Steatorrhea and azotorrhea are observed. Carbohydrate malabsorption is clinically not seen because salivary amylase is unimpaired. Pancreatic amylase is highly efficient and in fact would have to be reduced by 97% before carbohydrate malabsorption would develop.[61]

Insulin response to glucose is impaired in chronic pancreatitis. Overt diabetes mellitus will occur in most of these patients. The ability of the pancreas to release glucagon is also affected.

••••• Diagnostic Studies and Findings

Acute Pancreatitis

Amylase   Greater than 500 U/dl; highest levels 2 to 12 hours after onset, drop to normal (60 to 180 U/dl) within 48 to 72 hours

Lipase   Elevated; may remain elevated for 5 to 10 days

Hematocrit   Elevated secondary to dehydration; decreased secondary to abdominal blood loss

White blood count (WBC)   Greater than 12,000/mm³ with suppurative complications

Glucose   Greater than 180 mg/dl with no prior history of hyperglycemia

Bilirubin   Mildly elevated (<2 mg/dl)

Blood urea nitrogen (BUN) >45 mg/dl after fluid volume replacement

Chronic Pancreatitis

Amylase and lipase   Usually normal, increased in presence of pseudocysts and pancreatic ascites

Bilirubin   Possibly elevated

Alkaline phosphate   Increased five times normal for 4 weeks; indicates common bile duct stenosis

Glucose   Elevated

Urine   Glycosuria (diabetes mellitus)

Plain films of abdomen   Calcifications

Computerized tomography (CT)   Calcifications

Ultrasound   Calcification of pancreatic ducts

Endoscopic retrograde cholangiopancreatography (ERCP)   Ductal stones and irregularity with dilation and stenoses; rule out carcinoma and pseudocyst

Test of pancreatic exocrine function   Exogenous stimulation: Secretin-CCK; decreased stimulation of pancreatic enzymes greater than 45 mg/dl after fluid volume replacement

Calcium   Less than 8 mg/dl in severe pancreatitis

Albumin   Less than 3.2 g/dl

Urine amylase   Levels may remain elevated for 5 to 10 days

Arterial Po₂   Less than 60 mm Hg

Plain films of abdomen   Sentinel loop sign—isolated dilation of a segment of bowel; colon cutoff sign—gas distending the right colon that abruptly stops in the mid or left transverse colon

X-ray film   Left-sided pleural effusion

Upper gastrointestinal series   Widened duodenal loop, swollen ampulla of Vater

CT scan with IV contrast media   Necrosis, abscess, phlegmon (complications)

Endogenous stimulation: perfusion and feedings   Diminished function

Lundh test meal   Mean trypsin concentration decreased

Para-aminobenzoic acid (PABA) test   Urinary recovery of PABA low in pancreatic insufficiency

Fecal fat balance test $>25\%$ ingested fat indicates clinically significant steatorrhea

••••• Multidisciplinary Plan

Acute Pancreatitis

Surgery

Debridement of dead peripancreatic tissue in necrotizing pancreatitis

Surgical drainage of pancreatic pseudocyst may be indicated if it does not resolve spontaneously

Surgical drainage of pancreatic abscesses may be indicated

Laparotomy for common duct obstruction

Medications

Narcotic analgesics

  Meperidine (Demerol), 75-125 mg IM q4h or prn (hold analgesics until initial laboratory samples are drawn because many will cause elevations in serum amylase and lipase)

Antacids

  Aluminum-magnesium preparation, 30-40 ml (clamp nasogastric tube for 15 min after dosage)

Histamine H₂ receptor antagonists

  Cimetidine or ranitidine, 300 mg IV qid if any evidence of upper gastrointestinal bleeding

Antiinfective agents

  Cephalothin (Keflin), 2 g q6h IV or with peritoneal lavage

  For abscess, chloramphenicol (chloromycetin), 0.5 g q6h IV, and penicillin G, 5-10 million U/d IV, *or* cefoxitin, 1 g q6h IV (used before cultures are known)

Adrenergic agents

  For hypotension, dopamine (Intropin), 2-5 µg/kg/min, diluted in solution and titrated as needed or isoproteronol (Isuprel) may be used

General Management

Endoscopic sphincterotomy for biliary pancreatitis

Continuous hemodynamic and arterial blood gas monitoring; Swan-Ganz or CVP catheter

Nasogastric suctioning

Peritoneal lavage for persistent hypotension (removes pancreatic exudate, which contains large amounts of vasoactive kinins)

ARDS: endotracheal intubation and controlled ventilation with positive end-expiratory pressure (PEEP)

Restoration and maintenance of intravascular volume including human serum albumin, low–molecular weight dextran 40

Correction of electrolyte imbalances: hypocalcemia, hypomagnesemia, hyperglycemia, hyperkalemia, and metabolic acidosis

Nutritional support with TPN or feeding jejunostomy

Discontinue offending drugs associated with pancreatitis

Chronic Pancreatitis

Surgery

Not primary treatment but may be used to treat intractable pain and complications (e.g., pseudocysts or abscesses)

Drainage procedures

Longitudinal pancreaticojejunostomy (modified Puestow procedure)

Sphincteroplasty plus extraction of pancreatic calculi

Resection

Subtotal or total pancreatectomy

Pancreaticoduodenostomy (Whipple procedure)

To preserve islet cell function

Islet cell autotransplantation by infusion of islet cell preparations into portal system

Segments of pancreas autotransplanted

Insertion of closed-loop insulin infusion system

Medications

Analgesics

Acetaminophen or narcotics prn for pain

Pancreatic enzyme supplements (use one of the following)

Pancreatin (Viokase), 6 tablets with each meal

Pancrelipase (Cotazym), 5 capsules with each meal

Pancrelipase (Pancrease), enteric-coated, 2-3 capsules with each meal

Antacids and absorbents

Sodium bicarbonate or aluminum hydroxide antacids may be used with pancreatic enzyme supplements to improve results

Histamine H_2 receptor antagonists

Cimetidine, 300 mg po 30 min before meals (may be used to improve effects of pancreatic enzyme supplements)

Medium-chain triglycerides (MCT; Portagen) supplements

Insulin therapy: does vary with individual (remember that glucagon deficiency is present and patient may have hypoglycemic reactions easily)

General Management

Enteral nutritional support or TPN as indicated by nutritional status and weight loss

Discontinue alcohol intake

NURSING CARE

Nursing Assessment

Acute Pancreatitis

General

Fever of 38° C (100 ° to 101° F)

Abdominal Examination

Grey Turner's sign—bluish brown discoloration of flanks

Cullen's sign—bluish brown discoloration in periumbilicus area

Absent bowel sounds with intestinal ileus

Palpation: localized epigastric tenderness intensifies with deep palpation

Soft abdomen (retroperitoneal location of pancreas means that signs of peritoneal irritation, rigidity, and rebound tenderness will not be present initially)

Mild abdominal swelling and mild ascites

Abdominal mass with pseudocyst

Integumentary

Subcutaneous fat necrosis occurring as tender, red subcutaneous nodules

Jaundice in some patients; hyperbilirubinemia of 3 mg/dl

Spontaneous drainage of pancreatic abscess through an abnormal tract to skin or after surgical drainage of an abscess (pancreatic cutaneous fistula)

Pulmonary

Pleuritic pain; pleural rub; decreased breath sounds; increased respiratory rate

Cardiovascular

Tachycardia, hypovolemia, and hypotension may progress to circulatory shock and coma

Pain

Steady, dull, boring, severe pain in epigastrium or left upper quadrant: poorly localized; reaches peak intensity within 15 minutes to 1 hour; radiates to lower thoracic vertebral area; worsens in supine position; partially relieved by leaning forward; sometimes pa-tient has referred shoulder pain from irritation of diaphragm

Nutritional Status

Weight loss, if related to alcohol intake may show signs of chronic malnutrition from alcoholism

Chronic Pancreatitis

Pain

Intermittent or chronic pain; boring, dull, or sharp pain that is steady; epigastric, right or left subcostal region, periumbilical region, or lower abdomen; radiates to patient's back; patient observed sitting up and leaning forward to relieve pain

Nutritional Status

Weight loss, steatorrhea, voluminous diarrhea, nausea, and vomiting (associated with pain and with complications)

Endocrine

Signs and symptoms of diabetes mellitus; reactive hypoglycemia to insulin therapy

Nursing Dx & Intervention

Risk for fluid volume deficit related to fluid exudation in acute pancreatitis

- Assess for signs of impending cardiac failure *because circulatory shock is a possibility from the release of vasoactive peptides (kinin) from an injured pancreas (acute pancreatitis).*

- Assess for signs and symptoms of electrolyte imbalance.
- Assess intake and output, central venous pressure, Swan-Ganz catheter pressure, daily weights.
- Assess vital signs and blood pressure every 4 hours, more often if indicated.
- Monitor laboratory values, particularly hematocrit and hemoglobin, which will decrease after volume is restored.
- Provide fluid volume replacement as ordered; intravenous fluids, dextran, fluid expanders.

Ineffective breathing pattern related to pulmonary complications of acute pancreatitis

- Assess patient carefully for signs of respiratory distress: breath sounds, cough, sputum, fluid accumulation, elevated diaphragm, shallow breathing *because patients are candidates for ARDS.*
- Monitor arterial blood gases.

Risk for injury (complications) related to severe pancreatic inflammation

- Assess for signs of pseudocyst: upper abdominal pain, mass, tenderness, fever, a general deterioration or no improvement in patient's condition.

Risk for impaired skin integrity related to presence of pancreatic fistula

- Monitor output of any fistula.
- Provide skin protection for a pancreatic fistula with a clean pouch with skin barrier or with barrier ointments and dressings.

Pain related to acute or chronic inflammatory process

- Assess patient's pain: steady, dull, boring pain in epigastrium, worsens when supine.
- Allow patient to assume a comfortable position; usually sitting up and leaning forward will help relieve pain.
- Provide analgesics as ordered because pain may be severe and steady; analgesics before procedures alleviate or minimize discomfort.

Altered nutrition: less than body requirements related to pain and malabsorption

- Assess patient's nutritional status. Consult with the nutritionist.
- Give patient nothing by mouth during acute pancreatitis episodes *to eliminate unnecessary secretion of pancreatic enzymes.*
- Measure and record nasogastric output.
- Provide frequent mouth care.
- Monitor blood and urine glucose levels because damage to islet cells may result in mild transient hyperglycemia.
- Assess stools for diarrhea and steatorrhea, a sign of malabsorption of fats.
- Provide insulin as ordered for endocrine dysfunction in chronic pancreatitis (note possibility of reactive hypoglycemia to insulin therapy).

- When eating, provide small, frequent, low-fat meals that are high in protein and carbohydrates.
- Avoid coffee and spicy foods.
- Administer pancreatic enzyme supplements before meals as ordered.

Patient Education/Home Care Planning

1. Assist the patient in understanding the cause or causal relationships of pancreatitis with alcohol use or gallstones.
2. Plan an appropriate rehabilitation program if alcohol abuse is related to disease process.
3. Provide written dietary instructions.
4. Provide written medication instructions.
5. Provide the patient with information about diabetes mellitus: signs, symptoms, and insulin therapy.
6. Discuss with the patient ways to avoid another attack (abstain from alcohol; quit smoking; follow prescribed diet).

Evaluation

Nutritional and fluid status is stable Patient's hydration and electrolyte balance are adequate. Patient's nutrition is adequate. Patient's weight is stable. Patient does not experience steatorrhea or diarrhea. Patient's serum glucose is stabilized. Patient does not experience anorexia, nausea, or vomiting.

Respiratory function is normal Patient shows no signs of respiratory distress. Patient's arterial blood gas levels are within normal range.

Comfort level is achieved Patient shows a reduction or absence of guarding or protective behavior. Patient uses pain control strategies appropriately. Patient verbalizes increased control over pain.

Skin integrity is maintained Perifistular skin is effectively protected from enzymatic drainage

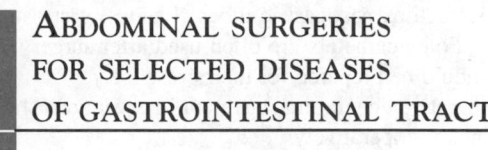

MEDICAL INTERVENTIONS AND RELATED NURSING CARE

ABDOMINAL SURGERIES FOR SELECTED DISEASES OF GASTROINTESTINAL TRACT

Description and Rationale

Abdominal surgeries involve an incision into the abdomen with the patient under general anesthesia. A variety of abdominal surgeries may be required under the broad scope of gastrointestinal diseases. Commonalities exist in the preoperative and postoperative patient care assessment and interventions that will be covered in this section. Examples of abdominal surgeries in which a portion of the gastrointestinal tract is surgically removed include appendectomy (appendix), cholecystectomy (gallbladder), colectomy (colon), and gastrectomy (stomach). An intestinal resection may be referred to as an ileotransverse colostomy (ileum is re-anastomosed to transverse colon with removal or bypass of the ascending colon: in this case there is no externalization of the bowel even though the term "colostomy" is used).

Laparoscopic surgical techniques are being used increasingly for abdominal surgeries. Laparoscopic cholecystectomies are now done routinely, and techniques are being developed for antireflux procedures, appendectomy, hernia repair, colectomy, vagotomy, and hysterectomy. Although laparoscopic surgeries may require increased intraoperative time, they often result in decreased hospitalization time, less discomfort and pain postoperatively, smaller scars, lower costs, and less time away from work and usual activities.

Surgery is indicated in many gastrointestinal diseases when medical management is ineffective or when complications develop. Surgery may be palliative, as in the case of Crohn's disease, or curative, as with ulcerative colitis and familial polyposis.

Contraindications and Cautions

1. Patients with signs and symptoms of an acute condition in the abdomen or an emergency situation will need to be quickly stabilized with fluid and electrolyte replacements.
2. The surgical intervention in an emergency may be considered a first stage, diverting the problem, with a required second operation for definitive treatment.
3. For patients with permanent colostomies, ileostomies, continent ileostomies, and ileoanal reservoirs, recommend medical alert card stating: "No rectal temperatures, no rectal enemas, no rectal suppositories: the rectum has been removed." Provide definition of above procedures.

Preprocedural Nursing Care

1. Thorough bowel preparation is required for many abdominal surgeries including oral cathartics, antibiotics, and enemas. The trend is toward eliminating the preoperative day and having the patient perform bowel preparation at home. Caution must be used not to deplete weakened or elderly patients with multiple tap water enemas.
2. Drains such as Penrose, silicone dual sump, Shiley sump, and tubes, such as nasogastric tubes, T tubes, gastrostomy tubes, and Foley catheters are often used after surgery, and patients should be prepared for their presence.
3. All postoperative general management interventions should be explained preoperatively.

•••••• Multidisciplinary Plan

Medications

Bowel preparation (for elective large intestinal surgery); nonabsorbable anitinfective agents (done preoperatively)
Neomycin, 1 g at 2 PM, 6 PM, and 11 PM
Erythromycin (base), 1 g at 2 PM, 6 PM, and 11 PM
Postoperatively, broad-spectrum antibiotic prophylaxis for 24-36 h

Narcotic analgesics given by intramuscular, subcutaneous injections q3-4h; by Patient-Controlled IV Analgesia (PCA); by epidural catheter

General Management

Pulmonary care: incentive spirometry, splinting, and coughing
Gastrointestinal decompression: nasogastric tube, gastrostomy tube
Early and progressive ambulation
Embolus prevention: thromboembolic disease support hose (TEDs) and pneumatic compression stockings
Pain management: Subcutaneous and intramuscular injections; patient-controlled analgesia (PCA); continuous epidural narcotics; transcutaneous electrical nerve stimulation (TENS)
Intravenous fluids with electrolytes (particularly potassium)
Nutrition: Enteral or intravenous feedings as supplement or maintenance

Respiratory Therapy

May be used to assist patient with pulmonary toilet

Physical Therapy

May be used to assist patient with progressive ambulation or mobility exercises

Nutritional Consultation

May be necessary to assist patient with postoperative dietary selections for well-balanced diet if surgery necessitates significant dietary changes; may be used to recommend formulations for enteral or parenteral therapy

NURSING CARE

Nursing Assessment

General

Low-grade fever first 24 to 48 hours common
Fever of 38° C (100° F) or fever that does not subside may indicate pulmonary complications, wound infection, urinary infection, or thrombophlebitis
Fever of 38.3° C (101° F) occurring suddenly and accompanied by chills, weakness, fatigue, rapid respiration, tachycardia, and sudden drop in blood pressure indicates septic shock

Gastrointestinal

Gas pains, passage of gas, bowel movement, hunger and appetite, constipation, diarrhea, nausea, vomiting

Pain

Assess intensity of pain using pain scale; note location, type, duration, intensity, pattern of pain occurrence, narcotic usage patterns, effectiveness of narcotics, and what makes the pain better or worse

Determine previous narcotic use or history of substance abuse (to plan for higher postoperative dosages)

Nutritional Status

Usual weight, percent change on admission, change in dietary habits

Assess patient for nutritional deficiencies; see nutritional assessment chart

Coping with Anxiety

Assess emotional reaction to surgery and consequences

Assess level of support and coping mechanisms

Assess health information needs

Ability for Self-Care

Determine usual activities and restrictions

Determine perception of responsibilities after surgery

Urinary Tract

Dehydration: urinary output <30 ml/h; urine specific gravity

Voiding problems after indwelling catheter removal, or secondary to temporary nerve damage after rectal manipulation

Abdominal Examination

Observations: distention (note shape and contour); presence of drains or tubes; staples, sutures, Steri-strips, dressing (dry or with drainage); incision (dry, draining, erythematous, indurated); presence of skin color changes (mottling, erythema, ecchymosis, rash, etc.)

Auscultation: presence or absence of bowel sounds; character (frequency and pitch) of bowel sounds

Palpation: soft, firm, location and intensity of pain, rigidity, rebound tenderness, and ascites

Percussion: dull, tympany (distinguish air from fluid from solid mass)

Integumentary

Assess nares for pressure from nasogastric tubes

Assess incision for erythema, induration, drainage, wound edge separation, and bleeding

Assess wounds healing by secondary intention: presence or absence of granulation tissue, necrotic tissue, exudate, odor, and evidence of contraction

Identify impairments to wound healing (steroids, malnutrition, obesity, sepsis, and so forth)

Assess patient's risk for developing pressure ulcers

Assess for skin breakdown from excess drainage, shearing tape, and pressure

Mental Status

Evaluation of effects of narcotics, anesthesia, and fatigue

Encephalopathy after surgery on patients with cirrhosis

Pulmonary

Decreased respiratory stimulus from respiratory depressants such as narcotics and anesthesia

Shallow breathing and inadequate coughing as a result of abominal pain

Oral Mucous Membranes

Hydration, presence of thrush, and cleanliness

Cardiovascular

Shock and circulatory failure associated with hemorrhage, sepsis, fluid, and electrolyte imbalance

Thrombophlebitis, pulmonary emboli: assess calves for tenderness, warmth, or cords, Homan's sign

Fluids and Electrolytes

Nausea, vomiting, diarrhea, and nasogastric and intestinal suctioning may affect fluid and electrolyte balance

Nursing Dx & Intervention

Pain related to surgical incision and manipulation and gas

- Assess the location, type, and duration of pain, as well as the pattern of pain occurrence and the effectiveness of medications.
- Assess and document the patient's pain in relation to eating, activity, medications, and the patient's emotional state.
- Discuss with the patient the importance of pain relief postoperatively *to prevent complications.*
- Provide analgesics as ordered for pain, keeping the physician informed of the patient's level of comfort and response to medication.
- Use adjunctive pain relieving strategies (massage, heat, or cool pads, relaxation techniques, and music). Document the effectiveness on the care plan.
- Premedicate the patient before ambulation, dressing changes, or other painful procedures.
- Reassure the patient and family that the usual postoperative patient does not become addicted to the narcotics.
- Evaluate the patient for side effects of the narcotics, and discuss with the patient respiratory depression, itching, nausea, and hallucinations.
- Be supportive of the patient while he or she is having pain; at the same time, evaluate the nature and location of the pain.
- Assist the patient in proper positioning.
- Gradually discontinue intravenous and intramuscular injections, and ease the patient on to oral analgesia when the patient is eating or able to tolerate it.

Anxiety related to change in body image, fear of the future, unfamiliar environment, feelings of lack of control, and separation from home and work roles

- Assess patient's and family's fears and concerns on a regular basis. Incorporate this information into the nursing care plan as necessary.

- Provide information related to patient's fears and concerns *so that he or she can gain understanding.*
- Set aside time to listen actively, allowing patient to sort out vague or anxious feelings. Help patient to verbalize and understand the feelings he or she is having.
- Provide for continuity in staffing or assign a primary nurse, if possible.
- Introduce patient to other patients who are in similar situations and can "buddy up," providing mutual support.
- Make a referral to a local support organization (United Ostomy Association; Crohn's and Colitis Foundation of America).
- Provide patient with quiet time alone or with significant others *to allow him or her uninterrupted time to sort through emotions.*
- Refer patient for psychiatric follow-up in the hospital or after discharge, if indicated.
- Talk with family and significant others, *to help them understand patient's situation better and to assist them in supporting patient.*

Altered nutrition: less than body requirements related to disease process, postoperative ileus, nausea, and vomiting

- Weigh patient every day and record the findings.
- Assess oral intake and record the findings.
- Assess abdomen for changes in symmetry, bowel sounds, evidence of gas or fluid, and tenderness.
- Monitor laboratory values that reflect nutritional status (albumin, prealbumin).
- Do calorie counts as needed.
- Request a consultation with the nutritionist.

Risk for infection related to perioperative contamination

- Ensure that all tubes and drains are well secured *to prevent accidental removal.*
- Assess wound during postoperative period for redness, pain, edema, unusual drainage, odor, and separation of the suture line.
- Observe wound dressing frequently for signs of bleeding.
- Monitor vital signs every 2 hours until patient is stable and then every 4 hours.
- Keep primary dressing intact for 48 hours.
- Reinforce if saturated.

Risk for altered renal, cardiopulmonary, gastrointestinal, and peripheral tissue perfusion related to postoperative fluid shifts and complications

- Assess patient for signs and symptoms of alterations in tissue perfusion associated with major abdominal surgeries for complications of pancreatitis, cholecystitis, ulcerative colitis, and other diseases, including shock, circulatory failure, intestinal ischemia, and renal failure.
- Monitor patient's vital signs and central venous pressure or Swan-Ganz cathether for changes in cardiac output and tissue perfusion.
- Encourage patient to do leg exercises, and measure and apply elastic hose *to facilitate venous circulation.* Provide pneumatic compression stockings, if indicated.

Ineffective breathing pattern related to narcotic use and abdominal pain

- Assess patient for shallow breathing, splinting with respirations, decreased breath sounds, and respiratory distress.
- Auscultate lungs every 2 to 4 hours.
- Encourage patient to turn, deep breathe, and cough every 2 hours.
- Encourage use of incentive spirometer *to promote maximal inspiratory maneuvers.*
- Provide pain medications and splint abdomen with pillow *to decrease abdominal pain associated with deep breathing and coughing.*
- Assist patient with early and progressive ambulation.
- Peripheral pulse oximetry may provide useful oxygen saturation levels.

Risk for fluid volume deficit related to postoperative fluid shifts

- Monitor intake and output, including all drainage from nasogastric, gastric, intestinal, and T tubes, as well as wound drainage or fistula output and urinary output.
- Weigh patient daily.
- Assess patient's hydration status by mucous membrane, skin turgor, blood pressure and pulse.
- Monitor color, consistency, amount, and odor of any drainage; test drainage (i.e., nasogastric aspirate, stool, urine, fistula) for blood or pH if indicated. Provide fluid replacement as ordered.

Risk for impaired skin integrity related to tissue ischemia; excessive wound drainage

- Assess patient for risks in developing pressure sores.
- Protect the nares when nasogastric tube is to be left in place several days.
- Change wound dressings frequently if output is high *to protect skin from moisture maceration.*
- Apply a pectin-based (Stomahesive, Hollihesive) wafer to the skin and tape to the wafer rather than applying tape on the skin. Montgomery straps can be applied on top of the pectin-based wafer. Keep in mind that drainage from the gastrointestinal tract continues to contain very irritating digestive enzymes (bile, gastric, pancreatic, intestinal).
- Evaluate patient with wound drainage for a wound pouching system to contain the drainage, protect the skin, allow for accurate measurement, and decrease cost of dressing changes (see box p. 783).
- Protect tubes from pulling by adequately taping and provide skin protection if there is leakage around a tube (see box p. 784).

POUCH METHOD

1. Premedicate patient if procedure will be painful.
2. Gather supplies:
   - Ostomy or wound pouch (with skin barrier attached) that will accommodate wound. The pouch should be designed to attach to a bedside bag.
   - Scissors, plastic film, marker.
   - Skin barrier paste (Hollister or ConVaTec, for example).
3. Make a pattern of the wound or fistula using a piece of plastic film. Carefully label the patient's left, right, head, and feet; pouch side and skin side.
4. Trace the pattern onto the skin barrier on the back of the pouch. be sure to match up the patient's right side, left side, head, and so forth so that the pouch will not be positioned backwards or upside down.
5. Cut the opening in the barrier following the pattern.
6. Cleanse the patient's skin with warm water, and pat dry. Fill in any folds or creases with paste.
7. Remove the paper backing from the back of the pouch, and apply a thin coat of paste around the cut opening.
8. Center the cut opening over the wound, pressing firmly at the wound edges. Cover any exposed skin with paste through the access cap or through the end of the pouch.
9. Close the spout, or apply a clamp. If the drainage is liquid, attach the spout to a bedside drainage bag.
10. Check the system each shift for signs of leakage; change when necessary.
11. If pouching sytem leaks consistently and you are unable to achieve an adequate seal, an enterostomal therapist consultation may be required to assess the need for a different pouching system.

SUCTION AND TRANSPARENT DRESSING METHOD

12. Premedicate the patient if the procedure will be painful.
13. Gather supplies:
    - Skin barrier, if the skin is intact; hydrocolloid wafer, if the skin has open ulcers or eroded areas near the wound
    - Paste
    - Powder (Stomahesive/ConVaTec or Premium/Hollister)—used if there are eroded, weeping areas near the wound
    - Transparent dressing or polyurethane film in the size that corresponds to the wound size
    - Catheters–soft, large lumen with hand-cut side holes; need 1 to 3 catheters, depending on the size of the wound and whether the wound is being irrigated
    - Connectors for catheters
    - Scissors, pattern, black marker, normal saline, if using flush and irrigation, razor, and washcloth
14. Turn off the wound irrigation before changing the pouch, if using irrigation.
15. Gently remove the old skin barrier/hydrocolloid and transparent film. Use a warm washcloth as needed.
16. Clean surrounding skin gently, and remove all accumulated pastes and so forth. To remove residual soft paste, use a dry facial tissue in a gentle, pinching and rolling motion. Shave any hair that will come into contact with the paste or barrier to make removal easier.

17. Let dry thoroughly.
18. Make a pattern of the wound opening using a black marker and clear piece of plastic, or use the existing pattern. If you are using an existing pattern, make certain it is still a good fit.
19. Trace the edges of the wound and any surrounding drains, ostomies, and so forth. Transfer your pattern to the skin barrier or hydrocolloid (it may have to be in two separate pieces). When in doubt where the skin edge lies, make the pattern slightly larger than the wound to avoid having the skin barrier on the wound surface.
    - Make sure you mark which is up and which is down or which is right and which is left; this will ensure that the pieces will not be upside down or backwards.
20. Place a bead of paste at the edge of the skin near the wound; place the cut barrier on the surrounding skin. Cover any exposed skin at the wound edge with the paste. Apply the paste with a slightly damp gloved finger. The paste seals the area between the skin barrier and the wound.
21. Now that the periwound skin is completely protected, squeeze a bead of paste about an inch away from the wound on the top of the skin barrier. This is the seal for the transparent dressing. If this bead of paste is too close to the edge, it will be sucked onto the wound when suction is applied.
22. If you are using irrigation, you will need two catheters. One at the top for the normal saline (NS) and the other at the bottom for suction of drainage. The dependent catheter can have side holes cut into it for better suction. Lay your catheters in the wound, with one in the superior portion of the wound and one in the most inferior portion of the wound. Lay them on top of the paste you have just applied. Apply another bead of paste over the top of each catheter. Make sure the tips of the catheters are not lying in paste, or they will clog.
    - You can bevel the tips of the catheters and lay them bevel down in the wound. If the suction is too high or the wound tissue friable, the tip should be placed on top of the skin barrier at the most dependent part.
23. Lay a piece of transparent dressing over the entire wound. If it is not big enough, lay it over the bottom of the wound first (this is where it is most likely to leak). *DO NOT remove the paper backing of the larger sizes before application because it becomes more difficult to apply the dressing.* Remove the paper backing after laying it over the wound. If there are still exposed areas on the superior aspect, cover them with an additional piece of transparent dressing. DATE the system!
24. Connect the lower catheter to suction (as low suction as possible to do the job); connect the upper cathether to the irrigant–usually NS.
25. Change the dressing on a regular schedule to prevent skin irritation. These systems can be patched by recaulking with the paste and applying more transparent dressing if the skin is still protected. The dressing can last for as long as a week.
26. If pouching system leaks consistently and you are unable to achieve an adequate seal, an enterostomal therapist consultation may be required to assess the need for a different pouching system.

■ GASTROSTOMY TUBE CARE

A variety of tube retention devices are manufactured and may be available at your institution. If not, the following steps may be taken to secure the tube and protect the skin around the tube from drainage:

1. Use a pectin-based wafer (skin barrier) around the tube. Cut a small opening in the wafer $\frac{1}{8}$ inch larger than the skin exit site.
2. Cleanse the skin with warm water and pat dry.
3. Apply the wafer, and seal to the skin.
4. Apply a thin coat of paste (Stomahesive) to any exposed skin around the tube.
5. Anchor the tube to the wafer with use of baby bottle nipple. Cut open the end of the nipple. Cut the end of the nipple large enough to accommodate the tube. Cut up through the side of the nipple (base to top), open the nipple, and wrap around the tube. Then tape the base of the nipple to the pectin-based wafer.
6. Tape the tube to the top of the nipple.
7. Remove the nipple daily and assess the exit site. If needed, gently cleanse around the tube exit site and dry, reapply paste, and replace nipple. If the skin barrier has drainage leaking under the seal, remove and replace. The wafer should be changed weekly otherwise.

Constipation; diarrhea related to altered bowel motility postoperatively

- Assess patient for first bowel movement after surgery.
- Assess dietary and fluid intake as it relates to normal stool consistency.
- Observe color, consistency, frequency, and amount of stools.
- Evaluate pattern change after gastrointestinal surgery (e.g., diarrhea related to bile in colon after cholecystectomy or small bowel resection).

Bathing/hygiene self-care deficit related to postoperative pain

- Assist patient with activities of daily living after surgery.
- Encourage patient to participate in self-care as tolerated.
- Encourage patient to assume primary responsibility for care as tolerated as nasogastric tube and IVs are removed.
- Provide regular mouth care to prevent problems associated with nasogastric tubes, limited oral intake for several days, and mouth breathing.
- Assist patient in brushing his or her teeth and rinsing the mouth with nonastringent solutions every 4 hours or more often for patient comfort.

Altered patterns of urinary elimination related to use of catheters or local trauma

- Asses for signs of urinary retention associated with anesthesia, pain, anxiety, removal of indwelling catheter, or local damage done to nerves (rectal surgery).
- Observe and record intake and output.
- Provide privacy and promote relaxation when patient needs to void.
- Palpate bladder for distention if patient has not voided for 6 to 8 hours or patient is voiding small amounts frequently (overflow voiding).
- Catheterize patient if ordered.

Patient Education/Home Care Planning

1. Ensure that patient understands that routine care follows major abdominal surgery: ambulate at regular times, rest frequently, and slowly increase activities as tolerated; report any signs of redness, pain, or drainage of incision; avoid heavy lifting for 6 to 8 weeks, and splint abdomen when coughing or sneezing. Ensure that patient understands that pain may accompany these activities and that pain medications are available, should be taken as necessary and as prescribed.
2. Explain medications and medication schedule to the patient.
3. Discuss with the patient the importance of regular followup care.
4. Review with the patient information related to primary diagnosis, type of surgery, and expected outcomes.
5. Review with the patient written instructions for any at-home care: wound, T tube, gastrostomy tube, and so on.
6. Arrange for home health nurses for the patient if needed.
7. Provide the patient with unit phone number and the physician's phone number in case questions or problems should arise after the patient's discharge.

Evaluation

Comfort level is achieved Patient has reduction or absence of guarding or protective behavior. Patient uses pain control strategies appropriately. Patient verbalizes increased control over pain. Patient is able increasingly to perform activities of daily living.

Anxiety is reduced Patient gains understanding of anxious feelings and is able to verbalize fears and concerns to the staff or to significant others.

Nutrition is adequate Patient tolerates recommended diet by the time of discharge. Patient passes gas and stool by the time of discharge. Weight is stable.

Fluid status is normal Vital signs at baseline, adequate intake and output reflect adequate circulation and tissue perfusion.

Pulmonary status returns to baseline Refer to patient's baseline functioning on admission assessment.

Bowel is functioning normally Patient is experiencing minimal or no diarrhea or constipation. Patient's abdomen is not distended; patient is without nausea or vomiting.

Patient returns to activities of daily living Patient is able progressively to do the things he or she was doing before surgery.

Bladder is functioning normally   Patient is able to void spontaneously and is able to completely empty the bladder. Patient shows no signs of urinary tract infections.

Integument is intact or healing   Patient's incision is free of erythema, drainage, and the edges are well approximated. If patient's wounds are healing by secondary intention, they are granulating without necrotic tissue or excess drainage. Patient's pressure areas are intact or are healing.

DIVERSIONS: COLOSTOMY AND ILEOSTOMY

Description and Rationale

A colostomy is a diversion involving the colon in which a segment of diseased or injured colon is bypassed or removed and an end or loop of colon is brought through a small opening in the abdominal wall and matured, forming a stoma. The anatomic location in the colon is an important description and influences the care. Ascending, transverse, and sigmoid colstomies may be performed. Transverse colostomies are most often loop ostomy stomas and are temporary. A loop means that the intact bowel has been brought through the abodminal wall, a rod placed under the bowel, the incision closed, and a cautery used to open the top wall of the bowel (the lower wall remains intact). The proximal opening will drain the stool while the distal opening may drain mucus and leads to the rectum. The patient may have bowel movements from the rectum that consist of stool remaining in the bowel before surgery, or the patient may continue to pass mucus. The stool is semiformed, odorous, and unpredictable.

The sigmoid colostomy is the most common permanent stoma and is indicated for cancer of the rectum. The stool from the sigmoid colostomy is similar to normal bowel movements. Generally, stool is evacuated once or twice a day. A regular pattern before surgery is used to predict the possibility of regulation of the sigmoid colostomy with diet or with colostomy irrigations.

For patients with a sigmoid colostomy a device that plugs the stoma is available. The two-piece system (Conseal) consists of a skin barrier flange or plate (which resembles the faceplate on several two-piece pouching sytems) and a plug made of a soft, pliable material that fits into the stoma and then snaps to the flange. The system is indicated for people who have four or fewer bowel movements a day or who are irrigating the sigmoid colostomy.

The removal of the entire colon and rectum (total proctocolectomy) results in the ileum being brought through the abdominal wall, forming an ileostomy stoma. The stool from the ileostomy is liquid to semiformed and contains residual digestive enzymes. The drainage from the ascending colostomy is similar, and the nursing intreventions are the same for both. Fluid and electrolyte imbalance is a potential problem with an ileostomy and may result in significant problems.

Contraindications and Cautions

1. Only a sigmoid colostomy should be irrigated to obtain regular bowel eliminations. The decision to do so is left up to the patient.

2. An ileostomy lavage for a food blockage refers to the insertion of 30 to 50 ml of normal saline through a small catheter using an Asepto syringe. *This is not a colostomy irrigation and should not be performed by patients.*

3. Laxatives should *never* be given to a patient with an ileostomy. The result can be severe fluid and electrolyte imbalance.

Preprocedural Nursing Care

1. Consultation with an enterostomal therapy (ET) nurse is arranged.

2. A preoperative visit by a United Ostomy Association (UOA) trained visitor (rehabilitated person with an ostomy) is recommended.

3. Stoma site selection is marked by ET nurse for the surgeon.

NURSING CARE

Nursing Assessment

Perineum

Perineal incision: redness, tenderness, drainage

Stoma

Color (necrosis)
Perfusion (moisture and color)
Protrusion (flush, retracted, prolapsed)

Peristomal Skin

Erythema
Erosion
Rash
Parastomal hernia

Sexual Functioning

Wide resections in perineal area for cancer of rectum may damage nerves responsible for erection, ejaculation, and orgasm in men; no impairment or one or a combination of all functions may be affected
Physiologic effects on women have been poorly studied

Self-Concept and Body Image

Adjustment and integration of ostomy require time and support from family and health care providers
Complications: prolonged use of defense behaviors, noninvolvement in physical care, social isolation

Nursing Dx & Intervention

Body image and self-esteem disturbances related to external abdominal stoma

- Assess patient's verbal and nonverbal responses to the alterations in bowel function and the physical change (presence of stoma).

- Provide patient and family an opportunity to express their feelings regarding the ostomy preoperatively and postoperatively.
- Remind patient that an ostomy is an alternative pattern of elimination, that it will take time to adjust to, both physically and emotionally, and that people are available to help.
- Provide consistent management of the ostomy, control odor, and prevent leaking, giving patient a sense of control over the stoma.
- Select a system that is invisible under clothing, is odorproof, and fits the body size.
- Encourage patient to return to all presurgical activities as soon as possible.
- Recommend a trained ostomy visitor of same age and sex as patient and preferably one who has had same type of ostomy procedure.
- Allow patient to grieve for the loss of a body part and the loss of control of elimination.
- Be realistic and positive: negative reactions will be picked up by patient and will make adjustment harder; most people adapt successfully to ostomy surgery.

Altered sexuality patterns related to external abdominal stoma

- Allow patient and significant other to discuss concerns and fears regarding sexual activities. Many patients fear rejection by the spouse or by a significant other. Many spouses and significant others worry about hurting the patient.
- Suggest fabric pouch covers; other patients have recommended crotchless panties for women and binders for men to hold pouch in place.
- Remind patient that he or she must first be comfortable with self. Spouse or significant other is most often kind, gentle, and caring. Communication between partners is extremely important.
- Refer men who have had nerve damage and are unable to obtain an erection to a urologist for information on penile prosthesis or vacuum erection devices.
- Refer to family and sexual counselors as indicated by poor coping or maladaptation.

Risk for impaired skin integrity related to improper pouch fit, allergic reaction, fungal infection, or folliculitis

- Assess the skin integrity with each pouch change.
- Protect the peristomal skin with skin barriers: pectin-based wafers and paste, skin sealant wipes or sprays.
- Change pouching system whenever the pouch first begins to leak (an early sign is odor); *do not* tape a leaking pouch seal and plan on changing it later.

Impaired skin integrity related to improper pouch fit, allergic reaction, fungal infection, or folliculitis

- Treat erythematous, noneroded skin reactions that are secondary to ileostomy drainage, stool, glue, solvents, and soaps as follows:

Remove the source of the irritation (frequently it is a too-large pouch opening or a sensitivity to adhesive).

Cleanse the skin with warm water and pat dry or use a hair dryer set on cool.

Cover all irritated skin with skin barrier; the opening in the skin barrier must be cut to the exact size and shape of the stoma.

Select a different pouch or adhesive if the patient shows an allergic reaction to a particular pouch.

- Treat skin that is eroded or ulcerated as follows:

Use normal saline to cleanse the skin (less painful).

Dust the eroded area with stoma powder; dust off the excess powder. Dab skin sealant wipe over powder to set powder.

If eroded areas are caused by diarrhea washing away the barrier, use stoma paste around the stoma or on the cut opening in the skin barrier; advise the patient ahead of time that it may burn for a few minutes.

Change pouch every 24 to 48 hours until erosion or ulceration heals, then resume usual pouching schedule.

- Avoid mechanical injury to the skin by gentle removal of tape and skin barriers.
- Empty pouches rather than changing and discarding pouches that are full.
- Observe for monilial *(Candida albicans)* reactions associated with antibiotics and changes in normal bowel flora. Skin appears bright red with weepy papulae, satellite lesions, and secondary crusting. Patients may complain of intense itching.
- Assess other sites for monilial infection: under arms, under breasts, around groin, and in mouth.
- Consult physician for order of nystatin (Mycostatin) powder. Rub into the affected area and dust off the excess. Dab skin sealant wipe over powder to set powder. Ointments will keep pouch from sealing.
- Prevent radiation dermatitis by not having any portion of the pouch or pouch adhesive in the field of radiation. If pouch must be removed daily for treatments use a Karaya-only backed pouch that is belted in place.

Altered bowel elimination related to necessity for external pouch

- Assess output for color, consistency, frequency, and amount. Colostomy patients may experience constipation.
- Select a pouching system that contains the stool, is easy to empty, is odorproof, and is invisible under the patient's clothing.
- Clean the spout after each emptying to eliminate odor from a dirty spout.
- Avoid pinholes in pouches that lead to constant odor release; either empty pouch of gas or use commercial gas release valves added or made into the pouching system.

Risk for fluid volume deficit related to postoperative diarrhea

- Assess patient for dehydration that may develop with high-volume ileostomy output.

- Observe patient with ileostomy for diarrhea: high-volume, watery, pouch emptied every 20 to 30 minutes.
- Monitor intake and output, vital signs, daily weights, and electrolytes.
- Replace fluids and electrolytes orally or intravenously as ordered.

Risk for altered nutrition related to food blockage

- Assess patient for sign of food blockage (ileostomy): history of high roughage in diet and not chewing well; no output and abdominal distention; nausea and vomiting.
- Perform an ileostomy lavage:

  Remove pouch; stoma will become edematous.

  Apply irrigation sleeve.

  Have patient assume knee-chest position and massage abdomen under stoma; if blockage is removed, stop here and reapply pouching system; if not, continue.

  Insert catheter gently into stoma to level of blockage (usually at fascia level).

  Irrigate with 30 to 50 ml normal saline using Asepto syringe; allow to return.

  Repeat instillation of 30 to 50 ml of saline.

  Procedure may take 1 to 2 hours; may try knee-chest position between irrigations if patient is stable.

  Assess for dehydration; fluid becomes trapped behind food blockage, which acts as an intestinal obstruction.

  Provide intravenous fluids as ordered.

  NOTE: This procedure is *not* taught to patients. However, patient should be taught to recognize early signs and symptoms and seek medical assistance. Assist patient in returning to regular diet, avoiding only foods that give that person problems.
- Instruct patient to chew food carefully and eat slowly.

Patient Education/Home Care Planning

1. Colostomy and ileostomy care involves the following:
   a. Stomal and skin assessment: stoma should be red and moist; skin should be free of irritation.
   b. Management of frequently encountered skin problems.
      (1) Usual causes include fungal infections, pouch opening cut too large, or an allergic reaction to barriers, paste, or tape. See interventions under "Impaired Skin Integrity" for management.
      (2) Remind patient that weeping skin may prevent a pouch or a skin barrier from adhering to the skin for long periods. If skin is severely irritated and weeping, it may be necessary to change pouch more frequently to prevent leakage and further damage until skin heals.
      (3) Remind patient that the hair under the barrier should be removed by an electric razor or a safety razor.

   c. Principles of changing a pouching system should be accompanied by several opportunities for practicing the procedure.
      (1) Instruct patient to assemble all equipment: tissues, toilet paper, wash cloths, towels, cut-to-fit stoma pouch; paste (if stool is liquid); pouch closure; tape or belt; and equipment for cleansing or disposing of used pouches.
      (2) A paper towel or template may be used to trace a pattern, which should hug the stoma but not ride up on it, and top should be labeled. Outer dimensions of the pattern (avoiding hip bones, pubic areas, ribs and folds at waist and navel) should be considered.
      (3) Instruct the patient to trace pattern on the paper side of the pouch, to cut out the hole using the pattern, and to remove paper backing from the pouch.
      (4) Empty and remove the pouch being worn. Cleanse and dry the skin.
      (5) Patient should note any changes in skin or stoma (color, size, ulcerations, irritations), center and apply skin barrier and pouch, close end, and tape edges (if necessary).
      (6) Instruct patient to check supplies and reorder as necessary.
   d. Dietary considerations should be discussed with the patient. Use a nutritionist, if one is available.
      (1) Foods associated with odor are fish, eggs, asparagus, onions, garlic, and some spices.
      (2) Foods associated with diarrhea are green beans, broccoli, spinach, raw fruits, highly seasoned foods, and beer.
      (3) Foods used to manage diarrhea (low-residue diet) are strained bananas, peanut butter (without nuts), rice, and applesauce.
      (4) Foods used to manage constipation are high-fiber foods (bran, celery), increased raw fruits and vegetables, and increased fluid intake (water, fruit juices).
      (5) Foods associated with gas are brussels sprouts, cabbage, beans, peas, mushrooms, carbonated drinks, onions, cucumbers, and beer.
      (6) Patients are encouraged to eat all above foods in moderation, chewing well, and adding one new food at a time to evaluate tolerance.
   e. Provide patient with written instructions for follow-up, and initiate home care referral if indicated.
2. Ileostomy patient teaching should include the following:
   a. Instruct patient about symptoms of food blockage and what to do if it occurs.
      (1) Discharge changes from semisolid to a thin liquid; lumen is blocked by food, but water passes around it.

(2) Total volume of output increases and functions almost constantly; water is drawn from bloodstream in attempt to rid the bowel lumen of blockage and intestines become hyperactive.

(3) There is an objectionable odor; bacterial overgrowth occurs at the blockage and causes fermentation of foodstuff.

(4) Cramping occurs, usually followed by increase in watery output; this is caused by increased bowel activity to rid itself of blockage.

(5) Abdomen is distended; the blockage traps gas and liquids in the bowel lumen.

(6) Vomiting occurs; this is a further attempt of body to rid itself of blockage by traveling in direction of least resistance.

(7) There is no ileostomy output because of complete blockage.

(8) Instruct patient to get into a knee-chest position for a few minutes or take a hot shower to relax and then try the knee-chest position.

(9) Many blockages relieve themselves; however, if the blockage persists more than 3 to 4 hours, contact physician.

b. Foods associated with blockage include celery, Chinese foods, corn, nuts, coleslaw, dried fruits, coconut, wild rice, popcorn, whole vegetable skins, and fibrous vegetables. Do not eliminate from diet. Eat in moderate amounts and chew well.

Evaluation

Patient begins to incorporate ostomy into self-concept Patient verbalizes feelings related to the ostomy and the external pouching system. Patient can care for the colostomy or the ileostomy.

Patient resumes normal patterns of sexuality and sexual activity Patient's and significant others' questions and concerns regarding sexuality and sexual changes have been discussed.

COLOSTOMY IRRIGATION

1. Explain procedure to the patient.
2. *Collect equipment:*
   a. Irrigation sleeve (either 2 ¼ or 2 ¾, depending on the size of the flange on the patient)
   b. Irrigation kit with cone or enema bag with Laird tip (do not use catheter for irrigations)
   c. Water-soluble jelly
   d. Disposable face cloths and toilet paper
   e. Disposable gloves
   f. Patient handout on colostomy irrigations to help the patient follow along
3. With the patient sitting on a chair facing the toilet (see note), remove pouch (leave skin barrier), and attach irrigation sleeve. Sleeve end will be in the toilet. (Have the patient wear something warm so that he or she does not get chilled.)
4. Fill the irrigation bag with lukewarm tap water. The extra water in the bag can be used to rinse the sleeve out. The first irrigation should only have 250 to 300 ml; gradually increase the amount. Never use more than 1500 ml.
5. Clear the tubing of air.
6. Hang the bag so it is about 18 inches above the stoma.
7. To determine the direction of the colon, insert a lubricated gloved finger into the stoma about 1 to 2 inches. Insert the cone in the direction of the colon. This only needs to be done with the first irrigation.
8. Lubricate the end of the cone with lubricant, and gently insert the cone into the colostomy. Do not force it. Hold the cone firmly in position.
9. Allow a little water to run into the intestine by releasing the clamp. If water leaks around the stoma, insert the cone in further.

10. The water must go in slowly. It should take at least 3 to 5 minutes (time it) for the water to enter the intestine. If the patient experiences cramping while the water is running in, clamp the tube and have the patient take several deep breaths. When the cramping subsides, allow more water to run in. *Do not* remove the cone until the irrigation is finished.
11. When all the water has run in, hold the cone in place 1 to 2 minutes to allow the fluid to remain in the colon to achieve good results. Gently remove the cone.
12. Clip or secure the top of the irrigating sleeve shut. NOTE: Expect returns of the first irrigation to be stool-colored water. As the patients diet and the amount of water increases, the irrigation will be more successful: the patient will expel soft stools after irrigation.
13. Most of the water and stool will be eliminated in 5 to 10 minutes. After that time, lift the sleeve out of the toilet, rinse the sleeve clean, and clip the bottom of the sleeve to the top of the sleeve. Have the patient walk around, go back to bed, or sit in a chair, to stimulate a better return from the irrigation.
14. After 20 minutes in the bathroom, use the remaining water in the bag to flush the sleeve clean; remove the sleeve. Wipe the skin barrier clean and attach a clean pouch and clip.
15. Wash the irrigation sleeve and bag with warm water, and store it in the bathroom. NOTE: If the patient is not able to perform the procedure at the toilet because he or she has had an abdominal perineal resection, or because he or she is debilitated, the procedure can be performed in bed. Protect the bed with disposable pads, and place the sleeve off the side of the bed. Keep the sleeve clamped and empty to prevent odors from escaping.

Peristomal skin is intact Patient has no redness or eroded areas near the stoma or under the pouch.

Nutrition and hydration are adequate Patient understands dietary principles and need for increased oral fluids (ileostomy; colostomy patients with diarrhea).

DIVERSION: CONTINENT ILEOSTOMY

Description and Rationale

The continent ileostomy or Kock pouch was first described by Nils Kock in 1969.[43] Other surgeons have developed adaptations of Kock's procedure. The procedure involves the creation of an internal pouch constructed of ileum and of a nipple valve that maintains continency of stool and flatus. The patient has a stoma flush with the skin located in the lower right quadrant, which is intubated with a large-bore tube several times a day to evacuate the stool and flatus. Most patients who have this procedure have already had their rectums removed at a prior operation.

The continent ileostomy is an alternative for people who do not want to wear an external pouch. Some patients also believe a flush stoma rather than a protruding stoma is an advantage. Patients do not find the intubation or catheterization procedure bothersome once the pouch capacity increases.

The advantages of the continent ileostomy include the following:[48]

No appliance required

No noise or odor from stoma except during emptying

No skin irritation

Improved psychosocial adjustment

The continent ileostomy has a higher risk of complications than conventional ileostomies. Long-term problems are common and may be associated with loss of continency.

The disadvantages of the procedure are associated with the high percentage of nipple valve dysfunction and the reoperative rate. Even with the high rate of reoperation, many patients who have converted to a continent ileostomy state that it is a more satisfactory procedure.

The continent ileostomy is constructed from a long segment of terminal ileum after the colectomy has been performed. The section of ileum is brought through the abdominal incision, maintaining the blood supply to the loop of small bowel. The end is left free and will ultimately be used to form the nipple valve. First, the surgeon loops the proximal segment back on itself. Then the loop is sutured along its antimesenteric border where the two segments touch. A long U-shaped incision is made around the loop close to the suture line. The ileum then can be opened up into a cuplike shape. The small flaps of tissue on either side of the suture line are sutured together, forming a double suture line. The double suture line produces a smooth internal surface of the reservoir and provides a safeguard against intestinal leakage from the pouch. The nipple valve is then constructed by one of several techniques. The pouch is then sutured closed and assessed for adequacy of the valve and

the suture line by filling it with a saline solution and air. If no signs of leakage are noted from the valve or from the sutures, the pouch is inserted into the abdominal cavity and anchored. The end portion of the distal ileum is brought through the abdominal wall, and a flush stoma is constructed. A catheter is placed in the reservoir during surgery and remains in the pouch for 3 to 4 weeks.

Complications of continent ileostomies include the following:

Leakage of nipple valve

Valve prolapse

Skin stricture

Pouch perforation

"Pouchitis": local crampy pain, diarrhea that may be bloody, fever, valve leakage, intubation difficulty

Contraindications and Cautions

1. The diagnosis must be familial polyposis or ulcerative colitis. This procedure is *not* performed for Crohn's disease due to the risk of ulcerations in and subsequent failure of the pouch.
2. The patient needs medical alert cards because the continent ileostomy is an uncommon procedure.
3. Obesity is considered a contraindication.

Preprocedural Nursing Care

1. There should be a preoperative consultation with an enterostomal therapist (ET) nurse to answer the patient's questions about possible surgical options: conventional ileostomy, continent ileostomy, and ileoanal reservoir.
2. If possible, a rehabilitated patient with a continent ileostomy should visit preoperatively.

NURSING CARE

Nursing Assessment

Body Image

Presence of stoma and no external pouch more positive; if valve leaks, requires external pouch (p. 783)

Peristomal Skin

Erythema, erosions from leakage, or excess mucus secretion

Nursing Dx & Intervention

Body image disturbance related to presence of abdominal stoma

- Assess patient's response to presence of stoma and intubation.
- Allow patient opportunity to explore feelings regarding surgery.
- Provide trained visitor for patient.
- Assist patient in getting used to intubating abdominal stoma.

Risk for impaired skin integrity related to leakage or mucus on the peristomal skin

- Protect peristomal skin with skin sealant (Bard Protective Barrier, Hollister Gel) from moisture in mucus.
- Cover stoma with small pad.
- Protect skin from ileostomy drainage if nipple valve leaks (p. 784).

Patient Education/Home Care Planning

1. Intubation and irrigation of continent ileostomy involve the following procedures (procedures vary with surgeon). The goal is to gently increase the pouch capacity without straining new suture lines.
   a. First 3 weeks (catheter in place)
      (1) Irrigate the internal continent ileostomy pouch; insert 30 ml water and allow to drain out by gravity; irrigate every 3 hours during day and once at night.
      (2) Attach bedside bag or leg bag.
      (3) Clean bedside and leg bags with soapy water; allow to dry; have two and alternate.
      (4) Eat a low-residue diet.
   b. Week 4
      (1) Catheter is removed in outpatient clinic, and the patient is taught to intubate the continent ileostomy.
      (2) Intubate and irrigate every 3 hours during day.
      (3) Intubate with catheter to straight drainage at night; irrigate once at night.
   c. Week 5
      (1) Intubate every 3 hours, and irrigate twice a day.
      (2) Connect to gravity drainage at night; irrigate once at night.
   d. Week 6
      (1) Intubate every 4 hours and irrigate twice during day.
      (2) Intubate at night only if sign of fullness or uncomfortable.
   e. Week 7 and thereafter
      (1) Intubate pouch four times each day.
      (2) Irrigate pouch once each day until return is clear.
2. The following procedure is used for emptying and intubating the continent ileostomy:
   a. The patient sitting on the commode inserts a well-lubricated catheter into the stoma and through the nipple valve. Stool and flatus will drain through the catheter directly into the toilet. If the stool is thick, water can be inserted through the catheter to loosen the stool. The catheter may need to be removed and flushed if the lumen becomes blocked with undigested residue. Grape juice and prune juice are often used by patients to keep their stool "thin."

   b. Several types of catheters are available (Marlen, Atlantic). The patient should have at least two catheters and should know how to order additional ones. It is important to discard catheters when they become old. Hard, brittle catheters are more likely to damage the valve or the pouch.
3. The patient should be provided with written instructions on the signs and symptoms of "pouchitis" and procedures if he or she experiences difficulty intubating pouch or leakage of nipple valve develops.
4. The patient should be given instructions on low-residue diet and advancing to a regular diet.

Evaluation

Patient begins to incorporate change in body image into new self-image   Patient verbalizes positive feelings related to the ostomy and the necessity for intubation. Patient can care for the new continent ileostomy.

Peristomal skin is intact   Patient has no redness or eroded areas near the stoma.

DIVERSION: ILEOANAL RESERVOIR

Description and Rationale

The ileoanal reservoir is the procedure performed for patients with ulcerative colitis and familial polyposis that provides the most normal mechanism for maintaining continency and the most natural method of evacuation. Factors that are assessed when evaluating a patient for this procedure include normal anorectal sphincter mechanism, absence of perianal disease, good physical conditions, motivation, and age. It is important that the patient understand that it is a one-, two- or three-stage procedure and that close follow-up is important throughout. A temporary ileostomy requires that the patient learn stomal care. The patient must also be aware that diarrhea may be a problem for 6 months to 1 year after the closure of the ileostomy. During this time, incontinence may occur but is usually minimal and is more common at night.[39]

Four types of procedures may be done to preserve normal bowel elimination. Each involves removal of the rectal mucosa. The first step in constructing the ileoanal reservoir is the mucosal stripping of the rectal segment to form a muscular cuff through which to bring the ileum. The rectal mucosectomy removes the mucosa and submucosa of the rectum for 2 to 3 cm above the dentate line. The rectal muscle layers and the anal sphincters are left intact while the primary disease is removed. During the abdominal colectomy, the rectosigmoid is removed with care to preserve the autonomic nerves on the posterior and lateral pelvic walls.

When no reservoir is constructed, diarrhea and incontinence are major problems. In 1978, Parks and Nicholls[52] added an ileoanal reservoir to the previously described rectal mucosectomy and ileorectal pull-through. The reservoir provided an important addition, a means by which the liquid effluent could be held until evacuation was appropriate. Thus the patient undergoing total colectomy also has rectal mucosectomy, construction of an ileal reservoir, ileoanal anastomosis, and a temporary ileostomy during the first stage of the procedure. During the second stage, the ileostomy is closed. The ileoanal reservoir may be constructed in three configurations. It is constructed from 30 to 50 cm of terminal ileum. In the S reservoir, three loops of ileum, approximately 12 to 15 cm in length, are aligned side by side. The reservoir is constructed by suturing the limbs and opening the segments, creating a pouch. A remaining 5 cm of ileum forms a spout that is sutured to the dentate line, completing the ileoanal portion of the procedure.

The J reservoir consists of two loops of ileum. The ileum is brought down to the rectal cuff and one limb is looped upward, creating a J shape. The loops are anastomosed in a side-by-side fashion by use of a stapler. The portion where the ileum curves upward is sutured to the anus and opened.

In the isoperistaltic reservoir, a single lumen of 25 to 30 cm of ileum is brought down and through the rectal cuff. The distal end is sutured to the anus, and the proximal end is closed. An ileostomy is performed. In the second stage the ileostomy is taken down and a lateral side-to-side ileal anastomosis is performed to create the reservoir.

The operation is done occasionally in one stage, avoiding an ileostomy. The patient should be in excellent health, and no tension should be on the rectal reservoir anastomosis during the operation. The adjustment period after a one-stage procedure is often more difficult (more frequency and incontinence) because of the diarrhea seen immediately after colectomy.

If a patient is very ill and malnourished, he or she will initially have a colectomy with end ileostomy. The patient returns in approximately 6 months for the creation of the ileal reservoir; at that time the end ileostomy is converted to a loop ileostomy. The third operation, the ileostomy takedown, restores bowel continuity.

The diverting loop ileostomy protects the ileal reservoir during the healing period—usually 6 to 8 weeks. The management of these loop ileostomies can be challenging and may require a convex pouch.

Because it is the most common approach, the nursing care plan focuses on the patient undergoing this operation in two stages.

The advantages of the ileoanal reservoir include the following:
Avoidance of a permanent abdominal stoma
Avoidance of repeated stomal catheterizations
Avoidance of body image alterations
Decreased incidence of sexual dysfunction
Provision of a near-normal pattern of defecation

The disadvantages of the procedure are as follows:
Possible residual rectal mucosa
Problems with differentiation of gas, fluids, and solids

Tenesmus or fecal urgency
Nocturnal incontinence
Diarrhea
Perianal skin denudation

Complications of the ileoanal reservoir include:
Anal stenosis
Ischemia of reservoir
Rectal cuff abscess
Nocturnal leakage
Fecal incontinence
"Pouchitis" (sudden onset of high-volume diarrhea, cramping, and bleeding)

Contraindications and Cautions

1. Crohn's disease or cancer of the rectum
2. Obesity
3. Short mesentery
4. Decreased sphincter control

•••••• Multidisciplinary Plan

Medications

Bulk-forming agents
  Psyllium (Metamucil), 1 tsp prn for diarrhea
Antidiarrheal agents
  Loperamide (Imodium), up to 8 capsules po per day for diarrhea
Dermatologic agents
  Balneol cleansing agent; skin barrier ointments
Antifungal agents
  Clotrimazole (Mycelex cream) 1%, prn for pruritus

General Management

Sitz bath
Meticulous skin care after each stool

Nutritional consultation

To advise patients regarding dietary management of diarrhea

NURSING CARE

Nursing Assessment

Perineum

Skin erosions from mucus, frequent bowel movements, incontinence, pruritus, and perianal pain

Fluids and Electrolytes

Urine output is decreased
Output is greater than input
Sudden weight loss
Hypotension

Nursing Dx & Intervention

Stage 1: Ileostomy; Ileoanal Reservoir Constructed

Fluid volume deficit related to postoperative diarrhea

- Assess patient for signs and symptoms of dehydration: dry mucous membranes, poor skin turgor, dry skin, decreased urinary output, hypotension, tachycardia.
- Monitor fecal output from ileostomy; 800 to 1200 ml is not uncommon.
- Replace fluid and electrolytes as ordered.
- Monitor daily weights.

Impaired skin integrity related to incontinence of mucus

- Assess perianal skin daily.
- Provide perianal skin care because mucus contains residual enzymes, is copious, and is odorous.
- Use skin sealants and moisture barrier creams before skin breaks down.
- Instruct patient in wearing absorbent pads at night.
- Protect peristomal skin and maintain pouch seal.

Stage 2: Ileostomy Closure; Ileoanal Reservoir Functioning

Impaired skin integrity related to stool frequency or incontinence

- Assess perianal skin frequently.
- Avoid irritants such as nylon underwear, harsh or deodorant soaps, and fragrant toilet papers. Have patient flush perianal area after each stool, Do not have the patient wipe with toilet paper.
- Protect skin with barrier ointments containing petrolatum or zinc oxide because of frequency of bowel movements and the residual enzymes present in the stool.
- Provide Sitz baths, Balneol cleansing agents, or Tucks pads *to help with perianal cleansing and to reduce pruritus.*

Diarrhea; bowel incontinence related to postoperative reservoir adaptation

- Assess frequency of bowel movements and consistency of stools.
- Expect 10 to 20 bowel movements per day in early postoperative period; frequency slows to 6 to 12 per day as diet increases and averages 3 to 4 per day after 1 year.
- Instruct patient in high-fiber diet *to decrease number of stools.*
- Provide psyllium (Metamucil) or loperamide (Imodium), as ordered and as needed for diarrhea.
- Provide consultation with nutritionist regarding dietary management of diarrhea.

Patient Education/Home Care Planning

The following list applies to stage 1.
1. Teach patient ileostomy management (p. 787). Wearing time is decreased with loop ileostomies.
2. Perianal skin care is essential. Mucous drainage through the anus is expected and may be irritating. The skin can be protected by the use of skin barrier ointments. Mini-pads may be worn at night to absorb the drainage.
3. Approximately 6 to 8 weeks after surgery, a Gastrograffin x-ray film is taken to assess the reservoir, ruling out anastomotic leaks and checking the anatomic position of the reservoir. Gastrograffin is water soluble and easier to evacuate from the reservoir than barium would be.

The following list applies to stage 2.
1. For perianal skin care:
   a. Avoid nylon underwear, harsh or deodorant soaps, and fragrant toilet papers.
   b. Cleanse the perianal skin with water and dry with hair dryer.
   c. Protect the skin with barrier ointments.
   d. Manage pruritus with Sitz baths. Balneol cleansing agents, or Mycelex cream.
2. Frequency of bowel movements will drop to 6 to 12 per day for first year and then decrease to 3 or 4 per day. Diarrhea associated with flu or viral infection will increase number and amount of bowel movements.

Evaluation

Patient maintains adequate fluid and electrolyte balance   Patient has balanced intake and output. Patient's vital signs are normal.

Perianal skin is normal   Patient's perianal skin is intact with no signs of irritation or pruritus.

LIVER TRANSPLANTATION

Orthotopic liver transplantation (OLT) has been performed since the early 1960s. Improved survival rates in the last decade have made it a more common therapeutic option for patients with liver failure. One-year patient survival rates are now 75% or better in many programs; that figure is up from 30% before 1980.[70] These improved statistics are the result of better surgical techniques and immunosuppressive medications, including cyclosporine (CSA), improved preoperative and postoperative care, and careful patient selection.[70] The procedure involves the removal of the recipient's liver (hepatectomy) and the transplantation of a donor liver. There are many more potential recipients than donors, especially in children, 25% of whom die while awaiting a transplant.[1]

Despite widespread publicity and availability of information about organ donation, many potential donors are lost. The Omnibus Budget Reconciliation Act of 1986 states that hospitals participating in Medicare programs must establish protocols to identify potential donors. Families of potential donors must be assured information about the options for donation of organs and tissue, as well as the right to refuse consent. The law also encourages discretion and sensitivity concerning the circumstances, views, and beliefs of the donor family. This law encourages organ and tissue donation when appropriate criteria are met.

A national organ sharing system was instituted in 1987. The system offers available livers first locally, then regionally, and then nationally until a suitable recipient is found. Improved techniques for preserving the liver graft allow for a day of safe storage,[70] thereby increasing the opportunity for a good match and making a more equitable distribution of donor livers.

Indications for liver transplantation vary somewhat from center to center, but generally they include (1) ascites refractory to medical management; (2) encephalopathy that significantly impairs the patient's lifestyle; (3) variceal hemorrhage refractory to sclerotherapy; (4) hepatorenal syndrome; (5) refractory pruritus (including primary biliary cirrhosis and extrahepatic biliary atresia); (6) severe metabolic bone disease with fractures (primary biliary cirrhosis); (7) recurrent cholangitis (primary sclerosing cholangitis and extrahepatic biliary atresia); (8) neurotoxicity (Wilson's disease); (9) correction of metabolic disease related to the impaired synthesis of a specific liver protein (e.g., familial hypercholesterolemia, tyrosinemia); (10) failure to thrive; (11) coagulopathy unresponsive to vitamin K therapy; and (12) progressive hepatic insufficiency.[70]

Once it has been determined that a patient is a candidate for liver transplantation they are listed by their weight and blood type. Only in cases of absolute emergency are ABO-incompatible donors used because of a decreased survival rate. Orthotopic liver transplantation in pediatric patients has been limited because of the size match needed between donor and recipient. Some surgeons now reduce the size of the donor liver for pediatric patients.[70]

Complications of liver transplantation can be divided into surgical and nonsurgical. Surgical complications are most commonly biliary in origin (12% to 13%), including disruption of the anastomosis and strictures. Other surgical complications include hepatic artery thrombosis (3% to 10%) and portal vein thrombosis (1.8%)—the former being very serious in the postoperative period, often necessitating retransplant. Nonsurgical complications include renal dysfunction most often related to cyclosporine; infections, including bacterial, viral, and fungal (40% to 50%); and rejection of the donor liver (70% to 80%). Rejection is diagnosed by percutaneous liver biopsy (performed weekly after transplant). When two biopsies in a row are normal, the biopsies are done yearly.

Contraindications and Cautions

1. An extensive workup and evaluation by the transplant team is required before transplantation. The workup includes a complete history and physical examination of the patient to establish a primary diagnosis and prognosis; an evaluation of the patient's psyche, financial status, and family situation; a determination of portal vein patency with ultrasound; chest x-ray, electrocardiogram, pulmonary function tests, and computed tomography scans of the abdomen to detect malignancies. Blood tests include ABO typing, HIV, hepatitis B, VDRL, and cytomegalovirus serologic screening; liver function tests, electrolyte, blood urea nitrogen, and creatinine panels; ammonia level; cholesterol and triglyceride levels; alphafetoprotein levels, and urinalysis.

2. Percutaneous transhepatic cholangiography with brushings may be used to rule out cholangiocarcinoma in patients with sclerosing cholangitis.

3. Patients and families should be provided with ongoing support and evaluations as they make the decision to undergo this major procedure. An evaluation of the educational needs is also made to provide the patient and family with the information needed to manage these life changes. Most transplant teams have nurse coordinators and social workers who monitor patients and families during evaluation and transplantation, as well as postoperatively.

4. Absolute contraindications may include (depending on the center) active infection or sepsis, extrahepatic malignancy, advanced cardiopulmonary or cerebrovascular disease, positive HIV test, and active alcohol or drug abuse. Relative contraindications include renal failure, age older than 60, positive test for hepatitis B surface antigen (HBsAg), hepatobiliary malignancy, previous portocaval shunt surgery, and portal vein thrombosis.

Preprocedural Nursing Care

1. Liver transplant patients usually are extremely ill and require expert nursing care to manage the primary diagnosis and any existing complications.

2. Inform the patient and family about the specific procedure and the rationale for the diagnostic procedure.

3. Inform the patient and family about general postoperative course and any drains and tubes that will be present after surgery. Encourage attendance at a transplant support group, if one is available.

•••••• Multidisciplinary Plan

Medications

Dosages and type vary by physician and center protocol
No one protocol or dosages will be referred to
Antibiotics
    Amipicillin or cephalosporin
    Trimethoprim or sulfamethoxazole (Bactrim), prophylaxis
        against *pneumocystis carnii* pneumonia
    Pentamidine puff, if allergic to Septra
Antivirals
    Acyclovir, prevent HSV infections
    Ganciclovir (DHPG), treat CMV infections for 5-7 d

Antifungals

Mycelex troche/Nystatin, or oral fluconazole prevent *Candida* infections

Immunosuppression

Maintenance to prevent rejection; dose based on blood level and renal function; cyclosporine A (CSA), may be given IV initially, then po; excreted in the bile; if patient has a T tube, it will need to be refed by a feeding tube or drunk po; azathioprine (Imuran); prednisolone or prednisone, often given IV, then po

Acute rejection (often based on biopsy)

Initial therapy: Corticosteroids given in large initial doses and gradually tapered; may be repeated if no improvement

Subsequent therapy

Polyclonal preparations (e.g., Minnesota antilymphocyte globulin [MALG]), for 5-14 d IV; antithymocyte globulin (ATG) for 14 d IV

Orthoclonal preparations (e.g., Orthoclonal OKT₃), for 5-14 d IV

Patients with chronic or irreversible rejection may be candidates for retransplantation

General Management

Mechanical ventilation for 24 to 48 hours, then oxygen by mask or nasal prongs

If patient has been encephalopathic preoperatively, intracranial pressure monitoring may be done until patient is awake

T tube

Jackson-Pratt drains

Intravenous fluids

Nasogastric drainage

Nasal feeding tube for bile after nasogastric tube discontinued

NURSING CARE

Nursing Assessment

Abdominal Examination

Assess surgical incision for drainage (note character, color, amount); monitor for signs and symptoms of infection

Abdominal girth measurements to monitor postoperative complications

Cardiovascular

Shock and circulatory failure associated with hemorrhage, sepsis, and fluid and electrolyte imbalance

Infection

Assess carefully for early signs of infection: fever, herpesvirus infections (oral, esophageal, or gastric), *Candida* or CMV, pulmonary infiltrate *(Pneumocystis)*, wound or urinary tract systems

Rejection

Malaise, fever, graft tenderness, diminished graft function as evidenced by decreased bile output

Increased bilirubin and transaminase levels

Monitor to evaluate liver function and evidence of increased cerebral pressure because intracranial bleeding is a major complication. Cyclosporine may also affect mental status. Notify physician of any of the following: Decreased intellectual function; altered state of consciousness; mild to moderate EEG abnormalities; altered behavior; asterixis; agitation; drowsiness; confusion

Coping and Anxiety

Assess emotional reaction to surgery and consequences

Assess level of support and coping mechanisms

Assess health information needs

Nursing Dx & Intervention

Altered renal, cerebral, cardiopulmonary, gastrointestinal, and peripheral tissue perfusion related to major surgical procedure with multiple anastomoses in compromised patient

- Monitor vital signs every 15 minutes until patient is stable and then every hour. Monitor intake and output every hour (include all drainage tubes: nasogastric, Jackson-Pratt [J-P], Foley, T tube).

- Monitor and document any incisional drainage.

- Monitor hourly central venous pressure, pulmonary artery pressure, pulmonary capillary wedge pressure, and right arterial pressure *because hemodynamic instability is a potential problem in the early postoperative period.* Intraoperative blood loss may be extensive.

- Observe carefully for signs of transfusion reactions because patients may receive multiple units of blood during and after surgery. Fresh frozen plasma may also be ordered.

- Assess for signs of shock: hypotension, tachycardia, peripheral vasoconstriction, oliguria.

- Weigh patient daily.

- Monitor serum electrolytes, CBC, prothrombin time, partial thromboplastin time, platelets, BUN, creatinine, bilirubin (total/direct) SGOT, SGPT, alkaline phosphatase, albumin, and CSA level.

- Assess patient in early postoperative period for signs of hyperkalemia (T-wave elevation and widening of QRS complex on ECG) and hypokalemia (U-wave on ECG, ectopic beats, leg cramps).

- Assess for signs of glucose shifts *resulting from the inability of the transplanted liver to control glucose metabolism in the early postoperative period and from steroid-induced diabetes and symptoms of hyperglycemia:* lethargy, decreased response to stimuli; hypoglycemia; glycosuria, osmotic diuresis, changes in mental status.

- Test urine for glucose and ketones.

- Monitor closely the urine output, serum creatinine level, and urine electrolyte levels *because a change in renal function is an early sign of nephrotoxicity associated with cyclosporine use.*

Risk for infection related to immunosuppressive medications

- Institute protective isolation *because patient is immunosuppressed and will be unable to combat infections.* Neutrophils are less than 500/mm^3.
- Provide meticulous care of the mouth, skin, and perineal area *to prevent breakdown.*
- Clean sites thoroughly with povidone-iodine when entering lines, especially central lines, *to prevent introduction of bacteria.*
- Monitor body temperature. Do not take rectal temperatures *because the mucous membranes are more fragile and can be irritated, leading to an infection* (although rectal probes may be used in some intensive care units).
- Routine cultures of body fluids may be ordered, including all drains, tubes, open wounds, and indwelling lines. Frequently the organisms cultured include cytomegalovirus, *Candida, Legionella,* or *Pneumocystis,* although any other viral or bacterial organism may be cultured.
- Additional diagnostic tests for signs of infection include lumbar puncture, transhepatic cholangiogram or ERCP, hepatitis screen, ultrasonography, CT scan, and an indium scan, with tagged white cells most commonly used.
- Observe wounds and tube sites for erythema, purulent drainage, and odor.
- Observe drains and tubes for increased or decreased drainage, changes in the type or color of drainage, and presence of odor.

Risk for rejection of donor organ related to patients' functioning immune system

- Assess for signs of rejection: malaise, fever, graft tenderness, and diminished graft function (increased transaminases, increased bilirubin, elevated clotting times, decreased platelet counts, and jaundice).
- Assess for signs of cyclosporine side effects: hypertension, hyperkalemia, decreased renal function, and gingival hyperplasia.
- Assess for signs of cyclosporine toxicity: tremulousness and nephrotoxicity.
- Monitor serum cyclosporine level every day to maintain a level of 250 to 350 mg/dl.
- Assess patient for signs and symptoms of side effects of OKT-3 or other drugs used to treat rejection (MALG, ATG, prednisone): chills, fever, development of ARDS and anaphylaxis, rigors, hypotension, chest pain, nausea, vomiting, diarrhea, pulmonary edema (if patient is fluid overloaded, no OKT-3 should be administered), joint pains, shortness of breath, and hypotension. If acute respiratory symptoms occur, discontinuation of the drug is necessary.
- Patient is maintained on a low dose of immunosuppressive drugs.

Risk for ineffective individual and family coping related to near-death experience before transplant, prolonged recuperation, mental status changes, medication regimen, rejection, or infection episodes

- Provide continuity of nursing care as able.
- Allow time for patient and family to verbalize fears and concerns.
- Refer patient to a psychiatrist or social worker for further support.
- If support group is available, encourage patient and family to participate.
- Encourage other transplant patients and their families to network and provide mutual informal support.
- Encourage the family to take breaks from the hospital.

Risk for mental status changes related to medications, intracranial hemorrhage, and encephalopathy

- Monitor small changes in mental status closely. Inform the transplant team.
- If cause is known, reassure the family about duration of changes and help them cope with changes.
- Minimize the number of people in the room at any one time if the patient is confused or combative.
- Reorient the patient frequently.
- Continue to explain and reassure the patient even though it may appear that he or she does not follow.

Patient Education/Home Care Planning

Patient education can be done effectively on a day-to-day or a group basis.

1. Instruct the patient on routine care after any major surgery; ambulate at regular times; rest frequently; increase activities slowly; keep incision dry; report any signs of redness, pain, or drainage; avoid heavy lifting; keep appointments for follow-up visits.
2. Provide written instructions on medication schedule and side effects.
3. Provide written instructions on signs and symptoms that should be reported to the physician.
4. Provide written instructions on any procedures for at-home care. Make sure that the patient has had an opportunity to practice the procedures before discharge.
5. Provide written instructions on the need for follow-up laboratory work and communication of laboratory values to the transplant program.

Evaluation

Tissue perfusion is within normal limits   Patient's blood pressure and pulse are normal. Laboratory values are within normal limits.

All efforts to prevent infection are taken   Cultures are negative.

Orthotopic liver transplantation is successful   There are no signs or symptoms of rejection of the transplanted organ.

Support is given to the patient and family through the patient's periods of infection, rejection, or changes in mental status   Patient and family coping mechanisms are intact.

Mental status changes are within normal limits for the patient   Patient is alert and oriented with appropriate responses and mood.

References

1. Alexander JW, Vaughn WK: The use of "marginal" donors for organ transplantation, *Transplantation* 51:135, 1991.
2. Aliberti LC: Managing esophageal achalasia: medical and nursing implications, *Gastroenterol Nurs* 16(3):126, 1993.
3. Barkin GJS, Rogers AL: *Difficult decisions in digestive diseases,* St Louis, 1994, Mosby.
4. Benacci JC et al: Epiphrenic diverticulum: results of surgical treatment, *Ann Thorac Surg* 55(5):1109, 1993.
5. Biel MA: Photodynamic therapy and the treatment of neoplastic diseases of the larynx, *Laryngoscope* 104(4):399, 1994.
6. Bolt RJ et al: *The digestive system,* New York, 1983, Wiley.
7. Bower TC: Ischemic colitis, *Surg Clin North Am* 73(5):1037, 1993.
8. Bowers AC, Thompson JM: *Clinical manual of health assessment,* ed 4, St Louis, 1992, Mosby.
9. Brastius TA, Sitrin MD: Intestinal malabsorption syndromes, *Annu Rev Med* 41:339, 1990.
10. Broadwell DC, Jackson BS: *Principles of ostomy care,* St Louis, 1982, Mosby.
11. Carpenito LJ: *Nursing care plan and documentation,* New York, 1990. Lippincott.
12. Coremans G et al: Diagnostic procedures in irritable bowel syndrome, *Digestion* 56(1):76, 1995.
13. Crissman JD, Visscher DW, Sakr W: Premalignant lesions of the upper aerodigestive tract: pathologic classification, *J Cell Biochem (Suppl)* 17F:49, 1993.
14. Department of Health and Human Services, *Organ transplantation, issues and recommendations,* Report of the Task Force on Organ Transplantation, United States, Washington, DC, 1986, US Government Printing Office.
15. Dixon MF. *Helicobacter pylori* and peptic ulceration: histological aspects, *J Gastroenterol Hepatol* 6:125, 1991.
16. Doherty MM, Carver DK: Transjugular intrahepatic portosystemic shunt: new relief for esophageal varices, *Am J Nurs* 93(4):58, 1993.
17. Doughty DB: *Gastrointestinal disorders,* St Louis, 1993, Mosby.
18. Dudrick SJ, Latifi R, Fosnoht DE: Management of the short bowel syndrome, *Surg Clin North Am* 71(3):625, 1991.
19. Everhart JE, Renault PF: Irritable bowel syndrome in office-based practice in the United States, *Gastroenterology* 100:998, 1991.
20. Everhart JE. Summary. In Everhart JE: *Digestive diseases in the United States: epidemiology and impact,* DHHS, PHS, NIH No 94-1447, Washington, DC, 1994, US Government Printing Office.
21. Fagniez PL, Rotman N, Pezet D: Severe acute pancreatitis: new insights in diagnosis and management, *Dig Dis* 9:165, 1991.
22. Falk GW: Current status of *Helicobacter pylori* in peptic ulcer disease, *Cleveland Clin J Med* 62(2):95, 1995.
23. Farmer RG, Achkar E, Fleshler B: *Clinical gastroenterology,* New York, 1992, Raven.
24. Fazio VW: Conservative surgery for Crohn's disease of the small bowel: the role of strictureplasty, *Med Clin North Am* 74(1):169, 1990.

25. Ferguson MK: Achalasia: current evaluation and therapy, *Ann Thorac Surg* 52:336, 1991.
26. Gitnick G: *Current gastroenterology,* vol II, St Louis, 1991, Mosby.
27. Goldenberg SP, Vos C, Burrell M, Traube M: Achalasia and hiatal hernia, *Dig Dis Sci* 37(4):528, 1992.
28. Goldstein JL, Watkins JL, Greager JA, Layden TJ: The esophageal mucosal resistance: structure and function of a unique gastrointestinal epithelial barrier, *J Lab Clin Med,* 123(5):653, 1994.
29. Greenberger NJ: *Gastrointestinal disorders,* St Louis, 1989, Mosby.
30. Guyton AC: *Textbook of medical physiology,* ed 8, Philadelphia, 1991, Saunders.
31. Guyton AC: *Human physiology and mechanisms of disease,* ed 5, Philadelphia, 1992, Saunders.
32. Hawkey CJ: Future treatments for arthritis: new NSAIDS, NO NSAIDS, or no NSAIDS?, *Gastroenterology* 109(2):614, 1995.
33. Hosoda S et al: Age-related changes in the gastrointestinal tract, *Nutr Rev* 50(12):374, 1992.
34. Jarvinen H, Franssila KO: Familial juvenile polyposis coli: increased risk of colorectal cancer, *Gut* 25:792, 1984.
35. Jeffcoat MK: Prevention of periodontal diseases in adults: strategies for the future, *Prev Med* 23(5):704, 1994.
36. Jewell DP, Snook JA: *Topics in gastroenterology 17,* Oxford, 1990, Blackwell Scientific.
37. Johnson LR, editor: *Gastrointestinal physiology,* ed 4, St Louis, 1991, Mosby.
38. Kahan BD, Ghobrial R: Immunosuppressive agents, *Surg Clin North Am* 74(5):1029, 1994.
39. Kelly KA, Pemberton JH, Wolff BG, Dozois RR: Ileal pouch-anal operation, *Curr Prob Surg* 29:64, 1992.
40. Kerber K: The adult with bleeding esophageal varices, *Crit Care Nurs Clin North Am* 5(1):153, 1993.
41. Kinney MD et al: *AACN's clinical reference for critical care nursing,* ed 2, New York, 1988, McGraw-Hill.
42. Knauer CM, Silverman S: *Current medical diagnosis and treatment,* Norwalk, Conn, 1993, Appleton & Lange.
43. Kock NG, Myrvold HE, Nilsson LO: Progress report on the continent ileostomy, *World J Surg* 4:143, 1980.
44. Kolokotronis A et al: Median rhomboid glossitis, *Oral Surg Oral Med Oral Pathol* 78(1):36, 1994.
45. Marotta RB, Floch MH: Diet and nutrition in ulcer disease, *Med Clin North Am* 75(4):967, 1991.
46. McMaster P: What's new in hepatobiliary surgery, *J R Coll Surg Edin* 36:1, 1991.
47. Mertz HR, Walsh JH: Peptic ulcer pathophysiology, *Med Clin North Am* 75(4):799, 1991.
48. Mullen P et al: Barnett continent intestinal reservoir: multicenter experience with an alternative to the Brooke ileostomy, *Dis Colon Rectum* 38:573, 1995.
49. Murphy D: Celiac sprue, *Gastroenterol Nurs* 18(4):133, 1995.
50. National Institute of Arthritis, Diabetes, and Digestive and Kidney Diseases (NIADDK): *Second annual report,* DHHS, PHS, NIH Pub N 83-2493, Washington, DC, 1988, US Government Printing Office.
51. Ormand JE, Talley NJ: *Helicobacter pylori:* controversies and an approach to management, *Mayo Clin Proc* 65:414, 1991.
52. Parks AG, Nicholls RJ: Proctocolectomy without ileostomy for ulcerative colitis, *BMJ* 2:85, 1978.
53. Pena AS et al: Genetic bases of gluten-sensitive enteropathy, *Gastroenterology* 75:230, 1978.
54. Pou AM, Johnson JT, Weissman J: Management decisions in parotitis, *Comprehensive Therapy* 21(2):85, 1995.
55. Rankin GB: Extraintestinal and systemic manifestations of inflammatory bowel disease, *Med Clin North Am* 74(1):39, 1990.
56. Ruderman WB: Newer pharmacologic agents for the therapy of inflammatory bowel disease, *Med Clin North Am* 74(1):133, 1990.
57. Schemelzeisen R et al: Sonography and scintigraphy in the diagnosis of diseases of the major salivary glands, *J Oral Maxillofac Surg* 49(8):798, 1991.
58. Schiff L, Schiff ER: *Diseases of the liver,* ed 7, Philadelphia, 1994, Lippincott.
59. Scholz FJ: Ischemic bowel disease, *Radiol Clin North Am* 31(6):1197, 1993.

60. Shanbour LL, Jacobson ED: Digitalis and the mesenteric circulation, *Am J Dig Dis* 17:826, 1972.
61. Sleisenger MH, Fordtran JS: *Gastrointestinal disease,* ed 5, Philadelphia, 1993, Saunders.
62. Sonis ST, Fazio RC, Fang L: *Principles and practice of oral medicine,* ed 2, Philadelphia, 1995, Saunders.
63. Spiro HM: *Clinical gastroenterology,* ed 4, New York, 1993, McGraw-Hill.
64. Starzl T et al: Homotransplantation of the liver in humans, *Surg Gynecol Obstet* 117:659, 1963.
65. Thompson WHF: The nature of hemorrhoids, *Br J Surg* 62:542, 1975.
66. Tolliver BA, Herrera JL, DiPalma JA: Evaluation of patients who meet clinical criteria for Irritable Bowel Syndrome, *Am J Gastroenterol* 89(2):176, 1994.
67. Way LW: *Current surgical diagnosis and treatment,* Norwalk, Conn, 1994, Appleton & Lange.
68. Whelan G: Epidemiology of inflammatory bowel disease, *Med Clin North Am* 74(1):1, 1990.
69. Wilson C, Imrie CW: Current concepts in the management of pancreatitis, *Drugs* 41(3):358, 1991.
70. Wood RP et al: Liver transplantation: the last ten years, *Surg Clin North Am* 74(5):1133, 1994.
71. Yamada T et al: *Textbook of gastroenterology,* ed 2, Philadelphia, 1995, Lippincott.
72. Zemel G et al: Percutaneous transjugular portosystemic shunt, *JAMA* 266(3):390, 1991.

Endocrine and Metabolic Systems

9

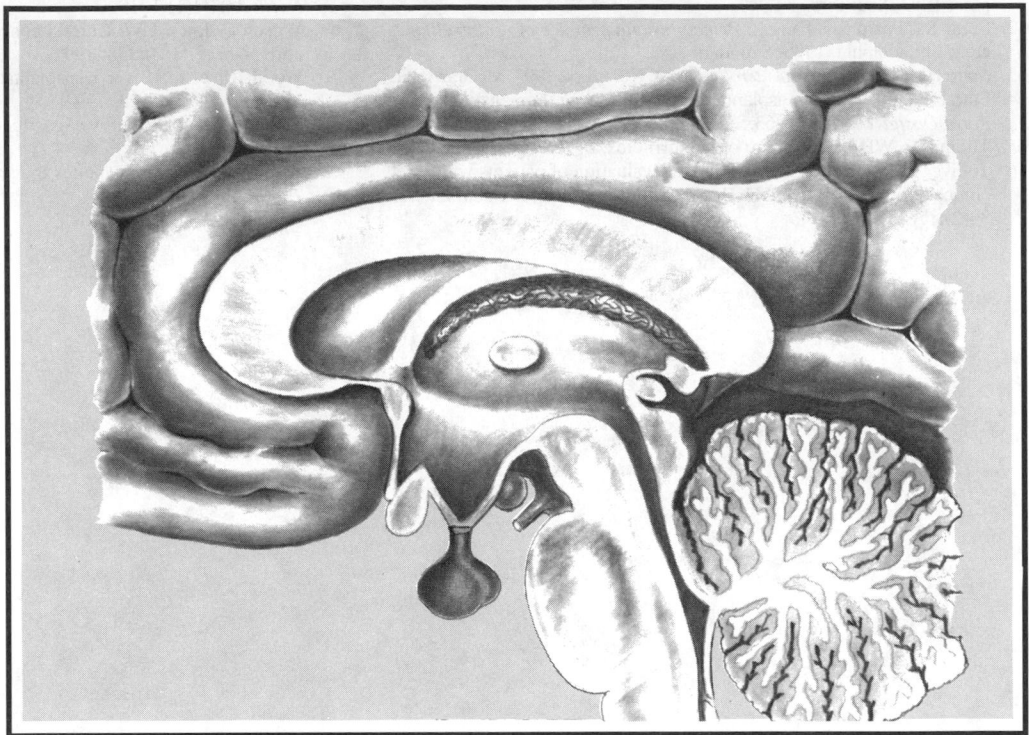

OVERVIEW

The endocrine–metabolic system is a widely diversified system of glands, hormones, intermediate metabolites, receptors, and ultimately cellular responses. The term endocrine refers to the secretion of biologically active substances secreted directly into the body. The substances being *released* are termed hormones which is derived from the Greek and means to "set in motion."[3] Usually, before hormones can exert an effect, they must attach to receptors. The hormones become keys opening the receptor doors for subsequent cellular and system responses. Metabolism, on the other hand, involves the biochemical control mechanisms such as gene expression or the modification, transformation, and degradation of biologic substances.

Although endocrine is thought of as a separate system, there is extensive overlap between the endocrine and every other body system. The most extensive of these overlaps occurs with the nervous system and has led to the new specialty of neuroendocrinology. The hypothalamus of the brain is a major source of hormones and a substance such as norepinephrine may be either a neurotransmitter or a hormone that acts through nervous system receptors. Other examples include atrial natriuretic factor from the atrium of the heart, insulin-like growth factors and somatomedin from the liver, and angiotensinogen, erythropoietin, and cholecalciferol (the active form of vitamin D_3) from the kidney.

Clinical problems in endocrinology were traditionally limited to whether there was an over- or under-production of a hormone from a particular gland. Today, clinical problems also encompass transport of hormone, hormone clearance, regulatory mechanisms to maintain hormone levels, ability of hormones to become unbound from carrier proteins and attach to receptors, and subsequent cellular responsiveness to the hormone. In addition, there is now the clinical distinction between adequate hormone production in a basal state and that amount of hormone required to meet physiologic needs is a stimulated, stressed, or maximal state.

Symptoms of endocrine problems are also as diverse as all tissues and organs in the body. They may vary from a general non-specific symptom like fatigue to a specific symptom like heat intolerance. Some symptoms such as atrial flutter/fibrillation may not be attributed to an endocrine problem until laboratory testing has been done, but it may be the only presenting symptom of thyrotoxicosis, particularly in the elderly.

Although the nursing care presented in this chapter addresses the patient with a newly diagnosed endocrine problem in the hospitalized setting, in today's managed care environment, initial diagnosis and management would most likely be conducted in the ambulatory arena. Patients might have very few symptoms or because of the interrelationship between hormones and behavior, they may have difficulty in performing their usual social roles as evidenced by mood swings, altered cognition, and altered family dynamics. The nursing care ideas presented in this chapter will need minor modifications, but can be equally applicable for ambulatory care. When a patient is hospitalized, it may be for surgical intervention or for an unrelated problem. In both cases, the goal of nursing care would be maintenance of hormone-related therapies. The information in this chapter can be used to prevent a patient from getting out of endocrine physiologic balance.

•••••• Anatomy, Physiology, and Related Pathophysiology

Hypothalamus and Pituitary Gland

The hypothalamus is located at the ventral portion of the diencephalon, beneath the thalamus and subthalamus. There are neural connections between the hypothalamus and the limbic system and thalamus above, and it is connected to the pituitary gland below by the pituitary stalk (Figure 9-1). Although most of the cells of the hypothalamus are involved in the functions of memory, temperature regulation, sleep, regulation of food intake, sexual behavior, cardiovascular function, and emotions, it secretes a number of hormones that directly stimulate or inhibit the release of hormones from the anterior pituitary gland.[65]

The hypothalamic stimulating hormones are corticotropin releasing hormone (CRH), growth hormone releasing hormone (GRH), thyrotropin releasing hormone (TRH), and gonadotropin releasing hormone (GnRH). The hypothalamic inhibiting hormones are melanocyte inhibiting factor (MIF), prolactin releasing inhibiting factor (dopamine), and growth hormone inhibiting hormone (somatostatin). These hormones travel down the pituitary stalk through a portal blood supply to the anterior pituitary gland.[19]

The pituitary gland rests in the sella turcica. Inferiorly, it is bounded by the sphenoid sinus and superiorly it is separated from the cranial cavity by the diaphragma sellae. The adenohypophysis (anterior pituitary) has no direct nerve supply with regulation being completely neurohumoral from the hypothalamus. The posterior lobe (neurohypophysis) is innervated through the hypophyseal stalk by the supraopticohypophyseal tract with hormone release by the magnocellular neurone of the supraoptic and paraventricular nuclei of the hypothalamus.[19]

The anterior pituitary releases luteinizing hormone (LH), follicle stimulating hormone (FSH), growth hormone (GH), prolactin (PRL), adrenocorticotropic hormone (ACTH), thyroid stimulating hormone (TSH), and melanocyte stimulating hormone (MSH). These hormones travel through the blood supply and cause subsequent release of hormones from specific glands called target organs (ACTH to the adrenal gland) as well as extraglandular cell-specific responses.

Hormones are released in a variety of temporal oscillations ranging from a few minutes to much longer. The most common pulsatile pattern is a circadian rhythm (also called a diurnal variation) that occurs within 24 hours and is linked to light-dark cycles. ACTH, TSH, PRL, and GH all increase during darkness. These variations provide an adaptive response to fluctuations in the environment and are associated with the rotation of the earth on its axis. FSH and LH are on an infradian rhythm with pulsatile changes occurring over more than 24 hours.

Pathology may occur when either the pulse amplitude or pulse frequency of a hormone is enhanced or restricted.

One of the major functions of the endocrine system is to help maintain body homeostasis in an ever-changing internal and external environment. This is done through a series of negative feedback loops. A negative feedback loop functions in a similar manner to the thermostat in a home, sending signals to the furnace about the temperature in a room or home. The feedback system between the hypothalamus and anterior pituitary gland is known as a short loop negative feedback mechanism. High levels of pituitary hormones cause the hypothalamus to decrease the release of its hormones, which in turn causes levels of the pituitary hormones to decrease. The target organs also communicate by a long loop negative feedback mechanism to regulate hormone release from the pituitary gland and the hypothalamus (Figure 9-2). The first step in the feedback mechanism is the amount of target organ hormone the body has circulating and functioning at the cellular level on a minute by minute basis. If there is not enough hormone, a message is carried by the bloodstream back to the pituitary gland and then to the hypothalamus that more hormone is required. In some instances such as thyroid hormone, the message may go to the hypothalamus directly in addition to the message being carried through the pituitary to the hypothalamus. Pathology may occur when there are problems with the body's ability to carry the hormone message in the proper sequence. In some instances,

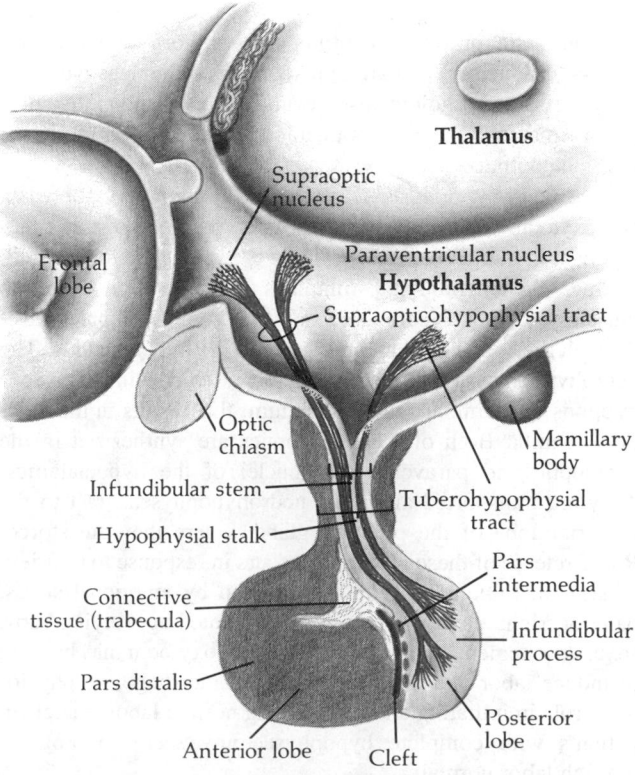

Figure 9-1 Anatomy of the hypothalamus and pituitary.

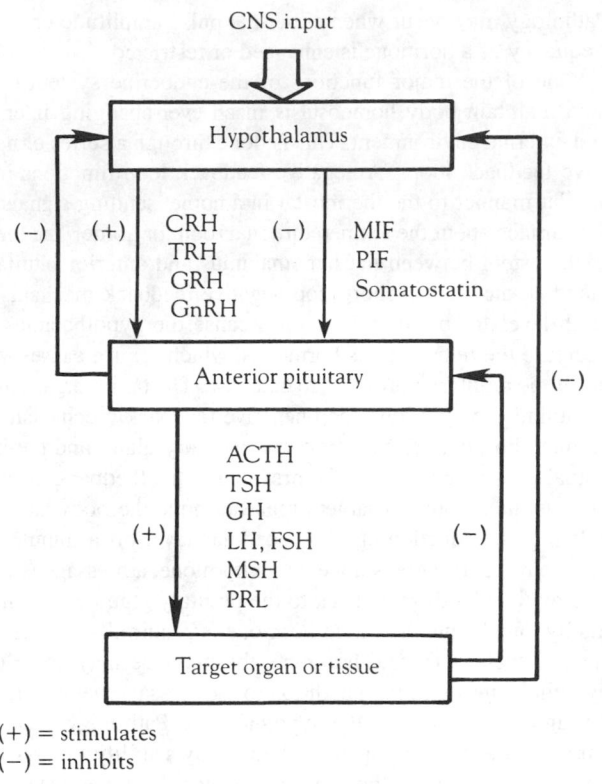

CNS input

Hypothalamus

(−)   (+)   CRH   (−)   MIF
TRH   PIF
GRH   Somatostatin
GnRH

Anterior pituitary   (−)

ACTH
TSH
GH
(+)   LH, FSH   (−)
MSH
PRL

Target organ or tissue

(+) = stimulates
(−) = inhibits

Figure 9-2 Negative-feedback mechanism.

hormones are produced continuously (tumors or extra loop stimulating factors) and are unresponsive to the negative feedback message. Pathology also occurs when a gland in the stimulatory message pathway is unable to respond with increased hormone output.

The neurohypophysis secretes two hormones: vasopressin and oxytocin. Vasopressin is the primary regulator of water metabolism in human beings. Oxytocin is responsible for the milk letdown phenomenon and stimulates the contraction of uterine muscles in labor. Neurogenic reflexes from the nipple travel through the spinal cord and midbrain to the hypothalamus. The neurohypophysis then releases oxytocin, which stimulates contractions of mammary myoepithelium; this results in the ejection of milk. Both of these hormones are synthesized in the supraoptic and paraventricular nuclei of the hypothalamus. They are transported along the neurohypophyseal tract to the posterior lobe of the pituitary gland, where they are stored. Rapid release of these hormones occurs in response to a variety of stimuli.[73] Oxytocin may be inhibited by emotional stress, pain, or fright. Oxytocin release is stimulated by a crying baby, sexual excitement, and orgasm. Although oxytocin may be used to induce labor and control obstetric hemorrhage, its physiologic role in initiating and maintaining normal labor is unclear. Patients with complete hypophysectomy seem to progress through labor normally.[73]

Vasopressin conserves water in the renal collecting duct; thus it is also known as the antidiuretic hormone (ADH). ADH causes an increase in the permeability of the renal collecting ducts to water, thereby increasing water retention and decreasing urine output. The production of ADH in the hypothalamus and the release of ADH from the posterior pituitary gland are determined by plasma osmolality and extracellular fluid volume. The secretion of ADH is regulated by three factors:

Osmoreceptors in the median eminence of the hypothalamus respond to changes in plasma osmolality. Increases in osmolality stimulate the release of ADH; decreases in osmolality inhibit ADH release. The osmotic threshold for ADH release is 284 mOsm/kg.

Volume receptors in the left atrium and great vessels inhibit ADH release when vascular volume is increased.

Baroreceptors in the carotid sinus and aortic arch stimulate ADH release when blood pressure is decreased.[4]

ADH secretion is stimulated by such factors as hemorrhage, a reduction in cardiac output, dehydration, and hypoalbuminemic states. The limbic system also plays a role in the stimulation of ADH during stress, trauma, heat, fear, and pain. Certain drugs also promote ADH secretion, such as morphine, nicotine, barbiturates, β-adrenergic agents, general anesthetics, vincristine, cyclophosphamide (Cytoxan), carbamazepine, and chlorpropamide. Inhibition of ADH occurs during states of hypervolemia and hypo-osmolality. Total body immersion in water and a sensation of cold also inhibit ADH secretion. Pharmacologic agents inhibiting ADH include morphine antagonists, α-adrenergic agents, and ethyl alcohol.[4]

Free water loss leads to concentration of the blood, and plasma osmolality rises. When plasma osmolality reaches about 288 mOsm/kg, two things occur. First, the osmoreceptors in the hypothalamus are stimulated and promote synthesis of ADH in the hypothalamic nuclei and release of ADH from the posterior pituitary gland. Second, a perception of thirst occurs, leading to the ingestion of water. ADH causes the kidney to increase water reabsorption, resulting in antidiuresis. As plasma osmolality returns toward normal, stimulation of osmoreceptors is reduced, and ADH secretion decreases. The sensation of thirst is reduced. Overhydration dilutes the blood, and plasma osmolality decreases. When it reaches about 282 mOsm/kg, the synthesis and release of ADH are inhibited. The kidneys decrease water reabsorption, and diuresis ensues. Serum osmolality returns toward normal.[77]

Thyroid Gland

The thyroid gland weighs 15-25 g in a healthy adult. It is composed of two encapsulated lobes positioned on either side of the trachea and joined by the isthmus. The right lobe is larger and more vascular than the left. The recurrent laryngeal nerves run in the grooves beside the trachea and behind the lobes of the thyroid gland. The thyroid gland is located anteriorly just below the cricoid cartilage (Figure 9-3).

Embryologically, the thyroid gland begins as epithelial tissue in the pharyngeal floor. Deviations in normal embryonic development may consist of failure of lobe development, development of a lingual thyroid gland from remnants of the thyroglossal duct, thyroglossal cyst formation from duct remnants,

ANTERIOR　　　　　　　POSTERIOR

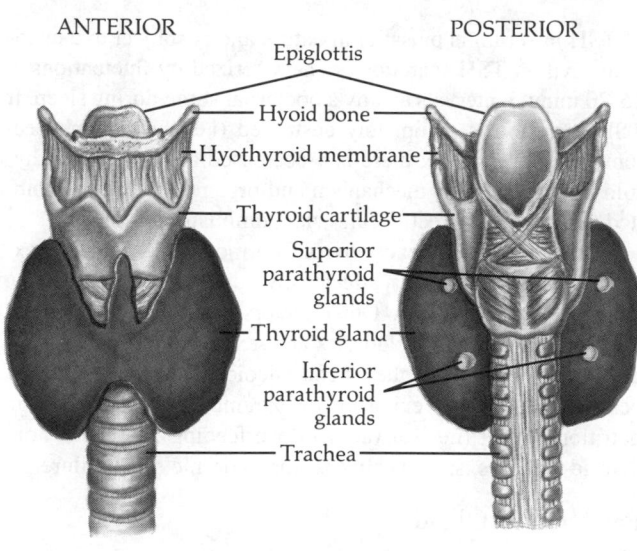

Figure 9-3 Thyroid anatomy.

or substernal goiter formation from resultant descent of the thyroid gland along the developmental path of the thymus into the thorax.[47]

Thyroid blood supply is greater than the kidney blood supply. This blood supply is furnished by two major pairs of arteries that account for the rich vascularity of the gland and for the increased risk of hemorrhage that may occur postoperatively. The presence of a palpable thrill or audible bruit over the gland or surrounding area is indicative of an increased blood flow.[47]

The thyroid gland is innervated by the adrenergic nervous system, from the cervical ganglia; the cholinergic nervous system, from the vagus nerve; and a network of adrenergic fibers that terminate near the basement membrane of the follicular walls.[47] Thyroid blood flow is regulated by neurogenic stimuli.

The thyroid is composed of follicular and parafollicular cells. The follicles are filled with proteinaceous colloid.[47] Colloid is the major constituent of total thyroid mass.

The function of the follicular cells is to secrete the two major thyroid hormones, thyroxine (T_4) and triiodothyronine (T_3). The parafollicular cells or C cells secrete a third hormone, thyrocalcitonin (calcitonin). Elevations in serum calcium stimulate calcitonin secretion, which is the most potent endogenous inhibitor of osteoclastic bone resorption. Parafollicular cells are located in the interfollicular connective tissue.[75]

The major component of thyroid hormones is iodine. Normal iodine balance depends on sufficient dietary intake. Seafoods and water are the major natural sources. Medications, diagnostic agents, dietary supplements, and the use of iodine by the food-processing industry and in the food given to animals have increased iodine ingestion in the more highly developed countries. Normal daily dietary intake of iodine varies widely throughout the world primarily because of the varying iodine content of soil and water and cultural food preferences. The minimum recommended daily requirement for iodine is about 150 μg (50 to 75 μg is required for adults to prevent goiter

caused by iodine deficiency).[75] However, dietary intake of iodine ranges from 300-1,000 μg daily in the United States.

Iodine is rapidly absorbed from the gastrointestinal tract, primarily as iodide, the form in which it is carried in the blood, and is largely confined to the extracellular fluid (ECF) compartment. When absorbed in organic form, iodine is converted to iodide in the liver. Small quantities of iodine are lost in stool, in expired air, and through the skin. During lactation, more notable losses occur. Removal from the ECF pool occurs by excretion of iodine into the urine and by transport of iodine into the thyroid gland.[75]

Renal clearance of iodide is important because it determines the availability of iodide to the thyroid gland. The kidneys are considered passive participants in iodide metabolism and are not a part of the body's defense mechanism for maintenance of thyroidal homeostasis.[75]

Biosynthesis of the thyroid hormones occurs in sequential stages: iodide trapping; oxidation of the iodide ion; organification of thyroglobulin; and coupling of iodotyrosines to form the active hormones T_4 and T_3.

The first step in synthesis is iodide uptake by the follicular cells. This step is referred to as iodide transport or the iodide pump. Iodide is transported from the ECF into the thyroid glandular cells and follicles. TSH stimulates iodide transport activity. In addition, iodide transport is depressed by excess iodide administration and increased by iodide deficiency.[75]

During the second phase of biosynthesis, the iodide ions are converted to an oxidized form of iodine capable of combining directly with tyrosine amino acids located within thyroglobulin. Thyroglobulin is a large glycoprotein molecule synthesized and secreted into the follicles.

Organification is the process by which iodide ions are oxidized before joining tyrosine residues of the thyroglobulin molecule. This process requires the enzyme thyroid peroxidase (TPO), which is the suspected antigen responsible for microsomal antibodies in patients with autoimmune thyroid disease. The organification process results in the formation of hormonally inactive iodotyrosine, monoiodotyrosine (MIT), and diiodotyrosine (DIT).

Coupling is the process by which the thyroid hormones are formed. Thyroxine (T_4) or tetraiodothryonine is the coupling of two DIT molecules, while triiodothyronine (T_3) is the coupling of one MIT with one DIT.

These hormones are released into the circulation through the process of exocytosis. During exocytosis, both T_4 and T_3 are cleaved from thyroglobulin and then quickly become attached to carrier proteins in the circulation. Inevitably some T_4, T_3, and thyroglobulin do not become bound to a protein (*free*) and are able to exert an immediate metabolic effect. The primary carrier proteins are thyroid binding globulin, transthyretin, and albumin. TSH actively stimulates each step of thyroid hormone synthesis and release.

There is more T_4 produced intrathyroidally than T_3, with a total daily production rate of 80 to 100 μg. The majority of T_3 is produced from extrathyroidal deiodination of T_4 with a total daily production rate of 30-40 μg and an extrathyroidal pool of

50 μg. The half life of T_4 is 6-7 days, and there are large stores in plasma allowing 10% turnover each day. It therefore takes 4 to 6 weeks for total thyroid hormone depletion to occur. T_3 on the other hand has a short half life with only 14% in plasma stores.

Regulation of thyroid function is achieved through the hypothalamic-pituitary-thyroid axis (Figure 9-4) and an autoregulatory mechanism within the gland. Thyrotropin-releasing hormone (TRH) is synthesized by neurons in the hypothalamus and is transported to cells of the anterior pituitary gland that contain specific cell membrane receptors for TRH binding. Thyroid-stimulating hormone (TSH) in the anterior pituitary gland is stimulated by the secretion of TRH. Most of the thyroid gland's metabolic processes are regulated by TSH. Although the primary action of TSH is the production and secretion of the thyroid hormones, it can also stimulate growth of the gland. The thyroid hormones, on the other hand, inhibit TSH secretion at the level of the anterior pituitary gland. Small alterations in serum T_4 and T_3 concentrations result in reciprocal changes in both TSH secretion and TSH response to exogenous TRH. Serum thyroid levels will override the pituitary gland's response to TRH if the T_4 and T_3 levels are high.[98]

Blockage or removal of TSH stimulation results in hypovascularity and atrophy of the thyroid gland. The reverse effects occur when stimulatory doses of TSH are produced. Secretion of TSH in serum is pulsatile in nature and is subject to a circadian rhythm. TSH secretion is characterized by fluctuations at 15-20 minute intervals and by a nocturnal surge during sleep. If TSH secretion is completely destroyed (i.e., by hypophysectomy or suppression), there is a decreased activity of the thyroid iodide transport mechanism and organic binding is inhibited. The reverse effect occurs with administration of TSH.[98]

Many factors influence thyroid hormone function. For example, TSH secretion is affected by somatostatin, dopamine, and the catecholamines. Other factors that influence thyroid hormone functioning include sex and sex hormones; pregnancy; the newborn state; age; the glucocorticoids; environmental temperatures, especially exposure to extreme cold; alterations in nutritional states (i.e., starvation or overfeeding); and other nonthyroid illnesses, such as cirrhosis and chronic renal failure.

Parathyroid Gland

The two pairs of parathyroid glands arise from the brachial pouches and descend along with the thymus until the embryo is approximately 18 mm in size.[91] Like the thyroid gland, the final location of any one of the parathyroid glands may be extremely variable. The position of the superior glands is usually behind the superior thyroid capsule while the inferior glands usually rest near the inferior poles of the thyroid. Inferior glands may be located in the mediastinum or the thyroglossal duct groove, and superior glands may reside near cervical vertebrae. In addition, the number of glands may also vary. Five percent of the population have only three glands, while 12%-15% may have five or more glands. The size and weight of the parathyroid glands varies between men and women and between caucasians and blacks. The average size of each gland is 2-7 mm in length, 2-4 mm in width, and 0.5-2 mm thick.[48] The glands are composed of chief, oxyphil, and clear cells. Oxyphil cells appear after puberty and increase in number with age. Clear cells are chief cells with increased cytoplasmic glycogen. Chief cells synthesize and secrete parathyroid hormone (PTH).

PTH is responsible for extracellular calcium homeostasis. It is under negative feedback regulation by ionized calcium in the extracellular fluid (ECF). It is secreted in a pulsatile interval of approximately 60 minutes with a peak circadian secretion at midnight.[91] The target cells for PTH are specialized calcium transport cells in the skeleton, intestine, and kidneys.

There is constant remodeling of bone that takes place between osteoclast (bone resorbing) and osteoblast (bone forming) cells. PTH increases osteoclastic activity while simultaneously inhibiting osteoblastic activity, yielding a net release of calcium from the skeleton into the ECF.

Calcium absorption from the intestine occurs as an active process and as passive diffusion. Passive diffusion relies on a concentration gradient and is responsible for the absorption of 10%-15% of dietary calcium. Active transport occurs by a carrier mechanism regulated by 1,25 dihydroxyvitamin D (1,25 $(OH)_2D$). Although 1,25 dihydroxyvitamin D is synthesized in the kidneys as well as by skin cells, lack of vitamin D (high SPF sunblock, poor dietary intake of dairy products) affects the amount of calcium the intestine will reabsorb.

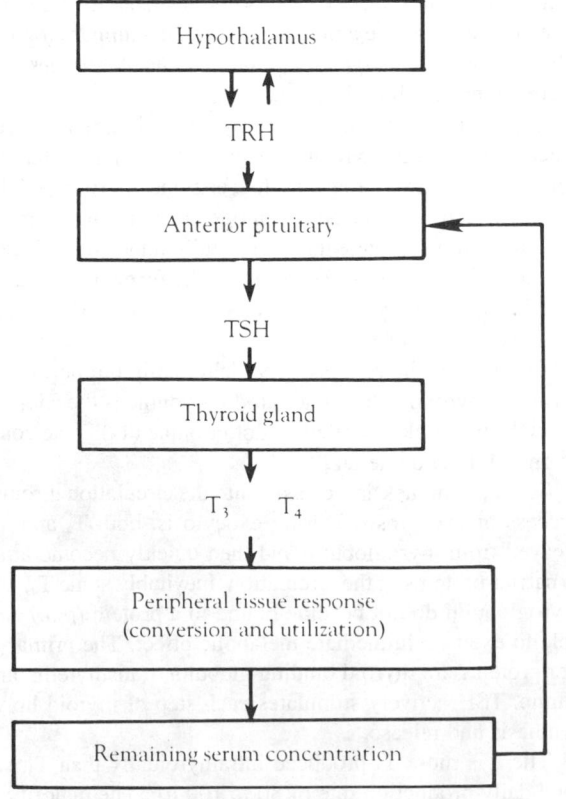

Figure 9-4 Thyroid negative-feedback mechanism.

The kidney filters about 10 g of calcium per day with approximately 65% of the calcium reabsorbed by the proximal tubule.[11] PTH will increase reabsorption of calcium in both the proximal and distal segments of the nephron by increasing transport from lumen to plasma. Vitamin D-dependent calcium binding protein in the distal tubule may also be modified by PTH. Along with renal calcium, PTH inhibits phosphate reabsorption from both proximal and distal sites and enhances 1,25 dihydroxyvitamin D in the proximal tubule. It also plays a role in the excretion or reabsorption of other ions and ion transporters.

Pathologic conditions arising within the parathyroid gland lead to alterations in skeletal, intestinal, and renal calcium homeostasis. Conversely, pathologic conditions arising in one of the three target areas will lead to altered calcium balance and will have secondary effects on the other two target areas and the parathyroid glands.

Adrenal Glands

The adrenal glands are located at the upper poles of the kidneys, on the posterior parietal wall on each side of the vertebral column and lateral to the eleventh thoracic and the first lumbar vertebrae. Each weighs 4-6 g, is 2 to 3 cm wide and 4 to 6 cm long.[64] Embryonically, the adrenal cortex (outer layer) is of mesodermic origin and comprises 90% of the total gland, whereas the adrenal medulla (inner layer) arises from primitive sympathetic nervous system cells derived from the neuroectoderm.[76]

The cortex has three distinct zones containing specific cell types responsible for the production of glucocorticoids, mineralocorticoids, and androgens. The zona fasciculata is the chief producer of glucocorticoids, while mineralocorticoids are from the zona glomerulosa and androgens from the zona reticularis.[106] The precursor of all steroid biosynthesis in the adrenal gland is cholesterol. Cholesterol (Figure 9-5), under the influence of two classes of enzymes (cytochrome P-450 and short chain dehydrogenases), is converted into the primary hormones of cortisol (glucocorticoid), aldosterone (mineralocorticoid), and testosterone and estradiol (androgens). All of the final products as well as the intermediary hormones of the adrenal steroid cascade can be measured in the peripheral circulation.

Cortisol production and secretion is regulated by ACTH. The negative feedback effects of cortisol are exerted at both the level of the pituitary and the hypothalamus. Cortisol is secreted in a diurnal variation. The level is higher in the morning than in the evening. The rhythm is maintained in people who work night shift and maintain a conventional schedule on weekends. The rhythm changes gradually over 2 to 3 weeks when light/dark cycles are permanently changed or when time zones are crossed. Increased production during periods of stress results from increased central nervous system activity possibly mediated by vasopressin.

Cortisol has multiple effects throughout the body with important roles in carbohydrate, protein, and lipid metabolism. Cortisol increases glucose production by increasing hepatic gluconeogenesis. It stimulates glycolysis, proteolysis, and

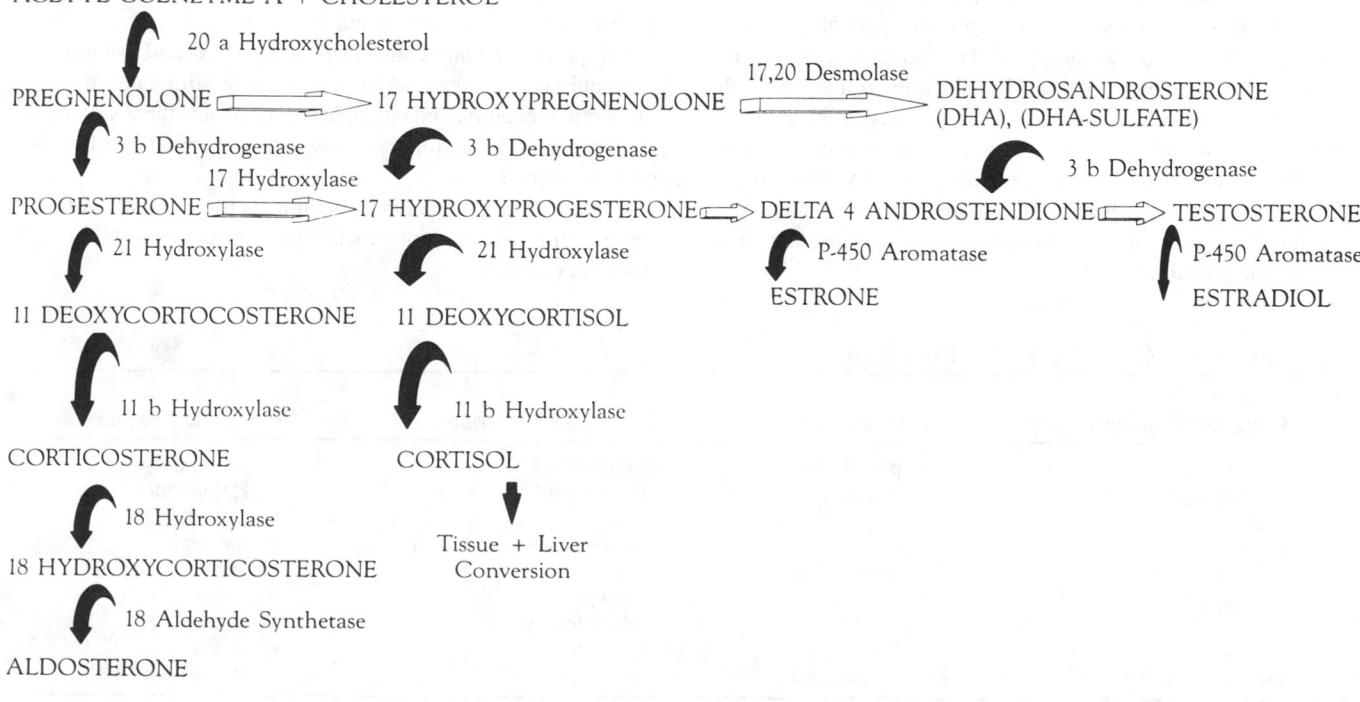

Figure 9-5 Adrenal steroid cascade.

lipolysis to provide more substrate for gluconeogenesis and increases cellular resistance to insulin. Free fatty acid levels are increased through lipolysis and decreased glycerol production. A catabolic effect is exerted on protein metabolism in fat, skeletal muscle, bone, lymphoid, and connective tissue. Glucocorticoids inhibit most immunologic and inflammatory responses. Other effects occur on connective tissues, calcium and bone metabolism, cardiac muscle, renal tubular excretion, growth and development, and central nervous system changes in mood.

Aldosterone is the most potent mineralocorticoid and accounts for 50% of plasma mineralocorticoid activity. The major function is to maintain intravascular volume by conserving sodium and eliminating potassium and hydrogen ions. Mineralocorticoids exert this effect in kidney, gut, salivary glands, sweat glands, vascular endothelium, and brain. The secretion of aldosterone is regulated by potassium ion concentration and the renin angiotensin system. When fluid-volume or intra-arterial volume is decreased, renin is released from the renal juxtaglomerular cells. This results in the formation of angiotensin I, which then converts to angiotensin II. Angiotensin II directly stimulates arteriolar vasoconstriction within seconds, stimulating the synthesis and secretion of aldosterone within minutes. The outcome is sodium reabsorption and potassium ion excretion. Increased plasma potassium stimulates aldosterone production; decreased plasma potassium decreases aldosterone production and may exhibit a blunted response to hyponatremia.[66]

Adrenal androgens are primarily under the control of ACTH, but the linking mechanism to the hypothalamic-pituitary-gonadal axis is not well understood. Adrenarche is the outcome of increased adrenal androgen secretion a few years before the onset of puberty. These androgens play a role in the development of some secondary sexual characteristics such as axillary and pubic hair growth. They decline with age in both men and women, although women tend to have higher levels than men for more years. The decline coincides with menopause in women and between ages 40-50 years in men. The physiologic effect is uncertain in men, but in women may account for testosterone effects seen after menopause (i.e., upper lip hair growth).[71]

Adrenal medullary tissue arises from pheochromoblasts that migrate from sympathetic ganglia and nest within adrenocortical tissue. These cells differentiate into chromaffin cells that are modified neuronal gland cells, not neurons. Central nervous system stimulation of the medulla is provided by the splanchnic nerve with acetylcholine the primary neurotransmitter. The blood supply is from the inferior phrenic artery, the aorta, the renal artery, and a corticomedullary portal system originating in the zona reticularis. The portal system provides a high level of adrenocortical steroids that influence catecholamine biosynthesis.[21]

The sympathetic nervous system innervates the adrenal medulla and stimulates the release of catecholamines. Catecholamines are hormones (chemical substances that are released into the circulation and elicit a response from a target organ) and neurotransmitters (chemical substances released from nerve endings that have local effects).[21] Catecholamines are biosynthesized from tyrosine, an amino acid that comes from dietary sources, or from conversion of phenylalanine to tyrosine in the liver. Tyrosine is acted on by enzymes to initiate the catecholamine pathway.

Norepinephrine and *epinephrine* are the main products of the pathway. Medullary catecholamine secretions are approximately 15% norepinephrine and 85% epinephrine. It is thought that the steroid-rich blood supply of the adrenal medulla maintains the enzyme phenylethanolamine N-methyl transferase (PNMT) and thus promotes the conversion of norepinephrine to epinephrine. The medulla is the primary source of epinephrine production, whereas norepinephrine is secreted almost exclusively by the central nervous system. Epinephrine is 5 to 10 times more potent than norepinephrine, although norepinephrine has a longer duration of action.[21]

Norepinephrine and epinephrine are both α- and β-adrenergic agonists, but norepinephrine primarily stimulates the α-adrenergic receptors, and epinephrine stimulates the β-adrenergic receptors. The actions of these catecholamines are briefly summarized in Table 9-1.

Urinary metabolites of catecholamines include epinephrine, norepinephrine, dopamine, metanephrine, and vanillyl mandelic acid (VMA).

■ TABLE 9-1 Catecholamine Functions

Class and Function	α-Adrenergic	β-Adrenergic	Dopaminergic
Agonist	Norepinephrine	Epinephrine	Dopamine
Antagonist	Phentolamine	Propranolol	Haloperidol
Actions			
Heart		Inotropic and chronotropic	Inotropic
Smooth muscle	Contracts	Relaxes	Mixed
Metabolic		Lipolysis	
		Glycogenolysis	
		Gluconeogenesis	
Molecular	Decreases cAMP	Increases cAMP	Increases cAMP

From Korenman.[41]

Pancreas

The pancreas lies behind the stomach to the left of the liver and is attached to the duodenum by ducts from the head and body section of the pancreas. It is through these ducts that the pancreatic digestive enzymes enter the small intestine.

Each islet of Langerhans consists of a grouping of several hundred cells. The islets are scattered over the entire gland, and the cellular composition of each varies with specific location within the pancreas. The islets contain at least four different types of cells. About 15% of islet cells are alpha (α) cells that produce glucagon; 60% are beta (β) cells that produce insulin; 10% are delta (δ) cells, producing somatostatin; and 15% are pancreatic polypeptide (PP) cells that produce pancreatic polypeptide.[28] Islets are organized with cells containing somatostatin, glucagon, and pancreatic polypeptide surrounding a core of insulin-producing cells. Biosynthesis of each of the islet cell hormones is similar. Prepropeptides give rise to propeptides that are packaged in secretory granules to provide bioactive hormone and a connecting or terminal peptide fragment.[33]

The islet cells have a large blood supply and the pancreas is the most highly innervated of all endocrine glands. The central nervous system is linked to the islets through sympathetic and parasympathetic nerves of the autonomic nervous system. Stimulation of the sympathetic fibers increases blood sugar through stimulation of glucagon production and inhibition of insulin. Parasympathetic stimulation increases insulin secretion.[18]

Glucagon is produced chiefly by the islet α cells and plays an important role in maintaining blood glucose homeostasis. Glucagon production is stimulated by decreased blood glucose, fasting, and exercise. The primary target organ of this hormone is the liver, where it attaches to hepatic glucagon receptors. Glucagon acts to raise blood glucose by trapping amino acids in the liver, and increasing gluconeogenesis, glycogenolysis, and ketogenesis. The fact that glucagon works in this manner to regulate glucose production is especially important in the fasting state. The secretion of glucagon and insulin are coordinated in a way that normally maintains blood sugar within a fairly narrow normal range. Glucagon and insulin have opposite actions, and the ratio, or relative concentration of both hormones, is important to blood glucose regulation.[28,97]

Insulin is synthesized in the endoplasmic reticulum of the beta cells under the direction of messenger RNA. After the terminal connecting C-peptide fragment is removed (Figure 9-6), the insulin molecule is folded and held together by disulfide bonds. Both insulin and C-peptide are secreted into the circulation along with small amounts of unchanged proinsulin. Since beta cell secretory granules contain equal amounts of C-peptide and insulin, C-peptide can be measured by radioimmunoassay to assess endogenous pancreatic β cell function. Insulin is the primary hormone controlling the storage and metabolism of ingested nutrients. Glucose is the main stimulus for insulin secretion, with fat and protein being less potent stimuli for insulin secretion. Once secreted, insulin travels in the portal circulation to the liver, and then through the general circulation. To be effective, insulin must bind to cell membrane receptors on target tissues (liver, fat, and muscle cells). The metabolic effects of insulin include: 1) increased glucose transport into insulin-dependent cells; 2) increased synthesis of protein, fat, and glycogen.[28,40]

In the fasting state, decreased insulin levels and increased glucagon levels allow glucose production by the liver through the processes of glycogenolysis and gluconeogenesis to maintain blood sugar levels and an adequate glucose supply to cells for energy. In the fed state, glucagon levels drop and insulin levels rise to 30-100 μU/ml to prevent severe elevations in blood sugar by both suppressing liver production of glucose, and stimulating glucose uptake by fat, muscle, and liver cells.[97] An estimated 25% of glucose ingested is used by non-insulin dependent cells (brain, eye, kidney, RBC) for energy.[28]

While blood glucose regulation is primarily controlled by insulin and glucagon, three other counterregulatory hormones

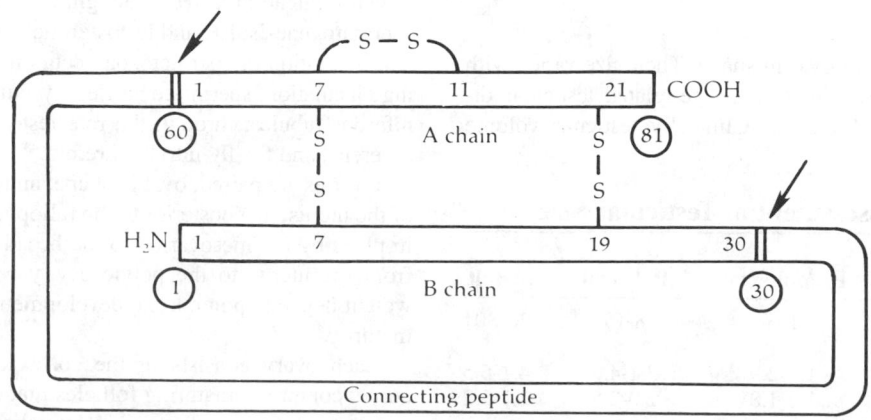

Figure 9-6 Formation of insulin and connecting peptide from proinsulin. (Reprinted with permission from Imagimedic Productions.[36])

interact with glucagon to raise blood glucose. Growth hormone, secreted from the anterior pituitary gland, increases blood sugar by decreasing cellular glucose uptake; cortisol decreases cellular glucose uptake and increases gluconeogenesis; and catecholamines decrease cellular glucose uptake and increase glycogenolysis. The secretion of counterregulatory hormones is stimulated by hypoglycemia, exercise, and stress.[28]

Somatostatin is widely distributed in the CNS, stomach, intestines, and pancreatic islets. It acts as an inhibitor of insulin and glucagon secretion through direct action (paracrine effect). In addition, somatostatin acts to inhibit GI hormones such as gastrin, secretin, and cholecystokinin, as well as pituitary hormones such as growth hormone and thyrotropin. Somatostatin secretion is stimulated by glucose, amino acids, and increased levels of extracellular calcium and potassium.[28,89]

Pancreatic polypeptide secretion is increased with protein ingestion, fasting, exercise, and hyperglycemia. Increased PP levels have been noted in persons with diabetes mellitus and pancreatic endocrine tumors. The secretion of PP is thought to be under vagal control and does not influence carbohydrate metabolism. Its main action is to regulate gastrointestinal function such as exocrine pancreas secretion and gall bladder emptying.[89]

Hormones produced by endocrine cells in the GI tract include somatostatin, gastrin, secretin, cholecystokinin, motilin, neurotensin, enteroglucagon, peptide YY, and glucose-dependent insulinotropic peptide. These hormones mediate a variety of absorptive, secretory, digestive, motor, and tropic actions in the GI tract and other organ systems that are essential to life.[28]

Gastrin is a peptide hormone that exists in three biologically active forms. It has a variety of effects on the GI tract including (1) stimulation of gastric acid secretion; (2) stimulation of water and electrolyte secretion; (3) stimulation of digestive secretions from the stomach and pancreas; and (4) promotion of growth of the gastric mucosa. Excessive secretion of gastrin is responsible for a number of disease states that may include the occurrence of non-β cell islet tumors (gastrinomas).[28]

Gonads

The testes are paired and oval in shape. Their size varies with age and degree of sexual maturity. Age-related testicular dimensions are found in Table 9-2. Clinically, testicular volume

■ TABLE 9-2 Assessment of Testicular Size

Method	Prepubertal	Pubertal	Adult
Orchidometer*	1-6	8-15	20-30†
Ruler measurement‡			
Length	1.6-2.9	3.1-4.0	4.1-5.5
Width	1.0-1.8	2.0-2.5	2.7-3.2

Modified from Sherins and Howards. From Santen RJ. In Felig P, Baxter JD, and Frohman LA.[78]
*Measured in milliliters;† 24 ± 4SD ml; *n* = 44;‡ measured in centimeters.

is measured with a Prader orchiometer in cubic centimeters. The testes are found within the scrotum, and are maintained at a temperature approximately 2 degrees lower than the abdomen.[78] Testes contain two functional areas, interstitial cells (Leydig cells) and seminiferous tubules (germinal and Sertoli cells).

Male gonadal hormone production in the testes is regulated by gonadotropin releasing hormone (GnRH) from the hypothalamus. Beginning at puberty, GnRH is secreted in a 24 hour pulsatile fashion. GnRH binds to receptors on anterior pituitary cells that subsequently produce and release leutinizing hormone (LH) and follicle stimulating hormone (FSH). LH binds to Leydig cell receptors and stimulates androgen production, mainly in the form of testosterone. About 7 mg of testosterone is released per day (in a pulsatile manner) by adult testes into the peripheral circulation via the spermatic vein.[43,78]

Testosterone circulates attached to testosterone binding globulin (TeBG) or albumin; 2% circulates unbound as free testosterone, the most biologically active form. The fractions of each are important in clinical evaluation.

Adrenal glands provide an additional source of testosterone in the amount of about 200 μg/day.[78] The hormonal effects of testosterone are direct in the testes (paracrine effect) and include the initiation of spermatogenesis. The peripheral effects of testosterone and a conversion product, dihydrotestosterone, are responsible for the masculinizing effects of androgens. The clinical actions of testosterone are summarized in the box below. After middle age, testosterone levels gradually decrease due to impaired hypothalamic control and Leydig cell attrition.

FSH binds to Sertoli cell receptors to stimulate the synthesis of proteins such as inhibin, transferrin, and androgen binding protein (ABP). Inhibin is thought to provide negative feedback to inhibit FSH secretion at the pituitary gland level. ABP is thought to play a role in maintaining high testosterone levels in the seminiferous tubules and testes. FSH is also thought to be necessary for the completion of spermatogenesis and maintenance of normal sperm counts.[43,78]

Sperm are produced by germinal cells through the process of cell replication. FSH is thought to be required for initiating spermatogenesis; LH and testosterone maintain the process. Final maturation of spermatozoa occurs in the epididymus. During ejaculation, sperm are carried by fluid flow from the seminiferous tubules, through the rete testes, epididymus and vas deferens, and finally into the urethra.[43]

Ovaries are paired, oval in shape, and situated on either side of the uterus, just posterior to the fallopian tubes. They are held in place by the mesovarian to the broad ligament that extends from the uterus to the pelvic cavity wall. Ovarian size and weight depend upon normal development and degree of sexual maturity.

Each ovary consists of the cortex and the medulla. The cortex comprises maturing follicles that contain oocytes (eggs) and steroidogenic cells, called interstitial cells, that produce and secrete androgens. The loose connective tissue of the medulla contains nerves and blood vessels that course towards the cortex.

Female gonadal hormone production is regulated by gonadotropin releasing hormone (GnRH) secreted in pulsatile fashion from the hypothalamus. GnRH binds to receptors on anterior pituitary cells that in turn produce LH and FSH in pulsatile fashion every 60-90 minutes beginning at puberty.

CLINICAL ACTIONS OF ANDROGEN

In utero
  External genitalia development
  Wolffian duct development
Prepubertal
  Possible male behavioral effects
Pubertal
  External genitalia
    Penis and scrotum increase in size and become pigmented
    Rugal folds appear in scrotal skin
  Hair growth
    Mustache and beard develop; scalp line undergoes recession
    Pubic hair develops
    Axillary, body, extremity, and perianal hair appears
  Linear growth
    Pubertal growth spurt
    Androgens interact with growth hormone to increase somatomedin C levels
  Accessory sex organs
    Prostate and seminal vesicles enlarge, and secretion begins
  Voice
    The pitch is lowered because of enlargement of larynx and thickening of vocal cords
  Psyche
    More aggressive attitudes are manifest
    Sexual potential develops
  Muscle mass
    Muscle bulk increases
    Positive nitrogen balance is demonstrable
Adult
  Hair growth
    Androgenic patterns are maintained
    Male baldness may be initiated
  Psyche
    Behavioral attitudes and sexual potency are maintained
  Bone
    Bone loss and osteoporosis are prevented
  Spermatogenesis
    Interaction with FSH to modulate Sertoli cell function and stimulate spermatogenesis
  Hematopoiesis
    Erythropoietin-stimulated
    Direct marrow effect on erythropoiesis

Modified from Bardin and Paulsen. In Williams, RD (ed), *Textbook of endocrinology*, ed 6, Philadelphia, 1981, Saunders.[78]
From Santen RJ. In Felig P, Baxter JD, and Frohman LA, editors: *Endocrinology and metabolism*, ed 3, New York, 1995, McGraw-Hill.

In response to LH and FSH secretion, females secrete 3 types of biologically active hormones in a process that depends on mixed function oxidase enzymes.[26] Steroidogenic cells convert cholesterol to pregnenolone, which is then converted enzymatically to progesterone, testosterone, and estrogen. FSH and LH control steroid metabolism enzymes and thus, the conversion rates and amounts of active hormone. The principle actions of these ovarian hormones are 1) stimulation of growth of female reproductive organs (uterus, vagina, breasts), and 2) development of secondary sex characteristics.[34]

Progesterone functions to (1) prepare the endometrium of the uterus for ovum implantation, (2) prepare the placenta, (3) prepare breasts for milk production, and (4) decrease uterine contractility. Estrogen affects the development and maturation of the breasts and genitalia. Androgens are responsible for the development of sexual hair. Table 9-3 summarizes the effects of these and other hormones.

Normal female reproductive function occurs when the hypothalamic-pituitary-ovarian axis is coordinated with uterine environment changes. LH and FSH levels follow a cyclic pattern of secretion each month beginning around puberty and continuing through the childbearing years, until menopause, with the exception of pregnancy and lactation. FSH plays a key role in controlling the growth of the primary follicle to maturation; estrogen production regenerates the uterine lining each month. A surge in LH and fall in estrogen follows, and causes the single follicle that reaches maturity to release an ovum

TABLE 9-3 Summary of Hormonal Effects

Areas of Concern	Hormonal Influence
Normal growth	Thyroid
	Insulin
	Growth hormone
	Gonadotropins
	Sex steroids
Metabolic rate	Thyroid
Protein, carbohydrate, and fat metabolism	Thyroid
	Glucagon
	Insulin
	Gastrin, glucocorticoids
Cardiac contractility	Calcium, epinephrine
Blood pressure; pulse rate	Glucocorticoids, mineralocorticoids
	Epinephrine, norepinephrine
Muscle mass and contractility	Glucocorticoids
	Insulin
	Growth hormone
	Androgens
Skin turgor	Mineralocorticoids, glucocorticoids
Secondary sex characteristics	Gonadotropins
	Sex steroids
Lactation	Calcium
	Prolactin, oxytocin
Skin pigmentation	Melanocyte-stimulating hormone

into the peritoneal cavity (ovulation). The ovum is swept up into the fimbrae of the fallopian tube, where it can potentially be fertilized, and then implanted in the uterus. After ovulation, the walls of the primary follicle form the corpus luteum, and secrete progesterone. If implantation does not occur, the corpus luteum deteriorates into dense connective tissue called the corpus albicans. A subsequent fall in progesterone causes spasm of the spiral arterioles, and the shedding of endometrium, menstruation, and the beginning of the next monthly cycle.

CONDITIONS, DISEASES, AND DISORDERS

DISORDERS OF THE ADRENAL GLAND

■ ADRENAL INSUFFICIENCY

Adrenal insufficiency is caused by inadequate function of the adrenal cortex. There are two types: primary and secondary.

In *primary* adrenal insufficiency (Addison's disease), destruction of the adrenal cortex prevents adequate production of glucocorticoid (cortisol) and mineralocorticoid (aldosterone). In *secondary* adrenal insufficiency, hypothalamic-pituitary dysfunction prevents the adequate secretion of ACTH by the pituitary gland and leads to a relative cortisol deficiency.[50]

•••••• Pathophysiology

Primary adrenal insufficiency can be insidious in onset; signs and symptoms appear after 90% of adrenocortical tissue has been destroyed.[70] Eighty percent of cases of Addison's disease are caused by autoimmune destruction of the adrenal glands. Other causes include infection (tuberculosis, fungus, HIV, syphilis), hemorrhage, metastases, drugs, and congenital adrenal disease. Bilateral adrenal hemorrhage should be considered in patients receiving anticoagulation.[14,17]

Primary adrenal insufficiency is the result of glucocorticoid and mineralocorticoid deficiency. Through negative feedback, low cortisol levels stimulate the pituitary gland to secrete increased amounts of ACTH. This compensatory overproduction of ACTH leads to the classical sign of primary adrenal insufficiency: hyperpigmentation. Hyperpigmentation is particularly obvious when examining scars, palmar surfaces, and skin creases. Other signs and symptoms include weakness and fatigue, anorexia, nausea, vomiting, diarrhea, weight loss, abdominal pain, muscle and joint pain, orthostatic hypotension, vitiligo, and changes in mentation.[17,49]

Secondary adrenal insufficiency occurs most commonly in patients recently withdrawn from exogenous glucocorticoid therapy. Recovery of a normal hypothalamic-pituitary-adrenal (H-P-A) axis can take months or years following this cessation

of steroid administration. Other causes include pituitary tumors, hypophysectomy, pituitary radiation, postpartum pituitary necrosis, tumors of the third ventricle, and optic glioma.[49]

The clinical manifestations of secondary adrenal insufficiency are caused by glucocorticoid deficiency. Mineralocorticoid production is not impaired because its regulation by the renin-angiotensin system is independent of pituitary ACTH. Hypotension and shock are less common, and less severe as a general rule.[70]

The central pathophysiologic alteration of adrenal insufficiency is cardiovascular: insufficient glucocorticoid reduces cardiac output, decreases vascular tone, and results in hypovolemia. This stimulates the release of vasopressin, causing water retention and hyponatremia. Cardiac contractility and output decrease, possibly leading to circulatory collapse. Reflex tachycardia results from a decrease in cardiac output. Free fatty acid mobilization is impaired, which reduces free fatty acid levels. This in turn leads to increased utilization of glucose, resulting in hypoglycemia. Decreased cortisol increases ACTH and MSH production causing hyperpigmentation, and there is a decrease in gastrointestinal enzymes. The loss of diurnal cortisol may cause a loss of vitality. Mineralocorticoid deficiency is reflected by hyperkalemia and hyponatremia.[49,50]

Adrenal crisis, or acute adrenal insufficiency, is characterized by an exacerbation of symptoms associated with adrenal insufficiency often precipitated by a major physiologic stress. It is usually associated with primary adrenal insufficiency, but can occur in secondary disease. Patients in adrenal crisis are usually dehydrated, hypovolemic, and hyponatremic. The hypotension resists volume repletion and requires glucocorticoid administration for rapid correction.[17] Vomiting and diarrhea contribute to volume depletion. Other symptoms include nausea, anorexia, weakness, and fatigue. Mentation ranges from lethargy to coma. Hallmark signs include abdominal pain and fever. Fever can be due to a precipitating infection or to the glucocorticoid deficiency itself. Hyperpigmentation and weight loss can be seen in patients with chronic adrenal insufficiency. Adrenal crisis can be caused by inadequate glucocorticoid replacement or failure to compensate for major stressors such as surgery, trauma, or infection. The prophylactic use of exogenous steroids in trauma has greatly decreased the occurrence of adrenal crisis.[49]

•••••• Diagnostic Studies and Findings[17,51]

Imaging PPD and/or chest x-ray: possible tuberculosis; abdominal CT scan: adrenal calcification or enlargement suggests infection, hemorrhage, or metastatic disease

Blood tests Hyponatremia, hyperkalemia (in primary disease), azotemia (if severe), hypoglycemia

Endocrine tests Plasma ACTH levels increased in primary disease, decreased or normal in secondary disease; short ACTH stimulation test (cortosyn test): baseline cortisol level is drawn, then cortosyn (ACTH) is administered; 30 minutes later, plasma cortisol level should rise; impaired response indicates adrenal insufficiency.[14]

•••••• Multidisciplinary Plan[49]

Hormone Replacement

Glucocorticoid replacement:
Hydrocortisone 12-15 mg/m^2
Mineralocorticoid replacement:
Fludrocortisone (Florinef) 0.05-0.1 mg/day

These medications are considered life-sustaining for the patient and cannot be discontinued. To avoid adrenal crisis, patients must be taught intramuscular self-injection of Solu-Cortef to be administered when oral medication cannot be taken. A family member or significant other should be included in intramuscular injection instruction.

Special considerations:

Over-treatment with glucocorticoids can result in symptoms of hypercortisolism (Cushing's syndrome). Excess mineralocorticoids can result in fluid overload and hypertension. Evaluation of dosage adequacy can be done by monitoring clinical signs and symptoms and measuring 24 hour urinary free cortisol.[14]

NURSING CARE

Nursing Assessment[52,53]

Circulation

Postural hypotension
Lightheadedness
Hypopyrexia or hyperpyrexia*
Shock*
Vital signs

Food and Fluid Needs

Salt craving
Weight loss
Nausea
Vomiting
Hyponatremia*
Hyperkalemia*
Skin turgor
Dietary intake

Elimination

Diarrhea
Renal shutdown*

Mobility

Tires easily
Muscle aches
Muscle wasting
Muscle weakness

*Characteristics of adrenal crisis.

Comfort and Pain

Severe headache*
Severe abdominal pain*
Severe leg pain*
Severe lower back pain*

Hygiene and Skin Care

Hyperpigmentation
Decreased body hair

Sexuality

Amenorrhea
Decreased libido

Nursing Dx & Intervention

Fluid-volume deficit related to mineralocorticoid deficiency

- Assess hydration status continuously.
- Monitor patient's skin turgor for signs of dehydration.
- Provide aggressive fluid replacement in adrenal crisis.
- Administer glucocorticoid and mineralocorticoid as ordered.
- Employ means to combat nausea, vomiting, and diarrhea *to maintain fluid and nutritional balance and to promote homeostasis.*
- Monitor patient's intake and output; be aware of the patient's high risk for renal shutdown in adrenal crisis.
- Monitor weight daily.
- Encourage high sodium, low potassium diet when tolerated.

Hypovolemia due to mineralocorticoid deficiency, and decreased cardiovascular tone from glucocorticoid deficiency

- Monitor patient's vital signs.
- Take patient's apical pulse *to detect dysrhythmias.*
- Recognize patient's early presyncopal signs: dizziness, lightheadedness, and visual changes.
- Have patient change positions gradually (from lying to sitting or standing positions) *to avoid fainting from orthostatic hypotension.*
- Administer IV fluids rapidly as ordered *to rehydrate patient,* but use caution *to avoid cardiovascular overload.*
- Explain rationale for IV fluid therapy to patient.
- Note that shortened PR interval on ECG can result from glucocorticoid deficiency.
- Hemodynamic monitoring may be indicated in adrenal crisis *to monitor atrial filling pressure and peripheral vascular resistance.*[53]

Pain related to biochemical factors (metabolic imbalance)

- Monitor patient for development of pain (headache; abdominal, leg, back pain); be aware that these signs may indicate adrenal crisis.
- Encourage the patient to report pain or discomfort.
- Provide hormonal replacement (hydrocortisone).
- Employ comfort measures for the patient as needed.

Impaired physical mobility related to decreased strength and endurance (or musculoskeletal weakness)

- Provide rest periods for patient between nursing activities.
- Assist patient with task analysis of daily activities.
- Allow patient to increase strength and endurance at own pace; muscle weakness will improve as hormone replacement is achieved.

Patient Education/Home Care Planning

1. Ensure that patient verbalizes the importance of taking medication and how to take it regularly and in emergency situations.
2. Discuss with the patient the steps to follow when early symptoms of insufficiency are noted.
3. Discuss with the patient the importance of regular medical follow-up and the wearing of medical identification.

Evaluation

Hydration and vital signs are normal   Patient's sodium and potassium blood levels are within normal limits. Patient's blood pressure is maintained within normal limits with no evidence of orthostatic hypotension. Patient makes no statements concerning syncope. Patient's peripheral pulses are adequate. Patient's output equals intake. Patient's urine output is greater than 40 ml/hour. Patient's skin is intact and turgor is normal. Electrolytes within normal range. Weight is stable.

Activity pattern is improved   Patient is able to independently perform daily activities.

Pain is relieved (in adrenal crisis)   Patient recognizes and reports onset of abdominal pain as a potential sign of acute adrenal crisis. Patient reports pain relief with cortisol replacement therapy.

■ PRIMARY ALDOSTERONISM

Primary aldosteronism is caused by the hypersecretion of aldosterone resulting in renal wasting of potassium and reabsorption of sodium. This leads to hypertension, usually accompanied by hypokalemia.[70]

Primary aldosteronism is an uncommon disease accounting for about 2% of patients with hypertension.[30] It must be distinguished from secondary aldosteronism which is a normal adrenal response to hyperstimulation of the renin-angiotensin system (diuretic therapy, hepatic insufficiency, congestive heart failure, nephrotic syndrome, and licorice ingestion). Edema rarely occurs in primary aldosteronism, but can be seen in secondary aldosteronism.

•••••• Pathophysiology

Primary aldosteronism is a disorder of the adrenal cortex. It is most commonly caused by adrenal adenoma and idiopathic bilateral adrenal hyperplasia. In rare cases, adrenal carcinoma and dexamethasone-suppressible hyperaldosteronism can also cause primary hyperaldosteronism.[30]

Primary aldosteronism is usually associated with asymptomatic hypertension and hypokalemia, but hypokalemia is not present in all cases. The diagnosis of primary aldosteronism should be suspected in all patients with spontaneous hypokalemia. Suppressed renin levels and aldosterone excess confirm the diagnosis.[59] Excess aldosterone results in increased sodium reabsorption, increased total body sodium, water retention, and hypervolemia. Edema rarely occurs because of an "escape" mechanism wherein proximal tubular sodium reabsorption is inhibited by renal hemodynamic changes.[70] Arterial hypertension results from volume expansion and increased vascular and sympathetic reactivity. The degree of hypertension ranges from mild to severe.[25]

Aldosterone causes potassium depletion, both intracellular and extracellular, by increasing renal tubular excretion of potassium.[70] The symptoms of muscle weakness, fatigue, and polyuria are related to the hypokalemia and thus are not seen in all cases. Hypokalemia can also cause altered electrical conductivity of the myocardium and diminished glucose tolerance.

Hydrogen ion secretion is increased, resulting in metabolic alkalosis. The alkalosis correlates to the degree of hypokalemia.[25] The ability to concentrate urine diminishes resulting in polyuria, and inappropriate excretion of potassium continues. Marked alkalosis is reflected by positive Chvostek's and Trousseau's signs.[70]

Plasma renin activity is suppressed. Laboratory values reveal suppressed renin levels after the patient is exposed to conditions that will cause elevated levels in normal patients.[30] Simultaneous elevation of aldosterone secretion is also observed in these patients.

•••••• Diagnostic Studies and Findings

Diagnosis of primary aldosteronism is suggested by hypertension, hypokalemia, suppressed renin levels, and an elevated aldosterone level.[14] Diuretics should be discontinued 2-4 weeks before diagnostic testing. The patient should be eating a normal sodium diet.[70]

Blood tests   Decreased potassium; decreased plasma renin activity (PRA). Note: If PRA is normal or elevated, secondary hyperaldosteronism is the probable cause of hypertension. Increased plasma aldosterone concentration (PAC); increased PRA:PAC ratio (>20-25)

Urine tests   24 hour collection: increased aldosterone

Imaging tests   CT scan used to define an adrenal mass; an adenoma is rarely too small to be seen on CT

Endocrine tests   Captopril test: 25-50 mg of captopril is administered orally to suppress renin activity; PRA and PAC are drawn 60 and 120 minutes later; the diagnosis of primary aldosteronism is reflected by the following results: decreased PRA, increased PAC, increased PAC:PRA ratio. Lying and standing renin and aldosterone levels: After confirming normal sodium diet, baseline renin and aldosterone levels are drawn after patient has been in a supine position for 30 minutes; normally, renin will increase with ambulation; decreased PRA in primary aldosteronism, PRA remains low post-ambulation; if resting and post-ambulation levels are high, secondary aldosteronism is implied; increased PAC, a post-ambulation decrease suggests an aldosterone-producing adenoma. Normal saline infusion test: to test the response of aldosterone (PAC) to extracellular fluid volume expansion; testing should be performed in the afternoon because the circadian pattern of PAC is to decrease in the morning; patient must be supine for 30 minutes prior to the test; obtain baseline PAC level, administer 2 liters saline over 4 hours, obtain PAC level following infusion; if aldosterone (PAC) level is greater than 10 ng/dL and does not fall below 10 ng/dL, the test is positive for primary aldosteronism; a negative test suggests renin essential hypertension.[70] Venous catheterization of adrenal glands with measurement of plasma cortisol and aldosterone: to distinguish between a unilateral and bilateral source of hyperaldosteronism.[30]

• • • • • • Multidisciplinary Plan[30,70]

Surgery

Unilateral adrenalectomy; to remove aldosterone-producing adenoma; preoperative spironolactone is administered for 2 weeks (200-400 mg/day)

Medications

Aldosterone receptor blockade: Aldactone, 200-400 mg/day
Antihypertensive therapy

General Management

Low sodium diet

NURSING CARE

Nursing Assessment[53]

Circulation

Moderate to severe hypertension
Hypokalemia
Hypernatremia

Food and Fluid

Polydipsia
Excessive ingestion of licorice[14] (mimics mineralocorticoid activity)
Tobacco chewing (licorice flavored tobacco)[14]

Elimination

Polyuria
Nocturia

Neurosensory Area

Positive Chvostek's sign
Trousseau's sign

Mobility

Muscle weakness

Nursing Dx & Intervention

Fluid-volume excess related to failure of regulatory mechanism—hypervolemia caused by sodium reabsorption due to overproduction of aldosterone

- Monitor patient's intake and output.
- Monitor patient's vital signs every 4 hours; watch for signs.
- Monitor patient's daily weight.
- Reinforce low-sodium diet *to decrease patient's fluid retention.*
- Monitor patient's serum electrolytes.
- Reassess Chvostek's and Trousseau's signs *to monitor patient for signs of alkalosis.*
- Monitor patient's respiratory status and quality of respirations *to monitor for early acidosis.*
- Administer spironolactone (Aldactone) to patient as ordered.

Patient Education/Home Care Planning

1. Preoperative education to help patient and family prepare for unilateral adrenalectomy to remove aldosterone-producing adenoma (see Adrenalectomy, p. 858).
2. Preoperative preparation includes spironolactone therapy for 2 weeks. Medication teaching should include discussion of side effects. Women can expect menstrual disturbances; men can experience gynecomastia, impotence, and decreased libido.
3. Ensure that the patient verbalizes the importance of compliance to the regimen, knows the importance of taking medication regularly, and knows the potential side effects to report.

Evaluation

Excess fluid is decreased or absent   Patient's aldosterone level is not elevated; it is within normal range. Patient's serum electrolytes are within normal limits. Patient's weight is within the normal range. Patient's vital signs are within the normal range; there is no evidence of dysrhythmias.

CUSHING'S SYNDROME (HYPERCORTISOLISM)

Cushing's syndrome is caused by excess glucocorticoid secretion by the adrenal cortex, or via the exogenous administration of glucocorticoids.

Cushing's syndrome is rare; its true incidence is not known.[69] Sexual predominance relates to cause; Cushing's disease occurs 4-6 times more often in women, but ectopic adrenocorticotropic hormone (ACTH) syndrome occurs more frequently in men. Occurrence is usually midlife.[69]

The etiologies of Cushing's syndrome are divided into two groups: ACTH-dependent and ACTH-independent causes. In ACTH-dependent disease, adrenal activation is caused by excessive ACTH production, as in pituitary adenoma (80%), ectopic ACTH syndrome (20%), and, rarely, ectopic CRH secretion. In ACTH-independent disease, adrenal hyperactivity is independent of ACTH stimulation, for example adrenal adenoma (40%-50%), adrenal carcinoma (40%-50%), and, less commonly, primary pigmented nodular adrenal disease (micronodular adrenal disease), McCune Albright syndrome, and macronodular adrenal disease.[69]

Seventy percent of all patients with Cushing's syndrome have Cushing's disease: hypersecretion of ACTH by a pituitary adenoma. Hypercortisolism can be caused by extra-pituitary sources of ACTH, such as oat cell carcinoma of the lung. Cortisol production correlates directly with ACTH secretion.[63] Hence, elevated ACTH levels result in adrenal hyperstimulation, hyperplasia, and hypercortisolism.[79]

Diseases of the adrenal cortex, such as adrenal adenoma (benign) and adrenal carcinoma (malignant) can lead to hypercortisolism.[80] When adrenal tissue becomes neoplastic, cortisol can be produced independently of ACTH stimulation.[69] This overproduction of cortisol leads to low levels of ACTH due to negative feedback effects of cortisol on the pituitary gland. Other conditions causing hypercortisolism include chronic alcoholism (alcoholic pseudo-Cushing's), depression, and the factitious administration of corticosteroid preparations.

The effects of glucocorticoid excess are reflected in changes in many tissue and organ systems. Early symptoms include weight gain, hypertension, and glucose intolerance.[80] The majority of these clinical effects result from the direct antagonism of insulin by glucocorticoids.[67] This leads to (1) impaired glucose tolerance and diabetes mellitus, and (2) altered fat distribution. Normally, insulin inhibits the breakdown of fat (lipolysis), but glucocorticoid alters the pattern of the process leading to central obesity. In this state of impaired energy metabolism, cells are deprived of this major energy source. Hence, specialized functions such as the elaboration of skin and bone matrix are sacrificed. The effects of cortisol on gluconeogenesis result in hyperglycemia, polydipsia, polyuria, and polyphagia. Diabetes mellitus occurs in 10% to 15% of patients.[70]

Weight gain is accompanied by a redistribution of fat, resulting in a protuberant abdomen, facial rounding (moon facies), supraclavicular fullness, dorsocervical fat pad (buffalo hump), and thinning of extremities (Figure 9-7).[80] Exophthalmos occurs in 6% of patients due to retro-orbital fat accumulation.[79] Weakness is associated with proximal muscle wasting, and patients can have difficulty rising from a squatting position, and in severe cases, getting up from a chair. Patients can experience a loss of height from severe osteoporosis.[80] Loss of subcutaneous tissue produces thin, fragile skin, characteristically, "cigarette paper" thin). Facial plethora and erythema is common. Violaceous striae are the result of thin, fragile skin being pulled across a grossly enlarged abdomen. Striae also can be found on breasts, hips, shoulders, and upper thighs, and are usually greater than 1 cm wide.[69,70]

Wound healing is slowed and immune function is suppressed. The normal sequelae of infection, fever and pain can be masked by hypercortisolism.

Cardiovascular complications are a major cause of morbidity and mortality in patients with Cushing's syndrome.[70] Hypertension is common and can be exacerbated by excessive production of mineralocorticoids. If mineralocorticoids are in excess, dependent edema also can be found. Congestive heart failure can result. Vessel fragility and loss of connective tissue leads to bruisability unrelated to trauma. Significant ecchymoses can occur with venipuncture.

Androgen excess from adrenal hyperfunction can cause menstrual irregularities, hirsutism (in females) (Figure 9-8), oily facial skin, acne, thinning scalp hair, and altered libido.[70] Cortisol excess can lead to loss of bone density and back pain, compression fractures, and, rarely, long-bone fractures. Hyper-

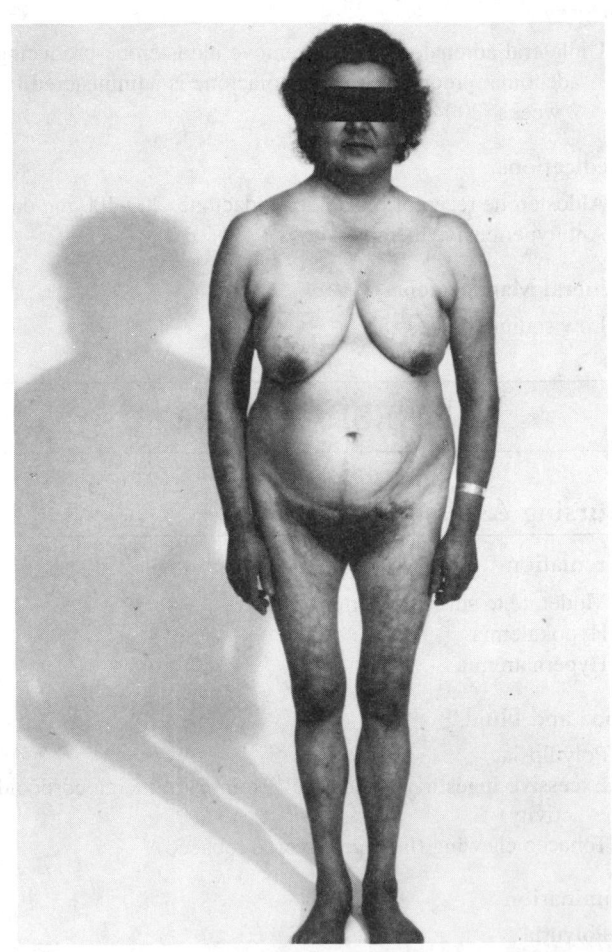

Figure 9-7 Forty-six-year-old woman diagnosed with Cushing's disease. Note classic cushingoid habitus with prominent supraclavicular fat pads and muscle wasting in extremities. (Courtesy National Institutes of Child Health, Bethesda, MD)

calciuria and renal calculi accompany the bone disease. This also explains the presence of polydipsia and polyuria.[70]

Emotional and cognitive changes from hypercortisolism can be severe. Effects include emotional lability, depression, impaired mentation and concentration, memory loss, irritability, anxiety, paranoia, and panic. Emotional and chemical depression may indicate the need for suicide precautions. Loss of the normal diurnal rhythm of cortisol has been associated with insomnia.

••••• Diagnostic Studies and Findings

The diagnosis of hypercortisolism can be difficult. Examining old photographs can help assess the progression of physical changes associated with Cushing's syndrome: central obesity with wasting of extremities, facial rounding and plethora, filling of supraclavicular areas and development of a "buffalo hump", thinning of hair, especially at scalp line, and onset of hirsutism.[69]

Blood tests Plasma cortisol: loss of diurnal rhythm (increased at night); plasma ACTH increased with ectopic syndromes; normal or slight increase with Cushing's disease; decreased with adrenal adenoma or carcinoma; potassium decreased; glucose increased; eosinophils decreased

Urine tests 24 hour collection: 17-hydroxysteroids (17-OH) increased; urinary free cortisol >200 g/day (This is the single best test for identifying endogenous hypercortisolism and diagnosing Cushing's syndrome.)

Imaging CT scan of sella to locate pituitary adenoma; CT scan of adrenal glands to locate adrenal adenoma, bilateral hyperplasia, macronodular hyperplasia; CT scan of chest to locate ectopic adenoma; MRI of pituitary gland to scan for adenoma

Endocrine tests Dexamethasone suppression test: Tests negative feedback of the hypothalamic-pituitary-adrenal (HPA) axis by administering dexamethasone (synthetic cortisol); normal response: glucocorticoids directly inhibit ACTH secretion from the pituitary; false positive results can occur with depression, alcoholism, and phenytoin or phenobarbital usage; low dose dexamethasone test, administration of 0.5 mg dexamethasone po q6h for 48 hours; normal response is decreased ACTH, decreased urinary 17-OH (24 hour urine);

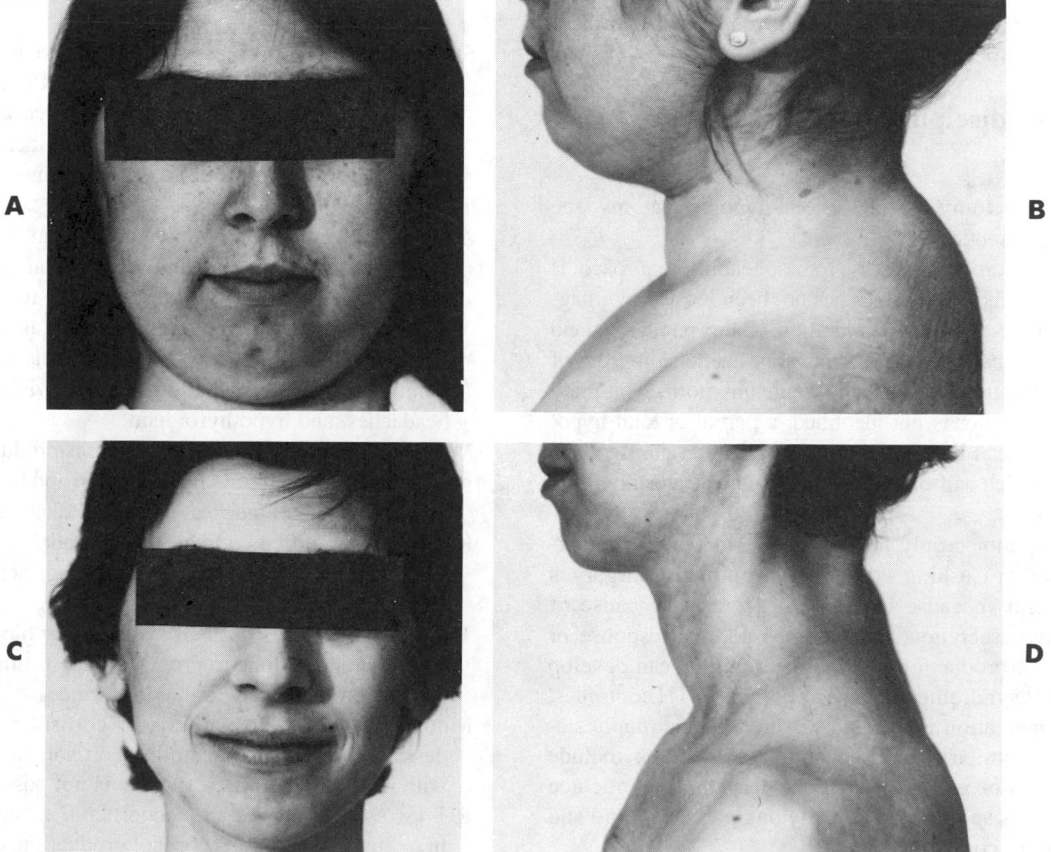

Figure 9-8 Preoperative and postoperative appearance of 23-year-old woman with adrenal carcinoma. Note moon facies, buffalo hump, supraclavicular fat pads, and mild hirsutism. **A,** Preoperative adrenal carcinoma with moon facies and hirsutism. **B,** Preoperative adrenal carcinoma with buffalo hump. **C,** Postoperative adrenal carcinoma with loss of moon facies and hirsutism. **D,** Postoperative adrenal carcinoma with loss of buffalo hump. (Courtesy National Institutes of Child Health, Bethesda, MD)

Cushing's disease: little or no effect; ACTH continues to be secreted despite attempts at negative feedback; high dose dexamethasone test: administration of 2 mg dexamethasone po q6h for 48 hours; normal response is same as low dose dexamethasone test; Cushing's disease: decreased urinary 17-OH by 50%; alternatives to standard dexamethasone suppression testing include the use of continuous intravenous infusion of dexamethasone (1 mg/hr × 7 hours), and an overnight high-dose (8 mg) dexamethasone test, but these have not been proven to be more reliable in diagnosing Cushing's disease. CRH stimulation test: CRH administration, 1 μg/kg as an intravenous bolus, is the best way to separate ACTH-dependent from ACTH-independent disease; ACTH-dependent illness always responds to CRH with an ACTH level greater than 10 pg/ml.[32] Inferior petrosal sinus sampling (IPSS):[24,92] Catheterization of the inferior petrosal sinuses (bilaterally) allows the measurement of ACTH secretion directly from the pituitary gland; ACTH levels from the petrosal sinuses ("central") and a peripheral venous site are compared; a pituitary adenoma is the likely cause of Cushing's syndrome if the ratio of central to peripheral ACTH is >2.0; if 1.0 μg/kg of ovine CRH is administered and the ratio is >3.0, the likelihood of pituitary adenoma is nearly 100%;[24,92] successful use of IPSS depends upon local experience and expertise.[62]

•••••• Multidisciplinary Plan

Surgery

Pituitary adenomectomy, partial, or total hypophysectomy (see hypophysectomy section p. 862)

   Removal of microadenoma by transsphenoidal approach is treatment of choice; if tumor has not been located by imaging techniques, surgical exploration of the pituitary gland can lead to localization and removal of adenoma in 90% of patients; this treatment usually maintains normal pituitary function; if tumor is not identified, a partial or total hypophysectomy can be undertaken; lateralization during IPSS indicates which half of the gland contains the adenoma[92]

Adrenalectomy

   Treatment of choice only for non–ACTH-dependent hypercortisolism or Cushing's disease when pituitary surgery is unsuccessful (because it does not address the cause of ACTH hypersecretion, it blocks the adrenal response of cortisol overproduction); a complication that can develop is Nelson's syndrome; hypersecretion of ACTH continues, hyperpigmentation is evident, and the clinical manifestation of a pituitary tumor occurs;[80] advantages include preservation of pituitary function; disadvantages include surgical risks and the need for lifelong glucocorticoid and mineralocorticoid replacement[69]

Ectopic tumor resection

   Ectopic ACTH-producing tumors should be surgically resected when possible, and may need to be followed with

radiation or chemotherapy;[80] if surgery is not possible, medications such as aminoglutethamide, metyrapone, and ketoconazole should be considered

Radiation

   Pituitary irradiation is a treatment alternative when pituitary surgery is unsuccessful or not desired; therapeutic response, however, is slow; side effects include hypothalamic-pituitary dysfunction, panhypopituitarism; efficacy is related to dosage, and higher dosages increase the likelihood of side effects, including radiation necrosis of the brain[80]

Medications

ACTH inhibitors

   Cyproheptadine: believed to exert an antiserotonin effect on hypothalamus; studies report successful treatment of symptoms in 60% of cases; symptoms usually recur when therapy is interrupted or discontinued; can be useful to treat metabolic imbalances while preparing for surgery, especially when impaired wound healing is anticipated from severe hypercortisolism[69]

   Bromocriptine: a dopamine agonist commonly used to treat prolactinoma-secreting pituitary tumors; not usually effective in treating Cushing's disease

   Sodium valproate suppresses ACTH secretion and lowers urinary free cortisol, 17-OH, and 17-KS levels; mechanism of action not known, but interference with ACTH response to CRH is suspected; not considered a standard treatment of Cushing's disease at this time

Adrenocortical inhibitors

   Aminoglutethamide: an anticonvulsant that suppresses cortisol secretion by blocking conversion of cholesterol to 5-pregnenolone; particularly useful to treat cortisol-secreting adrenocortical carcinoma; not an effective treatment for Cushing's syndrome; side effects include nausea, vomiting, lethargy, sedation, blurred vision, skin rash, headaches, and hypothyroidism

   Metyrapone: adrenal blockade decreases production of cortisol; side effects include hypertension and hypokalemic alkalosis, hirsutism, nausea, vomiting, dizziness

   Ketaconazole: inhibits adrenal and gonadal steroidogenesis; side effects include nausea, vomiting, abdominal pain, pruritis, and hepatoxicity

   Trilostane: decreases cortisol synthesis by blocking conversion of pregnenolone to progesterone; results in decreased production of cortisol and aldosterone

   Mitotane: inhibits biosynthesis of cortisol and chemically destroys adrenal cells secreting cortisol; can be combined with radiation therapy if surgery is not possible

   RU-486 (Mifepristone): a glucocorticoid antagonist effective in treating autonomous cortisol production, but as a receptor blockade, it can increase ACTH secretion thus counteracting its antiglucocorticoid effect; it is well tolerated, but remains investigational[80]

NURSING CARE

Nursing Assessment

Circulation

Mild to moderate hypertension
Blood vessel fragility: plethora and easy bruisability

Nutrition

Moderate weight gain
Fat distribution: truncal obesity, supraclavicular fat pads, buffalo hump, moon facies
Hyperglycemia
Increased appetite

Elimination

Glycosuria
Proteinuria
Hypercalciuria
Renal calculi

Neurologic Concerns

Impaired memory
Impaired concentration
Impaired cognitive function
Exophthalmos

Musculoskeletal Concerns

Fatigue
Muscle weakness: inability to rise from squat position
Muscle wasting in extremities
Activity intolerance
Pathological fractures
Osteoporosis

Pain and Discomfort

Back pain
Rib pain

Skin

Blood vessel fragility: plethora and easy bruisability
Thin, translucent skin
Hyperpigmentation
Poor wound healing
Hirsutism
Abdominal striae
Acne
Thinning of scalp hair

Psychosocial Concerns

Body image disturbance
Irritability
Emotional lability
Anxiety, panic
Paranoia
Depression
Insomnia
Suicidal nature

Reproductive

Amenorrhea
Hirsutism (women)
Decreased libido
Impotence

Nursing Dx & Intervention

Altered nutrition: more than body requirements related to excessive intake greater than metabolic need (state of hypercortisolism causes increased hunger, increased propensity to gain weight, and central obesity)

- Relate changes in patient's appearance to onset of disease (compare old photos with development of symptoms).
- Monitor patient's compliance to caloric restrictions.
- Encourage high-protein diet.
- Record patient's urine chemistry *to monitor metabolic balance.*
- Monitor patient's weight.

Activity intolerance; generalized weakness related to muscle atrophy

- Identify patient's priorities for energy expenditures.
- Plan activity and rest periods with patient *to maximize energy and minimize fatigue.*
- Discuss limitations with patient.

Impaired skin integrity related to altered metabolic and nutritional status

- Observe skin, especially areas of thinning and loss of integrity, *to identify areas of risk.*
- Instruct patient concerning good skin hygiene:
  Wash and dry thoroughly.
  Use lotions as needed.
  Use antifungal cream as needed.
  Perform aseptic care to minor lacerations and abrasions.
- Provide adequate pressure to venipuncture sites *to prevent subcutaneous hematoma.*
- Instruct patient to use caution during activities to avoid minor bumps and trauma.
- Keep patient's room clear of obstructions (excess furniture, etc.).
- Instruct patient in the use of protective clothing, especially shoes and socks, *to prevent trauma.*

Body image disturbance related to biophysical changes (central obesity), moon facies, hirsutism, facial plethora

- Assess degree of body image change since onset of disease *to determine what aspects of body image change are related to disease onset.*
- Discuss cushingoid features of the disorder with patient; give emotional support.
- Discuss palliative treatment for hirsutism (i.e., shaving or depilatories).
- Remind patient that symptoms are related to hypercortisolism and will resolve with treatment.

Altered thought processes related to impaired memory and cognitive functioning

- Assess patient's emotional factors related to disorder.
- Reassess patient's current stressors, as well as his or her effective and ineffective coping mechanisms.
- Give patient emotional support.
- Identify patient's sources of irritability and depression.
- Assist patient with problem-solving *to minimize anxiety and frustration.*
- Collaborate with mental health nursing specialist or psychiatrist.
- Explain effect of hypercortisolism on cognitive function and memory.

Risk for violence: self-directed related to depression (chemical) induced by hypercortisolism (see Risk for suicide, pp. 1383 to 1387)

- Assess presence of depression and suicidal ideation/intent.
- Establish supportive relationship to demonstrate concern and caring.
- Maintain close observation.
- Explain the relationship between depression and hypercortisolism, and that controlling disease state will also treat depression.

Patient Education/Home Care Planning

1. Ensure that patient verbalizes the importance of taking medication and knows to report side or toxic effects.
2. Discuss with the patient the importance of regular, lifelong medical follow-up.
3. Discuss with the patient the importance of wearing or carrying medical alert information.
4. Discuss with family the relationship between depression and hypercortisolism and the need for observation prior to treatment.

Evaluation

Nutrition is adequate   Weight is proportionate to height and stature. Urine chemistry levels are within normal limits. Blood sugar is within normal limits. Patient verbalizes use of appropriate dietary regimen.

Activity tolerance increases   Patient maintains maximum activity levels for physical limitations. Patient verbalizes realistic plan for alternating activities and rest based on limitations. Patient participates in recreational activities.

Skin is intact   Patient shows no breaks, cracks, ulcers, or ecchymosis. There is no infection. Patient's wound healing is normal. Patient verbalizes a method for maintaining hygiene.

Patient's self-concept improves   Patient uses realistic self-care methods to enhance physical features. Patient is not preoccupied with negative aspects of physical appearance. Patient participates in age-related activities and groups. Patient maintains peer relationships. Patient expresses realistic expectations concerning physical abilities and appearance. Patient demonstrates increased problem-solving ability with assistance from others. Patient functions at maximum level of independence based on limitations.

■ PHEOCHROMOCYTOMA

A pheochromocytoma is a tumor of the chromaffin cells of the adrenal medulla that produces excessive amounts of the catecholamines epinephrine and norepinephrine.

The incidence of pheochromocytoma is rare. Less than 0.5% of all patients with a recent diagnosis of hypertension have pheochromocytoma. The disorder is slightly more common in females, but has no age predominance. Tumors in children are usually associated with a familial tendency, are frequently bilateral, and are often malignant. Ninety percent of pheochromocytomas are sporadic; 10% are familial, inherited as an autosomal dominant trait. It is treatable when diagnosed, but if left untreated can be fatal. Pheochromocytomas are often linked with medullary carcinoma of the thyroid and multiple neoplasias (MEN II syndromes).[39]

•••••• Pathophysiology

Ninety percent of pheochromocytomas are found in the adrenal medulla. The remainder are extra-adrenal and are classified as paragangliomas; they usually are found in the abdomen. Most range in size from 3 to 5 cm. Multiple pheochromocytomas occur in approximately 20% of cases and often occur in patients possessing the inherited trait. Pheochromocytomas can occur in pregnancy and lead to increased morbidity and mortality for mother and fetus. Malignant pheochromocytomas are rare and occur in 5% of patients.[44]

Pheochromocytomas can vary in its clinical presentation from no symptoms to sudden heart attack, cerebral hemorrhage, or malignant hypertension. The hallmark sign is hypertension, occurring in 90% of patients. Hypertension is paroxysmal and characterized by a sudden and severe increase in blood pressure accompanied by a pounding headache, profuse sweating, palpitations, anxiety, pallor, nausea and possible vomiting, and abdominal or chest pain. Episodes can be spontaneous or induced by exercise, bending over, urination, defecation, abdominal pressure, or medications, but not usually by mental stress.[44] Many patients are asymptomatic or experience only mild symptoms. A majority of pheochromocytomas are diagnosed during autopsy.[38]

Pheochromocytomas produce excessive amounts of epinephrine and norepinephrine; however, norepinephrine is more prevalent and is responsible for most of the clinical manifestations. Norepinephrine, an α-adrenergic agonist, primarily causes the hypertensive effects of the disorder and is the principal hormone seen in extra-adrenal tumors. Epinephrine, a β-adrenergic agonist, is responsible for hypertensive as well as hypermetabolic and hyperglycemic effects of the disorder.[38]

Overproduction of norepinephrine causes paroxysmal hypertension, the most outstanding clinical sign. Excess epinephrine production can also bring about hypertension and postural hypotension. Blood pressure measurements can range from 200 to 300/150 to 175 mm Hg. Patients may have widely fluctuating blood pressures with or without paroxysmal hypertensive episodes. Hypertensive episodes can be provoked by stimuli such as palpation of the tumor, emotional stress, or increased abdominal pressure (i.e., micturition). Extreme cases of hypertension may lead to cerebrovascular accidents that can be life threatening. Nephrosclerosis and retinopathy may accompany severe sustained hypertension. Myocarditis, dysrhythmias, and congestive heart failure are seen in patients who develop cardiomyopathies related to the direct effect of high levels of catecholamines on the myocardium.[44]

Elevated levels of circulating epinephrine and norepinephrine can create a state of hypermetabolism similar to thyrotoxicosis. The patient can have tachycardia, tachyarrhythmias, weight loss, heat intolerance, tremors, and hyperreflexia. Sympathetic overstimulation can give rise to apprehension and emotional instability. Catecholamines suppress insulin secretion and stimulate the conversion of glycogen to glucose in the liver, resulting in hyperglycemia and glycosuria.[44]

•••••• Diagnostic Studies and Findings

Pheochromocytoma must be distinguished from essential hypertension, anxiety or panic attacks (blood pressure does not significantly increase), drug-induced states (amphetamines, cocaine, PCP, LSD, cold preparations, and diet aids containing phenylpropanolamine or PPA), myocardial infarction, or factitious administration of catecholamines.[38,39] The diagnosis can be made on the basis of a 24 hour urine collection.[44]

Urine tests 24 hour collections (during hypertension) for free catecholamines or their metabolites, metanephrines and vanillylmanedelic acid (VMA); refrigeration not necessary, but strong acid additive (20 ml 6N HCl) is required. The diagnosis of pheochromocytoma can be made on the basis of a 24 hour urine collection.

Endocrine testing Suppression tests, clonidine: Obtain baseline catecholamine levels; administer oral clonidine (0.3 mg/70 kg body weight); repeat blood sampling after 3 hours; normal response (and patients with essential hypertension): decreased catecholamines (into normal range or by 50%); pheochromocytoma: increased or same.

Provocative tests, (rarely done, potentially hazardous), glucagon: Obtain baseline catecholamine levels; administer 1.0 mg IV bolus of glucagon; repeat blood sampling 2 minutes later; monitor blood pressure and heart rate every 60 seconds; phentolamine (5 mg IV bolus) must be on hand for treatment of severe hypertension; pheochromocytoma is indicated if catecholamines levels triple.[39]

Imaging MIBG (metaiodobenzylguanidine) scan: tumor uptake for localization of extra-adrenal tumors; Effective, but expensive; Adrenal CT scan: tumor localization; MRI scan: tumor localization; Ultrasonography: after localized, to determine attachment to nearby organs (liver or kidney); PET (positron emission tomography) scan: localization of tumor

•••••• Multidisciplinary Plan

Surgery

Preoperative blockade with 7-10 days of phenoxybenzamine; dosage begins at 10 mg bid and increases to 0.5-1.0 mg/kg daily[31]

Excision of pheochromocytoma

Medications[39]

α-Adrenergic blocking agents used to lower atrial pressure and to increase vascular volume

Phentolamine (Regitine), 0.5-5.0 mg IV and/or by continuous infusion at a rate of 0.25 to 1.0 mg/min; short acting (carefully monitor blood pressure)

Phenoxybenzamine (Debenzyline), 10-60 mg/d po; long acting

Prazosin (Minipres), 2.0-5.0 mg, 2 or 3 times a day

β-Adrenergic blocking agents*

Propranolol (Inderal), 40 mg/d po; used for tumors that secrete epinephrine, which causes tachycardia and dysrhythmias

Tyrosine inhibitors

Metyrosine (Demser), 250 mg orally q6-8h up to 4 g/d; interferes with catecholamine synthesis and decreases the amount of circulating catecholamines; useful before and during surgery; causes sedation and reversible extrapyramidal signs in elderly patients; can cause frightening dreams

NURSING CARE

Nursing Assessment

Circulation

Increased heart rate

Palpitations

Postural hypotension

Sustained hypertension (one third of patients)

Paroxysmal hypertension (two thirds of patients)

---

*β-Adrenergic blocking agents should be added only *after* alpha blockade has been achieved. β-Adrenergic blockade alone may exacerbate hypertension.

Food and Fluid

Nausea

Vomiting (possible)

Neurosensory Concerns

Nervousness

Flushing sensation

Comfort and Pain

Headache (severe)

Abdominal or chest pain

Psychosocial Concerns

Anxiety

Sense of impending doom

Coping skills

Hygiene and Skin

Profuse sweating (excessive and inappropriate)

Pallor

Nursing Dx & Intervention

Altered tissue perfusion (total body) related to hypervolemia from excess catecholamines

- Monitor patient's blood pressure and pulse (use same arm; routinely take measurements lying and either sitting or standing).
- In hypertensive crisis:

    Notify physician.

    Have emergency cardiac drugs available (phentolamine, calcium channel blockers).

    Monitor patient's neurologic status frequently.

    Monitor patient's blood pressure and pulse electronically *to monitor for acute cardiovascular and neurologic changes.*
- Perform actions that minimize episode occurrence:

    Do not palpate abdomen.

    Assist patient to avoid constrictive clothing.

    Elevate head of bed.

    Restrict activity.

    Do not allow smoking.

    Eliminate patient's intake of beverages with caffeine.

    Assist patient to avoid Valsalva maneuver or straining at stools.

    Monitor frequency of episodes.

    Identify factor(s) that initiate an episode: coughing, micturition, any abdominal stimulation.

Ineffective individual coping related to situational crisis

- Assess patient's coping skills (especially the ability to tolerate episodic illness), support system, and adaptive skills that have been successful in the past.

- Collaborate with mental health nurse, specialist, or psychiatrist as necessary.
- Provide patient with opportunities to verbalize concerns and fears.
- Involve patient in plan of care *to decrease sources of feelings of powerlessness or loss of control.*

Pain related to sudden change in volume status

- Do not give patient pain medications—may exacerbate episode.
- Use supportive measures: dark room, cool cloth.
- Monitor patient's vital signs.
- Monitor duration of pain and relation to episodes.

Patient Education/Home Care Planning

1. Ensure the patient verbalizes an understanding about medication name, action, schedule, dose, and side effects.
2. Discuss with the patient the importance of regular visits to physician and the necessity of lifelong follow-up.
3. Discuss with the patient the need to carry or wear medical alert information.
4. Demonstrate to the patient how to measure and record blood pressure at home.
5. Ensure that the patient verbalizes an understanding of episode stimulators and how to reduce or eliminate them.

Evaluation

Tissue perfusion is normal   Blood pressure and pulse are within normal range, both lying and standing or sitting. There are no paresthesias, tremors, or palpitations.

Patient copes effectively   Patient identifies strengths and uses them in ADLs. Patient verbalizes ability to manage stressful situations or decrease their frequency. Patient maintains relationships with family and contemporaries. Patient participates in independent self-care.

Pain tolerance is improved   Patient able to tolerate pain without medications.

DISORDERS OF THE PITUITARY GLAND

◼ PITUITARY TUMORS

Pituitary tumors present two problems: intracranial mass and endocrine dysfunction. Tumors often go undetected until neurologic manifestations of the mass become evident. Associated endocrinopathies vary according to the hormone produced by the adenoma.

Pituitary tumors make up 15% of all intracranial tumors.[93] Epidemiologically, pituitary tumors are far more common than is suggested clinically. One autopsy series reported an incidence in the general population of 25%; the majority were undiagnosed.[16] Pituitary tumors are diagnosed more often in women, especially those of childbearing age, but autopsy results reveal an equal distribution between men and women. Prevalence increases with age, peak incidence being between 30 and 60. Rarely is the diagnosis made before puberty.[94] A hereditary predisposition exists for pituitary tumors; they can be part of the familial multiple endocrine neoplasia syndromes. Onset of disease can be slow and insidious making diagnosis difficult.

Recent scientific and technological advances have greatly improved the ability to diagnose and treat pituitary tumors. These advances include the development of (1) highly sensitive hormonal assays, (2) superior resolution imaging technology, (3) microsurgical transsphenoidal techniques, and (4) pharmacotherapeutic advances. Research continues to improve our understanding of the hypothalamic-pituitary interactions and target organ responses.

•••••• Pathophysiology

The origin of pituitary tumors is not fully understood. Two theories exist: some suspect that pituitary tumors result from hypothalamic dysfunction, while others believe tumors arise from an intrinsic pituitary defect.[94,96] Pituitary tumors can be classified functionally according to the hormone that is hypersecreted (Table 9-4).[93]

The pathophysiology of pituitary tumors depends on the size of the tumor and the hormone secreted in excess. In terms of size, tumors are classified as microadenomas (diameter less than 10 mm) or macroadenomas (diameter greater than 10 mm).[94] Larger tumors impinge on the surrounding tissue, including normal pituitary tissue, and can cause varying degrees of hypopituitarism. Other structures that can be affected by large tumors include the bony sella turcica, the optic chiasm, and the hypothalamus. Headaches due to intrasellar pressure are a common finding, regardless of tumor size,[60] although macroadenomas usually have marked symptoms related to pressure from the mass.[96] Pressure on the optic chiasm leads to visual field deficit, scotoma, and blindness. Compression of the pituitary stalk can cause hyperprolactinemia and impairment of portal circulation, leading to pituitary hypofunction. Cavernous sinus impingement can lead to defects of the 3rd, 4th, 5th, and 6th cranial nerves resulting in ptosis, diplopia, facial numbness, and ophthalmoplegia. If temporal and frontal lobes of the brain are invaded, seizures can occur. Hypothalamic involvement can cause disturbances in temperature regulation, appetite, thirst, sleep, and behavior.[61]

The second factor that affects pathophysiology is the hormon produced by the adenoma; physical manifestations vary according to the hormone secreted in excess. *Prolactinomas* represent 50% of all pituitary tumors found at autopsy. Women experience menstrual dysfunction, and men manifest decreased libido and impotence. Men usually do not seek treatment until

the tumor causes hypopituitarism.[93] Direct measurement of prolactin can adequately diagnose hyperprolactinemia; multiple (at least three) measurements should be drawn due to the pulsatile nature of prolactin secretion. Because prolactin is increased by stress, inserting a heparin lock one hour prior to sampling can help avoid false elevations caused by the stress of venipuncture.[104]

GH-secreting adenomas cause gigantism in children and acromegaly in adults. The clinical manifestations of acromegaly progress gradually. Symptoms relate to tumor growth (headache, visual disturbances, hypopituitarism—gonadal dysfunction, hypothyroidism, secondary adrenal insufficiency) or GH hypersecretion (in gigantism, excessive linear growth; in acromegaly, soft tissue thickening of face, lips, nose, scalp, vocal cords, hands and feet, and bony structures of skull, jaw, cheek bones; also arthralgias, backache, excessive sweating, and organomegaly; galactorrhea and mild hirsutism can occur in women; testicular enlargement can occur in men.)[96] GH suppression following oral glucose administration is the best diagnostic test. Other diagnostic tests include the TRH test and dopamine infusion. Tests for GH deficiency include direct measurement by radioimmunoassay, IGF I (Somatomedin C) measurements, insulin tolerance test, arginine stimulation test, L-dopa stimulation test, and clonidine stimulation test.[104] Patients with adenomas producing both GH and PRL often manifest acromegaly and galactorrhea. The galactorrhea responds well to bromocriptine therapy (see multidisciplinary plan).[94]

ACTH-secreting adenomas cause Cushing's disease or Nelson's syndrome (see hypercortisolism). Tests for ACTH production include the CRH stimulation test and the insulin tolerance test.[104] *TSH-secreting adenomas* are extremely rare and usually are accompanied by hyperthyroidism. TSH and gonadotroph secreting tumors are usually slow growing macroadenomas that present through the progressive growth of an intracranial mass, visual disturbance, and hypopituitarism.[93]

Two separate, yet related, disease entities deserve mention in a discussion of pituitary tumors. The first, Nelson's syndrome, is a rare disorder that occurs after bilateral adrenalectomy is performed to treat Cushing's disease. It is characterized by hyperpigmentation and is caused by excessive production of

TABLE 9-4 Incidence of Pituitary Tumors by Type

Type	Incidence
Growth hormone (GL) adenomas	17%
Prolactin PRL adenomas	30%
GH & PRL adenomas	10%
Corticotroph ACTH adenomas	14%
Gonadotroph GNRH adenomas	2%
Other (null cell, oncocytoma, unclassified)	25%

ACTH and melanocyte-stimulating hormone (MSH) by a pituitary tumor. It is believed that this tumor is the original cause of the Cushing's disease and that it enlarges after adrenalectomy because of a lack of negative feedback. Therefore, there is an increase in ACTH and MSH production. The second tumor occurs in the region of the pituitary but does not secrete hormones. This tumor is called a craniopharyngioma; it is important in the differential diagnosis of a sellar mass.

•••••• Diagnostic Studies and Findings

Imaging[108] MRI scan is preferred method for localizing pituitary adenomas; CT scan is an alternative when MRI is unavailable or contraindicated.

Physical examination Ophthalmologic examination for visual field deficits, decreased acuity; neurological examination for cranial nerve deficits associated with cranial nerves III, IV, V, and VI.

Endocrine tests Inappropriate baseline hormone levels in blood or urine; inability to suppress or stimulate hormone secretion normally

•••••• Multidisciplinary Plan

Surgery

Removal of pituitary tumor, preferably by transsphenoidal route; intracranial route may be necessary with large or inaccessible tumors

Medications

- Bromocriptine mesylate (Parlodel): a dopamine receptor antagonist useful for treating prolactinomas and, rarely, GH-secreting adenomas; usual dosage 2.5-10 mg/d for prolactinomas; GH secreting tumors require much higher doses with the upper limit usually determined by patient tolerance; side effects include nausea and vomiting[100]
- Octreotide (Sandostatin): a somatostatin analogue used to treat GH-secreting (acromegaly) and TSH-secreting tumors; 50-150 µg tid by subcutaneous injection; can be used in preparation for surgical tumor removal or after radiation[105]
- Hormone replacement therapy: thyroid, cortisone, estrogen, testosterone following radiation or surgery as needed to treat deficiencies

Radiation

- Radiation therapy, formerly a common treatment for pituitary tumors, has been replaced by microsurgical tumor removal and medications; currently used following incomplete tumor resection or in patients who cannot undergo surgery; side effects include hypopituitarism, damage to the optic chiasm or optic nerves and cranial nerves (resulting in visual deficits), cerebral ischemia, seizures, and development of malignancy;[96] incidence of complications increases in postsurgical patients, and varies among health care centers[96]

NURSING CARE

Nursing Assessment[53,54]

Macroadenomas

- Sensory and vision concerns
  - Bitemporal hemianopsia
  - Superior or bitemporal field defects
  - Loss of red perception
  - Decreased acuity
  - Scotoma
  - Papilledema
  - Blindness
- Neurologic concerns
  - Chronic headaches, intermittent or persistent of moderate intensity, and variably located; can be accompanied by nausea and vomiting
  - Possible neurologic changes, particularly those involving cranial nerves III, IV, V, VI (unequal pupil size, inappropriate reaction to light)
- Endocrine concerns
  - Signs and symptoms of hypofunction (in regard to hormones other than those produced by the tumor)

Growth Hormone–Secreting Tumors (Acromegaly)

- Musculoskeletal concerns
  - Coarse facial features (thick ears, nose)
  - Prognathism causing chewing difficulties
  - Thick fingers and toes with concomitant increase in shoe or glove size
  - Atrophied skeletal muscle
  - Laryngeal hypertrophy causing voice to deepen
  - Arthritis, arthralgia, backaches
  - Osteoporosis
  - Mobility difficulties related to pain, fatigue
- Hygiene and skin
  - Oily skin
  - Acne
  - Diaphoresis
- Psychosocial concerns
  - Irritability, hostility, and other psychologic manifestations
  - Body image disturbance
  - Difficulty with social interactions, including sex partner and family (acting fearful, hostile, withdrawn)
  - Incongruity between self-concept and current self-image

Prolactin-Secreting Tumors

- Gynecologic concerns
  - Galactorrhea involving one or both breasts
  - Irregular menses
  - Oligomenorrhea or amenorrhea
  - Infertility

Androgenic concerns
  Decreased libido
  Impotence
  Gynecomastia
Psychosocial concerns
  Anxiety about fertility, sexual performance, and self-image

Thyroid-stimulating hormone–secreting tumors (see hyperthyroidism)

Adrenocorticotropic hormone–secreting tumors (see Cushing's disease)

Nursing Dx & Intervention

Pain related to physical factors of excess hormones or tumor compression

- Monitor type, location, intensity, and frequency of patient's pain. Inquire about successful and unsuccessful measures patient used in the past to control pain.
- Monitor use and schedule of medications and other physical comfort measures: heat, cold, light massage.
- Discuss with patient factors that precipitate pain and restructure the environment accordingly *to decrease or eliminate these factors.*
- Assist patient to use relaxation techniques; deep breathing, selective focusing.
- Discuss with patient realistic expectations about pain control.

Body image disturbance related to biophysical changes

- See pp. 1685 to 1687.

Anxiety related to change in health status

- Reassess patient's coping behaviors, stresses, and adaptive skills.
- Discuss with patient and family the relationship of psychologic manifestations to the disease process *to increase family understanding and support.*
- Encourage family to avoid blaming patient for inappropriate behavior.
- See also pp. 1669 to 1673.

Sexual dysfunction related to altered libido, menstrual pattern, or fertility

- Establish trusting relationship with patient and sex partner.
- Encourage patient to verbalize feelings, with both health care provider and sex partner.
- Instruct patient and sex partner regarding relationship between disease process and sexual dysfunction.
- Provide patient and sex partner with information about various methods to obtain sexual gratification *to maximize skills of sexual expression.*

Activity intolerance related to generalized weakness

- Monitor patient's current activity levels and priorities for activity performance.
- Thoroughly evaluate patient's abilities and limitations at home and in the community.
- Discuss with patient alternate ways of performing limited activities.
- Help patient structure time to allow for rest periods throughout the day, especially after activities.
- Encourage patient to set realistic goals and prioritize activities *to maximize patient satisfaction.*

Patient Education/Home Care Planning

1. Discuss with the patient methods for modifying pain control program for use at home: structuring a supportive physical environment and appropriate self-administration of analgesics.
2. Discuss with the patient community mental health resources (support groups, individual therapists, and so forth).
3. Discuss with the patient methods for modifying activity program for use at home.
4. Ensure that the patient verbalizes understanding of medication administration and the need for follow-up examinations.

Evaluation

Comfort is increased   Patient verbalizes a decreased frequency and amount of pain. Patient verbalizes pain-precipitating factors and means of decreasing or eliminating these factors. Patient demonstrates relaxation techniques. Patient follows a pain control program.

Body image improves   Patient verbalizes acceptance of body changes. Patient maintains relationships with others. Behavior is appropriate during interactions. Patient maintains physical appearance appropriate to age. Patient verbalizes and expresses feelings and concerns about differences between ideal self and realistic self.

Anxiety is decreased   Patient can identify results of ineffective coping mechanisms. Patient used strengths in planning home care. Patient discusses alternate home care methods and makes positive choices.

Sexual functioning improves   Patient verbalizes feelings about sexual dysfunction. Patient expresses an understanding of the relationship between prolactinoma and sexual dysfunction or infertility. Patient verbalizes improvement in sexual functioning.

Activity tolerance improves   Patient identifies increased number of activities performed independently. Patient demonstrates active range-of-motion exercises and performs these three times daily. Patient demonstrates an ability to structure day, including all ADLs and appropriate rest periods.

DIABETES INSIPIDUS

Diabetes insipidus can be transient or permanent disturbance of water metabolism that results in the excretion of a large volume of dilute urine. It may be hypothalamic, nephrogenic, or psychogenic in nature.

Central (or hypothalamic) diabetes insipidus results from a failure of vasopressin synthesis or release from the neurohypophysis. Nephrogenic diabetes insipidus results from a deficiency of vasopressin action in the renal collecting ducts. Psychogenic diabetes insipidus (polydipsia) is the result of a large fluid intake that suppresses antidiuretic hormone (ADH) secretion.[5] All these causes result in the excretion of large volumes of dilute urine. The treatment of central diabetes insipidus is the administration of potent vasopressin analogues. The treatment of nephrogenic insipidus is confined to genetic counseling. The treatment of psychogenic polydipsia is psychiatric in nature.

•••••• Pathophysiology

The maintenance of water homeostasis is a function of the posterior pituitary gland and the kidney. The neurohypophysis secretes antidiuretic hormone (ADH), a polypeptide hormone with marked antidiuretic properties. ADH acts on the collecting duct of the nephron and regulates its permeability to water. In the absence of ADH, an average adult will produce 10 to 12 L of dilute (specific gravity = 1.001; osmolality = 100 mOsm/kg) urine daily. In the presence of maximal vasopressin concentrations, urine flow can be reduced to less than 0.5 L/day of very concentrated (specific gravity = 1.035; osmolality = 1000 mOsm/kg) urine.[53]

Central diabetes insipidus can be caused by head trauma, neurosurgery, hypothalamic tumors, or infiltrative diseases. Half of all cases are idiopathic. Diabetes insipidus is transient when the supraoptic hypophyseal tract is damaged below the median eminence, and it is permanent when damage is above the median eminence. Only 10% of the neurosecretory neurons need be present to prevent diabetes insipidus. It may be corrected by vasopressin replacement therapy.[5]

Nephrogenic diabetes insipidus can be acquired or inherited (rare, but severe). The inherited form is sex linked and usually is clinically manifest in infancy as severe polyuria, dehydration, and failure to thrive.[5] It can be acquired in association with disorders causing a decrease in glomerular filtration rate (chronic renal disease, electrolyte disturbances, pharmacologic agents, sickle cell disease, or dietary abnormalities) and prolonged polyuria (hypothalamic DI). Treatment of nephrogenic diabetes insipidus is directed toward the primary disorder and may involve the use of diuretics that can produce a paradoxical antidiuretic effect that enhances fluid reabsorption.

Psychogenic polydipsia results in the same clinical picture as central and nephrogenic diabetes insipidus. This disorder is dangerous only when intake exceeds renal capacity to excrete water. Treatment is directed at control of fluid intake.

•••••• Diagnostic Studies and Findings

The diagnostic triad of diabetes insipidus is serum hypotonicity (>300 mOsm/L) in association with a dilute urine in volumes inappropriate for the clinical state of the patient, that is, there is a net loss of free water.

Partial defects in ADH secretion can often be revealed with the dehydration test. Water is withheld until urine osmolalities stabilize, or 5% of body weight has been lost. Antidiuretic hormone is then administered. An increase in urine osmolality of >15% suggests central DI; <15% suggests nephrogenic DI.[5]

•••••• Multidisciplinary Plan

Medications

Desmopressin (DDAVP; synthetic arginine, vasopressin), 5-40 µg/d in 1-3 divided doses; administer by nasal insufflation (high in nose, not inhaled into throat); onset 1 h; duration of effects 8-20 h; drug of choice for chronic treatment because of its long duration and infrequent side effects

Lypressin nasal solution (Diapid Nasal Spray; synthetic lysine), 1 or 2 sprays in one or both nostrils qid; onset 1 h; duration 3-8 h; may be used alone or in conjunction with vasopressin tannate; if patient has nasal congestion, there will be decreased absorption of drug

Vasopressin (Aqueous Pitressin), 2-5 U 2-4 times daily IM, subcutaneously, or IV; duration of drug: 2-8 h; used in acute settings or for initial emergency treatment; for close monitoring during transient episodes; too short acting for chronic use; used for differential diagnosis of diabetes mellitus

NURSING CARE

Nursing Assessment

Thirst

Polydipsia
Unquenchable thirst
Preference for cold or iced water

Urinary Function

Polyuria (output greater than 2.5 L/24 hours × 2 days with ad lib fluid intake)[5]
Frequency
Nocturia
Low specific gravity (1.001 to 1.005)

Hydration Status

Poor skin turgor
Dry skin
Weight loss

Bowel Function

Constipation

Nursing Dx & Intervention

Fluid-volume deficit related to output greater than intake from loss of antidiuretic hormone

- Monitor for signs and symptoms of dehydration: dry mouth, poor skin turgor, soft eyes, low blood pressure, fast pulse, output greater than intake, and weight loss.
- Measure urine output. *With diabetes insipidus, urine output is usually greater than 4 L/day and may exceed 10 L/day if severe. Rule of thumb: patient voiding more than 200 ml/ hour of dilute urine indicates presence of diabetes insipidus.*
- Obtain accurate daily weight *to assess fluid loss.*
- Specific gravity measurement is not necessary *because urine excretion rates of this magnitude can occur only with dilute urine except in case of diabetes mellitus.*
- Measure urine glucose *to exclude diabetes mellitus as cause of polyuria* ("insipidus" means tasteless, "mellitus" means sweet).
- Measure plasma osmolality. *If thirst mechanism is normal, plasma osmolality will be in high normal range. If thirst mechanism is abnormal, plasma osmolality will be above normal.*

Patient Education/Home Care Planning

1. Demonstrate to the patient how to measure and record intake and output.
2. Demonstrate to the patient how to administer vasopressin; discuss with the patient side or toxic effects to report to physician and the parameters for as-needed administration based on output volume and characteristics.
3. Demonstrate to the patient how to check the urine's specific gravity.
4. Discuss with the patient the importance of wearing a medical alert bracelet to identify the disorder.

Evaluation

Hydration is adequate Adequate hydration is evidenced by moist mucous membranes, good skin turgor, firm eyes, normal vital signs, stable weight, and intake approximate to output. Urine output is less than 4 L/day. Plasma osmolality is normal (285 to 290 mOsm/L).

SYNDROME OF INAPPROPRIATE ANTIDIURESIS

The syndrome of the inappropriate secretion of antidiuretic hormone is the result of a continuous secretion of antidiuretic hormone when plasma osmolality is low, that is, at a time when ADH secretion should be inhibited. This results in a state of dilutional hyponatremia.[90]

The clinical criteria established by Bartter and Schwartz in 1967 include:[2]

1. Hyponatremia with low plasma osmolality.
2. Urine osmolality greater than plasma osmolality.
3. Excessive renal sodium excretion.
4. Absence of hypotension, hypovolemia, and edema.
5. Normal renal and adrenal function.

The syndrome of inappropriate antidiuresis (SIAD) is one of the most common causes of hyponatremia. Etiologies include head trauma, central nervous system neoplasms, pulmonary disease, certain endocrinopathies, and some pharmacologic agents such as morphine and barbiturates. The following outline provides a complete listing of conditions that may predispose a patient to SIAD.[101]

1. Central nervous system disorders
   Brain tumor
   Head injury
   Cerebral hemorrhage
   Infections:
      Meningitis
      Encephalitis
      Abscess
   Guillain-Barré syndrome
   Acute intermittent porphyria
   Cerebellar and cerebral atrophy
   Cavernous sinus thrombosis
   Neonatal hypoxia
   Rocky Mountain spotted fever
   Delirium tremens
2. Pulmonary disorders
   Pneumonia
   Tuberculosis
   Cystic fibrosis
   Cavitation (aspergillosis)
   Abscess
   Empyema
   Pneumothorax
   Asthma
   Positive pressure breathing
3. Hypovolemia and hypotension
   Sodium-losing renal disease
   Adrenal insufficiency
   Hemorrhage
4. Endocrinopathies
   Addison's disease
   Hypopituitarism
   Myxedema
5. Tumors producing ectopic ADH
   Mesothelioma
   Carcinoma of lung, duodenum, pancreas, ureter, bladder, prostate
   Thymoma
   Ewing's sarcoma
   Lymphoma, leukemia
   Hodgkin's disease
   Bronchial adenoma

6. Pharmacologic agents
   Drugs that increase tubular reabsorption of water:
   Vasopressin, oxytocin
   Drugs that stimulate the release of ADH:
   Vincristine, vinblastine, cisplatin
   Nicotine
   Morphine
   Barbiturates
   General anesthesia
   Drugs potentiating the action of ADH:
   Chlorpropamide
   Carbamazepine
   Thiazide diuretics
   Phenothiazides
7. Acute psychosis
8. Idiopathic causes

Antidiuretic hormone (ADH) also can be secreted by nonpituitary neoplasms such as oat cell carcinoma of the lung. The most common form of treatment is water restriction, but current research in the area is directed primarily at devising improved therapies. For example, lithium salts and demeclocycline can antagonize the effects of ADH and have found a place in the treatment of this syndrome.[101]

•••••• Pathophysiology

The syndrome of inappropriate antidiuresis occurs when there is continuous synthesis and release of ADH in the presence of serum hypo-osmolality. Normally, when plasma osmolality drops, production and release of ADH are reduced, resulting in a diuresis. In SIAD, antidiuretic hormone release continues in the face of a subnormal serum osmolality. This also results in a simultaneous urine osmolality that is greater than that of serum. Dilutional hyponatremia occurs in SIAD from an increase in tubular reabsorption of water. The retention of water causes an expansion of plasma volume. This increase in intravascular fluid causes an increase in the glomerular filtration rate, and the reabsorption of sodium and water in the renal tubules is inhibited. The expansion of the plasma volume also inhibits the release of renin and aldosterone. This further increases the loss of sodium in urine and intensifies the dilutional hyponatremia. Because SIAD results in the retention of free water and not salt, edema is not a feature of this disorder.[90]

•••••• Diagnostic Studies and Findings

Serum osmolality   Below normal (less than 285 mOsm/L)
Urine osmolality   Above normal (greater than the simultaneous serum osmolality)
Serum sodium   Below normal (less than 135 mEq/L)

•••••• Multidisciplinary Plan

Medications

Demeocycline (600-1200 mg daily) to block antidiuretic action of vasopressin[5]

Diuretics

Furosemide (Lasix), 40-80 mg/day in divided doses, or 20-40 mg/day IV with salt supplementation (3 g/day)
Hypertonic saline, dosage individually calculated

General Management

Fluid restriction (free water restriction) 500 ml/24 hours to increase sodium levels

NURSING CARE

Nursing Assessment

Fluids and Electrolytes

Euvolemia
Decreased volume of urine
Increased specific gravity of urine
Increased weight
Abdominal and muscle cramping

Neurologic Changes

Early sign: change in level of consciousness, confusion
Disorientation; uncooperativeness
Hostility
Increased deep tendon reflexes
Drowsiness
Lethargy
Headache
Increased seizure potential

Gastrointestinal Changes

Anorexia
Nausea and vomiting
Diarrhea (from water intoxication)
Constipation (from fluid restriction and hyponatremia motility)

Psychosocial Changes

Anxiety
Frustration
Irritability
Uncooperativeness
Hostility

Nursing Dx & Intervention

Altered thought processes related to fluid excess

- Check orientation to time, place, and person *to assess for confusion and level of consciousness.*
- Set limits as necessary *to maintain stable and safe environment.*
- Reduce confusing environmental stimuli.
- Explain rationale for disturbances in thought processes to family members.

Evaluation

Fluid volume is normal Intake is approximately equal to output. Specific gravity is within normal limits. Vital signs are within normal limits. Weight of patient is stable.

Thought processes are normal Patient is oriented to time, place, and person. There is no injury to self, others, or property. Statements are reality oriented. Patient performs ADLs, within physical limitations, independently.

DISORDERS OF THE THYROID GLAND

◼ THYROTOXICOSIS/HYPERTHYROIDISM

Thyrotoxicosis is the term used to mean the clinical syndrome that results when circulating concentrations of thyroxine (T_4) or triiodothyronine (T_3) are increased. Hyperthyroidism is the term used to mean sustained increases in thyroid hormone biosynthesis and release from the thyroid gland.[9] The terms are not directly interchangeable although many patients have both.

•••••• Pathophysiology

There are many causes of thyrotoxicosis with and without hyperthyroidism. Table 9-5 presents an outline of possible disorders, their incidence, and underlying causes. Also included is whether the disorder is thyrotoxicosis alone (T) or thyrotoxicosis accompanied by hyperthyroidism (T&H).

Graves' Disease

Graves' disease is the most common cause of thyrotoxicosis with hyperthyroidism. It occurs from two to ten times more frequently in women than in men.[15] Graves' disease is an autoimmune disorder in which thyroid stimulating hormone (TSH) receptor antibodies bind to the TSH receptors in the thyroid gland. These antibodies mimic pituitary TSH causing an increase in thyroid hormone synthesis and release that is unresponsive to the normal negative feedback signals. The receptor antibodies are from two families of immunoglobulins called thyroid stimulating immunoglobulins (TSIs) or thyroid binding inhibiting immunoglobulins (TBIIs), both of which can be measured in serum. There is a genetic preponderance for the development of Graves' disease, although it is unknown what specifically triggers the production of the antibodies. The genetic linkage may be with other autoimmune thyroid disorders such as Hashimoto's thyroiditis, which is an underlying cause of hypothyroidism, or it may be with other systemic autoimmune disorders such as rheumatoid arthritis, pernicious anemia, or lupus. TSH stimulates growth as well as hormone synthesis resulting in a diffusely enlarged thyroid gland (diffuse toxic goiter) with increased vascularity.

TSIs also have the ability to attach to TSH receptors outside of the thyroid gland and are the presumed causative agent for Graves' ophthalmopathy, which has been partially defined as T-lymphocyte infiltration and fibroblast proliferation of orbital connective tissue leading to edema and enlargement of eye muscles.[12] Infiltrative dermopathy called pretibial myxedema has also been described, but seems to occur less frequently than ophthalmopathy. The most rare complication is thyroid acropachy, which is a process of soft tissue swelling similar to localized myxedema, but is associated with clubbing of the digits and subperiosteal new bone formation.[102] These problems do not affect all patients with Graves' disease, although both an increased occurrence and severity of ophthalmopathy have been seen in people who smoke.[12]

There is no treatment that directly affects the presence or level of TSIs. They may increase and decrease over a person's lifetime. Treatment of Graves' disease is therefore directed to the target organ, the thyroid gland. This also means that TSIs may independently continue to affect a person's eyes or skin even years after the Graves' disease has been treated.

Clinical signs and symptoms may affect any body organ. The most common include tachycardia, heat intolerance, hyperkinesis, tremor, fatigue, increased sweating, conjunctivitis or chemosis, anxiety, restlessness, and irritability. These symptoms may be absent in the older person, who may experience atrial flutter/fibrillation alone. Laboratory tests usually show elevated levels of T_4 and T_3 with suppressed or undetectable levels of TSH. If TSH is in the normal range, than a TSH-secreting pituitary tumor must be suspected.

There are three general treatments available for Graves' disease. These are anti-thyroid medication, radioactive iodine, and surgery. Anti-thyroid medication lowers thyroid hormone levels by blocking synthesis of new thyroid hormone by the thyroid gland. They are usually combined with a beta blocker to aid in adrenergic-related symptom relief. If the patient has a small gland and is willing to have frequent blood tests and take medication for 12 to 18 months, then there is a 50% chance of remission of the Graves'. Recurrence could occur within the first year after treatment or at any time afterwards. Long term use of these agents is more frequently recommended in Europe or Japan than in the United States.[83]

A common goal of therapy is destruction of the thyroid gland so that the thyrotoxicosis cannot return. Although radioactive iodine is the usual treatment of choice in the United States, surgery may be recommended in special circumstances.[83] The usual outcome of both of these therapies is hypothyroidism so that the patient will require life-long thyroid hormone replacement therapy.

Toxic Nodule/Multinodular Goiter

A nodule is a lump in the thyroid gland; these lumps may be singular (solitary) or multiple (multinodular). Some of these

TABLE 9-5 Varieties of Thyrotoxicosis (T) and Hyperthyroidism (H)

Disorder	Incidence	Cause
Graves' disease (Basedow's disease; often referred to as toxic diffuse goiter)	More common in women during third and fourth decades of life; estimated to occur in 0.4% of U.S. population	An autoimmune disorder resulting from thyroid-stimulating immunoglobulins (T&H)
Subacute thyroiditis (granulomatous, giant-cell, or de Quervain's thyroiditis	Uncommon; more frequent in women; increased incidence during fourth and fifth decades; tendency for seasonal and geographic aggregations; mild hyperthyroidism in about 50% of cases	Probable viral infection of gland results in: Destruction of follicular epithelium Loss of follicular integrity Release of large quantities of preformed hormones and abnormal iodinated materials (T)
Painless thyroiditis/Post partum thyroiditis	Increasing in general population; occurs in 7% of pregnant women	Painless thyroiditis is a type of chronic autoimmune thyroiditis (T)
Toxic multinodular goiter (Plummer's disease)	Unknown: more frequent in women in the sixth or seventh decade; usually a long history of gradually increasing thyroid enlargement	Hyperfunctioning autonomous thyroid tissue (T&H)
Toxic nodule (solitary autonomous nodule)	Female/male ratio: 3:1 to 6:1; US incidence: 5% of hyperthyroid patients; adults: all ages, especially in younger age group in 30s and 40s; occasionally seen in children	Adenoma functions autonomously; with continued growth, the adenoma assumes a greater share of glandular function and ultimately results in atrophy and complete suppression of the remainder of the gland; adenoma may infarct, resulting in a change from hyperfunctioning to hypofunctioning nodule with relief from hyperthyroidism (T&H)
Exogenous hyperthyroidism, iatrogenic	Clinically has elevated hormone levels and symptoms; subclinical has suppressed TSH, normal T_4 and T_3, no symptoms	L-Thyroxine L-Triiodothyronine (T)
Factitious (thyrotoxicosis factitia)	More common in women with background of underlying psychiatric disease, paramedical personnel with access to thyroid hormone, or patients for whom thyroid medications have been prescribed in the past	Chronic ingestion of excessive quantities of thyroid hormone (T)
Iodide-induced hyperthyroidism (Jod-Basedow)	Iodide-deficient populations (usually in patients with underlying thyroid disorders) or in multinodular goiter)	Administration of supplemental iodine to individuals with endemic, iodine-deficiency goiters; hyperthyroidism may be induced in patients with nonendemic goiter when large quantities of iodine are administered in the form of expectorants, x-ray contrast media, medications containing iodine, or any other form (T&H)
Ectopic hyperthyroidism (struma ovarii)	Very rare, usually mild, no exophthalmos	Dermoid tumor or teratoma of ovary that contains a hyperfunctioning thyroid adenoma (T)
Pituitary thyrotropin (TSH)	Rare tumor, usually large and seen on CT scan	Excessive TSH secretion from a pituitary tumor or inappropriate TSH secretion caused by pituitary resistance to thyroid hormone (T&H)
Trophoblastic tumor	Hyperthyroidism occurs in 10%-20% of patients	Tumors of trophoblastic origin: hydatidiform mole, choriocarcinoma or embryonal carcinoma of the testis with very high levels of chorionic gonadotropin, lower ratios of T_3/T_4 than Grave's disease

nodules are considered non-functional (do not make thyroid hormone, cold on scintigraphy) or functional (make thyroid hormone; warm, hot on scintigraphy). A functional nodule that makes a continuous uninterrupted amount of thyroid hormone and is unresponsive to normal negative feedback signals is called autonomous. The symptoms tend to be mild without the eye or skin complications of Graves' disease. Surgery is usually recommended for these problems, although radioactive iodine may be used in patients at risk from surgery. Anti-thyroid drugs are used to lower thyroid hormone levels prior to surgery.

Thyroiditis

Postpartum thyroiditis is also an autoimmune thyroid disease. The antibodies involved (antimicrosomal, antithyroglobulin) are associated with lymphocytic infiltration of the thyroid gland, which may interfere with thyroid hormone synthesis or release. Pregnancy decreases immunologic responsiveness to all types of antibodies, whereas parturition is a trigger for increased immunologic responsiveness. These patients may have a hyperthyroid phase, with a return to normal or a hyperthyroid phase followed by a prolonged hypothyroid phase. They may eventually become euthyroid, or they may remain permanently hypothyroid. The chance of postpartum thyroiditis occurring increases with each subsequent pregnancy.[84] Graves' disease may also occur in the first six to nine months postpartum.

Subacute thyroiditis is a spontaneously resolving inflammation of the thyroid gland thought to be of viral origin. Like postpartum thyroiditis, it can have a hyperthyroid phase followed by a hypothyroid phase before the gland recovers with a return to normal thyroid hormone synthesis and release. Each phase may last from two to ten weeks. Unlike postpartum thyroiditis, antibodies are negative and the patient may experience fever or pain in the thyroid area that may radiate to the neck or jaw. Because the hyperthyroid phase is usually of short duration, beta blockers along with aspirin will provide symptomatic relief, although some patients may require corticosteroid therapy.

Subclinical Hyperthyroidism

Subclinical hyperthyroidism is defined as normal T_4 and T_3 levels with a suppressed or undetectable TSH level. It usually occurs as a result of exogenous thyroid hormone therapy. This may be purposeful as a goal of suppressive therapy for thyroid cancer, non-toxic multinodular goiter, or a solitary cold nodule. It may also occur inadvertently as a result of overzealous thyroid hormone replacement therapy. Hyperthyroidism is known to increase osteoclast activity of bone with a loss of bone mineral mass. The occurrence of fractures in postmenopausal women with hyperthyroidism, while no different in location, tend to occur about ten years earlier than in postmenopausal women with other types of thyroid disorders.[85] It has been postulated that subclinical hyperthyroidism may also decrease bone mass, increasing the risk of osteoporosis. This continues to be an area of controversy and ongoing research. Subclinical hyperthyroidism has recently been shown to be an independent risk factor for atrial fibrillation. A threefold higher risk was found in patients 60 years of age or older.[79] This may put the patient at a higher risk for embolic events that may result from the atrial fibrillation.

Thyroid Storm

Very severe hyperthyroidism is called thyroid storm. Its most common cause is Graves' disease, although it has occurred in people with toxic multinodular goiters. Thyroid storm may occur if the patient has delayed seeking medical treatment, has not been compliant with anti-thyroid drug therapy, or has not been responsive to anti-thyroid drug therapy. This condition may be life-threatening and is the usual reason a patient may be admitted to a hospital for hyperthyroidism or thyrotoxicosis (see Emergency Alert box).

EMERGENCY ALERT

THYROID STORM

A complex hypermetabolic decompensation with symptoms and signs such as high fever, agitation, tachycardia, tachyarrhythmias, congestive heart failure, and often a psychotic component. *Hyperthyroidism* is generally categorized into three types: overproducing thyroid gland, thyrotoxicosis with an increased amount of hormone in circulation (i.e., overside), and drug-induced hyperthyroidism (i.e., iodine, lithium). Thyroid storm does not occur at a specific hormone level threshold, but its onset appears to be precipitated by factors such as surgery, hospitalization, trauma, stress, cerebral vascular accident (CVA), diabetic ketoacidosis (DKA), congestive heart failure (CHF), infection, and other disorders.

Assessment

- Obtain history to rule out hyperthyroidism.
- Assess body temperature (often fever >100-105° F).
- Assess cardiovascular status: (often heart rate >200 beats/minute); increased systolic blood pressure, premature ventricular contractions (PVCs), congestive heart failure.
- Assess central nervous system, gastrointestinal, or cardiovascular system dysfunction.
- Assess neurosensory system for presence of fine tremors, restlessness, anxiety, labile mood, manic behavior, psychosis.
- Determine presence of diarrhea, nausea, vomiting, abdominal cramps, jaundice.

Interventions

- Aggressive intervention is important.
- Obtain IV access and provide fluid resuscitation.
- Administer high flow oxygen (10-15 L/minute) by mask.
- Reduce thyroid levels as rapidly as possible; possible therapies may include Tapazole, Lugol's solution, propranolol, dexamethasone, occasionally peritoneal dialysis, plasmapheresis or charcoal hemodialysis may be indicated.
- Provide supportive care and fever control.

• • • • • • Diagnostic Studies and Findings

Laboratory findings   Serum T_4 increased; serum T_3 increased; serum free T_4 and T_3 increased; thyroid radioiodine uptake and scan, increased uptake in most patients with hyperthyroidism except patients with subacute thyroiditis, painless thyroiditis, and exogenous hyperthyroidism.

3rd Generation TSH   Suppressed and does not respond to TRH; thyroid-stimulating immunoglobulins (TSI) present in Graves' disease

• • • • • • Multidisciplinary Plan

Surgery

Thyroidectomy (toxic multinodular goiter or toxic nodule, occasionally in Graves' disease)

Medications

Thiomides

Propylthiouracil (PTU), 50-800 mg/d in 3-4 doses po for adults; initially 300-600 mg/d; inhibits thyroid hormone synthesis but not release; inhibits extra thyroidal conversion of T_4 to T_3; used to lower thyroid hormone levels; agranulocytosis may occur in 1.4% of patients during first 2 mo of therapy; skin rashes occur in roughly 3% of patients

Methimazole (Tapazole) (MMI), 5-80 mg/d po in 2-3 doses for adults; initially 30-60 mg/d in either a single daily dose or 3-4 doses inhibits thyroid hormone synthesis but not release; similar to PTU; does not inhibit T_4 to T_3 conversion

Oral cholecystographic agents (Ipodate), adults: oral, 1.5-3 g; rapidly inhibits extrathyroidal T_3 production; may be useful for short-term therapy for the occasional patient in whom antithyroid drug treatment or ^{131}I is contraindicated

β-Adrenergic blockers (atenolol 50 mg po daily)

Propranolol (Inderal), 20-80 mg/d po in divided doses for adults; 5 mg or less IV at 1 mg/min or more slowly for adults; controls symptoms of hyperthyroidism but does not lower T_3 and T_4 levels; controls palpitations, tremor, sweating, proximal muscle weakness, and cardiac symptoms of hyperthyroidism by competitively blocking β-adrenergic receptors; bronchospasm may occur in asthmatics

Iodides

Potassium or sodium iodide (Strong Iodine Solution, SSKI, Lugol's Solution), 0.1-0.3 ml po tid for adults (SSKI 5-10 drops several times a day); IV 250-500 mg/d for adults in thyrotoxic crisis; produces short-term inhibition of thyroid hormone secretion; used as presurgical medication to reduce size of thyroid gland after thiomide therapy; used with thiomide and propranolol for hyperthyroid crisis

Radioactive iodine (^{131}I NaI)

Adults, up to 29.9 mCi as a single dose

Dose is calculated from uptake and gland size; smaller doses are used for diagnostic purposes; concentrated in the thyroid and release radiation, which destroys thyroid tissue; used to destroy thyroid tissue without surgery for control of hyperthyroidism; hypothyroidism ultimately develops in most patients

General Management

Treatment of Graves' disease ophthalmopathy (often no cure)

Palliative treatment

Corticosteroids

Surgical orbital decompression

Surgical correction of muscle imbalance

Radiation of orbit

0.5% methylcellulose eye drops for eye irritation and pain

Treatment of Graves' disease dermopathy (often no cure)

Palliative treatment for extensive bulbous or ulcerated lesions

0.2% fluocinolone or other corticosteroid cream

NURSING CARE

Nursing Assessment

Skin and Appendages

Warm and moist; smooth velvety texture; erythema

Increased body temperature (37.8° C or greater may indicate thyroid storm)

Increased sweating

Hyperhidrosis

Alopecia

Hyperpigmentation

Onycholysis

Acropachy

Pretibial myxedema

Urticaria

Puritis

Vitiligo

Eyes

Lid retraction and lag

Proptosis

Conjunctival irritation; lacrimation, chemosis

Characteristic bright-eyed, frightened, or startled look (exophthalmos)

Cardiovascular Status

Increased systolic blood pressure; wide pulse pressure

Tachycardia, palpitations

Presence of dysrhythmias

Shortness of breath

Gastrointestinal Status

Weight loss or modest weight gain (especially if large food intake; seen in younger patients)

Polyphagia; increased food intake

Hyperdefecation or diarrhea

Tremor of tongue

Increased thirst

Muscular Status

Generalized muscular wasting and weakness

Hyperactive deep tendon reflexes

Noticeable tremor

Nervous System Status

Fatigue

Restlessness; irritability

Insomnia

Heat intolerance

Mental and Emotional Status

Decreased ability to concentrate, memory loss, easily distracted
Emotionally labile; irritable
Manic behavior
Family members report changes in performance
Anxiety/depression

Nursing Dx & Intervention

Decreased cardiac output related to alteration in rate

- Monitor patient's pulse, blood pressure, color, and temperature to evaluate cardiovascular status and effectiveness of treatment.
- Measure and record patient's intake and output *to detect fluid overload and impending heart failure.*

Fatigue related to increased energy requirements

- Help patient identify work and home demands.
- Formulate with patient options for decreasing demands (delegating home tasks, reduction in work hours).
- Help patient plan a schedule that includes rest.

Hyperthermia related to increased metabolic rate

- Regulate environmental temperature; place patient in cool and quiet room.
- Have patient wear light clothing.
- Provide light bed linens (sheet only).

Altered thought processes related to physiologic changes and sleep deprivation

- Avoid discrepancies in timing, activities, and methods of performing procedures.
- Provide physically and emotionally safe environment for patient.
- Explain procedures slowly and carefully *to facilitate patient concentration.*
- Repeat instructions to patient and limit number of instructions. Provide written instructions.
- Limit number of caregivers *to facilitate routines and decrease distractions.*
- Decrease external stimuli *to minimize distractions and increase the hyperactive patient's ability to concentrate.*

Activity intolerance related to imbalance between oxygen supply and demand

- Monitor patient's ability to perform activities of daily living.
- Provide rest periods for patient between all activities.
- Reassess need for assisting patient after discharge.

Risk for injury (cornea and conjunctiva) related to inadequate tearing

- Monitor patient's eyes for symptoms of dryness.
- Give patient artificial tears frequently.
- Reassess patient's need for lubricated eye patch or gel.

Patient Education/Home Care Planning

1. Give patient a list of the signs and symptoms of hypothyroidism.
2. Patient verbalizes understanding of medication, name, dosage, action, frequency, and importance of taking medications on schedule.
3. Discuss with patient on outpatient follow-up visits whether plan needs modification after implementation.
4. Discuss with patient the importance of planned rest and avoidance of excessive exercise.
5. Discuss with the patient and family the possibility that the patient may have emotional outbursts and may need support.
6. Discuss with the patient the importance of follow-up evaluations.
7. Recommend patient and family read "Your Thyroid: A Home Reference."[109]

Evaluation

Cardiovascular function is normal Dysrhythmias are absent or less frequent. Patient's skin remains warm and dry.

Fatigue is managed Patient establishes a plan of rest and activity that enables fulfillment of role and energy demands.

Comfort is increased Patient identifies and uses several techniques to control heat intolerance.

Thought processes are normal Patient demonstrates increased problem-solving ability and judgement.

Activity tolerance is improved Patient is able to perform most activities of daily living independently.

Eyes have adequate protection Patient is able to self-administer artificial tears or lubricant.

■ HYPOTHYROIDISM

Hypothyroidism is the clinical and biochemical syndrome that results from deficient thyroid hormone production and is ameliorated by administration of exogenous thyroid hormone.

Hypothyroidism is a common disorder affecting both sexes from birth through old age. Overt hypothyroidism is a combination of low thyroxine (T_4) and low triiodothyronine (T_3) with increased TSH levels accompanied by easily identified physical signs and symptoms. Subclinical hypothyroidism denotes biochemical abnormalities without the presence of clinical signs or symptoms. Subclinical hypothyroidism may have normal T_4 and T_3 levels, with either a slightly elevated TSH level or a normal TSH level which rises to higher levels only at the time of provocative testing.

Hypothyroidism occurs two to eight times more often in women than in men with the incidence increasing with age. The reported frequencies vary widely depending on the population studied. Overt hypothyroidism may occur in from

1 to 2 per 1000 persons to as high as 18 per 1000 elderly persons. In persons seeking medical care 5 to 20 per 1000 have had overt hypothyroidism. Subclinical hypothyroidism has reportedly been found in 20 to 120 per 1000 persons in the community.[99]

The many causes of hypothyroidism are listed in Table 9-6. If the cause of the hypothyroidism is within the thyroid gland, it is called *primary hypothyroidism*. If the cause lies within the pituitary gland, it may be termed *secondary hypothyroidism*, while loss of TRH from the hypothalamus may be called *tertiary hypothyroidism*. These last two are also known as *central hypothyroidism*.

•••••• Pathophysiology

Hashimoto's Thyroiditis

Hashimoto's thyroiditis, also known as chronic lymphocytic thyroiditis or autoimmune thyroiditis, is the most common cause of hypothyroidism in the United States, while iodine deficiency is the leading cause of hypothyroidism worldwide. Hashimoto's thyroiditis is characterized by the presence of circulating antimicrosomal antibodies (antiperoxidase autoantibodies) and/or antithyroglobulin antibodies, which are often at very high levels. These antibodies lead to infiltration of the thyroid gland with lymphocytes, designated killer or K lympho-

▌ TABLE 9-6 Varieties of Hypothyroidism

Variety	Incidence	Cause
Chronic autoimmune thyroiditis Hashimoto's thyroiditis	Most common cause of spontaneously occurring hypothyroidism in both children and adults More common in older women Strong hereditary risk factor (thyroid autoantibodies are found in up to 50% of siblings of patients)[99] Patients and their relatives have a higher incidence of other associated autoimmune disorders	Autoimmune disorder; probably results from both cell- and antibody-mediated thyroid injury Characterized by antimicrosomal and antithyroglobulin antibodies in serum, often in very high titer; more prevalent in HLA-DR3 and DR5 haplotypes
Transient autoimmune thyroiditis	Most often occurs in postpartum period; rare in other populations Usually appears 3 to 6 months after delivery Recurrences following subsequent pregnancies are common	Autoimmune disorder; characterized by development of modest thyroid enlargement, hypothyroidism, and high titers of antithyroid microsomal antibodies may progress to permanent hypothyroidism
Hypothyroidism after radioiodine therapy and external neck radiation therapy	Common occurrence within a year after therapy with ^{131}I for hyperthyroidism (thereafter it occurs at a rate of 0.5% to 2% per year)	Radioiodine (^{131}I) therapy; external neck radiation therapy using doses of 2500 rad or more[83]
Postoperative hypothyroidism	Following total thyroidectomy: takes 3-4 wks Following subtotal thyroidectomy: less predictable, ranges from 2% to 75% in first few years after surgery Following thyroidectomy for hyperthyroid Graves' disease: 25% to 75% occurrence in first year	Surgery with loss of thyroid tissue or damage to it
Transient hypothyroidism from subacute painful thyroiditis	Several weeks or months following hypothyroidism	Part of recovery from initial viral insult
Thyroid dysgenesis (sporadic nongoitrous cretinism)	Most common cause of hypothyroidism in newborn; occurs in 1 of every 4000 to 5000 births)	Developmental defects of thyroid gland; cause is unknown
Hypothyroidism caused by iodine deficiency	Most common cause of hypothyroidism in many parts of world	Iodine deficiency resulting in decreased production of thyroid hormones; important contributing factors are dietary goitrogens, genetic factors, and water pollution
Hypothyroidism caused by drugs and iodide excess	Exact prevalence unknown;	Ingestion of compound with antithyroid potency Drugs: thiocyanate, perchlorate, rifampin nitroprusside, sulfonamides, sulfonylureas, iodides, lithium, paraaminosalicylic acid Antithyroid drugs: PTU, MMI Goitrin plants: rutabaga, white turnips, soybeans, cabbage, peanuts

■ TABLE 9-6 Varieties of Hypothyroidism—cont'd

Variety	Incidence	Cause
Hypothyroidism caused by hereditary defects in thyroid hormone biosynthesis	Rare	Defects caused by defective iodide transport Defective iodide organification caused by inadequate or defective thyroid peroxidase, thyroglobulin formation, or peroxide Defective or insufficient thyroglobulin biosynthesis and formation of abnormal iodoproteins Defective dehalogenation of iodotyrosines
Thyroid hormone resistance	Rare; also in some patients with pseudohypoparathyroidism	Autosomal recessive defects with point mutations of T_3 receptor
Hypothyroidism due to thyroid injury from other causes	Incidence unknown Occurs occasionally in patients with hemochromatosis, amyloidosis, sarcoidosis, scleroderma, cystinosis, and frequently in those with fibrous invasive thyroiditis (Riedel's thyroiditis)	Thyroid tissue damage
Pituitary hypothyroidism	Unknown, but common after pituitary surgery or radiation	Deficiency of TSH caused by destruction of pituitary tissue: functioning or nonfunctioning pituitary macroadenomas, surgery, pituitary radiation, postpartum pituitary necrosis (Sheehan's syndrome), pituitary cysts, craniopharyngioma, carotid aneurysm, trauma, hemochromatosis, and infiltrative diseases such as metastatic tumor, tuberculosis, histiocytosis
Hypothalamic hypothyroidism	Rare; occurs predominantly in children[83]	TRH deficiency caused by cranial irradiation; traumatic, infiltrative, and neoplastic diseases of hypothalamus; pituitary lesions that interrupt hypothalamic-pituitary portal circulation[83]
Spontaneous hypothyroidism following Graves' disease	Generally occurs following remission of Graves' disease; not associated with antithyroid drugs	May result from concomitant chronic autoimmune thyroiditis that frequently occurs with Graves' disease or may be an increase in TBII with a concomitant decrease in TSIs

cytes, and plasma cells causing follicular destruction, fibrosis, and colloid depletion. It is unknown when in a person's life these antibodies might become active, although iodine ingestion has been suggested to be a trigger.[82] There is a genetic predisposition for this type of hypothyroidism. Patients with HLA-DR5 antigen exhibit an increased incidence of goitrous hypothyroidism. The effects of these antibodies against the thyroid gland is an extended process that may take many years. This is why more hypothyroidism is seen in older women than in younger women. In addition, environmental factors such as iodide or viral exposures may modify an already genetically predisposed gland to begin developing thyroiditis and hypothyroidism. Like autoimmune hyperthyroidism, autoimmune hypothyroidism is associated with other organ-specific systemic autoimmune disorders such as idiopathic adrenal insufficiency, pernicious anemia, lupus, or rheumatoid arthritis.

An intermediary step in the development of hypothyroidism may be the formation of a goiter or nodules. As the thyroid gland begins to fail from destruction of individual follicles, feedback signals are sent to the pituitary gland, which increases its TSH output. TSH acts as a growth stimulator to increase the number of functional follicles. This may be adequate for a time until the antibodies cause more destruction.

When thyrotoxicosis occurs coincidentally with Hashimoto's thyroiditis, it is called *hashitoxicosis*. The patient's symptoms in this situation would be identical to that of any patient with thyrotoxicosis. These patients, however, have a greater chance of remission of their hyperthyroidism and are more prone to spontaneous hypothyroidism after treatment.

The clinical manifestations of hypothyroidism range from mild, with few signs or symptoms, to severe, culminating in life-threatening myxedema coma. The clinical manifestations depend on the degree and duration of thyroid hormone deficiency. Most of the signs or symptoms are a result of slowing of normal physical and mental activity and edema. The edema or myxedema is from increased interstitial glycosaminoglycan deposition, which is a highly hydrophilic substance. Although slight weight gain or an inability to lose weight while dieting may occur, morbid obesity does not occur from hypothyroidism. The skin, hair, nail, and voice changes are obvious in younger patients, but may be mistaken for normal aging in the older individual.

The treatment for hypothyroidism is levothyroxine. This is a synthetic preparation of only thyroxine. The T_4 is converted (deiodinated) to T_3 at peripheral cells. Therefore one medication is able to provide replacement of the two major thyroid hormones. The goal of treatment is called *replacement therapy*. This means that enough T_4 is prescribed to maintain the TSH level in a normal range without either the T_4 or T_3 levels being too high or too low. Levothyroxine has a long half life, therefore if a patient is unable to take medication by mouth because of another illness or surgery, it may be withheld for up to 7 days. After 7 days, however, intravenous levothyroxine should be substituted for the oral preparation. The specific brand of levothyroxine is also important since generic preparations do not always have the same bioavailability as the branded preparations.

Non Goitrous Chronic Autoimmune Thyroiditis

This was previously called idiopathic hypothyroidism, primary myedema, or primary thyroid atrophy. This form of hypothyroidism differs from Hashimoto's thyroiditis in that goiter does not develop. Pathologically, there is thyroid follicle atrophy, lymphocytic infiltration, and atrophy of the entire gland.[98] Genetically, patients with HLA-DR3 tend to exhibit this form of hypothyroidism. This form of hypothyroidism has the same clinical presentation, diagnostic test, and treatment as Hashimoto's thyroiditis.

Myxedema Coma

Myxedema coma is a life-threatening emergency. Long-standing, severe hypothyroidism compromises the patient's ability to withstand the trauma of an intercurrent illness. It occurs most often in the winter in older individuals. It may be precipitated by cold exposure, infection, cardiovascular or respiratory disease or inappropriate use of narcotic and analgesic agents.[98] Clinically, nearly all these patients have hypothermia and hypoventilation with a metabolic acidosis. Survival of the patient depends on vigorous treatment of the precipitating non-thyroidal illness. Since patients may also have idiopathic adrenal insufficiency, they should be treated simultaneously with glucocorticoids. This is the primary reason a patient with previously undiagnosed hypothyroidism would be admitted to a hospital.

•••••• Diagnostic Studies and Findings

TRH stimulation tests   Primary hypothyroidism: TSH increases above normal basal level; pituitary hypothyroidism: subnormal TSH response or no response to TRH; hypothalamic hypothyroidism: normal TSH, but retarded response to TRH
  RAIU   Below normal uptake
  Serum T_4   Decreased
  Serum T_3   Decreased; neither a specific nor a sensitive test for hypothyroidism
  Serum free T_4 and T_3   Decreased
  Serum TSH   Elevated (primary hypothyroidism, chronic autoimmune thyroiditis, after subtotal thyroidectomy, ^{131}I therapy) *normal or undetectable* (pituitary or hypothalamic hypothyroidism, nonthyroidal illnesses)

•••••• Multidisciplinary Plan

Medications

Synthetic thyroid hormones
  Levothyroxine sodium (Levothroid; Synthroid), dose depends on degree of hypothyroidism, age, and body weight of patient; may vary from 0.025 mg (25 μg) to 0.2 mg (200 μg) per day; each of these preparations are available in equivalent intravenous doses
Thyroid stimulating hormone (TSH)
  Thytropar is rarely used as a diagnostic agent to differentiate primary from central hypothyroidism; it comes as a lyophilized powder containing 10 IU of bovine pituitary and is given IM or SQ
Protirelin (thyrotropin-releasing hormone, TRH) (Relefact TRH; Thypinone) 400-500 μg IV for adults; synthetic preparation of natural hypothalamic tripeptide hormone; diagnostic agent to differentiate pituitary-induced hypothyroidism from other types of hypothyroidism; may transiently produce nausea, facial flushing, hypertension, and urge to micturate

General Management

Control of environment
Diet: high protein, high fiber, low calorie

NURSING CARE

Nursing Assessment

Skin and Appendages

Cool, pale, dry, coarse; yellowish tint
Rough, scaly skin
Puffy, masklike face
Periorbital edema
Brittle nails
Hypothermia
Myxedema

Cardiovascular Status

Bradycardia; mild hypertension to decreased blood pressure
Decreased exercise tolerance

Gastrointestinal Status

Modest weight gain
Constipation; fecal impaction
Abdominal distention; myxedema ileus
Nausea
Enlarged tongue

Muscular Status

Nonspecific fatigue; weakness
Slow muscle movement, muscle cramps
Delayed relaxation of deep tendon reflexes
Aches and stiffness of joints
Carpal tunnel syndrome

Nervous System Status

General slowing of all intellectual functions, including speech

Decreased hearing

Lethargy and somnolence

Impaired memory; inattentiveness

Loss of initiative

Harshness of voice

Sensitivity to narcotics, sedatives

Cerebellar ataxia

Mental-Emotional Status

Paranoia

Depression

Agitation

Apathy

Nursing Dx & Intervention

Decreased cardiac output related to alteration in rate (myxedema, coma only)

- Monitor pulse, blood pressure, color, and temperature *to determine cardiovascular stability.*
- Measure and record intake and output; weigh daily *to evaluate fluid balance.*
- Observe level of consciousness and orientation.
- Monitor for potentiating effects of drugs (use lower doses of sedatives, narcotics, etc.) *to identify cardiovascular depression caused by drug accumulation, resulting from lowered metabolic rate.*

Altered thought processes related to physiologic changes (myxedema, coma only)

- Assess level of orientation to person, place, and time.
- Provide tolerable activity schedule *to conserve energy.*
- Provide physically and emotionally safe environment.
- Explain procedures slowly and carefully *to support decreased concentration.*
- Assist family in accepting patient's dullness and slowness.
- Time nursing activities to patient's response level *to prevent further disorientation.*
- Explain procedures slowly and simply, reinforcing them repeatedly, *to support the patient with lethargy, impaired memory, and inattentiveness.*
- Schedule nursing activities around patient's activity cycles.

Hypothermia related to decreased metabolic rate (myxedema coma)

- Monitor patient's temperature.
- Use non–alcohol-containing, warmed lotions to protect the patient's skin.
- Use warmed blankets; however, do not increase the weight of the patient's clothing by using too many.
- Give patient warmed intravenous solutions slowly if ordered.

Activity intolerance related to generalized weakness

- Reassess patient's ability to perform activities of daily living.
- Help patient take measures to conserve body temperature (warm blankets, robes, socks, bed jacket) *to prevent further hypothermia.*
- Provide safe environment *to protect patient with hypoactive reflexes, lethargy, or impaired memory.*
- Provide scheduled, uninterrupted rest.

Constipation related to neuromuscular impairment

- Reassess patient's frequency, color, consistency, and amount of stool.
- Monitor effectiveness of anticonstipation aids.
- Provide high-protein, high-fiber, low-calorie diet in smaller, frequent meals.
- Encourage patient to increase fluid intake; record patient's I and O *to monitor dehydration.*
- Establish daily routine bowel training program.
- Avoid use of enemas *to prevent fluid retention in a patient with myxedema.*

Patient Education/Home Care Planning

1. Give the patient a list of the signs and symptoms of hypothyroidism and hyperthyroidism and encourage the patient to report occurrence of either to physician.
2. Discuss with the patient that thyroid hormones are essential for life and that treatment is therefore lifelong.
3. Discuss with the patient medication administration: name, dosage, frequency of taking, and side effects.
4. Discuss with the patient the importance of adequate rest alternated with increased periods of exercise.
5. Discuss with the patient the importance of and the necessity for follow-up evaluations.
6. Recommend the patient and family read "Your Thyroid: A Home Reference."[109]

Evaluation

Cardiovascular function is normal Patient demonstrates normal sinus rhythm. Skin remains warm and dry. Patient remains alert and fully oriented.

Thought processes are normal Patient is oriented to person, place, and time. Patient validates thought processes with staff. Statements are reality-oriented. Patient is interested in work, environment, friends, and family.

Activity tolerance is improved Patient is able to perform most activities independently.

Constipation is absent or decreased Bowel movements are regular and of normal consistency, color, and quantity. Patient verbalizes adherence to prescribed diet and fluid intake. Patient identifies high-fiber foods to use in diet plan.

Normothermia exists   Temperature is normal; skin is intact, warm, and dry.

Nutrition is adequate   Patient verbalizes adherence to dietary plan.

THYROID CANCER

Thyroid cancers are malignancies arising from cells normally found in the thyroid gland.

The incidence of thyroid cancer is about 12,000 new cases annually in the United States, with an estimated 1000 deaths per year. Papillary accounts for about 80% of cases with 5%-10% from follicular, 10% medullary, and 2% anaplastic. External radiation to the head or neck and environmental radiation exposure (nuclear reactors) increase the risk of thyroid cancer. An additional type of malignancy is thyroid lymphoma. Once thought to be rare, it now constitutes close to 8% of all thyroid malignancies.

All thyroid disorders, including thyroid cancer, are more common in women than in men. Thyroid cancer can occur at any age, with an increased incidence occurring 15 to 20 years after radiation exposure and a prevalence of lymphoma after age 50 (see the box). Papillary cancer (85%) is most often associated with radiation exposure.[56]

• • • • • • Pathophysiology

Thyroid tumors may be classified as epithelial (papillary, follicular, medullary, anaplastic) or nonepithelial (lymphoma). Some patients may have a mixed papillary-follicular pattern.

Epithelial Tumors

Papillary and follicular tumors specifically arise from the follicular cells of the thyroid gland and tend to be slow-growing. These tumors usually appear as hypofunctioning nodules within the thyroid gland, alone, as a dominant nodule within a multinodular gland, or as a hypofunctioning nodule in a Graves' thyrotoxic gland. Cancer is occasionally found within a hyperfunctioning nodule, or it may occur with an extrathyroidal mass. Papillary cancer is usually nonencapsulated and may extend beyond the thyroid gland. Recurrence and metastasis are usually to local lymph nodes within the cervical region; distant metastasis is rare.

Follicular cancers are usually encapsulated. Invasion of tumor through the capsule or local blood vessels or evidence of extrathyroidal involvement differentiates follicular cancer from the benign follicular adenoma. Distant metastasis is common; lung, lymph node, and bone are the common sites. This cancer may manifest as a lung or bone mass before any thyroidal abnormalities are found.

Medullary thyroid cancer arises from the calcitonin-secreting parafollicular or C-cells. It may occur in isolation (sporadic) or as part of Sipple's syndrome (multiple endocrine neoplasia [MEN Type II]). If MEN is suspected then the patient is also evaluated for the simultaneous presence of pheochromocytoma and hyperparathyroidism. Medullary thyroid cancer may also have both local and distant metastases.

Anaplastic thyroid carcinoma is rarely discovered as a primary diagnosis. These are infiltrative tumors that grow rapidly, invade the trachea and major blood vessels, and metastasize to distant areas (bone, liver) rapidly.

Prognosis of cancer survival varies with the type, the extent of involvement at the time of diagnosis, and the presence of distant metastases. Papillary cancer generally shows the best survival, even in the presence of lymph node involvement. Follicular cancer tends to be more aggressive in affecting vital organs; however, if it is discovered early, life expectancy may not be decreased. Medullary cancer has a mortality of 35% in 10 years. Anaplastic cancer is resistant to all known therapy, and death usually occurs within months. Either papillary or follicular cancer may change aggressively and become anaplastic-like.

Nonepithelial Tumors

The last type of cancer is a non-Hodgkin's lymphoma that occurs as a nodule or mass, usually within a multinodular gland that may have an autoimmune lymphocytic component (Hashimoto's thyroiditis). These masses grow rapidly; they may or may not have extrathyroidal metastases. Patients with Hashimoto's thyroiditis are treated with standard lymphoma therapy—unlike other patients with thyroid cancers.

The goal of therapy for papillary and follicular tumors is first and foremost surgical removal of the thyroid gland. The procedure recommended would be a total or near total thyroidectomy (see thyroidectomy). If local metastasis is identified at the time of surgery, a more extensive procedure may be required, including a modified radical neck dissection. Depending on the size of the cancer, and the presence of metastasis at presentation, the patient may or may not receive radioactive iodine to chemically kill any remaining thyroid tissue or microscopic cells (see radioactive iodine therapy). If the patient is to receive ^{131}I, an assessment of the amount of remaining tissue must be performed. This is done by a nuclear medicine ^{131}I uptake and whole body scan. Preparation for this procedure involves purposefully making the patient hypothyroid with a TSH greater than 40. This process usually takes 4 to 6 weeks. If the patient receives [131]I

 RISK FACTORS FOR THYROID CANCER

1. Nodule greater than 3 cm
2. Solitary solid rather than cystic nodule
3. Male sex
4. Age less than 20 or greater than 70 years
5. Extrathyroidal masses at initial presentation
6. A rapidly growing mass
7. A growing nodule within a multinodular gland during thyroid hormone-suppressive therapy
8. Known family history of medullary cancer or multiple endocrine neoplasia

that is ≥30 mCi then according to Nuclear Regulatory Commission guidelines, the patient must be placed in radiation isolation. The final step in treatment will be lifelong thyroid hormone therapy. Unlike the patient with hypothyroidism, however, the goal in these patients is *suppressive therapy*. This means that enough levothyroxine is prescribed to lower the TSH to extremely low levels, sometimes called undetectable levels. This is to reduce any growth-stimulating, or thyroid hormone production potential of any microscopic tumor cells that might remain. This amount of T_4 therapy may render the patient *subclinically hyperthyroid*, with all of the possible consequences to bone mass or cardiac abnormalities as endogenous subclinical hyperthyroidism (see thyrotoxicosis/hyperthyroidism).

The goal of therapy for medullary thyroid cancer is also a total or near total thyroidectomy as a first step. [131]I is not indicated in this type of cancer as uptake of iodine by medullary tumor cells is negligible. External beam radiation may be used particularly in an attempt to reduce tumor mass when metastasis is present.

•••••• Diagnostic Studies and Findings[87]

Fine needle aspiration An outpatient cytologic procedure to obtain cells from the thyroidal or extrathyroidal mass and determine cell type

Thyroid hormone levels Serum TSH, serum T_4, possibly serum T_3 to exclude hyper- or hypothyroidism

Serum antibodies Antimicrosomal, antithyroglobulin; may be positive in Hashimoto's thyroiditis and suspected lymphoma

Serum calcitonin Elevated in medullary thyroid cancer

Calcium/pentagastrin stimulation test A provocative test to further assess whether the patient may have medullary thyroid cancer; usually performed when baseline calcitonin level is in the normal range; elevated stimulated calcitonin levels may represent early medullary thyroid cancer

Serum thyroglobulin Used as a tumor marker after total thyroidectomy; elevated levels indicate persistence or recurrence of papillary or follicular tumors; may also be elevated if normal thyroid tissue remains after treatment

Technetium scan Used to identify whether presenting thyroidal mass is hypofunctioning (cold) or hyperfunctioning (warm, hot)

Thyroid ^{131}I uptake and scan Used after total thyroidectomy to help determine amount of remaining tissue and amount of radioactive iodine to give the patient for papillary, follicular, or anaplastic tumors; also used to determine if there is new recurrence or metastasis of papillary or follicular tumors beginning 6 months after initial therapy. How often this procedure is done varies with the type of tumor and initial presentation of the patient.

•••••• Multidisciplinary Plan[87]

Surgery

Total thyroidectomy as first therapeutic step
Recurrence or metastasis may require additional surgical intervention; modified radical neck surgery

For all types except lymphoma
Radioactive iodine (^{131}I) ablation—used primarily for epithelial tumors; dose is variable depending on patient presentation; may not be given if tumor ≤2 cm. If dose ≤30 mCi, given as an outpatient; if ≥30 mCi, hospitalization and radiation isolation are required.
Recurrence/metastasis—150-400 (mCi)
Maximum cumulative dose is 1000 mCi before bone marrow dysfunction occurs
External beam radiation—primarily used for recurrence of medullary and occasionally anaplastic tumor

Medications

Thyroid hormone to replace body requirement and to suppress possible cellular growth; long-term exposure to supraphysiologic doses of thyroid hormone may increase risk of osteoporosis

Chemotherapy

Adriamycin may be used in anaplastic tumors

NURSING CARE

Nursing Assessment

Psychosocial

Anxiety
All other assessment applies to posttreatment (see thyroidectomy, hypothyroidism, radioactive iodine)

Nursing Dx & Intervention

Anxiety related to change in health status

- Encourage patient to discuss feelings about diagnosis and planned therapies.
- Explore coping mechanisms with patient.
- Help patient identify a coping mechanism that will decrease anxiety.

Patient Education/Home Care Planning

1. Discuss with patient before and after thyroidectomy care.
2. Discuss with patient the need to become hypothyroid (by end of 6 weeks postoperative) in preparation for first ^{131}I treatment, including signs, symptoms, and ways to cope with symptoms.
3. Ensure that patient understands low-iodine diet in preparation for ^{131}I treatment and institution rules for radiation isolation.
4. Ensure that patient understands thyroid hormone suppressive therapy and the need for reevaluation for the rest of their life.

5. Discuss with patient the need to stop thyroid medication, start low-iodine diet, and become hypothyroid in preparation for ^{131}I neck and chest or whole body nuclear medicine scan, within the first 6 months postoperative.

Evaluation

Anxiety is decreased   Patient demonstrates one coping mechanism that decreases anxiety. Patient is able to discuss diagnosis.

DISORDERS OF THE PANCREAS

INSULIN-DEPENDENT AND NON–INSULIN-DEPENDENT DIABETES MELLITUS

Diabetes mellitus is a heterogenous group of disorders caused by a relative or absolute lack of insulin, and affecting carbohydrate, protein, and fat metabolism.

In 1993, the American Diabetes Association estimated that 13 million Americans had diabetes, including 6.5 million undiagnosed cases. About 5% have insulin-dependent diabetes mellitus (IDDM); 80%-90% have non–insulin-dependent diabetes mellitus (NIDDM).[28,46]

The guidelines for classifying diabetes mellitus were standardized by the NIH National Data Group. Their classification of diabetes mellitus is as follows[68]:
1. Insulin-dependent diabetes mellitus (IDDM)
2. Non–insulin-dependent diabetes mellitus (NIDDM)
3. Secondary diabetes (diabetes mellitus occurring with, or as a result of, other conditions or syndromes)
4. Impaired glucose tolerance

5. Gestational diabetes mellitus
6. Previous abnormality in glucose tolerance
7. Potential abnormality in glucose tolerance.

This discussion is limited to IDDM and NIDDM (see Table 9-7).

•••••• Pathophysiology

IDDM is a condition of absolute insulin deficiency. Genetic predisposition for insulin-dependent diabetes mellitus is conferred by a certain histocompatibility antigen, human leukocyte antigen (HLA), coded on chromosome 6.[6] Environmental factors can have a role in the development of insulin-dependent diabetes in the genetically susceptible individual. Viruses (coxsackie, mumps, rubella) can either cause direct destruction of the beta cells or induce an immunologic reaction to the beta cells of the pancreas.[6]

Autoimmunity plays a definitive role in IDDM. Autoantibodies directed against beta cells and insulin are present in IDDM and include islet cell antibodies (ICA), insulin autoantibodies (IAA), and anti-glutamic acid decarboxylase (anti-GAD). Several are present before the development of frank hyperglycemia. Why autoimmune destruction of the beta cells occurs, how it is activated, and whether or not the process of autoimmune beta cell destruction can be interrupted is under worldwide clinical investigation.[72]

Once beta cells are destroyed, metabolic compensation and the ability to maintain blood sugar within normal limits deteriorate steadily. Symptoms are the direct result of the lack of insulin and subsequent deterioration of body processes and metabolism associated with or requiring insulin.

Insulin deficiency disrupts normal nutrient metabolism and results in hyperglycemia. In the absence of insulin, glucose uptake by liver, muscle, and fat cells is inhibited; glucose production is promoted. Lack of restraining effect by insulin on the liver processes of glycogenolysis and gluconeogenesis cause the liver to overproduce glucose. Synthesis of protein, fat, and glycogen is impaired. Muscle and fat are actually broken down,

TABLE 9-7 Clinical, Genetic, and Immunologic Characteristics of Insulin-Dependent and Non–Insulin-Dependent Diabetes

	Insulin-Dependent Diabetes (Type I)*	Non–Insulin-Dependent Diabetes (Type II)†
Age of onset	Usually <30	Usually >40
Ketosis	Common	Rare
Body weight	Nonobese	Obese (80% of patients)
Prevalence	0.5%	4%-5%
Genetics	HLA-associated; 25%-35% concordance rate in twins	Non–HLA-associated; 95%-100% concordance rate in twins
Circulating islet-cell antibodies	65%-85%	<10%
Treatment with insulin	Necessary	Usually not required
Complications	Frequent	Frequent

From Felig P and Bergman M. In Felig P, Baxter JD, Frohman LA, eds.[28]
*Formerly "juvenile-onset" diabetes.
†Formerly "maturity-onset" diabetes.

freeing up more substrate for the liver to use in out-of-control gluconeogenesis. Although blood glucose levels are elevated, glucose is not available to cells as an energy source. If not corrected, lipolysis occurs to help provide cells with needed energy. However, by-products of lipolysis, called ketones, are overproduced, excreted in the urine, and build up in the blood. Symptoms of hyperglycemia including polydipsia, polyuria, polyphagia, fatigue, weight loss, and blurred vision may occur whenever IDDM is poorly controlled.[72]

NIDDM comprises a group of disorders of relative insulin deficiency. Individuals with NIDDM are usually over 30 years old at the time of diagnosis, may have a family history of NIDDM, and most are obese. Genetics, environment, and lifestyle factors play a role in the development of NIDDM. Although NIDDM is highly familial, a specific genetic marker has yet to be identified. The prevalence of NIDDM increases with age. African- and Mexican-Americans, as well as Native Americans, are at increased risk for developing NIDDM.[28,72]

Insulin resistance is a basic defect that occurs at the target cell. Both beta cell defects and target cell defects are present in NIDDM. Beta cell defects may include impaired insulin secretion due to the toxic effect of elevated glucose levels on the beta cell, or diminished insulin response to usual stimuli. Low, normal, or elevated insulin levels may be present. At the target cells, malfunctioning of insulin receptors on target tissues and/or intracellular postreceptor processes may be present. The ability to identify exactly what defect(s) are present in any one individual with NIDDM still needs investigation. Additionally, many experts believe that NIDDM, obesity, atherosclerosis, and hypertension may all be related to insulin resistance and hyperinsulinemia.[28,72]

The relative insulin deficiency of NIDDM also results in hyperglycemia. However, because some insulin is produced, hyperglycemia is insidious, and may be present for years before diagnosis. Symptoms of hyperglycemia including polydipsia, polyuria, polyphagia, fatigue, and slowed wound healing may be present. Often symptoms are attributed to a preexisting condition or the aging process.

The primary causal factor associated with the development of long term complications of diabetes is hyperglycemia. Initially, changes are reversible (like increased polyol pathway activity), but may be irreversible in the long term (like basement membrane thickening). Long term complications of diabetes include conditions associated with (1) microangiopathy (retinopathy, nephropathy, and neuropathy), (2) macrovascular disease (coronary heart disease, peripheral vascular disease), and (3) neuropathy.[28] Many other metabolic abnormalities associated with hyperglycemia may be present: dyslipidemia, hypertension, electrolyte abnormalities and volume depletion, as well as decreased leukocyte effectiveness and increased platelet aggregation. When present, complications do not occur in isolation, but may pose some complex diabetes management issues.[28,72]

Normalizing blood sugar control has been shown to decrease the risk of developing long term complications of diabetes. The Diabetes Control and Complications Trial (DCCT) found that tight control of blood sugar to near normal in persons with IDDM reduced the risk for development and progression of retinopathy, nephropathy, and neuropathy by approximately 60%.[68] Because hyperglycemia is the causal factor implicated in the development and progression of long term complications, diabetes management goals for persons with IDDM and NIDDM should include good blood sugar control. Glycosylated hemoglobin measurements are useful in assessing overall diabetes control over the 3 to 4 months before measurement.

•••••• Diagnostic Studies and Findings

Fasting blood sugar   Venous plasma >140 mg/dl × 2, or >200 mg/dl with polyuria, polydipsia, and weight loss

Glucose Tolerance Test   2 hour sample *and* one other sample between 0 and 2 hours must be 200 mg/dl or greater

Blood insulin levels   Absent to low in IDDM; low, normal or high in NIDDM

Plasma C-Peptide   Absent to low in IDDM; low, normal or high in NIDDM

•••••• Multidisciplinary Plan

Standards of care for persons with diabetes are outlined in detail by the American Diabetes Association[1] and include:

1. Regular medical evaluation and follow-up
2. Medical nutrition therapy (refer to dietitian)
3. Exercise prescription
4. Education/behavior change (diabetes educator, dietitian, exercise specialist)
5. Psychosocial coping and support (diabetes educator, mental health professional)
6. Medications

Insulin preparations—Four types available in human, pork, beef, and beef-pork sources; doses are individually adjusted

   Short-acting preparations—Regular and semilente
   Intermediate-acting preparations—NPH and lente
   Long-acting preparations—Ultralente
   Premixed—70/30 (NPH/regular)
Oral hypoglycemic agents
Sulfonylureas[57]
   First generation
      Tolbutamide (Orinase), 250 mg to 3 g/d in divided doses
      Chlorpropamide (Diabinese), 100-750 mg/d, in single or divided doses
      Acetohexamide (Dymelor), 250 mg to 1.5 g/d in divided doses
      Tolazamide (Tolinase), 100 mg to 1 g/d in divided doses
   Second generation
      Glipizide (Glucotrol), 2.5-40 mg/d, in single or divided doses
      Glyburide (Micronase, DiaBeta), 1.25-20 mg/d, in single or divided doses
   Oral antihyperglycemic drug
      Metformin (Glucophage), 500-2550 mg/d in single or divided doses[10]

Other General Management Plans

Alternative insulin delivery devices
Photocoagulation (see Chapter 6)
Kidney dialysis (see Chapter 11)
Assistive devices for low vision
Treatment for impotence (see Chapter 12)
Surgery (intervention for complications, i.e., CABG)

NURSING CARE

Nursing Assessment

Food and Fluid

Hunger, thirst, nausea
Weight loss or obesity

Elimination

Polyuria
Nocturia

Neurosensory Concerns

Decreased sensation to pain and temperature in feet
Blurred vision
Headaches, cataracts, halos around lights

Skin

Infection
Rubeosis; dermopathy
Foot ulcers

Sexuality

Impotence
Vaginal discharge/infection

Circulation

Cold extremities
Loss of hair on toes; skin shiny, thin, and atrophic
Orthostatic hypotension
Painful calves when walking
Numbness and tingling of lower extremities
Weak pedal pulse

Psychosocial Concerns

Verbalization of inability to cope
Non-compliance with treatment plan
Verbalization of change in life-style
Negative feeling about body

Teaching and Learning

Lack of exposure to diabetes if newly diagnosed
Lack of recall
Misinformation
Inadequate demonstration of skills required (urine and/or blood testing, injection technique)

Lack of interest
Unfamiliarity with survival level

Nursing Dx & Intervention

Fluid-volume deficit related to failure of regulatory mechanisms

- Encourage patient to drink noncaloric fluids for hyperglycemia *to replace fluid loss resulting from polyuria.*
- Discuss causative factors with patient and family.
- Monitor indicators of patient's fluid balance (intake and output, daily weights, signs of dehydration) during episodes of hyperglycemia.

Nutrition altered: less than body requirements related to inadequate intake of nutrients in diet (IDDM)

- Reassess patient for factors that may influence diet preferences.
- Arrange a dietary consultation for patient.
- Reinforce the patient's meal plan as ordered.
- Encourage patient to verbalize feelings about weight, body size, and eating behavior.
- Monitor patient's laboratory and self-monitored blood glucose (SMBG) data to monitor blood glucose control.
- Discuss causative factors with patient and family.
- Monitor patient's compliance with all aspects of the diabetes treatment regimen.

Nutrition altered: more than body requirements related to long-established eating habits (NIDDM)

- Reassess for psychosocial concerns that may be related to overeating.
- Arrange a dietary consultation.
- Reinforce the meal plan as ordered.
- Suggest support group such as Weight Watchers *to provide group and peer support.*
- Allow patient to verbalize feelings regarding weight.
- Positively reinforce patient's effort at weight loss.
- Discuss causative factors with patient and family.
- Help patient develop a pattern of rewards other than food for weight loss.
- Teach patient the use of a food diary for self-monitoring.
- Suggest techniques to change patient's eating behaviors.
- Monitor patient's laboratory and SMBG data to monitor blood glucose control and lipids.
- Help patient to identify, select, and participate in energy-expanding activities 3 times a week.
- Explore techniques to change eating behaviors.

Risk for impaired skin integrity related to internal factors (altered metabolic state, altered circulation, altered sensation)

- Initiate health instruction for patient related to risks and referral to health care professional, as needed.
- Minimize hazardous environmental factors.

- Provide assistive devices as needed.
- Discuss causative factors with patient and family.
- Keep patient's skin clean and dry.
- Monitor patient closely for signs and symptoms of infection.
- Observe patient performing daily foot care.
- Encourage measures to maximize patient's local circulation.

Ineffective individual coping related to multiple life changes

- Offer patient support and positive reinforcement.
- Assess personal strengths and weaknesses, current stressors, and stress-management skills.
- Emphasize that daily management can become as routine as personal hygiene.
- Encourage self-care to patient's maximum ability.
- Encourage participation in diabetic support groups through local American Diabetes Association (ADA) and Juvenile Diabetes Foundation (JDF).
- See pp. 1739 to 1744.
- Teach problem solving skills.

Noncompliance related to inadequate knowledge, motivation, conflict in values, complexity of regime

- Encourage and support patient's individual efforts.
- Give patient positive reinforcement for self-care efforts.
- Explore patient's feelings related to compliance.
- Provide patient with specific detailed instruction.
- Correct patient's misconceptions.
- Assist patient to use strategies to facilitate his or her behavior change.
- Use collaborative goal setting with patient.
- Assist patient in setting personal goals consistent with goals of treatment regimen.

Sexual patterns altered related to disordered metabolic function

- Encourage patient and partner to discuss sexual concerns.
- Acknowledge patient's feelings related to discussion of sexual concerns.
- Explore patient's knowledge regarding sexuality.
- Discuss causative factors with patient and partner.
- Offer patient some suggestions regarding alternative sexual expression.
- Provide patient with referrals to appropriate health care professionals.

Sensory/perceptual alterations (visual, kinesthetic, tactile) related to altered sensory reception

- Discuss causative factors with patient and family.
- Discuss patient's feelings about limitations.
- Assist patient to identify and to use assistive devices to minimize injury.

- Minimize hazardous environmental factors.
- Assist and support patient as needed to reduce chance of injury.
- Discuss injury prevention with patient and family.

Patient Education/Home Care Planning

1. Demonstrate to the patient how to administer insulin or oral hypoglycemics; teach the patient to report side effects or toxic effects.
2. Demonstrate to the patient the method for monitoring blood sugar: regular urine testing or SMBG.
3. Ensure that the patient verbalizes understanding of the prescribed diet and regular, routine exercise and activity needed to maintain blood sugar control.
4. Ensure that the patient verbalizes the early signs or symptoms and treatment of hypoglycemia and hyperglycemia.
5. Discuss with the patient sick day management.
6. Discuss with the patient personal hygiene, stressing specifics related to dental, foot, and skin care.
7. Discuss with the patient the methods of care to prevent complications.
8. Discuss with the patient the importance of regular medical care.
9. Discuss available community resources.

Evaluation

Fluid balance is maintained No signs of dehydration are present. Patient initiates fluid replacement during periods of hyperglycemia. Patient verbalizes causes of dehydration.

Intake of nutrients is adequate Patient's blood sugar control is within individual target values. Patient ingests recommended types and amounts of nutrients. Patient describes causative factors. Patient's weight is within range for height and age (IDDM). Patient's glycosylated hemoglobin is within individual recommended range. Patient's weight gradually reduces no more than 1 to 2 pounds per week (NIDDM). Patient participates in support group. Patient uses strategies to facilitate behavior change.

Skin is intact Patient performs daily foot, skin, and dental care correctly. Patient uses measures to minimize risk. Patient accepts referrals. Patient describes causative factors and rationale for measures to minimize risk. Patient has no infection present.

Patient copes effectively Patient uses appropriate coping strategies. Patient accepts support. Patient shows increased independence in self-care.

Compliance is increased Patient demonstrates accurate knowledge and skills for self-care. Patient demonstrates behaviors consistent with goals of treatment regimen. Patient accepts support. Patient identifies and uses strategies to facilitate behavior change. Patient sets personal goals that are consistent with goals of the treatment regimen.

Patient attains satisfying level of sexual functioning compatible with functional capability   Patient and partner verbalize concerns about sex. Patient and partner identify alternative expressions of sexuality. There is open communication about sexual concerns. Patient accepts referrals as appropriate. Patient resumes sexual activity.

Patient remains free of personal injury   Patient seeks assistance as needed. Patient uses assistive devices as needed. Patient verbalizes understanding of risk for injury with sensory/perceptual changes. Patient verbalizes cause of potential for injury. Patient recognizes environmental hazards and avoids them.

DIABETIC KETOACIDOSIS AND HYPERGLYCEMIC HYPEROSMOLAR NONKETOTIC SYNDROME

Diabetic ketoacidosis (DKA) is a condition of severe metabolic disturbance caused by an acute insulin deficiency characterized by severe hyperglycemia and metabolic acidosis from ketosis.

Hyperglycemic hyperosmolar nonketotic syndrome (HHNS) is a condition of severe metabolic disturbance characterized by severe hyperglycemia, hyperosmolarity, and dehydration with significant ketoacidosis.

DKA accounts for 9% of all diabetic hospital admissions.[55] (See Emergency Alert box.) It is estimated that 25% to 30% of all episodes of DKA occur during initial diagnosis, and 25% to 30% of all cases are related to illness or infection.[72] There are many predisposing factors possible in the development of DKA: failure to take insulin, insufficient amount of insulin taken, intercurrent illness or infection, or physiologic or emotional stress.

Currently, HHNS accounts for approximately 5% to 15% of all hospital admissions for diabetic coma.[55] Severe hyperglycemic hyperosmolarity has been observed in association with intravenous therapy with large amounts of glucose solutions; dialysis of hyperosmolar dialysate; acromegaly; drugs such as the thiazide diuretics, phenytoin, diazoxide, glucocorticoids, furosemide, propranolol, and cimetidine; and after the ingestion of large amounts of sugary beverages or high-protein gastric tube feedings.[55] Other additional precipitating factors for HHNS include acute pancreatitis, inadequate or limited access to fluids, impaired thirst, social isolation, massive fluid losses, or illness/infections.[55,72] About 80% of patients with HHNS have impaired renal function, a significant predisposing condition that contributes to the development of HHNS.[55] Most victims are elderly and infirm, institutionalized or mentally impaired, with mild or previous undiagnosed diabetes. The mortality rate for HHNS is much higher than DKA, 20% to 40%, due to misdiagnosis, or delay in diagnosis.

Unfortunately, both hyperglycemia and hyperosmolarity are present in the patient with DKA and HHNS. A continuum of severe hyperglycemia actually exists, with HHNS without ketosis on one end of the spectrum, and DKA on the other end with overlap in the middle.

•••••• Pathophysiology

The contribution of counterregulatory (stress) hormones to the extreme hyperglycemia of insulin deficiency can quickly cause the development of diabetic ketoacidosis (DKA). During stress, the secretion of these hormones (glucagon, catecholamines, growth hormone, and cortisol) increases. In the insulin-deficient individual the effects of these hormones are magnified because of both an exaggerated release and an enhanced responsiveness when insulin levels are below normal.[18] A deficiency of insulin and excess catecholamines, cortisol, and growth hormone increase hepatic glucose production, decrease peripheral glucose utilization, and increase fat mobilization and ketogenesis. Glucagon stimulates glycogenolysis, gluconeogenesis, and ketogenesis. Thus deficiency of insulin itself permits an out-of-control secretion and response to the secretion of counterregulatory hormones, which only serve to accelerate the development of DKA. Because the stress that precipitates the occurrence of DKA is prolonged, the effects of all four stress hormones are also prolonged. In addition, there appears to be a synergistic effect among all four stress hormones, which further increases blood sugar and causes a rapid deterioration of metabolic balance.[42]

The events of DKA are summarized in Figure 9-9. In the absence of adequate insulin, peripheral fat, muscle, and liver cells are unable to utilize glucose. Breakdown of fat and protein is accelerated, freeing up more substrate (fatty acids and amino acids) for use in gluconeogenesis and overproduction of glucose by the liver.

 EMERGENCY ALERT

DIABETIC KETOACIDOSIS (DKA)

This metabolic disturbance occurs in those with diabetes mellitus and is typically caused by insulin depletion.

Assessment

- Determine compliance with insulin regimen including (if applicable) pump malfunction.
- Assess for increased insulin demand from such factors as infection, stress, surgery, trauma, pregnancy, acute MI, or certain medications.
- Assess for the following:
    hyperglycemia, ketonemia, or acidosis
    hypervolemia or electrolyte imbalance
    nausea, vomiting, thirst, polyuria, abdominal pain, drowsiness
    tachypnea, hyperventilation, flushed skin, acetone odor of the breath

Interventions

- Obtain IV access and in collaboration with the physician provide fluid resuscitation using normal saline (NS) (may be as much as 1 L/hour).
- In collaboration with physician, administer insulin therapy by IV infusion.
- Monitor electrolytes and arterial blood gases and in collaboration with physician correct imbalances.
- Provide periodic and careful monitoring of vital signs, urine output, mental state, and pulmonary status.

Excessive amounts of fatty acids are used by the liver (under the control of glucagon) to overproduce ketoacids (ketone bodies, β-hydroxybutyric acid, and acetoacetic acid). Acetone, responsible for the characteristic fruity breath in DKA, is formed from acetoacetic acid. The ketone bodies are produced faster than they can be metabolized or excreted. Acetoacetic acid and β-hydroxybutyric acid cannot be metabolized in the absence of insulin; therefore their levels also increase in the plasma. These strong organic acids dissociate at body pH and provide 1 mEq of H^+ cation and a ketoacid anion. Metabolic acidosis occurs when the body's buffer system and respiratory compensatory mechanisms are unable to maintain normal pH.

Hyperglycemia results in glycosuria with a large osmotic water and electrolyte loss through the kidneys. Although glomerular filtration is increased initially, the development of hypovolemia is associated with decreased glomerular filtration

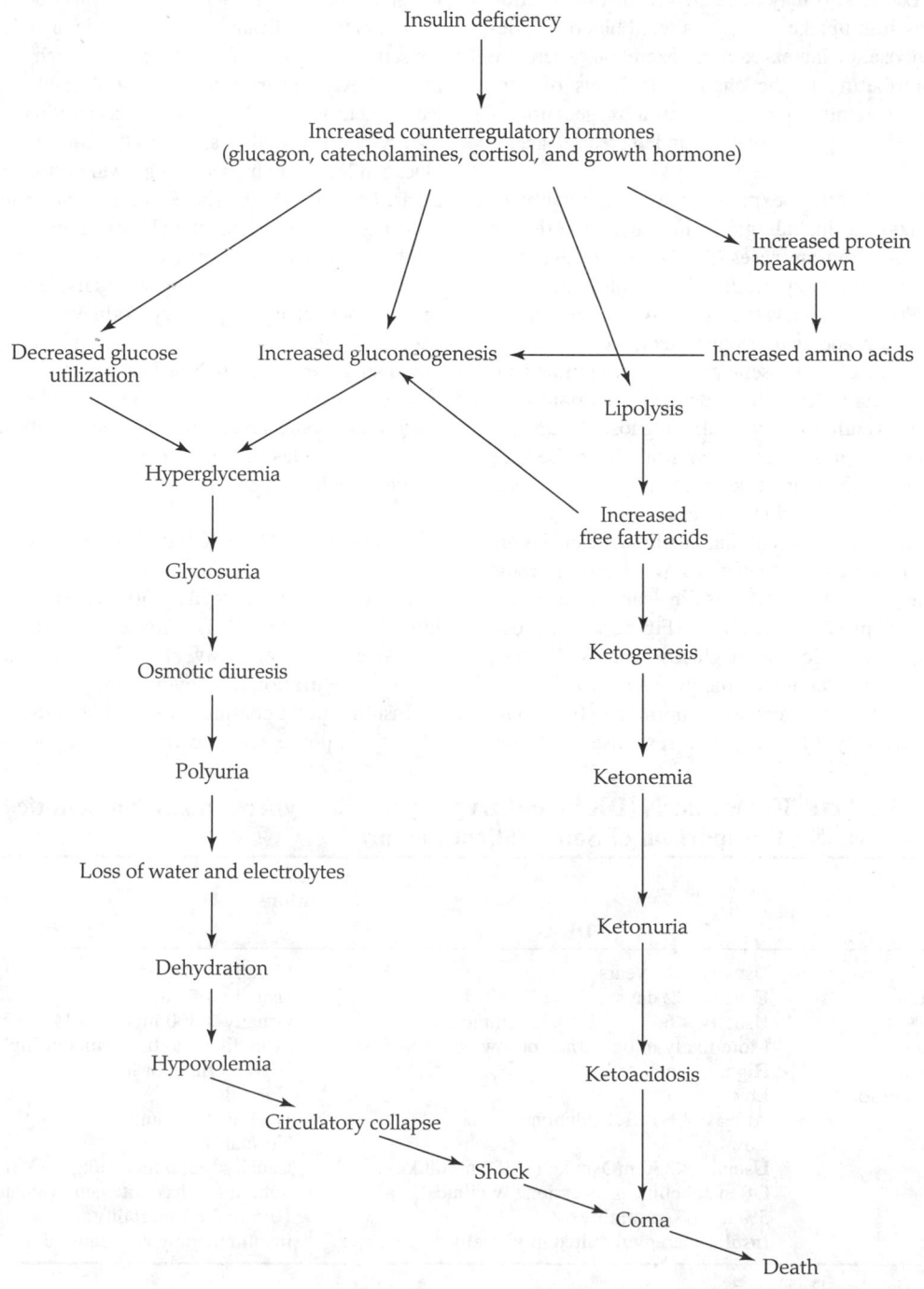

Figure 9-9 Diabetic ketoacidosis.

and worsening of hyperglycemia. In addition, the organic acids are excreted through the kidneys as anions, significantly decreasing potassium and sodium in the body. The acidotic state creates a shift in electrolytes; extracellular H^+ is exchanged for intracellular K^+. Therefore serum K^+ may be elevated as H^+ moves intracellularly. Hypovolemia may seem to increase the degree of hyperkalemia, but eventually the loss of potassium through the kidneys seriously depletes body potassium. There is a tendency towards a fairly rapid fall in potassium once therapy is started for DKA. This may be related to the direct action of insulin on potassium uptake by cells, altered blood pH, decreased serum glucose, or increased renal excretion. There are many factors contributing to the changes in levels of consciousness in DKA patients, such as decreased oxygenation of tissues, increased H^+, hyperosmolarity, and increased acetoacetic acid.

Many patients with DKA experience an abnormality of plasma serum enzymes including serum amylase, creatine phosphokinase (CPK), transaminases (AST or SGOT, and ALT or SGPT), and lysosomal enzymes.[42] Alkaline phosphatase is often increased. Normal or elevated electrolyte levels should not be misinterpreted as adequate. Depletion of body stores and severe deficiencies are often present with rehydration and insulin therapy. Potassium deficit is the most important, and recognition and intervention is essential. Diagnosis of DKA is made first by clinical impression, with confirmation of bedside testing (blood glucose and urine ketone); laboratory values must be obtained before therapy is initiated.

HHNS is similar to DKA except that insulin deficiencies are not as profound, and the condition evolves over a longer period of time (see Table 9-8). Decreased insulin leads to disrupted carbohydrate, fat, and protein metabolism (Figure 9-10). Blood sugar rises in response to decreased glucose use by the cells and increased glucose production by the liver due to insulin deficiency and increased counterregulatory hormone effects. Osmotic water and electrolyte loss begin in response to glycos-

uria. Extracellular volume depletion is more pronounced in the elderly due to decreased ability to concentrate urine, responsiveness to antidiuretic hormone (ADH), and conservation of body water. There is less total body water available to buffer losses. Hypovolemia and severe dehydration develop quickly, with concomitant mentation changes. Electrolyte losses include sodium, potassium, chloride, phosphate, magnesium, and calcium. Amino acid uptake and protein synthesis are halted. Breakdown of protein furnishes the liver with more substrate for gluconeogenesis. Increased lipolysis does not occur.[55]

The most significant factor differentiating HHNS from DKA is the serum level of the free fatty acids, which are lower in HHNS than in DKA. This may be the most plausible explanation for the lack of ketosis in HNNS. Serum concentrations of the counterregulatory hormones differ significantly from those in DKA: serum glucagon levels are higher, and growth hormone and cortisol levels are lower in HNNS. The elevated glucagon levels appear to be primarily responsible for the elevations in blood sugar, a direct result of stimulation of liver gluconeogenesis by glucagon.

Eighty percent of patients with HNNS have renal impairment, either related to primary (kidney) or secondary (volume depletion) disease. This plays a significant role in elevating blood sugar levels in HHNS. The kidneys are unable to rid the body of excess sugar or maintain water balance. Inability to replace body water results in hyperosmolality and dehydration. Increased solutes increase osmotic pressure. The effective serum osmolarity (Eosm) is calculated as follows[55]:

$$Eosm = 2(Na + K\ [in\ mEq]) + Glucose\ \frac{(mg/dl)}{18}$$

When this value exceeds 350 mOsm/L, severe hyperosmolarity is present.[55] The hyperosmolarity of HHNS is a direct result of excessive blood sugar and increasing sodium concentration in dehydration.

Insulin output continues to prevent ketosis. The steady loss of sodium, potassium, and water with hyperglycemia and gly-

TABLE 9-8   Diabetic Ketoacidosis (DKA) and Hyperglycemic Hyperosmolar Nonketotic Syndrome (HHNS): Comparison of Some Salient Features

Feature	Conditions	
	DKA	**HHNS**
Age of patients	Usually <40 years	Usually >60 years
Duration of symptoms	Usually <2 days	Usually >5 days
Glucose level	Usually <600 mg/dl (<33.3 mmol/L)	Usually >800 mg/dl (>44.4 mmol/L)
Sodium concentration	More likely to be normal or low	More likely to be normal or high
Potassium concentration	High, normal, or low	High, normal, or low
Bicarbonate concentration	Low	Normal
Ketone bodies	At least 4+ in 1:1 dilution	<2+ in 1:1 dilution
pH	Low	Normal
Serum osmolality	Usually <350 mOsm/kg (<350 mmol/kg)	Usually >350 mOsm/kg (>350 mmol/kg)
Cerebral edema	Often subclinical; occasionally clinical	Subclinical has not been evaluated; rarely clinical
Prognosis	3% to 10% mortality	10% to 20% mortality
Subsequent course	Insulin therapy required in virtually all cases	Insulin therapy not required in many cases

Modified with permission from Davidson.[22]
From Peragallo-Dittko V, Godley K, and Meyer J.[72]

cosuria exacerbates the hyperosmolar state and ultimately results in hypovolemia, hypotension, hemoconcentration, and increased blood viscosity, and may contribute to the development of vascular occlusion, the most important complication of HHNS.[55] Most of the abnormal and confusing abnormalities resolve following treatment; it is suggested that the neurologic examination be repeated 48 hours after homeostasis has been restored by fluid and insulin replacement therapy.

Like DKA, diagnosis of HHNS is made by clinical impression, bedside testing (blood glucose and urine ketones); initial laboratory values are obtained before treatment is initiated. Enormous fluid losses (up to 20 L) and deficits in sodium and potassium may be present. Other abnormal blood work findings may be present, such as elevated hematocrit, triglycerides, cholesterol, liver function tests, and a variety of serum enzyme values.[55]

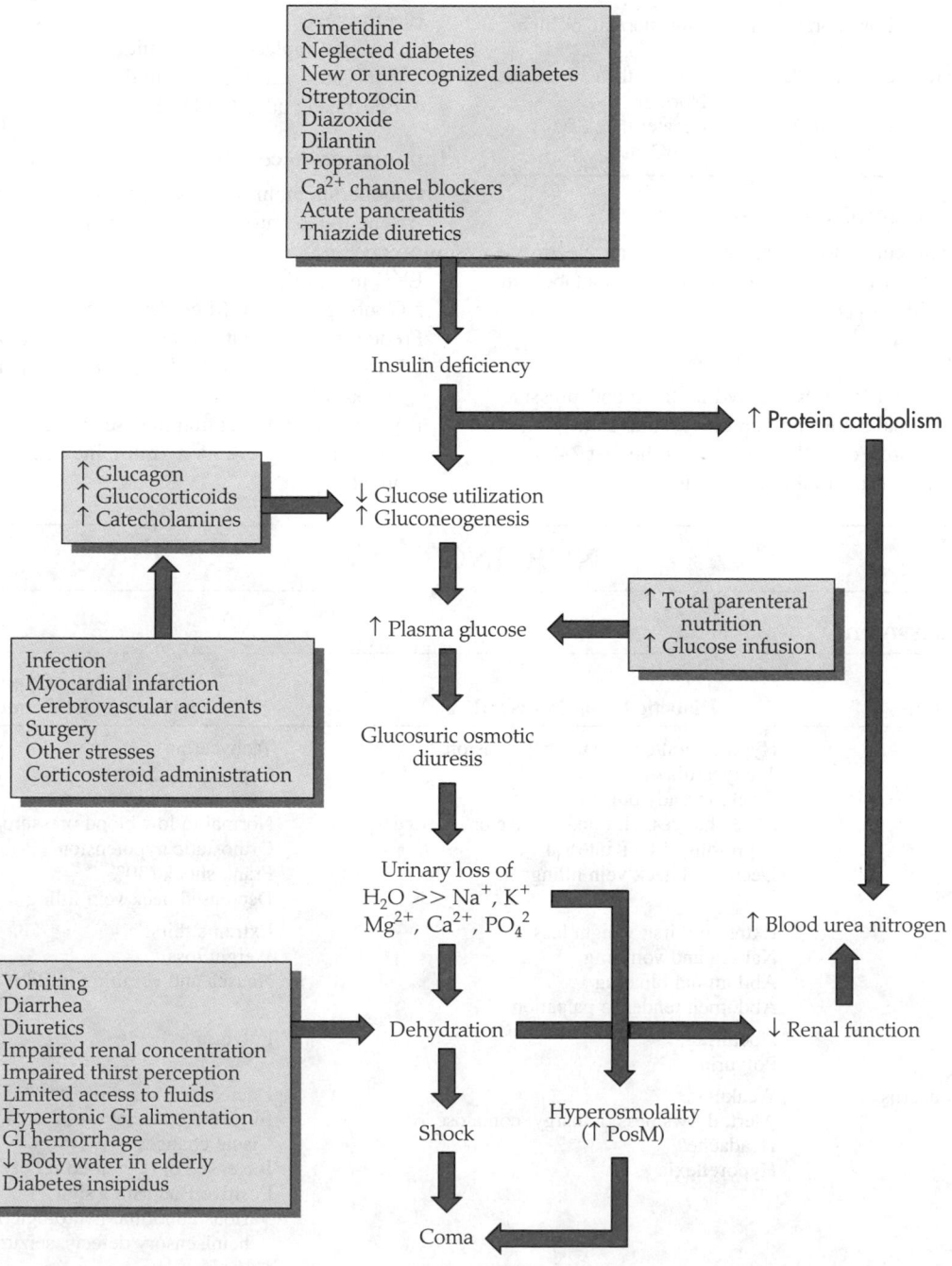

Figure 9-10 Pathogenesis of hyperosmolar nonacidotic uncontrolled diabetes.

Diagnostic Studies and Findings

Study	Diabetic Ketoacidosis (DKA)	Hyperglycemic Hyperosmolar Non-ketotic Syndrome (HHNS)
Blood sugar	High (300-600 mg/dl)	Over 800 mg/dl
Plasma ketones	Strongly positive	Not present (or only in small amounts)
Serum sodium	Low, normal, or high	Normal or high
Serum potassium	Low, normal, or high	Low, normal, or high
Serum bicarbonate	0-15 mEq/L	Greater than 16 mEq/L
Blood pH	6.8 to 7.3	Normal
Serum osmolarity	Less than 350 mOsm/L	Greater than 350 mOsm/L

Multidisciplinary Plan

The goal of treatment is to (1) replace fluid and electrolyte losses, (2) provide insulin to normalize nutrient metabolism, and (3) correct acidosis (DKA).

Medications[22,55,72]

Fluid replacement (depends on hydration, blood pressure, age, weight, renal status, and cardiovascular status)
0.9% normal saline or 0.45% saline over the first 2-4 hours (rate 1-2 L/h) for initial rehydration

Follow with 0.45% saline with rate adjusted on basis of clinical and laboratory findings
After blood glucose near 250-300 mg/dl range, 5% or 10% dextrose is added to IV infusion
Insulin
U-100 regular insulin given IM or IV; low dose continuous infusion by IV is the preferred route if method is available to regulate infusion; given at same rate for both DKA and HHNS, although less needed in HHNS
Electrolytes
Sodium: replaced as IV fluid
Potassium: added to IV fluid
Phosphate: added to IV fluid

Intravenous Access

Continuous monitoring with use of flowsheet to follow essential laboratory data and patient assessment areas of concern
EKG monitoring
NG tube placement (if comatose)
Frequent assessment and evaluation of the patient
Work-up for causes of DKA/HHNS (including infection work-up)
Psychosocial intervention in cases of recurrent DKA
Education for prevention (must include sick day management)

NURSING CARE

Nursing Assessment

Area of Concern	Diabetic Ketoacidosis (DKA)	Hyperglycemic Hyperosmolar Nonketotic Syndrome (HHNS)
Circulation	Hypotension/orthostatic hypotension Tachycardia Weak, thready pulse ECG changes: elevated P wave or inverted prolonged Q-T interval Decreased neck vein filling	Tachycardia Rapid, thready pulse Cool extremities Normal to low blood pressure Orthostatic hypotension Frank shock (30%)[48] Decreased neck vein filling
Food and fluid	Extreme thirst; weight loss Nausea and vomiting Abdominal bloating Abdomen tender to palpation	Extreme thirst Weight loss Nausea and vomiting (mild if present)
Elimination	Nocturia Polyuria	Polyuria
Neurosensory concerns	Weakness Alert, drowsiness; lethargy; comatose Headache Hyporeflexia	Decreased mentation Impaired consciousness (50%) Visual changes Increased or decreased reflexes Positive Babinski's sign Various abnormal neurologic findings (aphasia, hemisensory defects, seizures, hemiparesis)
Mobility	Decreased muscle tone Muscle wasting Muscle weakness	Muscle weakness

Area of Concern	Diabetic Ketoacidosis (DKA)	Hyperglycemic Hyperosmolar Nonketotic Syndrome (HHNS)
Hygiene and skin	Hyperthermia/hypothermia Dry mucous membranes Sunken eyeballs Hot, dry flushed skin Parched tongue Poor skin turgor	Hyperthermia Parched, dry lips and tongue Poor skin turgor Soft, sunken eyeballs Flushed face
Psychosocial concerns	Frightened Crying; restlessness Unable to care for self because of high levels of anxiety or decreased consciousness	Inability to care for self because of change in level of consciousness
Respiration	Hyperpnea (Kussmaul) Acetone breath	

Nursing Dx & Intervention

Fluid volume deficit related to failure of regulatory mechanism

- Reassess skin turgor *to determine fluid balance.*
- Reassess pulse, temperature, and blood pressure every 30 to 60 minutes.
- Monitor intake and output every hour and urine specific gravity as ordered *to assess changes in fluid balance.*
- Administer intravenous fluids, insulin, potassium, and other electrolytes as ordered.
- Report signs and symptoms of circulatory collapse immediately.
- Start and maintain patent peripheral IV line.
- Provide mouth care every hour *to maximize comfort.*
- Monitor for circulatory overload during fluid replacement.
- Continue to monitor and report worsening of fluid-volume deficit or electrolyte imbalance signs and symptoms.
- Record patient data on flowsheet.

Nutrition altered: less than body requirements related to inadequate intake of nutrients in diet

- Monitor patient's laboratory data *to assess fluid and electrolyte balance.*
- Encourage patient to ingest small amounts of ice chips frequently and sip clear, cool fluids as tolerated.
- Encourage patient to maintain good oral hygiene.
- Discuss causes of nausea, vomiting, and thirst with patient.
- Treat underlying problem with intravenous fluids, insulin, potassium, and other electrolytes as ordered.
- Monitor patient's blood glucose and urine ketones as ordered.
- Review patient's diet prescription with dietitian before discharge.

Coping, ineffective, individual: related to situational crisis

- Explain all procedures to the patient and family.
- Encourage the patient's participation in self-care *to maximum ability as soon as able.*
- See pp. 1739 to 1744.

- Discuss causes of situational stress with the patient.
- Assist patient to identify and use appropriate coping strategies.
- Offer support and positive reinforcement.

Risk for injury related to sensory dysfunction

- Assist and support patient as needed *to reduce chance of injury.*
- Provide assistive devices as needed.
- Minimize hazardous environmental factors.
- Discuss causative factors and prevention of injury with patient and family.
- Assess mental status frequently.

Patient Education/Home Care Planning

1. Ensure patient verbalizes understanding of the essential skills and concepts of diabetes mellitus education (p. 839), especially sick day rules.

Evaluation

Fluid balance is achieved Patient's blood pressure is within normal limits. Patient's pulse is within normal limits. Shock is not present. Patient's circulation to peripheral tissues is adequate. Patient has no dehydration. Patient's output equals intake. Patient's skin turgor is normal. Patient's electrolytes are within normal limits.

Intake of nutrients is adequate Patient's blood pH is normal and blood sugar is within normal limits. Patient is conscious and alert. Patient's respiratory rate and character are normal. Patient's electrolytes are within normal limits. Patient's ECG is at baseline. Patient's blood sugar is within normal limits. Patient has no ketonuria. Patient's weight is stable. Patient has ingested the recommended amounts and types of nutrients. Patient describes causative factors and rationale for treatment. Patient's fluid and electrolyte balance is normal. Patient has no nausea, vomiting, or thirst.

Patient copes effectively Patient verbalizes concerns and fears. Patient's behavior is calm and appropriate. Patient discusses potential causes of condition. Patient verbalizes methods to prevent recurrence. Patient uses appropriate coping strategies. Patient accepts support. Patient shows increased independence in self-care.

Patient remains free of personal injury　Patient seeks assistance as needed. Patient uses assistive devices as needed. Patient verbalizes cause of potential for injury. Patient recognizes environmental hazards and avoids them.

■ Hypoglycemia

Hypoglycemia includes conditions of excess serum insulin which causes a reduction in blood sugar and produces symptoms of hypoglycemia. These symptoms are generally relieved when normal blood sugar levels are restored. (See Emergency Alert box.) The presence of hypoglycemia, once proven, should be viewed as a marker of an underlying disorder, and the etiology determined.[81]

Hypoglycemia is classified as follows:

Fasting

Insulin-producing islet cell tumor (insulinomas)
Islet cell hyperplasia (nesidioblastosis)
Extra-pancreatic tumors
Hepatic disease
Gluconeogenic substrate defects
Insulin autoimmune syndromes

Reactive

Reactive hypoglycemia
Alimentary hypoglycemia
Early diabetes mellitus

Induced

Exogenous insulin or sulfonylurea use by persons with known diabetes
Factitious use of insulin or sulfonylureas by nondiabetic patients
Drug/alcohol-induced

The following discussion will be limited to conditions that are endocrine in nature, with hyperinsulinemia as a causative factor: insulinomas, islet hyperplasia, reactive, and induced hypoglycemia. Of all types of hypoglycemia, fasting is the most serious.

The true prevalence of each entity is uncertain. Insulinomas are uncommon, with episodic hypoglycemia occurring in the fasting state. Episodes become more frequent and severe in nature. Insulinomas are the most common islet cell tumors. They arise from pancreatic beta cells and produce insulin. Tumors vary in size, but no relationship exists between the size of the tumor and the severity of symptoms. Most insulinomas are benign, and 90% occur in individuals over age 30.[81] Insulinomas can occur with other endocrine abnormalities, such as in Type I multiple endocrine neoplasia (MEN-I), which is associated with adenomas of the pituitary and parathyroid tissue and with the occurrence of Zollinger-Ellison syndrome. Nesidioblastosis

is a rare disease causing persistent hypoglycemia. This condition was formerly believed to affect only newborns and infants; however, it has been reported recently in adolescents and adults. Nesidioblastosis results from diffuse proliferation of beta cells and inappropriate insulin release.

Reactive hypoglycemia is somewhat poorly defined and controversial. Hypoglycemia occurs as a result of excessive or delayed insulin secretion. Early diabetes mellitus and alimentary hypoglycemia are conditions sometimes associated with reactive patterns of hypoglycemia. True reactive hypoglycemia is rare, occurring primarily in individuals who consume high amounts of refined carbohydrate calories. It is well-documented that ingestion of large amounts of simple sugar often causes a transient drop in blood glucose. When meals contain a balance of complex carbohydrate, protein, and fat, the same degree of carbohydrate reactivity is not present.

Drug-induced hypoglycemia is commonly associated with diabetic persons who use blood sugar–lowering medication. Not only may the agent itself lower blood glucose, but also may interact with other agents in an additive or synergistic way to produce hypoglycemia. Common causes of hypoglycemia in persons with known diabetes who use blood sugar–lowering medications include (1) error in dosage, (2) poor comprehension of medication information, (3) increased activity/exercise, (4) lack of sufficient food intake, and (5) decreased insulin requirements.[45,81] In these cases, hypoglycemia occurs as a complication of medical therapy; however, factitious use of these same medications by nondiabetic patients is the result of a deliberate attempt to create the illusion of a hypoglycemic disor-

---

 EMERGENCY ALERT

HYPOGLYCEMIA

Dangerously low glucose levels that are classified as either fasting or reactive. This results from an underproduction of glucose, oversupply of insulin, or some drug interactions.

Assessment

- Determine history of diabetes and management.
- Assess for the following:

Sweating	Visual changes
Tachycardia	Confusion
Restlessness	Personality changes
Tremors	Seizures
Headache	Coma
Appearance of drunkenness	

Interventions

- Obtain IV access.
- In collaboration with physician, administer 50% dextrose by IV.
- Stop insulin pump (if applicable).
- In collaboration with physician, administer oral glucose as possible.
- Assist to determine the cause of the hypoglycemia.

der. Hypoglycemia induced by factitious use of insulin was first described in 1947. C-Peptide is useful in differentiating endogenous from exogenous hyperinsulinemia. The possibility of insulin self-injection in the nondiabetic patient (surreptitious insulin use) should be considered in all cases of fasting hypoglycemia, particularly in instances involving health professionals or persons who have contact with those who have diabetes. These persons can be ingenious in concealing their use of insulin and often display no psychologic disturbance. Sulfonylurea abuse has also been reported as a cause of factitious hypoglycemia, and together with surreptitious insulin abuse, factitious hypoglycemia may occur as frequently as insulinoma.[45] Many other drugs have been reported to cause hypoglycemia including pentamidine, quinine, and disopyramide.

• • • • • • Pathophysiology

Insulin is responsible for maintaining normal blood glucose levels in conjunction with counterregulatory hormones (epinephrine, glucagon, cortisol, and growth hormone) that oppose insulin action in the fasting and fed state. In hyperinsulinemia, excess insulin levels disrupt this balance by increasing glucose use and inhibiting hepatic glucose production. Negative feedback control over insulin secretion is lost; insulin secretion is not suppressed as plasma glucose levels decrease, and glucose utilization is increased. Disrupting this balance results in a decrease in serum glucose. The clinical severity of hypoglycemia is not well-correlated to specific blood glucose levels. The early symptoms of low blood sugar are associated with inhibition of glucose receptors in the ventromedial hypothalamic nucleus. This stimulates the sympathetic fibers of the autonomic nervous system to release epinephrine to restore blood glucose levels to normal. A decrease in blood glucose leads to an increased secretion of all four counterregulatory hormones. Glucagon plays the primary counterregulatory role by increasing hepatic glucose production. Catecholamines exert a major influence in counterregulation and are responsible for the appearance of early or adrenergic symptoms of hypoglycemia. These symptoms include sweating, palpitations, tachycardia, tremors, pallor, hunger, and nervousness. This adrenergic response serves as an early warning mechanism that precedes changes in cortical function occurring as a result of inadequate glucose to brain cells.

The brain is completely dependent on glucose as an energy source, and therefore, extremely sensitive to hypoglycemia. Neuroglycopenic symptoms follow as a result of an inadequate supply of glucose to maintain normal function, and include headache, fatigue, irritability, visual disturbances, decreased attentiveness, amnesia, confusion, paresthesias, paralysis, seizures, and loss of consciousness. These symptoms can be most severe and occur at a higher blood glucose level in the elderly than in the young.[45] Some irreversible brain damage can occur as the result of frequent or prolonged hypoglycemia, including a decrease in intellectual function, impaired nerve function, and personality changes.

Insulin-producing islet cell tumors (insulinomas; islet cell hyperplasia nesidioblastosis) and induced forms of hypo-

glycemia produce absolute elevations in plasma insulin levels that are not responsive to change in blood glucose. Hypoglycemia results from (1) elevated glucose uptake by insulin-dependent tissues and (2) inhibition of hepatic glucose production. Exercise intensifies hypoglycemic symptoms because of additional glucose uptake by muscle cells.

In contrast with fasting hypoglycemia, neuroglycopenic symptoms are not observed postprandially or in reactive patterns of hypoglycemia. In these cases, hypoglycemia is brief, mild, and accompanied by adrenergic and non-specific symptoms. Alimentary hypoglycemia is thought to be mediated by rapid gastric emptying, rapid early glucose absorption with excessive hyperglycemia and hyperinsulinemia, and/or vagal interruption. Increased gut hormone secretion may also play a causative role.[45,81] Reactive hypoglycemia resolves spontaneously with counterregulation, and does not require intervention with carbohydrate feeding.

Hypoglycemia is episodic; symptoms may recur, lasting for a few minutes to a few hours. If food ingestion does not occur to return blood glucose levels to normal, blood glucose will continue to decline, leading to loss of consciousness, seizures, or death.[24] In most cases, symptoms of hypoglycemia are reversible within minutes after euglycemia is restored.

• • • • • • Diagnostic Studies and Findings[22,23]

Insulinomas Blood sugar (low fasting or when symptomatic); plasma insulin (inappropriately elevated fasting or when symptomatic); plasma proinsulin and C-peptide (elevated fasting or when symptomatic); 72-hour supervised fast (elevated insulin, low blood glucose; most are symptomatic within 24 hours); tumor localization by CT scan, ultrasound, percutaneous transhepatic portal venous sampling, and/or selective arteriography.

Nesidioblastosis Blood sugar (low-fasting or when symptomatic); plasma insulin (inappropriately elevated fasting or when symptomatic); plasma proinsulin and C-peptide (elevated fasting or when symptomatic)

Exogenous insulin or sulfonylurea use by diabetic patients Plasma glucose (low when symptomatic)

Factitious insulin use Blood sugar (low when symptomatic); plasma insulin (elevated when symptomatic); plasma proinsulin and C-peptide (low levels); plasma insulin antibodies (may be present with use of nonhuman source insulin)

• • • • • • Multidisciplinary Plan

Surgery

Subtotal pancreatectomy (for nesidioblastosis)
Insulinoma resection

Medications[81]

Insulinoma and nesidioblastosis
  Diazoxide (Proglycem), 150-600 mg/d
  Phenytoin (Dilantin), 300-600 mg/d
  Propranolol (Inderal), 80 mg/d

Malignant insulinoma
    Antineoplastic agents: streptozocin, 5-fluorouracil, asparaginase, mithramycin, or adriamycin (see Chapter 16)
    Somatostatin analog (Octreotide) 200-675 μg daily
Unconscious hypoglycemia (all types)
    Glucagon 1 mg subcutaneously, IM, or IV
    50% dextrose, 25 g IV over 1-3 minutes

General Management

Diet
    Insulinoma and nesidioblastosis
        Increase number of feedings per day; may need to ingest food q 2 to 4 hours through day and night
        During symptomatic episodes: rapidly absorbable forms of simple carbohydrates
        Continuous intravenous administration of glucose by infusion for severe refractory hypoglycemia
    Exogenous insulin and sulfonylurea use by diabetic patients
        Medical nutrition therapy (individualized)
        During symptomatic episodes: 10-15 g of simple carbohydrate for mild (adrenergic symptoms) reaction; 20-30 g of simple carbohydrate for moderate (adrenergic and neuroglycopenic symptoms) reaction
        May need to follow with mixed snack (complex carbohydrate and protein) if next meal is more than 1 hour away after initial treatment
    Reactive
        Carbohydrate restriction, especially with simple sugars
        Decrease meal size
        Increase meal frequency
        Dietitian referral
    Factitious insulin and sulfonylurea use
        Before diagnosis, same as insulinoma and nesidioblastosis
    Psychiatric consultation (factitious insulin and sulfonylurea use)

NURSING CARE

Nursing Assessment

Food and Fluid

Relief of symptoms with food intake
    Hunger
    Weight gain

Circulation

    Tachycardia
    Palpitations

Neurosensory Concerns

    Tremor
    Headache
    Mental dullness
    Confusion
    Amnesia

    Seizures
    Unconsciousness
    Paralysis
    Paresthesias
    Dizziness
    Irritability
    Visual disturbance

Psychosocial

    Change in role performance
    Resents enforced dependence
    Unable to stay alone: related to episodes of loss of consciousness
    Past history of destructive behavior

Nursing Dx & Intervention

Nutrition; altered: more than body requirements related to excess intake for metabolic needs

* Assess for symptoms that patient normally experiences with hypoglycemia and whether or not patient is awakened by symptoms at night.
* Assess patient for symptoms of low blood sugar, and check blood glucose by fingerstick using bedside blood glucose monitoring (BBGM): fasting, before and 2 hours after meals, at bedtime, and at 3 to 5 AM.
* Check blood pressure, pulse, and respiration with occurrence of symptoms.
* Provide patient with 3 AM snack if needed *to prevent nocturnal hypoglycemia.*
* Arrange a dietary consultation.
* Identify symptoms of hypoglycemia experienced by patient.
* Provide prompt intervention for episodes of hypoglycemia.
* Monitor patient's blood sugar frequently (every 2 to 4 hours) including during the night.
* Discuss cause of weight gain.
* Discuss with the patient the importance of frequent meals and monitoring for prevention and early detection of hypoglycemia.
* After successful treatment of underlying cause, assist patient to set realistic goals related to weight management.

Coping, ineffective, individual: related to situational crisis

* Assess patient's personal strengths and weaknesses and coping skills.
* Remove potentially dangerous articles from patient's room (factitious use of insulin or sulfonylureas).
* Encourage patient toward maximum independence.
* Assist patient to communicate with others.
* Discuss need for restrictions and precautions related to potential loss of consciousness *to maintain patient's safety and prevent injury.*
* Give information about disease *to enhance feeling of control.*

- Encourage patient to consult with psychiatrist.
- Offer support to the patient.
- Discuss cause of situational stress with patient.
- Assist patient to identify and use appropriate coping strategies.
- See pp. 1739 to 1744.

Risk for injury related to sensory dysfunction

- Provide patient with consistent daily meal plan, including 3 AM snack.
- Limit patient's physical activity or mobility during episodes of hypoglycemia.
- Minimize hazardous environmental factors.
- Discuss causative factors with patient and family.

Patient Education/Home Care Planning

1. Explain to the patient the signs and symptoms of hypoglycemia, and importance of early recognition and prompt treatment.
2. Discuss with the patient a 24-hour diet plan and the importance of adhering to it.
3. Provide patient with information regarding amounts and types of foods/fluids to treat hypoglycemia.

Evaluation

Intake of nutrients is adequate Patient has no hypoglycemia, or hypoglycemia is detected early and managed adequately. Patient experiences no seizures or loss of consciousness. Patient ingests the recommended types, amounts of nutrients at desired times. Patient describes causative factors and rationale for treatment. Patient's weight gain is minimized until the problem is resolved.

Patient copes effectively Anxiety is decreased. Family verbalizes adapting to changes imposed by hypoglycemia. Patient accepts support from health professionals. Patient establishes and follows plan to minimize symptoms and maximize functioning. Maximum independence is maintained. Patient shows no self-destructive behavior. Patient complies with the precautions and restrictions imposed.

Patient remains free of personal injury Patient identifies and avoids factors that increase potential for injury. Patient uses preventive measures. Patient verbalizes cause of potential for injury. Patient complies with diet and monitoring prescription, as well as activity restrictions during episodes of hypoglycemia. Patient shows no seizures or loss of consciousness.

▌ ZOLLINGER-ELLISON SYNDROME (GASTRINOMA)

▌ Zollinger-Ellison syndrome (ZES) is a syndrome characterized by gastric acid hypersecretion and recurrent peptic ulcer disease, caused by excessive gastrin secretion from non-beta cell islet cell tumors, or gastrinomas.

Although ZES is uncommon, it is not rare. Approximately 20% to 25% of pancreatic endocrine tumors are gastrinomas.[107] Multiple endocrine neoplasia type I (MEN) is present in 25% to 30% of patients with ZES. Although most gastrinomas occur in the pancreas, extrapancreatic tumors may occur in the duodenum, stomach, spleen, ovary, and lymph nodes.

Gastrinomas vary in size and location, and approximately two thirds are malignant. Usual sites of metastasis are lymph nodes, liver, spleen, bone, skin, and peritoneum.

Before the development of potent antisecretory drug therapy, the mortality from ZES was high—not always from metastases of the malignant tumor, but often from the extreme effects of hypergastrinemia and complications of ulcers: perforation, fistula formation, and hemorrhage. Total gastrectomy was the only relatively successful treatment for ZES. The development of histamine H-receptor blocking agents and benzimidazole inhibitors of gastric acid secretion in 1990 represents a major breakthrough in the management of ZES.

•••••• Pathophysiology

ZES is characterized by recurrent and severe peptic ulcer disease. Gastrin has a variety of effects on the gastrointestinal tract. The major effect of gastrin is the stimulation of gastric acid secretion from parietal cells, possibly through stimulation of a histamine or cyclic AMP-mediated process. The secretion of gastrin by tumor tissue (gastrinomas) is not responsive to the normal inhibitory stimuli of low gastric pH and secretin; secretin paradoxically stimulates gastrin release. The continuous high serum gastrin levels found in ZES produce a state of constant gastric acid hypersecretion, which exceeds the duodenum's capacity to neutralize acid. This accounts for the upper gastrointestinal ulcerations found in sites as far distal to the stomach as the jejunum. Gastrin is also known to cause moderate stimulation of pepsin release from gastric chief cells. In the presence of low pH in the proximal and distal duodenum and jejunum, pepsin contributes to the development of mucosal erosions and ulceration at points as distal as the jejunum.[23] Gastrin also directly decreases salt and water absorption in the intestine, and results in the presence of large amounts of fluid in both stomach and duodenum even in the fasting state. Marked hyperplasia of parietal cells and mucosal cell proliferation with hypertrophy of the pyloric gastric mucosa is the direct result of high serum gastrin levels, ultimately causing the development of prominent rugal folds in the stomach.[74] The increased number of parietal cells in ZES is significant in the development of hyperacidity because a close relationship exists between the number of parietal cells and the amount of gastric acid secreted.[23,88]

The diarrhea and steatorrhea of ZES is caused by a number of factors:

1. Large amounts of hydrochloric acid irritate the gastrointestinal mucosa and increase peristalsis.
2. Gastrin increases intestinal motility.
3. Pancreatic lipase is inactivated in the presence of low intestinal pH and fat breakdown, and absorption is not accomplished.
4. Precipitation and inactivation of bile salts in the acid environment of the small intestine also prevents fat absorption.

5. The direct effect of gastrin stimulates gastric, pancreatic, liver, and intestinal secretion of water and electrolytes.

6. The malabsorption of a variety of substances is caused by inactivation of intestinal enzymes in the presence of acidity.

Diarrhea and steatorrhea are accompanied by severe losses of potassium and magnesium in patients with ZES.

Gastrin also stimulates intrinsic factor secretion. In ZES, malabsorption of vitamin B_{12} is thought to result from the low intestinal pH, which may interfere with the action of intrinsic factor in facilitating the absorption of vitamin B_{12}. This condition is not corrected by the administration of the intrinsic factor; only monthly vitamin B_{12} injections can ameliorate it.

•••••• Diagnostic Studies and Findings

Elevated serum gastrin   Level of 1000 pg/ml virtually diagnostic of ZES after exclusion of other disorders with hypergastrinemia[23]

Provocative testing   Secretin; serum gastrin rises by at least 200 pg/ml over basal value within 30 minutes of secretin injection; gastrin analysis[24]; basal acid concentration of greater than 15 mEq/hr in previously unoperated patient and greater than 5 mEq/hr in previously operated patients; ratio of basal/maximal acid output (BAO/MAO) is 0.6 or greater.[23]

Radiologic findings   Irregular thick gastric mucosal folds with ulcers at usual and unusual sites; pancreatic islet cell tumor demonstrated by angiography

Tumor localization   Abdominal CT scan; abdominal ultrasound; selective mesenteric arteriography; portal venous sampling

•••••• Multidisciplinary Plan

Surgery

Total gastrectomy (see Chapter 8)
Partial pancreatectomy (tumor excision)

Medications[23]

Histamine H_2 receptor antagonists
  Cimetidine, 300-600 mg q6h
  Ranitidine, 150 mg qid or qid and hs
  Famotidine, 20-160 mg q6h
Benzimidazoles
Omeprazole, 20-60 mg/d
Streptozoticin, 5-FU, doxorubicin (see cancer section) for treatment of metastatic gastrinomas
Miscellaneous
  Octreotide (Sandostatin) 220-675 μg daily[74]

NURSING CARE

Nursing Assessment

Circulation

Decreased blood pressure
Tachycardia
Cold, clammy skin

Food and Fluid

Burning, pain in epigastric region between meals
Coffee-ground or frank blood emesis
Thirst
Decreased appetite
Weight loss
Dry mouth

Elimination

Increased frequency of stools
Foul smelling, foamy stools
Abdominal cramping/pain

Comfort and Pain

Severe upper abdominal pain, may be referred to top of shoulders
Abdomen rigid and tender

Psychosocial

Feelings of helplessness
Decreased participation in outside-the-home activities because of diarrhea
Embarrassment

Nursing Dx & Intervention

Risk for fluid-volume deficit related to excessive loss through normal routes

- Assess fluid balance (intake and output, daily weights, vital signs, signs of dehydration) *to identify dehydration early.*
- Measure daily fluid loss in stools and drainage *to prevent undetected loss.*
- Replace fluids with water, tea, carbonated beverages, gelatin, popsicles, and broth.
- Have a dietary consultation to include foods high in potassium and magnesium *to replace losses in diarrhea.*
- Discuss causes of fluid loss with patient and family.
- Treat underlying cause as ordered.

Diarrhea related to inflammation, irritation, and malabsorption

- Assess fluid losses in diarrhea by daily measurement.
- Check with physician about medication for perianal irritation from frequent stools.
- Replace lost fluid and electrolytes *to prevent fluid and electrolyte imbalance.*
- Observe patient for signs and symptoms of dehydration, decreased potassium, and magnesium.
- Discuss causative factors with patient and family.
- Treat underlying cause as ordered.

Coping, ineffective, individual: related to situational crisis

- Assess patient's and family's coping skills and support systems, and adaptive skills successful in the past.
- Encourage open communication between patient and family members.

- Assist patient in identifying strengths and positive coping skills *to cope with current stressors.*
- Offer suggestions as to how patient can cope with problem areas and function away from home.
- Discuss causes of situational stress.
- Offer support and positive reinforcement.
- Assist with problem solving.

Pain (acute) related to injuring agent

- Discuss causes of pain with patient and family.
- Assist patient to use pain control measures.
- Treat underlying cause as ordered.
- Monitor pain and effectiveness of comfort measures.

Patient Education/Home Care Planning

1. Discuss with the patient the importance of fluid and electrolyte replacement for diarrhea to prevent dehydration and changes in electrolyte balance.
2. Ensure the patient understands the need for strict medication compliance to maintain the status of healed ulcers and avoid pain.
3. Ensure the patient understands the dose, schedule, action, and side effects of the medication ordered, to ensure safe and effective use of medication.

Evaluation

Fluid balance is achieved   Patient has no hemorrhage. Patient shows no changes in blood pressure or pulse. Patient verbalizes understanding of and complies with fluid and electrolyte (potassium, magnesium) replacement with diarrhea. Patient is not dehydrated.

Normal bowel elimination pattern   Patient has a more normal pattern of bowel elimination. Patient describes causative factors and rationale for interventions. Patient shows no perineal irritation.

Patient copes effectively   Patient uses appropriate coping strategies. Patient accepts support. Open communication exists between patient and family. Patient uses suggestions to increase independence and ability to function away from home.

Pain is resolved   Patient uses suggested comfort measures. Patient describes causative factors. Patient verbalizes increased comfort.

DISORDERS OF THE PARATHYROID GLANDS

PRIMARY HYPERPARATHYROIDISM (HPT)

Primary hyperparathyroidism (HPT) is caused by the excessive secretion of parathyroid hormone (PTH) from one or more of the four parathyroid glands.

Primary hyperparathyroidism is part of the differential diagnosis of hypercalcemia. It is the most common cause of hypercalcemia among non-hospitalized patients; malignancy accounts for the most common cause of hypercalcemia among hospitalized patients. The box below lists many of the causes of hypercalcemia. Only primary hyperparathyroidism will be discussed in this section.

HPT may be triggered by a benign adenoma isolated to a single gland (80% of all HPT); more than one adenoma in a patient (1-2%); hyperplasia of all four glands (15%); or parathyroid carcinoma (≤1% of all HPT). The incidence of HPT increased greatly in the early 1970s when multichannel screening

---

■ CAUSES OF HYPERCALCEMIA

PARATHYROID GLAND
Idiopathic
Associated with MEN Type 1 or 2a
Familial

MALIGNANCIES
Osteolytic hypercalcemia
Humoral hypercalcemia of malignancy
1,25 dihydroxyvitamin D-mediated hypercalcemia
Hematologic malignancies

OTHER ENDOCRINE DISORDERS
Thyrotoxicosis
Pheochromocytoma
Addisonian crisis
VIPoma syndrome
Acromegaly
Familial hypocalciuric hypercalcemia (FHH)

MEDICATIONS
Vitamin D and A intoxication
Lithium
Thiazide diuretics
Estrogen/antiestrogens, androgens
Theophylline
Milk alkali syndrome (excess calcium drugs)
Parenteral nutrition

GRANULOMATOUS DISORDERS
Sarcoidosis
Tuberculosis
Histoplasmosis
Coccidioidomycosis
Candidiasis

MISCELLANEOUS
Dehydration
Renal failure
Advanced chronic liver disease
Immobilization
Serum protein disorders
Hypophasphatemia
Pagets' disease

tests were first used. Today, the incidence has stabilized at about 1:1000 and approximates the prevalence. It can occur at all ages, but is unusual in children and peaks between ages 50 and 60 years. It is more frequent in women than men with a 3:2 ratio. A history of radiation to the neck may be a predisposing factor.[91]

Parathyroid hyperplasia occurs most frequently in conjunction with the multiple endocrine neoplasia (MEN) syndromes Type I and IIA. MEN I is an autosomal dominant disorder with a high degree of penetrance. These patients usually have tumors of the pituitary, parathyroid, and endocrine pancreas. MEN IIA is also autosomal dominant and involves medullary thyroid carcinoma, HPT, and pheochromocytoma.

• • • • • • Pathophysiology

Parathyroid hormone is usually regulated by the ionized calcium level. As ionized calcium decreases, it stimulates release of PTH. Conversely, as ionized calcium increases, it suppresses the release of PTH. In primary hyperparathyroidism, PTH continues to be secreted in the presence of an elevated ionized calcium. It has been theorized that either the parathyroid cells have developed an altered set point so that they can only respond to a higher than normal ionized calcium or the parathyroid cells have increased in number without an altered set point.[91] The altered set point means that the gland still has the ability to be suppressed, such as by increasing dietary calcium intake. Both of these mechanisms may be operational in an adenoma, while hyperplasia is more closely linked to an increased number of parathyroid cells without alteration of the set point. In about 4% of adenomas, there is also evidence of a rearrangement involving the PTH gene and the parathyroid adenoma gene (PRAD1). PRAD1 is a monoclonal oncogene that may supplant PTH in the adenoma leading to both growth of the cells as well as the altered set point. This rearrangement seems to be limited to the adenomatous gland and has not been found in the remaining normal parathyroid glands. In fact, the non-involved glands become suppressed by the adenomatous gland, which means they are hormonally inactive. Hyperplasia, on the other hand, appears to be a polyclonal process. In parathyroid carcinoma, there seems to be true autonomy of one of the glands, which means that the gland no longer responds to any feedback mechanism and continues to secrete PTH unabated.

Primary hyperparathyroidism at present is recognized most frequently as an asymptomatic disease. The diagnosis is arrived at as a result of an elevated serum calcium obtained on routine laboratory examination. If symptoms do occur, they have traditionally been described in relation to the primary target organs for PTH of bones and kidney. The patient may be predisposed to nephrolithiasis or to osteopenia, although it is rare for the patient to have both. The osteopenia may be seen as osteitis fibrous cystica on x-rays or as a decreased bone mineral density. Since HPT tends to occur in older postmenopausal women who may already have osteopenia, the onset of HPT may lead to osteoporosis. The gastrointestinal tract is the other major target organ. Peptic ulcer disease and acute pancreatitis have both been associated with HPT.

There are also a number of other systemic effects of hypercalcemia. Intracellular to extracellular calcium balance in neurotransmission seems to be altered leading to atrophy of type II muscle fibers and causing a proximal muscle weakness. Fatigue may be the nonspecific complaint voiced by the patient.

The area of greatest controversy today involves what has been termed the "psychic moans" of HPT. Distinct psychiatric manifestations of HPT have long included clinical depression, lethargy, stupor, and coma. The question remains whether, in mild HPT, the patients are truly asymptomatic, or whether there are more subtle psychological alterations that increase difficulty in completing activities of daily living and social responsibilities. Cognitive deficits have been described that include memory impairment and concentration difficulties. Just as in muscle cells, it has been postulated that the elevated PTH and calcium affect cerebral vascular adenyl cyclase and nerve conduction velocity. In addition to cognitive deficits, the following have also been described: obsessive-compulsive behavior, psychoticism, anxiety, and paranoia.[86]

The treatment for HPT varies from a wait and watch plan to surgical intervention. Some patients may have mild elevations in calcium and PTH levels that can remain unchanged over 5 or more years. These patients must be aware of symptoms of increasing calcium and be willing to have regular laboratory and physical reevaluations. Surgical intervention for an adenoma involves removal of the adenoma. The national consensus[20] criteria for surgery include (1) serum calcium above 12 mg/dl, (2) >400 mg calcium/g creatinine in the urine, (3) worsening creatinine clearance, (4) nephrolithiasis, and (5) substantially reduced bone mass (osteoporosis). After surgery, the patient is usually left with three healthy parathyroid glands that provide normal calcium/phosphorus metabolism. The surgical intervention for the patient with hyperplasia, however, involves removal of 3.5 to 3.75 glands. It is hoped that the remaining piece of a gland will eventually become hyperplastic and again provide normal calcium metabolism. If this does not occur, and some of the removed tissue was cryopreserved, then minced pieces of parathyroid tissue might be implanted into a muscle of a forearm.

• • • • • • Diagnostic Studies and Findings

Total serum calcium—greater than 11 mg/dl
Ionized calcium—increased (varies by assay method)
Parathyroid hormone (PTH)—increased (intact >65 pg/ml)
Intact PTH (1-84) better than C-terminal or N-terminal assay for differentiating primary hyperparathyroidism from renal disease and the hypercalcemia of malignancy
24-hr urine calcium—normal to high
Creatinine clearance—normal to high

• • • • • • Multidisciplinary Plan

Hyperparathyroidism is mild—wait and watch; may persist for months to years
Moderate/severe—parathyroidectomy
General—increased hydration 2-3 L/day
Possible low calcium diet
Psychologic/psychiatric evaluation

NURSING CARE

Nursing Assessment

No symptoms
Renal—polyuria, nephrolithiasis
Gastrointestinal—ulcer-type pain, constipation
Skeletal—demineralization, pain, activity intolerance
Psychosocial—depression, paranoia, mood swings, anxiety, obsessive-compulsive behavior
Neuromuscular—weakness, fatigue

Nursing Dx & Intervention

Fatigue related to altered metabolic balance

- Help patient plan a daily schedule that includes pacing leisure activities, rest, and exercise.
- Help patient identify excessive demands of role obligations.
- Encourage patient to keep a diary of the degree of fatigue, precipitating factors and specific symptoms that are perceived as fatigue.

Constipation related to musculoskeletal impairment and less than adequate intake

- Encourage patient to ingest fluids to 3000 ml/day.
- Administer stool softeners to patient as ordered.
- Encourage patient to ingest a high-fiber diet.
- Avoid giving the patient enemas or laxatives.

Activity intolerance related to generalized weakness

- Observe patient for steadiness of ambulation.
- Assist patient with ambulation when necessary.
- Help patient identify environmental hazards at home, and suggest alterations as necessary *to prevent injury.*

Ineffective coping, individual: related to personal identity vulnerability

- Help patient identify precipitating factors of stress.
- Help patient identify coping skills and adaptive behaviors used successfully in the past.
- Maintain a calm approach if the patient becomes agitated or irritable.
- Let patient know that the hormonal alteration reduces his or her ability to control his or her responses and that this is acceptable.

Patient Education/Home Care Planning

1. Discuss with patient the need to keep follow-up appointments and get calcium levels rechecked.
2. Demonstrate to the patient how to monitor and maintain adequate fluid intake.
3. Discuss with patient symptoms of kidney stones.
4. Discuss with the patient the importance of proper body alignment and mechanics and the need to gradually increase activity tolerance.
5. Ensure that the patient understands the importance of changing the home environment to prevent accidents.
6. Discuss with the patient the need for tolerance by family of patient mood swings, irritability, or decreased decision-making ability until therapy is completed.

Evaluation

Hydration is adequate   Patient's intake is at least 2 liters per day.

Comfort and activity level are increased   Patient's optimum level of mobility is maintained with little or no pain. Patient follows plan for using alternative pain-relieving methods. Patient uses pain medications infrequently. Patient verbalizes increased feelings of well-being. Patient participates in desired activities.

Coping is improved   Patient can identify one stimulus to decreased coping. Patient uses one coping technique successfully.

HYPOPARATHYROIDISM

In hypoparathyroidism, the parathyroid glands secrete an inadequate amount of parathyroid hormone (PTH) to maintain normal levels of serum calcium.

Hypoparathyroidism is manifested by hypocalcemia. This condition may occur at any age and is usually the result of damage to the parathyroid glands during parathyroid or thyroid surgery or purposeful removal of the parathyroid glands. It may also be from autoimmune destruction of the glands, either idiopathic or as part of a polyglandular autoimmune syndrome.

•••••• Pathophysiology

Although hypoparathyroidism is usually caused by damage to the parathyroid glands during surgical procedures, the disease may also be idiopathic. Idiopathic hypoparathyroidism is a rare autoimmune disorder that may occur before 15 years of age. It is sometimes one of several endocrine disorders included in a polyendocrine syndrome called HAM (hypoparathyroidism, Addison's disease, and moniliasis). Hypoparathyroidism has been acquired, in a few rare cases, following treatment with ^{131}I therapy. It has also been associated with metastases of malignant tumors to the parathyroid glands.[91]

The signs and symptoms of hypoparathyroidism are associated with hypocalcemia resulting from the decreased level of PTH. Neuromuscular irritability is the most common and recognizable feature of hypocalcemia, causing symptoms that range from mild paresthesias to tetany and hypocalcemic seizures. These symptoms are caused by a decrease in resting ability and increased excitability of nerve and muscle membranes.[29]

Bone resorption decreases in hypoparathyroidism, causing a decrease in osteoclastic activity. Bones remain normal or slightly more dense in adults. New growth is suppressed and may cause dwarfism in children. Calcification of the basal ganglion, another clinical manifestation of hypoparathyroidism, results in a Parkinson-like syndrome with bizarre posturing and dystonic choreoathetoid movements. Other characteristics of the disease include dental abnormalities caused by decreased calcium levels, cataracts resulting from a calcification of the lens, and hypotension caused by decreased cardiac contractility. Pseudohypoparathyroidism is a separate disease entity that is a familial disorder characterized by an atypical phenotype, chemical hypoparathyroidism, and increased circulating PTH levels.[91]

•••••• Diagnostic Studies and Findings

Serum calcium   Less than 8 mg/dl
Serum intact PTH   Less than 50 pg/μl

•••••• Multidisciplinary Plan

Medications

Calcium Salts—Requirement 1500-2000 mg elemental calcium/day
  Calcium carbonate, 400 mg elemental calcium/1000 mg tablet
  Calcium citrate, 210 mg elemental calcium/1000 mg tablet
  Calcium lactate, 130 mg elemental calcium/1000 mg tablet
  Calcium gluconate, 90 mg elemental calcium/10 ml IV push in 3-5 minutes
  Calcium glubionate, 115 mg elemental calcium/5 ml syrup
Vitamin D
  Ergocalciferol, vitamin D_2 50,000-100,000 U; 1.25-2.75 mg/day
  Dihydrotachysterol, 125-250 μg/day
  25,Hydroxyvitamin D_3, cholecalciferol, 50-250 μg/day
  1,25 Dihydroxyvitamin D_3, calcitriol, 0.5-1.0 μg/day

NURSING CARE

Nursing Assessment

Central Nervous System

  Personality disturbances
    Lassitude
    Depression
    Irritability
    Cognitive deficits
  Increased neuromuscular excitability
    Paresthesias
    Tetany
    Positive Chvostek's and Trousseau's signs
  Headache

Cardiovascular System

  Decreased contractility
  Decreased output

Skin

  Dry, coarse, flaky

Eyes

  Cataracts

Nursing Dx & Intervention

Altered nutrition: less than body requirements related to altered metabolism

- Identify food preferences that are high in calcium.
- Make high-calcium snacks available to patient at all times.
- Have the dietitian discuss dietary calcium supplements with the patient.
- Give calcium replacement medications on time *to enhance dietary intake of calcium.*
- Monitor Chvostek's and Trousseau's signs *to identify early loss of calcium.*

Ineffective coping individual related to personal vulnerability

- Assess patient's current coping skills, support systems, and history of adaptive behaviors that worked in the past.
- Maintain a calm approach if the patient is agitated or irritable.
- Observe for precipitating factors causing stress; intervene when possible *to decrease stressors.*
- Observe for changes in mood and thought processes *to identify psychologic changes that may require medical interventions.*
- See also pp. 1739 to 1744.

Decreased cardiac output related to alteration in conduction

- Assess vital signs, mental status, and urine output for symptoms of hypoperfusion.
- Check rhythm strip for Q-T interval changes and abnormal T wave and P wave changes *to identify hypocalcemia that is interfering with normal electrical activity of the myocardium.*

Patient Education/Home Care Planning

1. Ensure that the patient verbalizes an understanding of calcium and vitamin D supplements and the reasons for the treatment.
2. Give the patient a list of the early signs and symptoms of hypocalcemia and its treatment.
3. Suggest patient wear medic alert bracelet.

Evaluation

Nutrition is adequate   Patient routinely consumes high-calcium foods without difficulty. Chvostek's and Trousseau's signs are negative.

Patient copes effectively   Patient expresses feelings and uses effective coping mechanisms for problems surrounding illness. Patient is able to identify factors leading to increased stress and possible solutions to prevent these situations. Patient's affect is appropriate to the situation.

Cardiac output is normal   Cardiac rate and rhythm are normal.

METABOLIC DISORDERS

■ DYSLIPIDEMIA (HYPERLIPIDEMIA)

■ Dyslipidemia is a condition of abnormal metabolism of plasma lipids that is manifested as abnormally high levels of lipids in the blood.

Although in other disorders the term "abnormally high" refers to levels present in the upper 5% of the population (95th percentile), in most hyperlipidemias it refers instead to blood lipid levels associated with significantly increased risk of coronary artery disease.

The hyperlipidemias are a group of disorders of lipid metabolism. They vary in cause, severity, response to treatment, and prognosis. Hyperlipidemias occur in all ages and races and in both sexes. *Primary hyperlipidemias* are often hereditary disorders caused by deficiencies of certain mechanisms involved in lipid metabolism. *Secondary hyperlipidemias* occur in relation to other conditions or disorders. The majority of hyperlipidemias seen in Western society are related to other conditions, the most common being diet. The American diet often includes foods that are high in cholesterol, total fat, saturated fat, and excess calories. Of these, total fat and saturated fat have the most potent effect on cholesterol levels. Other common causes of secondary hyperlipidemia include (1) diabetes mellitus, (2) hypothyroidism, (3) renal disease, (4) bile duct obstruction, (5) excessive alcohol intake, and (6) drug-induced.

Various medications such as beta adrenergic blockers, retinoids, thiazide diuretics, corticosteroids, and oral contraceptives can cause blood lipid levels to increase significantly.

The most significant hyperlipidemias are those associated with an increased risk of coronary artery disease. Heart disease is the leading cause of death in the United States; it is responsible for more than 900,000 deaths per year—over 45% of all deaths in the United States. Elevated blood lipid levels are associated with the development of atherosclerosis and resultant coronary artery disease.[8] Over 50% of the adult population in the United States has elevated lipid levels.

Only a few types of hyperlipidemia do not carry an increased risk of coronary artery disease. In these specific disorders, recurrent severe pancreatitis tends to be the disease sequela.

Lipid Metabolism

Three major types of lipids circulate in the blood: cholesterol, triglycerides, and phospholipids. Cholesterol is absorbed from food and produced by the liver, and released from aging cells. It is used in the manufacture of cell membranes, hormones, vitamins, and bile salts. Triglycerides, also absorbed from food, are composed of fatty acids and glycerol. Fatty acid components are used by the cells for energy, or stored in adipose tissue. Excessive calorie intake and obesity encourage increased triglyceride synthesis by the liver and decreased removal from peripheral tissues. Phospholipids are synthesized mainly in the liver and intestines, although they can be made by most body tissues. Phospholipids form cell membranes and lipoproteins.[8,35]

Lipids are important components of body tissue, but must be transported by complex molecules called lipoproteins because they are insoluble in water. Lipoproteins contain an inner core of cholesterol and triglyceride, covered by a thin membrane of phospholipids, cholesterol, and protein. These membrane proteins are called apoproteins, and are made in the liver and intestines. To date, 11 apoproteins have been described, and genes responsible for their synthesis have been mapped.[8] They function to bind and transport lipids in the bloodstream, binding to specific receptors on peripheral tissues that include vascular endothelial cells. They also function as enzyme co-factors and inhibitors in lipid metabolism.

There are the major classes of lipoproteins: chylomicrons, very-low-density lipoproteins (VLDLs), low-density lipoproteins (LDLs), high-density lipoproteins (HDLs), and lipoprotein (a) [Lp(a)]. Chylomicrons, the largest lipoproteins, have a large triglyceride content, and are formed in the GI tract. Their primary role is to transport dietary fat from the intestines, in the plasma, to the liver. Normally they are rapidly cleared from the blood by lipoprotein lipase action. Remaining fragments are cleared by liver cell receptors. Chylomicrons are considered to be atherogenic, so any delay in clearance is potentially detrimental.

VLDLs are produced by the liver from fatty acids, triglyceride, and carbohydrate. They are the primary transporters for endogenous triglycerides, and go through plasma to peripheral tissue where fatty acids can be used for energy or stored as triglyceride. VLDLs are eventually converted to intermediate-density lipoproteins (IDL), and then to LDL. LDL contains 45% cholesterol by weight, and is the major carrier of cholesterol to nerve tissues, cell membranes, and other cholesterol-using cells.[8] LDL is usually formed from the breakdown of VLDLs. Most LDL is removed from the blood by receptor binding with internalization into cells.

HDL is produced by the liver and intestines, and by peripheral catabolism of chylomicrons and VLDLs. HDL carries cholesteryl ester, and is involved in the reverse transport of free cholesterol from peripheral tissues. One subfraction is associated with protection against premature atherosclerosis.

Lipoprotein (a) is present in the plasma as a minor lipoprotein. Although it is similar in structure to LDL, its specific physiologic function is not fully understood; lipoprotein (a) is an independent risk factor for CAD.[8,35]

After a meal, fat and cholesterol are absorbed from the gut. Ingested fat is transported in the blood as chylomicrons (containing triglycerides) and carried to the tissues. There apoprotein C-II activates an enzyme in the capillary endothelium, lipoprotein lipase, which leads to the removal of fatty acids from the triglycerides. These fatty acids are either used by muscle tissue for energy or stored as fat in the adipocytes. A chylomicron remnant containing apoprotein E is left over from this process and is transported to the liver. There apoprotein E interacts with hepatic cell surface receptors to facilitate the uptake of remnant particles from the plasma.

Cholesterol is synthesized by the liver at a rate regulated by the enzyme HMG CoA reductase, an enzyme that assists in the production of mevalonic acid which is, in turn, converted to cholesterol. Cholesterol from dietary sources also adds to the body's cholesterol pool. About 40% of dietary cholesterol is absorbed by the intestines. A number of factors encourage cholesterol synthesis by the liver: excessive caloric intake, excessive saturated fat in the diet, and high total dietary fat content.[35] Cholesterol-rich LDL is carried in the plasma to provide cholesterol to be used by cells for membrane synthesis, hormone production, bile acid synthesis, and production of vitamin D.

The second report of the NCEP expert panel continues to identify LDL as the target of cholesterol-lowering therapy. There is a strong positive correlation between elevated LDL cholesterol and increased risk for cardiovascular morbidity and mortality.[27] The liver is critical in regulation of LDL levels. LDL receptors on the liver cells recognize the apoprotein B component of LDL. Apoprotein B binds LDL to these receptors, permitting the liver cells to degrade LDL, which releases cholesterol. Excess LDL is also removed by circulating macrophages, or scavenger white blood cells. Despite these regulatory mechanisms, excess LDL may accumulate, depositing cholesterol into arterial walls to form atheromatous plaques.

•••••• Pathophysiology

Hyperlipidemias are classified based on plasma lipoprotein patterns, and not on etiology of the disorder. There are four basic patterns: (1) hypercholesterolemia (and elevated LDL) with normal triglycerides (Type IIa); (2) hypercholesterolemia (and elevated LDL) with triglycerides that are 1 to 3 times higher than cholesterol (Type IIb and III); (3) primary increase in triglycerides (and increased VLDL) with normal or slightly increased cholesterol (Type IV); and (4) moderate to marked hypercholesterolemia (>300 mg/dl) with markedly elevated triglycerides (>1000 mg/dl) in which plasma appears lipemic (and associated increases in VLDL and chylomicrons) (Type I and V). The risk for CAD rises significantly when plasma cholesterol is greater than 240 mg/dl, or LDL is greater than 160 mg/dl. A fifth category of dyslipidemia exists: very low HDL levels, which increase the risk for development of CAD.

Type IIa and IIb primary hyperlipidemias are associated with genetic disorders. Familial hypercholesterolemia (FH) is an inherited disorder caused by a deficiency in LDL receptors. As a result, LDL accumulates in the blood. Of all the different types of hyperlipidemias, familial hypercholesterolemia is characterized by premature atherosclerosis, CAD, and xanthomas (yellowish deposits of plaque in the skin) and corneal arcus (a white ring around the eye). Lipid profiles show elevated levels of LDL and cholesterol. Triglyceride levels may or may not be elevated.

The treatment of FH emphasizes a very low cholesterol, low fat diet and achievement of ideal body weight if needed. Cholestyramine, colestipol, or lovastatin therapy may be added since diet alone is usually insufficient in reducing blood levels of LDL and cholesterol.

Type IIa, IIb and IV are associated with familial combined hyperlipidemia, a common (1:300) hereditary disease that in its milder form is often associated with diabetes mellitus. For an as yet unknown reason, apoprotein B levels are elevated in this disorder, resulting in high levels of LDL and possibly VLDL, cholesterol, and triglycerides. Severe premature atherosclerosis is the result. Men with this disease have myocardial infarctions at the average age of 40 years. Cigarette smoking greatly increases the risk of myocardial infarction. Treatment includes very low cholesterol diets, avoidance of concentrated sweets, and achievement or maintenance of ideal body weight. Therapy with niacin, clofibrate, or gemfibrozil may be necessary.

Type IV is associated with Familial endogenous hypertriglyceridemia, which is the result of a metabolic defect that causes over synthesis of VLDL and triglyceride by the liver. This disorder is common (1:300 to 1:200) and usually does not present a problem before 20 years of age. Patients with familial hypertriglycerdemia also are predisposed to coronary artery disease although the risk is not clearly delineated. However, it can be worsened by poor diet and cigarette smoking as well as by obesity, alcohol, and drugs, which elevate triglyceride levels (estrogen, glucocorticoids). Asymptomatic persons do not require treatment but should avoid using drugs that increase triglyceride levels.

Type I is associated with familial lipoprotein lipaseitalils deficiency, a very rare lipid disease in which there is an abnormality in synthesis, storage or release of lipoprotein lipase. A deficiency in apoprotein C-II has been reported in several families. The deficiency results in inadequate breakdown of triglyceride. Patients with this disorder often show an intolerance to fatty foods in childhood. Additional symptoms are hepatosplenomegaly, abdominal pain, lipemia retinalis, and xanthomas, especially of the elbow, knees, and buttocks. Patients are at very high risk for pancreatitis. Treatment focuses on low fat and low cholesterol diets and abstention from alcohol. Drugs are ineffective.

Type III is associated with familial dysbetalipoproteinemia which is characterized by an increase of VLDL. It is an inherited deficiency of aproprotein E2. This deficiency results from incomplete catabolism of chylomicrons and VLDL particles. Familial dysbetalipoproteinemia is uncommon; estimate of its incidence are 1:10,000. Patients with this disease exhibit xanthomas on the palms, Achilles tendons, and patellae, as well as corneal arcus. Lipid studies can vary widely in the same patient but generally reveal markedly elevated levels of VLDL and elevated levels of cholesterol and triglyceride. In addition, hyperglycemia and hyperuricemia may occur in these patients. Patients with familial dysbetalipoproteinemia have accelerated atherosclerosis and pancreatitis. Weight loss (if indicated) and a low cholesterol, low fat diet are an important part of treatment. Therapy with niacin or clofibrate may also be required.

Chylomicronemia syndrome, LCAT deficiency, apolipoprotein B deficiency, and *Tangier disease* are rare lipid disorders. These disorders manifest themselves in unusual ways, such as in the accumulation of cholesterol esters in many body tissues (Tangier disease). They may cause pancreatitis rather than coronary artery disease and also may require drug and dietary therapy. Plasmapheresis may be used to remove excess chylomicrons from plasma.

····· Diagnostic Studies and Findings

Lipid profile "Normal" and "elevated" levels vary among laboratories; cholesterol, normal to markedly elevated: 200->1000 mg/dl; triglycerides, normal to markedly elevated: 150->1500 mg/dl (even up to 29,000 mg/dl); LDL, normal to elevated: 100-200 mg/dl; HDL, normal to low: 50-20 mg/dl; LDL/HDL ratio, normal to high: 2:1->4; VLDL, normal to elevated: 30->40 mg/dl. NOTE: Patient should be fasting for 12-15 hours before venipuncture to avoid postprandial elevation in plasma triglyceride concentrations.

Liver function tests To verify normal liver function before pharmacologic therapy; periodically thereafter to identify abnormalities necessitating discontinuation of medication.

Uric acid level To verify normal levels before pharmacologic therapy; periodically thereafter to identify abnormalities necessitating discontinuation of medication.

Glucose level To verify normal levels before pharmacologic therapy; periodically thereafter to identify abnormalities necessitating discontinuation of medication.

Ophthalmologic examination To establish baseline of lens opacity before pharmacologic therapy; periodically thereafter to identify abnormalities necessitating discontinuation of medication.

····· Multidisciplinary Plan

Guidelines established by the National Cholesterol Education Program (NCEP) provide information about the levels of LDL and total cholesterol above which diet and drug therapy is recommended.[27]

Dietary Management

Foundation of management of hypercholesterolemia

AHA Step I diet: Reduce total dietary fat to <30% of total calories

Reduce saturated fat in diet to <10% of total calories

Maintain polyunsaturated fats in diet up to no more than 10% of total calories

Reduce dietary cholesterol to <300 mg/day

AHA Step II Diet: Reduce total dietary fat to <30% of total calories

Reduce saturated fat in diet to <7% of total calories

Maintain polyunsaturated fats in diet up to no more than 10% of total calories

Reduce dietary cholesterol to <200 mg/day

Achieve and maintain ideal body weight

Regular, Moderate Physical Activity

Elimination or Management of Other Risk Factors

Cigarette smoking

Hypertension

Diabetes mellitus

Alcohol abuse

Medications[8,27,58]

Pharmacologic therapy usually employed only after dietary management has proven inadequate in reducing blood lipids to target levels; cholesterol-lowering medications are then added to dietary regime:

Bile acid sequestrants

Cholestyramine 12-24 g/d

Colestipol 15-30 g/d

Niacin (nicotinic acid) 3-6 g/d

Probucol 500-1000 mg/d

Fibric acids

Clofibrate 1-2 g/d

Gemfibrozil 600-1200 mg/d

HMG CoA reductase inhibitors 20-80 mg/d

Lovastatin

Pravastatin

Simvastatin

Omega-3 unsaturated fatty acids

Special medication precautions: Because bile acid sequestrants can greatly reduce the absorption of other drugs administered simultaneously, other drugs should be taken 1 hour before, or 4 to 6 hours after these antilipemic medications. Cardiac glycoside (digoxin) levels should be monitored carefully. If antilipemic drug therapy is stopped, cardiac glycoside absorption may greatly increase, resulting in toxicity. Antilipemic drugs also interact with other medications: oral contraceptives and rifampin may increase the effect of clofibrate. Probenecid antagonizes clofibrate's effect. Oral hypoglycemic agents may antagonize the response to colestipol. Fibric acid derivatives may increase the anticoagulant effect of Coumadin.

NURSING CARE

Nursing Assessment

Circulation

Signs and symptoms associated with coronary artery disease (CAD) (see Chapter 1)

Food and Fluid Needs

Gastrointestinal upset
Nausea/vomiting
Dyspepsia
Excessive ETOH intake
Obesity

Elimination

Constipation
Diarrhea
Flatulence

Psychosocial

Noncompliance with diet, medications, exercise

Nursing Dx & Intervention

Nutrition, altered: more than body requirements related to excessive intake

- Reassess patient for psychosocial concerns that may be related to overeating.
- Arrange a dietary consultation.
- Encourage patient to choose foods that are low in fat, especially saturated fat and cholesterol, *to maintain nutritional balance and avoid elevating lipid levels.*
- Reinforce meal plan as needed.
- Suggest that patient join a support group such as Weight Watchers *to provide group and peer support.*

Knowledge deficit related to lack of information

- Develop readiness for learning with patient.
- Provide information about disease, treatment, side effects, and reportable health changes.
- Include family in all instructions.

Health maintenance, altered related to ineffective coping

- Identify blocks to health maintenance.
- Support patient in organizing and using strengths for health maintenance.
- Collaborate with patient to determine and develop positive behaviors.

Patient Education/Home Care Planning

1. Ensure that the patient verbalizes an understanding of the dietary management of the disease.
2. Discuss with the patient the importance of achieving ideal body weight.
3. Discuss with the patient the importance of engaging regularly in moderate physical exercise.
4. Discuss with the patient the importance of eliminating other factors related to hyperlipidemia and coronary artery disease, such as cigarette smoking and hypertension.
5. Ensure that the patient understands the name, action, dosage, schedule, side effects, and reportable health changes of ordered medications.
6. Ensure that the patient understands the importance of regular reevaluations (follow-up medical care).

Evaluation

Nutrition is adequate Patient verbalizes understanding of dietary restrictions. Patient complies with ordered diet.

Patient is knowledgeable about disease cause, symptoms, and treatment Patient and family verbalize understanding of disease, cause, symptoms, and treatment. Patient complies with medication regimen.

Health is maintained Patient verbalizes one coping strategy. Patient demonstrates one positive health maintenance behavior.

MEDICAL INTERVENTIONS AND RELATED NURSING CARE

ADRENALECTOMY

Description and Rationale

Adrenalectomy is the removal of one or both adrenal glands. Unilateral adrenalectomy can be indicated for pheochromocytoma, primary aldosteronism, and benign adrenal adenomas involving one gland. Treatment of adrenal carcinoma requires bilateral adrenalectomy. Bilateral adrenalectomy can be performed to treat Cushing's disease when other therapies have failed or when an ectopic ACTH-secreting tumor cannot be localized.[70]

Contraindications and Cautions

1. Bilateral adrenalectomy dictates lifelong glucocorticoid and mineralocorticoid replacement. (See adrenal insufficiency.)
2. Patients undergoing unilateral adrenalectomy will be adrenally insufficient immediately postoperative and will require glucocorticoid (but not usually mineralocorticoid) replacement for 6 months to 2 years or until the remaining adrenal gland recovers. Preoperative glucocorticoids are indicated.
3. Hyperglycemia should be controlled before surgery.
4. Patients undergoing adrenalectomy can have hypoaldosteronism or hyperkalemia after surgery.
5. Preoperative alpha blockade is essential for hypertension control in pheochromocytoma.

Preprocedural Nursing Care

Administration of preoperative steroids

Postoperative Nursing Care[69]

Administer supraphysiologic dosage of glucocorticoids (hydrocortisone 300 mg) tapering over 3-4 days. Monitor blood and urine cortisol levels to assess potential onset of adrenal insufficiency. Later, administer replacement hormones.

Hydrocortisone (12-15 mg/m²) orally

Florinef 100 μg/day orally (follow plasma renin activity levels)

NURSING CARE

Nursing Assessment

Skin

Poor wound healing

Surgical incision

Complications

Adrenal insufficiency (potential)

Unresolved hypertension from primary aldosteronism or pheochromocytoma may require continued treatment with medication

Nursing Dx & Intervention

Impaired skin integrity

- Monitor the patient's wound for edema, redness, warmth, induration, and drainage *to observe for signs of healing or infection.*

Risk for infection

- Follow actions for adrenal insufficiency and for acute adrenal insufficiency when applicable.

Patient Education/Home Care Planning

1. Teach the patient wound care.
2. Give the patient a list of early signs and symptoms of adrenal insufficiency. Inform patient to expect flulike symptoms during remission of hypercortisolism following surgery.
3. Demonstrate to the patient how to use replacement steroids: the dangers of glucocorticoid withdrawal, the importance of compliance with medication administration, and the need to double the dosage for nausea, diarrhea, and fever.
4. Instruct the patient and family regarding emergency intramuscular injection of steroids during emesis, trauma, or severe stress. Medical follow-up should be pursued.
5. Discuss with the patient the need to wear or carry medical alert information about the need for glucocorticoid replacement.

Evaluation

The patient's wound is healed Patient's wound has closed without redness, edema, warmth, or drainage. Normal or subnormal plasma cortisol levels.

The patient is adrenally sufficient Patient displays no symptoms of adrenal insufficiency.

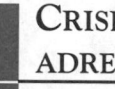

CRISIS INTERVENTION FOR ADRENAL INSUFFICIENCY

Description and Rationale

The patient experiencing adrenal crisis must receive adrenocorticosteroids (glucocorticoids and mineralocorticoids).

The response to IV cortisol can be dramatic. Nelson[50] has reported blood pressure response from an unobtainable diastolic reading to one of over 80 after the initial dose of cortisol was given. Therefore the patient must be treated with corticosteroids before other interventions, to enable the system to stabilize. The effects of corticosteroids on the electrolyte imbalance, hypovolemia, and blood pressure will become apparent quickly. An IV infusion of 5% dextrose in saline should be part of the therapy, because the patient will likely be hypoglycemic as a result of the vomiting, diarrhea, and lack of food. Dehydration also compounds the problem. Response to therapy is encouraging; in fact, within 24 hours most patients are able to resume an oral course of corticosteroids.

Since most glucocorticoids (such as hydrocortisone) exert some mineralocorticoid effect, additional mineralocorticoid is not always necessary. Also, the sodium present in IV fluid can be sufficient to restore a normal level. However, if mineralocorticoid replacement is necessary, desoxycorticosterone pivalate can be given intramuscularly.[50]

Antibiotic therapy may also be necessary if the underlying cause of the adrenal crisis is infection.

Volume expanders may or may not be used, depending on how effective the steroid treatment and IV fluid are.

There is controversy in the literature regarding use of vasopressors to treat hypovolemic shock. Response to initial glucocorticoid infusion and IV therapy should be evaluated before employing the use of vasopressors.

Contraindications and Cautions

1. Complications associated with IV therapy
2. Severe hyperkalemia and hyponatremia may be present and require treatment

NURSING CARE

Nursing Assessment

Circulation

Hypotension

Hypopyrexia or hyperpyrexia*

Shock*

---

*Characteristic of adrenal crisis.

Food and Fluid

Vomiting
Hyponatremia*
Salt craving
Hyperkalemia*

Elimination

Decreased urine output*
Diarrhea

Neurosensory Concerns

Confusion*
Dizziness
Coma*
Visual changes
Lightheadedness

Mobility

Muscle weakness

Comfort and Pain

Severe headache*
Severe abdominal pain*
Severe leg pain*
Severe lower back pain*

Psychosocial Concerns

Anxiety

Teaching and Learning

Lack of knowledge about medications and crisis

Nursing Dx & Intervention

Risk for infection related to lack of primary defense

- Reassess patient's understanding of the risk of infection.
- Keep patient in an environment as free from stress as possible (low lighting, warm temperature, reduced noise level) *to minimize environmental stress.*
- Encourage frequent rest.
- Reinforce importance of medications to patient.

Nutrition altered: less than body requirements; related to inability to absorb nutrients

- Monitor the patient's intake of electrolytes, especially potassium and sodium.
- Encourage patient to choose foods high in sodium and low in potassium.
- Take apical pulse *to detect cardiac dysrhythmias.*
- Employ means *to combat nausea.*
- Maintain intake and output records.

---

*Characteristic of adrenal crisis.

Altered peripheral tissue perfusion related to hypovolemia

- Reassess for early presyncopal signs (dizziness, lightheadedness, visual changes).
- Have patient change positions (from lying to sitting to standing) slowly *to prevent orthostatic hypotension.*
- Take lying and standing blood pressures and pulses *to compare orthostatic values.*
- Administer IV fluids as ordered.
- Monitor intake and output.
- Monitor vital signs frequently (every 15 to 30 minutes).
- Explain rationale for IV therapy to patient.

Impaired physical mobility related to pain

- Give the patient cortisol replacement as ordered.
- Do not give the patient pain medications.
- Monitor degree and location of the patient's pain.
- Use only comfort measures: cool cloth; do not turn on lights (headache); reposition patient (back pain).
- Assist the patient with daily activities as needed.

Anxiety related to threat of death

- Support patient with comfort measures until the patient is alert enough for verbal communication.
- Identify whether the crisis is within the patient's ability to control: the patient purposely stops taking cortisone replacement vs other precipitating factors, such as an infection.
- Obtain psychiatric consult if the patient's intent is purposeful.

Knowledge deficit related to new disease and medications

- Identify patient's readiness to learn.
- Identify precipitating factors.
- Discuss cause, signs, symptoms, and lifelong treatment with patient.

Patient Education/Home Care Planning

1. Discuss with the patient the steps to follow when early symptoms of adrenal insufficiency are noted.
2. Discuss with the patient the importance of regular medical follow-up and wearing medical identification.

Evaluation

Patient is free of infection Patient's temperature is within normal range. Patient has no signs or symptoms of infection. Serum cortisol and aldosterone levels are within normal range.

Electrolytes are within the normal range Patient's sodium and potassium blood levels are within normal limits.

Tissue perfusion is adequate Patient's hydration is normal. Patient's intake equals output. Patient's electrolytes are normal. Patient's vital signs are normal.

Patient is independently mobile Patient is able to perform self-care without discomfort, although some weakness may be present.

Patient has decreased anxiety Patient can verbalize precipitating factors for adrenal crisis and how these can be avoided. Patient agrees to continue counseling.

GONADOTROPIN REPLACEMENT THERAPY[26,57,78]

Description and Rationale

Approaches to treatment differ with individual clinical circumstances and preferences. Restoring gonadal function requires both gonadal steroid replacement and treatment of infertility for both men and women.[26] In general, the lowest dose that produces the desired clinical effect is used.

Contraindications and Cautions

1. Human chorionic gonadotropin (HCG) is generally not given in the presence of the following conditions:
   a. Prostatic carcinoma
   b. Prior allergic reaction to HCG (rare)
   c. Pituitary hypertrophy or tumor
   d. Undiagnosed vaginal bleeding
   e. Uterine fibroids or cyst
   f. Pregnancy
   g. History of thrombophlebitis
2. Estrogen and progesterone is generally not given in the presence of the following conditions:
   a. Thromboembolic disorders
   b. Breast, reproductive, or genital cancers
   c. Pregnancy
   d. Abnormal genital bleeding
   e. Patients with cardiac, renal, or hepatic disease
3. Testosterone is generally not given in the presence of the following conditions:
   a. Patients with prostatic cancer, breast cancer
   b. Patients with cardiac, renal, or hepatic disease
   c. Benign prostatic hypertrophy with obstruction
   d. Pregnancy, breast feeding

•••••• Multidisciplinary Plan

Medication

In postmenopausal women
  Estrogen replacement therapy can take one of the following forms:
    Ethinyl estradiol 5-20 μg/day
    Premarin 0.625-1.25 mg/day
    Estradiol transdermal patch (Estraderm) 50-100 μg/day
  Estrogen is given 20-25 days per month, and accompanied by
  Progesterone medication on the last 5-10 days each month
    Provera 5-10 mg/day or Estrogen daily with 2-2.5 mg Provera daily

Androgens may be given in small amounts (specifically for decreased libido)
  Testosterone enanthate 50 mg q 1-2 months, IM
  Fluoxymesterone 5-10 mg 1-2 times per week, po
Clomiphene citrate may be used to induce ovulation in women with hypothalamic gonadal deficiency; pergonal (menotropins) and HCG, or GnRH by intermittent infusion pump may be used to induce ovulation (restore fertility) in women with pituitary gonadal deficiency

In adult men
  Androgen replacement therapy:
    Testosterone enanthate or sypionate IM 200 mg q 2 weeks
    Testosterone transdermal system (Testoderm) 4 mg/d, 6 mg/d
    GnRH by intermittent infusion pump may be used to initiate spermatogenesis and restore fertility in men with hypothalamic gonadal deficiency
    HCG alone or with Pergonal (menotropins) may be used in men with pituitary gonadal deficiency

NURSING CARE

Nursing Assessment

Sexuality
  Development/maintenance of secondary sex characteristics

Musculoskeletal
  Bone density
  Strength/mass

Skin
  Injection sites

Psychosocial Concerns
  Increase in libido
  Increase in self-esteem
  Increased confidence with both male and female peers
  Improved body image

Nursing Dx & Intervention

Anxiety related to threat to self-concept

- Assess with the patient areas causing anxiety and usual coping mechanisms.
- Encourage open communication between patient and partner.
- Assist with problem solving.
- Explore alternative coping behaviors.
- Ask patient about any need for home health nurse visits for continued supervision of injections.

Sexual dysfunction related to lack of normal hormones

- Provide climate in which patient can openly discuss concerns and goals.

- Provide information and discuss length of time for improvement.
- Discuss expected changes in appearance, attitude, behavior.
- Discuss possible need for contraception.
- Stress importance of medication compliance.

Patient Education/Home Care Planning

1. Ensure that the patient verbalizes name, dosage, action, schedule, side effects, and proper storage of medications.
2. Demonstrate to the patient the procedure for intramuscular self-injection, including preparation and site rotation.
3. Discuss with the patient the importance of follow-up medical care.

Evaluation

Anxiety decreases   Patient discusses feelings about need for treatment. Patient continues open communication with partner regarding body changes. Patient complies with medical treatment program.

Patient complies with intramuscular injection of gonadotropins   Patient is able to prepare medication and perform self-injection without hesitance or difficulty. Partner demonstrates preparation of medication, injection, site rotation, and disposal of equipment.

HYPOPHYSECTOMY

Description and Rationale

Surgical resection of a pituitary adenoma is the preferred treatment for tumors of the pituitary gland (Cushing's disease, GH- and TSH-secreting adenomas). A hemihypophysectomy can be performed when an ACTH-secreting pituitary adenoma cannot be seen by CT or MRI scans, but inferior petrosal sinus sampling (IPSS) indicates lateralization to one half of the gland (excessive ACTH levels from the left or right half of the pituitary gland).[24] An adrenalectomy is usually preferred over a total hypophysectomy (to preserve pituitary function) if the tumor cannot be localized. Total hypophysectomy is performed if multiple tumors exist, or if the tumor is very large. Emergency hypophysectomy is occasionally required to treat pituitary apoplexy.

Surgical approach to the pituitary gland is by the transsphenoidal or transfrontal approach. The transsphenoidal route is preferred because it provides direct access to the contents of the sella turcica, is relatively safe, and avoids disruption of intracranial structures. It is a well-tolerated procedure that produces no visible scarring. The surgical goal is to remove as much tumor tissue as possible without impairing anterior pituitary function. Transsphenoidal adenomectomy or hypophysectomy is microscopic surgery performed with the patient in a semi-sitting position. A gum-line incision is made, a nasal speculum is introduced, and the surgeon accesses the pituitary gland through the sphenoid sinus and floor of the sella turcica. Transfrontal craniotomy may be indicated if the tumor is inaccessible by the transphenoidal route because of its geometry or if carotid arteries obstruct access to the pituitary gland. Following successful surgery, visual field deficits usually improve, and symptoms of hormone hypersecretion remit.[60]

Contraindications and Complications

Contraindications for transsphenoidal surgery include sphenoid or nasal infection, or vascular anatomy preventing access to the pituitary gland.

The incidence of postoperative complications increases with tumor size and difficulty of resection. Microadenoma resection rarely leads to permanent side effects. CSF leakage, transient diabetes insipidus, or hypopituitarism occur in up to 20% of patients. Permanent diabetes insipidus, cranial nerve damage, or visual deficits occur in up to 10% of cases. Meningitis is rare, and mortality occurs in 1% of cases.

Disease of the adrenal cortex, such as adrenal adenoma (benign) and adrenal carcinoma (malignant) can lead to hypercortisolism.[80] When adrenal tissue becomes neoplastic, cortisol can be produced independently of ACTH stimulation.[69] This overproduction of cortisol leads to low levels of ACTH due to negative feedback effects of cortisol on the pituitary gland. Other conditions causing hypercortisolism include chronic alcoholism (alcoholic pseudo-Cushing's), depression, and the factitious administration of corticosteroid preparations.

The effects of glucocorticoid excess are reflected in changes in many tissue and organ systems. Early symptoms include weight gain, hypertension, and glucose intolerance.[80]

Preprocedural Nursing Care

Provide explanations regarding diagnostic testing and procedures (CT and MRI scans, urine collection, blood work and endocrine tests). Preoperative teaching specific to transsphenoidal hypophysectomy includes:

Presence of nasal packing postoperatively (2 or 3 days)
Mouth breathing while nasal packing is in place
Moustache dressing
Graft site on thigh (muscle plug removed from thigh for packing dura)
Expected decrease in sensation of smell and taste (few months)
Fluid restrictions possibly necessary
Possibly sent to ICU, surgical ICU, or neurosurgical ICU (variable with institution)

NURSING CARE

Nursing Assessment

Neurologic Status

Postnasal drip (CSF rhinorrhea)

Fluid and Electrolyte Balance

Polydipsia
Polyuria
Decreased urine specific gravity

Gum Line Incision

Redness, swelling, drainage

Cardiovascular

Blood pressure, heart rate stable
Evidence of postsurgical hemorrhage

Graft Site (Thigh)

Redness, swelling, drainage

Respiratory

Difficulty breathing because of mouth breathing
Dry mouth

Nursing Dx & Intervention

Impaired oral mucous membrane related to mouth breathing and incision

- Reassess secretions from nasal drains; assess quality and quantity of drainage.
- Question the patient about postnasal drip.
- Perform frequent oral care with normal saline or half-strength H_2O_2 solution. Do not allow tooth brushing for 2 weeks, until sutures are healed.
- Apply petroleum jelly *to prevent the patient's lips from cracking as a result of mouth breathing.*
- Discuss with the patient the need to avoid sneezing, coughing, nose blowing, straining, and bending over *to protect muscle graft.*
- Monitor possible signs of infection of incision or graft sites.

Risk for fluid-volume deficit related to loss of regulatory mechanism (vasopressin) and leading to transient or permanent central diabetes insipidus

- Assess serum and urine osmolality and electrolytes.
- Check urine specific gravity *to identify early signs of diabetes insipidus.*
- Measure and record intake and output.
- Consider the need for vasopressin replacement therapy if serum sodium >150, serum osmolality >300 (and greater than urine osmolality).
- See diabetes insipidus, p. 822.

Patient Education/Home Care Planning

1. Provide instruction regarding hormone replacement therapy if indicated (glucocorticoids, thyroid hormone, LH, FSH, etc.).

2. Provide information regarding emergency medical alert identification if patient receives glucocorticoid replacement.
3. Provide instruction on emergency injection of hydrocortisone in the event of trauma, vomiting, or major stress.

Evaluation

Healing progresses normally Patient shows no signs or symptoms of infection at operative sites (gum line, thigh). Signs and symptoms of meningitis (i.e., nuchal rigidity, fever, headache) do not develop. There is no evidence of CSF leak (rhinorrhea or post nasal leakage). No evidence of postoperative hemorrhage exists.

Fluid balance is normal Patient's intake approximates output; weight is stable. Patient's urine output is less than 200 ml/hour. Patient's specific gravity is 1.005 to 1.015.

 ## PARATHYROIDECTOMY

Description and Rationale

Surgical removal of hyperactive parathyroid tissue is the treatment of choice. Surgical techniques vary with different etiologies. When an adenoma is evident, surgical removal of the entire gland is necessary (there may be more than one adenoma present). Hyperplasia usually affects more than one gland; therefore three glands are removed completely, and three fourths of the remaining gland is removed, leaving enough tissue to maintain normal serum calcium levels. Following parathyroidectomy, implantation of a portion of a gland may be done in hyperplasia, usually in a muscle of the forearm. Sometimes a gland is frozen for implantation in the future.

Contraindications and Cautions

1. Contraindications for surgery
   a. Inability to locate the glands
   b. Underlying medical conditions such as renal failure or severe cardiac disorders
   c. Hypercalcemia from nonparathyroid etiology
2. Complications
   a. Hypocalcemia—temporary (48 hrs) from "hungry bone syndrome" or permanent
   b. Edema
   c. Airway obstruction
   d. Paralysis of vocal cords

NURSING CARE

Nursing Assessment

Cardiovascular Concerns

Dysrhythmias
Bleeding

Respiratory Concerns

Obstruction of airway
Edema of incisional area

Neuromuscular Concerns

Paresthesias
Dysphagia
Laryngeal spasm
Positive Chvostek's and Trousseau's signs

Pain

Incision
Shoulder
Throat

Nursing Dx & Intervention

Risk for ineffective breathing pattern related to inflammatory process

- Keep a tracheostomy set at bedside.
- Elevate head of patient's bed 15 to 30 degrees.
- Monitor patient's vital signs and breathing pattern every 4 hours for first 48 hours.

Physical mobility impaired related to neuromuscular impairment

- Reassess patient for signs of pain during movement.
- Observe patient to assess steadiness on ambulation *to maintain patient safety.*
- Handle patient gently; allow patient to move slowly *to prevent injury.*

Pain related to physical factors

- Monitor type and degree of patient's pain.
- Administer pain medication to patient as needed.
- Provide ice chips to patient for pain from sore throat.
- Support the patient's neck when the patient is turning or sitting *to protect the incision and to promote healing.*
- If pathologic fractures are apparent, splint ribs while the patient turns or coughs *to limit pain or additions to fractures.*

Nutrition altered: less than body requirements; related to inability to absorb nutrients

- Reassess Chvostek's and Trousseau's signs *to identify symptoms of hypocalcemia.*
- Make high-calcium snacks available to patient at all times.
- Keep emergency calcium replacement medications available at bedside.
- Obtain a nutrition consultation for the patient.
- Monitor patient's serum electrolytes.

Patient Education/Home Care Planning

1. Give patient a list of the signs and symptoms of hypocalcemia (paresthesias, muscle cramps in extremities, and tingling in fingers and around the mouth) to report.

2. Demonstrate incisional care to the patient.
3. Demonstrate body mechanics and the importance of mobility (especially for patients with irreversible skeletal impairment).
4. Ensure the patient verbalizes understanding of calcium replacement medications: actions, uses, side effects, and measures to use in case of emergencies.

Evaluation

Comfort increases   Patient's incisional pain is minimal (can be tolerated without need for pain medication); sore throat is absent, and shoulder and posterior neck pain is minimal. Patient can perform a small neck and head circle movement.

Nutrition is adequate   Patient's electrolytes are in the normal range.

Patient tolerates increased activity   Patient resumes independent ADLs.

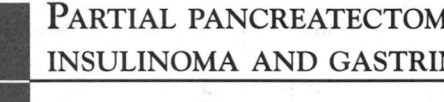

PARTIAL PANCREATECTOMY: INSULINOMA AND GASTRINOMA

Description and Rationale

Surgery is the treatment of choice for insulinoma and gastrinoma. Preoperative localization of the tumor by CT scan, venous sampling, or selective arteriography increases the chance of successful surgery; however, it is sometimes difficult. In the case of unsuccessful surgery or tumor metastasis, symptoms should be controlled by diet and medication. In nesidioblastosis an 80% pancreatectomy usually relieves the hyperinsulinemia. Usually no more than 85% of the pancreas is resected to prevent malabsorption problems.

Contraindications and Cautions

1. With gastrinoma, active bleeding ulcer

NURSING CARE

Nursing Assessment

Circulation

Decreased blood pressure
Tachycardia
Increasing abdominal girth

Food and Fluid

Dry mouth
Nausea
Abdominal pain

Comfort and Pain

Describes incisional pain
Splints, protects, or favors incisional area when moving
Abdomen rigid and tender

Skin

Redness, swelling at incision
Wound disruption
Drainage from incision

Nursing Dx & Intervention

Risk for fluid-volume deficit related to loss of fluid through abnormal routes

- Monitor blood pressure, pulse, and respiratory rate every 2 to 4 hours.
- Observe patient for signs or symptoms of bleeding or shock.
- Check dressing and drainage tube every 1 to 4 hours post-operatively *to identify early signs of hemorrhage.*
- Discuss causative factors with patient and family.
- Monitor indicators of patient's fluid balance (intake and output, daily weights, signs of dehydration) *to identify dehydration early.*
- Replace patient's fluids via intravenous line as ordered.

Nutrition altered: less than body requirements related to inability to ingest or digest nutrients

- Assess bowel sounds every shift postoperatively.
- Stop feeding if pain, vomiting, or nausea ocurs.
- Monitor laboratory data to assess patient's fluid and electrolyte status.
- Encourage the patient to eat ice chips and to take sips of cool, clear fluids as tolerated.
- Teach the patient to maintain good oral hygiene.
- Discuss cause of gas pain or nausea with patient and family.
- Review the patient's diet prescription with dietitian before patient's discharge.

Pain (acute) related to injuring agent

- Monitor type, location, character, and duration of patient's pain.
- Evaluate effectiveness of pain medication.
- Report sudden increase in patient's incisional pain or abdominal pain.
- Discuss cause of pain with patient and family.
- Assist patient to use pain control measures.

Skin integrity impaired related to external factors

- Monitor patient's incision site every shift for redness, swelling, and drainage.
- Report signs of wound infection or dehiscence immediately to physician.
- Perform prescribed dressing changes for the patient as ordered.
- Provide adequate nutrition for the patient as tolerated.

Patient Education/Home Care Planning

1. Demonstrate proper wound care to decrease the chance of infection.
2. Discuss with the patient the signs and symptoms and treatment of hypoglycemia (if surgery is unsuccessful) to ensure correct management and no loss of consciousness (insulinoma only).

Evaluation

Cardiac output is normal   Patient's vital signs are within normal limits.

Fluid balance is achieved   Patient's blood pressure is within normal limits. Pulse is within normal limits. Shock is not present. No signs of dehydration are present. Output equals intake.

Intake of nutrients is progressive   Patient ingests recommended amounts and types of nutrients. Patient describes causative factors. Patient's fluids and electrolytes are in balance. Patient has no nausea and no gas pain. Patient's bowel sounds return. Patient describes discharge diet planning.

Pain is relieved   Patient uses comfort measures and pain control measures. Patient describes causative factors. Patient verbalizes decreased pain.

Skin is intact   Wound healing is evident. Patient has no signs or symptoms of infection. Patient participates in prescribed dressing changes to promote wound healing.

RADIATION THERAPY FOR TREATMENT OF PITUITARY TUMORS

Description and Rationale

Conventional radiation therapy administers 4500 to 5000 rads of high voltage Cobalt-60 radiation to the region of the sella turcica.[80] It is used as an alternative or adjunct to surgical excision of the tumor. Indications include tumors with suprasellar extension, incompleted surgical removal of the tumor, regrowth of a surgically treated tumor, or when surgery is contraindicated. Typically, radiation therapy reduces tumor size, but hormone levels do not always return completely to normal. The best results are seen in patients less than 40 years of age.[80] It can take 6 to 18 months to see clinical results of radiation therapy.

Contraindications and Cautions

1. Optimally, radiation therapy is not used with tumors large enough to mandate treatment faster than radiation therapy can provide (e.g., pressure on the optic nerve with ensuing partial blindness).
2. Often there is an initial acute inflammatory response with subsequent possible hydrocephalus and exacerbation of symptoms.

3. Destruction of normal tissue (pituitary, hypothalamus, or cranial nerves) and radiation necrosis of the brain is possible up to 20 years following therapy.[80]
4. Pituitary tumors occasionally turn out to be radioresistant.[24]
5. Hypopituitarism occurs in 30%-50% of patients.[80]

NURSING CARE

Nursing Assessment

Pain

Headache

Psychologic Concerns

Level of anxiety initially and as therapy proceeds

Mobility

Decreased energy level

Nursing Dx & Intervention

Pain related to injuring agent

- Encourage patient to report headache immediately.
- Provide analgesics and other supportive measures for headaches (quiet environment, cool compresses, etc.) *to minimize increased intracranial pressure.*

Anxiety related to change in health status

- Assess patient frequently for psychosocial and physiologic manifestations of anxiety.
- Encourage the discussion of concerns and feelings regarding therapy, including the length of time needed to see the results of therapy, *to support realistic expectations.*

Activity intolerance related to generalized weakness

- Monitor patient's activity tolerance and limitations; identify the patient's priorities regarding rest and activity.
- Help patient to structure each day to include frequent rest periods.
- Encourage patient to limit activities during the period of radiation therapy.

Patient Education/Home Care Planning

1. Discuss the importance of returning consistently for follow-up examinations.

Evaluation

Pain is relieved   Patient reports no headache or worsening of headache if it is present at baseline.

Anxiety decreases   Patient verbalizes concerns regarding radiation therapy. Patient states general and specific facts about radiation therapy. Patient exhibits no observable signs of anxiety.

Activity tolerance improves   Patient uses stress-reducing methods routinely. Patient structures each day to allow for rest periods and desired activities. Patient performs ADLs within limitations imposed by underlying disease state. Patient's statements about "feeling tired" are reduced.

RADIOACTIVE IODINE THERAPY (RAI)

Description and Rationale

The goal of radioactive iodine (RAI) therapy is to chemically destroy functioning thyroid tissue. This is called ablation therapy. ^{131}I is the isotope of choice in the treatment of thyrotoxicosis and thyroid cancer.

Radioactive iodine is the preferred definitive therapy in the United States for Graves' disease.[83] It is considered less costly and less traumatic than surgery and avoids the complications of surgery. It may be used in the treatment of a toxic multinodular goiter when the patient is at risk from surgery. It may also be used to decrease the size of a large non-toxic substernal goiter, to reduce the mass effect of the goiter around the trachea. The desired consequence of radioactive iodine is complete thyroid gland destruction rendering the patient hypothyroid. This is usually achieved with a single dose, but in some patients with Graves' disease who have high TSIs and large glands, more than one dose may be required. It may take 3 to 6 months for ^{131}I to have its full destructive effect. Therefore, if a second dose is required it would not be given until 6 months after the first dose.

Theoretically, in thyrotoxic patients, ^{131}I may cause a sudden release of thyroid hormone from the gland into the bloodstream causing thyroid storm. Patients are required to stop their antithyroid medication 3-5 days before treatment since these drugs interfere with the uptake of the ^{131}I by the thyroid gland. They are then restarted on antithyroid medication 3 to 5 days after receiving treatment. On the other hand, stopping antithyroid drugs 3 to 5 days before radioiodine therapy has been found to increase thyroid hormone levels more than the RAI treatment itself.[13] Radioiodine is also given to patients without pre-treatment by antithyroid drugs without any untoward effects. This last option is usually reserved for relatively young patients who have adequate beta blockade. The doses of ^{131}I for Graves' disease are relatively small, ranging from 6-15 mCi. Doses for toxic multinodular goiters tend to be higher, toward the outpatient limit of 30 mCi.

Radioactive iodine use in the treatment of papillary and follicular thyroid cancer is quite variable. If the patient has a papillary tumor 2 cm or less without local or distant metastasis then 60% of physicians would recommend the patient receive ^{131}I after total thyroidectomy. The dose for this patient may range from 30 to 150 mCi. If the patient has a larger tumor, or local or distant metastasis then almost 100% of physicians would recommend the patient receive ^{131}I and at a higher dose.[87]

When a patient with thyroid cancer has been on thyroid hormone suppression for 6 months or more, a ^{131}I whole body scan may be requested to assess whether the patient has developed new recurrence or to identify metastasis previously unidentified. Scanning doses in thyroid cancer patients range from 1-10 mCi. Since levothyroxine has a very long half life, the preparation for this study takes 4 to 6 weeks. The patient usually stops taking levothyroxine and is placed on pure T_3 (Cytomel) for 2 to 3 weeks. This medication has a short half life and is usually prescribed at a dose of 25 μg three times per day. This allows the patient to stay relatively euthyroid while dissipating thyroxine stores. The patient then must stop the T_3 for the next 2 to 3 weeks. The goal is to have the patient become purposefully hypothyroid with a TSH level greater than 40. Because the TSH stimulates iodine uptake in thyroid tissue, when the scanning dose of ^{131}I is given, it should amplify any recurrent tissue. Another mechanism to enhance this effect is to have the patient follow a low iodine diet for the last 2 weeks before the test. Theoretically, this diet should enhance radioactive iodine uptake in both malignant and normal thyroid tissue, but this issue is still controversial. This diet is very difficult to follow because all water, except distilled water, has iodine added to it. Iodine is also in all processed flour and food products. As an alternative to this lengthy preparation, recombinant TSH is undergoing phase III clinical trials. The patient would self-administer the drug by IM injection for a specified number of days, raising the TSH above 40 just prior to the scan. The advantage to this newer investigational approach would allow the patient to continue taking thyroid hormone, eliminating the profound hypothyroidism and eliminating the need for the low iodine diet. If the results of the whole body scan indicate the presence of tissue, then the patient may require a second treatment dose of [131]I.

Contraindications and Cautions

1. [131]I crosses the placenta and can destroy the fetal thyroid. A pregnancy test should be performed on all women of childbearing age before treatment. Pregnancy is an absolute contraindication to its use.
2. Pregnant nursing personnel should be restricted from contact with patients receiving radiation therapy.
3. Complications associated with RAI therapy include parotitis, salangitis, radiation thyroiditis, exacerbations of hyperthyroidism, and thyroid crisis.
4. Antithyroid drugs may be given before radiation therapy. Drug therapy must be discontinued 3 to 7 days before the ^{131}I uptake is determined.
5. Iodides, iodide-containing drugs, and contrast agents should not be given before therapy.
6. After therapy, saliva, perspiration, urine, feces, vomitus, wound drainage, and breast milk, are radioactive.

7. Hyperthyroidism, increased swelling of the gland, pain, tenderness, and sore throat are signs of radiation thyroiditis. These signs may develop 1 to 2 weeks after therapy.

Preprocedural Nursing Care

1. Small doses of RAI are usually given on an outpatient basis. Special instructions are included in the section on patient education.
2. Large doses of radioiodine require hospitalization and radiation isolation.
   a. Private room at least 6 feet away from other patients or traffic flow
   b. Special protective measures for caregivers and visitors: gowns, gloves, booties, dosimeter, radiation badges, and consultation by radiation safety branch of hospital
   c. Special precautions regarding visitors (no children, or pregnant women)

NURSING CARE

Nursing Assessment

Thyroid Gland

Increased swelling
Tenderness and pain with pressure
Difficulty swallowing

Respiratory Status

Dyspnea
Difficulty breathing

Psychosocial Concerns

Social isolation
Fear
Anxiety

Nursing Dx & Intervention

Ineffective individual coping related to anxiety, fear, social isolation

- Reassess patient's coping skills, support systems, and history of the adaptive skills that were successful.
- Listen attentively and provide an atmosphere of acceptance.
- Reduce situations that might startle or frighten patient.
- Avoid discrepancies in timing, activities, and methods of performing procedures.
- Anticipate and provide for patient's needs.
- Encourage expression and discussion of feelings.
- Help patient clarify source(s) of anxiety.
- Help patient identify strengths and resources.
- Encourage patient to learn and use diversional activities.

- Encourage use of telephone to communicate with family and friends.
- Keep patient informed of daily reductions in radioactivity.
- Remind patient that isolation is limited.

Knowledge deficit related to radiation isolation procedures

- Provide private room away from traffic flow; keep door closed.
- Explain rationale for isolation and visitor limitations.
- Explain purpose of gowns, gloves, booties, dosimeter, and radiation badges.
- Explain all procedures for handling of secretions according to hospital radiation safety policies.
- Have patient handle own specimens if able.
- Explain rationale for rotation of nursing personnel assigned to patient.
- Instruct patient concerning signs and symptoms to report.
- Establish and practice procedures for communicating with nursing personnel.
- Check on patient approximately every 2 hours or more often as determined by his or her physical and emotional state *to reduce social isolation.*
- Establish patient's plan for diversional activities *to reduce boredom of isolation.*

Risk for ineffective breathing pattern or swallowing related to inflammation

- Monitor patient's ability to communicate verbally.
- Monitor patient's ability to eat and drink without difficulty.
- Have patient suck on sour candy to increase salivary flow and reduce parotitis.
- Have patient drink 1.5 to 2 liters fluids per day.

Patient Education/Home Care Planning

1. For an outpatient, discuss:
   a. The importance of a high fluid intake during the first 24 hours after dose
   b. The avoidance of contact with others (especially children) (Suggest sleeping alone for at least 2 nights following dose.)
   c. The avoidance of sharing eating utensils, kissing, and intercourse for at least 48 hours.
2. For an inpatient or outpatient, explain:
   a. Signs and symptoms of hypothyroidism and radiation thyroiditis
   b. Importance of follow-up care

Evaluation

Patient develops strategies for coping with anxiety, fear, or social isolation   Patient demonstrates ability to cope with restrictions imposed by isolation. Patient verbalizes fears and concerns regarding radiation isolation. Patient identifies source(s) of anxiety and fears. Patient verbalizes decrease in or absence of anxiety and fear. Patient uses strategies to reduce anxiety and fear.

Patient understands radiation isolation procedure   Patient verbalizes rationale for isolation, visitor restriction, and special radiation precautions. Patient verbalizes procedures for nursing personnel entering and leaving isolation room. Patient verbalizes or demonstrates procedures for handling of secretions. Patient verbalizes signs and symptoms to report. Patient verbalizes or demonstrates method(s) of communicating with nursing staff. Patient verbalizes fears or concerns regarding radiation isolation. Patient verbalizes diversional activities to be used during isolation.

 ## THYROIDECTOMY

Description and Rationale

Partial (lobectomy, isthmusectomy), near total (95%), or total thyroidectomy results in a decrease of thyroid hormones through permanent removal of thyroid tissue. Thyroidectomy may be used for patients with hyperthyroidism from a toxic adenoma or Graves' disease, large goiters, or nodules that suggest the presence of cancer.[37]

Contraindications and Cautions

1. Patients may be euthyroid or mildly hyperthyroid at the time of surgery. Preoperative treatment is accomplished by antithyroid drugs for 1 to 2 months to bring the patient into a euthyroid state, and with iodine preparations for 7 to 10 days to reduce excessive vascularity of the gland.
2. Inadvertent removal or damage to the parathyroid glands may result in hypocalcemia and tetany.
3. Damage to the recurrent laryngeal nerves during surgery may result in aphonia or dysphonia because of vocal cord paralysis.
4. Permanent hypothyroidism following near total or total thyroidectomy will occur in all patients.
5. Permanent or transient hypothyroidism may occur after lobectomy/isthmusectomy.
6. Discharge occurs on second or third postoperative day.

NURSING CARE

Nursing Assessment

Respiratory Status

Tachypnea
Abnormal breath sounds
Increased restlessness
Complaints of tightness in throat; inability to swallow; inability to get air; pressure or fullness in neck; dressing too tight
Change in level of orientation

Circulatory Status

Variations in pulse and blood pressure readings
Changes in skin condition: cool and clammy
Increased swelling in tissue surrounding incision
Decreased peripheral pulses
Excessive bleeding on surgical dressing
Hemorrhage

Electrolyte Imbalance

Dysphagia: laryngeal spasms
Headache
Positive Chvostek's or Trousseau's sign
Tetany: muscular twitching
Personality changes
Complaints of numbness and tingling of lips, fingers, and toes

Laryngeal Nerve Damage

Change in pitch and tone of voice
Aphonia
Hoarseness, weakness, "whispery" voice

Incision Site

Redness
Swelling
Drainage
Fever
Pain
Guarding behavior
Distraction behavior (restlessness, moaning)

Nursing Dx & Intervention

Risk for decreased cardiac output related to hemorrhage

- Monitor pulse, blood pressure, color, and temperature.
- Monitor level of consciousness and orientation.
- Check the dressing for evidence of excessive bleeding; watch for bleeding at the side of the neck and back of the head (immediately after operation, check every hour) *to identify signs of bleeding.*

Ineffective breathing pattern related to inflammation

- Monitor rate, depth, and character of respirations *to identify early signs of tracheal compression from edema.*
- Monitor level of consciousness.
- Monitor for apprehension, restlessness, and cyanosis.
- Keep suction equipment and tracheostomy set at bedside *to use in case of sudden tracheal compression.*

Sensory/perceptual alterations (kinesthetic) related to chemical imbalance

- Monitor patient's calcium levels.
- Check reflexes every 2 hours; check vital signs every 4 hours.
- Check Chvostek's and Trousseau's signs every 2 hours.

- Observe for changes in personality.
- Have a 10% solution of calcium gluconate and equipment for IV administration at the bedside or readily available *to treat hypocalcemia.*

Pain related to physical factors

- Place patient in semi-Fowler's position *to promote ease in breathing.*
- Monitor edema surrounding incision.
- Observe body language for evidence of pain *to ensure comfort despite impaired communication.*
- Log-roll patient's head and chest *to prevent strain on sutures.*
- Teach patient to support the head and neck with a folded towel during mobility *to support surgical site.*

Impaired verbal communication related to anatomic deficit

- Monitor pitch and tone of patient's voice every 1 to 2 hours postoperatively *to evaluate damage to recurrent laryngeal nerves (vocal cord paralysis).*
- Discourage talking *to prevent edema of vocal cords.*
- Monitor for edema of glottis and surgical incision.
- Establish alternate means of communication (i.e., pad and pencil).
- Reassure patient that hoarseness (from edema or pressure) will subside in a few days.

Patient Education/Home Care Planning

1. Discuss with the patient the name, action, dosage, schedule, route of administration, and side effects of thyroid hormone replacement if ordered.
2. Demonstrate to the patient the care of the surgical incision.
3. Demonstrate to the patient head and neck circle exercises.

Evaluation

Cardiovascular function is normal Patient's serum electrolytes, hemoglobin, and hematocrit are normal. Patient's skin remains warm and dry. Patient's vital signs remain stable.

Respiratory function is normal Patient demonstrates adequate respiratory depth and rate. Patient does not demonstrate cyanosis, dyspnea, or restlessness.

Electrolyte balance is normal Patient's serum calcium levels are normal. Chvostek's and Trousseau's signs are negative. Patient shows no signs of tetany.

Comfort increases Patient verbalizes decreased pain or relief from pain. Signs of edema at surgical incision are decreased or absent. Patient demonstrates adequate support of head and neck during rest and mobility.

Communication is normal or adequate Pitch and voice tone of patient are normal. Patient shows no voice changes (i.e., hoarseness). Patient uses alternate means of communication to preserve voice.

References

1. American Diabetes Association: American diabetes association: clinical practice recommendations 1995, *Diabetes care* 18 (Suppl 1):1, 1995.
2. Bartter FC, Schwartz WB: The syndrome of inappropriate antidiuretic hormone, *Am J Med* 42:790, 1967.
3. Baxter JD, Frohman LA, Felig P: Introduction to the endocrine system. In Felig P, Baxter JD, Frohman LA, editors: *Endocrinology and metabolism,* New York, 1995, McGraw-Hill.
4. Baylis PH, Thompson CJ: Diabetes insipidus and hyperosmolar states. In Becker KL et al, editors: *Principles and practice of endocrinology and metabolism,* ed 2, Philadelphia, 1995, Lippincott.
5. Baylis P: Vasopressin and its neurophysin. In DeGroot LJ, et al, editors: *Endocrinology,* ed 3, Philadelphia, 1995, Saunders.
6. Bennett PH: Epidemiology of diabetes mellitus. In Rifkin H, Porte D, editors: *Ellenberg and Rifkin's diabetes mellitus,* ed 4, New York, 1990, Elsevier.
7. Bononi PL, Robinson AG: Central diabetes insipidus: management in the postoperative period, *Endocrinologist* 1(3):180, 1991.
8. Braunwald E, editor: *Heart disease: a textbook of cardiovascular medicine,* ed 4, Philadelphia, 1992, Saunders.
9. Braverman LE, Utiger RD: Introduction to thyrotoxicosis. In Braverman LE, Utiger RD, editors: *Werner and Ingbar's the thyroid a fundamental and clinical text,* ed 6, Philadelphia, 1991, Lippincott.
10. Bristol-Meyers Squibb Company: *Glucophage (metformin HCL tablets) product monograph,* Wilton, CT, 1995, Medical Education Programs.
11. Brown EM: Physiology of calcium metabolism. In Becker KL, et al, editors: *Principles and practice of endocrinology,* ed 2, Philadelphia, 1995, Lippincott.
12. Burch HB, Wartofsky L: Graves' ophthalmopathy: current concepts regarding pathogenesis and management, *Endocr Rev* 14:747, 1993.
13. Burch HB, Solomon BL, Wartofsky L, Burman KD: Discontinuing antithyroid drug therapy before ablation with radioiodine, *Ann Intern Med* 121:553, 1994.
14. Burch WM: *Endocrinology,* ed 3, Baltimore, 1994, Williams and Wilkins.
15. Burman KD: Hyperthyroidism. In Becker KL, et al, editors: *Principles and practice of endocrinology,* ed 2, Philadelphia, 1995, Lippincott.
16. Burrow GN et al: Microadenomas of the pituitary and abnormal sellar tomograms in an unselected autopsy series, *New Engl J Med* 304:156, 1981.
17. Chodosh LA, Daniels GH: Addison's disease, *Endocrinologist* 3:166, 1993.
18. Cook DL, Taborsky GJ: B-cell function and insulin secretion. In Rifkin H, Porte D, editors: *Ellenberg and Rifkin's diabetes mellitus,* ed 4, New York, 1990, Elsevier.
19. Cooper PE, Martin JB: Physiology and pathophysiology of the endocrine brain and hypothalamus. In Becker KL et al, editors: *Principles and practice of endocrinology and metabolism,* ed 2, Philadelphia, 1995, Lippincott.
20. Consensus Development Conference Panel: Diagnosis and management of asymptomatic primary hyperparathyroidism: consensus development conference statement, *Ann Intern Med* 114:593, 1991.
21. Cryer P: Diseases of the sympathochromaffin system. In Felig P, Baxter JD, Frohman LA, editors: *Endocrinology and metabolism,* ed 3, New York, 1995, McGraw-Hill.
22. Davidson JK: Diabetic ketoacidosis and the hyperglycemic hyperosmolar state. In Davidson J, editors; *Clinical diabetes mellitus: A problem-oriented approach,* ed 2, New York, 1991, Thieme Medical Publishers.
23. DelVallen J: Zollinger Ellison syndrome. In Yamada T, editor: *Textbook of gastroenterology,* ed 2, Philadelphia, 1995, Lippincott.
24. Doppman JL: The search for occult ectopic ACTH-producing tumors, *Endocrinologist* 2:41, 1993.
25. Edwards CRW: Primary mineralocorticoid excess syndromes. In DeGroot LJ et al, editors: *Endocrinology,* ed 3, Philadelphia, 1995, Saunders.
26. Erickson GF: The ovary: basic principles and concepts A. physiology. In Felig P, Baxter JD, Frohman LA, editors: *Endocrinology and metabolism,* ed 3, New York, 1995, McGraw-Hill.
27. Expert panel on detection, evaluation and treatment of high blood cholesterol in adults: Summary of the second report on the national cholesterol education program (NCEP) expert panel on detection, evaluation and treatment of high blood cholesterol in adults, *JAMA,* 269:3015, 1993.
28. Felig P, Bergman M: The endocrine pancreas: diabetes mellitus. In Felig P, Baxter JD, Frohman LA, editors: *Endocrinology and metabolism,* ed 3, New York, 1995, McGraw-Hill.
29. Fitzpatrick LA, Arnold A: Hypoparathyroidism. In Degroot LJ et al, editors: *Endocrinology,* ed 3, Philadelphia, 1995, Saunders.
30. Gill JR: Primary hyperaldosteronism: Strategies for diagnosis and treatment, *Endocrinologist* 1:365, 1991.
31. Golub MD, Tuck ML: Diagnostic and therapeutic strategies in pheochromocytoma, *Endocrinologist* 2:101, 1992.
32. Grossman A: Corticotropin-releasing hormone: Basic physiology and clinical applications. In DeGroot LJ et al, editors: *Endocrinology,* ed 3, Philadelphia, 1995, Saunders.
33. Hoet JJ, Reusens B, Remacle C: Anatomy, developmental biology, and pathology of the pancreatic islets. In DeGroot LJ et al, editors: *Endocrinology,* ed 3, 1995, Philadelphia, Saunders.
34. Hsueh AJW, Billig H: Ovarian hormone synthesis and mechanism of action. In DeGroot LJ et al, editors: *Endocrinology,* ed 3, Philadelphia, 1995, Saunders.
35. Illingworth DR, Duell PB, Connor WE: Disorders of lipid metabolism. In Felig P, Baxter JD, Frohman LA, editors: *Endocrinology and metabolism,* ed 3, New York, 1995, McGraw-Hill.
36. Imagimedic Productions: *Practical diabetology* 2:3, 1983.
37. Kaplan EL, Ito K, Tanaka R: Surgery of the thyroid gland. In Becker KL et al, editors: *Principles and practice of endocrinology,* ed 2, Philadelphia, 1995, Lippincott.
38. Keiser HR: Pheochromocytoma and other diseases of the sympathetic nervous system. In Becker KL et al, editors: *Principles and practice of endocrinology and metabolism,* ed 2, Philadelphia, 1995, Lippincott.
39. Keiser HR: Pheochromocytoma and related tumors. In DeGroot LJ et al, editors: *Endocrinology,* ed 3, Philadelphia, 1995, Saunders.
40. Kitabchi AE, Duckworth WC, Stentz FB: Insulin synthesis, proinsulin and c-peptides. In Rifkin H, Porte D, editors: *Ellenberg and Rifkin's diabetes mellitus,* ed 4, New York, 1990, Elsevier.
41. Korenman et al: *Practical diagnosis and endocrine disease,* Boston, 1978, Houghton-Mifflin.
42. Kreisberg RA: Diabetic ketoacidosis. In Rifkin H, Porte D, editors: *Ellenberg and Rifkin's diabetes mellitus,* ed 4, New York, 1990, Elsevier.
43. Kretser DM, Risbridger GP, Kerr J: Basic endocrinology of the testis. In DeGroot LJ et al, editors: *Endocrinology,* ed 3, Philadelphia, 1995, Saunders.
44. Landsberg L, Young JB: Catecholamines and the adrenal medulla. In Wilson JD, Foster DW, editors: *William's Textbook of Endocrinology,* ed 8, Philadelphia, 1992, Saunders.
45. Lefebvre PJ, Scheen AJ: Hypoglycemia. In Rifkin H, Porte D, editors: *Ellenberg and Rifkin's diabetes mellitus,* ed 4, New York, 1990, Elsevier.
46. Lipsett L, Geiss L: Statistics: prevalence, incidence, risk factors, and complications of diabetes (memorandum), *Am Diabetes Assoc Bull* 1993.
47. Livolsi VA: Morphology of the thyroid gland. In Becker KL et al, editors: *Principles and practice of endocrinology and metabolism,* ed 2, Philadelphia, 1995, Lippincott.
48. Livolsi VA: Morphology of the parathyroid glands. In Becker KL et al, editors: *Principles and practice of endocrinology,* ed 2, Philadelphia, 1995, Lippincott.
49. Loriaux DL, McDonald WJ: Adrenal insufficiency. In DeGroot LJ et al, editors: *Endocrinology,* ed 3, Philadelphia, 1995, Saunders.
50. Loriaux DL: Adrenocortical insufficiency. In Becker KL et al, editors: *Principles and practice of endocrinology and metabolism,* ed 2, Philadelphia, 1995, Lippincott.

51. Loriaux DL: Tests of adrenocortical function. In Becker KL et al, editors: *Principles and practice of endocrinology and metabolism,* ed 2, Philadelphia, 1995, Lippincott.
52. Loriaux TC: Endocrine anatomy and physiology. In Kinney MR, Packa DR, Dunbar SB, editors: *AACN's clinical reference for critical-care nursing,* ed 3, St Louis, 1993, Mosby.
53. Loriaux TC: Endocrine data acquisition. In Kinney MR, Packa DR, Dunbar SB, editors: *AACN's clinical reference for critical-care nursing,* ed 3, St Louis, 1993, Mosby.
54. Loriaux TC, Drass JA: Endocrine and diabetic disorders. In Kinney MR, Packa DR, Dunbar SB, editors: *AACN's clinical reference for critical-care nursing,* ed 3, St Louis, 1993, Mosby.
55. Matz R: Hyperosmolar nonacidotic diabetes (HNAD). In Rifkin H, Porte D, editors: *Ellenberg and Rifkin's diabetes mellitus,* ed 4, New York, 1990, Elsevier.
56. Mazzaferri EL: Thyroid cancer. In Becker KL et al, editors: *Principles and practice of endocrinology and metabolism,* ed 2, Philadelphia, 1995, Lippincott.
57. McEvoy G, editor: *American hospital formulary service drug information 95,* Bethesda, MD, 1995, American Association Health System Pharmacists, Inc.
58. McKenney J: New guidelines for managing hypercholesterolemia, *Am Pharm* 33(7): 24, 1993.
59. Melby JC, Azar ST: Adrenal steroids and hypertension: new aspects, *Endocrinologist* 3:344, 1993.
60. Melmed S: General aspects of the management of pituitary tumors by surgery or radiation therapy. In DeGroot LJ et al, editors: *Endocrinology,* ed 3, Philadelphia, 1995, Saunders.
61. Melmed S: Tumor mass effects of lesions in the hypothalamus and pituitary. In DeGroot LJ et al, editors: *Endocrinology,* ed 3, Philadelphia, 1995, Saunders.
62. Meikle AW: A diagnostic approach to Cushing's syndrome, *Endocrinologist* 3:311, 1993.
63. Miller J, Crapo L: The biochemical diagnosis of hypercortisolism, *Endocrinologist* 4:7, 1994.
64. Miller WL, Tyrrell JB: The adrenal cortex. In Felig P, Baxter JD, Frohman LA, editors: *Endocrinology and metabolism,* ed 3, New York, 1995, McGraw-Hill.
65. Molitch M: Neuroendocrinology. In Felig P, Baxter JD, Frohman LA, editors: *Endocrinology and metabolism,* ed 3, New York, 1995, McGraw-Hill.
66. Mortensen RM, Williams GH: Aldosterone action: physiology. In DeGroot LJ et al, editors: *Endocrinology,* ed 3, Philadelphia, 1995, Saunders.
67. Munck A, Náray-Fejes-Tóth A: Glucocorticoid action: physiology. In DeGroot LJ et al, editors: *Endocrinology,* ed 3, Philadelphia, 1995, Saunders.
68. National Diabetes Data Group: Classification and diagnosis of diabetes mellitus and other categories of glucose intolerance, *Diabetes* 28:1042, 1979.
69. Nieman LK, Cutler GB: Cushing's syndrome. In DeGroot LJ et al, editors: *Endocrinology,* ed 3, Philadelphia, 1995, Saunders.
70. Orth DN, Kovacs WJ, DeBold CR: The adrenal cortex. In Wilson JD, Foster DW, editors: *William's textbook of endocrinology,* ed 8, Philadelphia, 1992, Saunders.
71. Parker LN: Adrenal androgens. In Degroot LJ et al, editors: *Endocrinology,* ed 3, 1995, Philadelphia, Saunders.
72. Peragallo-Dittko V, Godley K, Meyer J, editors: *A core curriculum for diabetes education,* ed 2, Chicago, 1993, American Association of Diabetes Educators and the AADE Education and Research Foundation.
73. Pickering BT: Oxytocin. In Degroot LJ et al, editors: *Endocrinology,* ed 3, Philadelphia, 1995, Saunders.
74. Redfern J, O'Dorisio T: Gastrointestinal hormones and carcinoid syndrome. In Felig P, Baxter JD, Frohman LA, editors: *Endocrinology and metabolism,* ed 3, New York, 1995, McGraw-Hill.
75. Reed L, Pangaro LN: Physiology of the thyroid gland I: synthesis and release, iodine metabolism, and binding and transport. In Becker KL et al, editors: *Principles and practice of endocrinology and metabolism,* ed 2, Philadelphia, 1995, Lippincott.
76. Rittmaster RS, Arab DM: Morphology of the adrenal cortex and medulla. In Becker KL et al, editors: *Principles and practice of endocrinology,* ed 2, Philadelphia, 1995, Lippincott.
77. Robertson GL: Physiology of vasopressin, oxytocin, and thirst. In Becker KL et al, editors: *Principles and practice of endocrinology and metabolism,* ed 2, Philadelphia, 1995, Lippincott.
78. Santen RJ: The testis. In Felig P, Baxter JD, Frohman LA, editors: *Endocrinology and metabolism,* ed 3, New York, 1995, McGraw-Hill.
79. Sawin CT et al: Low serum thyrotropin concentrations as a risk factor for atrial fibrillation in older persons, *New Engl J Med* 331:1249, 1994.
80. Schteingart DE: Treating adrenal cancer, *Endocrinologist* 2:149, 1992.
81. Shamoon H: Hypoglycemia. In Felig P, Baxter JD, Frohman LA, editors: *Endocrinology and metabolism,* ed 3, New York, 1995, McGraw-Hill.
82. Shapiro LE, Surks MI: Hypothyroidism. In Becker KL et al, editors: *Principles and practice of endocrinology,* ed 2, Philadelphia, 1995, Lippincott.
83. Solomon B, Glinoer D, Lagasse R, Wartofsky L: Current trends in the management of Graves' disease, *J Clin Endocrinol Metab* 70:1518, 1990.
84. Solomon B, Fein HG, Smallridge RC: Usefulness of antimicrosomal antibody titers in the diagnosis and treatment of postpartum thyroiditis, *J Fam Pract* 36:177, 1993.
85. Solomon BL, Wartofsky L, Burman KD: The prevalence of fractures in postmenopausal women with thyroid disease, *Thyroid* 3:17, 1993.
86. Solomon B, Schaaf M, Smallridge R: Psychological symptoms before and after parathyroid surgery, *Am J Med* 96:101, 1994.
87. Solomon BL, Wartofsky L, Burman KD: Current trends in the management of well differentiated papillary thyroid carcinoma, *J Clin Endocrinol Metab* 81:333, 1996.
88. Spiro H et al: *Clinical gastroenterology,* ed 4, New York, 1993, McGraw-Hill.
89. Steomer DF, Bell GI, Tagu HS, Rubenstein AH: Chemistry and biosynthesis of the islet hormones: insulin, islet amyloid polypeptide (amylin), glucagon, somatostatin, and pancreatic polypeptide. In DeGroot LJ et al, editors: *Endocrinology,* ed 3, 1995, Philadelphia, Saunders.
90. Streeten DHP, Moses AM: The syndrome of inappropriate vasopressin secretion, *Endocrinologist* 3:353, 1993.
91. Strewler GJ, Rosenblatt M: Mineral metabolism. In Felig P, Baxter JD, Frohman LA, editors: *Endocrinology and metabolism,* New York, 1995, McGraw-Hill.
92. Teramoto A: Selective venous sampling in Cushing's syndrome, *Endocrinologist* 4:412, 1995.
93. Thapar K et al: Pituitary adenomas: current concepts in classification, histopathology, and molecular biology, *Endocrinologist* 3:39, 1993.
94. Thapar K, Kovacs K, Horvath E: Morphology of the pituitary in health and disease. In Becker KL et al, editors: *Principles and practices of endocrinology and metabolism,* ed 2, Philadelphia, 1995, Lippincott.
95. The Diabetes Control and Complications Trail Research Group: The effect of intensive treatment of diabetes with insulin on the development and progression of long term complications in insulin-dependent diabetes mellitus, *New Eng J Med* 329:977, 1993.
96. Thorner MO, Vance ML, Horvath R, Kovacs K: The anterior pituitary. In Wilson JD, Foster DW, editors: *William's Textbook of Endocrinology,* ed 8, Philadelphia, 1992, Saunders.
97. Unger RH, Orci L: Glucagon. In Rifkin H, Porte D, editors: *Ellenberg and Rifkin's diabetes mellitus,* ed 4, New York, 1990, Elsevier.
98. Utiger RD: The thyroid: physiology, thyrotoxicosis, hypothyroidism, and the painful thyroid. In Felig P, Baxter JD, Frohman LA, editors: *Endocrinology and metabolism,* New York, 1995, McGraw-Hill.
99. Utiger RD: Hypothyroidism. In Becker KL et al, editors: *Principles and practice of endocrinology,* ed 2, Philadelphia, 1995, Lippincott.
100. Vance ML: When bromocryptine fails, *Endocrinologist* 1:119.

101. Verbalis JG: Inappropriate antidiuresis and other hyperosmolar states. In Becker KL et al, editors: *Principles and practice of endocrinology and metabolism,* ed 2, Philadelphia, 1995, Lippincott.

102. Volpe R: Graves' disease. In Braverman LE, Utiger RD, editors: *Werner and Ingbar's the thyroid a fundamental and clinical text,* ed 6, Philadelphia, 1991, Lippincott.

103. Wartofsky L et al: Differences and similarities in the diagnosis and treatment of Graves' disease in Europe, Japan and the United States, *Thyroid* 1:129, 1991.

104. Wass JAH, Besser M: Tests of pituitary function. In DeGroot LJ et al, editors: *Endocrinology,* ed 3, Philadelphia, 1995, Saunders.

105. Wenzel E, Comi RJ: Use of octreotide in clinical endocrinology, *Endocrinologist* 1:256, 1991.

106. White PC, Pescovitz OH, Cutler GB: Synthesis and metabolism of corticosteroids. In Becker KL et al, editors: *Principles and practice of endocrinology,* ed 2, Philadelphia, 1995, Lippincott.

107. Wilding JPH, Ghatei MA, Bloom S: Hormones of the gastrointestinal tract. In DeGroot LJ et al, editors: *Endocrinology,* ed 3, Philadelphia, 1995, Saunders.

108. Witte RJ, Mark LP, Daniels DL, Haughton VM: Radiographic evaluation of the pituitary and anterior hypothalamus. In DeGroot LJ et al, editors: *Endocrinology,* ed 3, Philadelphia, 1995, Saunders.

109. Wood LC, Cooper DS, Ridgway EC: *Your thyroid a home reference,* New York, 1995, Ballantine.

Female Reproductive System

10

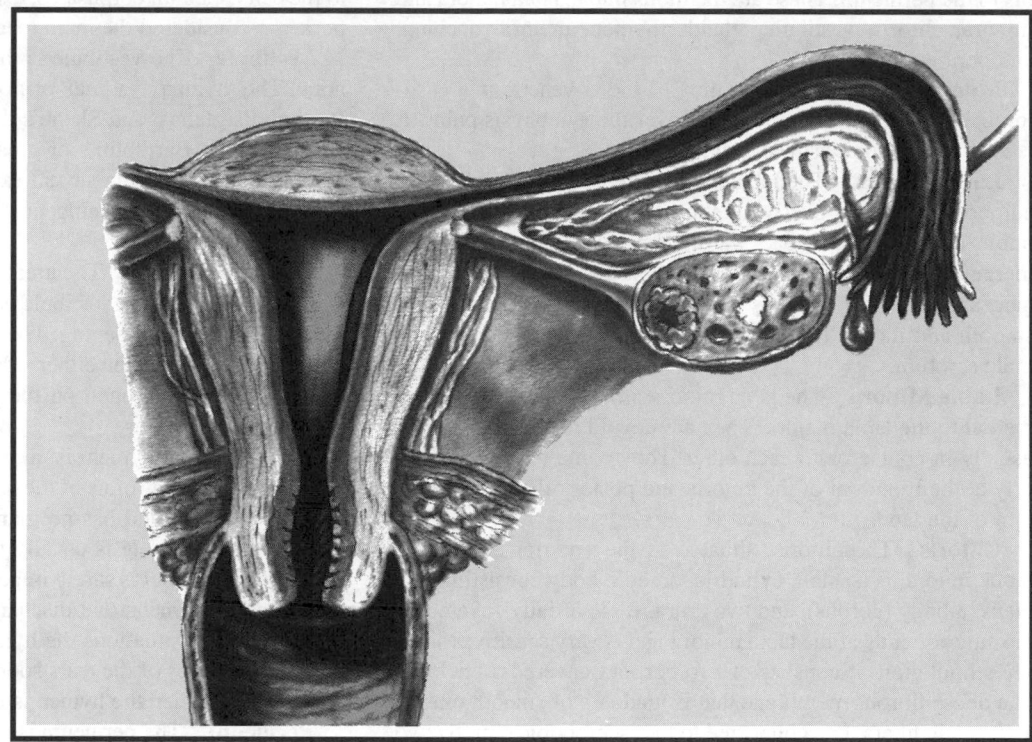

OVERVIEW

The major physiologic function of the reproductive system is the procreation of new life and perpetuation of the human species. This biologic process is primarily under endocrine control, but it is also influenced by neural and metabolic factors and human sexuality. Not merely a biologic phenomenon, human sexuality is the sum of physical, functional, and psychologic attributes that are expressed by a person's gender identity and sexual behavior. These factors interact when gynecologic and reproductive processes or conditions threaten, alter, or interfere with female sexual integrity.

The focus of this chapter is on the female organ system and includes those conditions for which patients are routinely hospitalized and those conditions that are most commonly managed in the outpatient or ambulatory care setting. A recent study quantifies the rate of hospitalization for gynecologic disorders among reproductive-age women (15 to 44 years old) in the United States.[50] This study was based on data from the National Hospital Discharge Surveys for 1988, 1989, and 1990 and included data collected annually by the National Center for Health Statistics. It was learned that based on average annual discharge rates for 10,000 women of reproductive-age, the five most frequent diagnostic groups were pelvic inflammatory disease (PID) (average annual rate 49.3), benign cysts of the ovary (average annual rate 32.7), endometriosis (average annual rate 32.4), menstrual disorders (average annual rate 31.4), and uter-

ine leiomyomas (average annual rate 30.4). The highest rates for PID were among women 25 to 39 years old and for women of races other than white. Highest rates for uterine leiomyomas were among women 40 to 44 years old and for women of races other than white. Highest rates for endometriosis were among women 40 to 44 years old and white women. Racial differences existed among all ages in the uterine leiomyoma and endometriosis groups. It was noted that the average annual rates of benign cysts and menstrual disorders increased with age, but there were no statistically significant differences according to race in these two diagnostic groups.[50]

Pelvic inflammatory disease, benign cysts of the ovary, endometriosis, menstrual disorders, and uterine leiomyomas are discussed in this chapter, as well as other selected female organ dysfunctions. After a review of anatomy and physiology, the pathophysiology of each condition is presented, as well as diagnostic studies and findings, multidisciplinary plan of care, nursing assessment, diagnosis, intervention, evaluation, and patient education/home care planning.

•••••• Anatomy, Physiology, and Related Pathophysiology

The female organ system consists of internal organs in the pelvic cavity and external organs in the perineum. The internal organs are the ovaries, fallopian tubes, uterus, and vagina. The external genitalia are the mons pubis, labia majora, labia minora, and the vestibule of the vagina (Figure 10-1).

External Structures

The vulva includes all externally visible structures from the pubis to the perineum. These are the mons pubis, labia majora and minora, clitoris, vestibular glands, hymen, urethral opening, and perineum.

Mons pubis   The mons pubis or mons veneris is a cushionlike elevation of adipose tissue over the symphysis pubis. It is covered by pubic hair after puberty.

Labia majora   The labia majora are two rounded folds of adipose tissue with overlying skin that extend from the mons pubis downward and backward, encircle the vestibule, and merge into the perineum. The outer surfaces are covered by hair, and the inner surfaces containing sebaceous follicles are smooth and moist. The labia majora are homologous with the male scrotum.

Labia Minora   The labia minora are two flat folds of skin medial to the labia majora. They are devoid of hair and fat and usually in contact with each other. They come together anteriorly at the frenulum of the clitoris and posteriorly at the frenulum of the labia.

Clitoris   The clitoris, situated at the anterior end of the labia minora, is a small, cylindric, erectile body consisting of a glans, a body (corpus), and two crura. It is partially covered by the anterior ends of the labia minora and is very sensitive to tactile stimulation. It consists of two corpora cavernosa enclosed in a dense fibrous membrane that is made up of smooth muscle and elastic fibers. It is connected to the ischiopubic rami by two crura. The clitoris, which corresponds to the male penis, rarely exceeds 2 cm in length even in a state of erection during sexual arousal. The glans of the clitoris is covered by stratified epithelium that is richly supplied with free nerve endings within the fibers, terminating in small knoblike thickenings in or adjacent to the cells. Genital corpuscles, distributed in the glans and corpora, are considered the main mediators of erotic sensation.

Vestibule   The vestibule is the area between the labia minora. The hymen, vaginal orifice, urethral orifice, ducts of Bartholin's glands, and Skene's ducts are contained within the vestibule. The Bartholin's or greater vestibular glands secrete mucoid material during sexual excitement. They are on either side of the vaginal opening posteriorly under the constrictor muscle of the vagina.

Urethral opening   The urethral opening or urinary meatus is in the midline of the vestibule posterior to the clitoris and anterior to the vaginal opening. The Skene's or paraurethral ducts open on the vestibule on either side of the urethra. Occasionally these openings are found on the posterior wall of the urethra just inside the meatus.

Hymen   The hymen is a fold of vascularized mucous membrane at the introitus of the vagina. It is not richly supplied with nerve fibers and has no glandular or muscular elements. The hymenal opening is usually very small in virgins who do not use tampons but is rarely imperforate, which would cause a retention of the menstrual discharge. During the first coitus or in certain other situations the hymen generally tears at several points. The edges of the tears soon cicatrize. Bleeding does not always occur when the hymen is ruptured.

Perineum   The perineum is a triangular area that is the inferior end of the trunk. It is situated dorsal to the pubic arch, superior to the tip of the coccyx, and lateral to the pubic and ischial rami. It supports and surrounds the distal portions of the

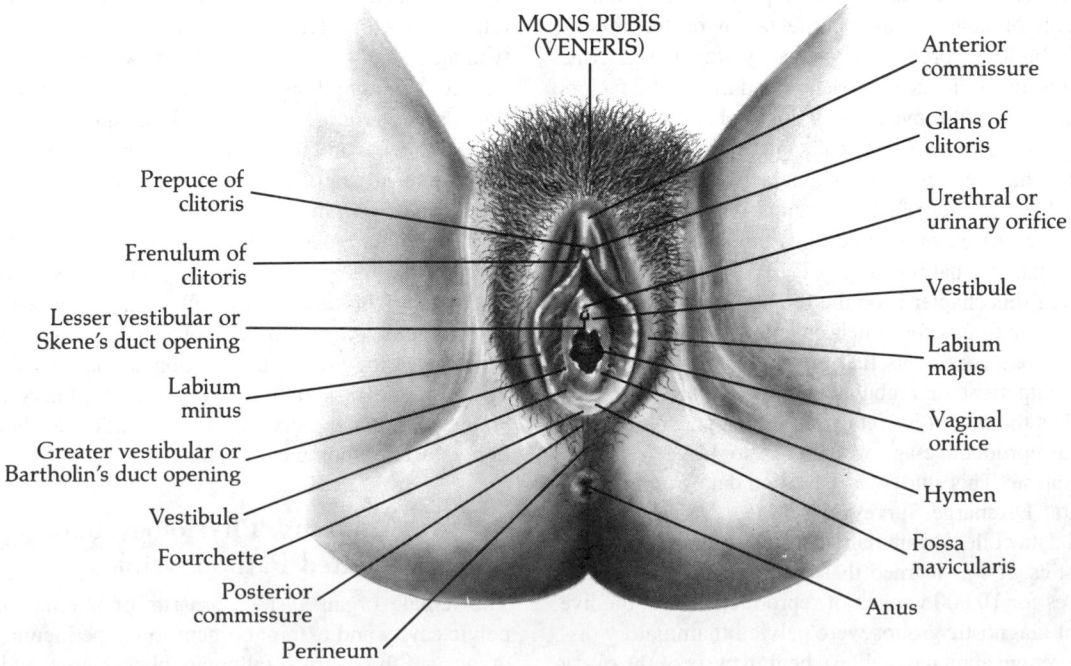

Figure 10-1 External female genitalia. (From Bobak.[9])

urogenital and gastrointestinal tracts of the body. The central fibrous perineal body between the vagina and the anus divides the perineum into a posterior anal triangle and an anterior urogenital triangle.

Internal Structures

The internal organs include the ovaries, uterine (fallopian) tubes, uterus, and vagina.

Ovaries   The ovaries are two oval structures in the upper part of the pelvic cavity, between the uterus medially and the lateral pelvic wall. They are suspended from the posterosuperior surface of the broad ligaments by the mesovarium. During the childbearing years each ovary is 2.5 to 5 cm in length, 1.5 to 3 cm in breadth, and 0.6 to 1.5 cm in thickness. After menopause the ovaries diminish markedly in size. In young women the ovary has a smooth, dull white surface through which glisten several small clear follicles. With advancing age the ovary becomes more corrugated, and in elderly women its exterior may appear convoluted. From the first states of development until after menopause, the ovary undergoes constant change. From birth to puberty an estimated 200,000 to 400,000 oocytes are present. It is evident that a few hundred ova suffice for reproduction because ordinarily only one ovum is cast off during a menstrual cycle. The glandular elements of the ovaries are described as interstitial, thecal, and luteal cells. The interstitial glandular elements are formed from cells of the theca interna of degenerating follicles. The thecal glandular cells are formed from the theca interna of ripening follicles. Luteal cells are derived from granulosa cells of ovulated follicles and from undifferentiated stroma surrounding them.

The ovarian cycle and its hormones are discussed in greater detail later in the chapter.

Uterine (fallopian) tubes   The uterine (fallopian) tubes are two flexible, trumpet-shaped, muscular tubes that extend from the uterine cornua to the ovaries and provide the ova with access to the uterine cavity. They are approximately 10 cm in length in an adult and are suspended by a fold of the broad ligament called the mesosalpinx. The isthmus end of the tube opens into the uterine cavity. The ampulla is the dilated central part of the tube that is continuous with the infundibulum, the fimbriated funnel-shaped opening of the distal end of the tube. This fimbriated portion of the tube, which is adjacent to the ovary, draws the ovum into the tube, where fertilization may occur. The tubal musculature undergoes rhythmic contractions that transport the ovum into the uterus, and the lining cells produce secretions essential for the fertilized ovum.

Uterus   (Figure 10-2) The uterus is a pear-shaped, thickwalled, muscular organ suspended in the anterior part of the pelvic cavity above and posterior to the bladder and in front of the rectum. It consists of two major but unequal parts: an upper triangular portion, the body or corpus, and a lower cylindric or fusiform portion, the cervix (Figure 10-3). The isthmus divides these two portions. The uterine (fallopian) tubes emerge from the cornua of the uterus at the junction of the superior and lateral margins. The convex upper segment between the cornua is the fundus uteri. Before puberty the length of the uterus varies

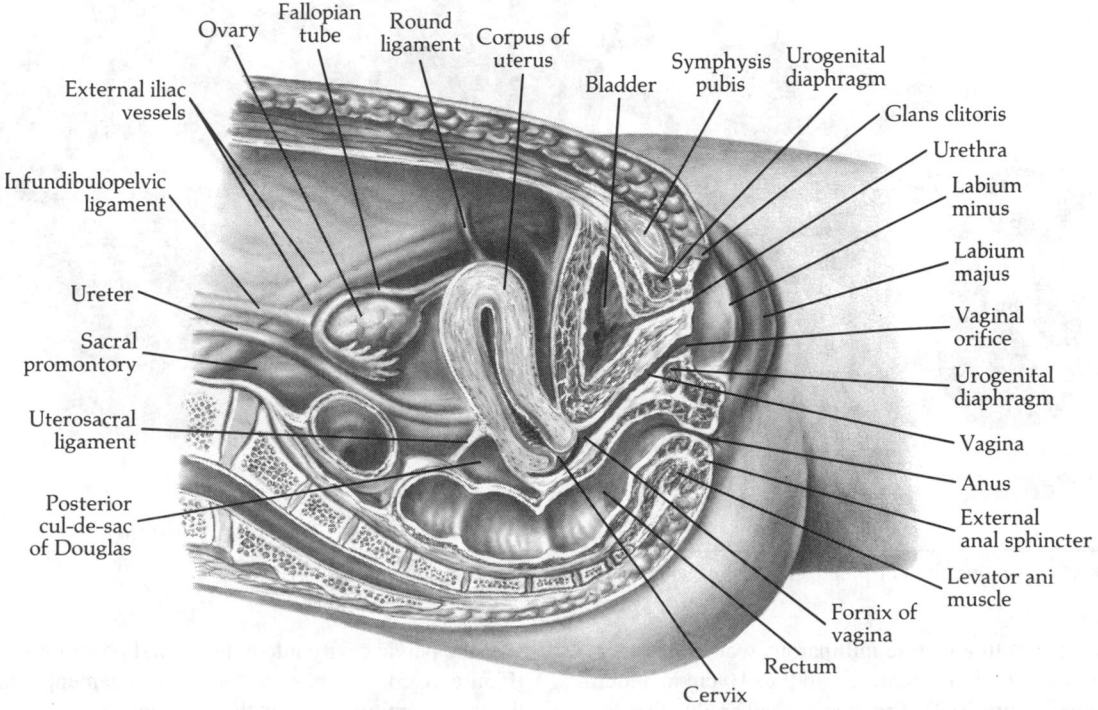

Figure 10-2 Midsagittal view of female pelvic organs, with woman lying supine. (From Bobak.[9])

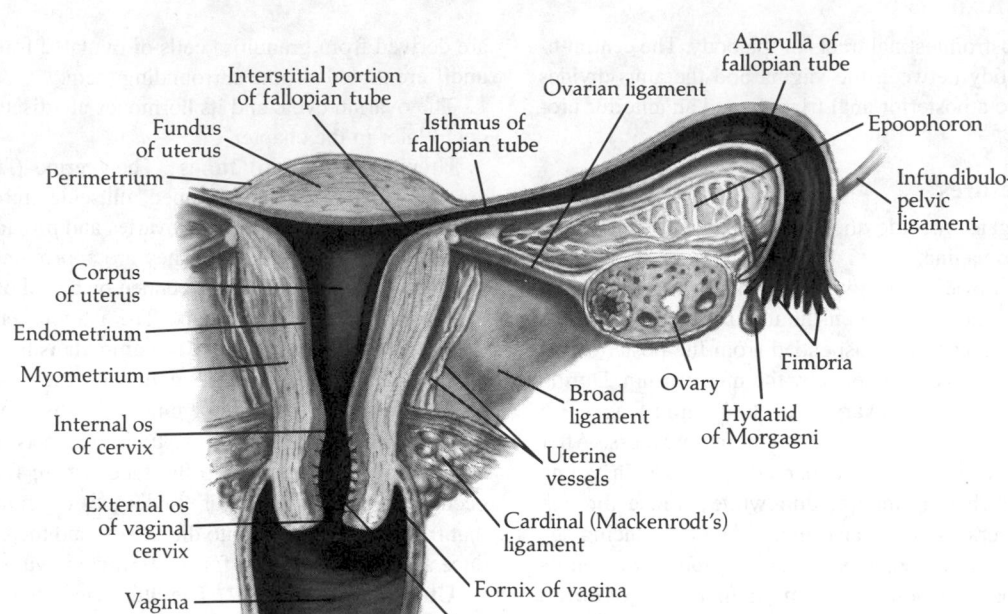

Figure 10-3 Cross section of uterus adnexa and upper vagina. (From Bobak.[9])

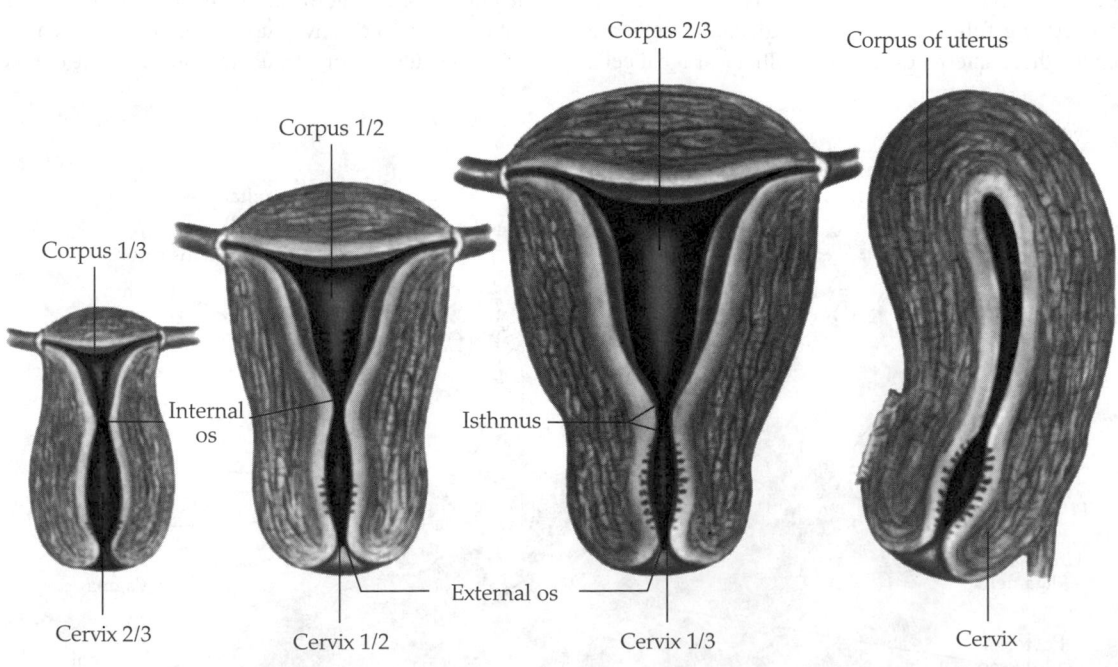

Figure 10-4 Comparative sizes of prepubertal, adult nonparous, and multiparous uteruses.

from 2.5 to 3.5 cm. In a mature nulliparous woman the uterus is 6 to 8 cm in length, as compared with 9 to 10 cm in a multiparous woman (Figure 10-4). The uterus is covered with a layer of peritoneum from which arise the broad ligaments that extend from the lateral margins of the uterus to the pelvic walls and di-

vide the pelvic cavity into anterior and posterior compartments (Figure 10-5). The base of the broad ligament, which is quite thick, is continuous with the connective tissue of the pelvic floor. The densest portion (cardinal ligament) surrounds the uterine blood vessels. The two round ligaments extend from

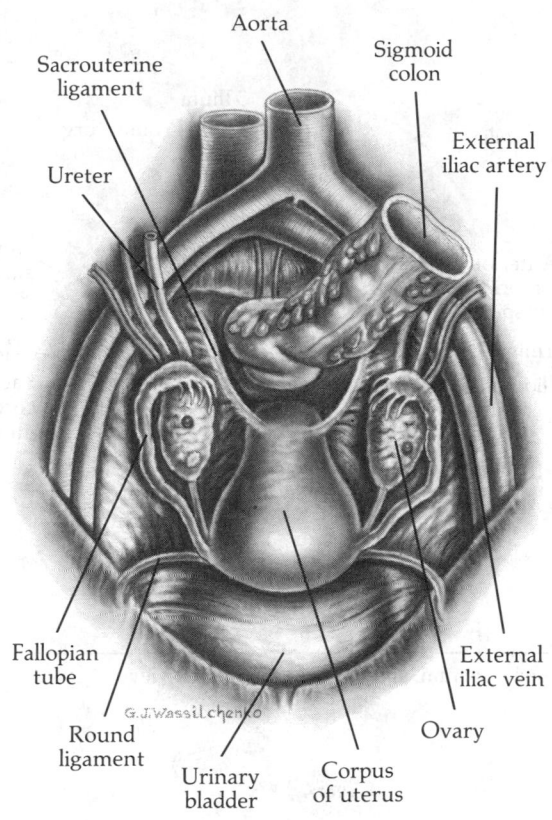

Aorta

Sacrouterine
ligament

Sigmoid
colon

Ureter

External
iliac artery

Fallopian
tube

External
iliac vein

G.J.Wassilchenko

Round
ligament

Ovary

Urinary
bladder

Corpus
of uterus

Figure 10-5 Female pelvic contents as viewed from above.

each side of the uterus below and anterior to the uterine tubes. During pregnancy the round ligaments undergo considerable hypertrophy and increase in both length and diameter. The uterosacral ligaments extend from the sacrum around the rectum to the cervix of the uterus. They help support the uterus and maintain its position. The uterosacral and cardinal ligaments are the most important ligaments of the uterus; without them the uterus would tend to pass through the vagina, or prolapse.

The wall of the uterus comprises three layers: serosal, muscular, and mucosal. The serosal layer is formed by the peritoneum covering the uterus. The muscular portion, or myometrium, consists of bundles of smooth muscle that are united by connective tissue containing many elastic fibers. During pregnancy the thickness of the myometrium increases markedly. This occurs because of hypertrophy (enlargement of existing fibers) and addition of new fibers derived from transformation and division of mesenchymal cells. The innermost or mucosal layer that lines the uterine cavity in the nonpregnant state is the endometrium. It comprises surface epithelium, glands, and interglandular tissue. The uterine glands extend through the entire thickness of the endometrium to the myometrium and secrete a think alkaline fluid that keeps the uterine cavity moist.

Two types of arteries supply blood to the endometrium. The straight basal arteries extend to the basal layer of the endometrium from the radial and arcuate arteries in the my-

ometrium. The coiled or spiral arteries, which are a continuation of the radial and basal arteries, supply the superficial layer of the endometrium. The coiled arteries play an important part in the mechanism of menstruation.

The cervix is the lower part of the uterus. The entrance of the uterus is the cervical os or opening, which changes in size and shape depending on pregnancy or previous deliveries. Hormonal changes influence mucus production by the endocervical glands.

Vagina   The vagina is a tubular canal 10 to 15 cm in length, directed backward and upward and extending from the vestibule to the uterus. It is located between the bladder anteriorly and the rectum posteriorly. It is the female organ of copulation, the birth canal, and the excretory duct of the uterus through which the menstrual flow escapes. In an adult the anterior wall of the vagina is approximately 8 cm long and the posterior wall is 9 to 10 cm long. The difference is because of the projection of the cervix into the anterior aspect of the superior end of the vagina. The anterior, posterior, and two lateral fornices are produced by the cervix projecting into the vagina. The fornices are of clinical importance because the internal pelvic organs can be easily palpated through the thin wall. The epithelium lining the vagina forms folds so that the vaginal walls are in contact with each other and kept moist by cervical secretions. The folds stretch with coitus and during the birth process.

Pelvis

The pelvis is composed of two innominate bones, the sacrum, and the coccyx (Figure 10-6). The innominate bones are formed by fusion of the ischium, ilium, and pubis and are joined to the sacrum and each other at the symphysis pubis. The pelvis has two parts: the shallow, upper, or false pelvis and the lower, smaller, or true pelvis. The false pelvis is bounded posteriorly be the lumbar vertebrae, laterally by the iliac fossa, and anteriorly by the abdominal wall. The true pelvis is bounded by the sacrum, the inner surface of the ischial bones, and the pubic bones. The shape and diameter of the true pelvis are important in obstetrics because it must accommodate the fetal head in a vaginal delivery.

Pelvic inlet   The pelvic inlet is bounded posteriorly by the sacral promontory, laterally by the linea terminalis, and anteriorly by the horizontal rami of the pubic bones and symphysis pubis. It has the following anterior-posterior diameters (Figure 10-7):

True conjugate (conjugata vera), the distance from the upper margin of the symphysis to the sacral promontory

Obstetric conjugate, the distance from the most convex posterior surface of the symphysis to the sacral promontory; this is about 0.5 cm less than the true conjugate and is the shortest anteroposterior diameter through which the fetal head must descend

Diagonal conjugate, the distance from the lower border of the symphysis to the sacral promontory; this is the only anteroposterior measurement that can be obtained by clinical examination

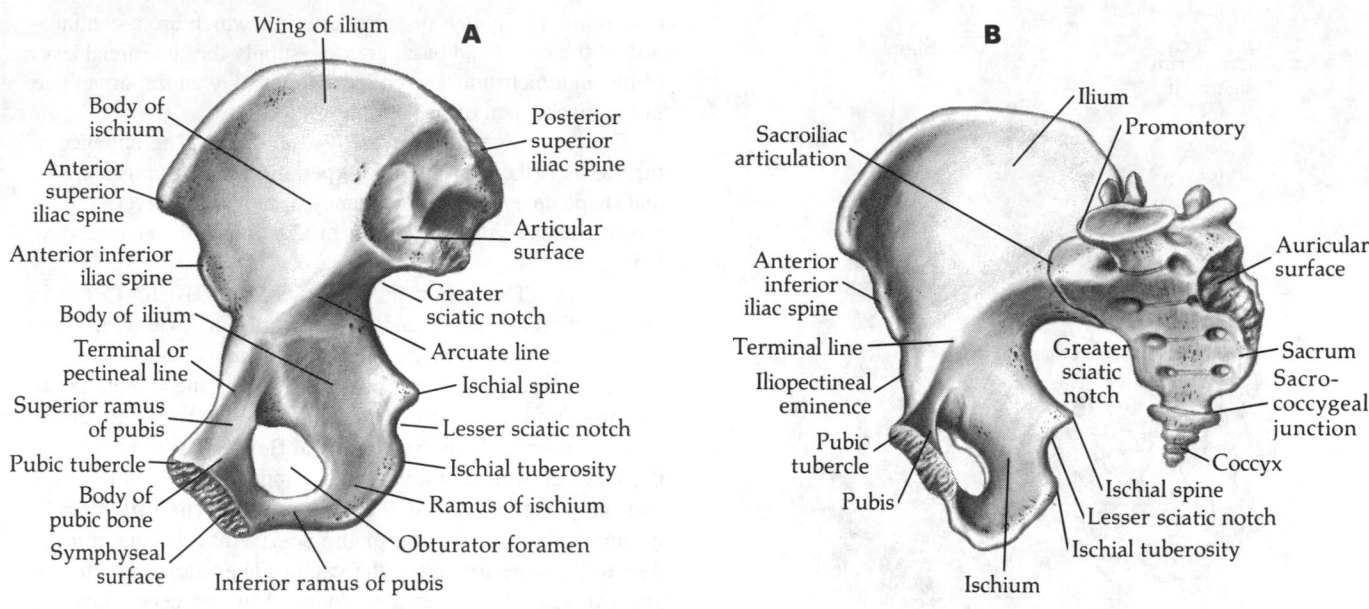

Figure 10-6 A, Right coxal bone, medial aspect. **B,** Articulated right coxal bone, sacrum, and coccyx, left oblique view.

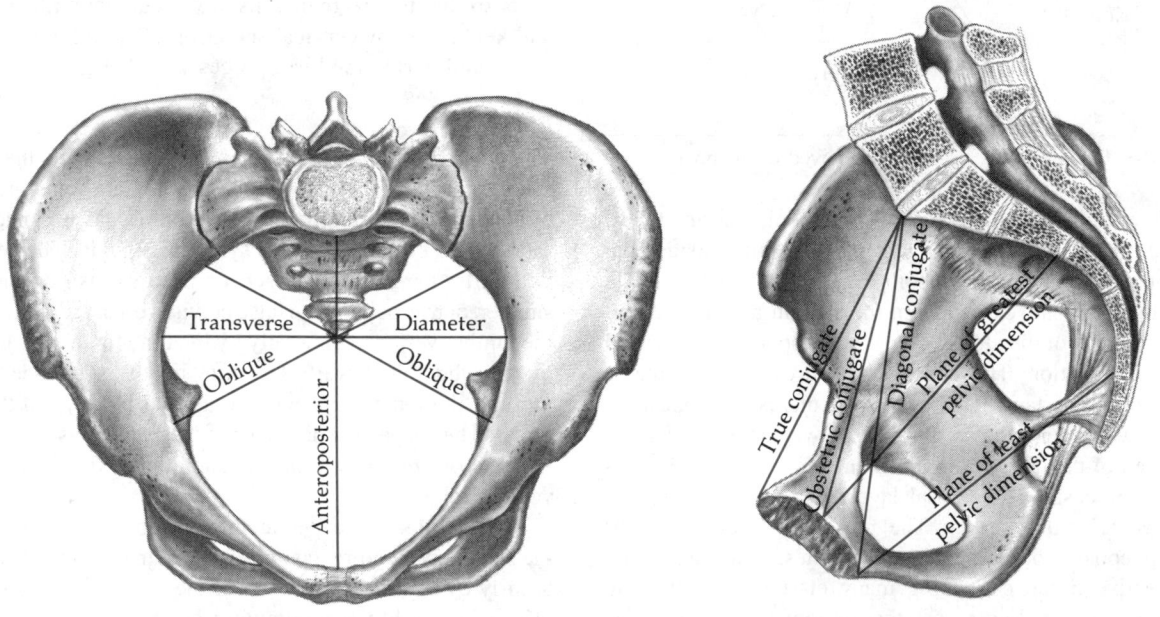

Figure 10-7 Planes of pelvic inlet.

The transverse diameter of the pelvic inlet is at a right angle to the obstetric conjugate and represents the greatest distance between the lineae terminales on either side. The oblique diameters extent from each sacroiliac synconodrosis to the opposite iliopectineal eminence.

Midpelvis   The midplane of the pelvis is the roomiest portion of the pelvic cavity. It extends from the middle of the symphysis pubis to the junction of the second and third sacral vertebrae and passes laterally through the ischial bones over the middle of the acetabulum. The interspinous (bispinous) diameter of 10 cm or slightly more in an adult is usually the smallest diameter of the pelvis. The anteroposterior diameter at the level of the ischial spines is normally at least 11.5 cm. The posterior sagittal diameter of the midpelvis is normally approximately 4.5 cm.

Pelvic inclination   In a woman who is standing, the upper portion of the pelvis is normally directed downward and backward and the lower portion is directed downward and forward.

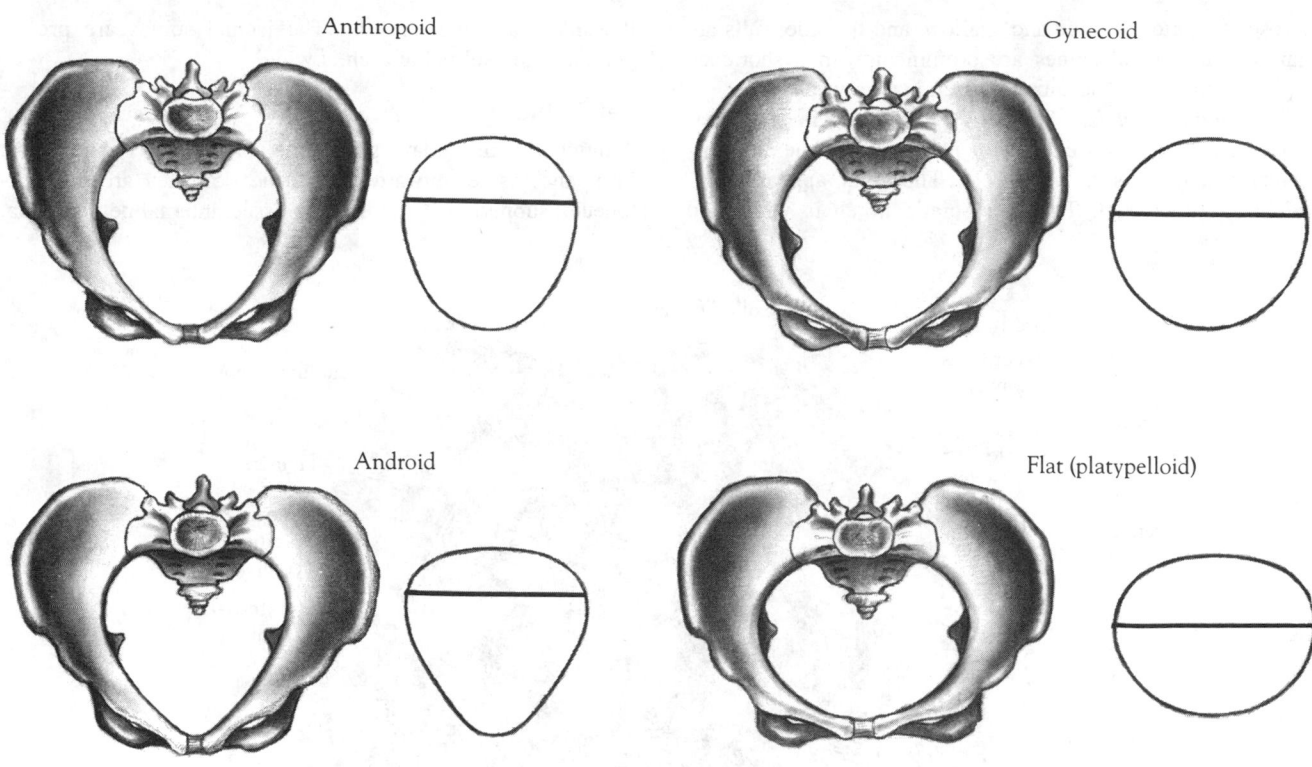

Anthropoid   Gynecoid

Android   Flat (platypelloid)

Figure 10-8 Female pelvis–pure types.

The tilt of the pelvis, or inclination, is altered with posture. Straightening of the lumbar curve reduces the pelvic inclination, and an exaggeration of the lumbar curve increases it. This tilt can influence the progress of labor.

Pelvic outlet   The outlet consists of two triangles having a common base at a line drawn between the two ischial tuberosities. The anteroposterior diameter extends from the lower border of the symphysis pubis to the tip of the sacrum. The transverse diameter is the distance between the ischial tuberosities. This is also called the intertuberous or bi-ischial diameter. The posterior sagittal diameter extends from the tip of the sacrum to a right-angled intersection with a line between the ischial tuberosities.

Pelvic classification   The pelvis is classified into four basic shapes: gynecoid, anthropoid, platypelloid, and android. The classification is based on the configuration of the inlet and the corresponding changes in the midpelvis and lower pelvis. The pelvis inlet is divided into a posterior segment behind a line of the widest transverse diameter and an anterior segment in front of it. The length of the transverse diameter and the anteroposterior length of each segment are assessed to classify the inlet.

The sacrosciatic notch is visualized laterally. A narrow notch indicates a reduced anteroposterior diameter because the sacrum lies forward. A wide notch means that the sacrum is displaced posteriorly. Evaluation of the midpelvis and outlet includes measurement of the bispinous diameter and observation

of shape of the spinous processes and the length, width, and curve of the sacrum. The subpubic angle and contour of the arch are noted. The degree of divergence or convergence of the lateral walls is also noted when classifying pelvic shapes.

The four basic types of pelvis are evaluated to assess the adequacy of the pelvic structures for a vaginal delivery. It is uncommon for a pelvis to conform exactly in every dimension to any one type; most pelves are mixed types showing combinations of various characteristics. (Figure 10-8).

Gynecoid pelvis.   The gynecoid pelvis is characteristic of the female and is associated with the lowest incidence of fetopelvic disproportion. The inlet is nearly round. The sacrum is well curved and has average inclination. The sacrosciatic notch is of average size. The side walls are straight, and the ischial spines are not prominent. The subpubic arch is wide, and the transverse diameter is about 10 cm.

Android pelvis.   The android pelvis is characteristic of the male. The posterior segment is wide and flat, and the anterior segment is narrow. The sacrum is straight and inclined forward. The sacrosciatic notch is narrow, and the side walls convergent. The ischial spines are prominent, and the subpubic arch is narrow. This is a typical "funnel pelvis."

Anthropoid pelvis.   The anthropoid pelvis has a reduced transverse diameter as compared with the gynecoid pelvis, making it a long narrow oval with an elongated anterior-posterior segment and a slightly narrowed forepelvis. The sacrum is long and narrow with an average curvature posteriorly. The sacrosciatic notch is wide and shallow, and the side walls are straight. The ischial spines are prominent with a shortened bispinous diameter. The subpubic arch is narrowed.

Platypelloid pelvis.   The platypelloid pelvis is similar to the gynecoid pelvis except for narrowing of the anterior-posterior diameters at all levels. The inlet appears as a wide transverse oval. The sacrosciatic notch is wide, and

the side walls are straight. The ischial spines are prominent, and the subpubic arch is wide.

Pelvic Floor

A number of tissue layers form the pelvis floor (Figure 10-9). From the inside outward toward the skin they are the peritoneum, subperitoneal connective tissue, internal pelvis fascia,

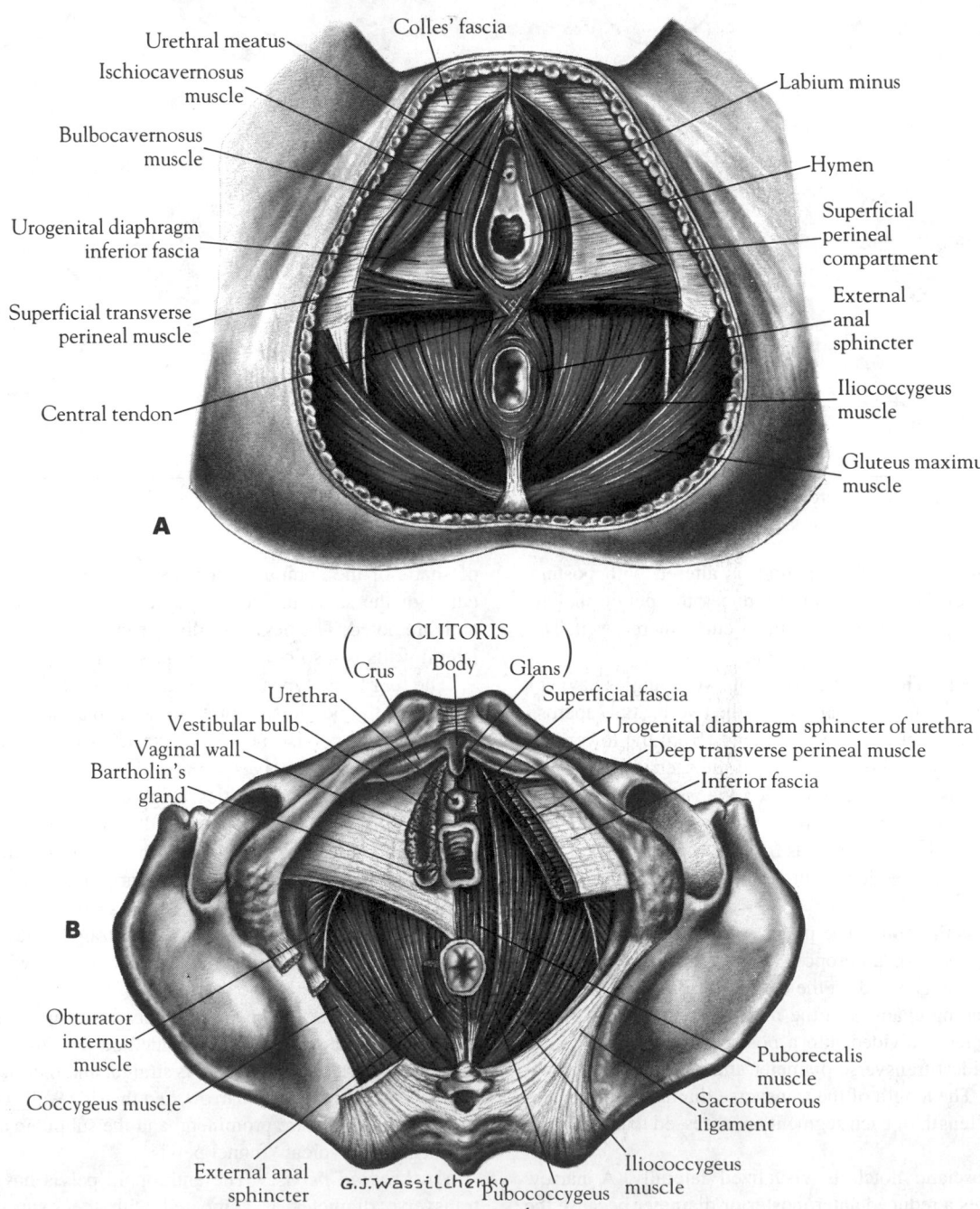

Figure 10-9 Perineum. **A,** Superficial components. **B,** Deep components.

levator ani and coccygeus muscles, external pelvic fascia, superficial muscles, subcutaneous tissue, and skin.

The levator ani and the fascia close the lower end of the pelvic cavity and diaphragm and present a concave upper surface. On both sides the levator ani consists of a pubic and iliac portion. The fibers pass backward to encircle the rectum, and a few fibers pass behind the vagina. The posterior and lateral portions of the pelvic floor not covered by the levator ani are covered by the piriformis and coccygeus muscles on either side.

Three layers of fascia fill out the triangular space between the pubic arch and a line joining the ischial tuberosities. This is called the urogenital diaphragm; it forms a compartment in which lie the superficial perineal muscles.

Breasts

The breasts, or mammary glands, are accessory organs of reproduction (Figure 10-10). They consist of a glandular epithelium and a duct system embedded in interstitial tissue and fat. They lie anterior to the pectoralis major muscle and are separated from it by a layer of fat that is continuous with the fatty stroma of the gland itself. They extend from the anterior border of the axilla to the lateral edge of the sternum. Each gland consists of a comma-shaped mass of fat and collagenous tissue. The tail of Spence extends toward the axilla. The position of the

breasts is maintained by suspensory (Cooper's) ligaments, which are condensations of connective tissue. They are easily stretched, especially if the breasts are large. Lymph drainage is mainly toward the axillary lymph nodes, with some drainage directed toward the substernal, diaphragmatic, and subclavicular nodes. Some women (as well as some men) have supernumerary nipples or breast tissue that develops along the longitudinal ridges extending from the axilla to the groin, which existed during early embryonic development. (Figure 10-11).

The center of the fully developed breast in an adult woman is the nipple, which is elevated anterior to the breast. Bundles of smooth muscle fibers in the nipple have erectile properties. The areola that surrounds the nipple has a diameter of 1.5 to 2.5 cm. Small sebaceous glands located under the areola give it a rough appearance. Arranged radially under the areola are 15 to 20 lactiferous ducts. In a lactating woman these ducts drain milk from the lobes of glandular tissue embedded in the adipose tissue of the breast. The ducts enlarge slightly before reaching the nipple to form the short lactiferous sinuses in which the milk may be stored. From the sinuses the ducts extend toward the chest wall, uniting various lobules or acinar structures of the breast. Each lobule contains 10 to 100 alveoli or acini, and 20 to 40 lobules compose each of the 15 to 20 lobes that are distributed in each breast. The alveolus is lined

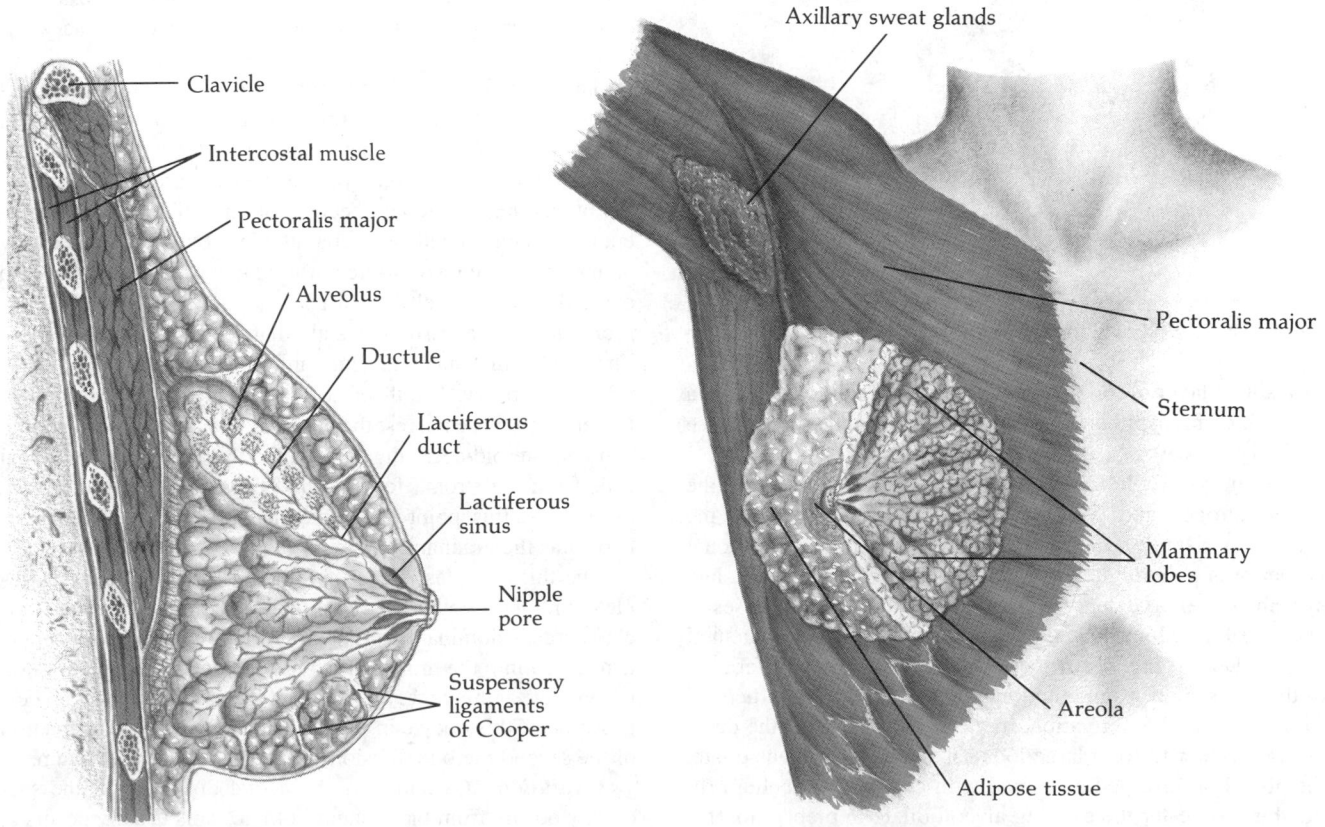

Figure 10-10 Anatomy of breast.

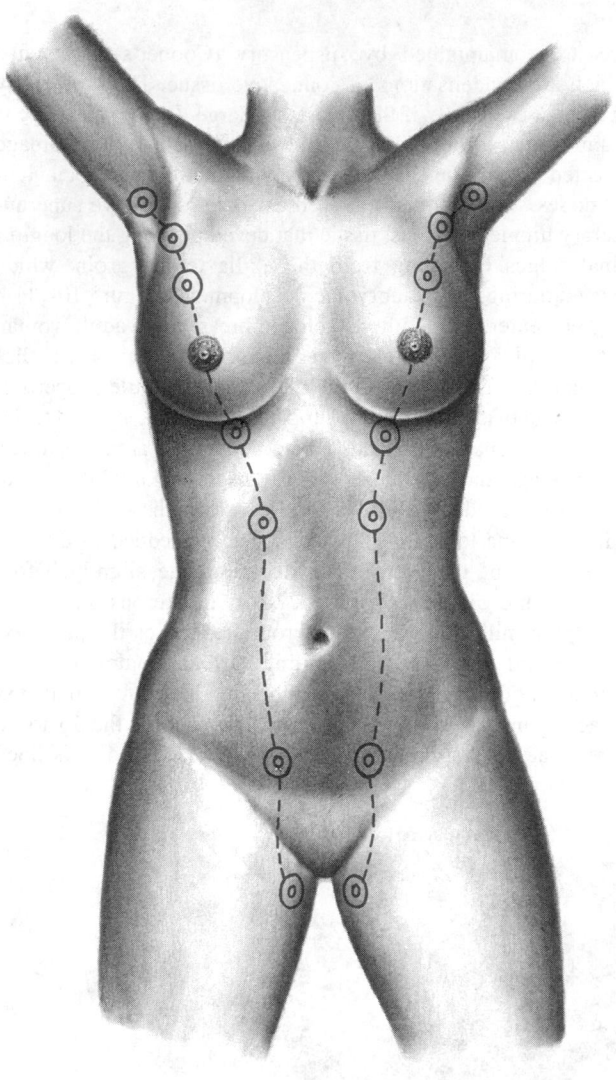

Figure 10-11 Supernumerary nipples.

by a single layer of milk-secreting epithelial cells, encased in a network of myoepithelial strands; it is surrounded by a dense capillary network.

Secretory alveoli develop in pregnancy as a response to the rising estrogen and progesterone levels. Before puberty the breasts consist mostly of lactiferous ducts. Under the hormonal influence of puberty there are branching and growth of the duct system, as well as extensive distribution of fat. Small masses of cells are formed at the ends of the ducts that are the potential alveoli. During the first trimester of pregnancy a proliferation of the ducts creates a maximum number of epithelial structures for future alveolus formation. In the second trimester the ducts group together to form large lobules, and as the lumens dilate, the alveoli are formed and lined with cuboidal epithelium. In the third trimester the existing alveoli dilate in preparation for lactation. As glandular and duct tissue proliferates during pregnancy, the adipose tissue appears to diminish.

Toward the end of pregnancy and until lactation begins 1 to 3 days after childbirth, the mammary glands form colostrum. It is produced at a much lower rate than milk and contains protein and lactose in amounts similar to milk but almost no fat.

Initiation and maintenance of lactation are achieved through a complex neuroendocrine process involving sensory nerves in the nipple and breast tissue, the spinal cord and hypothalamus, and the pituitary gland.

Ovarian Cycle and Hormones

The purpose of the ovarian cycle is to provide an ovum for fertilization, whereas the purpose of the endometrial cycle is to furnish a suitable site for the fertilized ovum to implant and develop.

Follicle development   Female primordial germa cells are derived from the germinal epithelium in the embryo. By mitotic division these form primitive ova, or oogonia, until the fifth or sixth month of gestation. Between the second month of gestation and the sixth month of life some oogonia become primary oocytes through the prophase of meiosis. At birth some 2 million oocytes are in the ovary, decreasing through attrition to about 300,000 by the onset of puberty.

The first stage of follicle development occurs slowly during the childbearing years. The cells of the follicle divide, creating several layers of granulosa cells around the oocyte. Mucopolysaccharides secreted from the granulosa cells form a protective halo or zona pellucida around the oocyte (Figure 10-12). The primary oocyte, the surrounding layers of granulosa cells, and the outer basal lamina membrane make up the primary follicle.

The second stage of development occurs more rapidly, requiring 2 to 4 weeks for completion. During an ovarian cycle, approximately 6 to 12 primary follicles undergo growth and development but usually only one reaches maturity and ovulates. All others degenerate and become atretic follicles. The proliferating granulosa cells are separated into two parts. The cavity or antrum is filled with follicular fluid that presses the oocyte to one side. Several cells known as the cumulus oophorus surround the oocyte, forming a stalk that projects into the antrum. The follicle distends with fluid and moves outward to the surface of the ovary. The theca cells surrounding the antrum proliferate, and those nearest the basal lamina are transformed into cuboidal steroid-secreting cells called the theca interna. Spinal cells from the stroma form around this, comprising the theca externa. At this point in development the entire complex is known as the graafian follicle.

The third and last stage of follicular development is complete within 48 hours. Before ovulation a single graafian follicle becomes dominant, and as the follicle ruptures, the oocyte is released into the fimbria. Because the initial meiotic division is complete at this time, this is called the secondary oocyte. Fertilization of this oocyte in the fallopian tube causes completion of the second meiotic division, resulting in a haploid ovum.

Ovulation   Ovulation is the actual discharge of the secondary oocyte from the graafian follicle. This usually occurs at the midpoint of both the ovarian and the menstrual cycle. The time from the first day of the menstrual period to ovulation is the follicular phase or preovulatory period. The postovulatory period is the luteal phase.

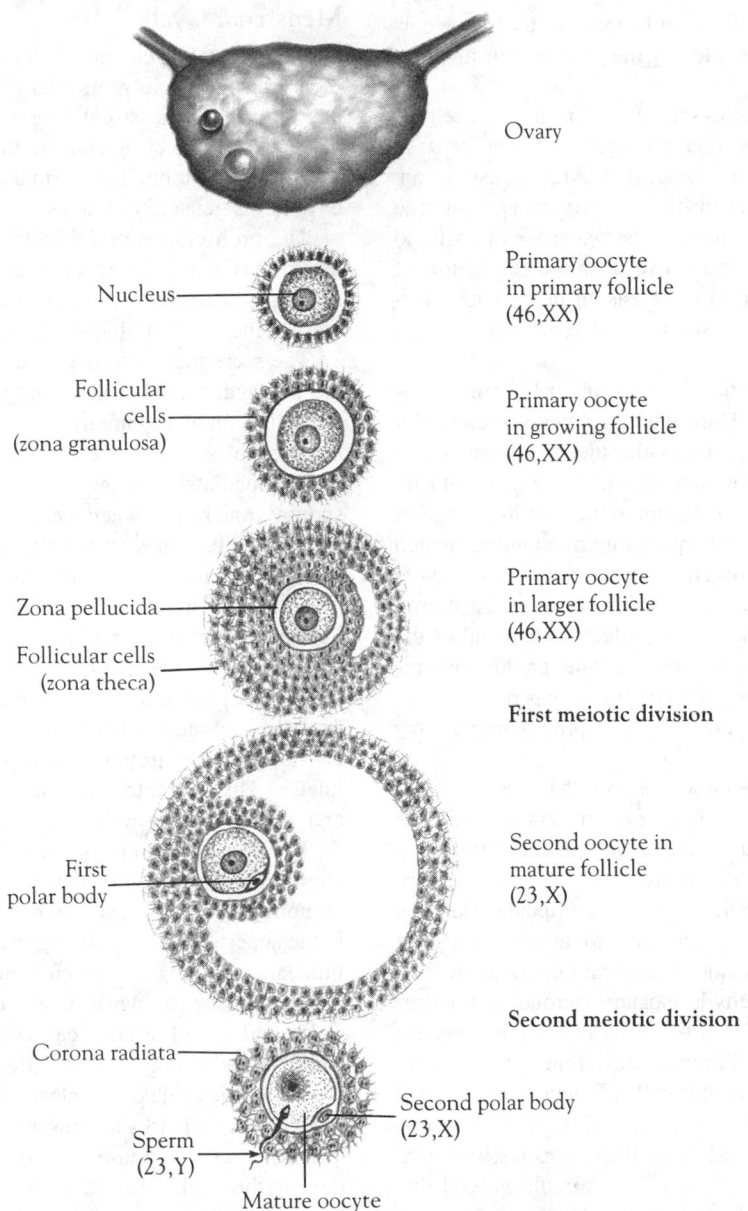

Ovary

Nucleus

Primary oocyte
in primary follicle
(46,XX)

Follicular
cells
(zona granulosa)

Primary oocyte
in growing follicle
(46,XX)

Zona pellucida

Follicular cells
(zona theca)

Primary oocyte
in larger follicle
(46,XX)

First meiotic division

First
polar body

Second oocyte in
mature follicle
(23,X)

Second meiotic division

Corona radiata

Second polar body
(23,X)

Sperm
(23,Y)

Mature oocyte

Figure 10-12 Oogenesis. Chromosome content of germ cell shown at each stage, including sex chromosome shown after comma.

Some women experience mittelschmerz, a lower abdominal discomfort at the time of ovulation. This is believed to be caused by peritoneal irritation from blood or follicular fluid that has escaped from the ruptured follicle. Another response to ovulation is an increase in basal body temperature caused by the thermogenic action of progesterone. Changes in the cervical mucus near the time of ovulation include decreases in viscosity and opacity, an increase in clarity, and an increase in sodium chloride content, which is demonstrated by arborization or ferning when mucus is allowed to dry on a glass slide. The signs and symptoms of ovulation are important both for women who wish to conceive during a particular cycle and for those who desire to avoid conception.

Corpus luteum　A yellow glandular mass formed at the site of the ruptured follicle is called the corpus luteum. It secretes large amounts of progesterone and lesser amounts of estrogen. If fertilization occurs, the corpus luteum increases in size, remains enlarged for about 3 months until the placenta takes over secreting functions, and then degenerates. If fertilization does not occur, the corpus luteum degenerates and shrinks. The yellow or "luteal" tissue then changes to a white fibrous tissue known as the corpus albicans.

Estrogens　Estrogen is a generic term for substances capable of producing the typical changes of estrus. The common estrogens are estradiol, estrone, and estriol. They are secreted by the developing ovarian follicle and subsequently by the corpus luteum. Estrogens are secreted by the placenta during pregnancy.

Estrogens are responsible for the development of the female secondary sex characteristics, increased growth of the uterus at puberty, and repair of the endometrium after menstruation. They tend to increase uterine sensitivity to oxytocin and uterine motility. In this respect the actions of estrogens are opposite to those of progesterone. Estrogens also decrease resorption of calcium from bones, secondarily increasing bone matrix formation and slightly increasing sodium and water reabsorption by the renal tubules.

Progesterone   Progesterone is the principal hormone secreted by the corpus luteum. During pregnancy it is secreted by the placenta. Progesterone prepares the uterine endometrium for the reception and development of the fertilized ovum by converting a proliferative endometrium to the secretory stage. It also inhibits the contractility of smooth uterine muscle, which is the opposite action of estrogen. Progesterone is responsible for the development of acini and lobules in the breast during pregnancy and inhibits the action of prolactin. Removal of the placenta, a source of massive progesterone production, removes the inhibitory effect on prolactin, thereby permitting lactation. Progesterone is also called luteo or progestational hormone.

Androgens   Androgens are substances that produce masculine characteristics such as hair growth, lowering of the voice, muscularity, and, in the male, development of the genital system. The major androgen secreted by the female ovary is androstenedione, a biologically weak compound but one that can undergo peripheral conversion to testosterone. The adrenal gland also secretes androgens, androstenedione and dehydroepiandrosterone (dehydroisoandrosterone). Dihydrotestosterone is formed in peripheral tissue by the action of an enzyme on testosterone. In addition, testosterone, which is secreted by the embryonic testicular cells of Leydig, is required in the male fetus for the differentiation of the genital tubercle, swellings, folds, and urogenital sinus into the penis, scrotum, penile urethra, and prostate. Testosterone stimulates fetal differentiation of the wolffian ducts into the epididymis, vas deferens, and seminal vesicles.

Pituitary gonadotropic hormones   The basophils of the anterior pituitary gland secrete follicle-stimulating hormone (FSH) and luteinizing hormone (LH). The acidophils secrete prolactin, which is also called lactogenic or luteotropic hormone (LTH).

Follicle-stimulating hormone stimulates ovarian follicle growth and maturation. The FSH level rises slightly before both ovulation and menstruation. This hormone is essential to the production of estrogen by the ovary. After menopause the level of FSH in the plasma and the amount excreted in the urine are increased.

Luteinizing hormone induces ovulation and stimulates formation of the corpus luteum and progesterone secretion.

Prolactin serves as a luteotropic hormone in helping to maintain the corpus luteum. This hormone stimulates the mammary glands to develop secretory alveoli and secrete milk.

Menstrual Cycle

The menstrual cycle begins at puberty and continues until menopause some 40 years later (Figure 10-13; Table 10-1). The day of onset of menstrual flow is considered to be the first day of the cycle. The cycle ends on the last day before the next onset of menstruation. The normal cycle can vary from 22 to 35 days but is generally 28 days.

The proliferative or follicular phase begins about the fifth day of the cycle and extends through ovulation. It is also known as the postmenstrual or estrogenic phase. During this phase the uterine endothelium thickens as estrogen secretion rises.

The secreting phase occurs after ovulation. It is also called the postovulatory, luteal, or progestational phase. During this phase the three endometrial zones become well defined. The basal zone is adjacent to the myometrium; the compact zone lies immediately below the endometrial surface; and the spongy zone lies between the compact and basal layers. The endometrium becomes extremely vascular and rich in glycogen, an ideal environment for implantation of the fertilized ovum. The uterine spiral arteries become more coiled, and tortuous during this period, growing almost to the surface of the endometrium. If implantation of a fertilized ovum does not occur, the corpus luteum loses functional activity and degenerates. If fertilization and implantation occur, the secretion of human chorionic gonadotropin by the placenta maintains the corpus luteum. This promotes the continued secretion of progesterone and estrogen and prevents menstruation.

The premenstrual phase occurs 2 to 3 days before menstruation with infiltration of the stroma by polymorphonuclear or mononuclear leukocytes. The reticular framework of the stroma in the superficial zone disintegrates, resulting in a loss of tissue fluid and thinning of the endometrium. Some 4 to 24 hours before the onset of menstruation, a vasoconstriction in the arterioles and coiled arteries causes anoxia and shriveling of the compact and spongy zones. After a period of constriction the coiled arteries relax and bleeding occurs from them or their branches. This marks the onset of menstruation.

The menstrual phase lasts from the first to about the fifth day of the cycle. As the coiled arteries rupture, hematomas form that distend and eventually rupture the superficial endometrium. Fissures develop in adjacent layers and tissues, become fragmented, and detach. The entire functional layer of the endometrium is eventually sloughed, leaving only the deep basal layer intact. Bleeding stops when the coiled arteries return to a state of construction.

Physiologic Female Sexual Response

Vasocongestion and myotonia are responsible for the phenomena observed during the cycle of sexual response. Vasocongestion is a congestion primarily of venous blood vessels and is the major response to sexual stimulation. Myotonia is a secondary response to stimulation characterized by an increase in muscular tension.

In their class work published in 1966 Masters and Johnson[29] describe the female sexual response cycle as divided into four physiologic phases: excitement, plateau, orgasm, and resolution.

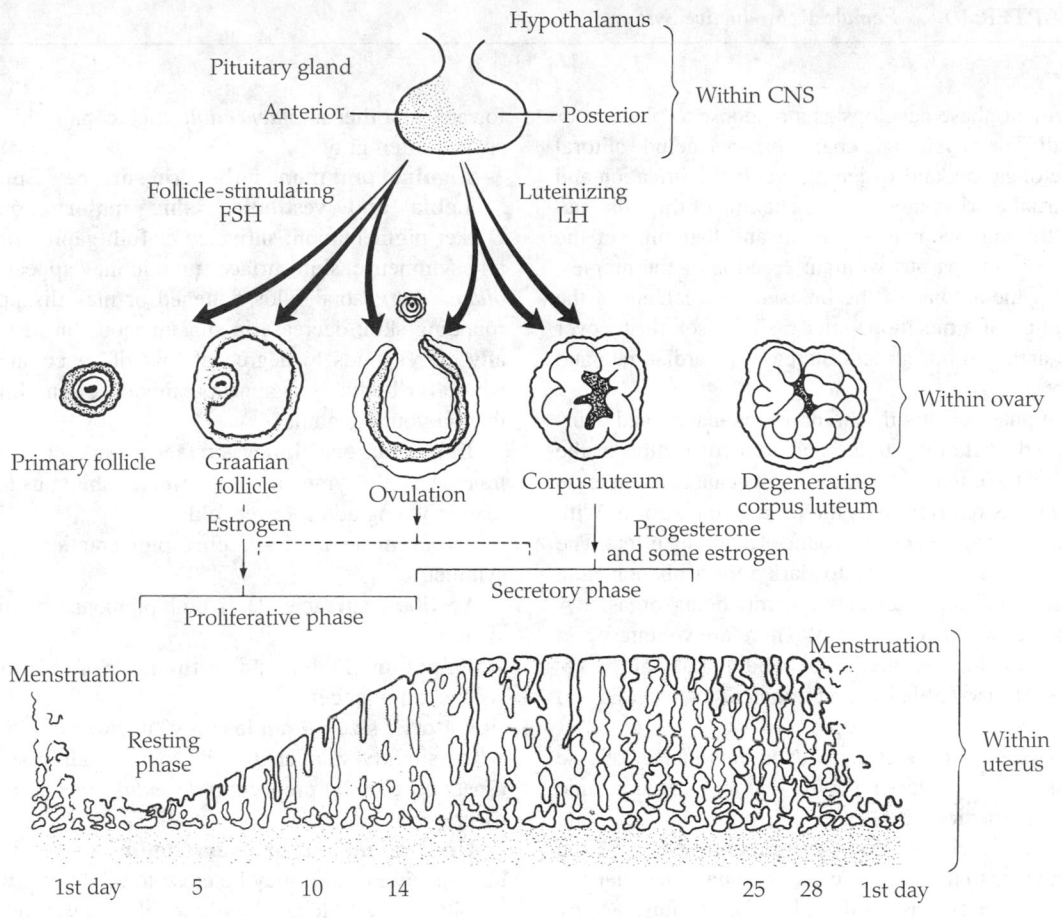

Figure 10-13 Interrelationships among cerebral hypothalamic, pituitary, ovarian, and uterine functions throughout menstrual cycle. (From Bobak.[9])

TABLE 10-1 Correlation of Ovarian and Endometrial Cycles (Ideal 28-Day Cycle)

	Menstrual (1-3 to 5 days)	Early Follicular (4 to 6-8 days)	Advanced Follicular (9 to 12-16 days)	Ovulation (12-16 days)	Early Luteal (15-19 days)	Advanced Luteal (20-25 days)	Premenstrual (26-32 days)
Ovary	Involution of corpus luteum	Growth and maturation of graafian follicle		Ovulation	Active corpus luteum		Involution of corpus luteum
Estrogen	Diminution	Progressive increase		High concentration	Secondary rise		Decreasing
Progesterone	Absent			Appearing	Rising		Decreasing
Endometrium	Menstrual desquamation and involution	Reorganization and proliferation	Further growth and watery secretion		Active secretion and glandular dilation	Accumulation of secretion and edema	Regressive
Pituitary secretion							
Follicle-stimulating hormone (FSH)	Fairly constant until just before ovulation			Moderate increase just before	Rapid decrease in previous levels		
Luteinizing hormone (LH)	Same as above			Marked increase just before	Same as above		

The excitement phase develops as a response to physical or psychic stimuli. The physiologic characteristics include clitoral tumescence, elongation, and widening; vaginal lubrication and expansion; partial uterine elevation; thickening of the labia majora in a multiparous woman; elevation and flattening of the labia majora in a nulliparous woman; erection of the nipples; engorgement of the areolae of the breasts; enlargement of the breasts; spreading of a maculopapular rash or "sex flush" over the epigastric area and breast; and increase in cardiac rate and blood pressure.

The plateau phase occurs if stimulation is maintained. During this period the clitoris retreats and vasocongestion in the labia majora and the outer third of the vagina causes an increase in their size. This is referred to as the orgasmic platform. With elevation of the uterus, the cervix produces a tenting effect. The labia minora changes from pink to dark red, a phenomenon known as "sex skin" that indicates an impending orgasm. A "sex flush" may cover the entire body. There are voluntary and involuntary contractions of the facial, abdominal, and intercostal muscles. Hyperventilation and transient tachycardia and hypertension occur during this phase.

The orgasm phase is characterized by an involuntary release of sexual tension. The primary response occurs in the orgasmic platform with contraction of the perineal, pubococcygeal, and bulbospongiosus muscles. Uterine contractions begin at the fundus and progress to the lower uterine segment. The intensity of the orgasmic experience is paralleled by the sex flush and by excursions of the contracting uterus. Respiratory rate, pulse rate, and blood pressure increase during this phase.

The resolution phase generally parallels the excitement phase in length. The uterus descends, the clitoris descends, and the vagina, labia majora, and labia minora return to their normal sizes. Normal coloring returns to the vaginal wall and the labia minora. The cervical os remains open for 20 to 30 minutes after orgasm. The nipples lose their erection, breast size decreases, and the sex flush disappears. Respiratory and pulse rates and blood pressure return to normal levels. Pelvic vasocongestion and myotonia decrease and eventually disappear.

Parallels between sexual response, birth, and breast feeding were described by Niles Newton in 1973.[31] Labor has been compared with the excitement phase of sexual response and orgasm with birth. In addition, a close resemblance between the emotions experienced during breast feeding and sexual arousal has been described. Birth, breast feeding, and sexual response are all based on neurohormonal reflexes, are sensitive to environmental stimuli, and appear to elicit care-taking behaviors.

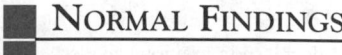

■ NORMAL FINDINGS

External Genitalia

Surface characteristic   Homogeneous

Hair distribution   Variable in adults; usually inverse triangle with base over pubis; some hair may extend up midline toward umbilicus; *older adult:* pubic hair thinned, perhaps sparse, often gray

Inguinal and mons pubis skin surface   Smooth; clear

Labia and vestibule; labia majora, outer surface   Darker pigmentation; shriveled or full; gaping or closed; usually symmetric; skin surface smooth; may appear dry or moist; *older adult:* labial folds flattened or may disappear into surrounding skin; decrease in subcutaneous fat in folds that usually corresponds to degree of loss of subcutaneous fat elsewhere on body; skin appears smooth, often shiny, and paler than in younger adult

Labia majora, inner surface   Dark pink pigmentation; moist; usually symmetric; *older adult:* shiny; usually dry; paler than in young adult; fewer folds

Labia minora   Dark pink pigmentation; moist, usually symmetric

Vestibule surface   Dark pink pigmentation; moist, usually symmetric

Palpation of labia and vestibule   Soft, homogeneous consistency; nontender

Clitoris; size   2 cm length visible; 0.5 cm diameter; *older adult:* slightly smaller than in younger adult; surface: medial aspect covered by prepuce; *older adult:* medial aspect covered by prepuce; pink

Urethral meatus and surrounding tissue surface   Irregular opening or slit; may be close to or slightly within vaginal introitus; usually located midline; *older adult:* relaxed perineal musculature may result in meatus being situated more posteriorly; very near or within vaginal introitus; milking of urethral duct: nontender; no discharge

Vaginal introitus and surrounding tissue   Surface: thin vertical slit or large orifice with irregular edges (hymenal caruncles); moist tissue; *older adult:* may be smaller than in younger adult; multiparous client may manifest gaping introitus with vaginal walls rolling toward opening

Palpation of lateral and posterior introitus   Nontender; no discharge; *older adult:* opening may be very narrow and admit only one finger

Vaginal tone   Nullipara: squeezes tightly around examiner's index and middle fingers; unipara or multipara: squeezes firmly but with less tone than nullipara; no bulging or urinary incontinence when bearing down or pushing; *older adult:* may be relaxed; client has difficulty squeezing examiner's finger with voluntary vaginal constriction; vaginal wall may roll slightly outward; no incontinence

Perineum   Surface: smooth; midline or mediolateral episiotomy scar may be visible; *older adult:* smooth; midline or mediolateral episiotomy scar may be visible; palpation between index finger and thumb; nontender; nullipara: thick, smooth; unipara or multipara: thin, rigid, scarring; *older adult:* thin; rigid

Anal surface   Increased pigmentation and coarse skin

Internal Genitalia

Cervix

Color   Pink color evenly distributed; bluish in pregnancy; symmetric, circumscribed erythema surrounding os may indicate normal condition of exposed columnar epithelium, but inexperienced examiners should consider any reddened appearance a problem for consultation; *older adult:* paler than in younger woman; color evenly distributed

Position Midline; cervix and os may be pointed in anterior or posterior direction; may project into vaginal tube 1 to 3 cm (resulting in 1 to 3 cm fornices surrounding cervix); *older adult:* cervix protrudes less into vaginal tube; may be flush against back of vaginal wall; surrounding fornices diminish or may disappear

Size Usually 2.5 cm diameter; *older adult:* cervix decreases in size with age

Surface Smooth; firm; occasional visible squamocolumnar junction (symmetric reddened circle around os); nabothian cysts (smooth, round, small, yellowish raised areas); *older*

adult: smooth; may appear paler than in younger woman; occasional visible squamocolumnar junction (symmetric reddened circle around os)

Contour Evenly rounded or slightly ovoid; *older adult:* Nabothian cysts (smooth, round, yellowish, raised areas) common

Os Nullipara: small, evenly round; unipara or multipara: slitlike, may be star shaped or irregular; *older adult;* often very narrow or stenosed; may be obliterated

Cervical discharge Mucus plug may be present at os; odorless; creamy or clear; thin, thick, or stringy; discharge often heavier at midcycle or immediately before menstruation; *older adult:* Often scanty; if present, should be clear or slightly opaque and odorless

Vagina

Length 10 to 15 cm

◼ PERTINENT BACKGROUND INFORMATION

An additional consideration in assessment of the female organ system is a review of pertinent background information, including the following:

Concurrent diseases or conditions
  Menstruation
    Age at onset
    Length of cycles (duration)
    Interval between cycles
    Regularity of cycles
    Amount and type of flow
      Number of tampons or napkins used
      Date of most recent douching
      Type of contraceptive used
    Date of last menstrual period (LMP)
    Associated symptoms (such as dysmenorrhea, menorrhagia, metrorrhagia, abnormal pelvic or abdominal pain)
    Premenstrual syndrome (PMS)
  Obstetric history
    Gravity, parity, abortions, number of living children
    Complications of pregnancy and delivery or abortion
  Infertility
    Length of time attempting pregnancy
    Knowledge of fertile period during menstrual cycle
    Partner factors
    Diagnostic evaluation studies to date
  Menopause
    When occurred
    Related symptoms
      Hot flushes
      Dry vaginal mucosa
  Gastrointestinal (GI) system
    Constipation
    Hemorrhoids
    Vaginal protrusion on straining
  Endocrine system
    Hypothyroidism
    Hyperthyroidism
    Stein-Leventhal syndrome

  Blood dyscrasias
  Hypertension
  Urinary system
    Frequency
    Nocturia
    Urgency
    Dysuria
    Incontinence (stress, urgency)
  Previous surgery or illness
    Gynecologic surgery
    Other major surgery or illness (e.g., of abdomen or endocrine system)
    Sexually transmitted diseases
    Pelvic inflammatory disease
  Family history
    Cancer
    Sickle cell disease
    Thyroid disorder
    Diabetes
    Other diseases
    Death from gynecologic-related condition
    Maternal diethylstilbestrol (DES) usage
  Social history
    Smoking, tobacco use, alcohol use
    Illegal drug abuse or prescription drug abuse
  Sexual history
    Age at first coitus
    Frequency of coitus
    Abnormal lesions or discharge in sex partner
    Satisfaction and orgasmic response
    Dyspareunia
    Use of contraceptives: type and duration
  Medication history
    Oral contraceptives
    Estrogen therapy
    Intrauterine contraceptive device (IUD)
    Phenothiazines
    Digitalis
    Diuretics

From Tucker[48] and Edge.[15]

Color Pink; *older adult:* shortens with aging: paler than in younger women

Surface Transverse rugae (diminish after vaginal deliveries); moist; smooth; *older adult:* less moisture; smooth (rugae diminish with aging); shiny

Consistency Smooth; homogeneous

Secretions Minimum to moderate amount; thin; clear or cloudy; odorless; *older adult:* May be absent or sparse; if present, should be clear or slightly opaque

Fornices Pliable; smooth; *older adult:* diminish and may disappear with aging; if palpable, should be pliable, smooth, and nontender

Uterus Mobile; nontender; *older adult:* diminishes greatly; often not palpable

Position Fundus anteverted; palpable at level of pubis; *older adult:* if palpated with internal hand, body of uterus should be smooth, firm, freely movable, and nontender

Contour of fundus Rounded

Uterine wall Firm consistency; smooth surface; pear shaped; 5.5 to 8 cm long

Ovaries May not be palpable; slightly tender on palpation; firm; smooth; ovoid; mobile; diameter about 4 cm (size of walnut); *older adult:* atrophy with age and rarely palpable in aged women; fallopian tube palpable

Breasts

Size Varies: *older adult:* increase in adipose tissue

Symmetry Bilaterally equal; slight asymmetry; breasts hang equally when woman is seated and leaning forward; breasts appear symmetric when woman is seated and pushing hands into hips or pushing palms together

Contour Smooth; convex; even

Skin color Even throughout

Skin texture Smooth; elastic; movable; striae

Venous patterns Bilaterally similar

Moles, nevi Long history of presence; nonchanging; nontender

Areolae

Size Bilaterally equal

Shape Round or oval

Surface characteristics Smooth; bilaterally similar; Montgomery tubules

Nipples

Direction Bilaterally equal in pointing direction

Size and shape Bilaterally equal; long-standing inversion (unilateral or bilateral)

Color Homogeneous

Surface characteristics Smooth or may be slightly wrinkled; skin intact

Discharge Absent

Suspensory ligaments Equal bilateral pull when woman is seated with arms abducted over head; *older adult:* relaxed; breasts may appear elongated or pendulous

Palpation of breasts

Tone Bilaterally firm and equal; sagging of breast tissue may occur with aging or poor bra support

Tissue qualities Smooth diffuse tissue bilaterally; nodular, bilateral granular consistency; premenstrual engorgement; elastic; nontender, firm mammary ridge along each breast at approximately 4 to 8 o'clock position; *older adult:* decrease in grandular tissue

Lymph nodes (including supraclavicular, infraclavicular, central and lateral axillary, pectoral, subscapular, scapular, brachial, intermediate, and internal mammary chains) Nonpalpable

CONDITIONS, DISEASES, AND DISORDERS

UTERINE AND OVARIAN DISORDERS

■ PELVIC INFLAMMATORY DISEASE

Pelvic inflammatory disease is an infectious process that may involve the fallopian tubes, ovaries, pelvic peritoneum, veins, or uterine connective tissue.

The incidence of PID is difficult to estimate because it is not a reportable disease and is not identified in a consistent manner; however, it is estimated that 1 million women are affected annually with one third of them less than 19 years of age.[24] It is not always treated, especially when symptoms are mild. It often occurs in sexually active women as the result of infection transmitted through sexual intercourse. It can also be associated with immunologic or renal disorders or through childbirth or abortion. In addition, frequent vaginal douching has been identified as a risk factor in predisposing women to PID.[40] It has been directly or indirectly linked to approximately one fifth of all gynecologic problems. Specific risk factors include teenager (10 to 19), multiple sex partners, single status, previous diagnosis of PID, and sexual contact with urethritis or gonorrhea.

Pelvic inflammatory disease may be confined to one structure or involve the entire pelvis. Infections may be acute, subacute, recurrent, or chronic. Pelvic inflammatory disease in the fallopian tubes (the most common site) is referred to as salpingitis. Sequelae of PID include ectopic pregnancy, infertility, chronic pelvic pain, salpingitis, hydrosalpinx, and tubo-ovarian abscess.[4]

•••••• Pathophysiology

Pelvic inflammatory disease begins in the vulva or accessory glands and spreads upward through the entire genital tract. One of the principal pathogens is *Chlamydia trachomatis,* but aerobic and anaerobic gram-negative bacilli and gram-positive cocci are also implicated as causative agents.[46] Salpingitis resulting from tuberculosis has become rare. If PID follows childbirth or an abortion, anaerobic streptococci, staphylococci, coliform bacteria, or *Clostridium perfringens* are usually involved. Infections can also be caused by actinomycosis, schistosomiasis, leprosy, and oxyurias. Sarcoidosis and foreign bodies (such as radiographic contrast media) can cause inflammation.

The second principal pathogen is *Neisseria gonorrhoeae.* Gonococcal disease is characterized by an acute suppurative reaction with subsequent copious discharge of yellow pus. Hyperemia, edema, and tenseness occur in the involved structures, which are often bilaterally involved. The organisms spread over the mucosal surfaces, eventually involving the tubes and tubo-ovarian region. In an adult the vagina is resistant to the inflammation, but vulvovaginitis may develop in a child because of the more delicate mucosa. As the lumen of the fallopian tube fills with purulent exudate, some leaks out of the fimbriae. Over the course of days or weeks the fimbriae may seal or become adherent to the ovary, causing salpingo-oophoritis. The collection of pus in the sealed tube causes distention of the tube and is referred to as pyosalpinx. In this form the infection may persist for months. The demise of the organisms and sterilization of the infection occur eventually owing to progressive anaerobiasis and increasing acidity. The pus then undergoes a slow proteolysis, and the exudate is transformed to a thin serous fluid in a condition known as hydrosalpinx.

Tubo-ovarian abscesses can occur when exudate collects where the tube is sealed against the ovary. This inflammatory process affects the most superficial layers of the ovary but spares the underlying ovarian tissue. Peritonitis resulting from spread of the exudate to the pelvic peritoneum is common. Infertility caused by mucosal destruction and tubal occlusion is a common sequel of salpingitis. Rupture of tubo-ovarian abscess and peritonitis can be life threatening.

•••••• Diagnostic Studies and Findings

Culture of purulent secretions From cervix or posterior cul de sac during surgery; identification of organism and sensitivity to antibiotics

White blood cell count Elevated, with increased differential

Erythrocyte sedimentation rate Elevated

Laparoscopic examination Visualization of pelvic inflammation; mild: erythema, edema, no obvious purulent exudate, tubes freely movable; moderate: gross, purulent material evident; marked erythema and edema; tubes not always freely movable; severe: pyosalpinx, severe inflammation, abscess

Gram stain of secretions Identification of gram-positive or gram-negative organisms

Ultrasonography Visualization of mass consistent with abscess or inflammation

Culdocentesis White blood cells or nonclotting blood; purulent material

•••••• Multidisciplinary Plan

Surgery

Hysterectomy with bilateral salpingo-oophorectomy—may be required for patients with abscesses, hydrosalpinx, and tubal obstruction if antibiotic therapy is unsuccessful

Laparotomy with incision and drainage of abscesses and lysis of adhesions

Colpotomy

Medications

Inpatient Treatment

Cefoxitin, 2 g IV every 6 hours, *or*

Cefotetan, 2 g IV every 12 hours, *plus*

Doxycycline, 100 mg every 12 hours orally or IV

This regimen is given for at least 48 hours after the patient clinically improves. Doxycycline, 100 mg orally two times a day, is taken after the patient is discharged from the hospital, to complete a total of 10-14 days of therapy.

Alternative regimen

Clindamycin, 900 mg IV every 8 hours, *plus*

Loading dose of gentamicin, 2.0 mg/kg IV, followed by a maintenance dose of 1.5 mg/kg IV every 8 hours

This regimen is given for at least 48 hours after the patient improves, following which the patient is discharged on doxycycline, 100 mg orally twice daily, to complete a total of 10-14 days of therapy.

Outpatient Treatment

Cefoxitin, 2 g intramuscularly (IM), with probenecid, 1 g orally, *or*

Ceftriaxone, 250 mg IM, *or*

Equivalent cephalosporin, *plus*

Doxycycline, 100 mg orally 2 times daily for 10-14 days

For patients unable to tolerate tetracyclines,[24] use

Ofloxacin 400 mg orally bid for 14 days, *plus*

Metronidazole 500 mg orally bid for 14 days, *or*

Clindamycin 450 mg four times daily for 14 days

General Management

Pain management

Bed rest in semi-Fowler's position

Parenteral fluids

Nasogastric suctioning if ileus is present

Removal of intrauterine device (IUD)

Social services support

Counseling and education (especially if sexually transmitted disease [STD] is precipitating factor)

NURSING CARE

Nursing Assessment

Subjective Data

Abdominal and pelvic pain (aching, burning, cramping and stabbing); low back pain; dyspareunia; menstrual irregularity; urinary discomfort (dysuria; frequency and urgency); constipation; malaise; nausea and vomiting; diarrhea; vaginal drainage (see Emergency Alert box on p. 890)

EMERGENCY ALERT

ABDOMINAL PAIN—FEMALE

Commonly, women seek treatment for lower abdominal and pelvic pain. Ovarian cysts and pelvic inflammatory disease (PID) are common causes of pelvic pain, although there are many others. Pelvic inflammatory disease is an infection that may involve the uterus, fallopian tubes, ovaries, and adjacent structures. It does not cause acute lower abdominal pain.

Assessment and Interventions

OVARIAN CYST

- Presentation is similar to ectopic, although pregnancy test is negative.
- Patient reports pain, often severe.
- Vaginal or intraperitoneal bleeding may be present, and surgical intervention may be indicated.
- Obtain IV access as indicated.
- Obtain order for laboratory tests.

PELVIC INFLAMMATORY DISEASE

- Assess for anorexia, fever, chills, nausea, and vomiting.
- Evaluate pain without pelvic examination with purulent vaginal discharge.
- Assess abdomen tenseness on palpation.
- In collaboration with physician's orders, obtain complete blood count (CBC), sedimentation rate, smears to rule out pregnancy, and urinalysis.
- Normal temperature, sedimentation rate, and white blood cell (WBC) count do not support PID as a diagnosis.
- Provide antibiotic therapy as ordered.
- Treat partner as indicated.
- Provide emotional support and education.

Abdomen

Rebound tenderness; normal bowel sounds progressing to ileus in untreated persons

Cervix

Pain with movement; copious purulent discharge

Vulva

Pruritus; maceration

Temperature

Elevated >100.4° (38° C)

Fluid balance

Nausea; vomiting; dry skin; poor skin turgor

Nursing Dx & Intervention

Pain related to inflammation

- Maintain complete bed rest; semi-Fowler's position may be most desirable *to prevent pus from pelvis moving to upper abdominal area.*
- Explain cause of pain *to allay any undue anxiety.*

- Instruct patient to request analgesic before pain becomes severe *to avoid inconsistent control of pain.*

Risk for impaired skin integrity related to drainage of purulent secretions on perineum

- Explain cause of vaginal discharge and pruritus if present.
- Assist and teach patient to perform perineal care every 3 to 4 hours or as needed *to maintain skin integrity.*
- Do not rub; blot skin dry *to prevent excoriation.*
- Prevent excessive warmth in room; lightweight covers over bed cradle may be indicated.

Risk for fluid volume deficit related to fever

- Explain need to increase fluid intake during infectious processes.
- Encourage fluid intake of 3000 ml daily unless contraindicated.
- Monitor intake and output as indicated.

Knowledge deficit related to lack of information about condition

- Explain importance of hand washing before and after contact with perineal area and of wiping from front to back after elimination *to prevent contamination of vaginal area with crosscontaminants from anal area.*
- Explain need to use perineal pads, which should be changed frequently according to amount of vaginal drainage. Instruct patient not to use tampons.
- Explain that a shower is preferable to a tub bath.
- Encourage patient to share concerns regarding sexual partner as probably source of infection *to promote health-seeking behaviors of partner.*
- Explain rationale for removal of IUD if this is ordered by physician.

Patient Education/Home Care Planning

1. Explain the need to avoid using tampons, having intercourse, or douching for at least 1 week after antibiotic therapy.
2. Explain methods to prevent venereal disease if the condition is caused by gonorrhea or *Chlamydia.*
3. Explain the importance of encouraging the patient's sex partner to be examined and treated.
4. Explain alternative methods of conception control if the condition is associated with an IUD.
5. Describe symptoms of recurrence that the patient should report to a physician.

Evaluation

Comfort is achieved; pain is controlled Patient reports that lower abdominal, low back, pelvic, or perineal pain is controlled.

Skin and mucous membrane color is good There is no vaginal drainage or pruritus, inflammation, or maceration of vulva. Patient is hydrated with balanced intake and output.

Hydration and body temperature are normal   There is no fever. Temperature is within normal limits. Intake and output are within normal limits.

Patient understands home care and follow-up instructions   Patient showers rather than taking tub baths. Patient verbalizes intent to prevent venereal disease if condition is caused by chlamydia or gonorrhea. Patient verbalizes intent to avoid douching, intercourse, or use of tampons for at least 1 week after completion of drug therapy. Patient wipes front to back after elimination. Patient verbalizes intent to have sex partner examined. Patient takes medications at time and dosage prescribed by physician. Patient describes symptoms of PID and expresses intent to notify health care provider in timely manner if they recur.

TOXIC SHOCK SYNDROME

Toxic shock syndrome (TSS) is an acute bacterial infection generally caused by a toxin from *Staphylococcus aureus* and most frequently associated with the use of tampons during menses.

National attention was not directed to TSS until the fall of 1980, when some 300 cases were reported to the Centers for Disease Control. Twenty-five deaths were reported in 285 women within a 9-month period. Toxic shock syndrome was most common in women who used high-absorbency tampons, but it has also occurred in newborns, children, and men. The incidence in women dropped precipitously in 1981 after widespread publicity and withdrawal of some ultra–high absorbency vaginal tampons from the market.[14]

Toxic shock syndrome continues to be associated with a variety of surgical situations unrelated to menses. It has been diagnosed in patients with surgical wounds, tubal ligation, hysterectomy, laparotomy, mastectomy, bladder suspension, orchidectomy, uterolithotomy, hip osteoplasty, and knee surgery. It has also been associated with septal reconstruction in which nasal packing was used. It apparently can occur in situations in which staphylococal infection can be harbored, including cellulitis, infected skin bites, burns, and hidradenitis.

•••••• Pathophysiology

Toxic shock syndrome initially causes a flulike illness with a high fever, vomiting, diarrhea, muscle weakness, and general malaise. Almost all cases of TSS have been caused by pyrogenic exotoxin-producing strains of phage group I *S. aureus.* The organism has been found in the nasopharynx, vagina, and trachea, as well as sequestered in empyema and abscess sites. It is thought that mechanical factors associated with use of high-absorbency tampons, including cotton and cotton/rayon tampons, by a woman with a preexisting *S. aureus* colonization of the vagina increases the risk.[39] As the outflow of menses is obstructed by the tampon, bacterial exotoxins are able to enter the bloodstream through a mucosal break. Adult respiratory distress syndrome (ARDS), which is manifested as pulmonary and

peripheral edema despite low central venous pressure, may be a cardiopulmonary complication of TSS.

In postsurgical cases, TSS symptoms appear within 48 hours. Exceptions occur when packing is used to control bleeding, such as in nasal surgeries, and with postpartum or dilation and curettage procedures. A common factor in all cases of TSS is a disruption of the normal skin or mucous membrane barrier, allowing a localized *S. aureus* infection to transmit toxins systemically.

Nursing and medical management focus on controlling or preventing potentially serious complications such as adult respiratory distress syndrome, renal failure, electrolyte imbalances, disseminated intravascular coagulation, encephalopathy, and cardiomyopathy.[14]

•••••• Diagnostic Studies and Findings

White blood cell count   Increased with shift to left; polys to bands

Blood urea nitrogen   Increased

Creatinine   Increased

Bilirubin   Increased

Aspartate aminotransferase (AST) [formerly SGOT]) Increased

Alanine aminotransferase (ALT) [formerly SGPT])   Increased

Creatinine phosphokinase (CPK)   Increased

Platelets   Decreased

Urine analysis with Gram stain

•••••• Multidisciplinary Plan

Medications

Antiinfective agents
  β-Lactamase resistant agents
    Nafcillin sodium (Nafcil, Unipen) 2-3 g IV or IM qd in divided doses
    Cefoxitin sodium (Mefoxin), 1-2 g IV or IM q6-8h
    Cefazolin sodium (Ancef), 250 mg to 1 g q6-8h IM or IV
    Cephalothin sodium (Keflin), 500 mg to 1 g q4-6h IV or deep IM
  Penicillinase-resistant agents
    Methicillin sodium (Staphcillin), 1-1.5 g IM q4-6h
    Oxacillin sodium (Bactocill), 500 mg q4-6h for at least 5 d
    Cloxacillin sodium (Cloxapen), 500-1000 mg q4-6h
  Antistaphylococcal agents
    Penicillin G (Bicillin), 600,000 U IM at various intervals
    Dicloxacillin sodium (Dycill, others), 125 mg po q6h
    Methicillin sodium (Staphcillin), 1-1.5 g IM q6h
  Corticosteroids
    Hydrocortisone sodium succinate (Solu-Cortef), 50-300 mg/d IV or IM

General Management

Cooling measures
Septic shock treatment if indicated
  Fluids and electrolytes
  Blood plasma expanders
  Packed RBCs and coagulation factors

CVP or PWP monitoring
Intake and output
Fluid intake of 3000 ml daily unless contraindicated
Respiratory support in presence of ARDS

NURSING CARE

Nursing Assessment

Subjective Data

Sudden onset of high fever (102° to 105° F [39° to 40.5° C]); myalgia; vomiting; profuse watery diarrhea; sore throat; headache; profound tiredness

Extremities

Edema; impaired perfusion

Palms and Soles

Erythematous rash (sunburnlike); desquamation and sloughing within 1 to 2 weeks

Level of Consciousness

Disorientation; intermittent confusion

Blood Pressure

Rapid hypotension (within 48 hours); orthostatic syncope

Renal System

Diminished urine output

Conjunctiva

Nonpurulent inflammation

Oropharynx

Hyperemia; edema

Vagina

Hyperemia
Fluid intake of 3000 ml daily unless contraindicated

Nursing Dx & Intervention

Altered tissue perfusion related to exchange problems associated with shock

- For complete list of nursing diagnoses and interventions, see care of patient in septic shock in Chapter 1 and adult respiratory distress syndrome in Chapter 2 if applicable.
- Instruct patient to use sanitary napkins rather than tampons during menses.

Patient Education/Home Care Planning

1. Explain to the patient the importance of the need to avoid using tampons until vaginal culture findings are negative

and clearance from a physician is obtained; to wash hands thoroughly before inserting a tampon; not to use high-absorbency, noncotton tampons; not to use tampons on light flow days *to avoid risk of abrasion* and not to use tampons overnight; to change tampons frequently during the day, to wear sanitary napkins at night, and to avoid prolonged use of a single tampon; not to use tampons if she has a concurrent skin infection *because there is a possibility of reinfection* with *S. aureus;* and to report signs of recurrence to a physician immediately.

Evaluation

Tissue perfusion is adequate   There are no symptoms of shock.

Absence of infection   Vaginal culture findings are negative for causative organism. Patient does not have fever; hyperemia of oropharynx, conjunctiva, or vagina; myalgia; vomiting; diarrhea; sore throat; headache; or malaise.

Patient education is effective   Patient demonstrates understanding of reasons for health education and expresses intent to maintain behaviors and health practices that will prevent reinfection.

 ## UTERINE BLEEDING

Dysfunctional Uterine Bleeding

Dysfunctional uterine bleeding (DUB) occurs during the reproductive years and is associated with neuroendocrine factors.

Abnormal Uterine Bleeding

Abnormal uterine bleeding can occur at any time and is associated with non-menstrual cycle factors, including tumors, inflammation, trauma, pregnancy, or exogenous hormone effects.

Abnormalities and variation in uterine bleeding are the most frequently encountered health care problems for women. Patients often think that abnormal uterine bleeding is life threatening or indicative of a major problem in reproductive or sexual functioning. Abnormal bleeding, varying from spotting to the passage of clots, may occur at any age and for a variety of reasons (see Emergency Alert box on p. 893).

Dysfunctional uterine bleeding (DUB), which is always anovulatory and usually painless (whereas dysmenorrhea is associated with ovulatory cycles), can occur at any age from puberty through menopause. It generally occurs at the extremes of menstrual life, when disturbances in ovarian function are common. About 50% of dysfunctional bleeding occurs in premenopausal women (age 40 to 50), about 20% during the adolescent years, and about 30% during the reproductive period.

! EMERGENCY ALERT

VAGINAL BLEEDING/HEMORRHAGE

Commonly, women seek treatment for vaginal bleeding, which can occur for a variety of reasons. It is essential to rule out life-threatening illness or injury, search for a cause, and rule out normal menstruation and pregnancy.

Assessment

- Obtain history.
- Monitor vital signs. Determine the quantity and quality of vaginal bleeding and the duration and regularity.
- Determine pregnancy status.

Interventions

- Direct interventions at stabilizing condition and managing the cause.
- Maintain airway, breathing, and circulation; oxygenization; and IV access as indicated.
- Obtain order for laboratory studies as relevant.
- Provide reassurance and support to the patient.

! EMERGENCY ALERT

ABORTION

In women of childbearing age, abortion is the leading cause of vaginal bleeding. Abortion occurs when the pregnancy ends before fetal viability, usually at 24 weeks, has been achieved. Abortions are classified as threatened, inevitable, incomplete, messed, septic, habitual, and therapeutic.

Assessment

- Determine signs of significant vaginal blood loss, shock.
- Determine pregnancy status, rule out ectopic pregnancy.
- Assess pain and cramping.

Interventions

- Monitor vital signs closely.
- Obtain serum HCG to verify pregnancy, HCG status.
- Obtain IV access, as needed.
- Assist physician during pelvic examination.
- Anticipate suction curettage.
- Administer medications as appropriate.
- Observe client for at least 2 hours after procedure.

The following terms are often used to describe variations in uterine bleeding:

dysfunctional uterine bleeding (DUB) uterine bleeding during the reproductive period from neuroendocrinologic factors.

abnormal uterine bleeding can occur at any time during the life cycle and is generally associated with tumor, inflammation, pregnancy, trauma, or exogenous hormonal effects.

hypomenorrhea abnormal amount of menstrual flow.

menorrhagia (hypermenorrhea) increased amount (≥60 ml each period) or duration of menstrual bleeding.

metrorrhagia intermenstrual bleeding.

metrorrhea any pathologic uterine discharge.

oligomenorrhea infrequent menstruation.

polymenorrhea increased frequency of menstruation (not consistently associated with ovulation).

postmenopausal bleeding bleeding from the reproductive tract occurring 1 year or more after menopause.

spotting small amounts of bloody vaginal discharge ranging from pink to dark brown.

Medical therapy should be the first line of treatment for premenopausal women who are found to have no obvious cause for their abnormal uterine bleeding. For those who do not respond to treatment or who are unable to tolerate it, a conservative surgical solution is hysteroscopic resection of polyps or submucous fibroids. Hysteroscopic endometrial ablation may be used to treat women suffering from intractable menorrhagia. A hysterectomy is the final course of action if symptoms are not controlled or corrected.[11,22,51]

•••••• Pathophysiology

The preceding terms used to describe abnormal bleeding do not indicate the cause of the abnormality or reason for bleeding. The following are the most common types of bleeding and their causes:

Midcycle spotting–midcycle estradiol fluctuation associated with ovulation

Delayed menstruation with excessive bleeding–anovulation or threatened abortion

Frequent bleeding–chronic pelvic inflammatory disease, endometriosis, DUB, or anovulation

Profuse menstrual bleeding–endometrial polyps, adenomyosis, DUB, submucous leiomyomas, or presence of intrauterine contraceptive device

Intermenstrual or irregular bleeding–endometrial polyps, DUB, uterine, or cervical cancer, or oral contraceptive use

Postmenopausal bleeding–endometrial hyperplasia, estrogen therapy, or endometrial cancer

Other causes of bleeding include foreign bodies, lacerations, and systemic diseases such as leukemia, hypothyroidism, and blood dyscrasias. In addition, precocious puberty may warrant consideration as a cause, as may vaginal adenosis in young women with prenatal exposure to the synthetic estrogen diethylstibestrol (DES).

Dysfunctional uterine bleeding is most common during the reproductive years and occurs as painless, irregular, heavy bleeding (menometrorrhagia), midcycle spotting, oligomenorrhea, or periods of amenorrhea. In most cases the cause is anovulation, but bleeding may reflect defects in the follicular or luteal phase of the ovulatory cycle.

With anovulation, the persistent unopposed estrogen stimulation may be endogenous from an ovarian tumor such as a granulosa cell tumor, polycystic ovaries (Stein-Leventhal syndrome), or abnormal metabolism of estrogen as in liver disease. Unopposed estrogen stimulation may cause endometrial hyperplasia; when the estrogen can no longer maintain the endometrium, sloughing and vaginal bleeding occur.

Follicular phase defects result from premature maturation of the ovarian follicle owing to pituitary hyperstimulation. The cycle is less than 22 days. Increased levels of follicle-stimulating hormone (FSH) and slightly elevated estradiol levels result in a progressively shortened proliferative phase that can cause spotting in perimenopausal women. Oligomenorrhea most commonly occurs in young women and may result from a prolonged proliferative phase.

Luteal phase defects may result in profuse and prolonged bleeding caused by delayed involution of the corpus luteum. A corpus luteum cyst or persistent corpus luteum can cause a delay in menses, with premenstrual spotting.

The endometrium of women with menorrhagia has been found to have higher levels of prostaglandin E_2 and prostaglandin F_2 when compared with women with normal menses. Prostaglandin E_2 is associated with vasodilatory effects that contribute to bleeding.

•••••• Diagnostic Studies and Findings

Complete blood count   To determine the degree of anemia and to detect abnormal leukocyte production

Thyroid function tests   To assess thyroid function

Dilation and curettage with cervical or endometrial biopsy   To assess endometrium and identify carcinoma or polyps

Hysterography   To identify presence of endometrial polyps, submucous myomas, adenomyosis, endometrial carcinoma, and adnexal lesions

Hysteroscopy   To identify intrauterine abnormalities such as submucous myomas, endometrial polyps, and foreign bodies

Endovaginal ultrasonography   To differentiate endometrial polyps, hyperplasia, and carcinoma[21]

Endocrine profile   To assess functioning of the adrenal glands, ovaries, and pituitary glands

Tests confirming luteinization   Endometrial biopsy to demonstrate secretory or menstrual endometrium; basal body temperatures: biphasic pattern is indicative of ovulation; examination of cervical mucus to determine presence of ferning; serum or urine progesterone levels to assess progesterone metabolites consistent with progestational phase of menstrual cycle

Measurement of blood loss   Weigh pads and tampons

•••••• Multidisciplinary Plan

The plan of medical care selected is contingent on the cause of the bleeding.

Medications

Oral contraceptive therapy
Progesterone or progestogen
    Medroxyprogesterone (Provera, others), 2.5-10 mg/d po or 100-400 mg/d IM (may be given if patient is anovulatory and infertility is not a concern)
Estrogens
    Conjugated estrogens (Premarin), 0.625-3.75 mg/d followed by high doses of estrogen-progestin combinations (given for excessive anovulatory bleeding)

    Clomiphene citrate can be used when excessive bleeding is caused by inadequate luteal phase or to anovulation
Prostaglandin inhibitors
    Meclofenamate sodium 100 mg po tid
Antigonadotropin
    Danazol (Danocrine), 100-800 mg/d in divided doses
Gonadotropin-releasing hormone (GnRH) agonists
    Nafarelin acetate (Synerel), 2 mg/ml nasal spray, 1 spray in nostril bid
Leuprolide acetate (Lupron), 3.75-7.5 mg IM once per month
Analgesics as indicated

Surgery

Dilitation and curettage (see p. 918)
Hysteroscopic excision of polyps/myomas
Endometrial ablation
    Done with a hysteroscopic resectoscope by applying a cauterizing current to the endometrium in women who are not candidates for hysterectomy, such as those with major medical diseases, severe heart disease, bleeding diatheses, and major respiratory difficulty
Abdominal or vaginal hysterectomy with partial or complete bilateral salpingo-oophorectomy (TAH/BSO) (see p. 919)

Psychosocial services and counseling as indicated

NURSING CARE

Nursing Assessment

Variations depend on the cause of the bleeding.

Bleeding

Heavy menstrual flow; bleeding between periods; infrequent menstruation; increased frequency of menstruation; spotting

Pain

Menstrual cramps or pain with menses; low abdominal pain at midcycle*; uterine cramps at midcycle*

Vaginal Secretions

Wet mucoid vaginal secretion at midcycle*

Other Complications

Altered sexual function; psychosocial concerns; anemia

Nursing Dx & Intervention

Powerlessness related to illness-related regimen

- Assess meaning of dysfunction for patient to explore *self-concept issues related to control over own activities.*

---

*Signs and symptoms suggestive of ovulation.

- Encourage patient to express her feelings *to increase understanding of individual coping style.*
- Consider nursing interventions associated with loss and grief if results of diagnostic studies confirm anovulatory cycles and infertility.

Pain related to uterine cramps

- Assist in and teach patient pain-relieving techniques *to promote self-sufficiency in managing pain.*

Sexual dysfunction related to altered body function associated with uterine bleeding

- Explain importance of sharing concerns with sexual partner *to come to an understanding of preferences, concerns, and behavior related to uterine bleeding.*

Patient Education/Home Care Planning

1. Explain the importance of recording dates, type of flow, and number of pads or tampons used.
2. Explain the importance of ongoing care.

Evaluation

Patient demonstrates adaptive responses related to self-concept Patient asks appropriate questions. Patient keeps record of bleeding, including type and date. Patient shows signs of grief if she learns of undesired infertility.

Comfort is achieved; there is no pain Patient uses pain-relieving techniques or medication as ordered.

Sexual adjustment is made Patient indicates that she has discussed concerns with partner.

■ DYSMENORRHEA

Dysmenorrhea is menstruation that is painful enough to limit normal activity or cause a woman to seek medical treatment.

Dysmenorrhea is a common gynecologic complaint. It occurs in approximately 10% of high school–age girls, keeping them home from school for 1 or 2 days, and it also affects many college students and young women in the workforce. More than 50% of menstruating women have some degree of dysmenorrhea with 5% to 20% of women being incapacitated. Dysmenorrhea is classified as primary or secondary. Primary dysmenorrhea is pain associated with menstruation during ovulatory cycles in the absence of organic disease. Secondary dysmenorrhea is due to an organic disease such as PID or endometriosis.

•••••• Pathophysiology

Primary dysmenorrhea usually develops 1 or 2 years after menarche, when ovulatory cycles are established. Increased amounts of prostaglandin are released from the endometrium under the influence of progesterone in the luteal phase of the cycle. Very little prostaglandin is produced during anovulatory cycles, which are almost never painful. Increased sensitivity of the myometrium and endometrium to prostaglandin F_2 can produce uterine contractions and ischemia, causing the cramping pain of dysmenorrhea.

Secondary dysmenorrhea is associated with pelvic disorders such as endometriosis, adenomyosis, or chronic pelvic inflammatory disease. It may appear after years of normal menstruation, and it is characterized by cramping. Dysmenorrhea caused by endometriosis is related to the number of endometrial implants.[34]

•••••• Diagnostic Studies and Findings

Pelvic examination To rule out or confirm underlying disorders in secondary dysmenorrhea

Laparoscopy To rule out or confirm underlying disorders in secondary dysmenorrhea

Dilitation and curettage/hysteroscopy To rule out or confirm underlying disorders in secondary dysmenorrhea

Hysterosalpingography To rule out or confirm underlying disorders in secondary dysmenorrhea

•••••• Multidisciplinary Plan

Surgery

Laparoscopic CO_2 laser uterine nerve ablation (for treatment of drug-resistant primary dysmenorrhea)[17]

Laser ablation or fulguration of endometriosis

Abdominal or vaginal hysterectomy and bilateral salpingo-oophorectomy (TAH/BSO)—may be indicated for disorder associated with secondary dysmenorrhea

Presacral neurectomy (severance of nerve trunks in hypogastric plexus)—performed in *rare* cases when no underlying disorder can be found and there is no response to medications

Medications

Nonsteroidal antiinflammatory agents

Ibuprofen (Motrin), 400-600 mg po q4-6h as prostaglandin synthetase inhibitor

Naproxen sodium 550 mg, po, then 275 mg q4-8h

GnRH agonists may be considered by the physician

Analgesic/antipyretic agents

Aspirin, 650 mg po q3-5h beginning 1-2 d before menses to control mild discomfort

Oral contraceptives—may be ordered for hormonal effect to relieve pain by suppressing ovulation

General Management

Adequate exercise

Balanced diet with increased consumption of complex carbohydrates, fruits, and vegetables, as well as a decreased consumption of salt, alcohol, sugar, and caffeine

Adequate rest and sleep

Attention to personal hygiene

No tobacco

NURSING CARE

Nursing Assessment

Comfort

Colicky and cyclic pain, infrequently nagging and dull in low pelvis and often with radiation toward vulva, perineum, rectum, and down back of thighs; may be experienced 24 to 48 hours before menses or with start of menstruation; may be associated with symptoms of premenstrual tension, including nausea, vomiting, diarrhea, urinary frequency, chills, abdominal bloating, and breast tenderness

Psychoemotional status

Irritability, depression

Nursing Dx & Intervention

Pain related to uterine cramping

- Identify and help patient use pain-reduction methods, including relaxation techniques, heating pad, effleurage (abdominal massage), and orgasm (relieves cramps in some women).
- Evaluate patient's use of pain control techniques and encourage use of those that reduce her pain.

Body image disturbance related to negative feelings about menses

- Encourage patient to express feelings about any self-perceptions, as well as how she believes she is viewed by others.
- Explore patient's role and behaviors when dysmenorrhea is present *to identify effects on lifestyle.*
- Evaluate support system and coping strategies *to determine their effects on body image.*

Patient Education/Home Care Planning

1. Explain the prescribed dosage and frequency of doses of prostaglandin antagonists or other medications.
2. Provide pain management information, including use of antiinflammatory and analgesic agents that should be taken every 4 to 6 hours instead of waiting for pain to peak before taking the next dose of medication.

Evaluation

Comfort is achieved   Patient uses pain-relieving techniques as ordered.

Pain is gone   Patient initiates suggestions for coping with condition.

Body image is intact   Patient applies learned behaviors in dealing with stressful feelings. Patient verbalizes understanding of dysmenorrhea process and treatment.

ENDOMETRIOSIS

Endometriosis is an abnormal growth of endometrial tissue outside the uterine cavity.

Endometriosis is a benign disease, but it has certain characteristics of a malignancy, including the ability to grow, infiltrate, and spread. The ectopic tissue is responsive to hormonal variations of the menstrual cycle and is subject to menstrual-like bleeding.

Endometriosis is estimated to affect 1% to 5% of women of reproductive age. A familial incidence of endometriosis has been documented. A female patient who has an affected first-degree relative has an approximately tenfold increased risk for developing the disease. Cervical or vaginal atresia and mullerian fusion defects with obstructed outflow are commonly associated with pelvic endometriosis; this represents another genetic or at least congenital mechanism.[3] Characteristic lesions are found in at least 20% of patients undergoing gynecologic surgery. Endometriosis is a significant finding in only about one third of these patients. Symptoms severe enough to require treatment generally occur between the ages of 25 and 35 years. Endometriosis is rare in women over 50 years of age. The greatest incidence of the disease seems to be in women who tend to marry later and have fewer children. The fertility rate of patients with endometriosis is about 66%, compared with 88% for the general population. Endometriosis occurs in young women with congenital obstructions of the vagina or cervix that are associated with reflux menstruation.

Endometriosis is associated with infertility, pregnancy wastage, decreased fertilization, pain, and decreased pregnancy rates with in vitro fertilization. Recent studies suggest that endometriosis is associated with polyclonal B cell activation, which is a classic characteristic of autoimmune disease.

A rare but important complication of endometriosis that can mimic ovarian cancer is ascites. Most cases have been reported in nulliparous young black women who have massive ascites. It is important that this rare complication be considered in the presence of ascites with abdominal or pelvic masses and weight gain because this otherwise indicates the presence of malignant disease. Treatment is effected by ablation of ovarian function by surgery, radiotherapy, or suppression of endometriosis by endocrine therapy, which is the preferred treatment in very young women.[44]

•••••• Pathophysiology

Endometriosis has been identified in unusual sites in the body, but the majority of lesions are limited to the pelvis. The most common pelvic sites, in order of frequency, are the ovary, peritoneum of the cul-de-sac or pouch of Douglas, uterosacral ligaments, round ligament, oviduct, and peritoneal surface of the uterus (Figure 10-14). Endometriosis of the cervix occurs infrequently but is associated with diagnostic and therapeutic traumatizing cervical procedures such as colposcopy. Isolated lesions in the appendix, bladder, ileum, cecum, cervix, or vagina are far less common. Endometriosis has been identified infrequently in laparotomy or episiotomy scars, in the umbilicus, and in distant sites (arms, legs, lungs, kidneys, and nose). There is a direct relationship between the number of endometrial implants and the severity of associated dysmenorrhea.[34]

Three major theories exist regarding the pathogenesis of endometriosis:

Transportation Endometrium is regurgitated throughout the fallopian tubes during a normal menses. After the retrograde flow, endometrial fragments implant on the ovary, on peritoneal surfaces, and on other areas.

Metaplasia or formation in situ Celomic epithelium differentiates to endometrial epithelium by inflammatory or hormonal influence and alteration.

Induction This is a combination of transportation and metaplasia in which regurgitated endometrium liberates chemical-inducing substances that activate undifferentiated mesenchyme to form endometrial epithelium. This is believed to be the most likely pathogenesis of endometriosis.

The appearance of the lesions varies depending on the stage of the disease and its duration. The foci of endometrial tissue are under hormonal influence and bleed periodically. The foci appear as bluish red to yellow-brown nodules implanted on or lying beneath serosal surfaces. They may be microsocpic or 1 to 2 cm in diameter. As individual lesions enlarge and coalesce, they can immobilize the affected structures and form adhesions. Endometriosis of the ovaries is characterized by endometriomas, cystic spaces 8 to 10 cm in size. Because they are filled with brown blood debris, they are also referred to as chocolate cysts.

• • • • • Diagnostic Studies and Findings

Laparoscopy To visualize foci and perform a biopsy of lesions (a conclusive diagnosis is based on surgical visualization)

Biopsy of lesions To confirm histologic diagnosis by presence of glands, stroma, or hemosiderin pigment (an insoluble form of storage iron that indicates bleeding)

• • • • • Multidisciplinary Plan

The treatment plan is directed toward producing maximum relief of symptoms and minimum interference with childbearing function in patients who desire children in the future.

Surgery

Laparoscopic removal of endometriotic implants, endometrioma capsules, and lysis of adnexal lesions surgically, using electrical or laser energy

Total abdominal hysterectomy and bilateral salpingo-oophorectomy

Resection or cautery destruction of visible lesions

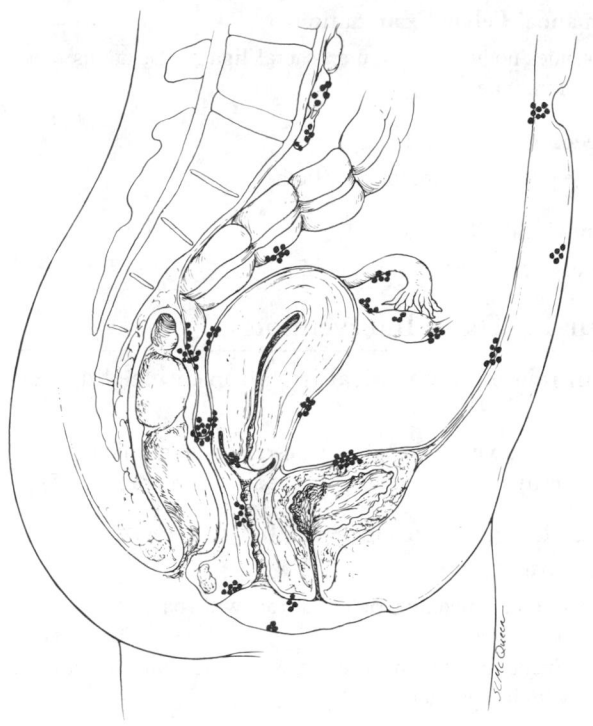

Figure 10-14 Common sites of endometriosis. (From Herbst.[18])

Medications

GnRH agonists

Goserelin acetate implant (Zoladex), 3.6 mg

Nafareline acetate (Synarel), 2 mg/ml nasal spray, 1 spray in 1 nostril bid

Leuprolide acetate (Lupron), 3.75-7.5 mg IM q1mo

Progestins

Medroxyprogesterone acetate (Provera), 2.5-10 mg po for 5 d q2mo

Hydroxyprogesterone (Delalutin), 125-250 mg IM q4wk; discontinue after 4 cycles as indicated

Antigonadotropic agents

Danazol (Danocrine), 100-800 mg/d in divided doses for 6-9 mo; produces hypoestrogenic state similar to menopause with eventual atrophy of endometrial lesions

Gestrinone, 2.5 mg 2-3 times wk or 1.25 mg/d

Psychosocial support services

NURSING CARE

Nursing Assessment

Comfort

Pelvic pain with menstruation; vague aching, cramping, or bearing-down sensation in pelvis or lower back; dyspareunia; pain with defecation

Bimanual Pelvic Examination

Tender nodules along uterosacral ligaments; uterus may be immobile

Bleeding

Menses excessive, long, or both

Behavioral Changes

Personality changes; depression

Nursing Dx & Intervention

Pain related to chemical irritation of bleeding in pelvic cavity

- Assist with and explain pain-relieving techniques.
- Instruct patient to take analgesics as ordered.

Body image disturbance related to altered body function

- Explore meaning of condition with patient *to establish plan of care.*
- Encourage patient to express feelings and to share these with her partner.

Anticipatory grieving related to potential infertility

- Encourage verbalization of fears, concerns, and other emotions.
- Determine current sources of emotional support such as spouse, mother, or sister *because this can influence the extent of self-care management and coping behaviors.*
- Refer to nursing interventions for specific surgical procedure if done.

> ### Patient Education/Home Care Planning
>
> 1. Instruct the patient about the importance of ongoing patient care.

Evaluation

Comfort is achieved   Intervention has relieved pain, ended abnormal bleeding, and preserved fertility if desired.

Body image is positive   Patient verbalizes increasing confidence in ability to cope with plan of care and verbalizes positive feelings about body.

Grief response is managed   Patient verbalizes fears and concerns and is able to cope in an adaptive manner with support of significant others.

■ LEIOMYOMAS

Uterine leiomyomas are well-circumscribed, nonencapsulated, benign tumors of the uterine musculature; they are also called myomas, fibromyomas, fibromas, or fibroids (Figure 10-15).

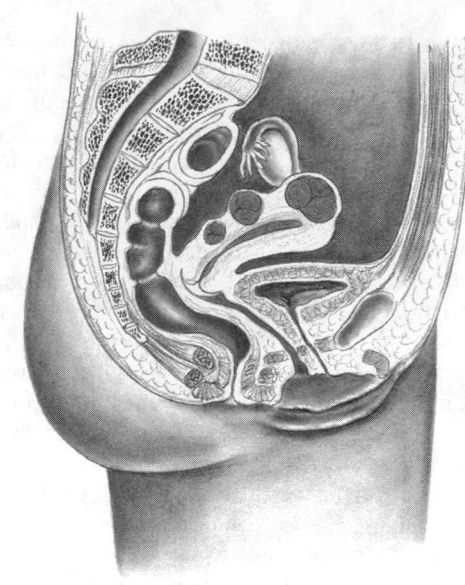

Figure 10-15 Myomas of the uterus (fibroids). (From Seidel.[41])

Uterine leiomyomas are the most frequently occurring uterine tumor and can be found in at least one third of all women past 30 years of age. Leiomyomas are the most common indication for hysterectomy among the approximately 600,000 women who have this procedure each year in the United States. Almost one third of women undergoing a hysterectomy have a diagnosis of leiomyoma. Most hysterectomies for uterine leiomyomas are performed for the relief of symptoms. Common complaints include abnormal uterine bleeding and pelvic pain or pressure. It has been determined that there is an increase in operative blood loss and postoperative morbidity, including urinary tract infections, vaginal cuff cellulitis, and febrile morbidity, when uterine weight exceeds 500 g. The use of GnRH agonists in the preoperative period to reduce the size of uterine leiomyoma is a preventive adjunct to surgical management. The benefits of a short course of GnRH agonists may also include the potential for conversion to a vaginal as opposed to an abdominal hysterectomy, reduction in preoperative bleeding accompanied by an increase in preoperative hematocrit, and decreased operative blood loss.[19]

• • • • • • Pathophysiology

Leiomyomas are classified according to their location in the uterus as follows:

Intramural—central portion of the uterine wall

Submucous—beneath the endometrium protruding into the intrauterine cavity; may become pedunculated with growth, protruding into the cervix or vagina

Subserous—beneath the peritoneal covering and projecting into the abdominal cavity; may become pedunculated with growth

Cervical—within the musculature of the cervix

Intraligamentous—lateral tumor growth between the leaves of the broad ligament

Wandering or parasitic—a subserous growth that has lost its connection to the uterus and receives blood from adjacent viscera, peritoneum, or omentum

Leiomyomas arise from smooth muscle within the myometrium, most commonly during the reproductive years. They increase in size during pregnancy, when estrogen production is high, and with the use of oral contraceptives. They generally regress after menopause. Symptoms occur in only 20% to 50% of women who have fibroids.[8]

As the tumor enlarges, the blood supply may not increase as quickly as needed, resulting in degenerative changes. The most common type of degeneration is hyalnization, in which fibrous and muscle tissue is replaced by hyaline tissue that is smooth and soft and lacks the whorled fascicular pattern. Less commonly, cystic degeneration occurs, with the hyaline material breaking down further and undergoing liquefaction owing to a further decrease in blood supply. Calcification of the leiomyoma may occur. In a large tumor, areas of yellow-brown or red softening, referred to as red or carneous degeneration, may develop because of aseptic necrosis associated with hemorrhage into the tumor. Necrosis may also occur because of twisting or torsion of a pedunculated leiomyoma. Fertility may be impaired when leiomyomas occlude the endocervical canal, the tubal ostia, or the endometrial cavity.

• • • • • • Diagnostic Studies and Findings

Bimanual examination   Enlarged, bulky, or nodular uterus

Pregnancy test   To confirm or rule out pregnancy as a cause of symptoms

Dilitation and curettage/hysteroscopy   To detect submucous leiomyomas

Hysterosalpinogram   To evaluate the endometrial cavity and fallopian tubes

Laparoscopy   To visualize subserous myomas

Ultrasonography   To distinguish between adnexal inflammatory masses and endometriosis from pedunculated or subserous leiomyomas

MRI   Useful in differentiating subserasal fibroids from ovarian masses

Laboratory studies   Leukocytosis with degenerating tumor

• • • • • • Multidisciplinary Plan

Medical Management

GnRH agonists

Leuprolide acetate (Lupron), 3.75 to 7.5 mg IM ql mo (to reduce size of myoma before surgery, which decreases operative blood loss and postoperative morbidity; or during short transition period before menopause in an effort to avoid surgery)[5]

Surgery

Hysterosopic or laparoscopic myomectomy to preserve uterus for potential future childbearing in young women

Total hysterectomy

General Management

Pelvic examinations at regular intervals to monitor status of leiomyoma

NURSING CARE

Nursing Assessment

Pain

Dull ache, soreness, or colicky pain; acute pain if torsion or twisting of pedunculated leiomyoma has occurred; bilateral pelvic discomfort if large tumor causes pressure on adjacent viscera; cramping pain if uterus attempts to expel submucous tumor; dysmenorrhea from intramural tumors; pelvic heaviness; feeling of bearing down; backache; dyspareunia

Elimination

Constipation from pressure on rectum; urinary frequency and urgency if leiomyoma causes pressure on bladder; nocturia, incontinence

Abdomen

Firm, irregular nodules palpated in lower abdomen; irregular abdominal contour; swelling

Bleeding

Profuse bleeding with flooding or clots; menses excessive, long, or both

Temperature

Elevated with degenerating tumor

Nursing Dx & Intervention

Body image disturbance related to body change

- Assess meaning of condition for patient.
- Encourage patient to express her feelings.

Pain related to pressure of tumor on adjacent structures

- Assist and teach patient to use pain-relieving methods, including relaxation techniques and analgesics as ordered.

Patient Education/Home Care Planning

1. Explain to the patient the importance of obtaining follow-up care and regular examinations to check for unusual growth or complications.

Evaluation

Patient's body image is positive   Patient verbalizes feelings demonstrating a positive image.

Comfort is achieved   There is no pain. Menses is normal if myomectomy was performed. There are no subjective or objective signs or symptoms of leiomyomas if hysterectomy was performed.

POLYPS

Polyps are benign neoplasms or protruding growths in the cervix or endometrium.

Cervical polyps are soft, red, pedunculated lesions protruding from the cervical os. Endometrial polyps are small, mostly sessile masses that project into the endometrium and may be pedunculated.

Polyps are usually asymptomatic and are often an incidental discovery during visual examination of the cervix, curettage, or hysterectomy. Because endometrial polyps may occur in association with leiomyomas and endometrial hyperplasia, specific symptoms are difficult to identify. The symptoms of cervical polyps are similar to those of chronic cervicitis with irregular bleeding. Polyps are the most common lesions of the cervix and occur most often during the reproductive years. Endometrial polyps can also occur at any age but are more common around the time of menopause. Polyps associated with the use of oral contraceptives tend to regress after the drug is discontinued.

Pathophysiology

Cervical polyps most commonly arise from the lower end of the endocervix and vary from a few millimeters to 2 cm in diameter. The base of the pedicle is usually small. Polyps may develop as a result of inflammatory hyperplasia of endocervical mucosa owing to hyperestrinism, chronic inflammation, or vascular congestion. Microscopic examination shows a surface covered by columnar epithelium with areas of metaplasia and ulceration. The stroma is often congested with blood and infiltrated by inflammatory cells. The polyps may bleed after trauma from coitus or douching.

Endometrial polyps develop as single or multiple soft tumors composed of endometrium. Most arise from the fundus or cornua, and some may protrude through the cervix. They are usually paler and firmer than cervical polyps. Most frequently the polyp is made up of endometrium similar to that of the basalis and therefore does not show secretory changes. Polyps protruding into the cervix may become necrotic or inflamed, particularly if they are long.

Diagnostic Studies and Findings

Endometrial polyps are usually an incidental finding with curettage or hysterectomy, but it is possible to diagnose an endometrial polyp from a hysterosalpingogram or endovaginal sonography. Cervical polyps are diagnosed by inspection of the cervix.

Multidisciplinary Plan

Surgery

   Curettage to remove endometrial polyps
   Hysteroscopic resectoscope to remove polyps

Removal and cauterization of base of cervical polyps; can be performed in outpatient setting
Cryosurgery for cervical polyps (see discussion of cervical conization on p. 1486)

UTERINE PROLAPSE

Uterine prolapse (pelvic relaxation, pudendal hernia) is an abnormal protrusion of the uterus through the pelvic floor and vaginal outlet (Figure 10-16).

Approximately half of all parous women have some degree of vaginal or uterine prolapse. One or two women in 10 have symptoms severe enough to warrant surgical intervention. Most cases of pelvic relaxation are associated with cystocele and rectocele. A cystocele is a herniation of the bladder base into the vagina. Uterine prolapse is often seen in multiparous women during the postmenopausal period. Some believe that childbirth causes nerve damage that results in decreased muscle strength.

Pathophysiology

Some authorities believe that probably all cases of vaginal or uterine prolapse are associated with some degree of endopelvic fascial weakness, neurologic impairment, and changes in the uterine axis secondary to childbirth. The aforementioned incidence of varying degrees of uterine prolapse presents a strong argument for this belief.

A more generally accepted belief is that the most common cause of uterine prolapse is childbirth trauma. Examples of trauma are an episiotomy extension, laceration of the vagina or cervix, or improper episiotomy repair. Pelvic support tissues are damaged by the normal stretching, tearing, and pressure of a vaginal delivery. Other precipitating factors include these:

Pregnancy. Hormonal changes and the increased weight of the uterus during pregnancy contribute to softening or relaxation of uterine support structures.

Menopause. Decreased hormone levels after menopause contribute to atrophy of uterine support structures. If prolapse is present premenopausally, it will progressively worsen during this time.

Chronic pressure. Pelvic structures that are exposed to chronic abdominal pressure from asthma, chronic bronchitis, or obesity are weakened.

It appears that many factors contribute to progressive relaxation of uterine support structures, which eventually leads to varying degrees of uterine prolapse.

The amount of uterine descent into the vagina is measured in degrees:

A first-degree prolapse occurs when the cervix is between the ischial spines (normal placement is at the level of the ischial spines) and the vaginal opening.

A second-degree prolapse occurs when only the cervix, not the entire uterus, protrudes through the vaginal opening.

A third-degree prolapse occurs when the entire cervix and uterus extend beyond the vaginal opening. This is sometimes referred to as a procidentia. Some authorities use total procidentia as a fourth-degree classification.

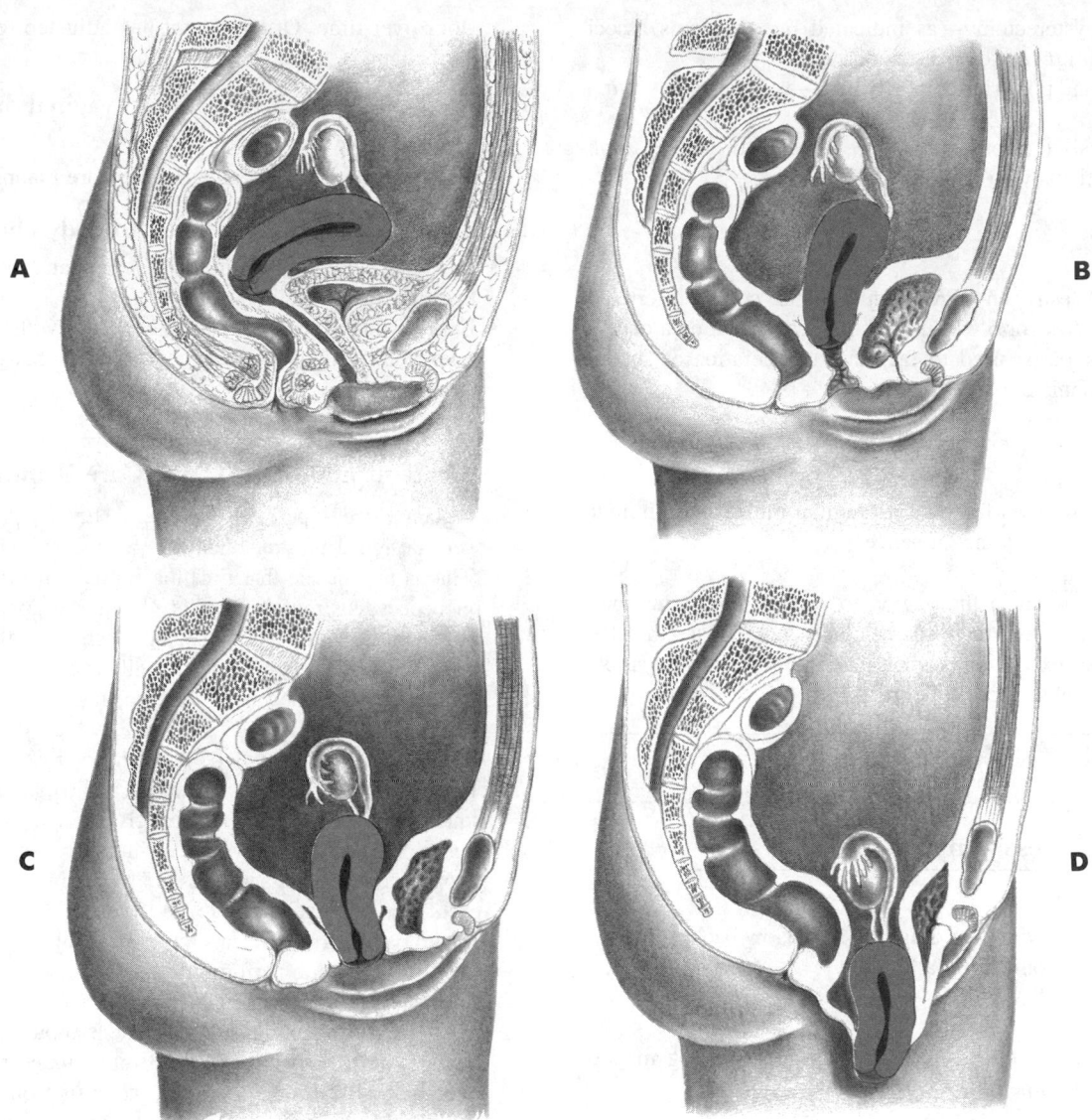

Figure 10-16 Uterine prolapse. **A,** Normal uterus. **B,** First-degree prolapse of the uterus. **C,** Second-degree prolapse of the uterus, **D,** Complete prolapse of the uterus. (From Seidel.[41])

Normally the pelvic floor supports the pelvic viscera and resists intraabdominal pressure from daily straining, lifting, and coughing. A narrow opening in the central anterior portion of the pelvic floor allows the urethra, vagina, and rectum to enter the pelvic floor, thus creating a weakened area. Certain members of the levator muscle group, puborectalis, pubococcygeal, and iliococcygeal, act as a control mechanisms for this narrow opening. The uterus usually forms an acute angle with the axis of the vagina, which prevents prolapse. When the cardinal or sacral ligaments relax, the relationship of the uterus to the vagina is altered, which contributes to prolapse. When the levator muscles or cardinal and sacral ligaments weaken or are injured, the uterus can descend through the weakened area, which leads to uterine prolapse, cystocele, and rectocele. Both cysto-celes and rectoceles can occur without uterine prolapse, depending on which pelvic support structures are weakened.

Diagnostic Studies and Findings

Pelvic examinations   To determine the degree of uterine prolapse, cystocele, and rectocele

Multidisciplinary Plan

Surgery

Retropubic cystourethropexy—associated with long-term results in maintaining urinary continence

Transvaginal sacrospinous suspension of the vaginal vault for uterovaginal prolapse and vaginal vault prolapse[33]

Vaginal hysterectomy—as indicated by symptoms associated with increased pelvic pressure

Anterior and posterior colporrhaphy—as indicated by symptoms

Colpocleisis (LeFort's procedure)—used for elderly, high-risk patients who are not sexually active

Medications

Hormones

Topical estrogen—Premarin vaginal cream inserted 2 times/wk for 6 wk; if effective, continued on a once-a-week basis; used to facilitate regeneration of support mechanism

General Management

Perineal exercise

Kegel exercises for relaxed vaginal outlet and minimum stress urinary incontinence

Pessaries

Devices worn in the vagina to support the uterus; once widely used, they are currently not the treatment of choice except for women who are poor surgical risks

Psychosocial services support

NURSING CARE

Nursing Assessment

Subjective Data

A sense of heaviness or dragging in the low back or pelvis, a feeling of something falling out

Vagina

Dyspareunia, excess vaginal mucus and bleeding in postmenopausal period

Cervix

Depending on degree of prolapse, may have constant irritation with tissue changes and cervical erosion

Bladder

Urinary tract infection, stress urinary incontinence

Bowel

Hemorrhoids from straining with constipation
Constipation

Behavior Changes

Disturbed body image

Nursing Dx & Intervention

Pain related to body change and pressure of protruding uterus

- Assess patient's degree of discomfort. Responses are varied and relate to the gradual relaxation of the pelvic

floor over time. Often patient has adjusted to the pressure changes.

Impaired skin integrity related to vaginal drainage on perineal area

- See under Patient Education/Home Care Planning.

Body image disturbance related to body change

- Assess meaning of dysfunction for patient. Encourage patient to express feelings.
- Explain importance of sharing concerns with sex partner to explore feelings that may contribute to changes in body image.

Patient Education/Home Care Planning

1. Explain Kegel's perineal exercises. The Kegel exercises were designed to strengthen the pubococcygeus muscle. (This is the muscle that rims the vagina.) To firm up the pubococcygeus muscle, do this: When you urinate, try to stop in midstream. Then start again. Then stop again. When doing the exercise correctly, you will have the sensation of "pulling up" into the vagina with the buttocks squeezed together. The pubococcygeus muscle, which controls the starting and stopping, will be strengthened by this exercise. The muscles surrounding the vagina and rectum should be squeezed off when doing this exercise, which will create a sensation of pulling everything up into the vagina. Hold for 3 to 5 seconds, relax, and repeat 15 to 25 times in sequence each time the exercises are performed. These exercises should be performed at least four times daily. Once the patient has learned to perform the exercises, she should perform them at times other than during urination.
2. Give written instructions to the patient about the need to change the pessary every 2 to 3 months and to douche once or twice a week to prevent vaginitis from the presence of the pessary.
3. Explain the importance of reporting any changes in vaginal secretions or elimination patterns to a physician.

Evaluation

Comfort is achieved   Discomfort is relieved, abnormal vaginal discharge has stopped, skin integrity is maintained, and normal elimination patterns are achieved.

Patient demonstrates progress toward acceptance of altered body image and self-concept   Patient shows adaptive response to changes in self-concept and movement toward acceptance of physiologic and psychologic changes associated with treatment regimen, whether it is exercise or surgical correction.

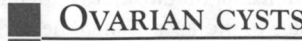

OVARIAN CYSTS

A cyst is a sac containing fluid or semisolid material. Ovarian cysts may develop at any time but are most common from puberty to menopause.

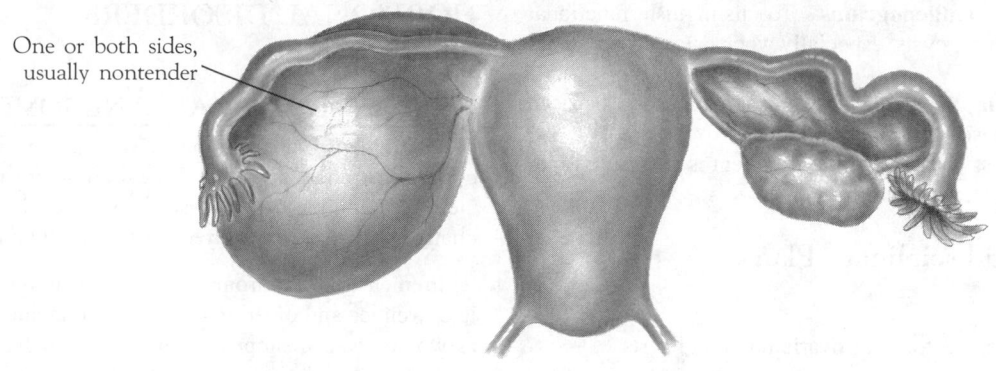

One or both sides,
usually nontender

Figure 10-17 Ovarian cyst. (From Seidel.[41])

The ovary is a frequent location of a pelvic mass (Figure 10-17). There are a variety of ovarian cysts, most being small and considered clinically unimportant. Only a few cysts require surgical removal. Most cyst enlargements disappear within a few months. However, malignancy must be considered when evaluating all pelvic masses.

Ovarian cysts are classified as follows[7]:

Functional cysts are follicle and corpus luteum cysts that are normal transient physiologic structures.

Follicle cysts. These are common and appear on the ovary surface. They are usually asymptomatic and disappear spontaneously within 60 days.

Lutein cysts

Granulosa lutein cysts are found within the corpora lutea. They are nonneoplastic enlargements of the ovary caused by an unexplained increase in fluid secretion by the corpus luteum after ovulation or during early pregnancy. They are 4 to 6 cm in diameter, raised, brown, and filled with tawny serous fluid. They may cause local pain and tenderness with either amenorrhea or delayed menses. Most cysts disappear within 2 months in nonpregnant women and gradually decrease in size during the third trimester of a pregnancy. A small percentage of cysts may rupture, requiring surgery.

Theca lutein cysts can vary in size from minute to several centimeters in diameter and are filled with straw-colored fluid. They appear in association with hydatidiform mole, choriocarcinoma, and gonadotropin therapy. Few abdominal symptoms are present, but the patient may feel a sense of pelvic aching or weight. Pregnancy signs and symptoms continue, especially hyperemesis and breast tenderness. A small percentage of cysts may rupture, requiring surgery, but most disappear spontaneously after removal of the causative factor.

Inflammatory cysts. Cysts of the fallopian tube and ovaries can form after an acute infection, such as gonorrhea. Pain is persistent and severe in the pelvis and accompanied by hypermenorrhea. The white blood cell count is elevated, and a pregnancy test will be negative. Surgery is generally not required unless an ectopic pregnancy or acute appendicitis is suspected.

Endometrial cysts. Patients with endometriosis may have endometrium implant on the ovary that will bleed with hormonal stimulation, thus forming a cyst through alternate oozing and healing. These cysts vary in size from microscopic to 10 to 12 cm in diameter. The cysts are filled with thick, chocolate-colored old blood. Large endometrial cysts should be surgically removed, leaving as much functioning ovary as possible. Endometrial cysts are sometimes referred to as "chocolate cysts," although not all chocolate cysts are endometrial in origin.

Inclusion cysts. These cysts are most often microscopic in size and located just beneath the surface of the ovary. The cysts are filled with a minute amount of serous fluid and cause no discomfort. They occur after menopause or after an inflammatory state. No treatment is required.

Parovarian cysts. These cysts are located between the fallopian tube and ovary and are rarely larger than 4 cm in diameter. Found only in postpubertal females, these cysts are generally asymptomatic unless they grow in size to become palpable.

The most important consideration in evaluating an ovarian cyst is the patient's age. Perimenopausal and postmenopausal women with palpable ovarian cysts stand a greater chance of having malignancy that are characterized by solid ovarian masses.

• • • • • • Diagnostic Studies and Findings

Pelvic and rectal examination To determine location and size of ovarian cyst

Ultrasonography To distinguish functional cysts from neoplastic cysts and to confirm findings of the pelvic examination

Laparoscopy Used when the diagnosis of endometriosis is uncertain

Abdominal roentgenograms   To distinguish functional cysts from neoplastic cysts, especially when calcified structures are present

Barium enema   To determine if an adnexal mass is caused by a colonic disease; not done routinely

Pregnancy test   To determine if patient is pregnant, especially with suspected lutein cysts

•••••• Multidisciplinary Plan

Surgery

Laparoscopic cystectomy of ovarian dermoid cysts[26]

Laparotomy to remove cysts, especially if they rupture, torse, and bleed, so as to control hemorrhage

Aspiration and tetracycline sclerotherapy for management of simple ovarian cysts[1]

General Management

Pelvic examinations at regular intervals to monitor reduction of cyst size

Suppression of activity of functional cysts

NURSING CARE

Nursing Assessment

Pain

Dull ache, severe pain, local pain and tenderness depending on the type of cyst; severe pain if cyst ruptures

Abdomen

Some cysts are palpable, bilaterally or unilaterally, in the lower abdomen

Bleeding

Menses can be excessive with inflammatory cyst

Nursing Dx & Intervention

Pain related to pressure of cyst on adjacent areas

- Assist with and teach patient to use pain-relieving methods, including relaxation techniques and analgesics as ordered.

Patient Education/Home Care Planning

1. Explain the importance of obtaining follow-up care and regular examinations to check for growth or reduction of cyst.

Evaluation

Comfort is achieved   There is no pain, and cyst has been reduced in size or removed.

HORMONAL DISORDERS

■ PREMENSTRUAL SYNDROME

Premenstrual syndrome (PMS) may be defined as the cyclic recurrence, during the luteal phase of the menstrual cycle, of a combination of physical, psychologic, and behavioral changes sufficient to interfere with normal activities.[2]

Premenstrual syndrome generally occurs in women in their late twenties and older and increases in incidence and severity as women near menopause. The various behaviors and symptoms described in epidemiologic studies can be placed in the three major categories of edema, emotionality, and headache. The symptoms generally appear 7 to 10 days before menses and sharply decrease with the onset of menses. The cause of PMS remains obscure. The highest incidence occurs in the late twenties to early thirties. PMS is rarely encountered in adolescents.

•••••• Pathophysiology

The exact cause of premenstrual tension is unknown. Progesterone stimulates the production of aldosterone, which increases sodium retention and edema formation. Interestingly, no distinct differences in aldosterone levels have been shown between women with and those without premenstrual syndrome. The decrease in brain levels of monoamine oxidase that occurs as estrogen production falls before menses probably accounts for the feeling of depression. Fluctuation of monoamine oxidase and catecholamine levels in the brain may result in the frequently observed symptom of irritability. Studies have shown that carbohydrate metabolism and the adrenal production of corticosteroids change before menses. Serotonin levels are significantly lower during the last 10 days of the menstrual cycle in women with PMS. Decreased serotonin is known to be associated with depression in humans. The treatment of PMS must be individualized for each woman, and practices vary. For example, there is concern that even low doses of vitamin B_6 may result in potentially toxic effects. Premenstrual tension may be caused by a variety of factors.

•••••• Diagnostic Studies and Findings

There are no specific tests for diagnosis of premenstrual syndrome. A personal log maintained by the woman can be helpful in diagnosis and efficacy of treatment.[25]

•••••• Multidisciplinary Plan

Medications

Hydrochlorothiazide, 50-100 mg/d po or spironolactone 25-100 mg/d po during 7-10 d before cycle or 24-36 h before onset of expected symptoms

Mefenamic acid, 550 mg po tid or qid, from symptoms to menses

Naproxen sodium, 550 mg po q12h during premenstrual period

Medroxyprogesterone (Provera), 10-20 mg/d po during last half of cycle

Alprazolam (Xanax), 0.25 mg po tid from cycle day 20 until second day of menstruation[16]

Danazol, 200 mg po qd from onset of symptoms, tapered dose until onset of menses

GnRH agonists

Naferelin acetate (Synarel) nasal spray, 1 spray in 1 nostril bid

Leuprolide acetate (Lupron), 3.75 mg to 7.5 mg IM qlmo

Antidepressants (serotonin uptake inhibitors), e.g., Doxepin HCl, Elavil[6]

Vitamins

Vitamin B, 50 mg to 500 mg/d

Vitamin E, 600 U/d

General Management

Limitation of intake of salt, refined sugars, caffeine, and animal fats

Emotional and psychologic support

Reflexology techniques of ear, hand, and foot to reduce somatic symptoms[32]

Exercise

NURSING CARE

Nursing Assessment

Hydration

Edema; weight gain; backache; breast tenderness; oliguria, palpitations; mastalgia

Gastrointestinal

Abdominal bloating; diarrhea or constipation; nausea; vomiting; food craving; compulsive eating

Affect and Behavior

Irritability; anxiety; lability; fatigue; depression; crying; lethargy; agitation; insomnia; hypersomnia; difficulty in concentrating; decreased interest in usual activities; mood swings; confusion; forgetfulness; tension; increased libido

Neurologic

Headache; vertigo, fainting; migraine; paresthesias of head and feet

Respiratory

Increase in colds, asthma, or allergic rhinitis

Urologic

Cystitis; enuresis; urethritis

Ophthalmologic

Conjunctivitis; styes

Breasts

Tenderness; enlargement

Dermatologic

Recurrence of herpes; acne; urticaria; boils; easy bruising

Nursing Dx & Intervention

Anxiety related to cyclical change in health status

- Reassure patient that her symptoms are temporary
- Assist to explore feelings about self-image, fears, and behaviors; clarify and correct misconceptions.

Altered and partially ineffective individual coping

- Help patient evaluate personal strengths and needs that affect health maintenance ability.
- Encourage participation in group therapy or sharing of feelings with family or significant other.
- Encourage patient to express her feelings and discuss or identify coping strategies to manage mood swings.
- Suggest that patient may wish to maintain a personal journal or diary *to describe feelings, strengths, and needs on a daily basis.* This should be reviewed on a regular basis *to identify any patterns or opportunities for changes in behavior or treatment regimen.*

Patient Education/Home Care Planning

1. Explain that fatigue exaggerates symptoms and that adequate rest and sleep are needed during the premenstrual period.
2. Engage in some form of moderate exercise, such as brisk walking 3 to 4 times a week.
3. Encourage the patient to avoid stressful activity during the premenstrual period.
4. Give printed instructions to patient to avoid glucose fluctuation by taking small frequent feedings of a high-protein, complex carbohydrate diet and by decreasing sugar intake to less than 5 tablespoons daily.
5. Discuss with the patient the need to reduce salt intake and to avoid foods with "hidden salts" such as soy sauce, salted crackers and bread, luncheon meats, dried meats, hot dogs, tomato juice, and cheeses. Discuss with the patient the need to avoid dairy products and animal fats, the need to restrict caffeine by decreasing intake of coffee, tea, cola, and chocolate, and the need to restrict alcohol.
6. Discuss with the patient the need to increase intake of leafy green vegetables, whole grain cereals, and complex carbohydrates.
7. Instruct the patient to take medications as prescribed and explain the reasons for taking specific medications. (For example, Vitamin B_6 is taken to increase blood progesterone and promote diuresis, and vitamin E is taken to reduce breast tenderness.)
8. Suggest and offer printed educational materials.

Evaluation

Comfort is achieved; there is little or no anxiety Patient describes feeling of well-being and absence of bloating, weight gain, edema, mastalgia, irritability, anxiety, and other symptoms of PMS.

Patient uses strengths to cope and comply with plan of care Patient recognizes personal strengths and needs that are directed toward elimination or reduction of symptoms.

Patient establishes appropriate coping with mood swings Patient verbalizes about mood and advises others of her particular sensitivities. Patient develops a support system with significant others. Patient demonstrates increased interest in social and occupational activities.

■ MENOPAUSE AND CLIMACTERIC

Menopause is the physiologic cessation of menses. The climacteric is the transitional period during which reproductive function diminishes and eventually ceases.

As the average life span has increased in the United States, so has the number of postmenopausal women. Of the 120 million women in the United States, 40 million are over 50 years of age. Postmenopausal women constitute one eighth to one sixth of the population. The average life span of women is 81 years, whereas that of men is only 72 years. As the ratio of men to women decreases with age, many women in the climacteric phase of life must cope with societal, as well as physical, changes.

The normal decrease in ovarian function begins during the fourth decade, and the majority of women cease to menstruate between the ages of 48 and 55. The average age at which menses disappears is 50 years, although some women cease to menstruate as early as 40 years and others continue until 55 years or older.

Induced or premature menopause is the cessation of ovarian function as a result of radiation, surgery, immunologic disease, or bacteriologic or viral agents. Although the signs and symptoms of natural and premature or artificial menopause are similar, the medical management may vary based on the patient's age.

•••••• Physiology

A notable event of the climacteric phase of life is menopause, the complete cessation of menses. Before the actual menopause there are usually gradual changes, such as a decrease in the amount of menses, lengthening of the interval between menses, periodic amenorrhea, and finally slight spotting. These events are due to a progressive decline in the ovarian secretion of estrogen. When too little estrogen is secreted to cause endometrial growth, bleeding stops permanently. Irregular menses followed by amenorrhea for more than 1 year is indicative of menopause.

With menopause the estrogen fractions change and estrone becomes more available than estradiol. Peripheral conversion of androstenedione, a product of the adrenal glands, to estrone

occurs principally in the fat. Some women produce enough estrone to cause endometrial growth and shedding or bleeding. Because obesity is a common factor in women with endometrial cancer, it has been hypothesized that production of estrone in the adipose tissue may contribute to the genesis of a tumor.

Changes in reproductive structures are related directly to decreased estrogen. Labial fat is reabsorbed; the labia majora become flattened and the labia minora may disappear. The vaginal epithelium becomes thinner, the vagina smaller, and the fornices shallower. The myometrium thins, causing the uterus to decrease in size until it resembles that of a prepubertal girl.

Hot flushes, the most characteristic symptom of menopause, result in a slight increase in core body temperature and a higher increase in skin temperature. The sensation of heat is often accompanied by tachycardia, vertigo, palpitation, and a feeling of faintness.

The atrophic changes that result from estrogen deprivation may lead to dyspareunia owing to decreased precoital lubrication or constriction of the introitus or vagina.

Nervousness and other psychologic symptoms are not a direct result of estrogen deficiency. The patient's personality and response to aging are the keys to promoting adaptation to the climacteric.

Anthropometric studies, including weight, body mass index (BMI), waist-to-hip girth ratio, and body composition (particularly percentage of body fat and water), show a significant increase in body weight and fat mass in early postmenopausal women (44 to 54 years of age). A shift from gynecoid to android fat distribution is more likely to be observed in women who do not take hormone replacement therapy.[35]

•••••• Diagnostic Studies and Findings

Papanicolaou smear Decrease in estrogen effect noted in vaginal mucosa

Blood chemistry Estradiol <5 ng/dl; follicle-stimulating hormone >40 mIU/ml

•••••• Multidisciplinary Plan

The use of hormonal therapy in the treatment of menopause is associated with a diminution of subjective complaints, a decrease in age-specific mortality for all categories of cause of death, including cardiovascular dysmenorrhea, and a decrease in osteoporosis.[27,36]

The decision to use hormone replacement therapy (HRT) should be made by the patient with full disclosure of the risk, side effects, and benefits by the physician. Cyclical bleeding, a common side effect associated with HRT, is unacceptable to most women who have looked forward to its absence, and this factor often contributes to the discontinuation of HRT in the long term.[10,36] Although there is a correlation between estrogen and breast cancer, which is not ameliorated by the inclusion of oral progesterone agents, clinical studies do not demonstrate that the use of HRT is a significant risk factor for breast cancer.[10,30,43] Most practitioners believe that the overall benefits (from menopausal symptoms, cardiovascular disease, and osteoporosis) outweigh any risks of HRT.[13,48]

Medications

Estrogens

Conjugated estrogen (Premarin), 0.3-2.5 mg/d po, or ethinyl estradiol (Estinyl, others), 0.05-0.2 mg/d po; initial doses should be lowest amount that will control symptoms; drug is taken for first 25 d of month; withdrawal should be gradual over several months to prevent recurrence of hot flushes

Indications: Treatment of hot flushes and senile atrophic vaginitis; prevention of osteoporosis

Contraindications: Presence or history of breast or genital cancer (except cervical cancer is some cases); history of thromboembolism; fluid retention due to cardiac, renal, or hepatic disease, abnormal liver function

Cautions: Administration is closely monitored in women with uterine fibroids, endometriosis, hypertension, familial hyperlipidemia, gallbladder dysmenorrhea, or insulin-dependent diabetes mellitus; annual endometrial biopsy needed for patient receiving long-term estrogen therapy

Transdermal estradiol (Estraderm), 0.05 mg transdermal patch changed twice weekly

Estrogen creams applied to vagina are more effective than oral estrogen in treatment of atrophic vaginitis

Progestins or progestogens

Medroxyprogesterone acetate (Provera), 2.5-10 mg/d po for the first 25 days of the month or in last 10 d of estrogen cycle

Indications: To prevent endometrial cancer, which may develop with unopposed estrogen stimulation

Cautions: May stimulate withdrawal bleeding; patients receiving long-term estrogen-only replacement therapy or those receiving progestogens on a quarterly basis should have annual endometrial biopsies

Bisphosphonates (as indicated for osteoporosis)

Fosamax 10 mg po QD, 30 min ac in AM

Psychosocial-educational Support Groups/Classes

NURSING CARE

Nursing Assessment

Subjective Complaints

Hot flushes; night sweats; diaphoresis; insomnia; headache; vertigo; syncope; numbness, tingling, or pain in joints; chilly sensation; lack of appetite or weight gain; constipation or diarrhea; nausea or vomiting; flatulence; fatigability; irritability; dyspareunia (resulting from vaginal atrophy); vaginal dryness, burning, and itching

Vulva

Decreasing labial fat; atrophy of muscle

Vagina

Decreased size with shallow fornices; dry appearance

Abdomen

Abdominal fat deposition

Cardiac Rate and Rhythm

Tachycardia; palpitations

Breasts

Reduction in size

Body hair

Loss of pubic and axillary hair; increase in facial and lip hair

Behavioral Changes

Anxiety; decreased tolerance level; body image change

Nursing Dx & Intervention

Knowledge deficit related to lack of information about self-care management

- Explain physiologic process of climacteric and menopause.
- Explain importance of keeping fit and eating well-balanced diet, getting adequate rest and sleep, avoiding stress and fatigue, and continuing contraception until health care provider indicates it is safe to stop.
- Inform patient about side effects of estrogen replacement therapy, need to report any vaginal bleeding occurring 6 months or more after last menstrual period, an availability of water-soluble lubricants if needed before coitus.

Body image disturbance related to body change

- Encourage patient to express concerns about femininity, sexuality, and aging.
- Reinforce correct information and provide factual information *to correct any misconceptions.*

Altered sexuality patterns relate to altered body function

- Encourage patient to express her concerns regarding sexuality.
- Encourage patient to discuss concerns with partner or significant other.
- Provide information for patient to access group or individual counseling and education.

Evaluation

Patient has acquired knowledge about climacteric   Patient expresses understanding of physiology and desired health behaviors. Patient relates understanding or prescribed medications including dosage, route of administration, frequency, and side effects.

Patient demonstrates progress toward acceptance of altered body image, self-concept, and sexuality Patient shows adaptive responses to changes in self-concept and movement toward acceptance of both physiologic and psychologic processes associated with climacteric.

■ FERTILITY CONTROL

■ Fertility can be controlled by natural, mechanical, chemical, hormonal, and surgical means.

Contraception has been identified as one of the most important issues facing the world today by the World Health Organization. The birth rate in the United States is approximately 15.9, reflecting a zero population growth; it is a phenomenon that is not occurring in many other countries. Continued population growth at current rates could have a negative impact on natural resources, food supply, and political stability, especially in Third World countries. The number of people the earth can sustain is unknown.

Fertility rates are higher among the poor and less educated, and the problem of teenage pregnancy remains unsolved. The goal of every pregnancy occurring as a result of an informed decision and resulting in a wanted child is far from being achieved.

Many factors affect the selection of a fertility control method, including the person's perception of the risk of pregnancy, knowledge of fertility control methods, and willingness and ability to use them; social pressures; the attitude of health care providers; desires of the partner; and the cost and effectiveness of various methods. The methods most widely used in the United States in order of popularity are oral contraceptives, condoms, intrauterine devices (IUDs), rhythm, foam, diaphragm, and coitus interruptus. The method of fertility control varies according to the duration of the relationship or marriage. Young couples often use oral contraceptives until their first child is born, between pregnancies until their family is complete, and then select sterilization.

There has been an increase in those selecting sterilization in the last decade. Approximately equal numbers of men and women have undergone sterilization. Approximately 1 million Americans are sterilized annually.

Induced abortion, although not a contraceptive technique, is a method of preventing unwanted children. In January 1973 the U.S. Supreme Court declared all restrictive abortion laws by individual states unconstitutional. As a consequence, abortion in both the first and second trimesters is legal in all states, with the decision made by the woman. Since the Supreme Court decision, the numbers of illegal abortions and abortion-related deaths have fallen precipitously.

The health care provider has a responsibility to provide information to women or couples choosing a method of contraception. The decision is a voluntary one based on explanation of the methods available, including their action, safety and effectiveness, expected effects, risks, and contraindications. The methods of fertility control can be divided into five major groups: natural or physiologic, mechanical, chemical, hormonal, and surgical.

Natural or Physiologic methods

Rhythm In the rhythm method, coitus is confined to phases in the menstrual cycle when conception is unlikely to occur. This can be determined by the calendar method, temperature method, or ovulation method. With the *calendar* method the fertile period is determined by recording the number of days of each menstrual cycle for a year, subtracting 18 days from the length of the shortest cycle to determine the beginning of the fertile period, and subtracting 11 days from the length of the longest cycle to determine the postovulatory safe period. The *temperature* method is based on abstinence from the end of the menses until 4 days after the rise in basal body temperature. The woman must take her temperature the first thing in the morning because the basal body temperature is the lowest temperature reached by the body during the waking hours. The *ovulation* method is based on the recognition of characteristic changes in cervical mucus. Initially after menstruation there is little mucus and the introitus is dry. The mucus becomes sticky and cloudy as estrogen stimulation increases, and as ovulation occurs it becomes abundant, clear, and slippery and stretches without breaking, the spinnbarkheit phenomenon. Following ovulation and an increase in progesterone, the mucus becomes opaque and sticky again, with the woman experiencing a sensation of dryness. Coitus should be avoided from first recognition of the sticky mucus until after the watery discharge disappears.

Coitus interruptus Withdrawal of the penis from the vagina before ejaculation is probably the oldest and most frequently used fertility control method throughout the world. It is associated with a fairly high failure rate because live sperm may be present in the seminal fluid that leaks from the urethra during coitus.

Mechanical Methods

Condom The condom or penile sheath must be applied over the erect penis, leaving space at the tip to contain the ejaculate. It must be removed before penile detumescence, with the rim held tightly to prevent leakage.

Diaphragm The diaphragm is a latex dome-shaped cup that must be fitted to the patient to ensure that the cervix is covered. The woman must be instructed in its use and be able to demonstrate its application.

Cervical cap The cervical cap is smaller than the diaphragm and made of thick rubber or plastic. It may be applied some time before intercourse and left in place for at least 8 hours after intercourse. It is more difficult to apply than the diaphragm, and some women object to the odor when it is left in place for a long time. Its use, except in a few research centers, is not approved by the Food and Drug Administration.

Intrauterine device (IUD) The IUD is a small plastic device connected to a string that protrudes into the vagina. IUDs are available in various sizes and shapes. A health care provider inserts the device into the uterus, usually during menses when the cervix is partially open.

Chemical Methods

Spermicidal jellies, creams, suppositories, or aerosol foams are placed in the vagina immediately before intercourse and act as a chemical barrier to the sperm. They are often used in conjunction with another method such as a natural or a mechanical method. The spermicidal sponge inserted deep into the vagina at the cervical os blocks, absorbs, and kills sperm.

Hormonal Methods

The most popular form of hormonal contraception is the oral contraceptive ("the pill"). This is most commonly a combination of estrogen and progestin that inhibits ovulation and changes in the endometrium, cervical mucus, and probably tubal function. Oral contraceptives are extremely effective in preventing pregnancy but are known to affect every body system and may produce significant dangers with long-term use. Generally the benefits and effectiveness outweigh the risk in healthy women below 30 years of age. See Table 10-2 for a summary of current agents.

Diethylstilbestrol (the "morning-after pill") is the postcoital agent most commonly used in the United States. It is not for routine use but should be considered an emergency measure to be taken as soon as possible but no later than 72 hours after unprotected midcycle intercourse. The possibility of an established pregnancy must be ruled out before this drug is administered because ingestion by the mother is known to cause vaginal adenosis and clear cell carcinoma in daughters. Other "morning-after" contraceptive agents include estrogens, progesterone, and the abortifacients methotrexate and RU486 (mifepristone), which are considered investigational drugs by the federal Food and Drug Administration (FDA).

Surgical Methods

Abortion   First-trimester abortion is done by dilitation and curettage, aspiration of intrauterine contents through a suction device, or menstrual extraction. Second-trimester abortion is achieved by dilation and evacuation, intrauterine drug instillation, or hysterotomy.

Dilation and curettage is a painful procedure requiring general anesthesia; a sharp metal curette is inserted into the uterus to remove products of conception. When this surgical method of abortion fails because of uterine or cervical anomalies, methotrexate and misoprostol can be used to induce abortion in pregnancies up to 8 weeks of gestation. The methotrexate is administered by IM injection and a misoprostol vaginal suppository is self-administered in 3 days.[28,38]

Vacuum aspiration can be done after a cervical block. The cervix is prepared by instillation of laminaria, an absorbent dried seaweed, into the cervix to expand the cervical canal. After the laminaria is removed, the aspiration curette is inserted and the products of conception are removed.

Menstrual extraction is the aspiration of endometrium and intrauterine contents through a polyethylene catheter that has been inserted into the uterus through the cervix. The procedure seldom requires cervical dilation and is performed not later than 8 weeks after the last menstrual period. Uterine injury and bleeding and continuation of pregnancy are the major risks associated with this procedure, which should not be considered a substitute for contraception.

The cervix must be more dilated for dilation and evacuation than for curettage. Dilation is usually effected with laminaria. The intrauterine contents are evacuated through a crushing instrument, followed by aspiration. The procedure is most frequently done in women who are 13 to 16 weeks pregnant.

Hypertonic saline solution is injected into the amniotic cavity to induce a second-trimester abortion. Complications are inadvertent infusion into the maternal bloodstream, producing salt intoxication; disseminated intravascular coagulation; and infection, especially if there is a long interval between instillation of the drug and uterine evacuation. Prostaglandin can be given by intramniotic or intravenous infusion or as a vaginal suppository. This method has virtually replaced use of hypertonic saline solution for abortion. Prostaglandins stimulate contractions of smooth uterine muscle and generally result in abortion within 24 hours. Side effects include nausea, vomiting, diarrhea, and abdominal cramping, which can be controlled with analgesics and antiemetics.

Hysterotomy is a surgical incision into the uterus for the removal of products of conception. It is associated with morbidity and is used only rarely for midtrimester abortions.

Text continued on p. 914.

 EMERGENCY ALERT

SEXUAL ASSAULT

Sexual assault affects an estimated 80 per 100,000 women each year and is one of the four most violent and frequent crimes in the United States. Sexual assault can affect people of any age and of either sex.

Assessment and Interventions

- Recognize and acknowledge the victim.
- Place patient in quiet area or room; ideally do not leave victim alone; call sexual assault team or counselors if available in your community.
- Assess for life-threatening injury; record vital signs and obtain a *thorough* history, with details such as time, location, use of weapons.
- Discuss forensic examination with patient and obtain consent. The forensic examination includes a battery of observations, specimen collecting, and historical information; the specific content varies from state to state so be familiar with local requirements.
- Protect patient from pregnancy and STD by administering medications, as appropriate.
- Arrange follow-up care.

TABLE 10-2 Summary of Methods of Conception Control

Method	Action	Safety-Effectiveness	Effects	Contraindications
Oral Contraceptive ("The Pill") Combination pill: each pill contains progestin and estrogen; schedule: one pill daily for 21 days, then discontinue for 7 days; placebo may be advised for last 7 days; pill cycle started and repeated on fifth day after onset of menstrual flow	Inhibits ovulation by suppression of pituitary gonadotropin Produces cervical mucus that is hostile to sperm Modifies tubal transport of ovum May have effect on endometrium to make implantation unlikely	Effective if taken accurately Failure results from failure to take pill regularly If woman forgets to take pill one day, she can "make up" by taking two pills next day Chances of pregnancy increased if pill is missed for even 1 day Highly acceptable to users; easy to take Linked with mortality caused by thromboembolus phenomena Does not alter fertility	Useful Relief of dysmenorrhea in 60% to 90% of cases Relief of premenstrual tension Regulation of menstrual cycles Relief of acne in 80% to 90% of cases Improved feeling of well-being Minor side effects (usually decrease after third cycle) Weight gain Breast tenderness Headaches Corneal edema Nausea Breakthrough bleeding Hypertension Major side effects Thromboembolus disorders CVA; MI May decrease lactation in breast-feeding women	Active thrombophlebitis Cerebrovascular or coronary artery disease Undiagnosed vaginal bleeding Breast or pelvic cancer Liver disease Use with caution if history of Epilepsy Multiple sclerosis Porphyria Otosclerosis Asthma Cardiovascular disease Renal disease Thyroid disease Diabetes Uterine fibroid tumors Smoker Age >40 years old Deep vein thrombophlebitis
Intrauterine Contraceptive Device (IUD or IUCD) Small objects of various shapes made of plastic, nylon, or steel inserted into uterus; medicated with copper or a progestational agent Most have nylon string attached that protrudes from cervix into vagina; inserted using aseptic technique; follow-up visits in 1 month, then individualized EXAMPLES ParaGard (Copper T380A) Progestesert	Unknown Copper may interfere with sperm transport Progestational agent causes progestin effects on cervical mucus and endometrial maturation	Easily inserted highly effective: 97% to 99% Can be inserted any time during cycle; presence of menstrual flow rules out early pregnancy Can be inserted immediately postpartum, but expulsion rate is higher Can be left in place indefinitely Effectiveness highly dependent on knowing IUD remains in place; women need to be taught to feel for string after each period Spontaneous expulsion occurs most often during menstruation (expulsion rates: 10% to 20%)	Uterine cramping Heavy menstrual flow Irregular menses Vaginal discharge NOTE: Usually disappear in 2 to 3 months Problems Infection: usually minor and occurs soon after insertion Perforation of uterus: varies with types of device; highest rates in first 6 weeks postpartum; usually occurs at time of insertion	Current infection of reproductive tract Uterine fibroids Undiagnosed vaginal bleeding Nulligravida Multiple sexual partners History of salpingitis (PID) Known or suspected pregnancy Uterine abnormalities with distortion Immunosuppressive disorders Known or suspected uterine or cervical malignancy Genital actinomycosis Allergy to copper (copper-containing IUDs)

TABLE 10-2 Summary of Methods of Conception Control—cont'd

Method	Action	Safety-Effectiveness	Effects	Contraindications
		Failure rate (pregnancy) 1.5% to 3% during first year of use; rate declines thereafter Does not alter fertility		
Diaphragm (with Spermicidal Foam, Cream, Jelly)				
Rubber dome attached to flexible metal ring; inserted into vagina to cover cervix; available in various sizes (require careful fitting; self-inserted by user; surfaces and rim of diaphragm coated with spermicide before insertion; inserted no more than 2 hours before intercourse and left in place at least 6 hours after intercourse	Provides mechanical barrier to sperm Spermicidal preparation destroys large number of sperm	97% to 98% effective if fitted properly and used correctly Requires sustained motivation for repeated insertion and removal Refitting necessary after childbirth, surgery of cervix and vagina, or weight change of 10 pounds or more	None	Severe uterine prolapse History of reaction to product History of toxic shock
Cervical Cap				
A flexible natural rubber device available in various sizes (requires careful fitting); self-inserted by user; inserted before intercourse and left in place at least 8 hours (but no more than 48 hours) after intercourse	Provides mechanical barrier to sperm	82.6% to 93.6% effective if fitted properly and used correctly Requires 30-90 minutes' education time to learn insertion procedure Requires sustained motivation for repeated insertion and removal	Potential for Papanicolaou test conversion from normal to abnormal Papanicolaou test conversion from normal to abnormal at 3 months' follow-up (use of cervical cap is discontinued if this occurs) Cervicitis	Cervical dysplasia with abnormal Papanicolaou test History of toxic shock syndrome Concurrent vaginal or cervical infection History of reaction to product
Condom ("Rubber," "Safe," "Prophylactic")				
Thin, flexible plastic worn over penis; available without prescription; does not require medical supervision	Provides mechanical barrier to prevent sperm from entering vagina Prevents spread of venereal diseases	Effectiveness increased with use of diaphragm by woman Effectiveness decreased by tearing or slipping of condom during intercourse and by use of condoms without a reservoir end Failure rate 10% to 15%	None	None

Continued.

TABLE 10-2 Summary of Methods of Conception Control—cont'd

Method	Action	Safety-Effectiveness	Effects	Contraindications
Natural Family Planning (Ovulation, Symptothermal, Billings Method)				
Periodic abstinence from intercourse during fertile periods of menstrual cycle; days 12 to 16 before expected date of menstruation are possible ovulating days; because sperm can survive up to 48 hours, days 11, 17, and 18 added to fertile period	Sexual abstinence around time of ovulation	Safe 65% to 85% effective Fertile period varies; precise time of ovulation not known Effectiveness increased with calculation of fertile period, high motivation to prevent pregnancy, determination of basal body temperature, and observation of mucous secretions' consistency	Frustration Lack of sexual gratification during period of abstinence	Irregular menstrual cycles Medical contraindications to pregnancy
Chemical Contraceptive (Jellies, Creams, Foams, Suppositories)				
Applied inside vagina by means of plunger-type applicator or aerosol spray	Contains spermicidal ingredients Partial barrier to entrance of sperm into cervix	Effectiveness increased when used with diaphragm or condom Easily available without prescription Effectiveness depends on dispersion of substance within vagina	None	History of reaction to product
Levonorgestrel Subdermal Implant (Norplant)				
Six capsules of Silastic are implanted in the patient's arm; each capsule contains 36 mg of crystalline levonorgestrel	Inhibits ovulation by suppression of pituitary gonadotropin Produces thick cervical mucus that is hostile to sperm	Contraceptive failure rarely occurs Pregnancy rate 0.8/100 users over 5 years	Irregular bleeding, spotting, or amenorrhea may occur in the first year Headache	Hypertension History of thromboembolism, valvular heart disease; first 6 weeks postpartum; same as for oral contraceptives
Injectable Medroxyprogesterone Acetate (Depo-Provera)				
Intramuscular injection of long-acting progestrogen of 150 mg every 3 months	Inhibits ovulation	Efficacy similar to surgical sterilization	Amenorrhea may occur in women after 1 year of use Headache	Should be used by women only for long-term deferral of pregnancy; takes average of 22 weeks to ovulate after injection
Emergency Contraceptive pill[2]				
Nordette, Levlen, Lo Ovral, Triphasil, Tri-Levlen, and Ovral	Inhibits ovulation May effect endometrium to make implantation unlikely	Reduces risk of pregnancy by at least 75% if treatment initiated within 72 h of unprotected intercourse	Nausea Headache Breast tenderness	Reproductive cancers Cerebral hemorrhage

TABLE 10-2 Summary of Methods of Conception Control—cont'd

Method	Action	Safety-Effectiveness	Effects	Contraindications
Vaginal Sponge				
	Sponge is inserted adjacent to cervix and releases spermicide	Water activates sponge and facilitates insertion; spermidice is released for 24 hours	At least 6 hours should elapse after last intercourse before removal of sponge. Sponge must be discarded after use and is not reusable	Irritation and allergic reactions in 2% to 3%; some increased risk of candidiasis; difficult removal reported in 6% of users	None
Vaginal Sheath (Female Condom)				
	Sheath is made of natural latex rubber with flexible rings at both ends; device is a combination of a diaphragm and condom; closed end of pouch is anchored around cervix, and open ring covers labia	Provides mechanical barrier to prevent sperm from entering vagina/cervix. Spermicide jelly, foam, or cream should be added before intercourse	Effectiveness in excess of condom and diaphragm. Failure rate of 15/100 (15%). May provide more protection than condoms against sexually transmitted diseases (STDs)	Relatively loose sheath provides heightened sensation for the man	None

Sterilization Sterilization is the ultimate method of fertility control, rendering a person unable to reproduce. This is accomplished by vasectomy in men and tubal ligation or hysterectomy in women.

Vasectomy is a procedure for male sterilization involving the bilateral surgical removal of a portion of the vas deferens. It is most commonly performed on an outpatient basis with the patient under local anesthesia.

Tubal sterilization is the disruption of tubal patency to prevent the union of the ova and spermatozoa. It can be achieved through the vagina or by an abdominal approach through an incision or with laparoscopic visualization. A variety of techniques can be used:

Irving procedure. The oviduct is severed, and the uterine end is buried in the myometrium posteriorly and the distal or ovarian end is placed in the mesosalpinx.

Pomeroy procedure. A loop of oviduct is ligated and excised.

Parkland procedure. A segment of the fallopian tube is separated from the mesosalpinx and ligated proximally and distally, and then the midportion is excised.

Fimbriectomy. The distal portion of the ampulla, including all of the fimbriae, is resected.

Tubal sterilization can be done at any time but is most convenient during the postpartum period because the uterine fundus is near the umbilicus and the fallopian tubes are readily accessible. Laparoscope sterilization is often referred to as "band aid" surgery because it can be performed in an ambulatory surgical center with general or occasionally local anesthesia. A pneumoperitoneum is produced with carbon dioxide, and the oviduct is ligated and most commonly electrocoagulated. In a vaginal tubal sterilization the peritoneal cavity is entered through the posterior vaginal fornix (culdotomy, colpotomy) and a Pomeroy procedure or fimbriectomy is performed. The care of women undergoing tubal ligation is discussed on p. xxx.

A summary of the common methods of conception control is provided in Table 10-2.

INFERTILITY

Infertility is the inability to conceive during a period of 1 year of unprotected intercourse. Primary infertility exists when there has been no prior conception. Secondary infertility follows at least one pregnancy.

Infertility affects 10% to 15% of couples in the United States. About 25% of women who do not use contraception and who have coitus regularly conceive within 4 months, more than 60% do so within 6 months, and about 80% within 1 year. The incidence of infertility shows a progression with advancing age of the woman. Fertility peaks between 20 and 25 years of age and decreases significantly after 40 years of age in women and 50 years of age in men.

It is estimated that male factors are responsible for about 30% of infertility problems. The cause of infertility is not identifiable in up to 15% of cases. Female factors are responsible for the remaining cases. Of these around 20% to 30% are the result of disorders of the fallopian tubes, 10% to 15% lack of ovulation, and 50% cervical factors. It is believed that endometriosis is responsible for 30% to 40% of female infertility.

About 40% of those who seek medical attention for infertility eventually conceive. The identified cause of infertility cannot be corrected in 40% of the couples and the cause of infertility in the remaining couples is never identified.

There are profound psychosocial effects of infertility on the couple. Nurses can play a crucial role in helping infertile couples cope by providing counseling and stimulating the adoption of strategies to manage the stress of infertility. Promotion of social support can also lead to a greater contentment over the course of time in infertile couples.[20]

•••••• Pathophysiology

Normal fertility is dependent on many factors, including normal ovarian function, endocrine preparation of the uterus for implantation of the fertilized ovum, cervical mucus favorable for transport of sperm, normal anatomic structures, lack of obstruction to sperm and ovum, and normally functioning fallopian tubes. The male partner must have a sufficient number of motile and mature sperm that can be ejaculated without any anatomic or physiologic obstruction and that are capable of penetrating the egg.

The causes of infertility are as follows[52]:

Female factors

Vaginal abnormalities

Rigid hymen or small hymenal orifice; psychogenic vaginismus; hyperacidity of vaginal secretions

Cervical abnormalities

Obstructive lesions such as polyps or congenital atresia; alterations in cervical mucus owing to bacteria or chemical agents; surgical destruction of endocervical glands

Uterine factors

Submucous myomas; structural malformations such as bicornuate or septate uterus; hypoplasia owing to endocrine disturbances; synechiae owing to endometritis; pelvic inflammatory disease

Uterine age >40 years increases pregnancy losses in ovum donation patients after implantation is completed[12]

Tubal and peritoneal abnormalities

Peritubal and periovarian adhesions following peritonitis; inflammatory damage owing to intrauterine devices, severe puerperal infections, and pelvic inflammatory disease; endometriosis

Ovarian abnormalities

Oligo-ovulation or anovulation owing to hypothalamic, pituitary, or ovarian deficits; hyperprolactinemia and galactorrhea associated with anovulation or luteal phase defects; faulty nutrition; metabolic dysfunction; luteal phase defects, which may be due to abnormal stimulation of the graafian follicle, hyperandrogen states, or increased prolactin levels; ovarian tumors (such as Stein-Leventhal syndrome)

Male factors
  Sperm-related factors
    Testicular hypoplasia; endocrine disorders such as hypopituitarism and hypothalamic disorders; cryptorchidism; varicocele; gonadal damage from trauma, surgery, or radiation; exposure of testicles to heat including wearing of tight shorts; systemic infections including mumps, tuberculosis, and syphilis; late descent of testicles; high viscosity of semen; autoimmunity as a result of trauma, vasectomy, or infection; low volume
  Ductal obstructions
    Resulting from epididymitis or infection of ejaculatory ducts; congenital absence of ducts
  Transport-related factors
    Hypospadias; ejaculatory problems; impotence
Factors affecting either male or female
  Stress
    Physical or psychic; long-term psychiatric problems
  Nutritional deficiencies
    Malnutrition such as anorexia nervosa and starvation; vitamin, mineral, or fat deficiencies
  Substances
    Exposure to toxins including alcohol, nicotine, metals such as lead, dyes such as aniline dyes, drugs such as narcotics, quinine, hormonal agents, and antineoplastic drugs, radiation
  Congenital anomalies
    Chromosomal abnormalities (such as Turner's and Klinefelter's syndromes)
  Disease processes
    Dysfunctions or disturbances of thyroid, adrenal, or pituitary gland; diabetes mellitus; anemia; chronic nephritis; severe cardiac disturbances; infections; immune responses
Causes of infertility in the couple
  Sexual problems
    Unconsumated relationships; infrequent intercourse; sexual dysfunction; vaginismus; suboptimum technique
  Other problems
    Discordant relationships; immunologic reaction

•••••• Diagnostic Studies and Findings

Semen analysis (split ejaculate) Standards for fertility are volume of 2 to 6 ml semen per ejaculation; semen liquefication ≤30 minutes; semen pH 7.2 to 7.8; 20 to 300 million sperm/ml; 60% to 80% of sperm actively motile; 60% or more of sperm normally shaped

Vaginal examination Cervical examination in midcycle; cervix not opened; lack of copious mucus; lack of spinnbarkheit and arborization

Tubal patency determination Hysterosalpingography may indicate obstruction of tube if radiopaque dye fails to spill into peritoneum

Diagnostic endoscopy Laparoscopy or culdoscopy: absence of direct observation of dye passing through fimbriated ends of fallopian tube; peritubal adhesions may be observed

Basal body temperature graph Absence of normal biphasic pattern with sustained rise of at least 1° F during last 2 weeks of cycle

Follicle-stimulating hormone (FSH) and Luteinizing hormone (LH) Elevated with ovarian failure; suppressed with pituitary or hypothalamic disorder

Serum progesterone Level less than 10 ng/ml indicative of abnormal luteal function; concentration of less than 3 ng/ml suggestive of anovulation

Endometrial biopsy Findings inconsistent with cycle; premenstrual biopsy can confirm ovulation

Ultrasound Observation of ovarian follicle rupture

Postcoital test (Sims-Huhner) Fewer than five highly motile sperm in mucus from upper cervix; inadequate spinnbarkheit and arborization suggestive of estrogen deficiency and secretory defect of cervical epithelium

Immunologic compatibility tests Evaluation of sperm aglutination and immobilization

Other tests (female) Hysteroscopy; karyotype; T_4 level

Other tests (male) Testicular biopsy; vasography; sperm penetration assay; mucus migration test; venography; transrectal ultrasound

•••••• Multidisciplinary Plan

Surgery

Removal of myomas
Polypectomy
Dilitation and curettage
Unilateral or bilateral tuboplasty
Salpingostomy
Ovarian wedge resection (for patients with polycystic ovaries)

Medications

Antiinfective agents
  Therapy based on culture findings
Ovulatory stimulants
  Clomiphene citrate (Clomid), 50-100 mg for 5-7 d
  Gonadotropin (Pergonal), 1 ampule IM for 9-12 d followed by 10,000 IU human chorionic gonadotropin 1 d after last dose of Pergonal
  GnRH (Factrel) as ordered to treat hypothalamic amenorrhea
Estrogens
  Estrone (Hormonin, others), 0.7-1.4 mg po qd cyclically
  Conjugated estrogens (Premarin), 0.625-3.75 mg qd po cyclically
Pituitary-related agents
  Bromocriptin (Parlodel), individually adjusted

Assisted Reproductive Technologies

Artificial insemination
In vitro fertilization (IVF)
Gamete intrafallopian transfer (GIFT)
Zygote intrafallopian transfer (ZIFT)
Embryo transfer (ET)

General Management

Counseling and psychotherapy

Improvement in coital technique

Comments

IVF: There is some maternal and neonatal morbidity associated with IVF. In vitro fertilization mothers have more multiple gestations, pregnancy-induced hypertension (PIH), premature labor, labor induction and preterm deliveries than their matched counterparts in clinical studies. Infants conceived using IVF have lower birth weights, shorter gestations, longer hospitalizations, more days of oxygen therapy, more days of continuous positive airway pressure, and an increased prevalence of respiratory distress syndrome (RDS), patent ductus arteriosus, and sepsis.[47]

GIFT: Hysteroscopic GIFT under local anesthesia (achieved by cannulating tubal ostia after hysteroscopic visualization) in patients with documented tubal patency at a previous diagnostic laparoscopy has demonstrated comparable results as laparoscopic GIFT under general anesthesia. This process can be achieved in a less costly outpatient setting and ensures advantages in terms of repeatability.[42]

NURSING CARE

Nursing Assessment

Couple

Name; age; occupation; religion; ethnocultural influences; years of marriage; previous marriages; duration of involuntary infertility; habits; diet; health status; exposure to alcohol, nicotine, narcotics, quinine, hormones, antineoplastic agents, metals, dyes, and radiation; physical or psychic stress

Female

Health history

Tuberculosis; venereal disease; endometriosis; tumors; signs of endocrine dysfunction, such as delayed deep tendon reflexes, galactorrhea, visual disturbances

Gynecologic history

Menarche; frequency, duration, and amount of menstrual flow; menstrual irregularities; evidence of dysmenorrhea; mittelschmerz; increased midcycle discharge; pelvic inflammatory disease; previous surgical procedure including pelvic operation and appendectomy

Obstetric history

Full-term deliveries; complications; abortions (reason, if elective) or premature deliveries

Conception control history

Type of contraceptives used and duration of use

Sexual history

Frequency of coitus; postcoital practices; libido; orgasm capacity; position during and after intercourse; use of lubricants; sexual involvement with other partners

Male

Health history

Tuberculosis; venereal infection; mumps; orchitis; varicocele; previous surgical procedure including orchiopexy and herniorrhaphy; hydrocele; injury to genitals

Sexual history

Frequency of coitus; technique and position; premature ejaculation; adequacy of erection; timing of coitus; sexual involvement with other partners

Male and Female Psychosocial Factors

Motivation for pregnancy; perception of and feelings related to inability to achieve conception; effect of sociocultural and familial factors related to desired pregnancy

NOTE: Because the couple-is-the-patient idea may serve to mask the very different responses, interests, and needs regarding infertility of the two people constituting the couple, it is important to dialogue with the individuals to identify important differences that may be present between the man and woman.[37]

Nursing Dx & Intervention

Knowledge deficit related to lack of information about optimum sexual technique; sexual dysfunction related to lack of knowledge

- Ensure that both partners are aware of practices that promote conception, including the following:
  - Intercourse every 2 days during fertile period
  - Woman in supine position with man astride
  - Woman's hips elevated on pillow with thighs flexed
  - Avoidance of commercial lubricants
  - Penis maintained in vagina without thrusting for short time after ejaculation
  - Woman remaining in bed with hips elevated for approximately 30 minutes after coitus
  - Woman not urinating or douching for at least 1 hour after coitus

Anticipatory grieving related to potential for loss of reproductive function

- Support couple's grief through listening and offering explanations about their reactions.
- Promote cohesiveness; avoid laying "blame" on one person.
- Help couple express their feelings when they find it difficult to do so.
- Help couple explore their feelings and eventually accept the normal ambivalence toward expectations of being a parent.
- Promote grief work with responses to grieving process of denial, isolation, depression, anger, guilt, fear, and rejection.

Ineffective individual coping related to situation crises

- Assess both partners' coping mechanisms.
- Explain consequences of prolonged stress

- Help couple problem solve in constructive manner.
- Discuss alternatives to treatment.
- See also p. 1739.

Body image disturbance related to perceived or actual change in body structure or function

- Encourage patient to express feelings about the way patient views himself or herself.
- Clarify misconceptions.
- Promote sharing of feelings with partner.
- Explore patient's personal strengths and resources.
- Promote discussion regarding resolution of altered body image.

Evaluation

Knowledge of sexual functions is increased Patient indicates practice of optimum sexual technique. Patient relates valid information about sexual function.

Grief is resolved Patient has expressed grief, shared concerns with partner, and planned constructively for future.

Patient uses adaptive coping behavior Patient verbalizes feelings about infertility and altered body image and can identify personal strengths. Patient follows through with decisions and appropriate actions.

Realistic self-concept is achieved Patient exhibits adaptive responses to altered body image through verbal statements.

BREAST DISEASE

■ CYSTIC BREAST DISEASE

Fibrocystic disease of the breast is the presence of singular or multiple cysts in the breast. NOTE: The College of American Pathologists formally abandoned the term *fibrocystic disease* as a histologic diagnosis in 1985.[2] Other descriptive names are used in association with cystic conditions, including benign mastopathy, chronic cystic mastitis, fibroadenosis, cystic mammary hyperplasia or dysplasia, cystic mastopathy, cyclic nodularity, blue dome cyst, Bloodgood's disease, and Schimelbusch's disease.

Fibrocystic breast changes are the single most common condition of the breast, accounting for more than half of all surgical procedures on the female breast. It affects 10% to 25% of all women, but it is not always clinically apparent and frequently is undiscovered until postmortem examination. Fibrocystic changes occur primarily in the menopause years and are a rare occurrence before adolescence and after menopause.

Controversy exists as to whether cystic changes in the breast constitute a disease process because the defining characteristics are estimated to be clinically present in 50% of women and histologically present in 90% of women.

•••••• Pathophysiology

Cystic breast changes are thought to be caused by hormonal imbalance in the reproductive years, principally because of estrogen excess and progesterone deficiency during the luteal phase of the menstrual cycle. They are characterized by pain and tenderness of one or both breasts immediately before menses. The cysts may be unilateral or bilateral, firm, regular in shape, and mobile and are most common in the upper outer quadrant of the breasts. Their size may fluctuate during the cycle.

A wide variety of morphologic changes can be found, ranging from an overgrowth of fibrous stroma to a proliferation of epithelium. Four patterns of morphologic change are distinguishable; fibrosis, cyst formation, sclerosing adenosis, and duct epithelial hyperplasia.

Fibrosis is characterized by an overgrowth of stromal fibrous tissue. This type is usually unilateral and occurs most often in women from 30 to 35 years of age. The breast becomes larger before menses and then regresses with a recurrence of pain and tenderness in the next cycle.

Cystic disease is also known as Bloodgood's disease, Schimmelbusch's disease, and blue dome cyst. It is characterized by the formation of cysts, usually over 3 mm in diameter. It is thought to be caused by dilation of ducts and hyperplasia of ductal epithelium concurrent with the menstrual cycle. This type of disease is more common in women between 45 and 55 years of age. Multiple bilateral cysts are readily palpable and usually distinguishable from the characteristic solitary focus of carcinoma.

The histologic characteristics of sclerosing adenosis are proliferation of small acini and intralobular fibrosis. It is most commonly unilateral and more common in women between 35 and 45 years of age.

Epithelial hyperplasia of the ducts are ill-defined masses found most commonly in women between 35 and 45 years of age. The more atypical the hyperplasia, the greater the risk of carcinoma.

Biopsy and examination of the tissue is the only method of specifically differentiating fibrocystic disease from carcinoma.

Women with fibrocystic disease have a nearly threefold greater risk of developing carcinoma than women without it.

•••••• Diagnostic Studies and Findings

Mammography

Ultrasonography

Stereotactic or ultrasound-guided percutaneous biopsy Fibrosis: collagenous stroma engulfing epithelial structures and obliterating periductal and myxomatous stroma; cysts: overgrowth of stroma with cystic dilation of ducts filled with serous opaque fluid; fibroadenosis: proliferation and compression of small ducts and gland buds; epithelial hyperplasia: proliferation of epithelium lining duct, sometimes with solid masses of hyperplastic cells encroaching into lumen of duct

Needle aspiration of cyst Varying histologic descriptions

•••••• Multidisciplinary Plan

Surgery

Subcutaneous mastectomy in lieu of multiple diagnostic biopsies and associated discomfort

Medication

Progestins or progestogens

Progesterone (Proluton, others), 5-50 mg IM during second half of cycle

General Management

Local heat

Support bra

Avoidance of foods with methylxanthines, including tea, coffee, cola, and chocolate, which tend to stimulate cyclic adenosine monophosphate (cAMP) and increase metabolic activity in breast

NURSING CARE

Nursing Assessment

Breast

Palpation of discrete or diffuse nodules; asymmetry; nipple discharge; irregular firmness; cyclic pain of cystic area during premenstrual period

Nursing Dx & Intervention

Anxiety related to uncertainty of final diagnosis

- Explain rationale for tests and procedures *to allay anxiety.*
- Encourage verbalization of concerns.
- Answer patient's questions and explain disease process.
- See also p. 1669.

Pain related to pressure of cysts on adjacent structures

- Encourage use of bra *to maintain adequate breast support.*

Patient Education/Home Care Planning

1. Ensure that the patient understands the method for breast self-examination (BSE) and can demonstrate this procedure.
2. Explain that only 10% to 15% of masses are malignant and that 90% of cancers confined to the breast are curable.
3. Outline a diet that avoids foods with methylxanthines.
4. Explain importance of maintaining appointments for clinical examination and mammography.

Evaluation

Anxiety is diminished   Patient demonstrates adaptive responses to knowledge about prognosis related to fibrocystic disease.

Patient understands and monitors condition   Patient demonstrates BSE and lists progression of signs and symptoms to report to health care provider, including increase in dimension of cyst, change in texture, lack of clearly defined margins, nipple discharge, severe pain, immobility of cysts, skin dimpling or retraction, and increasing asymmetry. Patient avoids foods with methylxanthines.

Pain is managed   Patient adjusts supportive bra *to achieve breast support.*

MEDICAL INTERVENTIONS AND RELATED NURSING CARE

DILITATION AND CURETTAGE; HYSTEROSCOPY

Description and Rationale

Dilitation and curettage is the expansion of the cervix and scraping of the uterine endometrium. It is performed for diagnostic or therapeutic purposes, such as the removal of products of conception after an incomplete abortion. Hysteroscopy is the visual inspection of the interior of the uterus through an endoscope. This procedure has not been found to be reliable in the diagnosis of tubal pathology.[45]

NURSING CARE

Nursing Assessment

Bleeding

Vaginal hemorrhage

Pain

Pelvic and low back pain

Signs of infection

Foul odor of vaginal drainage; fever; hematuria

Nursing Dx & Intervention

Risk for infection related to invasive procedure

- Administer perineal care after elimination as necessary.
- Explain importance of wiping from front to back after elimination.

- If vaginal packing was used, ensure that it is removed by the physician as indicated in the medical plan of care.

Pain related to uterine cramping

- Administer analgesics as ordered.

Patient Education/Home Care Planning

1. Explain that spotting and bleeding may last a week and may be accompanied by cramping.
2. Explain signs and symptoms of infection that should be reported to the physician.
3. Inform the patient that coitus and douching should be avoided for 2 weeks.
4. Explain that minimum activity is preferred for a day or two.

Evaluation

There are no signs of infection Color and amount of urine are normal. Vaginal drainage decreases in amount and is not purulent.

Comfort is achieved Patient says that she is comfortable and does not have uterine cramping.

■ SALPINGECTOMY
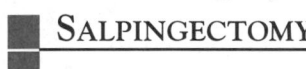

Description and Rationale

Salpingectomy is the removal of one or both fallopian tubes. It is performed for ectopic or tubal pregnancy (see Emergency Alert box), chronic salpingitis, and hydrosalpinx.

Nursing Care

The care of a patient undergoing salpingectomy is similar to that of a patient with a total hysterectomy, with a few exceptions:

Anti-Rh globulin should be administered to an Rh-negative woman after a unilateral salpingectomy for tubal pregnancy.

The patient should understand the importance of preventing pregnancy for at least 2 months or as indicated by the physician and that reproductive ability is usually diminished, especially if a tubal pregnancy occurred as a result of acute or chronic salpingitis.

Her partner should be included in the discuss of feelings of loss and grief, especially if pregnancy was desired.

■ HYSTERECTOMY AND BILATERAL SALPINGO-OOPHORECTOMY

Description and Rationale

Surgical removal of the uterus, both fallopian tubes, and the ovaries is most commonly done to treat malignant neoplastic

disease of the reproductive tract and chronic endometriosis. Other indications for hysterectomy are an enlarged myoma, adenomyosis, and hydrosalpinx. If possible, a portion of one ovary is left to prevent symptoms of sudden menopause. The patient is under anesthesia during the procedure.

Contraindication and Cautions

Abdominal hysterectomy is preferred to vaginal hysterectomy or laparoscopic hysterectomy when the diagnosis is in question and exploration is needed, when the uterus is excessively large, when an incidental appendectomy is to be done, and when there is a history of severe pelvic inflammatory disease.

Preprocedural Nursing Care

A douche with an antiseptic solution is usually ordered the evening before or the morning of surgery, or both.

NURSING CARE

Nursing Assessment

Perineum

Vaginal hemorrhage; vaginal discharge other than serosanguineous; vaginal discharge with foul odor

Temperature

Fever

! EMERGENCY ALERT

ECTOPIC PREGNANCY

Ectopic pregnancy occurs when the fertilized ovum implants anywhere except the uterine cavity. The ovum commonly implants in the fallopian tube (95%), abdominal cavity, ovary, or cervix. Rupture usually occurs after the twelfth week of pregnancy.

Assessment

- Assess client's last menstrual period and knowledge of pregnancy; pregnancy status is often unknown.
- Assess pain and rate from mild to severe.
- Determine presence of Kehr's sign, right shoulder pain suggesting peritoneal irritation.
- Assess for abdominal rigidity, which may indicate intraperitoneal hemorrhage, shock.
- Evaluate vaginal bleeding: absent, spotty, or profuse.

Interventions

- Obtain IV access; provide fluid resuscitation as indicated.
- Monitor vital signs; hypotension is common.
- Draw labs; prepare blood transfusion.
- Prepare for gynecologic consultation, surgery.

Abdomen

Diminished or absent bowel sounds

Redness, pain, swelling, or drainage at site of incision of abdominal or laparoscopic procedure

Pelvic Area

Congestion as evidenced by fullness, pain, or thrombophlebitis of legs

Urinary Output

Rention of urine, with or without overflow; burning, urgency, and frequency of urination; vaginal leakage of urine

Mental Status

Emotional investment in value of uterus; signs of depression; misconceptions about procedure

Potential Complications

Paralytic ileus; pneumonia; ligation of ureter during surgery

Nursing Dx & Intervention

Altered renal, cerebral, cardiopulmonary, gastrointestinal, and peripheral tissue perfusion related to invasive procedure

- Provide routine measures for postanesthesia recovery.
- Monitor blood pressure, temperature, pulse, and respiration every 4 hours for 24 hours, then four times a day for 2 days or as ordered.
- Avoid placing patient in high Fowler's position and placing pressure under knees *to promote venous circulation in legs.*
- Apply antiembolic stockings as ordered *to provide intermittent compression and to prevent thrombus formation in legs.*
- Auscultate abdomen for bowel sounds every 6 to 8 hours. permit nothing by mouth until bowel sounds are active *to prevent paralytic ileus.*
- Assist with initial ambulation as needed *to support if faintness occurs secondary to orthostatic hypotension.*

Risk for fluid volume deficit related to NPO status

- Administer parenteral fluids as ordered, progressing to 3000 ml of fluid orally daily.
- Monitor intake and output *to ensure appropriate hydration and fluid balance.*

Ineffective breathing pattern related to abdominal discomfort

- Assist with turning, coughing, and deep breathing every 2 hours or as needed, decreasing frequency as patient increases general activity *to prevent stasis of pulmonary secretions and risk of pneumonia.*
- Auscultate chest for breath sounds four times a day for 2 days and as needed thereafter *to ensure that breath sounds are clear.*

Impaired skin integrity related to invasive surgical procedure

- Observe for drainage or hemorrhage every 2 to 4 hours, decreasing frequency as indicated.
- Change or reinforce dressing as indicated.

Constipation related to decreased peristalsis associated with anesthesia

- Progress to high-protein or high-fiber diet as ordered *to promote adequate nutritional status for wound healing.*
- Give Harris flush or insert rectal tube *for gas as indicated.*
- Give stool softeners or mild laxatives as ordered *to prevent constipation and straining at stool.*

Altered patterns of urinary elimination related to neuromuscular impairment associated with anesthesia

- Maintain closed gravity drainage.
- Promote micturition when catheter is removed *to avoid the need for recatheterization.*
- Monitor for signs of urine retention, such as small amounts of urine voided or a distended bladder.
- Encourage voiding on commode rather than bed pan to promote complete emptying of bladder.

Bathing/hygiene self-care deficit related to discomfort and mobility

- Assist with bed bath, allowing patient to bathe or shower alone when indicated.
- Administer catheter care twice a day or as needed until removed.

Body image disturbance related to change in body structure and function

- Encourage patient's comments and questions about surgery, progress and prognosis *to encourage understanding of same.*
- Reinforce correct information and provide factual information *to correct any misconceptions.*
- Encourage patient to talk about feelings with significant others.
- Acknowledge the patient's feelings to support her in sharing this information with significant others.

Pain related to invasive surgical procedure

- Administer analgesics as ordered.
- Assist with moving and positioning *to promote comfort.*

Sexual dysfunction (risk for) related to altered body function

- Encourage patient to express any concerns in a private setting.
- Avoid premature responses and reassurances *to promote full expression of concerns.*

- Be aware of own values regarding sexuality and body image *to avoid transference or overidentification with the patient.*
- Consistently use terminology the patient understands.

Patient Education/Home Care Planning

1. Explain to the patient the importance of avoiding coitus or douching for 4 to 6 weeks or as indicated by physician to maintain integrity of the vaginal cuff, to maintain the healing process, and to prevent infection.
2. Explain to the patient the importance of walking at regular intervals and to avoid sitting for prolonged periods at home or when traveling.
3. Explain abdominal incision care and signs of infection to report to the physician, including redness, swelling, pain, or discharge at the incision site, increase in vaginal drainage, or presence of foul odor.
4. Emphasize the need to avoid heavy lifting and vigorous activities after surgery, as indicated by physician.
5. Instruct the patient to maintain regular outpatient gynecologic examinations.
6. If both ovaries have been removed, explain that surgical menopause will occur and that replacement estrogen may be ordered.
7. Explain that menstruation will no longer occur and that pregnancy is no longer possible.
8. Explain the importance of appropriate diet and exercise.

Evaluation

Body functioning is normal Wound healing is normal. Vaginal drainage decreasing over 2 to 4 weeks. Bowel and bladder elimination are adequate. Ventilatory pattern has returned to presurgical state. Fluid balance is evident.

Patient resumes activities of daily living Patient walks with erect posture. Patient avoids prolonged sitting and heavy work until physician permits them.

There is no infection; skin integrity is restored There is no evidence of inflammation, swelling, pain, or discharge at abdominal site, no fever, and no purulent or odorous vaginal discharge. Urinary elimination pattern is normal.

Patient demonstrates adaptive responses related to self-concept and body image Patient asks appropriate questions. Patient gives correct information related to procedure and prognosis. Patient speaks appropriately about body parts that are present or absent.

Comfort is achieved Patient says she has no lower abdominal, pelvic, or vaginal pain.

Patient makes sexual adjustment Patient indicates that she has discussed concerns with partner. Patient expresses sexual concerns and is working toward resolution of any related problems.

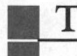

TUBAL LIGATION

Description and Rationale

Tubal ligation is tying of the fallopian tubes. Usually the procedure includes excision of a portion of the tubes to ensure that their continuity is disrupted. The procedure is done through the laparoscope with the patient under a general or local anesthetic. However, it can be performed through an abdominal incision, as is often done in the immediate postpartum period.

NURSING CARE

Nursing Assessment

Pain

Abdominal pain

Signs of Infection

Inflammation at site of incision; fever

Other Potential Complications

Abdominal distention; absence of bowel sounds; body image disturbances

Nursing Dx & Intervention

Impaired skin integrity related to invasive surgical procedure

- Observe site of incision for inflammation.
- Keep dressing dry; patient should not shower for at least 24 hours.

Pain related to altered bowel motility

- Auscultate bowel sounds *to confirm peristalsis before giving food or fluids by mouth.*
- Administer stool softeners as indicated.
- Give Harris flush or insert rectal tube *to relieve abdominal distention.*

Pain related to incision

- Administer analgesics as ordered.

Body image disturbance related to change in body structure and function

- Encourage patient to express feelings and concerns.
- Correct any misconceptions. Explain that hormonal therapy is not necessary *because ovaries are not affected by this procedure.*

Patient Education/Home Care Planning

1. Explain that sterility is considered permanent and is rarely reversible.

2. Explain that libido will not be diminished and is often increased by removal of fear of pregnancy.
3. Inform the patient that ovarian function will continue because the ovaries are not removed in this procedure.
4. Explain signs and symptoms of wound infection that should be reported to the physician.

Evaluation

Incision heals normally   Site of incision shows no sign of inflammation or infection.

Patient has normal body functioning   Vital signs are within normal limits. Bowel function is normal. Pain is controlled.

Patient has no disturbance in self-concept   Patient does not report adverse changes in body image.

References

1. AbdRabbo S, Atta A: Aspiration and tetracycline sclerotherapy for management of simple ovarian cysts, *Int J Gynaecol Obstet* 50(2):171, 1995.
2. American College of Obstetricians and Gynecologists: *Guidelines for Women's Health Care,* Washington, DC, 1996, College.
3. ACOG Technical Bulletin: Endometriosis: The American College of Obstetricians and Gynecologists 184:No. 184, September 1993.
4. Ault KA, Faro S: Pelvic inflammatory disease. Current diagnostic criteria and treatment guidelines, *Postgrad Med* (93)2:85, 1993.
5. Balasch J et al: Trial of routine gonadotropin releasing hormone agonist treatment before abdominal hysterectomy for leiomyoma, *Acta Obstet Gynecol Scand* 74(7):562, 1995.
6. Barnhart KT, Freeman EW, Sondheimer SJ: A clinician's guide to the premenstrual syndrome, *Med Clin North Am* 79(6):1457, 1995.
7. Benson R: *Handbook of obstetrics and gynecology,* Los Altos, Calif, 1983, Lange Medical.
8. Bernhard LA: Understanding fibroids, *Innovations Women's Health Nurs* 1(2):21, 1994.
9. Bobak IM, Jensen MD: *Essentials of maternity nursing: the nurse and the childbearing family,* St Louis, 1994, Mosby.
10. Boyd ME: The risks and benefits of hormone replacement therapy, *Can J Surg* 38(5):415, 1995.
11. Brill AI: What is the role of hysteroscopy in the management of abnormal uterine bleeding? *Clin Obstet Gynecol* 38(2):319, 1995.
12. Cano et al: Effect of aging on the female reproductive system: evidence for a role of uterine senescence in the decline in female fecundity, *Fertil Steril* 64(3):584, 1995.
13. Colditz GA et al: The use of estrogens and progestins and the risk of breast cancer in menopausal women, *N Engl J Med* 332:1589, 1995.
14. Creehan PA: Toxic shock syndrome: an opportunity for nursing intervention, *J Obstet Gynecol Neonatal Nurs* 24(6):557, 1995.
15. Edge V, Miller M: *Women's health care,* St Louis, 1994, Mosby.
16. Freeman EW et al: A double-blind trial of oral progesterone, alprazolam, and placebo in the treatment of severe premenstrual syndrome, *JAMA* 274(1):51, 1995.
17. Gurgan T et al: Laparoscopic CO₂ laser uterine nerve ablation for treatment of drug resistant primary dysmenorrhea, *Fertil Steril* 58(2):422, 1992.
18. Herbst AL et al: *Comprehensive gynecology,* St Louis, 1987, Mosby.
19. Hillis S, Marchbanks PA, Peterson HB: Uterine size and risk of complications among women undergoing abdominal hysterectomy for leiomyoma, *Obstet Gynecol* 87(4):539, 1996.
20. Hirsch AM, Hirsch SM: The long-term psychosocial effects of infertility, *J Obstet Gynecol Neonatal Nurs* 24(6):517, 1995.
21. Hulka CA et al: Endometrial polyps, hyperplasia, and carcinoma in postmenopausal women: differentiation with endovaginal sonography, *Radiology* 191(3):755, 1994.
22. Jennings JC: Abnormal uterine bleeding, *Med Clin North Am* 79(6):1357, 1995.
23. Kim MJ, McFarland GK, McLane AM: *Pocket guide to nursing diagnoses,* St Louis, 1995, Mosby.
24. Kottmann LM: Pelvic inflammatory disease: clinical overview, *J Obstet Gynecol Neonatal Nurs* 24(8):759, 1995.
25. Lewis LL: One year in the life of a woman with premenstrual syndrome: a case study, *Nurs Res* 44(2):111, 1995.
26. Lin P, Falcone T, Tulandi T: Excision of ovarian dermoid cyst by laparoscopy and by laparotomy, *Am J Obstet Gynecol* 173(3):769, 1995.
27. Lip GY, Beevers G, Zarifis J: Hormone replacement therapy and cardiovascular risk: the cardiovascular physicians' viewpoint, *J Internal Medicine,* 283(5):389, 1995.
28. Maiolatesi CR, Peddicord K: Methotrexate for nonsurgical treatment of ectopic pregnancy: nursing implications, *J Obstet Gynecol Neonatal Nurs* 25(3):205, 1996.
29. Masters W, Johnson V, Kolodny A: *Human sexuality,* Boston, 1988, Scott Foresman/Little, Brown
30. Newcomb PA et al: Long-term hormone replacement therapy and risk of breast cancer in postmenopausal women, *Am J Epidemiol* 142(8):788, 1995.
31. Newton N: Interrelationships between sexual responsiveness, birth and breastfeeding. In Zubin J, Money J, editors: *Contemporary sexual behavior: critical issues in the 1970s,* Baltimore, 1973, Johns Hopkins University Press.
32. Oleson T, Flocco W: Randomized controlled study of premenstrual symptoms treated with ear, hand, and foot reflexology, *Obstet Gynecol* 82(6):906, 1993.
33. Pasley WW: Sacrospinous suspension: a local practitioner's experience, *Am J Obstet Gynecol* 173(2):440, 1995.
34. Perper et al: Dysmenorrhea is related to the number of implants in endometriosis patients, *Fertil Steril* 63(3):500, 1995.
35. Reubinoff BE et al: Effects of hormone replacement therapy on weight, body composition, fat distribution and food intake in early postmenopausal women: a prospective study, *Fertil Steril* 64(5):963, 1995.
36. Rozenberg S et al: Compliance to hormone replacement therapy, *Int J Fertil Menopausal Stud* 40(suppl 1):23, 1995.
37. Sandelowski M: On infertility, *J Obstet Gynecol Neonatal Nurs* 23(9):749, 1994.
38. Schaff EA et al: Methotrexate and misoprostol when surgical abortion fails, *Obstet Gynecol* 87(3):450, 1996.
39. Schlievert PM: Comparison of cotton and cotton/rayon tampons for effect on producing toxic shock syndrome toxin, *J Infect Dis* 172(4):1112, 1995.
40. Scholes et al: Vaginal douching as a risk factor for acute pelvic inflammatory disease, *Obstet Gynecol* 81(4):601, 1993.
41. Seidel HM et al: *Mosby's guide to physical examination,* ed 2, St Louis, 1991, Mosby.
42. Seracchioli R et al: Gamete intrafallopian transfer: prospective randomized comparison of hysteroscopic and laparoscopic transfer techniques, *Fertil Steril* 64(2):355, 1995.
43. Shibata HR: Hormone replacement therapy: boon or bane? *Can J Surg* 38(5):409, 1995.
44. Spitzer M, Benjamin F: Ascites due to endometriosis, *Obstet Gynecol Surv* 50(8):628, 1995.
45. Swart P et al: The accuracy of hysterosalpingography in the diagnosis of tubal pathology: a meta-analysis, *Fertil Steril* 64(3):486, 1995.
46. Sweet RL: Role of bacterial vaginosis in pelvic inflammatory disease, *Clin Infect Dis* 20(suppl 2):S271, 1995.
47. Tallo CP et al: Maternal and neonatal morbidity associated with in vitro fertilization, J PediatrI 127(5):794, 1995.
48. Tucker SM et al: *Patient care standards,* St Louis, 1996, Mosby.
49. Udoff L, Langenberg P, Adashi EY: Combined continuous hormone replacement therapy: a critical review, *Obstet Gynecol* 86(2):306, 1995.
50. Velebil P et al: Rate of hospitalization for gynecologic disorders among reproductive-age women in the United States, *Obstet Gynecol* 86(5):764, 1995.
51. Wortman M, Daggett A: Hysteroscopic endomyometrial resection: a new technique for the treatment of menorrhagia, *Obstet Gynecol* 83(2):295, 1994.
52. Yes SSC, Jaffe RB: *Reproductive endocrinology,* Philadelphia, 1991, Saunders.

Renal System

11

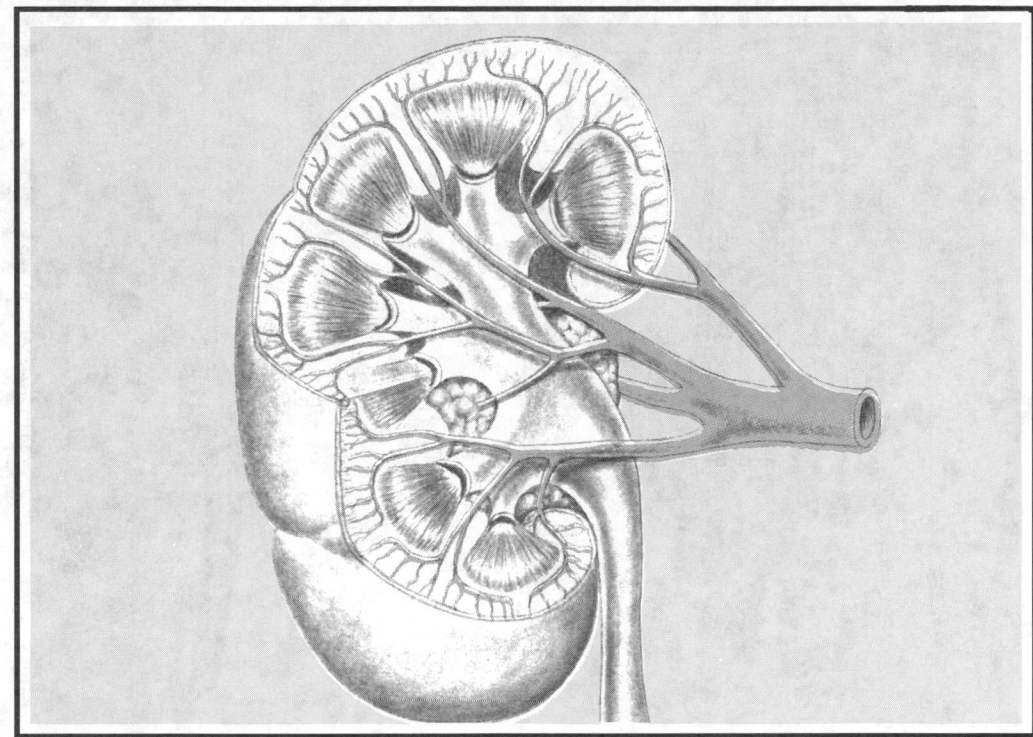

OVERVIEW

The renal system functions to excrete water-soluble waste products from the body and to maintain the homeostasis of plasma water, electrolytes, and pH.

Renal function depends on the normal and interrelated functioning of the cardiovascular, nervous, endocrine, and urinary collecting systems. The cardiovascular system delivers the blood to be filtered, sustains the hydrostatic pressure needed for filtration, and provides specialized capillaries that do the filtering. The nervous system helps regulate blood pressure, thus contributing to the first two functions.

The nervous system also controls the process of urination (see Chapter 12) and interacts with the activity of the endocrine system to affect renal function directly through aldosterone and antidiuretic hormone (ADH). The calyces, pelvis, ureters, urinary bladder, and urethra form the urinary collecting system. The urethra provides the exit for urine from the body.

Urine volume varies with food and fluid intake and extrarenal fluid losses through feces, perspiration, and respiration. A diurnal variation in volume that is associated with light-dark periods or sleep-wake patterns occurs.

The kidneys have excretory and nonexcretory functions vital to the regulation of substances essential to the human body.

Excretory functions are excretion of end products of metabolism (urea, creatinine, uric acid, phosphates, sulfates, nitrates, and phenols); excretion of excess normal fluid and electrolyte components (H_2O, Na^+, K^+, HCO_3^-, Cl^-, H^+), thus maintaining the volume, pH, and osmolality of the extracellular and intracellular fluids; and excretion of certain drugs and other substances (penicillin and metabolites of hormones).

Nonexcretory functions are secretion of renin, erythropoietin, kallikrein, and prostaglandins; metabolism of carbohydrates, lipids, plasma proteins, and peptide hormones such as insulin and glucagon; and regulation of vitamin D metabolism.

For additional information on the genitourinary system, see Chapter 12.

•••••• Anatomy, Physiology, and Related Pathophysiology

The kidneys are located in the posterior abdominal cavity in the retroperitoneal area to the right and left of the lumbar spinal column and are level with the T12 and the L1 to L3 vertebrae.

Each kidney is covered by a tough capsule, surrounded by a cushion of fat, and supported by fascia. Each kidney is partially protected by the ribs. The lower end of each kidney extends below the ribs; the right one is lower than the left (Figure 11-1). The kidneys move downward during respiration as the diaphragm contracts.

The renal artery, vein, nerves, lymph vessels, and ureters all enter or leave the kidney on the medial surface in the indented region called the hilum or renal sinus.

Each kidney has an outer cortex, an inner medulla, and a pelvis—the area in which urine is collected (Figure 11-2). The fluid filtered from the blood travels through the nephron to

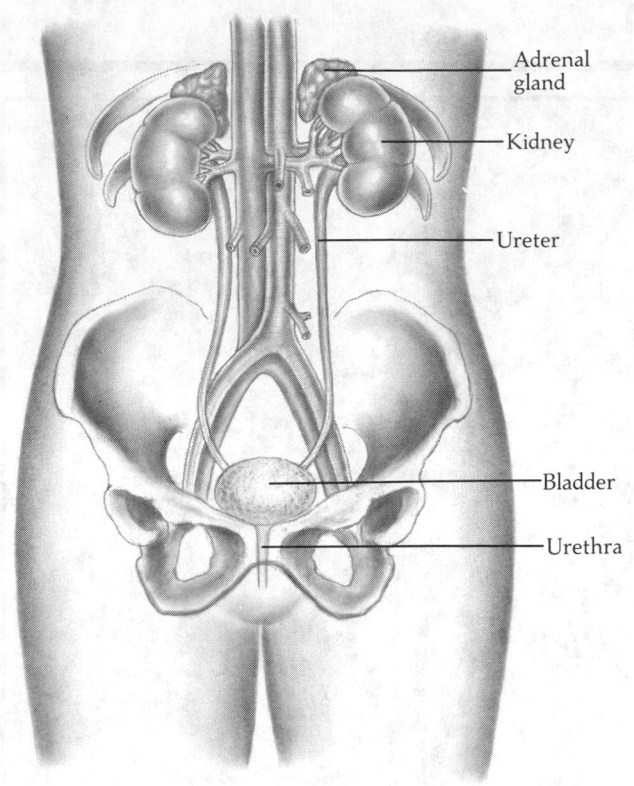

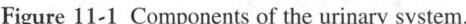

Figure 11-1 Components of the urinary system.

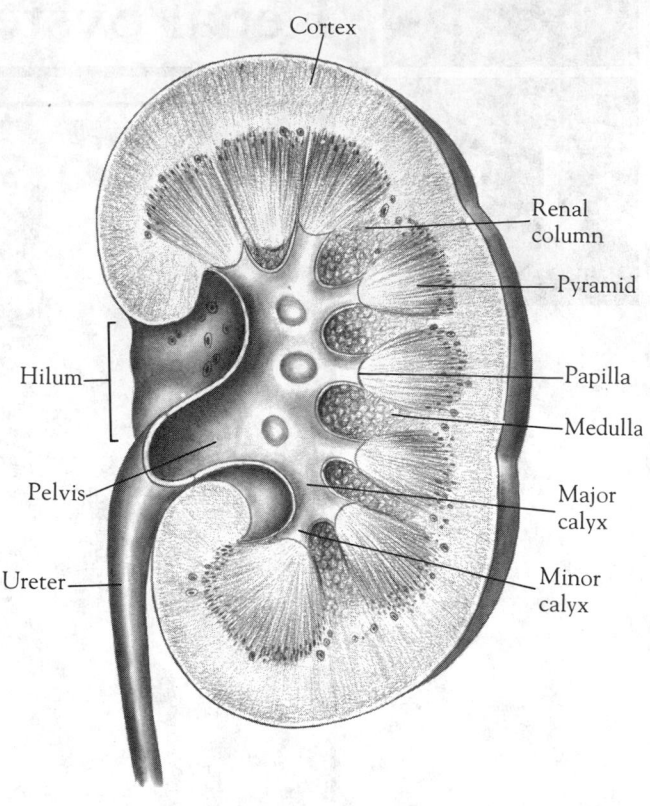

Figure 11-2 Cross section of kidney.

reach the large collecting ducts (ducts of Bellini) that form the renal pyramids in the medulla. The ducts empty into a calyx at the papilla. Interspersed between the pyramids is cortical tissue known as the "renal columns" (columns of Bertin). The glomerulus, proximal and distal tubules, and most of the loop of Henle and the collecting ducts are in the medulla.

Blood Supply to the Kidneys

The renal arteries are short and wide to ensure that 20% to 25% of the resting cardiac output (about 1200 ml/min) passes through the kidneys. This volume exceeds the amount needed to meet the kidneys' oxygen needs; it permits the formation of filtrate that is needed to maintain homeostasis of the blood.

Almost 90% of the blood flows rapidly through the cortex; the rest moves slowly through the medulla. The renal artery branches into interlobar, arcuate, and interlobular arteries (Figure 11-3). Veins draining the kidneys follow the same pattern as the arteries.

Nephrons are divided into superficial cortical and juxtamedullary nephrons. The efferent arteriole of the superficial cortical nephron divides to form a peritubular capillary network. The efferent arteriole of the juxtamedullary nephron branches to form a peritubular network and a series of vascular loops, the vasa recta, that form a capillary network around the collecting ducts and ascending limbs of the loope of Henle. Each nephron is perfused by

peritubular capillaries arising from the efferent arterioles of many different glomeruli.

Each nephron can control the amount of blood that enters and leaves the glomerulus by means of the afferent and efferent arterioles. Such autoregulation permits the kidney to respond to variations in blood flow and pressure.

Autonomic nerve fibers are found in the kidneys. They are thought to mediate renal vasoconstriction.

The lymph vessels that drain the kidney are located near the corticomedullary junction.

Nephron

The nephron is the functional unit of the kidney (Figure 11-4). Each nephron is composed of a glomerulus with afferent and efferent arterioles, Bowman's capsule, proximal (convoluted) tubule, loop of Henle, and distal (convoluted) tubule. The nephrons empty into the collecting ducts. The filtrate formed follows the course of the nephron from Bowman's capsule to the collecting ducts.

The major functions of the nephron components are (1) glomerulus: filtration; (2) proximal tubule: reabsorption of sodium, potassium, chloride, bicarbonate, phosphate, glucose, amino acids, urea, and water (ADH not required); secretion of hydrogen ions and some unwanted substances (toxins, drugs); (3) Henle's loop: countercurrent flow, concentration of urine; reabsorption of sodium (passively), chloride (actively), and cal-

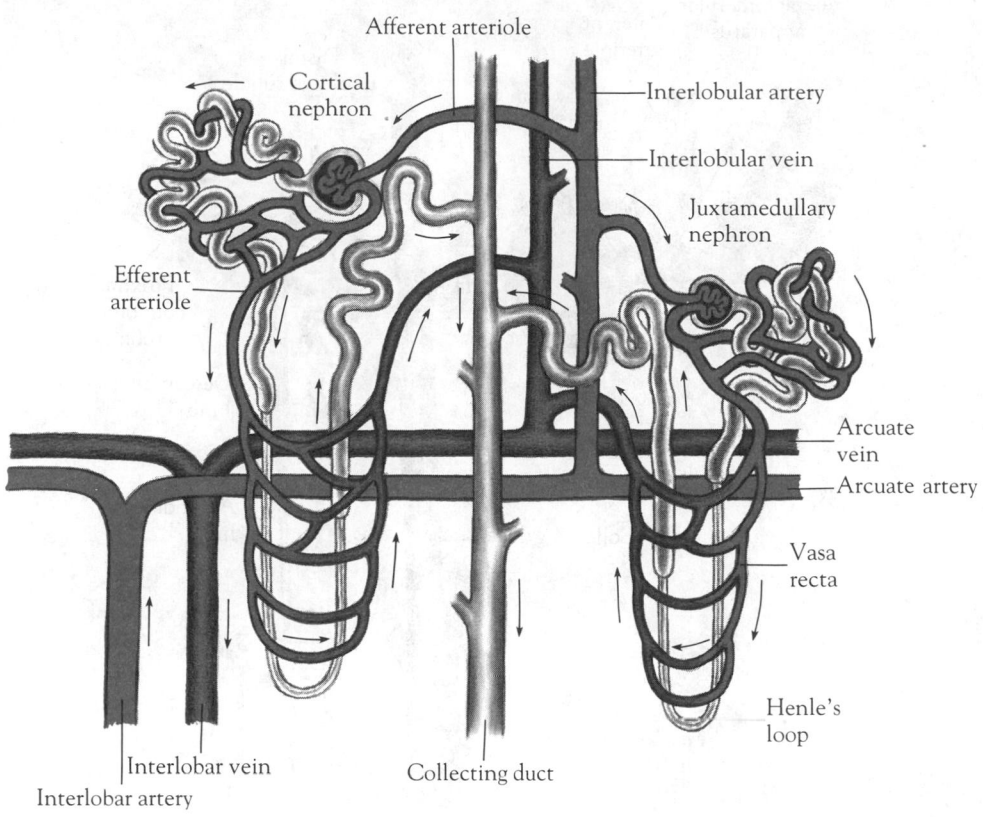

Figure 11-3 Blood supply of nephron.

cium; (4) distal tubule: reabsorption of sodium, potassium, chloride, bicarbonate, urea, and water (ADH required); secretion of hydrogen and potassium; and (5) collecting duct: sodium, potassium, hydrogen, and ammonia may be secreted or reabsorbed; aldosterone increases sodium reabsorption and potassium secretion.

Each nephron part has a distinctive location, histologic structure, and pattern of vascular network. The glomerulus is discussed in some detail because of its major role in renal disease.

Glomerulus The glomerulus, a tuft of capillaries invaginated in Bowman's capsule, serves as the filter. The urinary space in Bowman's capsule is continuous with the lumen of the proximal tubule. A parietal (outer) layer of cells and their basement membrane are continuous with the epithelium and basement membrane of the proximal tubule. The inner wall of the cup-shaped structure is lined with special epithelial cells called "podocytes" that cover the external surface of the glomerular basement membrane (GBM). The podocytes have many processes that extend from their surfaces to form foot processes or pedicles. The GBM has three layers: external, middle, and inner. Fenestrated endothelial cells are located on the inner side of the GBM (toward the capillary lumen). Also on this side of the GBM are the mesangial cells. These irregularly shaped cells embedded in

an amorphous matrix form a slender branching stalk of specialized connective tissue that supports the capillaries.

Thus the filtration barrier has numerous complex layers. Solutes and water move through the pores in the capillary endothelium, loose matrix of the GBM, and filtration slit membranes of the pedicle layer of the podocytes. Molecules are filtered by size and electrical charge. There are fixed anionic charges in various elements of the capillary barrier. Cationic particles have greater clearance than neutral or anionic particles.

All of these glomerular cells (epithelial, endothelial, and mesangial) can undergo pathologic changes: proliferation of epithelial cells may fuse the foot processes (nephrotic syndrome) or obliterate the space in Bowman's capsule and form the crescents of cellular-fibrous material found on microscopic examination associated with rapidly progressive glomerulonephritis. Proliferation of endothelial cells may occlude the capillary lumen such as in hemolytic uremic syndrome. Mesangial cell proliferation occurs as part of diabetic nephropathy and membranoproliferative glomerulonephritis, causing collapse of the glomerular vessels and damage to the GBM.

The GBM may be damaged by deposits of immune complexes in the mesangial, subendothelial, and subepithelial spaces, as well as by damage to the glomerular cells previously described.

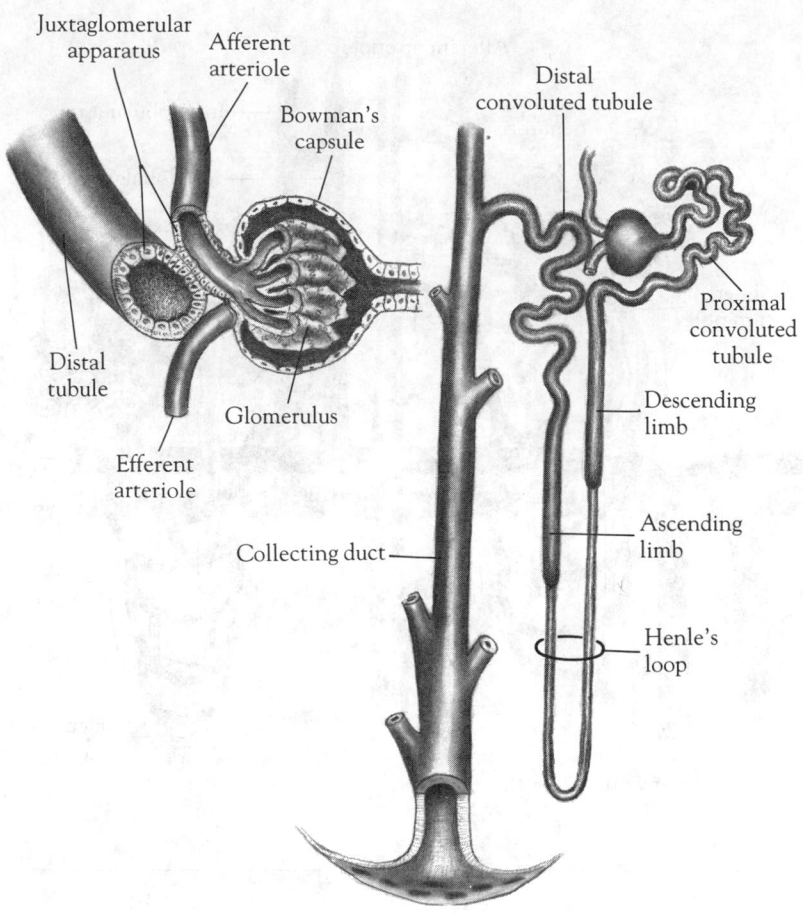

Figure 11-4 Components of nephron.

Tubules and collecting ducts   Since the filtering mechanism is nonspecific, provision is made for reabsorption of essential substances and the secretion of excess substances. The tubules and collecting ducts carry out these functions.

The proximal tubule is lined with cells that have interdigitations to increase their area and surfaces covered by microvilli. This segment has high transport capacity and low transepithelial resistance to the movement of molecules being reabsorbed.

The cells of the loop of Henle appear to be simpler, with cells in the thick limb having highly developed active transport properties. This limb can reabsorb sodium against a concentration gradient and is relatively water impermeable. The thin limb appears to lack the transport systems of the thick limb.

The distal tubule passes between the afferent and efferent arterioles of its glomerulus. In the region where the distal tubule lies near the arteriole, specialized cells, the macula densa, are found (see "Juxtaglomerular Apparatus," p. 928). After this segment the tubular cells become more complex. Cells here can absorb sodium ions without an equivalent amount of negatively charged particles. This segment develops both ionic and electrical gradients.

The collecting tubule has two well-defined cell types, light cells and dark cells. The light cells have sparse microvilli. The dark cells have conspicuous microvilli. As the duct descends to the papilla, the number of dark cells decreases until there are none in the papillary region. The significance of this histologic structure is not clear.

Renal interstitium   Cells that form the interstitium lie between the nephrons and their blood supply. More interstitial cells are found in the medulla than in the cortex. The function of these cells is unknown.

Urine Formation

Glomerular filtration   Total renal blood flow to both kidneys is approximately 1200 ml/min. Approximately 650 ml of this volume is plasma; of this amount about 125 ml filters through the glomerulus to Bowman's capsule. The renal arteries branch directly off the aorta. Therefore blood perfuses the glomerulus at a high pressure. The filtration force is the result of the pressure gradient between the glomerular capillary and Bowman's space, the permeability of the capillary wall, and the difference between the colloid osmotic pressure in Bowman's space and in the capillary lumen.

The rate of glomerular filtration is proportional to filtration pressure. When filtration pressure falls, the pressure receptors in the afferent arteriole activate the renin-angiotensin system of the juxtaglomerular apparatus, which functions to return the afferent pressure to its optimal level.

The glomerular filtrate is an isotonic ultrafiltrate of plasma. Large molecules of protein and the cellular elements of the blood are not filtered. The pH of the glomerular filtrate is about 7.4, or equal to that of plasma. The volume of the filtrate decreases with systemic hypotension, localized renal ischemia, urine outflow obstruction, and changes in the filtering surface. Moderate reductions in glomerular filtration also occur with exercise, pain, and dehydration. Extreme reductions in glomerular filtration occur with severe hypotension. Activation of the sympathetic nervous system can inhibit urine production completely.

Glomerular filtration remains fairly constant even with a marked increase in arterial blood pressure owing to the kidney's autoregulatory mechanisms.

Solute reabsorption and secretion Solutes and water move by active and passive membrane transport mechanisms. They include simple diffusion—electrochemical potential gradient; convection—hydrostatic or osmotic pressure gradient; and mediated transport—facilitated diffusion, electromechanical potential gradient, and active transport, which requires free energy from metabolism.

"Transport maximum" refers to the amount of a substance that can be reabsorbed per minute. It is a constant value, and when the amount of a substance filtered exceeds this value, the excess is excreted in the urine.

The solutes in the glomerular filtrate are threshold and nonthreshold substances. Urea, sodium, potassium, and others are nonthreshold substances, since the urine always contains at least some of each. Glucose and phosphates are threshold substances, since a certain serum level must be reached before the glomerular filtrate will contain enough that the transport maximum of the substance will be exceeded and the excess will be excreted in the urine.

As the glomerular filtrate moves through the tubules, selective reabsorption of water and solutes and selective secretion of solutes occur. A large volume of isosmotic glomerular filtrate is converted into a small volume of hyperosmotic urine. The composition of the glomerular filtrate triggers appropriate activities in the tubular cells. In the tubules about 87% of the water and electrolytes, all of the glucose, and almost all of the amino acids are reabsorbed in the proximal tubules. The proximal tubule preserves metabolically important components and resists the reabsorption of nitrogenous wastes. It secretes foreign substances. The remaining 13% of the glomerular filtrate passes through the loops of Henle and the distal tubules where variable amounts of the water and electrolytes remaining are absorbed. The exact amounts depend on the needs of the body. The final quantity of urine is about 1 ml/min. The pH of the urine may vary from 4.5 to 8.0, and the osmolality may range from one fourth to four times that of plasma (50 to 1200 mOsm/kg). Urine specific gravity may range from 1.001 to 1.030. The usual range is 1.003 to 1.029 with a normal fluid intake.

Urine concentration and dilution Obligatory water reabsorption occurs in the proximal tubule since active reabsorption of sodium is accompanied by passive reabsorption of water and anions. Facultative water reabsorption occurs in the distal tubule. Water and solutes are reabsorbed independently, depending on the body's needs. The urine becomes either concentrated, as water without solutes is reabsorbed, or dilute, as solutes without water are reabsorbed. Antidiuretic hormone controls the volume and concentration of the urine by regulating the reabsorption of water. Atrial naturetic peptide controls sodium reabsorption and excretion. ADH is secreted whenever osmoreceptors in the anterior hypothalamus are stimulated by an increase in osmolality of body fluids or whenever atrial receptors are stimulated by a fall in venous blood volume. ADH combines with receptors in the distal tubule and collecting ducts and increases their capacity to be permeated by water. When enough water has been reabsorbed to bring blood osmolality, volume, and pressure within the normal range, ADH secretion ceases. If ADH raises blood volume and pressure, atrial naturetic peptide decreases sodium reabsorption, which then inhibits ADH secretion and reabsorption of water until blood volume and pressure return to normal.

The medulla increases in hypertonicity with increasing distance from the cortex. The collecting ducts, the long capillary loops (vasa recta), the slower circulation in the medulla, and the impermeability to sodium of the ascending limb of the loop of Henle contribute to the countercurrent mechanism that permits the concentration of urine (Figure 11-5).

In the juxtamedullary nephrons, the loop of Henle serves as a countercurrent multiplier; that is, it returns sodium ions to the peritubular fluid of the medulla, creating hypertonic interstitial fluid. The back-diffusion of urea (possibly a legacy of an evolutionary stage) adds to the osmolality. The degree of hypertonicity depends on antidiuretic hormone, urine flow rate, and the amount and types of solutes in the tubular fluid in the loops of Henle. The osmotic concentration may become four times that of normal extracellular fluid. The vasa recta loops receive increasing amounts of sodium chloride as the blood flows downward and reaches 1200 mOsm/kg at the bottom of the loop. As the blood flows upward, sodium chloride diffuses into the interstitial fluid, thereby remaining in the medulla. The hypertonic interstitial fluid causes water to be absorbed by osmosis from tubular fluid in the presence of antidiuretic hormone by creating a concentration gradient. Normally, 500 ml of concentrated urine removes the day's solutes. More than 2 L of water would be needed to excrete the same solute load in isotonic urine. Failure of the concentrating mechanism causes polyuria and especially nocturia.

Acid or alkaline urine The kidneys excrete strong nonvolatile acids and excess alkali. They provide the third line of defense against changes in hydrogen ion concentration. Acid-base buffer systems in all body fluids and the respiratory system respond rapidly, while the kidneys require several hours to a day or more to readjust the balance. The kidneys excrete

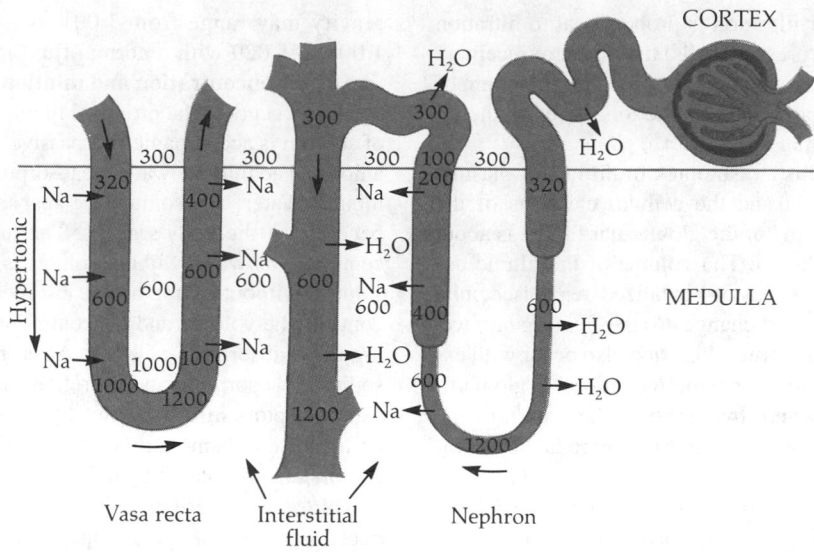

Figure 11-5 Countercurrent mechanism for concentrating urine. Numbers represent osmotic concentration (in mOsm/kg).

excess hydrogen ions and conserve bicarbonate ions. Chloride ions are excreted when bicarbonate ions are needed by the body. Almost all of the bicarbonate in the glomerular filtrate is reabsorbed. Excess bicarbonate ions are excreted when present, causing the urine to become alkaline.

Urine pH may range from 4.5 to 8.0. While the lungs remove the volatile acid, as in the following reaction

$$H^+ + HCO_3^- \rightleftharpoons H_2CO_3 \rightleftharpoons H_2O + CO_2 \uparrow$$

the kidneys excrete strong nonvolatile acids (sulfuric and phosphoric) and strong organic acids (ketone bodies). Hydrogen ions are buffered by bicarbonate ions. The anion base of the acid is balanced electrochemically by sodium ions (Na_2SO_4 and Na_2HPO_4). The tubular cells form bicarbonate ions that combine with the sodium ions of these salts and are reabsorbed. The tubular cell manufactures ammonia, which accepts a hydrogen ion and combines with the sulfate to form $(NH_4)_2SO_4$, which enters the urine. This mechanism permits excretion of hydrogen ions without lowering the urine pH. The Na_2HPO_4 accepts a hydrogen ion to become the acid salt, NaH_2PO_4, which is excreted. The other sodium ion is reabsorbed. Potassium and hydrogen ions compete for excretion in exchange for the reabsorbed sodium ions. The concentration of each ion is important. Acidosis and potassium depletion enhance hydrogen ion secretion. In chronic renal failure, the acid residues of nitrogen metabolism accumulate, and the tubules cannot meet the demand for hydrogen ion secretion. Since the tubular transport system is overwhelmed, potassium cannot be excreted and hyperkalemia results.

Juxtaglomerular Apparatus

The juxtaglomerular apparatus is composed of special epithelial cells (the macula densa cells) in the first part of the distal tubule and special myoepithelial cells in the renal afferent arteriole near the glomerulus (see Figure 11-4). These juxta-

glomerular cells respond to renal ischemia, low sodium concentration, and activity of the renal sympathetic nerves by secreting renin, which initiates the process that results in the formation of the vasopressor substance, angiotensin II.

Renin is an enzyme that acts on angiotensinogen, a glycoprotein made in the liver, to form angiotensin I. A converting enzyme formed in the lungs changes it to angiotensin II, which causes peripheral vasoconstriction and increased secretion of aldosterone. The first action elevates blood pressure by increasing peripheral resistance; the second action decreases salt and water loss and therefore increases extracellular fluid volume. Both actions cause an increase in arterial pressure, which relieves renal ischemia. The schema of the renin-angiotensin mechanism is outlined in Figure 11-6.

The juxtaglomerular apparatus appears to play a role in the autoregulation of renal blood flow and the glomerular filtration rate (GFR) by responding either to the concentration of sodium ions or to the osmolality of the urine in the distal tubule. The conditions of the distal tubule appear to control blood flow in the afferent arteriole.

Other Renal Functions

The kidneys produce erythropoietin, which promotes differentiation, proliferation, and maturation of precursors of red blood cells in the bone marrow. Erythropoietin is produced in response to decreases in oxygen tension and renal perfusion that may arise from anemia, hypoxia, or renal ischemia.

Renal prostaglandins are synthesized in the renal cortex and medulla. They appear to be produced in response to both renal ischemia and vasoconstriction. Observations suggest that they participate in the maintenance of renal vascular resistance and glomerular filtration rate especially when renal hemodynamics are altered. The complex relationships of renal prostaglandins are not yet clearly understood.

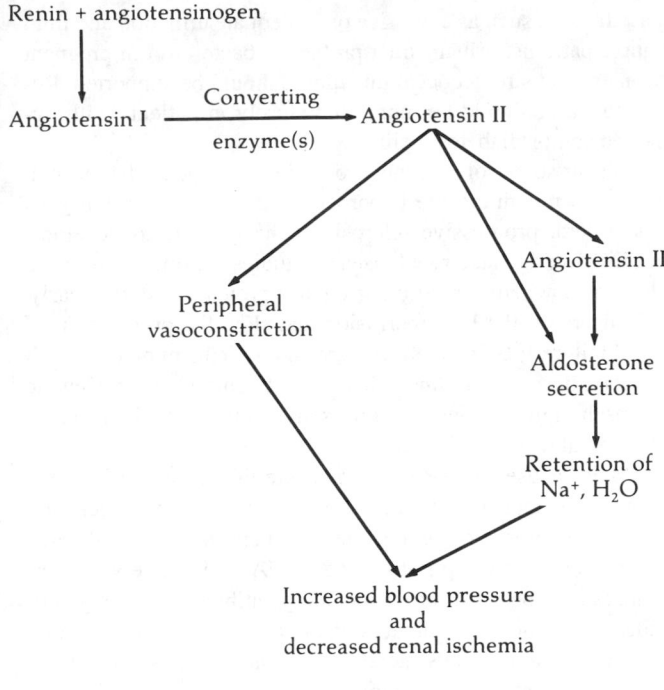

Renin + angiotensinogen

Angiotensin I —— Converting enzyme(s) ——→ Angiotensin II

Angiotensin III

Peripheral vasoconstriction

Aldosterone secretion

Retention of Na$^+$, H$_2$O

Increased blood pressure and decreased renal ischemia

Figure 11-6 Renin-angiotensin mechanism.

The kidneys have a role in the metabolism of vitamin D. Vitamin D$_3$ is formed in the skin, metabolized in the liver to 1-hydroxy D$_3$, and then metabolized by the kidney to an active form (1,25-dihydroxy D$_3$ and others). The 1,25-dihydroxy D$_3$ is produced in response to hypocalcemia or hypophosphatemia. It acts in conjunction with the parathyroid hormone to increase intestinal absorption of calcium and phosphate, mobilize calcium from bones, and increase renal tubular reabsorption of calcium and phosphate. The production of 1,25-dihydroxy D$_3$ is suppressed by hypercalcemia and hyperphosphatemia. Decreased production of 1,25-dihydroxy D$_3$ occurs in chronic renal failure and is considered significant in the development of renal osteodystrophy.

Concept of Clearance

Since the kidneys' functions include clearing the plasma of unwanted materials, the concept of renal clearance of a substance is helpful in evaluating renal function. The rate at which a substance is excreted in terms of its plasma concentration is the clearance of that substance.

Clearance of creatinine is used to monitor renal function since it is an endogenous product from muscle creatinine phosphate, and its production is relatively independent of protein anabolism and catabolism. The amount of creatinine produced depends on the lean body mass, and this variation is responsible for the differences in serum creatinine levels and creatinine clearances found in men and women. While a small part of the creatinine that appears in the urine is secreted by the tubules, the major portion is filtered by the glomerulus and is not reabsorbed. Creatinine clearance is a practical, clinically useful measure of glomerular filtration rate. Clearances show wide variations between subjects but are reproducible in the same subject. Serial clearance studies permit the following of a patient's clinical course. Creatinine clearance may be affected by the presence of high glucose concentration, acetone, acetoacetic acid, ascorbic acid, methyldopa, and levodopa in the urine. It may also be affected by a high-protein diet before the test and by strenuous exercise during the urine collection period.

Because the total urine for a specified period is required for accurate determination, patients and staff must understand the procedure: (1) empty the bladder and mark the time; (2) save all urine; (3) void exactly 24 hours later (or the period specified) and save the specimen; (4) measure total volume; and (5) collect serum creatinine once during the 24-hour period.

$$\text{Creatinine clearance (ml/min)} = \frac{\text{Urine creatinine (mg/dl)} \times \text{Urine flow (ml/min)}}{\text{Serum creatinine (mg/dl)}}$$

Inulin clearance is clinically useful as a measure of GFR. Inulin is freely filtered by the glomerulus and is not reabsorbed or secreted by the tubules so that the amount filtered is the amount secreted. Inulin clearance is used when an exact measure of GFR is required.

$$\text{Inulin clearance (ml/min)} = \frac{\text{Urine inulin (mg/dl)} \times \text{Urine volume (ml/min)}}{\text{Plasma inulin (mg/dl)}} = \text{GFR}$$

Age and Renal Function

Differences in age are associated with differences in renal function that become clinically significant when a young or aged individual has an illness that places excessive demands on the kidneys.

The kidney is immature at birth. Renal blood flow and the glomerular filtration rate of infants are low compared with those of adults. The ability to excrete sodium, potassium, water, and acid loads is limited. The kidneys continue to develop until 1 year of age. Their combined weight continues to increase beyond adolescence (24 g at birth, 140 g at 6 years, 183 g at age 12 years, and 300 g for adults).

Renal blood flow decreases with age, which is partly related to a decrease in cardiac output. The loss of renal mass and functioning nephrons also decreases the effective filtering surface and glomerular filtration rate. Creatinine clearance is stable until the fourth decade, when it begins to decrease. Serum creatinine decreases with the decrease in muscle mass associated with aging. Therefore serum creatinine levels may overestimate glomerular filtration rate. To avoid overdoses of drugs in the elderly, creatinine clearance rate is used when dosage of such drugs as digoxin is determined. Also of note is the slower rate of response in elderly patients to acute changes in fluid and electrolyte balances associated with illness. The renin-aldosterone system becomes less responsive with lowered renin levels and an associated reduction in plasma level of aldosterone. The ability to conserve Na$^+$ and excrete K$^+$ is decreased.

The decrease in renal response to antidiuretic hormone and in glomerular filtration rate contribute to the inability to conserve water and concentrate the urine. The maintenance of Na⁺, K⁺, and water balance becomes exceedingly important in elderly patients.

NORMAL FINDINGS

General   Temperature: normal range; blood pressure: normal range; weight: no marked increase (>2 kg); skin: warm, dry and normal turgor; no pallor, yellowish color, excoriations, uremic snow, edema, petechiae, ecchymoses, or purpura

Eyes   No periorbital edema, conjunctival redness, retinal hemorrhages, exudates, or papilledema

Ears   Hearing normal; no tophi in ear cartilages

Mouth   No odor of ammonia; no stomatitis: ulcers, exudate, or bleeding

Neck   Parathyroid glands not palpable

Chest   Normal breath sounds, rate, and rhythm; normal heart sounds, rate, and rhythm

Abdomen   Normal bowel sounds; no masses; no tenderness in flank, groin, or costovertebral angle on palpation or percussion; no bruit on auscultation

Neurologic examination   No change in cognitive function, level of consciousness, or behavior; no change in superficial or deep tendon reflexes; no change in muscle action or sensation

Extremities   No edema

CONDITIONS, DISEASES, AND DISORDERS

RENAL FAILURE

ACUTE RENAL FAILURE

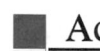

Acute renal failure (ARF) is a sudden, severe impairment of renal function, causing an acute uremic episode.

Changes in renal function may be considered on a continuum from impairment to failure. Renal impairment may be revealed only by specific urine concentration or dilution tests. Renal insufficiency is revealed when the kidneys cannot meet the extra demands of dietary or metabolic stress. Renal failure occurs when the normal demands of the body cannot be met.

Health professionals can help detect renal problems early and thus help prevent renal failure. Control of environmental factors, such as nephrotoxic substances (drugs, organic solvents, insecticides, and cleaning agents), is important. Safe use and disposal of such agents in industry, agriculture, and the home must be encouraged. Avoiding unnecessary urinary tract instrumentation could prevent infection. Elimination of predis-

ease factors, such as excessive or inadequate urination and fluid intake patterns, urinary tract problems, bacteriuria in pregnant women, and streptococcal infections, should be supported. Renal function should be monitored closely in patients with hypertension or diabetes mellitus.

When some of the nephrons are damaged, the normal nephrons remaining are hyperperfused. If this condition goes unchecked, progressive sclerosis of the glomerulus develops, leading to end-stage renal disease. Studies continue in order to determine whether restricting dietary protein, if started early, will decrease the hyperperfusion and slow the progression of renal failure.[11] Being alert to prerenal problems in patients with surgery, burns, or trauma helps prevent complications. Genetic counseling may be indicated for some families in which hereditary renal disorder surfaces.

Major causes of ARF include acute tubular necrosis, acute glomerulonephritis, acute urinary tract obstruction, occlusion of the renal artery or vein, acute pyelonephritis, bilateral cortical necrosis, and nephrotoxic agents. A wide variety of substances may be nephrotoxic including antibiotics (aminoglycosides), anesthetics, iodinated radiographic contrast medium, organic solvents, heavy metals, endogenous toxins, and abnormal concentrations of physiologic substances.

It is helpful to categorize the causes of ARF as prerenal, renal, or postrenal. Prerenal causes include dehydration, hemorrhage, shock, burns, and trauma and result from a decrease in renal blood flow. Renal causes include glomerulonephritis, acute pyelonephritis, occlusion of renal arteries or veins, bilateral cortical necrosis, nephrotoxic substances, and blood transfusion reactions. Postrenal causes include acute urinary tract obstruction.

Prerenal problems arise from inadequate perfusion of a normal kidney caused by pump failure, hypovolemia, loss of peripheral resistance, or altered renal hemodynamics. Renal causes stem from primary damage to the kidneys, intrinsic parenchymal damage, involving the nephron. Damage can result from acute tubular necrosis, such as that caused by ischemia of toxins, cortical necrosis, infection, major disorders of the blood supply, infiltration (e.g., leukemia), and intravascular coagulation. Postrenal causes involve obstruction of the urinary tract distal to the kidneys, resulting in interference with the flow of urine. Such causes may include intrarenal obstruction by crystals, pigments, or Bence Jones protein or extrarenal obstruction caused by stones, tumors, or hypertrophy of other structures, such as the prostate.

ARF has a high morbidity and a mortality rate of 40% to 60%. Nearly 5% of patients admitted to medical and surgical services have or develop ARF.[8] Mortality is high despite advances in preventing and treating ARF; a prime reason for the foregoing statistics is the changing population of hospital patients, who tend now to be older and generally much sicker.

The prognosis for ARF depends on the cause and extent of renal failure. The mortality rate goes up with sepsis, respiratory failure ventilatory support, and failure of additional organ systems. The very young and very old are particularly at risk. The box lists predisposing factors that indicate ARF is likely to occur.

PREDISPOSING FACTORS IN ACUTE RENAL FAILURE

Hypotensive episodes
Hypovolemia, renal ischemia from any cause
Sepsis, burns, jaundice
Advanced age
Recent surgery (especially cardiac or vascular)
Failure of several organ systems
Preexisting renal disease or diabetes mellitus
Drug therapy (multiple drugs, aminoglycoside antibiotics, angiotensin-converting enzyme blocking agents)

ARF frequently occurs in older patients because the typical inciting events are more common. Dehydration is more often a cause of ARF in the elderly or in very young persons than in middle-aged adults. Elderly patients with multiple-system problems or preexisting renal insufficiency are particularly at risk.

The five stages of ARF are (1) onset: usually a short time from precipitating event to onset of oliguria or anuria; (2) oliguric-anuric stage: the period during which output is less than 400 ml/day (usually 8 to 15 days; if longer, the prognosis is poor); (3) early diuretic stage: extends from the time daily output is greater than 400 ml/day to the time that the blood urea nitrogen (BUN) concentration stops rising; (4) late diuretic or recovery stage: extends from the first day BUN falls to the day it stabilizes or is in the normal range; (5) convalescent stage: extends from the day BUN is stable to the day the patient returns to normal activity and urine volume and BUN are normal. This may take several months, and during this time, chronic renal failure develops in some patients.

•••••• Pathophysiology

In prerenal azotemia, urinary osmolality is high (greater than 900 mOsm/kg) and urinary sodium concentrations are low (less than 20 mEq/L), which is consistent with renal hypoperfusion and well-preserved tubular function. These findings reflect the physiologic response to hypovolemia or ineffective circulating blood volume. Urinary findings with parenchymal disorders reflect glomerular damage and inability either to conserve sodium (urinary sodium greater than 27 mEq/L) or to concentrate the urine (urine osmolality less than 250 mOsm/kg). In postrenal problems urinary osmolality and sodium levels may be normal.

Generally, the ratio of the blood urea nitrogen to serum creatinine is 10:1. A higher ratio suggests dehydration, gastrointestinal bleeding, increased protein intake, decreased cardiac output, or antianabolic agents.

Damaged caused by nephrotoxins appears to affect the proximal tubular epithelium and leave the tubular basement membrane intact. Damage caused by renal ischemia is more widespread and involves patchy areas of epithelial necrosis. Whatever the damage, the glomerular filtration rate decreases, and urine formation is impaired.

The current explanations for the pathogenesis of ARF include leakage of tubular fluid from damaged tubules into the interstitial areas, tubular obstructions caused by accumulation of intratubular debris or casts, glomerular abnormalities, and changes in renal hemodynamics, primarily excessive vasoconstriction.

Carefully managing fluid volume before, during, and after surgery helps protect renal function; using crystalloid and colloid volume replacement products and blood products helps prevent volume depletion and renal ischemia.

Attempts to maintain renal blood flow (using a low dosage of dopamine) and urine flow rate (through forced diuresis by fluid bolus and diuretics) may prevent hypovolemia from advancing to acute renal failure. The increased urine flow helps to prevent casts and other debris from obstructing the tubules. When renal function is at risk, nephrotoxic agents such as the anesthetic methoxyflurane and the aminoglycoside antibiotics gentamicin or tobramycin, should be avoided.

•••••• Diagnostic Studies and Findings

Urine pH   Lowered

Urine osmolality   Hyperosmotic, hyposmotic, or isoosmotic in relation to serum osmolality

Urine specific gravity   Prerenal: high; renal: low; postrenal: normal

Urine sodium   Prerenal: low; renal: increased; postrenal: normal

Urine creatinine   Prerenal: normal; renal: increased; postrenal: normal

Urine sediment   Normal or hematuria; proteinuria; bacteriuria; pyuria, casts

24-hour urine output   Olguric: <400 ml; nonoliguric: 1 to 2 L; diuretic phase: 2 to 3 L; recovery phase: near normal volume

Hemoglobin (Hgb)/hematocrit (Hct)   Anemia; hemoconcentration with dehydration; hemodilution with hypervolemia

Platelets   Decreased adhesiveness

White blood cells (WBC)   Increased with infection

Serum pH   Low-acidotic

Serum bicarbonate   <22 mEq/L

Serum potassium   Hyperkalemia

Serum chloride   Normal or elevated

Serum sodium   Normal or low with hemodilution

Serum calcium   Low

Serum phosphate   High

Blood urea nitrogen (BUN)   Increased

Serum creatinine   Increased

Ratio BUN/serum creatinine   10:1-15:1; decreased urea concentration <10:1; decreased renal function >15:1

Serum osmolality   Increased

Creatinine clearance   Decreased with poor glomerular function; 50-84 ml/min (mild failure); 10-49 ml/min (moderate failure); <10 ml/min (severe failure)

Electrocardiogram (ECG)   Dysrhythmias possible with hyperkalemia or hypokalemia

Kidney-ureter bladder (KUB) x-ray examination   Kidney is normal size or slightly enlarged

Renal ultrasound   Kidney size or shape may be abnormal

Intravenous urogram (IVU)   Obstruction, strictures, or masses may be present

Renal scan   May reveal cysts, tumors, or impaired perfusion

Renal biopsy   May be necessary to determine cause and extent of injury

• • • • • • Multidisciplinary Plan

The goal of treatment is to prevent decreased renal perfusion from progressing to ARF. Fluids and diuretic agents may be used. The cause of the ARF is determined, if possible. Failing body systems are supported until recovery (see box below). Evaluation for dialysis or transplantation may be necessary if recovery is not complete.

The major complications of ARF in the oliguric-anuric stage are acidosis, hyperkalemia, infection, hyperphosphatemia, hypertension, and anemia. Hypovolemia and hypokalemia may be problems in the diuretic stage. Prompt and adequate management is essential to survival.

Medications

Alkalinizing agents (for acidosis)
    Sodium bicarbonate, po, IV, 1-4 g/d; 2-5 mEq/kg infused over 4-8h
    Sodium citrate and citric acid (Shohl's solution), po, 10-20 ml tid (1 mEq Na^+ /ml)

⚠ EMERGENCY ALERT

RENAL FAILURE—ACUTE

Acute or sudden renal failure (RF) is a life-threatening event that requires immediate and comprehensive intervention.

Assessment

• Known renal failure history
• History of drug overdose or toxic injection that precipitated renal failure
• Laboratory values indicating renal failure

Intervention

All intervention should be directed at maintaining maximum renal blood flow.
• Maintain airway, breathing, and circulation.
• Obtain IV access: fluid replacement must be based on laboratory results *unless* patient is in shock.
• In collaboration with physician, administer medications carefully with attention to volumes.
• Record meticulously intake and output.
• Renal dialysis may be indicated.

Treatment for hyperkalemia
    Sodium polystyrene sulfonate (Kayexalate, SPS), po or enema, 15 g qd-qid; give oral dose in 45-60 ml of water, syrup, or sorbital solution
    Calcium gluconate (Kalcinate), IV, 1 g (90 mg Ca^{++}) in 10 ml
    Sodium bicarbonate, IV, 2-5 mEq/kg infusion over 4-8h
    Glucose 50%, IV, 25-50 g, and insulin-regular, IV, 10-15 units
Antihypertensive agents
    Vasodilators
    Sodium nitroprusside (Nipride), IV, in emergency, continuous infusion, 0.5-10 µg/kg/min as required
Angiotensin antagonists
    Captopril (Capoten), po, initially 25 mg tid, slowly increase by 50 mg increments, maximum dose 150 mg tid
    Atenolol (Tenormin), po, initially 50 mg/d, may increase to 100 mg/d
Calcium channel blockers
    Diltiazem (Cardizem), po, initially 30-60 mg q6-8h, may be increased gradually to 180-480 mg in 3 or 4 equal doses; prolonged action forms are available
    Nifedipine (Procardia), po, initially 10 mg tid, may be increased slowly to 20-30 mg tid
Centrally acting agents
    Clonidine (Catapres, Dixarit), po, 0.1 mg bid or tid initially, then increase by 0.2-0.8 mg/d (maximum effective dose, 2.4 mg/d)
Diuretics
    Furosemide (Lasix, Uritol), po, 20-80 mg followed by second dose in 6-8 h up to 600 mg; IM, IV, 20-40 mg given slowly over 1-2 min; high dose by IV not more than 4 mg/min
    Hydrochlorothiazide (Hydrodiuril, Esidrix), po, 25-100 mg/d or bid initially, then maintenance 25-100 mg/d according to patient's response
Phosphate binders
    Calcium acetate (PhosLo); 2 tabs (667 mg each) with each meal to start; 3-4 tabs per meal are usually required
    Aluminum carbonate (Basaljel), po, 30-40 ml with meals and at bedtime (400 mg Al $[OH]_3$/5 ml); 15-20 ml 1 h with meals and at bedtime
    Aluminum hydroxide gel, dried (Amphojel tab, Alu-Cap), 8 tab with meals and at bedtime
H_2 receptor antagonist
    Cimetidine (Tagamet), po, 300 mg qid; IV, 300 mg q6h, maximum daily dose 2.4 g
    Ranitidine (Zantac), po, 150 mg bid; IM, slow IV, 50 mg q6-8h; maximum daily dose 400 mg
Antiinfective agents
    Infection is frequently a complication of ARF
    Agents specific to the microorganism cultured should be used
    Agents whose route of excretion is primarily renal should be omitted or used in smaller doses or at lengthened intervals depending on glomerular filtration rate

Agents excreted by only the liver require no change in dosage; when partial excretion occurs via the kidney, some adjustment is needed at low glomerular filtration rates

Particular care is needed in all drug administration: dosage, interval between doses, and recognition of increased sensitivity because of altered renal function[2]

General Management

Dialysis, either hemodialysis or peritoneal dialysis, is used to manage fluid volume and electrolyte imbalances (see p. 970); dialysis is particularly necessary with pulmonary edema, hyperkalemia, uremic pericarditis, and seizures; some nephrotoxic agents are dialyzable; hemodialysis is used in hypercatabolic patients to remove nitrogenous wastes and to control serum pH and potassium levels; peritoneal dialysis is not used in cases involving trauma, infection, immunosuppression, neutropenia, recent abdominal surgery, or severe liver disease

Continuous arteriovenous hemofiltration or continuous venovenous hemofiltration is used to remove fluid in an unstable patient, especially in oliguric-anuric patient (see p. 965)

Fluid intake must equal amount needed to replace measurable losses in urine, nasogastric drainage, wound drainage and estimated insensible losses; fluid overload must be avoided; daily weights reflect fluid gain or loss

Packed red blood cells may be needed if symptoms associated with anemia develop; Hgb levels should be higher than 10 g/dl

Nutritional support should include maintenance of body weight and positive nitrogen balance; a period of negative nitrogen balance and weight loss cannot be completely avoided

Calorie intake should include 100 g of glucose per day

Excess carbohydrate intake can contribute to respiratory acidosis

Protein intake may be maintained through parenteral infusion of essential amino acids (50 to 85 g/L solutions); oral intake is started as soon as possible; desired protein intake is 0.4 to 0.6 g/kg/day or 1 to 1.5 g/kg/day if on dialysis with 70% of high biologic value; high-biologic-value proteins are those that contain essential amino acids in the proportions needed to promote growth, such as milk, eggs, and meat; serum albumin levels of 3 to 3.5 g/dl or higher are desirable; excess protein intake contributes to metabolic acidosis and increased nitrogenous wastes

Sodium intake is 0.5 to 1.0 g/day or 40-90 mEq/day depending on blood pressure; potassium in diet is restricted to 1500 mg/day or 60 mEq/day if hyperkalemia is present

Vitamin supplements are needed, since a limited protein diet is deficient in calcium and folic acid and low in phosphorus and the B vitamins; water-soluble vitamins are lost in dialysis

NURSING CARE

Nursing Assessment

Renal

Urine volume normal, oliguria, or anuria; nocturia; change in color or odor

Cardiovascular

Hypotension; flat neck veins; dry mucous membranes; decreased skin turgor; hypertension; peripheral edema; jugular venous distention; tachycardia

Respiratory

Altered rate and rhythm (dyspnea, tachypnea, hyperventilation, Kussmaul breathing); altered breath sounds (rales, crackles, rhonchi); increased sputum production; urinelike odor to breath

Gastrointestinal

Nausea; vomiting; anorexia; hematemesis; melena; stomatitis; metallic taste in mouth

Hematologic

Pale mucous membranes; pallor

Skin

Bruises; pruritus; dry skin

Neurologic

Change in level of consciousness (somnolence or coma); change in cognitive function; change in behavior; asterixis; seizures

General

Fever; headache; pain in flank or costovertebral angle; muscle cramps; weakness; fatigue; short-term weight changes

Psychosocial

Change in family relationships; family expresses concern for outcome of illness

Nursing Dx & Intervention

Altered renal tissue perfusion related to damage to nephrons from hypovolemia, ischemia, toxins, or obstruction

- Assess for Chvostek's or Trousseau's sign; assess respirations *to identify tetany (hypocalcemia); and Kussmaul respirations (acidosis).*
- Monitor laboratory values: serum pH, sodium, potassium, calcium, bicarbonate, chloride, magnesium, BUN,

creatinine; *these reflect kidneys' ability to excrete nitrogenous wastes, excess fluids, and electrolytes.*

- Administer medications as ordered with care; monitor response to drugs. Dosages of medications may be less than usual, and intervals between doses may be lengthened; *monitoring determines the effectiveness of the drug and its dosage and timing and helps to identify adverse side effects.*
- Avoid nephrotoxic drugs; *kidneys are less able to excrete drugs they normally eliminate.*

Fluid-volume deficit related to decreased effective circulating blood volume resulting from active losses and failure of regulatory mechanisms

- Assess neck veins, capillary refill, oral mucous membranes, skin turgor; monitor weight daily, also 24-hour intake and output; assess lying and sitting or standing blood pressure, pulse, and respirations every 6-8 hr; assess central venous pressure and pulmonary artery pressures every 6 to 12 hours *to identify changes in fluid status.*
- Monitor laboratory data: serum sodium, potassium, chloride, and bicarbonate *to identify electrolytes lost through body fluid losses.*
- Administer medications as ordered (vasoconstrictors, fluids, and electrolyte replacements) *to increase systemic resistance and blood pressure and thus renal blood flow, and to replace losses and ensure adequate circulating volume.*

Fluid-volume excess related to sodium and water retention

- Assess weight daily, also 24-hour intake and output; assess blood pressure, pulse, respirations, including breath sounds every 6 to 8 hours; monitor edema, jugular venous distention and, if necessary, central venous pressure and pulmonary artery pressures *to recognize altered fluid status.*
- Monitor serum potassium level, which may be lowered by vigorous diuretic therapy. Monitor electrocardiogram; *increase or decrease in potassium may be associated with dysrhythmias.*
- Administer diuretics as ordered and monitor response *to determine effect of drug and observe for side effects such as hypokalemia and ototoxicity.*

Altered nutrition: less than body requirements related to gastrointestinal effects of azotemia and restricted dietary intake

- Monitor food intake and dry weight; encourage food intake as prescribed or administer enteral or parenteral feedings *to ensure adequate intake within limits prescribed;* weight is assessed *to determine if weight changes are related to fluid balance or to inadequate caloric intake and the loss of muscle mass.*
- Monitor for nausea, vomiting, and anorexia; *these conditions decrease intake of needed nutrients.*
- Provide oral hygiene regularly *to improve taste in mouth.*

- Monitor laboratory data: serum protein, lipids, potassium, and calcium *to determine if protein intake is adequate.* Refer complex problems to dietitian; a team approach to managing the renal diet is helpful to all concerned.

Risk for infection related to suppressed immune response associated with azotemia

- Monitor for signs and symptoms of infection in secretions, excretions, and exudates, and assess for fever *to detect any infection early.*
- Monitor laboratory data: white blood cell count; temperature every 4 to 6 hours; *levels may be only slightly increased in azotemia.*
- Wash hands thoroughly and consistently; avoid exposing patient to persons with infection; ensure aseptic technique for any invasive procedure or wound care *to decrease chances for infection.*
- Encourage regular oral hygiene, hand washing, bathing, adequate rest, and nutrition *to help prevent infections.*

Risk for confusion related to endogenous chemical abnormalities associated with azotemia

- Monitor orientation to time, place, and person; *this knowledge is lost as mental status is altered.* Orient patient to reality *to decrease the possibility that disorientation is caused by isolation and lack of information.*
- Maintain safety precautions: bedrails up, sharp objects out of reach, and call bell within reach *to provide a safe environment and to prevent injury.*

Risk for bathing/hygiene and toileting self-care deficits related to side effects of azotemia

- Assess need for assistance; assist with care as needed *to help patient return to self-care as appropriate.*
- Implement measures such as deep breathing, coughing, and turning *to prevent adverse side effects of bed rest, such as pneumonia.*

Risk for altered family processes related to health crisis in family member

- Assess family structure and role relationships; monitor family's response to the illness, treatment, and prognosis; encourage verbalization of needs and concerns; discuss impact on roles and adaptation required; identify family strengths; assist with problem solving; support family decisions; crisis intervention may be all that is needed.
- Refer patient and family to other services as appropriate *to help resolve problems requiring time and skills beyond the nurse's capabilities.*

Knowledge deficit related to ARF, its causes, manifestations, and treatment; need for medical follow-up; and the potential need for dialysis or transplantation in the future

- See box on p. 935.

Patient Education/Home Care Planning

1. Explain the cause of the episode of acute renal failure.
2. Explain the level of renal function after the acute phase is over.
3. Explain diet and fluid restrictions, which may continue or be lessened or discontinued.
4. Help patient practice self-observation skills, such as measuring temperature, pulse, respirations, blood pressure, intake and output, daily weight, and record keeping.
5. Explain good personal hygiene.
6. Explain how to avoid infections.
7. Explain exercise and rest in the amounts advised.
8. Describe medications, if any, with name, purpose, dosage, time interval, and adverse reactions (by discussion and in writing).
9. Explain the schedule of medical follow-up.
10. Explain renal dialysis and transplantation if they are likely options for the future.

Evaluation

Renal tissue perfusion is adequate Renal function tests are normal or stable.

Fluid balance is normal Urine volume is normal and balances intake; there is no sign of edema or postural hypotension.

Nutritional status is normal No restrictions are required on food or fluids.

No infection is present No signs or symptoms of infection are noted.

Skin is intact No skin breakdown is present; pruritus and dry skin are controlled.

There is no confusion Patient is oriented to time, place, and person.

Patient has resumed self-care Patient has no restrictions in activities of daily living (ADLs).

Family has adapted to patient's illness and recovery The family has dealt with the crisis constructively and can identify sources of help available.

Patient and family are knowledgeable about ARF Patient and family can explain ARF, its causes, manifestations, and treatment; the need for medical follow-up; and the potential need for dialysis or transplantation in the future.

CHRONIC RENAL FAILURE

Chronic renal failure (CRF) is a slow, insidious, and irreversible impairment of renal function. Uremia usually develops slowly.

Major causes of CRF include diabetic nephropathy, nephrosclerosis (hypertensive nephropathy), glomerulonephri-
tis, and polycystic kidney disease. CRF can arise as primary renal disease or secondary to other systemic diseases. Primary renal disease includes glomerulonephritis, pyelonephritis, polycystic kidneys, and renal cell carcinoma. Renal problems that develop secondary to systemic disease include lupus nephritis, renal amyloidosis, myeloma kidney, nephrocalcinosis, and hereditary nephropathy, as well as diabetic nephropathy and nephrosclerosis.

The levels of chronic renal failure are identified by changes in the glomerular filtration rate. In early renal failure the rate is 30 to 10 ml/minute; in late renal failure it is 10 to 5 ml/minute; in the terminal stage it is 5 ml/minute. Symptoms are prominent in later renal failure and life threatening in terminal renal failure or end-stage renal disease (ESRD). Because patients vary greatly in their clinical picture, renal function, and performance capabilities, criteria for evaluating the severity of established renal disease take into account the severity of the signs and symptoms, the level of impairment of the patient's renal function (glomerular filtration rate and serum creatinine), and the patient's performance level (what the patient says he or she is able to do).

•••••• Pathophysiology

The various causes of failing renal function eventually lead to a final common pathway. Often the specific, initial renal insult cannot be identified.

When the kidneys fail, a variety of substances accumulate that normally are excreted. These substances include nitrogenous wastes, the so-called uremic toxins, and normal substances, such as electrolytes that may alter cellular function (i.e., enzyme pathways).

A variety of pathogenic processes can cause chronic renal failure. Infections, for example, may be localized or may accompany systemic disease. Autoimmune disorders may be caused by antigen-antibody complexes and anti–glomerular basement membrane antibodies. Metabolic disorders such as renal tubular acidosis and calcium-phosphate abnormalities may cause renal calculi. Renovascular changes may arise from occlusion, stenosis, thrombosis, diabetes mellitus, or hypertension. Urinary obstruction, renal cancer, and congenital anomalies may end in chronic renal failure. These topics are discussed in some detail in this section.

Nephrons are permanently destroyed by various processes that occur in the course of renal disease, such as ischemia, inflammation, necrosis, fibrosis, sclerosis, and scarring. The normal nephrons remaining may respond with hypertrophy and hyperplasia. However, eventually a point is reached when renal deficits become manifest (as many as 50% of the nephrons may be lost before renal deficits are discovered). Such deficits include the inability to respond to excessive salt intake or decreased water or salt intake, a decreased synthesis of substances such as erythropoietin by the kidney, or the inability to excrete the end products of metabolism. All the organ systems are eventually affected by renal dysfunction (see box on p. 936).

Changes in renal function may be manifested by an increase or decrease in substances usually found in the body (e.g.,

COMPLICATIONS OF CHRONIC RENAL FAILURE

Anemia
Hypertension
Hyperkalemia
Congestive heart failure
Pulmonary edema
Pericarditis
Accelerated atherosclerosis
Bleeding diathesis
Peptic ulcer disease
Osteodystrophy
Metabolic encephalopathy
Peripheral neuropathy

hemoglobin, BUN, serum creatinine, sodium, potassium, calcium, and phosphate). The body's attempts to accommodate these changes may cause hypertension; pulmonary edema; altered protein, carbohydrate, and fat metabolism; and osteodystrophy. Mental status, peripheral nerve conduction time, and platelet adhesiveness also may be altered.

Diagnostic Studies and Findings

Urinalysis   pH: acidic; osmolality: low; specific gravity: fixed; sediment: may contain WBCs, RBCs, and granular, hyaline, broad, and waxy casts; 24-hr volume decreased or nonexistent; proteinuria

Complete blood count   Hgb/Hct lowered; decreased RBC survival time; platelets reduced in number with decreased adhesiveness

Blood chemistry   Decreased serum pH, bicarbonate; increased potassium, sodium, magnesium, hydrogen, phosphate, and calcium ions; increased serum uric acid, osmolality, BUN; decreased iron and total iron-binding capacity; creatinine clearance: decreased

Kidney-ureter-bladder (KUB) x-ray   Small, contracted kidneys

Renal ultrasound   Small, contracted kidneys

Multidisciplinary Plan

Conservative management of CRF is initiated when marked decreases in renal function are noted, and it is continued until the need for dialysis or transplantation is determined. The principles guiding management are (1) treat underlying renal disease; (2) prolong the life of the native kidneys; (3) identify and prevent causes of ARF in the presence of CRF; (4) treat the complications of CRF; and (5) relieve the symptoms of uremia.

Surgery

Renal transplantation (p. 979), creation of an internal arteriovenous fistula for hemodialysis or insertion of a Tenckhoff catheter for peritoneal dialysis

Medications

Modifications of drug dosages are required when renal function is decreased. The estimated renal function using creatinine clearance can be used to adjust dosages of drugs excreted by the kidneys. If only serum creatinine is available, the following formula may be used to estimate creatinine clearance in the patient with steady state renal function.

$$\text{Men: } \frac{\text{weight (kg)} \times (140 - \text{age})}{72 \times \text{serum creatinine (mg/dl)}} = \text{creatinine clearance (est.) in ml/min}$$

Women: $0.85 \times$ the above value

Treatment for acidosis
Sodium bicarbonate, po, 1-4 g/d; IV, 2-5 mEq/kg infused over 4-8 h
Sodium citrate and citric acid (Shohl's solution), po, 10-20 ml tid (1 mEq Na^+/ml)
Treatment for hyperkalemia
Sodium polystyrene sulfonate (Kayexalate, SPS), po or enema, 15 g qd-qid; give oral dose in 45-60 ml of water, syrup, or sorbital solution
Calcium gluconate (Kalcinate), IV, 1 g (90 mg Ca^{++}) in 10 ml
Sodium bicarbonate, IV, 2-5 mEq/kg infusion over 8 h
Glucose 50%, IV, 25-50 g, and regular insulin, IV, 10-15 units
Antihypertensive agents
Vasodilators
Sodium nitroprusside (Nipride), IV, in emergency, continuous infusion, 0.5-10 µg/kg/min as required
Angiotensin antagonists
Captopril (Capoten), po, initially 25 mg tid, slowly increase by 50 mg increments, maximum dose 150 mg tid
Atenolol (Tenormin), po, initially 50 mg/d, may increase to 100 mg/d
Calcium channel blockers
Diltiazem (Cardizem), po, initially 30-60 mg q6-8h, may be increased gradually to 180-480 mg in 3 or 4 equal doses; long-acting forms are available
Nifedipine (Procardia), po, initially 10 mg tid, may be increased slowly to 20-30 mg tid
Centrally acting agents
Clonidine (Catapres, Dixarit), po, 0.1 mg bid or tid initially, then increase by 0.2-0.8 mg/d (maximum effective dose, 2.4 mg/d)
Diuretics
Furosemide (Lasix, Uritol), po, 20-80 mg followed by second dose in 6-8 h up to 600 mg; IM, IV, 20-40 mg given slowly over 1-2 min; high dose by IV not more than 4 mg/min and repeat in 6-8 h
Antiinfective agents
Infection is frequently a complication of chronic renal failure
Agents specific to the microorganism cultured should be used

Agents whose route of excretion is primarily renal should be omitted or used in smaller doses or at lengthened intervals depending on glomerular filtration rate; agents excreted by only the liver require no change in dosage; if partial excretion occurs via the kidneys, some adjustment is needed at lower glomerular filtration rates

Anticonvulsant agents

Phenytoin (Dilantin, Novophenytoin), po, 100 mg tid up to 600 mg/d

Diazepam (Valium, Novodipam), po, 2-10 mg bid-qid

For status epilepticus, IM, IV, 5-10 mg initially; repeat if necessary at 10-15 min intervals, if necessary up to 30 mg; repeat in 2-4 h if necessary

Phenobarbital (Luminal, Barbita), po, 50-100 mg/d

Phenobarbital sodium, IV, 100-320 mg/d

Phosphate binding agents

Calcium acetate (PhosLo), po, 667 mg/tab, 2 tabs with each meal to start; 3-4 tabs per meal usually required

Aluminum carbonate gel (Basaljel), po, 30-40 ml (400 mg Al[OH]$_3$/5 ml) with meals and at bedtime

Aluminum hydroxide gel (Amphojel, Dialume), po, 40 ml with meals and at bedtime

Aluminum hydroxide gel, dried (Amphojel tab, AluCap), po, 8 tab with meals and at bedtime

H$_2$ receptor antagonist

Cimetidine (Tagamet), po, 300 mg qid; IV, 300 mg q6h, maximum daily dose 2.4 g

Ranitidine (Zantac), po, 150 mg bid; IM, slow IV, 50 mg q6-8h; maximum daily dose 400 mg

Antianemics

Recombinant human erythropoietin (r-hEPO) epoietin alfa (Epogen), initial dose 50-100 units/kg body weight 3 times a wk IV for hemodialysis patients; IV or subcutaneous administration for peritoneal dialysis patients and nondialysis CRF patients; maintenance doses are individually titrated

Androgenic agents

Fluoxymesterone (Halotestin, Android-F), po, 10-30 mg/d

Methandrostenolone (Dianabol), po, 5-20 mg/d

Nandrolone (Deca-Durabolin, Anabolin-LA), IM, up to 300 mg/wk

Antiemetic agents

Prochlorperazine (Compazine), po, 5-10 mg tid-qid

Trimethobenzamide (Tigan, Ticon), po, 250 mg tid or qid; IM, 200 mg tid or qid

Antihistamines (for antiemetic effect)

Cyproheptadine (Periactin, Cyprodine), po, 4 mg tid or qid, not more than 0.5 mg/kg/d

Phenothiazine (for antiemetic effect)

Trimeprazine tartrate (Temaril, Panectyl), po, 2.5 mg qid

H-1 receptor antagonists

Diphenhydramine (Benadryl), po, 25-50 mg q6-8h

Trimeprazine (Temaril), po, 5 mg q 12 h in sustained release form

Laxatives/stool softeners

Methylcellulose (Methulose, Cologel), po, 5-20 ml tid

Docusate sodium (Colace, DCS), po, 50-200 mg/d

Electrolytes, minerals, and nutritional replacements

Calcium supplements

Calcium carbonate (Titralac, Tums), po, 0.5-2 g 4-6 times daily

Calcium gluconate (Kalcinate), po, 1-5 g tid

Hematinic agents

Ferrous sulfate (Feosol), po, 300 mg-1.2 g/d

Ferrous fumarate (Chromagen), po, 325 mg bid

Polysaccaride iron complex (Niferex), po, 150 mg bid

Iron dextran injection, (InFeD), IM, IV, varies with weight and hemoglobin level

Vitamins

Multivitamin supplements (water-soluble vitamins), daily requirements: thiamine, 1.5 mg/d; riboflavin, 1.8 mg/d; niacin, 20 mg/d; pantothenic acid, 5 mg/d; pyridoxine, 5 mg/d; vitamin B$_{12}$, 3 μg/d; vitamin C, 100 mg/d

Folic acid (Folvite, Folate sodium), po, subcutaneously, IM, IV, up to 1 mg/d

Vitamin D

Calcitrol (1,25 dihydroxycholecalciferol) (Rocaltrol), po, 0.25 μg/d; maintenance is 0.5-1 μg/d

Dihydrotachysterol (DHT, Hytakerol), 0.2-0.4 mg/d

General Management

The goal is to maintain the ideal body weight—the weight at which the blood pressure is easily controlled without postural hypotension

Dialysis: peritoneal (see p. 975) or hemodialysis (see p. 970) may be needed

Fluid intake should balance output: about 400 to 600 ml (about the amount of insensible losses) plus an amount equal to 24-hour urine volume; avoid dehydration and volume overload

Diet modifications focus on providing vitamins and controlling the intake of protein, carbohydrate, fat, sodium, potassium, and phosphate; a high-protein diet increases the GFR and appears to accelerate the natural deterioration of renal function in patients with a variety of lesions[11]; this finding is the basis for proposing the use of a low-protein diet early in the course of renal disease, although this may not be effective

Protein: If nephrotic syndrome: .8-1.0 g/kg/day with 60% of protein of high biologic value; if on hemodialysis or peritoneal dialysis: 1.2-1.5 g/kg/day

Sodium: 2 g/day if on hemodialysis; 2-4 g/day if on peritoneal dialysis

Potassium: 2-3 g/day for hemodialysis; 3-4 g/day for peritoneal dialysis; no restriction is needed if urine output is at least 800 ml/day

Calories: >35 kcal/kg/day; sufficient to attain or maintain ideal body weight; calories from protein and nonprotein sources (50% from carbohydrate and the remaining from fat)

Vitamins: B complex, C, folate, but not A

Minerals: Calcium 1400 to 1600 mg/day; phosphate 8 to 17 mg/kg/day

NURSING CARE

Nursing Assessment

Renal

Oliguria; anuria

Cardiovascular

Edema; hypertension; tachycardia; jugular venous distention

Dermatologic

Pruritus; excoriations; yellow-tan or grayish color; pallor; uremic frost; bruises; petechiae; purpura; fragile, dry skin; thin, brittle nails

Gastrointestinal

Urinelike odor on breath; metallic taste in mouth; stomatitis and gingivitis; loss of sense of smell; anorexia; nausea; vomiting and hematemesis; hiccoughs; melena; diarrhea or constipation

Neurologic

Changes in cognitive function and behavior; altered levels of consciousness; changes in motor function and proprioception; peripheral neuropathy, nocturnal leg cramping; formication and other paresthesias of lower extremities; apathy, lethargy, and fatigue; headaches; insomnia

Ocular

Calcification of conjunctiva (red eyes); blurred vision

Reproductive

Impotence; amenorrhea; decreased libido; gynecomastia

Respiratory

Hyperventilation; Kussmaul breathing; apnea; altered lung sounds (rales, rhonchi, crackles); dyspnea; orthopnea

Skeletal

Bone pain; joint swelling and pain

General

Weight loss (muscle mass); weight gain (fluid accumulation); fever; chills

Psychosocial

Change in family relationships; family expresses concern about long-term implications of illness

Nursing Dx & Intervention

Altered renal tissue perfusion related to nephron destruction with inability to excrete metabolic wastes

- Monitor ECG for changes; respirations (rate and depth); Chvostek's and Trousseau's signs. *Peaked T waves, prolonged PR interval and widened QRS complex are associated with increased serum potassium; Kussmaul respirations are associated with acidosis; tetany may occur with low-calcium level. Increase or decrease in potassium may be associated with dysrhythmias; potassium may be lowered by vigorous diuretic therapy.*
- Monitor laboratory data: serum pH, potassium, bicarbonate, calcium, magnesium, phosphate; hemoglobin and hematocrit; BUN; serum creatinine. *Levels reflect kidneys' ability to excrete nitrogenous wastes, excess fluids, and electrolytes; values also indicate kidneys' nonexcretory functions (e.g., erythropoietin production).*
- Avoid nephrotoxic drugs; kidneys' ability to excrete drugs normally is reduced.
- Administer medications with care; monitor response to drugs. Doses of medications may be less than usual, and intervals between doses may be lengthened; *monitoring determines the effectiveness of drug, dosage, and timing and aids in identifying adverse side effects.*
- Monitor weight daily, also 24-hour intake and output; assess blood pressure (standing and sitting), pulse, and respirations (including breath sounds) every 6 to 8 hours; assess mental status; monitor edema, jugular venous distention, hepatojugular reflex, and, if necessary, central venous pressure and pulmonary artery pressures *to identify altered fluid status.*
- Monitor laboratory data: serum sodium, potassium, chloride, bicarbonate *to identify electrolyte accumulations.*
- Offer limited fluid intake over 24 hours *to avoid nocturnal dehydration,* since the kidneys' normal diurnal variation in urine output is lost; offer cool liquids that may help quench thirst.
- Administer diuretics as ordered; monitor response *to determine the effect of drugs and observe for side effects such as hypokalemia and ototoxicity.*

Altered nutrition: less than body requirements related to restricted dietary intake and gastrointestinal effects of uremia, which cause primarily protein-calorie malnutrition

- Assess for nausea, vomiting, and anorexia; *these conditions decrease intake of needed nutrients.*
- Monitor food intake and dry weight; monitor laboratory data: serum protein, lipids, potassium, and sodium *to determine how well the diet is being followed.*
- Encourage food intake as prescribed; postpone meals, if necessary; serve food the patient likes, and present it attractively *to ensure adequate intake within limits prescribed.*

- Provide oral hygiene before meals; offer gum or sour candy *to help remove bad taste from mouth.*
- Administer antiemetics and monitor response *to determine the effect of dosage and timing and to observe for adverse side effects.*
- Refer complex or problem situations to dietitian; using a team approach to managing the complex renal diet is helpful to all concerned.

Risk for infection related to suppressed immune responses associated with uremia

- Assess for signs and symptoms of infection in secretions, excretions, and exudates; assess for fever and chills *to detect any infection early.*
- Monitor temperature every 4 to 6 hours; monitor laboratory data: white blood cell count (WBC); blood, urine, and sputum cultures; serum potassium. *Uremia may mask the usual increase in temperature and WBC found with infection; a hypermetabolic state such as infection can cause a marked risk in serum potassium.*
- Wash hands thoroughly and consistently; avoid exposing patient to people with infections; ensure aseptic technique for any invasive procedure or wound care *to decrease chances of infection.*
- Encourage regular oral hygiene, hand washing, bathing, adequate nutrition, and rest; *good health habits help prevent infection.*

Risk for impaired skin integrity related to the effects of uremia

- Assess for dry skin, pruritus, excoriation, and infection; *such changes may be related to decreased activity of sweat glands or deposits of calcium or phosphate crystals in cutaneous layers.*
- Assess for petechiae and purpura; *bleeding abnormalities are related to decreased number and altered function of platelets in uremia.*
- Monitor skin folds and edematous areas *because these areas are easily injured.*
- Provide meticulous care to normal and injured areas of skin *to prevent infection and to help healing.*
- Administer antipruritic drugs; vinegar or starch baths; use bland soap sparingly *to relieve pruritus.*
- Keep fingernails trimmed *to decrease injury during scratching.*

Risk for confusion related to endogenous chemical abnormalities associated with uremia

- Assess neurologic status; orientation to person, place, and time; sleep pattern; level of consciousness; and seizure activity; *such changes reflect alterations in central autonomic nervous system function.*
- Assess premorbid personality *to identify changes associated with uremia.*
- Observe for changes in behavior and presence of peripheral neuropathy: restless legs, burning feet, muscle cramps, other paresthesias, and dysesthesias *because metabolic changes may cause cerebral and peripheral neurologic dysfunction; demyelination of large nerve fiber and axonal degeneration may occur.*
- Orient patient to reality *to decrease the possibility that disorientation is caused by isolation and lack of information.*
- Maintain safety precautions: bed rails up, bed in low position, sharp objects out of reach, call bell in reach; institute seizure precautions if needed *to provide safe environment and prevent injury.*
- Allow extra time for patient to respond to questions and to process new information; use a consistent, calm, nonargumentative approach; *short-term memory loss may occur.*
- Encourage normal daytime activities and presleep relaxation training; provide periods of rest *to maintain or encourage normal sleep-rest patterns; uremia can reverse sleep-wake patterns.*

Risk for bathing/hygiene, toileting self-care deficit related to uremia

- Assess fatigue and weakness, and assist with care as needed *to respond to need for assistance.*
- Implement measures such as deep breathing, coughing, and turning regularly *to prevent adverse effects of bed rest, such as pneumonia.*
- Increase activity as tolerated *to help patient return to self-care as appropriate.*

Risk for sexual dysfunction related to the effects of uremia

- Assess patient's and spouse's response to alterations *to determine presence of problems.*
- Allow patient and spouse or significant other to talk about their feelings; suggest the positive aspects of closeness and touching without intercourse *to help patient and spouse adjust to changes.*
- Refer patient and spouse for counseling when needed *to help resolve problems requiring time and skills beyond the nurse's training.*

Risk for body image disturbance related to altered renal function

- Assess for evidence that change in renal function or in appearance or the possibility of dialysis or transplantation is a problem; allow patient to talk about feelings; recognize defense mechanisms such as denial, guilt, aggression, fear, displacement, regression, resentment, disbelief, and anxiety; recognize losses in psychosocial aspects of patient's life; isolation, job loss, financial instability, dependency, and altered hopes for the future may be problems; *early intervention may prevent patient distress.*
- Explain skin changes to patient (in color, easy bruising); *pallor may be caused by anemia, yellowish cast by urochrome pigment deposits in skin; black patients become more deeply pigmented, and Hispanics and Asians show pallor.*

Risk for altered family processes related to CRF of family member

- Assess family structure and role relationship *to identify family strengths.*
- Monitor family's response to illness, treatment, and prognosis *to identify potential problems.*
- Encourage patient and family to discuss their needs and concerns; discuss impact of situation on roles and adaptation required *to help in adjustments indicated.*
- Assist with problem solving, and support family decisions; crisis intervention may be needed.
- Refer family to other services as appropriate *to help resolve problems requiring time and skills beyond the nurse's capability.*

Knowledge deficit related to chronic renal failure, its cause, manifestations, and treatment; the need for medical follow-up; and the potential need for dialysis or transplantation

- See box below.

Patient Education/Home Care Planning[5,8]

1. Explain the nature of chronic renal failure.
2. Explain the medical regimen and its rationale, including diet (restricted protein, sodium, and potassium intake), restricted fluid intake, and medications (purpose, dosage, interval, and adverse reactions).
3. Help patient learn self-observational skills (temperature, pulse, respirations, blood pressure, intake and output, and weight) and record keeping.
4. Explain avoidance of infection.
5. Explain personal hygiene, rest, and exercise.
6. Explain when to call the physician.
7. Explain the plan for medical follow-up.
8. Explain renal dialysis and transplantation.

Evaluation

Renal tissue perfusion is adequate Renal function tests are normal or stable.

Fluid balance is normal Urine output balances intake; there are no or minimum signs of edema.

Patient's nutritional status has improved and is maintained Food and fluid intakes are within the limits imposed by CRF; dry weight is maintained or increased if necessary.

No infection is present No signs or symptoms of infection are noted.

Skin is intact Patient has no areas of excoriation.

No confusion is present Patient is oriented to time, place, and person; alterations in sensation are not progressing; sleep pattern is normal.

Patient has resumed self-care Patient has no or few restrictions in ADLs.

Patient has accepted alterations in sexuality Patient has acceptable sexual relationships within the limits imposed by CRF.

Patient has adapted to changes in body image associated with CRF Patient demonstrates adjustment to altered renal function and any change in appearance.

Patient and family have adapted to patient's disorder Patient and family have dealt constructively with diagnosis and treatment regimen and can identify available sources of help.

Patient and family are knowledgeable about CRF Patient and family can explain CRF, its causes, and its manifestations; the need for medical follow-up; and the potential need for dialysis or transplantation in the future.

■ PYELONEPHRITIS

Pyelonephritis (PLN) is an infection of the kidney and renal pelvis. It is a major problem of the renal system.

Pyelonephritis is one of a group of conditions generally called urinary tract infections (the others are asymptomatic bacteriuria and cystitis). Urinary tract infections occur more frequently in women than in men, and the incidence of infection increases with age, instrumentation of the urinary tract, and urologic abnormalities, including vesicoureteral reflux or urinary tract obstruction.

Although urinary tract infections, including PLN, cause considerable morbidity, they do not progress to end-stage renal disease unless there is an underlying urinary tract problem such as obstruction. During pregnancy, women should be screened for bacteriuria and treated to prevent the development of PLN. Personal health habits should include adequate fluid intake (2500 to 3000 ml/day) and prompt emptying of the bladder.

•••••• Pathophysiology

The infection in PLN is caused by bacteria that spread by hematogenous or lymphatic routes or that (most commonly) ascend from the lower urinary tract.

The organisms most frequently involved are gram-negative bacilli and enterococci—bacteria that colonize the bowel. Such bacteria can proliferate and ascend to the kidneys. *Escherichia coli, Klebsiella pneumoniae, Proteus mirabilis* or *Proteus vulgaris, Pseudomonas aeruginosa,* and *Streptococcus faecalis* can cause urinary tract infection and progress to PLN.

Obstructive uropathy, glomerulonephritis, polycystic kidney disease, diabetes mellitus, renal calculi, and analgesic abuse appear to lower the kidney's resistance to infection. Without treatment, a significant number of pregnant women with asymptomatic bacteriuria will develop PLN.

The kidneys are damaged by the inflammation, fibrosis, and scarring caused by the infection. Chronic PLN causes tissue destruction and results in small, contracted kidneys. The medulla is susceptible to the ascending spread of bacteria because of its hypertonic environment and slow blood flow. Infection spreads through the collecting ducts to the interstitium. Papillary necrosis may be a complication of PLN, and detached pieces of tissue may block the ureters. Infection spreads to the cortex and eventually involves the nephron and blood vessels. Renal abscesses or septicemia may also develop.

Most infections are acute, although long-term, smoldering, chronic infection occasionally may occur. One or more of the factors previously mentioned contribute most often to a chronic kidney infection.

•••••• Diagnostic Studies and Findings

Urinalysis Antibody-coated bacteria (more often associated with PLN than with cystitis); bacteriuria; WBC casts, pyuria

Complete blood count Increased WBC

Intravenous urogram Small kidneys with an irregular outline and focal clubbing of the calyceal system

•••••• Multidisciplinary Plan

Medications

Antiinfective agents: parenteral
Carbenicillin (Geopen), IM, IV, 250-500 mg/kg/d in divided doses
Piperacillin (Pipracil), IM, IV, 8-18 g/d in 2-6 divided doses
Ampicillin (Omnipen), IM, IV, 1-12 g/d in 4-8 divided doses
Cefazolin (Ancef, Kefzol), IM, IV, 0.25-1.5 g/d q6-8h
Cefoxitin (Mefoxin), IM, IV, 1-2 g, q6-8h
Ceftazidime (Fortaz), IM, IV, 0.5-2 g, q8-12h
Gentamicin (Garamycin), IM, IV, 3-5 mg/kg q8h
Tobramycin (Tobrex), IM, IV, 3-5 mg/kg q8h
Amikacin (Amikin), IM, IV, 15 mg/kg/d in 2-3 doses
Co-trimoxazole IV (Septra IV), 8-10 mg/kg trimethoprim (with 40-50 mg/kg sulfamethoxazole) daily divided into 2-4 equal doses
Oral agents
Carbenicillin (Geocillin), po, 382-764 mg q6h
Ampicillin (Polycillin), po, 1-4 g/d in 4 divided doses
Amoxicillin-clavulanic acid (Augmentin) 250-500 mg q8h
Cephalexin (Keflex), po, 250-500 mg q6-12h
Cefaclor (Ceclor), po, 250-500 mg q8h
Cefixime (Suprax), po, 400 mg/d
Co-trimoxazole (Septra), po, 160 mg trimethoprim (with 800 mg sulfamethoxazole), q12h
Sulfamethizole (Proklar), po, 0.5-1 g/d in 3-4 divided doses (total 1.5-4 g)
Sulfisoxazole (Gantrisin), po, 2-4 g/d initially, then 4-8 g/d in 4-6 equally divided doses
Trimethoprim (Proloprim), po, 100 mg q12h or 200 mg/d
Nalidixic acid (NegGram), po, 1 g qid for 7-14 d
Ciprofloxacin (Cipro) po 250-750 mg q12h for 10-14 days
Norfloxacin (Noroxin), po, 400 mg q12h
Nitrofurantoin (Furadantin), po, 50-100 mg 4 qid for 7 d or more
Methenamine (Hexamine), po, 1 g qid after meals and at bedtime

General Management

The goals of treatment are to eradicate the infection and relieve the symptoms
High normal fluid intake (3500 to 4500 ml/day) is prescribed to dilute urine, decrease burning on urination, flush out the urinary tract, and prevent dehydration (with normal renal function)
Bed rest is commonly encouraged during acute phase

NURSING CARE

Nursing Assessment

General

Sudden onset of fever, chills, dull constant pain in flank

Renal

Hematuria; bacteriuria; pyuria; urine culture: significant growth; dysuria; nocturia; frequency; urgency; suprapubic tenderness occasionally

Nursing Dx & Intervention

Altered body temperature related to effects of infection

- Assess for diaphoresis and dehydration; assess temperature every 4 to 8 hours. *Water loss via the skin increases with fever; perspiration is part of the body's attempt to lower the temperature.*
- Administer antiinfective agents as ordered, and monitor response; monitor laboratory data: urinalysis and WBC *to determine effects of drugs and to watch for adverse side effects.*
- Encourage bed rest during acute phase of illness *to increase patient's comfort.*
- Encourage high-normal fluid intake unless contraindicated *to flush kidneys (but avoid lowering drug concentration to ineffective levels).*

Pain in flank related to distention of renal capsule by infectious process

- Assess need for analgesia; administer analgesics as needed. As swelling in the kidney decreases, pain lessens; *analgesics promote comfort.*
- Apply heat externally to painful area *to help relieve pain.*

Knowledge deficit related to pyelonephritis, its causes, signs, symptoms; treatment; follow-up care; and prevention

- See box on p. 942.

Patient Education/Home Care Planning

1. Explain pyelonephritis: its causes, signs, symptoms, and the need to have an intravenous urogram to rule out any structural defect.
2. Explain antimicrobial therapy: drugs, dosage, interval, side effects, and the need to complete the course of treatment.
3. Explain the possibility of relapse or reinfection.
4. Explain measures to prevent urinary tract infection, including adequate fluid intake (2000 to 2500 ml/day for adults) to avoid dehydration, regular emptying of bladder to avoid overdistention, and good perineal hygiene and postcoital elimination for women to prevent the entrance of microorganisms from the urinary tract.

Evaluation

Signs and symptoms of PLN have cleared   Patient's temperature is normal, pain is gone; urine is clear of bacteria or pus cells; problems in urination are gone.

Evaluation of urinary tract, if needed, has been completed   Intravenous urogram has determined whether there is any structural defect.

Patient is knowledgeable about PLN   Patient can describe the signs and symptoms of PLN and whether any further treatment is needed.

■ RENAL AND PERINEPHRIC ABSCESSES

A renal abscess is a localized infection within the cortex of the kidney; a perinephric abscess is a renal abscess that extends into the tissues surrounding the kidney.

Abscesses can arise in a normal or diseased kidney; they also can develop as a complication of subacute bacterial endocarditis and systemic infections. With perinephric abscess, delay in treatment results in a high mortality.

•••••• Pathophysiology

Renal abscess may be caused by diffuse pyelonephritis or hematogenous transport of bacteria in a systemic infection. Staphylococcal bacteremia, for example, may cause multiple cortical abscesses. Frequently abscesses are caused by gram-negative organisms such as *Proteus* species and *Escherichia coli*. When infection from the kidney spreads to the fatty and fascial tissues surrounding the kidney, the abscess is known as a perinephric abscess. Drainage collects at the lower pole of the kidney because of the effects of gravity. Such abscesses are frequently associated with renal calculi or urinary tract obstructions. The infection may extend through the fascia to nearby organs, such as the pancreas, duodenum, and colon.

•••••• Diagnostic Studies and Findings

White blood cell count   Elevated

Intravenous urogram   Renal mass, calyceal distortion, or renal displacement

Renal computed tomography (CT) scan   Differentiates between an abscess and a cyst

•••••• Multidisciplinary Plan

Medications

Antiinfective agents
   Sulfisoxazole (Gantrisin, Novosoxazole), po, 1-2 g initially followed by 1 g bid or tid
   Ampicillin (Omnipen, Polycillin), po, patients ≥20 kg: 250-500 mg q6h; patients <20 kg: 50-100 mg/kg/d in equally divided doses q6-8h
   Carbenicillin disodium (Geopen, Pyopen), IM, IV, 1-2 g q6h
   Gentamicin (Garamycin, Apogen), IM, IV, 3-5 mg/kg/d q8h
Antipyretics for fever
   Acetaminophen (Tylenol)

Surgery

Incision and drainage may be required if the renal abscess is localized; incision and drainage are usually required for perinephric abscesses
Intrarenal: percutaneous aspiration and then instillation of antibiotics; this procedure is less expensive and causes less discomfort than open drainage
Perinephric: percutaneous drainage, if possible; although open surgical drainage is more likely; the specimen is sent for culture and sensitivity determinations

General Management

Bed rest, adequate fluids (2500 to 3000 ml/day), and normal nutrition are important; a normal diet ensures protein, calories, and other nutrients sufficient to meet the needs of the individual's current stage of the life cycle; sterile dressing changes are needed after incision and drainage of abscesses

NURSING CARE

Nursing Assessment

Signs of Infection

Renal abscess: none with solitary abscess; otherwise chills and fever; flank tenderness; nausea; vomiting; anorexia; and malaise
Perinephric abscess: chills and fever; dull ache in flank; costovertebral angle tenderness on palpation; mass in flank; abdominal pain with guarding

Nursing Dx & Intervention

Impaired skin integrity related to percutaneous or open surgical drainage

• Assess condition of the incision and the nature and the amount of drainage *to determine extent of healing.*

- Monitor temperature every 6 to 8 hours; *body temperature rises with infection.*
- Administer antiinfective agents as ordered; *interruption in dosage can permit drug resistance to develop.*
- Encourage oral fluids (up to 3 L/day if not contraindicated) *to flush bacteria from urinary tract.*
- Change wound dressing using aseptic techniques *to promote healing and avoid introduction of additional organisms.*
- Monitor laboratory data: WBC *to follow body's response to infection and treatment.*

Pain related to drainage of abscess

- Assess need for pain relief; administer analgesic drug as ordered; monitor response to analgesic. Incisional pain is not unusual in the first 24 hours; *analgesic promotes patient comfort and monitoring determines effectiveness of drug, dosage, and timing.*

Knowledge deficit related to causes and treatment of a renal or perinephric abscess

- See box below.

Patient Education/Home Care Planning

1. Explain the side effects and adverse reactions of pharmacologic agents used.
2. Explain care of the incision and teach dressing changes if necessary.
3. Explain the relationship between perinephric abscesses and pyelonephritis, renal calculi, and urinary tract obstruction.

Evaluation

Infection has cleared   Temperature is normal; patient is free of pain; WBC is normal.

Incision has healed   No sign of infection is noted; wound is closed.

Patient is knowledgeable about renal or perinephric abscess   Patient can describe the cause and treatment of a renal or perinephric abscess.

◼ GENITOURINARY TUBERCULOSIS

◼ Infection caused by *Mycobacterium tuberculosis* can occur in the kidney and spread to the rest of the genitourinary tract.

Genitourinary tuberculosis is much less common today than in the past; however, 4265 new cases of extrapulmonary tuberculosis were reported in the United States in 1994. Of these cases, 340 (7.9%) were in the genitourinary system.[6] Prevention is important; about 15% of people with active pulmonary tuberculosis develop genitourinary involvement.

Contact with people with active tuberculosis should be avoided, and early diagnosis is important.

Genitourinary tuberculosis often occurs in older people and in immigrants from countries with high prevalence rates. Prophylactic care with isoniazid is important for susceptible individuals (e.g., household members of patients with tuberculosis and persons with positive reactions to the tuberculin skin test).

•••••• Pathophysiology

The tuberculosis organism is carried by the bloodstream from the lungs or gastrointestinal tract. Genitourinary tuberculosis is associated with concurrent primary pulmonary lesion, or it occurs many years later during reactivation of an infection that was previously seeded in the kidney. The renal lesion, initially in the glomeruli, causes inflammation, caseation, and rupture, thus spreading the infection to the rest of the nephron and resulting in a progressive destruction of the renal parenchyma.

Tuberculosis occurs more frequently in men; the bladder, prostate, epididymis, and testicle may also be involved. An abscess in the cortex may erode into a calyx, spreading infection to the pelvis and downward to the bladder. Early treatment of pulmonary tuberculosis may be reducing the number of patients who develop renal lesions.

The tuberculosis organism causes a low-grade inflammation and granuloma formation; healing causes fibrosis, calcification, and scarring, and thus destruction of renal tissue. Damage may obstruct the drainage system and impair blood supply, causing hypertension.

•••••• Diagnostic Studies and Findings

Routine urinalysis   Sterile pyuria; hematuria; early morning urine specimen 3 days in a row: acid-fast bacillus; urine culture: *M. tuberculosis* grown

Skin test (intradermal Mantoux)   Positive tuberculin reaction

Intravenous urogram   Cavity formation shown by irregular outline of kidney and calcification; impaired excretion of dye because of parenchymal destruction (tissue may appear "moth eaten"); ureteral stricture; decreased bladder capacity

Kidney-ureter-bladder (KUB) x-ray   Kidney enlarged because of granulomas or hydronephrosis, or shrunken because of fibrosis and atrophy

•••••• Multidisciplinary Plan

Treatment, such as for tuberculosis, takes more than 6 months to 2 years (see Chapter 13).

Medications

Antiinfective agents
  Isoniazid (INH, Isotamine), po or IM, 5 mg/kg/body weight up to 300 mg/d
  Rifampin (Rifadin, Rifampicin), po, 600 mg/d
  Streptomycin, IM, 1 g/d, reduce to 1 g 2-3 times/wk when sputum cultures become negative

Ethambutol (Etibi, Myambutol), po, 15 mg/kg body weight/d

Pyrazinamide (PZA) 15-30 mg/kg/d, maximum 2000 mg or 50-70 mg/kg twice weekly

Pyridoxine (Beesix, Vitabee-6), po, IM, or IV, for isoniazid-induced deficiency: 100-200 mg/d for 3 wk, then 25-100 mg/d maintenance

Surgery

May be necessary to remove nonfunctioning kidney, a continuing source of organisms or uncontrollable hypertension

Repair of sequelae, such as ureteral strictures, may be necessary

General Management

Bed rest may be prescribed at first; ensure adequate nutrition; observe isolation precautions if sputum or urine is positive for tuberculosis bacilli; proper disposal of urine (flushed down toilet, not bedpan flusher) and other infected material (double-bagged and incinerated) is part of the plan of care

NURSING CARE

Nursing Assessment

General

Fever; weight loss; flank pain; sweating

Urinary Tract

Urgency; frequency; flank pain; lethargy; malaise; NOTE: Far-advanced disease may manifest itself by renal failure or urinary tract obstruction; most cases show few or no symptoms

Nursing Dx & Intervention

Altered tissue perfusion related to effects of infection

- Assess body temperature every 4 to 6 hours; *body temperature increases during active infection.*
- Assess hydration status by examining skin turgor and mucous membrane; provide fluids; *water loss increases with fever; fluids help maintain normal balance and replace insensible losses.*
- Administer antiinfective drugs as ordered; *interruption in dosage can permit drug resistance to develop.*
- Monitor laboratory data: urinalysis (second voided early morning specimen), liver function tests; *acid-fast bacilli should disappear from urine within 2 to 4 weeks of effective therapy; if not, check for drug resistance and compliance; drugs given may alter liver function; rifampin may darken the urine.*

Altered pattern of urinary elimination related to urinary tract stricture, inflammation

- Assess frequency and urgency; *decreased bladder capacity and inflammation of the urinary tract lining may cause these symptoms.*
- Provide urinal or bedpan; patient may not be able to reach toilet in time.

Risk for bathing/hygiene and toileting self-care deficit related to bed rest

- Assess patient's compliance; assist with personal hygiene as needed; *bed rest may be ordered during acute phase of illness.*
- Remind patient to turn, cough, breathe deeply, and exercise legs several times a day *to prevent adverse effects of bed rest such as pneumonia and deep vein thrombosis.*

Knowledge deficit related to cause, spread, treatment, and follow-up care

- See box below.

Patient Education/Home Care Planning
1. Explain the nature of tuberculosis, its cause, spread, and treatment, including the need for follow-up care.

Evaluation

Infection is resolved   Urine culture is negative in 2 months; temperature is within normal range; follow-up x-ray examination reveals healing and no strictures.

Pattern of urinary elimination has improved   Patient experiences no urgency or frequency.

Patient has returned to independent physical activities and self-care   Patient has no limitations on ADLs.

Patient is knowledgeable about genitourinary tuberculosis   Patient can describe measures to prevent spread of tuberculosis, the rationale for drug treatment, and the side effects of the drugs taken.

OBSTRUCTIVE AND CONGENITAL DISORDERS

HYDRONEPHROSIS

Hydronephrosis is the dilation of the renal pelvis by the pressure of urine that cannot flow past an obstruction of the urinary tract.

Obstruction can be proximal to the bladder or occur below the level of the bladder. Hydronephrosis, which is usually on the right side, always occurs during pregnancy and for a time after delivery because of obstruction caused by the enlarged uterus.

Pathophysiology

Obstruction of the ureter that results in hydronephrosis may be caused by renal calculi, tumors, inflammation associated with infection, fibrous bands that obstruct the ureteropelvic junction, or prostatic urethral valves. The renal pelvis and ureters dilate and hypertrophy. The pressure of the urine, if prolonged, causes fibrosis and loss of function in affected nephrons. The duration and severity of the obstruction are significant. Compression causes ischemia and then atrophy of renal tissue. The kidney may be destroyed without pain.

Diagnostic Studies and Findings

Renal ultrasonography Dilation of collecting system
Intravenous urogram Calyceal clubbing is shown after injection of radiopaque dye

Multidisciplinary Plan

Surgery

Performed to relieve the obstruction and preserve renal function; pyeloplasty or repair of ureteropelvic junction may be indicated; nephrectomy may be necessary if the kidney is severely damaged (see "Other Kidney Surgery," p. 983)

Medications

Antiinfective agents if infection is present
Parenteral agents (IM or IV)
Gentamicin (Garamycin, Apogen), 3-5 mg/kg/d q8h
Cephalosporins
Cefazolin sodium (Ancef, Kefzol), 250-1000 mg q6-8h
Penicillins
Ampicillin sodium (Omnipen-N, Polycillin-N), patients ≥40 kg: 250-500 mg q6h; <40 kg: 25-50 mg/kg/d in equally divided doses q6-8h
Carbenicillin disodium (Geopen, Pyopen), 1-2 g q6h
Penicillin G potassium (Aqueous penicillin G), Penicillin G sodium, 1-20 million U/d
Oral agents
Sulfonamides
Sulfisoxazole (Gantrisin, Novosoxazole), 2-4 g initially, followed by 1-2 g q4-6h
Tetracycline (Achromycin, Tetracyn), 250-500 mg q6h
Penicillins
Amoxicillin (Amoxil, Amoxycillin), patients ≥20 kg: 250-500 mg q8h; <20 kg: 20-40 mg/kg/d in divided doses q8h
Ampicillin (Omnipen, Polycillin), patients ≥20 kg: 250-500 mg q6h; <20 kg: 50-100 mg/kg/d in equally divided doses
Erythromycin (Erythrocin, E-Mycin), 250 mg q6h
Sulfamethoxazole and trimethoprim (Septra, Bactrim), 2 tab q12h

General Management

Usually conservative if the condition is not severe

NURSING CARE

Nursing Assessment

Renal

Hematuria; pyuria

Abdomen

Kidneys may be palpable

General

Dull backache; fever with infection

Nursing Dx & Intervention

Risk for altered renal tissue perfusion related to increased pressure within the urine channel because of obstruction at some point in the urinary tract

- Assess blood pressure every 6 to 8 hours, 24-hour intake and output; weigh daily; monitor laboratory data: serum creatinine, BUN, serum sodium, potassium, bicarbonate. *Postobstruction diuresis may occur; acute renal failure may develop.*

Risk for infection related to urinary tract obstruction

- Assess for signs and symptoms of urinary tract infection (fever, increased WBC, pyuria, bacteriuria, foul-smelling urine). *Likelihood of infection is increased with obstruction.*
- Administer antiinfective agents as ordered; monitor response to drugs given *to treat any infection present and to determine response to drug.* Prepare for surgery (see "Other Kidney Surgery," p. 983).

Impaired skin integrity related to surgery

- After surgery, assess site of incision for drainage and signs of infection *to detect any complications promptly.* Keep area clean and dry *to avoid skin breakdown and promote healing.*
- Keep any drainage tubes patent, unkinked, and anchored *to maintain urine flow and to avoid inadvertent displacement.* Care for urethral catheter. Tubes may include a stent (a catheter inserted into the ureter), a nephrostomy tube, and a drain in the incision; drainage from the incision may continue for several days.

Pain related to surgical incision

- Assess for discomfort and give analgesics as ordered *to determine the need for pain relief and to relieve discomfort.* Monitor and record response to drug *to determine effectiveness of drug, dosage, and timing and to identify any side effects.* Report any pain that occurs after the immediate postoperative period; *pain with fever and decreased urine output may indicate obstruction or leakage of urine into the retroperitoneal space.*

Knowledge deficit related to hydronephrosis and follow-up care

- See box below.

Patient Education/Home Care Planning

1. Explain the kidney-ureter abnormality.
2. Explain possible problems: recurrent infection and obstruction.
3. Explain signs and symptoms of urinary tract infection and obstruction.
4. Explain measures to prevent urinary tract infection: adequate fluid intake to avoid dehydration, regular emptying of bladder to avoid overdistention, and good perineal hygiene to prevent entrance of microorganisms into the urinary tract.
5. Explain postoperative care, including care of the incision and self-monitoring skills as needed.
6. Explain plans for medical follow-up of renal function.

Evaluation

Obstruction is relieved; renal function is normal X-ray examination shows that hydronephrosis is lessened or has not increased; renal function tests are normal or stable.

No infection is present in the urinary tract Patient has no signs or symptoms of urinary tract infection.

Incision is healing No drainage, redness, swelling, or separation of incision is noted.

Patient is pain free Patient does not complain of pain.

Patient and family are knowledgeable about hydronephrosis Patient and family understand the condition and the need for follow-up medical care.

CONGENITAL ANOMALIES

A wide variety of anomalies related to the kidneys can occur. The abnormalities may be in number, volume, form, location, rotation, blood vessels, pelvis, or ureter. These errors in renal development result from failure to develop, abnormal division of the elements, fusion of the elements, or abnormal movement from the pelvis to the lumbar area. These anatomic deviations may range from minor to severe and from easily correctable to incompatible with life. Renal abnormalities are frequently associated with additional anomalies such as low-set ears, imperforate anus, genital anomalies, and abnormalities of the spinal cord and extremities.

KIDNEY DISPLACEMENT AND SUPERNUMERARY KIDNEYS

Kidney displacement occurs occasionally when the kidneys do not ascend to their normal position, or one may cross over, causing both kidneys to be on one side. A supernumerary, or extra, kidney, rarely occurs, although duplication of the renal pelvis is common.

Pathophysiology

The displaced kidneys may be normal except for their abnormal location or rotation. They have increased susceptibility to trauma because they are not protected as well as a kidney in its normal location. Obstruction may occur, as may infarction or infection if the normal blood supply and urinary channel are interrupted. The extra kidney may be small, dysplastic, and infected.

Diagnostic Studies and Findings

Intravenous urogram Abnormally located or rotated kidney; extra kidney(s)

Multidisciplinary Plan

Surgery

Correction of obstruction to blood supply or urine elimination in displaced kidney and removal of extra kidney(s) may be indicated; function of remaining kidney tissue must be adequate

---

NURSING CARE

Nursing Assessment

Urinary Tract

Asymptomatic; signs of infection or obstruction

Nursing Dx & Intervention

Risk for infection related to abnormality of blood supply or urine channel

- Assess for signs and symptoms of urinary tract infection; monitor temperature, nature of urine. *Abnormal urine channel or blood supply may increase susceptibility to urinary tract infection.*

Impaired skin integrity related to surgery

- Prepare patient for surgery (see "Other Kidney Surgery," p. 983). After surgery, assess site of incision for drainage and signs of infection *to detect complications promptly.*
- Keep area clean and dry *to avoid skin breakdown and promote healing.*
- Keep any drainage tubes patent, unkinked, and anchored *to permit continuous drainage and avoid inadvertent displacement.*

- Be alert to and report any foul-smelling urine, pus, or blood *to detect complications promptly.*

Pain related to surgery

- Assess patient's need for pain relief; administer analgesic as ordered; monitor response *to determine need for drug, promote patient's comfort, and determine effectiveness of drug, dosage, and timing; also to identify any side effects.*

Knowledge deficit related to patient's condition and follow-up care

- See box below.

Patient Education/Home Care Planning

1. Explain the location of the displaced or extra kidney(s).
2. Explain the signs and symptoms of possible problems (trauma to abdomen, urinary tract infection, or urinary tract obstruction).
3. Explain measures to prevent urinary tract infection: adequate fluid intake (to avoid dehydration), regular emptying of the bladder to avoid overdistention, and good perineal hygiene to prevent the entrance of microorganisms into the urinary tract.
4. Explain postoperative care, including care of the incision and self-monitoring skills (intake and output, weight, temperature).

Evaluation

No urinary tract infection is present Patient's temperature and WBC are normal; urinalysis has no bacteria or pus cells.

Incision has healed Wound is closed, and no infection is present.

Patient is pain free Patient does not complain of discomfort.

Patient and family are knowledgeable about patient's condition Patient and family can explain the signs of possible problems related to the location of the kidney, measures to prevent urinary tract infections, and any postoperative care needed.

Hypoplasia and Dysplasia of the Kidney

Hypoplasia is a condition in which fewer than the usual number of nephrons are present. Dysplasia is a condition in which areas of the kidneys have underdeveloped structures. When these defects occur together, the term used is hypodysplasia.

• • • • • • Pathophysiology

With hypoplasia, the kidneys are small but normal in structure. They may be dysplastic, with malformation of renal tissue. If both kidneys are severely malformed, death occurs in the neonatal period. One kidney usually has poorer function than the other.

• • • • • Diagnostic Studies and Findings

Intravenous urogram Small, malformed kidney(s)

• • • • • • Multidisciplinary Plan

Surgery

Elective surgical removal of the dysplastic kidney is usually performed. Careful assessment of the contralateral kidney is essential. If chronic renal failure occurs, renal dialysis or transplantation may be undertaken if technically feasible (see "Other Kidney Surgery," p. 983, "Renal Dialysis," pp. 970 to 975, and "Renal Transplantation," p. 979).

Medications

Antiinfective agents
  Parenteral agents (IM or IV)
    Gentamicin (Garamycin, Apogen), 3-5 mg/kg/d q8h
    Cephalosporins: Cefazolin sodium (Ancef, Kefzol), 250-1000 mg q6-8h
  Penicillins
    Sodium ampicillin (Omnipen-N, Polycillin-N), patients ≥40 kg: 250-500 mg q6h; <40 kg: 25-50 mg/kg/d in equally divided doses q6-8h
    Carbenicillin disodium (Geopen, Pyopen), 1-2 g IM q6h
    Penicillin G potassium (aqueous penicillin G), penicillin G sodium, 1-20 million U/d
  Oral agents
    Sulfonamides: Sulfisoxazole (Gantrisin, Novosoxazole), 2-4 g initially followed by 1-2 g q4-6h
    Tetracycline (Achromycin, Tetracyn), 250-500 mg q6h
  Penicillins
    Amoxicillin (Amoxil, Amoxycillin), patients ≥20 kg: 250-500 mg q8h; <20 kg: 20-40 mg/kg/d in divided doses q8h
    Ampicillin (Omnipen, Polycillin), patients ≥20 kg: 250-500 mg q6h; <20 kg: 50-100 mg/kg/d in equally divided doses
    Penicillin G, 200,000-500,000 U q6-8h
    Erythromycin (Erythrocin, Ilotycin), 250 mg q6h
    Sulfamethoxazole, trimethoprim (Septra, Bactrim), 2 tab q12h

General Management

Chronic renal failure may ensue (see "Chronic Renal Failure" and "Renal Dialysis," pp. 935 and 969 to 970)

NURSING CARE

Nursing Assessment

Renal Function

May be asymptomatic; bilateral: uremia; unilateral: infection, hypertension, or renal failure

Nursing Dx & Intervention

Impaired skin integrity related to surgery

- Prepare patient for surgery (see "Other Kidney Surgery," p. 983). After surgery, monitor site of incision for drainage and signs of infection *to detect any complications promptly.*
- Keep area clean and dry *to avoid skin breakdown and promote healing.*
- Keep any drainage tubes patent, unkinked, and anchored; care for urethral catheter *to permit continuous drainage and avoid inadvertent displacement;* tubes may include a drain in the incision.
- Report any foul-smelling urine, blood, or pus in drainage. *Such complications may follow surgery.*

Pain related to surgery

- Assess patient's need for pain relief; administer analgesic as ordered; monitor response *to determine need for analgesic, to promote comfort, to determine drug's effectiveness in timing and dosage, and to identify any side effects.*
- Assist with personal hygiene as needed after surgery *because pain may interfere with self-care.*

Risk for infection related to abnormality of urine channel

- Assess for signs and symptoms of urinary tract infection; monitor temperature, WBC, problems with urination, and urine (bacteriuria or pyuria). *Infection may occur in the urinary tract after surgery.*

Knowledge deficit related to the renal abnormality and its implications

- See box below.

Patient Education/Home Care Planning

1. Explain the kidney's abnormality.
2. Explain the possible problems, such as urinary tract infection, renal failure, and their signs and symptoms.
3. Describe measures to prevent urinary tract infection, such as adequate fluid intake to avoid dehydration, regular emptying of the bladder to avoid overdistention, and good perineal hygiene to prevent microorganisms from entering the urinary tract.
4. Explain postoperative care, including care of incision and any self-monitoring skills needed.
5. Explain that renal dialysis and transplantation are likely future options in the event of chronic renal failure.

Evaluation

Patient has recovered from surgery   Incision is healed.
Patient is free of pain   Patient does not complain of discomfort.

Patient has no infection   No signs or symptoms of urinary tract infection are noted.
Patient and family are knowledgeable about patient's condition   Patient and family can describe the renal abnormality and its implications.

■ POLYCYSTIC KIDNEY DISEASE

■ Polycystic kidney disease (PKD) is a disorder in which the kidney tissue is replaced by grapelike clusters of cysts.

Polycystic kidney disease is a genetically transmitted disorder (autosomal dominant in adults). An infant form (autosomal recessive) occurs, but these children rarely live more than a year. The adult form of the disease has a similar onset, clinical course, and manifestations within a family. Approximately 5% to 10% of patients on dialysis have the adult form of PKD. It is important that the cysts characteristic of PKD be differentiated from tumors. Fifteen percent of patients with polycystic kidney disease may have an associated berry aneurysm with the possibility of subarachnoid hemorrhage. The incidence of polycystic kidney disease is 1 in 1000.

•••••• Pathophysiology

In polycystic kidney disease, normal kidney tissue is replaced by grape-like clusters of cysts that enlarge over time and destroy the surrounding tissue by compression. Why cysts are formed is not clear. They may be associated with cysts in the liver. Cysts may occur anywhere along the nephron, and they are filled with a yellow or brown fluid that may be thick and cloudy and may contain urine components. Progressive fibrosis of the interstitial tissue occurs. Infection and renal stones often develop because of urinary stasis and compression. Ascending infection may become a persistent source of infection. These kidneys do not resist infection well and thus may harbor organisms; poor perfusion may prevent antibiotics from reaching pockets of infection. A perinephric abscess may form; septicemia may occur. In these cases a nephrectomy may be necessary. Hypertension and renal failure follow the onset of symptoms within 5 to 15 years.

•••••• Diagnostic Studies and Findings

Urinalysis   Intermittent hematuria; proteinuria; bacteria; pyuria; renal function tests (serum creatinine, blood urea nitrogen, creatinine clearance): function may be decreased
Kidney-ureter-bladder x-ray examination and renal ultrasonography   Enlarged kidneys
Intravenous urogram   Irregular outline and distortion of calyceal pattern; presence of cysts, nephrocalcinosis, or obstruction of the collecting system

•••••• Multidisciplinary Plan

No specific treatment is available for PKD. Medical goals concentrate on preventing hypertension and infection to preserve renal function. Instrumentation of the urinary tract, which is occasionally followed by a urinary tract infection, should be avoided. If patients do not have symptoms, creatinine clearance and urine cultures should be obtained twice a year. Genetic counseling may be suggested for families with PKD. Renal dialysis and transplantation may be indicated when chronic renal failure ensues.

NURSING CARE

Nursing Assessment

Urinary Tract

Urgency, frequency, and dysuria with infection

Abdomen

Palpable kidneys, dull ache in costovertebral or loin areas

Psychosocial

Acceptance or rejection of situation by patient; change in family relationships; concerns about long-term impact of illness

Nursing Dx & Intervention

Altered renal tissue perfusion related to replacement of normal tissue with cysts

- Assess and monitor intake, output, and weight if necessary *because renal insufficiency may develop.*
- Monitor blood pressure; administer antihypertensive drugs if ordered; *antihypertensives decrease effect of elevated blood pressure on already damaged kidneys.*
- Monitor laboratory data that reflect renal function *to follow any decrease in renal function.*

Risk for infection related to alterations of the collecting system by cysts

- Assess for signs and symptoms of urinary tract infection; cysts are prone to infection *because of changes caused in renal blood flow or urine flow.*
- Avoid inserting catheters or other instruments into urinary tract *to prevent nosocomial infections.*

Pain related to enlarged or infected cysts

- Assess patient's need for pain relief; *enlarged, infected cysts cause pain by increasing intrakidney pressure.*

Risk for altered family processes related to diagnosis of a genetically transmitted disease

- Assess how diagnosis of patient's condition affects others in the family *to determine need for family counseling.*
- Provide information about genetic counseling if appropriate; *some people do not want to know this information.*

Knowledge deficit related to PKD and plans for follow-up care

- See box.

Patient Education/Home Care Planning

1. Explain the nature of the kidney abnormality and the availability of genetic counseling.
2. Explain the need to monitor renal function and blood pressure.
3. Explain measures to prevent urinary tract infection: adequate fluid intake to avoid dehydration, regular emptying of the bladder to avoid overdistention, observation of urine, and good perineal care to prevent entrance of microorganisms into the urinary tract.
4. Explain signs and symptoms of urinary tract infections (see "Pyelonephritis," p. 940).
5. Explain renal dialysis and transplantation as options for the future.

Evaluation

Early decreases in renal function are recognized Urinalysis and blood chemistries are performed every 6 months, and any change is noted.

Infections are treated promptly Patient seeks medical help when signs and symptoms of urinary tract infection occur.

Patient is free from pain Patient has no complaint of pain.

Patient is knowledgeable and plans are made for long-term treatment Patient describes the anticipated course of the disease and the possible relationship of dialysis and transplantation for the future.

AUTOIMMUNE DISORDERS

GLOMERULONEPHRITIS

Glomerulonephritis (GN) may be a primary disease of the kidneys or may develop secondary to a systemic disease, such as lupus erythematosus. Glomerulonephritis is a disease primarily of the glomeruli caused by immunologically mediated damage (immune complex or autoantibody). The immune complexes (antibody-antigen) arise from antigens such as those from microorganisms, drugs, and autologous tissues. The major antibody involved is that against the glomerular basement membrane (GBM).

The clinical syndrome may include asymptomatic proteinuria, microscopic or macroscopic hematuria, or nephrotic syndrome. Nephrotic syndrome is characterized by proteinuria, normal or slightly decreased serum albumin levels, minimally decreased plasma lipid levels, marked hematuria, moderate edema, decreased urine volume and glomerular filtration rate, and hypertension.

A discussion of glomerulonephritis is difficult because of the confusion between older definitions (used before renal biopsy was introduced) and newer terms (used afterwards).

One classification uses clinical course (acute, rapidly progressive, and chronic), histopathology (e.g., membranoproliferative), and pathogenetic mechanism (immune complexes and antibodies against renal tissue).

The kinds of glomerulonephritis include acute poststreptococcal GN (APSGN) (immune complexes); Goodpasture's syndrome and rapidly progressive GN (anti–glomerular basement membrane or anti-GBM antibodies); and membranoproliferative GN. A renal biopsy is necessary to differentiate among the various kinds (see p. 1484). Only APSGN is discussed in this section.

Acute poststreptococcal glomerulonephritis

Acute poststreptococcal glomerulonephritis (APSGN) is an inflammation of the glomeruli that occurs after a streptococcal infection elsewhere in the body.

Glomerulonephritis can follow a respiratory or skin infection. Several strains of group A β-hemolytic streptococci that cause GN have been isolated. In temperate zones the most common nephritogenic strain causing pharyngitis is M-type. Only about 5% of such infections are followed by APSGN. Children and young adults are affected most frequently. The incidence of APSGN decreases with age because many children (especially in urban areas) develop immunities to M-type β-hemolytic streptococci before reaching adulthood. Renal problems occur abruptly 1 to 3 weeks after the infection. Most patients (95%) recover normal renal function within 2 months. The others have irreversible damage that causes long-term problems. It is not clear whether prompt treatment of streptococcal infections prevents renal complications of APSGN.

•••••• Pathophysiology

In acute poststreptococcal glomerulonephritis, antibodies of the host react with circulating antigens that appear to arise from the toxic products of the infecting organism; the antibodies and antigens form immune complexes that then become lodged in the glomeruli. Both kidneys are affected by an acute, diffuse, nonsuppurative inflammation that damages the glomerular basement membrane (GBM). The kidneys respond through GBM thickening, endocapillary proliferation, scarring, necrosis, and extracapillary proliferation. The damage causes an acute interference with renal function. Glomerulonephritis is a major cause of renal failure among patients on dialysis.

•••••• Diagnostic Studies and Findings

Routine urinalysis   Hematuria: >0-5 RBCs per high power field; proteinuria: >30-150 mg/24 hours; color change: red, red-brown; sediment: RBC casts

Serum albumin   <3.5-5 g/dl

Serum lipid   >400-800 mg/dl

Serum creatinine   >1.2 mg/dl (men); 1.1 mg/dl (women)

Blood urea nitrogen (BUN)   >5-20 mg/dl

Hemoglobin (Hgb)/hematocrit (Hct)   Hgb: <15.5 ± 1.1 g (men); 13.7 ± 1 g (women); Hct: <46 ± 3.1% (men); 40.9 ± 3% (women)

Complement (C3)*   <400-800 μg/ml

Circulating immune complex*   >25 μg/ml aggregated human gamma globulin

Cryoglobulins*   Present

Antistreptolysin O*   >25 Todd units

Creatinine clearance   <85-125 ml/min/1.73 mm³ (men); <75-115 ml/min/1.73 mm³ (women)

Culture of throat or skin lesion   Streptococcal organism may be present early in course of disease

Kidney-ureter-bladder (KUB) x-ray examination   Kidneys normal size, or slight bilateral enlargement

Renal biopsy   Diffuse endocapillary proliferation with many polymorphs in glomerular tuft; immunofluorescence reveals deposits of IgG, IgM, and C3

•••••• Multidisciplinary Plan

The medical plan includes treating the symptoms, attempting to prevent cerebral and cardiac complications, and supporting the patient through a period of decreased renal functioning.

Medications

Antihypertensive agents

Clonidine (Catapres, Dixarit), po, 0.1 mg bid or tid initially, then increase by 0.2-0.8 mg/d (maximum effective dose 2.4 mg/d)

Diazoxide (Hyperstat IV, Proglycem), IV, 300 mg by bolus in 30 sec or 1-2 mg/kg up to 150 mg at 5-15 min intervals

Hydralazine (Apresoline, Dralzine), po, 10 mg qid for 2-4 d; increase to 25 mg qid, then 50 mg qid; maintenance dose is lowest effective level; IM, IV, 10-40 mg repeated as needed (q4-6h)

Captopril (Capoten), 25-250 mg bid or tid, 1 hour before meals, (maximum 450 mg/d)

Diuretics

Furosemide (Lasix, Uritol), po, 20-80 mg followed by second dose in 6-8 h up to 600 mg; IM, IV, 20-40 mg given slowly over 1-2 min; high dose by IV not more than 4 mg/min

Hydrochlorothiazide (Hydrodiuril, Esidrix), po, 25-100 mg/d or bid initially; then maintenance of 25-100 mg/d according to patient's response

Spironolactone (Aldactone), po 25-200 mg/d in divided doses initially for 5 d, then adjust to maintenance level

Agents for treatment of hyperkalemia

Sodium polystyrene sulfonate (Kayexalate, SPS), po or enema, 15 g qd-qid; give po dose in 45-60 ml of water, syrup, or sorbital solution

Calcium gluconate (Kalcinate), IV, 1 g (90 mg Ca⁺⁺) in 10 ml

---

*Altered early in the course of the disease.

Sodium bicarbonate, IV, 2-5 mEq/kg infusion over 4-8 h

Glucose 50% IV, 25-50 g, and regular insulin, IV, 10-15 U

Antiinfective agents (if infection is still present)

Infection is frequently a complication of APSGN

Agents specific to microorganism cultured should be used

Agents whose route of excretion is primarily renal need to be used in smaller doses or at lengthened intervals depending on glomerular filtration rate; agents excreted by only the liver require no change; when partial excretion occurs via the kidneys, some adjustment is needed at low glomerular filtration rates

H$_2$ blockers

Cimetidine (Tagamet), po, 300 mg qid; IV, 300 mg q6h, maximum daily dose 2.4 g

Ranitidine (Zantac), po, 150 mg bid; IM, slow IV, 50 mg q6-8h; maximum daily dose 400 mg

Phosphate-binding agents

Calcium acetate (PhosLo), po, 667 mg/tablet, 2 tabs with each meal to start; 3-4 tablets per meal usually required

Aluminum carbonate (Basaljel), po, 30-40 ml with meals and at bedtime of regular strength (400 mg Al[OH]$_3$/5 ml) 15-20 ml with meals and at bedtime

Aluminum hydroxide gel (Amphojel, Dialume), aluminum hydroxide gel, dried (Amphojel tab, AluCap), po, 40 ml with meals and at bedtime; 8 tablets with meals and at bedtime

Other agents as dictated by complications: cardiac glycosides for congestive heart failure, antiinfectives if infection is still present, anticonvulsants for seizures

General Management

Goals are to control edema, preserve renal perfusion, treat hypertension while avoiding postural hypotension, and treat any intercurrent infection

Hemodialysis, peritoneal dialysis, CAVH or CVVH (see pp. 966, 970, 975)

Limit sodium intake to 2-4 g/day; variable with urine output

Limit fluids to 500-1000 ml plus amount equal to volume of urine for previous 24 hours

Limit potassium intake (if hyperkalemia) or if GFR <10 mL/min

Limit protein intake (if uremic) to 1-1.2 g/kg/day, with 50-60% of high biologic value

Provide 2500 to 3500 calories/day

Prescribe bed rest during acute phase of illness

NURSING CARE

Nursing Assessment

General Complaints

Headache; low back pain; malaise; fever, chills; weight gain

Cardiovascular

Hypertension; edema

Gastrointestinal

Nausea; vomiting

Urine

Decreased volume; dark brown or rust color

Nursing Dx & Intervention

Altered renal tissue perfusion related to immunologic injury to kidneys

- Assess blood pressure every 6 to 8 hours, 24-hour intake and output, and edema; monitor laboratory data: serum potassium, creatinine, carbon dioxide, phosphate; BUN, Hgb, Hct, and urinalysis. *Acute renal failure may develop with azotemia, anemia, hyperkalemia, hyperphosphatemia, acidosis, and seizures.*
- Administer antihypertensive agents as ordered; administer agents to lower potassium level if needed; administer agents to lower phosphate level if ordered; administer anticonvulsant agents if ordered *to control uremic symptoms and cardiovascular complications.*

Fluid-volume excess related to altered renal function

- Assess for peripheral edema; weigh daily at same time, using same scale and patient in same clothes; measure blood pressure, pulse, respirations every 6 to 8 hours; measure 24-hour intake and output *to determine the extent of fluid retention.*
- If volume excess is severe, assess pulmonary artery pressures and central venous pressure, jugular venous distention, breath sounds, and respiratory rate *to assess cardiac function and pulmonary status.*
- Limit sodium and fluid intake *to limit fluid retention.*
- Administer diuretic agents as ordered *to mobilize retained fluids.*
- Administer cardiac glycosides if ordered *to prevent congestive heart failure.*

Risk for altered nutrition, less than body requirements related to proteinuria

- Assess for weight loss; encourage protein intake of 0.8 to 1 g/kg body weight per day plus the amount lost in 24-hour urine output; *excessive protein losses may occur.*
- Monitor food intake; monitor for anorexia, nausea, and vomiting; offer small, frequent feedings *to ensure adequate caloric intake and thus prevent metabolism of tissue protein for energy.*
- Limit protein and potassium intake if uremic symptoms occur *to decrease excretory load on the kidneys and possible accumulation of potassium and hydrogen ions.*

Risk for infection related to altered immune state

- Assess for urinary tract infection; monitor temperature; monitor WBC; avoid exposure to individuals with infections. *Patients with GN are susceptible to urinary tract infection because of their altered immune status.*

- Administer antiinfective agents if ordered; a streptococcal infection may still be present.

Knowledge deficit related to APSGN, its treatment, and follow-up care

- See box below.

Patient Education/Home Care Planning

1. Explain APSGN, its signs, symptoms, and the course of the disease.
2. Explain the medical regimen, if any, for discharge.
3. Explain follow-up care: monitoring of blood pressure and urinalysis (hematuria and proteinuria).

Evaluation

Patient has normal or improved renal function Renal function tests are within normal limits.

Patient's fluid intake balances output Urine output balances with intake; urine is clear; edema is gone; blood pressure is in normal range; weight is stable.

Patient's nutritional intake is adequate Proteinuria has resolved; serum albumin and cholesterol levels are normal.

Patient is free of infection No signs or symptoms of infection are noted.

Patient is knowledgeable about acute poststreptococcal glomerulonephritis Patient can describe the signs, the symptoms, the course of the disease, the level of renal function, possible problems, and the medical regimen prescribed.

■ INTERSTITIAL NEPHRITIS

■ Interstitial nephritis (IN) is an acute, often drug-induced renal disease that involves inflammatory damage to interstitial tissue.

Damage to interstitial tissue is a frequent cause of chronic renal failure. Causes of IN include infection (e.g., streptococcal) and drug use, analgesics, antibiotics such as methicillin and ampicillin, sulfonamides, phenindione, and phenytoin). Such drugs may cause dose-related toxic reactions or non-dose-related allergic reactions.

Interstitial nephritis also may arise from idiopathic causes. Early detection of drug reactions, infection, and urinary tract obstruction is useful. It is important to be alert to the possibility that some patients may abuse over-the-counter analgesics, especially those containing acetaminophen.

• • • • • • Pathophysiology

Acute inflammation of the interstitium may cause scarring and a rapid decline in renal function. The inflammatory process is usually diffuse and accompanied by interstitial edema. An immune response appears to cause acute IN that may involve deposition of immune complex and anti–tubular basement membrane antibodies.

Chronic IN results in a shrunken kidney with an irregular outline caused by scarring and tissue destruction. It follows a slowly progressive course with few clinical manifestations. Changes in renal hormone activity may occur, and the production of renin, erythropoietin, and vitamin D may decline. The ability to concentrate urine also decreases. Common causes of chronic IN are anatomic abnormalities (e.g., obstruction in the urinary tract), analgesic overuse, hyperuricemia, and nephrosclerosis.

• • • • • • Diagnostic Studies and Findings

White blood cell count Eosinophilia if drug-induced

Urinalysis Eosinophilic casts; hematuria; dilute urine (low specific gravity)

Intravenous urogram Normal or slightly enlarged kidneys; immediate, dense nephrogram; with chronic interstitial nephritis: decreased size, irregular cortex, calyceal distortion

Renal biopsy Differentiates acute tubular necrosis from acute interstitial nephritis

• • • • • • Multidisciplinary Plan

The cause of IN can be removed by treating infection, discontinuing the drugs associated with acute IN, and relieving obstruction. Renal function may gradually improve. Chronic IN requires monitoring as renal function decreases. Changes in the function of the glomeruli and tubules occur as the interstitial inflammation and scarring progress (see "Chronic Renal Failure," p. 935).

Surgery

May be performed to relieve any obstruction

Medications

Antiinfective agents if needed

General Management

Dialysis if needed
Nutritional support, fluid limitations, vitamin supplements as needed
See "Acute Renal Failure," p. 930

NURSING CARE

Nursing Assessment

Renal

Polyuria; nocturia

Skin

May have an allergic skin rash

General

Headache, low back pain, weight loss or gain, fever, chills

Nursing Dx & Intervention

Altered renal tissue perfusion related to damaged interstitial tissue

- Assess blood pressure every 6 to 8 hours; 24-hour intake and output and edema; monitor laboratory data: Hgb, Hct, serum creatinine, BUN, serum potassium, phosphate, carbon dioxide; monitor mental state; *nonoliguric renal failure may develop with hypertension, azotemia, anemia, acidosis, and increased serum potassium and phosphate.*
- Administer antihypertensive agents if needed and agents to reduce serum potassium and to reduce phosphate absorption as ordered; monitor response *to control complications of uremia and to determine effectiveness of drug, dosage, and timing.*

Risk for fluid-volume deficit related to inability to concentrate urine

- Assess for dehydration: weigh daily; measure blood pressure, pulse, and respirations every 6 to 8 hours; measure 24-hour intake and output *to check for inability to concentrate urine and to determine the extent of fluid loss.*
- Administer fluids as ordered; monitor response *to prevent dehydration and further decrease in renal blood flow.*

Risk for fluid-volume excess related to acute renal failure associated with oliguria or anuria

- Monitor for edema and listen to breath sounds; if fluid excess is severe, monitor central venous pressure and pulmonary artery pressures *to identify hypervolemia.*

Risk for infection related to damaged interstitium

- Assess for signs and symptoms of urinary tract infection; administer antiinfective agents if ordered; monitor response to drug. *Renal failure alters immune response; monitoring determines effectiveness of drug, dosage, and timing.*

Knowledge deficit related to interstitial nephritis and follow-up care

- See box below.

Patient Education/Home Care Planning

1. Explain the nature of interstitial nephritis and the cause in the individual patient.
2. Explain the patient's level of renal function.
3. Explain the need for periodic medical evaluation with tests of renal function.
4. Explain the likelihood of dialysis or transplantation in the future.

Evaluation

Renal function has returned Electrolyte balances are within normal limits; serum creatinine and BUN levels are normal.

Patient's fluid intake balances output Urine output equals intake; polyuria ceases; blood pressure is normal; weight is stable.

Patient is free of infection No signs or symptoms of infection are noted.

Patient is knowledgeable about interstitial nephritis Patient and family can describe the nature and extent of interstitial nephritis, the need for follow-up care, and the implications for the future.

METABOLIC DISORDERS

■ NEPHROTIC SYNDROME

Nephrotic syndrome (NS) encompasses a group of symptoms: proteinuria (primarily albuminuria), hypoalbuminemia, generalized edema, hyperlipidemia, and lipiduria. NS occurs in both adults and children.

NS may occur in various conditions such as glomerulonephritis, glomerular lesions associated with systemic diseases and conditions such as diabetes mellitus, infections, circulatory diseases, reactions to allergens and drugs, pregnancy, and renal transplantation. NS is frequently idiopathic in children. Long-term studies are underway to determine the usefulness of corticosteroids and cyclophosphamide in children and adults.

•••••• Pathophysiology

Nephrotic syndrome results from increased glomerular permeability. The albuminuria causes hypoalbuminemia because the liver cannot replace the losses rapidly enough. The resulting drop in oncotic pressure permits water to escape from the vascular compartment. Adaptive responses to the contraction of fluid volume include increased secretion of antidiuretic hormone and aldosterone, which contributes to the problem of fluid retention. The liver is stimulated to increase the synthesis of many proteins and it also increases production of lipoproteins, thereby causing the hyperlipidemia characteristic of NS.

A renal biopsy in patients with NS may show either minimum changes or marked changes, including proliferation of endothelial cells (hypercellularity), changes in the epithelial cells (diffuse fusion of the foot processes), deposition of immunoglobulins and complexes along the capillary walls, tubular changes (fatty deposits and eosinophilic casts), and glomerular changes (epithelial crescents caused by irregular patches of sclerosis).

Most patients with NS who have minimum changes respond well to corticosteroid therapy. Patients with marked changes are usually unresponsive and progress to end-stage renal disease.

The decrease in plasma proteins may result in less binding proteins for drugs. The usual effect of a drug may occur with half the usual dose. The protein loss may also cause a decrease in vitamin D precursor, transferrin, T₃, and thyroid-binding globulin. Calcium may be required, but thyroid hormone usually is not. Iron may be needed if iron deficiency anemia occurs.

••••• Diagnostic Studies and Findings

Urine   Foamy, deeper in color; oval fat bodies; proteinuria that may be >3 g/day

Blood chemistry   Hypoalbuminemia: serum albumin <2.5 g/dl; hyperlipidemia: increased total serum cholesterol, phospholipids, triglycerides, low-density lipids, very-low-density lipids

Renal biopsy   To identify histologic features of lesion classified as: minimum change—podocytes of epithelial cells appear to be fused together on electron microscopy; membranous change—predominantly thickening of the basement membrane and visible by light and electron microscopy; proliferative change—glomerular cells appear hypercellular; membranoproliferative change—both hypercellularity and basement membrane thickening are noted

•••••• Multidisciplinary Plan

Immunosuppressive agents are used because they have been shown empirically to decrease or stop the proteinuria. Prednisone, the treatment of choice, is initially given as a single dose at breakfast and may be later given on alternate days. The other immunosuppressive agents are used if corticosteroids cannot be used. Diuretics are often used in conjunction with salt-poor albumin infusions to relieve massive edema. Thoracentesis or paracentesis may be needed if excess fluid accumulates in the chest or abdominal cavities. In minimum disease NS, corticosteroids are started and the responses noted. Often proteinuria clears rapidly. Repeat treatment with corticosteroids is indicated for those who have a relapse after therapy is discontinued.

Medications

Corticosteroids
    Prednisone (Deltasone, Orasone), po, 5-60 mg/d
Antineoplastic agents (used for immunosuppressive effect)
    Cyclophosphamide (Cytoxan, Neosar), po, 1-5 mg/kg/d; IV, 40-50 mg/kg/d initially, 10-15 mg/kg q7-10d, or 3-5 mg/kg twice wk, or 1.5-3 mg/kg/d maintenance
    Azathioprine (Imuran), po (highly individualized): 3-5 mg/kg/d initially; 1-2 mg/kg/d maintenance
    Chlorambucil (Leukeran), po, 0.1-0.2 mg/kg/d for 3-6 wk initially; 0.03-0.1 mg/kg/d maintenance
Plasma expanders and blood components
    Albumin human (Albuminate, Plasbumin), 5 g/dl or 25 g/dl, IV, 25 g initially; repeated in 15-30 min
Diuretics
    Furosemide (Lasix, Uritol), po, 20-80 mg followed by second dose in 6-8 h up to 600 mg; IM, IV, 20-40 mg given slowly over 1-2 min; high dose by IV not more than 4 mg/min

Hydrochlorothiazide (Hydrodiuril, Esidrix), po, 25-100 mg/d or bid initially; then maintenance of 25-100 mg/d according to patient's response
    Spironolactone (Aldactone), po, 25-200 mg/d in divided doses initially for 5 d; then adjust to maintenance level
Protein diet supplements
    Meritene, 8-10 oz bid or tid
    Citrotein, 8 oz bid or tid

General Management

Protein intake is increased to replace protein losses. If the glomerular filtration rate is normal, adults may have 1.5 to 2 g/kg body weight, with 50% to 60% of high biologic value. If the glomerular filtration rate is decreased, protein intake is lowered. Sodium intake is limited (500 to 1000 mg/day) to control edema. Caloric intake must be sufficient to prevent muscle catabolism and provide energy. The amount varies with height, weight, age, sex, and daily activity. Adults need 35 to 45 kcal/kg ideal body weight/day. The help of a dietitian and the use of exchange lists make implementing these complex diets easier.

Changes in vascular volume are monitored carefully to prevent hypovolemic shock, as well as the hypokalemia and ototoxicity that can accompany diuretic use. Hospitalization is avoided unless the patient has severe generalized edema with ascites, significant hypertension, severe infection, hypovolemic shock, or a persistently low glomerular filtration rate. Bed rest is advised if complications are present. The level of proteinuria is monitored.

NURSING CARE

Nursing Assessment

General Complaints
Weight gain; fatigue

Urine Output
Oliguria; foamy urine

Cardiovascular
Edema, soft and pitting (periorbital, external genitalia, peritoneal and pleural spaces, extremities); jugular venous distention

Gastrointestinal
Anorexia; nausea; vomiting

Nursing Dx & Intervention

Altered tissue perfusion related to altered glomerular cells causing proteinuria

- Assess blood pressure, pulse, and respirations every 6 to 8 hours; assess abdomen, back, and extremities for ascites, anasarca, or peripheral edema *to identify hypovolemia.*

- Monitor laboratory data: urine protein and specific gravity. Protein may vary with circadian rhythm (high, 4 PM; low, 3 AM).
- Monitor serum protein, albumin, calcium, and Hct *to help determine replacement needed; decreased serum protein means decreased protein-bound calcium.*
- Monitor sodium, potassium, chloride, and pH; *levels may be lowered by vigorous diuretic therapy;* monitor BUN and serum creatinine *to determine renal function.*
- Administer immunosuppressive agents as ordered; monitor response to drugs *to decrease protein excretion; to determine effectiveness of agent, dosage, and timing; and to observe for adverse side effects.*

Fluid volume excess related to decreased vascular oncotic pressure caused by proteinuria and inadequate protein replacement by the liver

- Assess weight daily; assess 24-hour intake and output; assess blood pressure (sitting and standing), pulse, and respirations; monitor edema, jugular venous distention, and, as necessary, central venous pressure and pulmonary artery pressures; monitor laboratory data: urine specific gravity and protein; serum albumin and calcium; Hct *to check for altered fluid status and orthostatic hypotension.*
- Monitor serum sodium, potassium, chloride, and pH *because levels may be lowered by vigorous diuretic therapy.*
- Administer drugs as ordered (i.e., diuretics and albumin); monitor response to drugs *to correct fluid imbalance, to determine effectiveness of drugs, and to observe for side effects such as hypokalemia and ototoxicity.*
- Limit sodium intake as ordered; *if serum sodium levels are high, edema will be worsened by fluid retention.*
- Restrict fluid intake as ordered. *Restrictions may be necessary in cases of hyponatremia; massive edema or ascites; respiratory distress; or pleural effusion.*

Altered nutrition: less than body requirements related to proteinuria, anorexia, nausea, and vomiting

- Assess food intake *to ensure adequate intake within the limits prescribed.*
- Monitor dry weight *to determine if weight changes are related to fluid balance or inadequate caloric intake and loss of muscle mass.*
- Monitor laboratory data: serum protein, lipids, potassium, and calcium *to determine whether protein intake is adequate.*
- Encourage food intake as prescribed. Prescribed diet may include increased protein *to increase protein synthesis and to avoid a negative nitrogen balance* and an adequate intake of carbohydrates *to prevent use of body proteins for energy;* include optimum levels of potassium, calcium, and calories as needed; no cholesterol or saturated fats as long as serum lipids are elevated.

- Provide palatable meals, considering patient's likes and dislikes; encourage small, frequent meals; provide oral hygiene before meals; offer hard candy *to increase intake of needed calories.*
- Administer protein supplements if ordered; *protein intake needed may be hard to achieve by foods alone.*
- Refer complex or problem situations to dietitian; *a team approach to managing the complex renal diet is helpful to all concerned.*

Risk for bathing/hygiene, toileting, and self-care deficit related to bed rest during acute phase of illness

- Assess need for assistance; assist with self-care as needed; encourage deep breathing, coughing, and turning; increase activity as tolerated *to prevent unwanted side effects of bed rest.*

Risk for infection related to altered immune response resulting from lowered serum albumin or immunosuppressive drugs

- Assess for signs and symptoms of infection in secretions, excretions, and exudates *to detect any infection early.*
- Monitor laboratory data: WBC; *level may be lowered in patients taking immunosuppressive drugs; level may not be elevated with infection.*
- Monitor temperature every 4 hours; *corticosteroids may mask usual temperature increase with infection.*
- Wash hands thoroughly and consistently; avoid exposing patient to individuals with infections; ensure aseptic technique for any invasive procedure or wound care *to decrease chances for infection.*
- Encourage regular oral hygiene, hand washing, and bathing and adequate rest and nutrition; *good health habits help prevent infections.*

Risk for impaired skin integrity

- Assess skin in edematous areas; provide meticulous care to these areas (skin folds, joint creases, genital areas, and back). *Such areas are easily injured, especially skin-to-skin areas.*
- Elevate edematous genitalia or extremities *to prevent excoriation, maceration, or infection.*

Risk for body image alteration related to excessive edema or the side effects of drugs

- Warn patient to expect alopecia or other drug side effects or changes caused by edema; *temporary side effects of drugs and recurrence of edema may change patient's appearance.*
- Assess for evidence that change in patient's appearance is a problem; *early intervention may prevent patient distress.*

Knowledge deficit related to nephrotic syndrome and follow-up care

- See box on p. 956.

Evaluation

Glomerular function is normal Patient has normal serum albumin and lipid levels and urine components.

Fluid balance is normal Urine volume is normal and balances intake.

Nutritional status is normal Patient has no restrictions on food or fluids.

Patient has resumed self-care Patient has no restrictions on ADL.

No infection is present Patient has no signs or symptoms of infection.

Skin is intact Patient has no areas of excoriation or maceration.

Patient has no problem with body image Patient has returned to previous appearance or has adjusted to alteration.

Patient is knowledgeable about nephrotic syndrome Patient can explain causes of nephrotic syndrome, possible relapse, need for long-term medical supervision, and possible need for dialysis or transplantation in the future.

◼ RENAL CALCULI

Renal calculi are stones formed in the kidneys, primarily in the pelvis. Stones may resemble gravel or may be formed in the shape of the pelvis (staghorn calculus).

Calculi that pass spontaneously without discomfort present no serious health threat. However, many calculi found in the urinary tract are extremely painful and can cause obstruction and infection. Urinary calculi occur more frequently in men than in women, and some geographic areas, such as the southeastern United States, have a particularly high incidence. The peak incidence of calculus formation is in the third to fifth decades of life.

Long-term ingestion of calcium carbonate, vitamin D, antacids, megadoses of vitamin C, acetazolamide, probenecid, or triamterene can lead to stone formation. The risk can be increased by anatomic abnormalities (medullary sponge kidney), biochemical influences (cystinuria), or environmental factors (diet and fluid intake patterns, climate, occupation).

⬤⬤⬤⬤⬤ Pathophysiology

The formation of a stone is a physicochemical process involving a nidus of crystals or organic material around which the stone components form. The pH, temperature, ionic strength, and concentration of the urine affect the solubility of the stone-forming substances. Supersaturation of poorly soluble substances, absence of crystalline inhibitors, and sources of seed crystals contribute to calculus formation.

The primary components of renal calculi include calcium salts (carbonate and oxalate), uric acid, cystine, and struvite (magnesium ammonium phosphate). The stones most frequently contain calcium or uric acid.

Hypercalciuria with or without hypercalcemia may be caused by hyperparathyroidism or osteoporosis or may be idiopathic. Calcium and phosphate are more soluble when pH is low. Bacterial infection by urea-splitting organisms causes the urine to become alkaline. Stones composed of struvite are called infection stones.

Hyperuricemia occurs with idiopathic gout, renal failure, blood dyscrasias, and the use of thiazide diuretics and alkylating agents. Uric acid is less soluble in high concentrations, low urine volume, and with low urine pH.

⬤⬤⬤⬤⬤ Diagnostic Studies and Findings

Kidney-ureter-bladder (KUB) x-ray examination Radiopaque stone

Renal ultrasound Stones identified

Intravenous urogram Filling defects; ureteral dilation; hydronephrosis

Analysis of stones Constituents such as cystine, calcium, oxalate, and uric acid

⬤⬤⬤⬤⬤ Multidisciplinary Plan

The goals of medical care are to remove calculi, relieve effects of the calculi (pain and infection), resolve any causative factors (obstruction, infection, and metabolic abnormalities), and prevent future calculus growth. The achievement of these goals should prevent permanent damage to the kidney and recurrence of calculi.

Surgery

Procedures used may include: pyelolithotomy, nephrolithotomy, ureterolithotomy, cystoscopy-basket extraction of calculi, and percutaneous fragmentation and extraction through a nephroscope; surgical intervention is a last resort with struvite stones because recurrence is so frequent

Additional procedures: extracorporeal shock wave lithotripsy, percutaneous lithotripsy (see p. 986)

Medications

Analgesics

Meperidine (Demerol, Pethadol), po, subcutaneously, IM, IV, 50-150 mg q3-4h

Codeine sulfate (generic), oral, subcutaneously, IM 15-60 mg qid

Morphine sulfate, po, subcutaneously, IM, IV, 5-15 mg q4h prn

Electrolytes (used to ensure alkaline urine)

Sodium bicarbonate, po, 300 mg to 1.8 g qd-qid not to exceed 16 g/d

Diuretics

Hydrochlorothiazide (Hydrodiuril, Esidrix) (to reduce idiopathic urinary calcium excretion), po, 25-50 mg bid

Other Drugs

Allopurinol (Zyloprim, Alloprin), decreases uric acid production, po, 200-800 mg in divided doses if more than 300 mg

Cellulose sodium phosphate (Calcibind), po, initially 15 g/d (5 g tid with meals) for urinary calcium >300 mg/d; reduced to 10 g/d (5 mg with main meal, 2.5 g with other two meals) when urinary calcium 150 mg/d

Penicillamine (Cuprimine, Depen), combines with cystine to form a soluble compound, po, 250 mg qid

Antiinfective agents, if infection present

General Management

Diet: modifications may be required, depending on stone type; low-calcium diets (<400 mg/day) and extra-high fluid intake (3500 to 4000 ml/day) are helpful but difficult to maintain; patients should avoid dehydration by drinking water rather than fluids that may be high in unwanted substances (such as tea with its high oxalate content); increased fluid intake should be spread out evenly over the 24-hour period, including once during the night; low-purine diets may help decrease uric acid output; foods extremely high in purines (>150 mg/100 g) are limited; oxalate intake is usually limited to less than 50 mg/day on low-oxalate diets

NURSING CARE

Nursing Assessment

Urinary Tract

Irritative voiding symptoms: dysuria, urgency, and urge incontinence

General

Fever (with urinary tract infection); pain associated with renal colic (in flank or costovertebral angle radiating to groin, labia, or testicle); tenderness in the flank or costovertebral angle; nausea; vomiting

Nursing Dx & Intervention

Pain related to presence of calculus

- Note pattern of pain, and assess need for analgesia. *Intensified pain may indicate impaction of calculus or obstruction of urine flow; sudden relief of pain may indicate stone has passed through a narrow junction (ureteropelvic or ureterovesicle); movement of calculus may be associated with colicky pain.*
- Administer analgesic agents as ordered; monitor response to drugs *to relieve pain* and *to determine effectiveness of drug, dosage, and timing; to identify adverse reactions.*
- Apply external heat to painful flank *to relieve discomfort.*
- Assist with walking as ordered *to help passage of stone.*

Altered nutrition: more than body requirements related to altered metabolism of calcium, purine, or oxalate

- For calcium stones, lower calcium intake (e.g., dairy products); for uric acid stones decrease purine intake (e.g., organ meats, meat extracts, shrimp, or dried beans); lower intake of foods containing oxalate (e.g., tea, chocolate, nuts, or spinach) *to prevent formation of renal calculi.*
- Avoid dehydration by encouraging high-normal fluid intake *to prevent high concentrations of unwanted substance in the urine.*

Risk for infection related to presence of calculus

- Assess for fever, chills, and irritative voiding symptoms; monitor laboratory data: WBC, bacteriuria; monitor temperature every 4 hours *to detect presence of infection.*
- Encourage high to normal fluid intake over 24-hour period *to help flush urinary tract to prevent urinary tract infection;* may also facilitate passage of calculus.

Knowledge deficit related to renal calculi and follow-up care

- See box below.

Patient Education/Home Care Planning

1. Explain the nature of renal calculi, their causes, and manifestations.
2. Explain medical management, including medications (purpose, dosage, interval, and side effects), diet (low calcium, purine, or oxalate), and fluid intake (amount, schedule, and kinds).
3. Explain medical follow-up to monitor the outcome of treatment.

Evaluation

Pain is gone   Patient reports being free of pain.

No signs or symptoms of urinary tract infection are noted   Temperature, urine, and WBC are normal.

Fluid intake is adequate, and unwanted substances are avoided in the diet   Fluid intake is high normal; diet restrictions are followed correctly.

Patient is knowledgeable about renal calculi   Patient can explain factors that contribute to calculi and the signs and symptoms of recurrence.

RENAL TUBULAR ACIDOSIS

Renal tubular acidosis (RTA) occurs when the kidneys are unable to excrete an acid urine because of a defect in the tubules. Hyperchloremic acidosis ensues.

Both infants and adults may have tubular defects in acid handling. The causes of RTA may be hereditary or associated with cystinosis and hyperparathyroidism.

•••••• Pathophysiology

The tubular defect in RTA may be in the proximal tubule or the distal tubule. In the former case the proximal tubule fails to conserve bicarbonate ions and the distal tubule, which is normal, cannot handle the increased bicarbonate load. Sodium and potassium are also lost, and hypokalemia and hypovolemia may result. In the latter case the distal tubule cannot maintain the hydrogen ion gradient across the tubular cell and either fails to secrete hydrogen ions or permits back-diffusion of the hydrogen ions secreted. The serum pH is lowered, the hydrogen-sodium exchange decreases, and the sodium-potassium exchange increases, with a resulting hypokalemia and hypovolemia.

The skeletal system becomes involved in buffering the acidosis; calcium carbonate is released, causing hypercalcemia and hypercalciuria. Renal function is otherwise normal. A third type of RTA involves defects in both parts of the tubule and a normal or elevated serum potassium. Renal calculi occur frequently in patients with distal RTA (see p. 956).

•••••• Diagnostic Studies and Findings

Blood chemistries   Lowered serum pH and potassium; elevated serum chloride and calcium

Urinalysis   Urine pH >6 in distal RTA; 4.5 to 8 in proximal RTA with increased potassium level and hypercalciuria

Kidney-ureter-bladder (KUB) x-ray examination   Decreased kidney mass; renal calculi or intrarenal calcification

•••••• Multidisciplinary Plan

Medications

Electrolytes (alkalinizing agents)
Sodium bicarbonate, Shohl's solution, or Polycitra; for distal RTA: po, 1-3 mEq/kg/d; for proximal RTA: po, 5-10 mEq/kg/d
The acidosis must be corrected slowly to avoid further lowering the potassium level
Diuretics (for proximal RTA)
Hydrochlorothiazide (Hydrodiuril, Esidrix) (to decrease Ca^{++} excretion), 1.5-2 mg/kg/d
Potassium supplement (for proximal RTA if serum K$^+$ <3 mEq/L) KCl (4 mEq K$^+$/5 ml), po, 20 mEq/kg/d in divided doses

General Management

There is no cure for renal tubular acidosis; therefore the major goal of therapy is to control the metabolic acidosis with moderate doses of bicarbonate

NURSING CARE

Nursing Assessment

General

Weakness; lethargy; anorexia; bone pain

Nursing Dx & Intervention

Risk for altered acid-base balance related to defect in renal tubule causing metabolic acidosis

- Monitor laboratory values: serum hydrogen, bicarbonate, calcium, potassium, and pH; urinary pH and calcium *to assess effectiveness of medical regimen.*
- Administer medications as ordered *to treat acidosis and prevent electrolyte losses.*

Knowledge deficit related to renal tubular acidosis and follow-up care

- See box below.

Patient Education/Home Care Planning

1. Explain the nature of renal tubular acidosis.
2. Explain the treatment regimen: alkalinizing agent with dosage, interval, and side effects.
3. Teach the patient to check urine for pH and calcium.
4. Explain medical follow-up.

Evaluation

Acid-base imbalance has been corrected; potassium level is normal, and nephrocalcinosis and renal calculi have been prevented   Urine pH is 4.5-8; urine calcium is 2 to 3 mg/kg/day; serum bicarbonate is 24 to 28 mEq/L; serum chloride is 97 to 107 mEq/L; serum potassium is 3.5 to 5 mEq/L; serum pH is 7.32 to 7.43. No renal calculi or calcifications are noted.

Patient and family are knowledgeable about RTA   Patient and family can describe RTA and medical management being instituted.

RENOVASCULAR ABNORMALITIES

DIABETIC NEPHROPATHY

Diabetic nephropathy (DN) is the renal manifestation of diabetes mellitus; it is glomerulosclerosis, caused by lesions of the arterioles and glomeruli and associated with pyelonephritis and necrosis of the renal papillae.

Diabetic nephropathy, or diabetic glomerulosclerosis, is an important complication of noninsulin-dependent diabetes mellitus and the most important complication leading to death in insulin-dependent diabetes. The changes are related to the duration of the diabetic state. Approximately 30% to 40% of patients with insulin-dependent diabetes develop DN.[12] Patients with non-insulin-dependent diabetes have variable courses and may or may not develop DN. Of new patients starting end-stage renal disease (ESRD) therapy in 1991, diabetes was the most frequent cause—surpassing both hypertension and glomerulonephritis.[16] Once proteinuria occurs, the renal changes invariably progress. Patients with diabetic nephropathy have increased morbidity and mortality. Although the survival of diabetic patients treated with dialysis or transplantation has improved somewhat in recent years, the outcomes are not nearly as good as in nondiabetic patients. Diabetic patients have particular problems with atherosclerosis, coronary artery disease, peripheral vascular disease, retinopathy, and neurologic deficits. The likelihood of their successful rehabilitation is limited but has increased in recent years.

······ Pathophysiology

The glomeruli are affected by diffuse sclerosis and thickening of the basement membrane and mesangial areas. Nodular glomerulosclerosis may also occur. Both afferent and efferent arterioles are affected by thickened walls and hyaline deposits. The glomerular filtration rate decreases and azotemia occurs. The diabetic patient may appear clinically uremic at levels lower than the nondiabetic patient. This may be related to the diabetic patient's systemic vascular changes.

Diabetic nephropathy may not manifest clinical symptoms for years after diabetes develops. Diabetic individuals vary considerably in their susceptibility to renal failure, possibly because of genetic defects or vascular changes related to metabolism of carbohydrates, fat, and protein. Poor control of blood pressure and glucose levels is an important factor.

······ Diagnostic Studies and Findings

Blood chemistries Increased serum creatinine and BUN; decreased albumin; increased cholesterol

Urinalysis Proteinuria, pyuria, or bacteriuria

Creatinine clearance Lowered values

Intravenous urogram Kidneys may be of normal size, swollen, or small and scarred (irregular cortical surface)

Renal biopsy Diffuse or nodular thickening of glomerular basement membrane and mesangial regions

······ Multidisciplinary Plan

Some authorities believe that control of blood pressure and fluctuations in blood sugar levels slows the deterioration of renal function. Others believe that diabetic nephropathy follows an inexorable downhill course.

Surgery

See "Renal Transplantation" (p. 979), diabetic patients who have a renal transplant have more complications, poorer rehabilitation, and a lower survival rate than nondiabetic patients with a renal transplant; the underlying disease process cannot be corrected by renal transplantation alone

Medications

Insulin requirements may decrease as renal degradation of the hormone decreases or may increase as resistance to insulin's effects increases; antihypertensive drugs and diuretics may be needed

For non-insulin-dependent diabetic patients, oral agents metabolized in the liver are used: tolbutamide (Orinase), glipizide (Glucotrol)

Alkalinizing agents (for acidosis)

Sodium bicarbonate, po, 1-4 g/d; IV, 2-5 mEq/kg infused over 4-8 h

Treatment for hyperkalemia

Sodium polystyrene sulfonate (Kayexalate, SPS), po or enema, 15 g qd-qid; give po dose in 45-60 ml of water, syrup, or sorbitol solution

Calcium gluconate (Kalcinate), IV, 1 g (90 mg Ca^{++}) in 10 ml

Sodium bicarbonate, IV, 2-5 mEq/kg infusion over 8 h

Glucose 50%, IV, 25-50 g, and regular insulin, IV, 10-15 U

Antihypertensive agents

Clonidine (Catapres, Dixarit), po, 0.1 mg bid or tid initially; then increase by 0.2-0.8 mg/d (maximum effective dose, 2.4 mg/d)

Diazoxide (Hyperstat IV, Proglycem), IV, 300 mg by bolus in 30 sec or 1-2 mg/kg up to 150 mg at 5-15 min intervals

Hydralazine (Apresoline, Dralzine), po, 10 mg qid for 2-4 d; increase to 25 mg qid then 50 mg qid; maintenance dose is lowest effective level; IM, IV, 10-40 mg repeated as needed (q4-6h)

Methyldopa (Aldomet, Dopamet), po, 250 mg bid or tid for 48 h; then increase or decrease q2d if needed; maintenance 500 mg to 2 g in 2-4 divided doses/d (maximum 3 g)

Prazosin (Minipress) (α-adrenergic blocker), po, 1 mg bid-tid initially; maintenance may be increased slowly to maximum of 20 mg/d in divided doses; up to 40 mg/d may be required

Propranolol (Inderal, Novopranol) (β-adrenergic blocker), po, 40 mg bid at 6-8 h intervals; increase if needed to 160-480 mg/d in divided doses; 640 mg/d may be needed*

Captopril (Capoten) (angiotensin converting enzyme inhibitor), po, 25 mg tid initially; increase to 50 mg tid in 2-3 wk if necessary; may be increased to 100 mg tid then to 150 mg tid*

Diuretics

Furosemide (Lasix, Uritol), po, 20-80 mg followed by second dose in 6-8 h up to 600 mg; IM, IV, 20-40 mg given slowly over 1-2 min; high dose by IV not more than 4 mg/min and repeat in 6-8 h

---

*Use cautiously, if at all in diabetics with ESRD.

Antiinfective agents

Infection is frequently a complication of nephropathy/chronic renal failure

Agents specific to the microorganism cultured should be used

Agents whose route of excretion is primarily renal need to be used in smaller doses or at lengthened intervals depending on glomerular filtration rate; agents excreted by only the liver require no change; if partial excretion occurs via the kidneys, some adjustment is needed at lower glomerular filtration rates

Phosphate-binding agents

Calcium acetate (PhosLo), po, 667 mg tab, 2 tabs with each meal to start; 3-4 tabs per meal usually required

Aluminum carbonate gel (Basaljel), po, 30-40 ml (400 mg Al[OH]$_3$/5 ml) with meals and at bedtime

Aluminum hydroxide gel (Amphojel, Dialume), po, 40 ml with meals and at bedtime

Aluminum hydroxide gel, dried (Amphojel tab, AluCap), po, 8 tab with meals and at bedtime

Antiemetic agents

Prochlorperazine (Compazine), po, 5-10 mg tid-qid

Antipruritic agents

Cyproheptadine (Periactin, Cyprodine) (antihistamine), po, 4 mg tid or qid not more than 0.5 mg/kg/d

Trimeprazine tartrate (Temaril, Panectyl) (phenothiazine), po, 2.5 mg qid

Laxatives/stool softeners

Methylcellulose (Methulose, Cologel), po, 5-20 ml tid

Docusate sodium (Colace, DCS), po, 50-200 mg/d

Electrolytes, minerals

Calcium (supplement): calcium carbonate (Titralac, Tums), po, 0.5-2 g 4-6 times daily

Calcium gluconate (Kalcinate), po, 1-5 g tid

Hematinic agents

Ferrous sulfate (Feosol, Fer-Iron), po, 300 mg-1.2 g/d in divided doses

Iron-dextran injection (InFeD), IV, IM, varies with weight and hemoglobin level

Vitamins

Multivitamin supplements (water-soluble vitamins)

Thiamine, 1.5 mg/d

Riboflavin, 1.8 mg/d

Niacin, 20 mg/d

Pyridoxine, 5 mg/d

Vitamin B$_{12}$, 3 μg/d

Vitamin C, 100 mg/d

Folic acid (Folvite), folate sodium, po, subcutaneously, IM, IV, up to 1 mg/d; maintenance: up to 0.3 mg/d

Vitamin D

Calcitriol (1,25-dihydroxycholecalciferol) (Rocaltrol), po, 0.25 μg/d; maintenance: 0.5-1 μg/d

Dihydrotachysterol (DHT, Hytakerol), 0.2-0.4 mg/d

General Management

See "Hemodialysis" and "Peritoneal Dialysis" (pp. 970 and 975); the underlying disease process cannot be corrected by dialysis; vascular complications of diabetes cause major problems in access to vascular system for hemodialysis

Fluid intake should balance output: about 400 to 60 ml (about amount of insensible losses) plus amount equal to 24-hour urine volume; avoid dehydration and volume excess; specific amount determined by patient's dry weight (weight at which, after dialysis, patient has normal volume relationship)

Nutritional modifications are made to achieve or maintain adequate nutritional status and to reduce work of diseased kidney

Weight reduction; intermediate levels of renal failure require low-protein diets with drugs to lower cholesterol; late in course of renal failure, insulin requirements decrease, but protein, carbohydrate, and fat intake must still be controlled

Protein, 0.6 g/kg body weight/day; glomerular filtration rate (GFR), 20 to 25 ml/minute—90 g/day; GFR, 10 to 15 ml/minute to 50 g/day; GFR, 4 to 10 ml/minute—40 g/day

Sodium, 1000 to 2000 mg/day; specific amounts depend on weight, blood pressure, serum creatinine, and 24-hour sodium excretion

Potassium, 1500 to 2000 mg/day; with normal urine output (at least 800 ml/day) no restriction is needed

Calories, 35 to 55 kcal/kg body weight/day; calories from fat and carbohydrate are used; adequate calories must accompany protein intake to prevent use of protein for energy and weight loss; control of protein intake takes priority in nutritional management; calories from fat and carbohydrates are increased

NURSING CARE

Nursing Assessment

Renal

Oliguria or anuria; urinary retention

Cardiovascular

Hypertension; postural hypotension; edema or dehydration

Gastrointestinal

Nausea; anorexia; thirst; weight loss

Nursing Dx & Intervention

Altered renal tissue perfusion related to diffuse and nodular glomerulosclerosis

- Assess vital signs, intake and output, and weight, as needed; monitor laboratory data: serum glucose, BUN, and serum creatinine *to reflect status of diabetes and renal function.*
- Administer medications as ordered with care *because dosages are given in smaller amounts or at longer intervals.*
- Determine insulin dosage by serum glucose level *because urine glucose level does not accurately reflect serum glucose level owing to altered renal handling of glucose.*
- Avoid nephrotoxic drugs *because kidneys are less able to excrete drugs.*
- Monitor response to drugs given *to determine effectiveness of drug, dosage, and timing and to identify adverse reactions.*

Altered nutrition related to changes in renal handling of glucose

- Assess food intake and dry weight; monitor laboratory data: serum glucose, urinary glucose; encourage food intake as ordered *to ensure adequate intake within prescribed limits*

Risk for fluid deficit related to osmotic diuresis

- Assess neck veins, capillary refill, oral mucous membranes, and skin turgor every 4 to 6 hours; monitor weight daily, also monitor 24-hour intake and output; assess blood pressure, pulse, respirations every 6 to 8 hours; assess central venous pressure and pulmonary artery pressures every 6 to 8 hours if needed *to identify changes in fluid status.*
- Monitor laboratory data: serum glucose, sodium, potassium, chloride, and bicarbonate *to identify electrolytes lost with fluid losses.*

Risk for infection related to increased susceptibility with diabetes and chronic renal failure

- Assess for signs and symptoms of infection in secretions, excretions, and exudates; assess for fever; monitor and record temperature every 4 to 6 hours; monitor laboratory data: WBC, *to detect infection early.*
- Ensure aseptic technique for any invasive procedure or wound care *to decrease chance of infection.*

Knowledge deficit related to diabetic nephropathy and follow-up care

- See box below.

Patient Education/Home Care Planning

1. Explain the nature of diabetic nephropathy and chronic renal failure (see p. 935).
2. Explain the medical regimen and its rationale, including diet (restricted protein, sodium, and potassium), restricted fluid intake, and medications (purpose, dosage, interval, and adverse reactions).
3. Help the patient learn self-observational skills (temperature, pulse, respirations, blood pressure, intake and output, and weight) and record keeping.
4. Explain avoidance of infection.
5. Explain personal hygiene, rest, and exercise.
6. Explain when to call the physician.
7. Explain the plan for medical follow-up.
8. Explain renal dialysis and transplantation.

Evaluation

Renal tissue perfusion is adequate Renal function test results are normal or stable.

Nutritional status is adequate Food restrictions are appropriate to level of renal function and diabetic needs.

Fluid balance is within normal limits Urinary output balances intake within fluid restrictions.

No infection is present No signs or symptoms of infection are noted.

Patient and family are knowledgeable about diabetic nephropathy Patient and family can explain diabetic nephropathy, its causes, manifestations, and treatment; medical follow-up care; and the possibility of dialysis or transplantation in the future.

■ NEPHROSCLEROSIS

Severe hypertension can cause deterioration in renal function. Nephrosclerosis is the damage to the renal arteries, arterioles, and glomeruli caused by prolonged elevated blood pressure.

Renal parenchymal disease is a major consequence of prolonged elevated blood pressure. Important factors in the development of such problems are the age at which hypertension occurs, its severity, and the presence of risk factors (e.g., race, family history of hypertension or cardiovascular disease, obesity, diabetes mellitus, smoking, and lack of exercise). Many people develop arteriosclerosis as they age; such changes are accelerated with hypertension.

•••••• Pathophysiology

A slow, variable progression of vascular changes can occur over the years. The process includes spasm, thickening, hypertrophy, and hyaline degeneration of the renal arterial system. In malignant hypertension, renal changes are rapid and include fibrinoid necrosis. The damaged kidney decreases or stops production of substances that lower blood pressure.

•••••• Diagnostic Studies and Findings

Urinalysis   Proteinuria; hematuria

Blood chemistries   BUN, serum creatinine above normal; serum potassium variable, serum calcium elevated

Kidney-ureter-bladder (KUB) x-ray examination   Small kidneys, bilaterally

Intravenous urogram   Small kidneys, bilaterally

Electrocardiogram   Left ventricular hypertrophy

•••••• Multidisciplinary Plan

Goals of therapy include aggressive control of blood pressure to slow renal deterioration, delay of end-stage renal disease by conservative management, and initiation of dialysis or performance of a renal transplant at the appropriate point in the course of the disease. Drug dosages and intervals must be modified when the kidney is involved in the drug's excretion. Rates of excretion and metabolism and sensitivity to drugs may be altered. Bed rest, sodium restriction, and antihypertensive drugs are basic.

Surgery

Transplantation of donor kidney as described on p. 979.

Medications

Antihypertensives
  Vasodilators
    Minoxidil (Loniten), po, initially 5 mg bid; increase gradually; usual dose 10-40 mg/d; maximum 100 mg/d
    Sodium nitroprusside (Nipride), IV, in emergency, continuous infusion, 0.5-10 μg/kg/min as required
  Angiotensin antagonists
    Captopril (Capoten), po, initially 25 mg tid, slowly increase by 50 mg increments, maximum dose 150 mg tid
    Atenolol (Tenormin), po, initially 50 mg/d, may increase to 100 mg/d
  Calcium channel blockers
    Diltiazem (Cardizem), po, initially 30-60 mg q6-8h, may be increased gradually to 180-240 mg in 3 or 4 equal doses
    Nifedipine (Procardia), po, initially 10 mg tid, may be increased slowly to 20-30 mg tid
  Centrally acting agents
    Clonidine (Catapres, Dixarit), po, 0.1 mg bid or tid initially; then increase by 0.2-0.8 mg/d (maximum effective dose; 2.4 mg/d)
Diuretics
    Ethacrynic acid (Edecrin), po, 50-100 mg initially; maintenance 50-100 mg/d or bid after meals (up to 400 mg) on continuous or intermittent schedule
    Furosemide (Lasix, Uritol), po, 20-80 mg followed by second dose in 6-8 h up to 600 mg; IM, IV, 20-40 mg given slowly over 1-2 min; high dose by IV not more than 4 mg/min and repeat in 6-8 h

General Management

Dialysis by home or in-center hemodialysis, home or in-center intermittent peritoneal dialysis, or continuous ambulatory peritoneal dialysis (CAPD) may be needed if chronic renal failure develops (see pp. 969 and 979).

Fluid intake to balance output: about 400 to 600 ml (about the amount of insensible losses) plus amount equal to 24-hour urine volume; patient should avoid dehydration and volume excess

Nutritional modifications to achieve or maintain adequate nutritional status and to reduce work of diseased kidney
  Protein: 0.6 g/kg body weight/day; glomerular filtration rate (GFR) 20 to 25 ml/min—90 g/day; GFR 10 to 15 ml/min—50 g/day; GFR 4 to 10 ml/min—40 g/day
  Sodium: 1000 to 2000 mg/day; specific amounts depend on weight, blood pressure, serum creatinine, and 24-hour sodium excretion
  Potassium: 1500 to 2000 mg/day; with normal urine output (at least 800 ml/day), no restriction needed
  Calories: 35 to 55 kcal/kg body weight/day; calories from fat and carbohydrates used; adequate calories must accompany protein intake to prevent use of protein for energy and weight loss

NURSING CARE

Nursing Assessment

Cardiovascular

Elevated blood pressure; tachycardia; fourth heart sound; forceful apical impulse (PMI)

Optic Fundi

Retinal blood vessel changes: narrowing, hemorrhages, and exudates

Renal

Nocturia; proteinuria; hematuria

General

Headache; dizziness; fatigue; palpitations; blurred vision

Nursing Dx & Intervention

Altered renal tissue perfusion related to damage to nephrons

- Administer medications as ordered; dosages may be reduced and time intervals may be lengthened for drugs excreted by the kidneys. Observe response to drugs *to determine effectiveness of drug, dosage, and timing and to identify adverse reactions.*
- Monitor laboratory data: serum potassium, calcium, uric acid, bicarbonate, pH, and glucose. These substances may be altered when taking diuretics and in chronic renal failure.
- Follow ECG changes; ECG changes associated with hyperkalemia are peaked T wave, prolonged PR interval, widened QRS complex, and cardiac standstill.

- Watch for Kussmaul breathing and Chvostek's or Trousseau's signs *to identify acidosis and hypocalcemia.*
- Assess standing and lying blood pressures and pulse every 4 to 6 hours; record weight daily; calculate 24-hour intake and output *to identify increased peripheral vascular resistance, postural hypotension, and fluid retention.*

Knowledge deficit related to nephrosclerosis and follow-up care

- See box below.

Patient Education/Home Care Planning

1. Explain the nature of chronic renal failure (see p. 935).
2. Explain hypertension and its care (see Chapter 1).
3. Explain the medical regimen and its rationale, including diet (restricted protein, sodium, and potassium), restricted fluid intake, and medications (purpose, dosage, interval, and adverse reactions).
4. Teach self-observational skills (temperature, pulse, respirations, blood pressure, intake and output, and weight) and record keeping.
5. Explain avoidance of infection.
6. Explain personal hygiene, rest, and exercise.
7. Explain when to call the physician.
8. Explain the plan for medical follow-up.
9. Explain renal dialysis and transplantation as future options.

Evaluation

Renal tissue perfusion is stable   Renal function findings do not worsen.

Patient and family are knowledgeable about nephrosclerosis   Patient and family can describe nephrosclerosis,

the medical plan of care, and future options for dialysis or transplantation.

RENAL ARTERY OCCLUSION OR STENOSIS AND RENAL VEIN THROMBOSIS

Renal artery occlusion is a sudden complete blockage of the renal artery or a branch of it. Stenosis is a narrowing of the artery. The renal vein or a branch of it can be blocked by an embolus or thrombus.

Renal artery problems frequently are associated with atherosclerosis (in older patients) and fibromuscular hyperplasia. Renal vein thrombosis is most frequently associated with nephrotic syndrome (NS). It also may accompany an aortic aneurysm, a hematoma, trauma, or a neoplasm that compresses the renal vein.

•••••• Pathophysiology

In renal artery occlusion, complete cessation of arterial blood flow causes an infarct, with coagulation necrosis in the kidney. If the person has a single kidney, acute oliguric renal failure ensues. Occlusion is most frequently the result of an embolism caused by mitral valve stenosis, subacute bacterial endocarditis, and mural thrombi after a myocardial infarction.

Severe stenosis caused by atherosclerosis leads to ischemic atrophy and fibrosis. Decreased pressure in the arterioles stimulates the juxtaglomerular apparatus to produce an increase in renin secretion and can lead to renovascular hypertension.

A sudden, complete occlusion of the renal vein causes an infarct; the kidney swells, pressing against the capsule. If an occlusion evolves slowly, however, collateral venous circulation may develop, resulting in less impairment of renal function. Renal vein thrombosis may be associated with dehydration, sepsis, or hypercoagulable states.

•••••• Diagnostic Studies and Findings

	Findings		
Diagnostic Tests	**Renal Artery Occlusion**	**Renal Artery Stenosis**	**Renal Vein Thrombosis**
Intravenous urogram	Affected kidney is smaller, calyces are smaller, nephrogram phase is delayed		Unilateral change in kidney function when radiopaque dye is injected: enlargement, poorly visualized
Renal arteriogram	Absence of function in all or part of the kidney as it filters radiopaque dye		
Renal venogram			Demonstrable clot
Laboratory tests			
Urine	Microscopic hematuria		Gross hematuria; proteinuria; foamy, deep yellow color
Complete blood count	Leukocytosis		
Blood chemistries	Increased lactic dehydrogenase (LDH)		Signs of nephrotic syndrome
Plasma renin activity		Increased level in renal vein	

•••••• Multidisciplinary Plan

Surgery

Embolectomies are not usually performed for renal artery occlusion, since renal damage usually has occurred by the time diagnosis is made; selected patients with renal artery stenosis may have surgical correction by percutaneous transluminal angioplasty; if a thrombus begins in the aorta and extends into the renal artery, percutaneous transluminal angioplasty is less successful than if only the renal artery is involved; aortorenal bypass; autogenous vascular graft; a nephrectomy may be needed in renal artery stenosis for renovascular hypertension that does not respond to drug therapy

Medications

Anticoagulants (used for renal artery occlusion or renal vein thrombosis)

Heparin sodium, IV, subcutaneously: 10,000-20,000 U initially (68 kg man); maintenance 8000-10,000 U q8h or 15,000-20,000 U q12h

Warfarin (Coumadin, Panwarfin), po, IM, IV, 10-15 mg/d for 2-3 days; then maintenance dose of 2-10 mg/d

Analgesics

Meperidine (Demerol, Pethadol), po, subcutaneously, IM, IV, 50-150 mg q3-4h

Codeine sulfate (generic), po, IM, subcutaneously, 15-60 mg qid

Morphine sulfate (generic), po, subcutaneously, IV, 5-15 mg q4h prn

Antihypertensive agents (used for renal artery stenosis)

β-Blockers

Propranolol (Inderal, Novopranol), po, 40 mg q6h or q8h initially; increased to 160-480 mg/d in divided doses; up to 640 mg/d

Captopril (Capoten), po, 25 mg tid initially; may be increased to 50 mg tid after 1-2 wk then to 100-150 mg tid as needed

General Management

Conservative approach; patients usually have serious cardiac disease; pain relief is major focus in occlusion; with stenosis, blood pressure must be controlled; with renal vein thrombosis, preventing pulmonary emboli is vital; underlying cause of nephrotic syndrome should be treated if possible (see "Nephrotic Syndrome" on p. 953, and other disease states must be treated; monitor contralateral kidney function; stabilize cardiac function; dialysis may be needed with any of these conditions

NURSING CARE

Nursing Assessment

Cardiovascular

In renal artery stenosis: hypertension; abdominal bruits

General

In renal artery occlusion: pain in flank or upper abdomen; few signs if infarct is small

In renal vein thrombosis: flank pain

Nursing Dx & Intervention

Altered renal tissue perfusion related to altered arterial or venous flow

- Assess vital signs every 4 to 6 hours; assess weight daily *to determine systemic effects of renal problem.*
- Assess neck veins, central venous pressure, and pulmonary artery pressures if appropriate; monitor blood pressure both standing and lying every 4 hours; monitor intake and output daily; monitor laboratory data: urine protein, BUN, serum creatinine, and clotting times *to determine effect on cardiovascular and renal function.*
- Give antihypertensive and anticoagulant agents as ordered; observe response to drugs *to determine effectiveness of drug and dosage and observe for adverse and toxic side effects.*

Pain related to altered arterial or venous flow

- Assess pattern of pain, and determine need for analgesia; administer analgesics as ordered *to promote comfort; to determine the effectiveness of drug, dosage, and timing, and to identify adverse reactions.* Observe response to drug given. A sudden increase in pain may mean extension of the problem.

Knowledge deficit related to renal artery occlusion or stenosis or renal vein thrombosis and follow-up care

- See box below.

Patient Education/Home Care Planning

1. Explain the nature of renal artery occlusion, renal artery stenosis, or renal vein thrombosis.
2. Explain the treatment regimen and rationale.
3. Explain follow-up medical care required.

Evaluation

Some function returns after renal artery occlusion Patient's renal function tests show improvement.

Medical therapy or surgery helps renal artery stenosis Hypertension is relieved or is under control.

Renal function returns completely or is now impaired in renal vein thrombosis Renal function test results are normal or reflect degrees of impairment.

CONTINUOUS RENAL REPLACEMENT THERAPIES[1,12,13,19]

Description and Rationale

Continuous renal replacement therapies (CRRTs) include continuous arteriovenous hemofiltration (CAVH), continuous arteriovenous hemodiafiltration (CAVHD), continuous venovenous hemofiltration (CVVH), and continuous venovenous hemodiafiltration (CVVHD). Hemofiltration therapies (CAVH, CVVH) are prescribed when fluid removal is the primary goal. Hemodiafiltration therapies (CAVHD, CVVHD) are prescribed when the goal is solute removal plus or minus fluid removal. The continuous nature of these therapies allows for a slow and gentle removal of plasma water and dissolved solutes (electrolytes, toxins, drugs) from critically ill patients with renal insufficiency or failure.

Indications for CRRTs include acute renal failure or insufficiency with uremia, abnormal electrolytes, acid-base imbalance, or fluid overload in critically ill patients. These are safe and efficient therapies for patients who cannot tolerate conventional hemodialysis because of hemodynamic instability, arrhythmias, or increased intracranial pressure (ICP). Patients may not tolerate conventional hemodialysis because of the significant extracorporeal volume or the rapid fluid, electrolyte or osmolality shifts over 2 to 4 hours. Patients who require large fluid volumes, such as parenteral nutrition, blood products, and medications, benefit from continuous fluid removal. Fluid restrictions are obsolete for patients on CRRTs. Nonrenal indications being studied include cytokine removal in sepsis and multiple organ dysfunction syndrome (MODS), fluid removal and neurohormonal changes in congestive heart failure (CHF), and myoglobin removal in rhabdomyolysis.

CRRTS involve a low-volume blood circuit with a hemofilter and an ultrafiltration collection bag. The hemofilters have semipermeable membranes that separate the blood compartment from the ultrafiltrate compartment. Either hollow fiber or flat plate hemofilters are used for CRRTs. Plasma water and mid-molecular-weight solutes (10,000 to 30,000 daltons) move from the blood compartment across the semipermeable membrane to form ultrafiltrate (UF), which drains from the hemofilter into a UF collection bag. This process is similar to the filtration process across the glomerular basement membrane in the kidney. The resulting ultrafiltrate is composed of plasma water and solutes (e.g., Na^+, K^+, Cl^-, HCO_3^-, H^+, urea, creatinine, Mg^{++}, PO_4^-, Ca^{++}, cytokines, certain drugs).

Fluid removal in CRRTs is determined by the transmembrane pressure gradient (TPG) across the hemofilter filter membrane. The TPG is the difference between the oncotic and hydrostatic pressure within the hemofilter system. Positive hydrostatic pressure is exerted by blood when it is pushed through the blood compartment of the hemofilter either by the patient's mean arterial pressure (MAP) in CAVH or by the set rate of blood pump (ml/min) in CVVH. Positive hydrostatic pressure pushes fluid across the hemofilter membrane. Negative hydrostatic pressure in the UF compartment, on the opposite side of the hemofilter membrane, is created by gravity of the UF collection bag in relation to the hemofilter. This pressure is important in determining the rate of ultrafiltration. Oncotic pressure created by RBCs, WBCs, and plasma proteins in the blood compartment prevents all of the plasma water from ultrafiltrating.

There are two mechanisms of solute removal in CRRTs: convective transport and diffusive transport. Convective transport is the movement of solutes along with fluid across a semipermeable membrane. This is the only mechanism of solute removal in CAVH and CVVH, and it is directly proportional to the amount of ultrafiltration. The larger the volume ultrafiltrated, the more solute is removed. Diffusive transport is the movement of solutes across a semipermeable membrane from an area of higher solute concentration to an area of lower concentration. In CAVHD and CVVHD, a dialysate solution is infused throughout the UF compartment, countercurrent to the blood flow compartment, to create a diffusion gradient to enhance solute removal. Both convection and diffusion are mechanisms of solute removal in CAVHD and CVVHD.

Peritoneal dialysis solutions were used as dialysate in CRRTs in the past. The high dextrose concentrations of these solutions often led to hyperglycemia and additional insulin infusion therapy. New premixed dialysates made specifically for CRRTs are currently available. These dialysates contain physiologic levels of sodium, potassium, calcium, magnesium, chloride, and dextrose with a lactate buffer. Common dialysate flow rates through the hemofilter are 1000 to 2500 ml/hour. There is a curvilinear increase in solute removal with increases in dialysate flow rates, which plateaus around 2500 ml/hour. Higher flow rates are used for hyperkalemia, drug intoxication or rapid removal of urea.

Replacement fluid (RF) is the solution infused to maintain the prescribed hourly fluid balance. The composition of RF is determined by the patient's metabolic and electrolyte needs. Hyperalimentation, normal saline, bicarbonate solutions, and potassium additives are frequently prescribed replacement fluids. The amount of RF administered is calculated on an hourly basis and is dependent on the hourly amount of UF output, IV intake, and desired fluid balance. The RF is generally administered into the CRRT circuit via a prehemofilter. Prehemofilter RF hemodilutes the blood, which helps decrease clotting in the hemofilter.

Anticoagulation is prescribed to prevent hemofilter/circuit clotting and to maximize the clearance capability of the hemofilter. The goal is to anticoagulate the hemofilter and circuit, yet systemic anticoagulation may occur. Existing thrombocytopenia or coagulopathies may obviate the need for heparinization. Some institutions do not use any anticoagulation in their CRRT circuits. Commonly used anticoagulants include heparin, trisodium citrate, and prostacyclin. Most protocols require priming the hemofilter and circuit with heparinized saline, administering a bolus dose, and initiating a low-dose heparin infusion through a prehemofilter port in the circuit. Monitoring clotting times is required during continuous infusions of anticoagulants.

CAVH/CAVHD

Large bore arterial and venous access sites are required for CAVH and CAVHD. The femoral artery and vein are frequently used for access, but brachial, jugular, and subclavian sites also may be used. Blood is propelled from the arterial catheter through the circuit and hemofilter and back to the patient via the venous catheter by the force of MAP created by the patient's cardiac output. CAVH/CAVHD circuits require MAPs of at least 50 to 60 mmHg for effective flow through the circuit and ultrafiltration.

CVVH/CVVHD

Venous access with a dual-lumen catheter is required for CVVH and CVVHD. Common access sites include the femoral, internal jugular, or subclavian veins. A pump is required for CVVH and CVVHD because arterial pressure is not available. Blood is pulled and pushed through the blood circuit and hemofilter via a roller pump (rates of 30 to 300 ml/min). The blood pump is capable of monitoring circuit pressures and has an air detector and circuit clamp for safety purposes (Fig. 11-7).

Indications

- Inability to tolerate conventional hemodialysis due to hemodynamic instability, dysrhythmias, increased ICP

- Acute renal insufficiency/failure with uremia, metabolic acidosis, abnormal electrolytes, symptomatic fluid overload
- Sepsis, congestive heart failure, multiple organ dysfunction syndrome (MODS), rhabdomyolysis

Relative Contraindications

- Inability to obtain and maintain adequate access
- Hypercoagulable state with contraindication to anticoagulation

Complications

- Air embolus
- Inadvertent fluid overload or fluid removal
- Rapid electrolyte or acid/base shifts
- Hypothermia
- Bleeding from circuit, access, or systemic
- Excessive hemofilter/circuit clotting

•••••• Multidisciplinary Plan

Medications

Additives to RF: sodium bicarbonate, potassium chloride, etc.
Additives to dialysate: potassium chloride
Anticoagulant

Heparin sodium: initial dose 10-20 units/kg; continuous infusion 5-10 units/kg; monitor partial thromboplastin time (PTT) or activated clotting time (ACT) every 4-6 h or as ordered.

General Management

An hourly UF rate goal is prescribed depending on the patient's hemodynamic condition and hemofiltration needs. Typical UF

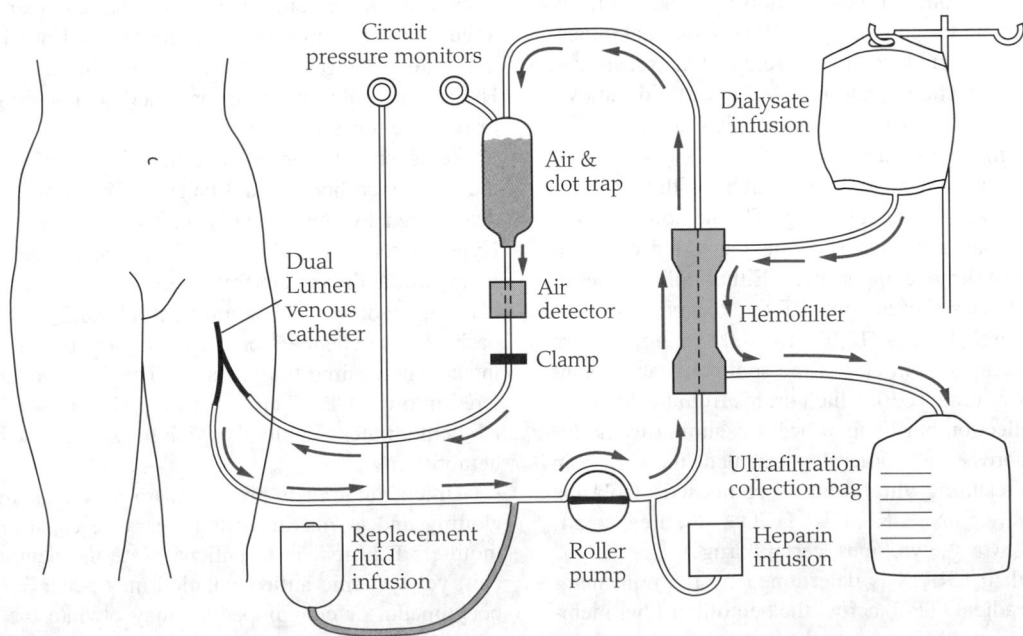

Figure 11-7 Continuous venovenous hemodiafiltration.

rates are 750 to 1500 ml/hour. The desired hourly fluid balance is prescribed based on the patient's volume status. Fluid balance orders can range from −400 ml/hour to +50 ml/hour. Replacement fluid solutions are prescribed based on the patient's metabolic and electrolyte needs. The calculation that determines the hourly RF infusion rate is:

$$RF = [net\ UF\ rate\ +\ other\ output)\ -\ (total\ intake)] - [desired\ fluid\ balance].$$

Monitoring the patient's pH, Na^+, K^+, Cl^-, CO_2, Mg^{++}, Ca^{++}, PO^{4-}, Cr, BUN, glucose and coagulation status is essential during CRRT. Hemodynamic monitoring required during CRRTs includes blood pressure (BP), heart rate (HR), and central venous pressure (CVP).

Safety goggles, mask, and gloves must be worn by staff to protect themselves from viruses and organisms that may be transmitted via the UF. For patient safety, hemofilter circuit, and access sites are monitored frequently (q1h minimum) for kinks, disconnects, leaks, and signs of clotting and air.

An assessment of the patient's nutritional needs and an understanding of the nutritional implications during CRRT help guide parenteral or enteral feeding prescriptions. Nutritional implications include vitamin, mineral, and protein losses via the UF and dextrose absorption from the dialysate.

Drug dosing for patients on CRRTs requires special attention. Guidelines for dosing take into account properties of the drugs and UF rates of the CRRT.

Mechanical Problems

Potential mechanical problems of CRRTs may involve the access catheter, hemofilter, circuit, or the blood pump (CVVH). The CRRT will not work if there is an obstruction to flow from a kink or obstruction (clot, vessel wall) in the catheter. The hemofilter and circuit are monitored for leaks, ruptures, and cracks, which may result in an air embolus or hemorrhage. In CVVH, the blood pump is tested and monitored to ensure that the air detector, blood leak detector, pressure transducers, and venous clamp are working.

Procedural Guidelines

Preparation for CRRTs

Assemble equipment and supplies. Prime hemofilter and circuit with heparinized saline to remove all air and filter preservatives. Ensure all connections are secure. Make sure the blood pump passes its self-test before use.

Before initiating therapy, monitor the patient's baseline temperature, HR, BP, CVP, weight, intake/output, creatinine, blood urea nitrogen, electrolytes, glucose, clotting times, platelet count, hematocrit and arterial blood gas. Review the CRRT orders for RF composition, dialysate additives, anticoagulation, UF rate goal, net fluid balance, blood pump rate, laboratory monitoring and parameters to notify the physician.

Assist with catheter insertion. Using sterile technique, check catheter patency and flow before connecting circuit to patient.

Initiation and Maintenance of CRRTs

Assemble supplies. Using sterile technique connect circuit to the access catheters. Monitor blood flow through the circuit for air bubbles and ease of flow. Begin dialysate, heparin and RF infusions. Establish ultrafiltration and monitor the patient's BP closely during the first 15 minutes of therapy. Secure the circuit to prevent an inadvertent disconnect or dislodgement. The blood circuit and blood pump should be kept visible at all times.

Monitor the patient's hemodynamic status and laboratory values closely. Monitor access sites for infection or bleeding. Check pulses distal to catheter sites. Monitor patient for bleeding if receiving anticoagulation.

Measure and regulate UF rate. Calculate RF rate based on the total output, total intake, and desired fluid balance hourly. Adjust height of the UF drainage bag appropriately to increase or decrease the hourly UF rate. Document accurate intake, output, and RF calculations every hour.

CVVH/CVVHD: Monitor and manage the blood pump circuit pressures. Identify and troubleshoot blood pump alarms.

Circuit Change or Discontinuation of CRRT

Discontinue infusions of dialysate, anticoagulant, and RF. Clamp UF tubing. If possible, return the blood in the circuit to the patient, then clamp the circuit tubings and the access catheters. Flush catheters with heparinized saline as ordered. Discard CRRT circuit and hemofilter in a biohazardous waste receptacle. Remove access catheters as ordered if the plan is to not restart therapy or convert to conventional hemodialysis.

NURSING CARE

Nursing Assessment

Cardiovascular

Hypervolemia: elevated central venous pressure. Jugular venous distention, extra heart sound (S3), lung sounds (crackles), frothy white or pink tinged sputum, dependent or generalized edema, weight gain

Hypovolemia: hypotension, tachycardia, low central venous pressure, flat neck veins, dry mucous membranes, thirst, weight loss

Metabolic

Acidemia: low arterial pH, Kussmaul respirations, hypotension

Alkalosis: high arterial pH, cardiac dysrhythmias, tetany

Skin

Pressure ulcers secondary to immobility/bedrest while on CRRT and critical illness

Musculoskeletal

Limited range of motion, stiff joints, foot drop, muscle atrophy related to immobility and critical illness

Nursing Dx & Interventions

Fluid-volume excess related to fluid accumulation caused by altered renal function or an inadvertent RF calculation error and infusion rate

- Monitor patient weight, intake and output, BP, HR, CVP, hourly UF rates and oxygenation *to determine fluid status.*
- Ensure accurate calculations to determine RF volumes every hour.
- Monitor trends in hourly UF rates to assess for clotting and hemofilter efficiency.
- Monitor laboratory values: BUN, creatinine, sodium, potassium, calcium, magnesium, and phosphate *to determine electrolyte balance, accumulation of nitrogenous wastes and solute removal efficiency.*

Potential for fluid-volume deficit related to too rapid removal of fluid (UF) caused by excess negative hydrostatic pressure in the UF bag or an inadvertent RF calculation error and infusion rate

- Monitor and record hourly intake and output; ensure accurate RF calculations and infusion rates *to prevent inadvertent hypovolemia.*
- Monitor BP, HR, CVP, intake and output and hourly UF *rate to determine fluid status and note changes.*
- Alter the level of the UF bag (raise the bag) *to decrease the negative hydrostatic pressure and decrease the rate of UF removal.*
- Administer intravenous fluid boluses as ordered *to treat symptomatic hypovolemia.*

Potential for infection related to invasive procedure

- Use sterile technique whenever the circuit is accessed including during connection and discontinuation *to protect the patient from nosocomial contamination.*
- Inspect access sites for redness, swelling, tenderness, drainage; monitor the patient's temperature and WBC *to detect infection.*
- Follow universal precautions for exposure to blood and body fluids *to protect patient and nurse from contamination.*
- Site care, dressing, and tubing changes per hospital policy *to prevent infection.*

Impaired physical mobility related to presence of large bore venous and/or arterial catheters and connection to the hemofilter circuit

- Physical therapy and range of motion activity with caution at least TID *to prevent stiff joints, muscle atrophy, and foot drop.*

- Turn frequently and encourage patient to assist; deep vein thrombosis prophylaxis as ordered; encourage coughing and deep breathing as appropriate and tolerated *to prevent atelectasis and other complications of bedrest.*
- Monitor skin at pressure points; float heels and elbows off pillows *to prevent skin breakdown.*

Potential for injury caused by bleeding related to inadvertent disconnect of circuit or anticoagulation therapy

- Monitor access sites and other potential sites for bleeding; no IM or SQ injections; monitor laboratory values: PT, PTT (or ACT), platelets, hemoglobin/hematocrit *to detect signs of bleeding.*

Potential alteration in perfusion related to large bore arterial and/or venous access catheters

- Monitor pulses and capillary refill distal to access catheters; note any increase in edema in limbs with access catheters and record circumference changes *to detect altered perfusion.*

Knowledge deficit related to CRRTs

- See box below.

Patient Education/Home Care Planning

1. Explain indications and purpose for the CRRT (i.e., to decrease the extra fluid in the patient's lungs or tissues); give a simple explanation of how the therapy works and what equipment is involved.
2. Explain that new catheter(s) will be inserted.
3. Explain that the therapy is continuous and will require bedrest and may limit movement of certain limbs.
4. Explain that the therapy is not painful.
5. Give the patient/family an idea of the probable/average duration of therapy if known.

Evaluation

Fluid status is within normal limits   Absence of signs and symptoms of fluid overload or dehydration.

No infection is present   Patient shows no signs or symptoms of infection related to the access sites or circuit.

No complications of immobility occur   Patient does not develop pneumonia, deep vein thrombosis, skin breakdown, decreased range of motion, or joint stiffness.

No complications of bleeding occur   Patient does not develop signs or symptoms of bleeding related to inadvertent disconnect or anticoagulation.

No complications of altered perfusion occur   Patient does not develop signs or symptoms of arterial or venous occlusion and altered perfusion.

RENAL DIALYSIS

Dialysis is the differential diffusion of permeable substances through a semipermeable membrane separating two solutions. Hemodialysis and peritoneal dialysis are two forms of dialysis used clinically to treat patients with acute or chronic renal failure. The dialysate fluid contains electrolytes similar to those in normal blood plasma to permit diffusion of electrolytes into or out of the patient's blood. Glucose is added to the dialysate fluid to raise the osmolality and remove water from the blood channel.

Dialysis replaces some, but not all, of the kidney's functions. Fluid volume, electrolyte balance, acid-base balance, and nitrogenous wastes are controlled. Adequacy of dialysis is measured by clinical factors: patient feels well, blood pressure controlled, stable weight, good fluid balance, and no uremic signs, as well as laboratory indices: individually determined serum creatinine levels, normal serum electrolyte levels, stable nerve conduction studies, and normal serum albumin levels.

Dialysis options include home or in-center hemodialysis, home or in-center intermittent peritoneal dialysis, continuous cycling peritoneal dialysis (CCPD), and continuous ambulatory peritoneal dialysis (CAPD). Dialysis plays an important role in renal transplant programs by providing a backup for failed transplants and a pool of potential transplant recipients.

According to the 1994 report of the United States Renal Data System, 138,277 patients were on dialysis at the end of 1991, the latest year for complete statistics.[16] In-center hemodialysis was used most frequently, but the use of home peritoneal dialysis (both CAPD and CCPD) is increasing. Home hemodialysis is much less frequently used currently.

Hemofiltration is an alternative to dialysis. This treatment uses a convective filtration process on a continuous rather than intermittent schedule. Pressure differences in the hemofilter force water and solutes through the highly permeable membrane in proportion to their concentrations in the blood. The ultrafiltrate formed is discarded, and depending on the patient's condition, most of the water and solutes removed are replaced. This procedure is used increasingly in the United States for acute renal failure; in Europe, it is used with a blood pump for patients with chronic renal failure. It is a simple system that uses a percutaneous access. A longer treatment time is required,

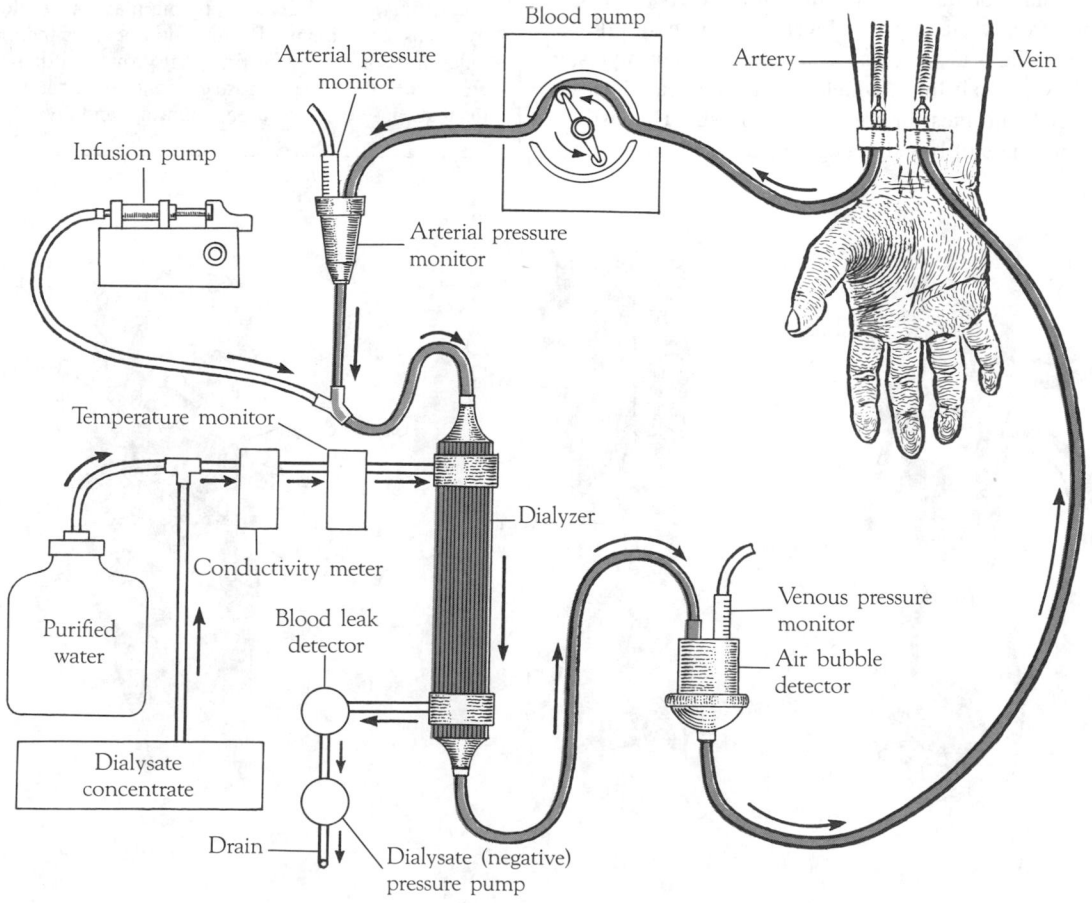

Figure 11-8 Components of a hemodialysis system. (From Thelan.[18])

thus avoiding peaks and valleys in blood chemistry values. Hemofiltration can be combined with hemodialysis in the process known as hemodiafiltration.

HEMODIALYSIS

Description and Rationale

Hemodialysis involves circulating the patient's blood through semipermeable tubing that is surrounded by a dialysate solution in the artificial kidney (Figure 11-8). It replaces part of the kidney's normal function.

The blood circuit includes an access device (cannula or internal arteriovenous fistula); arterial blood lines (with blood pressure monitor); a blood pump; a dialyzer, where diffusion, osmosis, and ultrafiltration occur; and venous lines with filter and monitors (for clots or air emboli and pressure), which return blood to the patient.

The dialysis circuit includes a supply of dialysate concentrate and a supply of treated water (see box), which are combined by a proportioning pump so that the desired concentration is delivered to the dialyzer; monitors that detect the pressure, concentration, and temperature of the dialysate and stop the flow of dialysate if preset levels are not met; a dialyzer, where the dialysate accepts wastes, excess electrolytes, and water; dialysate exit lines, which may have a leak detector (blood-in-effluent lines) or are monitored using Hemastix to detect the presence of blood; a negative pressure gauge on

the dialysate lines that controls ultrafiltration; and a bypass circuit (not shown in Figure 11-8) for diversion of dialysate that is not within the preset temperature, conductivity, or pressure limits.

The composition of the diluted dialysate solution is sodium, 130 to 145 mEq/L; potassium, 0 to 3 mEq/L; calcium, 2.5 to 4 mEq/L; chloride, 96 to 107 mEq/L; and acetate, 33 to 41 mEq/L. Bicarbonate can be used in place of acetate.

Blood access is achieved by means of an internal arteriovenous fistula created surgically with the patient's artery and vein, endogenous vein grafts, exogenous vein (bovine) grafts, or grafts made of artificial material such as expanded polytetrafluorethylene or by means of an external arteriovenous shunt or cannula (Figure 11-9).

WATER TREATMENT

Water must be treated to remove substances toxic to the patient or harmful to the machine. Methods include filtration, softening, deionization, reverse osmosis, and distillation. Substances removed are dissolved anions or cations (sodium, chloride, iron, magnesium, manganese, copper, nitrates, fluoride, iodide) and organic materials (chloramines, pyrogens, endotoxins). Bacteria do not cross the membrane unless a leak is present. Bacterial growth in dialysate may change pH, decrease glucose concentration, and release toxins that cause chills, nausea, vomiting, and fever.

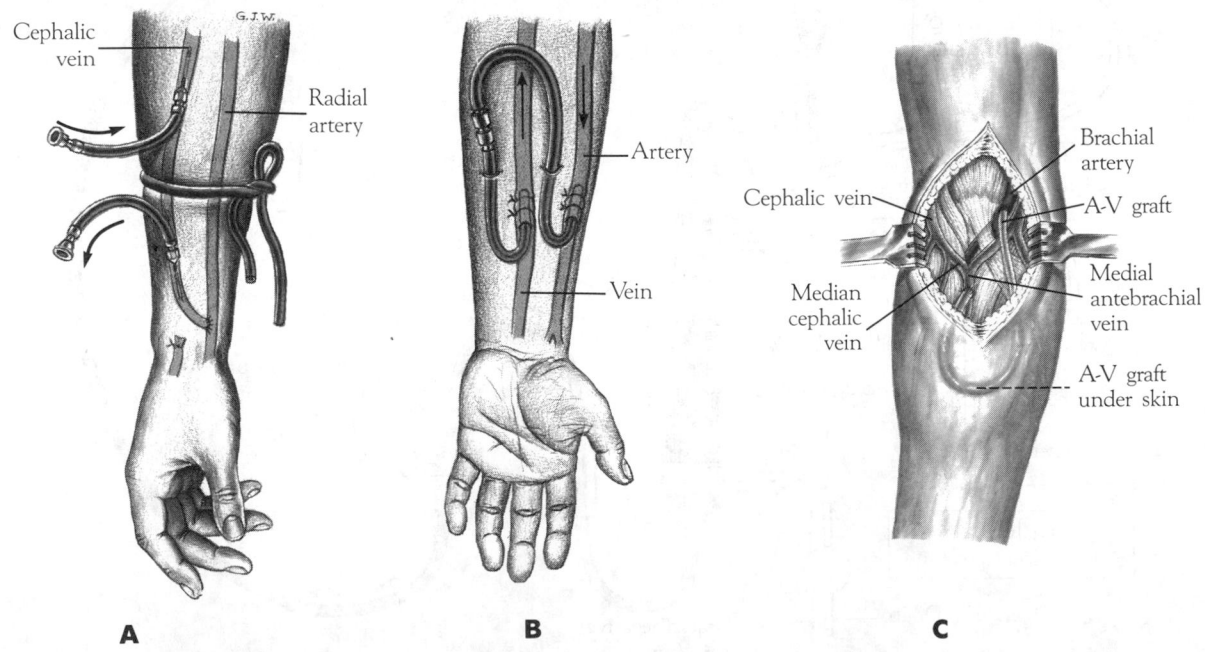

Figure 11-9 Circulatory access for hemodialysis. **A,** External (temporary) arteriovenous cannula (shunt). **B,** Internal (permanent) arteriovenous fistula. **C,** Internal (permanent) arteriovenous graft.

Hemodialysis treatment schedules vary with the kind of machine used and the patient's condition. Treatments are usually scheduled three times a week for 3 to 6 hours per treatment.

Major types of artificial kidneys are hollow fiber and flat plate. The hollow fiber kidney is increasingly used because it can be adapted to the size of the patient. In the hollow fiber kidney the blood flows through narrow filaments that are surrounded by dialysate (Figures 11-10 and 11-11). In the flat plate kidney the blood and dialysate flow in opposite directions in alternate layers.

Hemodialysis Monitors

Each machine has visible and audible alarms that signal problems outside the preset upper and lower limits and cause portions of the system to be shut off or bypassed.
    Dialysate compartment
        Temperature—measures and controls level
        Flow rate—reflects fluctuations in rate
        Conductivity—detects hyperosmolality or hypoosmolality
        Pressure—detects high or low levels
        Blood leak—detects blood in dialysate as it leaves the machine (membrane rupture)

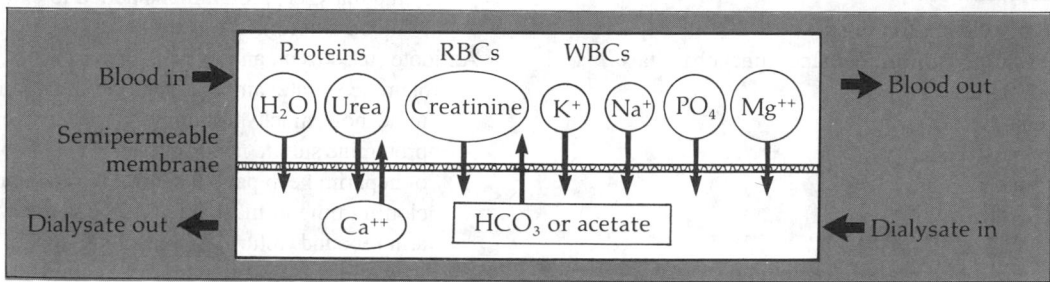

Figure 11-10 General scheme for dialyzer design. (Modified from Lancaster.[10])

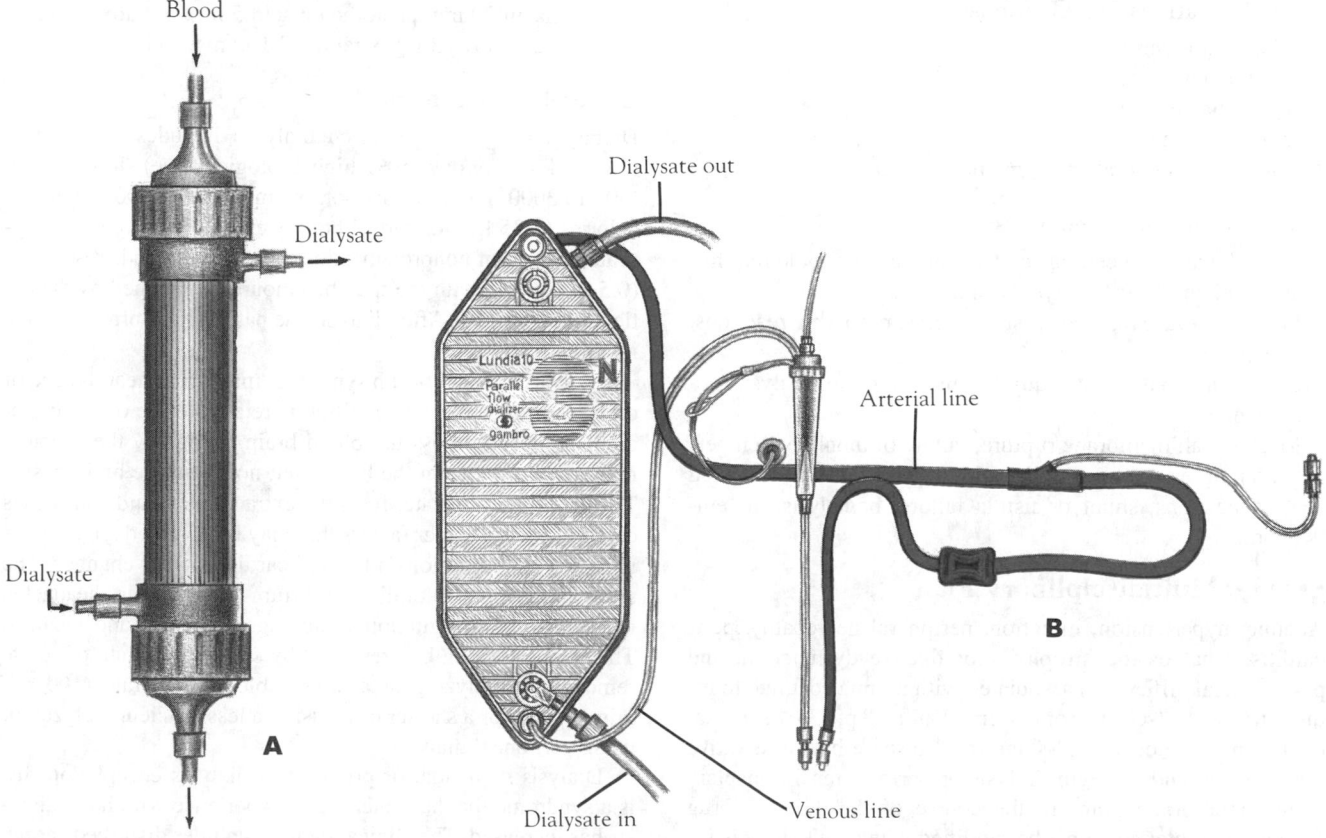

Figure 11-11 Kinds of dialyzers. **A,** Hollow-fiber. **B,** Flat plate.

Blood compartment

Pressure—arterial and venous lines (stops blood pump)

Air bubbles—detects air in venous line (stops blood pump and clamps venous line)

Blood Access Devices

External arteriovenous shunt

Internal arteriovenous fistula

Grafts

Subclavian vein catheter

Femoral vein catheter

Indications for Hemodialysis

Need for rapid, efficient treatment

Acute poisoning (aspirin, methanol, phenobarbital)

Acute renal failure

Chronic renal failure

Severe edema states

Hepatic coma

Metabolic acidosis

Hyperkalemia

Extensive burns with prerenal azotemia

Transfusion reactions

Postpartum renal insufficiency

Crush syndrome, rhabdomyolysis, and myoglobinuria

Contraindications and Cautions

Other major chronic illness

No vascular access

Hemorrhagic diathesis

Extremes of age

Inability to cooperate with treatment regimen

Complications of Hemodialysis

Hemodynamic: bleeding, clot formation, hypovolemia, hypervolemia, angina, dysrhythmias, anemia

Infectious: vascular access site abscess, pyrogenic reactions, hepatitis B

Metabolic: dialysis disequilibrium syndrome, dialysis dementia

Mechanical: membrane rupture, failure of monitors (temperature, pressure, osmolality, clot, and air bubble), loosened connections, shunt or fistula failure, hemolysis, air embolism

•••••• Multidisciplinary Plan

Anemia, hypertension, infection, peripheral neuropathy, pericarditis, renal osteodystrophy, reproductive dysfunction, and psychosocial difficulties associated with uremia continue to require treatment (see "Chronic Renal Failure," p. 935). The goal of therapy is to delay end-stage renal disease by conservative management and to begin dialysis or perform renal transplant at the appropriate point in the course of the disease. Drug dosages and intervals must be modified when the kidney is involved in the drug's excretion. Rates of excretion and metabolism and sensitivity to drugs may be altered.[2]

Surgery

Internal arteriovenous fistula created or shunt inserted to provide access to arterial and venous circulation

Medications

Anticoagulant agents

Heparin sodium, systemic: as determined by clotting time, which should be 30-60 min; via intermittent IV injection with priming dose 100 mg/kg body weight with additional doses as needed or continuous infusion by pump (1000-2000 U/h)

Regional: heparin is injected into blood line entering the dialyzer; protamine is added to exit blood line as blood is returned to patient

Antidote (used as an antiheparin agent)

Protamine sulfate: amount and kind of heparin used determine how much protamine is needed; each 1 mg of protamine sulfate neutralizes activity of about 90-115 U of heparin; keep patient's clotting time normal; monitor clotting time in machine and in patient; watch for heparin rebound (return of anticoagulation up to 10 h later) which may necessitate more protamine

Antihypertensive agents: omit dosage on day of dialysis if necessary to prevent excessive hypotension during treatment

Vitamins (water-soluble, lost in dialysis)

Daily requirements: thiamine 1.5 mg, riboflavin, 1.8 mg, niacin 20 mg; pantothenic acid 5 mg, pyridoxine 5 mg, vitamin B_{12} 3 μg, vitamin C 100 mg, folic acid 1 mg

General Management

Dietary management between dialyses includes low protein (1.2 to 1.4 g/kg/day, 50% high biologic value); low sodium (500 to 3000 mg/day); low potassium (2000 to 3000 mg/day); calories ($\geq$35 kcal/day ideal body weight, 50% from carbohydrate and rest of nonprotein calories from fat); fluids restriction (0.5 to 1 L/day, with the specific amount determined by the patient's dry weight). After dialysis the patient has normal volume relationships.

Dialysis disequilibrium syndrome may occur near the end of dialysis or after it. The condition is related to the osmotic gradient produced across the blood-brain barrier by the efficient removal of urea from the blood, but not from the brain tissue. The urea draws in water from the extracellular fluid and causes cerebral edema. Other factors that may be involved are changes in serum pH, rapid ion shifts, and cardiovascular changes. The signs and symptoms of disequilibrium syndrome are headache, nausea, vomiting, agitation, twitching, confusion, and seizures. This syndrome can be prevented by slowing the rate of solute removal by dialyzing at a slower blood flow rate (100 ml/minute) and for a shorter time, using a less efficient dialyzer, or using peritoneal dialysis.

Dialysis dementia, or progressive dialysis encephalopathy, is a syndrome that has emerged as experience with hemodialysis has increased. The clinical picture includes disturbed speech that occurs first during dialysis, myoclonus, dementia, or behavioral changes. It is a progressive condition that ends in death. A number of studies have implicated aluminum accumulation from the water supply or from aluminum hydroxide taken as a phosphate binder.

Dialysis-associated hepatitis B is a major concern for patients (often active carriers of the hepatitis B virus), staff (at risk because of frequent exposure to patient's blood), and families (at risk because of close contact, especially sexual, and from environmental surfaces). It should be noted that special precautions with blood and other bodily fluids are needed to prevent spreading the hepatitis B virus (HBV). Health care professionals and patients in dialysis units are particularly at risk, because a patient with chronic renal failure may receive transfusions and may have a subclinical case of hepatitis B infection owing to impairment of the immune system.

The hepatitis B surface antigen (Hb$_S$Ag) is a useful marker for active HBV infections.

Hepatitis B virus can be found in blood and secretions containing serum or derived from serum. Oozing skin lesions, saliva, semen, and vaginal secretions can be sources of the virus. Transmission can occur by introduction of the virus-containing fluid through (1) direct percutaneous inoculation (via needles, and so forth); (2) indirect percutaneous innoculation (through minute skin abrasions); (3) absorption through mucosal surfaces (mouth, eye, and during sexual contact); and (4) transfer from environmental surfaces.

Programs to prevent the spread of HBV infections focus on identifying persons who are Hb$_S$Ag positive. Screening of all dialysis unit personnel and patients is done regularly. Such programs also include hygienic measures: safe, reliable procedures for handling laboratory specimens; procedures for hepatitis B precautions for hospitalized patients, including safe care of disposable materials, food handling, and laundry service; segregation of dialysis equipment used for patients who are Hb$_S$Ag positive; vigilant handwashing practices; sterilization measures appropriate to the material involved; no eating, smoking, or other hand-to-mouth activity in the dialysis unit or laboratory; use of protective clothing, such as masks, goggles, gloves, aprons, shoe covers, gowns, and caps; and policy of reporting and recording any unusual exposure to HBV.

Hepatitis B vaccine is used for active immunization for preexposure prevention in high-risk populations, such as dialysis unit personnel. Hepatitis B immune globulin is used for passive immunization after exposure to HBV.

Procedural Guidelines
Prehemodialysis Care

Measure temperature, pulse, respirations, and blood pressure (both lying and standing) and record for baseline

Review pretreatment BUN; serum creatinine, sodium, and potassium levels; hematocrit; be aware of HBV and HIV status of patient, if known

Check electrical status of the dialysis machine; dialysate concentration as ordered; patent, sterile tubing with all air flushed out; removal of the sterilizing agent used (formaldehyde or chlorine bleach); secure all connections; set all monitors

During Hemodialysis

Wear mask and have patient wear mask during initiation and discontinuation of dialysis; wear protective garb, goggles, apron, and gloves; use sterile technique for needle insertions and shunt connections; anchor connections securely; precautions against infection for all concerned are mandatory

Check equipment for readiness, safety, and settings of gauges; monitor vital signs, intake and output, and equipment parameters (blood flow rate, pressures, temperature, osmolality, clots, air emboli, negative pressure for ultrafiltration, and blood leaks); monitor clotting times; watch for rapid shifts in volume or electrolytes that may result in hypovolemia, angina, dysrhythmias, nausea, or muscle cramps; minimize blood loss

After Hemodialysis

Measure and record vital signs and weight after discontinuing treatment; use precautions against infection; provide routine care to shunt or fistula; avoid trauma to sites; avoid blood pressure readings or needlesticks in arm with shunt or fistula; check circulation; palpate thrill or auscultate venous blood flow; record BUN, serum creatinine, sodium, and potassium levels to note effects of treatment

Care Between Treatments

Encourage patient to follow diet and fluid restrictions as ordered, to take medications as ordered, and to call nurse or physician as appropriate for problems; limit weight gain to 0.5 kg/day between treatments; regular shunt or fistula care is required

NURSING CARE

Nursing Assessment
Cardiovascular

Hypervolemia: hypertension, tachycardia, increased central venous pressure, jugular venous distention, extra heart sound (S3), lung sounds (crackles), postural edema, weight gain

Hypovolemia: hypotension, postural changes in blood pressure, tachycardia, flat neck veins, thirst, dry mucous membranes, weight loss, nausea, muscle cramps

Neurologic

Dialysis disequilibrium syndrome: headache, nausea, vomiting, agitation, twitching, confusion, and seizures

Dialysis dementia: disturbed speech, myclonus, dementia: confusion or personality changes

Psychosocial

Uncooperative, angry, depressed; patient expresses concerns about family problems

General

Redness, swelling, warmth, pain at shunt exit sites, fistula at puncture site or elsewhere, fever

Nursing Dx & Intervention

Fluid excess related to fluid accumulation since last treatment

- Assess weight, blood pressure, intake and output, respirations, and pulse *to determine fluid status as a basis for treatment parameters.*
- Monitor laboratory values: BUN; serum creatinine; sodium, potassium, calcium, magnesium, phosphate levels; hemoglobin and hematocrit *because nitrogenous wastes and electrolytes accumulate between treatments; anemia is a continuing problem with CRF and blood losses.*

Fluid-volume deficit related to too rapid fluid removal during treatment and potential blood loss

- Monitor intake and output, weight, blood pressure, pulse, and respiration *to recognize shifts in fluid balance.*
- Monitor blood clotting time *to monitor effect of anticoagulant therapy.*
- Minimize blood loss by careful blood sampling, return of all blood to patient, and pressure applied to fistula puncture sites at the end of treatment *to prevent worsening of anemia of CRF.*
- Avoid weight loss greater than 3 to 4 kg during treatment *to prevent hypovolemia.*

Risk for infection related to invasive procedure and blood transfusion requirements

- Follow universal precautions for exposure to blood and body fluids *to protect patient and nurse.*
- Use sterile technique to start and stop procedure and for shunt or fistula care *to protect patient from potential sources of infection during the procedure;* inspect shunt exit sites and fistula needle puncture sites for signs of infection *to detect infection promptly.*
- Monitor temperature and WBC; *small elevations may reflect significant infections.*

Altered thought processes related to dialysis disequilibrium syndrome or to dialysis dementia

- Assess during and toward the end of treatment for headache, nausea, vomiting, or agitation, *which are associated with too rapid removal of substances during dialysis.*
- Monitor speech during dialysis; observe for myoclonus or change in behavior *because these signs of dialysis dementia first appear during dialysis.*

Body image disturbance related to chronic renal failure requiring dependence on a machine

- Observe patient's response to chronic illness, altered renal function, other body system alterations, and the possibility of transplantation *because people vary greatly in their response to such life changes.*

- Recognize patient's response to having to depend on a machine *because the patient may feel helpless or hopeless, deny reality, personalize the machine, or accept it as necessary.*
- Support the patient's strengths: self-confidence, determination, and motivation to live, *since dialysis patients are not disabled in all aspects of life.*
- Be aware of changes in social involvement, and help patient develop or continue interests beyond dialysis *because the patient may participate in fewer social or recreational activities, experience life-style changes, or withdraw.*
- Be alert to excessive concerns with losses, to depression, to self-neglect, to noncompliance with medical regimen, and to the possibility of suicide; try to keep lines of communication open; encourage questions *because suicide is possible and the patient has access to several methods.*
- Be aware of the effect of the loss of libido, of impotence, and of decreased orgasm in the marital and sexual life of the patient *to refer patients as appropriate.*
- Try to help the patient develop realistic expectation of dialysis, *since hemodialysis does not reverse all the signs and symptoms of CRF.*

Altered family processes related to need for dialysis

- Recognize the impact CRF with hemodialysis has on the family, *since disruption, expense, and considerable alteration in time commitments may occur.*
- Help patient and family recognize the demands of illness on the patient's and the family's needs for emotional support.
- Recognize the spouse's fears.
- Support the family's cooperation in the patient's care, and discuss with them ways to reduce domestic tension and unhappiness; recognize the patient's inability to continue his or her family role, and help the patient toward acceptance through discussion of alternatives; in home hemodialysis treatment, recognize the stresses on the family, and support them in learning about dialysis and in carrying out treatments in the home; *patient outcomes affect the family's ability to cope and vice versa.*

Knowledge deficit related to hemodialysis and follow-up care

- See box below.

Patient Education/Home Care Planning

1. Explain function of normal and artificial kidney.
2. Explain principles of hemodialysis.
3. Explain aseptic technique for needle insertions or shunt care. Explain care of access sites.
4. Help the patient practice self-observation skills (temperature, pulse, respirations, blood pressure, intake and output, and weight) and record keeping.

5. Explain components of the system with preparation, operation, cleaning, and storage (repair and maintenance if home hemodialysis).
6. Explain initiating dialysis, monitoring during dialysis, and discontinuing dialysis.
7. Explain emergencies related to the machine and to the patient's medical condition.
8. Explain care while off the machine: diet, fluid restrictions, medical complications, care of blood access route, medications, and prevention of infection.
9. Explain medical supervision, including help available from medical center, and schedule of return visits, and assistance from the local physician.
10. Review education plan for chronic renal failure (see p. 940).

Evaluation

Weight gain between treatments is in desirable range Patient does not gain more than 0.5-1.0 kg/day.

Treatments are done safely without hypotension Patient does not have hypotension, nausea, or muscle cramps.

No infection occurs Patient does not have signs or symptoms of infection.

Thought processes are normal Patient does not develop the signs and symptoms associated with dialysis disequilibrium syndrome or dialysis dementia.

Changes in body image are accepted Patient and family adapt to the changes associated with CRF and hemodialysis.

Patient and family have adjusted to life on hemodialysis Patient and family have returned to work and social activities as much as possible. Family continues to use support of the health care team.

Patient and family understand chronic renal failure and hemodialysis Patient and family can discuss alterations and describe plans for adjusting to them.

PERITONEAL DIALYSIS

Description and Rationale

Peritoneal dialysis (PD) involves the introduction of dialysate fluid into the abdominal cavity, where the peritoneum acts as a semipermeable membrane between the dialysate and the blood in the abdominal vessels. A machine may be used, or the fluid may be instilled and drained manually from the peritoneal cavity.

Components of peritoneal dialysis solutions include varying amounts of glucose and electrolytes. Dextrose levels vary: 1.5% (15 g/L), 2.5% (25 g/L), and 4.25% (42.5 g/L). Electrolyte concentrations vary also: sodium—131-141 mEq/L, magnesium—0.5-1.0 mEq/l, chloride—94-102 mEq/L. Calcium is usually 3.5 mEq/L while potassium levels are 0. Any potassium needed in the dialysate must be added at the time of use.

Additions may include insulin and heparin, 500 to 1000 U/L.

Continuous ambulatory peritoneal dialysis (CAPD) is an alternative to intermittent peritoneal dialysis for chronic renal failure. A permanent peritoneal dialysis catheter is inserted into the abdomen; a Luer-Lok titanium connector joins the transfer set to the bag of fluid (Figures 11-12 and 11-13).

CAPD usually involves four exchanges of 1 to 2 L each in 24 hours and dwell times of 4 to 8 hours. Dialysate in plastic bags is used. When the solution is infused, the plastic bag is folded up and concealed under the person's clothes. When the fluid is drained, that bag is discarded and a new bag is attached, and its fluid is instilled for the next cycle. CAPD is self-administered and machine free.

Continuous cycling peritoneal dialysis involves connecting the peritoneal catheter to an automated peritoneal dialysis machine that performs three to seven cycles during the night while the patient sleeps. During the day one cycle of fluid is left in the abdomen. The person is free of dialysis activities during the day, and connections are less frequent than in CAPD.

Indications

Less rapid treatment needed
Unavailability of equipment and staff for hemodialysis
Severe cardiovascular disease
Inadequate access to vascular system
Shock after cardiovascular surgery
Refusal of blood transfusion
Internal hemorrhage or risk of bleeding

Contraindications and Cautions

Peritonitis
Abdominal adhesions
Recent abdominal surgery

Complications

Leakage and extravasation of dialysate
Drainage problems
Hyperglycemia, hypoproteinemia
Weight gain
Catheter exit site or tunnel infection
Peritonitis: bacterial or nonbacterial
Bowel adhesions
Respiratory embarrassment

•••••• Multidisciplinary Plan

Surgery

The peritoneal catheter is inserted into the peritoneal cavity, generally under local anesthetic in the operating room; if the catheter is permanent, it has an internal Dacron cuff that lies between the peritoneum and the abdominal muscles; it has an external cuff that is 1 to 1.5 cm below the skin at the other end of a 3 to 4 cm subcutaneous tunnel

Medications

Anticoagulants
Heparin may be added to dialysate to prevent fibrin formation and obstruction to the fluid flow

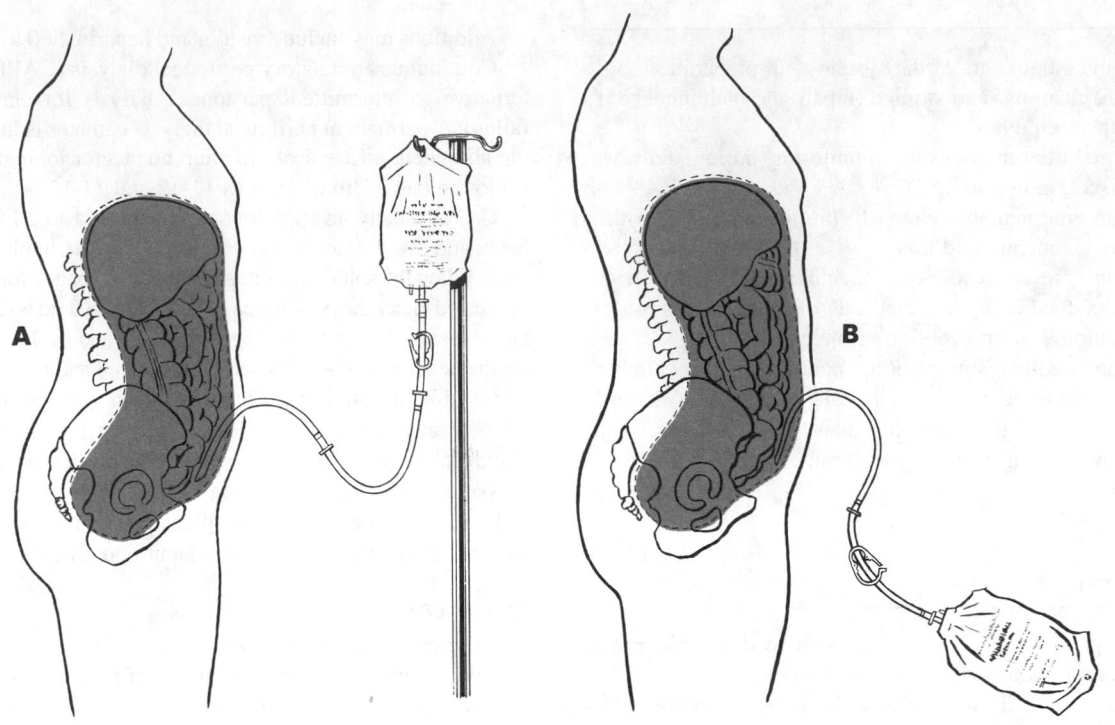

Figure 11-12 Peritoneal dialysis. **A,** Inflow. **B,** Outflow (drains to gravity).

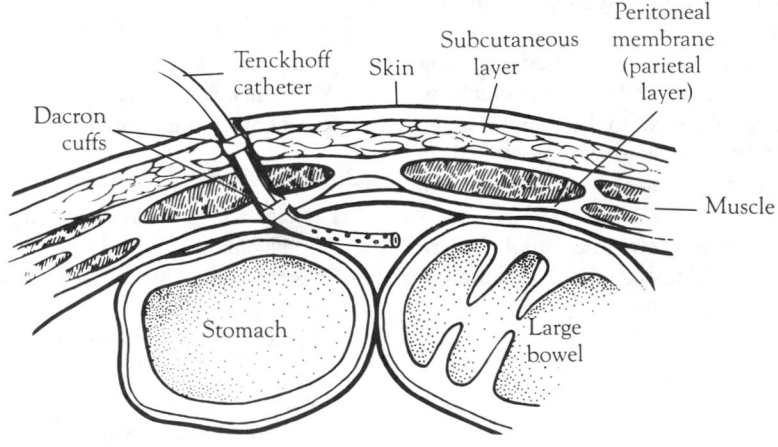

Figure 11-13 Peritoneal catheter. (From Lewis.[11])

Antimicrobials

Used when bacterial peritonitis is diagnosed and often given by both systemic and intraperitoneal routes

Vitamins (water-soluble) needed to replace those lost in dialysate

General Management

Medical management of the continuing uremic problems is discussed in the section on chronic renal failure (p. 935); the use of peritoneal dialysis causes an increased loss of blood proteins and amino acids with the fluid in the outflow; a more generous protein intake is indicated to replace these losses (suggested intake: 1.2 to 5 g/kg/day, 50% of high biologic value); restrictions continue in sodium (1500 to 2000 mg/day) and potassium (2500 to 3500 mg/day); caloric intake may be partly supplied by the glucose in the peritoneal dialysis fluid; patients need 35 kcal/kg ideal body weight/day; fluid restriction ranges from 0.5 to 1 L/day

Procedural Guidelines

Before Peritoneal Dialysis

Have patient empty bladder to avoid puncture during insertion of catheter

Measure and record as baseline data: weight, temperature, pulse, respirations, blood pressure (both lying and standing), abdominal girth

Review blood chemistry values (blood urea nitrogen; serum creatinine, sodium, potassium, and pH; and hematocrit); identify HBV and HIV status of patient, if known

Use sterile technique as temporary peritoneal catheter is placed in abdominal cavity; permanent catheters are inserted in the operating room; masks should be worn by patient, nurse, and physician; use sterile technique during subsequent connections of dialysis fluid to peritoneal catheter and for changing catheter dressings; observe for infection in catheter insertion site in temporary catheters and catheter tunnel site in permanent ones

After catheter insertion observe for perforation of bowel (dialysate outflow stained with feces or blood) or bladder (urine pink or blood tinged)

Dry warm (37° C) bottle of fluid before hanging it, or use plastic bags of solution warmed in a folded heating pad set on a low setting

Add medications to dialysate as ordered; flush tubing to remove air; connect to catheter; anchor connections and tubing securely; avoid having kinks in tubing

During Peritoneal Dialysis

Measure and record intake, output, weight, temperature, pulse, respirations, and blood pressure regularly; keep accurate records of dialysis cycles (inflow, dwell, and outflow times); record strength of solutions used, additions made, and fluid balance (amounts retained or lost)

Observe for peritonitis; collect samples of dialysate for culture and sensitivity tests if it is turbid, bloody, or has an odor, as well as when it is routinely ordered (see box below)

Observe for respiratory embarrassment (manifested by dyspnea and rales), resulting from the patient's abdomen being too full of fluid or leakage of dialysate into thoracic cavity through a defect in the diaphragm

---

CAUSES OF PERITONITIS

Peritonitis may be caused by gram-positive organisms (*Staphylococcus epidermis, Staphylococcus aureus*), enterococci, gram-negative organisms (*Escherichia coli, Pseudomonas*), anaerobes (*Bacteroides, Clostridium*), and fungi (*Candida albicans, Aspergillus fumigatus, Torulopsis glabrata*).

Usual Timing of an Hourly Cycle

Inflow time—10 minutes
Dwell time—10 to 30 minutes
Outflow time—20 to 30 minutes

Cycle-Related Problems

Inflow problems—obstructed catheter (clots, fibrin, omentum, or catheter malposition); leakage of fluid around catheter insertion site

Dwell time problems—prolonged time may cause water depletion or hyperglycemia

Outflow problems—kinks in tubing or catheter, catheter occluded by loops of bowel or by constipation

After Peritoneal Dialysis

Determine fluid balance; measure weight, temperature, pulse, respirations, blood pressure, and abdominal girth

Review postdialysis blood chemistries: blood urea nitrogen; and serum creatinine, sodium, and potassium

Care Between Peritoneal Dialysis Treatments

Encourage adequate protein intake (1.2 to 5 g/kg/day)

Restrict intake of sodium (1500 to 2000 mg/day) and potassium (2500-3500 mg/day)

Caloric intake at 35 kcal/kg ideal body weight should include the calories from the glucose in the dialysate solution

Fluid restrictions usually range from 0.5 to 1 L/day

Avoid constipation; consider use of stool softeners and laxatives as needed

Routine cleaning and dressing and avoidance of trauma at the exit site are essential to prevent infection

Manage continuing uremic problems (see "Chronic Renal Failure," p. 935)

NURSING CARE

Nursing Assessment

Cardiovascular

Hypervolemia: Hypertension, tachycardia, increased central venous pressure, jugular venous distention, extra heart sound (S3), lung sounds (crackles), postural edema, weight gain

Hypovolemia: Hypotension, postural changes in blood pressure, tachycardia, flat neck veins, thirst, dry mucous membranes, weight loss, nausea, muscle cramps

Abdominal

Rigidity, tenderness, cloudy dialysate drainage, decreased or no bowel sounds; redness, tenderness, swelling around catheter site

Neurologic

Headache, lethargy, confusion, coma

Respiratory

Tachypnea, dyspnea, rales

General

Fever, malaise

Psychosocial

Acceptance or rejection of situation by patient; change in family relationships; concerns about long-term impact of illness

Nursing Dx & Intervention

Fluid-volume excess related to fluid accumulation since last treatment

- Monitor weight and blood pressure.
- Monitor laboratory values: BUN, serum creatinine, sodium, potassium, and pH; hematocrit *to determine fluid status* as a *basis for treatment parameters;* nitrogenous wastes and electrolytes accumulate between treatments; anemia is a continuing problem of uremia.

Fluid-volume deficit related to too rapid removal of body fluid during treatment

- Monitor intake and output, weight, blood pressure, pulse, and respirations; note excess weight loss: markedly negative fluid balance as a result of dial-ysis *to recognize shifts in fluid balance and to pre-vent hypovolemia.*

Risk for infection (peritonitis) related to invasive procedure

- Follow universal precautions for exposure to blood and body fluids *to protect patient and nurse.*
- Use sterile technique to begin and end procedure and at access site *to protect patient from sources of infection during procedure.*
- Inspect catheter insertion site for signs of infection; monitor temperature, WBC in serum, and dialysate *to detect infection.*

Altered nutrition: less than body requirements related to protein loss through peritoneum into dialysate and decreased protein intake

- Assess serum protein and glucose regularly; monitor weight *to determine altered levels.*
- Ensure adequate protein intake (see p. 977) *to replace losses associated with peritoneal dialysis.*

Altered nutrition: high risk for more than body requirements related to caloric intake from glucose in dialysate fluid

- Limit caloric intake in diet and decrease glucose concentration in dialysate or decrease dwell time *if hyperglycemia or weight gain is a problem.*

Body image disturbance related to chronic renal failure requiring dependence on peritoneal dialysis

- Observe patient's response to chronic illness, altered renal function, other body system alterations, and the possibility of transplantation *because patients vary greatly in their responses to such life changes.*
- Recognize patient's response to dependence on peritoneal dialysis; try to keep lines of communication open; encourage questions *because the patient may feel helpless, hopeless, and deny reality; personalize the machine or accept it as necessary.*
- Support the patient's strengths: self-confidence, determination, and motivation to live: *dialysis patients are not disabled in all aspects of life.*
- Be aware of changes in social involvement; help patient to develop or to continue interests beyond dialysis *because patient may participate in fewer social or recreational activities, reject life-style changes, and withdraw.*
- Be alert to excessive concerns with losses, depression, self-neglect, noncompliance with medical regimen, and to the possibility of suicide; *suicide is possible and the patient has access to several methods.*
- Be aware of the effect that loss of libido, impotence, and decreased orgasm have on the marital and sex life of the patient, and be able *to refer the patient as appropriate.*
- Try to help the patient develop realistic expectations of dialysis, *since peritoneal dialysis does not reverse all the signs and symptoms of CRF.*

Altered family processes related to family member with CRF requiring peritoneal dialysis

- Recognize the impact of CRF with peritoneal dialysis on the family; *disruption, expense, and considerable alterations in time commitments may occur.*
- Help patient and family recognize demands of illness on family's and patient's need for emotional support; recognize family's fears. Support family's cooperation in patient's care, and help them look at ways to reduce domestic tension and unhappiness. Recognize patient's inability to continue his or her family's role, and help patient accept this through discussion of alternatives. In home peritoneal dialysis, recognize that the family is stressed, and support them in learning about dialysis in the home. Patient outcomes affect the family's ability to cope and vice versa.

Knowledge deficit related to chronic renal failure and peritoneal dialysis

- See box below.

Patient Education/Home Care Planning

1. Explain the nature of chronic renal failure.
2. Explain the medical regimen and its rationale, including diet (restricted protein, sodium, and potassium), restricted fluid intake, and medications (purpose, dosage, interval, and adverse reactions).
3. Explain the function of normal and artificial kidneys and the principles of peritoneal dialysis.
4. Explain and help patient practice aseptic technique.

5. Explain components of the system, preparation, operation, cleaning, and storage (repair and maintenance if home dialysis).
6. Explain initiating dialysis, monitoring during dialysis, and discontinuing dialysis.
7. Explain emergencies related to the machine, if used, and to the patient's medical condition.
8. Explain care while off the machine: diet, fluid restrictions, medical complications, care of peritoneal access route, medications, and prevention of infection.
9. Help patient learn self-observational skills (temperature, pulse, respirations, blood pressure, intake and output, and weight) and record keeping.
10. Explain ways to avoid infection.
11. Explain personal hygiene, rest, and exercise.
12. Explain when to call the physician.
13. Explain the plan for medical follow-up.

Evaluation

Weight gain between treatments is in desirable range Weight is maintained at or near ideal weight.

Treatment is done safely without hypotension Volume relationships and blood pressure are normal.

Peritonitis is avoided No signs or symptoms of peritonitis are present.

Protein and calorie intake meet body requirements Serum albumin and glucose levels are within normal limits; weight is stable.

Changes in body image are accepted Patient and family adapt to changes associated with CRF and peritoneal dialysis.

Patient and family have adjusted to life on peritoneal dialysis Patient and family have returned to work and social activities as much as possible. Patient and family continue to use support of health care team.

Patient and family understand CRF and peritoneal dialysis Patient and family describe chronic renal failure and medical plan of care. Patient and family describe principles of peritoneal dialysis, plan of care, and correct use of peritoneal dialysis equipment.

 ## RENAL TRANSPLANTATION

Description and Rationale

Renal transplantation (RT) is the surgical insertion of a human kidney from a living or cadaveric source into a patient with end-stage renal disease, thus replacing the lost renal function. A donor may be sought when the patient's serum creatinine is around 5 mg/dl, serum blood urea nitrogen is greater than 70 mg/dl, and creatinine clearance is 15 ml/minute. When successful, a transplant restores the recipient to a relatively healthy, useful life. If a transplant is unsuccessful, the patient can return to dialysis or have a second transplant.

The number of kidney transplants has increased each year since 1978. In 1991 there were 10,052 kidney transplants performed (7104 from cadaveric donors and 2122 from living, related donors) covered by Medicare. Patient survival and graft function have improved since 1983 when cyclosporine was introduced. By the end of 1991 there were 50,468 patients with end-stage renal disease who had functioning transplanted kidneys.[16]

The donated kidney is placed in the retroperitoneal area in the iliac fossa on the contralateral side. Thus a donated left kidney is placed in the recipient's right iliac fossa (Figure 11-14). The donor's artery is anastomosed end to end or end-to-side to the recipient's hypogastric artery.

The donor's vein is anastomosed to the recipient's internal iliac vein. The donor's ureter is implanted in the recipient's bladder.

The kidney from a living related donor is flushed with a cold solution and then placed in the recipient. A cadaveric kidney may be preserved by flushing followed by cold storage or by constant perfusion with a special solution.

Transplantation is usually the treatment of choice in children. Aging patients may have problems with transplantation because of atherosclerosis or other serious systemic disorders. Patients with diabetes are increasingly considered for transplantation, but the problems with the continuing diabetic condition increase complications such as infection. The use of corticosteroids exacerbates problems in glucose level control. Combined pancreas and kidney transplants are being used for the type I or insulin-dependent diabetic patient.

Indications

End-stage renal disease
Loss of a solitary kidney through trauma
Inability to adjust to dialysis

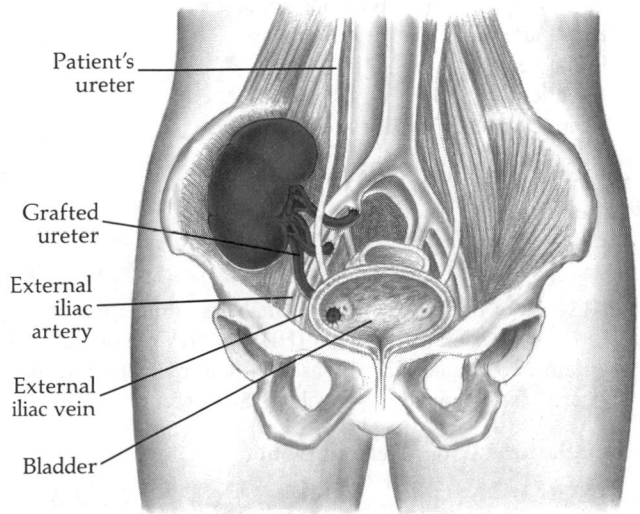

Figure 11-14 Renal transplant.

Contraindications and Cautions

Age younger than 1 years or older than 65 years
Malignancy
Acute uncontrollable infection
Hepatic disease
Presence of antikidney antibodies
Severe psychosis
Tuberculosis or peptic ulcer disease
Chronic respiratory insufficiency
Severe atherosclerosis
Severe myocardial dysfunction

Preprocedural Nursing Care

Assess preoperative status
Explain to the patient and family what to expect during the
   operative and early postoperative periods; refer to p. 982

Postprocedural Nursing Care

Assess vital signs and urine output q1h gradually lengthening interval; urine begins to flow in 2 to 10 minutes after
   revascularization at a rate of 5 to 10 ml/min; careful fluid
   replacement prevents overhydration or underhydration
Anchor catheters; do not clamp them, but connect them to a
   closed drainage system; measure urethral and ureteral volumes and record; urine may be bloody at first; cessation of
   urine flow may be caused by a clot; irrigation of the urethral catheter may be needed to dislodge it; if the ureteral
   catheter needs irrigating, extreme care is required to avoid
   damage to the ureteral anastomosis
Try to maintain patency of the blood access device in case
   dialysis is needed in the postoperative period

Complications

Acute tubular necrosis
Spontaneous rupture of graft
Organ rejection
Ureteral fistula or obstruction
Perirenal hematoma, lymphocele, or abscess
Renal artery stenosis or thrombosis
Renal vein thrombosis
Infection
Reappearance of primary renal disease

Criteria for Kidney Transplant

Criteria for Recipient

End-stage renal disease
Age 1 to 65 or 70
Absence of uncorrectable abnormalities of other major body
   systems, such as infection (HBV or HIV), urologic problems, severe cardiac disease, chronic pulmonary disease,
   preexisting cancer, or psychiatric disorder

Criteria for Living, Related Donor

Age 18 to 55
Excellent physical and mental health
Immunologic compatibility to recipient

Criteria for Cadaveric Donor

Age infant to 70 years
Normal renal function tests
Negative HBV and HIV
Immunologic compatibility to recipient
No systemic disease such as infection, cancer, advanced car-
   diovascular disease including hypertension, renal-urologic
   disorders, or diabetes
No hypoxia or hypotension

•••••• Multidisciplinary Plan

Surgery

The donor kidney is transplanted as described on p. 979; the
   patient is prepared with adequate dialysis for surgery (see
   "Hemodialysis," p. 970); the uremic problems are controlled before surgery

Medications

Antiemetics
   Prochlorperazine (Compazine), po, 5-10 mg tid or qid
   Trimethobenzamide (Tigan, Ticon), po, 250 mg tid or qid;
      IM, 200 mg tid or qid
Narcotic analgesics
   Meperidine (Demerol, Pethadol), po, subcutaneously, IM,
      IV, 50-150 mg q3-4h
   Codeine sulfate, po, subcutaneously, IM, 15-60 mg qid
   Morphine sulfate, po, subcutaneously, IM, IV, 5-15 mg
      q4h prn
Immunosuppressive agents
   Azathioprine (Imuran), po, 100-150 mg/d; 1.7-2.5
      mg/kg/d determined by white blood cell level
   Antilymphocyte globulin, IM, IV, 5-10 mg/kg depending
      on potency of preparation, qd for 5-21 d after surgery
      with intermittent doses for 4 mo
   Cyclophosphamide (Cytoxan, Neosar), po, 2 mg/kg/d as
      substitute for azathioprine in patients with liver dys-
      function
   Cyclosporine (Cyclosporin A, Sandimmune), po, IV, 8-17
      mg/kg/d
   Muromonab-CD3 (OKT3), IV bolus, 5 mg/kg/d for
      10-14 d
Corticosteroids (used as immunosuppressive agents)
   Prednisone (Deltasone, Orasone), po, 20-150 mg/d, 0.3-
      2.5 mg/kg decreasing to 10-15 mg/d by 4 mo; increase
      to 100-300 mg/d to treat rejection
Antirejection drugs
   Methylprednisolone (Solu-Medrol, A-MethaPred), IV,
      250-1000 mg/d or on alternate days for maximum dose
      of 3-5 g
   Muronab-CD3 (Orthoclone, OKT3), IV for 5-14 d, 5-
      mg/d by rapid injection
   FK 506 (Tacrolimus) [Investigational] po, 0.15 mg/kg qd
      or bid; IV, 0.075 mg/kg bid
Antacids (peptic ulcer disease may be a problem)
H_2 Blockers

Cimetidine (Tagamet) po, 300 mg qid; IV, 300 mg q6h, maximum daily dose 2.4 g

Ranitidine (Zantac) po, 150 mg bid; IM, slow IV, 50 mg q6-8h; maximum daily dose 400 mg

Insulin preparations (for hyperglycemia resulting from corticosteroid therapy): highly individualized according to blood and urine glucose determinations

Other drugs (antiinfectives or antihypertensives) as needed

Bactrim 1 single-strength tab qd (prophylaxis against pneumocystis pneumonia)

Acyclovir 200 mg to 800 mg tid (prophylaxis against CMV and herpes simplex virus)

Ganciclovir or Cytogam: prophylaxis for CMV

General Management

Dialysis may be needed

Fluid intake should balance output: about 400 to 600 ml (about the amount of insensible losses) plus amount equal to 24-hour urine volume; patient should avoid dehydration and volume excess

Nutritional modifications to achieve or maintain adequate nutritional status and to reduce work of diseased kidney

No dietary restrictions after gastrointestinal function returns; caloric intake may need to be restricted if appetite is increased by corticosteroids; if renal function is decreased or hypertension continues

Patient may need to restrict protein, sodium, and potassium and increase calories supplied by fats and carbohydrates

Routine cultures of likely places for infection (urinary tract, wound, throat, and blood) may be done, since immunosuppressive agents mask signs and symptoms of infection; all immunosuppressive agents currently in use affect phagocytosis, cellular immunity, or humoral immunity; liver function is monitored because azathioprine can cause cholestatic hepatitis; cyclosporine may damage the kidney and liver; muromonab-CD3 causes a flulike symptom complex (Table 11-1)

Signs and symptoms of rejection are monitored; if rejection occurs and is not reversed, graft is removed and patient is returned to dialysis

Most frequent complications are related to technical problems, effects of preexisting uremia, graft rejection, and side effects of immunosuppression

NURSING CARE

Nursing Assessment

Cardiovascular

Altered pulse, respirations, blood pressure, central venous pressure, weight, intake and output associated with excess or inadequate fluid replacement

TABLE 11-1 Selected Side Effects of Major Immunosuppresive Drugs

Drug	Side Effect
Cyclosporine (Sandimmune)	Renal and hepatic toxicity, hypertension, hirsutism, gingival hyperplasia, nausea, vomiting, diarrhea
Azathioprine (Imuran)	Nausea, vomiting, leukopenia, anemia, thrombocytopenia, hepatic toxicity
Tacrolimus (FK 506)	Renal and hepatic toxicity, hypertension, nausea, vomiting, diarrhea, diabetes
Prednisone	Depression, euphoria, hypertension, decreased wound healing, petechiae, ecchymoses, hirsutism, acne, adrenal suppression, muscle wasting, osteoporosis, redistribution of fat (moon face, buffalo hump)
Muromonab-CD3 (Orthoclone OKT 3)	Fever, chills, nausea, vomiting, diarrhea, chest tightness, dyspnea, pulmonary edema

 EMERGENCY ALERT

ORGAN REJECTION-RENAL

Organ rejection begins when the organ recipient's system begins to reject the transplanted organ.

Assessment

- Determine decreased urine output (cloudy/foul smelling urine), fever, anxiety, apathy, weight gain, proteinuria, hypertension.
- Perform physical assessment to determine tenderness and/or redness over graft area.
- Evaluate pain status.
- Monitor for altered vital signs.
- Assess for compliance and side effects of medications.

Interventions

- Maintain airway, breathing, and circulation.
- During all client encounters use adequate precautions to minimize risk of infection; patient is immunosuppressed.
- Determine nature of symptoms and manage accordingly.
- Carefully monitor intake and outflow; collect excreted urine.
- Obtain IV access; monitor fluids.
- Obtain laboratory specimens.
- Provide support and reassure patient and family.

Renal

Signs of rejection: decreased urine output, proteinuria, tenderness over graft area, fever, weight gain, hypertension, anxiety, apathy, lethargy (see Emergency Alert box)

Urinary Tract

Cloudy, foul-smelling urine

General

Fever, pain, changes in incision (red, swollen, draining, or tender)

Psychosocial

Patient expresses guilt, concern for donor; family expresses concern about what to expect of patient after surgery

Nursing Dx & Intervention

Risk for fluid-volume deficit or excess related to postoperative diuresis, altered renal perfusion (acute tubular necrosis, rejection)

- Monitor blood pressure, pulse, respirations, breath sounds, central venous pressure, cardiac output, intake and output, and weight *to determine fluid status;* patient is sensitive to changes in fluid volume.
- Monitor laboratory values: BUN, serum creatinine, uric acid, sodium, potassium, calcium, magnesium, and phosphate; hematocrit and hemoglobin; urine levels of creatinine, urea, uric acid, sodium, potassium, blood, and protein *to assess functioning of new kidney.*
- Balance fluid intake with output *to avoid hypervolemia or hypovolemia.*
- Monitor dialysis access device; take no blood pressure readings or venipunctures in that arm *because dialysis may be needed in the postoperative period.*

Pain related to surgical incision, bladder spasms

- Assess need for analgesic drugs; administer as needed; monitor response to *to control surgical pain.*
- When catheter is removed encourage patient to void frequently *to avoid overdistention of the bladder;* the unused bladder may spasm as it fills with urine.

Risk for infection related to surgery, catheter in urinary tract, and immunosuppression

- Use sterile technique for wound and catheter care *to protect patient who has increased susceptibility to infection because of antirejection drugs.*
- Inspect incision *to detect changes early;* little drainage is expected.
- Monitor temperature and assess laboratory values: WBC, urine for bacteria, pyuria, cloudy appearance, and culture results; *because signs and symptoms of infection may be masked by immunosuppression, even small increases are important.*
- Monitor visitors *to avoid exposure to persons with infections.*
- Encourage deep breathing, coughing, early ambulation *to prevent respiratory complications.*

Body image disturbance related to need to accept a new body part

- Be aware that patient may feel both guilty and concerned about the donor; *mixed feelings are not unexpected.*

- Explain side effects of immunosuppressive drugs that may change appearance. *Obvious changes may include alopecia, hirsutism, and redistribution of body fat* (Table 11-1).

Altered family processes related to change in patient's condition

- Keep lines of communication open; assist in patient-family communication. Family is used to a chronically ill person. *Return to health may require change in family patterns.* The recipient may be perceived as too independent or not independent enough.
- Recognize the feelings of the living, related donor; before the transplant the donor may have felt like a hero or heroine; after surgery all the attention may focus on the recipient.
- Inform family of changes possible when taking immunosuppressive drugs, especially prednisone; *emotional as well as physical changes may occur in patients taking prednisone.*
- Discuss the possible need for contraception, if appropriate; *potency may return in males; ovulation, menses, and libido may return in females.*
- If patient and family do not already know others who have experienced kidney transplant, introduce them to such a patient and family. *Family-to-family assistance is often useful.*
- Refer family to professional colleagues (social workers or psychologists) when other professionals can better meet family's needs (financial concerns, occupational problems, and the need for family counseling beyond the nurse's expertise). Professional colleagues can often be helpful in meeting family needs.

Knowledge deficit related to renal transplantation and follow-up care

- See box below.

Patient Education/Home Care Planning

1. Preparation for discharge includes teaching the following:
   a. Self-observational skills (temperature, pulse, respiration, weight, intake and output, urine collection, and record keeping)
   b. Medications: name, dosage, strength, schedule, purpose, and side effects
   c. Diet: restriction, if any (patient should avoid becoming overweight)
   d. Fluids: restriction, if any
   e. Signs and symptoms of rejection and infection
   f. Important laboratory values (serum creatinine, blood urea nitrogen level, white blood cell count, calcium, and phosphate); with an arteriovenous fistula, do not have blood pressure taken or blood drawn in that arm

2. Long-term follow-up care includes teaching the following:
   a. Medical appointment schedule for routine follow-up; plans for telephone communication between appointments
   b. Personal hygiene, prevention of infection, care of minor trauma, contraceptive device, and need for regular dental and eye examinations
   c. Body changes resulting from uremia and long-term antirejection therapy, including increased possibility of malignancies
   d. Physical activity levels (daily exercise, avoidance of contact sports, and avoidance of seat belts across the hips) and return to work and other activities
   e. Resources for rehabilitation (including vocational)

Evaluation

Fluid balance is within normal limits No signs or symptoms of fluid overload or dehydration are present. Renal function tests are within normal limits.

Patient is free of pain Patient has no complaints of pain.

Patient is free of infection Patient shows no signs or symptoms of infection in incision, urine, or elsewhere.

Body image changes are accepted Patient and family adapt to changes associated with transplantation and immunosuppression.

Patient and family adjust to life after transplant Patient and family return to work and social activities.

Patient and family understand the need for continuing care Patient and family demonstrate knowledge of home care and follow-up care.

■ OTHER KIDNEY SURGERY

Kidney surgery includes both open and closed (percutaneous) procedures. Open surgery of the kidney includes operations to obtain biopsy specimens, to remove all or part of a kidney, to repair traumatic injuries, or to implant a donated organ (Figures 11-15 and 11-16). Percutaneous procedures include removing renal calculi and establishing urinary drainage.

Open renal biopsy is used to obtain a specimen if the percutaneous approach is unsuccessful or if a person has a single kidney or severe hypertension or coagulopathy.

Nephrectomy is the surgical removal of the whole kidney or a part of the kidney. A partial nephrectomy usually involves the upper or lower poles of the kidney because they have well-defined blood supplies. In a simple nephrectomy the kidney (but not the adrenal gland, surrounding fat, or fascia) is removed. A radical nephrectomy refers to the removal of the kidney, adrenal gland, perirenal fat, upper ureter, and Gerota's fascia.

Nephrolithotomy is removal of a calculus through an opening in the renal parenchyma.

Pyelolithotomy is removal of a calculus through an opening in the renal pelvis.

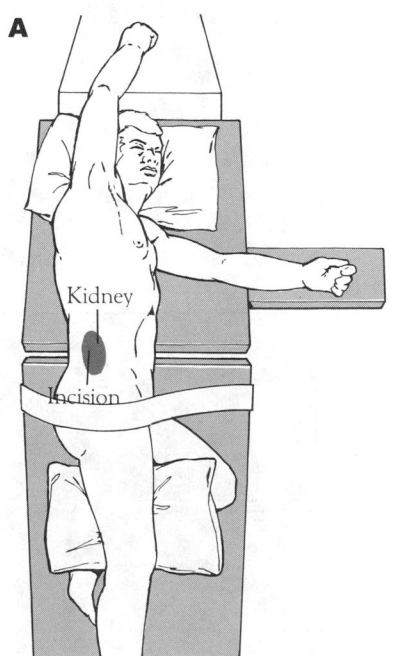 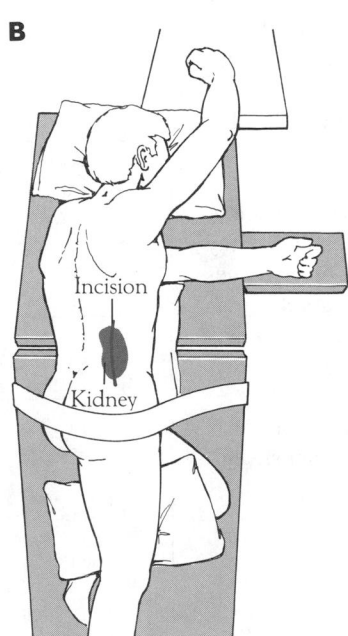 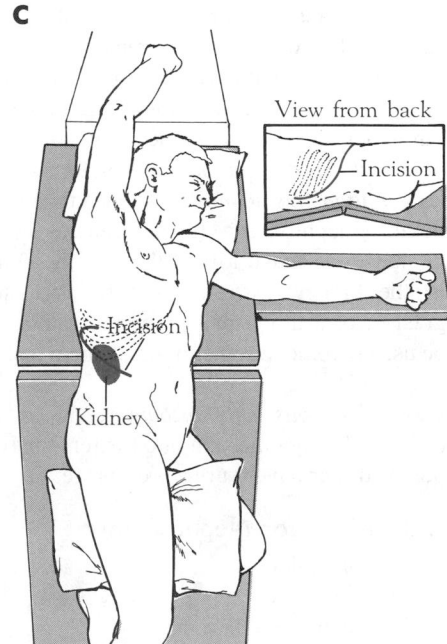

Figure 11-15 Types of incisions for kidney surgery. **A,** Flank approach. **B,** Lumbar approach. **C,** Thoracoabdominal approach. (From Brundage.[4])

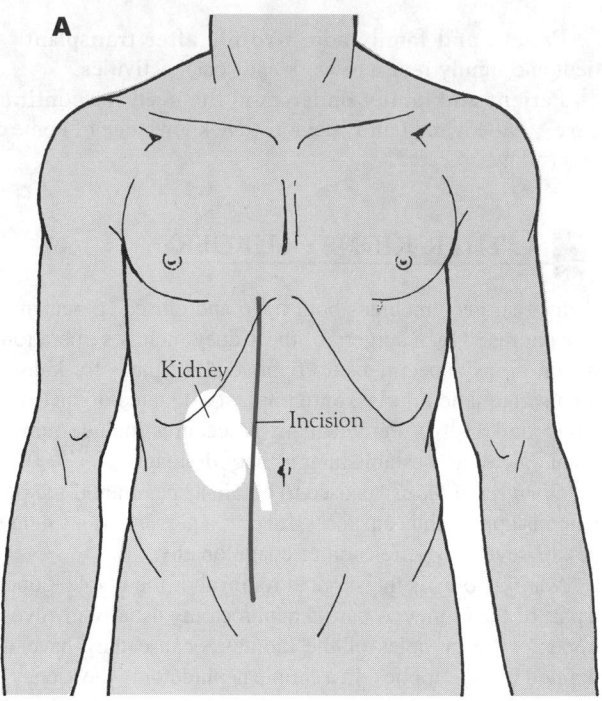 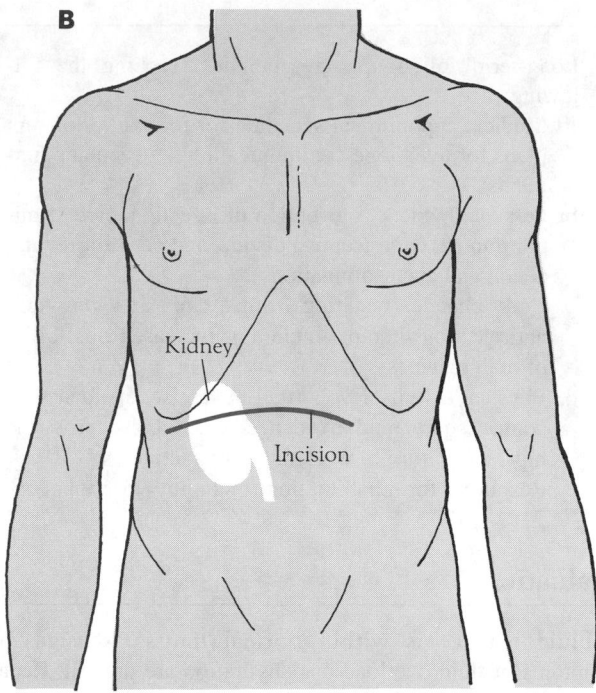

Figure 11-16 Abdominal approaches to kidney surgery, **A,** Vertical incision. **B,** Horizontal incision. (From Brundage.[4])

Pyeloplasty is the procedure used to repair the renal pelvis (after hydronephrosis, for example).

Nephrostomy (open) is the creation of an opening into the kidney to provide temporary or permanent drainage when a retrograde catheter is not possible. An incision is made into the renal pelvis and out through the renal parenchyma to place a catheter that will drain the renal pelvis. The catheter is anchored in the renal pelvis; the pelvis is sutured; the distal end of the catheter extends through the kidney and exits the skin through a stab incision in the flank.

Renal transplantation See p. 979.

Percutaneous nephrolithotomy refers to the use of a rigid or flexible nephroscope (under general anesthesia and x-ray guidance) to make a tract through the skin and other tissues to the kidney. Instruments such as a stone basket, stone grasper, or a lithotripter probe (percutaneous lithotripsy) may be used to remove stones or break them up before removal (Figure 11-17).

Percutaneous nephrostomy refers to the insertion of a catheter through the skin into the renal pelvis to establish temporary or permanent urinary drainage.

Indications for Nephrectomy

Staghorn calculus
Hemorrhage
Hydronephrosis
Renovascular hypertension
Neoplasms
Renal donation
Trauma
Vascular disease

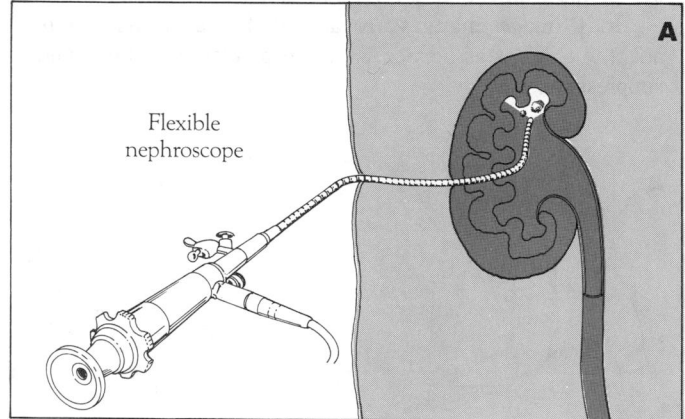

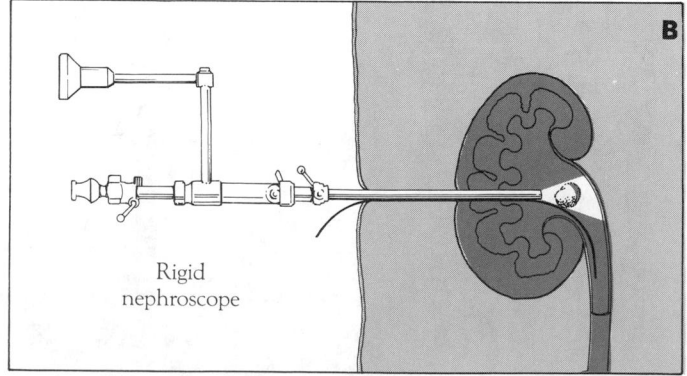

Figure 11-17 A, Flexible nephroscope. **B,** Rigid nephroscope. (From Brundage.[4])

Contraindications and Cautions

Nephrectomy
    Bilateral disease
    Single kidney
Percutaneous renal procedures
    Septicemia
    Urinary tract obstruction
    Caution is necessary before removing a diseased kidney (even if the other one is normal) if the disorder is likely to affect the remaining kidney in the future (urolithiasis, renal vascular disease, infection, inflammatory processes).

Complications

Nephrectomy
    Hemorrhage
    Infection
    Pneumothorax
Percutaneous renal procedures
    Hemorrhage
    Infection
    Urinary extravasation
    Perirenal hematoma

Types of Incisions Used

Flank
Lumbar
Thoracoabdominal
Abdominal
The type of incision used depends on the site of the defect
The approach may be retroperitoneal or transperitoneal

Procedural Guidelines

Prepare the patient and family for the operative procedure planned and the care that will follow it; discuss the location of the incision, tubes, stents, and drains, as well as routines for deep breathing, coughing, turning, and pain relief.

Determine functional level of each kidney; treat any urinary tract infection; bacteriuria impairs healing; leakage of infected urine into soft tissues may cause abscesses; obstruction may cause acute bacterial nephritis

Prepare the patient for surgery: bowel and skin preparation, as ordered; preoperative sedation is used

Tubes may include a stent (a catheter inserted into the ureter), nephrostomy tube, an incisional drain, and a urethral catheter; drainage may continue for several days; hematuria can be expected for 12 to 24 hours

NURSING CARE

Nursing Assessment

General

Fever, incisional pain, guarding behavior

Skin Incision

Redness; swelling; drainage of urine, blood

Urinary Tract

Urine output from each tube or catheter (amount, character); bleeding; absence of urine

Nursing Dx & Intervention

Impaired skin integrity related to surgical incision

- Assess incision site for signs of bleeding or infection *to detect complications promptly.*
- Note amount and kind of drainage from each tube; urine leakage is expected for several days after incision into the kidney.
- Keep area clean and dry *to prevent skin breakdown and to promote healing.*

Risk for fluid-volume deficit related to decreased intake by mouth; increased losses caused by diuresis and hemorrhage

- Measure intake, output, and weight every 24 hours
- Monitor vital signs, hemoglobin, and hematocrit *to identify alterations in fluid status promptly.*

Pain related to surgical incision

- Assess need for analgesic drugs; administer drug as ordered; record response *to determine patient's need for drug; determine the effectiveness of timing and dosage to identify adverse side effects.*

Altered patterns of urinary elimination related to use of tubes, catheters, or drains

- Keep drainage tubes patent, unkinked, and anchored *to maintain urine flow and avoid inadvertent displacement.*
- Monitor amounts of urine from each tube *to ensure adequate drainage, and to avoid tension on the suture lines, and to promote healing.*

Risk for infection related to a break in the skin barrier and to the presence of catheters

- Assess temperature, WBC, wound drainage, and urine for pyuria and bacteriuria *to detect any infection promptly.*

Knowledge deficit related to kidney surgery and follow-up care

- See box below.

Patient Education/Home Care Planning

1. Explain etiology of the problem requiring surgery.
2. Explain the posthospital care of incision, drains, or tubes as needed.
3. Explain techniques for preventing recurrence of renal problems.
4. Explain any need for follow-up medical care.

Evaluation

Skin integrity is unimpaired   Incision is healed.

Fluid balance is within normal limits   Fluid intake is adequate and balances output.

No pain is present   Patient has no complaint of pain.

Urinary elimination pattern is normal   All tubes, drains, and catheters are removed.

No infection is present   Patient is afebrile, with normal WBC and urinalysis.

Knowledge about the condition requiring surgery is increased   Patient and family understand the kidney problem, posthospital care, and the need for follow-up medical care.

EXTRACORPOREAL SHOCK-WAVE LITHOTRIPSY

Extracorporeal shock-wave lithotripsy (ESWL) is a noninvasive method used to treat renal calculi. Shock waves carefully directed into the body through a liquid medium surrounding the body disintegrate the calculus, and the pulverized material is flushed by the normal excretion of urine.

Fluoroscopy or ultrasonography is used to pinpoint the stone's location. Radiopaque stones are seen easily; radiolucent stones are visualized by using contrast media in the renal pelvis. The patient, under general anesthesia, is positioned in the lithotripter tub filled with treated water (degassed and deionized; Figure 11-18). After a series of 200 shock waves is delivered, fluoroscopy is used to determine the location and size of the stone fragments or gravel. The total number of shocks needed is related to the size of the stone; an average treatment is 1000 to 2000 shocks with a maximum of 2400 per treatment. If the gravel formed blocks the ureter, a percutaneous nephrostomy may be done to promote clearance of the particles.

Contraindications and Cautions

Pregnancy
Lower ureteral stones
Bladder stones
Cardiac pacemakers
Distal ureteral obstruction
Renal artery calcifications
Bleeding diathesis

Complications

Hematuria
Ureteral colic
Ureteral obstruction

Procedural Guidelines

Explain the nature of the procedure to the patient and the family

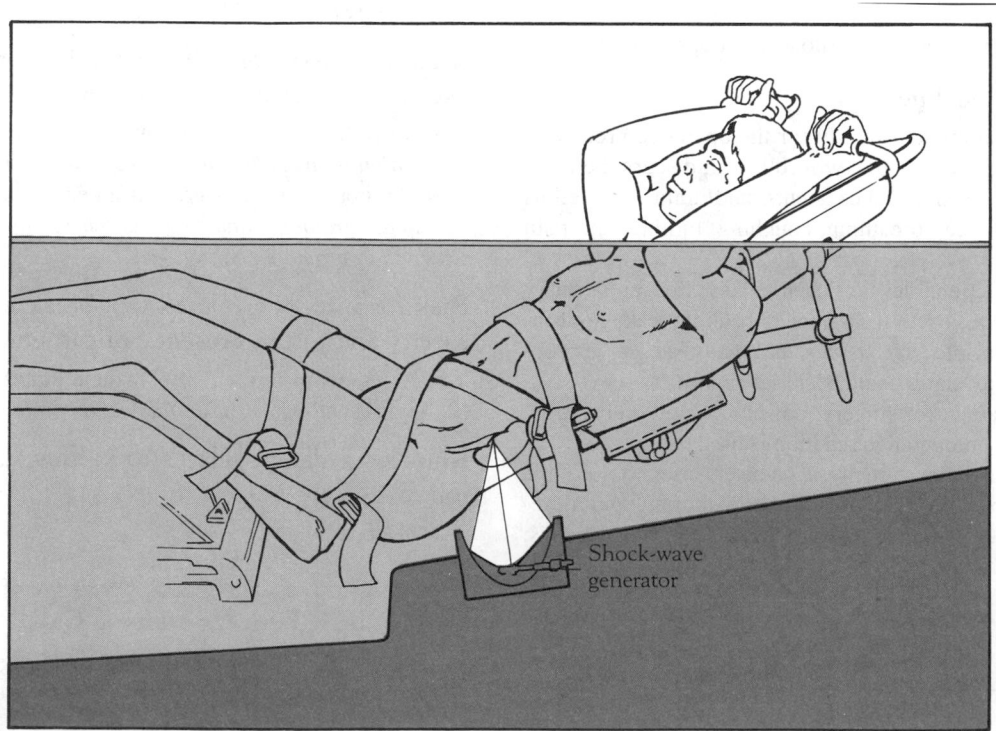

Figure 11-18 Patient positioned for shock-wave lithotripsy. Area of flank is exposed for efficient shock-wave conduction. (From Brundage.[4])

Prepare the patient for general anesthesia

Any urinary tract infection is treated, and preoperative antibiotics are given if an infected stone is to be pulverized

NURSING CARE

Nursing Assessment

Urinary Tract

Hematuria for 12 to 24 hours; passage of stone particles

General

Pain of passage of stone fragments (ureteral colic); fever, dysuria, pyuria, bacteriuria, increased WBC

Nursing Dx & Intervention

Altered pattern of urinary elimination related to passage of stone particles

- Assess intake and output and the nature of the urine *to identify urinary tract obstruction and to monitor the amount of hematuria.*
- Strain all urine *to observe the nature and size of particles being passed.*
- Ensure adequate fluid intake; *the extra fluid may be needed to help the passage of stone particles.*

Pain related to passage of stone particles

- Assess for pain; give analgesic drugs as ordered; monitor and record response; use nonpharmacologic methods, such as external application of heat, *to determine the need for analgesia, to provide relief, and to identify adverse side effects.*
- Help patient walk, if appropriate, *to help stones move by gravity.*

Risk for infection related to infected stone

- Assess temperature every 4 hours; monitor WBC and urinalysis for pyuria and bacteriuria *to identify urinary tract infection promptly.*

Knowledge deficit related to extracorporeal shock-wave lithotripsy and follow-up care

- See box below.

Patient Education/Home Care Planning

1. Explain the extracorporeal shock-wave lithotripsy procedure.
2. Explain the necessary preparation for general anesthesia.
3. Explain the postprocedure care and the possibility of hematuria for 12 to 24 hours, the passage of stone particles, the need to strain urine, and the need to drink extra fluids.
4. Explain how to prevent recurrence of the particular type of stone involved (see "Renal Calculi," p. 956).

Evaluation

Urinary pattern returns to normal Patient has no signs or symptoms of urinary tract infection or obstruction.

Pain is absent Patient is free of pain.

Infection is absent Patient is free of infection.

Knowledge about renal calculi and ESWL is increased Patient and family understand renal calculi and the need for postprocedural care and follow-up medical care.

References

1. Baldwin IC, Elderkin TD: Continuous hemofiltration: nursing perspectives in critical care, *New Horizons* 3:738-747, 1995.
2. Bennett WM et al: *Drug prescribing in renal failure: dosing guidelines for adults,* ed 2, Philadelphia, 1991, American College of Physicians.
3. Beto J: Which diet for which renal failure? Making sense of the options, *J Am Diet Assoc* 95:8, 898, 903, 1995.
4. Brundage DJ: *Renal disorders,* St Louis, 1992, Mosby.
5. Brundage DJ, Swearengen PA: Chronic renal failure: evaluation and teaching tool, *ANNA J* 21:265-270, 1994.
6. Centers for Disease Control: *Tuberculosis statistics, states and cities,* 1994, Atlanta, 1995, US Dept of Health and Human Services, Public Health Service.
7. Epstein M, Sowers JR: Diabetes mellitus and hypertension, *Hypertension* 19:403-418, 1992.
8. Hollingsworth AK: *Kidney failure: coping and feeling your best,* Atlanta, 1994, Pritchett & Hull.
9. Jacobson HR, Striker GE, Klahr S: *The principles and practice of nephrology,* ed 2, St Louis, 1995, Mosby.
10. Lancaster L: *Core curriculum for nephrology nurses: ANNA,* Pitman, New Jersey, 1995, Anthony J. Jannetti.
11. Lewis S, Collier I: *Medical-surgical nursing,* ed 2, St Louis, 1987, Mosby.
12. Lievaart A, Voerman HJ: Nursing management of continuous arteriovenous hemodialysis *Heart Lung* 20:152-160, 1991.
13. Mehta RL: Renal replacement therapy for acute renal failure: matching the method to the patient, *Semin Dial* 6:253-259, 1993.
14. Mitch WE, Klahr S, editors: *Nutrition and the kidney,* ed 2, Boston, 1993, Little, Brown.
15. Oberly ET, Compton A: Nursing interventions for rehabilitating renal patients, *ANNA J* 21:407-411, 1994.
16. Price CA: Continuous renal replacement therapy. In Burrows-Hudson S (ed): *American Nephrology Nurses' Association Standards of clinical practice for nephrology nursing,* Pitman, NJ, 1993, AJ Janetti.
17. Tanagho EA, McAninch JW: *Smith's general urology,* ed 14, Norwalk, Conn, 1995, Appleton & Lange.
18. Thelan LA, Davie JK, Urden LD, Lough ME: *Critical care nursing: diagnosis and management,* ed 2, St Louis, 1994, Mosby.
19. Strohschein BL, Caruso DM, Greene KA: Continuous venovenous hemodialysis, *Am J Crit Care* 3:92-101, 1994.
20. United States Renal Data System: *USRDS 1994 annual data report,* Bethesda, Md, 1994, National Institutes of Health, National Institute of Diabetes and Digestive and Kidney Diseases.

Genitourinary System

12

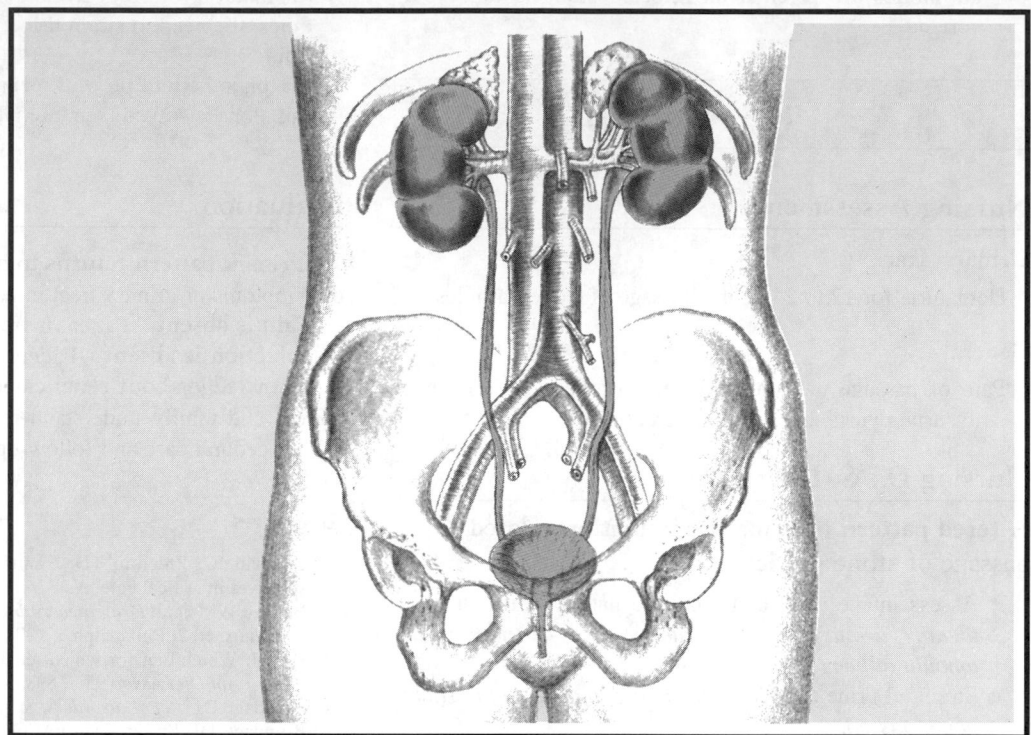

Genitourinary diseases affect the kidneys, ureters, bladder, urethra, or male genitalia. Urologic disorders may result from specific disease states such as infection, hyperplasia, or neoplasia. Other disorders, such as urinary incontinence or male sexual dysfunction, are symptoms rather than specific disease states but also cause significant health problems related to the genitourinary system. For information on the renal system, refer to Chapter 11.

• • • • • • Anatomy, Physiology, and Related Pathophysiology

Urinary Tract Structures

Kidneys The kidneys are a pair of reddish brown, symmetrically shaped organs located in the retroperitoneal space, adjacent to the vertebral column at spinal levels T12 and L1 to L3 (Figure 12-1). Because of the presence of the liver, the right kidney is lower than the left.[118] The lateral aspects of the kidneys are smooth and rounded; the medial aspects are marked by a concave surface known as the renal hilus. The renal veins, arteries, nerve plexus, and renal lymphatics are located at this hilus. The renal pelvis attaches to the kidney at the hilus before tapering into the ureters.[25,118]

The weight of the adult kidney varies from 115 to 175 g. Adult women have slightly smaller kidneys than do adult men. The kidney in the infant or young child is smaller than in the adult. However, a child's kidneys occupy a larger proportion of the child's body weight. The normal adult kidney is approximately 11 cm long, 5 to 7 cm wide, and 2 to 3.5 cm thick. The kidneys are remarkably symmetric in size and shape.[117]

A cross section of the kidneys (Figure 12-2) reveals two distinct sections: the renal pelvis and renal parenchyma. Within the renal parenchyma, a cortex and medulla are distinguished using the unaided eye. The renal medulla is characterized by pale, striated conical structures called pyramids. The bases of these pyramids are directed toward the periphery of the kidney; the apices face the renal hilus. The renal pyramids end in papillae that project into a minor calyx. The kidneys normally contain from eight to 18 renal pyramids that drain into four to 13 minor calyces. These minor calyces drain into two or three major calyces that open into the renal pelvis.[25,124]

The renal medulla is bounded by the renal cortex, which appears darker and has a granular rather than striated appearance. Cortical lobules arch over the pyramids within the medulla. Cortical columns dip between the pyramids. The renal cortex is bounded by the true renal capsule, a layer of dense connective tissue loosely adherent to the parenchyma. The kidneys are supported by the perirenal fascia and perinephric fat. The kidneys, along with the superiorly placed adrenals, are enclosed within Gerota's fascia.[25,124]

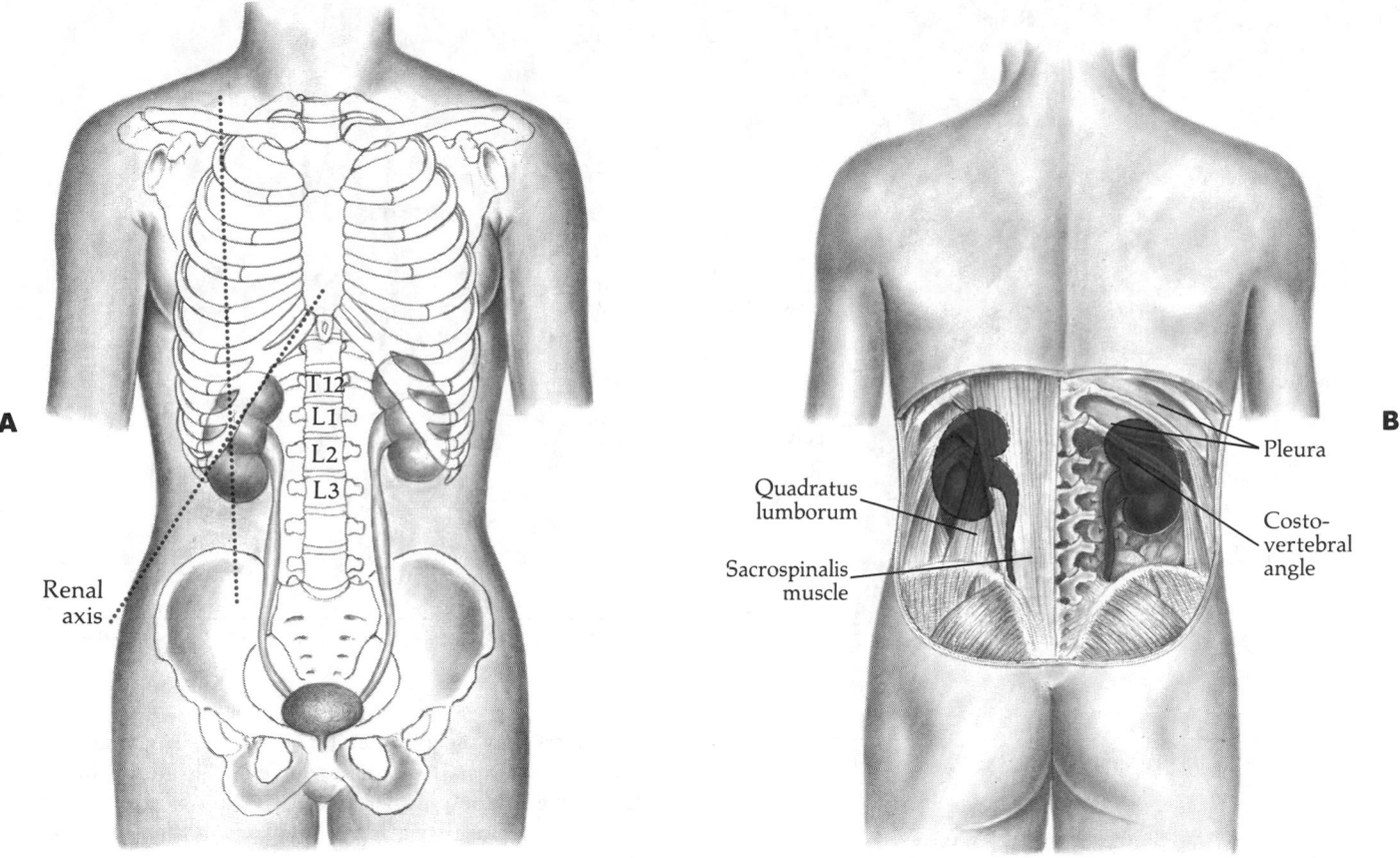

A **B**

Figure 12-1 Anatomic relation of kidneys to spinal column. **A,** Anterior view. **B,** Posterior view.

The renal fossa is bounded superiorly by the diaphragm, laterally by the abdominal musculature, and posteriorly by the quadratus lumborum muscle.

The blood supply of the kidneys arises directly from the abdominal aorta. Typically a single renal artery enters the kidney at the renal hilus. However, duplicate renal arteries may be found and are not considered pathologic. After entering the kidney, the renal artery bifurcates into superior and inferior branches, which further divide into the interlobular arteries. These vessels and their branches provide the substantial blood supply necessary for renal function.[118]

The veins that drain the kidneys are paired with arterial vessels. The renal veins exiting the kidney empty directly into the inferior vena cava, and their number corresponds to the number of renal arteries present.[108]

Lymphatics adjacent to the renal cortex and medulla drain into para-aortic and para–vena caval lymph nodes. The sensory and motor neurons that innervate the kidneys arise from the dorsal roots of T11 and T12. Autonomic neural control of the kidneys is mediated by fibers from the vagus nerve, splanchnic nerves, semilunar ganglia, and the celiac axis.[118]

The kidneys perform a number of essential functions related to the maintenance of internal homeostasis. These include maintenance of fluid and electrolyte balance and serum pH levels and excretion of the by-products of metabolism.

Renal pelvis and ureters The renal pelvis and ureters are continuous, thick-walled tubes that originate at the renal hilus and implant into the bladder wall, connecting the kidneys to the bladder. The renal pelvis is a funnel-shaped structure into which the major calyces empty urine for transport to the urinary bladder. After exiting the renal hilus the renal pelvis narrows inferomedially into the ureter.[108]

The ureters are approximately 24 to 30 cm long. The left ureter is slightly longer than the right. The course of the ureters forms an inverted S. After leaving the renal pelvis, the ureters pass medially over the psoas muscle. The ureters then progress medially to the sacroiliac joints before turning laterally to an area near the ischial spines of the pelvis. Finally, the ureters curve back laterally to insert into the bladder base at the trigone muscle.[12,108]

The internal diameter of the ureters varies from 2 to 10 mm. Three areas of anatomic narrowing have clinical

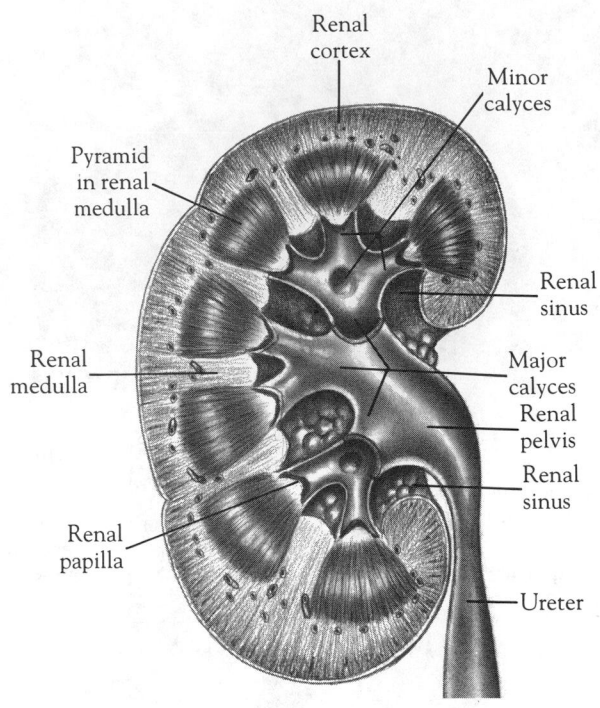

Figure 12-2 Cross section of kidney.

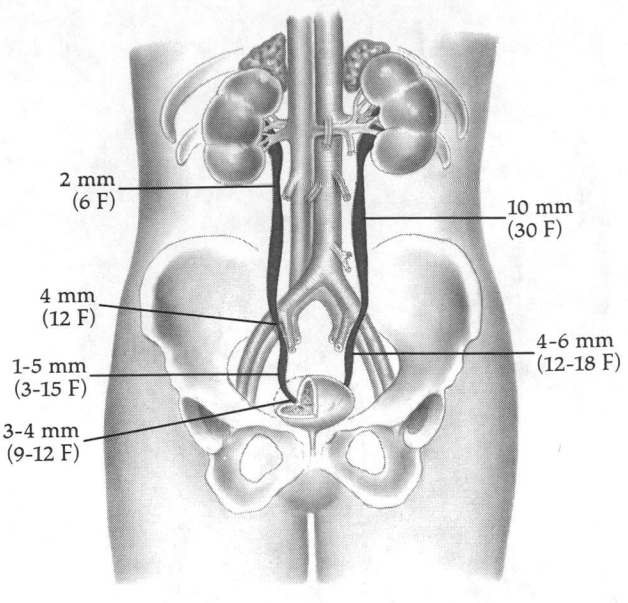

Figure 12-3 Course of ureter with its varying internal luminal sizes.

implications: the ureteropelvic junction, the area where the ureters cross the iliac arteries, and the ureterovesical junction (Figure 12-3).[108,118]

The ureters and renal pelvis share a common embryogenic origin and histologic makeup. The ureter and renal pelvis first appear during the fourth week of life. They arise from the mesonephric duct and grow cranially to meet the metanephric cap.[108]

The ureter and renal pelvis are composed of three histologically defined layers: the external adventitia, a smooth muscle coat, and an inner mucous membrane. The adventitia is a connective tissue sheath that encircles the renal pelvis and ureters to the level of ureterovesical junction. The adventitial layer blends into the surrounding retroperitoneal tissue, providing support for the ureters. The exact arrangement of these fibers is not known. Two layers of muscle fibers, an inner longitudinal layer and an outer circular layer, have been described.[127] However, histologic studies of ureteral smooth muscle have disputed this theory.[23] Tanagho[108] and Allen[4] describe the muscle fibers as arranged in bundles that are oriented in a helical or spiral fashion. The muscular tissue layer provides peristaltic activity needed to transport urine from the kidneys to the bladder. The mucous membrane lining the internal ureter is composed of transitional cell epithelium with a supportive lamina propria.[23]

The blood supply of the ureters is variable. The upper portion of the ureter and renal pelvis may receive arterial blood from branches of the renal, gonadal, or adrenal arteries. The pelvic ureters may receive arterial blood from the common iliac arteries, external iliac arteries, deferential arteries in the male, uterine arteries in the female, or the obturator artery. Blood enters the ureters via an arterial plexus located within the outer adventitial layer.[12]

Venous blood from the ureters drains into a venous plexus in the ureteral submucosa. This plexus drains into an adventitial venous plexus, which empties into veins closely paired with the arterial supply described previously.

Lymphatic drainage from the ureters is also variable. The upper ureteral and renal pelvic lymphatic channels empty into para-aortic or renal nodes. The middle and lower ureteral lymphatic channels drain into the common or external iliac nodes.[12]

The nerve supply of the ureters arises from the celiac plexus, mesenteric ganglia, and hypogastric plexus. Although the exact role of the autonomic nervous system in ureteral function remains unclear, the ureter is known to contain a rich supply of sympathetic and parasympathetic nerve receptors.[12]

The primary function of the renal pelvis and ureters is to transport urine from the kidney to the bladder. To accomplish this goal, the ureters must create a peristaltic muscular wave sufficient to drive a bolus of urine from the renal pelvis, through the ureters, and past the ureterovesical junction.[23]

Although the precise mechanisms of ureteral peristalsis remain unclear, it is influenced by mechanical, chemical, and neural stimuli. Generation of a peristaltic wave does not depend on specific neural firing. Like the muscle of the heart, ureteral smooth muscle will continue to rhythmically contract outside the body. In contrast to the heart, no specialized pacemaker has been clearly defined, although the existence of an intrinsic ureteral pacemaker is well established.[12] Multiple pacemaker cells regulating ureteral activity are thought to exist within the

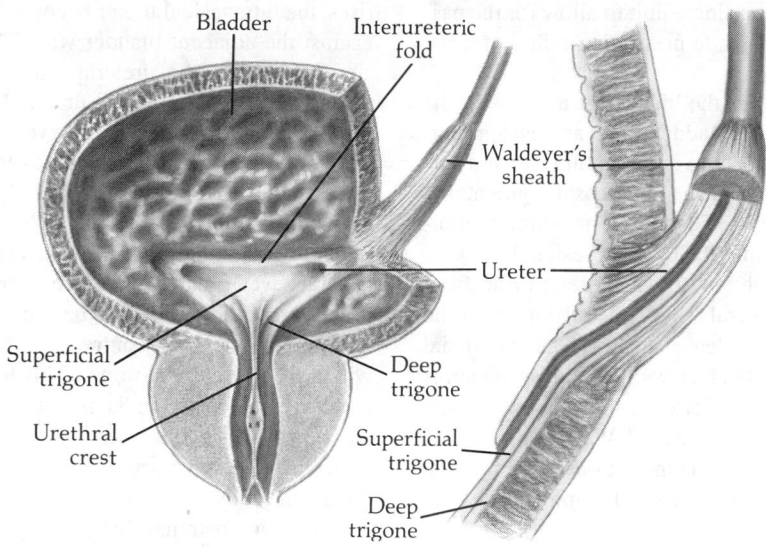

Figure 12-4 Normal ureterotrigonal complex.

renal calyces. The prolonged refractory period of the smooth muscle of the renal pelvis and ureters prevents all calyceal contractions from resulting in ureteral peristaltic waves. The renal pelvis and ureters average two to six peristaltic waves each minute.[12,118]

Ureteral peristaltic waves typically arise within the renal pelvis. They travel in an antegrade direction from the renal pelvis to the ureterovesical junction. During the resting phase, the renal pelvis assumes a conical shape with an area of narrowing at the pelvic-ureteral junction. At this time both the renal pelvis and ureters maintain a low intraluminal pressure of 2 to 5 cm H_2O. Urine enters the ureter from the renal pelvis passively during the resting phase. During a peristaltic wave the pressure rises to 20 to 60 cm H_2O, sufficient to force urine past the ureterovesical junction into the bladder. Only 5% of the total renal pelvic contents is evacuated from the renal pelvis during a peristaltic wave. Once the peristaltic wave is propagated into the ureters, urine is pushed ahead of the wave through the length of the ureter and past the ureterovesical junction into the bladder.[12,108]

An increase in renal output causes greater pelvic distention, which increases both the number of peristaltic waves generated per minute and the proportion of renal pelvic contents transported to the bladder with each contraction.[108]

The ureters are also affected by neural influences. Although it has been demonstrated that the normal ureter continues to contract when removed from the body, the autonomic nervous system does influence ureteral function. The ureters are extensively innervated with α- and β-adrenergic receptors. Stimulation of α-adrenergic receptors causes increased ureteral peristalsis. Stimulation of β-adrenergic receptors results in an inhibition of ureteral peristalsis. The role of the parasympathetic nervous system in ureteral and renal pelvic function is

not clearly understood. The parasympathetic nervous system is thought to potentiate ureteral peristalsis directly through the release of catecholamines.[12]

Ureteral peristalsis is also influenced by various chemical and pharmacologic agents. For example, the administration of epinephrine or catecholamines will, predictably, increase ureteral peristalsis. Increased histamine levels also stimulate ureteral peristalsis. However, the administration of serotonin, which enhances intestinal peristalsis, does not affect ureteral peristalsis. Upper ureteral dilation, which is commonly seen in pregnant women, was once attributed to fluctuations in the serum levels of the sex hormones. Recent investigation has demonstrated that this dilation was caused by mechanical factors rather than hormonal influences. This hypothesis is further supported by the observation that upper ureteral dilation is not seen in women taking oral contraceptives.[108]

Ureterovesical junction and trigone The ureterovesical junction is of particular interest in any discussion of genitourinary disease because of its importance in preventing vesicoureteral reflux and associated complications. The ureterovesical junction is located near the base of the bladder in the lateral aspects of the trigone muscle. The ureterovesical junction has three components important to its function: the intravesical ureter, the trigone, and the adjacent bladder wall (Figure 12-4).[108,118]

Embryologically, the ureterovesical junction is formed in the seventh week of gestation when the caudal end of the ureter opens into the urogenital sinus. The trigone muscle is formed from the same mesonephric tissue that forms the ureter. The intravesical ureter is further connected to the bladder by a continuous connective tissue sheath. Thus, although the intravesical ureter and trigone muscle have different embryogenic origins than the bladder, the ureterovesical junction in the fully developed human functions as a single unit to allow for the passage of urine into the bladder while preventing reflux of urine into the upper tracts.[107]

The intravesical ureter enters the bladder at a hiatus in the posterior, lateral aspect of the bladder base and is approximately 1.5 cm long. It is divided into an intramural section surrounded by the detrusor muscle and a submucosal segment that travels under the bladder mucosa. The intravesical ureter terminates at an orifice that opens into the bladder vesicle.[108,118]

The histologic features of the intravesical ureter differ from upper ureteral segments in several ways. The adventitia of the intravesical ureter contains two dense sheaths. The superficial sheath is continuous with the bladder wall. The deep sheath is derived from ureteral adventitia. Between these dense sheaths is a loose connective tissue plane called Waldeyer's sheath. This sheath allows for mobility of the intravesical ureter within the adjacent bladder wall and is of surgical significance when performing ureteroneocystostomy.[118]

The arrangement of smooth muscle fibers also differs in the intravesical ureter. Unlike the upper ureters, the intravesical ureter contains longitudinally arranged fibers and is easily collapsible. The ability of the intravesical ureter to seal itself by collapsing is an important mechanism in the prevention of reflux. Muscle fibers from the intravesical ureter decussate inferiorly to fuse with the superficial trigone and medially to form Mercier's bar.[58,118]

The trigone muscle is another essential component of the ureterovesical junction. The muscle is divided into two parts, the superficial trigone and the deep trigone. The superficial trigone is continuous with muscular fibers from the intravesical ureter. It continues along the bladder base and into the proximal urethra. In the male the trigone terminates at the verumontanum. In the female the superficial trigone terminates at the bladder neck.

The deep trigone is characterized by flat, tightly bound, smooth fiber groups. It is continuous with Waldeyer's sheath along the path of the intravesical ureter. The deep trigone is rolled into a tube that is incomplete on its anterior surface. The deep trigone terminates at the bladder neck and continues into the urethra as a layer of circular smooth muscle.[47,108]

The portion of the bladder wall adjacent to the ureterovesical junction is characterized by circular and longitudinal smooth muscle fibers that secure the ureters within the vesical wall. The outer, longitudinal smooth muscle layer is the strongest, most resilient segment of the bladder wall. This strength is vital to the maintenance of continuity between the upper and lower urinary tracts.[107]

The primary functions of the ureterovesical junction are to allow efflux of urine into the bladder and to prevent reflux of urine into the ureters. During bladder filling the ureterovesical junction maintains a relatively low closure pressure, between 8 and 15 cm H_2O. This closure pressure is adequate to prevent reflux of urine from the bladder, which also fills at low pressures. However, the closure pressure is easily overcome by a ureteral peristaltic wave, which generates pressure between 20 and 60 cm H_2O. As the bladder fills and intravesical pressure

rises, the intravesical ureter becomes progressively compressed against the adjacent bladder wall. The effect of this compression is to carry the ureteral hiatus outward, thus increasing pressure of the intravesical ureter. This compensatory mechanism prevents reflux of urine even when the bladder is filled with urine. At very high volumes the compression of the intravesical ureter becomes functionally obstructed and interferes with normal ureteral peristalsis.[108,118]

During the voiding phase the ureterovesical junction must generate even greater resistance to prevent reflux into the upper urinary tract. A few seconds before intravesical pressure rises in response to a detrusor contraction, there is a sharp pressure rise within the intravesical ureter. This high closure pressure at the ureterovesical junction is maintained throughout micturition and persists for a brief period after voiding is completed. The sharp increase in pressure was once attributed primarily to the contractile activity of the adjacent bladder wall. However, studies have demonstrated that the trigone is primarily responsible for the prevention of reflux during micturition. The marked pressure rise seen immediately before a detrusor contraction is caused by an increase in the tone of the trigone, which pulls the intravesical ureter tightly closed. The trigonal contraction is maintained for approximately 20 seconds after voiding is completed. As expected, no efflux of urine into the bladder occurs during voiding.[108]

Urinary bladder   The urinary bladder is a hollow muscular organ designed to store and expel urine produced by the kidneys. The size and shape of the bladder vary with its state of fullness and with age. When empty, the bladder assumes the shape of a tetrahedron and lies entirely within the lesser pelvis. As the bladder fills, it becomes more spheric in shape and moves upward and anteriorly toward the abdominal cavity.[102,124]

During infancy the bladder is located in the abdomen; even the bladder neck lies above the symphysis pubis. The bladder assumes its place in the pelvis shortly before puberty. The change in position is not caused by migration of the organ; rather, changes in the size and shape of the vesicle and maturation of the pelvic bone result in the change in relative location of the bladder.[118]

The bladder is characterized by two inlets and a single outlet located on the inferior aspect of the organ. Six anatomic areas are seen on gross inspection of the organ: the neck, the base or fundus, the apex, and the superior right inferolateral and left inferolateral surfaces (Figure 12-5).[102]

The bladder neck is the lower part of the organ and is several centimeters from the lower aspect of the symphysis pubis. The bladder neck is a relatively fixed structure regardless of the volume of urine present in the vesicle or the state of the adjacent rectum. The bladder neck is pierced by the internal urethral orifice. In the male it sits directly superior to the prostate gland; in the female it sits posterior to the vaginal wall.[102]

The base of the bladder is triangular and oriented posteriorly and downward from the bladder apex. Its borders are rounded and characterized by the junction of the intravesical ureters. In the adult male the bladder is superior to the seminal vesicles and adjacent to the rectum. Denonvilliers' fascia forms an

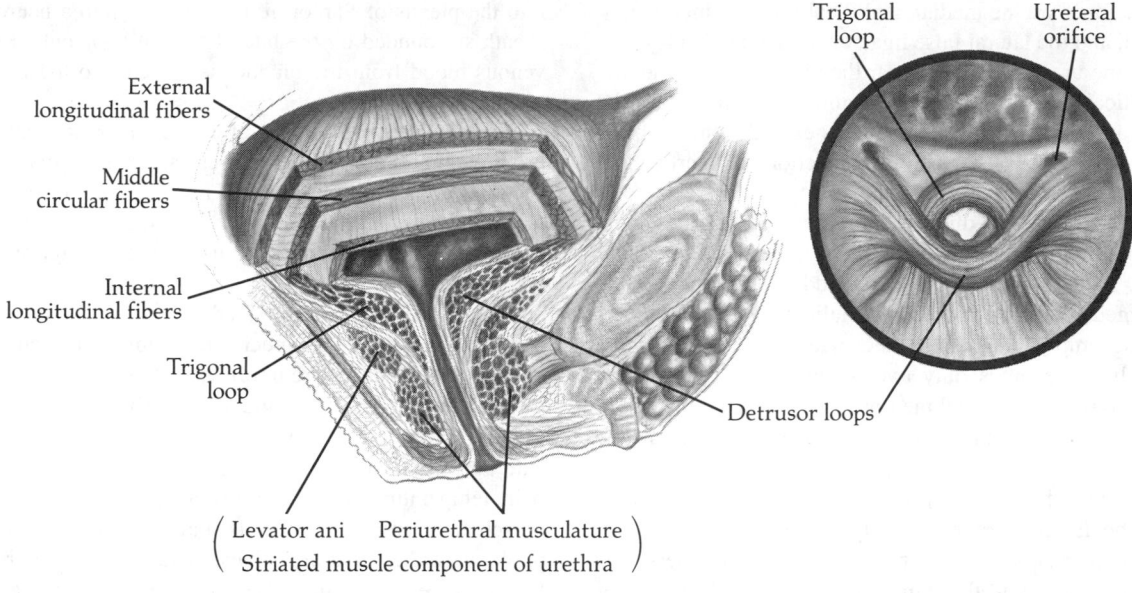

Figure 12-5 Common anatomy of urinary bladder.

anatomic barrier between the bladder base, rectum, and the vasa deferentia. In adult women the bladder base lies in close proximity to the anterior vaginal wall. Although the female lacks any fascial borders between the bladder and adjacent vagina, the two structures are separate at this point. In contrast, the lower urethra is anatomically continuous with the anterior vaginal wall.[102]

The apex of the bladder is the uppermost surface of the organ and is oriented anteriorly toward the abdominal wall. In the empty bladder of the adult, the apex lies within the pelvis. When the bladder is filled with urine, the apex is pushed upward and anteriorly so it enters the abdominal cavity. The apex is connected to the abdominal wall via the urachus.[102,108]

The superior surface of the empty bladder is bounded laterally by a line extending from the apex to the anterior borders of the intravesical ureters. The posterior border is formed by a line extending between the external borders of the intravesical ureters. In the adult male reflection of the peritoneum covers the superior surface. When filled, a prevesical pouch is formed that may contain a segment of the small bowel. In the adult female the superior surface of the bladder is separated from the ureters by the ureterovesical pouch.

The inferolateral surfaces of the urinary bladder can be distinguished primarily when the vesicle is empty. They lack any pelvic fascial covering and significantly change shape to accommodate bladder filling. When the bladder reaches capacity, the right and left inferolateral surfaces become a single, convex area lying adjacent to the abdominal wall.

The primary supportive structure of the urinary bladder is the pelvic floor. In addition, endopelvic fascia found adjacent to the bladder are presumed to provide additional support. The pelvic ligaments are thought to play a primary role in main-taining the bladder's position, and the additional reflections of the endopelvic fascia are presumed to play a lesser, supplemental role. The arrangement of this fascia varies between women and men.[102,124]

The "true" bladder ligaments are dense bands of fascia that arise from the tendinous arch of the peritoneum and connect it with the lateral aspects of the bladder wall. The tendinous arch is a condensation of endopelvic fascia that lies over the pelvic diaphragm and extends to the symphysis pubis and ischial spines. In the adult male the anterior aspect of this tissue forms the puboprostatic ligaments. The lateral puboprostatic ligaments extend from the anterior end of the tendinous arch to the upper aspect of the prostatic sheath. The medial puboprostatic ligaments extend from the tendinous arch to the back of the pubic bone, near the middle of the symphysis and the back part of the prostatic sheath, forming the retropubic space. In women the analogous structures are the pubovesical ligaments whose attachments are identical to those described in males except that the lower aspects of the ligaments attach to the bladder neck and proximal urethra in contrast to the prostatic sheath. From a neurological perspective the bladder neck may be divided from other bladder surfaces, which are collectively referred to as the bladder body.[102,124]

At the apex of the bladder, the allantois forms the median umbilical ligament or urachus, which is a fibrous cord extending to the umbilicus. Normally, the lower portion of the urachus is patent but does not communicate with the bladder vesicle. Occasionally, the inferior urachal remnant communicates with the vesicle of the bladder; this is not considered pathologic unless infection is present.[102,124]

In addition to the true ligaments, other reflections of peritoneum partially envelop the bladder. The three anterior endopelvic folds are the median umbilical fold, the medial umbilical fold, and the lateral false ligaments. The median fold extends over the urachal remnant near the bladder apex. The medial umbilical fold covers the remaining umbilical arterial remnants, and the lateral false ligaments extend from the bladder to the side walls of the pelvis. Reflections of sacrogenital peritoneum enfold the posterior bladder.[124]

The bladder wall is divided into four distinct histologic layers: urothelium, lamina propria, tunica muscularis, and outer adventitia. The urothelium of the bladder lines the vesicle and is formed of transitional cell epithelium six to eight layers deep in the empty bladder. As the bladder fills to capacity, the urothelium becomes only two to three layers deep. The urothelium has an associated membrane that is impermeable to water, thus preventing the reabsorption of urine stored in the bladder.[70,118]

Under the urothelium is the submucosal layer, or the lamina propria. The lamina propria is only loosely attached to the urothelium and rich with areolar tissues and elastic fibers. The lamina propria is found throughout the distensible portions of the bladder but is absent in the area of the deep trigone. Here, the mucosal lining of the vesicle is attached directly to the tunica muscularis in this nondistensible portion of the bladder.[118]

Unlike its loose connection with the urothelium, the lamina propria is firmly attached to the tunica muscularis of the bladder. The tunica muscularis is composed primarily of smooth muscle and is called the detrusor. Detrusor muscle cells are arranged in bundles and interspersed within a collagenous framework. A dense autonomic plexus provides autonomic innervation for the detrusor muscle cells. The detrusor muscle is variable in thickness; three layers (inner longitudinal, middle circular, and outer longitudinal) are described. The middle circular and outer longitudinal layers consist of relatively thick muscle cells. They are most prominent in the body of the bladder and terminate at the urethral orifice. Controversy exists whether detrusor muscle bundles of the inner longitudinal layer extend into the proximal urethra. Some investigators argue that the inner longitudinal layer continues into the urethra, forming an outer longitudinal layer of smooth muscle.[48] In contrast, others note that continuity between detrusor muscle bundles and urethral smooth muscle bundles is not seen in fetal histologic specimens. They conclude that vesicle smooth muscle and urethral smooth muscle are embryologically separate.[23]

The outermost histologic layer of the bladder is the adventitia. The adventitia is composed of fibroelastic tissue and is loosely connected to the various peritoneal coverings of the bladder described previously.[70]

The blood supply of the urinary bladder arises from several sources. Arterial blood reaches the bladder from the superior, medial, and inferior vesical arteries, which are branches of the internal iliac or hypogastric artery. Small branches from the obturator and inferior gluteal muscles also supply arterial blood to the bladder. Branches from the uterine and vaginal artery supply vascular nourishment to the bladder in the female. Unlike the veins of the kidneys, those of the bladder do not follow arterial routes. Venous drainage from the bladder exits anteriorly into the plexus of Santorini and laterally into a neurovascular sheath surrounded by the lateral vesical ligaments. From here venous blood from the bladder is routed into the inferior hypogastric vein.[108,117]

The lymphatic drainage of the bladder originates in the urothelium and drains into the vesical, external iliac, hypogastric, and common iliac nodes. The lymphatic channels in the urinary bladder are not clearly elucidated. Three areas of lymphatic drainage are postulated: the trigone, posterior wall, and anterior wall.[108,117]

The innervation of the bladder represents a deceptively complex discussion; the precise mechanisms of neural control of the urinary bladder are not fully understood. The sensory innervation of the urinary bladder is poorly understood. Sensory impulses from the urinary bladder are both proprioceptive and exteroceptive. Exteroceptive impulses from the bladder include pain, temperature, and touch. Proprioceptive impulses give the person an awareness of various states of vesical fullness. Morphologic studies in animals have demonstrated the presence of free nerve endings throughout the detrusor muscle with the greatest abundance in the trigone. Tension receptors and stretch receptors have also been noted in the detrusor muscle and presumably play an important role in the awareness of bladder filling. The impulses generated by the sensory receptors are thought to travel in the sensory portion of the pelvic plexus.[66,118]

The motor innervation of the bladder, like all smooth muscle, is provided by the autonomic nervous system. Parasympathetic receptors containing acetylcholine are abundant throughout the bladder body (detrusor muscle). Excitation of these receptors produces contraction of the detrusor muscle. Sympathetic receptors are also found in the bladder body and base. β-Adrenergic receptors containing norepinephrine are found principally in the body of the bladder. Excitation of these receptors causes relaxation of detrusor muscle bundles. α-Adrenergic receptors are abundant in the bladder base and proximal urethra. Unlike the β-adrenergics, they are excitatory when stimulated, causing contraction of smooth muscle bundles in the trigone and proximal urethra. Nonadrenergic, noncholinergic receptors are also found in the bladder body. They are postulated to be excitatory in nature, playing a yet undescribed role in contraction of the detrusor muscle.

Sympathetic neural signals are routed to the bladder via branches of the inferior hypogastric plexus. The spinal roots of the sympathetic component of the inferior hypogastric are at T12, L1, and L2. Parasympathetic neural signals are routed to the bladder via branches of the pelvic nerve. The spinal roots of the parasympathetic component of the pelvic plexus are located in the interomedial gray matter between the dorsal and ventral horns of spinal levels S2 to S4.

Urethra   The urethra extends from the bladder to an external meatus, serves as a conduit for urine expulsion during micturition, and aids in maintaining continence during bladder filling. In the male the urethra also serves as a conduit for semen expelled at ejaculation.[118,124]

The male urethra is approximately 23 cm long and is divided into two parts: anterior and posterior (Figure 12-6). The

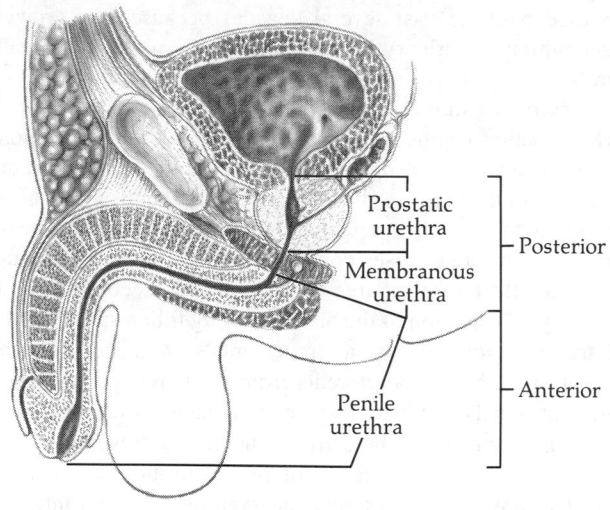

Figure 12-6 Male urethra.

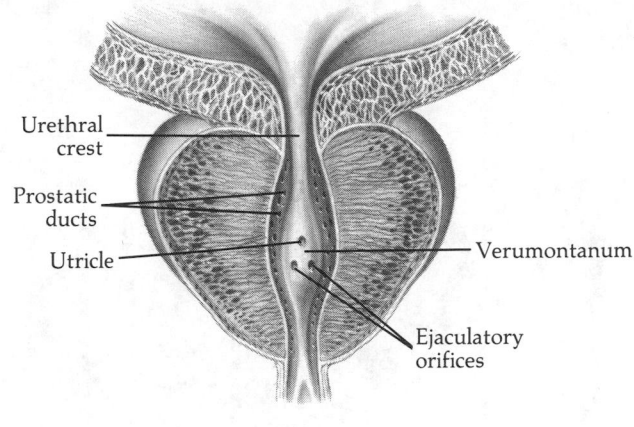

Figure 12-7 Prostatic (posterior) urethra.

posterior urethra is subdivided into the prostatic and membranous urethra. The prostatic urethra is approximately 3 cm long and extends from the bladder neck to the origin of the membranous urethral segment at the apex of the prostate gland. It runs through the prostate vertically, lying nearer the anterior surface of the gland. The posterior floor of the prostatic urethra is elevated at the verumontanum. It tapers inferiorly and superiorly to form the cristae, which are mucous membrane folds that form a depression on the posterior floor known as the prostatic fossa. Secretory ducts from the middle lobe of the prostate enter the urethra at this point (Figure 12-7).[118]

The membranous urethra is 2 to 2.5 cm long and extends from the apex of the prostate to the bulb of the penis. It pierces the area referred to as the urogenital diaphragm. Striated muscle fibers exist within the wall of the membranous urethra and significantly contribute to sphincteric function in the male. These muscle fibers are arranged in an omega-shaped pattern and are thinnest in the posterior midline. Periurethral striated muscle fibers from the pelvic floor also contribute to striated muscle sphincteric function of the urethra.[50,118] The membranous urethra is the least distensible segment, since it is anchored securely by the triangular ligament. It is the most susceptible to inflammatory urethral stricture.[118,124]

The anterior urethra tunnels the corpus spongiosum of the penis and is divided into the bulbous, pendulous, and glandular urethra. The bulbous and pendulous parts of the urethra together measure 15 cm long and extend from the distal border of the membranous urethra to the base of the glans penis. The suspensory ligament marks the border between these urethral segments. The bulbous urethra is distinguished by the orifices of the bulbourethral, or Cowper's, glands.[118]

The penile urethra is the most distal segment in the male and terminates at the external meatus. Immediately before the external meatus, the penile urethra is marked by a fusiform dilation called the fossa navicularis. It originates at the corona of the glans and is 2.5 cm long. The external meatus itself is a vertical slit approximately 8 mm in diameter that lies at the summit of the glans.[118,124]

The microscopic anatomy of the male urethra is characterized by an inner mucous membrane composed of columnar cell epithelium persisting throughout the posterior and anterior urethral segments to the level of the fossa navicularis. Here the urethral mucosa changes to a squamous cell epithelium near the external meatus. A submucosal layer composed of connective tissue and elastic fibers lies under the mucosa. The muscular layer of the urethra is composed primarily of smooth muscle fibers. In the prostatic urethra the smooth muscle fibers are indistinguishable from the adjacent musculature to the level of the verumontanum. Below the verumontanum, the urethral smooth fibers are arranged in an outer circular layer and an inner longitudinal layer. Striated muscle fibers have also been noted in the ventral wall of the prostatic urethra.[23,124]

The arterial blood supply of the male urethra arises from the urethral artery, which is a branch of the internal pudendal artery. Venous blood from the urethra drains into the deep vein of the penis and the pudendal plexus. The sensory innervation of the urethra is provided by branches of the pudendal nerve. Lymphatic drainage from the male urethra accompanies channels of the glans penis in the anterior segment and empties into the deep subinguinal nodes from the posterior segment.[124]

The female urethra forms a relatively short, straight path when compared with the male urethra (Figure 12-8). In nulliparous adult women the urethra measures 3.5 to 5.5 cm. The female urethra originates at the bladder neck orifice and travels at a 16-degree angle to its external meatus at the vestibule. Striated muscle fibers within the urethral wall are densest in the middle third of the female urethra and deficient in the posterior midline. Periurethral striated muscle fibers of the levator ani also contribute to sphincteric function in the female.[48,124]

Three histologic elements of the female urethra characterize its microscopic anatomy. The inner urethral lumen is lined by columnar epithelium that changes to squamous epithelium near the external meatus. The mucosal layer also contains numerous

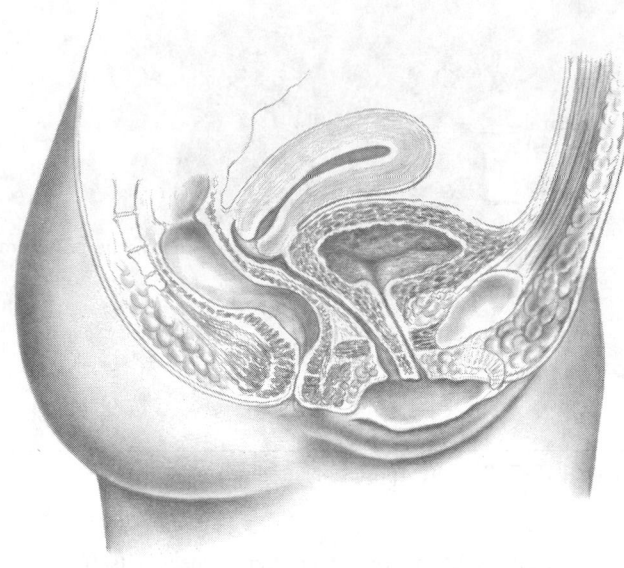

Figure 12-8 Anatomic relations of female urethra.

secreting glands. The muscular lining of the urethra contains an outer sheath of skeletal muscle fibers (the rhabdosphincter), an outer longitudinal layer of smooth muscle bundles, and inner circular layers of smooth muscle bundles. The lower two thirds of the female urethra is fused with the anterior vaginal wall so that the two layers of smooth muscle are indistinguishable. A spongy vascular cushion composed of an extensive venous network and arteriovenous communications lies between the urethral mucosa layer and the muscular layer of the urethral wall.[124]

Lower Urinary Tract Function

The bladder and urethra act as a coordinated unit under the influence of multiple centers of the central and peripheral nervous systems. Together with the pelvic floor musculature they form a single functional system called the urethrovesical unit. Lower urinary tract function is divided into two stages, filling and voiding. Bladder filling and storage is characterized by passive filling of the bladder vesicle in conjunction with urethral closure. Micturition is marked by relaxation of the urethral sphincteric mechanism in synchrony with contraction of the smooth muscle of the bladder wall. Knowledge of the two principal components that modulate function of the urethrovesical unit—the neural modulation of the bladder, urethra, and pelvic floor muscles and the components of the urethral sphincteric mechanism—is necessary to understand the factors that maintain continence and ensure complete urinary evacuation during micturition.

Neural Innervation of the Lower Urinary Tract

The neural control of micturition is modulated by three structures—the brain, spinal cord, and peripheral nervous system. Although our knowledge of the neural control of micturition remains incomplete, interest in this area of physiology has in-

creased over the past several decades because of a growing recognition of urinary incontinence as a worldwide health problem.

Brain   Central nervous system influence on lower urinary tract function begins in the cerebral cortex. A detrusor motor area is located in the superiomedial area of the frontal lobe and the genu of the corpus callosum within both hemispheres of the brain.[5] In the experimental animal model, stimulation of the detrusor motor area causes contraction of the bladder, although the net effect of this area in the human is considered inhibitory.[52] Distention of the bladder during filling stimulates the detrusor motor area via afferent signals from receptors that travel to the brain via afferents from the pelvic plexus. These afferent signals traverse the spinal cord via reticulospinal tracts. Efferent signals from the detrusor motor area travel to subcortical nuclei in the brainstem (pontine micturition center) to ultimately traverse spinal tracts and synapse on spinal interneurons in the conus medullaris (sacral micturition center).[117]

Volitional control and regulation of basal tone on the pelvic floor musculature and urethral rhabdosphincter also are influenced by the cerebral cortex. A pelvic floor muscle motor area is contained in the sensorimotor cortex and bilaterally in the medial aspect of the cortex.[52,118] The pelvic floor muscles are typical of other skeletal muscle structures in the human and are innervated via the pyramidal tracts of the central nervous system. They are further influenced by the extrapyramidal system.[52] Unlike many muscles of the human, the pelvic floor and rhabdosphincter consist of primarily slow-twitch muscle fibers that are particularly suited for prolonged periods of tone necessary for maintaining urethral closure during bladder filling.

The thalamus is the primary relay center for communication between the cerebral cortex and lower brain centers. Terminal synapses of proprioceptive sensory axons from the detrusor are located in nonspecific intraluminal nuclei of the thalamus. The exact location of the thalamic pathways of detrusor motor function is unclear.[118] The observable effect of the thalamus, then, on the function of the bladder in the human is participation in the brain's net inhibitory influence on micturition in the continent individual.

The basal ganglia are a well-known component of the extrapyramidal tracts and include the caudate nuclei, red nuclei, substantia nigra, putamen, and globus pallidus. Persuasive evidence demonstrates that the basal ganglia exert a direct inhibitory influence on the detrusor muscle.[17,74] Input to the neurons of the basal ganglia is provided by pyramidal cells of the detrusor motor area and pelvic floor muscle motor area in the cerebral cortex. Efferent messages from the basal ganglia are thought to be directed to the cerebral cortex and that area of the brainstem involved with lower urinary tract function.[74]

The limbic system modulates the autonomic nervous system via input to the reticular formation center of the brainstem and hypothalamus.[51] Direct stimulation of the limbic system alters the detrusor reflex,[36] although pathologic ablation of the temporal lobes (including the hippocampus and amygdala) has not been associated with clinically apparent voiding dysfunction in the human.[118]

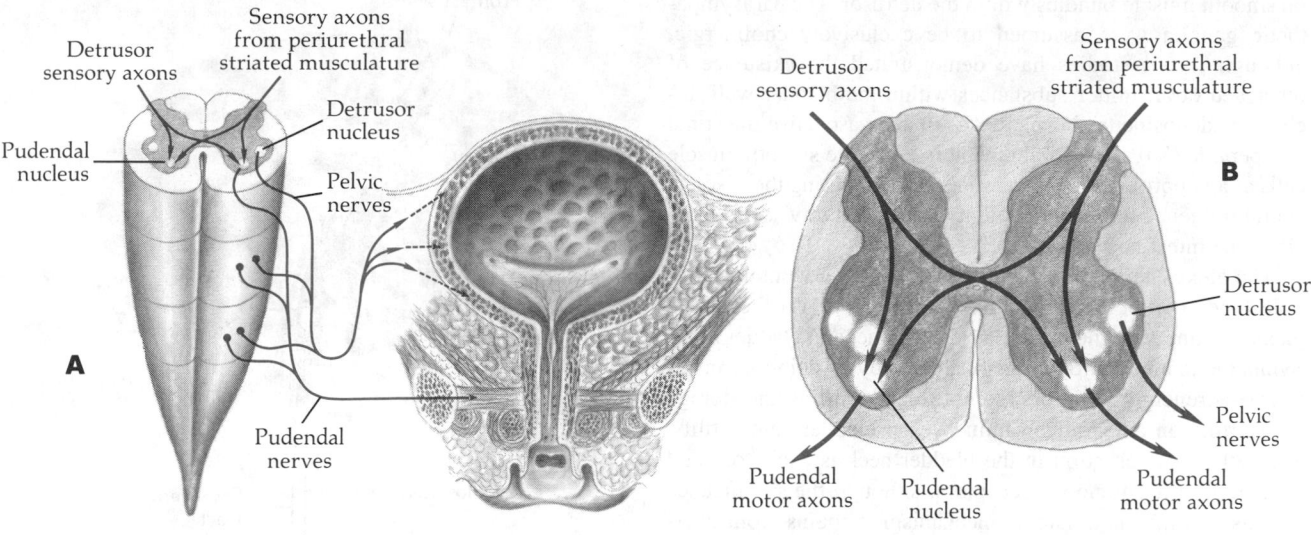

Figure 12-9 A, Sacral micturition center and peripheral bladder innervations. **B,** Loop III contains pelvic and pudendal nuclei and their interneurons.

The hypothalamus consists of a collection of nuclei that regulate the body's internal environment, including neuroendocrine functions and specific sexual behavioral responses. While the hypothalamus is not known to exert any direct influence on bladder function, it is known that bladder distention produces an effect on certain nuclei within the hypothalamus.[116]

The cerebellum is a significant component of the extrapyramidal tract and helps to coordinate voluntary movements and maintain the body's position in space. It affects bladder function by modulation of the detrusor reflex and pelvic floor muscular activity.[118] Cerebellar dysfunction in the clinical setting is associated with detrusor dysfunction.[69]

The brainstem is extremely important in lower urinary tract function. The gray matter of the dorsolateral pons and mesencephalon are the final common pathways to detrusor motor pathways in the spinal cord.[28] The pontine micturition center is of considerable clinical importance and is often referred to as the sphincter coordination center. This label is supported by observations that preservation of bladder and pelvic floor muscle activity is seen in neurologic lesions above the pons, while bladder striated incoordination (dyssynergia) is noted among persons with lesions below the pons and above the sacral micturition center.[13] The pontine micturition center plays a role in the initiation of the detrusor reflex, thus the reference to the act of micturition as a "brainstem reflex."[66]

Spinal cord The importance of the spinal cord to lower urinary tract function has been demonstrated in both animals and humans. Anatomically separate tracts provide communication between modulatory areas of the brain and pelvic and pudendal nuclei located within the conus medullaris.

The reticulospinal tracts of the lateral columns are involved with motor innervation of the detrusor.[96] Motor innervation of the pelvic floor muscles is mediated via corticospinal tracts.

The final synapse within the central nervous system for axons involved with both detrusor and pelvic floor muscle function is in the conus medullaris of the spinal cord. A reflexic inhibitory relationship exists between these systems so that stimulation of pelvic nuclei (involved with motor innervation of the detrusor muscle) results in inhibition of the pudendal nuclei (involved with motor innervation of the pelvic floor nuclei) and vice versa.[118]

In addition to the reticulospinal and corticospinal tracts, two specific areas of the spinal cord are significant to lower urinary tract function. Sympathetic outflow to the urethrovesical unit arises from spinal segments T10 to L1 or L2. Sympathetic outflow to the bladder body promotes relaxation of the detrusor, while sympathetic impulses at the bladder neck are noted to tighten the smooth muscle of the urethra. The significance of this neural modulation to urethrovesical function remains controversial.[52,118]

Spinal segments S2 to S4 are the location of both the pelvic nuclei, which provide motor innervation to the detrusor, and the pudendal nuclei, which provide innervation for the pelvic floor muscles. The pelvic nuclei are located within the intermediolateral portion of the gray matter, and the pudendal nuclei are found more dorsally in the ventromedial portion of the cord.[52] Injury to the sacral micturition center, which is necessary for the bladder to mount a contraction, results in loss of detrusor contractility.

Peripheral nervous system Two peripheral nerves are significant to urethrovesical function (Figure 12-9, *A*). The pelvic plexus exits the spine at S2, S3, and S4 to supply the bladder wall and proximal urethra with parasympathetic innervation. Stimulation of the pelvic plexus produces detrusor contraction and reflexic inhibition of the pudendal nerve and pelvic floor musculature.[118] Pelvic parasympathetic ganglia terminate on smooth muscle bundles within the detrusor. The parasympathetic ganglia were assumed to be exclusively cholinergic, although recent studies have demonstrated the existence of other neurotransmitter substances within the bladder wall, including adenosine triphosphate (ATP) and vasoactive intestinal polypeptide (VIP).[27] Neural receptors innervate smooth muscle cells at an approximately 1:1 ratio, thus explaining the discrete neural influence on bladder activity in contrast to visceral muscle in the intestine or stomach.[28]

The plexus nerve, like most peripheral nerves, contains multiple types of fibers. Sympathetic fibers travel via the pelvic plexus to innervate the bladder body, trigone, and bladder neck. Sympathetic innervation of the bladder body is inhibitory in nature; β-adrenergic receptors promote bladder filling and storage by exerting an antagonistic influence on bladder contractility. Sympathetic innervation in the bladder neck is excitatory and mediated by α-adrenergic receptors, although the significance of this neural modulatory mechanism remains controversial.[27,52,117] The termination of the pelvic autonomic fibers in the bladder form a microscopic forest that complicates any surgical procedure of the pelvis with the risk of denervation of the urethrovesical unit.

The pudendal nerve also arises from S2 to S4 and exits the spine via the greater sciatic foramen to run with the internal pudendal vessels. It provides somatic and sensory innervation to the pelvic floor musculature.[124]

Bradley's loop concept of innervation Bradley and his associates[18,118] have proposed a conceptual framework of the innervation of the lower urinary tract based on four reflex arcs or loops. Loop I consists of the cerebrocortical areas that modulate detrusor function (Figure 12-10). It originates with the detrusor motor area of the cerebral cortex and extends to the pontine micturition center. Loop II (Figure 12-10) consists of afferent and efferent spinal tracts between the pontine micturition center and detrusor nuclei in the sacral spinal cord. Loops I and II are essential for the maintenance of bladder stability in the human.

Loop III consists of the pelvic and pudendal nuclei and their interneurons (Figure 12-9, *B*). It controls the coordination between the detrusor and pelvic floor musculature. Interruption of loop III results in loss of coordination between detrusor and striated sphincteric activity, and is called detrusor/striated sphincter dyssynergia.

Loop IV consists of the supraspinal and spinal innervation of the pelvic floor musculature (Figure 12-11). Loop IV provides voluntary control of the striated sphincteric mechanism, which allows the individual to interrupt a urinary stream if desired. Loop IV begins in the sensorimotor cortex and extends to the pudendal nuclei of the conus medullaris. Interruption of spinal segments of loop IV occurs in conjunction with interruption of loops II and III and results in detrusor/striated sphincter dyssynergia.[18,118]

Other modulators of lower urinary tract function Prostaglandins also play a role in the modulation of urethrovesical function. The bladder produces PGE_2, PGE_1, and PGF_2-alpha. Among these prostaglandins, PGE_2 is predominant and enhances detrusor contractility in conjunction with inhibi-

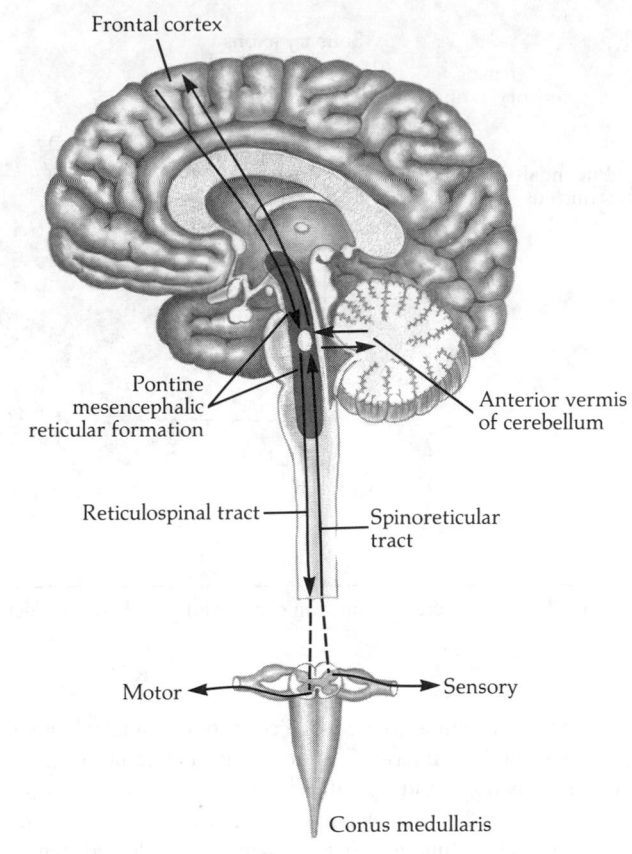

Frontal cortex

Pontine mesencephalic reticular formation

Anterior vermis of cerebellum

Reticulospinal tract

Spinoreticular tract

Motor

Sensory

Conus medullaris

Figure 12-10 Loops I and II extend from frontal cortex to pelvic nuclei in conus medullaris.

tion of urethral smooth muscle tone. PGF_2-alpha causes increased contractility of both bladder and urethral smooth muscle, but PGE_1 results in only modest increased contractility.[64]

Hormonal regulators of lower urinary tract smooth muscle have not been extensively investigated. Estrogens may exert an indirect influence on detrusor contractility by enhancing the production of prostaglandins.[18] Oxytocin receptors have been documented in the bladder wall of experimental animals and also may exert an influence on smooth muscle contractility in women.

Physiology of the Urethral Sphincter Mechanism

The urethral sphincter is a mechanism (rather than a discrete, circular muscle) that remains closed, preventing urinary leakage during bladder filling and storage, and it opens to allow an unobstructed flow of urine during micturition. Multiple components of the urethra and adjacent pelvis constitute the sphincter mechanism.

Two physiologic components of the sphincter mechanism contribute to urethral closure. Elements of compression form a watertight seal, preventing urinary leakage during passive filling. The softness of the urethral epithelium in conjunction with mucosal secretions produced by the urothelium produces a remarkably compliant structure that folds and deforms to produce

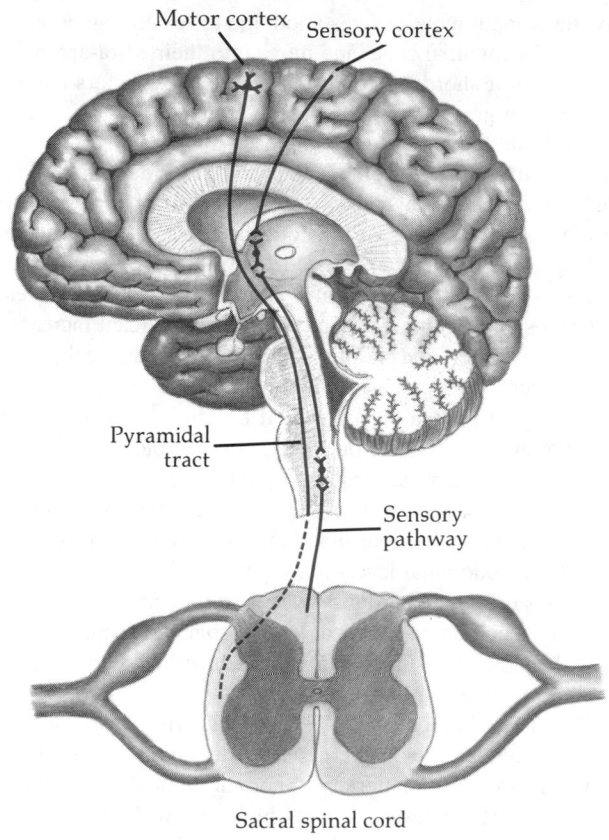

Motor cortex Sensory cortex

Pyramidal tract

Sensory pathway

Sacral spinal cord

Figure 12-11 Loop IV.

a watertight seal. The ability of the urethral lining to deform and maintain a watertight seal is evident when a rigid catheter is passed into the urethra. The urothelium conforms to the shape of the catheter without producing dribbling leakage.[100,112]

A vascular cushion formed by the rich submucosal venous plexus of the urethra also contributes to the urethral sphincteric mechanism. This cushion enhances the pliability of the urethral wall and serves as a transmitter of abdominal pressure along the course of the urethra. Transmission of this abdominal pressure is essential for the urethra to maintain a watertight seal in response to the stress produced by a sudden rise in pressure, for example, coughing, laughing, or physical exertion.[112]

Smooth and skeletal muscle cells within the urethral wall contribute to the sphincteric mechanism by producing active tone during bladder filling and storage. The smooth muscle of the bladder neck and proximal urethra and the fibers of the rhabdosphincter form an area of tension that is transmitted to the pliable urethral mucosa, thereby producing an efficient seal against urinary leakage.[126]

The pelvic floor musculature also contributes to active closure pressure of the sphincteric mechanism. The periurethral striated musculature is formed primarily by the levator ani. It acts as a sling; contraction of the pelvic floor elevates and compresses the proximal urethra and increases

urethral resistance to leakage in response to exertion that causes increasing abdominal pressure.[50]

The pelvic floor and its fascial coverings and the pubourethral ligaments in the male and female contribute indirectly to the sphincteric mechanism by maintaining the urethrovesical unit in its proper location in the pelvis. These structures form a hammock that supports the bladder in its proper abdominopelvic position and increases the efficiency of pressure transmission from abdomen to urethra.[50]

Male Genitalia

Scrotum The scrotum is a cutaneous, fibromuscular sac that is dependent below the pubis bone and houses the testes and lower portion of the spermatic cord. The skin of the scrotum is thin and deeply pigmented and contains abundant sebaceous glands, sweat glands, and hair follicles. The cutaneous layer of the scrotum is bisected by the median ridge or raphe, which extends from the base of the penis to the anus. The skin of the scrotum is further distinguished by rugae. The rugae are formed by parallel dermal muscle fibers and are more clearly seen on younger men, particularly when the testes have retracted because of a certain stimulus. Immediately under the skin is the dartos muscle, which is composed of smooth muscle fibers and elastic tissue. The dartos is a continuation of the suspensory ligament of the penis and superficial fascia of the abdominal, inguinal, and perineal fascia. It sends a sagittal reflection inward, creating an incomplete septum between the median ridge and the radix of the penis, which form the cavities in which the testes lie.[124]

The primary functions of the scrotum are to house the testes and provide an adequate environment for the production of sperm. The structure of the dartos allows for considerable variation of scrotal size in response to a variety of stimuli, such as external temperature, physical activity level, and emotions.[5]

Testes The testes are a pair of ovoid organs that lie in the scrotum. They receive vascular, neural, and lymphatic support from the spermatic cord; the scrotal ligament forms the single scrotal attachment for the testes. Each testis is approximately 4 to 5 cm long and 2.5 cm wide and weighs from 10.5 to 20 g. The left testis typically lies 1 cm lower than the right.[118,124]

The testes lie under three coverings: the tunica vaginalis, the tunica albuginea, and the tunica vasculosa. The tunica vaginalis arises from the peritoneum and forms a closed sac in which the testis is invaginated. The tunica albuginea is a white, fibrous covering for the testis that helps define the interior architecture of the organ. The posterior border of the tunica albuginea projects into the testis, forming an incomplete vertical septum called the mediastinum testis. From its front and lateral aspects, numerous fibrous projections extend toward the external border of the testis, dividing it into 200 to 300 lobules that contain multiple seminiferous tubules. The tunica vasculosa is the third testicular covering. It consists of a plexus of blood vessels within a framework of areolar tissue extending over the internal aspect of the tunica albuginea and covering its many septa, providing a vascular supply to each lobule.[118,124]

The functional unit of the testicular cortex is the seminiferous tubule. Each lobule of the testis contains one to three (or sometimes more) seminiferous tubules that are 30 to 60 cm of tortuous length with both ends terminating in a relatively short, straight segment called the canaliculus rectus. The seminiferous tubules occupy 75% of testicular mass; their combined length is almost 1 mile.[124]

A seminiferous tubule is formed of stratified epithelium four to eight cells thick with an identifiable internal lumen. The tubules contain Sertoli cells, spermatogenic cells, and an outer basement membrane with a fibrous tunica propria. The Sertoli cells are columnar in shape and extend radially from just within the outer basement membrane toward the tubular lumen. These interesting cells have indefinite cytoplasmic borders; spermatids and spermatocytes may be completely embedded within the cytoplasm of the Sertoli cells. The Sertoli cells are linked in tight junctions that divide the wall of the seminiferous tubule into two parts: a basal compartment containing spermatogonia and spermatocytes and a luminal compartment containing more advanced stages of testicular germ cells. The exact function of the Sertoli cells remains unclear. They are presumed to provide nourishment and succor for the germinal epithelium, help maintain the blood-testis barrier, secrete the testicular fluid seen in the lumen of the seminiferous tubules, and secrete an androgen-binding protein that promotes the accumulation of androgens in the immediate area of the germinal cell epithelium.[4]

The germinal cell epithelium of the seminiferous tubule is characterized by an ever-changing population of maturing stages of spermatic forms. The more primitive forms are found at the outer borders, and more mature forms are found nearer the inner lumen. Spermatogonia are the most immature cell form seen in the spermatic cycle. Other stages of germ cell epithelium seen in the wall of the seminiferous tubules are primary and secondary spermatocytes and spermatids.[4]

The interstitial tissue within the testicular lobules is composed of Leydig's cells, blood vessels, extensive lymphatic channels, and numerous macrophages. Leydig's cell are found in small groups of five to 20 and compose 12% of testicular volume. These are particularly significant because they secrete testosterone, which enters the bloodstream via interstitial capillary beds or goes directly into the seminiferous tubule without going through vascular routes.[4]

The structure and function of the testes in the adult male are significantly different from those during infancy and childhood. The germinal elements of the testes have a distinct embryologic origin from the other elements of the gonads. The nongerminal cell components of the testes arise as part of the mesodermic mass that will develop into the urogenital ridge; the germ cells of the testes arise from the entoderm lining the posterior aspect of the yolk sac. Development of both the germinal cell and somatic elements of the testes begins during the fourth week of life.[76]

From their retroperitoneal position, the testes must descend caudally to the scrotal sac to mature into viable structures away from the high temperature of the internal abdomen. During the third trimester they begin moving down the posterior aspect of the abdomen, bringing their neurovascular sheath with them.

By the seventh month of gestation, the testes enter the internal ring of the inguinal canal and move into their extra-abdominal position at or shortly after birth. The complex factors that regulate this migration are still not fully understood.[76]

At birth the testes are composed of small tubules with poorly differentiated components and few identifiable spermatogonia. Interstitial cells are present at birth but regress over the first several weeks of life to a baseline level that persists throughout the pubescent period. During the period between 4 and 10 years of age, the seminiferous tubules slowly increase in tortuosity. Beginning around age 10 a significant increase in the size, number, and mitotic activity of the germ cell epithelium occurs. This process continues until the onset of puberty around age 12 when the interstitial Leydig's cells mature and begin to produce testosterone levels comparable with adult values and active spermatogenesis begins.[4]

The blood supply of the testes is unique, since the temperature of arterial and venous blood must be cooled approximately 2° C from abdominal levels to support spermatogenesis. Cooling arises from interactions between arterial and venous vessels in which a countercurrent heat loss mechanism occurs. In addition, the slow, nonpulsating flow of the spermatic artery aids in cooling the vascular beds of the testes.[4]

The arterial blood supply of the testes arises from the internal spermatic artery, the cremasteric artery, and the deferential, or vasal, artery. The latter are important clinically as collateral circulation of the testes. Venous blood from the testes drains into the pampiniform plexus of the spermatic cord, which empties into the internal spermatic veins.[4]

Because of the unique embryologic origins of the testes, the lymphatic drainage is not into local inguinal or pelvic lymph nodes. Rather, the extensive lymphatic channels of the testes drain into the preaortic lymph nodes.[46,118]

Three adnexa of the testes are of clinical significance; all are composed of vestiges of the embryonic structures relevant to the formation and migration of the testes and spermatic cord. The appendix testis arises in the groove between the head of the epididymis and the testicular remnant of the müllerian duct. It is subject to torsion and must be differentiated from true testicular torsion, which constitutes a urologic emergency. The appendix epididymis is a pear-shaped body attached to the epididymal head, which is a remnant of epigenitalis tubules. The organs of Giraldes are a paragenitalis remnant sometimes noted in the lower spermatic cord anterior to the head of the epididymis.[46,118]

Epididymis and vas deferens   The epididymis and vas deferens are the efferent routes for sperm leaving the testes after completing the spermatogenic cycle. Along with the prostate and seminal vesicles, the epididymis and vas deferens provide transport, storage, and support for maturing sperm as they migrate toward the male urethra.[124]

The epididymis is a sausage-shaped structure approximately 5 cm long that is attached to the posterolateral aspect of the testis. Three anatomic regions of the epididymis are described: the head, or globus major; the body, or corpus; and the tail, or globus minor. The epididymis contains a single compartment, so injury is likely to entirely ablate the function of the organ. The epididymis is covered by the tunica vaginalis on all except the posterior border, where a fascial reflection forms the epididymal sinus.[118]

Inside the compartment of the epididymis is a long, tortuous canal with little muscular tone but abundant cilia lining the tubular lumen folded over on itself and tightly packed so that its total length is 4 to 5 cm. The head of the epididymis is directly connected to the efferent ductules, allowing sperm leaving the testis to enter the epididymal tubules via ciliary action. At the tail the tubules have more smooth muscle in their walls as the epididymis opens into the vas deferens.[124]

The vas deferens is a firm, elastic, cylindric tube extending from the termination of the epididymal tail to the ejaculatory duct located near the base of the prostate. The initial segment of the vas deferens is tortuous, although the part of the organ more distal to the testis is straight. From its origin at the epididymal tail, the vas deferens ascends along the posterior wall of the testis adjacent to the medial aspect of the epididymis. The vas then moves upward to the posterior part of the spermatic cord, traversing the inguinal canal to the level of the deep inguinal ring. At this point, the vas deferens leaves the spermatic cord, curves around the lateral aspect of the epigastric artery, and ascends several centimeters to the external iliac artery. The vas then crosses the external iliac obliquely and enters the false pelvis where it becomes a relatively fixed structure attached to the posterior abdominal wall. From this point the vas crosses the ureter and curves at an acute angle to traverse the prostatic base and terminate at the ejaculatory duct (Figure 12-12). The final segment of the vas deferens is characterized by a spindle-shaped dilation of the tube called the ampulla, which is approximately 10 cm long and contains several false pouches or diverticula that may or may not be clinically significant.[124]

The walls of the vas deferens comprise adventitial, muscular, and mucosal layers. The mucosa of the vas deferens comprises columnar epithelial cells, which, unlike the tubules of the epididymis, are not ciliated.[46,124] The smooth muscle of the vas deferens is divided into inner and outer longitudinal layers, separated by a middle circular layer of bundles. These smooth muscle bundles, like those of the ureter, contain gap junctions that allow rapid transmission of excitatory impulses and rapid contraction. The vas deferens serves as a conduit between the epididymis and ejaculatory duct, moving seminal fluid toward the prostatic urethra during emission. Relaxation of the circular smooth muscle of the wall of the vas deferens lengthens the vas, whereas contraction of the longitudinal smooth muscle lengthens the tube. As a result, seminal fluid is propelled in an antegrade fashion toward the prostatic urethra for ejaculation.[114] The adventitial layer of the vas deferens contains connective tissue and the neural, vascular, and lymphatic supply for the vas.[118,124]

The blood supplies of the vas deferens and the epididymis are closely related. The epididymis receives arterial blood from the internal spermatic artery or the deferential artery, and the vas receives arterial blood from the deferential artery. Venous blood from the epididymis and the lower segments of the vas

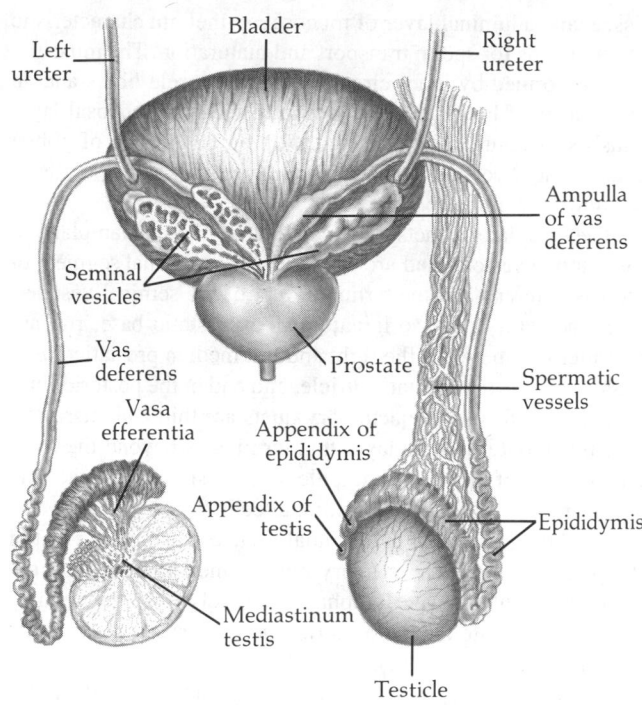

Figure 12-12 Anatomic relation of vas deferens to bladder (posterior view).

drain into the pampiniform plexus of the spermatic cord, which becomes the spermatic vein.[108,118]

The motor innervation of the vas deferens arises from pelvic ganglia near the seminal vesicle. Stimulation of sympathetic preganglionics causes contraction of the vas deferens and movement of seminal fluid. These adrenergic mechanisms are also responsible for contraction of smooth muscle in the bladder neck and posterior urethra, preventing the occurrence of retrograde ejaculation. Cholinergic mechanisms, mediated by parasympathetic pathways, may play an indirect or modulatory role in seminal emission and contraction of the vas deferens in the human. Other central neurotransmitters, such as gamma aminobutyric acid (GABA), prostaglandins, and bradykinins, also may play an as yet undefined modulatory role in contraction of the smooth muscle of the vas deferens.[114]

Seminal vesicles and ejaculatory ducts The seminal vesicles are a pair of saclike structures that lie between the posterior bladder and the rectum. Each vesicle is 4 cm long; they have a pyramidal shape with the superior end oriented laterally and backward from the base. The structure of the seminal vesicles is formed by a single coiled tube that gives rise to irregularly placed diverticula connected by dense fibrous tissue. The diameter of the tube of the seminal vesicle is 3 to 4 mm, and its length is 10 to 15 cm when uncoiled. The seminal vesicles are directed to the posterior bladder surface near the implantation of the ureters and lie in close proximity to the rectum.[75,124]

The walls of the seminal vesicle are composed of an outer areolar layer of connective tissue, a middle layer of muscular tissue, and a luminal layer of mucosal epithelium characteristic of the organs for sperm transport and maturation. The muscular tunic is formed by inner circular smooth muscle fibers and an outer layer of longitudinal smooth muscle. The mucosal layer consists of columnar epithelium with an abundance of goblet cells in the diverticula of the organ and small stellate cells of unknown significance.[124]

The ejaculatory ducts are located along the median plane of the seminal vesicles and are formed by the terminal segment of the vas deferens and the terminal duct of the seminal vesicles. The ejaculatory ducts originate at the prostatic base, run anteroinferiorly between the right and left median prostatic lobes, pass alongside the prostatic utricle, and end in the posterior urethra. The walls of the ejaculatory ducts are thin and characterized by an outer fibrous layer that terminates beyond the prostatic portion of the ducts, a middle layer of smooth muscle, and an inner layer of columnar epithelial cells.[124]

The blood supply of the seminal vesicles is similar to that of the prostate gland. The primary motor innervation arises from sympathetic fibers. The lymphatic channels from the seminal vesicles drain into the hypogastric, sacral, vesical, and external iliac nodes (Figure 12-12).[107]

Prostate   The prostate is a partly glandular, partly fibromuscular organ that lies at the base of the bladder and surrounds the initial 2 to 3 cm of posterior urethra. The prostate is conical with an anterior and posterior flattening; its average dimensions are 3.4 cm long, 4.4 cm wide, and 2.6 cm at its greatest thickness. The organ is securely anchored by the puboprostatic ligaments, Denonvillier's fascia, and the adjacent pelvic floor musculature. In addition, the resilient, strong prostatic capsule provides support.[118]

The structure of the prostate can be divided into lobes,[58] anatomic aspects,[124] and zones.[84] Williams and Warwick[124] conceptualized four anatomic aspects, the base, apex, posterior surface, and anterior aspect. The prostate base is adjacent to the bladder neck. The urethra pierces the prostate at the base, near its anterior aspect. The apex of the prostate faces away from the bladder and inferior to its base; its surface is contiguous with fascia covering the superior aspect of the periurethral muscles of the pelvic floor (sometimes called the urogenital diaphragm). The posterior surface of the prostate is transversely flat and vertically convex. It is separated from the rectum by the prostatic sheath. The superior surface of the prostate is analogous to its median lobe. Its inferior border is marked by a sulcus that defines the border between the right and left lateral lobes.

The prostate also can be divided into zones (Figure 12-13). This classification is based on examination of prostate tissue in different planes and on histologic and embryonic characteristics. There are the central zone, the peripheral zone, transitional zone, and anterior fibromuscular zone. Each of the zones has distinct histologic and embryonic characteristics, and each is prone to different pathologic changes with aging. The transitional zone and peripheral zone originate from the urogenital sinus, and they experience adenomas as the man ages. Frequently, these changes cause voiding dysfunction and obstruc-

tion, the cardinal symptoms of benign prostatic hyperplasia. The peripheral zone is also the site of malignant tumors (prostatic carcinoma), although the transitional zone is not the site of carcinoma. In contrast, the central zone of the prostate is morphologically and embryonically distinct from the peripheral and transitional zones. It is probably mesogenic in origin; and its primary function is thought to be occlusion of the urethral lumen during seminal emission, thereby preventing retrograde ejaculation into the bladder.[118] Although the concept of zonal anatomy of the prostate is not new,[58] ultrasonic examination of the prostate allows identification of the peripheral and transitional zones and the fibromuscular capsule in the clinical setting.

Primarily based on digital rectal examination, clinicians have divided the prostate into lobes.[58] Intraurethral lobes, right and left lateral, anterior, and subcervical lobes have been described. Posterior and median extraurethral lobes also have been described. Enlargement of the right and left lateral prostate lobes produces the symptoms of benign prostatic hyperplasia. In contrast, the presence of asymmetric enlargement, induration or discrete nodules on the posterior lobe is highly suspicious of prostatic carcinoma. While the division of the prostate into lobes may be clinically useful when describing the findings of digital rectal examination, this classification is not based on anatomically or histologically distinct segments of the gland.[118]

The microscopic anatomy of the prostate is characterized by glandular components and fibromuscular components. The fibromuscular capsule sends extensions into the interior of the organ, whose apices converge in the posterior urethral surface. The fibromuscular tissue is primarily nonstriated muscle with a relatively small area of skeletal muscle located ventral to and contiguous with the external urinary sphincter. The bulk of muscular tissue is located in the fibromuscular septa found throughout the gland.[124]

The glandular tissue is composed of numerous follicles with frequent papillary elevations that open into long canals seen throughout the organ. These follicles join to form 12 to 20 excretory ducts. The glandular tissue of the prostate is supported by extensions of muscular tissue and delicate areolar stroma that encapsulate a capillary plexus.

The motor and sensory innervation of the prostate gland arises from the lower segments of the inferior hypogastric plexus and the pelvic plexus. The tone of the bladder neck and prostatic smooth muscle is primarily controlled by α-1 receptors, which are 40 times more abundant in this area as compared to other aspects of the bladder.[72] These adrenergic receptors have been subdivided into α-1A -1B and -1C subtypes (which are predominant in the prostatic smooth muscle).[115] These subdivisions have potential clinical significance in the search to identify a medication that selectively inhibits prostatic smooth and bladder neck tone without producing side effects of postural hypotension and nasal congestion characteristic of current α-blocking medications.

The arterial blood supply of the prostate is derived primarily from branches of the inferior vesical artery, as well as from

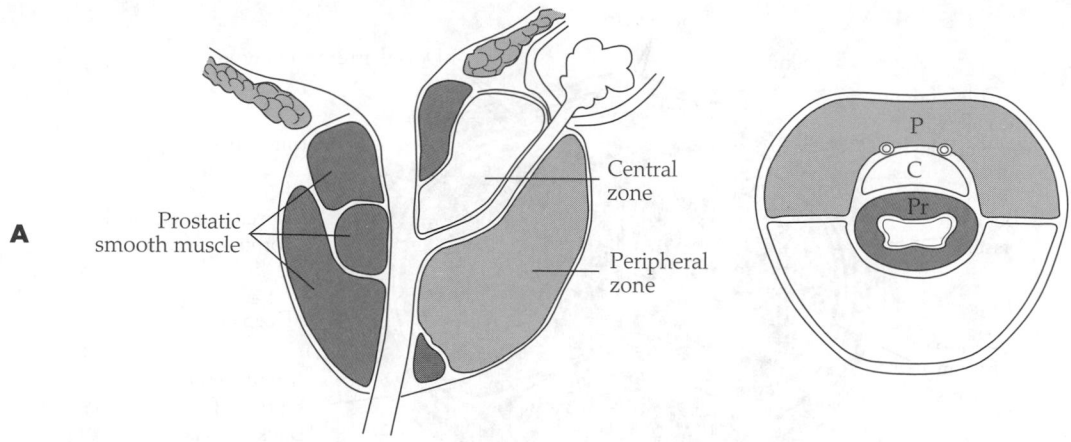

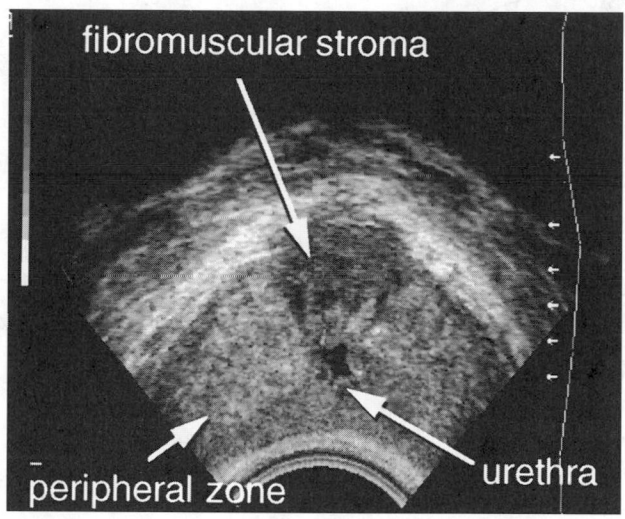

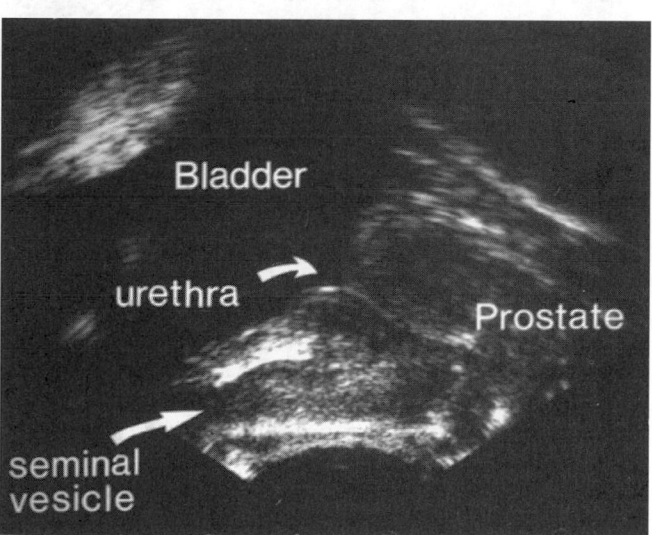

Figure 12-13 **A,** Zonal anatomy of the prostate gland. **B,** Ultrasonic image of a normal prostate in the transverse plane; the peripheral zone and fibromuscular stroma are indicated. **C,** Ultrasonic image of normal prostate in the longitudinal plane. Note the anatomic relations among the bladder, proximal urethra, prostate, and seminal vesicles.

the internal pudendal and middle rectal arteries. Venous blood from the prostate drains into the periprostatic space and the hypogastric vein. Lymphatic drainage exits from the periprostatic plexus located on the surface of the gland before emptying into the external, internal, and/or common iliac nodes.[46]

Penis The penis is a cylindrically shaped organ in its flaccid state that contains two portions: a root that attaches to the perineum and a pendulous portion called the corpus, or body. The root of the penis is attached to the pelvic floor via a continuation of Buck's fascia, the pubic rami (crura of the corpora cavernosa), and the suspensory ligament.[46,118]

The body of the penis contains three elongated bodies of erectile tissue that are capable of considerable enlargement when they become engorged with blood during tumescence (Figure 12-14). The left and right corpora cavernosa form the majority of the substance of the penile body and lie in close approximation to each other. They are surrounded by an extension of the tunica albuginea containing superficial and deep layers. The superficial layer is composed of longitudinally arranged fibers that surround the two corpora cavernosa as a unit; the deep layer is composed of circularly arranged fibers that encase each corpus separately via a fibrous septum that forms two median grooves of anatomic significance. The median groove houses the corpus spongiosum and pendulous urethra; the smaller median groove houses the deep dorsal veins. The corpora cavernosa do not reach the distal end of the penis; instead, they terminate in the proximal portion of the glans.[127]

The corpus spongiosum lies inferior to the corpora cavernosa and is pierced throughout its length by the urethra. It is smaller than the paired corpora cavernosa and is surrounded by a reflection of the tunica albuginea.[124]

The skin of the penis is characterized by its thinness, relatively dark color, and loose connection with the underlying fascia. At the distal portion of the penis, the skin is folded over on

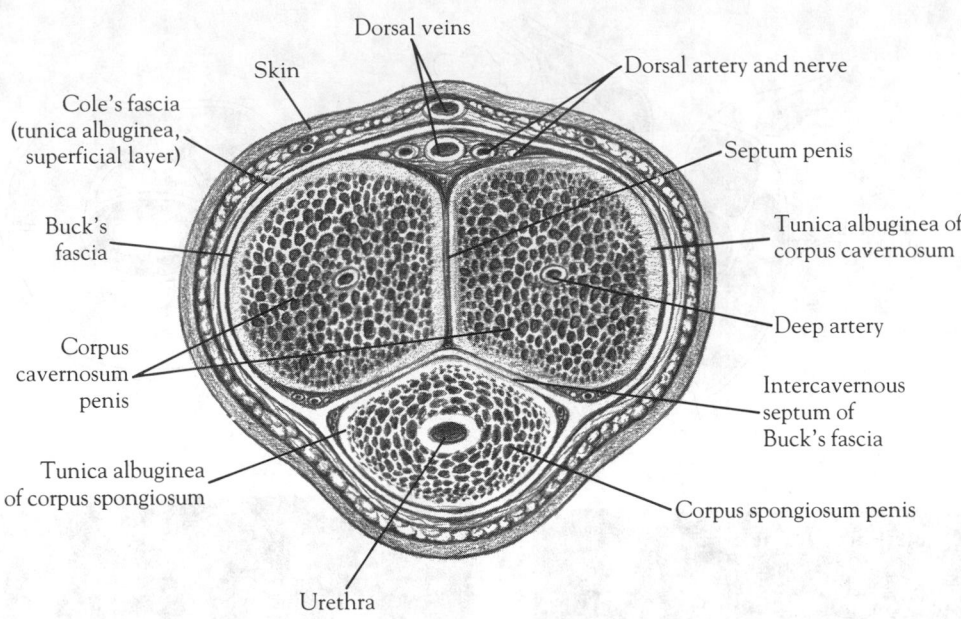

Figure 12-14 Cross section of human penis.

itself to form the foreskin covering the glans penis. The glans penis covers the distal portion of the corpora cavernosa and forms their terminal connection. It is pierced by the navicularis fossa of the urethra, which ends at a dorsal slit found on the interior surface of the glans.[124]

The superficial fascia of the penis is characterized by loose areolar tissue and is devoid of fat. A few fibers of dartos muscle from the scrotum are present, as are fibers from the fundiform ligament and the suspensory ligament.[124]

The arterial blood supply of the penis arises primarily from the internal pudendal artery, which branches into the dorsal arteries of the penis to supply the deep structures of the organ. The penile skin also receives arterial blood from the external pudendal and femoral arteries.[46,118]

The venous drainage of the penis can be divided into deep and superficial groups. The deep veins of the penis drain the erectile bodies via the deep dorsal veins, which empty into the plexus of Santorini and ultimately into the hypogastric vein. The superficial veins of the penis drain venous blood from the skin via the superficial dorsal penile veins that empty into the saphenous vein.[46,118]

The lymphatic drainage of the penis is also divided into deep and superficial groups. Deep lymphatic channels of the penis are drained by the subinguinal nodes and the external iliac nodes. Superficial lymphatic channels drain into the superficial inguinal nodes.[46,118]

The nerve supply of the penis has a somatic and an autonomic component. Sensory innervation of the penile skin arises from the pudendal nerve, which has its roots in spinal segments S2 to S4. Motor innervation to the corpus spongiosum and corpora cavernosa arises from the pelvic nerves, which also have their spinal roots at S2 to S4. Sympathetic fibers from the tho-

racolumbar spinal cord supply the penile vessels and are particularly evident in the vascular component of the corpus spongiosum.[67]

Male Reproductive Function

Spermatogenesis and hormonal regulation The testes, epididymis, vas deferens, seminal vesicles, and prostate gland function as a coordinated unit to ensure the production, maturation, and transport of sperm from the male urethra to the female vaginal tract necessary for propagation of the species. Male reproductive functions are regulated by a hormonal axis that consists of certain extrahypothalamic central nervous system centers, the hypothalamus, pituitary, testes, and gonadal-sensitive end organs.[60,118]

Extrahypothalamic central nervous system centers are assumed to play an inhibitory and augmentative role in reproduction. The precise interactions by which brain centers influence the male reproductive hormonal axis are unclear, but a correlation between reproductive function and testicular function is postulated.[118]

The more clearly elucidated hormonal axis governing male reproductive function originates in the hypothalamus, where a luteinizing hormone–releasing hormone (LHRH) is produced and travels to the median eminence of the adenohypophysis via a venous portal system. The presence of this releasing factor in the pituitary results in the direct stimulation of luteinizing hormone (LH) and is thought to stimulate the release of follicle-stimulating hormone (FSH).[46,118]

Both FSH and LH act at receptor sites in the testes to stimulate the gonadal androgens (primarily testosterone and dihydrotestosterone). LH directly stimulates the Sertoli cells to produce testosterone and stimulate spermatogenesis. FSH is not necessary for the production of testosterone, although it does play a role in spermatogenic testicular function. FSH and LH are released sporadically in response to feedback from the hypothalamic-pituitary-gonadal hormonal axis. When blood levels of the gonadal androgens increase, the production of LHRH in the hypothalamus is inhibited, which suppresses the production of LH by the pituitary. Conversely, decreased serum levels of gonadal androgens stimulate the hypothalamus to produce LRHR so that more LH is produced and excreted into the systemic circulation. The feedback loop for FSH production is not entirely understood; increased levels of testosterone and estradiol exert negative feedback on the production of FSH. In addition, a substance called inhibin, which is produced in the germinal epithelium of the testes, is postulated to inhibit FSH, although its physiologic significance is unclear.[24,60]

The gonadal androgens are essential to the genesis, support, and maturation of spermatozoa. In addition to this direct role in male reproductive function, certain androgens, primarily testosterone and dihydrotestosterone, cause the development and maintenance of the secondary male sex characteristics that characterize pubescence.[24,76]

The process of spermatogenesis occurs within the seminiferous tubule in the testis and is conceptualized in three phases. During the first phase the more primitive spermatogonia enlarge and undergo mitotic divisions into primary spermatocytes that contain 92 chromosomes. The second phase is characterized by two consecutive meiotic divisions accompanied by only one duplication of chromosomes so that the final product of this phase is four spermatids that contain a haploid number of chromosomes suitable for union with the ovum. The third phase of spermatogenesis—spermiogenesis—marks the transformation of spermatid to spermatozoon.[80]

The process of spermiogenesis is relatively slow; it requires 74 days to complete and is divided into four phases. The first phase is the Golgi phase when small granules of hyaluronidase, proteases, and other substances form a single large acrosomal granule enclosed within a vesicle that attaches to the nuclear membrane at the site of the future sperm head. During the second phase a cap appears around the acrosomal vesicle. The two centrioles of the spermatid now begin to move; the proximal centriole assumes a position at the posterior pole of the nucleus opposite the acrosomal sac and the distal centriole sprouts a flagellum consisting of two central microtubules and nine surrounding pairs of microtubules. The distal centriole will become the tail of the future spermatozoon. The third stage of spermiogenesis is the acrosomal phase, in which the developing sperm cell undergoes extensive metamorphosis so that the acrosome, nucleus, flagellum, and cytoplasm assume the characteristic appearance of the mature spermatozoon. During the acrosomal phase a mitochondrial sheath is formed to supply energy for the tail of the mature sperm when it becomes motile after ejaculation. The final stage of spermiogenesis is the maturation phase, which is characterized by the completion of the tail of the spermatozoon and the shedding of excess cytoplasm with the assistance of the Sertoli cells (Figure 12-15).[51,80]

Transport of the sperm from the seminiferous tubule occurs via the muscular activity of the tubules and fluid movement. Al-

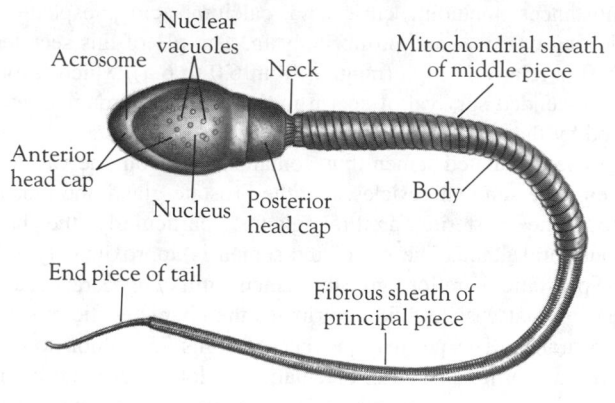

Figure 12-15 Mature spermatozoon cell.

though the sperm that enter the epididymis are mature in appearance, they are not yet capable of motility and not yet able to fertilize an ovum. Thus the epididymis also plays a necessary role in the maturation of sperm. The transit time of sperm through the relatively short epididymis is 12 days. The structure of the epididymis allows slow transit resulting from the slow peristaltic-like activity of the smooth muscle of the organ and the ciliary action of the efferent ductules. During the time spent within the epididymis, sperm gain the potential for motility, although a substance in the tubular fluid prevents sperm from becoming motile before ejaculation. Although the process by which this maturation occurs is not known, the epididymis is thought to play an active role under the influence of the gonadal androgens (primarily testosterone). The probable maturational functions provided by the epididymis are manipulation of the sodium ion, potassium ion, and chloride ion concentrations in the fluid in the epididymal tubule and the secretion of a variety of compounds such as glycerylphosphorylchlorine and glycoproteins, which are thought to enhance maturation of the spermatozoa.[51,118]

The epididymis also serves as a storage compartment for sperm. The cauda epididymis may store sperm for a period of several weeks, although the storage time in a man who is extremely sexually active is a matter of hours.[46,118]

After exiting the epididymis the sperm enters the vas deferens in response to smooth muscle contraction associated with ejaculation. Sperm is carried into the ejaculatory ducts where it is mixed with the nutritive secretions of the seminal vesicles. The seminal vesicles do not, as their name implies, serve as storage compartments for sperm; rather, they secrete a mucoid fluid rich with fructose and other nutritive substances into the ejaculatory duct after the vas deferens empties itself of sperm. In addition to their nutritive support, the seminal vesicles add prostaglandins to the ejaculate that are thought to aid in fertilization of the ovum.[51]

The prostate also supports the male reproductive act by adding its secretions to the ejaculate. During ejaculation the prostatic capsule contracts in synchrony with the vas deferens and secretes a thin, milky fluid that contains a variety of substances, including citric acid, calcium, acid phosphate, a clotting enzyme, and profibrinolysin. The pH of this secreted fluid is relatively high (ranging from 6.0 to 6.5), which favors the extended survival of sperm in the acidic environment created by the vaginal mucosa.[51]

The ejaculated semen thus contains fluid from the vas deferens, the seminal vesicles, and the prostate gland, the mucus from the posterior urethral glands, particularly the bulbourethral gland. The pH of the semen is approximately 7.5; the prostatic secretions give the semen a milky appearance, and the seminal vesicle fluid contributes the characteristic mucoid appearance. The normal ejaculate contains 75 million to 400 million sperm cells. After ejaculation a clotting enzyme in the semen interacts with profibrinolysin contributed by the prostate to form a weak coagulum. When this dissolves, the sperm gain their maximal motility as each seeks to fertilize an ovum. Although the sperm cell can survive several months in the male genital ducts, it can survive only 12 to 24 hours in the female genital tract after ejaculation. The relatively short life of sperm in the female genital tract is primarily the result of the acidic nature of the vaginal and fallopian mucosa.[51]

Physiology of penile erections   In addition to serving as a conduit for the expulsion of urine and semen, the penis is capable of generating an erection of sufficient duration and rigidity to penetrate the female's vagina and effect impregnation. Tumescence in the male is the direct result of neurovascular events and is modulated by central and peripheral nervous systems, as well as by the endocrine system.

The neurovascular events that produce an erection begin with an increase in arterial inflow through the arterioles of the cavernosal bodies. The vascular smooth muscle of these arterioles is controlled by the autonomic nervous system. Parasympathetic nerves originate from the spinal segments S2 to S4 and reach the penis via the pelvic plexus. Sympathetic input arises at spinal segments T11 to L2, and somatic signals travel via the pudendal nerve to sacral segments 2 to 4. The neurotransmitters that mediate penile erection are not entirely understood, but progress has been made toward resolving this question. Acetylcholine, released from muscarinic receptors in the corpus cavernosal bodies, plays a role in tumescence. Its effects, however, do not account for the process of erection or detumescence in the human.[113] De Tejada et al.[31] observed the effects of an endothelium-derived releasing factor that increases the inflow of blood into the corpus cavernosa. The biologic effects of this relaxing factor are probably mediated by the synthesis of nitric oxide and the presence of arachidonic acid, prostacyclin, and endothelin. In addition to these substances, the corpus cavernosum is capable of synthesizing prostaglandins that mediate the vascular response of local arterioles and sinusoids within the corpus cavernosum. Prostaglandin E_1 and E_2 act as vasodilators when injected into the corpus cavernosum of the penis. Prostaglandin I_2 enhances tumescence and arterial inflow by inhibiting adrenergic mechanisms.[113,117]

Detumescence is primarily mediated by α-adrenergic receptors that arise from the sympathetic nervous system. Alpha-adrenergic receptors are found in the cavernosal bodies of the penis. Excitation of these receptors produces contraction of the smooth muscle in the arteriolar wall, reduction of arterial inflow into the penis, and detumescence.[113]

Initially the increased volume will slightly enhance penile length and width as the compliant sinusoidal spaces in the corporal bodies are filled. Nonetheless, after the relatively small cavernous space is filled, penile rigidity and pressure increase rapidly as the engorged sinusoids press against the stiff, noncompliant fibrous covering of the corporal body. This rigidity is maintained by venous occlusion.

Three mechanisms of venous occlusion have been proposed. Active contraction of smooth muscle in the walls of the cavernosal veins may partially restrict outflow; the neurologic mechanisms that regulate this process remain uncertain. Valves have been observed in the veins of the corporal bodies; they may serve to prevent the rapid outflow of blood during tumescence. Mechanical occlusion of the veins also may contribute to the maintenance of an erection; as the sinusoidal spaces expand, venules in the corpora cavernosa are constricted, restricting venous outflow.[49]

Erectile function in the male relies on more than the neurovascular events that lead to a single episode of tumescence. Rather, penile tumescence requires the coordination of the central nervous system, peripheral nervous system, and neuroendocrine mechanisms. The motor activity of the corpora cavernosa is modulated by the autonomic nervous system, and stimulation of the pelvic nerve produces an erection. The pelvic plexus is only the preganglionic portion of the neural tract; thus infusion of atropine does not ablate an erection. The neurotransmitter substance at the postganglionic nerve in the corpora is unknown. Sympathetic fibers are present in the penile vasculature and are particularly prominent in the corpus spongiosum. Stimulation of sympathetic fibers produces vascular constriction but not erection. The significance of adrenergic fibers in the corpora cavernosa has not been fully appreciated, although they are thought to assume an active role in erectile activity.[67]

The spinal cord is important to male sexual function, since it is the origin of the autonomic outflow for the penis. Because both the sympathetic and parasympathetic nervous systems play a role in erections, injury to the spinal cord produces variations of erectile dysfunction. Injury to the sacral spinal cord is not always connected with impotence. Approximately one third of such patients are able to generate erections using psychogenic stimuli. If the spinal cord is injured, volitional erections are abolished but reflex erections are noted in response to local stimuli.[67]

The brain directly affects penile erections, as well as controlling male sexual behavior. A number of brain centers have been found to influence erectile activity, including the temporal lobes, the gyrus rectus of the cerebral cortex, the cingulate gyrus, the hypothalamus, the mammillary bodies, and the hippocampus. The hippocampus and cingulate gyrus influence emotional responses and communicate with the hypothalamus. The mammillary bodies and cingulate gyrus process visual stimuli; the gyrus rectus processes olfactory stimuli. The precise mechanisms through which the brain affects penile erections and human sexuality are complex and poorly understood.[67]

The neuroendocrine mechanisms that influence erectile activity are also poorly understood. Male sexual activity is decreased by serotonin activity and increased by dopamine activity. Male sexual activity is also affected by the presence of testosterone. Castration is connected with decreased sexual function, although it does not preclude the ability to produce an erection.[67,118]

Abosief and Lue[1a] have described six stages of an erection. Phase 1 is the flaccid state characterized by an equilibrium between arterial inflow and venous outflow that is sufficient to meet the metabolic and nutritional needs of local structures in the cavernous body. Concentrations of arterial blood gases in the corporal body are equivalent to those of other peripheral tissues during the flaccid stage. During the second (latent) phase of tumescence the smooth muscles of the penile arterioles relax, allowing an increased inflow of blood under the control of the autonomic nervous system that is influenced by the central nervous and endocrine systems. During this phase the intracavernous pressures remains unchanged; however, the volume of blood in the cavernous body increases, causing elongation of the penis. The third (tumescent) phase of tumescence begins when an increasing blood volume completely fills the cavernous body, compressing Buck's fascia. Pressure will rapidly rise and the penis will gain length, width, and rigidity. During the fourth (full erection) phase, intracavernous pressure rises to near mean arterial pressure, and the blood gases remain comparable to peripheral arterial levels. During the fifth (rigid erection) phase the ischiocavernous muscle contracts and cavernous pressure briefly exceeds mean arterial pressure, causing blood gases in the cavernous body to fall below systemic values. This phase is brief, causing no harm in the normally functioning system; however, prolonged, irreversible erection may be dangerous. The sixth (detumescent) phase is characterized by increasing sympathetic tone in the arteriolar smooth muscles that restricts blood flow to the penis. This initial fall in pressure is precipitous and followed by a more gradual decline and a return to the flaccid state.

■ NORMAL FINDINGS

Kidney Overlying skin: edema, bulges, and masses in abdomen absent; palpable only with deep inspiration; typically nonpalpable in obese or muscularly developed persons; smooth, nontender; costovertebral angle tenderness: absent; bruit over costovertebral area or upper abdominal quadrants: absent; transillumination with darkened room and fiberoptic light source: absent

Bladder Noted as bulge in abdomen when vesicle contains 500 ml or more urine; noted as dull area under suprapubic skin when vesicle is filled with 150 ml or more urine; inspection of voiding act: steady, straight stream, no spraying, no adominal straining; postvoid dribble absent; postvoid

residual: less than 20% of total bladder volume; *older adult:* decreased force of stream compared to younger adult years; absent split stream, spraying, and postvoid dribble

Penis Skin: may be darker than surrounding integument; ulcers, warts, indurated nodules: absent; foreskin: retractable over glans penis; absent in circumcised males; glans penis: hairless, sagittal slit near apex; penile shaft: absent nontender plaques beneath surface in flaccid state; erect state: even firmness and rigidity over both corpora cavernosa; straight line described between root of penis and glans penis; *older adult:* decreased rigidity to corpora cavernosa compared to younger adult years; lateral curvature: absent

Scrotum Skin: rugae; hair bearing and loosely mobile; sebaceous cysts: absent; testes: firm, nontender to gentle palpation; masses: absent; *older adult:* testes: softer to palpation than in younger adult years; epididymis: palpable as comma-shaped structure on posterior aspect of testes; no tenderness, masses, or nodules; spermatic cord: rolled between thumb and forefinger; vas deferens palpable but nontender; varicocele: absent; transillumination: no edema or solid masses that will transilluminate

Prostate Posterior aspect of organ accessible beneath anterior rectal wall; two firm, nontender, symmetric, rounded lobes separated by median sulcus (heart shaped and 2.5 cm long): projects into rectal lumen 1 cm or less; hard, irregular nodes: absent; *older adult:* increased bogginess noted on digital examination; seen with benign hypertrophy of organ; asymmetric changes in lobe size or discrete nodules: absent

CONDITIONS, DISEASES, AND DISORDERS

URINARY TRACT DISORDERS

■ CYSTITIS

Cystitis is an inflammation of the bladder wall. Many causative agents, including bacteria, viruses, fungi, chemical agents, and radiation exposure, may result in cystitis. The term is often used synonymously with urinary tract infection, although they are not strictly identical. Urinary tract infection is a nonspecific term that may be used to refer to infection anywhere in the urinary tract. Urethritis refers to inflammation of the urethra (see Chapter 15). Pyelonephritis refers to infection of the kidney and renal pelvis (see Chapter 11). Within the context of this discussion, cystitis is used in preference to the more vaguely defined concept of urinary tract infection.

The occurrence of infection in the urinary tract is second only to respiratory tract infections.[100] Infection of the urinary bladder is the most common focus of inflammation in the urinary tract. Women are particularly prone to symptomatic bacteriuria resulting in cystitis. A study of Jamaican women revealed that 2% of those between 15 and 24 years of age had bacteriuria on culture. Stamey[111] found that the prevalence of bacterial cystitis in women increased approximately 1% to 2% during each subsequent decade of life until reaching 10% among 54- to 64-year-old women. Gaymans and associates[43] corroborated these findings in a prospective study of 1758 Dutch women that revealed a 2.7% prevalence of bacteriuria among those 15 to 24 years of age and 9.3% among those 65 years of age and older. Among the general population, a woman can expect a 10% to 20% chance of having at least one episode of cystitis during her lifetime.[111]

Pregnant women and hospitalized women have an increased incidence of urinary tract infection. Among pregnant women the rate of cystitis is approximately 4% to 6%; studies have demonstrated an incidence of urinary tract infection as high as 30% among hospitalized women.[111]

In addition to a greater susceptibility to bacterial cystitis, women are more likely to have interstitial cystitis than are men. A study in Finland found that the prevalence of interstitial cystitis was 10.6:100,000 with a 10:1 preference of the disease for women.[53] Leach[69] and Raz[96] also report an incidence of 20:100,000 cases of interstitial cystitis among women, with a ratio of 10 cases in women for every case reported among men.

The incidence of cystitis among men has not been extensively studied but is generally thought to occur in only 10% as many men as women. Unlike in women, most cases of bacteriuria in men occur as a result of some known infectious focus such as bacterial prostatitis or urinary calculi.[46,118]

Clearly, the most significant rate of cystitis, resulting in an alarming incidence of associated morbidity and mortality, is that associated with nosocomial urinary tract infection in the presence of an indwelling catheter. In a prospective study of 1458 patients in the United States, 131 patients acquired 136 urinary tract infections during 1474 indwelling bladder catheterizations. Among those studied, 12 deaths may have been caused by acquired urinary tract infections, and another 10 patients died with a retrospective clinical picture compatible with serious infection, although no conclusive culture data were available. Thus the authors concluded that acquisition of a nosocomial urinary tract infection was associated with a three-fold increase in death rate (see Emergency Alert box).[94]

•••••• Pathophysiology

The pathogenesis of cystitis depends on the causative agent. In this discussion cystitis is divided into three categories:

Infectious cystitis
    Bacterial
    Viral
    Fungal
    Tubercular
    Parasitic
Chemotherapy- and radiation-induced cystitis
Inflammatory lesions of the bladder
    Cystitis cystica
    Cystitis glandularis

    Eosinophilic cystitis
    Cystitis emphysematosa
    Interstitial cystitis

Bacterial cystitis is the most common form of infectious cystitis. The most common causative pathogen in both women and men is *Escherichia coli.* Other common pathogens include strains of *Klebsiella, Enterobacter, Proteus, Pseudomonas,* and *Serratia;* gram-positive organisms such as staphylococci and streptococci are occasionally seen.[118]

The three routes of bacterial invasion into the bladder are ascension through the urethra, the hematogenous route, and via lymphatic channels; the most common is the ascending urethral pathway. Bacteria are commonly forced into the bladder without necessarily resulting in infection. The determinants of bacterial cystitis depend on the virulence and inoculum size of invasive bacteria and the adequacy of the host's defense mechanisms. Data concerning the number of bacteria needed to produce a bladder infection are based solely on animal studies, which show that an extremely large inoculum (over 1 million) is needed to produce cystitis if host defense mechanisms are not compromised. Fortunately, normal numbers of bacteria that enter the bladder through the urethra are considerably smaller (fewer than 100).[62]

The human body has two primary defense mechanisms that oppose the establishment of infection when bacteria enter the bladder. The first is the urine itself, which is bacteriostatic or bactericidal to the most common pathogens associated with cystitis, such as *E. coli* and a number of other anaerobic bacteria commonly found in urethral flora. The efficiency of this

EMERGENCY ALERT

Septic Shock

Septic shock is classified as a vasogenic shock in which severe vasodilation occurs. Commonly, septic shock results from overwhelming infection. Typically, blood volume is normal but fluids have shifted into dilated vessels. Mortality ranges from 30% to 50%.

Assessment

- Evaluate for decreased blood pressure, elevated pulse, and temperature.
- Evaluate for chills, tremors with warm, dry skin.
- Evaluate for nausea, vomiting, diarrhea.
- Evaluate decreased level of consciousness.
- Evaluate increased cardiac output, metabolic acidosis.

Interventions

- Maintain airway, breathing, and circulation.
- Administer high flow oxygen (10-15 L) by mask.
- Obtain IV access.
- In collaboration with physician, administer antibiotics and fluids.
- Collect laboratory specimens, including blood and fluid cultures.
- Administration of dopamine, naloxone, or corticosteroids as ordered.

antibacterial activity depends on the size of the bacterial inoculum, the osmolality of the urine, and the concentration of urea nitrogen and ammonium in the urine. A urinary pH of 6.0 or greater adversely affects antibacterial activity, but the presence of specific antibodies in the urine such as IgA and IgG has not been shown to cause significant effects.[62]

The bladder wall is the second line of defense for bacterial invasion from the urethra, bloodstream, or lymphatic route. Inflammatory changes within the bladder wall are apparent within 30 minutes of invasion when polymorphonucleocytes (PMNs) begin to migrate to the bladder mucosa. Within 2 hours the entire mucosal lining is injected by PMNs, and significant antibacterial activity is measurable by the fourth hour. Inspection at 24 hours reveals clumps of PMNs throughout the mucosal lining, and urine culture is negative.[62]

Perhaps the most important defense against bacterial cystitis is the unobstructed flow of urine throughout the urinary tract and regular, complete evacuation of the bladder. This important concept is the basis of the rationale for clean intermittent catheterization. Regular emptying of the bladder flushes bacteria that would ultimately colonize the urine if allowed to remain within the bladder.[62]

Abnormalities that interfere with natural host defenses against urinary tract infection include the presence of residual urine, which provides an opportunity for bacteria to reproduce and overwhelm other inherent antibacterial mechanisms. Vesicoureteral reflux also compromises the body's defense mechanisms by allowing the spread of bacteria from the urine into the upper tracts and possibly into the renal parenchyma. Urinary calculi are often obstructive to urinary outflow and serve as a nidus for infection during antibiotic therapy. In addition, any disease or circumstance that interferes with the body's immune system decreases the efficiency of the bladder wall's reaction to bacteriuria.[62]

Women are particularly susceptible to bacterial cystitis for a number of reasons. Stamey[111] studied the problem of bacterial cystitis in women and concluded that much of the nomenclature used to describe the condition does not adequately define this condition. He described four bacteriurial states in women: first infection, unresolved bacteriuria during therapy, bacterial persistence, and reinfection (recurrence).

The etiology of first infection is unclear but is presumed to be similar to reinfections. Unlike recurrent episodes of cystitis, bacteria from the first infection are typically sensitive to any antibiotic and are unlikely to recur within 2 to 3 years unless other predisposing factors are present.[118]

Unresolved bacteriuria during therapy may arise from several causes. The bacteria may be resistant to the antibiotic chosen for therapy, or selection of a secondary strain may become predominant as the primary form of bacteria is eliminated. In approximately 6% of patients treated, resistant, mutant bacteria develop and proliferate. Renal insufficiency may cause inadequate concentrations of antibiotic in the urinary tract, although the correct agent has been chosen. A staghorn calculus may be large enough to support a critical mass of bacteria too great for antibiotics to resolve.[118]

True bacterial persistence may arise after 5 to 10 days of therapy, resulting in culture-proven nonsterile urine from one of two causes. Men with chronic bacterial prostatitis have a persistent focus for ascending urethral infection from the prostatic ductal system. Women or men with struvite stones in the urinary tract have a site of persistent bacteria even after antibiotic therapy.[118]

Reinfection of the bladder accounts for the majority of occurrences of bacterial cystitis among women. The most common route for bacteria to gain access to the bladder is from the urethra. The colonization of the urethra arises from the vaginal introitus and vestibule rather than from the rectum, as is commonly assumed. Longitudinal studies show that cultures of the vaginal vestibule and distal urethral mucosa are more predictive of recurrent bacterial cystitis than analysis of rectal flora. Ascending infection in the female is particularly problematic because of the relatively short, straight course of the urethra and plentiful flora in the genital area. The relationship between vaginal flora and urethral bacteria is further supported by examining the close anatomic relationship of these two structures, which are confined by the distal labia minora.[111]

The role of sexual intercourse in recurrent urinary infections has been studied repeatedly. Sexual intercourse is associated with an increased incidence of recurrent urinary tract infections, and some women specifically correlate intercourse and recurrence. It is interesting to note that nuns have a 0.4% to 1.6% incidence of urinary tract infection, which is lower than the general population, and that married women have a higher incidence than single women. Although sexual intercourse does not cause bacterial cystitis, it does promote the milking of bacteria into the bladder and can cause inner urethral injury that may result in infection among women predisposed to the condition.[111]

Changes in the urinary tract unique to pregnancy also increase a woman's likelihood for having recurring urinary tract infections or experiencing a first infection of the bladder. The primary urologic change noted with pregnancy is the "physiologic hydroureter of pregnancy," which is the reversible dilation of the ureters and renal pelvis. This dilation often begins as early as the seventh week of gestation and progresses until delivery. The right ureter is more extensively affected than the left, and ureteral peristalsis is significantly slowed after the second month of gestation so that intraureteral volume may be as great as 25 times normal.[7]

Bacteriuria is more common among pregnant women than in nonpregnant women in the same age group. The presence of ureteral dilation may play a role in this increased incidence. It is known that pregnant women with bacteriuria are at a significantly increased risk (20% to 40%) for developing pyelonephritis and that this risk is dramatically reduced by treating the bladder infection. In addition, catheterization during pregnancy is associated with increased risk of subsequent bacterial cystitis. Although the association between premature delivery and pyelonephritis is well documented, no correlation exists between bacteriuria and premature delivery.[7]

Bacterial cystitis is likely to result in urinary frequency, urgency, and dysuria. Women in particular may complain of suprapubic discomfort and a feeling of pressure in the perineal area. Nocturia and low back pain are also caused by bladder infection. Urge incontinence may take the form of detrusor instability with subsequent painful bladder "spasms" and associated leakage, or it may occur as urethral instability allowing urine passage into the posterior urethra and causing a perception of intense urgency and urinary leakage. Gross hematuria, chills, fever, and flank pain occur only occasionally in the presence of cystitis unless it is also associated with pyelonephritis. Approximately half of patients with significant bacteriuria are asymptomatic. Women with dysuria and frequency who have no bacteriuria or a colony count of fewer than 10,000/ml are typically diagnosed as having an "acute urethral syndrome."[111]

Cystitis caused by fungal infection is much less prevalent than bacterial cystitis, but its incidence and recognition have greatly increased within the past 25 years. The most common fungal infection of the bladder is candidiasis. *Candida* is endemic to the human body and can often be found in the pharynx, stomach, intestinal tract, and vaginal vault (particularly in pregnant women). The increasing incidence of candidal overgrowth is related to the use of antibiotics. Administration of antibiotics is thought to stimulate the production of *C. albicans* by altering the pH of gastrointestinal mucosa, suppressing normal bacterial flora that competes with the fungus for food, and inhibiting polymorphonuclear phagocytosis, which helps the body guard against overgrowth.

The body's defenses against candidal infection of the urinary tract include the presence of normal bacterial flora that inhibit fungal growth and the presence of PMNs in the mucosa of the urethra and bladder, which have marked anticandidal effects. In addition, prostatic fluid in the male is fungicidal, which helps explain the relatively low incidence of candidal cystitis in males compared to females. Cell-mediated immunity and other white blood cells also help the body prevent candidiasis.[118]

Candidal cystitis often occurs in the presence of predisposing factors such as diabetes mellitus, obstructive prostatic enlargement, and pregnancy and is often noted after the patient has undergone antibiotic therapy for bacterial infection. Symptoms are similar to those of bacterial cystitis and include urgency, marked frequency, dysuria, suprapubic pain, and nocturia. Pneumaturia (the expression of gas or air through the urethra during or after micturition) may be seen. The mucosal lining of the bladder is marked by grayish white spots that result in mucosal bleeding if removed. The ureteral orifices may be affected so that cystoscopic findings may resemble tubercular infection of the bladder. In certain cases asymptomatic candidal colonization of the urine without inflammation of the bladder may be seen.[118]

Tuberculosis of the bladder results from the implantation of the tubercle bacilli into the wall, causing an uneven mix of inflamed areas interspersed with normal mucosal segments. The cystoscopic picture of the bladder may resemble interstitial cystitis or candidal infection with patches of inflamed tissue and reddened ureteral orifices. The anterior urethra is not affected by the infection, but the posterior urethra and prostate are heavily involved in men, representing progression from prostate to bladder. The trigone is relatively spared from inflammatory changes, but the dome of the bladder is extensively affected, resulting in a marked loss in capacity.[118]

The primary symptom of tubercular cystitis is marked frequency and urgency. Bladder volume rapidly decreases and may result in irreversible changes in advanced stages of the infection.[118] Urodynamic assessment in advanced cases may reveal poor compliance of the bladder wall and a functional capacity of 60 ml of urine or less.

Although schistosomiasis is relatively rare in the United States, it is relatively common elsewhere in the world. The ova of this parasite enter the bloodstream via penetration of the skin. The veins of the bladder are a popular breeding site for the parasites. The eggs are then extruded into the vesicle for further spread of the parasitic organisms. The healing of the affected areas of the bladder causes thickening and contraction of the bladder wall. Damage of the ureterovesical junction often occurs, resulting in vesicoureteral reflux. Contracted bands mar the bladder and may extend into the lower ureter. Urinary calculi may be present because of urinary stasis and presence of ova in the urine.[98]

Chemotherapy- or radiation-induced cystitis is characterized by inflammatory changes in the bladder wall in the absence of infection. The symptoms are similar to those of infectious cystitis and include urgency, frequency, and suprapubic pain. Detrusor instability and urge incontinence may occur.[57,109]

Although the bladder is relatively resistant to radiation, therapeutic doses greater than 6000 to 7000 rad over a 6- to 7-week period may result in cystitis. The bladder's tolerance to radiation is significantly compromised if schistosomiasis is present. Chemotherapy-induced cystitis may arise from systemic cyclophosphamide (Cytoxan) or intravesical antineoplastic drugs such as mitomycin. Diagnosis is made when symptoms of cystitis are reported in the presence of a normal culture and positive history of exposure to radiation or a chemotherapeutic agent.[57,109]

Cystitis cystica occurs as a result of chronic infection of the bladder or recurrent episodes of cystitis. It is characterized by cysts seen mostly near the base of the bladder and trigone. These cysts are approximately 1 cm in diameter, have a rounded shape, and may extend into the upper urinary tract. The lesions are benign, and the etiology of the condition is unknown. Because of the gross similarities between these lesions and malignancies of the bladder, biopsy is indicated to rule out cancer.[97]

Cystitis glandularis is a relatively rare, potentially premalignant lesion associated with adenocarcinoma of the bladder. This form of cystitis is particularly common among patients with a history of bladder exstrophy and pelvic lipomatosis. Biopsy is done to rule out malignancy, and follow-up examination for potential cancer of the bladder is recommended.[100]

Eosinophilic cystitis is a severe inflammatory lesion of the bladder that is thought to have an allergic etiology. The bladder mucosa is extensively invaded by eosinophils and exhibits multiple polypoid lesions. The associated signs and symptoms of cystitis are particularly severe.[97]

Cystitis emphysematosa is a rare form of bladder inflammation resulting from infection by gas-forming urinary bacteria or (more commonly) vesicoenteric fistula. The condition may also be observed after urologic instrumentation or urodynamic testing using carbon dioxide. Pneumaturia is associated with this form of cystitis.[97]

•••••• Diagnostic Studies and Findings

Urine culture and sensitivity Greater than 100,000 Colony Forming Units (CFU)/ml bacterial colonies on an agar culture plate or tube indicates clinically significant bacteriuria and associated cystitis; sensitivity discs indicate bacterial sensitivity, intermediate sensitivity, or resistance to a given antibiotic agent; urine culture negative in other forms of infectious cystitis and cystitis caused by chemotherapy and radiotherapy.

Urinalysis Color: dark yellow or pinkish red, cloudy with or without sediment; nitrate/nitrite: positive in bacterial cystitis; glucose oxidase: positive in bacterial infection; catalase: positive in bacterial cystitis; microscopic examination: positive for bacteria, fungus, and parasites in the various forms of infectious cystitis; positive for esoinophils in eosinophilic cystitis; greater than 7 WBCs per high-power field in infectious cystitis; red blood cells with or without gross hematuria

Cystoscopy Red, inflamed bladder wall; reddened, swollen trigone; ureteral orifices may be inflamed; hemorrhagic patches in urothelial lining; findings for specific inflammatory lesions of the bladder described under "Pathophysiology"

Biopsy Cystitis cystica: negative; cystitis glandularis: negative or positive for adenocarcinoma of bladder; eosinophilic cystitis: extensive infiltration of eosinophils into bladder tissues; interstitial cystitis: chronic inflammation with extensive invasion of lymphocytes and other white blood cells into submucosa of bladder wall

Urodynamics Infectious cystitis: urodynamic testing typically contraindicated; tubercular cystitis: decreased functional capacity with poor compliance of bladder wall; detrusor unstable or areflexic; sensory urgency present; chemotherapy- or radiation-induced cystitis: sensory urgency with decreased functional capacity; detrusor instability may be present; compliance of bladder wall may be normal or impaired

Voiding cystourethrogram (VCUG) Cystitis emphysematosa: lucent filling defect consistent with gas in vesicle of bladder with or without extravasation of contrast material into vesicoenteric fistula

•••••• Multidisciplinary Plan

Surgery

Tubercular cystitis: in cases of advanced tubercular cystitis when bladder contraction is irreversible, augmentation cystoplasty may be employed after infection is controlled; colocystoplasty (placing an isolated segment of colon onto the bladder dome in order to enlarge storage capacity) or ileocystoplasty (placing an isolated segment of small bowel on the bladder dome) may be used to restore reasonable bladder storage capacity

Cystitis glandularis: transurethral resection of lesion done because of its premalignant potential

Medications

Bacterial cystitis

Treatment of choice is oral antibiotic therapy guided by culture and sensitivity data (Table 12-1)

For first-time infections or recurrent infections, short-term therapy with oral antibiotics favored

In more severe cases or when resistant bacteria are identified, parenteral therapy is indicated

For recurrent infections, suppressive antibiotic therapy may be used for 6 mo to 24 mo; first choice for long-term antibiotic suppression among women with recurrent bacterial cystitis is nitrofurantoin or trimethoprim-sulfamethoxazole

Nitrofurantoin absorbed in upper intestinal tract so that it does not promote mutation of resistant

TABLE 12-1 Bacterial Pathogens Commonly Encountered in the Urinary Tract and Treatment Options

Pathogen	Commonly Effective Antibiotic Agents*
Escherichia coli	Trimethoprim-sulfamethoxazole, ampillicin, norfloxacin, amoxicillin clavulanate (Augmentin), nitrofurantoin, ciprofloxacin
Pseudomonas	Carbenicillin (Geocillin), gentamicin,† norfloxacin, ciprofloxacin
Klebsiella	Cephalexin, tetracycline, trimethoprim-sulfamethoxazole, norfloxacin
Proteus mirabilis	Ampicillin, tetracycline, trimethoprim-sulfamethoxazole, norfloxacin, amoxicillin clavulanate, nitrofurantoin
Morganella morganii	Trimethoprim-sulfamethoxazole, norfloxacin
Serratia	Trimethoprim-sulfamethoxazole, norfloxacin, carbenicillin
Group D *Streptococcus*	Ampicillin, nitrofurantoin, amoxicillin clavulanate
Staphylococcus	Cephalexin, tetracycline, trimethoprim-sulfamethoxazole
Staphylococcus saprophyticus	Cephalexin, trimethoprim-sulfamethoxazole, tetracycline

*Antibiotic therapy is guided by individual culture and sensitivity reports.
†Requires parenteral administration.

strains of bacteria in intestinal tract; exerts its antibacterial effects on bacteria that have reached bladder

Trimethoprim-sulfamethoxazole will kill pathogens in vaginal vestibule, preventing bacterial invasion of bladder but does alter intestinal flora, which can lead to selection of bacteria resistant to drug

Fungal infections

Two drugs, amphotericin B and 5-fluorocystine, are indicated in cases of nonmucocutaneous infection

Amphotericin B has disadvantages of requiring parenteral administration and significant side effects such as fever, chills, nausea and vomiting, headache, vertigo, and potential nephrotoxicity with prolonged use

5-Fluorocystine may be administered orally and is effective against *Candida;* side effects include bone marrow depression, potential nephrotoxicity, and eosinophilia

Production of resistant strains of fungi is problematic

Tubercular cystitis

Drug therapy must be long term (2 yr recommended), and multiple agents are often more effective than any single medication

Combination of isoniazid (INH), ethambutol, rifampin, streptomycin, para-aminosalicylic acid (PAS), cycloserine, or kanamycin is indicated

Parasitic cystitis

Drugs used for schistosomiasis have potentially dangerous side effects and are not approved by the U.S. Food and Drug Administration

Current drug of choice is nitrofurantoin given over a period of 5 to 7 d

Early treatment essential for prevention of irreversible urinary changes from drug

Other chemotherapeutic agents may be used to provide symptomatic relief from cystitis caused by infection, chemotherapy, or radiotherapy; anticholinergic agents or antispasmodics such as oxybutynin and propantheline may ameliorate sensory urgency and provide greater functional capacity

Eosinophilic cystitis

Antihistamines and oral steroid agents are indicated
Antibiotic therapy will control related bacteriuria[100]

General Management

Caffeine intake should be restricted because its mild irritative effect exacerbates frequency

Citrus juices should be restricted because its mild irritative effect exacerbates frequency

Citrus juices not effective in lowering urinary pH

Cranberry juice effective in lowering urinary pH only if taken in extremely large quantities

Plentiful fluid intake indicated to encourage movement of pathogens out of urinary tract

NURSING CARE

Nursing Assessment

Suprapubic Area

Tender on palpation

Costovertebral Angle

No tenderness

Voiding Behavior

Frequency, urgency, dysuria, nocturia

Nursing Dx & Intervention

Infectious Cystitis, Chemotherapy or Radiotherapy Cystitis, and Inflammatory Bladder Lesions

Altered patterns of urinary elimination related to bladder inflammation

- Assist the patient to attain adequate fluid intake 30 ml/kg of body weight per day.[87] *Fluids flush the urinary system, enhancing the removal of pathogens and toxins.*
- Instruct the patient to avoid limiting fluid intake in an attempt to reduce urinary frequency. *Limiting fluid intake will concentrate the urine, paradoxically increasing rather than alleviating frequency and discomfort.*
- Administer, or teach the patient to self-administer, anti-infective medications as directed. *Anti-infective medications reverse bladder inflammation by assisting the body to rid itself of infections.*
- Reassure the patient with instability (urge or reflex) urinary incontinence that any recurrence of leakage is temporary. *Instability incontinence often recurs with acute infection of the lower urinary tract; management of the inflammation will alleviate this condition.*
- Administer intravenous fluids as directed when the patient cannot tolerate oral beverages because of fever and nausea. *Infection of the upper urinary tracts may cause nausea and intolerance of oral beverages. Intravenous fluids are given until oral intake is tolerated.*

Pain related to inflammation

- Encourage the patient to take a warm Sitz bath with water above the waist. *The warm water will relieve lower back and suprapubic discomfort.*
- Encourage the intake of clear, caffeine-free fluids; discourage excessive intake of citrus beverages, coffee, or carbonated fluids. *Caffeinic, carbonated, or citrus beverages may cause mild irritation of the bladder wall, enhancing discomfort. Clear liquids may relieve this discomfort.*
- Provide external applications of heat to the lower back *to relieve discomfort.*

- Administer, or teach the patient to self-administer, urinary analgesics, as directed. *Urinary analgesics relieve bladder and urethral discomfort via unclear pharmacologic mechanisms.*
- Encourage the patient to urinate regularly and not to attempt to refrain for long periods when acute infection occurs. *Bladder filling increases discomfort and promotes bacterial replication by retaining urine.*
- Administer, or teach the patient to self-administer, nonsteroidal anti-inflammatory agents as directed. *Antiinflammatory agents relieve irritative symptoms and discomfort produced by certain inflammatory lesions.*
- Prepare the patient with a bladder inflammatory lesion for diagnostic cystoscopy and resection, if indicated. *Inflammatory bladder lesions may respond to fulguration or transurethral resection.*
- Administer, or teach the patient to self-administer, antispasmodic agents as directed. *Antispasmodic agents reduce detrusor contractility, irritative symptoms, and enhance capacity.*

Noncompliance (medical therapy) related to resolution of symptoms before complete eradication of bacteriuria

- Administer a one-time intramuscular dose or ongoing intravenous and intramuscular medications. *Urinary tract infection (UTI) recurrence or persistence is minimized by complete eradication of an existing infection.*
- Teach the patient who self-administers antiinfective medications to complete a 3- to 10-day course as prescribed. *UTI recurrence or persistence is minimized by complete eradication of existing infection.*
- Teach the patient the potential side effects of antiinfective medications and strategies to counteract or eliminate these effects. *Patients are likely to discontinue medications if unpleasant side effects occur. Simple strategies may relieve these effects or antibiotic agents may be switched when more serious untoward effects occur* (Table 12-2).
- Instruct the patient concerning signs and symptoms of hypersensitive reaction. Advise the patient to discontinue the drug immediately and contact his or her physician or nurse. *Hypersensitive reactions to a medication are potentially life threatening, warranting prompt treatment and a change in pharmacologic agent.*
- Advise the patient who undergoes resection or other management of inflammatory bladder lesion about the importance of follow-up examinations, including cystoscopic evaluation, as indicated. *Inflammatory lesions represent a variable risk for malignant degeneration; routine surveillance may be indicated until the lesion is resolved.*

Patient Education/Home Care Planning

1. Provide instruction concerning potential risk factors for cystitis, including altered urinary elimination patterns or urinary retention.
2. Provide instruction concerning prevention of recurrence of urinary tract infection, including increased fluid intake, strategies to acidify the urine, and choice of materials for undergarments.
3. Provide instruction concerning expected actions and potential side effects of medications used to treat infection or alleviate symptoms associated with cystitis.

Evaluation

Patterns of elimination are improved; bacterial cystitis is resolved Urine culture is negative 24 hours after completing antibiotic therapy.

Fungal cystitis is resolved Fungal culture is negative after completion of antifungal therapy.

Parasitic cystitis is resolved There are no ova or parasites in urine. There are no complications, or they have been surgically repaired.

Chemotherapy- or radiotherapy-induced cystitis is symptomatically improved Urgency and frequency are decreased. Functional capacity as measured by urodynamic assessment is increased. Nocturia is decreased or absent. Patient

---

TABLE 12-2 Common Side Effects of Urinary Antiinfective Drugs

Drug	Side Effect	Nursing Management
Trimethoprim/sulfamethoxazole (Bactrim, Septra)	Renal toxicity	Administer with water, maintain adequate fluid intake
Nitrofurantoin (Macrodantin)	Nausea, gastrointestinal upset	Administer with meals or snack
Carbenicillin (Geocillin, Geopen)	Diarrhea	Administer with Lactinex, 2 tablets, given with antibiotic
	Nausea related to medication odor, foul taste	Administer with iced water; advise patient to swallow rapidly and avoid smelling drug; drug may need to be discontinued if intolerance is marked
Cephalexin (Keflex)	Nausea, mild diarrhea	Administer with meals or snack

Modified from Gray.[49]

■ HYPERSENSITIVITY REACTIONS

SIGNS AND SYMPTOMS
Rash
Urticaria
Anaphylaxis
Diaphoresis
Wheezing or bronchoconstriction
Nausea or vomiting
Pounding headache
Stevens-Johnson syndrome (rare, potentially lethal sloughing of skin)

NURSING MANAGEMENT
Prevention
  Obtain careful history of drug allergies.
  Teach patient signs and symptoms of hypersensitivity response and their management.
Management of ongoing reaction
  Stop medication immediately.
  Seek emergency medical care if symptoms of wheezing or bronchoconstriction and anaphylaxis occur.
  Promptly contact health care professional for management of symptoms and alternate drug therapy.
  Administer steroidal anti-inflammatory drugs, antihistamines, and cardiorespiratory drugs as directed for severe response with anaphylaxis.
  Single-dose therapy is an alternative to short-term antibiotic therapy.
  Administer parenteral medications when oral drugs are not tolerated or when pathogens are resistant to oral agents.
  Administer parenteral fluids when oral fluids are not tolerated because of fever, nausea, and vomiting.
  Administer suppressive antibiotic drugs for 6 to 24 months for recurrent infections.

From Gray.[49]

subjectively reports decreased symptoms of suprapubic discomfort. Cystoscopic findings are normal.

Inflammatory lesion of the bladder is resolved Cystoscopic findings are normal.

Patient's comfort is improved Patient uses medication or other strategies effectively to decrease both low back pain and suprapubic discomfort.

Patient's compliance with treatment regimen is adequate Patient understands methods of treatment and follows prescribed regimen.

Patient copes with problem in a constructive manner Patient uses coping and support groups as necessary, maintains appropriate diversional and recreational activities, and understands the need for and acceptability of frequent toileting.

Patient's sex life is satisfactory Patient and significant other are comfortable with sexual activity and are aware of the availability of referral to sex therapist, if necessary.

■ INTERSTITIAL CYSTITIS

Interstitial cystitis (IC) is a chronic, idiopathic disorder of the urinary bladder that causes reduced bladder capacity, frequency of urination, nocturia, and discomfort associated with bladder filling. Because specific diagnostic criteria have not been defined, IC is diagnosed by the presence of characteristic symptoms and the absence of physical evidence for related disorders including acute urinary tract infection or inflammatory lesions of the bladder.[49]

The prevalence and incidence of interstitial cystitis are unknown. Approximately 20,000 to 90,000 individuals in the United States have been diagnosed with IC, but some researchers believe that as many as 450,000 Americans with the condition are undiagnosed or incorrectly diagnosed. Epidemiologic investigations are primarily limited by the lack of specific diagnostic criteria for this painful bladder condition. IC occurs most frequently in younger, white women. Its occurrence in children remains controversial, although several suspicious cases have been described.[49,61]

Several possible risk factors for IC have been identified; however, their role in the pathogenesis in the development of bladder wall inflammation remains speculative. These include sensitivities or allergic reactions to medications, rheumatoid arthritis, food allergies, asthma, and hay fever. These risk factors are based on an unproved supposition that IC has a significant autoimmune component. Additional risk factors, abdominal cramping, irritable bowel syndrome, and spastic colon assume a significant emotional distress component associated with IC.[65]

The etiology of IC remains unclear. IC shares certain characteristics with autoimmune disorders, and anti-inflammatory agents provide relief from pain in certain patients. Bladder wall biopsies and blood samples have demonstrated the presence of antibodies that may attack the bladder wall, producing the characteristic pain and voiding dysfunction of IC. Other research has focused on loss of integrity of the glycosaminoglycan (GAG) layer covering the bladder and urethral epithelium. This layer comprises the mucosal film that covers the epithelial cells of the bladder lining and contributes to the lower urinary tract's impermeability to the reabsorption of urinary constituents. Still others have speculated that IC may be caused by chronic ischemia, perhaps representing one form of a reflex sympathetic dystrophy.[49]

Occult infection has been implicated as a causative factor for IC. In this scenario, an acute urethritis leads to a secondary infection of the bladder mucosa, causing denudation of the GAG layer and chronic inflammation and mast cell invasion.[82] This secondary infection would be undetectable to urine culture, and certain patients have experienced relief from IC symptoms after a prolonged course of antiinfective medications.[85] Toxic agents or medications in the urine have been speculated to cause IC, but specific substances have not been identified. Psychologic factors have been associated with the etiology of IC, but it is more likely that psychologic distress represents a response to the condition, rather than its cause.[49,95]

• • • • • Pathophysiology

The primary symptoms of IC are pain and voiding dysfunction.[65] The pain is frequently described as a continuous burning pain located in the suprapubic area with moderate to intense severity. Others experience recurring episodes of pain, described as bladder spasms, localized to the suprapubic and right lower quadrant of the abdomen. Other symptoms associated with IC include pelvic discomfort and pressure, and an intolerance of restrictive clothing or abdominal compression. Typically, the pain of IC is transiently relieved by urination, but returns promptly as the bladder refills. In addition to bladder filling, emotional distress and sexual intercourse commonly exacerbate the pain. The pain produced by intercourse may persist for days. Acidic, caffienic, carbonated, or alcoholic beverages, as well as spicy or greasy foods or chocolates also exacerbate IC pain in certain patients.

The discomfort of IC is chronic in nature. Patients experience only temporary, incomplete relief from narcotic analgesics, non-steroidal anti-inflammatory drugs, urinary analgesics, or antispasmodics. In contrast, the burning pain of IC may respond to amitriptylene, an agent commonly used to relieve the chronic, burning pain produced by peripheral polyneuropathies. Like other forms of chronic pain, the discomfort of IC is cyclical. Patients frequently report exacerbation of their symptoms, lasting from weeks to months, followed by periods of reduced pain and urinary frequency. These acute exacerbations of IC symptoms are frequently referred to as "attacks" or "flares"[122] and are managed symptomatically by analgesics, narcotic agents, sleeping aids, dietary modifications (primarily avoidance of irritating beverages and foods), and assertive toileting behaviors.

The voiding dysfunction produced by IC is related to bladder inflammation and pain. Urinary frequency may be severe, and many patients report diurnal frequency exceeding every half hour. Nocturia also occurs, and chronic fatigue is a frequent component of the condition. Because bladder filling typically exacerbates the condition, patients with IC are unable to postpone urination, although urge incontinence and unstable detrusor contractions do not occur.

The natural history of IC remains unclear. The long-term clinical course of IC commonly begins with a sudden onset of bladder pain, followed by frustrated attempts at relief by short course anti-infective therapy. The pain associated with IC is particularly intense during the earlier course of the condition, which may last for months or years. Persons with IC over a period of years to decades may enter a later stage characterized by a small, contracted bladder with low compliance. In this stage, voiding frequency remains, but the bladder may become relatively insensitive to pain. Ironically, even bladder augmentation or cystectomy with urinary diversion may fail to adequately relieve the pain of IC, even though these procedures are effective in alleviating associated voiding dysfunction.[49]

• • • • • Diagnostic Studies and Findings

Urinalysis Negative
Urine culture Negative

Cystoscopy Frequently negative, punctate hemorrhagic lesions of the bladder lining may be noted (glomerulations); Hunner's ulcers (larger ulcerations surrounded by linear hemorrhagic lesions) are seen in some patients

Biopsy Absence of *carcinoma in situ,* other inflammatory lesions; mucosal denuding and evidence of chronic inflammation frequently observed

Urodynamics Small bladder capacity, bladder filling with pain and urgency; discomfort is associated with bladder filling, rather than unstable detrusor contractions

• • • • • Multidisciplinary Plan

Surgery

Open surgery Augmentation enterocystoplasty, urinary diversion with and without cystectomy, subtrigonal cystectomy and substitution cystoplasty may be used to treat IC. Surgical procedures are effective in reducing the voiding dysfunction of IC, but they have not uniformly ablated the pelvic or suprapubic pain.[40]

Endoscopic laser therapy Neodymium ablation of lesions of Hunner's ulcers may be used to relieve pain of IC.

Medications

Urinary analgesics, antispasmodics: increase bladder capacity; produce little effect on the pain of IC

Narcotic analgesics: transient relief from the pain of IC; the effectiveness of narcotics in managing the burning pain associated with IC is inconsistent

Nonsteroidal antiinflammatory drugs: transient relief of the pain of IC; the effectiveness of these agents in relieving the pain of IC is inconsistent

Amitryptilene (Elavil): reduces burning pain associated with IC with chronic administration; typically given before sleep to produce drowsiness and assist sleep patterns; anticholinergic side effect may increase bladder capacity[53]

Calcium channel antagonists (nifedipine, verapamil, diltiazem): relaxation of vascular smooth muscle may reduce ischemia-induced pain of IC; relaxation of detrusor muscle may increase bladder capacity, immunosuppressive actions may reduce autoimmune aspects of disorder

Hydroxizine: H_1 receptor antagonist may reduce IC associated pain by blocking neuronal actions of mast cells

Intravesical Therapies

Bladder hydrodistention/hydrodilation: transient relief from pain of IC (6 months to 1 year) and increased bladder capacity occur in some patients; bladder distention under endoscopic control; the patient is under general or epidural anesthesia and the bladder is passively filled with sterile saline to an intravesical pressure of 60-80 cm H_2O; or a balloon is inserted into the bladder and filled to the halfway point between diastolic and systolic blood pressure[101]

Silver Nitrate: Solution of 1:500 to 1%-2% instilled and retained in the bladder producing transient relief from pain of IC in some patients (up to 1 year); treatment is contraindicated in patients with vesicoureteric reflux; leakage of silver nitrate into pelvis, peritoneum, or retroperitoneum may cause death

Sodium oxychlorosene (Chlorpactin): 0.4% solution is instilled into the bladder, exerting "detergent" and antimicrobial effects; transient relief from pain and voiding dysfunction of IC in certain patients (relief may last from 6 to 12 months)

Dimethyl Sulfoxide (DMSO): intravesical solution instilled into the bladder provides transient relief from pain and voiding dysfunction of IC in some patients; has anti-inflammatory, analgesic, antispasmodic, and mast cell inhibitory effects[22]

Heparin: administered as intravesical or subcutaneous form; transient relief of pain and voiding dysfunction of IC in some patients (up to 1 year), possibly due to protective effects of bladder epithelium (palliating damage to GAG layer)[92]

NURSING CARE

Nursing Assessment

Primarily based on symptom assessment (Table 12-3)

Nursing Dx & Intervention

Pain, related to interstitial cystitis

- Administer intravesical agents as directed, assist patient to retain agent for 30 minutes or prescribed length *to relieve the chronic pain and urinary frequency of IC.*
- Teach patient to self-administer amitriptyline, calcium channel blocking agent or hydroxyzine as directed, teach patient importance of chronic administration *to alleviate the chronic, burning pain of IC, and to increase bladder capacity.*
- Administer transvaginal or transrectal electrical stimulation in consultation with physician, provide 10 Hz current for work period of 4 seconds, followed by 4 to 8 second rest period; to alleviate chronic pain of IC and enhance bladder capacity.
- Advise the patient to avoid or limit intake of bladder irritants: caffeine, alcoholic beverages, carbonated beverages, citrus juices, spicy foods or chocolates; teach the person to alleviate foods or beverages one at a time *to judge its effect on IC-related pain and urinary frequency.*
- Advise the patient to discontinue smoking *to alleviate vasoconstriction and bladder irritant effects that may exacerbate IC pain.*
- Advise the individual to avoid strenuous exercises that may exacerbate IC pain.
- Advise the patient to avoid tight fitting clothing *to reduce abdominal constriction and associated IC pain.*
- Advise the patient to apply local heat as tolerated *for temporary relief from IC pain.*

- Teach the patient self-care strategies *to alleviate and cope with IC-related pain including:*
  - biofeedback techniques to reduce emotional distress
  - biofeedback techniques to relax the pelvic muscles
  - assertive toileting during "attacks/flares" for temporary pain relief
  - supplementation of dietary vitamin intake as indicated
  - bladder retraining techniques (restricted to those with mild to moderate pain and significant urinary frequency)
  - nonvigorous, low impact exercise including walking, yoga, swimming to relieve stress and promote physical fitness within limitation of chronic IC

Altered urinary elimination, related to chronic IC

- Advise the patient to avoid prolonged, severe restriction of fluid intake; concentration of urine increases its irritating effect on the bladder, rather than relieving urinary frequency.

TABLE 12-3 Signs and Symptoms of Interstitial Cystitis[46,122]

Characteristic Signs and Symptoms	Exclusionary Signs and Symptoms
Urinary frequency more than 5 times during 12 waking hours	Age <18 years (suspicious cases in children have been described)
Nocturia more than twice	Absence of intense urge to void when bladder filled with 10 ml of CO_2 or 150 ml of sterile water or saline
Symptoms present more than 1 year	Unstable detrusor contractions associated with symptoms of discomfort
Urgency	Duration of symptoms <9 months
Pain with bladder distention or fullness	Absence of nocturia
Pain temporarily relieved by micturition	Symptoms relieved by antiinfectives, antispasmodics
Suprapubic, pelvic, vaginal and/or perineal discomfort	Diagnosis of bacterial cystitis or prostatitis within 3 months
Negative urine cultures	Current bladder or ureteral calculi
Cystoscopy/Endoscopy: glomerulations of bladder wall petechiae	Active genital herpes
Hunner's ulcer absent malignancies	
Bladder capacity <350 ml on urodynamic testing	Uterine, cervical, vaginal or urethral cancer
	Cyclophosphamide treatment; must rule out chemical cystitis
	Tubercular cystitis
	Radiation therapy of the pelvis or diagnosed radiation cystitis
	Active vaginitis

Data from Gillenwater and Wein[46] and Wein et al.[122]

- Teach the patient that transient restriction of fluids may be advisable when toilet access is limited.
- Teach person to identify potential bladder irritants and limit or eliminate them from the diet.
- Reassure the patient that assertive toileting is an appropriate and effective strategy to cope with IC-related pain.

Sleep pattern disturbance, related to pain and voiding dysfunction of IC

- Teach patient to schedule amitriptyline before sleep. Amitriptyline produces drowsiness, which assists with sleep.
- Assist patient to explore possibility of napping during daylight hours to supplement sleep. The pain and voiding dysfunction may prevent more than 2 hours of uninterrupted sleep, particularly during "attacks" or "symptom flares." Short naps during the day may be needed to supplement sleep and alleviate chronic fatigue.
- Counsel family and significant others concerning the need for napping as needed.
- Teach the patient to administer sleep aids as directed *to promote drowsiness and uninterrupted sleep.*

Ineffective individual coping, related to chronic pain, fatigue, voiding frequency of IC

- Provide the name and address of Interstitial Cystitis Association (see box below) and local IC support group *to strengthen the supportive network.*
- Encourage patient to identify and maintain diversional or recreational activities.
- Reassure patient that frequent voiding is necessary and acceptable.
- Counsel the patient's family and significant others of the need for frequent voiding, emotional support needed to cope with the chronic pain, fatigue and frequent voiding associated with IC.
- Encourage the patient to use humor and candor when coping with the chronic pain of IC. Expressions of humor assist others to understand the symptoms and distress of IC in a positive and easily acceptable manner.

■ INTERSTITIAL CYSTITIS ASSOCIATION

Goals
1. To share common experiences among those affected by the disease.
2. To provide information for interstitial cystitis patients and their families.
3. To foster research related to interstitial cystitis, its causes, care, and cure.

Address
PO Box 1553, Madison Square Station
New York, NY 10159

From Gray.[49]

- Reassure the patient that the expression of negative feelings is acceptable when coping with the symptoms of IC. The expression of negative feelings is appropriate when coping with the discomfort and frustrations caused by the symptoms of IC.
- Reassure the patient that assertive seeking of health care providers with expertise and compassion when managing persons with IC is both appropriate and necessary. Patients with IC are frequently misdiagnosed or undiagnosed, leading to frustration with health care providers and unnecessary suffering.

Sexual dysfunction, related to IC

- Advise the person that sexual intercourse, particularly when associated with prolonged pressure on the abdomen and suprapubic area may exacerbate IC pain in certain individuals under certain circumstances.
- Reassure the individual that the act of sexual intercourse is not the sole means to express intimacy. Alternate expressions of sexual intimacy provide satisfaction without aggravating bladder pain.
- Teach the patient that sexual intercourse is acceptable only when *both* partners consent. Assertiveness in avoiding sexual intercourse is necessary during intense IC-related pain.
- Consult a therapist as indicated. A reduced ability to engage in intercourse may cause distress in a marriage or intimate, sexual relationship. A therapist can assist the couple to explore alternatives in sexual expression and reduce estrangement related to the pain, voiding dysfunction, and chronic fatigue associated with IC.

Patient Education/Home Care Planning

1. Teach the patient nonpharmacologic methods to manage the pain of IC.
2. Teach the patient a variety of self-care strategies to manage the pain, chronic fatigue, and voiding dysfunction of IC.
3. Provide a written list of foods and beverages that may exacerbate IC pain, and instruct the person to eliminate these items one at a time to determine their influence on the bladder.

Evaluation

Patterns of urinary elimination are improved; the goal of diurnal frequency must be individualized   Persons with severe frequency may strive for micturition every 1/2 to 1 hour, while those with less severe symptoms may select a goal of every 1.5 to 2 hours. A bladder log (voiding diary) is recommended to evaluate changes in urine elimination patterns.

IC-related pain is alleviated   A visual analog scale for pain intensity may be used to evaluate changes in IC-related pain.

Patient identifies coping strategies to manage the pain, fatigue, and voiding dysfunction of IC

Intimate sexual relationships are maintained The patient and partner identify the impact of IC on their relationship and alternatives to sexual intercourse are recognized.

URINARY CALCULI

Calculi are stones that are formed in the urinary tract.

Calculi that pass spontaneously without discomfort present no serious threat to health. However, many urinary calculi are extremely painful, obstructive, and a focus of infection. The problem of urinary calculi must be addressed by both urologists and nephrologists, since stones have both medical and surgical implications. A detailed discussion of medical aspects of urinary calculi is presented in Chapter 11. This discussion focuses on the two primary urologic complications associated with urinary calculi, infection and obstruction, as well as the surgical and electromechanical therapeutic options available to patients.

The incidence of calculi varies significantly with a number of intrinsic factors, such as age, sex, and race, and extrinsic factors, such as geographic location and climate. In the United States the five most common types of urinary stones are calcium oxalate, magnesium-ammonium-phosphate (struvite), uric acid, cystine, and mixed element calculi.[46,118]

The peak incidence of calculus formation is the third to fifth decades of life. Many patients report an onset of symptoms associated with urolithiasis beginning in their twenties; surgical or medical interventions for urinary calculi are most commonly performed in the fifth decade of life. Men are three times more likely to have calculus formation in the upper urinary tract and bladder than are women.[49] The disease is relatively rare among American and African blacks, North American Indians, and native-born Israelis but relatively common among whites and Eurasians.[118]

Throughout the world those persons at greatest risk for urinary calculi live in mountainous areas (see box). The United States, a number of European countries, and Australia have a high incidence of urinary lithiasis, whereas the African and South American countries have a relatively low incidence. The southeastern and arid southwestern United States generally have a higher incidence of calculi than other regions.[118]

Sedentary occupations are associated with an increased incidence of urinary lithiasis. Intake of certain foods can also contribute to stone formation. The patient should be questioned concerning intake of foods containing calcium (dairy products), oxalate (green, leafy vegetables and certain fruits), and purines that are metabolized to uric acid (meat, fish, and poultry).[96] In rare instances medications are responsible for stone disease. Long-term ingestion of calcium carbonate, vitamin D, antacids, megadoses of vitamin C, acetazolamide, probenecid, or triamterene can lead to various types of stone formation.[99]

•••••• Pathophysiology

The etiology of calculi formation is complex and incompletely elucidated. Urinary calculi are approximately 97.5% crystalline

and 2.5% mucoprotein or glycoprotein matrix and are described by their predominant salt content. To understand the pathophysiologic process of stone formation in the urinary tract, it is necessary to understand basic principles of biologic crystallization. Calculi formation requires the following conditions in the urinary tract. A solution has a given solubility product that is constant. Once this product has been reached, adding further solute (such as calcium oxalate or other stone salt) will not raise its concentration within the solution. Supersaturation occurs when further solute is added to the solute (urine). At a formation concentration the supersaturated solute spontaneously precipitates from the solution, forming the beginning of a potential calculus. Unlike the solubility product, the formation concentration varies with circumstances. Calculus formation requires the initiation of a crystal from precipitation of a stone salt from the urine followed by crystal growth and aggregation. This process requires energy that is obtained from urine in a supersaturation.[36]

SPECIFIC RISK FACTORS FOR URINARY CALCULI

Although the cause of calculus formation remains unclear, the following specific risk factors increase the likelihood that an individual will form urinary stones:

1. Renal tubular acidosis (RTA) is a condition that occurs when the kidneys cannot excrete an acidic urine. As a result, systemic hyperchloremic acidosis ensues. Individuals with untreated renal tubular acidosis develop hypercalciuria and often form calcium stones.
2. Cystinuria is another risk factor for urinary calculi. Excessive cystine in the urine probably represents a metabolic abnormality that predisposes these individuals to the formation of cystine calculi.
3. Hypercalcemia, or excess calcium in the blood, predisposes an individual to hypercalciuria. The most common cause of hypercalcemia is hyperparathyroidism, or excessive secretion of the hormone parathormone, causing mobilization of calcium from body storage into the blood.
4. Xanthinuria, excessive excretion of xanthine in the urine, predisposes a person to urinary calculi. The condition may be an untoward effect of allopurinol administration or of a genetic deficiency.
5. Hyperoxaluria predisposes the affected individual to oxalate calculi. The condition may occur as the result of excessive dietary intake or a metabolic disorder.
6. Urinary infection may predispose a person to calculi, particularly when the pathogen can split urea molecules.
7. Immobility, neuropathic bladder dysfunction, and urinary retention also predispose an individual to urinary stones.

All of these conditions cause urinary stasis, which enhances the precipitation of stone-forming salts from the urine while slowing urinary transport, thus giving the potential stone nidus a greater chance of forming an obstructive latticework.

From Gillenwater and Wein.[46]

Two predisposing epidemiologic factors have been identified in association with an increased likelihood of stone formation: predisposing anatomic or biochemical factors, such as the inherited predisposition for cystinuria or medullary sponge kidney, and environmental factors, such as diet, climate, fluid intake patterns, and occupation.[6]

Several theories have attempted to explain calculus formation in the urinary tract. The *precipitation-crystallization theory* is based on the general principles of biologic crystallization; it delineates four necessary steps for stone formation. The first step is the nucleation phase in which the smallest unit of a crystal is formed in the urine. This nucleus may be of homogenous or heterogeneous form relative to the remaining portion of the calculus. In the second phase the crystal form grows and aggregates into a larger form. For this growth to occur, supersaturation of the urine persists and circumstances allowing a formation concentration to be attained continue. The greater the degree of supersaturation, the greater the rate of stone formation. The third stage of stone formation occurs when the crystal becomes entrapped in the upper urinary tract. Otherwise, the crystal is passed into the urine and no clinically apparent disease occurs. The final stage of the precipitation-crystallization process involves the continued growth of the trapped particle, resulting in clinically significant disease.[37,110]

The *inhibitor lack theory* attempts to explain why some persons form stones and others do not even though both groups excrete urine that is supersaturated with certain substances that inhibit crystallization and subsequent calculi. These substances have been identified as magnesium, pyrophosphate, citrate, mucoproteins, and various peptides.

The *matrix initiation theory* observes the finding that the matrices of calculi in certain persons are mucoproteins that typically act as crystal inhibitors. In this case mucoproteins are hypothesized to contain a qualitative defect that renders them dysfunctional; thus they predispose the person toward calculi formation rather than serve as a crystal inhibitor as they do in normal individuals.[36,118]

The *epitaxy theory* attempts to account for the presence of mixed urinary calculi and the process by which a crystal is formed with layers of different substances. The crystalline lattice of a specific substance is organized in a predictable manner that may closely resemble other crystalline lattices. Certain calculi may have an inner core of uric acid and an outer covering of calcium oxalate. Thus one crystal forms upon the lattice work of a similar substance, resulting in a mixed urinary stone.[37]

Which of these factors relevant to urinary stone formation will prove predominant and which will prove secondary remains to be elucidated. A *final theory* of stone formation will be based on elucidation of the process of biologic crystallization and the role of the kidneys and urinary transport organs for maintaining a crystal- and stasis-free system.[118]

The presence of a urinary calculus is typically discovered when the stone becomes entrapped, resulting in the abrupt onset of acute renal or bladder colic. The most common sites of entrapment are a calyx or calyceal diverticulum, the ureteropelvic junction, the segment of ureter at or near the pelvic brim adjacent to the point where the ureter crosses the iliac vessels, the posterior pelvic portion of the ureter in women, and the ureterovesical junction. Of all the areas of anatomic narrowing, the ureterovesical junction is the most difficult for a calculus to pass.

The renal colic typically occurs at night or during the early morning hours when the patient is sedentary. The pain begins in the flank and radiates to the groin and testes in men or the labia majora and broad ligament in women. As the stone moves to the midureter, the pain radiates to the lateral portion of the flank and lower abdomen. As the calculus moves toward the ureterovesical junction, the pain associated with the initial renal colic may recur, associated with irritable voiding symptoms of urinary urgency or urge incontinence. Colic is perceived most intensely as the calculus moves or if it implants at a certain site. Movement of the stone also causes localized pain resulting from obstruction.[46,118]

Bladder colic is characterized by bladder pain that crescendoes immediately after micturition. A stabbing pain may be felt when changing position, and urinary urgency and urge incontinence are commonly associated.[46,118]

Because visceral pain such as renal colic is mediated by the autonomic nervous system via the celiac ganglia, nausea and vomiting, intestinal stasis, and ileus may occur. Patients are typically restless as they change position to reduce discomfort. Grunting respirations signaling distress may be present. The pulse and blood pressure may be elevated in response to pain. Fever is rare unless a urinary tract infection is present.[46,118]

Many urinary calculi pass spontaneously and do not require urologic intervention, but others need prompt attention. The decision to intervene surgically, endoscopically, or via extracorporeal shock wave lithotripsy is based on prevention of the most significant complications of calculi: obstruction, loss of renal function, and infection.

Obstruction of the urinary tract in the presence of calculi results in adverse changes in renal and ureteral function associated with hydronephrosis. The adverse effects of acute hydronephrosis have been studied in laboratory animals and divided into the following stages. During the first 90 minutes after the onset of obstruction, ipsilateral renal blood flow is dramatically increased and intramural pressure in both ureters rises. In the second stage, lasting from 90 minutes to the end of the fifth hour, renal blood flow to both kidneys decreases while pressure in the ureters remains high in an attempt to compensate for and overcome the obstruction. From the fifth through the eighteenth hour following acute obstruction, renal blood flow in the affected side and intraureteral pressure decrease as compensatory mechanisms are overwhelmed. Intrarenal changes on the affected side include an early rapid redistribution of blood from the medullary to cortical nephrons during the initial period after obstruction. Later, the renal plasma flow, glomerular filtration rate, and tubular function are slowed as kidney function is impaired.[46,118]

Ureteral peristalsis is also adversely affected by obstruction. The creation of acute obstruction in animal models resulted in an initial rise in ureteral pressure and the frequency of peristaltic waves. However, these compensatory mechanisms were soon overcome, resulting in dilation of the ureters and loss of smooth muscle tone and fibrotic replacement in the ureteral wall.[118]

In humans progressive changes from hydronephrosis include renal pelvic dilation and an initial rise in kidney weight because of renal edema. Parenchymal mass decreases as a result of atrophy and adverse changes in the structure and function of the nephron. If hydronephrosis persists for 8 weeks or more, the parenchymal mass may be dramatically compromised with only a thin shell of tissue remaining around a hydronephrotic, distorted collecting system.[46,118]

Obstruction may be complicated by infection leading to pyelonephritis. In such cases the infection may become the dominant aspect of the disease, requiring immediate intervention before stone manipulation or surgical removal is attempted. Pyelonephritis is characterized by fever, chills, flank pain, and irritative voiding symptoms. Destruction of parenchymal mass by inflammatory changes and sepsis is a serious complication of the condition. Children with pyelonephritis are especially susceptible to renal scarring with subsequent loss of nephric function.[111,118]

Examination of a patient with calculous pyohydronephrosis may reveal a giant or intermediate-size hydronephrotic kidney or an atrophic kidney. The giant hydronephrotic kidney has a massively dilated collecting system with a thin shell of functioning parenchyma. The surface of the kidney is nodular and densely adherent to adjacent perirenal fat. An atrophic kidney is small because of extensive damage. Only a small mass of parenchymal tissue remains in this kidney, and progressive failure of function is likely. The intermediate-size hydronephrotic kidney is not as large as the giant kidney or as severely compromised in its function as the atrophic kidney. Microscopic examination of this type of kidney reveals more nearly normal nephrons than the other types of infected kidney, although inflammatory damage is present.[118]

Multiple factors influence the decision to attempt endoscopic manipulation or surgical removal of a urinary calculus. The patient's occupation must be considered when contemplating urologic intervention for a calculus. Persons in certain occupations (for example, a pilot) may subject themselves and others to danger if renal colic occurs during the performance of their jobs.[118]

A stone more than 4 mm in diameter is unlikely to pass through the ureter. Even smaller stones that are securely implanted into the wall of a calyx or ureter are less likely to pass and more likely to be obstructive or cause infection.

Aggressive removal of urinary calculi is considered for any patient who has a single kidney or significant renal insufficiency. Because of age and general health status, however, a patient may be a poor candidate for the anesthesia necessary for calculus manipulation.[118]

•••••• Diagnostic Studies and Findings

Kidneys, ureters, and bladder (KUB) Calcifications in urinary tract; calcium phosphate calculi are most densely radiopaque; uric acid stones are radiolucent

Intravenous pyelogram (IVP) Filling defects in conjunction with calculus; ureteral dilation on affected side if calculus is obstructive; hydronephrosis may be present with dilation of calyces and renal pelvis; clubbing of calyces in advanced cases of hydronephrosis; signs of pyelonephritis (parenchymal enlargement with impairment of excretion) if calculous pyohydronephrosis is present

Voiding cystourethrogram (VCUG) Of limited value in diagnosing bladder calculi, which are appreciated as intravesical filling defect

Retrograde pyelography Useful in cases of radiolucent calculi that cannot be localized by routine radiographic studies or when patient is hypersensitive to intravenous injection of contrast material[53]

Ultrasonography Presence of calculi

Analysis of stones Prominent constituents such as cystine, calcium, oxalate, and uric acid; provides guidance for medical therapy to prevent recurrence

Urine calcium Elevated in patients with calcium stones or renal tubular acidosis

Urine oxalate Elevated in patients with calcium oxalate stones

Urine uric acid Elevated in patients with uric acid stones

Urinary pH Acidic in patients with uric acid or cystine stones; alkaline in patients who form calcium phosphate, calcium oxalate, and struvite stones

Urine culture Bacteriuria if infection is due to presence of calculi

Antibody-coated bacteria Positive in pyelonephritis

Serum calcium Elevated in hyperparathyroidism

Serum parathormone Elevated in hyperparathyroidism

•••••• Multidisciplinary Plan

Surgery

Once the mainstay of urologic management of stones, surgical procedures are currently reserved for patients who fail to respond adequately to extracorporeal shock-wave lithotripsy or endoscopic manipulation

Medications

For calcium and calcium oxalate stones: sodium bicarbonate or citrate (inhibits urinary excretion of calcium), hydrochlorothiazide, trichlormethiazide (reduces urinary calcium excretion in patients with idiopathic hypercalciuria; may have some benefit among normocalciuric individuals), orthophosphate (decreases urinary calcium excretion), cellulose phosphate (binds calcium in the intestinal tract), potassium citrate (reduces incidence of stones in patients with hypocitriuria

For cystine stones: D-penicillamine, α-mercaptopropinoglycide, captopril (bind with cystine to enhance its solubility)

For uric acid stones: allopurinol (reduces urinary excretion of urinary acid), sodium bicarbonate or citrate (raises urinary pH, favoring solubility of uric acid)

For oxalate stones: pyridoxine (reduces urinary oxalate excretion in patients with primary hyperoxaluria), cholestyramine (binds oxalate in the intestine for fecal excretion)

General Management

Percutaneous removal of upper urinary tract stones using stone basket or by crushing stones via ultrasonic shock waves, electrohydraulic means, or laser techniques; avoids open surgery but does require invasive percutaneous access into the upper urinary tract

Extracorporeal shock wave lithotripsy uses shock waves to crush calculi into small fragments that can be passed through the urinary tract and expelled into the urine; technique is noninvasive

Chemolysis uses a chemical solution to dissolve urinary calculi by reversing environmental conditions favorable to calculi crystallization and aggregation; a percutaneous tract into the renal pelvis is established and chemolytic solution is used to dissolve calculi

Dietary restrictions for preventive therapy

To prevent all forms of stones: ensure adequate fluid intake

To prevent calcium stones: reduction of dietary calcium indicated only in certain patients with abnormal intestinal absorption of calcium (absorptive calciuria); a moderate restriction is recommended (400 to 600 mg/day)[91]

To prevent oxalate stones: reduce intake of foods high in oxalates, including asparagus, beets, plums, raspberries, rhubarb, spinach, almonds, cashew nuts, cranberries, cocoa, cranberry juice, grape juice, grapefruit juice, Worcestershire sauce

To prevent uric acid stones: reduce intake of foods high in purines such as organ meats, lean meats, and whole grains

NURSING CARE

Nursing Assessment

Pain

Renal colic or bladder colic; may be severe; flank pain noted with pyelonephritis

Voiding Behaviors

Irritative voiding symptoms

Fever

Elevated if infection is present

Nausea and Vomiting

Associated with renal colic

Nursing Dx & Intervention

Pain related to urinary obstruction

- Administer, or teach the patient to self-administer, narcotic pain medications as directed *to reduce discomfort.*
- Minimize environmental noises and activity *to enhance pain-relieving action of narcotics and to promote rest.*
- Apply warm compresses to the patient's flank *to relieve pain caused by renal colic.*
- Observe the patient for a sudden increase in the intensity of pain, *which may indicate acute obstruction of the urinary system with embedding of a stone.*
- Observe the patient for acute relief from pain, *which may indicate passage of a stone through a narrow segment of the system and relief from obstruction.*
- Advise the patient that "anticipatory watching" is necessary before invasive or extracorporeal procedures. Reassure the patient that aggressive pain management will be maintained throughout this procedure. *Approximately one half of all symptomatic stones pass spontaneously. Invasive or extracorporeal procedures are reserved for those calculi that produce significant obstruction and infection.*
- Encourage the patient to maintain adequate fluid intake (at least 30 ml/kg of body weight per day[87] and up to 3000 ml in special circumstances) *to promote flushing of the urinary system with passage of partially obstructing stones.*
- Encourage the patient to ambulate as feasible *to promote passage of urinary calculi and sediment from upper to lower urinary tract.*

Risk for infection (urinary system) related to urinary obstruction and stasis

- Perform urinalysis and urine culture studies as directed *to detect the presence of coexisting urinary infection.*
- Monitor vital signs and body temperature *to detect the presence of febrile urinary tract infection or urosepsis.*
- Administer, or teach the patient to self-administer, anti-infective medications as directed *to eradicate urinary infection.*
- Administer, or teach the patient to self-administer, prophylactic antiinfective medications as directed before invasive diagnostic or therapeutic procedures (such as percutaneous, nephroscopic or ureteroscopic stone manipulation) *to prevent the systemic spread of bacteria from the urine.*
- Encourage adequate fluid intake (at least 30 ml/kg of body weight per day[87] and up to 3000 ml in certain circumstances) *to promote stone passage and to flush the urinary system of pathogens and related toxins.*

Altered patterns of urinary elimination related to urinary obstruction

- Reassure the patient that irritative voiding symptoms are temporary. *Irritative symptoms (frequency, urgency, and nocturia) are related to obstruction and infection; symptoms are relieved as the stone passes or is removed and as the infection is eradicated.*

- Reassure the patient experiencing urge incontinence that this condition is expected to be temporary. *Passage of a urinary calculus through the ureterovesical junction into the bladder often produces unstable bladder contractions that are relieved as the stone is passed in the urine.*
- Advise the patient who has undergone removal of an obstructive stone that urinary urgency and frequency will persist for a brief period following manipulation of the urinary system. *Manipulating the urinary system produces transient inflammation with irritative voiding symptoms. Frequency and urgency are also affected by a postobstructive diuresis caused by stone removal.*

Altered tissue perfusion (renal) related to urinary obstruction

- Advise the patient that urinary calculi may recur, emphasizing the need for prompt prevention and prompt management. *Urinary calculi often produce obstruction and infection that compromises renal function unless rapidly managed.*
- Teach the patient to strain the urine when watching for a calculus to pass and to preserve the stone for analysis. *Stone analysis may provide clues to an underlying, treatable metabolic disorder amenable to treatment, preventing the recurrence of calculi with coexisting obstruction and infection.*
- Teach the patient to drink an adequate volume of liquids each day (30 ml/kg of body weight[87]). *Fluids dilute the urine, reducing the risk of urinary calculi formation.*
- Teach the patient to change his or her diet or to self-administer medications, as directed. *Specific medications or dietary modifications reduce the risk of stone recurrence in certain individuals.*
- Assist the patient to minimize or reverse specific risk factors for urinary calculi. *Specific risk factors for urinary stones, such as immobility or urinary retention, may be modulated or removed, reducing the concurrent risk for calculi in the urine.*

Patient Education/Home Care Planning

1. Provide explanation of analysis of stone, adjunct medical therapy aimed at prevention of recurrence, and associated dietary restrictions.
2. Provide instruction concerning options of treatment should manipulation of stones be indicated.

Evaluation

Pain is diminished   Patient receives adequate pain relief until stone has passed or been removed.

No urinary system infection develops   Patient understands the need for administration of antiinfective medications and maintains adequate fluid intake to promote hydration

and stone passage. No fever or other change in vital signs develops. Urinalysis is within normal limits.

Patterns of urinary elimination return to normal; renal tissue perfusion is normal   Irritative symptoms diminish, and urge incontinence improves. Patient understands the need to strain urine and to preserve stone for analysis. Measures are then taken to prevent further calculus formation; no obstruction or infection occurs.

■ URINARY INCONTINENCE

■ Urinary incontinence is the involuntary leakage of urine after the age of toilet training.

Incontinence is not a disease; it is a symptom that represents a significant health problem and may underlie a serious disease process. Urinary incontinence is a particularly appropriate area of intensive investigation and intervention for nurses who manage patients with genitourinary disease.

The problem of incontinence occurs throughout the life span and is particularly problematic for the elderly. In the United States the National Institutes of Health have estimated that at least 13 million adults experience urinary incontinence, creating an annual cost of $10.3 billion. As many as 55% of the institutionalized elderly in this country experience chronic incontinence,[3] and approximately 70% experience intermittent episodes of urinary leakage. Approximately 15% to 30% of community-dwelling, aged persons are incontinent. Many cases of incontinence are transient, caused by infection, acute immobility, or other factors; many cases represent a chronic condition that will persist for months, years, or a lifetime if left untreated.

A Welsh study of 1060 women 18 years of age and over revealed that 45% of these women had some degree of incontinence. Symptoms consistent with stress incontinence were reported by 22% of the women, and those of urge incontinence were reported by 10%. A combination of stress and urge incontinence was reported by 14% of those surveyed. In the majority of the women, urinary incontinence was assessed as mild, but 5% related severe enough symptoms to necessitate changing clothing daily. Over 3% of the women reported that urinary incontinence significantly interfered with their daily lives, yet less than half of these had sought medical treatment for the problem.

The prevalence of urinary incontinence in men is less well documented. In the Danish population, 2% of all adults have urinary incontinence severe enough to prompt them to seek medical help. Among men over 65 years of age, 5% suffer from incontinence; among men under 50 years approximately 20% to 25% develop symptoms of obstruction and dribble after voiding because of benign prostatic hyperplasia.[52,54]

Urinary continence in childhood is typically accomplished by 5 years of age. Incontinence most often takes the form of enuresis, which is seen in 15% of all 5-year-olds.[57]

For further information, see Part Four (Incontinence, Urinary Retention, and Altered Patterns of Urinary Elimination).

• • • • • Pathophysiology

Many classification schemes for urinary incontinence have been proposed. In this discussion, Wheatley's four types of incontinence[123] are used because they offer a simple, comprehensive conceptual framework for this condition. The four types of incontinence are stress urinary incontinence, instability incontinence, overflow or paradoxic incontinence, and constant or extraurethral incontinence.

Stress urinary incontinence occurs when bladder pressure exceeds urethral closure pressure, resulting in leakage of urine in the absence of a detrusor contraction. Although the condition is most common among women, it is also noted among males. The causes of stress urinary incontinence are pelvic relaxation, sphincteric incompetence, or a combination of these factors.[96,112]

Pelvic relaxation, most typically seen in women, occurs when the support structures of the pelvis lose their optimum competence, resulting in descent of pelvic organs. Cystocele describes the protrusion of the bladder into the vaginal space; rectocele describes protrusion of the rectum into the vaginal space. The often used term "urethrocele" is a misnomer; the condition typically refers to hypermobility of the urethra associated with increased abdominal pressure seen during physical examination. Uterine prolapse occurs when the uterus descends into the vaginal space as a result of a loss of normal support mechanisms.[50] Multiparity, aging, and menopause are associated with pelvic relaxation.[123]

Childbirth via vaginal delivery is associated with pelvic relaxation, at least partly because of traction placed on the pelvic ligaments during delivery and denervation of the pelvic floor musculature.[5,110] Other causes of pelvic floor relaxation are associated with pelvic floor muscle denervation. Peripheral neuropathy, as seen in diabetes mellitus, and traumatic and iatrogenic nerve damage resulting from extensive pelvic surgery can cause pelvic floor relaxation. Obesity may exacerbate the condition.[50,112]

Although a causal relationship between pelvic relaxation and stress urinary incontinence remains unestablished, the principal pathophysiologic mechanism is probably loss of normal urethrovesical anatomy. The urethra is no longer maintained in its normal position, resulting in inefficient transmission of abdominal pressures along the urethral length. As a result, a precipitous increase in abdominal pressure is not transmitted to the urethral sphincteric mechanism, resulting in a temporary condition when bladder pressure exceeds urethral closure pressure and urinary leakage occurs.

Intrinsic sphincter deficiency (ISD) also causes stress urinary incontinence. Damage to the neuromuscular components of the urethra results from any process that causes denervation of the pelvic floor musculature or smooth muscle of the proximal urethra. Iatrogenic damage resulting from radical prostatectomy or transurethral resection of the prostate may cause ISD and stress urinary incontinence. Multiple anti-incontinence procedures or Y-V plasty in men or women also may result in incontinence.[124] Pelvic trauma or metabolic conditions result-ing in peripheral neuropathy affecting the pelvis may result in stress urinary incontinence as a result of sphincteric incompetence.[50]

Stress urinary incontinence in a woman may represent a combination of ISD and pelvic relaxation. Stress incontinence in a man is caused by ISD alone.

Instability incontinence is the condition of urinary leakage that occurs when the detrusor contracts at inappropriate times. The concept of instability arises from Hodgkinson, Ayers, and Drukker's description of dyssynergic detrusor activity among women with urinary incontinence.[55] Other terms have been used to describe the condition. Detrusor hyperreflexia is often used synonymously with instability. Nonetheless, the term is defined by the International Continence Society as the occurrence of an uninhibited detrusor contraction in the presence of a known neurologic disease. Other terms, such as detrusor hyperactivity or overactivity, are less commonly used.

Detrusor instability is associated with disease or trauma of the central nervous system. Diseases of the brain typically result in loss of volitional control over detrusor activity with preservation of coordination between the striated sphincter mechanism and detrusor activity. Such diseases include cerebrovascular accidents, parkinsonism, and brain tumors affecting the frontal lobes or cerebellum. Incontinence is preceded by a feeling of urgency followed by an unstable bladder contraction with relaxation of the sphincteric mechanism and evacuation of the bladder. Bladder emptying often is efficient, so urinary tract infections are not typically associated with this condition. The nursing diagnosis associated with this form of incontinence is "Urge incontinence."

Instability incontinence also is associated with neurologic abnormality of the spinal cord above the level of the sacral micturition center (S2-4).[123] Spinal cord injury is the most commonly noted lesion. Nontraumatic lesion include those seen in multiple sclerosis or other demyelinating diseases. Incontinence is not preceded by any sensation of urgency. A detrusor contraction is triggered by bladder filling or other stimulus, and the person is aware of the incontinence via perception of urinary leakage. Detrusor contraction is often associated with contraction of the pelvic floor and rhabdosphincter. This condition is called detrusor-sphincter dyssynergia and is associated with urinary retention, urinary tract infection, and upper tract deterioration.[50] The nursing diagnosis for this form of instability incontinence is "Reflex incontinence."

Nonneuropathic conditions also are associated with detrusor instability. Bladder outlet obstruction has been associated with instability incontinence among men with benign prostatic hyperplasia. Irritative bladder disorders caused by bacterial, viral, fungal, or parasitic infection of the bladder have been labeled as a cause of instability incontinence.[123] While these conditions are associated with increased sensations of bladder filling, little evidence supports the supposition that they cause detrusor instability.[9] Instability incontinence is associated with bladder irritation caused by bladder calculi and carcinoma of the urothelial lining of the vesicle. The leakage of urine into the posterior urethra seen in stress urinary incontinence has been speculated to cause instability of the detrusor.[123] Indeed, detrusor instability is often seen among women with stress urinary incontinence, and the condition is often relieved by surgical correction of the stress incontinence. Nonetheless, other investigators have failed to confirm this association, and the relation between detrusor instability and urinary leakage into the posterior urethra remains unclear.[96]

The underlying cause of many cases of instability incontinence is unclear, and the condition is termed idiopathic. Such instability may arise from a psychogenic or behavioral source, or it may be due to subtle neuropathy yet to be elucidated.

Overflow or paradoxic incontinence is the leakage of urine in the presence of a large residual. The nursing diagnosis associated with this form of incontinence is Urinary Retention. The two causes of overflow incontinence are deficient detrusor function and bladder outlet obstruction.[124] Deficient detrusor function may result from a variety of causes. Neurologic lesions of the sacral micturition cord such as that noted in myelomeningocele cause an autonomous neurogenic bladder with detrusor areflexia, lack of sensations of urgency, and overflow incontinence. Other central nervous system disorders associated with overflow incontinence are cauda equina syndrome, multiple sclerosis, tabes dorsalis, and poliomyelitis. Peripheral nervous system trauma or abnormalities that compromise parasympathetic innervation of the detrusor muscle also result in overflow incontinence. Examples are herpes zoster, extensive pelvic surgery, pelvic trauma, and diabetes mellitus.[123]

Other factors that result in overflow incontinence and detrusor areflexia are the result of chronic overdistention. The "nurse's bladder," "teacher's bladder," or "librarian's bladder" arises from overdistention of the bladder because of perceived inability to interrupt work for micturition. Acute illness and immobility may also result in deficient detrusor function. Severe constipation or fecal impaction is associated with temporary detrusor failure and overflow incontinence. Certain patients may suffer from urinary retention because of hysterical conversions.

Patients with overflow incontinence may not be aware of their inability to empty the bladder. Symptoms of deficient detrusor function are urgency, frequency, nocturia, and a dribbling, intermittent stream. Urinary tract infection is commonly an associated condition. Low back pain and vague abdominal discomfort may be the result of bladder enlargement.

Bladder outlet obstruction is also a cause of overflow incontinence. Types of bladder outlet obstruction include prostatic enlargement owing to inflammation, benign hypertrophy, or adenocarcinoma. Internal sphincter dyssynergia, bladder neck hypertrophy, and bladder neck contracture are particularly prevalent in men with highly stressful life styles and may lead to overflow incontinence. Urethral stricture in a man or urethral distortion in a woman may obstruct normal bladder emptying and lead to incontinence.[123]

Patients with bladder outlet obstruction are acutely aware of their problem because of high pressures generated by the detrusor during micturition. Symptoms of bladder outlet obstruction include frequency, nocturia, and poor urinary stream. A dribble after voiding is often noted.

Constant or extraurethral incontinence results when the normal sphincteric mechanism is bypassed, causing failure of urinary storage that is continuous. The causes of extraurethral incontinence are urinary fistula, ectopia, or surgical creation of a conduit for evacuation of urine. Congenital ectopic defects of the urinary tract including urethral duplication, epispadias, and exstrophy are relatively rare and may be associated with severe urinary leakage that may persist even after surgical leakage.[49] Ureteral ectopia is a more common congenital defect and results in a continuous, dribbling discharge superimposed on a normal voiding pattern if the orifice bypasses normal sphincteric mechanisms.[123]

Urinary fistula is most commonly noted among adult women. A fistula is created when tissue between the bladder or urethra and an adjacent structure erodes; the normal sphincteric mechanism is bypassed, resulting in urinary leakage. A fistula between the bladder and vagina is termed vesicovaginal fistula; a fistulous tract between the urethra and vagina is termed urethrovaginal fistula. Symmonds reviewed 800 cases of urinary fistulas seen at the Mayo Clinic over a 30-year period and found that the leading cause of fistula was pelvic surgery. Hysterectomy was the most common procedure associated with the condition. Other causes of fistula include penetrating trauma, radiation therapy, and obstetric complications.[116a] In the Mayo Clinic study, only 5% of the patients reviewed developed fistula as a result of obstetric complications. Nonetheless, childbearing is thought to account for the largest incidence of fistulous tracts worldwide.[118]

••••• Diagnostic Studies and Findings

Voiding cystourethrogram (VCUG)   Stress incontinence: pelvic descent below pubis; urethral excursion and leakage of contrast material with abdominal strain; instability incontinence: normal or trabeculated narrowing of membranous urethra noted with micturition in presence of detrusor-sphincter dyssynergia; diverticulae, vesicoureteral reflux may be noted in presence of detrusor-sphincter dyssynergia; overflow/paradoxic incontinence: large capacity, poor filling of proximal urethra with bladder outlet obstruction; failure of bladder neck funneling with detrusor-sphincter dyssynergia; urethral narrowing with stricture; constant extraurethral incontinence: leakage of contrast material through fistulous tract or from ectopic structure

Urodynamic testing   Stress incontinence: normal capacity, sensations, and compliance; stable detrusor; explosive flow with low-pressure detrusor contraction during micturition; normal electromyographic (EMG) findings; instability incontinence: decreased functional capacity; early sensations; normal compliance; unstable detrusor and/or urethra; EMG findings normal or indicative of detrusor-sphincter dyssynergia; overflow incontinence with deficient detrusor function: large capacity, delayed sensations, abnormally compliant; with detrusor hypotonic or areflexic: urinary stream poor or absent, large residual present after voiding; bladder outlet obstruction: normal or enlarged capacity; sensations may be delayed; compliance normal or impaired owing to detrusor hypertrophy; detrusor contraction is high pressure with poor urinary flow; constant incontinence: normal or impaired urine storage with large fistulous tract

Intravenous pyelogram (IVP) Constant incontinence: ureteral duplication with ectopic opening below bladder neck or outside urinary tract; extravasation of contrast material in fistula

Retrograde urethrogram (RUG) Presence of urethral stricture

Cystoscopy-urethroscopy Stress incontinence: normal findings in pelvic relaxation or open bladder neck with sphincteric damage; overflow incontinence: large capacity in deficient detrusor function; localization of obstruction in some cases; constant incontinence: ectopia or fistulous tract

Urinalysis and urine culture Instability incontinence: normal findings or presence of bacterial infection

Bladder biopsy Instability incontinence: normal findings or presence of transitional cell carcinoma or carcinoma in situ

•••••• Multidisciplinary Plan

Surgery

For stress incontinence

Vesicourethral suspension; over 100 procedures described in literature; commonly performed types include Marshall-Marchetti-Krantz, Stamey or Raz needle suspension, Burch's culposuspension

Artificial urinary sphincter for stress incontinence caused by ISD; cuff of device placed at bladder neck or proximal urethra, abdominal reservoir positioned, pump mechanism placed in scrotum or fascia of labia

Suburethral sling surgery for stress incontinence caused by ISD and pelvic relaxation with urethral hypermobility

Suburethral GAX collagen injections for ISD without coexisting urethral hypermobility

For overflow incontinence

Transurethral resection of enlarged prostate; open prostatectomy or radical prostatectomy in certain cases

Correction of urethral stricture by internal urethrotomy or urethral dilation

Correction of female distortion by open surgical reconstruction

For constant extraurethral incontinence

Removal or repair of ectopic structures

Open surgical repair of urinary fistula

Medications

To affect detrusor contractility

Autonomic drugs

Propantheline, up to 150 mg/d in 3 divided doses

Oxybutynin, 5 mg bid or tid

Central nervous system drugs

Imipramine, 1.5-2 mg/kg in single dose at bedtime

Spasmolytic agents

Dicyclomine, 10-20 mg tid or qid

Hyoscyamine, 0.125-0.25 mg tid-qid

Drugs that increase detrusor activity and tone

Autonomic drugs

Bethanechol, 15-30 mg tid or qid

Drugs used to increase bladder neck tone

Autonomic drugs

Norephedrine or ephedrine (Sudafed S.A.), 1 tablet bid

Drugs used to decrease bladder neck tone

Autonomic drugs

Terazosin, 2-10 mg at HS

Doxazosin, 2-8 mg at HS

Drugs used to decrease external muscle tone

Central nervous system drugs

Baclofen, 5-20 mg tid

NURSING CARE

Nursing Assessment

Bladder

Suprapubic tenderness associated with cystitis; suprapubic and lower abdominal distention in overflow incontinence

Vaginal Vault

Bulge in anterior wall in cystocele associated with pelvic relaxation; discharge in vesicovaginal or ureterovaginal fistula or ureteral ectopia in the vagina or uterus

Pale, friable mucosa, tender to touch

Minimum Assessment for Urinary Incontinence[3]

History (including current patterns of urinary elimination, duration of urinary leakage exacerbating and alleviating factors, urologic, neurologic, reproductive systems review)

Focused physical examination (perineal inspection including vaginal rectal examination and integument, focused neurologic examination, functional assessment for mobility, dexterity, cognition)

Urinalysis (culture and sensitivity testing only when suspicion of urinary tract infection is raised by urinalysis)

Postvoid urinary residual measurement (strongly recommended)

Bladder log (voiding diary) for at least 24 hours (strongly recommended)

Nursing Dx & Intervention

Altered urinary elimination (general considerations) related to urinary leakage

• Provide the patient with an appropriate urinary containment system (pad, dribble pouch, continent brief, incontinent briefs, or other device) *to contain urinary leakage until a definitive management program can be instituted.*

- Encourage the patient to drink an adequate volume of fluids (30 ml/kg of body weight per day[87]) *to prevent concentration of the urine and intensification of irritative voiding symptoms.*
- Assist the patient to identify and modify the intake of food and beverages that aggravate irritative symptoms. *Caffeinic, carbonated beverages, and certain spicy foods or chocolates may produce mild bladder irritation, aggravating symptoms of urinary incontinence.*
- Encourage the patient who smokes to stop. *Cigarette smoke may act as a mild bladder irritant, aggravating symptoms of urinary incontinence.*

Stress incontinence related to pelvic descent

- Teach the patient to identify, isolate, and contract the pelvic muscles and to perform pelvic (Kegel) exercises using principles of physiotherapy[34] *to strengthen the periurethral striated muscles.*
- Perform electrostimulation therapy *to supplement the success of pelvic muscle exercises in the individual with profound weakness of the pelvic muscles.*
- Teach the female patient to use vaginal cones *to strengthen the periurethral muscles.*
- Administer, or teach the patient to self-administer, α-sympathomimetic agents or imipramine as directed (see box below). *Alpha-sympathomimetics increase urethral sphincter resistance, alleviating or ablating stress incontinence.*

■ DRUGS USED FOR STRESS INCONTINENCE

α-SYMPATHOMIMETICS: Ephedrine, pseudoephedrine, phenylpropanolamine

Over-the-counter preparations: Sudafed, Sudafed S.A. capsules, Dexatrim without caffeine capsules (preparations with antihistamines are avoided; generic substitutes are available)

Prescription preparations: Entex L.A., Ornade spansules

Action and administration: increases tone of urethral smooth muscle and rhabdosphincter; taken only during daytime hours and may be taken before physically demanding activities (exercise, walking) exclusively

Side effects: tachycardia, hypertension, anxiety, nervousness, insomnia

TRICYCLIC ANTIDEPRESSANT

Prescription preparations: imipramine (may be used with estrogens)

Action: α-sympathomimetic action increases tone of urethral smooth muscle and rhabdosphincter; anticholinergic effect relaxes detrusor and increases functional capacity in cases of SUI mixed with unstable detrusor

Administration: 10-25 mg PO, tid to qid; administered over a 24-hour period; individual is gradually withdrawn from drug using tapered doses

Side effects: drowsiness, urinary retention, dry mouth, constipation, mydriasis (mild), hypertension

From Gray.[49]

- Administer, or teach the patient to self-administer, topical or systemic estrogens as directed. *Estrogen replacement therapy may alleviate stress incontinence and related irritative bladder symptoms by its trophic effects on the urethral mucosa.*
- Place, or assist the physician or nurse specialist to place, a pessary, and teach the patient to care for the device. *A pessary device may alleviate or relieve stress incontinence by mechanically restoring more normal urethrovesical anatomy.*
- Prepare the patient for surgical repair of stress incontinence as indicated. *Surgical repair of stress incontinence restores urethrovesical anatomy to nearly normal.*
- Prepare the patient with stress incontinence caused by sphincter mechanism incompetence for periurethral injection of a bulking agent. *Urethral bulking agents alleviate stress incontinence by promoting coaptation of urethral surfaces.*
- Prepare the patient with stress incontinence caused by sphincter incompetence for implantation of an artificial urinary sphincter, as directed. *The artificial urinary sphincter is a mechanical device that performs a function similar to the intrinsic sphincter mechanism.*
- Prepare the female with sphincter incompetence causing stress incontinence for suburethral sling as directed. *The suburethral sling is a procedure in which a segment of fascia or synthetic material is placed around the urethra, promoting closure of the sphincter mechanism.*

Instability (urge) incontinence related to detrusor instability

- Institute a timed voiding schedule based on results of a voiding diary *to encourage voluntary bladder evacuation before unstable contractions cause leakage.*
- Administer, or teach the patient to self-administer, antispasmodic or anticholinergic medications as directed *to suppress unstable bladder contractions and to enhance bladder capacity.*
- Combine pharmacotherapy with a timed voiding schedule. *Pharmacotherapy for instability (urge) incontinence increases bladder capacity and suppresses unstable contractions. Nonetheless, these contractions will inevitably occur if the bladder is allowed to overfill.*
- Teach the patient to manipulate fluid intake. Ensure that the patient obtains an adequate daily fluid intake (30 ml/kg of body weight per day[87]), while avoiding intake of large volumes of fluids with meals or before bedtime *to avoid acute large intake of fluid and unstable contractions.*
- Institute a bladder drill therapy consisting of a regimen to increase the time interval between toiletings to a goal of every 3 hours. *Bladder drill therapy is a behavioral technique designed to gradually enhance capacity and diminish urge incontinence.*
- Institute electrostimulation therapy alone or in combination with bladder drill therapy. *Electrostimulation therapy is a technique that inhibits unstable bladder contractions*

and sensations of urgency and enhances capacity. Bladder drill therapy probably supplements this approach to therapy. Electrostimulation therapy may enhance bladder capacity and inhibit unstable contractions by reflex inhibition of the pelvic plexus or by other, unknown actions.

- Administer, or teach the patient to self-administer, antispasmodic medications, and teach the patient to perform self-intermittent catheterization using a clean technique, as directed. *Antispasmodic medications can be used to "pharmacologically paralyze" the detrusor muscle. Intermittent catheterization is used to ensure regular, complete evacuation of urine. Acceptance of this regimen is limited by the occurrence of side effects from relatively high doses of anticholinergic medications and the acceptability of intermittent catheterization among individuals with normal urethral and bladder sensations.*

- Insert an indwelling urethral or suprapubic catheter, as directed. Teach the patient to care for the catheter and drainage bags. *An indwelling catheter represents a "last option" for the patient with instability (urge) incontinence; however, it may be necessary for the patient with limited dexterity or with limited family or other ongoing caretakers.*

Instability (reflex) incontinence related to detrusor hyperreflexia with sphincter dysynergia

- Administer, or teach the patient to self-administer, antispasmodic medications, and teach the patient to perform clean, intermittent catheterization. *Antispasmodics are used to suppress all bladder contractions, and intermittent catheterization is used to provide regular, complete bladder evacuation. The acceptability of this program is enhanced by the absence of urethral and bladder sensations and is limited when upper extremity dexterity is compromised.*

- Apply a condom catheter to the male patient who is to be managed by a "reflex voiding program" for instability (reflex) leakage. Teach the patient and family to change the catheter routinely (daily or twice daily) and to inspect the penile skin for integrity with each change. *Condom drainage is a realistic option for males who are unable to perform self-catheterization. The long-term safety of a "reflex voiding" program is affected by the presence and severity of detrusor-sphincter dyssynergia.*

- Administer, or teach the patient to self-administer, α-sympathomimetic blocking agents *to reduce urethral resistance and obstruction caused by detrusor-sphincter dyssynergia; the condom is used to contain urinary leakage.*

- Prepare the male patient who is unable to perform self-catheterization for transurethral sphincterotomy, as directed. *Sphincterotomy is the incision of the striated sphincter mechanism providing relief of bladder outlet obstruction caused by detrusor-sphincter dyssynergia.*

- Prepare the patient for insertion of a urethral stent device, as directed. *Urethral stents are inserted under endoscopic guidance and used to reduce the urethral resistance caused by detrusor sphincter dyssynergia.*

- Prepare the patient with instability (reflex) incontinence, who is capable of self-catheterization, for augmentation enterocystoplasty or continent urinary diversion, as directed. *Augmentation enterocystoplasty is the surgical anastomosis of detubularized bowel or stomach with the bladder muscle. It reduces detrusor contractility and enhances bladder capacity; catheterization is required for bladder evacuation. Continent urinary diversion is the creation of a urinary reservoir and continence abdominal or stoma, using bowel or stomach. It is reserved for particularly small or hostile bladders not amenable to less extensive reconstruction. Continent urinary diversion also requires intermittent catheterization for evacuation of urine.*

- Insert an indwelling urethral or suprapubic catheter, as directed. Teach the patient to care for the catheter and drainage bags. *An indwelling catheter represents a "last option" for the patient with instability (reflex) incontinence; however, it may be necessary for the patient with limited dexterity and limited family or other ongoing caretakers.*

Urinary retention related to bladder outlet obstruction or deficient contractility

- Teach the patient the technique of double voiding. Instruct the patient to urinate and sit on the toilet for 3 to 5 minutes, followed by a second episode of urination. *Double voiding may relieve mild to moderate urinary retention caused by minimally compromised detrusor contractility.*

- Administer, or teach the patient to self-administer, a cholinergic agonist (such as bethanechol chloride) alone or in combination with an α-antagonist, as directed, *to stimulate bladder sensations, to enhance contractility, and to reduce urethral resistance. A cholinergic agonist is of limited therapeutic benefit for patients with compromised detrusor contractility. It is probably most helpful for patients with compromised contractility, coexisting with altered sensations of bladder filling.*

- Teach the patient with urinary retention to perform intermittent catheterization after consultation with the physician. *Intermittent catheterization provides regular, complete bladder evacuation, preventing bladder overdistention and urinary system distress.*

- Place an intermittent or long-term, indwelling urethral or suprapubic catheter, as directed, *to provide chronic urinary drainage.*

- Teach the patient with an indwelling catheter to care for the catheter and to routinely clean the collection bags used for drainage of urine. *Routine cleaning of drainage bags prevents overgrowth of pathogens, reducing the likelihood of symptomatic infection.*

Total (extraurethral) incontinence related to fistula or ectopia

- Assist the patient to select and apply a urinary containment device *to minimize the effects of continuous urinary leakage.*

- Provide the patient with extraurethral incontinence caused by a surgically-created stoma with a proper pouching system after consultation with the ET nurse.
- Prepare the patient for surgical correction of fistula or urinary ectopia *to provide a definitive repair of extraurethral leakage.*
- Administer, or assist the physician to administer, a sclerosing agent (such as tetracycline in a saline suspension) *to ablate extraurethral leakage by progressive scarring and closure of the fistulous tract.*

Functional incontinence related to limited mobility, dexterity, access to toilet or cognition deficit

- Assist the patient with compromised mobility to attain and use assistive devices, as indicated, *to minimize the time needed to ambulate to the toilet.*
- Assist the patient to remove any environmental barriers *to maximize access to the toilet.*
- Assist the individual with compromised dexterity to alter clothing to minimize the need for manipulating buttons, zippers, or similar devices, *minimizing the time required to remove the clothing for toileting.*
- Assist the individual with compromised dexterity to obtain and use assistive devices, as indicated, *to maximize the ability to manipulate the clothing for toileting.*
- Begin a prompted voiding program for the individual with impaired cognitive ability.

Altered skin integrity related to urinary leakage

- Teach the patient to perform routine skin care for all skin areas routinely exposed to urinary leakage. Routine care consists of daily washing, with thorough drying, and applying a skin barrier or moisture barrier. Skin that is exposed to particularly severe leakage or skin affected by ammonia contact dermatitis is dried under a blow dryer turned to the lowest (warm) setting for 10 to 15 minutes each day. *Routine skin care minimizes the risk of altered skin integrity.*
- Apply an antifungal cream to skin affected by monilial rash, as directed. *A monilial rash often compromises skin routinely exposed to urinary leakage.*

Social isolation (high risk for) related to shame, embarrassment

- Teach the patient that urinary incontinence is a treatable condition and that failure of one treatment strategy does not imply that leakage is "intractable" or "incurable." *Urinary incontinence is often defined as an insignificant problem that is untreatable or as an inevitable process of aging or certain surgical procedures. Social isolation and personal shame are encouraged by these misperceptions.*
- Provide the patient with the name and address or telephone number of a continence support group, such as Help for Incontinent People, Inc. (HIP). *Advocacy groups provide support, advice, and assistance for individuals learning to live with and overcome urinary incontinence.*

Patient Education/Home Care Planning

1. Provide instruction on technique of medication regimens and need for continuous therapy in neuropathic bladder cases.
2. Provide a list of signs and symptoms of urinary tract infection and other conditions requiring medical attention.
3. Provide instructions for intermittent catheterization technique or care of long-indwelling Foley catheter.
4. Provide instruction about the relationship of incontinence to fluid intake, various medications, and compliance with medical and nursing strategies for prevention.
5. Provide information on support groups (see box below).

Evaluation

Stress incontinence resulting from pelvic relaxation has been surgically corrected Continence is maintained. Residual after voiding is less than 25% of total bladder volume. There is no urinary tract infection.

Stress incontinence has been surgically corrected with placement of artificial urinary sphincter Continence is maintained. Sphincter device is functioning. There is no urinary tract infection.

Unstable bladder is adequately managed Continence is maintained.

Reflex incontinence is adequately managed Continence is maintained or patient is using condom device to collect urine.

Instability incontinence caused by irritative disorder is resolved Continence is maintained. Underlying irritative disorder is resolved.

 PATIENT ADVOCACY AND SUPPORT GROUPS FOR INCONTINENCE

CONTINENCE RESTORED, INC.

Co-directors:	Anne Smith-Young, C.U.T.
	Douglas Whitehead, M.D.
Address:	785 Park Avenue
	New York, New York 10021

HELP FOR INCONTINENT PEOPLE, INC. (HIP)

Director:	Katherine Jeter, Ed.D., E.T.
Address:	P.O. Box 544
	Union, South Carolina 29379

SIMON FOUNDATION FOR CONTINENCE

Director:	Cheryl Gartley
Address:	P.O. Box 835
	Wilmette, Illinois 60091

From Gray.[49]

Overflow incontinence in bladder with deficient detrusor function is adequately managed   Continence is maintained. Residual after voiding is less than 25% of total bladder volume.

Overflow incontinence caused by bladder outlet obstruction is resolved   Continence is maintained. Obstruction is resolved.

Constant incontinence is resolved   Continence is maintained. Fistula is closed or ectopia is repaired.

Skin integrity is maintained   Patient learns to perform skin care to prevent breakdown from exposure to urinary leakage. Antifungal cream prevents development of monilial rash.

Social isolation does not occur   Patients maintain normal activities and relationships and seek assistance from support groups, as needed.

PROSTATE DISORDERS

BENIGN PROSTATIC HYPERPLASIA

Benign prostatic hyperplasia (BPH) is the progressive enlargement of the prostate gland. The symptoms of BPH are caused by bladder outlet obstruction and its sequelae. In the majority of males, BPH is a quality of life disorder. In unusual cases, BPH produces a significant obstructive uropathy and compromised renal function.[2]

BPH is the most common neoplastic growth in men past the fifth decade of life.[53,55] Histologic evidence of BPH can be found in men as young as 25 to 30 years of age, and its incidence increases steadily, affecting 50% of men over age 60 years, and 90% of men 85 years and older. The prevalence of symptomatic BPH is not known, partially due to differences in evaluation of the symptoms that comprise the condition. In one study combining digital rectal examination and a symptom score,[42] the prevalence of symptomatic BPH was 138/100,000 among men in their fifties, and 400 per 100,000 among octogenarians.

No risk factors for BPH have been identified.[119,125] Sexual activity (or celibacy), cigarette smoking, alcohol use, or social factors have not been associated with an increased incidence in the development of BPH. A congenital absence of androgens, or the enzyme needed to convert testosterone to dihydrotestosterone, prevents normal prostate development and subsequent BPH.[115] Orchiectomy also prevents normal prostate development and BPH, and diabetes mellitus may or may not reduce the risk of prostatic enlargement.

Serious complications or death due to BPH are rare. The incidence of significant renal insufficiency is low, as is the presence of urinary infection or bladder calculi. The mortality rate directly attributable to BPH is approximately 1.8 per 100,000.[2] There is no clear relationship between BPH and prostate cancer.[45] Nonetheless, an increased risk for prostate cancer has been reported among men with BPH[8]; although this relationship may be limited to "atypical patterns" of hyperplasia, rather than classic, benign prostatic enlargement.[46]

As the number of elderly men living in the United States continues to grow, so will the prevalence of BPH. Approximately 1 in 4 men with symptoms of BPH will seek relief by the age of 80 years. More than 300,000 procedures are performed each year for BPH, and the condition produces an annual cost of approximately $4.5 billion.[2,56]

•••••• Pathophysiology

The etiology and natural history of BPH remain unclear, although significant progress has been made in understanding certain elements of the pathogenesis of prostate enlargement.[115] Prostatic hyperplasia is influenced by the presence of the hormones testosterone and dihydrotestosterone. The prerequisites for prostatic enlargement are aging, androgen receptors, and functioning testis capable of producing testosterone for conversion to dihydrotestosterone. Luteinizing hormone is released from the hypothalamus and acts on Leydig cells to produce testosterone. Ninety-five percent of testosterone is produced by the testes; 5% arises from the adrenal glands.

The majority of testosterone produced by the testes and adrenals is bound to an androgen-binding protein in the serum and remains physiologically inactive. A small portion of circulating testosterone (approximately 2%), however, remains unbound and can be converted to dihydrotestosterone by the prostate. An enzyme, 5 α-reductase, is required to convert testosterone to dihydrotestosterone. After diffusing into the prostate, testosterone is converted into dihydrotestosterone by this enzyme, resulting in release of local growth factors and proliferation of prostatic tissue. Testosterone ablation or inhibition of 5 α-reductase will arrest prostatic hyperplasia and reduce the size of the prostate gland.[115]

Nonetheless, the actions of the androgens testosterone and dihydrotestosterone and the enzyme 5 α-reductase, alone, do not explain the association of BPH with aging.[121] In the aging male, the serum concentrations of both bioavailable and bound testosterone is diminished, and these effects would be expected to hinder, rather than produce, hyperplasia of the prostatic stroma. The relation between prostatic hyperplasia and aging is partly explained by an increase in nuclear androgen receptors that compensates for the reduction in circulating androgens. In addition, other local factors, including epidermal growth factor, insulin growth factor, basic fibroblast growth factor, and nerve growth factor, influence prostatic hyperplasia by mechanisms that have not yet been defined.[115]

It is the presence of voiding dysfunction, rather than enlargement of the prostate gland per se, that causes men to seek treatment. The voiding dysfunction associated with BPH is divided into two symptom types, obstructive and irritative. Obstructive voiding symptoms related to BPH include a slow or intermittent urinary stream, hesitancy when initiating urination, post void dribbling, and feelings of incomplete bladder evacuation. Irritative voiding symptoms include the urgency to urinate, frequency of urination, and nocturia.[2,115]

The initial symptoms of BPH are primarily obstructive and include a slowing of the urinary stream, hesitancy to initiate urination, and a post void dribbling. This effect is partly explained by a reduction in the cross sectional area of the urethra as it passes through the prostate. Obstruction of the bladder outlet also arises from increased smooth muscle tone at the prostate and bladder neck, causing poor funneling of the proximal urethra during micturition. This smooth muscle of the prostate and proximal urethra is richly innervated by α_{1-c} receptors, and alpha antagonistic drugs partially block this tone. During the early stages of BPH, the detrusor muscle hypertrophies and the symptoms of BPH may subside. If the magnitude of bladder outlet obstruction increases, however, compensatory hypertrophy of the detrusor also causes trabeculation of the detrusor muscle, diverticulae, and hypertrophy of the trigone.[107,119]

When the hyperplasia of BPH progresses, obstructive symptoms are exacerbated, and the person is prone to episodes of acute urinary retention. Acute urinary retention is characterized by the inability to urinate. It is a relatively common complica-

tion of BPH, occurring in as many as 54% of a group of British men undergoing treatment for prostate enlargement. Acute urinary retention is a medical emergency and potent incentive for prompt management of prostatic hyperplasia.

The pathophysiology of the irritative symptoms associated with BPH is less well defined than the obstructive symptoms. The hypertrophic detrusor muscle may be more sensitive to the neurotransmitters responsible for bladder contraction, or the process of chronic obstruction may cause changes in the function of the sensory nerves of the bladder. Sensory nerve enlargement of the bladder has been noted in experimental studies of animal models and humans, and stimulation of nerve growth factor caused by obstruction may contribute to these neurologic changes in the bladder muscle.[115]

In some patients with BPH, irritative voiding symptoms may be related to unstable detrusor contractions. Denervation changes in the neuromuscular units of the detrusor muscle oc-

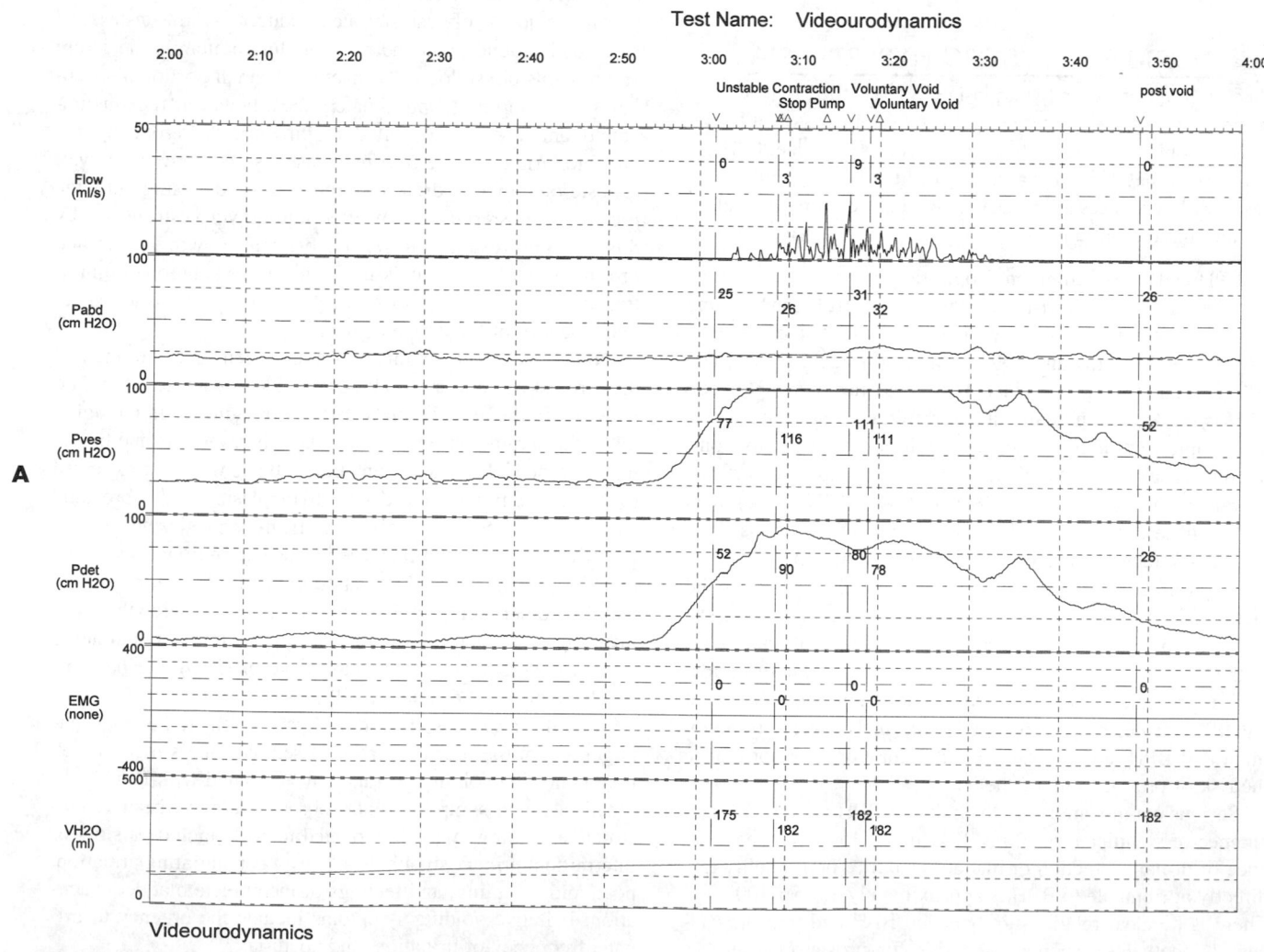

Videourodynamics

Figure 12-16 Voiding pressure study of prostatic outlet obstruction. **A,** Urodynamic tracing demonstrates high voiding pressure (maximum detrusor contraction pressure [Pdet] is 96 cm H_2O, but maximum flow is only 9 ml/second).

cur with obstruction, and there is some evidence that these changes cause hyperactive (unstable) contractions of the bladder.[26] An unstable contraction in a man with bladder outlet obstruction, and BPH is likely to cause an immediate urgency to urinate, frequency of urination, and nocturia. Nonetheless, because of the obstruction, the man is unlikely to experience urge incontinence. Rather, he is likely to experience the irritative symptoms (urgency, frequency, and nocturia) of BPH, as well as obstructive symptoms.

In some patients, severe, prolonged obstruction may lead to decompensation of detrusor muscle contraction strength. The bladder wall becomes increasingly noncompliant, and detrusor contractions become less efficient, causing larger post void urinary residual volumes, a high risk of urinary infection, vesicoureteral reflux, or compromised renal function.[107] Fortunately, these cases of severe obstruction and upper urinary tract decompensation are uncommon, and BPH remains primarily a disorder that affects the quality of life.

Diagnostic Studies and Findings

Prostate specific antigen Abnormally high values raise suspicion of prostate cancer.

Serum creatinine Abnormally high values indicate compromised renal function or renal failure.

Urinalysis/urine culture and sensitivity Nitrites and white blood cells on dipstick and white blood cells and bacteriuria and pyuria on microscopic examination raise suspicion of urinary tract infection. A urine culture is obtained when urinalysis raises suspicion of urinary tract infection.

Uroflowmetry Identifies abnormal voiding patterns; diminished maximum and mean flow rate indicate the possibility of bladder outlet obstruction. The uroflow does not differentiate abnormal flow caused by poor detrusor contraction strength from abnormal flow caused by obstruction.

Pressure-flow study Provides the best evaluation of bladder outlet obstruction; diminished maximum and mean flow rate with elevated intravesical voiding pressures indicate bladder outlet obstruction. Results from a voiding pressure study may be plotted on one or more voiding pressure nomograms allowing comparison with age-matched males with and without symptomatic BPH (Figure 12-16).

Post void residual volume Elevated post void residual volume is not diagnostic of BPH, but larger volumes may

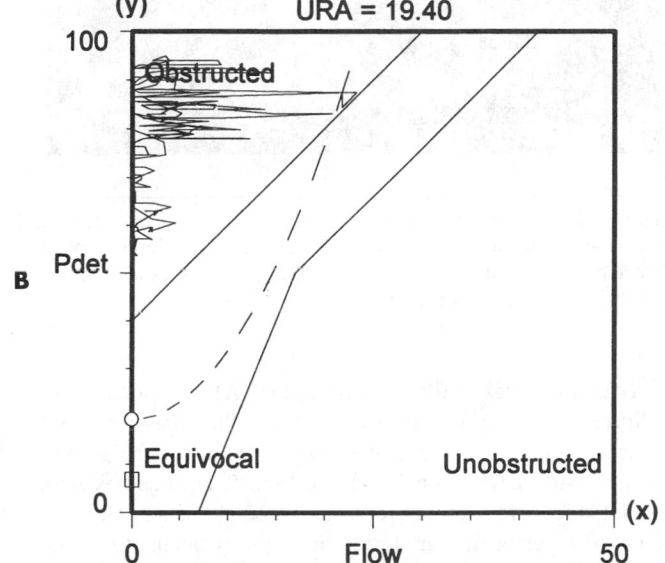

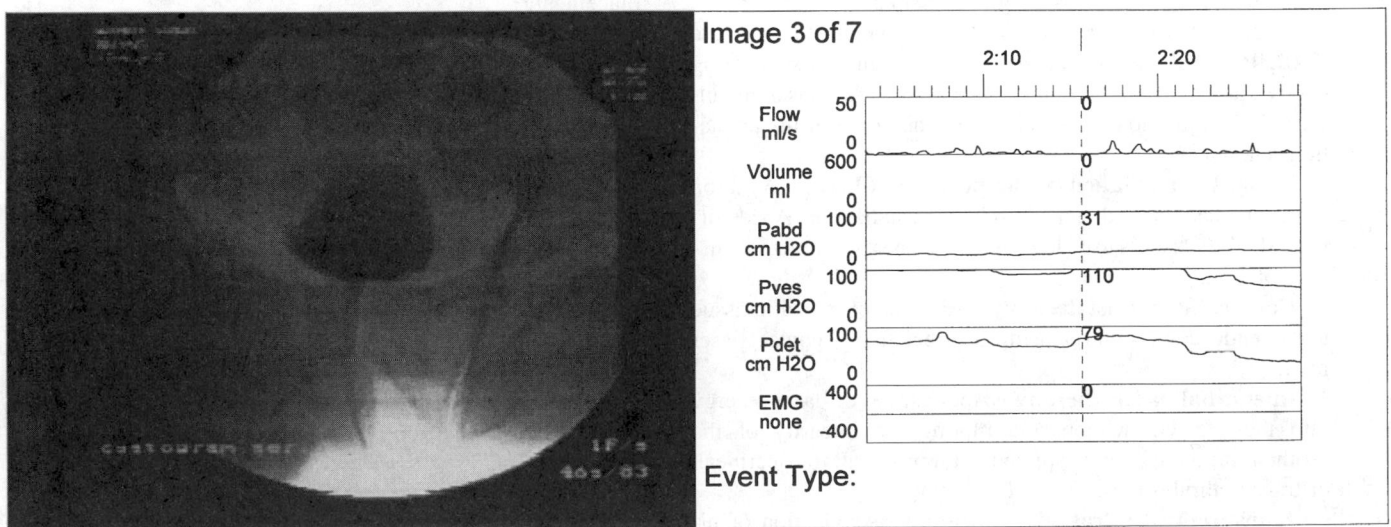

Figure 12-16—cont'd Voiding pressure study of prostatic outlet obstruction. **B,** Abrams-Griffith nomogram comparing detrusor contraction pressure (Pdet on Y axis) versus flow rate (flow on X axis) is consistent with bladder outlet obstruction. **C,** Fluoroscopic image with real time tracing shows high detrusor contraction pressure, with diminished flow. Note incomplete funneling of the bladder neck, poor filling of the prostatic urethra, and trabeculation of the bladder indicating significant obstruction.

indicate a greater need for treatment and reduction in residual volumes can be used to determine the effect of treatment[2]

Intravenous pyelogram   Not recommended for routine evaluation of BPH; occasionally helpful when prostatism is complicated by hematuria, calculi, urinary tract infection

Cystoscopy   Not indicated for routine evaluation of BPH, or to determine the need for treatment; used as an adjunctive modality during invasive endoscopic procedures (transurethral resection of the prostate gland, etc.)

Transrectal ultrasound of the prostate   Not indicated for the routine evaluation of BPH; used as an adjunctive modality to define the anatomy of BPH; presence of potentially malignant tumors, cysts, or other unexpected anatomic findings (Figure 12-17).

• • • • • • Multidisciplinary Plan

(See Table 12-5: Alternative Procedures for Prostate Tissue Removal, p. 1056)

Surgery and Transurethral Procedures

Open prostatectomy   Removal of the prostate from a suprapubic approach; the prostatic capsule is left intact; typically reserved for severe enlargement (glands >60-80 g).

Transurethral resection of the prostate (TUR-P)   Resection of prostatic tissue under endoscopic control. The outcomes for TUR-P are considered the "gold standard" for prostatectomy; the efficacy of all other modalities are compared to this technique.

Transurethral vaportrobe   Ablation of prostatic tissue using a "roller ball" type device with electrocautery energy.

Transurethral incision of the prostate (TUIP)   Incision of the prostatic capsule using electrocautery endoscopic knife; generally reserved for prostate glands <40 g.[115]

Transurethral ultrasonic laser incision of the prostate (TULIP)   Ablation of prostate tissue using a side firing neodymium Yttrium-aluminum-garnet (Nd:YAG) laser and ultrasonic imaging to ensure adequate penetration of the prostatic adenoma.[15]

Visual laser ablation of the prostate (VLAP)   Ablation of the prostate under direct endoscopic visualization. A side firing Nd:YAG laser is used to provide the energy for prostate tissue ablation.[15]

Contact laser prostatectomy   Ablation of prostatic tissue under endoscopic control using a direct firing, contact laser fiber.

Interstitial laser therapy   Application of laser energy into the prostate without interrupting the integrity of the urothelium; the energy is applied via transrectal, transperineal, or transurethral routes.

Transurethral ultrasonic aspiration   Application of ultrasonic energy fragmenting tissues high in water content (such as the prostate) while preserving tissues with greater collagen content (such as the bladder neck and membranous urethra) followed by aspiration of the fragmented tissue.[115]

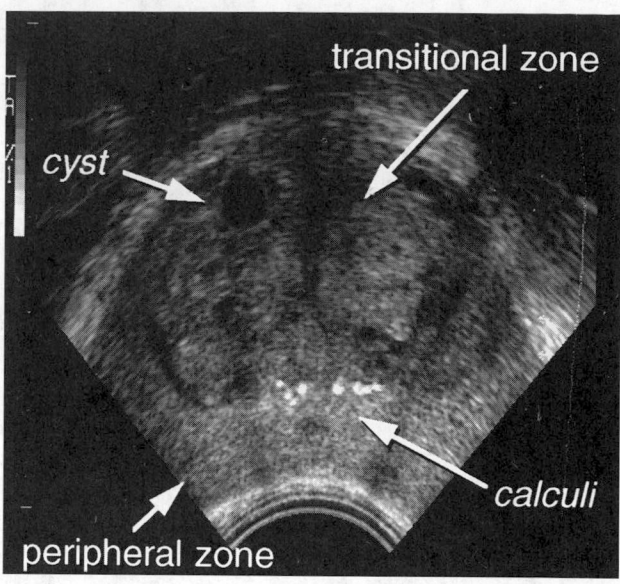

Figure 12-17 Ultrasonic image of the prostate demonstrating BPH. Note that the transitional zone has become enlarged and is detectable on this image, as is the peripheral zone. A cyst and prostatic calculi also are indicated.

Transurethral needle ablation (TUNA)   Application of radiofrequency energy (of lower level than laser energy) capable of ablating prostate tissue. The procedure is performed using a 22 French catheter and 2 cm needles with special shields to protect urethral and rectal tissues. The procedure is performed under endoscopic visualization and using ultrasonic imaging to determine the depth of needle placement.[32]

High-intensity focused ultrasound (HIFU)   Ablation of prostate tissue using focused ultrasonic energy applied via a transrectal probe surrounded by a condom and degassed water.[14]

Cryotherapy   Rapid cooling/freezing of prostatic tissue via a transurethral route; more commonly used for prostate cancer.[115]

Hyperthermia   Application of microwave energy via transurethral or transrectal routes to destroy prostate tissue.[68]

Intraurethral stent   Placement of a wire mesh stent under endoscopic control designed to mechanically open prostatic urethra.[49]

Transurethral balloon dilation   No longer recommended for BPH due to poor long-term efficacy[41]

Pharmacotherapy

Hormonal agents   Finasteride, a 5α-reductase inhibitor, is the principal endocrine agent used to manage BPH (see Table 12-4)

Alpha antagonists   Reduce smooth muscle tone at the bladder neck and prostatic urethra (see box on p. 1033)

TABLE 12-4 Hormonal Agents Used to Treat Benign Prostatic Hyperplasia[83]

Agent	Pharmacologic Action	Side Effects
Antiandrogen agents: Flutamide, Anandron, Casodex	Selectively block androgenic receptors	Gastrointestinal upset, impaired libido (uncommon), erectile dysfunction, gynecomastia
Progestins: Megestrol acetate, Hydroxyprogesterone caproate	Inhibits production of leutinizing hormone, production of testosterone, dihydrotestesterone	Gastrointestinal upset, heat intolerance, flushing, reduced libido, erectile dysfunction
5α-reductase enzyme inhibitors: Finasteride, Episteride	Inhibits conversion of testosterone to dihydrotestosterone without reduction in serum levels of testosterone	Loss of libido, erectile dysfunction (rare), gynecomastia (uncommon), decreased ejaculatory volume

Data from Grayhack JT, Kozlowski JM.[50a]

General Management

Watchful waiting Routine assessment of symptoms (every 6 months to 1 year) without intervention; appropriate for a majority of patients with mild to moderate symptoms and no complicating factors

NURSING CARE

Nursing Assessment

Minimum Evaluation of BPH[2]

History: including duration of symptoms, patterns of urine elimination, episodes of acute urinary retention, previous prostate evaluation, **all** patients should complete an AUA Symptom Index (see box on p. 1034), a voiding diary/bladder log is strongly recommended

Physical examination: including digital rectal examination for prostate size, symmetry between lateral lobes, evidence of induration, discrete nodules

Serum Prostate Specific Antigen (optional): to determine need for further evaluation for prostate cancer

Serum creatinine: to assess renal function

Urinalysis: to rule out presence of urinary infection (culture and sensitivity obtained only when history, physical assessment and/or urinalysis raises index of suspicion)

Nursing Dx & Intervention

Urinary retention, related to BPH

- Teach the patient the signs and symptoms of acute urinary retention. Acute urinary retention is a common complication of BPH and constitutes a medical emergency.
- Advise the patient of the risk factors for acute urinary retention including over-the-counter decongestants or diet pills, prescription antidepressants, anticholinergics, calcium-channel blockers, antispasmodics, antiparkinsonian agents, and antipsychotics. Decongestants and diet pills contain an α-adrenergic agonist that creates a risk of acute

---

α-ADRENERGIC BLOCKERS USED TO TREAT BPH

AGENTS

Nonselective α-adrenergic blockers (block α_1- and α_2-adrenergic receptors):
  Phenoxybenzamine 5-10 mg PO bid
Short acting, selective α_1 adrenergic blockers:
  Prazosin 1-5 mg PO bid*
  Alfuzosin 7.5-10 mg PO daily**
Long acting, selective α_1 adrenergic blockers:
  Terazosin 1-10 mg PO daily (at HS)
  Doxazosin 1-12 mg PO daily (at HS)
  Tamusulosin 0.1-0.4 mg daily (at HS)

PHARMACOLOGIC ACTION

Phenoxybenzamine blocks α_1- and α_2-adrenergic receptors in the bladder neck, prostatic urethra and distant sites; all other agents selectively block α_1 adrenergic receptors in the bladder neck, prostatic urethra and other sites

SIDE EFFECTS

General: Postural hypotension, tachycardia, drowsiness, prolonged fatigue, rhinitis, flulike syndrome
Specific: *Postural hypotension associated with prazosin administration may be intensified with hyponatremia, **the therapeutic dosage range of alfuzosin for BPH has not been established

From Lepor.[71]

urinary retention by increasing smooth muscle tone of the prostate, bladder neck, and proximal urethra. *The other agents listed increase the risk of acute urinary retention by relaxing detrusor muscle contractions.*

- Instruct the man with BPH to drink no more than 8 to 12 ounces with meals, to sip beverages throughout the day, and to avoid intake of large amounts of fluid over a short period of time. *Intake of a large bolus of fluid over a brief period of time will rapidly fill the bladder and increase the risk of an episode of acute urinary retention.*

1034   CHAPTER 12   *Genitourinary System*

■ **AUA SYMPTOM INDEX**

VOIDING DYSFUNCTION ITEMS:

1. Over the past month, how often have you had a sensation of not emptying your bladder completely after you finished urinating?
2. Over the past month, have you had to urinate again less than 2 hours after you finished urinating?
3. Over the past month, how often have you found you stopped and started again several times when you urinated?
4. Over the past month, how often have you found it difficult to postpone urination?
5. Over the past month, how often have you had a weak urinary stream?
6. Over the past month, how often have you had to push or strain to begin urination?

These questions are answered on a Likert type scale of 0-5; a response of 0 indicates not at all, 1 indicates less than 1 time in 5; 2 indicates less than half of the time, 3 indicates about half of the time, 4 indicates more than half of the time, and 5 indicates almost always

7. Over the past month, how many times did you most typically get up to urinate from the time you went to bed at night until the time you got up in the morning?

This item is answered on a scale of 0-5; 0 indicates no episodes of nocturia, and 5 indicates 5 episodes or more each night

QUALITY OF LIFE ITEM

If you were to spend the rest of your life with your urinary condition just the way it is now, how would you feel about that?

This item is answered on a scale of 0-6; 0 indicates that the respondent would be delighted with his condition and 6 indicates that the person would feel terrible about his condition

From AHCPR Guideline.[2]

- Advise the patient to warm up before attempting to urinate. *Micturition is more difficult when the body is coping with cold weather.*
- Advise the patient who is unable to urinate despite repeated attempts to drink a cup of warm tea or coffee, and to attempt urination while sitting in a tub of warm water, or while showering under warm water. Instruct the patient to ensure privacy while attempting to void, and to urinate while in the tub or shower, rather than attempting to transfer to the toilet. Drinking warm coffee or tea acts as a mild bladder irritant, increasing the desire to void. A warm sitz bath or tub bath assists the patient to relax the pelvic muscles and void. Transferring to the toilet is avoided since this action may jeopardize attempts at toileting.
- Counsel the patient who remains unable to void after 6 to 8 hours of attempts to seek immediate care from his primary health care provider, immediate care center, urologist, or local hospital emergency department. *Acute urinary retention is a medical emergency, requiring prompt care to avoid bladder rupture and subsequent infection.*
- Teach the patient with significant post voiding urinary residual volumes (typically greater than 100 ml or 25% of bladder capacity) to double void by urinating, resting on the toilet for 2 to 3 minutes, and voiding again. *Double voiding may promote more complete bladder evacuation.*
- Teach the patient to perform intermittent self-catheterization as directed. The role for self-catheterization in men with BPH is limited, primarily because of technical difficulties inserting a catheter past a significantly enlarged prostate. Nonetheless, self-catheterization is sometimes used as a temporary measure to ensure regular, complete bladder evacuation until more definitive treatment can be completed.
- Insert an indwelling catheter as directed. An indwelling catheter provides continuous urinary drainage for the individual who has experienced acute urinary retention. It is considered a temporary measure before definitive management of prostatic obstruction.
- Teach the patient to self-administer medications to reduce the obstruction associated with BPH as directed. Alpha-adrenergic blockers or 5 α-reductase enzyme inhibitors are used to inhibit smooth muscle tone at the bladder outlet or reduce prostate size, respectively. Both agents reduce the chronic obstruction and urinary retention associated with BPH and resulting risk of acute urinary retention.
- Prepare the patient for prostatectomy as directed. Consult the physician concerning the method of prostate tissue removal for this patient. Multiple methods of prostate tissue removal are being used to relieve the symptoms of BPH. (See Medical Interventions and Related Nursing Care, pages 1056 and 1057.)

Altered urinary elimination, related to bladder outlet obstruction

- Teach the patient with mild to moderate symptoms of BPH a fluid management program, emphasizing adequate intake of fluid (30 ml/kg of body weight per day). Avoiding fluids will concentrate the urine, exacerbating irritative voiding symptoms.
- Instruct the man with symptoms of BPH to avoid or limit intake of caffeinic beverages, alcoholic drinks, coffee, tea, aspartame, chocolates, or spicy foods. These substances act as mild bladder irritants, increasing irritative symptoms of BPH.
- Teach the patient with chronic urinary retention to perform intermittent catheterization as directed. Intermittent catheterization has a limited role in BPH, primarily due to technical difficulties catheterizing the man with significant BPH and the risk for infection and bleeding with difficult catheterization. Nonetheless, it may be used as a temporary measure to alleviate significant urinary retention in select patients.

Risk for infection, related to urinary stasis

- Teach the patient the signs and symptoms of urinary tract infection and pyelonephritis. Advise him to promptly seek care if urinary tract infection occurs. Although rare, significant urinary tract infection can occur in the patient with BPH and retention of urine.

Patient Education/Home Care Planning

1. Teach the patient to self-administer α-adrenergic antagonists, including dosage, administration, and special considerations when taking these medications for relief of symptoms of BPH.
2. Teach the patient to self-administer finasteride, including dosage, administration, and side effects.
3. Assist the patient who elects watchful waiting to design a program of routine evaluation in consultation with the physician. Emphasize the importance of follow-up care for this evolving condition.
4. Assist the patient who elects invasive removal of prostate tissue with a schedule for routine follow-up evaluation. Remind the patient that benign prostate tissue may recur over a period of years, necessitating reevaluation and, possibly, repeated treatment.
5. Counsel the person undergoing treatment for BPH to schedule routine follow-up evaluation of the prostate, including a digital rectal examination and prostate specific antigen test for prostate cancer.

Evaluation

Patterns of urinary elimination improve Diurnal urinary frequency and episodes of nocturia are reduced.

Episodes of acute urinary retention are avoided or promptly managed

Symptoms of BPH are diminished (evaluated using AUA Symptom Index)

PROSTATITIS

Prostatitis is the inflammation of prostatic acini and surrounding tissue that is particularly pronounced in the periurethral portion of the gland.

Inflammation of the prostate is commonly divided into four types: acute bacterial, chronic bacterial, nonbacterial, and prostatodynia. Each form of prostatitis has a distinctive clinical presentation and is managed differently.[111]

Prostatitis is most commonly observed in males after the onset of pubescence, but rare cases of the disease have been reported among children and infants. Nonbacterial prostatitis (also named prostatosis) is the most common form of the disease. Acute and chronic bacterial prostatitis is less commonly seen. Rarer forms include viral, fungal, parasitic, and allergic prostatitis.[57]

••••• Pathophysiology

Acute bacterial prostatitis is caused by the ascent of bacteria via the urethra or the hematogenous route. Acute infection may be precipitated by urethral instrumentation or prostatic massage in the presence of chronic bacterial prostatitis. Common causative pathogens include *E. coli, Proteus, Klebsiella, Pseudomonas,* and *Enterobacter.* An acute episode of prostatic infection is characterized by a sudden onset of fever, chills, myalgia, arthralgia, and general malaise. These symptoms rapidly progress to localized discomfort in the perineal area or low back associated with irritative voiding symptoms including urgency, frequency, nocturia, dysuria, and a persistent burning sensation in the urethra after micturition. Pain in the prostate results in varying degrees of functional bladder outlet obstruction that may cause significant urinary hesitancy or even acute urinary obstruction.[58,118]

Histologic examination of prostatic tissue will reveal diffuse glandular inflammation with edema and hyperemia of the stroma. Abscesses are common and may hemorrhage in severe cases. Polymorphonucleocytes, bacteria, and cellular debris are present within the acini of the gland. Rectal palpation of the prostate reveals an exquisitely tender organ. Vigorous massage is contraindicated because of the associated pain and the danger of bacteremia. Acute bacterial cystitis is typically associated so that urine culture provides an excellent clue to the causative prostatic pathogen. An objective diagnosis of acute bacterial prostatitis is made in the presence of evidence of inflammation on expressed prostatic secretions (over 10 leukocytes per highpower field), positive bacterial culture of this expressed prostatic secretion, positive bacterial cystitis, and an abnormal rectal examination.[58,118]

Chronic bacterial prostatitis commonly occurs as a result of ascending infection from the urethra. The condition may arise following an inadequately treated episode of acute bacterial prostatitis, or it may occur via hematogenous bacterial invasion. However, the precise etiology of chronic bacterial prostatitis remains unclear.[108]

The clinical symptoms of chronic bacterial prostatitis vary widely. Some men have no symptoms of prostatitis other than recurrent urinary tract infections or asymptomatic bacteriuria. More commonly, men with prostatitis note recurring irritative voiding symptoms such as urgency, frequency, dysuria, nocturia, and urethral irritation. Perineal pain, postejaculatory pain, hematospermia, and a mucoid urethral discharge may also be noted.[46,118]

Rectal palpation of the prostate may reveal the presence of prostatic calculi or may be unremarkable. Histologic examination of the prostate shows moderate inflammatory changes that are less localized than in acute infections. Objective diagnosis of chronic bacterial prostatitis requires the presence of inflammatory cells on microscopic examination of expressed secretions, a positive culture of these secretions, and a nontender gland on rectal examination.[46,118]

Unlike acute bacterial prostatitis, the chronically infected prostate is relatively resistant to antibiotic treatment because of the poor absorption of non-lipid-soluble substances into the prostatic fluid. The chronically infected prostate has deficient levels of prostatic antibacterial substance. Prostatic calculi may also lower antibiotic susceptibility by serving as a nidus for persistent infection. Thus even extended periods of oral antibiotics may not cure chronic bacterial prostatitis.[46,118]

Nonbacterial prostatitis is the most common form of symptomatic prostatic inflammation. Although the causative agent of nonbacterial prostatitis has not been identified, chlamydia has been implicated as a possible pathogen. Unfortunately, cultures are difficult to obtain so verification of this suspicion requires further investigation.[35]

The symptoms of nonbacterial prostatitis are similar to those of chronic bacterial prostatitis and include pelvic area pain and irritative voiding symptoms. Objective diagnosis is made by demonstrating the presence of inflammatory cells in expressed prostatic secretions in the presence of negative prostatic secretion and bladder urine cultures. Rectal examination will be normal.[35,118]

Prostatodynia is the presence of symptoms of prostatitis in the absence of physical findings. The etiology of this form of prostatitis is unknown. Objective diagnosis is made by demonstrating negative inflammatory cells in expressed prostatic secretions, negative bacterial culture of these secretions, negative urine cultures in the presence of recurrent perineal pain, and irritative voiding symptoms.[35]

Other forms of prostatitis occur rarely and include viral prostatic inflammation following an upper respiratory infection, tubercular prostatitis, or mycotic prostatitis from blastomycosis, coccidioidomycosis, histoplasmosis, and candidiasis. Symptoms are similar to bacterial prostatitis with the presence of perineal area pain and inflammation of the prostate associated with irritative voiding symptoms.[118]

Complications of prostatitis include acute urinary retention, bladder neck contracture, and obstruction in the presence of chronic inflammation. Cystitis is typically associated with the condition, and epididymitis is not uncommon. Pyelonephritis and bacteremia may be associated with acute infection.[35,118]

•••••• Diagnostic Studies and Findings

Intravenous pyelogram (IVP)   Normal or evidence of bladder neck obstruction with elevation of bladder base (owing to prostatic edema and large post void residual)

White blood cell (WBC) count   Acute bacterial prostatitis: 20,000/L

Urinalysis   Bacterial infection: bacteria and WBCs on microscopic examination

Culture: divided specimen   Patient is asked to void his first 10 to 15 ml in a sterile cup and switch to another cup without interrupting the urinary stream, where he will collect the next 50 to 100 ml; when voiding is completed, patient is cautioned not to squeeze out the last several drops; prostate is then milked for an "expressed prostatic secretion," or all residual urine is expressed by straining if no secretions are obtained; three portions are obtained from first container of urine (these represent "urethral discharge"): one portion examined microscopically, one portion used for culture, and remaining portion

used for dry mounting on a slide using alcohol; second container constitutes a midstream urine specimen and is used for routine urine culture and urinalysis; final specimen is expressed prostatic fluid and is examined microscopically for inflammatory cells and submitted for culture; bacterial prostatitis diagnosed by presence of more than 5000 bacteria/ml with less than 3000 bacteria/ml obtained from bladder and urethral specimens[35]

Urine culture and sensitivity   Acute bacterial cystitis: positive; chronic bacterial prostatitis: positive; nonbacterial prostatitis: negative; prostatodynia: negative

•••••• Multidisciplinary Plan

Surgery

Open prostatectomy a possible curative measure but generally contraindicated because of associated side effects, including urinary incontinence and impotence[118]

Transurethral resection of prostate effective if all of the affected prostatic tissue is removed; clinical results indicate that approximately one third of patients treated in this manner have complete resolution of symptoms; remaining two thirds have improvement of symptoms or remain the same[35,118]

Medications

Antiinfective agents guided by routine urine culture and sensitivity reports indicated in cases of acute bacterial prostatitis; 30-day course of trimethoprim (Trimpex) or trimethoprim-sulfamethosoxazole (Bactrim DS; 1 tablet po bid) given to prevent occurrence of chronic infection

Mild cases of acute infection may be treated with oral antibiotics

Severe cases require parenteral antibiotic therapy with gentamicin (Garamycin) or tobramycin (Nebcin) and ampicillin (Amcil) until culture sensitivity reports are available or patient is afebrile[118]

Chronic bacterial prostatitis treated by 30 days of double-strength tablets of trimethoprim-sulfamethoxazole (Bactrim DS or ciprofloxacin [Cipro]) given twice daily; tetracyclines may be substituted if patient is allergic to sulfonamides; combination of erythromycin and sodium bicarbonate may be used although results are not uniformly successful[57]

Antipyretics (ASA) often indicated in presence of acute bacterial prostatitis

Stool softeners may lessen discomfort associated with straining with a bowel movement[118]

General Management

Alcohol intake often causes exacerbation of symptoms in prostatitis; should be limited to 2 or 3 ounces per day or deleted from diet totally

Foods that contain chili powder or other "hot" spices are possibly associated with exacerbation of symptoms and are serially deleted from diet to assess their role in relief of symptoms

Dietary manipulation particularly important in management of prostatodynia

Placement of suprapubic catheter or suprapubic needle aspiration of urine indicated in cases of acute urinary retention from acute bacterial prostatitis[73,118]

NURSING CARE

Nursing Assessment

Prostate

Acute bacterial prostatitis: firm gland with asymmetry or focal area of enlargement; exquisitely tender to touch

Chronic forms of prostatitis: relatively nontender; may note presence of calculi[107]

Voiding Behavior

Frequency, urgency, dysuria, bladder irritability, difficulty initiating stream

Nursing Dx & Intervention

Pain related to prostate inflammation

- Force intake of fluid *to decrease irritative voiding symptoms.*
- Provide local heat such as Sitz bath as prescribed *for symptomatic relief of perineal pain and to encourage urination in patients experiencing discomfort from a distended bladder.*
- Note that gentle prostatic massage is contraindicated during acute infection *but may offer relief for chronic prostatitis.* (Massage should be performed no more than once a week.)
- Sexual activity may also afford relief in cases of chronic prostatitis.

Altered urinary elimination related to bladder outlet obstruction

- For acute bacterial prostatitis, monitor intake and output and percuss bladder *to assess for signs of overdistention.*
- Provide a warm bath *to encourage urination by helping relieve discomfort and to relax the pelvic floor musculature.*
- If a suprapubic catheter is placed, monitor intake and output *to assess patency of tube.* Securely tape tube to abdomen *to prevent kinking.*

Noncompliance (medical therapy) related to need for long-term therapy

- Advise patient to continue antibiotic therapy for the full 30 days *to achieve optimum therapeutic results.*

Patient Education/Home Care Planning

1. Provide information concerning the prostate's relative resistance to antibiotic therapy.
2. Assure the patient that prostatitis is not associated with an increased incidence of adenocarcinoma of the prostate and that prostatitis is not a form of venereal disease.
3. Provide anticipatory guidance on managing acute urinary retention.

Evaluation

Acute bacterial prostatitis is resolved There are no bacteria in expressed prostatic secretion. Bacteriuria is not present. Patient is afebrile. Irritative voiding symptoms are absent.

Chronic bacterial prostatitis is resolved There are no bacteria in expressed prostatic secretion. Bacteriuria is not present. Irritative voiding symptoms are absent. There are no complications; urinary flow is unobstructed.

Patient adheres to medical regimen Patient understands necessity of completing full course of antibiotic therapy to prevent recurrence of infection.

Nonbacterial prostatitis or prostatodynia is resolved There are no inflammatory cells in expressed prostatic secretions. Irritative voiding symptoms are absent. Perineal pain is absent.

SEXUAL FUNCTION DISORDERS

EPIDIDYMITIS

Epididymitis is defined as any inflammation of the epididymis; it may be caused by bacteria, viruses, parasites, chemicals, or trauma. Epididymitis is divided into three categories: nonspecific, specific, and traumatic. Complications from this condition include orchitis, testicular infarction, and sterility.[58,118]

Epididymitis is the most common of all intrascrotal lesions. It is almost always unilateral and must be differentiated from testicular torsion, tumor, or trauma. An estimated 600,000 cases occur in the United States each year. In men under 35 years of age, epididymitis is most often associated with sexually transmitted disease. It accounts for 20% of all inpatient admissions in military urology practices. In men over 35 years of age, gram-negative rods associated with some abnormality of the urinary tract or performance of some urologic procedure constitute the most common presentation of the condition. Epididymitis is rare in prepubertal boys.[59]

•••••• Pathophysiology

Epididymitis occurs most frequently as a result of reflux of urine or some pathogenic agent through the posterior urethra, prostatic ducts, or seminal vesicles. In rare instances the causative pathogen may reach the epididymis via retrograde lymphatic pathways from the wall of the vas deferens or via hematogenous or metastatic routes. In its earlier stage, epididymitis occurs as a type of cellulitis associated with local pain and edema. In the acute stage the entire hemiscrotum becomes a single erythematous, exquisitely painful mass often associated with an inflammatory hydrocele produced by the tunica vaginalis. Later changes include peritubular fibrosis and occlusion of the epididymis that may result in sterility.[89,108]

Nonspecific epididymitis refers to a group of common pathogens that typically gain access to the organ via urethral-vasal reflux in the presence of infected urine. Bladder outlet obstruction requiring the individual to strain in order to void is a predisposing factor to this condition. Nonspecific epididymitis is a common complication of prostatitis, urethral stricture disease, and seminal vesiculitis. Occasionally a nonspecific epididymitis arises from a septic focus such as a pharyngitis. Reflux of sterile urine into the epididymis has been reported to result in inflammation,[57,118] although others dispute this possibility.[47] Strenuous exercise has also been connected with non-pyrogenic epididymitis.[118]

Nonspecific epididymitis also occurs as a complication of certain urologic procedures, particularly transurethral resection of the prostate and urethral catheterization. Postprocedure epididymitis may occur as late as several months following instrumentation because of the persistence of subclinical amounts of bacteria in the urine. It is significant to note that the rate of epididymitis following transurethral resection of the prostate has dropped from 20% to 4% following the institution of routine prophylactic antibiotics after the procedure. Vasectomy has been advocated as a prophylactic measure for men undergoing prostatectomy, but the efficacy of this intervention remains unproven.[57]

Traumatic epididymitis (also referred to as epididymo-orchitis) arises from straining, with reflux of urine into the organ. The etiology of this form of epididymitis remains unclear. Some argue that the trauma only inflames an already present subclinical inflammation of the epididymis, while others propose that the trauma lessens resistance to some more distant foci of infection, allowing invasion of pathogens into the area.[46,118]

Specific epididymitis refers to a group of known pathogens that invade the epididymis from a urinary focus or via the hematogenous route. The causative organisms most commonly associated with sexually transmitted epididymitis are *Neisseria gonorrhoeae* and *Chlamydia trachomatis* among heterosexual males and *Escherichia coli* among homosexual males. Prompt, aggressive treatment of these sexually transmitted diseases helps curtail the incidence of subsequent epididymitis as demonstrated by the decreasing incidence of gonococcal epididymitis.[59]

Syphilitic epididymitis may occur more often than has been suspected. This form of epididymal inflammation is typically asymptomatic and connected with the second stage of the disease. Diagnosis of syphilitic epididymitis is presumptive and established when other evidence of syphilis is present while urinary tract infection, prostatitis, and urethritis are absent.[59,118]

Many forms of specific epididymitis have been reported that have spread to the organ via the hematogenous route. In cases of brucellosis, epididymitis may be the initial symptom of the condition. Meningococcal septicemia, pneumococcal pneumonia, *Haemophilus influenzae,* and other bacterial diseases have been associated with epididymal invasion. Various parasites such as amebae, schistosoma, and fungi are known to invade the epididymis.[59]

Tubercular epididymitis arises from involvement of the prostate and is one of the few painless forms of the disease. Tuberculosis of the epididymis produces a thickened, beaded organ on palpation and leads to occlusion of the epididymal lumen.

The most common complication of epididymitis is orchitis, so the term "epididymo-orchitis" is used. Infertility is a serious long-term complication of epididymitis. Sterility among men with chronic or recurrent bilateral epididymitis is 40%, and men with unilateral epididymitis have a 25% chance of infertility. Recurrences of epididymitis are particularly likely when the underlying disease process (e.g., prostatitis) remains unresolved.[57]

•••••• Diagnostic Studies and Findings

White blood cell count   Generally between 20,000 and 30,000 in an acute episode[99]

Urinalysis   Signs of infection may be present

Urine culture   Reveals associated bacterial cystitis if present

Urethral discharge culture   Reveals associated gonococcal or chlamydial urethritis

Prostatic secretion culture   Reveals associated prostatitis

Doppler stethoscope   Good blood flow rules out torsion of testis

Testicular radionuclide scan   Good blood flow rules out torsion of testis

•••••• Multidisciplinary Plan

Surgery

Epididymectomy rarely indicated as a therapeutic measure in chronic or tubercular epididymitis[34]

Medications

Mild to moderate cases: oral antiinfective agents, which may be guided by culture and sensitivity data when appropriate; analgesics (nonsteroidal antiinflammatory drug) used to manage pain and control fever

Severe cases: hospitalization and broad-spectrum antibiotics; combination of ampicillin and aminoglycoside given pending results of blood culture

Very severe cases: spermatic cord block with lidocaine or procaine hydrochloride; use of steroids has been advocated but any beneficial anti-inflammatory activity is outweighed by potential side effects[123]

Antiemetic agent may be required to control associated nausea and vomiting during acute epididymitis; antipyretics may be indicated for associated fever

Administration of antiemetics justified in order to prevent progression of nausea to a severe state that threatens fluid and electrolyte balance

General Management

Urethral discharge may be copious and is managed by regular cleansing of meatus with hydrogen peroxide[73]

NURSING CARE

Nursing Assessment

Scrotum

Initial stages of epididymitis: scrotal skin is reddened or normal in appearance; as infection progresses, scrotal skin becomes red and hot to touch

Varicocele a common finding

Moderate to severe cases: significant edema of epididymis and adjacent structures (including testis) causes a large mass in affected hemiscrotum so epididymitis cannot be distinguished; overlying skin dry, flaky, and without its normal rugose appearance; spontaneous rupture may occur; mass is exquisitely tender

Elevation of scrotum may result in relief from pain (Prehn's sign)[57]

Testis

Testis on affected side may be painful and enlarged

Masses or induration possible

Abdomen

Lower quadrant pain perceived on affected side

Nausea and Vomiting

Vomiting may be severe during acute period

Nursing Dx & Intervention

Pain related to inflammation of epididymis

- Assess and support the scrotum via an athletic support, a towel placed under the scrotum, or a Bellevue bridge *to relieve discomfort.*
- Provide analgesics as ordered *to relieve discomfort.*
- Use a Sitz bath, local heat, or ice pack as prescribed *to relieve discomfort.*
- Provide bed rest during the acute period *to prevent discomfort.*
- Inform patient that sexual activity or any strenuous physical activity is contraindicated in even mild cases *to prevent discomfort.*

Risk for fluid volume deficit related to vomiting

- Assess and curtail oral intake *to reduce potential for vomiting.*
- Maintain records of intake and output including frequency and amount of vomitus *to assess for fluid volume deficit.*
- Administer antiemetics as ordered.

Fear related to potential for malignancy

- Assess and reassure patient that epididymitis is not a malignant process and that the mass effect is caused by inflammation.

Patient Education/Home Care Planning

1. Provide instructions on the risk factors associated with epididymitis: prostatitis, urethritis (particularly gonococcal and chlamydial), cystitis, and unusually strenuous physical activity.
2. Emphasize the need for follow-up care aimed at identifying the underlying causes of epididymitis in certain cases.
3. Provide information on the signs and symptoms as well as the natural history of epididymitis and the importance of seeking care promptly.

Evaluation

Pain is resolved   There is no pain in affected epididymis. Hemiscrotum is not enlarged. Urethral, prostate, and blood cultures are negative. Underlying prostatitis, urethritis, cystitis, tuberculosis of the urinary tract, or septic hematogenous focus is resolved. Sperm count and motility are normal.

Fluid volume remains normal   Vomiting is curtailed; patient is able to tolerate fluid intake.

Fear is diminished   Patient is reassured that this is a treatable inflammatory process.

◼ ERECTILE DYSFUNCTION

◼ Erectile dysfunction (impotence) is the inability to produce an erection of the penis of sufficient duration and rigidity to engage in intercourse.

Both psychogenic and organic factors contribute to erectile dysfunction. Treatment is aimed at restoring normal erectile and orgasmic function or mimicking the erect penis by injecting a drug into the phallus or via mechanical or surgically implanted devices. Other forms of male sexual dysfunction manifested as loss of libido, premature ejaculation, or inability to achieve orgasm are discussed in Part Four, Pattern IX, Sexuality—Reproductive.

Sexual dysfunction in the male may be noted any time after the onset of puberty. The incidence of erectile dysfunction increases with age. The incidence of men who seek treatment for erectile dysfunction during the fourth decade of life is 1.5% of the general population; by the seventh decade of life the incidence has risen to 25% of all males.[70] Although the aging process does not inevitably lead to impotence, sexual activity does generally decrease with age because of a variety of social, cultural, and physical factors. A survey of men revealed that 88% of sexually active males under 20 years of age engage in intercourse at least once each week. During the fourth decade of life the proportion of men reporting intercourse at least once a week declined to 80%. During the sixth decade of life only 50% of the men surveyed reported intercourse on a weekly basis; by the seventh decade only 25% had intercourse each week.[75]

The relative incidence of impotence from psychogenic versus organic causes has received great attention. Some investigators have reported that 90% to 95% of cases of impotence are the result of psychogenic causes.[75,107] However, recent data using more sophisticated diagnostic techniques reveal a greater percentage of men whose erectile dysfunction has organic as well as psychogenic components.[75]

•••••• Pathophysiology

A wide variety of organic conditions may cause or be associated with impotence.[118] Within this discussion only some of the more commonly encountered organic causes of impotence are considered. An in-depth discussion of the psychosocial influences and ramifications of this condition is presented in Pattern X.

A number of disease processes are associated with erectile dysfunction. These medical disorders may affect the physiologic processes of erection directly, or they may suppress sexual drive without causing true impotence. The psychosocial implications of illness, particularly a chronic condition, may alter a man's self-image and profoundly affect his sexual identity and sexual behaviors. To understand and treat this complex problem, the nurse or physician must have an understanding of the underlying influences affecting erectile function in each individual.[75]

Endocrine problems may affect male sexual function by altering normal function of the hypothalamic-pituitary-gonadal hormonal axis. The typical result of this problem is hypogonadism, which is potentially reversible. The range of hypogonadism is significant and includes cases of mildly impaired libido and incidences of overt eunuchoidism requiring long-term hormonal replacement.[75,118]

The severity of impotence related to endocrine disorders is based on the age of onset and related symptoms that influence any medical decision to attempt to establish or restore potency in an affected male. Complete prepubertal gonadotropic failure may be expressed as hypogonadotropic eunuchoidism. Kallmann's syndrome is a specific luteinizing hormone–follicle-stimulating hormone disorder. In all of the above conditions a failure of the production and propagation of gonadotropins is noted prepubertally and persists throughout the patient's lifetime. Abnormal growth patterns, a high-pitched voice, and a lack of secondary sex characteristics are associated with hy-

pogonadism leading to impaired sexual function and infertility. Kallmann's syndrome is associated with significant mental retardation, which may affect the medical approach to treatment of impotence.[75,121]

Partial prepubertal gonadotropic failure produces symptoms similar to those of delayed puberty that actually do stem from an identifiable hormonal deficit rather than normal developmental processes. These males have significantly decreased testosterone levels arising from a deficiency in the production of FSH and LH, or LH only.[75]

Selective postpubertal hypogonadism is associated with a loss of testosterone production and a gradual loss of beard and body hair, declining libido, and resultant impotence and infertility. The eunuchoid aspects of this condition are not as prominent as those associated with prepubertal hypogonadism.[75]

Panhypopituitarism causes erectile dysfunction and a number of other hormonal imbalances. The condition is caused by a lesion that renders the pituitary or hypothalamus functionless or by surgical or traumatic ablation.[75,121]

Several congenital syndromes cause erectile dysfunction along with other medical problems. Prader-Willi syndrome causes neonatal hypotonia, mental retardation, obesity, and hypogonadism. Laurence-Moon-Biedl syndrome is an autosomal recessive disorder that results in retinitis pigmentosa, polydactyly, renal anomalies, cryptorchidism, and erectile dysfunction. Familial cerebellar ataxia is also associated with hypogonadism along with ataxic movements and neural deafness. Other syndromes associated with hypogonadism and impotence include Klinefelter's syndrome, Noonan's syndrome, and Ullrich's syndrome.[75]

Any disease or drug that produces hyperprolactinemia also interferes with the hypothalamic-pituitary-gonadotropic axis and causes erectile dysfunction. Medical conditions associated with hyperprolactinemia include certain hormone-producing tumors, endocrine disorders, and a number of drugs such as estrogen compounds and psychotropic drugs.[75]

Other endocrine-based disorders involving the thyroid or adrenal glands may affect erectile function. Castration has been used since antiquity to decrease libido and ultimately ablate normal male sexual function.[75,121]

Chronic heart disease has been associated with impotence, which may be attributed to the disease processes involved and to the use of certain antihypertensive drugs or digitalis preparations. Men with heart disease that is reasonably well controlled should consider sexual activity reasonably safe. In many of these men erectile dysfunction can be prevented by prudent counseling. Sexual dysfunction may be complicated by the use of antihypertensive or antidepressant medications. Digoxin may also adversely affect sexual function by reducing LH and testosterone levels in the body while raising estradiol. Among those men who undergo heart transplant, erectile dysfunction is a potential complication that may be associated with postoperative immunosuppressions.

Erectile dysfunction is relatively common among men who have chronic renal insufficiency and renal failure. Multiple factors contribute to the problem, related both to the disease process itself and to the use of dialysis as a treatment modality. Impotence is a result of Leydig's cell abnormalities with concomitant decreases in the production of testosterone. Hyperprolactinemia and hyperparathyroidism may further complicate the situation. Erectile dysfunction may worsen after the start of dialysis. Many problems in erectile dysfunction are resolved by renal transplantation, although transient impotence may be noted in patients who have ligation of the internal artery to provide a blood supply for the transplanted kidney.

Kass and his associates studied a group of men with chronic obstructive pulmonary disease and found that 19% had problems with sexual function. The incidence of impotence in these men was largely attributed to psychosocial aspects of the disease rather than primary organic sexual dysfunction.[61a]

Several neurologic conditions are associated with erectile dysfunction. The presence of erectile dysfunction in spinal cord injury is influenced by the level of the lesion, the presence of spinal shock, and the "completeness" of the injury. Following a traumatic injury to the spinal cord, all erectile activity of the penis is inhibited. The generation of posttraumatic erections is typically associated with cessation of spinal shock. The period of time after which erectile activity reappears following spinal cord injury is highly variable, ranging from 24 hours to 18 months.[75]

Two types of erection are observed in men with spinal cord injury: reflexogenic erections, which are mediated by spinal cord centers, and psychogenic erections, which are mediated by supraspinal sexual centers. The incidence of erections among spinal cord–injured men is 63.5% to 94%, but the incidence of consistently successful erections is 23% to 33%.[75] The relatively low rate of successful potency among men with spinal cord injuries is largely the result of the characteristics of reflexogenic erections, which are relatively brief and respond to a variety of tactile sensations, rendering penile response significantly altered from previous brain-centered control of sexual response.

Ejaculation is relatively rare among men with spinal cord injury. Ejaculation requires smooth coordination between autonomic and somatic impulses. The likelihood of orgasm among patients with complete spinal cord injuries is 3% to 19.7%. Lower spinal cord injury is correlated with an increased likelihood of ejaculation but a relatively low incidence of erections (24.2%).[75]

Multiple sclerosis is another neurologic condition associated with male sexual dysfunction. Demyelination of the lateral horns of the lumbar spinal cord is theorized to be the critical underlying organic explanation for impotence among these men. Approximately 91% of men with multiple sclerosis have significant sexual dysfunction.[75]

Epilepsy involving the parietal lobes of the brain is associated with a higher incidence of impotence than other forms of the disease. In most cases the relative contribution of antiseizure medications to sexual dysfunction is negligible. Many men experience continuing desire for sex with inability to sustain or maintain erections, and fewer experience a loss of libido.

Diabetes mellitus is a causative factor in the development of erectile dysfunction because of a complex interplay of psychologic and organic factors. Erectile dysfunction may be noted near the time a diagnosis of diabetes is established; the diagnosis contributes to psychosocial factors (alterations in self-image and anxiety related to chronic disease) and physiologic factors resulting from insulin deficiency. Sexual dysfunction is generally resolved after the condition is regulated with exogenous insulin.

Later problems related to sexual function in the diabetic male have an insidious onset and are generally progressive. Hormonal factors have been theorized but are not supported by objective evidence. Diabetic neuropathies are often implicated in the genesis of impotence among diabetic men based on indirect evidence linking autonomic nervous abnormalities. Vascular compromise associated with diabetic angiopathy may influence potency by affecting the arterial blood supply of the cavernous bodies of the penis.[75]

Vascular disorders also produce male sexual dysfunction when they compromise the arterial blood supply needed to *fill* the cavernosal bodies for an erection and when they compromise the venous structures needed to *sustain* this erection. Arterial insufficiency may arise as the result of large vessel disease. Aortoiliac occlusion leads to erectile dysfunction in approximately 70% of affected males, and arteriosclerosis of the pelvic or penile arteries will cause sexual dysfunction in 50% or more of affected males. Cigarette smoking also produces disease of the smaller arteries, often leading to compromised erectile function among chronic smokers.[46]

Venous insufficiency produces erectile dysfunction when the veins fail to occlude blood shunted to the corpora cavernosa. While the etiology of this venous incompetence remains uncertain, a history of pelvic injury is often noted.[46]

Many drugs have been associated with erectile dysfunction. Duration, frequency, and dosage of the drug affect the likelihood of impotence or loss of libido and secondary erectile dysfunction. It is essential to assess the use of all drugs including prescribed, over-the-counter, and recreational agents a man may be using.[75]

Endocrine drugs are used in a variety of hormonal abnormalities and may be used to treat cancer. Any exogenous estrogens or progestins ultimately result in impotence if given in sufficient dosages. Anabolic steroids may suppress endogenous steroid levels and cause impotence when the drug is discontinued.[75]

Antihypertensive drugs, particularly the α- and β-adrenergic blocking agents, are associated with impotence, although the exact mechanism of sexual dysfunction may be more closely related to a loss of libido than to lowering of systemic arterial blood pressure.[75] The following antihypertensive drugs are associated with male sexual dysfunction: clonidine (Catapres), guanethidine (Ismelin), hydralazine (Apresoline), monoamine oxidase inhibitors, methyldopa (Aldomet), phentolamine (Regitine), propranolol (Inderal), and reserpine (Serpasil).[75]

Two cardiac agents, digoxin and disopyramide, are commonly linked to male sexual dysfunction. The role of digoxin in erectile function was discussed in Chapter 1; disopyramide is an antidysrhythmic agent with parasympathetic properties that may contribute to erectile difficulties.[75]

The diuretic agents chlorthalidone and spironolactone may cause loss of libido and erectile dysfunction in a few instances. Hydrochlorothiazide is also linked to sexual dysfunction.[75]

Psychoactive drugs affect the central nervous system in many ways that are poorly understood. A significant number of these drugs, including sedatives, amphetamines, antidepressants, and antipsychotic agents, may cause impotence, presumably because of their effects on the central nervous system. The precise mechanisms by which this side effect occurs are not completely understood.[75] These drugs include weight reduction drugs (diethylpropion and phentermine hydrochloride), antidepressant agents (amitriptyline and monoamine oxidase inhibitors), antianxiety/sedative agents (benzodiazapines and glutethimide), and lithium carbonate.[75]

Anticholinergic agents such as propantheline are known to cause impotence as a side effect. Antiparkinson drugs are linked to erectile dysfunction and delayed ejaculation. The immunosuppressive agents are associated with impotence, but the underlying mechanism may be related to chemically induced psychogenic factors and general alterations in metabolism. Indomethacin is related to impotence arising from its antiprostaglandin effects. Metronidazole suppresses libido via some unknown process.[75]

A number of recreational drugs also affect male sexual function. Alcohol has been known to heighten desire while adversely affecting performance. Alcoholism is particularly associated with an increased incidence of impotence. Tobacco use has been linked to erectile dysfunction in several recent studies. Nicotine may cause impotence by causing vasoconstriction of the penile arteries, although the phenomenon requires further study to establish a causal link. Other drugs connected with male sexual dysfunction include amphetamines, barbiturates, opiates, cannabis (the active component of marijuana), and cocaine.[75]

A comprehensive discussion of the drugs that affect male sexual function is beyond the scope of this chapter. Inserts in packages of individual drugs are an excellent source for assessing sexual dysfunction as a causative agent when impotence is a problem. However, nurses must be aware that overzealous cautions regarding potential sexual dysfunction are not indicated, since such counseling may itself increase performance anxiety and exacerbate impotence.

Certain surgical procedures of the abdomen, thorax, and genital area may result in temporary failure of erectile function; prostatectomy and ileostomy or colostomy are particularly likely to result in alterations in male sexual function. Of all the forms of prostatectomy, open surgery using a perineal approach is the most likely to produce impotence. Transurethral resection of the prostate, the most common approach to prostatectomy, should not result in impotence but is associated with retrograde ejaculation. An open, communicative relationship with the patient including anticipatory guidance of expected postoperative potency is associated with a dramatically reduced likelihood of complaints of erectile dysfunction following the procedure.

Any extensive surgical procedure involving the lower abdomen may lead to the inadvertent destruction of nerves or blood vessels that supply the cavernous bodies in the penis. The incidence of erectile dysfunction is particularly high in men who undergo ileostomy or colostomy with the attendant alteration in body image. Thus sexual dysfunction in these men may have psychogenic and organic components.

Erectile dysfunction may also arise from local disorders of the penis such as priapism, Peyronie's disease, and abnormal leakage of blood from the corpora cavernosa. Priapism is a prolonged, painful erection caused by the blockage of blood flow from the corpora cavernosa. Underlying causes may be primarily traumatic, neurogenic, vascular, or neoplastic. Some men experience idiopathic episodes of priapism, although the condition has been tentatively linked to alcohol and drug use often noted among these men. Peyronie's disease is an abnormal lateral curvature of the penis that is most likely to occur during the fifth and sixth decades of life. There is also a known association with Dupuytren's contractures. The etiology is unclear; curvature is caused by fibroelastic plaques that form in the penis. The plaques may regress spontaneously, or they may persist despite various treatment methodologies. Impotence often accompanies Peyronie's disease and may be related to abnormal blood flow through the corpora cavernosa. Mechanical defects of the corpora cavernosa may result in low intracavernous pressure, which causes insufficient rigidity for penetration. Potency is restored by surgical repair of the defect.[75]

••••• Diagnostic Studies and Findings

Serum testosterone   Low in impotence with dysfunction of hypothalamic-pituitary-gonadal axis

Serum prolactin   High when testosterone is abnormally low

Serum FSH   Abnormal when impotence is result of abnormality of hormonal axis

Serum LH   Abnormal when impotence is result of abnormality of hormonal axis

Glucose tolerance test   Abnormal in cases of diabetes mellitus

Sacral evoked responses   Increased bulbocavernous latency in diabetic males with autonomic neuropathy

Urodynamic testing   Abnormal sensations of bladder filling on cystometrogram and abnormal urecholine supersensitivity test in males with autonomic neuropathy

Penile systolic blood pressure   Low in cases of vascular impotence

Penile pulse volume recording   Abnormal in cases of vascular impotence

Dynamic infusion cavernosometry and cavernosography   Presence of venous leakage (failure to sustain); presence of arterial insufficiency (failure to fill); presence of neuropathic or psychogenic disorders (failure to initiate an erection)

Nocturnal penile tumescence   Absent nocturnal erections when underlying cause of impotence is primarily organic rather than psychogenic[70]

Snap-gauge testing   Breakage of three pressure-sensitive plastic bands indicates sufficient pressure for penetration; inability to break bands during sleep study indicates erectile dysfunction

•••••• Multidisciplinary Plan

Surgery

Corrective surgery of arterial occlusion or venous drainage anomalies may correct erectile dysfunction

Revascularization of penis may be attempted by isolating epigastric artery and reanastomosing it directly to a corporal body[63]

Penile prosthesis may be implanted to produce sufficient rigidity for penetration and intercourse; semirigid and inflatable devices are available[39,86]

Medications

Testosterone replacement therapy indicated in cases of hypogonadism

Luteinizing hormone–releasing hormone (LHRH), LH, or FSH may be used in males with identifiable abnormalities of the hypothalamic-pituitary-gonadal axis; all other results of hormonal therapy in males with erectile dysfunction are caused by placebo effect

Bromocriptine, zinc, and glyceryl trinitrate have been used to treat erectile dysfunction in selected cases with variable results

Papaverine, phentolamine or prostaglandin E_1 may be injected into penis to produce a pharmacologically induced erection; the male patient is taught to self-inject these agents

General Management

Mechanical pump systems using a vacuum device such as the Erect-Aid or Correct-Aid may produce erections; a vacuum that encourages blood inflow into the penis is established external to the penis, and a restrictive device is used to discourage venous outflow and thereby produce tumescence

Discontinue use of any recreational drugs associated with erectile dysfunction, including illicit drugs, tobacco, ethanol, and anabolic steroids; alcohol consumption must be controlled to reestablish potency

NURSING CARE

Nursing Assessment

Minimum Assessment for Erectile Dysfunction[88]

History, including detailed review of sexual practices (frequency, technique, practices), sexual partner is included whenever possible

Physical examination (male secondary sex characteristics, femoral and lower extremity pulses, focused neurologic examination including perianal sensation, bulbocaver-nosus sensation, anal sphincter tone, scrotal examination including testicular size and consistency, palpation of penile shaft for Peyronie's plaques)

Laboratory evaluation: serum testosterone (preferably morning measurement), serum leuteinizing hormone, serum follicle-stimulating hormone, and serum prolactin (when indicated)

External Genitalia

Normal appearance of penis, scrotum, and perineal area

Normal hair distribution, normal phallic size, bilaterally descended testes except in males with endocrine disorders resulting in hypogonadism, in which cases penis will be small, testes small and abnormally soft or cryptorchid, and hair distribution abnormal or absent

Palpation of penis will reveal hard plaques in Peyronie's disease

Polaroid pictures of penile erection obtained by patient will show penile curvature[75]

Rectal Examination

Loss of anal sphincter tone with absent bulbocavernous reflex in local neuropathy

Absent saddle sensation with certain partial or complete spinal cord injuries[75]

Peripheral Pulses

Decreased or absent in vascular impotence

Neurologic Examination

Abnormal in men with underlying neurologic disease

Nursing Dx & Intervention

Sexual dysfunction related to neuropathic, metabolic, endocrine, or vascular factors

- Encourage the male patient to seek counseling and evaluation for perceptions of erectile dysfunction. *Erectile dysfunction is an embarrassing health problem with significant personal and interpersonal implications for affected individuals.*

- Assist the male patient to alter behaviors, such as cigarette smoking or illicit drug use, *that predispose toward erectile dysfunction.*

- Consult with the physician and assist the male patient to eliminate prescription medications whenever feasible that predispose to erectile dysfunction. *Prescription medications may predispose the male to erectile dysfunction. Altering the dosage or substituting a similar agent may reverse or relieve this side effect.*

- Teach the male patient to self-inject a vasodilating agent, as directed. Teach proper techniques for self-injection, dosage, frequency of injections, and potential side effects, including priapism. *Self-injection therapy has potentially harmful effects unless the correct dosage of drug is injected into the proper place on the body at safe intervals.*

- Teach any male patient who attains an erection using a self-injection technique to recognize and manage priapism. *Priapism, a prolonged painful erection, is a potential of pharmacologic erection therapy. Treatment of the condition is necessary to prevent tissue ischemia and damage.*
- Teach the male patient who performs self-injection therapy to wear a barrier device (condom) whenever engaging in intercourse with multiple partners. *Self-injection therapy subtly compromises skin integrity at the site of injection. A barrier device is used to prevent spread of sexually transmitted diseases.*
- Teach the patient to use a vacuum erection device as directed. *The vacuum erection device uses a vacuum to draw blood into the penis and a constricting device to trap the blood until intercourse is completed.*
- Teach the patient who uses a vacuum erection device to remove the restriction (tourniquet) device promptly after intercourse is completed *to prevent ischemia and tissue damage.*

Self-esteem disturbance related to sexual dysfunction

- Empathy and opportunities to express feelings are indicated as the patient reintegrates self-concepts following a change in body image.
- Male sexuality is deeply rooted in ideals of social, athletic, physical, and sexual performance. Any circumstance that significantly alters self-concepts and threatens self-esteem may adversely affect sexual function. Chronic disease, creation of a surgical stoma, and physical changes resulting from neurologic disease or spinal cord trauma significantly challenge any man's self-image.
- Psychologic or psychiatric counseling is often a useful adjunct and may be suggested to a patient after a sufficiently trusting relationship has been established *to reestablish positive, realistic self-concept.*

Patient Education/Home Care Planning

1. Provide instruction about various implantable prosthetic devices in suitable candidates after consultation with the physician.
2. Instruction of expectations of sexual abilities following specific surgical procedures will help prevent needless loss of sexual function resulting from anxiety.

Evaluation

Impotence is resolved   Patient reports increased satisfaction in sex life and adequate onset, duration, and rigidity of erections.

Penile prosthesis is successfully implanted   Patient has an operational semirigid or inflatable penile prosthesis. There is no local infection, pain, or erosion.

MEDICAL INTERVENTIONS AND RELATED NURSING CARE

■ BLADDER NECK SUSPENSION

Bladder neck suspension is a broad term used to describe more than 100 surgical procedures performed to correct stress urinary incontinence caused by pelvic descent and urethral hypermobility. Fixation of the urethrovesical junction can be accomplished through a suprapubic, vaginal, or combined approach. For the Marshall-Marchetti-Krantz procedure the surgeon approximates periurethral fascia to the cartilage of the posterior symphysis pubis. A retropubic colposuspension (Burch procedure) requires fixation of the urethrovesical junction to Cooper's ligament. The anterior urethropexy requires placement of absorbable sutures to anchor the urethrovesical junction to the periosteum of the symphysis bone.[34]

Needle suspensions are performed through the vagina. A U-shaped vaginal incision is made, and the vagina and urethra are carefully separated. The urethra is then moved to an intraabdominal position by ligature carriers that are inserted into the abdominopelvic cavity via two small (3 to 5 cm) incisions in the lower abdomen. The Stamey procedure requires mobilization of tissue lateral to the urethra to fixate the urethrovesical junction; the Raz procedure uses four sutures for fixation.[34,47]

The suburethral sling is used to correct stress incontinence caused by pelvic descent and urethral hypermobility and, in certain circumstances, to correct leakage caused by sphincter mechanism incompetence. A fascial sling (obtained from the rectis abdominis or fascia lata from the thigh) or a Goretex strip is placed around the proximal third of the urethra through a vaginal incision. The tension of the sling is minimized to avoid obstruction of the outlet.[34,47]

Contraindications and Cautions

1. Bladder neck suspension is indicated for stress incontinence caused by pelvic descent and urethral hypermobility. Detrusor instability may or may not be corrected by bladder neck suspension. Bladder neck suspension is contraindicated in cases of incontinence caused by intrinsic sphincter deficiency without coexisting urethral hypermobility.

Preprocedural Nursing Care

1. Teach all patients who undergo bladder neck suspension about the high risk for urinary retention (typically transient) or for infection following surgery.
2. Discuss with the patient who experiences stress and urge incontinence that detrusor instability may or may not resolve following surgery. Reassure the patient that persistent instability (urge) incontinence will be managed by medications, electrostimulation therapy, bladder drill, or other management techniques.

3. Inform the patient with an abdominal procedure or pubo-vaginal sling that hospitalization is required for approximately 5 days. Inform the patient undergoing a vaginal or needle procedure that hospitalization for approximately 3 days is required.

4. Advise the patient undergoing a vaginal procedure that a vaginal pack will be placed during surgery and removed approximately 24 hours following the procedure.

5. Consult with the surgeon concerning self-intermittent catheterization instruction before surgery. Explain to the patient that intermittent catheterization is used to provide regular, complete bladder emptying until postoperative urinary retention is resolved.

NURSING CARE

Nursing Assessment

Abdomen

Redness, edema, and drainage at wound site if abdominal approach used

Perineum

Vaginal discharge
Pain if wound infection present

Voiding Behaviors

Decreased force of urinary stream
Perceptions of incomplete bladder emptying or acute urinary retention

Pain

Dysuria
Pelvic pain
Incisional or abdominal pain

Nursing Dx & Intervention

Altered urinary elimination related to obstruction of urinary outflow

- Monitor indwelling catheter for patency *to prevent acute overdistention and disruption of delicate surgical repair.*
- Remove the indwelling catheter as directed (as early as the first postoperative day for certain patients and as late as 1 month postoperatively for others). Carefully monitor the patient for urination and urinary residual volumes. *Urinary retention may occur after catheter removal, possibly because of postoperative edema and inflammation.*
- Institute an intermittent catheterization program in consultation with the physician *to avoid overdistention for the patient with postoperative distention.*

Pain related to surgical trauma or bladder distention

- Assess the character, location, and duration of pain. *Incisional pain is perceived as a dull, boring, and prolonged pain, while bladder spasms produce a cramping pain with a sudden onset and relatively short duration.*
- Administer analgesics or narcotic medications as directed *to relieve incisional pain.*
- Administer anticholinergic or antispasmodic medications as directed *to relieve discomfort produced by bladder spasms.*
- Monitor the catheter for patency. *Catheter blockage produces bladder overdistention, bladder spasms, and suprapubic discomfort.*
- Minimize noise, bright lighting, and environmental distractions during the immediate postoperative period *to minimize pain.*

Patient Education/Home Care Planning

1. Reassure the patient that the urinary retention experienced following bladder neck suspension is expected to be temporary.
2. Patient teaching before surgery should include a specific plan to manage postoperative urinary retention.
3. Advise the patient to avoid heavy lifting or strenuous exercise for at least 6 weeks after surgery.

Evaluation

Altered urinary elimination patterns are improved Urodynamics are normal. Marshall test is negative. Post void residual is 20% of total bladder volume or less.

Pain is minimized Patient receives adequate relief of pain and spasms from medication.

 # SUBURETHRAL INJECTION OF GAX COLLAGEN

Description and Rationale

Glutaraldehyde cross linked collagen (GAX collagen) is a bulking substance comprising types I and III bovine collagen. In addition a very small amount of glutaraldehyde is added to inhibit the action of the enzyme collagenase, an enzyme that breaks down collagen in the body. Suburethral injections of GAX collagen may be used for women and men with stress urinary incontinence caused by intrinsic sphincter deficiency (ISD). Collagen is indicated for women who have ISD but no urethral hypermobility; those with both conditions are typically managed by a suburethral sling. All men with stress urinary incontinence are potential candidates for GAX collagen, since urethral hypermobility affects women exclusively.

GAX collagen is injected via transurethral or transperineal access, under endoscopic control (Figure 12-18). A cystoscope is used to identify the urethral sphincter mechanism, and a specially designed needle is advanced through the working port for injection of collagen. Several injection sites are identified, and collagen is injected until the urethral lumen is closed. Repeated injections may be required to gain continence. In some cases, a perineal approach may be used to inject collagen. The urethra is visualized, the sphincter mechanism is identified, and the needle is inserted until its movement just beneath the urethral mucosa is appreciated. GAX collagen is then injected until the urethral coaptation occurs.

Contraindications and Cautions

1. Hypersensitivity to GAX collagen may occur. A subdermal skin test is required before suburethral injection of collagen.
2. GAX collagen injections will not correct stress urinary incontinence caused by urethral hypermobility.
3. Repeated injections of GAX collagen may be required, particularly in males with urethral scarring following radical prostatectomy.
4. The long-term efficacy of GAX collagen (>7 years) has not been determined.
5. GAX collagen injections will not alleviate or cure urge incontinence.

Preprocedural Nursing Care

1. Inject 0.5 ml of Xyderm via a subdermal technique into the forearm to test for hypersensitivity to bovine collagen. Teach the patient the signs and symptoms of a positive response (local redness, itching, induration). Monitor the site after 72 hours and after 30 days.

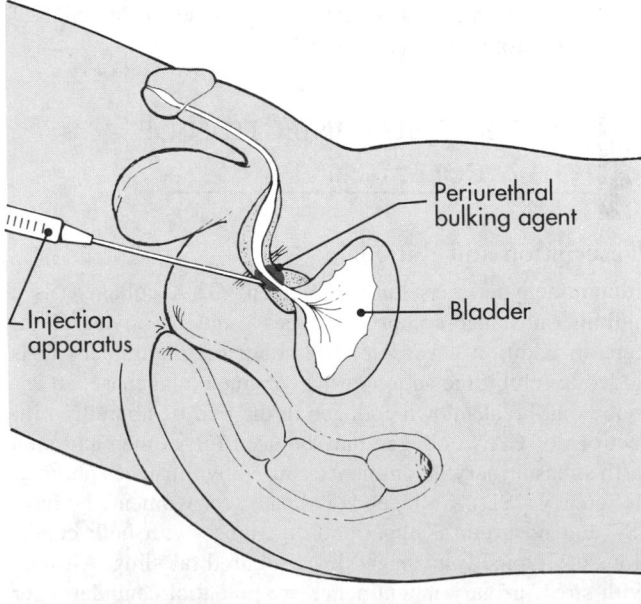

Figure 12-18 Transperineal injection of a urethral bulking agent in a male. (From Gray.[49])

2. Inform the patient that GAX collagen is injected under local, spinal, or general anesthesia. Consult the physician and anesthesiologist about the method of anesthesia for that patient.
3. Inform the patient that transient urinary retention may occur, but that prolonged retention is unlikely, unless she or he is experiencing retention requiring self-catheterization before the procedure, or unless the individual voids exclusively by abdominal straining.
4. Teach the patient to perform self-intermittent catheterization to manage transient urinary retention before the procedure.
5. Advise the patient that repeated injections of GAX collagen may be required.
6. Inform the patient that the long-term effectiveness of GAX collagen has not been established and that repeated injections may be required.

•••••• Multidisciplinary Plan

Medications

1. Antiinfective medications may be administered before and after collagen injection.
2. Analgesics may be administered after the procedure.

General Management

1. An indwelling catheter may be placed temporarily; other urologists avoid catheterization to reduce the risk of extrusion of the collagen through the injection sites.
2. Intermittent catheterization is preferred for management of transient urinary retention.

NURSING CARE

Nursing Assessment

Forearm

Redness, itching, induration indicating hypersensitivity to GAX collagen

Perineum

Urethral discharge

Voiding Behaviors

Decreased force of urinary stream
Acute urinary retention

Pain

Dysuria
Pelvic pain

Nursing Dx & Intervention

Altered urinary elimination, related to suburethral or transperineal injection of GAX collagen

• Monitor indwelling catheter for patency and urinary output. An indwelling catheter may be left in place for a brief period after collagen injection. *Occlusion of the catheter increases pain, and may increase the risk of urinary tract infection.*

- Remove the catheter as directed and monitor the patient for spontaneous voiding. *Transient urinary retention may occur after collagen injection.*
- Assist the patient who is unable to spontaneously urinate to perform self-catheterization. Prolonged urinary retention is rare, unless the individual has experienced this condition before the procedure.

Pain, related to endoscopic instrumentation and suburethral or transperineal injections

- Teach the patient to self-administer urinary or systemic analgesics as directed. Transient discomfort after collagen injection may occur.
- Advise the patient that a warm Sitz bath or warm shower may relieve the discomfort associated with collagen injection.

Patient Education/Home Care Planning

1. Remind the patient that repeated injections may be required. Reabsorption of the collagen may occur, or reduction of urethral edema may be associated with recurrence of urinary incontinence.
2. Teach the patient to recognize the signs and symptoms of urge incontinence, and to seek care for this condition if it occurs.
3. Advise the patient that repeated treatment may be necessary within 2 to 5 years. The long-term efficacy of collagen is not known, and recurrent urinary leakage has been noted within 2 to 5 years.

Evaluation

Stress urinary incontinence is alleviated or ablated
Transient urinary retention is resolved
Pain is minimized The patient receives adequate relief of urethral and pelvic discomfort from analgesics and warm Sitz baths or showers.

EXTRACORPOREAL SHOCK-WAVE LITHOTRIPSY

Extracorporeal shock-wave lithotripsy (ESWL) uses shock waves to reduce calculi to smaller particles capable of spontaneous transport and excretion from the urinary tract. Shock waves used for ESWL differ from ultrasonic waves in several significant aspects. Ultrasonic sound waves create a sinusoidal pattern with gentle peaks and valleys, whereas shock waves create a single positive-pressure front with several frequencies, a sharp onset, and a gradual decline. When transmitted through degassed water or water-containing viscera, these waves lose only a small portion of their original energy without producing significant tissue damage. As these shock waves pass through a urinary stone, the stone is shattered; with repeated application, the stone is pulverized into sand.

ESWL is performed in a specially designed stationary or mobile suite (the latter is usually situated in the cab of a large truck), containing a large reservoir of degassed water (bath) or other medium for the transmission of shock waves, fluoroscopic or ultrasonic imaging equipment capable of locating the stone within a three-dimensional perspective, and a mobile chair for placing a body in the bath.

Anesthesia is usually required for ESWL; the urinary calculus is located by ultrasound or fluoroscopy, and repeated applications of shock waves are used to pulverize the stone. A nephrostomy tube or ureteral catheter is often placed to prevent urinary obstruction as the fragments of the stone pass down the ureter to the bladder.

Advances in the technology of lithotripsy have led to second-generation units that use a minibath or membrane to deliver shock waves to a urinary stone. The spark gap generator used in the original ESWL units has also been modified so that shock waves can be generated from a piezoceramic (piezoelectric), a 10 mg lead azide pellet, or an electromagnetic shock wave generator (Figure 12-19).[46]

Contraindications and Cautions

1. Bleeding disorders, presence of a cardiac pacemaker, marked anatomic abnormalities that render correct positioning unfeasible, extreme obesity, and short stature constitute relative contraindications to ESWL. Greater experience with ESWL continues to limit or eliminate the application of these relative contraindications for treatment.

Preprocedural Nursing Care

1. Explain that while ESWL does not require an incision, sedation or anesthesia is often required because the procedure causes discomfort, requiring the patient to remain relatively motionless for a prolonged period.
2. Advise the patient that small fragments of urinary stones will be passed in the urine during the first week following ESWL. Teach the person to strain the urine for stone fragments as directed.
3. Advise the patient that renal colic (pain) may occur after ESWL, particularly when a large stone burden is pulverized.
4. Reassure the patient that aggressive pain management will be maintained until all stone fragments are passed.

NURSING CARE

Nursing Assessment

Urinary Output and Voiding Behavior

Passage of stone particles
Dysuria; bladder colic

Pain

Renal colic

Temperature

Fever

Nursing Dx & Intervention

Altered peripheral tissue perfusion (renal) related to urinary obstruction

- Question the patient concerning the use of any anticoagulant medications (including aspirin) before ESWL, and obtain any history of bleeding or clotting disorders. *ESWL causes trauma to renal tissue as the stone fragments are pulverized and transported to the bladder. Uncontrolled bleeding disorders may produce significant hematuria unless adequately managed before ESWL.*
- Monitor the patient for hematuria following ESWL *to prevent the occurrence of excessive bleeding.*
- Teach the patient to monitor the urine at home for resolution (or persistence) of hematuria. Instruct the patient to call the physician should persistent hematuria occur. *Since most patients undergo ESWL as an outpatient procedure, teach self-monitoring for potential complications.*

Pain related to urinary obstruction

- Assess pain for character, location, duration, and intensity. *Obstructing fragments produce a renal colic type of pain; bladder spasms produce a sharp cramping pain in the suprapubic area with dysuria.*
- Prepare the patient for additional endoscopic, ESWL, or percutaneous procedures, as directed, *to relieve obstruction and discomfort produced by residual fragments.*
- Administer, or teach the patient to self-administer, analgesic or narcotic medications, as directed, *to relieve discomfort of renal colic.*
- Administer, or teach the patient to self-administer, urinary analgesics or antispasmodic drugs, as directed, *to relieve discomfort produced by bladder spasms or inflammation.*

Altered urinary elimination related to urinary obstruction

- Encourage the patient to maintain an adequate intake of fluid (at least 1500 ml per day) *to assist in the elimination of stone fragments.*

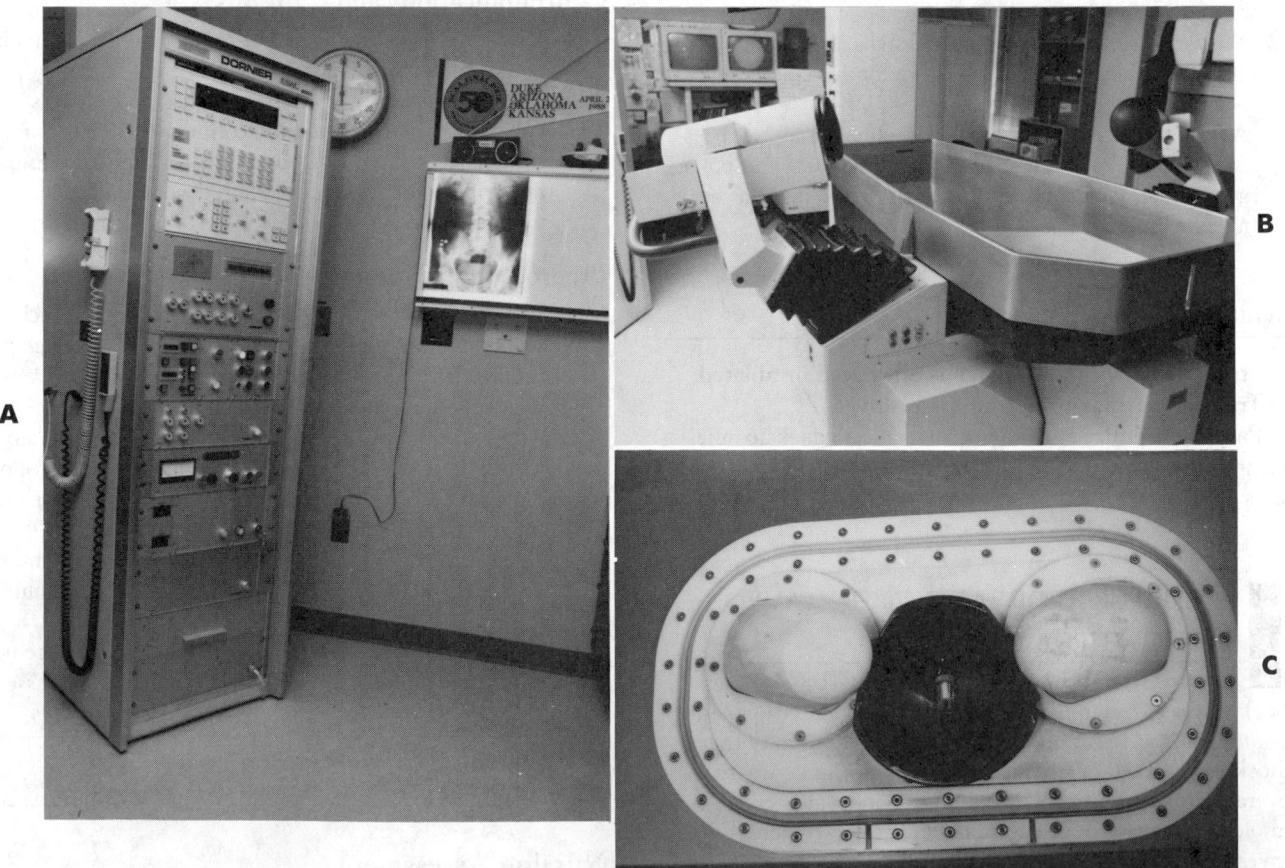

Figure 12-19 A, ESWL control panel and x-ray (see stones in left kidney and marker on right kidney). **B,** Tub for extracorporeal shock wave lithotripsy (ESWL). **C,** Source of impulse located in bottom of tub.

• Reassure the patient that irritative voiding symptoms and urinary frequency experienced after ESWL are transient. *The passage of stone fragments and relief of obstruction produce some urinary tract inflammation and diuresis.*

Patient Education/Home Care Planning

1. Discuss with the patient techniques for preventing recurrent stone formation, including drugs, diet, and fluid intake.

Evaluation

Renal tissue perfusion is improved X-ray of kidneys, ureters, and bladder (KUB) and intravenous pyelogram (IVP) are normal.

Comfort level is maintained Patient does not experience pain. Patient learns to self-administer medications to prevent pain or spasms as necessary.

Urinary elimination patterns return to normal Patient maintains fluid intake of at least 1500 ml per day. Irritative voiding symptoms subside.

■ INTRAPENILE PROSTHETIC DEVICES

Intrapenile prosthetic devices are used when pharmacologic treatment, vacuum device therapy, or vascular surgical procedures are inadequate or unacceptable for the patient seeking to restore erectile activity. Placement of the device relies on thorough investigation of the vascular, neurologic, endocrine, and psychogenic aspects of erectile dysfunction for a particular individual.

The choice of penile prosthesis is affected by the patient's and surgeon's preference and technical considerations. There are two general types of implants: semirigid and inflatable. The semirigid devices maintain a continuous state of tumescence (Figure 12-20). The Small-Carrion device has a silicone exterior and sponge interior and the Jonas prosthesis is composed of silicone with silver wires that can be positioned for better concealment beneath clothing.

The inflatable devices are capable of imitating the flaccid and tumescent penis. The Scott inflatable prosthesis consists of dual rods in the cavernosal bodies, an abdominal reservoir, and a pump mechanism (Figure 12-21). Fluid can be baffled into

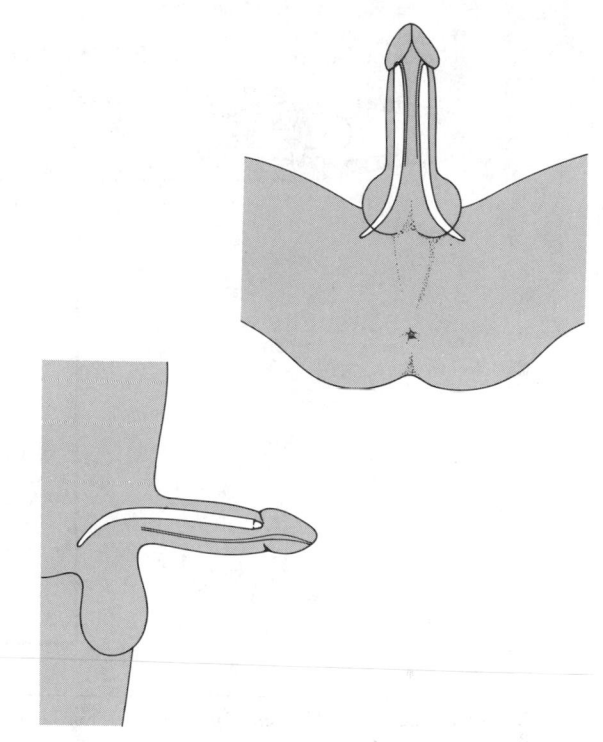

Figure 12-20 Semirigid intrapenile prosthesis. (From Beare and Myers.[10])

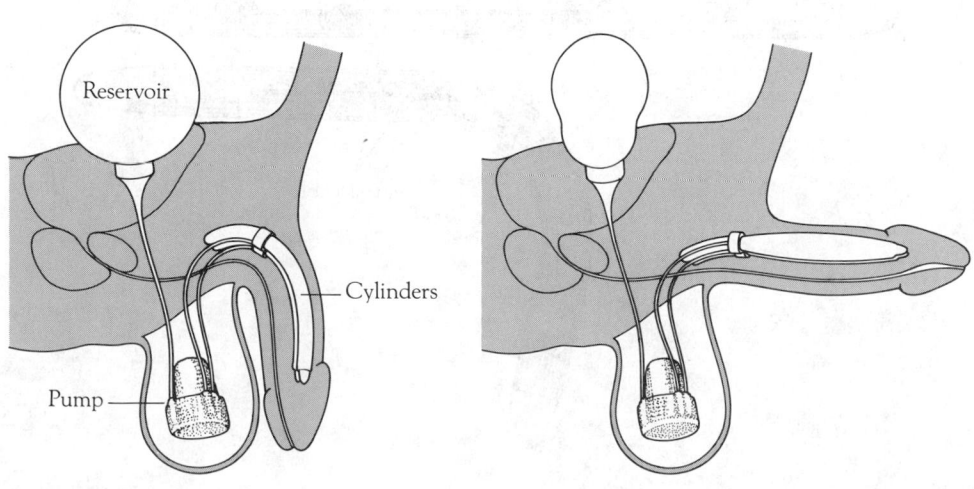

Figure 12-21 Scott inflatable penile prosthesis. (From Beare and Myers.[10])

the abdominal reservoir to mimic a flaccid state and into the rods to imitate an erection. The two-piece inflatable prosthesis uses the same principles as the Scott inflatable device by combining the pump and reservoir into a single piece, reducing the risk of mechanical complications. One-piece inflatable systems use a baffling system contained within each of the two rods (Figure 12-22). An alternate, one-piece device mimics an erection by shortening a cable that is surrounded by plastic bodies (Figure 12-23).

Contraindications and Cautions

1. Intrapenile prosthetic devices are contraindicated in patients with deep-rooted psychologic abnormalities underlying erectile dysfunction.

Preprocedural Nursing Care

1. Sexual counseling for the patient and his partner during preoperative and postoperative periods may be necessary.

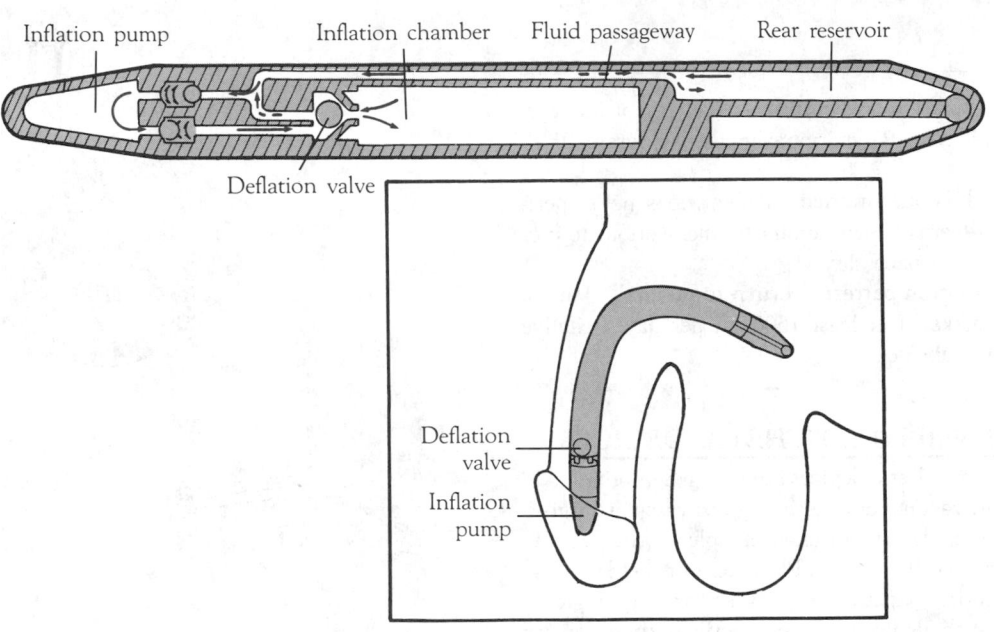

Figure 12-22 One-piece inflatable penile prosthesis. (From Gray.[49])

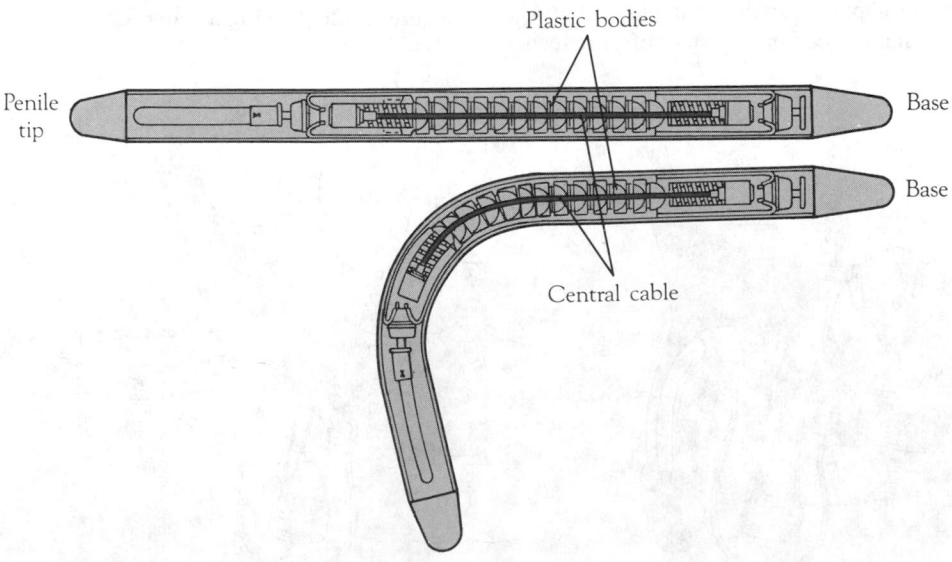

Figure 12-23 One-piece prosthesis with central cable that shortens plastic bodies to produce erection. (From Gray.[49])

2. Teach the patient and partner (when appropriate) to manipulate inflatable prosthetic devices before the procedure.

3. Advise the patient that the presence of an implant may carry a risk for infection during an invasive genitourinary procedure. Instruct the patient to discuss the need for antibiotic prophylaxis with his urologist before future procedures.

NURSING CARE

Nursing Assessment

Penis

Redness
Edema
Signs of erosion of prosthetic device

Scrotum and Perineum

Hematoma for 2 to 3 weeks; edema for 24 hours postoperatively
Discharge and hemorrhage from incision

Temperature

Fever

Urinary Output

Normal voiding patterns; catheter drainage rarely needed

Nursing Dx & Intervention

Pain related to surgical trauma

- Reassure the patient that scrotal discomfort is temporary, although bruising and some scrotal swelling will persist for approximately 2 weeks.
- Administer analgesic or narcotic agents, as directed, *to relieve pain.*
- Advise the patient to wear comfortable jockey-type underwear *to minimize excess jostling and discomfort of the penis and scrotum.*

High risk for infection related to implantation of prosthesis

- Administer antiinfective medications before the procedure, as directed, *to prevent infection.*
- Teach the patient to observe the penis for signs of infection following implantation. *Prompt treatment during the immediate postoperative period may prevent loss of the implant from intractable prosthetic device infection.*
- Advise the patient to check with his physician concerning the need for prophylactic antibiotics before any invasive procedures. *Infection of a penile prosthesis necessitates explaining to the patient about how to prevent persistent infection. Suppressive antiinfective medications may reduce this risk.*

Risk for impaired skin integrity related to presence of prosthesis

- Observe the penis for signs of prosthetic device erosion during the immediate postoperative period; teach the patient to observe for signs of erosion after discharge from the hospital. *Erosion (noted as pale, thinned-appearing skin near the glans penis) may occur after surgery. Reconstruction may be required.*

Self-esteem disturbance (high risk for) related to sexual dysfunction

- Provide reassurance concerning the device and its expected impact on erectile dysfunction.
- Refer the patient and his partner to a qualified counselor, as indicated. *Erectile dysfunction may produce significant discord in the individual and couple, requiring intervention by a qualified specialist.*

Patient Education/Home Care Planning

1. Inform patient to abstain from sex for 21 days after surgery to allow for adequate healing if semirigid device is used.
2. Discuss with the patient the need to inflate Scott inflatable penile prosthesis repeatedly before use to encourage formation of fibrous sheath around device.
3. Demonstrate to the patient techniques of concealing semirigid device in clothing.
4. Inform the patient about signs of erosion or infection.
5. Demonstrate to the patient *and partner* inflation and deflation of inflatable penile prostheses.
6. Discuss with the patient the need to avoid contact sports or lifting heavy objects for 21 days after prosthesis is placed.

Evaluation

There is no pain   Comfort level is maintained.

There is no infection   Patient is afebrile. Wound healing is normal.

There is no erosion   Size, color, and contour of penis are normal.

Patient makes an adequate adjustment to the prosthesis   Patient *and* partner give subjective report of satisfaction with device. Patient resumes sexual relations with partner. Patient can demonstrate correct technique for inflating and deflating Scott inflatable prosthesis.

■ OPEN PROSTATECTOMY

Description and Rationale

Open prostatectomy refers to removal of the prostate gland with or without the prostatic capsule. Several surgical approaches may be used including suprapubic, transvesical, retropubic, perineal, and transcoccygeal. In the suprapubic or transvesical procedures the prostate is removed through the cavity of the bladder. Retropubic prostatectomy is performed through a low abdominal incision without opening the bladder. The most radical of the open procedures for prostatectomy is the perineal approach in which the incision is made between the scrotum and rectum. The transcoccygeal approach allows better surgical access to the posterior lobes of the prostate. The perineal approach is usually associated with loss of erection, orgasm, and ejaculatory function. It is not uncommon for sexual dysfunction to occur when the prostatic capsule is removed.

The suprapubic and retropubic approaches may be used as open surgical approaches when the gland is too large for transurethral resection; they are not generally used for cancer. In these incidences the capsule is left intact.

Perineal prostatectomy is most often performed for cancer of the prostate when it is confined to the capsule. Some controversy exists regarding the use of radical prostatectomy when the tumor extends through the capsule.

Contraindications and Cautions

1. Small fibrous prostate
2. Presence of cancer (suprapubic, retropubic)

Preprocedural Nursing Care

1. Patient teaching is done, including potential sexual impairment if appropriate.
2. Perineum, external genitalia, abdomen, and upper halves of thighs are shaved the night before surgery.
3. Cleansing enemas are given until clear.

•••••• Multidisciplinary Plan

Medications

Laxatives (stool softeners)
    Docusate (Colace), 100 mg/d po
    Analgesics prn

General Management

Urethral catheter, suprapubic catheter, and Penrose drain
Intravenous fluids
Clear diet progressing to regular diet
Heat lamp; Sitz bath (perineal incision)

NURSING CARE

Nursing Assessment

Incision

Redness; pain; edema; drainage

Temperature

Fever

Pain

Postoperative pain

Urinary Output

Amount of urinary output through urethral catheter or suprapubic catheter
Presence of bright red blood
Stress incontinence (may last for a few days to 6 months)
Urethral stricture

Other Complications

Epididymitis

Sexual Dysfunction

Impotence
Retrograde ejaculation

Nursing Dx & Intervention

Risk for hemorrhage related to surgical resection

- Observe urine output for color, consistency, volume, and presence of blood clots *to assess for excessive bleeding.*
- Maintain catheter traction as directed *to prevent hemorrhage.*
- Monitor vital signs *to assess for systemic signs of hemorrhage.*

Risk for infection related to surgical trauma

- Maintain sterile urinary drainage system *to prevent infection.*
- Monitor vital signs *to assess for systemic signs of infection.*

Altered urinary elimination related to potential obstruction of urinary outflow

- Assess output through urethral or suprapubic catheter for volume *to prevent urinary retention.*
- Observe catheters for kinking and presence of blood clots *to prevent urinary retention.*

Body image disturbance related to altered erectile and fertility function

- Discuss implications of removal of prostatic capsule with patient and in consultation with urologist. *Likelihood of altered erectile dysfunction varies significantly with surgical techniques. Altered high risk for fertility is expected and must be discussed fully with patient.*
- Assist patient in exploring anxiety and fears related to procedure, provide factual information concerning implications of procedure as indicated. *Exploration of feelings of fear and anxiety with reassurance of objective facts related to procedure allows optimum opportunity for patient to regain positive body image.*
- Discuss alternative means of sexual expression, such as penile prosthesis, as indicated and in consultation with urologist *to reassure patient of realistic alternatives in cases where erectile dysfunction may occur.*

Risk for impaired skin integrity related to drainage from wound

- Change dressing frequently *to prevent skin irritation from damp dressing.*
- Cleanse skin gently and pat dry or use a hair dryer *to dry skin and prevent irritation.*
- Apply moisture barrier ointments and skin sealants (Brad Protective Barrier Film; Skin Prep) *to protect the skin.*

Patient Education/Home Care Planning

1. Discuss incisional care with the patient.
2. Discuss skin protection techniques with the patient if drainage is still continuing at time of discharge.
3. Urine color will not clear up for 4 to 8 weeks, but the patient should notify physician if it changes and becomes bright red with clots.
4. Provide teaching and counseling regarding sexual concerns.

Evaluation

No hemorrhage occurs   Urine remains clear and free of clots.

There is no infection   Patient remains afebrile and experiences no symptoms indicative of infection.

Urinary elimination is normal   Output is adequate. Color is clear. Patient does not experience pain, burning, or bladder spasms.

Sexual functioning resumes   Patient is able to obtain an erection. Retrograde ejaculation may occur. Patient is scheduled for or has had a penile prosthesis if indicated.

Skin integrity is maintained   No skin irritation or breakdown occurs.

■ OPEN UROLOGIC SURGERY

(Nephrectomy, partial nephrectomy, nephrolithotomy, pyelolithotomy, ureterolithotomy, cystectomy)

Description and Rationale

Open urologic surgeries include nephrectomy, partial nephrectomy, nephrolithotomy, pyelolithotomy, ureterolithotomy, and cystectomy. The care of the patient during these procedures is similar, and all involve an open surgical incision. Surgery of the kidney is accomplished through a flank incision, while the operative approach for bladder surgeries is an anterior incision.

Indications for nephrectomy include calculus, hemorrhage, hydronephrosis, hypertension, neoplasms, renal donation, trauma, and vascular disease.[43] Partial nephrectomy is performed to preserve as much renal function as possible in the same conditions that may require nephrectomy. A partial nephrectomy is important when contralateral renal function is impaired. Stones in the kidney, pelvis, or ureter may be re-

moved by an open urologic incision if newer techniques of extracorporeal shock wave lithotripsy (ESWL) and percutaneous ureteroscopic stone removal are ineffective.

Contraindications and Cautions

1. If the condition is bilateral, it is important to preserve total renal function.
2. Nephrostomy drainage may be required following open urologic surgeries through stents or tubes to allow for adequate healing when the potential for wound healing is suboptimal, scar tissue is significant, or reconstructive procedures require splinting.

Preprocedural Nursing Care

1. Preoperative teaching concerns the procedure, presence of catheter, and stents for surgery, and turning, coughing, and leg exercises following surgery.
2. Give nothing by mouth past midnight.

NURSING CARE

Nursing Assessment

Incision
Redness; pain; edema; drainage

Temperature
Fever

Urinary Output
Amount of urinary output through nephrostomy tube or catheter
Presence of bright red blood
Absence of urinary output through catheter

Pain
Incisional; postoperative

Hemorrhage
Incisional; through drains, tubes, or catheter

Nursing Dx & Intervention

High risk for hemorrhage or infection related to surgical trauma

- Assess patient for signs and symptoms of bleeding.
- Evaluate all tube drainage for amount, color, and consistency. *Persistent bleeding is noted as bloody or serosanguineous discharge through surgical drains.*
- Observe surgical wound for color, warmth, and discharge *to assess for signs of bleeding (bloody discharge through wound with or without separation of borders) and signs of infection (purulent discharge from wound, increasing redness, warmth at operative site).*

Risk for fluid volume deficit related to surgical manipulation of kidney

- Monitor intake and output, daily weights, and BUN and creatinine levels *to assess for hypovolemia; poor fluid intake, rising BUN and creatinine, and rapid weight loss are potential signs of fluid volume deficit that impair healing and may compromise renal function.*

Pain related to surgical trauma

- Provide analgesics as ordered.
- Provide medications to decrease detrusor contractility as ordered *to prevent bladder spasm associated with urethral or suprapubic catheterization and surgical manipulation of the lower urinary tract.*

Altered patterns of urinary elimination related to surgical manipulation

- Monitor urinary output through urethral catheter, nephrostomy tube, suprapubic catheter, or other drainage tube *to prevent urinary retention.*

Risk for impaired skin integrity related to drainage from wound

- Use skin barrier (pectin wafer) around Penrose drain or stab wound *to protect skin from potential irritation from discharge.*
- Use a sterile drainage wound collection system if drainage is copious *to protect skin from discharge and to assess output.*
- Maintain sterile dressing changes *to protect skin adjacent to surgical incision from discharge.*

Patient Education/Home Care Planning

1. Patient education varies with primary etiology; refer to specific discussions of urologic diseases.
2. The patient should be informed about incision care and management of any drains or tubes.

Evaluation

There is no hemorrhage No bleeding or excessive serosanguineous drainage occurs.

Urinary output is adequate; no retention occurs Urinary output is sufficient. BUN and creatinine levels are normal. Weight remains normal.

There is no infection There are no signs of redness, edema, or inflammation of incision.

Comfort level is maintained Patient experiences minimal pain.

Skin integrity remains intact No skin breakdown occurs.

▌ PERCUTANEOUS NEPHROSCOPIC STONE REMOVAL

Description and Rationale

Percutaneous nephroscopic stone removal is a nonsurgical technique to treat urolithiasis. A nephrostomy tube is placed percutaneously into the proper calyx under fluoroscopic monitoring, and a dilator system is used to allow insertion of a nephroscope with one or more working channels. Several methods may be used to remove calculi percutaneously. A stone basket may be used to retrieve relatively small calculi. Larger stones may be first broken via ultrasonic lithotripter, laser, or electrolysis. Remaining fragments are then removed via a stone basket or flushed from the collecting system mechanically or physiologically.

Contraindications and Cautions

1. Septicemia should be adequately controlled before percutaneous nephroscopic stone removal is attempted.
2. If obstruction is significant, a nephrostomy tube may be placed with the patient under local anesthesia to facilitate adequate pelvic drainage.

Preprocedural Nursing Care

1. Monitor for signs and symptoms of gram-negative septicemia and septic shock including increased fever, pulse, respirations, and blood pressure followed by hypotension and potential cardiovascular compromise.

NURSING CARE

Nursing Assessment

Pain

Renal colic
Acute flank pain

Temperature

Fever

Urinary Output

Oliguria or anuria in cases of bilateral obstruction

Other Complications

Nausea, vomiting, and ileus secondary to renal colic

Nephrostomy Tube

Hematuria
Frank bleeding

Nursing Dx & Intervention

Risk for hemorrhage related to manipulation of kidney

- Observe flank for mass and observe nephrostomy tube for amount and characteristics of discharge (color, consistency) *to assess for hemorrhage from affected kidney and urinary transport system.*
- Monitor pulse and blood pressure *to assess for systemic signs of hemorrhage.*

Pain related to urinary obstruction

- Administer analgesics as ordered.

Altered urinary elimination related to potential obstruction of urinary outflow

- Observe output through nephrostomy tube for color consistency and volume *to prevent urinary retention.*
- Monitor patency of tubes and irrigate tubes as directed *to prevent urinary retention.*

Patient Education/Home Care Planning

1. Teach techniques for preventing recurrent stone formation including drugs, diet, and fluid intake.

Evaluation

Hemorrhage is absent Urine drainage from nephrostomy tube is clear. Vital signs are within normal limits.

There is no obstruction Patient does not experience renal colic. Creatinine and BUN levels are within normal limits.

Infection is absent Patient is afebrile. Urine and blood cultures are negative.

Urinary elimination patterns return to normal No urinary retention occurs.

TRANSURETHRAL RESECTION OF THE PROSTATE AND ALTERNATIVE PROCEDURES FOR PROSTATE TISSUE ABLATION

Description and Rationale

Transurethral resection of the prostate (TUR-P) is the removal of prostatic tissue under endoscopic control. A rigid cystoscope is inserted into the urethra, and the prostatic urethra is identified. A resectoscope is inserted and tissue is removed by a small loop with electrocautery energy (Figure 12-24). Blood, tissue, and other debris are irrigated with a glycine or sorbitol solution. The resected prostate tissue is collected and sent for pathologic analysis. The glycine or sorbitol solutions allow electrocauteri-

zation of bleeding vessels in the prostatic bed without damage to adjacent tissue. The area of resection varies with each patient, but typically encompasses the bladder neck and prostatic urethra. The resection frequently extends to the urethra just above the verumontanum.[47,49]

Multiple alternative procedures for prostatic tissue ablation have been described. Some have gained relatively widespread use, whereas others are in earlier stages of clinical investigations. Table 12-5 summarizes alternative approaches of prostate tissue removal. It is important to remember that the nursing management of the majority of these alternative procedures has not been adequately defined, primarily because of a lack of clinical experience.

Because BPH is typically a quality of life condition, prostate tissue ablation is indicated when voiding dysfunction symptoms are significant, and the patient chooses this treatment rather than watchful waiting or pharmacotherapy. Prostatic tissue destruction also is indicated when BPH is associated with acute urinary retention, compromised renal function, or urinary tract infection.[2]

Contraindications and Cautions

1. Prostatic tissue ablation is contraindicated in the presence of a urinary tract infection, or when acute prostatitis is present.

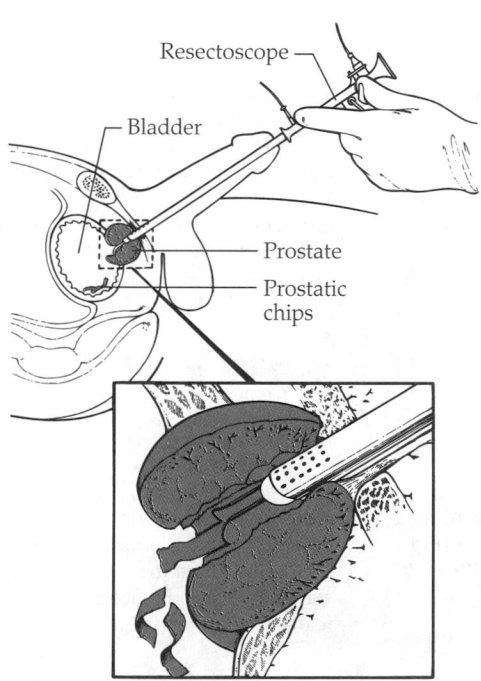

Figure 12-24 Continuous irrigation of the bladder requires a three-way Foley catheter that allows simultaneous infusion and drainage of an irrigating solution (normal saline) through the bladder. The solution is infused rapidly into the bladder, and the bedside drainage bag is assessed for evidence of excessive bleeding and then drained every 1 to 2 hours. (From Beare and Myers.[10])

TABLE 12-5   Alternative Procedures for Prostate Tissue Removal (All procedures are compared to TUR-P)*

Procedure	Description	Advantages	Disadvantages	Postprocedural Care‡
Transurethral vaportrobe (Figure 12-25)	Resection of prostatic tissue under direct, endoscopic visualization. Tissue is removed using a "roller ball", or "roller bar" and electrocautery energy.	• Superior visualization of prostate • Less risk of bleeding • Possibly less risk of TUR syndrome • Procedure may be performed as outpatient • Prostate tissue available for pathologic analysis to determine presence of prostate cancer • Additional equipment costs are relatively low	None yet identified	Indwelling catheter for 24 hours, patient may experience some hematuria for several days, passage of scabs with transient hematuria in 7-10 days
Transurethral incision of the prostate (TUIP)	Incision of the prostatic capsule under direct endoscopic visualization. A small cutting loop and electrocautery energy are used to incise the prostatic capsule.	• Local anesthesia may be used to reduce risk of spinal or general anesthesia • Reduced hospital stay (1-2 days shorter when compared to TUR-P) • Less risk of bleeding, retrograde ejaculation, bladder neck contracture • Lower risk of TUR syndrome • Additional equipment relatively inexpensive	• Limited to smaller glands • Marked enlargement of median lobe comprises relative contraindication • Risk of incontinence, erectile dysfunction similar to TUR-P • Prostate tissue not available for pathologic analysis	Brief hospital stay may be necessary; indwelling catheter for 24 hours, three way irrigation not typically required but catheter is placed under gentle traction
Laser prostatectomy (Laser prostatectomy, transurethral incision of the prostate, visual laser ablation of the prostate [VLAP])	Ablation of prostate tissue using laser energy (Nd:YAG). The visualization technique varies; VLAP is generally preferred because of the ability to visualize the prostate using direct endoscopy.	• Hospitalization not required • Low risk of bleeding • Less risk of retrograde ejaculation • Reduced mortality rate	• Prolonged period of tissue slough (7 days; may persist up to 30 days) • Post-operative discomfort and irritation occur with prolonged edema • Long-term efficacy as compared to TUR-P has not been established • Prostate tissue is not available for pathologic analysis • Additional equipment costs are significant	Indwelling (suprapubic or urethral) catheter for at least 7 days; postprocedure discomfort may occur during period of edema and tissue slough
Intraurethral stent insertion (Figure 12-26)	Placement of a medical grade steel in the prostatic urethra to widen the prostatic urethra and mechanically alleviate obstruction	• Less risk of bleeding • No risk of TUR syndrome • Procedure is reversible (limited window of opportunity)	• Does not correct bladder neck obstruction • Occasionally causes discomfort requiring removal • Urethral tissue may fail to reepithelialize around stent, necessitating removal	Performed as outpatient; suprapubic catheter up to 30 days after insertion; initial irritative voiding symptoms may require antispasmodic therapy
Interstitial laser therapy	Ablation of prostate tissue using a transurethral, transrectal or transperineal approach. Prostatic size and	• Similar to laser prostatectomy • Preservation of urothelium may reduce post-	• Degree of postprocedure discomfort has not been determined • Tissue not available for	Indwelling catheter, otherwise unknown

*References 15, 29, 30, 32, 49, 68, 77, 78, 103, 104, 115.
‡Refined nursing care plans may not be available, primarily due to a lack of clinical experience with these techniques.

TABLE 12-5 Alternative Procedures for Prostate Tissue Removal (All procedures are compared to TUR-P)*—cont'd

Procedure	Description	Advantages	Disadvantages	Postprocedural Care‡
Interstitial laser therapy—cont'd	location are determined using ultrasonic techniques. Laser energy used to ablate prostate tissue, without disrupting integrity of the rectal or urethral wall.	procedure discomfort, irritative voiding symptoms	pathologic analysis	
Transurethral ultrasonic aspiration	Destruction of prostate tissue, using ultrasonic energy (0-700 micron vibration) at an excursion rate of 39 kHz; maximum power 100 W. Prostatic size and location determined using ultrasound imaging.	• Lower risk for significant bleeding • Incontinence rate may be reduced • Impotence risk is comparable to TUR-P	• Procedure will not correct significant bladder neck hypertrophy obstruction	Indwelling catheter for 18-24 hours, in hospital stay 2-3 days
Transurethral needle ablation of the prostate (TUNA)	Ablation of prostatic tissue under indirect endoscopic visualization (the surgeon will see the prostatic urethra, but does not see the needles penetrate the prostatic capsule). Low level radiofrequency energy is used to heat the prostate, causing tissue destruction.	• Lower risk of significant blood loss • Lower risk of postprocedure irritative voiding symptoms • Lower risk of impotence • Lower risk of retrograde ejaculation	• Tissue not available for tissue analysis • Prolonged time for symptom improvement (>1 month) • Transient urinary retention, approximately 3 days (range 1-21 days) • Urethral stricture may occur	Hematuria and dysuria persist for 2-3 days. An indwelling catheter may be left in place for 7-10 days.
High intensity focused ultrasound (HIFU)	Coagulative destruction of prostate tissue using high intensity, focused ultrasonic energy. The ultrasonic energy is delivered via a transrectal route, and the prostate is localized using ultrasonic imaging techniques.	• Less risk of bleeding • Low postoperative discomfort • No risk of TUR syndrome	• Transient retention lasting 6 days (range 1-42 days) • Hematospermia, mild hematuria • Urinary tract infection • Moderate symptom improvement only	PSA values are transiently elevated (12-24 hours). Suprapubic catheter for 6-7 days. Symptom improvement generally requires 6 months.
Transurethral microwave thermotherapy (TUMT)	Microwave (radiating heat energy) is used to destroy prostate tissue while conductive cooling is used to prevent urethral injury. The microwave energy is delivered via a 20 French balloon type catheter and a temperature probe is then placed to measure anterior rectal wall temperature.	• Performed as an outpatient • Less risk of significant bleeding • No risk of TUR syndrome • Low risk of retrograde ejaculation	• Multiple treatments may be required • Rectal wall injury may occur • Long-term efficacy (>12 months postprocedure) has not been established • Effect of therapy on the bladder neck is not known	PSA values are transiently elevated following procedure (up to 3 months). Transient urinary retention occurs and suprapubic catheter drainage is required.
Cryotherapy	Prostate tissue is destroyed by rapid freezing. A cryotherapy probe is inserted into the prostate and the adjacent tissue is rapidly cooled to −180° to −190° C.	• Less risk of bleeding • Reduced risk of TUR syndrome	• Risk of impotence and incontinence may be significant when compared to TUR-P • Urethrorectal, urethrocutaneous fistulae may occur • Tissue not available for pathologic analysis	Indwelling catheter for several weeks, sloughing of tissue will occur during this period, primarily used for prostate cancer.

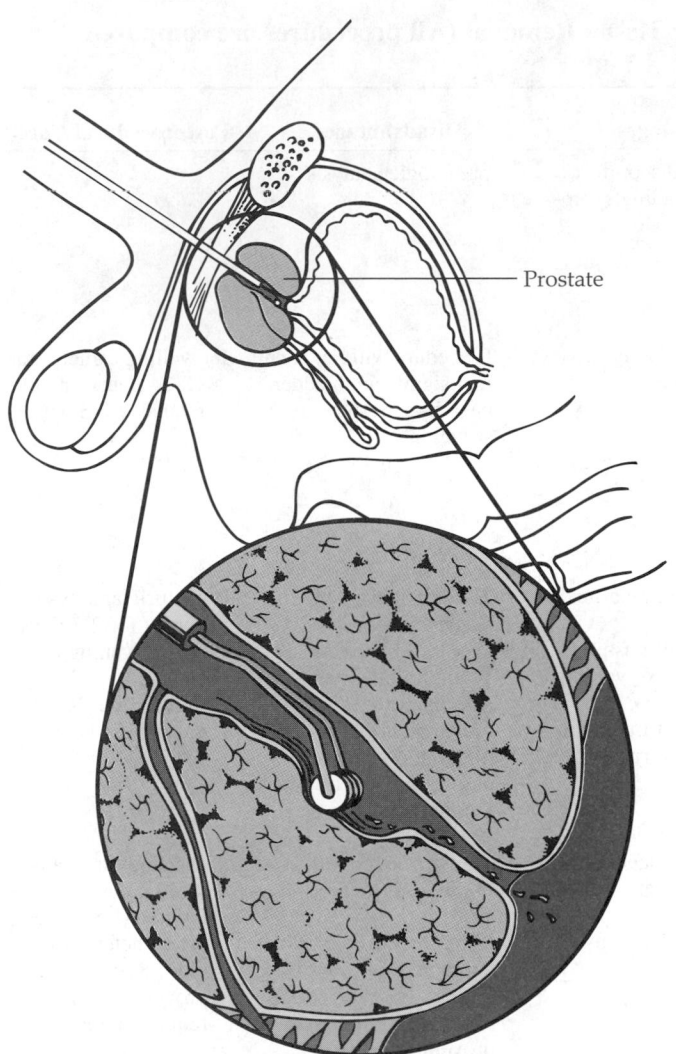

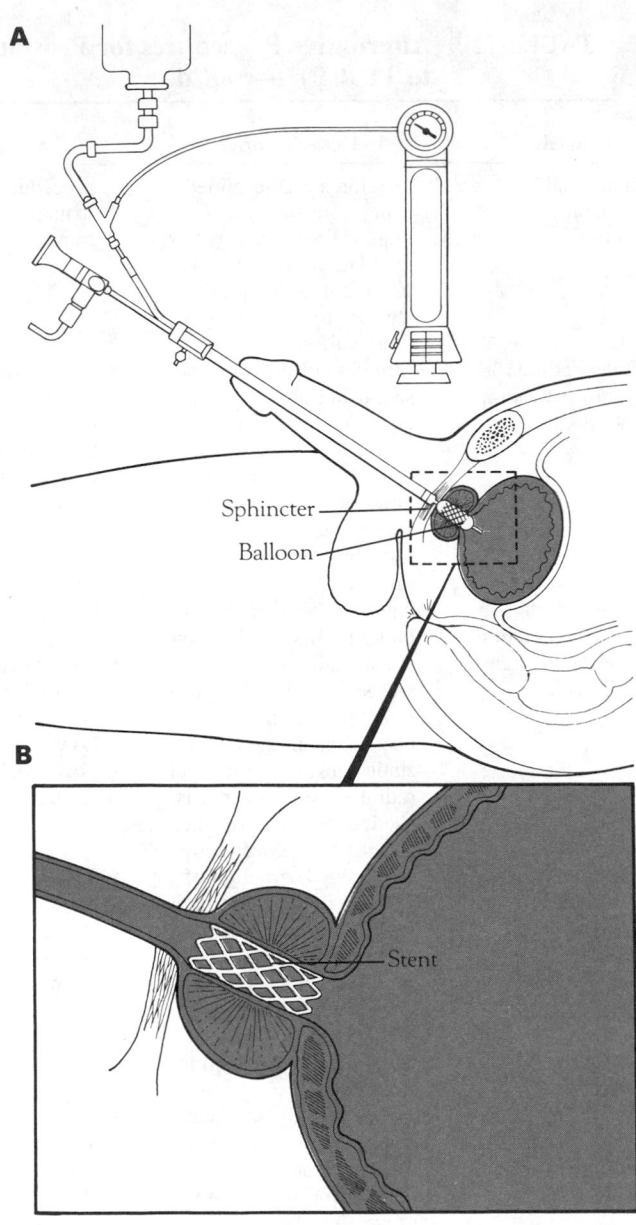

Figure 12-25 Prostatectomy using the vaportrobe uses the same energy source as the TUR-P but allows direct endoscopic visualization. A rollerball blade device is used to ablate prostatic tissue.

Figure 12-26 Prostatic stent. **A,** Placement of stent. **B,** Stent in place increases prostatic urethral lumen. (From Gray.[49])

2. Physical conditions such as ankylosis of the hip or irreversible scrotal hernia may interfere with positioning of the patient for TUR-P, and alternative procedures may be considered.

Preprocedural Nursing Care

1. Discuss the technique of prostatic tissue destruction with the urologist before the procedure. Advise the patient of the procedure and anticipated outcomes based on this discussion.

2. Advise the patient that prostate tissue destruction may affect aspects of sexual function including libido, antegrade ejaculations, erectile function, and fertility. Counsel him to consult his urologist to discuss specific concerns related to the incidence and nature of these potential complications.

3. Reassure the patient that the incidence of erectile dysfunction following prostate tissue destruction for BPH is relatively low. Advise the patient to discuss specific concerns with his urologist since the relative risk varies according to the technique used for prostatectomy.

•••••• Multidisciplinary Plan

Medications

1. Antiinfective medications are commonly administered before and after prostatic tissue ablation. An aminogly-

coside may be given intravenously before and for 12 to 24 hours after the procedure.

2. Systemic urinary analgesics, anticholinergics, or antispasmodics administered as indicated for pain.

General Management

1. A three-way indwelling catheter with continuous irrigation is required following TUR-P (Figure 12-27).
2. Variable periods of indwelling catheter drainage are required following alternative procedures (see Table 12-4).

NURSING CARE

Nursing Assessment

Bladder and Prostate

Urinary output, presence of clots

Flow rate of irrigation following TUR-P, character of output, volume of fluid in irrigating bags and catheter drainage bag

Significant Blood Loss (TUR-P Associated with Greatest Risk)

Changes in serum hematocrit and hemoglobin

Changes in vital signs; rapid pulse with increased blood pressure followed by declining blood pressure with severe loss

Presence of large quantities of bright red blood and clots in catheter drainage bag

Temperature

Fever

TUR Syndrome (TUR-P Carries Greatest Risk)

Acute confusion

Restlessness

Bradycardia, tachypnea

Hyponatremia

Nursing Dx & Intervention/TUR-P

(See Table 12-4 for differences in care with alternative procedures)

Altered tissue perfusion related to bleeding from prostatic urethra

- Maintain three-way indwelling catheter with continuous irrigation, to remove debris and clots from bladder, and prevent blockage of urinary outflow.
- Maintain gentle traction on the catheter, to prevent excessive bleeding from the operative site (Figure 12-28).
- Obtain a serum hemoglobin and hematocrit as directed; compare preoperative and postoperative values. Significant hemorrhage may occur from the prostatic bed following TUR-P.

- Remove the indwelling catheter as directed (typically 36 to 72 hours after TUR-P). Assist the patient to save urine from each voiding episode. The "string of bottles" obtained after catheter removal is used to monitor resolution of hematuria from the prostatic bed.
- Reinsert an indwelling catheter as directed if marked hematuria persists, or if significant hematuria occurs. Reinsertion of the catheter with gentle traction may be required to prevent persistent bleeding from the operative site.
- Reassure the patient that a pink tinged urine and flecks of dark blood may occur for 10 to 14 days. Dark flecks of blood and pink-tinged urine (indicating minimal bleeding mixed with urine) indicate spontaneous release of scabs from the operative site.

Risk for altered tissue perfusion, related to deep vein thrombosis of the lower extremities

- Assist the patient to apply antiembolic stockings before TUR-P, and to wear them for 1 week postoperatively. TUR-P requires prolonged positioning of the legs in stirrups increasing the risk of deep vein thrombosis of the legs; antiembolic stockings encourage venous return from the lower extremities.
- Raise the foot of the bed 20 to 30 degrees during the first postoperative day to encourage venous return from the legs.

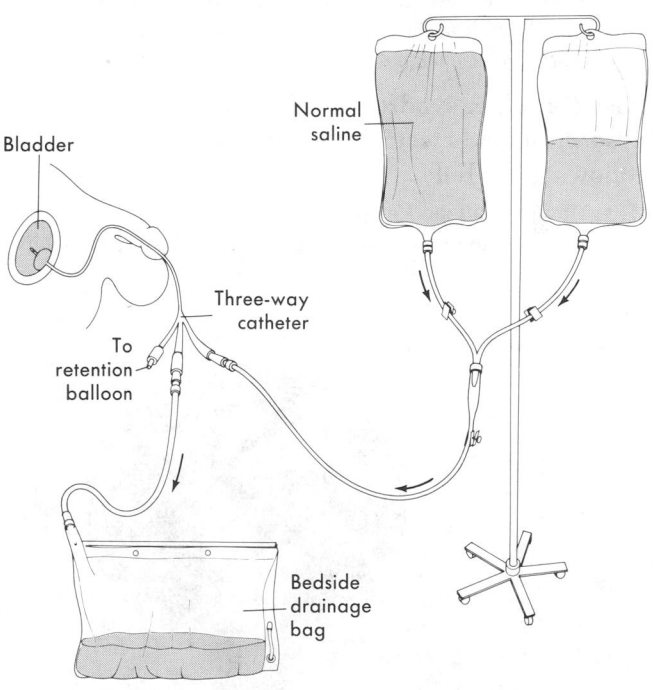

Figure 12-27 Continuous irrigation of bladder requires a three-way Foley catheter that allows simultaneous infusion and drainage of an irrigating solution (normal saline) through bladder. Solution is infused rapidly into bladder, and bedside drainage bag is assessed for evidence of excessive bleeding and then drained every 1 to 2 hours. (From Beare and Myers.[10])

- Teach the patient to perform passive leg exercises until the catheter is removed and he is able to walk. Contraction of the leg muscles before ambulation will encourage venous return.
- Maintain adequate fluid intake (30 ml/kg of body weight per day). Dehydration increases the risk of deep vein thrombosis of the legs.

Risk for urinary retention, related to debris and blood clots from operative site, scarring and contracture at operative site

- Maintain continuous irrigation with three-way catheter for 24 hours after TUR-P. Continuous bladder irrigation removes clots and debris from the bladder, preventing catheter occlusion and retention.
- Select a large drainage bag for the catheter (at least 2000 ml). The drainage bag will fill rapidly during irrigation.
- Empty the catheter drainage bag every 1 to 2 hours or more frequently as indicated. Continuous irrigation causes rapid filling of the catheter drainage bag, and frequent emptying is required to prevent retention.
- Irrigate the catheter gently with saline, or assist the physician to complete irrigation as indicated. Irrigation may be required to remove larger blood clots.
- Monitor urine elimination patterns after removal of the indwelling catheter. Urinary retention may occur after catheter removal, requiring prolonged catheter drainage.
- Advise patient of the importance of postoperative follow-up care. A urethral dilation may be indicated to correct or prevent bladder neck contracture and subsequent obstruction.

Risk for TUR syndrome, related to fluid absorption and electrolyte imbalance following TUR-P

- Monitor patient for signs and symptoms of TUR syndrome (acute confusion, restlessness, bradycardia, tachypnea, vomiting, dilutional hyponatremia) after transurethral surgery. TUR syndrome is an uncommon but potentially fatal complication of TUR-P.
- Maintain adequate fluid intake (30 ml/kg of body weight per day) using oral and parenteral fluid as available. Maintenance of adequate hydration may reduce the risk of TUR syndrome.
- Promptly consult the physician if signs or symptoms of TUR syndrome occur. TUR syndrome is managed with fluid replacement and supportive care; the condition can be fatal without prompt intervention.

Pain, related to prostatic tissue resection, endoscopic instrumentation

- Administer anticholinergic or antispasmodic medications as directed. These medications prevent unstable (hyperactive) bladder contractions or spasms may occur following TUR-P causing intermittent, cramping pain.
- Advise the patient that mild dysuria (discomfort with urination) may occur after catheter removal. Provide adequate fluid intake, a warm Sitz bath, warm shower, or urinary analgesics (as directed) to minimize dysuria.
- Administer systemic analgesics as indicated to reduce generalized pain and discomfort related to prostatectomy.

Altered urinary elimination, related to surgical resection of the prostate

- Advise the patient that transient urinary frequency and urgency is expected after catheter removal. Instruct him to maintain adequate fluid intake (30 ml/kg of body weight per day) and to avoid or limit intake of bladder irritants. Irritative voiding symptoms occur following TUR-P; these symptoms are related to surgical trauma, endoscopic instrumentation, and the indwelling catheter.

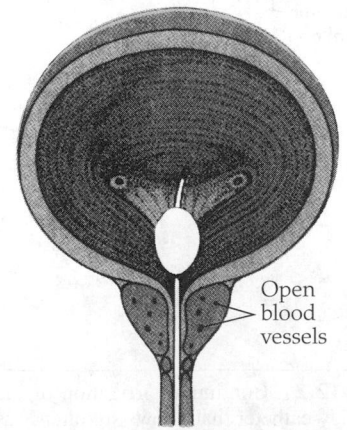 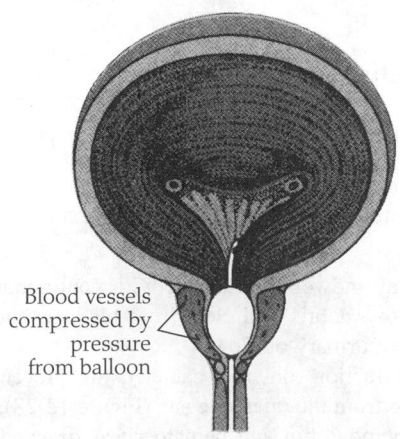

Open blood vessels

Blood vessels compressed by pressure from balloon

Figure 12-28 Gentle traction is maintained against prostatic vascular bed to prevent excessive bleeding after transurethral resection. (From Beare and Myers.[10])

- Teach the patient with stress incontinence following TUR-P to perform pelvic muscle exercises. Pelvic muscle exercises strengthen the periurethral muscles and minimize or ablate stress urinary leakage.
- Advise the patient to consult his urologist or a continence nurse specialist if stress incontinence persists for more than 6 months following TUR-P.
- Advise the patient with persistent urge (instability) incontinence to seek care from his urologist or a continence nurse specialist. Persistent urge incontinence requires aggressive behavioral or pharmacologic therapy if it does not resolve within 1 to 2 weeks after catheter removal.

Patient Education/Home Care Planning

1. Teach the patient the potential complications of TUR-P including urinary retention, urinary incontinence, persistent erectile dysfunction, and altered fertility potential.
2. Inform the patient of the potential for regrowth of BPH with subsequent symptoms (usually 10 years or more after a TUR-P). Emphasize the importance of routine prostate evaluations for recurrence of BPH, and for prostate cancer.

Evaluation

AUA symptom index indicates relief of bothersome symptoms of BPH

Significant bleeding is avoided or promptly managed

TUR syndrome is prevented or promptly managed

Urinary residual volumes and urinary flow variables indicate relief from obstruction

TRANSURETHRAL SURGERY (TRANSURETHRAL RESECTION OF BLADDER TUMORS [TUR-BT], TRANSURETHRAL SPHINCTEROTOMY, TRANSURETHRAL BLADDER NECK INCISION)

Description and Rationale

Transurethral resection of bladder tumors is the removal of superficial, malignant bladder tumors with a resectoscope, under endoscopic control. Postoperative bleeding may be significant when multiple tumors are resected, and the risk of TUR syndrome may be comparable to that for TUR-P. TUR-BT may or may not be combined with intravesical chemotherapy. Transurethral resection is initially preferred when managing a bladder tumor; laser ablation of the tumor may be performed following initial pathologic analysis of resected tissue, and bladder cancer staging.

Transurethral sphincterotomy is the incision of the striated urethral sphincter under endoscopic control. It is reserved for males with detrusor sphincter dyssynergia who agree to manage their bladders by condom catheter containment after the procedure. The incision required for an adequate sphincterotomy is significant, and life-threatening postoperative bleeding may occur. Women are not appropriate candidates for a transurethral sphincterotomy because there is no adequate condom device to contain the urinary leakage that inevitably occurs after transurethral sphincterotomy.

Transurethral incision of the bladder neck is a single incision of the circular smooth muscle at the bladder neck under endoscopic visualization. The incision is relatively small and the postprocedure bleeding is minimal, as is the risk of TUR syndrome.

Preprocedural Nursing Care

1. The role of transurethral resection of bladder tumors as a diagnostic and therapeutic measure is emphasized before initial treatment.
2. Patients are counseled that pathologic analysis will require several days.
3. Patients undergoing transurethral sphincterotomy are counseled that dribbling incontinence (stress urinary incontinence due to iatrogenic intrinsic sphincter deficiency) is expected to occur after the procedure, and a condom catheter will be required to contain urinary leakage.
4. Patients undergoing transurethral sphincterotomy or bladder neck incision are advised of the risk or retrograde ejaculation and altered fertility potential.

•••••• Multidisciplinary Plan

Medications

1. Preoperative and postoperative antibiotic agents as ordered.
2. Anticholinergic or antispasmodics may be required to manage bladder spasms.
3. Analgesic medications as needed.

General Management

1. An indwelling catheter is required following TUR-BT; a three-way irrigation system may be indicated in special cases.
2. A three-way irrigation system is required after transurethral sphincterotomy; typically for 2 to 3 days postoperatively.
3. An indwelling catheter is required after bladder neck incision.

NURSING CARE

Nursing Assessment

Bladder and Urethra

Urinary output, presence of clots and bright red bleeding in urine

Significant bleeding (particularly following transurethral sphincterotomy) with signs of hypovolemic shock (rapid pulse with increased pressure followed by falling blood pressure and bradycardia)

Temperature

Fever

TUR Syndrome (TUR-BT carries greatest risk)

Acute confusion
Restlessness
Bradycardia, tachypnea
Hyponatremia

Nursing Dx & Intervention

Altered peripheral tissue perfusion (bladder or urethral) related to transurethral surgery

- Maintain indwelling catheter as directed; assess urinary output for presence of blood and clots, and assess catheter for patency. Significant bleeding may occur after transurethral surgery causing hypovolemia and catheter obstruction.
- Maintain three-way irrigation as directed (required after transurethral sphincterotomy) with adequate flow rate to maintain pink-tinged urine for at least 24 hours. Do not reduce the irrigation to "keep open rate" for at least 24 hours after transurethral sphincterotomy. Significant bleeding frequently occurs after a transurethral sphincterotomy, and brisk irrigation is required to maintain catheter patency and prevent filling of the bladder with clots.
- Assist the patient to obtain adequate fluid intake, using parenteral or oral routes as indicated. Postoperative bleeding causes fluid loss from the body that must be replaced.
- Evaluate the patient's serum hematocrit and hemoglobin as indicated; promptly inform the physician if these values are significantly abnormal as compared to preoperative values.
- Monitor vital signs (blood pressure, pulse, respiration) for signs of significant blood loss or impending hypovolemic shock.

Risk for urinary retention, related to debris and blood clots from operative site, scarring and contracture at operative site

- Maintain continuous irrigation with three-way catheter or indwelling catheter as directed. Continuous catheter drainage with or without bladder irrigation provides drainage of clots or debris from the bladder, preventing catheter occlusion and retention.
- Empty the catheter drainage bag every 1 to 2 hours or more frequently as indicated when bladder irrigation is required after transurethral surgery. Continuous irrigation causes rapid filling of the catheter drainage bag, and frequent emptying is required to prevent retention.

- Irrigate the catheter gently with saline, or assist the physician to complete irrigation as indicated. Irrigation may be required to remove larger blood clots.
- Monitor urine elimination patterns after removal of the indwelling catheter. Urinary retention may occur after catheter removal, requiring prolonged catheter drainage.

Risk for TUR syndrome, related to fluid absorption and electrolyte imbalance following TUR-P

- Monitor patient for signs and symptoms of TUR syndrome (acute confusion, restlessness, bradycardia, tachypnea, vomiting, dilutional hyponatremia) following transurethral surgery. TUR syndrome is an uncommon but potentially fatal complication of transurethral surgery.
- Maintain adequate fluid intake (30 ml/kg of body weight per day) using oral and parenteral fluid as available. Maintenance of adequate hydration may reduce the risk of TUR syndrome.
- Promptly consult the physician if signs or symptoms of TUR syndrome occur. TUR syndrome is managed with fluid replacement and supportive care; the condition can be fatal without prompt intervention.

URINARY DIVERSION

Description and Rationale

A urinary diversion is any one of a number of surgical procedures that establish an unimpeded flow of urine, usually through a stoma. It is possible to divert the urine at any level in the urinary tract.

Supravesical diversions   Diverting the urine at the level of the kidney is done by nephrostomy or pyelostomy. A nephrostomy is a high urinary diversion involving the placement of a catheter through the renal pelvis and into the renal calyces. Indications for placement of a nephrostomy tube are complete obstruction of the ureter, bypassing a urinary fistula, or irrigation of the renal pelvis. A nephrostomy tube is placed intraoperatively during a pyeloplasty or as an emergency procedure for the relief of kidney or ureteral obstruction.[47] Percutaneous placement of a nephrostomy tube under radiographic or ultrasound control has largely replaced the more traditional method of placement. The Pezzer or mushroom catheter, the Malecot or batwing catheter, or a small-lumen Foley catheter with a 5 cc balloon are used as nephrostomy tubes.[93]

Because of the problems associated with long-term nephrostomy drainage (infection, stone formation, intermittent hematuria, frank renal hemorrhage, or accidental dislodgment of the tube), it is typically used only as a temporary method of diversion.[118]

A pyelostomy is an opening into the renal pelvis made by catheter placement or by the creation of a stoma. Tube pyelostomy diversion carries equal risk as a nephrostomy; therefore tubeless diversion is substituted whenever possible. A cutaneous pyelostomy is performed infrequently, but is designed for children requiring a high urinary diversion. Because children have less subcutaneous fat and a relatively mobile kidney, it is a comparatively simple technical procedure.

Ureterostomy, another type of supravesical urinary diversion, is done with a tube or stoma. A cystoscope may be used to pass a ureter catheter up the ureter into the renal pelvis if the ureter is unobstructed or only partially obstructed. A diversion where the ureter is anastomosed to the skin is called a cutaneous ureterostomy.[90] Ureterostomy is appropriate in a patient with thickened dilated ureters when more aggressive urinary diversion surgery is not feasible. A ureterostomy forms a small, flush, pale pink stoma. It is difficult to manage; urinary reflux and infections are common. One or two stomas may be present.[19]

Ureteroenterocutaneous diversions It is possible to isolate any segment of the healthy intestinal tract caudal to the jejunum for use as a conduit for urine. The isolated intestinal segment serves as a conduit to bridge the gap from ureter to skin when the bladder must be removed or bypassed. Invasive transitional cell carcinoma of the bladder is the most frequent reason for cystectomy in the adult patient.[47]

Urinary diversion using a segment of small intestine is the most common form of permanent urinary diversion (Figure 12-29). The Bricker ileal conduit was first described in 1950; it is used by isolating a 15 to 20 cm segment of the terminal ileum close to the ileocecal valve.[106] The distal end of the isolated segment is brought out through the right lower abdominal quadrant and everted to form a budded stoma. The ureters are excised from the bladder and implanted near the proximal end of the conduit, which is sutured closed. The conduit is

isoperistaltic; urine flows in the same direction as peristaltic waves of the intestine. The ileal conduit is not a storage area; urine passes through quickly without residual.[33]

Jejunum may be used for small bowel permanent diversion if the ileum has been damaged by radiation. Patients with jejunal conduits are prone to a particular electrolyte imbalance called jejunal conduit syndrome, which is characterized by hypochloremic metabolic acidosis with hyperkalemia and hyponatremia.

The principal indications for small bowel urinary diversion are bladder cancer and severe neuropathic bladder dysfunction.[47] Long-term complications of the small bowel diversions are particularly prevalent after the first 5 years. Upper tract deterioration is significant and is associated with the bacteriuria and reflux that characterize the ileal or jejunal conduit.

A segment of large bowel may be isolated to form a urinary conduit. The primary advantage of using a segment of large intestine rather than small is the ability to create a nonrefluxing ureterointestinal anastomosis by tunneling the ureters into the submucosa of the colon. Nonetheless, the large bowel conduit leaves the patient with a stoma and continuous urinary incontinence. In addition, because obstruction at the ureteroenteric anastomosis is a serious complication, the large bowel conduit is used only in select cases.[47]

The ideal urinary diversion has not been developed. It would be an antirefluxing, continent diversion without the electrolyte disturbances that result from urine in prolonged contact with intestinal mucosa. This ideal diversion would have a reservoir with a functional capacity requiring catheterization only two or three times daily.

Continent urinary diversion A continent urinary diversion provides the patient with an internal reservoir for urine and eliminates the need for an external appliance. There is an abdominal stoma and the patient performs clean intermittent catheterization through the stoma to empty the internal reservoir of urine.

A reservoir for urine constructed from the small intestine was first devised in the 1960s. The urinary Kock pouch involves isolating a 60 to 70 cm segment of the ileum (Figure 12-30). The mesentery and its blood supply to this isolated

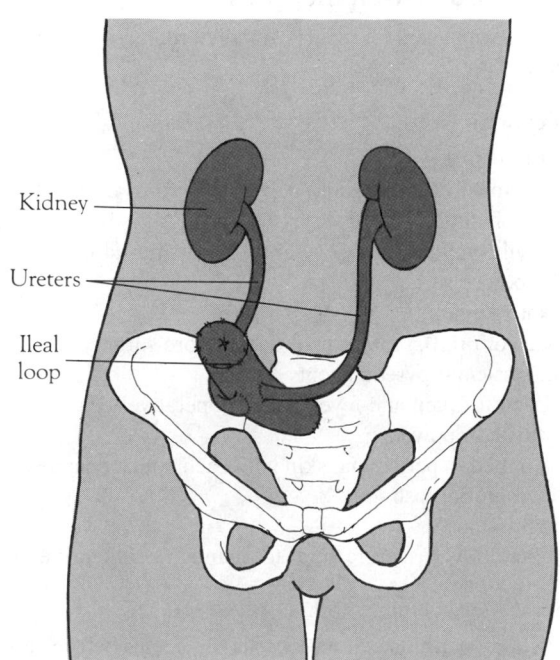

Figure 12-29 Urinary diversion (ileal conduit). (From Gray.[49])

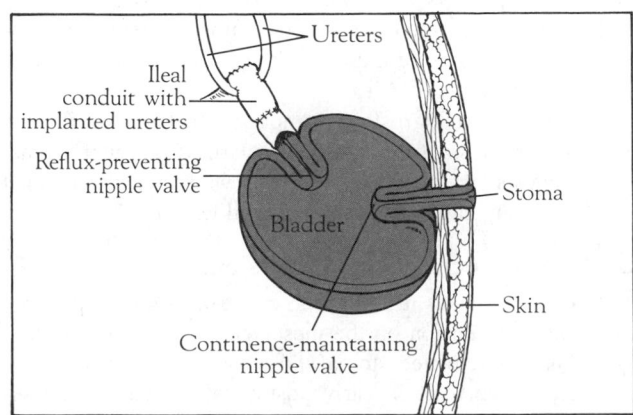

Figure 12-30 Kock pouch. (From Belcher.[11])

segment of ileum is left intact. The middle 40 cm of this segment is split open and folded back on itself to form a reservoir to hold urine. The entrance and exit to this reservoir have a nipple valve constructed by intussusception or telescoping back of the intestine on itself. The ureters are implanted into the proximal nipple valve in an attempt to prevent urine from refluxing up to the kidneys. The distal nipple valve ends in a right-sided abdominal stoma and makes the stoma continent of urine. The reservoir expands in volume with time, and the patient ultimately catheterizes the stoma four or five times a day using a no. 18 to 26 French catheter. The patient wears an absorptive pad or Band-Aid over the stoma to collect the mucus it secretes. In addition, reservoir irrigations are performed at least once daily using a 50 to 60 ml catheter tip or bulb syringe to remove the mucus that has accumulated in the reservoir.[20,38,44]

The ileocecal reservoir is another continent urinary diversion that was developed in the late 1970s. The distal 20 cm of ileum, a segment of the cecum, and part of the ascending colon are isolated, and continuity of the gastrointestinal tract is restored. The ureters are anastomosed into the ascending colon with an antirefluxing tunneling method similar to the one used in the construction of a sigmoid conduit. The ileum forms the outflow tract with a nipple valve for continence and a right lower quadrant abdominal stoma. The cecum and ascending colon form the reservoir for urine. The patient catheterizes the stoma and irrigates the reservoir as with the Kock reservoir.[81]

Continent urinary diversions are an attempt to provide the patient with a more acceptable form of urinary diversion and to make the adjustment to the presence of a stoma easier. Careful patient selection is important. Long-term consequences have yet to be studied.

Contraindications and Cautions
Supravesical Diversions

1. Nephrostomy or pyelostomy tube drainage is discouraged in patients with bilateral ureteral obstruction as a result of a malignant disease, because these patients are highly susceptible to serious complications.[47]
2. Cutaneous pyelostomy diversion can be done only in pediatric patients with a large extrarenal pelvis.
3. Adequate methods of securing tube diversions are important to prevent kidney damage or accidental tube dislodgment.
4. Cutaneous ureterostomy is not done if the ureters are of a normal size or poorly vascularized, because stomal stenosis may result. A large adult with a thick abdominal wall may have inadequate ureteral length.[93]

Ureteroenterocutaneous Diversions

1. Obesity makes it difficult to construct a good stoma because of tension on the mesentery, which can lead to a flush or retracted stoma and the development of either stomal necrosis in early postoperative phase or subsequent stomal stenosis.
2. A sigmoid conduit is avoided in patients with severe diverticulosis or inflammatory bowel disease.[118]

3. A sigmoid conduit is not advised for the patient needing radical cystectomy and irradiation for bladder cancer, since the altered blood supply to the rectum and the sigmoid colon may negatively affect healing.[47]

Continent Urinary Diversions

1. The noncompliant patient with a tendency toward psychologic or social problems or the patient with already compromised renal function should not have a continent urinary diversion.
2. The need for postoperative radiation therapy may be related to a higher rate of failure.
3. The patient must be highly motivated to avoid wearing an external appliance.
4. Nipple valve failures can render the diversion incontinent of urine and necessitate a second surgical procedure to revise the intussusception.
5. Electrolyte disorders may result from urine in prolonged contact with intestinal mucosal lining.
6. Risk of malignancy from urine in prolonged contact with intestinal mucosa has not been fully evaluated.

Preprocedural Nursing Care

1. Intensive bowel preparation is started 2 to 3 days before surgery.
2. Preoperative stoma site selection is done by an enterostomal therapy (ET) nurse.
3. Preoperative teaching and consultation with an ET nurse is important.
4. The patient talks to an ostomy visitor if appropriate.

•••••• Multidisciplinary Plan

The following medical plan is for ureteroenterocutaneous diversions.

Medications

Antiinfective agents
   Neomycin (Mycifradin), 1 g po q4h for 4 doses; then 1 g q6h until NPO for surgery (begins 3 days before surgery)
   Erythromycin base (Erythrocin), 1 g po q4h for 3 doses before surgery
Laxative agents
   Castor oil, 0.5 ml/kg po 3 days before surgery
Analgesic/antipyretic agents
   Used for pain and fever prn postoperatively
Mycostatin powder
   Applied to peristomal skin with each pouch change prn for monilial rash
Vitamin
   Vitamin C (ascorbic acid) to maintain acidic urine pH

General Management

Bowel preparation: saline enemas for 2 days before surgery; neomycin retention enemas (200 ml of a 1% solution) the night before and day of surgery if sigmoid conduit is to be performed

Low-residue diet 2 days before surgery
Clear liquid diet 1 day before surgery
Intravenous fluids during bowel preparation and postoperatively until patient can tolerate food

NURSING CARE

Nursing Assessment

Incision

Redness, pain, edema, drainage

Hemorrhage

Incisional drains, sumps
Urethral catheter (promotes drainage of operative site)

Urinary Output

Amount and color
Mucus normal in ileal/sigmoid conduit

Sexual Dysfunction (Male)

Erectile dysfunction
Ejaculatory incompetence—if prostate removed

Stoma

Viability
Mucocutaneous border
Edema

Peristomal Skin

Intact
Erythematous
Signs of monilial infection
Maceration

Intestine

Paralytic ileus, intestinal obstruction, abdominal distention, constipation
Nasogastric suctioning prolonged owing to intestinal anastomosis

Nursing Dx & Intervention

Altered urinary elimination related to diversion of urinary tract

- Assess stoma color and suture line, *to recognize any change in viability or mucocutaneous separation.*
- Provide an appropriate pouching system with an antireflux valve and a spout. Connect to bedside drainage and check frequently to prevent tubing from kinking *to prevent urine pooling on skin or refluxing from pouch to stoma.*
- Monitor amount and color of urine. If no urine is present, check all drainage sites (sumps, urethral catheter, Penrose drain) for urine *to determine if there has been an ileal-ureteral leakage or decreased renal function.*

- Arrange for enterostomal therapy (ET) nurse to assess stoma and drainage system and *to provide appropriate pouching system.*
- Obtain all urine specimens for urinalysis or culture and sensitivity by catheterizing the ileal stoma (exception: monitoring urine pH).

Altered peripheral tissue perfusion related to immobility

- Assess blood pressure every 4 hours for 5 to 6 days or until removal of nasogastric suctioning and intravenous fluids.
- Apply antiembolic stockings. Remove and reapply daily *to prevent venous stasis and thrombophlebitis.*
- Auscultate abdomen for bowel sounds; note any signs of abdominal distention.
- Assess stoma for color (i.e., blood supply). Ileal conduit stoma should be bright red and moist; ureterostomy stoma is pale or dark pink.
- Assist patient with progressive ambulation.
- Encourage patient to turn every 2 hours and to perform leg exercises.
- Observe all drains, sumps, and catheters for amount, color, and consistency of drainage.
- Monitor intake and output; weigh daily.

Risk for infection related to presence of incision

- Provide antibiotics as ordered.
- Observe incision for signs of infection: redness, edema, pain, and drainage. Assess patient's skin (under the arms and breasts, groin, perineum) *for monilial infections associated with prolonged antibiotics, intense bowel preparation, and moisture.*

Risk for hemorrhage related to surgery or surgical resection

- Observe incisional dressing *for color and amount of drainage.*
- Monitor color, consistency, and amount of drainage from nasogastric tube, sumps, urethral catheter, and stoma output *to prevent hypovolemic shock.*
- Monitor vital signs for shock.

Ineffective breathing pattern related to effects of general anesthesia

- Assist patient in turning, coughing, and deep breathing *to counteract effects of general anesthesia.*
- Auscultate chest for breath sounds four times each day.
- Provide analgesics and splinting of abdomen when encouraging patient to deep breathe and cough.

Constipation related to ileus or segmental resection and anastomosis in GI tract

- Monitor patient for first bowel movement.
- Auscultate abdomen for bowel sounds each shift.

- Observe for signs of paralytic ileus or intestinal obstruction.
- Monitor patient for signs and symptoms of peritonitis, which would indicate a leakage or failure of the intestinal reanastomosis: fever, abdominal pain, rebound tenderness, drop in blood pressure, or shallow respirations.

Pain related to surgical trauma

- Provide analgesics as ordered.
- Assist patient in finding comfortable positions.

Body image and personal identity disturbances related to presence of stoma and pouch

- Provide an opportunity for patient and partner to discuss the implications of the surgery, stoma, and external pouch.
- Explore the patient's and partner's feelings regarding the presence of the stoma and pouch.
- Discuss the presence of the pouch and the inability of detecting it under clothing and how to manage embarrassing leakages and odor.

Risk for impaired skin integrity related to creation of urinary stoma

- Change the pouch whenever it appears to be leaking under the faceplate or when there is an overt leakage.
- See pouch change procedure, p. 1067.

Impaired skin integrity related to effects of urine on peristomal skin

- Assess skin integrity frequently because *rash can occur under the tape or faceplate and on any part of the skin where the pouch lies. Causes of skin rashes may be a leaking appliance, perspiration, allergies to tape, or hair follicle irritation.*
- Use lamp with a 60-watt bulb 1 foot away from skin or hair dryer set on cool *to dry the skin.*
- Powder the skin on which the pouch lies. *Avoid cornstarch powders, which encourage the growth of monilia.*
- Advise patient to make or buy a pouch cover.
- Ulcerated area on stoma may occur if stomal opening of the pouch is too small or activities are causing the faceplate to rub or cut into stoma.
- Evaluate patient's activities: a different faceplate size or shape may be needed.
- Waterlogged skin between opening of the faceplate and the stoma can occur if too much skin is exposed between the stoma and the faceplate and the urine pools on unprotected skin.
- Decrease the size of stomal opening in faceplate; use skin sealant *to waterproof skin.*
- Urinary yeast infection on skin surrounding the stoma may extend beyond the faceplate.
- Apply nystatin (Mycostatin) powder to the area, blow off the excess powder, and seal this in with a thin coat of a skin sealant. Apply pouch in the usual manner.

- Advise patient to drink sufficient fluids and add buttermilk or yogurt to the diet *to help restore normal gut flora.*
- Urine crystals may form on the stoma or around the stoma base if the patient has alkaline urine and a predisposition for stone formation.
- Swab vinegar on the stoma when changing the pouch *to help dissolve crystals.*
- Insert vinegar into the pouch while patient is wearing it. For a minor formation, insert twice a day; for an excessive formation, insert four times a day.
- Remove antireflux valves *to allow the vinegar to come into contact with the stoma.*
- Monitor urine pH and provide instructions for maintaining an acid urine, including increased fluid intake and ascorbic acid (vitamin C).

Altered sexuality related to cystectomy and altered body image

- Assess patient and partner's readiness to discuss sexual matters.
- Discuss the sexual implications of the presence of the stoma, such as feelings of attractiveness, desirability, and worth.
- Explain separate nerve pathways for sexual excitement, erection, ejaculation, and orgasm *to point out the effect of cystectomy on erections only.*
- Mention sexual counseling, alternative methods of sexual expressions, and penile prosthesis or external devices to aid in achieving erections *to assist patient in resuming sexual activity that is fullfilling for him.*

Patient Education/Home Care Planning

1. Demonstrate to the patient how to empty the pouch when it is one-third to one-half full.
2. Show the patient the use of the bedside drainage bag at night.
3. Demonstrate to the patient pouch change procedure (see box below). This includes treatment of minor peristomal skin irritations and monitoring urine pH.
4. Explain fluid intake requirements—10 to 12 glasses a day to acidify urine.
5. Review dietary considerations in terms of urine odor; fish, eggs, asparagus, and spicy foods can cause a temporary increase in urine odor.
6. Define routine follow-up care for the patient with a urinary diversion, including correct method of obtaining urine for culture (see box on p. 1067).
7. Provide the patient with ostomy supply and supplier information and availability of community support groups, such as the United Ostomy Association.[33]

Evaluation

Tissue perfusion is normal   Stoma is red, healthy, moist, and viable. Blood pressure and pulse are within normal limits.

PROCEDURE FOR URINARY POUCH CHANGE

1. Assemble all supplies.
   a. To clean the skin, paper towels, washcloths, or towels may be used. Several of these should be rolled into "wicks" that can be placed on top of the stoma to absorb urine while keeping the peristomal skin unencumbered. Tampons can also be used as wicks. Premoistened towelettes should not be used.
   b. Pouch—a urinary pouch with a precut opening for stoma should be sized large enough to bypass any creases or dimples in the skin around the stoma. A pouch that needs to be cut out before application should be cut to avoid any creases or dimples in the immediate peristomal area. Check for creases or dimples while the patient is sitting and when he is lying down. The outer diameter of the pouch's adhesive faceplate may be trimmed to avoid umbilicus, rib cage, incisions, hip bones, pubic areas, or folds at the waist.
   c. Karaya powder
   d. Skin sealant—protects the skin from the macerating effects of urine and the stripping effects of tape or adhesive. Most skin sealants are a liquid copolymer with alcohol as the vehicle for spreading it. Skin sealants come in spray form, dab-on applicators, or wipes.
   e. Tape—such as Micropore or paper tape. Some patients prefer waterproof tape.
   f. Plastic bag for disposal of used pouches
2. Take off old pouch by unsticking the skin from the pouch's adhesive faceplate. Dispose of used pouch.
3. Wash the stoma and peristomal skin free of mucus and urine with warm water only and let dry.
   a. Soap may leave a residue on the skin and prevent the next pouch from adhering.
   b. Traces of cement or adhesives may be on the skin. Rough cleansing to remove these may do damage to the peristomal skin.
4. Examine the peristomal skin for any signs of redness or irritation. Apply a light dusting of karaya powder to irritated skin.
   a. If the peristomal skin needs to be shaved, use a dry razor over powdered skin. Brush away excess karaya powder.
   b. If irritation is severe, a skin barrier in wafer form may be added to the pouch's adhesive faceplate. Urine will melt the skin barrier and decrease the pouch's seal, but a pouch's adhesive faceplate should not be applied directly over severely irritated skin.
5. Apply a skin sealant to peristomal skin. Keep the stoma "wicked" to absorb urine.
   a. In the presence of skin irritation, a skin sealant will cause a momentary stinging sensation.
   b. If karaya powder was applied to irritated skin, the skin sealant will seal in the karaya powder and, once dry, will provide a skin surface to which the pouch can adhere.
6. Center pouch over stoma and apply to dry skin.
   a. Try to avoid creating any wrinkles or creases in pouch's adhesive faceplate that will encourage urine leakage.
   b. The pouch may be angled straight down or medially for an ambulatory patient to facilitate emptying.
7. Close the pouch's spout.
8. Use the tape to picture-frame the pouch's adhesive faceplate and increase the pouch's wearing time.
9. Check the pH of the urine from the first drops of urine in the freshly changed pouch.
   a. Do not touch the pH paper to the stoma or the skin, since this will give an inaccurate reading.
   b. An acidic urine pH should be maintained, since alkaline urine is more likely to have a foul odor, create crystals on or around the stoma, predispose the patient to kidney stone formation, and provide a medium for infection. An adequate fluid intake or ascorbic acid (vitamin C, 500 mg) four times a day will acidify urine. Acidic urine has a pH of 6.0 or less.

PROCEDURE FOR OBTAINING A URINE CULTURE FROM ILEAL-SIGMOID CONDUIT (SINGLE-LUMEN CATHETERIZATION)

1. Explain procedure to patient.
   a. Catheterizing the stoma is painless because ureteroenterocutaneous stomas have no sensory nerve endings.
   b. Patient should be aware that no urine for culture should be obtained from the pouch itself. This specimen needs to be obtained sterilely.
2. Assemble supplies for reapplying the pouch once the specimen is obtained.
3. Set up equipment for obtaining a urine specimen on a sterile field:
   a. Catheter (may be a no. 12 or 14 French straight catheter)
   b. Betadine swabs (three)
   c. Sterile, water-soluble lubricant
   d. Sterile urine cup
   e. Dry, sterile gauze
   f. Sterile gloves
4. Take off the old pouch.
5. Drape patient with Chux to keep him or her dry.
6. Wipe stoma free of mucus with gauze.
7. Put on sterile gloves.
8. Swab the stoma three times with the Betadine swabs.
9. Let urine run over the stoma to wash away Betadine *or* wipe stoma free of Betadine with dry, sterile gauze. Introducing Betadine into the specimen will kill the bacteria for which the culture is checking.
10. Lubricate the tip of the catheter with water-soluble lubricant.
11. Gently insert the catheter into the stoma about 1½ to 2 inches. Do not force or poke. It is desirable to pass catheter beneath fascia level if possible.
12. Wait until about 5 ml of urine passes through the catheter into the sterile urine cup. To facilitate obtaining specimen, instruct the patient to sit up or turn on one side.
13. Remove the catheter.
14. Reapply the pouch.

There is no infection or hemorrhage   Temperature is within normal range. There are no signs or symptoms of infection or bleeding. Incision is healed.

Breathing pattern remains normal   Patient's respiratory status is managed appropriately. Breath sounds remain clear.

Bowel elimination is normal   The patient experiences a return to presurgical bowel habits.

Body image is not disturbed   The patient adapts to the presence of the stoma and external pouch. The patient recognizes that adaptation is a continuous process.

Skin integrity is maintained   Peristomal skin is intact. There are no signs of irritation. Pouch seal is appropriate (3 to 5 days). Women return to presurgical sexual pattern. Men experiencing sexual dysfunction receive counseling regarding erectile dysfunction.

The patient resumes activities of daily living   The patient returns to presurgical activities including work and recreational interests. The patient does not change his style of dress.

References

1. Aboseif S, Lue TF: Hemodynamics of penile erection, *Urol Clin North Am* 15:1-18, 1988.
1a. Abrams P: Detrusor instability and bladder outlet obstruction. *Neurourol Urodyn* 4:317, 1985.
2. Agency for Health Care Policy and Research Benign Prostatic Hyperplasia Guideline Panel: *Benign prostatic hyperplasia: diagnosis and treatment*, Rockville Md, 1994, US Department of Health and Human Services.
3. Agency for Health Care Policy and Research Urinary Incontinence in Adults Guideline Panel: *Urinary incontinence in adults*, Rockville Md, 1992, US Department of Health and Human Services.
4. Allen TD: The non-neurogenic neurogenic bladder, *J Urol* 116:638, 1977.
5. Anderson RS: A neurogenic element to genuine urinary stress incontinence, *Br J Obstet Gynaecol* 91:41, 1984.
6. Andrew J, Nathan PW, Spanos NC: Cerebral cortical control of micturition, *Proc R Soc Med* 58:533, 1968.
7. Andriana RT, Carson CC: Urolithiasis, *Clin Symp* 38:3, 1986.
8. Armenian HK et al: Relationship between benign prostatic hyperplasia and cancer of the prostate: a prospective and retrospective study, *Lancet* 2:115, 1974.
9. Barrington FJF: The nervous mechanisms of micturition of the cat, *Q J Exp Physiol* 54:177, 1931.
10. Beare PG, Myers JL: *Principles and practice of adult health nursing*, St Louis, 1990, Mosby.
11. Belcher A: *Cancer nursing*, St Louis, 1992, Mosby.
12. Bergman H, editor: *The ureter*, New York, 1981, Springer-Verlag.
13. Blaivas JG: The neurophysiology of micturition: a study of 550 patients, *J Urol* 127:958, 1982.
14. Bihrle R et al: High intensity focused ultrasound for the treatment of benign prostatic hyperplasia: early United States clinical experience, *J Urol* 151:1271, 1994.
15. Boone TB, Gilling PJ, Husmann DA: Ureteropelvic junction disruption following blunt abdominal trauma, *J Urol* 150:33-36, 1993.
16. Borda E et al: Relationship between prostaglandins and estrogens on the motility of isolated rings from the rat urinary bladder, *J Urol* 129:1250, 1983.
17. Bors E, Comarr AE: *Neurological urology*, Baltimore, 1971, Williams & Wilkins.
18. Bradley WE, Timm GW, Scott FB: Innervation of detrusor muscle and urethra, *Urol Clin North Am* 1:3, 1974.
19. Broadwell DC, Jackson BS, editors: *Principles of ostomy care*, St Louis, 1982, Mosby.
20. Brogna L, Lakaszawaski M: Nursing management: in the continent urostomy, *J Enterostom Ther* 13:139, 1986.
21. Brundage E: *Renal disorders*, St Louis, 1992, Mosby.
22. Childs SJ: Dimethyl sulfone (DMSO) in the treatment of interstitial cystitis, *Urol Clin North Am* 21:85, 1994.
23. Chisholm GD, Williams ID, editors: *Scientific foundations of urology*, St Louis, 1982, Mosby.
24. Crockett AT, Urry DL, editors: *Male infertility: workup, treatment and research*, New York, 1977, Grune & Stratton.
25. Crouch JE: *Functional human anatomy*, ed 4, Philadelphia, 1985, Lea & Febiger.
26. Cucci A: Detrusor instability in prostatic obstruction in relation to urethral opening pressure, *Neurol Urodyn* 9:17, 1990.
27. Daniel EE, Cowan W, Daniel VP: Structural basis for neural and myogenic control of human detrusor muscle, *Physiol Pharmacol* 61:1247, 1983.
28. DeGroat WE: *CNS modulation of detrusor storage*, New York, 1986, Presented at Eighth Annual Urodynamic Society Meeting.
29. de la Rosette JJMHC, Froeling FMJA, Debruyne FMJ: Clinical results with microwave thermotherapy of benign prostatic hyperplasia, *Eur Urol* 23:68, 1993.
30. de la Rosette JJMHC et al: Transurethral microwave thermotherapy (TUMT) in benign prostatic hyperplasia: placebo versus TUMT, *Urology* 44:58, 1994.
31. de Tejada S et al: Impaired neurogenic and endothelium mediated relaxation of penile smooth muscle from diabetic men with impotence, *N Engl J Med* 320:1025, 1989.
32. Dixon CM: Transurethral needle ablation of benign prostatic hyperplasia, *Urol Clin North Am* 22:441, 1995.
33. Dobkin KA: Nursing care of a patient with ileal conduit, *J Urol Nurs* 4:340, 1985.
34. Doughty D, editor: *Urinary and fecal incontinence: nursing management*, St Louis, 1991, Mosby.
35. Drach GW: Prostatitis: man's hidden infection, *Urol Clin North Am* 2:499, 1975.
36. Finlayson B: Renal lithiasis in review, *Urol Clin North Am* 1:181, 1974.
37. Finlayson B, Hench LL, Smith LH, editors: *Urolithiasis: physical aspects*, Washington, DC, 1972, National Academy of Science.
38. Fowler JE: Continent urinary reservoirs and bladder substitutes in the adult. II. *Monogr Urology* 1987.
39. Furlow WL: Use of the inflatable penile prosthesis in erectile dysfunction, *Urol Clin North Am* 8:181, 1981.
40. Gallaway NTM, Irwin PP: Interstitial cystitis: surgical management of interstitial cystitis, *Urol Clin North* 21:145, 1994.
41. Ganabathi K et al: Prospective urodynamic evaluation of the efficacy of prostatic balloon dilatation, *Neurourol Urodyn* 11:483, 1992.
42. Garraway M, Collins G, Lee R: High prevalence of benign prostatic hyperplasia in the community, *Lancet* 38:469, 1991.
43. Gaymans R et al: A prospective study of urinary tract infections in a Dutch general practice, *Lancet* 2:674, 1976.
44. Gerber A: The Kock continent ileal reservoir: an alternative to the conventional urostomy, *J Enterostom Ther* 12:15, 1985.
45. Gillenwater JY et al: Doxazosin for the treatment of benign prostatic hyperplasia in patients with mild to moderate essential hypertension: a double blind, placebo controlled, dose-response multicenter study, *J Urol* 154:110, 1995.
46. Gillenwater JY, Wein AJ: Summary of the national institute of arthritis, diabetes, digestive and kidney diseases workshop on interstitial cystitis, *J Urol* 140:203, 1987.
47. Glenn JF: *Urologic surgery*, New York, 1991, JB Lippincott.
48. Gosling JA: The structure of the bladder and urethra in relation to function, *Urol Clin North Am* 6:31, 1979.
49. Gray ML: Genitourinary disorders, St Louis, 1992, Mosby.
50. Gray ML, Dougherty MC: Urinary incontinence: pathophysiology and treatment, *J Enterostom Ther* 14(4):152, 1987.
50a. Grayhack JT, Kozlowski JM: Benign prostatic hyperplasia. In Gillenwater JY, et al, editors: *Adult and pediatric urology*, ed 3, St Louis, 1996, Mosby.
51. Guyton AC: *Medical physiology*, Philadelphia, 1978, WB Saunders.
52. Hald T, Bradley WE: *The urinary bladder: neurology and dynamics*, Baltimore, 1982, Williams & Wilkins.
53. Hanno PM: Diagnosis of interstitial cystitis, *Urol Clin North Am* 21:63, 1994.

54. Hinman JF, editor: *Benign prostatic hypertrophy,* New York, 1983, Springer-Verlag.

55. Hodgkinson CP, Ayers MA, Drukker BH: Dyssynergic detrusor dysfunction in apparently normal females, *Am J Obstet Gynecol* 87(6):717, 1963.

56. Holtgrewe HL et al: Transurethral prostatectomy: practice aspects of the dominant operation in urology, *J Urol* 141:248, 1989.

57. Hurst JW, editor: *Medicine for the practicing physician,* ed 2, Boston, 1988, Butterworth.

58. Hutch JA, Rambo ON: A study of the anatomy of the prostate, prostatic urethra, and the urinary sphincter system, *J Urol* 104:443, 1970.

59. Ireton RC, Berger RE: Prostatitis and epididymitis, *Urol Clin North Am* 11:83, 1984.

60. Jenkins AD, Turner TT, Howards SS: Physiology of the male reproductive system, *Urol Clin North Am* 5:437, 1978.

61. Jensen H, Nielsen K, Fromodt-Moller C: Interstitial cystitis: review of the literature, *Urol Int* 44:189, 1989.

61a. Kass I, Updegraff K, Muffly RB: Sex in chronic obstructive pulmonary disease, *Med Aspects Hum Sex* 6:33, 1972.

62. Kay D: Host defense mechanisms in the urinary tract, *Urol Clin North Am* 2:407, 1975.

63. Kedia KR: Vascular disorders and male erectile dysfunction, *Urol Clin North Am* 8:153, 1981.

64. Klarskov P et al: Prostaglandin type E activity dominates in urinary tract smooth muscle in vitro, *J Urol* 129:1071, 1983.

65. Koizol JA: Epidemiology of interstitial cystitis, *Urol Clin North Am* 21:7, 1994.

66. Krane RJ, Siroky MB: *Clinical neurology,* Boston, 1979, Little, Brown.

67. Krane RJ, Siroky MB, Goldstein I, editors: *Male sexual dysfunction,* Boston, 1983, Little, Brown.

68. Laduc R, Bloem FAG, Debruyne FMJ: Transurethral microwave thermotherapy in symptomatic benign prostatic hyperplasia, *Eur Urol* 23:274, 1993.

69. Leach GE: Urodynamic manifestations of cerebellar ataxia, *J Urol,* 128:348, 1982.

70. Leeson CR, Leeson TS: *Histology,* ed 4, Philadelphia, 1981, WB Saunders.

71. Lepor H: Alpha blockade for the treatment of benign prostatic hyperplasia, *Urol Clin North Am* 22:375, 1995.

72. Lepor H, Shapiro E: Characterization of the alpha$_1$ adrenergic receptor in human benign prostatic hyperplasia, *J Urol* 132:1226, 1984.

73. Lerner J, Khan Z: *Manual of urologic nursing,* St Louis, 1982, Mosby.

74. Lewin RJ, Dillard GV, Porter RW: Extrapyramidal inhibition of the urinary bladder, *Brain Res* 4:301, 1967.

75. Libertino JA, editor: *International perspectives in urology,* vol 5, Baltimore, 1982, Williams & Wilkins.

76. Lipschultz LI, Howards SS, editors: *Infertility in the male,* ed 2, St Louis, 1991, Mosby.

77. Madersbacher S et al: Tissue ablation in prostatic hyperplasia with high-intensity focused ultrasound, *Eur Urol* 23:39, 1993.

78. Madersbacher S, Kratzik C, Susani M, Merberger M: Tissue ablation in benign prostatic hyperplasia with high intensity focused ultrasound, *J Urol* 152:1956, 1994.

79. Malloy TR et al: Bladder outlet obstruction treated with transurethral ultrasonic aspiration, *Urology* 37:512, 1991.

80. Mann R, Lutwak-Mann C: *Male reproductive function and semen,* Berlin, 1981, Springer-Verlag.

81. Mansson W: The continent caecal reservoir for urine, *Scand J Urol Nephrol* Suppl:8, 1985.

82. Maskell R: Are fastidious organisms an important cause of dysuria and frequency? The case for. In Asscher AW, Brumfitt W, editors: *Microbial diseases in nephrology,* London, 1986, John Wiley & Sons.

83. McConnell JD: Hormonal treatment, *Urol Clin North Am* 22:387, 1995.

84. McNeal J: Pathology of benign prostatic hyperplasia, *Urol Clin North Am* 17:477, 1990.

85. Messing E, Stamey TA: Interstitial cystitis: early diagnosis, pathology and treatment, *Urology* 12(4):381, 1978.

86. Narayan P, Lange P: Semirigid penile prosthesis in the management of erectile impotence, *Urol Clin North Am* 8:169, 1981.

87. National Academy of Sciences, Food and Nutrition Board: Recommended daily allowances, ed 9, Washington, DC, 1980, The Academy.

88. National Institutes of Health: (NIH) Consensus Statement Development Panel, *Impotence* 10:1, 1992.

89. Nistal M, Paniagua R: *Testicular epididymal pathology,* New York, 1984, Thieme Medical Publishers.

90. Noorgard JP, Pedersen EB, Djurhuus JC: Diurnal antidiuretic hormone levels in enuretics, *J Urol* 134:1029, 1985.

91. Pak CYP et al: Dietary management of idiopathic calcium urolithiasis, *J Urol* 131:850, 1984.

92. Parsons CL: The therapeutic role of polysaccharides in the urinary bladder, *Urol Clin North Am* 21:93, 1994.

93. Phipps WJ, Long BC, Woods NF, editors: *Medical-surgical nursing: concepts and clinical practice,* ed 4, St Louis, 1991, Mosby–Year Book.

94. Platt R et al: Mortality associated with nosocomial urinary-tract infection, *N Engl J Med* 307:637, 1982.

95. Ratliff TL, Klutke CG, McDougall EM: The etiology of interstitial cystitis, *Urol Clin North Am* 21:21, 1994.

96. Raz S, editor, *Female urology,* Philadelphia, 1983, WB Saunders.

97. Resnick MI, Older RA, editors: *Diagnosis of genitourinary disease,* New York, 1982, Thieme Medical Publishers.

98. Riley TW et al: Use of radioisotopic scan in evaluation of intrascrotal lesions, *J Urol* 116:472, 1976.

99. Rose BD: *Pathophysiology of renal disease,* ed 2, New York, 1987, McGraw-Hill.

100. Rud T et al: Factors maintaining urethral pressure in women, *Invest Urol* 17:343, 1980.

101. Sant GR, LaRock DR: Standard intravesical therapies for interstitial cystitis, *Urol Clin North Am* 21:73, 1994.

102. Sarma KP: *Tumors of the urinary bladder,* London, 1969, Butterworths.

103. Shulman CC, Vanden Bossche M: Hypothermia and thermotherapy of benign prostatic hyperplasia: a critical review, *Eur Urol* 23:53, 1993.

104. Shulman CC et al: Transurethral needle ablation (TUNA): safety, feasibility, and tolerance of a new office procedure for treatment of benign prostatic hyperplasia, *Eur Urol* 24:415, 1993.

105. Skidmore-Roth L: *Mosby's 1996 nursing drug reference,* St Louis, 1996, Mosby.

106. Slade DKA: Interstitial cystitis: a challenge to urology, *Urol Nurs* 9:5, 1989.

107. Smith AD: Causes and classifications of impotence, *Urol Clin North Am* 8:79, 1981.

108. Smith DR: *General urology,* ed 11, Los Altos, Calif, 1984, Lange Medical.

109. Smith PH, Prout GR, editors: *Bladder cancer,* London, 1984, Butterworth Publishers.

110. Snooks SJ et al: Perineal nerve damage in genuine stress incontinence, *Br J Urol* 57:522, 1985.

111. Stamey TA: *Pathogenesis and treatment of urinary tract infections,* Baltimore, 1980, Williams & Wilkins.

112. Staskin DR et al: Pathophysiology of stress incontinence, *Clin Obstet Gynaecol* 12:357, 1985.

113. Steers WD: Neural control of penile erection, *Semin Urol* 8:66, 1990.

114. Steers WD: Physiology of the vas deferens, *World J Urol* 12:281, 1994.

115. Steers WD, Zorn B: Benign prostatic hyperplasia, *Dis-Mon* 41:437, 1995.

116. Stuart PG et al: Hypothalamic unit activity: visceral and somatic influences, *Clin Neurophysiol* 16:237, 1964.

116a. Symmonds RE: Incontinence: vesicle and urethral fistulae, *Clin Obstet Gynecol* 27:499, 1984.

117. Tejada IS, Goldstein I, Krane RJ: Local control penile erection: nerves, smooth muscle and endothelium, *Urolog Clin North Am* 15:9-16, 1988.

118. Walsh PC, Retik AB, Stamey TA, Vaughan ED: Campbell's Urology, ed 6, Philadelphia, 1992, WB Saunders.

119. Walsh PC et al: Tissue content of dihydrotestosterone in human prostatic hyperplasia is not abnormal, *J Clin Invest* 72:1772, 1983.

120. Webster DC, Brennan T: Self-care strategies used for acute attack of interstitial cystitis, *Urol Nurs* 15:86, 1995.

121. Weidman CL, Northcutt RC: Endocrine aspects of impotence, *Urol Clin North Am* 8:143, 1981.

122. Wein AJ, Hanno PM, Gillenwater JY: Intersitial cystitis: an introduction to the problem. In Hanno PM, Staskin DR, Krane RJ, Wein AJ, editors: *Interstitial cystitis,* New York, 1990, Springer-Verlag.

123. Wheatley JK: Causes and treatment of bladder incontinence, *Compr Ther* 9:27, 1983.

124. Williams P, Warwick R: *Gray's anatomy,* ed 37, New York, 1989, Churchill Livingstone.

125. Wilson JD: The pathogenesis of benign prostatic hypertrophy, *Am J Med* 68:745, 1980.

126. Zinner NR, Sterling AM, Ritter RC: Role of inner urethral softness in urinary continence, *Urology* 16:115, 1980.

Infectious Diseases

13

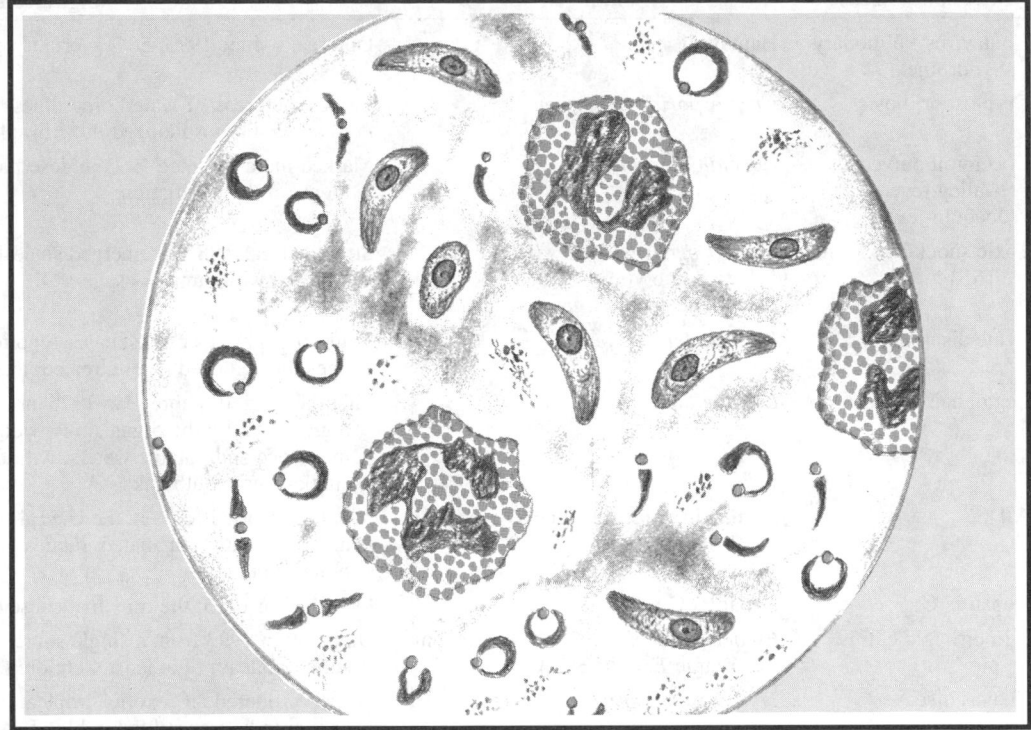

OVERVIEW

At the beginning of the nineteenth century, no infectious disease was controlled in America. Major efforts in environmental sanitation, advances in immunization and antibiotic therapy, and application of antimicrobial technology to disease agents have resulted in control of many of the dreaded infectious diseases of the past. Today, most health professionals in the United States never see cases of the major killers, such as yellow fever, cholera, typhus, smallpox, malaria, typhoid fever, and plague. They see, however, new killers, such as acquired immunodeficiency syndrome (AIDS) and increasing numbers of cases of hepatitis, tuberculosis, and sexually transmitted diseases. Vaccine-preventable diseases, such as measles and mumps, persist despite the availability of vaccines. Antibiotic-resistant organisms flourish, and new infectious disease agents are being identified (Table 13-1). Misuse of antimicrobial therapy has created new strains of pathogens that are resistant to previously effective therapy. Table 13-2 lists some of the documented drug-resistant pathogens and the body systems most often affected. In addition, many of the major killers, such as cholera and yellow fever, continue to cause death in other parts of the world, necessitating a vigilant attitude toward infectious diseases everywhere (see box on p. 1073).

Because all infectious diseases have characteristics in common, this overview discusses the following aspects:

Stages of Infection

The infection process, from transmission of a pathogenic agent to infectious disease, results from a complex interaction between organisms, an environment conducive to transmission, and a susceptible human host. Once transmission has occurred, more than one outcome is possible. The first is *contamination* of a body surface or object with a pathogenic agent. The process may stop there if host first-line defenses, such as intact skin and mucous membranes, block the infectious agent from invading host tissue; however, the organism may invade and begin replicating, a condition called *colonization*. This period is referred to as the *latent phase* (or incubation phase) in the infection process. Further host defenses, such as inflammatory and immune responses, may fight off the multiplying pathogens during the latent phase, before they have an opportunity to produce damage in host tissue. At the other extreme, the pathogen or its products may begin destructive action on undefended host tissue, resulting in a disease stage in the infection process. By definition, *infectious disease* is the pathophysiologic response of the host, resulting from the action of the pathogen (or its products) in host tissue or from the host responses to eliminate the pathogen. This pathophysiologic response is generally symptomatic. An asymptomatic response is called a *subclinical infection*.

TABLE 13-1 Emerging Infectious Disease in the United States

Infectious Disease	Pathogen	Significance
Hantavirus Pulmonary Syndrome	Hantavirii	Outbreaks since 1993; 50% mortality rate
Cryptosporidiosis	*Cryptosporidium parvum*	Largest outbreak of waterborne illness in US history; over 400,000 ill and 4400 hospitalized in Milwaukee, Wisconsin
Coccidioidomycosis (Valley fever, San Joaquin fever)	*Coccidioides immitis*	Marked increase since 1991 in desert areas of CA affecting all segments of the population
Toxic shock syndrome (TSS)	*Streptococcus pyogenes* (Group A beta-hemolytic streptococci) *Staphylococcus aureus*	Streptococcal TSS has emerged since 1987; Staphylococcal TSS associated with tampon usage
Lyme disease	*Borrelia burgdorferi*	Transmitted by deer ticks; cases reported in 47 states; disease often goes undiagnosed and untreated, leading to chronic disability
Legionnaires' disease	*Legionellae* spp.	First recognized outbreak in 1976 among attendees at a convention; high mortality; the organism is widespread in the environment in surface and potable waters, with the potential for producing single-source outbreaks
AIDS	Human immunodeficiency virus (HIV)	500,000 reported cases in the U.S. alone; almost 100% fatal; epidemic continues unabated; modes of transmission make prevention difficult.
Hepatitis C	Hepatitis C virus	Identified in 1975; the principal cause of transfusion-related hepatitis
Hemorrhagic colitis	*Escherichia coli* 0157:H7 (Enterohemorrhagic *E. coli*: EHEC)	Outbreak in 1993 from a single source undercooked hamburger resulted in death of at least 4 children
Chagas disease	*Trypanosoma cruzi*	Once considered an "exotic" tropical infection; the parasite is now known to be transmitted in blood donated from travelers to areas where the disease is endemic
Leishmaniasis	*Leishmania* spp.	12,000,000 people are infected worldwide with 400,000 new cases reported annually; has been diagnosed in military personnel returning from the Persian Gulf conflict

Data from Benenson,[3] Centers for Disease Control.[17]

*Emerging infectious diseases are diseases of infectious origin whose incidence in humans has increased within the past two decades or threatens to increase in the near future.

Symptoms of infectious disease need not be present for a host to transmit the pathogen. A person, with or without symptoms, may harbor an infectious agent in sufficient quantities to shed the organism in body secretions, excretions, or exudates. Organisms may be shed during the incubation phase before symptomatic disease, during the course of a subclinical infection, or during convalescence following symptomatic disease. In all cases a person who is capable of transmitting organisms in the absence of discernible infectious disease is called a carrier.

Pathogenic Agents

Most of the multitude of microorganisms in our environment are not harmful to the host with a normal immune system. These organisms have coexisted with humans in complex, mutually beneficial relationships. Nonetheless, many organisms are pathogenic (disease producing). Pathogens are parasites that maintain themselves at the expense of their human host, thus producing disease.

The microorganisms pathogenic to humans are classified, in order of decreasing size, as protozoa, fungi and yeasts, bacteria, rickettsiae, chlamydiae, mycoplasmata, and viruses. A larger group of organisms, also parasitic to humans, are the helminths, or worms.

The likelihood of a pathogen producing infectious disease and the type of disease elicited are influenced by characteristics of the organism. The first is the organism's *infectivity:* its ability to invade and multiply in the host. Invasiveness is promoted by a variety of pathogen-produced enzymes that either protect the pathogen from host defenses or dissolve connective tissue to facilitate spread in the host. The second characteristic refers to the organism's *pathogenicity,* or ability to produce disease. This in turn relies on the pathogen's speed of reproduction, extent of tissue damage, or production of a toxin. The third characteristic is its mode of action. Some pathogens cause direct cellular damage leading to cellular necrosis and death. Others, such as viruses, interfere with cellular metabolism. Still others produce toxins that stimulate local or systemic reaction. The fourth characteristic, *virulence,* refers to the potency of the pathogen in producing severe disease. Closely related to virulence is the toxigenicity of some pathogens. Agents vary in the amount and destructive potential of the toxins they produce. Some bacteria

TABLE 13-2 Super Bugs: New Strains of Pathogens Resistant to Therapy

Drug-Resistant Pathogens	Body System Affected
Mycobacterium tuberculosis (multidrug-resistant: MDR-TB)	Respiratory
Streptococcus pneumoniae (multidrug-resistant)	Respiratory
Staphylococcus aureus (methicillin-resistant: MRSA; vancomycin-resistant:VRSA)	Respiratory, circulatory, musculoskeletal, skin
Staphylococcus epidermidis (VRSE)	Skin
Bordetella pertussis	Respiratory (whooping cough)
Neisseria gonorrhoeae	Genitourinary
Salmonella spp.	Gastrointestinal, circulatory, urinary
Enterococcus spp. (multidrug resistant, including vancomycin-resistant: VRE)	Urinary, circulatory, wound, respiratory, central nervous system
Enterobacter spp.	Urinary, wound, respiratory, circulatory
Pseudomonas aeruginosa	Wounds, eye, ear, circulatory, musculoskeletal, respiratory
Klebsiella spp.	Respiratory, urinary, wound, circulatory
Acinetobacter spp.	Respiratory, urinary, wound, circulatory
Other gram-negative organisms developing drug resistance: *Citrobacter Freundii, Escherichia coli Morganella morgannii Providencia* spp., *Serratia* spp.	Multiple body systems

Data from Murray et al[27] and Centers for Disease Control.[19,24]

YOU CAN HELP PREVENT THE FURTHER DEVELOPMENT OF MULTIDRUG-RESISTANT ORGANISMS

Drug resistant organisms have developed from misuse/abuse of antimicrobial therapy. **How has this occurred?** Effective antimicrobial therapy eliminates or suppresses a significant proportion of microbes, thus allowing the body's natural defenses to control the remaining pathogens. Incomplete therapy merely exposes the microorganisms to the antimicrobial without eliminating or sufficiently suppressing them. Thus the surviving microorganism are those that have developed resistance to the drug. These survivors are able to transfer this resistance, not only to their progeny but to other adult microorganisms with similar cell structures. For example, vancomycin-resistant enterococci (VRE) can transfer the gene that confers high level resistance to other gram-positive bacteria such as *Staphylococcus aureus.*

What can you do to stop the proliferation of drug-resistant pathogens? Educate all of your patients and their families about the importance of taking antibiotics and other antimicrobial medications only when prescribed by a physician or a nurse practitioner. Instruct them verbally and in writing to take the medication exactly as prescribed for as long as prescribed, even if symptoms are resolved before the medication has been completed. The only acceptable reason for not completing the prescribed therapy is an adverse reaction to the medication, which should be reported to the physician at once. Further, instruct your patients to *never* share their medications with another person, even with a member of one's family, and to *never* take medication prescribed for a previous infection. In addition, instruct that antibiotics *should not* be taken for nonbacterial infections, such as the common cold. We are all responsible for controlling the escalating problem of drug resistance. We all will suffer if the "super bugs" continue to develop.

secrete water-soluble antigenic *exotoxins* that are quickly distributed by the blood, causing potentially severe systemic and neurologic manifestations. Diseases associated with exotoxins are tetanus, botulism, and diphtheria. *Endotoxins* make up the cell wall of some bacteria and cause local inflammation and destruction of host tissue. They are weakly toxic, are relatively stable, and are not antigenic. Diseases associated with endotoxins include staphylococcal food poisoning and cholera.

A final characteristic, *antigenicity,* is the ability of a pathogen to induce an antibody response in the host. Pathogens vary according to this characteristic. Some have intrinsic antigens (proteins, polypeptides, or polysaccharides) that cause the host to produce antibodies against the antigen.

Chain of Transmission

The ability of a pathogenic agent to produce infectious disease in humans depends on the agent's characteristics plus an intact chain of transmission. The chain includes a host reservoir, mode of escape from the reservoir, environment conducive to transmission of the pathogen, entry into a new host, and susceptibility of the new host to the infectious disease.

Reservoir A reservoir is a person, animal, plant, soil, or organic substance, alone or in combination, in which an infectious agent lives and multiplies. The agent depends on the reservoir for its reproduction and consequent survival. Humans are the only reservoir for some pathogens, whereas other pathogens require an intermediate animal or chain of animal or inanimate reservoirs. The human, as a reservoir for an infectious agent, may have a symptomatic infectious disease, may have a subclinical infectious disease, or may be a carrier of the agent.

Escape The organism escapes from the reservoir at the site of the multiplication of the organism. Portals of exit may be the genitourinary tract, the gastrointestinal tract, the oral cavity, the respiratory tract, open lesions, or mechanical escape of blood. There may be more than one portal of exit for any one disease process. The duration of escape coincides with the period of communicability and varies with each disease. Generally, there is an inverse relationship between the length of the communicable period and the infectivity of the organism. Highly infectious organisms such as the influenza virus have a short duration of escape, whereas the less infective *M. tuberculosis* has a long duration of escape.

The portal of exit of an organism determines its mode of transmission and is therefore an important consideration for health workers in contact with infectious agents.

Transmission   The organism may have a single or multiple routes of transmission. In general, the organism may be transmitted *directly* through person-to-person contact or *indirectly* through an animate or inanimate vehicle of transmission. Direct contact occurs when there is actual physical contact between the source and the victim as is the case with sexual, fecal-oral, or mucous droplet transmission. Indirect transmission requires that the organism survive outside the human on or in animate or inanimate vehicles. Animate vehicles include animals and vectors. Inanimate vehicles are air, food, water, milk, soil, fomites, or biologic materials. If an inanimate vehicle has the potential of infecting many persons, it is called a common vehicle.

Entry   Portal of entry into a new host corresponds frequently with the portal of exit from the reservoir. Entry may be by ingestion, by inhalation, by percutaneous injection, through the mucous membranes, or across the placenta. The duration of the exposure and the numbers of organisms necessary to start the infectious process in the new host vary with each disease.

Host susceptibility   Susceptibility refers to those host conditions that increase the probability that disease may develop in the host. Susceptibility is affected by specific resistance factors such as the immunologic responses and nonspecific body defenses against disease agents, both of which will be discussed in the next section. Host susceptibility is also affected by general human characteristics such as age, sex, ethnic group, and heredity; behaviors regarding eating and personal hygiene; geographic and environmental living conditions; and general health status, including nutritional status, hormonal balance, and the presence of concurrent disease. All of these factors either determine the type of pathogenic agent to which the person is exposed or determine the extent of the host response and resistance to the pathogens (Table 13-3).

Control   Control of infectious disease relies on procedures aimed at breaking the chain of transmission at one or more of its links. The point of the chain most amenable to control varies with the organism and its reservoirs, the disease process, and available technology. Control measures may be directed to killing or altering the virulence of the agent, destroying nonhuman reservoirs and vectors, isolating the infected persons, using precautions with infected body fluids and contaminated inanimate objects, and altering host resistance, defenses, and immunity.

Effective control is also based on monitoring of disease occurrence to facilitate early intervention (see box). Certain diseases must be reported to the local health authority. These are identified in the overview table presented for each disease discussed in this chapter.

▪▪▪▪▪▪ Anatomy, Physiology, and Related Pathophysiology

Physiology of the Human Response to Infection

Certain anatomic and physiologic characteristics of the human operate to increase resistance to infectious diseases and to fight

---

■ TABLE 13-3   Chain of Transmission of Infectious Disease

Transmission Chain	Factors
Agent (living parasite)	Bacteria, rickettsiae, fungi, chlamydiae, mycoplasmae, viruses, helminths, protozoa
Reservoir (where agent lives and multiplies)	Humans (frank cases, subclinical cases, carriers) Inanimate organic matter Animals
Portal of exit	Genitourinary tract, gastrointestinal tract, respiratory tract, oral cavity, open lesions, blood
Transmission	Direct: person to person (fecal-oral, sexual, droplet) Indirect: through a vehicle (animate: animal or vector; inanimate: food, water, soil, milk, air, intravenous therapy or catheters)
Modes of entry	Ingestion, inhalation, percutaneous injection, transplacental entry, mucous membranes
Susceptible host	Specific immune reactions Nonspecific body defenses Host characteristics: age, sex, ethnic group, heredity, behaviors Environmental and general health status

---

> **■ SPECTRUM OF DISEASE OCCURRENCE**
>
> Characteristics of the organism and mode of transmission are the two most important factors in how often a particular infectious disease occurs and how many people are affected.
> *Sporadic disease* is the occasional, irregular appearance of cases in a population over a given period.
> *Endemic disease* occurs at a constant rate, affecting about the same number of people in a population over a given period.
> *Epidemic disease* is a definite increase over its expected endemic pattern.
> *Pandemic disease* is an epidemic occurring over a very wide area and usually affecting a large proportion of the population.
> Some diseases also demonstrate predictable seasonal, yearly, or geographic variation in occurrence.

From Grimes.[26]

the infectious process once it occurs. These characteristics can be considered as lines of defense against pathogenic agents.

The first line of defense against infection is external and consists of mechanical barriers, chemical barriers, and the body's own population of microorganisms.

The two internal barriers come into play when the external line of defense is breeched. Operating as the second line of defense, the inflammatory response is aimed at preventing an invading pathogen from becoming established, reproducing, and invading other tissues. The third line of defense is the immune response, which is activated after the inflammatory response. Although inflammation and immune response are two events, they cannot always be easily separated because both events involve many of the same processes and cellular components. In addition to these defenses, the human characteristically responds to an infectious process with a change in body temperature.

First Line of Defense: Barriers

Every surface of the body that is exposed in any way to the environment is involved in first-line defense.

Mechanical barriers   Certain anatomic characteristics prevent the invasion of microorganisms. These include the intact skin and mucous membranes and oil and perspiration on the skin. Ciliary action in the respiratory tract, reflexes such as coughing and sneezing, and peristalsis in the gastrointestinal tract act to remove an organism before its penetration into tissue. The flushing action of body secretions such as tears, saliva, and mucus further protects against invasion. Compromise in any of these barriers increases susceptibility to invasion of infectious agents.

Chemical barriers   In addition to the mechanical barriers, the chemical composition of body secretions is protective. The pH of saliva, vaginal secretions, urine, and digestive secretions prevents or inhibits growth of some microbes. Bile acts to decrease the surface tension causing changes in the cell wall of some bacteria. This renders the organisms more digestible by other digestive enzymes. Oil and sweat secretions contain chemicals that are bactericidal to some microbes.

Normal flora   The normal flora of microorganisms on the skin and mucous membranes and in the intestinal and vaginal tracts protect against invasion of pathogenic agents through a mechanism termed microbial antagonism. The importance of this mechanism in controlling the replication of pathogenic organisms becomes evident when the normal flora are disturbed during antibiotic therapy. Extensive penicillin therapy, for example, may precipitate the growth of *Candida albicans,* normally controlled by the endogenous bacteria in the vaginal tract.

Some indigenous flora are themselves pathogenic under certain conditions. They can be responsible for infection when the immune system is impaired, the skin or mucous membranes are breeched, or the flora are displaced from their natural habitat to another area of the body. This latter event is explained by the fact that the normal flora are tissue specific—that is, a particular type of bacteria normally colonizes a particular type of tis-

sue, adhering to specific receptors on epithelial cells. As a result, the normal composition of flora varies from one part of the body to another.

Displacement of indigenous flora to another area is a common cause of nosocomial (hospital-acquired) infection, such as urinary tract infection from enteric bacteria following catheterization.

Components of Internal Defense

The second and third lines of defense (the inflammatory response and the immune system) share several components. These components include the lymphatic system, leukocytes, and a multitude of chemicals, proteins, and enzymes that facilitate the internal defense systems (see Chapter 14 for an in-depth review of these components).

Second Line of Defense: The Inflammatory Response

Once a microorganism penetrates the first line of defense and invades cells, the inflammatory response is initiated. Inflammation is a local reaction to cell injury of any type, whether from physical, chemical, or thermal damage or microbial invasion. As a response to microbial injury, inflammation is aimed at preventing further invasion by walling off, destroying, or neutralizing the invading organism. Repair is also an integral part of inflammation, and in "clean" injuries, which do not involve microbes, repair is the primary beneficial result.

The early inflammatory response is protective, but it can continue for sustained periods of time in some infections. The production of new leukocytes (particularly phagocytic leukocytes) may be stimulated for weeks or months in some infections, as reflected in an elevated white blood cell count (particularly neutrophils and monocytes) for prolonged periods. However, sustained inflammation can become chronic and result in the destruction of healthy tissues. Extensive necrosis from persistent inflammation can actually increase tissue susceptibility to the infectious agent or provide an ideal setting for invasion by other pathogens.

The inflammatory response is limited to vascularized tissues, since the molecular and cellular components of inflammation are delivered via blood vessels. Inflammation develops in a series of interrelated steps that involve blood vessels, fluid and cellular blood components, the lymphatic system, and the surrounding connective tissue.

Stages of inflammatory response   The complex mechanisms of the inflammatory response can be divided into three interdependent stages: cell response to injury, vascular response, and phagocytosis.

The cellular response to injury is the same regardless of the method of injury. A number of metabolic changes occur within the injured cell. The injured cell swells because it can no longer pump out sodium ions. Nearly all cells contain specialized sacs called *lysosomes* that contain a multitude of enzymes capable of digesting portions of the cell if its metabolic activity has been severely disrupted. The resulting cellular atrophy reduces metabolic demands on the cell. Cell death occurs if metabolism can no longer be maintained, and enzymes are released to dissolve the cellular contents and stimulate the inflammatory process in surrounding tissue.

The vascular response occurs shortly after injury. The arterioles, venules, and capillaries in the surrounding area dilate, producing a localized hyperemia. This increases the filtration pressure of the blood and capillary permeability, causing fluid exudate to leak from the blood vessels into the interstitial spaces. Proteins, enzymes, and other chemical components in the exudate attract more fluid into the interstitial spaces, producing edema in an effort to wall off the inflamed area from uninvolved tissues.

Inflammatory exudate serves the important function of transporting phagocytic cells into the injured area. As fluid leaks from the blood, blood flow in the area slows, allowing leukocytes to collect (marginate) along the vascular endothelium. Leukocytes, particularly neutrophils and monocytes, emigrate through the endothelium to the injured tissue, attracted by chemicals released by the injured cells.

Phagocytosis is the process of engulfing, digesting, and thus destroying infectious agents and other material. This is done primarily by circulating macrophages, the majority of which are neutrophils and monocytes that are dispatched to an injured area in fluid exudate. Some macrophages reside in tissue and are found in lymph nodes, bone marrow, lungs (alveolar macrophages), spleen, liver (Kupffer cells), and other organs. Phagocytes also perform the essential "housekeeping" chore of cleaning up dead cells and other debris.

Intracellular phagocytosis occurs at the site of tissue invasion, but it also extends into lymphatic and blood circulation if infection becomes systemic. The intracellular activity of phagocytosis stimulates release of chemicals that induce lysis of the leukocytes. These dead leukocytes, together with dead organisms and fluid from the blood, make up the inflammatory exudate.

Patterns of inflammation   Both local and systemic symptoms of inflammation can occur. Heat, redness, swelling, and pain are local reactions to inflammation that may vary considerably in severity. The first three characteristics result from response of the vasculature to injury. Pain is produced partly from pressure of the exudate against nerve endings in the surrounding tissue, but prostaglandins and possibly other chemicals also play some role in causing pain.

Several types of inflammatory exudates are produced. Serous exudate, which typically occurs in early inflammation, contains only plasma and proteins. Mucinous or catarrhal exudate contains increased secretions from inflamed mucous membranes and may include both live and dead organisms. Fibrinous exudate forms on tissue, particularly mucous membranes, when large amounts of fibrinogen are extravasated into the tissue. Purulent exudate, such as pus, contains both live and dead leukocytes, live and dead microorganisms, serous exudate, and liquefied digestive products of necrotic tissue. Some inflammatory conditions produce combinations of exudates. The characteristic fibrinopurulent exudate of diphtheria results from necrosis of the mucous membrane in the throat.

Inflammation and its exudates may remain localized, may permeate the tissue, or may spread throughout the body via the blood or lymph. An abscess is an example of a localized infection and inflammation with purulent exudate. Leukocytes form a wall around the organisms. The abscess deepens as more leukocytes are drawn into the area, more organisms are killed, and more necrotic tissue is dissolved. The exudate may eventually be autolyzed and resorbed by the body, in which case the inflammation and infection are resolved. Resolution may leave a cavity, ulcer, or scar tissue. Calcification around the exudate occurs in some instances, such as in tuberculosis, walling off the live infectious agents inside the tissue. Rupture of the abscess and drainage into other tissues can spread the infection to other areas of the body.

Systemic symptoms can include fever and chills, diaphoresis, malaise, and nausea and vomiting. The inflammatory process also causes changes in blood components, such as an increased number of leukocytes or a change in the type of leukocytes.

Chronic inflammation may result from a low-grade inflammatory response that fails to elicit an acute response. Agents most often responsible for chronic inflammation are those that cannot penetrate deeply or spread rapidly, such as *Mycobacterium tuberculosis,* the treponemata that cause syphilis, some viruses, fungi, and many helminths. Inadequate specific immune response or a hyperimmune response can also lead to chronic inflammation, such as occurs in autoimmune disorders.

Chronic inflammation is marked by tissue infiltration with macrophages, lymphocytes, and plasma cells rather than neutrophils. Exudates are not generally formed, although some types of chronic inflammatory disorders are characterized by certain types of exudates. Rheumatoid arthritis, for example, is accompanied by synovial effusions, an exudate into the joint. A proliferation of fibroblasts results in greater formation of scar tissue that sometimes replaces normal connective tissue or other tissue. Some chronic inflammations result in formation of granulomas, which are 1 to 2 mm lesions caused by the massing of macrophages surrounded by lymphocytes around an infectious agent. A dense membrane of connective tissue may encapsulate the lesion, as occurs in tuberculosis.

Several factors affect the outcome of the inflammatory process. Age, nutritional status, and general health greatly affect the individual's ability to mount an effective inflammatory response. Agent factors, such as virulence and size of inoculum, can overcome even an aggressive host defense and promote spread of the organism. In addition, some pathogens are effective intracellular parasites and are capable of surviving and multiplying in phagocytes. These include some viruses, *M. tuberculosis,* and *Rickettsia.* The immune response, the third line of defense, is activated to combat invaders that survive phagocytosis.

Third Line of Defense: The Immune Response

The first and second lines of defense are nonspecific—that is, they operate against all infectious agents in the same manner. In contrast, the immune system responds in a very specific manner to individual pathogens, as long as the organism has antigenic characteristics. Generally speaking, antigens are either proteins, large polysaccharides, or large lipoprotein complexes that stimulate antibody production. Not all microorganisms are antigenic, but some are bound by complement or other host-produced substances to form an antigen that elicits an immune response.

The immune system has several unique characteristics:

Self- or nonself-recognition. It normally recognizes host cells as nonantigenic and therefore responds only to foreign agents as antigens. In autoimmune diseases, there is a breakdown in this distinction, and the immune system attacks host cells as if they were antigens.

Antibody production. It produces specific antibodies that target specific antigens for destruction; it can produce new antibodies in response to new antigens.

Memory. It remembers antigens that have invaded the body in the past, allowing a quicker response to subsequent invasion by the same antigen.

Self-regulation. It monitors its own performance, turning on when antigens invade and turning off when infection is eradicated, preventing destruction of healthy tissue.

An immune response is triggered after foreign materials have been cleared from an area of inflammation. After phagocytes digest the pathogens, antigenic material appears on their surface. Phagocytes, primarily macrophages, serve as antigen-presenting cells to introduce the pathogen to lymphocytes. Recognition of the antigen as "nonself" by receptors on lymphocytes in blood, lymph, or tissue exudate sets up a chain of responses to destroy or neutralize the antigen. Two types of immune responses can occur; cell-mediated immunity and humoral immunity. These processes begin with the differentiation of lymphocytes into B or T cells. These two types of responses overlap and interact considerably, but the distinction is useful in understanding how the immune system is activated.

Cell-mediated immune response The cellular immune response is activated with the invasion of intracellular pathogens, such as viruses, mycobacteria, fungi, and protozoa, and it is a component of the host response to tumors and tissue transplants. Cell-mediated immunity, directed primarily by T cells, results from cell interaction with antigens expressed on phagocytes. T cell receptor binding to the antigen causes T cells to differentiate into subsets and proliferate. Helper T cells initiate the cell-mediated response by releasing interleukin-2, which stimulates the production of cytotoxic T cells. Cytotoxic T cells kill the antigen directly by releasing lymphokines, an event that also attracts more macrophages to the area. Suppressor T cells slow or halt the activity of other T cells.

Cell-mediated immunity is the basis for many skin tests, such as the tuberculin test. Cellular immunity cannot be transferred passively to another person.

Humoral immune response Humoral (antibody-mediated) immunity protects against many gram-positive and certain gram-negative bacteria. Antibody production also aids in neutralizing viruses, enhances phagocytosis, and activates the complement system. B cells, the antibody-producing lymphocytes, are responsible for humoral immunity.

Humoral immunity can be initiated in two ways. Some antigens are not recognized by T cells (T-independent antigens) and stimulate B cells directly. Most antigens, however, will bind to T cells (T-dependent antigens), and the helper T cells act to stimulate B cells. In either case, the stimulated B cells differentiate into antibody-producing plasma cells and memory B cells. Antibodies appear on the surface of plasma cells and bind to antigen. Once antigens are immobilized, cytotoxic T cells are activated and eradication of the pathogen begins. Suppressor T cells halt the humoral response after the infection is resolved.

The amount and type of antibody produced depend on the nature and amount of antigen present, the site of the antigen stimulus, and the number of previous exposures to the same antigen. The initial antibody production, the *primary response,* occurs the first time a particular antigen invades the body (from 1 to 7 days after initial exposure to the antigen). Depending on the nature of the antigen and the efficiency of antibody production, the response peaks in 1 to 10 weeks. Antibody titers can usually be detected within 10 days of exposure.

Memory B cells allow a more efficient humoral response on subsequent exposure to the same antigen (the *secondary response*). The memory cells generate more rapid, prolific, and sustained response, producing higher antibody titers that are usually detectable in a shorter period of time and for a longer duration.

The strength and persistence of the humoral immune response are determined by maintaining a correct balance between helper and suppressor T cells. Helper T cells must be present in sufficient numbers to stimulate B cell production of antibodies, and the correct proportion of T suppressor cells is needed to shut off the immune response. An imbalance can result in inadequate production of antibodies, leading to immune deficiency states, or the unchecked overstimulation of the immune response, resulting in autoimmune disorders. The normal helper to suppressor ratio is 2:1, whereas a 1:1 ratio is typical in AIDS patients.

The humoral immune response is more rapid than the cell-mediated response and is more frequently a factor in resistance to acute bacterial infections. Humoral immunity can be transmitted to another person, either by inoculation or by maternal transfer via the placenta or breast milk.

Immunoglobulins Immunoglobulins are the protein molecules that compose antibodies. There are five major classes of immunoglobulins that are able to combine in an endless number of ways to produce antibodies specific against a particular antigen. When the humoral immune response is initiated, more than one class may be activated. Table 13-4 summarizes the characteristics of the immunoglobulin classes.

Immunoglobulins perform four major functions:

1. Immunoglobulins directly attack antigens, destroying or neutralizing them through the processes of agglutination

(clumping the antigens together to inactivate them), precipitating the toxins out of solution, neutralizing antigenic substances, and lysing the organism's cell wall.

2. Immunoglobulins activate the complement system.
3. Immunoglobulins activate anaphylaxis by releasing histamine in tissue and blood.
4. Immunoglobulins stimulate antibody-mediated hypersensitivity.

Acquired immunity   Immunity refers to the presence of or acquisition of antibodies. Immunity can be acquired as a result of exposure to a specific antigenic agent or pathogen. Acquired immunity may be gained by natural means through inadvertent contact with an antigen (active) or antibodies (passive). Artificial immunity is intentionally induced through inoculation of antigen (active) or antibodies (passive) (Table 13-5). Active immunity, whether

naturally or artificially induced, produces physiologically identical immune responses (see Immunizations, p. 1162).

Body Temperature Response

A change in body temperature is a characteristic systemic symptom of infectious diseases. The causes of fever in infectious diseases are discussed here. Fever patterns associated with specific infectious diseases are described with each disease.

Causes of fever in infectious diseases   Body temperature is normally maintained within a range around 98.6° F (37° C) with predictable variations within any 24-hour period that coincide with metabolic activity. Fever, a sustained temperature above normal, can be caused by abnormalities of the hypothalamus, brain tumors, dehydration, or toxic substances affecting the temperature-regulating center of the hypothalamus. Certain protein substances and toxins can cause the "set point" of the

TABLE 13-4 Immunoglobulin Classes

Immunoglobulin	Characteristics	Functions
IgG	Accounts for about 80%-85% of antibodies in normal serum; most abundant in blood but also found in lymph, cerebrospinal, synovial, and peritoneal fluid and breast milk; the only immunoglobulin that crosses placenta and provides temporary immunity in neonate	Develops slowly during primary response, appearing about 1 wk or more after IgM, then reaches a peak in 1-3 wk or longer after IgM peaks; may persist for years; highest concentration during secondary immune response; activates complement system, involved in opsonization; attacks antigens directly
IgM	Accounts for about 5% of antibodies in normal serum	First antibody to form during viral or bacterial infection; usually peaks 1-2 wk after clinical symptoms appear; highest concentration during primary response; is increased in chronic infections; binds with viral and bacterial antigens in the circulation, which activates the complement cascade
IgA	Accounts for about 15% of antibodies in normal serum; found in blood and secretions (tears, saliva, colostrum, respiratory tract, and stomach and accessory organs)	Secretory antibody; increased in chronic infections and chronic inflammation
IgE	Accounts for <1% of antibodies in normal serum; found also in tissues	Sensitizing antibody; triggers release of histamine; involved with certain allergic disorders, especially atopic diseases; increased in parasitic diseases
IgD	Accounts for <1% of antibodies in normal serum	Function unclear, but increases in chronic infection

From Grimes.[26]

TABLE 13-5 Types of Acquired Immunity

Type of Immunity	How Acquired	Length of Resistance
Natural		
Active	Natural contact and infection with the antigen	May be temporary or permanent
Passive	Natural contact with antibody transplacentally or through colostrum and breast milk	Temporary
Artificial		
Active	Inoculation of antigen	May be temporary or permanent
Passive	Inoculation of antibody or antitoxin	Temporary

From Grimes.[26]

hypothalamic thermostat to rise. This results in activation of the hypothalamus to conserve heat and to increase heat production. Substances that cause these effects are called *pyrogens.* In infectious diseases the endotoxins of some bacteria and the extracts of normal leukocytes (interleukin) are pyrogenic. They act to raise the "thermostat" in the hypothalamus, thus raising the body temperature.

Fever is not a failure of the body to regulate temperature. During the fever response, temperature is merely regulated at a higher level than normal. Four stages of the fever process can be observed. The first is a prodromal period, with no notable change in temperature but with nonspecific symptoms of discomfort. A chill accompanies the second stage when the body temperature is being raised toward the higher thermostat setting. The third stage, flush, occurs when the temperature reaches the new setting and sweating occurs.

Distinct patterns of fever onset and resolution and characteristic temperature curves are associated with different infectious diseases. Fever onset may be abrupt or gradual. A persistent elevation may be maintained throughout the disease, or there may be remissions at specific times of the day or certain days in the illness. Fever associated with some diseases follows a "saddle back" curve with a high fever initially, followed by a few days of remission and then another high elevation. A habitual fever is a low-level fever present in some diseases for years. Intermittent fevers have predictable cycles of paroxysms and remissions. Relapsing fevers are those that recur after apparent recovery. Fevers may resolve suddenly by crisis or gradually by lysis.

For each degree Fahrenheit of temperature elevation there is a 7% increase in body metabolism, necessitating fluid and calorie supplements to meet metabolic needs.

A fever that goes too high may damage cells irreversibly. Temperature elevation to 104° F (40° C) may cause delirium and convulsions, particularly in children. Fever above 106° F (41.1° C) can cause irreparable damage, impairing regulation of the hypothalamic control center, which results in inability to lower temperature.

NORMAL FINDINGS

Refer to specific chapters in this book to obtain normal findings pertinent to each body system.

Diagnostic Procedures

Culture of specimen and direct examination of the culture to identify organism by its characteristics

Microscopic examination of specimen prepared through a variety of chemical or staining procedures to identify microscopic organisms

Examination of the specimen for antigen/antibody reactions to identify the antigen or toxin in the specimen

Serology Immunologic tests applied to serum to identify circulating antibodies to the organism.

CONDITIONS, DISEASES, AND DISORDERS

CENTRAL NERVOUS SYSTEM INFECTIOUS DISEASES

MENINGITIS

Meningitis is an inflammation of the meninges covering the brain and spinal cord. The inflammation may result from an acute infection of the meninges caused by the invasion of bacteria, viruses, fungi, or parasitic worms into the tissues or from the iatrogenic introduction of a substance that is irritating to the meninges. The forms of meningitis discussed in this section are those caused by bacterial and viral invasion (Table 13-6).

Meningococcal meningitis is an acute communicable inflammation of the meninges caused by *Neisseria meningitidis.* It frequently occurs in epidemic form.

Haemophilus meningitis is an acute communicable inflammation of the meninges caused by *Haemophilus influenzae.* It is the most common form of bacterial meningitis.

Pneumococcal meningitis is an acute inflammation of the meninges caused by *Streptococcus pneumoniae.* The meningitis frequently results from an extension of a primary infection in the upper respiratory tract. Patients infected with *S. pneumoniae* have a high risk of fatality.

Viral (aseptic or serous) meningitis is an acute meningeal inflammation that occurs as a sequela to many viral diseases. The condition is usually self-limited and benign.

Many bacteria are capable of producing a suppurative meningitis; the most common forms are *Haemophilus,* meningococcal, and pneumococcal meningitides. They are discussed together, since their pathologic manifestations and symptoms are similar. Viral meningitis is discussed as a separate disease entity regardless of the viral disease that preceded the meningitis.

Pathophysiology

Bacteria causing the type of meningitis being considered here are inhaled in mucous droplets from infected persons or carriers. The bacteria invade the respiratory passages and are disseminated by way of the blood to meninges of the brain and spinal cord. The respiratory phase is generally subclinical in meningococcal meningitis, although organisms present in respiratory secretions can be transmitted to another host. The respiratory phase is usually symptomatic in pneumococcal and *Haemophilus* meningitides. The bacteremia produced during dissemination causes toxic manifestations. In the case of meningococcus the organism penetrates and damages vascular endothelium. This results in petechial and purpuric lesions of the skin.

■ TABLE 13-6 Overview of Meningitis

	Meningococcal Meningitis	Pneumococcal Meningitis	*Haemophilus* Meningitis	Viral Meningitis (Aseptic)
Occurrence	Endemic and epidemic; worldwide; greatest during winter and spring; greatest in males, in children less than 5 yr, and in persons in crowded living conditions	Endemic; greatest in infants, elderly persons, and alcoholics; follows pneumococcal pneumonia	Worldwide; most common bacterial meningitis in children 2 mo to 3 yr	Worldwide; epidemics, seasonal outbreaks, and sporadic cases associated with other viral infections
Etiologic agent	*Neisseria meningitidis,* with many subgroups	*Streptococcus pneumoniae,* many serotypes	*Haemophilus influenzae,* six serotypes; type B (Hib) responsible for 90% of *Haemophilus* meningitis	Most viruses (e.g., mumps, herpes, and polio) produce the syndrome
Reservoir	Humans	Humans; many carriers	Humans	Humans
Transmission	Direct contact with droplets from respiratory passages of infected persons and carriers	Direct and indirect contact with discharges from respiratory passages	Direct contact with droplets from respiratory passages	Not transmitted at this stage
Incubation period	2-10 days; usually 3-4 days	Not well known	Unknown, probably 2-4 days	Depends on virus and associated viral disease
Period of communicability	Until organism is not present in discharges: within 24 hr of treatment with sulfonamides	Until organism is not present in respiratory discharges: 24-48 hr after antibiotic treatment	Prolonged; until organism is not present in nasal discharge Communicable 24-48 hr after beginning effectively	
Susceptibility and resistance	Susceptibility to clinical disease is low; many carriers; group-specific immunity of unknown duration follows infection	Infants and elderly most susceptible; immunity for specific type persists for years	Children most susceptible; otitis media may be a precursor; immunity of unknown duration follows infection	Children, elderly and immunocompromised patients, and those unimmunized against vaccine-preventable viral diseases
Report to local health authority	Mandatory case report	Only epidemics; no individual case reports	Yes, in certain endemic areas	Yes, in endemic areas

Data from Benenson.[3]

The invasion may produce a primary or secondary infection. Some bacteria produce a primary focal infection in the meninges. Such is the case with *N. meningitidis* and *H. influenzae,* which cause meningococcal and *Haemophilus* meningitides, respectively. Other bacterial and viral pathogens are capable of producing a secondary infection in the meninges following hematogenous dissemination from a primary focal infection elsewhere in the body. *H. influenzae, S. pneumoniae* (pneumococcal meningitis), many viruses, and other bacteria have this pathogenic potential.

Bacteria in the meninges elicit an inflammatory response and the production of an exudate, consisting of leukocytes, fi-brin, and bacteria in the subarachnoid space. Cerebrospinal fluid may be thin or thick and have plaque-like accumulations and high leukocytosis, with the majority of the leukocytes being neutrophils. In untreated disease the cerebrospinal fluid may achieve a thickness that interferes with its circulation and reabsorption. An internal or external hydrocephalus may result. Extension of the bacteria into brain tissue may produce a bacterial encephalitis.

Meningococcal infections may be so severe in the systemic stage that they produce an acute meningococcemia that leads to death or the initiation of therapy before meningeal involvement (see Emergency Alert box). Meningococcemia may become chronic, with toxic symptoms persisting intermittently for weeks or months. Recurrent meningitis is usually of the pneumococcal form and is frequently associated with an undetected skull fracture.

Complications of bacterial meningitis include internal hydrocephalus, deficits of cranial nerve function that lead to blindness and deafness, arthritis, myocarditis, pericarditis, and neuromotor and intellectual deficits. Symptomatic and asymptomatic infection with bacterial meningitis results in a protective immune response of unknown duration.

Aseptic (viral, serous, or nonsuppurative) meningitis is a syndrome generally associated with an existing systemic viral disease, the most common one being mumps. Inflammation and

EMERGENCY ALERT

MENINGITIS

An acute infectious process that is an inflammation of the meninges of the spinal cord and brain. The infection carries a mortality ranging between 10% and 30% for bacterial meningitis.

Assessment

- Assess for fever, headache.
- Assess for nuchal rididity.
- Assess for mental alterations, changes in behavior, level of consciousness.
- Assess for increased intracranial pressure.

Interventions

- Maintain airway, breathing, and circulation, intubation and ventilation may be indicated if respiratory status is inadequate.
- Obtain IV access; in collaboration with physician, administer antibiotics, anticonvulsants, and antipyretics as indicated.
- Manage shock.
- Assist physician with lumbar puncture to evaluate cerebrospinal fluid.
- Obtain laboratory studies, including blood cultures.

lymphocytic infiltration of the meninges occur with a wide gradient in clinical severity, depending on the infectious agent. Toxic and meningeal symptoms are usually less severe than in suppurative meningitis; cerebrospinal fluid leukocytes are fewer and consist primarily of lymphocytes. This form may also progress to clinical encephalitis. The disease is usually self-limited with complete recovery, although patients may experience muscle weakness and malaise during a prolonged convalescence.

Complications

Bacterial Meningitis

Internal hydrocephalus

Cranial nerve function deficits that lead to blindness and deafness, arthritis, myocarditis, pericarditis, and neuromotor and intellectual deficits

Aseptic Meningitis

Clinical encephalitis

Muscle weakness and malaise during prolonged convalescence

•••••• Diagnostic Studies and Findings[27]

Cerebrospinal fluid (CSF) examination

Gross appearance: bacterial: turbid; viral (aseptic): clear

Leukocytes: bacterial: 500 to 20,000/mm³; viral: 10 to 500/mm³

Cell types: bacterial: neutrophils; viral (aseptic): lymphocytes

Protein: increased for both

Glucose: bacterial: low to normal; viral (aseptic): normal

Culture and microscopic examination of specimen of CSF

Positive for bacteria

Negative: suggests viral origin

Serologic tests: Positive for antibodies to *N. meningitidis*

Gram's stain of scrapings from petechial skin lesions Positive for meningococci

Culture of respiratory secretions Positive for *H. influenzae, N. meningitidis,* or *S. pneumoniae*

Blood culture Positive for *H. influenzae* or *N. meningitidis* (meningococci)

Serology Antibody titers increase depending on the infecting virus with specific viral infections

•••••• Multidisciplinary Plan[3,27]

Medications

Antiinfective agents for bacterial meningitis

Initial therapy until organism is identified: Ampicillin, plus chloramphenicol if *H. influenzae* is suspected for patients >2 mo

Antiinfective agents for pneumococci: Penicillin, chloramphenicol, vancomycin

Antiinfective agents for meningococci: ceftriaxone, ciprofloxacin

Antiinfective agents for *H. influenzae*: Ampicillin ceftriaxone, cefotaxime or chloramphenicol. All of the above are administered by rapid IV infusion; therapy should continue for 5 d after temperature is normal and clinical signs have cleared. The patient may be given rifampin before hospital discharge

Analgesics prescribed for headache and muscle pain (nonnarcotic); barbiturates may be given for seizures

Immunologic agents prescribed for prevention of bacterial meningitides

Meningococcal polysaccharide vaccine used against group A C, Y, and W-135 for patients >2 yr at risk for epidemic disease; group A serotype given to children 3 mo to 2 yr; routine immunization of the public is not recommended

Pneumococcal polysaccharide vaccine given to patients at high risk for pneumococcal pneumonia and subsequent systemic complications such as immunocompromised and chronically ill persons

H. influenzae type B conjugate vaccine now recommended for all children >2 mo (see p. 1164)

Antiinfective agents for meningococcal contacts

Rifampin (Rifamycin, others), 600 mg bid (adults) for 2 d

Sulfadiazine, 1 g bid for 3 d for mass prophylaxis during meningococcal epidemics or for close patient contacts if strain is proved susceptible

Anti-infective agents for *H. influenzae* contacts—(e.g., household, adults and children in day care) (excluding pregnant women)

Rifampin, 20 mg/kg/d (maximum daily dose of 600 mg) for 4 d as soon as possible after contact

Osmotic agents (e.g., dexamethasone) for cerebral edema

General Management

Intratracheal intubation

Ventilatory assistance

IV therapy and dopamine if shock is present

Fluid restriction to two thirds of daily needs if excess secretion of antidiuretic hormone (ADH)

Control of intracranial pressure

Close monitoring for early diagnosis of patient contacts

NURSING CARE

Nursing Assessment

See nursing care for meningitis and encephalitis, p. 1084.

ENCEPHALITIS

Encephalitis is an inflammation of the tissues of the brain and spinal cord, resulting in altered function of various portions of these tissues. Encephalitis is frequently accompanied by signs of systemic infection. Clinical disease manifestations range from mild to severe to death, and disease may be followed by temporary or permanent neurologic sequelae or complete recovery.

Similar to meningitis, encephalitis may result from at least four causes: a toxemia accompanying an infectious disease, an allergic response to microbial antigens, direct invasion of central nervous system tissue by pathogens as a primary focal infection, or direct invasion of central nervous system tissue secondary to hematogenous dissemination from a primary focal infection elsewhere in the body. Direct invasion, either primary or secondary, is usually caused by a virus, a great many of which are capable of producing encephalitis.

The majority of viruses producing encephalitis as a primary focal infection are transmitted by mosquitoes and are discussed together. Encephalitides occurring secondary to other viral diseases are discussed as infectious encephalitis. A rarer form of meningoencephalitis caused by direct invasion of an ameba is also discussed (Table 13-7).

Infectious viral encephalitides are acute inflammations of the central nervous system that are associated with and sequelae to systemic viral infections; they are commonly caused by the genus *Herpesvirus*.

Mosquito-borne viral encephalitides are a group of acute inflammatory diseases of the brain, spinal cord, and meninges caused by a variety of viruses transmitted to humans through bites from infected mosquitoes.

Amebic meningoencephalitis is an acute and severe inflammation of the brain and meninges caused by invasion of the tis-

TABLE 13-7 Overview of Encephalitis

	Infectious Viral Encephalitis	Mosquito-Borne Viral Encephalitides (Equine and St. Louis Encephalitis)	Amebic Meningoencephalitis
Occurrence	Worldwide; epidemic and sporadic; associated with other viral diseases	Warm, moist climates; summer and early fall when mosquitoes are most common	Worldwide, but rare; greatest in young persons, in warm climates, and during summer
Etiologic agent	A variety of viruses, commonly the *Herpesvirus*	A variety of diseases, each caused by a different virus	*Naegleria fowleri; Acanthamoeba culbertsoni*
Reservoir	Humans	Birds, rodents, bats, reptiles, and amphibians; differing for each virus	Amebae that are free living in water and soil
Transmission	Direct contact with droplets from respiratory passages or other excretions harboring the virus	Bite of infective mosquitoes	Water infected with *N. fowleri* forced into nasal passages while swimming; *Acanthamoeba* enters a skin lesion
Incubation period	Depends on viral disease	5-15 days	3-7 days or longer
Period of communicability	Depends on viral disease	Not communicable person to person; mosquitoes are infective for life	Not communicable person to person
Susceptibility and resistance	Depends on viral disease	Highest susceptibility to clinical disease is infancy and old age; in endemic areas, adults are immune to local strains of virus because of subclinical infections	Unknown; immunosuppressed persons are susceptible to infection with *Acanthamoeba*
Report to local health authority	In select endemic areas	Mandatory case report	Only for means of surveillance

Data from Benenson.[3]

sues by a free-living ameba usually found in water, soil, and decaying vegetation. The disease is frequently fatal.

• • • • • Pathophysiology

Infectious Viral Encephalitis

A variety of directly transmittable viruses are capable of producing encephalitides either as a concomitant to or as a sequela of clinical viral diseases (e.g., measles, mumps, rubella, and chickenpox) or as a result of a subclinical viral infection, such as herpes. In both cases the pathologic manifestations of the encephalitis may result from a postinfection autoimmune response to the virus or from direct invasion of the central nervous system by the virus. Timing of the onset of central nervous system manifestations in relationship to the associated disease symptoms and the ability to isolate the virus from cerebrospinal fluid allow differentiation between postinfection and direct invasion encephalitis.

Disease onset may be acute or insidious, and disease severity may be mild to severe depending on the virus and the distribution, location, and concentration of the neuronal lesions. Mumps virus usually produces a more benign disease, whereas herpes encephalitis is frequently fatal. Permanent neurologic sequelae are also more common in herpes infections.

Mosquito-Borne Viral Encephalitis

A variety of viruses capable of infecting animals and birds can be carried to humans by vector mosquitoes that feed on infected animals. The virus, injected into humans from a mosquito bite, rapidly localizes in the central nervous system and produces congestion, edema, and small hemorrhages in the brain. Neuronal lesions with nerve cell necrosis and destruction and foci of cellular infiltration are widespread throughout the brain and spinal cord. Disease severity depends on the virus and on host resistance factors. Generally, older persons are more severely affected and have the highest fatality. Disease onset may be acute or insidious, depending on the virus involved. Infants generally have a more acute-onset encephalitis than do other age groups. Infants and children are also more likely to develop motor and mental disabilities (e.g., seizures, hydrocephalus, and mental retardation) as a sequela to mosquito-borne encephalitis.

An antibody response can be seen within 7 days. Duration of the disease is variable, depending on the virus. Blood leukocyte levels are generally normal or slightly elevated with some viruses. The virus cannot be recovered from blood, secretions, or discharges and is therefore not communicable from person to person.

Amebic Meningoencephalitis

Two types of ameba, *Naegleria* and *Acanthamoeba,* are capable of producing meningoencephalitis in humans. *Naegleria* infection is caused when water containing the pathogen is forced into the nasal passages, usually by diving or swimming in water containing large amounts of organic matter. The organism colonizes and invades the mucosa, travels along olfactory nerves to the meninges and brain, and produces a severe and rapidly fatal fulminating pyogenic meningoencephalitis, *Acanthamoeba* colonizes a skin lesion and travels to the central nervous system along peripheral nerves to produce a meningoencephalitis with a more insidious onset and prolonged course. Immunologic investigations have shown many people to have a natural antibody against these organisms, suggesting that more subclinical than clinical infections may occur.

Complications
Infectious Encephalitis

Permanent neurologic sequelae are more common in herpes infections

Mosquito-Borne Viral Encephalitis

Motor and mental disabilities (e.g., seizures, hydrocephalus, and mental retardation), more likely in infants and children

Amebic Meningoencephalitis

Severe and rapidly fatal fulminating pyogenic meningoencephalitis

• • • • • Diagnostic Studies and Findings[27]

Cerebrospinal fluid (CSF) examination Viral: 50-500/mm³ leukocytes (predominately lymphocytes), many RBCs, normal glucose, elevated proteins (50 to 150 mg/dl); mosquito-borne: 50 to 500/mm³ leukocytes (up to 1000/mm³ in infants) (usually lymphocytes), rare to have RBCs; normal to high glucose, elevated protein, amebic: polymorphonuclear leukocytes, RBCs, low to normal glucose, elevated protein

Culture and/or microscopic examination of CSF All: negative for bacteria; viral: virus can sometimes be isolated; mosquito-borne: virus can sometimes be isolated; amebic: mobile amebae can be visualized by microscopic examination

Serology Viral and mosquito-borne; fourfold increase in antibody titer between early disease and convalescence. (Immunofluorescent tests available from CDC for differentiating *Acanthamoeba* species).

Examination of biopsied brain tissue using immunofluorescent staining Viral: positive for specific viruses

Hematology (WBC) Mosquito-borne: range from 10,000 to 66,000/mm³, depending on virus

• • • • • Multidisciplinary Plan[3]

Medications

Anti-infective agents
  Amebic meningoencephalitis: combination of the following drugs (individual dose calculation)
    Amphotericin B (Fungizone), IV
    Miconazole (Monistat), IV
    Rifampin (Rifamycin, others), po
  Mosquito-borne: no specific treatment
  Infectious viral encephalitides: no specific treatment except for herpes infections; acyclovir, IV; acyclovir, po for prophylaxis

General Management
   Tracheostomy
   Assisted ventilation
   Suction
   Sedatives for hyperexcitability and seizures
   IV fluids and electrolytes
   Nasogastric tube feedings

NURSING CARE

Nursing Assessment

History

   Meningitis   Recent upper respiratory or ear infection; contact with person with rhinitis or meningitis; pneumonia and otitis media frequently precede pneumococcal and *Haemophilus* meningitis

   Encephalitis   Viral: systemic viral infection; mosquito-borne; exposure to mosquitoes; amebic: swimming and diving in fresh water

Subjective Symptoms

   Meningitis   Severe throbbing headache, muscle pains, stiff neck, backache, chills, expressions of fear; malaise and irritability in chronic meningococcemia

   Encephalitis   Severe frontal headache, nausea and vomiting, dizziness, fever and chills

Body Temperature

   Meningitis   38° to 41° C (100° to 106° F), starting in systemic phase; flushed, hot, dry skin; perspiration; intermittent low-grade fever in chronic meningococcemia

   Encephalitis   39° to 41° C (102° to 106° F); may be acute-onset fever accompanying CNS symptoms or a 1- to 4-day prodromal period with fever and chills before CNS symptoms

Vital Signs

   Meningitis   Pulse may be slow as intracranial pressure increases; BP increases with intracranial pressure

   Encephalitis   Tachypnea, tachycardia

Level of Consciousness

   Meningitis   Alert early in disease but may show delirium progressing to deep coma later

   Encephalitis   Alterations in consciousness—mild listlessness progressing to confusion, stupor, and eventual coma; may be extremely irritable; bizarre behavior with temporal lobe involvement of herpes encephalitis; seizures, particularly in infants with postinfectious encephalitis

Neurologic

   Meningitis   Reflex changes: absence of abdominal reflexes, absence of cremasteric reflexes in male, alteration of tendon reflexes; resistance to neck flexion; Brudzinski's sign positive (attempted flexion of neck will elicit flexion of knees and hips); Kernig's sign positive (limitation in angle at which a straight leg may be raised with patient supine); bulging fontanel in infants

   Encephalitis   Focal neurologic signs, aphasia, olfactory hallucinations; nuchal rigidity (if meningeal irritation); weakness, accentuated deep tendon reflexes, extensory plantar response; ataxia, spasticity, tremors; herpes encephalitis; may be a flaccid paralysis and depression of tendon reflexes with spinal cord involvement and bowel and bladder paralysis; postinfectious encephalitis: motor signs may not manifest

Fluids and Electrolytes

   Meningitis   Poor skin turgor; decreased urine output
   Encephalitis   Excess or deficient ADH secretion

Musculoskeletal

   Meningitis   Chronic meningococcemia: swelling and pain in large joints (especially knees and ankles)

Skin

   Meningitis   Meningococcemia: petechia and purpura lesions preceded by a rash resembling measles on trunk and extremities (recurring with chronic meningococcemia); large ecchymotic lesions on face and extremities in severe disease

Nursing Dx & Intervention

Risk for infection related to pathogen in CSF and respiratory secretions

- Assist in collection of CSF. Record amount and character of CSF. Administer anti-infective agents as soon as ordered *to provide for laboratory diagnosis of infectious agent and to prevent transmission.*
- Employ respiratory isolation for 24 hours after initiation of antibiotic therapy for bacterial meningitis. Treat urgently *to prevent complications of bacterial meningitis and amebic encephalitis.* Encephalitis is frequently fatal.
- Employ secretion precautions for duration of hospitalization for viral meningitis and viral encephalitis *to prevent transmission of pathogen during this highly contagious time.*
- Encourage patient contacts to be examined and immunized or treated *to prevent transmission of pathogen.*

Hyperthermia related to infection

- Monitor body temperature *to detect fever.*
- Administer antipyretics, as ordered.
- Bathe with tepid water or alcohol *to reduce high fever.*
- Adjust environmental temperature *for patient's comfort.*
- Remove excess clothing and bedding *to ensure heat loss.*
- Encourage adequate fluid intake to *compensate for fluid loss associated with elevated body temperature.*

Pain related to inflammation of meninges and brain

- Administer analgesics as prescribed. (Do not give narcotics or sedatives that will depress vital functions in patients with increased intracranial pressure.) Provide moist heat (in absence of high fever).

- Place blanket roll under knees (in absence of elevated intracranial pressure) *to relieve muscle aches and pains and to relieve pain in back and joints.*
- Darken room and provide ice pack for head *to relieve headache.*

Altered cerebral tissue perfusion related to inflammation and edema of brain and meninges

- Monitor patient carefully, particularly after lumbar puncture.
- Have patient lie flat for 4 to 6 hours or as ordered after lumbar puncture *to prevent headache associated with alterations in CSF pressure.*
- Monitor for signs of intracranial pressure throughout course of disease (e.g., slowing of pulse, increased BP, decreased level of consciousness [LOC], arrhythmic breathing, altered pupillary response, and facial weakness) *to detect signs of shock that must be reported to physician for early intervention.*
- Monitor vital signs and neurologic findings every 5 to 30 minutes for patient with intracranial pressure.
- Report changes to physician immediately. *These changes indicate alterations in intracranial pressure and necessitate early intervention.*
- Avoid bent leg positions or movement of patient; provide bed rest *to prevent increased intracranial pressure.*
- Elevate patient's head slightly. Prevent any sudden or unnecessary movements of head and neck and avoid neck flexion; use log roll to turn *to decrease intracranial pressure.*
- Assist patient with all activities and movements.
- Administer stool softeners as prescribed (avoid enemas).
- Instruct patient to exhale while turning or moving in bed.
- Position patient to avoid knee or hip flexion *to prevent muscle straining that leads to increased intracranial pressure.*
- Time nursing procedures to coincide with periods of relaxation or sedation; avoid unnecessary environmental stimuli *to prevent excitation that stimulates the already irritated brain and leads to seizures.*
- Administer hypertonic agents or steroids, as prescribed, *to lower intracranial pressure.*
- Give clear, concise explanations to confused patient; interpret environment to patient and reorient confused patient *to lessen disorientation and to clarify impaired sensory perceptions.*
- Evaluate during convalescence for motor, sensory, and intellectual impairment *to refer for rehabilitation.*

Altered peripheral tissue perfusion related to infection with meningococcus

- Monitor peripheral circulation, pulses, purpura *to detect increased vascular permeability.*

- Administer range of motion exercises to patients with no sign of elevated intracranial pressure; frequently change position *to prevent contractures and pressure on skin and to stimulate peripheral circulation.*

Ineffective breathing patterns related to altered LOC

- Monitor depth and rate of respiration, breath sounds, and blood gases *to detect altered oxygenation.*
- Oxygenate before suctioning, and limit suctioning to 10 to 15 seconds for apneic patients; employ mechanical ventilation if necessary.

Ineffective airway clearance related to altered LOC

- Continually monitor delirious or convulsive patient; maintain fully patent airway for patient with increased intracranial pressure; suction secretions; perform endotracheal care *to prevent aspiration.*

Risk for fluid volume deficit related to fever and vomiting

- Monitor intake and output, urine specific gravity, and weight loss accurately.
- Administer frequent oral or continuous IV fluids *to prevent dehydration.* (Administer IV fluids *carefully* to prevent overload if fluid retention is likely.)
- Monitor vital signs. *Decreasing BP may indicate bleeding.*

Risk for fluid volume excess related to excess secretion of ADH

- Monitor intake and output, serum electrolytes, and weight; restrict IV fluids to two thirds of needs if signs of fluid retention occur *to detect signs of fluid retention and prevent increasing intracranial pressure.*
- Test urine specific gravity. *Concentrated urine may indicate excess secretion of ADH.*
- Administer osmotic agents as prescribed *to decrease fluid overload.*

Fear related to severity of condition

- Allow patient and significant others to verbalize fears *to foster confidence in care.*
- Instruct patient and family regarding disease course, diagnostic procedures, and treatments. Inform patient that symptoms are temporary and recovery is usually complete *to relieve fear of unknown and provide a sense of comfort to patient and family.*

Risk for injury related to altered LOC

- Continually supervise patient who has convulsions or is delirious; pad bed and provide restraints for delirious patient; keep side rails up; prevent aspiration or injury during convulsions.
- Maintain quiet environment. *Excessive stimuli may induce seizures.*

Self-care deficit related to CNS alterations

- Provide all feedings and hygiene measures *to conserve energy*.
- Maintain indwelling catheter if necessary *to empty bladder of unconscious patient*.

Patient Education/Home Care Planning*

1. Inform the patient of the diagnostic procedures that may be performed:

   Neurologic assessment and eye examination

   Cultures of blood, CSF, and respiratory secretions to identify the causative organism

   Serologic tests of blood to identify viral antibodies

   Lumbar puncture to obtain spinal fluid for analysis

2. Instruct the patient to lie flat for 24 hours following lumbar puncture and to report change in symptoms.

3. Explain purposes of antibiotic therapy to patients receiving antibiotic therapy. Discuss dosage, time, rationale, route of administration, and side effects for each prescribed drug. Anti-infective therapy for bacterial meningitis must be continued as prescribed for 5 days after temperature returns to normal. Exacerbation of symptoms should be reported to the physician immediately.

4. Instruct patients who have positive sputum cultures about respiratory isolation procedures.

5. Explain to patient and family that convalescence is of variable duration, depending on the severity of the disease. Patients should allow adequate time for recovery before resuming full activities. Exacerbation of symptoms should be reported to the physician immediately.

6. Recovery is usually complete in meningitis; however, neurologic sequelae do occur. The patient should be evaluated during convalescence for functional and neurologic deficits and should participate in rehabilitation if prescribed.

7. Sequelae of encephalitis include mental deterioration, paralysis, and possible convulsive disorders, particularly in children. Families should be informed of the need for periodic evaluation and long-term physical therapy and of potential resources to help them cope with a handicapped family member.

8. Prophylactic measures should be initiated for close patient contacts. Patient contacts should be evaluated medically for early detection and treatment of bacterial meningitis.

9. Amebic meningoencephalitis can be prevented by swimming in chlorinated pools only. Mosquito-borne encephalitis can be prevented by environmental control of mosquitoes, particularly through elimination of stagnant pools of water (where mosquitoes breed), and by wearing protective clothing, screening living quarters, and using repellents.

*From Grimes.[26]

Evaluation

Patient is free of infection and complications of meningitis and encephalitis   CSF findings: <30 cells/mm³, glucose, protein, and pressures are normal; cultures are negative for bacteria; color is clear. Neurologic signs are normal. Pupils are equal and reactive to light. Neck flexion is unimpaired. Straight legs may be raised from the bed from a prone position. Abdominal, cremasteric, and tendon reflexes are normal. Patient is able to walk and perform all functions without residual weakness or impairment. No skin petechiae or purpura is present. Blood cultures are negative for bacteria. Patient is alert, responds appropriately to questions and environmental stimuli, is oriented to person and place, and has memory of recent and past events.

Infection is not transmitted to patient contacts   Hospital personnel and patient contacts are free of infection.

Body temperature is maintained within normal range; comfort and safety are maintained during fever   There is an absence of flushing, chills, and seizures. Body temperature is maintained 35.8° to 37.3° C. Vital signs are within normal limits for patient.

Relief from pain is obtained   Patient verbalizes relief, alternates periods of activity and rest, and sleeps 3 to 4 hours at a time.

Improved tissue perfusion and oxygenation are demonstrated   Vital signs are within normal limits; shock has been avoided. No petechiae or purpura is present. Patient is alert and oriented to person, place, and time and exhibits recall of recent and past events. Affect is appropriate to environmental stimuli. Adults demonstrate cognitive ability, ability to problem solve, concentration, and attentiveness.

Normal respiratory pattern and blood gases are demonstrated; secretions have not been aspirated   Breathing patterns are normal. Blood levels (O_2 saturation, CO_2 and Po_2) are normal. Skin is warm and a normal color. No signs of pneumonia are present.

Fluid and electrolyte balance is maintained   Patient shows no excessive thirst or weight loss; serum electrolytes are within normal limits. Input and output are balanced; urine specific gravity is within normal limits (1.01 to 1.025); skin turgor is good. Patient shows no restlessness or confusion.

Fear of disease and disability is reduced   Patient and significant others trust care providers, are participating in treatment, and have realistic expectations of recovery. Patient sleeps.

Activities of daily living have been performed for ill patient and will be managed after hospital discharge   Patient has not lost weight; skin is intact; urinary and bowel elimination are normal. If patient cannot manage ADLs at home, care has been arranged.

No injury is experienced   Seizures have been prevented, or no trauma has resulted from seizures.

Patient or family is aware of needs and able to use resources   Patient with a residual limitation in physical or mental function has been referred for appropriate therapy during convalescence. Family of disabled person has been given an opportunity to express concerns and has been referred for counseling and to support groups if necessary.

CHILDHOOD AND VACCINE-PREVENTABLE INFECTIOUS DISEASES

The infectious diseases presented in this section are preventable with routine immunization. Each is presented separately. An overview of all of the diseases is presented in Table 13-8.

■ CHICKENPOX

■ Chickenpox (varicella) is an acute, highly communicable viral disease common in childhood and young adulthood. It is characterized by a sudden-onset fever, mild malaise, and a skin eruption that is maculopapular for a few hours and vesicular for 3 to 4 days, leaving a granular scab.

•••••• Pathophysiology

The varicella-zoster (V-Z) virus, a herpesvirus, enters the body by way of the respiratory mucous membranes and produces systemic disease and skin lesions. The lesions are generally superficial unilocular vesicles. Lesions generally occur in successive crops with several stages of maturity present at one time. They are generally more abundant on covered areas of the body; however, they may appear everywhere including the scalp, conjunctivae, and upper respiratory tract.

Lesions have been found in the lungs, liver, spleen, adrenal glands, and pancreas. Complications include conjunctival involvement, secondary bacterial infections, viral pneumonia, encephalitis, aseptic meningitis, myelitis, Guillain-Barré syndrome, and Reye's syndrome. Disease is severe in those with deficiencies in cell-mediated immunity. After recovery the virus is believed to remain in the body in an asymptomatic latent stage, possibly localized in the dorsal root ganglia.

Reactivation of the infection with the V-Z virus can occur later in life or during time of altered immune status. It leads to the disease manifestation of herpes zoster, in which there is a localized eruption of vesicles with an erythematous base. The vesicles are restricted to the skin areas supplied by sensory nerves of a single or associated group of dorsal root ganglia.

Complications

Conjunctival ulcers
Secondary bacterial infections
Viral pneumonia
Encephalitis and meningitis
Myelitis
Guillain-Barré syndrome
Reye's syndrome

•••••• Diagnostic Studies and Findings

Microscopic examinations of specimen Electron microscopy of vesicular fluid: visualization of v-z virus during first 3 days after eruption

Giemsa-stained scrapings from lesions: multinucleated giant cells are visualized

Serology Not usually performed

•••••• Multidisciplinary Plan[3]

Medications

Acyclovir (Zovirax) or vidarabine (Ara-A) may be helpful for immunocompromised or older persons if administered early in the disease

Zoster immune globulin (ZIG) (for high-risk persons only), within 96 h of exposure

Varicella vaccine for prevention (see immunizations, p. 1164)

General Management

Relief of pruritus
Management of fever
Treatment of complications: encephalitis (see p. 1082), viral pneumonia (see Chapter 2)
Strict isolation of hospitalized patients until all lesions have crusted (see p. 1167)

NURSING CARE

Nursing Assessment

History

Exposure within past 2 to 3 weeks to person with chickenpox

Subjective Symptoms

Headache, anorexia, malaise, chills

Body Temperature

Fever: 38° to 39° C (101° to 103° F) during prodrome

Upper Respiratory Concerns

Coryza during prodrome

Skin and Mucous Membranes

Lesions in various stages of development; may have lesions on buccal mucosa, palate, or conjunctivae

Nursing Dx & Intervention

Risk for infection (patient contacts) related to virus in respiratory secretions

• Observe strict isolation of hospitalized patients until all lesions have crusted *to prevent transmission to others* (see p. 1167).

■ TABLE 13-8 Overview of Childhood and Vaccine-Preventable Infectious Diseases

	Chickenpox	Diphtheria	Mumps (Infectious Parotitis)	Pertussis (Whooping Cough)
Occurrence	Worldwide; in metropolitan areas 90% of the population has had chickenpox by age 15 yr, and 95% by young adulthood	Formerly a prevalent disease; rare in United States with immunization; affects unimmunized children under 15 yr and adults	Occurs commonly in winter and spring; one third of those exposed have subclinical infections; incidence decreasing with immunization	Common in children; worldwide; decline in incidence in areas with active immunization programs; cases increasing in United States in recent years
Etiologic agent	Varicella-zoster (V-Z) virus, a member of the *Herpesvirus* group	*Corynebacterium diphtheriae,* with many toxigenic strains	A type of paramyxovirus; antigenically related to parainfluenza viruses	*Bordetella pertussis,* the pertussis bacillus
Reservoir	Humans	Humans	Humans	Humans
Transmission	Direct and indirect contact with droplets from respiratory passages; an extremely contagious disease	Direct or indirect contact with exudate from mucous membrane lesions of infected persons or carrier; raw milk may also be a vehicle	Direct contact with saliva droplets from infected person	Direct contact with droplets from respiratory passages
Incubation period	2-3 wk; commonly 13-17 days	2-5 days; occasionally longer	12-25 days; commonly 18 days	6-20 days; commonly 7 days
Period of communicability	1-2 days before onset of rash and until lesions have crusted over (not more than 6 days after first appearance of vesicles)	Variable; until bacilli have disappeared from discharges and lesions (usually in 2 wk); a carrier may shed bacilli for 6 mo	6 days before parotid symptoms to 9 days after; most communicable 48 hr before parotid swelling	7 days after exposure to 3 wk after onset; highly communicable in early catarrhal stage before cough; not communicable after 3 wk for nonhousehold contacts even though cough may persist
Susceptibility and resistance	General; one attack confers long immunity; second attacks are rare; recurs as herpes zoster	Unimmunized children most susceptible; infants born of immune mothers have passive immunity for 6 mo; recovery from clinical disease confers temporary immunity	General; immunity is lifelong and develops after clinical and subclinical disease; placental transfer of antibodies occurs	General; nonimmunized children under 5 yr most susceptible; no passive immunity from mother, attack confers prolonged, but not lifetime immunity
Report to local health authority	Case report required in most states	Case report required	Case report required in some areas	Case report required

Data from Benenson.[3]

- Refer high-risk patient to physician for prophylactic treatment with zoster immune globulin *to lessen risk for infection.*

Impaired skin integrity related to lesions

- Bathe or encourage patient to bathe regularly *to remove exudate.*
- Apply calamine lotion or cornstarch *to relieve itching.*
- Caution patient against scratching lesions *to prevent spread of exudate and potential scarring and introduction of bacteria into lesions.*

Hyperthermia related to infection

- Monitor body temperature *to detect fever.*
- Administer antipyretics, as ordered.
- Bathe with tepid water or alcohol *to reduce high fever.*
- Adjust environmental temperature *for patient's comfort.*
- Remove excess clothing and bedding *to ensure heat loss.*
- Encourage adequate fluid intake *to compensate for fluid loss associated with elevated body temperature.*

Poliomyelitis	**Rubella (German Measles)**	**Measles (Rubeola)**	**Tetanus**
Worldwide; commonly in summer and early autumn; highest in children and adolescents but does affect nonimmune adults; U.S. incidence rare with immunization	Worldwide and endemic; most common in winter and spring; primarily a disease of children but does occur in unimmunized adolescents and adults	Worldwide; endemic and epidemic occurrences; seen more in adolescents and adults since routine immunization of children	Worldwide; occurs sporadically and affects all ages; rare in United States with immunization; common among agricultural workers, parenteral drug abusers, and elderly
Polio virus, types 1, 2, and 3; all are paralytogenic	Rubella virus	Measles virus, a type of paramyxovirus	*Clostridium tetani,* the tetanus bacillus (an anaerobic pathogen)
Humans, particularly children with subclinical infections	Humans	Humans	Intestines of humans and animals
Direct and indirect contact with respiratory discharges and feces; fecal-oral route more common than respiratory transmission	Direct or indirect contact with nasopharyngeal secretions of infected persons; transplacental transmission leads to congenital rubella syndrome	Direct or indirect contact with nasal secretions from infected persons; highly communicable	Tetanus spores enter body through a wound (usually puncture wound) contaminated with soil and feces; necrotic tissue favors the growth of the anaerobic bacillus
3-35 days: commonly 7-14 days	14-23 days: commonly 16-18 days	Commonly 10 days; 7-18 days until fever; 14 days until rash	3-21 days; commonly 10 days
Highly communicable during first days after onset of symptoms; virus is in throat secretions in 36 hr and in feces in 72 hr after infection and remains 1 wk in throat and 6 wk in feces	From 1 wk before and 4 days after appearance of rash; highly communicable; infants with congenital rubella syndrome may shed virus for months after birth	A few days before fever to 4 days after appearance of rash	Not directly transmitted
General; paralytic infections are rare and risk increases with age; infection confers long-term immunity; second attacks are result of another virus type	General; infants born with passive immunity from mother lasting 6-9 mo; one attack confers lifetime immunity for most, but reinfections (mostly asymptomatic) have been documented	General; acquired immunity from infection is permanent; artificial active immunity may not be permanent; infants, born to mothers with antibodies, retain immunity for 6-9 mo	General; recovery from tetanus does not confer permanent immunity; temporary active immunity provided by tetanus toxoid
Case report required	Case report required	Case report required in most states	Case report required

Patient Education/Home Care Planning*

1. Chickenpox is usually a benign condition with complete recovery. However, complications do occur. Report to physician any symptoms appearing during convalescence, such as a secondary rise in fever, headache, or respiratory or neurologic symptoms.
2. Chickenpox is communicable 1 to 2 days before onset of the rash until lesions have crusted over. The disease is transmitted by droplets of respiratory secretions. The incubation period is 2 to 3 weeks.
3. Avoid trauma or scratching of lesions to prevent secondary infection and scars. Daily bathing without irritating soaps is encouraged.
4. Manage fever by taking antipyretic agents and tepid sponge baths, wearing minimal clothing and maintaining a cool environment. Avoid giving children aspirin because it has been implicated in Reye's syndrome.

5. Manage itching with applications of calamine lotion or cornstarch. Avoid greasy lotions and creams. Maintain a cool environment to relieve itching associated with perspiration.
6. Encourage intake of foods and fluids as tolerated. Popsicles and soft drinks may appeal to young children.
7. Immunocompromised patient contacts should be referred to a physician for prophylactic treatment with zoster immune globulin.

*From Grimes.[26]

Evaluation

Infection has not been transmitted   Patient contacts and health personnel have not acquired chickenpox. Immunocompromised patient contacts have received zoster immune globulin.

Patient is free of secondary bacterial infection of skin and mucous membranes; skin is free of lesions and scars   Crusts are shed. Skin is warm and moist and natural color returns to skin and mucous membranes. Patient is not observed scratching lesions.

Body temperature is maintained within normal limits; comfort and safety are maintained   Body temperature is between 36° and 38° C (96.8° and 100° F) oral. Pulse and respirations are within normal limits. Skin is cool to touch and free of excess perspiration; patient's clothing and bedding are dry. Patient is free of headache and malaise associated with fever. Reye's syndrome is prevented.

■ DIPHTHERIA

Diphtheria is an acute communicable disease in which a bacterial toxin affects the mucous membranes of the respiratory tract. The disease is manifest as fibrinopurulent exudative membranes, commonly on the tonsils and pharynx but also on the larynx, nasal passages, skin, conjunctivae, and genitalia, and as systemic symptoms resulting from toxin dissemination.

•••••• Pathophysiology

Corynebacterium diphtheriae, widely available in the nasopharynx of carriers and persons with inapparent infection, invades and multiplies in the nasopharynx of susceptible persons. The pathogen produces a toxin that is disseminated by the blood and lymph throughout the body. The toxin first causes necrosis of the local tissue, resulting in a fibrinopurulent exudative membrane characteristic of this disease. The membrane appears as grayish membrane patches surrounded by a red zone of inflammation on the tonsils, pharynx, larynx, nasal mucosa, or skin. Edema is present in adjacent and underlying tissue and in the cervical lymph nodes. Laryngeal edema and the extension of the membrane into the trachea, bronchial tree, and alve-

oli may result in suffocation. Nasopharyngeal diphtheria and laryngeal diphtheria are the most severe types. Nasal diphtheria is mild and marked by one-sided nasal excoriations and discharge. Cutaneous diphtheria lesions are variable and may resemble impetigo.

Disseminated toxin inhibits protein synthesis primarily in the heart, peripheral nerves, and muscle tissue. Effects of toxin absorption appear early and include fatty degeneration, edema, and interstitial fibrosis in the myocardium and in the myelin sheath of peripheral nerves. Damage to peripheral nerves results in peripheral motor and sensory palsies. The spleen and kidneys also may be affected. Otitis media, peritonsillar abscess, and albuminuria are less severe complications. Severe toxemia may result in a life-threatening myocarditis, motor or sensory paralysis, pharyngeal and respiratory paralysis, and pneumonia.

Complications

Peripheral motor or sensory paralysis
Toxemia
Myocarditis
Pharyngeal or respiratory paralysis
Pneumonia
Diphtheria is completely preventable with active immunization (see p. 1163). No care plan is provided here because the disease is so rare today.

■ MUMPS
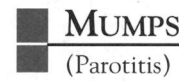
(Parotitis)

Mumps (parotitis) is an acute, communicable systemic viral disease characterized by localized unilateral or bilateral edema of one or more of the salivary glands, with occasional involvement of other glands.

•••••• Pathophysiology

The paramyxovirus invades and multiplies in the parotid gland or the superficial epithelium of the upper respiratory passages, enters the blood, and subsequently localizes in glandular or nervous tissue. Interstitial tissue edema and infiltration with lymphocytes occur in the affected gland. Cells of the glandular ducts degenerate, producing an accumulation of necrotic debris and polymorphonuclear leukocytes in the lumina, resulting in plugging of the ducts or tubules. The parotid and testes are the glands most frequently involved, but mumps may also affect the pancreas, other salivary glands, ovaries, breast, and thyroid. Testicular atrophy follows mumps orchitis, but sterility is rare. The intensity of symptoms in mumps is variable; at least 30% of infections are asymptomatic. Elevated cerebrospinal fluid protein concentrations are common even in the absence of clinical symptoms of meningoencephalitis. Glucose levels may be depressed.

Complications

Meningoencephalitis
Pericarditis

Deafness
Male sterility (rare)
Nephritis
Arthritis

•••••• Diagnostic Studies and Findings[27]

Cell cultures from saliva, urine   Saliva positive for virus up to 9 days after onset of infection; in urine up to 2 weeks after infection onset

Serology   Fourfold increase in antibody titer between acute and convalescent stages

Serum amylase determination   Elevated early in acute illness

CSF analysis   Protein: elevated; glucose: depressed

•••••• Multidisciplinary Plan

Medications

Steroids for treatment of orchitis
Analgesics for pain
Active immunization for prevention (see p. 1163)

General Management

Relief of pain with heat or cold applications
Fluid diet until patient tolerates solid food
Support of scrotum (small pillow or Alexander bandage)
Respiratory isolation of hospitalized patients for 9 days after onset of swelling (see p. 1167)

NURSING CARE

Nursing Assessment

History

Inadequate immunization for mumps; exposure within 2 to 3 weeks to person with mumps

Subjective Symptoms

Feeling hot or chilled; headache; pain in parotid glands, testes, or other glands (tender to touch); parotid pain is aggravated by eating

Body Temperature

38° to 39° C (100° to 103° F) for 3 to 4 days; higher if orchitis is present

Head and Neck

Variable parotid swelling lasting up to 1 week; severe parotid pain aggravated by eating, particularly sour substances; parotid gland (or other glands) tender to touch; hooked lobe of parotid gland (extending under ear lobe) can be palpated

Testes

Swollen and tender to touch; patient has severe pain

Breast

Inflammation and pain associated with mastitis

Abdomen

Pain from pancreatitis or oophoritis

Nursing Dx & Intervention

Risk for infection (patient) related to risk for secondary infection

- Monitor for signs indicating complications of mumps. Refer to physician *for early diagnosis and medical management.*

Risk for infection (patient contacts) related to virus in saliva

- If patient is hospitalized, employ respiratory isolation for 9 days after onset of swelling *to prevent transmission to others.*
- Ensure that patient contacts are immunized for mumps.

Pain related to glandular edema

- Administer analgesics, as prescribed, *to relieve pain.*
- Give liquid or soft diet, as prescribed, *to minimize pain with swallowing.*
- Apply warm or cold compresses, whichever is more comfortable to patient, *to relieve pain.*
- Support scrotum with small pillow or an adhesive tape bridge between the thighs (or nest of cotton for infant) *to relieve pressure on testes.*

Hyperthermia related to infection

- Monitor body temperature *to detect fever.*
- Administer antipyretics, as ordered.
- Bathe patient with tepid water or alcohol *to reduce high fever.*
- Adjust environmental temperature *for patient's comfort.*
- Remove excess clothing and bedding *to ensure heat loss.*
- Encourage adequate fluid intake *to compensate for fluid loss associated with elevated body temperature.*

Impaired swallowing related to infection in parotid gland

- Encourage liquid or soft, bland diet, as prescribed. Allow patient to drink from a straw *to minimize mouth movement, which is painful.*

Anxiety related to fear of sterility

- Inform patient that testicular atrophy does not result in impotence and that sterility is extremely rare *to allay anxiety regarding effects of orchitis.*

Patient Education/Home Care Planning*

1. Mumps is transmitted by direct contact with saliva of infected persons. It is communicable from 6 days before parotid swelling to 9 days after. Disease onset is between 2 to 3 weeks after exposure to infection.
2. Transmission of the infection to others can be prevented by handwashing and avoiding contact with respiratory secretions.
3. Mumps can be prevented by active immunization.
4. Manage fever with antipyretics, tepid sponge baths, minimal clothing, and a cool environment. Avoid chilling. Avoid giving children aspirin. Encourage intake of fluids and food as tolerated. Popsicles and soft drinks may appeal to young children.
5. Manage other symptoms with analgesics for pain, soft bland foods and liquid diet, scrotal support for testicular pain, and local application of warm or cold compresses.
6. Report the following complications to physician: headache, photophobia, hearing disturbance, stiff neck, joint pain, kidney pain, convulsions, or disturbance in gait.
7. Contacts should be referred to a physician for active immunization.
8. Convalescence is usually complete with no residual disability.

*From Grimes.[26]

Evaluation

Patient is free of infection and complications of mumps   There are no signs of glandular edema or pain. Body temperature is normal. There are no signs of complications.

Infection is not transmitted to patient contacts   Appropriate isolation procedures are implemented on hospitalized patients soon after infection is confirmed. Patient demonstrates behavior to prevent transmission of pathogens to others. Patient's contacts are adequately immunized for mumps.

Patient obtains relief from pain   Facial expression is calm and relaxed. Posture is normal. Muscles are relaxed when patient is resting and motionless. There is no pain in any glandular area. Patient has not developed distress mannerisms.

Body temperature is maintained within normal range; comfort and safety are maintained   Body temperature is between 36° and 38° C (96.8° to 100° F). Pulse and respiraton are normal. Skin is cool to touch and free of excess perspiration. Patient's clothing and bedding are dry. Patient is free of headache and malaise associated with fever.

Adequate fluid and nutrition intake is maintained; oral intake improves   Skin turgor is good. Elimination is adequate. Intake is adequate for needs.

Patient demonstrates reduction in fear of residual disability   Patient discusses any concerns about future sexual function.

■ PERTUSSIS (WHOOPING COUGH)

Pertussis (whooping cough) is an acute communicable bacterial infection of the mucous membranes of the tracheobronchial tree, characterized by paroxysms of repeated and violent coughing. Paroxysms are terminated by a prolonged, high-pitched inspiratory whoop and the expulsion of clear, tenacious mucus. This disease is most severe in children under 1 year of age and in persons living in poverty.

••••• Pathophysiology

The toxigenic *Bordetella pertussis* bacillus enters the respiratory passages by airborne droplets of respiratory secretions from persons with asymptomatic infections or with clinical disease. The organism reproduces in the mucous membranes of the trachea, bronchi, and bronchioles, producing a toxin that causes necrosis to the ciliated mucosa. There are three stages of the disease: catarrhal, paroxysmal, and convalescent. A serous exudate is produced initially in the catarrhal stage, lasting 1 to 2 weeks. This is followed by a viscid mucopurulent exudate that is irritating to the mucosa. The exudate, which is difficult to expel, initiates severe spasmodic coughing (paroxysms) that may persist for 1 to 2 months. Coughing may also be initiated by toxin stimulation to the central nervous system.

Local necrosis of the tracheal and bronchial epithelium is extensive, with an inflammatory infiltrate. Unexpelled mucous plugs may produce areas of atelectasis and emphysema. Paratracheal and bronchial lymphadenopathy may be present. Edema, congestion, and hemorrhage may occur in lung tissue, and edema and petechial hemorrhages are commonly found in brain tissue. These pathologic findings result from anoxia during the prolonged paroxysms of coughing. Paroxysms may also result in epistaxis, scleral hemorrhage, periorbital edema, vomiting, exhaustion, aspiration, and aspiration pneumonia. Also, umbilical and inguinal hernias and rectal prolapse may result from increased intra-abdominal pressure during paroxysms.

The convalescent stage is characterized by a cessation of whooping and vomiting with a gradual decrease in the number of paroxysms over a 2- to 3-week period. Some patients develop exacerbations of paroxysms of cough, whooping, and vomiting during subsequent respiratory infections.

Complications

Hernia
Rectal prolapse
Scleral hemorrhage
Secondary bacterial infection (otitis media, pneumonia)
Seizures

••••• Diagnostic Studies and Findings

Microscopic examination of stained nasopharyngeal secretions during catarrhal stage   Positive for *B. pertussis*
WBC count   Leukocytes: 15,000 to 40,000/mm³; may be as high as 175,000 to 200,000/mm³
Differential WBC count   90% lymphocytes

•••••• Multidisciplinary Plan[3]

Medications

Anti-infective agents (shortens the period of communicability but does not reduce symptoms unless given in incubation period)
  Erythromycin (Erythrocin)
Corticosteroids
  Hydrocortisone sodium succinate (Solu-Cortef)
Active immunization for prevention for those under 7 years of age (see p. 1163)
Prophylaxis for case contacts, erythromycin for 14 days

General Management

Suction of respiratory secretions
Ventilatory assistance, if needed
Oxygen administration
Parenteral fluid and electrolyte therapy
Small, frequent feedings
Postural drainage following paroxysms
Respiratory isolation for 3 weeks after onset of paroxysms or 7 days after antimicrobial therapy (see p. 1167)

NURSING CARE

Nursing Assessment

History

Inadequate immunization for pertussis; exposure to pertussis during past 3 weeks

Respiratory

Catarrhal stage: normal respirations: dry, hacking cough
Paroxysmal stage (after 1 or 2 weeks): paroxysms of cough (40 to 50 per 24 hours in severe cases), followed by high-pitched inspiratory whoop; vomiting frequently follows paroxysm
Convalescent stage: paroxysms and vomiting become gradually less frequent and prolonged

Mucous Membranes

Catarrhal stage: serous rhinorrhea, sneezing, lacrimation, conjunctivitis
Paroxysmal stage: tenacious mucus; epistaxis

Skin

Color may be cyanotic following paroxysms; loss of turgor because of dehydration

Body Temperature

Normal or low-grade fever; elevated in secondary infection

Head and Neck

Venous engorgement of face and neck during paroxysms; scleral hemorrhages and periorbital edema may be present

Neurologic

Anoxic convulsions

Activity Patterns

Exhaustion following paroxysms

Abdomen

Umbilical or inguinal hernia complications

Nursing Dx & Intervention

Risk for infection (patient) related to risk for secondary infection

- Collect nasopharyngeal specimen for examination. *Incorrect collection and handling of specimens may destroy the pathogen or contaminate the specimen with environmental organisms, interfering with accurate diagnosis and treatment. Improper handling can also contaminate the health care worker.*
- Administer anti-infective agents as soon as prescribed to prevent severe disease and death.
- Monitor temperature and respiratory status *to detect signs of secondary infection for early treatment.*

Risk for infection (patient contacts) related to pathogen in respiratory secretions

- Employ respiratory isolation for 3 weeks after onset of paroxysms or for 7 days after onset of antimicrobial therapy (see p. 1167) *to prevent transmission to health care workers, other patients, and patient contacts.*
- Refer patient contacts to physician to ensure that they are examined, treated, and immunized.
- Ensure that case of pertussis is reported to local health authority.

Ineffective airway clearance related to tenacity of mucus

- Place infant on lap with infant's head down during paroxysms *to drain secretions.*
- Suction pooled secretions if necessary *to maintain patent airway.*
- Provide moist air to *liquify secretions.*

Ineffective breathing pattern related to coughing spasms

- Assess patient's skin color and behavior *to detect symptoms of anoxia.*
- Provide oxygen by mask *to restore breathing after paroxysms.*
- Assist respiration, if necessary, *to maintain oxygen.*
- Monitor breathing for signs of atelectasis or pneumonia *to report to physician for intervention.*

Risk for fluid volume deficit related to severe vomiting and inability to swallow

- Assess skin turgor and urinary output *for signs of dehydration.*

- Give frequent, small liquid feedings or parenteral fluids if vomiting is excessive *to maintain adequate fluids.*

Activity intolerance related to coughing spasms and decreased O₂

- Provide for rest in a nonstimulating environment *to compensate for exhaustion from paroxysms.*

Risk for injury related to coughing spasms

- Provide convulsion precautions (padded bed, side rails, and tongue blade) *to prevent from trauma during convulsions.*
- Monitor for complications from excessive coughing *to report to physician for early intervention.*

Hyperthermia related to infection

- Monitor patient's body temperature *to detect fever.*
- Administer antipyretics, as ordered.
- Bathe patient with tepid water or alcohol *to reduce high fever.*
- Adjust environmental temperature *for patient's comfort.*
- Remove excess clothing and bedding *to ensure heat loss.*
- Encourage adequate fluid intake *to compensate for fluid loss associated with elevated body temperature.*

Patient Education/Home Care Planning*

1. Pertussis is transmitted by direct contact with droplets from respiratory passages. It is communicable from 7 days after exposure to 3 weeks after disease onset (highly communicable during early catarrhal stage). Disease onset is between 7 to 12 days from exposure to the infection.
2. Transmission of the infection to others can be prevented by handwashing, avoiding inhalation of respiratory secretions, and disinfecting items contaminated with respiratory secretions.
3. Pertussis can be prevented by active immunization.
4. Manage fever with antipyretics, tepid sponge baths, minimal clothing, and a cool environment. Avoid chilling. Avoid giving children aspirin. Encourage intake of fluids and food, as tolerated. Popsicles and soft drinks may appeal to young children.
5. Manage other symptoms: moist air in environment, frequent liquids and soft foods, and bed rest.
6. Report the following symptoms of complications to physician: convulsions, rise in fever, recurrence of respiratory symptoms, whooping, or vomiting.
7. Contacts should be referred to a physician for early diagnosis, treatment, and prophylaxis, with a booster dose of pertussis vaccine.
8. Convalescence is slow, with gradual cessation of whooping and vomiting over a 2- to 3-week period. Subsequent respiratory infections predispose to recurrence of symptoms.

*From Grimes.[26]

Evaluation

Patient is free of infection and complications of pertussis   Blood leukocyte count is normal. Bacterial culture is negative. Breathing patterns are normal. Body temperature is normal.

Infection is not transmitted   Patient contacts are free of infection. Children are immunized for pertussis. Infection is reported to local health department.

Airway is patent and aspiration of secretions is avoided   Patient does not aspirate secretions during paroxysms of coughing and returns to normal coughing and breathing patterns during convalescence.

Patient demonstrates normal respiratory pattern, oxygen intake, and blood gas levels   Skin, nails, lips, and earlobes are warm, with natural color. Breathing pattern, rhythm, rate, and depth are regular. Oxygen saturation, carbon dioxide, Po_2 and Pco_2 are normal.

Fluid and electrolyte balance is maintained   Skin turgor is good; secretions are thin. Urine output equals intake. Urine specific gravity is normal.

Patient achieves adequate rest and returns to preillness level of activity   Patient moves and cares for self at level of development. There is no weakness or malaise. Breathing during activity is regular.

Patient does not experience injury   Patient experiences no injury associated with seizures.

Body temperature is maintained within normal range; comfort and safety are maintained   Body temperature is between 36° and 38° C (96.8° to 100° F). Pulse and respiration are normal. Skin is cool to touch and free of excess perspiration. Patient's clothing and bedding are dry. Patient is free of headache and malaise associated with fever.

POLIOMYELITIS

Poliomyelitis is an acute communicable systemic viral disease affecting the central nervous system with variable severity ranging from subclinical infection, to a nonfebrile illness, to an aseptic meningitis, to paralytic disease, and possibly to death.

•••••• Pathophysiology

Three immunologically distinct polioviruses produce poliomyelitis, an infection that occurs 100 times more frequently in a subclinical form than in clinical disease. The polioviruses are all enteroviruses; that is, they multiply in the intestinal tract and can be recovered from the feces of cases and subclinical cases. Transmission of the virus is primarily by the fecal-oral route and sometimes by direct contact with respiratory secretions.

Once in a susceptible host, the virus multiplies in the lymphoid tissue of the throat and ileum, producing follicular necrosis. A transient viremia follows with subsequent viral invasion of the central nervous system producing cell damage primarily in the anterior horn cells of the spinal cord, in the medulla and pons, in the midbrain, and in the motor area of the precentral gyrus. Damage to the motor neurons results from destruction within the body of the cells. Damage may be reversible at this point, with complete recovery, or it may progress to necrosis and phagocytosis of the neurons, resulting in clinical disease concomitant with the extent and concentration of neuron destruction.

Clinical paralysis results when there is extensive damage to motor neurons associated with any one functional motor group. Skeletal muscle fiber groups atrophy rapidly from absence of innervation from associated destroyed motor neurons. Paralysis is characteristically asymmetric, involving the lower extremities and muscles of respiration and swallowing.

Clinical poliomyelitis may be seen in three phases: a systemic stage, a phase of central nervous system involvement, and the paralytic stage. The onset of the systemic phase is acute, with low-grade fever, headache, nausea, abdominal tenderness, occasional vomiting, and the presence of a mild tonsillitis or pharyngitis. These symptoms subside within 24 to 36 hours, and the infectious process is terminated for about 80% of patients.

A small percentage of patients manifest signs of the second phase within 1 to 4 days, with a higher fever, frontal headache, vomiting, strained anxious expression on the face, dermal hypersensitivity, and hyperhidrosis, particularly around the head and neck. The symptoms may end here or progress to the paralytic stage, with nuchal and spinal stiffness from spasm of back and hamstring muscles, positive spinal fluid findings, hypertension, and paralysis.

Paralysis may affect different parts of the body depending on the area of central nervous system damage, giving rise to the differentiation of types of paralysis as spinal, spinobulbar, bulbar, ataxic, encephalitic, or meningitic. Complications are associated with the areas of muscle paralysis or weakness and the effect on body functioning. They include intercostal and respiratory paralysis, pharyngeal, facial, and palatal paralysis, and paralysis of eye muscles and of the urinary bladder.

Complications

Motor paralysis
Poliomyelitis is completely preventable with active immunization (p. 1164). No care plan is provided here because of the rareness of this disease.

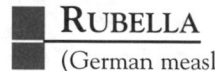

RUBELLA
(German measles)

Rubella (German measles) is a mild, febrile, highly communicable viral disease characterized by a diffuse punctate macular rash. Symptoms in the prodromal period include low-grade fever, coryza, malaise, headache, lymphadenopathy, and conjunctivitis. Infection during the first trimester of pregnancy may lead to infection in the fetus and may produce a variety of congenital anomalies: the congenital rubella syndrome.

Pathophysiology

Rubella is a usually mild disease caused by a specific virus that invades and is present in nasopharyngeal secretions, blood, urine, and feces. The virus is transmitted primarily through contact with nasopharyngeal secretions of persons with clinical and subclinical infections 7 days before to 5 days after the appearance of the rash. The virus may also be transmitted transplacentally, producing active infection in the fetus. This may result in death to the fetus or congenital damage (congenital rubella syndrome). Infants born with congenital rubella syndrome generally have the virus in their nasopharyngeal secretions, stools, and urine for up to 1 year after birth, indicating the presence of a chronic infection.

In acquired rubella the virus invades the lymph glands from the nasopharynx, producing a lymphadenopathy. It subsequently enters the blood, stimulating an immune response that is responsible for the development of the rash. Once the rash appears, the virus can no longer be found in the blood, and prodromal symptoms of a viremia subside. There may be a temporary leukopenia during acute infection. The disease is generally mild, particularly in children. Complications are rare. They include a transitory arthritis, an extremely rare encephalitis, and hemorrhagic manifestations that subside in 2 weeks. In the latter case there is a decrease in blood platelets and an increase in clotting time.

Congenital rubella syndrome is a much more serious manifestation, affecting about 25% of infants born to mothers who were infected with rubella virus during their first trimester. Infection later in the pregnancy carries a lesser risk for congenital damage. The syndrome is characterized by a variety of permanent or transitory defects including cataracts, microphthalmia, microcephaly, mental retardation, deafness, patient ductus arteriosus, arterial or ventral septal defects, congenital glaucoma, retinopathy, purpura, hepatosplenomegaly, neonatal jaundice, and bone defects. There is a high risk for death during the first 6 months, generally from congenital heart disease and sepsis.

The pathologic mechanisms producing the syndrome are not clear, but they appear to be the direct result of viral invasion and infection of developing tissue of the placenta and embryo. One hypothesis is that persistent infection with the virus may lead to mitotic arrest of cells, causing retardation in organ growth. Maternal infection may also result in placental and fetal vasculitis resulting in retarded growth of the fetus. Also, chromosomal breakage has been found in cultured cells from children with congenital rubella syndrome.

Complications

Transitory arthritis
Encephalitis
Hemorrhagic manifestations
Congenital rubella syndrome

Diagnostic Studies and Findings[3,27]

Culture of pharyngeal secretions (also blood, urine, or stool) Positive for rubella virus in pharyngeal secretions 7 days before rash in postnatal rubella; virus present up to 1 yr following birth in congenital rubella syndrome; decreasing with age

Acquired Rubella

Serology Fourfold increase in antibody titer between acute and convalescent stages indicates recent infection; one time elevated titers suggest immunity

Congenital rubella

Serology A constant IgG or IgM antibody titer within the first 6 months of life is diagnostic of congenital rubella; increase in antibody titer within 6 mo to 1 year indicates active immune response in infant

•••••• Multidisciplinary Plan

Medications—Acquired Rubella

Antipyretics for temperature control
Antibiotic treatment of otitis media, an infrequent complication
Active and passive immunization for prevention (p. 1163)

Medications—Congenital Rubella Syndrome

Treatment of sepsis
Treatment of congestive heart failure

General Management—Congenital Rubella Syndrome

Rehabilitation of children who survive infancy
Strict isolation of neonates with rubella until throat culture is free of virus

Surgery—Congenital Rubella Syndrome

Correction of various anomalies

NURSING CARE

Nursing Assessment

Acquired Rubella

History

Inadequate immunization for rubella; exposure to person with symptoms of rubella within the past 2-3 wks

Body Temperature

37° to 38° C (99° to 101° F) during 1- to 5-day prodrome in adult and adolescent; subsiding after rash appears
Elevated temperature with rash in children

Upper Respiratory

Coryza, sore throat, cough during prodrome

Head and Neck

Postauricular, postcervical, and occipital lymphadenopathy (small, shotty, and occasionally tender nodes can be palpated during prodrome and a few days after rash fades)
Mild conjunctivitis and headache possible later complication

Skin

Light pink to red, discrete macular rash, rapidly becoming papular; appearing on the first day of the rash on face and trunk and by the second day on the upper and lower extremities; rash fades within 3 days
Purpura is a rare complication, appearing several days to several weeks after the rash

Oral Cavity

Reddish spots, pinpoint or larger, on soft palate during prodrome or on first day of rash (Forchheimer spots)

Musculoskeletal

Self-limiting polyarthritis possible complication
Inflammation and pain in proximal interphalangeal and metacarpophalangeal joints of hand and knee and ankle joints (begins within 5 days of rash and persists for more than 2 weeks)

Neurologic

Symptoms of complicating encephalitis very rare; usually during first few days after rash

Congenital Rubella Syndrome

A variety of defects may be present. Some are listed here.

CNS

Encephalitis; psychomotor retardation

Head and Neck

Microencephaly; large anterior fontanelle

Cardiovascular

Patent ductus arteriosus; septal and aortic arch defects; pulmonary artery and valvular stenosis; myocardial necrosis

Eyes

Cataracts; retinopathy; corneal clouding; glaucoma

Ears

Deafness

Lungs

Interstitial pneumonitis

Hematopoietic

Anemia; hepatitis; thrombocytopenia

Skin

Purpura; jaundice

Abdomen

Inguinal hernia; hepatomegaly; splenomegaly

Lymphatic

Generalized lymphadenopathy

Skeletal

Metaphyseal rarefaction; growth retardation

Nursing Dx & Intervention

Risk for infection (patient contacts) related to virus in pharyngeal secretions

- For acquired rubella: isolate child from pregnant women. Select nursing personnel who are not at risk for rubella infection to care for patient *to prevent perinatal infections and their congenital sequelae.*
- If patient is hospitalized, employ contact isolation for 5 days after rash. For congenital rubella, employ contact isolation until three throat cultures after 3 months are free of virus *to prevent transmission of infection.*
- Ensure adequate immunization of patient contacts.
- Administer immune globulin, as indicated, for unimmunized persons exposed to rubella *to increase their resistance to these infections.*

Hyperthermia related to infection

- Monitor body temperature *to detect fever.*
- Administer antipyretics, as ordered.
- Bathe with tepid water or alcohol *to reduce high fever.*
- Adjust environmental temperature *for patient's comfort.*
- Remove excess clothing and bedding *to ensure heat loss.*
- Encourage adequate fluid intake *to compensate for fluid loss associated with elevated body temperature.*

Patient Education/Home Care Planning*

1. Rubella is transmitted by direct or indirect contact with nasopharyngeal secretions and transplacentally. It is communicable from 1 week before to 4 days after onset of rash; infants with congenital rubella may shed virus for months. Disease onset is between 14 to 23 days from exposure to the infection.
2. Transmission of the infection to others can be prevented by control of contact with respiratory secretions and by handwashing.
3. Rubella can be prevented by active immunization.
4. Manage fever with antipyretics, tepid sponge baths, minimal clothing, and a cool environment. Avoid chilling. Avoid giving children aspirin. Encourage intake of fluids and food as tolerated. Popsicles and soft drinks may appeal to young children.
5. Report the following symptoms of complications to a physician: inflammation and pain in joints, severe headache, altered consciousness, bleeding, or bruising.
6. Contacts should be referred to a physician for active or passive immunization.
7. Inform women patients that pregnant women should not be given rubella vaccine and that women should avoid pregnancy for 3 months after receiving rubella vaccine.
8. Convalescence should be uneventful.

*From Grimes.[26]

Evaluation

Patient is free of infection and complications of rubella Temperature is 37° C (98.6° F). Joints are not inflamed or tender. There are no signs of encephalitis or purpura. Lymph nodes are not palpable. Skin is free of rash. Infection has not been transmitted. Leukocyte and platelet counts and bleeding time are normal.

Infection is not transmitted Hospital personnel and patient contacts are free of infection. They are immunized for rubella or have received immune globulin.

Body temperature is maintained within normal range; comfort and safety are maintained Body temperature is between 36° and 38° C (96.8° and 100° F). Pulse and respiration are normal. Skin is cool to touch and free of excess perspiration. Patient's clothing and bedding are dry. Patient is free of headache and malaise associated with fever.

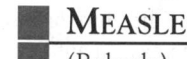

MEASLES
(Rubeola)

Rubeola (hard measles or red measles) is an acute, highly communicable viral disease manifest as a prodromal fever, conjunctivitis, coryza, bronchitis, Koplik's spots on the buccal mucosa, and a characteristic red blotchy rash. The rash appears on the third to seventh day on the face, becomes generalized, lasts 4 to 7 days, and sometimes ends in a branny desquamation.

•••••• Pathophysiology

The virus of rubeola (measles) is a paramyxovirus that can be found in the blood, urine, and pharyngeal secretions of infected persons. It is transmitted directly and indirectly through contact with respiratory secretions of infected persons during the catarrhal phase of the illness (from 4 days before to 5 days after the onset of the rash). The virus invades the respiratory epithelium and multiplies there. It spreads by way of the lymph system, producing a primary viremia. The virus then spreads in leukocytes to the reticuloendothelial system. The infected reticuloendothelial cells necrose, an increased amount of virus is released, and a reinvasion of leukocytes with a secondary viremia results. With the secondary viremia the entire respiratory mucosa becomes infected, producing upper respiratory symptoms. Edema of the mucosa may predispose to secondary bacterial invasion and complications such as otitis media and pneumonia.

Within a few days after the occurrence of generalized involvement of the respiratory tract, Koplik's spots appear on the buccal mucosa and a dermal rash develops. The virus appears to invade the cells of the epidermis and oral epithelium, producing histologic changes and stimulating a cell-mediated immune response manifested by the rash. The onset of the rash, following respiratory prodrome, coincides with the production of serum antibodies. Uncomplicated disease lasts 7 to 10 days. There are frequently leukopenia and lymphocytosis. Leukocytosis later in the disease occurs if there is a secondary bacterial infection.

Complications of measles involve the respiratory tract and central nervous system. Pneumonia may result from direct invasion of the virus or by secondary bacterial infection. Encephalitis resulting from direct viral invasion of the brain affects many persons subclinically. Gross evidence of edema, congestion, and petechial hemorrhages can be seen in the brain and spinal cord. Symptoms range from mild to severe. Many patients are left with neurologic sequelae. Rarely, a subacute sclerosing panencephalitis develops several years after infection.

Complications

Secondary bacterial infections (otitis, pneumonia)
Viral pneumonia
Encephalitis
Delayed subacute sclerosing panencephalitis

•••••• Diagnostic Studies and Findings[3,27]

Tissue culture of secretions from nasopharynx, conjunctiva, blood or urine   Positive for measles virus

Serology   Detects long-lasting antibodies; therefore useful for determining immune status; significant increase in antibodies between acute and convalescent stages is diagnostic of recent infection

Lack of antibodies indicates susceptibility

•••••• Multidisciplinary Plan

Medications

Anti-infection therapy for secondary infections only
Antipyretics for temperature control
Active immunization for prevention (p. 1163)
Passive immunization for high-risk contacts: immune globulin within 6 d of exposure

NURSING CARE

Nursing Assessment

History

Inadequate immunization status (see p. 1165 for update on assessing immunization status of those previously immunized for measles); exposure to person with measles (rubeola) during past 8 to 14 days

Subjective

Headache; feels hot or chilled

Body Temperature

Up to 40° C (104° F) during prodrome; decrease in 3 to 5 days (when rash appears)

Upper Respiratory

Hacking cough; coryza within 24 hours of fever, increasing in intensity until rash appears, gradually subsiding within 5 to 10 days

Eyes

Periorbital edema; conjunctivitis, subsiding with appearance of rash; photophobia

Head and Neck

Lymphadenopathy

Oral Cavity

Koplik's spots on buccal mucosa, most often opposite second molars; appear 2 to 4 days after onset of prodrome; resemble tiny grains of bluish white sand surrounded by inflammatory areola

Skin

Irregular macules appear on face and neck and in front of and behind the ears 3 to 4 days after onset of prodrome; rash rapidly becomes maculopapular, spreading to trunk and extremities within 24 to 48 hours; at this time it begins to fade from the face; rash is brownish pink and irregularly confluent; petechiae or ecchymoses may be present in severe cases; rash fades in 4 to 7 days, leaving a brownish desquamation; acute thrombocytopenic purpura with hemorrhage may be a complication

Neurologic

Symptoms of encephalitis, a rare complication, within 2 days to 1 week of onset of rash; secondary elevation of temperature; headaches; seizures, altered state of consciousness

Ears

Otitis media may result as a secondary infection

Abdomen

Symptoms of secondary acute appendicitis

Activity Level

Severe lethargy or prostration after onset of rash may indicate a secondary bacterial infection

Breathing Patterns

Dyspnea may indicate secondary bacterial infection

Nursing Dx & Intervention

Risk for infection (patient) related to risk for secondary infection

- Collect specimen. *Incorrect collection and handling of specimens may destroy the pathogen or contaminate the specimen with environmental organisms, interfering with accurate diagnosis and treatment. Improper handling can also contaminate health care workers.*
- Monitor systemic and local responses suggesting bacterial infection with a pathogen (elevated body temperature, localized inflammatory response, pain); report findings. *Early detection of bacterial infection and treatment with anti-infective agents may prevent dissemination of the pathogen, severe disease, and death.*

Risk for infection (patient contacts) related to virus in nasal secretions

- Initiate universal blood and body secretion precautions and other isolation procedures, as indicated. Dispose of contaminated equipment, body fluids, and dressings, as required. If patient is hospitalized, employ respiratory isolation for 4 days after onset of rash. *Isolation procedures should be initiated as soon as possible to prevent transmission to health care workers, other patients, and patient's contacts.*
- Use protective isolation procedures as indicated. Prevent patient exposure to infected visitors or staff. Limit visitors, if necessary, *to limit the exposure of patients to additional pathogens.*
- Participate in follow-up of patient contacts *to ensure that patient contacts are examined, treated, and immunized.*
- Report to the local health authority *as required by law to facilitate public health monitoring and control of outbreaks.*

Hyperthermia related to infection

- Monitor body temperature *to detect fever.*
- Administer antipyretics, as ordered.
- Bathe with tepid water or alcohol *to reduce high fever.*
- Adjust environmental temperature *for patient's comfort.*
- Remove excess clothing and bedding *to ensure heat loss.*
- Encourage adequate fluid intake *to compensate for fluid loss associated with elevated body temperature.*

Sensory-perceptual alterations (visual) related to viremia

- Assess patient for photophobia. Dim lights if photophobia is present *to prevent pain.*
- Cleanse eyelids with warm water *to remove crusts or secretions.*

Patient Education/Home Care Planning*

1. Rubeola is transmitted by direct or indirect contact with nasal secretions. Virus remains viable in air for more than 2 hours. It is communicable from a few days before fever to 4 days after appearance of rash.
2. Transmission of the infection to others can be prevented by avoidance of contact with respiratory secretions of infected persons.
3. Rubeola can be prevented by active immunization.
4. Manage fever with antipyretics, tepid sponge baths, minimal clothing, and a cool environment. Avoid chilling. Avoid giving children aspirin. Encourage intake of fluids and food as tolerated. Popsicles and soft drinks may appeal to young children.
5. Manage other symptoms: dim lights if photophobia is present; employ bed rest.
6. Report the following symptoms of complications to physician: secondary rise in fever, pain in ear, abdominal pain, nose bleeds, bruising, shortness of breath, coughing, headache, seizures, or alterations in alertness.
7. Contacts should be referred to a physician for active immunization within 72 hours of exposure or immune globulin up to 6 days after exposure.
8. Convalescence in uncomplicated disease lasts 7 to 10 days. Recovery is usually complete.

*From Grimes.[26]

Evaluation

Patient is free of infection and complications of measles Vital signs are within normal limits. Cultures of body secretions, excretions, and exudates are negative for colonized pathogens. WBC count is within normal limits. There are no signs of injury associated with complications.

Infection is not transmitted to patient's contacts Patient care staff members wash hands after providing care to each patient and follow universal blood and body secretions procedures with all patients. Appropriate isolation procedures are implemented on hospitalized patients soon after infection is confirmed. Patient or family describes transmission of pathogen, demonstrates proper procedures for handling infective materials, and demonstrates proper handwashing and other behaviors necessary to prevent transmission. All patient contacts are adequately immunized or examined and treated for infection.

Body temperature is maintained within normal range; comfort and safety are maintained Patient's body temperature is between 36° and 38° C (96.8° and 100° F). Pulse and respiration are normal. Skin is cool to touch and free of excess perspiration. Patient's clothing and bedding are dry. Patient is free of headache and malaise associated with fever.

Patient is not confused or frightened by environmental stimuli; visual function returns to normal Pupils are normal and reactive. Patient is calm and rests comfortably during acute illness. There is no startle response to environmental stimuli. During convalescence the patient correctly identifies letters on a Snellen eye chart at a distance of 20 feet.

■ TETANUS

Tetanus (lockjaw) is an acute neurointoxication induced by the tetanus bacillus growing anaerobically at the site of an injury. It is manifested as tonic rigidity and painful, intermittent tonic spasms of the masseter and cervical muscles and muscles of the trunk and extremities. Abdominal rigidity, a position of opisthotonus, generalized spasms induced by sensory stimuli, and a facial expression known as risus sardonicus are characteristic. Fatality is high.

•••••• Pathophysiology

Tetanus spores enter through a trivial or extensive injury to the skin. The anaerobic organism multiplies in the wound, even after the injury has healed, producing a lethal toxin. The toxin (tetanospasmin) reaches the central nervous system by the bloodstream or by centripetal passages along peripheral motor nerves. The toxin binds with central nervous system tissue and spinal motor ganglia. There it interferes with the release of an inhibitory transmitter and induces a hyperexcitability of motor neurons, resulting in tonic rigidity and spasms of facial, cervical, masseter, respiratory, abdominal, and extremity muscles. The bound toxin cannot be neutralized by an antitoxin.

The permanency of pathologic changes in the central and peripheral nervous system in patients who recover has not been determined. Neonatal tetanus generally leaves no permanent neurologic sequelae. Central nervous system findings in fatal cases range from mild congestion to definite hemorrhage, areas of demyelination, gliosis, and tissue necrosis in the cerebral hemispheres.

Complications

Pathologic changes in other parts of the body result from anoxia caused by respiratory impairment, asphyxial convulsions, toxic degeneration, and inanition. Pulmonary complications are frequent in tracheotomized patients. Changes in striated muscles such as hemorrhage and rupture also occur throughout the body. The risk for further pathologic change increases with duration of the disease. Cardiac, pulmonary, and musculoskeletal complications are common.

Tetanus is completely preventable with active immunization and passive immunization for wound management (see p. 1163). No care plan is provided here because of the rareness of this condition.

GASTROINTESTINAL INFECTIOUS DISEASE

A wide range of gastrointestinal (GI) infectious diseases are caused by pathogens that are ingested in contaminated food or water or by contact with feces from an infected person.

The following are presented in three sections:
1. Food poisoning caused by pathogens that have already multiplied in the food at the time of ingestion:
   Staphylococcal food poisoning
   Botulism
   Food poisoning: enteric infections
       Bacillus cereus
       Clostridium perfringens
       Vibrio parahaemolyticus
2. Acute gastroenteritis produced by bacteria and viruses that multiply in the gastrointestinal tract after ingestion:
   Campylobacter
   Escherichia coli
   Shigella
   Norwalk virus
   Rotavirus
3. *Salmonella* gastroenteritis (salmonellosis)

■ FOOD POISONING

Food poisoning is the generic term applied to illnesses acquired through consumption of food or water contaminated with chemicals, bacteria and bacterial toxins, or organic poisons naturally present in some edible substances.

The food poisonings caused by bacteria and bacterial toxins are discussed here. In all cases disease is produced in the host shortly after ingestion of food containing bacteria that have already multiplied in the food. These diseases are not directly communicable. If the bacteria have produced a toxin in the food, the resulting disease in the host is intoxication, as in staphylococcal food poisoning and botulism. If the bacterial cells are antigenic, they produce an infection in the host, such as those caused by *Clostridium perfringens* and *Vibrio parahaemolyticus* (Table 13-9).

■ STAPHYLOCOCCAL FOOD POISONING

Staphylococcal food poisoning is an enteric intoxication of acute onset. Symptoms are severe nausea, intestinal cramps, vomiting, diarrhea, prostration, and occasionally subnormal temperature and hypotension. The intensity of the disease depends on the quantity of the ingested toxin and host susceptibility. The duration of the illness is 1 to 2 days, and recovery is generally complete.

•••••• Pathophysiology

The ingested enterotoxin acts on the abdominal viscera, creating a sensory stimulus that reaches the vomiting center of the brain by way of the vagus and sympathetic nerves. The action of the enterotoxin on the gastric mucosa produces a patchy hyperemia, erosions, petechiae, and a purulent gastric exudate. Diarrhea results from inhibition of water absorption from the intestinal lumen and from increased transport of fluid into the lumen.

Complications

Dehydration—particularly in infants and older adults
Prostration—particularly in infants and older adults

■ BOTULISM

Botulism is a severe neurointoxication with a wide range of neurologic symptoms and severity of symptoms. In the United States 10% of cases under treatment result in death, primarily from respiratory failure. Three types of botulism have been recognized: foodborne, wound, and infant botulism.

•••••• Pathophysiology

Clostridium botulinum, a spore-forming anaerobe capable of withstanding boiling, produces a potent toxin in anaerobic conditions. A common source of botulinal toxin is improperly

▪ TABLE 13-9 Overview of Food Poisonings

	Staphylococcal Food Poisoning	Botulism	*Clostridium Perfringens*	*Vibrio Parahaemolyticus*	*Bacillus Cereus*
Occurrence	Widespread and frequent: one of the principal acute food poisonings in the United States	Worldwide; sporadic; family-grouped cases occur	Widespread and frequent in countries with cooking practices that favor growth of organism	Sporadic cases and outbreaks occur in warm months of the year	Worldwide; rare in the U.S.
Etiologic agent	Several enterotoxins of staphylococci; stable at boiling temperature	Toxins produced by *Clostridium botulinum* in anaerobic conditions; destroyed by boiling	Type A strains of *C. perfringens (C. welchii)*	*V. parahaemolyticus* (many types)	*B. cereus,* an aerobic spore former that produces two enterotoxins—one heat stable, causing vomiting, and one heat labile, causing diarrhea
Reservoir	Humans; cows with infected udders; dogs and fowl	Soil, marine sediments, and intestinal tract of animals and fish	Soil and gastrointestinal tract of humans and animals	Marine silt, coastal waters, fish, and shellfish	Soil; commonly found in raw, dried, and processed foods
Transmission	Ingestion of food containing staphylococcal toxin, which formed while food was held at room temperature	Ingestion of food in which toxin has formed; generally home-canned vegetables, fruits, and meats; also onions and potatoes cooked and held at room temperature	Ingestion of food, especially meat, contaminated by soil or feces; spores survive normal cooking temperatures, germinate, and multiply during cooking and reheating	Ingestion of raw or undercooked contaminated seafood; food contaminated with seawater and by handling seafood.	Ingestion of food that has been kept at ambient temperatures after cooking, permitting multiplication of the organism
Incubation period	30 min to 8 hr; usually 2-4 hr	12-36 hr	6-24 hr; usually 10-12 hr	4-96 hr; usually 12-24 hr	1-6 hr for disease causing vomiting; 6-24 hr for disease causing diarrhea
Period of communicability	Noncommunicable	Noncommunicable	Noncommunicable	Noncommunicable	Noncommunicable
Susceptibility and resistance	General; no immune response	General; no immune response	General; no resistance develops from exposure	General	Unknown
Report to local health authority	Prompt report of outbreaks	Report of cases and outbreaks	Prompt report of outbreaks	Report outbreaks	Report cases and outbreaks

Data from Benenson.[3]

processed canned foods. Less commonly, *C. botulinum* enters the body through a wound and produces toxin in traumatized, necrotic tissue. Ingestion of *C. botulinum* spores does not result in toxin production in adults and children but does cause toxin production in the bowel lumen of some infants, producing infant botulism.

The botulinal toxin is hematogenously disseminated to peripheral cholinergic synapses, where it becomes irreversibly bound. This action blocks the release of acetylcholine, producing impaired autonomic and voluntary neuromuscular transmission and muscular paralysis. Gradual recovery occurs over a period of weeks from the regeneration of terminal motor neurons to reinnervate noncontracting muscle fibers.

Intestinal stasis predisposes to the colonization of any ingested viable spores of *C. botulinum.* Additional toxin is produced in vivo, prolonging the course of the disease.

Complications

Complications in hospitalized patients with botulism are similar to those affecting other critically ill paralyzed persons who depend on mechanical support to sustain life, including death from respiratory failure.

FOOD POISONING: ENTERIC INFECTIONS

The three enteric infections discussed here are all caused by ingestion of food contaminated with specific bacteria that have already multiplied in the food. Disease occurs in the host shortly after ingestion of the food and manifests as symptoms of gastroenteritis.

C. perfringens generally causes a mild intestinal infection characterized by sudden onset of abdominal colic, nausea, and diarrhea. Fever and vomiting are rare.

V. parahaemolyticus is a moderately severe intestinal infection characterized by sudden-onset abdominal cramps and watery diarrhea lasting 1 to 7 days. Nausea, vomiting, fever, and headache may be present.

B. cereus food poisoning is a gastrointestinal infection characterized by sudden-onset nausea and vomiting or colic and diarrhea, lasting no longer than 24 hours.

•••••• Pathophysiology

C. perfringens, a spore former widely distributed in feces, soil, and water, multiplies rapidly in foods that have been cooled and reheated. The organism produces an enterotoxin in the intestinal tract within 6 to 24 hours after ingestion. The enterotoxin acts on the epithelial layer of the ileum, increasing the secretion of sodium, chloride, and fluid, and inhibiting the absorption of glucose.

V. parahaemolyticus multiplies in uncooked, contaminated seafood. When ingested, the pathogen directly invades intestinal tissue to produce necrosis, ulceration, possible hemorrhage, and granulocytic infiltration of the mucosa. Disease intensity ranges from asymptomatic to severe; duration ranges from 2 hours to 10 days.

The spores of *B. cereus* survive cooking and multiply in food held at room temperature. One type of enterotoxin that is heat stable attacks the gastric mucosa. Another type, which is heat labile, affects the intestinal mucosa. Thorough reheating of food destroys the heat-labile enterotoxin but not the enterotoxin that causes vomiting.

Complications

Dehydration, particularly in infants and older adults
Prostration, particularly in infants and older adults

•••••• Diagnostic Studies and Findings[3]

Culture of stomach contents, feces, or suspected food 10^5 enterotoxin-producing staphylococci per gram of specimen, positive for *C. botulinum;* $>10^5$ spores of *C. perfringens* or *B. cereus* per gram of specimen; or positive for *V. parahaemolyticus*

Serum Positive for botulinal toxins; circulating toxins found in about one third of hospitalized patients with botulism

•••••• Multidisciplinary Plan

Medications for Botulism

Trivalent (ABE) botulinal antitoxin (not used for infants) administered IV as soon as possible after onset of symptoms; obtained from CDC
Anti-infective agents
　　Penicillin for wound botulism; agent-specific, anti-infective agents for secondary bacterial infection

General Management

For botulism
　　Gastric lavage initially
　　Mechanical ventilation in the event of respiratory paralysis
　　Suction of secretions
　　Intubation of tracheostomy
　　Nasogastric feedings
　　IV fluid and electrolytes
　　Must be reported to local health authority immediately
　　All patient contacts known to have eaten the same food should have gastric lavage, high enemas, and cathartics and should be kept under close medical supervision
For staphylococcal poisoning and enteric infection
　　Oral fluids if tolerated; IV fluids and electrolytes if needed

NURSING CARE

Nursing Assessment

Assessment	Staphylococcal Food Poisoning	Botulism	Enteric Infections
History	May have eaten within past 7 hours at a picnic or large gathering where food has been sitting unrefrigerated	Consumption of home-canned food within past 36 hours	Ingestion within past 24 hours of high-risk food (e.g., raw seafood or cooked meat dishes held at room temperature)
Subjective symptoms Gastrointestinal	Weakness; prostration Acute-onset nausea, vomiting, intestinal cramps, and diarrhea	Vertigo and neurologic symptoms Vomiting, diarrhea, and constipation	Nausea and abdominal pain Acute-onset nausea, abdominal cramping, and diarrhea in *C. perfringens* infections Diarrhea may be watery and bloody and persist up to 7 days in *V. parahaemolyticus* infections Acute-onset nausea and vomiting or colic and diarrhea in *B. cereus* infections

Assessment	Staphylococcal Food Poisoning	Botulism	Enteric Infections
Vital signs	Subnormal temperature; hypotension	Normal	Usually normal
Head and neck		Abrupt onset, bilateral and symmetric: ptosis, blurred vision, diplopia, dry mouth, dysphagia, dysphonia, dysarthria, and nasal regurgitation	
Respiratory		Paralysis of muscles of respiration	
Large muscles		Symmetric flaccid paralysis; motor disturbances but no sensory disturbances	

Nursing Dx & Intervention

Fluid volume deficit related to vomiting and diarrhea

- Monitor fluid and electrolyte balance, intake and output, urine specific gravity, moisture of skin and mucous membranes, skin turgor, frequency of vomiting and diarrhea, vital signs, and weight loss. *Fluids, sodium, and potassium lost through diarrhea and vomiting must be replaced.*
- Encourage small amounts of oral fluids as tolerated. Administer IV fluids and electrolytes as prescribed *to maintain adequate intake and replace those lost in vomitus and diarrhea.*

Diarrhea related to pathogens and toxins in the intestinal tract

- Collect fecal specimen. *Incorrect collection and handling of specimens may destroy the pathogen or contaminate the specimen with environmental organisms, interfering with accurate diagnosis and treatment. Improper handling can also contaminate the health care worker.*
- Monitor frequency and characteristics of stool *to detect complications.*
- Provide air circulation and room deodorization.
- Wash hands and lubricate anal opening frequently *to prevent skin irritation.*

For botulism: ineffective airway clearance related to neurologic effects of botulinal toxins

- Monitor cough and gag reflexes *to detect and report loss of patency of airway.*
- Suction secretions *to prevent aspiration.*
- Have tracheostomy tray available for emergency use. Provide tracheostomy care *to maintain patent airway.*

Impaired swallowing related to neurologic effects of toxins

- Assess ability to swallow *to prevent aspiration of oral fluids or food.*
- Administer nasogastric tube feeding or alimentation as prescribed; offer frequent, small oral feedings as patient tolerates *to maintain adequate intake.*

Ineffective breathing pattern related to neurologic effects of toxins

- Monitor for signs of respiratory paralysis and oxygen insufficiency; initiate mechanical ventilation and oxygen as prescribed *to assist breathing; to ensure adequate oxygen intake.*
- Monitor patient on respirator for signs of hyperventilation or hypoventilation *to prevent or detect early signs of respiratory acidosis or alkalosis.*

Impaired physical mobility related to neurologic effects of toxins

- Position in proper body alignment *to prevent contractures and foot drop.*
- Assist with range of motion exercises *to prevent joint stiffness.*
- Turn every 2 hours *to prevent skin pressure sores and pooling of secretions.*
- Provide total hygienic care as needed *to prevent skin breakdown.*

Sensory/perceptual alterations (visual) related to neurologic effects of toxins

- Interpret environment and stimuli for patient whose vision is altered *to minimize injury.*
- Explain that condition is not permanent *to relieve fear associated with vision changes.*
- Minimize stimuli *to prevent confusion.*

Impaired verbal communication related to neurologic effects of toxins

- Anticipate patient's needs and provide necessary care. Explain that loss of speech is not permanent *to relieve anxiety of patient who cannot communicate.*

Patient Education/Home Care Planning*

Provide patient with the following instructions:
1. These conditions are transmitted by contaminated food and can be prevented by proper food handling.
2. Cooked foods should not be held at room temperature; they should be kept hot (140° F) or should be refrigerated. Reheating should be done rapidly and completely.

3. All seafood should be cooked at a temperature above 60° C (140° F) for 15 minutes.

4. Keep all seafood, raw or cooked, adequately refrigerated before eating.

5. Handle cooked seafood to avoid its contamination with raw seafood or with contaminated seawater.

6. All persons should wash hands thoroughly following defecation and before handling food.

7. Destroy all canned food and containers from same batch that contained the *C. botulinum* by burying deep in soil or boiling 3 minutes before discarding. Commercial canned foods should be submitted for laboratory examination. Contaminated cooking utensils should be sterilized by boiling for 3 minutes before reuse.

8. No questionable canned food should ever be tasted. Foods containing *C. botulinum* do not necessarily have "off" odors or a spoiled taste.

9. Recommended processing times and temperatures for home canning must be followed to ensure killing of all *C. botulinum* spores. This information is available through state agricultural extension services.

10. Home-canned vegetables and meats should be boiled for 3 minutes to destroy botulinal toxin.

11. Honey must not be given to infants under 1 year of age.

12. Fluids should be encouraged and food may be eaten when tolerated.

13. Report the following symptoms of complication to a physician: vomiting and diarrhea persisting beyond 1 to 2 days; alteration in consciousness; loss of skin turgor, particularly in infants and children; fever; absence of urination; and severe prostration.

14. Explain that food poisonings are self-limiting.

*From Grimes.[26]

Evaluation

Fluid and electrolyte balance is maintained   Patient's skin turgor is good. Urine output equals intake. Urine specific gravity is normal. Measurements of sodium, potassium, chloride, magnesium, and calcium in blood are normal.

Patient returns to normal pattern of bowel elimination   Patient's stools are soft, formed, and normal colored. Abdomen soft; bowel sounds normal. Patient tolerates regular diet. Weight returns to normal. Stool specimens are negative for any pathogen.

Patient has information to prevent further episodes of food poisoning   Patient discusses proper food-handling practices to prevent contamination of food.

Airway is patent and aspiration of secretions is avoided   Patient's airway is open. Secretions are thin and easily coughed up by patient. Patient swallows without difficulty. Breathing is quiet.

Adequate fluid and nutrition intake is maintained   Patient's skin turgor is good; secretions are thin. Urine output equals intake. Weight loss is avoided. Energy improves and patient eats regular diet during convalescence.

Patient demonstrates normal respiratory pattern, oxygen intake, and blood gas levels   Patient's respiratory rate is normal. Respirations are of normal depth. There is no dyspnea. Skin and mucous membranes are warm and moist with normal color. O_2 saturation, CO_2, Po_2 and Pco_2 are normal.

Patient maintains function, comfort, and skin integrity and demonstrates increasing strength and movement   Patient moves extremities and changes position in bed. During convalescence, patient sits, stands, and walks without signs of contractures, foot drop, or pain.

Patient is not confused or frightened by environmental stimuli; visual function returns to normal   There are no startle responses to environmental stimuli. During convalescence, the patient correctly identifies letters on a Snellen eye chart from a distance of 20 feet. Pupils are normal and reactive.

Patient communicates needs; speech returns to normal   Health care workers and visitors respond to patient's nonverbal cues. Patient speaks audibly during convalescence.

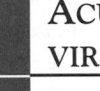

ACUTE BACTERIAL AND VIRAL GASTROENTERITIS

Many forms of acute gastroenteritis are caused by ingestion of food and water contaminated with pathogenic agents or by fecal-oral transmission directly or indirectly from an infected person. These infections differ from the food poisonings previously discussed in the following ways:

The pathogenic agents causing these diseases invade, colonize, and multiply in the human intestinal tract.

The incubation periods are slightly longer, ranging from 1 day to several weeks.

Direct and indirect fecal-oral transmission is possible.

Acquired immunity of varying duration results from many of these infections.

In addition, the predominant manifestation of these diseases is acute-onset diarrhea of varying intensity and duration. The bacterial- and viral-caused gastroenteritises discussed here are usually self-limited diseases (Table 13-10). This is not a complete list of all pathogens causing diarrhea.

Campylobacter enteritis is an acute bacterial enteric infection lasting from 1 to 10 days and is considered to be an important cause of "traveler's diarrhea." Prolonged illness may occur.

Escherichia coli diarrhea is an acute infection of the colon. Disease is severe or mild depending on whether the strain of *E. coli* causing disease is enterohemorrhagic, enterotoxigenic, enteroinvasive, or enteropathogenic.

Shigellosis (bacillary dysentery) is an acute bacterial infection of the large intestine with severity ranging from asymptomatic infection to fulminating diarrheal disease and death.

Epidemic viral gastroenteritis is usually a self-limited, mild gastric and intestinal infection lasting 24 to 48 hours. Disease often occurs in outbreaks.

■ **TABLE 13-10 Overview of Acute Bacterial and Viral Gastroenteritis**

	Campylobacter Enteritis	*Escherichia coli* Diarrhea	Shigellosis (Bacillary Dysentery)	Epidemic Viral Gastroenteritis	Rotavirus Gastroenteritis
Occurrence	Worldwide; common-source outbreaks occur; highest in warmer months; common cause of "travelers' diarrhea"	Worldwide; common-source-outbreaks occur; high in areas of poor sanitation and during warm months	Worldwide; highest in children under 10 yr old; outbreaks common in crowded living conditions, day care	Worldwide and common; epidemics and outbreaks occur; affects infants and adults	Worldwide; sporadic and in outbreaks; highest in infants and young children
Etiologic agent	*Campylobacter jejuni* and *C. coli*	Enterohemorrhagic (EHEC) Enterotoxigenic, invasive, or enteropathogenic strains of *E. coli*	Four different groups of *Shigella* bacteria, with many strains	Many viruses; Norwalk virus most common	Many types of rotaviruses
Reservoir	Domestic and wild animals and birds	Humans, who are often asymptomatic; cattle	Humans	Humans	Humans; pathogenicity of animal viruses undetermined
Transmission	Ingestion of water, food, or raw milk contaminated with organism from feces; contact with infected animals or infants; fecal-oral	Ingestion of food, including undercooked beef, water and baby formula contaminated with feces; transmitted to infant during delivery; fecal-oral, by hand	Direct or indirect fecal-oral transmission from infected person or carrier, usually by hand	Fecal-oral route; foodborne and waterborne transmission	Fecal-oral; possibly fecal-respiratory
Incubation period	2-5 days; range: 1-10 days	Enterohemorrhagic: 3-8 days (usually 3-4) Enterotoxigenic: 10 hrs-72 hr Enteroinvasive: 10-18 hr Enterpathogenic: 9-12 hr	12-96 hr; usually 1-3 days	Usually 24-48 hr; range: 10-50 hr	24-72 hr
Period of communicability	Several days to weeks throughout course of infection; usually 2-7 wk; carriers are rare	Duration of fecal excretion of organism, possibly weeks	During acute infection to 4 wk after illness; carrier state may persist for months	During acute stage and up to 48 hr after diarrhea stops	During acute stage and as long as virus is shed (up to 30 days)
Susceptibility and resistance	General; immune mechanisms not understood	Infants very susceptible; travelers to developing countries; duration of acquired immunity unknown	General; more severe in children and elderly and debilitated individuals; strain-specific antibodies develop	General; short-term (14 wk) immunity may follow infection with specific serotypes	By age 3 yr most individuals have acquired antibodies against most serotypes
Report to local health authority	Report cases	Report epidemic only	Report cases	Report epidemic only	Report epidemic only

Data from Benenson.[3]

Rotavirus gastroenteritis is a sporadically occurring gastric and intestinal infection of infants and young children ranging in severity from asymptomatic to severe disease and occasionally to death.

••••• Pathophysiology

Bacterial and viral agents that produce gastroenteritis produce pathologic conditions in one of four ways:

Toxigenic agents, such as some *Shigella* strains and enterotoxigenic *E. coli*, release an enterotoxin that acts on the small intestine to produce a local inflammation and a secretory diarrhea with rapid loss of electrolytes.

Invasive pathogens, such as *Shigella, Campylobacter,* and invasive strains of *E. coli,* penetrate the small or large intestine, producing cellular destruction, necrosis, and potential ulceration. The diarrheal stools in these conditions frequently contain leukocytes and erythrocytes.

Some pathogens, such as the rotaviruses and enteropathogenic *E. coli,* attach to the mucosal epithelium without invasion. They destroy cells of the intestinal villi, resulting in malabsorption of electrolytes and the potential for electrolyte imbalance.

Enterohemorrhagic strains of *E. coli* elaborate a toxin that can cause severe intestinal hemorrhage and, if absorbed, produces hemolytic uremic syndrome and thrombotic thrombocytopenic purpura.

The general effect of all of the above pathologic conditions is to increase gastrointestinal motility and to increase the secretory rate of fluids and electrolytes into the intestines. The result may be rapid dehydration, electrolyte imbalance, circulatory failure, and death. Fluid and electrolyte loss in other forms of gastroenteritis may develop more gradually or may not occur at all. Infants, small children, and debilitated individuals are at greater risk for severe dehydration.

The attachment of the pathogens to the mucosa may be altered by nonspecific resistance factors in the host:

The normal bacterial flora of the intestinal tract prevents attachment by competing for attachment sites or by production of volatile organic acids. If the normal flora is diminished as a result of antibiotic therapy or malnutrition, this host defense is ineffective.

The pH of the gastrointestinal tract impedes the growth of some microbes. Altering the pH through the ingestion of antacids reduces the effectiveness of this defense.

Normal gastrointestinal motility purges the intestinal tract of many pathogens, and interference with this function increases the risk for invasion of pathogens.

Specific immune responses of varying duration occur in the host following infection with *Shigella,* parvovirus-like agents, rotavirus, and *E. coli.*

Complications

Dehydration
Electrolyte imbalance
Circulatory failure and death

••••• Diagnostic Studies and Findings[27]

Diagnosis of these conditions relies on culture, isolation, and identification of the pathogen in a fecal specimen or a specimen obtained by a rectal swab.

Direction examination of bacterial colonies on plated agar media Used for identification of *Campylobacter, E. coli,* and *Shigella.*

Microscopic examination Visualization of motile *Campylobacter;* visualization of pus cells associated with shigellosis.

Biochemical tests to differentiate bacterial species

Serotyping differentiates serotypes of *E. coli* and *Shigella* spp.

Immunologic techniques that utilize antibody/antigen reactions applied to a specimen to identify rotavirus and Norwalk virus

Immunoelectron microscopy Used to identify Norwalk virus

••••• Multidisciplinary Plan[3]

Medications

Agents that suppress intestinal motility are not given for bacterial gastroenteritis
For shigellosis
    Anti-infective agents
    Trimethoprim-sulfamethoxazole (Septra, Bactrim), ciprofloxacin or ofloxacin
For *E. coli* diarrhea caused by entertoxigenic and enteroinvasive strains
    Anti-infective agents
        Trimethoprim-sulfamethoxazole or doxycycline, or ciprofloxacin or norfloxacin
Treatment for EHEC has not been determined

General Management

IV fluids and electrolyte replacement
For shock: rapid infusion of 20 to 30 ml/kg of Ringer's lactate, isotonic saline, or similar isotonic solution given within an hour
For complete rehydration after circulation is restored: glucose electrolyte solution (oral or IV hypotonic electrolyte solutions in amounts equal to estimated fluid loss)

NURSING CARE

Nursing Assessment

History

Travel to another country; ingestion of questionable food or water during past week; eating food contaminated by person with diarrheal disease during past week; eating undercooked beef

Subjective

Myalgia, headache, malaise, prostration

Gastrointestinal

Campylobacter: Days 1 and 2: nausea, vomiting, abdominal pain; days 2 to 4 (maybe 10): foul-smelling or liquid diarrhea; sometimes 20 to 30 stools per day; blood in stools after day 4; day 7: ulcerative colitis may occur

E. coli diarrhea: Day 1: vomiting; day 2 (lasting 7 to 10 days): mucous and bloody diarrhea or profuse watery diarrhea without blood or mucus

Infection with EHEC presents with bloody diarrhea, progressing rapidly to circulatory collapse and death

Shigellosis: Day 1: nausea, abdominal pain, colic, vomiting, painful diarrhea; days 2 to 5: stools contain blood, pus, and mucus; rectal irritation and tenesmus

Epidemic viral gastroenteritis: Day 1 (lasts 24 to 48 hours): nausea, vomiting, diarrhea, abdominal pain

Rotavirus gastroenteritis: Day 1: vomiting for 48 hours; days 2 to 8: watery diarrhea; rectal bleeding may occur

Fluids and Electrolytes

Campylobacter: anytime during disease: poor skin turgor, dry mucous membranes, faint pulse, hypotension

E. coli diarrhea: anytime during disease: poor skin turgor, dry mucous membranes, faint pulse, hypotension

Shigellosis: days 2 to 5: loss of turgor, oliguria, hypotension, weak pulse, shock

Epidemic viral gastroenteritis: usually no alteration in fluid balance

Rotavirus gastroenteritis: days 2 to 8: severe dehydration possible

Body Temperature

Campylobacter: 38° to 41° C (100° to 105° F); febrile convulsions

E. coli diarrhea: low-grade fever on day 1 or 2

Shigellosis: days 1 to 5: 38° to 41° C (101° to 105° F)

Epidemic viral gastroenteritis: low-grade fever

Rotavirus gastroenteritis: day 1: usually low-grade fever (up to 39° C [102° F])

Respiratory

Rotavirus gastroenteritis: pharyngeal exudate, cough, and rhinitis

Nursing Dx & Intervention

Risk for fluid volume deficit related to vomiting and diarrhea

- Monitor for symptoms of dehydration and electrolyte imbalance (e.g., oliguria and loss of skin turgor) *to detect early signs of dehydration for early intervention.*
- Measure all fluid output (emesis, urine, and diarrhea); measure all intake *to determine if intake compensates for output.*

- Monitor blood pressure, temperature, pulse, and respirations *to detect symptoms of circulatory collapse early.*
- Administer liquids frequently as tolerated *to maintain adequate intake.*
- Administer electrolytes as prescribed *to replace those lost during diarrhea.*
- Provide patient with oral glucose electrolyte solution as soon as patient can take oral fluids. *Oral fluids can usually be tolerated once electrolyte balance is corrected.*
- Gradually add clear fluids and soft foods (milk and cream products should be avoided at first; apple juice and clear soda [7-Up] are usually well tolerated). *Clear carbohydrates (fluids and foods) are easier to tolerate with nausea.*

Diarrhea related to pathogenic activity in GI tract

- Obtain stool specimens for culture *to identify pathogen.*
- Measure watery diarrhea output *to estimate rapidity of fluid loss.*
- Cleanse perianal area and lubricate after each diarrheal stool *to prevent irritation of skin.*
- Provide adequate air circulation, room deodorization, and privacy *to control odors and prevent embarrassment.*

Hyperthermia related to infection

- Monitor temperature *to detect fever.*
- Sponge with tepid water *to reduce temperature.*

Risk for infection (patient contacts) related to presence of pathogen in stool

- Collect fecal specimen. *Incorrect collection and handling of specimens may destroy the pathogen or contaminate the specimen with environmental organisms, interfering with accurate diagnosis and treatment. Improper handling of specimens can also contaminate the health care worker.*
- Use enteric precautions until three fecal cultures are negative for infecting *Shigella* organism; use enteric precautions for duration of illness for others *to prevent transmission to health care workers, other patients, and patient contacts.*
- Report shigellosis to local health authority; *reporting is required by law to facilitate public health monitoring and control of outbreaks.*

Patient Education/Home Care Planning*

Provide patient with the following instructions:
1. These conditions are transmitted by food or water contaminated with organisms from feces of infected person.
2. They are communicable while the organisms are in the feces (usually from onset of diarrhea until up to 7 weeks).
3. Disease onset is between 1 to 7 days from exposure to the infection.

4. Transmission of the infection to others can be prevented by thorough handwashing before eating and after bowel movements, changing diapers, or handling feces.
5. For patients cared for at home, teach the family:
   Signs of dehydration and the importance of prompt medical attention should dehydration occur
   Measurement of intake and measurement or estimation of output
   Maintenance of oral fluid intake equal to output
   Types of clear, high-glucose oral fluids that may be tolerated (apple juice; mildly carbonated beverages, such as 7-Up)
   Scrupulous handwashing; avoidance of food contamination
6. Persons with *Shigella* infections should not be permitted to handle food or provide child care until two successive fecal samples or rectal swabs are free of *Shigella* organisms.
7. Child day-care programs should provide for:
   Frequent handwashing of workers
   Separate areas for food preparation and diaper changing
   Separate rooms for children of different age groups
   Routine exclusion of children with diarrhea
8. Most acute gastroenteritis can be prevented by:
   Thorough handwashing after toileting, handling feces, or contact with animals
   Thorough cooking of all food derived from animals, and avoidance of recontamination within the kitchen after cooking
   Using pasteurized milk and chlorinated water
   Maintaining food at hot or cold temperatures
9. Report the following symptoms of complications to physician:
   Dry mucous membranes, loss of skin turgor, listlessness or change in level of consciousness, or absence of urination
   Continuation of diarrhea or blood in urine or stool
   Increase in colic or pain
   Increase in fever or convulsions
10. Food supplies should be protected from fly contamination. Travelers to areas when the water supply is not chemically treated or protected from sewage contamination should boil all water used in cooking, drinking, or making ice.

*From Grimes.[26]

Evaluation

Fluid and electrolyte balance is maintained Blood pressure and pulse are normal. Skin turgor is good. Mucous membranes are moist. Urine output is equal to intake. Blood levels of sodium, potassium, chloride, magnesium, and calcium are normal. Urine specific gravity is normal. Secretions are thin.

Patient returns to normal pattern of bowel elimination Stools are soft, formed, and brown. Abdomen is not distended. There is no cramping.

Body temperature is within normal range; comfort and safety are maintained Body temperature is between 36° and 38° C (96.8° and 100° F). Pulse and respiration are normal. Skin is cool to touch and free of excess perspiration. Patient's clothing and bedding are dry. Patient is free of headache and malaise associated with fever.

Infection is not transmitted to patient's contacts Patient care staff members wash hands after providing care to each patient and follow universal blood and body secretion procedures with all patients. Appropriate isolation procedures are implemented soon after infection is confirmed.

Patient has information to prevent further episodes of food-borne gastroenteritis Patient or family describes transmission of the pathogen. Patient or family demonstrates proper procedures for handling infective materials and proper handwashing and other behaviors necessary to prevent transmission.

 SALMONELLA GASTROENTERITIS
(Salmonellosis)

Salmonellosis is manifested by an acute gastroenteritis and sometimes a septicemia. It is frequently classified as a food poisoning because of the short incubation period following ingestion of food contaminated with *Salmonella*. The greater the number of organisms present in the food, the shorter the incubation period (Table 13-11).

•••••• Pathophysiology

Salmonella organisms ingested in contaminated food or water invade and multiply in deep mucosal layers of the stomach and small intestine, lodging in the lamina propria. An inflammatory response in the tissue with many polymorphonuclear leukocytes produces a gastroenteritis if the *Salmonella* is not *S. typhi* or *S. paratyphi*. The mesenteric lymph nodes become edematous, and the Peyer's patches show edema and superficial ulceration. The disease may be contained here, or the organism may invade beyond the lymph system and be disseminated into the vascular circulation, producing a septicemia or lesions in other organs.

Complications of gastroenteritis may include intestinal perforation and hemorrhage. Secondary infections such as otitis media, pneumonia, skin infections, and septicemia sometimes occur with all types of *Salmonella*.

A leukocytosis (10,000 to 15,000 WBC/mm^3) is generally present in the gastroenteritis form of *Salmonella* infections.

Several nonspecific host defenses affect the type and severity of clinical disease produced by *Salmonella*. Gastric acidity impedes *Salmonella* growth, and persons with hypochlorhydria or achlorhydria or who have had gastric surgery are more susceptible to infection. Normal intestinal peristalsis, intact mu-

TABLE 13-11 Overview of Salmonellosis

Occurrence	Worldwide; classified as a food borne disease; small outbreaks in institutions; 5 million cases per year in United States; increasing
Etiologic agent	2000 serotypes of *Salmonella,* a bacterium
Reservoir	Humans and domestic and wild animals, particularly chickens
Transmission	Ingestion of food contaminated with feces from an infected person or animal; ingestion of meat and animal products, including eggs; handling infected animals; fecal-oral contact
Incubation period	6-72 hr; usually 12-36 hr
Period of communicability	Throughout infection; days to weeks; temporary carrier state may continue up to 1 yr
Susceptibility and resistance	General; increased risk for those with achlorhydria, antacid therapy, gastrointestinal surgery, and immunosuppression
Report to local health authority	Mandatory case report

Data from Benenson.[3]

cous membranes, and the normal intestinal flora all act to prevent invasion. Anything interfering with these defenses increases the risk for more severe infection.

Cellular and humoral immunity appears also to interfere with invasion of *Salmonella,* and persons with an impaired immune system are more susceptible to systemic disease with *Salmonella.* In addition, systemic focal lesions most commonly appear in those tissues that are damaged or devitalized or in those persons with altered immune systems.

See box for another possible causal agent of chronic gastritis and duodenal ulcer disease.

Complications

Endocarditis
Meningitis
Pneumonia
Pyelonephritis
Osteomyelitis
Cholecystitis
Hepatitis
Intestinal perforation and hemorrhage
Septicemia

•••••• Diagnostic Studies and Findings

Culture, isolation, and identification of fecal specimen
Positive for *Salmonella* during first week
WBC count Salmonellosis: 10,000 to 15,000 WBC/mm³

UPDATE

Recently, a bacteria—*Heliobacter pylori,* has been implicated as a causal agent for chronic gastritis and duodenal ulcer disease. Eradication of the pathogen in its human host with antimicrobial therapy leads to remission of the gastritis and the duodenal ulcer disease. *H. pylori* is found worldwide in 20% to 50% of the adult population. Only a small portion of those infected develop either gastritis or an ulcer. The organism presumably is transmitted by oral/oral or fecal/oral routes. There is documentation of transmission occurring through incompletely decontaminated gastric scopes and pH electrodes.

•••••• Multidisciplinary Plan[3]

Medications

Anti-infective agents (used only if systemic disease is present)
 Ciprofloxacin, Chloramphenicol (Chloromycetin)
 Ampicillin
 Trimethoprim sulfamethoxazole (for organisms resistant to above drugs)
Corticosteroids
 Prednisone

General Management

IV fluids and electrolytes
Bed rest
Hyperalimentation
Treatment of complications such as perforation and hemorrhage
Avoidance of antispasmodics, laxatives, and salicylates

NURSING CARE

Nursing Assessment

Salmonellosis
History

Ingestion of undercooked meat or eggs

Onset

Acute abdominal symptoms

Gastrointestinal

Acute onset: abdominal pain, diarrhea, nausea, and vomiting, persisting for several days
Stool is greenish brown, slimy, watery, and foul; may contain mucus, pus, or blood
Bloody diarrhea more common in children

Body Temperature

Low-grade fever to 41° C (105° F); chills; lasting 2 to 7 days

Fluids and Electrolytes

Dehydration may be severe in infants: loss of skin turgor, dry mucous membranes, prostration, circulatory collapse, and death are possible

Skin

May have rose spots on trunk

Neurologic

Vertigo

Respiratory

Possible cough

Sensory

May have slight deafness or otitis media

Septicemia with Localized Infection

Symptoms depend on site of systemic lesions

Symptoms of appendicitis, cholecystitis, peritonitis, otitis media, meningitis, pneumonia, osteomyelitis, pyelonephritis, cystitis, and endocarditis

Septicemia without Localized Infection

Intermittent fever
Chills
Anorexia
Weight loss

Nursing Dx & Intervention

Risk for infection (patient contacts) related to presence of *Salmonella* in stool and urine

- Collect blood, stool, or urine specimen. *Incorrect collection and handling of specimens may destroy the pathogen or contaminate the specimen with environmental organisms, interfering with accurate diagnosis and treatment. Improper handling can also contaminate the health care worker.*
- Administer anti-infective therapy as ordered. Initiate universal blood and body secretion precautions and other isolation procedures as indicated. *Anti-infective therapy and isolation procedures should be initiated as soon as possible to prevent transmission to health care workers, other patients, and patient contacts.*
- Employ enteric precautions for duration of diarrhea with salmonellosis *to prevent transmission.*
- Use protective isolation procedures as indicated. Prevent patient exposure to infected visitors or staff. Limit visitors, if necessary *to limit the exposure of patients to additional pathogens.*
- Participate in follow-up of patient contacts *to ensure that they are examined and treated.*
- Report all *Salmonella* infections to the local health authority. *Reporting is required by law to facilitate public health monitoring and control of outbreaks.*

- Teach safe food handling practices, proper hygiene, nutritional and fluid requirements, and handwashing after defecating or handling raw foods or feces *to prevent recurrence of infection.*

Hyperthermia related to infection

- Monitor body temperature *to detect fever.*
- Administer antipyretics, as ordered.
- Bathe with tepid water or alcohol *to reduce high fever.*
- Adjust environmental temperature *for patient's comfort.*
- Remove excess clothing and bedding *to ensure heat loss.*
- Encourage adequate fluid intake *to compensate for fluid loss associated with elevated body temperature.*
- Do not administer aspirin. *High risk exists for GI hemorrhage with these conditions.*

Diarrhea related to infection in intestinal tract

- Measure output *to replace fluids equal to output.*
- Apply heating pad to abdomen *to help cramping (antispasmodic agents should be avoided).*
- Use room deodorizers and adequate ventilation.
- Obtain stool specimen for culture *to detect pathogen present.*
- Wash and lubricate skin around anal opening frequently *to prevent irritation and skin breakdown.*

Risk for fluid volume deficit related to vomiting and diarrhea

- Assess for symptoms of dehydration (e.g., oliguria and loss of skin turgor) *to intervene early.*
- Give oral fluids as tolerated *to maintain adequate intake.*
- Administer IV fluids and electrolytes as prescribed *to provide for rehydration.* (Once circulation is stabilized, the initial rate of IV infusion and type of IV electrolytes may be altered.)
- Measure all fluid output (emesis, urine, diarrhea). Measure all intake *to ensure that fluid intake compensates for output.*

Constipation related to invasion of *Salmonella* in intestinal mucosa

- Observe stool *to detect blood.*
- Monitor for signs of perforation and hemorrhage *for immediate medical intervention.*
- Check for and prevent abdominal distension. *Unresolved distention adds to the risk of perforation of the intestines.*
- Administer small low enema or glycerin suppositories, as ordered (do not give laxatives), *to relieve distention.*

Urinary retention related to *Salmonella* in urinary tract

- Monitor for bladder distention. Measure output *to detect urinary retention.*
- Catheterize if necessary *to empty bladder.*

Patient Education/Home Care Planning*

Provide patient with the following information:

1. This condition is transmitted by contaminated food or direct fecal-oral route.
2. This condition is communicable as long as the infective organism is in the feces or urine, which may persist for up to 1 year.
3. Transmission of the infection to others can be prevented by handwashing after defecating and urinating and through proper disposal of excretions so as not to contaminate food or water supply.
4. Follow enteric isolation procedures.
5. This disease can be prevented by eating thoroughly cooked food and shellfish, screening food from flies, and other methods listed below.
6. Manage fever with antipyretics, tepid sponge baths, minimal clothing, and by maintaining a cool environment. Avoid chilling and aspirin. Encourage intake of fluids and food as tolerated. Popsicles and soda may appeal to young children.
7. Manage other symptoms with bed rest; avoid laxatives or antispasmodics.
8. Report the following to a physician: signs of dehydration, any bleeding, or recurrence of symptoms.

Important:

9. Scrupulous handwashing after defecation and before preparing food is necessary.
10. Family and close contacts should be examined and treated if specimens from them are positive for any *Salmonella* bacilli.
11. All foods of animal origin, including eggs, must be thoroughly cooked; cross contamination of cooked and uncooked foods must be avoided; and foods must be refrigerated below 8° C (46° F) to avoid infection with *Salmonella*.
12. Frozen meat, particularly poultry, should be defrosted in the refrigerator.
13. All milk should be pasteurized, and water should be chlorinated.
14. Children should be protected from handling pet turtles and should be taught to wash hands after touching any animal.

*From Grimes.[26]

Evaluation

Patient is free of infection and complications of *Salmonella* Vital signs are within normal limits. Blood, stool, or urine cultures are negative for *Salmonella*. Blood count is within normal limits. Hemorrhage has been avoided.

Infection is not transmitted to patient's contacts Patient care staff members wash hands after providing care to each patient and follow universal blood and body secretion procedures with all patients. Enteric isolation procedures are implemented soon after infection is confirmed. Patient or family describes transmission of the pathogen and demonstrates proper procedures for handling infective materials and proper handwashing and other behaviors necessary to prevent transmission. Infection has been reported to local health department. Patient contacts have been examined and treated. Patient completes full course of anti-infective therapy.

Body temperature is maintained within the normal range; comfort and safety are maintained Body temperature is between 36° and 38° C (96.8° and 100° F). Pulse and respiration are normal. Skin is cool to touch and free of excess perspiration. Patient's clothing and bedding are dry. Patient is free of headache and malaise associated with fever.

Patient returns to normal pattern of bowel elimination Patient eats without nausea, vomiting, or abdominal distention. Stools are soft, formed, and brown. Abdomen is soft and nondistended. No cramping or pain occurs.

Fluid and electrolyte balance are maintained Skin turgor is good. Mucous membranes are moist. Urine output is normal. Secretions are thin. Blood levels of sodium, potassium, chloride, magnesium, and calcium are normal. Urine specific gravity is normal.

Patient experiences relief from constipation Patient has bowel movement at least every 3 days. Stools are soft and pass easily.

Urine is eliminated and patient resumes normal voiding pattern There is no bladder distention. Urine output equals fluid intake.

HEPATITIS

■ VIRAL HEPATITIS

Viral hepatitis refers to several distinct infections of the liver, each caused by a different hepatitis virus. Depending on the etiologic agent, the diseases differ in their mode of transmission and in their immunologic, pathologic, and clinical characteristics. Treatment is similar for each disease, but prevention and control vary greatly.

To date, five types of primary hepatitis viruses have been identified. These are hepatitis A, B, C, D, and E (Table 13-12). Hepatitis can also occur as a secondary infection during the course of diseases associated with cytomegalovirus. Epstein-Barr, herpes simplex, varicella-zoster, coxsackievirus B, and rubella viruses.

•••••• Pathophysiology

Although the etiologic agents, mode of transmission, and course of the disease vary with each type of hepatitis, the pathologic condition produced in the liver is similar with all types. The similarities in pathologic findings for each type are presented first, followed by the variations.

▪ TABLE 13-12 **Overview of Viral Hepatitis**

	Hepatitis A	Hepatitis B	Hepatitis C	Hepatitis D	Hepatitis E
Occurrence	Worldwide; sporadic and epidemic, with a tendency toward cyclic recurrence; outbreaks in institutions	Worldwide; endemic; highest in young adults, homosexual men, heterosexuals with multiple sex partners, parenteral drug users, and health care and public safety workers	Worldwide; 20% of cases of hepatitis; since screening of blood donors <5% associated with transfusions	Worldwide; occurs epidemically and endemically in populations at risk for HBV infection	Epidemic and sporadic cases, particularly in developing countries; highest in young adults; rare in children or elderly
Etiologic agent	Hepatitis A virus (HAV)	Hepatitis B virus (HBV)	Hepatitis C virus (HCV)	A viruslike particle (HDV, or the delta agent); coinfects with HBV	Viruslike particle (HEV)
Reservoir	Humans and captive primates	Humans and possibly captive primates	Humans; experimentally transmitted to chimpanzees	Humans, chimpanzees	Unknown; possible nonhuman reservoirs
Transmission	Person to person by fecal-oral route; contaminated food, water, shellfish	Direct and indirect contact with blood and serum-derived fluids such as vaginal secretions, saliva, and semen; sexual contact; perinatal	Parenteral; person-to-person and sexual and perinatal transmission have not been defined	Similar to HBV, including sexual contact	Contaminated water; person to person by fecal-oral route
Incubation period	15-50 days; average: 28-30 days	45-180 days; average: 60-90 days	2 wk to 6 mo; commonly 6-9 wk	2-10 wk	15-64 days; average: 26-42 days
Period of communicability	Latter half of incubation period to 1 wk after onset of jaundice	During incubation period and throughout clinical course of disease; carrier state may persist for years	From 1 or more wk before symptom onset, indefinitely during chronic and carrier states	Throughout acute and chronic disease	Not known; detected in stool 14 days after onset of jaundice
Susceptibility and resistance	General; usually affects children and young adults; immunity after infection probably lasts for life	All age groups; disease is mild in children; lifetime immunity follows infection if antibody to HBsAg develops and HBsAg is negative	General; all age groups; degree of immunity following infection is unknown	All persons susceptible to HB, HBV carriers; disease is severe in children	Unknown; no explanation for epidemics among young adults; pregnant women in third trimester susceptible to fulminating disease
Report to local health authority	Mandatory case report	Mandatory case report	Mandatory case report	Mandatory case report	Mandatory case report

Data from Benenson.[3]

The hepatitis virus, regardless of its type invades, replicates, and produces damage only in the liver. Inflammation and mononuclear cell infiltration in the parenchyma and portal ducts, hepatic cell necrosis, proliferation of Kupffer cells, cellular collapse, and accumulation of necrotic debris in the lobules and portal ducts all act to produce architectural changes in the lobules and portal ducts. The result is disturbance in bilirubin excretion.

Cellular regeneration and mitosis are usually concurrent with hepatocyte necrosis; complete regeneration usually occurs within 2 to 3 months. Failure of the liver cells to regenerate while the necrotic process progresses results in a severe, fulminant, frequently fatal hepatitis (Figure 13-1). This occurs more often in hepatitis B. Continuation of the inflammatory response and necrosis, also more common in types B and E, results in active chronic or persistent chronic hepatitis. In active chronic hepatitis the necrotic process, fibrosis, and architectural destruction continue throughout the hepatic lobes and portal ducts. In persistent chronic hepatitis the inflammatory process

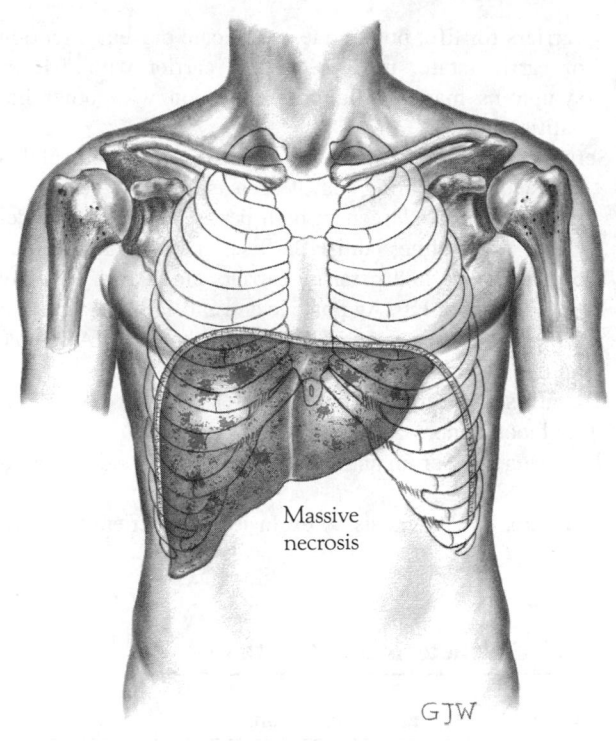

Massive
necrosis

GJW

Figure 13-1 Acute viral hepatitis (fulminant hepatitis).

is limited to the portal tracts with little or no evidence of hepatocellular necrosis. All types of hepatitis may be present with or without icterus and may have a clinical severity ranging from subclinical infection to acute fulminating disease. All types stimulate an antibody response specific to the type of virus causing the disease.

The identification of serologic markers for type-specific virus antigens and antibodies has been important in the diagnosis, prevention, and control of viral hepatitis. The standard nomenclature and abbreviation with characteristics and implications are presented here for easy reference (Table 13-13).

Hepatitis A virus (HAV) is acquired by ingestion of the HAV in food, water, or uncooked shellfish contaminated with feces containing the virus or by direct fecal-oral transmission. The virus localizes in the liver, replicates, enters the bile, and is carried to the intestinal tract where it is shed in the feces. Fecal shedding occurs late in the incubation period, usually before onset of clinical symptoms. Antibodies develop during acute disease and later during convalescence. Hepatitis A does not lead to chronic disease or the carrier state.

Hepatitis B virus (HBV) is viable in blood and in secretions containing serum (oozing cutaneous lesions) or derived from serum (e.g., saliva, semen, and vaginal secretions). Transmission may be by one of five routes: (1) direct percutaneous inoculation of infective serum or plasma by needle or transfusion of infective blood or blood products; (2) indirect percutaneous introduction of infective serum or plasma, such as through minute skin cuts or abrasions; (3) absorption of infective serum

or plasma through mucosal surfaces, such as those of the mouth or eye; (4) absorption of other potentially infective secretions, such as saliva or semen through mucosal surfaces, as might occur during vaginal, anal, or oral sexual contact; and (5) transfer of infective serum or plasma via inanimate environmental surfaces or possibly vectors. Fecal transmission of HBV does not occur. HBV may be transmitted transplacentally, or the infant may become contaminated at birth with the mother's infective blood.

HBV is composed of three antigens: the core antigen (HbcAg), an outer surface antigen (HbsAg), and a soluble antigen (HbeAg). HBV antigens infect the blood within 30 to 60 days of exposure to HBV and are at their peak before disease onset. They persist for varying lengths of time, and their presence is useful for determining the course of the disease and the carrier state. Antibodies specific for the antigens develop at different times during convalescence. Detection of serum antibodies is useful for predicting the course of the disease and for determining immune status.

A viruslike particle called the delta agent has recently been identified. This agent is pathogenic only with HBV, causing coinfection with the HBV or superimposing infection on an inapparent HBV carrier state. Prolongation or an increase in severity of an HBV infection may be attributable to the delta agent.

Hepatitis C virus (HCV) is a parenterally transmitted hepatitis virus causing a disease similar to hepatitis B (i.e., prolonged incubation period, insidious onset, and potential chronicity). A screening test for the antibody has recently been developed and is used for screening blood donors.

Hepatitis E virus (HEV) is an enterically transmitted hepatitis virus that causes disease with a clinical course similar to hepatitis A (i.e., shorter incubation period, acute onset, and complete recovery). Disease may be more severe in pregnant women, particularly in the third trimester. A serologic test for HEV antibodies has been developed, but is not currently available in the United States.

Complications

Fulminant, frequently fatal, hepatitis
Chronic hepatitis infection
Hepatic carcinoma

•••••• Diagnostic Studies and Findings[3,27]

Liver Function Tests

Serum enzymes Asparate aminotransferase (AST, SGOT) and alanine aminotransferase (ALT, SGPT): elevated during clinical disease, indicators of liver damage, peak at onset of jaundice and fall during recovery, persisting for months; alkaline phosphatase: elevated; lactic dehydrogenase (LDH): elevated; creatine phosphokinase (CPK): normal

Serum bilirubin Elevated

Prothrombin time Normal; elevated only in severe fulminating hepatitis

VDRL False positive

Hepatitis A

Examination of stool specimen (immune electron microscopy, radioimmunoassay, or enzyme immunoassay): positive for HAV 2 weeks before illness to several days after onset of symptoms, then is negative; HAV may be absent from stool by time patient is hospitalized

Serology: fourfold rise in anti-HAV antibodies between early disease and convalescence; identification of IgM antibodies during early disease indicates present infection; peak at 3 mo and then drop; IgG peaks after clinical disease and persists for life; high IgG levels indicate past infection and present immunity

Hepatitis B

Serum antigen tests: detect HBeAg and HBsAg in serum 1 to 2 weeks after exposure and 2 to 7 weeks before onset of clinical disease; peak and begin to drop during clinical disease; HBsAg remains in serum of chronic carriers for life; positive tests indicate present infection or carrier state; positive test in carrier with disease symptoms may misdiagnose infection with other hepatitis virii

Serum antibody tests: anti-HBe increases during clinical disease and peaks during convalescence; anti-HBe begins rising during convalescence; both persist and gradually decrease over time; anti-HBs rises rapidly during late convalescence and persists; carriers are always HBe-Ag positive and/or HBsAg positive and anti-HBs negative; for screening purposes: anti-HBs greater than 10 RIA sample ratio units indicates immunity

Hepatitis C   Serum antibody (EIA): used to detect anti-HCV in blood donors

Hepatitis D   Serum antibody (RIA or EIA): to detect anti-HDV

Hepatitis E   Diagnosis by exclusion of other etiologies of hepatitis

---

■ TABLE 13-13 Standard Nomenclature, Abbreviations, and Characteristics of Hepatitis

Abbreviation	Term	Characteristics and Implications
HAV	Hepatitis A virus	Etiologic agent with one serotype
Anti-HAV	Antibody to HAV	Detectable at onset of symptoms and persists for lifetime; probably confers lifetime immunity
IgM	Immunoglobulin M (antibody to HAV)	The anti-HAV is present early in the infection; it represents current infection and is used to establish the diagnosis; serum levels drop during convalescence and disappear in 4-6 mo
IgG	Immunoglobulin G (antibody to HAV)	The anti-HAV that develops late in the infection and persists for years; its presence in serum indicates past infection and present immunity
HBV	Hepatitis B virus	Etiologic agent of hepatitis B; also called Dane particle
HBsAG	Hepatitis B surface antigen	Previously known as Australian antigen; large quantities detectable in serum 2-7 wk before and during acute clinical disease, during chronic disease, and in carriers; its presence indicates infectious blood
HBeAg	Hepatitis B e antigen	Soluble antigen that correlates with HBV replication; indicates a high titer of HBV in serum and consequent infectivity of serum; it rises 2-7 wk before clinical disease onset and usually drops before acute disease; its persistence is associated with progression to chronic hepatitis; found only in HBsAg-positive serum
HBcAg	Hepatitis B core antigen	Found in liver cells; cannot be detected in sera with present technology
Anti-HBs	Antibody to HBsAG	Rises in serum during convalescence; its presence indicates immunity to HBV from past infection, passive antibody from HBIG, or active immune response from HBV vaccine
Anti-HBe	Antibody to HBeAg	Its presence in serum of person with continuing levels of HBeAg suggests chronic presence of HBV and infectivity of blood
Anti-HBc	Antibody to HBcAg	Appears at disease onset and increases during clinical disease, peaks during convalescence, and persists for years; presence indicates current or past infection with HBV
IGM anti-HBc	IGM antibody to HBcAg	Presence indicates current or recent infection with HBV; positive for 4-6 mo after infection
IG	Immunoglobulin	Formerly called immune serum globulin (ISG) or gamma globulin; given before and within 2 wk after exposure to HAV and NANB
HBIG	Hepatitis B immune globulin	Contains a higher titer of HB immune globulins than does IG; preferred for use after exposure to HBV
HB vaccine	Hepatitis B vaccine	Inactivated vaccine prepared from carriers of HBsAg; stimulates production of anti-HBs; series of three injections recommended for those at risk for hepatitis B
HDV	Hepatitis D virus	Etiologic agent of delta hepatitis; may only cause infection in presence of HBV
HDAg	Delta antigen	Detectable in early, acute delta infections
Anti-HDV	Antibody to delta antigen	Indicates past or present infection with delta antigen

From Centers for Disease Control.[3,8,11]

••••• Multidisciplinary Plan[3,11,23]

Medications

There is no direct chemotherapeutic treatment for acute viral hepatitis; however, supportive medications may be used for fulminating hepatitis

Alpha interferon is the only drug licensed for treatment of chronic hepatitis B

Hepatitis A Prevention: preventive medications may be used for <2 months for preexposure prophylaxis against hepatitis A (HAV) for those traveling to high-risk areas outside tourist routes

Immunologic agent Hepatitis A vaccine (Havrix) provides protection within 14 to 30 days of administration

Immunologic agent for rapid, but short-term protection
Immune globulin (IG), 0.02 ml/kg in a single dose IM
Immunologic agent for prolonged travel:

Immune globulin (IG), 0.06 ml/kg IM in a single dose q5 mo
Postexposure prophylaxis within 2 wk of close personal contact with hepatitis A infected person in the home, day-care center, institution for custodial care, or hospital

Immunologic agent:

Immune globulin (IG), 0.02 ml/kg in a single dose IM

Hepatitis B Preexposure prophylaxis against hepatitis B (HBV) for high-risk persons (e.g., health care workers, hemodialysis patients, multiple sexual partners, and household and sexual contacts of HBV carriers)

See Tables 13-14 and 13-15.

General Management

For nonfulminating hepatitis:

Hospitalization for those with bilirubin concentrations >10 mg/dl or >10 times normal and for those with a prolonged prothrombin time; bed rest until symptoms subside; diet as tolerated: small, frequent, low-fat, high-carbohydrate feedings may be better tolerated; symptomatic treatment for nausea (avoid chlorpromazine); symptomatic treatment for pain (acetaminophen preferred over aspirin); avoid all unnecessary medications, particularly sedatives

For fulminating hepatitis:

Hospitalization and bed rest; low-protein diet: 20 to 30 mg protein per day; enemas; discontinue any sedatives; IV fluids and electrolytes; central venous pressure line; nasogastric tube feedings; urinary catheter; fresh frozen plasma to correct coagulation defects

NURSING CARE

Nursing Assessment

History

Sexual contact with multiple or unknown partners; homosexual contact; household contact with person with hepatitis; IV drug abuse; unimmunized for HB

Disease Onset

Within 2 to 7 weeks of exposure for HA; within 6 weeks to 6 months for HB

Preicteric phase (3 to 10 days)
Subjective Symptoms

Malaise, weakness, dull headache, anorexia, intermittent nausea and vomiting, myalgias, chills; right, upper quadrant abdominal pain

Body Temperature

38° to 40° C (100° to 104° F) for hepatitis A; low-grade fever or normal for hepatitis B and C

Skin

For hepatitis B and non-A, non-B: urticarial pruritic hives, maculopapular lesions, or fleeting, irregular patches of erythema in some patients; multiple forearm pricks in drug users; exacerbation of acne; excoriations with severe pruritus

---

■ TABLE 13-14 **Recommended Doses of Currently Licensed Hepatitis B Vaccines**

Group	Recombivax HB*		Engerix-B*	
	Dose (µg)	(ml)	Dose (µg)	(ml)
Infants of HBsAg†-negative mothers and children <11 years	2.5	(0.25)	10	(0.5)
Infants of HBsAg-positive mothers; prevention of perinatal infection	5	(0.5)	10	(0.5)
Children and adolescents 11-19 years	5	(0.5)	20	(1.0)
Adults ≥20 years	10	(1.0)	20	(1.0)
Dialysis patients and other immunocompromised persons	40	(1.0)‡	40	(2.0)§

From Centers for Disease Control.[11]
*Both vaccines are routinely administered in a three-dose series. Engerix-B has also been licensed for a four-dose series administered at 0, 1, 2, and 12 months.
†HBsAg, Hepatitis B surface antigen.
‡Special formulation.
§Two 1.0-mL doses administered at one site, in a four-dose schedule at 0, 1, 2, and 6 months.

■ TABLE 13-15 Postexposure Prophylaxis Recommendations

Hepatitis B Prophylaxis Following Percutaneous or Permucosal Exposure

Exposed Person	HBsAg-Positive	HBsAg-Negative	Source Not Tested or Unknown
	Treatment When Source is Found to Be:		
Unvaccinated	HBIG × 1* and initiate HB vaccine†	Initiate HB vaccine†	Initiate HB vaccine†
Previously vaccinated known responder	Test exposed for anti-HBs 1. If adequate,‡ no treatment 2. If inadequate, HB vaccine booster dose	No treatment	No treatment
Known nonresponder	HBIG × 2 or HBIG × 1 + 1 dose HB vaccine	No treatment	If known high-risk source, may treat as if source were HBsAg-positive
Response unknown	Test exposed for anti-HBs 1. If inadequate,‡ HBIG × 1 + HB vaccine booster dose 2. If adequate, no treatment	No treatment	Test exposed person for anti-HBs 1. If inadequate,‡ HB vaccine booster dose 2. If adequate, no treatment

*HBIG dose 0.06 ml/kg IM.
†HB vaccine dose—see table, Recommended Doses and Schedules of Currently Licensed HB Vaccines.
‡Adequate anti-HBs is ≥10 milli-international units.

Hepatitis B Virus Postexposure

Exposure	HBIG		Vaccine	
	Dose	Recommended Timing	Dose	Recommended Timing
Perinatal	0.5 ml IM	Within 12 hr of birth	0.5 ml IM*	Within 12 hr of birth†
Sexual	0.06 ml/kg IM	Single dose within 14 days of last sexual contact	1.0 ml IM*	First dose at time of HBIG treatment†

From Centers for Disease Control.[8,11]
*For appropriate age-specific doses of vaccine, see table, Recommended Doses and Schedules of Currently Licensed HB Vaccines.
†The first dose can be given the same time as the HBIG dose but in a different site; subsequent doses should be given as recommended for specific vaccine.

Musculoskeletal Concerns

For hepatitis B and non-A, non-B: mild to moderate nondeforming polyarticular arthritis (migratory, affecting elbows, wrists, knees, and small joints of hands)

Abdomen

Bowel sounds normal; slightly enlarged, tender liver (9-13 cm), edges smooth, regular, and firm

Icteric Phase (bilirubin >2.5 mg/dl; lasts 1 to 3 weeks)
Subjective Symptoms

Nausea and vomiting frequently abate and appetite returns, but symptoms may worsen; malaise continues

Skin

Jaundice with or without pruritus may be present or absent; can be observed under the tongue

Eyes
Scleral icterus

Urine
Dark

Stools
May be clay colored

Vital Signs

Normal, although there may be a bradycardia with severe hyperbilirubinemia

Temperature
Normal or low-grade

Complications: Fulminant Hepatitis with Encephalopathy
Level of consciousness

Patient becomes lethargic and somnolent with personality changes; may show mild confusion, sexual or aggressive activity, loss of usual inhibitions

Lethargy may alternate with excitability, euphoria, or unruly behavior

Worsening of the condition leads to stupor and eventual coma

An early sign is asterixis (the irregular flapping of forcibly dorsiflexed, outstretched hands)

Circulatory system

Prothrombin time is prolonged: abdominal bleeding; epistaxis; prolonged bleeding from puncture sites; blood in vomitus, stool, or urine; easy bruising

Nursing Dx & Intervention

Risk for infection (patient contacts) related to presence of HAV in feces and HBV in blood, semen, and saliva

- Collect fecal or blood specimens as required. *Specimens must be handled correctly so as not to destroy or transmit the virus.*
- Employ enteric precautions for 7 days after onset of jaundice for hepatitis A. Employ universal precautions for all patients.
- Ensure that all patient contacts, including health care personnel, are protected against hepatitis.

Activity intolerance related to decreased energy metabolism by liver

- Maintain bed rest during acute symptoms *to conserve energy and avoid unnecessary stress to the liver.* (Patients need not be limited in their activity during convalescence.)
- Do necessary tests and procedures at one time *to allow for uninterrupted rest.*

Altered nutrition: less than body requirements related to anorexia, nausea and vomiting, and altered digestion of food

- Encourage frequent small feedings as patient tolerates; largest meal in AM. *Anorexia frequently worsens as day progresses.*
- Provide high-carbohydrate, low-fat feedings *to provide easily digested meals.*
- Administer nasogastric tube feedings for patients with hepatic encephalopathy and coma; administer IV fluids for patients with persistent vomiting or for those with hepatic encephalopathy, as ordered, *to avoid aspiration while ensuring adequate intake of food and fluids.*
- Offer hard candy *to soothe nausea.*

Fluid volume deficit

- Monitor fluid intake and output and laboratory values *to detect fluid and electrolyte imbalance.*
- Provide frequent high-carbohydrate fluids, as tolerated, during acute symptoms *to compensate for fluid loss with vomiting and diarrhea.*

Risk for patient problem: hemorrhage related to complications of hepatitis

- Monitor and report signs of bleeding. Provide care as warranted by bleeding *for early detection and intervention for coagulation and bleeding problems.*

Risk for encephalopathy related to complications of hepatitis

- Monitor and report signs of encephalopathy as were described under Nursing Assessment.
- Monitor and report progression of icterus.
- Provide care as warranted by patient's level of consciousness. *These are severe signs of the progression of the disease; these patients require protection from injury and may require life support.*

Patient Education/Home Care Planning

1. Educate patient about disease and disease transmission. Emphasize the self-limited nature of most episodes of hepatitis but the need for follow-up of liver function tests and serum HBsAg.
2. Follow-up serology in 1 or 2 months is necessary for all hepatitis B patients to determine the presence or absence of HBsAg.
3. Patients should follow precautions with blood and secretions until they are determined to be free of HBsAg. Close personal contacts should be examined and receive HBIG or HB vaccine.
4. HBV carriers should be aware that their blood and secretions are infectious. Close contacts of HBV carriers should receive HB vaccine. Carriers should not share razors or toothbrushes and must be cautious in handling cuts and lacerations. HBV carriers and patients with a history of HCV should not donate blood.
5. Patients caring for themselves at home during the acute stage of the disease should avoid alcohol and any nonprescribed medications, particularly sedatives and aspirin.
6. Severity of symptoms can determine patterns for bed rest and diet. Frequent, small feedings of low-fat, high-carbohydrate foods may be better tolerated; however, it is not necessary to limit the diet in any way.
7. Liver function tests should be monitored until normal.
8. Hepatitis A patients must wash hands thoroughly following toileting, must disinfect articles soiled with feces (boil 1 minute), and must not prepare foods for others during symptomatic disease. They should avoid sharing eating utensils, toothbrushes, toys, etc.
9. Sexual activity should be avoided during acute stage of hepatitis B and C. Ideally hepatitis B patients should not resume sexual activity until tests for HBsAg are negative or until partner has received HB vaccine or HBIG if HB vaccine is unavailable.

*From Grimes.[26]

Evaluation

Infection is not transmitted Patient returns for examination to determine when serum HBsAg and HBeAg tests are negative. Close, personal contacts of hepatitis B patients have received HBIG and HB vaccine or IG vaccine for hepatitis A.

Patient achieves adequate rest during active disease and returns to preillness level of activity during convalescence Extended periods of uninterrupted sleep are experienced. Patient has gradually increasing amounts of energy without relapses of extreme fatigue.

Adequate calorie intake and nutritional status are maintained; weight is stable Patient has full appetite and energy. Weight is at preillness state. RBCs are normal.

Fluid and electrolyte balance is maintained Fluid intake equals output. Urine is straw colored. Specific gravity, sodium, and albumin levels are within normal limits. Skin turgor is normal; no ascites or edema.

Patient is knowledgeable about need for follow-up, means of preventing transmission to others, and convalescent self-care Items listed in Patient Education/Home Care Planning are met.

Infection resolves without complications There is no icterus. Patient has full appetite and energy and has no right upper quadrant abdominal pain. Urine and stool are normal colored. There are no changes in personality or level of consciousness. SGPT (ALT), SGOT (AST), alkaline phosphatase, LDH, serum bilirubin, and prothrombin time are all within normal limits.

INFECTIOUS DISEASES OF THE HEMATOLYMPHATIC SYSTEM

The infectious diseases grouped here produce either primary pathologic findings in the lymphatic system or disseminated infection with lymphadenopathy as part of the clinical picture (Table 13-16).

■ MONONUCLEOSIS

Mononucleosis is an acute viral infectious disease that produces a generalized lymph node hyperplasia and is characterized by fever, exudative pharyngitis, lymphadenopathy, and splenomegaly.

•••••• Pathophysiology

The Epstein-Barr virus (EBV) is transmitted in saliva by prolonged direct contact, probably through kissing with salivary exchange. The pathogen invades B lymphocytes in lymphatic tissue and stimulates the development of a surface membrane antigen on the infected lymphocytes. T lymphocytes actively proliferate in response to the antigen and pro-

■ TABLE 13-16 Overview of Hematolymphatic Infectious Diseases

	Mononucleosis	Cytomegalovirus Infections	Toxoplasmosis
Occurrence	Worldwide; highest in adolescents and young adults in developed countries; asymptomatic infection in children	Worldwide; many asymptomatic infections; congenital infection may be severe	Worldwide; common in humans, mammals, and birds; many asymptomatic infections; congenital infection may be severe
Etiologic agent	Epstein-Barr virus (EBV), one of the herpesviruses	Cytomegalovirus (CMV)—one of the herpesviruses	*Toxoplasma gondii,* a protozoan
Reservoir	Humans and possibly primates	Humans	Cats; other mammals and birds are intermediate hosts
Transmission	Direct contact with saliva; through blood transfusions	Direct contact with secretions and excretions (blood, urine, saliva, semen, breast milk, and cervical secretions, and transplacentally	Transplacental if mother has active infection; eating infective meat; water contaminated with cat feces
Incubation period	4-6 wk	Unknown; 3-8 wk following transplantation or transfusion; in neonate, 3-12 wk following delivery-produced infection	Unknown; probably between 5-23 days depending on mode of transmission
Period of communicability	Prolonged; pharyngeal excretion may persist for years; 15%-20% of EBV antibody + adults are long term oropharyngeal carriers	Virus excreted in saliva and urine for months to years	Not directly transmitted except transplacentally; cysts in infected meat remain infective as long as meat is edible and uncooked
Susceptibility and resistance	General; infection confers a high degree of resistance	General; fetuses, immunosuppressed individuals organ allograft recipients and those with other chronic disease have more severe symptoms	General, but risk for infection increases with age; immunity after infection persists indefinitely
Report to local health authority	No	No	In some states

Data from Benenson.[3]

duce a generalized lymph node hyperplasia. Atypical T lymphocytes infiltrate the spleen, tonsils, lungs, heart, liver, kidneys, adrenal glands, central nervous system, and skin. The circulating T cells are not infective and therefore do not produce necrosis in these systems. Their infiltration causes enlargement, particularly of the spleen, and disturbs functioning of those organs.

The severity of the disease varies from asymptomatic disease (usually in children) to severe systemic and localized organ involvement. Lymphadenopathy, splenomegaly, and exudative pharyngitis are characteristic. More serious manifestations of the disease include hepatitis, pneumonitis, and central nervous system involvement.

Saliva remains infective for 18 months despite the development of EBV-specific antibodies early in the disease. The virus can be cultured from the throats of 10% to 20% of normal, healthy adults, suggesting that the disease may be contracted from asymptomatic viral shedders.

Complications

Splenic rupture
Hemolytic anemia
Agranulocytosis
Thrombocytopenic purpura
Pericarditis
Orchitis
Encephalitis
Hepatitis

•••••• Diagnostic Studies and Findings[3,27]

Differential white blood count Lymphocytes and monocytes greater than 50% with more than 10% being atypical lymphocytes

Leukocyte count Normal early in disease; rises to 12,000 to 20,000/mm³ in second week; occasionally rises to 50,000/mm³

Serology Elevated heterophile antibody titer (with compatible mononucleosis symptoms) is sufficient for diagnosis. Rapid forms of test are monospot, monoscreen, or monotest.

Liver function tests Serum transaminases (AST [SGOT], ALT [SGPT]): All elevated in hepatic involvement, bilirubin: elevated if there is hepatic involvement

•••••• Multidisciplinary Plan[2,3]

Surgery

For splenic rupture: surgical removal of the spleen

Medications

Corticosteroids
Prednisone 80 mg/d in divided doses, for 2-3 days decreasing over 2 wk, for severe neurologic complications, airway obstruction, thrombocytopenic purpura, or hemolytic anemia

General Management

Bed rest during acute stage
Saline throat gargle
Aspirin or acetaminophen for sore throat and fever

NURSING CARE

Nursing Assessment

See p. 1122.

■ CYTOMEGALOVIRUS INFECTIONS

■ Cytomegalovirus infections are extremely common viral infections that are ordinarily asymptomatic. Clinical disease in the adult resembles mononucleosis. Congenital and perinatal acquired infections are serious in the neonate and lead to irreversible central nervous system damage.

•••••• Pathophysiology

The cytomegalovirus (CMV), with several antigenically related strains, is a member of the herpesvirus group and has characteristics common to other herpesviruses. Like the Epstein-Barr herpesvirus, CMV produces a frequently asymptomatic mononucleosis-type infection in children and adults. CMV is similar to herpes types 1 and 2 in that it remains latent in body tissue and has the potential for producing recurrent infection. CMV, like herpes 1 and 2, also crosses the placental barrier and is shed in cervical secretions. Therefore it has the potential for producing congenital infection with severe congenital anomalies and perinatal infection acquired during vaginal delivery. Like herpes 2, the CMV is suspected of having oncogenic properties.

CMV can be found in all body secretions including saliva, blood, urine, semen, cervical secretions, and breast milk, even in the presence of CMV-specific antibodies. Transmission requires prolonged direct contact with secretions. Although the exact mechanism for postnatal transmission is not known, sexual, oral, and blood transfusion transmission is suspected in postnatal acquired infections.

Regardless of the mode of transmission, CMV may invade the cells of most tissues in the body. An inflammatory response with focal tissue destruction, areas of calcification, and hyperplasia of the reticuloendothelial system develops. Typical cellular lesions are characterized by enlarged cells containing intranuclear and cytoplasmic inclusion bodies. These lesions are disseminated widely, particularly in the brain, liver, lungs, kidney, and spleen.

A humoral and cell-mediated anti-CMV antibody response occurs. The response does not appear to alter the course of the spread of the virus from cell to cell or alter the presence of the virus in body secretions. Nor do circulating maternal antibodies in the fetus appear to impede the infectious process or the development of congenital anomalies.

Dependent on the mode of transmission, three different forms of the infection have been identified: congenital, perinatal, and postnatal acquired. All three forms can either be asymptomatic or occur as a mild or severe clinical disease.

Congenital CMV infection is acquired by transplacental transmission, usually resulting from a primary infection the mother acquired during pregnancy. Of infants with congenital infections, 95% are asymptomatic at birth. Maternal antibodies are present in cord blood at birth and the virus can be detected in the infant's urine until age 15 months. In utero viral invasion is most destructive to the developing fetal central nervous system, particularly the cerebellum and cerebral cortex. Neurologic defects such as microcephaly, psychomotor retardation, and severe mental retardation result. The infant born with symptomatic CMV infection also has evidence of a severe generalized infection plus symptoms of organ involvement of the liver, lung, kidney, or eye. This extraneural organ involvement is usually self-limited. If the child lives, there are invariably neurologic sequelae. Congenital CMV infections need to be differentiated diagnostically from toxoplasmosis, rubella, herpes, hemolytic anemias, and bacterial sepsis.

Perinatal infection is acquired at delivery from a serologic-positive mother who had either a primary infection during pregnancy or a reactivation of a latent infection. Cervical secretions of CMV are high during the last trimester, having increased as the pregnancy progressed. Perinatally infected infants develop signs of infection (virus in urine and an antibody response with or without clinical evidence of organ involvement) 4 to 8 weeks after birth. The long-term effects on neurologic development are unknown.

Postnatal acquired infection requires close contact with body secretions containing the virus, usually from an asymptomatic person. Blood transfusions and renal and bone marrow transplants (possibly because of immunosuppression) have been linked with CMV transmission. Sexual transmission and kissing are also suspected as modes of transmission. The disease may be asymptomatic, or there may be symptoms of liver and lung involvement or a mononucleosis-like syndrome. There is no evidence of chronic organ impairment in acquired CMV infections. Primary or reactivation infection can be severe and life threatening in the immunosuppressed individual.

Complications

    To immunocompromised: progressive pneumonitis, hemolytic anemia, purpura, GI ulceration, hepatitis, pericarditis, and retinitis
    To neonate infected in utero: neurologic defects (e.g., microcephaly, psychomotor retardation, and severe mental retardation)

•••••• Diagnostic Studies and Findings[27]

Culture of specimen of urine, saliva, throat washings, blood, or biopsy tissue (lung, kidney, spleen, liver, brain and retina) Positive for specific cytopathic effect of CMV; presence of CMV in infant's urine at birth suggests congenital infection

Microscopic examination of biopsy of liver tissue Histologic evidence of typical inclusion bodies

Serology (Complement fixation) Presence of IgG antibody in infant blood during first 6 months represents maternal antibodies; levels persisting after 6 months suggest congenital CMV infection; fourfold rise in titer in adult or child suggests current infection; very specific test with few false positive results

Indirect fluorescent antibody; immunofluorescence, anticomplement; immunofluorescent test Presence of IgM in cord blood at birth suggests congenital CMV infection; elevated titer in adult to child suggest current infection; these tests are more sensitive and detect antibodies earlier in infection

Serum transaminase (AST) Elevated in CMV hepatitis

Platelets May be as few as 5000/mm^3

Differential WBC count Increase in lymphocytes, many atypical

Differential diagnosis: heterophil agglutination Negative in CMV (positive in mononucleosis)

•••••• Multidisciplinary Plan[2]

Medications

    Ganciclovir, Foscarnet, Acyclovir (alone or in combination) for treatment of CMV retinitis and other severe disease manifestations. Dosages vary depending on the severity of the infection and the immune status of the patient.
    For bone marrow transplantation recipients: Ganciclovir plus CMV hyperimmune globulin

General Management

    Transfusion of sedimented RBCs for anemia
    Transfusion of platelet-rich plasma for thrombocytopenia
    Antipyretics for fever in CMV mononucleosis-like syndrome
    Experimental live CMV vaccines currently being evaluated for prevention
    Infants born of antibody-free mothers should not receive breast milk from a women serologically positive for CMV antibodies, since the virus may be in the milk

NURSING CARE

Nursing Assessment

See p. 1122.

■ TOXOPLASMOSIS

Toxoplasmosis is a systemic protozoan infection, ranging from subclinical to severe to chronic. Four different clinical syndromes can be identified, depending on where the pathogen localizes in the body. Transplacental transmission results in congenital toxoplasmosis, which may be fatal to the fetus or neonate.

•••••• Pathophysiology

Toxoplasmosis, like the cytomegalovirus (CMV) infections, may be congenital or acquired. Unlike CMV, there is not a risk for perinatal acquired toxoplasmosis. Both forms of toxoplasmosis may be present with clinical patterns ranging from subclinical infection to severe generalized infection (with neurologic and sensory sequelae) to death. Both may occur in latent or recurring forms under conditions of reduced host defenses.

The pathogen producing toxoplasmosis, *Toxoplasma gondii,* is a protozoan that is pathogenic to animals and humans. The pathogen can multiply only in living cells. This parasite exists in three forms: trophozoites, tissue cysts, and oocysts. Trophozoites are capable of invading, multiplying in, and necrotizing all host cells. Trophozoites can remain viable extracellularly in body secretions such as peritoneal fluid, breast milk, urine, saliva, or tears for a few hours to days. They cannot survive drying, heating, freezing, or contact with digestive juices.

Tissue cysts are formed within host cells. A surrounding membrane produced by the pathogen encapsulates up to 3000 organisms. This enables the parasites to maintain their viability for the life of the host in spite of circulating host antibodies. Tissue cysts are responsible for recurrent infection in humans and for transmission of the pathogen from animal reservoirs. Tissue cysts also cannot survive freezing, drying, or heating.

Oocysts are a form in the life cycle of *T. gondii* that occurs only in cats. Oocysts, a noninfectious form, aredischarged in the feces of infected cats. Oocysts sporulate in 1 to 21 days in environmental temperatures of 4° to 37° C (39° to 99° F). They can remain infectious in the soil for 1 year, given favorable environmental conditions.

Transmission of *T. gondii* can occur by one of two modes: by ingestion of tissue cysts in uncooked meat or ingestion of sporulated oocysts by hands or food contaminated with cat feces, or by transplacental transmission of trophozoites in maternal circulation during acute infection acquired by the mother during the pregnancy.

In ingestion-acquired toxoplasmosis the capsule surrounding ingested cysts is digested by gastric juices. This permits viable trophozoites to invade intestinal mucosa and to disseminate throughout the body by way of blood and the lymphatics. Organ cell invasion produces foci of necrosis surrounded by intense inflammatory reaction with mononuclear cell infiltration. The spleen, liver, brain, lung, myocardium, and eye are most frequently involved. The development of cysts and tissue calcifications may impair organ functioning.

An early antibody response destroys many parasites before they form tissue cysts and supports cyst formation by the remainder. Thus the infection is limited to its mild or subclinical form for the majority of infected persons. Failure of an immune response, as is the case with immunosuppressed patients or those with debilitating disease, is more likely to result in progressive, life-threatening infection with multiple organ involvement and extensive damage.

Transplacentally transmitted *T. gondii* is disseminated to every organ in the developing fetus, particularly in the brain, heart, lungs, adrenal glands, striated muscle, and eye. Focal necrotic and inflammatory lesions are produced with cyst formation and calcification. Extensive destruction may occur in the central nervous system, affecting the cortex, subcortical white matter, caudate and lenticular nuclei, midbrain, pons, medulla, and spinal cord. Obstruction of the foramina of Monro

or the aqueduct of Sylvius may result in an internal hydrocephalus. Microcephalus, hydrocephalus, or varying degrees of central nervous system impairment may occur.

Infection in the eye produces edema and necrosis of the retina, necrosis and disruption of the pigmented layer of the rods and cones, and infiltration of the retina and choroid with inflammatory cells. Granulation tissue and exudate may spread to the vitreous. This chorioretinitis may be manifested within weeks after birth or at some time later in life when the latent infection becomes reactivated.

Maternal infection early in the pregnancy is usually associated with fetal death or severe disease at birth. Infection later in pregnancy results in less severe or no manifestations at birth. Only 11% of maternal infections result in infants damaged at birth. The majority, 60% of infants, are not affected; 29% have subclinical infections that are manifest as neurologic or sensory defects as the infant develops.

Complications

Spontaneous abortion
Microcephalus, hydrocephalus, or other CNS impairment in neonate
Chorioretinitis
Multiple organ involvement in immunocompromised patients
Encephalitis

•••••• Diagnostic Studies and Findings[27]

Culture (mice or tissue culture) of specimen from lymph or muscle biopsy, blood or CSF during acute phase Identification of *T. gondii* cysts or trophozoites in 4-6 wk is presumptive evidence of current infection

Microscopic examination of tissue sections or smears Identification of trophozoites present during acute infection; identification of cysts does not differentiate between acute or chronic infection

Serology (Indirect fluorescent antibody) IgG antibodies (1:4) appear within 1 to 2 weeks after acute infection; reach high titers (over 1:1000) in 6 to 8 weeks; and then gradually decline over months or years to titers of 1:4-1:64; false positive results may follow blood transfusions; fourfold rise in titers or slow decline after the peak is diagnostic; may be false negative in immunosuppressed persons

•••••• Multidisciplinary Plan[3]

Medications

Treatment for initial infection during pregnancy or for active chorioretinitis, myocarditis, or other organ involvement
Pyrimethamine (paraprim) combined with sulfadiazine and folinic acid (to avoid bone marrow depression) for 4 weeks; dosages vary depending on age of patient, disease severity, and immune status

General Management

To prevent spread, reject leukocyte, or organ donors who are antibody positive

NURSING CARE

Nursing Assessment

	Mononucleosis	Cytomegalovirus Infection	Toxoplasmosis
History	Contact with person with mononucleosis	Immunosuppression	Exposure to cat feces; immunosuppression
Subjective symptoms	Fatigue, anorexia, chills, retroorbital headache, photophobia, dysphagia	Fatigue, nausea, myalgia, headache, photophobia	Fatigue and malaise 6 to 10 days preceding other symptoms; headache; photophobia
Body temperature	Marked elevation (1 to 2 wks) 38° to 41°C (100° to 105°F), peaks in afternoon	Low-grade fever lasting 2 to 5 wks	Fever up to 41° C (106°F)
Eye	Periorbital edema	Retinitis	Chorioretinitis: blurred vision, pain, loss of central vision
Throat	Painful, exudative tonsillitis (white or greenish gray), pasty membrane with bad odor; inflammation and tonsillar edema may be severe	No involvement	No involvement
Oral cavity	Bleeding gums, palatine petechiae	No involvement	No involvement
Lymph nodes	Cervical, submandibular, and axillary node discrete enlargement and tenderness	No involvement	Generalized lymphadenopathy: firm, smooth, discrete, movable enlarged nodes; tenderness, or may be painless
Abdomen	Splenomegaly; hepatomegaly	Splenomegaly; hepatomegaly	Splenomegaly
Skin	Jaundice, macular rash, or purpura	Rubelliform rash	Generalized bright red or pink maculopapular rash, blanching on pressure
Respiratory	Symptoms of pneumonia	Cough or symptoms of pneumonia	Coarse rales, cough, dyspnea, cyanosis
Neurologic	Meningitis or encephalitis	Sensory and motor weakness, pyramidal tract signs	Encephalitis: convulsions, ataxia, vomiting, confusion
Other		Myocarditis	Symptoms of myocarditis
Congenital		Jaundice, petechial rash; hepatosplenomegaly; lethargy; microcephaly; respiratory distress; retardation; chorioretinitis; seizures	Hydrocephalus or microcephalus; convulsions; pneumonitis; jaundice, purpura, petechial or maculopapular rash; bilateral chorioretinitis; hepatomegaly, splenomegaly

From Grimes.[26]

Nursing Dx & Intervention

Risk for infection (patient contacts) related to methods of transmission of CMV

- Employ secretion precautions for hospitalized infants known to be shedding CMV *to prevent transmission of CMV or mononucleosis.*
- Women of childbearing age or who are pregnant should wash hands thoroughly after handling diapers of neonates with congenital CMV *to prevent acquiring CMV infection.*

Hyperthermia related to infection

- Monitor body temperature.
- Bathe patient frequently *to lower body temperature and to remove perspiration.*

- Administer oral fluids freely *to compensate for increased needs.*
- Maintain comfortable environmental temperature with freely circulating air.

Pain related to inflammation and fever

- Administer analgesics per order or saline gargle for sore throat *to relieve pain.*

Activity intolerance related to fatigue

- Encourage bed rest during acute symptomatic disease *to conserve energy.*
- Assist patient in developing a realistic plan for returning to work or school during convalescence following mononucleosis. *Prolonged malaise accompanying these diseases may be unanticipated.*

Ineffective breathing pattern related to pneumonitis

- Assess ventilation to include evaluation of breathing rate, rhythm, and depth: chest expansion; presence of respiratory distress (e.g., dyspnea, shortness of breath, nasal flaring pursed-lip breathing, prolonged expiratory phase, use of accessory muscles, or adventitious sounds) *to detect pneumonitis, which is a potential complication of these infections, particularly in the immunocompromised.*
- Maintain patient in position that facilitates ventilation (head of bed in semi-Fowler's position or patient sitting and leaning forward on overbed table) *to facilitate lung expansion for improved air exchange.*
- Instruct patient in proper pulmonary hygiene routines *to promote easy effective breathing, facilitate removal of secretions from tracheobronchial tree, and minimize pulmonary congestion, which could lead to superinfections.*
- Assess patient for tiring in relation to attempts to breathe.
- Assist ventilation, if necessary. Administer O_2 *to provide adequate intake of O_2.*
- Protect patient from known sources of secondary infection, *which is common with these patients.*
- Administer antiinfectives as prescribed *to control progression of the pneumonitis.*

Risk for injury related to splenomegaly and to antiinfective agents prescribed for toxoplasmosis

- Monitor for signs of neurologic or purpuric complications *to detect splenic rupture.*
- Protect patient from activity *to reduce risk of splenic rupture.*

Sensory-perceptual alterations (visual) related to chorioretinitis of CMV and toxoplasmosis

- Provide a safe environment for patients with chorioretinitis. Assist patient with interpreting the environment, personal care, and ambulation as needed. Refer for rehabilitation for vision loss *to prevent injury.*

Patient Education/Home Care Planning*

Instruct patients with infectious mononucleosis or cMV:

1. Although complete bed rest is usually unnecessary during acute disease or convalescence, the patient caring for himself or herself at home should be encouraged to rest as symptoms dictate. Convalescence may be as long as 3 to 4 weeks.
2. The patient with splenomegaly should avoid heavy lifting, contact sports, or any activity that may increase the risk of injury to the spleen. Active children must be protected from injury.
3. Report to physician any jaundice, excess bruising or bleeding, or symptoms of abnormal central nervous system functioning.

4. EB virus is transmitted by contact with saliva; CMV is transmitted by contact with all body secretions and excretions.

Instruct patients with toxoplasmosis:

1. Patients treated with pyrimethamine (which depresses bone marrow) should have peripheral blood cell and platelet counts twice a week during therapy. Explain medication regimen, particularly the use of folinic acid or baker's yeast to counteract effects of pyrimethamine.
2. Immunocompromised persons and pregnant women can avoid exposure by cooking all meat to 60° C (140° F), washing fruits and vegetables, washing hands thoroughly after handling uncooked meat, wearing gloves while working in soil, and avoiding cat feces. Children's sandboxes should be kept free of cat feces.
3. Infants born with asymptomatic toxoplasmosis should be evaluated periodically for visual problems and developmental delays.
4. Refer families of infants with congenital toxoplasmosis to counseling, support, or rehabilitation resources as needed. Provide information about the resource and its services and how to access the resource.
5. The congenital anomalies do not represent a hereditary defect.
6. There is not a risk for congenital toxoplasmosis in subsequent pregnancies. The risk is present only when toxoplasmosis is acquired during the pregnancy.

*From Grimes.[26]

Evaluation

Infection will not be transmitted   Patient demonstrates behavior to prevent transmission of pathogens to others. Health care team washes hands after providing care to each patient and follows universal blood and body secretion procedures with all patients. Health care staff remain free of signs of infection.

Body temperature is maintained within normal range; patient comfort and safety are maintained   Patient's body temperature is between 36° and 38° C (96.8° and 100° F). Pulse and respiration are normal. Skin is cool to touch and free of excess perspiration. Patient's clothing and bedding are dry. Patient is free of headache and malaise associated with fever.

Patient obtains relief from pain   Patient swallows without pain. Patient's sleep is uninterrupted by pain. Patient rests in bed without overt signs of pain.

Patient achieves adequate rest to conserve energy during active disease and returns to preillness level of activity during convalescence   Patient maintains bed rest during acute disease, with gradual return of activity. No fatigue with exertion during convalescence.

Patient demonstrates normal respiratory pattern, oxygen intake, and blood gas levels   Bronchovesicular breath sounds are heard throughout patient's lungs. There are no areas of decreased breath sounds or consolidation. Respiratory rate is normal. CO_2, Po_2, and Pco_2 are normal.

Patient does not experience injury   Patient's spleen is nonpalpable and nontender. Leukocyte, lymphocyte, and platelet counts, billirubin level, and serum transaminase (SGOT, SGPT) levels are normal.

Patient is not confused or frightened by environmental stimuli during time of alteration in vision; visual function returns to normal   Persons with vision loss are aware of counseling, support, or rehabilitation resources and have phone numbers and names of people to contact at those services.

Patient self-administers anti-infective agents as prescribed   Patient completes full course of antiinfective therapy. No preventable drug interactions or allergic reactions are experienced. If untoward reactions are experienced, the patient discontinues the drug and contacts the physician immediately.

LYME DISEASE

Lyme disease is a multisystem disease caused by a spirochete that is transmitted by the bite of a tick. If untreated in early infection, the disease becomes chronic and mimics other rheumatic diseases. The disease was recognized in the early 1970s as a mysterious clustering of arthritis occurring among children in Lyme, Connecticut. It usually occurs in stages characterized by different clinical manifestations and by exacerbations and remissions (see box). The most common early sign is erythema migrans, an annular skin lesion that appears at the site of a tick bite. Systemic symptoms and neurologic, cardiac, or arthritic involvement occur in varying combinations over months to years.

•••••• Pathophysiology

The spirochete, *Borrelia burgdorferi*, is introduced into the skin by the bite of an ixodid tick. The spirochete produces an endotoxin, which causes initial vascular and cellular inflammation. Later pathologic changes appear to result from the immune response to the pathogen. The pathogen can remain localized in the initial lesion or can invade and replicate in any tissue. The spirochete has been cultured from blood, skin, CSF, and joint fluid and has been observed in specimens of skin, myocardial, retinal, and synovial lesions.

Complications

Aseptic meningitis or encephalitis
Chorea
Cerebellar ataxia
Cranial or peripheral neuropathies
Heart block
Congestive heart failure
Congenital infection

•••••• Diagnostic Studies and Findings[27]

Culture of specimen of blood into animal tissue   Positive for spirochete

Microscopic examination of stained (Warthin-Starry silver stain, direct and indirect immunofluorescence) specimen of skin taken from outside the periphery of EM   Positive for spirochete

Serology (IFA, ELISA, EIA)   Elevation of antibody titers. (Serologic tests are not reliable by themselves for diagnosis. They are not sensitive in early disease stages, leading to many false-negative results. In addition, the tests cross react with the antibodies to other pathogens with similar antigens, such as the spirochetes associated with syphilis, leptospirosis, and periodontal disease.)

•••••• Multidisciplinary Plan[3]

Medications

Doxycycline, 100 mg po bid or
Amoxicillin, 500 mg po qid
For children <9 years and pregnant and lactating women:
 Amoxicillin 50 mg/Kg/day in divided doses
For penicillin allergy: erythromycin or cefuroxime axetil
Duration of treatment with all of the above depends on the stage of disease

---

■ FACTS ABOUT LYME DISEASE

Occurrence: Most commonly reported vector-borne infectious disease in the United States; endemic foci according to geographic areas where the tick vectors occur; i.e., along Atlantic coast (MA to ME), upper Midwest (WI, MN), and west (CA, OR); also occurs in Canada, Europe, former Soviet Union, China, and Japan; seasonal variation depends on the life cycle of ticks in different geographic regions.

Etiologic Agent: Borrelia burgdorferi, a spirochete; three different subgroups have been identified in Europe.

Reservoir: Certain ixodid ticks that feed on deer and small mammals such as rats; tick genus varies with geographic location.

Transmission: Tick bite; experimental transmission in animals does not occur until the tick has been attached for 24 or more hours.

Incubation Period: 3-32 days until onset of erythema migrans; earlier stages may be asymptomatic.

Period of Communicability: No person-to-person transmission; rare reports of congenital transmission but no evidence of adverse pregnancy outcomes.

Susceptibility and Resistance: General; reinfection has occurred in those treated with antibiotics during early disease.

Report to Local Health Authority: Case report required in all states.

Data from Benenson.[3]

Treatment of localized EM is 2 weeks; for early disseminated disease 3-4 weeks; for arthritis-4 weeks

Other anti-infective regimens are suggested for neurologic and cardiac pathologies.

General Management

Anti-inflammatory drugs

Joint aspiration, surgical joint lining removal

NURSING CARE

Nursing care varies depending on the stage in the disease and the body system effected when the infected person presents to the health care providers. See related chapters in this book. Providing support during the diagnosis is important.

Patient Education/Home Care Planning

1. Instruct patient to take entire course of antibiotic as prescribed.
2. Instruct patient and the family that relapses may occur and recurrence of symptoms should be reported to the health care provider so that antibiotic therapy can be resumed immediately.
3. Instruct the public to avoid tick-infested areas and to check body surfaces every 3 to 4 hours for attached ticks if working or playing in infested areas.
4. Instruct the public to remove any ticks promptly and carefully without crushing. Apply tweezers or forceps close to the skin and, using gentle traction, remove tick from the skin. Protect hands with gloves or tissue. Swab the bite area with an antiseptic after removing the tick.

From Grimes.[26]

RESPIRATORY INFECTIOUS DISEASES

The respiratory infectious diseases discussed in this section are the acute and chronic respiratory pathologic conditions that are caused by a specific pathogenic agent that is transmitted by inhalation or by direct contact with infectious respiratory secretions. These include influenza, tuberculosis, histoplasmosis, and legionellosis (Legionnaire's disease).

Nonspecific lower respiratory infections such as pneumonia are discussed in Chapter 2. Nonspecific upper respiratory infections such as pharyngitis and tonsillitis are discussed in Chapter 7.

SIGNS AND SYMPTOMS OF LYME DISEASE

One or more of the following may be present at different times during the infection:

EARLY INFECTION

Rash: Erythema migrans (EM)
Migratory muscle and joint pain
Headache
Stiff neck
Significant fatigue/malaise
Fever
Facial paralysis (Bell's palsy)
Meningitis
Conjunctivitis (less common)
Myocarditis (less common)

LATE INFECTION

Arthritis
Central nervous system pathology, such as encephalitis, confusion (less common)
Skin pathology

Data from Grimes,[26] NIH.[28]

FACTS ABOUT INFLUENZA

Occurrence: worldwide in pandemics, epidemics, localized outbreaks, and sporadic cases; highest in winter in temperate zones

Etiologic agent: three types of viruses (A, B, and C), each with many strains

Reservoir: humans; some mammals suspected as sources of new strains of viruses

Transmission: direct transmission by inhalation of virus in airborne mucous discharge

Incubation period: 24 to 72 hours

Period of communicability: 3 days from onset of symptoms

Susceptibility and resistance: universal; infection produces immunity to a specific strain of virus, but duration of immunity depends on antigenic drift in strain

Mandatory case report to local health authority

Data from Benenson.[3]

INFLUENZA

Influenza is a generalized, acute, febrile disease associated with upper and lower respiratory infection; it is characterized by a severe and protracted cough, fever, headache, myalgia, prostration, coryza, and mild sore throat (see box above).

• • • • • • Pathophysiology

Influenza viruses A, B, or C, each with many mutagenic strains, are inhaled in aerosolized mucous droplets shed from infected persons. The viruses are deposited on and penetrate the surface of upper respiratory tract mucosal cells, producing cell lysis and destruction of the ciliated epithelium. Viral neuraminidase decreases the viscosity of the mucosa, thus facilitating the spread of virus-containing exudate to the lower respiratory tract. An interstitial inflammation and necrosis of the bronchiolar and alveolar epithelium result, filling the alveoli with a purulent exudate.

Regeneration of epithelium, following necrosis and desquamation, slowly begins after the fifth day of illness. Regeneration reaches a maximum within 9 to 15 days, at which time mucus production and cilia begin to appear. Before complete regeneration the compromised epithelium is prone to secondary bacterial invasion, resulting in bacterial pneumonia usually caused by *S. aureus.*

The initial invasion of the virus can be aborted at the portal of entry if virus-specific secretory antibodies (IgA) are present in mucous secretions and if virus-specific serum antibodies are adequate.

The disease is usually self-limited. Acute symptoms last 2 to 7 days and are followed by a convalescent period of about a week. The disease is important because of its cyclic epidemic and pandemic nature and because of the high mortality associated with pulmonary complications resulting from secondary bacterial pneumonia. This risk is highest in elderly and chronically diseased persons.

Complications

Primary viral pneumonia
Secondary bacterial pneumonia

····· Diagnostic Studies and Findings

Tissue culture of nasal or pharyngeal secretions Positive for influenza virus

Sputum culture Positive for bacteria in secondary infections

Antigen/antibody tests of secretions (fluorescent antibody) Direct identification of viral antigens

Serology (Hemagglutination inhibition or complement fixation) tests Fourfold increase in antibody titer between acute and convalescent stages

····· Multidisciplinary Plan[21]

Medications

Anti-infective agents: see Table 13-17 for recommended dosages for amantadine and rimantadine treatment and prophylaxis.

   Agent-specific anti-infective agents for bacterial complications or for patients with chronic pulmonary disease

Antipyretics: ASA, 600 mg po q4h for adults; acetaminophen for children

Adrenergic agents: Phenylephrine (Neo-Synephrine), 0.25%, 2 drops in each nostril for nasal congestion

Antitussive agents: Terpin hydrate with codeine, 5-10 ml po q3-4h for adults for cough

Active immunization: Vaccine must be repeated yearly in the fall for viral strain expected in the winter; recommended for any person over 6 mo who, because of age or medical condition, is at risk for complications of influenza. This

---

■ **TABLE 13-17 Recommended Dosage for Amantadine and Rimantadine Treatment and Prophylaxis**

Antiviral Agent	Age			
	1–9 yrs	**10–13 yrs**	**14–64 yrs**	**≥65 yrs**
Amantadine*				
Treatment	5 mg/kg/day up to 150 mg† in two divided doses	100 mg twice daily‡	100 mg twice daily	≤100 mg/day
Prophylaxis	5 mg/kg/day up to 150 mg† in two divided doses	100 mg twice daily‡	100 mg twice daily	≤100 mg/day
Rimantadine§				
Treatment	NA	NA	100 mg twice daily	100 or 200¶ mg/day
Prophylaxis	5 mg/kg/day up to 150 mg† in two divided doses	100 mg twice daily‡	100 mg twice daily	100 or 200¶ mg/day

From Centers for Disease Control.[21]
NOTE: Amantadine manufacturers include: Dupont Pharma (Symmetrel—syrup); Solvay Pharmaceuticals (Symadine—capsule); Chase Pharmaceuticals and Invamed (Amantadine HCL—capsule); and Copley Pharmaceuticals, Barre National, and Mikart (Amantadine HCL—syrup). Rimantadine is manufactured by Forest Laboratories (Flumandine—tablet and syrup).
*The drug package insert should be consulted for dosage recommendations for administering amantadine to persons with creatinine clearance ∪50 mL/min.
†5 mg/kg of amantadine or rimantadine syrup = 1 tsp/22 lbs.
‡Children ≥ 10 years of age who weigh <40 kg should be administered amantadine or rimantadine at a dose of 5 mg/kg/day.
§A reduction in dose to 100 mg/day of rimantadine is recommended for persons who have severe hepatic dysfunction or those with creatinine clearance <10 mL/min. Other persons with less severe hepatic or renal dysfunction taking >100 mg/day of rimantadine should be observed closely, and the dosage should be reduced or the drug discontinued, if necessary.
¶Elderly nursing-home residents should be administered only 100 mg/day of rimantadine. A reduction in dose to 100 mg/day should be considered for all persons ≥65 years of age if they experience possible side effects when taking 200 mg/day.
NA = Not applicable.

includes residents of nursing homes and chronic care fa-cilities and health care providers in contact with high-risk patients.

Children under 12 should receive only split virus vaccine

Age Group	Dosage	No. of Doses	Route
6-35 mo	0.25 ml	1 or 2	IM
3-8 yr	0.5 ml	1 or 2	IM
9-12 yr	0.5 ml	1	IM
>12 yr	0.5 ml	1	IM

General Management

Oxygen and IV fluid and electrolytes for complications

NURSING CARE

Nursing Assessment

History

Failure to receive influenza vaccine within the present sea-son; exposure to person with influenza

Subjective Symptoms

Prostration; myalgia (particularly in back and legs), anorexia and malaise, headache, photophobia, and retrobulbar aching

Body Temperature

Sudden-onset fever (38° to 39° C [102° to 103° F]) that grad-ually falls and rises again on the third day

Head and Neck

Conjunctivitis and anterior cervical lymphadenopathy may be present; flushed face

Respiratory Concerns

Initial (mild at first): sore throat, substernal burning; nonpro-ductive cough; coryza

Advanced: severe and productive cough; erythema of soft palate, posterior hard palate, tonsillar pillars, and posterior pharynx; increased respiratory rate

Complicating viral pneumonia: dyspnea, cyanosis, hemopty-sis, crepitant and subcrepitant rales

Complicating bacterial pneumonia: same as for viral pneu-monia plus purulent or bloody sputum

Nursing Dx & Intervention

Risk for infection (patient and patient contacts) related to presence of virus in nasopharyngeal secretions

- Collect pharyngeal specimen. *Incorrect collection and handling of specimens may destroy the pathogen or con-taminate the specimen with environmental organisms, in-*

terfering with accurate diagnosis and treatment. Improper handling can also contaminate the health care worker.

- Administer vaccine or antiviral agent as prescribed. *An-tiviral agents decrease severity of influenza.*
- Protect patient from exposure to bacteria. Monitor for a subsequent increase in temperature accompanied by chest pain, dyspnea, hemoptysis, purulent sputum, or ear pain; report findings. *Early detection of secondary infection and treatment with anti-infective agents may prevent dissemi-nation of the pathogen, severe disease, and death.*
- Initiate universal blood and body secretion precautions *to prevent transmission to health care workers, other pa-tients, and patient contacts.*
- Use protective isolation procedures as indicated. Prevent patient exposure to infected visitors or staff. Limit visi-tors, if necessary, *to limit the exposure of patients to addi-tional pathogens.*
- Participate in follow-up of high-risk patient contacts *to ensure that the patient receives flu vaccine or antiviral agent.*

Hyperthermia related to infection

- Monitor body temperature *to detect fever.*
- Administer antipyretics, as ordered.
- Bathe with tepid water or alcohol *to reduce high fever.*
- Adjust environmental temperature *for patient's comfort.*
- Remove excess clothing and bedding *to ensure heat loss.*
- Encourage adequate fluid intake *to compensate for fluid loss associated with elevated body temperature.*

Ineffective breathing pattern related to infectious process in respiratory epithelium

- Administer decongestants, as prescribed *to reduce edema in air passages.*
- Provide cool, humidified air *to liquify secretions.*
- Suction, if necessary, *to remove secretions.*
- Monitor for signs of viral or bacterial pneumonia *to inter-vene early with anti-infectives.*
- Provide oxygen, as prescribed; *to ensure an adequate sup-ply of oxygen.*
- Encourage as much fluids as patient can tolerate (3000 ml for adult) *to liquify secretions.*
- Administer IV fluids as prescribed, *to provide additional fluids required during infection.*
- Encourage bed rest *to decrease demands on respiratory system.*

Patient Education/Home Care Planning

1. Maintain bed rest for 2 or 3 days after temperature re-turns to normal.
2. Force fluids.
3. Continue to take antibiotics for duration, as prescribed for bacterial complications.

4. Report symptoms of secondary infection (e.g., ear pain, purulent or bloody sputum; chest pain, and increase in temperature) to physician.
5. High-risk persons should be encouraged to receive influenza vaccine before the start of the flu season.
6. Side effects of amantadine prophylaxis include nausea, dizziness, nervousness, insomnia, and impaired concentration. These disappear when the drug is stopped. These and other side effects, particularly in persons at risk for impaired renal function, should be reported to a physician.

Evaluation

Infection is prevented in persons experiencing risk factors   High-risk persons are vaccinated or are receiving antiviral agent. Patient's sputum cultures are negative; body temperature is normal; leukocyte count and sedimentation rate are normal.

Infection is not transmitted   All patient contacts are adequately immunized or examined and treated with antiviral agent.

Body temperature is maintained within the normal range; comfort and safety are maintained   Patient's body temperature is between 36° and 38° C (96.8° and 100° F) orally; pulse and respirations are between normal limits; skin is cool to touch and free of excess perspiration. Patient's clothing and bedding are dry.

Patient demonstrates normal respiratory pattern and blood gas levels   Patient's breathing patterns are normal; blood levels (O_2 saturation, CO_2, and Po_2) are normal; skin is warm and normal colored. Patient shows no signs of pneumonia, and secretions are clear and thin. There is no cough.

■ TUBERCULOSIS

Tuberculosis (TB) is a chronic pulmonary and extrapulmonary infectious disease acquired by inhalation of a dried-droplet nucleus containing a tubercle bacillus into the alveolar structure of the lung; it is characterized by stages of early infection, which may progress to active, infectious TB disease or to latency, and a potential for recurrent postprimary disease (see box).

•••••• Pathophysiology

Tuberculosis infection is different from tuberculosis disease (also called active tuberculosis). Tuberculosis infection is characterized by the presence of *Mycobacterium tuberculosis (M. tb)* and certain other mycobacteria in the tissue of a host. The other mycobacteria (e.g., *M. africanium, M. bovis*) are rare in developed countries. The term *tuberculosis disease* refers to the condition that results when invasion of tissue by the mycobac-

---

■ FACTS ABOUT TUBERCULOSIS

Occurrence: Worldwide; after a period of decline in the United States, incidence has increased; recent outbreaks have occurred among homeless, migrants, persons with HIV infection, health care workers and in correctional facilities.

Etiologic agent: *Mycobacterium tuberculosis* and, occasionally, other mycobacteria. Drug-resistant strains are an increasing problem.

Reservoir: humans; *M. bovis* in diseased cattle.

Transmission: inhalation of airborne droplets from the sputum of persons with tuberculosis disease; infrequently by ingestion or skin penetration.

Incubation period: An immune response can be demonstrated 4-12 weeks after exposure. Once one has been infected, disease can occur at anytime during one's lifetime.

Period of communicability: as long as bacilli are in sputum: some are intermittently communicable for years.

Susceptibility and resistance: All are susceptible; Highest is in children less than 3 years; adolescents, young adults, those over 65 years, the HIV infected, silicone and asbestos workers, the malnourished and other immunosuppressed individuals.

Mandatory case report to local health authority.

Data from Benenson.[3]

---

terium results in pathologic changes in tissue. *M. tb* is capable of remaining viable in host tissue for long periods of time. When tissue invasion has occurred but pathologic change has not occurred, individuals are considered to be tuberculosis infected. Tuberculosis disease occurs when that infection leads to pathologic changes (see Emergency Alert box).

Tuberculosis infection and disease occur in stages: (1) initial infection, (2) latency, and (3) active disease, which can either follow initial infection or recur as postprimary disease after a period of latency. The initial (primary) infection develops when tubercle bacilli invade tissue at the portal of entry (usually the middle or lower zones of the lungs), multiply there over 3 weeks, and create an inflammatory lesion. Transmission resulting in the initial infection is usually by inhalation of minute droplet particles coughed or sneezed into the air by a person whose sputum contains the tubercle bacilli. Less commonly, transmission may occur by ingestion or by invasion of the skin or mucous membranes. Once the bacteria have invaded, they enter the lymphatic system and are carried to the nearest group of lymph nodes where they also produce inflammatory lesions. In addition, hematogenous dissemination of the bacilli results in subclinical bacteremia and the production of inflammatory lesions throughout the body. Individuals who are in the initial stage of infection are not capable of transmitting the organism to others.

The sites and the extensiveness of the systemic lesions depend on the numbers of disseminated bacilli and the speed with which the host produces an immune response. These early lesions at the portal of entry and in the lymph nodes and hematogenously disseminated lesions are referred to as the primary complex.

The extent of inflammatory response at the sites of tissue invasion increases with the number of invading bacilli. Nonspecific cellular resistance permits some phagocytosis of tubercle bacilli, producing suppuration and necrosis in the central portion of the lesion. Bacilli continue to replicate at the periphery of the lesion. This initial or primary infection stage is generally symptomless.

Within 3 to 12 weeks a cellular and humoral immune response can be detected by a skin test. *Mycobacterium*-specific lymphocytes and antibodies stimulate a fibroblastic response at the periphery of the lesion, resulting in a dense connective tissue enclosure and the formation of a noncaseating granuloma. The focal lesions continue to harbor viable tubercle bacilli, with the potential for reactivation under conditions of decreased host resistance. This period is called latency.

The specific immune response results in successful encapsulation of the lesions in all but 5% to 10% of infected persons. All but about 5% of those who enter the latency stage will remain free of tuberculosis disease for the rest of their lives. However, the immune response does not preclude reinfection with subsequent exposure. Conversion from latency to the post-

primary stage of active disease is associated with HIV infection, other severe disease, age greater than 65 years, and immunosuppressive therapies. HIV infection is particularly likely to facilitate conversion from latency to tuberculosis disease. Individuals with latent *M. tb* infection who are co-infected with HIV are thought to convert to active tuberculosis at a rate of 7% to 10% a year.

Reactivated disease following latency accounts for most of the active tuberculosis diagnosed today. It occurs most frequently in aged persons, in the immunosuppressed, and in persons with chronic and debilitating disease. Although reactivation may occur in any of the focal lesions, it most commonly occurs in those in the upper lobes or at the apex of the lower lobes of the lungs, forming abscesses and tuberculous cavities at those sites. Untreated reactivated disease has a variable course with many exacerbations and remissions. Complications caused by excessive cavitation are common.

For 5% to 15% of infected persons, host responses are inadequate to contain the infection, and active disease progresses in the portal of entry lesion or in all lesions in the body. Necrosis and cavitation continue in the lesions, forming caseation. The lesions may rupture, spreading necrotic residue and bacilli throughout the tissue and throughout the body. Disseminated bacilli establish new focal lesions that progress through stages of inflammation, noncaseating granulomas, and caseating necrosis.

The disease symptoms vary with the body tissue affected. Extrapulmonary tuberculosis in the meninges, blood vessels, kidneys, bones, joints, larynx, skin, intestines, lymph nodes, peritoneum, or eyes is much less common than pulmonary tuberculosis.

Complications

Extrapulmonary disease

Cavitation and destruction of lungs

•••••• Diagnostic Studies and Findings[16,19]

Sputum culture   Positive for *M. tuberculosis* in active disease; will not be positive during latency.

Drug sensitivity studies   Reported as sensitive, intermediate and resistant indicating the effectiveness of the drug against the strain of *M. tb.*

Acid-fast with Ziehl-Neelsen stain smear of sputum (CSF or blood in extrapulmonary disease   Positive for acid-fast bacilli

Histologic examination or culture of tissue in extrapulmonary disease   Positive for *M. tuberculosis*

Skin tests: intradermal infection of antigen (Mantoux test: five tuberculin units of purified protein derivative [PPD] infected intradermally   Test is read in 48 to 72 hours. A positive reaction (see box) indicates past infection and presence of antibodies; does not indicate active disease; nonspecific reactions during first 48 hours can be overlooked; if reaction is negative and if person has not had a skin test in some time, a second test may be performed 1 week later, if the second test is negative, the patient is considered not infected. If the second

SUMMARY OF INTERPRETATION OF TB SKIN TEST RESULTS

1. An induration of ≥5 mm is classified as positive in:
   - persons who have human immunodeficiency virus (HIV) infection or risk factors for HIV infection but unknown HIV status;
   - persons who have had recent close contact* with persons who have active tuberculosis (TB);
   - persons who have fibrotic chest radiographs (consistent with healed TB).
2. An induration of ≥10 mm is classified as positive in all persons who do not meet any of the criteria above but who have other risk factors for TB, including:

   High-risk groups—
   - injecting-drug users known to be HIV seronegative;
   - persons who have other medical conditions that reportedly increase the risk for progressing from latent TB infection to active TB (e.g., silicosis; gastrectomy or jejunoileal bypass; being ≥10% below ideal body weight; chronic renal failure with renal dialysis; diabetes mellitus; high-dose corticosteroid or other immunosuppressive therapy; some hematologic disorders, including malignancies such as leukemias and lymphomas; and other malignancies);
   - children <4 years of age.

   High-prevalence groups—
   - persons born in countries in Asia, Africa, the Caribbean, and Latin America that have high prevalence of TB;
   - persons from medically underserved, low-income populations;
   - residents of long-term–care facilities (e.g., correctional institutions and nursing homes);
   - persons from high-risk populations in their communities, as determined by local public health authorities.
3. An induration of ≥15 mm is classified as positive in persons who do not meet any of the above criteria.
4. Recent converters are defined on the basis of both size of induration and age of the person being tested:
   - ≥10 mm increase within a 2-year period is classified as a recent conversion for persons <35 years of age;
   - ≥15 mm increase within a 2-year period is classified as a recent conversion for persons ≥35 years of age.
5. PPD skin-test results in health-care workers (HCWs)
   - In general, the recommendations in sections 1, 2, and 3 of this table should be followed when interpreting skin-test results in HCWs.

   However, the prevalence of TB in the facility should be considered when choosing the appropriate cut-point for defining a positive PPD reaction. In facilities where there is essentially no risk for exposure to *Mycobacterium tuberculosis* (i.e., minimal- or very low-risk facilities, an induration ≥15 mm may be a suitable cut-point for HCWs who have no other risk factors. In facilities where TB patients receive care, the cut-point for HCWs with no other risk factors may be ≥10 mm.

From Centers for Disease Control.[19]
*Recent close contact implies either household or social contact or unprotected occupational exposure similar in intensity and duration to household contact.

test is positive, the person should be considered to be positive, but not to have a recent infection.

Pleural needle biopsy   Positive for granulomas of tuberculosis; giant cells indicating caseation necrosis

Chest radiograph examination   Findings may show calcification at the original site, enlargement of hilar lymph nodes, parenchymal infiltrate representing extension of the original site of infection, or the appearance of pleural effusion or cavitation; not diagnostically definitive of TB

••••• Multidisciplinary Plan[16,19]

Medications

Certain individuals who have been infected with *M. tuberculosis,* are skin test positive, and who do not have active disease are candidates for prophylactic therapy utilizing isoniazid to prevent active disease. High priority candidates include the following individuals: (1) persons with known or suspected HIV infection, (2) close contacts of individuals with infectious TB, (3) persons who have chest radiographs suggestive of TB and who have received inadequate treatment, (4) persons who inject drugs, (5) recent tuberculin skin test converters, (6) persons under 35 years of age regardless of when their skin test conversion occurred, (7) foreign born persons from areas where TB is common, (8) medically underserved populations including high risk ethnic and ethnic groups, (9) residents of long-term care facilities, (10) children under 4 years of age, and (11) persons belonging to groups that have been identified by local health authorities as high prevalence groups (e.g., homeless, migrant workers). Isoniazid therapy is not recommended for persons over 35 years of age unless those people are at high risk of developing active tuberculosis because the risk of isoniazid-related hepatitis outweights the benefits of preventive therapy in this group.

The standard prophylactic dose is a single daily dose of 300 mg in adults and 10 to 15 mg/kg in children with the daily dose to not exceed 300 mg/dose. Therapy is maintained for 6 months in immunocompetent adults, 9 months in children, and 12 months in HIV-infected persons. Rifampin prophylaxis is sometimes used for close contacts of individuals with isoniazid-resistant *M. tuberculosis.*

The pharmacologic treatment of active tuberculosis is based on multidrug therapy for extended periods of time. The current recommendations for treatment are contained in Table 13-18. The success of these regimens is entirely dependent on patient compliance. If the patient does not adhere to the schedule, his or her infection will not be eliminated. In addition, the growth of drug-resistant strains of *M. tuberculosis* will be encouraged, making the eradication of the disease even more difficult. Unfortunately, because of the length and complexity of anti-TB drug therapy, noncompliance is widespread (up to 25%). Failure to follow the drug regimen is found in all population groups and social classes. The best method for assuring compliance with the drug regimen is directly observed therapy, a system whereby a public health representative is physically present while the patient takes each scheduled dose of the medications.

TABLE 13-18 Dosage Recommendations for the Initial Treatment of Tuberculosis in Children* and Adults

| | Dosage Schedule | | | | | |
| Drug | Daily Dose (Maximum Dose) | | Two Doses Per Week (Maximum Dose) | | Three Doses Per Week (Maximum Dose) | |
	Children	Adults	Children	Adults	Children	Adults
Isoniazid	10–20 mg/kg (300 mg)	5 mg/kg (300 mg)	20–40 mg/kg (900 mg)	15 mg/kg (900 mg)	20–40 mg/kg (900 mg)	15 mg/kg (900 mg)
Rifampin	10–20 mg/kg (600 mg)	10 mg/kg (600 mg)	10–20 mg/kg (600 mg)	10 mg/kg (600 mg)	10–20 mg/kg (600 mg)	10 mg/kg (600 mg)
Pyrazinamide	15–30 mg/kg (2 gm)	15–30 mg/kg (2 gm)	50–70 mg/kg (4 gm)	50–70 mg/kg (4 gm)	50–70 mg/kg (3 gm)	50–70 mg/kg (3 gm)
Ethambutol	15–25 mg/kg	15–25 mg/kg	50 mg/kg	50 mg/kg	25–30 mg/kg	25–30 mg/kg
Streptomycin	20–40 mg/kg (1 gm)	15 mg/kg (1 gm)	20–40 mg/kg (1.5 gm)	20–40 mg/kg (1.5 gm)	20–40 mg/kg (1.5 gm)	20–40 mg/kg (1.5 gm)

From Centers for Disease Control.[19]
*Persons ≤12 years of age.

Because of the cost of directly observed therapy, alternative drug regimens have been devised that involve taking higher docs less frequently. These alternative regimens are also shown in Table 13-19.

Multidrug-resistant tuberculosis (MDRTB), usually defined as resistant to both isoniazid and rifampin, is increasingly found in the United States. Often resistance is found to other antituberculosis drugs as well. Treatment of MDRTB is very complex and depends on number and nature of the drugs to which the organism is resistant. There are currently nine second line anti-TB drugs used in treating MDRTB. The treatment usually must be individually for the strain of the organism and for the patient's tolerance profile. It should only be treated by or in consultation with someone who is familiar with the treatment of multidrug resistant TB.

Corticosteroids: may be used in conjunction with the anti-infective agents for overwhelming and life-threatening disease.

Surgery

Intervention for complications

Resectional procedures for persisting cavitary lesions (less common since antimicrobial therapy)

Surgical intervention for massive hemoptysis, spontaneous pneumothorax, abscess drainage, intestinal obstruction, or ureteral stricture

General Management

After stabilization most patients can be effectively managed on an outpatient basis with monitoring for compliance with drug taking, drug side effects, and patient response to the drug therapy

AFB isolation until antimicrobial therapy is successfully initiated for sputum-positive patients to prevent spread to others (p. 1168)

Secretion precautions until wounds stop draining for patients with external TB lesions (p. 1168)

Skin testing: identify recent converters to TB skin tests; trace their contacts to identify persons with active disease; isoniazid therapy for 1 year for recent converters and for close household contacts of persons with active disease (not routine for those over 35); TB skin testing is recommended for children at school entry and again at age 14

BCG vaccine for children and infants who are at high risk for contact with active cases, who are skin test negative, and who are not immunosuppressed (benefits of BCG vaccine are controversial); receiving the vaccine results in a positive skin test

NURSING CARE

Nursing Assessment

History

Close contact with a person with TB or previous positive TB skin test; immunosuppression or chronic disease

Subjective Symptoms

History of weight loss, anorexia, and generalized weakness and fatigue

Body Temperature

Slight continued elevation with chills and night sweats

Respiratory

Initial: a nonproductive cough; later mucopurulent secretions
Advanced: hemoptysis; dyspnea on exertion and at rest; rales over apex of lung; chest pain with respiratory movement if pleura is involved; hoarseness with involvement of larynx; dysphagia with pharyngeal involvement; sibilant and sonorous rhonchi

TABLE 13-19 Regimen Options for the Treatment of Tuberculosis (TB) in Children and Adults

Option	Indication	Total Duration of Therapy	Initial Treatment Phase		Continuation Treatment Phase		Comments
			Drugs*	Interval and Duration	Drugs*	Interval and Duration	
1	Pulmonary and extrapulmonary TB in adults and children	6 mo	INH RIF PZA EMB or SM	Daily for 8 wk	INH RIF	Daily or two or three times wkly† for 16 wk‡	• EMB or SM should be continued until susceptibility to INH and RIF is demonstrated. • In areas where primary INH resistance is <4%, EMB or SM may not be necessary for patients with no individual risk factors for drug resistance.
2	Pulmonary and extrapulmonary TB in adults and children	6 mo	INH RIF PZA EMB or SM	Daily for 2 wks then Two times wkly† for 6 wk	INH RIF	Two times wkly† for 16 wk‡	• Regimen should be directly observed. • After the initial phase, EMB or SM should be continued until susceptibility to INH and RIF is demonstrated, unless drug resistance is unlikely.
3	Pulmonary and extrapulmonary TB in adults and children	6 mo	INH RIF PZA EMB or SM	3 times wkly† for 6 mos§			• Regimen should be directly observed. • Continue all four drugs for 6 mos.¶ • This regimen has been shown to be effective for INH-resistant TB.
4	Smear- and culture-negative pulmonary TB in adults	4 mo	INH RIF PZA EMB or SM	Follow option 1, 2, or 3 for 8 wk	INH RIF PZA EMB or SM	Daily or two or three times wkly† for 8 wk	• Continue all four drugs for 4 mos. • If drug resistance is unlikely (primary INH resistance <4% and patient has no individual risk factors for drug resistance), EMB or SM may not be necessary and PZA may be discontinued after 2 mo.
5	Pulmonary and extrapulmonary TB in adults and children when PZA is contraindicated	9 mo	INH RIF EMB or SM	Daily for 8 wk	INH RIF	Daily or two times wkly† for 24 wk‡	• EMB or SM should be continued until susceptibility to INH and RIF is demonstrated. • In areas where primary INH resistance is <4%, EMB or SM may not be necessary for patients with no individual risk factors for drug resistance.

From Centers for Disease Control.[19]

*EMB = ethambutol; INH = isoniazid; PZA = pyrazinamide; RIF = rifampin; SM = streptomycin.

†All regimens administered intermittently should be directly observed.

‡For infants and children with miliary TB, bone and joint TB, or TB meningitis, treatment should last at least 12 months. For adults with these forms of extrapulmonary TB, response to therapy should be monitored closely. If response is slow or suboptimal, treatment may be prolonged on a case-by-case basis.

§Some evidence suggests that SM may be discontinued after 4 months if the isolate is susceptible to all drugs.

¶Avoid treating pregnant women with SM because of the risk for ototoxicity to the fetus.

Note: For all patients, if drug susceptibility results show resistance to any of the first-line drugs, or if the patient remains symptomatic or smear- or culture-positive after 3 months, consult a TB medical expert.

Cardiovascular

Tachycardia

Extrapulmonary TB: depends on the system involved. The onset of symptoms is generally insidious, as is the onset of pulmonary TB

Cardiovascular

TB pericarditis: precordial chest pain, fever, and pericardial friction rubs, jugular venous distension, hepatic congestion, ascites, and peripheral edema

Gastrointestinal

TB peritonitis: Abdominal pain simulating that of appendicitis; abdominal distension; anorexia, vomiting, and weight loss; night sweats; abdominal tenderness when palpated; ascites

TB of GI tract: symptoms depend on area involved; may have GI bleeding, pain; constipation, or diarrhea; partial or complete obstruction

Systemic

Miliary TB: more severe symptoms of respiratory involvement: dyspnea, hyperventilation, and cough: hypoxemia; spontaneous unilateral or bilateral pneumothorax (manifested by sudden chest pain and breathlessness) and fever; painful, nodular cutaneous lesions (which may ulcerate) may be present

Neurologic

TB meningitis: headache, vomiting, fever, and anorexia; alterations in intellectual function, diminishing levels of consciousness, and neurologic deficits; CSF leukocytes of 100 to 400 cells/mm^3 and increase in protein

Lymphatic

TB lymphadenitis: palpable enlargement of supraclavicular and cervical lymph nodes

Musculoskeletal

Osteoarticular TB: pain in joints, aggravated by movement; swelling, minimal erythema, and tenderness to palpation; limitation of motion and gross deformities (most common in vertebral column, hip, and knee joints)

Genitourinary

TB of GU organs: urgency, frequency, dysuria, hematuria, and pyuria; salpingitis with lower abdominal pain and infertility; amenorrhea; abnormal vaginal discharge or bleeding

Nursing Dx & Intervention

Risk for infection (patient contacts) related to viable M. *tuberculosis* in respiratory secretions

- Obtain specimen for culture. *Incorrect collection and handling of specimen may destroy or contaminate specimen, thus interfering with diagnostic results.*

- Use AFB isolation until antimicrobial therapy is successfully initiated for sputum-positive patients *to prevent transmission of organism.*
- Use secretion precautions until wounds stop draining for patients with external TB lesions *to prevent transmission of organism.*
- Teach hospitalized patient to cough and sneeze into paper tissue and to dispose of tissues properly *to prevent transmission of organism.*
- Report to local health authority.

Risk for infection (chronic in patient) related to noncompliance with therapy

- Instruct patient regarding the prescribed therapy *to ensure that patient takes medication as prescribed;* see Patient Education/Home Care Planning.

Ineffective breathing pattern related to necrosis of lung tissue

- Monitor breathing *to detect dyspnea and signs of pneumothorax.*
- Initiate respiratory assistance as needed. Observe sputum for hemoptysis *to detect signs of complications.*
- Assist immobile patient to turn, cough, and deep breathe every 2-4 hours *to prevent pooling of secretions.*

Patient Education/Home Care Planning

1. Teach care of sputum if discharged patient still has positive sputum cultures.
2. Teach the patient handwashing and good hygiene.
3. Drug therapy must be continued uninterrupted for the designated time period. Explain dosage, frequency of administration, and purpose for prolonged treatment to the patient.
4. Explain medication's toxic and side effects:

   INH: infrequent toxic effects—peripheral neuropathy, convulsions, ataxia, dizziness, optic neuritis; older patients may experience a drug-related hepatitis with fatigue, malaise, and anorexia

   Ethambutol: reduced visual acuity with inability to perceive the color green

   Streptomycin: skin rash, fever, malaise, vertigo, and deafness; gastrointestinal disturbances and central nervous system symptoms

   PAS: toxic reactions more common with this drug and include symptoms of hypersensitivity, hepatic damage, gastrointestinal disturbances, and renal failure

   Rifampin: red-orange colored urine common, jaundice, nausea, anorexia, vomiting, diarrhea, cramps, occasional central nervous system disturbances, and hypersensitivity reactions; may interfere with actions of oral contraceptives

Ethionamide: gastrointestinal irritation and symptoms of hepatotoxicity

Pyrazinamide: hepatoxicity

Cycloserine: central nervous system effects, including seizures, somnolence, and muscle twitching

5. Discuss with the patient the need to report side effects to physician immediately.

6. Emphasize to the patient the need for periodic reculturing of sputum during period of therapy—monthly until cultures are negative, then every 3 months for duration of therapy.

7. Patient must report to the physician: hemoptysis, chest pain, difficulty in breathing, hearing loss, or vertigo.

8. Discuss with the patient the need to maintain adequate fluid and caloric intake.

9. Household and close contacts should be examined at time of treatment of the patient and again in 2 to 3 months.

From Grimes.[26]

Evaluation

Infection is not transmitted to patient's contacts Contacts do not convert to a positive skin test. Patient demonstrates behavior to prevent transmission of pathogens to others or to prevent contamination of the environment.

Patient is free of infection and complications of TB Sputum cultures are consistently negative. Chest roentgenograms show a reduction in the size of cavities and decrease in the thickness of cavity walls. Body temperature is normal. Patient does not experience chills or night sweats. Serum alkaline phosphatase levels, hematocrit, hemoglobin, and leukocyte count are normal. Urine does not contain erythrocytes. Patient does not manifest the extrapulmonary symptoms described under "Nursing Assessment."

Patient self-administers anti-infective agents as prescribed Patient completes full course on anti-infective therapy. No preventable drug interactions or allergic reactions are experienced. If untoward reactions are experienced, the patient discontinues the drug and contacts the physician immediately.

Patient demonstrates normal respiratory pattern, oxygen intake, and blood gas levels Patient does not experience dyspnea, cough, or pain on breathing.

■ HISTOPLASMOSIS

■ Histoplasmosis is a pulmonary and systemic infection, similar to tuberculosis, resulting from inhalation of the spores of *Histoplasma capsulatum*, which are frequently found in the soil. Infection is common, but overt clinical disease is rare. Five clinical forms of the disease have been recognized (see box).

■ FACTS ABOUT HISTOPLASMOSIS

Occurrence: worldwide; higher in eastern and central United States; increases with age to 15 years; no differences by sex; outbreaks in groups with common exposure

Etiologic agent: *Histoplasma capsulatum* (a fungus)

Reservoir: soil around chicken houses, caves harboring bats, and around starling, blackbird, and pigeon roosts and decaying trees

Transmission: inhalation of airborne spores

Incubation period: 3–14 days after exposure, commonly 10 days

Period of communicability: not transmitted from person to person

Susceptibility and resistance: general; inapparent infections are common and result in increasing resistance; this is an opportunistic infection in immunocompromised persons

Report to local authority in some states

Data from Benenson.[3]

•••••• Pathophysiology

Spores of *H. capsulatum,* a fungus, are inhaled when soil containing them is disturbed. A lesion is formed within the lung parenchyma where the spores convert to a yeast phase and are phagocytosed by macrophages. Lesions may also be formed in the hilar or mediastinal lymph nodes as a result of migration of yeast-laden macrophages to those areas. Dissemination and lesion formation may also occur in the spleen and liver. These primary lesions become necrotic at the center, build up a fibrotic capsule, and frequently calcify. In most cases where calcification occurs there is no reactivation of the infection and the host manifests no symptoms except an immune response to histoplasmin.

Four other clinical forms of the disease are possible: acute benign respiratory disease, acute disseminated disease, chronic disseminated disease and chronic pulmonary disease. In acute benign respiratory disease the primary pulmonary lesion remains active, resulting in a spreading infiltration pneumonia. In acute disseminated disease, inflammatory and necrotic lesions may result in septic-type fever, hepatosplenomegaly, severe prostration, and death. Chronic disseminated histoplasmosis results when there is extensive invasion by yeast-laden macrophages via the reticuloendothelial system to bone marrow, spleen, liver, and lungs. The inflammatory and necrotic reaction in those tissues is subacute but progressive and may eventually result in death. Chronic pulmonary histoplasmosis is manifest as a progressive emphysema. Fluid-filled cysts surrounded by chronic inflammation progress through stages of caseation necrosis and cavitation, continuing to disseminate the yeast through pulmonary tissue.

The clinical symptoms are quite varied but are generally more severe in infants, immunosuppressed persons, and chronically debilitated persons.

Complications

Pneumonia
Progressive emphysema
Septic type of fever
Hepatosplenomegaly
Severe prostration
Death

•••••• Diagnostic Studies and Findings[27]

Culture and examination of Giemsa- or Wright-stained smears of respiratory exudate, blood, bone marrow or exudate from ulcerated lesions Positive for *H. capsulatum;* results are frequently erratic, necessitating the culture of many specimens

Serology (Precipitation, complement fixation, agglutination test) Increase in antibodies within 3 to 4 weeks; fourfold increase suggests disease progression; agglutinins greater than 1:8 or 1:16 have suggestive diagnostic value

Chest roentgenogram Acute: transient parenchymal pulmonary infiltrates resembling lobar pneumonia; chronic; progressively enlarging areas of necrosis with or without cavitation

•••••• Multidisciplinary Plan[2,3]

Medications

Anti-infective agents
  Amphotericin B (Fungizone), 30-40 mg/kg IV for disseminated infection in immunocompromised
  Ketoconazole, 400 mg/day (up to 800 mg), po for 6-12 mos (approved for treatment of immunocompetent)
  Itraconazole, 200-400 mg/day, po for 6-12 mos
Corticosteroids
  Corticosteroids, may be mixed with the infusion to minimize the side effects of amphotericin B
Antihistamines
  Diphenhydramine (Benadryl), added to IV to control side effects

NURSING CARE

Nursing Assessment

History

Outdoor exposure to fungus; immunosuppression

Subjective Symptoms

Malaise, weakness; anorexia

Acute Pulmonary Histoplasmosis

Pleural and substernal chest pain
Dry or productive cough with metallic tone, suggesting tracheobronchial obstruction
Low-grade fever

Erythema multiforme, erythema nodosum
May have complicating symptoms of pericarditis

Chronic Pulmonary Histoplasmosis

Purulent sputum; hemoptysis; increasing signs of pulmonary insufficiency
Chronic low-grade fever
Erythema multiforme, erythema nodosum
May have complicating symptoms of pericarditis

Acute Disseminated Histoplasmosis

High fever
Enlarged liver or spleen

Chronic Disseminated Histoplasmosis

Symptoms of pneumonia
Purpura
Symptoms of endocarditis
Symptoms of GI ulcer, hepatitis, and peritonitis
Ulcerated lesions resembling epidermoid cancer in larynx, mouth, nose, or pharynx

Nursing Dx & Intervention

Risk for injury related to chemotherapeutic agent

- Monitor for cyanosis, change in pulse, respiratory rate, and signs of renal dysfunction *to detect signs of amphotericin toxicity.*
- Administer antihistamines and corticosteroids, as prescribed, *to prevent and control allergic reaction to amphotericin.*
- Encourage fluids high in potassium if nausea and vomiting persist *to replace lost potassium.*
- Use small-gauge needle for IV line. Agitate IV bag every 15 to 20 minutes while chemotherapeutic agent is administered *to evenly distribute drug and fluid in bag and in IV line.* Give infusion over 5 to 6 hours *to prevent phlebitis associated with amphotericin.*
- Reposition patient frequently during prolonged, painful IV infusions. Provide diversional activities *to promote patient comfort.*
- Administer analgesics before IV administration, as prescribed, *to decrease pain from drug therapy.*

Other related nursing diagnoses for progressive disease Ineffective breathing pattern, hyperthermia, decreased cardiac output, activity intolerance, and altered oral mucous membranes.

Patient Education/Home Care Planning

1. Inform the patient that medical follow-up for 1 year after treatment to prevent relapses is necessary.
2. Inform the patient that reinfection can be prevented by avoiding infected sites, wearing a protective mask, or sterilizing the site with 3% formalin solution.

Evaluation

Patient is free of signs of infection and complications of treatment Patient's sputum cultures are negative. Body temperature is normal. There is no cough, dyspnea, sputum, or hemoptysis. There are no lesions in mouth, larynx, pharynx, or nose. There is no purpura, erythema multiforme, or erythema nodosum. Patient has energy to carry out all daily activities. Patient does not have abdominal pain, is able to eat all desired foods, and is not jaundiced. There are no signs of phlebitis, renal dysfunction, electrolyte imbalance, pain, or neuritis.

Patient does not experience reinfection Patient states intent to see physician on a regular basis for 1 year after hospitalization. Patient states methods to use to avoid reexposure.

▮ LEGIONELLOSIS

▮ (Legionnaires' disease)

Legionellosis (Legionnaires' disease) is an acute bacterial infection so named because it caused an outbreak of pneumonia at a convention of American Legionnaires at a Philadelphia hotel (see box). The acute disease is a patchy pulmonary infiltrate and consolidation, with a high fever, malaise, myalgia and headache, nonproductive cough, and a high risk for respiratory failure and death.

•••••• Pathophysiology

Inhalation of *Legionella pneumophila* causes two distinct clinical syndromes: Pontiac fever, which resembles influenza, and Legionnaires' disease, with pathologic changes characteristic of lobar pneumonia. In the latter there is a cellular exudate consisting of polymorphonuclear leukocytes and macrophages with extensive necrosis of the exudate and alveolar septa. Bronchi are clear of the necrotic process. Rarely is a purulent sputum produced. The disease progresses rapidly during the first 4 to 6 days of clinical illness.

Complications

Renal failure, bacteremic shock, and respiratory failure resulting in death to 15% of patients

•••••• Diagnostic Studies and Findings[3,27]

Culture of blood, sputum, pleural fluid, and lung tissue Positive for *L. pneumophila*

Examination of stained (immunofluorescence) smear of respiratory secretions or involved tissue Positive for *L. pneumophila*

Antigen/Antibody (RIA) test of specimen of urine: Positive for *L. pneumophila* antigen

Serology (Indirect immunofluorescence) Fourfold or greater rise in antibody titer to 1:128 within 21 days of onset of illness

Chest radiograph examination Shows patchy pattern of pneumonia and small pleural effusions

WBC Slightly elevated

Sedimentation rate Markedly elevated

Others Hematuria, proteinuria, and laboratory evidence of liver dysfunction

•••••• Multidisciplinary Plan[2,3,5]

Medications

Anti-infective agents
Erythromycin (Robimycin), 0.5-1 g/6 h for adults (15 mg/kg/6 h for children) IV or po for 21 days
Rifampin (Rifomycin, others), as adjunct therapy

General Management

Assisted ventilation, oxygen therapy, temporary renal dialysis, and IV fluids and electrolytes

---

▮ FACTS ABOUT LEGIONELLOSIS
(LEGIONNAIRES' DISEASE)

Occurrence: Europe, United States, and Canada; first recognized in 1977; sporadic cases and outbreaks in summer and autumn; increases with age
Etiologic agent: *Legionella pneumophila* (a bacterial species with 18 serogroups; serogroup 1 associated with disease)
Reservoir: unknown but probably environmental; organism survives in hot and cold tap water and distilled water for months
Transmission: common source, airborne transmission suspected
Incubation period: 2 to 10 days, commonly 5 to 6 days
Period of communicability: no documented person-to-person transmission
Susceptibility and resistance: general; rare in those less than 20 years; greatest in males, smokers, immunosuppressed persons and persons >50 years of age
Report to local health authority in some states

Data from Benenson.[3]

▮ NURSING CARE

Nursing Assessment

Body Temperature

38° to 41° C (102° to 105° F) within a day

Subjective Symptoms

Anorexia, malaise, myalgia, chills, abdominal pain

Respiratory Concerns

Nonproductive cough, dyspnea, tachypnea, pluritic chest pain, and rales or rhonchi

Cardiovascular Concerns

Tachycardia, symptoms of shock

Digestive Concerns

Diarrhea, sometimes vomiting

Neurologic Concerns

Confusion, slurring of speech, and falling (infrequent symptoms)

Elimination

Renal insufficiency; hematuria

Nursing Dx & Intervention

Hyperthermia related to infection

- Monitor body temperature *to detect fever.*
- Administer antipyretics *as ordered.*
- Bathe with tepid water or alcohol *to reduce high fever.*
- Adjust environmental temperature *for patient's comfort.*
- Remove excess clothing and bedding *to ensure heat loss.*
- Encourage adequate fluid intake *to compensate for fluid loss associated with elevated body temperature.*

Ineffective breathing pattern related to pneumonia

- Assess ventilation to include evaluation of breathing rate, rhythm, and depth: chest expansion; presence of respiratory distress, such as dyspnea, nasal flaring, pursed-lip breathing, prolonged expiratory phase, and use of accessory muscles *to detect signs of respiratory failure for immediate intervention.*
- Assess patient for tiring from exertion in relation to attempts to breathe; assist ventilation, if necessary. Administer oxygen *to maintain circulating oxygen.*
- Maintain patient in position with head of bed in semi-Fowler's position or patient sitting and leaning forward overbed table. *These positions facilitate respiration by decreasing abdominal pressure on diaphragm.*
- Instruct patient in proper pulmonary hygiene routines such as postural drainage. *These will promote easy, effective breathing and facilitate removal of secretions from tracheobronchial tree and minimize pulmonary congestion, which could lead to superinfections.*

Patient Education/Home Care Planning*

To prevent reinfection:

1. Decontaminate implicated sources of infection by chlorination or super-heating of water supply.
2. Cooling water towers and misters should be drained and cleaned when not in use.

From Grimes.[26]

Evaluation

Body temperature is maintained within the normal range; comfort and safety are maintained Body temperature is between 36° and 38° C (96.8° and 100° F) orally. Pulse and respirations are within normal limits. Skin is cool to touch and free of excess perspiration. Patient's clothing and bedding are dry. Patient is free of headache and malaise associated with the fever. Patient experiences no injury associated with seizures. Body fluids are adequate. Serum electrolytes are within normal limits. Urine output and specific gravity are normal.

Patient demonstrates normal respiratory pattern, oxygen intake, and blood gas levels Bronchovesicular breath sounds are heard throughout lungs. There are no areas of decreased breath sounds or consolidation. Respiratory rate is normal. CO_2, Po_2, and Pco_2 are normal.

▌ STREPTOCOCCAL THROAT, SCARLET FEVER, RHEUMATIC FEVER

Streptococcal throat is an acute exudative tonsillitis or pharyngitis caused by group A β-hemolytic streptococci (GABHS). Coincident or subsequent otitis media or peritonsillar abscess may be present. Rheumatic fever, chorea, scarlet fever, and acute glomerulonephritis are possible sequelae (Table 13-20).

Scarlet fever is a group A β-hemolytic streptococcal disease characterized by a skin rash. It occurs when the infecting strain of streptococcus produces a toxin, causing a sensitivity reaction in the infected host. Clinical characteristics may include those of streptococcal sore throat plus enanthem, strawberry tongue, and exanthem.

Rheumatic fever is a sequela of group A streptococcal infection of the upper respiratory tract, occurring in about 2.8% of those having a streptococcal throat infection. The condition is thought to result from an altered immune reaction to the streptococcus organism. Rheumatic heart disease is a potential complication.

•••••• Pathophysiology

Infection with group A streptococci results in a number of related clinical disease entities, such as streptococcal throat, scarlet fever, and erysipelas, as well as nonsuppurative complications, such as nephritis and rheumatic fever. The type of disease resulting from group A streptococci depends on the site of tissue invasion, the antigenic characteristics of the infecting strain of streptococcus, and the immune status of the host. There are approximately 75 serologically distinct strains of group A streptococci, producing a variety of enzymes and at least three different erythrogenic toxins. These antigenic characteristics determine the type of enzyme-specific and toxin-specific antibodies produced by the host. A host with adequate antibodies against a particular serotype with or without antitoxic

■ TABLE 13-20 Overview of Streptococcal Throat, Scarlet Fever, and Rheumatic Fever

	Streptococcal Throat	Scarlet Fever	Rheumatic Fever
Occurrence	More common in temperate zones; may be endemic, epidemic, or sporadic in occurrence; highest in late winter or spring; ages 3-15 yr most often affected; no sex or racial difference		Increase in outbreaks since 1984
Etiologic agent	*Streptococcus pyogenes* (group A streptococcus of approximately 80 serologically distinct types)	Three erythrogenic toxins	Group A β-hemolytic streptococcus (GABHS)
Reservoir	Humans	Humans	Humans
Transmission	Direct contact with mucous droplets from patient or carrier; may follow ingestion of contaminated food	Sequela to streptococcal throat	Sequela to streptococcal throat
Incubation period	1-3 days	2-4 days (range: 1-7 days)	3-35 days after clinical strep throat (average: 19 days)
Period of communicability	Untreated, uncomplicated cases: 10-21 days; complicated: weeks to months; antibiotic treated: 24-48 hr	Not communicable	Not communicable
Susceptibility and resistance	General: many develop antitoxic and/or antibacterial immunity to one of the types of streptococci through inapparent infection	Permanent acquired immunity from active disease with type of toxin; second attacks due to different toxin	Persons who have suffered one attack are predisposed to a recurrent episode following group A streptococcal upper respiratory infections
Report to local health authority	Epidemics only	Epidemics only	Case report in some states

Data from Benenson.[3]

immunity may not develop clinical disease if reinfected with the same serotype. A person with antitoxic immunity resulting from previous group A infections but with no antibodies against a particular invading serotype may develop a clinical streptococcal throat. A person with no antitoxic immunity and no antibodies against an invading toxigenic group A streptococcus may develop clinical scarlet fever. In all clinical streptococcal disease a leukocytosis is present.

Streptococcal Throat

Streptococcal throat (septic sore throat) results when the streptococcus invades and remains in the lymphoid tissue of the oropharynx, rapidly producing inflammation with edema, erythema, and infiltration with polymorphonuclear leukocytes. The mucosal surfaces, particularly over the tonsils, become ulcerated, releasing a mucopurulent exudate. Cervical lymphadenopathy is present. Severity of symptoms increases with age. Untreated, uncomplicated disease lasts a few days to a week. The streptococcus may invade surrounding tissue producing suppurative complications.

Scarlet Fever

Scarlet fever results if the invading streptococcus releases an erythrogenic toxin stimulating a sensitivity reaction in the host. Dilation of small capillaries and toxic injury of the vascular epithelium may be widespread in the body, particularly in the liver, myocardium, and kidneys. The pathologic changes are most visible on the skin, with an erythematous rash and desquamation, and in the oral cavity, with the strawberry tongue and an enanthem. Hepatocellular damage and destruction of red cells may result in jaundice, increased bilirubin, mild anemia,

and increased number of reticulocytes. In rare situations, toxins may be disseminated in the bloodstream, producing a severe toxic illness. Streptococcus may invade adjacent tissue and the bloodstream, producing a severe septic scarlet fever.

In severe cases of scarlet fever, septic scarlet fever or toxic scarlet fever (also known as fulminating scarlet fever) may result. In septic scarlet fever the body temperature is elevated to 40° to 42° C (104° to 108° F), and the pulse becomes rapid and weak. Throat manifestations are more severe, with ulceration and perforation on the uvula, soft palate, and tonsils. Other findings include seropurulent or mucopurulent nasal discharge and excoriations on the lips, mouth, and nares. Breathing is labored because of swelling and occlusion.

In toxic scarlet fever the body temperature is 41° to 42° C (105° to 107° F) and the pulse is rapid. A bright punctate or erythematous hemorrhagic rash appears on the skin. Capillary fragility is evidenced by hematuria, epistaxis, and hematemesis. The oropharynx becomes edematous but without exudate. Other manifestations include intense headache and vomiting, symptoms of toxic myocarditis, and altered mental state (e.g., delirium, irrationality, or coma).

Rheumatic Fever

Rheumatic fever is a delayed complication of upper respiratory infection with group A streptococci, producing nonsuppurative inflammatory lesions in connective tissue of the heart, joints, subcutaneous tissues, and central nervous system. Symptoms may be present in all or some of those systems. The exact causal mechanism is not known. The following have been hypothesized: (1) there is direct tissue invasion by group A streptococci or by cell wall antigens of the microorganism; (2) streptococcal enzymes, particularly streptolysins S or O, induce tissue injury; (3) antigen-humoral antibody reactions localize in affected tissue; and (4) an autoimmune reaction is operative. The autoimmune theory is supported by the detection of heart-reactive antibodies (HRAs) in the sera of patients with rheumatic heart disease.

Cardiac connective tissue lesions show early fragmentation of collagen fibers, cellular lymphocytic infiltration, and fibrin deposits. These changes are followed by the development of the Aschoff nodule, a perivascular locus of inflammation with an area of central necrosis surrounded by large mononuclear and polymorphonuclear leukocytes. Cardiac findings include pericarditis, myocarditis, and left-sided endocarditis. Valvular lesions begin with edema and cellular infiltration of the leaflets and chordae with small verrucae forming along the closure lines. With healing the valves become thickened and deformed, the valve commissures become fused, and the chordae become shortened. These changes result in valvular stenosis and insufficiency, varying in extensiveness and severity. Carditis may result in long-term disability or death.

Joint lesions are characterized by a fibrinous exudate over the synovial membrane and a serous effusion without joint destruction. Subcutaneous nodules form that resemble the Aschoff nodules described previously.

A later neurologic sequela of rheumatic fever is Sydenham's chorea. The latent period for this condition may be so long as to occur in the absence of laboratory changes associated with rheumatic fever.

Complications

Streptococcal throat

Peritonsillar cellulitis and abscess
Retropharyngeal abscess
Sinus empyema
Otitis media
Mastoiditis
Meningitis
Cervical lymphadenitis
Pneumonia
Periorbital abscess
Toxin dissemination leading to rheumatic fever or nephritis

Scarlet fever

Severe disseminated toxic illness
Septicemia
Hepatic damage

Rheumatic fever

Valvular heart disease
Congestive heart failure
Persistent arthritis

•••••• Diagnostic Studies and Findings[3]

Culture of specimen of pharyngeal secretions on blood agar   Identification of β-hemolytic streptococci (GABHS) by colonial morphology and hemolysis of blood agar

Antigen/Antibody test on specimen of pharyngeal secretions (Rapid Strep Test)   Positive for streptococcal antigens in 1-2 hr

Serology (antistreptolysin O, antihyaluronidase, anti-DNA-ase B)   Rise in titers between acute and convalescent disease

Streptozyme test (a slide hemagglutination test)   Measures five different streptococcal enzymes; titers of 100 to 200 streptozyme units are equivocal; titers of 300 streptozyme units indicate recent streptococcal infection

C-reactive protein (CRP)   Normally not present in serum; presence of CRP in serum is diagnostic of rheumatic fever

Erythrocyte sedimentation rate   Elevated in rheumatic fever

Electrocardiogram   Elongation of PR interval in rheumatic fever

•••••• Multidisciplinary Plan[3,5]

Medications

Anti-infective agents

Benzathine penicillin G (Bicillin), 1,200,000 U IM one time for adults
Oral penicillin, 125-250 mg BID q10d, *or*
Procaine penicillin (Wycillin), 600,000 U IM q10d for severe scarlet fever
Erythromycin (Erythrocin, others), 250 mg po qid q10d for patients allergic to penicillin or Clindamycin 300 mg tid
Aminoglycocides for endocarditis

Antipyretic agents

Aspirin, for treatment of polyarthritis of rheumatic fever
Antipyretics for management of fever

Corticosteroids

Prednisone (Deltasone, others), 40-60 mg/d q2-3wk for treatment of carditis, *or*
Methylprednisolone sodium succinate (Solu-Medrol), IV, in severe cases; decrease to complete withdrawal in 3 wk

To prevent recurrent streptococcal infections in postrheumatic fever patients:

Anti-infective agents

Benzathine penicillin G (Bicillin), 1,200,000 U IM q4wk during and following convalescence for life (recommended duration is controversial), *or*
Erythromycin (Erythrocin, others) 250 mg bid po for those allergic to penicillin

General Management

Bed rest during febrile stage of all streptococcal diseases; bed rest for 3 weeks for patients without carditis; for an additional month after carditis is detected
Nonstimulating environment and sedation for patients with chorea
Fluid therapy as indicated
Treatment of heart failure with O_2, salt restriction, diuretics, and digitalis
To prevent transmission to others; secretion precautions of hospitalized patients with an upper respiratory streptococcal infection for 24 hours following initiation of antibiotic therapy

NURSING CARE

Nursing Assessment

Assessment	Streptococcal Throat	Scarlet Fever	Rheumatic Fever
History	Contact with person with sore throat	Contact with person with sore throat	Untreated sore throat within past month; previous episode or family history of RF
Subjective symptoms	Pain on swallowing, headache, anorexia, malaise, chills; abdominal pain in children	Pain on swallowing, headache, anorexia, malaise, chills; abdominal pain in children	Malaise, abdominal pain
Body temperature	38°-39° C (100°-103° F)	38°-39° C (100°-103° F)	Low-grade fever; 38° C (100° F)
Cardiovascular	Rapid pulse	Rapid pulse	Insidious onset of symptoms of carditis within 3 weeks: cardiac enlargement, pericardial friction rubs, congestive heart failure, signs of effusion, tachycardia, gallop rhythm, and diastolic and possibly systolic murmurs Three types of murmurs associated with acute carditis: (1) high-pitched blowing holosystolic apical murmur of mitral regurgitation, (2) low-pitched apical middiastolic flow murmur, (3) high-pitched decrescendo diastolic murmur of aortic regurgitation heard at the secondary and primary aortic areas Mitral and aortic stenotic murmurs associated with chronic rheumatic valvular disease
Head and neck	Enlarged, tender cervical lymph nodes; suppurative complications (mastoiditis, otitis media, periorbital abscess, sinus empyema)	Enlarged, tender cervical lymph nodes; suppurative complications (mastoiditis, otitis media, periorbital abscess, sinus empyema)	
Oropharynx	Edema, erythema (fiery red to dull red), and petechiae of uvula, tonsils, and posterior oropharynx Confluent, easily removable mucopurulent exudate May be suppurative complications	Edema, erythema (fiery red to dull red), and petechiae of uvula, tonsils, and posterior oropharynx Confluent, easily removable mucopurulent exudate May be suppurative complications	
Oral cavity		Tongue is inflamed and heavily coated at first; after the rash appears, the papillae become swollen and appear as red bumps on a gray background (strawberry tongue); within a few days the tongue peels, first at the tip and margins; by day 6 the tongue is complete denuded, beefy red, moist, and glistening (raspberry tongue); tongue returns to normal by the end of the second week Enanthem: for a few days around the time of rash's appearance on the skin there may be a hemorrhagic rash on the soft palate and anterior pillars of the fossae	

Assessment	Streptococcal Throat	Scarlet Fever	Rheumatic Fever
Respiratory	Complications: symptoms of pneumonia	Complications: symptoms of pneumonia	
Skin		Erythematous and punctate rash appearing within 2 days of streptococcal throat, becoming generalized rapidly; appearing first on upper chest and back and then on lower back, upper extremities, abdomen, and lower extremities	One to two dozen firm, painless, variable in size (3 mm to 2 cm), subcutaneous nodules; usually over bony prominences and tendons; lasting 1 to 2 weeks
		Extensiveness of rash is variable; it may be better felt (like sandpaper) than seen	Nonpruritic, erythematous macular eruption on the trunk or proximal extremities (erythema marginatum); lesions appear to be a vasomotor phenomenon, moving over the skin with a tendency to advance at the margins and clear at the center; individual lesions clear within hours, but the process persists intermittently for weeks or months
		Petechiae may precede rash on lower extremities; more common in skin folds	
		Desquamation may develop between 5 days and 4 weeks after appearance of the rash, starting on neck, upper chest, back, fingertips, or toes; skin peels in large sections, particularly on palms and soles	
		Flushing of cheeks with circumoral pallor	
Neurologic	Complications: symptoms of meningitis	Complications: symptoms of meningitis	Symptoms of chorea: involuntary, purposeless, rapid motions; irritability; emotional lability; weakness; restlessness or fretfulness, gradually increasing in intensity over 2 weeks, reaching a plateau, and gradually subsiding
Musculoskeletal		Tender, slightly inflamed; edematous joints possible	Acute onset of mild to severe symptoms of polyarthritis: heat, swelling, redness, and severe tenderness affecting mainly the knees, ankles, elbows, and wrists; migratory, with multiple joint involvement at one time; inflammation subsides in each joint in 1 to 2 weeks; entire episode subsides in 4 weeks
Abdomen		Liver may be slightly enlarged and tender	

From Grimes.[26]

Nursing Dx & Intervention

Risk for infection related to complications of streptococcal throat

- Collect pharyngeal secretions for culture *for diagnosis of Streptococcus organisms and proper interventions.*
- Administer antibiotics as prescribed, *to prevent progression to SF or RF.*

Risk for infection (patient contacts) related to GABHS in pharyngeal exudate

- Maintain respiratory secretion precautions of hospitalized patients for 24 hours after antibiotic therapy is initiated *to prevent transmission to others.*

Hyperthermia related to infectious process

- Monitor body temperature *to detect fever.*
- Administer antipyretics.
- Bathe with tepid water or alcohol *to reduce high fever.*
- Encourage adequate fluid intake *to compensate for increased demands associated with elevated body temperature.*

Activity intolerance related to cardiovascular complications of RF and SF

- Maintain complete bed rest for SF and RF patients. Provide all care, including hygiene and feeding *to conserve patient energy and prevent complications by relieving stress on the cardiovascular system.*

Altered oral mucous membrane related to exudative infectious process of GABHS and inflammatory response to toxin in SF

- Assess pharyngeal area *to detect hyperemia and exudate.*
- Provide frequent oral fluids and oral hygiene. Provide high humidity in room. Lubricate lips and nares *to promote comfort for patient.*

Patient Education/Home Care Planning

1. Oral antibiotics must be taken for prescribed length of time. Follow-up throat cultures may be necessary.
2. Compliance with prescribed long-term antibiotic therapy is necessary to minimize risk for recurrence of rheumatic fever with subsequent streptococcal infections.
3. Upper respiratory infections should be diagnosed and treated promptly in postrheumatic fever patients.
4. Continued rest during convalescence is necessary for postrheumatic fever patients.
5. Medical monitoring for cardiac complications is necessary after rheumatic fever.
6. Persons with residual rheumatic valvular disease must follow an antimicrobial regimen whenever they undergo dental or surgical procedures that would increase their risk for bacteremia.

From Grimes.[26]

Evaluation

Infection is not transmitted All patient contacts are examined and treated for infection.

Body temperature is maintained within the normal range; comfort and safety are maintained Patient's body temperature is between 36° and 38° C (96.8° and 100° F). Pulse and respiration are normal. Skin is cool to touch and free of excess perspiration. Patient's clothing and bedding are dry. Patient is free of headache and malaise associated with the fever.

Patient achieves adequate rest during active disease and returns to preillness level of activity during convalescence Patient maintains bed rest during acute disease with gradual return of activity. Patient does not experience fatigue on exertion.

Patient's mucous membranes return to prepathogenic state Patient's mucous membranes are moist, with natural color. There is no edema, inflammation, or exudate in oropharynx. Exanthem and enanthem of scarlet fever are not present.

Patient self-administers anti-infective agents as prescribed Patient completes full course of anti-infective therapy. No preventable drug interactions or allergic reactions are experienced. If untoward reactions are experienced, patient discontinues drug and contacts physician immediately.

Complications are prevented Patient's pulse rate is normal. ECG is normal. No murmurs are auscultated. There is no limitation of joint movement. Patient can move all joints without pain. Patient exhibits purposeful movement, indicating no signs of chorea.

SEXUALLY TRANSMITTED DISEASES

The term *sexually transmitted diseases (STDs)* refers to a large group of disease syndromes that can be transmitted sexually, irrespective of whether the disease has genital pathologic manifestations. STD is more encompassing than the previously used "venereal disease" categorization. The STDs, similar to other infectious diseases, can be classified as to their etiologic agent or according to their disease manifestations. The following pathogens are known or thought to be sexually transmitted:

Bacteria: *Neisseria gonorrhoeae; Chlamydia trachomatis; Mycoplasma hominis; Ureaplasma urealyticum; Treponema pallidum; Gardnerella vaginalis; Haemophilus ducreyi; Shigella; Calymmatobacterium granulomatis*

Viruses: herpes simplex virus; *Papillomavirus;* hepatitis A, B, and D viruses; molluscum contagiosum virus; cytomegalovirus; human immunodeficiency virus (HIV)

Protozoa: *Trichomonas vaginalis; Entamoeba histolytica; Giardia lamblia*

Fungi: *Candida albicans*

Ectoparasites: *Pthirus pubis; Sarcoptes scabiei*

The list of disease syndromes produced by the listed pathogens is equally extensive. Many pathogens produce multiple disease syndromes, and many of the disease syndromes may be caused by more than one pathogenic agent. The STDs are grouped in this section according to disease manifestations patients are most likely to present to health care providers (Table 13-21). It must be noted that patients with symptoms of a sexually transmitted disease frequently have multiple sexually transmitted diseases and should be evaluated accordingly.

■ GONORRHEA AND NONGONOCOCCAL URETHRITIS

Gonorrhea (clap, strain, gleet, dose, jack) is an inflammation of the columnar and transitional epithelium caused by the gonococcus. Symptoms, course of disease, and severity differ between males and females. Chronic and severe complications may result from untreated infections. *Nongonococcal urethritis* is a sexually transmitted urethritis in males (cervicitis and salpingitis in females) caused by an agent other than the gonococcus, most commonly *Chlamydia tracheomatis.*

The diseases discussed in this section are manifest as urethritis or cervicitis with an inflammatory pyogenic exudate. Salpingitis and other related sequelae may be present (Table 13-22).

•••••• Pathophysiology

In *gonococcal infections* the gonococcus attaches to and penetrates columnar epithelium, producing a patchy inflammatory response in the submucosa with a polymorphonuclear exudate. Affected areas in the male are the urethra, Littre's and Cowper's glands, the prostate, seminal vesicles, and the epididymis. Affected areas in the female include the glands of Bartholin and Skene, the urethra, the cervix, and the fallopian tubes. The

TABLE 13-21 STD Categories According to Disease Manifestations

Disease Manifestations	STD
Urethritis, cervicitis with an inflammatory pyogenic exudate, salpingitis, and related sequelae; proctitis	Gonorrhea; nongonococcal urethritis (*Chlamydia*)
Ulcerative lesions with systemic dissemination of pathogen	Syphilis; lymphogranuloma venereum; herpes
Ulcerative lesions only	Chancroid; granuloma inguinale (donovanosis)
Nonulcerative lesions	Molloscum contagiosum; condylomata acuminata
Vulvovaginitis	Trichomoniasis; candidiasis; bacterial vaginosis (*Gardnerella vaginalis vaginitis*)
Systemic infections without lesions	Cytomegalovirus; hepatitis; acquired immunodeficiency syndrome (AIDS)
Enteric infections	Giardiasis; *Campylobacter enteritis;* shigellosis; amebic dysentery; salmonellosis; *Mycobacterium avium intracellulare* (MAI); *Cryptosporidium; Isospora*
Pubic infestations	Scabies; pediculosis
Congenital and perinatal infections and anomalies	Syphilis; gonorrhea; *Chlamydia;* herpes; *Candida* infections; trichomoniasis; AIDS; cytomegalovirus; hepatitis B; genital warts; bacterial warts, bacterial vaginosis

Data from Centers for Disease Control, 1993.[15]

TABLE 13-22 Overview of STDs Manifested with Urethritis or Cervicitis

	Gonorrhea	Nongonococcal Urethritis, Cervicitis (*Chlamydia*)
Occurrence	Worldwide; highest in 15- to 30-yr-olds of both genders; decreasing in U.S.	Worldwide; 3 times more common than gonorrhea
Etiologic agent	*Neisseria gonorrhoeae,* the gonococcus	*Chlamydia trachomatis,* less commonly *urealyticum, Treponema vaginalis, Candida albicans*
Reservoir	Humans	Humans
Transmission	Contact with exudates from mucous membranes of infected persons, usually by direct sexual contact	Direct contact with exudates either sexually or during birth
Incubation period	2-7 days	Range 7-10 days for *C. trachomatis*
Period of communicability	Months, if untreated	Unknown
Susceptibility and resistance	Universal; antibodies are not protective against reinfection	Universal; no acquired immunity
Report to local health authority	Mandatory case report	Case report required in most states

Data from Benenson.[3]

stratified and transitional squamous epithelia are resistant to the gonococcus; therefore the bladder, upper urinary tract, preputial sac, vulva, vagina, and uterus are infrequently involved. The only exception is prepubescent girls who are susceptible to a gonococcal vulvovaginitis before changes in the vaginal epithelium that accompany puberty. In both sexes primary infections may also affect the pharynx, conjunctivae, and anus.

Direct extension of the infection occurs by way of lymph vessels. In the female, extension most frequently occurs unilaterally or bilaterally to the fallopian tubes, bypassing the uterus. It appears that some cell surfaces of gonococci have greater ability to attach to fallopian tube mucosa. Thus not all gonococcal cervicitis leads to salpingitis. Direct extension in the male most frequently occurs to the epididymis.

Localized infection in any of the above areas may produce cysts and abscesses. The infection may infrequently resolve without treatment if an adequate cellular immune response develops and if there is adequate drainage of the purulent exudate containing the organism. More commonly, the inflammatory exudate is replaced with fibroblasts, and fibrous tissue fills the inflamed tissue. Hardening of the fibrous tissue causes strictures of the lumen of the urethra, epididymis, or fallopian tubes. Complete or partial occlusion of the fallopian tubes results in sterility or increased risk for ectopic pregnancy.

Infection with gonorrhea does result in a short-lived cellular immune response and a longer-lasting humoral immune response, neither of which protects against future infections.

Nongonococcal urethritis and cervicitis are most frequently caused by strains of *C. trachomatis* that are pathogenic to columnar epithelium in a manner similar to *Neisseria gonorrhoeae*. Symptomatic manifestations are generally less severe than with gonorrhea, with many subclinical infections. Infection with *C. trachomatis* stimulates a cellular and humoral immune response, neither of which is protective against future infections.

Complications

Infection of the fallopian tubes with either organism may result in an acute pelvic inflammatory disease. Exudate may be released into the pelvic cavity, causing a severe peritonitis, or the pelvic inflammatory disease may become chronic, with recurrent inflammatory flare-ups that predispose to pelvic inflammation with normal flora organisms. Maternal infection during pregnancy can lead to chronic amnionitis and possible disseminated infection in neonates. Transmission of the pathogens during birth can result in ophthalmia neonatorum and pneumonia in the neonate.

Between 1% and 3% of gonococcal infections become disseminated in the blood, producing septicemia, arthritis, endocarditis, meningitis, or skin lesions. Most disseminated infections are asymptomatic before the dissemination. Occasionally, an extension of gonococcal or chlamydial salpingitis in a woman leads to perihepatitis.

Both organisms also cause postpartum endometritis in infected women.

•••••• Diagnostic Studies and Findings[3,27]

Culture of exudate from urethra, vagina, fallopian tubes, pharynx, or anus   Positive for *N. gonorrhoeae* or *C. trachomatis*.

Microscopic examination of exudate   Gonorrhea positive: Detection of gram negative diplococci: chlamydia positive: Detection of *C. trachomatis* in Giemsa- or fluorescent-stained specimen.

Enzyme-linked immunosorbent assay (ELISA)   Detects *C. trachomatis* antibody reaction in specimen and detects *N. gonorrhoeae* in urethral and voided urine specimens.

Serology   Fourfold rise in antibody titer between onset of infection and later disease for chlamydia. Titer of ≥1:16 is diagnostic.

All patients with gonorrhea or *Chlamydia* infection should be tested also for syphilis.

•••••• Multidisciplinary Plan[14,15]

Medications

Anti-infective agents: Uncomplicated gonococcal infections in adults and presumption of coexisting *Chlamydia* infection
Ceftriaxone, 125 mg IM single dose *or*
Cefixime 400 mg po single dose *or*
Ciprofloxacin 500 mg po single dose or
Ofloxacin 400 mg po single dose plus
Doxycycline hyclate (Vibramycin), 100 mg po bid for 7 d

If infection was acquired from source proven not to have penicillin-resistant gonorrhea
Amoxicillin (Amoxil; others), 3 g po, single dose with 1 g probenecid po, *or*
Ampicillin (Amcill; others), 3.5 g po, single dose with 1 g probenecid po, *or*
Aqueous procaine penicillin G, 4.8 million U IM at two sites with 1 g of probenecid po *plus* doxycycline 100 mg po bid for 7 d
Pharyngeal gonococcal infection
Ceftriaxone, 125 mg IM single dose *or*
Ciprofloxacin, 500 mg po once
During pregnancy
For gonorrhea: any recommended cephalosporin
For chlamydia: Erythromycin base 500 mg po qid for 7 d
Disseminated gonococcal infection (DGI)
Ceftriaxone, 1 g IM or IV, q24h, *or*
Ceftizoxime, 1 g IV, q8h, *or*
Cefotaxime, 1 g IV, q8h; continue all regimens for 24-48 h after improvement begins; then therapy is switched to Cefixime 400 mg po bid or Ciprofloxacin 500 mg po bid
Adult gonococcal ophthalmia
Ceftriaxone, 1 g IM single dose
Uncomplicated *Chlamydia* infection only
Doxycycline, 100 mg po bid for 7 d, *or*
Azithromycin 1 g po in a single dose
Ofloxacin 300 mg po bid for 7 days
Erythromycin base, 500 mg po qid for 7 d, *or*
Erythromycin ethylsuccinate, 800 mg po qid for 7 d, *or*
Sulfisoxazole, 500 mg po qid for 10 d

The above therapy, recommended by the Centers for Disease Control in 1993 (CDC), is not all inclusive. Consult CDC 1993 recommendations for treatment of infants and children and for alternative therapies. The recommendations are based on the increase in infections with antibiotic-resistant *N. gonorrhoeae,* such as penicillinase-producing *N. gonorrhoeae* (PPNG), tetracycline-resistant *N. gonorrhoeae* (TRNG), and strains with chromosomally mediated resistance to multiple antibiotics. They also consider the high frequency of concurrent *Chlamydia* infections with gonorrhea. All sexual partners of patients with gonorrhea or *Chlamydia* infection should be examined and treated. Doxycycline and azithromycin are contraindicated during pregnancy.

NURSING CARE

Nursing Assessment

For gonorrhea and nongonococcal urethritis and cervicitis (*Chlamydia*)

History

Unprotected sexual contact (vaginal, anal, or oral) with an infected person; multiple sexual partners or unknown partner; history of previous STD

Subjective Symptoms

Male: may be asymptomatic; dysuria; severe pain of epididymitis; urinary retention with prostatitis

Female: usually asymptomatic, dysuria or urinary frequency; pelvic inflammatory disease (pelvic pain, low back pain, dyspareunia, menstrual irregularity, constipation, malaise)

Male and female: rectal infection (anal pruritus, burning, or tenesmus); pain with defecation; pharyngeal infection, sore throat

Genitalia

Male: purulent yellow-white discharge from urethra (clearer discharge with *Chlamydia*); inflammation around meatus; swelling and severe pain in scrotum with epididymitis

Female: leukorrhea, usually goes unnoticed

Pelvis (with PID)

Female: Rebound tenderness; normal bowel sounds progressing to ileus in untreated persons; nausea and vomiting

Pharyngeal Infection

Usually asymptomatic or inflamed with visible exudate; red, dry tongue

Rectal Infection

Bloody or mucous diarrhea; purulent discharge

Eyes

Purulent discharge from conjunctiva

Systemic Manifestations of Disseminated Disease

Painful vesicular pustular skin lesions on an erythematous base; petechial skin lesions; symptoms of septicemia, endocarditis, meningitis, arthritis

Body Temperature

Low-grade fever, higher with systemic manifestations, PID, or epididymitis

See Nursing Dx & Intervention, p. 1155

■ SYPHILIS

Syphilis (lues) is a chronic systemic disease characterized by a primary lesion, a secondary eruption involving skin and mucous membranes, long latency periods, and late seriously disabling lesions of skin, bone, viscera, CNS, and cardiovascular system.

Syphilis is one of several sexually transmitted diseases that have both ulcerative lesions and systemic dissemination. Others are herpesvirus infections and lymphogranuloma venereum (Table 13-23).

•••••• Pathophysiology

Syphilis is a systemic infection of the vascular system characterized by five distinct stages: incubation, primary and secondary stages, latency, and late syphilis. Incubation begins with the penetration of *Treponema pallidum* into intact mucous membranes or abraded skin. Some of the pathogens remain at the site of invasion while others migrate, within hours, to regional lymph nodes, where some remain while others are disseminated throughout the body. *Treponema* can invade and multiply in any organ system, producing lesions wherever the concentration of the microorganism is the greatest. During this incubation period, blood containing the *Treponema* organisms is infectious.

Vascular pathologic manifestations are the consequence of treponemal tissue invasion at all stages. The inflammatory response in the endothelial tissue produces perivascular infiltration of lymphocytes and plasma cells, resulting in endothelial swelling and an obliterative endarteritis of terminal arterioles and small arteries. Concentric fibroblastic proliferative thickening occurs in the vessels, resulting in eventual foci of tissue necrosis.

The primary stage is characterized by a single lesion at the site of initial invasion containing the *Treponema* and appearing 10 to 90 days after infection. The lesion is firm and hard as a result of intense cellular infiltration accompanied by serum accumulation in connective tissue. The lesion heals spontaneously within 1 to 5 weeks (average of 2 to 3 weeks). A satellite lesion, or bubo, may develop in an inguinal lymph node.

The secondary stage begins as the primary lesion is resolving, lasts 2 to 6 weeks, and is manifested with parenchymal, systemic, and mucocutaneous symptoms that indicate treponemal pathologic manifestations throughout the body. *Treponema* can be recovered from all skin and mucous membrane lesions.

A period of latency, ranging from 1 to 40 or more years, follows the secondary stage. During the first year of latency there may be recurrence of secondary stage manifestations. Subclinical infection with progressive arterial damage continues for some number of infected persons.

About one third of infected, untreated persons manifest symptoms of late syphilis with clinical evidence of degenerative lesions of the cardiovascular and central nervous systems, the skin, and the viscera. These lesions, called gummas, may be the result of a hypersensitive cellular immune response to the *Treponema* in the tissue. Gummas are granulomatous lesions consisting of a necrotic, coagulated center with obliterative endarteritis of small vessels in the tissue. Lesions of late syphilis, including open gummas on the skin, do not contain *Treponema*. They are therefore not infectious.

Disease manifestations of late syphilis depend on the area of arterial lesions and the extent of circulatory insufficiency. Central nervous system disease may be asymptomatic, meningovascular, or parenchymatous. Parenchymatous neurosyphilis can be seen clinically as paresis (resulting from progressive cortical neuron degeneration) or tabes dorsalis (resulting from posterior column degeneration).

Cardiovascular symptoms frequently result from aortic necrosis with resultant aortic insufficiency.

The immune response in syphilis is not completely understood. Humoral antibodies develop early and persist in untreated persons, but they do not seem to alter the course of the

■ **TABLE 13-23 Overview of STDs with Ulcerative Lesions and Systemic Dissemination**

	Syphilis	Anogenital Herpes	Herpes Type 1	Lymphogranuloma Venereum
Occurrence	Worldwide; increasing in incidence; highest in persons 20-30 yr old of both genders; increasing in neonates	Worldwide; increasing rapidly; highest in persons 15-30 yr old; 20%-30% of U.S. adults have HSV-2 antibody	Worldwide; 70%-90% of adults have antibodies against herpes type 1; primary infection probably occurs by age 5 yr	Worldwide; higher in tropical and subtropical climates
Etiologic agent	*Treponema pallidum,* a spirochete	Herpes simplex virus 2;	Herpes simplex virus type 1	Several strains of *chlamydia trachomatis*
Reservoir	Humans	Humans	Humans	Humans
Transmission	Direct contact with exudates from lesions on skin and mucous membranes; body fluids and secretions (saliva, semen, blood, vaginal discharges) of infected people, usually during sexual contact; blood transfusion from infected donor during early disease; and congenital	Direct contact with saliva or secretions from mucous membranes and lesions; congenital	Contact with saliva of carriers and active lesions; may be transmitted sexually	Direct contact with open lesions
Incubation period	10 days to 12 wk; usually 3 wk	2-12 days; average of 6 days	2-12 days	3-30 days
Period of communicability	Variable; during primary and secondary stages and in mucocutaneous recurrences; 2-4 yr if untreated	Transient shedding of virus in absence of lesions probably occurs; 7-12 days with lesion	During lesions; virus in saliva found as long as 7 wk after recovery of lesions; transient shedding of virus is common	Variable; weeks to years as long as lesions are present
Susceptibility and resistance	Universal, although only 30% of exposures result in infection; no natural immunity; infection leads to gradually developing resistance to new infections	Universal; immune response does not prevent recurrence	Universal susceptibility	General suscpetibility; resistance is not clear
Report to local health authority	Mandatory case report	No	No	In some states

Data from Benenson[3] and CDC.[15]

disease. The cell-mediated immune response increases during latency. This may account for the lack of progression to late syphilis for a large portion of untreated persons. Antibody levels will gradually decrease in persons treated in primary and secondary stages.

Congenital transmission of *Treponema* may occur at any time during pregnancy, but the fetus does not develop an inflammatory response to the pathogen until around the fifteenth week of gestation. Treatment of infected pregnant women before the fifteenth week may prevent damage to the fetus. Evidence of congenital syphilitic damage includes early malformations, observed at birth or during the first 2 years of life, and later evidence of developmental deformities. Infants with congenital syphilis born to untreated or inadequately treated mothers will have active infection and must be treated.

Complications
Secondary and tertiary syphilis
Congenital syphilis

• • • • • • Diagnostic Studies and Findings[27]

Microscopic examination of specimen of exudate or cells from lesions or regional lymph nodes (Darkfield or phase-contrast microscopy) Positive for *T. pallidum* during primary and secondary stages

Detection of antigen in specimen through treponemal antigen/antibody tests (fluorescent treponemal antibody absorption [FTA-ABS]; microhemagglutination assay [MHA-TP]) Reported as nonreactive, borderline, or reactive; these tests become reactive earlier in primary stage

Serology (Venereal Disease Research Laboratory [VDRL]; rapid plasma reagin [RPR]) Increase in nonspecific antibodies 1 to 3 weeks after appearance of the chancre or 4 to 6 weeks after infection; tests become negative in 6 to 12 months after treatment of primary syphilis, 12 to 18 months after treatment of secondary syphilis; serologic tests may not revert to negative if treatment is delayed beyond 2 years.

Persons with early syphilis should be tested for other STDs and counseled to be tested for HIV.

• • • • • Multidisciplinary Plan[15]

Medications

Anti-infective agents

Primary, secondary, or early syphilis of <1 yr duration: benzathine penicillin G, 2.4 million U IM single dose

Of more than 1 yr duration: benzathine penicillin G (Bicillin), 7.2 million U total; 2.4 million U IM/wk for 3 successive wk

Patients allergic to penicillin

Tetracycline (Achromycin; others) 500 mg po qid for 15 d for infections of <1 yr and 30 d for infections of longer duration, *or*

Doxycycline, 100 mg po bid for 2 wk for infections of longer duration (pregnant women should not receive tetracycline or doxycycline)

Penicillin-allergic pregnant women should be skin tested and desensitized and then treated with penicillin in a hospital setting (no alternative drug therapies to penicillin are currently effective for treating syphilis in pregnancy, congenital syphilis, or neurosyphilis)

Neurosyphilis

Aqueous crystalline penicillin G, 12-24 million U/d administered 2-4 million U q4h IV for 10-14 d, *or*

Procaine penicillin, 2.4 million U IM/d plus Probenecid, 500 mg po qid, both for 10-14 d

NURSING CARE

Nursing Assessment

For syphilis

History

Unprotected sexual contact (vaginal, anal, or oral) with an infected person; multiple sexual partners or unknown partner, previous STD

Primary Stage: Within 10 to 90 Days After Exposure (Average of 21 Days); Lasts 1 to 5 Weeks

Genitalia

Single painless papule erodes to become a hard, painless, indurated chancre without an exudate; located at site of inoculation, usually on glans penis of male and on cervix or external genitalia of female; may be seen on scrotum, anus, rectum, lips, tongue, tonsils, nipples, and fingers; abraded ulcer exudes serous fluid teeming with *T. pallidum* organisms

Inguinal lymph nodes

Hard, nonfluctuant, painless, enlarged inguinal lymph nodes

Secondary Stage: Within 6 to 12 Weeks After Infection, Lasting a Few Days to 1 Year

Subjective symptoms

Malaise, headache, anorexia, nausea, aching in bones, fatigue, neck stiffness; fever; anemia; jaundice

Skin

Lesions, recurring local or generalized, papulosquamous, macular, papular, or pustular rash; bilateral and symmetric, beginning on trunk and proximal extremities, frequently on soles of feet and palms of hands; lesions are 3 to 10 mm, nonpruritic, and contain *T. pallidum* organisms

Condylomata lata: lesions on moist areas coalesce and erode to produce painless, moist, pink to grayish white, raised plaques

Alopecia: nonscarring, temporary hair loss in patches on head and eyebrows

Mucous membranes

Mucous patches: silver-gray superficial erosion surrounded by red periphery on mucous membranes

Gastrointestinal

Epigastric pain or vomiting associated with ulceration

Latent Stage: Lasts a Few Years to the Remainder of Person's Life

May have relapses of mucocutaneous symptoms of secondary stage early in latency; otherwise, no symptoms

Late Stages (Tertiary Syphilis): Benign Tertiary Syphilis of the Skin, Bone, and Viscera (3 to 10 Years After Infection)

Gumma lesions (a chronic granulomatous reaction, causing lesions, ulcers, or tumors); lesions are of varying sizes, appear anywhere on the body, and do not contain *T. pallidum;* they may occur in palate, nasal septum, and other submucosal tissue, causing disfigurement; gumma lesions in bones cause pain

Cardiovascular Syphilis (10 to 25 Years After Initial Infection)

Aortic valvular insufficiency, thoracic aneurysm, narrowing of coronary ostia

Neurosyphilis (May Be Asymptomatic or Symptomatic)

Meningovascular symptoms: focal neurologic signs depending on area of lesions; seizures; parenchymatous symptoms: paresis; personality changes, ranging from minor to severe psychosis; alteration in intellect and judgment; hyperactive reflexes; tabes dorsalis; ataxia, areflexia, paresthesias, bladder disturbance, impotence; sharp, tearing pain; trophic joint changes; optic atrophy with small, irregular pupils that are not reactive to light but respond normally to accommodation

Nursing Dx & Intervention

See p. 1155.

HERPESVIRUS INFECTIONS

Herpes simplex is a systemic viral infection characterized by a localized primary lesion, latency, and a tendency to localized recurrence. Two serologically distinct herpes viral agents, 1 and 2, generally produce distinct clinical syndromes. Herpes simplex virus type 2 (HSV-2) is most often implicated in genital herpes (see Table 13-22).

•••••• Pathophysiology

Two antigenically distinct herpes simplex viruses (HSV), types 1 and 2, are responsible for herpes infections. Both are capable of producing infection in epithelial tissue anywhere in the body, but HSV-1 is most often associated with oral, labial, ocular, or skin herpes above the waist, whereas HSV-2 is implicated in 90% of genital, anal, and perianal herpes or oral herpes associated with genital, oral, or sexual transmission. Infections caused by both types of HSV are discussed in this section because of the potential for sexual transmission of both agents and because both produce essentially the same pathologic findings.

All HSV infections have two characteristics in common: Once present in tissue, HSV produces a chronic infection initiated with active self-limiting tissue destruction. The lesions heal, but the organism continues to be viable in the body in the presence of circulating antibodies and in the absence of symptomatic disease.

There is a latent period during which the genome of the virus is present in tissue in a nondestructive form. Infectious virions cannot be recovered until the virus becomes reactivated and produces recurrent infectious disease. Active infection, either initial or recurrent, need not be symptomatic.

Initial infection refers to the first infection with the HSV type. Initial infection with HSV-1 usually occurs by age 4 years and is manifest as a clinical or subclinical gingivostomatitis. Initial infection with HSV-2 usually occurs during the ages of sexual activity and is usually manifested by clinical or subclinical genital herpes.

The organism is transmitted by close contact with saliva or genital secretions of persons with active clinical or subclinical infections either directly or by hand.

The transmitted virus invades and replicates in the parabasal and intermediate epithelial cells of mucous membranes or traumatized skin. Intracellular and extracellular edema and cell lysis cause the cells to lose their intercellular bridges and to undergo a ballooning degeneration. Polymorphonuclear cells infiltrate, forming a thin-walled intradermal vesicle on an erythematous base. Multiple grouped vesicles can be visualized at the sites of tissue inoculation. The superficial epithelium collapses and sloughs, leaving single shallow ulcers, or the vesicles may coalesce into large painful ulcers. Crusting may occur on nonmucous membrane ulcers. All ulcers spontaneously granulate without scarring in about 12 days in initial infections.

The virus may enter the lymphatic system, producing localized lesions there. Rarely, the virus is disseminated to visceral organs, particularly the liver, adrenal glands, lungs, or central nervous system, producing discrete focal areas of necrosis in epithelial tissues in those organs. The virus may also be spread to other external body sites by autoinoculation.

Cellular immune response and nonspecific host defenses appear to inhibit dissemination. Circulating humoral antibodies develop but do not appear to be protective against reinfection or recurrent infection.

After the primary infection, the HSV travels along sensory nerve pathways to a sensory nerve ganglion where it remains in a latent stage. The viral DNA is stored in ganglion neurons in the absence of other viral products. The virus is not pathogenic in this form. It appears that the transient viral shedding may occur during this stage.

The exact mechanism for reactivation of the virus to produce recurrence of lesions is not known. Recurrence of HSV lesions is generally in the area of initial inoculation. Genital recurrence is usually associated with HSV-2 and is usually less severe, lasting 4 or 5 days. Genital recurrence is common in women with asymptomatic cervical lesions. Oral HSV-1 infections frequently recur on the lips. Recurrence of either type may be triggered by another infectious disease, menstruation, emotional stress, and immunosuppression.

Complications

Potential complications of herpes infections include neuralgia, meningitis (HSV-1), encephalitis (HSV-2), ascending myelitis, urethral strictures, and lymphatic suppuration. In females there is the possibility of an increased risk for spontaneous abortion and cervical cancer. Neonates may become infected during vaginal delivery. Congenital herpes ranges from subclinical infections to severe infections of the skin, eyes, mucous membranes, visceral organs, or central nervous system. Congenital herpes has a high mortality. Many survivors have ocular or neurologic sequelae.

•••••• Diagnostic Studies and Findings[3,27]

Virus tissue culture of specimen from base of vesicles Identification of type 1 or type 2 viral cytopathogenic effect in tissue culture

Microscopic examination of stained smear from base of vesicles Direct identification of multinucleated giant cells with intranuclear inclusions

Serology Fourfold increase in antibody titer in paired sera; difficult to differentiate type 1 from type 2

Persons with a new infection with herpes should also be examined for syphilis, gonorrhea, and Chlamydia.

•••••• Multidisciplinary Plan[15]

Medications

Anti-infective agents

For first clinical episode of genital herpes: acyclovir 200 mg po, 5 times/d for 7-10 days, initiated within 6 d of onset of lesions

For severe infections: acyclovir 5-10 mg/kg q8h IV for 5-7 d or until clinical resolution

For proctitis: acyclovir 400 mg po 5 times/d for 10 d

Recurrent episodes: acyclovir 200 mg po 5 times/d for 5 d or acyclovir 800 mg po bid for 5 d or acyclovir 400 mg po tid 5 d

Suppressive therapy: acyclovir 200 mg po 3-5 times/d or acyclovir 400 mg po bid; discontinue after 1 yr

NURSING CARE

Nursing Assessment

See Nursing Care: Lymphogranuloma venereum.

■ LYMPHOGRANULOMA VENEREUM

Lymphogranuloma venereum is a systemic, disabling bacterial infection that begins with a small, painless evanescent erosion on the penis or vulva. Regional lymph nodes undergo suppuration, spreading the inflammatory process into adjacent tissue. The disease is disseminated further by the lymph system. There are usually systemic symptoms of lymphadenitis and serious complications in untreated individuals.

For an overview of lymphogranuloma venereum see Table 13-23 on p. 1146.

•••••• Pathophysiology

Lymphogranuloma venereum is a systemic infection produced by mucosal invasion of a number of closely related strains of *Chlamydia*. The disease has three stages: a primary lesion, regional and disseminated lymphadenitis, and late complications resulting from progression of the regional lymphadenitis.

A primary transient nodular or vesicular lesion forms at the site of inoculation. Dissemination of the organism to regional lymph nodes (primarily inguinal lymph nodes) results in lymph node lesions that are initially similar to the inoculation lesion. The lesions are composed of small masses of epithelioid cells with multinucleated cells scattered throughout and a necrotic center filled with polymorphonuclear leukocytes. Satellite lesions are formed in the lymph node, surrounded by a narrow layer of epithelioid cells. The nodes show hyperplasia with an inflammatory cellular infiltration consisting of plasma cells, polymorphonuclear leukocytes, large mononuclear cells, and lymphocytes. Spread of the inflammation throughout the nodes causes the nodes to become matted together and form a large abscess. These abscesses develop in one or more areas along the lymphatic system. Untreated, the abscesses may rupture through the skin or other epithelial surfaces to produce chronic draining sinuses or fistulas. If the condition is not treated, it progresses, producing complications resulting from the impaired lymph and draining sinuses.

Complications

Genital elephantiasis and perianal abscesses and fistulas result in eventual rectal stricture. Advanced stages of rectal stricture may be manifest as symptoms of painful ileus, distention, complete obstruction, perforation, and peritonitis.

•••••• Diagnostic Studies and Findings[3]

Cell culture of lesion exudate or bubo aspirate   Positive for *C. trachomatis*

Serology   Antibody titer 1:64 or higher within 1 to 3 weeks of infection; fourfold rise in titer between early infection and convalescence; nonspecific, since it detects antibodies against all *C. trachomatis* strains. A negative CF test rules out the diagnosis

These patients should be examined for other STDs, as well.

•••••• Multidisciplinary Plan[15]

Surgery

Aspiration of fluctuant lymph nodes as needed (incision and drainage or excision is contraindicated)

Strictures or fistulas may require surgery

Medications

Anti-infective agents

Doxycycline (Vibramycin), 100 mg po bid for 21 d; *or*

Erythromycin (Erythrocin; others), 500 mg po qid for 21 d; *or*

Sulfisoxazole, 500 mg po qid for 21 d; *or*

Equivalent sulfonamide course

NURSING CARE

Nursing Assessment

For herpes type 1, herpes type 2, and lymphogranuloma venereum (LV)

History

Herpes 2 and LV: unprotected sexual contact (vaginal, anal, or oral) with an infected person; multiple or unknown sexual partners; previous herpes lesions (herpes 2)

Subjective Symptoms

Herpes 1 and 2: burning or pruritus in areas of lesions; fever in initial infection; malaise

LV: fever, chills, headache, joint pains, anorexia, abdominal pain, urinary retention

Oral Cavity

Herpes 1 and 2: multiple vesicular and ulcerative lesions on labial and buccal mucosa, tongue, and larynx; erythema of gums; excessive salivation; infection heals in 7 to 10 days; recurrent infections rare in mouth

LV: may have lesions in mouth as described under genitourinary/rectal below

Lips

Herpes 1: recurrent "cold sore" or "fever blister" preceded by 1 or 2 days of paresthesia; lesions crust and heal within 3 to 10 days

Genitourinary/rectal

Herpes 2: asymptomatic or extensive vesicular lesions with deep ulceration and marked hyperplasia and erythema of cervix, labia, fourchette, and clitoris (sometimes vagina); may extend to anal area, buttocks, and thighs; dysuria, leukorrhea, and marked genital tenderness; scattered vesicles over glans, prepuce, and shaft of the penis (lesions heal in 10 days); urinary retention; urethritis may occur without genital lesions; anal lesions possible

LV: 2 to 3 mm painless, discrete, superficial vesicle or nonindurated ulcer at site of inoculation (frequently unnoticed); usually on glans or shaft of penis in males and on labia, vagina, or cervix in females; may be in rectum; rectal inoculation initially produces bloody discharge and tenesmus, and mucopurulent discharge, cramps, and diarrhea later; complications may include elephantiasis of prepuce, penis, scrotum, or vulva; perianal abscess; rectovaginal, rectovesical, and ischiorectal fistulas; rectal stricture 1 to 10 years after infection

Regional Lymph Nodes

Herpes 1: enlarged and palpable cervical lymph nodes
Herpes 2: bilateral lymphadenopathy of inguinal lymph nodes in 50% of initial genital infections
LV: 7 to 30 days after primary lesion: initially a firm, tender, discrete, movable inguinal lymph node, which later becomes indolent, fixed, and matted; may be unilateral or bilateral; may subside spontaneously or proceed to form an abscess that may rupture to produce a draining sinus or fistula; female lymph node involvement may be mainly in the pelvic nodes with extension to rectum and rectovaginal septum

Skin

Herpes 1 and 2: clustered vesicular lesions anywhere on body; deep burning; skin edema

Eyes

Herpes 1 and 2: keratitis and conjunctivitis (unilateral or bilateral); periauricular lymphadenopathy

See Nursing Dx and Intervention on p. 1155.

CHANCROID AND GRANULOMA INGUINALE

Chancroid, also called "soft sore" or "soft chancre," is an acute, localized, autoinoculable bacterial infection of the genitalia. Necrotizing ulceration occurs at the site of inoculation, frequently accompanied by suppuration of regional lymph nodes. Systemic dissemination does not occur.

Granuloma inguinale (donovanosis) is a mildly communicable, chronic and progressive, autoinoculable bacterial infection of the skin and mucous membranes, external genitalia, inguinal and anal regions, face, and oral cavity. Lesions first appear as small, painless papules or vesicles that become ulcerated and slowly develop into bleeding granulomatous masses. The disease may be difficult to differentiate from carcinoma (Table 13-24).

•••••• Pathophysiology

Although both chancroid and granuloma inguinale are manifest as ulcerative lesions, their pathophysiologies differ.

▪ TABLE 13-24 Overview of STDs with Ulcerative Lesions Without Systemic Manifestations

	Chancroid	Granuloma Inguinale (Donovanosis)
Occurrence	Most common in tropical and subtropical climates; more often diagnosed in males than in females	Most common in tropical and subtropical climates and in 20-40 yr old men
Etiologic agent	*Haemophilus ducreyi,* a bacterium	*Calymmatobacterium granulomatis*
Reservoir	Humans	Humans
Transmission	Direct sexual contact with exudate from lesions; autoinoculation to other areas	Direct sexual contact with lesions or with organism in rectum of nondiseased carriers
Incubation period	3-14 days	1-16 wk
Period of communicability	Until lesions heal (can be weeks)	Duration of open lesions
Susceptibility and resistance	General, but highest in uncircumcised males; no evidence of resistance, although women may have more subclinical infections	Susceptibility is variable; no evidence of immunity
Report to local health authority	Mandatory case report	Mandatory case report

Data from Benenson[3] and CDC.[15]

Chancroid

In chancroid the transmitted pathogenic bacteria initially invade genital skin or mucous membranes at sites traumatized by sexual contact. A preexisting abrasion facilitates invasion. A small papule is formed, surrounded by a zone of erythema. This erupts to form a shallow and painful ulcer.

A purulent exudate results from the extensive necrotic process. The ulcers may enlarge and continue to erode and destroy tissue, or they may become secondarily infected and produce even more rapid destruction of tissue. Fresh lesions may occur from autoinoculation. Extragenital lesions may occur on fingers, tongue, lips, breasts, and eyelids.

Lymphatic dissemination results in a unilateral or bilateral painful inguinal adenitis within 7 to 10 days of the primary lesion. The enlarged lymph gland (bubo) softens, becomes fluctuant, and may rupture spontaneously.

Granuloma Inguinale

The transmission of granuloma inguinale is less well understood. The pathogenic bacterium can be found in the rectum of nondiseased patients, suggesting that the organism may be part of the normal gastrointestinal flora of some persons. Lesions may result from autoinfection, possibly following trauma to the genitalia. The pathogen in the lesions is transmitted sexually, but repeated exposure seems to be necessary for transmission. The disease is rare in heterosexual partners of infected persons. Clinical disease is highest in homosexual males.

The organism invades endothelial cells and forms a small, painless papule or nodule at the site of dermal invasion. The epithelium overlapping the lesion softens, erodes, ulcerates, and then produces a gradually enlarging granulomatous ulcerating lesion that bleeds easily. Pronounced marginal epithelial proliferation may simulate early epitheliomatous changes of cancer. The raised mass of granulation tissue looks more like a tumor than an ulcer. Single or multiple lesions may coalesce, or lesions may spread to contiguous tissue. Lesions have variable clinical appearances depending on the area located, mode of spread, tissue resistance, and texture of the skin.

The lesions heal by fibrosis at the same time that tissue destruction is occurring in expanding lesions. Resultant scarring may produce urethral occlusion. The inguinal swelling that is sometimes seen with this disease is not a lymphadenopathy, but rather a subcutaneous granuloma.

Complications

Chancroid

Phimosis and urethral fistulas in males
Females frequently asymptomatic
Associated with increased risk for HIV infection

Granuloma Inguinale

Hematogenous spread of the pathogen to bones, joints, and liver is rare but has been reported
Lymphatic spread questionable
Secondary infection and expanding necrosis in untreated lesions may result in complete genital erosion

••••• Diagnostic Studies and Findings

Chancroid Culture or microscopic examination of exudate from bulbo or lesions; positive for *H. ducreyi* bacilli; tests to rule out other causes of ulcers, particularly syphilis and herpes

Granuloma inguinale Microscopic examination of scrapings from ulcer margins; Donovan bodies can be visualized; *tests to rule out carcinoma; examination for other STDs*

••••• Multidisciplinary Plan[3,15]

Surgery

Chancroid: fluctuant lymph nodes should be aspirated through adjacent normal skin (incision and drainage or excision of nodes is contraindicated)

Medications[15]

Anti-infective agents
  Chancroid
    Erythromycin (Erythrocin), 500 mg po qid 7 days, *or*
    Azithromycin 1 g po single dose
    Ceftriaxone, 250 mg IM once

NURSING CARE

Nursing Assessment

For chancroid and granuloma inguinale

History

Unprotected sexual contact (vaginal, anal, or oral) with an infected person; multiple or unknown sexual partners; history of previous STD

Subjective Symptoms

Chancroid: pain

Genitalia

Chancroid: one to 10 primary lesions; inflamed macule, papule, or pustule; irregularly shaped and of variable size (1 mm to 2 cm); surrounded by a zone of inflammation; erupts to produce a sharply circumscribed, nonindurated ulcer with a granulating base and ragged edges; abundant, purulent exudate; location: frenulum, prepuce, coronal sulcus, glans and shaft of penis, and urinary meatus in males; cervix, vagina, fourchette, labia, and perianal area in females
Variations in clinical appearance of lesions
  Follicular pustules rupture and form ulcers
  Dwarf chancroid lesions look similar to herpes lesions
  Transient chancroid lesion resolves quickly but is followed by an inguinal bubo
  Papular chancroid starts as an ulcer but becomes raised
  Giant chancroid frequently follows rupture of inguinal abscess and grows rapidly
  Phagedenic chancroid, a small lesion, rapidly extends and becomes necrotic and destructive

Granuloma inguinale: single or multiple, indurated, sharply defined but irregular papules or nodules; erode to form a beefy, exuberant granulomatous, heaped, clean ulcer, progressing slowly and coalescing with adjacent lesions; serous exudate; location: glans, prepuce, urethra, shaft of pcnis, and pcrianal area in males; labia and fourchcttc in females; lesions bleed easily; if secondarily infected, may have odorous necrotic exudate

Variations in clinical appearance

Oral lesions are painful and resemble malignancies

Vaginal and cervical ulcers produce profuse, purulent discharge and irregular bleeding

Cervical ulcers are soft, friable, irregular, and not well fixed to tissue; resemble cancer

Male genital ulcers may be hypertrophic and verrucose, destructive and necrotic, discoid (buttonlike), or chronic and indolent

Inguinal ulcers and ulcers on female genitalia are generally fleshy and exuberant

Anal ulcers are hypertrophic and verrucose or chronic and indolent

Inguinal Area

Chancroid: single, unilateral (can be bilateral), tender, and unilocular lymphadenopathy with overlying erythema; suppuration and rupture of fluctuant nodes in 5 to 10 days may occur, leaving a single, large ulcer

Granuloma inguinale: rarely any inguinal involvement; may have a subcutaneous granuloma that suppurates and mimics a lymphadenopathy

See Nursing Dx and Intervention on p. 1155.

MOLLUSCUM CONTAGIOSUM AND CONDYLOMATA ACUMINATA

Molluscum contagiosum is a viral disease of the skin that results in pearly pink to white papules with a central exudative pore. Multiple lesions appear on the genitalia and clear spontaneously in 6 to 9 months. Children develop lesions on skin elsewhere on the body.

Condylomata acuminata constitute one of the four major categories of virus-produced warts; this category occurs primarily on the genitalia or perineum. The warts appear as single or multiple, soft pink to brown, elongated lesions, usually in clusters and sometimes as large cauliflower-like masses (Table 13-25).

• • • • • Pathophysiology

The viruses of both these diseases invade superficial layers of the epidermis, and infect single epithelial cells and stimulate the cells to divide. In the case of condylomata there is excessive proliferation of the cells of the stratum spinosum, constituting the bulk of the wart. Microscopic examination of the infected cells shows aggregates of the virus particles. In the case of molluscum contagiosum, a central pore containing the virus and exudative material develops in the papules.

Both molluscum papules and genital warts appear as multiple lesions on the external genitalia. Genital warts may also be found in the vagina and cervix of females and anterior urethra of males. Perineal and anal warts in females are generally caused by spread, whereas anal warts in males are associated with anal coitus. Genital warts that resemble skin warts suggest hand-to-genital transmission of another category of skin warts.

The papules of molluscum contagiosum clear spontaneously in 6 to 9 months as a result of an immune response. Warts sometimes clear spontaneously, which suggests an immune response.

Laryngeal papillomatosis may develop in infants born to mothers with vaginal warts. Also, the enlarged size of some warts may lead to difficulty during a vaginal birth. Secondary infection and bleeding of warts are common. Enlarged or giant condylomata of the penis, although benign, may destroy large areas of the penis. Cancer must be ruled out in this situation. Malignant transformation, both invasive and intraepithelial, has been observed in some warts.

Complications

Secondary infection and bleeding of warts
Malignant transformation, particularly in cervix
Laryngeal warts in neonate

■ TABLE 13-25 Overview of STDs with Nonulcerative Lesions

	Molluscum Contagiosum	Condylomata Acuminata (Anogenital Warts)
Occurrence	Worldwide	Worldwide
Etiologic agent	A member of the poxvirus group	Human *papillomavirus* (HPV)
Reservoir	Humans	Humans
Transmission	Direct sexual contact and indirect contact	Direct sexual contact; childbirth
Incubation period	2-7 wk	1-20 mo (usually 2-3 mo)
Period of communicability	Unknown; probably as long as lesions persist	Unknown; probably as long as lesions persist
Susceptibility and resistance	Usually occurs in small children	General; increases in immunosuppressed
Report to local health authority	No	No

Data from Benenson.[3]

••••• Diagnostic Studies and Findings[3]

Microscopic examination of material in core of molluscum lesion Pathognomonic molluscum inclusion bodies can be visualized

Condylomata Biopsy necessary for definitive diagnosis to rule out malignancy; rule out condylomata lata of syphilis with serologic test for syphilis

••••• Multidisciplinary Plan[15]

Surgery

Alternative therapies for warts may include cryotherapy, electrosurgery, or surgical removal (scissors, curette, or carbon dioxide laser) no treatment should be initiated on cervical warts until results of a Papanicolaou smear are available

Molluscum lesions may resolve spontaneously or be removed by curettage after cryoanesthesia or cryotherapy or by the use of caustic chemicals

Medications

Keratolytic agents

Condylomata acuminata; podophyllin, 10%-25% in compound tincture of benzoin to wart only; to be washed off in 1-4 h; four weekly treatments (not to be used during pregnancy or with urethral, oral, cervical, or anorectal warts)

NURSING CARE

Nursing Assessment

For molluscum and condylomata

History

Sexual contact with infected person; multiple or unknown sexual partner; previous STD

Anogenital Area

Molluscum contagiosum: multiple, distinct, dome-shaped papules, 1 to 10 mm, pearly pink to white, with a central pore containing a cheeselike white exudate; may be surrounded by red or scaling skin

Condylomata (warts): multiple or single, soft pink to brown, elongated lesions, usually in cluster, may be in large masses; painless

See Nursing Dx and Interventions on p. 1155.

■ VULVOVAGINITIS

Vulvovaginitis is an inflammation of the superficial mucous membranes of the vulva and vagina caused by a number of microorganisms that are frequently part of the normal vaginal flora in adult women. The inflammation is accompanied by a purulent exudate with characteristics that differ with causative agents. The etiologic agents most frequently associated with vulvovaginitis are *Trichomonas vaginalis* (a protozoan), *Candida albicans* (a yeast form of fungus), and bacteria such as *Gardnerella vaginalis*, *Corynebacterium vaginale*, and *Haemophilus vaginalis*. They are responsible for trichomoniasis, candidiasis, and bacterial vaginoses, respectively (Table 13-26). In addition, the inflammation can be caused by mechanical irritants, contact allergens, and ectoparasites (pinworms, lice) (Table 13-27).

••••• Pathophysiology

The presence of estrogen in women supports a normal flora of microorganisms in the vagina and anterior urethra. Under certain conditions (alterations in hormonal levels during the menstrual cycle, pregnancy, antibiotic therapy, immunosuppression), imbalance occurs in the normal flora. Certain opportunistic organisms become pathogenic or may be sexually transmitted in large enough numbers to become pathogenic. They colonize on the superficial mucosal layers and produce patches of inflammation and exudate that contain large numbers of the pathogens. The infection rarely extends beyond the endocervix. There is a wide range in severity of infections. Many are asymptomatic. The organism may be transmitted to a male sexual partner who may or may not develop symptomatic urethritis. Reinfection of the female from untreated males is common.

The organisms may be transmitted to an infant during birth. Infections in newborns are generally temporary and are limited to the period before maternal estrogens are metabolized by the newborn.

Certain physiologic changes in the host support the pathogenic growth of different organisms. Trichomoniasis is exacerbated during and after menstruation, whereas bacterial infections such as *G. vaginalis* vaginitis are not associated with hormonal changes during the menstrual cycle. *G. vaginalis* vaginitis is associated with an altered vaginal pH; the organism usually does not grow in the normal acid secretions. Yeast infections, such as candidiasis, are greatly exacerbated preceding menstruation, during pregnancy, and in women taking oral contraceptives. Candidiasis is also exacerbated by the elimination of normal flora bacteria with antibiotic therapy or with any other condition that compromises skin or mucous membrane defenses.

Whereas *Trichomonas* and *Gardnerella* rarely extend beyond the vulvovaginal or anterior urethral area. *Candida* has the potential for producing infection anywhere in the body where normal defenses are altered. *Candida* is part of the normal gastrointestinal, oral, and cutaneous flora of many persons, and it may become pathogenic in those areas. Severe infection with invasion and abscess formation, particularly in the gastrointestinal tract, may lead to hematogenous dissemination of the yeast to other organs. The organism may also be introduced to internal organs through surgical procedures, catheters, or implanted devices and produce multiple microabscess in infected tissue. The areas most commonly infected are the central nervous system (particularly the meninges), lungs, peritoneum, heart

■ **TABLE 13-26   Vulvovaginitis Caused by a Pathogen**

	Trichomoniasis	Candidiasis	Bacterial Vaginosis
Occurrence	Worldwide; highest in females 16-35 yr; often accompanies other STDs	Worldwide; fungus is part of normal flora in 50% of women 15-45; most common cause of vaginitis	Worldwide; bacteria are part of normal vaginal flora in many asymptomatic women
Etiologic agent	*Trichomonas vaginalis,* a protozoan	*Candida albicans,* a fungus (yeast); occasionally other species of *Candida*	*Gardnerella vaginalis, Haemophilus vaginalis, Corynebacterium vaginale, Mycoplasma hominis*
Reservoir	Humans	Humans	Humans
Transmission	Direct and indirect contact with vaginal and urethral discharges	Direct and indirect contact with secretions from mouth, skin, vagina, and rectum of infected persons and carriers; transmitted to infant during vaginal delivery	Direct contact with vaginal and urethral discharges
Incubation period	4-20 days; average is 7 days	2-5 days in thrush in newborn	Variable
Period of communicability	Duration of infection; may last for years	Duration of lesions	Duration of infection
Susceptibility and resistance	General, but clinical disease is mainly in females; exacerbated during menstruation and pregnancy	Many persons have organism but few acquire infection; exacerbated during pregnancy, before menstruation, with oral contraceptives, and antibiotic therapy	General, but clinical disease is only in females; many women have the organism, but not all acquire symptomatic infections; results from changes in vaginal pH
Report to local health authority	No	No	No

Data from Benenson,[3] and CDC[15]

■ **TABLE 13-27   Vulvovaginitis of Nonpathogenic Origin**

Etiology	Epidemiology	Signs and Symptoms	Diagnostic Studies	Medical Plan
Postmenopausal vaginitis (atrophic vaginitis)	Occurs because of decreased estrogen levels	Thin watery discharge; burning and itching	Direct visual examination	Atrophic changes cannot be reversed but can usually be prevented with hormone therapy
Allergic or irritative vaginitis owing to thermal, chemical, and physical causes	Thermal sources: douching with excessively hot water, wearing nylon undergarments Chemical sources: douche solutions, hygiene sprays, soaps, detergents on undergarments, poor personal hygiene Physical sources: retained tampon, diaphragm, toilet paper, condom, or pessary	Redness, burning, and itching of excoriated skin Increase in type and amount of secretions; rash; burning and itching Foul-smelling, sero-sanguineous, or purulent discharge	Direct visual examination; wet smear; detailed history; bimanual examination	Avoidance of source; secondary infection should be treated according to etiology; oral antihistamines for allergic vaginitis, local cortisone ointment; wearing cotton undergarments

(myocardium, pericardium, and endocardium), endometrium, eyes, ears, joints, oral cavity, esophagus, skin, and nails. Deep tissue infection is more common in patients with neoplastic disease. Cutaneous infections are more commonly associated with skin injury or continual wetting of the skin. *Candida* infections may involve multiple organs and tissue simultaneously, a particular risk for immunosuppressed individuals.

Vaginal candidiasis may be transmitted to the infant during delivery. A common manifestation of such an infection in the newborn is thrush, an infection in the oral cavity. Creamy white, curdlike patches consisting of desquamated epithelial cells, leukocytes, bacteria, keratin, necrotic tissue, and food debris are formed on the oral mucosa. Scraping of the patches leaves a raw, bleeding, painful surface.

Complications

Candida hematogenous spread to CNS, lungs, peritoneum, heart, endometrium, eyes, ears, joints, a risk for immunocompromised persons; transmission to neonate at time of delivery

Bacterial vaginosis: may cause premature rupture of membranes in pregnant women (not proven)

••••• Diagnostic Studies and Findings[3,27]

Trichomoniasis Culture of vaginal secretions (urethral discharge): positive for *T. vaginalis;* microscopic examination of saline wet mount of vaginal secretions: visualization of motile protozoa

Candidiasis Culture of vaginal secretions: positive for *C. vaginale* in symptomatic women; because *Candida* is part of normal oral flora, culture is not useful in thrush; microscopic examination of Gram's stain or KOH wet mount preparation of vaginal secretions: visualization of yeast cells or pseudohyphae

Bacterial vaginosis Culture of vaginal secretions: positive for *G. vaginalis, mycoplasma hominis* or other bacteria in symptomatic women; microscopic examination of Gram's stain or KOH wet mount preparation of vaginal secretions: identification of "clue" cells; or vaginal pH ≥4.5

••••• Multidisciplinary Plan[15]

Medications

Anti-infective agents for trichomoniasis

    Metronidazole (Flagyl), 2 g po single dose, or

    Metronidazole, 500 mg bid for 7 d (contraindicated during the first trimester of pregnancy; asymptomatic women and their sexual partners should be treated to prevent sexual transmission)

Anti-infective agents for vulvovaginal candidiasis

    Miconazole nitrate (vaginal suppository 200 mg), intravaginally at HS for 3 d, *or*

    Clotrimazole (vaginal tablets 100 mg), 2 tablets intravaginally for 3 d, *or*

    Butaconazole (2% cream, 5 g), intravaginally at HS for 3 d *or*

    Terconazole 80 mg suppository or 0.8% cream 5g, intravaginally at HS for 3 d *or* 0.4% 5 g for 7 days

    Miconazole nitrate (vaginal suppository 100 mg or 2% cream 5 g), intravaginally at HS for 7 days, *or*

    Clotrimazole (vaginal tablets 100 mg or 1% cream 5 g) intravaginally at HS for 7 d or

    Clotrimazole 100 mg po bid 7 days or

    Tioconazole 6.5% ointment 5g intravaginally in a single application

    Nystatin and single-dose therapies not recommended; not necessary to treat male sexual partners unless *Candida balanitis* is present; treatment of candidiasis during third trimester of pregnancy is necessary to prevent oral thrush in newborn

Anti-infective agents for bacterial vaginosis

    Metronidazole (Flagyl), 500 mg po bid for 7 d (contraindicated during pregnancy), *or*

    Clindamycin, 300 mg PO, bid for 7 d (not necessary to treat male sex partners or asymptomatic women)

NURSING CARE

Nursing Assessment

For vulvovaginitis

History

Pregnancy or oral contraceptive use

Vulva and Vagina

Trichomoniasis: inflammation of vaginal walls and endocervix; punctate hemorrhagic lesions; painful coitus; copious loose "frothy" discharge with an odor; one third of patients have yellow-green discharge with bubbles

Candidiasis: severe perivaginal pruritus; pale or erythematous labia; labial excoriations; erythema extending into vagina and toward anus; tiny papulopustules beyond main area of erythema; discharge thick and adherent (containing curds) or thin and loose; no odor

Bacterial vaginosis: milder symptoms; less erythema; mild or moderate discharge; thin white or grayish white discharge; uniformly adheres to vaginal wall; 25% have gas bubbles in discharge; fishy or aminelike odor to discharge

Lymph Nodes

Trichomoniasis: may be inguinal lymphadenopathy

Urinary Concerns

Trichomoniasis: dysuria or frequency
Candidiasis: dysuria

Nursing Dx & Intervention

For gonorrhea and nongonococcal urethritis; syphilis; herpesvirus infections; lymphogranuloma venereum; chancroid and granuloma inguinale; molluscum contagiosum and condylomata acuminata; and vulvovaginitis.

Risk for infection (patient contacts) related to presence of pathogens in lesions or secretions or exudates from cervix, urethra, eyes, pharynx, or anus

- Collect specimen for laboratory examination; collect blood for serology for syphilis, herpes, or *Chlamydia for definite diagnosis and treatment.*
- Use universal precautions when handling specimens and examining patient; *lesions and mucous membrane exudates are infectious.*
- Examine and treat patient contacts *to prevent reinfection of patient.*
- Serologically screen all pregnant women for syphilis at least once during pregnancy. Rescreen high-risk women during third trimester and again at delivery (testing the mother's blood). Administer anti-infectives as prescribed. *Syphilis is transmitted to the fetus. Adequate treatment of the mother before the fifteenth week will prevent damage to fetus. High-risk women are at risk for reinfection during the pregnancy. Infants born of infected mothers are at risk for active infection and severe anomalies.*
- Reexamine and treat pregnant women with history of STDs before delivery.

- Examine newborn for symptoms and administer prophylactics for eyes. *A neonate may become infected on any mucous membrane during a vaginal delivery if mother has a cervical infection.*
- Ensure that pregnant women with *Candida* organism are treated during last trimester *to prevent transmission to neonate during vaginal delivery.*
- Report to local health authority if not previously reported by physician or laboratory; *it is required by law.*

Risk for infection (patient complications) related to extension or dissemination of disease if untreated or inadequately treated

- Administer anti-infectives or teach patient to take as prescribed. *Early treatment can prevent complications and transmission of STDs.*
- Counsel patient to return for follow-up *to ensure cure.*
- Monitor immunocompromised persons for signs of disseminated infection with herpes and *Candida. Immunocompromised persons are at greater risk for serious systemic disease.*
- Monitor body temperature and symptoms of PID and dissemination of gonorrhea and *Chlamydia. Early detection of infection and treatment with anti-infective agents may prevent dissemination of the pathogen, severe disease, and fertility problems.*
- Monitor for symptoms of complications of tertiary syphilis if patient has been infected over 1 year *to initiate supportive care, as needed.*

Patient Education/Home Care Planning*

General instructions

1. Sexual activity should be avoided until treatment is completed and follow-up examinations of secretion or exudates is negative for pathogens and when herpes lesions are present.
2. Sexual contacts must be examined and treated, even if asymptomatic.
3. Anti-infective agents must be taken for full prescribed course to avoid treatment failure, chronic infection, and complications.
4. If tetracycline is administered, it must be taken for the full prescribed course. It should be taken 1 hour before or 2 hours after meals. The patient should avoid dairy products, antacids, iron, other mineral-containing preparations, as well as sunlight.
5. Condoms may provide protection from future infections.
6. Counsel patients and their partners to be tested for HIV.

Specific instructions

7. For gonorrhea or *Chlamydia:* patients should return for reexamination 4 to 7 days after completion of treatment. Care should be taken with vaginal or urethral discharges to avoid contamination of eyes.

8. For syphilis: all sexual partners should be referred for examination and treatment (sexual contacts up to 3 months preceding primary infection, up to 6 months preceding secondary stage, and up to 1 year preceding latent stage). Treated patients should return for follow-up serologic tests 3 and 6 months after therapy (1, 2, 3, 6, 9, and 12 months, if HIV positive). A systemic reaction (e.g., fever, chills, headache, or tachycardia) 1 to 2 hours after onset of antibiotic treatment is attributable to endotoxin release from dying spirochetes. The condition is benign and self-limited. Bed rest and aspirin help.
9. For herpes: pregnant women should inform physician of history of genital herpes. Annual Papanicolaou smears are recommended. Recurrent episodes of lesions are less painful and less extensive than initial episode. The virus probably cannot be transmitted when there are no lesions present, but this is still being investigated. Proper handwashing following toileting is important to prevent autoinoculation.
10. For lymphogranuloma venereum: the sequelae of untreated lymphogranuloma venereum are serious. Patient must complete the prescribed antibiotic regimen and return for evaluation 3 to 5 days after treatment is begun and weekly or biweekly until the infection is entirely healed.
11. For chancroid: sex partners should be examined and treated as soon as possible. Sexual contacts 2 weeks before or after onset of chancroid lesions must be treated. Females may be asymptomatic; however, they should be treated. In chancroid the prepuce should remain retracted during therapy and the lesions should be cleaned three times daily. Retraction is contraindicated if there is preputial edema.
12. For granuloma inguinale: the patient should return for evaluation within 3 to 5 days of beginning therapy and weekly or biweekly thereafter until all lesions are healed. Total healing of granuloma inguinale takes 3 to 5 weeks. If treatment is stopped prematurely, lesions may become reactivated.
13. For molluscum and condylomata (warts): follow-up examination should take place 1 month after treatment for molluscum so new lesions can be removed. Follow-up examinations should be done weekly until all warts have been resolved. All women with anogenital warts should have a Papanicolaou smear. Patients should be informed of the recurrent nature of these conditions.
14. For vulvovaginitis: Recurrent infections are common. Patient should return for treatment if symptoms recur. Alcohol should be avoided until after 3 days following metronidazole therapy. See instruction number 4 regarding tetracycline. Vaginal suppositories for candidiasis should be stored in a refrigerator. Treatment should continue during menstruation. Sanitary pads can be worn to protect clothing. Teach the patient to wipe from

front to back when toileting. Instruct the patient not to douche routinely to avoid removal of normal vaginal flora. Instruct the patient to avoid using sprays, soaps, powders, and deodorants; to wear cotton undergarments to permit free airflow to the perineum and to avoid trapping moisture; to wash undergarments in mild detergent and to rinse them twice; to avoid sharing towels and washcloths with others; and to use water-soluble lubricants, if necessary, before intercourse.

From Grimes.[26]

Evaluation

Infection is not transmitted to others or back to patient after treatment Patient contacts are examined and treated. Newborn is free of signs of infection (no lesions, nonreactive serology and absence of other symptoms). Health care workers have used adequate precautions.

Infection is resolved before extension or dissemination Absence of signs of secondary or tertiary syphilis; CSF is normal. Follow-up serologic tests for syphilis indicate decreasing antibody titers. For gonorrhea or *Chlamydia:* body temperature, urination, and bowel movements are normal. Patient reports absence of nausea and vomiting, dysuria, pain, dysmenorrhea, abnormal menstrual bleeding, and other signs of complications. There is no exudate. Cultures are negative for gonococcus or *Chlamydia.* Patient has been tested for other STDs. For LV: lymph nodes are not swollen, hot, or tender. Mucopurulent exudate no longer drains from lesions or sinuses. Body temperature is normal. Rectum and anal opening are patent. There is no abdominal distention or cramping. Defecation is normal. For chancroid: lesions are healed without scarring. Patient verbalizes intent to return for follow-up. For herpes: no signs of CNS disease or infection of visual organs.

Patient has knowledge to self-administer anti-infectives as prescribed Patient describes medication regimen and intent to take anti-infectives for length of time prescribed.

Patient has information to prevent further episodes of an STD and to prevent transmission of this STD Patient verbalizes intent to avoid sexual contact until lesions are healed, describes correct use of condom, and verbalizes intent to return for follow-up.

NOSOCOMIAL INFECTIONS

Nosocomial describes infections that are hospital acquired in contrast to community acquired. An infection classified as nosocomial is not present nor is the microorganism incubating (unless the organism was acquired during a previous hospitalization) at the time of admission to an inpatient health care facility. Symptoms of the nosocomial infection need not be present during the hospitalization; however, the symptoms may become evident after discharge.

Any infectious disease that is transmitted directly or indirectly from person to person has the potential for becoming a nosocomial infection. Infections that develop in a hospital from microorganisms present in normal flora or from normally nonpathogenic microorganisms in the hospital environment and that invade and colonize in a susceptible patient are also considered nosocomial. Infections in newborns that are acquired during birth from an infected mother are also classified as nosocomial.

A community-acquired infection is one that is present or incubating at the time of hospital admission. The known incubation period of a disease is used to determine whether an infection that becomes symptomatic during or after hospitalization is hospital or community acquired. A disease occurring in the hospital with an unknown incubation period is generally classified as nosocomial.

Reported occurrences of nosocomial infections in the United States range from 5% to 10% of hospital discharges, depending on the type of hospital, type of patients, and completeness of the reporting system.[27] On the average, 5.7% of people who are admitted to a general hospital acquire a nosocomial infection.[29] The extent of nosocomial infections in hospital personnel is thought to be high, especially for TB and hepatitis.

Nosocomial infection studies report on body sites and the hospital services where infections occur most frequently. The National Nosocomial Infections Surveillance System reported that between 1990 and 1992, 33% of all nosocomial infections involved the urinary tract, 15% involved surgical wounds. 16% involved the lower respiratory tract, 13% were primary bacteremias, and 24% were other types. Most infections (64%) were caused by a single pathogen, with *E. coli, Pseudomonas aeruginosa,* enterococci, coagulase-negative staphylococci and *Staphylococcus aureus* most often implicated.[27]

Etiology

Certain interacting agent, host, and environmental characteristics of hospitals contribute to the risk for nosocomial infections. A large number of individuals (patients, families, and personnel) are brought together in one small environment. Some of these individuals have community-acquired, overt or subclinical infections. Taking care of patients requires close contact with body fluids and excretions, which increases the risk of transmission of pathogens from person to person and to the hospital environment. Thus a greater variety of microorganisms of greater virulence are likely to be present in hospitals. The increase in antibiotic-resistant strains of bacteria in hospitals is an example of this phenomenon. Hospitals also contain a wide range of potential reservoirs for microorganism growth such as infusion liquids, foods, biologic materials, and equipment.

Patients already weakened by existing disease or treatment are susceptible to invasion and infection by normal flora microorganisms, opportunistic organisms in the environment, and pathogens. Exposure to invasive diagnostic and treatment technologies further increases opportunities for microorganism invasion. Treatments that result in immunosuppression compromise patient resistance and further increase the risk for infection.

Nosocomial infections are transmitted according to the same chain of transmission as described on p. 1074.

Control

Control of nosocomial infections, as with community-acquired infections, relies on efforts to break the chain of transmission at one or more of its links. The point of the chain most amenable to control varies with the microorganism and disease process. (See the box below for general hospital procedures for control.)

Hospital infection control also requires systematic monitoring and complete reporting to the hospital infection control committee of *all* infections occurring in the hospital. In addition, select infections must be reported to the local health authority. These infections are identified in the tables in each disease section in this book.

The Joint Commission for the Accreditation of Healthcare Organizations requires that hospitals have an effective infection control program to qualify for accreditation. The program must contain the following components:

Infection control committee
Systematic surveillance of nosocomial infections

CONTROL OF NOSOCOMIAL INFECTIONS

AGENT

Sterilization and disinfection of inanimate reservoirs and vehicles of transmission

RESERVOIR

Antibiotic treatment of patients and employees
Limitation of visitors that may be infected
Policies that encourage ill employees to stay home

PORTAL OF EXIT AND MODE OF TRANSMISSION

Isolation procedures and secretion and excretion precautions
Handwashing between patients by personnel
Proper handling of specimens
Environmental air control, sanitation, proper waste disposal, and proper laundry practices

PORTAL OF ENTRY

Protective isolation of high-risk patients
Sterile techniques
Recommended procedures that minimize organism invasion (see recommendation for each body system discussed in this chapter)

SUSCEPTIBLE HOST

Nursing procedures that minimize stasis of body fluids (i.e., coughing, turning, ambulating), that prevent compromise in body defenses (i.e., skin and mucous membrane care, hydration, nutrition), and that improve immunologic status (i.e., active and passive immunization of patients and employees)

Employee health program
Isolation policies
In-service education on infection control for employees
Regular procedures for environmental sanitation
Microbiology laboratory
Implementation of accepted infection control procedures in patient care

URINARY TRACT INFECTIONS[1,4]

The urinary system, except for the distal urethra, is normally sterile. Endogenous or exogenous microorganisms enter the system from devices that enter it or have contact with it. Approximately 75% of nosocomial urinary tract infections have been preceded by urologic implementation, including catheterization. The organisms most frequently associated with urinary tract infections are gram-negative organisms usually found in the colon, including *E. coli, Klebsiella, Proteus, Enterobacter,* group D *Streptococcus, Pseudomonas,* and *Candida.* They are frequently introduced from the hands of health personnel at the time of catheterization. Bacteriuria increases the risk for septicemia and nephritis and should be treated.

Criteria for Classification

Urinary tract infections meeting the following Centers for Disease Control (CDC) criteria are classified as nosocomial:

Asymptomatic bacteriuria with colony counts greater than 100,000 organisms/ml urine where patient has had a previous negative culture at a time when the patient was not receiving antibiotics; or colony counts of a new organism greater than 100,000/ml even if patient had previous positive cultures of a different organism

Symptomatic urinary tract infection (fever, dysuria, costovertebral angle tenderness, suprapubic tenderness) with onset after admission and a prior negative urinalysis or a present urinalysis with one or both of the following: Colony counts greater than 10,000 microorganisms/ml of midstream urine specimen

Pyuria greater than 10 WBCs per high-power field in an uncentrifuged specimen

Urinary System Alterations That Increase Risk for Infection

Obstructions: urethral strictures, calculi, tumors, blood clots
Trauma: injury to abdomen, ruptured bladder
Congenital anomalies: polycystic kidneys, exstrophy of bladder, horseshoe kidney
Disorders of other symptoms: abdominal or gynecologic surgery, rectovesicular fistula, meningomyelocele, spina bifida
Acute or chronic renal failure
Postpartum state
Aging changes, particularly in the female

Procedures That Increase Risk

Urethral catheterization

Indwelling (continuous): risk increases greatly after 7 days; a closed system is superior to an open system in delaying colonization of urine. Disconnecting a closed system increases the risk

Straight catheterization: less risk than with indwelling catheter; intermittent urethral catheterization, using clean technique and performed by the patient, has less risk than indwelling catheterization

External (condom) catheter can cause urinary tract infections; however, the risk is less than with urethral catheterization

Suprapubic catheterization: risk for infection may be lower than for uretheral catheterization

Ureteral catheterization: microorganisms from urethral colonization or contaminated instruments increase the risk for urinary tract infection

Irrigations: irrigation equipment and solutions have great potential for contamination; frequent disconnection of system further increases risk for infection

Urethral dilation: the procedure may introduce bacteria and produce tissue trauma

Cystometrography: same risks as those with urethral catheterization

Cystoscopy: septicemia may result if urine is not sterile before the procedure

Transurethral resection of the prostate: bacteremia may result if urine is not sterile before the procedure

Operative procedures on the bladder and kidneys: microorganisms introduced at the time of the procedure or from a subsequent wound infection increase the risk for a urinary tract infection

Urinary diversion procedures: chronic infections are common as a result of colonization of bacteria at the stomal site

Recommendations for Prevention

1. Avoid unnecessary catheterization.
2. Use aseptic techniques for insertion of devices and for opening the drainage system.
3. Use closed indwelling catheter system in preference to an open system.
4. Decrease the duration of indwelling catheters.
5. Use external catheter for males who can empty bladder but cannot control micturition.
6. Use clean-catch midstream method of collecting urine specimens in preference to catheterization.
7. Use straight rather than indwelling catheter whenever possible.
8. Use smallest catheter possible to minimize trauma.
9. Avoid leg bags in acute care setting.
10. Obtain specimens by aspirating urine from catheter or sampling port rather than by disconnecting catheter from drainage tubing.
11. Use silicone catheters rather than latex for long-term catheterization.
12. Anchor the catheter to stabilize and reduce irritation of the urethra.
13. Maintain a continual downward flow of urine.
14. Routinely empty drainage bags, but do not change the drainage bag unless entire closed system is changed. (The addition of disinfecting agents in the bag is still controversial.)
15. Use a separate, clean measuring container for each patient.
16. Gently and regularly clean perineum. Meatal care with antimicrobial agents has not been found to be helpful and in some cases has produced infection.
17. Avoid irrigations unless obstruction is anticipated. Use continuous irrigation in a closed system in preference to intermittent irrigation in an open system.
18. Persons with chronic catheterization should receive antibiotic treatment only for clinically apparent pyelonephritis, epididymitis, or bacteremia.

SURGICAL WOUND INFECTIONS[1,25,30]

The intact integumentary system provides the first line of defense against the invasion of microorganisms; and any disruption in the integrity of the system increases the risk for infection. The risk is increased with the extensiveness and severity of the disruption of the skin integrity and the length of time until the disruption is repaired. Repair and healing are further influenced by host factors such as age, nutrition, and circulation status. Postoperative wound infections vary substantially by hospital, suggesting that hospital practices and surgical skill may also greatly affect the occurrence. The incubation period for surgical wound infections is 3 to 8 days after the operation, suggesting that many infections are acquired in the operating suite.

Criteria for classification   A surgical wound is classified as the site of a nosocomial infection if it drains purulent material with or without a positive culture for bacteria.

Surgical Variables That Increase Risk for Infection

Class of operation (The risk for infection increases from class I to class IV procedures)

Class I (clean wound): no break in sterile technique; no inflammation is encountered; the GI, respiratory, urinary, and genital tracts are not entered

Class II (clean-contaminated wound): GI, GU, or respiratory tract is entered with no spillage of contents; minor breaks in technique; operations involving the biliary tract, appendix, vagina, and oropharynx are included in this category

Class III (contaminated wound): acute inflammation without pus encountered; spillage from a hollow viscus occurs: trauma from a clean source

Class IV (dirty): pus or a perforated viscus is encountered; trauma from a dirty source; organisms causing infection were present before surgery

Duration of preoperative stay: prolonged presurgery hospitalization increases the risk for microbial colonization in or on the patient before the surgery

Location of the surgery: infection increases if surgery is in body areas with impaired circulation or in areas with microorganisms already present

Surgical technique: delayed wound closure, excess tissue trauma, improper suture tension, excess blood loss, and presence of a drain increase the risk

Presence of bacteria at closure: the single most common agent causing postoperative wound infection is *S. aureus,* which is part of the normal flora for some people and has been found in the respiratory passages of 21% of operating suite personnel; other gram-negative bacteria, accounting for 60% of infections, are transient on the hands of hospital employees and may be transmitted after surgery as well as in the operating suite

Alterations in the Host That Increase Risk for Infection

Impaired immune response

Age (newborns and elderly individuals)

Diabetes mellitus with accompanying degenerative blood vessel changes

Corticosteroids, which reduce inflammatory response

Chemotherapy, which decreases immune response

Neurologic deficits causing loss of sensation and potential tissue pressure and anoxia

Infection elsewhere in the host

Malnutrition resulting in inadequate nitrogen for tissue repair

Obesity

Presence of *S. aureus* on patient, particularly in the anterior nares

Recommendations for Prevention

1. Surveillance and classification: all surgical procedures should be classified and recorded; surveillance should be maintained on all postsurgical infections by classification. Surgeons should be apprised of their infection rates.

2. Preoperative preparation: the preoperative hospital stay should be as short as possible. Preexisting bacterial infections, excluding those for which the operation is performed, should be treated and controlled. Malnourished patients should receive oral or parenteral hyperalimentation before elective surgery. The patient should be bathed the night before elective surgery with an antiseptic soap. Hair should not be removed unless it will interfere with the procedure. If hair removal is necessary, it should be done immediately before surgery. Hair should be clipped or removed with depilatories rather than shaved. Skin preparation includes scrubbing with a detergent solution followed by application of an antiseptic solution.* The patient should be completely covered with sterile drapes.

3. Postoperative wound care: use aseptic technique in dressing changes. A drain for an infected wound should be placed in an adjacent stab wound and attached to a closed suction system. Dressings should be changed if wet or if patient has signs of infection. Exudate should be cultured. Personnel must wash hands before and after caring for a surgical wound.

4. Prophylactic antibiotics: parenteral antibiotic prophylaxis should be started immediately before operations that are associated with a high risk of infection. They should be discontinued promptly after the surgery.

Some Common Practices That Are Not Useful for Preventing Surgical Wound Infections

Routine microbiologic sampling of OR air and surfaces

Use of tacky or antiseptic mats at door entrances

 # BACTEREMIA AND SEPTICEMIA

Vascular System Alterations That Increase Risk for Infection

Thrombophlebitis caused by mechanical or chemical irritation from IV cannula or infusate

Decreased blood volume

Circulatory stasis caused by immobility or pressure

Immunosuppression of host

Vascular changes associated with diabetes, collagen diseases, and other chronic diseases

Procedures That Increase Risk for Cannula-Related Infection

Type of cannula used for IV therapy (plastic cannulas generally associated with higher rate of infection than steel "scalp vein" cannulas)

Method of insertion: cutdown has greater infection risk than percutaneous insertion

Duration over 48 to 72 hours

Purpose of the cannula: CVP lines are associated with high risk for infection

Microbial contamination of infusion fluid: rare and usually caused by gram-negative bacteria

Recommendations for Prevention of Secondary Bacteremia

1. Prevention of original underlying infection
2. Early recognition and treatment of underlying surgical wound, urinary tract, and pulmonary infections

Recommendations for Prevention of Primary Bacteremias Induced by Intravenous Catheters

1. Wash hands before insertion.
2. Use sterile gloves and antiseptic hand wash for cutdowns and central lines.
3. Use upper extremity veins; lower extremity veins develop phlebitis more readily.

---

*Tincture of chlorhexidine, iodophors, and tincture of iodine are among the preferred antiseptic solutions.

4. Use an antiseptic preparation before venipuncture (in declining order of preference: tincture of iodine, chlorhexidine, iodophors, 70% alcohol); avoid quaternary ammonium compounds and hexachlorophene.
5. Use plastic catheters for cannulation of central veins and steel needles for IV infusions.
6. Secure catheter and apply sterile dressing.
7. Inspect daily.
8. Insert new cannula every 48 to 72 hours.
9. Change dressing and apply antibiotic ointment every 48 hours.
10. Change IV tubing every 48 hours and after blood products or lipid emulsions.
11. Avoid irrigations or blood drawing.

LOWER RESPIRATORY TRACT INFECTIONS[1,4]

As many as 1% to 2% of hospitalized patients develop nosocomial bacterial pneumonias, with 30% of those infected persons dying even with adequate antimicrobial therapy. Certain factors contribute to the risk for pneumonia in hospitalized patients:

The integrity of normal respiratory defense mechanisms may be disrupted, thus permitting the invasion of oropharyngeal normal flora microorganisms into the lung alveoli.

Medical diagnostic and treatment procedures may introduce microorganisms from the oropharynx or from the equipment or solutions into the lower respiratory tract.

Ill persons with altered respiratory clearance mechanisms are susceptible to rapid oropharyngeal colonization of pathogens from the hospital environment, equipment, or the patient's normal flora; the pathogens that frequently colonize in hospitalized patients and are most often associated with nosocomial pneumonia are *Klebsiella, S. aureus, Pseudomonas, E. coli, Enterobacter, S. pneumoniae,* and *H. influenzae;* opportunistic organisms such as *Candida, Aspergillus,* cytomegalovirus, and *Pneumocystis carinii* cause pneumonia in immunocompromised hosts.

Microbial invasion of lung alveoli can occur from one of three routes:

Aspiration from the oropharynx

Inhalation of aerosolized droplets or gas containing suspended organisms

Lymphohematogenous spread

Aspiration is probably the most frequent route in nosocomial pneumonia.

Criteria for Classification

The criteria used by the Hospital Infections Branch of the Centers for Disease Control for classifying nosocomial pneumonia are as follows:

Purulent sputum developing 48 hours or more after admission, or increased production of purulent sputum with recrudescence of fever in a patient hospitalized with pulmonary disease; plus one of the following:

Cough, fever, and pleuritic chest pain, or

Infiltration seen on chest roentgenography or physical findings of infection

An infection present on admission can be classified as nosocomial if it is related to a previous hospitalization.

Host Factors That Increase the Risk for Nosocomial Pneumonia

Airway obstruction caused by tumors, foreign bodies, edema, fluid, or chronic obstructive pulmonary disease

Impairment of mucociliary defenses as a result of dehydration, inhalation of chemical irritants, viral infection, or anticholinergic drugs

Impaired immunologic function

Traumatic injury to respiratory tract or surgery to abdominal or thoracic cavity

Altered swallowing, clearing, or coughing caused by central nervous system disorders; alcoholism; depressed levels of consciousness; dysphagia; nasogastric tubes; anesthesia, sedation, or medications that alter the cough reflex; immobilization

Oropharyngeal colonization of bacteria; (colonization increases with length of hospital stay, prolonged intubation, and preceding antibiotic therapy)

Smoking

Procedures That Increase Risk for Infection

Large-volume nebulizers: the major source of aerosolized bacteria; humidifiers do not have the same risk

Any device or airway that may carry bacteria from the oropharynx to the lower respiratory tract including nasogastric tubes and endotracheal tubes

Ventilation equipment including intermittent positive pressure machines

Administration of oxygen or anesthesia

Pulmonary function testing

Bronchoscopy

Surgical procedures, including lung biopsy and tracheostomy

Recommendations for Prevention of Nosocomial Pneumonia Associated with Respiratory Care Equipment

1. Use sterile, adequately disinfected, or disposable breathing circuits (mouthpieces, tubing, cannulae) that come in contact with the patient.
2. Replace circuitry for patients on continuous assisted or controlled ventilation and on intermittent therapy every 24 to 48 hours. Remove fluid buildup in the tubing.
3. Use high-efficiency bacterial filters on ventilators and intermittent positive pressure machines between the machine and the patient. Use in-line filters to prevent contamination of internal parts of anesthesia machines and ventilators from patient's exhaled air.
4. Change, sterilize, or disinfect aerosol-producing equipment between patients and every 24 hours for the same patient. Do not use spinning disc nebulizers.

5. Use sterile solutions in fluid reservoirs, dispensed under aseptic conditions. Fill water reservoirs at the time needed; do not fill in advance. Unused portions should be discarded every 24 hours at the time the reservoir is sterilized or replaced.

6. Do not add to fluid levels in nebulizers or humidifiers. If additional fluid is needed, empty reservoir and fill with sterile water.

7. Use sterile medications in single-use vials for nebulization.

8. For suctioning, use sterile catheter and sterile glove. Change suction catheter after each use. Use intermittent rather than continuous suctioning.

Recommendations for Prevention of Nosocomial Pneumonia Associated with Patient Risk Factors

High-risk surgical patients and patients with impaired chest function should receive:

Preoperative and postoperative therapy to treat any underlying infection

Preoperative instruction to discontinue smoking

Preoperative and postoperative instruction and therapy to encourage and stimulate postoperative deep breathing, coughing, movement in bed, and early ambulation

Postoperative interventions to remove secretions and stimulate coughing (i.e., percussion, postural drainage)

Postoperative pain control

MEDICAL INTERVENTIONS AND RELATED NURSING CARE

IMMUNIZATIONS

Immunization is the action of artificially stimulating an immune response in a host. Two methods are available. The first method is active immunization, in which an antigen in the form of a vaccine is injected. The second method is passive immunization, in which antibodies, produced in another host, are injected in the form of immune globulins, antitoxins, or antisera. Clinical considerations for active and passive immunization, general recommendations for administration of vaccines, and a schedule for administration of vaccines for the diseases discussed in the section on vaccine-preventable infectious diseases will be presented here.

Clinical Considerations for Active and Passive Immunization

Active immunization   Vaccines used for active immunization are prepared from bacteria or viruses, or their derivatives, that have been modified to stimulate antibody production without causing disease. Modification is accomplished by inactivation or killing of the organism or by alteration of the organism so it retains its antigenicity while losing its virulence (attenuated).

Inactivated vaccines must be given in multiple first doses to stimulate an adequate antibody response, and a periodic booster must be given to maintain serum antibody levels. Attenuated vaccines stimulate lifetime antibody levels with one administration.

Routine immunizations are given according to a schedule that facilitates administration at a time earliest in life when the vaccine will be effective. The health care provider administering the immunization should fully inform the patient or parent of the reason for the immunization, the schedule, side effects that may occur, and actions to take in the event of side effects. Informed consent must be obtained (Tables 13-28 to 13-30).

Passive immunization   Active immunization is preferred to passive in most situations. Passive immunization with serum antitoxins prepared in animals or with human immune globulins is recommended only for those situations where active immunization procedures have not been developed; exposure has already occurred, leaving insufficient time for active immunization; or concurrent active and passive immunization is required for immediate and future protection.

The use of human immune globulins for passive immunization is preferred to use of serum antitoxins from animals. The risk for anaphylaxis-like reactions and serum sickness is greater when prepared animal sera are used. Anaphylaxis-like reactions affect principally the cardiovascular and respiratory systems, producing dyspnea, asthma, respiratory decompensation, and possible death. These reactions occur in minutes to a few hours after administration of the serum, and they range from mild to severe. The much more common serum sickness reactions develop in 7 to 12 days after injection of the serum, producing mild to severe symptoms of fever, urticaria, or arthralgia. The severity of the symptoms depends on the type of serum and the route of administration (IV administration leads to more severe reactions). Individuals previously sensitized to the serum may react within 1 to 3 days of receiving the serum.

Multiple-dose vaccines   Some vaccines must be administered in more than one dose for full protection. If the intervals between doses are longer than recommended, there is usually not a reduction in final antibody levels. It is therefore unnecessary to restart an interrupted series or to add extra doses.

Simultaneous administration of certain vaccines   Most of the widely used vaccines can be safely and effectively administered simultaneously. Inactivated vaccines can be administered simultaneously at different sites unless the person is known to have experienced past side effects to one or more of the vaccines. In that case the vaccines should be administered on separate occasions. An inactivated vaccine and a live attenuated virus vaccine can be administered simultaneously at different sites.

Hypersensitivity to vaccine components   Vaccine antigens produced in systems or with substrates that contain allergenic substances may cause hypersensitivity reactions and possible anaphylaxis. Antigens grown in eggs of chickens or ducks should not be given to anyone with a history (or questionable history) of allergy to eggs. Influenza vaccine antigens, although produced from viruses grown in eggs, are highly purified and are associated with only rare hypersensitivity reactions. Influenza vaccine should not be administered to anyone with a history of anaphylactic reaction to eggs.

TABLE 13-28 Clinical Considerations for Commonly Administered Immunizations

Disease	Vaccine/Route	Recommendation	Contraindications*	Adverse Reactions	Less Severe Reactions	Passive Immunization
Tetanus	Toxoid (detoxified toxin)/IM; administered with diphtheria and pertussis as DPT; given to those over 7 years as DT	Ideally begin first of 4 infant doses at 2-3 months of age; tetanus toxoid given every 10 years to adults; can be given to persons infected with HIV	Encephalopathy within 7 days of previous dose; anaphylactic reaction to vaccine	Rare neurologic reactions, including neuritis and transverse myelitis	Fever within 24-48 hours; soreness at injection site; urticaria, malaise	Immune globulin following injury for those without active immunization
Diphtheria	Toxoid/IM; same as tetanus	Same as tetanus	Same as tetanus	Same as tetanus	Same as tetanus	Antitoxin for unimmunized contacts with an active case
Pertussis	Killed vaccine/IM; same as tetanus	Same as tetanus; not given after 7 years of age	Same as tetanus	Rare CNS disturbances-convulsions	Thrombocytopenia	No longer recommended
Measles (Rubeola)	Live attenuated virus/subcutaneous; administered with mumps and rubella as MMR	First dose given after 12 mos. of age because of maternal antibodies; second dose at age 4 to 12 years	Anaphylactic reaction to egg ingestion or to neomycin; pregnancy; severe, symptomatic immunodeficiency	Rare CNS reactions-encephalitis	Anorexia, malaise, rash, fever within 7-10 days	Immune globulin for unimmunized contacts of active cases; given within 6 days of exposure
Mumps	Same as measles	Same as measles	Same as measles	Rare encephalomyelitis	Brief, mild fever	Not recommended
Rubella	Same as measles	Same as measles	Same as measles	Transient arthralgia and arthritis within 2 weeks in older children	Mild rash lasting 1 to 2 days	Not recommended

*Moderate or severe illness with or without fever is a contraindication for all immunizations.
Data from Centers for Disease Control.[10,13,18,22]

Continued.

TABLE 13-28 Clinical Considerations for Commonly Administered Immunizations—cont'd

Disease	Vaccine/Route	Recommendation	Contraindications*	Adverse Reactions	Less Severe Reactions	Passive Immunization
Polio	Live attenuated virus: Trivalent Oral Polio Vaccine (TOPV)/oral or inactivated vaccine (IPV)/subcutaneous	Ideally, begin first of 4 infant doses at 6 weeks of age; inactivated vaccine recommended for persons who are immune compromised	OPV: HIV or household contact of person with HIV; IPV: anaphylactic reaction to neomycin or streptomycin	Rare paralysis within 2 months	None	None
Influenza	Inactivated virus/IM	Vaccine must be readministered yearly; recommended for persons infected with HIV/AIDS	Anaphylactic reaction to ingested eggs	Hypersensitivity	Soreness at administration site; fever, malaise, myalgia persisting for 1-2 days	None
Haemophilus influenzae type b (Hib)	Bacterial polysaccharide conjugated to protein/IM	Ideally, begin primary series of 4 doses at 6 weeks of age	Previous anaphylactic reaction to the vaccine	None identified	None identified	None
Hepatitis B	Inactivated viral antigen/IM	Recommended for infants before hospital discharge and adults at risk for infection, including those with HIV	Anaphylactic reactions to common baker's yeast	Anaphylactic reactions	None identified	Hepatitis B Immune Globulin (HBIG) for post-exposure prophylaxis
Varicella	Attenuated live virus/subcutaneous	Single dose can be given anytime after 18 months of age; give to children and adults who have not had a prior infection	Not available at this time	None identified	None identified	Varicella Zoster Immune Globulin (VZIG) for post-exposure prophylaxis for immunocompromised persons, susceptible pregnant women and perinatally exposed infants

TABLE 13-29 Recommended Childhood Immunization Schedule*—United States, January 1995

Vaccine	Birth	2 Months	4 Months	6 Months	12† Months	15 Months	18 Months	4-6 Years	11-12 Years	14-16 Years
Hepatitis B‡	HB-1									
		HB-2			HB-3					
Diphtheria, Tetanus, Pertussis§		DTP	DTP	DTP	DTP or DTaP at ≥ 15 months			DTP or DTaP	Td	
H. influenzae type b¶		Hib	Hib	Hib	Hib					
Poliovirus		OPV	OPV	OPV				OPV		
Measles, Mumps, Rubella**					MMR			MMR or MMR		

*Recommended vaccines are listed under the routinely recommended ages. Shaded bars indicate range of acceptable ages for vaccination.
†Vaccines recommended in the second year of life (i.e., 12-15 months of age) may be given at either one or two visits.
‡Infants born to hepatitis B surface antigen (HBsAg)-negative mothers should receive the second dose of hepatitis B vaccine between 1 and 4 months of age, provided at least 1 month has elapsed since receipt of the first dose. The third dose is recommended between 6 and 18 months of age. Infants born to HBsAg-positive mothers should receive immunoprophylaxis for hepatitis B with 0.5 ml Hepatitis B Immune Globulin (HBIG) within 12 hours of birth, and 0.5 ml of either Merck Sharpe & Dohme (West Point, Pennsylvania) vaccine (Recombivax HB®) or of SmithKline Beecham (Philadelphia) vaccine (Engerix-B®) at a separate site. In these infants, the second dose of vaccine is recommended at 1 month of age and the third dose at 6 months of age. All pregnant women should be screened for HBsAg during an early prenatal visit.
§The fourth dose of diphtheria and tetanus toxoids and pertussis vaccine (DTP) may be administered as early as 12 months of age, provided at least 6 months have elapsed since the third dose of DTP. Combined DTP-Hib products may be used when these two vaccines are administered simultaneously. Diphtheria and tetanus toxoids and acellular pertussis vaccine (DTaP) is licensed for use for the fourth and/or fifth dose of DTP in children aged ≥ 15 months and may be preferred for these doses in children in this age group.
¶Three *H. influenzae* type b conjugate vaccines are available for use in infants: 1) oligosaccharide conjugate Hib vaccine (HbOC) (HibTITER®, manufactured by Praxis Biologics, Inc. [West Henrietta, New York], and distributed by Lederle-Praxis Biologicals, [Wayne, New Jersey]); 2) polyribosylribitol phosphate-tetanus toxoid conjugate (PRP-T) (ActHIB™, manufactured by Pasteur Mérieux Sérums & Vaccins, S.A. (Lyon, France), and distributed by Connaught Laboratories, Inc. [Swiftwater, Pennsylvania], and OmniHIB™, manufactured by Pasteur Mérieux Sérums & Vaccins, S.A., and distributed by SmithKline Beecham); and 3) *Haemophilus* b conjugate vaccine (Meningococcal Protein Conjugate) (PRP-OMP) (PedvaxHIB®, manufactured by Merck Sharp & Dohme). Children who have received PRP-OMP at 2 and 4 months of age do not require a dose at 6 months of age. After the primary infant Hib conjugate vaccine series is completed, any licensed Hib conjugate vaccine may be used as a booster dose at age 12-15 months.
**The second dose of measles-mumps-rubella vaccine should be administered EITHER at 4-6 years of age OR at 11-12 years of age.
Source: Advisory Committee on Immunization Practices, American Academy of Pediatrics, and American Academy of Family Physicians. CDC.[20,22]

TABLE 13-30 Recommendations for Tetanus Prophylaxis in Wound Management

	Clean Minor Wounds		All Other Wounds	
History of Tetanus Immunization	Toxoid (Detoxified Toxin; Td)*	Tetanus Immune Globulin (TIG)	Toxoid (Detoxified Toxin; Td)*	Tetanus Immune Globulin (TIG)
Uncertain history or <three doses	Yes	No	Yes	Yes
Three or more doses†				
Last dose within past 5 yr	No	No	No	No
Last dose 5-10 yr ago	No	No	Yes	No
Last dose over 10 yr ago	Yes	No	Yes	No

Data from Centers for Disease Control.[9]
*For children under 7 yr, administer DTP (or DT if pertussis vaccine is contraindicated).
†If only three doses of fluid toxoid have been administered, a fourth dose of toxoid, preferably an absorbed toxoid, should be given.

No hypersensitivity reactions have been reported from administration of live attenuated measles, mumps, or rubella (MMR) vaccine prepared from viruses grown in cell cultures.

Some vaccines that are derived from organisms grown in bacteriologic media frequently produce local or systemic reactions that are not allergenic. These vaccines—including cholera; diphtheria, pertussis, and tetanus (DPT); plague; and typhoid—should not be given to persons who have a history of serious side effects from the vaccine.

Vaccines that contain preservatives or trace amounts of antibiotics, as indicated on the package insert, should not be given to any person with a history of hypersensitivity to those substances.

Contraindications for immunization

1. Altered immunity: severely immunosuppressed persons should not receive live attenuated virus vaccines (MMR, TOPV) because of the risk for multiplication of the virus within those persons. MMWR should be given to asymptomatic HIV infected children. Also, individuals living in the same household with a severely immunocompromised person should not be given oral polio vaccine (OPV) because vaccine viruses are excreted and may be transmitted to other persons. These persons should be given Inactivated Polio Vaccine (IPV). Killed or Inactivated vaccines, such as the influenza vaccine, are safe for HIV infected persons.[13]

2. Severe febrile illnesses: although the presence of mild illnesses does not preclude vaccination, immunization should be deferred for those with severe febrile illnesses.

3. Pregnancy: attenuated virus vaccines, particularly measles, mumps, and rubella (MMR), should not be given to pregnant women or women who may become pregnant within 3 months of the vaccination. Oral poliovaccine (OPV) and yellow fever vaccines may be given if there is a high risk for acquired infection. There is no contraindication for administration of inactivated viral vaccines, bacterial vaccines, or toxoids to pregnant women. Influenza vaccine can be given safely.

4. Recent administration of immune globulin: live attenuated virus vaccines should not be administered within 3 months of passive immunization. Similarly, immunoglobulins should not be administered for at least 2 weeks after a vaccine has been given. These precautions reduce the risk that high serum levels of immunoglobulins would prevent the development of active acquired immunity.

5. All adverse reactions to vaccines must be reported to the local or state health authority since the passage in 1988 of the Vaccine Adverse Event Reporting System.[27]

6. DPT or single-antigen pertussis vaccine is contraindicated if any of the following events occurred after the patient received a vaccine containing pertussis antigen:

    Allergic hypersensitivity

    Fever of 40.5° C (105° F) or higher within 48 hours

    Collapse or shocklike state within 48 hours

    Persistent, inconsolable crying lasting 3 hours or more or an unusual, high-pitched cry occurring within 48 hours

    Convulsion(s) with or without fever occurring within 3 days of receipt of pertussis vaccine

    Encephalopathy (with generalized or focal neurologic signs or alterations in consciousness) occurring within 7 days

    Children with a history of seizure or other neurologic disorders should be evaluated before vaccine administration

7. Health care workers are at risk for many vaccine preventable diseases and should be protected. See box.

ISOLATION PROCEDURES

Isolation procedures are designed to prevent the spread of microorganisms among hospitalized patients, personnel, and visitors. Most of the infectious diseases discussed in this chapter have the potential for being transmitted to others. For infections that can be transmitted, the recommended hospital isolation category precautions are specified in this chapter under "Nursing Diagnoses and Interventions." These recommendations were published in 1983 by the Centers for Disease Control (CDC).[6]

The 1983 CDC guidelines provide for two isolation systems: one based on revised categories of isolation and a new system based on disease-specific isolation precautions. The disease-specific isolation system differs from the category system by specifying only the necessary precautions to interrupt the transmission of each disease (see box). Only a single instruction card is used, on which specific precautions may be checked or written.

The category system specifies seven categories of isolation based on the major modes of transmission of infectious diseases. Each disease has been assigned to one of the categories. Precautionary procedures have been specified for each category. Color-coded, category-specific instruction cards are available for use with this system.

Hospitals may choose one of these systems, modify one, or develop their own system. The CDC recommendations are not meant to restrict hospitals or medical and nursing personnel from requiring more stringent precautions. Nurses are advised to follow isolation procedures that are operative within their institution of employment and to use the material presented here for reference and clarification. The isolation precautions presented here may also require modification for patients who need constant care or require emergency intervention.

Hospital policy usually designates the personnel responsible for placing a patient on isolation precautions and the personnel who have ultimate authority to make decisions regarding isolation precautions when conflicts arise. All personnel are responsible for complying with isolation precautions to protect themselves, co-workers, patients, and visitors.

Research on AIDS transmission has led the CDC to publish recommendations for prevention of human immunodeficiency virus (HIV) transmission in health care settings. The CDC now recommends that all health personnel consistently use "universal blood and body-fluid precautions" with *all* patients, because the infection status of the patient is rarely known. Portions of these recommendations are reproduced in the box on p. 1169.

 IMMUNIZATION RECOMMENDATIONS FOR HEALTH CARE WORKERS

Hepatitis B	Rubella	Diphtheria
Measles	Poliomyelitis	Influenza*
Mumps	Tetanus	Pneumococcal disease*

From Grimes.[26]
*For those with chronic diseases or other personal risks.

CATEGORY-SPECIFIC ISOLATION SYSTEM

STRICT ISOLATION

Strict isolation is an isolation category designed to prevent transmission of highly contagious or virulent infections that may be spread by both air and contact.

Specifications for Strict Isolation

1. Private room is indicated; door should be kept closed. In general, patients infected with the same organism may share a room.
2. Masks are indicated for all persons entering the room.
3. Gowns are indicated for all persons entering the room.
4. Gloves are indicated for all persons entering the room.
5. Hands must be washed after touching the patient or potentially contaminated articles and before taking care of another patient.
6. Articles contaminated with infective material should be discarded or bagged and labeled before being sent for decontamination and reprocessing.

Diseases Requiring Strict Isolation

Diphtheria, pharyngeal
Lassa fever and other viral hemorrhagic fevers, such as Marburg virus disease*
Plague, pneumonic
Smallpox*
Varicella (chickenpox)
Zoster, localized in immunocompromised patient or disseminated

CONTACT ISOLATION

Contact isolation is designed to prevent transmission of highly transmissible or epidemiologically important infections (or colonization) that do not warrant strict isolation.

All diseases or conditions included in this category are spread primarily by close or direct contact. Thus, masks, gowns, and gloves are recommended for anyone in close or direct contact with any patient who has an infection (or colonization) that is included in this category. For individual diseases or conditions, however, 1 or more of these 3 barriers may not be indicated. For example, masks and gowns are not generally indicated for care of infants and young children with acute viral respiratory infections; gowns are not generally indicated for gonococcal conjunctivitis in newborns; and masks are not generally indicated for patients infected with multiply-resistant microorganisms, except those with pneumonia. Therefore, some degree of "over-isolation" may occur in this category.

Specifications for Contact Isolation

1. Private room is indicated. In general, patients infected with the same organism may share a room. During outbreaks, infants and young children with the same respiratory clinical syndrome may share a room.
2. Masks are indicated for those who come close to patient.
3. Gowns are indicated if soiling is likely.
4. Gloves are indicated for touching infective material.
5. Hands must be washed after touching the patient or potentially contaminated articles and before taking care of another patient.
6. Articles contaminated with infective material should be discarded or bagged and labeled before being sent for decontamination and reprocessing.

Diseases or Conditions Requiring Contact Isolation

Acute respiratory infections in infants and young children including croup, colds, bronchitis, and bronchiolitis caused by respiratory syncytial virus, adenovirus, coronavirus, influenza viruses, parainfluenza viruses, and rhinovirus
Conjunctivitis, gonococcal in newborns
Diphtheria, cutaneous
Endometritis, group A *Streptococcus*
Furunculosis, staphylococcal in newborns
Herpes simplex, disseminated, severe primary or neonatal
Impetigo
Influenza, in infants and young children
Multiply-resistant bacteria, infection, or colonization (any site) with any of the following:
1. Gram-negative bacilli resistant to all aminoglycosides that are tested. (In general, such organisms should be resistant to gentamicin, tobramycin, and amikacin for these special precautions to be indicated.)
2. *Staphylococcus aureus* resistant to methicillin (or nafcillin or oxacillin if they are used instead of methicillin for testing).
3. *Pneumococcus* resistant to penicillin.
4. *Haemophilus influenzae* resistant to ampicillin (betalactamase positive) and chloramphenicol.
5. Other resistant bacteria may be included if they are judged by the infection control team to be of special clinical and epidemiologic significance.
Pediculosis
Pharyngitis, infectious, in infants and young children
Pneumonia, viral, in infants and young children
Pneumonia, *S. aureus* or Group A *Streptococcus*
Rabies
Rubella, congenital and other
Scabies
Scalded skin syndrome, staphylococcal (Ritter's disease)
Skin wound or burn infection, major (draining and not covered by dressing or dressing does not adequately contain the purulent material) including those infected with *S. aureus* or group A *Streptococcus*
Vaccinia (generalized and progressive eczema vaccinatum)

RESPIRATORY ISOLATION

Respiratory isolation is designed to prevent transmission of infectious diseases primarily over short distances through the air (droplet transmission). Direct and indirect contact transmission occurs with some infections in this isolation category but is infrequent.

Specifications for Respiration Isolation

1. Private room is indicated. In general, patients infected with the same organism may share a room.
2. Masks are indicated for those who come close to the patient.
3. Gowns are not indicated.
4. Gloves are not indicated.
5. Hands must be washed after touching the patient or potentially contaminated articles and before taking care of another patient.
6. Articles contaminated with infective material should be discarded or bagged and labeled before being sent for decontamination and reprocessing.

Continued.

CATEGORY-SPECIFIC ISOLATION SYSTEM—cont'd

Diseases Requiring Respiratory Isolation

Epiglottitis, *H. influenzae*
Erythema infectiosum
Measles
Meningitis
   H. influenzae, known or suspected
   Meningococcal, known or suspected
Meningococcal pneumonia
Meningococcemia
Mumps
Pertussis (whooping cough)
Pneumonia, *H. influenzae,* in children (any age)

TUBERCULOSIS ISOLATION (AFB ISOLATION)**

Tuberculosis isolation (AFB isolation) is an isolation category for patients with pulmonary TB who have a positive sputum smear or a chest X-ray that strongly suggests current (active) TB. Laryngeal TB is also included in this isolation category. In general, infants and young children with pulmonary TB do not require isolation precautions because they rarely cough, and their bronchial secretions contain few AFB, compared with adults with pulmonary TB. On the instruction card, this category is called AFB (for acid-fast bacilli) Isolation to protect the patient's privacy.

Specifications for Tuberculosis Isolation (AFB Isolation)

1. Private room with special ventilation is indicated; door should be kept closed. In general, patients infected with the same organism may share a room.
2. Masks should be worn by every person entering the patient's room.
3. Gowns are indicated only if needed to prevent gross contamination of clothing.
4. Gloves are not indicated.
5. Hands must be washed after touching the patient or potentially contaminated articles and before taking care of another patient.
6. Articles are rarely involved in transmission of TB. However, articles should be thoroughly cleaned and disinfected or discarded.

ENTERIC PRECAUTIONS

Enteric precautions are designed to prevent infections that are transmitted by direct or indirect contact with feces. Hepatitis A is included in this category because it is spread through feces, although the disease is much less likely to be transmitted after the onset of jaundice. Most infections in this category primarily cause gastrointestinal symptoms, but some do not. For example, feces from patients infected with "poliovirus" and coxsackieviruses are infective, but those infections do not usually cause prominent gastrointestinal symptoms.

Specifications for Enteric Precautions

1. Private room is indicated if patient hygiene is poor. A patient with poor hygiene does not wash hands after touching infective material, contaminates the environment with infective material, or shares contaminated articles with other patients. In general, patients infected with the same organism may share a room.

2. Masks are not indicated.
3. Gowns are indicated if soiling is likely.
4. Gloves are indicated if touching infective material.
5. Hands must be washed after touching the patient or potentially contaminated articles and before taking care of another patient.
6. Articles contaminated with infective material should be discarded or bagged and labeled before being sent for decontamination or reprocessing.

Diseases Requiring Enteric Precautions

Amebic dysentery
Cholera
Coxsackievirus disease
Diarrhea, acute illness with suspected infectious etiology
Echovirus disease
Encephalitis (unless known not to be caused by enteroviruses)
Enterocolitis caused by *Clostridium difficile* or *S. aureus*
Enteroviral infection
Gastroenteritis caused by
   Campylobacter species
   Cryptosporidium species
   Dientamoeba fragilis
   Escherichia coli (enterotoxic, enteropathogenic, or enteroinvasive)
   Giardia lamblia
   Salmonella species
   Shigella species
   Vibrio parahaemolyticus
   Viruses—including Norwalk agent and rotavirus
   Yersinia enterocolitica
   Unknown etiology but presumed to be an infectious agent
Hand, foot, mouth disease
Hepatitis, viral, type A
Herpangina
Meningitis, viral (unless known not be caused by enteroviruses)
Necrotizing enterocolitis
Pleurodynia
Poliomyelitis
Typhoid fever *(Salmonella typhi)*
Viral pericarditis, myocarditis, or meningitis (unless known not to be caused by enteroviruses)

DRAINAGE/SECRETION PRECAUTIONS

Drainage/secretion precautions are designed to prevent infections that are transmitted by direct or indirect contact with purulent material or drainage from an infected body site. This newly created isolation category includes many infections formerly included in Wound and Skin Precautions, Discharge (lesion), and Secretion (oral) Precautions, which have been discontinued. Infectious diseases included in this category are those that result in the production of infective purulent material, drainage, or secretions, unless the disease is included in another isolation category that requires more rigorous precautions. For example, minor limited skin, wound, or burn infections are included in this category, but major skin, wound, or burn infections are included in Contact Isolation.

CATEGORY-SPECIFIC ISOLATION SYSTEM—cont'd

Specifications for Drainage/Secretion Precautions

1. Private room is not indicated.
2. Masks are not indicated.
3. Gowns are indicated if soiling is likely.
4. Gloves are indicated for touching infective material.
5. Hands must be washed after touching the patient or potentially contaminated articles and before taking care of another patient.
6. Articles contaminated with infective material should be discarded or bagged and labeled before being sent for decontamination and reprocessing.

Diseases Requiring Drainage/Secretion Precautions

The following infections are examples of those included in this category provided they are not (1) caused by multiply-resistant microorganisms, (b) major draining (and not covered by a dressing or dressing does not adequately contain the drainage) skin, wound, or burn infections, including those caused by *S. aureus* or group A *Streptococcus,* or (c) gonococcal eye infections in newborns. See Contact Isolation if the infection is one of these three.

Abscess, minor limited
Burn infection, minor limited
Conjunctivitis
Decubitus ulcer, infected, minor or limited
Skin infection, minor or limited
Wound infection, minor or limited

From Centers for Disease Control.[6]
*A private room with special ventilation is indicated.
**CDC Update.[19]

UNIVERSAL BLOOD AND BODY FLUID PRECAUTIONS

1. All health care workers should routinely use appropriate barrier precautions to prevent skin and mucous-membrane exposure when contact with blood or other body fluids of any patient is anticipated. Gloves should be worn for touching blood and body fluids, mucous membranes, or nonintact skin of all patients, for handling items or surfaces soiled with blood or body fluids, and for performing venipuncture and other vascular access procedures. Gloves should be changed after contact with each patient. Masks and protective eyewear or face shields should be worn during procedures that are likely to generate droplets of blood or other body fluids to prevent exposure of mucous membranes of the mouth, nose, and eyes. Gowns or aprons should be worn during procedures that are likely to generate splashes of blood or other body fluids.
2. Hands and other skin surfaces should be washed immediately and thoroughly if contaminated with blood or other body fluids. Hands should be washed immediately after gloves are removed.
3. All health care workers should take precautions to prevent injuries caused by needles, scalpels, and other sharp instruments or devices during procedures; when cleaning used instruments; during disposal of used needles; and when handling sharp instruments after procedures. To prevent needlestick injuries, needles should not be recapped, purposely bent or broken by hand, removed from disposable syringes, or otherwise manipulated by hand. After they are used, disposable syringes and needles, scalpel blades, and other sharp items should be placed in puncture-resistant containers for disposal; the puncture-resistant containers should be located as close as practical to the use area. Large-bore reusable needles should be placed in a puncture-resistant container for transport to the reprocessing area.
4. Although saliva has not been implicated in HIV transmission, to minimize the need for emergency mouth-to-mouth resuscitation, mouthpieces, resuscitation bags, or other ventilation devices should be available for use in areas in which the need for resuscitation is predictable.
5. Health care workers who have exudative lesions or weeping dermatitis should refrain from all direct patient care and from handling patient-care equipment until the condition resolves.
6. Pregnant health care workers are not known to be at greater risk of contracting HIV infection than health care workers who are not pregnant; however, if a health care worker develops HIV infection during pregnancy, the infant is at risk of infection resulting from perinatal transmission. Because of this risk, pregnant health care workers should be especially familiar with and strictly adhere to precautions to minimize the risk of HIV transmission.

Implementation of universal blood and body-fluid precautions for *all* patients eliminates the need for use of the isolation category of "Blood and Body Fluid Precautions" previously recommended by CDC for patients known or suspected to be infected with blood-borne pathogens. Isolation precautions (e.g., enteric, "AFB") should be used as necessary if associated conditions, such as infectious diarrhea or tuberculosis, are diagnosed or suspected.

PRECAUTIONS FOR INVASIVE PROCEDURES

In this document, an invasive procedure is defined as surgical entry into tissues, cavities, or organs or repair of major traumatic injuries 1) in an operating or delivery room, emergency department, or outpatient setting, including both physicians' and dentists' offices; 2) cardiac catheterization and angiographic procedures; 3) a vaginal or cesarean delivery or other invasive obstetric procedure during which bleeding may occur;

Continued.

UNIVERSAL BLOOD AND BODY FLUID PRECAUTIONS—cont'd

or 4) the manipulation, cutting, or removal of any oral or peri-oral tissues, including tooth structure, during which bleeding occurs or the potential for bleeding exists. The universal blood and body-fluid precautions listed above, combined with the precautions listed below, should be the minimum precautions for *all* such invasive procedures.

1. All health care workers who participate in invasive proce-dures must routinely use appropriate barrier precautions to prevent skin and mucous-membrane contact with blood and other body fluids of all patients. Gloves and surgical masks must be worn for all invasive procedures. Protective eyewear or face shields should be worn for procedures that com-monly result in the generation of droplets, splashing of

blood or other body fluids, or the generation of bone chips. Gowns or aprons made of materials that provide an effective barrier should be worn during invasive procedures that are likely to result in the splashing of blood or other body flu-ids. All health care workers who perform or assist in vaginal or cesarean deliveries should wear gloves and gowns when handling the placenta or the infant until blood and amniotic fluid have been removed from the infant's skin and should wear gloves during postdelivery care of the umbilical cord.

2. If a glove is torn or a needlestick or other injury occurs, the glove should be removed and a new glove used as promptly as patient safety permits; the needle or instrument involved in the incident should also be removed from the sterile field.

From Centers for Disease Control.[7]

References

1. Association for Practitioners in Infection Control: *The APIC curriculum for infection control practice,* Dubuque, Iowa, 1981, Kendall/Hunt.
2. Bartlett JG: *Pocket book of infectious disease therapy,* Baltimore, 1993, Williams & Wilkins.
3. Benenson AS, editor: *Control of communicable diseases manual,* ed 16, Washington, DC, 1995, American Public Health Association.
4. Bennett J, Brachman P, editors: *Hospital infections,* ed 2, Boston, 1986, Little, Brown.
5. Berkow R, Fletcher AJ, editors: *Merck manual of diagnosis and therapy,* vol 1, ed 16, Rahway, NJ, 1992, Merck Research Laboratories.
6. Centers for Disease Control: CDC guideline for isolation precaution in hospitals, HHS pub no (CDC) 83-8314, Atlanta, 1983, The Centers.
7. Centers for Disease Control: Recommendations for prevention of HIV transmission in health-care settings, *MMWR* 36(2S): 1987, 25-185.
8. Centers for Disease Control and Prevention: Protection against viral hepatitis: Recommendation of the Immunization Practices Advisory Committee (ACIP), *MMWR* 39(RR-2): 1990, 1-26.
9. Centers for Disease Control and Prevention: Recommendations of the Immunization Practices Advisory Committee (ACIP): Diphtheria, tetanus, and pertussis: Recommendations for vaccine use and other preventive measures, *MMWR* 40(RR-10): 1991, 1-28.
10. Centers for Disease Control and Prevention: Recommendations of the Immunization Practices Advisory Committee (ACIP): update on adult immunization, *MMWR* 40(RR-12): 1991, 1-94.
11. Centers for Disase Control and Prevention: Hepatitis B Virus: A comprehensive strategy for eliminating transmission in the United States through universal childhood vaccination: recommendations of the Immunization Practices Advisory Committee (ACIP), *MMWR* 40(RR-13): 1991, 1-25.
12. Centers for Disease Control: Public Health focus: Surveillance, prevention, and control of nosocomial infections, *MMWR* (42), 783, 1992.
13. Centers for Disease Control and Prevention: Recommendations of the Immunization Practices Advisory Committee (ACIP): Use of vaccines and immune globulins in persons with altered immunocompetence, *MMWR* 42(RR-4): 1993, 1-18.
14. Centers for Disease Control and Prevention: Recommendations for the prevention and management of chlamydia trachomatis infections 1993, *MMWR* 42(RR-12): 1993, 1-39.
15. Centers for Disease Control and Prevention: 1993 Sexually transmitted diseases treatment guidelines, *MMWR* 42(RR-14): 1993, 1-102.
16. Centers for Disease Control and Prevention: *Core curriculum on tuberculosis: what the clinician should know, ed 3,* Atlanta, 1994, US Department of Health & Human Services, Public Health Services.
17. Centers for Disease Control and Prevention: *Addressing emerging infectious disease threats: a prevention strategy for the United States,* Atlanta, 1994, US Department of Health and Human Services, Public Health Service.
18. Centers for Disease Control and Prevention: General recommendations on immunization: Recommendations of the Advisory Committee on Immunization Practices (ACIP), *MMWR* 43(RR-1): 1994, 1-38.
19. Centers for Disease Control and Prevention: Guidelines for preventing the transmission of *Mycobacterium tuberculosis* in health-care facilities, 1994. *MMWR* 43(RR-3): 1994, 1-132.
20. Centers for Disease Control and Prevention: Recommended childhood immunization schedule-United States, 1995, *MMWR* 43(51&52): 1995, 959-960.
21. Centers for Disease Control and Prevention: Prevention and control of influenza: Recommendations of the Advisory Committee on Immunization Practices (ACIP), *MMWR* 44(RR-3): 1995, 1-22.
22. Centers for Disease Control and Prevention: Recommended childhood immunization schedule-United States, 1995, *MMWR* 44(RR-5): 1995, 1-9.
23. Centers for Disease Control and Prevention: Licensure of inactivated hepatitis A vaccine and recommendations for use among international travelers, *MMWR* 44(29): 1995, 559.
24. Centers for Disease Control and Prevention: Recommendations for preventing the spread of vancomycin resistance, *MMWR* 44(RR-12): 1995, 1-13.
25. Garner J: CDC guidelines for prevention of surgical wound infections, 1985, *Infect Control* 7:193, 1986.
26. Grimes DE: *Infectious diseases,* St Louis, 1991, Mosby.
27. Murray PR et al: *Manual of clinical microbiology,* ed 6, Washington, DC, 1995, ASM Press.
28. National Institutes of Health: *Lyme disease: the facts, the challenge,* NIH Publication No. 92-3193, 1992.
29. Roizman B: *Infectious diseases in an age of change,* Washington, DC, 1995, National Academy Press.
30. Simmons B: Center for Disease Control guideline for prevention of surgical wound infection, *Infect Control* 3: 1982, 193-200.

Immunologic System

14

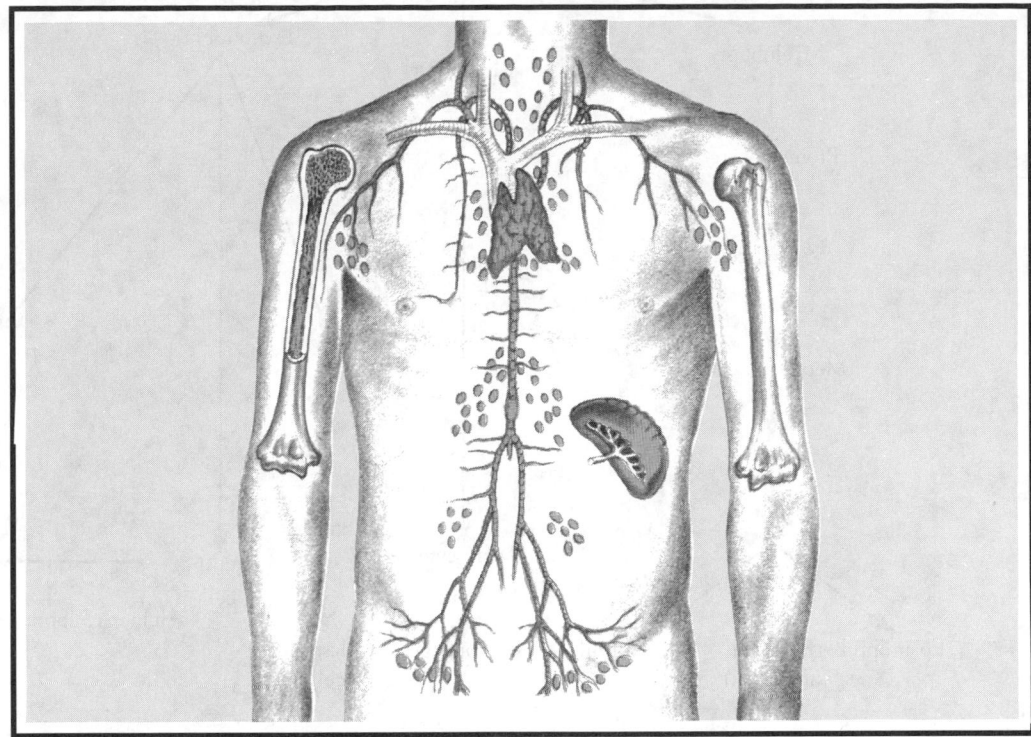

OVERVIEW

The immune system is a highly specialized group of cells and tissues that protects the internal milieu of the host. Immune responses are initiated when cellular components of the system recognize an agent as foreign and attempt to eliminate it. One role of the immune system is defense against invasive microorganisms. A second function is to maintain homeostasis by removing damaged cellular elements from the circulation. In addition, the immune system serves as a surveillance network to guard against the development, growth, and dissemination of tumor cells.

When the immune system responds appropriately to a foreign stimulus, the host's integrity is maintained. If the immune response is too weak or too vigorous, a derangement in homeostasis results. Certain hypersensitivity reactions and autoimmune diseases can occur when the regulatory cells of the immune system do not adequately control effector cell activities. Similarly, a depression in immune reactivity caused by regulatory or effector cell dysfunction can result in host susceptibility to recurrent infections and malignant disease.

Knowledge of basic immunology is increasing at a rapid rate and has had a profound influence on medical and surgical practice. Immunodulatory agents are being widely used to augment immune function in cancer patients and persons with immunodeficiency disease. Histocompatibility matching and the development of pharmacologic agents that selectively depress immune reactivity have had a major impact on organ transplantation. Since a number of diseases, such as cancer, rheumatoid disorders, and certain hematologic and gastrointestinal problems, have been associated with immunologic changes, therapies involving immunologic manipulation may soon play a pivotal role in all clinical specialty fields.

•••••• Anatomy, Physiology, and Related Pathophysiology

Cellular Components and Their Anatomic Organization

The cellular constituents of the immune system include granulocytes, mononuclear phagocytes, and lymphocytes (Figure 14-1). White cells have been grouped into these three general categories on the basis of cell morphology, functional activities, and stem cell derivation.

Cells of the granulocyte series, that is, basophils or mast cells, eosinophils, and neutrophils, are derived from a common bone marrow progenitor cell, the myeloblast. *Basophils* comprise 0.5% to 1% of the circulating white blood cell (leukocyte) population. *Mast cells,* tissue counterparts of the blood basophil, are found adjacent to smooth muscle in the perivascular and peribronchiolar tissues. Mast cells and basophils are important sources of mediators, such as histamine in allergic reactions. Eosinophils make up 1% to 3% of peripheral blood leukocytes. They accumulate at sites of anaphylaxis, may influence the host response to parasitic infections, and play a lesser

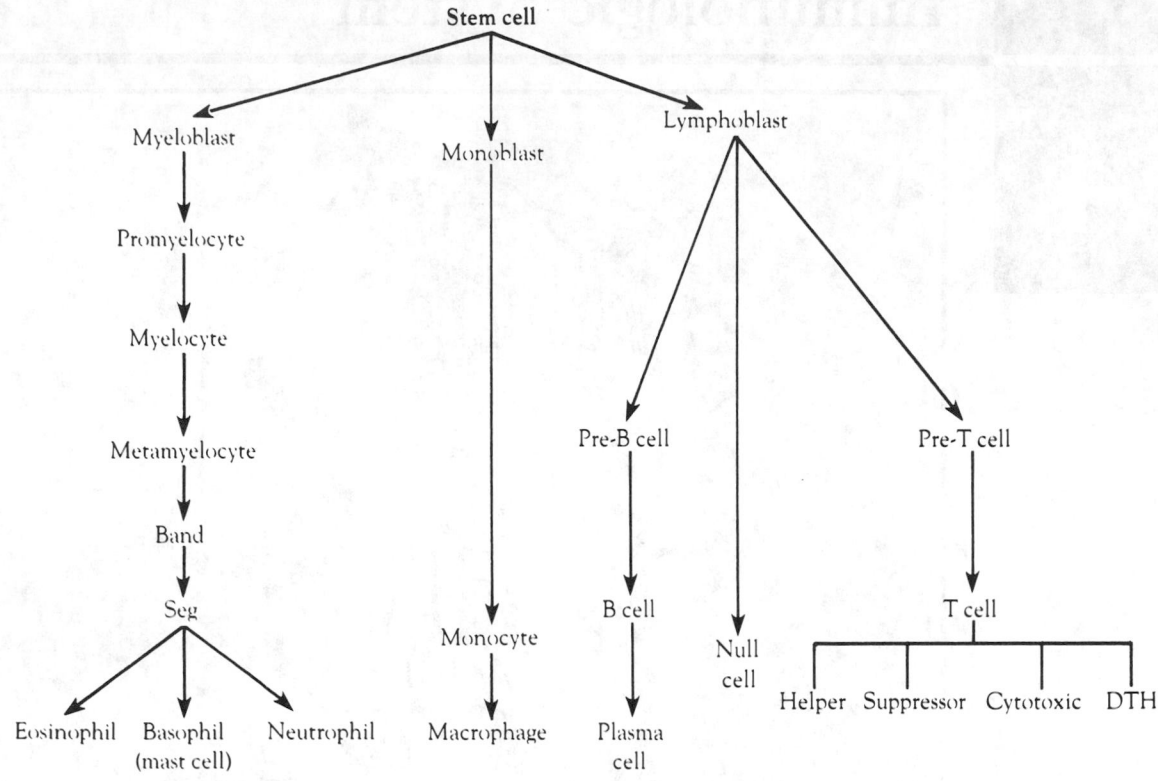

Figure 14-1 Leukocyte development. All peripheral white blood cells are thought to be derived from common pluripotent bone marrow stem cells that can differentiate into myeloblasts, monoblasts, or lymphoblasts. Replication of these differentiated stem cells serves to replenish blood and tissue leukocyte populations. Mature leukocytes protect host against invasive organisms, participate in removal of particulate material from circulation, and serve as a surveillance network to guard against development and dissemination of tumor cells. DTH, delayed-type hypersensitivity.

role in phagocytosis. Neutrophils make up as much as 70% of the blood leukocyte population. Neutrophils are actively phagocytic cells that leave the vascular compartment and rapidly accumulate within the tissue spaces at sites of inflammation.

Cells of the mononuclear phagocyte series, all originally derived from the bone marrow monoblast, are distributed throughout the body. *Monocytes* comprise approximately 5% of the circulating leukocyte population. Following a brief interval in the blood, monocytes migrate into the tissues where they mature into *macrophages,* the metabolically and functionally mature cells of this series. Macrophages are present in the brain (microglial cells), spleen, and lymphoid tissues. They also line the lung alveoli, the blood sinusoids of the liver (Kupffer cells), and most extravascular tissue spaces. Mononuclear phagocytes help protect the host from invasive organisms, clear tissue debris from sites of tissue injury, may serve as surveillance cells in antitumor host defense, and may be important in the recognition and processing of antigen; antigen may be necessary for induction of specific immunologic responses.

Cells of the lymphoid series play a key role in the development of acquired immunity. All *lymphocytes* (T, B, and null

cells, which do not have surface markers identifying them as either B or T lymphocytes) are derived from a common bone marrow progenitor cell. Certain immature lymphocytes leave the bone marrow and populate the thymus, where under the influence of thymic hormones they proliferate and differentiate into mature *T lymphocytes.* Other immature lymphocytes proliferate and differentiate into mature *B lymphocytes.* In birds this maturation takes place in an organ called the bursa of Fabricius. No mammalian bursal equivalent tissue has been identified. It is thought that B cell maturation in humans may take place in the bone marrow or in the lymphoid tissues lining the gastrointestinal tract.

After maturation, T and B lymphocytes, now capable of interacting specifically with foreign materials and participating in immune responses, are released into the circulation and populate the peripheral lymphoid tissues, including the spleen, lymph nodes, and tonsils. Mature lymphocytes are also localized in lymphoid tissues directly associated with the mucosal surfaces of the body. Such organized tissues comprise the appendix, Peyer's patches of the ileum, and bronchial-associated lymphoid tissue. The major organs housing the cellular elements of the immune system are illustrated in Figure 14-2.

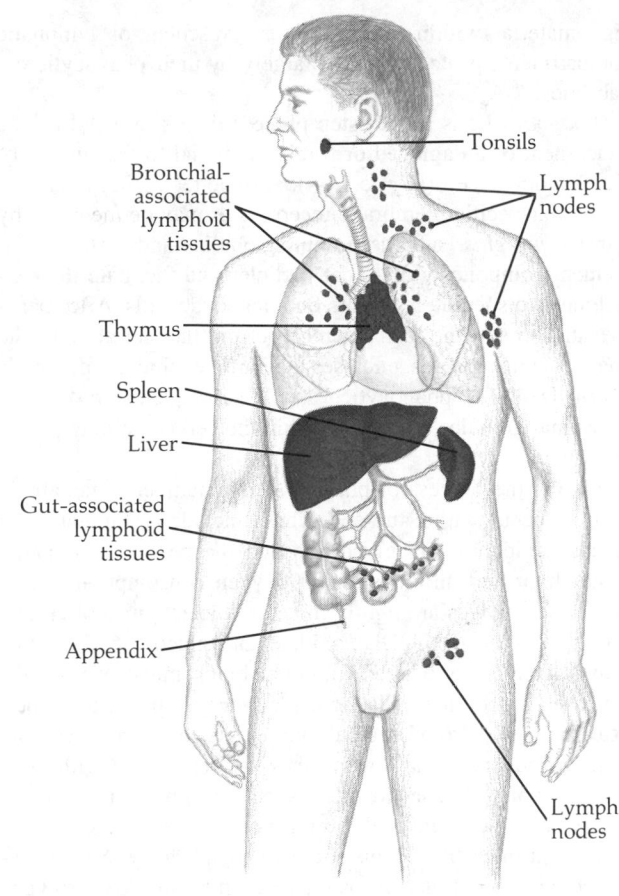

Bronchial-associated lymphoid tissues

Tonsils

Lymph nodes

Thymus

Spleen

Liver

Gut-associated lymphoid tissues

Appendix

Lymph nodes

Figure 14-2 Organization of immune system. Cellular constituents of immune system are derived from bone marrow stem cells. On maturation, these cells are released into peripheral blood and subsequently populate organized tissues of the lymphoreticular system.

Nonspecific Immune Mechanisms

Physical and chemical barriers   The first line of defense against invasive organisms is provided by intact skin and mucous membranes. These structures not only serve as a physical barrier to invasion but also provide a chemically unsuitable milieu to support microbial growth. Certain skin and mucosal secretions, such as lactic acid, gastric acid, and lysozyme, have bactericidal properties. Mechanical factors, such as ciliary action in the respiratory tract, also act to protect the host in a nonspecific manner.

Microbial factors   Resident normal flora of the skin and mucous membranes also provide a defense against colonization with pathogenic bacteria. These resident microorganisms suppress growth of infectious agents by competing for essential nutrients, producing growth-inhibiting substances, and altering pH. When normal flora are reduced by antibiotic treatment a person is more susceptible to infection with pathogenic microorganisms.

Inflammatory response   When a microorganism transcends the physical, chemical, and microbial barriers afforded by the host, or the body is injured by mechanical or chemical means, an inflammatory response is generated. At the onset of inflammation a rapid vasodilation occurs. Within minutes, blood neutrophils accumulate along the endothelial cells of vessels at the site of injury, migrate to the junctional zones between the vascular endothelial cells, and extravasate into the tissue spaces. Neutrophils within an inflammatory site represent the first line of cellular defense against invasive microorganisms.

If neutrophils do not neutralize (ingest and destroy) the inflammatory focus within a few hours, monocytes and lymphocytes begin to accumulate at the site of tissue injury. These cells attempt to localize the inflammatory response, providing a cellular barrier against the migration of the infectious organism into the lymphatic compartment, blood vessels, or neighboring tissues. When neutrophils, lymphocytes, and monocytes neutralize the inflammatory focus (phagocytose and respond with specific humoral and cell-mediated phenomena), granulation tissue is laid down and inflammation subsides. If the acute inflammatory response is unsuccessful at eliminating the infectious agent, or if tissue repair is incomplete, chronic inflammation results.

The persistence of an infectious agent during chronic inflammation results in granuloma formation. *Granulomatous lesions* are characterized by accumulations of lymphocytes and macrophages surrounding a central core of foreign material. Fibrotic tissue laid down on the periphery of the granuloma acts as a physical barrier that separates the lesion from surrounding normal tissues.

Accompanying the cellular responses that occur during inflammation are elevations in serum levels of certain proteins. These *acute phase proteins,* which include C-reactive protein and serum amyloid A protein, are used clinically to detect the presence of an infectious or inflammatory process. *C-reactive protein* may play a protective role by activating the complement pathway and influencing certain leukocyte responses. Large increases in the serum concentrations of globular proteins and fibrinogen may also accompany episodes of infection, inflammation, and tissue necrosis. In vitro, an elevation in the levels of these plasma proteins increases the aggregation and precipitation of erythrocytes suspended in plasma. This phenomenon, manifested in the laboratory as an elevation in *erythrocyte sedimentation rate* (ESR), is indicative of an ongoing inflammatory process.

Other serum proteins that play a major role in inflammation include the kinins, vasoactive amines, prostaglandins, and certain complement components (C3a, C4a, and C5a). These factors increase *vasodilation* and induce a widening of the junction between adjacent vascular endothelial cells, thus facilitating the exudation of fluid and cellular elements into the tissue spaces. *Chemotactic factors,* molecules that attract leukocytes toward an inflammatory focus, also contribute to the generation of inflammatory processes. These mediators include bacterial products, certain fluid phase components of the complement systems (C5a), and products of stimulated leukocytes.

Mononuclear phagocytic system When an infectious agent is able to permeate the barriers afforded by the local cellular response that occurs during acute or chronic inflammation, it enters the vascular compartment or the lymphatic channels. The lymphoreticular system, comprised of organs housing both tissue macrophages and lymphoid cells, functions to remove bacteria, tissue debris, or tumor cells from the lymph and blood.

When foreign materials enter the lymphatics, they are filtered by, and become lodged within, the lymph nodes (Figure 14-3). Within the nodes they may be engulfed and destroyed by fixed phagocytic cells or, alternatively, may activate a specific immune response. In a corresponding fashion, when a foreign agent enters the blood, it is phagocytosed by macrophages lining the blood sinusoids of the liver and spleen. If these macrophages do not completely destroy or neutralize the foreign material, they present it in a modified form to lymphoid cells, initiating a specific immune response.

Phagocytosis Granulocytes and mononuclear phagocytes are key cellular participants in the nonspecific immune response. Monocytes and neutrophils that have migrated into an inflammatory site and tissue macrophages that encounter foreign material within the respiratory, vascular, or lymphatic compartments protect the host largely by their phagocytic capabilities.

Phagocytosis is a multistep process that is initiated by the attachment of a damaged or foreign material to the surface of the phagocytic cell (Figure 14-4). Particle recognition may occur at nonspecific membrane receptors or may be mediated by *opsonic proteins,* such as immunoglobulins and certain complement components that coat particles and facilitate their attachment to specific receptors on phagocytic cells. After particle attachment the cell membrane on the surface of the phagocyte invaginates, encloses the particle, pinches off, and is internalized. The phagocytic vacuole subsequently fuses with lysosomal granules, vacuoles within the cell containing potent hydrolytic enzymes.

During the process of phagocytosis a number of metabolic changes occur within the cell. These include a stimulation in glucose oxidation via glycolysis and the hexose monophosphate shunt and an elevation in oxygen consumption. These metabolic changes are tightly linked to the activities of certain cellular enzymes, NADPH oxidase and glucose 6-phosphate dehydrogenase. Associated with these biochemical events is the increased production of lactic acid, hydrogen peroxide, superoxide anion, hydroxyl radical, and singlet oxygen. These oxidative products of the *respiratory burst,* in concert with lysosomal granule constituents such as myeloperoxidase, lysozyme, lactoferrin, and granular cationic proteins, are important antimicrobial agents employed by phagocytic cells. Under certain conditions, lysosomal enzymes and toxic oxygen

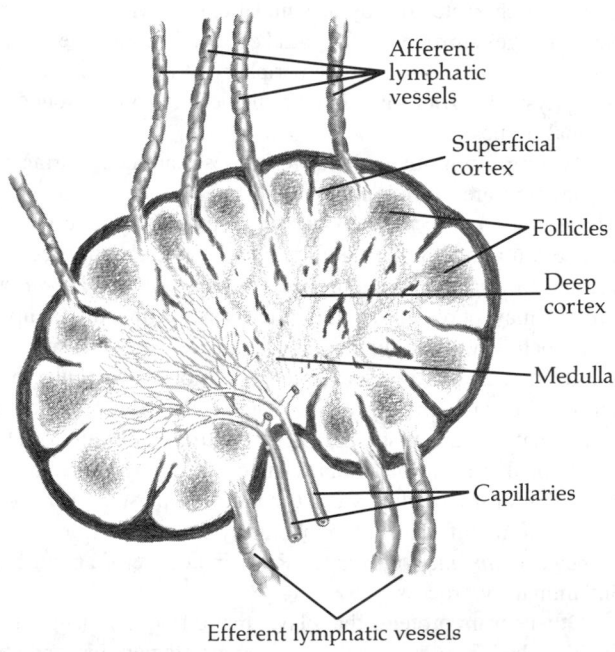

Figure 14-3 Lymph node structure. Lymph enters node via afferent lymph vessels, percolates through cortex and medulla, and leaves via efferent lymphatics. Foreign materials are trapped by macrophages in cortex, digested, and presented to lymphoid cells to initiate specific immune response. Superficial cortex is composed of B lymphocytes clustered into follicles. Interfollicular regions of superficial cortex and bulk of deep cortex are populated by T lymphocytes.

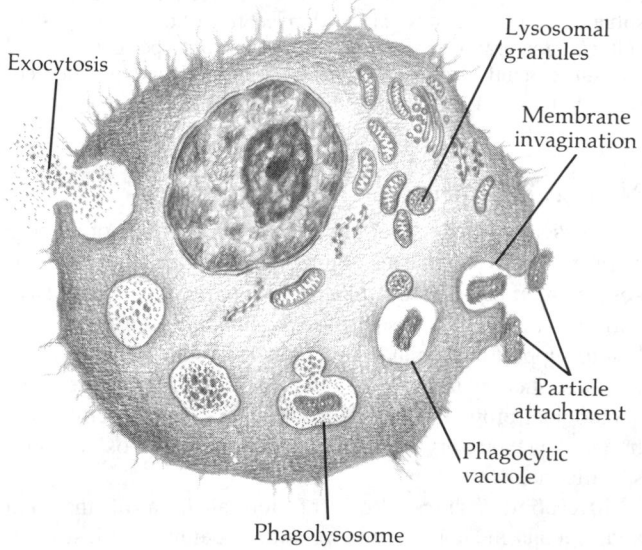

Figure 14-4 Phagocytosis. This multistep process is used by granulocytes, monocytes, and macrophages to remove foreign materials from the body. These materials come in contact with digestive enzymes and destructive oxygen metabolites within the phagocytic vacuole. Incompletely digested materials, lysosomal enzymes, and toxic oxygen products may be released from the cell.

products are released from the phagocytic cell. These events are responsible for much of the tissue damage that occurs in an ongoing inflammatory process.

Specific Immune Mechanisms

Antigenicity An *antigen* (or immunogen) is a substance capable of evoking an immune response. To qualify as an antigen a molecule must be recognized as foreign by the immune system. Antigens present on bacteria, viruses, molds, and pollens can induce a detectable immune response.

Similarly antigens found on mammalian cells and tissues can be immunogenic. *Autologous* antigens are tissue determinants that under normal conditions do not evoke an immune response. When these "self" antigens are altered by infectious or inflammatory processes, the immune system recognizes its own tissues as "foreign" and produces an autoimmune response. *Alloantigens* are genetically determined antigens that discriminate individuals within a given species. Red cells, for example, have on their surface a number of determinants, including A, B, and Rh antigens, that may precipitate an immunologic reaction following the transfusion of incompatible blood. Similarly human leukocyte antigens (HLA), present on the surface of all nucleated cells, have a profound influence on allograft survival. The human *major histocompatibility complex* (MHC) is a genetic region on chromosome 6 that codes for these human alloantigens. Gene products of the HLA-A, HLA-B, and HLA-C loci appear on all nucleated cells, whereas HLA-D region products are found primarily on lymphocytes, macrophages, epidermal cells, an sperm.

Induction of a specific immune response Antigen specific responses are designated as either humoral or cellular immunity (Table 14-1). *Humoral immunity* is mediated by B lymphocytes that synthesize and secrete γ-globulins in response to antigenic challenge. *Cell-mediated immune mechanisms* involve the partipation of effector T lymphocytes and macrophages. Humoral immunity can be transferred from an immune to a nonimmune host with cell-free globulin-bearing serum, whereas cellular immunity is transferred with sensitized cells. Although the body's response to an antigenic challenge usually involves both cellular and humoral immune mechanisms, one response may predominate.

A specific immune mechanism involves the participation of T and B lymphocytes that have been genetically programmed to recognize and interact with unique antigenic determinants on a foreign material. A specific immune response is triggered after the clearance of foreign materials from an inflammatory site, the lymph, or the vascular compartment by tissue macrophages. These phagocytic cells internalize and degrade the foreign antigens. The processed antigens are reexpressed on the macrophage surface in a highly immunogenic form for presentation to lymphocytes that continuously circulate through the lymphoid organs. Recognition of antigen by specific receptors on lymphocytes results in their stimulation and sequestration within the tissue.

Humoral immunity When confronted with an antigen, B lymphocytes synthesize and secrete specifically reactive γ- globulins called *antibodies* or *immunoglobulins*. On first exposure to a given antigen, a *primary humoral immune response* is evoked. This response occurs after a lag period of 1 to 7 days during which only trace amounts of specific antibody can be detected. During this induction period, antigen is processed and specific clones of B lymphocytes are stimulated to divide and differentiate ultimately into two different cell types. The first type, *plasma cells,* synthesizes and secretes antibodies. Other B lymphocytes, *memory cells,* remain quiescent until secondary exposure to a given antigen.

The *secondary,* or *anamnestic response* that occurs after subsequent exposure to a particular antigen has a short lag period, produces high levels of antibody, and is more sustained than the primary response. This memory property of the immune system increases resistance to infection in persons who have been immunized against, or previously infected with, a particular antigen.

The humoral immune response offers protection against many gram-positive and certain gram-negative organisms. Specific antibody generated during a humoral immune response facilitates viral neutralization, enhances bacterial ingestion and destruction by phagocytic cells, and results in activation of the complement system.

When a humoral immune response is generated against soluble antigens, small antigen-antibody complexes form. These *immune complexes* may be rapidly cleared from the circulation by fixed macrophages in the liver and spleen or, alternatively, may be deposited within tissues. Tissue-bound immune complexes can activate the complement system and provide inflammatory destruction of normal cells.

Regulation of the humoral immune response Certain antigens are capable of stimulating B cells directly or after presentation on the macrophage surface. These *T-independent antigens* have a primary structure of repeating identical units.

Most antigens, however, require the activation of a subpopulation of lymphocytes, *T-helper cells,* in addition to B lymphocytes, to effect an antibody response. The antibody response to a *T-dependent antigen* is initiated by macrophage presentation of antigen to T helper cells and secretion of

---

TABLE 14-1 Humoral and Cell-Mediated Immune Responses

	Humoral	Cell-Mediated
Effector cells	B lymphocytes	T lymphocytes and macrophages
Regulatory cells	T helper cells and T suppressor cells	T helper cells and T suppressor cells
Effector mechanisms	Elaboration of antibody	Generation of factors that are directly toxic to target cells
Host protection	Against many gram-positive and certain gram-negative bacteria	Against mycobacteria, fungi, protozoa, and tumors

interleukin 1, a T cell growth-promoting substance. T helper cells, stimulated in this way, interact with B lymphocytes and promote their growth and differentiation. B cell growth factor, derived from T cells, may play a role in B cell activation (Figure 14-5).

The antibody response to T-dependent antigen is under the control of the major histocompatibility complex (MHC). To interact with antibody-presenting macrophages, helper T cells have to recognize and bind "self" antigens, called Ia antigens, on the macrophage surface. These self antigens are coded for

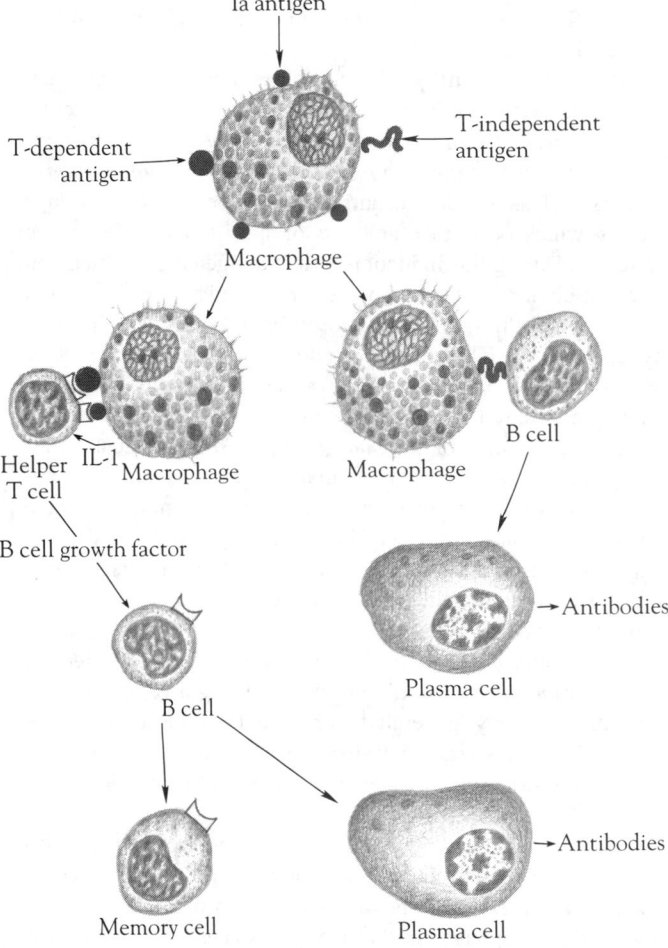

Figure 14-5 Humoral immune responses. Antibody response to T-dependent antigens involves interaction between macrophages, T cells, and B cells. Macrophages ingest foreign materials, reexpress processed antigen on their surface, and present it in context of Ia molecule to T helper cells. T helper cells facilitate B lymphocyte proliferation and differentiation. On primary exposure to given T-dependent antigen, memory cell generation occurs, although little antibody is generated. During anamnestic response, plasma cells synthesize large quantities of specific antibody. Humoral response to T-independent antigens may be a macrophage-dependent or independent process. This response generally produces only antibody of IgM class and has little or no memory. *IL-I*, Interleukin 1.

by genes of the HLA region. Similarly, T cell binding to B lymphocytes involves their recognition of a genetically determined marker on the B cell surface.

In addition to T lymphocytes that provide help in the induction of an immune response, certain other T lymphocytes depress immune reactivity. *Suppressor T cells* have an important role in homeostatic control, since they maintain the humoral immune response at a level appropriate for the stimulus. Suppressor T cells are activated during the generation of all immune responses. They limit the immune response by acting at the level of the helper T cell or B lymphocyte (Figure 14-6). The modulatory activity of suppressor T cells may be mediated by direct cell-to-cell contact or, alternatively, may involve the release of suppressor factors.

The relative numbers and functional reactitivities of helper and suppressor cells determine the strength and persistence of an immune response. When the delicate balance between T helper and T suppressor cell populations is disrupted, autoimmune or immunodeficiency disease may result. Since helper and suppressor T lymphocytes have distinct surface markers and can be readily discriminated in the laboratory, immune function can be estimated by measuring the T helper/T suppressor cell ratio. Normally a person has roughly twice as many T helper cells as T suppressor cells. In contrast, patients with acquired immunodeficiency syndrome (AIDS) frequently demonstrate a T helper/T suppressor cell ratio of 1:1 or less.

Biologic activities of immunoglobulins   The γ-globulin-bearing or antibody-bearing fractions of serum are referred to as *immunoglobulins.* The immunoglobulins are a highly heterogenous population of proteins, not a singular molecular species. Currently five physiochemical classes of immunoglobulins are recognized: IgG, IgM, IgA, IgE, and IgD.

Immunoglobulin molecules are made up of a four-chain polypeptide (protein) unit consisting of two identical high–

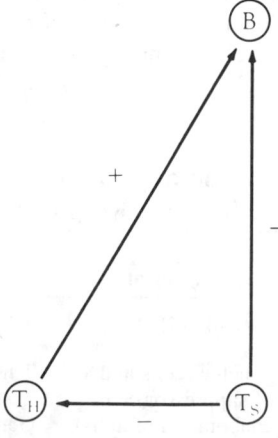

Figure 14-6 Regulation of humoral immune responses. Generation of humoral immune response is facilitated by interaction of T helper *(T_H)* lymphocytes with antigen-specific B cells. This response can be down-regulated by T suppressor *(T_S)* lymphocytes that act at the level of either the T helper or B lymphocyte.

molecular weight (heavy) chains and two identical low–molecular weight (light) chains. The immunoglobulins have been assigned to their respective classes on the basis of their heavy chains, gamma (γ), mu (μ), alpha (α), epsilon (ε), and delta (δ). There are two different light chain types, kappa (κ) and lambda (λ). A schematic representation of the five major immunoglobulin classes is shown in Figure 14-7.

When a humoral immune response is triggered, one or more classes of antibody may be elaborated The nature of the antibody response is dependent on the chemical and physical nature of the antigen, route of administration, and immunization history of the host.

IgG is the predominant serum antibody and represents a large proportion of the immunoglobulin found in internal secretions (for example, pleural, synovial, and peritoneal fluids). Specific IgG is produced only in small amounts late in the primary immune response, but it is the major antibody generated during a *secondary challenge* with antigen. The generation of IgG protects the host, since this class of immunoglobulin has a number of biologically significant properties. For example, IgG can neutralize toxins produced by various strains of bacteria and induces the agglutination of infectious organisms, facilitating their uptake by phagocytic cells. In addition, IgG has opsonic activity and can activate complement, resulting in the lysis of certain strains of bacteria. IgG is thought to play a crucial role in neonatal host defense, since it is the only immunoglobulin class to be transferred across the placenta.

IgM, comprising approximately 10% of the serum immunoglobulins, is the first antibody to appear during the *primary immune response.* Exposure to antigen via the respiratory or gastrointestinal tract results in the elaboration of IgM into the external secretions. IgM shares many of the biologic properties of IgG: it can neutralize bacterial toxins, can agglutinate certain microorganisms, and is a potent activator of the complement system.

IgA, comprising only a small portion of the serum antibody pool, is the predominant immunoglobulin in all *serous* and *mucous secretions.* Secretory IgA interferes with bacterial attachment to mucosal surfaces, impedes colonization, and virtually prevents bacterial penetration into the general circulation. In addition, IgA is capable of neutralizing certain bacteria toxins but does not have opsonic or complement-fixing properties. Secretory IgA in maternal milk affords protection to infants before maturation of their secretory immune system.

IgE antibodies, present in the serum in trace amounts, are found attached to mast cells and basophils. These immunoglobulins play a major role in the generation of anaphylactic reactions. When an *allergen,* a substance capable of inducing an allergic reaction, binds to IgE on the surface of basophils or mast cells, mediators such as histamine, serotonin, and leukotrienes are released. These products stimulate bronchial smooth muscle contraction and precipitate systemic vasodilation. Although IgE is generated in small amounts during conventional humoral immune responses, the physiologic significance of IgE production is not well understood. Evidence suggests that IgE may afford protection against parasitic infections by facilitating eosinophil recognition and destruction of the parasite.

IgD is only a minor component of the serum immunoglobulin pool and is not found in appreciable amounts in external or internal secretions. The biologic function of IgD has not been elucidated, but it may play a role in antigen-triggered lymphocyte differentiation.

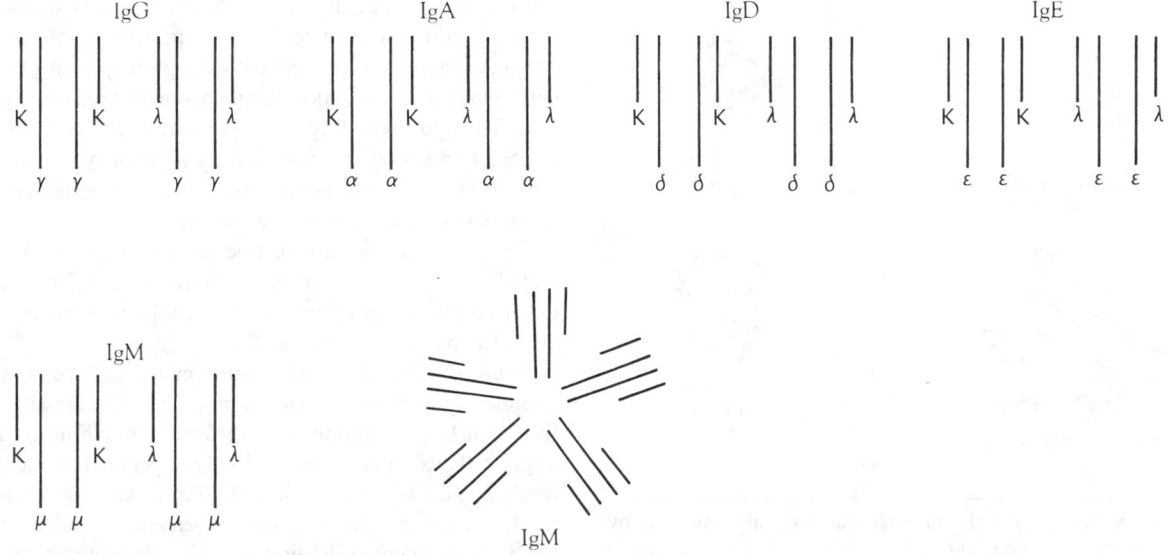

Figure 14-7 Antibody structure. All immunoglobulins are four-chain polypeptide units. Differences among immunoglobulin classes reside in heavy chain structure. IgM, found in serum and external secretions, is a pentamer consisting of five identical subunits. (Modified from Unaue.[24])

Cell-mediated immunity Whereas humoral immune mechanisms afford protection against many gram-positive and certain gram-negative organisms, *cell-mediated immunity is important during host infection with intracellular pathogens such as mycobacteria, fungi, viruses, and protozoa.* Cell-mediated reactions are also elicited as a component of the host response to *tumors* and *tissue transplants.*

Cell-mediated immune responses have been classically characterized as either *delayed-type hypersensitivity* (DTH) or *cytotoxic T lymphocyte* (CTL) reactions (Figure 14-8). CTL reactions play a major role in host defense against tumors, virally infected cells, and allogenic tissue transplants, whereas DTH reactions are activated by host infection with intracellular pathogens.

Generation of a DTH response involves the participation of macrophages, T helper cells, and DTH-effector T cells. During a primary infection the organisms are ingested by macrophages that process and reexpress antigen on their surface for presentation to helper cells. T helper cells, stimulated by antigen presentation and macrophage release of interleukin 1, induce proliferation of a pool of antigen-specific DTH-precursor T cells. The major portion of these cells remain quiescent until secondary challenge with antigen.

On secondary exposure an anamnestic response develops. Macrophages present processed antigen to antigen-specific T helper cells that rapidly stimulate large numbers of DTH-effector T cells, previously generated by clonal expansion. The activated DTH-effector cells release factors, called lymphokines, that stimulate other cells, particularly macrophages. Most tissue macrophages are incapable of killing intracellular pathogens; however, macrophages activated by exposure to lymphokines are avidly bactericidal.

The duration and magnitude of a DTH response are regulated by T suppressor cells. In general, a secondary DTH reaction can be demonstrated within a few hours of antigen challenge, peaks at 24 to 48 hours, and gradually recedes as the inflammatory focus is eliminated. A person's capacity to generate a secondary DTH response can be measured by intradermal injection with a battery of skin test antigens. If, for example, persons with normal immunity and a history of tuberculosis are tested with purified tuberculoid antigen (PPD), they demonstrate a classic wheal-and-flare reaction. This positive response is evidence of a functionally intact cell-mediated immune system.

CTL reactions are mediated by a subpopulation of T lymphocytes known as *cytotoxic T lymphocytes.* These lymphocytes have surface receptors that recognize genetically different MHC markers on allogeneic tissues and mediate tissue rejection. Similarly cytotoxic lymphocytes recognize tumor- and virus-infected host cells as foreign. On primary exposure to genetically different or altered cells, a population of cytotoxic T precursor cells is expanded with the participation of T helper cells. On secondary exposure an anamnestic response is generated. The cytotoxic T lymphocyte, once activated, attaches to its target and lyses it, through enzymatic or lymphokine reactions. CTL reactions, like all classic immune responses, can be downregulated by T suppressor cells.

The recognition and destruction of tumor- and virus-infected target cells are not limited to cytotoxic T lymphocytes. Other categories of effector cells include mononuclear phagocytes and natural killer cells.

Natural killer (NK) cells, often called null cells, are large granular lymphocytes that do not bear the classic markers found on B or T lymphocyte surfaces. They bind to and lyse target cells using either an antibody-dependent or independent mechanism. Target cell lysis by NK cells that requires antibody is described as an antibody-dependent cellular cytotoxic (ADCC) mechanism. Killing by NK cells occurs naturally and is not enhanced by immunization. Although NK cells do not have immunologic memory, their functional activities can be modified. Interferons, protein products of stimulated lymphocytes, increase NK killing of target cells. In contrast, certain prostaglandins depress NK function.

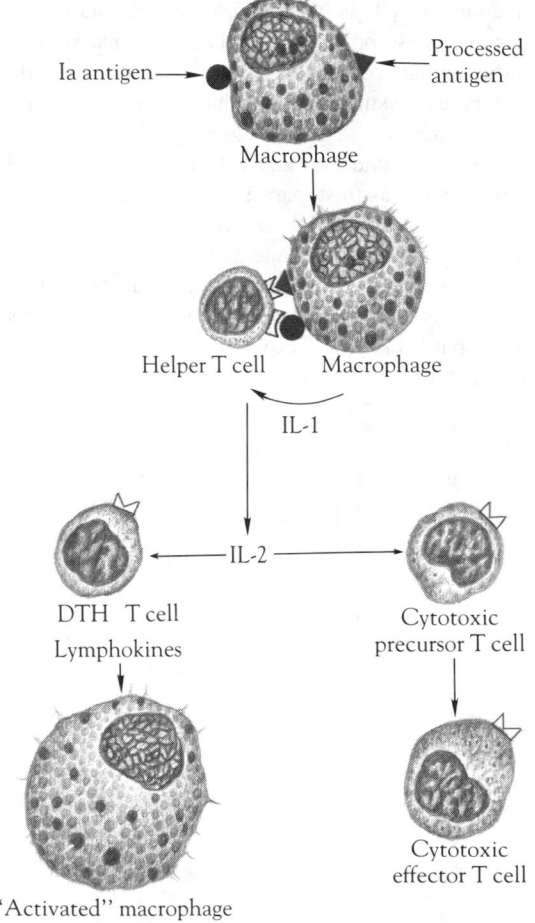

Figure 14-8 Cell-mediated immune reactions are initiated by macrophage presentation of processed antigen to helper T lymphocytes. Stimulated T helper cells release interleukin 2 *(IL-2)* that activates DTH and cytotoxic T lymphocytes. Targets, such as tumor or virus-infected cells, are lysed directly by cytotoxic T cells. Following infection with intracellular pathogens, activated macrophages are the major effector cell population generated *IL-1,* Interleukin 1.

Cells of the mononuclear phagocyte series can kill target cells directly or by an ADCC mechanisms. Peripheral blood *monocytes* and resident tissue *macrophages* exhibit low levels of antitumor activity. Following activation with T–lymphocyte–derived products such as γ-interferon, macrophage lysis of tumor- and virus-infected target cells increases.

Because immunization is not generally required for the activities of NK and mononuclear phagocytic cells, these populations are thought to play an important host defense role in early stages of infection and tumor growth, before CTL effector cells have been generated. Interferon, shown experimentally to increase both NK cell and macrophage cytotoxic activities, is being used in clinical trials to treat certain malignancies and immunodeficiency disorders.

Complement system   The complement system is comprised of a series of proteins that when activated serve to amplify an immune response. Activation of the complement system leads to the elaboration of potent inflammatory mediators, facilitates particle opsonization and clearance, and may result in the direct lysis of altered mammalian cells and certain bacteria. The complement system may be activated by a number of immunologic and nonimmunologic stimuli. Complement activation proceeds by two mechanisms, the classical and alternative pathways (Figure 14-9).

The *classical complement pathway* comprises 11 distinct proteins. The early-acting components are numbered according to the order of their discovery, and the later-acting components according to their order of reaction. Thus the sequence of action of these components is C1, C4, C2, C3, C5, C6, C7, C8, and C9. C1 is made up of three distinct proteins, C1q, C1r, and C1s.

The first step of complement activation through the classical pathway involves the interaction of C1 with immune complexes containing IgM or IgG or with antibody-coated particles. When activated, C1, the recognition complex of the classical pathway, cleaves C4 and C2. Two protein fragments subsequently combine and form an active enzyme (C4b2a) that cleaves C3 molecules. C3a generated in this way is a potent anaphylatoxin, a substance capable of stimulating basophils and mast cells and thus provoking release of vasoactive amines. A portion of the C3b fragments elaborated during this cleavage is deposited on the activating surface and facilitates particle attachment to phagocytic cells. Certain other C3b molecules combine with C4b2a to form an enzyme (C4b2a3b) that cleaves C5 into two fragments. C5a released into the fluid phase has both anaphylatoxic and chemotactic properties. C5b has an affinity for membranes and, when deposited on a surface, facilitates the binding of C6 and C7. This trimolecular complex (C5b67) provides a binding site for C8, the complement component responsible for initiating target cell lysis. Although some membrane damage occurs following the formation of the C5b-8 complex, lysis is accelerated by the binding of C9. C5b-9, on the surface of a target cell, is called the membrane attach complex.

Before the generation of specific antibody, the complement system can be activated via the *alternative pathway*. Known activators of the alternative pathway include bacterial lipopoly-saccharide, virus-infected cells, yeasts, fungi, and certain bacterial cell walls. The constituents of the alternative pathway include all the classical complement components except C1, C4, and C2. Two other proteins, factor B and factor D, contribute to activation of the alternative pathway.

The alternative pathway is activated with the formation of an enzyme that cleaves C3 molecules. This enzyme (C3bBb), distinct from the classical pathway enzyme (C4b2a), is generated following the spontaneous hydrolysis of C3, which in the

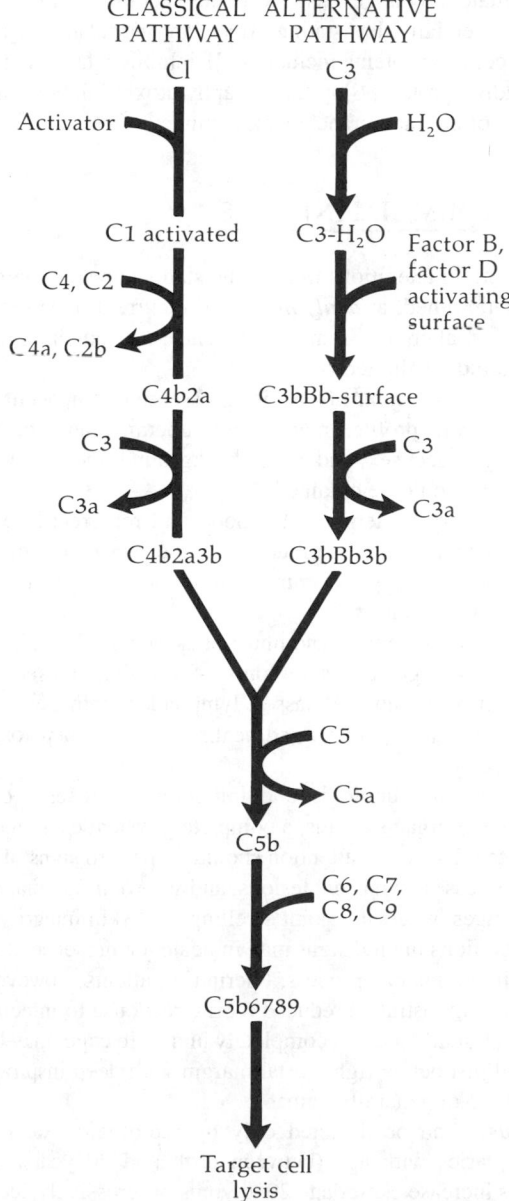

Figure 14-9 Complement activation. Complement activation can proceed by either classical or alternative pathway. Activation of these pathways results in generation of chemotactic factors (C5a), anaphylatoxins (C3a, C5a), and membrane attack complex (C5b6789).

presence of factor D cleaves factor B. C3bBb generated in this way and bound to an activating surface (such as a bacterium) is capable of cleaving many more C3 molecules, which results in the generation of C3bBb3b, an enzyme that cleaves C5 into C5a and C5b. The subsequent steps of the alternative pathway are identical to those of the classical pathway and lead to the elaboration of anaphylatoxins, chemotactic factors, and target cell lysis.

Although the complement system protects the host against infectious organisms and may play a role in tumor cell destruction, the uncontrolled activation of this system would result in inflammatory changes and lytic destruction of host tissues. These potentially devastating effects are modulated by a number of control proteins including C1 inhibitor, factors H and I, C4 binding protein, S protein, anaphylatoxin inhibitor, and inhibitors of the membrane attack complex.

 ## NORMAL FINDINGS

Since certain alterations in immune status appear to be genetically determined, a *family history* of recurrent infections, malignancies, allergies, immunodeficiency, and autoimmune disease should be elicited.

A detailed *patient history* is an essential component of the immune status profile. In addition to documentation of the patient's age, race, sex, and ethnic background, the following information should be obtained:

Past history—allergies, childhood and recurrent infections, malignancy, autoimmune disease, primary disorders known to suppress immune function, immunization profile, medications

Social, occupational, and nutritional habits

Abnormal signs and symptoms—fever, diaphoresis, rashes, joint pain, unusual masses, lymphadenopathy, overt signs of infection, poor wound healing, eczema, hepatosplenomegaly

Because immunologic and inflammatory disease can involve many organ systems, a complete physical examination is warranted. Particular attention should be paid to signs of infection (abscesses, persistent lesions, and so on), inflammatory tissue changes, wheezing, joint swelling, and skin integrity.

Alterations in vital signs may indicate the presence of an ongoing inflammatory process. (Geriatric patients, however, frequently demonstrate a reduced febrile response to infection.)

Liver   Usually located completely under rib cage; may be palpated just below right costal margin with deep inspiration

Spleen   Not generally palpable

Thymus   Can be detected only by radiologic examination; size varies with age (between birth and 20 years, thymic mass increases; after age 20, thymus progressively decreases in size until age 60, when thymic involution is complete)

Lymph nodes (head and neck, axillary, inguinal, epitrochlear)   Generally not palpable; small, nontender nodes may be found in cervical or inguinal chain of persons with history of local infection

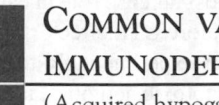 ## CONDITIONS, DISEASES, AND DISORDERS

IMMUNODEFICIENCY DISEASES

▌ COMMON VARIABLE IMMUNODEFICIENCY[7,23,24]

(Acquired hypogammaglobulinemia)

Common variable immunodeficiency (CVID) is an immune disorder of unknown cause that predominantly affects the B cell system. The clinical features include severe depression or absence of plasma cells.

The immunologic feature of acquired hypogammaglobulinemia that is shared with the X-linked form is the marked depression or absence of all five classes of globulin. Consequently, recurrent bacterial infections are observed in this disorder. Other common features include malabsorption syndromes (usually resulting from *Giardia lamblia* infestation) and an increased incidence of autoimmune and lymphoreticular malignancies. A predilection for autoimmune and neoplastic disease in first-degree relatives of these patients suggests a hereditary influence.

CVID is distinguished by the presence of defective B lymphocytes and a higher than normal incidence of abnormalities in T cell immunity. Also, patients with CVID may manifest hyperplasia of lymphoid tissue, including the tonsils, nodes, and spleen. In addition, acquired hypogammaglobulinemia occurs in both sexes equally and at any age, with symptoms appearing from age 15 to 35 years. Genetic studies have demonstrated an autosomal recessive mode of inheritance in certain families in which abnormal lymphocyte metabolism is inherited. However, in most cases no clear genetic transmission can be demonstrated.

•••••• Pathophysiology

The cause of acquired hypogammaglobulinemia is an intrinsic defect in B-cell antibody production. In addition, excessive suppressor T-cell activity may inhibit B-cell functioning. In some cases, helper T-cell activity may be inadequate to assist B-calls to make antibody.

•••••• Diagnostic Studies and Findings

B cell quantitation and function   B cells low, normal, or increased; cell clonally diverse and relatively immature; fail to respond to most antigens and mitogens by differentiating into plasma cells; in some patients B cells synthesize but do not secrete immunoglobulin

Immunoglobulin quantitation   Total less than 300 mg/dl; IgG less than 250 mg/dl

T cell studies   Levels may be normal or reflect increased numbers of T suppressor cells with decreased numbers of helper cells; B cells are unable to function without T helper cell feedback; generally T cell function deteriorates with time

Antibody response Absent following specific immunization

Lymphoid tissue biopsy Absence of plasma cell in B cell–dependent areas; hyperplasia of lymphoid tissue

Chest roentgenogram Chronic lung disease

Sinus roentgenogram Chronic sinusitis

Pulmonary function tests Findings abnormal

Malabsorption studies Blunting of villi on biopsy; abnormal findings on D-xylose absorption test; lack of normal intestinal enzymes

Stool examination for ova and parasites *Giardia lamblia* detected most frequently

Antinuclear antibody and other optional studies To detect presence of autoimmune disease or lymphoreticular malignancies; antinuclear antibody present in autoimmune disease

•••••• Multidisciplinary Plan

Medication

Gamma globulin, IM, 20-40 ml/mo; IV, 100-400 mg/kg/mo, for acute illness given daily or weekly

Fresh-frozen plasma, 1-2 U/mo

Antibiotics, often given continuously in various combinations

Metronidazole, 750 mg tid for 10 d for malabsorption associated with *Giardia* infection

General Management

Pulmonary physical therapy in presence of chronic lung disease

Chest x-ray examination and pulmonary function tests to determine adequacy of treatment

Dietary restriction for secondary enzymatic deficiencies resembling celiac disease

Treatment of associated autoimmune disorders (see specific condition)

NURSING CARE

Nursing Assessment

Recurrent Infection (Usually Chronic)

Sinusitis; pharyngitis; pneumonia; osteomyelitis; conjunctivitis; abscesses; otitis; chronic lung disease

Gastrointestinal Tract

Chronic diarrhea; malabsorption

Lymphatic System

Lymphadenopathy; splenomegaly

Presence of Concomitant Autoimmune Disease

Signs and symptoms associated with systemic lupus erythematosus; dermatomyositis; hemolytic anemia; rheumatoid arthritis–like disorder; idiopathic thrombocytopenic purpura; hypothyroidism; Graves' disease; pernicious anemia

Presence of Concomitant Neoplastic Disease

Signs and symptoms associated with leukemia, lymphoma, and gastric carcinoma

Nursing Dx & Intervention

Impaired gas exchange related to recurrent sinopulmonary infections and/or chronic lung disease

- Assess vital signs and respiratory status; monitor rate, rhythm, and quality of respirations, presence of cyanosis, adventitious breath sounds, and restlessness.
- Monitor results of pulmonary function studies, arterial blood gas studies, and chest roentgenograms.
- Position patient for optimal chest excursion, usually with head elevated 30 to 60 degrees. Resting arms on padded overbed table may increase comfort for patients with chronic lung disease.
- Remind patient to cough and deep breathe every 2 hours.
- Turn patient frequently to move secretions.

Diarrhea related to giardiasis or enzymatic deficiencies

- Monitor intake and output, weight, and electrolytes for imbalances.
- Assess frequency, volume, consistency, and pattern of bowel movements.
- Assist with toileting activities, as necessary, *to prevent skin breakdown.*
- Gradually increase intake, beginning with liquids and nonstimulating foods.
- Monitor stool for ova and parasites.

Altered nutrition: less than body requirements related to malabsorption

- Perform nutritional assessment.
- Provide gluten-free diet, when necessary.
- Provide small, frequent feedings as tolerated.
- Encourage family members to provide patient's favorite foods within diet parameters.
- Provide dietary supplements.
- Determine the need for parenteral nutrition if oral intake is deficient.

Risk for infection related to compromised immunologic system

- Assess for evidence of infection at sites of invasive procedures.
- Assess for breaks in skin integrity, particularly over pressure areas and oral mucosa.
- Assess pulmonary status; auscultate lung fields *to determine presence of adventitious breath sounds.*
- Maintain optimal nutritional status and fluid intake.

- Assess ocular integrity for evidence of conjunctivitis: erythematous, pruritic conjunctiva.
- Assess mentation for evidence of central nervous system infection: decreased level of consciousness, headache, and visual disturbances.
- Assess mobility and joint function for pain and swelling.
- Assess ears for pain, discharge, or diminished hearing.
- Assess for evidence of gastrointestinal infection: abdominal pain, fever, and diarrhea.
- Monitor temperature and vital signs for evidence of fever and sepsis.
- Maintain body hygiene.
- Limit environmental stress.
- Monitor laboratory data: white blood cell count and differential, erythrocyte sedimentation rate, C-reactive protein, urinalysis, and cultures.
- Promote pulmonary toilet: breathing exercises, postural drainage, and chest physical therapy.
- Maintain normal sleep and rest patterns.
- Protect patient from physical injury.
- Restrict contact with family and health care providers who have infectious diseases.

Patient Education/Home Care Planning

1. Discuss with the patient the techniques to prevent recurrent pulmonary infection: prophylactic antibiotics, breathing exercises, postural drainage, and chest physiotherapy.
2. Stress to the patient the importance of compliance with regular follow-up examinations for γ-globulin level and clinical evaluation.
3. Give the patient a list of risk factors associated with infection, and discuss signs and symptoms to report.
4. Explain to the patient the principles of gluten-free diet.
5. Explain to the patient the facts about the importance of prescribed medications.
6. Refer the patient for genetic counseling to explain the inheritance pattern and to the dietitian for a diet plan.
7. Stress to the patient the importance of wearing medical alert identification.

Evaluation

Respiratory status is within normal limits Patient's rates and rhythm are within normal limits; cyanosis, restlessness, and adventitious breath sounds are absent.

Laboratory data return to normal limits Patient's IgG, IgE, ILgD, white blood count, erythrocyte sedimentation rate, and C-reactive protein level are within normal limits. (IgA and IgM may not return to normal limits.) Culture findings are negative. Urinalysis findings are within normal limits.

Bowel pattern returns to normal Consistency and volume of patient's bowel movements are normal, intake and output are balanced, weight is stable, and electrolytes are within normal limits.

Nutrition is adequate Weight is within normal range for patient; patient chooses and consumes gluten-free diet.

Infection is decreased or absent Patient's vital signs are within normal limits; patient maintains mobility; patient remains alert and oriented; patient's skin is intact; patient shows no eye, ear, or gastrointestinal manifestations of infection.

■ SELECTIVE IgA DEFICIENCY[16,24]

Selective IgA deficiency is the presence of serum IgA in quantities less than 5 mg/dl while other immunoglobulins are present in normal amounts.

Selective IgA deficiency is the most common immunodeficiency disease. In the United States the incidence is approximately 1 in 700. Although the disease is most commonly detected during the first decade of life, patients often survive until the sixth or seventh decade. It cannot be diagnosed before 1 year of age because infants may not produce IgA until then.

As discussed previously, IgA is the predominant immunoglobulin of external secretions. Therefore bacterial infections of the respiratory, gastrointestinal, and urogenital tracts are the major clinical manifestations associated with this disorder.

Many affected persons are asymptomatic. Autoimmune disease develops in 25% of those affected. Recently IgG subclass deficiencies were reported in association with IgA deficiency.

Morbidity is associated with recurrent sinopulmonary infections, autoimmune disease, and rarely, neoplastic disease. Sprue-elike disease may also complicate the disease course.

•••••• Pathophysiology

The immunopathogenesis of this disorder is unclear. The presence of normal numbers of IgA B cells suggests that the underlying defect involves decreased synthesis or release of IgA. However, lymphocyte culture studies have demonstrated that IgA B cells synthesize but do not secrete immunoglobulin. Therefore the underlying defect probably occurs in the transformation of the IgA B lymphocyte to the plasma cell. T suppressor mechanisms may influence this process.[17] The presence of antibodies to IgA in as many as 44% of cases of IgA deficiency implies that an autoimmune process is involved as well. See p. 1177 for a description of the role of IgA.

A genetic predisposition has also been postulated. Autosomal recessive and autosomal dominant modes of inheritance have been implicated. IgA deficiency appears with greater than normal frequency in families with a variety of immunodeficiency diseases. In addition, the presence of HLA-A1, HLA-B8, and HLA-DW3 is associated with IgA deficiency and autoimmune disease.

Whatever the cause, the lack of secretory IgA antibody promotes the attachment of infectious microbes at the mucosal surfaces and explains the occurrence of gastrointestinal, urogenital, and sinopulmonary infections. In addition, IgA probably acts to prevent absorption of other foreign proteins such as those in the diet. Its absence may explain the spruelike syndrome associated with selective IgA deficiency.

The deficiency of IgA may not be primary. Instead it may follow the administration of certain drugs such as phenytoin or penicillamine. In this case the decreased serum levels may result from induction of T suppressor cells that interfere with B cell maturation.

•••••• Diagnostic Studies and Findings

Ig quantitation   IgA level less than 5 mg/dl; IgG, IgM, IgD, and IgE normal or increased
Immunization   Normal antibody response
B cell quantitation   Normal numbers of B cells, including IgA-bearing lymphocytes
T cell studies   Normal findings
Chest roentgenograms   Pneumonia
Sinus roentgenograms   Sinusitis
Pulmonary function tests   Findings abnormal
Gastrointestinal studies   Findings abnormal in celiac disease; abnormal D-xylose absorption in malabsorption
Antinuclear antibody   Positive findings in presence of autoimmune disease

Differential diagnoses that must be excluded include chronic mucocutaneous candidiasis, Nezelof syndrome, and drug-induced IgA deficiency

•••••• Multidisciplinary Plan

Since no replacement therapy is yet available, treatment is aimed at management of recurrent infections and serial assessment for the presence of autoimmune and neoplastic disease.

Medications

Antibiotic therapy according to system involved and culture results

General Management

Gluten-free diet for celiac disease
Chest physical therapy, breathing exercises, postural drainage, and oxygen therapy as prophylaxis or for treatment of chronic pulmonary disease
Serial sinus and chest roentgenograms and pulmonary function tests to follow the disease course and determine adequacy of treatment
Follow-up for, and treatment of, concomitant and autoimmune or neoplastic disease as needed
Administration of IgA-deficient blood products to prevent future antigen-antibody reaction

NURSING CARE

Nursing Assessment

Recurrent Infection

Sinusitis; pneumonia; gastrointestinal infections; genitourinary infections

Gastrointestinal Status

Symptoms of celiac disease

Presence of Concomitant Autoimmune Disease

Signs and symptoms associated with systemic lupus erythematosus, rheumatoid arthritis, dermatomyositis, pernicious thyroiditis, anemia, Sjögren's syndrome, allergic conditions

Nursing Dx & Intervention

The majority of IgA-deficient patients are asymptomatic; the rest may seek treatment for infections. See "Acquired Hypoglobulinemia," p. 1180, for sinopulmonary or gastrointestinal infections, and Chapter 13 for other infections.

■ DISORDERS OF COMPLEMENT

Primary deficiency or dysfunction of complement components in the classical pathway increases host susceptibility to infection. In acquired complement disorders, particularly immune complex disease, activation of complement and subsequent inflammatory mediator involvement may cause increased tissue damage.

The classical and alternative complement systems (see Figure 14-9) play an integral role in the amplification of nonspecific host defense mechanisms to invading organisms and in clearance of circulating immune complexes from the serum.

Complement proteins are present in the serum in inactive form, and activation leads to biologic activity. Activation occurs in a cascade fashion and is regulated by four complement proteins.

Certain complement components, when activated, generate chemotactic factors, enhancing the accumulation of leukocytes at an inflammatory site. Other components are deposited on the surface of bacteria, enhancing their ingestion of phagocytic cells (opsonization). The terminal components (C5 to C9) have the capacity to mediate direct lysis of certain bacteria. Complement attaches to circulating immune complexes, decreasing their solubility and thus increasing their removal from the serum.

Primary complement disorders account for less than 1% of primary immunodeficiencies. Deficiency or dysfunction has been identified for each of the classical complement components; none have been identified in the alternative pathway. Certain of these disorders, especially those late in the cascade, have a benign clinical course, but as many as 5% of these patients have severe *Neisseria* infections.

In contrast, defects involving key complement components that regulate the complement cascade or components early in the cascade may be associated with severe, recurrent infections or autoimmune diseases.

Secondary complement deficiencies arise when a disease process causes decreased synthesis or triggers increased consumption. With increased activation, as occurs in immune complex disease, tissue damage often occurs because of the inflammatory mechanisms modulated by complement.

• • • • • • Pathophysiology

A brief schema of the sequence of activation is shown in Figure 14-10.

With deficiency or dysfunction in one of the classical complement components, activation of the normal cascade can occur only to the deficient component. Activation of the remainder of the pathway theoretically should not occur. However, because the classical and alternative pathways share the same terminal components, activation through a different regulatory point in the cascade can compensate for the deficiency.

Deficiencies in the C1, C4, and C2 proteins are the most commonly reported. C2 deficiency occurs in 1 in 10,000 persons. Persons with these deficiencies may be in good health and usually do not have difficulties with recurrent infections. When infections do develop, bacterial rather than viral organisms are involved. In addition, as many as 50% of persons with C2 deficiency have autoimmune disease, particularly systemic lupus erythematosus and juvenile rheumatoid arthritis.

Clinically, C3 is one of the most important complement components because of its place in the complement cascade, and C3 deficiency is the most severe disorder identified. Patients with this abnormality have recurrent, fulminant, pyogenic bacterial infections. C3 deficiency may result from a genetic defect in production. Some persons, including those with nephritic factor, have serum factors that continuously activate and thus deplete C3. Other persons lack C3bI, a regulatory protein that prevents continuous consumption of C3 once the alternative pathway is activated.

Terminal complement component deficiencies (C5 through C9) have also been identified. Many affected persons are asymptomatic. Others may manifest an increased incidence of infection with *Neisseria gonorrhoeae* and *N. meningitidis*. Although persons with C9 deficiency have been identified, this abnormality has not been associated with clinical disease. These persons show normal resistance to infection with bacterial, viral, and fungal organisms.

In C5 dysfunction all levels of complement components including C5 are normal, but serum chemotactic and opsonic activities are reduced because of a defect in C5 activity. Clinical features of C5 dysfunction resemble those of C5 deficiency. Susceptibility to recurrent infections, particularly of the skin and gastrointestinal tract, is increased.

C1 inhibitor deficiency is also known as hereditary angioedema. C1 inhibitor is a regulatory protein that controls activation of C1. Continuous activation of C1 with resultant depletion of C2 and C4 may be due to a failure of this control protein to "turn off" primary pathway activation once initiated. Possibly deficiency of C1 inhibitor, which also inhibits kinin activation, allows kinin formation with subsequent vascular permeability and tissue edema, leading to angioedema.

Association of primary complement disorders with various autoimmune diseases is common (Table 14-2), although the cause is unknown.

TABLE 14-2 Complement Component Deficiencies and Associated Diseases

Component	Collagen-Vascular Diseases*	Infections‡	Other
C1q	+	+	Glomerulonephritis; immunodeficiencies
C1r	+	+	Glomerulonephritis
C1s	+	+	
C4	+	−	
C2	+	+	Glomerulonephritis
C3	+	+	Nephritis
C5	+	+	
C6	+	+	
C7	+	+	
C8	+	+	
C9	−	+	
I‡	−	+	
H‡	−	−	Hemolytic uremic syndrome
Properdin‡	−	−	
C1INH‡	+	+	Hereditary angioedema

*A variety of autoimmune diseases have been described.
†A variety of infective organisms have been identified.
‡Control proteins.

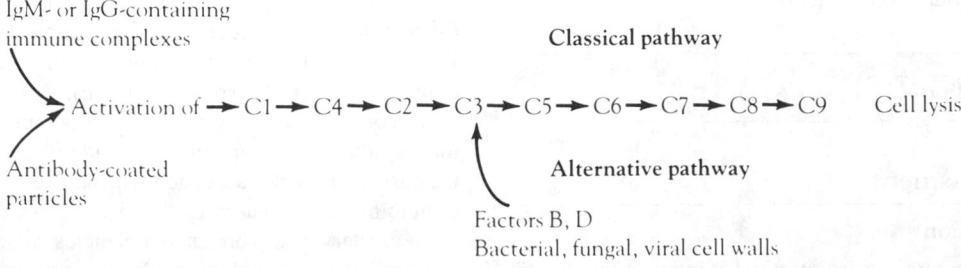

IgM- or IgG-containing immune complexes

Antibody-coated particles

Activation of → C1 → C4 → C2 → C3 → C5 → C6 → C7 → C8 → C9   Cell lysis

Classical pathway

Alternative pathway

Factors B, D
Bacterial, fungal, viral cell walls

Figure 14-10 Sequence of complement activation.

Secondary disorders of complement have multiple pathophysiologic mechanisms. The degree of complement disorder will vary with the severity of the underlying disease process. In extreme protein deficiency states, decreased synthesis results in overall depression of the total complement component quantities resulting in inadequate host defense.

Various disease states may result in increased complement consumption. In fulminant bacterial infections, complement is consumed and production cannot meet demand.

Complement activation is an integral component of the pathophysiology of diseases associated with circulating immune complexes. With involvement of complement, and resultant inflammatory response, tissue damage occurs. Degree of complement activation correlates with activity of disease and is often monitored as an indicator of disease activity or response to therapy.

The following are some of the factors associated with secondary disorders of complement:

Decreased synthesis
  Asplenia
  Sickle cell disease
  Protein-deficient states
    Cirrhosis
    Malnutrition
    Severe burns
    Anorexia nervosa
  Newborns (up to 6 months)
Increased consumption
  Acute nephritis
  Partial lipodystrophy
  Immune complex diseases, especially systemic lupus erythematosus
  Bacteremia, endotoxins
  Dialysis (renal, plasmapheresis, heart-lung)

•••••• Diagnostic Studies and Findings

History Recurrent bacterial infections, autoimmune disease
Physical examination Dependent on disease process
Laboratory findings Serum complement protein levels*
Classical pathway†
  C1q, 7 mg/dl
  C1r, 3.4 mg/dl
  C1s, 3.1 mg/dl
  C4, 50 mg/dl
  C2, 2.5 mg/dl
  C3, 160 mg/dl
  C5, 8 mg/dl
  C6, 7.5 mg/dl
  C7, 5.5 mg/dl
  C8, 8 mg/dl
  C9, 5.8 mg/dl

Alternative pathway
  Factor B, 20 mg/dl
  Factor D, 0.2 mg/dl
  Properdin, 1.5 mg/dl
Control proteins
  C1q inhibitor, 12.5 mg/dl
  C3b inactivator (factor I), 2.5 mg/dl
  Anaphylatoxin inactivator, 5 mg/dl
  C4 binding protein, 25 mg/dl
  S protein, 50 mg/dl
  Factor H, 50 mg/dl
CH50, 20 to 40 units/ml*

•••••• Multidisciplinary Plan

No therapy is available for direct treatment of complement disorders. With primary complement disorders, aggressive management of infections is indicated. Management of hereditary angiodema is discussed elsewhere in this text.

In secondary complement disorders, management of the disease process should restore normal complement levels. The reader is referred elsewhere in this text for management of individual diseases.

ACQUIRED IMMUNE DEFICIENCY SYNDROME[5,19]

Acquired immune deficiency syndrome (AIDS) is a condition characterized by dysfunction of cell-mediated (i.e., T-cell) immunity. The progressive decrease in the CD4 helper subset of T-lymphocytes results in the clinical manifestations of immunosuppression and susceptibility to numerous opportunistic infections (e.g., *Pneumocystis carinii* pneumonia) and neoplasms (e.g., Kaposi's sarcoma).

In 1981, the initial cases of AIDS were reported. By 1982, the syndrome was being identified in certain high-risk groups (i.e., homosexual men, IV drug users, hemophiliacs, and Haitians). In 1983, the human immunodeficiency virus (HIV-1) was discovered, and by 1985 a blood test was available that could identify individuals infected with the HIV virus before they developed AIDS. With the advent of the blood test, most clinicians began to think about the spectrum of HIV disease, which ranges from asymptomatic seropositivity to full-blown AIDS.

Infection with the HIV-1 virus has reached epidemic proportions worldwide. Recent estimated suggest that 5 to 10 million people worldwide are infected with HIV-1 or related retroviruses. Most of these individuals will develop symptomatic and progressive disease associated with profound immunosuppression. Two of the most common conditions associated with full-blown AIDS are Kaposi's sarcoma and *Pneumocystis carinii* pneumonia.

---

*C3, C4, and CH50 assays are available in most laboratories. Reference laboratories generally perform other assays. Numbers will be decreased in specific complement deficiency. With control protein abnormalities, succeeding component will be depressed.
†Detects quantity and not functional capacity. Ranges vary among laboratories.

---

*Indicative of classical pathway integrity; measures the dilution of serum required to lyse 50% of a standard number of antibody-coated sheep red blood cells; normal values determined within each laboratory.

Kaposi's Sarcoma

Kaposi's sarcoma (KS) is the neoplastic disease most frequently associated with AIDS. Kaposi's sarcoma is a malignant tumor of the endothelium, the layer of epithelial cells that lines the cavity of the heart, blood vessels, lymphoid tissues, and serous cavities. In its most benign form, KS is usually limited to the skin, particularly of the lower extremities. Until recently, this form affected only select populations, including Jewish and Italian men over 50 years of age, and severely immunocompromised persons such as organ transplant recipients and cancer patients receiving immunosuppressive drug therapy.

The incidence of KS is estimated to be 20,000 times greater among HIV-infected individuals than in the general population. Since 1989, the incidence of KS in HIV-infected individuals in the United States is approximately 15%. AIDS-associated KS is seen more frequently among homosexual or bisexual men with AIDS than in other groups infected with the virus. These data suggest that HIV infection itself is not sufficient to account for the increased incidence of KS, but that other factors may be important in the pathogenesis of the neoplasm.

Kaposi's sarcoma usually presents as a nonblanching red macule skin lesion. As the skin lesions increase in size, they become surrounded by ecchymosis and become more violet in color. Skin lesions may appear at multiple sites and can occur at any site on the skin. Lymphatic involvement is not unusual and KS may present as lymphadenopathy. Kaposi's sarcoma may also occur in the trachea, lungs, and gastrointestinal tract. Clinical symptoms associated with pulmonary involvement include dyspnea and fever. Gastrointestinal involvement is manifested as nonspecific abdominal complaints and low-grade blood loss. The most significant morbidity associated with KS is lymph node involvement with subsequent lymphedema of the lower extremities, groin, and head and neck.

Pneumocystis carinii Pneumonia

Pneumonia due to *Pneumocystis carinii* is the most common pulmonary infection in patients with HIV disease. In the United States, *Pneumocystis carinii* pneumonia (PCP) is the initial opportunistic infection in 50% to 60% of AIDS patients. Eventually 70% to 80% of AIDS patients will experience one or more episodes of PCP. Approximately 10% to 50% of the episodes of PCP are fatal, and PCP accounts for nearly 50% of the deaths caused by opportunistic infections in persons with AIDS.

P. carinii is a protozoan organism that is ubiquitous in the environment. Usually a benign flora in the healthy population, it is an aggressive pathogen in immunocompromised individuals. Until the advent of AIDS, PCP was considered a relatively rare complication in cancer patients receiving chemotherapy, transplant patients, and patients with congenital defects in cellular immunity.

This opportunistic infection produces fever, cough, and dyspnea. The organism assaults the pulmonary tissue and results in diffuse, bilateral interstitial infiltrates and alveolar infiltration by exudates of many clumped organisms or cysts.

Opportunistic Infections

Listed below are some of the ever-growing number of opportunistic infections associated with AIDS:

Protozoal
   Pneumocystis carinii pneumonia
   Toxoplasmosis
   Cryptosporidiosis
   Giardiasis
   Isospora belli
Fungal
   Candidiasis
   Coccidiodomycosis
   Cryptococcus neoformans
   Histoplasmosis
   Aspergillosis
Viral
   Cytomegalovirus (CMV)
   Herpes (HSV)
   Epstein-Barr virus
   Progressive multifocal leukoencephalopathy
Bacterial
   Mycobacterium avium-intracellulare
   Salmonella
   Shigella
   Clostridium difficile
   Mycobacterium tuberculosis

The occurrence of these opportunistic infections in patients with HIV disease is consistent with findings that the immune deficiency is characterized by T-cell dysfunction.

Populations at Risk

In 1993, the Centers for Disease Control and Prevention expanded the AIDS definition (see box below). Current estimates are that 1 million Americans are infected with HIV. The modes of transmission of HIV are similar to those of hepatitis B. The risk of sexual transmission varies with particular sexual practices; anal intercourse is associated with the highest risk.

In the United States, 63% of AIDS cases are reported in gay or bisexual men and 23% are intravenous drug users. The remainder of the cases occur in infants of infected mothers, heterosexual contacts of infected individuals, and recipients of contaminated blood or blood products.

The number of women with AIDS is increasing rapidly. The two major risk factors for women are intravenous drug use and heterosexual contact with an infected partner. The increased incidence of AIDS in women has been associated with an increase in the number of perinatally infected children.

The rate of progression to symptomatic disease is variable (see Emergency Alert box on p. 1188). Once clinical symptoms develop, outcomes are variable. With improvements in treatments, patients are living longer with the disease. Mean survival after the first episode of PCP is 18 to 24 months. Survival after diagnosis of HIV-related lymphomas is approximately 8 months.

■ CDC AIDS CASE DEFINITION FOR SURVEILLANCE OF ADULTS AND ADOLESCENTS

DEFINITIVE AIDS DIAGNOSES (WITH OR WITHOUT LABORATORY EVIDENCE OF HIV INFECTION)

1. Candidiasis of the esophagus, trachea, bronchi, or lungs.
2. Cryptococcosis, extrapulmonary.
3. Cryptosporidiosis with diarrhea persisting >1 month.
4. Cytomegalovirus disease of an organ other than the liver, spleen, or lymph nodes.
5. Herpes simplex virus infection causing a mucocutaneous ulcer that persists longer than 1 month; or bronchitis, pneumonitis, or esophagitis of any duration.
6. Kaposi's sarcoma in a patient <60 years of age.
7. Lymphoma of the brain (primary) in a patient <60 years of age.
8. *Mycobacterium avium* complex or *Mycobacterium kansasii* disease, disseminated (at a site other than or in addition to lungs, skin, or cervical or hilar lymph nodes).
9. *Pneumocystis carinii* pneumonia.
10. Progressive multifocal leukoencephalopathy.
11. Toxoplasmosis of the brain.

DEFINITIVE AIDS DIAGNOSES (WITH LABORATORY EVIDENCE OF HIV INFECTION)

1. Coccidioidomycosis, disseminated (at a site other than or in addition to lungs or cervical or hilar lymph nodes).
2. HIV encephalopathy.
3. Histoplasmosis, disseminated (at a site other than or in addition to lungs or cervical or hilar lymph nodes).
4. Isosporiasis with diarrhea persisting >1 month.
5. Kaposi's sarcoma at any age.
6. Lymphoma of the brain (primary) at any age.
7. Other non-Hodgkin's lymphoma of B cell or unknown immunologic phenotype.
8. Any mycobacterial disease caused by mycobacteria other than *Mycobacterium tuberculosis,* disseminated (at a site other than or in addition to lungs, skin, or cervical or hilar lymph nodes).
9. Disease caused by extrapulmonary *M. tuberculosis.*
10. *Salmonella* (nontyphoid) septicemia, recurrent.
11. HIV wasting syndrome.
12. CD4 lymphocyte count below 200 cells/μl or a CD4 lymphocyte percentage below 14%.

13. Pulmonary tuberculosis.
14. Recurrent pneumonia.
15. Invasive cervical cancer.

PRESUMPTIVE AIDS DIAGNOSES (WITH LABORATORY EVIDENCE OF HIV INFECTION)

1. Candidiasis of esophagus: (a) recent onset of retrosternal pain on swallowing; and (b) oral candidiasis.
2. Cytomegalovirus retinitis. A characteristic appearance on serial ophthalmoscopic examinations.
3. Mycobacteriosis. Specimen from stool or normally sterile body fluids or tissue from a site other than lungs, skin, or cervical or hilar lymph nodes, showing acid-fast bacilli of a species not identified by culture.
4. Kaposi's sarcoma. Erythematous or violaceous plaque-like lesion on skin or mucous membrane.
5. *Pneumocystis carinii* pneumonia: (a) a history of dyspnea on exertion or nonproductive cough of recent onset (within the past 3 months); and (b) chest x-ray evidence of diffuse bilateral interstitial infiltrates or gallium scan evidence of diffuse bilateral pulmonary disease; and (c) arterial blood gas analysis showing an arterial oxygen partial pressure of <70 mm Hg or a low respiratory diffusing capacity of <80% of predicted values or an increase in the alveolar-arterial oxygen tension gradient; and (d) no evidence of a bacterial pneumonia.
6. Toxoplasmosis of the brain: (a) recent onset of local neurologic abnormality consistent with intracranial disease or a reduced level of consciousness; and (b) brain imaging evidence of a lesion having a mass effect or the radiographic appearance of which is enhanced by injection of contrast medium; and (c) serum antibody to toxoplasmosis or successful response to therapy for toxoplasmosis.
7. Recurrent pneumonia: (a) more than one episode in a 1-year period; and (b) acute (new symptoms, signs, or radiologic evidence not present earlier) pneumonia diagnosed on clinical or radiologic grounds by the patient's physician.
8. Pulmonary tuberculosis: (a) apical or miliary infiltrates and (b) radiographic and clinical response to antituberculosis therapy.

•••••• Pathophysiology

The HIV-1 virus can infect all cells that express the CD4 antigen. Once the virus enters the cell, it causes cell death by an unknown mechanism. The cell primarily infected is the CD4 (helper-inducer) lymphocyte. The CD4 cell directs other cells of the immune system. Other immune cells are also infected by HIV including B-lymphocytes and macrophages. In addition to the immunologic effects of HIV, the virus can cause a variety of neurologic effects.

Clinical findings of HIV disease are consistent with profound immunosuppression. Because T-cell–mediated immunity is important in tumor surveillance and in defense against intracellular pathogens such as viruses, protozoa, mycobacteria, and fungi, deregulation within this component of the body's defensive network results in the development of characteristics of AIDS, such as:

Cutaneous anergy

Leukopenia

Lymphopenia

Decreased T-cell function and reactivity

Reduced or absent T-helper cells

Increased percentage of T-suppressor cells

Depressed natural killer cell activity

Depressed interferon production by peripheral blood leukocytes

Normal or increased immunoglobulin levels

! EMERGENCY ALERT

AIDS—ACQUIRED IMMUNODEFICIENCY SYNDROME

An infection caused by the human immunodeficiency virus (HIV) that is most commonly transmitted through sexual contact, IV drug use, and from mother to unborn child.

Assessment

- Verify or determine HIV status, AIDS status.
- Rule out opportunistic infections as patient is immuno-suppressed.
- Assess for change in level of consciousness, stability of vital signs and nutritional status.
- Rule out potentially life-threatening infections such as *Pneumosystis carinii,* cryptococcal meningitis, cerebral toxoplasmosis.
- Rule out thrombocytopenia, granulocytopenia.

Interventions

- Administer oxygen as indicated by either nasal cannula or mask.
- Obtain clinical evaluation and perform indicated intervention directed at determining cause(s).
- Obtain IV access; in collaboration with physician, administer fluids and medications as appropriate.
- Protect client with altered level of consciousness from injury.
- Provide support and reassure patient and family.

Abnormal immunoglobulin function in some cases
Normal phagocytic function

•••••• Diagnostic Studies and Findings

Enzyme-linked immunoabsorbent assay (ELISA)   Repeated reactivity with confirmation by a second assay such as Western blot
   Polymerase chain reaction (PCR)   Detection of HIV
   White blood cell count   Depressed
   Lymphocyte count   Depressed
   T cell studies   T cell numbers and function depressed; delayed hypersensitivity skin test shows decreased or absent response to cutaneous recall antigens (anergy); T helper/T suppressor cell ratio reversed (less than 0.5)
   Absolute CD4 lymphocyte count   Most widely used predictor of HIV progression. Risk of progression to AIDS high with CD4 <200 cells/μl.
   B cell studies   B cell numbers and function normal or increased; immunoglobulin levels normal or increased
   β₂-microglobulin cell surface protein   Indicative of macrophage-monocyte stimulation. Levels <3.5 mg/dl associated with rapid progression of disease.
   p24 antigen   Indicates active HIV replication
   Natural killer cell activity   Usually depressed
   Complement   Normal to increased
   Cultures   Polymicrobial (fungal, viral, protozoal, and bacterial) infections

Tissue biopsy   Kaposi's sarcoma; *Pneumocystis carinii* pneumonia; lymphoreticular malignancies
   Viral titers   Document exposure to herpes simplex, hepatitis, Epstein-Barr virus, cytomegalovirus; elevated titers may explain panhypergammaglobulinemia
   Chest roentgenogram   Used in initial evaluation of respiratory complaints; pneumonia, pneumonitis, pulmonary infiltrates detected (causative agents determined via culture, bronchoscopy with brushings, or biopsy)
   Gallium scan   Useful in early detection of interstitial pneumonias
   Stool for ova and parasites   Variety of parasites, including *Giardia lamblia* and *Cryptosporidium*
   Neurologic workup, cerebrospinal fluid analysis, brain CT scan, brain biopsy, electromyography, nerve conduction studies, ophthalmic examination, electroencephalogram, magnetic resonance imaging (MRI)   Indicated for evaluation of changes in mentation and fever of unknown etiology; variety of AIDS-associated disorders may be detected, including progressive multifocal leukoencephalopathy, cryptococcal meningitis, encephalitis, organic brain syndrome, and toxoplasmosis
   Staging workup for Kaposi's sarcoma   Skin: photographs and biopsies of representative lesions; nodes: biopsy of accessible nodes, CT scan of abdomen and pelvis; gastrointestinal tract: endoscopy, colonoscopy, and gastrointestinal contrast studies; lung: bronchoscopy (if chest roentgenogram shows abnormalities); liver: CT scan or radioisotope scan; bone: bone scan when alkaline phosphatase level is elevated; see Table 14-3
   Bronchoscopy   *Pneumocystitis carinii* pneumonia (PCP); cryptococcal pneumonia
   Sputum induction   *Pneumocystis carinii* pneumonia (PCP); cryptococcal pneumonia
   Pulmonary function tests   Useful in early detection of interstitial pneumonias
   Serologic antigen test   Cryptococcosis
   Bone marrow biopsy   Histoplasmosis disseminated in bone marrow
   AFB stain   Confirmation of *Mycobacterium tuberculosis*
   Endoscopy   Disseminated CMV in the gastrointestinal tract; *Candida* esophagitis
   Barium swallow   *Candida* esophagitis
   KOH preparation of yeast   Confirmation of oral thrush
   Lumbar puncture   Cryptococcal meningitis
   Ophthalmic examination   Disseminated CMV causing retinitis

•••••• Multidisciplinary Plan

The goals include rapid detection and treatment of opportunistic infections and neoplastic disease, management of signs and symptoms, and prevention of complications from treatment. The ultimate object for treatment of AIDS is reconstitution of the immune system. However, all attempts to correct the underlying immune defect, including bone marrow transplantation, have been unsuccessful.

TABLE 14-3 Staging System of Kaposi's Sarcoma

Stage	Description
I	Cutaneous, locally indolent
II	Cutaneous, locally aggressive with or without regional lymph nodes
III	Generalized mucocutaneous or lymph node involvement
IV	Visceral

Subtypes
A. No systemic signs or symptoms
B. Systemic signs: 10% weight loss or temperature greater than 100° F orally, unrelated to identifiable source of infection, and lasting more than 2 weeks

Generalized: more than upper or lower extremities alone; includes minimal gastrointestinal disease defined as more than five lesions and larger than 2 cm in combined diameters

From Friedman-Kien.[11]

Treatment for individual AIDS patients varies considerably and depends on the degree of immunosuppression and systemic involvement.

Surgery

Placement of a venous access device, such as a Hickman catheter, to facilitate frequent blood drawing, total parenteral nutrition, transfusions, and administration of chemotherapy

Surgical intervention for treatment of malignancies in certain cases

Medications

The development of antiretroviral therapy (i.e., drugs that suppress HIV infection itself) rather than its complications is an important development in the management of HIV disease. In addition, other medications are used to treat the opportunistic diseases associated with AIDS.

Antiretroviral therapy

Zidovudine (AZT), 500 to 600 mg, po, daily in three divided doses

Adverse reactions: anemia, neutropenia, nausea, malaise, headache, insomnia

Didanosine (ddI), 125 to 300 mg, po, twice a day

Adverse reactions: peripheral neuropathy, pancreatitis, dry mouth, hepatitis

Zalcitabine (ddC), 0.375 to 0.75 mg, po, three times a day

Adverse reactions: peripheral neuropathy, aphthous ulcers, hepatitis

Stavudine (d4T), 40 to 60 mg, po, daily (depending on weight) in two to three divided doses

Adverse reactions: peripheral neuropathy, hepatitis, pancreatitis

Antiretrovirals—protease inhibitors

Saquinavir (Invirase), 600 mg (in three capsules), po, three times a day taken within two hours of a meal

Adverse reactions: diarrhea, nausea, mouth ulcers

Ritonavir (Norvir), 600 mg (in six capsules) or 7.5 mL of oral solution, po, twice a day taken with meals; consider mixing the oral solution with chocolate milk or liquid dietary supplement (within one hour of taking the oral solution of the drug to mask the taste)

NOTE: Original po dose may be 300 mg (in capsules) and increasing dosage over time to 600 mg to avoid possible nausea

Adverse reactions: nausea, diarrhea, peripheral paresthesias, taste perversion

Indinavir (Crixivan), 800 mg, po, every 8 hours, taken without food (one hour before or two hours after a meal) but with water

Adverse reactions: nausea, abdominal pain, diarrhea, headache, nephrolithiasis

Kaposi's sarcoma

Interferon Alpha-2a (Roche), 18 to 36 million units, SC, daily for 8 weeks, then three times weekly

Interferon Alpha-2b (Schering), 30 million units, SC, three times weekly

Adverse reactions: nausea, anorexia, diarrhea, fatigue, myalgias, fever, chills, headache

Vincristine, 2 mg, IV, every 2 weeks with vinblastine, 4 to 8 mg, IV, on alternative weeks

Adverse reactions: (vincristine) neuropathic pain, paresthesias, muscle weakness, headache, constipation, leukopenia, alopecia; (vinblastine) bone marrow suppression, nausea, vomiting, anorexia, diarrhea, constipation, numbness, paresthesias, peripheral neuropathy

Prophylaxis against *Pneumocystis carinii* pneumonia (PCP)

Trimethoprim-sulfamethoxazole, 1 double strength tablet, daily or three times weekly

Adverse reactions: nausea, neutropenia, anemia, hepatitis, rash

Dapsone, 100 mg, po, daily

Adverse reactions: nausea, neutropenia, anemia, hepatitis, rash, methemoglobin

Treatment of PCP

Trimethoprim-sulfamethoxazole, 15 mg/kg/day, po or IV, for 14 to 21 days

Adverse reactions: see above

Pentamidine, 3 to 4 mg/kg/day, IV for 14 to 21 days

Adverse reactions: hypotension, hypoglycemia, anemia, neutropenia, pancreatitis, hepatitis

Trimethoprim, 15 mg/kg/day, po with dapsone, 100 mg/day, po, for 14 to 21 days

Adverse reactions: see above

Primaquine, 15 to 30 mg/day, po, and clindamycin, 600 mg, every 8 hours, po, for 14 to 21 days

Adverse reactions: hemolytic anemia in G6PD-deficient patients, methemoglobinemia, neutropenia, colitis

Atovaquone, 750 mg, po, three times a day with meals for 21 days

Adverse reactions: rash, fever, headache, nausea, diarrhea, elevated liver enzymes

Candidiasis

Oral *Candida:* Clotrimazole troches 10 mg, dissolved orally, 5 times daily or nystatin 100,000 swish and swallow, four times a day, or ketoconazole 200 to 400 mg, three times a week, or fluconazole 100 mg, three times weekly

Esophageal *Candida:* Fluconazole 100 to 200 mg, daily or ketaconazole 200 mg, twice a day for 14 to 21 days

Adverse reactions: (clotrimazole) nausea, vomiting; (nystatin) hypersensitivity (ketoconazole) hepatotoxicity, nausea, vomiting, diarrhea, abdominal pain, headache; (fluconazole) nausea, vomiting, diarrhea, abdominal pain, rash, increased liver enzymes, headache

Cryptococcus

Amphotericin, 0.5 to 1.0 mg/kg/day, IV, for 2 to 3 weeks, then fluconazole, 400 mg, daily for 8 to 12 weeks

Adverse reactions: (amphotericin) nephrotoxicity, fever, chills, nausea, vomiting, anorexia, headache, joint pain

Cryptosporidium

Paromomycin, 500 to 750 mg, four times a day, for 15 to 30 days, then 500 mg, twice a day

Adverse reactions: nausea, diarrhea, abdominal cramps

Cytomegalovirus

Ganciclovir, 5 mg/kg, IV, twice a day for 14 to 21 days followed with 6 mg/kg, daily, five times a week or Foscarnet 60 mg/kg, IV, every 8 hours for 14 to 21 days followed with 90 to 120 mg/kg, IV, daily

Adverse reactions: (ganciclovir) granulocytopenia, thrombocytopenia, skin rash, phlebitis, fatigue, nervousness; (foscarnet) nausea, diarrhea, anemia, thrombocytopenia, fever, acute renal failure, seizures, hyper/hypocalcemia, hypokalemia, hypomagnesemia, hyper/hypophosphatemia, genital ulcers

Herpes simplex

Acyclovir 200 mg, five times a day for 10 to 14 days

Adverse reactions: arthralgias, diarrhea, headache, nausea, vomiting, dizziness

Mycobacterium avium **complex**

Clarithromycin, 500 mg, twice a day and clofazamine, 100 to 200 mg, daily with or without ethambutol 15 to 25 mg/kg/day

Adverse reactions: (clarithromycin) headache, diarrhea, nausea, abnormal taste sensation, ototoxicity; (clofazamine) reversible discoloration of the skin, urine, sweat, and feces; abdominal pain, nausea, increased liver enzymes, skin dryness, rash, itching, diarrhea; (ethambutol) increased uric acid levels, increased liver enzymes, optic neuritis, peripheral neuritis, headache, dizziness, nausea, vomiting

Toxoplasmosis

Sulfadiazine 75 mg/kg loading dose followed by 100 mg/kg/day plus pyrimethamine 100 mg, daily for 2 days (loading dose) followed by 50 to 100 mg daily, plus folinic acid, 10 to 20 mg, daily for at least 6 to 9 weeks

Adverse reactions: (sulfadiazine) nausea, anorexia, diarrhea, headache, peripheral neuropathy, impaired folic acid absorption, leukopenia, thrombocytopenia, methemoglobinemia, crystalluria, photosensitivity; (pyrimethamine) megaloblastic anemia, thrombocytopenia, leukopenia, anorexia, vomiting, ataxia, tremors, increased liver enzymes, hypersensitivity reaction; (folinic acid) allergic sensitization

General Management

Chest physiotherapy, postural drainage, positioning, and oxygen therapy in conjunction with antimicrobial therapy if needed for pulmonary infections

Reduction of risk factors for infection: malnutrition, exposure to infectious sources or invasive procedures such as contaminated equipment, frequent venipuncture, or Foley catheterization

Maintenance of adequate hydration, particularly during acute febrile episodes and with administration of nephrotoxic medications or with individuals who have chronic diarrhea

Maintenance of optimal nutritional status with high-calorie, high-protein diet, use of supplemental feedings such as osmolite and Ensure if needed; total parenteral nutrition if necessary

Physical therapy for immobilized patients; regular program of rest and exercise for ambulatory patients

Administration of analgesics as needed to minimize discomfort and pain; assistance with alternative therapies and selection of distracting measures

Support services as appropriate: social workers, clergy, psychologist, psychiatrist, clinical nurse specialist, support groups, involvement of significant others (partner and family) in care

NURSING CARE

Nursing Assessment

As noted earlier, the signs and symptoms of AIDS vary greatly. Clinical manifestations depend on the degree of immunosuppression and the opportunistic infections and neoplasms that develop secondarily. Nonspecific complaints may also occur and are usually exacerbated as the disease progresses.

Assessment

The multiple problems associated with AIDS are included.

Pulmonary

Cough

SOB

Dyspnea

Wheezing
Tachypnea
Cyanosis
Hemoptysis
Intercostal retraction

Neurologic

AIDS dementia complex
  Cognitive
    Memory impairment
    Poor concentration
    Slowed thought processes
    Confusion
  Motor
    Unsteady gait
    Weakness, especially lower extremities
    Decreased hand coordination
    Tremors
    Seizures
  Behavioral
    Decreased animation
    Withdrawal
    Depression
    Emotional liability
    Psychosis
  Other
    Paresthesias
    Paralysis
    Headache
    Nuchal rigidity
    Altered consciousness
    Coma

Ophthalmological

Cotton wool exudate
Photophobia
Blurred vision
Papilledema
Diplopia
Proptosis
Visual field deficits
Blindness

Skin and Mucous Membranes

Oral/esophageal
  White to gray/white patches
    May appear hairy if dried
  Red to purple/brown lesions
    Macular, nodular, or plaque-like
  Gingivitis
Perioral or lips
  Corners of mouth; red fissures; crusted
  Hepatic vesicles
Skin
  Pink/purple to brown lesions
  May appear as bright red subconjunctival mass
  Vesicles

Diaphoresis
Rash
Dryness
Delayed wound healing
Lymphadenopathy: nodes not fixed or hard

Gastrointestinal

Loss of appetite
Difficulty chewing or swallowing: retrosternal pain
Nausea, vomiting
Unintentional weight loss, 10% in 1 to 2 months
Abdominal cramping/pain
Diarrhea, at least 2 stools/day for 1 month
  Intractable
Rectal: bleeding, fissures, itching, pain

Hematological

Splenomegaly
Petechiae
Purpura
Easy bruising
Epistaxis
Gingival bleeding

Systemic

Night sweats
Severe fatigue
Elevated temperature

History

Hepatitis
Sexually transmitted diseases
Frequent viral illnesses
Amebiasis
Exposure to contaminated needles
IV drug use
Recipient of blood or blood products (1978-1984)
Multiple sex partners
Sexual preference
Alcohol use
Support system
Work/productive activities
Fatigue
Stress factors
Previous losses
Coping patterns
Self-concept
Conceptualization of illness

Nursing Dx & Intervention

Impaired gas exchange related to altered alveolocapillary membrane changes caused by *Pneumocystis carinii*

- Assess respiratory status: rate, rhythm, and regularity of respirations; use of accessory muscles; adventitious breath sounds on auscultation, cough, and cyanosis.

- Maintain patent airway at all times.
- Encourage patient to report cough and progressive dyspnea on exertion.
- Obtain sputum specimens as needed *to determine appropriate antibiotic therapy.*
- Monitor results of pulmonary function studies.
- Provide preprocedural teaching before bronchoscopy, lung biopsy, CT scans, pulmonary function tests, and other procedures *to decrease anxiety and ensure informed consent.*
- Provide chest physiotherapy and postural drainage as indicated *to open the airways and mobilize secretions.*
- Instruct patient in breathing exercises such as pursed-lip or diaphragmatic breathing and encourage patient to perform them *to decrease respiratory effort required.*
- Instruct patient in relaxation techniques *to prevent hyperventilation from anxiety caused by shortness of breath.*
- Instruct patient in energy conservation measures during ADLs *to decrease respiratory effort required.*
- Encourage patient to stop smoking *to increase resistance to respiratory infections.*
- In collaboration with physician, determine need for mechanical ventilation if respiratory status worsens or if patient becomes uncomfortable.

Altered nutrition: less than body requirements related to protracted diarrhea, malabsorption, or anorexia

- Assess nutritional status: height and weight, caloric intake, total protein, serum albumin, hematocrit, and hemoglobin levels.
- Determine need for dietary changes, enteral feedings, and total parenteral nutrition.
- Provide vitamin supplements for deficiencies.
- In collaboration with physician, provide prescribed therapy such as antiemetic agents 30 to 60 minutes before meals *to alleviate nausea and aid patient's food tolerance.*
- Provide small, frequent, high-calorie, high-protein feedings *to help patient take in more calories, tolerate food, and regain and maintain weight.* Encourage patient to eat. Have favorite foods brought from home.
- Provide or encourage patient to perform frequent oral hygiene *to prevent oral infection and offer comfort.* Correct stomatitis.
- Monitor intake and output, daily weight, laboratory values, and skin integrity *to monitor nutritional status.*

Diarrhea related to chemotherapy or gastrointestinal infection

- Assess elimination pattern: quality, quantity, and frequency of stool and presence of gross blood, fat, or undigested food.
- Monitor intake and output and daily weight *to determine fluid deficit and weight loss.*
- Monitor vital signs for evidence of hypovolemia.
- Monitor for signs and symptoms associated with fluid and electrolyte imbalance *to determine appropriate replacement therapy.*

- Assess perianal skin condition and provide skin care after every stool *to prevent breakdown;* provide application of skin barrier or fecal incontinence bag if necessary.
- In collaboration with physician, administer and assess effectiveness of prescribed antibiotics and antidiarrheal agents *to determine whether treatment is adequate or changes in regimen are needed.*

Risk for impaired skin integrity related to malnutrition, Kaposi's sarcoma, frequent venipunctures, immobility, or side effects of chemotherapy

- Assess skin integrity: presence of lesions, texture, temperature, moisture, color, vascularity, and evidence of poor wound healing.
- Monitor lesions for signs of infection, desquamation, and other abnormal changes *to prevent further skin breakdown.*
- Provide or encourage patient to perform meticulous hygiene in involved areas *to maintain integrity.*
- For stomatitis: perform regular oral care, avoid acidic oral fluids, provide topical viscous anesthetic, and serve bland foods at medium temperatures *to alleviate pain and discomfort.*
- Provide or encourage use of mild, hypoallergenic, nondrying soaps for skin cleansing and massage with oils and lotions.
- Soak feet and hands in warm water and apply isopropyl alcohol afterward *to prevent or treat fungal infections.*
- If Kaposi's lesions are present, assess response to chemotherapy; note changes in size, color, and configuration *to determine if therapy is adequate.*
- Avoid trauma to the skin. Do not allow more than 2-hour periods of immobilization. Assist with position change *to prevent pressure sores.*
- Encourage mobility within functional limits to facilitate circulation to extremities and pressure points.
- Implement pressure sore care as indicated.
- Use appropriate beds and appliances such as egg-crate mattresses, *to allow pressure relief.*

Pain related to neoplasm, sites of infections, or peripheral neuropathy

- Assess pain: location, onset, duration, precipitating or alleviating factors, character, and frequency; have patient use pain rating scale.
- In collaboration with physician, provide appropriate antiinflammatory and analgesic agents. Assess effectiveness and note side effects *to determine whether therapy is relieving patient's pain.*

Altered thought processes related to memory deficits, impaired judgment or orientation

- Assess level of disruptions in cognitive process, interpretation of stimuli, and changes in attention, routine patterns, or emotions.
- Assess level of consciousness and orientation.

- Reorient as needed. Identify self when interacting with patient.
- Use clear, direct terms, giving one direction at a time.
- Redirect misinterpretations of stimuli. Keep conversation reality centered.
- Provide items in environment to maintain orientation.
- Post schedule of activities. Label and keep familiar objects, such as pictures, nearby.
- Give positive reinforcement for participation in activities.
- Assist family in dealing with changes. Enlist family's aid in maintaining reality-based behavior.
- Consider routine administration of analgesic agents *to prevent intolerable pain.*
- Give analgesics with the intent of relieving pain. Suggest that medication will be effective *to stimulate the placebo response.*
- Ensure calm environment and quiet, undisturbed rest periods *to allow patient the opportunity to relax.*
- Use alternative therapies such as massage, visualization, and meditation, and teach relaxation techniques *to minimize patient's perception of pain.*
- Provide diversional activities as tolerated.
- Provide thermal therapy for affected muscles and joints as needed *to promote vasodilation.*
- Consider placement of venous access device if frequent venipuncture is necessary.

Risk for activity intolerance related to weakness, fatigue, side effects of therapy, dyspnea, fever, malnutrition, or fluid and electrolyte imbalances

- Assess degree of activity intolerance.
- Assist with ADLs as needed.
- Encourage regular exercise and rest as tolerated. Confer with physical or occupational therapist *to determine optimal approach.*
- Teach patient energy conservation measures and evaluate response to instruction.
- Monitor tolerance for visits and phone calls. Suggest limits as appropriate *to conserve energy and reduce environmental factors of intolerance.*
- In collaboration with physician, provide appropriate treatment for underlying causes of activity intolerance such as pain, infections, sleeplessness, or malnutrition. Assess effectiveness *to determine if treatment is adequate.*

Anxiety related to diagnosis, poor prognosis, hospitalization, perception of unknown threat, knowledge deficit

- Assess level of anxiety in terms of behaviors and statements.
- Provide atmosphere of individual acceptance.
- Provide opportunities for patient to express feelings.
- Avoid false reassurances but encourage hope. Inform patient of current research findings to stimulate positive mental attitude.
- Engage in honest, consistent communication with patient.

- Provide accurate information about AIDS and related treatment. Include information about diagnostic procedures *to ease fear of the unknown.*
- Increase simplicity, concreteness, and repetitions in communications *to ensure that patient hears, absorbs, and understands information.*
- Explain features of immediate environment *to allow patient self-control.*
- Keep door open and light on at night, visit frequently, and use touch as appropriate *to decrease feelings of isolation and loneliness.*
- Assist patient in identifying signs and symptoms of anxiety. Discuss coping measures with the patient, and encourage the patient and significant others to use them.
- Encourage patient to participate in care as much as possible *to promote feelings of self-control.*
- Involve hospital and community resources *to assist patient and significant others where appropriate.*
- Encourage patient to use available resources *to decrease feelings of isolation.*
- Assess need and monitor effectiveness of psychopharmacologic interventions *to determine whether therapy is adequate.*

Body image disturbance related to weight loss, Kaposi's lesions, or side effects of chemotherapy

- Assess patient's self-concept in terms of statements and behavior.
- Provide atmosphere of acceptance, encourage expression of feelings, and refrain from negative criticism.
- Acknowledge change in body image but focus on identifying strengths and accomplishments. Praise appropriately and emphasize functions that have stabilized or improved.
- Provide accurate information as indicated *to correct myths and clarify controversial information the patient might have seen, heard, or read.*
- Strongly encourage participation in self-care to tolerance, even if tolerance is severely limited, *to enhance self-esteem.*
- Have family and significant others bring in clothes, pajamas from home, and personal toileting items and suggest use of makeup for Kaposi's sarcoma lesions, especially facial lesions.
- Direct patient to appropriate resources: clergy, social workers, psychologist, psychiatrist, or AIDS clinic counselor.
- Encourage patient to participate in AIDS support groups *to increase socialization and feelings of acceptance.*

Risk for infection related to immune deficiency, disease process, effects of chemotherapy, malnutrition, frequent venipunctures, immobility, and environmental pathogens

- Assess skin integrity including pressure areas, oral mucosa, rectum, invasive procedure sites (IVs) for evidence of infection or breakdown.
- Monitor vital signs, especially temperature, every 4 hours and as needed *to note evidence of fever and signs of infection.*

- Monitor laboratory data: WBC count and differential and shifts in these *to note acute stress on the bone marrow or severe bacterial disease.*
- Observe strict aseptic technique for all invasive therapies and procedures.
- Initiate neutropenic precautions per hospital protocol whenever necessary (usually when absolute neutrophil count <1000).
- Restrict contact with visitors and health care providers who have infectious diseases.
- Maintain thorough handwashing before and after patient contact.
- Provide clean environment.
- Protect patient from physical injury.
- Limit environmental stress.
- Promote hygiene and oral care measures.
- Maintain optimal nutritional status and fluid intake.
- Maintain normal sleep and rest patterns.

Risk for injury related to visual, auditory, or tactile changes caused by CNS, HIV, or opportunistic infection

- Assess level of consciousness, behavior, cognitive function, reflexes, vision, and hearing for deficits.
- Maintain needed items, and approach patient within the patient's field of vision.
- Protect eyes using patches and eye medication to prevent injury.
- Maintain objects, furniture, and materials required for self-care or feeding in same place if patient's vision is severely diminished or absent *to allow patient control over activities.* Assist as needed.
- Provide alternate method of communication if hearing is impaired.
- For patient with mental confusion:
  Reorient frequently and remind to call for assistance.
  Check status every 30 minutes and as needed.
  Restrain as appropriate.

Risk for injury related to decreased circulating hemostatic mechanisms

- Assess vital signs every 4 hours and as needed. Note tachycardia, hypotension, pallor, anxiety, and restlessness as signs of internal bleeding.
- Assess body surfaces for ecchymosis, petechiae, and hematomas every 8 hours. Monitor urine, stool, and emesis for heme.
- Implement safety precautions for patients with low platelet counts (<50,000) *to decrease risk of bleeding.*
  Avoid using toothbrushes, use electric razors, do not take rectal temperatures, use side rails and fall precautions, avoid IM injections, avoid use of aspirin, and use stool softeners to prevent rectal bleeding.
- Instruct patient, family, and significant others on safety precautions.

Patient Education/Home Care Planning

1. Explain to the patient the disease process, methods to prevent transmission, and the importance of obtaining current factual information.
2. Discuss with the patient the need to follow safe sex guidelines.
3. Give the patient information about and assist the patient with methods to observe for signs and symptoms of opportunistic infections and cancer complications.
4. Discuss with the patient the risk reduction (see box on p. 1195):
   Maintenance of home environment
   Avoidance of persons with infections
   Prevention of injury to skin
   Promotion of personal hygiene measures
   Management of activity, rest, stress, and nutrition
   Avoidance of high-risk sex behaviors, use of recreational drugs, use of alcohol and tobacco products
5. Provide the patient with information about financial resources and community support: self-help groups, psychologic or psychiatric referrals, home aid, hotlines, or legal resources.
6. Discuss with the patient the importance of regular follow-up care, the need to inform all health care givers about diagnosis, and the need to refrain from donating blood.
7. Stress to the patient the need to wear medic alert identification.
8. Demonstrate to the patient and have the patient and significant other care giver demonstrate the necessary procedures, such as TPN, IV, or aerosol medication administration.

Evaluation

Optimal respiratory status is maintained Arterial blood gases are within normal range. There are no symptoms associated with respiratory distress.

Optimal nutritional status is maintained Albumin and total protein are within normal limits. Weight is approaching normal for patient's height and build.

Frequency and consistency of stools are within normal limits for patient Frequency of stools is reduced and soft consistency returns.

Dermatologic signs and symptoms are improved or controlled Skin integrity is intact. Circulation to affected part is uncompromised.

Pain is managed or minimized Patient reports that pain is reduced to a tolerable level or resolved. Patient can now perform activities, since pain is controlled.

Activity tolerance is increased Patient participates in ADLs. Patient uses energy conservation measures.

Anxiety level is diminished Patient verbalizes understanding of own anxiety and demonstrates methods to manage it.

■ BODY SUBSTANCE ISOLATION (BSI) PRECAUTIONS

All patients are considered infected.

IN HOSPITAL

1. The door to the patient's room need not be closed.
2. Gloves must be worn only if in *direct* contact with specimens, linen, and items or surfaces exposed to blood or body fluids. Gloves need *not* be worn if one is merely conversing with the patient or walking into the room.
3. A mask must be worn if secretions may be aerosolized onto the face during suctioning, oral hygiene, and other procedures. A mask should be worn if a health care worker with a respiratory infection must enter the room of a severely immunosuppressed patient.
4. Protective eyewear should be worn if aerosolization of secretions or blood may contact the conjunctiva (as during suctioning or blood drawing).
5. A moisture resistant gown must be worn if clothing is likely to become contaminated with blood or body fluids, as during bathing of the patient, linen changes, some specimen collections, or dressing changes.
6. Proper isolation technique must be used. Gown and gloves must be removed in the room when used.
7. Specimens must be bagged.
8. Special care in handling contaminated needles is essential. Attempts to recap needles must be avoided, since most needle-stick injuries occur this way. Needles must be disposed of in a puncture-resistant container, which should be sealed before being taken from the room.
9. Handwashing must be performed in the room before and after contact with the patient.
10. Contaminated nondisposable items must be cleaned with soap and water and bagged for autoclaving, wearing personal protective equipment. Items that cannot be auto claved must be washed with soap and water, 10% bleach solution, or other solution recommended in the hospital procedure manual.
11. A private room may be given to patients unable to maintain scrupulous hygiene (those with intractable diarrhea, incontinence, or central nervous system infections leading to altered sensorium).
12. Usually no precautions are needed when handling food trays.
13. Disposable resuscitation equipment (Ambu bags, airways, and so on) must be available at all times.
14. Postmortem handling of the body must include the use of personal protective equipment.

AT HOME

1. Disposable gloves must be worn by family members who come in direct contact with the patient's blood and body fluids.
2. Linen and clothing soiled with secretions or excretions should be washed separately with 10% bleach solution (¼ cup bleach to 1 gallon of water).
3. Dishes and eating utensils do not require separate handling but should be washed in hot, soapy water.
4. Dry waste contaminated with blood or body fluids must be disposed of in a separate container and bagged securely.
5. Any needles used for the administration of medication must be placed in an impervious container before disposal.
6. Meticulous handwashing before and after contact with the patient is essential.

Self-image is improving   Patient participates in own hygiene and grooming. Patient verbalizes realistic expectations. Patient acknowledges personal strengths.

Knowledge is acquired through individual learning experiences   Patient verbalizes accurate information about diagnosis, treatment, and home care; patient demonstrates skills in performing procedures required for home care.

New infectious processes are prevented or minimized   There is no WBC elevation or shift in differential. Sites of infection are stable or healing as evidenced through assessment.

Optimal care is managed at home   Patient demonstrates knowledge of local support systems and resources. Patient completes plans for adequate living arrangements.

Injury is prevented or minimized   There are no falls or other injuries. Patient requests assistance with movement when needed. Patient uses visual and hearing aids appropriately.

Bleeding episodes are prevented or minimized   There are no ecchymoses, petechiae, hematomas, or signs of internal bleeding.

INFLAMMATORY DISEASES

■ WEGENER'S GRANULOMATOSIS[1,8,23,24]

Wegener's granulomatosis is a multisystem disorder of unknown cause characterized by diffuse granuloma formation and vasculitis primarily involving the respiratory tract.

Wegener's granulomatosis occurs in a male to female ratio of 3:2. It may appear at any age, with a peak incidence in the fourth and fifth decades of life.

Signs and symptoms may be widespread but usually occur in the upper or lower respiratory tract and the kidneys. Other manifestations include hearing loss (resulting from recurrent otitis), pericarditis, myocarditis, polyneuropathy, ocular inflammatory disease, arthralgias, and some dermatologic manifestations associated with vasculitis.

Once considered a fatal disease, Wegener's granulomatosis now has a good prognosis when detected early and treated with cyclophosphamide, which is capable of inducing prolonged remission in most cases. However, extensive renal disease is indicative of a poor prognosis.

Pathophysiology

Any organ may become involved with granuloma formation and vasculitis. Although the immunopathogenesis remains an enigma, these manifestations suggest that delayed-type hypersensitivity or cell-mediated reactions may be involved. Immune complex deposition may also occur.

Histologic features include widespread necrotizing vasculitis of small arteries, venules, arterioles, and some capillaries, together with granuloma formation. Almost all patients have pulmonary involvement. Paranasal sinuses and the nasopharynx demonstrate granuloma formation. Pansinusitis may result in erosion of adjacent bones and septum perforation. Sinuses often become secondarily infected with bacteria. Saddle-nose deformity may be observed as well. Diffuse, bilateral, nodular lesions that tend to cavitate are found in lung tissue. Renal findings include necrotizing angiitis, focal glomerulonephritis with thrombosis of glomerular capillaries, crescent formation, glomerular and interstitial necrosis and granuloma formation, progressing to renal failure.

Diagnostic Studies and Findings

Biopsy of affected tissue Granuloma formation; vasculitic lesions

Complete blood count Mild anemia (normochromic, normocytic); lymphocytosis in presence of superimposed infection

Erythrocyte sedimentation rate Elevated during active disease

Serum protein electrophoresis Mild hypergammaglobulinemia (especially IgA)

Renal status Proteinuria, hematuria, and granular or cellular casts

Differential diagnoses include other vasculitides, connective tissue diseases, infectious and noninfectious granulomatous diseases, pulmonary neoplasia, and lymphomatoid granulomatosis.

Multidisciplinary Plan

Medications

Antineoplastic agents (used as immunosuppressant)
Cyclophosphamide (Cytoxan), 1-2 mg/kg/d po; dosage adjusted to maintain total WBC at >3000/mm^3, treatment continued 1 yr after remission is achieved

Corticosteroids
Prednisone; may be added to above regimen if disease course is fulminant; 60 mg recommended as starting dose and should be continued until cyclophosphamide produces therapeutic effect (within 14 d); prednisone should then be tapered and eventually discontinued unless disease course accelerates

---

NURSING CARE

Nursing Assessment

Respiratory Status

Paranasal sinus pain; purulent or blood rhinorrhea; nasal mucosa ulceration; septal perforation; saddle-nose deformity; serous otitis media; epistaxis; chronic cough, pleurisy; dyspnea; chest pain; hemoptysis

Ocular Integrity

Mild conjunctivitis; episcleritis; granulomatosis sclerouveitis; ciliary vessel vasculitis, proptosis

Skin Integrity

Vasculitis dermatitis

Renal Status

Hematuria; abnormal urinalysis findings; intake and output imbalance

Nursing Dx & Intervention

Impaired gas exchange related to alveolar capillary membrane changes

- Assess degree of impairment; monitor blood gases, note presence of cyanosis or respiratory distress, auscultate lungs for presence of adventitious sounds, monitor chest roentgenograms, and note presence of hemoptysis, epistaxis, and sinus pain; report significant abnormal findings to physician.
- Position patient for optimal chest excursion *to facilitate ventilation.*
- Encourage deep breathing and coughing *to move secretions.*
- Assist with ADLs *to conserve patient's energy.*
- In collaboration with physician, institute other interventions (such as oxygen therapy) for related conditions. Assess effectiveness.

Pain related to sinusitis, headache, ocular inflammation, or dermatitis

- Assess pain: location, onset, duration, and precipitating or alleviating factors. Have patient use pain rating scale.
- In collaboration with physician, administer appropriate analgesic and antiinflammatory agents. Assess effectiveness and note side effects.
- Use warm or cold compresses as patient desires *to increase eye or sinus comfort.*
- Maintain low lighting and noise level *to reduce stimuli.*
- Provide soothing baths and application of lotion *to promote increased skin comfort.*

Altered renal tissue perfusion related to exchange problems

- Assess renal status: blood urea nitrogen, serum creatinine, blood pressure, urinalysis results, presence of edema, intake and output balance, and rapid weight gain *to detect and prevent renal compromise.* NOTE: Hypertension is usually *not* present.
- Provide fluids of choice to amount allowed.
- Monitor dietary intake. Provide six small feedings *to meet caloric needs when food tolerance decreases.*
- In collaboration with physician, institute appropriate interventions related to treatment of glomerulonephritis (diet; fluids); assess effectiveness.

Sensory/perceptual alterations (visual) related to altered status of eyes caused by conjunctivitis, episcleritis, or proptosis

- Assess degree of visual impairment.
- Orient patient to location of personal items and furniture; maintain these items in the same position.
- Remind patient to call for assistance with ambulation or unfamiliar activities *to prevent accidents.*
- Arrange food and liquids so spillage does not occur.
- Institute safety precautions *to prevent falls.*

Risk for impaired skin integrity related to altered circulation

- Assess skin integrity: texture, lesions, temperature, moisture, color, and vascularity.
- Monitor lesions for signs of infection and other abnormal changes.
- Provide or encourage patient to maintain meticulous hygiene in involved areas.
- Turn and reposition every 2 hours. Use devices to reduce pressure.

Patient Education/Home Care Planning

1. Provide and discuss with the patient information about cyclophosphamide and steroid therapy.
2. Stress to the patient the importance of regular follow-up visits with a physician and the importance of regular eye examinations.
3. List significant changes for the patient to report: visual impairment, hematuria, oliguria, pyuria, sinusitis, hemoptysis, dyspnea, and vasculitis.
4. Remind the patient of the importance of medical alert identification.

Evaluation

Respiratory status is within normal limits Lungs are clear on auscultation; no respiratory distress or sinusitis is observed.

Pain is controlled Patient states comfort is increasing and appears relaxed.

Renal status is stable Patient's intake and output are balanced. Patient's vital signs and weight are stable. Patient takes diet and fluids allowed.

Vision is normal Patient states vision has returned to normal. No presence of infection is observed. No injuries occurred.

Skin is intact Patient's skin color and turgor are good. No lesions are present.

■ POLYARTERITIS NODOSA[17,24]
■ (Periarteritis nodosa)

Polyarteritis nodosa, a multisystem inflammatory disorder of unknown cause, is characterized by necrotizing inflammation of segments of small arteries.

Polyarteritis nodosa occurs from infancy to old age and affects two to three men for every woman. The onset and clinical presentation of this disorder vary greatly depending on the location of the arteries affected and the severity of the involvement. Widespread lesions may involve arteries of the heart, abdominal mesentery, kidneys, muscles, and vasa vasorum. Involvement of the central nervous system and pulmonary tissue is unusual.

Although the cause remains an enigma, some evidence suggests that this type of vasculitis may result from immune complex deposition in tissues following exposure to an infectious antigen. The findings of hepatitis B surface antigen (Hb_SAg) in the sera of 30% to 40% of these patients further suggests that this may be true.

Drugs have been implicated as causes. Suspected agents include sulfonamides, penicillin, phenytoin, arsenicals, thiouracil, iodides, thiazides, and parenteral methamphetamine.

The prognosis of polyarteritis nodosa is guarded. Renal involvement denotes rapid disease progression. Death often occurs from renal failure, myocardial infarction, heart failure, infection, or gastrointestinal bleeding. However, with early diagnosis and treatment, the 5-year survival rate is 80%.

•••••• Pathophysiology

The inciting agent that leads to inflammation within the blood vessels is unknown. The inflammatory process is characterized by early infiltration of polymorphonuclear leukocytes. New lesions are often surrounded by older lesions characterized by cells that respond late in the inflammatory reaction—monocytes, lymphocytes, and plasma cells. This suggests that the inflammatory process involved in polyarteritis is chronic, although subjected to repeated insults, perhaps by antigen that is continuously available.

Chronic inflammation within the vessel walls leads to obliteration and ischemia of involved tissues as the lesion evolves. Finally, the vessel is replaced by fibrous tissue. Blood supply to major organs and other structures diminishes. Tissue ischemia and infarction are the notable outcomes.

●●●●● Diagnostic Studies and Findings

No specific laboratory tests exist for polyarteritis nodosa. The abnormalities observed depend largely on the organ systems affected. Differential diagnoses include systemic lupus erythematosus, trichinosis, heart failure, and infection.

White blood count   Elevated owing to neutrophilia

Erythrocyte sedimentation rate   Elevated during acute phase

Angiography   Detects characteristic aneurysms at bifurcation points of arteries in kidneys, mesentery, liver, pancreas, and so on (acute), or narrowing and thrombosis of involved arteries (late)

Tissue histologic studies   Necrotizing inflammation of segments of medium and small arteries; aneurysms at areas of arterial bifurcation; invasion of tissue by polymorphonuclear leukocytes and monocytes

●●●●● Multidisciplinary Plan

Medications

Corticosteroids
  Prednisone, 40-60 mg to start; tapered gradually
Antineoplastic agents
  Used as immunosuppressants; use controversial (e.g., cyclophosphamide, 2 mg/kg/d) but has been successful in some cases, particularly when corticosteroid therapy has failed

NURSING CARE

Nursing Assessment

Nonspecific Manifestations

Fever; weakness; anorexia; weight loss

Kidneys

Glomerulitis; glomerulosclerosis; progressive renal failure; hypertension

Gastrointestinal Tract

Abdominal pain; anorexia; nausea and vomiting; mucosal ulceration and hemorrhage; appendicitis; cholecystitis; hepatitis; bowel infarction or perforation; pancreatitis

Heart

Coronary arteritis; myocardial ischemia or infarction; pericarditis; congestive heart failure

Lungs

Asthma: bronchitis; pneumonia

Cutaneous

Subcutaneous nodules (5 to 10 mm) along course of arteries in extremities; purpuric, urticarial exanthemata; subcutaneous hemorrhage; ulcerations; livedo reticularis; ischemic changes of distal digits

Muscles

Muscle weakness; myalgias

Central Nervous System

Headache; seizures; papillitis; meningeal irritation; peripheral neuropathy

Testes

Pain; edema

Genitourinary

Hemorrhagic cystitis, dysuria

Nursing Dx & Intervention

Altered Tissue Perfusion Related to Interruption of Flow or Exchange Problems:

Renal, related to glomerulonephritis, glomerulosclerosis, or failure

- Assess for development of glomerulonephritis, renal failure, and hypertension. Monitor blood urea nitrogen, creatinine, hemoglobin, hematocrit, blood pressure, urinalysis results, presence of edema and rapid weight gain, and symptoms associated with hypertension (headache and visual disturbances). Report significant findings to physician.
- Monitor intake and output.
- Provide restricted diet and fluids as allowed.

Gastrointestinal, related to ulceration, hemorrhage, infarction, perforation, or cholecystitis

- Assess for presence of abdominal pain, anorexia, nausea, vomiting, and findings compatible with gastrointestinal ulceration or hemorrhage, appendicitis, cholecystitis, hepatitis, or pancreatitis.
- Palpate abdomen *to detect areas of tenderness or pain.*
- Perform Hemoccult or guiaic test of stool *to check for gastrointestinal blood loss.*
- Report significant findings to physician.

Cardiopulmonary related to myocardial ischemia infarction, congestive heart failure, or bronchitis

- Assess for myocardial and pleural changes:
    Monitor serial electrocardiograms and chest roentgenograms.
    Auscultate chest for presence of pericardial friction rub or adventitious breath sounds.
    Monitor serial cardiac enzymes.
- Monitor vital signs.
- Report significant findings to physician.
- Position patient for optimum chest excursion and comfort.
- Teach and assist patient with stress-reducing measures.

- Plan care with patient to schedule periods of rest. Assess response to increasing activities.

Peripheral, related to muscle and subcutaneous changes

- Assess skin for presence of ecchymosis, purpura, ulcerations, gangrene, and vasculitic lesions.
- Monitor lesions for signs of infection and other abnormal changes.
- Provide meticulous skin care using mild, nondrying hypoallergenic soaps for cleansing.
- In collaboration with physician, provide appropriate treatment for lesions as ordered. Assess effectiveness.
- Protect skin from further injury: use paper or cloth tape; apply dressings loosely; avoid venipunctures.
- Gently massage skin *to promote circulation to area.*

Cerebral, related to occlusion and sclerosis

- Assess for development of headache, changes in sensorium, seizures, and papilledema *to determine presence of cerebral edema, anoxia.*
- Perform mental status examination *to assess level of consciousness and overall mentation.*
- Perform ophthalmic examination of fundus and disc *to determine presence of cerebral edema.*
- Provide for patient's safety *to prevent injury.*

Impaired physical mobility related to muscle weakness

- Assess degree of physical limitations: perform neuromusculoskeletal assessment.
- Provide progressive physical and occupational therapy. Encourage patient's participation.
- Provide for patient's safety *to prevent injury.*
- Assist with activities of daily living as needed.

Pain related to tissue and organ ischemia resulting from vasculitis

- Assess pain: location, onset, duration, and precipitating and alleviating factors. Have patient describe intensity, using rating scale.
- In collaboration with physician, provide appropriate analgesic agents. Assess effectiveness and note side effects.
- Teach and assist patient with alternative pain-relieving techniques: visual imagery or music therapy.
- Position patient for comfort, using pressure-reducing or support materials.

Patient Education/Home Care Planning

1. Teach the patient methods of self-assessment, and emphasize the importance of reporting significant changes to the physician. Teach the patient to monitor the patient's blood pressure, pulse, weight, proteinuria, edema, intake, and output. Instruct the patient to report dyspnea, unexplained weight gain, proteinuria, oliguria, hematuria, hypertension, abnormal changes in the eyes, paresis, new pain, and melena.
2. Give the patient information about medications, and stress the importance of not stopping medications without the physician's knowledge.
3. Outline diet for the patient to follow. Arrange consultation for the patient when needed.
4. Provide the patient with information about needed rest, alternating with increasing activity as tolerance improves.
5. Teach the patient alternative methods for pain relief: relaxation techniques, biofeedback, and guided imagery.
6. Teach the patient to keep a log of the disease course, the treatments, and the other disease-related information. Stress to the patient the importance of keeping follow-up medical appointments.
7. Teach the patient to carry medical identification (especially if the patient is taking steroids).

Evaluation

Renal function is maintained Patient's intake and output are balanced. Weight and blood pressure are within patient's normal limits; patient follows restricted dietary and fluid plan.

Gastrointestinal function is maintained Nausea and vomiting are absent; no presence of bleeding is noted; normal bowel pattern is achieved.

Cardiopulmonary status is within normal limits Patient's vital signs are stable; no ectopic rhythms are present; heart and breath sounds are normal.

Peripheral circulation is normal Patient's skin is warm and dry, with good turgor. No lesions or discoloration are present.

Central nervous system is intact Patient is alert and oriented, without complaints of headache or visual disturbances.

Mobility is maintained Patient performs ADLs without limitation.

Pain is controlled Patient's body posture and face are relaxed; patient states that comfort is achieved.

 ## GIANT CELL ARTERITIS[24,28]

(Temporal arteritis)

Giant cell arteritis is an inflammatory disorder of unknown etiology that affects large and medium-sized arteries, especially those branching from the proximal aorta that supply the neck and the extracranial structure of the head and arms.

Giant cell arteritis affects persons of both sexes usually older than 50 years of age. It is twice as common in women as men. This disease is rarely seen in blacks. Any artery or the aorta may be involved, but the diagnosis is often made through biopsy of the temporal artery. Patients initially show nonspecific systemic signs, including fever. Morning headaches are frequent. Other clinical findings are related to the arteries involved.

Although the etiology is unknown, the disease may have some basis in immunologic dysfunction similar to that of other vasculitides such as polyarteritis nodosa. Cellular and humoral mechanisms reactive against elastic arterial tissue may play a role.

The prognosis for giant cell arteritis is good, particularly when major vessels are uninvolved. The disease tends to be self-limited in 2 to 5 years, but the threat of blindness makes treatment imperative. Patients respond dramatically to corticosteroid therapy with remission of clinical manifestations and lowering of the erythrocyte sedimentation rate, which can be serially monitored for recurrence of inflammatory episodes.

•••••• Pathophysiology

Giant cell arteritis is distinguishable from other vasculitides because small vessels such as arterioles and capillaries are not involved. Histologic characteristics include the accumulation of histiocytes, epithelioid cells, multinucleated giant cells, lymphocytes, and plasma cells in the interna and media adjacent to the internal elastic lamina of medium-sized arteries. The elastic lamina is fragmented and may be absent in some areas. In large arteries and the aorta the media tends to be inflamed, with fragmentation of the elastic fibers. The intima is thickened more than would be expected from age alone. The lesions are spotty and do not involve long stretches of arteries. Thrombosis may occur at inflammation sites.

•••••• Diagnostic Studies and Findings

Giant cell arteritis should be suspected in any elderly person who has a fever of unknown origin and an elevated erythrocyte sedimentation rate. It is often associated with polymyalgia rheumatica.

Erythrocyte sedimentation rate   Greater than 50 mm/hour

Temporal artery biopsy   Positive; demonstrates lymphocyte infiltration and giant cells in vessel wall

Muscle enzyme   Normal

Electromyography   Normal

Muscle biopsy   Normal

Complete blood count   Anemia, normochromic, normocytic

Gammaglobulin   Diffuse increased, α-globulin increased

•••••• Multidisciplinary Plan

Medications

Corticosteroids

Prednisone, 60 mg po tapered for 2-4 wk until symptoms abate and erythrocyte sedimentation rate returns to normal; maintenance dose 10 mg or less po qd until disease is controlled clinically; alternate-day therapy

not successful; can be discontinued eventually in most patients; monitor for side effects associated with steroid therapy

Vitamin D

Calcium

NURSING CARE

Nursing Assessment[43]

Temporal Artery

Warm, tender, red, with or without nodules

Ophthalmic

Intermittent blurring, diplopia to visual loss (insidious or sudden onset)

Cerebrovascular

Transient ischemic attacks, stroke, cranial nerve palsies

Cardiovascular

With aorta involvement—myocardial ischemia, peripheral claudication

Systemic Signs and Symptoms

Fever; malaise; anorexia; morning headache

Nursing Dx & Intervention

Altered tissue perfusion related to interruption of arterial flow

Cerebral

- Assess temporal artery for warmth, redness, tenderness, or diffuse headache. Assess visual acuity, mental status, level of consciousness, and motor function. Monitor vital signs and visual acuity.
- Position for comfort. Usually the head is elevated 30 to 60 degrees on bed rest.
- Assess effectiveness of administered analgesics.
- Encourage and assist with ambulation as needed.

Peripheral

- Assess quality of pulses, skin color, temperature, and turgor.
- Encourage ambulation and range of motion exercises.
- Discourage activities that decrease blood flow, such as crossing the legs, or activities that may cause injury.

Cardiopulmonary

- Assess for myocardial ischemia and infarction: monitoring for angina, monitoring of serial electrocardiograms, monitoring of chest roentgenograms, auscultation of heart to determine rate, rhythm, and regularity of pulse, monitoring of cardiac enzymes, monitoring of vital signs.

- Position patient for comfort *to ease respirations and chest pain.*
- Assist patient with learning stress-reducing activities.

Risk for sensory/perceptual alteration: visual related to altered status of the ophthalmic and retinal arteries

- Assess visual acuity and report negative changes immediately.
- Familiarize patient with immediate surroundings.
- Maintain safety precautions *to prevent injuries.*
- Encourage self-care. Assist with only those activities that patient is unable to perform because of other incapacities.

Patient Education/Home Care Planning

1. Provide patient with information about steroid therapy. Stress to the patient the importance of not stopping medications without notifying physician.
2. List signs and symptoms that the patient must report to the physician concerning recurrence of disease process, especially any eye changes.
3. Discuss with the patient the self-limiting aspect of the disease process.
4. Stress to the patient the need to wear medical alert identification, to inform all health care workers about treatment, and to keep appointments for follow-up care.

Evaluation

CNS status is stable   Patient has no redness, warmth, or tenderness over temporal artery site; patient reports no headache, is alert, and is oriented, with good motor activity and coordination.

No peripheral claudication is present   Patient's peripheral pulses are palpable, regular, and of good quality. Patient's skin is warm, dry, and intact, with good turgor.

Cardiopulmonary status is stable   Patient reports no chest pain; ECG shows no ectopy; vital signs are stable.

Visual acuity is normal   Patient reports no blurring of vision, diplopia, or diminished vision; patient uses safety precautions in presence of diminished vision.

■ POLYMYALGIA RHEUMATICA

Polymyalgia rheumatica is a well-defined inflammatory disorder of the proximal muscles that usually affects women more than men older than 50 years of age. It is a self-limiting condition.

Polymyalgia rheumatica is accompanied by a highly elevated erythrocyte sedimentation rate and is often diagnosed on the basis of a rapid clinical response to corticosteroid therapy. The onset may be acute or insidious and is associated with pain and morning stiffness in the back and neck, as well as in the pelvic and shoulder girdles.

•••••• Pathophysiology

The origin and pathogenesis of polymyalgia rheumatica are unknown. Although elevation of the erythrocyte sedimentation rate is indicative of an inflammatory process, and despite the severe pain associated with the muscle involvement, findings of muscle examinations are normal.

•••••• Diagnostic Studies and Findings

Erythrocyte sedimentation rate   Elevated (often greater than 100 mm/hour)

Red blood cells   Anemia (normochromic, normocytic)

Corticosteroid challenge   Rapid, dramatic response

Creatine phosphokinase   Normal; to distinguish from polymyositis

Muscle biopsy   Normal; to distinguish from polymyositis

Serum protein electrophoresis   Normal; to distinguish from myeloma

Rheumatoid factor   Normal; along with absence of synovitis, to distinguish from arthritis

•••••• Multidisciplinary Plan

The goal of the treatment plan is to induce a remission of the disease using low-dose corticosteroid therapy.

Medications

Corticosteroids

Prednisone, 10 mg/d, or equivalent low-dose corticosteroid; although some patients are able to discontinue drug after several months, most require prolonged maintenance therapy with small doses

Nonsteroidal anti-inflammatory drugs

May be added to control mild discomfort that may occur while corticosteroids are being tapered

---

NURSING CARE

Nursing Assessment

Musculoskeletal System

Bilateral pain and stiffness to pectoral and pelvic girdles, increasing at night and in the early morning; muscle weakness

Systemic

Fever, fatigue

Nursing Dx & Intervention

Pain related to proximal muscle involvement

- Assess pain: location, onset, duration, and provocative and palliative factors. Have patient indicate intensity, using pain rating scale.

- Administer hot or cold thermal therapy to affected muscles.
- Perform limited range of motion exercises as tolerated *to combat stiffness and prevent atrophy from immobilization.*

Patient Education/Home Care Planning

1. Give the patient information about prednisone; discuss its importance and side effects, as well as the need to continue medication.
2. Teach the patient that temporal (giant cell) arteritis may be a complication of the disease. Alert the patient to associated symptoms to report, including headache, scalp tenderness, and any vision changes.
3. Teach the patient the importance of medical alert identification.

Evaluation

Laboratory findings are within normal limits   Patient's erythrocyte sedimentation rate is within normal limits.

Pain is relieved or minimized   Patient reports increasing ability to use shoulder and pelvic muscles without pain.

SARCOIDOSIS[21,24]

Sarcoidosis is a multisystem granulomatous disorder of unknown cause.

In the United States approximately 34 cases of sarcoidosis per 100,000 persons are diagnosed each year. Cases are equally distributed between both sexes. Although all races and age groups may be affected, sarcoidosis occurs most commonly in adults, especially blacks younger than 40 years of age.

The prognosis of sarcoidosis varies depending on the degree of systemic involvement and the intensity of steroid therapy. Sarcoidosis may be staged according to international standards that are based on chest roentgenograms of patients with pulmonary involvement, the major clinical finding (Table 14-4).

The disease is fatal in about 5% of patients. Current research focuses on determining the immunologic pathogenesis of the disease through detailed studies of immune function of cells derived from sarcoid tissue.

• • • • • • Pathophysiology

Recent data suggest that the pathophysiology of sarcoidosis involves a process in which macrophages initiate cellular responses to some unknown antigen. The macrophage releases various factors (e.g., interleukin 1) that cause accumulation and proliferation of helper T-cells. In addition, B lymphocytes are stimulated to produce immunoglobulins, fibroblasts proliferate, and suppressor T-cells predominate. These immunologic responses result in the formation of granulomas in affected organs, depression of delayed hypersensitivity reactions to common antigens, and an increased synthesis of immunoglobulins.

• • • • • • Diagnostic Studies and Findings

Differential diagnoses include tuberculosis, mediastinal lymphoma, and other granulomatous lung diseases.

T cells   Decreased circulating cells

Bronchoalveolar lavage fluid   Increased macrophages and helper T cells

Delayed-type hypersensitivity skin test   Absence of response (anergy)

Chest roentgenogram   Varies from prominent hilar lymphadenopathy to diffuse pulmonary infiltrates with fibrosis

Serum protein electrophoresis   Polyclonal hypergammaglobulinemia: usually increased IgG, but IgA and IgM may also be elevated

Kviem test   Intradermally injected saracoid tissue suspension; positive in 60% to 80%

Tissue biopsy   Noncaseating granulomas

C-reactive protein   Elevated in associated acute arthritis

Erythrocyte sedimentation rate   Elevated in associated acute arthritis

• • • • • • Multidisciplinary Plan

Medications

Corticosteroids
  Prednisone in doses adjusted to relieve symptoms and reverse fibrosis of pulmonary tissue
Optic agents
  Methylcellulose eye drops and assorted ophthalmic ointments to treat ocular manifestations
Antidysrhythmic agents
  For ventricular ectopy

■ TABLE 14-4 Staging, Prognosis, and Treatment of Sarcoidosis

Stage	Chest Roentgenogram	Prognosis	Corticosteroid Therapy
1	Bilateral hilar adenopathy	Resolves in 60% of cases	None
2	Bilateral hilar adenopathy with parenchymal pulmonary infiltration	Resolves in 46% of cases	Yes, to decrease pulmonary fibrosis and relieve symptoms
3	Advanced parenchymal pulmonary infiltration with nodular densities	Resolves in 12% of cases	Same as stage 2

Treatment of arthritis manifestations varies depending on their severity; salicylates used first, followed by non-steroidal anti-inflammatory agents, and finally corticosteroids, including intra-articular injections

General Management

Chest physiotherapy, breathing exercises, postural drainage, and oxygen therapy as necessary for prophylaxis or as treatment for chronic pulmonary disease

Serial sinus and chest roentgenograms and pulmonary function studies as necessary to follow disease course and determine adequacy of treatment

See arthritis (p. 377)

NURSING CARE

Nursing Assessment

Constitutional Signs and Symptoms

Fatigue

Pulmonary Status

Parenchymal lesions (in asymptomatic patients or associated with dyspnea and nonproductive cough); pulmonary fibrosis; cough; superinfection; restrictive disease; decreased vital capacity

Skin and Mucous Membrane Integrity

Small skin nodules over face, neck, and extremities; vitiligo; alopecia; erythema nodosum

Ocular Integrity

Blurred vision; lacrimation; ocular pain; conjunctival infection; uveitis; Sjögren's syndrome; iritis

Reticuloendothelial System Status

Lymphadenopathy; bilateral hilar adenopathy; mediastinal or peripheral lymphadenopathy; splenomegaly with or without anemia, leukopenia, and thrombocytopenia

Cardiovascular Status

Dysrhythmias: bundle-branch block or ventricular ectopy
Congestive heart failure; angina pectoris; pericardial effusion

Nursing Dx & Intervention

Impaired gas exchange related to pulmonary fibrosis, infection, restrictive disease, or parenchymal lesions

- Assess respiratory status: note respiratory rate, rhythm, and quality, presence of hemoptysis, cough, adventitious breath sounds, or dyspnea *to prevent respiratory compromise.*

- Monitor results of pulmonary function studies.
- Obtain sputum specimens for culture *to determine presence of secondary pulmonary infection(s).*
- Reinforce teaching related to proper positioning, body mechanics, and breathing exercises.
- Institute chest physiotherapy.

Risk for decreased cardiac output related to dysrhythmias or congestive heart failure

- Assess for signs and symptoms associated with decreased cardiac output: hypotension, dyspnea, edema, jugular venous distention, rales, and pulse irregulatories.
- Monitor electrocardiograms for rate, rhythm, and ectopy.
- Report significant electrocardiographic irregularities and other abnormal assessment data to physician.
- Position for increased comfort, usually with head elevated.
- Adjust patient's activity *to reduce oxygen demands and provide rest periods.*
- Assess response to oxygen therapy and other interventions.

Pain related to ocular discomfort, arthralgias

- Assess pain: location, quality, onset, duration, and provocative and palliative factors. Have patient indicate pain intensity using a pain rating scale.
- In collaboration with physician, institute appropriate interventions and administer analgesics based on underlying cause of pain. Assess effectiveness, and note side effects.

Body image disturbance related to skin nodules, alopecia

- Assess perception of change and effect on life-style.
- Assess hygiene and grooming.
- Discuss measures to enhance appearance.
- Comment on positive accomplishments and abilities. Assist patient in recognizing these.

Patient Education/Home Care Planning

1. Give information to the patient about, and discuss the importance of, prescribed medications.
2. Provide information related to system involvement: assessment and reporting of signs and symptoms.
3. Teach the importance of chest physiotherapy.
4. Teach signs and symptoms of infections.
5. Teach about the avoidance of risk factors associated with infection.
6. Teach the principles of good nutrition.
7. Teach the importance of medical alert identification.

Evaluation

Pulmonary involvement is stabilized Patient's chest roentgenogram shows clear or improved lung fields. Patient's respiratory pattern and breath sounds are within normal limits.

Laboratory findings are within normal limits Patient shows a positive response to cutaneous recall antigens (anergy is reversed). Patient's serum protein electrophoresis findings return to normal. Kviem test-findings are negative.

Cardiac status is stable Patient's ECG shows no ectopy. Vital signs are within patient's normal limits.

Pain is controlled Patient reports no eye, muscle, or chest discomfort. Patient's position and face are relaxed.

Patient accepts physical changes Patient uses grooming techniques to enhance appearance. Patient recognizes strengths and abilities.

■ REITER'S SYNDROME[14]

Reiter's syndrome is a relatively common, chronic, multisystem inflammatory disease characterized by the development of seronegative arthropathy that affects the lower extremities and may be associated with urethritis, conjunctivitis, or mucocutaneous disease involving the penis, oral mucosa, palms, and soles.

Reiter's syndrome has been a subject of worldwide research since the discovery of its link with HLA-B27 in 80% of patients in 1973. This finding suggested a genetic predisposition. A search for the environmental factor or factors that act as inciting agents ensued. Although such an agent remains elusive, current data suggest that enteric infection may play a role. Microbes that have been implicated include *Shigella flexneri, Shigella dysenteriae,* and *Yersinia enterocolitica.* Venereal infections with *Chlamydia* and *Mycoplasma* have also been associated with Reiter's syndrome.

Based on this evidence it is theorized that patients with a specific genetic background (HLA-B27) may develop Reiter's syndrome following infestation by a variety of microbes. Research continues with the goals of improving its recognition, defining etiologic factors, and ultimately, finding a cure.

The incidence of Reiter's syndrome is difficult to assess for a variety of reasons. Current research indicates that this disease occurs primarily in white males throughout the world. Although it may be detected at any age, it is usually diagnosed in the third decade. Reiter's syndrome may be the most common inflammatory arthropathy detected in young men. The pathogenesis of Reiter's syndrome is unknown.

•••••• Diagnostic Studies and Findings

Differential diagnoses include infective arthritis, psoriatic arthropathy, and ankylosing spondylitis.

History Recent history of dysentery or venereal disease combined with inflammatory of monarthropathy or oligoarthropathy, urethritis, cervicitis, and ocular and cutaneous inflammatory changes

Roentgenograms of musculoskeletal system Fluffy periosteal proliferation of lower extremity joints

Leukocytosis Mild

Erythrocyte sedimentation rate Variable from 1 to 130 mm/hour

HLA typing HLA-B27 (this test is costly and unnecessary and is usually performed only as an academic endeavor)

•••••• Multidisciplinary Plan

The goals of the treatment plan include management of signs and symptoms and early detection of disabling complications. This disease has no cure, and current treatment is empiric and inadequate.

Medications

Nonsteroidal antiinflammatory agents

To treat synovitis and arthralgias; any agent may be tried; one clinician reports success with indomethacin (Indocin), 25-50 mg tid, and phenylbutazone (Butazolindin), 100 mg tid or qid

Corticosteroids

Methylprednisolone (Medrol), 40-80 mg intralesionally for arthropathy, tendinitis, etc.

Steroid eye drops or subconjunctival ointments for conjunctivitis

Antineoplastic agents

Azathioprine (Imuran), 0.75-2.5 mg/kg body weight qd for immunosuppression until symptomatic improvement, usually 2-12 wk, then tapered dosage

Methotrexate may be used in cases of severe illness but is not warranted in majority of patients

Analgesics and nonsteroidal antiinflammatory agents

To reduce pain associated with arthritis and ocular inflammation

Optic agents

Methylcellulose eye drops for symptomatic relief of ocular discomfort

General Management

Physical therapy for arthritis complications

NURSING CARE

Nursing Assessment

Musculoskeletal Involvement

Arthritis, particularly of weight-bearing joints; tendinitis, especially of Achilles tendon; plantar fasciitis; back pain such as sacroiliitis and ankylosing spondylitis; costochondritis, often manifested as pleuritic chest pain; dactylitis

Genitourinary Involvement

Urethritis; cervicitis; cystitis; balanitis

Ocular Involvement

Conjunctivitis; uveitis

Skin Integrity

Keratoderma blennorrhagica (thick keratotic lesions of palms and soles); balanitis circinata: painless, superficial lesions of coronal margins of prepuce and adjacent glands; nails: subungual, corny material that accumulates under and may lift nail plate, which becomes yellow and thickened

Cardiovascular Status

Electrocardiogram: increased PR interval, heart block, ST segment changes, abnormal Q waves; palpitations; transient murmurs; pericardial rub; aortic regurgitation

Nursing Dx & Intervention

Impaired physical mobility related to arthritis

- Assess degree of physical immobility resulting from arthritis.
- In collaboration with physician, provide nonsteroidal antiinflammatory agents. Assess effectiveness.
- Encourage patient to rest joints during periods of acute inflammation. Otherwise, encourage program of regular exercise, including range of motion exercises, as tolerated. Confer with physical or occupational therapist *to determine other beneficial interventions.*
- Provide assistive devices as needed.

Pain related to inflammatory conditions of eye, genitourinary tract, and joints

- Determine location of pain.
- Assess degree of discomfort using a 0 to 10 numeric rating scale.
- In collaboration with physician, provide analgesic agents as ordered. Assess effectiveness and note side effects.
- In collaboration with physician, institute other appropriate measures relative to system involved. Assess effectiveness.

Risk for impaired skin integrity related to mucocutaneous manifestations

- Assess skin for presence of lesions and hyperkeratotic areas.
- Monitor lesions for signs of infection, dissemination, and other abnormal changes.
- Provide or encourage patient to perform meticulous hand and foot care with special attention to nail integrity.
- Provide mild, nondrying, hypoallergenic soaps for skin cleaning and encourage their use.
- Assess effectiveness of treatment of lesions.

Altered patterns of urinary elimination related to urethritis or cystitis

- Assess for signs and symptoms associated with urethritis or cystitis: dysuria, pyuria, hematuria, and fever.
- Monitor intake and output.

- In collaboration with physician, administer appropriate anti-infective agents. Assess effectiveness and note side effects.

Risk for decreased cardiac output related to carditis

- Assess patient for presence of palpitations, murmurs, and pericardial rub.
- Assess electrocardiogram for prolonged PR interval, heart block, ST segment changes, and abnormal Q waves.
- In collaboration with physician, institute appropriate measures based on assessment. Assess effectiveness of specific interventions.

Patient Education/Home Care Planning

1. Teach the importance of reporting symptoms associated with significant complications of Reiter's syndrome: spondylitis, uveitis, and cardiopulmonary disease.
2. Teach that the use of a condom during sexual activity will limit exposure to venereal disease, which could exacerbate Reiter's syndrome.
3. Teach the importance of physician follow-up to monitor the disease course. The physician should also be consulted for management of acute episodes.
4. Teach facts about and the importance of prescribed medications.
5. Teach the importance of keeping a log of the disease course, treatments, and other disease-related information.
6. Teach the importance of using medical alert identification.

Evaluation

Mobility is improved   Patient performs ADLs without difficulty. Patient uses assistive devices as necessary to maintain mobility. Patient maintains daily exercise program.

Pain is controlled   Patient has relaxed body posture and facial expression; patient verbalizes no eye or other pain.

Skin integrity is maintained   Patient's skin is warm, with good color and turgor; patient performs daily skin care and maintains nails.

Urinary elimination pattern is within normal limits   Patient's intake and output are balanced; patient reports no frequency, burning, or urgency.

Cardiac function is maintained   Patient's vital signs are stable, and ECG pattern exhibits normal sinus rhythm.

■ SJÖGREN'S SYNDROME[10,20]

Sjögren's syndrome is a chronic autoimmune disorder of unknown etiology that affects primarily the lacrimal and salivary glands.

The major symptoms of Sjögren's syndrome are keratoconjunctivitis and xerostomia, which result from decreased lacrimal and salivary gland secretion, respectively. The syndrome is often associated with other connective tissue diseases, especially rheumatoid arthritis, systemic lupus erythematosus, and progressive systemic sclerosis (scleroderma). Raynaud's phenomenon is manifested by 20% of patients with Sjögren's syndrome. Middle-aged women with a mean age of 50 years constitute 90% of Sjögren's syndrome patients. All races may be affected. There is evidence that sex hormones play an etiologic role in the disease, and research in this area continues.

•••••• Pathophysiology

Biopsy specimens from glandular lesions demonstrate infiltration by lymphocytes, plasma cells, and macrophages, which replace secretory acinar tissue. Anti-salivary duct antibodies have been observed. The factors precipitating such autodestruction of host tissue are unknown. Destruction of tissue results in decreased secretion by involved glands. In addition, dryness of the nose, pharynx, and tracheobronchial tree may occur.

•••••• Diagnostic Studies and Findings

Differential diagnoses include Felty's syndrome, Raynaud's phenomenon, chronic thyroiditis, hepatomegaly, chronic active hepatitis, gastric achlorhydria, acute pancreatitis, adult celiac disease, polymyositis, drug-induced xerostomia, irradiation xerostomia, diabetes, sarcoidosis, salivary duct stones, and mumps.

Salivary scintigraphy   Decreased uptake, concentration, and excretion of intravenous ^{99m}Tc pertechnetate by major salivary glands; measured by means of sequential scintiphotographic technique

Sialography   Dilations and other changes such as atrophy within intrasalivary duct system

Labial salivary gland biopsy   Infiltration of tissue by lymphocytes, plasma cells, and macrophages; replacement of acinar tissue

Schirmer test   Decreased tear production; less than 15 mm of filter strip wetted

Complete blood count   Mild anemia; leukopenia

Erythrocyte sedimentation rate   Elevated

Serum protein electrophoresis   Hypergammaglobulinemia

Rheumatoid factor   Elevated (90%)

Antinuclear antibody   Greater than 1:80 (70%) anti-salivary duct antibodies, thyroid antibodies, gastric-parietal cell autoantibodies

•••••• Multidisciplinary Plan

The goals of the treatment plan are to provide palliatative measures and prevent complications of this chronic disorder.

Medications

Corticosteroids
  Prednisone; dose titrated for relief of *severe* symptoms; usually administered only late in course of disease when symptoms are unrelieved by supportive approaches

Antineoplastic agents
  Cyclophosphamide; success varies and use is controversial in massive lymphocytic infiltration of vital organs
Artificial saliva preparations
Optic agents
  Artificial tears (0.5% methylcellulose eye drops) as needed

General Management

Avoidance of sour or sweetened drinks or candies
Mouth rinses of 1% methylcellulose
Oral hygiene with frequent brushing, flossing, and fluoride rinses
Regular dental examinations
Regular conjunctival cultures to detect ocular infections

NURSING CARE

Nursing Assessment

Oral Cavity

Xerostomia: dental caries (multiple), oral candidiasis, dysphagia, difficulty chewing, changes in phonation, adherence of food to buccal mucosa, hoarseness, fissures and ulcerations of tongue, buccal mucosa, and lips, frequent ingestion of liquids with meals

Eyes

Conjunctivitis: foreign body sensation, "grittiness," burning, accumulation of thick, ropy strands at inner canthus, decreased tearing, redness, photosensitivity, eye fatigue; pruritus; filmy sensation that interferes with vision; (late) corneal ulceration, vascularization, and opacification

Vagina

Dry membranes, dyspareunia

Ears

Recurrent otitis media

Respiratory Tract

Nasal mucosal dryness; epistaxis; bronchitis; pneumonia

Nursing Dx & Intervention

Risk for impaired tissue integrity related to irritants

Eyes

- Assess condition of the eyes, observing for presence of foreign bodies and infection.
- Administer 0.5% methylcellulose eye drops as needed *to maintain moisture at conjunctival surface.* Observe effect.

- Obtain regular cultures of eye *to determine presence of infection.*
- Stress importance of wearing protective glasses, especially out-of-doors, *to prevent tissue injury.*
- Instruct in use and care of contact lenses, if ordered, *for protection.*

Mouth and Nose

- Assess condition of mouth and nose; assess ability to breathe nasally and to chew and swallow food.
- Provide items for frequent oral hygiene: for brushing, for flossing, and for rinsing.
- Stress importance of regular mouth care and the use of artificial saliva.
- Provide fluids and sugarless gum or candies *to stimulate salivary secretion.*

Vagina

- Avoid use of tampons during menstrual period.
- Use water-soluble lubricant to relieve dyspareunia.

Patient Education/Home Care Planning

1. Provide information and discuss with patient the use of artificial tears or saliva and vaginal lubricants.
2. Stress to the patient the need for routine oral hygiene throughout the day.
3. List and demonstrate for patient the method of assessing for signs and symptoms of increasing severity of condition.
4. Discuss with patient the need for regular follow-up care.
5. Discuss with patient the use of protective eye covering and the use of nighttime humidification.

Evaluation

No tissue injury occurs   Patient's eyes are clear. Patient uses medication appropriately. Patient reports increased eye comfort. Patient's oral cavity is pink, moist, and clean. Patient breathes nasally without discomfort. Patient reports no dyspareunia.

■ AMYLOIDOSIS[12]

■ Amyloidosis is a syndrome characterized by deposition of amyloid (proteinaceous material) in tissues.

Amyloidosis occurs as an acquired or hereditary disorder and may be a primary disease or be associated with a variety of other illnesses. Although its etiology is unknown, at least two observations suggest that amyloidosis represents immunologic dysfunction: the presence of immunoglobulin proteins in amyloid deposits and the syndrome's increased incidence in inflammatory, infectious, and neoplastic diseases.

The term "amyloid," which means starchlike, is a misnomer. The syndrome is actually characterized by the diffuse deposition of insoluble proteinaceous material in the extracellular matrix of one or more organs. The accumulation of amyloid encroaches on parenchymal tissues and compromises organ function. Clinical manifestations of amyloidosis vary widely and depend on the organs involved and the severity with which they are affected. Specific immunotherapy to treat the underlying cause of organ failure is lacking, so treatment is restricted to management of signs and symptoms. For this reason amyloidosis is usually fatal. Renal failure and cardiac diseases are the most frequent causes of death.

Types of Generalized Amyloidosis

Primary generalized amyloidosis (PGA) occurs in the absence of associated diseases, although most patients exhibit some type of plasma cell dyscrasia. PGA accounts for 50% to 60% of all cases of amyloidosis. Deposits of amyloid are found in mesenchymal tissues of the heart, tongue, carpal tunnel, gastrointestinal tract, peripheral nerves, skin, joints, and skeletal muscle. Although this type of amyloidosis may occur as early as the second decade, the mean age at diagnosis is approximately 60 years. Men are affected more often than women, and whites more than nonwhites. Virtually all patients with classic PGA demonstrate a monoclonal immunoglobulin in their serum or urine and bone marrow plasmacytosis.

Multiple myeloma-associated amyloidosis (MMA) accounts for approximately 30% of cases. In roughly 15% of myeloma patients, clinical findings are consistent with a diagnosis of amyloidosis.[23] Serum and urine paraproteins are found. The clinical symptoms, age at diagnosis, and sexual predilection are similar to PGA. Amyloidosis contributes to early morbidity in myeloma disease.

Secondary generalized amyloidosis (SGA), detected in 10% of the patients, occurs as a result of a variety of long-term or poorly controlled inflammatory, infectious, or neoplastic diseases. Adult and juvenile rheumatoid arthritis may be the most frequent predisposing factor. SGA is also reported in other inflammatory conditions, including ankylosing spondylitis, Reiter's syndrome, psoriatic arthritis, chronic rheumatic heart disease, dermatomyositis, scleroderma, Behçet's disease, and systemic lupus erythematosus.

Neoplastic diseases associated with the development of amyloidosis include gastrointestinal, pulmonary, and genitourinary carcinomas, non-Hodgkin's lymphomas, malignant melanomas, and most frequently, hypernephroma and Hodgkin's disease. Chronic, systemic infections are a significant factor associated with worldwide distribution. Such infectious diatheses include tuberculosis, pyelonephritis, osteomyelitis, inflammatory bowel disease, and chronically infected burns.

In addition to the above types, amyloidosis is also described as a hereditary illness detected with increased frequency in various countries and some well-defined areas of the United States. Neuropathic, nephropathic, and cardiopathic syndromes have been described.

• • • • • Pathophysiology

Only limited insight has been gained into the pathogenesis of this syndrome. Histologic staining techniques and electron microscopy have provided some clues. Fibers formed from laterally aggregated protein fibrils have been detected in amyloid deposits. Some of these fibrils are apparently derived from free immunoglobulin light chains. In addition, amyloid deposits are further constructed of globular glycoprotein subunits (pentagonal, or "P" components) absorbed from the serum into the fibrillar units.

An explanation for the deposition of the proteinaceous substance has not yet been found. Whatever the reason, accumulation of amyloid in extracellular spaces results in pressure atrophy and eventual necrosis and destruction of underlying tissue. Organ dysfunction and failure are responsible for clinical manifestations. Amyloid deposition occurs in the following area:

Articular
  Glenohumeral junction
  Synovial villi
Neurologic
  Dural blood vessels
  Autonomic ganglia
  Spinal nerve roots
  Peripheral nerves
Renal
  Glomeruli
  Arteriolar walls
  Tubular basement membranes
Cardiac
  All layers of the cardiac walls (predominantly myocardium)
  Conduction tissue
  Intramural coronary arterioles
Pulmonary (any area)
  Upper nasal passages
  Vocal cords
  Tracheobronchial submucosa
  Parenchyma
Gastrointestinal (any area)
  Gingiva
  Tongue
  Oropharyngeal muscles
  Liver
  Voluntary muscles of upper third of esophagus
  Diffuse esophageal infiltrates
  Small bowel
Integumentary
  Face
  Upper trunk

• • • • • Diagnostic Studies and Findings

Tissue biopsy   Apple-green birefringence of Congo red–stained tissue specimens under polarization microscopy; tissue from organ suspected to be infiltrated with amyloid preferred, but rectal biopsy findings positive in approximately 80% of cases of generalized amyloidosis

Serum and urine electrophoresis   Paraproteins detected in presence of associated plasma cell dyscrasia

Bone marrow aspiration and biopsy   Plasmacytosis in presence of associated multiple myeloma

• • • • • Multidisciplinary Plan

The goals of therapy in amyloidosis are to prevent further deposition of amyloid material and to promote or accelerate its resorption.

Surgery

Serial biopsies to determine regression of amyloid deposition

Medications

Antineoplastic agents
  May be used to reduce the serum concentration of amyloid precursor light chains if underlying B cell dyscrasia is present
Colchicine, dimethyl sulfoxide (DMSO), and corticosteroids have met with some success, although their use remains controversial; corticosteroids are used primarily to treat underlying inflammatory or neoplastic disorder

General Management

Plasmapheresis may interrupt dissemination of amyloid precursor light chains (see p. 1241)
Family and patient counseling to assist in coping with fatal illness
Supportive approaches for complications
  For congestive heart failure: conservative management; avoid use of digitalis unless closely monitored in hospital setting (usually cardiac amyloid is unresponsive to treatment with digitalis)
  For neuropathic hypotension: elastic stockings
  For malabsorption syndromes: broad-spectrum antibiotics
  For macroglossia: supplemental Keo-Feed gastrostomy feeding; tracheostomy for upper airway obstruction
  For respiratory tract amyloidosis: bronchoscopy with curettage of amyloid deposits
  For renal failure: dialysis

NURSING CARE

Nursing Assessment

Neurologic Status

Idiopathic, sensorimotor, peripheral neuropathy with autonomic neuropathy; depressed pain and temperature sensation, and motor dysfunction of lower extremities

Cardiovascular Status

Restrictive cardiomyopathy with low-voltage electrocardiogram; chest pain; myocardial infarction; conduction disturbance in absence of other recognized causes

Skin Integrity

Waxy, indurated papules and purpura; skin thickening; "orange-peel" skin; alopecia; periorbital purpura

Renal Status

Proteinuria; idiopathic nephrotic syndrome

Pulmonary Status

Nasal lesions; vocal cord nodules; bronchiectasis; airway obstruction; wheezing; dyspnea; hilar adenopathy

Gastrointestinal Status

Macroglossia: dysphagia, impaired esophageal peristalsis: gastric accumulation, motility disturbances, hemorrhage, obstruction achlorhydria, and vitamin B_{12} deficiency; small bowel impairment: diarrhea, constipation, malabsorption, hemorrhage, protein-losing enteropathy, perforation, and ischemic necrosis; hepatomegaly without portal insufficiency or hypertension

Nursing Dx & Intervention

Impaired gas exchange related to amyloid deposition in pulmonary tissue

- Assess degree of respiratory distress: note rate, rhythm, and quality of respirations, auscultate lung fields for presence of adventitious breath sounds, and note use of accessory muscles.
- Maintain open airway at all times.
- In collaboration with physician, institute appropriate interventions, relative to type and severity of pulmonary compromise. Assess effectiveness.
- Be prepared to institute measures for respiratory arrest as symptoms increase.

Decreased cardiac output related to amyloid deposition in cardiac structures and subsequent myopathy and ischemia

- Assess for signs and symptoms associated with decreased cardiac output: hypotension, dyspnea, edema, jugular venous distention, rales, and pulse irregularities.
- Monitor electrocardiogram for rate, rhythm, and ectopy. Note in particular presence of ischemia, infarction, and conduction abnormalities.
- Report significant electrocardiographic changes and other abnormal assessment data to physician.
- In collaboration with physician, institute appropriate interventions (such as oxygenation) relative to type and severity of cardiac compromise. Assess effectiveness and note side effects of medications.
- Adjust patient's activity and provide rest periods *to reduce oxygen demands.*

Altered renal tissue perfusion related to amyloid deposition in kidneys

- Assess for renal insufficiency: monitor blood urea nitrogen and creatinine, 24-hour urine for creatinine clearance, blood pressure, urinalysis result, presence of edema and rapid weight gain, and intake and output.
- Report significant abnormal findings to physician.
- Institute dialysis in event of renal failure.

Altered nutrition: less than body requirements related to amyloid deposition in gastrointestinal tract

- Assess degree of malnutrition: note presence of hypoalbuminemia, hypoproteinemia, negative nitrogen balance, protein and calorie deficit, and weight loss.
- Assist physician in determining underlying cause of malnutrition, such as malabsorption, dysphagia, and impaired esophageal peristalsis.
- Provide and encourage patient to maintain nutritionally balanced diet. Determine need for parenteral nutrition *to maintain nutritional balance.*
- Weight patient weekly *to detect weight loss.*

Pain related to arthritis, cardiac ischemia, or gastrointestinal distress

- Assess pain: location, onset, duration, and provocative and alleviating factors. Have patient describe intensity on scale of 0 to 10.
- In collaboration with physician, administer appropriate analgesics. Assess effectiveness and note side effects.
- Position for maximum comfort.

Sensory/perceptual alterations (tactile) related to peripheral neuropathy

- Assess degree of sensory impairment: perform sensory neurologic examination.
- Provide for patient's safety *to prevent injury.*
- Discuss loss or alteration with patient and provide appropriate measures to prevent injury.

Risk for impaired skin integrity related to amyloid deposition in dermis

- Assess skin integrity: color, temperature, moisture, and presence of lesions.
- Protect skin from injury or infection.

Patient Education/Home Care Planning

1. Teach patient facts about the importance of managing signs and symptoms and frequent physician follow-up.
2. Teach patient care and methods of self-assessment relative to the systems involved.
3. Refer the patient and family for counseling to assist in coping with this potentially fatal illness.
4. Teach patient the importance of medical alert identification.

Evaluation

Respiratory status is stable Patient's rate, rhythm, and pattern of respirations are within normal limits. Patient's breath sounds are normal.

Cardiac status is stable Vital signs are within patient's normal limits. ECG reveals no ectopy.

Renal system is not compromised Patient's intake and output are balanced. Patient weight is stable. No edema is reported.

Nutrition is maintained Patient takes diet and fluids without difficulty. Patient has no nausea, diarrhea, or constipation.

Pain is relieved or minimized Patient reports increased comfort level. Patient's body posture and face are relaxed.

Laboratory findings improve Patient's paraprotein level detected in serum and urine electrophoresis is decreased.

Skin appears normal Patient's skin is warm and dry, with good turgor. Lesions are present but are without induration.

◼ SYSTEMIC LUPUS ERYTHEMATOSUS[2,3,22]

Systemic lupus erythematosus (SLE) is a chronic, multisystem, autoimmune disorder characterized chiefly by antibody formation directed against autologous tissues and serum factors.

SLE has no cure. Although its origin remains elusive, increasing evidence suggest that multiple factors—genetic, hormonal, immunologic, and possibly viral—may play a role in the onset and perpetuation of the disease.

In the United States approximately 500,000 persons have this disease. Although virtually anyone may be affected, SLE has a predilection for women of childbearing age. Nine times more women than men are affected. Three times as many blacks as whites have SLE. Late-onset (sixth decade or later) SLE accounts for 12% of cases.

SLE was once considered a fatal illness of young women, but 85% of patients now survive longer than 15 years after diagnosis. This improved prognosis reflects advances in the diagnosis and treatment of the disease. Patients with central nervous system involvement and renal failure have poorer prognoses. Complications, especially infections, associated with the long-term use of steroids used to control the disease also significantly contribute to early mortality.

Despite the significant improvements in the treatment of SLE, it can be a serious and potentially life-threatening illness. Because of this, as well as the recognition that SLE is a prototype of autoimmune disease, it has been a subject of worldwide research.

The cause of SLE remains unknown, but several etiologic factors have been proposed. It is unlikely that any single factor is the cause. Most researchers conclude that SLE is probably caused by an unknown inciting agent coupled with a genetic "lupus diathesis."

Drugs

During the past 30 years many drugs have been implicated in the development of a reversible lupuslike syndrome that includes elevated antinuclear antibody (ANA) titers and well-defined clinical features. Perhaps certain drugs alter tissues to such a degree as to make them act as immunogenic stimuli. Both hydralazine and procainamide can bind to and alter the physical properties of DNA, perhaps enhancing its immunogenicity. There may also be some correlation between an individual's ability to metabolize certain drugs and a predisposition for SLE.

The following outline lists drugs thought to induce lupuslike syndromes. Once these drugs are discontinued, clinical manifestations disappear:

Definite
  Hydralazine
  Procainamide
  Isoniazid
  Chlorpromazine
  Methyldopa
  Quinidene
Possible
  Dilantin
  Captopril
  Cimetidine
  Propranolol
  Penicillamine
  Propylthioracil
  Practolol
  Acebutolol
  Lithium carbonate
Unlikely
  Griseofulvin
  Phenylbutazone
  Oral contraceptives
  Gold salts
  Allopurinol
  Reserpine
  Penicillin

•••••• Pathophysiology

The pathogenesis of SLE is characterized by the development of antibodies directed against "self" tissues, cells, serum proteins, or all of these. The presence of autoantibodies reflects a loss of tolerance, or autoimmunity, and constitutes a serious defect in the regulatory components of the immune system. The T lymphocytes are the primary group of white cells responsible for control of the immune response. In SLE the number of T suppressor cells is decreased. In addition, T suppressor cell activity is inhibited. Polyclonal hypergammaglobulinemia occurs as a result, since B cells proliferate unrestrained by normal suppressor mechanisms.

In most SLE patients, antibodies develop directed against native, double-stranded DNA, as well as other antigens. The combination of autoantibodies and autoantigens, or immune complexes, may circulate or be deposited within capillary plexuses, near basement membranes, and in other tissues such as glomeruli, renal interstitia, serosal (pleural, pericardial, or peritoneal) membranes, the choroid plexus, and the vasculature of the lungs. Immune complex formation triggers the inflammatory response, which is the primary mechanism by which tissue destruction and subsequent clinical disease occur. Chronic deposition of immune complexes leads to chronic destruction of the host tissue. *The intensity and location of the inflammatory process dictate the severity of the clinical response and organ involvement, respectively.*

•••••• Diagnostic Studies and Findings

A variety of autoantibodies may be detected by serologic assay. Some of these are listed in Table 14-5.

Antinuclear antibody (ANA)   Positive in titers greater than 1:80

Anti–double-stranded DNA antibody (ds-DNA)   Positive in titers greater than 1:80

Rapid plasma reagin (RPR) test   Falsely positive

Fluorescent treponemal antibody absorption (FTA-ABS) Negative

Complement (C3 and C4)   Decreased during flares, indicative of acute inflammation; otherwise within normal limits

Skin or muscle biopsy   Evidence of inflammation with or without tissue necrosis; deposits of immunoglobulin and complement at dermal-epidermal junctions

Kidney biopsy   Focal or diffuse proliferative nephritis; also membranous or interstitial disease

Complete blood count   Pancytopenia or selective deficits; lymphopenia during flare

C-reactive protein   Elevated during flares, indicative of acute inflammatory state

Erythrocyte sedimentation rate   Elevated during flares, indicative of acute inflammatory state

Coombs' test   Positive in presence of hemolytic anemia because of autoantibody production against erythrocytes

Coagulation profile   Prolonged prothrombin time and partial thromboplastin time if circulating anticoagulant antibodies are present

▇ TABLE 14-5 Autoantibodies in SLE

Autoantibody	Clinical Manifestations
Antinuclear	Nephritis; vasculitis; pleuritis; peri-
Anti-double-stranded DNA (ds-DNA)	carditis; synovitis; peritonitis
Antineuronal	Cerebritis; organic brain syndromes; peripheral neuropathies
Anticoagulant	Coagulopathies
Anti-RBC	Anemia
Anti-WBC	Leukopenia; lymphopenia; immunosuppression; infection
Antiplatelet	Thrombocytopenia
Anti-basement membrane	Dermatitis; nephritis

Rheumatoid factor (RF) (anti-IgG antibody)   Usually positive in titer greater than 1:40

Circulating immune complexes   Present during flares

Urinalysis   Abnormal casts and sediment associated with renal damage

Antibodies to single-stranded DNA (ss-DNA)   May be present in ANA-negative lupus and associated with congenital heart block in lupus patients' neonates

The 1982 revised classification of SLE is based on the 11 criteria defined below. For the purpose of identifying patients in clinical studies, a person should be said to have SLE if any four or more of the 11 criteria are present, serially or simultaneously, during any interval of observation.

Malar rash: fixed erythema, flat or raised, over malar eminences, tending to spare nasolabial folds

Discoid rash: erythematous raised patches with adherent keratotic scaling and follicular plugging; atrophic scarring may occur in older lesions

Photosensitivity: skin rash as result of unusual reaction to sunlight, based on patient history or physician's observation

Oral ulcers: oral or nasopharyngeal ulceration, usually painless, observed by physician

Arthritis: nonerosive arthritis involving two or more peripheral joints, characterized by tenderness, swelling, or effusion

Serositis: pleuritis—convincing history of pleuritic pain or rub heard by a physician or evidence of pleural effusion—or pericarditis—documented by electrocardiogram, rub, or evidence of pericardial effusion

Renal disorder: persistent proteinuria greater than 0.5 g/day or greater than 3+ if quantitation not performed or cellular casts—may be red cell, hemoglobin, granular, tubular, or mixed

Neurologic disorder: seizures in absence of offending drugs or known metabolic derangements (such as uremia, ketoacidosis, or electrolyte imbalance) or psychosis in absence of offending drugs or known metabolic derangements

Hematologic disorder: hemolytic anemia with reticulocytosis or leukopenia—less than 4000/mm³ total on two or more occasions or lymphopenia—less than 1500/mm³ on two or more occasions or thrombocytopenia—less than 100,000/mm³ in absence of offending drugs

Immunologic disorder: positive LE cell preparation or anti-DNA—antibody to native DNA in abnormal titer or anti-Sm—presence of antibody to Sm nuclear antigen or false positive serologic test for syphilis known to be positive for at least 6 months and confirmed by *Treponema pallidum* immobilization or fluorescent treponemal antibody absorption test

Antinuclear antibody: abnormal titer of antinuclear antibody by immunofluorescence or equivalent assay at any point in time and in absence of drugs known to be associated with "drug-induced lupus" syndrome

•••••• Multidisciplinary Plan

The goals of the treatment plan include management of signs and symptoms, induction of remission, prevention of untoward complications of therapy, and early recognition of "flares."

Surgery

Joint replacement may be indicated if chronic synovitis and pain have been problematic.

Medications

Nonsteroidal antiinflammatory agents Acetylsalicylic acid (aspirin) may be given in a daily oral dosage of 3 to 6 g for adults. Indomethacin (Indocin) is given orally, 25 to 50 mg three or four times a day for adults. The patient should be monitored for evidence of gastrointestinal bleeding.

Antiinfective agents Hydroxychloroquine (Plaquenil), 200 to 400 mg orally twice a day for adults, or chloroquine, 250 mg orally daily to twice weekly for adults, is given. The patient should be started on therapy slowly. Gastrointestinal intolerance may occur when full doses are used initially. The beneficial effect of these drugs is usually demonstrated within a month or two. Nonsteroidal anti-inflammatory agents should be continued until this time. Retinal toxicity may occur at higher doses, so patients should receive pretreatment and annual ophthalmic examinations.

Corticosteroids Prednisone (Orasone, Deltasone, Meticorten) is given orally in low doses (15 mg/day), moderate doses (16 to 40 mg/day) or high doses (41 to 120 mg/day). The amounts listed above may be given in divided doses to provide more sustained anti-inflammatory action. Alternative-day dosage may be instituted as maintenance therapy (see p. 1240).

Methylprednisolone (Solu-Medrol, A-methaPred) is given intravenously for acute crisis in a dosage of up to 1000 mg/day for adults. Central nervous system involvement (psychosis, grand mal seizures) requires 35 to 40 mg methylprednisolone intravenously every 6 hours. The dose should be doubled if no response is attained in 48 hours.

Topical steroids include hydrocortisone (Cortaid), fluocinonide (Lidex), betamethasone dipropionate (Diprosone), flurandrenolide (Cordran), betamethasone valerate (Valisone), and fluocinolone acetonide (Synalar).

Antineoplastic agents Azathioprine (Imuran) is given in an oral dosage of 150 mg/day to 25 mg thrice weekly for adults. The patient should be monitored for pancytopenia, gastrointestinal distress, skin rash, hepatic toxicity, and hyperuricemia. Cyclophosphamide (Cytoxan, Neosar) is given at 150 mg/day to 25 mg thrice weekly for adults. The patient should be monitored for pancytopenia, cardiotoxicity, gastrointestinal distress, hemorrhagic cystitits, and hyperuricemia. Chlorambucil (Leukeran) is given orally as 10 mg/day to 2 mg thrice weekly for adults. The patient should be monitored for pancytopenia, exfoliative dermatitis, and hyperuricemia.

Other medications A variety of anti-infective agents may be used to treat infections associated with SLE or immunosuppressive therapy. Treatment of renal disease includes the use of antihypertensive agents and aluminum derivatives. Raynaud's phenomenon may respond to biofeedback or sympatholytic drugs such as guanethidine, nifedipine, reserpine, and tolazoline. Intra-articular steroid injections may prove useful in the alleviation of synovitis and joint pain.

General Management

Plasmapheresis (see p. 1241) has been shown to decrease circulating immune complexes and autoantibodies. To circumvent a rebound effect, a brief course of cytotoxic medication, often cyclophosphamide intravenously, may be administered after the plasmapheresis series.

Peritoneal dialysis or hemodialysis may be indicated in the treatment of renal insufficiency or failure.

A balanced diet with salt restriction should be followed

NURSING CARE

Nursing Assessment

General

Fever, malaise; weakness; history of lupus-inducing drugs

Skin and Mucous Membrane

Facial erythema; butterfly dermatitis; alopecia; photosensitivity; oral and nasal ulcers; vasculitis lesions

Gastrointestinal System

Dysphagia; nausea, vomiting; weight loss

Hematologic Status

Autoimmune hemolytic anemia

Cardiovascular Status

Diffuse vasculitis; pericarditis; dysrhythmias; murmurs; cardiomegaly

Pulmonary Status

Pleurisy; interstitial fibrosis

Renal Status

Hypertension; hematuria; cellular casts; proteinuria; edema; azotemia

Neuropsychiatric Status

Slowed cognitive function; depression, psychoses; neuritis; headache; seizures

Musculoskeletal Integrity

Arthralgias; nondeforming arthritis; diffuse myalgias
See Table 14-6.

Nursing Dx & Intervention

Because of the multiple systemic effects of SLE, nursing care must be structured to cope with the patient's individual requirements. Therefore nursing care often varies greatly, ranging, for example, from minor application of topical steroids to aggressive pulmonary toilet for an intubated patient. The following is meant to provide a generalized perspective. Refer to other chapters for a detailed approach to systems involved.

Ineffective breathing pattern related to fatigue and pulmonary involvement

- Assess respiratory status, monitor respiratory rate and rhythm, auscultate lungs for presence of adventitious breath sounds, and monitor for subjective distress (chest pain; dyspnea) *to detect or prevent respiratory compromise.*
- Maintain bed rest with head elevated during acute phase *to conserve oxygen.*
- Provide chest physiotherapy and postural drainage *to treat or prevent pneumonia.*
- Teach deep breathing exercises and encourage patient to perform exercises as often as needed to increase pulmonary function.
- Monitor chest roentgenograms and sputum culture *to detect pneumonia.*

Decreased cardiac output related to alterations in mechanical/electrical factors caused by disease

- Assess cardiac status. Auscultate apical pulse for irregularities, presence of murmurs, tachycardia, and bradycardia.
- Auscultate for pericardial friction rub. Monitor for subjective distress: syncope, palpitations, and dyspnea.
- Monitor electrocardiographic results.
- Monitor for presence of peripheral edema.

Altered tissue perfusion: cerebral related to exchange problems

- Assess changes in neurologic status: orientation, judgment, and intellectual function.
- Assess patient's ability to cope.
- Assess for suicidal ideation.
- Work with patient to identify resources for support and coping mechanisms that have proved helpful in past.
- Provide emotional support and attempt to limit patient's fears through frequent explanations of tests and procedures.
- Encourage visits by family and friends.
- If orientation is a problem in the hospital, provide familiar articles from home. Provide clock and calendar *to orient patient to time.*
- Maintain patient's safety.
- Encourage participation in local chapter of Lupus Foundation.

Altered renal tissue perfusion related to exchange problems

- Assess renal status. Monitor for presence of dyspnea, hypertension, edema, weight gain, anorexia, and nausea. Monitor urinalysis results, blood urea nitrogen, serum cre-

atinine, hemoglobin, hematocrit, and urine and serum electrolytes *to detect or prevent compromise.*
- Monitor specific gravity *to determine ability to concentrate urine.*
- Modify diet as indicated *to prevent azotemia.*
- Monitor for symptoms of electrolyte and intake and output imbalance.

Impaired physical mobility related to general weakness and joint involvement

- Assess degree of limitation: range of motion, joint integrity, presence of pain (location, duration, quality, severity, and precipitating or alleviating factors), deformity, and muscular atrophy.
- Perform range of motion exercises as tolerated *to maintain joint integrity.*
- In collaboration with physician, administer analgesics according to appropriate and regular time schedules. Assess patient's response.
- Administer thermal therapy to muscles and joints *for pain control.*
- Confer with physical or occupational therapist *to determine other beneficial interventions.*

TABLE 14-6 Frequency of Clinical Symptoms in SLE

Symptom	Percent
Fever	83
Weight loss	62
Arthritis, arthralgia	90
Skin	74
Butterfly rash	42
Photosensitivity	30
Mucous membrane lesions	12
Alopecia	27
Raynaud's phenomenon	17
Purpura	15
Urticaria	8
Renal	53
Nephrosis	18
Gastrointestinal	38
Pulmonary	47
Pleurisy	45
Effusion	24
Pneumonia	29
Cardiac	46
Pericarditis	27
Murmurs	23
Electrocardiographic changes	39
Lymphadenopathy	46
Splenomegaly	15
Hepatomegaly	25
Central nervous system	32
Psychosis	15
Convulsions	15
Cytoid bodies	11

From Schur.[22]

Impaired skin integrity related to integumentary manifestations

- Assess skin and mucous membranes: Inspect and palpate noting color, vascularity, lesion size, configuration, and distribution, edema, moisture, temperature, texture, thickness, mobility, and turgor.
- Monitor skin lesions *for signs of infection.*
- In collaboration with physician, administer topical steroidal or antiinfective creams and ointments as indicated. Assess response.
- Provide hypoallergenic, nondrying soaps and mild shampoos.
- Encourage use of sunscreen products if patient is photosensitive.

Altered nutrition: less than body requirements, related to anorexia, electrolyte imbalance, or chemotherapy side effects

- Assess nutritional status: Monitor serum protein and albumin values; monitor for evidence of poor wound healing; determine weight loss and compare to ideal body weight.
- Encourage balanced diet with supplements if indicated.
- Encourage weight reduction diet for patients who have gained weight while taking steroids.
- Low-sodium, high-potassium diet may be indicated for patients receiving steroids.
- Encourage intake of vitamin supplements for patients who are pregnant or dieting.

Risk for activity intolerance related to flare, chronic anemia, arthralgias, and other effects of SLE

- Assess degree of activity intolerance.
- Encourage balance between rest and exercise.
- Flares warrant temporary rest.
- During periods when disease is quiescent, encourage program of regular, aerobic exercise that places as little stress on joints as possible (such as swimming).

Risk for infection related to altered immune system or steroid therapy

- Assess for evidence of infection at sites of invasive procedures.
- Assess for breaks in skin, particularly over pressure areas and oral mucosa *to prevent infection.*
- Assess pulmonary status: auscultate lung fields to determine presence of adventitious breath sounds *to detect or prevent pneumonia.*
- Maintain optimum nutritional status and fluid intake.
- Assess ocular integrity for evidence of conjunctivitis; erythematous, pruritic conjunctiva.
- Assess mentation for evidence of central nervous system infection: changes in level of consciousness, headache, and visual disturbances.
- Assess for evidence of gastrointestinal infection: abdominal pain, fever, and diarrhea.

- Monitor temperature and vital signs for evidence of fever or sepsis.
- Maintain body hygiene.
- Promote pulmonary toilet: breathing exercises, postural drainage, and chest physical therapy.
- Maintain normal sleep and rest patterns.
- Protect patient from physical injury.
- Provide clean environment.
- Restrict contact with family and health care providers who have infectious diseases.
- Wash hands thoroughly before and after contact with patient.

Patient Education/Home Care Planning

1. Teach patient the side effects of medications.
2. Teach the patient the importance of avoiding contact with persons who may expose the patient to infection.
3. Teach the patient the importance of frequent assessment for signs and symptoms associated with infection. While steroids are being given, many of these findings are masked, so the slightest change in temperature, wound characteristics, or other parameters should be reported immediately.
4. Teach the patient the importance of skin care. Tell the patient to avoid dryness and use of irritant soaps, shampoos, chemical coloring, or permanent waving of hair. Encourage use of hypoallergenic makeup and wearing wig if there is hair loss. Teach photosensitive patients to avoid sun exposure: limit outdoor activities between 10 AM and 4 PM, wear long sleeves, pants, and hats, and use sunscreen products with a sun protection factor of at least 15.
5. Teach the patient methods to cope with arthralgias and myalgias: range of motion exercises, balance between rest and exercise, use of analgesics and nonsteroidal anti-inflammatory agents, joint supports at night, contacting Arthritis Foundation.
6. Teach the patient the importance of regular follow-up by a physician and the need for blood tests.
7. Teach the patient the importance of recognizing factors that lead to a flare: psychologic and physical stress, use of drugs that induce a lupuslike syndrome (see p. 1210), abrupt cessation of medications, and photosensitivity.
8. Teach the patient warning signs of a flare: fever, chills, excessive fatigue and malaise, nausea, muscle weakness, increased joint pain, chest pain, oliguria, and dysuria—essentially, exacerbation of an old symptom or development of a new one.
9. Teach the patient the importance of maintaining a balanced diet; include restrictions associated with medications.
10. Teach family planning. Pregnancy is usually allowed during remissions with close monitoring. Barrier contraceptives such as a condom or diaphragm are recommended.

11. Teach the patient the importance of keeping a log of the disease course, treatments, and other disease-related information.
12. Teach the patient the importance of obtaining up-to-date information about SLE.
13. Teach the patient to carry medical alert identification.
14. Direct the patient to available resources.

Evaluation

Respiratory status is stable   Patient's respiratory pattern and breath sounds are within normal limits. Patient performs respiratory toilet.

Cardiac status is stable   Patient's vital signs are normal. No ectopy is noted on ECG. Patient is alert and oriented; judgment, mental acuity, and behavior are within patient's normal parameters.

Renal status is stable   Patient's intake and output are balanced. Findings of kidney function studies are within normal limits.

Patient maintains independence in activities of daily living   Patient returns to baseline ability to perform ADLs. Patient reports decreased fatigue and no discomfort with movement.

Skin integrity is maintained   Patient's skin is warm and dry, with good turgor and color.

No infection occurs   Patient shows no signs or symptoms associated with infection.

Patient complies with treatment   Patient verbalizes understanding of importance of compliance and adheres to prescribed regimens and methods of symptoms control.

ALLERGIC DISORDERS

ATOPIC DISEASE

The term "allergy" was initially used to describe "altered reactivity" and has evolved over the years to refer broadly to any immunologic reaction for a foreign substance that produces detrimental consequences to the body. It is often used interchangeably with atopy.

Atopy is an abnormal immune response mediated by IgE antibody produced against substances that normally occur in the environment. Atopic diseases include anaphylaxis, allergic rhinoconjunctivitis, allergic asthma, atopic dermatitis, gastrointestinal allergy, and occasionally urticaria or angioedema. Allergy to a drug or an insect bite or sting can cause anaphylaxis or hives by an immunologic IgE mechanism in persons with or without other allergic symptoms (atopic or nonatopic).

Atopy appears in approximately 20% of the population and is thought to be inherited through genes linked to HLA antigen haplotypes. The expression of atopy has been linked to multi-ple factors including hormonal changes, antigen exposure, and concurrent illness. Expression of symptoms can occur at any time during life and varies from mild to life threatening in severity.

Pathophysiology

The genetic defect is thought to be in T suppressor cell modulation, which allows increased or unmodulated production of IgE antibody.

The antigens precipitating the IgE response are restricted to either complete protein antigens with specific carrier and antigenic determinants or low–molecular weight substances that function as haptens by combining with serum or tissue proteins to form a complex. Antigens may be inhaled (tree, grass, or weed pollens, mold spores, dust, animal proteins), ingested (food, drugs), injected (venom, drug), or touched.

On initial exposure the antigen (allergen) is processed by a macrophage and then presented to the appropriately responsive T lymphocyte. Interaction then occurs with B lymphocytes, which, when stimulated, develop into mature plasma cells and secrete the antigen-specific IgE antibody.

Only a very small amount of IgE antibody circulates in the serum. Most IgE is found fixed to the surface of mast cells (fixed in tissue) or basophils (circulating). There may be 5000 to 500,000 IgE molecules on a single mast cell. A mast cell may have a large variety of antigen-specific IgE antibodies on its surface.

Mast cells and basophils contain several potent chemical mediators of inflammation, including histamine, arachidonic acid metabolites such as prostaglandins and leukotrienes C, D, or S, eosinophil chemotactic factors of anaphylaxis (ECF-A), and platelet-activating factor (PAF). Mediators may exert a direct pharmacologic effect or release or activate other mediators potentiating the response. Mediators initiate a sequence of physiologic events in various organ systems that result in such responses as vasodilation, enhanced vasopermeability, smooth muscle contraction, and increased mucus production (Figure 14-11).

On reexposure and entry the antigen binds to IgE antibodies. This causes degranulation of the mast cell and release of the mediators that initiate the pathophysiologic responses. Symptoms of atopic disease are the result of tissue response to the mediators. Symptoms may be generalized (anaphylaxis) or localized (for example, in bronchi, conjunctiva, nasal membranes, skin, or gut). This mechanism of tissue reaction occurs immediately on exposure to the antigen and is identified as a type I anaphylactic or immediate hypersensitivity reaction by the Gell and Coombs nomenclature.

Mast cell mediators are responsible for both the well-known "class" allergic response, in which symptoms occur immediately upon exposure, as well as the less well-known late phase response in which symptoms begin hours after allergen exposure and result from tissue inflammation and damage.

Anaphylactoid reactions mimic allergic reactions and clinically may be identical to IgE-mediated responses. However, no IgE is involved and symptoms result from direct action on mast

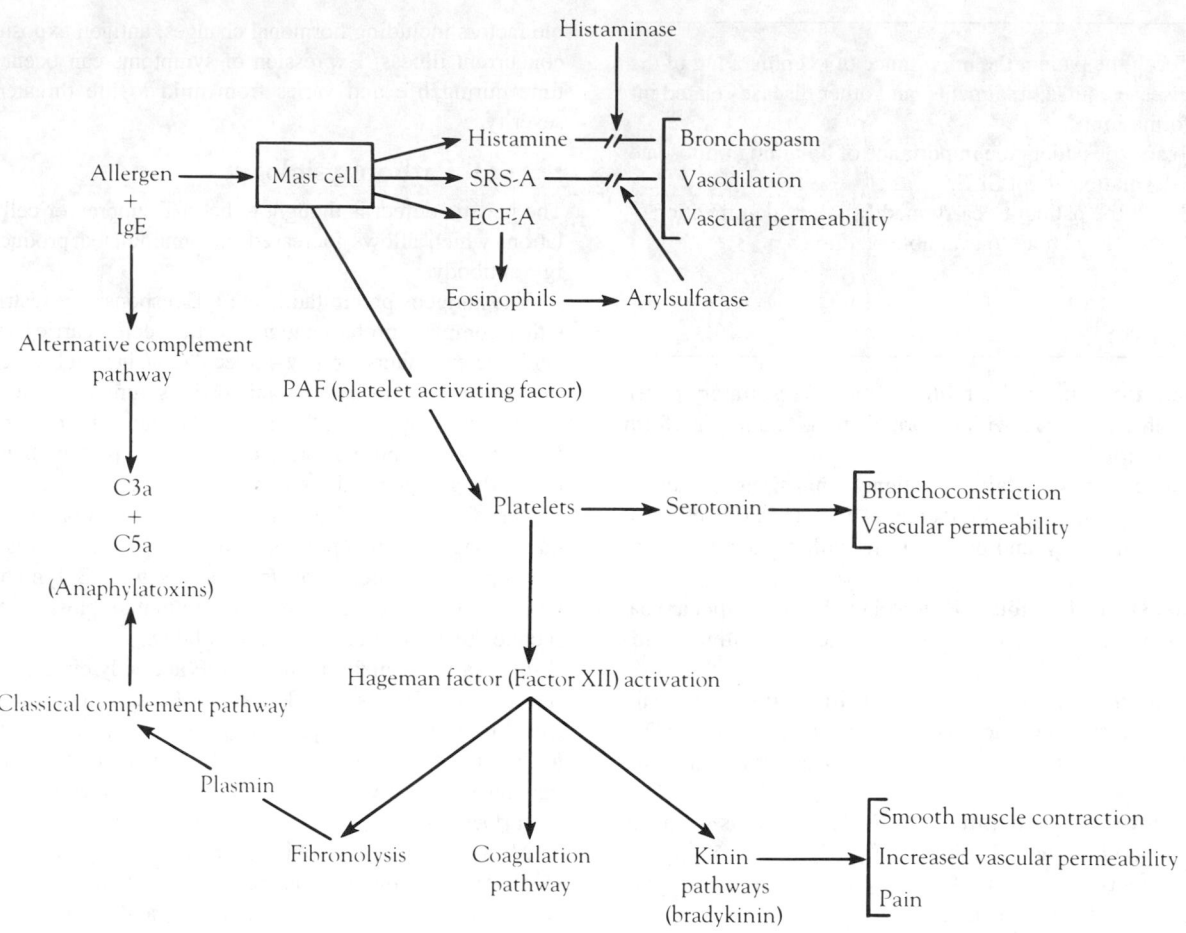

Figure 14-11 Mediators of immediate hypersensitivity. Interaction of allergen-antibody reaction, complement system, clotting system, and kinin system (→ indicates stimulation; // indicates inhibition.) (From Lawlor.[15])

cells that causes release of chemical mediators (occurs with dextran and radiocontrast media), prostaglandin activation (occurs with acetylsalicylic acid and some nonsteroidal antiinflammatory agents), or complement activation (occurs with aggregated IgG). The exact trigger mechanism and pathways of inflammatory responses are not fully understood. However, these reactions are treated in the same manner as anaphylactic reactions. The only clinical difference is that, since IgE is not involved, skin testing is of no value and reactions can occur with the first exposure; prior sensitization is not required.

•••••• Diagnostic Studies and Findings

A thorough history is by far the most important diagnostic tool. The physical examination focuses on all areas of potential atopic manifestations. Laboratory studies may be useful in supporting the diagnosis and in monitoring response to therapy but are not in themselves diagnostic.

History

Onset, nature, and progression of symptoms; aggravating and alleviating factors; frequency, time, and duration of symptoms; complete environmental history including occupational, chemical, smoking, animal, and hobby exposures; household description including heating and cooling systems, pets, and bedding; past medical history; medications; family history including atopic history

Physical Examination

Skin; external ear canal and tympanic membrane; conjunctiva; nasal membranes; naso-oropharynx; chest

Laboratory Studies

Complete blood count
  Within normal limits
Differential
  May have eosinophil percentage, up to 5%
Eosinophil count
  Within normal limits or increased up to 10% (up to 700 cells/mm³), but range of normal is wide and increases may also occur in other diseases that have similar symptoms

Smears for eosinophils
  Generally predominate in secretions (up to 90% of total) during symptomatic periods
Total serum IgE levels
  Within normal limits or increased (up to 700 U/ml), but there is wide range of normal and increases can also occur in other diseases
Skin testing
  Demonstrates presence of specific IgE antibody; most reliable test for allergy; reliable correlation for inhalants, much less reliable for foods; false positive findings may result from irritant response; false negative findings may result from poor skin response or antihistamines; findings must correlate with history; drug may be hapten or metabolite; testing currently limited to penicillin, horse serum, insulin, and egg-based vaccines
Radioallergosorbent test (RAST)
  Demonstrates presence of specific circulating IgE antibody; less reliable than skin testing (not as sensitive; difficulty in standardization of test and reproducibility of tests among reference laboratories)
Provocative testing
  Specific antigen challenges performed under controlled conditions to demonstrate clinical reactivity
Elimination testing
  Demonstration of clinical sensitivity to antigen by removing and then reintroducing it while monitoring clinical symptoms

•••••• Multidisciplinary Plan

The goals of the treatment plan include symptom management through medications, environmental control, and immunotherapy. Specific plans are discussed with each disease.

Medications

Medications are used to prevent the tissue response and resultant symptoms. The choice of medication is to some extent organ specific, since the tissue response differs in specific organ systems, and these are discussed with the specific allergic disease.

Antihistamines
  Six classes of older antihistamines are available as well as newer H_1 antihistamines; topical preparations should be avoided because of potential for sensitization; they may be given orally or intramuscularly depending on preparation and with dose adjustments to any patient older than 3 mo, including pregnant women (who may receive selected antihistamines, including chlorpheniramine)
Cromolyn sodium
  Intal, via Spinhaler or metered dose inhaler, q6h or as needed before exposure for adult and child older than 6 yr
  Nebuluzer solution, 1 ampule via nebulizer q6h or as needed before exposure for adult and child older than 2 yr

Nasalcrom 1 spray q4-6h or as needed before exposure for adult and child older than 6 yr
Opticrom, 1 drop in each eye as above
Immunotherapy recommended for inhalant antigens (e.g., tree, grass, and weed pollens) and venoms, but not for foods
Desensitization for insulin and penicillin requires special protocols performed under close supervision and is done only when medically indicated

Environmental Control

Environmental control is the preferred method of treatment because complete avoidance of the offending allergen affords total relief of symptoms. The following is a representative list of allergens and possible measures:

Tree, grass, and weed pollens—air-conditioning, closing bedroom or car windows during pollen season (times of pollination depend on geographic area)
Mold spores—removal of source (such as plant dirt), application of mold retardant solutions for damp areas (for example, crawl spaces, bathrooms), air filtration by a high-efficiency particulate-arresting (HEPA) filter or electrostatic air cleaner.
House dust and mites—plastic mattress casing, removal of carpets, damp dusting and face masks while dusting, air filtration
Epidermals (feather, animal protein)—removal of source
Foods—avoidance
Drugs—avoidance
Stinging or biting insects—avoidance

NURSING CARE

Nursing Assessment

Allergic responses may involve one or more organ systems, and symptoms may range from mild to severe. Symptoms may be episodic or perennial depending on exposures. Assessment must also discriminate among possible concurrent diseases. Specific assessment is discussed with each allergic disease.

Nursing Dx & Intervention

Because of the variable expression of atopic disease, the following is included as part of the comprehensive overview of the disease. Specific interventions are addressed with discussion of each disease.

Risk for injury related to exposure to antigen

- Obtain complete allergy history and record in appropriate places.
- Emphasize potential harm of repeat exposure.
- Identify and teach patient the measures to institute if patient is reexposed to antigen.
- Emphasize need for medical alert identification.

Risk for activity intolerance related to medication side effects

- Modify activity prescriptions based on current symptoms status, including fatigue.
- Encourage full activity schedule for growth and developmental age. Make appropriate medication adjustments and apply environmental control measures.

Risk for infection related to depressed immune system

- Assess for signs and symptoms of concurrent infection.
- Maintain optimal nutritional intake.
- Maintain appropriate rest patterns.
- Monitor use of medications *to control or eliminate symptoms.*

Body image disturbances related to perceived chronic illness

- Assess patient for current restrictions in life-style and work, adjustment to illness, self-management behaviors, and family's adjustment to illness.
- Coordinate with physician and patient modifications in medical, therapeutic prescriptions as indicated.

Altered health maintenance related to lack of knowledge

- Assess patient's and family's knowledge of disease process, relationship to symptoms, and methods of preventing or controlling symptoms.
- Provide education *to achieve optimum level of health.*

Patient Education/Home Care Planning

1. Review the disease process with the patient to assess the accuracy of the patient's understanding.
2. Review with the patient medication use and expected response to therapy.
3. Teach the patient self-responsibility for allergen identification and avoidance measures.
4. Direct the patient to support and educational groups.

Evaluation

Specific criteria are identified with discussion of each atopic disease. The following are general outcome measures for any atopic disease.

Symptoms are resolved in response to therapeutic measures   There are no symptoms associated with individual system involvement.

Normal activity and exercise are maintained   Patient performs activities appropriate for growth and developmental age.

Patient is knowledgeable about allergy and its treatment   Patient and family describe allergy, medical plan of care, environmental control, and other self-care measures.

ALLERGIC RHINITIS/ALLERGIC RHINOCONJUNCTIVITIS

Allergic rhinitis/allergic rhinoconjunctivitis is a complex of symptoms resulting from an antigen–IgE antibody reaction occurring in the nasal membranes, conjunctiva, or nasopharynx. The antigen is generally inhaled and deposited on the mucous membrane surface. Symptoms may also result from injected or ingested antigen transported to the site.

Approximately 18.6 million infants, children, and adults in the United States have seasonal or perennial allergic rhinitis. An estimated $224 million is spent annually for physician services and $300 million for medications, and some 28 million days each year are lost because of restricted activity or absence from school or work.

Symptoms may develop as early as infancy but can occur at any time throughout the life span. A positive family history may be obtained in the majority of cases. Without intervention, symptoms may remain constant, increase, or diminish over time.

•••••• Pathophysiology

With antigen-antibody linkage, mast cell degranulation and chemical mediator release occur, resulting in slower ciliary action, stimulation of mucosal glands, vasomotor instability, leukocyte infiltration (primarily eosinophilic), and tissue edema because of vasodilation and capillary permeability. Histamine is the major mediator of the inflammatory response, although other mediators such as eosinophil chemotactic factor of anaphylaxis (ECF-A), prostaglandins, and leukotrienes participate.

With prolonged exposure, basement membrane destruction and foamy cell formation occur. More chronic and irreversible changes include hyperplasia and thickening of the mucosal epithelium, mononuclear cellular infiltration, and connective tissue proliferation.

Symptoms generally result from inhalant allergen exposure or occasionally, especially in infants, from food ingestion. The inflammatory response may be confined to the nasal membranes or extend to the conjunctiva or oropharynx. Symptoms begin immediately on exposure and may be prolonged because of the late phase reaction.

•••••• Diagnostic Studies and Findings

See p. 1216.

Skin tests   Positive responses that correlate with history

Sinus roentgenogram   Within normal limits; may be necessary to rule out other diseases such as cysts, nasal polyps, infective rhinitis, and structural defects

CT scan of sinuses   Rules out other diseases and structural defects

•••••• Multidisciplinary Plan

The goal of the treatment plan is to block symptoms, maintain optimum function, and prevent sequelae such as fatigue, infections, serous otitis, and restricted activity.

Medications

Antihistamines

May be used prn or round the clock; long-acting compounds generally best; tolerance avoided by using different antihistamines; often combined with decongestants

Cromolyn sodium, prn before known antigen exposure (cat, dog, dusting) but more effective round the clock; short half-life often requires doses q4-6h or concomitant nocturnal antihistamine

Sympathomimetic agents

Topical decongestants: over-the-counter; should not be used for more than 3 consecutive days; useful for severe acute symptoms until other medications take effect

Oral decongestants: agents available (phenylephrine, phenylpropanolamine, pseudoephedrine); may be obtained over-the-counter or by prescription; age-dependent dosage; may be used from 3 mo of age; often used in combination with antihistamines and in long-acting preparations for decreased dosage schedule; must be used with caution in patients with hypertension or glaucoma; blood pressure monitoring needed

Corticosteroids

Topical: excellent for controlling more severe symptoms; must be used on regular basis

Flunisolide (Nasalide), 1 spray q8h for adult or child older than 6 yr

Beclomethasone (Vancenase, Beconase), 2 sprays q8h for adult or child older than 12 yr

Decadron (Decadron Turbinaire), 2 sprays q8h for adult; 1-2 sprays bid for child older than 6 yr

Oral: rarely used since advent of topical agents; should be considered only when symptoms are severe and other measures have failed

Ocular: because of side effects, even short-term use severely restricted and closely monitored

Antiinfective agents

Used for secondary bacterial infections; synthetic penicillins, sulfa, or erythromycin generally recommended and should be used for 10 d to 2 wk

Analgesic agents

Used to reduce symptoms of pressure headache until appropriate medications achieve symptom control

Environmental Control

Allergic rhinitis responds dramatically to removal of allergen; see p. 1217 for control of antigen exposure

Immunotherapy

Allergic rhinitis responds well to appropriately designed immunotherapy program

General Management

Increased fluid intake to liquefy secretions and counter loss from obligatory mouth breathing

Steam or topical nasal saltwater solutions to decrease irritability and help loosen secretions

---

NURSING CARE

Nursing Assessment

The goal of assessment is to confirm the extent and severity of organ involvement and establish a baseline for later evaluation.

Conjunctival Inflammation

Hyperemia; edema (chemosis) involving either palpebral or bulbar membranes; secretions in palpebral fissures; superficial keratitis; edema; hyperplasia of papillae

Facial Changes

Dark discoloration in orbital-palpebral groove beneath lower eyelids ("allergic shiners"); adenoidal facies consisting of elongated maxilla, narrow chin, gaping expression, possible dental malocclusion, and transverse crease across top of nose

Nasal Membrane Inflammation

Swollen, wet, pale turbinates; mucosal edema; glistening, clear, watery or serous drainage; more variability in chronic disease

Oropharyngeal Inflammation

Nasal secretions; erythema; edema; high-arched palate; overbite

Tympanic Membrane Involvement

Bulging or retracted; prominent bony landmarks or none present; membrane thick, dull, or wrinkled, with gray, pink, amber, slightly yellow, or deep blue color; injected; evidence of fluid levels or bubbles

Nursing Dx & Intervention

Ineffective breathing pattern related to inflammatory response

- Assess for obligatory mouth breathing, paroxysmal nocturnal dyspnea, snoring, or sleep apnea that may contribute to "allergic fatigue."
- Elevate head of bed to 45 degrees *to facilitate mucus drainage.*
- Humidify air as needed.
- Monitor medication schedule *to block symptoms adequately.*
- Assess environment for presence of offending allergens and remove if possible.
- Emphasize importance of nasal breathing.

Impaired home maintenance management related to lack of knowledge

- Discuss chronicity of disease process and reinforce need to prevent symptoms through medications and environmental control.

Risk for injury related to autoimmune response

- Emphasize importance of avoiding antigens known to cause severe reactions, and explain potential for severe reactions to people who are likely to have contact with patient.
- Adhere strictly to immunotherapy protocols, and monitor patient for 20 minutes after injections.

Risk for activity intolerance related to sedentary life-style

- Explain that normal work, exercise, and recreation activities can and should be maintained through medications and environmental control.

Risk for infection related to inadequate primary defense

- Assess for signs and symptoms of infective rhinitis, infective otitis, and infective conjunctivitis.
- Maintain adequate nutritional intake and appropriate rest.
- Discuss rationale for adequately controlling symptoms and self-monitoring for secondary infections.

Patient Education/Home Care Planning

1. Assess the patient's current knowledge of the disease process and reinforce the concept of self-care and self-management of the disease.
2. Assess the patient's current knowledge of medications, side effects, and rationale for the use of medications, and reinforce the concepts of prophylaxis and prevention of symptoms.
3. Teach the patient the importance of environmental control measures and the patient's responsibility for implementing recommended measures.
4. Teach the patient the importance of monitoring symptom response to therapies, recording any difficulties, new symptoms, and untoward effects, and communicating this on an ongoing basis to those prescribing the therapies.

Evaluation

Symptoms are resolved in response to therapeutic measures   There are not symptoms associated with inflammatory response or infective process.

Health is maintained at optimum level   Patient can identify all recommended therapies and provide information related to self-management.

Optimum functional levels are maintained   Patient engages in normal work, school, or recreational activities without restrictions.

■ ANAPHYLAXIS

Anaphylaxis results from a systemic IgE-mediated antigen-antibody response. It is an immediate and often life-threatening event in which massive release of mediators triggers a sequence of events in target organs throughout the body, resulting in a variety of symptoms that may include respiratory embarrassment or circulatory collapse.

As with other IgE antigen-antibody reactions, prior sensitization to the antigen must have occurred for anaphylaxis to take place. Anaphylactoid reactions and blood transfusion reactions are mediated by a non-IgE mechanism with the same final common pathway as IgE-mediated reactions. Reactions must be differentiated from vasovagal reactions, syncopal attacks, myocardial infarctions, insulin reactions, hysterical reactions, and shock or respiratory obstruction from other causes.

A systemic reaction is any organ involvement away from the site of antigen deposition. Reactions are classified as mild, moderate, or severe and may involve the respiratory tract, cardiovascular system, gastrointestinal tract, or skin (Table 14-7). Symptoms may progress in minutes from mild to severe, or severe reaction may occur without warning. Reactions may occur up to 2 hours after exposure. Reactions that occur immediately are the most life threatening. Resolution of symptoms may be immediate or take several days. Resolution depends on the severity of the reaction, the promptness of medical intervention, and any complications occurring during the reaction. Early recognition and rapid intervention may prevent progression to severe reactions.

•••••• Pathophysiology

A history of atopic disease is often not elicited from patients with anaphylaxis. Previous exposures to the offending antigens may or may not have caused an untoward reaction.

Anaphylactoid reactions, through direct mast cell destabilization, immune complex aggregation, or prostaglandin-activating mechanisms, may also cause the release of mediators that results in a systemic reaction clinically similar to anaphylaxis (see Emergency Alert box). The following are some mechanisms that have been proposed for anaphylactoid reactions:

Direct mediator release (agents such as dextran and radiopaque dyes)

Immune complex aggregation (agents such as γ-globulin administered intramuscularly or intravenously)

Cytotoxic antibody transfusion reactions (agents such as whole blood and cryoprecipitate)

Prostaglandin-induced (agents such as aspirin and nonsteroidal anti-inflammatory agents)

Anaphylaxis may result from injection of antigen (subcutaneous, intravenous, or intramuscular drugs or venom stings), although enough antigen may be absorbed from the gut (ingested food or drug) or from the respiratory tract (inhaled antigen) to precipitate the reaction. The antigen is distributed via the blood stream and fixes to IgE antibody on mast cells and basophils, triggering mediator release. On reexposure to antigen and its subsequent linkage with IgE antibody, mediator release occurs and affects the end organ responses (Table 14-8).

■ TABLE 14-7 Potential Symptom Complex of Anaphylaxis

Target Organ	Mild	Moderate	Severe
General status (prodromal)	Malaise; sense of illness	Greater malaise and sense of illness	Deep malaise and strong sense of illness
Skin	Hives; erythema; tingling; warm sensation; itching	Generalized urticaria; flushing; generalized pruritus; periorbital edema	Cyanosis; pallor
Upper respiratory tract	Nasal congestion; sneezing; rhinorrhea; conjunctivitis	Profuse congestion and rhinorrhea	Periorbital edema; obligatory mouth breathing
Upper airway	Fullness in mouth or throat	Edema of tongue, larynx, and pharynx; hoarseness	Stridor; completely occluded airway
Lower airway	Cough	Bronchospasm; dyspnea; cough; wheezing; air trapping	Severe dyspnea; hypoxia; respiratory arrest
Gastrointestinal tract	Cramping	Nausea; vomiting; increased peristalsis	Dysphagia; intense abdominal cramping; diarrhea
Cardiovascular system	Tachycardia	Hypotension; syncope	Coronary insufficiency; cardiac dysrhythmias; shock; circulatory collapse
Central nervous system	Anxiety	Intense anxiety; confusion	Seizures; coma

---

! EMERGENCY ALERT

ANAPHYLACTIC SHOCK

Anaphylactic shock is classified as a vasogenic shock where severe vasodilation occurs. Anaphylactic shock is an antigen-antibody reaction where a sensitized person is exposed to an antigen. Common allergies are to stings, shellfish, and medications. A relative hypovolemia results from intervascular fluid shifting.

Assessment

- Signs of respiratory distress, bronchospasm, wheezing airway obstruction, respiratory arrest.
- Edematous tongue.
- Skin may be warm and dry or present with urticaria or edema.
- Dysrhythmias or cardiopulmonary arrest may occur.

Interventions

- Maintain airway, breathing, and circulation.
- Administer high flow oxygen (10-15 L) by mask.
- Obtain IV access; in collaboration with physician administer epinephrine 0.1-0.5 ml of a 1:10,000 solution; may repeat as indicated.
- If further medication is indicated, in collaboration with physician administer aminophylline, benadryl, and/or corticosteroids.

TABLE 14-8 Physiologic Response to Mediators

Mediator	Effect	End Organ Response
Histamine	Vascular permeability	Edema of larynx, gut, and airways; urticaria
Leukotrienes	Vascular smooth muscle relaxation	Decreased peripheral volume; decreased peripheral resistance
Kallikrein	Vasodilation and vascular engorgement	Decreased blood pressure; bronchospasm
Platelet-activating factor	Increased bronchial smooth muscle tone	Rhinorrhea; bronchorrhea
Others	Mucous gland secretion; irritability of peripheral nerve endings; intestinal smooth muscle tone	Pruritus; gut motility; rhinorrhea; bronchorrhea

Drugs
　Proteins (presumably complete antigens)
　Foreign serum
　Vaccines
　Allergen extracts
　Enzymes
Nonprotein drugs (presumably haptens)
　Penicillin and other antibiotics
　Sulfonamides
　Local anesthetics
　Hormones
Venoms
　Hymenoptera (honeybee, wasp, hornet, yellow jacket)
　Deerfly
　Fire ant

Almost any drug may precipitate an anaphylactic reaction. Subcutaneous, intramuscular, and intravenous routes provide sufficient antigen for overwhelming systemic reactions. Anaphylaxis produced by insect venom may account for more than 100 deaths annually. Foods may generate an anaphylactic reaction, particularly in adults, although this is not common. The following are some common antigens of anaphylaxis:

Foods
  Legumes (especially peanuts)
  Nuts
  Berries
  Seafood
  Egg albumin

•••••• Diagnostic Studies and Findings

The diagnosis is based on a history of signs and symptoms of anaphylaxis immediately after exposure to a likely offending agent, as well as supportive laboratory data.

Complete Blood Count

Within normal limits or increased hematocrit value resulting from hemoconcentration

Blood Chemistries

Within normal limits unless myocardial or renal damage has occurred owing to circulatory collapse

Chest Roentgenogram

Normal appearance or hyperinflation with or without atelectasis; pulmonary edema

Electrocardiogram

Normal unless myocardial damage or hypoxemic changes are present

Skin Tests

Must be done at least 4 weeks after anaphylactic episode to ensure adequate repopulation of IgE antibody; requires extreme caution; usefulness limited to egg-based vaccines, venom, foods, horse serum, insulin, and penicillin

•••••• Multidisciplinary Plan

The goal of the treatment plan is swift, aggressive management of symptoms. Establishment of an airway and maintenance of blood pressure are crucial. Therapy is individualized based on organ involvement and severity of reaction.

Medications

Medications used to counteract effects of mediator release, block additional mediator release, and protect organ system involved; continued until all symptoms have completely resolved; given over sufficient time to prevent further symptoms development; withdrawn with careful monitoring

General Management

Maintained until all symptoms of anaphylaxis are resolved
  Airway with suctioning as appropriate
  Endotracheal tube or tracheostomy if indicated
  Arterial blood gas monitoring
  Treatment of acidosis
  Volume replacement and vasopressors

Intake and output
Monitor electrocardiograms
Treat dysrhythmias if present
Complete drug allergy history before administration of any new drug
Human serum preparations preferred, if antiserum indicated
Skin testing for vaccines, venoms, antivenoms, insulin, and penicillin
Use of pretreatment protocols and close monitoring required in the special circumstances when patients at risk must be exposed (to radiologic contrast media, insulin, or penicillin)

NURSING CARE

Nursing Assessment

Because of multisystem involvement, anaphylactic or anaphylactoid reactions may initially have a variety of manifestations.

Laryngeal Involvement

Hoarseness; stridor; use of accessory muscles; difficulty in speech

Respiratory Status

Dyspnea; substernal tightness; use of accessory muscles; cough

Bronchospasm

Mucus production; rales; wheezing; decreased breath sounds; anxiety; inability to lie supine; evidence of air trapping or atelectasis on chest roentgenogram

Pulmonary Edema

Wet rales at base; frothy clear or blood-streaked secretions

Respiratory Arrest

No air movement

Circulatory Status

Hypotension; weak, thready pulse; tachycardia; oliguria; mental confusion

Cardiac Status

Dysrhythmias; tachycardia; cardiac arrest

Central Nervous System Status

Anxiety; malaise; sense of illness; mental confusion; obtundation; coma

Dermal Status

Pruritus; erythema; flushing; urticaria; angioedema; cyanosis; pallor

Gastrointestinal Status

Nausea; vomiting; diarrhea; gastrointestinal cramping

Upper Respiratory Status

Rhinorrhea; congestion; sneezing; conjunctivitis; tearing

Nursing Dx & Intervention

Risk for ineffective breathing pattern related to tracheobronchial obstruction

- Maintain endotracheal tube or tracheostomy, if instituted. Suction carefully.
- Assess and record ventilation pattern, including rate, rhythm, use of accessory muscles, and length of expiratory phase.
- Monitor for mouth breathing and rhinorrhea.
- Maintain 45-degree elevation of patient's head if possible.
- Assess for laryngeal involvement, including stridor, hoarseness and difficulty in swallowing or speech.
- Be prepared for respiratory arrest management.

Impaired gas exchange related to alveolar-capillary membrane changes

- Monitor blood gases.
- Administer oxygen at indicated rate.
- Assess breath sounds; report rales, rhonchi, or wheezing.
- Assess for shortness of breath, dyspnea.
- Monitor fluid replacement and assess for pulmonary overload.

Altered tissue perfusion: cardiopulmonary, cerebral related to exchange problems

- Monitor vital signs, CVP, level of consciousness, chest pain, intake and output, and ECG pattern.
- Assess for symptoms of anxiety, confusion, obtundation, or coma.
- Report signs of hypotension.
- Place in supine position to promote venous return.
- Use safety measures if confused.
- Monitor parenteral fluids carefully to prevent overload.
- Be prepared to institute cardiopulmonary resuscitation.

Altered gastrointestinal tissue perfusion related to exchange problems

- Monitor for nausea, vomiting, abdominal cramping, and diarrhea. Record findings.
- In conjunction with physician, administer antihistamines as indicated.

Altered peripheral tissue perfusion related to exchange problems

- Monitor for cyanosis, pallor, and pulse abnormalities. Record findings.
- In conjunction with physician, administer epinephrine, fluids, or vasopressors as indicated.

Risk for injury: anaphylaxis related to exposure to inciting agent

- Obtain complete drug allergy history before administering new drug.
- Put label noting allergic drug history in all appropriate places.
- Closely monitor patient for 30 minutes after administering new drug.

Patient Education/Home Care Planning

1. Reassure patient during procedures.
2. Explain to the patient the reason for each procedure.
3. Explain to the patient the relationship of symptoms to anaphylactic reaction.
4. Explain to the patient the absolute necessity of avoiding causative agent.
5. Discuss with the patient the need for follow-up care and for allergy testing when indicated.
6. Explain to the patient the need to carry or wear medical alert identification and to inform other health care personnel.
7. Stress to the patient the importance of avoiding any medications without first checking with the physician.
8. Teach the patient self-administration of epinephrine and subsequent measures, including oral administration of antihistamine and seeking immediate medical care.

Evaluation

Symptoms resolve in response to therapeutic measures Patient is symptom free. Patient expresses feeling of well-being. There is no evidence of urticaria or angioedema or subjective complaint of pruritus or swelling. There is no evidence of rhinoconjunctivitis, asthma, pulmonary edema, or laryngeal edema. Blood pressure and pulse rate are normal. There is no evidence of hypoxia.

Recurrence is prevented Patient can identify triggering agent and explain all appropriate avoidance measures.

■ FOOD ALLERGY

Food allergy is an IgE-mediated hypersensitivity disease. It may be manifested in the respiratory, integumentary, or gastrointestinal system as rhinitis, asthma, atopic dermatitis, urticaria, nausea, vomiting, diarrhea, or cramps or may result in anaphylaxis. An adverse food reaction is any untoward symptom complex resulting from food ingestion.

Adverse reaction to food is a complex diagnostic problem. There are various causes for adverse food reactions. True food allergy is mediated by IgE antibody (type I hypersensitivity reaction) in sensitized individuals on exposure to the offending antigen. Antibody-antigen linkage occurs and results in mediator release and symptoms.

Food intolerance is any abnormal physiologic response to an ingested food or food additive that is nonimmunologic in nature. Other immunologic mechanisms have been identified in adverse food reactions, including IgA deficiency, cytotoxic responses (type II), immune complex formation (type III), and cell-mediated reactions (type IV). Adverse reactions to food may have multiple origins, with a variety of nonimmunologic mechanisms resulting in a clinically abnormal host response. An idiosyncratic response in an individual may result in an anaphylactoid reaction, as with ingestion of monosodium glutamate. A metabolic defect such as lactose enzyme deficiency may cause foods to be improperly digested, or a metabolic problem such as diabetes may result in an abnormal response. Toxic responses to spoiled food are well known. Pharmacologic properties such as those of caffeine may exert a direct untoward effect. All these reactions are well documented and reproducible in controlled settings.

Other clinical syndromes are ascribed to foods or food additives, but this cannot be substantiated by reproducible, objective studies. While anecdotal evidence exists to support a relationship between food ingestion and behavior, other causal relationships have not been adequately ruled out. Tension-fatigue syndrome, hyperactivity syndrome, and psychiatric disorders such as mood swings are among the many disorders identified as being linked to food. Similar reports linking foods to rheumatoid arthritis or vasculitis and other physical syndromes also have not been substantiated. Other causes of vomiting, diarrhea, and stool abnormalities must also be excluded.

The prevalence of food allergy is unknown. Estimates range from 0.1% to 7% of the population, with a male/female ratio of approximately 2:1. If one sibling has a documented food allergy, a 50% probability of food hypersensitivity exists in other siblings. Anaphylactic episodes are most common in adults but may occur at any age. Nonimmunologic-mediated adverse food reactions have a much higher prevalence than immunologic reactions.

In exquisitely sensitive persons merely inhaling the antigen in cooking odors can precipitate a massive allergic reaction. Reactions are often dose related and may vary with time in the same individual. The foods most commonly associated with allergic reactions are milk, eggs, wheat, and soybeans in children, and fish, shellfish, peanuts, nuts, and seeds in adults, although virtually any food may cause an allergic response. Families of foods may share allergenic features, and thus cross-reactivity among those foods (for example, shellfish) is more common. Because of absorption characteristics, the reaction may be immediate or delayed up to 2 hours after ingestion.

•••••• Pathophysiology

As with other antigen–IgE antibody-mediated responses, prior exposure with sensitization in the atopic individual must occur. On reexposure, antigen-antibody linkage occurs with resultant mediator release. For reasons unknown, one end organ may be affected with a localized response, as in urticaria, or loss of sensitivity may occur with time.

Why different individuals become sensitized to particular food is also unknown. Allergenicity of the protein correlates with its heat-labile or enzyme-resistant properties. Although cooking or digestion may alter the protein, rendering it less allergenic, the altered protein may still precipitate an allergic response. An alteration in the original protein may contribute to false negative skin test findings if the unaltered food is used as the test antigen.

The gastrointestinal tract plays an important role in food allergy. The gut normally reaches maturity by 2 years of age. Before maturation there is a greater likelihood of absorption of food protein prior to complete digestion. Increase in absorption of potentially antigenic substances may also occur in IgA deficiency, malabsorption disease, and chronic inflammatory bowel diseases and after viral, parasitic, or bacterial diseases when the normal protective barriers have been damaged. These clinical syndromes may also contribute to adverse food reactions by decreasing normal flora, decreasing digestive enzymes, bile salts, and other secretions, reducing peristalsis, and interfering with cell renewal.

When the gut mucosal wall is damaged, protein may be absorbed and may precipitate IgE and IgG involvement or immune complex formation. Increased immunologic reactivity involving IgG and immune complex formation may result in enteropathies. Aspiration of milk in infancy may stimulate an IgE host defense response.

Genetic factors, amount of food ingested, food-drug interactions, contaminants, infections, pharmacologic properties, and nonimmunologic mechanisms have all been identified as contributing to adverse food reactions (Table 14-9).

Because of the multiple pathophysiologic mechanisms involved, clinical manifestations of adverse food reactions are widely variable (see Table 14-9). Depending on the mechanisms, amount, and duration of exposure, symptoms may vary from episodic to chronic and from mild to severe, and consequences may be reversible or irreversible.

•••••• Diagnostic Studies and Findings

Diagnostic studies are chosen based on the presentation of the adverse food reaction. The history is by far the most important diagnostic tool. The physical examination focuses on the clinical presentation.

Laboratory tests are chosen based on the suspected mechanisms of the adverse food reaction. Cytotoxic testing, sublingual testing, and red blood cell lysis have no proven efficacy in diagnosis and should not be employed.

History Frequency, duration and seasonality of symptoms; onset, severity, progression, and nature of symptoms; timing between ingestion and symptom onset; amount and nature of provoking food; concomitant illnesses; nutritional history; drug history; atopic history; infectious disease history.

Physical examination Skin; upper and lower respiratory tract; gastrointestinal tract; oropharynx; weight and height; growth and development; general appearance; vital signs; muscle mass and amount of subcutaneous tissue; texture and amount of hair; hepatomegaly

TABLE 14-9 Adverse Reactions to Foods

Type	Mechanism	Food (Examples)	Host Response
Type 1 Hypersensitivity			
Food allergy	IgE antibody—antigen linkage	Shellfish; nuts	Urticaria; angioedema; rhinitis; bronchospasm; nausea; vomiting, diarrhea; anaphylaxis
Metabolic Reactions			
Enzyme deficiencies	Lactase deficiency	Milk	Bloating; diarrhea; cramps
	Glucose 6-phosphate dehydrogenase (G6-PD) deficiency	Fava beans	Hemolytic anemia
	Phenylketonuria	Nutrasweet	Central nervous system changes
Severe chronic inflammatory bowel disease	Loss of enzymes through diarrhea and decreased production	Saccharides	Bloating; diarrhea; cramps; malabsorption
Medication interactions	Monoamine oxidase inhibitors	Cheese	Hypertensive crisis
Celiac disease	Probable type IV reaction	Wheat	Bloating; diarrhea; malabsorption
Gallbladder disease	Decreased bile salts	Fats	Bloating; indigestion; diarrhea; cramping
Diabetes	Decreased insulin	Sugar	Hyperglycemia
Cystic fibrosis	Inadequate pancreatic function	Fats; proteins	Fatty, foul-smelling stools; malabsorption
Natural Pharmacologic Agents			
Psychoactive agents	Direct sympathetic stimulation	Caffeine; theobromine	Central nervous system stimulation
Vasoactive amines (e.g., tryptamine, tyramine)	Direct action on end organ or autonomic stimulation	Cheese; chocolate	Headaches
Food Contamination by Infectious Agents, Microbes, and Toxins			
Bacteria; viruses; parasites; fungi	Endotoxins; neurotoxins; toxic alkaloids; damage to gut wall	Contaminated foods	Nausea; vomiting; diarrhea; bloating; weight loss; liver dysfunctions; headaches; fever; chills
Natural Toxic Agents			
Licorice	Sodium retention	Licorice	Hypertension
Glycoalkaloids	Probable direct blood vessel effect	Green potatoes; lima beans	Angioedema; urticaria
Anaphylactoid Reactions			
Chemical mediator release	Direct action on mast cell	Strawberries; tomatoes	Urticaria; angioedema; diarrhea
Nonimmunologic	Unknown	Tartrazine (FD & C yellow #5)	Urticaria; angioedema; rhinitis; asthma
	Unknown	Sodium metabisulfite	Urticaria; angioedema; rhinitis; asthma; anaphylaxis
	Unknown	Monosodium glutamate	Headache; flush; asthma
Types II, III, and IV Hypersensitivity			
Immune complexes with food antigen	Complement activation	After acute viral gastroenteritis	Diarrhea; cramping
Weiner's syndrome	IgG-antigen complexes; also type IV reaction	Milk	Respiratory symptoms; failure to thrive
Enteropathies	IgG precipitating antibodies	Milk; soy	Gastrointestinal bleeding; malabsorption; diarrhea; cramping
IgA deficiency	Failure to regulate antigen absorption	Variable	Malnutrition; diarrhea; increased with severity of disease

Laboratory tests

Type I hypersensitivity

Skin tests

May have false positives or negatives; not diagnostic; must be used in conjunction with challenge tests

Radioallergosorbent test (RAST)

May be less sensitive and has more limited panel than skin tests; may also have false positives or negatives; not diagnostic; must be used in conjunction with challenge tests

Total serum IgE
  Not specific indicator, not helpful
Eosinophil count
  Not specific indicator, not helpful
Elimination diets
  Aid in diagnosis by symptom response; used in conjunction with rechallenge; strict elimination diets difficult and cannot be used for more than 7 days
Food rechallenge
  Confirms diagnosis; not to be used if there is history of anaphylaxis
Types II, III, and IV hypersensitivity
  Biopsy of involved tissue
    Demonstrates presence of IgG, IgM, complement activation, or T cell involvement
  Hemagglutination
    May be present in persons without disease or absent in persons who have disease
  IgA deficiency
    IgA level
      Wide range of normal (80 to 350 mg/dl); may be low normal or depressed
Natural pharmacologic agents
  Diet diary and elimination diet
    Correlates symptoms with suspected agents
  Food rechallenge
    Confirms diagnosis
  Food contamination by infectious agents
    Stool cultures
      Document infectious agent
Natural toxic agents
  Diet diary and elimination diet
    Correlate symptoms with suspected agent
  Food rechallenge
    Confirms history
Anaphylactoid reactions
  Diet diary and elimination diet
    Correlate symptoms with suspected agent
  Food rechallenge, unless systemic reaction
    Confirms history

Metabolism
  Disease-specific workup (refer to discussion of specific disease elsewhere in text)

• • • • • Multidisciplinary Plan

The goal of the treatment plan is to eliminate the offending food, thus preventing recurrence of symptoms. Types I, II, III, and IV hypersensitivity reactions to natural pharmacologic agents and natural toxic agents, and anaphylactoid reactions respond completely to elimination of the offending food. Often symptoms are time limited and resolve without therapy.

Medications

Based on severity and nature of symptoms, organ system involved, and mechanisms of reaction (Table 14-10).

General Management

Based on nature and severity of symptoms and mechanisms of adverse drug reactions; goal of supportive therapy is to facilitate healing process
Restriction of activity while symptoms are acute
Use of anaphylaxis kit
Breast feeding with some maternal dietary restriction and delay in introduction of new foods to prevent or minimize food allergy in infants

NURSING CARE

Nursing Assessment

Response to therapy is based on the underlying mechanism, degree, and length of exposure. The symptom complex may vary among individuals

Type I Hypersensitivity, Anaphylactoid Reactions, Reactions to Glycoalkaloids

Laryngeal involvement
  Hoarseness; stridor; use of accessory muscles; difficulty in speech

---

■ TABLE 14-10 **Medications Used in Treatment of Adverse Food Reactions**

Mechanism	Potential Organ Involvement	Class of Medication
Type I hypersensitivity	Skin	Antihistamines
Anaphylactoid reactions	Upper respiratory tract	Sympathomimetic agents
Penicillin, drug contamination	Lower respiratory tract	Bronchodilators
Glycoalkaloids	Upper airway; gastrointestinal tract; multiorgan	Corticosteroids
Types II, III, and IV hypersensitivity (IgG-mediated, immune complex, and T cell sensitization, respectively)	Gastrointestinal tract Skin; respiratory tract	Topical or oral corticosteroids Nonsteroidal anti-inflammatory agents
Infectious agents (bacterial, fungal, parasitic, viral)	Multisystemic response; gastrointestinal tract	Anti-infective agents
Metabolic reactions (enzyme deficiencies [cystic fibrosis], chronic inflammatory bowel disease)	Gastrointestinal malabsorption; protein-calorie deficiencies	Enzyme replacement; see specific therapy for disease process

Respiratory involvement
  Dyspnea; substernal tightness; use of accessory muscles; cough
Bronchospasm
  Mucus production; rhonchi; wheezing; decreased breath sounds; anxiety; inability to lie down; evidence of air trapping or atelectasis on chest roentgenogram
Dermal involvement
  Pruritis; erythema; flushing; urticaria, angioedema; cyanosis; pallor
Upper respiratory involvement
  Rhinorrhea; congestion; sneezing; tearing; conjunctivitis
Gastrointestinal involvement
  Nausea; vomiting; bloating, diarrhea; cramping; distention
Anaphylaxis
  All the above

Immunogenic (Type II [IgG], Type III [Circulating Immune Complexes], Type IV [T Cell Sensitization] IgA Deficiency)

Gastrointestinal involvement
  Nausea; vomiting; bloating; distention; diarrhea; cramping; gastrointestinal bleeding; malabsorption; failure to thrive; hepatomegaly
Dermal involvement
  Vasculitic lesion; contact dermatitis; hair thinning
Musculoskeletal involvement
  Muscle mass loss; subcutaneous tissue loss
See IgA deficiency assessment

Infective Agents

Gastrointestinal involvement
  Nausea; vomiting; bloating; distention; diarrhea; cramping; gastrointestinal bleeding; malabsorption
Systemic
  Fever; arthralgias; malaise

Reactions to Natural Pharmacologic Agents

Psychoactive agents
  Central nervous system stimulation
    Palpitations; anxiety; tachycardia; irritability
Vasoactive amines
  Central nervous system
    Vascular headaches; migraines

Metabolic Reactions (Cystic Fibrosis, Diabetes, Phenylketonuria, Glucose 6-Phosphate Dehydrogenase Deficiency, Chronic Inflammatory Bowel Disease, Celiac Disease, Gallbladder Disease)

See specific disease process
Gastrointestinal involvement
Nausea; vomiting; diarrhea; cramps; bloating; flatulence; fatty, foul-smelling stools; presence of occult blood in stool; failure to thrive; malnutrition; hepatomegaly; protuberant abdomen

Dermal involvement
  Sparse hair; lanugo
Musculoskeletal
  Loss of muscle mass; subcutaneous tissue

Nursing Dx & Intervention

The nursing diagnosis and interventions are based on the mechanism of the adverse food reaction and the severity of symptoms.

Altered nutrition (less than body requirements) related to inability to digest food or absorb nutrients

- Obtain complete history of adverse food reactions, and put labels specifying history in appropriate places.
- Maintain elimination diet.
- Assess dietary intake for caloric and nutritional requirements.
- Teach alternative choices for balanced diet.
- Arrange dietary consultation.
- Monitor intake, output, and weight.
- Provide fluid supplementation.
- Teach patient self-care measures, such as reading labels, alternative choices, and his or her role in management of disease process.

See anaphylaxis for altered cardiopulmonary and cerebral tissue perfusion (p. 1121).

Patient Education/Home Care Planning

1. Assess the patient's current knowledge of the disease process and reinforce the concept of self-care and self-management of the disease.
2. Explain to the patient that the disease is a chronic one, and reinforce the need to prevent symptoms through avoidance of foods that cause them.
3. Teach the patient the importance of monitoring the response of symptoms to therapies, recording any difficulties, new symptoms, and cause-effect relationships noted, and communicating this on an ongoing basis to those prescribing the therapies.
4. Emphasize to the patient the importance of carrying appropriate identification and sharing information with significant others.
5. For patients at risk of anaphylaxis, teach self-administration of epinephrine and subsequent measures to take.

Evaluation

Symptoms resolve in response to therapeutic measures Patient is symptom free. Patient's intake, output, and weight are stabilized.

Recurrences are prevented Patient can identify causative food and explain appropriate measures to avoid it.

DRUG ALLERGY

An adverse drug reaction is any noxious or unintended effect of a drug. True drug allergy is mediated by IgE antibody–antigen interaction. Adverse reactions may also be mediated by other immunologic mechanisms.

Adverse drug reactions have steadily increased with the increase in available pharmacologic preparations. Drug allergy is one of the most common itarogenic problems.

The incidence of adverse reactions is unknown. Three percent of hospitalizations are attributed to adverse drug reactions, and approximately 15% to 30% of hospitalized patients have an adverse drug reaction. Hospitalized patients sometimes receive 10 or more drugs, which obviously increases the risk of adverse drug reaction. The contribution of most additives or contaminants in adverse reactions is unclear, although idiosyncratic responses to tartrazine, sodium metabisulfite, and sodium benzoate have been well described.

Symptoms may affect any organ system of the body and may have a short or protracted course. Symptoms may range from mild to severe, and resolution of symptoms depends on the initiating mechanisms, amount of drug, and host response.

Drug and host factors can influence the development of an adverse drug reaction:

Drug factors
  Nature of drug—class; weight; size; metabolites; ability to bind as hapten to protein (generally low molecular weight [500-1000])
  Route of administration—IV, IM, subcutaneous, oral, topical (in descending order or risk)
  Degree of exposure— prolonged course, high doses, and intermittent exposures increase risk; risk increases in first 2 to 3 weeks of therapy
Host factors
  Age—adult at greater risk than child, probably because of total exposure and greater need for drugs
  Sex—no difference except that women at greater risk with muscle relaxants and chymopapain
  Atopic history—no greater incidence but appears to be associated with more severe reactions
  Genetic—may contribute by influencing metabolic pathways or increased mediators
  Prior drug reactions—increased tendency with new drugs
Underlying disease state—may compromise immunologic mechanisms or alter metabolic pathways

•••••• Pathophysiology

Adverse drug reactions may be classified according to mechanisms of reaction (Table 14-11).

TABLE 14-11 Adverse Drug Reactions

Reaction	Mechanism	Example
Non-Drug Related (symptoms dissimilar to expected pharmacologic effects)		
Psychogenic	Vasovagal	Syncope; anxiety
Coincidental symptoms	Disease process itself	Viral rash with antibiotics
Drug-Related in Any Patient (symptoms similar to expected pharmacologic effects)		
Overdose	Increased intake, lowered metabolism, overdose, decreased liver excretion, toxic pharmacologic effect	Digoxin toxicity in elderly
Side effects	Undesirable pharmacologic effect of drug, often unavoidable with normal dose	Sleepiness with antihistamine
Secondary effects	Indirectly related to primary pharmacologic action	Vaginal infection after orally administered antibiotics
Drug interactions	Alter normal physiology of host, e.g., changes in absorption, metabolism, excretion; additive effects	Erythromycin changes liver metabolism and thus slows metabolism of theophylline
Disease-associated effects	Decreased absorption, metabolism, excretion; alteration in metabolic pathways	Digoxin toxicity
Drug-Related in Susceptible Patients (symptoms, except for intolerance, dissimilar to expected pharmacologic response)		
Intolerance	Quantitatively greater effect at normal dosages	CNS excitation with pharmacologic dose of adrenergic drug
Idiosyncracy	Qualitatively abnormal response that is different from pharmacologic effects (nonimmunologic)	Adverse response to local anesthetics
Genetic	Lack of enzyme or metabolic pathway	Hemolytic anemia in G6-PD deficiency
Anaphylactoid	Nonimmunologic	Aspirin-induced bronchospasm
Allergy	IgE antigen-antibody	Penicillin allergy
Cytotoxic	Cytotoxic antibody-mediated against cell membranes with involvement of complement, IgG, and IgM	Coombs' test-positive hemolytic anemia
Immune complex	Drug–IgG, IgM–drug immune complexes, complement	Serum sickness, drug-induced lupus
Cell-mediated	T lymphocyte sensitization	Fixed drug eruption, photosensitivity eruptions

Non-drug-related reactions of the psychogenic type generally occur only with fear of pain, as with the intramuscular or subcutaneous route of administration. Coincidental symptoms are more easily distinguished with knowledge of disease symptoms.

Adverse drug reactions that any patient may experience are the most common and most predictable. Overdosage results in toxic pharmacologic effects of the drug and occurs most commonly in pediatric or geriatric populations with dosage miscalculations or with failure to recognize concurrent drug or host factors that delay the metabolism and excretion of the drug.

Side effects vary among patients and with drugs. They are most commonly seen with drugs that directly or indirectly affect the central nervous system or gastrointestinal system.

Drug interactions are complex, and thoughtful analysis is required before administration of more than one drug. Drug interactions may potentiate, decrease, or negate the desired therapeutic effects and may place the patient at risk of overdose.

Disease-associated effects generally result in toxic overdose as a result of decreased metabolism or excretion. In gastrointestinal diseases, drugs may be poorly absorbed, resulting in lack of therapeutic response.

Intolerance is a common problem. Many patients exhibit increased side effects or gastrointestinal sensitivity to numerous drugs at normal doses.

Idiosyncratic responses of an anaphylactoid nature are nonimmunologic. Direct action on mast cells resulting in release of chemical mediators, prostaglandin activation, or IgG aggregation result in clinical symptoms similar to IgE antibody hypersensitivity. The following are some mechanisms of anaphylactoid reactions:

Mast cell degranulation (for example, codeine, morphine, radiocontrast media)

Prostaglandin-induced reactions (for example, dextran and other plasma expanders, aspirin, nonsteroidal anti-inflammatory agents, tartrazine)

Immune complex aggregation (for example, intramuscular or intravenous γ-globulin)

Cytotoxic antibody transfusion reactions (for example, mismatched blood transfusions)

In anaphylactoid reactions, prior exposure is not required, the host response may be variable over time, reactions can be produced with minute quantities, and the reaction resolves after the drug is discontinued.

Allergic, IgE antibody mechanisms account for a large proportion of adverse drug reactions because of the frequency with which drugs that fall in this category are prescribed. Some examples are penicillin and synthetic penicillins, sulfonamide antibiotics, sulfonylurea hypoglycemics, thiazide diuretics, carbonic anhydrase inhibitors, insulin and other hormones, egg-based vaccines, enzymes including chymopapain, antitoxins, and allergen extracts. The drug may act directly, it may bind with serum or tissue protein as a hapten, or a metabolite of the drug may be the offending antigen.

The allergic response requires prior exposure, can be reproduced by agents with cross-reacting structures, and can be produced by minute quantities. The reaction resolves after the drug is discontinued.

In cytotoxic or type II hypersensitivity, IgG or IgM antibody activates complement that results in damage to cell membranes. A drug may act as a hapten by binding to a cell surface, a drug-antibody complex may be absorbed to the cell surface, or a drug may change or modify a cell membrane leading to cell destruction.

In circulating immune complex or type III hypersensitivity, drug or drug hapten bound to protein may bind with antibody, forming circulating immune complexes.

In cell-mediated reactions or type IV hypersensitivity, T lymphocytes are sensitized, resulting in skin or organ damage. A drug may elicit symptoms through more than one mechanism, for example, penicillin allergy or serum sickness.

In allergic, cytotoxic, immune complex and cell-mediated reactions the evolution of symptoms often suggests an immunologic mechanism, although the exact mechanism may be impossible to establish and the diagnosis is commonly made on clinical grounds.

Certain medications have been associated with induction of antinuclear antibody (ANA). This may lead to a clinical picture of rashes or arthritis-like symptoms.

······ Diagnostic Studies and Findings

There are no simple, rapid, and predictable in vitro tests, nor is there safe and reliable in vivo testing for most adverse drug reactions. Demonstration of IgE antibody is limited to selected cases. No test is available for non-drug-related reactions, drug-related intolerance, or anaphylactoid adverse drug reactions. The clinical history is the most important tool in diagnosing adverse drug reactions.

Drug history All drugs taken by patient within last 2 weeks, including over-the-counter preparations; time between exposure and symptom onset (delay of 7 to 10 days is common); route of administration and duration of treatment; prior drug exposure; onset, progression of severity, and nature of symptoms; clinical course after drug is discontinued; concomitant diseases; infectious disease history

Skin testing Limited because of lack of knowledge of true antigen-inducing response; available only for penicillin, toxoids, antisera, insulin, ACTH, egg-based protein; must be done under strict protocol with close supervision

Patch testing Useful in diagnosing contact sensitivity to topical preparation only

Radioallergosorbent test (RAST) Not generally useful for drug allergy; useful for chymopapain

Enzyme assays See specific enzyme deficiency disease, G6-PD

Eosinophil levels May be elevated in inflammatory tissue response

Anti-DNA (12%) May be elevated (single stranded) in certain drug-induced reactions

Antinuclear antibody (ANA) (1:20) Speckled or homogeneous pattern

Complete blood count with differential Leukocytosis in serum sickness

Erythrocyte sedimentation rate May be elevated in inflammatory tissue response

Direct challenge Can confirm suspected drug but is generally not done because of potential morbidity and mortality

Multidisciplinary Plan

The goal of the treatment plan is to eliminate the offending drug and thus prevent further symptoms. Most symptoms respond quickly to removal of the offending drug and resolve without therapy. Choice of medications and supportive therapy is dependent on the nature and severity of symptoms, organ system involved, and mechanism of the reactions.

Medications

See Table 14-12

General Management

Forcing fluids to increase renal clearance of drug

Plasmapheresis to remove circulating immune complexes

Hemodialysis or peritoneal dialysis in severe overdose to remove drug rapidly

Emesis or stomach lavage to remove drug in overdose

Patient with allergic drug reaction should not receive that drug or cross-reacting one, if possible

If drug must be given, informed consent and administration under strict protocol necessary

Always check history before administering a new drug

NURSING CARE

Nursing Assessment

Adverse drug reactions have multiple mechanisms. Coincidental symptom assessment varies, since it is based on manifestations of the disease process. Drug-related reactions of overdose toxicity, side effects, intolerance, and secondary effects are related to specific drugs, and knowledge of the drug mechanisms makes it possible to identify potential symptoms. In immunologic mechanisms, organ system involvement may also be variable. The reader is referred elsewhere in this text for specific organ assessment.

Type I Hypersensitivity, Anaphylactoid Reactions

See section on anaphylaxis

Type II, Cytotoxic

Hematologic involvement

See assessment for hemolytic anemia, thrombocytopenia, agranulocytosis

Renal involvement

See assessment for interstitial nephritis

Type III, Immune Complex

Serum sickness

Drug fever

Systemic

Low-grade fever, malaise

Drug-induced lupus

See lupus assessment

Vasculitis

See vasculitis assessment

Type IV, Cell Mediated

Contact dermatitis

Photosensitivity eruptions

Nursing Dx & Intervention

Nursing interventions are based on the mechanisms and the organ involved. The reader is referred to the discussion of the specific organ involved for the nursing diagnosis and nursing interventions.

Risk for injury related to adverse antibody–antigen interaction

- Obtain complete drug allergy history before administering new drug.
- Put labels concerning allergic drug history in appropriate places.
- Closely monitor patient for 30 minutes after administering new drug intramuscularly, subcutaneously, or intravenously.
- Maintain emergency equipment and drugs and be prepared to use them.
- Maintain high index of suspicion with patients receiving any medications.
- Monitor patient for development of new symptoms during course of medication therapy and for 2 weeks after drug administration ends.

TABLE 14-12 Medications Used in Treatment of Adverse Drug Reactions

Mechanism	Potential Organ Involvement	Categories of Medications
Type I hypersensitivity, anaphylactoid reactions	Skin Upper and lower respiratory tract Upper airway Gastrointestinal tract	Antihistamines Sympathomimetic agents Bronchodilators Corticosteroids
Type II, cytotoxic	Gastrointestinal tract, skin	Rarely immunosuppressive agents, e.g., azothiaprine, cyclophosphamide, nonsteroidal antiinflammatory agents
	Renal	Corticosteroids
	Hematologic	Oral corticosteroids
Type III, immune complex	Vascular, skin, kidney, heart, liver	Nonsteroidal antiinflammatory agents
Type IV, cell-mediated	Skin	Antihistamines, topical corticosteroids

Evaluation

Symptoms resolve in response to therapeutic measures Patient is symptom free.

Recurrence is prevented Patient can identify causative drug and explain appropriate avoidance measures.

■ ANGIOEDEMA (AND URTICARIA)[18]

■ Angioedema is soft tissue swelling in submucosal or subcutaneous tissues as the result of increased local vascular permeability and serum transudation. Urticarial lesions occur in the upper stratum corneum of the dermis, whereas angioedema lesions occur in the deeper subcutaneous tissues.

Urticaria (discussed in detail in Chapter 5) and angioedema have the same pathophysiologic features. Urticaria is more common; angioedema may be associated with urticaria or may occur independently. Why some patients have urticaria and others have angioedema is not known.

Angioedema may occur anywhere on the skin, but the periorbital area, lips, throat, tongue, larynx, area around joints, and tips of the extremities are the most common sites. Urticaria and angioedema may occur at any age, and as much as 20% of the population may be affected with acute, self-limited episodes. Episodes greater than 6 weeks in duration are defined as chronic. Symptoms may be mild or life threatening, and death may result from laryngeal involvement.

•••••• Pathophysiology

With antigen-antibody linkage, mast cell or basophil degranulation and chemical mediator release occur. Histamine and other mediators interact with receptors along the lymphatic, capillary, and venule walls, resulting in dilation, engorgement, and increased capillary permeability with a perivascular mononuclear cell infiltrate in which eosinophils may predominate. This inflammatory response usually resolves within 6 hours after insult, although in soft tissues nonpitting edema may be more diffuse and reabsorption of fluid may take up to several days. Complaints of burning pain or tightness are more commonly associated with angioedema than is pruritus.

Other immunologic mechanisms may precipitate the same pathophysiologic response.

Physical or environmental factors may also trigger or exacerbate urticaria and angioedema (Table 14-13). In addition,

■ TABLE 14-13 **Mechanisms of Angioedema**

Mediator	Example	Proposed Mechanism
Immunologic		
Circulating immune complexes	Autoimmune phenomena	Activation of complement cascade
Cytotoxic antibodies	Transfusion reactions	Activation of complement cascade
Antigen-antibody complexes	Serum sickness reactions; malignancies	Activation of complement cascade
Drugs—directly or as haptens	Opiates; muscle relaxants; dextran	Direct mast cell degranulation
Foods—directly or as haptens	Tomatoes; strawberries; citrus fruits	Direct mast cell degranulation
Chemicals—directly or as haptens	Radiocontrast media; thiamine; bile salts	Direct mast cell degranulation
Drugs	Aspirin; indomethacin	Alteration of arachidonic acid metabolism
Chemical additives	Tartrazine	Alteration of arachidonic acid metabolism
Nonimmunologic		
Pressure	Tight garments; sitting	Unknown
Vibratory	Electric shavers; steering wheels	Unknown; autosomal dominant; genetically transmitted
Solar (five types)	Exposed areas	Unknown except for type IV, production of erythrocytic protoporphyria
Aquagenic	Water contact, regardless of temperature	Unknown
Heat	Direct contact	Unknown
Cholinergic	Heat exposure; emotional stress; vigorous exercise	Release of acetylcholine from cholinergic sympathetic nerve fibers
Cold	Delayed onset (30 minutes to 4 hours)	Autosomal dominant inheritance
	Exposed areas, immediate response	Unknown
	Associated with underlying disease	Presence of abnormal proteins with cold-dependent properties: cold hemoglobins, cryofibrinogens, cold agglutinins, cryoglobulins

urticaria and angioedema may occur in different disease states (Table 14-14). In as many as 60% of cases, no causative agent can be identified.

•••••• Diagnostic Studies and Findings

History Exceptionally important onset; distribution; aggravating and ameliorating factors; time sequencing; food history; past, current, and infective history; contactant or insect exposures; family and atopic history; occupational, hobby, and environmental history; travel.

Drug history Any medications, including over-the-counter and oral contraceptive preparations, may precipitate urticaria and angioedema

Clinical examination All areas of potential involvement: periorbit, oropharynx, joints, tips of extremities

Tests See Table 14-15

•••••• Multidisciplinary Plan

The goal of the treatment plan is to prevent symptoms of angioedema. Obviously, with removal of the causative agent, no further therapy is necessary.

Medications

Antihistamines are the drugs of choice

Drugs used in hereditary angioedema

Hormones

Danazol (Danocrine), 200 mg tid; androgen derivative; contraindicated in children and pregnancy

Hemostatic agents

Aminocaproic acid, 3.5 mg qid for adults; antifibrinolytic agent, plasminogen inhibitor

---

TABLE 14-14 Diseases Associated with Angioedema

Type	Proposed Mechanisms
Systemic mastocytosis	Accumulation of mast cells that spontaneously or easily degranulate in dermis, bone marrow, and gastrointestinal tract
Infections: viral parasitic (infectious mononucleosis, hepatitis), rarely bacterial	Circulating antigen–antibody complexes with activation of complement cascade
Endocrinopathies: hyperthyroidism, pregnancy, menses	Unknown
Hereditary angioedema	Autosomal dominant, genetically inherited deficiency or malfunction of C1 esterase inhibitor with activation of complement cascade
Malignancies	In addition to antigen–antibody complexes, interference with C1 esterase inhibitor and resultant activation of complement cascade
Psychogenic	Rarely primary but may be exacerbating factor through hormonal and neural secretory mediators

---

Transexamic acid, 1 g tid for adults before dental procedures etc.

Blood products

Fresh-frozen plasma during acute attacks

Drugs used in urticaria and angioedema

Antihistamines*

Cyproheptadine (Periactin), 4-8 mg po q6h

Chlorpheniramine (Chlor-Trimeton), 2 mg/kg/24 h po in 4 divided doses

Clemastine (Tavist), 1.34 or 2.68 mg po q8-12h

---

*Available in syrup form; dosage calculated by patient's weight.

TABLE 14-15 Diagnostic Tests for Urticaria and Angioedema

Condition Suspected	Test*
Atopic: food or drug (inhalent or contactant) sensitivity	Elimination of offending agent; daily symptom diary; challenge with suspected foods; skin tests to food or selected drugs; total serum IgE determination; eosinophil count; skin tests or radioallergosorbent tests of suspected antigens
Cutaneous vasculitis or systemic collagen vascular disease	Immunoglobulin analysis; antinuclear antibody; rheumatoid factor; cryoglobulins; cryofibrinogens; complete complement profile; skin biopsy with immunofluorescence
Hereditary angioedema	C4; C2; C3; total hemolytic complement (CH50); C1-esterase inhibitor (immunochemical and functional assays)
Physical urticaria Dermatographia Cold	Firm stroke on skin with tongue blade Ice cube test; cryoglobulins; cryofibrinogens; VDRL test
Cholinergic urticaria	Exercise challenge; methacholine skin test
Solar urticaria	Exposure to various wavelengths of light; protoporphyrin and coproporphyrin determinations
Pressure urticaria and angioedema	Application of pressure with weights for 10 minutes
Vibratory angioedema	Vibratory stimulation of skin for 4 minutes
Aquagenic urticaria	Tap-water challenge at various temperatures
Infections	Appropriate cultures and x-rays; stool for ova and parasites; hepatitis B antigen and antibody
Urticaria pigmentosa	Test for dermatographia; skin biopsy
Malignancy with angioedema	Total hemolytic complement (CH50); C1; C1-esterase inhibitor
Idiopathic urticaria	Skin biopsy with immunofluorescence

From Fineman.[9]
*General screening consists of complete blood count, urinalysis, and erythrocyte sedimentation rate determination.

Diphenhydramine (Benadryl), 25-100 mg po q6h or 5 mg/kg/d

Doxepin (Sinequan), 10-30 mg po q8-12h

Histamine receptor antagonists*

Cimetidine (Tagament), 300 mg po q6h

Ranitidine (Zantac), 150 mg po q12h

Famotidine (Pepcid), 20 mg po q12h

Hydroxyzine (Atarax), 25 mg po q6h to maximum total of 400 mg

Adrenergic agents

Appear to be of limited value in long-term therapy but may be employed for control of acute symptoms

Epinephrine

Aqueous (Adrenalin), 0.2-0.3 ml subcutaneously q30 min or 0.01 mg/kg

Long-acting (SusPhrine), 0.1-03. ml subcutaneously q4-6h or 0.005 mg/kg (maximum dose 0.15 ml)

Ephedrine (Bronkaid), 20-50 mg q4h or 3 mg/kg/24 h in 4 divided doses

Corticosteroids

May be used if symptoms are unresponsive to above therapy but should be limited to lowest possible dose and alternate-day therapy with monitoring of side effects

Prednisone (Deltasone, Orasone, Liquid Pred), 2 mg/kg/d up to 100 mg

Topical agents

Sun blockers with sun protection factor of at least 15 (Total Eclipse [15-18], Super Shade [15], Coppertone [15], Pre Sun [20]); used to block ultraviolet light in solar urticaria

Mild analgesics for pain associated with swelling

General Management

Cool compresses to reduce periorbital edema

Restricted activity during acute episodes

Endotracheal tube placement or tracheostomy for extensive laryngeal involvement

NURSING CARE

Nursing Assessment

Because angioedema may have multiorgan involvement, careful assessment should be made of all potential organ systems.

Laryngeal Involvement

Hoarseness; stridor; use of accessory muscles; difficulty in speech

Dermal Status

Concurrent urticaria

---

*Available in syrup form; dosage calculated by patient's weight.

Ocular Status

Periorbital edema

Gastrointestinal Status

Nausea; vomiting; diarrhea; gastrointestinal swelling

Oropharyngeal Status

Swelling of lip, tongue, and uvula

Articular Status

Swelling at tips of extremities, in soft tissue, and around joints

Nursing Dx & Intervention

Ineffective breathing pattern related to allergic response

- Maintain endotracheal tube or tracheostomy if instituted.
- Assess and record ventilation pattern including rate, rhythm, and use of accessory muscles.
- Assess for presence of laryngeal involvement, including stridor, hoarseness, and difficulty in speech or swallowing. Record if present.

Risk for injury related to allergic response

- Obtain complete history of drug allergies before administering new drug.
- Put labels indicating allergic drug history in all appropriate places.
- Closely monitor patient for 30 minutes after administering each new drug.

Patient Education/Home Care Planning

1. Explain to the patient the relationship between symptoms and exposure to the causative agent.
2. Explain to the patient the necessity of avoiding use of the causative agent.
3. Explain to the patient the need, if appropriate, to carry appropriate identification and to share information when necessary.
4. Provide the patient with information on medical alert identification.
5. Teach the patient self-administration, if appropriate, of epinephrine and subsequent measures including oral administration of antihistamine and seeking immediate medical care.

Evaluation

Symptoms resolve in response to therapeutic measures Patient is symptom free, with no evidence of soft tissue swelling, joint restriction or subjective feelings of tightness or swelling, hoarseness, or difficulty in swallowing, speech, or air movement. Bowel sounds and elimination pattern are normal.

Recurrence of symptoms is prevented Patient can identify triggering agent and explain appropriate avoidance measures. Patient can identify appropriate medications to use, dosage, and length of therapy if symptoms occur. Patient can identify nondrug therapeutic measures to institute if symptoms occur.

MEDICAL INTERVENTIONS AND RELATED NURSING CARE

 ## BONE MARROW TRANSPLANTATION

Description and Rationale

Bone marrow transplantation (BMT) is the treatment of choice for patients with severe aplastic anemia who are younger than 50 years of age and have a compatible donor. Marrow transplantation is also a treatment modality for severe immunodeficiency disorders, and is being used with increasing success in the treatment of patients with leukemia, lymphoma, and selected solid tumors.

Bone marrow is harvested in the operating room with the donor under general or spinal anesthesia. Multiple aspirations from the posterior iliac crests are performed; if necessary toe anterior iliac crests and sternum may be used. A small volume of bone marrow is collected with each aspiration and placed into tissue culture medium containing heparin. This solution is filtered through stainless steel screens to remove bone chips, fat globules, and clots and then is transferred to a blood transfusion bag.

The amount of bone marrow aspirated depends on a number of factors: the donor's weight, the concentration of cells in donated marrow, and the processing procedures employed before the marrow is transfused. If no special processing is done, the volume of marrow obtained is approximately 10 to 15 ml/kg of the recipient's body weight. In the typical adult a volume of 500 to 750 ml of blood and marrow contains 10 to 20×10^9 nucleated marrow cells.

After harvesting, the marrow is either administered intravenously to the recipient through a central venous access device such as a Hickman or Raaf catheter or is cryopreserved and stored for future use. In the latter case, which occurs only with autologous bone marrow transplantation, the harvested marrow may be treated before cryopreservation to eliminate any occult tumor cells that may be present, especially in lymphohemopoietic malignancies. Ex vivo treatment with 4-hydroperoxycyclophosphamide (4-HC), an analog of cyclophosphamide, is one method used to treat the marrow. More recently, immunologic approaches using monoclonal antibodies are being tested in clinical trials for diseases such as T cell lymphoma and common acute lymphocytic leukemia (ALL).

Until recently most marrow transplants have involved donors of two types, an identical twin or an HLA-matched,

mixed lymphocyte culture (MLC)–compatible sibling. A syngeneic transplant, using marrow from an identical twin, is ideal because the donor is matched with the recipient at all genetic loci.

Transplantation using marrow from anyone other than an identical twin or the patient himself is called an allogeneic transplant. In most allogeneic bone marrow transplants a sibling who matches at HLA-A, -B, -C, and-D loci is the donor. The HLA loci are on a small chromosomal region of the sixth chromosome; these loci are usually inherited as a unit known as a haplotype. Each parent has two haplotypes, and a child inherits one haplotype from each parent. A 25% probability exists that two siblings will be HLA identical.

A partially matched donor (such as a sibling, parent, or uncle) may be selected when no HLA-identical sibling is available, or an HLA-identical unrelated donor may be used. The chances of finding an unrelated HLA-identical donor are 1:50,000. Preliminary reports using partially matched or unrelated identical donors are encouraging, but further investigation in this area is needed.

A third form of bone marrow transplantation, the autologous graft, involves use of the patient's own marrow. As with the identical twin situation, in this circumstance no clinically significant graft-versus-host disease will occur. However, with autologous grafts, tumor cells may be present in marrow harvested during remission; therefore attempts to purge marrow of occult tumor cells before cryopreservation are being investigated. Autologous bone marrow transplants are now being completed on a regular basis. The results from this type of transplant are encouraging.

The rationale for bone marrow transplantation is to replace defective or missing host hemopoietic stem cells with healthy stem cells. In the treatment of neoplasm the transplant is done after therapy designed to rid the patient of the tumor. The patient's normal bone marrow is destroyed with high-dose therapy, and the transplant is designed to repopulate the patient's hemopoietic system.

Graft-Versus-Host Disease

Graft-versus-host disease (GVHD) presumably results from the attack of host tissue by immunocompetent donor T lymphocytes. In acute cases the peak onset occurs 30 to 50 days after the transplant. In chronic cases the onset occurs 100 days after the transplant. Tables 14-16 and 14-17 give two systems for the clinical staging of GVHD.

Conditioning Regimen

Pretransplant conditioning regimens include high-dose chemotherapy with or without radiotherapy. The purposes of conditioning are to eliminate defective stem cells, to provide immunosuppression to minimize the possibility or rejection, and to eliminate any residual malignant cells.

The conditioning regimen used before bone marrow transplantation varies depending on the disease being treated. The use of multiple-day chemotherapy may or may not be preceded or followed by local or total body irradiation (TBI).

TABLE 14-16 Proposed Clinical Stage of Graft-Versus-Host Disease According to Organ System

Stage	Skin	Liver	Intestinal Tract
+	Maculopapular rash over 25% of body surface	Bilirubin 2-3 mg/dl	Greater than 500 ml diarrhea/day
++	Maculopapular rash over 25%-50% of body surface	Bilirubin 3-6 mg/dl	Greater than 1000 ml diarrhea/day
+++	Generalized erythroderma	Bilirubin 6-15 mg/dl	Greater than 1500 ml diarrhea/day
++++	Generalized erythroderma with bullous formation and desquamation	Bilirubin greater than 15 mg/dl	Severe abdominal pain with or without ileus

From Thomas.[25]

TABLE 14-17 Overall Clinical Grading of Severity of Graft-Versus-Host Disease

Grade	Degree of Organ Involvement
I	+ to ++ skin rash; no gut involvement; no liver involvement; no decrease in clinical performance
II	+ to +++ skin rash; + gut involvement or + liver involvement (or both); mild decrease in clinical performance
III	++ to +++ skin rash; ++ to +++ gut involvement or ++ to ++++ liver involvement (or both); marked decrease in clinical performance
IV	Similar to grade III with ++ to ++++ organ involvement and extreme decrease in clinical performance

From Thomas.[25]

Preprocedural Nursing Care

Immediate concerns are related to the conditioning regimen using chemoradiotherapy. The patient, family, donor, and significant others are instructed on the procedure, its course, and complications.

Radiation Dosage varies, in general from 800 to 1200 cGy. For example, 1000 cGy may be given in fractionated doses (250 cGy per day). Single-dose whole body irradiation may be used. Typical side effects include nausea, vomiting, diarrhea, erythema of the skin, and parotitis. These side effects are usually of short duration when moderate fractionated radiotherapy is used. With the exception of erythema of the skin, they usually resolve within 7 days.

Chemotherapy Side effects are usual after administration of chemotherapeutic agents. These side effects will vary with the agent used but may include nausea, vomiting, stomatitis, diarrhea, electrolyte imbalances, renal dysfunction, and pancytopenia. Symptoms of side effects specific to each agent must be known, observed for, reported, and treated.

•••••• Multidisciplinary Plan

Infusion of bone marrow is used to restore defective or missing stem cells. For autologous marrow, blood bags containing approximately 50 ml of cryopreserved marrow are thawed quickly, one at a time, in a basin of warm water at approximately 100° F. The contents of the blood bag are removed using a 50 ml syringe with a 16-gauge needle and then adminis-

tered rapidly through a central line (double-lumen Raaf catheter or Hickman catheter). A solution of 0.9 normal saline is infused during the procedure. Epinephrine, diphenhydramine, and hydrocortisone are kept at the bedside.

For a syngeneic or allogeneic donation, a standard-type blood bag containing fresh bone marrow just obtained from a donor is transported from the operating room. The donated marrow is administered slowly (over a period of 4 hours) through a right atrial catheter without a filter.

NURSING CARE

Nursing Assessment

Fluid Overload

Increased respiratory rate; dyspnea; rales, rhonchi

Micropulmonary Emboli

Shortness of breath; chest pain; increased heart rate

Reaction to White Cells in Marrow

Chills; fever; urticaria; chest pain

Hematuria

Hemastix-positive urine normal for first 24 hours after bone marrow transplant

Bacterial Contamination of Marrow

Hypotension; fever; shaking chills

Engraftment

No evidence of hematologic recovery 2 to 4 weeks after bone marrow transplant

Infection

Fever; pain; redness; swelling of any site; wound drainage; cough; dyspnea; sore throat; headache; dysuria; frequency; urgency; positive blood culture findings; change in mental status

Anemia

Decreased red blood cell count, hematocrit, and hemoglobin level; excessive fatigue

Stomatitis

Oral soreness; dryness; burning or tingling; taste changes; erythema; ulcerations or patches on oral mucosa

Thombocytopenia

Petechiae; purpura; bleeding from any body orifice or site of catheter; hemoptysis; hematemesis, hematuria; hematochezia; seizures; change in mental status

Nutritional Status

Anorexia; decreased weight; nausea; vomiting; diarrhea

Psychosocial Status

Anger, depression; frustration; anxiety

Graft-Versus-Host Disease (GVHD)

Mild maculopapular rash; generalized erythroderma with desquamation; increase in serum bilirubin, serum glutamic oxaloacetic transaminase (SGOT), or alkaline phosphatase; abdominal cramping; diarrhea (green, watery); hematochezia

Veno-Occlusive Disease (VOD)

Sudden weight gain; right upper quadrant pain; jaundice; hepatomegaly; ascites; encephalopathy

Nursing Dx & Intervention

Risk for fluid volume excess related to marrow infusion

- Assess baseline hemodynamic status before marrow infusion.
- Monitor rate of infusion carefully to decrease incidence of overload and to ensure completion of administration within 4 hours *to prevent destruction of cells.*
- Assess vital signs and response to administration of marrow every 5 to 10 minutes during infusion, then every 30 minutes for 2 hours *to detect early signs of volume excess.*

Altered nutrition: less than body requirements related to nausea, vomiting, or inability to ingest nutrients because of chemotherapy

- Assess amount and types of foods and liquids tolerated; maintain calorie count, intake and output, and weight record *to ensure required nutrients are taken* (33 to 38 kcal/kg, 1.5 g protein/kg and 2500 to 3000 ml fluid).
- Assess onset, frequency, duration, and factors that predispose to nausea or vomiting.
- Eliminate predisposing factors when possible; collaborate with physician to determine best time and type of medication most effective *to prevent onset of symptoms.*
- Arrange dietary consultation *to adjust dietary and fluid intake.*
- Consider use of behavioral relaxation techniques.
- Provide frequent oral hygiene.
- Instruct patient to avoid quick movements while nauseated.

- Encourage patient to eat or drink when not nauseated regardless of the time.
- Encourage patient to eat slowly and chew thoroughly.
- Suggest high-protein, high-calorie diet.
- Suggest small, frequent, low-fat meals.
- Encourage patient to drink liquids (clear, cool beverages or soups) slowly through a straw before, not during, meals.
- Provide patient with beverages or foods that may curb nausea; carbonated beverages such as cola or ginger ale; dry crackers or toast; tart foods such as lemons or sour pickles; ice pops and gelatin desserts.
- Instruct patient to avoid favorite foods during periods of nausea.
- Instruct patient to avoid lying flat for at least 1 hour after eating.
- Administer total parenteral nutrition (TPN) when ordered if the patient is unable to ingest food or fluids; monitor electrolytes, urine glucose, proteins, and ketones.

Risk for infection related to leukopenia

- Maintain protective environment. (Reverse isolation protocols vary among centers from simple protective isolation to sterile laminar airflow rooms.)
- Monitor white blood cell count and absolute granulocyte count daily.
- Monitor vital signs every 4 hours.
- Check skin and mucous membranes.
- Inspect all body orifices daily *for redness, swelling, and pain.*
- Auscultate lungs every 8 hours *for increased or decreased breath sounds, rhonchi, and rales.*
- Inspect site of insertion of venous access device for redness, swelling, and pain.
- Assess patient for complaints of dysuria and frequency.
- Note any change from patient's baseline vital signs, behavior, or appearance.
- Encourage turning, coughing, and deep breathing exercises.
- Maintain integrity of skin and mucous membranes. (Skin care measures vary among centers from use of povidone-iodine to use of antibacterial soap.)
- Maintain meticulous mouth care. (Mouth care varies among centers.)
- Use strict aseptic technique when changing dressings.
- Use strict aseptic technique in intravenous preparation and administration.
- Avoid bladder catheterization.
- Avoid administering enemas and suppositories and taking rectal temperatures.
- Encourage patient to use deodorant rather than antiperspirant. (Axillary sweat glands are blocked by antiperspirants, which may promote infection.)
- Obtain surveillance cultures of throat, urine, stool, skin, and other areas as ordered. (Need for surveillance cultures to detect colonization before infection is controversial.)

- Maintain dietary restrictions as ordered. (Efficacy of low-bacteria diets has not been established.)
- Eliminate stagnant water in patient's room.
- Do not allow fresh-cut flowers or plants in patient's room.
- Limit number of visitors, and screen them for infection, recent vaccinations, or exposure to communicable diseases.
- Provide mask, gloves, and gown for patient when patient leaves room.
- Obtain culture and sensitivity tests and Gram's stain of all potential sites of infection per physician's order.
- Administer antibiotics on schedule per physician's order.
- Control fever with tepid sponge baths and acetaminophen.
- Maintain adequate nutrition and hydration of patient.
- Administer colony-stimulating factors as ordered.

Altered tissue perfusion (bladder) related to local effect of cyclophosphamide

- Begin intravenous hydration 4 hours before cyclophosphamide administration and continue for 24 hours after therapy. Intravenous fluids should be administered 1½ to 2 times maintenance rates.
- Perform continuous bladder irrigations using three-way Foley catheter if ordered. If patient can void every hour to eliminate toxic products of cyclophosphamide that irritate bladder lining, catheter is unnecessary.
- Monitor urine for blood every 4 hours.
- Maintain accurate intake and output records.

Risk for decreased cardiac output related to effects of cyclophosphamide

- Check results of electrocardiogram (ECG) for decreased voltage and transient changes. ECG is taken daily while patient is treated with high-dose cyclophosphamide.
- Monitor heart function continuously during drug administration *to check for cardiotoxicity.*

Risk for injury related to thrombocytopenia

- Monitor platelet count regularly. Risk of bleeding is high when platelet count is less than 10,000 cells/mm³.
- Inspect skin and mucous membranes daily. Monitor for increased bruising tendencies, petechiae, bleeding gums, and epistaxis.
- Test stool, urine, and emesis for occult blood.
- Note any changes in patient's vital signs or behavior. Changes may indicate intracranial hemorrhage.
- After invasive procedures such as bone marrow aspiration and biopsy, monitor site frequently for any oozing of blood.
- Avoid giving intramuscular or subcutaneous injections.
- Avoid taking rectal temperatures and administering rectal suppositories and enemas.
- Encourage adequate fluid intake and use of stool softener to prevent constipation and straining.
- Avoid invasive procedures.
- Place sign indicating bleeding precautions over patient's bed.

- Administer medroxyprogesterone acetate as ordered to control menses.
- Instruct patient to avoid cutting, bruising, or bumping self. Eliminate sharp objects in environment.
- Instruct patient to use electric razor rather than hand razor.
- Instruct patient to wear shoes or slippers—no bare feet while walking.
- Instruct patient to use soft-bristled toothbrush. If platelet count is less than 20,000/mm³, use toothette rather than a toothbrush.
- Flossing may be contraindicated. Instruct patient to discontinue if bleeding occurs.
- Instruct patient to avoid use of toothpicks.
- Teach patient to avoid use of aspirin and products containing aspirin.
- Teach patient to avoid use of all beverages containing alcohol.
- Instruct patient to avoid blowing the nose forcefully or sneezing forcefully.
- If epistaxis occurs, keep patient in sitting position. Application of ice helps to constrict small vessels. Local application of pressure may control bleeding. Nasal packing may be indicated if these measures fail.
- Bleeding in oral cavity may be controlled with iced saline mouth rinses.
- Administer irradiated platelet transfusions rapidly as ordered. (Families are encouraged to find donors for blood products.) Monitor posttransfusion platelet counts.

Activity intolerance related to anemia, disruption of sleep, or anxiety

- Administer irradiated red blood cell transfusions as ordered.
- Monitor hemoglobin levels and hematocrit values regularly.
- Arrange nursing care so patient has uninterrupted periods of rest and sleep, especially during the night.
- Encourage progressive activity program as tolerated.
- Encourage patient to verbalize feelings and concerns.
- Explain reasons for fatigue.

Altered oral mucous membrane related to conditioning regimen or infection

- Implement nursing care for stomatitis based on assessment using grading system developed by Capizzi.[4]
  - Grade 1—generalized erythema of oral mucosa
  - Grade 2—isolated small ulcerations or white patches
  - Grade 3—confluent ulcerations with white patches covering more than 25% of oral mucosa
  - Grade 4—hemorrhagic ulcerations
- For grade 1 or 2 stomatitis:
  1. Perform oral hygiene regimen every 2 hours while awake and every 6 hours during night, as follows:
     a. Use normal saline mouthwash if crusts are absent. (One teaspoon of salt in 1 L of sterile water may be used.) If crusts and debris are

present, use *either* one part hydrogen peroxide* diluted† with three parts water‡ *or* sodium bicarbonate solution (1 teaspoon mixed in 8 ounces of water.‡). Perform mouth care every 2 hours while patient is awake. Alternate *either* hydrogen peroxide or bicarbonate solution with normal saline. Rinse with normal saline after the use of either.

    b. Floss gently with unwaxed dental floss every 24 hours; discontinue if bleeding occurs.

    c. Brush using soft toothbrush and nonabrasive toothpaste, after each meal and before sleep.

    d. Remove dentures or partial plates. Replace only for meals. Keep meticulously clean.

    e. Apply water-soluble lip lubricant four times a day and as needed.

2. Use measures for oral pain per physician's order. Suggestions are:

    a. Dyclonine (Dyclone) 0.5% or 1% (available in spray or gargle), 5 to 10 ml every hour

    b. Viscous lidocaine (Xylocaine) 2%, 10 ml every 2 hours

    c. Hydrocortisone (Orabse) or carbamide peroxide (Gly-Oxide) applied to affected sites

    d. "Stomatitis cocktail"—equal parts viscous lidocaine (Xylocaine), diphenhydramine (Benadryl) elixir, and magnesium and aluminum hydroxide mixture (Maalox), 30 ml every 2 to 4 hours

    e. One part diphenhydramine (Benadryl) elixir mixed with one part kaolin and pectin (Kaopectate), every 2 to 4 hours

3. Implement dietary measures including the following:

    a. Instruct patient to avoid abrasive foods such as toast, apples, and celery.

    b. Encourage intake of pureed, bland foods.

    c. Instruct patient to avoid tart or acid foods, hot beverages, or iced drinks.

    d. Instruct patient to avoid spices and vinegar.

    e. Instruct patient to avoid alcohol.

    f. Arrange for dietary consultation.

4. Discourage smoking.

5. Recommend use of artificial saliva for xerostomia. No comparative research of various agents is available.

- For grade 3 or 4 stomatitis:

    1. Obtain samples from suspicious area and culture—one culture for bacteria and one for fungus—per physician's order.

2. Institute oral hygiene regimen:

    a. Alternate antifungal or antibacterial suspension with warm saline mouthwash every 2 hours while patient is awake and every 4 hours during night.

    b. Do not floss.

    c. Brush gently using toothettes or cotton-tipped applicators.

    d. Remove dentures or bridge. Do not replace for meals.

    e. Apply lip lubricant every 2 hours.

3. In addition to local measures as indicated for grade 1 and 2 stomatitis, systemic analgesics may be indicated, especially before eating.

4. Liquid diet may be indicated. If not, use pureed diet. See other measures as indicted in no. 3 for grade 1 and 2 stomatitis.

5. Discourage smoking.

Diarrhea related to effects of total body irradiation on gastrointestinal mucosa or GVHD

- Administer antidiarrheal agents as ordered.
- Maintain adequate hydration.
- Suggest bland, low-residue diet that is high in potassium.
- Instruct patient in meticulous perianal skin care.
- Apply soothing lubricant to perianal area after each bowel movement.

Risk for altered skin integrity related to chemoradiotherapy or GVHD

- Assess skin integrity every 8 to 24 hours.
- Assess level of pain and pruritus and administer analgesics and antihistamines as needed.
- Provide meticulous skin care, including daily bath with povidone-iodine and normal saline or other antibacterial solution. Oatmeal baths may be indicated for pruritus.
- Apply creams or lotions on intact skin *to minimize breakdown.*
- Explain need to prevent scratching. Use mittens if necessary on infant or child.
- Use gowns and linens washed in nondetergents *to prevent skin reactions.*
- Use flotation-type bed for patient with extensive skin involvement.
- Use bed cradle to prevent linens from touching skin if patient has extensive skin involvement.
- Assist patient frequently with turning and active or passive range of motion exercises.
- Provide meticulous perianal skin care.
- Observe and record frequency, amount, character, and presence of frank or occult blood for all stools.
- Teach patient to perform perianal care after each stool.
- Monitor closely for dehydration, electrolyte imbalance, and weight change.
- Administer replacement fluids containing electrolytes as ordered.
- Auscultate bowel sounds every 8 hours to monitor for development of ileus.

---

*Hydrogen peroxide should not be used if the patient has fresh granulation tissue.

†Hydrogen peroxide solutions should be prepared immediately before use, since hydrogen peroxide decomposes rapidly in water.

‡Sterile water or normal saline should be used for mouthwash or dilution of agents when patients are immunosuppressed. Whether using non-sterile solutions for dilution increases the number of infections is unknown.

- Monitor bilirubin and serum glutamic oxaloacetic transaminase (SGOT) levels daily.
- Measure abdominal girth twice a day.
- Position patient on left side to decrease pressure on liver.
- When ordered, permit nothing by mouth to allow bowel to rest.
- Reinstate oral feedings with iso-osmotic, low-fat, lactose-free beverages, as ordered, increasing to allowed diet when tolerated.

Risk for fluid volume excess related to venoocclusive disease

- Assess for sudden weight gain, right upper quadrant pain, ascites, jaundice, and disorientation.
- Measure abdominal girth twice a day at level of umbilicus with patient supine.
- Restrict sodium intake as ordered.
- Administer all intravenous medication in minimum volume of fluid.
- Monitor urine sodium levels.
- Monitor blood pressure for orthostatic change daily.
- Monitor patient closely for toxic side effects of medications *because of impaired liver function.*
- Monitor blood urea nitrogen levels frequently.

Body image disturbance related to alopecia, weight loss, sterility

- Encourage patient and significant others to verbalize feelings and concerns.
- Explore perceived meaning of loss with patient and significant others.
- Help patient and significant others recognize that alopecia and weight loss are temporary.
- Assist patient to identify methods to improve appearance (such as use of clothing, scarves, hats, or hairpieces).
- Assist patient to identify strengths.
- Convey attitude of acceptance and understanding.
- Emphasize that negative reactions to altered body image are normal and expected.
- Consult other health care providers in planning comprehensive approach to patient.

Anxiety related to uncertain outcome of treatment or severity of responses to chemoradiotherapy

- Encourage patient and significant others to express feelings and concerns and to ask questions *to dispel misconceptions.*
- Assist patient to use relaxation techniques, such as visual imagery, *to reduce anxiety.*
- Reinforce and restate information given to patient and significant others *to promote understanding.*
- Encourage patient and significant others to discuss hopes for positive outcome.
- Reassure that patient will not be alone and that care and treatment will be given when needed.
- Recognize and discuss use of positive coping methods.

Patient Education/Home Care Planning

1. Teach the patient self-care procedures: central line care, heparin flush, administration of TPN, and use of volumetric pump, when required; oral hygiene and skin care measures; handwashing technique; use of incentive spirometer; temperature-taking; urine and stool testing method for presence of blood; use of safety measures; and measurement of weight, intake, and output.
2. Teach the patient to assess for signs or symptoms of infection, GVHD, veno-occlusive disease, renal involvement, anemia, and bleeding; teach the patient when to report signs or symptoms.
3. Explain to the patient the diet for optimum nutritional status. (Ideally the patient must be able to tolerate 1000 calories a day to be discharged.)
4. Teach the patient measures to prevent the occurrence of infection. Precautions are more rigid during the first 3 months after bone marrow transplantation and are relaxed as the year progresses.
   Wear face mask when outside home.
   Avoid contact with young children who attend school.
   Avoid contact with anyone who has a cold or illness.
   Avoid crowds; go to grocery stores, theaters, restaurants, and other public places when they are not crowded.
   Avoid restaurant food for the first 3 months.
   Wear a mask. (Walks can be taken without wearing a mask, but one should be carried in case of contact with other pedestrians.)
   Wash hands well before eating, after using the toilet, and after contact with someone who has a cold.
   Avoid contact with any pets in living quarters for the first 3 months. Do *not* clean litter boxes or come in contact with animal feces.
   Avoid contact with plants and flowers.
   Do not swim in private or public pool for the first year after bone marrow transplant.
   Maintain good dental hygiene.
   Do not have immunizations without the physician's approval.
   Take prophylactic antibiotics as prescribed.
5. Discuss with the patient the routine measures for him or her to practice daily to minimize occurrence of complications.
6. Discuss with the patient the daily maintenance of home environment, equipment, and supplies.
7. Emphasize to the patient the importance of ongoing health and mental health care.

Evaluation

Fluid volume is within normal limits Patient's vital signs remain stable; lung sounds are clean on auscultation.

Optimal nutrition status is maintained Patient's weight is maintained or loss is less than 5% of original body weight; patient takes required nutrients and fluids, or patient maintains TPN without difficulty—no nausea, vomiting, or diarrhea is present.

No presence of infection is noted   Patient's vital signs are within normal limits; skin and mucous membranes are clear, warm, and with good turgor; lungs are clear; patient remains oriented.

Renal function is maintained   Patient's intake and output are balanced; patient voids without difficulty; urine is clear, light yellow.

Cardiac function is maintained   Patient's ECG shows normal sinus rhythm without changes; cardiac rate and rhythm is within normal range.

Hematologic function is maintained   Patient shows no evidence of bruising, petechiae, or bleeding; platelet count is normal; patient remains infection free.

Skin and mucous membranes are intact   No lesions or breaks are present; patient demonstrates skin and oral care.

Anxiety and feelings about self-concept are controlled Patient discusses feelings and responses freely. Patient remains relaxed, participates in care, and uses grooming techniques to enhance appearance. Patient makes plans to effect life-style changes.

CORTICOSTEROIDS

Synthetic corticosteroids are pharmacologic agents that mimic the effects of the major endogenous glucocorticoid, cortisol. They are used in the treatment of many immunologic diseases because of their potent anti-inflammatory and immunosuppressive effects. Corticosteroids exert their widespread effects by initially binding to a specific cytoplasmic receptor protein that is present on most cells. This complex then enters the nucleus where alteration in the rate of synthesis of specific proteins occurs.

Synthetic corticosteroids should be used with caution in persons with hepatic disease or hypoalbuminemia or in patients who are receiving phenytoin, barbiturates, or rifampin. Lower-dose therapy is recommended in these cases. In addition, care should be exercised in prescribing steroid therapy for persons who are predisposed to or have known histories of diabetes, osteoporosis, peptic ulcer disease, infections, hypertension, psychosis, or coronary artery disease.

A major concern with the use of corticosteroid therapy is suppression of the hypothalamic-pituitary-adrenocortical axis (HPAA) (Table 14-18). Exogenous steroids provide negative feedback to this mechanism, which promotes total body homeostasis via the regulation of cortisol production. Therefore suppression of the HPAA results in widespread systemic manifestations. To limit this untoward effect, steroids are administered in as low a dosage as possible to control the disease for which they are being prescribed. However, to control acute exacerbations of many inflammatory disorders, corticosteroids are usually prescribed initially in relatively high doses (greater than 40 mg daily), so HPAA suppression is unavoidable. Once the disease is under control, the dosage is lowered at a rate of 2.5 to 5 mg per week. *Gradual* tapering of the dosage of corticosteroids is necessary, since the body cannot respond quickly to changes in cortisol levels owing to the initial suppression of the natural HPAA feedback mechanisms. It may take as long as 12 months for adaptation to occur when the patient has received high-dose therapy for a month or more. Although useful in controlling many clinical manifestations, steroid therapy is not without inherent dangers. Because these agents exert such widespread systemic effects, their adverse effects are diverse and often complicate the course of the disease for which they are being used.

The type and severity of side effects are dose dependent and related to the duration of therapy. Although alternate-day therapy (single doses every other day) has been associated with fewer side effects, it is not recommended for control of acute disease.

γ-GLOBULIN THERAPY[5]

γ-Globulin administration is indicated as replacement therapy for immunodeficiency diseases affecting the humoral or antibody-mediated immune system. Recurrent, severe, sinopul-

TABLE 14-18   **Comparison of Various Glucocorticoids with Hydrocortisone**

Glucocorticoid	Anti-Inflammatory Potency	Equivalent Potency (mg)	Sodium-Retaining Potency	Duration of HPAA Suppression (Hours)
Hydrocortisone	1.0	20	2	12
Cortisone	0.8	25	2	12
Prednisolone	4.0	5	1	24-36
Prednisone	3.5	5	1	24-36
Methylprednisolone	5.0	4	0	24-36
Triamcinolone	5.0	4	0	24-36
Paramethasone	10.0	2	0	24-36
Betamethasone	25.0	0.60	0	More than 48
Dexamethasone	30.0	0.75	0	More than 48

monary infections are hallmark clinical manifestations of the humoral immunodeficiency diseases. The frequency and severity with which these infections occur assist the clinician in evaluating the effectiveness of γ-globulin therapy. γ-Globulin is also used to provide passive immunity against a variety of infectious agents, such as the hepatitis virus.

For the past 30 years, human immune serum globulin (HISG) has been available for intramuscular administration. Its use has effectively limited both the severity and frequency of infections in antibody immune deficient patients. The usual dose of HISG ranges from 100 to 200 mg/kg/month. Only IgG is present in significant quantities in HISG.

Although untoward side effects are uncommon, rare anaphylactic reactions to the intramuscular injections have been reported. Patients who have such reactions should be treated immediately with epinephrine and antihistamines. Later, therapy may resume, but HISG from a different manufacturer should be used following a skin test of HISG from the new lot.

Long-term monthly injections produce local pain. HISG is slowly degraded within the injection sites. The risk of entering the intravenous compartment in infants and malnourished patients is high. In addition, large doses of γ-globulins require multiple injections.

Recently, modified preparations of intravenous immune serum globulin (Gamimmune, Intraglobin) are available. Data indicate that these products are effective as replacement therapy. Larger doses of γ-globulin may be delivered with greater efficacy. Serum levels of IgG are reached early and maintained longer. In addition, minimum side effects are associated with its administration.

Doses of intravenous γ-globulin preparations range from 100 to 300 mg/kg/month to maintain IgG serum levels at a minimum of 200 mg/dl. The therapy is usually well tolerated, although chills, fever, and transient leukopenia have been reported. Several researchers indicate that intravenous γ-globulin therapy is highly superior, in terms of clinical efficacy, to intramuscularly administered immunoglobulin. Intravenous γ-globulin therapy appears to be useful for the treatment of patients who require large doses of immunoglobulin, debilitated patients who might not tolerate monthly intramuscular injections, and Wiskott-Aldrich patients who are prone to hemorrhage. It is used routinely in all bone marrow transplant patients and in all patients who have immunoglobulin deficiencies. Research to prolong platelet half-life is underway.

γ-Globulin is used for passive immunization in bone marrow transplant patients to provide passive immunity against a variety of infectious and viral agents. It is also used to protect against the hepatitis virus in the immunocompetent host.

IMMUNOTHERAPY[5,12]

Immunotherapy has a role in the treatment of allergic and immune deficiency diseases, some autoimmune disorders, and cancer. In allergic diseases immunotherapy is used to hyposensitize the patient. (Desensitization is discussed elsewhere.) In immunodeficiency disease the aim is to restore absent or deficient products; for example, in X-linked hypogammaglobulinemia, treatment involves administration of γ-globulin. Patients with autoimmune disorders such as systemic lupus erythematosus may benefit from therapeutic plasmapheresis (a type of immunotherapy), with removal of circulating immune complexes. (Immunodeficiency and autoimmune disorders are discussed elsewhere.) Immunotherapy in the treatment of cancer, whether it is the sole form of treatment or used as adjunct therapy, is currently being investigated. There are now some forms of immunotherapy available for the oncology patient. Cancer immunotherapy is manipulation of the immune system to control or eliminate the growth of neoplastic cells.

PLASMAPHERESIS

Apheresis is the separation of the whole blood into its various components by passage through automated centrifugation devices or membrane filters. After fractionation, certain blood constituents are discarded, while others are returned to the donor. Apheresis can be performed as a therapeutic protocol or to obtain donor blood products.

Plasmapheresis is the procedure by which plasma is selectively removed from whole blood. This experimental therapeutic manipulation is employed in certain diseases to remove an abnormal constituent from the plasma or replenish a deficient plasma factor. During therapeutic plasma exchange, patient plasma is removed and the cellular elements of the blood are reinfused following reconstitution with normal plasma or a suitable colloidal substitute.

Although not many well-controlled scientific studies concerning the therapeutic efficacy of plasmapheresis have been performed, it is being employed to treat a number of immunologic and nonimmunologic disorders. Conditions commonly treated with plasma exchange are outlined in Table 14-19.

Patients treated with plasmapheresis may expect to experience only temporary clinical improvement. Since therapeutic

TABLE 14-19 Disorders Treated with Therapeutic Plasma Exchange

Disorder	Rationale
Autoimmune hemolytic anemia	Removal of antiplatelet antibodies
Myasthenia gravis	Removal of antibodies directed at acetylcholine receptor
Goodpasture's syndrome	Removal of anti–basement membrane antibodies
Multiple sclerosis	Removal of putative anti-myelin antibodies
Systemic lupus erythematosus	Removal of circulating immune complexes
Amyloidosis	Removal of immunoglobulin
Thrombotic thrombocytopenic purpura	Replenishment of plasma factor

TABLE 14-20 Complications of Therapeutic Plasma Exchange

Complication	Nursing Care
Trauma or infection at site of vascular access	Keep entry site clean and dry; inspect regularly for signs of infection
Disequilibrium syndrome (nausea, diaphoresis, light-headedness, tachycardia, and hypotension resulting from hypovolemia)	Monitor fluid balance and vital signs closely; administer fluids as needed; offer patient orange juice or saltines
Hypokalemia, hypocalcemia (which may predispose to cardiac irregularities)	Monitor electrolyte balance and replace electrolytes as needed
Bleeding owing to temporary depletion of platelets and clotting factors	Maintain safe environment; observe for signs of bleeding or bruising
Temporary pareshtesias, muscle twitching, nausea, and vomiting owing to administration of citrated plasma	Provide comfort measures and reassurance; add calcium gluconate to replacement fluids
Anemia owing to hemolysis	Replace erythrocytes in combination with fluids or plasma
Increased risk of infection owing to depletion of certain plasma proteins	Observe for signs of infection
Transient peripheral edema owing to fluid shifts	Symptoms are transient and no further treatment is warranted
Hypothermia owing to infusion of cool fluids	Provide extra blankets; prewarm replacement fluids

plasma exchange is designed to relieve the manifestations of a clinical disease process without affecting the underlying disorder, repeated treatments are usually indicated. Patients undergoing therapeutic plasma exchange to remove plasma antibodies of circulating immune complexes are treated concomitantly with immunosuppressive drugs to retard the recovery of immunoglobin levels.

Although plasmapheresis is generally believed to be a benign procedure, a number of complications are associated with this treatment. These untoward effects and suggested patient management are described in Table 14-20.

References

1. Ataman M et al: Wegener's granulomatosis: case report and review of the literature, *Rhinology* 32:92, 1994.
2. Boumpas DT et al: Systemic lupus erythematosus: emerging concepts. part 2: Dermatologic and joint disease, the antiphospholipid antibody syndrome, pregnancy and hormonal therapy, morbidity and mortality, and pathogenesis, *Ann Intern Med* 123:42, 1995.
3. Boumpas DT et al: Systemic lupus erythematosus: emerging concepts. part 1: Renal, neuropsychiatric, cardiovascular, pulmonary, and hematologic disease, *Ann Intern Med* 122:940, 1995.
4. Capizzi RL et al: Methotrexate therapy of head and neck cancer: improvement in therapeutic index by the use of leucovorin "rescue," *Cancer Res* 30:1782, 1970.
5. Carmichael CG et al: *HIV/AIDS primary care handbook,* Norwalk, CT, 1995, Appleton & Lange.
6. Dorr RT, Von Hoff DD: *Cancer chemotherapy handbook,* Norwalk, CT, 1994, Appleton & Lange.
7. Eisenstein EM, Sneller MC: Common variable immunodeficiency: diagnosis and management, *Ann Allergy* 73:285, 1994.
8. Fauci AS, Wolff SM: Wegener's granulomatosis: studies in 18 patients and a review of the literature, *Medicine* 73:315, 1994.
9. Fineman S: Urticaria and angioedema. In Lawlor GJ et al, editors: *Manual of allergy and immunology,* Boston, 1981, Little, Brown.
10. Foster HE et al: The treatment of sicca features of Sjögren's syndrome: a clinical review, *Brit J Rheumatol* 33:278, 1994.
11. Friedman-Kein AE, Laubenstein LS, editors: *AIDS: the epidemic of Kaposi's sarcoma and opportunistic infections,* New York, 1984, Masson.
12. Gertz MA, Kyle RA: Amyloidosis: prognosis and treatment, *Arthritis Med* 24:124, 1994.
13. Hansen F: Hematopoietic growth and inhibitory factors in treatment of malignancies. A review, *Acta Oncol* 34:453, 1995.
14. Hughes RA, Keat AC: Reiter's syndrome and reactive arthritis: a current view, *Semin Arthritis Rheum* 24:190, 1994.
15. Lawlor G et al, editors: *Manual of allergy and immunology,* Boston, 1981, Little, Brown.
16. Liblau RS, Back JF: Selective IgA deficiency and autoimmunity, *Int Arch Allergy Immunol* 99:16, 1992.
17. Lightfoot RW, Jr: Churg-Strauss syndrome and polyarteritis nodosa, *Curr Opin Rheumatol* 3:3, 1991.
18. Megerian CA et al: Angioedema: 5 years' experience with a review of the disorder's presentation and treatment, *Laryngoscope* 102:256, 1992.
19. Muma RD et al: *HIV manual for health care professionals,* Norwalk CT, 1994, Appleton & Lange.
20. Oxholm P: Primary Sjögren's syndrome—clinical and laboratory markers of disease activity, *Semin Arthritis Rheum* 22:114, 1992.
21. Pollack CV, Jr, Jorden RC: Recognition and management of sarcoidosis in the emergency department, *J Emerg Med* 11:297, 1993.
22. Schur P, editor: *The clinical management of systemic lupus erythematosus,* New York, 1983, Grune & Stratton.
23. Sneller MC et al: New insights into common variable immunodeficiency, *Ann Intern Med* 118:720, 1993.
24. Tierney LM, Jr et al: *CURRENT Medical Diagnosis and Treatment,* Norwalk, CT, 1995, Appleton & Lange.
25. Thomas ED: Bone marrow transplantation, *New Engl J Med* 292:896, 1975.
26. Tucker SM et al: *Patient care standards: collaborative practice planning guides,* ed 6, St Louis, 1996, Mosby.
27. Unaue ER, Benacerraf B: *Textbook of immunology,* Baltimore, 1984, Williams & Wilkins.
28. Weinberg DA et al: Giant cell arteritis: corticosteroids, temporal artery biopsy, and blindness, *Arch Fam Med* 3:623, 1994.

Hematolymphatic System

15

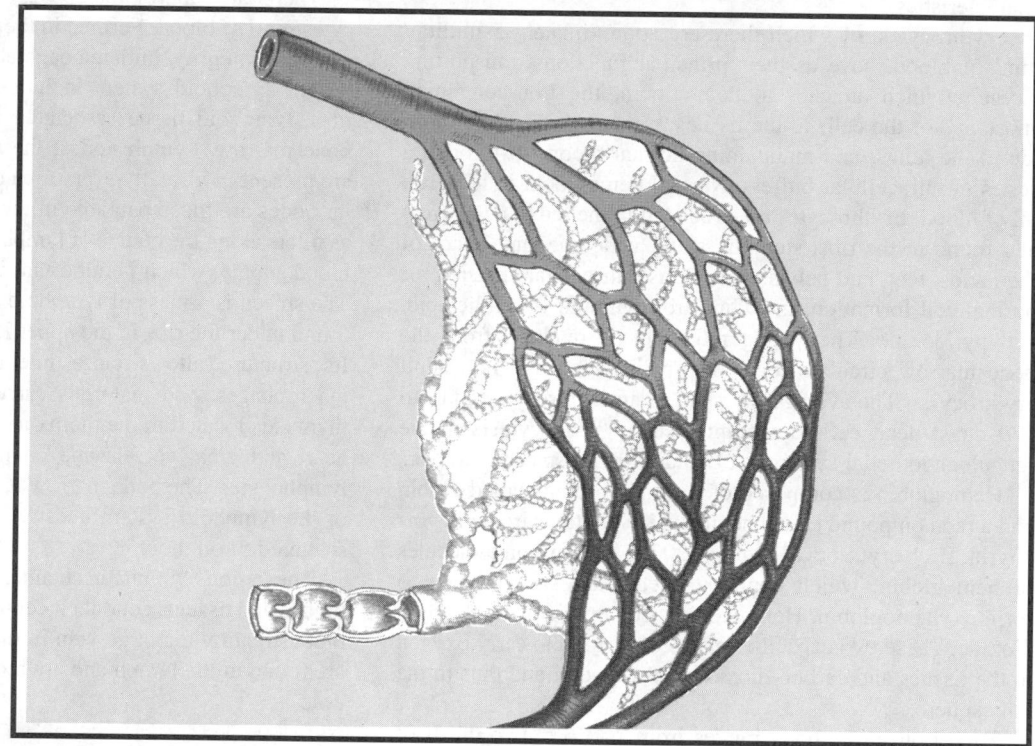

OVERVIEW

The hematolymphatic system is composed of blood and blood-forming organs, the bone marrow, spleen, liver, and the lymphatics.

Blood, which circulates continuously through the heart and vascular system, performs numerous vital functions, such as (1) transporting oxygen and absorbed nutrients to cells and waste products, including carbon dioxide, to the kidneys, skin, and lungs; (2) transporting hormones from their origin in the endocrine glands to other tissues; (3) protecting the body from life-threatening microorganisms; and (4) regulating body temperature by heat transfer.

Major characteristics of blood include color (arterial blood is bright red; venous blood is dark red); viscosity (blood is three to four times thicker than water); reaction (the pH is 7.35 to 7.4); and volume (adults have approximately 70 to 75 ml/kg of body weight, or 5 to 6 L).

The four physiologic disturbances likely to occur in the hematologic system are decreased number of cells, overproduction of normal or abnormal cells, defects in the clotting mechanism, and disorders of the spleen. Causative factors may be idiopathic (unknown) or one of the following: dietary deficiencies, malabsorption, drug toxicity, metabolic disorders, hemorrhaging, infection, malignancy, genetic predisposition, or immunologic defects.

The lymphatic system also has numerous functions, including transporting lymph; producing lymphocytes and antibodies; phagocytosis; and absorbing fats and fat-soluble matter from the intestine.

The major characteristics of the lymphatic system are that the formation of lymph is regulated by exchange of fluid between capillaries and tissue spaces; that the muscle pump is responsible for the movement of lymph; and that the amount of lymphoid tissue and the distribution of lymph nodes are related to age. The lymphatic system includes peripheral lymphatics, regional nodes, main lymphatic ducts, and the thoracic duct.

The two basic physiologic disturbances that can occur in the lymphatic system—enlargement and swelling of soft tissues—are usually caused by infection, inflammation, neoplasm, or obstruction.

•••••• Anatomy, Physiology, and Related Pathophysiology

Blood, a suspension of particulate matter in an aqueous solution of colloid and electrolytes, serves as a medium of exchange for body cells between themselves and the exterior. It also has protective properties that benefit the body and the blood itself. The liquid portion, plasma, is a suspension of colloid, electrolytes, proteins, and numerous other substances. The particulate matter includes red blood cells (erythrocytes), white blood cells of several types (leukocytes), and platelets (thrombocytes). All of these cells are believed to be derived from a single stem cell, which divides and matures to produce three distinct types of cells with different functions, properties, and characteristics.

Erythrocytes, of which there are approximately 5 million/mm³ of blood, have as their principal functions transporting oxygen (which attaches to hemoglobin, the iron-containing substance of the cell) to the tissues; transporting carbon dioxide to the lungs; and maintaining normal blood pH through a series of intracellular buffers. Normal hemoglobin is 15 g/100 ml of blood. Erythrocytes are produced in the red bone marrow and found in the ribs, sternum, skull, vertebrae, and bones of the hands, feet, and pelvis. Numerous nutrients are needed for normal cell formation, including iron, vitamin B₁₂, folic acid, and pyridoxine. The young reticulocytes released from the bone marrow circulate for 4 days while maturing into adult erythrocytes. The average life span of an erythrocyte is 115 to 130 days; dead cells are eliminated by phagocytosis in the reticuloendothelial system, particularly in the spleen and liver.

Hemoglobin is composed of a simple protein called globin and a red compound called heme, which contains iron and porphyrin. Each erythrocyte contains 200 to 300 million molecules of hemoglobin, which combine chemically with oxygen to form oxyhemoglobin. Hemoglobin also combines with carbon dioxide. These two capacities enable the blood to carry oxygen to the tissues and carbon dioxide to the alveoli and thus to the atmosphere.

Total iron in the body ranges from 2 to 6 g, two thirds of which is contained in hemoglobin; the rest is stored in the bone marrow, spleen, and liver. Iron is obtained from such rich dietary sources as liver, oysters, lean meats, kidney beans, green leafy vegetables, apricots, and raisins.

When hemoglobin is phagocytosed in the liver or spleen, it breaks down into its heme and globin factors. The heme's iron is reused by the liver to make fresh hemoglobin, whereas the porphyrin is converted into bilirubin that is excreted by the body in feces and urine.

Leukocytes, of which there are approximately 5000 to 10,000/mm³ of blood, are divided into three major categories: granulocytes, lymphocytes, and monocytes. Granulocytes, which make up 70% of all white blood cells, are produced by the bone marrow and function according to the type of granule: (1) polymorphonuclear leukocytes (PMNs or neutrophils), whose main function is to fight bacterial infections through a process of phagocytosis (foreign particulate matter, or breakdown products from cells, is also digested); these cells are present during the early, acute phase of an inflammatory reaction; (2) eosinophils, which have a similar phagocytic function and are particularly important in digesting bacteria; they appear to play a role in combating allergic reactions; and (3) basophils, which contain many enzymes believed to play a role in combating acute systemic allergic reactions.

Lymphocytes, which are mainly produced in the lymph nodes, make up about 25% of the leukocytes. They are primarily concerned with producing antibodies and maintaining tissue immunity. Monocytes, which are derived from components of the reticuloendothelial system, are responsible for the phagocy-

tosis of dead erythrocytes and leukocytes in the blood. They are also important in the processing of antigenic information.

There are approximately 250,000 to 500,000 thrombocytes/mm³ of blood. Formed in the bone marrow, they maintain capillary integrity, initiate coagulation, and retract clots.

The lymphoid system includes lymph nodes, spleen, thymus, lymphoid tissue associated with mucosal surfaces, and bone marrow. Lymph nodes, the most numerous component, are present in virtually every area of the body. The most familiar nodes are those palpable in the neck and groin. They serve as filters along the course of lymphatic channels and have a rich blood supply, which is important in transporting lymphocytes. The spleen is a mass of lymphoid and reticuloendothelial cells found under the ribs in the upper left quadrant of the abdomen. Its structure allows close interaction among lymphocytes, macrophages, and materials carried in the bloodstream. The thymus is located in the thorax anterior to the upper part of the heart and great vessels and contains lymphatic follicles and lymphocytes. The bone marrow is considered an important part of the lymphoid system because millions of lymphocytes are scattered throughout it.

The various lymphatic channels in the body drain fluid from organs and tissues, conduct it centrally, and introduce it into the bloodstream via a large vein in the thorax. Many lymphocytes are found in the lymph and are recycled for variable periods of time.

NORMAL FINDINGS[1]

Blood

Erythrocyte   Biconcave disk when viewed laterally; appears to have lighter center and to be thicker on outer perimeter

Reticulocyte   Young, nonnucleated cells formed in bone marrow; stain gray-blue

Granulocyte   Neutrophil (PMN): faint, pink, acidophilic granules; Eosinophil: refractive, eosinophilic granules; Basophil: large blue granules

Lymphocyte   Single, round nucleus; cytoplasm has faintly basophilic, heavily clumped nuclear chromatin pattern

Monocyte   Folded or indented nucleus; often looks lobulated; has clumped nuclear chromatin pattern; cytoplasm is bluish gray or light sky blue

Thrombocyte   Nucleate, disk-shaped fragments of megakaryocytes of the lymphoid system

Lymph nodes   Not normally palpable in adults

Spleen   Located in the left upper outer quadrant; not normally palpable

Thymus   Reticular framework densely infiltrated with lymphocytes arranged in pattern of cortex and medulla

Lymphoid tissue associated with mucosal surfaces—that is, gastrointestinal and respiratory tracts   May be distributed diffusely or in nodular aggregates

Bone marrow   Myeloid tissue located only in the ribs, sternum, and at the ends of long bones

CONDITIONS, DISEASES AND DISORDERS

ERYTHROCYTIC DISORDERS

Two basic pathophysiologic processes can be used to classify all disorders of red blood cells: inadequate numbers of circulating cells (anemia) and increased numbers of circulating cells (polycythemia). Anemias result from insufficient production or defective synthesis, increased destruction, or loss of erythrocytes. Polycythemia results from idiopathic causes or as a compensatory mechanism in response to tissue hypoxia.

Although not a disease per se, anemia is the primary manifestation of many abnormal states, including dietary deficiencies of iron, vitamin B_{12}, and folic acid; hereditary disorders; bone marrow damaged by toxins, radiation, or chemotherapy; renal disease; malignancy; chronic infection; overactive spleen; or bleeding from a tract or organ. The incidence of anemia is high; as much as 50% of the world's population suffers from anemia at any one time.

The major physiologic effect of anemia is to reduce the oxygen-carrying capacity of the blood; thus the symptoms of anemia are the result of tissue hypoxia.

■ POSTHEMORRHAGIC ANEMIA

Posthemorrhagic anemia is a disorder of decreased hemoglobin in the blood caused by traumatically induced hemorrhage.

Acute posthemorrhagic anemia develops as the result of the rapid loss of large quantities of erythrocytes during a hemorrhage, that is, traumatic severance of blood vessels, rupture of an aneurysm, or arterial erosion by a cancerous or ulcerative lesion. The severity of symptoms and the prognosis depend on the rate of bleeding, site of bleeding, and volume of blood loss. The rapid loss of less blood is more dangerous than is the slower loss of more blood.

In general, a 20% loss of total blood volume results in vascular insufficiency; a 30% loss causes circulatory failure, shock, and coma; and with a 40% loss, death is imminent, unless there is immediate and extensive blood value replacement.

•••••• Pathophysiology

During the first 24 to 48 hours after hemorrhage, vasoconstriction and loss of plasma volume distort the erythrocyte count, hemoglobin, and hematocrit, which appear high when they are actually quite low. These laboratory tests more accurately reflect the patient's status after intravenous fluids are infused and extracellular fluid moves into the blood vessels. The red blood cell count and hemoglobin usually return to normal in 4 to 6 weeks, with many reticulocytes observed in the blood.

Chronic blood loss anemia, which is caused by bleeding peptic ulcers, menstrual disorders, bleeding hemorrhoids, or gastrointestinal neoplasms, results in continuous loss of erythrocytes and iron. Symptoms and laboratory findings are identical to those of iron deficiency anemia.

•••••• Diagnostic Studies and Findings

Erythrocytes $6.1/mm^3$ (initial); $4.7/mm^3$ (after fluid volume increase)

Hemoglobin 16.5 g/dl (initial); 14.5 g/dl (after fluid volume increase)

Hematocrit 50% (initial); 40% (after fluid volume increase)

Coagulation time Decreased

•••••• Multidisciplinary Plan

Surgery

If indicated to control source of bleeding

Medications

Hematinic agents

Iron supplements when dietary therapy is insufficient: ferrous sulfate (Feosol), 200 mg tid po with meals

General Management

Initial intravenous fluids are noncolloid, contain electrolytes; followed by plasma, packed red blood cells, or both as needed to correct cell deficit

Whole blood may be administered, after typing and cross-matching, to correct fluid volume and cell deficit as needed

Oxygen by nasal catheter or mask to maintain sufficient oxygenation of circulating blood volume

Sedation and rest to reduce patient's energy expenditure

Oral fluids as tolerated to maintain adequate tissue hydration and renal perfusion

Diet high in protein and iron as basis for erythropoiesis

NURSING CARE

Nursing Assessment

Cardiovascular Function

Rapid, thready pulse

Hypotension

Sensory Function

Restlessness, dizziness, syncope, severe headache

Mental Status

Disorientation

Appearance of Skin

Pallor, diaphoresis, coolness

Respiratory Function

Rapid, deep respirations; later become shallow

Fluid and Electrolyte Balance

Thirst
Decreased urinary output

Nursing Dx & Intervention

Decreased cardiac output related to decreased circulating blood volume

- Provide rest and anticipate patient's needs *to reduce cardiac workload.*
- Monitor apical pulse, heart sounds, orthostatic blood pressure, and respirations *to assess cardiopulmonary function.*
- Monitor central venous pressure, breath sounds, and pulmonary artery pressure as indicated *to assess fluid volume and cardiopulmonary function.*
- Monitor erythrocyte count, hemoglobin, and hematocrit *to determine effectiveness of blood component therapy and body's compensatory mechanisms.*
- Avoid stress (e.g., strong emotions, overexertion, fatigue, coughing, and straining at stool) *to reduce cardiac workload.*

Altered peripheral tissue perfusion related to decreased blood volume and vasoconstriction

- Place patient on bed rest in semi-Fowler's position *to reduce cardiac workload and enhance systemic circulation.*
- Maintain warm environment *to prevent shivering and vasoconstriction.*
- Inspect trunk and extremities *for adequacy of circulation.* Skin should be pink, dry, and warm.
- Palpate for arterial pulses *to determine patency of peripheral arterial circulation.*
- Protect patient from injury (e.g., put up side rails) *to prevent further blood loss.*
- Assess level of consciousness and orientation *to determine adequate cerebral circulation.* Patient should be alert and oriented to time, place, and person.
- Discourage smoking, *which causes vasoconstriction of peripheral vessels and increased cardiopulmonary activity.*
- Encourage exercise, including range of motion exercises, *to promote peripheral circulation.*

Fluid volume deficit related to blood loss

- Apply ice bag and manual pressure or dressing over site of blood loss *to constrict damaged vessel or tissue and prevent further loss of blood.*
- Elevate and immobilize affected body part *to promote blood return to the heart and reduce blood loss at site of damage.*
- Estimate blood loss *to determine need for volume replacement.*
- Administer intravenous fluid, including blood components, as ordered *to replace lost fluid volume.*
- Monitor for transfusion reaction if blood is administered.

- Assess patient's response to fluid therapy (i.e., check breath sounds, pulse, and blood pressure) *to avoid circulatory overload.*
- Measure intake and output *to determine adequacy of renal function.* Output should be at least 30 ml/hour.
- Increase oral fluid intake as tolerated *to maintain tissue hydration and renal perfusion.*
- Observe for recurrent bleeding, which may result from dislodgment of clot, increased vascular pressure, or further pathophysiologic conditions.

Patient Education/Home Care Planning

1. Encourage the patient to avoid overexertion, fatigue, and emotional states because they place a strain on the cardiovascular system that may result in respiratory distress, cardiac damage, or impaired peripheral arterial circulation.
2. Discuss the need to report to the physician serious symptoms, such as pain, dyspnea, extreme fatigue, and blood in urine or feces, because they may signal recurrent internal bleeding.
3. Support the patient in maintenance of normal bowel elimination to avoid strain on the cardiovascular system.
4. Discuss the importance of regular exercise to maintain adequate peripheral circulation and cardiac and respiratory tone.
5. Plan with the patient how to maintain a diet high in iron and protein, with adequate fluid intake, to promote production of erythrocytes and ensure adequate fluid volume.

Evaluation

Vital signs are within normal limits Respirations, blood pressure, and pulse are within normal limits.

The patient's vitality is maintained The patient is mentally alert, with good concentration and attentiveness. The patient experiences no malaise, fatigue, or weakness.

Color of the skin and mucous membranes is good The skin, nails, lips, and ear lobes are warm and moist and have a natural color.

Body hydration is normal There is no edema or thirst. Urinary output balances with fluid intake.

■ IRON DEFICIENCY ANEMIA

Iron deficiency anemia is caused by an inadequate supply of iron needed to synthesize hemoglobin.

Iron deficiency anemia, which is high in incidence worldwide and the most prevalent anemia, is caused by inadequate absorption or excessive loss of iron. The disease occurs most frequently in women, young children, and the elderly in underdeveloped countries.

The principal cause of iron deficiency anemia in adults is acute or chronic bleeding secondary to trauma; excessive menses; gastrointestinal tract bleeding (usually chronic and occult) caused by peptic ulcer, hiatal hernia, diverticulosis, or cancer; or blood donation. Another cause is inadequate dietary intake of foods high in iron. A third cause in defective absorption caused by malabsorption syndromes, clay eating (pica), chronic diarrhea, high intake of cereal products with low intake of animal protein, and partial or complete gastrectomy.

Pathophysiology

Iron deficiency anemia is a chronic, microcytic, hypochromic anemia; in other words, the erthrocytes are small and pale because of a low hemoglobin level. Although the total erythrocyte count is only moderately reduced, the serum iron level may drop dramatically.

Diagnostic Studies and Findings

Hemoglobin level   As low as 3.6 g/dl
Total erythrocyte count   Rarely below 3 million cells/dl
Mean corpuscular hemoglobin (MCH)   <27 pg
Mean corpuscular hemoglobin concentration (MCHC) 20 to 30 g/dl
Serum iron level   As low as 10 μg/dl
Hematocrit   Male: <47 ml/dl; female: <42 ml/dl
Iron binding capacity   Increased
Serum ferritin level (one of the forms in which iron is stored in the body)   Decreased

Multidisciplinary Plan

Medications

Hematinic agents (to increase iron available in the blood)
  Ferrous sulfate (Feosol), 0.2 g tid with meals
  Ferrous gluconate (Fergon), 0.3 g bid
  Iron-dextran (Imferon), 100 to 250 mg/dl
Ascorbic acid (as indicated)

General Management

Diet high in iron-rich foods to correct nutritional deficiency—including red meats, organ meats, kidney beans, whole-wheat products, spinach, egg yolks, carrots, and raisins

NURSING CARE

Nursing Assessment

In a mild case the patient generally has no symptoms.

Sensory, Neural, and Motor Function

Dizziness
Irritability
Numbness and tingling in limbs
Fatigue

Decreased concentration
Headache

Cardiovascular Function

Tachycardia

Respiratory Function

Dyspnea on exertion

Condition of Skin, Hair, and Nails

Sensitivity to cold
Brittle hair and nails (spoon shaped)

Gastrointestinal Function

Atrophic glossitis (tongue inflamed and smooth)
Stomatitis
Dysphagia

Nursing Dx & Intervention

Sensory/perceptual alterations (kinesthetic) related to nervous system tissue hypoxia

- Provide safe environment *to prevent injury.*
- Assist patient with ambulation and changing position because patient's sense of balance, sensation, and position may be altered.

Fatigue related to decreased tissue oxygenation, impaired cardiovascular and respiratory function

- Help patient plan balance between rest and activity *to reduce cardiac workload.*
- Monitor pulse and respirations *to identify signs of increased cardiopulmonary workload, such as tachycardia or dyspnea on exertion.*
- Assess patient for headache and decreased concentration, *which may indicate inadequate cerebral oxygenation.*
- Help patient and significant others understand the physiologic basis for fatigue and that it will diminish on improvement or correction of the iron-deficient state.
- Encourage patient to discuss feelings related to fatigue.
- Encourage patient to identify behaviors associated with fatigue, such as emotional lability or irritability, and *to understand that they are temporary, caused by the anemic condition.*

Impaired skin integrity related to decreased tissue perfusion

- Maintain warm, clean environment *to decrease sensitivity to cold.*
- Wash hair with care *to avoid breaking and other damage.*
- Provide nail care *to avoid damage.*

Altered nutrition: less than body requirements related to inadequate or unbalanced diet

- Remove dentures if present *to prevent infection.*
- Provide soft food and nonirritating fluids *to decrease discomfort and irritation.*

- Provide frequent mouth care *to remove secretions.*
- Initiate dental consultation *to correct caries and other sources of irritation or infection.*
- Administer iron medication as ordered *to correct deficiency.*
- Monitor laboratory reports *to determine effectiveness of medication.*
- Encourage diet high in iron *to correct deficiency.*
- Observe for difficulty in swallowing *to determine need for changes in diet or nutritional support.*
- Provide small, frequent feedings as indicated by patient's condition.

Patient Education/Home Care Planning

1. Discuss the need for correct oral hygiene, including regular dental care, to prevent irritation and infection of the oral cavity.
2. Assist the patient in the maintenance of a diet high in iron to promote the production of healthy erythrocytes.
3. Discuss factors in ongoing self-medication wtih iron supplements, including proper timing, dilution, and awareness of change in stool color.
4. Discuss the importance of continuing all prescribed therapy, even when the patient is feeling well.
5. Discuss general hygienic measures (e.g., proper care of hair and nails) to prevent damage and loss.
6. Discuss general safety precautions to prevent injury from dizziness.

Evaluation

Patient can easily ambulate Patient avoids contact with stable and moving objects. There is no reported dizziness. Activities of daily living are accomplished without fatigue.

Daily intake includes the essential food groups Patient's diet includes foods high in iron.

General body cleanliness and health are maintained Hair and nails are clean and not brittle. Mouth is clean, with no ulceration or other oral irritation. Skin is dry and warm to touch, without evidence of damage or irritation.

Patient has sufficient energy to carry out activities of daily living Patient participates in regular exercise as tolerated.

◼ PERNICIOUS ANEMIA

◼ Pernicious anemia is a progressive anemia caused by a lack of intrinsic factor essential for the absorption of vitamin B_{12}.

Pernicious anemia is the most prevalent type of vitamin B_{12} deficiency anemia in the United States. Caused by a deficiency of the intrinsic factor, it is a chronic, progressive, macrocytic anemia that affects adults, mainly men and women over 50 years of age, and blue-eyed people of Scandinavian origin.

•••••• Pathophysiology

Atrophy of the glandular mucosa of the gastric fundus results in a lack of intrinsic factor. Why this occurs is unknown, but there are several popular explanations: heredity (the disease tends to "run in families"); prolonged iron deficiency, which can cause gastric atrophy; or an autoimmune disorder (90% of patients have autoantibodies that react against gastric cells, and 40% of patients react against the intrinsic factor).

Other anemias in this category result from a lack of vitamin B_{12}, which is caused by inadequate dietary intake and corrected by daily oral administration and a more balanced diet, or caused by poor absorption, which is treated with vitamin B_{12}.

Anemias caused by a deficiency in folic acid are quite common and usually the result of a poor diet, especially one lacking in green leafy vegetables, liver, citrus fruits, and yeast; malabsorption syndromes; or the increased need during the third trimester of pregnancy. Parenteral or oral therapy with folic acid is required. Vitamin C may be used supplementally. The symptoms of this anemia resemble those of pernicious anemia except for the absence of neurologic signs and symptoms.

•••••• Diagnostic Studies and Findings

Erythrocyte count Below 3 million/dl; elevated mean corpuscular volume (MCV) and mean corpuscular hemoglobin concentration (MCHC), decreased white blood cell count (WBC) and mean corpuscular hemoglobin (MCH)

Bone marrow biopsy Increased number of megaloblasts

Bilirubin Unconjugated forms; usually elevated

Serum vitamin B_{12} Deficient

Serum folate Low

Gastric analysis Scanty secretions, elevated pH, and no free hydrochloric acid

Therapeutic trial with parenteral vitamin B_{12} Large numbers of reticulocytes in blood 4 to 5 days after injection

Hemoglobin Decreased to 4 to 5 g/dl

•••••• Multidisciplinary Plan

Medications

Lifelong maintenance therapy

Vitamin derivatives (to correct nutritional or metabolic deficiency)

    Cyanocobalamin (Berubigen, Hemocyte, vitamin B_{12}, and others), 100 mg IM 2 to 3 times/wk until 10 doses are given and remission is obtained

    Cyanocobalamin, 200 mg IM monthly or 100 mg IM every 2 wk (maintenance therapy)

    Folic acid (Folvite), up to 1 mg/d po

Hematinic agents (to correct nutritional deficit)

    Ferrous sulfate (Feosol) or ferrous gluconate (Fergon), 0.3 g tid with meals po as needed

Digestants (to enhance metabolism of vitamins)

Hydrochloric acid (HCl), 4 to 10 ml po well diluted in water tid with meals during first weeks of vitamin B_{12} therapy

General Management

Blood transfusions to correct anemia

Nutritious diet, including fish, meat, milk, and eggs to enrich diet deficient in vitamins

Bed rest as needed for rest, recovery, and safety

Physical therapy to prevent complications from impaired motor function

NURSING CARE

Nursing Assessment

Sensory and Motor Function

Tingling, numbness of hands and feet, weakness, fatigue

Disturbed coordination (i.e., wobbly legs, poor balance)

Mental Status

Irritability, depression

Poor memory, impaired judgment

Appearance of Skin

Pallor and jaundice, waxy

Petechiae, purpura

Gastrointestinal Function

Weight loss, indigestion, constipation, or diarrhea

Anorexia

Sore mouth

Smooth, beefy red tongue

Respiratory Function

Dyspnea

Cardiovascular Function

Tachycardia

Wide pulse pressure

Palpitations

Nursing Dx & Intervention

Risk for injury related to sensory and motor losses, alteration in mental status

- Use bed rest with side rails up as needed *to prevent patient fatigue and falls caused by weakness.*
- Assist with ambulation *to avoid falls.*
- Use bed cradle or footboard *to prevent pressure on lower extremities.*
- Apply heat with extreme caution *to avoid burning the skin.*

- Support patient with patience and reassurance *to reduce irritability and depression.*

Risk for impaired skin integrity related to capillary fragility

- Observe skin color, warmth, texture, moisture, and intactness.
- Apply heat with extreme caution *to avoid burning.*
- Maintain skin with proper hygiene *to prevent irritation or damage.*

Altered nutrition: less than body requirements related to sore mouth and tongue, diarrhea, and/or constipation

- Administer vitamin B_{12} and other medications as prescribed *to promote erythropoiesis.*
- Encourage diet high in vitamins, iron, and protein *to promote production of healthy erythrocytes.*
- Provide rigorous and frequent oral hygiene *to promote nutrition and prevent infection.*
- Offer small, frequent feedings *to prevent digestive overload.*
- Observe for diarrhea or constipation and treat as prescribed *to avoid fluid and electrolyte imbalance and discomfort.*

Impaired gas exchange related to inadequate numbers and impaired functioning of erythrocytes

- Provide bed rest, with side rails up, *to decrease cardiopulmonary workload.*
- Monitor pulse, blood pressure, and rate and quality of respirations *to assess adequacy.*
- Observe mood, appropriateness of behavior, and orientation *to determine mental status.*
- Ask patient to report dyspnea and palpitations.
- Monitor laboratory reports *to determine oxygenation of blood.*

Patient Education/Home Care Planning

1. Discuss precautions in the use of heat-therapy devices such as heating pads or hot compresses (patient may have impaired sensitivity to heat and pain), as well as general safety measures.
2. Emphasize general hygiene, that is, skin and oral care.
3. Practice physical therapy activities and general exercise (patient may have possible neurologic damage as a result of the disease).
4. Discuss the importance of a diet high in vitamin B_{12}, the use of maintenance therapy with vitamin B_{12}, and the need to maintain this lifelong treatment.

Evaluation

There is no evidence of physical injury   There is no evidence of skin damage or physical sign of an injury. Patient is oriented, calm and able to provide self-care. Patient participates in regular exercise as tolerated.

Color of the skin and mucous membranes is good   The skin, nails, lips, and ear lobes are warm and moist and have a natural color. There is no discoloration.

Daily intake includes the essential food groups   Patient's diet is high in iron, protein, and vitamins. Mouth is clean and free of irritation.

Vital signs are within normal limits   Respirations, pulse, and blood pressure are within normal limits. Patient has sufficient energy to carry out activities of daily living.

▋ APLASTIC ANEMIA

Aplastic anemia is the term most frequently used to describe a decrease in the number of circulating erythrocytes caused by a failure of the bone marrow. It is usually accompanied by agranulocytosis and thrombocytopenia, in which case the condition is referred to as pancytopenia.

•••••• Pathophysiology

In half of all diagnosed cases of aplastic anemia, the cause is unknown; in the other half, it results from exposure to a specific toxin. The myelotoxins are (1) agents that always cause damage when given in large doses: radiation (e.g., x-rays, radium, and radioactive isotopes), benzene and its derivatives, alkylating agents, and antimetabolites; (2) agents that sometimes cause failure: chloramphenicol (Chloromycetin), sulfonamides, phenytoin, and others; and (3) suspicious agents such as streptomycin, chlorophenothane (DDT), and carbon tetrachloride. The disease also may be immunologic in origin or the result of a severe disease, such as liver failure. There is some evidence that this anemia may be a sequela of viral infection such as Epstein-Barr virus, cytomegalovirus, or hepatitis B.

•••••• Diagnostic Studies and Findings

Erythrocyte count   Usually less than 1 million/mm³; reticulocyte count also low

Leukocyte count   May be less than 2000/mm³

Serum iron   Elevated

Total iron-binding capacity   Normal or slightly reduced

Platelet count   <30,000/mm³

Bone marrow biopsy   Marrow fatty with few developing blood cells

•••••• Multidisciplinary Plan

General Management

Immediate removal of the causative agent
Blood transfusions as needed to replace cells
Prevention and treatment of complications such as infection and bleeding with such therapies as antibiotics, corticosteroids, and bone marrow transplantation

NURSING CARE

Nursing Assessment

Energy Level

Progressive fatigue, lassitude, and dyspnea
Intolerance to activity

Possibility of Infection

Fever, "sniffles," sore throat, severe anorexia, ulcerations on mucous membranes, pain and burning with urination

Vascular Status

Petechiae or ecchymosis
Bleeding from gums, injection sites, or nose; hematuria; occult or frank blood in feces

Nursing Dx & Intervention

Activity intolerance related to inadequate tissue oxygenation

- For hypoxia: Place the patient in a sitting position; observe respiration rate, pulse, and dyspnea; observe skin color and temperature; assist with care; plan rest periods; administer oxygen as needed; monitor laboratory values to improve gas exchange.
- Assist with activities of daily living as necessary.
- Encourage patient to engage in activities on a progressive basis as fatigue decreases in response to therapy.
- Help patient explore feelings associated with fatigue.

Risk for infection related to increased susceptibility

- Maintain reverse isolation *to avoid exposure to pathogens.*
- Observe for increases in temperature, pulse, and respirations *as signs of infection.*
- Observe the patient for "sniffles," sore throat, anorexia, pain on urination, and so on.
- Administer antibiotics as needed *to combat specific pathogens.*
- Encourage mobility, turning, coughing, deep breathing, and increased fluids *to reduce susceptibility to infection.*

Risk for fluid volume deficit related to inadequate platelet count and impaired clotting

- Handle the patient gently *to avoid trauma.*
- Give injections only if necessary and apply pressure afterward *to prevent extravasation.*
- Observe for changes in vital signs and for bleeding (e.g., urine, stool, gums, or nose) *to identify internal blood loss.*
- Avoid constipation *to prevent tissue irritation and possible bleeding.*

- Apply ice bag or manual pressure *to promote vascular constriction and clotting.*
- Monitor blood studies *to determine status of intravascular volume.*
- Observe for petechiae and ecchymosis *as signs of intradermal bleeding.*

Patient Education/Home Care Planning

1. Assist the patient to maintain a balance between rest and activity.
2. Discuss with the patient how to avoid infection, especially of the respiratory or urinary tract.
3. Discuss with the patient how to avoid trauma (e.g., use soft toothbrush and electric razor) to prevent bleeding.
4. Plan with the patient a self-assessment for bleeding, what signs and symptoms to report, and first aid for bleeding.

Evaluation

The physical appearance of the patient indicates sufficient rest and activity   Patient has good concentration and coordination. Patient walks, bicycles, or performs some other type of exercise. Patient carries out activities of daily living.

Patient's surroundings are safe   Patient uses safety precautions and avoids trauma.

There is no evidence of physical injury   Patient does not have cuts, abrasions, or other signs of injury. No petechiae or ecchymoses are found.

Patient does not have an infection   Oral temperature is 37° C (98.6° F). There is no evidence of inflammation, purulent drainage, pain, or aching.

Vital signs are within normal limits   Respirations, pulse, and blood pressure are within normal limits.

Color of the skin and mucous membranes is good   The skin, nails, lips, and ear lobes are warm and moist and have a natural color.

■ HEMOLYTIC ANEMIA

■ Hemolytic anemia is a disorder in which the rate of erythrocyte destruction is greatly accelerated.

•••••• Pathophysiology

Hemolytic anemia is the result of either an intracorpuscular defect or an extracorpuscular factor. This causes a shortened life span for the erythrocytes, abnormally large numbers of erythrocytes being destroyed by reticuloendothelial cells, and inadequate replacement of lost cells by the bone marrow.

Intracorpuscular defects include a deficiency in glucose 6-phosphate dehydrogenase (G6-PD) and hereditary spherocytosis. Extracorpuscular factors include trauma, such as burns or surgery; chemical agents or drugs, such as lead poisoning; immune response; infectious organisms, such as infectious hep-

atitis, mononucleosis, miliary tuberculosis; systemic diseases, such as Hodgkin's disease, leukemia, systemic lupus erythematosus; isoimmune reactions, such as fetalis erythroblastosis; autoimmune disorders; and paroxysmal hemoglobinurias.

Hemolytic anemia may be acute or chronic; hemolytic crises can occur in either form, both of which have the particular danger of acute renal failure.

•••••• Diagnostic Studies and Findings

Red blood cell count   Normocytic anemia
Reticulocyte count   Increased
Red blood cell fragility   Increased
Erythrocyte life span   Shortened
Bilirubin level   Increased
Fecal and urinary urobilinogen   Increased
Bone marrow biopsy   Hyperplasia
Ultrasound/gallbladder studies   Cholelithiasis

•••••• Multidisciplinary Plan

Surgery

Splenectomy if steroids fail to arrest erythrocyte destruction by the spleen

Medications

Corticosteroids to suppress extracorpuscular factors, such as inflammation
  Prednisolone (Delta-Cortef, Meti-Derm, others), 10 to 20 mg qid (used if autoimmune disease is present)
Osmotic diuretics to prevent acute tubular necrosis (mannitol, urea)

General Management

Eliminate causative factors
Maintain fluid and electrolyte balance for fluid volume
Maintain renal function, using sodium bicarbonate or lactate to alkalize the blood to prevent overload and failure
Combat anemia and shock with careful administration of blood component therapy

---

NURSING CARE

Nursing Assessment

Fluid and Electrolyte Balance

Decreased urinary output
Fluid loss or overload

Gastrointestinal Function

Nausea and vomiting
Enlargement of liver or spleen

Skin Integrity

Jaundice
Fever and chills

Mobility

Weakness and fatigue

Comfort

Back or abdominal pain

Nursing Dx & Intervention

Fluid volume deficit related to blood cell hemolysis, impaired renal blood flow

- Increase oral fluid intake *to maintain intravascular fluid volume.*
- Give small but frequent drinks *to prevent distention or cardiac overload.*
- Monitor intake and output *to determine fluid therapy needs.*
- Observe for adequate renal function: color, specific gravity, volume, and pH of urine *to detect failure early.*
- Administer intravenous fluids as ordered *to correct volume deficit.*
- Administer urine alkalizers as ordered *to promote renal function.*
- Administer blood transfusions as ordered *to correct volume deficit.*
- Assess skin turgor *to determine adequacy of hydration.*
- Encourage exercise as tolerated *to increase patient's strength.*

Altered nutrition: less than body requirements related to decreased appetite

- Provide balanced diet rich in iron and protein *to enhance erythropoiesis.*
- Give small, frequent feedings *to prevent distention or satiation.*
- Avoid fatty foods *to decrease discomfort and stress on gallbladder.*
- Measure body weight *to monitor nutritional status.*
- Observe and record food intake *to assess patient's appetite.*
- Palpate liver and spleen *to assess for enlargement.*
- Observe urine color *to assess liver function; mahogany color indicates dysfunction.*
- Monitor laboratory values, especially bilirubin, *to assess liver function.*

Impaired skin integrity related to impaired circulation

- Provide skin care, such as cool water and lubrication, *for patient's comfort.*
- Maintain cool room temperature with adequate humidity *to enhance patient's comfort.*
- Expose skin to sunlight *to promote warmth and circulation.*
- Advise patient not to scratch skin *to avoid irritation and abrasions.*

Impaired physical mobility related to tissue hypoxia

- Assist with mobility *to compensate for patient's weakness.*
- Provide walker, wheelchair, or cane as needed *to assist patient with mobility.*
- Observe for weakness and fatigue *to pace exercise and rest.*

Pain related to back or abdominal discomfort and distention

- Provide warmth, analgesia, and other pain relief measures as needed and prescribed *to relieve discomfort or at least increase patient's tolerance.*
- Administer antipyretics as needed *for temperature control.*
- Have blankets, extra clothing, and external sources of warmth such as a heating pad or lighted bed cradle available *to warm patient when chilling occurs.*
- Offer antiemetics, carbonated beverages, oral care, and other measures of patient's choice *to reduce incidence of nausea and vomiting.*

Patient Education/Home Care Planning

1. Assist the patient in finding a balance between rest and exercise.
2. Discuss with the patient the need for a well-balanced diet.
3. Help the patient to identify comfort measures.

Evaluation

Skin and mucous membranes have good color The skin, nails, lips, and ear lobes are warm and moist and have a natural color.

Body hydration is normal Skin turgor and color are good. Patient has thin secretions. Balance between intake and output is maintained.

Daily intake includes essential food groups Patient's diet is especially high in iron and protein.

Patient maintains general body cleanliness Patient's skin is clean, and patient does not complain of itching.

Patient activity level is normal Patient exercises regularly, uses assistive devices as needed, and rests when tired.

Patient reports absence of pain No complaints of back or abdominal pain.

■ SICKLE CELL ANEMIA

Sickle cell anemia is a severe incurable anemia that occurs in people who are homozygous for hemoglobin S (Hb S).

•••••• Pathophysiology

Sickle cell anemia is the result of a genetic mutation that is transmitted from parent to child. Between 45,000 and 75,000 black people in this country have the disease, and 2.5 million carry the trait (Figure 15-1). The incidence of the trait is less than 1% in nonblacks and the disease is nonexistent.

The erythrocytes of patients with sickle cell anemia contain more Hb S than Hb A, which causes them to assume a sickle or crescent shape when exposed to decreased oxygen tension. These "sickled" cells are then easily destroyed as they enter smaller blood vessels in the body. The sickle cell trait is usually a mild condition found in heterozygous carriers, who have few or no symptoms.

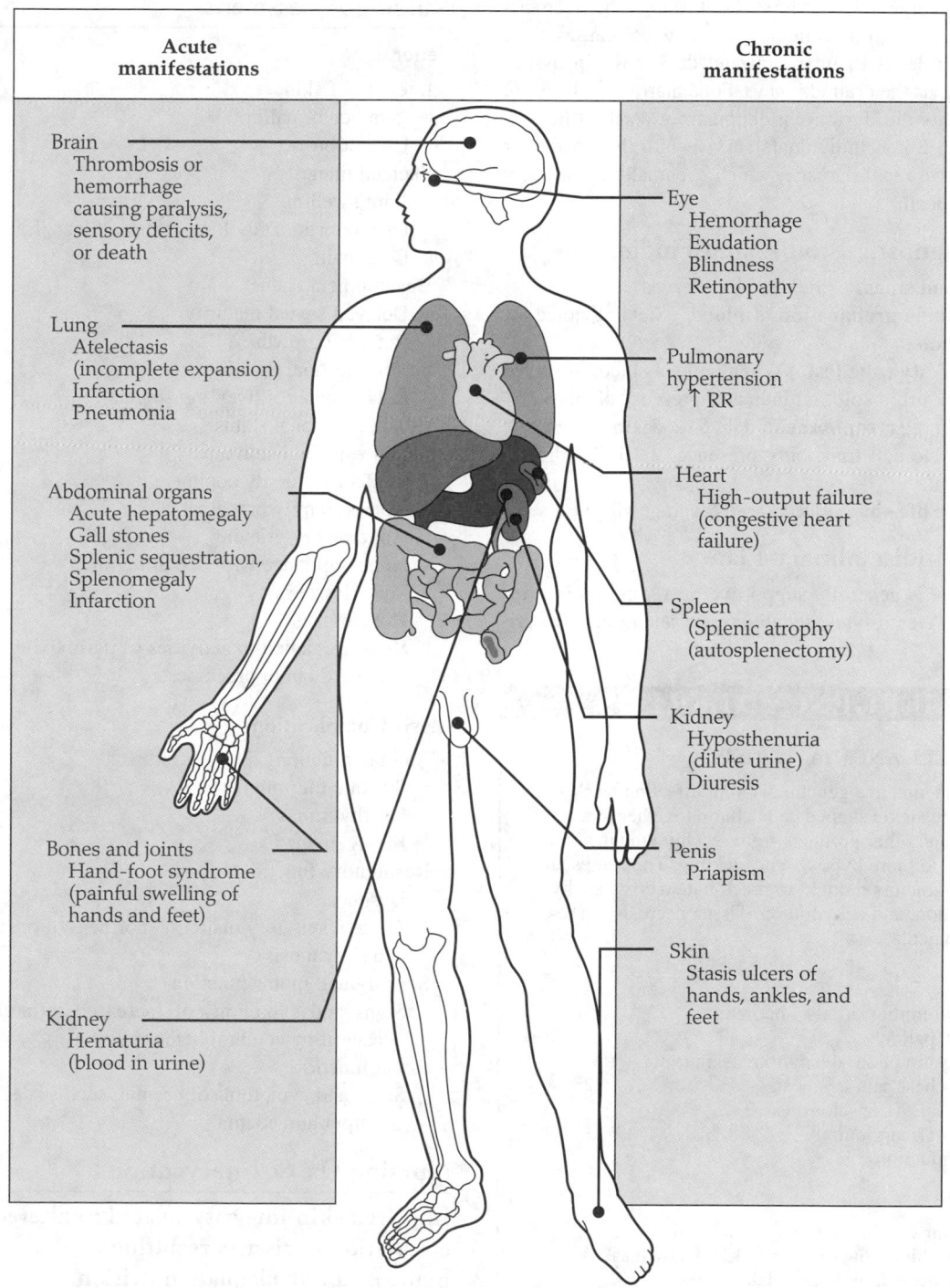

Acute manifestations

Brain
  Thrombosis or hemorrhage causing paralysis, sensory deficits, or death

Lung
  Atelectasis (incomplete expansion)
  Infarction
  Pneumonia

Abdominal organs
  Acute hepatomegaly
  Gall stones
  Splenic sequestration, Splenomegaly
  Infarction

Bones and joints
  Hand-foot syndrome (painful swelling of hands and feet)

Kidney
  Hematuria (blood in urine)

Chronic manifestations

Eye
  Hemorrhage
  Exudation
  Blindness
  Retinopathy

Pulmonary hypertension
  ↑ RR

Heart
  High-output failure (congestive heart failure)

Spleen
  (Splenic atrophy (autosplenectomy)

Kidney
  Hyposthenuria (dilute urine)
  Diuresis

Penis
  Priapism

Skin
  Stasis ulcers of hands, ankles, and feet

Figure 15-1 Clinical manifestations of sickle cell disease. (From Belcher.[1])

The exact cause of sickling crises is unknown, but two factors have been identified: hypoxia caused by low oxygen tensions (such as climbing to high altitudes, exercising strenuously, or inadequate oxygenation during anesthesia) and elevated blood viscosity caused by a concentration of cells and dehydration resulting from such factors as vomiting, diarrhea, diaphoresis, or diuretics (see Emergency Alert box). Occlusion of the microcirculation then occurs, with resultant hypoxia, which causes more sickling. Anoxia leads to infarction and thrombosis in tissues and organs such as the brain, kidneys, bone marrow, and spleen.

Many patients die during childhood from cerebral hemorrhage or shock. Some individuals survive into their fifties or older. Progressive renal damage, which eventually causes uremia, results in death.

• • • • • • Diagnostic Studies and Findings

Stained blood smear   Sickle cell observed

Sickle cell slide preparation of blood   Sickling noted after deoxygenation

Sickle-turbidity tube test   When patient's blood is mixed with Sickledex, turbid solution indicates presence of Hb S

Hemoglobin electrophoresis   Hb S and Hb A indicate presence of sickle cell trait; only presence of Hb S indicates sickle cell anemia

Erythrocyte life span   Decreased (average 20 days)

• • • • • • Multidisciplinary Plan

The plan of care is generally supportive: rest, oxygen, intravenous fluids and electrolytes, sedatives, and analgesics. Experi-

---

! EMERGENCY ALERT

SICKLE CELL ANEMIA—CRISIS

Sickle cell anemia is a genetic disorder affecting black people, where sickle shaped cells clump together preventing oxygen and other products from reaching microcirculation, leading to more hypoxia and sickling. The causes are unknown but factors thought to precipitate a crisis are hypoxia, infection, and dehydration. Tissue necrosis can result if prolonged.

Assessment

- Pain in extremities, joints, abdomen
- Weakness, pallor
- Cardiac dysfunction: dysrhythmias, murmurs
- Dyspnea, chest pain, cyanosis
- Altered level of consciousness
- Decreased urinary output
- Signs of infection

Interventions

- Maintain airway, breathing, and circulation.
- Administer high flow oxygen (10-15 L) by mask.
- Obtain IV access, hydration, lab studies.
- Manage pain with medications, and positioning for comfort.
- Provide rest environment for patient.
- Monitor intake and output.

---

mental use of antisickling agents (urea, cyanate, carbamoyl phosphate); oral maintenance therapy with folic acid and/or iron

NURSING CARE

Nursing Assessment

General

Integrity of skin
   Jaundice or pallor
   Ulceration
Skeletal integrity
   Joint swelling
   Disproportionately long arms and legs, fragility
   Bone pain
Development status
   Delayed sexual maturity
   Retarded growth
Gastrointestinal function
   Enlargement of liver and spleen
Psychoemotional status
   Self-esteem disturbance
   Ineffective family coping
   Altered family processes
   Anticipatory grieving
   Noncompliance with health regimen
   Powerlessness
   Hopelessness
   Self-care deficit in activities of daily living (ADLs)
   Altered thought processes

Crisis Complications

Cardiac function
   Systolic murmurs
   Dysrhythmias
   Enlargement
Respiratory function
   Dyspnea
   Acute respiratory distress (shortness of breath, chest pain, and cyanosis)
Sensory and motor function
   Signs and symptoms of increased intracranial pressure caused by cerebral hemorrhaging
Renal function
   Signs and symptoms of uremia, such as decreased urinary output and edema

Nursing Dx & Intervention

Impaired skin integrity related to altered circulation to tissues resulting in hypoxia and inadequate nutrition

- Remove constrictive clothing *to enhance circulation.*
- Maintain room and body warmth *to avoid discomfort or chilling.*

- Initiate range of motion exercises; support joints at rest and with movement *to stimulate circulation.*
- Inspect extremities *for adequate circulation.*
- Palpate for arterial pulses *to assess patency of arterial circulation.*
- Monitor blood studies for gas exchange and hematology *as indicators of adequate tissue perfusion.*
- Place patient on bed rest *to decrease resistance to peripheral circulation.*
- Elevate affected part *to enhance venous return.*
- Implement cleaning procedure (use hydrogen peroxide or saline solution) *to remove drainage and necrotic tissue.*
- Apply sterile dressing or expose affected area to air *to promote healing.*
- Apply heat with lamp or cradle *to enhance circulation and healing.*
- Observe response to therapy *to evaluate its effectiveness.*
- Cut patient's nails and discourage scratching to avoid injury.

Risk for injury related to joint swelling and bone fragility

- Change the patient's position frequently with joint support *to avoid trauma.*
- Initiate range of motion exercises and physical activity *to maintain muscle tone.*
- Encourage the patient to eat foods high in calcium, protein, and vitamins *to enhance bone integrity.*
- Observe for pain, swelling, or abnormal alignment *as signs of trauma such as fracture.*

Pain related to increased intraabdominal pressure and discomfort

- Place the patient in a sitting position *to increase intraabdominal space.*
- Remove constrictive clothing *to relieve pressure.*
- Change the patient's position frequently *to relieve pressure and enhance comfort.*
- Give small, frequent feedings *to avoid distention.*
- Auscultate for abdominal bowel sounds *to assess gastric motility.*
- Monitor for physical dependency on analgesics.

Altered cardiopulmonary tissue perfusion related to dysrhythmias and occlusion of pulmonary circulation

- Encourage the patient to rest and avoid strenuous activity *to decrease cardiac workload.*
- Advise the patient to avoid oral stimulants, such as smoking, *to avoid vasoconstriction.*
- Auscultate apical pulse *to detect dysrhythmias.*
- Monitor blood pressure *to assess peripheral circulation.*
- Monitor blood studies, especially of enzyme and electrolyte levels, *to evaluate cardiac status and tissue perfusion.*

- Monitor respiratory status *to detect respiratory distress early.*
- Auscultate for breath sounds, rate, rhythm, *to assess cardiopulmonary status.*
- Monitor blood pressure and pulse *to assess cardiovascular function.*
- Monitor blood studies for gas exchange *to determine pulmonary function.*
- Observe for headache, nausea, confusion, dyspnea, cyanosis, *as signs of decreased tissue perfusion.*

Altered cerebral tissue perfusion (potential) related to increased intracranial pressure

- Place the patient on complete bed rest with the head elevated *to reduce energy expenditure.*
- Decrease environmental stimuli *to promote rest.*
- Change the patient's position slowly *to avoid trauma or excessive energy use.*
- Discourage oral stimulants, such as smoking, *to avoid increasing vasoconstriction.*
- Monitor neurologic signs, such as level of consciousness, pupillary response, and reflexes, *to detect changes in status.*
- Observe for changes in pulse, blood pressure, and behavior *to detect changes in status.*

Altered renal tissue perfusion related to cell sickling

- Inspect for edema *as sign of impaired renal function.*
- Measure body weight and intake and output *to assess renal status.*
- Monitor blood studies for abnormal electrolytes, hematology, and renal function.
- Monitor urine studies *for indications of renal function failure.*
- Monitor temperature and blood pressure *for signs of infection or fluid retention.*
- Observe urine for abnormal color, content, and odor *for signs of infection or bleeding.*
- Test urine for protein; *its presence in the urine is a sign of renal failure.*
- Maintain adequate fluid intake (oral, intravenous) *to maintain fluid balance and enhance renal perfusion.*

Patient Education/Home Care Planning

1. Alert the patient to the need for family testing to determine the presence of Hb S; genetic counseling is available for carriers.
2. Explain how to avoid sickle cell crises: avoid high altitudes, flying in unpressurized planes, dehydration, cold temperatures, iced liquids, and vigorous exercise; use stress-reduction methods.
3. Explain to the patient that young pregnant women have a high risk for developing pulmonary and/or renal complications.

4. Practice range of motion exercises and encourage regular physical activity to prevent bone demineralization. Explain the need for balance between rest (physical and mental) and activity, such as range of motion and isometric exercises.

5. Discuss principles of good nutrition, such as the importance of protein, calcium, vitamins, and adequate fluids; the patient should not have oral stimulants, such as cigarettes.

6. Alert the patient to the signs and symptoms of increased intracranial pressure, to the need to blow the nose gently, to avoid coughing, and to avoid straining on elimination.

7. Demonstrate to the patient how to monitor his or her oral intake, urinary output, and urine protein.

8. Advise the patient to avoid trauma and extremes in temperature; patients should not smoke and should protect extremities from injury because of impaired circulation.

Evaluation

Tissue perfusion is adequate   The skin, nails, lips, and ear lobes are warm and moist and have a natural color. Vital signs, blood gas values, hemoglobin level, and hematocrit are within normal limits. Electrocardiogram shows a normal tracing.

Activity and exercise are adequate   Patient changes position and body movement frequently (walking, sitting, and standing). Patient participates in daily physical exercise, such as walking, and in range of motion and isometric exercises; patient avoids strenuous exercise. Patient carries out activities of daily living.

Patient has physical appearance of comfort   Posture is normal. Patient has freedom of body movement and expresses comfort. Patient does not complain of pain.

The patient's energy and vitality levels are good   Patient is mentally alert and has good concentration and attentiveness. Malaise, fatigue, and weakness are absent.

Waste elimination is adequate   Daily fluid output is equal to fluid intake. Blood urea nitrogen and serum creatinine levels are within normal limits. Results of urine protein test are negative. Results of urine specific gravity, creatinine level, and creatinine clearance studies are within normal limits.

Skin and mucous membranes are intact   Patient does not complain of itching.

■ THALASSEMIAS

Thalassemias, another group of chronic hemolytic anemias, are caused by an insufficient number of hemoglobin polypeptide chains, which are necessary for production of hemoglobin.

•••••• Pathophysiology

The thalassemias are inherited disorders most frequently affecting people of Mediterranean or Southern Chinese ancestry, as well as American blacks and individuals from Southern Asia

and Central Africa. Thalassemia major and intermedia, the more serious anemias, appear in homozygotes; thalassemia minor is milder and appears in heterozygotes. The deficiency in hemoglobin polypeptide chains results in extremely thin, fragile erythrocytes called "target cells." People with thalassemia major do not reach adulthood, whereas those with the intermedia or minor disorder respond to supportive care. Persons with these disorders may develop a mongoloid appearance and cranial bone hyperplasia and may experience delayed puberty.

•••••• Diagnostic Studies and Findings

Blood smear   Target cells and other strangely shaped erythrocytes observed; pale, nucleated red blood cells (RBCs)

Red blood cell count   Decreased

Serum bilirubin   Greatly elevated

Fecal and urinary urobilinogen   Greatly elevated

Fetal hemoglobin (Hb F) via electrophoresis   Elevated; may be as high as 90%

Hemoglobin A (Hb A) via electrophoresis   Elevated

•••••• Multidisciplinary Plan

The plan of care is supportive, such as transfusions of packed red cells on a monthly, bimonthly, and/or "as needed" basis. Splenectomy is necessary if transfused cells are rapidly destroyed by the spleen.

Chelating agents such as diethylenetriamine pentaacetic acid (DTPA) may be used if iron overload results from multiple transfusions.

NURSING CARE

Nursing Assessment

Integrity of Skin

Jaundice

Leg ulcers

Pallor

Gastrointestinal Function

Enlarged spleen and liver

Intolerance of fatty foods and abdominal discomfort

Cardiovascular Function

Dysrhythmia

Heart failure

Bleeding tendency

Nursing Dx & Intervention

Risk for impaired skin integrity related to peripheral hypoxia

- Assess skin color, tone, temperature, and moisture.
- Provide skin care, using cool water and lubrication, *to promote hygiene and moisture.*
- Place the patient on bed rest *to rest the affected part(s).*

- Elevate the affected part *to enhance peripheral circulation.*
- Implement cleaning procedure, such as with hydrogen peroxide or saline solution, *to remove drainage and necrotic tissue.*
- Apply sterile dressing or expose affected area to air *to promote healing.*
- Apply heat with lamp or cradle *to promote healing.*
- Observe the patient's response to therapy *to evaluate its effectiveness.*
- Advise patient not to scratch skin *to avoid injury.*

Altered nutrition: less than body requirements, related to enlarged liver and spleen and altered metabolism

- Help patient into semi-Fowler's or Fowler's position for eating *to lessen abdominal pressure.*
- Provide low-fat, high-calorie diet.
- Offer antiflatulence medication.
- Assist patient with oral hygiene and washing face and hands before eating.
- Remove constrictive clothing *to relieve pressure.*
- Change the patient's position frequently *to relieve pressure and enhance comfort.*
- Give small, frequent feedings *to avoid distention.*
- Auscultate for abnormal bowel sounds *to assess gastric motility.*

Altered cardiopulmonary tissue perfusion related to dysrhythmia and bleeding tendency

- Encourage patient to rest and avoid strenuous activity *to reduce cardiac workload.*
- Avoid oral stimulants, such as smoking, oral tobacco, or coffee *to prevent vasoconstriction.*
- Auscultate apical pulse *to assess cardiac function.*
- Monitor blood pressure and respirations *to assess peripheral blood flow and pulmonary function.*
- Monitor blood studies (i.e., enzymes, electrolytes, and gas exchange) and electrocardiogram *to determine cardiac status.*

Patient Education/Home Care Planning

1. Assist the patient to maintain skin cleanliness and integrity and to minimize potential damage from jaundice or stasis ulcer.
2. Discuss the value of a diet low in fat and high in calories.
3. Explain to the patient the need to avoid trauma, extremes in temperature, and smoking to protect the extremities from injury caused by impaired circulation.
4. Advise the patient to seek genetic counseling.

Evaluation

Color of the skin and mucous membranes is good The skin, nails, lips, and ear lobes are warm and moist and have a natural color. Skin is intact. No complaints of itching.

Patient's nutrition is adequate Patient eats a balanced diet, avoiding foods high in fat. No complaints of abdominal discomfort.

The patient's cardiovascular function is normal Vital signs are within normal limits. No evidence of bleeding is present.

■ POLYCYTHEMIAS

Polycythemia is a term used to describe an increase in the number of circulating erythrocytes and the concentration of hemoglobin in the blood.

•••••• Pathophysiology

The three forms of polycythemia are:

Polycythemia vera, a myeloproliferative disorder ("overgrowth of bone marrow"), which usually develops in middle age, particularly among Jewish men; the cause is unknown, but the overproduction of erythrocytes and thrombocytes results in increased blood viscosity, blood volume, and congestion of tissues and organs with blood

Secondary polycythemia, a compensatory response to tissue hypoxia in the presence of chronic obstructive lung disease, congenital heart disease, and prolonged exposure to high altitudes (10,000 feet or more)

Relative polycythemia, which is a relative increase in erythrocyte concentration in the presence of plasma loss caused by fluid loss and dehydration; specific causes may include insufficient fluid intake, diarrhea, vomiting, burns, or excessive diuretics

•••••• Diagnostic Studies and Findings

Erythrocyte count   As high as 8 million to 12 million/mm^3
Mean corpuscular hemoglobin concentration (MCHC) Decreased
Leukocytes   Increase in polycythemia vera
Thrombocytes   Increase in polycythemia vera

•••••• Multidisciplinary Plan

Medications

Antineoplastic agents (to suppress bone marrow function)
Busulfan (Myleran), 4 to 8 mg/d po
Chlorambucil (Leukeran), 4 to 10 mg/d po
Radioactive phosphorus P32 (Phosphotope), 6 μCi po; 3 to 5 μg IV
Mechlorethamine (Nitrogen mustard), 200 to 600 μg/kg IV in a single or divided dose

General Management

Venesection (phlebotomy) with emergency removal of 500 to 2000 ml of blood until hematocrit reaches 45%, then 500 ml every 2 to 3 months to reduce circulatory overload
Activity and ambulation to prevent circulatory stasis
Pheresis therapy

NURSING CARE

Nursing Assessment

Cardiovascular Function

Ruddy complexion

Dusky redness of mucosa

Hypertension with dizziness, headache, and sense of fullness in head

Congestive heart failure (e.g., shortness of breath and orthopnea)

Thrombus formation, leading to cerebrovascular accident, myocardial infarction, or gangrene of the feet

Signs and symptoms of bleeding and hemorrhage in gastrointestinal tract, oropharynx, or brain

Gastrointestinal Function

Enlargement of liver and spleen

Signs and symptoms of peptic ulcer

Skeletal Integrity

Signs and symptoms of secondary gout

Nursing Dx & Intervention

Altered cardiopulmonary tissue perfusion related to increased arterial pressure

- Encourage rest and quiet *to decrease cardiac workload.*
- Discourage oral stimulants, such as smoking, *to prevent vasoconstriction.*
- Avoid emotional situations, *which tend to increase systemic blood pressure.*
- Administer medication as ordered *to promote vasodilation, diuresis, or both.*
- Monitor blood pressure *to assess effectiveness of therapy.*
- Avoid sodium-rich foods *to reduce fluid retention.*

Altered cardiopulmonary tissue perfusion related to inadequate pulmonary ventilation

- Change the patient's position frequently; sitting is considered best *to enhance lung expansion.*
- Encourage coughing and deep breathing *to promote removal of secretions.*
- Ambulate as soon as possible *to enhance cardiopulmonary function.*
- Observe respiratory rate and ausculate breath sounds, among others, *to assess pulmonary function.*
- Monitor for cyanosis *as a sign of pulmonary decompensation.*
- Assess breath sounds.

Ineffective breathing pattern related to thrombus formation in lungs

- Encourage patient to perform range of motion and isometric exercises *to promote circulation.*

- Administer anticoagulants as ordered *to reduce incidence of clotting.*
- Observe for chest pain; dyspnea; coughing; hemoptysis; changes in pulse, respirations, blood pressure, pupillary response, reflexes, and level of consciousness, *which are signs of a pulmonary or cerebral embolism.*

Altered peripheral tissue perfusion related to bleeding

- Place patient on complete bed rest in a low Fowler's position *for patient comfort and decreased energy use.*
- Monitor level of consciousness and pupillary response.
- Observe for bleeding from gastrointestinal tract and oropharynx.
- Maintain warm environment with room temperature and clothing *to avoid vasoconstriction.*
- Initiate range of motion exercises *to enhance circulation.*
- Avoid applying heat or cold, tight clothing, and pressure under the knee, *which can impair circulation.*
- Inspect extremities for adequate circulation *to assess need for further intervention.*
- Monitor blood studies for hematology and gas exchange *as indicators of pulmonary status.*
- Monitor peripheral pulses.

Pain related to abdominal distention and ulceration

- Ausculate for abnormal bowel sounds *to assess gastric motility.*
- Monitor feces *for evidence of bleeding.*
- Assess patient complaints of abdominal pain.
- Intervene if pain is present: elevate head of bed, apply heat, offer analgesics as prescribed, and provide antacids at bedside.
- Place the patient in a sitting position *to promote comfort and increase intraabdominal space.*
- Remove constrictive clothing *to relieve pressure.*
- Change the patient's position frequently *to relieve pressure and enhance comfort.*
- Give small, frequent feedings *to avoid distention.*
- Observe for evidence of favorable response to therapy *to determine need for same or modified intervention.*
- Discourage smoking *to avoid vasoconstriction.*
- Decrease acidic and gas-forming foods *to avoid distention and flatus.*
- Give bland foods, carbonated beverage, and antacids *to relieve gastric distress.*

Impaired physical mobility related to inflammation of the joints

- Prescribe bed rest and joint rest *to reduce inflammation and irritation.*
- Administer medications as ordered, such as analgesics and antigout drugs, *to promote comfort.*
- Provide soft diet *to reduce necessity of chewing.*
- Provide compresses according to patient's tolerance *to reduce swelling and pain.*

Patient Education/Home Care Planning

1. Encourage the patient to protect extremities from injury, such as heat, cold, or pressure.
2. Assist the patient to do range of motion and isometric exercises safely and correctly.
3. Advise the patient to avoid trauma and protect body parts, to use safety precautions, and to use a soft toothbrush.
4. Encourage the patient to handle stress in a healthy way and to balance rest with exercise.
5. Advise the patient of the need to stop smoking and to avoid other oral stimulants.
6. Advise the patient of the need for dietary modification, that is, to use low-sodium, low-acid, and low–gas-forming foods, foods high in alkaline, and foods low in purines.
7. Discuss with the patient the signs and symptoms of bleeding and thrombus formation, as well as interventions and the need to report findings.

Evaluation

Vital signs are within normal limits Respirations, blood pressure, and temperature are within normal limits.

Color of the skin and mucous membranes is good The skin, nails, lips, and ear lobes are warm and moist and have a natural color. There is no evidence of bleeding.

Patient has physical appearance of comfort Patient is calm, contented, and relaxed. Posture is normal, and patient has freedom of body movement.

Patient frequently changes position and body movement Patient walks, sits, stands, and performs range of motion and mild exercises.

Patient reports well-balanced diet No complaints of distention, bowel irregularities, or abdominal pain.

LEUKOCYTIC DISORDERS

■ AGRANULOCYTOSIS

Agranulocytosis, also referred to as granulocytopenia or malignant neutropenia, is an acute, potentially fatal blood disorder characterized by (1) agranulocytic angina, a severe, painful, ulcerative infection of the oral mucosa and throat, with symptoms of high fever and severe weakness and (2) severe neutropenia.

Agranulocytosis is a worldwide disorder that affects women more often than men. The onset is usually rapid, and prompt treatment is required. The condition may develop slowly based on drug dosage and duration of effect, such as in response to cancer chemotherapy.

•••••• Pathophysiology

Agranulocytosis is most frequently caused by drug toxicity or hypersensitivity from large-dose, long-duration drugs such as nitrogen mustard, radiation, and benzenes and drugs that produce individual sensitivity such as certain tranquilizers (chlorpromazine HCl [Thorazine]), antithyroid agents (propylthiouracil), anticonvulsants (phenytoin), and antibiotics (chloramphenicol). It may also develop during the course of diseases such as tuberculosis, uremia, aplastic anemia, multiple myeloma, and overwhelming infection.

•••••• Diagnostic Studies and Findings

Leukocyte count Leukopenia (500 to 3000 WBCs/mm^3 with extremely low polymorphonuclear [PMN] cell count of 0% to 2%)

Bone marrow biopsy Absence of PMN leukocytes; maturational arrest of young developing cells

Cultures of urine and blood; ulcerative lesions in throat and mouth Positive for bacteria

•••••• Multidisciplinary Plan

Medications

Agent-specific antiinfective agent (to treat infection)

General Management

Monitoring of patient's blood cell count to evaluate status
Observation for infection to initiate therapy
Reverse isolation to reduce exposure to pathogens
Bed rest and high-protein, high-vitamin, high-calorie diet to conserve energy and enhance resistance to infection
Granulocyte transfusions to replace deficient cells
Colony-stimulating factors to boost immune system

NURSING CARE

Nursing Assessment

Energy Level

Severe fatigue and weakness
High fever, severe chills, tachycardia, and prostration
Weak, rapid pulse

Gastrointestinal Function

Sore throat, ulcerative lesions of pharyngeal and buccal mucosa, and dysphagia

Nursing Dx & Intervention

Activity intolerance related to effects of infection on metabolism and cardiopulmonary function

- Anticipate the patient's needs *to avoid excess energy expenditure.*
- Encourage rest and adequate activity *to maintain energy level.*

- Place objects within reach while patient is on bed rest *to decrease need for getting out of bed.*
- Observe for increasing weakness and dyspnea *to assess need for further intervention, such as oxygen therapy.*
- Assess pulse and respirations *to monitor cardiopulmonary function.*

Risk for infection related to decreased antibodies

- Place the patient on bed rest *to conserve energy.*
- Enforce reverse isolation *to protect patient from pathogens.*
- Provide high-protein, high-vitamin, high-calorie diet *to maintain nutritional status.*
- Encourage patient to take fluids *to promote hydration.*
- Monitor heart rate, respirations, blood pressure, and temperature *to assess for signs of infection.*
- Observe for restlessness and irritability *as possible signs of infection.*
- Observe the patient for extreme fatigue, sore throat or mouth, and fever *as signs of infection.*
- Observe white blood cell count *because a marked increase indicates infection.*
- Use cooling measures (alcohol rub and tepid baths) *to reduce fever if present.*
- Administer antibiotics as ordered *to combat specific pathogens.*
- Use enemas and stool softeners as needed *to prevent intestinal stasis as site for infection.*
- Provide perineal care *to maintain hygiene and prevent infection.*

Altered oral mucous membrane related to ulceration

- Give frequent mouth care; irrigate every 1 to 2 hours *for hygiene and patient comfort.*
- Apply ice collar to reduce pharyngeal swelling.
- Offer anesthetic lozenges, analgesics, and sedatives as ordered *to provide comfort.*
- Offer soft, bland foods and protein concentrates *to reduce buccal irritation and increase ease of swallowing.*

Patient Education/Home Care Planning

1. Discuss with the patient the use of frequent, thorough oral hygiene to treat or prevent mouth and pharyngeal infection.
2. Explain the need for a diet high in protein, vitamins, and calories with soft, bland foods.
3. Discuss the need to avoid self-medication because of the danger of hypersensitivity.
4. Encourage a balance between rest and activity to prevent fatigue and generalized weakness.
5. Explain the need to avoid crowds, people with infectious diseases, and cold or hot environments; also teach signs and symptoms of infection and appropriate interventions.

Evaluation

The patient's vitality is maintained Malaise, fatigue, and weakness are absent. Patient performs activities of daily living.

Patient consumes daily intake of essential food groups Patient consumes diet high in protein, vitamins, and calories and eats soft, bland foods as needed; patient drinks adequate fluids. Patient's mouth is clean and free of ulceration.

Patient's body functions are normal Vital signs are within normal limits.

LEUKEMIA

Leukemia ("white blood") is a usually fatal cancer that involves the blood-forming tissues of the bone marrow, spleen, and lymph nodes. It is characterized by the neoplastic proliferation of leukocytes and their precursors.

Leukemia represents about 3% of cancers detected each year and causes about 4% of cancer deaths, or about 16,000 people annually. Although survival rates have improved since the 1950s, mortality is still high, especially for those with acute leukemias, that is, acute lymphocytic leukemia (ALL), which is responsible for half of all cancer deaths among children.

Although leukemia is considered a disease that strikes children, most cases occur in adults over 55 years of age, except in blacks, whose median age for leukemia ranges from 35 to 54 years. Men develop leukemia slightly more often than do women.

For reasons as yet unknown, the incidence of leukemia is rising. However, several factors have been implicated: chronic, repeated exposure to relatively small doses of radiation; use of chloramphenicol; exposure to certain chemicals, such as benzene; presence of primary immune deficiency diseases; possible viral etiologic factors; and a genetic predisposition, such as among siblings or in children with Down syndrome.

•••••• Pathophysiology

Leukemia's major effects on the body are proliferation of large numbers of abnormal, immature leukocytes, accumulation of these cells within the lymph nodes, and eventual infiltration of these cells into tissues all over the body. All organs are eventually involved in the leukemic process.

Leukemias are classified according to the following criteria: *Type of cell and tissue involved:* The major types of cells are lymphocytes (lymphocytic leukemia: acute and chronic) and granulocytes (myelocytic: acute and chronic; monocytic: acute and chronic). The acute leukemias are sometimes classified as lymphoblastic, myeloblastic, or monoblastic because of the prevalence of immature cell forms. Lymphocytic leukemia causes hyperplasia of the lymphoid tissue, whereas myelocytic leukemia causes hyperplasia of the bone marrow and spleen. Ninety percent of all leukemias are lymphocytic.

Course and duration of disease: Acute forms have a rapid onset, with progression to death within days or months. The large numbers of leukocytes produced are immature and rapidly cause organ malfunction. Chronic forms have a gradual onset and a slower course. The cells are more mature and function more effectively. Acute leukemia occurs more frequently in children, whereas chronic leukemia is more prevalent in people 25 to 60 years of age.

Number of leukocytes in blood and bone marrow: If the patient has a normal or lower than normal leukocyte count, the disease is called aleukemic or subleukemic leukemia.

Acute leukemia has its peak incidence in children who are 1 to 5 years of age. There is usually a prodromal period when the child experiences fatigue, headache, sore throat, night sweats, and shortness of breath. These symptoms are followed by severe tonsillitis, ulcerations in the mouth, bleeding from the gums and rectum, bleeding into the skin, and joint and bone pain. The lymph nodes, liver, and spleen enlarge, and severe anemia develops. The patient dies from overwhelming infection or severe hemorrhaging. With treatment the patient may survive 5 years or longer.

Chronic myelocytic leukemia, which is usually found in people 25 to 40 years of age, is characterized by a massive spleen, enlarged liver, and severe pain in the long bones. The onset is usually insidious, with the patient complaining for months or years of weight loss and weakness. Initial signs of disease may be a heavy sensation in the abdomen, a sense of extreme abdominal distention after meals, sternal tenderness, and mild enlargement of the lymph nodes.

Chronic lymphocytic leukemia is found most often in people 50 to 70 years of age, many of whom do not have symptoms for years. Early signs and symptoms are chronic exhaustion, anorexia, swollen lymph nodes, and a slightly enlarged liver and spleen. Anemia, fever, increased susceptibility to infections, and mild bleeding tendencies occur as the disease progresses. Visual disturbances, skin lesions, deafness, otitis media, or Ménière's syndrome may develop. Pain and paralysis result from lymph node pressure on the nerves. Respiratory symptoms result from enlargement of the mediastinal lymph nodes. Late complications include hemolytic anemia and hypogammaglobulinemia.

• • • • • • Diagnostic Studies and Findings

During its early stages, leukemia may be accidentally found during a routine physical examination that includes blood work.

Leukocyte count Elevated (15,000 to 500,000/mm³ or higher); "shift to the left" (presence of large numbers of immature neutrophils); one type of white blood cell predominates

Bone marrow biopsy Massive number of white blood cells in blast phase

Blood smear Numerous blast cells

Red blood cells, hemoglobin and hematocrit Decreased

Platelets Decreased

Tumor markers Present or absent based on type of leukemia

• • • • • • Multidisciplinary Plan

The goal of treatment is to stop the proliferation and infiltration of abnormal and immature leukocytes and to obtain as long a remission as possible.

Medications

Dosages are based on body surface area; the following are examples of drugs in use

Acute lymphoblastic leukemia

    Antineoplastic agents

        Methotrexate (Amethopterin, Mexate)

        Mercaptopurine (Purinethol, 6-MP)

        Cyclophosphamide (Cytoxan)

        Vincristine sulfate (Oncovin, VCR)

        Asparaginase (Elspar, L-asparagine)

        Daunorubicin (Daunomycin, DNR)

        Cytosine arabinoside (Cytosar-U, Ara-C)

    Corticosteroids

        Prednisone (Meticorten)

Acute myeloblastic leukemia

    Antineoplastic agents

        Cytosine arabinoside (Ara-C)

        Thioguanine (6-TG)

        Daunorubicin

        Prednisone

        Vincristine

        Doxorubicin

Chronic lymphocytic leukemia

    Corticosteroids

        Prednisone (Deltasone, Meticorten)

    Antineoplastic agents

        Chlorambucil (Leukeran)

        Cyclophosphamide (Cytoxan)

        Vincristine

        Doxorubicin

Chronic myelocytic leukemia

    Antineoplastic agents

        Busulfan (Myleran)

        Hydroxyurea (Hydrea)

        Cytosine arabinoside (Ara-C)

General Management

Radiation therapy for the entire body or focused on liver and spleen to suppress bone marrow and reduce organ size

Bone marrow transplant or peripheral blood stem cell transplantation to provide healthy tissue

Transfusions (whole blood, platelets); reverse isolation techniques; antibiotics to treat bleeding and infection

Parenteral fluids to maintain hydration

Medications such as analgesics and hypnotics to relieve patient's discomfort, fear, and pain

Colony-stimulating factors such as G-CSF and GM-CSF may be ordered to be given subcutaneously or intravenously

NURSING CARE

Nursing Assessment

Susceptibility to Infection

Ulcerations of mouth and throat
Signs and symptoms of pneumonia
Signs and symptoms of septicemia
Recurrent infections

Susceptibility to Bleeding

Gum bleeding, ecchymoses, petechiae, and retinal hemorrhages
Epistaxis

Renal Function

Pain in area of kidneys
Decreased urinary output

Cardiac Function

Tachycardia
Palpitations
Fatigue, weakness, and pallor
Shortness of breath

Sensory and Motor Function

Headache and disorientation
Hemiplegia, aphasia, and other deficits caused by cerebral vascular accident
Lethargy
Convusions (late)

Comfort

Bone and joint pain
Abdominal pain

Gastrointestinal Function

Anorexia, nausea, and vomiting
Weight loss

Nursing Dx & Intervention

Risk for infection related to inadequate numbers and immature leukocytes

- Place patient in reverse isolation (may use laminar air flow environment) *to protect from pathogens.*
- Encourage rest and limited activity *to prevent fatigue.*
- Maintain warm, clean environment *to avoid chilling and exposure to pathogens.*
- Encourage increased intake of foods high in protein and fluids *to enhance antibodies and prevent dehydration.*

- Teach patient and family proper handwashing, and screen visitors with infections *to prevent exposure to pathogens.*
- Maintain oral hygiene *to avoid infection.*
- Monitor vital signs: temperature, pulse, respirations, and blood pressure because *changes may signal infection.*
- Observe the patient for restlessness, temperature elevation, sore throat, "sniffles," chills, skin lesions, and *other signs of infection.*
- Check blood studies *for evidence of specific pathogens.*
- Administer antibiotics as ordered *to treat infection.*
- Use cool sponge baths, alcohol rubs, and antipyretic drugs as needed *to reduce fever.*
- Administer granulocyte transfusions as ordered *to replace defective WBC and to fight infection.*
- Administer γ-globulin as ordered (for chronic lymphocytic leukemia) *to provide protein for antibody formation.*
- Administer colony stimulating factors G-CSF (granulocyte-colony stimulating factor) or GM-CSF (granulocyte-macrophage colony stimulating factor) SC or IV as ordered *to stimulate formation of granulocytes/macrophages, increase level of circulating neutrophils, and improve neutrophil function in order to fight infection.*

Altered peripheral tissue perfusion related to decreased platelets and bleeding

- Handle patient carefully *to avoid injury and possible bleeding.*
- Avoid use of injections, constrictive clothing, or other agents *that impair circulation or cause trauma.*
- Protect the patient from falls and other injuries *to avoid bleeding.*
- Apply pressure over an injection site *to prevent extravasation.*
- Prevent constipation; use stool softener, fiber in diet, and fluids *to avoid anal trauma.*
- Assess pulse, respirations, blood pressure, level of consciousness, skin color, and so on *to detect signs of internal bleeding.*
- Observe the skin for petechiae and ecchymosis *as signs of bleeding.*
- Observe for signs of bleeding from mouth, nose, and rectum *to assess need for intervention.*
- Monitor blood studies *to detect decreased hematocrit, hemoglobin, and platelets, which indicate actual or potential bleeding.*
- Administer transfusions as ordered, such as whole blood and platelets *to replace loss and enhance clotting.*

Altered patterns of urinary elimination (potential) related to inadequate perfusion

- Ambulate patient as tolerated *to enhance circulation and elimination.*
- Change patient's position frequently *to enhance circulation.*
- Encourage patient to take fluids such as carbonated beverages and urine-alkalinizing juices *to maintain normal pH and prevent crystallization.*

- Inspect for bleeding and flank pain *as signs of possible obstruction.*
- Test pH of urine *to assess effectiveness of fluids and medication.*
- Administer allopurinol as ordered *to inhibit uric acid biosynthesis.*
- Observe urine studies *to assess renal function.*
- Observe blood studies *to detect elevated levels of minerals.*

Altered cardiopulmonary tissue perfusion related to blood loss and side effects of chemotherapy

- Encourage alternate rest and activity as tolerated *to reduce cardiopulmonary workload.*
- Count pulse and respirations and auscultate breath sounds and blood pressure *to monitor function.*
- Observe for signs of fatigue, restlessness, and dyspnea *as indications of inadequate tissue perfusion.*

Altered cerebral tissue perfusion related to diffusion of leukocytes into central nervous system

- Place the patient on bed rest in a quiet, dim environment *to reduce stimulation.*
- Provide safety (e.g., side rails up) *to protect patient from injury.*
- Provide emergency equipment, such as padded tongue blade, *in case of convulsion.*
- Observe for increased intracranial pressure; monitor vital signs, pupillary response, level of consciousness, reflexes, and orientation *to assess need for intervention.*
- Observe the characteristics of the convulsion if it occurs *to aid in diagnosis of irritation site.*
- Assess range of motion, strength, and communication abilities *to detect cardiovascular accident.*

Pain related to infusion of leukocytes into joints, bones, liver, spleen, and lymph nodes; and to use of colony stimulating factors

- Position patient comfortably in semi-Fowler's position *to decrease abdominal pressure.*
- Remove constrictive clothing *to relieve pressure.*
- Handle gently *to avoid irritation or injury.*
- Discuss possible pain and ways to relieve it with patient *to individualize intervention.*
- Administer analgesics as prescribed and per the patient's request *to control discomfort.*
- Observe effectiveness of pain relief measures *to determine need for further or different interventions.*

Altered nutrition: less than body requirements related to increased metabolic rate and anorexia

- Provide balanced diet, with emphasis on protein, vitamins, and calories, *to restore nutritional balance.*
- Monitor caloric intake *to ensure sufficient intake.*
- Give small, frequent feedings; snacks should be soft, bland, and cold *to enhance appetite and prevent distention.*

- Encourage patient to make specific food requests *to increase intake.*
- Balance rest with exercise *to stimulate appetite.*
- Discourage smoking and oral stimulants *that may alter taste or appetite.*
- Measure body weight *to monitor nutritional status.*
- Use oral anesthetic or antiemetic before eating *to decrease buccal irritation and nausea.*
- Encourage patient to take fluids *to maintain hydration.*
- Provide oral hygiene *to maintain patient comfort.*

Patient Education/Home Care Planning

1. Advise the patient to avoid situations in which he or she is likely to contract infection, such as inclement weather or crowds.
2. Plan with the patient a well-balanced diet especially high in protein, fiber, and fluids.
3. Instruct the patient to observe for and report signs and symptoms of infection, bleeding, and anemia.
4. Encourage the patient to take antibiotics as prescribed.
5. Discuss ways to avoid tissue damage (e.g., use soft toothbrush, blow nose gently, and avoid constipation).
6. Encourage the patient to drink large volumes of fluid, especially carbonated beverages and urine-alkalizing juices.
7. Discuss nonaddictive pain relief measures; pain will increase with progression of the disease and is likely to increase in amount, intensity, types, and locations.
8. Encourage the patient to avoid smoking and oral stimulants to stimulate appetite and maintain tissue perfusion and to deal with stress and fear in constructive, healthful ways.
9. Be sure that the patient is aware of support resources available: financial, treatment related, and psychosocial.

Evaluation

Patient's body functions are normal Vital signs are within acceptable limits. Elimination is adequate, and healing is prompt. Daily weight is stabilized at normal level for body build.

Infection is absent There is no evidence of inflammation, purulent drainage or secretions, or pain or aching. Oral temperature is 37° C (98.6° F), and blood leukocyte count is 5000 to 10,000/mm³. There are no red blood cells, white blood cells or hemoglobin casts in urine. Results of the bacterial culture of γ-globulin are negative: 20% or 0.7 to 1.6 g/dl.

Color of skin and mucous membranes is normal Skin, nails, lips, and ear lobes are warm and moist and have a natural color.

Patient prevents accidents, physical injury, deformity, infection, and hypersensitivity response There is no evidence of physical injury or that accidents have occurred. There is no evidence of deformity resulting from treatment.

Patient maintains vitality   Patient is mentally alert, has good concentration and attentiveness, and experiences less malaise, fatigue, or weakness.

Patient has physical appearance of comfort   Patient is calm and contented and has relaxed facial expression. Posture is normal, and patient has freedom of body movement. Patient expresses comfort and uses pain control methods effectively.

Daily intake includes essential food groups   Protein, vitamins, and calories are emphasized.

Patient has normal pattern of urinary elimination

■ MULTIPLE MYELOMA

Multiple myeloma, a neoplastic disease, strikes men over the age of 40 years twice as often as it does women.

•••••• Pathophysiology

Multiple myeloma used to be a relatively rare disorder, but the incidence is increasing. The characteristics of the disease are an abnormal malignant growth of plasma cells; development of single or multiple abnormal plasma cell tumors within the bone marrow; destruction of bone throughout the body; and later dissemination of the disease into the lymph nodes, liver, spleen, and kidneys.

The onset of the disease is usually gradual and often insidious. Many patients experience a presymptomatic period for 5 to 20 years, during which some people experience recurrent bacterial infections, especially pneumonia. This increased susceptibility to infection is believed to be related to disturbed antibody formation caused by plasma cell abnormalities.

Symptoms usually involve the skeletal system, especially the pelvis, spine, and ribs, and produce backache or bone pain that worsens with movement. Some patients sustain a pathologic fracture that causes severe pain. As skeletal destruction increases, the deformities in the sternum and rib cage may develop, with some people losing stature (5 or more inches). Diffuse osteoporosis with a negative calcium balance is also present. As the diseased bones become demineralized, renal stones develop, especially if the patient is on bed rest.

In addition, impaired production of erythrocytes, leukocytes, and thrombocytes occurs, with resultant anemia, bleeding tendencies, and increased danger of infection.

Complications may also be neurologic, such as spinal cord compression and/or renal dysfunction caused by convoluted tubules' blockage by coagulated protein particles.

•••••• Diagnostic Studies and Findings

Roentgenograms and scanning   Diffuse bone lesions, demineralization, and osteoporosis

Bone marrow biopsy   Large numbers of immature plasma cells (30% to 95% of cell population)

Blood studies   High concentration of serum globulin, particularly m-type globulin called Bence Jones protein; decreased hemoglobin and red blood cells; increased sedimentation rate; increased calcium level; increased total protein; elevated serum uric acid and creatinine

•••••• Multidisciplinary Plan

Medications

Antineoplastic agents (to suppress bone marrow function)
  Melphalan (Alkeran; L-PAM), 6 mg po for 2 to 3 wk; maintenance 2 mg/d
  Cyclophosphamide (Cytoxan), 40 to 50 mg/kg IV in divided doses over several d, then adjusted to lower maintenance dosage
  Corticosteroids

General Management

Reduction of tumor mass by radiation to relieve pressure and pain

Control of pain to enhance patient's comfort

Promotion of adequate ambulation to maintain mobility

Treatment of complications: anemia, infection, hypercalcemia, and spinal cord compression to increase patient's comfort and longevity

Bone marrow transplantation

NURSING CARE

Nursing Assessment

Skeletal Integrity

Backache or bone pain that worsens with movement
Signs and symptoms of pathologic fractures

Sensory and Motor Function

Loss of sensory and motor function caused by spinal cord compression

Renal Function

Signs and symptoms of calculi (flank pain, renal colic)

Energy Level

Weakness, fatigue, dyspnea, bleeding, and infection

Fluid and Electrolytes

Lethargy, polyuria, polydipsia, and other symptoms related to hypercalcemia

Nursing Dx & Intervention

Pain related to bone fragility resulting from destruction

- Position the patient for comfort *to lessen pain.*
- Change the patient's position slowly *to prevent trauma.*
- Maintain the patient's body alignment *to prevent injury.*

- Apply heat *to reduce muscle spasm and swelling.*
- Massage gently *to reduce muscle spasm.*
- Use firm mattress *to support skeletal structure.*
- Encourage rest *to reduce stress on skeletal structure.*
- Work with patient on ways to reduce pain, including analgesics, *to intervene most effectively.*
- Assess for evidence of fracture *to detect and treat early.*

Impaired physical mobility related to musculoskeletal impairment

- Assist with ambulation *to prevent injury.*
- Mobilize as necessary using a walker, cane, or wheelchair *to prevent injury.*
- Provide range of motion exercises and assistance with turning *to maintain mobility.*
- Decrease environmental barriers, such as chairs, tables, or rugs, *to prevent injury.*
- Limit distance patient ambulates *to avoid fatigue and injury.*
- Observe patient's gait, coordination, and stability *to assess changes in musculoskeletal function.*
- Assess body alignment and complaints of pain *as signs of injury.*
- Provide trapeze *to assist with movement in bed.*
- Help patient turn in bed every 1 to 2 hours *to prevent pulmonary-circulatory stasis and to promote mobility.*
- Encourage increased protein and vitamin intake *to enhance mineralization and muscle tone.*

Impaired physical mobility (potential) related to spinal cord compression

- Maintain body alignment *to prevent injury to vertebrae.*
- Support the spine with brace or traction *to avoid injury.*
- Place the patient on bed rest as needed *to protect from falls.*
- Log roll the patient *to maintain alignment.*
- Observe respiratory rate and rhythm *to assess for cervical cord compression.*
- Assess motor function, sensation, and reflexes; report findings to physician if abnormalities occur *to detect early signs of compression.*

Altered patterns of urinary elimination (potential) related to calcium nephropathy, severe proteinuria, and hyperuricemia

- Provide adequate hydration of 3000 to 4000 ml of fluid per day *to prevent urinary stasis.*
- Maintain adequate urinary output *to prevent urinary stasis.*
- Ambulate the patient as much as possible *to enhance elimination.*
- Encourage a diet low in calcium and phosphorus *to prevent formation of calculi.*
- Give urine-acidifying juices *to maintain urinary pH.*
- Avoid bicarbonates and carbonated beverages *to maintain slightly acid urine.*

- Monitor output, frequency, and urgency; report findings to physician *to detect retention, inflammation, and infection.*

Fluid volume excess; potential fluid volume deficit related to renal calculi and failure

- Monitor intake and compare with output *to identify fluid deficit or excess.*

Activity intolerance related to weakness, fatigue, and dyspnea

- Place patient in sitting position *to enhance cardiopulmonary function.*
- Observe respiration rate and dyspnea *to assess respiratory status.*
- Observe skin color and temperature *to assess oxygenation and circulation.*
- Assist with care *to provide rest and reduce fatigue.*
- Plan rest periods *to control fatigue.*
- Monitor laboratory values *to detect inadequate cardiopulmonary function.*

Altered peripheral tissue perfusion (potential) related to bleeding

- Handle the patient gently *to avoid trauma.*
- Give injections only if necessary; apply pressure afterward *to prevent extravasation.*
- Observe for change in vital signs or for blood in urine, stool, gums, nose, or skin *because these are signs of internal bleeding.*
- Avoid constipation *to prevent anal irritation and bleeding.*

Risk for infection related to decreased leukocytes

- Maintain reverse isolation *to protect patient from pathogens.*
- Observe for increases in temperature, pulse, and respirations *to assess for infection.*
- Observe the patient for "sniffles," sore throat, anorexia, pain on urination, and so on *to assess for infection.*
- Administer antibiotics as ordered *to treat specific pathogens.*
- Help patient to turn, cough, and deep breathe *to maintain respiratory function.*
- Provide oral, skin, and perineal hygiene *to prevent development of irritation and infection.*

Altered nutrition: high risk for more than body requirements related to hypercalcemia

- Encourage a decrease in intake of foods with calcium, and encourage an increase in fluid intake *to correct imbalance.*
- Monitor blood studies *to determine effectiveness of interventions.*
- Observe for complaints of constipation, headache, nausea, thirst, weakness, bone pain, and fatigue; report findings to physician because *these are signs and symptoms of hypercalcemia.*

> ## Patient Education/Home Care Planning
>
> 1. Discuss the need for good body balance, good body mechanics, and mechanical support, such as a cane or brace.
> 2. Plan with patient methods of pain control: pain-reducing measures and medications.
> 3. Discuss the importance of drinking adequate fluids, controlling intake of high-calcium foods, and the need for a diet high in protein and vitamins.

Evaluation

There is no evidence of physical injury   There is no evidence of pathologic fractures.

Patient verbally expresses comfort   Patient expresses comfort and uses analgesics effectively.

Patient frequently changes position and body movement   Patient walks, sits, and stands using assistive devices as needed.

Patient has physical appearance of comfort   Patient is calm, contented, and has relaxed facial expression. Posture is normal, and patient has freedom of body movement. Patient relaxes muscles when resting and motionless.

Body hydration is normal   Skin turgor is good, mucous membranes are moist, and patient is not thirsty.

Daily fluid output is equal to fluid intake   Urine output is 1500 to 3000 ml. Patient's diet includes foods high in protein and vitamins.

Color of the skin and mucous membranes is good   The skin, nails, lips, and ear lobes are warm and moist and have a natural color.

Vital signs are within normal limits   Respirations, pulse, and blood pressure are within normal limits.

Infection is not present   There is no evidence of inflammation, pain, or aching.

Patient carries out activities of daily living without difficulty

Patient maintains adequate nutrition

THROMBOCYTIC DISORDERS

■ THROMBOCYTOPENIA

Thrombocytopenia is a term used to describe a platelet count below 100,000/mm³, which causes (1) spontaneous bleeding into the skin, mucous membranes, internal cavities, and organs, and (2) oozing of blood for long periods of time from lacerations and punctures.

•••••• Pathophysiology

The major types of thrombocytopenia are idiopathic thrombocytopenic purpura (ITP) and secondary thrombocytopenic purpura. In ITP platelets are prematurely destroyed (survival decreases from 8 to 20 days to 1 to 3 days). It is believed to be caused by an autoimmune process. The acute form is found mostly in children, whereas the chronic form is found among patients of all ages; it is more common among women. Secondary thrombocytopenic purpura results from diseases such as viral infections, bone marrow failure, infectious mononucleosis, and drug hypersensitivity.

•••••• Diagnostic Studies and Findings

Platelet count   <100,000/mm³
Bleeding time   Prolonged
Coagulation time   Normal
Capillary fragility   Increased

•••••• Multidisciplinary Plan

Surgery

Splenectomy

Medications

Corticosteroids
    Prednisone (Deltasone, Meticorten), 10 to 20 mg po qid

General Management

Platelet transfusions

NURSING CARE

Nursing Assessment

Vascular Integrity

Petechiae, ecchymosis, and easy bruising
Epistaxis
Bleeding from gums and nose

Female Reproductive Function

Heavy menses and bleeding between periods

Sensory and Motor Function

Signs and symptoms of increased intracranial pressure caused by cerebral hemorrhage
Nerve pain and anesthesia of extremities and/or paralysis

Gastrointestinal Tract

Hematemesis
Melena

Renal Function

Hematuria

Cardiac Function

Tachycardia

Respiratory Function

Dyspnea
Tachycardia

Nursing Dx & Intervention

Impaired skin integrity related to intradermal bleeding

- Apply ice bag and/or manual pressure over any bleeding site *to control bleeding.*
- Handle gently *to avoid trauma.*
- Avoid injections or use of straight razor, *which may cause bleeding.*
- Observe for petechiae, ecchymoses, or frank bleeding.
- Protect patient from injury by assisting with ambulation and avoiding environmental barriers.

Impaired tissue integrity (nasal mucous membrane) related to bleeding

- Observe amount, color, and consistency of discharge *to monitor blood loss.*
- Position the patient with the head forward and elevated *to stop bleeding.*

Altered oral mucous membrane related to bleeding

- Remove dentures *to avoid irritation.*
- Provide mouth care with soft toothbrush *to minimize tissue trauma.*
- Give soft foods and iced liquids *to avoid trauma.*
- Observe for bleeding.

Impaired tissue integrity (vaginal mucous membrane) related to bleeding

- Provide perineal hygiene *to promote comfort.*
- Count pads used *to determine amount of bleeding.*
- Observe amount, color, consistency, and frequency of discharge *to monitor blood loss.*

Altered cerebral tissue perfusion related to bleeding

- Observe for signs of increased intracranial pressure— level of consciousness, pupillary response, and reflexes and intervene based on findings *to prevent permanent alterations.*
- Instruct patient to avoid Valsalva maneuver (e.g., coughing and straining at stool) *to decrease potential for bleeding.*

Pain related to pressure and altered sensations or loss of sensation in extremities

- Position patient comfortably *to minimize pain and pressure.*
- Handle patient gently (massage) *to relax muscles.*
- Apply bed cradle, lightweight clothing, and blanket *to relieve pressure.*
- Apply heat lamp, cradle pad, hot water bottle, warm or cold compress bag; do what the patient thinks will make him or her comfortable.
- Give analgesics as ordered *to relieve pain.*

Impaired tissue integrity (gastrointestinal mucous membrane) related to bleeding

- Observe amount, color, consistency, and frequency of discharge *to monitor blood loss.*
- Maintain perianal hygiene *for patient comfort.*
- Avoid use of rectal thermometer, enema tube, or other instruments *that might cause bleeding.*
- Encourage high-fiber foods and increased fluids *to prevent constipation.*
- Test stool for occult blood.
- Measure emesis and test for occult blood.

Altered cardiopulmonary tissue perfusion related to bleeding

- Place patient on bed rest in a low Fowler's position *to enhance cardiopulmonary function.*
- Dress patient warmly and maintain warm room temperature *to enhance vasodilation.*
- Remove constrictive clothing *to facilitate chest expansion.*
- Discourage smoking and oral stimulants, *which cause vasoconstriction and dyspnea.*
- Monitor vital signs and laboratory studies *to determine adequacy of function.*
- Observe pulse rate and rhythm, respiration rate and depth, and blood pressure *to determine need for intervention.*

Altered renal tissue perfusion related to bleeding

- Observe color, amount, and presence of red blood cells in urine, report to physician *for early intervention.*

Patient Education/Home Care Planning

1. Explain the need to stop smoking to avoid impairment of arterial circulation.
2. Assist the patient to avoid mechanical trauma:
   a. General safety precautions
   b. Soft toothbrush
   c. Gentle nose blowing
   d. Stool softeners and maintenance of diet high in roughage and fluids
3. Discuss with the patient the need to detect and report signs and symptoms of bleeding.

Evaluation

Vital signs are within normal limits Respirations, pulse, blood pressure, and temperature are within normal limits. Mucous membranes are intact.

Bowel and bladder elimination are normal Stools are soft, and there is no evidence of bleeding in stool or urine.

Patient is mentally alert Patient has good concentration and is oriented to time, place, and person.

Patient has physical appearance of comfort Posture is normal, and patient has freedom of body movement. Patient changes position and body movement frequently (i.e., walks, sits, and stands). Patient makes no complaints of pain.

Patient's surroundings are safe   Patient uses safety precautions; room temperature and humidity are appropriate.

There is no evidence that an accident or physical injury has occurred   There are no signs of injury or bleeding.

Patient's skin is intact   There is no evidence of intradermal bleeding.

DISSEMINATED INTRAVASCULAR COAGULATION SYNDROME

Disseminated intravascular coagulation (DIC) syndrome is a bleeding disorder that results from the blood's increased tendency to clot.

DIC syndrome causes the transformation of fibrinogen to fibrin clot and is often associated with acute hemorrhage. States of physiologic disequilibrium that precipitate this syndrome include hemorrhagic shock, crush syndrome, leukemia, carcinoma, abruptio placentae, septic abortion, incompatible blood transfusion, and endotoxic shock.

•••••• Pathophysiology

The result of the physiologic disequilibrium caused by the factors cited previously is a systemic activation of coagulation and fibrinolysis, with diffuse intravascular fibrin formation and deposition of fibrin in the microcirculation. As a consequence of these processes, clots accumulate in the body's capillaries, which are more than 100,000 miles in length. Clotting factors are used at a rate that exceeds their replenishment, with circu-lating thrombin waiting in the intravascular space for fibrinogen. The excessive thrombin formation greatly decreases the availability of the inhibitor antithrombin III.

Activation of the fibrinolytic system results in fibrin degradation products, which interfere with both platelet function and fibrin clot formation. As a consequence, the patient has a simultaneous, self-perpetuating combination of thrombosis and bleeding (Figure 15-2).

The kallikrein and complement systems also are activated, resulting in arterial hypotension. Clotting activity is enhanced by kallikrein's activation of factor XII to XIIa. Kallikrein also releases kinins, which increase vascular permeability and vasodilation, thereby further increasing the arterial hypotension.

Activation of the complement system causes not only increased vascular permeability but also lysis of erythrocytes, granulocytes, and platelets; this produces phospholipids, which activate factor XII.

Arteriolar vasoconstriction and capillary dilation result in shunting of blood to the venous side, leaving the dilated capillaries with stagnant blood, which produces metabolic waste and resultant acidity. This results in three concurrent, procoagulating effects in the capillary blood: blood stagnation, the presence of coagulation-promoting substances, and acidosis.

The patient with DIC syndrome bleeds because of increased fibrinolysis, diminished antithrombin III, and consumption of clotting factors. Antithrombin III cannot keep pace with the excessive production of thrombin, which continues to activate the conversion of plasminogen to plasmin, exacerbating the bleeding (see Emergency Alert box).

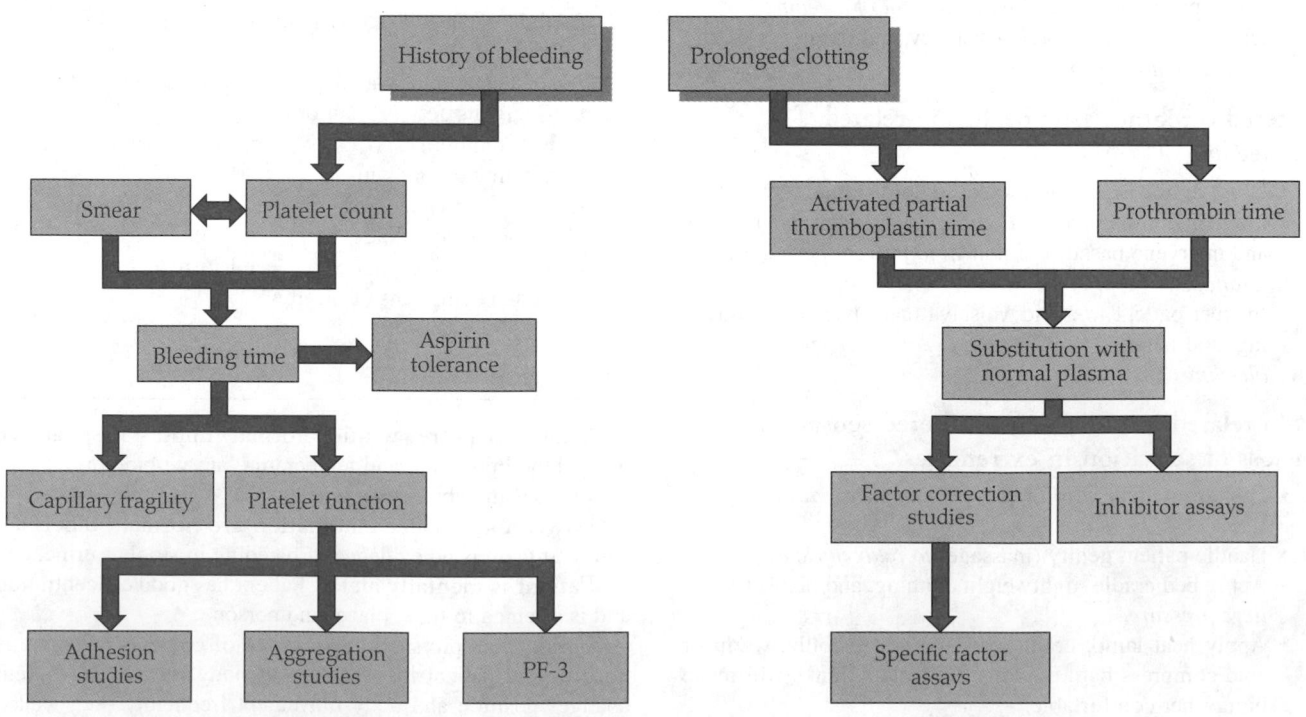

Figure 15-2 Laboratory study algorithm for bleeding disorders. (From Belcher.[1])

••••• Diagnostic Studies and Findings

Prothrombin time INR (PT/INR) Prolonged
Activated partial thromboplastin (PTT) Prolonged
Platelet count <100,000/mm³
Fibrinogen level Decreased
Antithrombin III level Decreased
Thrombin time Prolonged
Fibrin degradation products Elevated
Plasminogen levels Decreased

••••• Multidisciplinary Plan

Medications

Heparin therapy, 30,000 U IV in 24 hours; 2500 to 5000 U q
 4 to 8 hours subcutaneously
Chemotherapy for irradiation of tumor
Antibiotics for control of infection

General Management

Elimination of the cause
 May require correction of hypovolemia, hypotension, hypoxia and acidosis, or hemostatic deficiencies
 Physiologic disequilibrium, such as septic shock, must
 also be treated
Administration of depleted factors such as whole blood or
 fresh-frozen plasma, which contain fibrinogen; platelets

NURSING CARE

Nursing Assessment

Vascular Integrity

Bleeding from the nose, gums, and infection sites
Petechiae, purpura, and ecchymosis

 EMERGENCY ALERT

**DISSEMINATED INTRAVASCULAR
COAGULATION (DIC)**

A serious complication in which the blood clotting mechanism is accelerated resulting in diffuse intravascular fibrin
formation that settles in microcirculation.

Assessment

- Obtain patient's history. DIC is generally precipitated by
 acute hemorrhage as in shock, abruptio placentae, incompatible blood transfusion, leukemia, carcinoma.

Interventions

- Maintain airway, breathing, and circulation.
- Administer high flow oxygen (10-15 L) by mask.
- Obtain IV access, laboratory studies, and fluid resuscita-
 tion as indicated.
- Prepare to provide replacement of clotting factors,
 platelets, fresh frozen plasma, packed cells.
- In collaboration with physician, administer heparin therapy.

Respiratory Function

Tachypnea, dyspnea
Cyanosis or pallor
Basilar rales

Cardiac Function

Dysrhythmias, tachycardia
Hypotension
Gallop rhythm

Renal Function

Decreased urinary output

Sensory and Motor Function

Altered level of consciousness, orientation, and pupillary reaction
Decreased movement and strength of extremities

Mental Status

Fear, anxiety
Restlessness

Nursing Dx & Intervention

Fluid volume deficit related to bleeding

- Monitor vital signs and level of consciousness *for evidence of acute hemorrhage.*
- Administer blood component and intravenous fluids as ordered *to replace fluid loss.*
- Apply ice pack and manual dressing over site of blood
 loss *to promote clotting and slow or stop bleeding.*
- Place patient in semi-Fowler's position *to prevent respiratory distress caused by nasal bleeding.*
- Avoid using injections or razor *to prevent further
 bleeding.*
- Assess amount, consistency, and frequency of bleeding *to
 determine need for replacement therapy.*
- Monitor laboratory tests *to determine degree of blood loss
 and effect of treatment.*
- Administer heparin as prescribed; apply pressure to injection site for at least 5 minutes *to avoid seepage.*
- Assess skin for presence, size, and color of petechiae, purpura, and ecchymosis *to determine degree of bleeding into
 tissues.*
- Check stool, urine, emesis, and sputum for presence of occult and observable blood *to identify presence of gastrointestinal or renal hemorrhage.*
- Provide gentle care to skin, oral mucosa, fingernails, and
 toenails *to avoid further bleeding.*

Impaired gas exchange related to arterial hypotension

- Position patient to facilitate breathing, that is, in semi-
 Fowler's position, *to reduce pressure on diaphragm and
 promote chest expansion.*
- Encourage patient to take deep breaths *to reduce hyperventilation.*

- Provide oxygen therapy as prescribed *to reduce cardiopulmonary workload and to enhance tissue oxygenation.*
- Help patient maintain a balance between rest and activity *to decrease oxygen requirement.*
- Maintain warm environment *to avoid shivering.*
- Monitor respiratory rate and breath sounds *to identify increasing difficulty and assess effectiveness of treatment.*
- Assess skin color and temperature *to determine adequacy of tissue oxygenation.*

Decreased cardiac output; altered cardiopulmonary tissue perfusion related to arterial hypotension

- Maintain patient in semi-Fowler's position with legs elevated *to enhance cardiac output and venous return.*
- Administer antidysrhythmic drugs as prescribed *to correct dysrhythmias, slow the heart rate, and increase cardiac output.*
- Monitor apical, brachial, carotid, radial, femoral, and tibial pulses *to determine pumping action of heart and adequacy of tissue perfusion.*
- Administer cardiotonic and vasoconstricting drugs as ordered *to strengthen pumping action of the heart and increase vascular tone.*
- Help patient avoid stress as much as possible *to decrease cardiac workload* (e.g., balance rest and activity, avoid straining at stool, use relaxation exercises).
- Assess skin color *to determine adequacy of tissue perfusion.*
- Monitor laboratory tests, especially blood pH studies, *to detect acidosis.*

Altered patterns of urinary elimination related to decreased output

- Monitor fluid intake and output, color and consistency of urine, and frequency of voiding *to assess renal function.*
- Use Foley catheter and drainage bag as prescribed *to monitor urine production.*
- Monitor laboratory studies, including electrolytes, *to determine adequacy of renal function.*
- Monitor intravenous and oral fluids *to detect early signs and symptoms of fluid overload, such as shortness of breath, restlessness, confusion, hypertension, and abnormal breath sounds.*

Sensory/perceptual alterations related to arterial hypotension

- Place patient on bed rest with the head elevated *to reduce intracranial pressure and unnecessary activity.*
- Decrease environmental stimuli *to lessen stress and distraction or confusion.*
- Discourage use of oral stimulants, such as caffeine, *which might increase intracranial pressure.*
- Monitor neurologic signs, such as level of consciousness, orientation, pupillary responses, and reflexes *to detect changes early.*

- Assess range of motion and strength of extremities *to monitor neurologic status.*
- Monitor vital signs for alterations *that would indicate increasing intracranial pressure.*
- Report to physician any change in pupillary response, projectile vomiting, or decrease in level of consciousness.

Fear related to cerebral hypoxia, dyspnea, tachypnea, and bleeding

- Encourage patient to talk about specific fears, *so that each can be dealt with.*
- Have patient describe his or her perception of danger and coping skills as a basis *for identifying specific interventions.*
- Deal with distorted perceptions of danger, isolation, and so on *to reduce degree of fear.*
- Orient patient to environment, including such equipment as drainage tubes, IV lines, hemodynamic monitoring equipment, and mechanical ventilator *to reduce fear of the unfamiliar.*
- Assure patient of observation and monitoring by health care providers *to reduce fear of abandonment.*
- Avoid startling patient by telling him or her what to expect and when.
- Teach patient ways of maintaining some degree of control, such as having access to the call light or bell and asking about his or her status and test results, *to reduce fear of dependence.*

Patient Education/Home Care Planning

1. Discuss with the patient and family signs and symptoms of the syndrome, which should be reported immediately to the nurse or physician.
2. Have patient learn to administer heparin therapy subcutaneously.
3. Assist the patient and family to avoid mechanical trauma such as from a hard toothbrush, blade razor, rough nose blowing, or contact sports.

Evaluation

Vital signs are within normal limits   Pulse, respirations, blood pressure, and temperature are within normal limits.

Bowel and bladder elimination are normal   There is no evidence of bleeding. Urinary output is sufficient.

Skin integrity is within normal limits   There are no open wounds. There is no evidence of discoloration, and the skin is warm, dry, and natural in color.

Neurologic function is within normal limits   Patient is oriented, alert, and calm. Pupillary responses are equal and normal. Patient has adequate movement and strength of extremities.

Patient is able to express fears and deal with them realistically

HEMOPHILIA

Hemophilia is a disorder characterized by impaired co-agulability of the blood and a tendency to bleed.

The classic disease is hereditary and limited to males; thus it is an X-linked recessive disease. All daughters of hemophiliac males become carriers, and the son of a female carrier has a 50% chance of being a hemophiliac. Homozygous females with hemophilia (father a hemophiliac, mother a carrier) are extremely rare.

•••••• Pathophysiology

Two of the major types of hemophilia are clinically identical: classic hemophilia, or hemophilia A, in which anti-hemophilic, factor VIII activity is deficient or absent, and Christmas disease, or hemophilia B, in which factor IX activity is deficient or absent. The degree of bleeding experienced by the patient is related to the amount of factor activity and the severity of the injury. When factor activity levels are below 1%, spontaneous bleeding, hemarthrosis (joint bleeding), and deep tissue bleeding occur (see Emergency Alert box). When levels are 5% or higher, bleeding usually results from trauma or surgical procedures, such as at circumcision.

Other less common forms of hemophilia include hemophilia C, a hemorrhagic susceptibility transmitted as an autosomal dominant trait and caused by a lack of clotting factor XI; calipriva, a bleeding tendency caused by a serum calcium deficiency; vascular hemophilia, also called angiohemophilia; and von Willebrand's disease, an autosomal dominant trait in both males and females with factor VIII_{VWF} and VIII_{AHC} deficiency and a platelet adhesion defect (see box).

! EMERGENCY ALERT

HEMOPHILIA

Hemophilia is a genetic disorder affecting males that causes bleeding that results from the absence of a clotting factor.

Assessment

- Bleeding gums, epistaxis
- Hemarthrosis causing joint immobility
- Severe bruises with minor trauma
- Bleeding history
- Other pain

Interventions

- Monitor vital signs.
- Administer oxygen as needed to maintain comfort and adequate oxygen saturation.
- Elevate any affected joint, apply gentle pressure to bleeding site, immobilize the area, and apply ice.
- Obtain IV access and provide hydration.
- Prepare to administer fresh frozen plasma.
- Aspirate joint if needed.

•••••• Diagnostic Studies and Findings

Prothrombin time INR (PT/INR)   Normal
Partial thromboplastin time (PTT)   Prolonged
Bleeding time (platelet function)   Normal; prolonged in von Willebrand's disease

•••••• Multidisciplinary Plan

General Management

Replacement of deficient factor
    For hemophilia A, cryoprecipitate containing 8 to 100 U of factor VIII per bag at 12-hour intervals until bleeding ceases
    For hemophilia B, plasma or factor IX concentrate (Konyne or Proplex), given every 24 hours until bleeding ceases
Treatment for the development of antibody inhibitors against the specific coagulation factor
Immunosuppressive agents
Plasmapheresis to remove the inhibitor
Prothrombin complexes, which bypass the inhibitors
Synthetically produced DDAVP (1-deamino 8-D arginine vasopressin) administered IV can induce a threefold to sixfold increase in factor VIII activity level

---

NURSING CARE

Nursing Assessment

Vascular Integrity

Hypotension, tachycardia, hyperpnea
Bleeding from nose, gums, lips, tongue, and infection sites
Petechiae, purpura, and ecchymosis
Menorrhagia
Hemarthrosis with pain and deformity
Hematuria
Melena

PLASMA CLOTTING FACTORS

    I. Fibrinogen: precursor of fibrin
   II. Prothrombin: precursor of thrombin
  III. Thromboplastin: activator of prothrombin
  IV. Calcium
   V. Plasma accelerator globulin
 VII. Serum prothrombin conversion accelerator
VIII. Antihemophilic globulin (AHG)
  IX. Christmas factor
   X. Stuart-Prower factor
  XI. Plasma thromboplastin antecedent (PTA)
 XII. Hageman factor
XIII. Fibrin-stabilizing factor
     Fletcher factor
     Fitzgerald factor

Sensory Function and Mental Status

Disorientation, confusion

Convulsions

Decreased reflexes, including pupillary

Nursing Dx & Intervention

Fluid volume deficit related to bleeding

- Monitor vital signs and level of consciousness *for evidence of acute hemorrhage.*
- Administer blood component therapy as ordered *to control bleeding:*

    Cryoprecipitate—observe for reactions such as urticaria or hives; administer diphenhydramine (Benadryl) to counteract reaction. Use normal saline to flush cryoprecipitate from bag to remove it from plastic. Include number of bags and amount of solution in intake and output records.

    Plasma thromboplastin component (PTC) and antihemophilic factor (AHF)—must be refrigerated until use; shake gently for up to 10 minutes and administer over a 5-minute interval; reactions are rare.

    Prothrombin complexes—high risk for hepatitis; dosage depends on patient's condition.

- Apply ice pack to affected joint or traumatized area *to control bleeding.*
- Casting may be used *to protect and rest affected joints.*
- Administer analgesics *to relieve joint pain.*
- Assess amount, consistency, and frequency of bleeding *to determine need for replacement therapy:*

    Nose, gums, lips, and tongue

    Joints

    Skin

    Stool and urine

    Pad counts

- Measure abdominal girth *to detect occurrence of deep bleeding.*
- Monitor laboratory tests *to determine degree of blood loss and effect of therapy.*
- Avoid trauma, such as falls, bumps, or injections.
- Observe for signs and symptoms of hepatitis, such as jaundice, clay-colored stool, mahogany-colored urine, nausea, and abdominal distention.

Sensory/perceptual alterations (potential) related to intracranial bleeding

- Place patient on bed rest with head elevated *to reduce intracranial pressure and unnecessary activity.*
- Protect head with helmet, and use padded side rails if patient is restless.
- Discourage oral stimulants, such as caffeine, *which might increase intracranial pressure.*
- Monitor neurologic signs, such as level of consciousness, orientation, pupillary response, and reflexes *to detect changes early.*

- Monitor vital signs *for evidence of increasing intracranial pressure.*
- Report changes in pupillary response, projectile vomiting, or decrease in level of consciousness to physician.

Patient Education/Home Care Planning

1. Practice with the patient self-administration of blood factor(s).
2. Discuss the need to avoid injury, such as that caused by contact sports or use of sharp instruments.
3. Discuss the need to report signs and symptoms of bleeding to a nurse or physician.
4. Encourage the patient to seek genetic counseling if he or she has a hereditary form of hemophilia.

Evaluation

Vital signs are within normal limits   Pulse, respirations, blood pressure, and temperature are within normal limits.

Gastrointestinal function is normal   There is no evidence of bleeding, and there are no signs or symptoms of hepatitis.

Renal function is normal   There is no evidence of bleeding.

The skin and skeletal structure are within normal limits   There is no evidence of bleeding or discoloration and no swelling of the joints; the skin is warm and dry.

Neurologic function is within normal limits   The patient is oriented, alert, and calm. Pupillary responses are equal and within normal limits.

■ MALIGNANT LYMPHOMAS

■ Malignant lymphomas are neoplasms of the lymphoid tissue.

Malignant lymphomas include lymphosarcoma, reticulum cell sarcoma, and Hodgkin's disease. Although the cause of these cancers is unknown, a viral etiologic factor is believed responsible for several types, particularly Burkitt's lymphoma (a childhood disease) and Hodgkin's disease. There may also be a genetic factor in Hodgkin's disease.

Non–Hodgkin's lymphomas may be further categorized as follows:

Lymphocyte malignancies

    Lymphocytic lymphosarcoma

    Lymphoblastic lymphosarcoma

    Reticulum cell sarcoma

    Burkitt's lymphoma

    Stem cell lymphoma/immunoblastoma

    "Mixed" lymphoma

Histiocytic lymphoma

······ Pathophysiology

Lymphosarcoma and reticulum cell sarcomas account for about 40% of malignant lymphomas; the incidence increases with age, primarily striking middle-aged people. Early widespread dissemination is common, with oropharyngeal lymphoid tissue, the gastrointestinal tract, and bones frequently affected. The earliest sign is painless lymphadenopathy, usually unilateral and in the neck. The disease spreads via lymphatic channels to other nodes and, in the case of lymphosarcoma, invades the bone marrow. Other organs that may be involved are the skin and nervous system. Pressure and organ obstruction produce symptoms such as abdominal pain, nerve pain, and paralysis. Other patient problems include anemia, fever, sweating, pruritus, weight loss, and malaise. Diagnosis and treatment of these lymphatic malignancies are similar to those for Hodgkin's disease.

▌ HODGKIN'S DISEASE

A chronic and progressive cancer, Hodgkin's disease primarily affects adults between 20 and 40 years of age. Men are affected twice as often as women and boys five times more than girls.

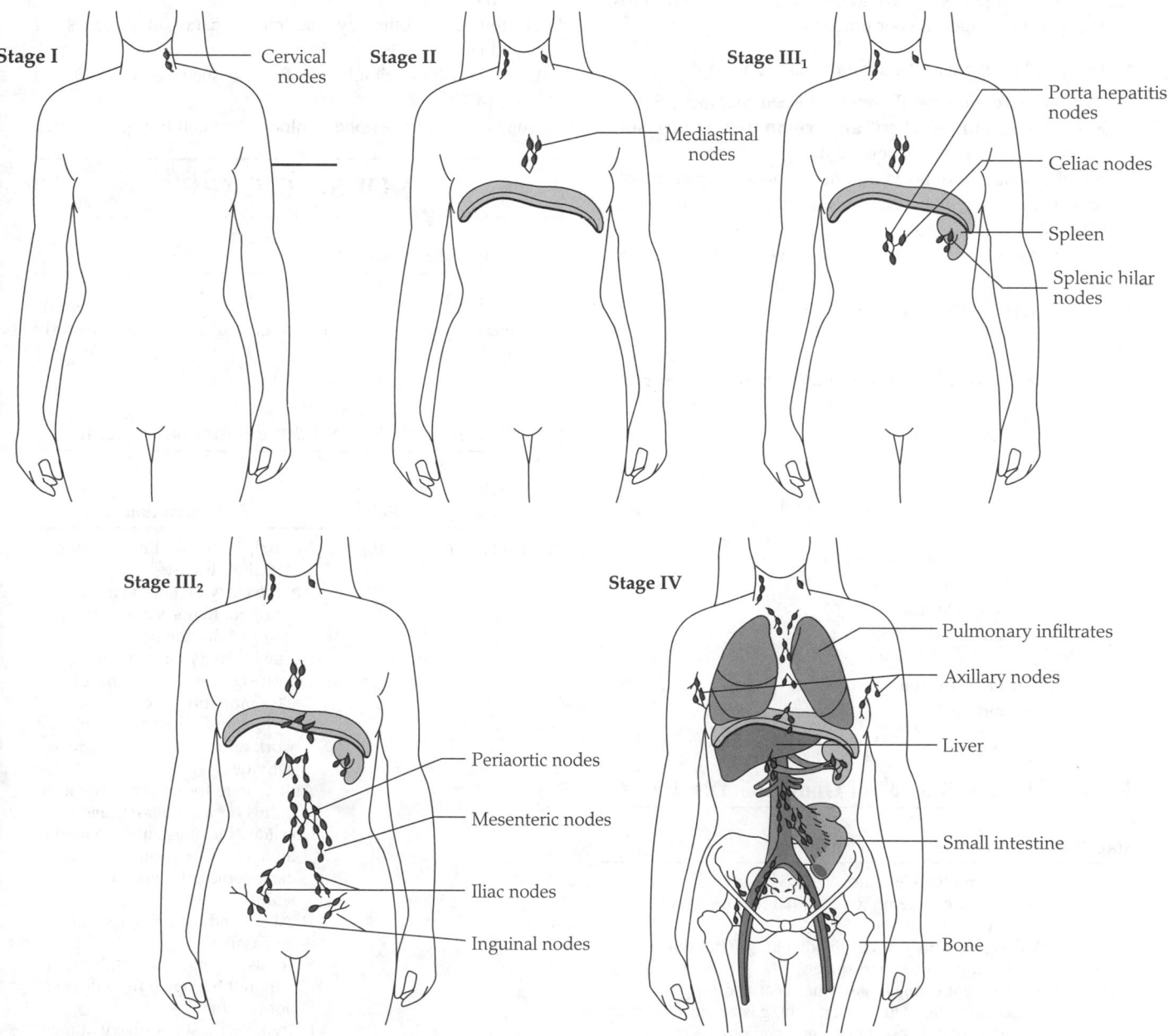

Figure 15-3 Nodal involvement by stage in Hodgkin's disease. (Based on modified Ann Arbor staging system.) (From Belcher.[1])

The disease is characterized by the abnormal proliferation of histiocytes called "Reed-Sternberg cells," which eventually replace the normal cellular structure of the lymph nodes and cause areas of necrosis and fibrosis to develop. Malignant reticulum cells are also present.

Hodgkin's disease initially affects one lymph node and then travels by lymphatic channels to nodes throughout the body; it may also appear in the liver and spleen, vertebrae, ureters, and bronchi. Staging of the disease is based on microscopic appearance of the lymph nodes (Figure 15-3), extent and severity of the disease, and prognosis. Table 15-1 shows one method of staging.

The prognosis for untreated patients is about 5 years; those diagnosed in stage I or II have a 95% cure rate, whereas those in stages III or IV have a poor prognosis.

•••••• Diagnostic Studies and Findings

Lymph node biopsy Presence of Reed-Sternberg cells
Roentgenogram of chest and computed tomography Mediastinal or hilar lymphadenopathy
Blood studies Normocytic normochromic anemia; neutrophilic leukocytosis; lymphopenia; eosinophilia; hemolytic anemia
Bipedal lymphangiography Abnormal nodes
Radiologic studies Vertebral compression; fractures

•••••• Multidisciplinary Plan

Surgery

The tumor that is causing pressure on an organ or nerve is excised
Therapeutic splenectomy

Medications

Antineoplastic agents in combination therapy, for example,
MOPP
*M*echlorethamine (Nitrogen mustard)
Vincristine (*Oncovin*)
*P*rednisone (Deltasone)
*P*rocarbazine (Matulane)
ABVD
Doxorubicin (*Adriamycin*)
*B*leomycin

■ TABLE 15-1 Staging of Hodgkin's Disease

Stage*	Definition
I	Single lymph node region
II	Two or more node regions limited to one side of the diaphragm
III	Disease on both sides of the diaphragm but limited to the lymph nodes and spleen
IV	Involvement of the bones, bone marrow, lung parenchyma, pleura, liver, skin, gastrointestinal tract, central nervous system, renal, and other sites

From Belcher.[1]
*All stages are subclassified as A or B to describe the absence (A) or presence (B) of systemic symptoms.

*V*inblastine
*D*acarbazine
No specific drug dosages are given for the chemotherapy combinations because (1) doses may change when used in combination; (2) doses differ depending on the patient's physical status, such as white blood cell and platelet counts and Karnofsky scale rating (Table 15-2); and (3) individual drug protocols differ from one institution to another.

General Management

Wide-field megavoltage radiation (3500 to 4000 roentgens over a 4- to 6-week period can be curative for stages I or II)
Combined radiotherapy and chemotherapy for stages III and IV
Use of colony-stimulating factors such as G-CSF and GM-CSF
Bone marrow or peripheral blood stem cell transplantation

NURSING CARE

Nursing Assessment

Skin Integrity

Painless swelling of lymph nodes, usually cervical (early sign)

■ TABLE 15-2 Karnofsky Performance Scale

Activity Status	Point	Description
Normal activity	10	Normal, with no complaints or evidence of disease
	9	Able to carry on normal activity but with minor signs or symptoms of disease present
	8	Normal activity but requiring effort; signs and symptoms of disease more prominent
Self-care	7	Able to care for self but unable to work or carry on other normal activities
	6	Able to care for most needs but requires occasional assistance
	5	Considerable assistance required, along with frequent medical care; some self-care still possible
Incapacitated	4	Disabled and requiring special care and assistance
	3	Severely disabled; hospitalization required but death from disease not imminent
	2	Extremely ill; supportive treatment and hospitalized care required
	1	Imminent death
	0	Dead

Severe pruritus
Jaundice
Edema and cyanosis of face and neck
Irregular fever, night sweats

Sensory and Motor Function

Bone pain, paraplegia, and nerve pain
Fatigue, malaise

Respiratory Function

Cough, stridor, dyspnea, chest pain, and pleural effusion
Recent upper respiratory infections
Laryngeal paralysis

Gastrointestinal Function

Splenomegaly and hepatomegaly, with resultant abdominal distention and discomfort
Weight loss, anorexia

Immune Function

Increased susceptibility to infection

Nursing Dx & Intervention

Impaired skin integrity related to swelling of lymph nodes and impaired function

- Bathe the patient in cool water or apply cool, moist compresses *to enhance comfort.*
- Apply calamine lotion, cornstarch, sodium bicarbonate, and medicated powder *to relieve itching.*
- Use a bed cradle and lightweight blankets and clothing *to relieve pressure.*
- Lubricate skin with baby oil, bath oil, body lotion, or petrolatum *for comfort.*
- Maintain adequate humidity and cool room *to decrease itching.*
- Avoid adhesive, alkaline soap, and local heat, *which irritate the skin.*

Impaired physical mobility (potential) related to fracture, vertebral compression, and nerve damage

- Maintain body alignment *to enhance mobility and comfort.*
- Move body as a single unit *to prevent injury.*
- Provide mechanical support during ambulation *to enhance mobility.*
- Observe motor function in extremities; monitor complaints of numbness and tingling; report findings to the physician.

Pain related to disease progression to bones and nerves

- For bone pain: position the patient comfortably, change position gradually, and handle the patient gently and in an unhurried manner *to avoid trauma.*
- Support affected body part *to prevent pressure.*

- Encourage adequate rest *to reduce incidence of pain related to activity.*
- Provide pain relief measures based on patient's choice.
- Give analgesics as ordered.
- For intraabdominal pressure: place patient in a sitting position; remove constrictive clothing; change patient's position frequently; give small, frequent feedings.

Ineffective breathing pattern related to airway edema

- Place patient in a sitting position *to increase chest expansion.*
- Remove constrictive clothing *to relieve pressure on the chest.*
- Encourage deep breathing *for alveolar expansion.*
- Administer oxygen as needed *to provide tissue oxygenation.*
- Provide standby emergency equipment *to relieve airway obstruction.*
- Inspect chest for respiratory rate and rhythm and symmetric expansion.
- Auscultate lungs for abnormal breath sounds, aeration, rales, and rhonchi.
- Observe for hoarseness, cough, stridor, pain, and change in skin color (cyanosis).
- Monitor blood studies *for abnormal gas exchange.*
- Plan rest periods *to avoid hyperventilation.*

Altered nutrition: less than body requirements related to disease progression to gastrointestinal tract

- Provide small feedings of high-calorie, high-protein foods and fluids *to increase nutritional intake.*
- Assist with oral care, general hygiene, environmental control (temperature, appearance, odors) *to enhance appetite.*
- Identify food preferences and provide them as often as possible *to promote adequate nutritional intake.*
- Place the patient in a sitting position after meals *to decrease feeling of fullness.*

Risk for infection related to impaired immunologic function

- Have the patient turn, cough, and deep breathe at regular intervals *to prevent respiratory tract infection.*
- Encourage fluids and balanced diet *for maintenance of general well-being.*
- Maintain reverse isolation *to protect patient from microorganisms.*
- Observe the patient for "sniffles," sore throat, anorexia, pain on urination, and increases in temperature, pulse, and respirations, *which indicate infection.*
- Administer antibiotics as ordered *to treat infection.*
For hyperthermia:
- Apply cool, damp cloth to the patient's face *for comfort.*
- Bathe the patient in cool water and apply ice bag or alcohol *to reduce fever.*

- Cover with lightweight blankets and clothing *to avoid chilling.*
- Maintain cool room temperature *for patient's comfort.*
- Increase fluid intake, especially iced liquids, *for hydration.*
- Monitor oral temperature level and pattern *to determine need for antipyretics, cooling blanket, or other interventions.*

Patient Education/Home Care Planning

1. Discuss the need to avoid scratching and to correctly care for skin to reduce susceptibility to infection and mechanical skin damage.
2. Practice with the patient correct maintenance of body alignment and use of body mechanics and ambulatory aids, and discuss the early symptoms of vertebral compression and paralysis to report to physician or nurse.
3. Plan ways to relieve pain without the use of medications as often as possible; bone, nerve, and abdominal pain is chronic in nature and increases with pressure of disseminated disease.
4. Emphasize the importance of respiratory therapy to prevent or decrease severity of symptoms of mediastinal lymph node enlargement, involvement of lung parenchyma, and invasion of pleura.

Evaluation

Color of the skin and mucous membranes is good The skin, nails, lips, and ear lobes are warm and moist and have a natural color. Skin is intact.

Vital signs are within normal limits Respirations, pulse, blood pressure, and temperature are within normal limits.

Patient's nutritional intake is adequate

Body hydration is normal Skin turgor is good; mucous membranes are moist.

Patient has physical appearance of comfort Patient is calm and relaxed. Posture is normal, and patient has freedom of body movement. Patient verbally expresses comfort and ceases previous complaining. Patient uses medications effectively.

There is no evidence of physical injury There is no evidence of complications arising from drugs, treatment, disease process, or nursing care. The patient uses ambulatory aids effectively.

There is no infection There is no evidence of inflammation, pain or aching, or purulent secretions.

MEDICAL INTERVENTIONS AND RELATED NURSING CARE

BLOOD TRANSFUSIONS

Infusion of blood may be lifesaving for the patient with anemia caused by acute blood loss whose hemoglobin is less than 10 g. The transfusion immediately increases the body's ability to re-ceive oxygen and avoid severe tissue damage. Transfusions are used less frequently for patients with severe chronic anemia (hemoglobin <6 g) because of potential complications.

Contraindications and Cautions

1. Hemolytic reaction is caused by the administration of mismatched blood.
2. Bacterial reactions are usually caused by contaminated blood.
3. Allergic reactions can occur. Their exact cause is unknown, although in some cases the donor may have ingested drugs or food to which the recipient is allergic.
4. Circulatory overload results from too rapid an infusion or too great a quantity.
5. Transmission of infectious agents such as hepatitis virus can occur.

•••••• Multidisciplinary Plan

General Management

Medications and other interventions are administered as needed in response to reactions to transfusions.

NURSING CARE

Nursing Assessment

Hemolytic Reaction

Chills and fever
Tachycardia
Nausea and vomiting
Hematuria or oliguria
Headache
Backache
Dyspnea
Cyanosis
Chest pain

Bacterial (Febrile) Reaction

Fever, chills, lumbar pain, headache, malaise, bloody vomitus, diarrhea, or red shock (skin warm, dry, and pink)

Allergic Reaction

Mild edema, hives, bronchial wheezing, or anaphylaxis

Circulatory Overload

Cough, dyspnea, edema, tachycardia, hemoptysis, and frothy pink-tinged sputum
Distended neck veins

Nursing Dx & Intervention

Risk for injury related to hemolytic reaction

- Discontinue blood transfusions immediately.
- Notify the physician and laboratory.

- Send remaining blood and sample of the patient's blood to the laboratory *for repeat type and cross-matching.*
- Administer intravenous fluids *(to maintain patency of line),* oxygen, and drugs—such as vasopressor agents, epinephrine, sedatives, and mannitol—as ordered *to manage hemolytic reaction.*
- Monitor vital signs.
- Insert Foley catheter *to monitor urinary output.*
- Provide analgesics, antiemetics, and massage *for patient comfort.*

Risk for injury related to bacterial reaction

- Discontinue blood transfusion; notify the physician.
- Send remaining blood and sample of the patient's blood to the laboratory *for repeat type and cross-matching.*
- Monitor vital signs.
- Use cooling measures as needed.
- Administer intravenous fluids *(to maintain patency of line).*
- Insert Foley catheter *to monitor urinary output.*
- Administer medications as ordered, such as vasopressors, corticosteroids, broad-spectrum antibiotics, analgesics, and antiemetics, *to manage bacterial reaction.*

Risk for injury related to allergic reaction

- Decrease transfusion flow if mild reaction occurs (mild edema, hives, or bronchial wheezing).
- Stop blood transfusion if severe reaction occurs (bronchospasm or severe dyspnea) and administer intravenous fluids *(to maintain patency of line).*
- Give medications as ordered, such as bronchodilators or epinephrine.
- Provide oxygen therapy as needed.

Fluid volume excess related to rapid or excessive infusion

- Slow rate of transfusion, and notify the physician.
- Give digitalis as ordered *to enhance cardiac output.*
- Prepare for venesection or rotating tourniquets as ordered *to decrease circulating volume.*
- Monitor pulse, respirations, blood pressure, and central venous pressure.

Evaluation

Color of the skin and mucous membranes is good The skin, nails, lips, and ear lobes are warm and moist and have a natural color.

Vital signs are within normal limits Respirations, pulse, and blood pressure are within normal limits. Breathing pattern is regular.

Laboratory studies are within normal limits The hemoglobin level, hematocrit, and leukocyte count are within normal limits.

Patient has normal body hydration Secretions are thin and mucous membranes are moist. There is no edema.

Daily fluid output is equal to fluid intake Urine output is 1500 to 3000 ml daily or equivalent to intake. Patient feels neither hot nor cold.

There is no evidence of physical injury There is no evidence of complications arising from drugs, treatments, or nursing care.

There are no signs of infection There is no evidence of inflammation, purulent drainage or secretions, or pain or aching.

 ## BONE MARROW TRANSPLANTATION

For a discussion of bone marrow transplantation, see p. 1234.

SPLENECTOMY

Description and Rationale

Although it serves various important functions, the spleen can be surgically removed from adults without harm. Hypersplenism, the destruction of excessive numbers of blood cells by the spleen, is a major reason for its surgical removal. Another frequent indication is splenic rupture with severe hemorrhage, often caused by trauma. The procedure is relatively simple unless the spleen is greatly enlarged or surrounded by adhesions.

•••••• **Multidisciplinary Plan**

Surgery

Removal of the spleen

General Management

Parenteral therapy

Analgesia

NURSING CARE

Nursing Assessment

Vascular Function

Signs and symptoms of hemorrhaging and shock

Gastrointestinal Function

Abdominal distension and discomfort

Gastric discharge

Metabolic Activity

Elevated temperature

Pulmonary Functions

Decreased breath sounds

Splinting with respirations

Tachypnea
Evidence of atelectasis

Immune Function

Infection secondary to wound contamination

Comfort

Pain at surgical site

Nursing Dx & Intervention

Risk for fluid volume deficit related to intravascular hypovolemia

- Administer intravenous fluids, including blood, as ordered *to maintain adequate fluid volume.*
- Measure intake and output *to assess balance.*
- Increase oral fluid intake as tolerated.
- Monitor pulse, respirations, and blood pressure.

Altered peripheral or gastrointestinal tissue perfusion (potential) related to hemorrhaging

- Check surgical incision *to determine its condition.*
- Apply ice bag and manual pressure or dressing over surgical site *to control bleeding.*
- Estimate blood loss *to determine need for replacement.*

Risk for fluid volume deficit related to fever

- Monitor oral temperature and notify physician *if patient becomes febrile.*
- Apply cool, damp cloth to the face of febrile patient *to promote heat loss by evaporation.*
- Bathe the patient in cool water, apply ice bag or alcohol, and cover with lightweight blankets and clothing *to reduce fever.*
- Maintain cool room temperature.
- Encourage rest.
- Increase fluid intake, especially iced liquids.

Risk for fluid volume deficit related to nasogastric drainage and paralytic ileus

- Monitor amount, color, and consistency of drainage.
- Replace fluids as necessary by intravenous infusion as ordered.
- Assess for bowel sounds and abdominal distention.
- Ambulate when possible *to promote gastric motility.*

Risk for infection related to wound contamination

- Monitor temperature, pulse, respirations, and breath sounds *for early indications of infection.*
- Have patient turn, cough, and deep breathe and use incentive spirometry at regular intervals *to maintain ventilatory function.*

- Change dressing, using sterile technique.
- Encourage fluids, monitor intake and output, and assess urine *to prevent urinary tract infection.*

Pain related to surgical incision

- Identify the patient's preferred pain relief measures; implement when feasible.
- Apply abdominal binder *for support of dressing and wound.*
- Apply warmth, such as with a heating pad, to abdominal area.
- Administer medications, such as neostigmine (Prostigmin) and mild analgesics, as ordered *to relieve distention.*
- Observe for increased complaints of pain, nausea, vomiting, diarrhea, and abdominal distention, *which indicate dehiscence and obstruction.*
- Evaluate effectiveness of pain relief measures.

Patient Education/Home Care Planning

1. Demonstrate to the patient care of the surgical incision.
2. Discuss the importance of gradually increasing the level of activity.
3. Emphasize the importance of a well-balanced diet, exercise, rest, and other healthful behaviors.

Evaluation

Color of the skin and mucous membranes is good The skin, nails, lips, and ear lobes are warm and moist and have a natural color.

Vital signs are within normal limits Respirations, pulse, blood pressure, and temperature are within normal limits.

Patient has the physical appearance of comfort Patient has calm, relaxed facial expression. Posture is normal, and patient expresses comfort.

References

1. Belcher A: *Blood disorders,* St Louis, 1993, Mosby.
2. Belcher A: *Cancer nursing,* St Louis, 1992, Mosby.
3. Cain J, Hood-Barnes J, Spangler J: Myelodysplastic syndromes, *Oncol Nurs Forum* 18(1):113, 1991.
4. *Cancer facts & figures, 1995,* Atlanta, 1995, The American Cancer Society.
5. Kim M, McFarland G, McLane A: *Pocket guide to nursing diagnoses,* St Louis, 1995, Mosby.
6. McCance K, Huether S: *Pathophysiology: the biologic basis of disease in adults and children,* ed 2, St Louis, 1994, Mosby.
7. Otto S: *Oncology nursing,* St Louis, 1994, Mosby.
8. Powers LW: *Diagnostic hematology: clinical and technical principles,* St Louis, 1989, Mosby.
9. Schneiderman E: Thrombocytopenia in the critically ill patient, *Crit Care Nurs Q* 13(2):1, 1990.

Neoplasia

16

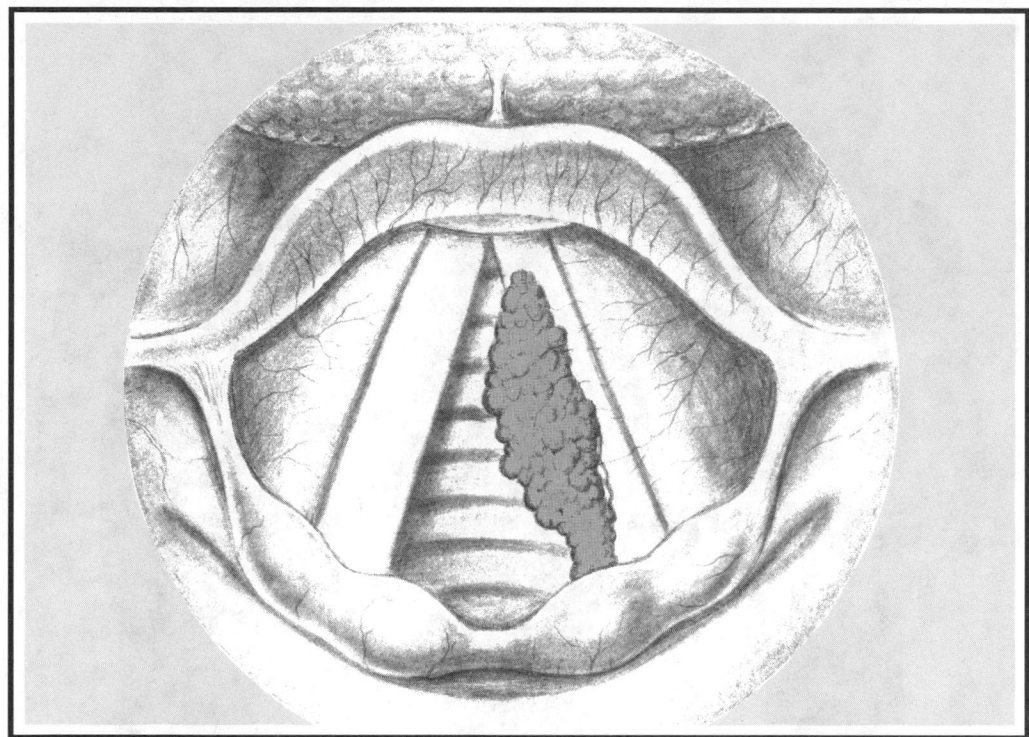

OVERVIEW

Cancer is the second most common cause of death in the United States, killing about 547,000 people annually. It is estimated that 1,252,000 new cases of cancer are diagnosed in Americans every year and this number does not include carcinoma in situ and basal and squamous cell skin cancers. Earlier diagnosis and treatment of certain cancers and better health practices have improved the outlook for people with cancer. Four out of ten people whose cancer was diagnosed in 1995 will be alive 5 years later.

Cancer is a universal disease that affects people without regard to race, sex, socioeconomic status, or culture; however, different forms of cancer strike specific age, racial, and sexual groups. For example, cancer mortality increases rapidly with aging; some researchers believe that anyone who lives long enough will eventually develop cancer. Social and environmental factors are thought to explain racial differences in cancer. Both incidence and mortality are higher in blacks than in whites. Although women are more likely than men to develop cancer, more men die of the disease. The sites in men that are associated with the greatest mortality are the lung, colon and rectum, and prostate. In women the leading sites are the breast, lung, colon, and rectum (Figure 16-1). Another interesting variable is heredity. Certain cancers, such as those of the stomach, breast, colon and rectum, uterus, and lung, occur in a familial pattern. In addition, certain diseases that are cancer precursors, such as multiple familial polyposis and Gardner's syndrome, seem to be hereditary.

Cancer is probably caused by many interacting factors (initiators and promoters) rather than by a single one, and its development appears to be a multistep process. Some causative agents have been found, and others are suspected. One predisposing factor is chronic irritation, such as frequent, prolonged exposure to sunlight or sustained alcohol consumption. Some benign lesions, such as leukoplakia of the oral cavity, colon and rectal polyps, and pigmented moles, may undergo malignant transformation. People whose cancer is already diagnosed are at risk for later development of the disease at the same or another site. Environmental carcinogens that have been identified include cigarette smoke, asbestos, uranium, asphalt, and aniline dye. Iatrogenic factors that have been implicated are radiation and drugs, for example, diethylstilbestrol (DES), certain cancer chemotherapeutic agents, radioisotopes such as phosphorus (^{32}P) and radium, and immunosuppressive drugs.

Among the factors theorized to cause cancer are (1) oncogenes that are normally dormant but may be activated by external agents and (2) viruses, such as the Epstein-Barr virus (EBV) and hepatitis B virus, which are associated with neoplasms and with impaired immune surveillance.

•••••• Anatomy, Physiology, and Related Pathophysiology

In describing the nature and possible causes of cancer, it is important to understand that cancer cells, unlike normal cells,

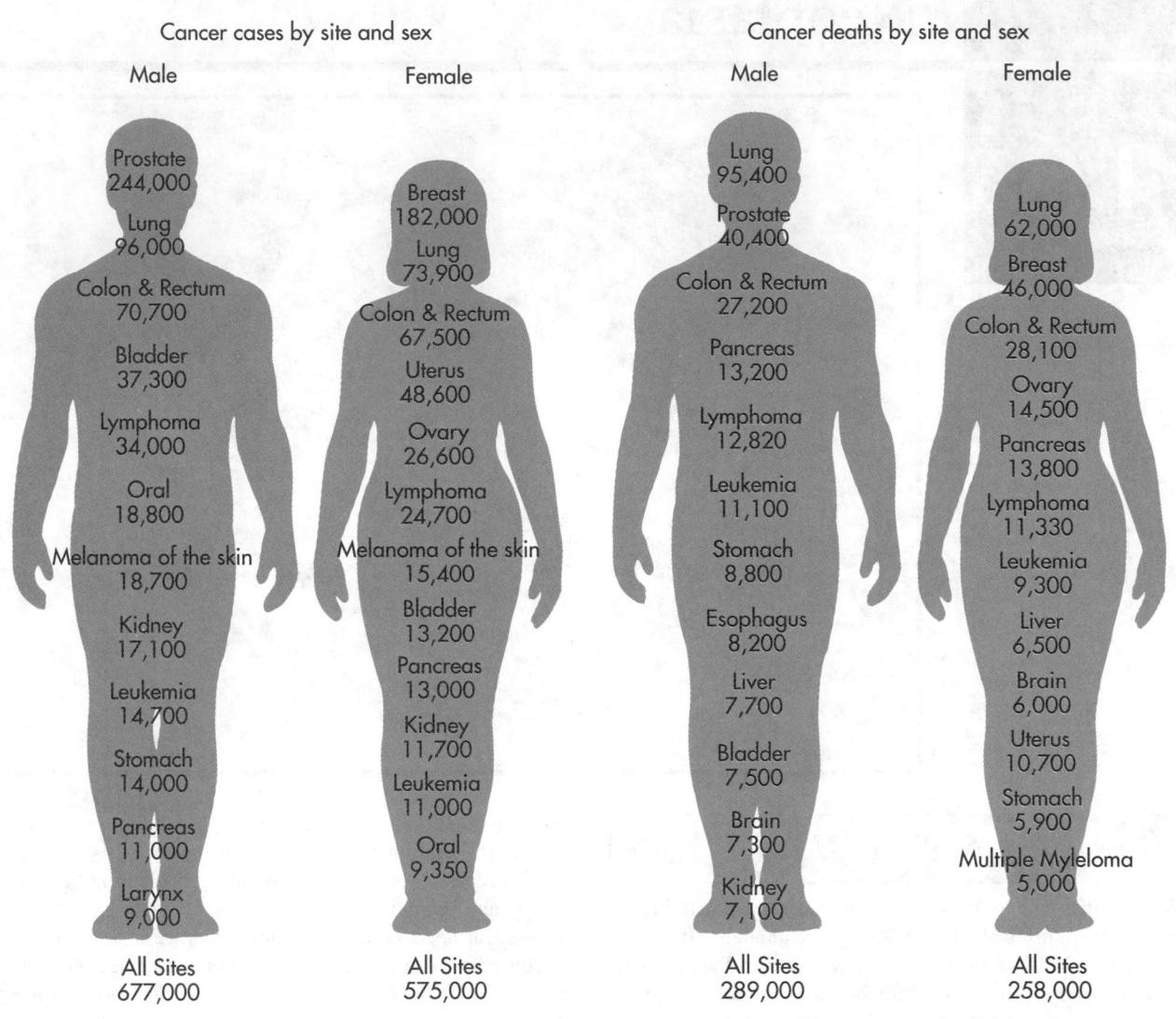

Figure 16-1 Cancer incidence and deaths by site and sex—1995 estimates. (*Excluding basal squamous cell skin cancer and carcinoma in situ.) (Data from American Cancer Society.[1])

proliferate without organization and often without differentiation. Certain stimuli are believed to initiate this process, which subsequently overpowers the normal control mechanism. The results are uninhibited growth (autonomy), uncontrolled function (anaplasia), and uncontrolled motility, permitting spread to other parts of the body (metastasis) via blood or the lymphatic system.

Normal cell division occurs in a pattern of sequential events referred to as the cell cycle. The stages of this cycle are mitosis and interphase. Mitosis, the actual growth phase, involves the cytoplasmic and nuclear separation within the cell, which results in two identical daughter cells containing the full complement of genetic information found in the parent cell. The interphase is the "resting stage" between cell divisions.

Neoplasia, a group of "new growth" cells, is the result of cells' unresponsiveness to the normal mechanisms of growth control. Cancer cells exhibit changes in the cytoplasm, including enzyme alterations, chromosome changes, and the produc-

tion of new proteins via an active anabolic process; mitochondrial changes, increased energy production to meet the neoplasm's increased rate of glucose utilization and lactic acid production; and nuclear changes in which DNA is altered.

Unique characteristics of neoplasms include their having more cells in active reproduction at a given time than do normal tissues, a shorter cell cycle time, and increased doubling time.

Neoplasms are described as benign or malignant. Benign tumors have little or no invasive activity, are generally encapsulated, usually grow more slowly, and are rarely fatal. Malignant tumors not only invade surrounding tissues but also produce metastases. If untreated, these tumors usually result in death.

The primary site of a malignant neoplasm is its place of origin, which is sometimes discovered after a secondary or metastatic site has been identified and diagnosed. The secondary site has characteristics similar to those of the primary site. Some people have additional primary sites, which may be

TABLE 16-1 Summary of American Cancer Society Recommendations for the Early Detection of Cancer in Asymptomatic Persons at Average Risk

Examination	Sex	Age	Periodicity
Sigmoidoscopy	M and F	50 yr and older	1 examination every 3 to 5 yr
Stool blood test	M and F	50 yr and older	Annual
Digital rectal examination	M and F	40 yr and older	Annual
Papanicolaou (Pap) and pelvic examinations	F	Women who have been sexually active or are age 18 yr or older	Annual. After 3 or more satisfactory, consecutive, normal annual examinations, the Pap test may be performed less frequently at the discretion of the physician
Endometrial tissue sample	F	At menopause; women at high risk*	At menopause
Breast self-examination*	F	20 yr and older	Monthly
Clinical breast examination	F	20-39 yr	Every 3 yr
		40 yr and older	Annual
Mammography	F	35-39 yr	Baseline
		40-49 yr	Every 1 to 2 yr
		50 yr and over	Annual
Health counseling†	M and F	20-40 yr	Every 3 yr
Cancer checkup‡	M and F	40 yr and older	Annual

From Holleb AI, Fink DJ, Murphy GE.[18]
*History of infertility, obesity, failure to ovulate, abnormal uterine bleeding, or estrogen therapy.
†To include counseling about tobacco control, sun exposure, diet and nutrition, risk factors, sexual practices, and environmental and other occupational exposures.
‡To include examination for cancers of the thyroid, testicles, prostate, ovaries, lymph nodes, oral cavity, and skin.

different types of cancer presenting different signs and symptoms at the same time (e.g., breast and ovarian cancers).

The malignant neoplasm's ability to invade surrounding tissues and to colonize distant sites is called metastasis. This may occur via direct extension, wherein the neoplasm expands, invades, and destroys normal adjacent tissue. The most frequent route is penetration of the lymphatic system and bloodstream, which enables cancer cells to disseminate throughout the body. Another less common route is penetration of body cavities, for example, dissemination through the cerebrospinal fluid or transabdominal spread within the peritoneal cavity.

There are numerous theories regarding the process of cancer invasion and metastasis. Some of these are (1) the mechanical theory, that the incidence and number of metastases are a function of the number and size of cells and cell groups gaining access to the circulation; (2) the "soil" theory, that metastasis is determined by the environment of the organs and tissues in which cancer cells arrive; (3) the intrinsic cellular factors theory, that tumor cell populations contain cell subpopulations with a high metastatic potential; and (4) the immunologic surveillance theory, that the formation of cancers and their spread is a result of a defect in the body's immunologic defense system.

The four types of cancer are carcinomas, usually solid tumors that arise from epithelial cells; sarcomas, derived from muscle, bone, and fat and other connective tissues; lymphomas, originating in lymphoid tissue; and leukemias, cancers of the hematologic system.

Some cancers can be prevented; for example, the risk of lung cancer can be virtually eliminated if a person stops smoking, and skin cancer can be prevented by avoiding overexposure to direct sunlight. These are both examples of primary preven-

CANCER'S SEVEN WARNING SIGNALS

1. Change in bowel or bladder habits
2. A sore that does not heal
3. Unusual bleeding or discharge
4. Thickening or lump in breast or elsewhere
5. Indigestion or difficulty in swallowing
6. Obvious change in wart or mole
7. Nagging cough or hoarseness

If you have a warning signal, see your doctor.

From American Cancer Society.[1]

tion, a process by which people avoid carcinogens. Secondary prevention is a process used to diagnose a cancer or its precursor as soon as possible after it develops. Breast self-examination and testicular self-examination are examples of secondary prevention (Table 16-1).

The American Cancer Society provides a list of persistent changes in normal physiologic functions that may indicate cancer; these changes are called cancer's seven warning signals (see box). Alterations in eating habits, loss of appetite, difficulty in swallowing, or increased constipation or diarrhea should be evaluated. The presence of a lump or nodule anywhere in or on the body (especially if it is painless and slowly increasing in size), bleeding from orifices, unexplained recurrent pain or fever, steady weight loss, and repeated infections are typical signs and symptoms of cancer that must be assessed. The nurse must stress primary and secondary prevention through public education, screening, and early detection activities.

····· Psychosocial Aspects of Cancer

Cancer evokes deep fears of pain, suffering, dependence, disfigurement, and death. Indeed, the fear of the disease is often so strong that a person may delay examination and diagnosis in hopes that the signs or symptoms will go away. This lag time between awareness of a problem and seeking medical attention can affect the impact of therapy and the prognosis. Thus awareness of attitudes toward cancer and efforts to influence them in a more hopeful direction through education are an important part of the nurse's role.

Variables that have been identified as shaping attitudes toward cancer are life experiences, especially those related to this disease; parental and cultural values and attitudes toward illness; society's emphasis on youth, health, and beauty; social pressures for early sexual experience, smoking, and other harmful behaviors; and portrayals of people with cancer in the mass media. Positive experiences and hopeful presentations of cancer and its treatment will give the individual, group, or community a clear perspective on the value of prevention, early diagnosis, and treatment.

Myths and Erroneous Beliefs

The following myths regarding cancer should be dispelled or at least clarified:

"Cancer is contagious." There is no clear evidence that this is true, although a human leukemic virus has been identified and some cancers do seem to occur with greater frequency in family members.

"All cancer patients have pain." Pain is highly variable and is related to the type, size, and location of the malignancy and the patient's pain tolerance.

"The treatment is worse than the disease because of disfiguring surgery and side effects of chemotherapy." This may be true in patients who are asymptomatic or relatively free of symptoms at the time of diagnosis.

"Sexual activity and other aspects of normal life must be forfeited." This is certainly not true if the patient and significant others are willing to consider modifications in lifestyle.

"Cancer is a death sentence." There are hundreds of thousands of cured cancer patients (almost 50% of people with cancer) in the United States today. With early diagnosis and treatment, most people with cancer could live long and productive lives.

The most common concerns of cancer patients are fear of alienation from family, friends, or health care providers; mutilation, particularly if surgery is the treatment of choice; vulnerability, dependence, or lack of control; and mortality. The emotional responses of a patient to these and other concerns related to the disease may be feelings of hopelessness, helplessness, guilt, denial, apathy, hostility, self-blame, withdrawal, and a sense of unreality. The nature and severity of these behaviors depend on the patient's usual behavior, attitudes toward illness in general and cancer in particular, the site of the disease, therapeutic options, and the expected outcome. All of these factors must be recognized as influencing the response of the patient and family.

Basic Needs and Responses

All people with cancer have certain basic needs that transcend their individual responses to cancer. These are:

To know what is happening and talk about its reality with someone who will listen

To participate in decisions affecting how they will live and die

To experience the pain of "feeling bad" rather than having to hide feelings from others

Not to be ignored are the effects of employability and insurability, potential loss of support systems, and the unfamiliarity of terms, procedures, drugs, and other aspects of therapy.

The ways in which patients cope with cancer are as varied as their reactions to the diagnosis. Some of the more positive coping strategies that have been identified and described by researchers include the following:

Seeking more information about the disease and its treatment

Using humor to lighten the situation

Using various distraction techniques

Sharing concerns with others, for example, in self-help groups

Negotiating feasible alternatives, such as treatment options

These coping strategies are generally considered less positive:

Reducing tension and anxiety with excessive drinking, drugs, or dangerous activities

Withdrawing into isolation

Blaming others, the situation, or a Supreme Being

Becoming fatalistic

Blaming self and expressing guilt feelings

Coping Strategies

The nurse and other health care providers should assess the patient's coping style, evaluate its effectiveness, and intervene when there is increasing distress or a continuing problem.

General nursing interventions that have been identified as helpful to cancer patients during the various stages of the illness include maintaining hope while avoiding false optimism, using a gentle, unhurried manner, expressing caring and concern, and focusing on the patient's strengths rather than weaknesses.

Many patients find self-help groups useful in dealing with the effects of cancer and its treatment. The value of receiving help from another person who has undergone a similar experience is well documented. The functions of such groups are to provide special information and successful coping techniques to people with similar problems, encouragement to maintain prescribed regimens, normalization of a behavior, and education of health care professionals and the public about cancer patients' special needs. The most useful aspects of this approach to coping are believed to be the modeling aspects ("You can do it—I did!") and the observation that helping someone else benefits the helper.

The family of the cancer patient may also need the assistance of health care team members. Factors to be assessed when determining the impact of cancer on the family include the age of the patient and other family members, family dynamics, communication style, family background, and practical matters of concern to the patient and family. Specific nursing interventions that are of value to the family are:

Giving the patient quality care

Communicating frequently with the family

Listening to the family

Making the family comfortable, such as by orientation to the institutional setting and policies

Referring the family to other members of the health care team as appropriate

Using touch to comfort family members as appropriate

Preparing the family for home care of the patient

Doing small things that are important to the family, such as rearranging a mealtime to permit a special dinner from home

Additional coping strategies that patients and their families may wish to learn about and use include relaxation exercises, meditation, imagery, self-hypnosis, music therapy, and humor. The nurse may serve as teacher or provide referral to resources for instruction in these techniques.

As previously mentioned, disfigurement is a particular concern of cancer patients. A change in body image may be actual (as with mastectomy) or perceived (as with hysterectomy). The visibility of the alteration may not affect the patient's reaction to it; perhaps of more significance is the function of the part or system and the patient's emotional attachment to it.

Patients may react to a change in body image in a variety of ways:

Denying the existence of the change, minimizing its presence, or deemphasizing its importance

Increased perception of phantom sensations

Use of unrealistic goal-setting

Use of inappropriate defenses, such as denial, inappropriate dress, self-imposed isolation, aggression, or dissociation

The nurse should help the patient develop more realistic responses to the change in body image. Some suggestions that may be beneficial to the patient include:

Resumption of prealteration life-style

Confinement of the effect of the disability to the area of loss

Emphasis on assets rather than liabilities

Solicitation of support from others

Reevaluation of personal and professional goals

Another area of concern to patients and their families that may be less readily discussed is sexuality and feelings regarding gender and gender role identity. Many beliefs (cultural, religious, personal, and societal) affect a person's ability to deal with an alteration in sexuality. These have been identified as especially influential:

The duty of a man to satisfy a woman and vice versa

The man as the aggressor and the woman as the passive recipient

The obsession of both sexes with performance

The use of sexual intercourse for procreation

These beliefs, as well as the other attitudes regarding masculine and feminine behaviors, may confuse and depress both the patient and partner. In addition, the symptoms of cancer, such as fatigue, malaise, fever, discharge, and odor, may ad-

versely affect libido and the patient's general view of his or her sexuality. This is further complicated by hospitalization, with the resultant lack of privacy.

The nurse's role in this sensitive area is to assess the patient's readiness to discuss sexual concerns, identify appropriate resources, provide oral and written information that will assist the patient in understanding sexual concerns and possible solutions, and respect the patient and partner's need for privacy.

Unproven Treatment Methods

Unproven methods of cancer treatment pose special challenges for both patient and nurse. These methods, which are touted as providing a high probability of cure, include a variety of machines and devices, drugs and chemicals, nutritional approaches, and psychologic techniques. The characteristics of unproven methods include a promoter with suspect credentials; no controlled studies of the treatment; an unscientific data base; the illusion of classified information; and an emphasis on the patient's freedom of choice and the availability of emotional support. The nurse's role in this domain includes assessing the presence of feelings of helplessness and hopelessness in the patient and pressure from family and friends to "keep trying," providing open communication with the patient and family regarding these issues, and providing information about and opportunities to discuss alternative therapies.

Informed Consent

The issue of informed consent often presents dilemmas for both the patient and nurse, especially if experimental therapy is being recommended. The nurse should serve as both teacher and advocate for the patient, who may need further explanation of the proposed procedure or protocol, answers to specific questions, or an opportunity to "think out loud." The consent process should include, at the least, the basic steps of explanation of the medical condition, explanation of the nature and purpose of the procedure or protocol, and explanation of the risks, alternatives, and consequences of the procedure or protocol.

If consent is to be informed there must be a patient of legal age and sound mind; a patient capable of cognition and reason; voluntariness; lack of coercion, deceit, or fraud; the right to refuse; comprehensible language; satisfactory answers to the patient's questions; and assurance of privacy and confidentiality.

Whatever the issue, the nurse should assess the patient's comprehension of the consent form, notify the physician if the patient is confused or ambivalent (unless a nursing procedure or protocol is being proposed), respect the individual's freedom of choice, and promote the patient's autonomy and independence in decision making.

Dying and Death

This section has included a few of the psychosocial issues confronting the cancer patient. Not discussed here but of equal concern is the experience of dying, which is faced by many cancer patients and their families. The nurse's support during this phase of the illness is invaluable. The hospice movement has been particularly useful to patients and their families who desire terminal care at home.

Meeting the psychosocial needs of the cancer patient and family is one of the greatest challenges facing the nurse. The roles of counselor, teacher, consultant, and resource person are used to their maximum to enhance the patient's and family's coping with this complex of diseases and therapies.

■ NORMAL FINDINGS

For assessment of a specific body system, see that chapter.

Area of Concern	Normal Adult Findings	
Respiratory rate	16-20 breaths/min	
Pulse rate	70-82 beats/min	
Blood pressure	18-44 yr	140/90 mm Hg
	45-64 yr	150/95 mm Hg
	65 yr and older	160/95 mm Hg
Temperature	36°-37.5° C (96.8°-99.5° F)	

CONDITIONS, DISEASES, AND DISORDERS

■ PRIMARY CARCINOMA OF THE LUNG

Carcinoma of the lung is an uncontrolled growth of anaplastic cells in the lung. Types are epidermoid (squamous cell), adenocarcinoma, small cell undifferentiated (oat cell), and large cell undifferentiated.

Carcinoma of the lung is the leading cause of death from cancer in men and women in the United States.[1] The incidence among women is steadily increasing, and more blacks than whites develop the disease. More than 90% of people with lung cancer will die of it.

Approximately 80% of lung tumors are linked to cigarette smoking. The people at highest risk began smoking in their teens, inhale deeply, and smoke at least half a pack a day. People who quit smoking have a gradual decline in risk, eventually reaching levels similar to those of nonsmokers. Passive smoking or side stream smoke contains as many, if not more, carcinogens than does inhaled smoke.

Another etiologic factor in the development of carcinoma of the lung is occupational exposure to such substances as asbestos, uranium, nickel, and chromate. Air pollutants have not yet been proved a cancer risk factor, but the incidence of the disease is higher in urban populations (see box).[3]

•••••• Pathophysiology

The length of time from a person's initial exposure to a carcinogen to the onset of lung cancer ranges from 10 to 30 years. A lesion detected by sputum cytologic study and found by fiberoptic bronchoscopy can be surgically resected and is potentially curable. This is not generally true of a lesion first found on a chest roentgenogram; the smallest detectable tumor on a roentgenogram is 1 cm.

The major histologic types of lung cancer are divided into two categories.

Non–small cell lung cancers (NSCLC) are usually not as aggressive as small cell lung cancers. However, for surgery, they have a limited potential response to treatment.

1. Squamous cell (epidermoid) tumors are the most common, comprising 35% of all lung tumors. Ninety percent occur in men. These tumors tend to be centrally located and often produce bronchial obstruction.
2. Adenocarcinoma is often located peripherally; it is a common scar carcinoma that arises in an area of fibrosis at the site of previous pulmonary damage. This cancer is less often associated with smoking than are the other types. These tumors frequently spread through the submucosal lymphatics to regional lymph nodes and often metastasize to the brain and other distant organs by vascular invasion.
3. Large cell undifferentiated tumors may appear in any area of the lung. This type tends to disseminate early in

---

■ FACTS ABOUT LUNG CANCER

Incidence: An estimated 169,900 new cases among men and women during 1995. While the incidence rate in men has been steadily declining to the present rate of 80 per 100,000, the rate is increasing in women to 42 per 100,000. Increased smoking among women is believed to be the major contributor to the rising incidence.

Mortality: An estimated 157,400 deaths in 1995. Since 1987, lung cancer in women has surpassed breast cancer as the leading cause of cancer death.

Warning Signals: Persistent cough, hemoptysis, chest pain, recurring pneumonia or bronchitis.

Risk Factors: Cigarette smoking remains the strongest risk factor. Exposure to certain industrial substances, such as arsenic, certain organic chemicals and asbestos, particularly for persons who smoke; radiation exposure from occupational, medical, and environmental sources. Risk increases further for cigarette smokers exposed to radon. Nonsmokers exposed to sidestream cigarette smoke are at an increased risk.

Early Detection: Due to the asymptomatic nature of early lung cancer, only 15% is detected in its initial stage. If smokers stop smoking when early precancerous cellular changes have occurred, damaged bronchial lining tissues frequently return to normal. Smokers who continue to smoke may form abnormal cell growth patterns leading to cancer. Diagnosis is made based on the findings of the chest x-ray, analysis of the types of cells contained in sputum, and fiberoptic examination of the bronchial passages.

Treatment: The type of lung cancer and its particular stage determines the treatment modality. Surgery is the treatment of choice for localized cancers. When the disease has spread, radiation and chemotherapy are often used in combination with surgery. Chemotherapy alone or in combination with radiation therapy is used in small cell lung cancer with a large percentage of patients experiencing remission.

From American Cancer Society.[1]

its course and is associated with a poor prognosis. Giant cell and clear cell carcinomas are subtypes.

Small cell lung cancer (SCLC), also called oat cell cancer, comprises 10% of lung tumors. It is the most aggressive cancer, with lymphatic and distant metastases usually present at the time of diagnosis. Paraneoplastic syndromes are more common with this type. It tends to be highly sensitive to both chemotherapy and radiation therapy.

All types have lymphatic metastasis early in the course of the disease, beginning in the bronchial and mediastinal nodes and extending upward to supraclavicular nodes and downward to nodes below the diaphragm and to the liver and adrenal glands. Distant metastasis via the bloodstream to brain, bones, and contralateral lung may occur.

A chronic cough and wheezing are the most common early symptoms; other symptoms are fatigue, chest tightness, and aching joints. Late but clinically significant signs include hemoptysis, clubbing of the fingers, weight loss, and pleural effusion. Invasion of the superior vena cava causes edema of the neck and face. Phrenic nerve involvement results in paralysis of the diaphragm. A superior sulcus tumor involving the brachial plexus may manifest as shoulder and arm pain and paresthesias.

The chest lesion may be relatively asymptomatic, with the chief complaint caused by metastatic disease. Metastasis to the brain may result in headache, unsteady gait, and other neurologic signs. Weight loss, jaundice, or anorexia may occur with liver involvement. Localized bone pain or pathologic fractures may accompany skeletal involvement.

Paraneoplastic syndromes may be associated with lung cancer. For example, inappropriate antidiuretic hormone (low serum sodium) or Cushing's syndrome from ectopic adrenocorticotropic hormone production occurs in some patients with small cell cancer. Other syndromes include hypercalcemia, resulting from production of ectopic parathormone-like substance (squamous cell cancer); carcinomatous neuropathy and myopathy; dermatomyositis; and hypertrophic pulmonary osteoarthropathy (see box).

Diagnostic Studies and Findings

Sputum cytologic study   Positive for malignant cells

Chest x-ray examination   Presence of tumor; invasion of chest wall or mediastinum

Computed tomogram of chest   Precise delineation of nodule, its density, and presence of calcium; invasion or compression of vascular structures; abnormal mediastinal lymph nodes

Computed tomogram of upper abdomen   Metastatic disease in liver or adrenal glands

Magnetic resonance imaging   Invasion or compression of vascular structures by tumor

Fluoroscopy   Paralysis and phrenic nerve involvement

Barium esophagram   Extension of tumor into central mediastinum

Bronchoscopy with bronchial brushing and biopsy   Presence of malignant cells

Mediastinoscopy and mediastinotomy   Presence of malignant cells in mediastinal lymph nodes

Transthoracic or transbronchial fine-needle aspiration Presence of malignant cells

Thoracentesis   Presence of malignant cells

Scalene or supraclavicular node biopsy   Presence of malignant cells in palpable lymph nodes

Bone marrow biopsy   Presence of malignant cells in centrally located small cell tumor

Pulmonary function tests   Reduction of 50% in predicted forced vital capacity (FEV_1), maximum voluntary ventilation (MVV), or vital capacity (VC)

Arterial blood gas analysis PaO_2 under 65 torr; $PaCO_2$ over 45 torr

Ventilation and perfusion radionuclide scanning   Little or no function in lung tissue to be resected

Abdominal computed tomography or ultrasound Metastatic disease to liver

Computed tomography or magnetic resonance imaging of brain   Metastatic disease to brain

Bone scan   Metastatic disease to bone

Multidisciplinary Plan

Surgery

Thoracotomy: an exploratory surgical incision of the chest wall during which a biopsy specimen is collected; ribs are spread and pleura is opened

Limited pulmonary resection (segmental, wedge)

Lobectomy: removal of a lobe of the lung and regional node dissection

---

PARANEOPLASTIC SYNDROMES ASSOCIATED WITH LUNG CANCER

Endocrine
  Antidiuretic hormone excess
  Cushing's syndrome
  Hypercalcemia
  Carcinoid syndrome
  Ectopic gonadotropin
Neuromuscular
  Myasthenia-like syndrome
  Subacute cerebellar degeneration
  Peripheral neuropathy
  Myopathy
Dermatologic
  Acanthosis nigricans
  Dermatomyositis
Skeletal
  Hypertrophic pulmonary osteoarthropathy
  Clubbing
Hematologic
  Anemia
  Intravascular coagulopathy
  Leukocytosis
  Red cell aplasia
Vascular
  Thrombophlebitis
  Nonbacterial endocarditis

From Holleb AI, Fink DJ, Murphy GP.[18]

Pneumonectomy: surgical removal of an entire lung

Extended resection: en bloc removal of portions of the chest wall, vertebral body, left atrium, and/or diaphragm

Resection of subcarinal, lobar, and mediastinal nodes

Surgical excision of solitary metastatic disease to brain

Review Thoracic Surgeries in Chapter 2

Radiation Therapy

External beam

Interstitial/endobronchial bradytherapy with ^{131}I

Chemotherapy

For Advanced Non–Small Cell Lung Cancer

VdP: vindesine, cisplatin (Platinol)

VbP: vinblastine, cisplatin (Platinol)

CAMP: cyclophosphamide, doxorubicin (Adriamycin), methotrexate, procarbazine

MVbP: mitomycin, vinblastine, cisplatin (Platinol)

PtVP-16: etoposide [VP-16] cisplatin

CAP: cyclophosphamide, doxorubicin (Adriamycin), cisplatin (Platinol)

CBP: cyclophosphamide, bleomycin, cisplatin (Platinol)

FOMi: 5-fluorouracil, vincristine (Oncovin), mitomycin-C

For Small Cell Lung Cancer

CAV: cyclophosphamide, doxorubicin (Adriamycin), vincristine

CEA: cyclophosphamide, etoposide, doxorubicin (Adriamycin)

CEV: cyclophosphamide, etoposide [VP-16], vincristine

EVAC: etoposide [VP-16], vincristine, doxorubicin (Adriamycin), cyclophosphamide

Hansen's: cyclophosphamide, lomustine, vincristine, methotrexate

Hansen's VP: cyclophosphamide, lomustine, vincristine, etoposide [VP-16]

VP-16 + P: etoposide [VP-16], cisplatin (Platinol)

Biological Response Modifiers

Monoclonal antibody KC4 for non–small cell lung cancer

Endobronchial Laser Therapy

Photodynamic Therapy (PDT)

Sclerosis

For the Treatment of Malignant Pleural Effusion

The prognosis for people with lung cancer is correlated with tumor cell type. Those with well-differentiated squamous cell cancer have the best chance of survival; those with undifferentiated small cell cancer have the poorest. Peripheral tumors are more curable than central lesions. The presence of lymph node and distant metastases reduces the chance of cure. The stage of disease, patient's performance status, and immunologic state of the patient are important prognostic signs. Patients with gross supraclavicular adenopathy, a malignant pleural effusion, mas-

sive local extension, or distant metastases usually survive less than 1 year.

NURSING CARE

Nursing Assessment

Respiratory Function

Chronic cough, nonproductive or productive; wheezing; chest tightness; hemoptysis; dyspnea; hoarseness; change in sputum amount or odor; orthopnea; tachypnea; hemoptysis, frequent upper respiratory tract infections

Comfort Level

Clubbed fingers; chest pain; chest tightness; shoulder and arm pain with paresthesia

Systemic Function

Fatigue; weight loss; edema of neck and face; anorexia; fever; activity intolerance

Psychosocial

Fear

Nursing Dx & Intervention for Untreatable Tumors (see also section on Metastatic Disease and Terminal Stage of the Disease)

Ineffective airway clearance related to bronchial obstruction secondary to tumor invasion

- Place patient in sitting position and change position frequently *to enhance breathing.*
- Encourage coughing and deep breathing with splinting of chest *to relieve congestion.*
- Ambulate patient as soon as possible *to increase circulation and chest expansion.*
- Encourage fluids *to liquefy secretions.*

Ineffective breathing pattern related to discomfort and lack of pulmonary expansion

- Administer oxygen therapy as prescribed *to maintain adequate tissue oxygenation.*
- Anticipate patient's needs *to decrease unnecessary energy expenditure.*
- Inspect chest for respiratory rate and rhythm and symmetric expansion *to determine adequacy of pulmonary function.*
- Auscultate for abnormal breath sounds, lung aeration, rales, and rhonchi *to detect ventilatory problems.*
- Percuss chest for abnormal resonance or decreased diaphragmatic descent *to detect ventilatory problems.*
- Monitor blood studies for abnormal gas exchange *to detect inadequate oxygenation.*
- Observe for cyanosis and change in amount or character of sputum *as signs of respiratory failure or infection.*

- Discourage smoking *to decrease pulmonary workload.*

Altered nutrition: less than body requirements related to fatigue and dyspnea

- Assess dietary habits and needs *to help individualize the patient's diet.*
- Weigh patient weekly *to note any weight gain, an indication of improved nutrition.*
- Auscultate bowel sounds *to document gastrointestinal peristalsis.*
- Assess psychologic factors (e.g., depression, anger) *to identify the effect of psychologic factors that may decrease food and fluid intake.*
- Monitor albumin and lymphocytes *to determine if visceral protein needed for the immune system is adequate.*
- Measure mid-arm circumference and triceps skinfold *to determine protein and fat stores, which indicate presence of malnutrition.*
- Provide oxygen to patient while eating as ordered *to reduce dyspnea by reducing the work of breathing.*
- Encourage oral care before meals *to remove taste of sputum that may reduce appetite.*
- Position patient *to facilitate breathing thereby improving appetite.*
- Provide frequent small feedings *to lessen fatigue.*
- Administer antiemetics before meals *to reduce nausea that may interfere with eating.*
- Provide soft foods and liquids *to lessen energy required to eat, thereby reducing oxygen requirement.*
- Provide high-protein diet *to support immune system.*
- Administer vitamins as ordered *to supplement diet.*

Activity intolerance related to generalized weakness

- Provide progressive increase in activity as tolerated *to slowly increase the number of and endurance of activities (as tolerance allows) to promote as much independence as possible.*
- Provide oxygen as needed *to decrease work of breathing during activity.*
- Instruct patient and family in use of equipment *to ensure proper use and decrease frustration of users.*
- Keep frequently used objects within reach *for patient's convenience and to decrease oxygen demand.*
- Problem solve with patient to determine methods of conserving energy while performing tasks (e.g., sit on stool while shaving; dry skin after bath by wrapping in terrycloth robe instead of drying skin with a towel *to use less oxygen thereby producing less carbon dioxide.*

Patient Education/Home Care Planning

1. Discourage smoking by the patient and family or significant others.
2. Explain how to cough productively and to perform breathing exercises and other respiratory therapy as prescribed to maintain pulmonary function.

3. Help the patient ambulate, and instruct the patient in the use of assistive devices such as canes and walkers to maintain mobility.
4. Explain how to self-administer medication for pain to maintain comfort.
5. Inform the patient of the need for adequate nutrition (high-calorie, high-protein diet) to maintain energy.
6. Inform the patient of the signs and symptoms of complications or adverse reactions to chemotherapy, radiation therapy, or both so that they can be treated immediately.
7. Help the patient identify resources and support systems to help in rehabilitation and maintenance of quality of life.
8. Alert the patient to the signs and symptoms of recurrence or metastatic disease, such as shoulder or arm pain, superior vena cava syndrome, liver disease, and central nervous system changes, so that they can be treated as soon as possible.

Evaluation

Airway is patent   Airways are clear and breathing occurs without secretions; clear breath sounds; on chest x-ray examination, lungs are clear; cough is subsided.

Nutritional status has improved   Weight gain is present; patient is eating a balanced diet; albumin equals 3.2-4.5 g/dl, lymphocytes equal 2100 or 35%-40% per mm³ blood; triceps skinfold equals 12 mm for men or 23.0 mm for women; midarm circumference equals 32.7 cm for men or 29.2 cm for women.

CANCERS OF THE COLON AND RECTUM

Cancer of the colon and rectum is an uncontrolled growth of anaplastic cells in the colon or rectum. Types are adenocarcinoma, carcinoid tumor, leiomyosarcoma, and lymphoma (see box on p. 1288).

•••••• Pathophysiology

The most common symptom of colorectal cancer is rectal bleeding, followed by changes in bowel pattern (constipation or diarrhea), excessive flatus, distention, cramps, obstruction, and unexplained anemia. The presence of symptoms depends on the location of the tumor. Left-sided colonic lesions present as altered bowel habits, decreased stool caliber (pencil-like), urgency to defecate, vague abdominal pain, and hemorrhoids. Right-sided colonic lesions may manifest as unexplained iron deficiency anemia and gastrointestinal tract bleeding. Tumors of the sigmoid are characterized by obstruction from napkin ring growth. Rectal tumors are evidenced by gross rectal blood and tenesmus with a feeling of incomplete evacuation.

The majority of colorectal cancers are adenocarcinomas; others are carcinoid tumors, leiomyosarcomas, and lymphomas. Regional lymph nodes are involved in at least half of

COLORECTAL CANCER

Incidence: An estimated 138,200 new cases among men and women during 1995. Of these new cases, 100,000 will be colon cancer and 38,200 rectal cancer.

Mortality: An estimated 47,500 from colon cancer and 7,800 from rectal cancer in 1995. For women, the mortality rate from colorectal cancer has dropped 29%, and for men 7% over the past 30 years.

Warning Signals: Rectal bleeding, blood in the stool, changes in bowel habits (constipation or diarrhea).

Risk Factors: Familial polyposis of the colon or rectum, chronic ulcerative colitis, diverticulosis, and villous adenomas of the colon. A high fat and/or low-fiber diet may play some role in increasing the risk to develop colorectal cancer.

Early Detection: The American Cancer Society recommends a yearly digital rectal examination after age 40; beginning at age 50, a yearly fecal occult blood testing and a sigmoidoscopy every three years are recommended. Should these tests identify abnormalities, flexible colonoscopies and barium enemas may be required.

Treatment: Surgery remains the mainstay of therapy for colorectal cancer. In some cases, adjuvant radiation therapy may be employed. Chemotherapy, either alone or in combination with surgery and/or radiation therapy, for advanced disease is presently under study. Postoperative patients with cancerous lymph nodes have benefitted from combinations of chemotherapy and immunologic agents.

From American Cancer Society.[1]

the patients. Most colon cancers spread to periaortic nodes. Anal carcinomas spread into perineal nodes. Distant metastasis is most often to the liver and lungs.

The 5-year survival rate for patients with localized disease is 88% for colon tumors. This rate is reduced by half with regional or distant involvement. The earlier the diagnosis and treatment, the more curable the cancer. Even with a large tumor and invasion of adjacent structures, the prognosis is favorable if appropriate treatment is provided. Only the presence of distant metastases precludes the possibility of cure.

•••••• Diagnostic Studies and Findings

Digital rectal examination Palpation of suspect lesion

Fiberoptic colonoscopy Visualization and biopsy of suspect lesion

Barium enema Visualization of suspect lesion

Testing of stool for occult blood Presence of blood may be indicative of ulcerating malignancy

Carcinoembryonic antigen Elevated

Hematocrit Lower than normal as the result of blood loss

•••••• Multidisciplinary Plan

Surgery

Local excision of well-differentiated rectal cancers

Resection of primary colon lesion with all mesentery that contains lymph nodes to which tumor is likely to spread; end-to-end anastomosis (is only curative treatment)

En bloc resection of colon, small bowel, bladder, uterus, and/or ovaries

Surgical bypass for inoperable obstructing tumors, with creation of fecal stoma

Review Abdominal Surgeries for the Gastrointestinal Tract in Chapter 8

Radiation Therapy

Intraoperative radiation therapy

Radiation seeds

External beam therapy for inoperable obstructing rectal tumors

Transanal irradiation

Postoperative adjuvant therapy with radiation sensitizers for tumors dissecting the bowel wall or with positive lymph nodes

Palliation

Chemotherapy

Adjuvant regimen of 5-fluorouracil (5FU) with Levamisole

Radiation sensitization with 5-fluorouracil and metronidazole

Endoscopic Laser

For inoperable obstructing rectal tumors

NURSING CARE

Nursing Assessment

Gastrointestinal Function

Right colon—anemia, weight loss, abdominal pain, nausea, vomiting

Sigmoid—bleeding, obstruction

Left colon—mucous stool, constipation, intermittent abdominal pain

Rectal—bleeding, diarrhea, abdominal and/or low back pain, incomplete evacuation

Psychosocial

Fear

Nursing Dx & Intervention for Untreatable Tumors (see section on Metastatic Disease and Terminal Stage of the Disease)

Constipation related to colorectal obstruction by tumor

- Ambulate patient frequently, and encourage moderate physical exercise *to enhance gastrointestinal (GI) motility.*
- Encourage increased intake of high-bulk foods and fluids; give fresh fruits, prune juice, hot coffee, and warm liquids *to increase GI motility.*

- Place patient in sitting position *to relieve abdominal pressure.*
- Give stool softeners and laxatives *to enhance elimination.*
- Administer enemas *top cleanse bowel.*
- Measure intake and output *to monitor hydration and quantity of feces.*

Diarrhea related to colorectal obstruction by tumor

- Provide fluids so intake equals output *to prevent dehydration.*
- Cover patient with warm blankets *to prevent loss of body heat.*
- Encourage adequate rest *to decrease energy expenditure.*
- Discourage oral stimulants, *which increase GI motility.*
- Discourage intake of high-bulk foods, *which increase GI motility.*
- Give tea, carbonated beverages, clear-liquid or full-liquid diet *to maintain hydration.*
- Administer antidiarrheal drugs as ordered *to control diarrhea.*
- Refrain from giving hot or iced liquids, enemas, or laxatives, *which irritate bowel.*
- Refrain from inserting rectal tube or taking rectal temperatures, *which irritate bowel.*
- Check for impaction; employ caution with pancytopenic patients *to prevent bleeding.*
- Auscultate abdomen for abnormal bowel sounds *to assess GI status.*
- Measure body weight and intake and output *to monitor hydration and nutrition.*
- Monitor blood studies for acid-base and electrolyte abnormalities resulting from loss of electrolytes and acid *caused by diarrhea.*
- Be alert for complaints of pain caused by abdominal cramping or anal irritation, *which may be precursors to diarrhea.*

Pain related to abdominal distention

- Change patient's position frequently; increase movement if tolerated *to relieve distention.*
- Discourage smoking, *which may increase distention.*
- Give small, frequent feedings *to prevent further distention.*
- Encourage decreased intake of gas-forming foods *to prevent further distention.*
- Restrict liquids at mealtime; give warm liquids after meals *to relax abdomen.*
- Refrain from giving iced liquids and carbonated beverages, *which increase cramping.*
- Avoid use of straws and swallowing air *because this causes gas formation in GI tract.*
- Give nonprescription drugs, such as simethicone, *to relieve flatus.*
- Encourage moderate physical activity *to relieve pressure on abdomen.*
- Remove restrictive clothing *to relieve pressure on abdomen.*

- Inspect abdomen for distention *to determine need for further intervention.*
- Auscultate abdomen for abnormal bowel sounds *to assess effect of therapy.*

Pain related to cramping

- Encourage decreased intake of fatty foods *to decrease formation of flatus.*
- Give bland foods *to relieve GI irritation.*
- Apply heat to abdomen *to relax abdomen and relieve cramping.*
- Involve patient in selection of other pain measures *to enhance comfort and patient's participation in care.*
- Evaluate effectiveness of pain relief measures *to determine need for further intervention.*

Pain (rectal) related to pressure/irritation from tumor

- Position patient comfortably *to relieve pressure.*
- Apply warm, moist compress to rectal area, or provide Sitz bath *to relax anal sphincter.*
- Increase fluid intake to 2000 ml daily *to maintain soft stool.*
- Encourage decreased intake of high-bulk food *to relieve GI distention.*
- Involve patient in selection of pain relief measures *to enhance comfort.*
- Evaluate pain for duration, intensity, and quality *to determine intervention needed.*
- Evaluate effectiveness of pain relief measures *to determine need for further intervention.*

Fluid volume deficit related to blood loss through rectum

- Apply ice bag to rectal area *to enhance vasoconstriction.*
- Change patient's position slowly *to avoid vascular trauma.*
- Cover patient with warm blankets *to maintain warmth and comfort.*
- Maintain complete bed rest if bleeding is severe *to avoid excessive blood loss.*
- Elevate foot of bed *to maintain blood flow to vital organs.*
- Refrain from giving enemas or laxatives, inserting rectal tube, or taking rectal temperature *to avoid tissue trauma and bleeding.*
- Estimate blood volume loss *to determine replacement need.*
- Monitor blood pressure and blood studies *to determine blood volume.*

Patient Education/Home Care Planning

1. Inform the patient of the need to maintain adequate gastrointestinal function.
2. Instruct the patient in pain relief measures.

3. Explain bowel changes (such as bleeding) the patient should report.
4. Instruct the patient in the care of an ostomy if present.
5. Help the patient plan an adequate and appropriate diet.
6. Help the patient contact resources and support groups, such as the United Ostomy Association.

Evaluation

Bowel elimination is normal Stools are soft and formed. Abdomen is soft and not distended. Patient reports regular bowel movements.

Pain is not reported Patient expresses comfort and freedom from pain.

There is no evidence of rectal bleeding Vital signs are within normal limits. Stool occult blood test results are negative. Blood counts are within normal limits. Patient reports usual energy and activity levels.

■ CARCINOMA OF THE BREAST

Carcinoma of the breast is an uncontrolled growth of anaplastic cells in the breast. Types include ductal, lobular, and nipple adenocarcinomas.

Although lung cancer is increasing in prevalence, the breast is the most common site of cancer in women between 25 and 75 years of age. Each year breast cancer is diagnosed in approximately 150,000 women in the United States, and it is the leading cause of death in women 40 to 44 years of age. One of every nine women will be diagnosed with breast cancer during her lifetime. Elderly women (those over 65 years of age) have twice the incidence of breast cancer of younger women. Breast cancer also develops infrequently in men. Symptoms and treatment are the same for men and women.

Most breast lesions are first detected by a woman during breast self-examination (see illustration) or by her sexual partner. The possibility for cure is 85% for women with localized disease at the time of diagnosis. Half of breast cancers are in the upper outer quadrant, 20% in the central portion, 20% in the medial quadrants, and 10% in the lower outer quadrant.

Risk factors that have been cited in the incidence of breast cancer include previous breast cancer, a family history of breast cancer, nulliparity, or a first pregnancy after 30 years of age. Irradiation, particularly as therapy for postpartum mastitis or as multiple chest fluoroscopies, is believed to contribute to breast cancer development. Obesity and total fat content in the diet, especially animal fat, may be factors. Total lifetime exposure to endogenous estrogen is a major risk factor. This disease is more common among white women, but the incidence among blacks is rising (see the box for general information on breast cancer).

■ FACTS ABOUT BREAST CANCER

Incidence: An estimated 182,000 new cases among women in the United States during 1995. Approximately one of every nine women will develop breast cancer during her lifetime. Breast cancer occurs rarely in men. Breast cancer incidence rates have increased about 2% a year since 1980, going from 84.8 per 100,000 in 1980 to 109.5 in 1988. Some of this increase is believed to be due to screening programs detecting tumors before they become clinically apparent. Other reasons for the increase are not fully understood.

Mortality: An estimated 46,240 deaths (46,000 women; 240 men) in 1995; in women, the second major cause of cancer death. Although incidence rates are increasing, early detection and improved treatment have kept mortality fairly stable over the past 50 years.

Warning Signals: Breast changes that persist, such as a lump, thickening, swelling, dimpling, skin irritation, distortion, retraction, scaliness, pain, or tenderness of the nipple.

Risk Factors: Over 50 years of age; personal or family history of breast cancer; never had children; first childbirth after 30 years of age.

Early Detection: The American Cancer Society recommends a mammogram every year for asymptomatic women 50 years of age and older; women should have a screening mammogram by 40 years of age; women 40 to 49 years old should have a mammogram every 1 to 2 years. In addition, a clinical physical examination of the breast is recommended every 3 years for women 20 to 40 years of age and every year for those over 40 years of age. The Society also recommends monthly breast self-examination as a routine good health habit for women 20 years of age or older. Most breast lumps are not cancer, but only a physician can make a diagnosis.

Besides its effectiveness in screening asymptomatic women, mammography is recognized as a valuable diagnostic technique for women who do have findings suggestive of breast cancer. Once a breast lump is found, mammography can help determine if there are other lesions too small to be felt in the same or opposite breast. All suspicious lumps should undergo biopsy for a definitive diagnosis, even when the mammography findings are described as normal.

Treatment: Taking into account the medical situation and the patient's preferences, treatment may require lumpectomy (local removal of the tumor), mastectomy (surgical removal of the breast), radiation therapy, chemotherapy, or hormone manipulation therapy. Often, two or more methods are used in combination.

From American Cancer Society.[1]

••••• Pathophysiology

Most breast malignancies occur in the upper outer quadrant. More than 75% of breast cancers are invasive ductal carcinomas, usually presenting as a single, unilateral, solid, irregular, poorly delineated, nonmobile, painless mass. This type grows as a fibrotic, stellate mass with long tentacled extensions that radiate from a central dense core, invading and distorting surrounding breast structures.

The mean diameter of a lesion detected by a woman on self-examination is 3 to 3.5 cm, a size associated with a greater than 50% incidence of occult axillary lymph node metastases.

• • • • • Diagnostic Studies and Findings

Clinical examination Palpation of lesion(s), usually a painless mass or thickening; restricted mobility of lesion; changes in skin texture (i.e., dimpling, orange peel); skin edema; discoloration of skin; dilated superficial blood vessels; change in breast size, shape, contour; nipple discharge; nipple retraction

Mammogram Solid nodule with ill-defined borders; clustered microcalcifications

Thermography Thermal "hot spot"

Biopsy

Lesion: Evidence of malignant cells

Axillary lymph nodes: Evidence of malignant cells

Estrogen receptors and progestin receptors <3 fmol/mcp receptor negative tumor; >10 fmol/mcp receptor positive tumor

Carcinoembryonic antigen (CEA) Elevated in metastatic liver disease

S phase index >5%-8%

Ploidy Aneuploid DNA

• • • • • Multidisciplinary Plan

Surgery

Lumpectomy: wide excision and removal of tumor and margin of healthy tissue

Partial mastectomy: simple excision of tumor and wider margin of healthy tissue

Quadrantectomy: removal of one quarter of breast

Mastectomy

  Subcutaneous: removal of all breast tissue while preserving overlying skin and nipple-areolar complex

  Total (simple): complete removal of breast tissue and tail of Spence

  Modified radical: removal of breast and axillary lymph nodes

  Radical: removal of breast, underlying pectoral muscles, and axillary nodes

  Superradical: removal of internal mammary lymphatic chain with breast, pectoral muscles, and axillary lymph nodes

Breast reconstruction

Radiation Therapy

Brachytherapy: implantation of radioactive sources

Teletherapy: use of external beam (photon or electron)

Regional node irradiation

Adjuvant Therapy

Combination chemotherapy

  CMF: cyclophosphamide, methotrexate, 5-fluorouracil

  CMFVP: CMF with vincristine and prednisone

  CA: cyclophosphamide, doxorubicin (Adriamycin)

  CAF: cyclophosphamide, doxorubicin (Adriamycin), 5-fluorouracil

Antiestrogen therapy (ablative)

  Tamoxifen citrate

Estrogens (additive)

  Diethylstilbestrol

  Ethinyl estradiol

Androgens (additive)

  Fluoxymesterone

  Testosterone

  Methyltestosterone

Progestins (additive)

  Megestrol acetate

  Medroxyprogesterone acetate

Patients with stage I tumors and no involvement of axillary nodes have a 10-year survival rate of greater than 80%; those with stage II tumors have greater than 60% 10-year survival rate; if the lymph nodes are involved, the 10-year survival rate is 30% to 40% in the absence of adjuvant chemotherapy. Recent studies have shown that patients whose cancers are estrogen receptor protein negative have a much poorer prognosis. Patients with stage IV disease have a 10-year survival rate of less than 10%.

Follow-up care includes early detection of second primary breast cancers and recurrent disease. Breast self-examination, annual mammography, and physician's examination of the intact breast and nodes are important. Rehabilitation is an essential intervention after primary treatment.

NURSING CARE

Nursing Assessment

Skin

Presence of redness, warmth

Open wound

Tenderness

Drainage—serous, serosanguineous

Flaking, peeling

Swelling, such as in the arm on the affected side

Vital Signs

Tachycardia; hypertension; altered respiratory rate

Psychosocial

Fear; anxiety; withdrawal; avoidance of physical intimacy; restlessness; fight or flight behavior; increased alertness; indecision

Pain

Localized at site of surgical incision or radiation

Nursing Dx & Intervention

Risk for impaired skin integrity related to surgery, node dissection, or radiation therapy

- Cleanse skin frequently *to prevent infection.*
- Apply warm, moist compresses *to promote circulation and drainage.*
- Apply antibiotic ointment and sterile dressing *to prevent infection.*
- Expose draining area to air (depending on patient's immunocompetence) *to promote healing.*
- Elevate arm *to enhance venous return.*
- Observe for increased or change in drainage character, skin changes (color, dimpling), swelling, or skin lesions *to detect infection or further breakdown of skin.*

Pain related to surgery or node dissection

- Administer analgesic as prescribed *to relieve pain.*
- Monitor pain character, intensity, and frequency *to evaluate effect of analgesic and determine need for change in amount, route, or frequency of administration.*
- Teach patient to use relaxation, guided imagery, and diversional activities *to enhance analgesic effect or to decrease need for analgesic.*
- Use massage, heat, or cold as appropriate *to increase comfort.*

Body image disturbance related to alteration in or loss of breast

- Help patient to identify personal meaning of loss of breast *to clarify fears, concerns, and needs.*
- Encourage patient to discuss change in body with husband or significant other *to use social support.*
- Refer patient to appropriate resources (i.e., health care providers, support group) *to provide external support.*

Decisional conflict related to treatment options

- Give nonjudgmental explanation of alternatives *to enable patient to select option consistent with values and expectations.*
- Use objective, factual materials such as reports *to enable patient to select option consistent with values and expectations.*
- Encourage patient to discuss options with family or significant others *to enable patient to select option consistent with values and expectations.*
- Provide sufficient time for making decisions.

Fear related to nature of cancer

- Encourage patient to talk about specific fears and feelings about fears *to help patient clarify what fears are.*
- Help patient identify previously helpful coping skills *to use in present situation.*
- Teach patient newer coping skills *to add to choices.*
- Deal with distorted perceptions and misinformation *to dispel misconceptions.*
- Encourage patient's use of such comfort measures as music, religious practices, and presence of family and friends *to distract self from focusing on fears.*

Patient Education/Home Care Planning

1. Explain how to care for skin overlying breast to prevent infection and ulceration.
2. Explain how to assess the body for further breast disease or evidence of spread by performing breast self-examination.
3. Explain use of nonpharmacologic interventions for coping with pain and fear.
4. Provide information about resources and support systems, such as Reach to Recovery of the American Cancer Society.

Evaluation

Skin is intact and free of infection in the area of disruption   Skin is clean, dry, and warm, with normal color and turgor.

Patient is free of pain   Patient's facial expression is calm, relaxed. Patient expresses comfort. Vital signs are within normal limits.

Patient accepts change in body image   Patient expresses acceptance of altered body image and altered self-concept.

Course of action is selected and implemented   Patient expresses that informed decision is consistent with personal values.

Fears have been resolved   Patient acknowledges fears of suffering and dying. Patient is able to focus on need for further treatment and/or follow-up.

CANCERS OF THE URINARY TRACT

■ RENAL TUMORS

Renal cancer is an uncontrolled growth of anaplastic cells of the kidney. Types include hypernephroma, parenchymal tumors, papillary tumors, and nephrotic carcinomas.

Renal cancer usually occurs in people over 40 years of age. It is twice as common in men as in women. Signs and symptoms develop late in the course of the disease; the most common sign is painless, intermittent hematuria.

•••••• Pathophysiology

Hypernephroma, or adenocarcinoma of the renal parenchyma, is the most common renal neoplasm in adults. It grows slowly but may metastasize at any stage. Metastasis via the bloodstream results in spread to the lungs, bone, regional lymph nodes, liver, and other visceral organs. Parenchymal tumors infiltrate more rapidly than hypernephroma and have a poor prognosis. Papillary tumors of the renal pelvis (transitional cell, squamous cell, adenocarcinoma) are usually multiple, involving the ureter and often the bladder and lymphatics.

Nephrotic carcinomas are usually large and encapsulated; as many as 50% may perforate the apparently intact capsule. Hematogenous metastasis results from early invasion of renal venules. The neoplasm often extends into the renal vein and vena cava. Distant metastases occur in the lung, lymph nodes, liver, bone, adrenal gland, opposite kidney, brain, and heart.

The kidney is the site of more metastatic than primary tumors. The most frequent sites of origin are the lung and breast.

The etiologic factors are unclear. Some studies have suggested a relationship between smoking and renal pelvis carcinoma. Persons with acquired cystic disease caused by renal failure are also prone to renal cell cancer. The autosomal dominant hereditary von Hippel-Lindau disease is frequently associated with renal carcinoma. Some renal pelvic tumors may occur as a result of chronic inflammation and irritation secondary to renal calculi. Hormones and radiation may also play a role in the development of renal cancer.

•••••• Diagnostic Studies and Findings

Urinalysis   Red blood cells

Excretory urography   Space-occupying mass with pelvocalyceal displacement and alteration of renal contour; filling defect in pelvocalyceal system

Nephrotomography   Presence of solid tumor

Retrograde pyelogram   Filling defect

Renal ultrasound   Presence of solid tumor

Renal computed tomogram   Presence of solid tumor, enlarged regional lymph nodes

Renal magnetic resonance imaging   Renal vein or vena caval involvement

Selective renal arteriography   Neovasculature

Venacavography   Shows extent of lesion in renal vein or vena cava

Fine-needle aspiration of avascular cystic masses, with cytologic studies and use of contrast medium   Presence of malignant cells; space-occupying mass

Abdominal computed tomography   Shows density and size of tumor, extent of local invasion, vena caval or renal vein involvement, metastases

•••••• Multidisciplinary Plan

Surgery

Radical nephrectomy (abdominotransperitoneal or thoracoabdominal approaches)

Lymphadenectomy (controversial)

Palliative nephrectomy for bleeding and pain control

Resection of solitary metastatic site, such as in brain or liver

Bilateral tumors

Nephrectomy of larger tumor and partial nephrectomy for smaller lesion in bilateral disease

Bilateral nephrectomies and chronic hemodialysis or peritoneal dialysis; later transplantation

Nephroureterectomy for renal pelvis carcinomas

Refer to Other Kidney Surgery on p. 983

Radiation Therapy

Used in treatment of local recurrences or symptomatic bony tumor

Postoperative irradiation for residual or recurrent tumor

Chemotherapy

Hormonal therapy with progesterone (Depo-Provera, Megace), testosterone, antiestrogens

Vinblastine

Biologic Response Modifiers

Alpha interferon, interleukin 2 (IL-2) with lymphokine-activated killer (LAK) cells

Autolymphocyte therapy with supernumerary lymphormones

Improved survival rates (5-year survival of 65% for early hypernephroma) have been attributed to thoracoabdominal nephrectomy with node dissection and earlier diagnosis of "incidental" carcinomas. Reports of spontaneous regression prompted investigational therapy with biologic response modifiers.

NURSING CARE

Nursing Assessment

Urinary Function

Painless hematuria; urinary retention

Comfort

Chronic aching pain; renal colic; nerve pain

Nursing Dx & Intervention for Untreatable Tumor (see also section on Metastatic Disease and Terminal Stage of the Disease)

Fluid volume deficit related to renal irritation by tumor as evidenced by gross hematuria

- Observe characteristics (particularly color) and amount of urine *to determine need for fluid and blood component replacement.*
- Monitor vital signs at frequent intervals during episodes of gross hematuria *to detect shock early.*
- Encourage patient to drink large volumes of fluid *to prevent dehydration.*
- Monitor input and output and urine specific gravity *to detect renal function and to monitor its progression.*
- Administer IV fluids as prescribed *to replace lost fluid volume.*
- Monitor laboratory reports *to detect development of anemia.*

- Observe for signs and symptoms of worsening fluid volume deficit, including decreased urine output, concentrated urine, output greater than intake, weakness, and changes in mental status *to determine the need for rapid infusions of large volumes of IV fluids and blood components.*

Pain related to progressive disease in kidney, such as passage of blood clots or obstruction of the ureteropelvic junction as evidenced by complaints of flank pain, palpable mass

- Assess patient's pain history, including previous analgesic use, *to determine previously effective medications.*
- Assess location, onset, duration, radiation, and intensity of pain *to determine appropriate interventions.*
- Provide prescribed medications for pain as needed *to decrease patient's discomfort.*
- Teach patient self-care strategies, such as relaxation exercises, imagery, and application of heat or cold, *to manage pain.*
- Demonstrate use of pillow to support flanks, exercises to relax muscles, and massage *to relieve discomfort.*

Patient Education/Home Care Planning

1. Emphasize need for balanced diet, adequate fluid intake, and high-calorie, high-protein diet.
2. Explain pain-relieving measures, such as exercise, warmth, and analgesics.

Evaluation

Hydration is normal Patient is able to maintain adequate intake by mouth, and electrolyte levels are within normal limits.

Patient is comfortable Facial expression and body are relaxed; denies presence of pain.

CARCINOMA OF THE BLADDER

The bladder is the most common site of urinary tract malignancy.

Cancer of the bladder occurs most often in men between 50 and 70 years of age. The incidence in women and in both younger men and women has increased. The most frequent sign of bladder cancer is hematuria, although some patients are asymptomatic until urethral obstruction occurs. Women are more likely to have been treated for urinary tract infection with antibiotics for hematuria believed to be hematuric cystitis.

The second most common symptom complex is marked urgency, dysuria, and frequency with small volumes of urine. Low back pain may be indicative of sacral or lumbar metastases.

Occupational exposure to dust or fumes of dyes, rubber, leather and its products, paint, and organic chemicals such as benzidine may be factors in bladder cancer development, with a 6- to 20-year latent period from the time of exposure to tumor transformation.

Cigarette smoking is associated with as much as a six times greater incidence of bladder cancers. Reducing the use of tobacco and tobacco products, especially among young people, would likely lower the incidence of this cancer as aging occurs (see box below).

•••••• Pathophysiology

Ninety percent of bladder tumors are transitional cell carcinoma, 6% to 7% are true squamous cell carcinoma, and only 1% to 2% are glandular cancer. Some of these tumors are undifferentiated. Depth of invasion (stage) is more important than grading in predicting prognosis.

Lymph node involvement is present in half of the patients with deep muscle infiltration and has a poor prognosis. The disappointing long-term survival rate of patients with deeply invasive tumors has led to an integrated form of therapy in which irradiation is followed by cystectomy.

The bladder is also the site for contiguous spread of cancer from lesions of neighboring viscera, especially the uterine cervix and the prostate.

•••••• Diagnostic Studies and Findings

Urine culture Sterile urine in patient with symptoms of cystitis

Excretory urography Tumor or evidence of ureteral or urethral obstruction

Cystoscopy with selected bladder biopsies and urinary tract cytologic studies Tumor visualization; presence of malignant cells

---

FACTS ABOUT BLADDER CANCER

Incidence: An estimated 50,500 new cases among men and women during 1995. Of these new cases, 37,300 will be men and 13,200 will be women, a four times greater incidence among men.

Mortality: An estimated 11,200 deaths in 1995. If detected early, the 5-year survival rate is 92%.

Warning Signals: Hematuria followed by marked urgency and dysuria.

Risk Factors: Smokers are two times more likely to develop bladder cancer than nonsmokers. Among men, 47% of the bladder cancer death rates and 37% among women can be attributed to smoking.

Early Detection: Cystoscopy is the primary method for detecting bladder cancer.

Treatment: In over 90% of bladder cancer cases, surgery, either alone or in combination with chemotherapy and/or radiation therapy is used.

From American Cancer Society.[1]

Bimanual abdominal examination Firm or hard nodularity

Cystoscopic retrograde ureteropyelography Tumor visualization; evidence of obstruction

Flow cytometry More than 15% of cells above diploid level or clearly aneuploid tumor cell line with greater or less than half the number of chromosomes usually found

Renal arteriography Evidence of obstruction or increased tumor vascularization

Renal ultrasound Local extent and degree of bladder wall involvement by tumor

Computed tomograms and magnetic resonance imaging of abdomen and pelvis Extent of local tumor; identification of pelvic lymph node metastases

Chest and skeletal x-ray examinations, bone scan, liver function studies Evidence of metastatic disease

Carcinoembryonic antigen (CEA) Elevated

Autocrine motility factor (AMF) Increased in widely metastatic disease

•••••• Multidisciplinary Plan

Surgery

Noninvasive Bladder Cancer

Endoscopic resection and fulguration; laser therapy

Invasive Bladder Cancer

Radical cystectomy with urinary diversion
Refer to Urinary Diversion in Chapter 12, p. 1062

Radiation Therapy

Preoperative, before radical cystectomy
Control of hemorrhage and bony metastases

Chemotherapy

Noninvasive Bladder Cancer

Intravesical instillation with bacillus Calmette-Guérin (BCG), thiotepa, doxorubicin, mitomycin C, interferons

Invasive Bladder Cancers

CMDV: cisplatin, methotrexate, doxorubicin, vinblastine
MVC: methotrexate, vinblastine, cisplatin
Single agents: methotrexate with or without leucovorin, doxorubicin, vinblastine
Neoadjuvant: before radiation therapy

NURSING CARE

Nursing Assessment

Urinary Function

Hematuria; urgency; dysuria; frequency; azotemia; pelvic mass

Comfort

Low back pain; pelvic pain; leg edema

Psychosocial

Fear of incontinence, altered sexuality and fertility, pain, death

Nursing Dx & Intervention for Untreatable Tumors (see section on Metastatic Disease and Terminal Stage of the Disease)

Altered patterns of urinary elimination related to tumor in bladder

- Measure intake and output *to monitor adequacy of elimination.*
- Inspect urine for blood; check with Hemoccult *to detect bleeding.*
- Inspect abdomen for swelling and distention *to determine presence of urinary retention.*
- Encourage adequate rest and exercise *to avoid stress-related distention.*
- Increase patient's fluid intake *to enhance renal circulation and flush bladder.*
- Apply heating pad or hot water bottle to abdomen as ordered *to relax abdominal muscles.*
- Catheterize patient only if necessary *to avoid infection associated with catheterization.*
- Monitor blood studies—acid-base balance, hemoglobin level, hematocrit value, blood urea nitrogen (BUN), and creatinine levels—*to assess renal function.*
- Monitor urine studies—acid-base balance, creatinine level, specific gravity, and protein level—*to assess renal function.*

Pain related to pressure of tumor or metastases

- Change patient's position slowly *to avoid injury or strain.*
- Place patient in whirlpool bath or apply heat *to relax muscles.*
- Administer bladder antispasmodics as ordered *to relieve bladder spasms.*
- Discuss possible pain-relieving measures with patient; use those possible, such as heat, cold, and massage *to promote self-care.*
- Evaluate effectiveness of pain relief measures *to determine need for further intervention.*

Fear related to loss of control of urinary function, impotence, infertility, pain, and possible death

- Validate sources of fear with patient *to guide therapeutic intervention.*
- Assist patient to identify coping and to facilitate problem-solving skills used successfully in the past.
- Encourage patient to ask questions and express feelings *to relieve anxiety and help patient put thoughts into perspective.*

Patient Education/Home Care Planning

1. Emphasize the need for adequate fluid intake, exercise, and rest.
2. Encourage oral fluids and foods that cause alkaline urine such as fruits, vegetables, and milk. Avoid tobacco and foods and fluids that irritate the bladder, such as alcohol, tea, and spices.
3. Explain that, to reduce the incidence of urinary tract infections, female patients should:
   a. Void after sexual intercourse to reduce the number of bacteria that may be introduced into the urethra.
   b. Avoid bubble baths.
   c. Wear cotton undergarments.
4. Discuss pain-relieving measures, such as exercise, warmth, safety, and medication.
5. Instruct the patient in self-care if the patient has undergone urinary diversion.
6. Provide the patient with information and referrals as needed for sperm banking, sexual counseling, and reconstructive/implant surgery.

Evaluation

Urinary function is normal   Patient does not complain of urgency, frequency, or dysuria. No evidence of hematuria is present.

Patient experiences no pain   Patient has no complaints of low back or pelvic pain. Patient able to carry out self-care activities.

Fears have been reduced   Patient acknowledges fears of loss of control of urinary function, impotence, sterility, pain, and death. Concerns are refocused toward resuming activities of daily living.

CANCERS OF THE MALE REPRODUCTIVE SYSTEM

■ CANCER OF THE PROSTATE

■ Cancer of the prostate is a malignant tumor arising from the parenchyma of the prostate gland.

The prostate is the most common site of cancer in men, accounting for 21% of all male cancers. The incidence and mortality of this cancer are increasing, especially in blacks. In men over 85 years of age, the incidence may be as high as 89% (see box).

Most prostatic cancers are adenocarcinomas discovered by a physician during rectal examination, which should be done yearly on all men over 50 years of age. These slow-growing tumors arise in the posterior portion of the prostate and eventu-

■ FACTS ABOUT PROSTATE CANCER

Incidence: An estimated 244,000 new cases during 1995. Black men have a 32% higher incidence rate than white men. Improved detection methods, particularly the use of the prostate-specific antigen screening test, have resulted in a 50% increase in incidence rates.

Mortality: Prostate cancer is the second leading cause of cancer death in men with an estimated 40,400 deaths in 1995.

Warning Signals: The signs and symptoms of prostate cancer often mimic benign prostatic hypertrophy. These include weak or interrupted urine flow, nocturia, dysuria, and hematuria.

Risk Factors: Age remains the strongest risk factor with over 80% of all prostate cancers diagnosed in men over age 65. There appears to be a geographic distribution of prostate cancer. Northwestern Europe and North America have a higher incidence and the disease is considered rare in the Near East, Africa, Central America, and South America. The role of dietary fat as an etiologic factor is under study.

Early Detection: The American Cancer Society recommends a yearly digital rectal exam for every man 40 and over. Beginning at age 50, an annual prostate-specific antigen screening test is recommended. Should either test reveal any abnormalities, a transrectal ultrasound should be performed.

Treatment: There are a number of options under study and available to men diagnosed with prostate cancer. These include surgery, radiation therapy, and/or endocrine manipulation.

From American Cancer Society.[1]

ally involve the entire gland. They spread via the lymphatics throughout the pelvic region and into the pelvic bones.

The influence of endogenous hormones, especially dihydrotestosterone, is the only factor clearly associated with the promotion and development of prostate cancer. Other possible etiologic factors include genetic influences; dietary fat; exposure to certain viruses, pathogens, or industrial chemicals; and urbanization.

•••••• Pathophysiology

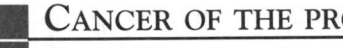

Most prostatic cancers are adenocarcinomas. These slow-growing tumors arise in the posterior portion of the prostate, are usually multifocal, and eventually involve the entire gland. They spread via the lymphatics throughout the pelvic region and into the pelvic bones. Hematogenous spread involves the lungs, liver, kidneys, and bones (vertebrae, pelvis, femur, and ribs). By the time of diagnosis, most of these cancers already have invaded the base of the bladder, seminal vesicles, or perivesicular fascia or have moved laterally into the levator ani muscles.

The rest of these tumors are ductal (transitional and squamous cell carcinoma, endometroid cancer, and sarcoma). Acinar dysplasia has been characterized as prostatic intraepithelial neoplasia (PIN), a premalignant lesion.

Grading of the tumors—as well, moderately, or poorly differentiated—correlates with the prognosis. Early symptoms resemble those of benign prostatic hypertrophy and include weak urinary stream, urinary frequency, dysuria, and difficulty in starting and stopping urination. Some patients initially report pain in the lower back, pelvis, or upper thighs. Bilateral ureteral obstruction with renal insufficiency is not uncommon at the time of diagnosis.

•••••• Diagnostic Studies and Findings

Digital rectal examination Fifty percent of palpable prostatic nodules are cancer

Excretory urogram Bladder outlet involvement; ureteral obstruction or displacement

Closed or open fine-needle biopsy via perineal or transrectal route Presence of malignant cells

Transrectal ultrasonography Prostatic lesions seen

Pelvic computed tomography Local extensions; nodal involvement

Magnetic resonance imaging Capsular penetration; seminal vesicle involvement

Lymphangiography Paraaortic and pelvic node involvement

Prostate specific antigen Elevated in localized disease; clinical recurrence

Prostatic acid phosphatase Elevated in localized disease

•••••• Multidisciplinary Plan

Surgery

Transurethral resection
Radical prostatectomy
Bilateral orchiectomy
Refer to Chapter 12 on p. 1051 for care of patient with open prostatectomy

Radiation Therapy

External beam
Interstitial implant

Chemotherapy

Single agents: cyclophosphamide, 5-fluorouracil, doxorubicin, methotrexate, cisplatin, mitomycin, dacarbazine (DTIC)
Hormonal therapy
Diethylstilbestrol (Stilphostrol), conjugated estrogens (Premarin), estradiol, estramustine phosphate
Medical adrenalectomy: aminoglutethimide, ketoconazole, spironolactone, glucocorticoids
Antiandrogens: cyproterone acetate, flutamide, megestrol acetate
GnH agonist: leuprolide

NURSING CARE

Nursing Assessment

Urinary Function

Weak urinary stream; frequency; dysuria; difficulty starting and stopping urination; renal insufficiency as evidenced by decreased output

Comfort

Pain in lower back, pelvis, or upper thighs

Psychosocial

Expressed fears of incontinence, altered sexuality, pain, death

Nursing Dx & Intervention for Untreatable Tumors (see section of Metastatic Disease and Terminal Stage of the Disease)

Altered patterns of urinary elimination related to presence of tumor surrounding urethra

- Weigh patient daily and measure intake and output *to monitor renal function and adequacy of elimination.*
- Monitor blood studies—blood urea nitrogen, creatinine, acid-base balance, hemoglobin, and hematocrit—and urine studies—acid-base balance, creatinine, and specific gravity—and test urine for protein *to monitor renal function.*
- Inspect patient for edema *as indication of fluid retention.*
- Monitor patient's blood pressure *as indication of fluid retention.*
- Be alert for patient's complaints of frequency, pain, and urination difficulties *to monitor the presence of infection or obstruction.*
- Encourage adequate rest and activity *to decrease stress on urinary system.*
- Increase patient's fluid intake *to flush renal system.*
- Catheterize patient only if necessary *to eliminate urine retention.*

Pain related to metastases to spine or pelvis

- Change patient's position slowly *to avoid injury and strain.*
- Place patient in whirlpool bath or apply heat *to relax muscles.*
- Provide safety measures (e.g., physical support when patient moves in bed or walks, use of assistive devices such as a walker) *to avoid injury.*
- Administer analgesics as needed *to relieve pain.*
- Offer massage *to provide muscle relaxation.*
- Evaluate effectiveness of pain relief measures *to determine need for further intervention.*

Fear related to incontinence, altered sexuality, pain, and death

- Validate sources of fear with patient *to guide therapeutic interventions.*
- Assist patient to identify coping skills used successfully in the past *to facilitate problem-solving.*
- Encourage patient to ask questions and express feelings *to relieve anxiety and help patient put thoughts into perspective.*
- Provide accurate information about control of urinary function, sexuality, control of pain, prognosis *to decrease patient's fears.*

Patient Education/Home Care Planning

1. Emphasize the need for adequate fluid intake, exercise, and rest.
2. Explain the use of alternative pain-relieving measures such as exercise, warmth, and medication.
3. Tell the patient to notify the physician or nurse if signs and symptoms of renal insufficiency appear (provide instructions in writing).
4. Discuss alternate expressions of sexuality, the value of sexual counseling, and the possibility of recovering some or all of sexual function after treatment ends.

Evaluation

Urinary function is normal   Patient has no complaints of urgency, frequency, or dysuria. Patient able to start and stop urine stream.

No pain is present   Patient has no complaints of lower back, pelvic, or upper thigh pain. Patient able to carry out self-care activities.

Fears have been reduced   Patient acknowledges fears of loss of control of urinary function, impotence, pain, and death. Concerns are refocused toward resuming activities of daily living.

■ TESTICULAR CANCER

Testicular cancer is a rare form of cancer but is the most common cancer in young men 15 to 35 years of age. With the advent of tumor markers (indicating the presence of disease and enabling the physician to monitor its response to treatment), refined surgery, and effective chemotherapy, the cure rate is as high as 90%.

The etiologic factors of testicular cancer are unknown, although its occurrence is higher in men with cryptorchidism (undescended testis) or atrophic testis. Men with either of these conditions have a 40 times greater likelihood of developing cancer than do those with normal testes. When orchiopexy (surgical descent of the cryptorchid testis) is performed on the male child before the age of 2 years, the likelihood of his developing cancer is virtually eliminated. Testicular cancer is more common in white males than in black males in the United States. There is also a higher incidence in the higher socioeconomic classes. Men whose mothers took exogenous hormones during pregnancy also have a higher incidence of testicular cancer.

The first sign of the disease is usually a small, hard, painless lump in the testicle. Symptoms reported include a sensation of heaviness in the testicle, sudden fluid accumulation in the scrotum, and perineal pain or discomfort.

Some men report a history of trauma, mumps, or orchitis; episodic testicular pain; low back, groin, or abdominal ache; and breast enlargement or tenderness. If symptoms persist after antibiotic therapy for suspected epididymitis, the physician should suspect testicular cancer.

•••••• Pathophysiology

Most testicular tumors are of germ cell origin and are malignant. The basic categories are the seminoma and heterogeneous, nonseminomatous germ cell tumor. Paraaortic lymph node involvement, ureteral obstruction, and pulmonary metastases may be present at diagnosis.

Dramatic responses to single agent and combination drug chemotherapy have made even advanced cases of testicular cancer curable. Radiation therapy is still used for seminomas but has been replaced by chemotherapy for nonseminomatous tumors. Tumor markers (α-fetoprotein [AFP] and human chorionic gonadotropin [hCG]) are useful not only in early diagnosis but also in follow-up monitoring for recurrent disease.

•••••• Diagnostic Studies and Findings

Palpation of testes   Presence of mass
Transillumination   Detection of intrascrotal lesion
Excretory urography   Displacement of ureters or kidney
Abdominal computed tomography and ultrasound and lymphangiogram   Areas of abnormality seen
Serum α-fetoprotein (AFP)   Elevated
Human chorionic gonadotropin (hCG)   Elevated
Chest x-ray examination, computed tomogram, and whole-lung computed tomogram   Evidence of metastatic disease
Radical inguinal orchiectomy (biopsy)   Presence of malignant cells

•••••• Multidisciplinary Plan

Surgery

Inguinal exploration and orchiectomy
Bilateral retroperitoneal lymph node dissection

Radiation Therapy

External beam

Chemotherapy

Seminomas: cyclophosphamide
Nonseminomas: cisplatin (Platinol), vinblastine, bleomycin

NURSING CARE

Nursing Assessment

Scrotum

Small, hard painless lump in testis; sensation of heaviness; swelling

Breasts

Enlargement or tenderness

Comfort

Perineal pain or discomfort; low back, groin, or abdominal ache

Psychosocial

Fear of altered sexuality, infertility, pain, death

Nursing Dx & Intervention Related to Untreatable Tumor, Orchiectomy

Body image disturbance related to changes in scrotum from tumor or surgery

- Assess patient's perception of impact of scrotal mass and/or breast enlargement on spouse or partner *to clarify severity of problem as perceived by patient.*
- Respect patient's need for period of denial *to allow patient to cope.*
- Respect patient's individual coping style because *patient may have used his coping style to deal effectively with other crises.*
- Assist patient in expressing such feelings as anger *to allow patient to "defuse" some of his anxiety.*
- Encourage patient to talk about alterations when he is able to do so *to help patient view problem realistically.*
- Explore patient's feelings about impact of alterations on personal appearance *to determine need for disguising the change.*
- Provide information about treatment options *to enable patient to make realistic and individualized decisions.*

Pain related to pressure of tumor or metastases on perineal, groin, or abdominal regions or orchiectomy

- Handle patient gently *to avoid further discomfort.*
- Apply heat as ordered with heating pad, hot water bottle, warm moist compress, or warm water bath *to promote circulation and decrease swelling and irritation.*
- Discuss pain-relieving measures such as scrotal support, analgesics, and massage. Implement (as feasible) patient preferences *to further patient comfort.*
- Evaluate effectiveness of pain-relieving measures *to determine need for further intervention.*

- Review care of post-operative pain, Part 2, Perioperative Nursing.

Fear related to altered sexuality, pain, and death

- Validate sources of fear with patient *to guide therapeutic interventions.*
- Assist patient to identify coping skills used successfully in the past *to facilitate problem solving.*
- Encourage patient to ask questions and express feelings *to relieve patient's anxiety and help patient put thoughts into perspective.*
- Provide accurate information about sexuality, control of pain, and prognosis *to decrease patient's fears.*
- Provide accurate information about sexuality (removal of testicles during adulthood has no impact on sexuality), control of pain, and prognosis *to decrease patient's fears.*

Risk for impaired skin integrity related to surgery

- Review care plan in Part Two, Perioperative Nursing on p. 1431.

Patient Education/Home Care Planning

1. Explain about the availability of testicular implants.
2. Discuss the testes' ability to compensate for loss of function in one testis so that male characteristics are not adversely affected.
3. Provide information about sperm banking and sexual counseling.
4. Stress the importance of follow-up evaluation for the rest of the patient's life.

Evaluation

Healthy body image is described by patient Patient able to look at and touch scrotum. Patient able to describe self as person with unique body configuration.

Patient expresses no pain Patient makes no complaints of perineal, groin, or abdominal pain.

Fears have been reduced Patient acknowledges fear, but concerns are refocused toward resuming activities of daily living.

GYNECOLOGIC CANCERS

Cancer of the uterus, both endometrial and cervical (including in situ), accounts for 15% of all female cancers. Although increasing in incidence, cancers of the female genital organs—uterus, ovaries, vulva, and vagina—also have an increasing rate of survival.

CANCER OF THE CERVIX

Cancer of the uterine cervix is a neoplasm that can be detected in the early, curable stage by the Papanicolaou (Pap) test.

Cancer of the uterine cervix has its highest incidence in women who are 35 years of age or older, began sexual activity in puberty, and have had multiple partners. Other risk factors include low socioeconomic status, poor prenatal and postnatal care, and in utero exposure to diethylstilbestrol (DES). Women in urban, industrialized areas and white or Jewish women have a lower incidence of the disease than do those in rural, underdeveloped areas and nonwhites. Celibate women and those in religious groups that encourage male circumcision and monogamy also have a lower incidence. Women with multiple genital infections such as herpes, *Trichomonas* infection, and gonorrhea are at greater risk. Beta carotene or some related aspect of a diet rich in carrots and green vegetables is believed to be protective against invasive cervical cancer. Vitamins C and A, types of barrier contraception, and partner vasectomy are also protective (see box).

Improved general and genital hygiene and cytologic screening with the Pap smear have contributed to decreased mortality of invasive cervical cancer. However, the incidence of carcinoma in situ is increasing and is affecting a younger population.

Changes in cells of the cervical epithelium may be present for 10 years before invasive cancer develops. However, a Pap smear can detect even the earliest changes, so regular Pap tests, as well as manual pelvic examinations, are the most important means of reducing mortality from cervical cancer.

••••• Pathophysiology

Abnormal bleeding is the most common sign of cervical cancer. The bleeding initially may be a thin, watery, blood-tinged vaginal discharge that progresses to spotting and frank bleeding. Other signs and symptoms include prolonged or intermittent menstrual periods, "contact" bleeding after intercourse, and anemia in the presence of chronic blood loss. Advanced disease is evidenced by odor; pain in the lower back, legs, and groin; lower extremity edema; difficulty voiding, urgency, or hematuria (invasion of the bladder); and rectal tenesmus and rectal bleeding (invasion of the rectum). Cervical cancer rarely occurs during pregnancy but should be ruled out in the presence of unexplained bleeding.

When symptoms appear, the cancer has usually progressed beyond its early stages. Squamous cell carcinoma accounts for 95% of all invasive tumors diagnosed, and adenocarcinomas account for most of the rest. Clear cell carcinoma develops in the cervix and vagina of women exposed in utero to DES. Invasive carcinoma of the cervix spreads by direct extension to the vaginal wall, laterally into the parametrium toward the pelvic wall, and anteroposteriorly into the bladder and rectum. Metastases to the pelvic lymph nodes are more common than those to distant nodes.

••••• Diagnostic Studies and Findings

Cervical examination and biopsy via colposcopy Presence of visible mass, malignant cells, or both

Computed tomography of the abdomen Involvement of retroperitoneal lymph nodes

Magnetic resonance imaging Estimated tumor volume

Lymphangiography followed by fine-needle aspiration biopsy Presence of malignant cells

Supraclavicular node biopsy Presence of malignant cells

Chest x-ray examination, excretory urography, cystoscopy, and proctosigmoidoscopy Evidence of spread of tumor

Complete blood cell count Anemia

••••• Multidisciplinary Plan

Surgery

Conization

Cryotherapy or laser ablation

Abdominal or vaginal radical hysterectomy and pelvic node dissection

Pelvic exenteration

Refer to Chapter 10, Female Reproductive System, on p. 873 for medical interventions and related nursing care

---

■ FACTS ABOUT CERVICAL CANCER

Incidence: An estimated 15,800 invasive and 65,000 carcinoma in situ in 1995. For the past decade the incidence rate of invasive cervical cancer had been dropping, but recently an increase has been noted in women under 50. Considered a precancerous condition, cervical carcinoma in situ is now more frequent than invasive cancer among women under 50.

Mortality: Black women are twice as likely as white women to succumb to cervical cancer. In 1995, an estimated 4,800 women will die.

Warning Signals: Watery vaginal discharge, abnormal uterine bleeding or spotting. In advanced disease, the woman may complain of pain in the pelvis, hypogastrium, flank, or leg.

Risk Factors: First intercourse at an early age; multiple sex partners; cigarette smoking; and genital infections with human papillomavirus.

Early Detection: The American Cancer Society recommends a yearly PAP test with a pelvic examination in women who are, or have been, sexually active or who have reached age 18 years. When three or more consecutive exams reveal no abnormalities, the PAP test may be performed less frequently at the discretion of the physician.

Treatment: Surgery, alone or in combination with radiation, is the treatment for invasive cancer. Cryotherapy, electrocoagulation or local surgery can be used for carcinoma in situ.

From American Cancer Society.[1]

Radiation Therapy
External beam
Intracavity

Chemotherapy
Cisplatin, carboplatin, cyclophosphamide, melphalan, 5-fluorouracil, vincristine, methotrexate, hydroxyurea

---

NURSING CARE

Nursing Assessment

Perineal Area
Unusual bleeding or vaginal discharge
Prolonged or intermittent menstrual periods
"Contact" bleeding after intercourse
Skin irritation or excoriation
Malodorous discharge

Hematologic
Anemia; fatigue

Renal
Difficulty voiding, urgency, hematuria

Intestinal
Rectal tenesmus, bleeding

Comfort
Pain in lower back, legs, and groin
Lower extremity edema

Nursing Dx & Intervention for Untreated Cancer, Pre-Surgical Status or Concurrent Care with Radiation or Chemotherapy

Impaired skin integrity related to vaginal discharge
- Change dressings or pads frequently; maintain dry, clean linen and dry skin; provide clean clothing *to maintain cleanliness and enhance patient's comfort.*
- Observe skin for irritation *to determine need for further intervention.*
- Observe quality and quantity of drainage *to determine status of infection.*
- Administer antibiotics as ordered *to combat infection.*
- Administer perineal care as indicated *to promote comfort and remove drainage from skin.*

Pain related to pressure of tumor on adjacent structures
For pressure in the abdominal area
- Change patient's position frequently *to relieve pressure.*
- Give small, frequent feedings *to avoid abdominal distention.*
- Place patient in sitting position *to relieve abdominal pressure.*
- Remove constrictive clothing *to relieve pressure.*
- Insert rectal tube as indicated *to relieve flatus.*
- Auscultate abdomen for abnormal bowel sounds *to assess gastrointestinal status.*

For back pain, leg pain, or lymphedema caused by pressure
- Position patient comfortably, and change position slowly *to avoid injury and increased pain.*
- Maintain body alignment *to avoid injury or muscular stretching.*
- Apply heating pad, hot water bottle, or warm, moist compress *to relax muscles and increase circulation.*
- Bathe patient in warm water *to relax muscles.*
- Massage gently *to promote circulation and relax muscles.*
- Encourage adequate rest *to decrease energy expenditure.*
- Provide pain relief measure of patient's choice *to promote self-care.*
- Be alert for complaints of pain, and assess duration and radiation of pain *to determine need for further intervention.*

Fatigue related to blood loss and anemia
- Help patient and significant others understand the physiologic basis for fatigue and that it will diminish on improvement or correction of the anemia *to help patient better tolerate the fatigue.*
- Encourage patient to discuss feelings related to fatigue *to relieve patient's anxiety (which can cause fatigue).*
- Encourage patient to identify behaviors associated with fatigue, such as emotional lability and irritability, *to help patient distinguish these temporary behaviors that are caused by the anemic condition.*
- Help patient plan periods of rest and activity *to achieve adequate levels of energy for activities of daily living.*

Altered patterns of urinary elimination related to pressure of tumor on urethra
- Measure patient's intake and output *to monitor for fluid balance.*
- Inspect urine for bleeding; check with Hemoccult *to detect urinary tract bleeding.*
- Encourage adequate rest and exercise *to maintain general well-being.*
- Encourage patient to ambulate often *to promote circulation and urinary elimination.*
- Apply heating pad or hot water bottle *to relax bladder musculature.*
- Catheterize only if necessary *to avoid infection.*

Body image disturbance related to actual or potential alteration in female structure
- Encourage patient to discuss feelings and concerns with health care providers and significant others *to alleviate anxiety.*
- Help patient identify, label, and express feelings about the significance of the female genitals, treatment modalities,

and anticipated prognosis *to allow patient to deal with specific issues.*

- Promote acceptance of a positive, realistic body image *so patient can resume pre-illness life-style.*

Patient Education/Home Care Planning

1. Emphasize the need to maintain perineal hygiene.
2. Explain the use of alternative nonpharmacologic comfort measures, such as the use of heat, positioning, relaxation exercises, guided imagery, and distraction.
3. Assist the patient in planning periods of activity and rest, which will enable her to accomplish activities of daily living and recreational activities.
4. Explain the importance of drinking large quantities of water and nonacidic fluids, of voiding when she feels the urge, and of using warmth and other individually effective techniques to stimulate voiding.
5. Refer the patient to support groups, sexual counselors, and other community programs that will be helpful to her in maintaining a positive self-image.

Evaluation

Perineal area is clean and odor-free   Perineal area is clean, free of odor, and normal in color. Patient reports feeling of cleanliness and comfort in perineal area.

Patient expresses no pain   Patient's facial expression is calm and relaxed; body appears relaxed; patient states she is without pain.

Patient expresses no fatigue   Patient is able to coordinate rest and activity so that she can carry out activities of daily living and enjoy recreational activities.

Urinary function is normal   Patient maintains a balance between intake and output. Patient voids without difficulty.

Patient's body image is realistic   Patient verbalizes realistic sense of self and body.

◼ OTHER GYNECOLOGIC CANCERS

Malignant diseases occur in all parts of the female reproductive system. They include cancers of the uterine endometrium, the vagina, the vulva, the ovaries, and the fallopian tubes, as well as gestational trophoblastic neoplasms.

Endometrial cancer   Endometrial cancer is the most common gynecologic cancer in women, occurring primarily in postmenopausal women. Etiologic factors include infertility, late menopause (after 52 years of age), obesity, diabetes, and hypertension. Long-term diethylstilbestrol (DES) therapy may also be a factor. Other etiologic factors are endometrial hyperplasia, polycystic ovarian disease, history of irregular menses, and a history of breast, colon, or ovarian cancer. Cancer of the endometrium occurs with higher frequency in urban, white, and Jewish women. The benefits of maintaining an ideal weight and careful management of estrogen therapy for menopause should be emphasized.

The most common initial symptom is intermenstrual or postmenopausal bleeding. The diagnosis of endometrial cancer is based on histologic tissue examination.

The usual treatment for cancer limited to the fundal portion of the uterus is preoperative intracavity radiation therapy followed by total hysterectomy and bilateral salpingo-oophorectomy. External radiation is added to the treatment plan when the cancer extends beyond the fundus.

The 5-year survival rate for patients with early endometrial cancer is greater than 85%. The cure rate drops to 50% when the cancer has metastasized.

Vaginal cancer   Vaginal carcinoma is rarely a primary lesion, although it does occur in both menopausal and postmenopausal women. It is related to in utero DES exposure in younger women. Vaginal cancer is rare in black and Jewish women. The primary signs and symptoms are vaginal spotting and discharge, pain, groin masses, and changes in urinary pattern.

Radiation therapy consists of intracavity irradiation combined with total pelvic external irradiation. Radical surgery includes complete vaginectomy, pelvic node dissection, and anterior exenteration as indicated. Grafting may be used to avoid vaginal stenosis, especially in younger patients.

Vulvar cancer   There is an increasing incidence of vulvar intraepithelial neoplasia (VIN) and carcinoma in situ (CIS) in older women. Vulvar cancer occurs most commonly in women who are between 50 and 70 years of age and in lower socioeconomic strata. Symptoms include vaginal discharge, pruritus, and bleeding.

The leukoplakic changes (whitish, plaquelike, or ulcerated lesions) that precede carcinoma can be eliminated by simple vulvectomy. Once carcinoma develops, invasion of the inguinal nodes and the lower vagina is common.

Surgery for this form of cancer may be preventive to remove precancerous lesions (hemivulvectomy or local excision with a wide margin of normal tissue), curative (radical vulvectomy), or palliative (extent depends on the patient's symptoms).

The 5-year survival rate is greater than 80% for women with early, localized lesions but is much lower when nodal or distant metastasis is present.

Ovarian cancer   Ovarian cancer has replaced cervical cancer as the leading cause of death from genital cancer. Its development is closely linked to breast cancer, which suggests abnormal endocrine activity. The peak incidence is between 60 and 80 years of age.

These tumors do not usually produce symptoms until intraabdominal metastasis has occurred, with outward signs such as ascites. Therefore the mortality is high; only 34% of patients survive the disease. When symptoms do occur, they include increasing abdominal girth, weight loss, abdominal pain, dysuria or urinary frequency, and constipation.

Treatment of ovarian cancer consists of hysterectomy and bilateral salpingo-oophorectomy. Radiation therapy and chemotherapy may be used in conjunction with surgery or when the cancer is inoperable.

Cancer of the fallopian tube Fallopian tube cancer is the rarest of the gynecologic malignancies. It is difficult to diagnose, and diagnosis is usually made at time of surgery. Most are adenocarcinomas. Patients are usually in their midfifties when fallopian tube cancer is detected. The most common symptoms are pelvic pain, abnormal vaginal bleeding, and a heavy, watery vaginal discharge. Colicky pain may be associated with bleeding.

Removal of the uterus, fallopian tubes, ovaries, and omentum is the usual treatment. Radiation and chemotherapy have been used postoperatively with some success. Survival rates are as high as 90% with early disease, although the overall 5-year survival rate is 38%.

Gestational trophoblastic neoplasms The gestational trophoblastic neoplasms include hydatidiform mole, invasive mole (chorioadenoma destruens), and choriocarcinoma. Molar pregnancy, the most common of these tumors, occurs in approximately 1 in 1500 live births in the United States; locally invasive disease develops in 16% of these patients and metastatic disease in 31%. These neoplasms can also develop after abortal, ectopic, and term gestations.

The measurement of human chorionic gonadotropin (hCG) by the β subunit radioimmunoassay test is essential for diagnosis, monitoring of therapy, and follow-up. Early diagnosis is facilitated by amniography and ultrasonography.

Hydatidiform mole is treated with suction curettage when preserving fertility is desirable. Actinomycin D, given prophylactically, reduces the incidence of sequelae when the uterus is larger than the fruit dates, the serum hCG titer is over 100,000 mU/dl, and the ovaries are cystic. Postevacuation monitoring of hCG levels is done weekly for 3 consecutive weeks and then monthly for 6 months or until hCG is undetectable. During this time pregnancy should be avoided. If fertility is not desired, total abdominal hysterectomy is the treatment of choice when the mole is in situ.

Locally invasive mole or choriocarcinoma is diagnosed by elevated hCG level, pelvic angiography, ultrasonography, and curettage. If fertility is desired, intermittent courses of single agent chemotherapy, such as methotrexate with citrovorum rescue or actinomycin D, yield a cure rate of 100%. When fertility is not desired, hysterectomy is the treatment of choice.

Metastasis is most common with choriocarcinoma; the most frequent sites are the lung, vagina, oral cavity, gastrointestinal tract, central nervous system, and liver. The treatment of choice is chemotherapy with a single agent or a combination of drugs. Surgery or adjunctive radiation therapy may be required. The overall survival with metastasis is still good, although the prognosis is poor with metastases to the liver or brain.

NURSING CARE

Nursing Assessment

Vaginal Bleeding

Excessive or prolonged; serosanguineous discharge

Pain

Back, abdominal, and pelvic pain; guarding of abdominal or pelvic area

Fear

Depression, anger, withdrawal, expressions of fear

Nursing Dx & Intervention for Untreatable Tumors (see section on Metastatic Disease and Terminal Stage of the Disease)

Nursing Care of the Woman With Endometrial Cancer

Fluid volume loss related to postmenopausal bleeding

- Observe characteristics and amount of blood loss *to determine need for fluid and blood component replacement.*
- Monitor vital signs at frequent intervals during episodes of heavy bleeding *to detect shock early.*
- Encourage patient to drink large volumes of fluid *to prevent dehydration.*
- Monitor patient's input and output and urine specific gravity *to detect renal dysfunction.*
- Administer IV fluids as prescribed *to replace lost fluid volume.*
- Monitor laboratory reports *to detect development of anemia.*
- Observe patient for signs and symptoms of worsening fluid volume deficit, including decreased urine output, concentrated urine, output greater than intake, weakness, and change in mental status *to determine need for large volumes of IV fluids and rapid infusion of blood components.*

Pain related to pressure of tumor on lumbosacral, hypogastric, and/or pelvic areas

- Assess patient's pain history, including previous analgesic use, *to determine previously effective medications.*
- Assess location, onset, duration, radiation, and intensity of pain *to determine appropriate interventions.*
- Provide prescribed medications for pain as needed *to decrease patient's discomfort.*
- Teach patient self-care strategies with which to manage pain, such as relaxation exercises, imagery, and application of heat or cold.
- Demonstrate exercises and use of pillow to splint abdomen *to relax back and pelvic muscles.*

Fear related to diagnosis, anticipated treatment, impact of disease and treatment on sexuality, and prognosis

- Assess patient's appetite, weight loss, sleep patterns, and activity level *to detect signs and symptoms of depression.*
- Assess presence and quality of support system *to determine if there are persons available to assist patient.*

- Monitor changes in patient's communication with others (e.g., silence or withdrawal), *which may indicate anger or depression.*
- Encourage patient to use physical expression of fears *because physical activity can be used as a way of expressing fears and anger.*
- Assist patient in identifying information, support groups, and other resources of value *to solve problems that cause her to be fearful.*

Evaluation

Laboratory findings are normal   Hematocrit and albumin levels are within normal limits.

Patient is comfortable   Facial expression is calm and relaxed. Patient expresses comfort.

Patient is calm and without fear   Patient discusses concerns in realistic and rational manner.

Nursing Care of the Woman With Vaginal Cancer

Altered sexual patterns related to presence of tumor or alterations in structure and lubrication related to treatment

- Assist patient to identify current and potential changes in sexual structure and function.
- Encourage patient to identify and use support systems for exchange of thoughts and feelings with significant other and with other women who have the same or similar experiences.
- Encourage patient to vent her feelings about potential loss of uterus and resultant sexual dysfunction.
- Assess the patient's understanding and level of comprehension regarding the function of the uterus in relation to sexual response cycle and the potential impact of therapy on sexual function.

Fear related to diagnosis, anticipated treatment, impact of disease and treatment on sexuality, and prognosis as evidenced by depression, anger, withdrawal, and expressions of fear

- See nursing care of the person with endometrial cancer on p. 1303.

Evaluation

Sexual function is normal   Patient has satisfactory libido and has identified alternate methods of achieving sexual satisfaction.

Nursing Care of the Woman With Vulvar Cancer

Impaired skin integrity related to pruritus, presence of a lump or mass, and bleeding or discharge

- Cleanse patient's skin *to prevent infection.*
- Apply warm, moist compress *to promote circulation and drainage.*

- Apply antibiotic ointment and sterile dressing if indicated *to prevent or treat infection.*
- Expose draining area to air if possible *to promote healing.*
- Observe for increased discharge, skin changes, swelling, and lesions *to detect complications early.*

Fear related to diagnosis, anticipated treatment, possible impact of disease and treatment on sexuality and body image, and prognosis as evidenced by depression, anger, withdrawal, and expressions of fear

- See nursing care of the person with endometrial cancer on p. 1303.

Evaluation

Skin is intact and free of infection in area of disruption   Skin is clean, dry, and warm, with normal color and turgor.

Nursing Care of the Woman With Ovarian Cancer

Altered nutrition: less than body requirements related to pressure of tumor on gastrointestinal tract as evidenced by abdominal discomfort, dyspepsia, indigestion, flatulence, eructations, loss of appetite, and nausea

- Assess patient's caloric intake—kinds, amounts, and percentages of protein, carbohydrate, and fat—*to determine needed changes in diet.*
- Observe the patient for evidence of weight loss and dehydration *to intervene quickly with foods, nutritional supplements, and fluids.*
- Assess whether patient is experiencing abdominal discomfort, dyspepsia, indigestion, flatulence, loss of appetite, or nausea *as evidence of tumor pressure and possible disease progression.*
- Provide palpable meals based as much as possible on patient likes and dislikes *to increase caloric consumption.*
- Offer dietary supplements as needed *to maintain adequate nutritional balance.*
- Offer medications that relieve abdominal distention and flatulence *because these symptoms tend to adversely affect appetite.*

Altered patterns of urinary elimination related to pressure of tumor on bladder as evidenced by urinary frequency, dysuria, incontinence, infection, and/or retention

- Measure patient's intake and output *to monitor for fluid balance.*
- Inspect urine for bleeding *to detect evidence of infection or bladder wall irritation.*
- Inspect abdomen for distention *to determine effectiveness of bladder emptying.*
- Encourage patient to ambulate as tolerated *to promote urinary elimination.*

- Apply heating pad or hot water bottle to patient's abdomen *to relax bladder.*
- Catheterize only as necessary *to avoid infection.*

Fear related to diagnosis, anticipated treatment, impact on sexuality, and prognosis as evidenced by depression, anger, withdrawal, and expressions of fear

- See nursing care of the person with endometrial cancer on p. 1303.

Evaluation

Nutritional status has improved   Weight gain is present; patient is eating a balanced diet.

Urinary function is normal   Patient does not complain of urgency, frequency, or dysuria. No evidence of hematuria.

CANCERS OF THE HEAD AND NECK

Cancers of the head and neck are neoplasms characterized by the uncontrolled growth of anaplastic cells in the larynx, oral cavity, pharynx, or salivary glands.

Although less than 5% of all cancers are neoplasms of the head and neck, they are important to understand because surgical treatment may result in extensive cosmetic deformities and may impair such vital functions as eating and speaking.

The most common site is the larynx, followed by the oral cavity, pharynx, and salivary glands. Etiologic factors for oral and laryngeal cancers include wood dust (nasal cavity cancer), chronic irritation, poor oral hygiene, prolonged heavy use of alcohol, snuff, or tobacco, and Epstein-Barr virus (associated with nasopharyngeal cancer).

•••••• Pathophysiology

Most head and neck cancers grow as malignant ulcerations on surface mucosa. The infiltrative, endophytic lesions are more aggressive and difficult to control than the less common elevated, fungating, exophytic growths. The signs and symptoms depend on the location and are as follows:

Oropharynx—"silent" area; dysphagia; local pain, pain on swallowing, referred pain to ear, enlarging cervical mass

Hypopharynx—another "silent" area; dysphagia, painful swallowing of food, referred ear pain, or neck mass

Nasopharynx—bloody nasal discharge, obstructed nostril, neurologic problems such as facial pain, diplopia, or hoarseness, conductive deafness

Nose and sinuses—bloody nasal discharge, nasal obstruction, diplopia, facial pain or swelling

Parotid and submandibular glands—painless local swelling, hemifacial paralysis

Larynx—persistent hoarseness, pain, referred ear pain, dyspnea, stridor, dysphagia

•••••• Multidisciplinary Plan

The goals of treatment for head and neck cancers are eradication of both clinically demonstrated disease and microscopic subclinical disease; maintenance of adequate physiologic function by reversal dysfunction and posttreatment dysfunction in the special senses, chewing and swallowing, respiration, and speech; and socially acceptable cosmesis, including sufficient surgical, radiation, plastic surgical, and prosthesis rehabilitation.

Treatment decisions involve a multidisciplinary approach with emphasis on such factors as age, general physical condition, other morbidity (such as extensive dental disease, premalignant mucosa, leukoplakia, erythroplasia, or second primary lesion), habits and life-style, occupation, and the patient's desires.

Surgery and radiation therapy (see p. 1306) are the major curative modalities. Chemotherapy is employed as adjuvant therapy or sequentially before radiation or surgery (see p. 1306). Speech therapy is used for speech and swallowing rehabilitation.

More than 75% of head and neck cancer patients whose treatment fails have the first recurrence in areas above the clavicles. The most common failure pattern is recurrent primary tumor with neck metastasis and subsequent carotid erosion or rupture. Distant metastasis to the lung, bone, and elsewhere occurs in long-term survivors of local or regional disease. Intercurrent disease such as alcoholism or chronic lung disease, accidents, and suicide account for 10% to 30% of deaths.

CANCERS OF THE ORAL CAVITY

Cancers of the oral cavity are neoplasms that may invade the tongue, buccal mucosa, and hard palate.

Although easily detected, oral cancers are generally discovered late; 80% to 90% are 2 cm or more in diameter at the time of diagnosis.

•••••• Pathophysiology

Identified carcinogens in oral cancer include cigarettes, ethyl alcohol, snuff, chewing tobacco, and products of the textile industry and of leather manufacturing. Other factors causing oral cancer are syphilis and vitamin deficiencies (see box).

Although relatively accessible to self-examination, dental evaluation, and routine physical examination, delays in the diagnosis of oral cavity cancer result from lack of unique symptomatology (painless lesion); confusion with traumatic, inflammatory, or infectious lesions; or patient delay because of fear and the false hope that the tumor will eventually disappear. The oral cavity and oropharynx are, after the larynx, the most common sites for squamous cell carcinoma of the head and neck. Patients tend to be males in their fifties and sixties, but the number of females is growing. There is also a downward trend in the age group most affected as chewing tobacco and snuff dipping have become more common practices among women in rural areas and among young boys. Use of any kind of tobacco and alcohol consumption are significant factors in the

FACTS ABOUT ORAL CANCER

Incidence: An estimated 28,150 new cases in situ in 1995. It is most frequently seen in men over age 40 and the incidence is more than twice as high in men as in women.

Mortality: An estimated 8,370 deaths in 1995.

Warning Signals: An easily bleeding, nonhealing oral sore; a lump or thickening; a red or white patch that persists. Dysphagia, difficulty in chewing or moving tongue or jaws are often signs of advanced disease.

Risk Factors: Smoking cigarettes, cigars or pipes as well as using smokeless tobacco; excessive use of alcohol.

Early Detection: The dental community has taken a major role in the early detection of oral cancer by including a screening exam in routine visits.

Treatment: Surgery, alone or in combination with radiation, is the treatment of choice. For advanced cases, chemotherapy is under study as an adjunct to surgery.

From American Cancer Society.[1]

development of these cancers. Oral cancers are almost always squamous cell carcinoma. The oropharynx, which includes the lymphoid tissue of the palatal and lingual tonsils, can also be the site of lymphoma.

These lesions tend to be poorly delineated, often spread submucosally, and are not confined by the anatomic midline. Deep muscle involvement of the tongue or pterygoid musculature is an ominous finding. The invasion of bony structures—that is, mandible, palate, maxilla, maxillary sinus, or spine—is serious in terms of both prognosis and treatment morbidity. Surgical treatment of a primary tumor that extends across the midline is much more debilitating than one that has remained localized.

Nodal metastases are relatively uncommon with oral cancer but are more frequent when the site of the primary lesion extends farther into the oropharynx or when the lesion grows toward the midline. To some extent this feature (along with a higher incidence of poorly differentiated lesions) accounts for oropharyngeal tumors having a worse prognosis than that of oral cancer.

Early lesions have a good chance for cure, whereas second primary lesions are a problem, especially in oral cancer. The addition of nodal disease, an advanced primary lesion, or a recurrence after previous treatment significantly decreases the chance for survival and adds a substantial risk for distant (usually pulmonary) metastasis. The overall 5-year survival rate for oral cavity tumors is in the 50% range; for oropharyngeal cancers it is about 35%. Tumors at the base of the tongue and pharyngeal walls and those that involve bone are particularly deadly. More than 80% of persons with oral cancer who die of their disease die of uncontrolled local disease rather than distant metastasis.

The most common sign of oral cancer is the presence of a lesion, often a white spot or sore in the oral cavity or oropharynx that is slow healing. Other complaints include difficulty with dentures, persistent ulcerations, and blood-tinged sputum. Complaints of difficulty in swallowing or in speech indicate more extensive disease.

Fissures, ulcers, or areas of induration in patches of leukoplakia may reflect malignant changes in the mucosa. Erythroplasia or well-defined red patches with velvety consistency among tiny areas of ulceration may be the earliest sign of malignancy.

An enlarged cervical node may be the first sign of oral cancer. Posterior tongue lesions should be suspected when there is hypoglossal nerve paralysis. Numbness over the chin may signal invasion of the inferior alveolar ridge and compression of the mandibular nerve.

•••••• Diagnostic Studies and Findings

Biopsy of areas of redness or inflammation lasting longer than 2 weeks Presence of malignant cells

Mandible x-ray examination and/or bone scan Presence of bone involvement

Computed tomography Parapharyngeal, spinal, carotid artery, or pterygoid muscle involvement

Endoscopy and examination under anesthesia Evaluation of the extent of primary lesion site and possibility of synchronous second primary lesions

•••••• Multidisciplinary Plan

Surgery

Transoral, intraoral, or transcervical resection and reconstruction
Total laryngectomy
Modified or radical neck dissection
Mandibular resection and reconstruction
CO_2 laser excision

Radiation Therapy

External beam
External and interstitial implant

Chemotherapy

Controversial role as adjunctive therapy

NURSING CARE

Nursing Assessment

Oral Cavity Appearance and Function

Leukoplakia (white patch); erythroplasia (red patch); chronic, nonhealing ulcer; localized pain; dysphagia; excessive secretions

Lymphatic Function

Enlarged nodes

Nutritional Status

Weight loss
Dehydration

Pain

Localized or referred

Nursing Dx & Intervention

Altered nutrition: less than body requirements related to difficulty/inability in swallowing

- Provide and teach patient thorough oral hygiene—such as frequent brushing with soft toothbrush and baking soda and use of oral gavage or Water Pik and non–alcohol-based mouthwashes—*to prevent halitosis and prevent infection of surgical site.*
- Offer artificial saliva for the patient who experiences decreased production of saliva.
- Assess patient's caloric intake—kinds, amounts, and percentages of protein, carbohydrate, and fat—*to determine needed changes in diet.*
- Observe patient for evidence of weight loss and dehydration *to intervene quickly with nutritional supplements and fluids.*
- When oral feeding is begun, assess for swallowing and gagging abilities.
- Provide palatable meals based as much as possible on patient likes and dislikes *to increase caloric consumption.*
- Monitor patient's electrolyte profile *to detect serious nutritional imbalances early.*
- Refrain from offering the patient hot or iced fluids, *which may irritate the mucous membranes.*
- Have suction equipment available *to remove excessive secretions.*

Pain related to pressure of tumor on surrounding structures as evidenced by difficulty expectorating and clearing secretions from oral cavity or pharynx, dysphagia, sore gums, sore throat, and sinus headaches

- Assess location, onset, duration, radiation, and intensity of patient's pain *to determine appropriate interventions.*
- Provide prescribed medications for pain as needed *to decrease patient's discomfort.*
- Apply ice or cold compress to nose, face, or throat *to relieve irritation.*
- Provide frequent oral hygiene, including warm saline throat irrigations, *to decrease mucosal dryness because patient often breathes through mouth.*
- Instruct patient not to blow nose because *this may trigger bleeding.*
- Place basin nearby so that patient will spit out secretions rather than swallow them *to avoid further irritation of mucosa.*
- Instruct patient to request analgesic before pain becomes severe *to avoid inconsistent control of pain.*
- Apply heat to face, particularly over sinuses, *to relieve sinus headache pain.*

Patient Education/Home Care Planning

1. Emphasize the need for adequate oral hygiene and dietary management.
2. Discuss signs and symptoms of progressive disease or side effects of treatment that should be reported to the physician.

Evaluation

Nutritional status has improved Weight loss has diminished and patient demonstrates adequate intake to improve nutritional status.

Mucous membrane color is normal Mucous membrane is warm, moist, and of natural color.

Body hydration is normal Mucous membranes are moist. Patient is not thirsty.

Body functioning is normal Digestion is adequate.

Patient is comfortable Facial expression is calm and relaxed. Patient expresses comfort.

▮ CANCER OF THE LARYNX

Cancers of the larynx arise from the epithelial lining of the laryngeal mucous membrane.

Carcinoma of the supraglottic larynx (epiglottis, aryepiglottic folds, arytenoids, and false cords) has a lower incidence than glottic carcinoma; 60% to 65% of laryngeal carcinomas occur in the glottic larynx (true vocal cord). Ninety percent occur in men, with highest incidence in those between 60 and 70 years of age. The early warning sign of progressive hoarseness, caused by a change in the phonating edge of the vocal cord, has led to 5-year survival rates of nearly 80% for localized lesions.

Early cancer can be treated by radiation therapy or surgery. Extensive lesions, which cause necrosis of cartilage or glottic extension, require total laryngectomy.

•••••• Diagnostic Studies and Findings

Indirect mirror examination Presence of lesion on larynx

Direct laryngoscopy and biopsy Presence of tumor, vocal cord fixation, occult extension, malignant cells

Anterior-posterior laryngeal tomography Subglottic extension of disease

Pulmonary function studies Assessment of preoperative pulmonary status

Chest x-ray examination Identification of associated pulmonary functional disease, coexistent lung cancer

•••••• Multidisciplinary Plan

Chemotherapy

Radiation therapy

External beam

Surgery

Total laryngectomy—removal of the entire larynx, hyoid bone, cricoid cartilage, 2 or 3 tracheal rings and strap muscles connected to larynx; requires permanent opening in neck for trachea and laryngectomy tube inserted (Figure 16-2)

Hemilaryngectomy—usually one true and one false vocal cord removed (Figure 16-3); temporary tracheostomy is performed; patient's voice returns, although sounds hoarse

Supraglottic laryngectomy—Epiglottis or false vocal cords removed; permanent tracheostomy is performed (Figure 16-4); patient retains voice

NURSING CARE

Nursing Assessment

Respiratory Function

Dyspnea; stridor; hemoptysis; excessive secretions

Comfort

Pain referred to ear (otalgia); dysphagia

Communication

Hoarseness; loss of speech

Nursing Dx & Intervention for Untreatable Tumors or Laryngectomy Procedures

Ineffective breathing pattern related to airway obstruction by tumor

- Place patient in sitting position *to enhance chest expansion.*
- Encourage deep breathing *to ensure effective ventilation.*
- Inspect chest for respiratory rate, rhythm, and expansion *to monitor respiratory status.*
- Auscultate for abnormal breath sounds and lung aeration *to monitor respiratory status.*
- Palpate and percuss chest *to assess pulmonary function.*
- Monitor blood studies *to determine adequacy of gaseous exchange.*

Ineffective airway clearance related to tumor and upper airway secretions or laryngectomy tube

- Suction airway as necessary *to remove secretions.*
- Provide standby emergency equipment (oxygen and tracheostomy tray) *in case of acute obstruction.*

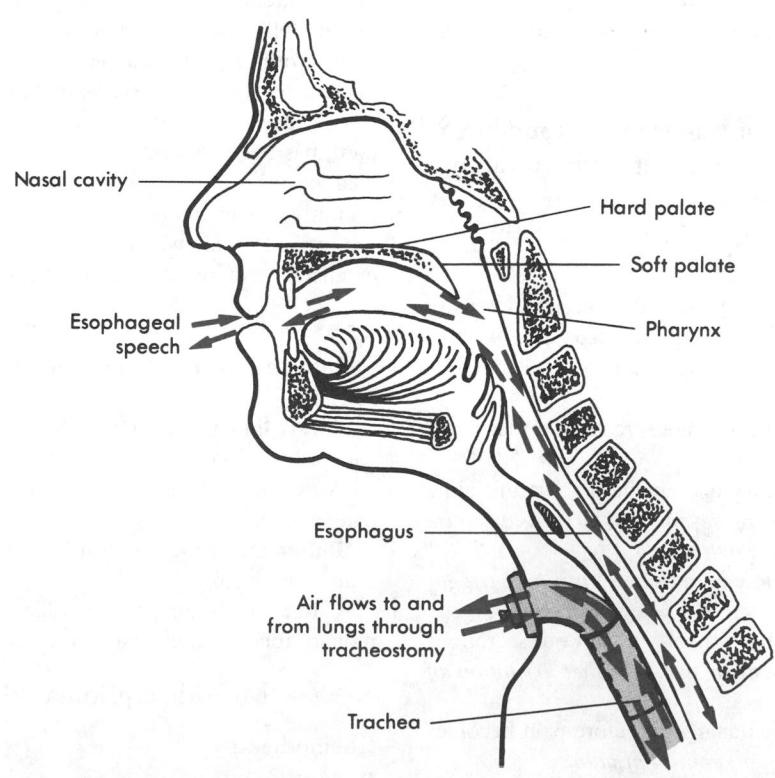

Nasal cavity

Hard palate

Soft palate

Esophageal speech

Pharynx

Esophagus

Air flows to and from lungs through tracheostomy

Trachea

Figure 16-2 Permanent tracheostomy: no connection exists between trachea and esophagus. (From Phipps et al.[26])

- Provide tracheostomy care as indicated (see Chapter 7).
- Feed patient slowly with small, frequent feedings *to avoid choking.*
- Give clear-liquid, full-liquid, pureed, or soft foods as tolerated *to avoid choking.*
- Have suction equipment available *in case of aspiration.*

Altered home maintenance related to need for permanent laryngectomy care

- Review convalescent care of tracheostomy patient (Chapter 7).
- Refer to local chapter of American Cancer Society for recommending vendors who supply laryngectomy appliances.

Pain related to pressure of tumor on esophagus, referred to ear or surgical procedure

- Apply heating pad, hot water bottle, or warm, moist compress *to relieve pain.*
- Maintain warm room temperature *to avoid irritation caused by cold air.*
- Provide pain relief measure of patient's choice *to enhance self-care.*
- Evaluate effectiveness of pain relief measures *to determine need for further intervention.*

- Be alert for complaints of pain, and assess duration and radiation of pain *to determine effectiveness of intervention or progression of problem.*
- Provide postoperative analgesics.

Impaired verbal communication related to altered anatomy and/or function because of the presence of tumor or response to therapy

- Maintain open communication by call light in patient's reach at bedside and use of pad and pencil or Magic Slate.
- Ask questions that require a "yes" or "no" answer.
- Wait for patient to write responses.
- Assist with use of artificial larynx if applicable.
- Support activities of speech therapist to develop esophageal speech.
- Recommend support group.

Patient Education/Home Care Planning

1. Explain methods of maintaining respiratory function, such as deep breathing, coughing, and use of oxygen; provide a list of emergency resources.
2. Discuss the value of speech therapy, and put the patient in touch with support groups, such as the Lost Cord Club.
3. Explain the use of various methods of managing pain.

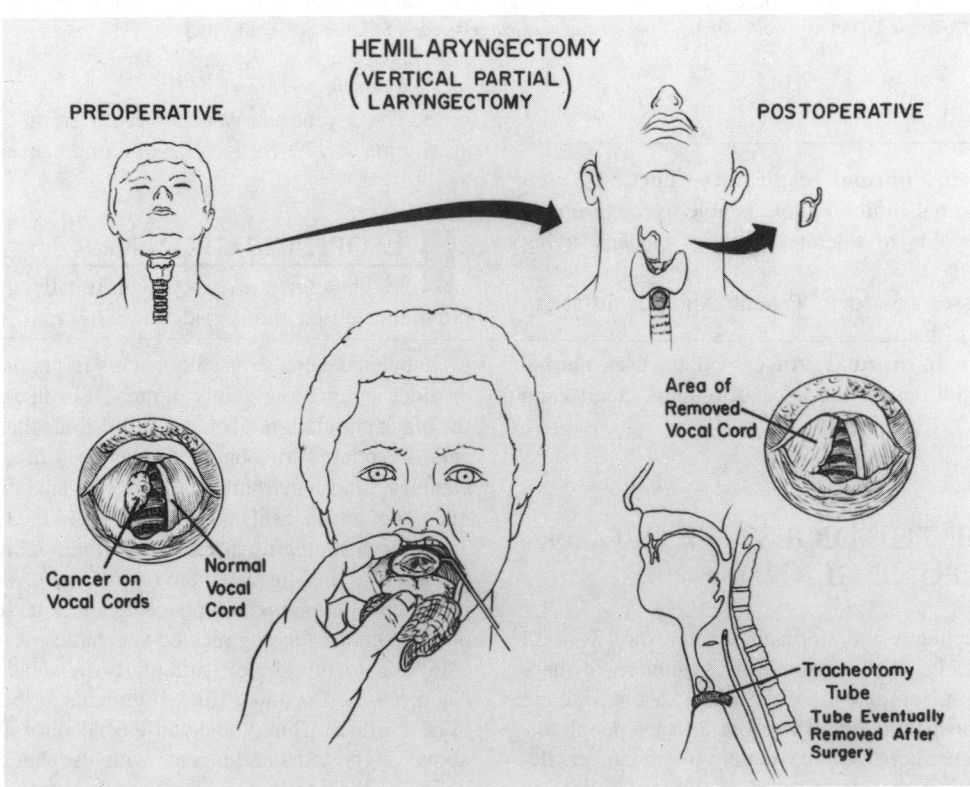

Figure 16-3 The technique of vertical partial laryngectomy. (From DeWeese DD et al: *Otolaryngology—head and neck surgery,* ed 7, St Louis, 1988, Mosby.)

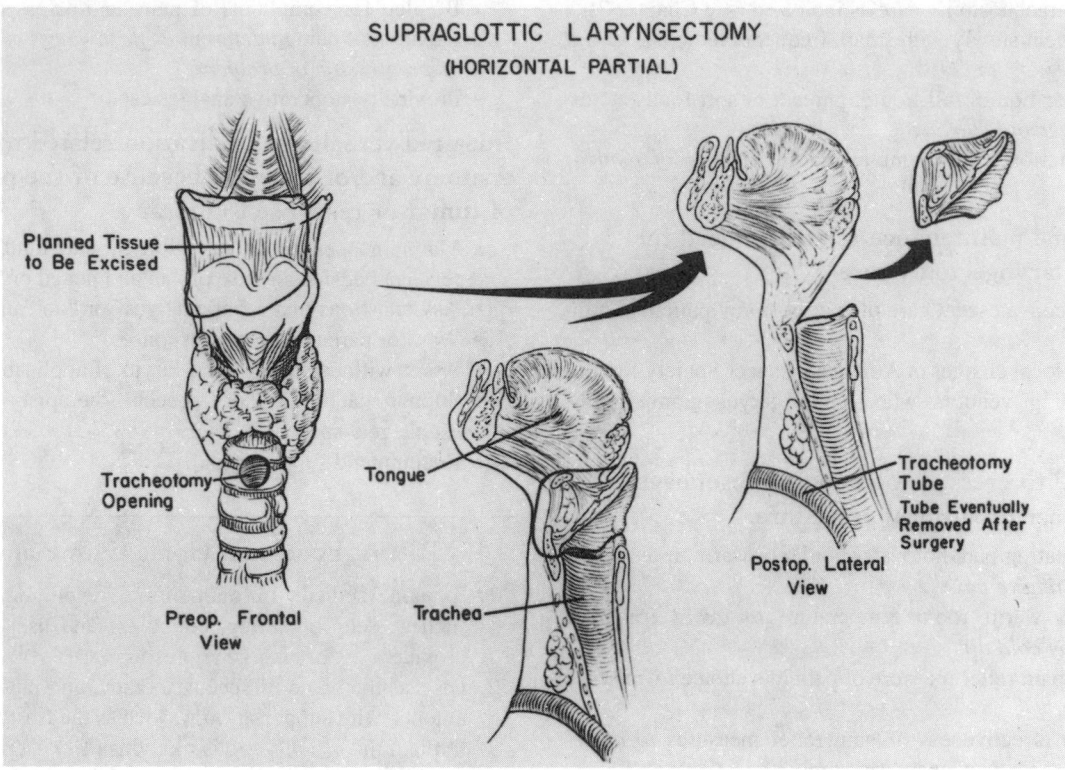

Figure 16-4 The technique of supraglottic laryngectomy. Removal of the endolaryngeal structures from tip of epiglottis down to laryngeal vertical. (From DeWeese DD et al: *Otolaryngology—head and neck surgery,* ed 7, St Louis, 1988, Mosby.)

Evaluation

Patient maintains normal respiratory function Vital signs are within normal limits. Patient is able to cough up secretions. Patient is able to tolerate activities of daily living without dyspnea.

Patient expresses comfort Patient expresses no verbal or nonverbal signs of pain.

Patient speaks in normal voice Patient uses normal structures or artificial devices as needed to speak clearly and distinctly.

CANCERS OF THE DIGESTIVE ORGANS AND ENDOCRINE GLANDS

Cancers of the esophagus and stomach account for 4% of all cancers. Unfortunately, many of the early symptoms of these diseases (dysphagia, epigastric discomfort, anorexia, and weight loss) are nonspecific, and therefore affected people often delay seeking treatment. Approximately 6% of cancers detected in the United States affect the digestive and endocrine glands. Some are easily detected because of their location and secretory patterns, whereas others are more difficult to diag-

nose. The 5-year survival rate varies from 1% for pancreatic carcinoma to 95% for localized thyroid cancer.

ESOPHAGEAL CANCER

Malignancy of the esophagus usually arises from squamous epithelium and is epidermoid in type.

Esophageal cancer usually occurs in people 50 years of age or older and predominantly in men. It is also more common in the black population. There are indications that esophageal cancers are related to tobacco and alcohol use, nutritional deficiencies, and environmental carcinogens. The highest frequency of esophageal cancers is found in the Caspian Sea area, Transkei in southern Africa, and northern China.

Some of the suggested environmental or nutritional factors in the development of esophageal cancer include nitrosamines or fungi contaminating pickled vegetables or in grains; chronic addiction to morphine, particularly in areas where opium is eaten; tobacco residue; silica fragments associated with millet bran (northern China); and abuse of alcohol. In associating the above suggested carcinogens with esophageal cancer, alcoholism is the one that has a clear relationship with epidermoid carcinoma of the esophagus. Chronic inflammation of the esophagus is also associated with a higher incidence of carcinomas. There is also an association between cancer of the esophagus and squamous cell carcinoma of the oropharynx or larynx, which is probably a result of exposure of the oral cavity, respiratory tract, and esophagus to the same carcinogenic factors. An increased incidence of esophageal cancer occurs among persons with achalasia.

•••••• Pathophysiology

Approximately 50% of esophageal cancers are at the esophagogastric junction (these cancers are generally adenocarcinoma and arise from the stomach rather than the esophagus); 25% are in the upper thoracic esophagus; 17% are in the lower esophagus; and 8% are in the cervical esophagus. Two thirds of these are squamous cell carcinomas. Adenocarcinomas are the second most common type.

Squamous cell carcinoma begins as a small mucosal patch that eventually grows, ulcerates, and protrudes into the lumen. Local extension to the recurrent laryngeal nerve or tracheobronchial tree is common. Unfortunately, local extension of the cancer is often present at the time of diagnosis. Metastasis to the local lymph nodes includes those around the hilum of the lung and in the neck. Metastases to the abdominal lymph nodes of the celiac axis occur. Metastases to the liver, lungs, kidney, and bone occur with decreasing frequency. Submucosal spread of the carcinoma does occur. Satellite lesions occur several inches away from the primary lesion.

Carcinoma of the bronchus or stomach often metastasizes to the esophagus. Mediastinal lymph node metastasis from other organ carcinomas may lead to esophageal involvement and symptoms of obstruction. Breast carcinomas may metastasize to the esophagus. Primary adenocarcinoma of the esophagus is rare and should be considered the result of Barrett's esophagus or of spread from an adenocarcinoma of the stomach cardia.

Dysphagia is the most common complaint of persons with esophageal cancer. It is usually first noticed with the ingestion of bulky foods, later with soft foods, and finally with liquids. Weight loss, regurgitation, and aspiration pneumonitis may also be noted. The most prevalent symptoms in persons without dysphagia are odynophagia (pain on swallowing) and symptoms of gastroesophageal reflux.

Signs and symptoms of advanced disease include cervical adenopathy; chronic cough; choking after eating; hemoptysis, hematemesis, or both; and hoarseness. Pain is an unusual symptom and indicates local extension.

•••••• Diagnostic Studies and Findings

Esophageal x-ray examination Irregular ragged mucosal pattern with luminal narrowing

Esophagoscopy with brush biopsy Presence of lesion with malignant cells in biopsy specimen

•••••• Multidisciplinary Plan

Surgery

Esophagogastrectomy
  Left chest for lesions in lower esophagus

Laparotomy and right thoracotomy or transhiatal approach for higher lesions

Transhiatal approach for lesions at thoracic inlet and cervical esophagus; stomach as esophageal replacement

Radiation Therapy

External beam for squamous cell lesions above aortic arch
Palliation for obstructive symptoms, pain control

Chemotherapy

Preoperative cisplatin-based chemotherapy alone or in combination with radiation therapy

Used alone for palliation with locally recurrent or metastatic disease

Used with radiation therapy (without surgery) for palliation of dysphagia

NURSING CARE

Nursing Assessment

Nutritional Status

Dysphagia, initially with solids and progressing to liquids; difficult or painful swallowing; sensation of food taking longer to go through segments of the chest (i.e., to reach the stomach) described by the patient; anorexia; weight loss; regurgitation

Comfort

Odynophagia

Nursing Dx & Intervention for Untreatable Tumor (see also section on Metastatic Disease and Terminal Stage of the Disease)

Esophageal Cancer

Altered nutrition: less than body requirements related to obstruction of esophagus by tumor

- Assess patient to determine those foods patient can and cannot swallow *to select and prepare edible foods.*
- Provide a diet that omits alcohol, spices, or foods at extreme temperatures and includes bland foods *to prevent irritation of the esophageal mucosa.*
- Teach the patient to eat slowly, chew food thoroughly, and arch back while swallowing *to increase amount ingested.*
- Have patient eat while sitting in the upright position and remain sitting after meal *to avoid regurgitation or aspiration.*
- Have patient avoid eating 1 to 2 hours before bedtime *to avoid heartburn or reflux esophagitis.*
- Have patient sip half a glass of water after each meal *to cleanse the esophagus.*

Pain related to esophageal irritation by tumor

- Place the head of the patient's bed on 4-inch blocks *to prevent reflux esophagitis.*
- Provide antacids at bedside *so that patient can medicate self when indigestion occurs.*
- Assess patient for evidence of mouth filling with fluid refluxing from esophagus, for dysphagia, and for heartburn (which increases when the patient lies down) as evidence of esophagitis, *which requires aggressive medical management.*
- Administer solution of meat tenderizer to relieve food impaction, which may be a cause of pain.
- Observe for evidence of gastrointestinal bleeding, such as hematemesis or melena, *which indicates severe esophageal irritation.*

Evaluation

Nutritional status has improved Patient is able to maintain weight and has made progress toward normal weight.

Patient is comfortable Facial expression is calm and relaxed. Patient expresses comfort.

■ GASTRIC CANCER

Gastric carcinoma refers to malignant neoplasms and tumors found in the stomach. Adenocarcinomas that arise from normal or metaplastic mucosa cells are the most common. Benign neoplasms of the stomach are rare and include leiomyomas and polyps.

The incidence of gastric cancers has significantly decreased in western Europe and the United States. The American Cancer Society[3] estimated that approximately 23,000 new cases occurred in 1990 (2.3% of all new cancer cases). In the 1940s gastric cancer was the most common malignant disease in the United States. No apparent change in the incidence of gastric cancer has occurred in Japan, where it accounts for 60% of all cancers in men and 40% of all cancers in women.

Many questions exist about the decline in gastric cancer. The answers to those questions would provide valuable clues in the early diagnosis, treatment, and ultimately prevention of gastric carcinomas. In addition, interesting geographic variations exist. Gastric cancer is higher in the north central and northeast regions of the United States. It is more common in urban than rural areas in England, but this is not true in the United States. Although it is very common in Japan, gastric cancer is less common in Japanese persons in Hawaii and the incidence decreases with each generation.

Genetic factors may play a role in the development of gastric cancer. Gastric cancers are more frequent in certain families and in persons with type A blood. In the United States, gastric cancer is more common in blacks than whites and in men than women. In Israel the incidence of gastric cancer is two and a half times higher in Jews of northern European backgrounds than Jews of Mediterranean or Asian descent.

The role of dietary factors has been studied to identify foods or soil contaminants that may lead to gastric cancers. Starches, pickled vegetables, and salted fish and meats have been associated with gastric cancers. However, whole milk, fresh vegetables, vitamin C, and refrigeration are inversely associated with gastric cancers. Increased salt consumption is also seen in patients with gastric cancers. Nitrates, which are converted into nitrites, are commonly found in the diet. Compounds formed with nitrites (nitrosamines and nitrosamides) have been carcinogenic in animals. Although not confirmed as a carcinogen in humans, nitrite-forming bacteria are increased in the upper gastrointestinal tract in people with hypochlorhydria and achlorhydria following gastric surgery. Hypochlorhydria and achlorhydria are often found in patients with pernicious anemia and atrophic gastritis. The reduced acid appears to support or allow colonization of the stomach by the bacteria.

Cold temperatures inhibit the conversion of nitrates to nitrites. Better refrigeration and decreased use of nitrates as food additives might explain the decreased incidence of gastric cancers.

Gastric cancer appears to be higher in individuals with late-onset immunoglobulin deficiency. Patients with celiac sprue with reduced IgA are at greater risk for gastric cancer. Other factors associated with gastric cancer are gastric ulcers, atrophic gastritis, gastric polyps, and pernicious anemia.

•••••• Pathophysiology

The carcinoma found in the stomach is epithelial growth arising from the mucosal membrane. Microscopically the cells resemble intestinal metaplasia and contain goblet cells characteristic of the intestines. The parietal and chief glands of the stomach are seldom seen in gastric tumors. Adenocarcinomas in the stomach have been classified in several ways.

First, according to cellular or extracellular characteristics, carcinomas are referred to as papillary, colloid or mucinous, medullary, and signet ring. Papillary refers to cells forming glandular structures in a papillary form. When excessive mucin secretion and extracellular aggregates are present, the adenocarcinoma is referred to as colloid or mucinous. Medullary is a solid band or a mass of undifferentiated cells. The signet ring adenocarcinoma refers to a well-differentiated adenocarcinoma with large amounts of intracellular mucinous material that compresses the nucleus to an unusual location.

Second, an adenocarcinoma of the stomach may be classified histologically according to the degree of cell differentiation—from well differentiated to poorly differentiated.

Unfortunately, the preceding two classifications and their parts are not mutually exclusive. Various cellular characteristics and degrees of differentiation may occur within a tumor. The third classification system reflects the biologic behavior of the tumor and defines gastric carcinomas as intestinal or diffuse. The intestinal type is a glandular tumor, and the diffuse type is composed of single cells or small groups of cells.

The fourth system is an expansion of the intestinal and diffuse definitions and classifies cancers in the stomach as expanding or infiltrating. The expanding (intestinal) type is characterized by a group of cells that are similar, maintain a coherent relationship, and push aside other cells as they grow. The infiltrative (diffuse) class is characterized by deep, wide infiltration by individual tumor cells.

The intestinal type of gastric cancer is associated with intestinal metaplasia and gastritis. The carcinoma tends to be circumscribed, and spread of the disease is through the bloodstream. The liver is a common site of metastasis. The diffuse type of carcinoma is less circumscribed, spreads by way of the lymphatics, and may take the form of linitis plastica, which is a diffuse fibrosis and thickening of the gastric wall.

The most common site of carcinomas is the lower half of the stomach. An exception occurs when gastric atrophy is a precursor to the cancer, and then the lesion tends to be in the upper portion of the stomach.

In early gastric cancers the disease is confined to the mucosa and submucosa. The symptoms with early gastric cancers may be vague and nonspecific and include complaints of epigastric discomfort or indigestion and occasional vomiting, belching, or postprandial fullness. The only observation that can lead to an early diagnosis is a positive stool occult blood test result.

Advanced gastric cancer denotes involvement of the muscular layer of the stomach with invasion of the pancreas, esophagus, colon, duodenum, gallbladder, liver, or the adjacent mesenteries. Metastases, local and distant, are common.

Gastric ulcers have been associated with gastric cancers. This may be a diagnostic issue. Previously radiologically diagnosed gastric ulcers have later been found to be carcinomas. Occasionally a benign gastric ulcer has a focal carcinoma at a margin. Also, malignant cells may be found at the base of the ulcer and at the margin. Most physicians routinely perform a biopsy of gastric ulcers during endoscopy to rule out the presence of gastric carcinoma.

Gastric atrophy and pernicious anemia are associated with achlorhydria. Achlorhydria is a precursor of gastric cancer. Gastric polyps are often found in atrophic mucosa. A polyp may be benign or malignant, and the recommended treatment is removal through an endoscope and histologic examination. Approximately 10% of gastric polyps are malignant.

•••••• Diagnostic Studies and Findings

Hematocrit   Slightly below normal; patient may have macrocytic or microcytic anemia secondary to decreased iron or vitamin B_{12} absorption

Stool for occult blood   Positive for blood

Upper gastrointestinal series (barium swallow)   Polypoid mass; ulceration surrounded by mass; thickened, fibrosed gastric wall

Computed tomography   Thickness of gastric wall; presence of metastasis (may assist in differentiating between benign and carcinogenic lesion)

Endoscopy and cytologic studies   Biopsy and cytology specimens examined for cancer cells; can visualize lesion

Liver function studies   Abnormal findings may indicate metastasis

•••••• Multidisciplinary Plan

Surgery

Exploratory celiotomy: initial intervention in all patients with gastric cancer except those with peritoneal metastases, documented liver metastases, or other distant metastases; if tumor is regionally localized, resection of primary tumor, as well as actual and potentially involved regional lymph nodes, is done; postoperative staging of the tumor is completed and further treatment decisions are made

Distal subtotal gastric resection

Proximal subtotal gastric resection

Total gastrectomy: includes resection of adjacent organs involved by local extension, such as body and tail of pancreas, portion of liver, transverse colon, or duodenum and head of pancreas

Palliative resection

Radiation Therapy

Palliation of obstruction, particularly in the cardia, or of chronic bleeding

Chemotherapy

Single agent palliation with 5-fluorouracil

Combination chemotherapy

5-fluorouracil, nitrosourea, mitomycin C, doxorubicin

FAM: 5-fluorouracil, doxorubicin (Adriamycin), mitomycin C

5-fluorouracil, semustine (methyl CCNU)

The prognosis for patients with gastric cancer is poor because almost two thirds have findings at the time of diagnosis that limit the possibility of survival. Nodal involvement is a significant prognostic factor. Those patients with a short history of symptoms have a poorer prognosis than do those with a longer history. Patients with ulcer syndrome do better than those with the more common symptoms of indigestion.

NURSING CARE

Nursing Assessment

Nutritional Status

Loss of appetite; anorexia

Feeling of fullness with minimum intake

Distaste for meats

Weight loss

Persistent midepigastric pain

Dysphagia

Vague epigastric discomfort

Vomiting; hematemesis

Belching

Postprandial fullness

Physical Examination

Tenderness in midepigastrium

Rebound tenderness

Abdominal guarding

Mass in epigastrium (late stage)

Enlarged liver

Positive supraclavicular nodes

Ascites (loss of albumin into gastric lumen)

Acanthosis nigricans (rare)

Signs of metastasis: myeloid metaplasia or primary central nervous system (CNS) disease

Nursing Dx & Intervention for Untreatable Tumor (see section on Metastatic Disease and Terminal Stage of the Disease)

Altered nutrition, less than body requirements related to gastric obstruction by tumor

- Assess patient's caloric intake—kinds, amounts, and percentages of protein, carbohydrate, and fat—*to determine needed changes in diet.*
- Observe the patient for evidence of weight loss and dehydration *to intervene quickly with nutritional supplements, and fluids.*
- Assess whether patient is experiencing discomfort or indigestion, vomiting, belching, postprandial fullness, or weakness as evidence of tumor pressure and obstruction.
- Provide palpable meals based as much as possible on patient likes and dislikes *to increase caloric consumption.*
- Offer dietary (liquid) supplements as needed *to maintain adequate nutritional balance.*
- Offer medications that relieve abdominal distention and flatulence because *these symptoms tend to adversely affect appetite.*
- Provide frequent small feedings each day.

Fluid volume deficit related to gastric obstruction or perforation

- Observe characteristics and amount of emesis and stool *to determine need for fluid and blood component therapy.*
- Monitor vital signs at frequent intervals during episodes of bleeding *to detect shock early.*
- Monitor patient's input and output and urine specific gravity *to detect renal dysfunction.*
- Administer IV fluids as prescribed *to replace lost fluid volume.*
- Monitor laboratory reports *to detect development of anemia.*
- Observe for signs and symptoms of worsening fluid volume deficit—including decreased urine output, concentrated urine, output greater than intake, weakness, change in mental status, blood in emesis or stool, severe and diffuse abdominal pain, rebound tenderness, and guarding—*to determine need for large volumes of IV fluids and rapid infusion of blood components.*

Patient Education/Home Care Planning

1. Ensure that patient understands the rationale for combination therapies of surgery, chemotherapy, and radiation therapy in the treatment of gastric cancers. Provide written information in the form of do's and don'ts during chemotherapy and radiotherapy, sequence of treatment, and potential side effects.
2. Explain the importance of regular follow-up endoscopies.

Evaluation

Patient can manage pain   Patient is comfortable and able to relieve pain and symptoms effectively.

Patient adapts to or accepts disease and prognosis   Patient has mobilized available resources to assist him or her and family in handling the emotional, social, and financial stressors of having cancer. Patient attends "I Can Cope" groups.

Patient complies with medical regimen   Patient has regular appointments with physician, maintains treatment sequence of drugs and radiotherapy, and reports signs of side effects. Patient uses home care (visiting) nurses to evaluate progress, reinforce teaching, and provide physical care as needed.

Laboratory findings are normal   Hematocrit and albumin levels are within normal limits. Stools have no occult blood. There is no cancer on repeat endoscopy.

Nutritional status is adequate   Caloric intake is maintained at level patient can tolerate. Weight loss is minimized.

■ DIGESTIVE GLAND TUMORS

Carcinomas of the digestive glands are neoplasms that may involve the pancreas, liver, or gallbladder.

Carcinoma of the gallbladder, with its insidious onset, may be diagnosed only during surgery for presumed acute cholecystitis. The only possibility of cure is with complete removal of the gallbladder; often a partial hepatectomy is also required because of early liver invasion. Mortality is as high as 75%; the 5-year survival rate is about 4%.

Carcinoma of the liver is usually metastatic; primary tumors constitute only 1% of hepatic cancer. One primary tumor, hemangiosarcoma of the liver, is a rare disease thought to be caused by vinyl chloride exposure. The risk of hepatocellular carcinoma is about 40 times greater in patients with ethanol-induced cirrhosis. Early signs and symptoms of hepatic cancer are often absent or insidious and slow to localize (Figure 16-5). The most common complaints are vague upper abdominal pain and generalized weakness. Other indications of liver involvement are anemia, anorexia, jaundice, weight loss, pain, and respiratory distress. Obstruction of the portal vein, sometimes occurring suddenly, may cause splenomegaly, esophageal varices, and ascites. Patients may also have fever of unknown origin and dependent edema. Diagnosis is based on laboratory data obtained from a liver profile, scanning, angiography, and biopsy.

The only possibility for cure is lobectomy to remove the diseased tissue. In some major medical centers, liver transplantation is being used as an alternative procedure for eligible patients. If surgery is contraindicated by the extent of the disease or the patient's condition, radiation therapy and chemotherapy via implantable infusion pump may be used. The prognosis is poor, and few patients are alive 5 years after the initial diagnosis.

The incidence of carcinoma of the pancreas has increased more than 20% in recent years. The reason for this is unknown, although cigarette smoking and dietary fat may be causative factors. As in liver and gallbladder disease, the onset is insidious and the diagnosis is made late in the course. Clinical signs indicating the tumor's location include the following:

Head of the pancreas—obstructive jaundice resulting from blockage of the common bile duct.

Body and tail of the pancreas—vague abdominal or back pain, progressive weight loss, anorexia, and a variety of gastrointestinal symptoms

Islet cells—hypoglycemia and insulin-shock syndrome, resulting from production of large quantities of insulin

As many as half of these patients have occult blood in the stools. The pain is steady, dull, and aching and unrelated to digestive activity. Because of the vagueness of the signs and symptoms, few pancreatic tumors are diagnosed at a curable stage. The diagnosis is usually based on tomographic scanning, ultrasonography, and biopsy.

Pancreatoduodenectomy (Whipple's procedure) is the standard surgical procedure for cancer of the head of the pancreas. Palliation may be effected with radiation therapy or chemotherapy. The prognosis is extremely poor; only 10% of patients are still alive 1 year after diagnosis.

Nursing Dx & Intervention for Untreatable Tumor (see section on Metastatic Disease and Terminal Stage of the Disease)

Altered nutrition: less than body requirements related to anorexia with weight loss, constipation, bloating or flatulence, recent onset or unstable diabetes, and weight loss

- Assess caloric intake—kinds, amounts, and percentages of protein, carbohydrate, and fat—*to determine needed changes in or additions to diet.*
- Observe the patient for evidence of weight loss and dehydration *to intervene quickly with foods, nutritional supplements, and fluids.*
- Ask patient if he or she is experiencing anorexia, constipation, bloating, flatulence, or other signs and symptoms of gastrointestinal distress *as evidence of tumor pressure and possible disease progression.*
- Provide palatable meals based as much as possible on patient likes and dislikes *to increase caloric intake.*
- Encourage the patient to eat frequent small meals *to increase intake.*

- Offer medications that relieve abdominal distention and flatulence because *these symptoms tend to adversely affect appetite.*

Pain related to tumor pressure and irritation of tissues in close proximity as evidenced by midepigastric pain that is steady, dull, boring, and usually worse at night, by back pain aggravated by lying flat, or by pruritus

- Assess location, onset, duration, radiation, and intensity of pain to determine appropriate interventions (e.g., back pain is often relieved by sitting up and bending forward or lying curled in a fetal position).
- Provide prescribed medications for pain as needed *to decrease patient's discomfort.*
- Teach patient self-care strategies such as relaxation exercises, imagery, and application of heat or cold *to manage pain.*
- Monitor diet *to determine if certain foods increase or decrease patient pain or gastrointestinal discomfort.*
- Offer patient frequent baths, lotions, and ointments *to soothe skin and decrease itching.*

Salivary gland tumors grow slowly and are often diagnosed late. Complete excision, although difficult to accomplish without producing facial nerve damage, is important to prevent recurrence. If the tumor cannot be removed surgically, radiation therapy may be used to shrink it.

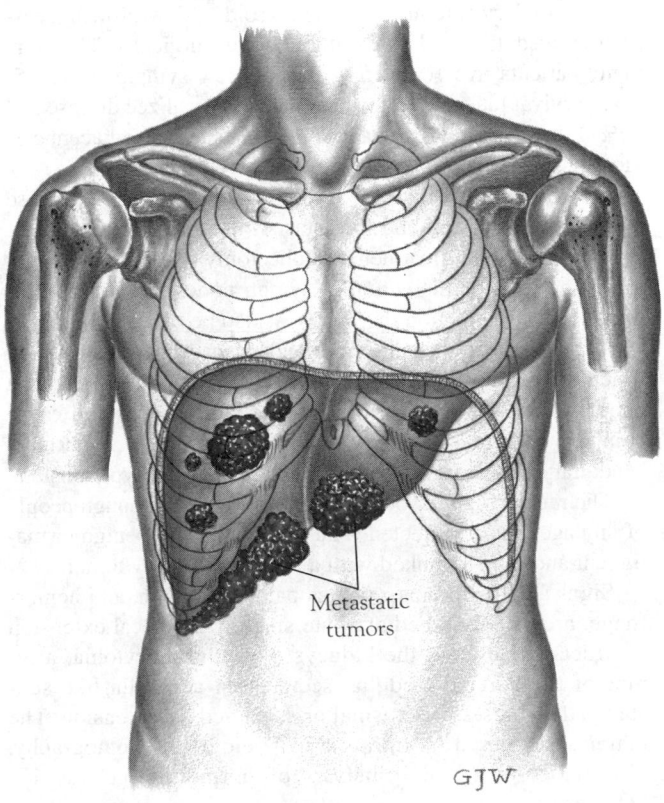

Figure 16-5 Hepatic carcinoma (liver cancer).

Evaluation

Nutritional status is adequate Caloric intake is maintained at level patient can tolerate.

Patient is comfortable Patient has a relaxed facial expression and verbally confirms feeling comfortable.

■ ENDOCRINE GLAND TUMORS

■ Endocrine gland tumors may occur in the parathyroid, thyroid, or adrenal glands.

Parathyroid tumors are rare. When they do occur, they produce excessive amounts of parathyroid hormone, which causes bony deformities and renal calculi. These tumors are treated by surgical excision.

Carcinoma of the thyroid has its highest incidence (37% of endocrine cancers) in people 25 to 44 years of age. It occurs most frequently in women and in whites. Those at high risk are people who as children received radiation therapy to the neck for such conditions as hypertrophy of the tonsils, adenoids, or lymphatic tissue, enlarged thymus gland, or skin disorders such as acne.

The initial sign of a thyroid tumor is a lump in the gland, which may first be palpated during a routine physical examination. More extensive local involvement causes hoarseness, dysphagia, or dyspnea. Thyroid scanning, ultrasonography, and biopsy are used to diagnose the lesion, which is most commonly papillary carcinoma of the thyroid, a slow-growing, easily removed tumor. Even without total surgical eradication, many patients live 10 to 15 years with few symptoms. The 5-year survival rate is 97% for patients with localized disease and 86% if the disease has spread. Spread is usually to adjacent cervical lymph nodes.

Undifferentiated thyroid cancers are more likely to cause tracheal compression and metastasis to cervical lymph nodes. For these patients treatment is lobectomy or total thyroidectomy and en bloc dissection of lymph nodes. Radioactive iodine (^{131}I) and radiation therapy may also be used.

Neoplasms of the adrenal glands cause changes in body functioning, depending on the affected component. Cortical neoplasms may alter the body's sex characteristics and cause complex steroidal changes, such as Cushing's syndrome. Medullary neoplasms may precipitate attacks of hypertension.

The median age for occurrence is 40 years, although people of any age may be affected. The tumors may be benign or malignant and may be linked with a specific pituitary tumor.

Signs and symptoms, such as pain, distention, and hemorrhage, are usually noted at a late stage, when local extension obstructs or destroys the kidneys. Pheochromocytoma, a tumor of the adrenal medulla, secretes an adrenalin-like substance that causes paroxysmal or sustained hypertension. The diagnosis is based on intravenous pyelography, tomography, ultrasonography, and urinalysis of hormones such as 17-ketosteroid.

Surgical excision, the treatment of choice, necessitates temporary or permanent cortisone replacement therapy. Radiation and chemotherapy may also be used, but because the diagnosis is rarely made before extension of the tumor has occurred, the prognosis is poor.

Ovarian and testicular tumors are discussed elsewhere in this chapter.

CANCERS OF BONE AND CONNECTIVE TISSUES

Sarcomas of bone and soft tissue, although relatively uncommon, are of particular interest because of their tendency to occur in young people, their generally poor prognosis, and the major surgery usually required. The prognosis has been improved in recent years by the combination of local surgery and chemotherapy. In addition, in many patients the primary can be successfully treated by more conservative surgical procedures combined with high-dose radiation therapy. However, 60% to 65% of bone cancers are metastatic from other primary lesions and thus are more difficult to treat successfully. In 1987 there were approximately 7400 new cases of these cancers and 4200 deaths.

■ BONE SARCOMAS

■ Bone cancer is a skeletal malignancy occurring as a primary sarcomatous tumor in an area of rapid growth.

People at high risk for development of bone sarcomas are those with Paget's disease of bone, Ollier's disease, multiple exostoses, retinoblastoma, or previous high-dose radiation therapy to bone. Osteosarcoma and Ewing's sarcoma occur most commonly in people under the age of 20 years. This is in contrast to reticulum cell sarcoma, fibrosarcoma, and chondrosarcoma, which occur later in life but with a much wider age distribution.

•••••• Pathophysiology

The patient's complaints are initially subtle and intermittent, with gradually increasing severity. An initially painless mass is the most common symptom; others include pain, functional deficit, or pathologic fracture. The pain is usually described as mild and brief and is often associated with a minor injury. It may increase in severity but is often reported as being a localized, dull ache. It usually does not increase with activity or decrease with rest but may be greater at night. This pain rarely responds to simple analgesic medication but requires narcotics for relief.

There may not be any symptoms; if they are present, they are dependent on the size, site, and patterns of local infiltration. The site and extent of pathologic fractures dictate the severity of symptoms. Metastases to regional lymph nodes are uncommon, but systemic illness may be related to pulmonary, visceral, and subcutaneous tissue involvement.

•••••• Diagnostic Studies and Findings

Roentgenograms of involved bones and soft tissues Visualization of suspect lesion

Chest roentgenogram Evidence of metastasis

Bone scan Evidence of primary lesion or metastasis

Computed tomography Evidence of cortical bone destruction

Blood studies Increased alkaline and acid phosphatase; increased calcium indicative of bone disease and demineralization

Urine study High calcium excretion secondary to hypercalcemia

•••••• Multidisciplinary Plan

Surgery*

Amputation with limb salvage to degree possible

Foot and ankle—below-knee amputation or knee disarticulation

Proximal tibia—thigh amputation

Distal femur—hip disarticulation

Proximal end of femur—modified hemipelvectomy

En bloc resection for low-grade malignant lesions; reconstruction with bone autografts, cadaver hemografts, or metal or plastic devices

Medications

Antineoplastic agents

Preoperative and postoperative systemic chemotherapy for osteogenic sarcoma; high-dose methotrexate (Amethopterin; Mexate) with leucovorin rescue; doxorubicin (Adriamycin) by intraarterial perfusion; dosages individually determined

Systemic chemotherapy for metastatic disease

Biologic response modifiers (interferon)

Radiation Therapy

For treatment of Ewing's sarcoma

Disease-free survival rates for patients whose osteogenic sarcoma is treated with surgery and chemotherapy appear to be greater than 50% at 5 years. Among patients with localized Ewing's sarcoma, the disease-free survival at 5 years is 50% following chemotherapy and radiation therapy.

NURSING CARE

Nursing Assessment

Musculoskeletal Function

Presence of mass; functional deficit; pathologic fracture

Pain

Mild and fleeting; dull and aching; increased at night; not affected by activity or rest; need for narcotics to obtain relief

Systemic Function

Fever; malaise, easy fatigability; anorexia; weight loss

Nursing Dx & Intervention for Untreatable Tumors (see also section on Metastatic Disease and Terminal Stage of the Disease)

Impaired physical mobility related to pressure of tumor, pain

- Assist patient with ambulation; control distance *to avoid injury and fatigue.*
- Have patient use walker, cane, or wheelchair as needed as assistive devices *to promote mobility.*
- Minimize environmental barriers *to avoid falls.*
- Encourage use of involved limb *to maintain function.*
- Observe for deficits, weakness, or abnormal gait *as indications of further impairment of mobility.*

Pain related to pressure of tumor

- Change patient's position slowly *to avoid stretching and pressure.*
- Provide whirlpool, or use heat applications *to promote relaxation and healing.*
- Provide safety *to avoid further injury to patient.*
- Discuss possible pain-relieving measures with patient; use those measures *to involve patient in self-care.*
- Observe for increasing pain and dysfunction *to determine need for further intervention.*
- Discuss "phantom" pain with patient (amputee) and significant other.
- Assist with and teach use of patient-controlled analgesic device if ordered.
- Administer morphine solution via continuous drip as ordered according to facility policy.

Activity intolerance related to systemic effects of disease and treatment

- Ambulate patient, or seat patient in armchair *to promote circulation.*
- Encourage moderate physical exercise, adequate rest, and performance of range of motion exercises *to maintain activity level and avoid immobility.*
- *Balance nutritional intake; supplement protein* to increase strength.
- *Observe for increased nutritional requirements and weakness* as indications of advancing disease.

Patient Education/Home Care Planning

1. Discuss the principles of safe ambulation: wide supportive stance; well-fitting, low-heeled shoes; good body mechanics; and weight bearing on unaffected side.
2. Plan pain relief measures with activities to enhance patient self-care.

---

*See Chapter 4 for postoperative nursing diagnoses and interventions.

Evaluation

Patient is mobile and able to tolerate activity   Patient walks independently or with assistive device. Patient can tolerate activities of daily living.

Patient is free of pain   Patient uses pain relief measures as needed.

■ SOFT TISSUE SARCOMAS

Soft tissue sarcomas are neoplasms that arise in soft tissue, parenchymatous organs, or hollow viscera and include fibrosarcoma, malignant fibrous histiocytoma, liposarcoma, rhabdomyosarcoma, leiomyosarcoma, angiosarcoma, synovial sarcoma, mixed mesenchymal sarcoma, Kaposi's sarcoma, and unclassified or spindle cell sarcoma.

Only among children are soft tissue tumors, especially rhabdomyosarcoma, relatively frequent.

•••••• Pathophysiology

A painless mass is the most common initial symptom. Masses in the thigh area are suspect because of the high number of sarcomas occurring there. Advanced local disease is rare except for large tumors arising in the retroperitoneal or pelvic areas. Lymph node metastases are uncommon except in patients with rhabdomyosarcoma, high-grade synovial sarcoma, and epithelioid sarcoma.

Rhabdomyosarcoma arises from the embryonic mesenchymal cells that form striated muscle. It may develop in almost any body site; the most common primary sites are the head and neck, extremities, genitourinary tract, trunk, and orbit. The prognosis depends on the primary site and the stage of the disease (histologic grade), which is in turn based on extent of disease and resectability. Genitourinary lesions generally have the most favorable prognosis, and extremity tumors have one of the worst prognoses.

Kaposi's sarcoma (KS), the malignancy most frequently associated with AIDS, is recorded as the syndrome's initial clinical manifestation in approximately 25% of cases. The epidemic form (EKS) affects primarily homosexual men and may be of greater incidence than noted above because subsequent malignant and infectious complications (after initial diagnosis) are not reported to the Centers for Disease Control.

The initial manifestations of EKS include nodular, macular, or papular lesions on the skin and mucosal surfaces; fever; weight loss; malaise; anorexia; and diarrhea. The lesions are frequently located on the trunk, arms, head, neck, and oral cavity. Lesions on the head and neck can be especially disfiguring and can cause symptoms of obstruction or compression. Fifty percent of patients with EKS have visceral involvement, particularly of the gastrointestinal tract. Pulmonary involvement can lead to progressive respiratory dysfunction and failure. Lymph nodes are often affected; involvement in the brain, liver, pancreas, adrenal glands, spleen, heart, and testes has been noted.

Therapy for EKS remains experimental and controversial, with chemotherapy, radiotherapy, and immunotherapy used with varying degrees of success.

•••••• Diagnostic Studies and Findings

Radiographic study of affected part (computed tomography, xerography, arteriography)   Visualization of suspect lesion and vasculature

Chest tomography or chest computed tomography   Evidence of metastasis

Excisional, incisional, or needle biopsy   Histologic evidence of malignancy

•••••• Multidisciplinary Plan

Surgery

Radical surgical excision—amputation, muscle group resection, radical local excision

Medications

Antineoplastic agents

Vincristine sulfate (Oncovin), 2 mg/m² for children, 1.4 mg/m² for adults

Doxorubicin (Adriamycin), 60 to 75 mg/m² at intervals of 21 d or 30 mg/m² on each of 3 successive d repeated q4wk

Cyclophosphamide (Cytoxan), 40 to 50 mg/kg IV or individual doses over several days, then adjusted to lower maintenance dosage; po 1 to 5 mg/kg qd

Cisplatin (Platinol), 50 to 80 mg/m² IV q3wk or by individually determined dosage

Radiation Therapy

External beam

NURSING CARE

Nursing Assessment

Pain in Area of Tumor
Body Contours

Painless mass

Sensory and Motor Function

Peripheral neuralgia; paralysis

Nursing Dx & Intervention for Untreatable Tumors (see also section on Metastatic Disease and Terminal Stage of the Disease)

Impaired physical mobility related to peripheral neuralgia, paralysis

- Assist patient with ambulation; control distance *to avoid stress and fatigue.*

- Use walker, cane, or wheelchair as needed *for added support.*
- Minimize environmental barriers *to prevent injury.*
- Encourage use of involved limb *to maintain tone.*
- Observe for deficits, complaints of weakness, and abnormal gait *as evidence of further dysfunction.*
- Test for impaired coordination *as evidence of further dysfunction.*

Pain related to pressure of tumor, ischemia

- Change patient's position slowly *to avoid additional discomfort.*
- Support affected part(s) *to prevent strain.*
- Place patient in whirlpool or use heat applications *for muscle relaxation.*
- Provide safety measures *to avoid injury.*
- Discuss possible pain-relieving measures with patient; use those measures.
- Monitor effectiveness of pain relief methods.
- Administer analgesics as ordered.
- Observe for increases in pain and dysfunction *as signs of need to reevaluate interventions.*

Patient Education/Home Care Planning

1. Explain the principles of safe ambulation.
2. Discuss the management of disease-related pain.

Evaluation

Patient is mobile and able to tolerate activity   Patient walks independently or with assistive device.

Patient is free of pain   Patient can tolerate activities of daily living. Patient uses pain relief measures as needed.

▌ CANCERS OF THE CENTRAL NERVOUS SYSTEM

Tumors of the central nervous system are neoplasms of the brain or spinal cord.

Tumors of the central nervous system (CNS) account for more than 2% of annual cancer deaths. Eighty percent of CNS tumors involve the brain, with as many as half of these metastatic from primary cancers of the lung, breast, kidney, melanoma, and gastrointestinal tract; the other 20% involve the spinal cord.

•••••• Pathophysiology

The majority of CNS tumors are gliomas, which are peculiar because they rarely spread beyond the CNS. There are no known etiologic factors, although childhood tumors are believed to be developmental in origin.

Spinal cord tumors are gliomas (23%), meningiomas or schwannomas (56%), or miscellaneous other forms such as epi-

dermoid and dermoid cysts, hemangioblastomas, and chordomas. These tumors produce symptoms in the body below the level of tumor location in the cord: difficulty in walking, postural disturbances, back pain, and changes in sensation and muscle power. The pain of a spinal cord tumor is worse at night.

Brain tumors in adults are categorized as follows:
Olioma
1. Glioblastoma—occur predominantly in the cerebral hemispheres; are highly invasive and malignant
2. Oligodendroglioma—most common in frontal lobes deep in the white matter; may arise in brainstem, cerebellum, and spinal cord; tend to be encapsulated

Astrocytoma: found anywhere in the brain; slow growing; invasive

Ependymoma: located in wall of ventricle; may arise in caudal tail of spinal cord

Neuronal cell medulloblastoma: found in posterior cerebellar vermis, roof of fourth ventricle; rapid growing

Mesodermal tissue meningioma: located in parasagittal falx of frontal and parietal lobes, sylvian fissure region, olfactory groove, wing of sphenoid bone, superior surface of cerebellum, cerebellopontine angle, spinal cord; slow growing; circumscribed; encapsulated; compressive nature

Neurilemoma (schwannoma): occur in cranial nerves, most commonly in vestibular division or cranial nerve VIII; slow growing

Pituitary adenoma: occurs in pituitary gland; may extend to invade floor of third ventricle; age linked; slow growing

Spinal tumors in adults are divided as follows:
Intramedullary
1. Ependymoma and astrocytoma: most common; usually extend over many spinal cord regions; most have slow, progressive onset with sensory loss of pain and temperatures; caudal region tumors may result in bowel, bladder, and sexual dysfunction
2. Oligodendroglioma
3. Hemangioblastomas

Extramedullary
1. Intradural tumors: include meningioma, neurofibroma, and congenital lesions; thoracic spine is frequent site; slow, gradual onset; local and radicular pain may be present
2. Extradural tumors: include metastic carcinoma, lymphoma, and multiple myeloma; rapid onset of symptoms; local pain at area of tumor and along spinal nerve dermatomes; increased pain with bed rest, movement, and straining

•••••• Diagnostic Studies and Findings

Brain Tumors

Brain scan   Increased uptake of isotope in the tumor

Pneumoencephalogram   Tumor localization; contraindicated if increased intracranial pressure suspected

Cerebral angiography Increased or obstructed cerebral blood flow

Positron emission tomography (PET) Details sites of glucose metabolism in the brain under various conditions

Skull x-ray examination Erosion of posterior clinoid process or presence of intracranial calcifications

Computed tomogram and magnetic resonance imaging Identification of vascular tumors, shifts in midline structures, changes in cerebral ventricular sizes

Electroencephalogram (EEG) Marked focal slowing; rhythmic, periodic, and high-voltage slowing

Dural sinus venography May indicate narrowed sinuses and interference with cranial drainage

Echoencephalogram Shifts in midline structures

Stereotaxic biopsy Identification of cell type

Ophthalmoscopic examination Papilledema

Spinal Tumors

Spinal x-ray examination Presence of vertebral column lesions and bony destruction

Myelography (with contrast medium) Identification of size, boundaries, and level of tumor

Cerebrospinal fluid (CSF) sampling Elevated protein levels; Froin's syndrome (xanthochromatic CSF with large amounts of protein, rapid coagulation, and absence of an increased number of cells)

Electromyogram (EMG) Useful in differential diagnosis

Queckenstedt test Positive finding

Computed tomogram Location of lesion

Spinal angiograms Differentiation of vascular lesions from tumors

Positron emission tomography (PET) Location of lesion

•••••• Multidisciplinary Plan

Brain Tumors
Surgery

Craniotomy for supratentorial tumor excision

Craniectomy for infratentorial tumor excision

Transsphenoidal for excision of pituitary tumor

Shunting procedures to treat secondary complications of hydrocephalus

Implantation of Ommaya reservoir for administration of intraventricular chemotherapy

Radiation Therapy

External beam

Brachytherapy, with implantation of radioactive seeds by stereotaxic techniques directly into tumor bed

Chemotherapy

Corticosteroids (dexamethasone, 10 to 20 mg/d po IV)

Agents dependent on type of tumor; must be able to cross blood-brain barrier

Spinal Cord Tumors
Surgery

Laminectomy

Radiation Therapy

Postoperative external beam

Palliative relief of cord compression

Chemotherapy

Corticosteroids (dexamethasone, 10 to 20 mg IV qid)

Despite therapeutic advances, CNS tumors have high morbidity and mortality. About 40% of people with brain tumors can return to a useful life, and another 30% gain good palliation. The neoplasms vary in their aggressiveness and consequently their prognosis. The earlier the diagnosis, the better the patient's chances for maximum restoration of function.

NURSING CARE

Nursing Assessment

Increased Intracranial Pressure

Early headache; nausea and vomiting; decreased level of consciousness; failing vision; changing pupillary response

Localizing Signs and Symptoms of Brain Tumors

See Table 16-2.

 TABLE 16-2 Localizing Signs and Symptoms of Brain Tumors

Frontal lobe	
Anterior portion	Disturbances in mental function
Posterior portion	Motor system dysfunction; convulsions; aphasia (dominant hemisphere)
Parietal lobe	Sensory deficits (contralateral); paresthesia; hyperesthesia; astereognosis; loss of two-point discrimination; finger agnosia; convulsions; visual field defects; defects in speech and recognition (dominant hemisphere)
Temporal lobe	Psychomotor convulsions; visual field defects; auditory disturbances; Wernicke's aphasia (dominant hemisphere)
Occipital lobe	Headaches; convulsions with visual aura; visual field deficit
Cerebellar tumors	Nystagmus; ataxia; unsteady gait; dysmetria; problems with rapid alternation movements
Brainstem and cranial nerve tumors	Hemiparesis; nystagmus; extraocular nerve palsies; facial paralysis; depressed corneal reflex; hearing loss, tinnitus; problems swallowing, drooling; vertigo, dizziness; ataxia; vomiting

Localizing Signs and Symptoms of Spinal Cord Tumors

See Table 16-3.

Nursing Dx & Intervention for Untreatable Tumor (see also section on Metastatic Disease and Terminal Stage of the Disease)

Sensory/perceptual alterations (visual) related to brain tissue compression

- Arrange environment *to minimize barriers and avoid injury.*
- Illuminate room adequately *to enhance visibility.*
- Place objects within site and reach *to facilitate self-care.*
- Provide frequent patient contact *to monitor needs.*
- Encourage expression of feelings, listen attentively, and offer feedback *to lower anxiety.*
- Reduce demands placed on patient *to avoid added stress.*
- Observe for irritability or unusual behavior *as evidence of difficulty with coping.*

Risk for injury related to increased intracranial/cord pressure and subsequent effects on balance, gait

- Maintain complete bed rest *to avoid falls.*
- Provide quiet *to reduce stimulation.*

TABLE 16-3 Localizing Signs and Symptoms of Spinal Cord Tumors

Cervical tumors	
C4 and above	Sensory: vertigo Motor: quadiparesis, atrophy of sternocleido-mastoid muscles; dysphagia; dysarthria; tongue deviation; respiratory insufficiency and/or failure Other: occipital headaches; nuchal rigidity; down-beat nystagmus; papilledema
C4 and below	Sensory: paresthesia; Horner's syndrome (ipsilateral pupillary constriction, ptosis, and anhidrosis) Motor: weakness, muscle fasciculation; muscle atrophy Other: shoulder and arm pain
Thoracic tumors	Sensory: hyperesthesia band immediately above level of lesion Motor: spastic paresis of lower extremities; positive Babinski's sign; lower motor neuron deficits Other: sphincter impairment
Lumbar tumors	Sensory: localized loss in legs and saddle area Motor: footdrop; diminished or absent patellar and Achilles reflexes Other: severe low back pain with radiation down legs; perianal and bladder discomfort; decreased libido; impotence; bladder disturbances

- Lower bed height *to avoid injury if patient leaves bed.*
- Subdue room lighting *to reduce stimulation.*
- Elevate patient's head, and change position slowly *to avoid increased intracranial pressure.*
- Discourage oral stimulants *to avoid increased intracranial pressure.*
- Refrain from jarring bed and performing nonessential procedures *to keep patient calm.*
- Place padded side rails up; place airway or padded tongue blade on bed for use in case of seizure *to avoid injury.*
- Inspect eyes for pupillary response, and observe for papilledema *as evidence of increasing intracranial pressure.*
- Monitor blood pressure and intracranial pressure as ordered *for early detection of increase.*
- Observe for confusion, lethargy, restlessness, vomiting, and complaints of headache and nausea *as signs of increasing pressure.*
- Palpate pulse rate and rhythm, and monitor volume *to determine adequacy of cardiovascular function.*

Risk for alteration in urinary elimination related to urinary sphincter disturbances

- Assess voiding patterns, palpate bladder, and monitor input and output *to determine the need for intermittent catheterization.*
- Measure postresidual voids *to determine need for more frequent catheterization.*
- Encourage fluid intake with even distribution throughout the day, and decrease patient's fluid intake at night *to maintain renal function and prevent infection.*
- Discourage intake of caffeinated beverages *to avoid bladder irritation.*

Risk for constipation related to disruption of innervation to bowel

- Assess bowel sounds and palpate abdomen *to determine extent of peristalsis and motility.*
- Monitor bowel elimination, noting frequency, consistency, and amount of stool *to detect constipation and prevent fecal impaction.*
- Encourage fluids *to facilitate formation of soft stool.*
- Encourage a diet high in fiber and roughage *to maintain soft stool.*
- Administer stool softeners as prescribed *to facilitate elimination.*
- Stimulate rectal sphincter with digital stimulation and/or suppository *to initiate reflex peristalsis and evacuation.*

Patient Education/Home Care Planning

1. Explain ways of adjusting to potential visual changes.
2. Emphasize the need to avoid injury.

3. Emphasize need to maintain adequate fluid and fiber in the diet.
4. Refer patient and family to appropriate community resources.

Evaluation

Patient compensates for altered visual perception Patient has environment arranged to facilitate mobility, self-care, and safety.

Patient compensates for alterations in balance and gait Patient rests quietly in bed as necessary. Patient's vital signs and neurologic status remain stable.

Patient demonstrates normal urinary elimination Intake and output are stable. Bladder is nondistended. Postvoid residual catheterization is less than 100 cc.

Patient demonstrates normal bowel elimination Bowel evacuation pattern is regular. No evidence of constipation or fecal impaction is present.

CANCERS OF THE SKIN

■ BASAL CELL AND SQUAMOUS CELL CARCINOMA

Basal cell carcinoma is a malignant, epithelial cell tumor that begins as a papule and enlarges peripherally. Squamous cell carcinoma is a slow-growing malignant tumor of squamous epithelium.

Skin cancer is the most common human malignancy. An estimated 800,000 cases are discovered each year. The vast majority are the highly curable basal cell and squamous cell carcinomas. Malignant melanoma, the most serious skin cancer, is diagnosed in about 34,100 persons annually, with the incidence increasing at the rate of 4% per year. The reason for the increasing incidence of all skin cancers is believed to be a widespread change in life-style, with greater exposure of successive generations to sunlight, specifically ultraviolet radiation (see box).

Other less common but clinically significant skin cancers include Bowen's disease (squamous cell carcinoma in situ), Kaposi's sarcoma, lymphangiosarcoma, dermatofibrosarcoma protuberans, leiomyosarcoma, and mycosis fungoides.

•••••• Pathophysiology

Basal cell and squamous cell cancers are more common among persons with lightly pigmented skin and those living at latitudes near the equator. Basal cell carcinoma is more common in men than women, and its incidence is higher in persons over 40 years of age. Squamous cell carcinoma is also more common in men, with the average age of onset at 60 years. Additional risk factors are excessive exposure to the sun and occupational exposure to coal, tar, pitch, creosote, arsenic compounds, and radium. Black persons, because of their heavy skin pigmentation, are at low risk for developing these skin cancers.

Basal cell carcinoma often presents as a single, small, firm, dome-shaped, flesh-colored nodule with raised edges and pearly white borders. Small, red, focal lesions (telangiectatic vessels) are often prominent and seen through the thin epidermis. The lesion may resemble a pimple that has failed to heal, with an ulcerated and bleeding center. The most common form, noduloulcerative cancer, occurs frequently on the face, especially the cheeks, forehead, eyelids, and nasolabial folds. Invasion is usually local, although metastatic disease may occur rarely. Untreated, the tumor will invade such vital structures as blood vessels, lymph nodes, nerve sheaths, cartilage, bone, lungs, and the dura mater. The histologic appearance of the tumor is that of small undifferentiated basal cells with minimum nuclear atypia. Recurrence indicates initial incomplete tumor destruction; however, 90% to 95% of patients are considered cured after surgery or radiation therapy.

Squamous cell carcinoma is a scaly, slightly elevated lesion with or without a cutaneous horn. This tumor occurs frequently on the hands and forearms, as well as on the head and neck region, especially the ears, lower lip, scalp, and upper

---

■ FACTS ABOUT CANCERS OF THE SKIN

Incidence: Over 800,000 cases per year of basal cell or squamous cell cancer. Both of these cancers are highly curable. An estimated 34,100 new cases of melanoma, a more virulent skin cancer, will be diagnosed in 1995 and its incidence has been increasing about 4% per year since 1973. Whites are 10 times more likely to develop skin cancer.

Mortality: Of the 9300 estimated deaths, 7200 will be attributed to malignant melanoma.

Warning Signals: This is considered a highly preventable disease by avoiding the sun's ultraviolet rays between 10 AM and 3 PM. In addition, protective clothing should be worn and sunscreens should be used. A change in size or color of a mole, bump, or nodule or other darkly pigmented growth or spot. A bump or nodule that scales, oozes, or bleeds. A change in sensation, itchiness, tenderness, or pain.

Risk Factors: Fair complexion (blonde hair, blue eyes) and overexposure to ultraviolet radiation, occupational exposure to coal tar, pitch, creosote, arsenic compounds, or radium.

Early Detection: The American Cancer Society recommends monthly skin self-examination for all adults, and suspicious lesions should be promptly evaluated.

Treatment: Surgery is used in 90% of early skin cancers. Other therapies for basal and squamous cell skin cancers are radiation therapy, electrodesiccation and cryosurgery. Surgery, including lymph node removal, is often the treatment for malignant melanoma.

From American Cancer Society.[1]

face. It is found most often in sun-damaged skin previously affected by actinic keratoses. These are erythematous, scaly lesions found especially on the face, shoulders, and dorsa of the hands. With complete tumor destruction, the prognosis is excellent. Tumors more difficult to treat are those arising in an old, unstable thermal burn scar (Marjolin's ulcer); a chronically ulcerated area at the site of a chronic sinus tract (such as that caused by osteomyelitis); or a site of prior radiation damage. Squamous cell carcinoma can metastasize, with 2% to 3% spreading to regional lymph nodes or to the lung. Primary tumors of the lip metastasize at a rate greater than 10%. The cure rate for this cancer is 75% to 80% when treated with surgery or radiation therapy.

• • • • • • Diagnostic Studies and Findings

Physical examination Careful inspection, particularly of lesions showing biologic activity, such as change in size, shape, or color; bleeding and ulceration seen in more advanced lesions

Incisional or total excisional biopsy For histologic confirmation of malignancy

• • • • • • Multidisciplinary Plan

Surgery

Scalpel excision with wide margin of skin and subcutaneous tissue; may be supplemented with split-thickness graft, adjacent flaps, distant pedicles, or free graft

Chemosurgery (Moh's procedure)

Cryosurgery

Electrodesiccation and curettage

Medications

Antineoplastic agents

Fluorouracil (5-FU), topical application to skin bid for several weeks

General Management

Radiotherapy by beam electron and superficial x-rays, especially for cancers around face (see p. 1336)

Lesions greater than 20 cm in diameter, those in such critical areas as the central third of the face, recurrent lesions, and lesions with histologic signs of sclerosis are associated with a poor prognosis. Treatment for cure at the time of initial therapy and frequent examination for at least 2 years are essential.

NURSING CARE

Nursing Assessment

Skin Integrity

Raised, hard, red or red-gray, pearly lesion on forehead, eyelid, cheek, nose, preauricular fold, or lip; scaly, slightly elevated lesion with irregular border; ulceration

Nursing Dx & Intervention for Untreatable Tumor (see also section on Metastatic Disease and Terminal Stage of the Disease)

Impaired skin integrity related to presence of tumor

- Bathe patient in warm water or apply warm, moist compress *to maintain cleanliness.*
- Clean skin with agents appropriate to therapy *to prevent infection.*
- Maintain dry skin *to avoid irritation and infection.*
- Use paper or transparent tape over dressings *to avoid irritation.*
- Observe lesions for change in shape, size, and color and bleeding.

Patient Education/Home Care Planning

1. Explain the importance of having regular physical examinations and self-examination.
2. Explain about the need for careful protection of the skin with use of sunscreens, avoidance of excessive exposure to sun, and limited exposure to ionizing radiation.

Evaluation

Skin is healed Skin integrity is maintained without infection or ulceration.

◼ MALIGNANT MELANOMA

◼ Malignant melanoma is a skin cancer that is composed of melanocytes.

Seventy-five percent of deaths from skin cancer, an average of 5500 deaths a year, are caused by malignant melanoma. This skin cancer is more common in whites and in persons over the age of 60 years. The incidence is equal between men and women. This cancer develops from melanocytes that migrate into the skin, eye, central nervous system, and mucous membranes during fetal development. Only 40% of melanomas develop from nevi; the majority arise de novo from melanocytes.

The exact cause of malignant melanoma is unknown. A hereditary factor is involved in 10% of patients. Other theories suggest possible hormonal factors, ultraviolet light exposure, or an autoimmunologic effect.

Malignant melanoma is easily recognized in its early stages and should be suspected in any patient with a history of change in a preexisting nevus or with a new pigmented lesion that has irregularities such as the following:

Various shades of brown and black plus red, white, or blue and the half tones of pink or gray

Notching or indentation of the border and pigment streaming from the lesion's edge

Loss of skin markings or development of a nodule, especially with erosion or ulceration

Bleeding of mole or change in color, size, or thickness

• • • • • • Pathophysiology

The four distinct forms of malignant melanoma, in order of decreasing incidence, follow:

Superficial spreading melanoma (70%) occurs anywhere on the body surface. The average patient age is 50 years. The lesion has a haphazard combination of colors and irregular shapes.

Nodular melanoma (15%) also occurs anywhere on the body surface and has a wide age distribution. It may be small and usually is darkly pigmented. Invasion is usually into the dermis, with resultant lymph node metastasis.

Acral (extremity) lentiginous melanoma (10%) occurs on palms, soles, nail beds, and mucous membranes. It is usually flat to slightly raised with an irregular pigment pattern and border.

Lentigo malignant melanoma (5%) is a slowly evolving lesion occurring on exposed surfaces (especially face and hands) of elderly people. It usually undergoes many color changes.

• • • • • • Diagnostic Studies and Findings

Total excisional biopsy   Deep margin to include subcutaneous fat preferred; performed to determine presence, type, and stage of malignancy

The prognosis is poorer with increased depth of invasion, lymphatic and vascular invasion, high number of mitotic figures per high-power microscopic field, little or no lymphocytic infiltration at the tumor base, and ulceration. The overall prognosis is better in women.

• • • • • • Multidisciplinary Plan

Surgery

Wide, deep excision of primary lesion

Regional lymph node dissection

Medications

Antineoplastic agents

Dacarbazine (DTIC), 2 to 4.5 mg/kg/d IV for 10 d or 250 mg/m²/d IV for 5 d

Tamoxifen citrate (Nolvadex), 10 to 20 mg bid (morning and evening)

Diethylstilbestrol (DES)

Nitrosourea (BCNU), cisplatin, methotrexate

Antiinfective agents

Bacille Calmette-Guérin (BCG) vaccine, active specific forms used as investigational drug

Biologic response modifiers (interferon, interleukin)

Radiation Therapy

For palliation of metastases

NURSING CARE

Nursing Assessment

Skin Integrity

Dark brown or black pigmentation; scaliness; oozing, ulceration, and bleeding of nevus; spread of pigment beyond normal border; change in sensation; itchiness; tenderness or pain; enlarged regional lymph nodes

Nursing Diagnosis & Intervention for Untreated Tumor

Impaired skin integrity related to presence of lesion

- Bathe patient in warm water or apply warm, moist compresses *to maintain cleanliness.*
- Apply sterile dressings with antibiotic ointments as prescribed *to prevent infection.*
- Observe lesion(s) for change in shape, size, color, and presence of bleeding *to detect progressive disease.*

Patient Education/Home Care Planning

1. Emphasize the need for regular physical examinations and self-examination (see box below).
2. Inform the patient of the need for meticulous skin care and assessment and the importance of avoiding ultraviolet light.

 ABCD RULE FOR EARLY DETECTION OF MELANOMA

Asymmetry
Most true moles tend to be symmetric. Melanomas tend to be asymmetric (one half does not match the other half).

Border
Most true moles have a clear-cut border. Melanomas tend to have a notched, scalloped, or indistinct border.

Color
True moles may be dark or light, but they usually are uniform in color. Early melanomas have an uneven or variegated color (may range from various hues of tan and brown to black, with red and white intermingled).

Diameter
Most melanomas, once they have A, B, and C characteristics, have a diameter greater than 6 mm. Moles tend to be smaller. A sudden or continued increase in the size of a mole should be reported.

Evaluation

Patient's skin is healed   Skin integrity is maintained.

Patient is calm and without fear   Patient discusses concerns in realistic and rational manner.

ONCOLOGIC EMERGENCIES

Oncologic emergencies arise from the impact advanced cancer has on body functioning. As many as 20% of patients develop one or more of these emergent conditions in the course of their illness. Among the most serious but most treatable acute conditions that can occur are hypercalcemia, obstruction of the superior vena cava, spinal cord compression, and cardiac distress. Other oncologic emergencies include pleural effusions, sepsis, disseminated intravascular coagulation, syndrome of inappropriate antidiuretic hormone (SIADH), and tumor lysis syndrome.

Hypercalcemia   Hypercalcemia occurs when the bones release more calcium into the extracellular fluid than can be excreted in the urine. This occurs most frequently in patients with multiple myeloma or cancer of the breast, lung, or prostate. In addition, some tumors produce parathyroid hormone or a substance with the same physiologic effects, which include increased resorption of calcium from bone, increased intestinal absorption of calcium, and reduced renal excretion.

The most common cause of hypercalcemia is thought to be bone destruction by invasive metastases. Other causes are tumor production of vitamin D—like substances and osteoclast-activating factors, dehydration, and immobilization.

Excessive calcium can cause bradycardia, increased cardiac contractility, depression of the central and peripheral nervous system (mild lethargy that may progress to coma), fatigue, muscle weakness, anorexia, nausea and vomiting, confusion, or irritability. Interference with reabsorption of water from the distal tubules leads to nocturia, polyuria, dehydration, polydipsia, and pruritus.

Acute hypercalcemia is treated initially with intravenous saline. Furosemide may also be given intravenously to encourage diuresis. Careful recording of intake and output, monitoring of electrolyte levels, and frequent cardiopulmonary assessment are necessary. Mithramycin inhibits bone resorption of calcium; given as a rapid intravenous infusion at 25 µg/kg body weight, it can lower serum calcium levels in 48 hours. Calcitonin and IV phosphorus are currently less frequently used because gallium nitrate (Ganite) is available.

Steroid administration and restriction of dietary calcium are thought to be of little therapeutic value. Orally administered phosphates and calcitonin injections may be used. Use of vitamin D, thiazides, absorbable antacids, and estrogens should be avoided.

External compression of the superior vena cava   Compression of the superior vena cava can occur slowly or quickly, owing to pressure from an adjacent tumor mass or enlarging lymph node. Most patients with superior vena cava syndrome have bronchogenic cancer; other causes of this syndrome are lymphoma, breast cancer, and gastrointestinal tract metastases.

Prompt diagnosis and treatment are needed to relieve the distressing symptoms, which are progressive shortness of breath, cough, distention of neck veins, and edema of the face and hands. Dilated veins may appear on the upper chest wall. The patient may complain of headache and visual disturbances.

The patient must be kept in the Fowler's position. Diuretics may be of some help. However, the obstruction must be relieved to prevent cerebral anoxia, hemorrhage, or strangulation. Radiation therapy is the treatment of choice for this. If the obstruction is not accessible, chemotherapeutic agents such as cyclophosphamide (Cytoxan) can produce good results.

Spinal cord compression   Compression of the spinal cord is extremely dangerous because of the possibility of a permanent neurologic deficit. The usual cause of compression is a tumor, such as lymphoma or cancer of the breast, lung, or prostate, that metastasizes to the bony vertebral body and grows into the epidural space.

Pain, localized in the spinal region or radicular, is almost always an early symptom. The pain may be constant and aggravated by movement or coughing. Relief is usually obtained with morphine, meperidine (Demerol), or an analgesic agent. Bed rest is recommended, and transfer and position change should be done by multiple personnel.

A careful neurologic examination should be performed to check motor and sensory function and the autonomic nerve tracts. Roentgenograms or myelograms should be done immediately to localize the destruction and determine its extent. The prognosis appears to be related to the patient's ability to walk at the time of diagnosis; if he or she is unable to do so, motor function is not recoverable, even with emergency radiotherapy or laminectomy.

Severe or prolonged cord compression can lead to extremity paralysis and loss of sphincter control, which is manifest as difficulty starting urination or as bowel incontinence.

Treatment must be prompt. Corticosteroids, such as dexamethasone, in high doses reduce swelling and inflammation around the cord. Surgical decompression or radiotherapy may be required. Early diagnosis is important for recovery.

Cardiac tamponade   Cardiac tamponade results from excessive amount and pressure of fluid on the pericardial sac, which is a response to metastasis or direct invasion by tumor. The normal diastolic filling is impaired, and stroke volume is reduced. If tamponade is untreated, circulatory collapse occurs.

Signs and symptoms depend on how quickly the fluid accumulates. Frequent signs of tamponade include rapid and weak pulse, distended neck veins during inspiration (Kussmaul's sign), pulsus paradoxus (inspiratory decrease in arterial blood pressure of greater than 10 mm Hg from baseline), ankle or sacral edema, pleural effusion, lethargy, and altered consciousness.

The diagnosis is confirmed with echocardiography and pericardiocentesis; the latter also provides immediate symptomatic relief. Palliative measures, such as surgical construction of a pericardial window, must also be taken; total pericardectomy is usually not practical. Newer techniques include catheter drainage of fluid and instillation of a sclerosing agent, such as tetracycline or bleomycin. Radiation therapy with an external beam is effective with sensitive tumors.

Pleural effusion   See Chapter 2.

Sepsis   This serious condition is exemplified by inadequate tissue perfusion, which results from bacterial invasion of the circulatory system. The most common causative agents, gram-negative bacteria, release an endotoxin from their cell walls, which causes increased capillary permeability and leakage. This in turn causes stagnation of blood, lactic acidosis, a decrease in the circulating blood volume, and decreased cardiac output. Sepsis is the most common cause of death in neutropenic patients. Signs and symptoms of sepsis include fever, chills, restlessness, confusion, tachycardia, hypotension, decreased pulses, cool clammy skin, decreased urinary output, and bleeding from one or more sites, which may be caused by disseminated intravascular coagulation (DIC).

The diagnosis is confirmed by positive blood culture findings, the presence of infiltrates on chest roentgenogram, depressed or elevated white blood cell level, metabolic acidosis via arterial blood gas analysis, and a prolonged prothrombin time and partial thromboplastin time. Interventions include monitoring of vital signs, arterial blood gas values, and hemodynamic stability; performance of blood cultures as needed; administration of antibiotics; temperature reduction with such measures as antipyretics, ice packs, and hypothermia blanket; and fluid volume replacement.

Disseminated intravascular coagulation (DIC)   This imbalance of normal coagulation is always secondary to an underlying cause, such as the release of tissue thromboplastin from tumor cells (e.g., lung and prostate leukemia); sepsis; infection, hemolytic transfusions, or hepatic failure. The pathophysiology is based on the uncontrollable triggering of the internal or external pathway of the clotting cascade, resulting in accelerated coagulation and the formation of excessive thrombin. As long as coagulation occurs, the fibrinolytic system is activated, so that clotting and bleeding continue at a life-threatening pace. Signs and symptoms of DIC include systemic bleeding, ranging from petechiae to hematuria to an acute gastrointestinal hemorrhage; organ dysfunction (e.g., pulmonary emboli, thromboemboli in the extremities, renal failure); decreased blood pressure and pulse; cool, clammy skin; anemia; pallor; and shortness of breath. A diagnosis of DIC is confirmed by the presence of prolonged thrombin time, prothrombin time, and partial thromboplastin time; decreased platelets; decreased fibrinogen; and elevated fibrin-split products. Appropriate interventions include such medical therapies as antibiotics, chemotherapy, heparin, and blood products. The nurse should continuously monitor sites and amount of bleeding and laboratory values, assess adequacy of tissue perfusion, and prevent or minimize bleeding.

Syndrome of inappropriate antidiuretic hormone (SIADH)   Antidiuretic hormone, which is normally released from the posterior pituitary in response to increased plasma osmolarity or decreased plasma volume, may be abnormally produced or stimulated as a result of tumor secretion (e.g., small cell lung cancer, lymphoma, and pancreatic and prostate cancers); stimulation by such drugs as vincristine and cyclophosphamide; viral or bacterial pneumonia; or neurologic trauma. The results of this abnormal production or stimulation are excessive water retention and hyponatremia. Signs and symptoms of SIADH include confusion, irritability, weakness, lethargy, headache, hyporeflexia, nausea, vomiting, anorexia, diarrhea, and weight gain without edema. Diagnosis is confirmed by a serum sodium level of less than 130 mEq/L, serum osmolarity of less than 280 mOsm/kg H_2O, and a urine sodium level of more than 20 mEq/L. Medical interventions may include chemotherapy, antibiotics, hypertonic saline (3% to 5% sodium chloride), diuretics, demeclocycline, and discontinuation of the causative agent. The nurse should also maintain an accurate intake and output record, restrict fluids as necessary, monitor laboratory reports of fluid and electrolyte balance, and provide safety measures for weak and confused patients.

Tumor lysis syndrome   This metabolic imbalance is caused by the rapid release of such intracellular components as potassium, phosphorus, and uric acid. The patient's risk of developing tumor lysis syndrome increases with the presence of bulky tumors that have a high growth fraction. The syndrome usually begins 1 to 5 days after the initiation of chemotherapy for non-Hodgkin's lymphomas and leukemia. Signs and symptoms include oliguria, anuria, urine crystals, flank pain, hematuria, cardiac dysrhythmias, muscular cramps, tetany, and confusion. The diagnosis is confirmed by elevated serum blood urea nitrogen (BUN), creatinine, potassium, phosphorus, and uric acid levels and by decreased serum calcium levels. Medical orders may include administering allopurinol and calcium supplements, giving intravenous fluids with sodium bicarbonate for 3 to 5 days after initiating chemotherapy, and preparing the patient for peritoneal dialysis or hemodialysis.

METASTATIC DISEASE AND TERMINAL STAGE OF THE DISEASE

Metastases are the major cause of death from cancer. The likelihood of a person with cancer developing metastatic disease is increased by the presence of a primary tumor of extended duration; high mitotic rate; trauma, such as tumor biopsy; dead tumor cells; heat; radiation; and chemotherapeutic agents. A metastasis is a tumor that is distant from the primary tumor and occurs as a result of seeding throughout a body cavity, such as the peritoneal or thoracic cavity; mechanical transport via instruments or gloved hands; lymphatic spread; and hematogenous spread. The most common sites of metastases follow:

The lung, from such primary sites as the colorectum, breast, renal system, testes, and bones

The liver, from such primary sites as the lung, colorectum, breast, and renal system

The central nervous system, from such primary sites as the lung and breast

Bone, from such primary sites as the lung, breast, renal system, and prostate

NURSING CARE

Nursing Assessment

Respiratory Function

Cough; hemoptysis; wheezing; fever; dyspnea; chest pain; hoarseness; enlargement of neck with venous distention; clubbing of fingers

Metabolic Function

Nonspecific abdominal complaints, such as increasing distention, right upper quadrant mass; weight loss; anorexia; nausea and vomiting; signs and symptoms of cirrhosis such as spider angioma and gynecomastia

Central Nervous System Function

Headaches; nausea and vomiting; disturbances in mental, motor, and/or sensory function; focal or generalized convulsive activity; visual field, speech, or auditory defects; vertigo; dizziness; ataxia; nystagmus; depressed corneal reflex; facial paralysis (Table 16-2)

Musculoskeletal Function

Pain; disturbances in sensory and/or motor function; urinary urgency, difficulty initiating urination, retention and overflow incontinence; contralateral loss of temperature and pain sensation; ipsilateral loss of motor function, touch and position sense (Table 16-3)

Communication

Difficulty with speech and hearing

Psychosocial

Expressions of fear regarding disease progression and prognosis; anxiety; depression; anger

The nurse should include in her ongoing assessment of a person with cancer an emphasis on early detection of signs and symptoms of metastatic disease (see Emergency Alert box). This requires a knowledge of usual sites of spread for specific cancers, as well as sensitivity to patient complaints, changes in laboratory values, and observable alterations in function that indicate metastatic spread.

Nursing diagnoses and interventions appropriate to each of the common metastatic sites follow.

Nursing Dx & Intervention

Altered cardiopulmonary and peripheral tissue perfusion related to pulmonary metastases

- Observe patient for hoarseness *to detect involvement of recurrent laryngeal nerve.*
- Observe for signs and symptoms of pleural effusion; have access to chest drainage equipment *to detect involvement of viscera or parietal pleura.* Thoracotomy may be needed *to prevent or treat pneumothorax.*

! EMERGENCY ALERT

ADVANCED DIRECTIVE

An advanced directive is a legal document executed by a competent person, which designates durable power of attorney for health care decisions when the person is no longer competent. Laws govern specific procedures for each state.

Assessment

- Determine if a living will or durable power of attorney exists and for what situations.
- Be aware that items such as CPR, intubation, use of medications, and heroic procedures may be included in the document, and therefore withheld from the patient.
- Generally supportive care, pain management, and nutritional support are not included in living wills and are to be provided.

- Observe for fever, hemoptysis *to detect and report to physician pneumonitis or abscess formation in lung.*
- Administer medications as needed with analgesics *to relieve chest pain.*
- Provide oxygen therapy as needed *to relieve dyspnea.*
- Observe for enlargement of neck with venous distention *to detect and report to physician compression or invasion of superior vena cava.*
- Observe for clubbing of fingers *to assess hypertrophic pulmonary osteoarthropathy.*
- Position patient comfortably with head elevated *to promote chest expansion.*
- Encourage coughing and deep breathing *to clear and maintain patent respiratory tract.*
- Administer vaporized air *to moisten secretions* and oxygen *to ensure adequate tissue perfusion.*
- Suction airway as needed *to relieve obstruction caused by secretions.*
- Encourage adequate rest *to decrease respiratory workload.*
- Remove constrictive clothing *to relieve pressure on chest.*
- Discourage smoking *to decrease respiratory distress.*
- Inspect chest symmetric expansion. Auscultate for abnormal breath sounds, voice sounds, rales, and rhonchi *to assess respiratory status and pulmonary function.*
- Monitor blood studies *to determine adequate oxygenation.*
- Be alert for complaints of cyanosis, dyspnea, wheezing, confusion, and fatigue *to monitor increasing respiratory distress.*
- Monitor respiratory rate and rhythm and pulse *to assess for adequacy of cardiopulmonary function.*

Altered nutrition: less than body requirements related to liver metastases

- Offer antiemetics as prescribed *to provide relief from vomiting and nausea.*
- Arrange pleasant surroundings; provide appealing selection of foods; encourage family and friends to bring in

food of patient's choice; and provide attractive meal tray *to enhance patient's appetite.*

- Postpone feeding when patient is fatigued; *patient is more likely to eat when rested.*
- Give patient small, frequent feedings *to avoid distention.*
- Feed patient slowly and provide rest periods *to avoid tiring patient.*
- Observe and record food intake, and measure body weight daily *to monitor nutritional status.*
- Elevate patient's head *to promote comfort.*
- Encourage deep breathing *to relieve feeling of nausea.*
- Give bland food or carbonated beverages or hot tea *to relieve nausea.*
- Observe for spider angioma and gynecomastia, *which indicate hormonal and circulatory alterations caused by liver damage.*

Risk for injury related to central nervous system metastases

- Raise and pad side rails and tape padded tongue blade to head of bed *to protect patient during convulsion.*
- Maintain patient on bed rest *to avoid falls or other trauma.*
- Provide quiet environment with subdued lighting *to relax patient.*
- Remove furniture, rugs, and other barriers *to minimize environmental danger.*
- Inspect patient for abnormal body movements *to monitor seizure activity.*
- Observe for confusion, decreased pupillary response, and reduced level of consciousness *to detect increased intracranial pressure.*

Pain related to bone and/or central nervous system metastases

- Observe for patient grimacing, holding head, or guarding extremity or specific area of trunk *to assess nonverbal signs of pain.*
- Maintain body alignment *to prevent muscular stretching.*
- Position patient with support (e.g., pillows), change position slowly, and support joints *to avoid fractures and decrease pressure.*
- Apply heating pad, hot water bottle, warm, moist compress, whirlpool bath, or mentholated ointment *to provide relaxation and relieve pain.*
- Exercise patient's limbs gently in range of motion *to maintain muscle tone.*
- Massage gently *to relax muscles.*
- Be alert for complaints of pain, and assess its duration and radiation *to intervene early.*
- Provide pain relief measure of patient's choice, such as relaxation therapy, diversion, or distraction *to enhance effect of medication.*
- Administer pain medications as ordered and evaluate pain for intensity and quality *to control pain and determine need for further intervention.*

Impaired physical mobility related to central nervous system or peripheral nervous system metastases

- Provide patient support when ambulating (e.g., walker, three-point cane) *to maintain mobility.*
- Provide range of motion exercises (active and/or passive) *to avoid muscle contractures.*
- Assess patient for altered gait and position sense *to determine need for further assistance.*
- Observe for signs of thrombophlebitis (i.e., calf pain, calf redness, Homans' sign, swelling, and warmth) *to detect and report to physician this common complication of immobility.*
- Use antiembolic stockings *to prevent venous stasis.*
- Reposition patient every 2 hours if on bed rest *to prevent skin breakdown.*

Altered patterns of urinary elimination related to central nervous system or peripheral nervous system metastases

- Assess voiding pattern, palpate bladder, and monitor intake and output *to determine need for intermittent catheterization.*
- Devise intermittent catheterization schedule *to avoid incontinence.*
- Encourage fluid intake with even distribution during the day and decreased intake at night *to maintain renal function while avoiding nighttime incontinence.*
- Discourage use of caffeine beverages *to avoid their diuretic-like effect.*

Impaired verbal communication related to central nervous system metastases

- Listen carefully and speak clearly to patient *to enhance ability to communicate.*
- Provide paper and pencil, chalk board, or erasable board *to provide alternate methods of communication.*

Activity intolerance related to generalized weakness

- Observe response to activity *to determine extent of tolerance.*
- Identify factors contributing to intolerance (e.g., stress, side effects of drugs) *to plan interventions to counteract their effect.*
- Assess patient's sleep patterns *to document a causative factor of weakness.*
- Plan rest periods between activities *to reduce fatigue by providing additional rest.*
- Perform activities for patient until he or she is able to perform them *to meet patient's need without causing fatigue.*

Fear related to evidence of metastases and terminal stage of the disease

- Encourage patient to discuss fears related to disease *to clarify specific fears and their basis in reality.*

- Provide factual information as requested by patient *to relieve anxiety.*
- Encourage participation in support group or in one-to-one relationship *to share experiences with others or with an experienced therapist.*
- Assess appetite, weight loss, sleep patterns, mobility, and constipation *to determine if depression is present.*
- Assess presence and quality of support system *to determine if persons are available to patient and if they are supportive, ambivalent, or disruptive.*
- Monitor changes in communication patterns with others *to determine presence of depression.*
- Monitor expressions such as of worthlessness, anxiety, powerlessness, abandonment, or exhaustion *to assess patient's state of mind and guide the nurse's communication with patient.*
- Monitor ongoing coping such as withdrawal, denial, rationalization, compliance, dependency *to assess patient's current coping strategies.*
- Encourage a balanced diet, regular sleeping habits, active or passive exercise, and comfort measures *to ensure that patient's physiologic needs are met while patient is unable to do so independently.*
- Accept patient's behavior at current level *to develop trust as the basis for all other interventions.*
- Listen and accept verbalized anger without personalizing reaction *to foster constructive expression of anger and negative feelings.*
- Assist patient to use physical expression geared to his physical capabilities (e.g., walking, punching a pillow) *to teach patient to use physical activity to express anger.*
- Encourage patient to keep a "gripe list"; discuss list with patient if patient agrees *to allow patient to write and verbalize anger.*
- Encourage patient to identify and redefine situations; to obtain needed information on, generate alternatives for, and focus on solutions *to support coping, problem solving, and decision making.*
- Respect patient's need for privacy *to allow patient and others to grieve together.*
- Use humor with patient as appropriate *to improve patient's mood and self view.*
- Administer antidepressants as ordered *to improve patient's depressed mood.*

Anticipatory grieving related to actual or perceived death

- Assess patient and family's reaction to diagnosis *to determine their stage of grieving.*
- Encourage patient to verbalize feelings *to reduce anxiety and fear.*
- Anticipate the patient's feelings of anger and fear *to be most supportive as needed arises.*
- Encourage patient to participate in activities of daily living *to reduce feelings of powerlessness.*

- Refer patient and family to support groups, counseling services, and hospice programs as needed *to provide financial, physical, and emotional support.*

Patient Education/Home Care Planning

1. Teach patient and family to avoid stress, exposure to environmental pollution, and others' infections.
2. Plan for periods of activity, balanced with rest.
3. Alter environment as necessary to enhance patient safety.
4. Provide a varied, attractive, and balanced diet.
5. Explain alternative nonmedication pain management strategies, such as guided imagery, relaxation, and distraction.
6. Encourage patient to ambulate, using assistive devices as needed.
7. Enhance communication with active listening and assistive devices as needed.
8. Explain ways of adjusting to potential visual changes.
9. Emphasize the need to avoid injury.
10. Emphasize need to maintain adequate fluid and fiber in the diet.
11. Refer patient and family to appropriate community resources.
12. Use bladder training strategies as needed to avoid incontinence.
13. Encourage continued expression of fears and use of problem-solving techniques to deal with patient's fears in a realistic manner.

Evaluation

Patient maintains optimal cardiopulmonary and peripheral tissue perfusion Skin, nails, lips, and earlobes are warm, moist, and of natural color. Respirations, pulse, blood pressure, and temperature are within normal limits.

Patient maintains optimal nutrition Diet is balanced and adequate; fluid intake equals output. Weight is maintained within normal limits.

Patient is free of injury Patient does not complain of pain. Patient's facial expression and body are relaxed.

Patient ambulates frequently Patient uses assistive devices as needed.

Patient compensates for any altered visual perception Patient has environment arranged to facilitate mobility, self-care, and safety.

Patient compensates for alterations in balance and gait Patient rests quietly in bed as necessary. Patient's vital signs and neurologic status remain stable.

Patient demonstrates normal urinary elimination Intake and output are stable. Bladder is nondistended. Postvoid residual catheterization is less than 100 cc.

Patient demonstrates normal bowel elimination Bowel evacuation pattern is regular. No evidence of constipation or fecal impaction is present.

Patient is able to communicate   Patient speaks without difficulty or uses assistive devices effectively. Patient is able to hear those speaking to him or her.

Patient is able to deal with fears   Patient discusses fears openly. Patient uses appropriate problem-solving techniques to deal with disease progression and prognosis.

Patient performs usual activities without fatigue or dyspnea   Patient performs self-care activities.

Patient expresses realistic perspective of diagnosis, treatment, and prognosis   Patient describes illness and its probable outcome in realistic terms. Patient participates in activities of daily living as physical condition permits. Patient and family use resources appropriately.

MEDICAL INTERVENTIONS AND RELATED NURSING CARE

BLOOD COMPONENT THERAPY

The goal of blood component therapy is to administer only the component needed by the patient. This minimizes transfusion reactions and increases the number of patients who can benefit from a single unit.

Granulocytes are used to treat patients with granulocytopenia with severe infection, particularly those in whom severe bone marrow depression develops during chemotherapy. Granulocytes are collected from a single donor by means of a machine that withdraws donor blood, removes the granulocytes, and returns the rest of the blood to the donor. This procedure, called leukopheresis, requires several hours. Administration of steroids before donation can increase the cell yield.

Although granulocytes can be stored up to 24 hours, immediate transfusion is recommended. Because of the short posttransfusion cell life, frequent transfusions are usually needed—for example, daily for at least 4 days, administered slowly over a 2- to 4-hour period.

The most common untoward reactions are shaking, chills and temperature elevation, which are treated symptomatically with acetaminophen 30 minutes before subsequent transfusions and with reduction of the flow rate. Hives are another minor reaction and are usually treated with an antihistamine. Life-threatening reactions include hypotensive response, anaphylactic response, and respiratory reaction. Emergency intervention is necessary.

Platelets are usually given to patients with thrombocytopenia and bone marrow depression resulting from chemotherapy or radiation therapy. Platelet concentrates are obtained through platelet pheresis of a single donor or prepared from units of platelets collected from as many as four to ten donors. Blood is removed from the donor into a machine with a centrifuge bowl, where platelets are separated, and red blood cells and plasma

are then returned to the donor. The procedure takes 1½ to 2 hours. Pheresis donors may give as many as 12 units of platelets at a time. The platelets should be administered within 24 hours.

The nurse is an essential member of the team involved in this therapy; it is often the nurse who identifies the patient's need for blood components, recruits donors, obtains the blood components from the donors, and administers the therapy to the patient.

CHEMOTHERAPY

Description and Rationale

Chemotherapy is a relatively new cancer treatment modality; the first patient was treated with nitrogen mustard in 1942. The use of chemical agents is especially important in the treatment of systemic disease. Researchers continue to discover drugs that kill cancer cells without causing extensive damage to normal tissues. In addition, combinations of chemotherapeutic agents and the combination of chemotherapy with other treatment modalities have increased the cancer cure rate.

Chemotherapy is used to cure patients, prolong life, increase the disease-free interval, and palliate symptoms, thus improving the quality of life.

Chemotherapeutic agents are highly toxic, attacking all rapidly dividing cells, both normal and malignant. Thus the contraindications and cautions are a reflection of the patient's pretreatment condition, stage of disease, response to therapy, and allergies or sensitivities. The nurse involved in drug administration and monitoring of the patient's responses must have a comprehensive baseline assessment to use in evaluating the patient's condition and ability to tolerate the treatment.

The most commonly used chemotherapeutic agents are listed in Table 16-4. Many others are being developed and tested for possible therapeutic value.

Depending on the drug's pharmacodynamics, chemotherapy may be administered by a variety of routes: intravenous, oral, central venous catheter, venous access via an implantable access device, intraarterial, intraperitoneal, intrapleural, intrathecal, or via ventricular reservoir. The intramuscular and subcutaneous routes are rarely used. In recent years use of intraarterial and venous access lines (i.e., Hickman catheter) has become important because of the ease of access to the arterial or venous system for drug delivery, increased patient comfort, and the addition of external or internal pump systems for more continuous infusion of drugs.

NURSING CARE

Nursing Assessment

Gastrointestinal

Nausea and vomiting; diarrhea; constipation; stomatitis; esophagitis; anorexia

■ TABLE 16-4 Cancer Chemotherapeutic Agents

Classification	Agents	Mechanism of Action
Alkylating agents	Mechlorethamine (nitrogen mustard); cyclophosphamide (Cytoxan); phenylalanine mustard (Alkeran, L-PAM, Melphalan); chlorambucil (Leukeran); bulsulfan (Myleran); dacarbazine (DTIC); thiophosphoramide (Thiotepa); cisplatin; carboplatin; ifosfamide	Produce breaks in DNA module and cross-linking of strands and thus interfere with DNA replication
Nitrosoureas	Bis-chloroethyl nitrosourea (BCNU); lomustine (CCNU), carmustine/BCNU (BiCNU); streptozocin	Action similar to that of alkylating agents
Antimetabolites		
Folic acid analog	Methotrexate (MTX)	Competitively inhibit enzymes necessary for cell function and replication
Pyrimidine analogs	5-Fluorouracil (5-FU); floxuridine (FUDR); cytosine arabinoside (Cytosar)	
Purine analogs	6-Mercaptopurine (6-MP); 6-thioguanine (Thioguanine)	
Plant alkaloids	Vinblastine (Velban); vincristine (Oncovin); etoposide (VP-16)	Bind to substances needed for formation of mitotic spindle and thus prevent cell division
Antibiotics	Doxorubicin (Adriamycin); daunorubicin (Daunomycin); bleomycin (Blenoxane); dactinomycin (actinomycin D); mithramycin (Mithracin); mitomycin C (Mutamycin); plicamycin	Bind with DNA to inhibit DNA and RNA synthesis
Hormonal agents		Alter cellular environment
Corticosteroids Estrogens Antiestrogens Androgens Progestins	Prednisone; prednisolone; methylprednisolone (Solu-Medrol); hydrocortisone (Solu-Cortef); dexamethasone (Decadron)	
	Ethinyl estradiol (Estinyl); fosfestrol (Stilbestrol); diethylstilbestrol (DES); diethylstilbestrol diphosphate (Stilphostrol); conjugated estrogens (Premarin); chlorotrianisene (TACE)	
	Clomiphene; nafoxidine; tamoxifen (Nolvadex)	
	Testosterone; calusterone; fluoxymesterone (Halotestin); nandrolone; testolactone	
	17-Hydroxyprogesterone (Delalutin); medroxyprogesterone acetate (Provera); megestrol acetate (Megace)	
Biologic response modifiers	Interferon Alfa-2b; interleukin-1 (IL-1), IL-2, IL-4; granulocyte colony-stimulating factor (G-CSF); granulocyte-macrophage CSF (GM-CSF); erythropoietin	Immune modulation
Miscellaneous agents	Hydroxyurea; L-asparaginase; procarbazine (Matulane); aminoglutethimide (Cytadren); estramustine (Emcyt); mitotane; dacarbazine (DTIC); levamisole	

Dermatologic

Alopecia; dermatitis; changes in skin color; extravasation; hyperpigmentation of nail beds; rash; jaundice; pruritus

Hematologic

Fatigue and dyspnea (anemia); petechiae; ecchymoses; frank bleeding (thrombocytopenia); fever; chills; hypotension (leukopenia)

Reproductive

Sterility; amenorrhea; decreased libido

Urinary

Hemorrhagic cystitis, as evidenced by hematuria, burning during urination, backache; nephrotoxicity, as evidenced by renal failure (decrease or absence of urinary output)

Neurologic

Ototoxicity (vertigo, tinnitus, loss of hearing); peripheral neuropathies, as evidenced by muscle weakness; numbness and tingling; jaw pain; absence of deep tendon reflexes

Musculoskeletal

Myalgia; muscle weakness; osteoporosis; gout

Respiratory

Pulmonary fibrosis, as evidenced by dyspnea, chest pain, or cyanosis

Cardiac

Congestive heart failure as evidenced by exertional dyspnea, cough, rales, electrocardiogram changes

Psychosocial

Fear; depression; anger; anxiety

Nursing Dx & Intervention

Fluid volume deficit related to nausea and vomiting

- Administer antiemetic (prochlorperazine, thiethylperazine, trimethobenzamide, mitoclopramide, intravenous dexamethasone, or δ-9 tetrahydrocannabinol [THC]) prophylactically before chemotherapy and on a regular schedule after therapy per physician order *to decrease incidence of nausea and vomiting.*
- Withhold food and fluids for 4 to 6 hours before treatment *to decrease gastric irritation.*
- Provide small feedings and increase fluids *to maintain nutrition and hydration.*
- Provide frequent mouth care *to promote patient's comfort.*
- Provide clean environment with fresh air and no odors *to reduce noxious stimuli.*
- Monitor intake and output, weight, and electrolytes *to avoid dehydration.*
- Administer intravenous therapy as ordered *to maintain fluid and electrolyte balance.*
- Use relaxation techniques, guided imagery, self-hypnosis, and distraction as indicated *to reduce nausea.*

Constipation related to impaired intestinal motility

- Offer fluids and foods high in fiber and bulk *to stimulate motility.*
- Offer stool softener or laxatives *to stimulate motility.*
- Avoid enemas *because they may traumatize the intestinal mucosa.*

Diarrhea related to intestinal irritation

- Offer clear liquids *to prevent dehydration.*
- Offer antidiarrheal agent, such as Kaopectate or diphenoxylate (Lomotil), per physician's order *to control diarrhea.*
- Maintain good perineal care *to avoid irritation and discomfort.*
- Test stools for occult blood *to identify evidence of blood.*
- Record number and consistency of stools *to monitor need for further intervention.*
- Observe for dehydration and electrolyte imbalance *to avoid complications.*

Altered oral mucous membrane related to poor oral hygiene, preexisting dental disorders, or drug-induced irritation

- Encourage good oral hygiene *to promote comfort and prevent infection.*
- Discourage spicy or hot foods *to avoid irritation or pain.*
- Offer topical agents for relief of pain (lidocaine or dyclonine) per physician's order *to soothe irritated membranes.*
- Apply K-Y jelly to lips *to maintain moisture.*
- Offer popsicles *for hydration and comfort.*

- Use oral assessment guide to monitor changes in voice, ability to swallow, and condition of lips, tongue, mucous membranes, gingiva, teeth, and saliva *to evaluate response to interventions.*
- Discourage alcohol, tobacco, difficult-to-chew foods, and highly acidic beverages *to avoid irritation of mucous membranes.*
- Administer nystatin oral suspension or suppository or clotrimazole (Mycelex) troche per physician's order *to combat infection.*
- Have patient postpone dental work if possible, brush teeth gently, and use toothettes *to avoid further trauma.*

Altered nutrition: less than body requirements related to increased body requirements and gastrointestinal irritation

- Offer bland or pureed foods *to facilitate swallowing.*
- Have patient avoid spicy foods, alcohol, and tobacco *to decrease irritation.*
- Offer antacids *to counteract gastric acid.*
- Identify food preferences *to increase patient's interest in eating.*
- Encourage patient to eat *by explaining need to maintain strength.*
- Offer small, frequent feedings *to avoid distention.*
- Do not rush meals, *so that patient will increase intake.*
- Keep room free of odors and clutter *to reduce noxious stimuli.*
- Provide meticulous mouth care *to enhance appetite.*
- Use enteral feeding tube or total parenteral nutrition if necessary *to maintain nutritional balance.*
- Weigh daily *to monitor nutritional status.*

Impaired skin integrity related to drug-induced changes, extravasation

For alopecia
- Help patient plan for wig, scarf, or hat before hair loss *to maintain self-esteem.*
- Offer tourniquet or ice cap preventive therapy based on policy and diagnosis *to decrease hair loss.*
- Have patient wash and comb remaining hair gently *to decrease hair loss.*
- Reassure patient that hair will grow back after therapy *to lessen patient anxiety and worry.*

For dermatitis
- Use cornstarch, Alpha Keri, calamine lotion, or other agent *to relieve itching.*
- Warn against overexposure to sun *to avoid further irritation.*
- Keep skin clean and dry *to avoid infection.*

For changes in color of skin or nail beds
- Assure patient that discoloration will fade with time *to lessen patient anxiety and worry.*
- Use nail polish according to patient's wishes *to mask discoloration.*

For jaundice
- Monitor hepatic enzymes *to determine liver function.*

- Assess skin and sclera daily for evidence of increase or decrease in discoloration.

For extravasation

- Observe for early signs—including pain or burning sensation at or above IV site (as reported by patient), blanching, redness, swelling, slowing of infusion, and absence of blood return—*to detect problem before tissue damage occurs.*
- Stop infusion, aspirate remaining drug from needle, inject antidote, apply topical ointment, heat, or cold as dictated by protocol *to prevent tissue damage.*

Impaired gas exchange related to anemia, pulmonary fibrosis, cardiotoxicity

- Have patient change position slowly *to conserve energy.*
- Encourage adequate rest *to conserve energy.*
- Observe patient for dyspnea and increased weakness *as evidence of further dysfunction.*
- Administer oxygen therapy as needed *to increase oxygenation of tissues.*
- Monitor hemoglobin and hematocrit *to determine effect of therapy.*
- Administer transfusions as ordered *to increase RBC count.*
- Monitor respiratory function with pulmonary function test *to detect changes in status.*
- Note limitation of lifetime dosage of bleomycin *to prevent irreversible toxicity.*
- Assist with pulmonary function studies *to detect changes in status.*
- Observe for dyspnea; report to physician as ordered *for further interventions.*
- Monitor heart rate, blood pressure, and ECG *to detect cardiac dysfunction.*
- Limit cumulative dosage of doxorubicin *to prevent irreversible toxicity.*

Risk for infection related to leukopenia/bone marrow suppression

- Warn patient to avoid crowds and people with cold, flu, or cold sore *to prevent exposure to pathogens.*
- Use sterile technique whenever needed *to prevent infection.*
- Initiate reverse isolation as indicated *to protect patient from pathogens.*
- Monitor temperature and leukocyte count; observe skin temperature, color, and odor *to detect signs of infection.*
- Encourage careful hygiene *to prevent infection.*
- Discourage fresh-cut flowers, *which may carry microorganisms.*
- Avoid using indwelling catheters or performing rectal procedures or examination *to prevent infection.*
- Administer antibiotics as prescribed *to treat infection.*

Altered peripheral perfusion related to bleeding

- Protect patient from injury (e.g., use precautions when shaving with razor blade, do not permit cluttered environment, and do not administer rectal suppositories) *to avoid trauma.*
- Have patient avoid using aspirin and aspirin products, *which increase clotting time.*
- Avoid giving injections; if they are necessary, apply pressure at site for 3 to 5 minutes afterward *to prevent bleeding.*
- Use toothettes for oral care *to avoid trauma to mucosa.*
- Monitor petechiae, ecchymoses, and stools *for blood.*
- Evaluate neurologic status *to identify intracranial bleeding.*
- Have nasal packing available should bleeding occur.
- Administer platelet transfusions as necessary *to control bleeding.*
- Monitor vital signs *to detect bleeding early.*
- Support patient in ambulation *to prevent injury related to weakness.*

Sexual dysfunction related to drug-induced changes in hormonal status

- Help patient explore alternatives for sterility, such as sperm banking, hormonal therapy during treatment, and postponement of conception and childbearing *to be proactive in dealing with changes in sexuality.*
- Refer to sexual counselor as needed *to deal with dysfunction.*

Altered patterns of urinary elimination related to drug-induced nephrotoxicity

- Force fluids *to maintain renal blood flow.*
- Monitor blood urea nitrogen, serum creatinine, creatinine clearance, and electrolytes *as indicators of renal function.*
- Monitor intake and output and presence of edema *to detect renal dysfunction.*
- Administer diuretics as ordered *to enhance renal excretion.*
- Encourage foods high in potassium *to prevent diuretic-related hypokalemia.*
- Administer normal saline and mannitol before cisplatin therapy per physician's order *to maintain fluid and electrolyte balance.*
- Administer allopurinol as prescribed with high fluid intake *to prevent uric acid accumulation in kidneys.*
- Encourage patient to empty bladder frequently, especially at night, *to avoid stasis, inflammation, and infection.*
- Provide adequate hydration *to maintain renal function.*

Sensory/perceptual/tactile alterations (auditory) related to drug-induced neurotoxicity

- Monitor hearing with baseline and periodic audiograms *to detect early hearing loss.*
- Speak clearly and in normal tone of voice *to enhance hearing.*
- Assess patient for numbness and tingling in extremities *to detect paresthesias.*
- Prohibit smoking and have patient observe placement of feet and hands *to promote safety.*

Impaired physical mobility related to drug-induced gout, osteoporosis, myelotoxicity

- Monitor calcium level *to determine bone status.*
- Provide safety measures *to prevent injury.*
- Be alert for complaint of pain over bony area; if patient has such a complaint, maintain bed rest until roentgenograms are taken for fracture *to detect injury.*
- Use assistive devices for ambulation *to enhance tolerance of activity.*
- Encourage range of motion exercise *to maintain mobility.*
- Position patient in proper anatomic alignment *to avoid stretching, pressure, or fracture.*

Ineffective individual coping related to stress of dealing with treatment

- Assess coping behavior; determine its effectiveness for patient *to determine need for new strategies.*
- Reassure patient that mood changes are temporary and dose related *to reduce anxiety.*
- Allow independence in self-care *to maintain patient self-esteem and promote effective coping.*
- Maintain supportive, nonjudgmental attitude *to foster patient coping.*
- Encourage use of resources, such as support groups, *to assist patient in coping.*

Patient Education/Home Care Planning

1. Encourage maintenance of adequate nutrition and hydration.
2. Emphasize the need for self-regulation of medication to control nausea, vomiting, constipation, diarrhea, itching, urinary distress, and oral irritation.
3. Discuss the warning signs of bleeding and infection that the patient should report to a physician.
4. Discuss the need for thorough personal hygiene and oral care.

Evaluation

Hydration is adequate   Patient experiences no nausea or vomiting; intake and output are balanced; patient is at normal weight; electrolyte levels are within normal limits.

Bowel elimination is normal   Patient experiences no constipation, diarrhea, or distention.

Oral mucous membranes are healthy   Mucous membranes, lips, tongue, and gingiva are of normal color and moisture. Patient has clean teeth, moist saliva, ability to swallow, and a normal voice.

Nutrition is adequate   Patient expresses no complaints of anorexia or unusual taste sensations. Patient is able to eat and swallow without pain. Patient is at normal weight.

Skin is healthy and intact   Patient expresses no complaints of itching. There is no evidence of rash or changes in pigmentation. Patient's hair is healthy.

Gas exchange and peripheral tissue perfusion are adequate   Patient expresses no complaints of fatigue or weakness. Patient has warm, pink skin and normal respirations, pulse, and blood pressure. There are no signs or symptoms of bleeding or cardiac dysfunction. The ECG findings are normal.

Infection is absent   Patient has normal temperature, normal WBC count, and cool, dry skin.

Sexual function is normal   Patient has satisfactory libido and has made plans for dealing with possible sterility.

Urinary elimination is normal   Patient expresses no complaints of urinary distress. Intake and output is balanced.

Hearing and sense of touch are normal   Patient is able to hear speaker and is aware of body sensations.

Physical mobility is normal   Patient is able to ambulate without assistance.

Patient is able to cope with stress of therapy   Patient discusses fears, anger, and sadness. Patient has made progress in problem solving.

■ BIOLOGIC RESPONSE MODIFIERS

Description and Rationale

Biologic response modifiers (BRMs) are still considered an investigational treatment for cancer. Their usefulness in treating a wide variety of tumors is being studied, but their value in improving long-term survival will require many years of evaluation.

The rationale for the use of BRMs in cancer care is based on animal studies and clinical observations such as the following:

Postoperative patients are often found to have malignant cells in circulating blood and in operative wound washings but may never receive a diagnosis of cancer.

Among transplant patients who receive immunosuppressant therapy, cancer occurs at a rate at least 80 times that of the general population.

Rapidly progressive recurrent cancer sometimes appears 10 to 20 years after cure.

Patients with congenital or acquired immunologic deficiencies have a greater incidence of cancer than does the general population.

People with faulty immune systems cannot be sensitized to certain chemicals, such as 2,4-dinitrochlorobenzene (DNCB), and are thus classified as anergic. An anergic cancer patient usually has a rapidly growing tumor and a poor prognosis.

The types of immunotherapy are classified as active and passive. Active therapy involves administration of an antigen to stimulate the patient's immune system, with subsequent development of immunity (antibody). The response may be specific or nonspecific (see the box on p. 1335).

Specific active immunotherapy stimulates an immune response to a tumor-associated antigen.

Nonspecific immunotherapy stimulates the immune response to a wide variety of antigens, including tumor-associated antigens.

Passive immunotherapy involves the direct transfer of transient immunity from person to person and may also be specific or nonspecific.

Nonspecific Active Immunotherapy

One group of nonspecific active immunologic agents are the cytokines, which include interferon, interleukin-2 (IL-2), and tumor necrosis factor. Interferon has three major types—alpha (derived from leukocytes), beta (derived from fibroblasts), and gamma (immune- or lymphocyte-derived). Interferons have been observed to inhibit viral replication and produce a possible direct antiproliferative effect on the tumor. This effect may be augmentation or induction of host-effector mechanisms such as natural killer cell activity or the induction of membrane antigens on tumor cells, which produces immune recognition. The tumors most responsive to interferon are hematologic, including non-Hodgkin's lymphomas, cutaneous T-cell lymphoma, and chronic myelogenous and hairy cell leukemias.

Lymphokines such as interleukin-1 (IL-1) and IL-2 cause T cell proliferation, activation of the lytic mechanisms of lymphokine-activated killer (LAK) cells, emigration of lymphoid cells from the peripheral blood, and the release of other lymphokines, such as tumor necrosis factor (TNF) and gamma interferon, and of other hormones, such as corticotropin, cortisol, and growth hormone. Toxicity is a major deterrent to the use of IL-2; the patient may experience chills and fever, nausea and vomiting, diarrhea, cutaneous erythema, weight gain, anemia, hypotension, tachycardia, and hepatic and renal dysfunction. IL-2 has demonstrated responses in renal cell cancer and malignant melanoma.

Nonspecific Passive Immunotherapy

The nonspecific passive immunologic agents include the cytokines and lymphokine-activated killer (LAK) cells. LAK cells lyse the tumor (e.g., natural killer cells).

Specific Passive Immunotherapy

Monoclonal antibodies are the result or the genetic fusing of cancer cells with leukocytes to produce specific antibodies, which provide passive immunity and serve as carriers of cytotoxic agents to malignant cells. For example, they are labeled with such isotopes as ^{131}I to seek occult tumor deposits throughout the body. Monoclonal antibodies may also activate complement, a stage in the immune response that leads eventually to cell death.

Colony-Stimulating Factors

One of the most exciting and promising developments of recent years in the area of supportive care has been the identification and use of hematopoietic colony-stimulating factors (CSFs). It is believed that CSFs could ameliorate or even eliminate the major hazard of cancer treatment, including neutropenia and thrombocytopenia. CSFs are involved in all aspects of hematopoiesis, including proliferation, differentiation, maturation, and functional activation. They may be categorized by (1) the number of blood cell lines affected (e.g., multilineage, such as IL-3 and hemopoietin-1, or single lineage, such as erythropoietin) or (2) biologic function.

The major endogenous human CSFs are produced in the hematopoietic microenvironment of the bone marrow by T lymphocytes, monocytes and macrophages, endothelial cells, and fibroblasts. Each CSF binds to and activates its unique, high-affinity protein receptor on the surface membrane of target cells. Receptors for granulocyte CSF (G-CSF) are found predominantly on the mature elements of the neutrophil line, whereas receptors for granulocyte-macrophage CSF (GM-CSF) are found predominantly among early cells. Macrophage

CSF (M-CSF) receptors predominate on the mature cells of the monocyte and macrophage series.

Both G-CSF and GM-CSF sustain the viability and potentiate the functions of neutrophils. GM-CSF also stimulates production of such cytokines as tumor necrosis factor and interleukin-1. M-CSF enhances the production of monocytes of colony-stimulating activity, interferon, and tumor necrosis factor (TNF). IL-3 may regulate the functions of mature eosinophils and monocytes.

CSFs have been studied in leukopenic persons with AIDS, in cancer patients receiving chemotherapy, and in bone marrow transplant patients. Side effects of CSF therapy include fatigue, fever, myalgias, loss of appetite, transient bone pain, rash, edema, and weight gain.

Nursing management of patients receiving CSF therapy includes pretreatment assessment, patient and family education, monitoring for side effects and toxicities, and implementing specific instructions depending on the treatment protocol.

 # RADIATION THERAPY

Description and Rationale

The goal of radiation in the treatment of cancer is the local destruction of malignant cells or their reproductive capability, with minimum damage to normal tissue. This treatment modality is used in the prevention, treatment, and palliation of cancer, either alone or with chemotherapy or surgery. Radiation therapy can be administered either externally or internally.

Ionizing radiation is the form used in cancer treatment because it causes cellular damage or alteration. Some examples of such radiation are x rays, gamma rays, electrons, and beta particles. Cells exposed to ionizing radiation undergo the following stages of reaction:

Physical stage—the cells' molecules become agitated and excited

Physiochemical stage—the agitated molecules break into stable molecules and chemically active substances

Chemical stage—chemical reactions take place inside the cell, causing changes in nuclear DNA

Biologic stage—DNA alterations occur, with consequent cell death

The substances used most for radiation therapy include:

X rays—the higher the voltage, the deeper the penetration; for example, high voltage is used for bladder cancer, and low voltage is used for superficial tumors such as skin cancers

Radioactive elements, such as radium and cobalt, which occur in nature

Radioactive isotopes, such as iodine, gold, and phosphorus, which are produced in atomic reactors

External radiation, the treatment of choice for such cancers as early laryngeal cancer, early retinoblastoma, and some brain tumors, is delivered by x ray or radioisotope via sophisticated equipment with refined delivery, such as the linear accelerator.

External radiation is also used as adjuvant therapy and for palliation through reduction of tumor mass.

Internal radiation may include temporary or permanent implants, intracavitary or interstitial instillation, or parenteral or oral administration. Specific uses for these forms of therapy are:

Implants (such as radon, iodine, and gold seeds) sutured into the tumor via tubes or needles for cancers of the tongue, lip, breast, and vagina and for small bladder tumors

Intracavitary or interstitial instillation via "seeding" with radioactive gamma ray–emitting beads such as radium or cesium for localized but inoperable lung cancers and invasive tumors of the uterus; "afterloading" with an applicator that provides channels through which to place the radioisotope may be used to reduce exposure

Radioactive isotopes administered orally or parenterally for thyroid cancer, chronic leukemia, or myeloma

The nurse involved in the care of patients receiving internal irradiation should avoid radiation damage by adhering to the principles of time (by being efficient but brief), distance (by standing as far as possible from the source), and shielding (by wearing a lead apron or using other precautions as determined by the radiation safety officer).

Radiosensitive cells—those most likely to be adversely affected by radiation—include relatively undifferentiated and rapidly dividing cells such as those of genes, the mucosa of the gastrointestinal tract, and lymphoid tissue. The most radioresistant cells are those originating from the connective tissue. At the cellular level the degree of sensitivity is related to the degree of cell differentiation, rate of mitosis, and mitotic potential. The degree of vascularity and oxygenation are also important in determining tissue responsiveness.

The side or toxic effects of radiation therapy depend on the site of irradiation, the volume of tissue irradiated, the total dosage delivered, and the time frame within which it is administered. Although newer technology has increased the therapist's ability to treat the cancer more precisely, surrounding or underlying healthy tissue may still be damaged.

The dose of radiation that can be delivered to any tumor is limited by the radiation tolerance of the adjacent normal tissues. One method of improving the therapeutic ratio is fractionation of treatment, or dividing the total dosage of radiation into multiple doses. This allows four processes to occur: repair of sublethal tissue damage, repopulation of clonogenic cells, reassortment of cells in the cell cycle, and reoxygenation of hypoxic cells. The best results are achieved with predetermined doses given five times a week for 4 to 6 weeks.

Before initiating therapy the therapist may localize the treatment portals with a stimulator, such as an x-ray machine that produces the geometric factors of actual therapy or computed tomography scanning that defines both the tumor-bearing volume and critical normal structures. The information obtained is used to produce, with computer assistance, an individualized treatment plan.

In combining surgery with radiation, the relative merits of preoperative or postoperative radiation for many cancers are still a matter of controversy. The use of chemotherapy with radiation requires careful monitoring of peripheral blood counts and observation for exacerbation of drug-induced disorders, such as severe dysuria (cyclophosphamide), enhanced mucositis (methotrexate), or carcinogenesis, such as leukemia. Actinomycin D and doxorubicin produce a recall phenomenon in which reactions appear in previously irradiated tissues when the drug is given as late as 1 year after the patient's radiation exposure.

NURSING CARE

Nursing Assessment

Gastrointestinal Tract

Nausea and vomiting; anorexia; taste changes; esophagitis; diarrhea; xerostomia; mucositis; radiation tooth decay; perianal irritation

Genitourinary

Urinary frequency; vaginal discharge; amenorrhea; impotence

Skin

Hair loss; dry desquamation; reddened area; dry, itchy feeling; moist desquamation—blistering and sloughing of skin surface

Central Nervous System

Headache; irritability; confusion; restlessness

Neuromuscular

Transient paresthesia; paresis or paralysis; fatigue

Cardiovascular

Pneumonitis—dry, hacking cough; dyspnea; pericarditis; chest pain; ECG changes; myocarditis; friction rub

Hemopoietic

Anemia; infection; bleeding

Nursing Dx & Intervention

Risk for fluid volume deficit related to nausea and vomiting

- Administer antiemetic as needed *to control incidence of nausea and vomiting.*
- Plan rest periods before and after meals *to enhance patient's appetite.*
- Provide small, bland feedings and increased fluids *to maintain nutrition and hydration.*
- Offer frequent mouth care *to promote comfort and appetite.*
- Provide clean environment with fresh air and no odors *to decrease noxious stimuli.*

- Administer intravenous therapy as ordered *to maintain hydration.*
- Monitor intake and output, daily weight, and electrolytes *to determine need for further intervention.*

Altered nutrition: less than body requirements related to gastrointestinal irritation and increased body requirements

- Encourage patient to eat high-calorie, high-protein diet *for maximum nutrition.*
- Offer small, frequent feedings *to increase intake.*
- Do not rush meals *to increase intake.*
- Keep room free of odors and clutter *to reduce noxious stimuli.*
- Provide meticulous mouth care *to increase comfort and appetite.*
- Use enteral feeding tube or total parenteral nutrition if necessary *to maintain nutritional balance.*
- Monitor weight daily *to detect nutritional imbalance.*

Diarrhea related to gastrointestinal irritation

- Encourage clear liquids and low-residue diet *to increase comfort.*
- Offer antidiarrheal agents per physician's order *to control intestinal irritability.*
- Maintain good perineal care *to prevent pain, infection, and patient's fear of eating caused by painful bowel movement.*
- Test stools for occult blood *to identify intestinal bleeding.*
- Record number and consistency of stools *to monitor effect of therapy.*
- Observe for dehydration and electrolyte imbalances *to determine need for further intervention.*

Altered patterns of urinary elimination related to bladder irritation

- Force fluids *to maintain renal and bladder hydration.*
- Encourage patient to empty bladder completely *to avoid distention.*
- Administer urinary antiseptics as prescribed *to reduce inflammation.*
- Observe for signs of infection, such as burning, cloudy urine, hematuria, and fever, *to determine the need for antibiotics and other interventions.*

Sexual dysfunction related to treatment-induced changes in hormonal status

For sterility
- Help patient explore alternatives such as sperm banking and hormonal therapy *to counteract sterility.*
- Refer patient to sexual counselor as necessary *to treat impotence.*

For vaginal discharge
- Encourage patient to douche as needed and to perform thorough perineal care *to maintain hygiene.*
- Observe for redness, tenderness, discharge, or drainage, *which may require further intervention.*

Altered oral mucous membrane related to mucositis, xerostomia, or radiation tooth decay

- Encourage good oral hygiene with use of dental floss or Water Pik *to prevent infection and promote healing.*
- Discourage spicy or hot foods and dry, thick foods, *which increase discomfort.*
- Offer topical relief of pain with lidocaine ointment, Aspergum, or ice chips *to promote comfort.*
- Apply K-Y Jelly to lips *to maintain moisture.*
- Offer popsicles *to increase comfort and hydration.*
- Offer artificial saliva *to moisten mucosa.*
- Encourage increased fluid intake with meals *to maintain hydration.*
- Use mouth irrigations or sprays, such as half-strength hydrogen peroxide and saline, *for oral hygiene.*
- Encourage use of sugarless lemon drops or mints *to promote feeling of freshness.*
- Discourage smoking, alcohol, and ginger ale, *which irritate mucosa.*
- Assess mouth for dryness, lesions, bleeding, discharge, and tooth decay *to determine need for specific interventions.*
- Consult with dentist as needed for dental care, including fluoride therapy, *to prevent further irritation and infection.*

Impaired skin integrity related to treatment-induced changes

For alopecia
- Help patient plan for wig, scarf, turban, or hat before hair loss *to avoid scalp damage.*
- Have patient gently wash and comb remaining hair *to avoid further hair loss.*
- Reassure patient that hair will grow back after therapy unless whole brain radiation used.

For dermatitis
- Observe irradiated area daily *to monitor for inflammation or other reactions.*
- Apply baby oil or ointment as prescribed: lanolin or Aquaphor *to maintain moisture.*
- Keep reddened area dry and aerated *to avoid infection.*
- Use cornstarch, A & D Ointment, or hydrocortisone ointment *to relieve dryness and itching.*

For moist desquamation
- Provide saline soaks, exposure to air, topical vitamins, steroids, or antibiotic ointments *to enhance healing.*
- Avoid the use of adhesive tape, *which irritates the skin.*
- Assist patient with bathing *to maintain markings.*
- Have patient avoid excessive heat, sunlight, tight, restrictive clothing, and soap, *which further irritate damaged skin.*
- Provide special skin care to tissue folds such as buttocks, perineum, groin, and axilla, *which may be sites of infection.*
- Avoid application of deodorant or after-shave lotion to treated area, *as these may irritate the skin.*

Pain (headache) related to increased intracranial pressure

- Assess presence and characteristics of headache *to monitor need for intervention.*
- Administer medications such as steroids and analgesics as prescribed *to relieve pain.*
- Offer patient other pain relief measures, if desired, *to encourage self-care.*
- Monitor pupillary response and changes in vital signs, irritability, confusion, and restlessness, *which indicate increasing intracranial pressure.*

Impaired physical mobility related to fatigue and impaired motor function

- Plan frequent rest periods *to avoid fatigue.*
- Assist with ambulation and remove environmental barriers *to avoid injury.*
- Assess reflexes, tactile sensation, and movement in extremities, and report abnormal findings *to detect complications.*
- Observe for Lhermitte's sign (sensation of electric shock running down back and over extremities), *which is indicative of cervical cord compression.*

Altered cardiopulmonary tissue perfusion related to pneumonitis, pericarditis, myocarditis, anemia, bleeding

- Auscultate lungs, and report signs of pleural rub *to assess pulmonary status.*
- Observe for cough, dyspnea, and pain on inspiration *as evidence of respiratory dysfunction.*
- Treat with antibiotics and steroids as prescribed *to reduce irritation and treat infection.*
- Auscultate heart, and report signs of friction rub, dysrhythmias, or hypertension *to detect complications.*
- Observe for chest pain and weakness, *which are indicative of cardiac dysfunction.*
- Monitor ECG reports *to monitor cardiac status.*
- Administer drugs as prescribed *to counteract dysrhythmias.*
- Encourage adequate rest; alternate rest and activity periods *to avoid stress on respiratory system.*
- Observe patient for dyspnea and increased weakness *as signs of further anemia.*
- Administer oxygen therapy as needed *to increase oxygenation of tissues.*
- Monitor hemoglobin and hematocrit *to determine effectiveness of therapy.*
- Administer transfusions as ordered *to increase circulating RBCs.*

Patient Education/Home Care Planning

1. Discuss the need for skin care such as maintenance of dye markings, avoidance of soap and other ointments, and avoidance of sunbathing or heat applications.

2. Emphasize the need to avoid injury to the skin.
3. Explain the maintenance of adequate nutrition.
4. Explain the patient's "radioactive state," if present, and precautions to be taken.
5. Discuss the management of fatigue and the maintenance of mobility.

Evaluation

Hydration is adequate Patient experiences no nausea and vomiting. Intake and output is balanced. Electrolyte levels are within normal limits.

Nutrition is adequate Patient makes no complaints of anorexia or unusual taste sensations. Patient is able to eat and swallow without pain. Patient is at normal weight.

Bowel elimination is normal Patient has no diarrhea.

Urinary elimination is normal Patient makes no complaints of urinary distress. Intake and output is balanced.

Sexual function is normal Patient has satisfactory libido and has made plans for dealing with possible sterility, absence of vaginal discharge, and erectile ability.

Oral mucous membranes are healthy Mucous membranes, lips, tongue, and gingiva are of normal color and moisture. Patient has clean teeth, moist saliva, an ability to swallow, and a normal voice.

Skin is healthy and intact Patient makes no complaints of itching. There is no evidence of rash or blistering or redness.

Patient is free from pain Patient makes no complaint of headache.

Physical mobility is normal Patient is able to ambulate without asisstance.

Cardiopulmonary tissue perfusion is adequate Patient makes no complaints of chest pain, cough, or dyspnea. Complete blood cell count is within normal limits.

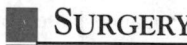

SURGERY

(Biopsy/staging, resection, and reconstruction)

Surgery has historically been the treatment of choice for most cancers. A decision to use this therapy is based on analysis of a variety of data, including a thorough history and physical examination; laboratory, radiologic, and other specialized procedures; and biopsy-obtained proof of cancer.

A radical surgical approach to operable tumors is no longer routinely used because of an increased variety of surgical procedures and more sophisticated disease staging. The current treatment of choice is excision of the primary tumor and enough surrounding tissue and lymph nodes to offer maximum protection against local recurrence. These are termed curative resections. Palliative resections may be done when there is spread to distant, previously (preoperatively) undetected sites.

A tumor is considered inoperable if it is large or in a difficult-to-reach place or if there is evidence of extensive local growth or metastasis.

Staging operations such as laparotomy may be performed to determine appropriate therapy. Secondary operations may be done for local recurrence. "Second look" operations may be performed in the absence of chemical evidence of recurrent disease, but the effectiveness of this procedure for finding recurrent disease is questionable.

Distant metastasis (e.g., pulmonary or hepatic) may respond to direct surgical resection. Indirect ablative procedures such as adrenalectomy and hypophysectomy may be useful in the palliation of hormonally sensitive cancers of the breast or prostate. Other indirect palliative procedures include cordotomy for relief of intractable pain and ostomy to relieve gastrointestinal obstruction.

Reconstructive surgery of the head and neck, breast, and extremities has become an important aspect of cancer rehabilitation in recent years. For example, the development of maxillofacial prosthodontics has enabled people treated with radical neck dissection to regain cosmetic appearance and the ability to eat and drink in a more natural manner. Breast reconstruction is an option for women whose disease and treatment enable the surgeon to implant a prosthesis or to transplant tissue from other areas of the body.

Whatever the surgery, the patient's nutritional status, both preoperatively and postoperatively, has been found to be significant in the amount of surgery that can be tolerated, recovery from the surgical procedure, and wound healing.

PHOTODYNAMIC THERAPY

Photodynamic therapy (PDT) involves injecting the patient with intravenous dihematoporphyrin ether (DHE) or other photo-sensitizing agent, waiting 48 to 72 hours for the drug to clear healthy tissues and concentrate in malignant cells, and then exposing the cancerous area to laser light delivered through a scope (cystoscope, bronchoscope).

PDT is used as a possible cure for early stages of skin and bladder cancers and for palliation of advanced lung, esophageal, and pelvic cancers. The patient selected for this therapy may have had previous treatment or may be currently undergoing conventional therapy or be newly diagnosed.

Although all cells absorb the photosensitizing agent, retention is higher in malignant tissue, the liver, spleen, kidneys, and skin. The laser emits a powerful red light that penetrates tissue and activates the photosensitizer in the malignant cells. A superoxide, which results from the chemical reaction between the laser beam and the photosensitizer, changes the cell membrane and thus destroys the malignant cells.

The procedure is painless because no tissue is burned or cut. However, because the photosensitizer causes profound photosensitivity, patients must avoid sunlight for up to 6 weeks after treatment. Similar to the laser, sunlight contains red light that easily penetrates the skin; thus exposure to sunlight could cause severe swelling and redness.

If PDT is used in the treatment of bladder cancer, the patient may have postsurgical complaints of severe urinary frequency and urgency caused by edema and hemorrhage. Bladder capacity may be decreased after the procedure; edema, the high energy source, or overdistention of the bladder during the procedure may cause the decrease. The bladder usually returns to normal capacity within 3 months after treatment. Oral analgesics, antispasmodics, and prophylactic antibiotics may be prescribed.

Palliation of symptoms caused by obstructive primary or secondary cancer can also be achieved with PDT. Debulking of the tumor can relieve bleeding, infection, pain, and symptoms of obstruction.

NUTRITIONAL SUPPORT

Patients with cancer must deal not only with the metabolic effects of the disease on their nutritional status, but also with the effects of treatment. In addition, an inability to eat or difficulty with eating may affect the patient psychologically because nutrition is not only a basic human need but often a source of social interaction. Patients with cancer who experience anorexia, nausea and vomiting, stomatitis, changes in taste, and difficulty swallowing face the challenge of eating when they least want to or are least able yet have the greatest need to do so. It has been shown through numerous research studies that a poor nutritional status adversely affects the patient's ability to tolerate both cancer and its treatment.

The body of the person with cancer responds to the increased demand for glucose, which is required by both normal and cancer cells by the increased rate of gluconeogenesis. This is the synthesis of glucose by the liver and renal cortex from noncarbohydrate sources such as lactate and amino acids. When protein is broken down to provide amino acids for gluconeogenesis, muscle wasting is the result. Progressive muscle wasting is called cachexia and gives the patient a characteristic appearance of emaciation.

Fat metabolism is also adversely affected in persons with cancer. Fat stored in the form of fatty acids is mobilized from adipose tissue and released into the bloodstream for use as fuel. This process, which is controlled by the inhibitory effects of insulin, is compromised in persons with cancer, so that body stores of fat are depleted as the disease progresses.

Persons with cancer also exhibit deficiencies in such vitamins as A, C, and thiamine. Iron deficiency may also occur. Fluid and electrolyte imbalances include hypercalcemia, hyperuricemia, hyperphosphatemia, and hyperkalemia. These alterations result from either the direct or indirect effects of tumors, such as paraneoplastic syndromes.

Poor nutrition also adversely affects immunocompetence, by decreasing the size of the lymphoid tissues, including the spleen, lymph nodes, and thymus. There is a resulting decreased function of B- and T-cell lymphocytes, which is directly correlated with the degree of malnutrition and which produces a delayed hypersensitivity response.

Local effects of cancer, such as the presence of tumors that adversely affect chewing, swallowing, and peristalsis, can alter the patient's nutritional status. Obstruction, pain, and distention affect the patient's ability to digest and metabolize food.

As discussed earlier, the treatment modalities—surgery, chemotherapy, radiation therapy, and BRMs—also compromise the patient's nutritional status. Thus the nurse must assess the patient's nutritional status at frequent intervals to obtain a baseline measure and to identify the need for aggressive intervention. Clinical observation, including the identification of concurrent health problems (diabetes, hypertension, malabsorption), psychosocial factors (home environment, methods of food preparation, patient's body image), and physical assessment provide the data needed to monitor the patient's nutritional status. Examination of the patient's hair, teeth, gums, and general muscle tone can provide early signs of nutritional deficiencies.

Dietary evaluation is also useful and includes a 24-hour food diary, a complete dietary history with food allergies and preferences, direct observation of dietary intake, and evaluation of nutrient composition. Biochemical measurements include such laboratory values as serum albumin, serum transferrin, and urine urea nitrogen levels and total lymphocyte count. Anthropometric measurements include the patient's midarm muscle circumference (MAMC), triceps, skin fold thickness (SFT), subscapular skin fold thickness (SST), and weight for height measurements.

Nutritional interventions for the person with cancer have been shown to decrease the morbidity and mortality of cancer by preventing weight loss, increasing response to therapy, minimizing the side effects of treatment, and improving quality of life. The type of nutritional support required by the patient is based on his or her functional abilities and limitations, severity of the nutritional deficiency, potential for complications, duration of therapy, cost, and psychologic effect.

Nutritional support may include oral, enteral, and parenteral nutritional management. The oral route is preferred because it is more natural and least invasive. Oral nutritional support may range from the addition of sauces and gravies to foods to more complex interventions such as dietary supplements. The patient with anorexia may benefit from frequent small meals and snacks. Foods high in protein and calories are recommended, such as cheese, fish, poultry, milkshakes, peanut butter on crackers, and prepackaged puddings.

If the patient has stomatitis or taste alterations, a high-calorie bland diet may be helpful. The patient should avoid seasoning and liquids with high acidity such as orange and lemon juices. Use of a topical analgesic, good mouth care, and avoidance of commercial mouthwashes reduces oral discomfort. Cold foods such as popsicles and ice cream have a numbing effect, which patients tolerate better than warm or hot foods.

Psychosocial support is also critical. Both the patient and family should be encouraged to try a variety of strategies and to be supportive of one another because this is a difficult and challenging problem. The patient's appetite can be enhanced by occasionally eating at the table with family and friends in an attractive environment. Using small plates, eating more often, and decreasing exposure to strong food odors may also be helpful. Antiemetics and artificial saliva can be used to control the symptoms of gastrointestinal irritation.

High-calorie high-protein supplements such as Isocal, Poly-cose, and Vivonex may be helpful to the patient; however, they are not well tolerated by patients with lactose intolerance.

The enteral route via a feeding tube may be needed by patients who are anoretic, hypermetabolic, or unconscious and by those who have a mechanical impairment. Parenteral feeding is indicated only for patients with totally nonfunctioning gastrointestinal tracts, those who require bowel rest, or those who cannot tolerate enteral nutritional support.

Patients with functioning gastrointestinal tracts who are not able to ingest adequate nutrients to meet their metabolic demands should be considered candidates for enteral feeding. These include patients with anorexia; cachexia; cancers of the head or neck, esophagus, stomach; central nervous system disease, which impairs swallowing; and intractable diarrhea.

Tube feedings may be administered by the nasogastric, nasoduodenal, nasojejunal, esophagostomy, gastrostomy, and jejunostomy routes (Figure 16-6). The most common routes involve passage of a small, flexible feeding tube through the nose into the stomach or intestine. Feeding ostomies such as the gastrostomy usually require surgical percutaneous insertion and are preferred for long-term nutritional support. The cervical esophagostomy is a surgically created, skin-lined canal extending from the border of the neck to the area below the cervical

esophagus; the feeding tube is passed through this opening to the stomach for each feeding and then removed.

Aspiration may occur more often with gastric feedings because only the gastroesophageal sphincter is functioning to prevent gastric reflux, whereas the intestinal feedings use both the gastroesophageal and pyloric sphincters to prevent reflux. When feedings are improperly selected or administered, nausea, diarrhea, and cramps can occur.

The volume and concentration of the nutriment provided by tube feeding should meet the needs of the individual patient and should be compatible with the size of the tube, the location of the tube, and the patient's tolerance of formula strength and rate of administration. Feedings may be delivered by bolus or gravity, as well as via enteral pump. The position of the tube and gastric residual should be checked frequently. The patient should be monitored for the development of dumping syndrome, aspiration, weight loss, and diarrhea; each of these conditions require evaluation of the formula and infusion rate for changes.

The patient may also complain of thirst, taste deprivation, and the inability to satisfy the appetite, as well as a sense of altered body image. The patient may be permitted to chew gum or suck on hard candies, drink fluids, and eat soft, bland foods. Referral to a support group may help the patient to accept the alterations in the social and aesthetic aspects of eating.

Complications of tube feedings may be mechanical, such as nasal irritation and erosion, esophagitis or pharyngitis, or tube dislocation or occlusion; gastrointestinal, such as abdominal distention, nausea and vomiting, constipation or diarrhea; respiratory (aspiration pneumonia); or metabolic, such as hyperglycemia, hypokalemia, hyperkalemia, hypernatremia, and dehydration. The nurse and patient should monitor the feedings to identify problems early and intervene before serious alterations occur. Because many patients receive enteral feedings in the home, a care giver and the patient should be taught general care of the patient and the tube to ensure safe and effective therapy.

Parenteral nutrition (also called hyperalimentation) supplies all of the essential nutrients by intravenous infusion. Total parenteral nutrition (TPN) supplies all of the daily requirements for protein and calories directly into the patient's bloodstream and is indicated for such patients as those with cancers of the gastrointestinal tract, other obstructions, radiation enteritis, and intractable diarrhea.

TPN is delivered via peripheral veins, most often those of the arm or the external jugular vein. Limitations of peripheral infusion include provision of limited calories, vein irritation, and limited usefulness for long-term therapy. Use of a central line into a major vein such as the superior vena cava provides for a large amount of calories and protein, high dextrose and amino acid concentrations, and usefulness for long-term therapy. Central lines used for TPN include ports, triple-lumen catheters, Broviac, Hickman, and Groshong catheters (Figure 16-7). When central infusion is used, the solution must be tapered down by rate and concentration to discontinue therapy without inducing profound hypoglycemia.

TPN contains glucose, amino acids, and fats for the provision of both immediate and long-term energy. Patients

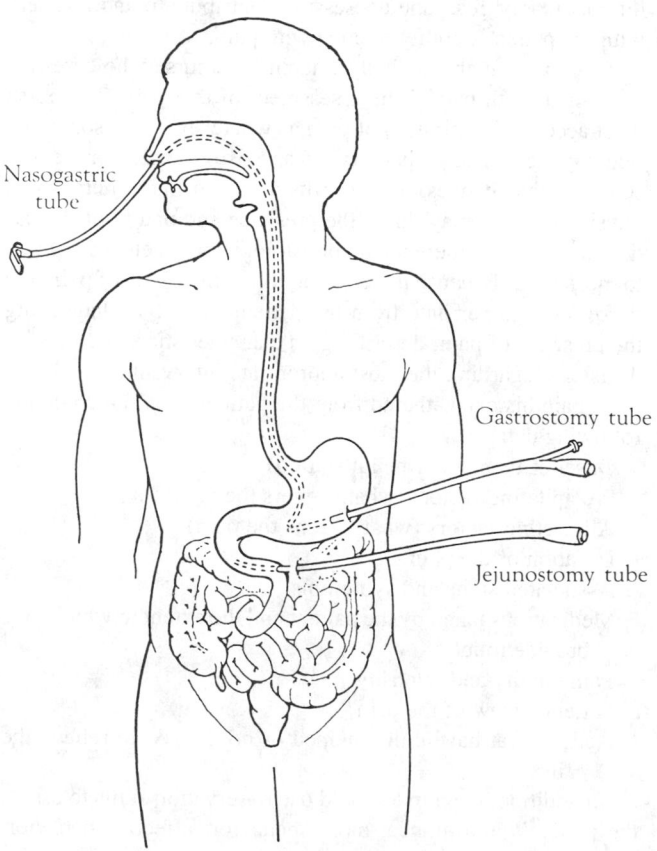

Nasogastric tube

Gastrostomy tube

Jejunostomy tube

Figure 16-6 Three routes for tube feeding.

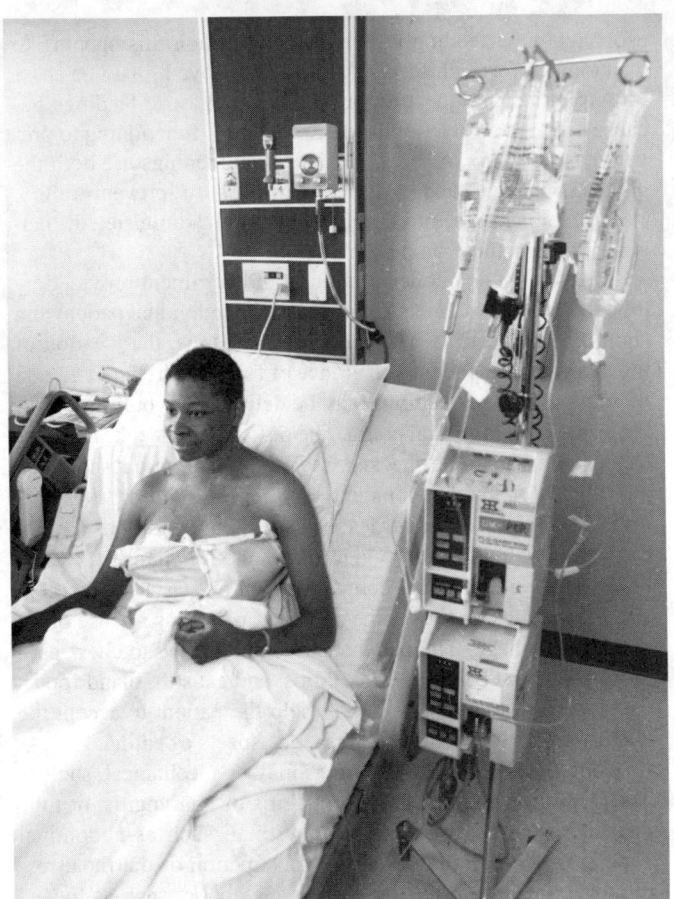

Figure 16-7 Hickman-Broviac catheter. This patient has a Hickman-Broviac catheter for venous access. Note the catheter's lift over the right breast, with a protective dressing and tape to prevent dislodgement. The patient is receiving multiple intravenous infusions via the catheter.

receiving TPN usually have a multilumen central venous catheter inserted so that there is access for the administration of medications and blood drawing.

TPN may be given continuously or by cycling, with cycling at night used most often for patients receiving TPN at home. Cycling enables the patient to be mobile during the day but does require an ability to tolerate a high-volume load. Programmable pumps are used to prevent or minimize hypoglycemia and hyperglycemia. Ambulatory patients benefit from the use of the portable pump, which is worn as a backpack-like carrying bag.

The nurse should assess the patient's life-style, home environment, family and support systems, body image, and perceptions about TPN to plan for the optimal acceptance of and adaptation to the therapy. Daily monitoring of vital signs, weight, and laboratory values enables the nurse to determine the need for adjustment of formula or rate of administration before the patient's discharge. Follow-up visits in the home are important and ensure the patient's compliance and tolerance of TPN.

The nurse's role in nutritional support is a critical one and includes comprehensive assessment, monitoring, and patient education to maintain the person with cancer in optimal nutritional status.

PAIN MANAGEMENT

Persons with cancer may experience pain at any point in time during the course of their disease and its treatment. Of the 4 million people throughout the world who die from cancer each year, 70% experience pain as a primary symptom. Unfortunately, many persons believe that pain is an early symptom of cancer and do not seek diagnosis until pain occurs. Pain is (almost without exception) a late symptom of cancer and indicates the presence of tumor obstruction, pressure on nerves, invasion of bone, phantom sensation, peripheral neuropathy, postherpetic neuralgia, mucositis, or incisional irritation.

It is estimated that 85% of patients with cancer pain can be managed effectively with appropriate therapy. The American Cancer Society, the American Pain Society, the World Health Organization, the Oncology Nursing Society, and many other organizations consider pain control to be a major issue in the management of the person with cancer. If not relieved, pain contributes to nausea, vomiting, anorexia, and insomnia. In addition, anxiety, fear, and depression contribute to and interfere with the patient's ability to cope with pain.

One of the many challenges facing the nurse who cares for the patient with pain is the assessment of that pain. The nurse must accept the definition of pain as whatever the person experiencing the pain says that it is and as existing wherever the person says that it does. This is frustrating to many nurses and physicians, who may doubt the presence and nature of the patient's pain when there are no physiologic parameters by which to measure it. Because there are no direct measures of pain, the nurse must gather data from the patient for use in diagnosing the presence of pain, describing its characteristics, and making decisions regarding the most appropriate interventions.

A pain history gathered from the patient should include the following data:

Onset of the pain (when it started)
Precipitating factors (what triggers the pain)
Alleviating factors (what lessens the pain)
Location of the pain
Associated signs and symptoms
Medications taken by the patient and the extent to which they provide relief
Pain quality and intensity
Patient's view of the pain
Actions that have either helped or not helped to relieve the pain

In addition, the nurse should use observation skills to assess the patient's appearance; motor behavior; affective behavior; verbal behavior; brainstem automatic responses, such as increase in heart rate, respirations, and blood pressure; spinal cord reflex responses; and nonverbal pain clues. The psychosocial dimensions of the pain must also be explored. These include personality, cultural, and religious factors; the patient's interpretation of pain; the patient's prior experience with pain; and the physical environment in which the patient is experiencing the pain.

General guidelines for the use of pain relief measures are:

1. Use a variety of pain relief measures.
2. Use pain relief measures before the patient's pain becomes severe.
3. Include pain relief measures that the patient believes will be helpful.
4. Determine the patient's ability or willingness to participate actively in the use of pain relief measures.
5. Rely on patient behavior that indicates pain severity rather than on known physical stimuli.
6. Encourage the patient to try a pain relief measure at least two times before abandoning it as ineffective.
7. Keep an open mind about what may relieve the patient's pain, including nonpharmacologic measures.
8. Keep trying to relieve the pain; do not become discouraged and stop working with the patient.

Chemical means of pain management include the use of narcotics and nonnarcotics. Nonnarcotic analgesics of value in the treatment of cancer pain are acetaminophen; aspirin; and nonsteroidal antiinflammatory drugs (NSAIDs) such as ibuprofen, indomethacin, and naproxen. One potential drawback of aspirin is its antiplatelet effect, which can create problems in the myelosuppressed patient. Acetaminophen may be a problem in patients with impaired liver function. Both aspirin and the NSAIDs are generally well tolerated but have the potential of causing gastrointestinal ulceration, renal toxic effects, and inhibition of platelet aggregation. If a nonnarcotic agent does not have a therapeutic effect initially, the dose should be increased before trying another type of drug. When a ceiling is reached with a nonnarcotic agent, a moderately potent narcotic such as oxycodone or codeine can be added. Some persons with cancer require such a combination from the initiation of treatment.

Narcotics (opioids) used in the management of cancer pain include morphine (the prototype), hydromorphone, and methadone. Sustained-release morphine in an oral form, such as MS Contin or Roxanol SR, has been found to be of particular value in the management of the terminally ill person with pain. The administration of narcotics via intravenous drips, both intrathecally and epidurally, has enhanced the analgesic effect of the opioids. Avoiding the peaks and valleys of pain relief experience with bolus injection has provided a more constant analgesic effect for the patient with cancer pain. The need for around-the-clock dosing has been noted, so that fixed dosing schedules with adequate doses for pain relief provide more constant blood levels and predictable pain relief. Some patients experience break-through pain that requires additional dosing, but the fixed dosing schedule should be maintained. Side effects of the narcotics that require nurse monitoring and intervention include constipation, vomiting, and respiratory and central nervous system depression.

Another category of drugs that may be used for pain management are the narcotic agonists and antagonists such as nalbuphine (Nubain), butorphanol (Stadol), pentazocine (Talwin),

and buprenex. Analgesic potentiators include the phenothiazine derivatives such as promethazine (Phenergan), prochlorperazine (Compazine), chlorpromazine (Thorazine), hydroxyzine pamoate (Vistaril), diazepam (Valium), lorazepam (Ativan), and diphenhydramine (Benadryl). Also used are stimulants such as cocaine, methylphenidate (Ritalin), dextroamphetamine, and caffeine; tricyclic antidepressants such as amitriptyline (Elavil), imipramine (Tofranil), and doxepin (Sinequan); the butyrophenones such as droperidol (Inapsine) and haloperidol (Haldol).

Patient self-control methods include distraction, massage, relaxation, biofeedback, hypnosis, and imagery. Many patients respond positively to the opportunity for self-care in the management of their pain and perceive such self-control measures to enhance the effectiveness of other prescribed pain interventions.

Pain technology includes the use of:

1. External pumps for the intravenous, epidural, and intrathecal administration of narcotic analgesics
2. Implantable pumps for the intravenous, epidural, and intrathecal administration of narcotic analgesics
3. Patient-controlled analgesia, particularly for the management of acute pain, such as postoperative pain
4. Transcutaneous electrical nerve stimulation (TENS)
5. Continuous subcutaneous infusion (CSCI) with an ambulatory infusion pump

In each instance, the nurse must develop the technical skills needed to initiate and monitor the therapy and to teach the patient and family the use and maintenance of the system. Each of these technologies has expanded the options for the patient with pain and has increased the degree of self-control experienced.

Other interventions for pain include (1) anesthetic procedures such as nerve blocks, trigger point injections, and the use of nitrous oxide; (2) neuroaugmentive therapies such as counterirritation, rubbing, TENS, and percutaneous nerve stimulation; (3) neuroablative procedures such as cordotomy; and (4) physiatric supportive measures such as the use of a prosthesis, physical therapy, and occupational therapy.

The nurse's unique contributions to pain management are placement as the key link between the patient and the health care team, the amount of time spent with the patient, the ability to assess the patient's response to the pain and its management, and the role of patient and family educator. In addition, the nurse has the ability to articulate a concise pain assessment, use equianalgesic charts for dosage guidelines, and anticipate and address patient, family, and health care provider misconceptions about pain management. For instance, many patients and their families experience opioid phobia, the irrational and undocumented fear that the appropriate use of narcotics causes addiction. This fear of addiction among both health care providers and the public seems to be a major reason for the undertreatment of pain. The nurse must understand and be able to articulate the differences between addiction, tolerance, and physical dependence to use pain management strategies appropriately and to enable patients and their families to accept the therapeutic value of drugs such as the narcotics.

References

1. American Cancer Society: *Cancer facts and figures, 1995,* Atlanta, 1995, The American Cancer Society.
2. Baird SB, McCorkle R, Grant M: *Cancer nursing: a comprehensive textbook,* Philadelphia, 1995, Saunders.
3. Belcher, AE: *Cancer nursing,* St Louis, 1992, Mosby.
4. Brundage, DJ: *Renal disorders,* St Louis, 1992, Mosby.
5. Cannobbio MM: *Cardiovascular disorders,* St Louis, 1992, Mosby.
6. Carter LW: Influences of nutrition and stress on people at risk for neutropenia: nursing implications, *Oncol Nurs Forum* 20(8):1241, 1993.
7. Chipps E, Clanin NJ, Campbell VG: *Neurological disorders,* St Louis, 1992, Mosby.
8. Di Saia PJ, Creasman WT: *Clinical gynecologic oncology,* ed 3, St Louis, 1989, Mosby.
9. Doogan RA: Hypercalcemia of malignancy, *Cancer Nurs* 4:299, 1981.
10. Duigan A: Anticipatory nausea and vomiting associated with cancer chemotherapy, *Oncol Nurs Forum* 13(1):35, 1986.
11. Ellerhorst-Ryan J: Complications of the myeloproliferative system: infection and sepsis, *Semin Oncol Nurs* 1(4):244, 1985.
12. Grimes DE: *Infectious diseases,* St Louis, 1991, Mosby.
13. Groenwald SL et al: *Cancer nursing: principles and practice,* Boston, 1993, Jones & Bartlett.
14. Gullatte M, Graves T: Advances in antineoplastic therapy, *Oncol Nurs Forum* 17(6):867, 1990.
15. Haeuber D: Future strategies in the control of myelosuppression: the use of colony-stimulating factors, *Oncol Nurs Forum* 18(2):16, 1991.
16. Hassey K: Care of patients with radioactive implants, *Am J Nurs* 85(7):788, 1985.
17. Heinrich-Rynning T: Prostatic cancer treatments and their effects on sexual functioning, *Oncol Nurs Forum* 14(6):37, 1987.
18. Holleb AI, Fink DJ, Murphy GP: *American Cancer Society textbook of clinical oncology,* Atlanta, 1991, The American Cancer Society.
19. Jenkins B: Patients' reports of sexual changes after treatment for gynecological cancer, *Oncol Nurs Forum* 15(3):349, 1988.
20. Kim MJ, McFarland CK McLane AM: *Pocket guide to nursing diagnoses,* ed 6, St Louis, 1995, Mosby.
21. Loescher LJ, editor: Skin cancers, *Semin Oncol Nurs* 7(1):1, 1991.
22. Lotze MT, Rosenberg BA: The immunologic treatment of cancer, *CA* 38(2):68, 1988.
23. Mayer, DK: Biotherapy: recent advances and nursing implications, *Nurs Clin North Am* 25(2):291, 1990.
24. McCance KL, Huether SE: *Pathophysiology: the biologic basis for disease in adults and children,* ed 2, St Louis, 1994, Mosby.
25. Mourad LA: *Orthopedic disorders,* St Louis, 1991, Mosby.
26. Otto SE: *Oncology nursing,* St Louis, 1991, Mosby.
27. Phipps WJ et al: *Medical-surgical nursing,* ed 5, St Louis, 1994, Mosby.
28. Poe C, Taylor L: Syndrome of inappropriate antidiuretic hormone: assessment and nursing implications, *Oncol Nurs Forum* 16(3):373, 1989.
29. Smith DB: Sexual rehabilitation of the cancer patient, *Cancer Nurs* 12(1):10, 1989.
30. Strohl RA: Radiation therapy. Recent advances and nursing implications, *Nurs Clin N Amer* 25(2):309, 1990.
31. Tootla J, Easterling A: PDT: destroying malignant cells with laser beams, *Nurs 89* 19(11):48, 1989.
32. Valentine AB, Stewart JA: Oncologic emergencies, *Am J Nurs* 83:1281, 1983.
33. Welch-McCaffrey D: When it comes to cancer, think family, *Nursing 83*:32, 1983.
34. Wickham R: Managing chemotherapy-related nausea and vomiting: the state of the art, *Oncol Nurs Forum* 16(4):563, 1989.
35. Wilson, SF, Thompson JM: *Respiratory disorders,* St Louis, 1990, Mosby.

Mental Health

17

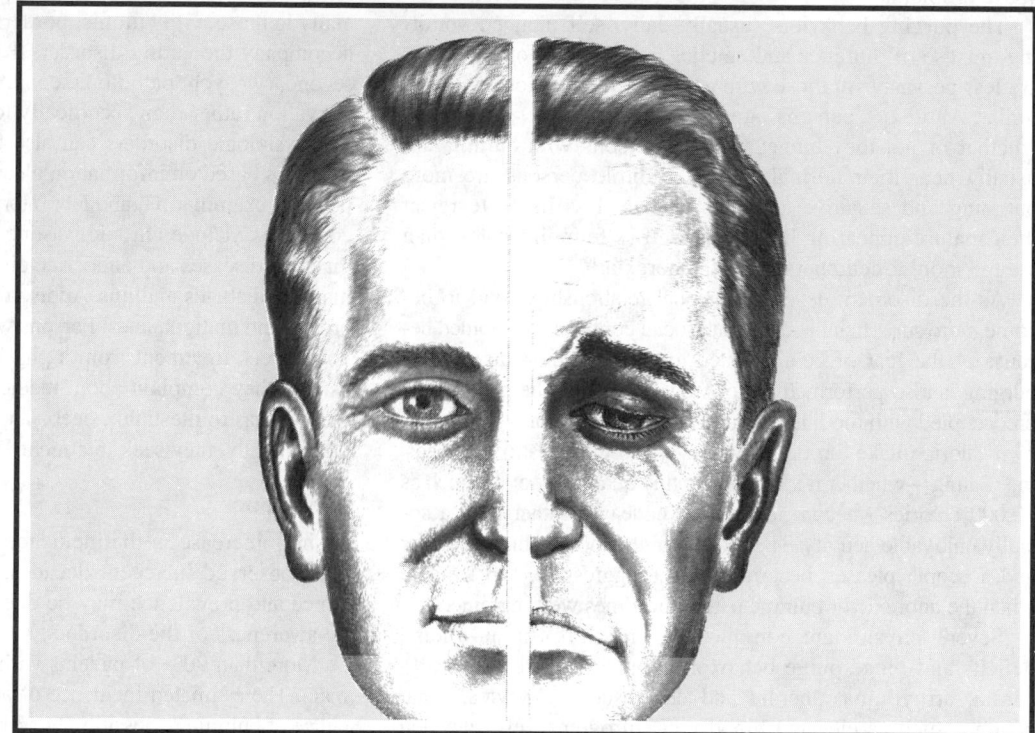

OVERVIEW

Mental health is an elusive concept with diverse definitions. Not all theorists identify the same personality traits as indicators of healthy functioning, but their definitions are not necessarily contradictory. The diversity is related to the complexity of human beings and the beliefs each theorist has about human nature. Theorists recognize that biologic, social, and psychologic influences all contribute to healthy personality functioning, but each theorist emphasizes one dimension over the others.

Characteristics of healthy personality functioning compiled from psychoanalytic, interpersonal, and cognitive theories are listed below. The list is not exhaustive and is not in order of importance, but all characteristics are indicators of mental health.

Positive self-identity

Awareness of oneself as a psychologically separate individual

Responsibility for oneself and one's own actions

Acceptance of emotions and ability to correct faulty ones

Constructive use of cognitive processes

Achievement of satisfying interpersonal relationships

Autonomy, which includes use of self-supports

Flexibility to adapt to change

When personality growth and development go awry because of psychologic, social, cultural, or biologic influences, the person may become mentally ill. This chapter describes major mental health problems nurses are likely to encounter.

CONDITIONS, DISEASES, AND DISORDERS

ANOREXIA NERVOSA AND BULIMIA NERVOSA

Anorexia nervosa is a formidable eating disorder characterized by a determination to lose weight mainly by restricting food intake even when emaciated. Bulimia nervosa is characterized by eating binges followed by maladaptive or inappropriate reparative behaviors, such as dieting and purging, occurring at least two times each week for three or more months.[2]

Anorexia nervosa and bulimia nervosa are eating disorders that generally occur in young adults with distorted views of their body shape, weight, and selves. A major issue in these conditions is attaining a sense of control of the self and of the environment.[2,13] Through dieting and weight loss these persons believe they will experience control, autonomy, and competence.

Eating is a source of anxiety for anorexic or bulimic persons. Some persons with anorexia never engage in binge eating and purging because of a strong self-discipline; those with binge/purging behaviors are more likely to exhibit impulse, out-of-control, and chaotic behaviors and some have substance abuse problems.

The purging behaviors (usually daily, self-induced vomiting, misuse of diuretics and emetics, and overuse of laxatives) are less pervasive in those with anorexia than in those with bulimia. Anorexic persons are likely to become emaciated, whether or not they binge; whereas persons with bulimia are usually near their normal weight. Bulimic persons are more outgoing and sensitive to others and are less likely to reject their mature-appearing bodies, as well as feminine roles, than are the more ascetic persons with anorexia.[40]

As the disorders develop, personal relationships tend to become more superficial and distant. Social contacts are avoided because of the fear of being invited to eat and being discovered; purging is also performed out of view of others. The patients are preoccupied with food, meal planning (especially for others), their own caloric intake throughout the day, and methods to avoid eating. Eating—whether it is normal, in tiny quantities, or as much as 20,000 calories—becomes a private endeavor rather than a socially enjoyable activity. The model child, who is a high achiever and a people pleaser, becomes defiant, aggressive, and irritable when the anorexic or bulimic pattern becomes well ingrained.

Severe physiologic complications result from nutritional deficits and binge-purge behaviors. Some of these are bradycardia, arrhythmia, anemia and decreased leukocytes, renal changes such as elevated blood urea nitrogen levels, elevated liver function tests, electrolyte imbalance such as hypokalemia, hypochloremic alkalosis, and hypomagnesemia, dental problems usually resulting from vomiting, and thyroid hormone level changes such as decrease in triiodothyronine (T_3). In females, a decrease in serum estrogen leads to amenorrhea and, in males, there is reduced testosterone.[2,40] Skeletal maturation is delayed especially in the adolescent when a starvation diet is tenaciously maintained.

Brain imaging techniques identify changes that occur in anorexia and bulimia, but findings are not specific to eating disorders. Ventricular enlargement is secondary to starvation but also sometimes occurs in those with bulimia nervosa at normal weight.[54] Metabolic encephalopathy may be related to fluid and electrolyte imbalance. Convulsions may be another neurologic complication.

Researchers have found that disturbances in brain neurotransmitters such as serotonin, dopamine, norepinephrine, and the endogenous opioids play a role in anorexia and bulimia. Impaired functioning of neurotransmitters can affect behavior; some neurotransmitters have a strong influence in eating disorders.[54] It is unknown whether some disturbances in the neurotransmitters and other hormonal and neuroendocrinologic abnormalities reflect an underlying biologic pathology or are secondary to the eating disorders.

Eating disorders, such as anorexia nervosa and bulimia nervosa, should be differentiated from other mental disorders, such as depression, schizophrenia, hysteria, obsessive-compulsive disorders, and substance abuse disorders. In these disorders weight loss does not involve a fundamental drive for thinness; instead, weight loss occurs because the person has a lack of in-terest in food, has a fear of germs, or experiences delusions. However, secondary psychopathologic factors, such as depression, anxiety, and obsessive-compulsive disorders, and, especially in those with bulimia, borderline personality disorder, can accompany the eating disorders.[40] It is also possible that some secondary psychopathologic conditions are due to the effects of starvation rather than specifically to bulimia or anorexia.

Physiologic disorders can also be differentiated from eating disorders based on information gleaned from the patient's history, physical examination, and laboratory and other tests. Physiologic conditions include chronic wasting caused by tumors and hypothalamic diseases and endocrine disorders such as thyroid abnormalities, diabetes mellitus, Addison's disease, gastrointestinal disorders, and malignancies. Persons with eating disorders generally do not seek treatment from a physician concerning weight loss; usually they complain about medical disorders such as amenorrhea or gastrointestinal, sleep, and concentration disturbances. Occasionally, they seek treatment for emotional disorders.

Prevalence

A sharp increase in the incidence of anorexia and bulimia has been observed in recent decades. This increased rate in incidence and prevalence may be due to greater medical and public awareness of the disorders.

More than 90% of patients with anorexia and bulimia are female. The estimated incidence of anorexia is 0.5%-1%; the incidence of bulimia is possibly 2 to 3 times as great as anorexia. The mean age of onset of anorexia is at 17 years.[2] Bulimia nervosa is more difficult to identify because patients may be at normal weight or slightly overweight. On the other hand, persons with anorexia will lose 15% or more of their normal weight. Also, persons with bulimia can hide their binge-purge behaviors more easily than those with anorexic behaviors. The mortality rate for anorexia is over 10% and often "results from starvation, suicide, or electrolyte imbalance."[2] The long-term outcome of bulimia is unknown.

Population at Risk

The onset of anorexia nervosa and bulimia nervosa occurs primarily in adolescents and young adults and rarely in persons over 40 years of age. The disorders occur predominantly in industrialized societies such as Europe, Japan, Australia, and the United States where food is abundant and thin bodies are ideal.[2] The conditions occur mainly in Caucasians, formerly almost exclusively in the upper social classes; now they also occur in other ethnic groups and other socioeconomic levels. Women and men such as models, dancers, and gymnasts are at greater risk because they are expected to restrict their weight.[2]

Persons who have first degree biologic relatives with eating disorders are at greater risk for the disorders. They are also at greater risk for mood disorders when they have close relatives with eating disorders, especially the binge-eating and purging type.

Identical twins are at significantly higher risk for anorexia than fraternal twins.[2] Persons with bulimia experience a high degree of depression, especially dysthymic disorder and major depression disorder and anxiety symptoms that may precede the eating disorders. Substance abuse may also present a problem, especially the use of stimulants to control appetite.

Hospitalization

Hospitalization is recommended when a person with anorexia nervosa or bulimia nervosa shows evidence of severe medical complications, such as weight loss of 15% or more of normal body weight, severe fluctuations in weight, electrolyte imbalances resulting from starvation and binge-purge behaviors, and gastrointestinal disturbances (see Emergency Alert box). The patient may deny being in any physical danger or deny the need for hospitalization, even when emaciated. The fear of losing control looms large in the patient's mind. To decrease resistance, the protective nature of and the reasons for hospitalization should be emphasized.

Patients need to believe that the staff is interested in helping them deal with problems in their lives other than the eating disorder alone. Abnormal diagnostic test results need to be addressed and treated by the health care professional. Because the initial therapy focuses on steady weight gain or on stabilization of weight, the staff must cultivate supportive and trusting relationships that help patients experience a sense of security.

Involving the patient in the treatment and informing her about the criteria for discharge will encourage her cooperation. Gaining weight to normal body weight or stabilizing weight (for a nonemaciated patient) should be part of the discharge criteria.

If weight gain does not occur or if eating is resisted, high-protein, high-calorie nasogastric tube feedings may be prescribed. If the patient begins to drink a liquid diet, tube feedings may be discontinued.[12,26] A desirable target weight should be discussed with the patient. Daily weight gains of $\frac{1}{4}$ to $\frac{1}{2}$ pound are generally acceptable for the emaciated patient, and weight stabilization (without gorge-purge behaviors) is expected for the bulimic patient.

A dietitian discusses food preferences, provides nutritional counseling, and plans a well-balanced diet with the patient. The patient is taught how to eat slowly and chew the food well to experience tasting it. A nurse usually monitors the patient's food intake during meals. The nurse, being cognizant of the patient's anxiety about eating and about gaining weight, reassures the patient that weight gain is being controlled to prevent obesity. Especially in anorexia nervosa, patients need an explanation about the nausea and abdominal pain and distention they experience after eating. One explanation is related to gastrointestinal motor dysfunction as a consequence of malnutrition due to severe food restrictions; this condition is reversible.[11] Assisting the patient to interpret weight gain or stabilization of weight as a sign of being in control can decrease the patient's feelings of powerlessness and impotence.

The nurse challenges the patient's misconceptions about the illness and the self by questioning the patient's assumptions and irrational conclusions. As the nurse-patient relationship develops, the nurse helps the patient increase her self-awareness and self-acceptance by encouraging the patient to clarify thoughts and to trust her own thought processes and self-evaluations.

•••••• Psychopathology

Psychoanalytic Theory

From a psychoanalytic perspective, eating disorders stem from the oral phase of development. Affected persons frequently have anxious, compulsive mothers and throughout life continue to have disturbed relationships with the parents.[40] Food is used as the vehicle for obsessive-compulsive control of their bodies and their lives.

During the developmental phases the child is expected to disengage from the mother to become a person who is psychologically separate and who has clear ego boundaries, autonomy as a person, and reality testing abilities.[29] However, in anorexic or bulimic persons, some mechanisms in the developmental processes go awry; what leads them to become anorexic or bulimic as opposed to some other pathology is unclear.

The early developmental failures may be related singly or jointly to constitutional inadequacies, a chaotic environment, or an unresponsive, controlling primary caretaker. When spontaneous behaviors of children are contrary to parental wishes, the children may be rejected emotionally if not physically. These children have difficulty developing an identity of self and, may instead, become confused biologically, emotionally, and interpersonally. Being filled with self-doubt, the persons hide these evaluations with perfectionistic and self-controlling behaviors. Maintaining extreme control over bodily functions including food intake and thoughts is central in the person's attempts to overcome self-doubt and to feel powerful.

Interpersonal Theory

Interpersonal theorists believe the eating disorders arise because of family relationships. They view the family as dysfunctional in its relationships with one another. Parents avoid dealing with their own tensions and conflicts by focusing on the child. The self-identity of the person with future eating disorders becomes blurred and self-esteem is low.[36] As the child

---

 EMERGENCY ALERT

EATING DISORDERS: ANOREXIA NERVOSA AND BULIMIA NERVOSA

Anorexia nervosa is characterized by a determination to lose weight, mainly by restricting food intake. Bulimia nervosa is characterized by eating binges followed by purging.

Assessment

- Weight loss below 85% of that expected for individual
- Extremely restricted food intake, binges, and/or purges
- Fear of weight gain even if thin and holds distorted perception of body size
- Excessive exercise
- Abnormal laboratory test findings, e.g., serum electrolytes

Interventions

- Treat medical complications of eating disorders.
- Encourage patient to collaborate actively in treatment to increase sense of control and decrease resistance, especially initially during the restoration of normal nutritional state.
- Assist patient to correct misconceptions about self, abilities, and performance.

moves into adolescence and begins to seek independence and autonomy, the parents are unwilling to give up their accustomed pathologic interpersonal patterns of behavior. They become more overcontrolling and demanding, which foils the adolescent's efforts to achieve autonomy.

The parents expect selfless conformity from the child but are emotionally inaccessible; they demand that the child deny and mistrust perceptions that are incongruent with theirs. As the adolescent responds to the parents by offering support and strength, she perceives herself as loved for what she gives rather than for herself. The adolescent overorganizes her life to become perfect in her parents' eyes and to assume responsibility for her own physical and emotional safety. These dynamics within the family prohibit maturation of the adolescent and discourage achievement of the elevated goals parents establish.[36]

Although family characteristics predispose to the development of eating disorders, environmental, constitutional, and psychologic factors also enter into the determination of whether persons develop these conditions.

Cognitive Theory

Cognitive and behavioral theorists say that the behaviors of persons with eating disorders are learned. The glorification of thinness in industrial societies where food is abundant influences individuals to conform to cultural ideals of physical appearance.[2,36,40] Models resembling prepubertal girls in high-fashion magazines are considered beauties. These magazines and other media bombard women with reduction diets, exercises, and recipes; at the same time the same media also display advertisements for high-fat, high-calorie foods.

The future anorexic or bulimic person, who may be slightly overweight, is told by her parents, teachers, or friends that she would look much better if she lost a little weight. The positive reinforcement she receives from dieting and losing weight and the pleasure she experiences in her new shape encourage her to lose more. If she happens to eat more than she deems correct, she learns from peers to purge her body by vomiting and misusing laxatives and diuretics. The elation of controlling caloric intake and losing weight leads her to compete with others to be the thinnest in her peer group. She devotes herself to activities related to food, weight, and exercise, with no time or energy left for social relationships and activities. The young woman has irrational cognitions of herself and her body so that fatness is viewed negatively and thinness is viewed positively as increasing self-esteem and self-worth.[2,36]

•••••• Diagnostic Studies and Findings

Computerized tomography (CT scan), magnetic resonance imaging (MRI)   To screen for intracranial tumors and other brain lesions

Complete blood count   To screen for anemia and infections

Sequential multiple analyzer with computer (SMAC)   To screen for abnormalities; if electrolytes are abnormal, repeat electrolyte tests once a day until stable

Serum thyroid-stimulating hormone (TSH), serum thyroxine (T$_4$), and serum triiodothyronine (T$_3$)   To rule out abnormal thyroid function

Electrocardiogram   To screen for anomalies

Chest x-ray   To assess lung and heart conditions

Urinalysis   To screen for urinary and systemic abnormalities

•••••• Multidisciplinary Plan

Medications[38,52]

Fluoxetine (Prozac) 20 mg po each AM for bulimia nervosa even without depression; may increase to 60 mg

Amitriptyline 50 mg, po, qhs or clomipramine 25 mg, po, bid with meals for anorexia nervosa; medicine may or may not be used initially; responses to medicine for persons with anorexia have been inconclusive

General Management

Consult with dietitian; for severely emaciated client, 1200 calorie liquid diet in divided feedings; gradually (e.g., weekly) change to soft and regular diet with increases to 3000 calorie diet; for patient near normal weight or as a maintenance diet 1600-2000 calorie diet

Occupational therapy and recreational therapy after patient's nutritional status stabilizes

NURSING CARE

Nursing Assessment

Signs and symptoms of anorexia and bulimia vary from individual to individual; no one experiences all of those listed

Emotional

Anxiety; depression; lability of mood; irritability; anger

Thought Processes

Denial of hunger; fear of eating and weight gain; mistrust of self and others; low self-esteem; shame at being discovered binging and purging; sense of failure even when successful; perfectionism; rejection of feminine role; fear of psychosexual maturation; fear of physical changes, especially the development of secondary sexual traits; lack of interest in sex and opposite sex; impairment in concentration and cognition

Nursing Dx & Intervention

Nursing care should be implemented selectively based on severity and type of symptoms and behaviors.

Altered nutrition: less than body requirements related to distorted drive for thinness and distorted body image

- Assess patient's eating patterns and food preferences and concerns about eating. Have dietitian discuss nutritional plan and rationale and body's nutritional needs. Encourage patient (as able) to assume responsibility for planning well-balanced meals *to increase sense of control and decrease anxiety about eating.*

- If patient has been on starvation diet, be alert for gastric dilation if re-feeding is rapid. *To prevent this, a 1200-1500 calorie, liquid diet (e.g., Ensure), divided into frequent feedings, may be prescribed initially.*
- Inform patient that abdominal discomfort or bloating will be experienced with increased food intake and symptoms will disappear. Encourage patient to eat slowly *to learn to taste and enjoy food.*
- *To allow more supervision,* have patient eat alone rather than in unit dining room. When patient develops control over eating, encourage eating in dining room with others.
- *To prevent vomiting,* permit patient's use of bathroom only if accompanied by staff for 1 to 2 hours after eating.
- Explain nasogastric feedings and rationale in matter-of-fact yet sensitive, supportive manner *to decrease loss of control feelings.* (Nasogastric feedings may be prescribed if patient does not gain or electrolyte balance is viewed as unsafe.) After each instillation of high-protein, high-calorie fluid (such as Ensure), observe patient for at least 30 minutes *to prevent vomiting.* If patient is willing, allow drinking of feeding instead of instilling in tube.
- As patient begins to gain weight or stabilize her weight, help her deal with anxiety (which sometimes reaches panic level). Remain with patient (especially when eating) and demonstrate slow, deep relaxation breathing *to decrease anxiety.* Reinforce relaxation technique.
- Administer medication as prescribed. Explain purpose of medication and its effects and side effects *to increase compliance with treatment.*
- *To allay patient's fears of becoming obese,* explain that uncontrolled weight gain is not the goal. With assistance of dietitian, review with patient weight-maintenance diet.
- Explain that, as caloric intake is increased, the amount will not make patient fat *to assure her that metabolism is slowed as protective mechanism during a starvation diet.*
- Avoid power struggles over food *to prevent reenactment of food struggles at home.*
- Encourage good oral hygiene *to prevent oral disease from vomiting and malnutrition.*
- Begin to help patient identify role low weight plays in patient's life (e.g., as way of avoiding dealing with frightening adolescent and adult issues). Continue to explore meaning of weight loss, expectation and reality of weight loss, and restrictions in areas of life resulting from preoccupation with food *to increase self-awareness.*
- Monitor patient's weight as prescribed, but prevent patient from indiscriminate frequent self-weighing. Remain nonjudgmental about weight gains and losses. (Weight monitoring will continue with less frequency.)
- When appropriate, encourage participation in occupational therapy *to develop skills and learn to view tasks as enjoyable.*
- Encourage patient to drink at least 2000 ml of fluid per day *for proper hydration.* Monitor and record intake and output.

Ineffective individual coping related to dysfunctional cognitions and maladaptive behaviors

- Assess previous and current coping skills including substance abuse for dealing with events and relationships.
- Begin to develop safe, trusting relationship with patient *to promote security.* Continue to develop relationship through working and termination phases.
- Explain treatment plan explicitly *to allay anxiety and decrease resistance.* Review plan with the patient and invite participation at regular intervals.
- Assist patient to identify emotions that precede binging and past alternatives to binging and fasting.
- Assist patient to identify and participate in healthy coping strategies—such as relaxation techniques, reinterpretation of thoughts and emotions, problem-solving, and diversionary activities (e.g., watching television, listening to the radio, talking with friends, reading)—*to develop alternatives to dysfunctional eating and to develop enjoyable, relaxing behaviors.*
- If patient denies she has eating problem, encourage her to examine difficulties in other areas of life and eventually to relate these to preoccupations with eating *to deal with less anxiety-provoking areas than eating.*
- Begin to help patient identify fears associated with starving, binging, and purging *to eventually identify issues dealing with loss of control.*
- Correct misconceptions about binging-purging behaviors (e.g., laxatives will not prevent absorption of calories). Assist patient to use problem-solving approach *to examine issues and to assess possible consequences of choices.*
- Encourage patient to implement and evaluate new behaviors *to determine appropriateness of choices.*
- Discuss with patient how to get needs met by herself *to develop self-support* and how to ask others to meet her needs rather than meeting only theirs *to develop social support.*
- As patient is physically able, encourage participation in occupational therapy *to learn skills and to engage in enjoyable activities.*
- Begin to assist patient to identify and reinforce strengths. Help patient assess abilities and accomplishments realistically using problem-solving approach. Encourage acceptance of abilities and choices patient makes *to begin to feel positive about herself and to develop realistic self-expectations, including an acceptance of limitations and mediocre performance.*

Body image disturbance related to cognitive perception

- Assess patient's feelings about self and body.
- Encourage patient to wear loose clothing *to avoid focus on body size and weight.* Encourage patient to give "skinny" wardrobe away *to avoid longing for thinness and relapsing.* Suggest new lifestyle for patient in nonthreatening way.

- Begin to correct patient's distorted perceptions about body size. Assist patient to perceive body size correctly and accept appearance.
- Encourage patient to accept positive self-appraisals and take pride in appearance.
- As patient gains more mature-appearing body or stabilization of weight, explore meaning of sexuality and feminine role *to assist in dealing with sexual identity issues including menses.* Encourage self-acceptance.

Powerlessness related to lifestyle of helplessness

- Assess patient's sense of lack of control about treatment plan and sense of helplessness in relation to her life.
- Convey to patient that treatment plan is developed *to help and protect and not to control her.*
- Encourage patient, when able, to make decisions about her treatment regimen *to provide a sense of control and to increase self-confidence.*
- Begin to role-play with patient about how to become assertive with others and, as able, with parents *to share needs with others.* Emphasize that patient can assume responsibility for herself and that she is not responsible for others' happiness or discomfort.
- Help patient to practice assertiveness skills and critique them together *to learn how to assess her behavior realistically.*
- As patient is physically able, encourage participation in recreational therapy *to learn social skills in group-type activities.*
- Help patient identify her wants and needs and choose not to binge-purge or starve.
- Assist patient to develop beginning skills in how to function in ambiguous situations *to learn how to deal with conflict and unclear situations* (e.g., by negotiating, assessing importance of issue, or clarifying issue with others).

Altered family processes related to inability to accept or express needs of members

- Assess family's knowledge of eating disorder and interaction patterns with patient.
- Discourage family from discussing patient's dietary intake, bringing in food, or phoning during mealtimes *to avoid power struggles about eating.*
- Assist parents to understand illness without blaming each other.
- In family sessions help parents and patient become aware of unhealthy interaction.
- Begin to help family members alter their interactional patterns (e.g., by speaking for self only and not for others and by responding to one another's messages) *to foster relationships that encourage autonomy of family members.*

Other related nursing diagnoses   Risk for fluid-volume deficit related to altered nutrition and purging behaviors; risk for impaired skin integrity related to malnutrition; constipation related to laxative abuse and inadequate fiber intake; anxiety related to self-concept; sleep pattern disturbance related to malnourishment; social isolation related to discomfort with others.

Patient Education/Home Care Planning

1. Ensure that the patient verbalizes knowledge of problem-solving techniques to correct misconceptions of self and performance.
2. Discuss with the patient the need to continue practice of assertiveness skills and techniques to increase a sense of control.
3. Review the patient's social and physical activity plans for the time after discharge.
4. Ensure that the patient verbalizes an understanding of well-balanced, weight-maintenance diet and of the need for continued contacts with a dietitian regarding diet.
5. Review with the patient the adverse effects of starving, binging, and purging behaviors.
6. Encourage the patient to comply with the medical regimen and with the continued psychotherapy after discharge.
7. Encourage the patient to participate in a self-help eating disorder group.

Evaluation

Patient establishes healthy eating habits to achieve normal body weight   Patient verbalizes knowledge of maintenance diet and expected average weight. Patient states that preoccupation with food has decreased.

Patient begins to implement problem-solving approach to increase coping ability   Patient practices problem-solving approach to deal with issues such as the feminine role, sexuality, and social interactions with others.

Patient demonstrates a beginning acceptance of her body image   Patient verbalizes her body size accurately and states a beginning acceptance of a more mature-appearing body. Patient wears clothing that is appropriate for body shape.

Patient verbalizes an increased sense of control over self   Patient practices beginning assertive behavior skills. Patient views weight-maintenance diet as evidence of self-control.

Patient and family demonstrate increased efforts to clarify and resolve issues   Patient and family verbalize increased satisfaction in interactions. Patient and family develop beginning skills in identifying and resolving issues.

SUBSTANCE USE DISORDERS

The diagnostic category "psychoactive substance use disorders" was changed to "substance use disorders" in the latest diagnostic manual.[2] These disorders are characterized by exposure to chemical substances that include drugs that lead to abuse (such as alcohol), dosage and side effects of medications (such as analgesics, antidepressants, and corticosteroids), and toxic substances (such as lead, antifreeze, and glue). The chemical substances can be taken by any route of administration and affect cognition and mood and adversely affect health. Some substances are obtained legally such as over-the-counter and medically prescribed drugs; others are obtained illicitly such as cocaine and marijuana.[43]

Substance use disorders are divided into two general groups: *substance abuse* and *substance dependence*.[2] Substance abuse is a residual category in which the person experiences physical impairment (e.g., when operating machinery) or social difficulties because of substances used at any time during a 12 month period. Substance abuse does not reach the criteria for dependence. In substance dependence, the person continues use while experiencing a "cluster of cognitive, behavioral, and physiological symptoms"[2] and has an impaired ability to control use. Excessive time and energy may be spent obtaining the substance and recovering from the consequences with limited ability or an inability to fulfill social and occupational responsibilities. Some additional criteria for substance dependence include the following:[2]

Intoxication—occurs in both abuse and dependence due to exposure to a substance that impairs the person's ability to function psychologically and physically

Tolerance—drug dosage must be increased progressively to reproduce the initial desired physical and psychologic effects

Withdrawal—when the substance(s) is decreased or discontinued abruptly especially after prolonged heavy use, the person develops adverse physiologic and cognitive consequences

Compulsivity—although persons set limits on usage, they are unable to discontinue use even though intoxicated, that is, they develop behavioral or psychologic changes directed toward obtaining the substance(s) that affect the central nervous system

The person recognizes the difficulties caused by the chemical substances, but he fails to abstain from continued use.

If the person abstains from use for at least one month, he may be designated as being in early remission; if he abstains for 12 months or more, he is designated as being in sustained remission. The remission may be "full" meaning he has met none of the criteria for dependence or abuse or it may be "partial" meaning he has not met the full criteria for remission.[2]

Substance abuse and dependence most commonly begin during adolescence and young adulthood. Vulnerability to abuse is greater among the drugs that have the greatest addictive power (such as cocaine, heroin, and morphine) than the least addictive drugs (such as caffeine). However, the least addictive chemicals can also become severe problems.[19] The reasons for becoming involved with chemical substances are many and include influence of peers, rebellion against parents and society, and attempts to bolster self-esteem. Most young adults are able to discontinue use as they take on the responsibilities of adulthood, but some may become chronic abusers and often engage in polydrug abuse.

Substance use disorders may also be associated with relief of pain, especially when pain is severe and chronic, among immature, easily frustrated persons, those with psychic disorders, and those with countercultural life-styles. Viewing substances as a way of coping with life stresses and experiences is a factor in brief, limited episodes of abuse to continued chronic abuse and dependence.[2,43]

Because chemical substances affect the central nervous system, abuse and/or dependence may cause transient or permanent brain dysfunction and other medical problems. Deterioration of physical health is caused in part by malnutrition, poor personal hygiene, and inattention to signs and symptoms of illnesses. Infections such as hepatitis, tetanus, septicemia, and abscesses can occur from substances administered with contaminated needles and syringes. In addition, the transmission of acquired immunodeficiency syndrome (AIDS) has become an increasing threat to substance users. Because the potency and purity of illicitly obtained substances are seldom known, fatal overdoses and toxic reactions occur.[19,43]

The mood-altering effects of substances may cause erratic, impulsive, aggressive, violent, and other irresponsible behaviors that cause problems and injury to the user or to others (see Emergency Alert box). Relationships with family and friends become disturbed and are sometimes severed. Drug habits, including alcohol, drain the financial resources of families. The user may also engage in criminal behaviors to support the substance dependency or violate laws when in an intoxicated drug state (e.g., burglaries, automobile accidents).

 EMERGENCY ALERT

SUBSTANCE USE DISORDERS

Substance use disorders are characterized by exposure to chemical substances (by any route of administration) that affect cognition and mood and adversely affect health.

Assessment

- Suicidal ideation
- Abuse of depressants, such as alcohol
  Intoxication evident, e.g., by slurred speech, unsteady gait, impaired judgment and memory, transient amnesia, tremors, delirium tremens, and agitation
- Stimulants, such as cocaine
  Euphoria, irritability, impaired concentration and judgment, cardiac dysrhythmias, respiratory distress, "track" marks from IV injections, inflammation of nasal mucosa, necrosis of nasal septum, and other symptoms.
- Positive blood and/or urine test findings for alcohol/drugs
- Compromised immune system and presence of infections
- Much time and energy expended obtaining and/or using substances and problems with law

Interventions

- Treat physiologic complications as medical emergencies.
- Administer medications as needed to reduce toxic effects of substances and to control withdrawal symptoms.

Changes in occupational, social, interpersonal, and academic functioning occur with substance abuse. The person loses interest in current activities and is less able to perform in expected roles.[19,43]

Table 17-1 lists some commonly used types of chemical substances, their uses, and their intoxication and withdrawal effects.[1,19,43]

Almost 20% of the population in the United States has abused alcoholic beverages and drugs.[19] Alcohol abuse affects an estimated 10% of adults, and an estimated 14.5 million people have used illicit substances.

Substance abuse costs individuals, families, and society a great deal, yet fewer than 10% of addicted persons receive treatment from the health care system or self-help groups. Projected costs of alcohol and other substance abuse are expected to continue to rise in the future. Current estimates of costs include 50% of the annual automobile deaths, 75% of the robberies and felonies, and 50% of the homicides

TABLE 17-1 Effects of Intoxication and Withdrawal of Substances

Drug	Usual Route of Administration	Use
Opiates		
Opium	Oral; sniffed; smoked	Analgesic, antidiarrheal
Morphine	Oral; injected	Analgesic
Diacetylmorphine (heroin)	Injected; sniffed; smoked	Analgesic (illegal)
Hydromorphone (Dilaudid)	Oral; injected	Analgesic
Meperidine (Demerol)	Oral; injected	Analgesic
Propoxyphene (Darvon)	Oral; injected	Analgesic
Codeine	Oral; injected	Analgesic; antitussive
Methadone	Oral; injected	Detoxification of opiates
Depressants		
Alcoholic beverages (e.g., liquor, beer, wine)	Oral	Tension relief; analgesic
Sedative-hypnotics		
Barbiturates		Anesthetic; anticonvulsant; sleep
Amobarbital (Amytal)	Oral; injected	
Secobarbital (Seconal)	Oral; injected	
Pentobarbital (Nembutal)	Oral; injected	
Other		
Meprobamate (Equinal, Miltown)	Oral	Antianxiety; sedation
Diazepam (Valium)	Oral; injected	Antianxiety; anticonvulsant
Glutethimide (Doriden)	Oral	Hypnotic
Chloral hydrate (Noctec and others)	Oral	Hypnotic
Stimulants		
Cocaine	Oral; smoked; sniffed; injected	Local anesthetic
Amphetamine (Benzedrine, Dexedrine)	Oral; injected	Narcolepsy; attention deficit disorder, weight control
Methylphenidate (Ritalin)	Oral	Attention deficit disorder with hyperactivity
Phenmetrazine (Preludin)	Oral	Weight control
Hallucinogens		
Lysergic acid diethylamide (LSD)	Oral	None
Phencyclidine (PCP)	Oral; smoked; injected	Animal tranquilizer
Mescaline	Oral	None
Psilocybin	Oral	None
Cannabis Sativa		
Marijuana, hashish	Oral; smoked	Stimulant and sedative (illegal drug)

and accidents. Decreased productivity and worker absenteeism are also among society's problems. Health care costs for abusers of alcohol are twice as much as health care costs for those who do not drink alcohol.[19] In addition to the physical and mental damage resulting from the use of such substances, the families of addicted persons are often severely stressed because they experience abuse in the form of violence or other destructive behaviors perpetuated by the substance abusers.

ALCOHOL ABUSE/ALCOHOL DEPENDENCE

Alcohol abuse consists of a pattern of use that leads to impairment in social, legal, and occupational performance experienced from continued alcohol consumption or from actual intoxication. Evidence of alcohol intoxication is impaired ability to function physically and psychologically with signs such as slurred speech, unsteady gait, emotional

Intoxication Effect	Withdrawal Effect
Opiates	
Euphoria with tranquility; emotional lability; drowsiness; clouding of consciousness; psychomotor retardation; slow, shallow respirations; constricted pupils; decreased muscle tone; with circulatory collapse and cyanosis, dilated pupils; coma; possible death	Runny nose; watery eyes; severe anxiety to panic; gooseflesh; hot and cold flashes; yawning; irritability; loss of appetite; muscle cramps; tremors; nausea and vomiting; tachycardia; hypertension; increased respirations and temperature; insomnia; after 24 hours, diarrhea and dehydration; symptoms peak 48 to 72 hours after last dose
Depressants	
Slurred speech; lack of coordination; unsteady gait; talkativeness; euphoria or depression; emotional lability; impaired attention or memory	Hyperactivity; tremors; psychomotor agitation; hypertension; tachycardia; irritability or depression; impaired attention and memory; illusions (misinterpretation of stimuli); hallucinations, auditory, tactile, or visual; disorientation; delusions; delirium; orthostatic hypotension; convulsions
Slurred speech; irritability; impaired attention, memory, and judgment; emotional lability; talkativeness; lack of coordination; confusion; tremors; cold, clammy skin; dilated pupils (with barbiturates, constricted pupils)	Nausea and vomiting; weakness; hypertension; tachycardia; orthostatic hypotension; gross tremors; agitation; disorientation; anxiety; nightmares; visual hallucinations; hyperthermia; delirium; convulsions; coma
Stimulants	
Euphoria; psychomotor agitation; mood lability; hypervigilance; chest pain; tachycardia; hypertension; dilated pupils; perspiration or chills; impaired judgment; psychotic symptoms; insomnia; tremors; confusion; convulsions; possible death	Fatigue; depression; disturbed sleep; apathy; cravings; possible agitation after prolonged use
Hallucinogens	
Tachycardia; hypertension; hyperthermia; dilated pupils; hyperreflexia; nausea; visual hallucinations; extreme emotional lability; poor time perception; feeling of depersonalization; psychic numbness; psychosis; violent outbursts; amnesia; convulsions; possible death	None reported; flashbacks occur episodically long after use of PCP, with catalepsy, agitation, and unpredictable violent outbursts
Cannabis Sativa	
Panic; depression; disorientation; hallucinations; delusions; flashbacks; psychotic symptoms; apathy; impaired attention, judgment, and coordination; increased appetite	Uncertain if clinically significant; irritability; insomnia; loss of appetite; tremors; perspiration; nausea

outbursts, impaired judgment and memory, transient amnesia or "blackouts," and in higher doses, coma and death.

Alcohol dependence is more serious and includes the criteria for substance dependence such as tolerance, withdrawal, ingesting more than intended, and continued use despite its harmfulness to self; patient may deny having a drinking problem.

This discussion focuses on alcoholism which includes alcohol abuse and alcohol dependence because it is the third largest health problem after heart disease and cancer.[36] Use of alcohol is accepted at social gatherings and business meetings and as part of cultural and religious celebrations such as marriages and births. About 70% of the adult population consumes at least one drink during a 1-year period, but 1 in 10 will become problem drinkers.[2,19]

•••••• Prevalence and Sociocultural Factors

Alcohol dependency is estimated to affect 14% of adults at some time in their lives. There are five times as many men who are dependent as women. Nearly identical rates of alcoholism are found in Caucasians and African-Americans.[2] Those at higher risk for alcoholism than the general population include Native Americans, African-American women, and Eskimos. The reasons for this vulnerability are not known exactly.[36] Of emergency department visits and medical-surgical division admissions to hospitals, 30% or more are persons with health problems related to alcoholism. Each year 5% of all deaths are caused by or related to alcohol.[4] The typical heavy drinker is probably male, with less education, and from a lower socioeconomic class than moderate drinkers. However, alcoholism is also present among the upper socioeconomic classes, and was found to be higher among certain occupational groups, such as physicians.[36]

•••••• Alcoholic Family

Some families may be dysfunctional before a member becomes alcohol-dependent; in others, dysfunction may be the effect of alcoholism. Drinking alcoholic beverages (e.g., beer, wine, spirits) and occasional drunkenness may be accepted initially by family members as normal social behavior. As the frequency and amount of use increases, problem drinking begins to have detrimental effects on the drinker and family members. The drinker's personality changes with severe mood swings; he or she may be arrested for driving while intoxicated (blood alcohol levels above 0.05 g/dl with legal definitions ranging from 0.08 to 0.10 g/dl in various states) or other infractions of law, and engage in mental and physical abuse, especially of family members. The person with an alcohol problem may eventually change employment behavior with decreased productivity, mistakes and accidents, and frequent absences or tardinesses.[4,36] Family relationships deteriorate, and family members feel trapped between the sober and intoxication phases of the alcoholic. They experience shame, anger, confusion, and guilt. Family conversations are increasingly focused on the alcohol-dependent behavior and issues related to it. Family members

unconsciously engage in enabling behaviors to protect the family reputation and keep the family secret. Such behaviors include making excuses to friends and employers, attempting to keep the alcoholic out of trouble, and sometimes buying liquor for the alcoholic. The person with a drinking problem offers alibis for his or her behavior or is unwilling to discuss it. If the spouse threatens to leave or no longer make excuses, the alcohol-dependent person may promise never to touch another drop. These promises are usually broken. The family members may be locked into dysfunctional behaviors including denial or may sever their relationship with the drinker.

Chemical Dependency Among Nurses

Chemical dependency among health professionals is estimated as two to three times greater than that of the general population, with 14% of registered nurses (one in seven) being impaired by alcohol, drugs, or both.[14] Drug-related disciplinary cases referred to state boards of nursing annually average 62%, with some states being much higher. Nurses with above average performance succumb to substance-related disorders given certain life conditions, such as role-overload from stresses at work, within the family, and in other areas of their lives.

State nurses' associations began to develop peer assistance programs for nurses in about 1980.[14] Before the assistance programs, impaired nurses were abandoned by employers through dismissals or forced resignations, without referrals for treatment. Formal assistance programs have been developed in many states to serve as a confidential alternative to the usual disciplinary procedures.[24] The programs serve to guide impaired nurses into treatment and to provide professional and public understanding of the disease through education. Generally, dedicated volunteer nurses assist their colleagues through the phases of recovery and with continued support in return-to-work programs for the recovering nurse.[14,24]

•••••• Psychopathology

Countless theories attempt to conceptualize the alcoholic, for example, as an oral personality or as a person with a harsh superego who uses alcohol to decrease self-punishment.[36] Although some alcoholics may fit these descriptions, it is difficult to know if the psychologic factors came first or if they are due to the alcoholism.

Among the many reasons for dependence on alcoholic beverages are low self-worth, feelings of inadequacy, stress, family- and work-related problems, economic difficulties, and feelings of social inadequacy. In some instances alcohol is secondary to mental disorders such as early behavioral problems in children, personality disorders (e.g., antisocial personality disorder), anxiety disorders (e.g., panic disorders, social phobias), schizophrenia, and major depression. In primary alcoholism, depression may be the result rather than the cause.

Genetic factors have been implicated in the development of alcoholism.[2] Close relatives of alcohol-dependent persons have a three to four times greater risk for alcoholism than those with no close alcohol-dependent relative. The risk for alcoholism is higher for identical twins than fraternal twins or same sex siblings in families with alcoholism.[2,43] If the child with alcoholic parents is adopted by nonalcoholic parents, the risk to the child for developing an alcohol problem is related to the alcoholism of the biologic parents. The opposite was found in that a child of nonalcoholic parents adopted into the home of alcoholic parents was unlikely to show increased alcohol use as an adult. Persons with a genetic predisposition for developing alcoholism may not necessarily do so because of environmental influences on their behaviors. Because women have lower percentages of body water, greater body fat, and slower metabolization of alcohol, they tend to have higher blood alcohol levels than males after drinking the same amount of alcohol.[2,36] Depressant effects of alcohol are greater in the elderly because of physiologic changes such as slowed liver metabolism.

Although the precise processes in intoxication and withdrawal are not known, some research findings are interesting. Alcohol seems to at least partially suppress brain function by activating an inhibiting neurotransmitter, gamma-aminobutyric acid (GABA). This substance slows and "eventually paralyzes cognitive and motor function."[36] Strangely in low doses, alcohol (ethanol) impairs reticular function, which seems to result in excitability of the cortex. However, thinking and motor coordination become disordered rather than actually stimulated.

Computed tomography (CT) and magnetic resonance imaging (MRI) permit visualization of brain changes in alcoholism. Cortical and cerebral atrophy is a major change observed with enlarged ventricles occurring in some instances.[54] These changes are partly reversible in many persons who abstain from alcohol.

A careful assessment of the drinking patterns and use of other chemicals by all patients, including those being treated for other conditions, is essential.[2,43] Attention must be given to the abuse of multiple drugs, because a person found to be dependent on one substance is probably also dependent on others that potentiate or inhibit the effects of the first. Although it is common for patients to deny use or minimize the amount they consume, a nonjudgmental attitude will help the nurse elicit the necessary information. Obtaining accurate information on the use of legal and illegal substances is important in all inpatient and outpatient settings, such as medical-surgical, pediatric, and psychiatric settings.

A person who abstains from alcohol use or who decreases alcohol use (usually following chronic intake) is likely to experience withdrawal symptoms that occur after 6 hours and peak at 24 to 48 hours. The early symptoms include slight tremors, nervousness, a slight increase in heart rate and blood pressure, nausea, and restless sleep.[19,43] A person who consumes large amounts of alcohol over a long period is likely to develop a more severe withdrawal syndrome characterized by tremors, agitation, tachycardia, hypertension, nausea and vomiting, abdominal cramps, sweating, flushed face, insomnia, dilated pupils, visual or tactile misperceptions, and mild disorientation. Memory lapses (blackouts) about events that happen while the person is drinking may occur.

Delirium tremens (DTs), another phenomenon of alcohol withdrawal, occurs (in a minority of persons) from 48 to 96 hours and up to 7 days after the last alcoholic drink. Persons who have been heavy drinkers (often more than 750 ml per day) for a week or more, and those who have experienced DTs before, are more susceptible to DTs than others.[19] Symptoms of DTs include confusion, disorientation, tremulousness, agitation, frightening hallucinations that are usually visual or tactile, diaphoresis, hyperpyrexia, tachycardia, and grand mal seizures.

The mortality for persons with DTs, especially if they are not treated, is 10% to 15%; the cause of death is usually hyperthermia or cardiovascular collapse. If adequate preventive treatment is instituted during the early signs and symptoms of alcohol withdrawal, DTs are unlikely to develop.

A majority of medical disorders in alcohol abusers develop approximately 5 years after heavy imbibing begins. The following are some physiologic problems of chronic alcoholism:[19]

Cardiovascular system
  Anemia
  Hypertension
  Tachycardia
  Dysarrhythmias
  Cardiomegaly
  Edema
Liver
  Hepatomegaly
  Edema
  Ascites
  Cirrhosis
Gastrointestinal (GI) system
  Gastritis
  Esophagitis and/or esophageal varices
  Duodenal and gastric ulcers
  Nausea
  Malabsorption syndrome
  Colitis
  Cancer of GI system
Neurologic system
  Fatigue
  Unsteady gait
  Depression
  Irritability
  Memory and learning deficits
  Severe head trauma from falls
  Tremors
  Polyneuropathy that typically begins in feet
  Degeneration of cerebellum
  Wernicke-Korsakoff syndrome
Decreased testosterone levels and erectile dysfunction
Immune impairment and infection
Fetal alcohol syndrome or spontaneous abortion

•••••• Diagnostic Studies and Findings

Sequential Multiple Analyzer with Computer (SMAC)
To screen for abnormalities:
  Complete blood count
  Prothrombin time

Blood alcohol level

Urinalysis

Urine toxicology   For other drugs of abuse

CT scan   To screen for head trauma

Chest x-ray   To screen for pulmonary infection and cardiac disease

Electrocardiogram   To screen for cardiopathy

Stool   For occult blood

•••••• Multidisciplinary Plan

Medications[41]

Antianxiety agents

Chlordiazepoxide (Librium): adults—25 to 50 mg po, stat and q4h during the acute stage; elderly persons or adolescents—25 mg po, stat and q4h during the acute stage to prevent or decrease serious alcohol withdrawal symptoms including grand mal seizures; intramuscular administration is generally avoided because of the slow and erratic absorption; the antianxiety drug is gradually discontinued within a short time in favor of nonpharmacologic approaches to rehabilitation; the drug acts to reduce anxiety and seizure level and promote drowsiness and hypotension

Vitamins

Megadose, multivitamin and multimineral supplement, 1 tablet po with meals; because of malnutrition generally seen in alcoholism, improvement in nutritional status is essential to prevent or decrease chronic medical disorders

General Management

Bland diet; introduction of regular diet as able to tolerate

NURSING CARE

Nursing Assessment

Emotional

Anxiety; emotional lability; depression

Thoughts

Denial of alcoholism; guilt; shame; sense of inadequacy; impairment of judgment and memory; suicidal ideation (correlation exists between alcoholism and suicide)

Physical

Type of drinking pattern established; duration and amount of last alcohol consumed; irritability to psychomotor agitation; demanding behavior; memory lapses (blackouts); tachycardia; hypertension; increased respirations; tremors; fatigue; nausea and vomiting; anorexia; abdominal cramps; insomnia; elevated temperature; illusions; hallucinations (most frequently visual, sometimes auditory); seziure potential

Social and Occupational*

Argumentativeness with family, friends, and co-workers; aggressiveness with others; tardiness at work; work absences because of "not feeling well"; sensitivity to criticism; mistakes at work

Nursing Dx & Intervention

*Alcohol withdrawal** related to decreased intake of alcohol following chronic use

- Assess patient's average alcoholic beverage intake and other chemicals used; time and amount of last alcohol consumed and kinds of other chemicals used; and the potential for seizures, such as tremors, elevated vital signs, and agitation.
- Minimize the number of people attending the patient *to prevent excitement;* provide quiet environment *to decrease stimuli and decrease possibility of agitation, anxiety, and belligerence caused by central nervous system (CNS) stimulation during withdrawal.*
- Administer chlordiazepoxide as prescribed (because of patient's tolerance to sedative effects of alcohol, larger doses are needed than for nonalcoholic patients) *to prevent agitation and seizures.*
- Explain to the patient reasons for and effects of medicine *to increase the patient's acceptance of the treatment.*
- Evaluate the effects of medicine.
- Provide physical protection in bed, such as side rails, bed in low position, and mechanical restraints, if needed, *to protect patient from harm.*
- Explain to patient the psychologic and physiologic effects of alcoholism and the effects alcohol has on patient's relationships with self and others *to help patient become aware of harmful effects in all areas of his or her life.*
- Correct patient's misconceptions about physiologic, psychologic, and social effects of alcoholic beverages.
- If suicidal ideation exists, assess its seriousness.
- Maintain light in the room, especially at night, *to decrease the possibility that the patient might misinterpret environmental stimuli.*

Fluid-volume excess related to effects of alcoholic beverages

- Assess and record fluid intake and output.
- Avoid forcing fluids *to prevent overhydration,* because alcohol initially exerts antidiuretic effects.
- Monitor blood pressure, pulse, and respirations every 15 minutes until stable and then as ordered *to detect changes resulting from agitation and other complications of withdrawal.*

---

*Non-NANDA Nursing Diagnosis

- Monitor temperature every 4 hours *to detect signs of infection.*
- Observe for infection (e.g., of respiratory tract) resulting from impaired immune system.

Altered nutrition: less than body requirements related to lack of interest in food

- Assess nutritional intake.
- Help to ensure adequate nutritional diet in collaboration with the physician and dietitian *to counteract the effects of inadequate diet and malabsorption of nutrients.*
- Offer bland food for gastric distress. Antacids may be prescribed *to decrease distress.*
- Administer vitamins as ordered with meal *to decrease nutritional deficits.*
- Explain to the patient the essentials of a nutritionally balanced diet, the adverse effects of alcohol on the digestion and absorption of food, and the importance of compliance *to prevent or alleviate malnutrition and the effects of alcoholism.*

Ineffective individual coping related to maladaptive behaviors of alcoholism

- Assess types of situations and interactions that trigger the patient's alcohol intake. Assess coping strategies that the patient uses and reinforce healthy ones.
- Establish a supportive, nonjudgmental relationship *to promote a decrease in the patient's denial and guilt about excessive drinking of alcohol.*
- Assist the patient to identify feelings of anxiety and relate them to stress-producing situations *to encourage the patient's awareness of his or her maladaptive coping mechanisms.*
- Help patient identify healthy methods for coping with anxiety instead of relying on alcohol. Methods include problem-solving, relaxation techniques (such as slow, deep breathing), and diversionary activities (such as physical exercise and watching television).
- Explain and practice assertiveness skills and evaluation of effects of skills *to increase patient's self-esteem.*
- Encourage patient to learn to ask for support and to deal with positive and negative responses.
- Assist the patient in developing skills to refuse alcohol in social situations *to help in learning to socialize without the use of alcohol.* Refer patients to Alcoholics Anonymous *to obtain support for nondrinking behavior and to prevent relapse.*
- Correct patient's misconceptions about physiologic, psychologic, and social effects of alcohol.
- Encourage patient to examine consequences of drinking behavior on self, family, and social and work functioning and to identify alternative behaviors *to increase patient's sense of adequacy when engaged in nondestructive behaviors.*

Altered family processes related to alcoholism

- Assess the knowledge the patient's family has about the patient's alcoholism and the family's enabling behaviors.

- Explain that alcoholism is a disease and describe the psychologic, physiologic, and social effects of alcoholism.
- Assist patient and family to identify interaction patterns to discuss the expectations each has, and to discuss each family member's willingness to meet these expectations.
- Assist each family member to begin identifying differences and to learn to negotiate disagreements *to accept conflicting views among family members.*
- Help family members to understand the disease *so that they will not blame themselves, believing that they caused the abuse and the alcoholism.*
- Refer family for counseling, if indicated.
- Recommend attendance at Al-Anon for spouse and Al-Ateen for children *to help them deal with painful feelings, such as guilt, anger, and despair, and to help them accept responsibility only for their own behaviors and not those behaviors of the problem drinker.*

Other related nursing diagnoses Impaired physical mobility related to cognitive and perceptual impairment; bathing and hygiene self-care deficit related to depressed mood.

Patient Education/Home Care Planning

1. Review with the patient that alcoholism is a chronic disorder and that recovery is a lifelong endeavor.
2. Ensure that the patient accepts responsibility for his or her own behavior and sobriety.
3. Reinforce the patient's active participation in Alcoholics Anonymous and other aftercare programs.
4. Ensure that the patient understands the need to practice healthy coping behaviors for dealing with anxiety and life problems related to family, friends, and work.
5. Elaborate on the need for social supports and the development of self-supports.

Evaluation

Recovery from withdrawal symptoms of alcohol is uncomplicated Patient has minimal signs or symptoms of alcohol withdrawal with no agitation or seizures. Patient recovers with no physical harm to self. Patient verbalizes knowledge of the physical, psychologic, and social effects of consuming alcoholic beverages.

Patient evidences normal fluid balance and vital signs Patient has adequate intake and output with normal electrolyte balance. Patient maintains stable vital signs with no evidence of infection.

Patient is cognizant of well-balanced diet Patient lists essentials of nutritionally balanced diet and acknowledges the adverse effects of alcohol on nutrition. Patient participates in choosing meals.

Patient is aware of healthy coping strategies for stress-producing situations Patient practices relaxation techniques and engages in physical exercise. Patient practices assertiveness skills and evaluates their effects on self and others. Patient practices refusal of alcoholic beverages in social situations. Patient begins to attend Alcoholics Anonymous meetings and lists dates, times, and places of meetings, as well as the name and phone number of his or her sponsor in the program.

Family demonstrates ability to obtain support from community agencies and verbalizes knowledge of alcoholism and of enabling behaviors   Patient and family verbalize knowledge of alcohol and its adverse effects on their relationships. Family expresses knowledge of enabling behaviors and responsibilities related to alcoholism. Spouse attends Al-Anon meetings, and the children attend Al-Ateen meetings.

COCAINE ABUSE/COCAINE DEPENDENCE

Cocaine abuse and cocaine dependence are the use of any of several types of preparations from the coca plant, which is an appealing illicit stimulant. Cocaine abuse is episodic use, such as around special celebrations, that results in neglected responsibilities and interpersonal problems. Cocaine dependence includes tolerance and compulsive behavior with intense cravings for the drug.[2]

Prevalence

In a 1991 survey, 12% of the population had used cocaine one or more times during their life, 3% used it in the past year, and 1% or less used it in the past month.[2] In 1988, hospital emergencies related to cocaine use increased an estimated fivefold over the emergencies recorded in 1984, and emergency department deaths increased approximately 2.4 times during that time period.[19]

Population at Risk

Cocaine use is prevalent among all socioeconomic levels and races and is used equally by men and women.[2] Although it is used by persons of all ages, it is most commonly used among 18 to 30 years olds.

•••••• Pathology

Although classified as a narcotic, cocaine is a central nervous system stimulant similar in action to amphetamine and has almost the same criteria for a clinical disorder. The euphoria with persistent cravings produced by cocaine makes it very appealing and can lead to tolerance in hours to days. The level of response varies with differences in genetics, and with previous experience with cocaine or similar drugs.[43]

Cocaine affects neurotransmitters in the brain such as dopamine, norepinephrine, serotonin, and acetylcholine by either blocking or releasing their reuptake. The pleasurable effect is usually ascribed to cocaine's "blockade of dopamine reuptake."[36] Cocaine is mainly metabolized by the liver. Whether physical dependence exists is questionable because it does not produce severe symptoms experienced with other substances; however, the psychologic cravings for the substance are strong.

Patterns vary from occasional to episodic to chronic or almost daily use, with low to high doses of cocaine.

Depending on the type of preparation, cocaine may be chewed, smoked, inhaled intranasally, or injected intravenously. Since the mid-1980s, crack, a combination of cocaine, baking soda, and water, has become the cocaine preparation of choice because of its low cost and ease of administration.[53] The name is due to the "cracking" sound made when it is heated and then smoked or inhaled. Intravenous and inhaled cocaine have an immediate euphoric effect, but the effect of the intravenously-administered form is short lived (30 minutes or less). The longest-lasting effects result when it is "snorted" or inhaled. The substance may remain in the nasal mucosa for 3 or more hours.

Suspicion of polydrug abuse and dependence must be entertained, since other drugs are also self-administered, such as alcohol in an estimated 60% to 80% of cocaine users.[43] Additional drugs are used to relieve the agitation, insomnia, and depression associated with cocaine or to prolong its euphoric effects.

Aside from the euphoria in which feelings of inferiority disappear, other effects of the drug are psychomotor agitation, confusion, anxiety, paranoid ideation, impaired judgment, and impaired social or occupational functioning. Physiologic symptoms include headache, tachycardia, palpitations, hypertension, tremors, pupillary dilation, diaphoresis or chills, and nausea. Especially with high doses, the person may experience chest pain, convulsions, small strokes that cause brain damage from high blood pressure, myocardial infarctions, and death, often from cardiac arrhythmias or respiratory paralysis. Convulsions can occur within 90 minutes of ingestion.[43]

Because the quality and purity of the cocaine are seldom known, serious consequences are possible from any street sample. For instance, the purity level of illicitly purchased cocaine may be between 0% and 17% (or more) with fillers of glucose and/or other substances.[43] Some medical complications from contaminated needles are hepatitis, abscesses, septicemia, and acquired immune deficiency syndrome (AIDS). Snorting or inhaling cocaine injures nasal mucous membrane with ulceration and bleeding, and when minute particles of cocaine remain on nasal tissue, erosion of the nasal septum may occur, requiring surgical repair. Damage to the vocal cords with permanent hoarseness and lung impairment occurs when cocaine is inhaled, especially with chronic use.

Some psychologic changes are loss of ambition and drive and deterioration of relationships, with all energies directed toward obtaining more cocaine. Malnutrition with severe weight loss results from not eating, and self-care activities such as bathing and grooming deteriorate with chronic use.

Few thorough studies have been performed to determine with clarity the withdrawal effects of cocaine. Depression, suicidal ideation, insomnia, irritability, confusion, anxiety, and paranoid features may be evident along with changes in brain neurotransmitters after abstinence with mild symptoms occurring for a long period of time. Cravings for cocaine decrease with time, but may last several months to one year or more.[43]

It is essential that medical conditions such as hyperthyroidism and mental disorders such as schizophrenia, bipolar disorders, depression, and antisocial personality disorders be identified and treated.[43] Difficulties with self-concept, interpersonal relationships, sense of identity, and feelings of emptiness are some motivations for cocaine use, although it is a maladaptive coping strategy.

Reasons for hospitalization include the inability to terminate cocaine use, the presence of severe symptoms such as severe depression and medical problems, the absence of an adequate support system in the community, and repeated outpatient failures.

Tolerance for this powerfully addicting, illicit substance causes users to increase the dose, thereby creating an extremely expensive habit to maintain.[19] To support the habit, many persons engage in illegal activities, such as violent crimes, robberies, prostitution, and drug dealing.

•••••• Diagnostic Studies and Findings

SMAC   To screen for systemic abnormalities

Thyroid-stimulating hormone, T_4, T_3   To rule out thyroid disorder

Chest x-ray   To screen for cardiopulmonary disease

Electrocardiogram (ECG)   To screen for substance-induced heart disorder

Urinalysis   To screen for urinary and systemic abnormalities

Urine toxicology   To screen for substance abuse

•••••• Multidisciplinary Plan

Medication[43]

Antidepressant such as desipramine (Norpramin) 50 mg po bid to treat severe symptoms of depression or chlordiazepoxide (Librium) to decrease anxiety; if bipolar disorder exists, lithium may be prescribed to counter the euphorigenic effects of cocaine and the disorder

General Management

Group therapy

Recreational therapy

NURSING CARE

Nursing Assessment

Emotion

Depression, anxiety, sense of worthlessness, irritability, sense of emptiness

Physiologic

Cardiac dysrhythmia, hypertension, elevated temperature, insomnia or disturbed sleep, fatigue, confusion, malnutrition, nausea

Thoughts/Activities

Suicidal ideation, denial, impaired concentration and judgment, psychomotor agitation

Social and Occupational

Deterioration in social behavior, interpersonal difficulties, impairment in occupational or student role

Nursing Dx & Intervention

*Cocaine withdrawal** related to decreased intake of cocaine after long-term use or overdose

- Assess physical and mental condition. Assess pattern and amount of cocaine use including type of cocaine, route of administration, and time of last dose. Assess use of other street drugs and prescribed and over-the-counter drugs. If experiencing physiologic complications, treat as a medical emergency.
- If suicidal ideation exists, assess its seriousness.
- Restrict visitors during the first week of hospitalization *to prevent stimulation and possible stresses associated with visitors and to prevent reintroduction of drugs.*
- Obtain urine specimens at intervals, as ordered, for drug testing.
- Administer medication as ordered *to decrease severe symptoms associated with termination or overdose of cocaine.* Evaluate the effects. As patient is able to comprehend, provide patient with information of effects and adverse effects of medicines.
- Encourage patient to identify negative experiences with drug use rather than only euphoric, positive aspects *to begin self-awareness of problems arising from abuse.*
- Provide information on cocaine and other substances as indicated *to increase patient's knowledge of effects and adverse consequences and to correct misconceptions.*

Ineffective individual coping related to maladaptive reactions to life experiences

- Assess types of discomforts patient has in various social and occupational or school situations and strategies used to cope.
- Establish supportive, nonjudgmental relationship *to promote trust and comfort.*
- Assist patient to identify stress-provoking situations *to help increase awareness of areas of discomfort.* Help patient identify healthy coping strategies *to reinforce strengths.*
- Practice assertiveness skills with patient, rather than reliance on cocaine, *to increase patient's self-confidence and comfort in social and work situations.* Techniques include role-playing and confrontation with feedback in group therapy setting.

---

*Non-NANDA Nursing Diagnosis

- Encourage patient to ask for help from others in group therapy *to begin reaching out to others for help.*
- Demonstrate relaxation techniques, such as muscle relaxation and slow, deep breathing *to manage stress.*
- Encourage participation in recreational therapy *to expend energy, decrease stress, and develop leisure-time interests.*
- Encourage patient to anticipate postdischarge stressors *to begin to develop strategies for managing them.*
- Because termination of substance abuse increases patient's free time, assist patient to develop a schedule of enjoyable nondrug-related activities *to prevent a sense of emptiness and anxiety related to free time.*
- Connect patient with self-help groups such as Cocaine Anonymous while in hospital *to act as transition for continuation after discharge.*
- Assist patient to learn how to deal with person who may pressure him or her to use cocaine, how to say no to use, and how to avoid places where drugs are available *to develop a lifestyle free of drugs and to increase self-supports.*

Altered nutrition: less than body requirements related to lack of interest in food

- Assess nutritional intake and observe for signs of malnutrition.
- Ensure adequate nutrition in collaboration with physician and dietitian *to counteract effects of inadequate diet.*
- Provide a bland diet and antacids as ordered *to decrease gastric discomfort.*
- Explain essentials of a nutritionally balanced diet *to prevent or alleviate malnutrition.*

Altered family processes related to effects of substance abuse

- Assess family's knowledge of patient's drug use and quality of family relationships.
- Talk with family about cocaine and its consequences *to provide information and correct misconceptions.*
- Help patient and family members to identify and discuss problem areas, including feelings of anger, and help them begin to resolve difficulties *to improve relationships and develop realistic expectations of each other.*
- Refer family members for counseling, if indicated, and self-help groups such as Al-Anon or Nar-Anon *to learn how to deal with effects of patient's substance abuse.*

Patient Education/Home Care Planning

1. Encourage the patient to follow through with medical treatment.
2. Ensure that the patient verbalizes understanding of healthy coping strategies for dealing with stress.
3. Reinforce use of self-supports and supports from others, including active participation in self-help groups such as Cocaine Anonymous.
4. Support the patient's plans to implement a relapse-preventive lifestyle.

Evaluation

Patient has an uncomplicated termination from cocaine   Patient demonstrates drug-free state verbally, and urine tests during hospitalization are drug-free.

Patient demonstrates knowledge of effects and consequences of cocaine dependence   Patient describes psychologic and physiologic effects and consequences of cocaine use. Patient discusses effects of cocaine use on self and significant others.

Patient demonstrates evidence of practicing healthy coping techniques for dealing with stress-producing situations   Patient practices relaxation techniques. Patient practices assertiveness skills and evaluates their effects on self and others. Patient practices techniques for avoiding cocaine-related situations. Patient develops an enjoyable non–drug-related activity schedule to manage free time.

Patient participates in meal planning and eats regular, well-balanced meals   Patient verbalizes knowledge of good nutrition. Patient chooses and eats nutritionally balanced meals.

Patient demonstrates participation in relationships with family   Patient participates in dealing with conflicts in the family and in shared activities.

SCHIZOPHRENIC DISORDERS

A diagnosis of schizophrenia is made if the person exhibits continuous signs of marked behavioral impairment in the areas of work, social relationships, and self-care activities for at least 6 months including a minimum of 1 month of psychotic symptoms such as delusions, hallucinations, grossly disorganized affect, and disorganized speech. The subtypes of schizophrenia identified in the DSM-IV are disorganized, paranoid, catatonic, undifferentiated, and residual. When the symptoms are similar to schizophrenia except for a duration of 1 month to less than 6 months with no "decline in functioning," the condition is diagnosed as schizophreniform disorder.[2]

The symptoms the person develops are the best solutions he or she is capable of at the time to restore a sense of equilibrium. The presentation of schizophrenia that follows is not specific to a diagnostic type but deals with dysfunctional behaviors that are common to persons with schizophrenia.

■ SCHIZOPHRENIA

■ Schizophrenia is a disorder in which a person exhibits psychotic symptoms, including disturbances in perceptions, thought, affect, and psychomotor behaviors during an acute phase. The person's social and psychologic abilities are impaired.[2,5]

Schizophrenia is characterized by the following:
Thoughts
    Associations—irrational, illogical, and bizarre
    Delusions—false beliefs that are usually negative, persecutory, and injurious; may be grandiose

Ideas of reference—belief that events or conversations are related to the individual or have special significance to him (e.g., that others are making negative comments about him)

Thought broadcasting—belief that others can hear the person's thoughts

Loosening of associations—irrational, illogical, and bizarre thoughts (e.g., shifts from one to another unrelated or obliquely related idea)

Incoherence—incomprehensibility, inability to think or express thoughts in a clear, orderly manner

Poverty of content—paucity of ideas and thoughts; vague, repetitive, overly concrete ideas

Information processing and attention—limited ability to process incoming information with slow reaction time; impaired ability to select relevant from irrelevant aspects of communication

Projection—disowning perceived or actual attributes of self while attributing them to someone or something in the environment

Perception

Hallucinations—false sensory perceptions with no external stimulus; auditory is most frequent form of perceptual disturbance; voices may be negative, insulting, or commanding; especially in chronicity, voices may be friendly and helpful; visual hallucinations occur occasionally in acute phase and involve seeing nonexistent things such as insects or people; smell (olfactory), taste (gustatory), and touch (tactile) are less common

Illusions—misidentification or distortion of stimulus

Affect

Blunting—reduction of affective, emotional expression

Flatness—impoverishment of emotional reactivity; emotionally dull, cold, colorless; monotonous voice

Apathy—apparent absence of emotions

Inappropriateness—incongruence between emotions and content or ideas (e.g., laughing in response to news of death of significant other)

Activity level

Psychomotor activity—decreased reaction to environment; stereotypic, purposeless movement such as rocking or pacing

Spontaneity and activity—markedly decreased activity to withdrawal; repetitive, stereotypic activity; apathy; immobility

Posture—rigid, inappropriate, manneristic

Other

Self-identity—impairment or loss of ego boundaries; impairment of self-identity

Volition—impaired ability to will self to act; disturbance in goal-directed activities

Role behaviors—impairment in work and social roles; lack of social skills

Personal appearance—neglect

The characteristics of schizophrenia are also dichotomized into positive and negative symptoms.[22] Examples of the positive are delusions, hallucinations, disorganized speech, and dis-organized or bizarre behavior; examples of the negative are apathy, poverty of speech, flat and blunted affect, and anhedonia, all leading to withdrawal and social isolation.

The onset of schizophrenia may be slow and insidious or sudden. In some persons the onset is preceded by a significant external event such as loss of a friend, marriage, or leaving home; in others the onset is not related to an identifiable external event. External events, if identified, are insufficient to evoke a psychosis if the internal processes such as relatedness to self and environment are not impaired.

Psychotic symptoms are present during the active phase. The person loses contact with reality.[3] Behaviors are unpredictable, in part because the person responds to internal processes such as hallucinations and delusions. He may hear voices that order him to protect himself from an evil and harmful world. Projection, the externalization of rejected, undesirable thoughts, feelings, and behaviors onto others, is a common defense mechanism. The secondary processes of mental integration that is based on logic and the reality principle deteriorate and give way to the primary processes of illogical, disorganized mental activity of the unconscious system that is normal during infancy.

Although some persons recover completely, a majority have residual effects of the schizophrenic process. Among this majority group, some have acute relapses, some maintain a stable course, and others gradually worsen with severe disabilities. Vulnerability caused by biologic and personality deficits and environmental stressors such as excessively stimulating environment and fault-finding, critical family relationships remain and may trigger relapses.[33] Impairments reduce the person's ability to cope with social and psychological experiences, such as processing information received from others and social problem-solving. Vigorous rehabilitation programs are needed to assist patients in making stable adjustments to living in the community.[3] Involving patients' families in psychoeducational and support groups increases their ability to cope with the stresses and stigma of having a mentally ill family member and decreases the patient-relapse rate.

It is important to differentiate the symptoms of schizophrenia from medical conditions and reactions to prescribed medicines and substance abuse. Medical conditions that may result in psychotic symptoms include syphilis, endocrine and metabolic disorders, tumors of the brain, temporal lobe epilepsy, vitamin deficiencies such as Vitamin B_{12}, and toxic reactions to noxious fumes and heavy metals.[2,22]

Substance abuse is a major concern with schizophrenic patients regardless of whether or not they are taking antipsychotic medications. It is not known with precision how or if substance abuse causes persistent psychosis or alters the course of the illness. Alcohol is frequently abused, and marijuana is a commonly used nonalcoholic drug. Among those abusing substances, 78% are involved in polydrug use.[46] Although many patients used drugs "to get high," many others abuse drugs to escape painful psychiatric problems such as depression and anxiety and to relieve the adverse effects of antipsychotic medications. Some patients who smoke cigarettes may be alleviating the symptoms of Parkinsonism by decreasing the levels of antipsychotic drugs in the blood. Important issues in counseling patients with dual diagnoses of schizophrenia and substance abuse are not to expect abstinence as a precondition for treatment and not to use highly confrontational techniques of counseling generally used by chemical dependency counselors.[46] While consistently discouraging patients from using drugs, caregivers should provide intensive treatment.

Prevalence

The United States has the highest reported prevalence of schizophrenia when compared with other countries. In part this is related to poor reliability of the diagnostic criteria used.[22] Researchers of some large U.S. studies have estimated the prevalence of schizophrenia to be between 0.2% to 2.0%. However, the overall prevalence rate is estimated to be 1% of the population in the United States.[2]

The person with schizophrenia has a shorter life expectancy than others in the population, and a suicide rate of about 10%. Some risk factors for suicide include being under 30 years of age and male, experiencing depressive symptoms, and being unemployed.

Population at Risk

The onset of schizophrenia typically occurs during late adolescence to the mid-30s, but has occurred in younger and older persons. The disease is almost equally distributed between males and females; however, the mean age for first psychotic break in males is 21.4 and in females is 26.8.[2,22] Genetic transmission of schizophrenia has been found, so that children with first degree biologic relatives have a ten times greater risk for schizophrenia than the general population.[22] A consistent finding is the relationship of social class and schizophrenia—the prevalence is greatest in lower socioeconomic groups and in poor neighborhoods.[36] Whether schizophrenia-prone persons are products of these environments or drift toward inner cities when they lose economic and social status is unknown.

Responses of Nurses to Schizophrenics

Schizophrenia is a chronic disorder in which the person appears cold, distant, and apathetic. Response to therapy is extremely slow, and obvious signs of success are few. The schizophrenic is emotionally unnourished and is unnourishing to the nurse and others around him. Nurses often find it easier to withdraw from the withdrawn schizophrenic than to experience a sense of helplessness, hopelessness, and inadequacy in dealing with the patient. The nurse needs to establish small goals with the patient such as having the patient speak to her, share an activity, or ask to have a need or want met. If unrealistic goals are established, the nurse is bound to experience frustration and hopelessness. If the goal is attainable, specific, and immediate, the nurse's frustration is reduced (see Emergency Alert box).

Family Caregivers

Family members experience anger, shame, and guilt about having an ill member. Having the patient in the home generally re-

sults in severe stress and conflict in relationships among the family as they attempt to cope with the dysfunctional behaviors.

The family members have been given primary responsibility for supporting and protecting the patient so that he remains in the community. Patients and families also need active community mental health services to provide information, support, and rehabilitation for the patient.

•••••• Psychopathology

Many neurochemical, neurophysiologic, and psychosocial explanations and theories exist for understanding the schizophrenic disorder. Although many anomalies are present, no characteristic pathology of schizophrenia clearly exists and no abnormal laboratory findings are predictable.[22] The history and mental status examination are important for a diagnosis of schizophrenia.

One explanation for the transmission of schizophrenia is found in the gene theory. Although researchers have been unable to identify a specific gene, they suspect that polygenes or the mutation of one or several genes are etiologic factors in schizophrenia.[27] Strong evidence of genetic transmission of schizophrenia has been identified in twin studies.[37] In European and U.S. samples of twins with schizophrenic parents, monozygotic pairs had a median rate of occurrence of 46% and dizygotic pairs 14%. When the monozygotic twins of schizophrenic parents were adopted by non-schizophrenic parents, they were

EMERGENCY ALERT

SCHIZOPHRENIC DISORDERS

Persons with schizophrenic disorders exhibit continuous signs of marked behavioral impairment in all areas of their lives for at least 6 months.

Assessment

- Loss of contact with reality: psychotic delusions, hallucinations, and/or other distortions of reality
- Agitated, aggressive, danger to self or others
- Evidence of neuroleptic malignant syndrome
- Extrapyramidal symptoms (EPS) due to antipsychotic medicine, e.g., dystonia, akathisia, Parkinsonian symptoms, and/or tardive dyskinesia
- Abuse of substances, e.g., prescribed, illegal, over-the-counter, and/or alcohol

Interventions

- If patient is psychotic and is increasingly agitated, administer medications as ordered.
- Provide safe environment, e.g., patient's room or quiet area to decrease stimuli. Make frequent, brief contacts with patient.
- If side effects such as EPS are present, treat according to type, e.g., administer antiparkinson drug, decrease or discontinue antipsychotic medicine, and/or substitute a different medication in collaboration with physician.

more likely to develop schizophrenia than adoptees from non-schizophrenic biologic parents. While genetic vulnerability to schizophrenia does exist, the environmental and psychosocial influences should not be ignored.

Computed tomography and other imaging techniques identified structural brain abnormalities, although the evidence has not been consistent or discrete.[20,22] The most consistent abnormality is ventricular enlargement in the brain and is likely to occur more often in males than females. A frequent change is atrophy of the cortical lobes or abnormal brain development with abnormalities being noted especially in those with chronic schizophrenia or with many negative symptoms. Decreased blood flow and reduced metabolic rate in the lobes have been observed with imaging techniques. The left temporal abnormalities are observed in many studies of schizophrenia and often related to positive symptoms.[20,36]

One major theory about neurotransmitters in the brain of schizophrenics is that an abnormal amount of dopamine is present. The evidence is that an excess of dopamine activity is associated with psychotic or positive symptoms of schizophrenia.[31,38] Support for this is that antipsychotic drugs block the postsynaptic dopamine receptors. On the other hand, hypodopaminergic activity is associated with negative symptoms. A minority of patients, possibly 30%, may have a different kind of pathophysiology and do not respond favorably to the usual antipsychotic medicines. Newer drugs, such as Clozaril (Clozapine), are dopamine and serotonin blockers, are effective against positive and negative symptoms, and are often effective when other antipsychotic medication has failed. Adverse effects include excessive salivation (which could lead to aspiration especially when sleeping), postural hypotension, lowered seizure threshold, hyperthermia (which may be an initial reaction to the drug or a sign of infection or severe blood disorder), and agranulocytosis which has caused deaths.[25] Agranulocytosis is thought to occur in about 1%-2% of patients, and most often during the first six months of therapy. Weekly monitoring of white blood cell count is essential as well as reporting flu-like symptoms or other signs of infection immediately. Clozaril is unlikely to cause tardive dyskinesia and rarely causes neuroleptic malignant syndrome. However, Clozaril and other atypical antipsychotic medications are not a panacea since they are effective in only about 30% of patients resistant to the older antipsychotic drugs. In addition, the cost of Clozaril with weekly blood tests becomes very expensive compared to the older medications.[22]

Some researchers believe that schizophrenia may be related to viral infections, autoimmune disturbances, and other pathophysiologic factors. Although the evidence for pathophysiologic causes is compelling, it does not provide all the answers. Social and environmental stressors are factors that must also be examined to assess whether stressors interact with genetic and biologic susceptibilities to produce the disorder. Because the boundaries of the schizophrenic spectrum are blurred, identification of the parameters of the disorder clearly is essential for an accurate diagnosis.

Psychoanalytic Theory

The functions of the ego include the ability to differentiate the self from objects in the environment, reality testing, organization of affect, and development of cognitive processes, such as perception, thinking, remembering, and learning. The organizing processes operate in integrating the id, ego, and superego and in differentiating the self from objects outside the self.

Because the functions of the ego develop in stages, traumatic experiences do not affect all functions adversely. Those functions affected negatively are subject to regression to an earlier phase of development and reflected in symptoms. Because the secondary processes of cognition that are reflected in abstract, logical thinking develop later in the person's development, these are among the first to be lost. The person regresses to the earlier primary processes of cognition, a simpler period of life, when fantasy and reality are not well differentiated, integration of new experiences is limited, language is concrete rather than abstract, and is partly autistically derived.[36]

The ego, as mediator of the id's instinctual drives, libido, and aggression (death instinct), neutralizes the aggressive energy and puts the energy into the service of itself. The ego uses the energy to maintain the various ego functions. If aggression is not neutralized, disorganization occurs when the person experiences angry thoughts and fears of acting on them. The patient attempts to defend against the aggression through projection, withdrawal, and regression of the ego, sometimes to the point of disintegration of the self.[36] The ego functions are not able to be maintained because of the regression to an instinctual drive; this consequently plays a role in the initiation of schizophrenic symptoms.

Interpersonal Theory

Interpersonal theory stresses that the personality develops through relationships with others. Sullivan[51] assumed that the mother of the future schizophrenic is more intensely anxious than the average mother. Because she transmits anxiety to the infant, severe anxiety experienced as dread and terror is evoked in the infant. To avoid overwhelming panic and with few resources, the infant attempts to get rid of the discomfort by dissociating from it as a "not-me" experience. The infant with excessive "not-me" experiences is vulnerable to future excessive anxiety.[51] Although dissociation serves to protect the person from extremely uncomfortable experiences, it also prevents him from recalling, examining, and correcting perceptions of these experiences and limits his capacity to deal with future ones. To avoid the sense of terror, the person urgently gets rid of situations that may evoke anxiety without determining whether the event is frightening and what aspect of it is. No learning can take place when the person is busy defending against anxiety.

Regression occurs when the feelings of self are compromised and weakened. The self-system is actively warding off or decreasing anxiety, and the dissociated experiences are no longer available for learning. Because complex cognitive processes of thinking, learning, and remembering are compromised, the person reverts to earlier modes of experiencing such as the momentary reverie of infancy or the distorted thinking of the young child in which illogical connections are made between experiences. The severity of the schizophrenic processes is related to the strength of the self-system and the degree of regression to more primitive functioning of the infant or young child.[5,51]

Cognitive Theory

Although all human beings are biologically predisposed to think illogically at times, to be self-destructive, and to experience inappropriate feelings, a seriously ill person may have a greater predisposition to disordered thinking. The person underestimates his abilities and emphasizes problems. Because past traumatic events are exaggerated, the person overreacts to even minor problems.[7] Even when new information makes possible a different perspective, the person resists and continues to think about the self and others illogically.

Thinking and emotional disturbances are also related to social learning. The child is taught to please his parents even when the directive appears illogical and begins to accept directives without thinking. When told often enough that he is worthless to himself and to others, he accepts the idea. Self-defeating beliefs are rigidly held and become strongly habituated patterns of thinking, feeling, and acting.[7]

•••••• Diagnostic Studies and Findings

SMAC   To screen for systemic abnormalities
Thyroid function tests
Syphilis serology
Electrocardiogram   To rule out cardiopathy
Computed Tomography scan   To rule out brain abnormalities
Routine urinalysis
Urine toxicology screen   To rule out substance abuse

•••••• Multidisciplinary Plan

Medications

Haloperidol (Haldol)
  For severely disturbed patient: 5 mg bid by tablet or concentrate to manage symptoms of psychotic disorders; for acute agitation: 2 mg IM prn; for elderly disturbed patient: 2 mg bid by tablet or concentrate; major initial side effect is orthostatic hypotension; in addition to the adverse effects of extrapyramidal symptoms, neuroleptic malignant syndrome (NMS), a potentially fatal disorder, has been reported with antipsychotic medicines; major clinical manifestations of NMS are muscular rigidity, tachycardia, diaphoresis, labile blood pressure with hypotension and hypertension, cardiac dysrhythmia, dyspnea, hyperpyrexia, and coma

General Management

  Occupational therapy to provide opportunities for participating in activities of daily living
  Recreational therapy for development of skills in group activities and for learning leisure activities

NURSING CARE

Nursing Assessment

Thoughts

  Disturbance in orientation to person, place, and time; retarded thought processes; impaired ability to process incoming information; blocking of thoughts; autistic thinking (i.e., inability to distinguish between reality and fantasy); suspiciousness; distorted, illogical thinking; false beliefs, such as of being persecuted or poisoned; projection (i.e., disowning aspects of self while ascribing them to something or someone in environment); poor judgment; fear of rejection and of interpersonal and physical closeness; lack of trust; vulnerability to stress

Perception

  Appearance of listening to voices observed as movement in vocal cords and lips, and head and facial movement

Affect

  Anxiety; loneliness; depression; apathy; colorless speech and monotonous voice; incongruity between emotional responses and idea; hostility

Activity

  Withdrawal from relationships and contact with others; impairment in goal-directed activity; purposeless movement such as pacing and mannerisms; unpredictable behavior that may be related to delusions or hallucinations; agitation; impairment or absence of social skills; poor work history

Self-Care

  Neglectfulness; lack of motivation; impairment in bathing, grooming, and hygiene

Nutrition

  Unawareness of hunger or thirst; apathy to food at mealtime; fear of eating (e.g., belief that food is poisoned)

Sleep

  Disturbed sleep patterns; reluctance to go to bed at night or inability to awaken in morning

Nursing Dx & Intervention

Social isolation related to alterations in mental status

- Assess degree of withdrawal and types of preoccupations patient has.
- Begin to establish a trusting relationship *to provide sense of security for patient.*
- Maintain appropriate physical distance when with patient *to decrease any sense of terror of physical closeness.*

- Speak slowly to patient, using brief statements *to increase patient's ability to process information and understand.*
- Visit patient frequently for brief time periods *to demonstrate concern and to decrease fears of interpersonal closeness.*
- Tell patient when you are leaving and let him or her know when you will return.
- Avoid pushing a nonverbal patient to respond to questions *to prevent further withdrawal.*
- Comment on neutral subjects, such as patient's immediate environment (e.g., items in the room, activities of others in the room, pictures in a shared magazine).
- As you and patient are able to tolerate longer time periods together, increase time gradually *to help patient begin working on issues.*
- If patient becomes increasingly agitated and distracting techniques are unsuccessful, medication may be administered in collaboration with physician *to decrease agitation.* Briefly explain reason for medication and its major effects and side effects to the extent that patient is able to comprehend.
- Assist patient to develop social skills *to help patient interact, initiate a conversation, or make requests* because these skills are often impaired.
- Explain to patient that others have responsibilities for interactions and that patient is responsible only for his or her own behavior. Assist patient to elaborate on and build on strengths *to encourage patient to identify and accept skills.*
- Assist patient to develop assertiveness skills and encourage practice of them; examine attempts to be assertive *to help patient become aware of successes,* even if attempts were awkward.
- Help patient to attend and participate in occupational therapy as prescribed *to promote skills and interests.*
- As patient is able to tolerate interactions with others, encourage recreational therapy *to gain skills in various activities, to expend energy through exercise, and to learn leisure activities.*

Altered thought processes related to non-reality based thinking

- Assess level of distractibility, delusional thinking, and ability *to process incoming stimuli.*
- Assess for substance abuse.
- Orient patient, as needed, to person, place, and time *to correct disorientation.*
- Listen attentively to patient, listening for themes, feeling tones, or reality-oriented phrases or thoughts *to increase patient's willingness to relate to another human being.* Do not pretend understanding, but comment on understandable conversation.
- Assist patient, as able, to elaborate on reality-oriented ideas.
- Assist patient *in correcting misconceptions about environment, self, and experiences* through recall of events and use of problem-solving.

- Do not encourage patient to repeat false beliefs by arguing or agreeing with him or her, *to avoid reinforcing ideas of reference and delusions.* "I find that hard to believe" may be appropriate comment.
- Assist patient to examine what he or she was experiencing before delusional thoughts began. Attempt to assist patient to identify thoughts and feelings toward himself or herself *to determine if patient was feeling threatened.* Gradually assist patient *to recognize and correct delusional content of thoughts and feelings.*
- When patient shows signs of anxiety or expresses discomfort, change topic *to decrease anxiety.* If patient is able to discuss an anxiety-provoking topic, help him or her identify his or her feelings (awareness of feelings will evolve slowly).
- Administer medication as ordered. If you suspect patient is not swallowing tablets, concentrates may be administered in collaboration with physician.
- Briefly explain reason for medication, as well as its effects and side effects. Inform patient of possible sleepiness and dizziness, especially when standing up. Caution patient to stand up slowly *to prevent falling.*
- Observe patient closely *to detect effects and side effects of medication,* and report to physician for dose adjustments as needed. Check vital signs four times a day initially.
- As patient is able to comprehend, describe effects and side effects of medication and reasons for medication *to increase potential for compliance.*

Sensory/perceptual alterations (auditory) related to mental illness

- Assess for perceptual distortions such as hallucinations.
- When patient is observed moving lips and vocal cords or cocking head as if listening, ask him or her, "Do you hear voices?" or "Who is talking to you?" Use distractive techniques such as involving patient in conversation or activity if patient is unable to examine reality of voices. If "voices" are chronic, teach patient to hum or whistle to prevent him or her from using vocal cords for "voices" *to increase his or her sense of control.*
- Gradually assist patient to examine thoughts and feelings just before hallucinations. Help patient recognize eventually that he or she expects to hear voices. Accept patient's protests and denials as his or her current understandings. Slowly encourage patient to accept a connection between thoughts or feelings and expectation of voices *to be aware that he or she has ability to control his or her experiences and correct thoughts and feelings about himself.*

Altered nutrition: less than body requirements related to psychologic factors

- Assess nutritional intake and misconceptions about food.
- When patient is suspicious of food, emphasize that food is nutritious and has not been tampered with; have patient participate in choosing foods and liquids *to decrease suspiciousness.*

- Obtain patient's attention and suggest eating *to decrease preoccupations or hallucinations.* If necessary, direct patient to take each mouthful (e.g., "Take a spoonful. Now eat it.")
- Offer fluids between meals *to maintain hydration.*
- Explain the ingredients and importance of good nutrition when patient is able to process information.

Sleep pattern disturbance related to psychologic factors

- Assess sleep patterns and fears about sleeping.
- If patient has fears of going to sleep, assist him or her to talk about them *to begin to correct misconceptions.*
- Offer warm milk *to assist sleeping.*
- Encourage slow, deep breathing while focusing on number "I" *to promote relaxation.*
- If helpful, turn the radio to soothing music at low volume *to decrease panic or fears.*
- Discourage naps during the day *to enhance restful sleep at night.*

Other related nursing diagnoses Bathing and hygiene and dressing and grooming self-care deficits related to alterations in mental status; altered family processes related to mental illness.

Patient Education/Home Care Planning

1. Reinforce beginning skills in the use of problem-solving techniques and social skills.
2. Ensure that the patient can identify and verbalize strengths.
3. With a community health worker, assist the patient to make contact with a continuing care program in a community mental health center and encourage participation.
4. Give a list of signs and symptoms of medications to report to the physician, and encourage compliance with the medication regimen.
5. Ensure that the patient verbalizes understanding of the need for continued care with the physician and community mental health center.

Evaluation

Patient participates in social activities with staff and other patients Patient spends less time alone in unit. Patient states he enjoys participating in some planned and unplanned activities.

Patient no longer has psychotic symptoms Patient is oriented to person, place, and time. Patient begins to use problem-solving methods to correct misconceptions. Patient verbalizes knowledge of effects and side effects of medicine and plans to comply with medication regimen.

Patient no longer hallucinates Patient states he or she no longer hears voices.

Patient participates in choosing well-balanced meals Patient is no longer suspicious of food and eats food at mealtime. Patient verbalizes knowledge of nutritionally balanced food.

Patient sleeps through the night Patient practices relaxation techniques before bedtime. Patient verbalizes that he or she is sleeping well during the night and is awakening refreshed.

Patient plans to continue treatment plan after discharge Patient makes appointment with psychiatrist for counseling and medication supervision. Patient develops a system to keep track of self-administration of medications. Patient visits a community mental health center and plans to attend regularly after discharge.

MOOD DISORDERS

Mood is an emotional reaction that is sufficiently intense to affect the person's entire psychic state. The two major moods are manic and depressive patterns of disturbance. Another way of classifying mood disorders is as bipolar or unipolar. A person with a bipolar disorder has experienced one or more manic and depressive episodes, whereas a person with a unipolar disorder has experienced at least one or more episodes of depression with no manic phase. The manic and depressive manifestations of the disorders are compared in Table 17-2.[2,6]

 TABLE 17-2 Comparison of Manic and Depressive Phases

Mania	Depression
Elation, expansiveness, irritability	Melancholia, sense of despair
Inappropriate laughing, joking, punning	Tearfulness, crying
Accelerated, sharpened thinking, flight of ideas	Retarded thinking, impaired attention and concentration
Unlimited self-confidence	Lack of self-confidence
Overoptimism	Pessimism, hopelessness
Loquacity	Decreased talkativeness
Exhibitionism	Inhibition
Extroversion to environment	Introversion
Rapid shift to aggression toward environment	Self-destructiveness
Gregariousness	Social withdrawal
Hedonism	Limited or absence of pleasure
Licentiousness	Limited or absence of sexual interest
Reduced need for sleep	Insomnia or hypersomnia
Unlimited energy	Fatigue, psychomotor retardation
Appetite ravenous but "no time" to eat	Appetite decreased or lost
Flight from superego	Submission to superego

The bipolar disorders are discussed here first with a focus on manic behavior. This is followed by a presentation of depression.

BIPOLAR DISORDERS

In the bipolar disorders, the manic phase is characterized by grandiosity, excessive excitement, flight of ideas, and psychomotor overactivity; the depressive phase is characterized by a sense of despair, retarded thinking, and psychomotor retardation or agitation.[2]

The *bipolar I disorder* has at least one or more frank manic to psychotic or mixed episodes and usually one or more major depressive episodes. *Bipolar II disorder* has one or more major depressive periods and at least one hypomanic episode. When the bipolar disorder episodes occur at least four times within a one year period, the diagnosis includes the specifier of *rapid-cycling*.[2] The phases must be separated by either a period of remission or by a distinct switch to the opposite polarity. For a *mixed episode,* the time period must be for at least one week with rapidly alternating moods of depression and mania occurring nearly every day.

In the hypomanic episode the mood is elevated, grandiose, very talkative and the person has flight of ideas, pressured speech, and decreased need for sleep. This distinctly observable period lasts for at least 4 days.

In *cyclothymic disorder,* numerous fluctuating symptoms of mania and depression are present for at least 2 years, but the severity does not achieve the criteria of a major depressive or manic episode.[2]

•••••• Manic Behaviors in Bipolar Disorders

Manic behavior is excessive mental and physical activity.[2] Thought is accelerated and expansive; mood is labile with rapid sequences of euphoria, irritability, depression, elation, and rage; and physical activity is excessive with boundless energy, little need for sleep, constant motion, and assaultiveness in response to limit setting. Persons in manic states have pressured speech and flight of ideas and are self-indulgent, impatient, humorous, extroverted, friendly, impulsive, and distractible. They appear to have unlimited self-confidence and self-assurance as they propel their energy outward into the environment. The levels of mood disturbance vary from mild to severe with psychotic features (see Emergency Alert box).

Prevalence

The prevalence of bipolar disorders is underestimated in the population because of inconsistencies in the diagnostic classifications used among investigators and clinicians in the same or between countries. Without a detailed history of the patient's previous symptoms, caregivers will be unable to accurately identify the chronic, cyclic nature of the disorders. The lifetime prevalence rate for bipolar disorders is estimated to be between 0.4% and 1.60% in the adult population. Cyclothymia is re-

ported to occur in 0.4% to 1.0% of the population.[2] Aside from focusing on the current acute episode, the history of the illness must be considered.

Population at Risk

No significant difference was found in the gender distribution of persons with bipolar disorders in the United States and several other countries, including Taiwan, Puerto Rico, and New Zealand.[35] The disorders occur equally in both sexes.

First degree biological relatives of persons with bipolar I disorder have a 4% to 24% greater chance of developing mood disorders than does the general population. Relatives of persons with bipolar II disorder have a 1% to 5% greater risk of developing the disorder.[2] Some early researchers found bipolar disorders to be overrepresented in the upper socioeconomic class; however, more recent researchers do not consistently corroborate those findings. In a large and diverse sample, no significant differences were found in "occupation, income, or education categories."[35]

In 20% to 30% of patients the first episode of the disorder is likely to occur before the age of 20, and the incidence rises

 EMERGENCY ALERT

MOOD DISORDERS

Persons with mood disorders exhibit emotional reactions so intense that their entire psychic state is affected.

Bipolar Disorders: Manic Phase

ASSESSMENT

- Loss of contact with reality/psychotic, delusions, hallucinations, and incoherent speech
- Grandiose, hyperactive, unlimited energy, loquacious, emotionally labile, impulsive, aggressive to intensely hostile, and poor judgment
- Adverse effects of medicine, e.g., diarrhea, vomiting, polyuria, tremors, ataxia, weakness, and extrapyramidal symptoms

Unipolar or Bipolar Disorders: Depressive Phase

ASSESSMENT

- Hopelessness, helplessness, paucity of thoughts, morbid thoughts, suicidal ideation, unworthy, immobility or agitation, inability or limited ability to think, and/or catastrophic expectations without external threat
- May be out of contact with reality/psychotic and delusional
- Suicidal ideation and/or attempts

INTERVENTIONS

- After completing blood work, administer medications as prescribed for severe mood disturbance.
- If patient is psychotic, highly agitated, and/or destructive to self and others, provide safe, protected environment. Contact patient frequently for brief periods.

until age 35. The highest prevalence is with persons between the ages of 18 and 44, with women having an earlier onset than men.[21] The onset of each phase can be sudden, especially in mania; symptoms can escalate within a few hours. However, both phases can have slower onsets. The episodes in bipolar disorders often occur irregularly but may also alternate regularly, such as with seasonal patterns of mania in the spring and summer and with depression in the fall and winter.[2] Episodes may be separated by symptom-free periods or may follow each other with no appreciable interval between them. The average duration of episodes in bipolar disorders ranges from 4 to 13 months (the longer duration generally occurred before the availability of current medications). Modern treatment methods, including medications, have obscured the phases and blurred the development of symptoms.[21]

Levels of Manic Mood Disturbances

Hypomania is a pathologic state that is less severe than mania. The person has intensified energy, a stable elated mood, self-indulgence, distractibility, pressured speech, poor judgment, and increased motor activity.[6] Hypomanic persons radiate good health, appear tireless, and are humorous and friendly to the point of being unacceptably personal with others. Their intolerance to limit setting is observed as irritability or anger.

Mania or acute mania is a more intense and disturbed level in which propriety and discretion are absent. Persons in this state tease and joke, often making others the butt of their jokes. Their good humor can change rapidly to vicious anger. They flit from one activity to another without completing anything. They may talk incessantly because impulses are expressed in words with flight of ideas proceeding to incoherence and clang association (mental association between dissociated ideas made because of similarity of sounds of words used to describe the ideas). These persons have delusions of grandeur concerning their wealth and power and have lost control of their behavior, but they do not have severe disturbances of self-identity as in schizophrenia.

Persons with delirious mania or psychosis evidence all of the symptoms of the previous levels plus loss of contact with reality. Speech is incoherent, activity is constant and purposeless, and delusions and hallucinations are present. At times incontinence of urine and feces occurs.[6]

Interactions with manics, and less so with hypomanics, are stressful to others because of their exploitative behaviors, which include the following:

Manipulating the self-esteem of others by praise and deflation

Striking exploitatively at vulnerable areas

Projecting responsibility onto others

Testing limits of rules by trying to extend them

Alienating others, especially family members

Family Issues

Family members often view the person in the manic phase as willful and spiteful because he or she embarrasses the spouse and children, is manipulative and argumentative, uses poor judgment, creates financial problems, and acts out sexually. Family life is very stressful. The spouse is more likely to seek divorce from the ill member immediately after a manic episode.[35]

Family members need knowledge about the chronic, cyclic nature of bipolar disorders, the symptoms, and treatment. They also need support and coping skills to lessen the stressfulness of family life. When able, the patient should participate in family sessions to help correct communication difficulties and to develop problem solving skills. Patients with supportive, knowledgeable families are more likely to comply with the treatment regimen than those with no families or nonsupportive ones.

•••••• Psychopathology

Biologic factors contribute to the development of bipolar disorders; however, the complex interactions in the brain and other body systems make it difficult to clearly delineate causes. The high prevalence of bipolar disorders among relatives suggests that the condition is inheritable. Genes, such as the X chromosome, have been implicated as a causative factor; however, research findings have not been consistently confirmed.[35]

Many biologic hypotheses currently being pursued in bipolar disorders seem promising, and yet raise many more questions. For example, one hypothesis posits that neurotransmitter metabolism, such as norepinephrine, serotonin, and dopamine, regulates the mood and behavior of individuals and is altered.[21,36] The electrolytes that have been implicated as abnormal are sodium, calcium, and magnesium, which are thought to be needed for lithium salts to work. Hypothyroidism is found in bipolar disorders especially in rapid cyclers. Other theories suggest that hormones, such as steroids, and circadian biologic rhythms may play a role in bipolar disorders.

Brain imaging techniques showed an abnormally lower metabolism rate in the frontal cortex of bipolars than normals. Electroencephalogram (EEG) findings are found to be abnormal in the left brain hemisphere.[36] The rate of temporal lobe epilepsy in mania is well above that in the general population.[28] The role of biologic disturbances is supported by the effectiveness of lithium in preventing the recurrence of symptoms. Persons who do not respond to lithium, and this is especially true of rapid cyclers, are likely to respond to anticonvulsive medications such as carbamazepine (Tegretol). However, the contribution of psychosocial or physical stress, especially to the onset of the first few episodes, cannot be dismissed. Such stressors may interact with biologic and genetic predispositions in the development of symptoms.[21]

Behaviors associated with the manic phase overlap with those of other psychiatric conditions and, when mild, those of nonpathologic deviations of normal behavior. Bipolar disorder should be differentiated from schizophrenia (especially the paranoid type), personality disorders, unipolar depressions, schizoaffective disorder, attention-deficit/hyperactivity disorder, and medical conditions (such as multiple sclerosis, Huntington's disease, and Cushing's syndrome). Prescribed medications such as cortisone and amphetamines and illicit drugs such as cocaine may precipitate a manic-type episode that must be distinguished from bipolar disorders.[2]

Psychoanalytic Theory

Persons with bipolar disorders have an oral-dependent character and the basic psychopathologic characteristics of unipolar depressives: the introjection of anger and hostility. Depression is repressed hostility, and mania, a defensive behavior, is a massive denial of depression. Manic behavior is a flight from the superego with an abatement of ego restraints, whereas depressed persons submit to the superego.

The apparent warmth and social responsiveness of persons with bipolar disorders may be related to satisfying early relationships with their mothers. However, these persons experience defective nurturing that inhibits their ability to master the intrapsychic separation-individuation processes of development. They do not become psychologically separate individuals with a sense of self-identity. The inability to develop close relationships with others or to recognize the needs of others is related to the absence of an integrated self. Psychoanalysts recognize that biologic and genetic factors are responsible for the patient's vulnerability to some psychologic and social influences that operate in the bipolar disorders.[21]

Interpersonal Theory

The family environment is extremely important in the development of manic depression. The mother enjoys her relationship with the helpless, dependent infant but attempts to control the independent and rebellious strivings of the toddler with threats of abandonment. As the young child develops, the mother or both parents expect compliance and conformity to extremely high standards of behavior and achievements to improve the family's social position and reputation rather than to instill a sense of self-achievement and pride in the child. The child receives favoritism and special attention because of either his or her superior ability to achieve or his or her greater effort to please and to remain dependent. The child grows into adulthood learning to use others for unlimited help and support, yet fears competitiveness and confrontation because he or she is afraid to alienate others. Mania is an escape from the burdens of the duty-bound self into superficial liveliness and freedom. Although these persons appear warm and sincere in interpersonal relations, they are shallow and nonempathetic.[6]

Cognitive Theory

According to cognitive theory, which is ahistorical, people process information by taking it in, evaluating their efforts, and then reacting to it. In mania and hypomania, the evaluations of the person are positive and their accomplishments impressive. These responses and reactions to the stimulus or event become automatic thoughts, i.e., are no longer evaluations based on the evidence of the specific event.[36,44] The euphoria they experience because of their inflated evaluation of their superiority and superb performance drives them into uninterrupted motion. When questioned about their inaccurate self-appraisals, they become inappropriately angry or belligerent.

••••• Diagnostic Studies and Findings

SMAC To rule out abnormalities in various systems including serum electrolytes. Repeat serum electrolytes after lithium is started. In addition repeat other tests when clinically indicated.

Complete blood count To rule out infections before lithium and follow-up to assess elevated white blood cell count due to lithium or infection.

Thyroid function tests To assess for abnormal thyroid. Repeat after beginning lithium q6-12 mo.

Lithium levels To obtain baseline before lithium treatment (normal values $\cong\varnothing$), and after therapy is initiated.

Electrocardiogram To obtain baseline level and to rule out cardiac disease, and after lithium treatment to assess changes due to lithium.

Pregnancy test in women during childbearing years To rule out pregnancy before initiating lithium to prevent abnormality in fetus, especially in the first trimester.

Urinalysis To screen for infection or systemic abnormalities.

Urine toxicology To screen for substance abuse.

••••• Multidisciplinary Plan

Medications

Lithium carbonate (Lithane, Eskalith),* 300 mg po qid or 600 mg po tid to treat manic symptoms and prevent recurrence; lithium citrate syrup may be ordered initially instead of tablets *to ensure that medicine is swallowed*

General Management

Occupational therapy as condition permits
Recreational therapy as condition permits
Regular diet with normal sodium intake; sometimes high-carbohydrate supplements are ordered

NURSING CARE

Nursing Assessment

The mental and physical activities of manic persons vary with the severity of the mood disturbance.

Physical Activity

Hyperactivity (moving rapidly from one activity to another, bustling about, restlessness, pacing, fidgeting); limited ability to complete tasks owing to distractibility; eyes bright;

---

*Serum lithium level determination is made before initiating lithium therapy, especially if the patient was formerly receiving medication. Normally no lithium is present without medication. After therapy is initiated, serum levels are examined frequently (e.g., every other day until level has stabilized and just before a lithium dose). Therapeutic serum lithium levels are 0.6 to 1.2 mEq/L. Toxic symptoms may occur at slightly more than or even at therapeutic levels. Early signs of lithium intoxication are diarrhea, vomiting, drowsiness, polyuria, and weakness. If hypothyroidism occurs with lithium treatment, thyroid supplement eliminates the condition.

face flushed; head erect; animated facial expression; increased metabolism; unrestrained playfulness and mischievousness; uninhibited activity (singing, dancing, and so on); expansive gesturing; dramatic self-expression in movement; colorful appearance (wearing bright colors, jewelry); telephone abuse (calls at all hours); acting out of impulses; sexual acting out without discretion; alcohol abuse; giving money and possessions away; assaultiveness, especially when requests are denied and limits are set; violation of rules; abusiveness; destruction of belongings or bedclothes; violent motor excitement in severely disturbed patients

Thought Processes

Enhanced sensory acuity (stimulated by other people, objects, and environment); flight of ideas (skipping from one idea to another without completing any); distractibility; expansive, vivid, intense thoughts; impaired judgment; intact memory and orientation to person, place, and time (except when severely disturbed); lack of motivation to change based on feeling well; self-confidence, self-centeredness; enthusiasm; self-will; overvaluing of abilities and performance; projection of responsibility onto others; loose associations evidenced in incoherence; paranoid ideation (emerges from anger); arrogance; haughtiness; vengeful ideas; criticism of others; delusions of grandeur (false beliefs of power, wealth, achievements; wish-fulfilling type); clang association of thoughts (words with similar sounds but no relation of meaning, such as ring, ding, and ling); loss of contact with reality; clouded consciousness; visual and auditory hallucinations when severe

Communication

Loquacity to logorrhea; pressured rapid speech; speaking with vigor, excitement, animation, emphasis; flowery, witty, loud, lewd, or pompous speech; superficial content; manipulativeness (pleas and threats, praise and deflation, ingratiating manner, excuses, bargaining, demanding, deception, verbal abuse, trying to extend limits)

Affect

Labile mood (elation, euphoria, exhilaration, irritability, anger, laughter, cheerfulness, tearfulness, tremulousness, depression, sadness)

Social Interactions

Appearance of warmth and likability; entertaining, humorous affect; joking, making others the butt of joke; fear of interpersonal intimacy; meddling; interference with and intrusion in others' interaction; attempts to dominate others; exploitation of others' vulnerable areas; destructiveness in group interactions

Self-Care

Obliviousness concerning infections and other physical illness as disturbance increases; neglect of personal needs and grooming

Nutrition

Decrease in appetite but no major weight loss; dehydration possible with hyperactivity

Family Processes

Promises to partner made and broken; demeaning of family with anger and blame; family conflicts and instability; spouse perceives patient as spiteful, lacks understanding and knowledge of condition, and has diminished self-esteem

Nursing Dx & Intervention

Nursing care should be implemented selectively based on severity of symptoms and presenting behaviors. Nurses need to be alert to their own responses to these patients and their behavior. These patients can evoke frustration and anger in nurses because of their hyperactivity, verbal abuse, and attempts to manipulate staff.

*Hyperactivity** related to psychologic and social influences and biochemical factors

- Assess degree of hyperactivity and factors that influence it.
- Assess for abuse of substances.
- Provide quiet, nonstimulating environment *to prevent escalation of excitement.*
- If patient is highly excited, restrict him from the general patient population areas *to avoid stimulation and the possibility of aggression toward others and abuse by other patients.*
- Explain restrictions simply and make use of distractibility.
- Permit patient on unit for brief periods as excitement decreases *to adapt to stimulation and less structure.*
- Begin to develop a supportive relationship through consistent, frequent interpersonal exchanges.
- Administer medication as prescribed *to begin treatment of mania.*
- Be certain patient swallows oral medication; *to set limits,* do not allow patient to bargain to take medication later.
- Monitor for effects and possible adverse reactions to medication *to prevent toxicity.*
- Explain the effects and the side effects of medication when condition stabilizes and patient is able to hear instruction *to increase compliance.*
- Discuss the importance of maintenance dose of medication and ongoing compliance (be aware that patient is concerned about losing sense of well-being).
- As excitement begins to decrease, involve patient in gross motor activities such as walking and exercise. Be aware that activities often increase excitement rather than produce tranquility and fatigue.
- *To set firm, consistent limits on behavior,* give short explanation as needed. Staff members need to understand

---

*Non-NANDA Nursing Diagnosis

and conform to uniform limits. Encourage patient, when he or she is able, to set his or her own limits on behavior, consistent with treatment goals.

- Allow patient opportunity to express anger about restriction in an appropriate way; if anger is inappropriate, use distraction *to change focus.*
- Gradually help integrate patient into general unit milieu; be alert for overstimulation.
- As patient is able, assist him or her to identify frequency, duration, and type of patient's mood changes *to learn to detect subtle changes and patterns indicating mood disturbances.*
- Explain illness and treatment to patient *to deal with chronicity and cyclic nature of illness and to increase self-awareness and compliance with treatment regimen.*

Risk for violence: self-directed or directed at others related to manic state excitement

- Assess potential for aggressiveness and suicide potential.
- Be alert for possible physical aggression against other patients and staff. If patient is in general unit area, remove him from situation, giving short, firm directions *to provide a "time out."*
- Use distraction before aggressiveness escalates.
- Protect patient from other patients' aggressiveness and pranks *to prevent him from being verbally or physically abused.*
- If necessary, obtain an order for medication as needed (e.g., haloperidol) *to decrease aggressiveness.*
- Evaluate patient for suicide potential. If patient is suicidal, institute precautions.
- Encourage patient, when able, to identify and accept angry feelings *to increase self-understanding.*
- Encourage use of a problem-solving approach *to relate feelings to events that evoked them and develop appropriate ways to resolve issues.*
- Help patient to attend occupational therapy activities and recreational activities when ready and as prescribed.
- Provide opportunities to talk about activities *to resolve problem areas.*
- Encourage patient to identify enjoyable activities.
- Direct patient to appropriate activities, such as punching bag or exercise, *to discharge energies.*

Impaired verbal communication related to flight of ideas

- Assess patient's communication patterns and content.
- When patient's speech is pressured, rapid, and loud, respond in soft, assertive voice, make short statements, and speak slowly *to help calm patient.*
- Respond to appropriate humor, but be careful not to escalate excitement and hostility.
- When patient is able, explore inappropriate humor. For example, when humor is inconsistent with content, assist patient to express himself directly.

- Let patient know what you will do and will not do in interactions and in the treatment plan when patient makes requests *to maintain consistent limits.*
- Maintain limits even when requests appear reasonable *to be firm and consistent.*
- Schedule frequent brief sessions with patient during an acute phase (e.g., 15 minutes) *to begin to develop a relationship.* Increase length of sessions as excitement decreases and patient is able to respond.
- When patient verbally strikes out at you, help patient identify underlying feelings. If patient continues, communicate your discomfort and let patient know that you will leave if abuse continues. Leave if patient does not stop.
- Practice assertiveness skills *to give patient sense of control and influence.*

Altered nutrition: less than body requirements related to hyperactivity

- Assess eating patterns and food and fluid intake.
- When patient is highly excited, provide food in small unbreakable containers or finger foods *to eat while standing or pacing.* If necessary, provide food in liquid form.
- Ensure that patient's fluid intake is more than 1000 ml *to prevent lithium toxicity.*
- Explain to patient the importance of good nutrition with normal sodium and fluid intake.
- If oral intake of fluids is to be restricted before medical treatments, such as surgery or laboratory tests, inform physician so intravenous fluids can be given *to prevent dehydration and lithium toxicity.*
- Have dietitian provide additional information on diet as needed.

Other related nursing diagnoses Altered thought processes related to altered mental status; ineffective individual coping related to labile mood; self-care deficit (bathing and hygiene and dressing and grooming) related to labile mood; sleep pattern disturbance related to excessive excitement; altered family processes related to family's lack of understanding of the illness.

Patient Education/Home Care Planning

1. Ensure that the patient verbalizes understanding of the chronic, cyclic nature of the illness and the importance of complying with the medical regimen.
2. Give the patient a list of the effects and adverse effects of medication and the need for regular assessment of serum lithium (e.g., at 1- to 2-month intervals when stabilized). Explain to the patient the signs and symptoms that should be reported to the physician, and provide the patient with phone number(s) of the provider.
3. Give a list of the signs and symptoms of increasing mood disturbances in depressive and manic behaviors to report to the physician.
4. Explain to the patient the importance of a normal diet and adequate daily fluid intake.

Evaluation

Patient attains persistent mood level nearing healthy state for self Patient sits quietly for periods of time. Patient accepts realistic limits and delays. Patient verbalizes knowledge of illness and treatment and makes plans to continue treatment regimen after discharge. Patient states major effects and adverse effects of medications.

Patient demonstrates decrease in aggressiveness Patient verbalizes beginning awareness of angry feelings and beginning skills in resolving issues.

Patient carries on normal conversations with others Patient speaks in a well-modulated manner. Patient practices assertiveness skills to deal with events and to communicate needs directly. Patient continues to work on listening skills with others.

Patient demonstrates knowledge of adequate nutrition Patient verbalizes accurate information on good nutrition. Patient identifies importance of adequate daily sodium and fluid intake.

■ DEPRESSIVE DISORDERS

Depression is an abnormal mood state in which a person characteristically has a sense of hopelessness, helplessness, worthlessness and despair, morbid thoughts, and psychomotor retardation or agitation.

Depression may occur as the polarity of mania in the bipolar disorder. It frequently occurs as a unipolar disorder, in which the person experiences depressive symptoms with no manic episodes.

The common diagnostic categories of unipolar depression identified in the DSM-IV[2] are listed below:

Major depressive disorder, single episode—severe symptoms of depression and loss of interest and pleasure in self and environment nearly every day for most of the day for at least 2 weeks. Loss of energy, feelings of worthlessness and hopelessness, decreased ability to think or concentrate, and psychomotor retardation or agitation are some symptoms that are present. The person has no manic episode and has only one major depressive episode with a return to premorbid functioning. Untreated depression typically lasts for 6 months or more.

Major depressive disorder, recurrent—the person has two or more major depressive episodes with a separation between episodes of at least 2 months, and with no previous manic states.

Dysthymic disorder—the adult has a chronic, milder depressive disturbance than the above almost every day for most of the day for at least 2 years (duration for children or adolescents is at least 1 year).

Some specifiers for the most recent disorder include moderate, severe with psychotic features, severe without psychotic features, in partial or full remission, and chronic.

For those with recurrent seasonal depressive episodes or bipolar disorders, the specifier "with seasonal pattern" may be included. The time of year is a feature of this, with depression most frequently occurring in the fall or winter and alleviating in spring.

Prevalence

Depression is the single most frequently occurring psychiatric condition in the general population. Because of social and occupational discrimination, people are resistant to seek treatment for depression and other psychiatric conditions; therefore, many go undiagnosed and untreated.[15] The incidence of major depression in women ranges from 20% to 25%, and in men from 5% to 12%; the milder form, dysthymia, is approximately 6%.[2,38] The suicide rate is approximately 15%. The onset of depression occurs usually in the twenties, but it may begin in childhood, in infancy, or in old age.

Population at Risk

Some groups are more susceptible to depression than others. Women are commonly at greater risk, by 2 to 1, for depression than men, although in prepubertal children the incidence may be equal among both sexes. The disorder is one and one-half to three times more common among first-degree biologic relatives than it is in the general population.[2]

The increased prevalence of depression in females is partly caused by traditional socialization practices for girls, such as reinforcement of dependency and passivity; males more often are trained to be self-reliant and active. In addition to the traditional roles of mother and wife, many women are expected to work outside the home. However, the role of mother and wife are frequently deprecated, and achievements at work are generally given fewer rewards than those of men.[45]

Depressive symptoms in the elderly are often missed and incorrectly attributed to organic disorders. Because mild depression evidenced in sulkiness, withdrawal from social activities, and restlessness is common among adolescents because of maturation crises, the more severe depressions may not be identified.[2]

Types of Depression

Two subtypes of depression are exogenous or reactive, and endogenous.[35,38] Reactive depression, also referred to as secondary depression, is precipitated by something outside the person. Reactive depressions can range from mild to severe and may be in response to stressors such as loss of a loved one, environmental catastrophe, divorce, or a medical condition such as stroke, chronic fatigue syndrome, chronic pain, myocardial infarct, or cancer. Some drugs, such as benzodiazepines, oral contraceptives, some antihypertensives, alcoholic beverages, and cocaine withdrawal, may also cause depression.[15,38]

The second subtype is endogenous, primary, or biological. It arises from within the person and may emerge seemingly spontaneously. The endogenous type may be caused by genetic or biochemical factors such as altered neurotransmitter functioning.[35,38] Depressions of this type may be more severe than reactive depressions.

When depressions are divided into exogenous and endogenous, few identifiable symptoms are distinguishable. Patterns of symptoms and life experiences were related only slightly. Because most persons can identify some past trauma or unhappy event, deciding if a depression had a precipitant may be difficult if not impossible.[35] However, these subtypes have broad but controversial support even with problems in distinguishable differences.

Degrees of Depression

Mild depression is often undiagnosed. Those with severe depression are easier to identify. Some symptoms of mild and severe depression, differentiated by Arieti and Bemporad,[6] are listed below:

Mild
- Unpleasant feelings about self and the environment
- Self-sacrificing, especially in relation to giving to others
- Inhibition of normal pleasurable activities
- Inhibition of spontaneous behavior
- Extra effort needed to concentrate
- Preoccupation with trivial failures and underestimating ability
- Pessimistic outlook toward life
- Self-reproach and irritability for not living up to an ideal standard
- Dependence on others for gratification
- Somatic symptoms

Severe
- Utter despair and hopelessness
- Sense of emptiness
- Unrelieved sense of guilt and feeling of worthlessness
- Severe immobility or agitated behavior that is purposeless and lacks conscious control
- Catastrophic expectations
- Lack of interest in self and environment
- Retarded thought processes to process and respond to stimuli
- Retardation of bodily processes
- Preoccupation with bodily functions
- Delusional thinking that becomes severe when contact with reality is greatly impaired or lost

Family Issues

Family members may feel sympathy and be supportive of the depressed person, but as the depression continues and even deepens, the family may become discouraged. All of their help does nothing to lift the person's mood. Because the depressed person makes known his or her feelings of helplessness, despair, and emptiness, family members may begin to experience similar feelings that may turn into anger and resentment. Family members require knowledge about depression and their ill member in particular. They also need emotional support and guidance through family therapy including the patient to learn to communicate with each other and cope with their concerns.

•••••• Psychopathology

Biochemical abnormalities are found in depressed persons, but none are specific for diagnosing major depressive disorder. There are changes in structural brain images, reduced metabolism in the frontal cortex, abnormalities in sleep electroencephalogram (EEG) in 40% to 60% of outpatients and 90% of inpatients, and alterations in the neurotransmitters. Some of the neurotransmitters that are deficient include norepinephrine and serotonin. Other changes found include acetylcholine, dopamine, noradrenaline, and gamma-aminobutyric acid. Changes in corticotropin in 50% to 60% of persons with major depression are significant so that no suppression of dexamethasone, a form of cortisone, occurs in the dexamethasone suppression test.[35,38]

Some of the newer class of antidepressants, the selective serotonin re-uptake inhibitors (SSRI), such as fluoxetine (Prozac) and sertraline (Zoloft), are especially noted for increasing the serotonin level, with a response rate of about 85%. Imipramine (Tofranil), one of the first antidepressants, may increase norepinephrine and serotonin to a lesser degree and has about a 57% response rate.[21,35] Caution is necessary with all depressive patients because of the possibility of suicide, especially as the depression deepens and as it begins to lift. These are times when the patient has enough energy to carry out a suicide plan.

Psychoanalytic Theory

Psychoanalysts theorize that persons experience ambivalent feelings of love and hate toward a former love object. Psychic energy (libido) is withdrawn from the lost object; hate or aggression felt for the love object is turned inward toward the self. The person then feels worthless, guilty, and depressed.[18]

Interpersonal Theory

Interpersonal theorists believe that depressive patterns develop within an interpersonal context and may begin in childhood. The child introjects an exaggerated sense of duty and responsibility. The duty and responsibility along with dependence on others are often emphasized by parents so that the child is unaware of self and his or her own resources. The inability to live up to parents' expectations provokes anxiety in the child; the anxiety becomes guilt, self-criticism, and lowered self-esteem. The child may experience many mild episodes of depression throughout life with no identifiable major stressor.[6]

Cognitive Theory

Cognitive and behavioral theorists hold similar beliefs that depression is a consequence of faulty logic. Persons blame themselves for actual or perceived loss of an object and become self-critical and self-rejecting. They generalize their feelings of self-blame and view themselves as failures, inferior, and helpless and as having bleak futures. Successes and achievements are disowned. Behaviorists view depression as a consequence of negative reinforcement or no reinforcement of positive, successful behavior.[9]

•••••• Diagnostic Studies and Findings

SMAC To screen for general medical causes for depression

Thyroid function tests To rule out abnormal thyroid, especially in depressed women 50 and over

Dexamethasone Suppression Test (DST) Dexamethasone, 1 mg administered orally at bedtime, and on the following day specimens obtained for serum cortisol at 4 PM and 11 PM (if outpatient, 4 PM specimen only); serum cortisol greater than 5 µg/100 ml at either 4 or 11 PM is indicative of depression (administration of dexamethasone, a synthetic steroid similar to cortisol, suppresses the adrenal corticotropin hormone in most normal persons); NOTE: This test is experimental, with false-negative and false-positive findings; positive DST findings have also been present in other mental disorders[35,41]; weakness and nausea may occur as mild side effects from dexamethasone

Electrocardiogram To rule out cardiopathy; this is particularly important with most antidepressant medications

Urinalysis To rule out urologic problems and other medical disorders

•••••• Multidisciplinary Plan

Medications

Fluoxetine (Prozac) 20 mg initially, po, qAM. If no reduction in symptoms after several weeks, dosage may be increased.

Fluoxetine (Prozac) 10 mg initially, po, qAM, for the elderly. May increase dosage in a few weeks if symptoms do not begin to abate.

Full antidepressant effect may take 4 weeks or more.

If depression is part of a bipolar disorder, the antidepressant may be prescribed with the addition of:

Lithium carbonate, 300 mg, tid, po; serum lithium levels must be assessed frequently until stable, then at 1 to 2 month intervals, to determine therapeutic serum levels before administration of next lithium dose; therapeutic serum lithium levels are 0.6 to 1.2 mEq/L; if bipolar disorder, observe closely to identify rapid switch to manic phase.

If patient has a psychotic depression, combined antipsychotic and antidepressant medications are much more effective than an antidepressant alone.[38]

General Management

Electroconvulsive therapy, *only* if patient does not respond to antidepressant or if suicidal risk is severe

Occupational therapy

Recreational therapy

NURSING CARE

Nursing Assessment

The severity and types of symptoms vary with each patient, with no one symptom experienced by all with depression.

Affect

Extreme sadness; despair; painful dejection; tearfulness; irritability; anxiety; feeling of emptiness

Activities

Low energy; fatigue; lack of ability or motivation to perform tasks; slow movements; eyes downcast and avoidance of eye contact; agitated, purposeless behavior evidenced by pacing and restlessness; substance abuse (e.g., alcohol)

Self-Care

Lack of interest and energy to perform activities of daily living such as bathing, dressing, and hygiene

Nutrition

Lack of appetite or interest in food (occasionally increased appetite); indigestion; weight loss, usually not critical but may be when condition is very severe or psychotic

Bowel Elimination

Constipation

Sleep Pattern

Inability to fall asleep, especially with anxiety, or waking early in morning; restless sleep; hypersomnia, occasionally through most of the day, owing to fatigue or withdrawal

Power

Sense of lack of power or control; hopelessness, usually greatest when awakening in the morning; helplessness; feeling that nothing the patient can do will make a difference

Self-Harm

Seriousness of suicidal risk: suicidal thoughts and threats, previous self-harming behavior, statements indicating intent and development of a plan

Thought Processes

Morbid thoughts; worry; narrow and repetitive range of thoughts; forgetfulness and inability to concentrate; self-rejection and criticism of self and others; somatic complaints; delusions about body and environment, especially bizarre in severe depression; negative view of self, environment, and the future; failures exaggerated; achievements disowned; paranoid ideation

Communication

Impaired ability to process and respond to verbal stimuli; slow thinking; slow speech; low voice; monotonous tone; limited ability to concentrate

Social Interactions

Withdrawal from social interactions and activities because of sense of unworthiness; limited social skills; loneliness; apathy concerning others

Nursing Dx & Intervention

Nursing care should be implemented selectively based on severity of symptoms and presenting behaviors.

Risk for violence: self-directed or directed at others related to sense of hopelessness and depression

- Assess for suicidal thoughts and self-destructive behaviors.
- Institute suicide precautions: safe environment, removal of harmful objects, and close observation *to prevent suicide attempts.*
- Begin to establish trusting, supportive relationship *to let patient know you care and are concerned.*
- Schedule frequent, brief therapeutic periods daily so they are tolerable to patient and nurse; schedule longer sessions as depression lifts and patient is able to tolerate more *to develop relationship.*
- Speak slowly, using short sentences *to increase patient's ability to attend to and comprehend words.* As patient is able, assist patient to identify abilities and communicate hopes for the future *to reinforce resources.*
- Continue close observation as depression lifts or as depression deepens because patient has energy to attempt suicide; observe for verbal and nonverbal clues to self-harm.
- Administer medication as ordered.
- Briefly describe the medicine's effects and side effects initially.
- When patient has improved, teach effects of medications and importance of compliance *to counteract depressive symptoms.*

Ineffective individual coping related to inadequate coping method

- Assess strengths and coping strategies.
- When patient is agitated, accept pacing and inability to sit still.
- *To let patient know of your presence,* say, for example, "I am here and want to help you."
- Discuss and assist patient with diversionary techniques when restless, such as an activity *to decrease emotional discomfort;* encourage patient to practice the techniques *to help strengthen patient's healthy strategies for dealing with inappropriate feelings.*
- Practice relaxation exercises, such as slow, deep breathing while focusing on number 1, *to promote relaxation and sense of control.*
- Help patient to identify positive attributes about self and about achievements *so that patient can begin to accept self realistically and develop a positive self-view.*
- Identify patient's own resources and social support system of family, friends, and community resources *to reinforce strengths.*
- Assist patient in developing interests and social skills *to increase self-confidence.*
- Practice with patient how to ask for and accept help *to increase sense of control.*

- Practice with patient how to accept others' refusals to give help without the patient's feeling rejected, guilty, or self-critical *to reinforce the idea that refusals are not rejection of patient.*
- Role-play assertiveness techniques *to give patient sense of control and to let others know needs and desires.*

Altered thought processes related to psychologic conflicts and psychomotor retardation

- Assess thought processes and quality of cognition.
- *To interrupt ruminations,* suggest diversionary activities if attempts fail to help patient appropriately focus on topics.
- Assist patient in monitoring subject change *to make decisions about changing subject a conscious choice.*
- Encourage patient to think about self and experiences realistically *to identify and accept positive attributes.*
- Assist patient to identify relationship between incorrect thoughts and feelings of depression.
- Help patient identify the stimulus or event *to examine inappropriateness of faulty thinking about behavior and self to correct misinterpretations and negative views of self.*
- Discuss and practice role-playing and problem-solving approach to problematic events and evaluate the possible consequences of alternative solutions *to learn effective methods to resolve issues.*
- Help patient to anticipate problems that may be encountered after discharge *to identify possible responses to issues and consequences of each solution.*

Other related nursing diagnoses Impaired verbal communication related to delusional thinking; self-care (bathing and hygiene and dressing and grooming) deficit related to lack of interest in self; altered nutrition: less than body requirements related to lack of appetite; constipation related to retarded body processes; altered patterns of urinary elimination related to retarded body processes; sleep pattern disturbance related to severe depression; powerlessness related to lack of interest in self or environment; social isolation related to sense of worthlessness; altered family processes related to depression

---

Patient Education/Home Care Planning

1. Give the patient a list of major effects and adverse effects of medications to report to the therapist or physician and phone number of provider.
2. Ensure that patient verbalizes understanding of his or her depression and the importance of adhering to the treatment plan after discharge.
3. Reinforce the use of formal and informal social support systems for help (e.g., write down the crisis center's name and telephone number, as well as the names of significant others to call for help).
4. Encourage the continued use of problem-solving techniques to examine and correct faulty thinking and reinforce self-supports and resources.

Evaluation

Patient demonstrates relief of symptoms of depression and hopelessness Patient verbalizes sense of hope about the present and future and the decline of depressive symptoms. Patient lists major effects and adverse effects of medications and describes the self-administration procedure he or she will use after discharge. Patient has made plans to continue treatment regimen after discharge.

Patient demonstrates increased coping skills Patient practices increased ability to identify needs, to ask others for help, and to use self-support procedures in a more self-confident manner. Patient uses increased social skills in interactions with others.

Patient demonstrates increased ability to correct impaired thinking Patient expresses an increased awareness of the relationships among experiences, thoughts, and depressive feelings. Patient practices use of problem-solving approach to correct misconceptions about self and the future.

■ ANXIETY DISORDERS

Anxiety disorders are a group of disturbances in which anxiety is the predominant symptom experienced or defended against by avoiding the anxiety-provoking object or developing a mechanism such as a compulsion to protect the self against anxiety.

Anxiety is a subjective experience that can be inferred by observing the person's behavior and physiologic responses and by subjective reports. Apprehension, dread, and intense alertness to an unspecified source of danger are symptoms of anxiety. It may be a mild to severe response to an unmet expectation. In mild anxiety the person becomes alert and is able to observe more of himself or herself and of his or her environment. In moderate anxiety, the person is selectively inattentive to stimuli outside a narrow field. Learning can occur in these levels of anxiety.[34] When a person experiences severe anxiety or a state of panic, no learning occurs unless anxiety is reduced because of reduced perception of stimuli and because of responses that are mainly automatic relief behaviors (see Emergency Alert box). Unlike fear, which is a response to an actual object or event, anxiety is a response to no specific source or actual object.

Prevalence

Normal anxiety is common in the general population; in fact, without it people would be unlikely to be productive or creative. It is proportionate to a given threat and is used constructively to alter a situation or object. The incidence of pathologic anxiety, which is disproportionate to a threat and can paralyze a person, is estimated at about 3%.[2]

Population at Risk

Gender differences occur among the various types of anxiety disorders. In generalized anxiety disorders women are somewhat more frequently diagnosed than men. Women are three times more likely to have panic disorder with agoraphobia than men. Obsessive-compulsive disorder is equally common in men and women.[2]

Some anxiety disorders have an onset in childhood and adolescence and others in late adolescence to mid-30s, with some occurring after age 45.

The biology of anxiety disorders is mainly obscure, although it appears that heterogeneous factors are involved. First degree biologic relatives of people with an anxiety disorder have a greater chance of developing an anxiety disorder than those without such a relative.[2] Biochemical factors, including neurotransmitters, appear to play a role in anxiety disorders. For example, an excess of serotonin is found in persons with obsessive-compulsive disorder.[48] Brain imaging techniques suggest increased metabolism in the orbitofrontal regions in patients with obsessive-compulsive disorder (OCD).[36] Hormones and other biochemicals such as cortisone seem to be involved, but specifics are often lacking or inconsistent.

Psychologic and interpersonal factors that predispose a person to anxiety disorders include early psychic trauma such as separation anxiety in childhood, pathogenic parent-child relationships, pathogenic family patterns, disturbed interpersonal relationships, and loss of social supports. Other experiences that may contribute to the disorders include threats to one's values, stressors that interfere with achievement of important goals, and exhaustion of adaptive coping resources.[2]

The person may experience chronic anxiety that is punctuated at intervals by acute anxiety attacks—that is, panic states.

! EMERGENCY ALERT

ANXIETY DISORDERS

Persons with anxiety disorders experience anxiety as the predominant reaction when confronted with a particular object or situation and develop compulsive mechanisms to avoid the anxiety-provoking object or situation.

Assessment

- Apprehension greatly disproportionate to external risk; dread; terror; blocking; panic; incapacitation; immobilizing fear; impaired memory, attention, and concentration; irrational fear with avoidance of a dreaded activity, event, and/or object
- Physiologic reactions with no functional pathophysiology, e.g., heart palpitations, tachycardia, dyspnea, gasping for air, heartburn, lightheadedness, tremors, generalized weakness, nausea, vomiting, insomnia, elevated blood pressure and pulse, urinary frequency

Interventions

- Stay with patient during a severe anxiety/panic attack. As patient is able to listen, suggest slow, deep breathing to increase oxygen supply and energy. Breathe with patient to demonstrate technique.
- Administer medication as prescribed to decrease anxiety and sense of helplessness.

These panic attacks are sudden and intense and may subside in a few minutes or last an hour or more. The person may have them several times a day, once a week, or less than once a month. The attacks occur during the day or night. The person may awake from a sound sleep with intense apprehension or terror. During the attack the person has fears of imminent death or physical catastrophe. Other fears include humiliation or appearing foolish or stupid. The fears arise in the absence of any apparent cause such as marked physical exertion or a life-threatening event.

Having obsessive-compulsive behavior is not necessarily pathologic. This behavior provides the person with the energy to accomplish tasks and responsibilities. When the behaviors become time-consuming and interfere with routine activities of daily living and occupational and social activities, they are no longer normal. Obsessions are persistent, intrusive, and inappropriate ideas and thoughts; and compulsions are repetitive behaviors that reduce anxiety, are time-consuming, and interfere with normal activities.[2,36] Persons may have more obsessions than compulsions or may be compelled to carry out an activity such as handwashing with the obsession of germs on their hands after touching a doorknob. "Checking" behavior is another type of compulsion, e.g., the obsession may be that the person did not disconnect a kitchen appliance which compels him to return to the kitchen to "check" or to check by visualizing the act of disconnecting the appliance. Anxiety will be experienced until the compulsion is performed.

Perceptions and interpretations of threatening situations influence how a person responds. Some react disproportionately to the threat by panicking or use nonadaptive defenses such as repression, denial, displacement, and somatization. Some use chemicals such as alcohol. The response is related in part to the person's ego strengths and the types of coping strategies used.

In addition to anxiety disorders, anxiety occurs in other mental disorders such as somatization disorders, schizophrenic disorders, psychophysiologic conditions, and various depressive disorders.[2]

Medical disorders must be ruled out because symptoms of these disorders can be confused with symptoms of anxiety. For example, in cardiopulmonary disorders, symptoms may include angina pectoris, palpitations, and breathing difficulties. Endocrine disorders such as hyperthyroidism are characterized by rapid pulse, perspiration, tremors, and restlessness. Some medicines such as epinephrine, antidepressants, thyroid tablets, and dextroamphetamine produce symptoms associated with anxiety.

•••••• Psychopathology

Psychoanalytic Theory

In psychoanalytic theory, anxiety, an intrapsychic phenomenon, develops as an automatic response to the ego's perception of a traumatic situation—that is, the ego's inability to master or discharge the overwhelming influx of stimuli. It initially develops in infancy when the ego is too weak and immature to deal with the stimuli. As the young child learns to anticipate dangerous stimuli that originate usually from the id (drives) but also from external situations, he or she reacts to avoid trauma. The maturing ego uses psychic energy (libido) to cope with dangerous events. The dangers and concomitant anxiety are characteristic of situations children face, particularly during the first 6 years of life, and persist throughout life in varying degrees and to an excessive degree in psychoneurotic conditions. Unconscious conflicts are present in all pathologic anxiety.[36]

The ego, the reality principle of the personality, attempts to neutralize the energy of the dangerous id by dealing with anxiety rationally and by developing healthy adaptive strategies, including identification and sublimation. When the ego is unsuccessful in dealing with anxiety adaptively, it overuses defense mechanisms. Less healthy defenses and their overuse require continuous expenditure of psychic energy and decrease the ego's strength. Since repression is part of all defense mechanisms, experiences that are repressed continue to operate unconsciously by distorting reality.

Interpersonal Theory

In interpersonal theory, anxiety is viewed as developing within an interpersonal context. It is transmitted from the mother in infancy; later it is a response to real or imagined threats to the person's self-system. Anxiety is experienced as apprehension and discomfort, which the person attempts to avoid by developing defensive strategies.[50] The self-system begins to develop to protect the person by excluding painful, threatening experiences from awareness. However, as the organization of the self-system becomes more complex in late childhood, experiences that provoked severe anxiety are out of awareness of or dissociated from the rest of the personality. The person is unable to examine dissociated experiences, correct distortions, and integrate these experiences into the personality. The dissociated material impairs the person's ability to perceive, remember, and think rationally. Although difficult, persons can recall, under certain conditions, significant aspects of situations that provoked anxiety to increase awareness of themselves and their environment.[50]

Cognitive Theory

Severe anxiety or panic is a sudden, overwhelming reaction to a perceived threat that is viewed as overpowering. Unlike depression, which is related to actual or perceived loss, anxiety is related to anticipated loss.

At the core of severe anxiety are faulty cognitive patterns that evoke a sense of vulnerability and helplessness because the person magnifies weaknesses and catastrophizes actual or imaginary threats to the self.[8] An anxious person has an impaired ability to examine repetitive, dangerous thoughts logically and evaluate them objectively. He or she may generalize dangers to almost any other stimulus or perceived changes in his or her world. Anxiety evoked in response to an initial danger is also evoked in response to the generalizations. The person responds automatically to dangerous thoughts and their generalizations without examining their validity, which leads the person to feel trapped in overwhelming situations. Correction of faulty thinking initiates appropriate emotional responses to perceived dangers that do not negate feelings about the self.[8]

••••• Diagnostic Studies and Findings

SMAC   To screen for various medical conditions
Complete Blood count   To rule out infection and other medical disorders
Thyroid function tests   To screen for thyroid dysfunction
Electrocardiogram (ECG)   To screen for cardiopathy
Routine urinalysis   To screen for urologic problems and other medical conditions

••••• Multidisciplinary Plan

Medications

Alprazolam (Xanax), 0.5 mg po tid as an initial dose that may be increased cautiously to maximum total daily dose of 4 mg, in divided doses for severe anxiety; 0.25 mg po bid for elderly patients; the action of the medication, a central nervous system depressant, is to decrease symptoms of anxiety; when anxiety levels decrease, dosage is decreased gradually because convulsions may occur after abrupt discontinuation, especially of high doses. Patients with an obsessive-compulsive disorder may be more successfully treated with a selective serotonin re-uptake inhibitor (SSRI), such as fluoxetine (Prozac), or an antiobsessional medication such as clomipramine (Anafanil), a tricyclic antidepressant.[38]

General Management

Occupational therapy
Recreational therapy

NURSING CARE

Nursing Assessment

Not all dysfunctional responses are experienced by all anxious persons.

Affect

Apprehension; dread; terror; tearfulness; sobbing; irritability; anger; helplessness; frustration; sometimes laughter; nervousness

Thoughts

Scattering of thoughts or focus on details; preoccupation with self, behavior, and bodily functions; lack of confidence in abilities; low self-esteem; worry; anticipation of adversity; jealousy; envy of others; lack of control to effect or influence outcome; impaired sense of responsibility for self and behavior; sense of worthlessness and rejection by others; distractibility; indecisiveness; vacillation, especially in conflict; forgetfulness; somatization

Communication

Stuttering; blocking; rapid, pressured speech; selective inattention to messages; frequent requests (e.g., in hospital, for water, medication, information on physician's visit, or laboratory tests); repetitive questioning about treatments, procedures, activities, and so on; petty complaining

Physical

Dizziness; light-headedness; hyperventilation; chest pain; difficulty breathing; palpitation; perspiration; weakness; heartburn; flushing or pallor of face; tachycardia; muscle ache, especially in the neck and back; jitteriness; tremulousness; restlessness to agitation; pacing; dry mouth; dilated pupils; blurred vision; darting eyes; headache; accident proneness; impaired sexual functioning

Nutrition

Increased (occasionally decreased) appetite; nausea; belching

Bowel and Bladder Elimination

Diarrhea or occasionally constipation; urinary urgency and frequency

Sleep Pattern

Insomnia; difficulty falling asleep; restless or interrupted sleep

Social Interactions

Discomfort interacting with others because of fear of rejection or humiliation; decreased social activities because of fear of failure, especially in competitive activities

Nursing Dx & Intervention

Before severely anxious patients can learn, anxiety levels must be reduced. Anxiety is contagious, affecting others by increasing their anxiety. Nurses need to be aware of their responses to anxiety and how they deal with their own feelings to be able to intervene therapeutically with patients. They can use changes in their anxiety level as indicators of changes in a patient's anxiety.

Anxiety related to unmet needs and threat of a loss or change

- Assess anxiety level and how it is manifested.
- Provide a nondemanding, comfortable environment *to decrease stressors.*
- Begin to establish a supportive, safe relationship *to prevent threats to self-esteem.*
- Allow temporary dependence.
- Remain with patient during panic attack *to decrease terror.*
- Acknowledge painfulness of patient's feelings *to convey understanding of his or her sense of helplessness.*
- Listen to patient's somatic complaints initially and slowly help patient relate it to anxiety level *to connect somatic symptoms with anxiety.*
- Inhibit patient's ventilation of feelings if escalation to a nonconstructive level occurs; change focus (e.g., to comfort measures, such as offering juice) *to decrease overwhelming discomfort.*

- Assist patient in breathing slowly and deeply; breathe with patient as needed *to demonstrate technique.*
- Briefly explain that breathing slowly at regularly scheduled times and when anxiety increases will help patient *to learn to relax and increase the oxygen supply and energy.*
- Administer medication as ordered. Elaborate on effects and side effects of medication including need for gradual discontinuation of medication *to promote informed participation in and compliance with medical regimen.*
- Encourage patient to monitor his or her own restlessness and engage in diversionary activities such as exercise, walking, and table tennis, *to decrease anxiety and to develop a sense of control over feelings.*
- Encourage patient to identify and realistically accept strengths and weaknesses *to develop self-supports.*

Altered thought processes related to psychologic conflicts

- Assess cognitive abilities and effects of anxiety on thought processes.
- Speak calmly, using patient's name frequently *to obtain patient's attention.*
- Give clear, concise directions *to ensure that patient is able to comprehend.*
- Assist patient to identify any thoughts he or she had just before anxiety experience *to connect cognitions to anxiety.*
- Begin to help patient to correct misconceptions about experiences before anxiety using problem-solving approach *to alter emotional reaction of anxiety.*
- Encourage patient to become aware of automatic thoughts when anticipating negative experiences and to examine evidence *to learn to monitor own thoughts.*
- Invite patient to reframe events (e.g., to think of his or her boss as a "purring kitten" instead of a "growling lion" and to redefine anxiety as a pleasant, exciting sensation) *to learn to think positively and decrease anxiety.*
- Help patient to anticipate realistically possible negative and positive outcomes of anxiety-evoking events *to learn how to implement remedial actions, as needed.*
- Assist patient to accept abilities *to influence events.*
- Assist patient in setting realistic goals *to prevent a decrease in self-confidence by failure to achieve unrealistic goals.*
- Encourage patient to ask for help in work and home situations *to prevent patient from viewing self as weak or incompetent.*

Impaired verbal communication related to psychologic barriers

- Assess skills and type of impaired communication.
- Initially answer repetitive questions simply and concisely *to help patient decrease anxiety.*
- Inform patient of plans and schedules and write them down so patient can refer to the paper *to assist in remembering, thereby increasing a sense of security.*

- As patient is able, help identify anxiety when patient questions repetitively, has petty complaints, stutters, and blocks *to increase awareness of emotional state.*
- Suggest that patient speak more slowly when stuttering. Encourage patient to breathe slowly and deeply *to increase energy, decrease stuttering and blocking, and be able to complete sentences.*
- Inform patient that saying "I stutter when I get excited or uncomfortable" to others may help him or her *to decrease stuttering and embarrassment.*
- State matter-of-factly that patient will remember blocked material later *to acknowledge patient's strength and abilities.*
- Practice assertiveness skills with patient through role-playing *to increase self-confidence in interactions and social activities.*
- Assist patient to accept positive feelings about interactions with others, and help patient examine interactions in which he or she expects rejection or disapproval *to identify evidence and correct misperceptions.*

Other related nursing diagnoses Altered nutrition: high risk for more than body requirements related to overeating when tense; altered patterns of urinary elimination related to anxiety; diarrhea or constipation related to anxiety and stress; sleep pattern disturbance related to anxious state; social isolation related to dread of social interactions.

Patient Education/Home Care Planning

1. Ensure that patient verbalizes knowledge of disorder and major effects and side effects of antianxiety medications, especially the effects that impair alertness and the dangers of abrupt discontinuation of medication.
2. Ensure that patient understands and practices self-management strategies for decreased anxiety, such as problem-solving methods, relaxation techniques, and diversionary activities, including various physical and social activities.
3. Assist patient to anticipate and deal realistically with potential issues to be faced immediately after discharge.
4. Encourage patient to continue treatment plan after discharge.

Evaluation

Patient evidences relief of severe symptoms Patient verbalizes relationship between anxiety and physical sensations. Patient lists major effects and side effects of medication, including danger of abrupt discontinuation. Patient develops system to ensure accurate self-administration of medication as prescribed after discharge. Patient practices relaxation techniques and engages in diversionary activities to relieve anxiety. Patient schedules appointment with provider to continue treatment plan after discharge.

Patient demonstrates use of problem-solving methods to correct faulty thoughts   Patient practices problem-solving approach to resolve issues and correct automatic, incorrect thoughts. Patient verbalizes a beginning awareness and acceptance of strengths.

Patient evidences increased confidence in communicating with others   Patient practices assertiveness skills and realistically evaluates consequences of interactions. Patient can express self and verbalizes feeling less anxiety when interacting with others.

PERSONALITY DISORDERS

Personality disorders are a category of conditions in which a person evidences enduring personality traits that are inflexible and maladaptive. These traits are stable patterns of perceiving, thinking, and relating to the person's world and self.[2] The inflexibility of the personality may remain unnoticed until adaption to environmental changes are expected of or subjective pressures are experienced by the person. The ten personality disorders are divided into three groups on the basis of their similarities: odd or eccentric, dramatic or erratic, and anxious and fearful.

The borderline personality disorder, one in the erratic or emotional group, is discussed here because its occurrence is increasing; its prevalence among clinic populations with personality disorders is 30% to 60%; and its management creates difficulties for health professionals in all settings.[2]

■ BORDERLINE PERSONALITY DISORDER

Borderline personality disorder is a condition in which the person exhibits enduring patterns of behavior that do not change with experiences.[2] The person may appear to function adequately until exposed to personal or environmental stressors.

Behaviors associated with borderline personality disorder are intolerance to frustration and to being alone, impulsivity in which the person acts destructively toward self and others, abuse of substances, unstable self-image, and instability of affect, with anger or rage the prominent expression rather than anxiety or depression. Anger and hostility are expressed as irritability, sarcasm, demandingness, and projection of feeling onto others. The borderline personality is vulnerable to brief, mild psychotic episodes that are triggered by stress.

Although the person forms intense relationships, he or she has difficulty with intimacy and maintaining close relationships; he or she shifts from idealizing to devaluing others. Being unable to hold an integrated view of self and others with degrees of good and bad, the borderline personality splits objects and thus holds fragmented, polarized views of self or others as either "all good" or "all bad" at any one time.[36] Because of feelings of emptiness, the borderline person avoids being alone and

spends most of his or her time in the presence of others. When alone the person experiences dread, rage, and a sense of abandonment.[39] Through manipulation the person attempts to exploit others to gain control without being rejected.[36]

Distorted perceptions are related to self-centeredness and an inability to empathize with others. Denial is a common ego defense against uncomfortable feelings and relevant past experiences.

When the person is questioned about or confronted with his or her contradictory actions and feelings, he or she uses denial and projection to avoid awareness of himself or herself and his or her behavior.

Hospitalization

The decision to hospitalize a person with a borderline personality disorder is usually based on a crisis, severe anxiety or panic, self-destructive acts including suicidal threats, or transient psychosis (see Emergency Alert box).

While in the hospital the patient evokes contradictory views among the staff of the patient, his or her behavior, and the treatment plan. The strong emotional reactions experienced by staff members are due to their countertransferrence of the patient.[47] Because of the patient's split-object view of self and others, he or she projects different identifications onto each person. Some staff members receive positive projections from the patient and may react in a nurturing, permissive way; other staff members receive negative projections from the patient and may react in a punitive, controlling, and hostile manner. It is important for staff to examine the feelings evoked in them by patients in general, and especially by those with borderline pathology.[47] The staff needs to be aware that the idealizations and denigrations

---

 EMERGENCY ALERT

BORDERLINE PERSONALITY DISORDER

Persons with borderline personality disorders exhibit enduring patterns of behavior that do not change with experiences.

Assessment

- Impulsive, emotionally labile mainly with hostility and rage, shifting polarized views of self and others as idealized or denigrated, demanding, uses projection and denial, and/or intolerance for stress/frustration
- Brief psychotic episodes often triggered by stress, self-mutilation, acts out sexually, abuses substances, engages in illegal behavior
- Suicidal ideation and/or attempts

Interventions

- If patient is acting out destructively, provide a quiet, safe environment.
- Involve patient in methods to control his/her own impulsive behaviors.
- Administer prescribed medication as needed to help decrease severely stressful behavior.

are ego defenses used by these patients in their shifting projections of the self onto others and not changed behaviors of staff.[30]

An understanding of the dynamics of the condition and open communication among staff members with regular staff meetings are essential to implement consistent care.

The hospital structure can provide the patient with a sense of security and protection. However, care must be taken not to overwhelm the borderline personality with too much nurturing and closeness because this evokes feelings of suffocation from which the patient needs to escape. Setting limits consistently and nonpunitively establishes expectations of responsibility and accountability for the patient. Because the borderline personality's tolerance for frustration is low, he or she responds to limit setting with hostility and rage. The nurse helps the patient examine the factors leading to the hostility, explore alternative responses, and handle feelings. The nurse clearly communicates the patient's behaviors that will and will not be permitted; for example, verbal expressions of anger may be allowed but not physical ones.

Prevalence

The prevalence of borderline personality disorder in the general population is estimated to be 1.6% to 4%.[30] The mental health outpatient population is 10% with about 20% in psychiatric inpatient units.[2] Some health professionals think the prevalence of borderline pathology is increasing, possibly because society is becoming less structured and there is increasing emphasis on individualism and violence.

Population at Risk

The borderline personality disorder begins in childhood or adolescence; however, the diagnosis is not applicable before the age of 18, with a clearer picture of the borderline personality emerging in middle or late adolescence.[2] About 75% of those diagnosed with the disorder are female. The suicide rate is estimated to be between 10% and 15%.[38] Because they feel bored and empty, borderline persons seek stimulation such as drug abuse, self-mutilation, or acting out sexually to "feel alive" or relieve tension.

There is considerable variation in the degree of impairment and instability during the course of the illness. As the persons move toward middle age they become more stable and less impulsive in relationships and in work situations.

Symptoms frequently overlap with other disorders, especially those within the personality disorder classification. Borderline personality disorder is most difficult to differentiate from the histrionic, narcissistic, and antisocial personality disorders because they are all characterized by impulsivity, dramatization, and emotionalism.

Motivation for psychotherapy is low, and dropout rates are high. When the patient's stress decreases, motivation for continuing in therapy frequently declines until the next crisis. Expected outcomes of therapy are increased adaptability in interpersonal relationships and to environmental events and increased openness in communications with others.

Family Issues

Parents of future borderlines are often neglectful of or underinvolved with the child, although some researchers characterize families as overinvolved. As children, borderline persons experience more parental separations or losses than the non-borderline person. Their families are viewed as less stable, less available, and less predictable; yet youngsters need stable and available parents to develop inner psychologic structures to function autonomously as adults.[47]

•••••• Psychopathology

The presence of organicity in the borderline personality disorder remains unclear; however, data exist showing it is five times more common in "first-degree biological relatives" among those with the disorder than the general public.[2] Some researchers have found deficiencies in serotonin metabolism that could be a factor in the impulsivity and mood lability of persons with the disorder. Other neurochemicals may also be abnormal in borderline pathology.[36,38]

Conceptualizations of the borderline personality disorder have been developed most clearly and extensively by psychoanalytic theorists. The interpersonal and cognitive theorists have not specifically addressed this disorder. Without an understanding of the dynamics of the borderline personality, it is difficult to intervene therapeutically to interrupt the psychopathologic condition.

Psychoanalytic Theory

The borderline personality has impaired development of object relations that have been conceptualized in the separation-individuation process. In this process, which occurs from 4 to 36 months of age, the child develops a sense of self as a psychologically separate object with clear boundaries differentiating him or her from other objects in the environment. In the identity of self the child has integrated stable inner images of himself or herself and other objects as having both good and bad qualities. He or she has the ability to function independently—that is, without his or her mother's presence.[29]

In the borderline personality the separation-individuation process is arrested during the rapprochement phase, which occurs between 16 and 24 months of age. The rapprochement phase occurs concomitantly with the anal phase of development during which aggression and ambivalence are experienced in response to the powerful parent figures. Issues of dependence and independence and control are intertwined with fears of abandonment, loss of love, or engulfment (being "swallowed up") by the mother.[30,36] The toddler with his or her growing autonomy experiences conflicts between the desire to be separate and omnipotent and the wish to have needs magically fulfilled. His or her feelings and wishes are still poorly differentiated from what he or she perceives as his or her mother's; he or she believes his or her thoughts and feelings are similar to his or her mother's as evidenced by the mother meeting his or her needs. The mother's empathetic understanding is viewed by the toddler as reading his or her mind.[30]

The anger and aggression of this period are unstructured and outside of ego control; no cohesive, integrated mental images of self and others have emerged within the personality. The split in mental images of good or bad precludes the development of evocation of memories and past experiences. In the borderline personality the images of self and others are predominantly bad. The arrest in this developmental phase in the borderline personality is generally attributed to the mother who rewards clinging, regressive behaviors and withdraws and is unavailable when the child shows healthy development. Constitutional and other environmental factors may contribute to the arrest of the child's development in this phase.[38]

• • • • • Diagnostic Studies and Findings

SMAC   To screen for systemic abnormalities
Complete blood count   To rule out medical condition
Routine urinalysis   To screen for urologic problems and other medical problems
Urine toxicology   To screen for abuse of drugs

• • • • • Multidisciplinary Plan

Medications

Fluoxetine (Prozac) 20 mg, po, qAM initially to reduce symptoms of depression and impulsivity; has a low degree of toxicity when overdose is taken. Fluoxetine is a selective serotonin re-uptake inhibitor (SSRI) that has fewer side effects than many of the older classes of antidepressants.[38] It may take 4 weeks for the patient to feel the full effects of the medicine. Choice of medication may vary according to the presenting symptoms.

NURSING CARE

Nursing Assessment

Signs and symptoms vary in type and severity among patients.

Emotions

Anger; hostility; depression; anxiety; emptiness; loneliness; emotional shallowness

Thoughts and Actions

Denial of contradictory feelings; denial of responsibility for behavior; intolerance of stress and frustration; demandingness; acting out of tensions and feelings; poor judgment; projection of hostile feelings onto others; misinterpretation of stimuli; impaired problem-solving; sense of inadequacy and insecurity; ambivalence; polarized views of others as good or bad; sense of specialness; masochistic and sadistic behavior; destructive behavior toward self and others; substance abuse

Communication

Demanding; sarcasm; criticism; verbally striking out at others' vulnerabilities; manipulativeness by evoking rescue fantasies in some individuals or hostility with subsequent counterattacks from others; evoking disagreements and competitive behaviors among others

Nursing Dx & Intervention

Nursing care should be implemented selectively based on severity and type of behavior. Because hospitalization is likely to be brief and change is slow, usually interventions only begin to have positive effects on the patient's healthy adaptation.

Ineffective individual coping related to destructive behavioral patterns

- Assess level of functioning and coping strategies, including abuse of substance.
- Begin to develop trusting relationship with patient without being too nurturing or overinvolved *to prevent fears of engulfment.*
- Involve patient in treatment plan by having him or her identify how he or she wants you and other staff members to help him or her *to avoid trying to anticipate needs and meeting them magically.*
- Communicate routines and expectations in a matter-of-fact way *to provide structure for patient.*
- Encourage patient to describe events that lead to impulsive behaviors, including thoughts and actions in events, *to help patient become aware of personal contributions in events.*
- Be alert to patient's omissions of own behaviors and focus on others *to prevent patient from projecting difficulties onto others.*
- Help patient correct distortions in perceptions, thought process, and definitions of an event *to begin using problem-solving approach.*
- Encourage patient to identify and evaluate consequences of impulsive behaviors *to learn, for example, how they achieved or did not achieve desired outcome.*
- Assist patient to examine and evaluate possible alternative behaviors *to achieve a satisfying outcome.*
- Ask patient what help he or she wants in controlling or preventing impulsive behaviors *to increase self-responsibility.*
- If patient is unable to control impulsivity, use diversionary techniques (such as escorting patient to quiet area, taking him or her for a walk, or changing subject) *to prevent or interrupt unacceptable behaviors.*
- After patient is calmer, encourage discussion of details of both issue and patient's feelings *to use problem-solving approach for dealing with situation and to examine possible consequences of alternative responses.*
- Inform patient about which behaviors are permitted and set limits consistently to provide a sense of security *to communicate clearly to patient what behaviors will not be permitted.*

- Be alert to self-destructive acts; take suicide threats and minor suicidal acts seriously, even if manipulative. If indicated and if in collaboration with physician, institute suicide precautions.
- Administer any medication ordered by physician *to decrease disturbing symptoms;* observe for adverse reactions such as an increase in hostility; explain to patient the medication's effects and possible side effects.
- Be alert to potential substance abuse.
- Encourage patient to use relaxation techniques, such as slow, deep breathing and focusing on breathing or the number "1" *to decrease panic and promote sleep and relaxation.* Listening to quiet, "easy-listening" music on the radio can have a hypnotic effect.
- Avoid an empathetic understanding of patient's thoughts and feelings. Because patient may conclude that you can read his or her mind; ask him or her to tell you his or her thoughts *to help him or her recognize the reality of his or her psychological separateness.*
- Matter-of-factly point out inconsistencies or contradictions in patient's actions and expressions of thoughts and feelings *to increase patient's awareness of his or her behavior.*
- Keep in mind that patient's negative and positive appraisals of others are his or her defenses *to be alert to patient's playing one staff member against another.*
- When patient complains about another staff member, encourage him or her to talk with that person *to work his problems out rather than tell you.*
- Hold regular staff meetings *to clarify or modify treatment plans, reinforce need for consistency, and support one another.*
- Assess whether patient is able to accomplish requested task; assist him or her as needed, to complete task.
- Assist the patient in evaluating his or her own behaviors realistically *to encourage patient to accept his or her strengths.*
- Encourage patient to continue self-administration of medication as prescribed and counseling after discharge *to prevent relapse of symptoms and to learn adaptive coping strategies to deal with encountered issues.*

Patient Education/Home Care Planning

1. Ensure that the patient verbalizes knowledge of major effects and adverse effects of medications and of accurate self-administration of medications and that he or she understands the importance of compliance with the entire treatment plan after discharge.
2. Give the patient the name and phone numbers of health professional(s) who will provide continued care after discharge.
3. Encourage the patient to continue to apply problem-solving approaches to issues encountered, rather than to act out impulsively.

Evaluation

Patient evidences reduction in symptoms and an increased ability to use adaptive coping strategies   Patient verbalizes a decrease in uncomfortable feelings and an increase in sense of control. Patient states major effects and adverse effects of medications and a knowledge of accurate self-administration of medications. Patient makes plans to comply with treatment plan after discharge. Patient begins to practice problem-solving approach and decreases impulsive behaviors.

ADAPTIVE AND MALADAPTIVE BEHAVIOR

Two conditions—high risk for suicide and crisis—are presented in this section. Although these related conditions are not classifications of mental disorders, they have serious implications for mental health. Crisis intervention began in World War II in the 1940s when the goal of the military was to treat distressed members of the military at the front lines whenever possible and return these members to duty.[23] Services for suicide prevention and crisis intervention for the general population began to evolve in the 1950s. Preventive strategies are emphasized in both. In high risk for self-harm the immediate goal is prevention of suicide; in crisis intervention a primary goal is the prevention of the maladaptation of mental illness. Alternative effective coping responses are sought when intervening in these conditions.

Psychosocial and environmental problems may play a part in the development of dysfunctional responses. DSM-IV[2] takes into account such problem categories as primary support group, health problems or loss of family members, occupational or housing problems, extreme poverty, and legal system difficulties, e.g., arrests. These factors may exacerbate a mental disorder or may be caused by a disorder. Therapeutic interventions are directed toward fostering adaptive rather than maladaptive responses. Adaptation is the ability to mobilize the resources needed to make changes in the self or in the external environment to cope effectively with stress. Maladaptation is the inability to mobilize the necessary resources to manage stress.

■ RISK FOR SUICIDE

Suicide is a self-harming act intended to terminate one's life. The term can be broadly categorized to include completed suicide, suicide attempt, and suicide ideation.

Completed suicide is the cessation of life resulting from self-destructive behavior; suicide attempt refers to an unsuccessful self-destructive act that is apparently intended to result in death.[10] Persons with suicide ideation are preoccupied with thoughts of terminating their lives without acting on the thoughts. They may indicate these wishes directly or indirectly by behavior such as making a final will or saying such things as, "Others would be better off without me." The term *suicide* does not explain the cause of death but only the mode of death or the presence of life-threatening thoughts and acts.

The seriousness of suicidal acts and thoughts is related to the lethality and intent. Lethality of an act or contemplated act is ranked from zero to high depending on its destructiveness and reversibility. Suicide attempts by firearms and hanging are highly lethal, whereas ingesting 15 aspirin is not. Sometimes ignorance of the consequences of a method enters into the lethality—that is, persons who lack information may incorrectly choose a method that is or is not fatal.[23]

Intent to commit suicide is a determination by the person to end his or her life. Extremes of intent range from absolute determination to none. The degree of intent is difficult to assess accurately because people exaggerate or deny their intent to kill themselves. Some persons may state a strong desire to commit suicide to manipulate others, with no intention of committing suicide. Others deny their intentions even though they have well-formulated plans and a serious intent to kill themselves. All threats and attempts must be taken seriously.

Families are often reluctant to admit that a member engaged in self-destructive acts or intended suicide because of the stigma attached to such behaviors. Religious beliefs and cultural norms in many countries prohibit self-destructive behaviors, viewing them as sinful or disgraceful.[23]

Accidental suicides occur for a variety of reasons. A suicidal gesture used as a manipulative ploy to gain favors or influence others may inadvertently result in death. Conditions that cloud consciousness such as chronic pain, organic disease, dysfunctional states (panic, severe depression, psychosis, and high stress), and drugs may lead to unintentional self-destructive behavior. For example, persons with severe pain may take repeated doses of analgesics until they no longer remember if or how much medicine was ingested. Psychotic suicides in depression or schizophrenia may be responses to delusional ideas or hallucinatory orders to punish the self through self-destructive behaviors.[6]

Some people after appraising their situation may consciously and logically decide that life is less desirable than death.[32] Because they have no hope that their life circumstances will change and believe they have no alternatives, they rationally plan and carry out their suicides. Some experts suggest that increases in suicides may be related to changes in the availability of support systems and close-knit families, in values related to living, and in having a purpose in life.

Health professionals must take the perspective of the person with suicidal ideation and behaviors rather than superimpose their own beliefs on the person, regardless of whether the behaviors are manipulative ploys or serious attempts in response to mild or severe stressors. All suicidal thoughts and acts must be taken seriously and responded to appropriately (see Emergency Alert box).

Prevalence

The official statistics on attempted and completed suicides are unreliable and underreported because of the cultural taboo and stigma associated with suicides in the United States. Unless the evidence clearly points to suicide, other causes are stated on medical record, insurance forms, and death certificates. A reported suicide figure for all ages is approximately 12 per 100,000, with an estimated 300,000 attempted or completed suicides each year in the United States.[23] This figure has remained relatively constant for several decades. An estimated 10 suicides are attempted for every completed act in the general population. In recent years suicide is ranked as the eighth leading cause of death in the United States.

Population at Risk

Many people have had at least fleeting thoughts of killing themselves at some point in their lives or know someone who has attempted self-harm. Women attempt suicide an estimated 20 to 50 times more frequently than men; however, more men commit suicide.[23] Suicide is the second leading cause of death for the age group between 15 and 24, and older white men commit suicide twice as often as younger white men.[23,42] Black males of all ages have a higher rate of suicide than white males.

Separation from or the death of a loved one, divorce, and the loss of health, money, or a job are powerful factors in suicide. Persons who come to believe that life has no meaning or who believe there is no longer a purpose in their lives are at risk for suicide.[23]

 EMERGENCY ALERT

POTENTIAL FOR SELF-HARM: SUICIDAL BEHAVIOR

A self-harming act intended to terminate one's life is termed *suicide*. Suicidal persons are preoccupied with thoughts of terminating their lives.

Assessment

- Preoccupation with suicidal thoughts; strong intent to end his/her life; hopelessness
- Develops highly **lethal** plan to end his/her life and has means to execute plan, e.g., with firearms, hanging, purposeful automobile accident
- Overdoses, accidently or intended, on prescribed, over-the-counter, and/or illegal drugs severe enough to lead to death
- Psychotic suicide in response to delusions and hallucinations and in other mental conditions
- Consciously and logically decides that life is less desirable than death, e.g., severe illness or deformity, absence of support system, isolated, elderly, and alone
- Family member or friends who have previously attempted or completed suicide

Interventions

- If risk for suicide is assessed to be high, institute suicide precautions to ensure safety of patient. Begin to establish a supportive relationship while instilling a sense of hope in patient's abilities to cope with events.
- Administer medication to patient as instructed by physician to decrease disturbed thoughts and feelings.

According to the Center for Disease Control and Prevention statistics, the suicide rate for those age 65 and older has risen 9% between 1980 and 1992 in the United States. The elderly make up approximately 13% of the population, but they account for 20% of all suicides.

Persons whose significant others have committed suicide or who have attempted suicide themselves in the past are more prone to suicide. The suicide may be related to a significant date such as an anniversary, a birthday, or becoming the same age as the lost person. A history of previous suicide attempts is an important predictor of future suicidal behavior; many of those who successfully complete a suicide have attempted suicide previously.[23]

Family disruptions affect younger family members more than older ones. Conflicts and arguments within the family create suicidal pressures on members. The potentially suicidal member is often isolated within the family and becomes the scapegoat.

Sequelae in the Family

Family members including children, loved ones, and friends of those who commit suicide are survivor-victims of suicide. They torture themselves by feeling guilt, shame, hatred, and confusion for years after the suicidal episode. Obsessional thoughts about the death and a search for reasons are often attempts to relieve self-blame. Family members and other relatives often deny that the cause of death was suicide despite the evidence and may continue to believe that the death was accidental or as a consequence of natural causes.[23]

Because children are especially vulnerable when they lose a loved one by suicide, adults may attempt to hide the facts by incorrectly thinking they are protecting the children from pain.[23] The children usually fantasize frightening stories, such as that they caused the death.

Survivors need help to alleviate their emotional distress and prevent the development of maladaptive coping techniques, such as suicide or abnormal grief responses, for years after the death. Crisis counseling for survivor-victims needs to be available to prevent or reduce the harmful effects of a suicide.[23]

•••••• Psychopathology

Psychoanalytic Theory

Psychoanalytic theorists view suicide from the psychopathology of depression. Ambivalent feelings of love and hate experienced toward the lost love object are withdrawn from the object, and the hate or aggression are turned inward toward the self. Suicide is the extreme response of self-hatred. The self-destructive act is carried out as self-punishment with the hope of gaining forgiveness from the sadistic component of the developing superego.[18]

Interpersonal Theory

In interpersonal theory, suicide stems from depression; the person believes that it is better to die than to suffer emotional pain and emptiness. Through self-punishment the person hopes to gain relief from guilt, feelings of helplessness, and failure. Often through self-destructive behavior the person gains relief from negative self-feelings and, if he or she survives, may begin to improve.[6]

Suicide in children is markedly different from that in adults. Before 9 years of age, children have no concept of the permanence and irreversibility of death. The rarity of suicide in children is caused by their cognitive immaturity to plan and implement it. When suicide occurs, it may be related to fears of punishment, especially by parents. Adolescents attempt suicide because of self-hatred and losses, especially of love objects; some do so as a desperate cry for help, often to others beyond their family. In some adolescents, coercive manipulation is involved to obtain revenge or peer approval.[6]

Delusions and hallucinations in psychotic persons reinforce and support self-redemption and forgiveness through the self-punishment of suicide.

Cognitive Theory

In studies done to determine the risk factors for suicide, hopelessness, not depression per se, is an important indicator of suicidal behavior.[17] Studies support Beck's findings that persons experiencing hopelessness and negative views of the future are at high risk for suicide. Depressed persons with hope are less likely to engage in suicidal behavior. Hopeless persons see no escape from their unbearable feelings and situation. The sense of no escape gives rise to suicidal ideas and behavior as the only solution and as an end to emotional distress.

Beck and others[9] state that realistic problems related to environmental factors such as work and school performance, loss of job by the head of the family, and unsatisfying interpersonal relationships may contribute to a person's hopelessness and wish to end it all. It is true that the expectation of regaining a lost loved one, wealth, status, or health is unrealistic unless the person is able to accept alternative solutions. Persons who view suicide as the only solution may carry it out in a logical, rational manner or may perform it as a highly illogical response to a situation.

The nurse should be aware that the tranquility and peacefulness observed in a formerly distressed or agitated person might not be a sign of improvement but rather a sign of having made a decision and plans to commit suicide.

•••••• Diagnostic Studies and Findings

SMAC   To screen for systemic abnormalities

Complete blood count   To rule out infection and other medical disorders

Thyroid function tests   To screen for thyroid abnormalities

Electrocardiogram (ECG)   To screen for cardiopathy

Urinalysis   To rule out urologic disorders and other medical conditions

•••••• Multidisciplinary Plan

Medications

Fluoxetine (Prozac) 20 mg po qAM initially for depression to decrease symptoms of hopelessness and suicidal ideation;

10 mg po qAM initially for elderly patients or adolescents; if there is suspicion that patient is not swallowing pills or is hoarding them, liquid medicine can be substituted

Chlorpromazine (Thorazine) 25 mg po qid for adults; 25 mg po bid for elderly and adolescent patients for psychotic disorders; IM or syrup may be substituted if patient is not swallowing pills

General Management

Suicide precautions

Seclusion if deemed necessary for patient's protection

Electroconvulsive therapy may be necessary to prevent completion of suicide act if the threat of suicide is strong and the patient does not respond to antidepressive medication

NURSING CARE

Nursing Assessment

Signs and symptoms will vary among individuals.

Violence

Instability or changes in life situation; thoughts that life is not worthwhile; presence, duration, and strength of self-harm thoughts; contemplation of ways of harming or killing self; development of well-formulated plans; strength of motive or serious intent to follow through with plans; availability of chosen suicide method; factors, such as family, religion, and additional stress, that may push person toward or deter suicide; previous thoughts and attempts of suicide along with intent and lethality of attempts or ideas; loss of significant other through suicide

Power and Control

Hopelessness; inability to influence or alter interpersonal or life situation

Affect

Sadness or depression; inappropriate feelings such as laughter; anger; distress; tranquility once decision and plan are finalized

Thoughts

Negative view of the future; humiliation (e.g., feeling of being a failure); perceived or actual recent losses, stressors, or changes; ambivalence; fantasies about how others may react (e.g., "They'll be sorry"); vengeful thoughts; delusions or auditory hallucinations of sin, self-punishment, and atonement

Communication

Comments such as saying good-bye instead of good night, "I won't be seeing you again," or "Next time you see me, I'll be riding in a hearse"; informing family or spouse of whereabouts of important papers, such as insurance papers, bankbooks, and will; threats of suicide as a cry for help or to manipulate interactions

Activities

Making or changing will; increasing life insurance; visiting or phoning relatives and friends for intense conversations; giving away prized possessions; demonstrating increased concern or care for others; buying tools needed to implement suicide, such as a gun, rope, or prescription refills; acting out behavior; writing a farewell note

Social Interactions

Perceived or actual lack of support from others; loss of valued relationships through separation, divorce, death, or romantic breakups

Family Process

Dysfunctional patterns of interactions such as conflict, arguments, and blaming; others not perceiving and responding to needs or wishes

Nursing Dx & Intervention

Although the environment should be made as safe as possible by removing any materials suicidal patients might use to harm themselves, it is not possible to make the environment completely suicide proof. The importance of developing a concerned, supportive interpersonal relationship with the patient cannot be overemphasized.

When working with suicidal patients, even when they are manipulative, nurses need to be aware of and manage their own feelings while empathizing with the patients' point of view. Nursing care should be implemented selectively based on seriousness of symptoms and presenting behaviors.

Risk for violence: self-directed related to despair and hopelessness

- Assess level of hopelessness and seriousness of suicidal ideations and intent.
- Begin to establish supportive relationship with patient *to demonstrate respect, concern, and worth of patient.*
- Institute precautions such as removing all harmful objects from environment (e.g., glass containers, drugs, belts, shoe laces), and closely observe patient (initially one-to-one observation day and night if necessary; later, observation every 15 minutes and frequent interactions while awake; and eventually hourly checks) *to decrease opportunities for self-harm and ensure safety of patient.*
- Allow patient to keep more possessions as deemed safe and as precautions become less stringent *to provide reasonable restrictions that promote the well-being of patient.*
- Continue close observation with knowledge of patient's whereabouts when on unit.

- While suicide precautions are in effect, engage patient, as able, in simple activities, such as exercises or looking at magazines, *to promote the relationship and encourage interest in the environment.*
- Convey a sense of hope in patient's abilities and in his or her future.
- Evaluate patient's condition frequently at first and at least once a day *to determine his or her mood and potential for self-harm.*
- Observe for changes in patient's mood, such as calmness or tranquility, as a possible prelude to suicide.
- Administer medication with a simple explanation, including a description of possible side effects, such as orthostatic hypotension and drowsiness. When condition improves, explain to the patient the effects and side effects of medication, and leave the patient opportunities to ask questions *to encourage knowledgeable participation in treatment plan during and after hospitalization.*

Altered thought processes related to psychologic conflicts

- Assess patient's abilities to think logically and to problem solve.
- Assist patient to identify meaning of suicide threats (or attempts) and what patient expected to happen to himself or herself and others *to help patient become aware of experiences that led to self-harm behaviors.*
- Examine losses and stressors that evoked self-harm behaviors *to begin a problem-solving approach to correct illogical thoughts and to identify alternative behavior.*
- Help patient recall and identify reasons for living *to examine experiences when life was better than it is currently.*
- Avoid reinforcing delusions and hallucinations; assist patient to examine experiences before delusions or hallucinations *to help patient gradually connect thoughts and feelings with development of false beliefs and perceptions.*
- Assist patient in anticipating future issues and in developing methods other than suicide for handling them.

Ineffective individual coping related to inadequate coping method

- Assess patient's coping strategies to deal with stressors and life situations.
- Examine appropriateness of patient's emotional responses to events, using a problem-solving approach *to reinforce healthy adaptive behavior.*
- When patient shows signs of increased tension, encourage slow, deep breathing *to help decrease tension.* Encourage patient to practice relaxation techniques daily.
- Explain and practice assertiveness skills *to begin to increase patient's confidence in self and to learn how to let others know of his or her needs.*
- Encourage patient to identify his or her social skills.

- Help patient deal with uncomfortable feelings in social situations *to begin to develop healthy coping strategies.*
- Assist patient in identifying social inadequacies, and encourage patient to begin to correct these; provide names of community resources *to assist with correcting social inadequacies after discharge and to increase social supports.*

Other related nursing diagnoses   Powerlessness related to perceived lack of control over environment; impaired verbal communication related to lack of willingness to discuss personal concerns; social isolation related to feelings of unease when interacting with others; altered family processes related to multiple conflicts among members.

Patient Education/Home Care Planning

1. Encourage the patient to verbalize knowledge and understanding of methods other than suicide for coping with his or her feelings of hopelessness and problems (e.g., problem-solving approach, community resources, including family and friends, and assertiveness techniques).
2. Encourage continued counseling after discharge, and emphasize that this is a sign of strength.
3. Give the patient a list of the major effects and the adverse effects of medications to report to health care provider and the phone number of the provider.
4. Write down names, addresses, and phone numbers of the local suicide prevention center and 24-hour help lines for the patient. Encourage the patient to use the numbers day or night to obtain support or to talk with a supportive person when his or her therapist is unavailable.
5. Review methods for dealing with social situations after discharge. Help the patient learn how to share or how to avoid sharing information about the suicide attempt, problems, and hospitalization that he or she wants to tell or wants not to tell others.

Evaluation

Patient evidences reduced potential for self-harm   Patient makes no suicide attempts and verbalizes the desire to live and reasons for living. Patient states accurate information about actions of medications and treatment plan and knowledge of self-administration after discharge.

Patient demonstrates increased ability to think logically about problem areas   Patient states beginning knowledge of experiences contributing to hopelessness. Patient begins to demonstrate constructive behaviors and is using problem-solving techniques to correct misconceptions and to consider alternative solutions.

Patient demonstrates coping skills   Patient develops skills and practices appropriate coping strategies for dealing with issues. Patient practices assertiveness behaviors and evidences increased self-assurance.

CRISIS

A crisis is an extreme emotional state of disequilibrium when a person's habitual problem-solving methods that worked previously are inadequate.[1] As anxiety and tension increase, the ability to find a solution decreases and the sense of helplessness increases. It is accepted generally as a normal response produced by a threatening event rather than a pathologic state.

The person may be in a vulnerable state because of efforts to deal with hazardous events before the crisis reaction. Despite being in a state of moderate anxiety or depression, the person is able to mobilize resources to cope, although possibly at a reduced level, with the initial stressors.[23] However, when an overpowering experience (the precipitant) occurs, it produces the disorganizing effect of a crisis reaction. For example, the initial stressor may be a surgical procedure that produces a vulnerable state, and the crisis-precipitating event may be the knowledge that the excised tumor was cancerous. Sometimes a person experiences just one stressor of sufficient force to precipitate the crisis.

An acute crisis is a subjective state of psychologic and physical disorganization in which the person experiences a temporary loss of control. This is called a panic state. Because emotional reactions to the stimulus are overwhelming and nonintegrated, the cognitive processes such as assessing, thinking, decision making, and judging are inoperative.[34] Thinking is scattered, with no ability to attend to anything or fix on one narrow point; affectional ties to others are severely disrupted or severed so that the person feels isolated. The person is immobilized or moves about aimlessly.

Two types of crisis have been differentiated on the basis of the person's previous life experiences: an exhaustion and an acute crisis.[49] In exhaustion crisis the person has coped effectively under emergency conditions for a long time and reaches a point of exhaustion when all energy and resources have been spent. In acute crisis the person is overwhelmed by an explosive release of emotions in response to a sudden external change. Too much has happened unexpectedly and rapidly for the person to assimilate and integrate the excess stimuli. Nursing interventions for these two types of crisis differ. A person in exhaustion crisis is unable to gain control over emotions and is apathetic to interpersonal contact or intervention techniques. A benign, supportive environment is essential for the person to regain energy slowly before attempting to deal with the crisis. A person in acute crisis is open to change and highly motivated to accept help in resolving it.

Although theoretically it is possible to isolate the phases in crises—vulnerable state, precipitating event, acute crisis, and reorganization—they overlap in reality. A crisis is conceived as lasting 4 to 6 weeks but may be much longer or shorter depending on the type of precipitating event, the level of stress experienced, the person's coping repertoire, and the adequacy of social supports (see Emergency Alert box).[1]

Prevalence

Crisis situations occur episodically throughout a person's lifetime because of normal developmental stages and the demands associated with anticipated life situations. In addition, unanticipated crisis situations occur during the life span. Many crises do not come to the attention of health professionals but are resolved with the help of family, friends, or the clergy. Because crises are time limited, the person may successfully deal with them or maladaptively resolve them so that precrisis functioning level is not regained.[23]

Population at Risk

From birth to death a person is exposed to crisis situations that are anticipated and predictable or unanticipated and accidental. Anticipated crises, which are described as maturational or developmental, are somewhat inconsistent with the assumptions of crisis theory that threatening events are external rather than internal. Unanticipated crises are unexpected traumatic events that may occur at any stage of life.[23]

According to Erikson[16] the eight developmental phases are basic trust versus mistrust; autonomy versus shame and doubt; initiative versus guilt; industry versus inferiority; identity versus role confusion; intimacy versus isolation; generativity versus stagnation; and ego integrity versus despair. The identity crisis of adolescents has been given considerable attention because of their rapid physiologic and cognitive changes and high vulnerability to stress. Parents who have difficulty dealing with their children in this age group may themselves be experienc-

 EMERGENCY ALERT

CRISIS

A person experiencing a crisis is in an extreme emotional state of disequilibrium in which habitual problem-solving methods are found to be inadequate.

Assessment

- Emotional state of disorganization, scattered thinking
- Failure of previously used problem-solving methods with perceived loss of control
- Exhaustion attempting to deal with emergency conditions over a long time
- Catastrophic event, e.g., untimely death of a loved one especially a child, irreversible physical disability, serious illness, economic disaster
- Paralysis of cognitive processes related to stress/severe anxiety

Interventions

- Assist patient to decrease severely disorganized feelings and cognitions by providing a supportive, accepting relationship.
- Encourage patient to review details of crisis events. Assist patient to correct misconceptions while giving factual information when appropriate.

ing midlife crises in the generativity versus stagnation phase of development. The elderly, who are in the ego integrity versus despair phase of development, are particularly susceptible to crisis because of decreases in physical and cognitive functioning, roles, and sense of purpose.

A person who has not resolved the conflicts engendered in previous phases of development may find the expectations of the current phase fraught with stress and may have a greater predisposition in crises.[23]

The expected transitional life crises, such as toilet training, beginning or changing schools, entering or retiring from the work force, marriage, parenthood, the "empty nest" syndrome when children leave home, and the death of parents, produce upheavals in roles and status and necessitate adaptation to new conditions.

Unanticipated events may affect individuals, communities, and countries.[23] They include natural catastrophic events, such as tornadoes, floods, and earthquakes, and man-made catastrophes, such as economic depressions, unemployment, and bank failures. Loss of a job and money creates a crisis not only for the person experiencing the loss but also for the family members, who are suddenly faced with changes in lifestyle and status.

Loss or threatened loss of a loved one through an untimely death or reduced capacity to function because of an accident or illness creates havoc for all involved. Although death of any loved person is stressful, the loss of a child or young adult is especially shocking to survivors. Unanticipated traumatic stress occurs in "victim crisis," in which physically or emotionally aggressive acts are perpetrated on a person. These include persecution of an individual or group and violent crimes such as assault, rape, and murder. The crisis situation can have a life-long effect because of the intense emotional trauma and possible irreversible physical disability such as paralysis or loss of an extremity. The person may have flashbacks in which the violence or aggressive-ness of the precipitating event is reexperienced. This can happen in persons who have successfully resolved the crisis issues.

In some instances a preexisting psychopathologic condition, such as schizophrenia or anxiety disorder, in a person or family is a contributing variable to a crisis reaction. The person's lowered tolerance to stressors, personal and social resources, and inadequate coping skills impair his or her ability to resolve crises successfully.

Approaches to Crisis Intervention

Generally persons experiencing crises have healthy personalities, and interventions are focused on the current crisis situation. Even when an underlying psychopathologic condition exists, interventions remain issue oriented to alleviate the crisis situation; the patient can be referred later to other resources for further help. If treatment is continued to deal with problems other than those related to the crisis, interventions are no longer viewed as crisis ones.[1]

General goals of crisis intervention are to reinforce interpersonal assets, to resolve the crisis event, to connect with social supports in the family or in the community, and to integrate the crisis experience into the personality. A minimum expectation of crisis intervention is the person's return to a precrisis level of functioning.

There are two general approaches in crisis intervention: generic and individual. The generic approach involves the use of brief, supportive interventions focused on the characteristic phases (such as that of grief) of the crisis experience. Little or no attention is directed toward the patient's personality dynamics. Nonprofessionals or paraprofessionals, such as trained volunteers at a 24-hour hotline or crisis center, usually use the generic approach. Although this approach is effective for some persons, dangers may exist when individual personality differences are not considered.

The individual approach is also focused on the current issues but has a more in-depth view in which the personality of the individual is considered. Stressors before the precipitating event, previous coping behaviors, and reactivated conflicts that contribute to the current reactions are identified, and how the individual's behavior contributed to worsening a threatening situation is evaluated. Resolution includes not only relief of symptoms but also development of effective coping skills to deal with similar situations in the future.

Three general approaches useful in crisis intervention are presented.[49] The first is the free discharge of emotions such as despair, anxiety, and anger. If anger is the only emotion expressed, it may be nonconstructive when used to deny fear and emotional pain, but it is constructive when it counteracts the feelings of helplessness. A second approach is the enhancement of the patient's cognitive processes, thus providing a sense of control. The patient is helped to remember details of the event, including painful ones, and to correct misconceptions. A third approach allows the patient to experience security and hope through a supportive relationship to reduce anxiety (which leads to increased disorganization of the personality). The supportive approach is particularly useful in exhaustion crisis, when the person must regain energy before beginning to deal with the crisis. These approaches overlap to some extent, and all three are useful with a given patient depending on his or her needs at different phases of crisis intervention.[49]

Because a crisis has built-in time limits, the nurse takes an active role to discover what kind of help the patient wants, to establish concrete, achievable goals. The nurse assists the patient in acute crisis in the following ways:

Allows the patient to be dependent initially, satisfying basic needs such as directing the patient to a chair, giving a drink, and providing a damp washcloth for face

Provides the patient with opportunities to express emotions in his or her own way (as long as they are nondestructive) within a safe, supportive relationship

Increase use of cognitive processes by helping the patient review details of stressful events and, if appropriate, by providing factual information related to the event to correct misperceptions and to expand the patient's perspective

Assists the patient to examine alternative choices and possible consequences of each choice

Encourages the patient to identify social supports in the family and community

Helps the patient deal with initial reactions to the crisis situation such as emotional upsets and to accept and integrate the crisis experience into his personality

Family Relationships

When one person experiences a crisis episode, family and friends who have a close relationship with that person are likely to share in the crisis reactions. Since a crisis often loosens close relationships, each person may suffer alone rather than support each other.

Nurses are valuable resources for helping the patient and family to open up communication with each other. This may be done by providing support to the patient and by assisting him or her to reconnect with close family and/or friends. With the patient's permission, the nurse may help the patient talk with family members about the crisis event and provide factual information about the episode to correct misconceptions when appropriate.

Support for Nurses Involved in Crisis Intervention

Because of their intense involvement with patients in crisis, nurses experience high levels of pressure and stress. The need for a fast, accurate assessment and rapid intervention requires a great expenditure of energy and can be emotionally and cognitively exhausting. Nurses continually involved in crisis interventions with patients need their own support system to deal with their responses to emotion-laden situations and to receive emotional nourishment.

•••••• Psychopathology

Psychoanalytic Theory

In psychoanalytic theory crisis is viewed as occurring in persons who have been unsuccessful in resolving conflicts of early development. Not having a crucial foundation in infancy and early childhood, the person has difficulty discharging repressed emotions and working through the conflicts related to the crisis situation.[1] During the intensive, long-term psychotherapeutic relationship, the patient rebuilds and strengthens healthy defenses.

Interpersonal Theory

According to interpersonal theory, persons are influenced by others and their environment throughout their lives. Persons who have excluded a significant number of anxiety-provoking experiences from awareness are less able to respond to events because these dissociated processes are no longer accessible to consciousness. These persons may have a decreased ability to assess new situations, especially stressful ones, and respond to them adequately. The goals of therapy are helping the patient to perceive the situation accurately, resolve reactivated conflicts, and develop skills to deal with the situation and future stressful events. Therapy is a growth-producing experience for the patient.[5,6]

Cognitive Theory

In cognitive or learning frameworks crisis is considered to be a result of sensory overload that interrupts the cognitive processes of perceiving, thinking, decision making, and evaluating. The overload may be related to a perceived or actual bombardment with stressful stimuli the person is unable to process logically. The person's definition of the situation determines whether it is interpreted as a crisis or as a challenging, exciting experience. Thus the person's definition also determines the person's response and methods of dealing with the situation. Intervention is directed toward correcting cognitive distortions, learning new skills to resolve the problem, unlearning inappropriate thinking patterns, and reinforcing gratifying patterns of behavior.[9]

•••••• Diagnostic Studies and Findings

SMAC   To screen for general medical conditions

Complete blood count   To screen for infection and other medical conditions

Thyroid function tests   To rule out thyroid disorders

Urinalysis   To screen for urologic disorders and other medical conditions

Note   Various laboratory tests were probably ordered and completed if the patient was hospitalized for a medical condition

•••••• Multidisciplinary Plan

Medications

Trazodone (Desyrel) for depression; 50 mg tid po; has high sedative action and low anticholinergic action to manage depressive symptoms such as guilt, worthlessness, and despair

or

Alprazolam (Xanax) for anxiety; 0.5 mg tid po for adult patients; 0.25 mg tid po for elderly patients; belongs to benzodiazepine class of drugs; to decrease symptoms of severe anxiety, anxiety associated with depression, or both; abrupt discontinuation may cause convulsions

General Management

Occupational and recreational therapy after initial acute phase if patient is hospitalized and if there are no contraindicating medical conditions

NURSING CARE

Nursing Assessment

Persons may seek help 1 to 2 weeks after the precipitating event; however, some do so immediately after the onset of an acute crisis. These persons ask for assistance in a variety of health care facilities such as hospital emergency rooms, community agencies, including mental health centers, and private physicians' offices. Acute crisis often affects hospitalized patients and their families as the result of a change in the seriousness of an illness, discovery of a poor prognosis, family responses to the patient's illness or death, or family difficulties unrelated to the ill member.

In crisis, rapid assessment is necessary and intervention often begins before the assessment has been completed. Each person responds to crisis in an individual way.

Affect

Severe anxiety to panic; depression; anger; apathy; tearfulness to convulsive crying; feeling of alienation; emptiness; motionless state; temporary lowered self-esteem

Thoughts

Paralysis of cognitive processes; impaired recall of crisis event; misinterpretation of events; forgetfulness; blocking; confusion; indecisiveness; frustration; conflicting thoughts; denial; guilt; psychophysiologic symptom complaints; suicidal or homicidal thoughts

Power and Control

Helplessness; hopelessness; vulnerability; lack of control

Activities

Paralysis or aimless, automatic behavior; agitation; tremors; stiffness of body as if trying to hold self together; clenched fists; contorted facial features; limpness of body, sometimes with impaired balance; impaired performance of tasks; regressive childlike behaviors such as tantrums

Sleep Patterns

Impaired sleep; inability to sleep; restless sleep; hypersomnia

Nutrition

Change in eating pattern, such as overeating or inability to eat; picking at food; nausea; vomiting

Social Interactions

Withdrawal from social support network; loosening of ties with loved ones

Nursing Dx & Intervention

Nursing care should be implemented selectively based on seriousness of symptoms and presenting behaviors. Because of the time limits of crisis, patients may be seen for only one or as many as 10 sessions.

Anxiety related to situational or maturational crises

- Assess emotional state rapidly to determine level of anxiety.
- Observe patient closely for appearance, dress, general demeanor, and muscle tightness *to identify signs of distress and comfort.*

- Provide quiet, calm environment *to avoid increasing anxiety.*
- Convey concern and caring through temporarily taking charge of activities (e.g., direct patient to comfortable chair and provide comfort measures such as drink and tissues) *to reduce panic and loss of control.*
- Address patient by name and speak calmly in concise sentences *to obtain patient's attention.*
- If exhaustion crisis is present, be supportive and giving *to help patient regain energy.*
- Encourage patient to express feelings *to discharge emotions rather than to keep them inside.*
- If patient is crying, help to identify and clarify feelings (such as despair, anger, or hopelessness) during or after this expression; for example, say "Tell me what you're feeling as you're crying" *to become aware of meaning of emotions.*
- Administer medication if ordered and as needed *to relieve emotional discomfort.* Briefly inform patient of effects and side effects, such as drowsiness and lightheadedness. More fully discuss effects and side effects when patient is calm if medication is to be continued. Emphasize the need for medical follow-up care.
- Acknowledge physical signs of discomfort and ask patient to identify emotional experience *to connect bodily sensation with feeling state.*
- When patient is able, identify previous painful emotions and successes in dealing with them *to reinforce positive coping techniques.*
- Encourage the use of relaxation techniques, such as slow, deep breathing, diversionary activities, and sharing feelings with others, *to help patient develop ways to deal with current feelings.*
- If patient is in hospital, encourage participation in occupational therapy as ordered *to provide diversionary activity and learn new skills.* (If there is no physical or emotional contraindication, recreational therapy may also be ordered *to reduce anxiety, expend excess energy, and teach new skills.*)

Ineffective individual coping related to situational or maturational crises

- Assess type of crisis (e.g., anticipated or unanticipated), precipitating event, duration of crisis and coping abilities.
- Assess for suicide ideation; if needed, institute suicide precautions.
- Clarify perceptions of issues and events before the crisis.
- When the patient with exhaustion crisis is able, identify various stressors along with their patterns, and explore coping strategies used in the past. Reinforce healthy methods for dealing with those stressors *to support successful behaviors and increase patient's confidence in his or her abilities.*
- If crisis is developmental, identify specific issues and assist patient to resolve them *to learn to deal with developmental tasks and accept self.* If crisis was unanticipated,

assist patient to begin to resolve issues related to both crisis and underlying conflict reactivated because of crisis events *to understand meaning of current crisis and integrate this new understanding into the personality.*

- In problem-solving, help patient explore possible consequences of various choices *to evaluate potential impact of decisions.*
- Provide factual information as appropriate (e.g., knowledge of crisis phases, tasks of developmental stage, and factors related to crisis situation) *to alter and broaden patient's perspective on issues.*
- Assist patient in identifying behaviors that contributed to or exacerbated the threatening situation (e.g., accumulation of large debts before loss of employment) *to help patient become aware of noneffective forms of behavior.* Help patient anticipate similar future events and identify ways of coping *to increase a sense of security and decrease apprehension about recurrence of crisis.*
- Assist patient to begin to deal with long-term impact of crisis events, such as cancer, changes in body image (e.g., facial disfigurement and mastectomy), and birth of an imperfect baby.
- Assess whether basis exists for physical complaints such as headache and abdominal pain. Medication, such as an analgesic or antacid, may be ordered for symptomatic relief.
- Help patient identify relationship between physical symptoms and emotional state *to increase understanding of his or her maladaptive coping strategies.*

Powerlessness related to overwhelming situation

- Assess level and source of helplessness and aspects of events that provoked those feelings.
- Convey to patient a realistic sense of optimism and hope that alternative ways of viewing and dealing with issues exist.
- Assist patient to recall and accept previous and current successful coping strategies *to increase confidence in his or her abilities and a sense of control over self.*
- Explain use of assertiveness skills and practice these with patient *to increase self-concept and abilities to be direct in making requests of others.*

Social isolation related to alterations in mental status

- Assess interpersonal assets and current state of social supports.
- Help patient identify persons viewed as supportive *to begin to reconnect with significant others.*
- Discuss how supportive person(s) can be helpful now and how patient can share problems *to encourage patient to use available resources.*
- If useful, ask patient to role-play, sharing problems and asking for help, *to increase confidence in asking for support.*
- If patient is in an emergency room or a community agency and alone, arrange to have someone drive him or her home

(if he or she will not be hospitalized). If patient lives alone, encourage staying at someone else's home or having someone stay with patient *to alleviate fears of being alone and to reduce stress.*
- Identify community resources, write down names, addresses, and phone numbers, and encourage patient to use them *to obtain immediate emergency services, as needed.*

Other related nursing diagnoses Sleep pattern disturbance related to high level of anxiety; altered family processes related to crisis

---

Patient Education/Home Care Planning

1. Give the patient a list of effects and side effects of medicines and of symptoms to report to physician. Include phone number of health care provider.
2. Encourage the patient to practice relaxation techniques each day.
3. Reinforce the use of assertiveness techniques and problem-solving approaches to increase self-supports and support from significant others and to resolve issues in a constructive manner.

Evaluation

Patient experiences reduction in anxiety level Patient participates in treatment plan during hospitalization. Patient expresses knowledge of effects and side effects of medications. Patient verbalizes decrease in anxiety and demonstrates skill in relaxation methods.

Patient demonstrates adaptive coping skills Patient uses problem-solving skills to examine issues and to promote adaptive behaviors.

Patient experiences increased sense of control over self-abilities and activities Patient expresses sense of hope and realistic view to deal with issues. Patient practices assertiveness techniques to tell others of needs and to request help from others.

Patient demonstrates decrease in social isolation Patient initiates contact with and receives support from significant others. Patient makes initial contact for assistance from community agency.

MULTIDISCIPLINARY INTERVENTIONS AND RELATED NURSING CARE

The major therapeutic interventions for psychiatric disturbances are counseling and drug therapy. Counseling techniques have been discussed in detail throughout this chapter. Specific pharmacologic interventions have been presented with each disorder. The specific categories and classes of pharmacologic agents used for psychiatric disturbances include antidepressants, tranquilizers, and sedative-hypnotics.

References

1. Aguilera DC: *Crisis intervention: theory and methodology,* ed 7, St Louis, 1994, Mosby.
2. American Psychiatric Association: Diagnostic and statistical manual of mental disorders, ed 4, Washington, DC, 1994, American Psychiatric Association.
3. Andreasen NC: Assessment issues and cost of schizophrenia, *Schizophr Bull 17:*475, 1991.
4. Antai-Otong D: Helping the alcoholic patient recover, *Am J Nurs 95*(8):22, 1995.
5. Arieti S: *Interpretation of schizophrenia,* ed 2, New York, 1974, Basic Books.
6. Arieti S, Bemporad J: *Severe and mild depression: the psychotherapeutic approach,* New York, 1978, Basic Books.
7. Beck AT: *Cognitive therapy and the emotional disorders,* New York, 1976, New American Library.
8. Beck AT, Emery G: *Anxiety disorders and phobias: a cognitive perspective,* New York, 1985, Basic Books.
9. Beck AT et al: *Cognitive therapy of depression,* New York, 1979, Guildford Press.
10. Buchanan DM: Suicide: a conceptual model for an avoidable death, *Arch Psychiatr Nurs 5:*341, 1991.
11. Buchman AL et al: Reversal of megaduodenum and duodenal dysmotility associated with improvement in nutritional status in primary anorexia nervosa, *Dig Dis Sci 39:*433, 1994.
12. Cahill, C: Implementing an inpatient eating disorders program, *Perspect Psychiatr Care 30*(3):26, 1994.
13. Conrad N, Sloan S, Jedwabny J: Resolving the control struggle on an eating disorder unit, *Perspect Psychiatr Care 28*(3):13, 1992.
14. Daun SM: When nurses need help: the Ohio peer assistance program for nurses, *Addiction Recovery 10*(3):35, 1990.
15. Depression Guideline Panel: *Depression in primary care: Volume I detection and diagnosis,* No 5, Rockville, MD, 1993, US Department Health and Human Services, Public Health Service (AHCPR Public No 93-0550).
16. Erikson, E: *Childhood and society,* ed 2, New York, 1963, Norton.
17. Farran CJ, Popovich JM: Hope: a relevant concept for geriatric psychiatry, *Arch Psychiatr Nurs 4:*124, 1990.
18. Fenichel O: *The psychoanalytic theory of neurosis,* New York, 1945, Norton.
19. Frances RJ, Miller SI, editors: *Clinical textbook of addictive disorders,* New York, 1991, Guilford Press.
20. Freeman T, Karson CN: The neuropathology of schizophrenia, *Psychiatr Clin North Am 16:*281, 1993.
21. Goodwin FK, Jamison KR: *Manic-depressive illness,* New York, 1990, Oxford University Press.
22. Hales RE, Yudofsky SC, Talbott J, editors: *The American psychiatric press: textbook of psychiatry,* ed 2, Washington DC, 1994, American Psychiatric Press.
23. Hoff LA: *People in crisis: understanding and helping,* ed 4, San Francisco, 1995, Jossey-Bass.
24. Hughes TL, Smith LL: Is your colleague chemically dependent? *Am J Nurs 94*(9):30, 1994.
25. Jaretz N, Flowers E, Millsap L: Clozapine: nursing care considerations, *Perspect Psychiatr Care 28*(3):19, 1992.
26. Krahn DD et al: Changes in resting energy expenditure and body composition in anorexia nervosa patients during refeeding, *J Am Diet Assoc 93:*434, 1993.
27. Levinson DF, Mowry BJ: Defining the schizophrenia spectrum: issues for genetic linkage studies, *Schizophr Bull 17:*491, 1991.
28. Lyketsos CG, Corazzini K, Steele C: Mania in Alzheimer's disease, *J Neuropsychiatr Clin Neurosci 7:*350, 1995.
29. Mahler MS, Pine F, Bergman A: *The psychological birth of the human infant,* New York, 1975, Basic Books.
30. Maxmen JS, Ward NG: *Essential psychopathology and its treatment,* ed 2, New York, 1995, Norton.
31. Meltzer HY: The mechanism of action of novel antipsychotic drugs, *Schizophr Bull 17:*263, 1991.
32. Moore SL: Rational suicide among older adults: a cause for concern? *Arch Psychiatr Nurs 7:*106, 1993.
33. O'Connor FW: Symptom monitoring for relapse prevention in schizophrenia, *Arch Psychiatr Nurs 5:*193, 1991.
34. O'Toole AW, Welt SR, editors: *Interpersonal theory in nursing practice: selected works of Hildegard E. Peplau,* New York, 1989, Springer.
35. Paykel ES, editor: *Handbook of affective disorders,* ed 2, New York, 1992, Guilford Press.
36. Pies RW: *Clinical manual of psychiatric diagnosis and treatment: a biopsychosocial approach,* Washington DC, 1994, American Psychiatric Press.
37. Prescott CA, Gottesman II: Genetically mediated vulnerability to schizophrenia, *Psychiatr Clin North Am 16:*245, 1993.
38. Preston J, O'Neal JH, Talaga MC: *Handbook of clinical psychopharmacology for therapists,* Oakland, CA, 1994, New Harbinger.
39. Ricci MS: Aloneness in tenuous self-states, *Perspect Psychiatr Care 27*(2):7, 1991.
40. Rothenberg A: Adolescence and eating disorder: the obsessive-compulsive disorder, *Psychiatr Clin North Am 13:*469, 1990.
41. Schatzberg AF, Cole JO: *Manual of clinical psychopharmacology,* ed 2, Washington DC, 1991, American Psychiatric Press.
42. Schepp KG, Biocca L: Adolescent suicide: views of adolescents, parents, and school personnel, *Arch Psychiatr Nurs 5:*57, 1991.
43. Schuckit MA: *Drug and alcohol abuse: a clinical guide to diagnosis and treatment,* ed 4, New York, 1995, Plenum.
44. Schuyler D: *A practical guide to cognitive therapy,* New York, 1991, Norton.
45. Seligman MEP: *Learned optimism,* New York, 1991, Knopf.
46. Selzer JA, Lieberman JA: Schizophrenia and substance abuse, *Psychiatr Clin North Am 16:*401, 1993.
47. Silver D, Rosenbluth M, editors: *Handbook of borderline disorders,* Madison, CT, 1992, Universities Press.
48. Simoni PS: Obsessive-compulsive disorder, *J Psychosoc Nurs Ment Health Serv 29*(4):19, 1991.
49. Specter GA, Claiborn WL, editors: *Crisis intervention,* vol 2, New York, 1973, Behavioral Publications.
50. Sullivan HS: *The interpersonal theory of psychiatry,* New York, 1953, Norton.
51. Sullivan HS: *Schizophrenia as a human process,* New York, 1962, Norton.
52. Walsh BT, Devlin MJ: *The pharmacologic treatment of eating disorders,* Psychiatr Clin North Am 15:149, 1992.
53. Weddington WW: Cocaine: diagnosis and treatment, *Psychiatr Clin North Am 16:*87, 1993.
54. Yudofsky SC, Hales RE, editors, *The American Psychiatric Press textbook of neuropsychiatry,* ed 2, Washington DC, 1992, American Psychiatric Press.

Mental Health Disorders in the Elderly

18

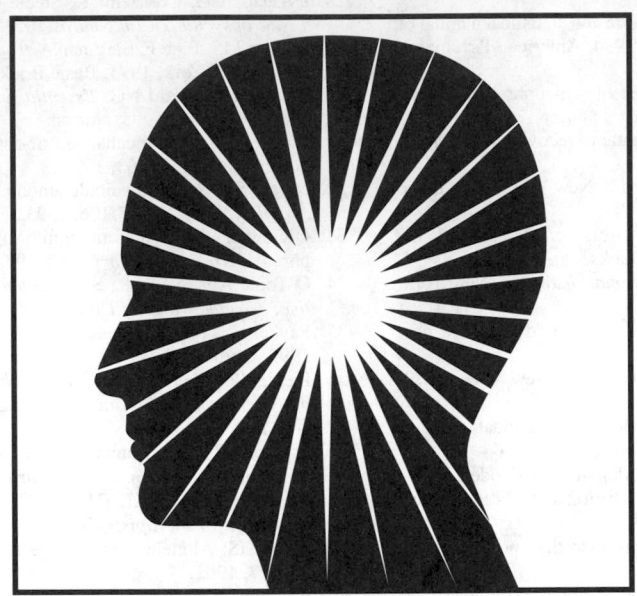

OVERVIEW

It is estimated that the population of the elderly, persons older than 65 years of age, will increase 117% between 1990 and 2050; and, the older old, those older than 85 years of age, will increase from about 10% of those older than 85 in 1990 to about 22% in 2050.[71, p. 6] Women experience different mortality rates than men. For example, "the ratio of women to men in 1990 climbs steadily from approximate parity at about age 50 to over 2:1 by age 85, and approaching and exceeding 3.5:1 at the most advanced ages."[71, p. 6] Elderly women are at greater economic risk and are more likely to be widowed and living alone than elderly men.

Normal aging is a process that eventually leads to noticeable changes in the body. Not all changes, however, are due to the normal aging process. Sloane[141, p. 25] states that "of changes in physiological function observed with advancing age, approximately one third is due to disease, one third to disuse, and one third to normal aging." Although the underlying mechanisms of the aging process are poorly understood, a number of theories have been proposed.[141] It has been theorized that aging is due to autoimmune processes, gene mutations, or protein degradation. Another theoretical position posits that the aging process is a result of toxic substance accumulation as from cell metabolism, whereas another view attributes the aging process to genetics (i.e., aging is viewed as a phenomenon that is genetically programmed).

Modest cognitive losses have been identified with advanced age.[20] Researchers have identified specific cognitive capabilities that are subject to age-related decline. These cognitive capabilities include higher intelligence requiring flexible reasoning, new learning where there is minimal structured support, decline in secondary memory as delayed visual or verbal recall, and reduced cognitive flexibility and speed in information processing. Primary memory (e.g., attention and registration, language skills, verbal intelligence) do not change in normal aging.[20] Although a cumulative degeneration of brain tissue exists with normal aging, the effects are not noticeable in most persons under ordinary circumstances unless other stressors are added.[151]

A number of theoretical perspectives address and attempt to explain psychologic aging. Chapter 17 lists characteristics of mental health. The elderly are confronted with a number of issues, losses, and transitions with which they have to cope and to which they have to adapt and thus contribute to preserving mental health. Issues faced by elderly persons include dealing with aging and perceiving oneself as old; alterations in autonomy and self-control; maintaining intimacy with significant others; major life transitions, such as retirement; death of significant others; changes in body; physical illness; meeting sexual needs; engaging in meaningful activities; using available resources maximally; and dealing with one's own impending death.[163]

A number of theoretical perspectives of psychological aging have been proposed.[168] Disengagement theory views aging as inevitable disengagement and mutual withdrawal with decreasing interactions of the older persons with others. Activity theory, on the other hand, espouses that those elderly who are active, socially involved, and productive will remain the most satisfied. Continuity theory proposes that elderly people will continue engaging in behavior patterns established in younger years. In symbolic interactionism the social world and subjective reality is constructed by means of interacting with other persons. The concept of beneficial attachments places significance on the ability of the elderly person to maintain attachments with others that are mutually beneficial. Developmental theory addresses stages of life with the last stage centering on ego-integrity or despair. Life review is viewed as the progressive return to past experiences. Most elderly, despite facing losses, transitions, and issues, remain psychologically robust. As Waters[162, p. 186] states, "We can use our understanding of this history to help older adults see their longevity not in association with rigidity but rather as a track record of coping skills. We also can acknowledge . . . working to come to terms with finitude is neither morbid nor eccentric but necessary to good mental health as we become old."

CONDITIONS, DISEASES, AND DISORDERS

MOOD DISORDERS IN THE ELDERLY

Mood disorders[6] are comprised of (a) depressive disorders, (b) bipolar disorders, and (c) mood disorder based on etiology.

Depressive disorders include (1) *major depressive disorder* characterized by the presence of one or more depressive episodes (includes five or more of the following symptoms—depressed mood, diminished pleasure in activities, suicidal ideation, difficulty concentrating or thinking, psychomotor retardation or agitation, weight loss, sleep disturbance, fatigue, feelings of worthlessness and guilt, symptoms that can cause impaired occupational and social functioning), with at least 2 weeks of depressed mood or loss of pleasure or interest but no evidence of manic, mixed, or hypomanic episodes; (2) *dysthymic disorder* characterized by presence of depressed mood for 2 years and other symptoms of depression but not of a major depressive episode and no evidence of manic, mixed, or hypomanic episodes; and, (3) *depressive disorder not otherwise specified* characterized by depressive features but does not meet, for example, criteria for major depressive disorder, dysthymic disorder, and no evidence of manic, mixed, or hypomanic episodes.

Bipolar disorders[6] include (1) *bipolar I disorder* characterized by one or more manic episodes (elevated mood, talkative, flight of ideas, grandiosity, psychomotor agitation, reduced need for sleep, involvement in pleasurable activities with potential adverse outcomes, impaired occupation and/or social functioning) or mixed episode (has characteristics of both de-

pressive and manic episodes, impaired occupational and/or social functioning) along with major depressive episodes; (2) *bipolar II disorder* characterized by one or more than one major depressive episodes and one or more hypomanic episodes (similar to manic episodes except that social and occupational functioning are not as markedly impaired); (3) *cyclothymic disorder* characterized by 2 years of hypomanic and depressive symptoms but not actual manic episodes or major depressive episodes; and, (4) *bipolar disorder not otherwise specified* characterized by bipolar features that do not meet criteria for bipolar I, bipolar II, or cyclothymic disorders.

Mood disorder based on etiology[6] includes (1) *mood disorder due to a general medical condition* characterized by mood disturbance caused by a general medical condition; (2) *substance-induced mood disorder* characterized by mood disturbance caused by drug abuse, a medication, or a toxin; and, (3) *mood disorder not otherwise specified* characterized by mood disturbance not readily meeting criteria or other diagnosis.

◼ DEPRESSION

Depression can be a mood state (characterized by feelings of disappointment, discouragement, sadness, and withdrawal from others), symptom, syndrome, or disease.[51]

In the elderly, lack of interest in usual activities may be one of the first signs, along with lack of energy and depressed mood. Other common signs and symptoms of depression in the elderly include more dependence on others such as family members; exclusive focus on the past; difficulties in concentration; numerous somatic complaints as of neck, back, head, abdomen, and gastrointestinal tract disturbances; sleep disturbances (i.e., insomnia, hypersomnia); refusal to eat or drink; apathy; loss of weight; psychomotor retardation or agitation; feelings of worthlessness; and paranoid symptoms.[28,68,69] In patient's with Alzheimer's disease, the presence of depression and its severity contribute to further deterioration of the ability to perform the activities of daily living.[53]

•••••• Pathophysiology/Psychopathology

Depression is considered to be among the most common emotional disorders among the elderly:[22,158] The rates of depression vary from 1% to 29%, depending in part on how the problem is defined with mild depression being more common.[28,68,69] According to the NIH Consensus Conference[119] 15% of community elderly manifest depressive symptoms and 3 percent manifest major depression. In primary care clinics, 5% of the elderly have minor or major depression, whereas among those in nursing homes it is 25 to 25%. More than 50% of elderly seen in psychiatric clinics have a diagnosis of depression.[17,18] Depression will increase in magnitude as the elderly population increases. Depression is more common in women and those living in urban areas.[28,98,158]

Biochemical abnormalities found in depressed persons are discussed in the psychopathology of depression in Chapter 17, Mental Health, as are three psychologic theoretical perspectives—

psychoanalytic theory, interpersonal theory, and cognitive theory. "Deficiencies in the concentrations of neurotransmitters, such as dopamine, norepinephrine, serotonin, and acetylcholine, and elevated cortisol, sodium, and monoamine oxidase levels have been suggested as possible etiologic factors."[22, p. 48] Dopamine, for example, likely contributes significantly to depression.[21] Genetically, late life depression may be different from early life depression and psychologic, physiologic, and psychosocial factors may play a more important role in the elderly.[22]

Bodily functions may slow down with age, and, although speculative, biochemical balances of amines, hormones, and electrolytes can be affected.[105] Medications used by the elderly can alter biochemical levels. As aging proceeds, the amount of neurotransmitters and hormones change.[105] A relationship is noted between depression and the neurobiologic nature of stress. The concept of stress system "failure" or dysregulation is being investigated.[132]

In discussing causes for depression in the elderly, the psychosocial perspective points to multiple losses and/or incapacitation and environmental stressors along with adaptive lifelong coping and adaptive strategies.[22,68,69]

Suicide is a great risk in depressed elderly: about 25% of all suicides occur in those older than age 65, with one in two suicide attempts in the elderly being successful.[22] Particularly vulnerable to suicide risk among the elderly are white men; those suffering from a chronic debilitating disease; those acutely ill with some physical disability and one or more ADL impairments[46]; those widowed, divorced and/or isolated; those engaging in drug or alcohol abuse; and those who are hopeless or impulsive.[28,68,69] The elderly also have a much higher rate of suicide completion.[28] Most persons visit their primary care physician within the month before the suicide with their depressive symptoms being unrecognized and untreated.[119]

•••••• Diagnostic Studies and Findings

Diagnosis and recognition of depression in late life may be more difficult than earlier in life because (a) symptoms of depression may be attributed to the aging process; (b) the actual symptoms of depression may be different from those in younger persons (i.e, more somatic complaints), and the elderly are less likely to acknowledge depressed mood; (c) there may be more concern over the presence of actual medical conditions; (d) the presence of dementia and stroke may compromise accurate reporting of symptoms; (e) there may be a lack of understanding of depression; and, (f) fear of expense of treatment can be present.[119] In fact, because the symptoms of dementia and depression have some similarity, differential diagnosis can be very problematic.[109,174]

Comprehensive interview and complete physical and mental examination[51]   To determine (a) presence of depression occurring secondarily to physical illness (either as a direct physiologic effect or as the medical condition acting as a psychologic precipitant of depression, or due to both of these processes[76] e.g., conditions of the cardiovascular system such as—congestive heart failure, cardiac arrhythmias, myocardial infarction; conditions of the central nervous system—cerebrovascular accident, multiinfarct dementia in

which 19% to 27% of the patients have depression,[90] Alzheimer's disease, Parkinson's disease, Huntington's disease, AIDS dementia, tumors especially abdominal malignancies, trauma of the neurologic system, meningiomas, epilepsy; autoimmune conditions—rheumatoid arthritis; conditions of the endocrine system—hyperparathyroidism, hypoparathyroidism, Addison's disease, diabetes mellitus; other conditions—anemias, infectious disease, malnutrition, hypothyroidism, systemic lupus erythematosus, chronic pain syndrome*; (b) to determine presence of depression that may be masked by somatic ailments or a single symptom as insomnia[22]; (c) to determine presence of depression occurring as a result of use of medications that can precipitate depression such as cardiovascular medications—digitalis, reserpine, clonidine, propranolol; analgesics—phenylbutazone, opiates; central nervous system medications—benzodiazepines, barbiturates, alcohol, cocaine withdrawal, amphetamine withdrawal; antimicrobials (that can also cause delirium)—sulfonamides, quinolones, ciprofloxacin; hormones—estrogen, progesterone, corticosteroids; other medications—heavy metals.

Survey of medications   To determine both over-the-counter and prescribed medication use.[89]

Nutritional survey

Routine diagnostic procedures   To determine presence of coexisting medical condition. This includes ECG, blood count, urinalysis, B_{12} level, liver function tests, folate level, T_4, thyroid-stimulating hormone, glucose, electrolytes, BUN, creatinine, VDRL.[89]

Neuropsychologic testing[51]   To differentiate conditions such as depression and dementia (e.g., dementia syndrome of depression [pseudodementia]), syndrome of depression as part or organic process in dementia of the Alzheimer's type.

Electrophysiologic and psychometric evaluation[51]   To differentiate depression (with early morning awakening) from sleep disorders of the elderly such as primary insomnia.

Psychometric assessment for depression[51]   Self-report tools can be used to determine presence of depression (e.g., Beck Depression Inventory, Geriatric Depression Scale, Zung Self-Rating Depression Scale, Profile of Mood States, Multiscore Depression Inventory); structured interview tools can be used to determine presence of depression (e.g., Structured Interview Guide for the Hamilton Rating Scale for Depression, Diagnostic Interview Schedule); projective tests can be conducted by psychologists to determine presence of depression (e.g., Rorschach, Thematic Apperception Test).

Symptom inventory   To detect elevated levels of depression and anxiety in the elderly.[106]

•••••• Multidisciplinary Plan

Surgery/other Treatment

Electroconvulsive therapy (ECT)   To treat elderly not responsive to other treatments including pharmacotherapy, especially patients who are catatonic or psychotically depressed.[27,28]

---

*References, 40, 51, 68, 69, 98, 99, 124.

Medications*

It should be noted that "As a result of . . . pharmacokinetic changes, psychotropic drugs achieve a higher blood level per dose and are metabolized and excreted more slowly in elders than in younger patients. At the same time, loss of nerve cells and receptor sites in the central nervous system contributes to relatively greater concentration and increased sensitivity to medications and their side effects. However, there is no uniformity in the aging process and an enormous amount of variability exists among elders in their response and sensitivity to medications."[28, p. 561] In general, however, the elderly may be more vulnerable to the side effects of medications (e.g., orthostatic hypotension, sedation).[164]

Because major depressions are often recurrent, maintenance drug treatment may be necessary after remission of the depression. After the first episode of major depression, medications should be maintained for 6 months; after the second episode or more, 12 months.[119]

It should also be noted that in relation to the treatment of emotional problems and mental conditions of the elderly in nursing facilities that the Omnibus Budget Reconciliation Act (OBRA) regulations must be observed: OBRA regulations refer especially to neuroleptic use. Psychosocial interventions are the preferred choice of intervention over use of medications, with psychotropic medications to be used minimally, unless the diagnosis is major depressive disorder, in which case drug therapy is initiated (i.e., unnecessary use of medications [chemical] and physical restraints should be avoided).[164] Before initiating drug therapy with antidepressants in the elderly, a very careful assessment is necessary along with regular evaluation for efficacy when treatment is prolonged.[5]

Selective serotonin reuptake inhibitors (SSRIs)   For example, fluoxetine 5 to 40 mg, sertraline hydrochloride 25 to 100 mg, also paroxetine, venlafaxine, fluoxetine. SSRIs are being more commonly used in treating depression in the elderly. Side effects include occasional gastrointestinal upset, sexual dysfunction, insomnia, and overstimulation, but minimal sedation, anticholinergic, or cardiovascular effects.[11,27,28]

Tricyclic antidepressants (TCAs)   For example, desipramine 25 to 150 mg; nortriptyline 10 to 100 mg. Nortriptyline is still a significant risk for orthostatic hypotension albeit less than amitriptyline. SSRIs are preferable in apathetic lethargic patients and are the first first-line drug of choice.

Nontricyclic antidepressants   For example, bupropion hydrochloride 75 to 150 mg; trazodone hydrochloride 50 to 400 mg. Trazodone is used in the elderly because there are no anticholinergic effects, for suicidal patients, and for those with insomnia, but it can cause sedation and orthostatic hypotension; bupropion can be used in the elderly; few anticholinergic, sedative, or cardiovascular effects; can cause insomnia, agitation, nausea, seizures.[27,28]

Monoamine oxidase inhibitors (MAOI)   For example, phenelzine 15 to 90 mg, to treat primary mood disorders and atypical depression; however, side effects include orthostatic hypotension that is very common among the elderly and insomnia; severe hypertensive reaction occurs if patient ingests tyramine found in certain foods as aged cheese or wines; major drug interactions can also occur with other medications such as tricyclic antidepressants, selective serotonin reuptake inhibitors, sympathomimetics, and opioids; to be used with great care by experts in psychopharmacology and needs of the elderly.[22,27,28]

Psychostimulants   For example, methylphenidate 5 to 20 mg. Psychostimulants are used to treat depression in elderly not candidates for ECT or other medications and usually those with extreme psychomotor retardation or who are medically ill.[27,28] Effects are seen within 2 to 3 days. They are often used as an adjunct to other antidepressants.

General Management

Individual therapy   To convey to the elderly patient that he or she can master the present through therapy that is time-limited, structured, and goal-oriented[68,69]

Individual insight psychotherapy   To resolve previous intrapsychic and interpersonal conflicts and fear of dependence for elderly with a mild depression[68,69]

Supportive psychotherapy   To provide support, specific directives, and counseling for elderly patients with severe depression[68,69]

Group therapy   To provide support and counseling. The elderly patient observes that others share similar experiences

Day treatment   To provide a structured daytime treatment milieu

Music, dance, art therapy   To focus thoughts and feelings on something other than despair, to permit interpersonal interactions, and to foster expression of feelings[79]

Focus treatment on symptoms in mixed anxiety-depression states common in elderly patients[156]

NURSING CARE

Nursing Assessment

Assess for risk factors for depression in the elderly.
  Physiologic factors
    Chronic illness
    Chronic pain[78]
    Alcoholism[39]
    Use of multiple medications[22]
  Psychosocial stressors and factors
    Absence of hardiness[30]
    Negative attitude toward death/death experience[30]
    Previous suicide attempts
    Loss of significant other
    Recently bereaved

---

*References 17, 18, 27, 28, 68, 69.

Strained family relationships
Family stress
Retirement
Loss of social network
Inadequate social support
Extreme isolation
Marital breakdown
Living alone[99]
Being a caregiver of cognitively-impaired dependent[31]
Economic stressors
    Lack of adequate finances
    Low socioeconomic status[99]
Loss of environmental and social stability
    Loss of neighborhood, home, familiar people/activities[165]
    Institutionalization
Presence of multiple concurrent crisis
Assess for symptoms of depression[157]
    Depressed mood
    Expressions of helplessness, worthlessness, hopelessness
    Feelings of failure
    Loss of interest in life
    Lack of interest in activities that were a source of pleasure
    Lack of motivation
    Withdrawal from others
    Multiple somatic complaints
    Lack of appetite
    Loss of weight
    Change in sleep patterns
    Fatigue
    Restlessness
    Irritability
    Low self-esteem
    Anxiety
    Diminished ability to concentrate
    Thoughts of suicide

Assess for denial of presence of depression: the elderly may deny depressed feelings and not seek mental health care readily.[17,18] Dysphoria may be a less prominent symptom of depression in the elderly than symptoms such as sleeplessness.[65] The elderly may also not discuss suicidal thoughts readily.[157] People of some cultures (e.g., Hispanics, Asians, African-Americans) may find it more acceptable to discuss somatic complaints rather than admit to emotional problems and signs of mental illness.[157]

Nursing Dx & Intervention

Risk for violence (self-directed) related to depression

- Assess for presence of depression in elderly client regardless of setting *because early diagnosis, referral, and treatment is critical in resolving this condition: depression in the elderly is generally responsive to treatment and lack of treatment can lead to lethal consequences.*[22]

- Assess for suicide potential *because the elderly have the highest suicide rate and are at a very high risk for completed suicide.*[10,27,28,68,69]
    Assess events (e.g., losses, abuse/use of medications, illness, spousal or elderly abuse).
    Assess behavioral changes (e.g., grooming, eating, sleeping).
    Assess feelings and thoughts (e.g., hopelessness, anger, ability to concentrate).
    Determine presence of suicidal thoughts and presence of suicidal plan, resources, and time frame.

- Collaborate with the interdisciplinary team to maintain a safe environment free of the potential of self-harm: one-to-one observation may be required when the patient is preoccupied with thoughts of suicide.

- Stress importance of medication regimen in hospital and compliance with medication regimen after hospitalization.

- Develop a supportive and nurturing therapeutic relationship with patient *because this will become the basis for future social integration.*[22]

- Be an empathetic listener, present a sense of optimism, and convey hope.

- Help patient examine alternative actions to his or her problems *to overcome a sense of hopelessness and ineffectuality.*

- Have patient engage in meaningful activities within his or her level of coping and capabilities *because such activities can distract from problems and be therapeutic.*[22]

- Alleviate isolation and reduced independence caused by immobility and/or sensory deprivation.[109]

Ineffective individual coping related to depression

- Use cognitive therapy strategies[68,69,175] *to help patient view situation in an alternative, more positive manner and to replace faulty perceptions with more valid ones.*
    Assist patient in examining thoughts for distortions.
    Discuss basic assumptions behind beliefs.
    Help patient change thoughts from negative to positive.
    Systematically reinforce positive input thought patterns.
        Have patient record daily pleasant and unpleasant thoughts in a daily diary.
        Have patient record sleep time and other activities.
        Discuss diary with patient commenting on performance, encouraging expression of feelings, identifying thoughts leading to depression, assisting in accepting conditions that cannot be changed and problem solving to solve problems that can be changed, supporting hope and hopefulness.[24]

- Facilitate grief work *to assist patient in resolving emotions related to multiple and major losses so frequently experienced by the elderly.*

- Assist patient in examining remaining relationships after the death of a significant person and develop new relationships *to maintain social contacts for companionship, support, love, and intimacy.*[105]

- Increase patient's self-esteem:

   Engage patient in life review reminiscence *that can be a useful tool in having elderly patient experience pleasures of previous life experiences by recalling them: this can actually combat depression and build self-esteem.*[22,146]

   Acknowledge progress made.

- Use humor, when appropriate, in interpersonal interactions and therapy with the elderly patient *because humor can reduce stress, is interactive, facilitates cohesion, and is life-affirming.*[130]
- Encourage social contacts *to reduce social isolation and develop sense of self-worth.*[157]
- Help patient focus on the here and now.

   Explore present situation and problems.

   Assist patient in forming alternative, more positive views.

   Engage patient in problem-solving, setting realistic expectations.

- Explore reality with patient and strategies to deal with stressors. *Aims of counseling should be limited and focus on coping with reality.*[22]

   Examine patient's strengths and potential.

   Examine current life stressors.

   Explore coping strategies previously used by patient.

   Assist patient to examine alternative coping strategies to deal with current stressors.

   Have patient try out new behavior in a supportive environment.

- Use behavioral strategies *to help patient focus on present behavior that can be changed and thus foster a sense of self-control and hope.*[68,69]

   Use role play to have patient model new behavior.

   Develop verbal contract with patient to try out new behaviors.

- Have elderly patient examine own goals to determine whether too much is expected of self.
- Have elderly patient compare self with others of same age to help him or her realize that they are not alone in what is being experienced.
- Instill hope by assessing and intervening with variables in an interactive model of hope *so that patient will once again feel that there is the prospect of regaining power over his or her life.*[49,79]

   Assess presence and meaning of stress life events.

   Examine with patient coping strategies used in past to deal with stressors and those that could be currently applied.

   In collaboration with interdisciplinary team, assess and treat medical problems.

   Assess meaning of medical condition for patient.

   In collaboration with interdisciplinary team, assess and treat mental disorders.

   Promote social support: identify adequacy of patient's social support system; determine functioning of social support system.

   Increase patient's sense of personal control.

   Determine ability to perform ADLs.

   Determine patient's spiritual and religious strengths.

- Engage the elderly patient in group therapy *because this form of therapy can assist the elderly patient to deal with stressors and solve problems such as adjusting to retirement, dealing with loneliness, and coping with insecurity, and can enhance self-esteem, especially when integrated into an overall interdisciplinary treatment plan.*[37]
- Use cognitive-behavioral group therapy or focused visual imagery group therapy *to decrease cognitive impairments in elderly depressed patients because these group therapies have shown promise with nursing home residents who are depressed and have mild to moderate cognitive limitations.*[1]
- Encourage healthy lifestyle habits *because improved self-care can restore a sense of mastery and assist in managing depression:*[17,18]

   Encourage balanced diet.

   Encourage use of good sleep habits.

   Encourage balanced rest/sleep and activity/exercise pattern.

- Encourage the family and significant others to be involved in elderly patient's recovery from depression. *Family and significant others can offer social support that has been found to protect elderly from depression.*[99]
- Engage the elderly patient and family in family therapy *to help the patient strengthen social support and enhance social networks and resources.*
- Engage the elderly patient in family therapy/marital therapy *because depression can have a negative impact on marital relationships.*[171]
- Work with the patient to develop or restore a social network by linking patient to various community activities and groups.

Patient Education/Home Care Planning

1. "Teach patient about nature, symptom, causes, and treatment of depression, including medications and their side effects.
2. Teach importance of continuing prescribed medication regimen and self-monitoring for occurrence of side effects.
3. Teach patient self-help strategies in coping with depressed mood and depression. For example, 'Do not set yourself difficult goals or take on a great deal of responsibility.'

   - Break large tasks into small ones, set some priorities, and do what you can as you can.
   - Do not expect too much from yourself too soon as this will only increase feelings of failure.
   - Try to be with other people; it is usually better than being alone.
   - Participate in activities that may make you feel better.

- Try mild exercise, going to a movie, a ballgame, or participating in religious or social activities.
- Don't overdo it or get upset if your mood is not greatly improved right away. Feeling better takes time.
- Do not make major life decisions, such as changing jobs, getting married or divorced, without consulting others who know you well and who have a more objective view of your situation. In any case, it is advisable to postpone important decisions until your depression has lifted.
- Do not expect to snap out of your depression. People rarely do. Help yourself as much as you can, and do not blame yourself for not being up to par.
- Remember, do not accept your negative thinking. It is part of the depression and will disappear as your depression responds to treatment."[121, pp. 3-4]

Evaluation

Risk for violence, self-directed   Patient will not harm self and partial or complete remission of symptoms of depression will occur.

Ineffective individual coping   Patient will experience partial or complete remission of characteristics of depression, achieve optimal functioning, engage in activities of daily living, experience enhanced functioning in social and occupational roles, and experience an increase in quality of life. Hope and a sense of optimism about the future will be restored and the patient achieves a sense of pleasure from living.

DELIRIUM, DEMENTIA, AND AMNESTIC AND OTHER COGNITIVE DISORDERS IN THE ELDERLY

Delirium, dementia, and amnestic and other cognitive disorders are comprised of (a) delirium, (b) dementia, (c) amnestic disorders, and (d) other cognitive disorders.[6,8,137,147]

Delirium is characterized by rapid onset (usually over a few hours to a few days) and lasts a few hours to several weeks. Signs and symptoms of delirium include altered consciousness; reduced attention span and/or ability to shift attention; altered awareness; reduced awareness of environment; changed cognition; some memory deficits especially for recent events; disorientation to time, place, and person; disorganized thinking; incoherent speech; altered perception; delusions; hallucinations, often visual; asterixis; multifocal myoclonus; sleep disturbances; and altered behavior. Symptoms develop rapidly over a short period of time and often fluctuate. Symptoms are often worse at night. The patient can be either drowsy and lethargic or restless, agitated, or irritable. In acute delirium the patient may be combative, appear flushed, have dilated pupils, sweat, experience a rapid heart rate and elevated blood pressure, and

manifest a fever. In severe delirium, there is multiple level impairment in nervous system metabolism. Stupor and coma can follow extreme drowsiness. Other signs and symptoms associated with delirium can include fear and anxiety, irritability, anger, euphoria, apathy or depressed mood, and labile emotions. Overall, the hallmark of the syndrome of delirium is "the relatively rapid development of global cognitive impairment combined with disorientation and confusion."[8, p. 179] Delirium can be caused by certain medical conditions, substance use, medication use, or toxin exposure that create a general upset in brain metabolism.[73] Delirium is a commonly encountered cognitive disorder and is as high as 80% on acute geriatric inpatient units. It is a common and more frequent psychopathologic condition in later life, after age 60.[133,147] After the age of 80, it is even more common.[8]

It is critical that delirium be recognized and properly diagnosed in the elderly because it is often one of the first signs of an underlying medical problem that, if not treated, can lead to irreversible brain damage or even death.[133,147] "An older individual becoming abruptly and acutely confused constitutes a medical emergency, and a rigorous diagnostic and therapeutic approach should be implemented."[73, p. 264] Up to 50% of elderly patients with delirium have been reported to die within 1 year.[8] Delirium can be difficult to diagnose from other conditions such as cognitive disorders and chronic dementia. Delirium must be differentiated from dementia: this can be difficult because demented patients can also be delirious, and delirious patients may have some underlying dementia. Misdiagnoses also occurs commonly in patients with delirium who present with symptoms of depression.[50] Delirium must be differentiated from mental disorders presenting with a functional confusional state.[8] With proper diagnosis and treatment, however, there can be full recovery from delirium.

Delirium include (1) delirium due to a general medical condition characterized by delirium resulting from the physiologic effects of a general medical condition; (2) substance-induced delirium characterized by delirium resulting from the effects of substance withdrawal or substance intoxication, (3) delirium due to multiple etiologies characterized by delirium caused by more than one etiology; and, (4) delirium not otherwise specified characterized by delirium that does not meet diagnostic criteria of other diagnostic categories of delirium.

Dementia (characterized by multiple cognitive deficits including impaired memory and one or more of the following—disturbed executive functioning, agnosia, apraxia, aphasia, impaired occupational or social functioning, caused by a medical condition, substance use, or a combination of these etiologies)[6] includes (1) dementia of the Alzheimer's type (See Chapter 3, Neurologic System, for information); (2) vascular dementia characterized by multiple cognitive deficits including memory impairment; one or more of the following cognitive disturbances—disturbed executive functioning, agnosia, apraxia, aphasia; impaired occupational or social functioning; and evidence of cerebrovascular disease. Vascular dementia, caused by cerebral blood flow disruption, is less common than dementia of the Alzheimer's type;[151] (3) dementia due to HIV disease characterized by dementia resulting from HIV; (4) dementia due to head trauma characterized by dementia from head trauma; (5) dementia due to Parkinson's disease (See Chapter 3, Neurologic System, for information); (6) dementia due to Huntington's disease characterized by dementia resulting from the effects of Huntington's disease; (7) dementia due to Pick's disease characterized by dementia resulting from the effects of Pick's disease; (8) dementia due to Creutzfeldt-Jakob disease characterized by dementia from the physiologic effects of Creutzfeldt-Jakob disease; (9) dementia due to other general medical conditions characterized by dementia from the physiologic effects of medical conditions other than those listed in this section; (10) substance-induced persisting dementia; (11) dementia due to multiple etiologies; and (12) dementia not otherwise specified characterized by a dementia that does not fit criteria of any of the other categories of dementia.

Amnestic disorders[6] include (1) amnestic disorder due to a general medical condition characterized by memory impairment with the inability to learn new information or recall information already learned, impaired social or occupational functioning, and caused by the physiologic effects of a medical condition, (2) substance-induced persisting amnestic disorder characterized by memory impairment with the inability to learn new information or recall information already learned, impaired social or occupational functioning, and caused by substance use, (3) amnestic disorder not otherwise specified characterized by memory disturbance and that does not meet criteria of the other amnestic disorders.

Other cognitive disorders[6] include cognitive disorder not otherwise specified characterized by cognitive dysfunction caused by physiologic effect of a general medical condition that does not readily fit into any of the above diagnostic categories.

DELIRIUM

Pathophysiology/Psychopathology

Psychological/Cultural Theories[147]
Environmental and psychologic factors can be contributing factors in delirium.

Biological/Genetic Theories[8,133,137,147,151]
Delirium can be caused by (a) a number of medical conditions and disorders (fever; septicemia; infections, e.g., pulmonary, urinary tract; HIV; viremias; encephalitis; myocardial infarction; arrhythmia; congestive heart failure; hypoxia; transient ischemia attack; acute stroke; seizure disorders; meningitis; subdural hematoma; brain tumors; organ failure, e.g., renal, hepatic, cardiac, pulmonary; organ transplantation; hypothyroidism; hyponatremia; hypoglycemia; hypercalcemia; thiamine deficiency; dehydration; burns; sleep deprivation; sensory overload or underload; (b) substance use (substance withdrawal, e.g., alcohol, sedatives, hypnotics); (c) medications, especially anticholinergic medications (anticholinergic toxicity; lithium toxicity; bromide toxicity; digoxin toxicity; low potency antipsychotics; polypharmacy); or, (d) toxins. Prescription drug intoxication is a very common cause of delirium in the elderly.[133] The most important causes are infections, cardiovascular disease, and medication effects.

The elderly are more vulnerable to delirium for a number of reasons. Age-related cell loss may occur, for example, in brain centers. Age-related physiologic changes can occur, such as decreased cerebral blood flow. Sensory changes can also occur in the elderly (e.g., hearing impairment). Finally, the elderly tend to suffer from more chronic medical conditions and are often prescribed medications or self-medicate themselves.

Diagnostic Studies and Findings

Complete Physical Examination
Critical examination of focal neurologic signs
Frontal lobe release signs
Papilledema
Global deficit state
Thyroid function tests
Laboratory tests such as blood counts, blood levels of ammonia, glucose, urea nitrogen
Electrolytes
Urinalysis
X-ray, especially chest x-ray because pneumonia is a common cause
CT scan
MRI
ECG
Lumbar puncture (selectively)
Blood gas studies
EEG
Toxin screen: To determine etiology for delirium[8,137] Urinalysis, chest x-ray, medication review, ECG, CBC, and chem are most important.

Multidisciplinary Plan

Surgery/Other Treatment
Treat etiology of delirium (e.g., treat infection, correct cardiovascular disease, and remove or adjust medications; treat other medical conditions, substance-related disorders; remove exposure to toxins, or correct effects of medication)
Remove noxious medication, substance of abuse, and/or toxins
Treat comorbid psychiatric symptoms[20]

Medications
High potency antipsychotics (haloperidol): To treat highly agitated delirious patients
Short-acting benzodiazepines (e.g., oxazepam; lorazepam): To treat delirious patients who require sedation

General Management
Avoid polypharmacy
Avoid sedative-hypnotics, if possible, except benzodiazepines to treat withdrawal symptoms

NURSING CARE

Nursing Assessment

Assess nature of and speed of symptom onset.

Assess level of awareness and presence of any fluctuation in awareness.

Assess level of consciousness and any fluctuation.

Assess cognitive impairment and any fluctuation.

Determine presence of delusions or hallucinations.

Evaluate emotional state (i.e, presence of fear, anxiety, anger, depressed mood, labile mood).

Note nature of speech and verbal ability.

Determine presence of any motor symptoms.

Obtain information from family and significant others regarding: (a) changes in physical health; (b) medications currently taken, including over-the-counter medications; (c) any history or current substance abuse; (d) any exposure to toxins; (e) patient's usual lifestyle; (f) any change in behavior; and (g) any assistance needed currently.

Nursing Dx & Interventions[8,81,133,137,147]

Acute confusion related to delirium

Maintain patient's safety.

   Use safety mechanisms such as call lights, safety rails as needed.

   Clear clutter in patient's environment.

   Provide constant observation as needed.

   Provide constant reorientation.

   Administer medications, being aware of potential effects.

   Use restraints if absolutely necessary: observe frequently while restraints are used.

   Ascertain that patient's visual or hearing impairments are corrected.

Maintain patient's health.

   Monitor laboratory values and observe for signs and symptoms of physical illness or effects of medications to assist in determining cause of delirium.

   Monitor carefully all medications prescribed or taken on own by patient.

   Assist with ADLs as needed.

   Give simple, clear instructions to patient *to aide in meeting ADLs.*

   Have family assist patient with ADLs when possible.

   Maintain adequate fluid intake.

   Provide for adequate nutrition.

   Implement strategies to help patient sleep: keep interruptions during night-time at minimum.

Create safe, comfortable, consistent environment *to minimize stress, augment patient's psychologic coping mechanisms, help patient remain oriented, and reduce potential for self-harm. Because patient experiences changed cognition and perception, level of consciousness, and/or con-fusion, it is very important to use interventions to help patient remain oriented as much as possible.*

   Provide moderate lighting; avoid high-intensity lighting or low lighting.

   Reduce noise in environment.

   Provide calendars, night lights, clocks, schedule for the day.

   Keep patient in same surroundings.

   Have family bring in familiar objects and possessions.

   Decorate with seasonal decorations.

   Assign consistent staff to patient.

   Offer one-to-one contact.

   Convey warmth as well as kind firmness.

   Call patient by name and refer to self and others by name.

   Explain necessary information in a simple way: repeat as necessary.

   Use nonverbal communication to reinforce speech (e.g., pointing to object).

   Make every effort to understand patient's communications.

   Speak very slowly, enunciating words carefully.

   Keep choices at a minimum: present only one task at a time.

   Clarify perceptions and validate accurate perceptions.

   Orient to time, place, person as often as needed.

   Offer orientation at beginning of each interaction with patient.

   Consistently reinforce reality.

   Use statements that are simple and direct.

Deal with irritability and agitation calmly and with use of distraction to prevent escalation rather than confrontation or argument.

Acknowledge patient's feelings.

Encourage patient to verbalize feelings.

Encourage family members, friends, and other persons familiar to patient to visit. *Significant others can have a calming influence as for example on the anxious or agitated delirious patient. They can support the patient's communication, provide orientation, and offer support.*[81,151]

Refer patient to community resources, such as a community health nurse.

Patient Education/Home Care Planning

1. Explain to patient and family reason(s) for delirium, stressors that may have contributed to the delirium, and any planned ongoing treatments.

2. Teach patient and family to seek health care from a consistent primary health care provider who is familiar with patient's needs for medication, to monitor medications prescribed and taken, to observe for side effects of medications, and to discard old medications when no longer needed.

3. Teach patient and family to monitor changes in cognition, level of awareness, or consciousness and report them to medical personnel immediately.

Evaluation

Acute confusion related to delirium   The patient will exhibit less confusion, sustain no injury, maintain physical health, manifest improved cognition, level of awareness, and level of consciousness.

ANXIETY DISORDERS IN THE ELDERLY

Anxiety disorders[6] are comprised of the following.

Panic disorder without agoraphobia is characterized by recurring panic attacks (period of sudden intense apprehension, terror, or fearfulness, often along with sense of doom); anxiety sensitivity (AS), or fear of anxiety-related sensations, is believed to play a role in panic attacks and panic disorders.[152]

Panic disorder with agoraphobia is characterized by recurrent agoraphobia (anxiety about or avoidance of situations/places where escape is difficult or help is not available in case of panic attack) and panic attacks.

Agoraphobia without history of panic disorder is characterized by panic-like symptoms but no actual panic attacks along with agoraphobia.

Specific phobia is characterized by clinically significant anxiety provoked by a specific feared situation or object often along with avoidance.

Social phobia is characterized by extreme anxiety provoked by exposure to social situation often along with avoidance.

Obsessive-compulsive disorder is characterized by obsessions causing significant anxiety and compulsions designed to neutralize the anxiety.

Post-traumatic stress disorder is characterized by reexperiencing a very traumatic event.

Acute stress disorder is characterized by reexperiencing a very traumatic event but occurring right after that event.

Generalized anxiety disorder is characterized by 6 months of excessive persistent anxiety; often a chronic condition with periodic remissions followed by exacerbations with a situational stressor as trigger.

Anxiety disorder is due to a general medical condition characterized by anxiety due to physiologic effect of a general medical condition.

Substance-induced anxiety disorder is characterized by anxiety caused by a physiologic effect of drug abuse, medication, or toxin exposure.

Anxiety disorder not otherwise specified is characterized by anxiety and that cannot be categorized into any of above diagnoses.

■ ANXIETY

Anxiety is a subjective feeling of dread or apprehension about something in the future. It is characterized by (a) cognitive symptoms—apprehension, distractability, fearfulness, irritability, nervousness, worry; (b) behavioral symptoms—hyperkinesis, phobias, pressured speech, repetitive motor acts, startle response avoidance; (c) physiologic—chest tightness, hyperventilation, light-headedness, muscle tension, palpitations, paresthesias, sweating, and urinary frequency.[140] Anxiety occurs on a continuum, ranging from mild to moderate to severe to panic. The characteristics of the different levels of anxiety—mild, moderate, severe, extreme/panic—are described in the Nursing Diagnosis Anxiety in the Self-Perception/Self-Concept Functional Health Pattern on p. 1669. Anxiety can be adaptive (mild to moderate levels), which can prepare the person for, or help the person to avoid, noxious situations. Or, anxiety can be maladaptive ranging from severe to extreme panic.

Types of anxiety include:

Situational anxiety—short-lived anxiety to a stressful stimuli that can also be affected by the elderly patient's self-esteem

Phobic anxiety—situational anxiety to a stressful stimuli in which avoidance is used as the method of coping

Anticipatory anxiety—anxious apprehension or worry occurring before the dreaded object or situation is encountered often associated with panic attacks

Free floating anxiety—pattern of indiscriminate anxiety with no close temporal link to precipitating stimuli and often a part of generalized anxiety disorder

Traumatic anxiety—anxiety occurring in persons who survive tragic or unanticipated experiences

Anxious depression—anxiety in which patients exhibit both anxiety and depression. About one third of patients with anxiety disorders suffer from clinical depression, and about two thirds of patients with a depressive disorder suffer from an anxiety disorder[142]

Anxiety secondary to medical conditions—anxiety is an overt symptom of these conditions[136]

Anxiety can also be classified as state anxiety (anxiety associated with a specific stimulus that remits once the stressor is reduced or eliminated) and trait anxiety (a persistent feature of the person's personality).[126]

•••••• Pathophysiology/Psychopathology

Many elderly experience a high quality of life in their later years. For others, old age becomes fraught with anxiety and feelings of loneliness and worthlessness. Real life problems, the loss of significant others, diminished financial resources, isolation, diminishing physical and/or mental health, and vulnerability to crime can be challenging and take their toll. Self-esteem and a sense of security can be threatened, resulting in anxiety.[142]

Some authors[55] claim that actual anxiety disorders are less common in the elderly than they are in younger persons. However, anxiety symptoms in the elderly (older than 65 years of age) are quite common and appear to range from 10% to 20%.[15] Symptoms of anxiety are common in more than half of the elderly patients seen in physician's offices, in nursing homes, and in acute care hospitals because anxiety is associated with many medical conditions, drug reactions, and dementia.[52] Markovitz[108, p. 64] notes that: "Although the overall level of anxiety is high in the elderly, pure anxiety disorders without co-morbid psychiatric or medical problems account for only a small portion of all cases of clinical anxiety." Anxiety disorders occur in more than 5% of the elderly living in the community. Generalized anxiety disorders and phobias are the most common anxiety disorders in the elderly.[55] Among the anxiety disorders, phobias appear to be the most common disorder in elderly women and the second most common in elderly men.[15] Panic disorders occur more frequently in women than in men, whereas generalized anxiety disorders occur slightly more frequently in women.[137,142] Overall, "it appears . . . that anxiety symptoms and disorders are among the most common psychiatric afflictions experienced by the elderly."[15 p. 413] And, "estimates of the prevalence of anxiety among elderly patients may be spuriously low because of lack of recognition or misdiagnosis as organic illness."[109 p. 1000] "Anxiety in its fully expressed form, or as a syndrome or symptom, reduces quality of life and, as with any chronic condition, may increase the risk of depression."[164 p. 7] A level of anxiety that interferes negatively with ADLs can lead to hospitalization.[15]

Psychologic Models: (See also Chapter 17)

Psychoanalytic/psychodynamic theory views anxiety as signaling danger and as a defense against unacceptable impulses; anxiety can also be viewed as originating during a child's separation from the mother, which in later life can reemerge when a satisfying person is not available

Classical conditioning theory proposes that phobias arise because of conditioning and relief of anxiety by avoidance, which serves as a reinforcer.

Cognitive-behavioral theory, the most accepted theory today, combines cognitive and conditioning paradigms. According to this theory, patients misinterpret sensations as those in normal anxiety responses and create catastrophic thoughts about these sensations, such as panic attacks.[15,142]

Biological Models

Four neurotransmitter systems appear to be involved in the biochemistry of anxiety disorders and anxiety states—the serotonergic system, the γ-aminobutyric acid system, the noradrenergic system, the mesocortical dopaminergic system. There may be a physiologic basis, for example, for panic attacks (i.e., the locus ceruleus is implicated, increased parahippocampal activity has been documented); panic disorders may be linked to a mendelian gene; the serotonergic neurotransmitter system is implicated in obsessive-compulsive disorder.[15,27,28,142]

•••••• Diagnostic Studies and Findings

Comprehensive history and physical examination   To determine presence of physical illnesses often presenting with prominent symptoms of anxiety (e.g., drug intoxication, drug toxicity, caffeinism, use of medications as stimulants, withdrawal from CNS depressant drugs, withdrawal from recreational drugs, caffeine-related disorder, cerebral arteriosclerosis, angina pectoris, cardiac arrhythmias, pain, con-

gestive heart failure, epilepsy, hyperinsulinism, hypoglycemia, asthma, obstructive pulmonary disease, pulmonary embolism, hyperthyroidism, premenstrual tension, monosodium glutamate allergy.[15,136] Anxiety is sometimes the first symptom of an impending medical disorder (e.g., anemia, hypoglycemia, hyperthyroidism).[41] However, in the elderly, somatic complaints are often the presenting symptom of anxiety.[164]

ECG, blood gas studies or pulse oximetry, computed tomographic scanning, serum electrolytes, urinalysis, thyroid function studies   To rule out CNS or acute cardiovascular diseases and other medical conditions and to assist in determining origins of anxiety disorder.[109]

Comprehensive mental examination   To determine presence of anxiety disorder; acuteness or chronicity of anxiety disorder; degree of impaired functioning from anxiety disorder;[136] to carefully differentiate, for treatment purposes, between anxiety and depression in the elderly, which can be very difficult. The mixed anxiety-depression syndrome is quite frequently seen in the elderly, presenting diagnostic difficulties.[15,156]

History of mental illness and conditions   To determine previous episodes of anxiety disorders because a number of these can be recurrent.

•••••• Multidisciplinary Plan

Surgery/Other Treatment[15]

Electroconvulsive therapy   To treat selected elderly with obsessive compulsive disorder who are not responsive to pharmacotherapy, although this is controversial.[27]

Psychologic treatment   Cognitive behavioral therapy to decrease avoidance, reduce anxiety, and rebuild self-confidence.

Relaxation training to reduce anxiety through progressive relaxation

Cognitive restructuring and activity structuring to manage anxiety

Psychotherapy to enable patients with situational anxiety to explore fears

Medications[136]

Careful prescription of correct (minimal) dose needed for reduction of anxiety and careful monitoring of anxiolytic medications in the elderly is required.[109]

Benzodiazepines   They are the most frequently used anxiolytics in the elderly for treatment of generalized anxiety disorder (GAD) (e.g., diazepam has sustained drug effect during the day but with the potential side effects of fatigue, drowsiness, impaired performance, and amnesia in the elderly; clonazepam use has increased; oxazepam (15 to 30 mg/day); and lorazepam (0.5 to 3 mg/day), which are short-acting, appear preferable in the elderly, especially those with liver disease. Use of benzodiazepines can result in tolerance; long-term use can result in CNS depression, ataxia, confusion, and falls in the elderly.[109] Benzodiazepines are the choice for treatment of panic disorders (e.g., alprazolam [0.25 to 1.5 mg/day]), although tricyclic antidepressants and MAOIs may also be used. Benzodiazepines can interact with other medications (e.g., alcohol, antihistamines, β-adrenergic blockers, sinemet).[41] There is less drug interaction with clonazepam, oxazepam, lorazepam.

Buspirone To treat GAD. Buspirone (20 to 30 mg/day) is an azapirone anxiolytic, with slower onset of action, and little dependence, memory, or motor impairment. Side effects include nausea, light-headedness, stimulation, and may cause increase in anxiety at first.[164] This medication is often not as effective in patients previously treated with benzodiazepines.

Antipsychotic agents (neuroleptics) To treat GAD-like state in elderly patients who are nonpsychotic but who are anxious and agitated and show signs of delirium or have dementia.

Cyclic antidepressants and serotonin selective reuptake inhibitors To treat anxiety in patients with panic episodes or with anxiety and depression; but it should be noted that some patients become more anxious on these medications.[109] SSRIs also useful for post traumatic stress disorder (PTSD).

For medically ill elderly patients with anxiety[148]

Benzodiazepine prescription must consider the functional capacity of the liver, which is involved in metabolism and becomes less efficient with aging. The nurse must be alert to signs of drug accumulation. Chronic heavy use of sedative-hypnotics can lessen effect of dose given. "In elderly patients, many aspects of brain functioning are more vulnerable to the adverse effects of benzodiazepines because of advanced age."[148, p. 28] These drugs can cause depressed mood, lability, memory disturbances, disorientiation, lessened awareness, drowsiness, gait impairment, and cause falls and lead to hip fractures.

Buspirone, an azapirone, is useful in reducing anxiety in medically ill elderly because of minimal sedation and lack of cognitive effects. It is the drug of choice in treating anxiety in patients with pulmonary disease because it is a mild respiratory stimulant rather than depressant. It is also useful in reducing anxiety in patients with dementia and brain injuries.

General Management

Physical therapy To teach muscle relaxation techniques.[109]

Music therapy To help patient deal with anxiety when faced with the unknown, as in prior to surgery.[36]

NURSING CARE

Nursing Assessment

Assess for presence of risk factors or causes of anxiety.
  General loss of health
  Impending surgery
  Chronic pain
  Diet (e.g., caffeine intake)

  Prescribed or over-the-counter medications (e.g., neuroleptics, amphetamines, bronchodilators, theophylline, sympathomimetics such as pseudoephedrine hydrochloride)
  Alcohol withdrawal
  Recreational drug withdrawal[41]
  Sedative-hypnotic withdrawal
  Financial stressors
  Environmental stressors
  Adaptation stressors (e.g., relocation to nursing home)
  Salient role stressors[95]
  Loss of friends, family
  Impaired role performance caused by major illness (e.g., cancer)[102]
Patient's description of current symptoms and life circumstances, changes, stressors
Assess for defining characteristics of anxiety. (For list see Nursing Diagnosis, Anxiety, p. 1669).
Beck Anxiety Inventory: a self-administered tool that can be used to detect anxiety.[41]
Assess for complaints of physical symptoms.
Identify level of anxiety (i.e., mild, moderate, severe, extreme/panic). (For characteristics see Nursing Diagnosis, Anxiety, p. 1669).
Assess effect of anxiety on daily functioning.
Strategies used by patient to avoid anxiety (e.g., to what degree is avoidance used?)
Resources available to patient such as significant others, spiritual resources, problem-solving skills.

Nursing Dx & Interventions

Severe anxiety related to perceived threats to self-esteem and personal sense of security

Use therapeutic listening skills to demonstrate acceptance of patient as he or she describes the experience of anxiety. *Elderly patients may prefer somatic descriptors for their feelings of anxiety and may see emotional problems or mental illness as stigmatizing.*[142]

Develop supportive relationship with patient *because providing reassurance to patient and providing assurance that patient will not be abandoned are important strategies to reduce anxiety: the reduction of severe anxiety to a lesser more manageable level is the first goal.*[109]

Assist patient in identifying and recognizing sources of threat. *Unexaggerated appraisal of potential or actual sources of threat are important in anxiety reduction.*

Assist patient in exploring link between source of threat, manifestations of anxiety, and consequences of anxious state.

Determine with patient whether there are any secondary gains from anxious state.

Assist patient in exploring ways to remove or manage source of threat.

Help patient develop an action plan to deal with anxiety.

Teach relaxation techniques (e.g., breathing exercises, diaphragmatic breathing, exercise, back rubs, massage, imagery, meditation, prayer, relaxation therapy, therapeutic touch).[64]

Use less stress technique.[136]

Have patient list goals and eliminate nonattainable goals. Subdivide tasks into manageable parts.

Have patient establish a priority list of tasks, including realistic time requirements to accomplish them.

Have patient begin with tasks that can readily be achieved.

Have patient look at ways his or her work environment can be organized.

Encourage patient to learn to say "no" to additional tasks.

Teach patient to break up stressful projects/tasks by doing something relaxing and use imagery to envision peaceful places.

Encourage patient to discuss anxiety-provoking situations with others.

Instruct patient in importance of balancing work, exercise, recreation, sleep.

Encourage support from clergy or other spiritual advisor *because prayer and spiritual beliefs can be a very supportive resource for the elderly patient.*[142]

Use cognitive-behavioral therapy strategies *to correct faulty appraisal of threat, restore self-esteem, decrease tension and anxiety, and decrease avoidance.*[136]

Use reengagement strategies, such as reexposure or desensitization, especially in patients with phobias *to assist patient in coping with sources of threat. Anxiety can usually be overcome with gradual and repeated exposure to the source of threat.*[41,136]

Encourage development and maintenance of strong social support system. *Stressors in roles that are salient to the elderly can erode feelings of control and lead to stress and anxiety. Social support can be a buffer to reduce the impact of stressors on well-being.*[96]

When appropriate, refer patient to group psychotherapy or family therapy.

Have patient exercise regularly. *Aerobic forms of exercise are associated with reduction in anxiety, with exercise duration needing to be at least 21 minutes to reduce state and trait anxiety.*[123]

Ask patient to limit intake of caffeine-containing beverages and other stimulants such as diet pills.

Patient Education/Home Care Planning

1. Teach patient about cause, manifestation, and treatment of anxiety. Refer to self-help books on coping with anxiety such as Lesman TL: *Healing the anxiety diseases.* New York, 1992, Plenum.[41]
2. Teach patient to monitor self for signs and symptoms of anxiety.
3. Teach patient about both positive and negative aspects of anxiety. On the one hand, anxiety is a normal emotion serving useful arousal in helping person cope with

a dangerous threat.[126] On the other hand, it can become maladaptive and self-defeating if the person repeatedly avoids experiences that do not need to be avoided or has such intense feelings and thoughts that interfere with daily living. Explain to patient that "Pessimistic or helpless thoughts may lead to more anxiety and more avoidance behavior and, thus, to still more negative thinking."[41 p. 164]

4. Teach patient self-control strategy for worry[41 p. 164] "(1) Closely observe your thinking during the day and learn to identify the antecedents of worry; (2) establish a daily half-hour worry period that takes place at the same time and in the same place; (3) postpone worrying until your worry period, but jot down the worries beforehand if necessary; (4) use the daily worry period to think intensively about your current concerns and to generate possible solutions, and (5) replace worrisome thoughts with focused attention on a task at hand or on anything else in your immediate environment."

Evaluation

Severe anxiety related to perceived threats to self-esteem and personal sense of security   Defining characteristics of severe anxiety (e.g., severe apprehension, severe worry, painful sense of helplessness and worthlessness, severe feeling of diffuseness, purposeless activity, reduced range of perception, lack of clear comprehension of immediate situation, ineffective functioning, tachycardia, hyperventilation, urinary frequency, nausea, dizziness, headache, insomnia) will be reduced or eliminated.

SLEEP DISORDERS IN THE ELDERLY

Sleep disorders[6] include four major categories: (1) primary sleep disorder, (2) sleep disorder related to another mental disorder, (3) sleep disorder due to a general medical condition, and (4) substance-induced sleep disorder. Primary sleep disorders include both dyssomnias—disturbances in the quality, the amount, or the timing of sleep that are not caused by a medical diagnosis, substance abuse, or another psychiatric diagnosis. Examples of dyssomnias include primary insomnia, primary hypersomnia, narcolepsy, breathing-related sleep disorder, circadian rhythm sleep disorder; and parasomnias—disturbances in physiologic or behavioral events that are associated with sleep, sleep stages, or sleep wake transitions that are not caused by a medical diagnosis, substance abuse, or another psychiatric diagnosis. Exmples of parasomnias include nightmare disorder, sleep terror disorder, and sleepwalking disorder. *Dyssomnia: primary insomnia* is characterized by difficulties in starting or maintaining sleep, inadequate/insufficient sleep, or by nonrestorative sleep and daytime fatigue that lasts minimally 1 month and causes changes in mood or concentration level, distress, or impaired functioning in such areas as occupational or social roles.[6,8,42,110] Primary insomnia is not due to the physiologic effects of a medical condition, substance use or abuse nor does it occur solely during the course of a mental disorder or another sleep disorder. *Dyssomnia: breathing-related sleep disorder* is characterized by sleep disruption with insomnia or excessive sleepiness caused by a sleep-related breathing condition, such as central sleep apnea syndrome, obstructive sleep apnea syndrome, *and* is not caused by substance abuse, medical condition, or mental disorder. The incidence of sleep apnea is estimated to be 20% to 40% in the elderly and is often missed. The repetitive partial of complete closure of the upper airway during continued efforts to breathe, along with repetitive arousals and oxygen desaturation, can result in extreme sleepiness, insomnia, irritability depression, memory impairment, hypertension, decreased concentration, fatigue, sexual dysfunction, and headaches.[170] *Sleep disorder due to another mental disorder* includes both insomnia related to another mental disorder and hypersomnia related to another mental disorder. Insomnia related to another mental disorder is a condition directly caused by a mental disorder other than substance abuse and is characterized by difficulty in falling and staying asleep during the night that lasts at least a month and results in feelings of daytime fatigue and impaired functioning. These mental disorders include major depressive disorder, anxiety disorder, borderline personality disorder, or dementia in the elderly.[110] Increased severity of dementia is associated with an increase in sleep disturbance.[16] *Sleep disorder due to a general medical condition* is a sleep disturbance caused by a physiologic consequences of a medical condition that results in impaired daytime functioning. Insomnia type is predominantly characterized by insomnia. *Substance-induced sleep disorder* is characterized by a sleep disturbance caused by physiologic effects of a substance (toxin, medication, drug abuse) resulting in impaired daytime functioning. Insomina type is predominantly characterized by insomnia.

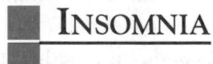

INSOMNIA

• • • • • • Pathophysiology/Psychopathology

Sleep is important biologically and clinically: it is essential for health, well-being, and for a satisfactory quality of life. Most persons sleep between 4 to 12 hours per night, with those sleeping less than 4 to 5 hours considered short sleepers and those requiring more than 9 to 10 hours, long sleepers, with the average adult requiring 7 to 8 hours of sleep.[8,32,138] Whether the person's sleep is adequate can be determined by whether he or she feels rested and refreshed when waking up.[138] The normal sleep cycle includes[93,138,139] (a) alert/wakeful state; (b) readiness for sleep, (c) alpha state, (d) nonrapid eye movement phase of sleep (NREM), including stage 1—characterized by light sleep, being easily aroused, having fleeting thoughts; stage 2—characterized by transitional sleep, having fragmented and short

thoughts, being unaware of environment; stage 3—characterized by deeper sleep, relaxed muscles, decreased and stable pulse, deeper and more regular breathing, decreased temperature; stage 4—(physically restorative sleep) characterized by deep sleep, difficulty in being awakened; few body movements; and rapid eye movement phase of sleep (REM)—(ocurs after about 45 minutes of movement through previous phases) (mentally restorative sleep, important for memory, adaptation, problem solving, and learning) characterized by bursts of CNS activity and aroused state of body; muscle and eye movements; irregular and often increased heart rate, breathing, and blood pressure; and dreaming. One sleep cycle usually takes about 90 minutes to complete.[169] Generally, the sleep wake cycle occurs over 24 hours and is part of the circadian rhythm of the body.[169] During sleep, the brain waves become slower and higher, becoming their slowest (deep slow wave sleep) during stage 3 and 4, whereas during REM sleep the brain waves become more shallow and are of mixed frequency.[138,139] Noradrenergic systems are primarily involved in controlling REM sleep, whereas serotonin-containing nuclei and pathways are key in regulating NREM sleep.[8] If primary insomnia represents a lifetime disorder or a trait characteristic, the pathophysiology may be "secondary to a neurochemical or structural disorder involving neural networks governing sleep-wake states. . . . Other patients develop primary insomnia following a period of severe stress."[118, p. 836]

Sleep disturbances/disorders affect about one third of the adults in the United States, with insomnia (insufficient, inadequate and/or nonrestorative sleep resulting in daytime fatigue and impaired functioning in general activities of daily living) being the most common complaint. For persons older than 64, almost 50% report poor sleep such as insomnia.[45] The incidence of poor sleep is even higher among institutionalized elderly, with up to 94% experiencing disturbed sleep.[45] Sleep pattern disturbances are so common among the elderly that often the misperception exists that poor sleep is part of the "normal aging process"; however, factors, such as chronic or acute illness and biologic and social routine changes, play a role, and chronologic age per se is not necessarily correlated highly with poor sleep.

In the elderly, changes affecting the sleep-wake cycle/pattern tend to result in some fragmentation, and instability in sleep.[57] The total sleep time, which does not appear to change much with age, is dispersed over a 24-hour cycle with a decrease in consolidated sleep time.[45,110] The older person may spend more time in bed with more time being awake in bed, but less time sleeping in one stretch without waking up, may be fatigued, and be less alert and/or nap during the daytime.[52,56,57] The type of sleep may change with advancing age (e.g., greater number of sleep stage shifts, increased number of awakenings, more transitional sleep [stage 1]), lighter sleep (i.e., less slow wave deep sleep [stage 3 and 4]), less tolerance for phase shifts in the sleep wake schedule and shortened rapid eye movement (REM) sleep latency but unchanged percentage of REM sleep, increase in abnormal breathing events, increase in frequency of leg movements, and report of poorer subjective quality of sleep.[45,56,57,110] In a research study by Floyd[57, p. 76] older people identified the following most bothersome sleep characteristics: "I have to get up in the middle of the night." "I can't fall back asleep if awakened." "It is too noisy where I sleep." "I awaken too easily." "I move around too much during sleep." "I have aches and pains when trying to sleep." "I am too drowsy during the day." "I sleep too much." Overall, the elderly retire to bed earlier, wake up earlier, wake up more frequently during the night, and find it harder to go back to sleep. Ineffective sleep or lack of adequate sleep in the elderly[93] can lead to apathy, decreased facial expression, depression, reduced attention span, lack of coordination, fatigue, burning of eyes, muscle tremor, and skeletal muscle weakness. It is important to understand that sleep is a very complex phenomenon and can be affected by numerous factors, esecially other psychiatric disorders.

•••••• Diagnostic Studies and Findings

Personal and family history of sleep disorders

Chief complaint: onset, duration, severity, and characteristics of sleep problem

Complete physical examination: To determine presence of any medical condition, sleep-related breathing conditions, use of medications or drugs that may be the cause of insomnia[52]

Blood alcohol, toxin, or medication levels: To determine presence of substance potentially causing insomnia[52]

Complete mental status examination: To determine presence of any psychiatric disorder (e.g., mood disorders, substance abuse, anxiety disorder, cognitive disorders as dementia, substance-related disorders) that may be causing insomnia

Nocturnal polysomnography or ambulatory polysomnography: To assess both the nature and the severity of the insomnia; assesses the discrepancy between subjective complaints and actual sleep problems experienced[116]

•••••• Multidisciplinary Plan

Surgery/Other Treatment

Referral to sleep disorder center especially for sleep-related breathing disorders. Surgery may be useful in treating certain sleep-related disorders (e.g., obstructive sleep apnea [OSA]).[161]

Continuous nasal-positive airway pressure (CPAP): To treat central sleep apnea along with having the patient quit smoking and lose weight

Medications

Pharmacologic approaches to treatment of sleep disturbances in the elderly is affected by age-related drug kinetics and dynamic changes: they may experience altered drug distribution, slowed drug metabolism caused by decreased liver function, reduced drug elimination caused by reduced renal function, and thus longer half-lives of medications.[45]

Pharmacologic Management of Insomnia[170]

Sedatives: Untoward side effects seen in elderly and potential development of tolerance and dependence with use of certain sedativs (e.g., barbiturates and SSRI antidepressants suppress REM sleep; benzodiazepines suppress Stage 3 and 4 sleep and REM; flurazepam and other long-lasting sedatives can lead to impaired cognition and increased risk of falls in elderly and should be avoided); tolerance can develop toward barbiturates; rebound insomnia after withdrawal of short half-life benzodiazepines can occur.

Minimal usage is recommended in elderly because chronic use can lead to chronic sleep disturbance.

Sedatives may be prescribed for 2 months (the ideal use, however, is 14 days or less) then gradually discontinued by one quarter the dose every 2 weeks.

Useful Sedatives/hypnotics in Elderly[170]

Initiate sleep rapidly.

Maintain sleep during normal sleeping hours.

Result in little sedative activity or other side effects during normal waking hours.

No hypnotic available that has no risk in elderly patients.[118]

Antidepressants: trazodone—useful as a hypnotic in the elderly: no tolerance or anticholinergic effects but with side effect of hypotension, daytime sleepiness, and increased risk for falls;[118] amitriptyline, should generally not be used in elderly to initiate and maintain sleep: it has side effects of anticholinergic delirium, daytime sedation, and increased risk for falls;[118] nortriptyline—tricyclic antidepressant (a medication that is alright for elderly for sleep) is given at bedtime to initiate and maintain sleep in the elderly.[45,52]

Benzodiazepines: triazolam 0.125 mg—a short-acting benzodiazepine, useful in elderly for sleep onset insomnia, with no daytime sedation but with side effect of rebound insomnia, also controversial because it may cause memory impairment,[118] there is significant interaction with cytochrome p450 system so lorazepam may be recommended instead; estazolam 0.5 mg—has an intermediate half life and is useful in elderly for sleep onset and maintenance insomnia but with side effects of daytime sedation and performance decrements.[118]

Antipsychotics; thioridazine—no tolerance but extrapyramidal side effects and increased risk for falls and anticholinergic delirium[118]; this medication should not be used for sleep in the elderly per se, only for sundowning in dementia patients.

Miscellaneous medications: zolpidem—an imidazopyridine without the usual benzodiazepine side effects, little disruption of sleep stages, no tolerance, but may mildy impair daytime performance.[118]

Discontinue use of offending medications or caffeine if insomnia linked to medication use.

Analgesics (aspirin or Motrin, for example) for pain control and management.[111]

Reduction/alteration in use of stimulants.

General Management

Treatment of underlying etiology of insomnia based on accurate assessment is critical in care of elders (i.e., treatment of medical condition, psychiatric disorder [especially mood disorders, anxiety disorders], substance abuse disorder)

Dementia management

Relaxation therapy for anxiety management

Elimination of toxic substances

Treatment of fecal incontinence

Urinary incontinence care

Aromatherapy[25]

Regular exercise program

Biofeedback: To increase patient's awareness of internal state of arousal that allows for a degree of influence over his or her own level of arousal[118]

Nasal continuous positive airway pressure (CPAP): To treat obstructive sleep apnea[161]

NURSING CARE

Nursing Assessment[52,110]

Quality/amount of sleep

Complaints of insufficient nighttime sleep

Meaning of sleep/wake experience for the patient (patient often bases this on actual length of nighttime sleep, number of awakenings, and quality or depth of sleep)[57]

Degree of difficulty in falling asleep at bedtime

Difficulty in staying asleep during the night

Number of interruptions with consequent incomplete sleep cycles

Arousability from sleep

Daytime fatigue

Daytime napping

Degree to which amount and quality of sleep results in feeling refreshed or not refreshed on awaking

Daytime distress/impairment in occupational role functioning

Daytime distress/impairment in social functioning

Daytime distress/impairment in performing other activities of daily functioning

Duration of sleep difficulty (Primary insomnia lasts over 1 month. Transient insomnia may last only a few nights and is linked to psychologically stressful events.)[8]

Risk factors/etiologic factors

Use of and timing of medication administration (e.g., diuretics, SSRIs)

Amount and timing of caffeine intake before bedtime

Alcohol use before bedtime

Type, duration of pain, or discomfort (e.g., gastrointestinal discomfort, musculoskeletal pain)[57]

Degree of immobility caused by physical illness

Lifestyle patterns including degree of regular physical exercise

Presence of nocturia or incontinence (fecal or urinary)[57]

Unnecessary awakening for vital signs, medications, blood draws, etc.

Late life events that are stressors (e.g., loss of significant other)

Emotions/emotional discomfort: presence of depression or anxiety; worries such as finances or health; disturbing dreams[56,57]

External environmental factors: noise, uncomfortable temperature, sleep partner's snoring

Sleep difficulty as described by bed partner

Structured sleep history questionnaire,[56] sleep questionnaire,[138,139] Pittsburgh Sleep Quality Index,[118] and two-week sleep-wake log[118] can be used to obtain information about sleep history

Sleep pattern disturbance

Assess for major defining characteristics: complaints of difficulty in falling asleep; early awakening; sleep latency; difficulty in staying asleep at night/interrupted sleep; patient complaint of not feeling well-rested.[91,167]

Assess for other minor defining characteristics: agitation; mood alteration; napping during day or daytime sleepiness; frequent yawning; thick speech; physical signs as slight hand tremor, mild nystagmus, ptosis of eyelid, expressionless face; irritability; listlessness; lethargy; disorientation.

Nursing Dx & Interventions[111]

Sleep pattern disturbance related to emotional state and poor sleep hygiene practices (for patient with DSM-IV diagnosis of primary insomnia)

Have patient record sleep-rest-activity pattern over a period of 1 week: use of such tools as the modified sleep chart[56] to record information may be useful. *Baseline information is critical in determining potential factors causing sleep pattern disturbance because underlying problems such as a psychiatric disorder should be treated by the interdisciplinary team.*

Examine sleep record to determine factors interrupting sleep.

Have patient monitor daytime napping *to assess personal effects on nighttime sleep and daytime quality of life. Napping does not seem to disturb a number of aspects of nighttime sleep and findings regarding sleep latency (time it takes to fall asleep at night) and number of awakenings during the night are not conclusive.*[56]

Encourage patient to describe personal meaning of sleep. *The meaning of sleep to an individual will affect his response to its disruption and must affect the approach of the nurse in effectively promoting sleep and rest.*[145, p. 255]

Explain normal sleep pattern and changes that can be expected with increasing age and condition(s) present. *In times of high stress, illness, or in hospitalization, for example, the need for sleep may increase.*[47]

Control environment in order *to facilitate uninterrupted, quality sleep,* for example:

Reduce noise level.

Maintain consistent temperature: avoid extreme temperatures.

Reduce bright lights.

Work through attitudes viewing sleep as a chore or struggle.

Reduce level of anxiety experienced by patient: *anxiety has been identified as a factor contributing to sleep disturbance and loss.*[128]

Determine presence and nature of stressor(s) and assist patient in coping with stressor(s) and stress level. *Stressors may be present in patients with recent-onset insomnia and the nature of the stressor will have a critical effect on the duration and severity of the sleep disturbance and its management.*[97]

Carefully monitor intake of stimulants/other substances *because such substances can affect sleep,* for example:

Do not offer caffeinated beverages past afternoon.

Instruct patient to avoid drinking alcohol at home close to bedtime because it can interfere with sleep maintenance.

Avoid patient drinking excessive fluids in the evening and encourage patient to void before going to bed *to decrease need to void during night.*

Administer diuretics minimally 4 hours before betime *to decrease need to void during night.*

Use behavioral treatment approaches as:[110]

Stimulus control *to avoid pairing anxiety on the part of the patient with either the bedtime ritual or the sleep environment.*

Teach patient that sleep (besides sexual activity that is conducive to sleep) is the only behavior allowed in bed.[139]

Teach patient not to go to bed until sleepy.

Teach patient not to stay in bed very long (i.e., over 10 minutes) after waking up during the night, but to get up and then do something boring and/or relaxing, and return to bed only when sleepy again.

Sleep restriction *to decrease sleep-onset time and wakings in the night while increasing overall sleep time.*

Do not vary time in going to bed.

Do not spend excessive time in bed per night (e.g., over 8 1/2 hours).

Do not vary time getting up in the morning.

Do not sleep-in/sleep late as a way to make up for a poor night's sleep.

Do not stay in bed a long time after waking up from sleep even if during the middle of the night.

Teach patient good sleep habits and practices[82] *to increase restorative nighttime sleep,* such as:

Engage in a regular bedtime routine. *A regular bedtime routine will help patient feel calm, fall asleep more quickly, awaken less often, feel more refreshed in the morning, and feel more satisfied with their sleep.*[82]

Avoid heavy exercise close to bedtime, but daily regular exercise is helpful.

Go to bed to sleep only when sleepy.

Do not stay in bed a long time after waking up from sleep even if during the middle of the night.

Do not view sleep as a struggle.

Avoid clock watching: remove clock if necessary *to reduce performance anxiety.*

For elderly with cognitive impairments, it is especially important to provide a regular and predictable bedtime routine and cues.[45]

Encourage patient to maintain social network and receive social support from significant others. *Social support can serve as a buffer from the negative effects of emotionally charged and negative events and thus lessen the impact of these events on patient's sleep.*

In collaboration with physician, administer medications (e.g., pain medication for pain for example before bedtime, nitroglycerine for angina, bronchodilators for bronchospasm, tricyclic antidepressants for depression in elderly).

For institutionalized elderly patients, selectively use techniques to promote relaxation and thus promote sleep, for example:

Offer calming music.

Offer taped ocean sounds[54] or other white noise.

Have patient engage in deep breathing.

Promote environment conducive to meditation.

Collaborate with spiritual advisor to encourage prayer or meditation.

Offer back rubs.

Assist with personal hygiene at bedtime.

Autogenic training: *the linking of relaxing somatic sensations as for example warmth and visual images can promote deep relaxation.*[139]

Examine the hospital environment for possible causes of nightime awakenings (e.g., noise, discomfort or pain, urinary/fecal incontinence, health alterations, interruptions from caregivers). *The number of times elderly patients wake up during the night increases during hospitalization.*[82]

For surgical patients preoperatively: (a) enhance patient's knowledge about surgery and postoperative experience, (b) encourage verbalization of fears and anxiety, (c) enhance patient's coping skills such as how to cope with confusion should it occur. *Preoperative psychiatric interventions play a part in preventing postoperative psychosis.*[114]

For surgical patients, both preoperatively and postoperatively: (a) protect patient's sleep patterns,[114] (b) group nursing care interventions to coincide with patient's wakefulness, (c) eliminate unessential caregiver interventions during sleep time, (d) control factors in environment that can disrupt sleep such as noise, uncomfortable bedding, etc.,[144] (e) build on patient's own personal sleep routines and practices, (f) understand particular patient's physiologic and psychologic state *because underlying physical and mental illness can impact sleep.*[169] *Sleep disturbances are associated with the development and duration of post-*

operative psychosis. Sleep disturbances can also delay tissue repair and recovery.[54] Patients are found to be most frequently disturbed during the most immediate postoperative period by caregivers so it is very important to protect the patient's sleep patterns during this period.[169]

Patient Education/Home Care Planning

1. Increase awareness of patient and family of importance of sleep and increased need for sleep during times of stress.[169]
2. Instruct patient to try to avoid tobacco, alcohol, and caffeine[139] if at all possible: if patient does drink alcohol at home, for example, have patient avoid drinking close to bedtime because it can interfere with sleep maintenance.
3. Assist the patient in developing program of balance in daytime activities (e.g., social activities, exercise).
4. Instruct patient in use of progressive relaxation (tensing and relaxing of muscle groups) and other techniques that help patient relax at home. *Progressive relaxation, for example, has been found to decrease time for sleep onset and nocturnal awakenings, increase sound sleep, feeling more refreshed, increase subjective feelings of experiencing more satisfactory sleep.*
5. Have family assist patient in ensuring that the home environment can be made secure for nighttime (e.g., use of security system).

Evaluation

Sleep pattern disturbance Patient states that he or she falls asleep easily, does not experience early awakening, or have difficulty in staying asleep at night. Patient feels energetic and well rested on waking up from sleep.

SCHIZOPHRENIA AND OTHER PSYCHOTIC DISORDERS IN THE ELDERLY

Schizophrenia and *other psychotic disorders* include[6,131]: (1) *schizophrenia* characterized by active-phase symptoms (disorganized speech, negative symptoms, disorganized behavior, hallucinations, delusions) lasting minimally 1 month with the disturbance itself lasting at least 6 months. (See Chapter 17 for details). Types include: residual type, undifferentiated type, catatonic type, paranoid type, and disorganized type. About 30% of patients with schizophrenia manifested at an early age will experience remission and a marked improvement in late life[84]; (2) *schizophreniform disorder* characterized by symptoms similar to schizophrenia but lasting only from 1 to 6 months with less decline in functioning; (3) *schizoaffective disorder* characterized by both mood

episodes and active-phase schizophrenic symptoms; (4) *delusional disorder* characterized by nonbizarre delusions lasting at least 1 month; (5) *brief psychotic disorder* characterized by psychotic disturbance with a short duration of at least 1 day and no more than 1 month; (6) *shared psychotic disorder* characterized by delusions similar to those suffered by someone else; (7) *psychotic disorder due to a general medical condition* characterized by psychotic symptoms especially prominent delusions and/or hallucinations caused by physiologic effects of a medical condition; (8) *substance-induced psychotic disorder* characterized by psychotic symptoms caused by medications, toxins, or drug abuse; and (9) *psychotic disorder not otherwise specified* characterized by psychotic disturbance that cannot be classified into any of the above categories.

Overall, the number of elderly patients with schizophrenia is expected to increase because of increasing longevity. "As newer generations of schizophrenic patients are cared for in the community, they often need special help when the problems of old age are added to their underlying illness."[163, p. 61] Late-life schizophrenia[83] falls into two groups. First, is the group of patients with schizophrenia manifested early in life who are now elderly. The second group are those patients who developed late-onset schizophrenia, sometimes after the age of 45. Although the onset of schizophrenia is typically early in life (late teens to mid-30s), late-onset schizophrenia,[2,6,29,172,173] after age 45, has also been documented. An annual incidence rate of 12.6 per 100,000 or half that of the 16 to 25 age group has been reported for late-onset schizophrenia.[29] About 13% of all persons with schizophrenia begin to manifest symptoms in their 50s, 7% in their 60s, and 3% at a later age. Women have a higher rate of late-onset schizophrenia. These patients also tend to have a better work history and more have been married compared with patients with early-onset schizophrenia. Signs and symptoms include a higher frequency of hallucinations that are often auditory. There are also visual, tactile, olfactory, and paranoid delusions that are often bizarre and less disorganization and negative symptoms, although there can be some first-rank and negative symptoms. Addonizio[2, p. 337] found that "persecutory delusions, organized delusions and running commentary, and abusive auditory hallucinations were more common in late-onset cases." In those with late-onset schizophrenia who are older than 60 years of age, sensory deficits appear to play a role. Often the patient manifests a paranoid or schizoid premorbid personality and eccentricity. Many lead socially isolated lives.[129] The condition is often chronic with frequent admissions. Many elderly patients with chronic schizophrenia may require long-term hospitalization or protective living arrangements. Risk of fatalities in the elderly persons with schizophrenia includes suicide (the incidence is higher than in the general population), infection (often attributed to poor hygiene), and accidents (elderly patients with schizophrenia have more lethal accidents than younger patients.[72]

Schizophrenia, paranoid type[6,131] does tend to manifest itself later in life with delusions (often centered around a theme) of the persecutory or grandiose type being the most common symptom. Mistrust, anger, hostility, anxiety, and aloofness are common in the patient who is paranoid.

Paraphrenia* refers to late-onset persecutory delusions, often after the age of 60. This condition is common in elderly women. Patients are often of lower socioeconomic status, are often socially isolated, often unmarried, and living alone. A British journal[66] reports that about 10% of elderly psychiatric clients, 40% of whom have hearing deficits or other sensory deficits, admitted to psychiatric hospitals have late-onset paraphrenia. Paranoid symptoms, including well-organized delusions, that are usually nonbizarre and paranoid in nature, are present, as well as poorly systematized hallucinations, often auditory, schizoid traits, and social isolation. The patient often shows symptoms of misinterpretation and misidentification, delusions of reference, delusions of persecution, delusions of control, or delusions of forces controlling mind or body.[80] Deterioration of intellect, personality, and affect is minimal. Formal thought disorders are not as common.[80] The course is chronic and often nonresponsive to treatment. (Paraphrenia no longer appears in the DSM-IV as a separate diagnostic category. However, much literature addresses this type of schizophrenia.)

For those elderly patients for whom schizophrenia has been a life-long chronic condition,[131] stressors encountered in late life may lead to exacerbations of the illness with the person becoming more noncommunicative, withdrawn, and paranoid. They may also exhibit problems with affect and orientation. Furthermore, their life-long social support system may decline in old age, leaving them more vulnerable to becoming institutionalized or homeless. On the other hand, the outcome of the schizophrenic process in late life can be variable, with the potential for improvement and in some elderly patients, complete remission.[12]

Although psychotic disorder due to a general medical condition can occur at any age, the elderly are more prone to medical illnesses and chronic medical conditions. Examples of medical conditions[6] in which the pathophysiology can lead to psychotic symptoms include cerebrovascular disease, deafness, hyperthyroidism, renal disease, hepatic disease, and neoplasms.

■ SCHIZOPHRENIA

•••••• Pathophysiology/Psychopathology

(See also Chapter 17)

Psychological, Sociocultural Theories and Factors

Childhood trauma, female gender, premorbid schizoid and paranoid traits, adverse factors such as living alone and being socially isolated, as well as deafness, are thought to play a role in late-onset paraphrenia.[4,66]

---

*References 2, 3, 66, 80, 131, 172.

Biological/genetic Theories

Much effort is being put on researching a genetic link for schizophrenia.[131] "Changes in dopamine receptor site sensitivity or changes in the availability of dopamine at the receptor site" may be linked to the onset of schizophrenia.[13, p. 98] Some organic changes have been noted in patients with paraphrenia (e.g., larger cerebral ventricles, sulcal widening, and more cognitive impairment).[66] The very late life appearance of late-onset paraphrenia is suggestive of a largely neurodegenerative etiology.[80] A vulnerability is reported for elderly patients with chronic schizophrenia to develop Alzheimer's disease (AD) or histologic changes that are commonly found in AD.[127] Nonspecific brain pathology has been noted on brain imaging in patients with late-onset paranoid disorders.[2] However, Goldberg[67] points out that the course of schizophrenia is that of a static encephalopathy and that no evidence for an active degenerative process with progressive and relentless decline of cognitive functioning exists. Walker[160] notes that, "it is likely that many of the cortical and subcortical abnormalities that have been linked with schizophrenia are secondary manifestations of a neuropathology in which the critical (schizophrenic) feature is a specific dysfunction of neural circuitry" [p. 472]. Gender differences have been attributed in part to biologic factors. The higher rate in women of late-onset schizophrenia may be influenced by the "protective" effect of antidopaminergic effect of estrogens in younger women.[29] Gender differences may also be related to men and women being differently prone to subtypes. Neurodevelopmental deviance leads to increased frequency in young males of the neurodevelopmental form (type A). The paranoid form (type B) is equal in men and women. The schizoaffective form (type C) is mostly found in females.[29] An association has been reported between visual and hearing impairments and late-life schizophrenia and paranoid disorder.[2,125] Visual impairments have been found to be associated with visual hallucinosis.[80]

•••••• Diagnostic Studies and Findings

Computed tomographic (CT) scans: To detect brain tumors that may present with schizophrenia-like psychosis[2]

Physical examination and laboratory tests (e.g., TSH, T_4, serologic tests for neurosyphilis): To rule out any physical condition that may present with schizophrenia-like psychosis

Mental status examination/neuropsychologic assessment (e.g., Hierarchic Dementia Scale, Paired Associate Subtest of the Wechsler Memory Scale): To evaluate presence of symptoms indicative of mental illness and to evaluate cognitive functioning[172,173]

Hearing tests: To detect hearing impairment

Vision screening: To detect visual impairment

Abnormal involuntary movement scale: To detect presence of movements indicative of tardive dyskinesia[85]

Diagnostic criteria and tools (DSM-IV, ICD-10, Carpenter, Research Diagnostic Criteria (RDC), Schneider, Langfeldt, New Haven Schizophrenia Index, Feighner,

Taylor and Abrams, PSE9-CATEGO4): To assess for presence of symptoms indicative of schizophrenia

•••••• Multidisciplinary Treatment Plan

(See also Chapter 17)

Medications

For late-life schizophrenia, neuroleptics are relatively effective but lower dosages are used.[83,84] The selection of a specific neuroleptic is based on the patient's previous response to the medication, potential adverse affects from drug interactions with the preexisting medication regimen, and the side effect profile of medications.[83,84] Trifluoperazine 10 to 100 mg po can be used, for example, as can fluphenazine enanthate, 5 mg once every 2 weeks, or haloperidol, 2 to 20 mg/day po.[2] Clozapine, 100 to 900 mg qd, an atypical antipsychotic, is used for the treatment of otherwise treatment-resistant patients with chronic schizophrenia[83,84] or for those with existing tardive dyskinesia. However, agranulocytosis may occur in about 1% to 2% of patients, so this necessitates a weekly CBC check before more drug is dispensed. In addition, anticholinergic effects, hypotension, and sedation are common. So there is limited use in the elderly, but the drug can be used if given in much lower dosages, especially for patients unable to tolerate side effects of neuroleptics.

General Management

Psychosocial interventions: To treat elderly patients with schizophrenia, especially because of high risk of medication side effects and drug-drug interactions[113]

Psychiatric inpatient treatment: To treat psychotic decompensation or acute psychotic phase of illness, provide safety to patient, and stabilize symptoms[117]

Brief hospitalization: To conduct psychologic assessment, stabilize symptoms, identify precipitating factors, adjust environment[117]

Extended hospitalization: To provide care to patients with treatment-resistant chronic schizophrenia who may be a danger to self or others and unable to care for self[117]

Room and care homes: To provide private rooms, meals, supervised medications for long-term support and maintenance[113]

Day treatment

NURSING CARE

Nursing Assessment

Obtain history from family members if patient is too paranoid to be cooperative.

Listen for underlying feelings as delusions and hallucinations are described during initial interview.

Assess degree of insight.

Assess for presence of sensory deficits.

Conduct medication inventory to assess for adverse drug effects, drug interactions, proper dosages, etc.

Assess level of social interactions and available social network.

Assess patient's strengths.

Nursing Dx & Interventions[70,94,131]

Altered thought processes related to perceptual alterations, psychologic conflicts, anxiety (patient with late-onset schizophrenia)

In collaboration with psychiatrist, administer neuroleptic medications to relieve symptoms such as hallucinations and paranoid delusions.

Monitor medication regimen for therapeutic effect and side effects (e.g., extrapyramidal symptoms, anticholinergic effects, tardive dyskinesia).

Monitor for any changes in functioning to determine responsiveness to medication treatment and any signs or symptoms of drug interactions or any physical illness. *Patients with schizophrenia tend to underreport medical symptoms and overestimate physical well-being. They are more likely to manifest physical illness by behavioral changes such as mood changes and exacerbations of symptoms and changes in performance of ADL.*[94]

Ascertain that any sensory deficits are referred to the appropriate professional and corrected.

Create a therapeutic milieu that is safe, predictable, and not overly stimulating but with enough sensory stimulation *because elderly patients with schizophrenia have reported phantom sights and sounds if not enough sensory stimulant is present.*[131]

Explain all procedures and schedule changes.

Provide feedback to patient as how she or he begins to assume responsibilities for ADL.

Assist with ADL if patient is too withdrawn to care for self.

Build trust with patient. *Building trust is critical because the patient is not inclined to want help, blames others for problems, is angry and often noncooperative.*

Use consistent one to one interactions.

Use same staff to work with patient initially.

Be honest in all interactions with patient.

Keep appointments made with patient.

Use active listening skills.

Use communication technique.

Keep communication simple.

Communicate empathy.

Use short, frequent contacts with patient.

Accompany patient on walks without making demands for conversation.

After initial assessment, avoid frequently focusing and asking the patient questions about his or her delusions.

Listen to patient without comment.

Do not communicate disapproval of him or her as a person.

Do not confront patient about the validity of his or her thinking.

Do not debate validity of delusions with patient.

Raise doubts and questions about patient's perspective.

Point out reality when appropriate.

Set parameters on behaviors based on altered perceptions.

Validate reality based aspects on delusions.

Evaluate what need the delusions are meeting.

Provide feedback on feelings generated by the delusions.

Do not personalize accusations.

Evaluate stressors that triggered the delusions. *These strategies will avoid reinforcing the delusions and minimize threat and avoid increasing anxiety.*

Allow patient to express feelings as anger within acceptable parameters (e.g, no injury to self or others), *recognizing that such feelings are often reactions to perceived threat. It is important to have patient learn to describe feelings with words.*

Use a kind, firm, matter-of-fact approach *to allow patient to set pace for development of relationship.*

Avoid being too friendly or to reassuring *because closeness may be perceived as very threatening by the patient.*

Allow the patient to set the limits on degree of closeness in relationship *because this will reduce the threat that he or she may perceive from the interaction. Isolation is often used by the patient to cope with fear of closeness or to keep from being flooded with too much stimulation. Patients are often unable to deal with too much intimacy. As trust increases, the ability to tolerate interpersonal closeness will increase.*

Do not invade the patient's personal space.

Avoid lengthy interactions with patient.

Watch for cues to determine tolerance of patient for length and frequency of interaction.

Use interventions to decrease anxiety. (See Part Four Nursing Diagnosis, Anxiety) *It is very important that the patient is not threatened in any way and that confrontational efforts are not used to remove delusions and hallucinations because that will only increase the patient's reliance on them.*

Recognize and build in patient's strengths.

Enhance self-esteem.

Permit patient to make as many decisions as capable because this will enhance cooperation and constructive behavior.

Build on and expand well-part of social functioning.[94]

Engage in reality-based activities that focus on the here and now.

Offer opportunity to engage in group activities but do not force patient to do so.

Offer opportunities to get involved in predictable activities.

Offer support to family in their attempts to interact with patient.

Assist patient in setting realistic goals and acquiring skills needed to meet them (e.g., social interaction skills, communication skills, assertive behavior skills, problem-solving techniques).

Develop with patient a satisfactory structure of daily activities that can be followed when he or she is living in the community.

Patient Education/Home Care Planning

1. Teach patient and family about importance of need for medication compliance. *Medication compliance and outpatient follow-up by a community psychiatric mental health nurse have been shown to increase a good response to medication treatment.*[66]

2. Teach patient and family about the risk of relapse in late-life schizophrenia if neuroleptic medications are suddenly withdrawn, along with such other effects as increased motor restlessness and social withdrawal. If decreased dosage or elimination of neuroleptic medication is desired, careful supervision by a health professional will be needed, as a graduated taper of the neuroleptic will be required and only in those elderly outpatients with a stable chronic condition.[83,84]

3. Teach elderly patient on neuroleptics and significant others to observe for signs of tardive dyskinesia (TD). *This is very important because being elderly, and especially female and diabetic, is one of the risk factors for developing TD.*[129]

4. Teach elderly patient on neuroleptics and significant others to observe for extrapyramidal side effects.[129]

5. Teach patient not to discuss delusions openly with persons other than close friends *to prevent negative reactions from others.*

Evaluation

Altered thought processes related to perceptual alterations, psychologic conflicts, anxiety The patient will exhibit and feel less conflicted and anxious. Patient will live in least restrictive community setting and function as optimally as able.

SOMATOFORM DISORDERS IN THE ELDERLY

Somatoform disorders* are disorders in which patients have multiple bodily complaints that cannot be explained on a physiologic basis. There are frequent visits to physicians with demands for attention and requests for physical examinations and treatment. There is a resistance on the part of these patients that there might be a psychologic basis for the symptoms. Somato-

---

*References 6, 14, 38, 44, 122, 163.

form disorders are comprised of (a) *somatization disorder,* or *hysteria,* characterized by sexual, gastrointestinal, pseudoneurologic symptoms and pain beginning before 30 and extending over a number of years. The physical symptoms that are expressed often involve multiple body systems, and an early onset, usually before the age of 30 and a chronic course. Health care is sought from many physicians and specialists but no actual physical signs can be determined for the complaints nor is there evidence of structural or laboratory abnormalities. Yet, these patients often undergo invasive procedures, treatment with medications, hospitalization, and/or surgery. Along with the vague physical symptoms there is a frequent history of psychiatric symptoms—drug abuse, depression, anxiety, suicidal attempts; (b) *undifferentiated somatoform disorder* characterized by physical complaints over 6 months or more that are unexplained but cannot be diagnosed as another somatization disorder; (c) *conversion disorder* characterized by unexplained symptoms related to sensory functions or voluntary motor functions; (d) *pain disorder* characterized by the symptom of acute or chronic pain with an important role being played by psychologic factors in the onset, severity, and maintenance of the pain. The pain leads to occupational, social, and/or other distress or impairment in daily functioning; (e) *hypochondriasis* characterized by fear of and preoccupation with having a serious illness based on misinterpretation of one or more bodily functions or bodily signs or symptoms; the fear continues for at least 6 months despite medical evaluation and support; the complaint is not delusional but the patient is unaware of the underlying conflicts represented by the symptoms; anxiety and depression are often present; distress or impaired social, occupational, and other daily functioning exists; (f) *body dysmorphic disorder* characterized by preoccupation with an exaggerated or an imagined defect in one's physical appearance; and (g) *somatoform disorder not otherwise specified* characterized by somatoform symptoms but not meeting criteria of any disorders above.

•••••• Pathophysiology/Psychopathology

Psychologic/Cultural Theories

Although older persons are more likely to suffer from actual physical symptoms than younger persons, they are also more likely to complain about physical symptoms than talk about emotional distress. The physical symptoms over which the patient has no conscious control are real for the patient. They function to relieve or to prevent anxiety, serve to achieve a primary gain, and/or serve to achieve a secondary gain in that expected role responsibilities may be temporarily waived and attention may be given by others to the patient.[44] Somatoform disorders, such as hypochondriasis, are more frequently identified in the elderly.[131]

Psychosocial factors can play a part in somatization disorder with the families of these patients often being dysfunctional. In these families, members find it difficult to express feelings and conflicts openly. In times of stress, a child may become ill with the focus of the family then shifting away from the stressor or conflict and onto the child's illness.[154] The expression of physical symptoms in response to stress in patients with somatization disorder may be also a learned pattern within their families of origin.[87, 155] There can also be the presence of physical abuse and sexual abuse. "Somatic symptoms may be an expression of underlying psychological pain as well as representing a symbolic means to express emotions and ask for care."[87 p. 315] Psychosocial stressors often precipitate the symptoms.[87, 122] For example, hypochondriasis is frequently precipitated by a major life event. Selective attention and excessive concern about an organ system by patients with hypochondriasis leads to more anxiety that can lead to physical signs and symptoms. In those with conversion disorder, the symptoms may be a means of social communication, precipitated by life stressors that activate intrapsychic conflicts.[87]

Cultural factors may also play a role. In some cultures, emotional states, such as depression, are primarily manifested through physical symptoms.[166]

Biological/Genetic Theories[122]

Recent studies of somatization disorders point to a possible biologic basis: abnormalities in cortical functioning and electroencephalographs have been noted. A familial pattern seems evident in somatization disorder, but whether this is a genetic or a learned pattern is not clear.[87] "Conversion Disorder may be an amplification of neurological disorder . . ."[87, p. 318] because the prevalence of neurologic disorders in these patients is as high as 50%.

•••••• Diagnostic Studies and Findings

Medical and psychiatric history[122]   A thorough and complete history is imperative because somatoform disorders are diagnosed, in part, in retrospect. This should include interviews with family members, friends, and an examination of old medical records. It should be noted that it is not uncommon for physical complaints to be attributed to a somatoform disorder, only to later be found to have a physical basis; therefore the patient's physical complaints should not be lightly dismissed.

Complete medical examination[122,136]   To rule out any general medical condition, or new symptoms of an actual chronic condition that could account for the person's complaints of physical signs or symptoms and fear of having a disease, which is especially important in the elderly. Tests must be scheduled and then not postponed because that can increase the patient's sense of not being taken seriously and increase insecurity.

Neurologic examination and testing   To differentiate between neurologic condition and conversion disorder.

Complete mental examination[122]   To rule out any other major psychiatric disorder and to differentiate among the types of somatoform disorders. In patients with hypochondriasis, fear of illness is more prominent than actual physical complaints, the latter being more frequent in somatization disorder. Mood disorder and anxiety disorders are frequently associated with hypochondriasis, especially in the elderly.[87, 163]

••••• Multidisciplinary Plan

Surgery/Other Treatment[87,122,136]

Treatment of specific physical or mental disorder (e.g., mood disorder) that may actually occur along with the somatoform disorder.

Invasive diagnostic or treatment procedures are avoided unless an actual objective physical basis exists.

Regular office visits not based strictly on the basis of a new complaint are scheduled.

Partial physical examination for each new symptom, but large-scale workups and referrals to subspecialists are avoided unless actual physical basis exists.

Hospitalizations avoided unless, for example, to special psychiatric units for treatment of somatization disorders.

Hypnosis or Intravenous Amobarbital-Assisted Interview: To treat symptoms of patients with conversion disorders along with posttreatment suggestion and the treatment of any actually existing physical illnesses. This treatment, however, is rarely used.[61,87,136]

Faradic Stimulation: To treat patients with conversion disorder with a low amperage electrical current used to cause a placebo effect in the patient or the use of stronger shocks for aversive conditioning.[61]

Medications[92,122,136]

Pharmacologic Treatment: To treat specific comorbid psychiatric disorders (e.g., use of anxiolytics for patients with symptoms of anxiety or anxiety disorders; use of antidepressants for patients with symptoms of depression or mood disorders; use of opioid analgesics, nonsteroidal antiinflammatory drugs, antidepressants, benzodiazepines, corticosteroids, anticonvulsants, clonidine, and/or ergotamine to treat patients with pain disorder; and use of trazodone to treat sleep disorders associated with somatoform disorders).

General Management[87,104,122]

Cognitive-Educational Approach: To treat with hypochondriasis by providing reassurance about the benign nature of their symptoms and correcting myths and misperceptions about the actual anatomy and physiology of the body

Cognitive-Behavioral Interventions: To treat patients with hypochondriasis by assisting them in reducing reliance on physical symptoms for control and coping with emotions and learning new ways of processing perceptions. Such behavioral techniques can be used as exposure to feared event, thought stopping, desensitization, implosion, imaginal flooding. According to the cognitive model, the patient "perceives bodily signs and symptoms as more dangerous than they really are and believes a particular illness to be more probable than it actually is. Treatment based on this model has two major components: (1) identifying and modifying automatic dysfunctional assumptions about health by demonstrating testable alternative explanations for symptoms (e.g., hyperventilation) experienced by the patient, and (2) identifying and modifying abnormal illness behavior by preventing certain behaviors (e.g., compulsive reassurance seeking) as a basis for helping the patient develop reattribution of illness assumptions".[104, p. 179] Also used to treat patients with pain disorder by focusing on "identifying and correcting patients' distorted attitudes, beliefs, and expectations. The goal of this therapy is to make patients more aware of factors that exacerbate and diminish pain and to modify their behavior accordingly. A variety of therapeutic techniques may be used to achieve this goal, including biofeedback, relaxation training, and hypnosis"[92, p. 1765]

Operant Conditioning: To assist patients with pain disorder to reduce focus on pain and engage in activities that they have avoided because of the pain[92]

Group Therapy: To help patient reduce the need to rely on somatic complaints

Supportive self-help groups: To provide social support

Specific focused groups: To teach patient about somatoform disorder and to provide mutual support

Psychotherapy: To help, for example, patients with somatization disorders, become aware that psychologic factors are playing a role in the illness, understand the basis for the condition, and resolve underlying emotional distress and problems

Supportive brief psychotherapy: To treat, for example, patients with conversion disorder

NURSING CARE

Nursing Assessment[44]

Health history: To obtain health-related information that is relative to current health concern.

Ongoing monitoring of physical symptoms and laboratory tests conducted: To determine emergence of any physical evidence of symptoms described and actual illness.

Ongoing monitoring of mental status: To determine emergence of any emotional problem or potential psychiatric disorder.

Assess for signs and symptoms indicative of somatoform disorders.

Assess attitudes about physical illness. Do physical symptoms interfere with ADLs and social or occupational functioning?

How long have these physical symptoms persisted?

Are there any environmental stressors that precipitated the physical symptoms?

Assess patient's social network and presence of strengths.

Assess patient's family's strengths and any evidence of dysfunctional interactions.

Assess presence of emotional themes. Examine patient's ability to express dependency needs and feelings of anger, for example.

Assess stressors and life circumstances that occurred before the beginning of the physical illness.

Assess strengths, strategies for coping with stressors, and interpersonal resources. What are the patient's limitations?

Does patient have any understanding of connection between physical symptoms and emotions or intrapsychic stress?

What happened to the patient as a consequence of physical illness on ADLs, social functioning, or family functioning?

Nursing Dx & Interventions

Ineffective individual coping related to inadequate coping skills along with use of physical symptoms to deal with underlying conflict, dependency needs, and anxiety

When first establishing a relationship with the patient, permit him or her to ventilate about the physical complaints *to prevent patient from becoming defensive and looking to someone else to describe the physical symptoms to, and to establish rapport with the patient so that he or she feels understood. It is important to accept the patient's feelings.*[44,122]

Encourage patient to remain with one primary physician or psychiatrist.

Respect and follow the primary physician's medical treatment guidelines for the patient.[122]

Be alert for overmedication or drug interactions because the patient may have been followed by several physicians.[131]

Be alert to the emergence of physical symptoms indicative of actual physical illness.

Initially, have patient use chart to document both stressful life events and occurrence of physical symptoms.[136]

Do not imply to patient that it is all in "his or her head". *Disregard for the patient's physical complaints impedes development of interpersonal trust and the establishment of a therapeutic relationship.*

Determine the nature of the secondary gains, such as obtaining attention or avoidance of need to deal with actual life demands or stressors, from the physical symptoms expressed by the patient.

Initially, provide nurturing and support *to initially meet patients dependency needs.*[44]

Gradually withdraw attention and time given to the patient's complaints of physical symptoms and encourage patient to become less dependent and more independent.

Model open communication when interacting with patient *to encourage patient to express feelings and concerns. It is essential that the patient learn to identify feeling states and be able to express feelings to others.*[149]

Teach patient assertive communication skills *to help patient express needs without relying on physical symptoms.*

Teach patient conflict resolution skills.[149]

Interact with patience and acceptance *so that fears of rejection and abandonment are minimized and the patient is free to express such emotions as anger.*[44]

Set and adhere to time limits for one-to-one interaction *so the ability to bring up new complaints at the close of the session is minimal.*

Matter-of-factly state that symptoms will be reported to the physician. *A determination of an organic basis for the complaint should always be made to assure patient's health and safety.*[154]

Explore with family and significant others impact of patient's illness and strategies for dealing with it.

Use behavior therapy techniques:[122]

Have staff and significant others consistently reduce reinforcing the physical symptoms by, for example, not rushing the patient to the doctor each time there is a complaint.

Do not reward continual complaining.[131]

Teach and encourage the patient to use self-help treatments for symptoms so that control of the symptoms is in the hands of the patient (e.g., use of heating pads).

Have the patient begin to focus on actual psychosocial problems that are currently faced.

Encourage more open and appropriate expression of emotional distress.

Use praise for movement away from physical complaints and more functional expression of emotional distress.

Teach patient to use techniques such as meditation, relaxation techniques, exercise, imagery *to deal with emotions such as fear and anxiety.*

Help patient link physical symptoms with actual emotions felt. The patient, for example, can be taught about the physiologic aspects of anxiety.[122]

Help patient reframe the physical complaints and focus on the link of the symptoms with real stressors currently being faced.[122]

Give feedback to patient about how overuse of complaints about physical symptoms can impact negatively on relationship with others and teach patient to use social skills if necessary.

Use positive reinforcers when patient is not ruminating about physical symptoms and for the actual use of adaptive coping skills.

Use anticipatory guidance in working with patient *to help patient prepare for potential changes and the related stress.*[44]

Use role play for patient to gain actual experience with use of adaptive techniques when faced with stressful situations.

Patient Education/Home Care Planning

1. Teach patient and family members patterns of interactions that do not rely on physical symptoms to deal with stress and anxiety.[44] *It is critical to involve family and significant others in examining patient's lifestyle and helping him or her achieve more adaptive coping skills.*[149]

   Encourage caring and supportive family atmosphere.

   Encourage family members to communicate openly and honestly, including expression of feelings.

Encourage respect among patient family members for differences of opinion.

Teach patient and family members conflict resolution strategies.

Teach patient and family flexible problem-solving strategies.

Discuss with patient and family the need for balance between needs for belonging and needs for separation.

Help patient and family identify community resources that may be helpful when faced with multiple stressors.

2. Teach patient and family strategies to adapt to ongoing life changes.

Evaluation

Ineffective individual coping   The patient will be able to recognize and express feelings.[149] Reliance on physical symptoms to cope with stressors and anxiety is minimized. Patient recognizes link between stressors, emotions, and expression of physical symptoms and demonstrates use of more adaptive coping strategies to meet personal needs and to deal with life stressors.

SUBSTANCE-RELATED DISORDERS IN THE ELDERLY

Substance-related disorders include two groups, *substance-use disorders* and *substance-induced disorders.* (See also Chapter 17.)[6]

Substance use disorders include (1) *substance dependence* characterized by a pattern of substance use that is maladaptive, leads to clinically significant distress or impairment, and is manifested by three or more of the following criteria within 12 months—tolerance; withdrawal; much time spent on obtaining, using, and recovering from substance; substance taken in larger amounts over longer time periods; unsuccessful efforts to reduce or stop use of substance; altered or reduced social, recreational, and/or occupational roles and activities resulting from substance use; continued use of substance despite recognition of negative physical or psychologic effects; and (2) *substance abuse* characterized by a pattern of substance use that is maladaptive, leads to clinically significant distress or impairment and is manifested by one or more of the following criteria within 12 months—major occupational, social, and/or academic role failure caused by recurrent substance use; engaging in activities that are physically hazardous when impaired by substance use; legal problems related to substance use; continued substance use despite major interpersonal or social problems linked to substance use.

Substance-induced disorders include (1) *substance intoxication* characterized by substance-specific syndrome caused by ingestion of or exposure to substance that is reversible; effect on CNS caused by the substance during or shortly after its use and leading to maladaptive psychologic or behavioral changes; and (2) *substance withdrawal* characterized by substance-specific syndrome caused by the reduction of or cessation of a specific substance after long-term, heavy use; maladaptive psychosocial changes resulting from the substance-specific syndrome. Mild withdrawal symptoms from alcohol, sedatives, hypnotics, and anxiolytics include anxiety, sleep disturbance, depressed mood, difficulty concentrating, psychomotor agitation, and periods of panic, with some patients also manifesting tachycardia, tachypnea, transient diastolic or systolic hypertension, and increased temperature.[143] Severe withdrawal syndrome can be life-threatening (e.g., seizures, delirium tremens). A postwithdrawal syndrome may present in patients detoxified from abuse of benzodiazepines.

The term "substance" as used in the DSM-IV refers to drugs of abuse, as well as medications and toxins.[63] Therefore substance-related disorders[6] include those disorders that are related to either (1) exposure to toxic substances, as for example, heavy metals, carbon monoxide, antifreeze, nerve gas, or rat poison; (2) over-the-counter or prescribed medications, as for example, corticosteroids, anesthetics, muscle relaxants, or chemotherapeutic agents; and, (3) 11 classes of substances described in detail in the DSM-IV[6] that include (a) alcohol, (b) sedatives, hypnotics, and anxiolytics; (c) cocaine; (d) amphetamine or similarly acting sympathomimetics; (c) hallucinogens; (f) opioids; (g) nicotine; (h) inhalants; (i) cannabis; (j) phencyclidine (PCP) or similarly acting arylcyclohexylamines; and, (k) caffeine. Similar features are shared by (a) and (b). Similar features are also shared among (c) and (d).

The medical complications of alcohol-related disorders (the cost is as much as heart disease according to Medicare data) in the elderly include pancreatitis, peptic ulcers, gastritis, gastrointestinal bleeding, peripheral neuropathy, hepatitis, cirrhosis, malnutrition, anemia, increased infections, hypercortisolemia, delirium tremens, and seizures. Other problems in elderly linked to substance-related disorders include impaired driving ability. (Small amounts of alcohol can result in motor impairment, deficits in visuospatial problem-solving, and confusion, which can all impair driving ability,[100] falls, cognitive impairment, depression, increased mental aging, delirium, cerebellar degeneration, peripheral or autonomic neuropathies, muscle weakness, malnutrition, hypocalcemia, hypokalemia, hypomagnesemia, orthostatic hypotension, hypertension, sexual dysfunction, incontinence, suicide, and risk of cancer (especially of the esophagus, head, or neck).[60,100,143] "When-ever a patient develops unexpected disturbed behavior and perse cutory symptoms within a week or so of admission, the possibility of drug or alcohol withdrawal should be investigated." [163, p. 161] Alcoholism in the elderly can be a life-threatening illness.[86]

"There is a demonstrable morbidity associated with long-term hypnotic and sedative use by the elderly." [150, p. 809]. The complications of hypnotic- and sedative-related disorders can include acute confusion, delirium, incontinence, restlessness, emotional distress, falls, immobility, and hip fractures.[150]

Polypharmacy is also a danger in the elderly. Drug interactions with alcohol occur. For example, the duration of benzodiazepines and meprobamate is affected because of the competition for metabolism in the hepatic microsomal enzyme system. The therapeutic effect of tolbutamide, diphenylhydantoin, and warfarin are decreased because with alcohol use the degradation rates of these medications are reduced. The CNS effects of sedative-hypnotic medications are potentiated.[60]

•••••• Pathophysiology/ Psychopathology[107,112,143]

(See also Chapter 17)

The incidence of chronic illnesses increases in the elderly (more than 80% have a chronic condition[s])[101,105] along with increased treatment with prescribed medications, as well as use of over-the-counter medications by the elderly themselves. Thus the use of multiple medications either concurrently or intermittently is common in the elderly. This increases the potential for either inadvertent or intentional misuse of medications and the potential for the emergence of substance-related disorders in the elderly.[115] Frequently misused drugs that can lead to substance-related disorders in the elderly include alcohol, tobacco, medications that have an addictive potential such as opioid analgesics, barbiturates, and benzodiazepines. Polypharmacy is also a problem.[143] Alcohol is the substance most abused.[86] From 7% to more than 12% of persons older than 65 are reported to suffer from alcohol problems, whereas 10% to 20% of elderly actually seeking health care suffer from alcohol problems.[107,143] Elderly persons with substance-related disorders are more likely to be male.[143] Gender differences occur across culture with elderly men having a higher incidence of alcohol-related disorders than women.[134] More alcohol abuse is reported among elderly of lower socioeconomic status.[86] Alcohol use in the elderly may be conceptualized as a lifestyle factor that can be used to reduce the effects of those events in roles that are perceived as less important by the elderly person. On the other hand, alcohol use may increase the noxious impact of those events or stressors when they are connected with highly salient roles.[95]

Three major types of elderly alcoholics have been identified.[86] The elderly person with early-onset alcoholism has abused alcohol most of their adult lives and is a survivor; many of their cohorts have died. These patients manifest symptoms of chronic alcoholism and are often physically ill. Personality disturbances, difficult interpersonal relationships, and diminished support systems are common. The elderly person with late-onset alcoholism generally begins drinking past the age of 40, often in response to a stressor, like the death of a loved one. Social drinking may develop. Late-onset alcoholism is often due to depression, loneliness, or boredom. The elderly person with intermittent alcoholism uses alcohol to relieve stress with binges during high-stress periods. In general, alcohol use tends to decline after the age of 60.[86]

Little data are available on the illicit use of drugs other than alcohol among the elderly. Opiate abuse, for example, is often not visible because it occurs among a group of urban elderly who are often isolated.[86] Elderly persons are much more likely than younger persons to abuse prescription drugs, for example, sedatives and hypnotics, and much less likely to abuse illicit drugs.[150] "Although the elderly rarely abuse illicit drugs, chemical dependence on alcohol and illicit drugs does occur in this age group due to the careless treatment of symptoms or as a result of psychological addiction."[115, p. 143] In institutionalized elderly, for example, the rate of use of hypnotics and long-acting benzodiazepines is greater than in the general population of elderly.[150] One study[143] reported that in their sample of addicts who were elderly, 35% abused benzodiazepines, 12%, oral opiates, and 4%, marijuana.

The problem of substance-related disorders is often underestimated[112] in the elderly because (a) the elderly may use small but frequent quantities of the substance, (b) may present with nonspecific physical complaints that can obscure the symptoms, and (c) can be misdiagnosed because of similar symptom presentation. There can also be present a lack of awareness among healthcare providers regarding the possibility of substance-related disorders in the elderly; some health care providers may not want to intervene in what is perceived by them to be long-term habits of the elderly person. The elderly often are not working, driving, and may live alone so are less likely to be noted.

Similar stages of addiction occur regardless of the drug abused.[143] Stage 1 is characterized by patient euphoria, bingeing, attempts to reduce or cease use of drug, and some shame. The patient's family seeks opinions from friends and other family members. Stage 2 is characterized by patient resentment, alternating times of use and abstinence, and unwillingness to travel places without a sure supply of the drug. The patient's family engages in enabling behaviors. Stage 3 is characterized by patient engaging in unreasonable behaviors; blaming others; paranoia; beginning interpersonal, legal, and/or occupational problems. The patient's family often isolates the patient. Stage 4 is characterized by the patient demonstrating a high degree of resentment and blame, withdrawing emotionally, guilt, depressed mood, anger, physical illness, suicidal behavior, and increasing social problems. Family members become increasingly angry and depressed. Marital separation may occur. Stage 5 is characterized as the stage of addiction. The patient feels hopeless, is continuously intoxicated, and admits defeat. The family basically gives up on the patient. Stage 5 is either death or "the bottom" in which case the patient is willing to try anything to get better.

Psychological, Sociocultural Theories and Factors

A number of psychosocial and cultural factors[107,143] and stressors can contribute to the occurrence of substance-related disorders in the elderly. These include cultural attitudes toward aging, burden of caregiving, multiple losses such as loss of income, death of spouse and/or significant others, loss of permanent home with relocation of residence, retirement, and other role changes. Social isolation, depression, and boredom can lead to drinking and alcohol-related disorders. Alcohol abuse can occur in patients with major depression or dementia.[9] Social learning theory suggests that behavioral patterns of alcohol consumption are learned in families and thus transmitted across the generations.[19]

Biological/Genetic Theories

Physiologic changes and risk factors occurring in the elderly can contribute to the occurrence of substance-related disorders.[107,143] These changes include increased susceptibility to drug-drug interactions and increased biologic sensitivity leading to toxic effects. Slower biotransformation and excretion of substances can occur as a result of altered substance absorption, distribution, and/or elimination. In the elderly, for example, there is a smaller volume of distribution for a substance like alcohol; thus after ingesting the same amount as a young person, the elderly one demonstrates a higher blood level.[143] Also, the ability to metabolize alcohol can be lowered in those elderly patients who use sedatives or hypnotics at the same time as alcohol.[143] The rate of both elimination and absorption is decreased in the elderly, so more CNS effects from, for example, barbiturates, that also last longer, result.[143] In the elderly, there is an increasing neuropharmacodynamic effect resulting from alcohol abuse, as well as the fact that in the elderly with chronic alcoholism, neuropsychologic deficits are magnified.[9] Decreased absorption and metabolism can lead to the accumulation of medications such as benzodiazepines. In relation to opioid analgesics, the elderly experience slower onset of action because the absorption rate is lowered, longer action because of a reduction in liver function, and more adverse effects because of receptor sensitivity changes.[143] If an elderly person is prescribed a potentially addictive medication over time, tolerance, withdrawal, and substance-related disorder can result. A biologic vulnerability to addiction and a strong genetic component have been noted as a cause for substance-related disorders.[143] Finally, other factors that can contribute to the occurrence of substance-related disorders include physical illness, chronic pain, decreased mobility, sensory deficits, and short-term memory deficits. Studies suggest that elderly addicts frequently have another mental health disorder that is affected by the substance-related disorder, as well as affecting the substance-related disorder.[143]

•••••• Diagnostic Studies and Findings

Drug use history (from patient and others): To determine type and amount of the substance being consumed and effects of substance use

Addiction history (from patient and others): To obtain information about the patient's drug addiction from a variety of persons

Family history: To determine presence of history of substance-related disorders among family members

Complete physical examination: To determine signs and symptoms of substance-related disorder; to determine presence of other physical conditions

Liver function studies (e.g., serum gammaglutamyl-transferase [SGOT] or transpeptidase): To determine

presence of hepatic damage caused by substances such as long-term alcohol use, as well as to monitor abstinence[34]

Serum toxicologic studies and urinary drug screen: To determine presence of substance-related disorders caused by toxin exposure

Complete blood count: To determine presence and any effects from substance abuse. Elevated MCV often suggests alcohol abuse and heavy alcohol use can result in anemia and/or suppression of blood lines

Complete mental examination: To determine signs, symptoms, and effects of substance-related disorder (the presenting symtoms of a substance-related disorder may mimic other mental disorders); to determine presence of other mental disorders[143]

Methadone maintenance program: To treat the elderly opiate user

CAGE (a mnemonic for 4 questions—"Have you ever felt you should *cut* down on your drinking? Have people *annoyed* you by criticizing your drinking? Have you ever felt bad or *guilty* about your drinking? Have you ever had a drink first thing in the morning to steady your nerves or get rid of a hangover (an *eye opener)?*" [34, p. 182]: To screen for an alcohol-related disorder

MAST (Michigan Alcoholism Screening Test): To assist in diagnosing presence of alcohol-related disorder

Chemical dependency screening tools (e.g., Manitoba Drug Dependency Screen): To detect presence of chemical dependency[103]

•••••• Multidisciplinary Treatment Plan[35,107,143]

(See also Chapter 17)

In-patient treatment of alcohol withdrawal (symptoms include increased prodromal symptoms of tremor, tachycardia, agitation, diaphoresis; delirium; hallucinations including auditory, tactile, or visual that are often threatening; delusions that are often paranoid; generalized seizures)[35]

Thiamine 100 to 200 mg IM or IV immediately

Sedative-hypnotics: Used prn to prevent or treat withdrawal

Parenteral fluid: To treat dehydration

Potassium chloride: To treat potassium deficit and prevent cardiac arrhythmias

Magnesium sulfate: To treat magnesium depletion

Elemental phosphorus: To treat hypophosphatemia

Vitamin K: To treat increased prothrombin time

Folic acid

Water-soluble vitamin supplement

Valium or Librium: As a prophylactic anticonvulsant

Treatment of complications of alcohol withdrawal[35]

Determine origin of and treat fever

Free water restriction of hypertonic sodium chloride solution: To treat hyponatremia

5% Dextrose: To treat hypoglycemia

Sedation and potassium and magnesium supplements: To treat alkalosis

Prednisone: To treat alcoholic hepatitis

Folic acid: To treat folate deficiency

Treat underlying etiology of hematologic disorders

Thiamine, folic acid, niacin: To treat patients with alcohol-related disorder who have history of poor nutrition

Supportive emergency measures (1 g ascorbic acid IV, IV ephedrine sulfate and antihistamines): To maintain blood pressure and treat shock in severe alcohol-disulfiram reactions

Clonidine: To aide in withdrawal from oral opioids[143]

Desipramine: To treat withdrawal from cocaine

Antidepressants: To treat persistent depressive symptoms in alcoholics (Note that suicide can be a serious problem in the elderly depressed alcoholic patient)[34]

Benzodiazepines: To support detoxification and treat withdrawal symptoms

Anxiolytics: To treat symptomatic anxiety in patients with alcohol-related disorders

General Management[107]

Detoxification programs: To manage withdrawal phase of substance-related disorder

Inpatient treatment program: To provide a structured program, free from access to substance, designed to assist patient to cease use/abuse of substance(s)

Structured supervised environment: To provide alcohol free facility for elderly alcoholics with cognitive disorders

Outpatient treatment program: To provide treatment and counseling to patient on an outpatient basis

Self-help groups (e.g., AA [12-step model]): To obtain support from other persons recovering from alcoholism

Long-term residential treatment program (e.g., half-way house): To provide ongoing shelter, support, and counseling

Individual psychotherapy: To help patient focus on the here-and-now, deal with problems resulting from substance abuse, help develop insight, and prevent relapse

Family therapy: To assist patient and family in developing insight into the process of substance-related disorders and family interactions

Group therapy: To assist patient in confronting problem, to enhance self-esteem, to instill hope, to build interpersonal skills, and to enhance knowledge about substance abuse

Disulfiram (Antabuse): To treat chronic alcoholism by deterring patient from ingesting alcohol; used with great care in the elderly. Antabuse interferes with normal metabolism of alcohol and is given to deter further drinking because even a small amount of alcohol while on Antabuse can result in an unpleasant reaction. Antabuse is contraindicated in patients with selected psychosis or myocardial disease. Also, the patient must be reliable to avoid alcohol even in disguised forms (e.g., cough and cold mixtures, after-shave lotions, sunscreens, back rub lotions, sauces, mouthwashes, certain medications), must be motivated and socially stable, and must not be depressed or suicidal[34]

| NURSING CARE |

Nursing Assessment[103,107,143]

History of substance-related disorder(s)

Presence of social contexts in which there is access to substance (primarily alcohol) and its use is accepted. For some elderly alcohol abusers, the tavern is the only social outlet

Presence of social isolation, loneliness, loss, and/or boredom

Low self-esteem

History of falls or accidents

Current physical symptoms and conditions

History or current use of over-the-counter and/or prescribed medications

Presence of and causes for polypharmacy and potential or actual drug misuse[115]

Assess patient for:

Accuracy in reporting current medications, medication side effects

Use of multiple refills, different pharmacies, multiple physicians without checking with primary health care provider

Self-medicating by use of over-the-counter drugs or borrowing medications from friends or family

Impairment in sensory functions

Characteristics of health care being provided to patient (i.e., Was patient given clear instructions about prescribed medications and their side effects? Was adequate follow-up provided to patient?)

Psychosocial changes or impairment (The elderly often do not exhibit the degree of social disturbances as younger persons)

Degree of social isolation

Housing problems

Legal problems

Martial problems

Social problems

Changes in physical health or patterns

Poor nutrition

Poor hygiene and self-care

Unexpected reaction to medications

Sleep problems

Tremors

Peripheral neurologic damage

Lack of exercise

Nonadherence to prescribed health care regimen

Gastrointestinal disturbances

Pain

Difficulty in performing activities of daily living

Falls

Chest pain

Changes in emotions and mental health

Loss of motivation or ambition

Conflicts about dependency needs after loss of love object[143]

Hostility toward and subsequent guilt related to loss of love object[143]

Labile mood

Personality changes

Irritability

Threats of violence

History of actual violence

Depressed mood

Anxiety

Phobias

Cognitive changes

Memory loss

Confusion

Paranoid ideation

Hallucinations (auditory, visual)

Suicidal ideation

Degree of denial of presence of substance-related disorder or misinformation provided about alcohol or drug use[143]

Social network available to patient

Attitudes of significant others toward presence of substance-related disorder

It is important to note that the elderly alcohol abuser is unlikely to ask for direct help in coping with alcohol problem, but will indirectly present with medical problems (falls, seizures, trauma, chest pain, malnutrition), psychologic problems (aggression, depression, hallucinosis). Legal problems (offensive behavior, assault), or social problems (family disturbances, self-neglect)[153]

Nursing Dx & Interventions[7,34,60,107,143]

Ineffective individual coping related to biopsychosocial symptoms/problems secondary to substance-related disorder.

Monitor for suicide potential.

Establish caring, trusting therapeutic relationship with patient. *This is critical in structuring interventions to help the elderly patient increase awareness of problem, achieve behavioral change, and enhance coping skills.*[7]

Determine degree of social impairment or impairment in ADLs. *The elderly often do not exhibit the degree of social disturbances as younger persons nor engage in criminal behaviors or drive while intoxicated. They are often no longer employed in an occupation and may live alone. Therefore their use and abuse of substances may be more difficult to detect.*

Determine impact of substance-related disorder on the physical health of the patient and provide corrective interventions, for example:

Provide for and teach importance of adequate nutrition (e.g., Meals on Wheels).

Assist patient in coping with sleep disturbances.

Assist patient in dealing with concerns about sexual dysfunction.

Assess presence of and level of anxiety and assist patient in decreasing anxiety present. *Anxiety is frequently present in the patient with a substance-related disorder and is often the reason the substance was prescribed and used in the first place. A cycle of tolerance-withdrawal-increased dosage occurs.*[143]

Assess presence and level of anger and assist patient in developing more adaptive strategies to express anger (e.g., participation in sports, exercise, verbal expression).

Determine extent to which patient is using denial, minimizing the substance-related disorder, rationalizing, and defocusing. *These symptoms very commonly are present in addiction.*

Assist patient in working through defenses as denial and accepting presence of substance-related disorder. *Patients with substance-related disorders often deny existence of problem and refuse to seek or accept treatment. They often complain about a number of psychiatric symptoms but do not complain about being an addict. Overcoming denial is the first step in treatment.*

Involve multidisciplinary team and patient's social network.

Refer patient to alcohol counselor and AA *to assist patient to confront substance abuse problem. The recovered alcoholic is an invaluable asset to the treatment team to assist patient in recognizing existence of problem and that recovery is possible.*[34]

Begin by using the least intrusive way of confronting the patient with the problem, relying on more intrusive measures if there is no change in recognition of problem and willingness to engage in treatment.[103]

Encourage assistance from the elderly patient's social network in helping patient recognize existence of problem and becoming motivated to change his or her lifestyle. *"The purpose of the intervention is to have all involved individuals recognize the dependency or potential dependency, identifiable negative consequences, complications of continued or habitual substance use, and enabling and codependency behaviors."* [103, p. 7]. *It is also very important to confront and work through enabling and co-dependency behaviors in significant others.*

Identify factors such as stressors contributing to substance-related disorder.

Assist patient in eliminating or altering these stressors.

Maximize patient's motivation for abstinence.[135]

Educate patient and family about substance-related disorders by lectures, counseling, videotapes, literature.

Assist patient to develop more adaptive coping strategies to deal with these stressors.

Build on patient's strengths, such as recreational skills, in identifying and developing more adaptive coping skills.

Place great emphasis on the patient for assuming responsibility for self.

May need such treatment as guardianship, conservatorship, and/or hospitalization.

Assist patient in rebuilding a lifestyle that is free of substance abuse.[135]

Explore with patient the constructive use of free time.

Encourage patient to develop friendships with persons that do not abuse substances.

Explore with patient ways to deal with mundane tasks of life on a regular basis.

Encourage family members to interact with patient and reestablish positive relationships.

Offer social skills training to help patient deal more effectively with environment (e.g., communication skills, assertive communication skills, problem solving, refusal skills).[159]

Refer to appropriate therapies (e.g., alcohol counselor, individual counseling, family counseling, cognitive therapy, individual supportive psychotherapy, group psychotherapy, family therapy).

Refer to community services (e.g., AA, Al-Anon, Ala-Teen, social services, Adult Children of Alcoholics, Senior Citizens Center). *Community services and groups can offer the elderly patient the support needed to abstain from substance abuse. Self-help groups can help patient learn more adaptive ways to handle stress, maintain sobreity, and incorporate adaptive coping skills into lifestyle.*[7]

Patient Education/Home Care Planning

1. Teach patient, family, and significant others about causes, course, and effects of substance use. Use printed matter to reinforce content taught (e.g., AA literature).
2. Teach patient and family changes that occur in normal aging and their impact on the effect of alcohol abuse.
3. Teach patient and significant others about the importance of compliance with the prescribed medical regimen.
4. Teach patient and significant others about potential drug interactions with substance that is abused, such as alcohol-drug interactions.
5. Teach patient and significant other importance of outpatient treatment recommendations such as the importance of attending AA meetings.
6. Teach patient and significant other the importance of prevention (e.g., avoid requesting long-term prescriptions of hypnotics or sedatives).[150]
7. Teach patient the importance of good nutrition.

Evaluation

Ineffective individual coping related to biopsychosocial symptoms/problems as a result of substance-related disorder   The patient will accept the fact that a substance-related disorder is present, develop self-awareness related to the problem, abstain from use of substance, develop coping skills to deal with stressors, increase quality of life, and lead a healthier lifestyle.

SEXUAL DISORDERS IN THE ELDERLY

Sexual disorders include *sexual dysfunctions, gender identity disorders,* and *paraphilias. Sexual dysfunctions*[6] are disorders in which patients experience a disturbance in the processes and changes that are part of the sexual response cycle—desire (phase of fantasies and sexual desire), excitement (phase of subjective sexual pleasure and physiologic changes), orgasm (peaking of sexual pleasure with release of sexual tension), and resolution (phase of muscle relaxation and sense of wellbeing)—or in which the patient experiences pain during sexual intercourse, and that leads to interpersonal or other distress. Subtypes of sexual dysfunctions, indicating etiologies, for ex-ample, include: (a) due to psychologic factors in which the onset, severity, and maintenance of the sexual dysfunction is due to psychologic factors only; (b) due to combined factors in which the onset, severity, and maintenance of the sexual dysfunction is due to psychologic factors *and* a medical condition or substance use.

Sexual dysfunctions[6] include: (1) *sexual desire disorders—* (a) hypoactive sexual desire disorder—characterized by lack of desire or fantasies for sexual activity causing interpersonal and/or personal distress; (b) sexual aversion disorder—characterized by active avoidance of sex with partner and causing interpersonal and/or personal distress; (2) sexual arousal disorders—(a) female sexual arousal disorder—characterized by inability to maintain lubrication-swelling sexual excitement responses and causing interpersonal and/or personal distress; (b) male erectile disorder—characterized by inability to attain or maintain an adequate erection and causing personal and/or interpersonal distress; (3) orgasmic disorders—(a) female orgasmic disorder—characterized by delay or absence of orgasm and causing personal and/or interpersonal distress; (b) male orgasmic disorder—characterized by delay or absence of orgasm and causing personal and/or interpersonal distress; (c) premature ejaculation—characterized by onset of ejaculation and orgasm with little sexual stimulation before penetration and causing personal and/or interpersonal distress; (4) sexual pain disorders—(a) dyspareunia—characterized by genital pain during coitus and causing personal and/or interpersonal distress; (b) vaginismus—characterized by involuntary perineal muscle contraction on penetration of vagina and causing personal and/or interpersonal distress (5) sexual dysfunction due to a general medical condition—characterized by sexual dysfunction caused by physiologic effects of a medical condition and causing personal and/or interpersonal distress; (6) substance-induced dysfunction—characterized by sexual dysfunction caused by effects of a substance and causing personal and/or interpersonal distress; (7) sexual dysfunction not otherwise specified includes those sexual dysfunctions that cannot be classified into any of the above categories.

•••••• Pathophysiology/Psychopathology

Psychologic, Cultural, or Environmental Theories and Factors

A number of psychologic factors[74] can contribute to sexual dysfunction in the elderly. Untreated depression can be an element as can the negative withdrawal from pleasurable activities by those elderly who become bored with life and/or their partner. Self-esteem can be lowered as a result of a negative body image as a result of the aging process especially in elderly women: the lowered self-esteem can lead to feelings of being sexually unattractive. Fear of illness during intercourse can also be a deterrent in pleasurable sexual encounters and intercourse in the elderly. A distressing relationship with the partner can lead to sexual dysfunction. Sexual activity, especially in women, may be restricted because of the lack of available partners. In restricted environments, such as nursing homes, inappropriate sexual behaviors may be exhibited especially by men because often no normal outlets exist to fulfill sexual needs, and there is usually a lack of privacy in institutions.

Biological/Genetic Theories

Elderly men and women, if they are in good health, have been sexually active earlier in life, and have an interested partner, maintain an interest and capacity for being active sexually into their seventies or longer. In general, however, there is a steady decline in sex.[141,167] "It is clear that age alone is not a barrier to sexual fulfillment in men or women. However, physical changes in both sexes can be inhibitory, and health professionals need to understand them."[74 p. 445] Physical changes do occur in the reproductive system of elderly men and women: and some elderly couples entirely give up sexual intercourse and display their physical affection in other ways.

In elderly men,[33,74] there is a decline in testicular mass, but increase in size of prostate gland; decline of testosterone production along with reduced secondary sexual characteristics, muscle loss, lowered aggressiveness; reduced size of penis and compromised erectile tissue; reduced sperm production; and reduced prostate secretions. The most common sexual complaint of elderly men is impotence, which may have a psychologic basis in part, but is often due to loss of vascular function or loss of neurologic function. This loss of function can be the result of medical conditions such as diabetes, thyroid disease, or drugs such as alcohol, nicotine, or antihypertensive drugs. As noted by Christiansen[33, p. 229], "All men over 70 and most men at an earlier age suffer some loss of sexual function short of impotence. Elderly men require a longer period of stimulation to produce an erection. The penis tends to be less firm when erect as well as less sensitive. More time is required to build to the climax that causes ejaculation. The amount of semen produced is less than in the earlier years; the intensity of the pleasure generated also is usually reduced. Speedier detumescence occurs. The recovery period following ejaculation increases: up to 24 hours may be needed before ejaculation can occur again and this may contribute to decreased sexual activity. The decrease in sexual activity may, in turn, contribute to further loss of function." In general, in elderly men[59] a longer time period is needed during the excitement phase, as well as more direct stimulation of the genitals. There is a decrease in the firmness of the erection. In the orgasm phase, the ejaculatory experience is reduced in intensity, ejaculation is not felt to be needed in each sexual encounter, but feelings of stimulation and satisfaction remain. The resolution phase does lengthen as age increases.

In elderly women,[33,59,74] menopause and menopausal-related symptoms occur around the age of 45 to 50. Estrogen levels become nearly depleted over time, the ovaries and breasts atrophy, the vagina and external genitals become smaller, the vaginal wall thins as well as loses elasticity, becoming more lax. During intercourse, variation in vaginal size is diminished. Along with a decline of vaginal secretions and stickier secretions, these changes can cause vaginal discomfort and painful intercourse. Vaginismus is also a common problem in elderly women. Atrophic vaginitis can also occur, with tender vaginal walls becoming raw and bleeding with the possibility of infection and dyspareunia present. In elderly women, orgasm itself is often shorter and less intense, and for some, can even be painful. In general, elderly women experience less vasocongestion of the breasts during the excitement phase, as well as less vaginal expansion and lubrication. In addition, they need a longer period to be stimulated. In the resolution phase, multiorgasmic ability does continue.

The use of certain medications[13,70,74,94] can result in sexual dysfunction in the elderly. For example, tricyclic antidepressants and monoamise oxidase inhibitors can decrease libido, alter sexual functioning, and can result in impotence. SSRIs can impede sexual functioning such as becoming anorgasmic, decrease libido, and decrease sexual response. The adverse effects of antipsychotic drugs (e.g., chlorpromazine, haloperidol include ejaculation inhibition, male impotence, and changes in libido). Opioids can cause reduced libido or potency. Chronic alcohol use can lead to impotence. Other medications that can alter the sexual response include antihypertensives, antihistamines, nicotine, and anticarcinogenics.

The physiologic effects of certain medical conditions can lead to sexual dysfunction in the elderly. Examples include diabetes, peripheral vascular disease, hypertension, diseases of the neurologic system such as Alzheimer's disease, sexually-transmitted diseases such as AIDS and gonorrhea, carcinomas of the reproductive system, and diseases such as tuberculosis. Conditions such as dyspnea, osteoarthritis, and rheumatoid arthritis can interfere with sexual activity and may require altered sexual techniques. Surgery on sexual organs can also impact sexual functioning. In addition, medical conditions in the elderly, can negatively impact the elderly person's body image and lead to feeling less attractive sexually.

•••••• Diagnostic Studies and Findings

Development, psychosocial, health history, sexual history: To determine nature and basis for sexual dysfunction

Evaluation of endocrine factors: To determine part played by hormones in sexual dysfunction; includes testosterone, follicle-stimulating hormone, luteinizing hormone, prolactin[77]

General medical and gynecologic examination: To rule out presence of medical conditions or substances that cause sexual dysfunction

•••••• Multidisciplinary Plan

Surgery/Other Treatment

Plastic surgical intervention: To correct physical changes that occur in some women after a period of abstinence and assist them in becoming able to be sexually active again[74]

Dilation procedure: Use of graduated series of dilators to treat vaginismus in some women[77]

Penile prosthetic implant or new tumescence techniques for men: To correct, for example, neurogenic impotence caused by such conditions as diabetes mellitus and treat male erectile disorder[74,77]

Vacuum constriction device: To treat male erectile disorder[77]

Corrective surgery for venous leaks: To treat male erectile disorder[77]

Medications

Dose reduction or discontinuation of medications causing sexual dysfunctions. Also, switching of medications or special dosing strategies can be useful[120]

Estrogen creams: To treat vaginal discomfort in elderly women

Vasoactive intracavernous pharmacology: Medications such as papavarine or a combination of phentalomine and prostaglandin E to treat irreversible male erectile disorder

Alprostadil: Intrapenile injection to treat impotence secondary to neuropathy, vasculogenic, psychogenic, and mixed etiology

Depo-injections of testosterone or testosterone patches (Testdoderm) patches to the scrotum: To treat hypoactive sexual desire disorder in men[13,77]

Trazodone: Reported to increase erections

Clomiphene: To treat some patients with erectile impairment[13]

Selegiline (Deprenyl): To treat some patients with reduced libido[13]

Neuroleptics or benzodiazepines or trazodone: To control inappropriate sexual behaviors—such as public genital exposure, attempts to fondle other's sexual organs, masturbation, and coitus in inappropriate places—in patients with dementia[81]

Medroxyprogesterone acetate: To suppress libido in elderly male patients[81]

General Management

Treatment of medical conditions known to cause sexual dysfunction

Sex therapy: To enhance communication and knowledge about sexual function and activity between two partners and enhance their ability to enjoy sexual pleasure; includes simple counseling; individual therapy; couples therapy; group therapy[23]; or, coaching patient to take advantage of various stimuli (i.e., physical and mental to assist engaging man's mind and in attaining erection)

Forced ejaculation, counterbypassing, or body work therapy: To treat male orgasmic disorder[77]

Stop-start technique and/or bibliotherapy: To treat premature ejaculation[77]

Standard sex therapy techniques or combined sex therapy and masturbation approach: To treat female orgasmic disorder[77]

Psychotherapy: To treat sexual dysfunctions that have no organic basis or have a combined etiology (i.e., organic and psychosocial)

Individual therapy or couples therapy: To treat hypoactive sexual desire disorder and other sexual dysfunctions in men or women where the causes are psychosocial (e.g., in the elderly, retirement, lowered self-esteem and self-worth caused by the psychologic effects of aging)[77]

Psychotherapy and cognitive imagery: To identify psychologic factors such as developmental factors, traumatic events, or relationship issues and treat dyspareunia[77]

NURSING CARE

Nursing Assessment

Identify presence of physical factors(s) or medical condition(s) that can impact on sexual functioning.

Assess knowledge about aging process and effect on reproductive system and sexual activity.

Identify present medication uses that can impact on sexual functioning.

Assess for evidence of current substance abuse.

Assess amount of caffeine or alcohol consumed.

Assess for any evidence of sexual abuse (e.g., fear or refusal of pelvic or rectal examination, hematomas on inner thighs, diminished rectal or vaginal sphincter tone, sexually transmitted disease. Note that the abuser is often a family member. Particularly at risk are women with dementia who are physically and/or financially dependent.[19,24]

Obtain sexual history.[23]

How learned about sex

Early sexual experiences

History of sexual trauma

Attitudes, values, beliefs, and feelings about sex

Importance of sexual activity to patient

Sexual relationships

Expression of sexual needs and preferences in the relationship

Level and type of sexual activity desired

Previous sexual problems

Current sexual habits and patterns

Assess for presence of life changes and/or stressors.

Nature of family interactions and ways of dealing with stressors and crisis.

Assess interpersonal relationship with partner.

Assess self-image, self-esteem, body image.

Nursing Dx & Interventions

Sexual dysfunction related to psychosocial factors and aging process

Examine own sexual attitudes and prejudices toward sexual activity in the elderly and become professionally informed about the subject of sexuality among the elderly. *"Societal prejudice and professional ignorance lead many health care professionals to avoid the subject of sexuality in old people. Simple advice can relieve much potential suffering from sexual dysfunction in both men and women."*[74 p. 445]

Have patient express sexual difficulties and dysfunction in own words along with own interpretation of experience.

Listen nonjudgmentally to patient discuss own values, beliefs, religious beliefs, and cultural and environmental factors that influence his or her perspective about human sexuality.

Encourage expression of feelings such as fear and anxiety.

Encourage communication between patient and partner about sexual concerns when they are ready to do so.

Involve partner of patient in plan of care, where appropriate.

Dispel myths that sexual activity in the elderly is abnormal. *"Unfortunately, prevailing ageism in American society has fostered an insensitivity to the intimacy and relationship needs of older persons. Sexuality of older persons in particular is viewed negatively. Sexual activity of older persons has received recent attention, but prevailing myths and attitudes are difficult to change. Sexually active older persons are often judged to be practicing aberrant behavior. Sexual practice is often denied or ignored by society at large, and concerns by older adults remain unspoken and unanswered."*[75 p. 36]

Use active listening to provide a trusting, nonthreatening, nonjudgmental atmosphere *to help patient freely talk about sexual problems that may be somewhat embarrassing.*

Dispel any myths or misinformation about sexual functioning in the elderly: tailor information to needs of patient.

Teach patient about the physical changes and changes that take place throughout the sexual response phases as one gets older.

Discuss ways to minimize the effects of these changes (e.g., use of lubricants, use of different sexual techniques, and other ways to express intimacy and love).

Encourage elderly female to use estrogen creams to reduce vaginal discomfort during intercourse.

Enhance patient's self-esteem.

Identify psychosocial stressors that may impact on patient's sexual functioning and activity.

Teach elderly patient that intercourse does not have to result in ejaculation to be "complete."[33]

Encourage patient and partner to use tactile stimulations and close physical contact and intimacy to enhance sexual pleasure even if orgasm is not achieved.

Encourage patient and partner to rely on patience and affection to increase pleasure during the prolonged period of stimulation.[33]

Refer patient to other members of the multidisciplinary team for specific therapy as needed (e.g., couples therapy, sex therapy, group therapy).

Refer to appropriate community resources.

Patient Education/Home Care Planning

1. Teach the patient about the aging process and changes in the reproductive system and in the phase of sexual intercourse.
2. Teach patient the importance of regular self-examination.[43]
3. Teach elderly women that lubrication can be a very important sexual aid.[74]
4. Teach patient to refrain from such substances as alcohol and high caffeine intake, both of which can diminish sexual performance.[74]
5. Teach elderly patient strategies to enhance sexual pleasures and alternate ways to express intimacy.
6. Teach patient communication skills so as to increase ability to express self assertively to partner about sexual needs and preferences.

Evaluation

Sexual dysfunction related to psychosocial factors and the aging process   The patient understands factors contributing to the sexual dysfunction, describes ways to enhance relationship and sexual pleasure with partner, experiences an improved sexual relationship with partner, experiences less sexual dysfunction, feels sexually more attractive to partner, and enjoys more sexual pleasure.[48]

References

1. Abraham IL, Neundorfer MM, Currie JL: Effects of group interventions on cognition and depression in nursing home residents, *Nurs Res* 41(4):196, 1992.
2. Addonizio GC: Late paraphrenia. The Psychiatric Clinics of North America, 18(2):335, 1995.
3. Almeida OP, Howard RJ, Levy R, David AS: Psychotic states arising in late life (late paraphrenia): psychopathology and nosology, *Br J Psychiatry* 166:205, 1995.
4. Almeida OP, Howard RJ, Levy R, David AS: Psychotic states arising in later life (late paraphrenia): the role of risk factors *Br J Psychiatry.* 166:215, 1995.
5. Amar KA, Wilcock GK: Antidepressant medicines for the elderly: are we using them appropriately? *Gerontology* 40:314, 1994.
6. American Psychiatric Association: *Diagnostic and statistical manual of mental disorders, DSM-IV,* ed 4, Washington DC, 1994, American Psychiatric Association.
7. ANA: *Standards of addictions nursing practice with selected diagnoses and criteria,* Kansas City, 1988, ANA.
8. Andreasen NC, Black DW: *Introductory textbook of psychiatry,* ed 2, Washington, DC, 1995, American Psychiatric Press.

9. Atkinson RM, Ganzini L, Bernstein MJ: Alcohol and substance use disorders in the elderly. In Birren JE, Sloane RB, Cohen GD, editors: *Handbook of mental health and aging,* San Diego, 1992, Academic Press.

10. Badger TA, Cardea JM, Biocca LJ, Mishel MH: Assessment and management of depression: an imperative for community-based practice, *Arch Psychiatric Nurs* 4:(4):235, 1990.

11. Ballenger J: Using SSRIs to treat depression in the elderly, *Geriatrics* 48(2):9, 1993.

12. Belitsky R, McGlashan TH: The manifestations of schizophrenia in late life: a dearth of data, *Schizophrenia Bull* 19(4):683, 1993.

13. Bernstein JG: *Handbook of drug therapy in psychiatry* ed 3, St Louis, 1995, Mosby.

14. Bienenfeld D: Nosology and classification. In Copeland JRM, Abou-Saleh MT, Blazer DG: *Principles and practice of geriatric pyschiatry,* New York, 1994, Wiley.

15. Birren JE, Sloane RB, Cohen GD, editors: *Handbook of mental health and aging,* San Diego, 1992, Academic Press.

16. Bliwise DL, Hughes M, McMahon PM, Kutner N: Observed sleep wakefulness and severity of dementia in an Alzheimer's disease special care unit, *J Gerontology* 50A(6):M303, 1995.

17. Blixen CE, Wilkinson LK, Schuring L: Depression in an elderly clinic population: findings from an ambulatory care setting, *J Psychosocial Nurs Ment Health Serv* 32(6):43, 1994.

18. Blixen CE, Wilkinson LK: Assessing and managing depression in the older adult: implications for advanced practice nurses, *Nurse Practitioner* 19(7):66, 1994.

19. Bloch S, Hafner J, Harari E, Szmukler GI: *The family in clinical psychiatry,* Oxford, 1994, Oxford University Press.

20. Breitner JCS, Welsh KA: Diagnosis and management of memory loss and cognitive disorders among elderly persons, *Psychiatric Services* 46(1):29, 1995.

21. Brown AS, Gershon S: Dopamine and depression, *J Neural Transm* 91:75, 1993.

22. Buschmann MBT, Dixon MA, Tichey AM: Geriatric depression, *Home Healthcare Nurse* 13(3):47, 1995.

23. Byers S: Sexuality and sexual concerns. In Johnson BS: *Psychiatric-mental health nursing: adaptation and growth,* ed 3, Philadelphia, 1993, Lippincott.

24. Campbell JM: Treating depression in well older adults: use of diaries in cognitive therapy, *Issues Ment Health Nurs* 13:19, 1992.

25. Cannard G: On the scent of a good night's sleep, *Nursing Standard* 9(34):21, 1995.

26. Capezuti E: Preventing elder abuse and neglect. In Lavizzo-Mourey R, Day SC, Diserens D, Grisso JA: *Practicing prevention for the elderly,* St Louis, 1989, Mosby.

27. Casey DA, Davis MH: Obsessive-compulsive disorder responsive to electroconvulsive therapy in an elderly woman, *South Med J* 87(8):862, 1994.

28. Casey DA: Depression in the elderly, *South Med J* 87(5):559, 1994.

29. Castle DJ, Murray RM: The epidemiology of late-onset schizophrenia, *Schizophrenia Bull* 19(4):691, 1993.

30. Cataldo JK: Hardiness and death attitudes: predictors of depression in the institutionalized elderly, *Arch Psychiatric Nurs* 8(5):326, 1994.

31. Chiu E, Ames D: Functional psychiatric disorders of the elderly. Cambridge, 1994, Cambridge University Press.

32. Chokroverty S: *Sleep disorders medicine: basic science, technical considerations, and clinical aspects,* Boston, 1994, Butterworth-Heinemann.

33. Christiansen JL, Grzybowski JM: *Biology of aging,* St Louis, 1993, Mosby.

34. Ciraulo DA, et al: *Alcoholism and its treatment.* In Shader RI, editor: *Manual of psychiatric therapeutics,* ed 2, Boston, 1994, Little, Brown.

35. Ciraulo DA et al: The treatment of alcohol withdrawal. In Shader RI, editor: *Manual of psychiatric therapeutics,* ed 2, Boston, 1994, Little, Brown.

36. Cirina CL: Effects of sedative music on patient preoperative anxiety, *Today's OR Nurse* 16(3):15, 1994.

37. Clark WG, Vorst VR: Group therapy with chronically depressed geriatric patients, *J Psychosocial Nurs Ment Health Serv* 32(5):9, 1994.

38. Cloninger CR, Yutzy S: Somatoform and dissociative disorders: a summary of changes for DSM-IV. In Dunner DL: *Current psychiatric therapy.* Philadelphia, 1993, Saunders.

39. Copeland JR, Abou-Saleh MT, Blazer DG: *Principles and practice of geriatric psychiatry,* New York, 1994, Wiley.

40. Cummings JL: Depression in neurologic diseases, *Psychiatric Annals* 24(10):525, 1994.

41. Danton WG, Altrocchi J, Antonuccio D: Nondrug treatment of anxiety, *Am Fam Physician* 49(1):161, 1994.

42. Diagnostic Classification Steering Committee: *International classification of sleep disorders—diagnostic and coding manual.* Rochelle, NY, 1990, American Sleep Disorders Association.

43. Doenges ME, Moorhouse MF: *Nurse's pocket guide: nursing diagnoses with interventions,* ed 3, Philadelphia, 1991, FA Davis.

44. Doscher MS: Psychophysiologic disorders. In BS Johnson: *Psychiatric-mental health nursing,* Philadelphia, 1993, Lippincott.

45. Dowling G: Part 5. Sleep problems in older adults, *Am Nurse* 27(3):24, 1995.

46. Dunham NC, Sager MA: Functional status, symptoms of depression, and the outcomes of hospitalization in community-dwelling elderly patient, *Arch Fam Med* 3:676, 1994.

47. Duxbury J: Avoiding disturbed sleep in hospitals, *Nursing Standard* 9(10):31, 1994.

48. Dyer JG, Sparks SM, Taylor CM: *Psychiatric nursing diagnoses.* Springhouse, 1994, Springhouse Corp.

49. Farran CJ, Popovich JM: Hope: a relevant concept for geriatric psychiatry, *Arch Psychiatric Nurs* 4(2):124, 1990.

50. Farrell KR, Ganzini L: Misdiagnosing delirium as depression in medically ill elderly patients, *Arch Intern Med* 155(Dec 11/25):2459, 1995.

51. Fernandez F, Levy JK, Lachar BL, Small GW: The management of depression and anxiety in the elderly, *J Clin Psychiatry* 56(suppl2):20, 1995.

52. Ferri F, Fretwell M: *Practical guide to the care of the geriatric patient,* St Louis, 1992, Mosby.

53. Fitz AG, Teri L: Depression, cognition, and functional ability in patients with Alzheimer's disease, *JAGS* 42(2):186, 1994.

54. Fitzsimmons L, Verderber A, Shively M: Enhancing sleep following coronary artery bypass graft surgery, *J Cardiovasc Nurs* 7(2):86, 1993.

55. Flint AJ: Epidemiology and comorbidity of anxiety disorders in the elderly, *Am J Psychiatry* 151(5):640, 1994.

56. Floyd JA: Another look at napping in older adults, *Geriatr Nurs* 16(3):136, 1995.

57. Floyd JA: The use of across-method triangulation in the study of sleep concerns in healthy older adults, *Adv Nurs Sci* 16(2):70, 1993.

58. Fontaine KL, Fletcher JS: *Essentials of mental health nursing,* ed 3, Redwood City, 1995, Addison-Wesley.

59. Forbes EJ, Fitzsimons VM: *The older adult: a process for wellness,* St Louis, 1981, Mosby.

60. Forciea MA: Nutrition, alcohol, and tobacco in late life. In Lavizzo-Mourey R, Day SC, Diserens D, Grisso JA: *Practicing prevention for the elderly,* St Louis, 1989, Mosby.

61. Ford CV: Conversion disorder and somatoform disorder not otherwise specified. In Gabbard GO, editor: *Treatment of psychiatric disorders,* Vol. 2, Washington, DC, 1993, American Psychiatric Press.

62. Foreman MD, Wykle M: Nursing standard-of-practice protocol: sleep disturbances in elderly patients, *Geriatr Nurs* 16(5):238, 1995.

63. Frances A, First MB, Pincus HA: *DSM-IV guidebook,* Washington DC, 1995, American Psychiatric Press.

64. Gagne D, Toye RC: The effects of therapeutic touch and relaxation therapy in reducing anxiety, *Arch Psychiatric Nurs* 8(3):184, 1994.

65. Gallo JJ, Anthony JC, Muthen BO: Age differences in the symptoms of depression: a latent trait analysis, *J Gerontol* 49(6):251, 1994.

66. Gannon MA, Wrigley M: Late paraphrenia, *Br J Hosp Med* 53(4):128, 1995.

67. Goldberg TE, Hyde TM, Kleinman JE, Weinberger DR: Course of schizophrenia: neuropsychological evidence for a static encephalopathy, *Schizophrenia Bull* 19(4):797, 1993.

68. Gomez GE, Gomez EA: Depression in the elderly, *J Psychosocial Nurs Ment Health Serv* 31(5):28, 1993.

69. Gomez GE, Gomez EA: The use of antidepressants with elderly patients, *J Psychosocial Nurs Ment Health Serv* 30(11):21, 1992.

70. Gorman LM, Sultan D, Luna-Raines M: *Psychosocial nursing handbook for the nonpsychiatric nurse,* Baltimore, 1989, Williams & Wilkins.

71. Greene VL, Monahan D, Coleman PD: Demographics. In Ham RJ, Sloane PD: *Primary care geriatrics: a case-based approach,* ed 2, St Louis, 1992, Mosby.

72. Hafner H, Hambrecht M: The elderly with schizophrenia. In Chiu E, Ames D: *Functional psychiatric disorders of the elderly,* Cambridge, 1994, University Press.

73. Ham RJ: Confusion, dementia, and delirium. In Ham RJ, Sloane PD: *Primary care geriatrics: a case-based approach,* ed 2, St Louis, 1992, Mosby.

74. Ham RJ: Sexuality. In Ham RJ, Sloane PD: *Primary care geriatrics: a case-based approach,* St Louis, 1992, Mosby.

75. Hamilton GP: Promotion of mental health in older adults. In Hogstel MO, editor: *Geropsychiatric nursing,* ed 2, St Louis, 1995, Mosby.

76. Harnett DS: Psychopharmacologic treatment of depression in the medical setting, *Psychiatric Annals* 24(10):545, 1994.

77. Heiman JR: Sexual dysfunctions. In Dunner DL: *Current psychiatric therapy,* Philadelphia, 1993, Saunders.

78. Herr KA, Mobily PR: Geriatric mental health: chronic pain and depression, *J Psychosocial Nurs Ment Health Services, 30(9):7, 1992.*

79. Hogstel MO: *Geropsychiatric nursing,* ed 2, St Louis, 1995, Mosby.

80. Howard R, Almeida O, Levy R: Phenomenology, demography and diagnosis in late paraphrenia, *Psychol Med* 24:397, 1994.

81. Jenike MA: *Geriatric psychiatry and psychopharmacology: a clinical approach,* St Louis, 1989, Mosby.

82. Jensen DP, Herr KA: Sleeplessness, *Nurs Clin North Am* 28(2):385, 1993.

83. Jeste DV et al: Treatment of late-life schizophrenia with neuroleptics, *Schizophrenia Bull* 19(4):817, 1993.

84. Jeste DV: Late-life schizophrenia: editor's introduction, *Schizophrenia Bull* 19(4):687, 1993.

85. Karch AM: *1996 Lippincott's nursing drug guide,* Philadelphia, 1996, Lippincott.

86. Kashka MS, Tweed SH: Substance-related disorders. In Hogstel MO: *Geropsychiatric Nursing,* St Louis, 1995, Mosby.

87. Katon W: Somatization disorder, hypochondriasis, and conversion disorder. In Dunner DL: *Current psychiatric therapy,* Philadelphia, 1993, Saunders.

88. Kellett J: Psychosexual disorders. In Chiu E, Ames D: *Functional psychiatric disorders of the elderly,* Cambridge, 1994, University Press.

89. Kennedy GJ: The geriatric syndrome of late-life depression, *Psychiatric Services* 46(1):43, 1995.

90. Kim E, Rovner BW: Depression in dementia, *Psychiatric Annals* 24(4):173, 1994.

91. Kim M, McFarland G, McLane A: *Pocket guide to nursing diagnoses,* ed 6, St Louis, 1996, Mosby.

92. King SA, Stoudemire A: Pain disorders. In Gabbard GO, editors: *Treatments of psychiatric disorders,* Vol. 2, Washington DC, 1995, American Psychiatric Press.

93. Knapp M: Night shift: the restorative sleep specialists, *J Gerontol Nurs* 19(5):38, 1993.

94. Krach P: Nursing implications: functional status of older persons with schizophrenia, *J Gerontol Nurs* 19(8):21, 1993.

95. Krause N: Stress, alcohol use, and depressive symptoms in later life, *Gerontologist* 35(3):296, 1995.

96. Krause N: Stressors in salient social roles and well-being in later life, *J Gerontology* 49(3):137, 1994.

97. Kupfer DJ, Buysse DJ, Nofzinger EA, Reynolds, CF: Sleep disorders. In Widiger TA, et al: *DSM-IV sourcebook,* Vol. 1, Washington, DC, 1994, American Psychiatric Association.

98. Kurlowicz LH: Depression in hospitalized medically ill elders: evolution of the concept, *Arch Psychiatric Nurs* 8(2):124, 1994.

99. Kurlowicz LH: Social factors and depression in late life, *Arch Psychiatric Nurs* 7(1):30, 1993.

100. Kyomen H, Liptzin B: Alcohol abuse. In Copeland JRM, Abou-Saleh MT, Blazer DG, editors: *Principles and practice of geriatric psychiatry,* Cichester, England, 1994, Wiley.

101. Lacro JP, Jeste DV: Physical comorbidity and polypharmacy in older psychiatric patients, *Biological Psychiatry* 36(3):146, 1994.

102. Lancee WJ, et al: The impact of pain and impaired role performance on distress in persons with cancer, *Can J Psychiatry* 39(10):617, 1994.

103. Lindblom L, et al: Chemical abuse: an intervention program for the elderly, *J Gerontol Nurs* 18(4):6, 1992.

104. Lipsitt DR: Hypochondriasis and body dysmorphic disorder. In Gabbard GO, editor: *Treatments of psychiatric disorders,* Vol 2, Washington DC, 1995, American Psychiatric Press.

105. Lum TL: An integrated approach to aging and depression, *Arch Psychiatric Nurs* 2(4):211, 1988.

106. Mackinnon A, et al: A latent trait analysis of an inventory designed to detect symptoms of anxiety and depression using an elderly community sample, *Psychol Med* 24(4):977, 1994.

107. Marcus MT: Alcohol and other drug abuse in elders, *J ET Nurs* 20(3):106, 1993.

108. Markovitz PJ: Treatment of anxiety in the elderly, *J Clin Psychiatry* 54(5 suppl):64, 1993.

109. Martin LM, Fleming KC, Evans JM: Recognition and management of anxiety and depression in elderly patients, *Mayo Clin Proc* 70:999, 1995.

110. McCall WV: Management of primary sleep disorders among elderly persons, *Psychiatric Services* 46(1):49, 1995.

111. McCloskey JC, Bulechek GM: *Nursing interventions classification (NIC)* ed 2, St Louis, 1996, Mosby.

112. McInnes E, Powell J: Drug and alcohol referrals: Are elderly substance abuse diagnoses and referrals being missed? *BMJ* 308:444, 1994.

113. Miller NE: The fate of schizophrenia with advancing age: research findings and implications for clinical care. In Copeland JRM, Abou-Saleh MT, Blazer DG, editors: *Principles and practice of geriatric psychiatry,* New York, 1994, Wiley.

114. Mirka T: Understanding post operative psychosis and sleep deprivation: a case approach, *CJCN* 3(4):3, 1993.

115. Montamat SC, Cusack B: Overcoming problems with polypharmacy and drug misuse in the elderly, *Clin Geriatr Med* 8(1):143, 1992.

116. Morin CM: Insomnia: psychological assessment and management. New York, 1993, Guilford Press.

117. Munich RL, Sledge WH: Treatment settings: providing a continuum of care for patients with schizophrenia or related disorder. In Gabbard GO, editor: *Treatments of psychiatric disorders,* Vol. I, ed 2, Washington DC, 1995, American Psychiatric Press.

118. Neylan TC, Reynolds CF, Kupfer DJ: Sleep disorders. In Hales RE, Yudofsky SC, Talbott JA, editors: *The American Psychiatric Press textbook of psychiatry,* ed 2, Washington DC, 1994, American Psychiatric Press.

119. NIH Consensus Development Panel on Depression in Late Life: Diagnosis and treatment of depression in late life, *JAMA* 268(8):1018, 1992.

120. Nitenson NC, Cole JO: Psychotropic-induced sexual dysfunction. In Dunner DL: *Current psychiatric therapy,* Philadelphia, 1993, Saunders.

121. Office of Scientific Information: Plain talk about depression. Bethesda, 1994, National Institute of Mental Health.

122. Parker PE, Ford CV: Somatization disorder. In Hersen M, Ammerman RT, editors: *Handbook of prescriptive treatments for adults,* New York, 1994, Plenum.

123. Petruzzello SJ, et al: A meta-analysis on the anxiety-reducing effects of acute and chronic exercise: outcomes and mechanisms, *Sports Med* 11(3);143, 1991.

124. Pies RW: Medical "mimics" of depression, *Psychiatric Annals* 24(10):519, 1994.

125. Prager S, Jeste DV: Sensory impairment in late-life schizophrenia, *Schizophrenia Bull* 19(4):755, 1993.

126. Pratt JA: The neuroanatomical basis of anxiety, *Pharmacol Ther* 55:149, 1992.

127. Prohovnik I, Dwork AJ, Kaufman MA, Willson N: Alzheimer-type neuropathology in elderly schizophrenia patients, *Schizophrenia Bull* 19(4):805, 1993.

128. Pulling C, Seaman S: Sleep: a reality or dream for the hospitalized adult? *Can J Cardiovasc Nurs* 3(4):7, 1993.

129. Rabins PV: Schizophrenia and psychotic states. In Birren JE, Sloane RB, Cohen GD, editors: *Handbook of mental health and aging,* ed 2, San Diego, 1992, Academic Press.

130. Richman J: The lifesaving function of humor with the depressed and suicidal elderly, *Gerontologist* 35(2):271, 1995.

131. Riley B. Schizophrenia, paranoid, anxiety, and somatoform disorders. In Hogstel MO, editor: *Geropsychiatric nursing,* St Louis, 1995, Mosby.

132. Rossen EK, Buschman MBT: Mental illness in late life: the neurobiology of depression, *Arch Psychiatr Nurs* 9(3):130, 1995.

133. Saul RW, Keltner NL: Cognitive disorders. In Keltner NL, Schwecke LH, Bostrom CE: *Psychiatric nursing,* St Louis, 1995, Mosby.

134. Saunders PA: Epidemiology of alcohol problems and drinking patterns. In Copeland JRM, Abou-Saleh MT, Blazer DG, editors: *Principles and practice of geriatric psychiatry,* Chichester, England, 1994, Wiley.

135. Schuckit MA: Goals of treatment. In Gabbard GO, editor: *Treatments of psychiatric disorders,* Vol 1, ed 2, Washington DC, 1995, American Psychiatric Press.

136. Shader RI, editor: *Manual of psychiatric therapeutics,* ed 2, Boston, 1994, Little, Brown.

137. Shader RI: Delirium and dementia. In Shader RI, editor: *Manual of psychiatric therapeutics,* ed 2, Boston, 1994, Little, Brown.

138. Shaver JLF, Landis CA: Part 1, Understanding the behavior of sleep, *Am Nurse* October, 1994.

139. Shaver JLF, Landis CA: Part 3, Helping people manage primary insomnia, *Am Nurse* 27(1):22, 1995.

140. Sheikh JI. Clinical features of anxiety disorders. In Copeland JRM, Abou-Saleh MT, editors: *Principles and practice of geriatric psychiatry,* New York, 1994, Wiley.

141. Sloane PD: Normal aging. In Ham RJ, Sloane PD: *Primary care geriatrics: a case-based approach,* ed 2, St Louis, 1992, Mosby.

142. Smith SL, Sherrill KA, Colenda CC: Assessing and treating anxiety in elderly persons, *Psychiatric Services* 46(1):36, 1995.

143. Solomon K, Manepalli J, Ireland GA, Mahon GM: Alcoholism and prescription drug abuse in the elderly: St. Louis University grand rounds, *J Am Geriatr Soc* 41(1):57, 1993.

144. Southwell MT, Wistow G: Sleep in hospitals at night: are patient's needs being met? *J Adv Nurs* 21(6):1101, 1995.

145. Spenceley SM: Sleep inquiry: a look with fresh eyes, *Image* 25(3):249, 1993.

146. Stevens-Ratchford RG: The effect of life review reminiscence activities on depression and self-esteem in older adults, *Am J Occup Ther* 47(5):413, 1993.

147. Stolley JM, et al: Clients with delirium, dementia, amnestic disorders, and other cognitive disorders. In Antai-Otong D, Kongable G, editors: *Psychiatric nursing: biological and behavioral concepts,* Philadelphia, 1995, Saunders.

148. Stoudemire A, Moran MG: Psychopharmacologic treatment of anxiety in the medically ill elderly patient: special considerations, *J Clin Psychiatry* 54(5 suppl):27, 1993.

149. Stuart GW, Sundeen SJ: *Principles and practices of psychiatric nursing,* ed 4, St Louis, 1991, Mosby.

150. Sullivan CF: Hypnotic and sedative abuse. In Copeland JRM, Abou-Saleh MT, Blazer DG, editors: *Principles and practice of geriatric psychiatry.* Chichester, England, 1994, Wiley.

151. Sundeen SJ: Cognitive responses and organic mental disorders. In Stuart GW, Sundeen SJ: *Principles and practice of psychiatric nursing,* ed 5, St Louis, 1995, Mosby.

152. Taylor S: Anxiety sensitivity: theoretical perspectives and recent findings, *Behav Res Ther* 33(3):243, 1995.

153. Ticehurst S: Substance use and abuse. In Chiu E, Ames D, editors: *Functional psychiatric disorders of the elderly,* Cambridge, 1994, University Press.

154. Townsend MC: *Nursing diagnoses in psychiatric nursing,* ed 3, Philadelphia, 1994, FA Davis.

155. Townsend MC: *Psychiatric mental health nursing concepts of care,* Philadelphia, 1993, FA Davis.

156. Tucker GJ: Part I. Treatment approaches to anxiety, depression, and aggression in the elderly, *J Clin Psychiatry* 55(2 suppl):3, 1994.

157. Valente SM: Recognizing depression in elderly patients, *AJN* 94(12):19, 1994.

158. Wade B: Depression in older people: a study, *Nursing Standard* 8(40):29, 1994.

159. Walitzer KS, Connors GJ: Psychoactive substance use disorders. In Husen M, Ammerman RT, editors: *Handbook of prescriptive treatment for adults,* New York, 1994, Plenum Press.

160. Walker EF: *Developmentally moderated expressions of the neuropathology underlying schizophrenia,* Schizophrenia Bulletin 20(3):453, 1994.

161. Walsh JK, Hartman PG, Kowall JP: Insomnia. In Chokroverty S, editor: *Sleep disorders medicine: basic science, technical considerations, and clinical aspects,* Boston, 1994, Butterworth-Heinemann.

162. Waters E: Let's not wait till it's broke: interventions to maintain and enhance mental health in late life. In Gatz M, editor: *Emerging issues in mental health and aging,* Washington DC, 1995, American Psychological Association.

163. Wattis J, Martin C: *Practical psychiatry of old age,* ed 2, London, 1994, Chapman & Hall.

164. Weiss KJ: Management of anxiety and depression syndrome in the elderly, *J Clin Psychiatry* 55(2 suppl):5, 1994.

165. Whall AL: What is the nursing treatment for depression? *J Gerontol Nurs* 20(1):42, 1994.

166. Whitney JD: Somatization. In McFarland GK, Thomas MD: *Psychiatric mental health nursing application of the nursing process,* St Louis, 1991, Mosby.

167. Wieseke A, et al: A content validation study of five nursing diagnoses by critical care nurses, *Heart & Lung* 23(4):345, 1994.

168. Williams S: A developmental psychology of old age. In Chiu E, Ames D: *Functional psychiatric disorders of the elderly,* Cambridge, 1994, University Press.

169. Wood AM: A review of literature relating to sleep in hospital with emphasis on the sleep of the ICU patient, *Intens Crit Care Nurs* 9(2):129, 1993.

170. Wooten V: Sleep disorders in geriatric patients, *Clin Geriatr Med* 8(2):427, 1992.

171. Wright LK: Mental health in older spouses: the dynamic interplay of resources, depression, quality of the marital relationship, and social participation, *Issues Ment Health Nurs* 11:49, 1990.

172. Yassa R, et al: The prevalence of late-onset schizophrenia in a psychogeriatric population, *J Geriatr Psychiatry Neurology* 6:120, 1993.

173. Yassa R, Suranyi-Cadotte B: Clinical characteristics of late-onset schizophrenia and delusional disorder, *Schizophrenia Bull* 19(4):701, 1993.

174. Yesavage J: Differential diagnosis between depression and dementia, *Am J Med* 94(suppl 5A):23, 1993.

175. Zerhusen JD, Boyle K, Wilson W: Out of the darkness: group cognitive therapy for depressed elderly, *J Psychosocial Nurs Ment Health Serv* 29(9):16, 1991.

PART TWO

Perioperative Nursing

OVERVIEW

The purpose of this chapter is to outline the important aspects of nursing care in the perioperative period. Rather than focusing on specific invasive procedures and/or surgical interventions that have already been covered in this text, this chapter will define general principles that guide the care of patients during the perioperative phase of their care.

Patient care during the perioperative phase demands knowledge of and skill in perioperative care and also requires an in-depth understanding of related disease processes that have brought the patient to seek treatment.

With the advances in surgical and anesthetic technology, and improved intraoperative monitoring techniques such as mass spectrometry, pulse oximetry, transesophageal echocardiography, hemodynamic monitors, EEGs, cell savers, and pharmacologic advances, virtually all patients are candidates for intervention regardless of their preexisting health status. Perioperative nursing must encompass all specialties in order to meet the needs of this diverse patient population.

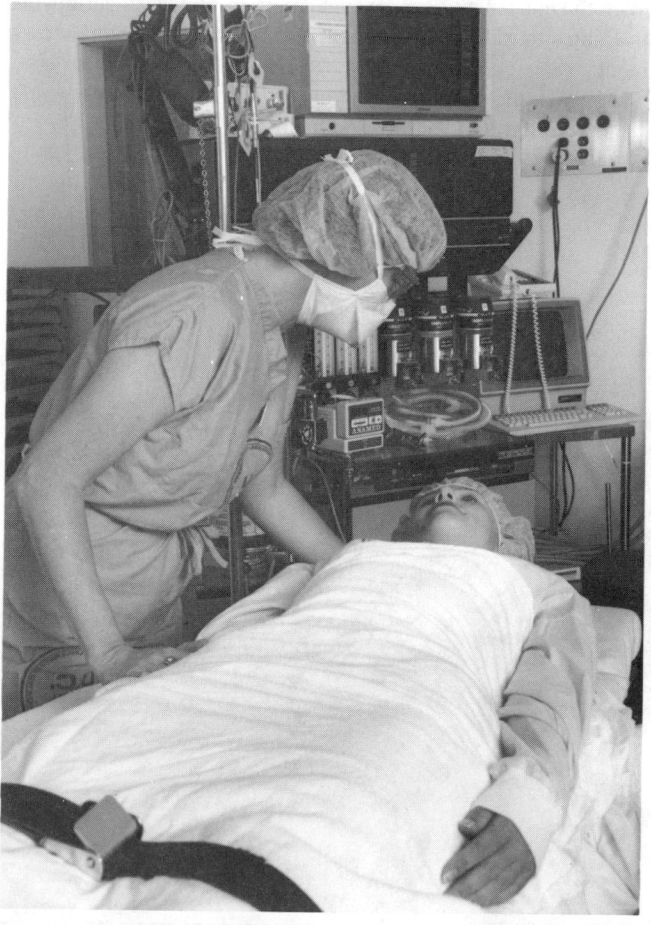

Nurse eases patient's anxiety before the procedure begins.

Operating room nurses *do practice nursing*. The Association of Operating Room Nurses defines the perioperative nurse in the following statement:

> *Perioperative nurse* is defined as the registered nurse who, using the nursing process, designs, coordinates, and delivers care to meet the identified needs of patients whose protective reflexes or self-care abilities are potentially compromised because they are having operative or other invasive procedures. Perioperative nurses possess and apply knowledge of the procedure and the patient's intraoperative experience throughout the patient's care continuum. The perioperative nurse assesses, diagnoses, plans, intervenes, and evaluates the outcome of interventions based on criteria that support a standard of care targeted toward this specific population. The perioperative nurse addresses the physiological, psychological, sociocultural, and spiritual responses of the individual that have been caused by the prospect or performance of the invasive procedure.[5]

Perioperative nurses should be familiar with the American Hospital Association Bill of Rights and the interpretation pertinent to the agency,[1] as well as the tenets of the American Nurses Association Code for Nurses.[2]

The ongoing coordination and organization of resources to provide a consistent response to fiscal realities and patient needs is known as case management. It reflects a dynamic process that focuses on the patient and the clinical system. Case management goals include the achievement of measurable, cost-effective, intraoperative resource utilization; the redesign of delivery systems; and the promotion of informed decision-making by the patient and all healthcare providers.[6]

As with the nursing process in other nursing arenas, there are overlapping steps of the perioperative nursing process. Intervention, evaluation, and discharge planning occur during the assessment and planning phases. Ongoing assessment and planning occur during the intervention phases, ensuring optimal outcomes for each patient.

Perioperative nursing not only incorporates the assessment, planning, implementation, and evaluation steps of the nursing process, but also allows for multiple nursing roles. Perioperative nurses may function as clinical practitioners, educators, managers, consultants, and/or researchers. They may practice in hospitals, clinics, ambulatory surgery centers, physicians' offices, or other patient environments.[20] The practice of perioperative nurses may be less visible than other specialties to patients and nursing colleagues, but it is still the practice of nursing.

PREOPERATIVE NURSING ASSESSMENT AND CARE

The primary function of preoperative nursing assessment is to ensure that all pertinent medical and psychosocial data regarding each patient are available to perioperative personnel before the induction of anesthesia. Data necessary for each procedure may include an informed consent, documentation of specific drug allergies, documentation of the patient's medical history and physical examination, and results of pertinent laboratory studies. Prior to general anesthesia for elective procedures, the perioperative nurse confirms that the patient has had nothing to eat or drink during the previous 6 to 8 hours.

The nursing diagnosis most pertinent to preoperative care is anxiety related to the situation. A preoperative assessment reveals the patient's concerns, which frequently include fear of death, disfigurement, or permanent injury; fear of pain and unknown outcome; and the possibility of impaired mobility postoperatively. Interventions include providing a calm environment and the opportunity to be with significant family member(s). Additionally, it is essential that the perioperative nurse convey a caring concern while completing routine preoperative checks (Figure II-1). Addressing the physical and emotional needs of the patient's spouse, family, and friends includes providing factual information regarding the impending invasive procedure and anesthesia and estimating the length of the procedure and the recovery period. Nursing intervention related to family members provides them with additional information about whom to call in the PACU after the procedure, the PACU visiting policy, the location of the family waiting areas, and the location of the hospital cafeteria or nearest restaurant. The preoperative nurse answers questions from the patient, friends, and family.

From the outset, an important goal of preoperative teaching is to return the patient to his/her environment with the skills and abilities to achieve optimal outcomes. Preoperative teaching is designed to reinforce the importance of postoperative pulmonary toilet and early postoperative ambulation; it is also designed to provide information about postoperative pain management alternatives. In the immediate preoperative period, explanations should be brief and easily understood. The nursing objective is to eliminate or minimize anxiety related to the impending procedure and to the postoperative period.

Before each procedure the perioperative nurse ensures the patient's safety:

1. Consult the schedule to determine the procedure to be performed.
2. Consult the preference cards to determine the surgeon's specifications: patient position, instruments, draping materials, sutures, special equipment, and supplies.
3. Collaborate with the scrub nurse on the patient's plan of care.
4. Proceed to the preoperative holding area to review the patient's chart. Check for informed consent for anesthesia and the procedure; laboratory results on blood and urine; results of electrocardiogram and chest x-ray examination, if ordered; current history and physical examination; availability of ordered blood; and any other data ordered by the physician.

With the concepts of case management in mind, the perioperative nurse introduces him/herself and begins the patient assessment:

1. Ask the patient to state his or her name.
2. Verify the identification band.

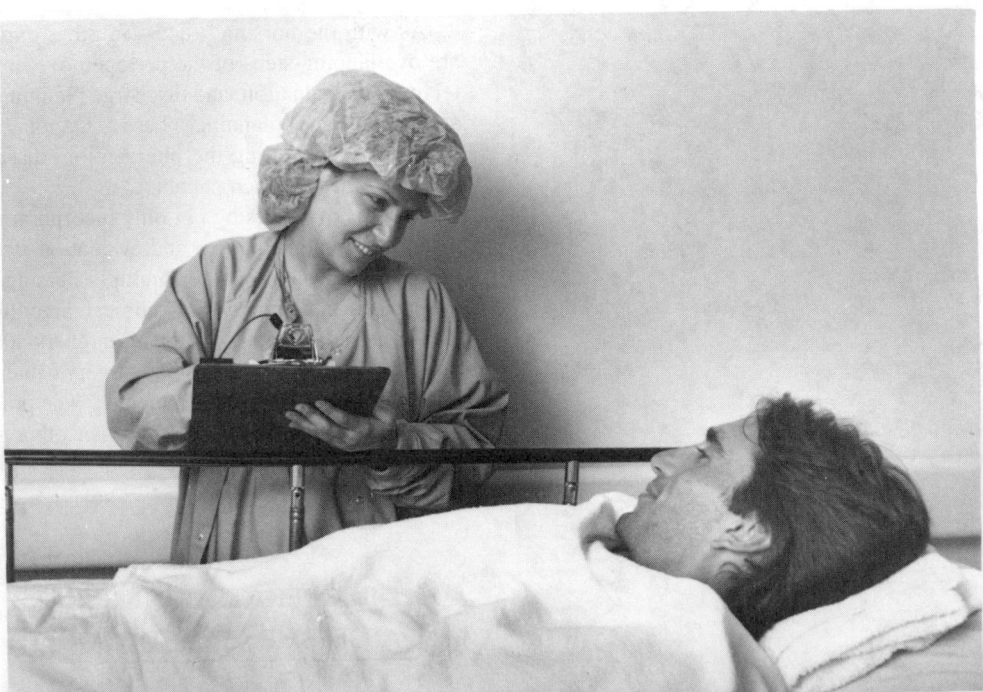

Figure II-1 Circulating nurse talks to patient before procedure and performs preoperative documentation.

3. Check for consistency between the patient's description of the procedure on the consent form and the procedure listed on the physician's notes.

4. Observe the patient's skin condition at the operative site and over the rest of the patient's body. Note any bruises, lacerations, or abrasions. Inspect incisions from previous procedures, and verify these with the patient.

5. Consult with the patient regarding his or her usual activity level.

6. Evaluate for limitation of motion, deformities, or other musculoskeletal considerations.

7. Note previous implants or prostheses on the perioperative record.

8. Document congenital anomalies or missing extremities.

9. Assess sensory functions, and note any impairments.

10. Consult with the patient regarding his or her surgical history.

11. Discuss with the patient any necessary accommodations to be made after discharge and initiate referrals as necessary.

Review patient data, and ascertain whether the values are within normal limits:

1. Review the patient's chart, and note deviation from the standard in laboratory values, x-ray examination, electrocardiogram, or other studies, as ordered.

2. Obtain vital signs, either on the nursing unit before transporting the patient to the preoperative holding area or in the preoperative area.

3. Document the patient's blood pressure, temperature, pulse, and respiration.

4. Report any deviations or abnormal findings to the appropriate physician.

Evaluate the cardiovascular status of the patient:

1. Check the patient's pulse for rate, rhythm, and irregularities (Figure II-2).

2. Review the electrocardiogram, and report any abnormalities to the physician.

3. Document the location of arterial and central lines on the perioperative record.

Evaluate the respiratory status of the patient:

1. Note the patient's skin color.

2. Assess the patient's breath sounds.

3. Review the patient's laboratory values of arterial blood gases, and report any abnormalities to the physician.

4. Document the location of chest tubes, if present.

Evaluate the renal status of the patient:

1. Note the patient's urinalysis and renal function studies. Review the results of input and output documentation for balance.

2. Check the patient's weight, and document the weight on the chart.

3. Verify that the patient has had nothing to eat during the previous 6 to 8 hours.

4. Document total parenteral nutrition line, if present.

Question the patient regarding allergies:

1. Elicit the details of the patient's allergic reaction to certain medications.

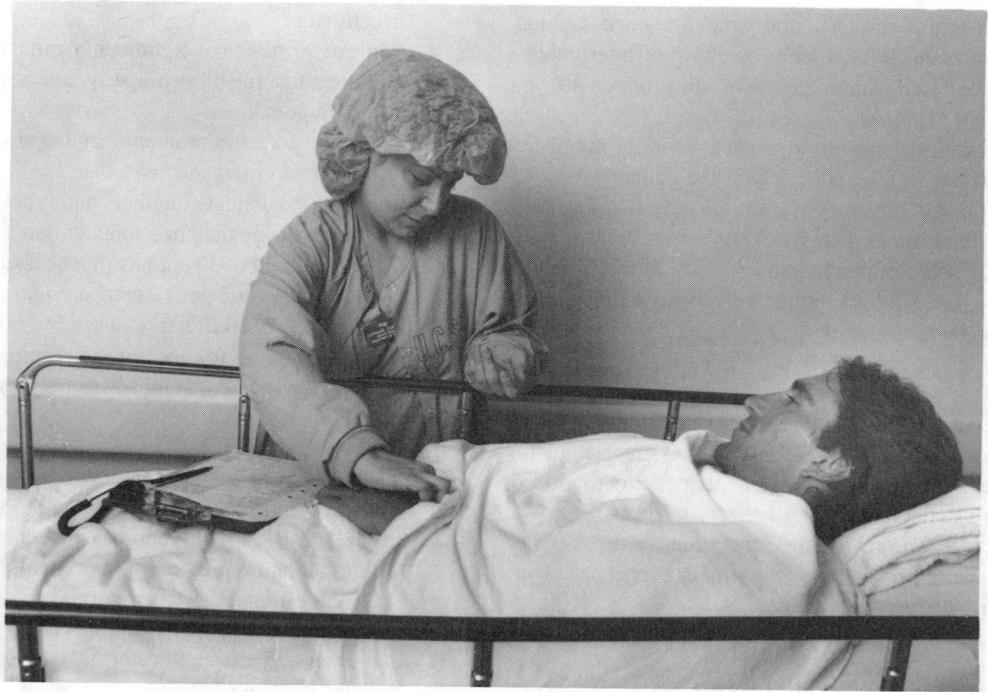

Figure II-2 Circulating nurse checks patient's pulse as part of preoperative assessment.

2. Ask the patient about side effects after ingesting foods.

3. Evaluate the patient's environmental allergies.

4. Incorporate allergies to chemicals (such as iodine) into the plan of care.

Ascertain details of any controlled substance use or abuse:

1. Question the patient about the use of drugs, alcohol, or tobacco products.

2. Observe the patient for skin integrity.

3. Review the patient's medical record.

4. Check the patient's laboratory studies and admission assessment.

Observe the psychosocial status of the patient during interaction with patient, family, and care givers:

1. Question the patient regarding his or her perception of the surgery.

2. Communicate any overreaction or inappropriate response to the surgeons and anesthesia personnel.

3. Question the patient about his or her expectations for the intraoperative period.

4. Reassure the patient that optimal care will be given and that he or she will not be left alone.

5. Address the concerns of the patient, and give additional information, as needed.

Analyze the patient's knowledge of the proposed intervention:

1. Incorporate the patient's verbal and nonverbal communication skills and hearing status into the nursing care plan.

2. Estimate the patient's level of knowledge as the prospective procedure is being discussed, and assist the patient to obtain more information if the patient's knowledge is not adequate.

3. Arrange for an interpreter if the patient's understanding is hampered because of a language barrier. Interpreters may often be family members, operating room staff, or other hospital personnel.

4. Elicit information from the designated family member, guardian, or agent, who is acting on the patient's behalf, if the patient demonstrates a lack of understanding because of mental impairment.

Ascertain the religious preference and ethnicity of the patient:

1. Discuss the wishes of the patient and family members regarding ceremonies and clergy.

2. Document specific requests on the patient's chart and care plan.

3. Clarify any other cultural beliefs that may influence care.

4. Assess own cultural and religious values in relation to those of the patient, and modify the plan of care to reflect the patient's beliefs.

Formulate nursing diagnoses to guide the patient's care (Table II-1 provides a generic perioperative nursing care plan based on the most frequent nursing diagnoses):

1. Interpret and prioritize assessment data to meet the needs of the patient.

2. Select the diagnoses based on scientific knowledge, current nursing practice, and interaction with the patient and family.

3. Document the diagnoses on the perioperative record and communicate this information to members of the health care team.[30]

Develop realistic outcome statements for the patient, including maintenance of skin integrity and freedom from infection:

1. Take into account the behavior patterns and physical status of the patient.

2. Address the patient's education needs, as well as his or her comfort and safety.

3. Develop criteria for measurement of goals based on laboratory data, vital signs, and symptom alleviation or improvement.

4. Identify tasks and procedures to be used in achieving outcomes.

5. Document goals on the perioperative record, and inform other members of the health care team.

6. Prioritize goals with the patient, considering Maslow's hierarchy of needs.[18]

7. Organize priorities in a logical sequence, taking into account the immediate and the long-term goals.

8. Interact with other departments to provide needed services to support the patient after discharge.

Anticipate and procure equipment and supplies before they are needed:

1. Consider the availability of instruments and potential scheduling conflicts affecting equipment and supplies.

2. Obtain necessary equipment from the appropriate departments.

3. Check and operate electrical equipment and powered surgical instruments according to the manufacturers' instructions.

4. Remove any piece of equipment from the operating room that does not function properly, and report it to the appropriate personnel.

5. Know the location, contents, and operation of the defibrillator and emergency cart.

6. Ensure that adequate numbers and types of personnel are available for the patient's transfer and care.

7. Use equipment and supplies in a cost-effective manner.

8. Document the judicious use of supplies and equipment to demonstrate cost-effective and appropriate patient care, thereby allowing for accurate reimbursement.

Direct professional and paraprofessional personnel to assist with implementation of patient care:

1. Take into account the preparation level of each person when assigning patient care responsibilities.

2. Maintain certification in cardiopulmonary resuscitation in the event that intervention is needed, and to meet institutional and regulatory requirements.

Control the environment to ensure optimal patient care:

1. Decrease sensory stimuli, especially during induction and emergence from anesthesia. The room should be as quiet as possible.

2. Decrease the risk for infection by limiting traffic to a minimum.

TABLE II-1 Expected Patient Outcomes

Diagnoses Labels	Interventions	Expected Outcomes
Preoperative		
Self-concept, alteration in body image, and role performance	Therapeutic communication Refer to appropriate person Assess for nonverbal cues Include physical or environmental changes in teaching Encourage patient participation (transfer, positioning, and conversation)	The patient demonstrates knowledge of the rehabilitation process.
Activity intolerance or immobility (actual and high risk for)	Assess range of motion, contributing factors (emotional and/or physical) Encourage patient participation Allow for ventilation of feelings (frustration)	The patient demonstrates knowledge of the rehabilitation process.
Intraoperative		
Infection (actual and high risk for)	Implement and maintain principles of aseptic technique Determine wound classification Assess contributing factors Follow hospital policy and procedure for room preparation	The patient is free from signs and symptoms of infection.
Hypothermia (high risk for)	Minimize patient heat loss by conduction (eg, contact with cold surfaces); convection (eg, through air currents); evaporation (eg, via wet solutions); radiation (eg, environmental temperature) Assess determinants (age, weight, dehydration) Compare baseline and intraoperative vital signs	The patient is free from injury related to exposure to heat loss.
Fluid and electrolyte deficit or excess (actual or high risk for)	Assess baseline lab values Note solutions being administered Note changes in monitoring equipment values Document urine/blood loss	The patient's fluid and electrolyte balance is maintained.
Impaired tissue or skin integrity	Assess for contributing factors (allergies, nutrition, disease process, extremes in age or weight) Assess areas at risk during positioning Implement safety measures (pads, safety straps, supports)	The patient's skin integrity is maintained.
Injury, high risk for foreign body	Implement procedures for (correct or incorrect) counts Document results	The patient is free from injury related to extraneous objects and physical hazards.
Injury, high risk for burn	Place ground pad close to incisional site in an area that is dry, free of scars, hair, skin folds, and lesions Select pad appropriate for patient's age and machine Be sure site is not in contact with spilled fluids or other metal objects Follow departmental procedure for assembly and use of electrosurgical unit	The patient is free from injury related to chemical, physical, and electrical hazards.
Injury, high risk for hemorrhage	Assess baseline data of personal history, previous surgeries, and lab values (Hg, Hct, PT) Provide sufficient equipment for estimated blood loss (sponges and suction canisters) Monitor patient intake and output status during surgery (blood loss, IV solutions, and irrigations) Coordinate care with staff	The patient's fluid balance is maintained.
Injury, high risk for neuromuscular trauma related to positioning	Assess for contributing factors (allergies, nutrition, disease process, extremes in age or weight) Assess areas at risk during positioning Implement positioning safety measures (pads, safety straps, supports) Position patient for procedure according to hospital policy and procedure	The patient is free from injury related to positioning hazards.
Injury, high risk for fall or trauma	Implement hospital procedures for surgical position Coordinate all patient transfers with sufficient number of personnel	The patient is free from injury related to positioning, extraneous objects, or physical hazards.

Continued.

◼ TABLE II-1 Expected Patient Outcomes—cont'd

Diagnoses Labels	Interventions	Expected Outcomes
Intraoperative—cont'd		
	Maintain patient alignment during transfer and positioning	
	Ensure OR bed accommodates patient size and age	
Injury, high risk for emboli or thrombi formation	Assess baseline data for coagulopathy	The patient is free from injury related to positioning, extraneous objects, or physical hazards.
	Assess activity level, determinants, and positioning requirements	
	Avoid dependent positioning without cardiovascular supports	
Anxiety, fear, and alteration in comfort related to local or regional procedure only	Assess baseline emotional and physical status	The patient demonstrates knowledge of the physiological and psychological responses to surgical intervention.
	Relate sequence of events intraoperatively and postoperatively	
	Provide emotional support through therapeutic communication	
	Monitor vital signs, oxygen saturation, reported patient pain level; report deviations from baseline	
Postoperative		
Alteration in comfort, pain (actual)	Assess location, duration, and intensity of pain	The patient demonstrates knowledge of the physiological and psychological responses to surgical pain.
	Change position as allowed	
	Therapeutic communication (touch and SOLER)	
	Relate complaints of pain to primary nurse	
Infection, high risk for	Maintain aseptic technique and good handwashing practices	The patient is free from signs and symptoms of infection.
	Assess dressing and incision site for infection	
	Review chart for vital signs and lab results	
Injury, high risk for hemorrhage or emboli	Review chart for recent vital signs and lab results	The patient is free from injury related to fluid loss, positioning, extraneous objects, or physical hazards.
	Assess dressing and drainage site where applicable	
	Assess for skin irritation because of prep solutions	
	Check electrosurgical conductive electrode	
	Analyze the effect of surgical position on pressure areas and gross sensory-motor activity	
	Assess patients at risk for circulatory compromise (Homan's sign, respiratory status, consciousness level)	
Anxiety related to postoperative care	Assess for nonverbal cues (diaphoresis, restlessness) and emotional status	The patient participates in the rehabilitation process.
	Therapeutic communication (SOLER and touch)	
	Identify and include family and significant others	
	Refer to support systems	
	Allow patient to ventilate feelings	
Ineffective airway clearance and breathing (actual or high risk for), aspiration (high risk for)	Assess breathing sounds and respiratory status	The patient is free from respiratory injury related to positioning, extraneous objects, or hypoxia.
	Have patient demonstrate turn, deep-breathing exercises, and use of incentive spirometer, if applicable	
	Note productive cough	
	Encourage fluids as clinically indicated	
Activity intolerance or immobility (actual)	Identify limitations and compare with preoperative baseline	The patient participates in the rehabilitation process.
	Validate knowledge of self-care	
	Assess effects of immobilizing devices applied during surgery (neurovascular checks and pressure areas)	
Grieving, actual related to loss of body part or postoperative surgical diagnosis	Encourage ventilation of feelings	The patient participates in the rehabilitation process.
	Encourage patient participation within limitations	
	Identify and include support systems	
	Refer to other professionals as clinically indicated	

From Association of Operating Room Nurses; perioperative nursing process.[3]

3. Maintain appropriate temperature and humidity of the room where care is administered.
4. Know the disaster plan evacuation routes, and procedures for removing the patient from the room while the intervention is in progress.
5. Keep the corridors free from obstructions at all times.

Collaborate with biomedical personnel to contain hazards:

1. Verify initial safety testing, performance testing, and routine preventive maintenance on all equipment.
2. Follow standard procedures for care and use of electrical hazards: check plugs, cords, and connections; observe delicate handling of cords and connections, secure cords to prevent tripping; avoid passing heavy equipment over cords; and remove and repair defective equipment.
3. Follow standard procedures for use of volatile liquids, ionizing radiation sources such as x-rays, and nonionizing radiation sources such as lasers.
4. Properly dispose of biohazardous waste in clearly marked containers.
5. Confine sharp objects and syringes to prevent injury.
6. Define maintenance and cleaning programs.
7. Verify regular inspections of the steam, electrical, vacuum, hydraulic, ventilation, plumbing, and emergency generator systems.
8. Report any situations requiring intervention between inspections.
9. Use good body mechanics and application of work-simplification principles to decrease the chance of personal injury.

Transport the patient in a safe and timely manner into the procedure room:

1. Confirm the patient's identity, both by verbal response and by comparison to the identification bracelet. If the patient cannot identify himself or herself, the identification should be provided by a family member or the health care professional accompanying the patient.
2. Select the appropriate mode of transport based on the patient's condition. The patient may be transported in a bed, on a gurney, in a wheelchair, or may walk into the room.
3. Document the mode of transport on the patient's record.
4. Determine the number and qualifications of transport personnel.
5. Reassure the patient and provide any comfort measures needed during transport.

Assess the needs of the patient and the family regarding protocols:

1. Explain the routine procedures to the patient and to the family, if they have not been previously instructed. Determine the complexity of the teaching based on the patient's attention span and anxiety level.
2. Instruct the patient in coughing and deep breathing. Give suggestions for enhancing the patient's comfort while the patient is performing those activities.
3. Question the patient about his or her understanding, and ask for a return demonstration.

4. Review the routine of the postanesthesia care unit, and address relevant discharge questions.
5. Document patient and family teaching on the perioperative record.

Record Keeping

Records and forms are established by the facility to safeguard patient confidentiality, to document informed consent for surgical and invasive procedures, and to provide for communication among health care personnel.[20]

The Joint Commission for the Accreditation of Healthcare Organizations requires that records be kept of each operation, including preoperative diagnoses, procedures performed, a description of the findings, the number and types of specimens removed, the postoperative diagnoses, and the names of participating personnel (see box).[15]

■ AORN 1995 STANDARDS AND RECOMMENDED PRACTICES

DOCUMENT THE FOLLOWING:

- Identification of persons providing care; name, title, and signature of the person responsible for the entry
- Evidence of a patient assessment upon arrival to the perioperative suite, including the level of consciousness, psychosocial status, and baseline physical data
- Patient's overall skin condition on arrival and discharge from the perioperative suite
- Presence and disposition of sensory aids and prosthetic devices accompanying the patient to surgery
- Patient's position, supports, and/or restraints used during the surgical procedure
- Placement of the dispersive electrode pad and identification of the electrosurgical unit and settings
- Placement of temperature control devices and identification of the unit, recording time and temperature
- Placement of electrocardiographic or other monitoring electrodes
- Medications, irrigations, and solutions administered or dispensed by the registered nurse
- Specimens and cultures taken during the procedure
- Skin preparation, solutions, area prepared, and any reactions that may have occurred
- Placement of drains, catheters, packings, and dressings
- Placement of tourniquet cuff and person applying the cuff, pressure, time, and identification of the unit
- Placement of implants, manufacturer, lot number, type, size, and other identifying information
- Occurrence and results of surgical item counts (Figure II-3)
- Time of discharge, disposition of patient, method of transfer, and patient status
- Intraoperative x-rays, fluoroscopy
- Wound classification
- Other direct patient care issues that are pertinent to patient outcomes

INTRAOPERATIVE NURSING CARE

Asepsis

The perioperative nurse is knowledgeable in the principles and practices of infection control. According to *Alexander's Care of the Patient in Surgery:*

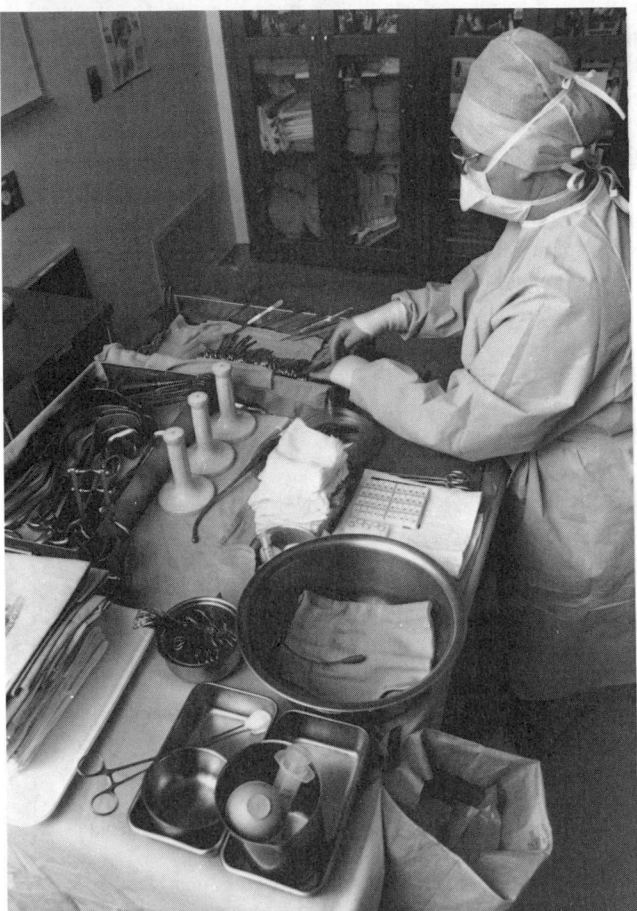

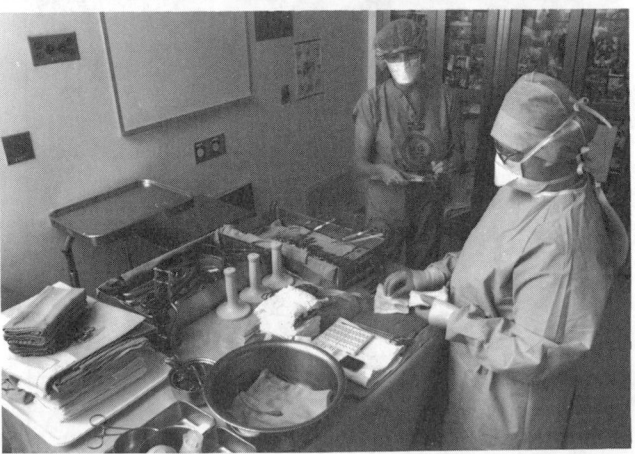

Figure II-3 A, Scrub nurse sets up instrument table. **B,** Scrub nurse and circulating nurse count sponges, instruments, and needles before surgical procedure begins.

Infection control practices should focus on prevention. Transmission of infection involves a chain of events, which include a pathogenic agent, reservoir, portal of exit, transmission, portal of entry, and host susceptibility. Prevention occurs when there is a break in the chain of transmission.

Infection control practices also involve personal and administrative measures. Personal measures include personal fitness for work, skin disinfection (patient and personnel), preparation of personnel hands, surgical attire, and personnel technique (surgical conscience). Administrative measures include provision of adequate physical facilities, appropriate surgical supplies, and operational controls.[20]

Each facility determines policies for proper operating room attire and universal precautions to comply with infection control practices (Figure II-4).[24] The principle of "confine and contain" protects personnel and prevents cross-contamination.

To ensure consistent, high-quality care for all surgical patients, regardless of the venue in which the care is rendered, principles of disinfection and sterilization must be followed. Instruments are decontaminated after use, mechanically washed, ultrasonically cleaned (to decrease the bioburden), and reassembled. The perioperative nurse is aware of preventive maintenance of equipment and of regular testing of equipment with chemical and biologic indicators. Sterilization may be ac-

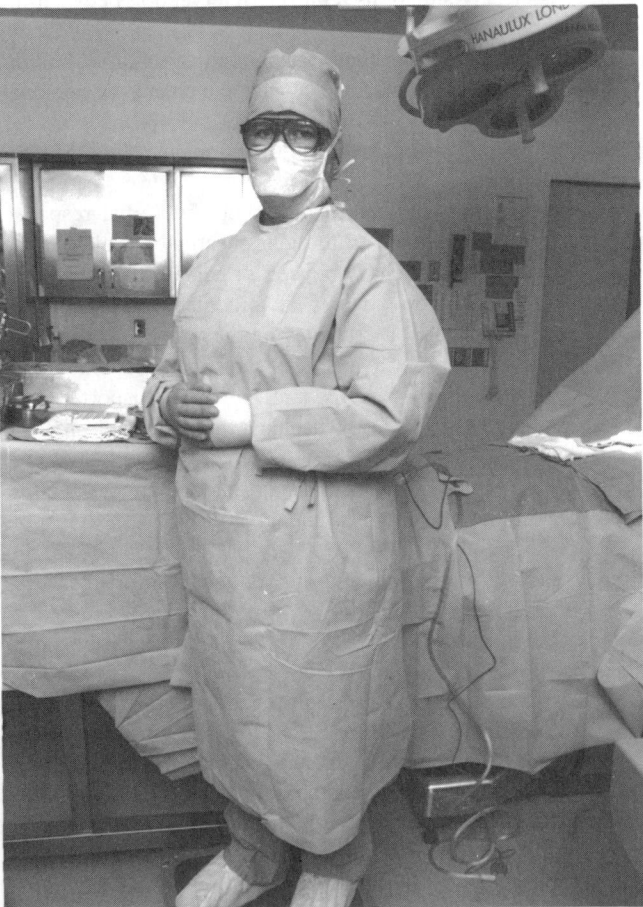

Figure II-4 Scrub nurse is properly attired for surgical procedure.

complished by dry heat, by steam under pressure, by plasma, or by chemical means. Disinfection may be used for those items that are not suitable for the sterilization process. Selection of a disinfectant is based on the need for high-, medium-, or low-level action. Various compounds are used for different surfaces and purposes. Activated glutaraldehyde is commonly used for disinfection and sterilization of heat-sensitive items. Phenols and hypochlorites are often used on operating room surfaces.[20] These recommended practices include rationale and interpretive statements that serve as a foundation for the practice of aseptic technique in the operating room.[5] *Alexander's Care of the Patient in Surgery* states that "the goal of each aseptic technique is to optimize primary wound healing, prevent surgical infection, and minimize the length of recovery from surgery."[20]

Surgical wounds can be classified as clean, clean-contaminated, contaminated, or infected. Wound types consist of those with no tissue loss, those with tissue loss, and those caused by underlying disease. Wounds with no tissue loss are primary closures and heal by first intention. Wounds with tissue loss, such as burns or traumatic injuries, heal by second intention or granulation.[21] Conditions that contribute to delayed wound closure are heavy contamination of the wound or removal of an inflamed organ.

The three phases of wound healing begin with an inflammatory response lasting 1 to 4 days. Vasoconstriction and clot formation maintain hemostasis and provide protection from contamination. During this edematous phase, leukocytes, macrophages, and basal cells migrate into the area. When fibroblasts are formed, the second stage of wound healing begins. This reconstructive phase lasts from 5 to 20 days, while collagen forms fibers that strengthen the connective tissue. The maturation phase of the wound may last for month or years. Complications of wound healing, if they should occur, include fistulas, hematomas, infections, wound disruptions, adhesions, or keloids. Wound healing is influenced by patient factors, such as nutritional status, weight, and the presence or absence of underlying disease, as well as environmental asepsis (see box) and

surgical tissue-handling technique. The selection of needles, sutures, and suturing techniques affects wound approximation and healing, as does the judicious use of intraoperative antibiotics.[17]

According to Kneedler and Dodge:

A surgical conscience means attention to aseptic principles during the perioperative period. It involves constant inspection, monitoring, and regulation of the surgical patient, environment, personnel, and equipment. The nurse anticipates the patient's and the surgical team's needs and gives unselfish, vigilant care to the patient.

A surgical conscience can be considered fully developed when the operating room nurse's attention to sterile technique and aseptic practices becomes automatic. It requires awareness of what is occurring at all times during the intraoperative period, even when attention is directed to other activities (see box).[17]

The skin of the patient and the members of the surgical team requires disinfection before the surgical procedure begins. The selection of an antimicrobial agent is made to remove dirt and transient microorganisms from the skin, reduce the number of resident microorganisms, and leave an antimicrobial residue on the skin surface, while minimizing skin irritation. Commonly used agents include povidone-iodine, chlorhexidine, alcohol, and hexachlorophene. Before the chosen agent is used, the patient's skin is prepared, if necessary, by clipping, by using depilatories, or by shaving. The skin of the surgical team is scrubbed, using a brush and nail cleaner for the length of time determined by the facility.[17]

Prepare the sterile field using the principles of asepsis:
1. Comply with operating room attire policy.
2. Procure the sterile supplies and equipment for each operative procedure.

AORN 1995 STANDARDS AND RECOMMENDED PRACTICES

SEVEN BASIC TENETS OF ASEPSIS
1. Scrubbed persons should wear sterile gowns and gloves.
2. Sterile drapes should be used to establish a sterile field.
3. Items used within a sterile field should be sterile.
4. All items introduced onto a sterile field should be opened, dispensed, and transferred by methods that maintain sterility and integrity.
5. A sterile field should be constantly monitored and maintained.
6. All personnel moving within or around a sterile field should do so in a manner to maintain the integrity of the sterile field.
7. Policies and procedures for basic aseptic technique should be written, reviewed annually, and readily available within the practice setting.

REQUIREMENTS FOR DEVELOPING A SURGICAL CONSCIENCE

1. Knowledge of the principles of asepsis.
2. The nurse's self-discipline in inspecting and regulating his or her hygiene, dress, and nursing practice, always giving attention to breaks in technique.
3. Ability to anticipate the need for services based on knowledge of the patient, the procedure being performed, the preferences of the surgical team, and where and how to obtain necessary supplies.
4. Good communication skills to determine the needs of patients and team members and to identify and correct breaks in technique.
5. Maturity to overcome personal preference and prejudice to provide optimum patient care, regardless of the surgical procedure, the patient's circumstances, or other surgical personnel.

From Kneedler and Dodge.[17]

3. Inspect supplies for package integrity and evidence of sterilization (Figure II-5).
4. Distribute supplies to the field aseptically.
5. Create a sterile operative field by using appropriate draping materials.
6. Monitor and correct aseptic practice during the procedure.

Positioning the Patient

Positioning has five major effects on the surgical patient: it affects respiration, circulation, peripheral nerves and vessels, musculoskeletal structures, and skin. Respiratory changes include disturbance of the ventilation-perfusion ratio, decreased stretchability of lung tissue, redistribution of inspired air, and mechanical restriction of lung expansion. Anesthesia is the primary cause of circulatory changes. Major vessels are dilated, lowering the blood pressure and leading to dependent pooling and decreased circulatory return. The medulla is depressed, compensatory mechanisms are hindered, and muscle tone is decreased. Effects on peripheral nerves from poor positioning include compromised blood supply or ischemia from stretching, hyperextending, compressing, or twisting. Because anesthesia reduces or eliminates the patient's normal defense mechanisms, care must be taken to safeguard the patient against inadvertent injury. Even patients who have normal range of motion can be compromised because of overzealous movement of extremities during positioning. Two factors to consider in relation to skin integrity are the location of bony prominences and the duration of pressure (Figure II-6). Decreased tissue perfusion can lead to ischemia, and shearing forces can lead to patient injury. Patients frequently cross their legs in the moments just before the induction of anesthesia; limbs should be checked for proper alignment after induction. Factors to be considered include the patient's age, weight, general health status, distribution of weight, blood pressure, nutrition, and duration of immobility.

Supine or dorsal recumbent position, with the patient lying on his or her back, is the position most commonly used. Careful placement of the extremities is important to avoid injury. The most common injury occurs to the brachial plexus when the arm is abducted greater than 90 degrees. Special attention must be paid to the elbows and fingers to prevent their contact with hard surfaces, and padding is essential to prevent pressure on bony prominences. Both the vital capacity and tidal volume are decreased, and obese patients experience a 40% to 50% increase in respiratory effort. Circulation is affected less in the supine position than in the other positions; however, the mean arterial pressure is decreased, and there is an increased volume of blood in the heart and lungs, when compared to sitting or standing.[17]

Trendelenburg's position is a variation of the supine position, with the patient's head positioned down. More respiratory changes occur; tidal volume and vital capacity are further decreased. Shift of the abdominal viscera impedes free movement

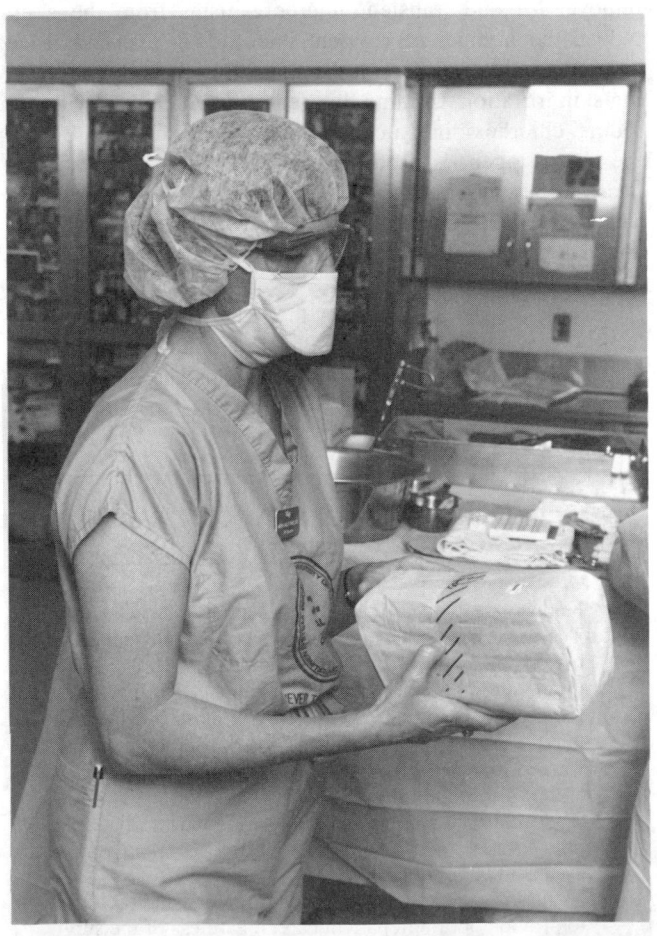

Figure II-5 Circulating nurse checks the integrity of the package of towels.

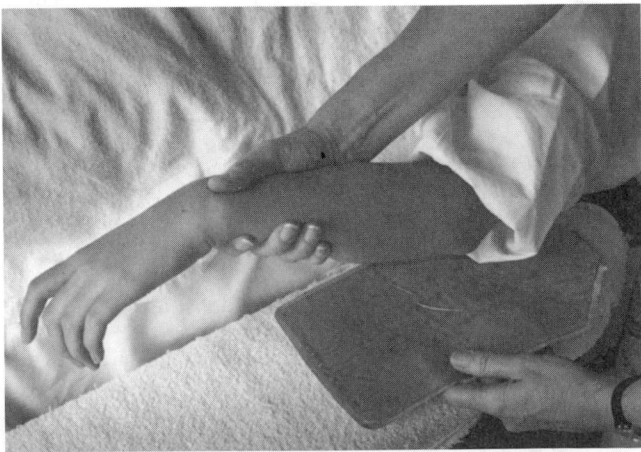

Figure II-6 Placement of gel pad to prevent injury during intraoperative period.

of the diaphragm, and intrathoracic pressure is increased. The patient should be moved slowly from supine to Trendelenburg's position to allow for gradual changes. The perioperative nurse must be constantly vigilant to prevent pressure on the patient's toes from the Mayo stand or instrument table.[17]

Reverse Trendelenburg's position, with the head up, must also be accomplished slowly. The respiratory function is affected less; however, circulation is affected more. The legs may be wrapped to prevent pooling of blood; however, it is important to avoid compression of the peroneal nerve at the head of the fibula.[20]

Lithotomy position, lying on the back with the legs flexed, decreases respiratory effectiveness because the diaphragm is restricted. Pulmonary blood volume is increased and vital capacity and tidal volume are decreased. Pressure from thigh flexion causes circulatory pooling in the lumbar area. The effects of this position are exacerbated if the patient is placed into Trendelenburg's position as well. The leg supports must be carefully chosen and applied securely to the operating room bed. The hands should be positioned across the chest or on armboards to prevent digital damage when the foot of the bed is lowered. The timing of leg movement is coordinated with the anesthesiologist. Two members of the surgical team move the legs simultaneously to prevent sacroiliac dislocation, and special consideration is given to patients with hip prostheses. Padding is applied to the knee area to prevent peroneal nerve damage.[17]

Modified Fowler's, or *sitting, position* is physiologically best for respiratory function. Venous pooling, sometimes leading to hypotension, is the primary systemic circulatory effect. The ischial tuberosities bear the majority of the patient's weight, creating the potential for pressure areas and sciatic nerve damage. Judicious use of padding can help to prevent such occurrences.[21]

Side-lying or lateral position decreases respiratory efficiency because the body's weight is on the lower chest. This position interferes with intercostal breathing and results in decreased respiratory efficiency, vital capacity, and tidal volume.[31] Pooling in the dependent limbs occurs when the abdominal vessels are compressed. Peripheral nerve injuries can occur when scrupulous attention is not given to arm position. If the legs are allowed to lie in contact with each other during the operation, there is a potential for skin abrasions or friction injuries. Lateral position is best accomplished by a team of four health care workers. The patient's flank is positioned over the kidney rest (bridge) on the operating room bed, and then the bridge of the operating bed is raised slowly. The bottom leg is flexed, while the top leg remains straight. Padding is placed between the legs, around the ankles, and elsewhere if deemed necessary. The arm on the bottom is positioned at an angle slightly less than 90 degrees from the body, and the elbow, wrist, and hand are padded and secured to the armboard. A soft roll is placed at the apex of the scapula to prevent brachial compression. The arm on the top is secured to a padded support or to an elevated armboard. The body is secured with tape, braces, or sandbags.

Prone or face-down position requires the patient to be anesthetized on the stretcher before being turned over on the abdomen. Respiration is restricted because of the weight of the body on the abdomen; the blood pressure may fall. Body rolls that support the patient from the acromioclavicular joint to the iliac crest are placed on the operating room bed. The move is accomplished using four health care workers and turning the patient in a logroll manner. Careful attention to the endotracheal tube and to the monitoring devices is essential during turning. Arms may be secured at the sides of the operating room bed or to padded armboards extending alongside the head. Care is taken to move the arms down and forward to avoid hyperextending the shoulder joints. The body rolls are adjusted to provide support, to allow full excursion of the lungs, and to prevent encroachment on the female breasts. The male genitalia are checked for impingement. The knees are padded, and a pillow is placed under the ankles to prevent the toes from coming in contact with the mattress.

Jackknife or Kraske position is the most precarious surgical position. Because of reduced negative intrathoracic pressure, the respiratory system is severely compromised. Blood pooling in the extremities is the most common circulatory effect and is caused by obstruction at the break in the operating room bed. Other concerns are the same as those for the patient in prone position.[17]

Determine the position of the patient by the need for adequate exposure of the operative site, accessibility to the patient's airway and monitoring devices, and considerations for the patient's safety.

1. Employ the four components: knowledge, forethought, teamwork, and housekeeping, when positioning the patient.[21]
2. Understand the consequences of improper positioning and body alignment, using your knowledge of anatomy and physiology.
3. Before moving, lock both the operating room bed and the stretcher for patient safety.
4. Identify equipment used for patient positioning.

Monitoring the Patient

The perioperative nurse is responsible for maintaining an awareness of the physiologic monitoring devices used during the procedure:

1. Observe the electrocardiogram, the pulse oximeter, and the patient's skin color. Note and document any changes.
2. Watch the patient for behavioral changes, such as restlessness or a change in the level of consciousness. Communicate this information to the appropriate personnel.
3. Monitor fluid intake and calculate blood loss.
4. Operate patient monitoring devices according to manufacturer's instructions.

5. Complete documentation of the patient intervention (Figure II-7).

Conclusion of the Procedure

The steps taken to conclude any operative or invasive procedure must be followed closely to ensure a smooth transition to recovery. Call the appropriate postoperative care unit to give a preliminary report on the patient's status before completion of the procedure.

Control materials used on the patient:
1. Count sponges, sharps, and instruments as delineated in the policy and procedure manual of the agency.
2. Relate result of counts to the surgical team.
3. Implement corrective actions if the counts are incorrect, including notifying the surgeon and the x-ray department and filling out the risk management report.

Administer medications to the patient:
1. Document drug, dosage, and route of administration on the perioperative record.
2. Observe the patient for reactions, complications, side effects, and efficacy.

Reassess the patient during the postoperative evaluation:
1. Correlate changes in the health status of the patient to the nursing diagnoses.
2. Review laboratory data and patient signs and symptoms.
3. Revise the patient care plan to reflect this evaluation.

4. Reevaluate patient outcomes.
5. Measure and document patient responses to the interventions.

Conclude the procedure and transfer the patient to the stretcher for transport:
1. Provide clean gown to maintain the patient's dignity and privacy.
2. Perform a skin assessment, giving special attention to areas that are dependent or are under the dispersive electrode pad.
3. Keep the safety strap in place until all personnel are ready to transfer the patient to the stretcher.
4. Place the stretcher adjacent to the bed with the wheels locked.
5. Determine the patient position on the stretcher after assessing patient for responsiveness.
6. Determine airway maintenance, proper body alignment, and availability and security of tubes, drains, lines, and monitoring devices.
7. Transfer the patient slowly and smoothly to the stretcher with concern for patient safety, good body mechanics, and coordination of team members.

ANESTHESIA

The anesthesiologist reports on the surgical procedure and anesthetic management. The perioperative nurse adds, vali-

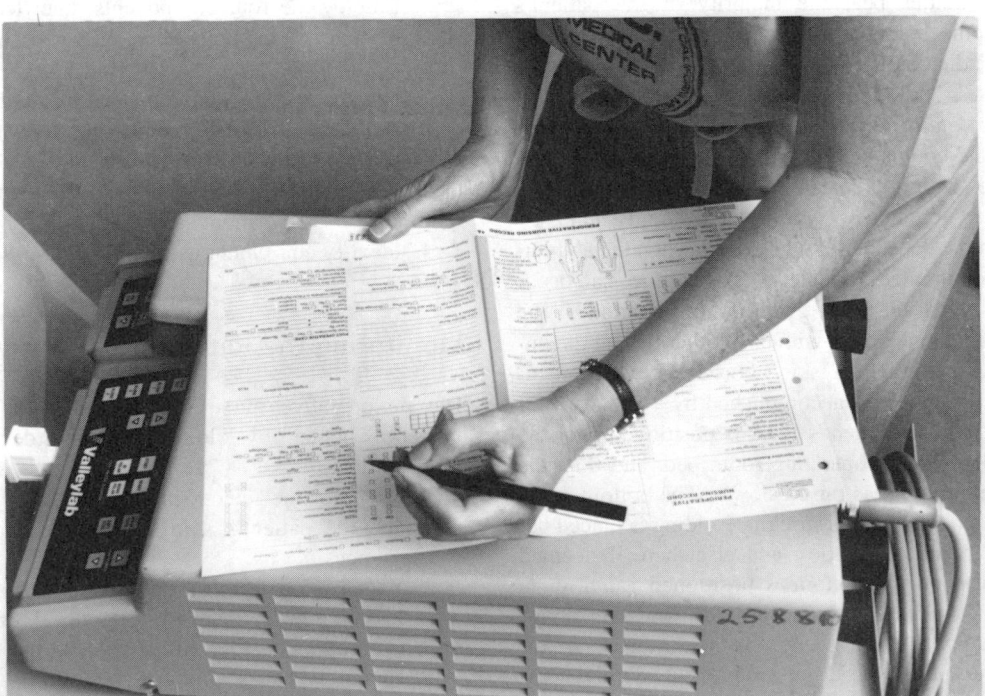

Figure II-7 Circulating nurse performs intraoperative documentation.

dates, and verifies important information for the postoperative care of the patient. Baseline data included in the report are the patient's name; age; preoperative and postoperative diagnoses; surgical procedure; anesthesia agents and technique; intraoperative information; primary language; preoperative level of consciousness; medical history; allergies; airway status; catheters, drains, lines; blood loss; nursing considerations; and special symptoms that are observed.[11]

Inhalation Anesthetics and Their Physiologic Effects

Inhalation anesthetic agents are used to render patients unconscious and insensible to noxious stimuli. Generally, these agents are used in conjunction with intravenous sedative or narcotic agents to achieve surgical anesthesia. This concept of "balanced" anesthesia uses the lowest effective dose of inhalation agents, which reduces the possibility of administering an overdose. The physiologic effects of inhaled anesthetics, besides producing anesthesia, are important considerations for the nurses providing care to postoperative patients because all organ systems are affected by these agents.

The four major inhalation anesthetic agents that are used alone to create surgical anesthesia are halothane, enflurane (Ethrane), isoflurane (Forane), and desflurane (Suprane). Nitrous oxide is also used as an anesthetic gas; however, it cannot be used alone because it is less potent than the other three. To anesthetize an average person for surgery, the partial pressure of nitrous oxide necessary in the alveoli (and therefore in the blood and brain) is 105%—enough to eliminate oxygen from the mixture of the inspired gases used to deliver anesthesia. Therefore nitrous oxide is used in conjunction with another inhalational agent or with narcotics. Although the exact mechanism by which inhalation agents produce the anesthetic state is not completely understood, all of them produce known physiologic effects that often last into the recovery period; these effects may be observed in the PACU.

Respiratory Effects

Inhalational anesthetics alter gas exchange, affecting both $Paco_2$ and Pao_2, and they also affect the muscles of respiration and airway protection.

Gas Exchange

The overall respiratory effect of the inhalation agents is profound respiratory depression. This occurs in a dose-dependent way, eventually producing respiratory arrest if the inspired concentration becomes high enough. Tidal volume is greatly reduced, predisposing the patient to respiratory acidosis via alveolar hypoventilation. All inhalation agents cause tachypnea during induction of anesthesia, and during any increase in delivered concentration to increase anesthetic depth if patients are allowed to breathe spontaneously. Even though the respiratory rate is increased, it does not compensate for the decrease in tidal volume because the dead space ventilation does not change. The effect of this respiratory depression re-

sults in increased $Paco_2$. In the central nervous system, inhalation agents depress the ventilatory response to increases in $Paco_2$. The combined effects result in (1) "resetting" to a higher level the $Paco_2$ necessary to stimulate breathing and (2) a decreased response to additional CO_2 that may occur during surgery.

Oxygenation is impaired (Pao_2 may decrease) during anesthesia from a number of effects of the inhalation anesthetics. First, there is alveolar hypoventilation, as described previously. In addition, the regular resting breathing pattern is altered. When a person is awake, there is a periodic "sigh" that entails taking a breath two to three times the normal tidal volume. This serves to reexpand any alveoli that have collapsed because of immobility. If this were not done, eventually the atelectasis would cause an increase in the blood "shunted" past nonventilated alveoli, which decreases overall oxygenation and results in a fall in Pao_2. This sigh mechanism is eliminated by inhalational anesthetics in patients who are breathing spontaneously, further predisposing to atelectasis and hypoxemia. All patients who are anesthetized, whether being ventilated mechanically or breathing spontaneously, are prone to atelectasis due to the fact that they are either supine or in other positions even less favorable to adequate alveolar expansion. Normally, in the awake state, the response to atelectasis (besides the sigh) is pulmonary vasoconstriction, which diverts pulmonary capillary blood away from the atelectatic portion of the lung. Inhalational anesthetics blunt this response also, further creating a right to left pulmonary shunt, thereby increasing arterial hypoxemia. Effects that work to decrease oxygenation explain why it is important to increase the inspired oxygen concentration during and after surgery, until all of the effects of the inhalation anesthetics have resolved.

Mechanics of Breathing

Inhalation anesthetics affect the muscles of breathing and those used for airway protection. As the muscles of the tongue become anesthetized, patients tend to develop upper airway obstruction. Maintaining a patent airway during recovery from anesthesia not only is necessary for efficient gas exchange, but also facilitates the elimination of anesthetic gases. As the anesthetic concentration is increased during the induction of anesthesia, use of the accessory muscles to assist ventilation progressively decreases—an event that normally occurs in unanesthetized individuals as hypoventilation is sensed. The diaphragm continues to function unless very high concentrations (anesthetic overdose) are reached. As patients recover from anesthesia, they recover their ability to use accessory respiratory muscles if necessary.

Inhalation anesthetics also depress the airway protective reflexes; if patients vomit during anesthesia they may not be able to cough efficiently enough to clear any material that enters the trachea. Pulmonary aspiration of the gastric contents, if allowed to occur, remains a serious consequence of the unprotected airway.

The mechanisms used by the body to clear secretions from the tracheobronchial system, particularly the cilia, are impaired by the use of inhalation anesthetics. Patients who produce sputum preoperatively often require tracheal suctioning during surgery and into the postoperative period in the PACU.

Special Respiratory Considerations

Halothane is the inhalation agent most commonly used in children because it is least irritable to the airway. This is an important consideration as it is generally easier to induce anesthesia in children by having them breathe an inhalational agent through a mask than it is to start an intravenous line. In addition, halothane, unlike the other inhalation agents, appears not to stimulate respiratory secretions, making its use valuable in patients with obstructive pulmonary disease who are prone to produce sputum. Isoflurane and desflurane, on the other hand, cause the greatest airway irritation, and induction with these agents may occasionally be characterized by coughing, breath holding, and laryngospasm. While halothane is often chosen, all inhalation anesthetics are bronchial smooth muscle dilators and are effective in reducing wheezing from asthma during anesthesia and surgery.

Cardiovascular Effects

Inhalation anesthetics affect each of the following parameters of the cardiovascular system: myocardial contractility, blood pressure, peripheral vascular resistance, coronary artery blood flow, and heart rate. They do not, however, have equal effects on each parameter at the same anesthetic dose. In patients with preexisting myocardial disease these effects are more pronounced.

All inhalation agents are myocardial depressants. In addition, they all produce hypotension (in the absence of surgery), and all decrease coronary blood flow. Both enflurane and isoflurane cause a larger fall in peripheral vascular resistance than halothane. Fortunately, myocardial oxygen consumption during anesthesia is reduced so that the coronary blood flow, although reduced, is sufficient to meet the metabolic needs of the myocardium. As with the respiratory effects, these cardiovascular effects are dose-dependent. The higher the anesthetic concentration, the lower the blood pressure and the more profound the myocardial depression.

Enflurane, isoflurane, and particularly desflurane, often cause an increase in heart rate while halothane does not. When enflurane and isoflurane are combined with small doses of intravenous narcotics, the increase in heart rate associated with these agents is not as great. The increased heart rate associated with increasing the inspired concentration of desflurane is often accompanied by a slight increase in blood pressure. The mechanism of these changes is not yet understood.

Halothane "sensitizes" the myocardium to the effects of catecholamines, an effect not shared by the other inhalation anesthetics.

Cardiovascular reflexes, including tachycardia in response to hypotension and bradycardia in response to vagal or baroreceptor stimulation, remain intact; however, these reflexes are reduced or depressed during anesthesia with any of the inhalation agents.

Because patients are brought to the PACU before all the inhalation agents have had time to be eliminated from the body, many of the effects on the cardiovascular system described above may be seen in the PACU. It is particularly important to remember that during the early postoperative period, patients' compensatory cardiovascular reflexes remain depressed. Hypotension will need early intervention because the patients' sympathetic nervous system may be unable to respond appropriately if inhalation agents remain in their bodies—even if they remain in minimal concentrations.

Circulatory Effects on Other Body Systems

Cerebral

All of the inhalational agents blunt the ventilatory response to rising P_{CO_2}. Carbon dioxide is a potent cerebral vasodilator, and its presence in the circulation in higher than normal concentrations increases cerebral perfusion. In addition, inhaled anesthetic gases tend to inactivate the cerebral metabolic control (autoregulation) of its own circulation; therefore no compensation is made for the increased cerebral perfusion secondary to hypercarbia. These agents also act directly on cerebrovascular smooth muscle. The combination of all of these effects increases the intracranial blood volume and the intracranial pressure of the patient under anesthesia.

Gastrointestinal

Hepatic blood flow is reduced when patients are anesthetized with inhalational agents. The reduced hepatic blood flow affects the metabolism of all other drugs given during the anesthetic period and the initial recovery phase. This is an important consideration for nurses in the PACU because dosages of analgesics must be titrated, keeping in mind the patient's preexisting sedation and impaired ability to metabolize drugs effectively.

Renal

Inhalational anesthetics increase renal vascular resistance and decrease renal cortical blood flow. Consequently the glomerular filtration rate is decreased and the urine output volume is reduced during anesthesia, perhaps by as much as 60% to 70%. The decrease in renal blood flow and the fall in blood pressure seen during inhalation anesthesia combine to activate the renin-angiotensin system. In addition, stimulation of the sympathetic nervous system is associated with release of antidiuretic hormone (ADH), contributing further to a decrease in urine volume during anesthesia.

Skeletal Muscles

All inhalation anesthetics cause skeletal muscle relaxation. If muscle relaxation is required for optimal surgical conditions (i.e., for abdominal surgery), however, intravenous muscle relaxants are used. The concentration of inhaled anesthetics necessary to create surgical relaxation is in the lethal dose range and would likely cause severe cardiovascular depression or collapse.

Cutaneous Circulation

Inhalation agents cause cutaneous vasodilation. This direct effect interferes with temperature regulation because heat loss through the skin is increased. As a result of this effect, and from surgical incisions that expose body cavities to the ambient environment, most patients have some degree of hypothermia when they are admitted to the PACU. Interestingly, patients in whom finding venous access preoperatively may be difficult will usually exhibit many potential intravenous sites soon after inhalation anesthesia is started because of peripheral vasodilation.

Balanced Anesthesia

As mentioned previously, inhalational anesthetics are almost always used in conjunction with other agents to achieve optimal surgical conditions. This concept of "balanced anesthesia" uses the minimal dose of each agent to achieve the desired surgical conditions. Other than the inhalation agents, almost all of the additional anesthetic agents are administered intravenously. Barbiturates, narcotics, benzodiazepines, and neuromuscular blocking agents are the classes of drugs used most often in combination with inhaled gases to produce balanced anesthesia.

Barbiturates

The most commonly used drug in this class is sodium thiopental. It is administered intravenously at the beginning of surgery to induce anesthesia. Thiopental is an ultra-short acting barbiturate that depresses the central nervous system, producing hypnosis and anesthesia without analgesia. The peak effect of an induction dose is achieved within 1 minute after intravenous administration, and the effect is gone after 5 to 10 minutes. This, like all barbiturates, is a potent respiratory depressant. Methohexital (Brevital) is another commonly used IV barbiturate whose clinical profile is similar to sodium thiopental.

Propofol

Propofol (a substituted isopropylphenol) is an intravenous induction agent that may have some advantages over thiopental and other barbiturates. Like thiopental, it is rapidly cleared from the plasma so the duration of action is short. The clearance of propofol from the plasma exceeds hepatic blood flow, so metabolism of the drug occurs to some extent in the plasma itself, and is therefore not dependent on liver and renal function. Clinical experience indicates that propofol causes less nausea than barbiturates and its rapid elimination prevents the feeling of a "hangover" that often accompanies recovery from anesthesia induced by thiopental. In addition, propofol can be used as an anesthetic itself when given by continuous infusion. When used in this manner, recovery from general anesthesia is accomplished more quickly and without the unpleasant side effects (nausea, vomiting and residual sedation) that often accompany recovery from other agents. Propofol has gained popularity in recent years and is frequently used in outpatient surgical settings to facilitate rapid recovery in patients who are going home the day of surgery.

Narcotics

Morphine sulfate, fentanyl, and sufentanil are the narcotic agents most commonly used to supplement general and regional anesthesia. All are analgesics, and that is the main reason for their use. All narcotics cause respiratory depression in a dose-related manner. Morphine is longer acting than fentanyl and sufentanil. Morphine and fentanyl are commonly used postoperatively for pain relief and intraoperatively as part of a balanced anesthetic.

Benzodiazepines

Diazepam (Valium) and midazolam (Versed) are the most commonly used drugs in this class; recently, however, the use of midazolam has exceeded that of diazepam because it is shorter acting and because it is an excellent amnestic agent. These agents are also anticonvulsant. The dose of these agents should be decreased in the elderly or debilitated patient. These agents are respiratory depressants and when used in combination with narcotics, severe respiratory depression may occur.

Neuromuscular Blocking Agents

Neuromuscular blocking agents are used in surgery as an adjunct to general anesthesia to provide an optimal surgical environment and to minimize the need for other potent anesthetic agents. Skeletal muscle relaxation is essential during abdominal and thoracic procedures and is often used during a variety of other surgeries to eliminate patient movement.

Muscle relaxants are divided into two general categories: depolarizing and non-depolarizing (competitive) agents. The most commonly used depolarizing muscle relaxant is succinylcholine (Anectine). After IV injection, succinylcholine binds with the acetylcholine receptor site at the neuromuscular junction, causing depolarization, then muscular contraction—seen clinically as fasciculations. Unlike acetylcholine, however, succinylcholine is not metabolized by acetylcholinesterase. The motor endplate remains depolarized and so is unable to accept subsequent stimuli until succinylcholine is eventually metabolized by serum pseudocholinesterase. The duration of action of a standard dose of succinylcholine is approximately 3 to 5 minutes. The primary use for succinylcholine is to facilitate tracheal intubation immediately after induction of anesthesia. Because succinylcholine is not metabolized by acetylcholinesterase, its effects cannot be reversed. Competitive blocking agents can be reversed pharmacologically. The commonly used blocking agents are pancuronium, *d*-tubocurarine, and vecuronium. After IV injection these agents combine with acetylcholine receptors; however, they do not cause depolarization of the motor endplate. When enough receptor sites are blocked, the normal neurotransmitter, acetylcholine, cannot activate enough receptors to raise the endplate potential for excitation and so neuromuscular blockade ensues. Generally the duration of action of nondepolarizing muscle relaxants varies between 30 to 60 minutes depending on the dose and the specific agent used. The onset of action of these agents is approximately 3 to 5 minutes, depending on the dose. They are primarily used for surgical relaxation rather than intubation. They can, however, be used for tracheal intubation when succinylcholine is contraindicated.

Nursing considerations in the immediate postoperative period for patients who have received neuromuscular blocking agents primarily concern the evaluation of respiratory function. Incomplete recovery from the effect of neuromuscular blocking agents is manifested as discoordinated breathing, that is, asymmetric chest movement resulting in inadequate tidal volumes. The patient may complain of "weakness" and an inability to breathe. A reliable test to determine whether the effects of the neuromuscular blocking agents have been fully reversed is to ask the patient to lift his or her head off the bed and keep it elevated for 5 seconds. A person with normal muscle tone, in the absence of neck injury, will be able to perform this maneuver. If it is determined that the patient is still experiencing the effects of neuromuscular blockade, an anticholinesterase agent may be administered.

Reversal Agents

Anticholinesterase agents are given to reverse the effects of neuromuscular blockers. The two most commonly used drugs in this class are edrophonium (Tensilon) and neostigmine (Prostigmin). The action of these drugs is to combine with cholinesterase to prevent the metabolism of acetylcholine. The acetylcholine plasma level increases, which allows the acetylcholine to compete with the neuromuscular blocker and bind with its receptor sites. The muscarinic effects of the increased plasma levels of acetylcholine include bradycardia, bronchospasm, and excessive salivation. Because the bradycardia may be hemodynamically significant, anticholinergic agents are administered in conjunction with the anticholinesterase agent. Atropine and glycopyrrolate are the anticholinergic agents most frequently used to avoid bradycardia when reversing the effects of neuromuscular blockers. The nurse in the immediate postoperative phase must be able to assess the adequacy of the patient's breathing and to recognize the need for airway support if the patient is still suffering from the effects of neuromuscular blocking agents.

Regional Anesthesia

Regional anesthesia includes a variety of techniques that use local anesthetic drugs. They can be used on any part of the CNS and every type of nerve fiber. Local anesthetics affect the nerve cells by preventing the transport of sodium across the cell membrane, which prevents depolarization and impulse conduction.

Local anesthetics are pharmacologically classified as amides or esters (Table II-2). Esters are rapidly metabolized in the plasma; their half-life is short. One of the metabolic degradation products is *p*-aminobenzoic acid, which is associated

TABLE II-2 Centroneuraxis Narcotic Bolus

Drug	Bolus Dose (mg)	Onset (min)	Duration (hr)
Epidural Route			
Morphine	1-10	30-60	6-24
Fentanyl	0.025-0.15	4-20	2.6-4
Demerol	20-200	5	6-8
Subarachnoid Route			
Morphine	0.1-0.5	15	8-24
Demerol	10-30	5	10-30

with allergic reactions in sensitive individuals. Amides are metabolized by the liver and have longer half-lives. Patients with severe liver dysfunction are at greater risk for adverse reactions. Adverse reactions are manifested as CNS toxicity, cardiovascular toxicity, or hypersensitivity reactions.

Central Nervous System Reactions

Early symptoms of blurred vision, nystagmus, and numbness of the tongue may progress to seizures and CNS depression. Treatment is supportive and includes airway management, hyperventilation, and intubation, if necessary. Intravenous diazepam is indicated if seizures do not respond to supportive measures.

Cardiovascular Reactions

Myocardial depression and hypotension may occur. Toxic doses slow the myocardial conduction as evidenced by prolongation of the PR interval and duration of the QRS and sinus bradycardia. Cardiac dysrhythmias are usually short lived; however, they may progress to life-threatening situations that require CPR. Hypotension is treated with the administration of intravenous fluids, Trendelenburg position, and if the patient is not responsive, the IV administration of phenylephrine or ephedrine.

Hypersensitivity Reactions

Allergic reactions are rare. The treatment for anaphylactic reactions is symptomatic and supportive. Bronchoconstriction is treated with epinephrine. Hypotension is treated with the administration of fluids and vasopressor support, as indicated. Urticarial reactions respond to the administration of diphenhydramine; with severe or prolonged reactions the administration of steroids may be necessary.

Methods of Regional Administration

Local infiltration is the injection of a local anesthetic drug, either intradermally or subcutaneously, which produces anesthesia within the site of injection.

Intravenous regional is the IV injection of an anesthetic solution into a limb (usually the arm). Before injection the limb is exsanguinated using an Esmarch bandage, and the vein is occluded with a tourniquet. The effects of the anesthetic last until the tourniquet is deflated. Maximum recommended tourniquet time is 2 hours. After deflation of the tourniquet the local anesthetic is flushed into the venous system. At this time the patient is at risk for toxic reactions; however, such reactions are rare.

In peripheral nerve blocks the local anesthetic is injected at the proximity of a peripheral nerve. The onset of anesthetic effect is rapid and, depending on the drug used, can last for several hours.

Plexus nerve blocks are the injection of a local anesthetic near a nerve plexus. The most common sites are the brachial plexus, the lumbar plexus, and the cervical plexus.

Central nerve blockade includes subarachnoid (spinal) and epidural, including caudal blocks. It is useful to review the anatomy of the spinal cord and meninges. The subarachnoid space contains the cerebrospinal fluid, spinal nerves, and blood vessels that supply the spinal cord. The epidural space that surrounds the dura mater contains spinal nerve roots, fat, lymphatics, and blood vessels. Caudal blocks use the sacral canal, which contains the terminal portion of the dural sac and a venous plexus—a part of the valveless vertebral venous plexus (Figure II-8).

Physiologic Effects of Centroneuraxis Blocks

Centroneuraxis blocks cause sympathetic blockade, as well as motor blockade and sensory analgesia. With pharmacologic sympathetic blockade the normal physiologic compensatory response to changes in blood pressure is obliterated. Venous dilation of the affected blood vessels results in a decrease in blood pressure. The block also interferes with autoregulation of blood pressure, heart rate, myocardial contractility, and vascular resistance. It is important to remember that sympathetic blockade is present at higher levels than sensory blockade—which is higher than motor blockade.

Sensory and motor blocks can be anxiety-provoking for patients. High thoracic motor blocks can interfere with movement of the intercostal muscles. Cervical motor blocks interfere with the movement of the diaphragm, and that leads to use of the accessory muscles of respiration. Cervical sensory blocks of C3-5 interfere with phrenic innervation, which can block cardiac accelerator fibers.

Spinal anesthesia is the administration of local anesthetic drugs into the subarachnoid space. The drug may be given as a single injection or, with the use of subarachnoid catheters, as a continuous spinal injection. Contraindications to the use of spinal anesthesia include allergy to local anesthetics, increased intracranial pressure, coagulopathy or anticoagulation therapy, sepsis, infections at or near the site of injection, and chronic back pain or deformities.

Complications of spinal anesthesia include hypotension secondary to the sympathetic block. This is self-limiting because the blood pressure returns to normal as the block recedes.

Spinal headaches can result from a small leak of the CSF through the dura. The headache is usually resolved by increasing fluid intake (intravenously or by mouth), by bed rest, and by analgesics. Occasionally the use of an epidural blood patch is necessary to stop the leak.

Epidural anesthesia consists of the administration of local anesthetics into the epidural space. These can be given as a bolus; however, usually they are given through a catheter for repeated injections. The added advantage is that the catheters may be left in place postoperatively for pain management in the form of continuous narcotic infusions or narcotic infusions combined with local anesthetic (Table II-2, II-3, and II-4).

Contraindications are the same as for spinal anesthetics. The most serious complication is the inadvertent injection of the drug into the subarachnoid space. Because more drug is needed for epidural anesthesia, this could lead to an unintentional total spinal block. The treatment is supportive until the block recedes. The patient may require intubation with ventilatory support and treatment of the accompanying hypotension. Hypotension secondary to sympathetic blockade is usually less severe than with spinal anesthesia.

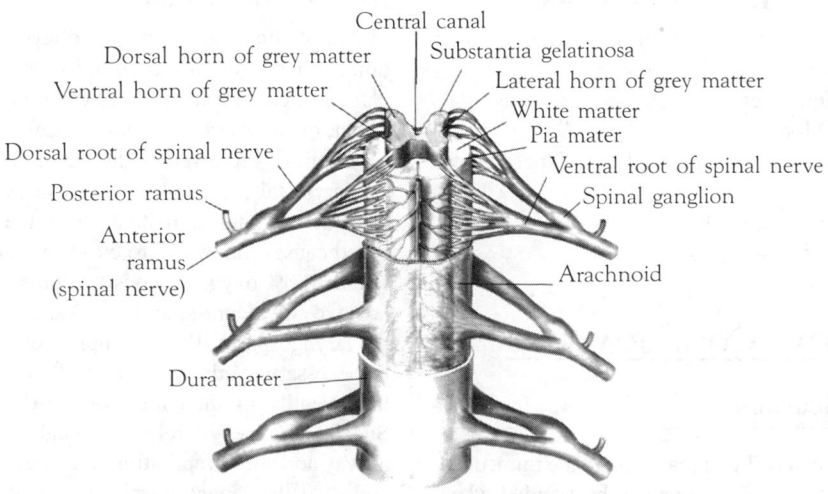

Figure II-8 Cross section of spinal cord showing attachments of spinal nerves. (From McCance.[19])

TABLE II-3 Side Effects of Epidural Opioids and Local Anesthetic Agents

Side Effect	Spinal Opioids	Local Anesthetics

Cardiovascular	Minor heart rate changes	Low block (below T_{10})
		    Sympathetic blockade
		    Postural hypotension

	Usually not postural hypotension	High block (above T_4)
		    Sympathetic blockade
		    Postural hypotension

	Vasoconstrictor response intact	Cardio-accelerator block ↓ heart rate, inotropic drive
Respiratory	Respiratory depression may occur 30 minutes to 16 hours (can be as long as 24 hours) after the injection or after discontinuing the infusion	Respiratory depression may occur immediately after injection
Central nervous system sedation	May be marked	Mild or absent depending on agent or dose
Nausea and/or vomiting	Yes	Yes (usually accompanies hypotension)
Urinary retention	Yes	Yes
Pruritis	Yes	No
Motor blockade and/or weakness	No	Yes, depending on concentrations used

From Fulk et al.[13]

TABLE II-4 Differences Between Local Anesthetic Analgesia and Opioid Analgesia

	Opioid Analgesics	Local Anesthetics
Mechanism	Opioid receptors	Nerve roots c fibers A-delta fibers
Pathways	Mu pain modulation	Pain Sensory Sympathetic Motor

SOURCES OF LARYNGEAL STIMULATION CAUSING LARYNGOSPASM

Blood
Secretions
Vomitus
Chemical mucosal irritation
Attempted intubation with insufficient anesthesia
Attempted extubation under light anesthesia
Suctioning
Surgical stimulation

From Fetzer-Fowler.[12]

Nursing Assessment for Regional Anesthesia

Assessment of the level of motor and sensory block
Hemodynamic monitoring
High risk for fluid volume deficit secondary to venous dilation of sympathetic block
Psychosocial or anxiety secondary to fear of permanent damage
Skin integrity secondary to immobility
Safety related to decreased sensation

POSTOPERATIVE COMPLICATIONS

Pulmonary Complications

Pulmonary complications can be life threatening in the immediate postoperative period. Many complications can be avoided when the care is approached in a collaborative manner with the anesthesiologist. Communication of intraoperative report and preexisting medical conditions may help prevent many complications.

Airway Obstruction

The most common and easily relieved cause of airway obstruction is pharyngeal obstruction by the tongue in an unconscious patient. It can usually be relieved by a chin lift or modified jaw thrust, or by inserting either a nasal or an oral airway until the obstruction is relieved as the patient arouses.

Laryngeal spasm also causes airway obstruction. The presence of mechanical irritants near the glottis by secretions or blood causes the larynx to close. Initial treatment is administration of 100% oxygen by positive-pressure mask. This continuous positive airway pressure (CPAP) is usually sufficient to terminate the laryngospasm. If the complete obstruction continues, it may be necessary to administer a small dose of succinylcholine while hand ventilating the patient by CPAP mask with 100% oxygen. Succinylcholine will relax the vocal cords sufficiently to open the airway and allow ventilation. If an adequate airway cannot be established, the patient must be intubated, using direct laryngeal visualization. If the larynx cannot be visualized and the trachea cannot be intubated, an emergency cricothyroidotomy will relieve the obstruction and permit ventilation (see the box).

Airway swelling may also be a cause of postoperative airway obstruction. Glottic edema may be caused by irritation from traumatic intubation, surgical manipulation, excessive coughing on the endotracheal tube, or allergies to the materials used in the endotracheal tube. Subglottic edema is seen in small children because of anatomic differences in their airway. In small children the larynx is made up of loose areolar tissue and the cricoid ring is the narrowest part of the larynx.

The treatment of both glottic and subglottic edema is administration of warm humidified oxygen by mask, nebulized racemic epinephrine, and, if edema is unrelieved, dexamethasone intravenously or by inhaler.

Hypoxemia

Hypoxemia can be defined as decreased arterial oxygen tension. With the advent of pulse oximetry it is easy to identify; however, the cause may be difficult to find. Common causes of hypoxemia in the postanesthetic period are low concentrations of inspired oxygen, hypoventilation, and ventilation-perfusion mismatch, including intrapulmonary right to left shunts.

As a rule all patients who have had general anesthesia should have supplemental oxygen; in rare instances, oxygen is contraindicated.

Hypoventilation is defined as reduced alveolar gas exchange, resulting in an increase in arterial carbon dioxide levels. Causes include the respiratory depressant effects of anesthetics and narcotics, poor respiratory muscle function secondary to inadequate reversal of muscle relaxants, or previous pulmonary disease. Postoperative respiratory depression, resulting from narcotics, can be reversed with small doses of Narcan without affecting the pain-relieving properties of the narcotics.

Respiratory muscle function may be affected by incomplete reversal of neuromuscular blocking agents. Muscle relaxants may need to be pharmacologically reversed. Factors that interfere with reversal of neuromuscular blocking agents include inadequate renal excretion of the drug secondary to renal failure; use of antibiotics, such as gentamicin, neomycin or clindamycin, which potentiate the neuromuscular blockade, and respiratory acidosis, which limits or prevents the antagonism of the neuromuscular blocking agent.

Surgical causes for hypoventilation include incisions of the upper abdomen or thorax, gastric dilation, or tight restrictive dressings. Obesity is also indicated in hypoventilation because total lung volume and functional residual capacity are reduced. Treatment is directed toward the underlying cause for the hypoventilation. If pain is the cause for splinting in patients with upper abdominal or thoracic incisions, regional nerve blocks or small doses of narcotics may be warranted.

Patients with preexisting pulmonary disease are at high risk for postoperative pulmonary complications.

By its nature the physiologic process of respiration is not static but dynamic. Oxygenation of venous blood is accomplished by ventilation of the alveoli with air and perfusion of the pulmonary capillaries with blood. Oxygen diffuses from the alveoli into the pulmonary circulation. Carbon dioxide diffuses from the capillaries into the alveoli and is exhaled. In normal healthy individuals there are physiologic variations of ventilation and perfusion. Disease states can alter this ratio in different ways. Right to left shunts occur when blood reaches the arterial system without passing through ventilated areas of the lung. At rest, normal physiologic shunting is between 2% to 5% of cardiac output.

Postoperatively the most common cause of increased right to left shunting is atelectasis. Atelectatic portions of the lung are perfused; however, they are not ventilated because of the alveolar collapse. Atelectasis may be caused by secretions and hypoventilation.

Pneumothorax may be caused by central line placement, incidental surgical manipulation, or tears in the pleura or regional anesthesia (i.e., intercostal nerve blocks). Pneumothorax causes hypoxemia because of atelectasis and intrapulmonary shunting. A small pneumothorax of less than 20% (in a healthy individual with no mechanical ventilation) usually resorbs spontaneously. A pneumothorax of greater than 20%, or a pneumothorax in any patient who is mechanically ventilated, should be treated with the insertion of chest tubes.

Postoperative pulmonary edema is a rare but life-threatening complication of general anesthesia. Causes may be cardiac or noncardiac. Treatment for cardiac pulmonary edema is directed toward improving left ventricular function. Noncardiac pulmonary edema is related to injury of the capillary membrane. In the postanesthetic period it may be caused by aspiration, blood transfusion reaction, or upper airway obstruction (see the box). Pulmonary edema following upper airway obstruction is probably caused by reduction in interstitial hydrostatic pressure. A dramatic pressure difference between the interstitium

---

■ DISEASE STATES ASSOCIATED WITH NONCARDIAC PULMONARY EDEMA (NCPE)

Sepsis
Fat or air embolism
Smoke inhalation
Pancreatitis
Oxygen toxicity
Inhaled chemical-induced lung injury
Near drowning
Transfusion reaction
High-altitude rapid ascent
Post reexpansion of lung
Uremia
Post radiation of pulmonary system
Aspiration of gastric contents
Drug ingestion
Interstitial viral pneumonia
Disseminated intravascular coagulation
Craniocerebral trauma
Traumatic pulmonary contusion

From Fetzer-Fowler.[11]

and capillary causes transudation of fluid through the membrane. Unilateral pulmonary edema may be present postoperatively if, during surgery, the patient has been placed in a lateral position. The dependent lung receives most of the perfusion while the superior lung receives most of the ventilation. The increase in hydrostatic pressure of the dependent lung causes unilateral pulmonary edema. Treatment for non-cardiac pulmonary edema is directed at supporting gas exchange across the interstitium until the alveolar-capillary membrane can be stabilized.

Pulmonary embolism caused by either thromboemboli or fat emboli are rare postoperative complications. The thrombi block the pulmonary artery, which leads to areas of the lung that are ventilated but are not perfused. This increases physiologic dead space and shunting (see pulmonary embolism on p. 181).

Aspiration of gastric contents is prevented in the normal, awake individual by the gastroesophageal and pharyngoesophageal sphincters. General anesthetics and narcotics may depress these protective mechanisms, putting patients at risk for aspiration. The degree of injury to the lung parenchyma is related to the pH of the fluid and the volume aspirated. Gastric pH of less than 2.5 causes chemical pneumonitis, local edema, and inflammation. Preventive measures include maintenance of NPO status, use of H_2 blockers, and antacids. Patients at high risk for aspiration include those with intestinal obstruction, increased intraabdominal pressure, pregnancy, obesity, hiatal hernia, and emergency surgery when NPO status cannot be verified.

Pain

Virtually all patients undergoing surgical manipulation have acute pain afterward. Postsurgical cellular and tissue damage excites nociceptors (pain-sensitive nerve fibers). Injury is believed to stimulate the release of neurotransmitters that serve as algesic substances. They include prostaglandins, histamine, serotonin, bradykinin, and arachidonic acid. Prostaglandins lower the nociceptive threshold.

After stimulation of the nociceptors, pain impulses are relayed via the afferent nerve fibers through the dorsal horn of the spinal cord. Thinly myelinated A delta and unmyelinated C fibers transmit to the neuraxis. A delta nociceptive fibers transmit sharp pain. A delta fibers transmit impulses that pass to the anterior and anterolateral horns to provoke segmental reflex responses. These responses are responsible for increased muscle tone, skeletal muscle spasm, increased oxygen consumption, and lactic acid production. C nociceptive fibers transmit burning, dull aching types of pain.

Other impulses are transmitted to higher centers via spinothalamic and spinoreticular tracts that initiate suprasegmental and cortical responses. Suprasegmental reflex response further increases oxygen consumption, sympathetic tone, and endocrine function. Cortical responses are concerned with integration and perception of pain. The individual psychologic response of increased apprehension and anxiety further increases

hypothalamic stimulation. These emotional responses appear to facilitate nociceptive transmission in the spinal cord and lower the pain threshold.

High-dose narcotics may delay the transmission of stimuli through A delta and C fibers. The reflex phenomena of muscle spasm associated with pain are not modified by narcotics.

Many complex theories of pain perception have been suggested. The current belief is that pain has a sensory and a reactive component. Three current theories on pain perception involve specificity, pattern, and gate. The specificity theory suggests that specific fibers conduct specific sensations that terminate at specific sites in the CNS. Pattern theory suggests that after initiation of painful impulses a pattern-generating mechanism can be established in the dorsal horn, causing pain perception even though no stimuli are present. The gate theory suggests that pain impulses can be modulated in the brain or spinal cord.

Opioid receptors are located in the midbrain and dorsal horn. The highest concentrations are found in the limbic system, substantia gelatinosa, and laminae I, II, and V of the dorsal horn. The term "opioid" refers to drugs that are derivatives of opium or are synthetically made to produce similar effects. Opioids are used primarily for analgesia; they react with specific opioid receptors. Opioids are chemically similar to the naturally occurring peptides, the enkephalins, the endorphins, and the dynorphins.

There are four major categories of opioid receptors in the CNS. Mu receptors mediate supraspinal analgesia, feelings of well-being, morphinelike physical dependence, and respiratory depression. Kappa receptors are responsible for sedation with minimal respiratory depression. Sigma receptors cause dysphoric states with rapid thoughts and altered visual and auditory perceptions. Delta receptors cause alterations in affective behavior.

Drugs can interact with opioid receptors in different ways. Opioid agonists are drugs that stimulate the opioid receptors, causing analgesia. Opioid antagonists are drugs that reverse the effects of the opioid agonists. Opioid agonist-antagonists are drugs that act as agonists at some receptors and antagonists at other sites.

Morphine remains the standard by which all analgesics are measured (see Table II-5).

Fentanyl and its derivatives, sufentanil and alfentanil, are frequently used during anesthesia. The onset of action following IV administration is very rapid, and the incidence of incomplete amnesia, hypotension, and hypertension is less than with morphine. Fentanyl and its derivatives are sometimes used postoperatively when rapid control of pain is warranted. Fentanyl can also be used via the epidural route for patients allergic to morphine.

Adverse Effects of Pain
Cardiovascular System

The increased stimulation of sympathetic neurons causes tachycardia, increased stroke volume, and increased cardiac

▪ TABLE II-5 Equipotency of Narcotics

Morphine (mg)	Demerol (mg)	Dilaudid (mg)	Fentanyl (micrograms)
1			12.5
1.33	10		
2			25.0
2.5		0.5	
3.325	25		
4			50.0
5		1.0	
6			75.0
6.65	50		
7.5		1.5	
8			100.0
10	75	2.0	125.0

▪ TABLE II-6 Pediatric Pain and Discomfort Scale

Observation	Criteria	Points
Blood Pressure	±10% preop	0
	>20% preop	1
	>30% preop	2
Crying	Not crying	0
	Cries, but responds to TLC*	1
	Cries, but does not respond to TLC	2
Movement	None	0
	Restless	1
	Thrashing	2
Agitation	Patient asleep or calm	0
	Mild	1
	Hysterical	2
Posture	No special posture	0
	Flexing legs and thighs	1
	Holding scrotum and groin**	2
Complains of pain (where appropriate by age)	Asleep, or states no pain	0
	Cannot localize	1
	Can localize	2

From Wilson et al.[36]
TLC, tender loving care.
**Used to assess analgesic effectiveness following orchiopexy.

work, increasing myocardial oxygen consumption. Hypercoagulation and decreased mobility increase the risk of deep vein thrombosis and pulmonary embolism.

Respiratory System

Pain associated with upper abdominal or thoracic surgery causes spasm and splinting of the abdominal and intercostal muscles, decreasing the ability to cough and breathe deeply. It also decreases the vital capacity and inspiratory capacity, as well as the functional residual capacity. Surgery on peripheral parts of the body does not appear to alter lung volumes.

Nursing Assessment of Pain

Pain is a subjective experience for patients. NANDA defines pain as "a state in which an individual experiences and reports the presence of severe discomfort or an uncomfortable sensation." It is sometimes difficult for the nurse to understand the severity and quality of the patient's pain. To objectify the pain as much as possible, it is helpful to obtain as much objective data as possible. In all cases it is important to determine the site of the pain, as well as its type. Using a visual analog scale or verbal integer scale of 0 to 10, with 0 being no pain and 10 being the worst pain imaginable, gives a clear picture of the intensity of the pain, and determining the effects of pain management therapy. Objective signs of pain are the sympathetic responses of tachycardia, hypertension, diaphoresis, and pallor, as well as grimacing facies and a splinting respiratory pattern. In the immediate postanesthetic period, these signs may be the first indication of the patient's pain. Judicious use of narcotics at this time can stall the deleterious sympathetic effects of pain. To objectify pain levels for infants, toddlers, and children, see the pediatric pain and discomfort scale (see Table II-6).

The traditional method of pain management postoperatively is intramuscular or IV narcotic administration. Narcotics are administered at the request of the patient or when objective assessment deems it necessary. However, this method is frequently inadequate because the pain may be too intense or the treatment may come too late. Following intramuscular administration, the absorption of the drug is variable, which delays the effectiveness of the drug. Following IV administration of narcotics, the uptake of the drug is more rapid and more predictable. However, intermittent boluses of narcotic will result in peaks and troughs of plasma concentration. At peak levels, pain perception may be obliterated; however, an increased risk for respiratory depression exists. At trough levels, the plasma concentration may be too low for analgesia.

With patient-controlled analgesia (PCA), patients can administer a small dose of narcotic when pain occurs. PCA pumps can be programmed to deliver narcotics at a basal rate hourly, as well as allowing the patient to self-administer predetermined doses at set time intervals. Studies have shown that patients using PCA maintain plasma concentrations at a consistent level. Patient acceptance and satisfaction are high with PCA.

Epidural and subarachnoid narcotics have a significant advantage over other types of pain management. They produce prolonged, intense segmental analgesia without the deleterious side effects of respiratory depression or sympathetic disturbance. These narcotics affect the nociceptive pathways in the dorsal horn by interacting with the mu opiate receptors. They do not affect proprioception or motor and sensory function. Epidural narcotics can be administered in a bolus, a continuous drip, or a combination of both; they also can be mixed with local anesthetics. Following administration of a narcotic into the epidural space, epidural narcotics cross into the spinal fluid and into the epidural veins where vascular absorption occurs.

Subarachnoid narcotics are administered as a bolus injection. Analgesia tends to be more profound; however, this route is also associated with a higher incidence of side effects. The incidence of respiratory depression peaks between 6 and 10 hours post-injection. Pruritus occurs in approximately 10% of patients receiving spinal narcotics. Naloxone (Narcan) is the narcotic antagonist of choice to reverse these unwanted side effects. With doses of 1 to 2 μg/kg there is little effect on the analgesia. Narcan has a high affinity for all opioid receptors; however, its affinity for mu receptors is generally higher than for kappa or delta receptors. The incidence of nausea, vomiting, and urinary retention is similar to that for patients receiving parenteral narcotics (see Table II-3).

Cardiovascular Complications

Hypotension

Hypotension is frequently seen in the immediate postoperative phase of recovery. The most common cause is hypovolemia secondary to fluid volume depletion. This can be the result of blood loss, third space fluid shifts, or unreplaced insensible fluid losses. The treatment consists of replacement of the fluid volume losses, institution of the Trendelenburg position, and, if the patient is unresponsive, small doses of a vasopressor, such as ephedrine or Neo-Synephrine, administered IV.

Hypotension may also be secondary to residual myocardial depression from the anesthetic or, more seriously, from perioperative myocardial ischemia or infarction. Prompt differential diagnosis and treatment are essential because hypotension leads to hypoperfusion of vital organs. Cardiac hypoperfusion leads to further ischemia and damage. Patients at risk for cardiac disease, or those who have had myocardial infarctions in the past, are at greater risk than the general population for perioperative myocardial infarction. Patients who have had infarctions more than 6 months previously have reinfarction rates of 1.9% to 8%. Patients with a more recent history—less than 3 months since infarction—have reinfarction rates as high as 37%. Patients having perioperative myocardial infarctions have mortality rates from 36% to 70% (see box).

Surgical causes of hypotension include bleeding at the surgical site or at sites of central venous catheter insertion. Inadvertent puncture of the pleura can lead to pneumothorax or hemothorax.

Hypertension

Hypertension is common in the early postanesthesia phase. The most common causes are pain, hypercapnia, hypoxemia, or fluid volume overload. Treatment of these causes usually resolves the hypertension. If the condition is unresolved, the administration of antihypertensive medications is necessary. Hypertension is usually transient and drug therapy is necessary for a few hours. Drugs frequently used are short-acting beta blockers, such as propranolol, labetalol, and esmolol. Nitroprusside is used because it is fast acting and because its results are rapidly reversed after the drug is discontinued. If the patient is at risk for myocardial ischemia, nitroglycerin may be administered IV or nifedipine may be given sublingually. Hydralazine is sometimes used; however, its onset of action is slow com-

PATIENTS AT RISK FOR PERIOPERATIVE MI

History of myocardial infarction within the last 6 months
Preexisting coronary artery disease or diffuse multivessel disease
History of disabling angina
Congestive heart failure
Severe preoperative myocardial ischemia
Fluid and electrolyte imbalance
Debilitated health
Elderly
Undetected medical problems
Diabetes
Obesity
Emergency surgery
Abdominal, intrathoracic, and vascular surgery
Prolonged anesthesia time

pared to that of newer antihypertensive drugs, and it causes a reflex tachycardia that may be detrimental to patients with increased cardiac risk factors.

Hypothermia

The incidence of iatrogenic hypothermia is between 60% and 80% of all postoperative patients. Hypothermia is defined as a core body temperature of less than 36 degrees centigrade. Metabolic heat production and thermoregulation are depressed with general anesthetics. Regional anesthetics can cause hypothermia by depressing regional thermal sensations, vasoconstriction, and shivering. Shivering-like activity occurs in approximately 40% of postanesthesia patients. However, not all patients who shiver are hypothermic, suggesting that hypothermia is just one cause of the mechanism of shivering. Shivering increases the metabolic rate and therefore increases oxygen consumption, as well as carbon dioxide production. If the patient also has some degree of respiratory depression, the deficit in oxygen supply may lead to anaerobic metabolism and lactic acidosis. This is especially dangerous for patients at risk for cardiac ischemia.

Shivering also exacerbates pain. Treatment is preventive, as well as supportive. Patients who shiver should have supplemental oxygen and external warming. Meperidine in small doses (25 to 30 mg) is helpful in decreasing shivering.

Hyperthermia

Malignant hyperthermia (MH) is a rare but potentially fatal complication of general anesthesia. The onset of symptoms usually occurs during the induction of anesthesia but in rare instances may occur in the PACU. It is an inherited disorder which is triggered by anesthetic agents. In patients that are genetically predisposed to MH, the triggering agent interferes with the reentry of calcium into the sarcoplasmic reticulum.

This hypercalcimic state activates metabolic pathways which deplete adenosine triphosphate, causing metabolic acidosis, membrane destruction, and cellular death. Dantrolene sodium is given intravenously as soon as a diagnosis of MH is made. Dantrolene sodium acts by decreasing the amount of calcium released from the sarcoplasmic reticulum. Treatment is supportive, correcting hypoxemia and acidosis, reducing fever, monitoring electrolytes, assessing renal function for acute tubular necrosis secondary to myoglobinuria.

Nausea and Vomiting

Postoperative nausea and vomiting can be caused by anesthetics and opioids that affect the vestibular portion of the inner ear, the chemoreceptor trigger zone (CTZ), and vomiting centers in the brain. Other causes for postoperative nausea and vomiting include increasing intracranial pressure, severe dehydration, and fluid and electrolyte imbalance. Factors that influence the incidence of postoperative nausea and vomiting include the use of general anesthesia by mask technique, patient history of motion sickness, or previous postoperative nausea and vomiting, intra-abdominal surgery, prolonged anesthesia, and obesity.

Treatment is preventive, supportive, and pharmacologic (Table II-7). Patients at high risk for aspiration are pretreated with drugs that increase the pH of gastric contents or that facilitate gastric motility. Nasogastric tubes can be used to empty gastric contents. The use of antiemetics intraoperatively and postoperatively reduces the incidence of nausea and vomiting. Vigilant nursing observation is the primary means of preventing aspiration in the PACU.

NURSING CARE FOR THE POSTANESTHESIA PATIENT

Nursing Assessment

Respiratory Status

Assess for signs of upper airway obstruction, stridor, retractions, asynchronous or asymmetric chest movement

Laryngospasm, high-pitched squeaky respirations with partial to total airway obstruction

Diminished breath sounds, evaluate inspiratory and expiratory wheezing, rales, rhonchi, or any abnormality

Residual neuromuscular blockade; weak inspiratory effort; inability to lift head; or inadequate muscle strength

Cardiovascular Status

Cardiac output has returned to baseline as indicated by blood pressure, cardiac rate and rhythm, and, if present, central venous pressures, and pulmonary artery pressures

Neurologic Status

Arouses easily to name; follows simple instructions; mobility at preoperative level

Pain and Discomfort

Level of pain or discomfort tolerable to patient

Gastrointestinal Status

Abatement of nausea or vomiting

■ TABLE II-7 **Antiemetics Used After Anesthesia**

Drug	Adult Dose (mg)	Action	Side Effect/Contraindications
Compazine (Prochlorperazine)	5-10 IM	Antiemetic Neuroleptic	Increased incidence of dystonia Contraindicated for patients with bone marrow depression
Droperidol (Inapsine)	0.625-1.25 IV	Antiemetic Neuroleptic Antagonizes emetic effect of opioids that act on CTZ	Drowsiness Extrapyramidal symptoms Potentiates other CNS depressants
Phenergan (Promethazine HCl)	25-50 IM, IV, or po	Antihistamine Antiemetic Thought to depress CTZ in medulla	CNS depression Disturbed coordination
Reglan (Metoclopramide)	10 IV over 1-2 min	Cholinergic Antiemetic Increased CTZ threshold enhances gastric emptying	Contraindicated in seizure disorders
Scopolamine patch	Transdermal patch releases 0.5 mg over 3 days Applied to skin preoperatively	Anticholinergic	CNS depression Disorientation Urinary retention

Genitourinary Status

Absence of bladder distention

Musculoskeletal

Absence of sensory, motor, or perceptual deficits

Primary Disease States

Evaluation and maintenance of therapy for primary medical disease

Nursing Dx & Intervention

Ineffective breathing pattern

- Assess upper airway for signs of obstruction.
- Assess rate and depth of respirations, as well as chest movement; note air exchange at nose and mouth.
- Continuously monitor oxygen saturation; administer oxygen per physician's order *to maintain saturation greater than 95%.*
- Suction oropharynx, as necessary, *to prevent potential aspiration of gastric contents.*
- Position patient *to maximize respiratory pattern;* if patient is awake, raise head of bed to 30 degrees; if there is partial airway obstruction or high risk for aspiration, place the patient on his or her side.
- Identify factors contributing to airway obstruction, such as inhalational anesthetics, narcotics, and muscle relaxants.
- Identify surgical interventions that may alter breathing pattern and contribute to upper airway obstruction.
- Maintain patient in proper alignment *to facilitate opening of the upper airway:* chin lift, jaw thrust, and hyperextension of the head; if obstruction is unrelieved by these measures, insert nasal or oral airway; if obstruction remains unrelieved, notify physician; patient may need to be endotracheally intubated.
- If mechanical ventilation becomes necessary, provide care and monitoring consistent with accepted guidelines.

Impaired gas exchange

- Observe closely because patients are at risk for atelectasis and right to left shunt, secondary to anesthetic agents; immobility during prolonged surgical procedure; physiologic splinting caused by pain, especially high abdominal or thoracic surgical sites; and preexisting disease states (see atelectasis, Chapter 2).
- Assess breath sounds to determine areas of hypoventilation and the possibility of interstitial pulmonary edema; if endotracheal tube is present, determine that the tube is in the correct position; *absence of breath sounds on the left side may indicate right mainstem intubation.*
- Position patient *to maximize expansion of the lungs.*
- Encourage patient to deep breathe and cough; begin use of incentive spirometry *to facilitate maximum expansion of the lungs.*
- Administer narcotics *to decrease splinting and anxiety.*

- Identify primary disease states that may contribute to impaired gas exchange; initiate treatment according to prescribed orders.
- Monitor arterial blood gases *to assess level of hypoxia and hypercarbia.*
- Monitor end-tidal carbon dioxide levels *to follow course of hypercarbia.*
- Anticipate potential ventilation problems by having emergency equipment at hand to mask ventilate patient with positive pressure.

Ineffective airway clearance

- Assess patient to determine if patient is able to mobilize secretions; if patient is unable, assist patient to cough by splinting the area of surgery with pillows or blankets; note characteristics of cough and secretions; suction if necessary.
- Turn patient *to mobilize secretions;* provide chest physical therapy, as needed.
- Administer nebulized medications as prescribed by the physician *to dilate bronchioles; assist with expectoration of secretions.*

Decreased cardiac output

- Monitor vitals signs at least every 15 minutes *to assess for signs of left ventricular failure, secondary to ischemia; fluid volume deficit; fluid volume overload; primary disease state; hypoxia; and myocardial depression, secondary to inhalational agents;* continuously monitor ECG rhythm for tachycardia, bradycardia, dysrhythmias, and signs of cardiac ischemia.
- Assess for symptoms of decreased cardiac output, including hypotension, tachycardia, pallor, or diaphoresis.
- Monitor hemodynamic parameters, if present, *to evaluate the patient's clinical status.*
- Review patient's preoperative history and ECG *to determine level of preexisting cardiac disease;* note if patient has taken routinely prescribed medications the morning of surgery.
- Evaluate urine output hourly if Foley catheter is present; if there is no Foley catheter present, palpate bladder *to check for bladder distention.*

Fluid volume deficit

- Monitor vital signs at least every 15 minutes *to assess for hypovolemia secondary to blood loss, insensible fluid loss, or relative hypovolemia caused by vasodilation secondary to autonomic nerve blocks.*
- Monitor intake and output, mindful of the type of surgical procedure; crystalloid, colloid, and blood replacement; surgical drains; and wound dressings.
- Administer crystalloids and colloids, as ordered, *to maintain cardiac output, as well as renal, cerebral, and all other tissue perfusion.*
- Initiate Trendelenburg position *to increase preload.*
- Administer vasoactive drugs, as ordered, *to improve cardiac contractility and peripheral vascular resistance.*

- Monitor electrolytes and hematocrit *to evaluate blood and fluid loss and the effectiveness of replacement therapy.*
- Monitor urine output hourly if Foley catheter is present; note specific gravity of urine *to determine concentration of urine.*

Pain

- Assess location of pain *to differentiate surgical pain from other types of pain, including cardiac, bladder, headache, spasm, pressure areas from surgical positioning, or restrictive dressings.*
- Using a visual or verbal analog scale (VAS), ask patient to rate the pain from 0 to 10 *to objectify the level of pain;* this allows the nurse to assess the effectiveness of pain-relieving medications.
- Provide medications *to alleviate the pain.*
- Provide a calm, nurturing atmosphere for the patient.
- Assure the patient that you will continue to provide pain medications until the pain is at a tolerable level.
- Position the patient in a comfortable position.
- If using patient-controlled analgesia, teach the patient to administer medications whenever he or she has pain; assure the patient that he or she will not be able to overdose because of the safety features programmed into the computer.
- Observe patient for nonverbal signs of pain, including restlessness, agitation, grimacing, hypertension, tachycardia, and diaphoresis; keep in mind that these signs can indicate hypoxia or hypercarbia; sedating a patient who is hypoxic or hypercarbic is contraindicated.
- Determine if the patient has been taking pain-relieving medications preoperatively; if so, this may increase the patient's tolerance to narcotics, causing him or her to require higher than average doses of narcotics.

Evaluation

Airway is patent Patient's respirations are normal; no signs of upper airway obstruction. Patient's breathing is coordinated between the thorax and the abdomen; accessory muscles of respiration are not used. Patient's breath sounds are clear to auscultation. Oxygen saturation is greater than 95% when breathing room air; if not, supplemental oxygen is administered.

Cardiovascular function has returned to preoperative level Patient's blood pressure has returned to within 20 mm Hg of baseline for at least 30 minutes. There are no changes in the ECG readings, and there is an absence of dysrhythmias. Patient's heart rate is between 60 and 100 bpm. For children, the heart rate should be + or −20 bpm from the preoperative baseline. Patient's skin is warm and dry, peripheral pulses are present at preoperative level, and capillary refill time is less than 3 seconds. Patient's urine output is greater than 30 ml per hour for adults and 0.5 ml/kg/hr for children. Patient's sensory and motor blockade has receded following regional anesthesia.

Comfort and pain levels are satisfactory for patient Patient shows an absence of nonverbal signs of pain: restlessness, anxiety, and grimacing. Patient verbalizes comfort level. If using patient-controlled analgesia for pain management, patient is able to correctly self-administer and understands mechanism for use. If using conventional pain management, patient is able to identify when to request pain medications.

References

1. American Hospital Association: *Patient's bill of rights,* Chicago, 1972, The Association.
2. American Nurses Association: *The code for nurses with interpretive statements,* Kansas City, 1979, The Association.
3. Association of Operating Room Nurses: *Perioperative nursing process.* Denver, 1990, The Association.
4. Association of Operating Room Nurses: *Perioperative nursing process,* Denver, 1991, The Association.
5. Association of Operating Room Nurses: *1995 Standards and recommended practices,* Denver, 1995, The Association.
6. Botsford J: *Care trac-ing: case management in the OR,* presented at the 42nd Annual AORN Congress, Atlanta, Georgia, March 8, 1995.
7. Capuano TA: Clinical pathways: practical outcomes, *Nurs Management* 26:1, 1995.
8. Drain CB, Shipley CS: *Recovery room: a critical care approach,* Philadelphia, 1987, Saunders.
9. Drasner K, Katz JA, Schapera A: Control of pain and anxiety. In Wood (editor): *Principles of critical care medicine,* New York, 1991, McGraw-Hill.
10. Dripps RD, Echenhogg JE, Vandam LD: *Introduction to anesthesia,* ed 8, Philadelphia, 1989, Saunders.
11. Fetzer-Fowler SJ: Managing sympathetic blockade in the post anesthesia care unit, *J Post Anesth Nurs* 9(1):34, 1994.
12. Firestone LL: *Clinical anesthesia procedures of the Massachusetts General Hospital,* ed 3, Boston, 1988, Little, Brown.
13. Fulk C, Hadely JC: Something new for pain: new trends in epidural analgesia, *J Post Anesth Nurs* 5:1, 1990.
14. Goodman AG, Gilman LS: *The pharmacological basis of therapeutics,* ed 8, New York, 1990, Macmillan.
15. Joint Commission of Accreditation of Healthcare Organizations: *1995 Comprehensive accreditation manual for hospitals,* Oakbrook Terrace, Illinois, 1994, The Commission.
16. Kleinbeck SVM: Developing nursing diagnoses for a perioperative care plan: a classroom research project, *AORN J* 49:1613, 1989.
17. Kneedler J, Dodge G: *Perioperative patient care,* ed 3, Boston, 1994, Jones & Bartlett.
18. Maslow AH: *Motivation and personality,* New York, 1970, Harper & Row.
19. McCance KM, Huether S: *Pathophysiology: the biologic basis of disease in adults and children,* ed 2, St Louis, 1994, Mosby.
20. Meeker MH, Rothrock JC: *Alexander's care of the patient in surgery,* ed 10, St Louis, 1994, Mosby.
21. Miller RD: *Anesthesia,* ed 4, New York, 1994, Churchill Livingstone.
22. Miller RD, Stoelting RK: *Basics of anesthesia,* ed 3, New York, 1994, Churchill Livingstone.
23. Morgan GE, Mikhail MS: *Clinical anesthesiology,* Norwalk, Conn, 1992, Appleton & Lange.
24. Rothrock JC: *Perioperative nursing care planning,* St Louis, 1990, Mosby.
25. Stein RS: The perioperative nurse's role in anesthesia management, *AORN J* 62:794-804, 1995.
26. Thelan LA, Davie JK, Urden LD: *Textbook of critical care nursing: diagnosis and management,* St Louis, 1994, Mosby.
27. Thompson JM et al: *Mosby's clinical nursing,* ed 3, St Louis, 1993, Mosby.
28. Way LW: *Current surgical diagnosis and treatment,* ed 8, Norwalk, Conn, 1988, Appleton & Lange.
29. Wilson R: Evaluation of the Plazlyte™ sterilization system, *J Healthcare Material Management* 12:4, 1994.

PART THREE

Diagnostic and Laboratory Procedures

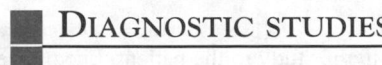

DIAGNOSTIC STUDIES

Visualization Studies

Direct ophthalmoscopy

Description Examiner uses an ophthalmoscope to view the retinal surface and inner structures of eye. Pupils are usually dilated, and examination takes place in dark room. Retinal structures and vessels are magnified 15 times.

Indications Used for diagnosis and visualization of the optic disk, arteries, veins, retina, choroid, and media and for evaluation of significant ocular and systemic disease. About half the fundus may be seen.

Complications Caution should be used when dilating the pupil of a patient with a shallow anterior chamber to avoid precipitating an attack of angle-closure glaucoma. Soft contact lenses should be removed before pupil dilation, and dilation should not be performed if an implanted intraocular lens was placed during cataract surgery.

Nursing care Indicate both the duration of effect of the medication used to dilate the pupil and the limitation in vision. Instruct patient to wear sunglasses if going outside after pupils are dilated.

Indirect ophthalmoscopy

Description Examiner wears a head-mounted binocular instrument. The patient is supine, usually with dilated pupils. The examiner stands 30 inches away and holds a convex lens over the patient's eye for focusing. The image is magnified four to five times; a greater visual field can be viewed than with direct ophthalmoscopy. A scleral depressor (blunt rod) may be used to compress the eyeball so ora serrata (tissue behind the iris) can be viewed.

Indications Permits detection and evaluation of minimal elevations of the sensory retina and retinal pigment epithelium, which are not evident with direct ophthalmoscopy. Useful in the detection of opacities in the media.

Complications None.

Nursing care Assure the patient that mild or no discomfort will be experienced if a scleral depressor is used. Inform the patient about side effects of the medication.

Gonioscopy

Description A corneal contact lens (goniolens) is placed over an anesthetized cornea to permit viewing of anterior chamber angles with a microscopic lens, mirror, or contact lens combined with a prism, since the opaque sclera and corneoscleral limbus prevent direct inspection of the angle of the anterior chamber.

Indications Assists in distinguishing between angle-closure glaucoma and open-angle glaucoma. It has also been used in the development of an effective surgical procedure for congenital glaucoma and in the diagnostic and therapeutic evolution of many types of secondary glaucoma.

Complications None.

Nursing care Explain the procedure to the patient.

Slitlamp examination

Description The examiner views corneal layers, anterior chamber, lens, and anterior vitreous through a microscope that magnifies these structures up to 20 times. A thin slit of light permits scrutiny of anterior structures for lesions or trauma.

Indications Used to detect the depth of the abnormality.

Complications None.

Nursing care Explain the procedure to the patient.

Pupil dilation

Description Short-acting, topical medication is used for pupil dilation to facilitate examination of the fundus with direct or indirect ophthalmoscopy. Mydriatic (adrenergic) drugs such as phenylephrine 2.5% (Neo-Synephrine, Mydfrin) dilate the pupil but do not inhibit accommodation. Mydriatic drug may be combined with cycloplegic drug (which inhibits accommodation) such as tropicamide 0.5% (Mydriacyl) to enhance and maintain pupil dilation.

Indications Diagnosis and evaluation of significant ocular and systemic disease.

Complications May be contraindicated for patients with shallow anterior chamber, certain intraocular lens implants, or vascular hypertension or who are taking MAO inhibitors or tricyclic antidepressants.

Nursing care Remove contact lenses before instillation. Warn the patient that blurred vision and photophobia may last for 3 to 6 hours after examination. Instruct patient to wear sunglasses if going outside during this period.

Lacrimal system testing

Description

Basic secretion test. Topical anesthetic is administered to the eyeball before filter paper is placed in the lateral portion of the lower eyelid. The anesthesia reduces lacrimal output to allow measurement of the tear production of accessory glands in eyelid.

Dacryocystography. A radiopaque medium such as Pantopaque is injected through the punctum and canaliculus into the lacrimal sac, and is followed by roentgenography.

Dacryoscintigraphy. Sodium pertechnetate (^{99m}Tc) in a dilute solution is instilled in each conjunctival sac, followed by a scintigram taken with a gamma camera to indicate its passage through the lacrimal drainage system.[21]

Dye disappearance. A dye, 0.25% to 2% fluorescein in alkaline solution or rose bengal, is instilled topically into the conjunctival sac to stain the Bowman's membrane and the stroma of the cornea. The stain can be intensified if a 2% cocaine ophthalmic solution is instilled into the eye or if the eye is illuminated with a cobalt blue filter to stimulate fluorescence.

Rose bengal staining. A drop of 1% or 2% solution is placed in conjunctival sac. The 2% solution demonstrates loss of corneal and conjunctival epithelium in keratoconjunctivitis sicca; the 1% solution is valuable in demonstrating conjunctival and corneal epithelial cell loss and degeneration. Patients with a deficiency of the aqueous portion of tears have punctate staining of the lower two thirds of the cornea and bright red staining of bulbar conjunctiva in the area corresponding to the palpable aperture.

Schirmer's test. A strip of filter paper, 3.5 × 0.05 cm, is placed in the conjunctival cul-de-sac of the lower lid for 5 minutes. A 10- to 15-mm length of paper wetted with tears is considered normal. More than 25 mm of moistened paper indicates excessive tearing.

Indications Used to determine the adequacy and patency of the lacrimal system; it can demonstrate obstruction or overproduction of tears.

Fluorescein is instilled in the eye for a variety of diagnostic tests. It demonstrates breaks in the epithelium and the dilution that occurs when anterior aqueous humor escapes from a postoperative fistula, penetrating wound, or conjunctival bleb following glaucoma surgery. It is also used to demonstrate areas of contact between the lens and the cornea and sclera in the fitting of contact lenses. The rate of disappearance through the nasolacrimal passages (normally 1 minute) estimates their patency.

Rose bengal dye is usually used to demarcate devitalized conjunctival epithelium in keratoconjunctivitis sicca, since it stains devitalized cells better than fluorescein does.

Complications Dyes stain soft contact lenses, so the lenses should be removed before the dye is instilled; lenses should not be reinserted until all evidence of dye is gone. Because it is possible for fluorescein to become contaminated with *Pseudomonas* spp., it should be instilled with either a single-dose container or a strip of sterile filter paper saturated with the dye.

Nursing care Explain the procedure to the patient.

Provocative testing

Description Used for patients with mildly elevated intraocular pressure (IOP), those who have optic nerve changes or field defects without elevated IOP, and those with shallow anterior chambers and compromised anterior angles. Their results are not definitive but may distinguish potentially glaucomatous persons from others.

Water drinking test. In the morning, the fasting patient drinks approximately 1 L of water as fast as possible (within 2 to 4 minutes). The IOP is measured before and at 15-minute intervals for 45 minutes. Normal eyes show an IOP increase of 3 to 5 mm Hg. An increase of 8 mm Hg is indicative of glaucoma.

Dark room test (for narrow-angle glaucoma). The patient sits in a dark room for 60 minutes to dilate pupils. An IOP increase of 7 to 8 mm Hg is indicative of iris bunching into and blocking of anterior angle flow.

Mydriatic testing. One eye is dilated at a time (under careful supervision), and the pupil is constricted when the test is ended. IOP increase of 8 mm Hg is indicative of glaucoma.

Indications These tests are indicated in patients with an intraocular pressure of 21 mm Hg or more, a coefficient outflow of less than 0.18, a ratio of intraocular pressure to coefficient outflow facility greater than 100, optic nerve changes suggestive of glaucoma, and field changes suggestive of glaucoma.[21]

Complications None.

Nursing care Explain the study to the patient. Encourage patient to have eyes tested periodically for glaucoma.

Visual field screening

Description
Central field tangent screen. Central vision covers approximately 50 degrees of patient's central vision, 25 degrees in each direction from the central fixation point. A black screen (1 m²) is placed 1 m from eye. Blind spots are outlined by using a 1- to 3-mm white target placed on a board. A normal blind spot is 13 to 18 degrees temporal from central fixation. Abnormal isolated spots (scotomas) or confluent areas can be identified. Nasal areas are usually lost first.

Automated perimetry. Various automatic machines (such as Goldmann perimeter) measure both central and peripheral fields.

Indications Method of assessing function of retinal periphery by measuring the peripheral field of vision. It is indicated as part of a routine vision screening or as part of a diagnosis of visual problems or deterioration.

Complications None.

Nursing care Explain the study to the patient.

Otoscopy

Description Inspection of the external auditory canal and middle ear. The largest speculum that will fit comfortably in the patient's ear is inserted to a depth of 1 to 1.5 cm to inspect the auditory canal from the meatus to the tympanic membrane.

Indications Any discharge, scaling, excessive redness, lesions, foreign bodies, or cerumen can be noted. The tympanic membrane is inspected for landmarks, color, contours, and perforations. The direction of the light can be varied to see the entire tympanic membrane and anulus.[28]

Complications None.

Nursing care Explain the procedure to the patient.

Rhinoscopy

Description Inspection of the nasal cavity using a nasal speculum and a light. The patient's head should be held erect to examine the vestibule and inferior nasal turbinate, and tilted back to visualize the middle meatus and turbinate.[28]

Indications Color, discharge, masses, lesions, and swelling of the turbinates may be noted, and the septum inspected for alignment, perforation, bleeding, and crusting.

Complications None.

Nursing care Explain the procedure to the patient.

Rigid endoscopy of pharynx

Description An instrument producing bright illumination is held in the patient's mouth to visualize nasopharynx when the instrument is turned upward, and hypopharynx and larynx when turned downward.

Indications Detection of abnormalities of the oropharynx or nasopharynx, and evaluation of symptoms of infection or abscess.

Complications None.

Nursing care Explain the procedure to the patient.

Laryngoscopy (direct, suspension, indirect)

Description

Direct laryngoscopy. Direct examination of the larynx under local or general anesthesia, performed by introducing a laryngoscope into the patient's mouth over the tongue; the tongue is raised, the patient's neck is slowly extended, and the laryngoscope is passed over the posterior portion of the epiglottis and raised to expose the vocal cords. Method can be used for biopsy or excision of polyp.

Suspension laryngoscopy. Essentially the same as direct laryngoscopy, but an attachment holds the laryngoscope so the examiner can use both hands; usually used in conjunction with a microscope, which provides magnification and binocular vision.

Indirect laryngoscopy. The most common way to examine the larynx; usually performed in the physician's office; the patient sits upright in a chair, and a laryngeal mirror is used to visualize the larynx.

Indications Hoarseness, burning in throat, dysphagia, dyspnea, muffled voice.

Complications None except that the gag reflex is abolished. The usual care must be taken to prevent aspiration.

Nursing care Explain procedure to patient. Observe the patient for respiratory distress for the first 2 to 4 hours. If the patient had a local (topical) anesthetic administered before the procedure, be aware that the gag reflex may be absent until the anesthetic wears off, so fluids should be withheld until gag reflex returns. Humidified oxygen provides additional moisture to the patient's airway.

Videolaryngoscopy

Description Videolaryngoscopy is the standard of practice when laryngeal pathology is suspected. A rigid 90-degree telescope is used to perform a transoral exam of the larynx, and a flexible fiberoptic scope is used to perform a transnasal examination. The rigid scope is used more frequently because it offers greater ease of examination and produces a video image of higher resolution. It provides the luxury of repeated reviews and closer scrutiny of the laryngeal examination without repeated manipulation of the patient and may enhance the identification of less obvious laryngeal lesions. This study may also assist with identification of decreased subtle vocal cord mobility that may otherwise be missed.

Indications Hoarseness, burning in throat, dysphagia, dyspnea, muffled voice.

Complications None except that the gag reflex is abolished. The usual care must be taken to prevent aspiration.

Nursing care Explain procedure to patient. Observe the patient for respiratory distress for the first 2 to 4 hours. If the patient had a local (topical) anesthetic administered before the procedure, be aware that the gag reflex may be absent until the anesthetic wears off, so fluids should be withheld until gag reflex returns. Humidified oxygen provides additional moisture to the patient's airway.

Fiberoptic bronchoscopy

Description This procedure, performed with the patient under local anesthesia, permits direct inspection of the larynx, trachea, and bronchi. The flexible fiberoptic bronchoscope is the preferred instrument because it is better tolerated by patients and permits improved visualization of distal subsegmental airways. The fiberoptic bronchoscope, which has an external diameter between 3 and 6 mm, is inserted through the patient's nose or mouth. General anesthesia may be used for this procedure if necessary.

Indications Collection of secretions for cytologic or bacteriologic examination; tissue biopsy for examination; cells and secretions via a brush biopsy technique that involves using a small brush inserted through the bronchoscope to brush the tissue walls. Location and biopsy of tumors; bleeding locations; removal of foreign bodies or heavy, blocking, mucous plug secretions; implantation of radioactive gold seeds for tumor treatment.

Complications Bronchospasm, increased sputum production, productive mild bronchitis, sore throat, hoarseness.

Nursing care The patient should receive nothing by mouth for 8 hours before the procedure and is usually given a pre-procedure sedative medication. Any dental prostheses should be removed. In the examination area, the patient's mouth, throat, and tongue will be sprayed with a topical anesthetic. An oxygen catheter is placed and remains in one nostril throughout the procedure. Lidocaine jelly is generally used as the bronchoscope lubricant; this helps to decrease the patient's cough and gag reflexes. After the procedure the patient should be carefully watched and positioned until the full gag and swallowing reflexes return. Patency of the patient's airway and the swallowing reflex should be evaluated, and the patient should be assessed for severe complications such as bronchospasms.

Mediastinoscopy, mediastinotomy, thoracoscopy

Description Surgical endoscopy procedures in which a biopsy is taken from a tumor in the upper mediastinum, the pleura, or the lung. They are also used to determine if metastasis has occurred.

Mediastinoscopy. The incision is made in the suprasternal notch, and the scope is passed through that incision to biopsy tissue from the upper mediastinum.

Mediastinotomy. The incision is made above the third rib along the sternal border. Lung biopsy may also be done by this technique.

Thoracoscopy. Done to obtain a biopsy from a peripheral lesion of the lung or pleura. The incision site, along the lateral or anterior chest wall, depends on the location of the lesion.

Indications Diagnosis of primary or secondary mediastinal disease; evaluation of metastasis to mediastinal nodes in primary lung carcinoma.

Complications Hemorrhage, pneumothorax, infection, left recurrent laryngeal nerve damage.

Nursing care For all procedures the patient receives a general anesthetic; therefore all preoperative procedures apply (see Part Two on p. 1433). Postoperatively the patient should be observed for pneumothorax, cardiac dysrhythmias, and bleeding. A drainage chest tube is frequently used after the thoracoscopy procedure.

Esophagogastroduodenoscopy (EGD)

Description   Permits visual examination of the esophagus, stomach, and upper duodenum. Dentures are removed. A local anesthetic is sprayed into the mouth and throat. An endoscope is passed through the mouth and swallowed. Saliva may need to be suctioned if it doesn't flow out the side of the mouth adequately. A mouth guard should be used to protect the teeth. The patient's head is repositioned throughout the procedure to facilitate movement of the endoscope.

The procedure is contraindicated in patients with recent ulcer perforation, large aortic aneurysms, cardiac disease or a recent myocardial infarction, and Zenker's diverticulum.

Indications   Useful in diagnosing inflammatory disease, ulcers, tumors, structural abnormality, and Mallory-Weiss tears.

Complications   Complications include the following perforations: cervical esophagus perforation (pain on swallowing and neck movements); thoracic esophagus perforation (substernal or epigastric pain that increases with respirations and trunk movements); diaphragmatic esophageal perforation (shoulder pain and dyspnea); gastric perforation (abdominal or back pain, cyanosis, fever, or pleural effusion).

Other signs of complications include difficulty in swallowing, persistent pain, fever, black stools, or hematemesis.

Nursing care   Give nothing by mouth for 6 to 12 hours before the procedure; during an emergency procedure a nasogastric tube is used to aspirate gastric contents. Explain the procedure to the patient and ensure that a signed consent form is obtained. Before the procedure, have the patient remove any dentures or partial plates. Monitor pain, blood pressure, pulse, temperature, and respirations. Anxiety and fear of procedure are expected, and the patient should be given emotional support before and throughout the procedure; sedatives and analgesics may be used to help the patient relax. Fluids and foods should be withheld until the gag reflex returns.

Endoscopy

Description   Direct visualization of the lining of a hollow viscus via an endoscope—a long, flexible tube with cable-like cluster of glass fibers that transmits light and returns an image to the scope's optical head; used to diagnose a variety of gastrointestinal disorders and allowing for biopsy of lesions through the scope.

Indications   Useful in diagnosing inflammatory disease, ulcers, tumors, structural abnormality, and Mallory-Weiss tears.

Complications   Complications include cervical esophagus perforation (pain on swallowing and neck movements); thoracic esophagus perforation (substernal or epigastric pain that increases with respirations and trunk movements); diaphragmatic esophageal perforation (shoulder pain and dyspnea); and gastric perforation (abdominal or back pain, cyanosis, fever, or pleural effusion). Other signs of complications include difficulty swallowing, persistent pain, fever, black stools, or hematemesis.

Nursing care   Give nothing by mouth for 6 to 12 hours before the procedure; during an emergency procedure a nasogastric tube is used to aspirate gastric contents. Explain the procedure to the patient and ensure that consent is signed. Before the procedure, have the patient remove any dentures or partial plates. Monitor blood pressure, pulse, and respirations before, during, and after procedure until patient is fully awake and effects of any sedative drugs have worn off. Anxiety and fear of the procedures are expected, and the patient should be given emotional support before and throughout them; sedatives and analgesics may be used to help the patient relax (usually midazolam or diazepam) (see box). Fluids and foods should be withheld until the gag reflex returns. Explain to patient about midazolam's amnestic effect.

Colonoscopy

Description   The patient is placed in the left lateral decubitus position, and a well-lubricated colonoscope is inserted through the anus. Air is inserted to help the physician visualize the mucosa and to facilitate advancement of the colonoscope. Occasionally position changes are required to assist advancement of the scope at the descending-sigmoid colon junction and splenic flexure. Barium studies should be made after the colonoscopy; thorough bowel preparation is required for good visualization of mucosa. Specimens for cytology and histology may be obtained as well as for biopsy.

Contraindications to the procedure include pregnancy, ischemic bowel disease, acute diverticulitis, peritonitis, toxic megacolon of ulcerative colitis, fulminant granulomatous colitis, and irradiation colitis.

Indications   Used to examine the colon and rectum to diagnose inflammatory bowel disease, including ulcerative colitis and granulomatous colitis. Polyps can be removed through the colonoscope. The colonoscope is also helpful in diagnosing or locating the source of lower gastrointestinal bleeding. A biopsy of lesions suspected to be malignant may also be performed; biopsies may also be advisable for patients with ulcerative colitis or Crohn's disease.

Complications   Complications include perforation of the bowel. Signs and symptoms include abdominal pain and distention, rectal bleeding, fever, and mucopurulent drainage. If the bowel is fixed—secondary to irradiation, surgical adhesions, or inflammatory disease—the physician may have difficulty during the procedure.

Nursing care   Bowel preparation is required for visualization of the mucosa. Colon electrolyte lavage preparations (Colyte, Go-lyte) may be used.

Patients need instructions for mixing the solution. Avoid all solid food and sugar the day of the prep. Alternatively, the bowel should be cleansed with laxatives and enemas; be careful in patients with ulcerative colitis and granulomatous colitis because laxatives can exacerbate the disease (special protocols are required for this patient group). Avoid soapsuds enemas in all

GUIDELINES FOR CONSCIOUS SEDATION

DEFINITION

Conscious sedation is the condition produced by the administration of a drug or combination of drugs to relieve pain or anxiety during diagnostic or therapeutic procedures. The patient receiving conscious sedation has an altered level of consciousness, but should retain the ability to maintain and protect a patent airway as well as to respond appropriately to verbal commands and physical stimuli. Because the administration of drugs to produce conscious sedation can have the unintended effect of compromising a patient's protective reflexes, these guidelines are intended to ensure the performance of safe and effective diagnostic and therapeutic procedures. These guidelines do not apply to the use of "deep sedation" or in the routine management of postoperative pain. *Deep sedation* is a medically controlled state of depressed consciousness or unconsciousness from which the patient is not easily aroused. Deep sedation may be accompanied by a partial or complete loss of protective reflexes, including the inability to maintain a patent airway independently and to respond purposefully to physical stimulation or to verbal commands. The state and risks of deep sedation may be indistinguishable from those of general anesthesia.

REQUIREMENT FOR ALL PATIENTS RECEIVING CONSCIOUS SEDATION
Personnel

A physician and a registered nurse/licensed vocational (LVN/LPN) nurse, who are familiar with basic life support and emergency airway management including bag and mask ventilation, must be in attendance or immediately available until the procedure is completed. One health care provider should have the primary responsibility of monitoring the patient's vital signs and level of consciousness and must remain with the patient until there is satisfactory recovery from the acute effects of the sedation agents (i.e., vital signs and level of consciousness have returned to *baseline*). In case of an airway emergency, a clearly defined plan for obtaining assistance with airway management must be activated.

In circumstances where a painful dressing change procedure is routinely performed by the nursing staff, the personnel requirement can be met by a single registered nurse and either a second registered nurse or a licensed vocational nurse, provided the responsible physician (or physician designee) is *immediately available.*

Equipment (required and immediately available)

1. Oxygen source
2. Equipment for oxygen administration (nasal cannula, masks)
3. Self-inflating resuscitation bag
4. Functioning suction source
5. Crash cart
6. Emergency airway equipment (masks, airways, and laryngoscopes with blades)
7. Telephone
8. Electrical outlet connected to emergency power supply
9. Monitoring equipment, including electrocardiogram, pulse oximeter, sphygmomanometer, and cuff and/or automated blood pressure monitor

Other Requirements

1. Supplemental oxygen should be administered to all patients during conscious sedation unless pulse oximetry data indicate satisfactory oxygenation.
2. Intravenous access should be secured in all adult patients. For pediatric patients, the skilled personnel and equipment to start an IV should be immediately available.
3. Agents to reverse effects of drugs immediately available (naloxone and flumazenil).

MEDICATIONS FOR CONSCIOUS SEDATION

The following sedatives and narcotics may be administered for the purpose of conscious sedation only by a physician, or by a registered nurse under the direct supervision of a physician, in the manner prescribed. The agents listed below shall be titrated to effect in accordance with the monitoring standards described below. The following schedule can be modified according to the judgment and practice of the prescribing physician. All routes of administration are intravenous unless otherwise specified.

Medications
Adults

Agents	Dose	Frequency
Diazepam	1-2 mg	q 3-10 min
Midazolam*	0.25-1 mg	q 1-5 min
Fentanyl	Loading dose up to 1 mcg/kg then 12.5-50 mcg	q 5-10 min
Morphine	1-3 mg	q 2-15 min
Meperidine	12.5-25 mg	q 2-15 min
Droperidol	0.625-1.25 mg	q 5-10 min

Continued.

GUIDELINES FOR CONSCIOUS SEDATION—cont'd

Pediatrics

Agents	Dose	Frequency
Diazepam	0.05-0.1 mg/kg (max dose 0.25 mg/kg)	q 3-10 min
Midazolam*	**IV** 0.04-0.08 mg/kg **PO** 0.3-0.5 mg/kg **Intranasal** 0.25 mg/kg **Rectal** 0.3-0.5 mg/kg	q 3-5 min
Fentanyl	0.5 mcg/kg	q 5-10 min
Morphine	0.05 mg/kg	q 5-10 min
Meperidine	0.5 mg/kg (max dose 2 mg/kg)	q 5 min
Pentobarbital	**IV** 1-2 mg/kg (max dose 6 mg/kg)	q 5 min
	IM 2-6 mg/kg	one time
	PO/PR 5 mg/kg	one time
Chloral Hydrate	50 mg/kg PO or PR	25 mg/kg prn once

*See midazolam guidelines in hospital formulary

In pediatric sedation, note that benzodiazepines may be associated with disinhibition. Pentobarbital occasionally can produce paradoxical excitement. Small doses of opiates can ameliorate these effects.

Conscious Sedation Antagonists (reversal agents)

Adults

Agents	Dose	Frequency
Naloxone	40-400 μg	q 5-10 min
Flumazenil	0.2 mg	q 1 min up to 1 mg

Pediatrics

Agents	Dose	Frequency
Naloxone	2-10 μ/kg	q 5-10 min

Any patient receiving reversal agents should be monitored for at least two hours after administration of reversal agent to detect potential resedation. Flumazenil is not approved for pediatric patients (over-sedation is not commonly associated with benzodiazepine administration in pediatric patients).

RESTRICTION ON AGENTS TO BE ADMINISTERED

The following medications, when administered intravenously, are for the provision of deep sedation and general anesthesia and are not appropriate for conscious sedation. Furthermore, they should only be administered by a physician trained in airway management, including endotracheal intubation and/or under the direct supervision of an anesthesiologist:

1. Neuromuscular blocking agents (e.g., succinylcholine, vecuronium)
2. Intravenous anesthetics
   a. Sodium thiopental
   b. Methohexital
   c. Propofol
   d. Ketamine
   e. Alfentanil
   f. Sufentanil
3. Fentanyl oralets

GUIDELINES FOR CONSCIOUS SEDATION—cont'd

NPO STATUS

The following are the guidelines for NPO status for otherwise healthy patients:

1. Patients less than 2 years old: NPO for 2 hours; clear liquids up to 2 hours before procedure; solids up to 6 hours before procedure.
2. Patients greater than 2 years old: NPO for 4 hours; clear liquids up to 4 hours before procedure; solids up to 6 hours before procedure.

PRE-PROCEDURE PATIENT EVALUATION

An appropriate medical history and physical examination must be performed and written in the chart prior to the procedure. An assessment of the patient's pre-procedure responsiveness to verbal and physical stimuli and vital signs should be performed. For the patient who is scheduled for an elective procedure, the availability and appropriateness of transportation following the procedure should be verified prior to the administration of conscious sedation. Prior to the procedure, patients must be given written discharge instructions, including the names and phone numbers of medical center staff to contact in the event of an emergency.

MONITORING DURING THE PROCEDURE

The objective of monitoring the patient during conscious sedation is to ensure the adequacy of ventilation, oxygenation, and circulatory function. The following guidelines for monitoring are considered a minimum standard that is required for any patient receiving conscious sedation. Departments and units where conscious sedation is performed may develop their own specific guidelines that delineate requirements for monitoring of special patient populations that exceed the minimum standards below.

1. Electrocardiographic monitoring should be available and used in selected patients (e.g., with cardiac and pulmonary disease) if clinically possible.
2. Blood pressure every 5 minutes (manually or with automated device) if clinically possible; heart rate and respiratory rate every 15 minutes.
3. Continuous pulse oximetry (SpO_2).
4. Assessment of adequacy of ventilation (observation of chest excursion, measuring respiratory rate, or, if possible, the detection of end-tidal carbon dioxide) at least every 15 minutes.
5. Responsiveness to verbal and physical stimuli should be assessed 5 minutes after administration of any agent and at least every 15 minutes thereafter.

DOCUMENTATION DURING PROCEDURE

Valid consent must be obtained and documented in the medical record as required by Medical Center policy prior to the beginning of the procedure and the administration of any sedative agents. The record should contain:

1. Procedure performed
2. Personnel involved
3. Record of vital signs and responsiveness to verbal and physical stimuli at least every 15 minutes or more frequently if indicated (heart rate or ECG rhythm, if used, BP, SpO_2, respiratory rate)
4. Time and dosage of medications administered
5. Documentation of any abnormal ECG rhythm, blood pressure 30% below or above baseline, SpO_2 of less than 90%, or respiratory rate less than 10 breaths per minute and any other complications

POST-SEDATION MONITORING AND RECOVERY CRITERIA

Following completion of the procedure, the patient must be monitored and vital signs assessed using the same parameters and protocol as described in *Monitoring During the Procedure* until the patient meets the following recovery criteria.

1. All patients should be monitored until their vital signs and responsiveness to verbal and physical stimuli have returned to their pre-procedure baseline.
2. Outpatients undergoing procedures with conscious sedation, including those in the emergency department, should be stable enough to safely return home.
3. Outpatients undergoing elective procedures and who are discharged home must be accompanied by a responsible adult.
4. Inpatients must be able to return to their pre-procedure level of care and monitoring.

For pediatric and neonatal patients, age-specific recovery criteria should be established by each group of practitioners involved in conscious sedation.

Evidence that the patient has met recovery criteria must be clearly documented in the patient's medical record.

REPORTING OF ADVERSE EVENTS

All cases in which the following events occur will be reported by the physician and/or nursing staff using the Confidential Report of Incident and, if appropriate, the Adverse Drug Reaction Report form.

1. All cases in which naloxone or flumazenil is administered
2. All cases in which *new* assisted ventilation is required

Continued.

■■ GUIDELINES FOR CONSCIOUS SEDATION—cont'd

_____

3. All unanticipated hospital admissions or increased level of care
4. All cases in which the oxygen saturation (SpO_2) is <90% for more than 5 minutes, including recovery period, or 80% at any time
5. All cases in which there is hemodynamic instability defined as a 30% change from baseline in blood pressure or heart rate and/or the occurrence of new atrial or ventricular dysrhythmias

EVALUATION OF NEW AGENTS FOR CONSCIOUS SEDATION

When a new agent for conscious sedation is added to the hospital formulary, the guidelines for its use will be established by the Pharmacy and Therapeutics Committees following the basic principles set forward in this document.

Courtesy University of California, San Francisco Pharmacy and Therapeutics Committee and the Drug Information Analysis Service.

patients, since this irritates the mucosa. Fluid and electrolyte problems may occur in elderly patients who receive high volume enemas; ensure that patients are alerted to potential effects.

The procedure is uncomfortable and embarrassing, so be supportive. Let the patient know that flatus is from air inserted during the procedure and cannot be controlled. A sedative may be given to help the patient relax; because midazolam or diazepam may be used, ensure that the patient is appropriately monitored during the procedure.

Proctosigmoidoscopy

Description Examination of the sigmoid colon, rectum, and anal canal. The sigmoidoscope and proctoscope may be rigid metal instruments or flexible scopes inserted to visualize the mucosa; a biopsy may be performed. Examination usually includes a digital examination of anus and anal canal.

Patients often dread the proctosigmoidoscopy examination because of the embarrassing and uncomfortable positioning and the discomfort caused by the rigid instrument. Patients are placed in a knee-chest position on a tilting table. Although the procedure can be done with the patient in a left lateral position, it is important to elevate the right buttock; most physicians prefer to use a tilting table and the knee-chest position for best visualization.

A proctoscope may be used to examine the rectum and anus, but when a sigmoidoscope is removed slowly, the rectum and anal canal can be viewed, thereby eliminating the need for a proctoscope.

Indications Changed bowel habits, rectal bleeding, weight loss, anemia, stools positive for occult blood.

Complications Complications include possible bowel perforation (see the discussion of colonoscopy); decreased blood pressure, pallor, diaphoresis, and bradycardia are signs of vasovagal stimulation and require immediate notification of the physician.

Nursing care Preparation varies with the expected diagnosis; clear liquid diets for 48 hours and a small sodium biphosphate enema may be used. Tell patient what to expect.

Cystoscopy and panendoscopy

Description The cystoscope and panendoscope are instruments that allow direct visualization of the bladder and urethra.

Cystoscopy and panendoscopy may be performed while the patient is under general or spinal anesthesia; in other cases, a local anesthetic, consisting of a lubricant jelly impregnated with lidocaine, is used.

The patient is placed in the lithotomy position. Sterile equipment is used; surgical gowns, gloves, and masks are typically worn. A single sheath through which both cystoscope and panendoscope will be passed is inserted into the bladder via the urethra, with adequate lubrication. A telescope is then passed through the sheath while the bladder is being filled with fluid. Using a fiberoptic system within the cystoscope, the urologist visualizes the internal architecture of the bladder including the bladder neck, urothelial lining, and ureteral orifices. Bladder tumors, trabeculation, and inflammatory changes within the internal mucosa are assessed via cystoscopy. A panendoscope is used to view the bladder neck, prostatic urethra (in a male), external urinary sphincters, and anterior urethra.

Fluid is infused into the bladder throughout the procedure. Infusion is stopped and the bladder drained when it becomes filled with 300 to 500 ml of fluid.

Cystoscopic and panendoscopic examination may be combined with radiographic diagnostic studies such as a retrograde pyelogram or with therapeutic procedures, such as transurethral resection of bladder tumor or prostate.

Indications Hematuria, dysuria, tumor or polyp removal or biopsy.

Complications Mild dysuria and transient hematuria should disappear within the first 48 hours post-procedure. The patient usually should be able to void normally after a routine cystoscopic examination, although some burning may be experienced.

Nursing care If a general or spinal anesthetic is used the patient will be sent to the postanesthesia care unit after the procedure and should be closely monitored for potential postanesthesia complications, such as a low-grade fever (≤38° C [101° F]). This may occur for 24 to 48 hours after the procedure. Instruct the patient to notify the physician if this occurs, as sepsis may occur. If patient experiences burning with urination, suggest sitz baths and increased fluid intake, unless contraindicated. Explain to the patient that only minimal discomfort will be experienced following the procedure if it is performed gently and with adequate lubrication.

Pelvic endoscopy

Description Visualization and examination of pelvic and abdominal viscera with a high-intensity fiberoptic or video light source inserted via a laparoscope through the abdominal wall and into the peritoneum.

Indications The procedure is performed when a hysterosalpingography suggests tubal abnormality and the patient does not become pregnant. It is also performed before certain surgical procedures, such as a tuboplasty, and may reveal the presence of unsuspected tubal or ovarian disease, such as peritubal adhesions and endometriosis.

Complications Bowel perforation; bleeding.

Nursing care Because a general anesthetic is used, the patient will be sent to the postanesthesia care unit after the procedure and should be monitored for potential complications.

Colposcopy

Description Examination of the cervix and vagina with a colposcope—a stereoscopic binocular microscope with various levels of magnification.

Indications Dysplasia; to elevate the vascular pattern, intercapillary distance, surface pattern, color, tone, opacity, clarity, demarcation, and extent of a lesion. To differentiate between inflammatory atypia and neoplasms or between invasive and noninvasive cervical lesions, and to enable follow-up.

Complications None.

Nursing care Prepare the patient (in the lithotomy position) for a vaginal examination. Show her the colposcope and explain that it will not be inserted into the vagina. A vaginal speculum is used to expose the vagina and cervix, and the colposcope then focuses on the cervix, allowing careful examination, outlining of the lesion, and biopsy and specimen removal. Inform the patient that she may have slight vaginal bleeding if specimens were taken, and suggest that she wear a sanitary pad until the bleeding subsides. Provide emotional support and allow patient to voice any concerns related to procedure or findings.

Culdoscopy

Description Visual examination of female pelvic viscera by means of an endoscope inserted through the posterior vaginal fornix. The patient is usually sedated, but a general anesthetic is not used. The procedure is performed with the patient in the knee-chest position. If necessary, CO_2 may be instilled into the peritoneal cavity to allow better visualization of the pelvic organs.

Indications Investigation of infertility. It determines gross anatomic and pathologic conditions, i.e., congenital abnormalities or the sequelae of traumatic or inflammatory processes.

Complications None.

Nursing care Tell the patient that once the endoscope is removed, she will be required to exhale as forcefully as possible to push out intraperitoneal air; this maneuver will minimize shoulder pain caused by trapped CO_2 when she sits up.

Hysteroscopy

Description Direct visual examination of the cervical canal and uterine cavity through a hysteroscope, a fiberoptic instrument; procedure most often performed with the patient under spinal anesthesia.

Indications To examine the endometrium, secure a specimen for biopsy, remove an intrauterine device, or excise cervical polyps.

Complications Perforation of the uterus (usually at the fundus), bleeding, infection.

Nursing care The patient should be maintained in a flat position for 8 hours after the procedure to recover fully if spinal anesthesia is used. Provide routine postanesthesia care, and advise the patient to rest during the next 24 hours and to avoid heavy lifting to prevent uterine hemorrhage.

Laparoscopy

Description With the patient under general anesthesia, the abdominal and pelvic organs are visualized and examined with a laparoscope inserted through a small incision in the abdominal wall; the abdomen is insufflated with carbon dioxide to enhance visualization. The procedure usually lasts 10 to 15 minutes.

Indications Therapeutic procedures may also be performed, including removal of peritubular adhesions, sterilization through fulguration of oviducts, laser treatment for endometriosis, cholecystectomy and appendectomy.

Complications Bleeding from a puncture injury, misplacement of gas, thermal burns.

Nursing care Provide routine presurgical and postanesthetic care. Inform the patient that he or she may experience a sore throat from intubation and a sore chest from insufflation of the abdomen. These sensations usually disappear within 48 hours. Shoulder pain caused by trapped CO_2 may also be experienced.

Arthroscopy

Description Insertion of a specially designed endoscope through an incision at a certain joint, often the knee. By means of lenses and lights on the scope, the tissues are examined. The arthroscope also permits the removal of loose bodies, pieces of torn cartilage, and biopsy of the synovium if desired. The procedure is performed in an outpatient surgical or operative suite, often as a 23-hour stay procedure.

Indications To determine the condition of the joint, tissues, cartilage, meniscus (of knee), and ligaments. It is most frequently performed on the knee and shoulder, and less often on the hip, elbow, ankle, and other joints.

Complications Possible joint swelling after the procedure and at times some bleeding into the joint. Infection is also possible.

Nursing care Explain to the patient about the skin preparation, application of a tourniquet to decrease blood flow, sterile draping, and administration of a local anesthetic to one or more areas before insertion of the arthroscope into the joint. After the procedure, instruct the patient about applying a compression dressing and ice around the joint to lessen bleeding and edema. Caution the patient to avoid excessive joint use for 24 to 48 hours, but explain that weight bearing is permitted after knee arthroscopy. Use of other joints varies with the purpose and extent of the arthroscopic repair or procedure done. Instruct the patient about signs of infection, restrictions or limitations of joint use, and the return physician's appointment. Mild analgesics (no aspirin) may be prescribed for postprocedural discomfort or pain.

Body Fluid Examination

Sputum examination (direct method)

Description   The microbiologic evaluation of sputum is vitally important in the evaluation of the respiratory system. The two laboratory procedures commonly performed with sputum examination are microscopic Gram stain and culture and sensitivity.

Direct method.   Voluntary coughing to produce sputum specimen. With this procedure, early morning specimens are sent on three consecutive days if TB is suspected. Ensure that a sputum and not a saliva specimen has been obtained.

Sputum induction.   This technique may be used if voluntary coughing does not produce a specimen. With this technique the patient is instructed to breathe for several minutes using a heated, nebulized mist of distilled water or a sodium chloride solution. Following this nebulization the sputum collection technique as described is performed.

Indications   Evaluation of pneumonias, suspected malignancies.

Complications   None.

Nursing care   The sputum should be collected in a wide-mouthed, sterile container with a tightly fitting lid and should be transported immediately to the laboratory.

Instruct the patient to brush teeth and gargle before the collection of the specimen. Instruct the patient to spit out any postnasal secretions. Instruct the patient to take a deep breath to the lungs' full capacity and then to exhale the air with an expulsive deep cough. The specimen should be coughed directly into the sterile, wide-mouthed container. Instruct patient not to touch inside the sputum container or cover. Note and document the color, consistency, odor, and amount of the sputum. Number the specimens serially for each of the 3 days.

Sputum examination (indirect method)

Description   One of two indirect methods may be used.

Nasotracheal suctioning.   This technique is used to obtain specimens from the trachea via a catheter that has been passed transnasally. Causes some patient discomfort.

Endotracheal suctioning.   Used to obtain specimen from trachea via a catheter that has been passed through an endotracheal tube.

Indications   Evaluation of pneumonias or suspected malignancies.

Complications

Nasotracheal suctioning.   Hypoxemia; dysrhythmias; BP changes.

Transtracheal aspiration.   Subcutaneous or mediastinal emphysema and cervical infections at the site of the aspiration.

Nursing care   For both types, ensure that emotional support is provided, and that appropriate pre- or post-procedure care is given.

Nasotracheal and endotracheal suctioning.   Assist the patient to a sitting position. The nurse, physician, or respiratory therapist passes a catheter through the patient's nose into the trachea to suction tracheobronchial secretions. Oxygen may be administered during the procedure. Cardiac response and the patient's oxygenation should be monitored.

Pleural fluid examination (diagnostic thoracentesis)

Description   A needle is inserted through the chest wall into the pleural space to remove pleural fluid.

Indications   May be performed therapeutically to drain fluid and relieve lung congestion, and also diagnostically to collect pleural fluid for examination in patients with symptoms of inflammation, infection, or malignancy.

Complications   Hemothorax, pneumothorax, air embolism, subcutaneous emphysema, hypotension, hypoxemia, acute fluid shifts.

Nursing care   Instruct the patient regarding the procedure. Advise the patient not to move suddenly, cough, or breathe deeply during the procedure. Record baseline vital signs. Assist with positioning the patient comfortably, and provide emotional support during the procedure. After the procedure, monitor the patient's vital signs and respiratory status for any complications.

Gastric analysis (basal gastric secretion test)

Description   Measures basal secretion under fasting conditions; stomach contents aspirated through a nasogastric tube, with the patient in supine, left lateral decubitus, and right lateral decubitus positions.

Histamine may be injected to stimulate flow. Normal values of gastric secretions are 0.2 to 3.8 mEq/hr for females; 1 to 5 mEq/hr for males. High values may indicate a duodenal or jejunal ulcer; depressed values may indicate gastric carcinoma or benign gastric ulcer; absence of gastric secretion indicates pernicious anemia; markedly high levels indicate Zollinger-Ellison syndrome.

Indications   Indicated for patients with anorexia, weight loss, and epigastric pain.

Complications   Dysrhythmias may develop during intubation.

Nursing care   The patient must be relaxed and isolated from sensory stimulations of foods. (Gastric acid secretions are increased by external factors, including the sight and smell of food and psychologic stress.) The patient should have nothing to eat for 12 hours and not smoke for 8 hours before the test. The following drugs should be withheld for 24 hours: antacids, anticholinergics, cholinergics, alcohol, H_2 blockers, reserpine and adrenergic blockers. Adrenocorticosteroids should be held for approximately 12 hrs before the test.

To prevent contamination of gastric contents with saliva, the patient should be instructed to expectorate excess saliva rather than swallow it.

Check the location of the nasogastric tube for placement by aspirating gastric contents. Paroxysms of coughing or cyanosis may indicate a tube in the trachea. Clamp the tube during removal to prevent aspiration from fluids in the lumen. Sore throat following intubation may be treated with soothing lozenges, viscous lidocaine (Xylocaine), or benzocaine (Cetacaine) spray.

Gastric acid stimulation test

Description Normally follows basal gastric secretion test. A drug, usually pentagastrin, is given to stimulate gastric acid output; specimens are collected every 15 minutes for 1 hour. Normal values are 11 to 21 mEq/hr for females and 18 to 28 mEq/hr for males.

Indications Clinical diagnosis of the following is indicated by certain results of gastric acid secretion:

Duodenal ulcers: high values

Zollinger-Ellison syndrome: markedly high values

Gastric carcinoma: low values

Pernicious anemia: achlorhydria (low acid levels are considered normal in patients over 60 years of age)

Complications Side effects of pentagastrin include abdominal pain, nausea, vomiting, flushing, transitory dizziness, faintness, and numbness of extremities. Check the patient's history for hypersensitivity to pentagastrin.

Nursing care Same as for gastric analysis. Tell the patient that the q 15 min specimen collection is normal.

Gastric lavage

Description The procedure includes an early morning suctioning of gastric contents after a nasogastric tube has been properly placed. The timing of the procedure is early morning because it is assumed that the patient swallows sputum at night while sleeping and in the early morning with morning coughing. The gastric contents are sent to the laboratory for sputum analysis.

Indications This technique, although infrequently used, may be helpful in the diagnosis of patients with suspected tuberculosis or lung cancer.

Complications None.

Nursing care The patient should be given nothing by mouth after midnight. In the early morning, a nasogastric (NG) tube is inserted through the patient's nose. Suction is applied to the NG tube with a large syringe, and the gastric contents are removed. The contents are placed in a specimen container and are sent immediately to the laboratory. The NG tube is removed.

Peritoneal fluid analysis

Description Examines a sample of peritoneal fluid obtained by paracentesis. Normally, peritoneal fluid is sterile, odorless, clear to pale yellow, and less than 50 ml in volume, with no red blood cells, bacteria, or fungi. Normal values: white blood count—less than 300 mg/μl; protein—0.3 to 4.1 g/dl; glucose—70 to 100 mg/dl; amylase—138 to 404 U/L; ammonia—less than 50 μg/dl. Alkaline phosphatase: male

over 18 years—90 to 239 U/L; female under 45 years—76 to 196 U/L; female over 45 years—87 to 250 U/L.

Indications To determine the composition of ascitic fluid, to assist in diagnosis of hepatic or other systemic disease, or to detect abdominal trauma.

Complications Perforation of abdominal organs or vessels. Signs include those for hemorrhage and shock, increasing pain, and abdominal tenderness.

Patients with severe hepatic disease should be observed for signs of hepatic coma. Observe the patient for mental changes, drowsiness, and stupor.

Nursing care Record baseline vital signs, weight, and abdominal girth measurement for comparison with posttest results. Consent forms are generally required. The patient should void immediately before the procedure to prevent injury to bladder when the trocar is inserted. The patient is usually sitting with feet flat on the floor or on a foot stool and the back supported; if the patient cannot tolerate this, use a high Fowler's position.

Provide emotional support to the patient before and during the procedure.

Check vital signs every 15 minutes during the procedure and compare with baseline values; note signs of dizziness, pallor, perspiration, and increased anxiety. Rapid aspiration of peritoneal fluid may induce hypovolemia and shock; in such a case, slow the rate of aspiration.

After the test has been completed, monitor vital signs frequently (every 30 minutes for 2 hours; every hour for next 4 hours; every 4 hours for 24 hours). Weight and abdominal girth should be measured and compared with baseline.

Cover the site with a sterile dressing. If the site continues to drain, requiring frequent dressing changes, consider application of a skin barrier and a pouch for collection of drainage and accurate measurement of output.

Monitor urinary output for 24 hours and observe for hematuria. Observe the patient closely for signs of hypovolemic shock if large amounts were aspirated. Assess aspiration site for signs of infection.

Cytologies

Description Body secretions collected and examined for cells, which are stained and evaluated; examples are the Papanicolaou smear and examinations of cervical discharge, sputum, gastric washings, pleural fluid, and urinary washings.

Indications Suspected malignancies, infection, inflammation.

Complications None, usually.

Nursing care Explain purpose of test and tell patient what to expect. Assist with individual procedures.

Cerebrospinal fluid studies

Description

Lumbar puncture. Insertion of needle into the lumbar subarachnoid space to obtain cerebrospinal fluid for examination and to detect spinal subarachnoid block. The needle is inserted in the L3-L4 interspace.

Lateral cervical puncture. Insertion of a needle into the C1-C2 interspace through to the subarachnoid space to obtain cerebrospinal fluid. The needle is inserted perpendicular to the neck with the patient in a supine position.

Cisternal puncture. Insertion of a short-beveled needle immediately below the occipital bone into the cisterna magna to obtain cerebrospinal fluid. It can be inserted simultaneously with lumbar puncture to demonstrate subarachnoid block.

Ventricular puncture. Insertion of a ventricular needle (in adults and older children) through burr holes into the lateral ventricle.

Indications The lumbar puncture, or spinal tap, is a common neurologic test performed to measure cerebrospinal fluid pressure, remove cerebrospinal fluid for visualization and laboratory analysis, inject medications (i.e., spinal anesthesia, intrathecal injection of antibacterial agents) or contrast media, and determine the degree of subarachnoid block by means of spinal dynamics.

A cisternal puncture may be performed if a subarachnoid block is present, if a lumbar puncture is contraindicated, to reduce intracranial pressure, to perform encephalography, and to introduce air or a contrast medium for myelography.

A ventricular puncture is indicated if a lumbar or cisternal puncture is contraindicated, for injection of contrast medium into an infant's ventricles to determine the type of hydrocephalus, for removal of cerebrospinal fluid, for injection of air or oxygen to localize a tumor, and as a preliminary to ventricular drainage.

Complications Infection, leakage of cerebrospinal fluid, dysuria, headache, nausea, and vomiting. Signs of meningeal irritation are increased intracranial pressure and convulsions.

Nursing care Position the patient on a firm surface and maintain the spine in a horizontal position. Assist in obtaining a manometer reading of cerebrospinal fluid pressure. A sterile manometer is attached to the needle used in lumbar puncture and the pressure is measured. A pressure above 200 cm H_2O is considered abnormal.

If a subarachnoid block is suspected, a Queckenstedt test is performed. Place a blood pressure cuff around the patient's neck and inflate to 20 mm Hg pressure (or compress jugular veins) for 10 seconds. Obtain manometer pressure readings at 10-second intervals until the pressure stabilizes. Keep the patient flat in bed (or on side) for 4 to 6 hours after procedure. Force fluids, unless contraindicated. Monitor vital signs and neurologic signs frequently. The procedure should be performed with *extreme* caution when intracranial pressure is elevated. Provide emotional support to patient as indicated. Provide pain medication as necessary if headache develops.

Vaginal smears

Description Vaginal examination is performed, and vaginal secretions are placed on a slide with 1 drop of normal saline

placed on one side and 1 drop of 10% to 20% potassium hydroxide (KOH) on the other side.

Indications *Trichomonas vaginalis* can be observed at the saline end of the slide, and *Candida albicans* at the KOH side; other organisms can also be identified with this procedure.

Complications None.

Nursing care Prepare the patient for a vaginal examination and assist with the procedure. Provide emotional support as patient may fear results.

Fecal examinations

Fecal fat

Description Qualitative (random sample) and quantitative (72-hour collection) tests are used. Qualitative tests identify undigested muscle fibers and various fats, and quantitative tests can confirm steatorrhea. Fecal lipids normally are less than 20% of excreted solids or less than 7 g/24 hours.

A sudan stain can be made on a sample to test for presence of fat.

Indications Steatorrhea—excessive secretions of fecal lipids—may be observed in some malabsorption syndromes.

Complications None.

Nursing care Have the patient avoid alcohol ingestion for 72 hours before and during stool collection, and maintain a high-fat diet, 100 g/day for 72 hours before and during collection.

Avoid use of waxed collection containers because wax can become incorporated into the stool and distort results. Each specimen should be labeled appropriately and sent to the lab as soon as collected.

During the test, inform patient to avoid use of azathioprine, kanamycin, bisacodyl, cholestyramine, neomycin, colchicine, aluminum hydroxide, calcium carbonate, potassium chloride, and mineral oil because they inhibit absorption of fats or affect chemical digestion, producing inaccurate results.

Fecal urobilinogen

Description Determines the amount of urobilinogen (result of breakdown of bilirubin by intestinal flora) excreted in urine and feces.

Random stool specimen required. Normal values are 50 to 300 mg/24 hours. Low levels may indicate hepatocellular jaundice from cirrhosis or hepatitis or extrahepatic disorders such as tumors obstructing bile flow. Low levels are also seen in aplastic anemia with depressed erythropoiesis. Elevated levels are found in hemolytic jaundice, thalassemia, and hemolytic pernicious anemia.

Indications May be used as an indicator of hepatobiliary and hemolytic disorders.

Complications None.

Nursing care May be a 2-hour afternoon specimen or a 24-hour collection. If possible avoid the following for 2 weeks before stool collection: broad-spectrum antibiotics, which inhibit bacterial growth in the colon and may inhibit fecal urobilinogen levels; sulfonamides, which react with the reagents used in the test; salicylates, which in large doses can raise fecal urobilinogen levels. Stool container must be light-resistant because urobilinogen breaks down to urobilin on exposure to light.

Fecal occult blood

Description Procedure consists of a patient collecting small samples from three separate stool specimens. Their color may indicate the site of bleeding (e.g., melena is common with esophageal or gastric bleeding; a dark maroon color may indicate a lesion below the ligament of Treitz; and bright red may be from a low rectal carcinoma or hemorrhoids).

Indications Used to detect gastrointestinal bleeding and as a screening test for colorectal cancer.

Complications None.

Nursing care With guaiac-impregnated pad tests (Hemoccult, HemoFec, Colo-Screen), discuss with the patient how to collect the stool specimen. Have the patient avoid red meats, poultry, fish, turnips, and horseradish for 48 to 72 hours before the test begins and throughout the collection period.

Withhold iron preparations, bromides, iodides, rauwolfia derivatives, indomethacin, colchicine, salicylates, and phenylbutazone for 48 hours before collection begins and throughout the test. If the patient is taking steroids, accuracy of the test may be affected. Do not collect during menses because false positive results may be obtained. Ascorbic acid can interfere with the accuracy of the test and should be withheld 48 hours before the collection period begins.

With HemoQuant tests, explain to the patient how to use the collection device included in HemoQuant kits. Have the patient avoid ingesting aspirin and red meat for 48 to 72 hours before the test begins and during the collection period.

Roentgenograms

Chest roentgenogram (x-ray)

Description Gives information regarding the anatomic location and abnormalities of the heart, great vessels, and lungs. Routine views in a cardiac series are posterior-anterior (PA), lateral, right anterior oblique (RAO), and left anterior oblique (LAO). Roentgenograms are also used to determine the position of the heart (normal is situs solitus: left thoracic heart); cardiothoracic size (normal is less than 50% of the internal dimensions of the thorax); cardiac silhouette (thorax, aorta, ventricular chambers, atrial chambers, pulmonary artery); presence of calcifications (visualized in great vessels and on valves); lung fields (used to determine normal distribution of pulmonary blood flow); increase in pulmonary congestion; presence of pulmonary hypertension; and presence of pleural effusions.

The normal chest roentgenographic examination includes PA and lateral views (as shown in Figure III-1). In young, healthy individuals or in asymptomatic persons only the PA view is used for screening. A lateral view should be obtained if disease is suspected or if the individual is over 40 years old.

Chest roentgenograms in the upright position are preferred over those taken in the supine position so that the abdominal viscera does not push up on the diaphragm.

Indications Chest roentgenograms are evaluated for normal structure, position, and outlines, the presence of fluid lines, foreign bodies, infiltration, and abnormal shadows. An anterior oblique view may be used to visualize the thymus in patients with immune disorders.

Complications None.

Nursing care Explain the procedure. Inquire if the patient is or may be pregnant. All neck jewelry or garments containing metal clasps, buttons, or ornaments must be removed. The patient should be wearing a hospital gown.

Musculoskeletal films

Description Examination of musculoskeletal tissues by means of roentgenographic exposure.

Indications To determine injury, fracture, degeneration, inflammation, or neoplasm in one or more musculoskeletal tissues.

Complications None.

Nursing care Explain to the patient the purpose of the examination. Caution radiologic technicians to move the patient carefully and to support the joints above and below the affected tissues to prevent additional discomfort or trauma.

Sella turcica/skull films

Description Simple roentgenographic study of the skull. AP and lateral views are most frequently ordered to detect configuration, density, and vascular markings of skull. Initial roentgenographic evaluation of the pituitary gland begins with high-quality skull films that focus on the sella turcica, the bony structure in which the pituitary gland is located.

Indications Skull films provide important data about vascular abnormalities, the shape and size of the cranial and facial bones, the presence of fractured skull bones, degenerative changes (i.e., bone erosion), unusual calcifications (e.g., tumors or chronic subdural hematomas), the position of the pineal body, investigation for cranial masses, Cushing's disease workup, hypopituitary workup, and precocious puberty.

Complications None.

Nursing care Instruct the patient regarding the procedure.

Spinal films

Description Simple roentgenographic study of different spinal regions: cervical, thoracic, lumbar, or sacral. Anterior, posterior, and lateral views are most common.

Indications Spinal roentgenograms are taken when there has been trauma, pain, or sensory or motor impairment to the back or vertebral column. Roentgenograms of the spine usually include anterior, posterior, and lateral views to pinpoint fractures of the irregularly shaped vertebrae. Abnormal findings of spinal roentgenography include vertebral dislocation or fracture, bone erosion, unusual calcification, collapsed vertebrae and wedging, spondylosis, and spurs.

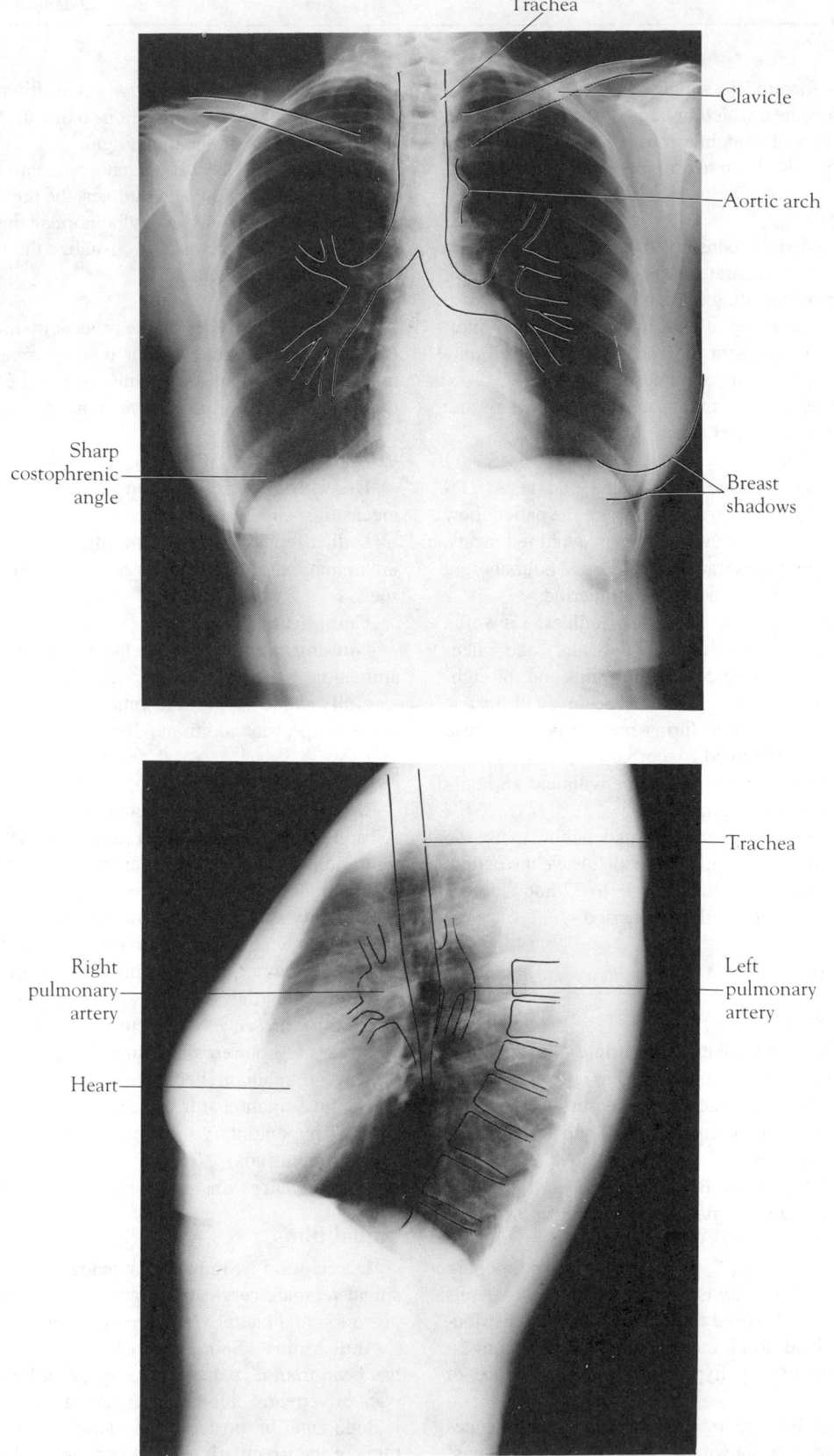

Figure III-1 Normal PA and lateral chest roentgenogram. Note no abnormal bony prominences, heart of normal size, sharp costophrenic angles, lung fields clear, diaphragms visible throughout except against heart border, mediastinum midline with bronchial structures visible, and breast shadows. (Courtesy R. Keith Wilson, M.D., Baylor College of Medicine, Houston, Texas.)

Complications None.

Nursing care Instruct the patient regarding the procedure.

Mastoid films

Description Roentgenograms of temporal bone. If mastoiditis is present, characteristic findings are clouding of the mastoid air cells and decalcification of bony walls between the cells.

Indications A thick purulent discharge from the ear, low-grade temperature, a dull ache behind the ear.

Complications None.

Nursing care Instruct the patient regarding the procedure.

Sinus films

Description Roentgenograms taken to diagnose sinusitis by determining clouding or possible fluid levels in sinuses. The usual views include Waters' view (orbits, frontal and maxillary sinuses, and nasal septum); Caldwell view (frontal sinuses, ethmoid air cells between each orbit, nasal septum, and petrous portion of temporal bone); and the lateral view (sphenoid sinus and posterior wall of frontal sinuses).

Indications Headache, facial pain, low-grade temperature, a feeling of fullness or pressure in the face or sinus area.

Complications None.

Nursing care Instruct the patient regarding the procedure.

Mammography, xeromammography

Description Mammography is soft tissue roentgenography of the breast with low-energy roentgenographic and high-contrast film. Xeromammography is the use of a dry photoelectric process to make roentgenograms of soft tissues of the breast. The roentgenographic image is recorded on an electrostatically charged plate. The image is transferred to plastic-coated paper by pressing the plate and the paper together and exposing them to heat. All of this is performed automatically in a commercial processor.

Indications The American Cancer Society's guidelines (1996) recommend that a woman get her first mammogram between the ages of 35 and 40; between the ages of 40 and 50, mammograms are recommended every other year, depending on the advice (and annual breast examination) of a physician; and annual mammograms are recommended after the age of 50. If a breast has been resected, the woman should have an annual mammogram of the other breast regardless of age.

Complications None.

Nursing care Ensure that the patient does not have powder, lotion, or ointment on her breasts. Explain the procedure and provide information to decrease anxiety about outcome of test.

Kidneys, ureters, bladder (KUB)

Description Roentgenographic film of kidneys, ureters, and bladder without contrast material. It is important as a scout film when performing an intravenous pyelogram and as a diagnostic study to determine the presence of radiopaque calculi, or to evaluate lower intestinal obstruction, soft tissue masses, or bowel perforations.

Indications To determine the size and location of kidneys and radiopaque stones; to detect abnormal gas patterns in the GI tract.

Complications None.

Nursing care Preparation is not standardized. An IVP prep is used when KUB is performed as part of this extensive roentgenographic study. In other situations, no preparation is indicated.

Contrast Studies

Contrast radiography

Description Examination of an area of the body with a contrast medium during a roentgenographic study. Barium sulfate is one form of a contrast medium given by mouth or rectum for intestinal studies; meglumine diatrizoate is another form and can be injected or given intravenously or through a tube or catheter. Other commercial agents are available.

Single-contrast intestinal studies use barium alone, whereas double-contrast studies use barium and air.

In addition to roentgenography (passage of radiation through the patient to create a roentgenogram), cineradiography, fluoroscopy, and video are used in many of these procedures. Cineradiography is a rapid-sequence roentgenographic procedure that films motion; fluoroscopy is the projection of roentgenograms onto a screen or fluoroscope, permitting continuous observation of motion.

Indications Examination of soft and bony tissues of the body; diagnosis of certain pathologic conditions that requires the visualization of details not revealed by plain film radiography.

Complications Barium retained in the intestine may harden and cause an obstruction or fecal impaction. Before giving meglumine diatrizoate, check for hypersensitivity to iodine, seafood, and contrast media. Symptoms of an allergic reaction include nausea, vomiting, flushing, urticaria, sweating, and (rarely) anaphylaxis. An intraductal injection may be accompanied by tachycardia and fever.

Nursing care Barium as a contrast material precludes effective use of fiberoptic endoscopy for several hours and of arteriography for 24 to 48 hours.

For most patients, clear liquids before and forced fluids after a barium procedure, along with ambulation, are sufficient to clear the barium from the intestine. Healthy patients may take a mild laxative. Inform the patient of the need to clear all the barium. The nurse may need to examine the patient's stools to ensure this is happening, especially if the patient is debilitated. Inform patients that stools will initially be very light in color, darkening as the barium is eliminated.

The patient with a colostomy should be instructed to irrigate after the barium procedure is concluded and to repeat the irrigation the next morning. If upper gastrointestinal series or small bowel follow-through has been performed, the patient should irrigate after the last delayed spot film (approximately 6 hours after ingestion). The patient with an ileostomy should never receive a laxative or an enema before or after a barium study.

Ventriculography

Description A ventriculogram depends on the injection of air or positive contrast medium via a ventricular puncture directly into the lateral cerebral ventricles. The procedure is performed in the operating room under strict aseptic technique. Following the ventricular puncture, cerebrospinal fluid is gradually removed and replaced with air or a positive contrast medium, and roentgenograms are taken.

Indications Indications for a ventriculogram include determination of patency of the ventricular system, localization of a brain tumor, and detection of cerebral anomalies.

Complications Nausea and vomiting, headache, increased intracranial pressure, respiratory distress, seizures, air embolus, shock.

Nursing care General anesthesia may be required for young pediatric patients. Observe for signs and symptoms of intracranial or subdural hematoma (especially in patients with noncommunicating hydrocephalus). Frequently monitor vital signs and neurologic signs. Keep the patient flat in bed for 24 to 48 hours after the procedure. Encourage fluids. Keep accurate intake and output records. Institute seizure precautions for 24 hours after the procedure.

Barium swallow

Description Examination of the pharynx and esophagus on a fluoroscope after barium sulfate ingestion.

Indications Used to diagnose or detect hiatal hernia, achalasia, diverticulum, varices, strictures, ulcers, tumors, motility disorders, and polyps.

Complications Retained barium may harden and cause an impaction or obstruction.

Nursing care Required fasting after midnight. Once the mixture is ingested, the patient is placed in various positions. The esophagus is also examined fluoroscopically during swallowing of the solution. Barium swallow is contraindicated in patients with an intestinal obstruction. Ensure evacuation of barium, as described previously.

Upper gastrointestinal and small bowel series (UGI and SB series)

Description Fluoroscopic examination of the esophagus, stomach, and small intestine after ingestion of barium sulfate; as barium passes through the system, fluoroscopy outlines mucosal contours. Spot films are used to record significant findings. Follow-up spot films after 6 hours can provide some evaluation of gastrointestinal motility. The procedure is contraindicated in patients with intestinal perforations and intestinal obstructions.

Indications Useful in detecting or diagnosing hiatal hernias, diverticulum, varices, ulcers, strictures, tumors, regional enteritis (also called granulomatous ileitis or Crohn's ileitis), and motility disorders.

Complications Retained barium may cause a fecal impaction or obstruction.

Nursing care The patient is given nothing by mouth past midnight, and a mild laxative may be ordered. The patient should also increase fluid intake and maintain a low-residue diet for 2 to 3 days before test. Smoking should be avoided from midnight before the test and throughout procedure. Anticholinergics and narcotics are withheld for 24 hours before the study if intestinal motility is of concern. Ensure evacuation of barium as described.

Oral cholecystography (OCG)

Description Roentgenographic examination of the gallbladder. Contrast medium is given the evening before the test. Iopanoic acid is usually used, but other commercial contrast media are available. The abdomen is examined fluoroscopically to evaluate gallbladder opacification. Spot films are taken of significant findings. Fat stimulus may also be used during the roentgenographic procedure. Fluoroscopy is then used to observe emptying of the gallbladder. Spot films are taken, as indicated.

The procedure is not performed in the presence of severe renal or hepatic disease or jaundice.

Indications Evaluation of gallbladder disease.

Complications Diarrhea commonly occurs; nausea, vomiting, and abdominal cramps, or dysuria occurs in rare cases.

Nursing care The diet before the test includes a lunch meal containing fats and a fat-free evening meal. Check the patient for allergies to iodine, seafood, or contrast media before giving tablets—iopanoic acid, 3 g, given as one tablet with a total of 240 ml (8 oz) of water. Check any emesis or diarrheal stools for undigested tablets.

Barium enema

Description Instillation of barium sulfate or barium sulfate and air through the anus into the large intestine. A barium enema should precede a barium-swallow upper gastrointestinal series with small bowel follow-through. Once this was the most effective means of identifying colon carcinomas above the level of sigmoidoscope; colonoscopy examinations are now effectively used for visualization of the entire large intestine.

Barium enemas are contraindicated in patients with fulminant inflammatory bowel disease, toxic megacolon, suspected perforations, and suspected obstructions. Caution should be used for patients with acute inflammatory bowel disease, ischemic bowel disease, acute fulminant bloody diarrhea, and pneumatosis cystoides intestinalis.

Indications Used as one method of diagnosing colorectal cancer and inflammatory bowel disease. It will also detect polyps, diverticula, and other changes in the colon and rectum.

Complications Retained barium may cause fecal impaction or obstruction.

Nursing care Careful bowel preparation is necessary to cleanse the bowel of fecal material. An ileostomy patient has no large intestine and requires only clear liquid for 24 to 48 hours as a "bowel" preparation; the site of the colostomy will determine the preparation.

Patients with suspected inflammatory bowel disease (ulcerative colitis or granulomatous colitis) should not be given a routine preparatory kit for barium enemas. The condition can be greatly exacerbated by irritants and may require surgical intervention; check with the physician.

Evacuation of barium from the bowel should be ensured, as previously described.

Intravenous cholangiography (IVC)

Description   Provides better visualization of the biliary ducts than does oral cholangiography, which is useful in gallbladder disease. IVC involves roentgenographic and tomographic studies after intravenous infusion of a contrast medium. Fluoroscopy spot films are made every 10 minutes until visualization of the bile ducts is satisfactory, which may take 25 to 40 minutes; tomograms are then made. Films and tomograms are repeated 2 to 2½ hours later, when maximal opacification of the gallbladder has occurred. (This would be unnecessary in patients with cholecystectomies.) Delayed films of the gallbladder may be taken at 4 and 24 hours. IVC should precede any barium studies, since retained barium clouds roentgenograms.

Indications   Generally indicated in patients with right upper quadrant or epigastric pain after cholecystectomy. Pain suggests biliary tract disease.

Complications   Hypersensitivity reactions.

Nursing care   The diet should be low residue the day before the test with an evening meal high in simple fats (milk, cream, eggs, butter); the patient should be given nothing to eat after midnight. Mild cathartics may be ordered. Check with the patient for a history of hypersensitivities to iodine, seafood, and contrast media. A fatty meal may be given so that, with fluoroscopy, emptying may be viewed.

Hypotonic duodenography

Description   Barium sulfate and air instilled through an intestinal catheter for fluoroscopic examination of the duodenum. Intravenous infusion of glucagon or intramuscular injection of propantheline bromide is used to induce duodenal atony. A catheter is inserted through the nose and into the stomach while the patient is sitting; in a supine position under fluoroscopy, a catheter is advanced into the duodenum.

Administration of anticholinergics is contraindicated in the presence of severe cardiac disorders or glaucoma.

Indications   Demonstrates small duodenal lesions and tumors at the head of the pancreas.

Complications   Retained barium may cause fecal impaction or obstruction.

Nursing care   Explain the procedure to the patient. Ensure the evacuation of barium from the bowel as described.

Percutaneous transhepatic cholangiography

Description   Fluoroscopic examination of biliary ducts after the injection of iodinated contrast medium directly into the biliary tree. The liver is punctured by a thin, flexible needle, and contrast medium is injected as the needle is slowly withdrawn. Contrast medium slowly flows through the biliary ducts, outlining the biliary tree. The catheter used to inject the dye is sometimes left in place to drain the biliary tree.

Percutaneous transhepatic cholangiography is contraindicated in patients with cholangitis, severe ascites, uncorrectable coagulopathy, and hypersensitivity to iodine.

Indications   Helps to distinguish between obstructive and nonobstructive jaundice. The procedure helps to determine the location, the extent, and often the cause of mechanical obstruction of the biliary tree.

Complications   Hypersensitivity reactions, peritonitis, bleeding.

Nursing care   Check with the patient for a history of hypersensitivity to iodine, seafood, or contrast media. Check the patient for normal bleeding, clotting, prothrombin times, and platelet count.

The patient should remain in bed for 6 hours after the procedure. Check vital signs frequently (every 15 minutes for 1 hour, every 30 minutes for the next 2 hours, every hour for 4 hours after that, and then every 4 hours). Check the injection site for bleeding, swelling, and tenderness. Check for signs of peritonitis: chills, a temperature of 38° to 39° C (102° to 103° F), abdominal pain, tenderness, distention.

Postoperative cholangiography or T-tube cholangiography

Description   Contrast medium is injected through a T-tube, and the flow of medium outlining biliary tree can be visualized with fluoroscopy. This is performed 7 to 10 days following a cholecystectomy or common bile duct exploration in which a T-tube has been left in the common bile duct to facilitate drainage.

Indications   To evaluate the patency and size of ducts and to identify calculi, strictures, neoplasms, or fistulas in the ductal system.

Complications   Sepsis, hypersensitivity reactions.

Nursing care   Some physicians have the T-tube clamped for 24 hours before the procedure to eliminate air bubbles in the tube. A cleansing enema to evacuate large intestine may be ordered. Check with the patient for allergies to iodine, seafood, and contrast media.

The T-tube may be removed after the procedure if no stones are obstructing the common duct. A sterile dressing is applied. Note the amount and characteristics of any drainage. If frequent dressing changes are required, consider application of a sterile skin barrier and drainable pouch. Monitor the patient for signs and symptoms of peritonitis.

Endoscopic retrograde cholangiopancreatography (ERCP)

Description   Fluoroscopic examination of the pancreatic duct and hepatobiliary ductal system by injection of a contrast medium into the duodenal papilla. Endoscopy is performed, and the duodenal papilla located. A cannula filled with contrast medium is passed through the endoscope, into the duodenal papilla and ampulla of Vater. The pancreas is visualized first with injection of dye and then fluoroscopically; then the cannula is repositioned for injection of additional contrast medium, allowing for visualization of the hepatobiliary tree. Tissue biopsy or fluid for histology may be obtained before the endoscope is removed. Some centers are able to perform sphincterotomy and to snare and remove stones.

ERCP is contraindicated in patients with acute pancreatitis, pancreatic pseudocysts, strictures or obstruction of the esophagus or duodenum, cholangitis, infectious disease, or cardiorespiratory disease.

Indications   To diagnose cancer of the duodenal papilla, pancreas, or biliary ducts; to detect calculi or stenosis of ducts; and to evaluate obstructive jaundice.

Complications   Cholangitis and pancreatitis may develop. Signs of cholangitis include fever, chills, and hyperbilirubinemia; late symptoms may include hypotension and gram-negative septicemia. Pancreatitis may be indicated by upper left quadrant pain, tenderness, elevated serum amylase, and transient hyperbilirubinemia.

Nursing care   Assess the patient for a history of hypersensitivity to iodine, seafood, or contrast media.

Frequent vital sign checks are indicated when the procedure is completed (every 15 minutes for 4 hours; every hour for the next 4 hours; and then every 4 hours for 48 hours). Check for voiding, since urinary retention may be a side effect of anticholinergics. Monitor the patient for bleeding after the procedure, and for signs and symptoms of cholangitis or pancreatitis.

Splenoportography (transsplenic portography)

Description   Cineradiographic study of the splenic veins and portal system. It generally provides a cleaner definition of the venous system than does superior mesenteric arteriography (which offers the advantage of outlining the splenic and portal veins during reverse blood flow and has fewer complications). Splenoportography may result in excessive bleeding, requiring transfusions and occasionally a splenectomy.

Splenic pulp pressure is measured before the dye is injected by attaching a spinal manometer filled with normal saline to a sheath inserted in the spleen. Normal splenic pulp pressure is 50 to 180 mm H_2O (or 3.5 to 13.5 mm Hg). Contrast medium is injected into the splenic pulp.

This procedure is contraindicated in patients with ascites, uncorrectable coagulopathy, splenomegaly secondary to infection, hypersensitivity to iodine, or markedly impaired liver or kidney function.

Indications   Used to diagnose or assess portal hypertension and to stage cirrhosis.

Complications   Hypersensitivity reactions, bleeding.

Nursing care   Assess the patient for a history of allergies to iodine, seafood, or contrast media. Frequent assessment of vital signs is required after the procedure (every 15 minutes for 1 hour, every 30 minutes for the next 2 hours, and then every hour for 4 hours). Check for bleeding, swelling, and tenderness at the site of injection.

The patient should remain on the left side for 24 hours to minimize risk of bleeding. An additional 24 hours of bed rest is recommended. Hematocrit levels may be obtained every 8 to 12 hours until values have stabilized.

Intravenous pyelogram (IVP), intravenous urogram, excretory urogram

Description   Contrast-enhanced roentgenographic study that provides detailed anatomic information about the urinary tract. Clues to kidney function are provided by assessment of the organ's ability to concentrate and excrete contrast material. Information concerning the transport of urine through the ureters is provided by use of sequential films after a contrast medium is injected. Compression over ureters may be used to provide additional detail. Assessment of bladder function is made by obtaining films of the vesicle filled with contrast material (after asking the patient to void). IVP is performed after adequate preparation and after a KUB is done.

The patient is placed in a slight Trendelenburg's position or supine, and contrast material is injected intravenously. Serial films of kidneys, ureters, and the bladder are obtained over a period of time. The entire examination requires approximately 30 minutes. A nephrotomogram may be performed as part of the IVP to provide a more detailed reproduction of anatomic detail by focusing on a specific plane of the kidney rather than a nonspecific picture of the entirety of the kidneys.

Because of the risk of hypersensitivity reactions and potential renal failure secondary to IVP, a number of relative contraindications should be considered before completing the study. These include (1) a history of allergic reaction when given intravenous iodine-bound contrast material and (2) patients at higher risk for dehydration, including elderly persons and patients with severe diabetes mellitus, multiple myeloma, renal insufficiency, or only one functioning kidney.

Indications   Evaluation of renal masses, cysts, ureteral obstruction, retroperitoneal tumors, renal trauma, and bladder abnormalities; evaluation of renal disease and hypertension.

Complications   Hypersensitive reactions and acute renal failure. Observe for allergic reactions such as urticaria, rhonchi, and shortness of breath. Acute renal failure is a rare but serious complication of IVP. Observe urinary output (at least 30 ml/hour) while ensuring adequate fluid intake.[14]

Nursing care   Explain procedure to patient, and tell him or her that sequential or serial films are normal. Ensure that patient has no allergies to iodine. After procedure, encourage increased fluid intake to ensure excretion of contrast.

Whitaker and Pfister tests

Description   The Whitaker test is performed by placing a nephrostomy tube percutaneously into the pelvis of the affected kidney. A urethral catheter is also placed to measure bladder pressure. Sterile water, saline, or radiographic contrast material is perfused through the nephrostomy tube via a pump at a specific rate. Continuous-pressure monitoring is used to detect the presence of ureteral obstruction with the bladder empty and full.

The Pfister test is similar to the Whitaker test, except that a 20-gauge spinal needle is used in place of a nephrostomy tube, and intermittent rather than continuous pressure monitoring is used to assess ureteral obstruction.

Indications   Performed to assess ureteral obstruction when other methods (IVP, Lasix-enhanced renogram) fail to diagnose clearly or to rule out any obstruction.

Complications   Bleeding and infection.

Nursing care   Vital signs should be monitored regularly for the first 24 hours after testing. Temperature is an important parameter in the assessment of febrile urinary tract infection.

Elderly patients may not become febrile with a UTI and should have other vital signs monitored carefully.

Retrograde pyelogram (RPG)

Description   Provides a detailed anatomic description of the ureter and renal pelvis. It is performed in conjunction with cystoscopy because it requires placement of a 4 or 5 French ureteral catheter within the ureter to be studied. Radiographic contrast material is then injected into the collecting system via gravity infusion or by syringe, and roentgenographic images are obtained.

Indications   Evaluation of renal disease, obstruction, trauma, or in patients who are not candidates for IVP due to insufficient blood flow.

Complications   Pyelonephritis and overdistention of renal collecting system, which may result in extravasation of contrast medium leading to pain and fever. The reaction is typically transient; effects should disappear within 48 hours.

Nursing care   The patient should be closely observed for signs of infection (flank pain, fever, chills) for a 24- or 48-hour period after testing.

Retrograde urethrogram (RUG)

Description   Provides a detailed description of urethral anatomy. It is made by injecting contrast material in a retrograde manner into the urethra via a catheter-tipped syringe or a Brodny clamp. The patient is typically placed in a supine position, and oblique films are taken.

Indications   Evaluation of trauma or stricture.

Complications   Urethritis, cystitis.

Nursing care   The patient should be encouraged to force fluids for a 24-hour period after testing. Mild dysuria should cease within 24 hours of testing. Inform patients that sitz baths may help. Watch for signs of infection.

Cystogram, voiding cystourethrogram (VCUG)

Description   Provides a detailed picture of bladder anatomy; also, vesicoureteral reflux is assessed by visualizing the area over the ureters and right and left renal pelves. A voiding cystourethrogram provides information given by a cystogram along with images of the urethra during the voiding phase of bladder function. A cystogram is performed by infusing a roentgenographic medium intravesically under fluoroscopic monitoring. A voiding cystourethrogram is made in the same manner. Urethral images during voiding are obtained by removing the catheter and asking the patient to void while under the fluoroscope.

Indications   Assessment of bladder function.

Complications   Because cystogram and VCUG require placement of an indwelling catheter, cystitis is a potential complication.

Nursing care   The patient should be encouraged to force fluids for 24 hours following testing. Urinary frequency or mild dysuria should disappear completely within 24 hours.

Hysterosalpingography

Description   Injection of radiopaque contrast material, such as ionized oil or water-soluble material, through the cervix so that it fills the cervical canal and body of the uterus, flows through the fallopian tubes, and spills into the peritoneal cavity. The procedure should be performed no sooner than 6 weeks after delivery, abortion, or dilation and curettage.

The patient should be screened for contraindications to the procedure, including active pelvic inflammatory disease, vaginitis, cervicitis, or severe systemic illness.

Indications   Most commonly, to determine whether infertility is caused by an anatomic defect. It can also be used to confirm tubal occlusion and investigate the cause of dysmenorrhea, postmenopausal bleeding, or repeated abortion.

Complications   None.

Nursing care   The patient may experience pelvic pain resulting from spillage of contrast material; manage, as indicated, with pain medication. If indicated by the physician, assist the patient to walk for 30 minutes after the procedure until another film is taken.

Myelogram

Description   A roentgenographic procedure in which a needle is inserted into a disc space below the spinal cord, and 2 to 6 ml of spinal fluid is removed. A radiopaque solution is injected and distributed to the various tissues and structures to be examined, and roentgenograms are taken frequently. A water-soluble radiopaque solution is absorbed into the cerebrospinal fluid rather rapidly, but an oil-based solution must be removed by tilting the patient while observing the image monitor until the solution moves to the needle tip, from which it is withdrawn into a syringe. It is important that all or most of the solution be removed because even small amounts of retained solution may lead to persistent postmyelogram headaches and possibly adhesive arachnoiditis.

Indications   Aids in the diagnosis of spinal stenosis or obstruction within the spinal canal caused by a ruptured or herniated nucleus pulposus. It also detects distortion of spinal cord, spinal nerve roots, and the subarachnoid space.

Complications   Complications vary depending on whether a water-soluble agent, metrizamide (Amipaque), or an oil agent, iophendylate (Pantopaque), is used. With metrizamide, the patient may have nausea, vomiting, or headache and possible seizures, chest pain, dysrhythmias, and speech disorders. With iophendylate, common complications include headache, meningeal and nerve root irritation, and adhesive arachnoiditis.

Nursing care   The patient is allowed a clear liquid breakfast and then is given nothing by mouth. Any possible allergy to iodine is determined, and a mild sedative (diazepam, 10 mg) may be given. The patient must lie flat in bed for 8 to 12 hours if oily iophendylate was used, and fluids are forced to replace the cerebrospinal fluid. After the use of metrizamide the head of the patient's bed may be raised and fluids forced. If the patient complains of a headache, lowering the bed to the flat position is usually sufficient to relieve the pain. Mild analgesics may be ordered for persistent pain. Observe the patient for the other side effects already described.

Discogram

Description   A roentgenographic procedure similar to a myelogram, in which radiopaque solution is injected into a disc space (L3-L5 areas) and roentgenograms are taken.

Indications   To determine the condition of the disc spaces.

Complications   Possible development of discitis.

Nursing care   Explain to the patient that a radiopaque solution will be injected into the disc and roentgenograms will be taken. After the procedure, neurologic checks are performed, and mild analgesics may be required for pain. Monitor vital signs frequently.

Arthrogram

Description   Through use of a radiopaque solution, fluoroscopy, and multiple roentgenograms, any tissues not normally seen by roentgenograms are visualized. A needle is inserted into the joint; its position is verified by fluoroscopic examination. A radiopaque solution is injected into the joint, and the needle is removed. The site is sealed with collodion. The patient is asked to move the joint through its range of motion while roentgenograms are taken. The radiopaque solution is usually rapidly absorbed into the joint fluids.

Indications   To outline the structures of the joint capsule being studied and to aid in the diagnosis of injuries to the joint muscles, ligaments, cartilage, or bursa.

Complications   Joint swelling after the procedure, soreness or pain, and crepitus (noise on joint movement).

Nursing care   Explain to the patient that skin around the joint will be cleansed with an antiseptic and that a local anesthetic will be administered. After the procedure, instruct the patient in applying a compression bandage and ice around the joint to lessen edema. Explain that the joint should be held at rest for 12 or more hours and that use is then dependent on the findings of the arthrogram. Mild analgesics can be prescribed for pain.

Electrodiagnostic Studies

Electrocardiogram (ECG, EKG)

Description   Electrical representation of myocardial activity. It is used to determine the presence of abnormal transmission of heart impulses through the conduction tissue of heart muscle (see Chapter 1 for normal findings).

Indications   Chest pain; to evaluate cardiac disturbance; for routine diagnostic study during physical examinations and preoperatively.

Complications   None.

Nursing care   Explain the procedure. Ensure electrical safety measures, and provide privacy during the procedure.

Ambulatory electrocardiography (Holter monitor)

Description   A portable recorder, worn by the patient, magnetically records cardiac activity continuously while the patient is going about usual activities. The tapes are scanned by electrocardioscanners, and areas of interest can be printed out in real time.

Indications   Used to detect ECG rhythm disturbances that may occur over an extended period of time, to evaluate effectiveness of antidysrhythmic drug therapy, and to evaluate chest pain episodes. It is also capable of recording ECGs over a 24- to 48-hour period.

Complications   None.

Nursing care   Explain the procedure. Instruct the patient in the care of electrodes at home and about the importance of keeping a diary of symptoms or activities at times designated by the physician.

Electrophysiologic studies (bundle of His)

Description   Involves insertion of a catheter via a peripheral vein into the right atrium and right ventricle (right heart catheterization).

Indications   To detect atrioventricular conduction disturbances, diagnose syncope, and assist in selection of antidysrhythmic agents.

A-V interval (atrioventricular): conduction time from the low right atrium through the AV node to the His bundle. Normal is 60 to 125 msec.

H-V interval (His-ventricle): conduction time from the proximal His bundle to the ventricular myocardium. Normal is 35 to 55 msec.

P-A interval: conduction time from the beginning of the P wave to the beginning of the A defection. Normal is 20 to 40 msec.

Sinus node disease: sinus node exit block; depression of sinus node automaticity.

Atrioventricular block: Mobitz II.

Intraventricular block: bifascicular block.

Tachycardias: supraventricular tachycardia with a rate of more than 200 beats per minute associated with symptoms, or with recurrent bouts that are refractory to therapy.

Accessory pathway tachycardias: Wolff-Parkinson-White syndrome.

Ventricular tachycardia: tachycardia caused by irritable ventricular foci firing repetitively.

Unexplained syncope: cardiac arrest patients resuscitated from sudden cardiac death.

Contraindications include dysrhythmias that will be difficult to treat because of an underlying cardiac disorder, e.g., acute myocardial infarction, class IV heart failure, severe aortic stenosis.

Complications   Dysrhythmias, phlebitis, pulmonary emboli, hemorrhage, cardiac perforation.

Nursing care   Ensure that informed consent is obtained. Explain that the procedure will last 1 to 3 hours and that the patient will be awake and may feel slight pressure. Instruct the patient to report any discomfort. Permit nothing by mouth for 6 hours before the procedure. After the procedure, check vital signs every 15 minutes for 1 hour, then every 4 hours for 24 hours. Check the insertion site for bleeding every 30 minutes to 1 hour for 8 hours.

Electroencephalogram (EEG)

Description   An electroencephalogram (EEG) provides a graphic record of brain wave activity. Generally, between 17 and 21 electrodes are attached with collodion to the patient's head at corresponding areas over the prefrontal, frontal, temporal, parietal, and occipital lobes. After the electrodes are attached, the patient is instructed to remain quiet with the eyes closed and is informed of the need to refrain from talking or moving unless otherwise required (the patient is asked to hyperventilate for a short period during the test to accentuate abnormalities).

The brain waves recorded during an EEG are called alpha, beta, delta, and theta rhythms. *Alpha* rhythms occur in the adult at 8 to 13 cycles/sec and are most prominent in the occipital leads. Apprehension and anxiety can decrease the frequency of the alpha waves. *Beta* wave forms are prominent in the frontal and central areas and occur at a rate of 18 to 30 cycles/sec. Beta rhythm indicates normal activity, when an individual is alert and attentive with the eyes open. *Delta* wave forms indicate serious brain dysfunction or deep sleep. This rhythm occurs at a rate of less than 4 cycles/sec. *Theta* wave forms occur at a rate of 4 to 7 cycles/sec and come primarily from the temporal and parietal areas. Theta rhythm indicates drowsiness or emotional stress in adults.

Complications None.

Nursing care Stimulants such as coffee, tea, chocolate, cola, and smoking are not permitted for 8 hours before the procedure. The adult patient should have minimal sleep (i.e., 4 to 5 hours) the night before the procedure. Explain to patient that if taking anticonvulsant medications, the medications should be continued. Hair should be washed before test. Post-test ensure that paste is removed from patient's hair; some paste is water-soluble, but some requires acetone for removal.

Electromyogram (EMG)

Description Surface electrodes or monopolar electrodes measure and record electrical properties of skeletal muscle and nerve conduction. Electrical activity is picked up by a needle electrode inserted into the muscle and displayed on a cathode-ray oscilloscope. For example, EMG needles, hooked wire electrodes, and pediatric ECG surface electrodes may be placed directly into the external urinary sphincter, or they may be placed over the perianal sphincter to measure the activity of pelvic floor musculature, including the response of the urinary sphincter to bladder filling and storage and to micturition.

Indications The diagnosis of myopathies and muscle responses to electrical stimuli may be performed in the patient's room, depending on the number of muscles to be studied.

Complications None.

Nursing care Explain to the patient that a small needle will be inserted into one or more muscles to be studied and that the muscle will be stimulated with a small electrical impulse. The results will be recorded on a graph. Explain to the patient that the procedure may cause some minor discomfort when the needle is inserted but otherwise is not painful.

Nerve conduction velocity determination

Description Study of nerve conduction velocity calculated by division of the distance between proximal and distal points by the time required for the electrical stimulus to travel between those two points.

Indications To diagnose neuromuscular problems.

Complications None.

Nursing care Explain that this study may be performed in conjunction with the electromyogram (EMG) and uses the same machine.

Electrocochleography

Description Permeatal transtympanic electrode placement in contact with the promontory of the cochlea to record acoustically evoked potentials from the cochlea. Three distinct evoked potentials can be recorded: cochlear microphonic potential, summating potential, and vestibulocochlear nerve compound action potential.

Indications Measures auditory function; aids in the differential diagnosis of auditory disorders (i.e., vestibulocochlear nerve disorders); provides the prognosis for auditory disorders.

Complications Potential vertigo, middle ear infection, perilymph leak.

Nursing care Explain the procedure to the patient.

Electronystagmography

Description Graphic recording and measuring electrical potentials of eye movements during spontaneous, positional, or calorically-evoked nystagmus. Intensity, frequency, and speed of the fast and slow components of nystagmus are recorded.

Indications To assess and evaluate neurologic disorders.

Complications None.

Nursing care Patient's eyes must be open during the procedure.

Plethysmography

Description Measures venous flow in limbs by recording changes in volume and vascular resistance. There are two types: digital plethysmography (to evaluate digital pulse volume) and venous occlusion plethysmography (to evaluate arterial responses to temporary block of the venous system). A pneumatic cuff is applied to a limb to occlude venous return. Two electrodes are applied to the limb, and a very weak electrical current is passed through it. The resistance of the limb to the current is measured and recorded on graph paper.

Indications Used to detect deep vein thrombosis in the leg and to screen patients at high risk for thrombophlebitis.

Complications None.

Nursing care Explain the procedure, and assist the patient into a position to promote venous drainage of the limb to be studied.

Ultrasound

Ultrasonography

Description The ultrasound machine uses high-frequency waves (5000 to 20,000 Hz) to detect vibrations reflected from soft tissues of varying density. The vibrations (echoes) are converted into electrical potential and displayed on an oscillograph. The A-scan machine registers varying acoustic densities as spikes on linear tracing; the B-scan registers a two-dimensional "picture."

Ultrasonography is a painless procedure that is useful in evaluating soft tissues and does not involve the use of roentgen rays. A transducer, which is able to transmit and to receive high-frequency sound waves, is placed against the patient's body. The sound waves, which cannot be heard by the human ear, are bounced off the tissues inside the body. Tissues of different densities echo the sound in different ways. The echoes are received by the machine and are translated into an image on a TV screen.

In dehydrated patients, ultrasound can fail to define boundaries between organs and tissue structures because of a deficiency of body fluids.

Indications   Ultrasonography is useful for assessment of almost all body systems.

Head and neck.   For the eye ultrasonography is useful for diagnosing intraocular tumors, retinal detachment, and fibrous tissue proliferation. The examiner holds the probe (attached to machine) over the patient's eyelid. For the thyroid, ultrasonography reveals diffuse or localized enlargements of the gland and differentiates between cystic or solid lesions.

Chest.   Ultrasound has limited usefulness in evaluation of the lungs because sound beams are not transmitted well by air-containing tissue. Ultrasonographic examination is useful to detect pericardial effusion and fluid-containing or solid tissue lesions.

Gastrointestinal

Gallbladder and biliary system.   Ultrasonography of the gallbladder and biliary system can be used if cholecystography is inconclusive or does not adequately visualize the gallbladder. It is useful in confirming cholelithiasis, diagnosing acute cholecystitis, and distinguishing between obstructive and nonobstructive jaundice. Sincalide, a hormonal analogue, may be given to cause the gallbladder to contract and expel bile. It allows an evaluation of gallbladder function.

Liver.   Ultrasonography of the liver is indicated for patients with jaundice of unknown cause, since it helps to distinguish between obstructive and nonobstructive jaundice. It can be used in a screening or diagnostic test for hepatocellular disease and hepatic metastases. It can also be used after abdominal trauma to detect a hematoma and define cold spots found on liver scans in the presence of severe ascites. Ultrasonic examination may be combined with placement of a biopsy needle to evaluate masses or obtain specimens for culture.

Spleen.   Ultrasonography of the spleen is used to demonstrate splenomegaly, to evaluate changes in splenic size, to evaluate the spleen following abdominal trauma, and to clarify cold spots found on scans of the spleen. CT scans often provide more information on splenomegaly than ultrasonography does.

Pancreas.   Ultrasonography of the pancreas is used to detect anatomic abnormalities such as pseudocysts and pancreatic carcinomas. It detects alterations in size, contour, and parenchymal texture of the pancreas.

Renal and genitourinary tracts.   Ultrasonography of these tracts is a noninvasive way to identify a dilated collecting system, calculi, cysts, perirenal collections of blood, pus, lymph, or urine, solid masses, and kidney size.

Ultrasonography of kidneys.   The patient is placed in the prone position. An outline of the kidneys is obtained and marked on the skin. Serial scans are made 1 to 2 cm apart perpendicular to the longitudinal axis. Obtaining additional views with the patient in a supine position helps elucidate the kidneys' position relative to other abdominal organs.

Ultrasound-guided biopsy of kidney.   Ultrasonic examination may be combined with placement of a biopsy needle to define makeup of a renal or juxtarenal mass. Routine ultrasonographic examination of the affected kidney is completed first. The mass is then located and marked on the skin. With use of sterile drapes, gloves, and a local anesthetic, the biopsy needle is placed into the mass, and a tissue sample is withdrawn. Aspiration of a renal cyst may be performed the same way.

Ultrasonography of bladder and ureters.   Ultrasonography of a distended bladder provides some detail of vesical outline and may be used to evaluate the diverticulum. Abdominal ultrasound detects the presence of ureteral dilation, although normal ureters may not be completely visualized. It is typically combined with examination of the kidneys.

Ultrasonography of testes.   This is used to differentiate solid and cystic masses. In addition, torsion of the testes is assessed by Doppler ultrasound techniques, which assess both testicular morphology and blood flow.

Ankle pressure.   Doppler ultrasound is used to measure systolic blood pressure in distal arteries, to amplify audible sounds of peripheral pulses, and to measure blood flow velocity along the course of an artery. Ankle systolic pressure should be equal to or greater than brachial systolic pressure—0.45 to 0.75 mm Hg (ankle/brachial index).

Complications   Bleeding with ultrasound-guided biopsies.

Nursing care   Explain the procedure to the patient. For gastrointestinal ultrasonography, the patient is allowed nothing by mouth 8 to 12 hours before the procedure to reduce bowel gas. For gallbladder ultrasound give the patient nothing to eat for 8 to 12 hours before the procedure. The patient should have a fat-free meal the evening before the test (which allows bile to accumulate in the gallbladder). For ultrasound-guided biopsy of solid organs, the patient is kept NPO for 8 to 12 hours before the procedure.

Side effects of sincalide include abdominal cramping, tenesmus, nausea, dizziness, sweating, and flushing; sincalide should not be given during pregnancy.

For bladder ultrasound, because of the necessity of distending the bladder to evaluate it, the patient will wish to void immediately after the examination, or unclamp Foley if appropriate.

Echocardiogram

Description   Noninvasive method of evaluating internal structures and motion of heart. The ultrasound beam penetrates cardiac structures, which reflect "echo" waves that travel back to the transducer to form images.

There are several modes: M-mode, or one-dimensional; two-dimensional, cross-sectional, real-time motion; and Doppler, in which continuous wave combined with pulse ultrasound gives an image of heart pulse and indicates the direction of blood flow within the heart.

Indications Echocardiograms are used to determine internal dimensions of ventricles, the size and motion of intraventricular septum and posterior wall of left ventricle, valve motion and anatomy, the presence of pericardial fluid, the direction of blood flow, and the presence of blood clots and myomatous tumors.

Complications None.

Nursing care Explain the procedure to the patient.

Biopsies

Brain biopsy

Description Removal of a small brain tissue sample, usually accomplished during intracranial surgery.

Indications Useful in the evaluation of neurologic disorders.

Complications Bleeding, infection.

Nursing care Frequent monitoring of vital signs and neurologic signs.

Thyroid biopsy

Description Sterile aspiration of thyroid tissue. It is often performed to help determine if surgery is needed because it is a relatively simple, effective way of ascertaining if a thyroid nodule is malignant.

Indications Differentiates between benign and malignant nodules; assists in the diagnosis of subacute thyroiditis in atypical cases, Hashimoto's disease, or multinodular goiter.

Complications Puncture of the esophagus or trachea.

Nursing care Support during procedure; assessment for esophageal or tracheal puncture post-procedure.

Lung biopsy

Description and indications Lung biopsy may be performed in one of four ways. The purpose of all techniques is to obtain a tissue sample for histologic evaluation.

Transbronchial biopsy. This biopsy is taken with the fiberoptic bronchoscope from the bronchial area of concern.

Nursing care. See the discussion under fiberoptic bronchoscopy, p. 1463.

Percutaneous needle biopsy with aspiration. In this procedure fluids and cells are aspirated into the syringe through a long, 18- to 20-gauge needle inserted percutaneously under fluoroscopic control into the suspected lesion. When the needle is in the lesion, the syringe is generally rotated to obtain a tissue specimen. This procedure is used most often if malignancy is suspected. A contraindication to needle aspiration is a patient who cannot hold his or her breath when required.

Nursing care. The procedure is performed with the patient under local anesthesia after the skin has been disinfected and a sterile field has been prepared. The patient is instructed to hold his or her breath for 15 to 30 seconds during the procedure. The aspirated material is sent for cytologic examination and for stains and cultures of microorganisms. The major postprocedural complication is pneumothorax. Therefore careful respiratory assessment is indicated.

Percutaneous biopsy with a cutting needle. Three procedure options are possible: a punch biopsy with a Vim-Silverman needle; a high-speed drill biopsy with trephine-lung biopsy drill; a suction excision biopsy with an Abrams needle or a modification of the Abrams needle. The cutting needle procedure is indicated when the patient has diffuse pulmonary infiltrates. These techniques have significant complications and therefore are not usually done until other diagnostic procedures have failed to identify the problem.

Nursing care. These procedures are performed with the patient under local anesthesia and after a sterile field has been prepared. Major complications include hemorrhage and pneumothorax. Careful postprocedural assessment is indicated.

Open lung biopsy or exploratory thoracotomy. This is an invasive procedure used to confirm a suspected diagnosis of lung or chest disease by obtaining lung specimens. The chest is opened through a standard thoracotomy incision, and the lung is inspected and biopsied. An open lung biopsy is indicated only after other investigative procedures have not clearly identified the patient's problem.

Nursing care. General anesthesia is used. Ensure that consent is obtained. A chest tube connected to water-seal drainage is used for 1 to 2 days after surgery because of the surgically induced pneumothorax. Several days of postprocedural chest roentgenograms are normally ordered. The procedure may have several major complications, including postoperative respiratory failure, emphysema, and chronic bronchopleural fistula.

Pleural biopsy

Description A small tissue sample is taken by special biopsy needle from the parietal pleura. It may be necessary to collect tissue samples from several different spots. Although some authorities advocate pleural biopsy every time a thoracentesis is performed, others claim that it should be done only when granulomatous disease or malignancy is suspected.

Indications Evaluation of pulmonary disease.

Complications Rare, but include pneumothorax, hemothorax, and intercostal nerve injury.

Nursing care Position the patient as for thoracentesis and provide support during the procedure. Monitor vital signs and assess the patient for symptoms of complications.

Lymph node excision and scalene node biopsy

Description Excision of peripheral lymph node or biopsy of a palpable scalene node. The incision and biopsy are performed in the supraclavicular scalene region.

Indications Performed to assess immunologic function in suspected immunodeficiency diseases and to stage certain malignancies.

Complications Bleeding, erythema, infection at site.

Nursing care Provide an occlusive dressing. Check the surgical site for bleeding, erythema, or purulent drainage.

Bone marrow aspiration and biopsy

Description Needle biopsy of marrow performed after entering marrow cavity of sternum, iliac crest, posterosuperior iliac spine, spinous process, rib, or tibial head. Bone marrow cellularity is determined.

Indications Evaluation of the immune and hematolymphatic systems, useful in differential diagnosis of thrombocytopenia, leukemia, granulomatous disease, and aplastic, hypoplastic, or megaloblastic anemias.

Complications Bleeding, infection, or pain at site.

Nursing care Exert immediate pressure over the biopsy site. Apply an occlusive dressing. Check the biopsy site for bleeding, erythema, or purulent drainage. Maintain bed rest for 1 hour. Administer analgesics as needed.

Muscle and nerve biopsy

Description Removal of a small muscle or nerve tissue sample for histologic, histochemical, ultrastructural, or biochemical studies.

Indications Aids in the dignosis of myopathies, such as muscle atrophy, degeneration, or inflammation, and determines the extent of damage to myelinated and unmyelinated nerve fibers.

Complications Mild soreness or stiffness of muscle or nerve that has undergone biopsy.

Nursing care Explain to the patient that the procedure will be performed with the patient under local anesthesia in the operating suite. After the procedure, encourage the patient to move the affected area and to walk (if the leg or foot is involved) to prevent stiffness. Provide analgesics, if required. Monitor for bleeding or infection at the site. If sutures are used, remove them in 7 to 10 days.

Synovial biopsy

Description Biopsy of the synovium by means of a special needle. The biopsy specimen is sent for histologic examination.

Indications Aids in the differential diagnosis of various forms of arthritis.

Complications Joint effusion or hemorrhage into the joint.

Nursing care Explain to the patient that the biopsy is performed after the skin is cleansed with antiseptic solutions and a local anesthetic is administered (occasionally a synovial biopsy is taken during open surgery). After the procedure, apply a small compression dressing and an elastic bandage around the joint. Caution the patient to restrict joint use for 24 hours to prevent hemorrhage or effusion.

Bladder, prostate, urethra biopsies

Description Biopsy specimens from a bladder, urethra, or prostate may be obtained with a cystoscopic/panendoscopic system. A resectoscope, which uses an electrically activated wire loop or a tubular cold knife, is positioned over the lesion, and a specimen is obtained. The bladder must be relatively full when a specimen is obtained to prevent inadvertent damage to normal mucosal folds. Transrectal or transperineal needle biopsies are often taken in conjunction with cystoscopic examination.

A transperineal biopsy is performed by injecting a local anesthetic into the skin of the perineum, over the area where the needle will enter. A finger in the rectum is used to guide the needle toward the area in question. The procedure may be repeated several times to ensure an adequate biopsy.

A transrectal biopsy requires no anesthesia. Preparation includes cleansing enemas to decrease the likelihood of introducing intestinal bacteria into the bloodstream or prostatic tissue. Prophylactic antibiotics are also indicated. When obtaining the specimen, the tip of the needle is placed on the examining finger and advanced gently to an area over which the biopsy is to be obtained. The needle is then pushed, and a biopsy is taken. The procedure may be repeated several times.

Indications Hematuria, pain, suspected malignancy.

Complications Hematuria. The primary complication of transrectal biopsy (the more commonly performed of the two techniques described) is sepsis from perforation of the bowel.

Nursing care Postprocedural care is similar to that of routine cystoscopic examination. Mild dysuria may be seen with hematuria during the first 48 hours following the procedure. If a general anesthetic is used, low-grade fever may occur over the first 24 to 48 hours after the procedure. Hematuria may recur 5 to 7 days after the procedure. The patient should be assured that the lesion is healing and that such hematuria is normal; the patient should not experience dysuria or a significant frequency of urination at this time. Fever and chills must be reported to the physician at once. A prophylactic antibiotic regimen must be adhered to after the transrectal needle biopsy.

Renal biopsy

Description In a renal biopsy a small piece of tissue is obtained via a special needle (percutaneous) or through a surgical incision (open). Roentgenography of the kidney, ureter, or bladder, intravenous urography, and ultrasonography may be used to locate the kidney for biopsy.

The absolute contraindications to renal biopsy are a solitary kidney (except posttransplant, when a transplanted kidney must be biopsied to evaluate for rejection) or for irreversible hemorrhagic tendencies. The relative contraindications are an uncooperative patient, a suspected renal tumor or cysts, gross sepsis, very small kidneys, horseshoe kidney, ectopic kidney, severe hypertension, massive obesity, severe spinal deformity, and pregnancy.

Indications Indications include persistent proteinuria, nephrotic syndrome, unexplained hematuria, controlled therapeutic trials of new drugs, evaluation of rejection transplant.

Complications Bleeding from the biopsy site, i.e., microscopic or gross hematuria, perirenal hematoma, retroperitoneal hematoma, arteriovenous fistula in the kidney, passage of clots, ureteric colic from a clot; hypotension; anemia; local infection; pain; perforation of other nearby structures.

Nursing care   Before the procedure, prepare the patient for the possibility of pain during the procedure. The patient should cooperate by holding his or her breath, on command. Explain that 24 hours of bed rest is needed after the biopsy, and that some hematuria is normal in the first 24 hours.

Record baseline vital signs. Review the chart for hemoglobin and hematocrit levels, platelet count, prothrombin time, and bleeding and clotting times. Review the type and cross-match report for two units of blood. Review the outcome of any test for pregnancy.

Explain the reason for the biopsy and the need for observation after the biopsy. Explain that for several days the patient should avoid contact sports, lifting or heavy exercise, and swimming. Normal activities can be resumed gradually after 48 to 72 hours. Explain the need to call the physician if there is any hematuria after the first 24 hours, draining from the biopsy site, persistent fever, or pain.

Measure output carefully and collect the voidings individually. Watch for hematuria. Check for microscopic hematuria, which is invariably present in the first two specimens. The urine may appear pink. Report profuse or persistent hematuria. If no hematuria occurs in the first 24 hours, bathroom privileges can be instituted for the next 24 hours.

A tight dressing is applied to the biopsy site. Check the dressing for bleeding. Apply external pressure for 30 minutes by having the patient lie prone with a sandbag placed directly on the biopsy site. Measure blood pressure, pulse, and respirations every 15 minutes for 4 hours and then every 4 hours for 24 hours.

Ensure adequate hydration of 1000 to 2000 ml to ensure a good urine flow. Monitor the hematocrit 3 to 6 hours after biopsy. Any decrease from the prebiopsy level suggests perirenal bleeding.

Give a nonaspirin analgesic agent for mild pain after the anesthesia wears off, as ordered by the physician. Report severe loin pain.

Brush biopsy of renal pelvis and calyces

Description   A ureteral catheter with a steel guide wire is placed using a cystoscope as a guide. The catheter is then removed, and a steel or nylon brush is inserted to the level of lesion to obtain a biopsy. The specimen is then smeared on slides and prepared with a 95% ethanol solution. After the specimen is obtained, the renal pelvis is irrigated with normal saline.[9]

Indications   Allows urologist to obtain a tissue biopsy from the renal pelvis or calyces without an open surgical incision to assist in the diagnosis of renal disease.

Complications   Irritation of the renal system because of manipulation.

Nursing care   Postprocedural care is similar to that of routine cystoscopic examination. A low-grade fever may be noted. Flank pain secondary to ureteral manipulation is not uncommon and should disappear within 48 hours. Fever greater than 38° C (101° F) and severe flank pain should be reported to

physician. Remember that elderly patients may not become febrile even with sepsis.

Skin and tissue biopsy

Description   The lesion is marked, and the area is infiltrated with lidocaine. A small circular punch or scalpel is used to obtain tissue to determine cell histology.

Indications   For evaluation of abnormal lesions or tissue. The biopsy can be incisional (surgical excision of tumor section), excisional (removal of entire growth), or aspiration (removal of small tumor plug or fluid). Frozen section involves freezing questionable tissue removed during surgery for microscopic study.

Complications   Infection, bleeding at site.

Nursing care   Cleanse the site with an antibacterial solution. Give the patient information regarding the procedure. Apply direct pressure over the area to stop the bleeding (sutures may be used for areas larger than 3 cm). Apply a bandage.

Liver biopsy

Description   Percutaneous biopsy of liver tissue. With the patient lying down, a needle is inserted into the liver, and a small amount of tissue is withdrawn to establish a pathologic and microscopic picture of the liver cells.

Indications   Abnormal liver function; hepatomegaly or hepatosplenomegaly of unexplained origin; suspected malignancy of the liver; suspected systemic or infiltrative disease, such as sarcoidosis; routine evaluation for rejection in a transplanted liver.

Complications   Hemorrhage.

Nursing care   Permit nothing by mouth after midnight before the biopsy. Have the patient void before the biopsy. Record baseline vital signs. Review the chart for hemoglobin and hematocrit levels, platelet count, and bleeding and clotting times. After the biopsy, instruct the patient to lie on the right side to keep pressure on the site. Monitor the vital signs frequently for 4 to 6 hours. Postbiopsy protocols regarding bed rest and activity vary; ensure familiarity with institutional procedures.

Cervical biopsy

Description   Biopsy of cervical epithelium and shallow layer of underlying stroma to diagnose malignant invasion.

Indications   Suspicious Pap smear.

Complications   Bleeding.

Nursing care   Prepare the patient for a vaginal examination. After the procedure, give the patient a perineal pad, and inform her that spotting will occur for 24 hours or so.

Endometrial biopsy

Description   Biopsy of endometrial uterine lining. It is generally performed on the first day of menses of premenopausal patients and anytime in postmenopausal patients. A tissue specimen may be obtained by a Gravlee jet washer (isotonic saline solution is forced through an intrauterine cannula, flushing endometrial cells into an external collecting reservoir) or a Nova curette (a curette attached to a syringe scrapes the endometrium, and cell samples are drawn into the syringe).

Indications Suspected endometrial carcinoma.

Complications None.

Nursing care Prepare the patient for a vaginal examination. Explain that she may experience cramping because of dilation of the cervix during the procedure. Teach and assist her with relaxation and breathing techniques. Give the patient a perineal pad after the procedure. Ensure that menstrual data are noted on the laboratory specimen slip for the pathologist.

Cervical conization (cone biopsy)

Description Surgical removal of cervical tissue in the shape of a cone for diagnosis or for treatment of cervical infection or carcinoma in situ. It is performed by a physician with a cold knife scalpel. The procedure is frequently called cold knife conization (CKC) or cryosurgery.

Indications Treatment of cervical infection or carcinoma in situ.

Complications Bleeding.

Nursing care After the procedure assist the physician with removal of vaginal packing, usually within 24 hours. Give perineal care with an antiseptic solution and change the perineal pad every 4 hours and as needed. Instruct the patient to avoid coitus, douching, or tampons for 6 weeks or until directed by the physician; report excessive bleeding (if it lasts longer than 7 to 10 days); avoid constipation; maintain good perineal hygiene; and report signs of infection to physician.

Radioisotope Studies and Scans

Brain scan

Description Intravenous injection of a small amount of radioactive substance (e.g., technetium-99). The head is then scanned with a special sensing device to pick up areas of concentrated uptake.

Indications Assessment of neurologic disease, brain tumors, headache, coma, intracerebral hemorrhage.

Complications None.

Nursing care Obtain a careful history regarding any existing allergies, particularly to iodine. Assure the patient that the procedure is painless, the radioactive substance is harmless, and there will be no aftereffects.

Cisternography

Description Injection of a radioisotope into the subarachnoid space through a cisternal or lumbar puncture. The head is then scanned at regular intervals to determine the amount of time it takes for the radioisotope to clear from the circulating cerebrospinal fluid.

Indications To assess the circulation of the cerebrospinal fluid.

Complications As for cisternal or lumbar puncture.

Nursing care As for cisternal or lumbar puncture.

Thyroid uptake and scan

Description Tracer doses of ^{131}I, ^{123}I, or ^{99m}Tc pertechnetate are given. A scanner is then passed over the gland to record graphically the amount of radioactive iodine taken up by the gland over a period of time (e.g., 6, 8, or 24 hours). Pregnancy is a contraindication.

Indications Not used for routine screening, but rather to answer specific questions regarding the localization of functioning or nonfunctioning thyroid tissue; it gives evidence of gland size and function.

Complications None.

Nursing care Assess for dietary intake of iodine, for administration of iodine-containing medications, and for the use of antithyroid drugs before the test, since test results may be affected by any ingestion of these.

Ventilation/perfusion lung scan

Description A scanning device records the pattern of pulmonary radioactivity after the inhalation or intravenous injection of gamma ray–emitting radionuclides (such as xenon-133), thus providing visual images of the distribution of blood flow in the lungs.

Indications The major indications for this procedure are to evaluate whether patient has pulmonary thromboembolism and to study preoperative lung function.

Complications None.

Nursing care Explain the procedure to the patient.

Radionuclide imaging of breast

Description Evaluation of breast image after intravenous injection of radioactive substance.

Indications Breast masses or tissue abnormalities.

Complications None.

Nursing care Explain the procedure to the patient, and reassure concerning potential findings.

Bone scan (scintigraphy)

Description Roentgenographic procedure in which a radioisotope, usually technetium-99 (^{99}Tc–sodium pertechnetate) is injected intravenously. The radioisotope is picked up on a special scanning camera as it is passed over the musculoskeletal tissues of the body from head to foot, and a picture of the isotope's distribution in the bony tissues is produced. The scan takes about 1 hour and is painless.

Indications Aids in the diagnosis of bony metastatic lesions and traumatic, inflammatory, or infectious conditions of musculoskeletal tissues. The scan will show the injured or diseased tissues as darker or "hot" areas on the scan pictures as much as 3 to 6 months earlier than roentgenograms can reveal the condition.

Complications None usually, although infrequently a hematoma, redness, or edema may develop at the site of the injection.

Nursing care Explain to the patient that the radioisotope will be injected intravenously 1 to 3 hours before the scan is to be performed and that he or she will be required to drink several glasses of water or tea during the waiting period to aid in excreting the radioisotope that is not absorbed by bone tissue. After the procedure, check the injection site for redness or edema, and inform the patient to check it at home if procedure is performed as outpatient.

Liver or spleen scan

Description Injection of a radioactive colloid (e.g., technetium-99m), which concentrates in the reticuloendothelial cells through phagocytosis. Kupffer cells in the liver take up 80% to 90%, spleen takes 5% to 10%, and bone marrow takes 3% to 5%.

Indications Used to screen patients for hepatic metastases, cirrhosis, and hepatitis. It also assists in identifying focal lesions such as tumors, cysts, and abscesses, and may demonstrate splenic infarct, hepatomegaly, and splenomegaly. It is also used to evaluate liver and spleen following abdominal trauma.

Complications None.

Nursing care The patient will need to know he or she will be asked to lie very still and placed in several positions. The patient also should know that the procedure will not be painful, with the exception of the intravenous injection.

Some patients will have a reaction to a stabilizer added to the colloid; observe for anaphylaxis or for pyogenic response.

Do not schedule the patient for more than one radionuclide scan on one day. Radionuclides administered in other studies may interfere with liver-spleen imaging.

Renal scans (DTPA, DMSA)

Description Provides a functional assessment of glomerular filtration rate (GFR) and effective renal plasma flow (ERPF). The DTPA scan also provides an assessment of the ureters and bladder. Renal scans expose patients to less radiation than does IVP. A DMSA scan provides an assessment of individual kidney function.

Other radionuclides such as hippurate and radioxenon have been used for renal scans,[12] but are no longer widely used.

The DTPA scan is used primarily to assess upper urinary tract obstruction. Radionuclide is injected in an intravenous bolus and sequential images are obtained. A 30-second film is taken to assess cortical blood flow; a 1-minute image and two images are obtained at 5, 10, 15, and 20 minutes. The bladder and ureters are included in the DTPA scan. It assesses GFR and ERPF and provides differential renal function.

Indications To assess urinary tract obstruction. Because the radionuclide used is affected by diuretics, furosemide is typically given, and the change in renal excretion rate is quantified. Delays in excretion indicate obstruction.[12]

The DMSA scan is useful in assessing functional renal cortical mass,[12] the radionuclide used in DMSA scanning is taken up by renal tubule so that functional cortical mass can be quantified. As with the DTPA scan, an intravenous bolus of radioisotope is administered, and delayed images are obtained. It is indicated in cases of suspected renal scarring, assessment of segmental renal ischemia, and suspected intrarenal mass.

Complications None.

Nursing care Requires no preparation. Patients exposed to significantly less radiation than required by IVP; however, since a radioisotope is injected and excreted by the kidneys, the patient may continue to excrete radionuclide after the study is completed. Pregnant caregivers are advised not to empty or measure waste products during the initial 24 hours after testing.

Nuclear cystogram (radionuclide cystogram)

Description Performed in a manner similar to roentgenographic cystography except that normal saline with a dose of a pertechnetate radionuclide is used instead of an iodine-bound contrast solution. Like roentgenographic cystography, the study requires no preparation.

An indwelling catheter is passed into the bladder via the urethra. Normal saline is infused into the bladder, and radionuclide is injected into the solution during bladder filling. It may be performed in place of a roentgenographic cystogram because the patient is exposed to less radiation; however, a nuclear cystogram does not provide the anatomic detail seen with standard cystography.

Indications Measures certain parameters of bladder function.

Complications Cystitis.

Nursing care The patient should be encouraged to force fluids for a 24-hour period following the test and informed that mild dysuria and urinary frequency should disappear completely within this time period.

^{125}I fibrinogen uptake (radioactive fibrinogen uptake, RFU)

Description A noninvasive procedure involving the injection of a small amount of a radioisotope and then the passing of a scanning camera over the involved area beginning 2 hours later. The procedure is used to detect the presence or enlargement of a deep vein thrombosis. Serial readings are taken on successive days following administration of the radioisotope, at 24 hours, but patients can be studied daily for 7 to 14 days. A 20% increase in uptake in one area over a 24-hour period is considered positive.

Indications Deep vein thrombosis.

Complications None.

Nursing care Explain the procedure to the patient.

CT and MRI Scans

Computerized tomography (CT)

Description Computerized tomography (CT) scanning was introduced in the early 1970s. CT scans use a roentgen ray beam and a computer to provide very accurate images of thin cross sections (0.8 to 1.3 cm) of the body.[3]

The CT scanner has many advantages: it is safe and painless; there is a very small amount of radiation exposure; data can be collected in early stages of the dysfunction; and it reduces the need for more invasive diagnostic procedures.

During the CT scan procedure the patient lies on a table with the body part to be studied inside the scanner's opening. The scanner then is moved to various angles and rotated slowly around the patient's body as repeated roentgenograms are taken. This information is recorded on a computer printout, and film prints (i.e., hard copy) of these visual images are taken. The scan usually is completed in 10 to 45 minutes. Cross-sectional, horizontal, or sagittal plane roentgenographic images are translated by a computer and displayed on an oscilloscope. These images are much sharper, more sensitive, and clearer than conventional roentgenograms. The CT scan takes pictures of small layers or "slices" of the tissues being examined (Figures III-2 and III-3).

CT scanning is contraindicated during pregnancy.

Indications   Useful in diagnosing disorders of multiple body systems.

Brain.   Head trauma, cerebrovascular disturbances, hydrocephalus, abnormal brain development, identification of space-occupying lesions, metastatic tumors, and brain abscesses.

Endocrine.   CT of sella turcica, adrenal glands, and abdomen is indicated in the following: presence of adrenal adenoma, diabetes-related tumors, Cushing's disease workup, hypopituitary workup, and precocious puberty workup.

Eye.   Diagnosis of eye disorders. It contrasts orbital contents and tumors because of difference in tissue density.

Respiratory system.   Identifies exact morphologic characteristics of a chest lesion.

Renal and genitourinary systems.   Determines kidney size, cysts, abscesses, masses, hematomas, and collecting system dilation. It is particularly valuable in defining abnormalities of the renal parenchyma. It provides an estimate of the density of masses and has the potential to differentiate solid tissue masses from cystic or hemorrhagic structures. Varying densities are displayed as Hounsfield units: normal renal parenchyma measures 80 to 100 Hounsfield units, and density of a cyst is lower whereas solid tumors have a density similar to that of renal parenchyma. CT scanning is also used in evaluation of adrenal masses. It is a useful technique for evaluating masses (tumors) of pelvic contents and lymphatic enlargement that may be the result of metastatic invasion. Pelvic abscesses may be elucidated by CT scanning of that area; it may elucidate any mass effect that causes distortion of bladder.

Gastrointestinal system.   In the biliary tract and liver CT scanning can be used to identify focal points found on nuclear scans as solid, cystic, inflammatory, or vascular. A biopsy may be necessary to distinguish between metastatic or primary tumors or to rule out malignancy. CT scanning can also identify hematomas after abdominal trauma. It is used to determine if the cause of jaundice is obstructive or nonobstructive.

CT scanning and ultrasound are both effective in biliary tract and liver diagnosis. A CT scan proves to be better in obese

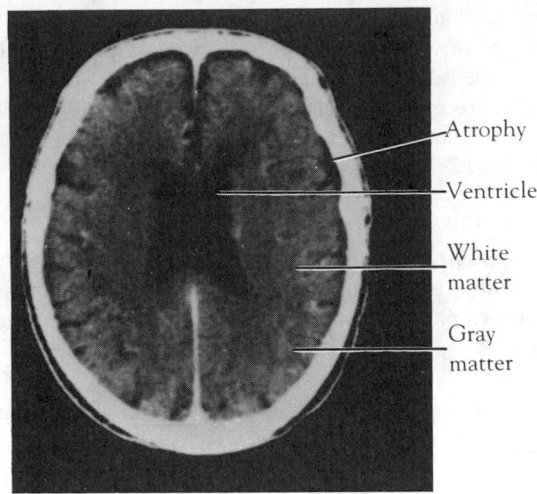

Figure III-2   CT scan printouts. CT brain scan differentiates between gray and white brain matter. (From Ballinger.[2])

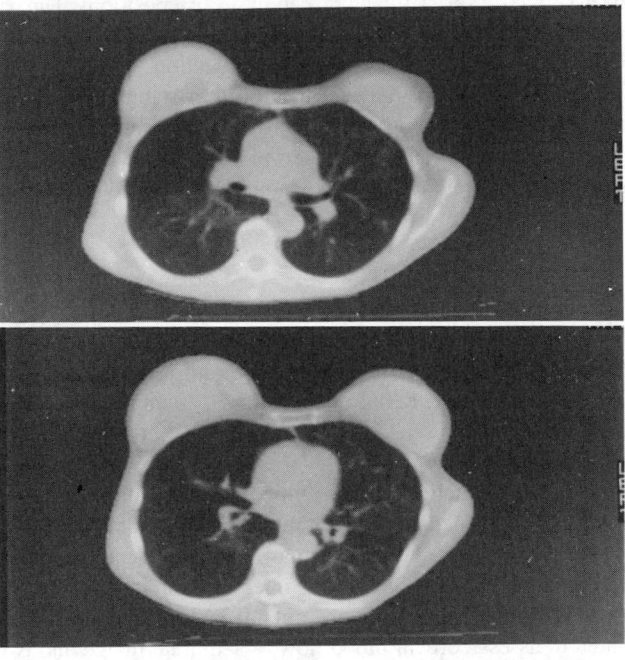

Figure III-3   CT scan of female patient. On this transverse scan through upper chest, bilateral breast shadows are evident. Heart, pulmonary arteries, and main bronchi are also visible. (Courtesy R. Keith Wilson, M.D., Baylor College of Medicine, Houston, Texas.)

patients or patients whose liver is located high under the rib cage because bone and excessive fat hinder ultrasound transmission. Contrast medium is also used during CT scanning to intensify vascular structures and liver parenchyma, aiding in visualization of the biliary tract. A general CT scan of the abdomen is valuable in defining the relationship of organs and identifying the presence of tumors. In the pancreas, CT scanning is used to diagnose pancreatic carcinoma and pancreatitis and to distinguish between pancreatic disorders and disorders of the retroperitoneum.

Complications   None, unless patient experiences reaction to contrast.

Nursing care   Explain to the patient that he or she will lie flat on a narrow table, which will be moved inside a round opening of the scanner. The scanner will make a loud clicking sound as it moves around and along the patient. The scan will take 10 to 60 minutes, depending on whether or not some parts only or the entire body is scanned. The patient must lie still without moving during the scan. A radiopaque solution may be given to outline the blood vessels more clearly if needed, although the majority of CT scans are made without such an agent. Occasionally a sedative may be required to calm a nervous or restless patient.

If contrast medium is to be used, assess the patient for allergies to iodine, seafood, or contrast media. Barium studies should be made at least 4 days before the CT scan or barium obscures the film. The contrast media excreted in bile used in earlier diagnostic studies may interfere with biliary tree detection.

The patient is given nothing to eat past midnight before the test, depending on hospital procedure.

Positron emission tomography (PET)

Description   Intravenous injection of deoxyglucose with radioactive fluorine. The head is scanned, and a color-composite picture is obtained. Various shades of colors indicate levels of glucose metabolism.

Indications   Assists in the diagnosis and differentiation of neurologic disorders.

Complications   None.

Nursing care   Same as for a CT scan.

Magnetic resonance imaging (MRI)

Description   Magnetic resonance imaging (MRI), also termed nuclear magnetic resonance (NMR) imaging, is a technique of tomography based on the magnetic behavior of protons (hydrogen nuclei) in body tissues.[7,10] The scanner produces images when protons are placed in a strong external magnetic field and then are subjected to short computer-programmed pulses of additional energy in the form of radio frequency waves. When placed in the magnetic field, positively charged nuclei and negatively charged electrons align uniformly. Short pulses of radiofrequency waves are then applied, which tip the atoms out of their magnetic alignment, causing uniform spinning (resonance) of the nuclei. When the radiofrequency wave is stopped, the atoms realign uniformly with the magnetic field and emit tissue-specific signals that are based on realignment time and the relative proton density (water content) of nuclei. These signals are then monitored, processed, and displayed as a high-resolution image by the MRI computer.

Indications   MRI is indicated for detecting a variety of neurologic disorders, including central nervous system (CNS) malignancies, CNS degenerative disorders (e.g., Alzheimer's disease), brain edema, spinal cord edema, spinal lesions, is-

chemic-infarcted areas of the CNS, arteriovenous malformations, congenital anomalies, and hemorrhagic areas of the CNS and spinal cord.[15]

MRI is an excellent aid for the diagnosis of musculoskeletal conditions because MRI clearly differentiates various types of tissues such as bones, fat, and muscles. It produces clear images of soft tissues such as tumors, nucleus pulposus, and blood vessels. Individual cells may be defined. It also aids in the detection of renal masses, especially in distinguishing simple cysts from those complicated by hemorrhage. It is used to detect and stage neoplasms.

Complications   None.

Nursing care   The patient should be instructed that MRI is a painless and noninvasive procedure with no known risks. Explain to the patient that he or she will lie flat on a narrow table inside a round opening of a large magnet and should lie still during the scan. Many patients find the MRI to be claustrophobic. The nurse can prepare the patient for this, and explain the use of imagery, which may help the patient tolerate the examination better. A description of the equipment and procedure should be given. The patient also should be informed that a soft humming sound and the on-off pulses of the radiofrequency waves will be heard. The patient should be instructed to remove all metal objects because the strong magnetic field may damage jewelry and watches.

A careful assessment of any existing ferromagnetic implants (e.g., pacemakers, metallic orthopedic devices) or known foreign bodies (e.g., metallic splinters or fragments) must be made before the procedure because these objects produce image deformation. MRI also may move some metallic devices (e.g., metal intracranial aneurysm clips); therefore patients with such implants or foreign bodies cannot be exposed to MRI.

Skin Assessment/Testing

The following studies are commonly used for diagnostic purposes.

Scrapings

Description   The area is cleansed with alcohol and air dried so that superficial fine dry scale is apparent. The scale is scraped with a sharp scalpel and gathered on a glass slide or in a blood collection tube. Nail and hair clippings are also used. Scrapings are covered with 10% KOH (potassium hydroxide) and examined microscopically for the presence of mycelia in fungal infections. The fungus appears as branching, threadlike elements.

Indications   Fungal conditions of skin.

Complications   None.

Nursing care   Explain the procedure to the patient.

Diascopy, side lighting, Wood's light, Gram stain, culture, electron microscopy, cytology

Description

Diascopy.   The lesion is covered with a glass slide or piece of clear plastic to determine whether dilated capillaries or extravasated blood is causing redness of lesion.

Side lighting. A beam of light is directed from the side over the lesion to reveal minor elevations or depressions in the lesion. This helps determine the configuration and degree of eruption.

Wood's light. The skin is viewed in a darkened room under ultraviolet light with wavelength of 360 nm ("black light"). Certain disease-producing fungi and bacteria show a characteristic color.

Gram stain. Exudate from the lesion is smeared onto a glass slide and stained with gentian or crystal violet. The violet is washed off, and the smear is flooded with iodine solution, which is then washed off. The smear is then flooded with 95% alcohol and counterstained with safranin red dye. The stain will differentiate gram-negative from gram-positive bacteria based on their ability to pick up one or both of the two stains.

Culture. For pustular lesions a swab sample is placed in a broth culture media. For chronic bacterial and fungal infections, a biopsy specimen is used for culturing. Cultures are incubated or refrigerated and observed for fungal or bacterial growth.

Electron microscopy. A glass slide smear of vesicular fluid or crusted tissue is viewed under an electron microscope to determine the presence of a virus.

Cytology. Cellular material is scraped from the base of the vesicle and stained with Wright's or Giemsa stain, or a clean glass slide is touched to the surface of the lesion so the cells can adhere to it. The cells are sprayed with a fixative and viewed microscopically after staining. Multinucleated giant cells are present in herpes simplex, herpes zoster, and varicella. Pemphigus is diagnosed by the presence of typical acantholytic cells.

Indications   Dermatologic lesions.
Complications   None.
Nursing care   Explain the procedure to the patient.

Patch test

Description   The suspected allergen is applied to the skin under a nonabsorbent adhesive patch and left for 48 hours. A positive test consists of erythema with some induration and occasional vesicle formation. Some reactions do not occur until after the patch is removed from the site.
Indications   Sensitivity to allergens.
Complications   None, although itching or burning may occur.
Nursing care   Instruct the patient to leave the patch on, to keep the area dry, and to return for site inspection in 48 hours. Instruct the patient to remove the patch if itching or burning develops before 48 hours and to return for inspection of the site. Reinspect at 72 hours.

Thermography

Description   Measures and plots areas of localized elevation of skin temperature over inflammatory or malignant lesions; takes photographs of infrared radiation (heat) coming from any part of the body. For breast thermography the patient is placed in a draft-free room at a temperature of about 20° C

(68° F). Clothing above the waist is removed, and the patient waits for about 15 minutes until the skin cools before infrared photographs are taken.
Indications   Presence of dermatologic lesions that are inflamed or suspected of being malignant.
Complications   None.
Nursing care   Explain to the patient that the room will be cool. Provide reassurance, especially if test is being done due to suspected malignancy.

Allergy skin testing

Description   An antigen is introduced by scratching or pricking the skin surface or by intradermal injection.
Indications   Sensitivity to allergens.
Complications   Erythema at site; hypersensitivity, including anaphylaxis.
Nursing care   Check for erythema at the site of antigen introduction 20 minutes after administration. Observe for potential anaphylactic reactions following antigen introduction. Antihistamines may be administered as a comfort measure.

Schick test

Description   This is a test to determine the presence or absence of a significant quantity of diphtheria antitoxins in the blood. The presence of these antitoxins indicates an immunity to diphtheria.
Indications   For susceptibility to diphtheria.
Complications   None.
Nursing care   Draw 0.1 ml of purified diphtheria toxin dissolved in human serum albumin into a tuberculin syringe. In a second syringe draw up 0.1 ml of inactivated diphtheria toxoid to be used as a control in the other arm (to rule out any sensitivity to culture proteins). Attach 26- or 27-gauge 1.25 cm (½ inch) needles to both syringes. Clean the volar surfaces of both forearms. Intradermally inject the toxin in one forearm and the toxoid in the other forearm. Carefully record which was injected in each arm. Examine the areas at 24 and 36 hours.

A positive reaction is indicated when the site of the toxin injection begins to redden in 24 hours. The redness, swelling, and tenderness continue until it reaches maximum size—usually 3 cm in diameter at the end of 1 week. The skin at the injection site may flake, and the center may appear as a dark pigmented spot. The area of the toxoid injection should show no reaction. With a negative result there is no flaking or erythema at either injection site.

Tuberculin skin testing

Description   Two types of tuberculin are currently being used for testing: old tuberculin (OT) and purified protein derivative (PPD). The PPD is the preferred tuberculin preparation because its strength is standardized and tests with the same dose are comparable.

Contraindications for testing include patients with known active TB infection, and previous BCG vaccine, because they will demonstrate a positive reaction to the PPD.

Indications   Provides evidence of whether the tested individual has been infected, either past or present, with *Mycobacterium tuberculosis* or has had contact with someone who has TB.

Complications   None.

Nursing care   Each type of multiple puncture unit is slightly different; usually an intradermal injection is administered. Carefully read the manufacturer's instructions regarding the administration of the test. A positive reaction for all brands consists of the formation of separate papules at each of the puncture sites or a large papule over the entire area. Refer to the manufacturer's instructions regarding specific interpretation, reading of results, and documentation.

Testing for fungal diseases

Description   For patients suspected of having coccidioidomycosis, skin tests are available from lysates of both the mycelial (coccidioidin) and the spherule (spherulin) forms. Skin tests with either form are highly specific and become positive 3 to 4 weeks after infection and 12 to 20 days after the onset of clinical illness. An intradermal injection is given.

Indications   Respiratory or other systemic symptoms that may indicate infection with coccidioidomycosis.

Complications   None.

Nursing care   Explain the purpose of the test to the patient. Observe the injection site for a reaction: erythema, swelling, or hardening at the site.

Delayed-type hypersensitivity (anergy) testing (cell-mediated immunity testing)

Description   Measures the capacity to generate a delayed-type hypersensitivity (DTH) response. The patient is injected intradermally with four common soluble recall antigens (for example, PPD, *Candida* spp., *Trichophyton* spp., and tetanus) and examined for induration and erythema after 48 hours. Most young, healthy persons respond positively to at least one antigen. Reactivity may decline with age and with protein- and calorie-deficiency states.

Indications   Suspected immunodeficiency or protein-calorie deficiency.

Complications   None.

Nursing care   Check for local erythema and induration at 48 hours.

Arteriographic (Angiographic) and Venographic Studies

Arteriography or venography consists of the infusion of a radiopaque substance into the arterial or venous system, followed by a series of roentgenograms that allow visualization of the vessel systems and assist in the diagnosis of any abnormalities.

Arteriography and venography may be used in many body systems. In addition to those described here, selective arteriography may also be performed to localize possible tumors of the parathyroid, adrenal, and pancreatic glands, and a procedure similar to arteriography may be used to perform serial venous sampling to obtain hormone levels.

Cerebral arteriography

Description   Cerebral arteriography requires the infusion of a radiopaque substance into the cerebral arterial system; during infusion of the contrast medium, a series of roentgenograms is taken for visualization of the extracranial and intracranial vessels. To outline the anterior, middle, and posterior cerebral arteries and returning venous circulation, the injection is made into the carotid system. If visualization of the vertebral-basilar system in the posterior fossa is needed, the injection is made into the vertebral artery.[3]

There are two approaches (open or closed) to performing the arteriography. The *open* method is performed in the operating room and involves the surgical exposure of the internal carotid before injection of the contrast substance. After the procedure, the incision is sutured and dressed. The actual procedure and aftercare are the same as those for the closed method. The *closed* method involves injection of the contrast medium directly into the carotid or vertebral arteries or indirectly (injection of the carotid or vertebral vessels by way of the femoral, brachial, subclavian, or axillary artery).[3] Following the injection a series of roentgenographs is taken for visualization of arterial and venous circulations.

Contraindications include the following: anticoagulant therapy, age, recent embolic or thrombotic occurrences, sensitivity to the contrast medium, and severe liver, thyroid, or kidney disease.

Indications   Identification of cerebral circulatory anomalies (e.g., aneurysm, hematoma) and their site and size, and visualization of cerebral arteries and veins.

Complications   Complications generally occurring during or shortly after the procedure include seizures, stroke, allergic reactions (to dye), thrombosis, hemiparesis, visual disturbances, pulmonary emboli, and dysphasia.

Nursing care   Observe the puncture site for hematoma or hemorrhage. Frequently monitor vital signs and neurologic signs during and after procedure. (Make sure that baseline neurological data and vital signs are documented before the procedure.) Observe for signs of allergic dye reactions.

Fluorescein arteriography (and photography)

Description   A 10% solution of sodium fluorescein injected into the antecubital vein is relayed to retinal arteries in 10 to 16 seconds and to veins in 25 seconds. The pupils are dilated with short-acting cycloplegics in combination with a mydriatic. An ophthalmoscope with a blue filter can show the entire diameter of vessel, whereas ordinary ophthalmoscopy provides only a surface view.

Photography.   Black and white film with appropriate filters should be used in a camera that takes rapid-sequence photographs from 9 to 30 seconds after injection of fluorescein. The patient and examiner are seated at a table opposite each other, each looking into the camera.

Indications   Eye disorders.

Complications Subcutaneous leakage of dye causes local burning. A patient may experience a brief hot flash or nausea. A temporary yellowish discoloration of sclera may occur until the dye is excreted in the urine (within 48 hours).

Nursing care Inquire about previous allergies to fluorescein (the allergic response is usually hives and itching). Inform the patient what to expect in terms of the effects of mydriatic or cycloplegic medications. Inform patient about possible scleral discoloration.

Cardiac catheterization

Description An invasive procedure involving insertion of a radiopaque catheter via the peripheral artery or vein into the heart. It is used to determine the anatomy of heart chambers, valves, great vessels, and coronary arteries; ventricular wall thickness and motion; hemodynamic functions of the heart by pressure recordings of heart chambers and great vessels and pressure gradients across the valves; ventricular function and cardiac output; degree of valve competence; and intracardiac oxygen saturations. It also selectively visualizes the heart, coronary arteries, and great vessels by recording serial roentgenograms (angiograms). It is usually performed as an outpatient procedure; the patient should recover for 6 to 8 hours post-procedure.

Indications Symptoms of angina pectoris, myocardial infarct, or other cardiac dysfunction.

Complications Myocardial infarction, dysrhythmias, hematoma, or hemorrhage at the insertion site. Vascular obstruction distal to insertion site secondary to thrombus or hematoma formation; reaction to contrast medium, infection, pulmonary edema, cardiac tamponade.

Nursing care Ensure that informed consent is obtained. Explain that the procedure will last 2 to 4 hours, that the patient may feel pressure during insertion of the catheter and a hot flushing sensation or nausea with injection of contrast medium, the patient may also experience a salty taste when dye is injected, that the patient should cough when instructed by the physician, and that the patient will receive medication if chest pain occurs and may be given nitroglycerin to dilate coronary vessels. Determine any allergies or hypersensitivity to shellfish, iodine, or other contrast media. Obtain baseline vital signs and peripheral pulses. After the procedure check the vital signs every 15 minutes for 1 hour, every 30 minutes for 2 hours, and every hour for 4 hours or until stable. Keep the patient flat in bed for 6 to 8 hours with a pressurized dressing over the puncture site. Check the dressing and surrounding area for bleeding, pain, and swelling. Check the peripheral pulses, color, warmth, and feeling of the extremities distal to the insertion site. Give pain medication as indicated. Encourage fluid intake for first 6 to 8 hours to assist in the elimination of contrast medium.

Digital vascular imaging (DVI) (digital subtraction arteriography)

Description An invasive procedure using a computer system and fluoroscopy with an image intensifier to permit complete visualization of the arterial supply to a specific area.

Indications Carotid and renal artery disease, pulmonary embolism, aneurysms, thrombotic and embolic disease of the great vessels, coarctation of the aorta.

Complications Dysrhythmias, reaction to contrast medium, infection, bleeding at site.

Nursing care Ensure that informed consent is obtained. Explain that the procedure will last 1 to 2 hours and that the patient will be requested to hold his or her breath for 10-second intervals. Digital vascular imaging can be done on an outpatient basis, and may cause certain sensations. After the procedure, check the vital signs immediately and as ordered. Check site for bleeding. Instruct the patient to observe the site for infection and/or bleeding and to drink a minimum of 1 L of fluid on the day of the procedure.

Scintigraphy
Radionuclide Arteriography

Description Gives information regarding myocardial perfusion and contractility through the use of radionuclide imaging. The procedure involves injecting a radioisotope and passing a scanning camera over the patient repeatedly.

Indications Poor myocardial perfusion or contractility.

Complications None.

Nursing care Explain the procedure. Ensure that informed consent is obtained. Reassure the patient that the radiation exposure involved is less than with a chest roentgenogram; caution the patient to remain quiet and still during the study. Encourage the patient to use imagery if it helps them.

Technetium-99m Pyrophosphate Myocardial Imaging

Description Tracer isotope is injected 2 to 3 hours before the procedure, and scanning takes 30 to 60 minutes, during which time a scanning camera is passed repeatedly over the patient in several positions: anterior, left anterior oblique, right anterior oblique, and left lateral.

Indications To detect recent myocardial infarction and the extent of its damage; "hot spots" appear within 12 hours of the infarct and disappear after 1 week.

Complications None.

Nursing care Explain the procedure. Ensure that informed consent is obtained. Inform the patient that he or she may eat lightly before the study but should not smoke or drink alcoholic or caffeine-containing beverages for 3 hours before the test.

Thallium-201 Imaging

Description "Cold spot" myocardial imaging used in conjunction with a bicycle ergometer or treadmill stress ECG test to diagnose ischemic heart disease.

Indications To assess myocardial perfusion (myocardial blood flow) and to evaluate the patency of grafts after bypass surgery; also used in conjunction with exercise stress testing (EST) in the diagnosis of coronary artery disease (stress imaging).

Complications None.

Nursing care If performed in conjunction with EST, instruct the patient to avoid tobacco, alcohol, or unprescribed medication for 24 hours before the study and to take nothing by mouth for 3 hours before the test. NOTE: If chest pain, shortness of breath, or a drop in blood pressure develops, stress imaging should be stopped.

Scintigraphic blood pool imaging (multiple-gated blood pool)

Description   Involves injection of human serum albumin or RBCs tagged with the isotope technetium-99m pertechnetate. A scintillation camera records several pass images of the isotope as it passes through the ventricle. Imaging can be "gated" to systolic and diastolic events of the cardiac cycle. The normal left ventricular ejection fraction is 55% to 65%. The procedure is contraindicated in pregnancy.

Indications   Used to evaluate regional and global ventricular performance and to detect aneurysms of the left ventricle and areas of hypokinesis and dyskinesis.

Complications   None.

Nursing care   Explain the procedure. Ensure that informed consent is obtained. Determine if the patient is pregnant. The patient may eat and drink before the procedure. Inform the patient that the blood-labeling agent is given intravenously.

Pulmonary arteriography

Description   A radiopaque dye is injected rapidly into the pulmonary circulation by various routes: one or more systemic veins, or the chambers of the heart, or directly into the pulmonary arteries. After the rapid injection a series of roentgenograms is taken.

Indications   To detect pulmonary emboli and a variety of congenital and acquired thromboembolic lesions.

Complications   Hematoma development; occasionally, frank hemorrhage or thrombus formation; infection at the catheter insertion site.

Nursing care   Before the procedure, determine any allergies to radiopaque dye. After the procedure the patient must be observed for hematomas or inflammation around the injection site, absence of peripheral pulses, or complaints of numbness or pain.

Vena caval catheterization

Description   In vena caval catheterization a radiopaque catheter is introduced into the vena cava through the femoral vein. The catheter is guided into the vena cava with fluoroscopic assistance. Venous samples are obtained from different sites along the vena cava for catecholamine determination.

Patients with pheochromocytoma should receive alpha blockers before the procedure to prevent catecholamine release and hypertensive crisis.

Indications   The procedure is performed to assist the surgeon to localize the pheochromocytoma, and rule out bilateral or multiple tumors.

Complications   Pulmonary embolus, hematoma formation at catheter insertion site.

Nursing care   Before the procedure, give alpha blockers as prescribed. Have a cardiac arrest cart available. A physician or nurse should accompany the patient with a supply of intravenous phentolamine.

After the procedure, assess vital signs every 15 minutes for an hour, every 30 minutes for another hour, and every hour twice after that. Observe the affected extremity for color, temperature, edema, and pedal pulses to observe for post-operative loss of perfusion, and compare with unaffected extremity. Observe for hematoma formation, and notify the physician if any occur or if pulses disappear. Keep the patient flat in bed for 4 hours with no hip flexion.

Celiac and mesenteric arteriography

Description   Contrast medium is injected into the celiac, superior mesenteric, or inferior mesenteric artery for visualization of the vasculature. Superselective arteriography permits a detailed visualization of a particular area. As the contrast medium is injected, serial roentgenograms outline abdominal vessels in arterial, capillary, and venous phases of perfusion.

A radiologist inserts a needle into the femoral artery. A guide wire is passed through the needle into the aorta, and the needle is then removed. An arteriographic catheter is inserted over the guide wire, and placement is checked roentgenographically and fluoroscopically before the guide wire is removed. The catheter, under fluoroscopy, is advanced into one of the three arteries; placement is checked, and an automatic injection of contrast medium is attached. A rapid sequence of serial films is taken as the medium is injected. The catheter is repositioned for superselective visualization.

Indications   Can be used for locating gastrointestinal bleeding and for treating bleeding by either infusion of vasopressin at the site or injection of embolic material to form a clot. The embolic material includes aminocaproic acid (Amicar) clot or gelatin sponge (Gelfoam). It is also used to evaluate cirrhosis and portal hypertension, vascular damage after abdominal trauma, intestinal ischemia, and vascular abnormalities. It may be used in evaluating tumors (distinguishing between benign and malignant) when other tests are inconclusive.

Complications   Bleeding, hematoma formation, or infection at the catheter's insertion site.

Nursing care   Assess the patient for sensitivities to iodine, seafood, and contrast media. Blood work should include hemoglobin, hematocrit, clotting time, prothrombin time, activated partial thromboplastin time, and platelet count. The patient should remain flat in bed for at least 12 hours. Check the puncture site frequently for bleeding and hematoma; a sandbag may be used for 2 to 4 hours to provide some pressure.

Monitor the vital signs as ordered—usually every 15 minutes for 1 hour, every 30 minutes for 2 hours, and then every hour for 4 hours or until the patient is stable. Depending on the patient's reactions to the test and the potential problems of bleeding, this pattern may change. Monitor the peripheral pulses by observing vital signs. Compare pulses in each foot. Also observe the leg (of the puncture site) for color and temperature and compare with the alternate leg.

Notify the physician about continued or excessive bleeding, changes in the peripheral pulse and temperature, and color changes. Also notify the physician if vital signs change significantly, or if there is stinging pain or sensation at femoral site. This may mean that blood is irritating subcutaneous tissues. Check thigh for swelling.

Renal arteriography and venography

Description   Provides information concerning arterial and venous blood supply to the kidneys.

Arteriography.   A preprocedure antianxiety or narcotic injection is given. The patient is taken to a radiologic suite, and an additional local anesthetic is given in the area over the femoral artery. The patient is placed in a supine position, and a femoral puncture is performed. An opaque catheter is then passed from the femoral artery to the aorta and into the desired renal artery under fluoroscopy. A radiopaque contrast material is then injected into the renal artery. (If passage into the aorta via the femoral artery is not feasible, the axillary artery may be used as an alternative.)

Rapid roentgenographic images are used to assess the three phases of the arteriogram: the arterial phase lasts 2 to 4 seconds and provides a detailed outline of the principal renal arteries; the nephrogenic phase is seen as a marked opacification of the renal parenchyma, lasting 15 to 20 seconds; and the venous phase is of limited value because of the kidney's ability to extract and excrete contrast material (principally useful in assessing arteriovenous shunting).

Digital subtraction arteriography (DSA) is a new method of imaging that allows visualization of the kidney's arteries using a significantly smaller dose of contrast material than does the standard technique. It has the advantage of being rapid and relatively noninvasive compared with standard techniques, so it can be performed on an outpatient basis with an IVP. Limitations include poorer visualization of peripheral renal artery branches.[31]

Venography.   To perform this procedure, a percutaneous catheter is placed into the right femoral vein and advanced to the opening of the renal vein. Contrast material is injected, and the catheter is then directed upward to enter the contralateral (right) renal vein. The procedure is repeated. Imaging may be enhanced by injecting 6 to 10 μg of epinephrine into the renal artery followed by renal venography 10 seconds later.

Indications   Indications for arteriography include palpable renal masses, potential renovascular hypertension, and renal trauma; it is also used to determine the suitability of renal donors.[9]

Indications for venography include renal vein thrombosis, renovascular hypertension, elucidation of renal cell carcinoma, and various congenital abnormalities of the renal veins.

Complications   The two major complications are bleeding at the site of the arterial puncture and allergic reactions to the contrast material.

Nursing care   Pedal pulses and capillary filling of the nail beds of the foot should be assessed before the procedure. After

the renal arteriogram is completed, the femoral puncture site should be assessed regularly (every 1 to 2 hours) for hematoma or external bleeding. Assessment of capillary refill and the affected foot's appearance is indicated; compare to unaffected side. Vital signs and signs of allergic reaction to the contrast material should be assessed frequently (every 1 to 2 hours). Signs of allergic reaction include pruritus, wheezing, dyspnea, and flushed skin.

Phlebography (venography)

Description   Invasive procedure used to identify and locate venous thrombi. It involves injection of a radiopaque dye (technetium-99 microaggregated albumin) into the venous system of the affected extremity followed by serial roentgenograms. Abnormal filling of the vein indicates a positive finding that thrombosis exists.

Indications   Deep vein thrombosis.

Complications   Reaction to the contrast media, subcutaneous infiltration of dye, embolism caused by dislodgment of the thrombus.

Nursing care   Explain that the procedure may take from 30 minutes to an hour and that a warm flushed sensation may be felt with the injection of the dye. No preprocedure fasting is required.

Lumbar venography

Description   Injection of contrast medium to visualize epidural venous plexus. The catheter is inserted percutaneously into the femoral vein and then guided into the internal iliac vein or ascending lumbar vein.

Indications   When performed for neurologic or musculoskeletal conditions, lumbar venography aids in outlining the blood supply to or through a tumor or other structure under study and thereby aids in the preoperative assessment and determination of possible operative treatment. The study can be made as an outpatient procedure.

Complications   Bleeding, hematoma formation, infection at the catheter's insertion site.

Nursing care   Monitor the site for signs of hemorrhage or infection. Immobilize the affected extremity for 12 hours after the procedure.

Lymphangiography

Description   Radiopaque medium introduced via a tiny catheter into the peripheral lymphatics to allow visualization of the deep femoral, iliac, and periaortic lymph nodes. Dye is injected locally into the hands and feet via small incisions, and roentgenograms are taken immediately after the injection and 24 hours later.

Indications   Swelling of lymph nodes; suspected malignancy, such as lymphoma, Hodgkin's disease.

Complications   Hypersensitive reaction to the contrast material; inflammation at the infection sites.

Nursing care   Inform the patient about the procedure. Ensure that informed consent is obtained. Have patient void prior to procedure and alert patient that procedure will take several hours. Encourage fluids after the procedure to flush the dye. Inform the patient that a bluish tint to the skin and urine will disappear within a few weeks.

Blood Studies

Blood studies are key diagnostic indicators and are used to assist in the diagnosis of almost every body system. Following are some descriptions of blood studies that require special nursing care utilized for hematolymphatic, immune, and neoplastic disorders. Also included is a discussion of arterial blood gas analysis.

The following blood studies are used to diagnose a wide variety of disorders:

Red cell count determines the number of red blood cells (RBCs) in 1 mm³ of blood

White cell count determines the number of white blood cells (WBCs) in 1 mm³ of blood

Differential count determines the percentage of various types of WBCs

Platelet count determines the number of platelets in 1 mm³ of blood

Hemoglobin concentration determines the amount of hemoglobin in a given volume of blood

Hematocrit determines the percentage of blood composed of RBCs

Mean corpuscular volume (MCV) determines the size and volume of each RBC

Mean corpuscular hemoglobin (MCH) determines the hemoglobin content in RBCs of average size

Mean corpuscular concentration (MCHC) determines the amount of hemoglobin in packed RBCs (hemoglobin of 100 ml RBCs)

Reticulocyte count determines the effectiveness and speed of RBC production and the responsiveness of bone marrow to decreased circulating RBCs

Erythrocyte life span determination estimates the rate at which RBCs tagged with chromium-51 disappear from circulation; the patient and a normal subject with comparable blood type are injected with tagged cells

Erythrocyte fragility test measures the rate at which RBCs burst in hypotonic solutions of varied concentrations

Direct Coombs' test detects autoantibodies against RBCs, which can cause cellular damage. The patient's RBCs are mixed with Coombs' serum, which is a solution containing antibodies against human antibodies. If the RBCs are not coated with the patient's antibodies against RBCs, agglutination (clumping) does not occur

Indirect Coombs' test is used to identify antibodies to RBC antigens

Serum iron level is the amount of iron found in a sample of blood

Bleeding time is measured by making a small stab wound in the earlobe or forearm; the time it takes for the bleeding to stop is noted, and a measurement is made of the rate at which a clot is formed; the patient must not take aspirin

for at least 5 days before the test; the patient is also advised not to drink alcoholic beverages before the test

Coagulation time is the time required for blood to form a solid clot on a foreign surface such as glass test tube

Capillary fragility is determined by the tourniquet test; positive or negative pressure is applied to various areas of the body, and the relative number of petechiae is noted

Therapeutic trial with parenteral vitamin B₁₂ requires that the patient be given intramuscular injections of vitamin B_{12} for 10 days; blood work and the patient's subjective feeling of well-being are evaluated

Schilling test measures the absorption of radioactive vitamin B_{12} before and after parenteral administration of intrinsic factor; it may be a three-staged procedure, and involves 24-hr urine collection

Bilirubin test requires that a venous sample be collected for measuring the total amount of bilirubin; differentiation of conjugated and unconjugated levels can also be determined

Serologic tests are frequently used to help determine the causative pathogens in fungal diseases and atypical pneumonia; the outcome of the test depends on the development of antibodies to the organism in the patient's serum that can be detected by agglutination, complement fixation, or precipitation reactions when the serum is exposed to a specific antigen; examples are the fungal antibody tests that detect coccidioidomycosis, blastomycosis, and histoplasmosis

HLA typing requires that a venous blood specimen be collected for use in the identification of HLA-A, HLA-B, HLA-C histocompatibility antigens; it is used for screening patients and potential donors for tissue transplantation

Immunofluorescence (IF) is measured after the serum or tissue specimen is viewed microscopically; an indirect IF test demonstrates that the serum of a patient with pemphigus or bullous pemphigoid contains specific antibodies that bind to different areas of the epithelium; in the direct IF test, a skin sample shows characteristic patterns for specific diseases

In vitro leukocyte function tests are used to evaluate patients with recurrent infections and suspected immunodeficiency diseases; normal values are determined in each laboratory

Lymphocyte stimulation requires that lymphocytes be incubated with a particular antigen or mitogen (polyclonal activator), and the cell proliferation determined; alterations may be seen in genetic or acquired immunodeficiency states

Cytotoxicity Lymphocytes are incubated with tumor cells or virally infected cells, and target cell lysis is measured; in the absence of any antibody, natural killer (NK) cell function measured; if the donor has been sensitized to a target cell in vivo, a secondary cytotoxic T lymphocyte (CTL) response can be determined

Chemotaxis Phagocytic cells are incubated in a chamber that permits cells to migrate through a filter toward a chemoattractant; when samples from the patient are incubated with standard chemotactic factors, chemotactic capabilities of phagocytic cells are assessed; alternatively one can incubate normal phagocytes with patient serum to test the ability of that serum to generate chemotactic factors

Phagocytosis　Particle uptake assays measure phagocytic cell function or the opsonizing capacity of the patient's serum; to assess phagocyte function, the patient's monocytes or neutrophils are incubated with test particle in the presence of normal human serum; to examine opsonization, normal phagocytic cells are incubated with particles in the presence of the patient's serum; phagocytosis can be assessed by direct visualization or use of radiolabeled particles

Bactericidal activity　Phagocytic cells are incubated with appropriately opsonized bacteria and then washed and lysed; the number of live intracellular bacteria is then determined

NBT dye reduction　Phagocytic cells are incubated with particles in the presence of oxidized nitroblue tetrazolium (NBT); on stimulation of respiratory burst activity, reducing equivalents are generated and NBT is converted into deep blue insoluble precipitate; NBT dye reduction does not occur in certain patients with genetic phagocytic cell defects

Chemiluminescence　Phagocytes are incubated with opsonized particles, and light emission is measured in a spectrophotometer; during phagocytosis, normal monocytes and neutrophils generate highly unstable oxygen intermediates that emit light during decay to the ground state; chemiluminescence is reduced in patients with certain phagocyte dysfunctions

Tumor Markers

Acid phosphatase
　Increased in prostatic cancer
　Increased in some primary bone malignancies, multiple myeloma
Alkaline phosphatase
　Increased in metastatic cancer to bone and liver, osteogenic sarcoma, myeloma, and Hodgkin's lymphoma with bone involvement
Alpha-fetoprotein (AFP)
　Increased in hepatocellular cancers; choriocarcinoma; teratoma; embryonal cell tumors of testis and ovary; some pancreatic, stomach, colon, and lung tumors
Carcinoembryonic antigen (CEA)
　Increased in colon cancer
　Also seen in lung, pancreas, hepatobiliary, stomach, breast, head and neck, and prostate cancers
Chorionic gonadotropin (beta subunit) (B-HCG)
　Increased in hydatidiform mole, choriocarcinoma, testicular teratoma
　Ectopic HCG production by some cancers of pituitary gland, stomach, pancreas, lung, colon, and liver

Pancreatic oncofetal antigen (POA)
　Positive in large percentage of pancreas tumors
Placental alkaline phosphatase (PAP)
　Increased in a variety of tumors
　Prostate-specific antigen (PSA) increased in prostate cancer

Hormones

Adrenocorticotropic hormone (ACTH)
　Increased in ectopic-ACTH producing tumors (especially small cell lung cancer), adrenal carcinoma, adenoma
Androstenedione
　Increased in ectopic ACTH-producing tumors, ovarian tumors
Antidiuretic hormone (ADH)
　Increased in brain tumors, systemic malignancies with ectopic ADH production
Calcitonin
　Increased in medullary carcinoma of thyroid, some lung and breast tumors, colon cancer, and GI malignancies
Estrogens, total
　Increased in estrogen-producing ovarian tumors, some testicular tumors, and adrenal cortical tumors
Estrogen (Estradiol) receptor assay
　60% of breast cancer characterized by estrogen receptors
Glucagon
　Decreased in some pancreatic tumors
Growth hormone (LGH)
　Increased in ectopic secretion by some stomach and lung tumors
Parathyroid hormone (LPTH)
　Increased squamous cell or epidermoid lung cancers and renal cell
Progesterone
　Increased in some ovarian tumors
Progesterone receptor assay
　May be useful in predicting tumors likely to respond to hormonal manipulations
17-Ketogenic steroids
　Increased in adrenal adenoma and carcinoma, ectopic ACTH syndrome
17-Ketosteroids
　Increased in adrenal tumors, testicular tumors, interstitial cell tumors, androgenic ovarian tumors
Testosterone
　Increased in some adrenocortical tumors, gonadotropin-producing extragonadal tumors

Enzymes

Amylase
　Increased in some lung and ovarian tumors
Amylase isoenzymes
　Increased in some bronchogenic or serous ovarian tumors
Lactic dehydrogenase (LDH) and LDH isoenzymes
　Increased in extensive carcinomatosis and malignant processes; acute leukemia

TABLE III-1 Hormone Tests

Hormone	Stimulation	Suppression
Antidiuretic hormone (ADH)	Water deprivation	Saline infusion
	Nicotine	Pitressin
Growth hormone (GH)	Insulin tolerance test	Glucose tolerance test
	Arginine tolerance test	
	Levodopa	
	Exercise stimulation test	
Thyroid-stimulating hormone (TSH)	Thyrotropin-releasing hormone (TRH)	Triiodothyronine
		Thyroxine
Prolactin (PRL)	Insulin tolerance test	Levodopa
	Chlorpromazine	
	TRH	
Adrenocorticotropic hormone (ACTH)	Insulin tolerance test (hypoglycemia will occur)	Dexamethasone
	Corticotropin-releasing hormone (CRH)	Metyrapone
Luteinizing hormone (LH)	Luteinizing-releasing hormone (LRH)	Testosterone
		Estrogen
Follicle-stimulating hormone (FSH)	Clomiphene	
Triiodothyronine (T_3)	TSH	T_3
Thyroxine (T_4)		T_4
Cortisol	ACTH	Dexamethasone
	CRH	Metyrapone
	Insulin tolerance test	
	Arginine tolerance test	
Aldosterone	ACTH	Salt loading/volume expansion
		Spironolactone
Norepinephrine	Histamine	Phentolamine
	Tyramine	
	Glucagon	
Progesterone	Human menopausal gonadotropin (HMG)	Provera
	Human chorionic gonadotropin (HCG)	Progesterone
Testosterone	HMG	Testosterone
	HCG	
Parathyroid hormone (PTH)	PTH infusion	Calcium infusion
Glucose	Glucagon	Insulin tolerance test
		Tolbutamide
Insulin	Glucose tolerance test (GTT)	Prolonged fast
	Leucine	
	Fructose	
Gastrin	Pentagastrin	Cimetidine
	Calcium infusion	
	High-protein, high-carbohydrate meal	

Leucine aminopeptidase (LAP)
  Increased in pancreatic cancer with liver metastases
Lysozyme
  Increased in acute monocytic or myelomonocytic leukemia and chronic myeloid leukemia
Serum gamma glutamyl transpeptidase (SGGT)
  Increased in some cases of renal cell cancer and liver metastases
Serum aspartate aminotransferase (AST)
  Increased in liver metastases
Serum alanine aminotransferase (ALT)
  Increased in some liver cancers

Proteins (immunoglobulins produced by lymphocytes and plasma cells)

IgA
IgO
IgE
IgG
IgM

Endocrine studies of hormones

Provocative endocrine testing is classified as either stimulation or suppression studies. Evaluation of secretory reserve by a *stimulation* test is useful for diagnosing hypofunction and for detecting impaired secretory reserve. *Suppression* tests are useful for diagnosis of hyperfunction because the hyperfunctioning gland by definition is not operating under normal control mechanisms.

Table III-1 lists tests according to the hormone being evaluated. These tests are associated with specific procedures de-

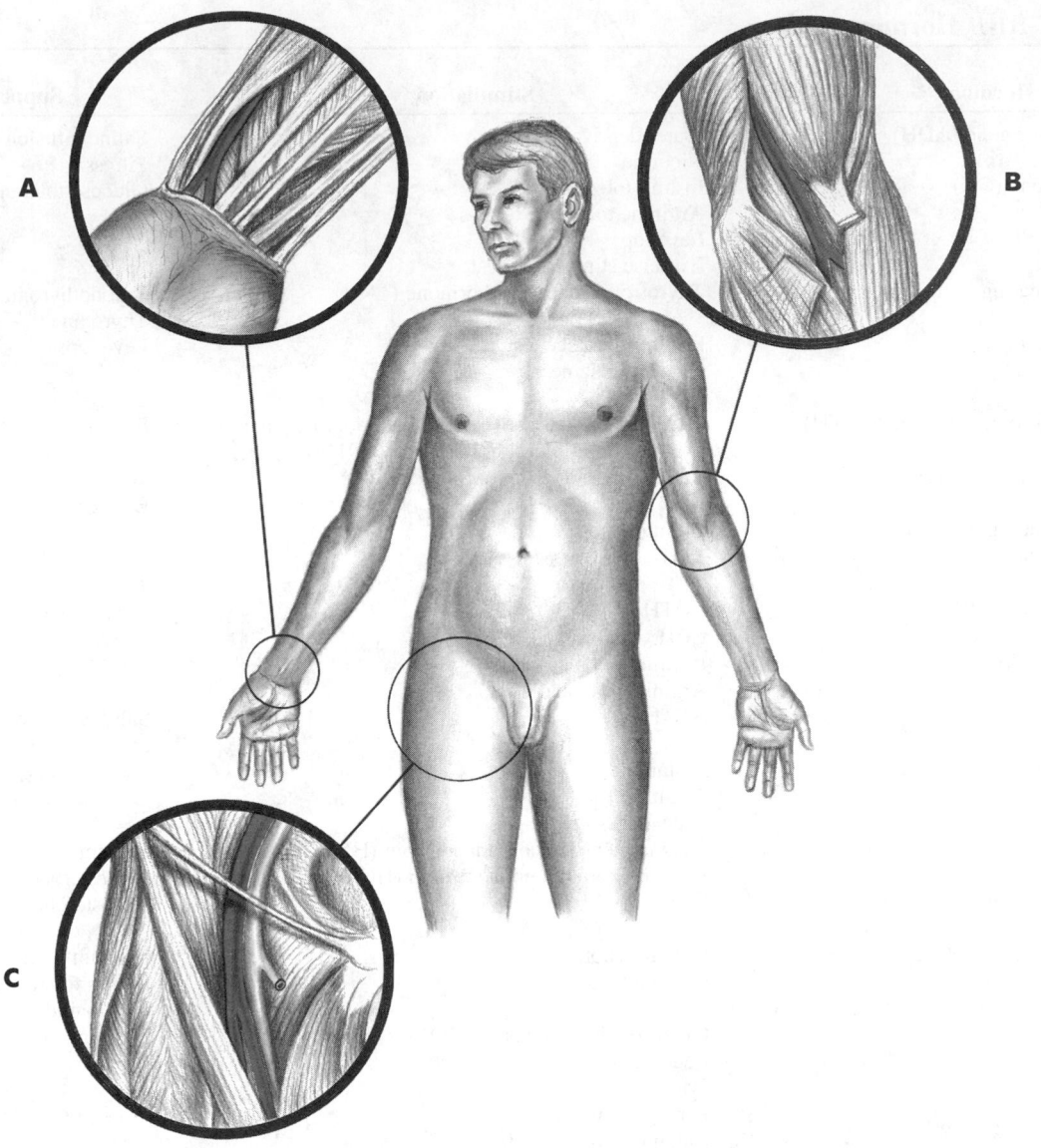

Figure III-4 Arterial blood gas sites. **A,** Radial artery. **B,** Brachial artery. **C,** Femoral artery.

pendent on the laboratory capabilities of the institution. Injection of some hormones (e.g., TRH) may produce a warm, flushed feeling. The nursing care includes education of the patient about the purpose, procedure, and possible side effects and support of the patient during the procedure. The insulin tolerance test will cause profound and purposeful hypoglycemia, requiring a nurse in attendance at all times. When the physician terminates the test, intravenous glucose (10% D/W; 20% D/W; 50% D) is infused immediately and is followed by a high-protein meal.

Arterial blood gas analysis

Description Arterial blood gas analysis is the most direct method to assess the patient's oxygen and blood gas status.

Indications The procedure is indicated for any patient who is seriously ill or injured, whose respiratory status and metabolic balance are in question. Most commonly, arterial blood gases are required for patients with hypoxemia or desaturation secondary to altered ventilatory patterns from any cause.

Arterial blood gas collection procedure

1. Gather the equipment: an ABG syringe with dry heparin with a 20- or 21-gauge needle (21- or 23-gauge for children); rubber stopper or Luer-Lok cap, alcohol swab or iodophor prep, gauze pads, and basin with crushed ice and water.
2. Position the patient in either a sitting or supine position and explain the procedure.
3. Locate the arterial puncture site: possible sites include the radial artery, brachial artery, and femoral artery (Figure III-4). Vessel criteria include the following:

a. Collateral blood flow: the radial artery has excellent collateral flow; the brachial artery has reasonable collateral flow; and the femoral artery has no collateral blood flow.

b. Vessel accessibility; it is easier to palpate, stabilize, and puncture superficial vessels than it is to work with deep ones. The more distal an artery, the more superficial it is.

c. Periarterial tissue: muscles, tendon, and fat are reasonably insensitive to pain. Bone periosteum and nerves are very sensitive. Therefore choose a site that avoids close sensitive structures or parallel veins. The sites of choice are first, radial; second, brachial; third, femoral.

4. When using the radial artery, perform the Allen test. This will evaluate the collateral blood supply. The technique is as follows:

a. Instruct the patient to close his fist tightly.

b. Obliterate both radial and ulnar arteries simultaneously.

c. Instruct the patient to relax his hand (not fully); watch for blanching of palm and fingers.

d. Remove obstructing pressure from only the ulnar artery and observe for capillary refill and flush of hand (within 15 seconds). This refill response, which is a positive Allen test, verifies that the ulnar artery alone is capable of supplying the entire hand.

e. If the Allen test is negative, do not use the radial artery for arterial puncture.

f. If the patient is unconscious or uncooperative, a similar response to the closed fist can be obtained by placing the patient's hand up in the air until blanching occurs; obliterate the arteries, lower the hand, and release pressure over the ulnar artery.

NOTE: The remaining procedure assumes that the radial artery has been chosen for arterial puncture:

5. Donning gloves, palpate the radial artery to locate a spot where maximum pulsation is felt.

6. Clean the area with iodophor prep, then with alcohol swab.

7. With one hand locate the radial pulse proximal to the area cleaned. This will provide landmark information. Keeping the fingers of one hand on the pulse, insert the heparinized needle and syringe into the radial artery distal to the palpating fingers. The angle between the needle and the artery should be approximately 45 degrees. This makes the hole through the arterial wall oblique so that the muscle fiber will seal the hole as soon as the needle is removed.

8. When the artery is punctured, the pulsating blood will push up the hub of the syringe. Do not make more than two attempts at any one site.

9. Obtain a sample of approximately 3 to 5 ml.

10. After the blood is obtained, remove the needle, apply gauze, and use firm and continuous pressure over the site for a minimum of 5 minutes. If the patient is on anticoagulants, pressure must be maintained for a much longer period of time.

11. Remove all air bubbles from the syringe (this will affect blood gas results).

12. Place the syringe in an iced container and send it to the laboratory. The ice will decrease the alterations of the true pH, oxygen, and carbon dioxide levels of the specimen.

Blood Gas Analysis[19,26]

Step by step analysis

1. pH (hydrogen ion concentration): assess patient's acid-base status

   Normal = 7.35 to 7.45

   Acidosis = Less than 7.35

   Alkalosis = Greater than 7.43 (when pH is normal, but when $Paco_2$ and HCO_3^- are both abnormal, compensation is probably occurring)

2. $Paco_2$ (carbon dioxide tension): evaluates the patient's ventilation

   Normal = 35 to 45 mm Hg

   Hyperventilation (hypocarbia) = Less than 34 mm Hg; this means that there is excessive loss of carbon dioxide

   Abnormal value indicates there is no respiratory compensation for a metabolic problem

   Decreased values may be caused by hyperventilation or ventilation-perfusion inequality

   To evaluate for respiratory acidosis and alkalosis and for compensation caused by metabolic acidosis and alkalosis

3. $Paco_2$ in relation to pH

   $\uparrow Paco_2 + \downarrow pH$ = Acidemia of respiratory origin

   $\uparrow Paco_2 + \uparrow pH$ = Respiratory retention of carbon dioxide to compensate for metabolic alkalosis

   $\downarrow Paco_2 + \uparrow pH$ = Alkalosis of respiratory origin

   $\downarrow Paco_2 + \downarrow pH$ = Respiratory elimination of carbon dioxide to compensate for metabolic acidosis

4. Bicarbonate (HCO_3^-): This is the metabolic component

   Normal = 16 to 24 mEq/L (infant), 21 to 28 mEq/L (arterial, children and adults), 22 to 27 mEq/L (venous, children and adults)

   Alkalosis = Greater than 26 mEq/L

   Acidosis = Less than 22 mEq/L

   A normal value indicates that there are no primary metabolic problems and that there is no metabolic compensation for a respiratory problem

5. HCO_3^- in relation to pH: To evaluate for metabolic acidosis and alkalosis and for compensation caused by respiratory acidosis and alkalosis

   $\downarrow HCO_3^- + \downarrow pH$ = Acidemia of metabolic origin

   $\downarrow HCO_3^- + \uparrow pH$ = Renal retention of hydrogen ion or elimination of HCO_3^- to compensate for respiratory alkalosis

   $\uparrow HCO_3^- + \uparrow pH$ = Alkalosis of metabolic origin

   $\uparrow HCO_3^- + \downarrow pH$ = Renal retention of HCO_3^- or elimination of hydrogen ion

6. PaO_2 and O_2 saturation

PaO_2 saturation: Normal = 80 to 95 mm Hg: 60 to 70 mm

Hg (newborn)

O_2 saturation: Normal = 95% to 99%

These values may be abnormal because of hypoventilation, shunting, ventilation-perfusion inequality, or a reduction of inspired oxygen

Acid-base imbalance[25]

Alkalosis

Respiratory

$\downarrow Pa_{CO_2}$ + $\downarrow HCO_3^-$ = Patient attempting to compensate

$\downarrow Pa_{CO_2}$ + Normal HCO_3^- = No patient compensation

Metabolic

$\uparrow HCO_3^-$ + $\uparrow Pa_{CO_2}$ = Patient attempting to compensate

$\uparrow HCO_3^-$ + Normal Pa_{CO_2} = No patient compensation

Clinical signs of alkalosis: dizziness, tingling of fingers and toes, muscle weakness or muscle spasm, muscle twitching, sweating, cardiac dysrhythmia, shallow respirations, nausea or vomiting, tachypnea, tremor, or convulsion

Fluid and electrolyte imbalances (contributing to alkalosis)

$\downarrow$ Serum sodium

$\uparrow$ Serum chloride

$\downarrow$ Serum chloride (if alkalosis is caused by gastric suctioning)

$\downarrow$ Potassium

Acidosis

Respiratory

$\uparrow Pa_{CO_2}$ + $\uparrow HCO_3^-$ + Patient attempting to compensate

$\uparrow Pa_{CO_2}$ + Normal HCO_3^- = No patient compensation

Metabolic

$\downarrow HCO_3^-$ + $\downarrow Pa_{CO_2}$ = Patient attempting to compensate

$\downarrow HCO_3^-$ + Normal Pa_{CO_2} = No patient compensation

Clinical signs of acidosis: headache, slowness in responding to questions, hand tremor when patient is instructed to extend arms, confusion, drowsiness, Kussmaul respirations, nausea or vomiting, tremor, confusion, tachycardia, coma

Fluid and electrolyte imbalances (contributing to acidosis)

$\downarrow$ Serum sodium

$\downarrow$ Serum chloride

$\uparrow$ Serum potassium

Complications[11] Hematoma from multiple attempts at puncture or from inadequate pressure to the site after arterial stick; ischemia of an extremity secondary to thrombus after the procedure; adjunct nerve damage secondary to incorrect technique.

Nursing care Explain the procedure fully before attempting technique. Assist the physician in administering a local anesthetic if indicated before obtaining arterial blood gases. Following procedure, apply direct pressure over the puncture site for at least 5 minutes to prevent hematoma or bleeding into the tissues. Carefully and systematically analyze the blood gas results according to the assessment guidelines. Monitor the patient's response to actual or potential blood gas acid-base imbalances to include the following:

Mental state: depression or stimulation of the central nervous system

Respiratory status: breathing pattern and depth and quality of respiration

Cardiovascular response: pulse rate, rhythm, and quality

Fluid and electrolyte status: disorders, such as vomiting and diarrhea, that could cause the imbalance; the patient's responses secondary to fluid and electrolyte imbalances

Urodynamic Studies

Uroflowmetry

Description Determines the rate, time, and volume of urinary flow. This study requires no catheterization; the patient voids into a device that measures the characteristics of bladder elimination. Results are displayed in graph form.

Indications Aids in the diagnosis and description of ureteral, urethral, and bladder function.

Complications None.

Nursing care The patient should force fluids and refrain from voiding for 2 hours before testing in order to have at least 300 ml of urine in the bladder.

Urethral pressure studies

Description These studies measure urethral resistance to urinary outflow. The catheter is pulled through the urethra at a given rate while water or carbon dioxide is infused through several side ports. A specialized catheter may be placed at the external urinary sphincter to measure the urethral response to bladder filling/storage and micturition.

Indications Aids in the diagnosis of bladder disorders.

Complications Cystitis.

Nursing care Instruct the patient to watch for signs of cystitis (frequency of urination and mild dysuria), which should disappear within the first 24 hours after testing.

Cystometry

Description Evaluates the two phases of bladder function: filling/storage and expulsion/micturition. One or more catheters is placed in the bladder urethrally or suprapubically. The bladder is then filled with liquid contrast material (water or a roentgenographic material) or carbon dioxide. The patient is asked to report sensations of an urgency to void or a bladder fullness. The study is completed by asking the patient to void voluntarily.

Indications Bladder, micturition disorders.

Complications Cystitis.

Nursing care Instruct the patient to watch for signs of cystitis (frequency of urination, dysuria), which should completely disappear within the first 24 hours after testing.

Cystometry with pharmacologic testing

Description Two comparative cystometrograms are performed before and 30 minutes after administration of a certain drug. The most commonly used drugs are bethanechol chloride (Urecholine) and propantheline bromide (Pro-Banthine).

Indications Bethanechol is used to assess "denervation" (neuropathic changes in bladder function) as opposed to functional voiding abnormalities. Propantheline is used to assess the clinical response of detrusor overactivity to an anticholinergic agent.

Complications Bethanechol may cause nausea and vomiting, hypotension, and shock. Atropine is given subcutaneously as an antidote if needed. Propantheline may cause hypotension, hypertension, tachycardia, angina, and atrial or ventricular fibrillation; physostigmine salicylate is given parenterally as an antidote if needed.

Nursing care Vital signs should be monitored every 15 to 30 minutes for a 2-hour period after testing.

Loopogram

Description Water-soluble contrast material is instilled into the urostomy stoma via a small catheter and observed under fluoroscopy; a roentgenogram is taken. The loop is then drained and the catheter removed: a 10-minute procedure.

Indications Assesses length and emptying ability of the ileal/sigmoid conduit; also assesses presence of stricture, reflux angulation, or obstruction.

Complications None.

Nursing care Provide the patient with a replacement urinary pouch, since it will be removed during the test.

Miscellaneous Studies

Echoencephalogram

Description An echoencephalogram is a noninvasive diagnostic technique that records sonic pulses from cerebral structures by reflection of ultrasonic impulses directed through the patient's skull and back toward the source. These pulses are then recorded and projected onto an oscilloscope screen.[3]

The procedure is performed by placing an ultrasonic transducer on the skull's midaxis in the temporoparietal region. The waves produced are called M-echos, which then are recorded and projected on a screen to provide a graphic representation of the distance from the reflecting surface to the source of the ultrasonic beam.[32] Pictures of these M-echo waves may become a permanent part of the patient's record. The procedure takes only several minutes, and the reliability of the results depends on the skill of the technician. Abnormal shifts of the midline structures are recorded in millimeters, and a shift of 3 mm or more in the adult is considered abnormal.

Indications Useful in determining ventricular size and cerebral midline shifts.

Complications None.

Nursing care Explain the procedure to the patient.

Tonometry

Description Several types of instruments (tonometers) measure intraocular pressure; all of them indent the globe and measure the force (or weight) necessary to cause the indentation.

Schiötz tonometer. This hand-held instrument has a curved footplate that is rested on the cornea. A local anesthetic is instilled into each eye. The patient lies supine and is asked to stare straight ahead. The examiner holds the lids open. As the tonometer is placed on the corneal surface, a scale reading is taken from the instrument and converted with a chart to pressure in mm Hg.

Applanation tonometer. This machines measures the force required to flatten rather than indent the central cornea. It is more accurate than the Schiötz tonometer. A spring tension knob records the pressure, and a local anesthetic is used.

Noncontact tonometer. This machine uses a rapid puff of air to exert and register pressure. It does not require any anesthetic and is very accurate except in higher-pressure ranges. It cannot be used for patients with corneal edema or those with irregular optic interface.

Indications For measurement of intraocular pressure; for routine screening of glaucoma and diabetes; for assessment of penetrating injuries.

Complications None; a risk of cross contamination exists if the tonometer is not sterilized between patients.

Nursing care Sterilize the tonometer before each use. Inquire about corneal injuries or abrasions. Assure the patient that no discomfort will be experienced.

Caloric test

Description Stimulation of the semicircular canals by introduction of either water or air (above or below body temperature) into the external auditory canal. Water below body temperature causes endolymphatic fluid to flow in a downward direction when directed against the tympanic membrane. The injection of cold water into the ear causes maximal stimulation of the semicircular canals and causes nystagmus and falling reactions in 10 to 20 seconds in the normal individual. Warm caloric tests have given reactions opposite to those induced by cold water tests. Specific tests include the following:

Caloric test for vestibular function. Cold or hot water is injected into the external auditory canal with the patient lying down and the head elevated at 30 degrees. The patient is observed for nystagmus.

Hallpike caloric test. Hot or cold water is injected into the external auditory canal. The time interval from the beginning of water flow to the end of visible nystagmus is recorded.

Nelson caloric test. Small amounts of ice water are injected into the external aural canal while the patient is in a supine position with the head tilted 30 degrees forward or in a sitting position with the head tilted 60 degrees backward. The patient is observed for nystagmus.

Indications The caloric test indicates whether the labyrinth is reacting normally and is hypoactive or hyperactive, or whether no labyrinthine response is present.[16] In patients who complain of dizziness, vertigo, unsteadiness, or nystagmus, it is important to know whether the labyrinth is functioning normally.

Complications None.

Nursing care Maintain bed rest, with the head of the bed elevated 20 to 30 degrees until subjective symptoms disappear. The patient is given nothing by mouth 6 hours before the procedure.

Specific audiometric and hearing testing

Description The following are some of the tests used to determine hearing loss.

Weber's test. The handle of a lightly vibrating tuning fork is placed in the middle of the forehead. Tones should normally be heard equally in both ears.

Rinne's test. When a softly struck tuning fork is placed alternately behind the ear on the mastoid process, and then in front of the same ear, the normal ear hears a tuning fork about twice as long by air conduction as by bone conduction.

Schwabach test. The examiner and patient hear tones equally when a tuning fork is alternately placed on the patient's and the examiner's mastoid processes.

Pure tone test. A series of tones is volume calibrated at different frequencies (400 to 3000 Hz). The speech threshold represents the loudness at which a person with normal hearing can perceive a tone. Both air and bone conduction are measured for each ear, and the results are graphed. With normal hearing, the line is plotted at 0 dB.

Speech audiometry. A normal-hearing person hears and correctly repeats 95% of words spoken by the examiner.

Impedance audiometry. Disorders of the middle ear are detected, thereby determining the degree of tympanic membrane and middle ear mobility. An impedance audiometer is used. One end is a probe with three small tubes inserted into the external canal, and the other end attaches to an oscillator. One tube delivers a low tone of varying intensity, the second contains a microphone, and the third has an air pump. A normal tympanic membrane reflects minimal sound waves and produces a low-voltage curve on the graph.

Tympanometry. A tympanometer, with the impedance audiometer, measures the tympanic membrane's compliance with air pressure variations in the external canal and determines the degree of negative pressure in the middle ear.

In addition to these tests, patients may be tested to differentiate sensory (cochlear) hearing losses from neural (acoustic nerve) hearing losses. These tests include recruitment, sensitivity to small increases in intensity, and pathologic adaptation.

Recruitment is the ability to hear loud sounds normally despite a hearing loss or an abnormal increase in the perception of loudness. This is absent in neural hearing losses and present in sensory hearing losses. It can be demonstrated by having the patient compare the loudness of sounds in the affected ear with the loudness of sounds in the normal ear. In sensory hearing losses the sensation of loudness in the affected ear increases more with each increment in intensity than it does in the normal ear. In neural hearing losses the sensation of loudness in the affected ear increases less with each increment in intensity than in the normal ear. This is called *decruitment.*[17]

Sensitivity to small increments in intensity can be determined by having a patient listen to a continuous tone of 20 dB and then briefly and intermittently increasing the intensity. Patients with neural hearing losses, as well as those with normal hearing, cannot detect small changes in intensity. On the other hand, a patient with a sensory hearing loss can easily perceive these changes.

Pathologic adaptation, or tone decay, is found when a person cannot continue to hear a constant tone above the hearing threshold. The findings are mildly abnormal with sensory losses and severely abnormal with neural losses.

Indications To diagnose hearing impairment.

Complications None.

Nursing care Explain the procedure to the patient.

Pulmonary function testing (see Table III-2)

Simple Spirometer

Description The simple spirometer is a basic office tool used to measure the presence and severity of disease in large and small airways and to distinguish between obstructive and restrictive patterns. It is most commonly used to measure VC, IC, ERV, V_T, IRV, $FEF_{200-1200}$, and $FEF_{25\%-75\%}$. There are two types of spirometers: volume and flow. Both types are usually computerized. Two of the most common are the water seal and dry rolling seal spirometers. The volume measurement spirometer is most common. This type works so that as the individual exhales or inhales into the mouth-piece, water or air already in the spirometer is displaced, causing the pen to touch the rotating drum and record the pattern. The presence and severity of respiratory dysfunction are determined by comparing observed values with those predicted for a normal person considering age, gender, height, weight, and race.

Spirometer with Gas Dilution

Description The spirometer with gas dilution is used to measure the following:

FRC (functional residual capacity)

RV (residual volume)

RV/TLC ratio (residual volume/total lung capacity)

$D_{L}CO$ (oxygen diffusing capacity of the lung)

The purpose of the technique is to measure the rate of diffusion. The measurement of lung volumes is by either the helium-dilution technique or the nitrogen-washout technique. In the *helium-dilution technique* the patient rebreathes a known concentration of diluted helium through the spirometer mouthpiece until the helium concentration in the spirometer and the

Text continues on p. 1506

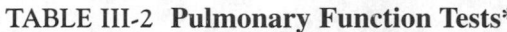

TABLE III-2 Pulmonary Function Tests*

Test	Description	Significance
Lung Volume Test†		
VC = Vital capacity (VC = ERV + V$_T$ + IRV)	This capacity test combining more than one lung volume is the maximum amount of air that can be expired slowly and completely following a maximum inspiration. Response values of this test, as well as all other pulmonary function tests, are directly dependent on patient's effort. From VC other pulmonary function values may be calculated, including ERV, IRV, V$_T$, and IC.	A decrease in VC may be caused by a loss of distensible lung tissue, as seen in bronchiolar obstruction, pulmonary edema, pneumonia, atelectasis, pulmonary restriction, surgery, pulmonary congestion, or by depression of the respiratory center in the brain.
FRC = Functional residual capacity (FRC = ERV + RV)	This capacity test combining more than one lung volume is the volume of air remaining in the lungs at the end of normal expiration. Open- or closed-circuit techniques of body plethysmography are used to measure concentration of a gas (either helium or nitrogen); from this the FRC can be calculated. This is actually calculated measurement of airway resistance.	The values help to differentiate obstructive from restrictive diseases. An increased FRC represents hyperinflation, which is seen with bronchiolar obstruction, emphysema, or asthma. An increased FRC results in muscular and mechanical inefficiency. A decreased FRC may be seen in diseases that occlude the alveoli such as pneumonia, and in fibrosis, asbestosis, or silicosis.
ERV = Expiratory reserve volume	This single-volume calculation is the maximum amount of air that can be exhaled following a resting expiratory level.	Although the ERV (approximately 25% of VC) has no diagnostic value, it must be calculated so that the RV can be calculated.
IRV = Inspiratory reserve volume	This single-volume calculation is the maximum amount of air that can be inspired following a normal inspiration.	
RV = Residual volume (RV = FRC − ERV)	This single-volume measurement is the volume of air remaining in the lungs at the end of maximal expiration. This is measured indirectly by subtracting the ERV from the FRC.	This value helps to differentiate restrictive from obstructive diseases. An increased RV indicates that despite maximal expiratory effort the lungs still contain an abnormally large amount of air. This may be seen in patients with emphysema or chronic bronchial obstruction. The RV usually decreases with restrictive lung disease.
IC = Inspiratory capacity (IC = V$_T$ + IRV)	This calculated measurement is a capacity test involving more than one lung volume. It is the largest volume of air that can be inspired in one breath from the resting expiratory level.	IC normally composes approximately 75% of the VC. Changes in the IC usually parallel increases or decreases in VC. Other than its use in postoperative care, this value is not commonly measured.
TLC = Total lung capacity (TLC = FRC + IC) or (TLC = VC + RV)	This capacity test combining more than one lung volume is the volume of air contained in the lung at the end of a maximal inspiration. The TLC is a derived calculation.	TLC differentiates obstructive from restrictive diseases. It may be decreased in pulmonary edema, atelectasis, neoplasms, pulmonary congestion, pneumothorax, or thoracic restriction. TLC may be increased in bronchiolar obstruction with hyperinflation and in emphysema.
RV/TLC Ratio = Residual volume/Total lung capacity ratio (RV/TLC × 100)	This is a statement of the fraction of the TLC that can be defined as RV, expressed as a percentage.	Values greater than 35% are seen in patients with emphysema or chronic air trapping.
Ventilation Tests		
V$_T$ = Tidal volume	This single-volume measurement is the volume of air inspired or expired during each respiratory cycle. This is measured at the bedside by a simple spirometer for 1 minute. The total is then divided by the rate (the number of breaths per minute) to determine the average V$_T$.	Decreased or increased V$_T$ may occur in various pulmonary disorders. V$_T$ should be considered in relation only to arterial blood gases and respiratory rate and minute volume.
V$_E$ = Minute volume	This is the total volume of air inspired or expired in 1 minute. It is determined by measuring the inspired or expired air over several minutes and dividing by the number of minutes. It may also be measured easily at the bedside by simple spirometry.	This value must be considered in conjunction with arterial blood gases. V$_E$ increases in response to hypoxia, hypercapnia, acidosis, and exercise. It is most commonly used in exercise testing.

Continued.

TABLE III-2 Pulmonary Function Tests*—cont'd

Test	Description	Significance
V_D = Respiratory dead space	This is the volume of the lungs that is ventilated but not perfused by pulmonary capillary blood flow. This includes the conducting airways, or anatomic dead space, and the nonfunctioning alveoli, or alveolar dead space.	The measurement of V_D provides important information regarding the status of the functional lung capacity. It is used primarily for exercise testing.
V_A = Alveolar ventilation $V_A = (V_T - V_D)\, f$ f = respiratory rate	This is the volume of air that participates in gas exchange in the lungs.	The adequacy of V_A can be determined only by arterial blood gas studies. It is used primarily for exercise testing.

Pulmonary Spirometry Tests

Test	Description	Significance
FVC = Forced vital capacity	This is the volume of air that can be expired forcefully and rapidly after maximal inspiration. The measurement is made directly by spirometer.	The FVC is normally equal to the VC. FVC may be reduced in chronic obstructive diseases, whereas the VC may appear close to normal. The FVC is decreased in restrictive diseases also. The test's validity depends largely on the individual's effort and cooperation.
FEV_T = Forced expiratory volume timed	This is the volume of air expired over a given interval during the performance of an FVC. The interval (T) is stated as a subscript to FEV. For example, $FEV_{0.5}$ indicates the interval is 0.5 second, and in FEV_1 the interval is 1 second. FEV_T is a calculated measurement by spirometer. After 3 seconds, FEV should equal FVC.	FEV_T is the most common screening test for detection of obstructive airway disease, in which the finding is a reduced response.
FEV% = FEV_T/FVC ratio × 100 (usually FEV_1/FVC%)	This is the percentage of the measured FVC that a given FEV_T represents.	By measuring the expiratory flow over time the severity of obstruction can be assessed. FEV% or a reduced ratio is decreased in obstructive lung disease. It usually remains within normal limits for persons with restrictive disease unless there is some type of secondary problem.
$FEV_{25\%-75\%}$ = Forced expiratory flow, 25% to 75% or MMEF = Maximum mid-expiratory flow rate	This is the average flow during the middle 50% of an FEV. It was previously known as the maximum midexpiratory flow rate (MMEF or MMF). Its reported value provides a picture of peripheral airway resistance. This value is then compared with the VC.	This measures the average flow rate over a given interval. It is an index of the status of the medium-sized airways. Decreased flow rates, when compared to the VC, are seen in early stages of obstructive diseases such as emphysema.
PEFR = Peak flow	This is the maximum flow rate attainable at any time during an FEV.	This measurement is of questionable diagnostic value. Children with asthma have a decreased PEFR.
F-V loop = Flow-volume loop	This is a graphic analysis of the maximum forced expiratory flow volume (MEFV) followed by a maximum inspiratory flow volume (MIFV). This technique uses a forced expiratory vital capacity followed by a forced inspiratory vital capacity. It is actually another way to display the forced vital capacity. Curves, reported as continuous loops on spirometric graphs, have distinctive sizes and shapes.	The inspiratory flow may show evidence of upper airway obstruction. With obstructive disease the flow is reduced out of proportion to the volume. In restrictive disease the flow and volume are proportionally decreased, or the flow may be better than would be expected for the volume. As the flow-volume loop is examined, the shapes of the inspiratory and expiratory sides are analyzed.
MVV = Maximum voluntary ventilation	This is the largest volume of air that can be breathed per minute by voluntary effort. The actual testing period lasts 10 to 15 seconds.	The MVV measures the status of respiratory muscles, the resistance offered by airways and tissues, and the compliance of the lung and thorax. This measurement depends greatly on the individual's effort.

TABLE III-2 Pulmonary Function Tests*—cont'd

Test	Description	Significance
Gas Exchange		
DL_{co} = Diffusing capacity of CO	The diffusing capacity rate of the lung provides a measure of the lung's gas exchange mechanism. It assesses the amount of functioning pulmonary capillary bed in contact with functioning alveoli. A common way to measure this is the *single-breath Krogh method:* the patient deeply inhales (from the residual volume level) a mixture of air containing 0.3% carbon monoxide and 10% helium gas, holds his breath for 10 seconds, and then exhales. The carbon monoxide levels are then remeasured.	The test is used primarily to differentiate various disease processes and for patient care monitoring.
R_{aw} = Airway resistance G_{aw} = Airway conductance	R_{aw} is the pressure difference required for a unit flow change. G_{aw} is the flow generated per unit of pressure drop in the airway. It is the reciprocal of R_{aw}. Measurements are made with a body plethysmograph. They are taken at the same time as FRC.	R_{aw} increases in an acute asthmatic attack, emphysema, or other obstructive diseases. The calculations are most useful in evaluation of the qualitative response to various bronchodilators.

*Normal values for pulmonary tests vary depending on the patient's age, gender, weight, and race.
†To best interpret these tests see Figures III-5 and III-6.

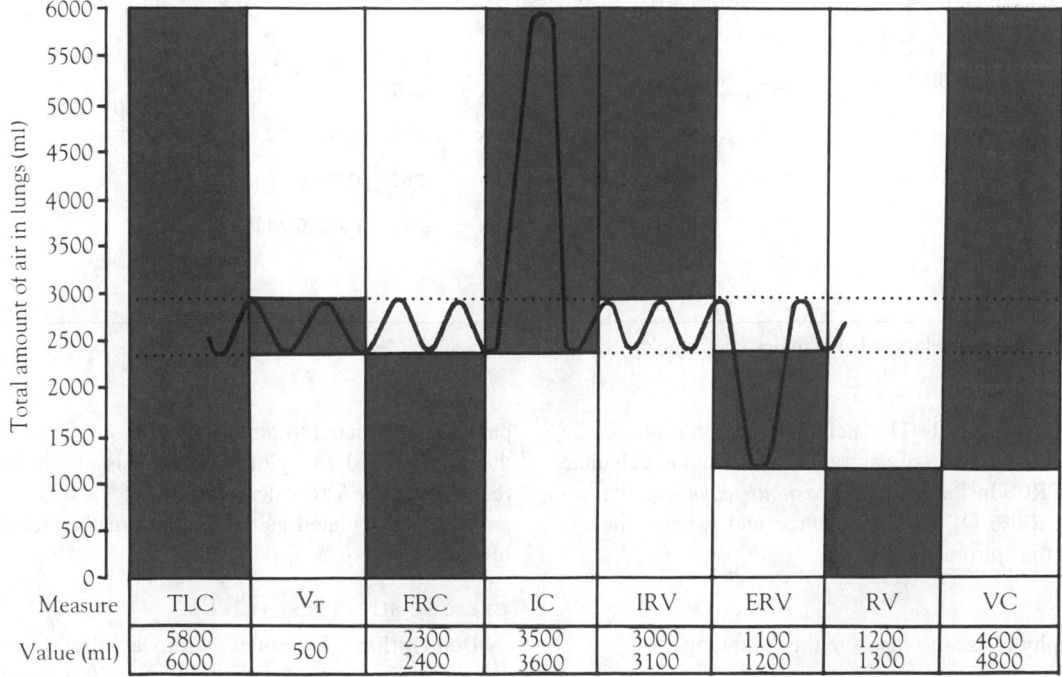

Measure	TLC	V_T	FRC	IC	IRV	ERV	RV	VC
Value (ml)	5800 6000	500	2300 2400	3500 3600	3000 3100	1100 1200	1200 1300	4600 4800

Figure III-5 Lung volume measurements. All values are approximately 25% less in women. *TLC,* Total lung capacity; *V$_T$,* tidal volume; *FRC,* functional residual capacity; *IC,* inspiratory capacity; *IRV,* inspiratory reserve volume; *ERV,* expiratory reserve volume; *RV,* residual volume; *VC,* vital capacity.

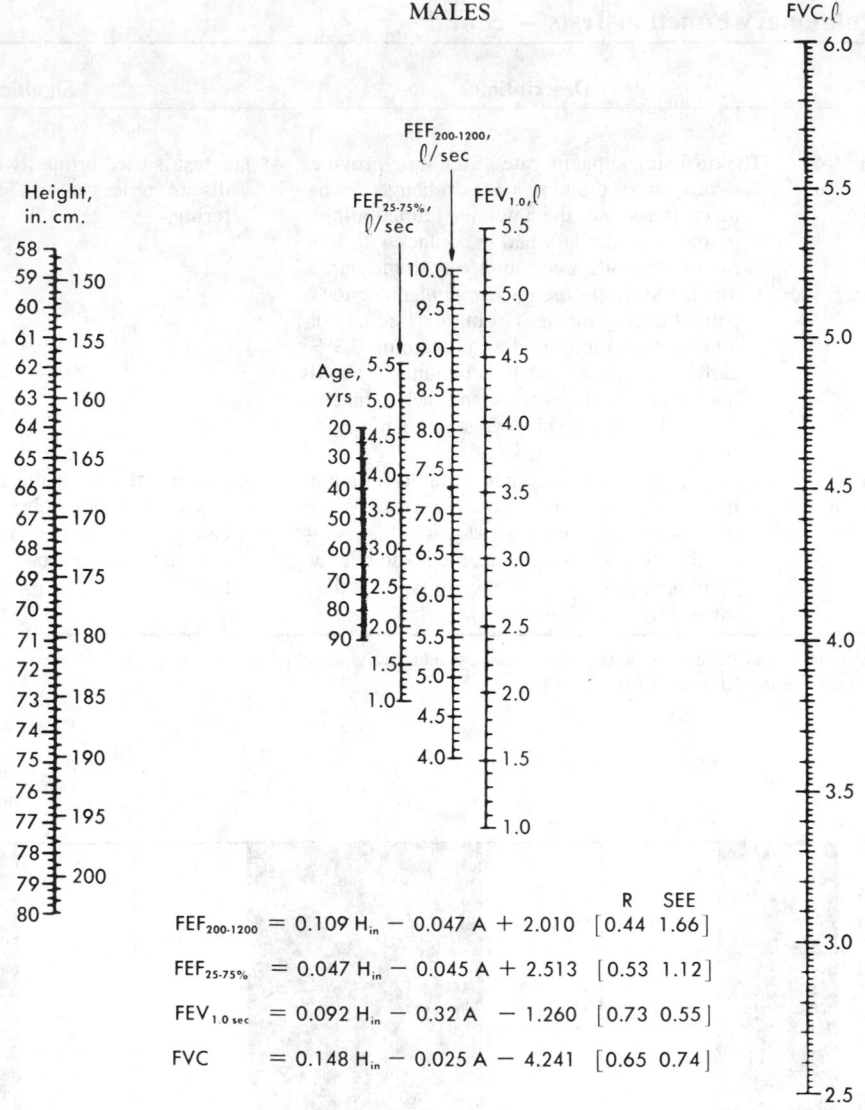

MALES

$$FEF_{200-1200} = 0.109\,H_{in} - 0.047\,A + 2.010 \quad [0.44 \quad 1.66]$$

$$FEF_{25-75\%} = 0.047\,H_{in} - 0.045\,A + 2.513 \quad [0.53 \quad 1.12]$$

$$FEV_{1.0\,sec} = 0.092\,H_{in} - 0.32\,A - 1.260 \quad [0.73 \quad 0.55]$$

$$FVC = 0.148\,H_{in} - 0.025\,A - 4.241 \quad [0.65 \quad 0.74]$$

Figure III-6 Spirometric standards for males and females. (From Morris.[17])

patient's lungs are equal. The helium concentration in the spirometer and the volume of gas can then be used to calculate the patient's FRC. In the *nitrogen-washout technique* the patient breathes 100% O_2 from one source and exhales the expired gas into the spirometer.

Description

Plethysmography is used to measure the following:

R_{aw} (airway resistance)
G_{aw} (airway conductance)
FRC (V_{TG} = FRC shutter is closed at end of expiration)

The plethysmograph is an air-tight chamber in which the patient sits. The patient is seated in the air-tight chamber, is fitted with nose clips, and is instructed to breathe through the mouthpiece, which is connected to a transducer. To calculate V_{TG}, the patient is instructed to pant into the mouthpiece while keeping the cheeks rigid and glottis open. This provides the pressure readings for the V_{TG} calculator. The R_{aw} and G_{aw} may be mathematically calculated as the patient breathes rapidly and shallowly.

Exercise stress test (EST)

Description Examines cardiovascular response to exercise. It is also used to detect and quantify ischemic heart disease, to determine patients considered at risk, and to determine cardiovascular fitness preceding exercise programs. The test consists of raising, in gradual increments, the exercise level on a motorized treadmill while the ECG is being monitored. Blood pressure and heart electrical activity are also measured, and expired gases can be collected, O_2 consumption and saturation

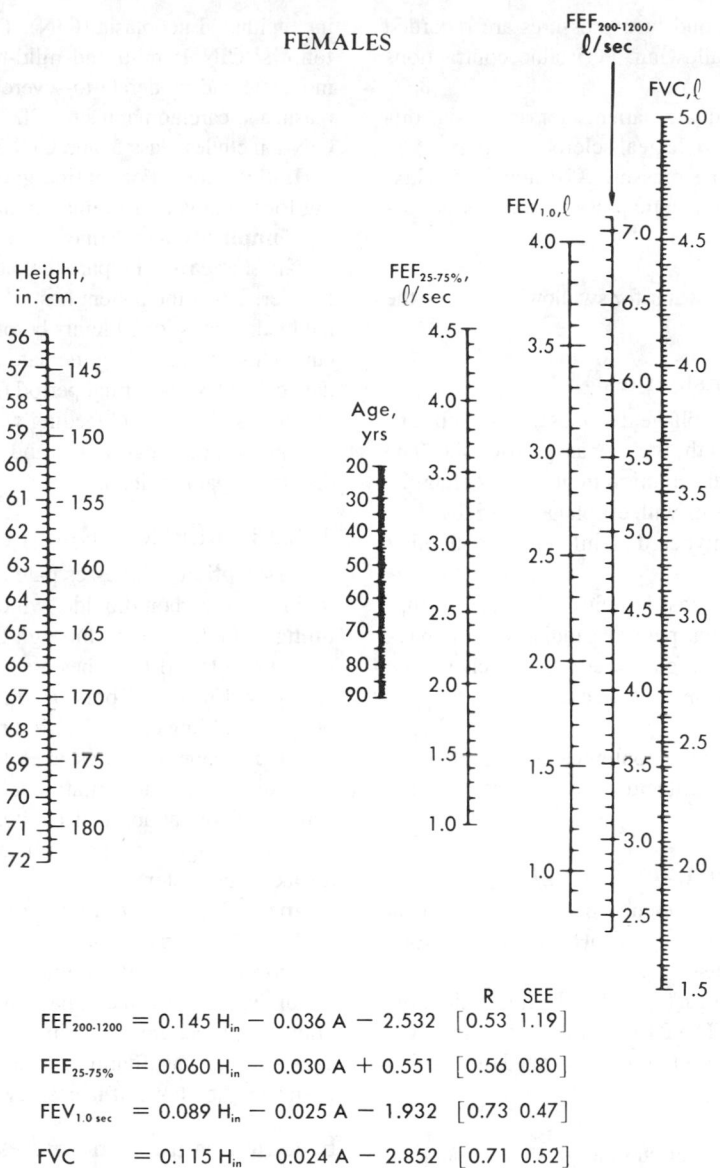

FEMALES

$$FEF_{200-1200} = 0.145\,H_{in} - 0.036\,A - 2.532 \quad [0.53\ 1.19]$$

$$FEF_{25-75\%} = 0.060\,H_{in} - 0.030\,A + 0.551 \quad [0.56\ 0.80]$$

$$FEV_{1.0\,sec} = 0.089\,H_{in} - 0.025\,A - 1.932 \quad [0.73\ 0.47]$$

$$FVC = 0.115\,H_{in} - 0.024\,A - 2.852 \quad [0.71\ 0.52]$$

Figure III-6, cont'd. Spirometric standards for males and females. (From Morris.[17])

monitored, and samples collected for blood gas determinations. Key end points during exercise may define physiologically the causes of the patient's symptoms.

Indications Differential diagnosis of chest pain; determination of workload level (exercise) when symptoms of ischemia occur; evaluation of therapy for angina; evaluation of patients who have multiple risk factors for coronary artery disease; evaluation of exercise-induced dysrhythmias.

Complications Recent myocardial infarction (4 to 6 weeks) (but such patients may perform submaximal EST before discharge from hospital); rapid ventricular or atrial dysrhythmia; heart failure; severe aortic stenosis; blood pressure greater than 170/100 mm Hg before the onset of exercise; complete A-V block.

Nursing care Explain the procedure, stressing the need for the patient to report any symptoms during and after the procedure. Instruct the patient to dress comfortably in shorts or gym clothes and tennis shoes. Instruct the patient not to eat for 1 hour before the test. During the procedure, monitor blood pressure, heart rate, ECG changes such as ST elevation or depression and dysrhythmias. Observe for symptoms such as chest pain or pressure, shortness of breath, fatigue.

Esophageal manometry

Description Measures upper and lower esophageal sphincter pressure. The patient swallows a manometric catheter containing a small pressure transducer along its length. Baseline measurements are taken, and then pressures are recorded before, during, and after swallowing. Peristaltic contractions are recorded.

Indications   Used to evaluate patients for achalasia, diffuse esophageal spasm, and esophageal scleroderma.

Normal values are: baseline pressure—20 mm Hg; relaxation pressure—18 mm Hg. Peristaltic pressure appears as a series of high-pressure peaks.

Complications   None.

Nursing care   Provide ice water for swallowing during the procedure.

Acid perfusion test (Bernstein test)

Description   Evaluates esophageal mucosa. Two solutions (saline and acidic) are dripped through a nasogastric tube. The presence of pain with the acidic solution indicates esophagitis. Test is contraindicated in patients with esophageal varices, congestive heart failure, acute myocardial infarction, and other known cardiac disorders.

Indications   Patients with gastric reflux often have symptoms of epigastric or retrosternal pain that radiates to the back or arms. The test is used to distinguish between the chest pain of esophagitis and the chest pain of cardiac disorders.

Complications   None.

Nursing care   If the patient continues to complain of pain or burning after the test, antacids may help relieve discomfort.

Esophageal acidity test (pH monitoring)

Description   Evaluates competence of lower esophageal sphincter by measuring intraesophageal pH with an electrode attached to a manometric catheter.

Indications   Will indicate gastric reflux. Normal value: pH of esophagus is 6.0 or higher. The 24-hour monitoring involves the patient writing down all the activities performed during that period.

Complications   None.

Nursing care   Antacids, anticholinergics, cholinergics, adrenergic blockers, H_2 blockers, and reserpine should be withheld for 24 hours before the test. If these medications are not withheld, note this on the laboratory request sheet.

Papanicolaou test (Pap test)

Description   Simple smear method of examining exfoliative cells, particularly malignant and premalignant conditions of the cervix. Desquamated cells from the cervical epithelium are obtained during a pelvic examination, stained, and examined under a microscope. Histologic classification includes class 1 through class 5.

Class 1—normal cells
Class 2—atypical cells
Class 3—mild dysplasia
Class 4—severe dysplasia, suspicious cells
Class 5—carcinoma cells

Recently, Pap smear reporting has changed to recognize the continuum of cervical dysplasia. Reports are in terms of cervical intraepithelial neoplasia (CIN). These subclasses are defined as follows: CIN 1: mild and mild-to-moderate dysplasia; CIN 2: moderate and moderate-to-severe dysplasia; CIN 3: severe dysplasia and carcinoma in situ. CIN 1 incorporates classes 2 and 3, CIN 2 includes class 3, and CIN 3 includes classes 4 and 5.

Indications   For routine gynecologic examination screening for malignant or premalignant conditions of the cervix.

Complications   None.

Nursing care   Prepare the patient for a vaginal examination and verify that the patient has not douched or inserted any vaginal medications for 24 hours before the procedure. Obtain an accurate history, including the date of the last Pap test and results; date of the last menstrual period (LMP); frequency and duration of periods; amount of bleeding with the periods; method of contraception; hormonal drugs; and presence and color of vaginal discharge, pain, or itching.

Tubal insufflation (Rubin test)

Description   Assesses patency of fallopian tubes by insufflation with carbon dioxide, which is introduced through tight-fitting cannula inserted through the cervical os at pressures up to 200 mm Hg. If the tubes are open, gas enters the abdominal cavity, and recorded pressure falls below 180 mm Hg. High-pitched bubbling can be heard through the abdominal wall with the stethoscope as gas escapes from the tubes. Shoulder pain from diaphragmatic irritation also indicates that gas has escaped into the abdominal cavity. Kymographic tracing shows pressure changes and may indicate tubal obstruction, spasm, or a leak in the system.

Indications   Inability to conceive.

Complications   None.

Nursing care   Be prepared to assist the patient with the cramping pain, dizziness, nausea, and vomiting that may occur after the procedure. Explain that shoulder pain (if present) is caused by an insufflation of gas and will subside. Mild analgesics may be taken if necessary.

Erectile dysfunction studies

Description and indications   Monitors nocturnal penile tumescence; snap-gauge devices are designed to determine whether cases of erectile dysfunction are caused by psychogenic or organic disease and to assess the efficiency of an erection. Endocrine disorders that may affect erectile activity are investigated by determining serum levels of FSH, LH, and testosterone and by physical examination. Vascular disorders are diagnosed via dynamic infusion cavernosgraphy, and cavernosometry, which reproduces an erection via mechanical means, or by vascular studies of the arterial or venous supplies of the penis—including internal pudendal arteriography, venography, or penile blood pressure or pulse volume assessment. Neurologic disorders that may contribute to erectile dysfunction are diagnosed by a variety of methodologies including physical examination, electromyography, nerve conduction, and evoked potential studies. The effect of drugs on erectile dysfunction may be determined by altering drug regimens and observing the effects on tumescence.

Complications None.
Nursing care Provide a supportive atmosphere and explain the procedure to the patient.

 NORMAL LABORATORY VALUES

Cerebrospinal Fluid Studies

Appearance: crystal clear, colorless
Pressure (lateral recumbent): 50 to 180 mm H_2O
Protein
    Lumbar
        6 months and up: approximately 15 to 50 mg/dl
        Ventricular CSF protein is generally lower
    Cisternal: 15 to 25 mg/dl
    Ventricular: 6 to 15 mg/dl
Cell count
    No RBCs
    0 to 5 WBCs
    0 to 10 cells/mm³ (all lymphocytes and monocytes)
Glucose
    50 to 80 mg/dl (60% to 70% of plasma glucose)
A/G rates: 8:1 (albumin to globulin)
Serologic studies
    Complement fixation: nonreactive
    Treponema pallidum immune adherence: nonreactive
    Treponema immobilization test: nonreactive
Gram stain: negative for organisms
Culture and sensitivity: no growth of organisms
Electrolytes
    Sodium: 141 mEq/L
    Potassium: 3.3 mEq/L
    Chloride: 110 to 125 mEq/L
Bilirubin: negative
Cholesterol: 0.2 to 0.6 mg/dl
Creatinine: 0.5 to 1.2 mg/dl
Urea: 7 to 15 mg/dl
Urea nitrogen: 10 to 15 mg/dl
Uric acid: 0.5 to 4.5 mg/dl
pH: 7.32 to 7.35
Specific gravity: 1.007
Glutamine: 6 to 15 mg/dl (enzymatic)
IgG index: 0.3 to 0.7
IgG: 0% to 11% of total protein
Lactic acid
    Control group with no CNS disorder: 0.6 to 2.2 mEq/L
        (0.6 to 2.2 mmol/L; 10 to 20 mg/dl)
LDH
    Fluid LDH activity normally much less than plasma LDH
        activity; normal spinal fluid LDH levels are about 10%
        of serum levels
Myelin basic protein: <4 ng/ml CSF is normal
Oligoclonal bands: normal CSF: no demonstrable oligoclonal bands

Protein electrophoresis (normal range depends on methodology)
    Gamma: 3% to 13%
    Beta: 7.3% to 17.9%
    Alpha₂: 3% to 12.6%
    Alpha₁: 1.1% to 6.6%
    Albumin: 56.8% to 76.9%
    Prealbumin: 2.2% to 7.1%
    CSF albumin: 13.4 to 23.7 mg/dl
    Total protein: 15 to 50 mg/dl
    Beta-gamma ratio: 1.67 to 2.3
    Oligoclonal bands: absent
FTA-ABS: nonreactive
Cryptococcal antigen titer: negative
VDRL: nonreactive
Mycobacteria culture: no growth
Counterimmunoelectrophoresis: negative
India ink preparation: no *Cryptococcus* identified

Blood Studies

Following are some descriptions of blood studies for which patients may require special nursing care utilized for hematolymphatic, immune, and neoplastic disorders. Also included is a discussion of arterial blood gas analysis.

CBC

RBC
    Male: 4.7 to 6.1 million/mm³
    Female: 4.2 to 5.4 million/mm³
Hemoglobin (Hgb)
    Male: 14 to 18 g/dl or 8.7 to 11.2 mmol/L (SI units)
    Female: 12 to 16 g/dl or 7.4 to 9.9 mmol/L
    Elderly: values may be slightly decreased
Hematocrit (Hct)
    Male: 42% to 52%
    Female: 37% to 47% (pregnancy >33%)
    Elderly: values may be slightly decreased
RBC indices
    MCV: 80 to 95 μm³
    (mean corpuscular volume)
    MCH: 27 to 31 pg
    (mean corpuscular hemoglobin)
    MCHC: 32 to 36 g/dl
    (mean corpuscular hemoglobin concentration)
WBC and differential
    Total: 5000 to 10,000/mm³
    Differential
        Neutrophils: 55% to 70%
        Lymphocytes: 20% to 40%
        Monocytes: 2% to 8%
        Eosinophils: 1% to 4%
        Basophils: 0.5% to 1%
Platelets
    150,000 to 400,000 mm³ or 150 to 400 × 10⁹/L

Reticulocyte Count

0.5% to 2%

Prothrombin Time (PT)

11 to 12.5 seconds; 85% to 100%
(should include use of international normalized ratio [INR]
value to ensure uniform results)

Partial Thromboplastin Time (PTT)

60 to 70 seconds

Activated Partial Thromboplastin Time (APTT)

30 to 40 seconds

Erythrocyte Sedimentation Rate (ESR) (Westergren Method)

Males age <50: 0 to 15 mm/hour
Males age >50: 0 to 20 mm/hour
Females age <50: 0 to 25 mm/hour
Females age >50: 0 to 30 mm/hour

Zeta Sedimentation Ratio

age <50: <55%
age 50 to 80: 40% to 60%

Fibrinogen (Plasma)

200 to 400 mg/dl

Fibrin Split Products

<10 μg/ml

Erythrocyte Fragility Test

Hemolysis starts at 0.45% to 0.39% saline solution
Hemolysis complete at 0.33% to 0.30% saline solution

Erythrocyte Life Span Determination

Approximately 120 days
Half-life 27 to 86 days

Lymphocyte Populations (%)

Total B cells: 5% to 11%
Total T cells: 75% to 90%
T helper cells (T$_4$ positive): 40% to 58%
T suppressor/cytotoxic cells (T$_8$ positive): 19% to 30%

Bone Marrow Differential Cell Counts (%)

Erythroblasts: 22.5%	Eosinophils: 4.0%
Myeloblasts: 1.0%	Basophils: <0.5%
Promyelocytes: 3.0%	Monocytes: 2.0%
Myelocytes: 15.0%	Lymphocytes: 7.5%
Metamyelocytes: 15.0%	Reticular cells: 6.5%
Stab cells: 15.0%	Plasmacytes: 1.0%
Segmented cells: 7.0%	Megakaryocytes: <0.5%

Chemistry

Acid phosphatase
0.11 to 0.6 μg/L

Albumin
Serum quantitative (age 1 to 31): 3.5 to 5 g/dl with A/G ratio greater than 1; after age 40, normal range gradually decreases
4 to 5.5 g/dl (electrophoresis)
Aldolase
3.0 to 8.2 Sibley-Lehninger μg/dl or 22 to 59 mU at 37° (SI units)
Alkaline phosphatase
30 to 85 International milliunits (ImU) ml
Ammonia
Varies somewhat between laboratories; 11 to 35 μmol/L
Amylase
56 to 190 IU/L (may be slightly increased in normal pregnancy and in the elderly)
Bile acids
Whole blood, serum, or plasma
Positive: >10 cholesterol monohydrate or calcium bilirubinate crystals per slide
Suspicious: 1 to 9 cholesterol monohydrate or calcium bilirubinate crystals per slide
Bilirubin
Direct (conjugated): up to 0.4 mg/dl
BUN
Age 1 to 40: 5 to 20 mg/dl; gradual slight increase subsequently occurs
Calcium
Serum
Ionized: 3.9 to 4.8 mg/dl for one formula available
Total (up to age 30): 8.2 to 10.5 mg/dl; decreases very slightly in older years
Creatinine
Serum
Men: up to 1.2 mg/dl
Women: up to 1.1 mg/dl
Electrolytes
Sodium: 135 to 145 mEq/L
Potassium: 3.5 to 5 mEq/L
Chloride: 97 to 107 mEq/L
Bicarbonate: 22 to 29 mEq/L
Folate
>2 mg/ml
Glucose
60 to 115 mg/dl (normal range increase with age over 50)
Oral glucose tolerance (serum or plasma)
Fasting: 60 to 115 mg/dl (normal range increases with age over 50)
30 min: 30 to 60 mg/dl above fasting
60 min: 20 to 50 mg/dl above fasting
120 min: 5 to 15 mg/dl above fasting
180 min: fasting level or below
2-hour postprandial
age 0 to 50: 70 to 140 mg/dl
age 50 to 60: 70 to 150 mg/dl
age 60 and up: 70 to 160 mg/dl

Haptoglobin
40 to 180 mg/dl (values are method dependent)
Iron
Total: 42 to 135 mg/dl
Binding capacity: 218 to 385 mg/dl
Saturation: 20% to 50%
Lactose
Lactic acid (lactate)
Venous: 5 to 20 mg/dl
Arterial: 3 to 7 mg/dl
Lactose intolerance
Increase of blood glucose <20 mg/dl over fasting level, with symptoms, is considered abnormal; evidence for lactase deficiency: >30 mg/dl is normal
Lipase
Method dependent
Lipid profile
Total: 400 to 800 mg/dl
Cholesterol: 100 to 210 mg/dl
Triglycerides (at 95th percentile)
White men
age 25 to 29: up to 250 mg/dl
age 35 to 54: up to 320 mg/dl
age 55 to 64: up to 290 mg/dl
age 65 and older: up to 260 mg/dl
White women
age 35 to 39: up to 195 mg/dl
age 55 to 64: up to 250 mg/dl
Lipoproteins
High density (HDL)
Men, age 15 to 34: 30 to 65 mg/dl
Women: 35 to 80 mg/dl
Low density (LDL)
White men, age 35 to 39: up to 190 mg/dl
Phospholipids: 150 to 380 mg/dl
Fatty acids: 9 to 15 mmol/L
Magnesium: 1.2 to 1.9 mEq/L
Mucoprotein: 80 to 200 mg/dl
Osmolality: 280 to 300 mOsm/kg H_2O
Phenylalanine: >3 mg/dl
Phosphorus: 2.5 to 4.5 mg/dl
Protein
Serum
Total: 6 to 8 g/dl
Albumin: 3.5 to 5 g/dl with A/G ratio >1
Globulin: 2.3 to 3.5 g/dl
Electrophoresis
Albumin: 58% to 74%; 4 to 5.5 g/dl
Alpha-1: 2% to 3.5%; 0.15 to 0.25 g/dl
Alpha-2: 5.4% to 10.6%; 0.43 to 0.75 g/dl
Beta: 7% to 14%; 0.5 to 1 g/dl
Gamma: 8% to 18%; 0.6 to 1.3 g/dl
Prostate specific antigen (PSA): <4 ng/ml
Uric acid
Serum
Male: 3.4 to 7 mg/dl or slightly higher
Female: 2.4 to 6 mg/dl or slightly higher

Vitamins
Vitamin A
Serum
15 to 60 μg/dl
Vitamin A tolerance: fasting 3 hours or 6 hours after 5000 μg: 15 to 60 μg/dl
Vitamin A/kg/24 hr: 200 to 600 μg/dl; fasting values are higher
Vitamin B_{12}
Serum
160 to 950 pg/ml
Unsaturated vitamin B_{12} binding capacity: 1000 to 2000 pg/ml
Vitamin C
Serum or plasma: 0.2 to 2 mg/dl
Zinc
Whole blood, serum, or plasma: 0.66 to 1.1 μg/ml

Blood Enzymes

Cardiac enzymes
Creatine phosphokinase (CPK)
Males: 55-170 U/L
Females: 30-135 U/L
CPK-MB (isoenzyme): 0 to 7 U/L
AST: 5 to 40 IU/L
Lactate dehydrogenase (LDH)
Isoenzymes (method dependent)
LDH_1: 22% to 36%
LDH_2: 35% to 46%
LDH_3: 13% to 26%
LDH_4: 3% to 10%
LDH_5: 2% to 9%
LDH (specific for heart, kidney, blood cells): 0.17 to 0.27 of total LDH
Glucose-6 phosphate dehydrogenase (G6PD): 140 to 280 U/billion cells
Gamma glutamyltransferase serum: 5 to 40 IU/L
ALT: 5-35 U/L

Blood Gas Values

Whole blood
pH
Arterial range: 7.35 to 7.45 (average 7.4)
Venous range: 7.32 to 7.35
Mixed venous: 7.36
PCO_2
Arterial range: 35 to 42 mm Hg (average 40 mm Hg)
Venous range: 35 to 50 mm Hg
Mixed venous: 46 mm Hg
PO_2
Arterial range: 80 to 95 mm Hg (average 95 mm Hg)
Mixed venous: 40 mm Hg
HCO_3^-
Arterial range: 24 to 28 mEq/L
Venous range: 24 to 28 mEq/L
Mixed venous: 24-28 mEq/L

So_2
   Arterial range (average 97%): 95% to 99%
   Venous range (average 75%): 70% to 75%
   Pulmonary artery: 75%
   Mixed venous: 75%
O_2 content
   Arterial range: 17 to 21 ml/dl or 17 to 21 vol%
   Venous range: 10 to 16 ml/dl or 10 to 16 vol%
   Mixed venous: 15 ml/dl
CO_2 content
   Arterial range: 22 to 29 mEq/L
   Venous range: 23 to 30 mEq/L
   Mixed venous: 26 mEq/L

Plasma

CO_2 content
   Arterial range: 21 to 30 mEq/L
   Venous range: 24 to 34 mEq/L

Hemoglobin

CO saturation (carboxyhemoglobin)
   Nonsmoker: 0% to 2%
   Smoker: 3% to 5%
   Heavy smoker: 9% to 10%

Drug Levels

Digoxin
   Therapeutic: 1 to 2 ng/ml
   Toxic: 3 ng/ml
   Underdigitalization: <0.5 ng/ml
Digitoxin
   Therapeutic: 10 to 30 ng/ml
   Toxic: >35 ng/ml

Endocrine and Hormonal Studies

Blood or serum

Adrenocorticotropic Hormone (ACTH)
   8 AM: <140 pg/ml
   4 PM: 10 to 50 pg/ml
Aldosterone
   Normal salt diet
      Supine: 5.4 to 9.8 ng/dl
      Upright: 8.9 to 58 ng/dl
   Low salt diet: 2 to 4 times above values
Androstenedione: <250 ng/dl
Calcitonin: <150 pg/ml; usual basal fasting level is about 20
   to 100 pg/ml, depending on assay
Catecholamines
   Supine
      Epinephrine: 0.5 to 20 μg/24 hours
      Norepinephrine: 15 to 80 μg/24 hours
      Dopamine: 65 to 400 μg/24 hours
      Metanephrine: 24 to 96 μg/24 hours
      Normetanephrine: 75 to 375 μg/24 hours

VMA: 1.8 to 7 mg/24 hours
   Standing
      Epinephrine: 20 to 109 pg/ml
      Norepinephrine: 169 to 515 pg/ml
C-peptide
   Fasting: 0.9 to 4.2 ng/ml
   Nonfasting: 1.5 to 9.0 ng/ml
Dehydroepiandrosterone (11-Deoxycortisol) (DHEA)
   Adult male: 270 to 1400 mg/dl
   Adult female: 200 to 800 ng/dl
DHEA sulfate (serum)
   Adult male: 130 to 550 μg/dl
   Premenopausal female: 60 to 340 μg/dl
   Postmenopausal female: <130 μg/dl
17-Hydroxysteroids
   Male: 3 to 10 mg/24 hours
   Female: 2.5 to 10 mg/24 hours
Free thyroxine
   Approximately 0.7 to 1.8 ng/dl (varies among laboratories)
Gastrin
   Fasting: 50 to 170 pg/ml
   Postprandial: 95 to 140 pg/ml; usually <250 pg/ml
Glucagon: 20 to 100 pg/ml
Growth hormone: <10 ng/ml
Human chorionic gonadotropin: <3 mIU/ml (nonpregnant)
Insulin
   Fasting level: up to 25 μU/ml with slight differences in
      upper limit of normal among laboratories
Karyotyping: Sex chromosomes: XX or XY
Luteinizing hormone
   Male: 7 to 24 mIU/ml; normal ranges vary among laboratories
   Female:
      Follicular phase: 6 to 27 mIU/ml
      Midcycle: 35 to 154 mIU/ml
      Luteal: 5 to 17 mIU/ml
      Older adult: postmenopausal women: 29 to 96 mIU/ml
Parathyroid hormone
   Dependent on individual laboratory, calcium result; the
      calcium value is related to the parathyroid hormone
      value by some laboratories on a two-dimensional graph
      or nomogram to ascertain abnormality
Phenylalanine: <20 mg/dl
Progesterone
   Male: 13 to 97 ng/dl
      Older adult: 7 to 33 ng/dl
   Female:
      Follicular: 95 ng/dl
      Luteal: 1130 ng/dl
Progesterone receptor assay: <5 fmol/mg protein is negative
Prolactin: 2 to 37 ng/ml
Hydroxyprogesterone
   Adult female
      Early cycle 100 ng/dl
      Late cycle 80 to 300 ng/dl

Renin
  Age 20-39: 0.1-4.3 ng/ml/hr
  Upright: Age >40: 0.1-3.0 ng/ml/hr
Somatomedin C: 0.4 to 2.0 U/ml
Somatostatin: 10 to 80 pg/ml
Testosterone
  Male: 300 to 1100 ng/dl
  Female: 20 to 100 ng/dl
Triiodothyronine
  Approximately 80 to 200 to 230 ng/dl with some variation among laboratories; increase occurs in pregnancy
Thyroglobulin
  About 1 to 20 ng/ml; mean values of 5.1 to 9.5 ng/ml
Thyroid-stimulating hormone (TSH)
  Upper limit of normal varies among laboratories from about 5.4 μU/ml to approximately 10 μU/ml
Thyroxine
  5.5 to 11.5 μg/dl
  Pregnancy: approximately 5.5 to 16 μg/dl
Thyroxine-binding globulin
  Variability among laboratories exists; 10 to 28 μg/ml; increased in pregnancy
Transferrin
  Approximately 200 to 360 mg/dl with some variation among laboratories
α_1-Fetoprotein
  Up to approximately 40 ng/ml for serum (interlaboratory differences exist); maternal serum increases to maximum of 500 ng/ml at week 32, and ranges are stratified by weeks of gestation
Chorionic somatomammotropin
  Varies with duration of gestation; may reach 10 μg/ml
Creatine: 0.2 to 0.8 mg/dl; increased in pregnancy
Creatinine
  Adult female 0.8 to 1.8 g/24 hours; creatinine excretion decreases with advanced age as muscle mass diminishes
Creatinine clearance
  Male: 85 to 125 ml/min/1.73 m^2
  Female: 75 to 115 ml/min/1.73 m^2
Dihydrotestosterone: None detectable
Estradiol
  Menstruating female
    Early cycle: 20 to 170 pg/ml
    Midcycle: 70 to 500 pg/ml
    Late cycle: 45 to 340 pg/ml
  Patient taking oral contraceptives: 12 to 50 pg/ml
  Postmenopausal female: 1 to 5 ng/dl
  Adult male: 13 to 42 pg/ml
Estriol
  Nonpregnant female less than 0.5 ng/ml; pregnant female—estriol increases until term and then decreases:
  30 to 32 weeks: 2 to 12 ng/ml
  33 to 35 weeks: 3 to 19 ng/ml
  36 to 38 weeks: 5 to 27 ng/ml
  39 to 40 weeks: 10 to 30 ng/ml

Estrogens, total
  Menstruating female: 15 to 80 μg/24 hours
  Postmenopausal female: less than 20 μg/24 hours
  Male: 6 to 40 ng/ml
Estrone
  Menstruating female
    Early in cycle: 50 to 300 pg/ml
    Midcycle: 100 to 600 pg/ml
    Late cycle: 80 to 450 pg/ml
  Menopausal female: 0 to 30 pg/ml
Calcium
  Varies with diet; based on average calcium intake of 600 to 800 mg/24 hours, excretion may be 100 to 250 mg/24 hours
  On a diet of 400 to 800 mg of calcium daily, others set the upper limit at 200 mg calcium in a 24-hour urine collection
Free cortisol
  Male: 11 to 84 μg/24 hours
  Female: 10 to 34 μg/24 hours
FSH
  Male: 3 to 11 IU/24 hours
  Female: 5 to 50 IU/24 hours
  Older adult: postmenopausal women: 2 to 3 times adult values
Hydroxyprolines
  See individual laboratory reference ranges; excretion on meat-free, gelatin-free diet is approximately 10 to 50 mg/24 hours
Follicle-stimulating hormone
  Follicular phase: 5 to 20 IU/24 hours
  Luteal phase: 5 to 15 IU/24 hours
  Midcycle: 15 to 60 IU/24 hours
  Menopause: 50 to 100 IU/24 hours
Luteinizing hormone
  Follicular phase: 2 to 25 IU/24 hours
  Ovulatory phase: 30 to 95 IU/24 hours
  Luteal phase: 2 to 20 IU/24 hours
  Postmenopausal: 40 to 110 IU/24 hours
Pregnanediol
  Proliferative phase: 0.5 to 1.5 mg/24 hours
  Luteal phase: 2 to 7 mg/24 hours
  Menopause: 0.2 to 1 mg/24 hours
  10 to 12 weeks pregnant: 5 to 15 mg/24 hours
  12 to 18 weeks pregnant: 5 to 15 mg/24 hours
  18 to 24 weeks pregnant: 15 to 33 mg/24 hours
  24 to 28 weeks pregnant: 20 to 42 mg/24 hours
  28 to 32 weeks pregnant: 27 to 47 mg/24 hours

Immunologic Studies

Serum immunoglobulin levels
  IgG: 600 to 1600 mg/dl
  IgM: 50 to 250 mg/dl
  IgA: 80 to 350 mg/dl

IgE: <125 ng/dl
IgD: 0 to 30 mg/dl
Macroglobulins, total
    Whole blood, serum, or plasma: 53 to 375 mg/dl
Autoantibody titers
    Anti-DNA
        Low levels of antibody or none; units and reference range
            depend on laboratory and method
    Antinuclear antibody (ANA): Negative at 1:20 dilution
    Rheumatoid factor (RF): Negative
    Sjögren's antibody: Negative
Nonspecific indicators of inflammation
    C-reactive protein (CRP): <6 μg/ml
    C3 complement (serum): 800 to 1800 μg/ml
Circulating immune complexes
    C1q binding assay
        <25 μg/ml aggregated human γ-globulin (AHGG) equivalents
    Raji cell assay: 0 to 12 μg/ml AHGG equivalents
    Gamma globulin
        Serum: 0.5 to 1.6 g/dl
    Globulins (total)
        Serum: 2.3 to 3.5 g/dl

Urine Studies

Urinalysis
    Albumin: <20 mg/dl
    Bilirubin: negative
    Color: clear, golden yellow
    Glucose: negative
    Hemoglobin: negative
    Ketones: negative
Microscopic urinalysis
    Bacteria: negative
    Casts: 0 to 4 hyaline casts per low-power field
    Crystals: interpreted by physician
    Mucous threads: negative
    Red blood cells: 0 to 5 per high-power field
    Squamous epithelial cells: seen on voided specimen in females; negative on voided specimen in males; negative for catheterized specimens
    White blood cells: 0 to 5 per high-power field
    Calcium
        24 hours: 100 to 250 mg/day (diet-dependent; based on average calcium intake of 600 to 800 mg/24 hours)
    Chloride: 110 to 250 mEq/24 hours
    Creatinine: men: 1 to 2 g/24 hours; women: 0.8 to 1.8 g/24 hours
    Glucose: up to 100 mg/24 hours
    Osmolality: 250 to 900 mOsm/kg
    Protein: 30 to 150 mg/24 hours (method dependent)
    pH: 4.5 to 8.0
    Phosphorus: 0.9 to 1.3 g/day (diet-dependent)
    Potassium: 26 to 123 mEq/24 hours (markedly intake-dependent)

Sodium: 27 to 287 mEq/24 hours (diet-dependent; output is lower at night)
Specific gravity: 1.003 to 1.029 (range in SI units)
Urea nitrogen: 6 to 17 g/24 hours
Cystine: random sample negative
Fructose: 30 to 65 mg/24 hours
Galactose: 10 mg/dl
Uric acid: 250 to 750 mg/24 hours
Urea nitrogen: 6 to 17/24 hours
Mucin: 100 to 150 mg/24 hours

References

1. Anderson KN, Anderson LE, Glanz WD, editors: *Mosby's medical, nursing, and allied health dictionary,* ed 4, St Louis, 1994, Mosby.
2. Ballinger PW: *Merrill's atlas of radiographic positions and radiologic procedures,* ed 8, St Louis, 1995, Mosby.
3. Bates B: *A guide to physical examination and history taking,* ed 6, Philadelphia, 1995, Lippincott.
4. Davis JE, Mason CB: *Neurologic critical care,* New York, 1979, Van Nostrand Reinhold.
5. Emmett JL, Witten DM: *Clinical urography,* Philadelphia, 1990, Saunders.
6. Fishman AP, editor: *Pulmonary diseases and disorders,* ed 2, New York, 1988, McGraw Hill.
7. George RB, Light RW, Matthay MA, Matthay RA, editors: *Chest medicine, essentials of pulmonary and critical care medicine,* ed 2, Baltimore, 1990, Williams & Wilkins.
8. Harrison JH et al: *Campbell's urology,* ed 6, Philadelphia, 1992, Saunders.
9. Hickey J: *The clinical practice of neurological and neurosurgical nursing,* ed 3, Philadelphia, 1992, Lippincott.
10. Kelalis PP, King, LR, Belman AB: *Clinical pediatric urology,* ed 3, Philadelphia, 1992, Saunders.
11. Kendall AR, Karafin R: *Urology: Goldsmith's practice of surgery,* Philadelphia, 1983, Harper & Row.
12. Kim MJ, McFarland GK, McLane AM: *Pocket guide to nursing diagnoses,* ed 6, St. Louis, 1995, Mosby.
13. Kintzel K, editor: *Advanced concepts in clinical nursing,* ed 2, Philadelphia, 1977, Lippincott.
14. Lerner J, Khan Z: *Mosby's manual of urologic nursing,* St Louis, 1982, Mosby.
15. Merritt HH: *A textbook of neurology,* ed 6, Philadelphia, 1979, Lea & Febiger.
16. Miller LG, Kazemi H: *Manual of clinical pulmonary medicine,* New York, 1983, McGraw-Hill.
17. Morris JF, Roski WA, Johnson LC: Spirometric standards for healthy nonsmoking adults, *Am Rev Respir Dis* 103:57, 1971.
18. Newell FM: *Ophthalmology: principles and concepts,* ed 7, St Louis, 1992, Mosby.
19. Pagana KD, Pagana TJ: *Diagnostic testing and nursing implications: a case study approach,* ed 4, St Louis, 1994, Mosby.
20. Pagana KD, Pagana TJ: *Mosby's diagnostic and laboratory test reference,* ed 2, St Louis, 1995, Mosby.
21. Robinson S, Russo P, editors: *Providing respiratory care: nursing photobook,* Springhouse, PA, 1979, Intermed Communications.
22. Sanderson RG, Kurth CC: *The cardiac patient,* ed 2, Philadelphia, 1983, Saunders.
23. Seidel HM et al: *Mosby's guide to physical examination,* ed 3, St Louis, 1995, Mosby.
24. Stell PM: *Stell and Maran's head and neck surgery,* ed 3, Boston, 1993, Oxford.
25. Tucker SM et al: *Patient care standards: collaborative practice planning guides,* ed 6, St Louis, 1995, Mosby.
26. Williams ID, Johnston JH: *Paediatric urology,* ed 2, London, 1982, Butterworth.
27. Wilson JD et al, editors: *Harrison's principles of internal medicine,* ed 13, New York, 1994, McGraw-Hill.
28. Youmans JR, editor: *Neurological surgery,* ed 3, Philadelphia, 1990, Saunders.

PART FOUR

Nursing Diagnoses and Interventions

I

Health Perception— Health Management

HEALTH-SEEKING BEHAVIORS (SPECIFY)

Health-seeking behaviors is the state in which a person in stable health is actively seeking ways to alter personal health habits and/or the environment to move toward optimum health. (*Stable health* status is present when the person has achieved age-appropriate illness prevention measures and reports good or excellent health and when signs and symptoms of disease, if present, are controlled.)

Motivation for the maintenance or expansion of a person's state of wellness manifests itself at different levels. Illness prevention motivation occurs when individuals in a health state are aware of personal, public, or environmental risks that jeopardize their state of well-being. Others are concerned about such public threats as sexually transmitted diseases, infectious diseases, criminal assaults, or bombardment by modern life stressors. They seek community services and education for assistance. The mass media have increased public awareness of certain prevalent problems such as alcoholism, AIDS, family violence, and some forms of cancer, and people want to know what they can do to prevent such afflictions. Still others are concerned about industrial pollution, nuclear waste products, and ultraviolet rays. They are motivated to prevent exposure and illness for themselves, as well as the general population. People are generally motivated to change their self-care habits when they are convinced that the effort will deter or eliminate a specific threat.

Beyond the prevention of illness, people wish to maintain their present satisfactory health state to ensure that they can continue to function successfully in their daily activities. Functional capacity incorporates physical, emotional, cognitive, spiritual, and social performance. Individuals engage in health-seeking behaviors to enhance their self-esteem, their appearance, or their physical capacity to work; to avoid discomfort and pain; and to re-create or maintain independence. Aging individuals are often concerned about dietary or exercise efforts that will help them maintain an independent functional status. People frequently engage in activities that promise to raise their participation level so that they can work, relate to other people, and live to their satisfaction. Still others wish simply to improve or excel in the physical, psychosocial, or spiritual realm. They are directed toward a level of mastery or self-actualization and are willing to explore greatly different or vigorous approaches to attain a peak level of wellness and fulfillment. Variables that typically affect motivation to seek and carry through with health improvement behaviors are the perceived threat of a particular disease or problem; the perceived benefits of taking action; the lack of interference with a present lifestyle; situational barriers (real or imagined) that might impose on a person; public (e.g., mass media campaigns) or private support for taking action; sense of self-efficacy (i.e., a sense of confidence that a person can complete the proposed actions successfully); and the individual's personal definition of health.

Individuals or groups in a health-seeking mode may exhibit a variety of behaviors. They may ask for information, outright assistance, advocacy, or support. They may exhibit frustration with present circumstances, fear of the future, or confusion about a specific concern. They may express concern about themselves, a loved one, or their entire community. They may display great self-confidence or exhilaration with the idea of impending change or self-improvement.

Related Factors*

Fear of disease or illness
Desire to maintain functional status
Cultural beliefs and norms; personal and family values
Increased awareness through public education (media, magazines) for optimum health state
Professional prescription, advice, or encouragement
Fear of pain

Defining Characteristics*

Expressed or observed desire to seek a higher level of wellness
Stated or observed unfamiliarity with wellness community resources
Verbalized or observed lack of knowledge in health promotion behaviors
Expressed or observed desire for increased control of health practices
Expressed concern about current environmental conditions on health status

*Adapted from North American Nursing Diagnosis Association, 1995.

Expected Patient Outcomes & Nursing Interventions

Clarification of health goals for the individual will be accomplished by assessment and restatement of the goals

- Assess the patient for:
    Definition of health
    Perceived threat(s) to health
    Description of goals the patient wishes to attain
    Perceived barriers to goal(s)
    Perceived benefits of taking action
    Perceived benefits or private support
    Sense of self-efficacy
    Any incapacities or barriers to health-seeking behavior
- Review assessment information with patient.
- Restate patient goal(s) with patient.

New knowledge will be integrated with existing knowledge to expand the patient's level of understanding of a given topic

- Assess patient for present level of knowledge on given subject.
- Identify supplemental areas for learning, and share them with patient.
- Review new material with patient, and request patient's evaluation of the usefulness of the new information.

Strategies will be identified for meeting stated goals

- Assess patient's perception that goal is attainable.
- Review any incongruities between nurse's and patient's perception(s).
- Identify specific strategies (behaviors) patient must enact to attain goal(s).
- Establish a schedule or time frame for goal attainment (goal attainment may be identified in increments over a time).
- Describe goal attainments in measurable or behavioral terms (e.g., Mrs. M will lose 3 pounds by *[date]*; Mr. G will identify three specific stressful incidents at work on his next visit).
- Identify specific behaviors that will precede or accompany each increment and review them with patient.
- Review nurse's and patient's perceptions about attainability of goal(s).

Monitoring of self-directed plans and strategies will be achieved

- Assess patient's comprehension of goal attainments.
- Assess patient's motivation to follow specific attainments.
- Work with patient to design a record-keeping system or a means of describing/reporting progress to self, support system, and nurse.

The patient will engage in self-rewarding behaviors

- Review benefits of health-seeking activity with patient and include possible side benefits (e.g., feeling more energetic, improved sleeping).
- Urge patient to note benefits during progress.

- If patient wishes, devise a "reward" as increments are attained.

Identification of social supports for reinforcement of health-seeking behaviors will be achieved

- Review family, loved ones, and peer support for patient's activities (e.g., purchasing prepared food for diet, transportation to exercise facility).

Self-behavior will be monitored as evidenced by ability to differentiate between negative and positive influences and factors on self

- Ask patient to monitor negative/positive influences, and discuss them with family or significant others.
- Continue education about potential negative factors.

Expand involvement in state of well-being as evidenced by expanding health-seeking opportunities and engaging in healthful living

- Continue education and discussion about healthful life patterns that extend beyond patient's current interests (goals).
- Assess patient's motivation to expand health-seeking concerns.
- Assist patient with translating wishes into options for healthful living.

Principles and Rationale for Nursing Interventions

A person who expresses or exhibits health-seeking behaviors may wish to pursue an urgent, short-term issue (e.g., acquisition of knowledge about AIDS prevention) or an elaborate long-term plan for high-level wellness. Nursing interventions rest heavily on careful assessment of the patient's goals, perceptions, and values. It is important to recognize incongruities between the nurse's wishes for the patient and the patient's own wishes. Carrying out a health care activity requires commitment and well-entrenched convictions from the patient. The patient will be more receptive to education and support when it is clear that his goals and the nurse's goals are not in conflict.

Goal attainment is best acquired in small increments (e.g., weight loss, stress reduction). The patient is rewarded with more immediate and frequent accomplishments if assisted in breaking down ambitious goals into small ones. Once the short-term, more immediate goals have been attained and the patient is feeling confident, further education and encouragement may lead to other health-seeking behaviors.

■ ALTERED HEALTH MAINTENANCE

■ Altered health maintenance is the inability to identify, manage, and/or seek out help to maintain health.

Health maintenance within this nursing diagnosis encompasses those health behaviors and prevention practices that maintain or protect the health of the individual and that are to be carried out by the individual. Health maintenance includes behaviors related to nutrition, rest, exercise, medical and dental care, hygiene, sexual activity, and other lifestyle choices such as tobacco, alcohol, and illicit drug use.[15,33] Altered health maintenance is diagnosed when the client's health is potentially or actually threatened by current health behaviors in any or all of the functional health patterns.[38,44] The diagnosis can apply to an asymptomatic person who is at risk, a patient with chronic illness with the potential for a higher level of wellness, or a patient with an acute problem who is also at risk for other health problems.[11] Because health maintenance incorporates such a broad range of behaviors, it may be useful to specify the particular functional area of alteration, e.g., condom use or eating patterns. *Altered health maintenance* describes a status of health at risk and must be differentiated from the nursing diagnosis *self-care deficit,* which applies to clients with actual health or self-care alterations who are unable to perform acts of daily living. Altered health maintenance can be caused by a variety of physical, psychological, social, and situational factors.[33] This diagnosis may be encountered in persons with altered cognitive function, e.g., dementia, mental retardation, or any condition causing altered level of consciousness, with sensory deficits or any condition affecting mobility, with emotional disorders including chemical addictions, with chronic diseases, inadequate financial or social resources, inadequate information, and in persons consciously choosing not to engage in primary or secondary health prevention behaviors.[15,36] *Healthy People 2000*[25] identified the elderly, persons living in rural areas, and ethnic minorities as vulnerable populations facing barriers in accessing and utilizing the health information and services they need to manage their health.[1,3,24,42,48] Research has demonstrated marginalized groups, e.g., elderly women,[47] lesbian women,[23,51] the homeless,[12,38] and migrant farm workers,[45] to be vulnerable. Males with high masculinity gender identification have been shown at risk for poor health practices such as ignoring symptoms and delaying help-seeking.[29] Altered health maintenance may also be diagnosed in the primary caretakers of family members requiring home care.[4,30]

The 1980 ANA Social Policy Statement clearly identified health maintenance as a responsibility of the nursing profession.[2] This responsibility affects every nurse-patient encounter. As such, the nursing diagnosis Altered health maintenance transcends disease-related categories and requires development by nurses in all facets of nursing practice. By definition, this diagnosis views health maintenance behaviors as the responsibility of the individual client; identifying, managing, and seeking out help are applicable to families and communities as well as clients.[3,4,15,36] Because the diagnosis encompasses such an extensive population, the remainder of this chapter focuses specifically on failure to assume responsibility for primary prevention.

Related Factors[44]

Lack of or significant alteration in communication skills (written, verbal and/or gestural)
Lack of ability to make deliberate and thoughtful judgments
Perceptual or cognitive impairment (Complete/partial lack of gross and/or fine motor skills)

Ineffective individual coping
Dysfunctional grieving
Lack of material resources
Unachieved developmental tasks
Ineffective family coping
Disabling spiritual distress

Defining Characteristics[44]

Reported or observed inability to take responsibility for meeting basic health practices in any or all functional pattern areas
Demonstrated lack of knowledge regarding basic health practices
Demonstrated lack of adaptive behaviors to internal or external environmental changes
History of lack of health-seeking behavior
Expressed interest in improving health behaviors
Reported or observed lack of equipment, financial, and/or other resources
Reported or observed impairment of personal support system

Expected Patient Outcomes & Nursing Interventions

General Public
Receive consistent, accurate information as evidenced by:

Public health goals met
- Use mass media (TV, electronic media, newspapers), printed material, closed circuit television, and patient interactive teaching methods *to reach diverse populations and accommodate different learning styles, educational levels.*[9,18]
- Encourage primary health care providers to provide verbal reinforcement to public in health care visits *to maximize effectiveness of media presentations and increase motivation to act.*[3,4,13,16,48]
- Engage target population, community leaders in needs assessment activities *to clarify community's perceptions of health and illness, identify unmet needs, and assist in tailoring of education, programs to local needs and resources.*[3,31]
- Include indigenous care providers and local health experts in rural or cultural communities in the planning and implementation of programs *to enhance community acceptance and facilitate consistency of information and approach.*[20,35]
- Provide health education/teaching in the primary language of target group *to increase understanding and utilization of information.*[45]
- Provide health teaching in culturally-acceptable formats, e.g., use elders, older health care providers for teaching, health counseling in American Indian groups where age confers respect, leadership roles, *to bridge cultural barriers.*[16,45,55]
- Make health information/service available where large numbers of target population gather, e.g., AIDS information and condoms in colleges, *to maximize exposure and decrease access barriers.*[7,30,40,51]

- Use social marketing techniques for promotion, e.g., payroll stuffers, invitations, or contests, *to motivate individuals to participate.*[9]

High-risk individuals*
Assume responsibility for primary health maintenance, as evidenced by:

Personal health goals identified
Factors contributing to altered health maintenance identified
Specific plan to alter targeted behavior
Multiple personal reinforcers identified
Community resources used

- Use health appraisal techniques that elicit client's perceptions of health *to facilitate identification of personal health values and goals.*[15,36,39,46]
- Use pertinent health risk appraisal/inventory to assist patient to identify personal health risks related to lifestyle, family history, ethnicity, gender, and age, *to increase awareness of personal vulnerability, which motivates health behavior change.*[8,14,36,46]
- Assist client to list factors they perceive are interfering with their ability to meet personal health goals *to identify the factors most significant to the client.*[8,46,56]
- Help patient identify personal strengths and resources *to establish foundation for planning and enhance perceptions of ability to make desired changes.*[6,15]
- Engage client in "brainstorming" of possible strategies to effect desired behavior change *to increase creativity and avoid tendency for repetition of unsuccessful strategies.*[8,15,39]
- Negotiate setting of both short-term and long-term goals *to provide opportunity for observable successes and strengthen competence in self-regulation of behavior.*[8,46,52]
- Have patient list perceived benefits and disadvantages for specific behavior(s) targeted *to clarify outcome expectations which influence motivation.*[8,46]
- Break the complexities of the behavior(s) desired into smaller, more manageable parts *to enhance perceptions of efficacy and avoid overwhelming patient.*[8,28,46]
- Ask client to rank-order target behaviors according to their beliefs that they can carry them out and sequence behaviors beginning with ones client feels most confident with *to increase probability that client will incorporate changes.*[6,37,50,52]
- Develop written contract with patient for behavior change using patient-identified rewards and consequences *to promote patient control, provide self-reinforcements, and increase commitment to plans.*[8,21,46]
- Schedule health maintenance counseling with other primary care appointments where possible *to decrease inconvenience and financial barriers to patient.*[48,51]
- Make audiovisual educational materials available where patient uses other primary care services *to convenience patient and increase perceived validity of information being offered.*[49,51]

- Include lay or traditional healers in planning where appropriate *to ensure development of a culturally acceptable plan and provide another professional source of encouragement, reinforcement for plan.*[20,55]
- Consider relaxation training for anxiety if present *to reduce unpleasant physiologic arousal which inhibits self-efficacy.*[46,52]
- Use small group discussion and support groups *to provide support and verbal persuasion.*[27]
- Encourage participation in reference groups where client can align with perceived powerful individuals, institutions *to enhance own sense of control and provide vicarious success.*[52]
- Follow up with telephone calls and letters *to provide verbal encouragement for plan and provide visual reminders which increase chances for behavior change.*[8,16,53]

Principles and Rationale for Nursing Interventions

Nursing interventions that approach altered health maintenance from a personal responsibility perspective are based on theories of health behavior change. Two key theoretical constructs of social cognitive theory, outcome expectations/response efficacy and perceived self-efficacy, have been shown to be powerful determinants of behavior change.[52] Outcome expectancies describe beliefs that certain behaviors will lead to certain outcomes that may be positively or negatively valued and influence one's motivation to carry out the behavior. Outcome expectancies are a key component of the health belief model and include one's expectations that they are vulnerable to negative outcomes of disease.[8,52] Perceived self-efficacy describes an individual's belief that they are capable of the specific behaviors. Past experiences with the desired behaviors, vicarious experience through observation of performance of others, verbal persuasion about one's capability with the behavior, and physiologic states, e.g., anxiety, associated with performance of the behavior, determine or inform one's sense of self-efficacy.[52] The theory of reasoned action looks at two factors, attitude and social norms, that influence a person's intention to carry out behaviors over which they have control.[10,34] Attitude is a function of outcome expectancies and social norm describes the individual's beliefs about what other people think they should do and their desire to comply with those wishes. In summary, adoption of health maintenance behaviors according to social cognitive theories is directly linked to attitudes and beliefs about health and health behaviors, and nursing assessment of those factors is essential to planning.[8,46] Nursing interventions that enhance self-efficacy beliefs and support positive, valued outcomes will be most effective. An important caveat to programs that focus on individual-level behaviors is the risk for "victim blaming" if the larger political economy of health and illness is not considered as context.[17,22,32,41,47]

The concept of sick-role behavior, now recognized to describe a powerless patient in an unequal provider-client relationship,[54] nonetheless provides a description of the traditional role assumed during an acute period of illness and, with minor modification, chronic illness. The concept does not adequately

---

*See section on noncompliance for additional interventions.

explain the behavior of persons who are at risk of developing an illness. Baric[5] compared and contrasted the concept of sick-role behavior to the at-risk role (Table IV-1). The current health care system exploits the traditional exempted status of the illness role and limits access to health care by demanding illness before services are rendered.[1,40] Provider services are usually scheduled when otherwise well persons at risk are fulfilling expected social roles, and health maintenance care is often not recognized for reimbursement by third-party payers.[49,51] Interventions that address those barriers to health maintenance increase the client's chance for success.

Social support is a vital component of programs to improve health maintenance. Interventions that strengthen social support facilitate behavior change by tapping into the accessible, affordable informal network of family, neighbors, and friends. These persons are most likely to understand the social and cultural context of the individual and to encourage realistic problem solving.[1,19,35,42,46]

The primary goal for an individual with altered health maintenance is to establish behavior patterns that maintain health. Nursing interventions are designed to provide large numbers of individuals with a cue or message identifying the behaviors necessary to maintain health and to provide individuals at high risk, with specific counseling on how to modify the behavior.

Messages appropriate for the general public need to be kept simple, identifying a global theme while avoiding complex, specific behavior.[9] Research supports increased effectiveness of the message with professional reinforcements.[3,7,8,48]

Primary prevention is the responsibility of the "healthy individual" who generally has limited contact with the health care system. A large percentage of health information is acquired from mass media, sources known for persuasive messages, fictionalization, and opinion. Personal encounters with a health care professional may take place, but they are infrequent, irregular, and generally during an acute health crisis. Receptiveness to information not directly related to the acute crisis is limited; it may be the only access for some populations, however.[3,38]

Nursing interventions to assist the general public in health maintenance should communicate clear, concise, and meaningful information. In addition, positive reinforcement of health information by a nurse validates the significance of the health message.[3,7,8,26,43] Such positive reinforcement could occur during routine activities, such as contact with visitors by nurses in acute care facilities, with families by nurses in home health care agencies,[30] at work and school settings by occupational and school health nurses, and by professionals speaking to lay groups.

In addition to providing information and positive reinforcement, nurses can identify persons at high risk for specific diseases related to lifestyle, family history, ethnicity,[24] and gender. For example, persons who smoke are at high risk for developing both cancer and heart disease; American Indians have a 10-fold greater probability of developing diabetes than the general population.[24] These high-risk individuals require general information and counseling related to methods of behavioral alteration. They need encouragement and assistance to strengthen their social support. Persons with altered health maintenance and those with noncompliance require changes in their behavior. Many of the nursing interventions listed are discussed in the section on noncompliance as well.

INEFFECTIVE MANAGEMENT OF THERAPEUTIC REGIMEN (INDIVIDUALS)

Ineffective management of therapeutic regimen (individuals) is "a pattern of regulating and integrating into daily living a program for treatment of illness and the sequelae of illness that is unsatisfactory for meeting specific health goals."[14]

Individuals experiencing illness or a change in health that requires a program of treatment must integrate the health status changes, as well as the therapeutic regimen, into self-awareness, activities of living, and life-style.[8-10,18]

The nurse must assess the individual's response to the impact of the health status change and the demands of the therapeutic regimen to determine if there are any behavior patterns, attitudes, perceptions, or knowledge deficits that negatively affect the individual's performance in meeting specific goals to improve health.[8,10,16-18]

Determining categories of responses is useful in developing approaches that will enhance the individual's achievement of health goals. Major categories of responses may include illness-related factors, perception of stress, level of motivation, physical and social environmental factors, coping behaviors, health beliefs, cognitive state, and lifelong experience.*

Basic to any plan to improve health is a clear definition of the problems the individual must face to set realistic goals. Assessment and intervention should be comprehensive and include

---

*References 3, 5, 10-12, 15, 16, 18.

TABLE IV-1 Comparison of Sick Role and At-Risk Role

Sick Role	At-Risk Role
1. Duties—must want to get well, try to get well, and seek and follow medical advice. Advantages—exempt from social responsibilities; it is legitimate to expect help from others.	1. Duties—must continue to fulfill social obligations; must change some existing behavior without help or social recognition.
2. Sick role is legitimized by society.	2. At-risk role is not formally recognized by society; behavior change depends on the individual.
3. Payoff (return to usual role) will occur in limited time.	3. Payoff (possibility of avoiding or minimizing disease) in distant future and often unrecognized.
4. Positive reinforcement for sick-role behaviors.	4. New behavior not formally reinforced by medical profession or society; rather, society is a continual source of stimuli to revert to prior behavior.
5. Symptoms decrease with sick-role behaviors.	5. Symptomless—relies on abstract beliefs or statistical probability.
6. Person not held responsible for illness.	6. Person held responsible for behavior.

Modified from Baric L: *Recognition of the "at-risk": a means to influence health behavior,* 1969, International Seminar on Health Education, 1970, Hamburg, Federal Republic of Germany.

environmental and financial areas that may directly affect the individual's ability to manage a therapeutic regimen.[8,10]

Building on a clear definition of the problem is a determination of the individual's perception of stress and level of motivation to deal with the illness and therapeutic regimen. Included in this category are factors such as the individual's emotional state, levels of stress, anxiety, fear, and grieving responses.[1-3,12,15]

The category of physical and social environmental factors focuses on how the individual views the illness, how the individual perceives the benefits from an effective therapeutic regimen, and which barriers are identified. Collaboration with the individual, his or her social support network, and the health care team is essential in developing approaches.[3,8,15,17,18]

Assessment of the individual's coping behaviors, as well as the coping behaviors of the family and significant others, may include previous life experiences and experiences with illness, coping mechanisms used by the individual and the family when confronted with stressful situations, and knowledge of ways to enhance coping skills and abilities in stressful situations. Developing strategies in this area promotes the individual's self-awareness of accomplishments in other stressful situations and may have an impact on the individual's desire to manage more effectively the individual's treatment of his or her illness.[3,4,6,7,12]

Assessment of the individual's values and belief systems and spiritual resources is essential for the full integration of illness and health status changes and therapeutic regimen in an individual's life-style. Successful integration is measured by changed behaviors and beliefs resulting in management or deceleration of illness symptoms.[3,8,15,16,22]

Related Factors[1-3,14]

Powerlessness
Perceived susceptibility
Decisional conflicts
Perceived lack of competency about therapeutic regimen
Knowledge deficits
Negative life experiences regarding illness and health care
Inadequate number and types of cues to action
Perceived seriousness
Perceived barriers
Perceived benefits
Social support deficits
Family conflict
Excessive demands made on individual or family
Economic disabilities
Mistrust of regimen or health care personnel
Disabling or inadequate components of the rehabilitative program
Complexity of health care system
Complexity of therapeutic regimen
Lack of readiness or desire for self-care management
Inadequate spiritual resources
Health beliefs

Defining Characteristics[14]

Major

- Choices of daily living ineffective for meeting the goals of a treatment or prevention program

Minor

- Acceleration of illness symptoms (expected or unexpected)
- Verbalized difficulty with regulation and integration of one or more prescribed regimens for treatment of illness and its effects or prevention of complications
- Verbalized that did not take action to include treatment regimens in daily routines
- Verbalized that did not take action to reduce risk factors for progression of illness or sequelae
- Verbalized desire to manage the treatment of illness and prevention of sequelae

Expected Patient Outcomes & Nursing Interventions*

Make appropriate daily choices for effectively meeting goals of the treatment program, as evidenced by:

Management of illness symptoms
Taking actions to integrate treatment regimen into daily routine
Verbalizing ways that can integrate, without difficulty, treatment regimen into daily routine and life-style

- Assess patient's perception of and knowledge about the illness, the severity of the illness, potential complications, the long-term impact on life-style, and the treatment regimen resources needed to manage illness; *illness-related factors can influence the outcomes of an illness crisis; a baseline is needed for intervention.*[12,15,17,18]
- Teach patient about nature of illness and the related treatment regimen, including expected outcomes and any potential complications.
- Teach patient about and/or refer patient to appropriate community resources in regard to: equipment needs, transportation needs, services, housing needs and adaptations, and financial support available, *to maximally match patient's needs with what is available in the community to meet the health care needs.*
- Encourage patient to identify strengths *that will promote adherence to treatment regimen.*[12,16,18]
- Encourage patient to identify barriers that impact adherence to treatment regimen and then approach barriers specifically.[1,17]
- Assess patient's emotional response to illness and treatment regimen: level of anxiety, degree of stress, level of depression, level of anger, and phase of grieving; *degree of emotional response can have an impact on learning and adaptive functioning and can influence the energy level needed to deal with the illness and engage in the therapeutic treatment regimen.*[12,15,17,18]
- Assist patient to work through emotional responses *to reduce emotional response levels so patient can use energies to cope with illness and with the demands of the therapeutic treatment regimen.*
- Assess how patient views the illness, the benefits that can be achieved from the treatment regimen, and the barriers to engaging in the treatment regimen.

---

*References 1, 3, 6, 12, 13, 15, 17, 18.

- Discuss with patient outcomes/consequences of non-adherence to treatment regimen.
- In collaboration with the interdisciplinary team and the patient, plan a comprehensive but realistic treatment regimen that takes into account the patient's individual situation.
- Encourage patient to draw from resources available: family, friends, neighbors, health care professionals, support groups, and community financial and health care resources; *social and environmental factors can facilitate the management of illness-related symptoms and the participation in treatment regimen.*[12,15,17,18]
- Assess patient's (1) previous life experiences, including any experience with illness and the health care system; and (2) coping strategies used by the patient and his or her family and significant other in dealing with stressful situations; *previous coping strategies can be useful in dealing with current illness and treatment regimen demands.*
- Have patient list coping strategies used previously and current strengths useful in dealing with stressful situations.
- Encourage patient to use coping strategies and strengths in dealing with current illness demands.
- Teach patient new coping strategies, such as stress management techniques.
- Assess patient's values and beliefs especially as related to current illness and its meaning for patient.
- Assess patient's spiritual resources; *spiritual resources can be useful in helping patient understand meaning of illness situation for self and in developing strengths in coping with the illness and its impact on his or her life-style.*
- Use behavioral contracting interventions/contracts for patients *to achieve selected outcomes.*[13]

Principles and Rationale for Nursing Interventions

Nursing interventions for the diagnosis ineffective management of therapeutic regimen are designed based on categorization of responses to illness and are related to the individual's perception of stress and level of motivation, physical and social environmental factors, coping behaviors, and ultimately lifestyle experiences. Outcomes are determined by effective management or deceleration of illness symptoms, as measured by observations of and verbalizations of ability to integrate regimen into lifestyle and activities of daily living.*

▌ EFFECTIVE MANAGEMENT OF THERAPEUTIC REGIMEN (INDIVIDUALS)

Effective management of therapeutic regimen (individuals) is a pattern of regulating and integrating into daily living a program for treatment of illness and its sequelae that is satisfactory for meeting specific health goals.

Effective management of acute and chronic health problems is the goal of health care. Individuals seek health care assistance to solve health problems and increase their sense of well-

being. Successful management of a therapeutic regimen is possible when individuals are highly motivated, are capable of engaging in self-care, have adequate economic and social resources, and make the deliberative decisions required to integrate prescribed behaviors into daily living. Orem's concept of self-care agency and the power components that enable individuals to engage in self-care provide a theoretical explanation for effective management of a therapeutic regimen.[1,2]

Defining Characteristics

Appropriate choices of daily activities for meeting goals of a treatment or prevention program
Illness symptoms within a normal range of expectation
Verbalized desire to manage the treatment of illness and prevention of sequelae
Verbalized intent to reduce risk factors for progression of illness and sequelae

Expected Outcomes and Nursing Interventions

Interact with health care personnel to develop a realistic plan of care as evidenced by:

Expresses desire to establish self-management behaviors
Expresses willingness to learn regimen-specific tasks
- Assist patient with identification of benefits of following prescribed therapeutic regimen.
- Determine the existence of potential barriers to integration of regimen into daily living.
- Help patient identify values and preferences in the process of developing goals and strategies.

Implement therapeutic regimen in daily living program as evidenced by:

Demonstrates ability to perform regimen-specific tasks
Monitors symptoms related to illness and/or treatment
Reallocates personal and economic resources to manage demands of therapeutic regimen
- Evaluate self-management skills and provide feedback.
- Teach self-monitoring of symptoms and response to treatment, e.g., teach use of daily log.
- Provide written information about availability and access to community resources.

Principles and Rationale for Nursing Interventions

Effective management of a complex therapeutic regimen may require a daily struggle with economic, social, and emotional components. Diet, exercise, taking medications, and monitoring bodily sensations and symptoms require attention and vigilance. Decision-making within a self-care frame of reference increases self-confidence in one's ability to engage in self-management tasks. Recording decisions and the outcomes of decisions provides an ongoing record of success and feedback with respect to adequacy of resources, identified self-care systems, and self-care actions.

---

*References 1, 3, 5, 8, 10, 12, 13, 15, 16, 18.

INEFFECTIVE MANAGEMENT OF THERAPEUTIC REGIMEN (FAMILIES)

Ineffective management of therapeutic regimen (families) is a pattern of regulating and integrating into family processes a program for treatment of illness and the sequelae of illness that is unsatisfactory for meeting specific health goals.[4]

Ineffective management of a therapeutic regimen (families) may be prevented by identifying families at risk. Families at risk include those in which a member has a new diagnosis, a member's regimen has become increasingly complex, the family's resources are already overburdened, and/or family members have little confidence in their ability to perform specific tasks. Confidence in one's ability to perform therapeutic tasks has been shown to influence the consistent practice of self-management behaviors. Social support is another factor associated with self-management, and regimen-specific support has a stronger correlation with self-management than social support.[3]

Related Factors

Complexity of health care system
Complexity of therapeutic regimen
Decisional conflicts
Economic difficulties
Excessive demands made on individual or family
Family conflict

Defining Characteristics

Major

Inappropriate family activities for meeting the goals of a treatment or prevention program

Minor

Acceleration (expected or unexpected) of illness symptoms of a family member
Lack of attention to illness and its sequelae
Verbalized desire to manage the treatment of illness and prevention of the sequelae
Verbalized difficulty with regulation/integration of one or more effects or prevention of complications
Verbalizes that family did not take action to reduce risk factors for progression of illness and sequelae

Expected Outcomes & Nursing Interventions

Family will assist with integration of regimen-specific tasks into daily living as evidenced by:

Participates in development of a plan to engage in required activities
Expresses willingness to learn regimen-specific tasks
Expresses desire to help establish self-management behaviors
- Provide verbal and written regimen-specific instructions to interested family members.
- Use formal teaching sessions *to increase confidence in ability to perform regimen-specific tasks.*
- Teach patient and family members to keep a written record of patient's response to regimen.
- Teach family members to include patient with problem-solving.
- Discuss with patient and family consequences of not adhering to prescribed regimen.

Family will provide opportunities for patient to engage in usual life experiences as evidenced by:

Participates in school, family, and community activities appropriate for developmental and ability level
Demonstrates same parenting expectations for affected family member as for well members
Maintains usual family routine and rituals
- Promote normalization, i.e., assist parents/siblings with provision of normal life experiences.
- Help affected family member communicate special needs to persons outside family who require information *to provide safe supervision.*
- Assist family with advocacy for affected family member in school system and health care system.

Principles and Rationale for Nursing Interventions

Expected outcomes and nursing interventions must be regimen-specific and individualized. Knowing a family, understanding the meaning of the therapeutic regimen to a patient and family members, and using their values and preferences in developing and selecting individualized care strategies provide a foundation for family success in meeting the day-to-day challenges of integrating a complex regimen into daily living. Self-efficacy has been positively associated with self-management, meaning that individuals with a strong sense of confidence in their ability to manage regimen-specific tasks were more likely to do so.[3]

The concept of normalization has been used by researchers to describe a common strategy used by families to facilitate an ill member's adaptation to a chronic illness, such as epilepsy or diabetes. Normalization includes acknowledgement of the abnormality and denial of its social significance. Knafl and Deatrick[5] reviewed the research of developers of the concept of normalization and identified five broad categories of behavior used by parents and family members to convey an impression of normalcy to others. The categories include engaging in usual parenting and family activities, limiting contacts with similarly situated others, making the family member appear normal, avoiding potentially embarrassing situations, and controlling information.[5]

NONCOMPLIANCE (SPECIFY)

Noncompliance is a person's informed decision not to adhere to a therapeutic recommendation.

Depending on the setting outcome, health behavior change has been termed *compliance; alliance; adherence; prevention or life-style modification;* or *recovery or cure.*[41] Characteristically, the term *compliance* is used when behavior change prescribed by a health care professional as primary or secondary disease prevention is adhered to. The three types of behavior changes are *removal, replacement,* and *addition.*[44] Removal refers to behaviors to be eliminated (e.g., tobacco use, street drug use, uncontrolled alcohol use); replacement refers to behaviors to be substituted (e.g., dietary); and addition refers to the inclusion of new behavior (e.g., exercise, regular use of medications). The term *noncompliance* is typically used when an individual is unable to alter habitual behaviors or adopt new behaviors necessary to a prescribed therapeutic regimen. The *nursing* diagnosis of noncompliance requires both that the health behaviors in question have been chosen by an informed and competent patient in a treatment plan mutually negotiated with the health care provider,[9,24,25] and that the patient desires to carry out the behaviors but is unable to do so because of restraining factors. (Where noncompliance is part of a strategy to maintain quality of life or protect oneself from perceived errors in clinical decisions,[16,44] for example, the criteria for the nursing diagnosis are not met.) The diagnosis must specify the particular behavior(s) the patient is unable to comply with; this recognizes the aspects of the treatment plan the patient is adhering to in addition to focusing nursing and patient interventions on the behavior(s) of concern. Noncompliance is not the appropriate diagnosis when factors restraining compliance would be more accurately addressed with other nursing diagnoses such as knowledge deficit, when the patient and/or family lack understanding of the treatment plan or are unable to read instructions; Altered Family Processes, when significant thers do not perceive support of the treatment plan as part of their role responsibilities; or Altered Thought Process, when impaired memory and conceptual and reasoning abilities preclude informed consent or recall of information.[9,25]

Numerous theories have been proposed to explain compliance and health behavior change. Three major themes that appear in a number of theories and studies of health behavior change are (1) personal meaning and perceptions, (2) social factors, and (3) deficiencies in the health care system.

Personal meaning and perceptions include knowledge, values, beliefs, attitudes, feelings, relative worth, self-efficacy and outcome expectations, quality of life, and past experiences. The Health Belief Model emphasizes the patient's perceptions of the seriousness of the potential or actual health problem, of his/her susceptibility to the disease or complications, and of the benefits and costs/barriers to treatment, and the cues that motivate patient action(s) as determinants of compliance.[1] Self-efficacy theory considers patients' beliefs about their capabilities of performing specific behaviors in particular situations.[43] Outcome expectations or response efficacy describe patients' beliefs that the behaviors will achieve the desired results.[43] High self-efficacy and beliefs in response efficacy are associated with compliance and positive outcomes.[6,23,38] Factors that inform one's self-efficacy beliefs and outcome expectations include personal performance experience, vicarious observation of others, and verbal encouragement.[43] The concept of health locus of control applies to compliance in that an internal locus of control is likely to enhance patients' valuing of shared or increased control in health care decisions/processes whereas patients' difficulty in setting and attaining mutual treatment goals may reflect a belief that what happens to them is ultimately outside, external to their

control and efforts.[23,39] Belief in the "powerful other" health care provider is also influenced by health locus of control.[5,23]

Age, gender, and culture have been minimally factored into theories to date considering health behavior change.[47] These factors are strong determinants of patients' values, attitudes, and beliefs, affecting their personal meaning and perceptions of both illness and treatment and their participation in the provider/patient relationship. The elderly in today's society, for example, are likely to have matured in a patriarchal, power-oriented health care system where the health care provider was considered to know best[2] and to have the authority; it was neither the traditional patient's sick role nor right to question or take part in decision making.[2,5,9,45] Health care providers are predominantly white and middle-class, corresponding with the predominant culture and ethnocentrism in Western countries.[14] The patient's culture may dictate beliefs in different etiologies and treatment for disease than those recognized by Western medicine requiring cultural assessment and cultural bridging in negotiation of the treatment plan.[4,28,46] Race and ethnicity have been shown to affect plasma concentrations and therapeutic response to different medications[4,27] (e.g., side effects may be experienced more severely by Asian patients at commonly prescribed doses of psychotropic drugs).[27] Definition of family and who should be included in care planning and caregiving are largely determined by cultural mores.[14,31]

Personal shame, humiliation, and stigma (e.g., public pill taking),[10,33] related to illness and its treatment arc factors likely to be overlooked but which may result in avoidance or denial behaviors affecting compliance.[30] Both illness and the consequent treatment may jeopardize social roles that give meaning to people's lives.[16,30] While health care providers may be concerned with noncompliance in that failure to adhere jeopardizes the patient's *life,* the patient's personal meaning may revolve around the *quality of life* afforded by compliance with the prescribed regimen.[30,44,47]

Social factors influencing behavioral change include the environmental context, social relationships and social support, societal norms, and macrosocial factors (e.g., economic resources, worksite, community, communications media).[42] Failure of social support, for example, significant others who do not possess accurate information, believe in the efficacy of therapy, or have the necessary time, energy, or resources, influences compliance.[6,9,15,19,32] Societal norms at macro and micro levels may be at variance with treatment goals; cultural beliefs may be opposed to prescribed regimens.[46] Inadequate resources,[22] such as lack of money, inadequate transportation, and lack of proper materials or equipment in the home are common obstacles and ones to which the elderly are particularly vulnerable.[19,32]

Transactional aspects of the patient-health care provider relationship have been shown to be a determinant of compliance.[8,21,34,35] Collaborative interactions that empower patients to share decision making according to their health locus of control and recognize the multidimensional nature of compliance are most successful.* Common health system barriers include access hours,[9] financial costs, prolonged waiting times for scheduled provider services, ethnocentric and monolingual

---

*References 8, 13, 19, 23, 25, 29.

services,[14,17,31] perceived disrespectful or demeaning treatment,[30] lack of confidence in the health care professionals,[10,15] and prescription of complex treatment regimens or equipment.[9,20,25,40] Education needed for successful implementation of regimens may be rushed or poorly timed.

Related Factors

Patient's value system
  Health beliefs
  Cultural influences
  Spiritual values
Patient-provider relationship

Defining Characteristics

Behavior indicative of failure to adhere by direct observation or statements by patient or significant others
Objective tests (physiologic measures, detection of markers)
Evidence of development of complications
Evidence of exacerbation of symptoms
Failure to keep appointments
Failure to progress
Inability to set or attain mutual goals

Expected Patient Outcomes & Nursing Interventions

Engage in behaviors consistent with goals of therapeutic regimen, as evidenced by:

Goals and priorities consistent with therapeutic regimen
Accurate performance of specific health-related behavior(s)
Identification of barriers to carrying out desired health behavior(s)
Verbalization of plan to deal with restraining factors/situations
Identification of sources of support, resources

- Assist the patient and family to identify barriers to compliance *so that barriers can be altered or regimen revised respectively.*
- Engage patient in values clarification strategies *to identify motivation and to increase consistency between beliefs and actions.*[6,11]
- Encourage the patient and family to discuss the solutions they believe will be most effective *to recognize family competence and avoid stereotypical interventions.*[7,18,29]
- Encourage self-monitoring *to make specific behavioral patterns and the antecedent variables more observable.*[26,37]
- Assess patient's and family's beliefs about their ability to carry out the required behaviors *to assess self-efficacy and identify where competence may be augmented.*[3,6,23,38,43]
- Adjust prescribed regimen and interventions to patient's life-style, value system, and circumstances where possible *to decrease the lifestyle changes being requested of the patient and to demonstrate that their needs are recognized.*[22]
- Provide opportunities to patient and family to discuss their concerns about therapeutic regimen *to validate feelings and provide verbal encouragement.*[12,16]

- Include patient designated support persons in treatment planning *to improve communication and increase motivation for support and involvement in implementation of plan.*[19,29,31,36]
- Sequence strategies from the easiest to more complex, setting short and long-term goals *to avoid overwhelming patient and provide for successes to enhance self-efficacy.*[7,9,19]
- Develop written contract with patient and support persons for specifics regarding therapeutic plan *to signify importance of plan and to provide a written reminder.*[9]
- Assist patient to make a list of relevant, accessible resources in the community *to provide support for implementation of treatment.*[9,19,29,36]
- Inform patient and family about relevant lay support groups *to provide opportunity for vicarious performance information and to access the expertise of others living with chronic illness.*[16,30]
- Devise a graphic representation of results, such as a chart, *to provide visual reinforcement of success and enhance positive outcome expectations.*[9,23]
- Ensure that patient education is provided in the client's primary language *as primary language is most influential in processing information.*[17,31]

Report that the health care system recognizes and provides for individual needs and abilities, as evidenced by:

Active participation in negotiation of goals, priorities, regimen
Free expression of feelings, beliefs, requests
Keeps appointments
Use of available resources
Noncompliance reported, with expectation of further negotiation or assistance
Verbalizes satisfaction with health care providers

- Ascertain which family members or significant others patient wants to include in treatment decision making *to empower patient and recognize cultural norms.*[14]
- Ask the patient what assistance he/she requires to enhance compliance *to encourage involvement in treatment decision making and to promote congruence of perceptions, goals in the patient-provider relationship.*[28]
- Offer patient and support persons training in assertive techniques which can be used in interactions with health care providers *to increase input to treatment decisions and make needs known to providers.*
- Collaborate with other health care providers involved with patient to coordinate and simplify medication regimens and treatment plans *to ensure consistency in approach, avoid contradictory advice, and decrease complexity.*[9,20]
- Schedule follow-up or home health care opportunities with same provider *to ensure continuity in care and increase opportunity for tailoring of interactions.*[3,21,23,34,35]
- Assess cultural preferences and beliefs *to ensure negotiation of therapeutic regimen that accommodates patient's cultural norms.*[14,28,46]
- Assess patient's beliefs in the efficacy of the therapeutic plan, that desired outcomes are indeed contingent upon

adherence *to determine outcome expectations, correct misinformation, and align nurse-patient perceptions.*[3,23,43]

Principles and Rationale for Nursing Interventions

Noncompliance should be approached from the multifactorial perspective that it may be as much a result of provider characteristics or health system deficiencies as of patient characteristics. Nursing interventions for noncompliance begin with determining that the behaviors of concern are ones which the patient values and wishes to comply with; assisting the patient to identify the factors preventing their compliance; and collaborating with the patient to modify or eliminate those factors or to renegotiate the treatment plan to more accurately fit the patient's beliefs and resources. Acknowledgement of the patient's personal meaning and resources, cultural norms, and lived experience with the illness may empower them to participate in decision making and planning. Consideration of the patient's self-efficacy and outcome expectations provides information about motivation. Nurse-patient interactions tailored to patient characteristics and goals increase chances of success. Strategies that strengthen social supports and involve support persons in planning are correlated with higher compliance.

■ RISK FOR INFECTION

Risk for infection is the state in which a person or group is at increased risk for being invaded by pathogenic organisms.

The risk of infection results from the state of the individual's resistance to potentially invading environmental and normal flora organisms and from increased exposure to pathogens in the environment. This diagnosis also applies when a potential exists for transmitting pathogens from an infected person to others.

Risk Factors

These risk factors either alter resistance to infection or increase the risk for environmental exposure. Combinations of risk factors are likely to increase the potential for infection.
Pathophysiologic risk factor
  Inadequate primary defenses
    Broken or burned skin
    Traumatized tissue
    Decreased ciliary action
    Stasis of body fluids
    Decreased secretions or changes in pH of secretions
    Altered enzyme activity
    Altered peristalsis
    Altered cough, blink, or sneeze reflex
    Alterations in protective normal flora organisms
  Inadequate secondary defenses
    Decreased hemoglobin
    Leukopenia
    Suppressed inflammatory response
    Immunosuppression
    Agranulocytosis
    Dysfunction of the thymus and lymphatic system
  Inadequate acquired immunity
  Tissue destruction caused by existing infectious process, altered circulation, or trauma
  Chronic disease
  Malnutrition or dehydration
  Premature rupture of amniotic membranes
  Spinal cord injury
  Loss of consciousness
  Impaired oxygenation
Developmental risk factors
  Age (infancy, childhood, older ages)
  Menarche, childbearing, postpartum period, menopause
Behavioral risk factors
  IV drug abuse
  Unsafe sexual practices
  Inadequate knowledge to avoid exposure to pathogens
  Poor hygiene practices
  Inadequate food and fluid intake
  Smoking practices
  Alcohol abuse
Treatment-related risk factors
  Invasive procedures
  IV infusions
  Pharmaceutical agents
  Inadequate or prolonged use of antibiotics
  Forced immobility
  Contaminated equipment used for respiratory therapy
  Artificial rupture of amniotic membranes
  Fetal monitoring
  Immunosuppression
  NPO status
  Radiation therapy
  Dialysis
  Chemotherapy
  Organ transplant
Environmental risk factors
  Environmental exposure to pathogens resulting from foreign travel, occupation, or living situation
  Contamination of food, water, hard surfaces, or any vector for transmission
  Inadequate control of vectors in the environment
  Inadequate sanitation and control of sewage, solid wastes
  Behaviors of others in the environment that increase the risk for transmission of the pathogens
  Inadequate community immunization levels

Defining Characteristics

The actual presence of pathogens or symptoms of infection indicates infection. These are the defining characteristics for risk for infection for the patient's contacts and include the following:
  Detection of viable pathogens or their eggs in body secretions, excretions, or exudates (urine, feces, blood, mucous secretions, mucous membrane or dermal lesion exudates, semen, gastric contents, cerebrospinal fluid)
  Systemic responses suggesting infection with a pathogen: elevated body temperature, leukocytosis, increase in serum antibodies

Expected Patient Outcomes & Nursing Interventions

Infection will be prevented in persons experiencing pathologic, developmental, behavioral, or environmental risk factors, as evidenced by:

Individuals describing the risk that they experience

Receiving recommended immunizations for their ages

Describing health behaviors that increase their resistance to infections or decreases their exposure to environmental pathogens

The incidence of infection decreases in the community

- Assess for the presence of risk factors. Host susceptibility for infection increases with impaired defenses, altered immune response, disease, extremes of age, and lack of immunization. Host behaviors, such as unsafe sexual practices, sharing needles, and unsafe food handling, increase the risk for exposure to pathogens.
- Instruct person on the risks associated with the altered life state or life stage and discuss behaviors to increase resistance to infection. Adequate nutrition, hydration, rest, stress reduction, personal and environmental hygiene, cessation of smoking, control of alcohol use, and cessation of drug use may improve host resistance.
- Discuss behaviors to reduce exposure to environmental pathogens. These include safe sexual practices, avoidance of sharing needles, proper food handling, and avoidance of vectors in the environment.
- Provide community education for safe food handling, water purification, and avoidance of vectors that normally carry pathogens.
- Support public health programs aimed at environmental sanitation; report to public health officials any infractions against sanitation codes. Control of the environment is the most expedient way of preventing transmission of pathogens to large numbers of people.
- Immunize persons of all ages who are inadequately immunized. Participate in community immunization programs to provide immunizations to high-risk populations. Even distribution of immunized persons in the community decreases risk for outbreaks and epidemics of vaccine-preventable diseases.

Infection will be prevented in persons experiencing treatment/hospital-related risks, as evidenced by:

Patient demonstrating behavior that will reduce risk for infection during and after treatments

Vital signs and WBC being within normal limits

Cultures of body secretions, excretions, and exudates being negative for pathogens

Patient self-administering antiinfective agents, as prescribed

Patient free of drug interactions or allergic reactions

Surgical wounds healed without signs of infection

Invasive lines discontinued as soon as possible

Patient discharged from the hospital in a timely manner

- Provide preprocedure instruction and postprocedure assistance to encourage deep breathing, coughing, ambulation, bladder emptying, and asepsis of invasive site. *Infection is associated with pooling of respiratory secretions, alterations in blood circulation, distention of the urinary bladder, and contamination of sites of invasion.*
- Turn frequently, and provide skin care to immobilized patients *to ensure circulation to compromised tissue.*
- Monitor vital signs, changes in WBC, and body secretions, excretions, and exudates for signs of infection. Obtain specimens as ordered. Report abnormalities to physician for early intervention.
- Monitor hydration and electrolyte balance, and ensure adequate fluid and food intake *to improve resistance to infection.*
- Teach patient and caregiver signs and symptoms of infection *in order for them to report the signs and symptoms. Delay in treatment can result in severe and life-threatening disease.*
- Administer antiinfectives as ordered and instruct patient or caregiver on the proper use of antiinfective agents. *Some foods and beverages alter the effectiveness of some antibiotics. Therapeutic drug levels are maintained with proper timing of drug administration.* Antiinfective agents must be taken for the recommended time *to prevent the development of drug-resistant organisms.*
- Instruct patient or caregiver on symptoms of adverse reactions to antiinfectives *because allergic reactions are common and life-threatening with some of these drugs.*
- Observe and report signs of superinfection in patients receiving antimicrobial therapy. *These drugs may destroy protective normal flora organisms, thus facilitating the growth of opportunistic organisms.*
- Avoid invasive procedures, if possible, *because they interfere with primary defenses.*
- Use strict aseptic technique when performing invasive procedures and when caring for the sites of invasion *to decrease the risk of introducing pathogens from the hospital environment.*
- Discontinue invasive lines in a timely manner *to decrease risk for colonization of pathogens at the insertion site.*
- Wash hands before and after contact with patient *to remove organisms before they can colonize the skin.*
- Prevent contamination of dressings and casts with urine or feces *to prevent transfer of normal flora organisms to a compromised part of the body.*
- Use protective isolation procedures as indicated. Prevent patient exposure to infected visitors/staff. Limit visitors, if necessary. Ensure that patient care staff do not work when they have an infectious disease. Discharge patient as soon as possible from the hospital. *All of the above are necessary to prevent hospital-acquired infections.*

Infection will not be transmitted to patient's contacts, as evidenced by:

Patient care staff practicing universal precautions and handwashing and remaining free of signs of infection

Appropriate isolation procedures implemented on hospitalized patients soon after infection is confirmed

All patient contacts adequately immunized or examined and treated for infection

Patient demonstrating behavior to prevent transmission of pathogens to others or to the environment

In addition, reportable infections reported to the local health department and the incidence of communicable infections decreasing in the hospital and in the community

- Monitor all patients for signs of infection and report findings so that prompt treatment can be initiated. Use universal precautions and other isolation procedures as indicated. *Both interventions will decrease opportunity for transmission of pathogens.*
- Participate in follow-up of patient contacts *so that they can be treated or counseled to take appropriate preventive measures.* Administer immune globulin, as prescribed, to unimmunized persons exposed to hepatitis B *to decrease the severity of the infection, if transmitted.*
- Instruct patient or caregiver in precautions for handling infective secretions, excretions, or exudates *to prevent transmission.* Discuss with patient the behaviors necessary to prevent transmission of STDs and foodborne infections.
- Report to the local health authority those infections that must be reported by law.
- Protect pregnant nursing personnel from contact with selected infections (rubella, cytomegalovirus, toxoplasmosis, herpes).
- Ensure that high-risk patient care staff have been immunized against hepatitis B virus, rubella, tetanus, and other vaccine-preventable conditions.
- Participate in educating patient care staff regarding pathogen transmission *to ensure that staff will protect themselves adequately while caring for all patients.*
- Educate pregnant women to prevent or seek early treatment for infections that can be transmitted to the fetus *to prevent fetal infections and their sequelae.*
- Participate in public education programs regarding safer sexual practices to help prevent the spread of AIDS and other sexually transmitted diseases.

■ RISK FOR INJURY

(Risk for trauma; Risk for poisoning; Risk for suffocation)

Risk for injury is a state in which an individual is at risk of injury as a result of environmental conditions interacting with the individual's adaptive and defensive resources.

Risk for trauma is an accentuated risk of intentional or unintentional tissue injury (e.g., wound, burn, fracture).

Risk for poisoning is an accentuated risk of intentional or unintentional exposure to or ingestion of drugs or dangerous products in doses sufficient to cause poisoning.

Risk for suffocation is an accentuated risk of intentional or unintentional suffocation (inadequate air available for inhalation).

The diagnostic label *risk for injury* includes three sub-components accepted by the North American Nursing Diagnoses Association (NANDA): trauma, poisoning, and suffocation. However, these are merely examples of the broader label. Therefore the discussion that follows is presented from a theoretic perspective and does not specifically include trauma, poisoning, and suffocation.

The injury process requires interaction of human factors (the host), energy sources (the agents), and physical and sociocultural factors (the environment).

Host, or human, factors include variables that pertain specifically to the person being considered. Examples include the individual's age, physical condition, eyesight, muscle strength, mental ability, fatigue level, growth and development, personal habits and values, stress level, blood alcohol level, and dexterity. Host factors also include the individual's ability to cope with an unexpected energy souce that may cause harm. These factors are essentially the individual's resistance characteristics.

Agent factors are the energy sources that challenge the individual's resistance characteristics and actually cause the injury. These include mechanical and gravitational (e.g., falls), thermal (e.g. burns), radiant (e.g., sunburn), chemical (e.g., poisoning), electrical (e.g., electrical shock), and lack of oxidation (e.g., drowning or suffocation).

Environmental factors may be divided into two areas: physical and sociocultural. Examples of physical environmental factors are defective or unsafe equipment, hazardous road conditions, and exposure to solid, liquid, or gaseous poisons. Sociocultural environmental factors include unsupervised small children, lack of knowledge to establish a safe environment, family stress, and lack of knowledge regarding developmental ability.

To establish the nursing diagnosis *risk for injury,* one must consider the collective interrelationship of host, agent, and environmental factors. The diagnosis may then be defined as the interaction between the individual (the host), the energy source (the agent), and the environment (physical and sociocultural) that imposes a risk for physical harm to the individual.

One should also consider the situation before the injury (preevent), during the impact (event), and after the injury has occurred (postevent). See table below.

Injury Model

	Human Factors (Host)	Energy Sources (Agents)	Physical-Sociocultural Factors (Environment)
Preevent Phase			
Event Phase			
Postevent Phase			

Preevent: Those events and factors before the injury; the interaction of these factors leads to the injury.
Event: During the injury process; the physical response, the intensity of the energy, and the environmental situation.
Postevent: After the injury; the body's response to the energy source, the final energy dose, and the emergency care provided by those in the environment.

Risk Factors[7]

Host Human Factors

Biologic and physiologic
   Age (under 40 years, over 60 years)
   Gender (males more than females)
   Chronic diseases
   Current disabilities, especially musculoskeletal, visual, hearing, and sensory
   Metabolism and nutritional status, especially calcium deficiency
   Fatigue
   High chemical substance or alcohol blood level
Mental/psychologic
   Mental disorders
   Orientation
   Temperament/mood
   Irritability, anger
   Emotional state/lability
   Personal stresses
   Social adjustment
   Altered levels of consciousness
   Aggressiveness/social deviance
Psychomotor
   Developmental level inappropriate for task or environment
   Skill/performance capabilities
   Muscle strength and coordination
Cognitive
   Experience
   Judgment
   Education (safety and general)
Behavioral
   Attitude
   Beliefs
   Habits
   Motivation
   Preoccupation

Agents (Energy Sources)

Physical factors
   Mechanical
      Defective or unsafe vehicle
      Excessive speeds
      Nonuse or misuse of safety belts
      Nonuse or misuse of headgear for bicycle or motorcycle riders
      Unsafe road or road-crossing conditions
      Play near vehicle pathways (driveways, laneways, railroad tracks)
   Dangerous machinery and appliances
   Sharp-edged toys
   Slippery floors (wet or highly waxed)
   Furniture with sharp edges, projections, or glass
   Unanchored rugs
   Bathtub without hand grip or antislip equipment
   Unsteady furniture
   Inadequately lit rooms
   Unsturdy or absent stair rails

   Unanchored electrical wires
   Litter or liquid spills on floor or stairways
   Unprotected open windows or stairs
   Use of cracked dishes or glasses
   Knives stored uncovered
   Guns or ammunition stored unlocked
   Fireworks or gunpowder
   Absence of designated play areas
   Shoes without traction
Thermal
   Playing with matches, candles, or cigarettes
   Highly flammable children's toys or clothing
   Smoking in bed or near oxygen
   Grease waste collected on stoves
   Contact with intense cold
   Pot handles facing toward front of stove
   Hot water heater set higher than 54.5° C (130° F)
   Lack of smoke detectors
   Potential igniting gas leaks
   Delayed lighting of gas burner or oven
   Experimenting with chemicals or gasoline
   Unscreened fires or heaters
   Improperly stored combustibles or corrosives (matches, oily rags, lye, gasoline)
Chemical
   Large supply of drugs in home
   Medicines stored in unlocked cabinets accessible to children
   Hazardous products placed or stored within reach of young children
   Lack of childproof caps
   Products not stored in properly labeled storage container or space
   Availability of illicit drugs potentially contaminated by poisonous additives
   Flaking, peeling paint or plaster
   Chemical contamination of food or water
   Unprotected contact with heavy metals or chemicals
   Paint, lacquer, etc., in poorly ventilated areas or without effective protection
   Presence of poisonous vegetation
   Presence of atmospheric pollutants
   Contact with acids or alkalies
Radiant
   Overexposure to sun, sunlamps, or radiotherapy
Electrical
   Overloaded fuse boxes
   Lack of safety plugs or appliance outlets
   Unused extension cords plugged in
   Worn electrical cords
   Electrical appliances and cords near water
   Overloaded electrical outlets
Lack of oxidation
   Household gas leaks
   Fuel-burning heaters not vented to outside
   Pacifier hung around infant's neck
   Pools without structural barriers
   Toys with cords
   Pillow or plastic sheet placed in infant's crib

Propped bottle placed in an infant's crib

Vehicle running in closed garage

Children playing with plastic bag or inserting small objects into mouth or nose

Discarded or unused refrigerators or freezers without doors removed

Environment (Physical-Sociocultural Factors)

Physical factors

Unsafe highways

No breakaway telephone poles

No air bags in cars

Sociocultural factors

Lack of parental awareness of hazards

Lack of safety education

Fatalistic attitude about injuries

Lack of knowledge of developmental stages

Negligent, abusive, or overprotective childrearing practices

Lack of parental supervision

Lack of resources to establish safe environment (knowledge, finances)

Presence of family stress (marital, financial, health)

Inadequate community emergency medical services response

Lack of public education (first aid, CPR)

Lack of community safety programs (water safety, lifeguards, crossing guards, building codes)

Expected Patient Outcomes & Nursing Interventions

Host Factors

Accurate appraisal of susceptibility factors, as evidenced by:

Valid appraisal of age and gender factors that indicate increased risk of injury

Appropriate steps to protect self or patients at risk from injury

- Teach and counsel patient about strategies and countermeasures to prevent injury.

   Prevent the creation of the hazard.

   Reduce the amount of energy source created.

   Prevent the release of the energy source that already exists.

   Modify the rate or spatial distribution of the energy from its source.

   Separate, in time or in space, the hazard or energy source and person or object to be protected.

   Separate the energy source by physical barrier.

   Modify the basic qualities of the energy source.

   Increase resistance to damage from energy source.

   Counter damage already done by energy source.

   Repair and rehabilitate injured individual.

- Inform that injury is more likely to occur in individuals under 40 or over 60 years of age.
- Inform that injury is more likely to occur in males than in females.

Appropriate recognition of biologic and physiologic factors that increase risk of injury, as evidenced by:

Identification of chronic diseases or physiologic conditions that increase risk of injury

Protective strategies to alter risk potential

Modification of environment to increase safety potential

- Perform assessment.
- Provide information regarding disease processes or physiologic conditions that increase risk of injury.
- Provide alteration strategies to adapt physical environment to the patient's physiologic state.

Appropriate assessment of psychomotor variables that increase risk of injury, as evidenced by:

Appropriate assessment of developmental capabilities and recognition of injury risk

Protective steps to prevent injury

Accurate assessment of skill competence and performance ability

Strategies to increase skill performance or to protect self from injury potential

Exercise or training program to meet task demand

Protective devices to separate self from potential injury source

Accurate recognition of fatigue state, which may lead to potential injury

Appropriate steps to prevent injury

- Conduct assessment of developmental level of individual.
- Provide educational information regarding safety strategies appropriate for individual.
- Assess skill competence and performance capabilities of individual.
- Assess muscle strength and coordination capabilities.
- Provide strategies to protect individual from potential injury.
- Assess and provide alteration strategies to increase self-protective capabilities for individual.

Accurate assessment of mental and psychologic variables that increase risk of injury, as evidenced by:

Recognition of variables (mental mood, temperament, stress, irritability, hostility) that may increase risk of injury

Seeking new methods to express emotions that will not increase injury potential

Demonstration of methods to decrease risk of injury

- Assess mental impairment or decision-making ability that may interfere with individual's ability to protect self from injury.
- Provide protective interventions that will protect individual from injury.
- Monitor mood and temperament, which may increase risk of injury.
- Assess individual's stress patterns, which may increase risk of injury.
- Assess personal and social adjustments, which may increase risk of injury.
- Provide protective interventions if necessary to prevent injury.

Appropriate behavioral response pattern to decrease risk of injury, as evidenced by:

Recognition of habits, aggressive behavior, and motivations that may increase injury potential

Seeking new knowledge and skill to decrease potential risk

Demonstration of methods that decrease risk of injury

- Identify individual's habits or aggressive acts that place the individual at higher risk for injury.
- Assess social deviance or effect of TV violence, which may place individual at risk for injury.
- Attempt to identify variables that affect individual behavior.
- Provide education and passive protection that will protect individual from injury.
- Assess for lack of motivation regarding injury protection.
- Where possible, provide passive protection.

Accurate assessment of cognitive ability to decrease risk of injury, as evidenced by:

Accurate assessment of the client's own ability, experience, judgment, and education to reduce injury risk

Does client seek new information and skill to decrease deficit areas?

Use of new knowledge and skill to decrease injury risk

- Assess experience and judgment in individual's ability to determine and maintain adequate injury prevention strategies.
- Assess educational needs in area of safety and injury prevention.

Agent Factors

Appropriate use of countermeasures to protect self from injury, as evidenced by:

Knowledge of countermeasures to reduce potential of injury

Use of appropriate countermeasures

Knowledge and use of safety devices and approved products that decrease risk of injury

- Provide education relevant to strategies and countermeasures.
- Provide prevention strategies that will protect individual from injury.

Appropriate identification of risk factors

- Provide information regarding product design and characteristics: restraining devices, safety caps, barriers separating the individual from the hazard (stairs, windows, pools, streets).

Environmental Factors

Ability to reduce environmental physical risks of injury, as evidenced by:

Accurate assessment of exposure to environmental risks, such as home products, hazardous materials, hazardous surfaces, and unprotected areas

Knowledge to reduce environmental physical risk

Altering physical environment to reduce risk of injury

- Assess physical risks in the environment.
- Provide education and structural recommendations to decrease injury risk.

- Assess task demand and provide protective intervention where necessary.
- Provide education regarding home hazards and methods to decrease injury potential.

Ability to reduce environmental social risks of injury, as evidenced by:

Recognition of social variables, such as childbearing practices, child supervision, and discipline practices, that may increase risk of injury

Seeking instruction to modify childrearing practices where appropriate

Seeking support to intervene when stress or lack of knowledge limits adult's ability to provide safe environment for childrearing

Acknowledgement of own limitations regarding ability to cope with social environmental stress

Seeking new knowledge and skill to cope with environmental social stress

- Assess parental expectations for child's behavior. Where appropriate, provide educational information congruent with growth and developmental level.
- Perform assessment of parental attitude toward injury prevention strategies.
- Where appropriate, provide information regarding injury potential and alternative prevention strategies.
- Assess components of family socioeconomic status that may place family in stress situation and thus increase injury risk.
- Assess child-rearing practices and provide alteration strategies to assist parents.
- Assess potential for family abusive behavior (see further intervention strategies under Risk for Violence: Self-Directed or Directed at Others).

Principles and Rationale for Nursing Interventions

The nursing care for this nursing diagnosis is directed toward host, agent, and environmental factors that potentially lead to injury. The intent of the interventions is preventive, not curative. Because of this, many of the interventions are either educational or include strategies to alter the environment or the individual's position in the environment. Injury prevention is a very complex process that takes place in an equally complex environment. Attention to prevention requires careful evaluation of the individual, the environment, and the agents with which the individual may come in contact.

Host Factors

Host factors deal with the human aspects of the injury process. Specific physiologic, biologic, psychomotor, psychologic, and behavioral factors must be considered as goal statements of risk for injury. The condition of the individual as it relates to each of these variables is assessed and determined if an area of risk is present.

Agent Factors

The injurious agent first must be identified. Thus the countermeasures may be determined. The patient needs instruction to protect himself or herself from the injury agent. Countermeasures may be passively or actively applied; their purpose is to protect the patient from the injury mechanism.

Environmental Factors

Injury may also be caused by factors in the environment, such as the physical environment, social environment, and family. Each of these factors requires a special assessment to determine areas of stress or concern. Often injury occurs because the demand for performance outweighs the individual's ability to perform. In such cases the environmental factors must be readjusted to meet the individual's ability to perform the tasks.

RISK FOR PERIOPERATIVE POSITIONING INJURY

Risk for perioperative positioning injury is the state in which the client is at risk for injury as a result of the environmental conditions found in the perioperative setting.

The patient's age, level of consciousness, state of general health, medications, nutritional status, and blood pressure are important considerations when assessing the risk for perioperative positioning injury. A careful documentation of the patient's preoperative condition establishes a baseline for further assessments, provides a focus for nursing interventions, and assists in the evaluation of postoperative outcomes.

Five areas to be considered when positioning the surgical patient are respiration, circulation, peripheral nerves and vessels, musculoskeletal structures, and skin. Distribution of the patient's weight may be altered with each specific position. Documentation of the patient's position and any special strategies used should be performed per institutional protocol.

Risk Factors

Disorientation
Immobilization
Muscle weakness
Sensory/perceptual disturbances due to anesthesia
Obesity
Emaciation
Edema

Expected Patient Outcomes & Nursing Interventions

The patient is free from respiratory injury related to positioning or hypoxia

- Preoperatively, have patient demonstrate turning, deep-breathing exercises, and the use of the incentive spirometer if applicable.
- Note presence of cough.
- When placing the patient in lithotomy, position the legs to cause minimal restriction of diaphragmatic movement.
- When placing the patient in lateral position, assure that the location of the upper arm contributes to proper intercostal breathing.

- When placing the patient in prone or jackknife position, assure that the selection and location of body rolls allow for proper chest expansion.

The patient is free from circulatory compromise as a result of positioning

- Assess baseline data for coagulopathy.
- Determine patient activity level and positioning requirements.
- Provide cardiovascular supports to prevent pooling of blood in dependent extremities and to aid in enhancing circulatory return.

The patient is free from injuries to nerves or peripheral vessels resulting from compromised blood supply or ischemia from stretching, hyperextending, compressing, or twisting

- Based on patient condition, select appropriate safety measures such as pads and supports.
- Ensure there are adequate personnel to move the patient safely.
- Move the patient with careful attention to proper body alignment.
- Avoid overextension of joints.
- Pay scrupulous attention to arm positioning to avoid peripheral nerve injuries.
- Place padding at knee area in lithotomy to prevent compression damage to the peroneal nerve.
- Place a soft roll at the apex of the scapula to prevent brachial compression when in lateral position.

The patient is free from musculoskeletal trauma related to positioning

- Assess preoperative range of motion.
- Encourage patient participation in positioning and elicit comfort level prior to the induction of anesthesia.
- Assure proper alignment of the limbs after induction.
- Avoid overzealous movement of the extremities during positioning.
- Give special consideration while moving patients with prostheses.
- Pad ischial tuberosities when in lithotomy or modified Fowlers to prevent pressure on sciatic nerves.
- Move legs simultaneously into and out of lithotomy to prevent sacroiliac dislocation.
- Pay careful attention to the fingers when adjusting the foot of the operating room bed for lithotomy position in order to prevent digital damage.
- When positioning the patient prone, avoid hyperextending the shoulder joints when moving the arms.
- When positioning the patient prone, the knees are padded and a pillow is placed under the ankles to prevent pressure on the toes from the mattress.
- Adjust body rolls for prone position to prevent encroachment on the breasts.
- Assure there is no impingement on the male genitalia when in prone position.

The patient is free from impaired tissue or skin integrity

- Assess for contributory factors such as allergy, nutrition, and existing disease processes.
- Consider duration of pressure and location of bony prominences and/or other areas at risk.
- Lift, rather than slide, the patient in order to prevent shearing force injuries.
- In order to prevent skin abrasions or friction injuries, position the legs so they are not in contact with each other when in lateral position.

Principles and Rationale for Nursing Interventions

The overall principle of the nursing interventions is one of causing no injury while positioning the patient, at the same time allowing for adequate surgical access. In addition, the administration of anesthesia reduces or eliminates the patient's normal defense mechanisms. Care must therefore be taken to safeguard the patient against inadvertent injury.

Rationales for the peripheral nursing interventions are as follows:

- To promote maximal respiratory movement while the patient is in the position required for the operative procedure.
- To promote efficient peripheral circulation and return of blood to the central circulation.
- To preserve the integrity of the neurovascular system.
- To provide support for the patient's musculoskeletal system to restore the patient to the preoperative level of function.
- To maintain the patient's preoperative tissue status and skin condition.

■ ALTERED PROTECTION

Altered protection is the state in which an individual experiences a decrease in the ability to guard the self from internal or external threats, such as illness or injury.

Protection involves processes that include defending, guarding, and safekeeping. Defending is resistance, guarding is watching over, and safekeeping is cherishing and ministering. The mechanisms involved in these processes are the systems of immune, hematopoietic, integumentary, and sensorimotor.[11] Protective nursing behaviors as defined by the American Nursing Association[1] are surveillance, assessment, and intervention in support of adaptive capabilities and developmental function of person.

The need for a diagnosis of protection was identified in clinical practice. Concerns that needed to be addressed involved infection and bleeding, as well as effects of drugs and therapies, such as biotherapy and radiation therapy. Identification studies and validation studies were conducted. The diagnosis was reviewed through the Diagnosis Review Cycle and revised to encompass a broader view.[13] This was consistent with Lunney,[10] who described protection as a broad diagnosis that could be specified. The diagnosis *altered protection* was presented and subsequently accepted.

The goals for altered protection can generally be outlined as maintaining protective defenses, restoring protective defenses, and promoting protective defenses. To maintain protection, strategies that are implemented include personal and environmental cleanliness, monitoring of vital signs and laboratory values, and incorporating safety precautions.[11] To restore protection, strategies to rebuild defenses include adequate nutrition and fluid intake, energy conservation, and comfort measures.[2] To promote protective defenses, relaxation exercises, stress management techniques, coping, and communication are used to enhance the immune system.[6] Providing nurse presence is an additional intervention that promotes protection.[5]

Interventions can generally be categorized to include, but are not limited to, surveillance, education, and relaxation. Surveillance includes those activities of assessment and monitoring of aseptic technique, cleanliness, vital signs, laboratory values, dietary intake, rest, and exercise. Education includes the patient's/significant other's ability to demonstrate safety measures, to recognize and report symptoms, and to learn health behaviors to maintain, restore, and promote protection. Relaxation includes interventions to assist with stress management and coping.

The nursing diagnosis *altered protection* encompasses a broad area and, for usefulness in clinical practice, the diagnosis can be specified according to type (e.g., altered protection [deficient immunity]; altered protection [altered clotting]). The nursing diagnosis is further specified by identifying the related factor (e.g., altered protection [impaired healing] related to inadequate nutrition). In some circumstances, the broad diagnosis without specification is preferred. For example, in home care, a community spectrum of protection may be needed. Interventions may include screening of visitors, review of immunization status, and environmental control (e.g., of plants).

Related Factors[9]

Altered protection may be associated with various diseases, treatments, and conditions.

Diseases

Cancer (e.g., hematologic cancers such as leukemia, lymphoma, multiple myeloma)

Immune disorders (e.g., acquired immune deficiency syndrome; autoimmune disorders, such as multiple sclerosis)

Coagulation disorders (e.g., hemophilia, disseminated intravascular coagulation)

Treatments

Radiation therapy

Surgery

Drugs (e.g., antineoplastics, corticosteroids, immunosuppressants, biologic response modifiers, anticoagulants, thrombolytic enzymes, antibiotics)

Invasive devices/procedures (e.g., intravenous catheters, urinary devices)

Conditions
  Infection
  Chronic, maladaptive stress
  Extremes of age (e.g., elderly, newborn)
  Inadequate nutrition
  Inadequate sleep
  Alcohol abuse
  Graft rejection
  Graft versus host disease

Defining Characteristics[9]

Deficient immunity
Impaired healing
Altered clotting
Maladaptive stress response
Neurosensory alterations
Chilling
Perspiring
Dyspnea
Cough
Itching
Restlessness
Insomnia
Fatigue
Anorexia
Weakness
Immobility
Disorientation
Pressure sores

Expected Patient Outcomes & Nursing Interventions

Patient and significant other demonstrate measures to maintain protective defenses, as evidenced by:

Measures for cleanliness and safety
Vital signs and laboratory values within normal limits
Reduced symptoms of infection, bleeding, chills, fever, headache, or discomfort
  • Assess for risk factors and side effects of disease and therapy.
  • Assess protective mechanisms (e.g., immune, hematopoietic, integumentary, sensorimotor).
  • Teach strategies to promote personal and environmental cleanliness.
  • Monitor vital signs and laboratory values.
  • Institute safety precautions.
  Injury must be avoided because of compromised protective mechanisms.

Patient and significant other demonstrate measures to restore protective defenses, as evidenced by:

Balanced diet
Normal rest/sleep/activity pattern
Reduced discomfort
  • Monitor weight.
  • Monitor dietary and fluid intake.

  • Teach measures to conserve energy (e.g., pacing of ADLs).
  • Provide comfort for symptoms (e.g., chills, fever, myalgias).
  Immune function is supported through sleep, nutrition, and energy conservation and avoidance of discomfort.

Patient and significant other demonstrate measures to promote protective defenses, as evidenced by:

Stress management
Report of increased well-being
  • Initiate stress management techniques (e.g., relaxation exercises, coping strategies, exercise).
  Stress may depress immune function.
  • Provide nurse presence.
  Presence nurtures and supports.

Principles and Rationale for Nursing Interventions

The patient outcome of maintaining protective defenses involves interventions of safety measures and monitoring. Monitoring laboratory values is an important intervention. A decreased white blood cell count, for example, is inversely proportional to the risk and severity of infections. Vital signs are important, especially temperature. Fever may be the only indication of infection because of lack of inflammatory response.[14] Strategies of personal and environmental cleanliness that maintain the integrity of the skin and mucous membrane ensure effective barriers that are the frontline of defense. Asepsis in patients, caregivers, and techniques, especially invasive procedures, decreases exposure to microbes. Safety precautions, including bleeding precautions, can prevent hemorrhage that may occur with decreased platelet counts.[11] Injury must be avoided when the immune system is compromised.

The patient outcome of restoring protective defenses involves interventions that rebuild strength. Stressors that increase the metabolic rate and nutritional requirements include infection, neoplasm, and medications such as corticosteroids. Immune function is supported by intake of adequate nutrition. Wound healing and recovery from illness may be delayed in the malnourished person. Protein and calorie malnutrition can alter immune responses (e.g., diminished ability to form circulating antibodies; reduction in the secretory antibody response in the respiratory, gastrointestinal, and genitourinary tracts). Protein energy-starved patients experience a higher incidence of morbidity and mortality during infections than well-nourished individuals. The elderly are at high risk due to age-related immune impairment and require in-depth and specialized assessment.[2] Adverse environmental events may influence susceptibility to infection, growth of tumors, and immunologic function. Stressful events may include life changes (e.g., divorce, death of a spouse) or sleep deprivation. Interventions of effective energy use and conservation can assist in restoring protective defenses. These interventions include good nutrition, stress management, maintenance of energy reserves through conservation and restoration of energy reserves through comfort, rest, and sleep.[4]

The patient outcome of promoting protective defenses involves interventions based on the principles of psychoneuroimmunology. Just as stress may depress the immune function, emotional and cognitive influences may enhance the immune system.[7] Interventions that reduce stress (coping, relaxation, stress management) may promote immune system function. In addition, nurse presence, touch, listening, and a caring attitude may be interventions that have a protective effect on patients.[7,8] As the knowledge of the mind-body connection increases, there is an increased responsibility for health care professionals to become aware of strategies and interventions in addition to medical treatment.[12] Cultural influences and healing practices must be recognized as a form of mind-body medicine in a holistic framework.[3]

ENERGY FIELD DISTURBANCE

Energy field disturbance occurs when there is a disruption of the flow of energy surrounding a person's being, which results in a disharmony of the body, mind, or spirit.[2]

Energy fields have been described by nursing theorists for many years. Myra Estrin Levine wrote about holism and conservation principles, which are energy, structural integrity, personal integrity, and social integrity, to keep the holism of the individual balanced. Martha E. Rogers characterized the life process by wholeness, openness, unidirectionality, pattern and organization, sentence and thought. She described energy fields as constituting the fundamental unit of both the living and the nonliving, in an infinite and open universe of open systems. Rogers described principles of dimensionality as: (1) complementarity—mutual and simultaneous movement of human and environmental fields; (2) resonancy—wave patterns that change from lower frequency to higher frequency patterns; (3) helicy—continuous, innovative, probablistic and increasing diversity of human and environmental field patterns characterized by nonrepeating rhythmicities. Other nursing theorists Joyce Fitzpatrick, Margaret Newman, and Rosemary Parse, have been inspired by Rogers to formulate similar descriptions of the individual as a unified whole with the rhythmical patterns of the environment of time, space, and consciousness.[5]

In addition to the reference of energy fields by nursing theorists, there are other aspects related to the flow of energy and equilibrium. Rooted in Eastern philosophy is the ancient art of "laying on of hands," which is based on the principle that from the universal flow of energy comes the life-giving healing energy that is present in all living systems. The use of therapeutic touch can facilitate the repatterning of an individual's environmental energy field processes. Nurses using therapeutic touch can facilitate the flow of healing energy when there is a disruption of the flow of energy due to a deficit, blockage, or disequilibrium.[3,4]

A specialized instruction and supervised practice is needed before the nurse engages in therapeutic touch to ensure that the desired changes are obtained. The nurse must have the intention and motivation to help the patient who must be open and receptive to accept the change. Dimensions of positive effect are the desired response to therapeutic touch and include relaxation, decrease in pain, contentment, joy, and vigor with a release of anxiety, guilt, depression, and hostility.[3,4,6,7]

Related Factors

Physiologic changes, including illness, injury, pain, trauma, or pregnancy

Situational and maturational experiences, including anxiety, fear, grieving, perioperative and perinatal experiences, and age-related developmental difficulties

Defining Characteristics[2]

Temperature change (warmth or coolness)
Visual changes (image or color)
Disruption of the field (vacant/hold/spike/bulge)
Movement (wave/spike/tingling/dense/flowing)
Sounds (tone or words)

Expected Patient Outcomes & Nursing Interventions[3,4,6,7,8,9]

The patient experiences a multidimensional effect as evidenced by:

Verbalized descriptions of a sense of physiological, emotional, and spiritual well-being

The nurse prepares the patient and environment for therapeutic touch.

- Provide privacy.
- Give preparatory explanation of therapeutic touch to the patient, emphasizing the patient's ability to discontinue at any time.
- Await the verbalization of understanding and acceptance by the patient before commencing therapeutic touch.
- Assist the patient to a position of comfort.

The nurse makes a determination as to the status of the person's energy field.

- Focus initially on self-centering and own internal energy.
- Scan the patient's body from head to feet with palms of hands about 3 inches away from the body.
- Sense variations indicative of energy imbalance including temperature variations, heaviness, lightness, tingling, absence of feeling.

The nurse stimulates a rhythmic flow of energy.

- Perform vigorous hand movements from head to toe over the patient.

The nurse repatterns imbalanced areas.

- Move hands in a sweeping motion from head to feet.
- Shake hands to remove congestion from field.
- Validate that energy is flowing over legs and feet; if not, continue to move hands to facilitate energy flow.
- Place hands at rest over the solar plexus (just above the waist) upon completion of therapeutic touch while focusing on the flow of healing energy to the patient.
- Provide a period of rest for the patient.

Patient provides positive feedback.
- Patient exhibits a slower and deeper respiratory pattern.
- Patient may sigh or demonstrate another audible response of relaxation.
- Voice volume decreases.
- Peripheral flush may occur in the face.
- Patient verbalizes relaxation, comfort, and sense of well-being.

Principles and Rationale for Nursing Intervention[1,3,8]

Nursing interventions are derived from the nurse's understanding of energy field disturbances and the skill used in the application of therapeutic touch. Specialized training is required in order for the nurse to develop the skill to enter into a meditative state that facilitates the nurse to enter the energy field of the patient. It is recommended that the nurse should have at least six months' experience in an acute-care setting and receive guided learning by another nurse who has at least two years' experience in therapeutic touch. This preparation would be in addition to 30 hours of instruction in the theory and practice of therapeutic touch, as well as 30 hours of supervised practice with relatively healthy individuals.[6]

During the process of applying therapeutic touch the nurse focuses on creating a state of balance and harmony while sensing or passively visualizing the free flow of energy to the patient with the intent of facilitating healing. This process takes a great deal of energy and concentration of the nurse, who must have a great degree of self-awareness, sensitivity, and skill. The healing process is one of balancing or centering and "unruffling" or clearing the energy field and directing the transfer of energy to the patient. An important part of the specialized training is knowing when to discontinue the energy flow in order to achieve the best outcome for the patient. The effects of therapeutic touch on the patient are a sense of relaxation and balance.

References

Health-seeking behaviors

1. American Nurses' Association: *Nursing: a social policy statement,* Kansas City, MO, 1980, ANA.
2. Brubaker BH: Health promotion: a linguistic analysis, *Adv Nurs Sci* 5:1, 1983.
3. Bruhn JG et al: The wellness process, *Community Health* 2(3):209, 1977.
4. Butler RH: Minority wellness promotion: a behavioral self-management approach, *J Gerontol Nurs* 13:22, 1987.
5. Duffy ME: Determinants of health promoting lifestyles in older persons, *Image* 25(1):23, 1993.
6. Duffey ME: Health promotion in the family: current findings and directives for nursing research, *J Adv Nurs* 13:109, 1988.
7. Dunn HL: *High level wellness,* Thorofare, NJ, 1977, Charles B Slack.
8. Hall BA, Allen JD: Sharpening nursing's focus by focusing on health, *Nurs Health Care* 7:315, 1986.
9. Horgon PA: Health status perceptions affect health-related behaviors, *J Gerontol Nurs* 13:30, 1987.
10. Kim MK, McFarland GK, McLane AM: *Pocket guide to nursing diagnosis,* ed 6, St Louis, 1995, Mosby.
11. Maslow AH, editor: *New knowledge in human values,* New York, 1959, Harper & Bros.
12. McCloskey JC, Bulechek GM: *Iowa Intervention Project: Nursing Interventions Classification (NIC),* ed 2, St. Louis, 1996, Mosby.
13. Pender NJ: *Health promotion in nursing practice,* ed 2, Norwalk, Conn, 1987, Appleton & Lange.

Altered health maintenance

1. Alford DM, Futrell M: Wellness and health promotion of the elderly, *Nurs Outlook* 40(5):221, 1992.
2. Nursing: a policy statement, Kansas City, Mo, 1980, author. American Nurses' Association.
3. Anderson J, Yuhos R: Health promotion in rural setting: a nursing challenge, *Nurs Clin North Am* 28(1):145, 1993.
4. Archbold PG et al: The PREP system of nursing interventions: a pilot test with families caring for older members, *Res Nurs Health* 18:3, 1995.
5. Baric L: Recognition of the "at risk" role: a means to influence health behavior, 1969, International Seminar on Health Education, *Behavior change through health education: problems of methodology: reports on fundamental research in health education,* Hamburg, Federal Republic of Germany, 1970.
6. Becker H, Stuifbergen A, Soo Oh H, Hall S: Self-rated abilities for health practices: a health self-efficacy measure, *Health Values* 17:42, 1993.
7. Bigbee JL: The uniqueness of rural nursing, *Nurs Clin North Am* 28(1):131, 1993.
8. Blair JE: Social learning theory: Strategies for health promotion, *AAOHN J* 41(5):245, 1993.
9. Blair JE: Social marketing: Consumer focused health promotion, *AAOHN J* 43(10):527, 1995.
10. Blue CL: The predictive capacity of the theory of reasoned action and the theory of planned behavior in exercise research: an integrated literature review, *Res Nurs Health* 18:105, 1995.
11. Carpenito LJ: *Nursing diagnosis: application to clinical practice,* ed 2, Philadelphia, 1987, Lippincott.
12. Carter KF, Green RD, Green L, Dufour LT: Health needs of homeless clients accessing nursing care at a free clinic, *J Community Health Nurs* 11(3):139, 1994.
13. Conn V: Self-care actions taken by older adults for influenza and colds, *Nurs Res* 40(3):176, 1991.
14. Connell CM, Sharpe PA, Gallant MP: Effect of health risk appraisal on health outcomes in a university worksite health promotion trial, *Health Education Res* 10(2):199, 1995.
15. Cox HC: *Clinical applications of nursing diagnosis: Adult, child, women's, psychiatric, gerontic and home health considerations,* ed 2, Philadelphia, 1991, FA Davis.
16. Dellasega C, Brown R, White A: Cholesterol-related health behaviors in rural elderly persons, *J Gerontol Nurs* 21(5):5, 1995.
17. Donahue JM, McQuire MB: The political economy of responsibility in health and illness, *Soc Sci Med* 40(1):47, 1995.
18. Elkamel F: The use of television series in health education, *Health Education Res* 10(2):225, 1995.
19. Felton GM, Parsons MA: Factors influencing physical activity in average-weight and overweight young women, *J Community Health Nurs* 11(2):109, 1994.
20. Goeppinger J: Health promotion for rural populations: partnership interventions, *Family Community Health* 16(1):1, 1993.
21. Goeppinger J et al: From research to practice: The effects of the jointly sponsored dissemination of an arthritis self-care nursing intervention, *Applied Nurs Res* 8(3):106, 1995.
22. Graham H: *When life's a drag: women, smoking and disadvantage,* Her Majesty's Service Office, London, 1993, HMSO.
23. Hall JM: The experiences of lesbians in Alcoholics Anonymous, *West J Nurs Res* 16(5):556, 1994.
24. Harper MS: Aging minorities, *Healthcare Trends Transition* 6(4):9, 1995.
25. *Healthy people 2000,* The Surgeon General's report on health promotion and disease prevention objectives, DHHS Publication No. 91-50212, Washington, DC, 1990, US Government Printing Office.
26. Hollis JF et al: Nurse-assisted smoking counseling in medical settings: minimizing demands on physicians, *Prev Med* 20:497, 1991.
27. Hollis JF et al: Nurse-assisted counseling for smokers in primary care, *Ann Intern Med* 118(7):521, 1993.

28. Jemmott LS, Jemmott JB: Increasing condom-use intentions among sexually active Black adolescent women, *Nurs Res* 41(5):273, 1992.
29. Kaplan MS, Marks G: Appraisal of health risks: the roles of masculinity, femininity, and sex, *Social Health Illness* 17(2):206-211, 1995.
30. Keating S: Health promotion and disease prevention in home care, *Geriatric Nurs* 16(4):184, 1995.
31. Kelly MP: Health promotion in primary care: taking account of the patient's point of view, *J Advanced Nurs* 17:1291, 1992.
32. Kendall J: Fighting back: promoting emancipatory nursing actions, *Adv Nurs Sci* 15(2):1, 1992.
33. Kim MJ, McFarland GK, McLane AM, editors: *Pocket guide to nursing diagnoses,* ed 4, St. Louis, 1991, Mosby.
34. Lierman LM, Young HM, Kasprzyk D, Benoliel JQ: Predicting breast self-examination using the theory of reasoned action, *Nurs Res* 39(2):97, 1990.
35. Long KA: The concept of health: Rural perspectives, *Nurs Clin North Am* 28(1):123, 1993.
36. Maas M, Buckwalter KC, Hardy M: *Nursing diagnoses and interventions for the elderly,* Redwood City, CA, 1991, Addison-Wesley Nursing.
37. Maibach E, Murphy DA: Self-efficacy in health promotion research and practice: conceptualization and measurement, *Health Education Res* 10(1):37, 1995.
38. May KM, Evans GG: Health education for homeless populations, *J Community Health Nurs* 11(4):229, 1994.
39. McKie L: Women's views of the cervical smear test: implications for nursing practice—women who have not had a smear test, *J Advanced Nurs* 18:972, 1993.
40. Melnyk KA: Barriers to care: Operationalizing the variable, *Nurs Res* 39(2):108, 1990.
41. Minkler M, Wallace SP, Mcdonald M: The political economy of health: a useful theoretical tool for health education practice, *Int Q Community Health Education* 15(2):111, 1995.
42. Moore P, Hepworth JT: Use of perinatal and infant health services by Mexican-American Medicaid enrollees, *JAMA* 272(4):297, 1994.
43. Morse EV, Simon PM, Besch CL, Walker J: Issues of recruitment, retention, and compliance in community-based clinical trials with traditionally underserved populations, *Appl Nurs Res* 8(1):8, 1995.
44. North American Nursing Diagnosis Association: Taxonomy I, Revised 1990. St Louis, 1990, Author.
45. Poss JE, Meeks BH: Meeting the health care needs of migrant farmworkers: The experience of the Niagara County Migrant Clinic, *J Community Health Nurs* 11(4):219, 1994.
46. Redland AR, Stuifbergen AK: Strategies for maintenance of health-promoting behaviors, *Nurs Clin North America* 28(2):427, 1993.
47. Sharpe PA: Older women and health services: Moving from ageism toward empowerment, *Women & Health* 22(3):9, 1995.
48. Sitzez CR: A community-based breast cancer education and screening program for elderly women, *Geriatric Nurs* 16(4):151, 1995.
49. Skinner CS, Zerr AD, Damson RL: Incorporating mobile mammography units into primary care: focus group interviews among inner-city health center patients, *Health Education Res* 10(2):179, 1995.
50. Smith SM, Wallston KA, Smith CA: The development and validation of the perceived health competence scale, *Health Education Res* 10(1):51, 1995.
51. Stevens PE: Marginalized women's access to health care: a feminist narrative analysis, *Adv Nurs Sci* 16(2):39, 1993.
52. Strecher VJ, DeVellis BM, Becker MH, Rosenstock IM: The role of self-efficacy in achieving health behavior change, *Health Ed Q* 13:73, 1986.
53. Wagner EH et al: Preventing disability and falls in older adults: a population-based randomized trial, *Am J Public Health* 84(11):1800, 1994.
54. Weaver SK, Wilson JF: Moving toward patient empowerment, *Nurs Health Care* 15(9):480, 1994.
55. West EA: The cultural bridge model, *Nurs Outlook* 41:229, 1993.
56. Yen P: What elders think about food, *Geriatric Nurs* 16(4):187, 1995.

Ineffective management of therapeutic regimen (individuals)
1. Bakker R et al: An analysis of the nursing diagnosis ineffective management of therapeutic regimen compared to noncompliance and Orem's self care deficit theory of nursing, *Nurs Diag* 6(4):161, 1995.
2. Cox C: Health self-determinism index, *Nurs Res* 34(3):177, 1985.
3. Freen M et al: Life style change in a cardiac rehabilitation program: the client perspective, *J Cardiovasc Nurs* 3(2):43, 1989.
4. Germain C, Nemchik R: Diabetes self-management and hospitalization, *Image* 20(2):74, 1988.
5. Kavanagh D et al: Prediction of adherence and control in diabetes, *J Behav Med* 16(5):509, 1993.
6. Kulik J, Mahler H: Emotional support as a moderator of adjustment and compliance after coronary artery bypass surgery: a longitudinal study, *J Behav Med* 16(1):45, 1993.
7. Laffrey S, Crabtree M: Health and health behavior of persons with chronic cardiovascular disease, *Int J Nurs Stud* 25(1):41, 1988.
8. Lubkin I: *Chronic illness: impact and interventions,* Boston, 1990, Jones & Bartlett.
9. Lunney M: Concept of management of therapeutic regimen: validation of four nursing diagnoses, unpublished paper submitted to NANDA, 1991.
10. Lunney M: Ineffective management of therapeutic regimen. In McFarland G, McFarlane E, editors: *Nursing diagnosis and intervention: planning for patient care,* ed 2, St Louis, 1993, Mosby.
11. MacLeod P, Stewart N: Predictors of participation in a peer-led exercise program for senior women, *Can J Nurs Res* 26(1):13, 1994.
12. Miller P et al: Regimen compliance two years after myocardial infarction, *Nurs Res* 39(6):333, 1990.
13. Neale A: Behavioural contracting as a tool to help patients achieve better health, *Fam Pract* 8(4):336, 1991.
14. North American Nursing Diagnosis Association: *Nursing diagnosis: definitions and classifications,* Philadelphia, 1994, NANDA.
15. Powers M, Jalowiec A: Profile of the well-controlled, well-adjusted hypertensive patient, *Nurs Res* 36(2):106, 1987.
16. Robertson D, Keller C: Relationships among health beliefs, self-efficacy, and exercise adherence in patients with coronary artery disease, *Heart Lung* 21(1):56, 1992.
17. Whetstone W, Reid J: Health promotion of older adults: perceived barriers, *J Adv Nurs* 16(11):1343, 1991.
18. Wilson B: Promoting compliance: the patient-provider relationship, *Advances in Renal Replacement Therapy* 2(3):199, 1995.

Effective management of therapeutic regimen (individuals)
1. Anderson JM: Home care management in chronic illness and the self-care movement: an analysis of ideologies and economic processes influencing policy decisions, *Adv Nurs Sci* 12(2):71, 1990.
2. Gast HL et al: Self-care agency: conceptualizations and operationalizations, *Adv Nurs Sci* 12(1):26, 1989.
3. Hartweg DL: Self-care actions of healthy middle-aged women to promote well-being, *Nurs Res* 12(1):221, 1993.
4. Jeng C, Braun LT: Bandura's self-efficacy theory: a guide for cardiac rehabilitation nursing practice, *J Holistic Nurs* 12(4):425, 1994.
5. Keller MI, Ward S, Baumann IJ: Processes of self-care: monitoring sensations and symptoms, *Adv Nurs Sci* 12(1):54, 1989.
6. Kim MJ, McFarland GK, McLane AM: *Pocket guide to nursing diagnoses,* ed 6, St Louis, 1995, Mosby.

Ineffective management of therapeutic regimen (families)
1. Austin JK: Family adaptation to a child's chronic illness, *Ann Rev Nurs Res* 9:103, 1991.
2. Bakker RH, Kastermans JC, Dassen TWN: An analysis of the nursing diagnosis ineffective management of therapeutic regimen compared to noncompliance and Orem's self-care deficit theory of nursing, *Nurs Diagnosis* 6(4):161, 1995.
3. DiIorio C, Faherty B, Manteuffel B: Epilepsy self-management: partial replication and extension, *Res Nurs Health* 17(3):167, 1994.
4. Kim MJ, McFarland G, McLane AM: *Pocket guide to nursing diagnoses,* ed 6, St Louis, 1995, Mosby.
5. Knafl KA, Deatrick JA: How families manage chronic conditions: an analysis of the concept of normalization, *Res Nurs Health* 9(3):215, 1986.
6. McCloskey JC, Bulechek GM: Normalization promotion. In *Nursing Interventions Classification (NIC),* ed 2, St Louis, 1996, Mosby.
7. Radwin LE: Knowing the patient: a process model for individualized interventions, *Nurs Res* 44(6):364, 1995.

Noncompliance (specify)

1. Becker MH: Perceptions and health. In Sackett DL, Haynes B, editors: *Compliance with therapeutic regimes,* New York, 1976, Appleton-Century-Crofts.
2. Beckingham AC, DuGas BW: *Promoting healthy aging: a nursing and community perspective,* Markham, Ont, 1993, Mosby.
3. Brown SJ: Tailoring nursing care to the individual client: empirical challenge of a theoretical concept, *Res Nurs Health* 15:39, 1992.
4. Campinha-Bacote J: Cultural competence in psychiatric mental health nursing, *Nurs Clin North Am* 29(1):1, 1994.
5. Champion V: Relationship of age to mammography compliance, *Cancer* 74(suppl 1):329, 1994.
6. Charlton MR: A cardiac rehabilitation compliance tool, *Rehab Nurs* 18(3):179, 1993.
7. Conn VS, Taylor SG, Messina CJ: Older adults and their caregivers: the transition to medication assistance, *J Gerontol Nurs* 21(5):33, 1995.
8. Cox CL: The interaction model of client health behavior: application to the study of community-based elders, *Adv Nurs Sci* 9(1):40, 1986.
9. Cox et al: *Clinical applications of nursing diagnosis: adult, child, women's, psychiatric, gerontic and home health considerations,* Philadelphia, 1993, FA Davis.
10. DeGeest S, Abraham I, Gemoets H, Evers G: Development of the long-term medication behavior scale: qualitative study for item development, *J Adv Nurs* 19:233, 1994.
11. Dennis K: Patients' control and the information imperative: clarification and confrontation, *Nurs Res* 39:162, 1990.
12. Downe-Wamboldt BL, Melanson PM: Emotions, coping, and psychological well-being in elderly people with arthritis, *West J Nurs Res* 17(3):250, 1995.
13. Eisenthal S, Emery R, Lazare A, Udin H: "Adherence" and the negotiated approach to patienthood, *Arch Gen Psychiatry* 36:393, 1979.
14. Eliason MJ: Ethics and transcultural nursing care, *Nurs Outlook* 41:225, 1993.
15. Eliopoulus C: *Gerontological nursing,* ed 3, Philadelphia, 1993, Lippincott.
16. Forsyth GL, Delaney KD, Gresham ML: Vying for a winning position: management style of the chronically ill, *Res Nurs Health* 7:181, 1984.
17. Francis CK: Hypertension, cardiac disease, and compliance in minority patients, *Am J Med* 91(suppl 1A):295, 1991.
18. Friedemann M-L: Evaluation of the congruence model with rehabilitating substance abusers, *Int J Nurs Studies* 31(1):97, 1994.
19. Funnell MM, Merritt JH: The challenge of diabetes and older adults, *Nurs Clin North Am* 28(1):45, 1993.
20. Gravely E, Oseasohn C: Multiple drug regimens: medication compliance among veterans 65 years and older, *Res Nurs Health* 14:51, 1991.
21. Hanna KM: Effect of nurse-client transaction on female adolescents' oral contraceptive behavior, *Am J Obstet Gynecol* 25(4):285, 1993.
22. Haynes RB, Taylor DW, Sackett HD, editors: *Compliance in health care,* Baltimore, 1979, Johns Hopkins University Press.
23. Johnson M: Interactional aspects of self-efficacy and control in older people with leg ulcers, *J Gerontol Nurs* 21(4):20, 1995.
24. Kahn DL, Steeves RH, Benoliel JQ: Nurses' views of the coping of patients, *Soc Sci Med* 38:1423, 1994.
25. Keeling A, Utz SW, Shuster GF, Boyle A: Noncompliance revisited: a disciplinary perspective of a nursing diagnosis, *Nurs Diagnosis* 4(3):91, 1993.
26. Keller ML, Ward S, Baumann LJ: Processes of self-care: monitoring sensations and symptoms, *Adv Nurs Sci* 12:54, 1989.
27. Keltner NL, Folks DG: Culture as a variable in drug therapy, *Pers Psychiatr Care* 28(1):33, 1992.
28. Kleinman A, Eisenburg L, Good B: Culture, illness and care, *Ann Intern Med* 88:251, 1978.
29. Kontz M: Compliance redefined and implications for home care, *Holistic Nurs Pract* 3:54, 1989.
30. Lazare A: The suffering of shame and humiliation in illness. In Starck PL, McGovern JP, editors: *The hidden dimension of illness: human suffering,* New York, 1992, NLN Press.
31. Martinez NC: Diabetes and minority populations, *Nurs Clin North Am* 28(1):87, 1993.
32. Monane M et al: Noncompliance with congestive heart failure therapy in the elderly, *Arch Intern Med* 154:433, 1994.
33. Morse EV, Simon PM: Using experiential training to enhance health professionals' awareness of patient compliance issues, *Acad Med* 68(9):693, 1993.
34. Morse J: Negotiating commitment and involvement in the nurse-client relationship, *J Adv Nurs* 16:455, 1991.
35. Oakley D: Rethinking patient counseling techniques for changing contraceptive use behavior, *Am J Obstet Gynecol* 170(5, part 2):1585, 1994.
36. Prescott PA, Soeken KL, Griggs M: Identification and referral of hospitalized patients in need of home care, *Res Nurs Health* 18:85, 1995.
37. Richardson A: The health diary: an examination of its use as a data collection method, *J Adv Nurs* 19:782, 1994.
38. Robertson D, Keller C: Relationships among health beliefs, self-efficacy and exercise adherence, *Heart Lung* 21:56, 1992.
39. Rotter JB: *Social learning and clinical psychology,* Englewood Cliffs, NJ, 1954, Prentice Hall.
40. Rudd P et al: Issues in patient compliance: the search for therapeutic sufficiency, *Cardiology* 80(supp 1):2, 1992.
41. Ryan P: *Behavior change: a concept analysis,* Unpublished manuscript, 1990, University of Wisconsin-Milwaukee.
42. Ryan P: Facilitating behavior change in the chronically ill. In Millar JF, editor: *Coping with chronic illness: overcoming powerlessness,* Philadelphia, 1992, Davis
43. Stretcher VJ, DeVillis BM, Becker MH, Rosenstock IM: The role of self-efficacy in achieving health behavior change, *Health Ed Q* 13(1):73, 1986.
44. Thorne S: Constructive noncompliance in chronic illness, *Holistic Nurs Pract* 5:62, 1990.
45. Weaver SK, Wilson JF: Moving toward patient empowerment, *Nurs Health Care* 15(9):480, 1994.
46. West EA: The cultural bridge model, *Nurs Outlook* 41(5):229, 1993.
47. Wuest J: Removing the shackles: a feminist critique of noncompliance, *Nurs Outlook* 41(5):217, 1993.

Risk for infection

1. Association for Practitioners in Infection Control: *The APIC curriculum for infection control practice,* Iowa City, IA, 1981, Kendall/Hunt.
2. Beneson AS, editor: *Control of communicable diseases manual,* ed 16, Washington, DC, 1995, American Public Health Association.
3. Bennett J, Brackman P, editors: *Hospital infections,* ed 2, Boston, 1986, Little, Brown.
4. Carpentino LJ: *Nursing Diagnosis: Application to clinical practice,* ed 2, Philadelphia, 1987, Lippincott.
5. Centers for Disease Control: *CDC guideline for isolation precaution in hospitals,* HHS pub. no. (CDC) 83-8314, Atlanta, 1983, CDC.
6. Centers for Disease Control: Recommendations for prevention of HIV transmission in health-care settings, *MMWR Morb Mortal Wkly Rep* 36(2S):1987.
7. Centers for Disease Control: General recommendations on immunization: recommendations of the Advisory Committee on Immunization Practices (ACIP), *MMWR Morb Mortal Wkly Rep* 43(RR-1):1994.
8. Centers for Disease Control: Guidelines for preventing the transmission of Mycobacterium tuberculosis in health-care facilities, 1994, *MMWR Morb Mortal Wkly Rep* 43(RR-3):1994.
9. Centers for Disease Control: Recommendations of the Immunization Practices Advisory Committee (ACIP): update on adult immunization, *MMWR Morb Mortal Wkly Rep* 40(RR-12):1991.
10. Centers for Disease Control: Recommendations of the Immunization Practices Advisory Committee (ACIP): use of vaccines and immune globulins in persons with altered immunocompetence, *MMWR Morb Mortal Wkly Rep* 42(RR-4):1993.
11. Centers for Disease Control: Recommended childhood immunization schedule-United States, 1995, *MMWR Morb Mortal Wkly Rep* (51-52):1995.
12. Centers for Disease Control: Recommended childhood immunization schedule-United States, 1995, *MMWR Morb Mortal Wkly Rep* 44(RR-5):1995.
13. Garner J: CDC guidelines for prevention of surgical wound infections, 1985, *Infect control* 7(3):193, 1986.
14. Grimes D: High risk for infection. In Thompson J et al, editors: *Mosby's clinical nursing,* ed 3, St Louis, 1993, Mosby.
15. Grimes DE: *Nursing diagnosis: Potential for infections, and potential for transmission of infectious agents to others,* 1984, Unpub-

lished manuscripts submitted to NANDA Diagnosis Review Committee.

16. Grimes DE: *Infectious diseases,* St Louis, 1991, Mosby.
17. Murray PR et al: *Manual of clinical microbiology,* ed 6, Washington, DC, 1995, ASM Press.
18. Simmons B: Centers for Disease Control guideline for prevention of surgical wound infection, *Infect Control* 3(3):1992.

Risk for injury (risk for trauma; risk for poisoning; risk for suffocation)

1. Baker S, O'Neil B, Karpf R: *The injury fact book,* ed 2, Lexington, MA, 1991, Heath.
2. Benner L Jr: Accident theory and accident investigators, *Hazard Prevention* 13:18, 1977.
3. Gordon J: The epidemiology of accidents, *Am J Public Health,* 39:504, 1949.
4. Haddon W: On the escape of tigers: an ecological note, *Am J Public Health* 60:2229, 1970.
5. Haddon W: Advances in the epidemiology of injuries as a basis for public policy, *Public Health Rep* 95:411, 1980.
6. Kim MJ, McFarland G, McLane A, editors: *Classification of nursing diagnosis: proceedings of the seventh conference,* St Louis, 1986, Mosby.
7. Kim MK, McFarland GK, McLane AM: *Pocket guide to nursing diagnosis,* ed 6, St Louis, 1995, Mosby.
8. Last JM, Wallace RB, editors: *Maxcy-Rosenau: Public health and preventive medicine,* ed 13, Norwalk, CT, 1992, Appleton & Lange.
9. McCloskey JC, Buelechek GM: *Iowa intervention project: nursing interventions classification (NIC),* ed 2, St Louis, 1996, Mosby.
10. National Safety Council: *Accident facts,* Chicago, 1995, National Safety Council.
11. Robertson L: *Injuries: causes, control strategies, and public policy,* Lexington, MA, 1993, Lexington Press.
12. Spiker JA, Semonin-Holleran R: Injury, potential for, related to sensory or motor deficits: using the stroke scale to validate defining characteristics of this nursing diagnosis. In Kim MJ, McFarland G, McLane A, editors: *Classification of nursing diagnosis: proceedings of the seventh conference,* St Louis, 1986, Mosby.
13. Sullivan LW: *Healthy difference program guide,* Washington, DC, 1991, U.S. Department of Health and Human Services.
14. United States Public Health Service: *Healthy People 2000. Midcourse review and 1995 revisions,* Hyattsville, MD, 1995, U.S. Public Health Service: Department of Health and Human Services.
15. Walker BL: *Injury prevention for the elderly: a research guide,* Westport, CT, 1995, Greenwood Press.
16. Whitefield R, Zador P, Fife D: *Expected mortality from injuries,* Washington DC, 1984, Insurance Institute for Highway Safety.
17. Wintemaute G, Mohan D, Teret S, editors: *Injury prevention in developing countries,* Baltimore, 1984, Johns Hopkins University Press.

Risk for perioperative positioning injury

1. McEwen DR: Intraoperative positioning of surgical patients, *AORN Journal* 63:1059, 1966.

Altered protection

1. American Nurses Association: *Nursing: a social policy statement,* Kansas City, MO, 1980, ANA.
2. Beare PG, Myers JL: *Principles and practice of adult health nursing,* ed 2, St Louis, 1994, Mosby.
3. Begley SS: Tibetan Buddhist medicine: a transcultural nursing experience, *J Holistic Nurs* 12(3):323, 1994.
4. Brophy L, Sharp EJ: Physical symptoms of combination biotherapy: a quality-life issue, *Oncol Nurs Forum* 18(1):25, 1991.
5. Bulechek GM, McCloskey JC: *Nursing interventions: treatments for nursing diagnoses,* Philadelphia, 1985, Saunders.
6. Dossey B: Awakening the inner healer, *Am J Nurs* 91(8):31, 1991.
7. Groer M: Psychoneuroimmunology, *Am J Nurs* 91(8):33, 1991.
8. Kiecolt-Glaser JK, Glaser R. Psychoneuroimmunology: can psychological interventions modulate immunity? *J Consult Clin Psychol* 60(4):569, 1992.
9. Kim MJ, McFarland GK, McLane AM: *Pocket guide to nursing diagnoses,* ed 6, St Louis, 1995, Mosby.
10. Lunney M: Nursing diagnosis: refining the system, *Am J Nurs* 82(3):456, 1982.
11. McNally JC, Somerville ET, Miaskowski C, Rostad M: *Guidelines for cancer nursing practice,* ed 2, Philadelphia, 1991, Saunders.
12. Pelletier KR: Mind-body health: research, clinical and policy applications, *Am J Health Promotion* 6(5):345, 1992.
13. Sheppard KC: Altered protection: a nursing diagnosis. In Carroll-Johnson R, editor: *Classification of nursing diagnoses: proceedings of the Ninth Conference,* Philadelphia, 1991, Lippincott.
14. Volker D: Neoplasia. In Beare PG, Myers JL. *Principles and practice of adult health nursing,* ed 2, St Louis, 1994, Mosby.

Energy field disturbance

1. Beare PG, Myers JL: *Adult health nursing,* St Louis, 1994, Mosby.
2. Kim MJ, McFarland GK, McLane AM: *Pocket guide to nursing diagnosis,* St Louis, 1995, Mosby.
3. Krieger D: *The therapeutic touch,* Englewood Cliffs, NJ, 1979, Prentice-Hall.
4. Macrae J: *Therapeutic touch: a practical guide,* New York, 1988, Knopf.
5. Marriner A: *Nursing theorists and their work,* St Louis, 1986, Mosby.
6. Meehan TC: Therapeutic touch. In Bulecheck G, McCloskey J, editors: *Nursing interventions: Essential nursing treatments,* Philadelphia, 1991, Saunders.
7. Quinn J, Strelkauskas A: Psychoimmunologic effects of therapeutic touch on practitioners and recently bereaved recipients: a pilot study, *Adv Nurs Sci* 15(4):13, 1993.
8. Samarel N: The experience of receiving therapeutic touch, *J Advanced Nurs* 17(6):651, 1992.
9. Tiernan PJ: Relaxation and guided imagery in critical care, *Crit Care Nurs* 14(5):47, 1994.

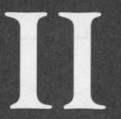

Nutritional—Metabolic

ALTERED NUTRITION: MORE THAN BODY REQUIREMENTS[14]

Altered nutrition: more than body requirements is a state in which an individual is experiencing an intake of nutrients that exceeds metabolic needs.

Related Factors

Excessive intake in relationship to metabolic need

Defining Characteristics

Weight 10% to 20% over ideal for height and frame
Triceps skinfold greater than 15 mm in men and 25 mm in women
Sedentary activity level
Reported or observed dysfunctional eating patterns
  Pairing food with other activities
  Concentrating food intake at the end of day
  Eating in response to external cues (e.g., time of day, social situation)
  Eating in response to internal cues other than hunger (e.g., anxiety)

Expected Patient Outcomes & Nursing Interventions*

Attain optimum weight for age, height, and gender

- Weigh patient *to establish a baseline against which the outcome can be measured.*
- Determine patient's desire to reduce body weight, *because this is a strong motivating factor.*
- Assess patient's knowledge of the hazards of obesity, and provide information as necessary.
- Determine patient's recommended body weight for age, height, and gender *so that a realistic outcome can be established.*

*References 1, 8, 12-14, 17, 20, 27, 30.

- Assess patient's triceps skinfold measurements, *which indicate fat stores.*
- Establish with the patient a realistic plan to include reduced food intake and increased energy expenditure. A goal of 1 to 2 pounds per week weight loss is a suggested starting point.
- Analyze with the patient reasons for past failures at attempting to lose weight *so that these might be avoided or reduced.*
- Ask the patient to keep a diary of what, when, where, and with whom he or she eats as well as the hunger level and feelings at the time, *to evaluate changes that need to be made in life-style.*
- Ask the patient to post the goal for weight loss in a strategic location so that it will be remembered. The refrigerator or pantry door is a common location selected, *so the persons can be reminded of the goal when tempted to eat additional calories.*
- Discuss eating a balanced diet using as a guide the Food Guide Pyramid or counting calories or fat grams, *so that nutritional needs can be maintained during weight loss.*
- Reward patient for attaining short-term goals, and encourage patient to use an internal reward system when goals are accomplished.
- Ask patient to identify people from whom support can be sought, and provide a list of support groups for weight loss.

Communicate what is required to maintain optimum body weight, as evidenced by:

Reason for obesity
Dietary plan for weight reduction
Exercise plan for weight reduction
Plans for follow-up care

- Discuss ways to maintain optimum weight by evaluating the life-style changes that have occurred and strategies to maintain them.
- Set a plan for follow-up monitoring of weight maintenance.

Principles and Rationale for Nursing Interventions*

Attain Optimum Weight

Comparing the patient's current weight with the recommended body weight provides baseline data from which realistic goals can be set. Triceps skinfold thickness provides data about the body's fat stores. Motivation for weight reduction comes from within the person. The person must want to lose weight before a program can be successful. Learning the hazards of obesity may be a motivator. These hazards include atherosclerosis, hypertension, and diabetes mellitus. The patient should write down realistic goals and post them in strategic places, such as on the refrigerator door, pantry door, or bathroom mirror.

Goals can be written based on following the Food Guide Pyramid or counting calories or fat grams (Fig. 1). The Food Guide Pyramid suggests 6 to 11 servings of bread, cereal, rice, and pasta; 3 to 5 servings of vegetables; 2 to 4 servings of fruits; 2 to 3 servings of milk, yogurt, and cheese; and 2 to 3 servings of meat, poultry, fish, dry beans, eggs, and nuts.[30] When calorie counting is used, a goal of 1 to 2 pounds weight loss per week frequently is suggested as a starting point. This goal is based on the fact that 1 pound of adipose tissue has the energy potential of 3500 calories. Reducing caloric intake by 500 calories for 7 days theoretically yields a weight loss of 1 pound. When counting fat grams, a goal of less than 30% of daily calories from fat, less than 10% of daily calories from saturated fat, and less than 300 mg from cholesterol per day is suggested.[30]

To monitor goal attainment, a food diary is kept by writing down everything the patient eats, the time, with whom he or she eats, the activity while eating, the hunger level prior to eating (using a scale of 0-4), and the patient's feelings at the time. Keeping a food diary is highly recommended because it raises the patient's awareness of what, where, and how much he or she eats, and the feelings at the time of the food choices. The diary is analyzed daily to determine whether goals were met and to identify where changes in eating habits can be made.[13] To decrease food intake, a person can drink an 8-ounce glass of water before eating and use a smaller than usual plate so that the smaller serving will not look small. The person should eat slowly, chew thoroughly, and think about the taste and smell of the food. While eating, the patient should avoid any other activity, such as reading or watching television. Recommended low-calorie snacks are carrots, celery, and apples, which satisfy the oral need for chewing and provide needed vegetables and fruits. Water and low-calorie soft drinks also are recommended.

When a person eats is important as well. One person may skip breakfast, work through lunch, snack while preparing dinner, and eat dessert while watching television. The caloric intake should be subdivided throughout the waking hours. Instead of eating while watching television, the person can do something else with the hands and chew sugar-free gum. Where a person eats includes the type of restaurant, as well as

*References 1, 8, 13, 14, 17, 20, 27, 30.

which room at home. Fast-food restaurants provide filling food quickly, but the food often is high in fat and carbohydrates. Excessive consumption of foods from fast-food restaurants may contribute to obesity. The room where a person chooses to eat is important when reducing caloric intake. Eating in only one place, such as the dining room table or kitchen, is helpful.

The circumstances around which the person eats pose the most difficult data collection problem. These include the motivation for eating and the external and internal cues, such as anxiety, stress, fear, anger, peer pressure, loneliness, and depression. Some overeating problems are due to psychologic factors. Discuss strategies to deal with feelings and stress instead of overeating. Psychologic counseling or support groups may be needed to identify and deal with the problem. Behavior modification is another strategy used for reinforcement and cue elimination.

In conjunction with decreased food intake, the patient needs to begin an exercise program and work toward a goal. The goal may be *minutes* of exercise or *activity or distance* (walking, jogging, or swimming). For weight loss it is better to exercise moderately for long periods rather than in short bursts (i.e., walk for 60 minutes rather than jogging for 30 minutes). Keeping an exercise log is beneficial to keep track of goal attainment, in addition to a record of feelings be-fore and after exercise and whether it is done alone or with someone.

Surgical procedures may be considered for an obese person who is unsuccessful in repeated weight reduction attempts or whose health is jeopardized by the obese state. An intestinal bypass (jejunoileal bypass) decreases absorptive surfaces of the jejunum. Preoperatively the patient requires counseling about causes of obesity and the consequences of this type of surgery. Postoperative care is similar to that for patients undergoing abdominal surgery.

Maintain Optimum Body Weight

Once goals for weight reduction are attained, the patient benefits from analyzing what behaviors, feelings, and circumstances led to the increase in weight and those that have led to weight reduction. Patients need to determine how they can maintain the weight reduction behaviors and develop an individualized follow-up plan.

ALTERED NUTRITION: POTENTIAL FOR MORE THAN BODY REQUIREMENTS[14]

Altered nutrition: potential for more than body requirements is a state in which an individual is at risk of experiencing an intake of nutrients that exceeds metabolic needs.

Risk Factors

Hereditary predisposition
Excessive energy intake during late gestational life, early infancy, and adolescence
Frequent, closely spaced pregnancies

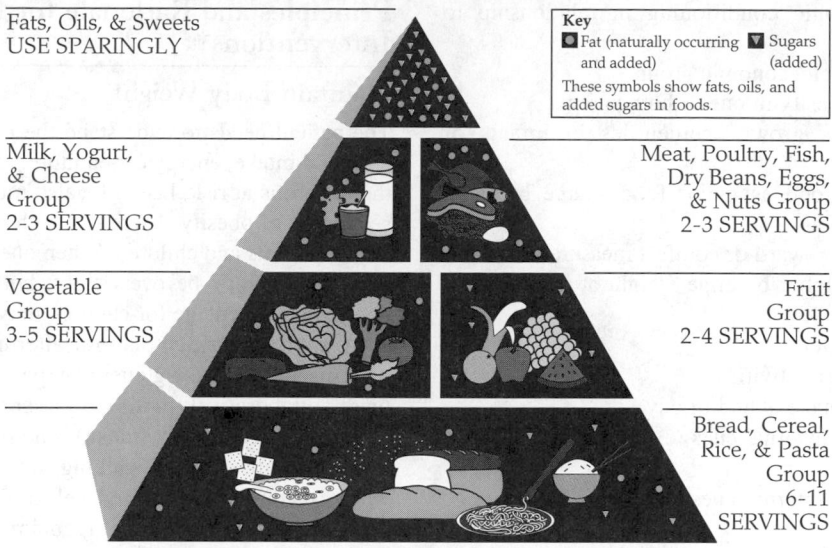

FOOD GUIDE PYRAMID

A Guide to Daily Food Choices

Fats, Oils, & Sweets
USE SPARINGLY

Key
■ Fat (naturally occurring   ▼ Sugars
and added)   (added)
These symbols show fats, oils, and
added sugars in foods.

Milk, Yogurt,
& Cheese
Group
2-3 SERVINGS

Meat, Poultry, Fish,
Dry Beans, Eggs,
& Nuts Group
2-3 SERVINGS

Vegetable
Group
3-5 SERVINGS

Fruit
Group
2-4 SERVINGS

Bread, Cereal,
Rice, & Pasta
Group
6-11
SERVINGS

Food Group	Suggested Daily Servings	What Counts as a Serving?
Breads, cereals, and other grain products Whole-grain Enriched	**6–11** servings from entire group *(Include several servings of whole-grain products daily.)*	• 1 slice of bread • ½ hamburger bun or english muffin • a small roll, biscuit, or muffin • 3 to 4 small or 2 large crackers • ½ cup cooked cereal, rice, or pasta • 1 ounce of ready-to-eat breakfast cereal
Fruits Citrus, melon, berries Other fruits	**2–4** servings from entire group	• a whole fruit such as a medium apple, banana, or orange • a grapefruit half • a melon wedge • ¾ cup of juice • ½ cup of berries • ½ cup cooked or canned fruit • ½ cup dried fruit
Vegetables Dark-green leafy Deep-yellow Dry beans/peas (legumes) Starchy Other vegetables	**3–5** servings from entire group *(Include all types regularly: use dark-green leafy vegetables and dry beans and peas several times a week.)*	• ½ cup of cooked vegetables • ½ cup of chopped raw vegetables • 1 cup of leafy raw vegetables, such as lettuce or spinach
Meat, poultry, fish and alternates (eggs, dry beans and peas, nuts and seeds)	**2–3** servings from entire group	Amounts should total 5 to 7 ounces of cooked lean meat, poultry, or fish a day. Count 1 egg, ½ cup cooked beans, or 2 tablespoons peanut butter as 1 ounce of meat.
Milk, cheese, and yogurt	**2** servings from entire group *(3 servings for women who are pregnant or breast-feeding and for teens; 4 servings for teens who are pregnant or breast-feeding)*	• 1 cup of milk • 8 ounces of yogurt • 1½ ounces of natural cheese • 2 ounces of process cheese
Fats, sweets, and alcoholic beverages	Avoid too many fats and sweets. If you drink alcoholic beverages, do so in moderation.	

Figure 1 Food guide pyramid.

Dysfunctional psychologic conditioning in relationship to food

Membership in lower socioeconomic group

Reported or observed obesity in one or both parents

Rapid transition across growth percentiles in infants or children

Reported use of solid food as major food source before 5 months of age

Observed use of food as reward or comfort measure

Reported or observed higher baseline weight at beginning of each pregnancy

Dysfunctional eating patterns

    Pairing food with other activities

    Concentrating food intake at end of day

    Eating in response to external cues (e.g., time of day or social situation)

    Eating in response to internal cues other than hunger (e.g., anxiety)

Expected Patient Outcomes & Nursing Interventions[1,8,9,17,20,27,30]

Maintain recommended body weight for age, height, and gender

- Measure weight and height to calculate body mass index [wt/(ht)^2] to obtain a baseline from which to plan strategies for meeting goals.
- Calculate growth percentiles for infants and children.
- Discuss the relationship between food intake, exercise, and obesity *so that the patient can understand how decreasing intake and increasing exercise can reduce obesity.*
- Discuss the risks of obesity—increased incidence for diabetes mellitus, hypertension, and atherosclerosis—*so that the patient can learn the potential long-term consequences of being overweight.*
- Determine the patient's motivation for changing eating habits *to help in selecting positive rewards for meeting goals to maintain recommended body weight.*
- Determine patient's recommended weight *so that realistic goals can be set.*
- Develop a method for patient to keep daily record of intake *to track progress toward the goals set.*
- Determine with the patient desirable, realistic weekly weight loss goals, *because patient participation improves compliance.*
- Encourage patient to write down realistic weekly goals for food intake and exercise and to display where they can be reviewed frequently.
- Encourage patient to identify support persons in his or her environment who can give encouragement and support in attaining these goals.
- Determine stressors (job, finances, family, school) and coping mechanisms, sources of social support, and relaxation techniques.

Principles and Rationale for Nursing Interventions*

Maintain Body Weight

The patient needs to understand the relationships among food and fluid intake, energy expenditure, and weight gain. Because the patient is at risk, he or she also must comprehend the consequences of obesity. There is a high correlation between obesity of parents and children. When one parent is obese, 40% of the children may be overweight, but when both parents are obese, the percentage for children may double.[10]

A realistic, written plan for altering food and fluid intake patterns and increasing energy expenditure needs to be developed collaboratively with the patient (See Table IV-2 of the Recommended Energy Intake). The American Heart Association recommends brisk walking for 20 minutes three times a week as a minimal exercise level for fitness. Begin the plan by determining the patient's recommended weight for age, height, and gender (See Table IV-3). Next, a review of the patient's typical day is helpful to identify what food and fluid patterns can be altered and when exercise can be planned. Patient needs to reduce food and drink that provide calories without nutrition (e.g., alcohol, corn and potato chips). A plan is derived with weekly goals for the patient to meet. A reward system also is included in the plan for use when goals are accomplished.

The growth and development of the patient should be considered. For example, an expectant mother needs a diet adequate in nutrients for herself and the fetus. For a breast-fed infant, parents use weight gain as the criterion for adequacy of feeding. For a bottle-fed infant, parents use this same criterion rather than whether the infant finishes all feedings. Infants and children should not be forced to eat, since this may contribute to overeating. Children should be offered well-balanced meals in an environment free from distractions such as television and be encouraged to eat at their own pace. Food should not be used as reward or punishment for children because this practice may cause compulsive eating. While growing up, the child needs to learn the foods in a balanced diet, as well as the importance of physical activity. When the child becomes an adolescent and begins taking responsibiilty for foods eaten, he or she will have a sufficient knowledge base about nutrition and exercise from which to make decisions. Adolescents and adults also need to balance food intake with physical activity. The hormonal change that occurs during puberty requires a change in eating and activity patterns. Likewise, after 50 years of age hormonal changes again necessitate reassessment of one's food intake and activity balance. Caloric needs decline as lean body mass is lost and replaced by body fat that is less metabolically active. Women especially experience an increase in body fat composition. Increases in body fat can be slowed by exercise and strength training to maintain lean body mass. After age 50,

---

*References 1, 8, 10, 17, 20, 27, 30.

TABLE IV-2 Median Heights and Weights and Recommended Energy Intake, 10th Edition RDA

Category	Age (years) or Condition	Weight (kg)	Weight (lb)	Height (cm)	Height (in)	REF[a] (kcal/day)	Average Energy Allowance (kcal) Multiples of REE	Average Energy Allowance (kcal) Per kg	Average Energy Allowance (kcal) Per day[b]
Infants	0.0-0.5	6	13	60	24	320		108	650
	0.5-1.0	9	20	71	28	500		98	850
Children	1-3	13	29	90	56	740		102	1300
	4-6	20	44	112	44	950		90	1800
	7-10	28	62	132	52	1130		70	2000
Males	11-14	45	99	157	62	1440	1.70	55	2500
	15-18	66	145	176	69	1760	1.67	45	3000
	19-24	72	160	177	70	1780	1.67	40	2900
	25-50	79	174	176	70	1800	1.60	37	2900
	51+	77	170	173	68	1530	1.50	30	2300
Females	11-14	46	101	157	62	1310	1.67	47	2200
	15-18	55	120	163	64	1370	1.60	40	2200
	19-24	58	128	164	65	1350	1.60	38	2200
	25-50	63	138	163	64	1380	1.55	36	2200
	51+	65	143	160	63	1280	1.50	30	1900
Pregnant	1st Trimester								+0
	2nd Trimester								+300
	3rd Trimester								+300
Lactating	1st 6 months								+500
	2nd 6 months								+500

[a]Resting energy expenditure (REE); calculation based on FAO equations, then rounded. This is the same as RMR.
[b]Figure is rounded.
From Grodner, Anderson, DeYoung.[10]

TABLE IV-3 Metropolitan Life Insurance Company Height-Weight Data, Revised 1983

Height-Weight Tables for Adults (1983)

Height Ft	Height In	Women Frame* Small	Women Frame* Medium	Women Frame* Large	Height Ft	Height In	Men Frame* Small	Men Frame* Medium	Men Frame* Large
4	10	102-111	109-121	118-131	5	2	128-134	131-141	138-150
4	11	103-113	111-123	120-134	5	3	130-136	133-143	140-153
5	0	104-115	113-126	122-137	5	4	132-138	135-145	142-156
5	1	106-118	115-129	125-140	5	5	134-140	137-148	144-160
5	2	108-121	118-132	128-143	5	6	136-142	139-151	146-164
5	3	111-124	121-135	131-147	5	7	138-145	142-154	149-168
5	4	114-127	124-138	134-151	5	8	140-148	145-157	152-172
5	5	117-130	127-141	137-155	5	9	142-151	148-160	155-176
5	6	120-133	130-144	140-159	5	10	144-154	151-163	158-180
5	7	113-136	133-147	143-163	5	11	146-157	154-166	161-184
5	8	126-139	136-150	146-167	6	0	149-160	157-170	164-188
5	9	129-142	139-153	149-170	6	1	152-164	160-174	168-192
5	10	132-145	142-156	152-173	6	2	155-168	164-178	172-197
5	11	135-148	156-159	155-176	6	3	158-172	167-182	176-202
6	0	138-151	148-162	158-179	6	4	162-176	171-187	181-207

Based on a weight-height mortality study conducted by the Society of Actuaries and the Association of Life Insurance Medical Directors of America, Metropolitan Life Insurance Company, revised 1983.
*Weights at ages 25 to 59 based on lowest mortality. Height includes 1-in heel. Weight for women includes 3 lb for indoor clothing. Weight for men includes 5 lb for indoor clothing.
From Grodner, Anderson, DeYoung.[10]

daily energy needs drop from 2200 to 1920 calories for women and from 2900 to 2300 calories for men. The Recommended Daily Allowances, however, remain constant after age 51 for both men and women. What does change is the body's ability to either process or synthesize certain nutrients.[10]

Instruction on how to implement the plan to prevent overweight and obesity is facilitated when all family members are present to discuss eating patterns and the meaning of food to them. The plan must be developed with active participation of all family members so that it is realistic, practical, and individualized for the family, considering cultural and religious food preferences as well as the family's schedule for eating. Instruction on stress reduction may be needed if this is a cue for eating. A written plan with guidelines for daily eating habits promotes compliance and attainment of goals.

ALTERED NUTRITION: LESS THAN BODY REQUIREMENTS[14]

Altered nutrition: less than body requirements is a state in which an individual experiences an intake of nutrients insufficient to meet metabolic needs.

Related Factors

Inability to ingest or digest food or absorb nutrients because of biologic, psychologic, or economic factors

Defining Characteristics

Loss of body weight with adequate food intake
Body weight 20% or more under ideal for height and frame
Reported inadequate food intake less than Recommended Daily Allowance
Weakness of muscles required for swallowing or mastication
Reported or evidence of lack of food
Lack of interest in food
Perceived inability to ingest food
Aversion to eating
Reported altered taste sensation
Satiety immediately after ingesting food
Abdominal pain with or without pathologic conditions
Sore, inflamed buccal cavity
Excessive hair loss
Lack of information; misinformation
Misconceptions
Decreased triceps skinfold
Decreased midarm circumference
Decreased midarm muscle circumference
Alteration in smell
Chronic sputum production
Decreased appetite
Dysphagia
Self-care deficit
Electrolyte imbalance

Decreased serum albumin
Decreased serum transferrin or iron-binding capacity
Decreased lymphocyte count
Dry, scaly, inelastic skin
Social isolation

Expected Patient Outcomes & Nursing Interventions*

Attain Adequate Nutrition, As Evidenced By:

Recommended weight for age, height, and gender
Expected bone and tooth development
Clear skin and eyes
Firm muscles
Triceps skinfold: men, 12.5 mm; women, 16.5 mm
Midarm circumference: men, 29.3 cm; women, 25.8 cm
Serum albumin: 3.5-5 g/dl or 53% of total protein
Lymphocytes: 1800-3000/mm^3 or 30% of leukocyte
Midarm muscle circumference: men, 26.2 cm; women, 19.7 cm
Prompt healing
Growth of 3-5 inches annually for children
Energy to perform activities of daily living

- Weigh patient *to establish a baseline against which the outcome can be measured.*
- Auscultate bowel sounds *to determine the presence of peristalsis.*
- Assess for possible causes of inadequate nutrition: nausea, vomiting, fatigue, mouth pain, tooth decay, loose teeth, bleeding gums, sores in mouth, dry mouth, ill-fitting dentures, inability to taste or swallow. Make referrals as needed for evaluation and treatment.
- Monitor daily calorie count *to determine calorie intake.*
- Assess skinfold measurements: *triceps skinfolds reflect fat stores, and midarm circumference reflects protein stores.*
- Monitor serum albumin and leukocytes: *low values may be indicators of malnutrition.*
- Reduce nausea and pain as ordered before eating.
- Determine number and type of medications patient takes.
- Provide nutrients: proteins (including albumin, carbohydrates, and fats), vitamins (A, B complex, C, and K), and minerals (iron, zinc, and copper).
- Provide foods in the form appropriate for patient: general diet, mechanical soft, blenderized, formula via nasogastric or gastrostomy tube, or total parenteral nutrition via subclavian vein as ordered by physician.
- Consider patient's food preferences as governed by personal choices and cultural and religious preferences.
- Provide oral care before meals *to moisten and refresh mucous membranes and tongue.*
- Provide rest before meals when fatigue interferes with eating.
- Ensure patient is in a sitting position before eating or feeding *to prevent aspiration.*

---

*References 1, 6, 8, 10, 12-14, 16, 17, 20, 27, 30.

- When patient feeds self:
  - Serve food at its appropriate temperature.
  - Ensure patient is comfortable and can reach necessary utensils for eating.
  - Provide adaptive/assistive devices.
- When patient is fed by mouth:
  - Serve food at its appropriate temperature.
  - Ensure patient is comfortable.
  - Allow patient sufficient time between bites.
  - Talk with patient during the meal.
- When patient is fed by nasogastric (NG) or nasoduodenal tube:
  - Ensure proper placement of tube.
  - Add blue or green food coloring to feeding *to detect aspiration.*
  - Ensure feeding at room temperature.
  - Flush tube periodically with full-strength cranberry juice or cola followed by water *to prevent obstruction.*
- When nasogastric tube is used:
  - Aspirate gastric contents *to determine the amount of the last feeding still in stomach.*
  - If aspirated contents is less than 50 ml, proceed with the feeding.
- When continuous feeding is used:
  - Refill feeding bag every 4 hours.
  - Check gravity drip rate or pump rate every hour.
- When patient is fed by total parenteral nutrition:
  - Check infusion rate every hour or infusion pump rate every hour.
  - Monitor blood glucose and urinary glucose and acetone every 6 hours *to detect hyperglycemia:* treat hyperglycemia with insulin as ordered.
  - Change dressing daily using sterile technique *to prevent infection;* inspect insertion site for redness and edema.
  - Monitor temperature every 4 hours *to detect fever.*

Identify factors that contribute to inadequate nutritional intake, as evidenced by:

Identify strategies to improve nutrition
Use referrals to health team members as needed

Socioeconomic

- Problem-solve with patient and family to identify socioeconomic factors contributing to inadequate nutrition.
- Determine with patient and family appropriate strategies to use to solve problems, e.g., lack of money or transportation.
- Use referrals to others members of the health care team as needed (dietitian, social worker, community health nurse).

Psychologic

- Discuss with patient perceptions of factors interfering with ability or desire to eat.
- Assess for eating disorders (e.g., anorexia nervosa and bulimia nervosa).

- Assess for depression.
- Discuss with patient strategies useful to improve nutrition.
- Refer patient for additional therapy as needed.

Gain knowledge of nutritional needs, as evidenced by:

Patient and family explaining:
  Reason for altered nutrition
  Actions to avoid it
  Types of menus to be used
  Any necessary dietary alterations (food to include and avoid)
  Community agencies to be contacted for assistance
  Medication program to be followed: state dosage, action, and side effects of prescribed drugs; over-the-counter drugs to avoid

- Assess learning needs of patient and family.
- Determine their understanding of the reason for altered nutrition.
- Teach types of menus to be used.
- Teach foods to avoid.
- Determine their understanding of the plan for follow-up treatment.
- Teach them reason for vitamin and mineral supplements to be taken.
- Provide them with names and phone numbers of personnel in community agencies.

Principles and Rationale for Nursing Interventions*

Attain Adequate Nutrition

The patient's height and weight are compared with tables of recommended weight for the height. Bowel sounds are assessed to determine if peristalsis is present. Physiologic causes of altered nutrition are ruled out as possible causes of inadequate nutrition. These include difficulty in chewing, swallowing, or metabolism.

Nausea and vomiting can be lessened with small amounts of cool liquids (cola, ginger ale, flavored gelatin, water). Cleaning the mouth and blowing the nose after vomiting eliminates nauseous tastes and smells. Alteration of medicines should be considered to prevent nausea and vomiting. Rectal administration of medication rather than oral may help. The vomiting center stimulation is decreased by slow deep breathing through the mouth, removal of unpleasant sights and smells, and eating and drinking slowly.

Skinfold measurements include triceps skinfold and midarm circumference. Triceps skinfold thickness gives data about fat stores, and arm circumference provides data about protein stores. The site measured for both the skinfold thickness and arm circumference is at the midpoint between the shoulder (acromial process) and the elbow (olecranon) of the nondominant arm. The average of three measurements is recorded. Measurement is made by pinching the skin and measuring its thickness with calipers. The arm circumference is measured at

---

*References 1, 6, 8, 10, 12-14, 16, 17, 20, 30.

the same place on the arm. Midarm muscle circumference (cm) = mean arm circumference (cm) − (0.314 × triceps skinfold thickness [mm]). The standards for these anthropometric measurements are listed in Expected Patient Outcomes & Nursing Interventions Section on p. 1546 to 1547. Serum albumin values are no longer useful after an infusion of albumin to maintain intravascular pressure. Visceral protein depletion is indicated when total lymphocyte count falls below 1500 cells/mm³ (Table IV-4).

Poor nutritional status can alter drug absorption, metabolism, or utilization. Also, medication side effects can cause symptoms that interfere with eating. For example, they may affect the gastrointestinal system directly resulting in dry mouth, decreased appetite, or nausea. Drugs may alter the central nervous system causing drowsiness, dizziness, or nervousness. They may also affect the cardiovascular system causing anemia, tachycardia, or postural hypotension. The more medications the patients takes, the more likely a drug side effect, drug-to-drug interaction, or drug-to-food interaction may occur.

For patients who eat a general diet, the nurse considers cultural or religious food preferences. Offering patients some selection in the food gives them a feeling of control in their lives. When meals are served, patients need to feel as comfortable as possible, which may require oral hygiene, position change, or medication to enhance appetite. They need to be able to reach their food, and some patients may require assistance with cutting food or opening containers. A pleasant eating environment free from unpleasant aromas enhances eating, as does an appropriate temperature for the food.

Before eating, the patient must be comfortable and in the optimum position. The patient also is encouraged to rest, receives medications for nausea or pain, and is offered oral care as needed before eating. Regardless of whether patients feed themselves or are fed, they need to be in an upright position. Offer high-protein, high calorie supplements such as milk shake or custard to provide calories and prevent body protein breakdown. When the feeding is accomplished via nasogastric (NG) or nasoduodenal tube, the nurse adds food coloring to the formula so that any aspiration of the feeding can be detected quickly. The feeding tubing is flushed with full-strength cranberry juice to prevent protein buildup in the tube. Flushing the tube with water is necessary to provide water to the patient, as well as to flush the tube. Before NG tube feedings, the nurse aspirates gastric contents to determine the amount of feeding left in the stomach. When more than 50 ml is obtained, the feeding should be delayed. After consultation with the physician, the nurse administers all the nutrients through the subclavian vein via total parenteral nutrition (TPN). TPN is used when the gut cannot be used. TPN contains 50% glucose, protein, electrolytes, vitamins, and trace elements. When a high concentration of glucose is given, the nurse must monitor blood glucose; also, urinary glucose and acetone must be monitored to determine the possible presence of glycosuria. Regular insulin is given in consultation with the physician to move the glucose into the cells when blood glucose or urinary glucose is found to be high. Because sepsis is a complication of TPN, the patient's temperature is monitored every 4 hours.

Factors that Interfere with Nutrition

Identifying socioeconomic factors that interfere with nutrition allows identification of community agencies that may assist the patient and family.

Psychologic factors may include eating disorders or depression. Eating disorders include anorexia nervosa and bulimia nervosa. *Anorexia nervosa* is characterized by refusal to maintain normal body weight through self-imposed starvation and obsession with body weight and shape and may include binge eating episodes. Amenorrhea may occur due to insufficient fat for estrogen function. *Bulimia nervosa* is referred to as the binge and purge syndrome. Binging is defined as feeling out of control when eating resulting in the consumption of excessive amounts of food in a short period of time. An average of two binges per week for 3 months accompanied with other psychological characteristics suggests bulimia. Weight gain is prevented by self-induced vomiting, misuse of laxatives or enemas, fasting, or excessive exercise. Frequent vomiting may result in yellowing of teeth or tooth decay from hydrochloric acid. Amenorrhea may occur as in anorexia nervosa.[6,10]

Assess for depression; patient may report sadness, pessimism, sense of failure, dissatisfaction, guilt, self-dislike, work difficulty, apathy, or anorexia. Depression may contribute to disinterest in eating.

Gain Knowledge of Nutritional Needs

To maintain weight gain, patients and families need a follow-up plan that will support their independence in making appropriate life-style changes to maintain adequate weight. Interactive teaching styles that encourage active participation of patients and family contribute to more positive outcomes.

■ IMPAIRED SWALLOWING[14]

Impaired swallowing is a state in which an individual has decreased ability to voluntarily pass fluids and/or solids from the mouth to the stomach.

Related Factors

Neuromuscular impairment (e.g., decreased or absent gag reflex, decreased strength or excursion of muscles involved in mastication, perceptual impairment, facial paralysis)

■ TABLE IV-4 Serum Assessments in Malnutrition

	Serum Albumin (g/dl)	Lymphocytes (per ml³)
Mild deficit	3.0-3.5	1500-1800
Moderate deficit	2.1-3.0	900-1500
Severe deficit	2.1	900

Mechanical obstruction (e.g., edema, tracheotomy tube, tumor)

Fatigue

Limited awareness

Reddened, irritated oropharyngeal cavity

Defining Characteristics

Observed evidence of difficulty in swallowing (e.g., stasis of food in oral cavity, cough/choking)

Evidence of aspiration

Expected Patient Outcomes & Nursing Interventions*

Patient swallowing food and fluids safely without gagging

- Consult with speech therapist, dietitian, patient, and family to develop a plan for improving swallowing.
- Assess mental status, concentration, orientation.
- Auscultate breath sounds.
- Inspect oropharynx for inflammation, altered oral mucosa, adequacy of oral hygiene.
- Assess gag and couch reflexes. (If reflexes are absent, use food tube or parenteral route for food and fluids.)
- Assess ability to swallow by observing patient swallow own saliva; then water.
- Collaborate with speech therapist and dietitian in planning management of swallowing difficulties.
- Progress slowly from clear liquids, to full liquids, to pureed food, to soft diet, to regular diet.
- Avoid mixing food textures.
- Ensure temperature of food and fluid is appropriate.
- Position patient in a 90-degree sitting position during meals.
- Have suction equipment at bedside ready for use if needed.
- When feeding liquids, add green or blue food coloring during initial feedings.
- Minimize distractions while eating or drinking.
- Encourage patient to chew food completely before attempting to swallow and to wear properly fitting dentures when applicable.
- When one side of the patient's face is paralyzed, food is placed in the unaffected side. Check affected side of mouth for food lodged in cheek during and after eating.
- When fatigue impairs swallowing, provide rest periods before and during meals as needed.
- If swallowing appears difficult, massage throat.
- Observe for signs of swallowing problems, e.g., coughing, choking, spitting up food, drooling, watering eyes, nasal discharge, gurgling voice.
- Perform Heimlich maneuver as needed.
- Monitor for signs of aspiration, such as obstruction of upper airway, fever, crackles, or decreased breath sounds.

Maintain adequate nutrition and hydration as evidenced by:

Stabilization of weight

Fluid intake of 2000 ml daily, elastic skin turgor, moist mucous membranes

- Weigh patient.
- Measure intake.
- Consult with dietitian, patient, and family regarding daily caloric requirements and food and fluid preferences.
- Provide small frequent meals.
- Provide for or perform oral care before and after meals.
- Record amount of food and fluids taken.
- Praise patient and family for attaining goal.

Demonstrate ability to assist with eating and take action when swallowing difficulties arise, as evidenced by:

Patient and family members selecting nutritious foods

Family members demonstrating Heimlich maneuver and stating their plan of action if patient chokes

- Teach patient and family about food selection and preparation.
- Supervise family members feeding patient.
- Teach Heimlich maneuver to family members for use in an emergency.
- Teach use of suction when necessary.

Principles and Rationale for Nursing Interventions†

Swallowing Safely Without Gagging

Before the patient with impaired swallowing eats or drinks, the nurse makes several assessments. Assess patient's mental status for alertness. Auscultate breath sounds before patient eats or drinks to document baseline respiratory status. Inspect oropharynx to detect any problems that may hamper swallowing, such as inflammation. Test gag and cough reflexes because these are protective reflexes to help prevent aspiration. However, even if the patient has a gag reflex, aspiration is possible.[2]

If these reflexes are absent, the patient should not be fed by mouth at this time; alternative routes such as feeding tubes or parenteral nutrition should be used. Ask the patient to swallow saliva so that the musculature can be observed.

Collaborate with a speech therapist, who has expertise in diagnosing and managing swallowing difficulties, and the dietitian, who can plan for appropriate foods to meet patient preferences and proper consistency to facilitate swallowing. Including patient and family in choice of foods improves cooperation.

For meals the patient should be seated at a 90-degree angle to allow gravity to assist in the peristaltic motion. A suction machine is ready for use at the bedside to remove food or fluids if patient chokes. Food coloring is added to liquids to help determine if aspiration has occurred (if patient's sputum is the color

*References 1, 2, 8, 14, 20, 27, 32.

†References 1, 2, 8, 14, 20, 27, 32.

of the liquid). Distractions are minimized so that the patient can concentrate on swallowing. Patient should be encouraged to chew food completely to facilitate swallowing. Food is placed on the unaffected side of the mouth to facilitate movement to the back of the mouth. Food may become lodged on the affected side and should be removed. Some patients benefit from the placement of food on the back of the tongue to assist in swallowing. Fatigue should be prevented as it may interfere with swallowing. When the patient begins eating, he or she may need several rest periods during meals. Serving small frequent meals is advisable in these cases. Massaging the throat may be necessary to stimulate the laryngopharyngeal muscles during swallowing. Tilting the head forward 45 degrees keeps the esophagus patent to facilitate swallowing. As feeding progresses, observe for difficulties so that aspiration can be prevented. Perform the Heimlich maneuver as needed to dislodge particles of food caught in the esophagus. After an incident of potential aspiration, assess breath sounds for changes from baseline.

Adequate Nutrition and Hydration

Monitoring weight changes is an objective way to determine if nutrition is sufficient. The dietitian confers with the patient and family to create meal plans that meet preferences and textures appropriate for patient's ability to swallow. Small frequent meals will prevent fatigue, both mental and physical. Oral care before meals is refreshing and enhances appetite and after meals ensures removal of any food remaining in the mouth. It also provides an opportunity to assess the moisture of mucous membranes, an indicator of adequate hydration. The amount of fluid drunk and percentage of food eaten are recorded to monitor adequacy of nutritional intake and evaluate the progress toward swallowing goals. Adequate intake prevents weight loss and decreases risk of muscular wasting.

Family Demonstrates Skills and Knowledge for Home Care

The patient and family need knowledge of how to assist the patient to eat at home. When the patient requires feeding, the family should practice in the hospital. To prevent choking, the family members must know how to perform the Heimlich maneuver on the patient. If a suction machine will be required at home, the family members will need instruction on how to use it. The family may require instruction on what foods to serve and how to prepare them. Finally, they need to know the plan for follow-up care.

◼ RISK FOR ASPIRATION

Risk for aspiration is a state in which an individual is at risk for entry of gastric secretions, oropharyngeal secretions, or exogenous food or fluids into tracheobronchial passages because of dysfunction of protective mechanisms.[15]

Aspiration of gastric content results in severe chemical burn of the lung, resulting in potential aspiratory pneumonia or other severe complications. The normal pH of the lung is above 2.5. If the individual aspirates, the pH of the lung may decrease to 1.5 or below. If this happens, damage to the lung occurs. The initial response to aspiration of acid is an intense bronchospasm. This leads to decreased pulmonary compliance and to pulmonary edema. The loss of intravascular volume into the alveoli and bronchi results in hemoconcentration, hypotension, and shock.[1]

Aspiration occurs most often when the patient is in an altered state of consciousness resulting from seizure, drugs, alcohol, anesthesia, or acute infection, or when the patient is debilitated. Feeding tube location and endotracheal tube cuff placement and cuff inflation result in the most common mechanical causes of potential aspiration.[3,4,13] Poor suctioning technique is another cause of risk for aspiration.[7,8]

Related Factors/Risk Factors[15]

Reduced level of consciousness
Depressed cough and gag reflexes
Presence of tracheostomy or endotracheal tube
Underinflated tracheostomy or endotracheal tube cuff
Presence of nasogastric feeding tube
Presence of gastrointestinal tube
Bolus tube feedings or medication administration
Situation hindering elevation of upper body
Supine position
Esophageal disease; hiatal hernia
Increased gastric residual
Decreased gastric motility
Impaired swallowing
Facial, oral, or neck surgery or trauma
Wired jaws
Impaired mastication
Inattentiveness to process of selecting, chewing, and swallowing food

Defining Characteristics[15]

Reduced level of consciousness
Depressed cough and gag reflexes
Impaired swallowing
Impaired mastication

Expected Patient Outcomes & Nursing Interventions

Does not aspirate food, fluid, or other substances into the tracheobronchial passages, as evidenced by:

Clear airway and lungs
Lung aspirate pH above 2.5
Absence of air hunger
Blood gases within normal limits
  • Monitor patient closely for respiratory rate, effort, and quality. Vesicular breath sounds should be heard over distal lung fields.

- Avoid triggering gag mechanism when performing care activities, especially mouth care. *Gagging may stimulate emesis.*
- Confirm that patient has received nothing by mouth for several hours before surgery. *Fluid or foods may compromise the anesthesia process.*
- For patients with diminished swallowing reflex, elevate head of bed when giving oral fluids and encourage patient to take only small sips. Semi-Fowler's position is best *to prevent aspiration.*
- Assess and document amount of secretions present, patient's level of consciousness, and ability to handle (swallow) secretions effectively *to prevent airway obstruction and potential aspiration.*
- Test patient's gag reflex to identify whether it is diminished.
- Identify contributing factors, such as oral surgery with jaw wiring or facial trauma.
- Instruct patient with wired jaws to avoid the use of alcohol and mind-altering substances.
- Instruct patient or significant other how to cut wires in the event of vomiting or if jaw is wired. Keep wire cutters at patient's bedside.
- Provide suction equipment at patient's bedside.
- Suction as often as necessary to remove secretions and maintain patent airway.
- If secretions are thick or inspissated, ensure adequate humidification to help liquify them.
- If patient is confused, monitor him or her closely when eating for evidence of adequate swallowing with no gagging or emesis. Also, remind patient to chew and swallow.

Tracheotomy

- Ensure that the cuff of the tube is inflated when patient eats or receives ventilatory assistance.
- Clean tube according to hospital protocol *to ensure that tube mucus and crusting is not aspirated.*

Endotracheal Tube

- Ensure that cuff is inflated to adequate 18 to 20 mm Hg *to avoid air leakage against tracheal wall.*[8]
- Suction according to hospital protocol *to avoid blockage of airway or aspiration of mucus.*
- Place blue food coloring on back of patient's tongue. Then suction. *If mucus is tinted blue, the nurse knows that cuff of tube is not adequately inflated. Aspiration of secretions may occur.*

Tube Feedings

- Carefully monitor placement of gastric feeding tubes before each feeding by using bubble technique: place end of feeding tube into glass of water; if bubbles appear, assess placement of tube.
- Elevate head of bed during tube feedings and for at least 30 minutes after tube feeding is stopped.
- Add food coloring to tube feeding; when suctioning, aspiration of tube feeding may be detected.

Public Education

- Participate in public education about the risk of aspirated food, and teach the Heimlich maneuver.
- Perform the Heimlich maneuver when appropriate.

Principles and Rationale for Nursing Interventions

The goal of the nursing interventions for normal lung and breathing function is that the patient's blood gases are within normal limits. Vesicular breath sounds should be present over the peripheral lung fields. The patient should not show signs of air hunger. Presence of bronchial breath sounds or bronchovesicular breath sounds over distal lung fields may indicate that aspiration has occurred. The nurse should take appropriate actions to reinstate normal breathing.

■ ALTERED ORAL MUCOUS MEMBRANE

Altered oral mucous membrane is a state in which an individual experiences disruptions in the tissue layers of the oral cavity.

Related Factors

Pathologic conditions—oral cavity (radiation to head and/or neck)
Dehydration
Trauma
   Chemical (e.g., acidic foods, drugs, noxious agents, alcohol)
   Mechanical (e.g., ill-fitting dentures; braces; tubes—endotracheal, nasogastric; surgery in oral cavity)
NPO instructions for more than 24 hours
Ineffective oral hygiene
Mouth breathing
Malnutrition
Infection
Lack of or decreased salivation
Medication

Defining Characteristics

Coated tongue
Xerostomia (dry mouth)
Stomatitis
Oral lesions or ulcers
Lack of or decreased salivation
Leukoplakia
Edema
Hyperemia
Oral plaque
Oral pain or discomfort
Desquamation
Vesicles
Hemorrhagic gingivitis

Carious teeth
Halitosis

Expected Patient Outcomes & Nursing Interventions*

Oral mucosa will be intact, as evidenced by:

Moist oral mucous membranes
Coral color
Ability to chew and drink without discomfort
Lack of halitosis

- Inspect patient's gums, oral mucosa, lips, and tongue for moisture, color, texture, and presence of edema or redness.
- Inspect oral cavity daily for inflammation, lesions, discolorations, bleeding, dryness.
- Ask patient to describe usual oral care habits and date of last dental visit. Encourage brushing or cleaning of dentures after meals, daily flossing, and annual dental visits.
- Determine patient's ability to provide own oral care. When providing oral care for patient, avoid use of hydrogen peroxide and lemon and glycerine swabs. Recommended solutions are normal saline or sodium bicarbonate (1/2 tsp, sodium bicarbonate, 1/2 tsp salt in 1 qt warm water).[28] Oral care for the unconscious patient is performed with the patient in a side-lying position and the head of the bed elevated at least 30 degrees. Rinsing is done using a large syringe and oral suction. Change position of oral airway or orotracheal tube every 8 hours.
- Monitor patient's nutritional and fluid status to determine adequacy.
- Determine if medication (e.g., anticholinergics) side effects could be contributing to dry mouth.
- Discourage smoking and use of alcohol.
- Stimulate saliva with chewing gum or hard candy.
- Keep lips well-lubricated using lanolin or vitamin A and D ointment.
- If patient's platelets are low or if patient takes an anticoagulant drug, use a soft bristle brush or toothette to clean teeth.
- If mouth is severely inflamed use frequent, gentle mouth care.
- Topical anesthetic agent (viscous lidocaine) may be needed to reduce pain. Also modify diet to soft, pureed, or liquid to prevent trauma or pain to mouth.

Explain knowledge of self-care, as evidenced by:

Patient and family stating reasons for alteration in oral mucous membrane
Plan for dental hygiene for all family members
Medications and treatment for home use
Plan for follow-up care

- Assess what the patient and family already know.

---

*References 1, 8, 14, 19, 27, 28.

- Provide information about:
  Reasons for alteration in oral mucous membrane
  Importance of dental hygiene for all family members
  Review of medications and treatments ordered for home use
  Plan for follow-up care

Principles and Rationale for Nursing Interventions[1,8,14,19,28]

Oral Mucosa Intact

Systematic assessment of patient's oral cavity and oral care habits can identify impending problems early. Determining patient's usual oral care habits will identify instruction needed. Regular oral care is needed to remove bacteria and food particles from the teeth and gums to prevent tooth decay, halitosis, and to promote comfort. Rinsing cleanses the mouth, reduces microscopic flora, soothes and relieves local discomfort, and provides moisture. Patients who are unable to complete their own care will need assistance. Hydrogen peroxide can damage oral mucosa, is distasteful,[28] and may promote bacterial growth.[14] Lemon in swabs can decalcify teeth and glycerin contributes to tooth decay. The unconscious patient is positioned side-lying for oral care to prevent aspiration. When an oral airway is needed, it must be removed and cleaned every 8 hours to remove secretions and increase patient comfort. The orotracheal tube should be repositioned to the opposite side of the mouth every 8 hours to prevent pressure ulcers in the mouth from the tube.

Malnutrition and dehydration predispose patient to altered oral mucous membranes. Side effects of many medications, smoking, and alcohol can cause dry mouth requiring increased efforts to keep mouth moist, such as chewing gum or hard candy. Keeping lips moist may prevent drying and promote comfort.

For patients who have low platelets or are taking anticoagulants, prevent bleeding or gums by using a soft bristle brush or sponge-type toothbrush (toothette).

Fluid and food intake decrease when they cause pain. Relief of the pain can be accomplished by changing the temperature of the fluid or food to tepid or warm, or the texture of the food to soft or pureed. Foods to avoid include fried foods, spicy foods, citrus fruits, crusty foods, and foods of extreme temperature. Topical anesthetics, per physician's orders, are useful before mealtime to provide temporary pain relief to increase intake. These include lidocaine (Xylocaine) viscous 2%; 0.5 aqueous Benadryl solution and Maalox; or equal parts of 0.5 aqueous Benadryl solution and Kaopectate. The patient swishes the solution and then swallows or expectorates. When lidocaine is swallowed, however, it may affect the gag reflex.

Knowledge of Self Care

The nurse assesses the patient's and family's knowledge to determine what content to teach. Prevention of alteration of oral mucous membranes is very important. The patient and family need to review their dental hygiene practices. Children benefit from visits to the dentist every 6 months after the age of 2 years. Fluoride supplements are helpful for children. They will need help brushing their teeth until age 6, but it is important for children to develop the recommended dental hygiene practices. Infants who are put to bed with a bottle should receive a bottle of water rather than juice or milk. The infant who is teething needs safe objects to put in the mouth. Adults require annual visits to the dentist. Sufficient fluids, adequate nutrition, and daily brushing and flossing will help prevent dental caries.

◼ FLUID VOLUME DEFICIT*

◼ Fluid volume deficit is a state in which an individual experiences vascular, cellular, or intracellular dehydration related to failure of regulatory mechanisms.

Related Factors

Actual loss
Failure of regulatory mechanisms

Defining Characteristics

Dilute urine†
Concentrated urine‡
Increased urine output†
Decreased urine output‡
Sudden weight loss
Output greater than intake‡
Increased sodium levels‡

Other Possible Defining Characteristics

Possible weight gain†
Hypotension
Decreased venous filling
Increased pulse rate
Decreased skin turgor
Decreased pulse volume and pressure
Increased body temperature
Dry skin
Dry mucous membranes
Hemoconcentration
Weakness
Edema†
Thirst
Change in mental status‡

---

*At the Eighth Conference on Nursing Diagnosis, NANDA combined the diagnoses of *fluid volume deficit (1)* (regulatory failure) and *fluid volume deficit (2)* (active loss).[3]
†Present when failure of regulator mechanisms occurs.
‡Present when active loss occurs.

Expected Patient Outcomes & Nursing Interventions[1,7,14,19,22]

Maintains adequate fluid and electrolyte balance, as evidenced by:

Elastic skin turgor
Moist mucous membranes
Absence of thirst
Balanced intake and output
Clearing of mentation
Blood pressure:
   160/95 (over 65 years)
   150/95 (45-65 years)
   140/95 (18-44 years)
Pulse: 70-80/min
Blood (see Risk for Fluid Volume Deficit)
   Serum osmolality: 280-300 mOsm/kg H_2O
   Hemoglobin (g/dl):
      Men 15.5 ± 1.1
      Women 13.7 ± 1.0
   Hematocrit (%):
      Men 46.0 ± 3.1
      Women 40.9 ± 3
Urine
   Specific gravity: range of 1.001-1.035; adult on normal fluid intake, 1.016-1.022; specific gravity decreases with increasing age
   Osmolality: 250-900 mOsm/kg for random specimens

- Measure vital signs. Observe for hypotension, including postural hypotension; *pulse will be elevated.*
- Measure central venous pressure or pulmonary capillary wedge pressure. *These reflect the pressure of the circulating blood volume and will be decreased.*
- Assess capillary refill time. *Refill time will be >5 sec, indicating the reduced blood volume requiring more time for the capillaries to fill.*
- Measure intake and output to monitor the fluid balance.
- Weigh patient to monitor fluid balance.
- Measure abdominal girth when ascites is present.
- Monitor electrolytes, especially potassium, sodium, calcium, and magnesium.
- Measure urine specific gravity.
- Monitor hemoglobin (Hgb) and hematocrit (Hct).
- Assess oral mucous membranes.
- Assess skin turgor.
- Administer intravenous or oral fluids as ordered by physician.
- Administer electrolytes as ordered.
- Administer regulating hormones as ordered (e.g., insulin, vasopressin) *to retain fluids. Insulin is given to counteract polyuria associated with diabetes mellitus. Vasopressin is given to replace antidiuretic hormone to treat diabetes insipidus.*
- Orient patient when confusion or disorientation occurs.
- Maintain safety when patient is sitting or standing. Observe for postural hypotension or confusion.

- Provide oral care.
- Provide skin care.

Communicate knowledge of self-care, as evidenced by:

Patient and family explaining reasons for fluid deficit

Foods and fluids consumed to prevent recurrence

Purpose, dosage, and side effects of medications ordered by physician; plan for follow-up care

- Assess what patient and family already know.
- Provide information concerning:

  Cause of this fluid deficit and how to prevent recurrence

  Reasons for treatments

  Foods and fluids to consume

  Purpose, frequency of administration, and side effcts of medications ordered by physician for patient to take at home

- When patient is going home to receive total parenteral nutrition as ordered by physician, have family demonstrate how to change tubing and fluid bags, as well as what to do when problems arise.
- Review the plan for follow-up *to ensure their understanding.*

Principles and Rationale for Nursing Interventions[1,7,14,19,22]

Assessment interventions provide data on the effect of the fluid deficit on other body systems and allow determination of the extent of deficit. The lack of fluid volume in the intravascular space is reflected in vital signs by an increased heart rate and a decreased blood pressure. Peripherally the reduced fluid volume causes blood flow slower, creating a prolonged capillary refill time. Because the fluid volume deficit results from output being greater than intake, these parameters must be monitored as indicators of whether the fluid balance is being reestablished. Body weight will reflect rapidly the changes in fluid balance. A loss of 1 pound represents a loss of 500 ml of fluid. Whereas weight *loss* usually occurs with a fluid volume deficit, a weight *gain* may occur with fluid deficit when the cause is ascites. The status of ascites can be evaluated by measuring abdominal girth at the iliac crests. Often electrolytes are lost with the fluid, particularly sodium, potassium, calcium, and magnesium. Symptoms of sodium deficit include the same vital signs, skin turgor, and mental status changes seen with fluid volume deficit. Potassium deficit manifestations are often gradual in onset and include skeletal muscle weakness, and loss of smooth muscle tone resulting in anorexia, nausea, vomiting, and paralytic ileus. Calcium deficit can be determined by skeletal muscle cramps, tetany, and hyperreflexia. Magnesium losses cause muscle weakness, hyperreflexia, and dysrhythmias such as premature ventricular contraction or t wave flattening. An increase in urine specific gravity indicates concentrated urine from lack of fluid. Likewise, hemoglobin and hematocrit values are abnormally high because of hemoconcentration. As the fluid is lost from the intravascular space, it is replaced by fluid from the interstitial space, leaving the mucous membranes and skin dry.

Therapeutic interventions begin with replacement of fluids and electrolytes either orally or intravenously as ordered by the physician. Intravenous fluids include crystalloids, colloids, and/or blood. When long-term therapy is needed, total parenteral nutrition is used as ordered to provide concentrated glucose and proteins for calories and a positive nitrogen balance, respectively. Regulatory hormones are replaced as ordered to regain fluid balance. For example, insulin is given to prevent fluid loss from polyuria from diabetes mellitus, and vasopressin (antidiuretic hormone) is used to treat polyuria from diabetes insipidus. When patient's mental status changes, they benefit from reorientation periodically. Inadequate fluid to brain cells can cause shrinkage of cells, resulting in a change in mental status. Patients also require a safe environment if they are confused. Safety is a primary concern when patients begin to sit and ambulate. If postural hypotension is occurring, the patient should be encouraged to rise slowly and to remain sitting until the blood pressure has stabilized. Oral care is valuable therapeutic intervention to replace moisture to the membranes, just as skin care is important to replace moisture to the skin.

■ RISK FOR FLUID VOLUME DEFICIT[14]

Risk for fluid volume deficit is a state in which an individual is at risk for experiencing vascular, cellular, or intracellular dehydration.

Risk Factors

Extremes of age

Extremes of weight

Excessive losses through normal routes (e.g., diarrhea)

Loss of fluid through abnormal routes (e.g., indwelling tubes)

Deviations affecting access to, intake of, or absorption of fluids (e.g., physical immobility)

Factors influencing fluid needs (e.g., hypermetabolic states)

Knowledge deficiency related to fluid volume

Medications (e.g., diuretics)

Increased fluid output

Urinary frequency

Thirst

Altered intake

Expected Patient Outcomes & Nursing Interventions[1,7,8,14,19]

Maintain fluid and electrolyte balance as evidenced by:

Stable weight

Vital signs within normal limits

Elastic skin turgor

Moist mucous membranes

Balanced intake and output

Blood:

Sodium: adult, 135-145 mEq/L

Potassium: 3.5-5.0 mEq/L; add approximately 0.2 to normal range if serum is sampled rather than plasma; pediatric ranges sometimes reported as slightly higher than adult levels

- Weigh patient and compare with previous values.
- Measure vital signs. Observe for hypotension including postural hypotension, elevated pulse, and fever.
- Measure intake and compare with output.
- Monitor electrolytes, especially potassium, sodium, and magnesium.
- Assess oral mucous membranes which may become dry from fluid loss.
- Assess skin turgor (skin may lose its elasticity and become tented with fluid loss).
- If patient can have oral fluids, keep fluids at the bedside within patient's reach and encourage fluid intake.
- If patient is unable to take oral fluids, use other routes: intravenous (crystalloids, colloids, or total parenteral nutrition), nasogastric, or gastrostomy.
- Provide oral care to moisten the mucous membranes.
- Provide skin care to replace moisture to the skin.
- Administer medications (e.g., antiemetics, antidiarrheals, or antipyretics) as ordered to prevent fluid loss.
- Evaluate therapeutic, side and adverse effects of medications.

Communicate knowledge of fluid balance, as evidenced by:

Patient and family explaining:

Actions to prevent actual loss

Foods and fluids to consume

Foods and fluids to avoid

Medications and treatments for home use

Plan for follow-up care

- Assess what patient and family already know.
- Provide information to prevent a fluid deficit:

Over-the-counter antiemetics or antidiarrheals

Actions to use to prevent actual deficit

Reasons for treatments

What foods and fluids to consume

What foods and fluids to avoid

Principles and Rationale for Nursing Interventions[1,7,14,19]

Assessment interventions provide data on patients' status so that fluid volume deficits can be prevented.

Fluid deficit will be detected first with a reduction in weight. A loss of 1 pound represents a loss of about 500 ml fluid. Changes in vital signs expected in a potential fluid volume deficit are a gradual increase in the pulse as the heart pumps faster to circulate blood and a gradual decrease in blood pressure as fluid is lost from the intravascular spaces. Measuring

intake and output documents fluid balance. The amount of intake from all sources (oral, enteral, and intravenous) should approximate the output from all sources (urine, feces, drainage tubes, insensible loss, and perspiration). Dry oral mucous membranes may indicate fluid movement from the interstitial spaces to the intravascular spaces as occurs in dehydration. Loss of skin turgor also occurs as fluid moves from the interstitial spaces.

Therapeutic interventions reduce abnormal fluid losses and replace fluids and electrolytes. Potassium, sodium, and magnesium are lost through vomiting, diarrhea, and gastrointestinal drainage.

If oral fluids are tolerated, they should be kept within the patient's reach. Intravenous fluids can provide water, glucose, electrolytes, and vitamins. Albumin may be given intravenously, per physician's order, to provide protein to maintain oncotic pressure. Total parenteral nutrition is frequently ordered by the physician when prolonged fluid therapy is required, because it supplies additional calories in the form of 50% dextrose, as well as proteins, electrolytes, vitamins, and water. Nasogastric tube feeding is another means of providing fluids along with nutrients.

The patient needs not only replacement fluids, but also treatment for the source of the fluid loss. Loss from vomiting can be lessened by discontinuing oral intake of fluids and food, in addition to changing medications that cause vomiting as a side effect. When medications causing vomiting cannot be discontinued, administration of antiemetics as ordered by the physician should be considered. Drainage from abnormal routes is difficult to stop. At times the drainage is necessary and must be replaced with fluids. Profuse diaphoresis also requires fluid replacement until the cause can be treated and fluid balance regained. Diarrhea is arrested by discontinuing oral intake and administering drugs as ordered to slow peristalsis.

The second goal is to communicate knowledge of fluid balance. Family members need to know the types of fluid replacements to use. For example, milk and milk products should be withheld from individuals with diarrhea. Clear liquids, such as ginger ale, apple juice, beef broth, and Popsicles, are the fluids of choice. Family members need to know the purpose, frequency of administration, and side effects of medications to be taken. They can keep a record of the intake and output to evaluate fluid balance.

▌ FLUID VOLUME EXCESS[14]

Fluid volume excess is a state in which an individual experiences increased fluid retention and edema.

Related Factors

Compromised regulatory mechanism

Excessive fluid intake

Exessive sodium intake

Defining Characteristics

Edema
Effusion
Anasarca
Weight gain
Shortness of breath, orthopnea
Intake greater than output
Third heart sound
Pulmonary congestion on x-ray film
Abnormal breath sounds: crackles (rales)
Change in respiratory pattern
Change in mental status
Decreased hemoglobin, hematocrit levels
Blood pressure changes
Central venous pressure changes
Pulmonary artery pressure changes
Jugular venous distention
Positive hepatojugular reflex
Oliguria
Specific gravity changes
Azoturia
Altered electrolytes
Restlessness and anxiety

Expected Patient Outcomes & Nursing Interventions[1,7,8,14,19]

Regain fluid balance as evidenced by:

Stable weight
Absence of edema
Intake equals output
Clear breath sounds
Vital signs within normal limits
- Measure vital signs. Observe for hypertension and a full bounding pulse.
- Measure central venous pressure or pulmonary capillary wedge pressure; note increases in pressures.
- Weigh patient to monitor fluid balance, note weight gains which may represent fluid excess.
- Measure intake and output; note increase in intake or decrease in output.
- Assess mental status; confusion, irritability, depression, and restlessness result from decreased sodium; ensure safety of patient.
- Auscultate lungs for breath sounds; crackles indicate fluid in alveoli, which may be caused by left-sided heart failure. Dyspnea also may be observed.
- Auscultate heart sounds for S3, ventricular gallop.
- Assess for ascites by measuring abdominal girth, presence of shifting dullness on percussion of the abdomen, or fluid wave on palpation of abdomen.
- Palpate for edema in feet and lower legs when patient is sitting or walking, and sacral area if patient is on bedrest; observe for jugular vein distention; these may be indications of right-sided heart failure.

- Monitor laboratory data for lowered values from hemodilution, e.g., hemoglobin, hematocrit, sodium, potassium, magnesium, albumin, blood urea nitrogen, creatinine, serum osmolarity, urine osmolarity.
- Restrict fluids and sodium as ordered.
- Alleviate thirst with tart-flavored candy or chewing gum.
- Administer diuretics, inotropics, or colloids as ordered.
- Encourage range of motion exercises, either passive or active.
- Assist patient to change positions, and provide skin care.
- Apply elastic stockings and support edematous extremities with pillows.
- Position patient in semi-Fowler's position and administer oxygen as ordered when breathing becomes labored as a result of fluid in the lungs.
- Assist with activities of daily living to conserve energy.

Communicate knowledge of self-care, as evidenced by:

Patient and family explaining reasons for fluid volume excess and symptoms of recurrence
Dietary alterations; medications and treatments for home use
Plan for follow-up care
- Assess knowledge of patient and family regarding cause, treatment, and prevention of fluid volume excess.
- Provide instruction as needed related to:
    Preventing further fluid volume excesses
    Reasons for any dietary alterations and how to implement them
    The therapeutic use of medications, along with dosage, time of administration, and side effects
    Symptoms to watch for indicating a recurrence of the fluid volume excess
    Plan for follow-up care

Principles and Rationale for Nursing Interventions[1,7,8,14,19]

Assessment interventions provide data on the effect of the fluid excess on other body systems and allow determination of the extent of excess. The excess of fluid volume in the intravascular space is reflected in vital signs by an increased blood pressure and full, bounding pulse. An excess of fluid returning to the heart will be reflected in an increased central venous pressure. An increase in pulmonary artery pressures will reflect excess fluid in the pulmonary vasculature. Body weight will reflect rapidly the changes in fluid balance. A gain of 1 pound represents 500 ml of fluid retention. The balance of intake and output are indicators of whether the fluid balance is being reestablished.

Excess fluids in the brain can cause cells to swell, resulting in confusion, depression, irritability, and possibly seizures. The nurse should provide a safe environment when the patient is confused and should reorient the patient as needed. When the patient appears depressed or irritable, verbalization of feelings should be encouraged and the nurse should provide explanations of treatment strategies.

Excess fluid in the pulmonary vasculature can move into alveoli causing crackles or decreased breath sounds. Fluid in alveoli impairs oxygen transport into the arteries resulting in dyspnea. The S3 heart sounds may indicate decreased compliance of the ventricle or increased ventricular diastolic volume. To compensate for fluid excess, some fluid may move into the abdominal cavity causing ascites. Ascites is identified by a fluid wave in the abdomen or as shifting dullness on percussion. It can be measured with the abdominal girth measuring around the patient at the iliac crests. The excess fluid moves into interstitial spaces causing dependent edema. Ambulatory patients may have edema in the feet, ankles, and lower legs, whereas patients on bedrest may have sacral edema.

Hemoglobin (Hgb) and hemocrit (hct) values are abnormally low because of hemodilution. Serum electrolytes, particularly sodium, potassium, calcium, and magnesium, may be low because of hemodilution, or they may be elevated when the fluid excess is the result of urine retention, such as renal failure. Symptoms of sodium deficit include the low blood pressure and rapid pulses, poor skin turgor, and mental status changes seen with fluid volume deficit. Potassium deficit manifestations are often gradual in onset and include muscle weakness, paralytic ileus, hypotension, and dysrhythmias, such as depressed ST segment. Calcium deficit can be determined by skeletal muscle cramps, tetany, and hyperreflexia. Magnesium losses cause muscle weakness, hyperreflexia, and dysrhythmias such as premature ventricular contraction or t wave flattening. Sodium excess symptoms include weight gain, edema, and hypertension. Potassium excess manifestations include muscle weakness, increased muscle irritability resulting in restlessness, intestinal cramping, and diarrhea. Calcium excess can be determined by fatigue, lethargy, anorexia, nausea, and constipation. Magnesium excess will be manifested by depressed skeletal muscle contraction and nerve function as evidenced by muscle weakness, bradycardia, and respiratory depression.

Therapeutic interventions for fluid volume excess are based on the cause of the problem. Fluids and sodium are restricted so that additional fluid does not accumulate. When fluids are restricted, the patient becomes thirsty even though his or her body has excessive fluids. Gum and tart-flavored hard candy stimulate saliva to moisten the mouth. In accordance with physician's orders, diuretics are given to remove excess fluids, and albumin is given to provide protein to pull fluid from the interstitial space into the intravascular space so that it can be excreted by the kidneys. Inotropic drugs are given to increase force of the ventricular contraction when heart failure is the causative factor. Active or passive range of motion exercises are performed to prevent contractures and improve venous return. The patient's position is changed every 1 to 2 hours to prevent pressure on edematous areas. Skin is inspected for redness or blanching to detect pressure ulcers at an early stage. Application of elastic stockings provides support to veins and prevents venous stasis. When the respiratory effort is compromised, place the patient in semi-Fowler's position to move the abdominal contents away from the diaphragm to improve chest expansion. Supplemental oxygen may be necessary when fluid in alveoli prevents transport of oxygen into the arteries. To conserve the patient's energy; assist him or her with activities of daily living.

To communicate a knowledge of self-care, the nurse determines what the patient and family already know. They need to understand the cause of the fluid volume excess. Many patients require dietary alterations of low sodium or altered protein intake. Persons who buy the food and prepare the meals need written information on appropriate menus. They need to read labels of food for sodium content. Information about medications to be taken includes the purpose, frequency of administration, and side effects. The patient needs to know how to support peripheral circulation. This includes applying elastic stockings before rising and avoiding crossed legs and standing for long periods. The feet and legs should be inspected daily for edema and redness to prevent pressure sores.

RISK FOR IMPAIRED SKIN INTEGRITY[14]

Risk for impaired skin integrity is a state in which an individual's skin is at risk of being adversely altered.

Risk Factors

External (Environmental)

Hypothermia or hyperthermia
Chemical substance
Mechanical factors
    Shearing forces
    Pressure
    Restraint
Radiation
Physical immobilization
Excretions and secretions
Humidity

Internal (Somatic)

Medication
Alterations in nutritional state (obesity, emaciation)
Altered metabolic state
Altered circulation
Altered sensation
Altered pigmentation
Skeletal prominence
Developmental factors
Alterations in skin turgor (change in elasticity)
Psychogenic
Immunologic

Expected Patient Outcomes & Nursing Interventions*

Maintain intact skin, as evidenced by:

Skin dry with natural color

Moist, adequate turgor with intact skin

Intake of balanced diet reported

Behaviors required to maintain skin integrity verbalized by patient and family

- Assess patient using a risk assessment scale or by determining the presence of the following risk factors: incontinence, immobility, inactivity, poor nutrition, edema, or diminished sensation.
- Inspect skin daily for reddened areas, bruises, blisters, excoriation, changes in tactile sensation, edema.
- Palpate skin for elastic turgor and moisture.
- Monitor lab data (e.g., hemoglobin, hematocrit, albumin, glucose, blood urea nitrogen, creatinine, liver enzymes) for evidence of malnutrition or chronic conditions that could affect the skin.
- Monitor drugs (e.g., corticosteroids) taken by patient for effect on skin integrity.
- Keep skin clean and dry.
- Use underpads to absorb moisture and change as needed to keep moisture away from skin.
- Lubricate dry skin with lotion.
- Provide balanced diet and adequate fluids including sufficient calories and proteins for tissue growth.
- When itching is a problem, encourage individuals not to scratch; pressing the area or applying ice decreases the sensation and does not damage skin. A cool environment is soothing as opposed to a warm environment. Other soothing measures include lubricating the skin with oil or lotion and taking a tub bath containing oatmeal powder, potassium permanganate, or cornstarch at 32° to 38° C (89.6° to 100.4° F). When other methods are unsuccessful, give antihistamine as ordered by physician.
- Inform individuals with altered pigmentation to wear long-sleeved shirts or blouses and hats to shield the sun.
- Instruct children and adults playing and working in the sun to wear protective clothing, to apply sun screen, and to limit exposure time.
- Inform individuals receiving radiation to blot their skin rather than rub it.
- Teach patient and family to inspect skin daily and to take actions when abnormalities are noted; such actions may include keeping pressure off the involved area, keeping area clean and dry, and proving a balanced diet or one high in protein.
- Ask family to return demonstrate proper skin care.
- Teach patient and family when to call physician if symptoms worsen.

Maintain circulation to the skin as evidenced by:

Warm skin

Strong peripheral pulses

- Inspect skin for color, palpate peripheral pulses and skin temperature, and assess capillary refill.
- Encourage patient to ambulate if possible.
- Have patient perform active range of motion, or have family perform passive range of motion when active is not possible.
- Keep pressure off skeletal prominences by positioning patient with pillows or mattress overlays.
- Prevent head of bed from being elevated 30 degrees (semi-Fowler's position) for long periods.
- Provide extra protection for heels such as foam or sheep skin boots. Remove boots at least three times daily to inspect skin.
- When patient is in bed, reposition him or her every 2 hours using lateral, dorsal, and prone positions if possible.
- Use lifting devices when repositioning to avoid shearing of skin against linens.
- Teach patient and family members how to reposition patient.
- Avoid massaging skin over bony prominences.
- Avoid use of donuts or rubber ring around areas of skin that become reddened.
- When feet and ankles swell, use support stockings and periodic leg elevation. Reduction in sodium and fluids may also be indicated to decrease swelling.
- *Do not massage legs; this practice can dislodge a thrombus and create an embolus.*

Principles and Rationale for Nursing Interventions†

The assessment tool used should be a validated risk assessment tool such as the Norton Scale or the Braden Scale to identify patients at risk for immobility-related skin breakdown.[21] Inspect skin daily to identify potential areas of skin breakdown early. Laboratory values are monitored to detect abnormalities such as renal failure, liver failure, anemia, diabetes mellitus, that might affect the skin or perfusion. Certain drugs, (e.g., corticosteroids) make the skin more susceptible to impairment. Patients taking these drugs need to be especially protective of their skin.

The skin is kept clean and dry to remove bacteria and prevent maceration from excessive moisture. Monitor the patient's continence status and minimize exposure of skin to moisture from incontinence, perspiration, and drainage. If the patient is incontinent, implement an incontinence management plan to prevent exposure to chemicals in urine and stool that can erode skin; refer patient to physician for incontinence diagnosis and treatment.[29] Moisture of the skin is maintained internally by intake of at least 2 liters of fluids daily, unless contraindicated,

---

*References 1, 3, 4, 8, 11, 14, 21, 25, 29, 31.

†References 1, 3, 4, 11, 14, 21, 25, 29, 31.

and externally by lubricating the skin with lotion. Eating an adequate diet following the food pyramid provides protein, vitamins, and minerals for tissue growth.

Protection of the skin includes wearing clothing appropriate for the outdoor temperature and humidity. Patients should avoid behaviors that constrict circulation; e.g., they should not smoke because tobacco causes vasoconstriction, and they should not wear constrictive clothing. When itching is a problem, the patient should be in a cool environment to decrease the perception of itching. The patient should be encouraged to press the area that itches rather than scratching to decrease itching without damaging the skin. Keeping the patient's nails short will limit the damage to the skin when scratching does occur. The patient and family can be active participants when they are taught to maintain the skin and prevent skin impairment.

Palpating peripheral pulses and assessing capillary refill time provide data on the adequacy of circulation to the tissues. Blood flows through capillaries at pressures between 22 and 32 mm Hg. When more than 32 mm Hg pressure is exerted on capillaries, blood flow is obstructed resulting in hypoxic tissue damage.[11] Circulation to the skin is maintained by moving, turning, and exercising. Circulation is maintained when the patient can ambulate or perform active range of motion. When this is not possible, passive range of motion exercises and periodic turning are needed to stimulate circulation and relieve pressure areas. The use of pillows, foam wedges and pressure-reducing devices in the bed are recommended.[21] Conclusions drawn from several studies indicate that (1) the standard hospital mattress exerts high pressures in all pressure-prone sites (sacrum, trochanter, and heel) and all positions and should not be used for patients at risk for pressure ulcers; (2) higher sacral pressures are created when the patient is in the semi-Fowler's position than the supine position, thus prolonged semi-Fowler's position must be avoided even though a special mattress or overlay is in use; and (3) despite the use of special mattresses or overlays, additional pressure-relieving devices may be needed to protect heels from pressure ulcers.[11,21,25,31] When additional protection is used for heels, the skin over the heels and lateral and medial malleoli should be inspected for red areas and excessive moisture from perspiration.

Massage over bony prominences formerly was recommended, however, scientific evidence for using massage to stimulate blood and lymph flow and avert pressure ulcer formation is not well established, whereas there is preliminary evidence suggesting that it may lead to deep tissue trauma.[21] The legs of a patient who is confined to bed are *not* massaged because the massage may dislodge a blood clot, creating an embolus. Applying elastic bandages facilitates venous return and is useful to prevent swelling of the feet.

◼ IMPAIRED SKIN INTEGRITY[14]

Impaired skin integrity is a state in which an individual's skin is adversely altered.

Related Factors

External (Environmental)

Hyperthermia or hypothermia
Chemical substance
Mechanical factors
  Shearing forces
  Pressure
  Restraint
  Radiation
  Physical immobilization
  Humidity

Internal (Somatic)

Medication
Altered nutritional state: obesity, emaciation
Altered metabolic state
Altered circulation
Altered sensation
Altered pigmentation
Skeletal prominence
Developmental factors
Immunologic deficit
Alterations in turgor (change in elasticity)
Excretions/secretions
Psychogenic
Edema

Defining Characteristics

Disruption of skin surface
Destruction of skin layers
Invasion of body structures

Expected Patient Outcomes & Nursing Interventions*

Intact skin as evidenced by:

Skin lesion clean and healing

- Assess wound (Stage I-IV) and surrounding skin as a baseline. (Stages I and II relate to *skin* integrity; Stages III and IV relate to *tissue* integrity.)
- Assess skin for color changes, redness, swelling, warmth, pain, sensation, signs of infection.
- Note odors from skin lesion.
- Monitor patient's continence status and minimize exposure of the site of skin impairment and other areas to moisture from incontinence, perspiration, or wound drainage.
- Monitor laboratory data (e.g., hemoglobin, hematocrit, albumin, glucose, blood urea nitrogen (BUN), creatinine, liver enzymes, arterial blood gases) for evidence of malnutrition or chronic conditions that could affect the skin.
- Note drugs (e.g., corticosteroids) taken by patient and their effect on wound healing.

*References 1, 3, 4, 11, 14, 16, 21, 25, 29, 31, 33-35.

- Determine attitudes and reactions of patient and significant others to skin lesion.
- Encourage verbalization about feelings and discuss effect of lesion on self-esteem.
- Provide wound treatment based on stage and drainage, using gauze, polyurethane film, hydrocolloid, foam, adsorptive dressing, hydrogel, or enzymatic therapy.
- Debride and clean wound as ordered.
- Ambulate patients if possible.
- When in bed turn every 2 hours, use lateral, prone, and dorsal sides if possible.
- Have patient perform active range of motion or instruct family to perform passive range of motion.
- Position off pressure ulcer.
- Use pressure-relieving therapy bed.
- Keep pressure off skeletal prominences by positioning patients with pillows and/or foam devices, or pressure-relieving mattresses.
- Use lifting devices and/or sheets to position patients to prevent shearing force on skin.
- Do not massage skin over bony prominences.
- Prevent head of bed from being elevated more than 30 degrees (semi-Fowler's position) for long periods.
- Use underpads or briefs that absorb moisture and leave quick drying surface toward skin if continuously moist.
- Avoid use of donuts or rubber rings.
- Provide adequate nutrition with increased calories and proteins, supplemental iron and vitamin C, and increased fluids (2-3 liters per day).

Communicate care of impaired skin after discharge and action to prevent recurrence, as evidenced by patient and family explaining:

Cause and prevention of altered skin integrity
Medications and treatment for home use
Dietary intake to promote wound healing
Plan for follow-up care

- Assess what patient and family need to learn.
- Provide information concerning:
    Prevention of skin integrity alterations
    How to change dressing and apply topical medication
    Purpose, frequency of administration, and side effects of medication
    Dietary intake to promote wound healing
    How to achieve comfort and relieve pain
    Notification of physician if skin impairment continues

Principles and Rationale for Nursing Interventions*

Skin integrity is regained by protecting the skin from further damage and by promoting wound healing. The stage of the wound (I to IV) provides the basis for treatment. The size and

---

*References 1, 3, 4, 11, 14, 16, 21, 25, 29, 31, 33-35.

color of the area of impairment are documented to evaluate healing. Skin integrity can be impaired by infections, as indicated by elevated leukocyte count, foul odor, and purulent drainage from the wound.

Covering the areas of impaired skin and giving antiinfective agents as ordered will treat existing infections by interrupting microorganism growth. The skin is kept clean and dry to remove bacteria and prevent maceration from excess moisture. Monitor the patient's continence status and minimize exposure of skin to moisture from incontinence, perspiration, and drainage. If the patient is incontinent, implement an incontinence management plan to prevent exposure to chemicals in urine and stool that can erode skin; refer patient to physician for incontinence diagnosis and treatment.[29]

Laboratory data are monitored to detect abnormalities (e.g., renal failure, liver failure, anemia, diabetes mellitus) that might affect the skin or perfusion. Certain drugs, (e.g., corticosteroids) make the skin more susceptible to impairment. Patients taking these drugs need to be especially protective of their skin.

Adequate tissue oxygenation can be determined by hemoglobin, hematocrit, and oxygenation from arterial blood gases. Adequate nutrition is reflected in a normal serum albumin. High glucose might indicate diabetes mellitus, which interferes with wound healing. Elevated liver enzymes may indicate liver disease, which decreases albumin production, contributes to fluid retention, and slows drug metabolism. Elevated BUN and creatinine may indicate renal disease, which contributes to fluid retention.

A positive mental attitude can improve immune function and increase motivation for healing. Thus, discussions of feelings toward skin lesions can further the wound healing efforts.

Circulation to the skin is maintained by moving, turning, and exercising. Circulation is maintained when the patient can ambulate or perform active range of motion. When this is not possible, passive range of motion exercises and periodic turning are needed to stimulate circulation and relieve pressure areas. The use of pillows, foam wedges and pressure-reducing devices in the bed are recommended.[21] Conclusions drawn from several studies indicate that (1) the standard hospital mattress exerts high pressures in all pressure-prone sites (sacrum, trochanter, and heel) and all positions and should not be used for patients at risk for pressure ulcers; (2) higher sacral pressures are created when the patient is in the semi-Fowler's position than the supine position, thus prolonged semi-Fowler's position must be avoided even though a special mattress or overlay is in use; and (3) despite the use of special mattresses or overlays, additional pressure-relieving devices may be needed to protect heels from pressure ulcers.[11,21,25,31] When additional protection is used for heels, the skin over the heels and lateral and medial malleoli should be inspected for red areas and excessive moisture from perspiration.

Massage over bony prominences formerly was recommended, however, scientific evidence for using massage to stimulate blood and lymph flow and avert pressure ulcer formation is not well established, whereas there is preliminary evidence suggesting that it may lead to deep tissue trauma.[21]

Healing is promoted by adequate oxygen and blood supply along with nutrients to support tissue growth. These nutrients include protein and carbohydrate to maintain a positive nitrogen balance. Iron and vitamins A, B complex, C, D, and E also are required. The age of the patient is a factor in wound healing because children normally heal more rapidly than adults. Elderly persons often heal more slowly because of decreased fibroblastic activity and impaired circulation. Patients receiving corticosteroids have delayed wound healing because these drugs depress the inflammatory response, which occurs before wound healing.

The nurse instructs the patient and family on actions to prevent skin impairment and to continue treatment of the impaired skin after discharge. Time should be made for the family and patient to perform return demonstrations on dressing changes and to ask questions about the treatment schedule.

IMPAIRED TISSUE INTEGRITY[14]

Impaired tissue integrity is a state in which an individual experiences damage to mucous membrane or corneal, integumentary, or subcutaneous tissue. See also Altered Oral Mucous Membrane.

Related Factors

Altered circulation
Nutritional deficit/excess
Fluid deficit/excess
Knowledge deficit
Impaired physical mobility
Irritants
  Chemical (including body excretions, secretions, medications)
  Thermal (temperature extremes)
  Mechanical (pressure shear, friction)
  Radiation (including therapeutic radiation)

Defining Characteristics

Damaged or destroyed tissue (cornea, mucous membrane, integumentary, or subcutaneous)

Expected Patient Outcomes & Nursing Interventions*

Regain tissue integrity, as evidenced by:

Subcutaneous tissue intact
Skin color and temperature consistent with unaffected tissue
For cornea, vision returned to previous status, without photophobia
- Inspect area of impaired integrity for redness, edema, purulent exudate, granulation tissue.

*References: 1, 3-5, 11, 14, 16, 21, 25, 29, 31, 33-35.

- Assess peripheral pulses and capillary refill supplying affected area.
- Assess sensation of affected area.
- Assess lesion for depth and classify pressure ulcers into Stage II or Stage IV. Stage III is full thickness skin loss involving damage to and necrosis of subcutaneous tissue that may extend down to but not through the underlying fascia. The ulcer appears as a deep crater with or without undermining of adjacent tissue.[1]
- Stage IV is full thickness loss with extensive destruction, tissue necrosis, or damage to muscle, bone, or supporting structures.[1]
- Monitor patient's continence status and minimize exposure of the skin impairment site to moisture of incontinence, perspiration, and wound drainage.
- Monitor laboratory data (e.g., hemoglobin, hematocrit, albumin, glucose, blood urea nitrogen [BUN], creatinine, liver enzymes, arterial blood gases) for evidence of malnutrition or chronic conditions that could affect the skin.
- Determine attitudes and reactions of patient and significant others to skin lesion.
- Encourage verbalization about feelings and discuss effect of lesion on self-esteem.
- Provide wound treatment based on stage and drainage, using gauze, polyurethane film, hydrocolloid, foam, adsorptive dressing, hydrogel, or enzymatic therapy.
- Debride and clean wound as ordered.
- Ambulate patients if possible.
- When in bed turn every 2 hours, use lateral, prone, and dorsal sides if possible.
- Have patient perform active range of motion exercises or instruct family to perform passive range of motion.
- Position off pressure ulcer.
- Use pressure-relieving therapy bed.
- Keep pressure off skeletal prominences by positioning patients with pillows and/or foam devices, or pressure-relieving mattresses.
- Use lifting devices and/or sheets to position patients, to prevent shearing force on skin.
- Do not massage skin over bony prominences.
- Prevent head of bed from being elevated more than 30 degrees (semi-Fowler's position) for long periods.
- Use underpads or briefs that absorb moisture and leave quick drying surface toward skin if continuously moist.
- Avoid use of donuts or rubber rings.
- Provide nutrients: proteins, including albumin; carbohydrates; fats; vitamins A, B complex, C, and K; and minerals: iron, zinc, and copper.

Corneal Tissue
- Examine the cornea.
- Maintain patches over eyes when there is no drainage from the eye.
- Administer atropine or scopolamine as ordered *to dilate pupil, thereby resting ciliary body and iris.*

- Administer topical or systemic steroids and antibiotics as ordered *to reduce inflammation.*

Communicate care of impaired tissue after discharge and action to prevent recurrence, as evidenced by patient and family explaining:

Causes and prevention of impaired tissue integrity
Medications and treatments for home use
Dietary intake to promote wound healing
Plan for follow-up care
- Instruct patient and family on the following:
    Care of the lesion
    Purpose and side effects of medications
    How to prevent tissue damage
    Plans for follow-up care

Principles and Rationale for Nursing Interventions*

Assess circulation to determine adequacy of blood supply to affected area. Absence of sensation allows injuries to go undetected due to absence of pain. The stage of the wound (e.g., III or IV) provides the basis for treatment. The size and color of the wound are documented to evaluate the healing process. Tissue integrity can be impaired by infection as indicated by elevated leukocyte count, foul odor, or purulent exudate from the wound.

The skin is kept clean and dry to remove bacteria and prevent maceration from excessive moisture. Monitor the patient's continence status and minimize exposure of skin to moisture from incontinence, perspiration, and drainage. If the patient is incontinent, implement an incontinence management plan to prevent exposure to chemicals in urine and stool that can erode skin; refer patient to physician for incontinence diagnosis and treatment.[29] Moisture of the skin is maintained internally by intake of at least 2 liters of fluids daily, unless contraindicated, and externally by lubricating the skin with lotion.

Adequate tissue oxygenation can be determined by hemoglobin, hematocrit, and arterial blood gases. Adequate nutrition is reflected in a normal serum albumin. High glucose may indicate diabetes mellitus, which interferes with wound healing. Elevated liver enzymes may indicate liver disease, which decreases albumin produced, contributes to fluid retention, and slows drug metabolism. Elevated BUN and creatinine may indicate renal disease, which contributes to fluid retention.

A positive mental attitude can improve immune function and increase motivation for healing. Thus, discussions of patient's feelings toward skin lesions can further the wound healing efforts.

Topical treatments act to stimulate tissue granulation, debride the wound, and prevent loss of plasma and fluids from the wound, while systemic antiinfectives treat or prevent infection of the wound.

Circulation to the skin is maintained by moving, turning, and exercising. Circulation is maintained when the patient can ambulate or perform active range of motion. When this is not possible, passive range of motion exercises and periodic turning are needed to stimulate circulation and relieve pressure. The use of pillows, foam wedges and pressure-reducing devices in the bed are recommended.[21] Conclusions drawn from several studies indicate that (1) the standard hospital mattress exerts high pressures in all pressure-prone sites (sacrum, trochanter, and heel) and all positions and should not be used for patients at risk for pressure ulcers; (2) higher sacral pressures are created when the patient is in the semi-Fowler's position than the supine position, thus prolonged semi-Fowler's position must be avoided even though a special mattress or overlay is in use; and (3) despite the use of special mattresses or overlays, additional pressure-relieving devices may be needed to protect heels from pressure ulcers.[11,21,25,31] When additional protection is used for heels, the skin over the heels and lateral and medial malleoli should be inspected for red areas and excessive moisture from perspiration. Massage over bony prominences formerly was recommended, however, scientific evidence for using massage to stimulate blood and lymph flow and avert pressure ulcer formation is not well established, whereas there is preliminary evidence suggesting that it may lead to deep tissue trauma.[21]

Nutrients promote collagen synthesis. Collagen fibers create cross-links and overlapping to fill the gaps of wounds and increase the strength of wounds. Protein aids in neovascularization, collagen synthesis, lymph formation, and fibroblast proliferation that improves resistance to infection and tissue granulation. Albumin controls osmotic pressure to reduce edema that slows oxygen diffusion and transport of vitamins and minerals. Proteins aid in cell proliferation and phagocytic activity of white blood cells to increase resistance to infection. Carbohydrates also provide energy for tissue granulation. Fat is essential as a source of cellular energy.[16]

Vitamins A, B complex, and C are needed. Vitamin A facilitates collagen synthesis and epithelialization. The B vitamins facilitate antibody and white blood cell formation and form enzymes necessary for metabolism of protein, fat, and carbohydrate and increases resistance to infection. Vitamin C improves capillary formation and decreases capillary fragility, is essential for neutrophil production, and facilitates epithelialization of tissue.[16]

Minerals include iron, zinc, and copper. Iron is needed for collagen synthesis and prevention or treatment of anemia. Adequate iron stores are needed to make heme to carry oxygen to tissues. Zinc promotes collagen formation and epithelialization. Copper also promotes collagen formation.[16]

When the cornea is damaged, the nurse assesses the eye for drainage, photophobia, and reports of pain. Patches are not used when the eye is draining because if the drainage remains in the eye, it could become infected. A patch may be placed over the eye when no drainage is noted, especially when the patient reports photophobia. Atropine or scopolamine is given to dilate the pupil to rest the ciliary body and iris. Antibiotics and steroids are given as ordered to treat the inflammatory processes.[13]

---

*References 1, 3-5, 11, 14, 16, 21, 25, 29, 31, 33-35.

The nurse instructs the patient and family on actions to prevent tissue impairment and to continue treatment after discharge. Time is needed for the family and patient to perform return demonstrations of dressing changes and to ask questions about treatment schedules, nutrition, administration of medications, and side effects.

RISK FOR ALTERED BODY TEMPERATURE[14]

Risk for altered body temperature is a state in which an individual is at risk for failure to maintain body temperature within normal range.

Risk Factors

Extremes of age
Extremes of weight
Exposure to cold/cool or warm/hot environments
Dehydration
Inactivity or vigorous activity
Medications causing vasoconstriction/vasodilation, altered metabolic rate, sedation
Inappropriate clothing for environmental temperature
Illness or trauma affecting temperature regulation

Expected Patient Outcome & Nursing Interventions[1,14,19,27]

Maintain normal body temperature, as evidenced by:

Body temperature within normal limits
Demonstration of behaviors for monitoring and maintaining expected body temperature

- Monitor vital signs: temperature, pulse, blood pressure, and respiratory rate.
- Monitor laboratory data (e.g., leukocytes) suggestive of infection or inflammation.
- Determine cause of risk for altered temperature.
- Assess patient for signs of hypothermia: cool skin, piloerection, pallor, slow capillary refill, cyanotic nailbeds, decreased mentation.
- Assess patient for hyperthermia: visual disturbances, headache, nausea and vomiting, muscle flaccidity, hot dry skin, delirium.
- Adjust bedding and clothing as appropriate for patient's temperature.
- Administer antipyretics as ordered.
- Apply external cooling measures, cooling blankets, ice packs to groin and axilla.
- Provide adequate nutrition and fluid. Administer intravenous fluids at room temperature.
- Teach family members how to recognize signs of changing temperature and interventions to maintain expected temperatures.

Principles and Rationale for Nursing Interventions[1,14,19,27]

For patients at risk, the nurse collects data to determine the adequacy of the patient's autoregulatory system. This is accomplished by monitoring temperature, pulse, blood pressure, and respiration for changes over time. Signs of hypothermia or hyperthermia may help to determine the cause of the alteration. Hypothermia is associated with decreases in vital signs, and hyperthermia is associated with increases. Elevations in leukocytes may indicate infection or inflammation that may increase body temperature. Adjustments in sheets and blankets as well as clothing are performed to facilitate warming or cooling to maintain expected body temperature. Interventions to lower elevated temperatures include antipyretics, such as aspirin, which alter the hypothalamus to lower temperature; external cooling blankets and ice packs facilitate loss of heat created by fever. Fluid administration is important to maintain a normal balance and prevent fluid loss from fever due to increased insensible loss and perspiration. Consult principles for the nursing diagnoses of hypothermia and hyperthermia.

Consider the age of the patient; premature infants and neonates have more difficulty maintaining body temperature due to rapid metabolism for body size. Older adults have difficulty maintaining body heat due to less subcutaneous fat to maintain body heat and a slower metabolic rate.

Family members need instruction on how to attain goals set to maintain normothermia, both how to recognize changes in temperature and how to maintain desired body temperature of patient.

INEFFECTIVE THERMOREGULATION

Ineffective thermoregulation is a state in which an individual's temperature fluctuates between hypothermia and hyperthermia.

Related Factors

Trauma or illness
Immaturity
Aging
Fluctuating environmental temperature

Defining Characteristics

Fluctuations in body temperature above or below normal range
See also defining characteristics of hypothermia and hyperthermia.

Expected Patient Outcomes & Nursing Interventions[1,14,15,23,24]

Maintain normothermia as evidenced by:

Temperature within expected range

- Assess neurologic status: level of consciousness, mental status, motor and sensory status.

- Assess vital signs: temperature, pulse, blood pressure, and respirations.
- Assess for signs of hypothermia: difficult arousal, irritability, lethargy, cyanotic nailbeds, slow capillary refill time, pallor, cool skin, bradycardia. Additional signs for premature infant: poor feeding, increase or decrease in spontaneous activity, weak cry, decreased muscle tone.
- Assess for signs of hyperthermia: visual disturbances, headache, nausea and vomiting, muscle flaccidity, hot, dry skin, and delirium.
- Adjust bedding and clothing as appropriate for patient's temperature.
- Adjust environmental temperature to infant's needs using an incubator or radiant warmer; avoid drafts and cold environments; keep infant clothed in undershirt, diaper, gown, and hat.
- Administer intravenous fluids at room temperature.
- Administer electrolytes and medications as ordered to restore or maintain body function.
- Teach family members how to recognize signs of changing temperature and interventions to maintain expected temperatures.

Principles and Rationale for Nursing Interventions[1,14,15,23,24]

Changes in neurologic status may be evident as thermoregulation changes, with lethargy associated with hypothermia and delirium associated with hyperthermia. Likewise, changes in vital signs reflect the body temperature with a decrease in heart rate, blood pressure, temperature, and respiration during hypothermia and an increase in vital signs during hyperthermia. Monitoring of signs of hypothermia and hyperthermia may help to determine the cause of the thermoregulatory imbalance.

Adjustments in sheets, blankets, and clothing are performed to facilitate warming or cooling to maintain expected body temperature. For example premature infants have an immature hypothalamus, which impairs thermoregulation. Head covers are particularly important in premature infants because 60% of heat loss occurs through the head. Other clothing prevents heat loss by evaporation and radiation for adults and infants. Fluids are important to maintain normal fluid and electrolyte balance. Fluid at room temperature prevent cooling caused by entry of cool fluid into the vascular system.

Family members need instruction on how to recognize changes in temperature, and how to maintain desired body temperature of patient.

■ HYPERTHERMIA[14]

Hyperthermia is a state in which an individual's body temperature is elevated above his/her normal range.

Related Factors

Exposure to hot environment
Vigorous activity

Medications/anesthesia
Inappropriate clothing
Increased metabolic rate
Illness or trauma
Dehydration
Inability or decreased ability to perspire

Defining Characteristics

Increase in body temperature above normal range
Flushed skin
Warm to touch
Increased respiratory rate
Tachycardia
Seizures/convulsions

Expected Patient Outcomes & Nursing Interventions[1,14,15,22,23]

Regain normal body temperature, as evidenced by:

Normal body temperature
- Measure core body temperature.
- Assess for shivering and complaint of chills.
- Assess neurologic status: level of consciousness, mental status, motor and sensory status.
- Assess for signs of hyperthermia: visual disturbances, headache, nausea and vomiting, muscle flaccidity, hot, dry skin, delirium, seizures.
- Assess heart rate and rhythm for abnormalities.
- Monitor respirations. Hyperventilation may occur initially, but ventilation may be impaired by seizures and hypermetabolic state.
- Inspect and palpate skin for color and temperature.
- Monitor complete blood count especially leukocyte, hemoglobin, and hematocrit.
- Administer antipyretics as ordered.
- Promote surface cooling by removal of clothing and use of fans.
- When fever is over 104° F (40° C) use alcohol, tepid baths, immersion, or local ice packs to groin and axilla.
- Use hypothermia blanket when patient's temperature is greater than 105° F (40.5° C) or when fever is caused by hypothalamic dysfunction.
- Administer medication (e.g., diazepam, chlorpromazine) to control shivering and seizures.
- Administer supplemental oxygen as ordered.
- Administer medications (e.g., antibiotics for infections, dantrolene for malignant hyperthermia, beta blockers for thyroid storm) to treat underlying conditions.
- Administer fluids and electrolytes orally or parenterally.
- Encourage frequent rest periods.
- Provide a high calorie diet.
- Provide frequent oral hygiene.
- Teach patient and family the value of fever (up to an oral temperature of 104° F [40° C]) in increasing immune system function.

- Teach use of antipyretics as most effective way to reduce fever to below 104° F (40° C) caused by infection or inflammation.
- Teach use of non-drug methods to reduce fever.
- Discuss importance of adequate fluids to prevent dehydration.
- Review signs and symptoms of hyperthermia and when to call physician.

Principles and Rationale for Nursing Interventions[1,14,15,22,23]

Rectal and tympanic temperatures more closely approximate core temperature; however, abdominal temperature monitoring may be used in premature neonates. Shivering and chills indicate a rising body temperature. For every degree of temperature elevation up to 104° F (40° C), there is a proportional increase in immune system function.[15] Heart and respiratory rates are elevated because the metabolic rate increases during fever. Heart rate and rhythm may change due to electrolyte imbalance, dehydration, specific action of catecholamines, and direct effects of hyperthermia on blood and cardiac tissue. The skin is warm and may appear flushed due to vasodilation of peripheral blood vessels. An increased leukocyte count may indicate infection or inflammation as a cause of fever. Hemoglobin and hematocrit may be elevated due to dehydration from fluid lost through perspiration. Antipyretics (aspirin, acetaminophen, ibuprofen) are effective in lowering fever by direct action on the hypothalamus. Remove extra bedding and clothing so that body heat will not be retained. A fan in the patient's room increases air circulation, which reduces body heat by convection. When the temperature is greater than 104° F (40° C) ice bags to the groin and axilla facilitate heat loss by conduction. A tepid bath reduces fever by evaporation of heat. A cooling blanket is used when fever is over 105° F (40.5° C), cannot be reduced by antipyretics, or is neurologically related.

Oxygen is given to offset increased demands of fever. Fluids are given to replace those lost by insensible water loss and perspiration. Rest is encouraged to prevent increased metabolic need and to facilitate function of immune system. A high calorie diet is provided to meet the increased metabolic needs during fever and the healing process. Oral hygiene is important because the oral mucous membranes easily become dehydrated during fever.

Family and patient education are important to actively engage them in care and to prepare them for care at home. Education should include recognizing signs of fever, ways to treat fever using both non-drug methods and antipyretics, importance of fluids to prevent dehydration, and when to call physician.

■ HYPOTHERMIA[14]

Hypothermia is a state in which an individual's temperature is reduced below normal range but not below 96.1° F (35.6° C; rectal 97.5 °F (36.4 ° C; rectal, newborn).

Hypothermia has been arbitrarily defined as a core body temperature of less than 95° F (35° C) and can be considered mild, moderate, or severe. Mild hypothermia ranges from 91.4° to 96.8° F (33° to 36° C) moderate hypothermia from 86° to 91.4° F (30° to 33° C) and severe hypothermia from 80.6° to 86° F (27° to 30° C).

Although used historically as a treatment modality for a variety of disorders because of the resultant decrease in metabolic rate and endocrine functions, hypothermia as discussed here relates to accidental or unintentional hypothermia and the need for its prompt recognition and treatment.

Related Factors

Exposure to cold environment
Illness or trauma
Inability or decreased ability to shiver
Malnutrition
Inadequate clothing
Consumption of alcohol
Medications causing vasodilation
Evaporation from skin in cool environment
Decreased metabolic rate
Inactivity
Aging

Defining Characteristics

Shivering (mild)
Cool skin
Pallor (moderate)
Slow capillary refill
Tachycardia
Cyanotic nail beds
Hypertension
Piloerection

Expected Patient Outcomes & Nursing Interventions[1,14,15,18,26]

Regain normal body temperature

- Assess temperature using low-recording thermometer if necessary.
- Monitor heart rate, respiration, and blood pressure for increases as the patient's temperature rises.
- Monitor signs of hypothermia: shivering, cool skin, piloerection, pallor, slow capillary refill, cyanotic nail beds, decreased mentation.
- Monitor arterial blood gases for respiratory acidosis.
- Auscultate lungs for crackles and rhonchi.
- Control shivering when patient has cerebral edema.
- Perform passive warming (e.g., set room temperature between 70° and 75° F (21.1° C to 24.0° C), layer clothing and blankets, cover patient's head with a cap or towel); allow patient to rewarm at his or her own pace.

- Perform active rewarming: cover patient with warmed cotton blankets or a forced warm air blanket; use radiant heat lights as available. As ordered, apply hydrothermic blankets, administer heated and humidified oxygen, and carefully administer heated intravenous fluids.
- Perform active core rewarming techniques as ordered (e.g., colonic lavage, hemodialysis, peritoneal lavage, extracorporeal blood rewarming, bladder irrigations).
- Make referral to social service as needed to locate shelter and food for patient.

Principles and Rationale for Nursing Interventions[1,14,15,18,26]

Vital signs are decreased during hypothermia. Monitoring temperature is an objective way to evaluate therapeutic outcomes of interventions. The circulating blood volume slows, causing decreased cardiac output and reduced tissue oxygen delivery. Hypoxia, metabolic acidosis, and intrinsic irritability of the myocardium result in various dysrhythmias. Arterial blood gases are monitored for hypoxia, metabolic acidosis from hypoxia, and respiratory acidosis from depression of the medulla oblongata. Lungs are auscultated because bronchopneumonia is a common complication of hypothermia. Shivering increases intracranial pressure and must be controlled when the patient has cerebral edema.

Passive rewarming prevents heat loss via radiation and evaporation. Head cover is important because 60% of heat is lost through the top of the head. Gradual rewarming limits complications associated with hypothermia. Active rewarming enhances heat gain by radiation, conduction, convection, and evaporation, while active core rewarming techniques increase heat gain by conduction.

Hypothermia is often unrecognized and appropriate treatment is delayed, because the thermometer may be incorrectly used or may not register the patient's actual temperature if it is below the lowest number on a standard thermometer. However, recognition of the scope of the problem is increasing and new advances in therapy are being discovered, such as core rewarming. The aging of the population and the increase in the number of homeless persons, as well as the popularity of winter sports, are factors that necessitate a thorough understanding of the symptoms of hypothermia. Trauma victims also frequently become hypothermic, since treatment rooms are kept cool and the victim is uncovered while being treated.

The most obvious consequence of hypothermia is a decrease in the basal metabolic rate, falling to 50% of normal at 28° C (82.4° F). Shivering, which is the most obvious early symptom of the lowering of the core temperature, is an attempt by the muscles to provide a large amount of heat, with associated vasodilation, increased blood flow, and delivery of warmed blood to the core.[12] Partly in response to shivering in the early stages of hypothermia and partly because of sympathoadrenal stimulation, early symptoms are tachycardia with a gradual decline in heart rate and cardiac output as temperature falls. A lowered body temperature causes an increased affinity of hemoglobin for oxygen, impairing the release of oxygen to tissue. The principles governing heat loss are critical to the understanding of hypothermia: conduction, convection, radiation, and evaporation of water.

References

Nutritional-metabolic

1. Ackley BJ, Ladwig GB: *Nursing Diagnosis Handbook: A Guide to Planning Care,* ed 2, St Louis, 1995, Mosby.
2. Baker DM: Assessment and management of impairments in swallowing, *Nurs Clin North Am* 28:793, 1993.
3. Bergstrom N et al: The Braden scale for predicting pressure sore risk, *Nurs Res* 36(4):205, 1987.
4. Bergstrom N et al: Treatment of pressure ulcers, Clinical Practice Guidelines, No 15, Rockville, MD, December, 1994, Agency for Health Care Policy and Research, Public Health Service, US Department of Health and Human Services (AHCPR Publication No. 95-0652).
5. Bryant R: *Acute and chronic wounds,* St Louis, 1993, Mosby.
6. Chitty KK: The primary prevention role of the nurse in eating disorders, *Nurs Clin North Am* 26:789, 1991.
7. Cullen L: Interventions related to fluid and electrolyte balance, *Nurs Clin North Am* 27(2):569, 1992.
8. Doenges ME, Moorhouse MF: *Nurse's pocket guide: nursing diagnoses with interventions,* ed 5, Philadelphia, 1996, FA Davis.
9. Giota MP: Nutrition during pregnancy: reducing obstetric risk, *J Perinat Neonat Nurs* 6(4):1, 1993.
10. Grodner M, Anderson SL, DeYoung S: *Foundation and clinical applications of nutrition: A nursing approach,* St Louis, 1996, Mosby.
11. Hedrick-Thompson J, Halloran T, Strader MK, and McSweeney M: Pressure-reduction products: making appropriate choices, *J Enterstomal Therapy Nurs* 20(6):239, 1993.
12. Himes JH, Dietz WH: Guidelines for overweight in adolescent preventive services: recommendations from an expert committee, *Am J Clin Nutr* 54:307, 1994.
13. Karvetti R, Knuts L: Validity of estimated food diary: comparison of 2-day record and observed food and nutrient intake, *J Am Diet Assoc* 92(5):580, 1992.
14. Kim MJ, McFarland GK, McLane MA: *Pocket guide to nursing diagnoses,* ed 6, St Louis, 1995, Mosby.
15. Kluger MJ: The adaptive value of fever. In Mackowiak PA, editor: *Fever: basic mechanisms and management,* New York, 1991, Raven Press.
16. Konstantinides NN, Lehmann S: The impact of nutrition on wound healing, *Crit Care Nurs,* 13(5):25, 1993.
17. Kostas GG: *The balancing act: nutrition and weight guide,* Dallas, 1993, Cooper Clinic.
18. Lawson L: Hypothermia and trauma injury: temperature monitoring and rewarming strategies, *Crit Care Nurs Q* 15(1):21, 1992.
19. Metheny NM: *Fluid and electrolyte balance: nursing considerations* ed 2, Philadelphia, 1992, JB Lippincott.
20. *Nutrition intervention manual for professionals caring for older Americans,* Washington, DC, 1929, Nutrition Screening Initiative.
21. Panel for Prediction and Prevention of Pressure Ulcers in Adults: *Pressure ulcers in adults: prediction and prevention. Clinical Practice Guidelines, No. 3,* Rockville, Md, May, 1992, Agency for Health Care Policy and Research, Public Health Service, US Department of Health and Human Services (AHCPR Publication No. 92-0047).
22. Porth A, Erickson M: Physiology of thirst and drinking: implications for nursing practice, *Heart Lung* 21(3):273, 1992.
23. Roberts NJ: The immunological consequences of fever. In Mackowiak PA, editor: *Fever: basic mechanisms and management,* New York, 1991, Raven Press.
24. Roncoli M, Medoff-Cooper B: Thermoregulation in low birth weight infants, *NAACOG's Clin Issues* 3(1):25, 1992.
25. Sideranko S, Quinn A, Burns K, Froman R: Effects of position and mattress overlay on sacral and heel pressures in a clinical population, *Res Nurs Health* 15:245, 1992.

26. Stevens T: Managing post-operative hypothermia, rewarming and its complications, *Crit Care Nurs Q* 16(1):60, 1993.
27. Thompson J, Wilson S: *Health assessment for nursing practice,* St Louis, 1996, Mosby.
28. Tombs MB, Gallucci B: The effects of hydrogen peroxide rinses on the normal oral mucosa, *Nurs Res* 42(9):246, 1993.
29. Urinary Incontinence Guideline Panel: *Urinary incontinence in adults: Clinical Practice Guidelines.* Rockville, Md, March, 1992, Agency for Health Care Policy and Research, Public Health Service, US Department of Health and Human Services (AHCPR Publication No. 92-0038).
30. US Department of Agriculture, US Department of Health and Human Services: *Nutrition and your health: dietary guidelines for Americans,* ed 3, Home and Garden Bulletin No. 232, 1990, Washington, DC, US Government Printing Office.
31. Whittemore R, Bautista C, Smith C, Bruttomesso K: Inter-face pressure measurements of support surfaces with subjects in the supine and 45-degree Fowler positions, *J Enterstomal Therapy Nurs* 20(3):111, 1993.
32. Williams MJ, Walker GT: Managing swallowing problems in the home, *Caring* 11:59, 1992.
33. Wound, Ostomy, and Continence Nurses Society: *Standards of care: dermal wounds: pressure ulcers,* Costa Mesa, CA, 1992, WOCN.
34. Wound, Ostomy, and Continence Nurses Society: *Standards of care: patient with fecal incontinence,* Costa Mesa, CA, 1994, WOCN.
35. Wound, Ostomy, and Continence Nurses Society: *Standards of care: patient with urinary incontinence,* Costa Mesa, CA, 1992, WOCN.

Risk for aspiration

1. Bartlett JG: Aspiration pneumonia. In Baum GL, Wolinsky E, editors: *Textbook of pulmonary diseases,* ed 4, Boston, 1989, Little, Brown.
2. Bockus S: Trouble shooting your tube feedings, *Am J Nurs* 91(5):24, 1991.
3. Bresilin EH, Lery MJ: Prevention and treatment of aspiration pneumonitis secondary to massive gastric aspiration, *Crit Care Q* 6:73, 1983.
4. Cherniack RM: *Pulmonary testing function,* ed 2, Philadelphia, 1992, Saunders.
5. Goodnough SC: Reducing tracheal injury and aspiration, *Dimens Crit Care* 7(6):324, 1988.
6. Gorback MS: What we still don't know about the risk of aspiration, *Curr Rev Nurs Anesth* 14(6):43, 1991.
7. Hudack CM, Gallo BM: *Critical care nursing: a holistic approach,* ed 6, Philadelphia, 1994, Lippincott.
8. Ibanez J et al: Gastroesophageal reflux in intubated patients receiving enteral nutrition: effect of supine and semi-recumbent positions, *JPEN* 16;419, 1992.
9. Kim MK, McFarland GK, McLane, AM: *Pocket guide to nursing diagnosis,* ed 6, St Louis, 1995, Mosby.
10. McCloskey JC, Buelechek GM: *Iowa intervention project: nursing interventions classification (NIC),* ed 2, St Louis, 1996, Mosby.
11. Montecalvo MA et al: Nutritional outcome and pneumonia in critical care patients randomized to gastric versus jejunal tube feedings, *Crit Care Med* 20(10):1377, 1992.
12. Mullan H et al: Risks of pulmonary aspiration among patients receiving enteral nutrition support, *JPEN* 16(2):160, 1992.
13. Potts RG et al: Comparison of blue dye visualization and glucose oxidase test strip methods for detecting pulmonary aspiration of enteral feedings in intubated patients, *Chest* 103(1):117, 1993.
14. Saleh KL: Practical points in understanding aspiration, *J Post Anesth Nurs* 6(5):347, 1991.
15. Waugaman WR, Jordan LM, Tallman RD Jr, Burckner TA: Does the employed technique of endotracheal extubation reduce the risk of aspiration? *Nurse Anesth* 1(1):5, 1990.
16. Wooldridge J: Nursing diagnosis: Potential for aspiration. In Carroll-Johnson RM, editor: *Classification of nursing diagnoses: proceedings of the eighth conference,* Philadelphia, 1989, Lippincott.

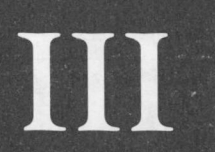

Elimination

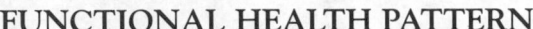

COLONIC CONSTIPATION

Colonic constipation is the state in which an individual's pattern of elimination is characterized by a hard, dry stool that results from a delay in passage of food residue.

The term "colonic constipation" reflects the importance of etiologic factors in making a diagnosis and in designing specific nursing interventions. It is generally accepted that etiologies are inferred from subjective and objective data and that etiologies influence the selection of interventions. The use of the term "colonic constipation" captures a difference between closely related phenomena; it is more functional than the all-purpose label "constipation."[9,11,13]

Colonic constipation is the result of a delay in the passage of food residue in the gastrointestinal tract (decrease in transit time). Low fiber in the daily diet, inadequate liquids (less than six glasses per day), and a sedentary life-style delay the transit time of the products of digestion. Transit time may also be prolonged by mechanical obstruction, defective innervation, iatrogenic effects of drugs, metabolic disorders, depression, and perhaps the physiologic effects of aging. The effect of normal aging on the transit time in the entire large bowel has not been demonstrated.[9,11,13]

Related Factors[6]

Inadequate fluid intake
Changes in dietary intake
Inadequate fiber in diet
Missed meals, change in mealtimes
Inadequate physical activity
Immobility
Lack of privacy
Emotional disturbances
Chronic use of medications, laxatives, and enemas
Stress
Change in daily routine
Metabolic problems (e.g., hypothyroidism, hypocalcemia, hypokalemia)

Defining Characteristics[6]

Decreased frequency of bowel elimination
Hard, dry stool
Straining at stool
Painful defecation
Abdominal distention
Palpable mass
Rectal pressure
Headache; appetite impairment
Abdominal pain
Blood with stool

Expected Patient Outcomes & Nursing Interventions

Describes health behaviors that prevent constipation in relation to diet, fluid, exercise; contributing factors, when known; and methods to reduce contributing factors, as evidenced by:

Explaining importance of well-balanced diet, including importance of eating breakfast
Describing importance of bulk in diet through ingestion of dietary fiber and bran
Naming six readily available foods high in fiber
Discussing importance of including eight to ten glasses of fluid in daily intake
Recognizing and integrating daily exercise into life-style (15-minute walk per day minimum amount)
Describing individual stimulus behaviors (e.g., warm fluids on arising; prune juice) that are helpful in initiating bowel movement
Expressing the importance of responding to defecation urge when it arises naturally
Understanding the physiology of defecation
Naming conditions that promote normal bowel functioning as well as those that contribute to development of constipation
  • Provide instruction for:
     Appropriate use of bulk in diet
     Adequate daily fluid intake
     Appropriate level of exercise for age and physiologic status
     Fiber provides bulk and keeps stool soft through mechanism of water absorption.
     The mechanism decreases transit time of stool and decreases water absorbed in large intestine.

Initiate a bowel repatterning program to establish normal bowel functioning, as evidenced by:

Elimination of regular use of laxatives or enemas

Attending to defecation urge when it arises naturally

Consumption of well-balanced diet, including sufficient fiber and laxative foods

Relating following process of bowel repatterning:

Eats high-fiber breakfast; sits on toilet 10 minutes

Establishes a relaxing environment (diversional activities, reading, listening to music)

When defecation urge occurs, responds to it so it does not weaken

- Provide instruction for understanding:

Role of stimulus behaviors

Recognition and attention to stimulus behaviors (e.g., warm fluids on arising)

Drinking warm liquids sets in motion gastroduodenal and defecation reflexes.

Importance of immediate response to defecation urge

Effective position for defecation

- Assist with implementation of new health behaviors relative to good bowel habits, including diet, fluids, exercise, and emotional equilibrium.

Use appropriate therapy to produce a bowel movement within 12 to 24 hours, as evidenced by:

Taking oral laxative correctly

Understanding the desired effects of medication

Making the correct decision, if prescribed therapy is no longer effective

- Provide instruction for appropriate use of oral laxatives (see Table IV-5).
- Assess and monitor side effects of medications.
- Assess and monitor laxative and enema use.

Principles and Rationale for Nursing Interventions

Careful assessment of dietary, medication, fluid consumption, and exercise patterns and potential must precede any intervention. Long-standing habits of eating and mobility must be altered slowly with full commitment from the patient to be effective. Both nurse and patient must be aware of changes that cannot occur and ready to work for an improved life-style within the constraints of chronicity.[3] Dietary bulk should include about 6 to 10 g of fiber each day, but fiber must be added slowly to avoid abdominal cramping and flatus.[9,10] Adequate fluids (2500 ml per day) must accompany fiber intake. Fluids that stimulate diuresis (e.g., coffee, colas) should not be included as part of the required intake. The purchasing and preparation of food must be explored, in addition to consideration of the patient's preferences, before changes can be planned. Sedentary individuals can begin an exercise program by walking 15 to 20 minutes every day. Walking with other people increases physical activity and may be a social stimulus.

Multiple stressors or emotional disturbances that result in life-style upheavals may require referral or prolonged counseling before a routine can be reestablished. Medical intervention may be needed to stabilize endocrine disorders or other illnesses that disrupt daily routines, mobility, or dietary practices. When the patient is irreversibly impaired, the nurse and patient must work together to plan for a bowel retraining program that incorporates abdominal exercises, positioning techniques, and constant elimination monitoring and supervision. Laxatives and enemas may have to be used for some patients to assist with regulation of elimination.

■ PERCEIVED CONSTIPATION

Perceived constipation is the state in which an individual makes a self-diagnosis of constipation and ensures a daily bowel movement through use of laxatives, enemas, and suppositories.[6]

Individuals develop a set of expectations regarding their bowel evacuation patterns based on their past experiences, as well as on family beliefs and practices. Failure to evacuate on a daily basis is the most common contributor to perceived or imagined constipation. Many individuals expect to have a bowel movement on arising or immediately after breakfast. This physiologic and emotional ritual signals the beginning of a healthy day. Concern over the failure to evacuate may result in regular concerted efforts to defecate (straining), and a growing preoccupation with the failure. Use or abuse of laxatives is a typical solution for this concern. Laxatives may be consumed until the person has established a satisfactory elimination pattern and is convinced that regular laxative intake is mandatory. The person may discover that constipation only worsens because chronic laxative abuse may lead to an atonic colon musculature, decreased awareness of the presence of stool in the rectum, and finally authentic constipation.

If a careful assessment has established that real constipation does not exist, further assessment of beliefs, life-style changes, self-treatment measures, and the degree of concern must precede any nursing intervention.

Related Factors[6,13]

Cultural or family health beliefs

Lack of information about normal processes or faulty appraisal

Impaired thought processes

Long-term expectations and habits

Defining Characteristics[6]

Expectation of daily bowel movement with resulting overuse of laxatives, enemas, and suppositories

Expected passage of stool at same time every day

■ TABLE IV-5 Nonprescription Drug Therapy to Relieve Constipation

Generic (Trade) Name	Dosage and Administration	Comments
Bulk-Forming Agents		
Karaya gum	Oral: 5-10 g daily, taken with water	Nonprescription
Methylcellulose, carboxymethylcellulose (Cologel, Hydrolose)	Oral: 4-6 g daily	Nonprescription
Mantago (psyllium) seed	Oral: 2-5 to 30 g daily; add to water and drink rapidly	Nonprescription
Polycarbophil	Oral: 4-6 g daily	Nonprescription
Psyllium hydrocolloid (Effersyllium) Psyllium hydrophilic (Konsyl) Pscilloid (L A Formula, Metamucil, Modane Bulk)	Oral: 1 round tsp (7 g) or 1 packet; add to glass of water and drink rapidly and then follow with second glass of water; repeat 1 or 2 times daily if necessary	Nonprescription
Stimulant (Irritant) Cathartics		
Blacodyl (Biscolax, Dulcolax, various others)	Oral: 10 mg, up to 30 mg may be given to clear gastrointestinal tract Rectal: 10 mg	Nonprescription; initial response in 6 to 12 hr; do not take within 60 min of milk or antacids; rectal administration effective in 15 min
Cascara sagrada (Bileo-Secrin, Cas-Evac)	Oral: 200-400 mg of extract; 0.5-1.5 ml of fluid extract or 5 ml of aromatic extract	Nonprescription; one of the mildest of the stimulant cathartics
Castor oil	Oral: 15-60 ml	Nonprescription; castor oil is degraded to ricinoleic acid, which is the active drug
Castor oil, emulsified (Neoloid)	Oral: 30-60 ml	Nonprescription; mint flavored; turns alkaline urine pink
Damron (Anavac, Danvac, Dorbane, Modane, Weslax)	Oral: 75-150 mg	Nonprescription; turns alkaline urine pink
Glycerine suppositories	Rectal: 3 g	Nonprescription; effective in 15 to 30 min
Phenolphthalein (Chocolax, Exlax, Feen-A-Mint)	Oral: 30-270 mg daily	Nonprescription; turns alkaline urine pink
Senna, whole leaf	Oral: 0.5-2 g or 2 ml of senna fluid extract	Nonprescription
Sennosides A and B (Glysennid)	Oral: 12-24 mg at bedtime	Nonprescription
Saline Cathartics		
Magnesium hydroxide (Milk of magnesia)	Oral: 10-15 ml (concentrated) or 15-30 ml (regular)	Nonprescription
Magnesium sulfate (Epsom salt)	Oral: 15 g in glass of water	Nonprescription
Monosodium phosphate (Sal Hepatica)	Oral: 5-20 ml with water	Nonprescription
Sodium phosphate	Oral: 4 g in glass of warm water	Nonprescription
Sodium phosphate with sodium biphosphate (Phospho-Soda)	Oral: 20-40 ml in glass of cold water	Nonprescription
Lubricants		
Mineral oil (Agoral, Plain; Kondremul, Plain; Neo-Cultol; Petrogalar, Plain)	Oral: 15-30 ml at bedtime	Nonprescription; to ease strain of passing hard stools; should not be used regularly because the fat-soluble vitamins (A, D, E, and K) are not absorbed; response in 1-3 days
Fecal Softeners		
Dioctyl calcium sulfosuccinate (Surfak)	Oral: 50-360 mg daily	Nonprescription
Dioctyl sodium sulfosuccinate (Colace, Comfolax, D-D-S, various others)	Oral: 50-360 mg	Nonprescription

From Clark.[3] (See references for Constipation).

Expected Patient Outcomes & Nursing Interventions

Modify belief about need for daily evacuation, as evidenced by:

Identifying normal variations in bowel elimination

* Help patient identify beliefs and convictions about present bowel habits. Confrontation of erroneous beliefs may confuse patient if health beliefs and convictions are not fully explored.
* Clarify with patient what is viewed as a normal pattern.

Expresses acceptance of present bowel habits, as evidenced by:

Comfort with new elimination pattern.

* Support patient's efforts to monitor difference between real and perceived constipation.

Decrease reliance on laxatives, as evidenced by:

Reporting the taking of laxatives rarely

Describing variety of bulk and fiber foods eaten daily to support regular bowel habits

* Suggest substituting natural bulk and fiber from fruits, grains, and vegetables for laxative being consumed.
* Acknowledge possibility that reduction in use of a laxative may be gradual if there is heavy consumption at present or if patient needs time to relinquish or alter convictions.
* If gradual reduction of laxative use is necessary, establish a schedule with patient.
* Be prepared to provide support in future to review patient's concerns and progress.

Experiences regular, comfortable bowel movements, as evidenced by:

Attainment of previously identified normal elimination schedule

Noting absence of discomfort and straining at defecation

Reporting absence of distention, flatus, or intense feelings of rectal fullness before defecation

Reporting that stools are soft, brown, and regular in caliber

* Assess patient's willingness and interest in altering eating, fluid intake, mobility, or exercise habits.
* If numerous alterations are needed, proceed slowly and establish priorities according to patient's wishes.
* Acknowledge possibility that life-style changes and ensuing elimination routines may alter slowly.
* Enlist support of family or peers to assist patient with change (if agreeable with patient).

Principles and Rationale for Nursing Interventions[3,10,11]

An appraisal of the patient's beliefs and degree of concern about bowel habits is as important as any intervention that follows. Concern about bowel habits may be coupled with other concerns about aging, illness, or physical deterioration. A preoccupation with defecation might be an indicator of boredom or mental alterations that lead to a fixation of this daily event. A mere confrontation with facts and a new regimen may leave the patient confused, suspicious, and ultimately noncompliant if his or her beliefs and convictions about the body and its functions are not fully explored and acknowledged. Patient and nurse must accept the idea that change occurs slowly. The patient needs to believe that control of his or her body is being maintained and that giving up an ingrained habit will not be a health risk.

■ CONSTIPATION

Constipation is the state in which an individual experiences a change in normal bowel habits characterized by a decrease in frequency and/or passage of hard, dry stools.

Since constipation may be a symptom of some underlying disease as well as a functional health problem, a medical evaluation, including abdominal and rectal examinations, should be done to exclude organic causes. Patients with constipation associated with weight loss, abdominal pain, or fresh rectal bleeding, should be referred for medical evaluation. Patients with constipation of recent onset, sudden aggravation of existing constipation with recent abdominal pain, or the passage of blood and mucus in the stools should also be evaluated for organic disease.

Although patients usually diagnose constipation themselves, its true nature is very elusive. Five categories and eight subcategories of indicators reflect the complexity of normal elimination and constipation.[5,9]

    I. Signs and symptoms
      A. Description of constipated stool
        1. Character: qualities of the stool, color, consistency
        2. Amount: amount of stool
        3. Frequency: lapse of time between stools
      B. Feelings and sensations: physical feelings and sensations associated with constipation, e.g., stomachache, bloating
   II. Etiology: contributing factors, e.g., diet, fluids, inadequate exercise, medications, change in routine
  III. Attending behaviors: consistent use of measures for the express purpose of alleviating or preventing constipation
      A. Treatment: measures taken to relieve constipation
      B. Prevention: measures taken to prevent constipation
  IV. Health behaviors: behaviors influencing normal elimination, diet, fluid intake, exercise
   V. Patterning: behaviors related to the production of a bowel movement, including toilet routine
      A. Expected frequency of bowel movement(s)
      B. Time of day of bowel movement(s)

C. Stimulus behaviors
   1. Actions taken to stimulate a bowel movement, short term, within the hour, e.g., drinking hot water
   2. Actions in daily routine that result in a bowel movement, e.g., eating breakfast
D. Response to reflexes: behaviors in response to the urge to defecate

Related Factors[6]

Less than adequate fluid intake
Less than adequate dietary intake and bulk
Less than adequate physical activity; immobility
Personal habits
Lack of privacy
Pregnancy
Emotional status
Chronic use of medication and enemas
Pain on defecation
Diagnostic procedures
Neuromuscular impairment
Musculoskeletal impairment
Weak abdominal musculature
Chronic obstructive lesions
Decreased activity level
Use of laxatives

Defining Characteristics[6]

Frequency less than usual pattern
Hard formed stool
Palpable mass
Reported feeling of pressure in rectum
Reported feeling of rectal fullness
Straining at stool
Abdominal distention
Abdominal pain
Appetite impairment
Back pain
Headache
Interference with daily living (consequence)
Decreased bowel sounds
Less than usual amount of food

Expected Patient Outcomes & Nursing Interventions[10]

Describes health behaviors that prevent constipation in relation to diet, fluid, exercise; contributing factors, when known; and methods to reduce contributing factors, as evidenced by:

Explaining importance of well-balanced diet, including importance of eating breakfast
Describing importance of bulk in diet through ingestion of dietary fiber and bran
Naming six readily available foods that are high in fiber

Discussing importance of including 8 to 10 glasses of fluid in daily intake
Recognizing and integrating daily exercise into life-style (15-minute walk per day minimum amount)
Describing individual stimulus behaviors (e.g., warm fluids on arising, prune juice) that are helpful in initiating bowel movement
Expressing importance of responding to defecation urge when it arises naturally
Understanding physiology of defecation
Naming conditions that promote normal bowel functioning as well as those that contribute to development of constipation
   • Provide instruction for:
      Appropriate use of bulk in diet
      Adequate daily fluid intake
      Appropriate level of exercise for age and physiologic status

Initiate a bowel repatterning program to establish normal bowel functioning, as evidenced by:

Elimination of regular use of laxatives or enemas
Attending to defecation urge when it arises naturally
Consuming well-balanced diet, including sufficient fiber and laxative foods
Relating proces of bowel repatterning:
   Eats high-fiber breakfast; sits on toilet 10 minutes
   Establishes relaxing environment (diversional activities, reading, listening to music)
   When defecation urge occurs, responds to it so it does not lessen
   • Provide instruction for understanding:
      Role of stimulus behaviors
      Recognition and attention to stimulus behaviors (e.g., warm fluids on arising)
      Importance of immediate response to defecation urge
      Effective position for defecation
   • Assist with implementation of new health behaviors relative to good bowel habits, including diet, fluids, exercise, and emotional equilibrium.

Use appropriate oral drug therapy to produce bowel movement within 12 to 24 hours, as evidenced by:

Taking oral laxative correctly[3]
Understanding desired effects of medication
Making the correct decision, if prescribed therapy is no longer effective
   • Provide instruction for appropriate use of oral laxatives (see Table IV-5).
   • Assess and monitor effects of medications.
   • Assess and monitor laxative and enema use.

Principles and Rationale for Nursing Interventions

Health behaviors, such as a well-balanced diet, adequate fluid intake, and exercise, are essential to the promotion of normal bowel functioning. A diet adequate in dietary fiber provides bulk and keeps the stool soft through the mechanism of water absorption. The fiber acts as a bulking agent through its water-binding properties. This mechanism increases the speed at which the stool passes through the intestines. The increased speed decreases the amount of water absorbed by the large intestine, and the stool remains soft and bulky. Some high-fiber foods are whole-grain cereals and breads, leafy vegetables, and raw and cooked fruits. Fruits, such as bananas, prunes, dates, and figs, and rhubarb, are good laxatives and are high in fiber.[10,11]

A healthy person's body fluids (water and electrolytes) are constantly being metabolized and must be replaced to maintain normal processes. Normal fluid intake should be about 2500 ml per day. Of this amount approximately 1000 ml is obtained from water in food, 300 ml from oxidation, and 1200 ml as liquid. These fluids enter the intestines each day, along with saliva, gastric secretions, pancreatic juices, and bile, to comprise total body fluids of 9 to 10 L for absorption of nutrients and electrolytes. The healthy person reabsorbs most of this fluid; only about 100 ml of water is excreted in feces.

Exercise in any form is essential for total body functioning and well-being. Normal defecation depends on adequate muscular strength in the abdominal and pelvic muscles. People who are sedentary, immobile, or debilitated from illness benefit from conditioning exercises to strengthen the muscles of the abdomen and pelvic floor. Lack of tone in abdominal muscles can be corrected by doing sit-ups. These should be done with knees bent and arms flexed behind the head, so as not to put undue strain on the back. Isometric contraction of perineal muscles and the pelvic tilt strengthens muscles of the pelvic floor. Walking briskly for at least 15 minutes a day is the easiest overall exercise.[2] Exercise in the form of strenuous activity is related to preventing an incidence of constipation.

Persons can be educated to use health behaviors for maintaining bowel function that are familiar and have proved helpful, such as drinking a cup of hot liquid before breakfast, drinking prune juice, or using other measures. Many of the measures are based on stimulating physiologic processes and have sound bases for their effectiveness. The practice of drinking warm fluids on arising, for example, sets in motion the duodenocolic, gastrocolic, gastroileal, enterogastric, and defecation reflexes.

When feces are forced into the rectum, the process of defecation is normally initiated, including reflex contraction of the rectum and relaxation of anal sphincters.[10] However, before actual defecation occurs, the conscious mind takes over voluntary control of the external sphincter and either inhibits it to allow the process to occur or further contracts it if the moment is not convenient. When contraction of the external sphincter is maintained, the defecation reflex stops after several minutes and will not return until an additional amount of feces enters the rectum, which may not happen for several more hours.

When the time is more convenient for the person to defecate, defecation reflexes can usually be initiated by taking a deep breath to force the diaphragm downward and then contracting the abdominal muscles to increase abdominal pressure, thereby forcing feces into the rectum to initiate new reflexes.

However, it should be noted that reflexes initiated this way are never as effective as those that arise naturally. For this reason, people who inhibit their natural reflexes often become severely constipated.[10]

Stress and tension can interfere with normal bowel elimination, especially in an already stressful hospital environment. Stimulation of the sympathetic nervous system inhibits gastrointestinal activity, slowing the peristaltic waves yet innervating the internal anal sphincter at the same time. Therefore, during a time of stress, movement is delayed temporarily, but incontinence can occur. Thus, in addition to including measures to decrease stress and ensuring adequate privacy, it is important to provide enough time for a bowel movement. In the acute care setting, treatments and tests are frequently scheduled so closely that the person has no relaxed uninterrupted time for a bowel movement. This situation can be very serious for a person with constipation who has succeeded in developing a satisfactory schedule of elimination, only to have it thoughtlessly disrupted during a hospitalization. This problem can be minimized by making sure that hospitalized patients participate in decision making and planning related to their care.

The most physiologically effective position for defecation is a squatting position in which the pressure of the thighs increases the intraabdominal pressure and thus aids expulsion of the stool. Most adults can achieve this position by leaning forward while sitting on the toilet, but children and short people may find it comfortable to use a footstool to raise their thighs when using the toilet. Some elderly people who find it difficult to use a low seat use an elevated toilet seat to get off the toilet without assistance. A higher toilet seat often means that their feet barely touch the floor; they may therefore need a footstool to flex knees and hips for effective defecation.

Enemas are used when lower bowel and rectal evacuation are indicated in the management of a fecal impaction or to prepare a patient for endoscopic and radiographic tests and surgery. Enemas should not be used regularly for the treatment of constipation. The normal saline enema is the safest, most effective, and best tolerated. Large volumes of normal saline solution, when correctly administered, cleanse the rectum and sigmoid colon with little mucosal irritation or disturbance in fluid and electrolyte balance. Disposable oil-retention enemas are frequently used in small volumes to soften a fecal impaction. Removal of the impaction is easily achieved if the oil-retention enema is followed by a normal saline enema after 4 to 6 hours. Disposable hypertonic saline solution enemas (Fleet) are safe and frequently used. They contain a mixture of sodium phosphates and citrates. They are easy to self-administer and are disposable. They act by drawing water into the lumen from the body in significant quantities so that adequate fluid and electrolyte balance is maintained.[17]

DIARRHEA

Diarrhea is the state in which an individual experiences a change in normal bowel habits characterized by the frequent passage of loose, fluid, unformed stools.

Consistency is a more reliable indicator of diarrhea than frequency, since there is general agreement that loose or watery stools are abnormal. Diarrhea is defined as the passage of over 200 g of stool per day containing 70% to 90% water. Normal stool is 60% to 80% water. An increase in daily rectal water excretion of 100 to 200 ml will markedly alter the frequency and consistency of bowel movements. Acute diarrhea is usually self-limiting, lasting 24 to 48 hours, whereas chronic diarrhea persists for several weeks or is intermittently present for several weeks.

The volume of diarrhea fluid is an important indicator of the mechanism of the diarrhea. Stools of high volume, often exceeding 1 L per day, suggest a small intestinal origin for the diarrhea, whereas a small stool volume suggests a colonic origin, as does the presence of bright blood and mucus.

Related Factors[6]

Acute Diarrhea

Diet alteration
Improper cooking
Spoiled food
Drug reaction
Infection
Ingestion of toxins

Chronic Diarrhea

Lactase deficiency
Laxative abuse
Stress and anxiety
Inflammatory bowel disease
Irritable bowel syndrome
Cancer of colon
Chemotherapeutic agents
Radiation
Gastrointestinal surgery
Malabsorption diseases

Defining Characteristics

Abdominal pain
Cramping
Increased stool frequency
Increased frequency of bowel sounds
Loose, liquid stools
Urgency
Change in color of stool

Expected Patient Outcomes & Nursing Interventions

Achieve relief of symptoms, evidenced by:

A decrease in number of stools; no more than three bowel movements per day
Stool is formed and easy to pass

Free of abdominal pain
- Administer antidiarrheal medication, as prescribed.
- Monitor consistency and frequency of stools.
- Provide instruction for perirectal skin care; use Desitin ointment in affected areas.

Take prescribed medication correctly, as evidenced by:

Schedule taking medications as part of daily activities
Verbalize actions and correct dosage of medication
Report side effects of medication to health professionals
- Provide instruction for use of antidiarrheal medications.
- Assist patient with integration of taking medications as part of daily routine.

Understand mechanism of diarrhea, as evidenced by:

Describe factors associated with diarrhea (infection, side effects of antibiotics, tube feedings, and lactose intolerance)[2]
List two changes in own health practices that affect elimination pattern
- Provide instruction to assist the patient and family with understanding the mechanism of the diarrheal episode.

Ingest adequate fluids and foods, as evidenced by:

Urinary output that is >30 ml/hr
Body weight that stabilizes within normal limits
- Monitor body weight, hydration, and intake and output.

Principles and Rationale for Nursing Interventions

The goals of nursing care include prevention, treatment, health teaching, and repatterning of bowel elimination. Prevention begins with a determination of the etiology or mechanism of the diarrhea; maintenance of fluid, electrolyte, and nutritional status; and assessment of the need for health teaching.

Treatment of acute diarrhea is focused on management of symptoms, elimination of the offending agent, and physician referral, when indicated.[3,4] Antidiarrheal drugs are not recommended for routine use in acute infectious diarrhea because they may delay the natural eradication of the infection.[4] Physician referrals should be made when specific drug therapy is needed, when the diarrhea persists for more than 3 days, when the stool contains blood or has the appearance of steatorrhea, and when patients admit to fecal incontinence. Diarrhea associated with the use of antiinfective agents is normally alleviated when the offending agent is withdrawn. However, some persons continue to have diarrhea associated with cramps, tenderness, and fever because of an overgrowth of anaerobic organisms or the presence of their toxins. Physician consultation is suggested because the individual may have developed pseudomembranous colitis. Tube feeding–induced diarrhea can be controlled by the use of Metamucil or by adjusting the type of tube feeding. Metamucil (1 tbs) may also be used 1-3 times daily to help relieve medication-induced diarrhea and diarrhea associated with irritable bowel syndrome (IBS). Equalactin may help relieve symptoms of IBS by equalizing water balance in the bowel. Physician consultation is strongly recommended prior to using Equalactin for more than 2 days. Lactose-intolerant individuals will experience immediate relief when all lactose is removed from their diet. Although this may seem a simple solution, the actual implementation of a lactose-free diet is complicated by the presence of powdered whey and nonfat dry milk in many medications and food products, including crackers, cookies, cereals, and sausages. Maintaining an adequate fluid and caloric intake may be difficult in more severe cases of diarrhea, and hospitalization for intravenous replacement of fluid and electrolytes might be required.

The type of health teaching required is unique to the situation and to the patient. Initially, sufficient information should be given to the patient and family to help them understand the nature of the problem, treatment objectives, and rationale for laboratory studies, drugs, and supportive care. The patient's history and results of microbiologic studies provide a guide for other patient education programs designed to improve safe handling of food, handwashing techniques, and understanding of the mechanisms of disease transmission at home and when traveling in foreign countries.

Persons with chronic diarrhea associated with irritable bowel syndrome may benefit from individual and group counseling and from learning stress reduction techniques, such as systematic relaxation. It is important to remember that an individual's bowel elimination pattern is a reflection of the total life process and is not comprised of isolated physiologic events.

■ BOWEL INCONTINENCE

Bowel incontinence is the state in which an individual experiences a change in normal bowel habits characterized by involuntary passage of stool.

Persons at high risk for becoming incontinent are the elderly, persons with a low level of awareness, patients with a long-standing dependence on suppositories, individuals with neurologic abnormalities regardless of age, diabetic patients with neuropathy, patients with chronic diarrhea, persons with a history of rectal surgery, especially hemorrhoidectomy and those with a history of trauma to the lumbosacral area.[1,3]

Fecal incontinence is often functionally disabling.[5,8] Social isolation and depression may occur as individuals attempt to cope with odor and continence aids by remaining at home. Patients in long-term care agencies also tend to withdraw from social interaction as they attempt to deal not only with the incontinence but also with the reactions of personnel who continually face the unpleasant task of "cleaning up."

Related Factors[1]

Autoimmune diseases such as myasthenia gravis
Central nervous system disruptions such as stroke
Cognitive-perceptual impairment
Demyelinating diseases

Depression
Diarrhea
Fecal impaction
Loss of sphincter control
Musculoskeletal involvement
Neuromuscular involvement
Severe anxiety
Spinal cord injuries (transient or permanent)

Defining Characteristics[1]

Involuntary passage of stool
Embarrassed conduct
Fecal odor
Stained clothing
Stained bed linens
Decrease in social interaction
Washed underwear

Expected Patient Outcomes & Nursing Interventions

Decrease episodes of incontinence, as evidenced by:

Evacuation of bowel contents regularly, usually every other day
Ingestion of foods and fluids consistent with bowel elimination program, usually high-fiber diet
Maintenance of a log of defecations and episodes of incontinence

- Reduce or eliminate contributing factors, when possible.
- Implement bowel retraining program when bowel sounds return and ileus is resolved, if cord-injured patient.
- Establish evacuation schedule consistent with patient and family preferences.
- Teach patient and family use of laxatives and stool softeners *to aid timing of defecation.*
- Teach use of elimination log *to monitor pattern of defecation.*
- Teach pelvic floor exercises. Pelvic floor exercises are repetitive contraction and relaxation of the anal sphincter and puborectalis muscles; contractions should be maintained for only 3 to 4 seconds because sphincters tend to fatigue. Contraction and relaxation exercises should be performed 25 to 30 times—three times a day.[1,4]

Perirectal skin is normal in appearance, as evidenced by:

Absence of areas of redness, itching, and irritation in perirectal area

- Wash, rinse, and dry area after each incontinent episode.
- Use Desitin Ointment on affected area to relieve itching or pain and to toughen skin.

Reestablish patterns of social interaction, as evidenced by:

Engaging in social activities
Engaging in planning future goals

Free of odor
  • Use continence aids temporarily until elimination pattern is established.
  • Change clothes immediately after an incontinent episode.

Principles and Rationale for Nursing Interventions

Bowel management programs are designed to reduce the unpredictability of fecal incontinence and provide individuals with more security from episodes of incontinence. Reestablishment of continence through a successful bowel training program and the assistance of supportive, understanding nurses who provide privacy and an unhurried atmosphere are the key elements in the treatment of incontinence. The type of bowel retraining program selected for a patient depends on the cause of the incontinence and the preferences of the patient and family. Retraining a cord-injured patient is delayed until bowel sounds have returned and paralytic ileus is resolved.[2,4]

■ ALTERED URINARY ELIMINATION

Altered urinary elimination is the state in which the individual experiences a disturbance in the patterns of urine storage or elimination.

The diagnosis of altered urinary elimination is a broad, nonspecific description of voiding dysfunction. Altered urinary elimination states include specific types of urinary incontinence, urinary retention, sensory disorders of the urinary bladder such as acute or interstitial cystitis, and other dysfunctional voiding conditions. Altered urinary elimination may predate a more specific diagnosis, such as stress or urge incontinence. It also may be used to describe a condition not covered by more specific nursing diagnoses, such as altered patterns of urinary elimination (frequent or infrequent voiding), and sensory disorders of the bladder such as acute cystitis, or the urethral syndrome. Following the diagnosis, the phrase "related to. . . ." is advised to provide a more specific description of altered urinary elimination.

Related Factors[3,14,23]

Incontinence (see specific diagnoses)
  Functional
  Reflex
  Stress
  Urge
  Total
  Stress urinary
  Overflow/paradoxic
  Instability
  Extraurethral/continuous
  (See Chapter 12)
Urinary retention
Urinary tract infections
  Bacterial cystitis
  Fungal cystitis
  Parasitic cystitis
  Chemotherapy-induced cystitis
  Radiotherapy-induced cystitis
  Interstitial cystitis
  Cystitis glandularis
  Cystitis cystica
  Eosinophilic cystitis
  Cystitis emphysematosa
  Pyelonephritis
Inflammation of testis/epididymis
Inflammation of prostate
  Acute bacterial prostatitis
  Chronic bacterial prostatitis
  Nonbacterial prostatitis
  Prostatodynia
Inflammation of urethra
  Gonococcal urethritis
  Nongonococcal urethritis
Urethral syndrome
Bladder outlet obstruction
  Prostatic enlargement
    Benign prostatic hyperplasia
    Prostatic cancer
  Urethral stricture
  Female urethral distortion
Bladder diverticula
Paraurethral diverticula
Urinary fistulas
  Vesicovaginal
  Urethrovaginal
  Vesicoenteric
  Vesicocutaneous
  Ureterovaginal
Urinary ectopia
  Bladder exstrophy
  Hypospadias
  Epispadias
  Ureteral ectopia
Neuropathic bladder dysfunction
  Autonomous neurogenic bladder
  Reflex neurogenic bladder
  Motor paralytic neurogenic bladder
  Sensory paralytic bladder
  Uninhibited neurogenic bladder
Urinary calculi
  Ureteral
  Bladder
Psychogenic states
  Depression
  Attention seeking
  Regression
  Anxiety
  Confusion
  Disorientation
  Hysterical conversions

Constipation
Fecal impaction
Impaired physical mobility
Fluid volume state
  Fluid volume deficit: dehydration
  Fluid volume excess
    Water intoxication
      Syndrome of inappropriate antidiuretic hormone secretion
Polyuria

Defining Characteristics[23]

Failure to store urine (incontinence)
Failure to eliminate urine (urinary retention)
Diurnal urinary frequency (voids more often than every 2 hours)
Urinary infrequency (voids less often than every 6 hours during waking hours)
Dysuria
Strangury
Split stream or spraying stream
Urinary urgency
Urinary hesitancy
Nocturia
Nocturnal enuresis

Expected Patient Outcomes & Nursing Interventions[17,34,36]

(See nursing interventions for Functional Reflex, Stress, Urge, and Total Incontinence)

Patient exhibits behaviors that promote optimal bladder health as evidenced by:

Adequate hydration is maintained.

- Assess the patient's current fluid intake using a record or log.
- Calculate the patient's Recommended Daily Allowance, based on the formula: 30 ml/kg of body weight.[32]
- Advise patients of potential bladder irritants; those at risk of urinary incontinence or sensory disturbances of the bladder should avoid or limit intake of these substances.

Constipation is avoided.

- Assist the patient to maintain adequate hydration as outlined above.
- Advise the patient of dietary sources of fiber and its role in the prevention of constipation.
- Assess the patient's current bowel elimination strategies and remind the patient with recurrent constipation to heed the urge to defecate to promote effective bowel elimination.

Smoking is stopped or never begun.

- Advise the patient to discontinue use of tobacco products to reduce the risk of bladder cancer and urinary incontinence.

Patients at risk for stress urinary incontinence perform pelvic muscle exercises three to seven times per week.

- Advise women at risk for developing stress urinary incontinence that a regular pelvic muscle regimen *may* help to prevent the onset of stress urinary incontinence.
- Advise women who experience stress incontinence that pelvic muscle exercises is expected to alleviate or resolve urinary leakage.
- Advise men who undergo radical prostatectomy for prostate cancer that pelvic muscle exercises *may* alleviate or prevent stress urinary incontinence following surgery.

Resolves incontinence; contains incontinence; maintains skin integrity; reestablishes normal voiding pattern, as evidenced by:

Diurnal voiding patterns: 2 to 4 hours during waking hours
Nocturia limited to two times or less nightly
Fluid intake: 30ml/kg of body weight

- Assess patient's current fluid intake and urinary output.
- Ask patient to keep voiding diary for 7-day period.
- Determine symptoms associated with this alteration of urinary elimination patterns: incontinence, dysuria, stangury, urinary urgency, urinary hesitancy, feelings of incomplete bladder emptying.
- Assess patient's medications that affect urinary elimination.
- Assess strategies patient is currently employing to cope with altered urinary elimination patterns.
- Institute a timed voiding schedule with fluid volume control.
    Have patient void by the clock every 2 to 4 hours, as appropriate.
    Ask patient to keep voiding diary at intermittent periods after initiation of timed voiding schedule, including fluid intake.
- Assist the patient to maintain adequate fluid intake.
- Teach the patient to identify and avoid foods or beverages that intensify urinary urgency and predispose toward incontinent episodes. Instruct the patient to eliminate potential irritants from the diet (coffee, citrus juices, spicy foods, or carbonated beverages) singly *to evaluate their effect on voiding patterns.*
- Consult a continence nurse specialist, urologist, gynecologist, or other continence specialist *to determine the cause of altered patterns of urinary elimination.* Reassure the patient that bladder control problems are *not* a part of normal aging, that they will respond to treatment, and that they may be alleviated or cured with proper care.
- Consult physician concerning referral to mental health care professionals for altered urinary elimination patterns secondary to behavioral or psychogenic causes.
- Consult physician concerning referral to endocrinologist for altered urinary elimination patterns secondary to inappropriate antidiuretic hormone secretion or other fluid electrolyte imbalance caused by hormonal abnormality.

Prevent or resolve urinary tract infection, as evidenced by:

Sterile urine in urine culture

No symptoms of urinary tract infection

- Assess types of urinary tract infections patient experiences and presence of pain and burning on urination.
- Determine if infection is associated with hematuria; fever; testicular, perineal, or scrotal pain; or vaginitis.
- Assess identifiable factors that place patient at increased risk for urinary tract infection: feelings of incomplete bladder emptying, sexual activity, history of urinary calculi, or history of known neurogenic bladder dysfunction or incontinence.
- Assess coping strategies, including medically prescribed regimens, patient uses to deal with urinary tract infections.
- Assess type of infections patient is currently experiencing. Determine if this is first infection or one of several recurrent infections. (See Chapter 12 on p. 988.)
- Establish voiding routine of every 2 hours as needed. Postponing voiding is contraindicated in presence of active bacterial, fungal, or parasitic cystitis.
- Advise the patient with a urinary tract infection to maintain an adequate intake of fluids (30ml/kg of body weight), and to avoid dehydration, which may intensify irritative symptoms, or overhydration, which may reduce the urine's defense mechanisms toward pathogens.
- Provide patient with appropriate expectations for reduction and ablation of symptoms after antiinfective medications are begun. Counsel patient concerning appropriate time to contact physician (typically 72 hours after antiinfective medication is begun) for possible alteration of medication regimen if symptoms persist.
- Advise patient of importance of adherence to antiinfective medication regimen to reduce likelihood of recurrence or persistence of infection.
- Teach patient principal side effects of antiinfective medications: nausea and diarrhea. Advise patient to take antibiotics with meals to reduce nausea and to ingest yogurt, buttermilk, or other appropriate dairy products with active cultures to restore normal intestinal flora.
- Teach patient to recognize allergic reactions to medications (rash, urticaria) and when to consult physician concerning discontinuing medication.
- Teach women proper perineal hygiene: wipe from urethral meatus to anal area rather than the opposite.
- Contact physician if symptoms of infection occur.
- Consult physician concerning appropriateness of self-start therapy for recurrent urinary tract infections.
- Consult physician for appropriateness of postcoital therapy for recurrent urinary tract infections.

Principles and Rationale for Nursing Interventions

All patients should be taught the general principles intended to promote bladder health.[30] Mainaining an adequate fluid intake avoids the deleterious effects of dehydration, including irritation of the bladder wall with concentrated urine, and a possible reduction in the risk of bacteriuria. Bladder irritants should be limited or eliminated from the diet of those with sensory disorders of the bladder including interstitial or acute cystitis, urinary frequency and urge urinary incontinence. Constipation should be managed and prevented, because of its potential association with recurrent urinary tract infections, and urinary retention.

Altered urinary elimination patterns arise from excessively frequent or infrequent episodes of urination. Abnormal bladder function, such as that seen in incontinence and urinary retention, abnormal fluid intake, or altered bladder sensory states, may produce an altered pattern of micturition. Chronic bladder overdistention may predispose the individual to delayed perceptions of bladder filling and ultimately to urinary retention and deficient detrusor muscle function.[10] Prolonged urinary frequency predisposes the individual to early perceptions of bladder filling and decreased functional capacity.

The causes of urinary frequency are inflammation of the lower urinary tract, frequent micturition as a behavior, excessive fluid intake, and endocrine disorders, including diabetes mellitus and diabetes insipidus, that produce polyuria and polydipsia.[14] The causes of infrequent micturition are behavioral postponement of urination, urinary retention because of lower urinary tract dysfunction, or diseases producing oliguria or anuria.[14] A voiding diary that includes fluid intake and urinary output assists the health care professional in the assessment of the cause of altered urinary elimination patterns.[22] Establishing a routine of controlled fluid intake and timed voiding habits in conjunction with care for the physiologic or psychogenic causes of the voiding dysfunction is the best approach to this often persistent condition.

Urinary tract infections alter urinary elimination patterns by producing inflammation of the urinary tract. The most common form of urinary tract infection is cystitis; in addition, the condition is often associated with infection of the upper urinary tract and ureters (see Chapters 11 and 12 on pp. 923 and 988). Postponement of urination is not recommended in this condition because routine, complete bladder evacuation is a useful defense mechanism against microbial invasion of the urinary system.[28] Adequate fluid intake promotes regular bladder evacuation and serves to flush the urinary system of pathogens and associated debris.[28,29]

Antiinfective therapy remains the cornerstone of care for urinary tract infection. Patients are taught side effects and allergic reactions of medications. Certain antiinfective medications may be taken with meals to reduce nausea or stomach upset. Diarrhea occurs with antiinfective medications because of a reduction in normal intestinal flora. Use of yogurt or other dairy products with active cultures containing common intestinal flora assists in resolving diarrhea.

Recurrent urinary tract infections are managed by strategies designed to prevent recurrences, as well as measures designed to ablate a current infection. Using proper perineal cleansing and choosing rapid-drying undergarments are advocated in the prevention of recurrent infections.[25] Ingestion of cranberry juice or oral intake of ascorbic acid has been tentatively recommended as a strategy to lower urinary pH. An acidic urine is advocated because it exerts an antibacterial effect against certain strains of bacteria. The ingestion of cranberry juice alone is of limited value because of the large quantities required to produce significant urinary pH reduction.[13]

Alternate forms of antiinfective medication therapy may be used when recurring urinary tract infections occur. Prophylactic medication is used for recurrent urinary tract infections, whereas suppressive medications are used when pathogenic persistence occurs. A single dose is typically given at bedtime so that the highest serum level is attained while the patient experiences prolonged retention of urine during sleep.[28]

Self-start therapy offers two advantages. The strategy allows the patient to begin therapy quickly after recognizing symptoms of urinary tract infection and reduces the cost of multiple visits to a physician's office or clinic. The patient is provided with a home urine collection system for cultures and a prescription that allows him to begin antiinfective agent therapy immediately. The principle limitations of the strategy are the need for meticulous follow-up placed on the patient and for reasonable accuracy in recognizing the symptoms of infection.[29]

Postcoital therapy for urinary tract infections is used for women who experience cystitis following coitus. These women are provided with adequate antibiotics for a prophylactic dosage of medications after coitus. Successful therapy requires a well-established correlation between coitus and urinary tract infection occurrences and meticulous compliance with the medication regimen.[29]

▮ FUNCTIONAL INCONTINENCE

▮ Functional incontinence is the state in which an individual experiences an involuntary, unpredictable passage of urine.

The diagnosis functional incontinence may be a distinct entity or a complicating factor associated with other forms of urinary incontinence. As a distinct entity, functional incontinence may exist in an individual who is unable to reach the toilet or to manipulate clothing for successful toileting, despite a normally functioning lower urinary tract. These persons may suffer from impaired mobility, impaired dexterity, or a combination of these factors. Functional incontinence is exacerbated by a hostile environment that renders the toilet inaccessible to the individual or by barriers that impede access.

Functional incontinence may coexist with other forms of voiding dysfunction. For example, an individual with limited mobility and instability (urge) incontinence may be unable to move rapidly enough to a relatively distant toilet in an unfamiliar setting, causing urinary incontinence, even though he or she is able to maintain continence in the home, where the bathroom is readily accessible and urges to urinate can be acted on promptly.

In other instances the distinction between functional and other forms of incontinence is less clear. For example, the individual with significantly impaired cognitive function may be defined as having an unstable (overactive) detrusor muscle because the International Continence Society definition of the term assumes that the person undergoing testing is attempting to inhibit micturition during filling cystometry.[8,14]

Establishing the diagnosis functional incontinence is complex because of interaction between cognitive, locomotor, and environmental factors and the pathophysiologic aspects of incontinence remains unclear.[8] For example, the relationship between cognitive impairment and detrusor muscle instability still is not clear because the International Continence Society's definition of instability implies that the person being tested is attempting to inhibit micturition.[19] No such statement can be made with confidence if the individual undergoing testing has significant short-term memory loss and dementia. Thus, it is best to apply the diagnosis of functional incontinence most often in conjunction with other forms of incontinence unless urodynamic data exist to rule out physiologic bladder dysfunction contributing to urinary leakage.

Related Factors[23]

Acute confusion
Chronic confusion
Impaired environmental interpretation syndrome
Altered environment
Activity intolerance
Impaired adjustment
Anxiety
Impaired memory
Impaired verbal communication
Ineffective individual coping
Urge incontinence
Stress incontinence
Total incontinence
Urinary retention
Impaired physical mobility
Sleep pattern disturbance
Social isolation
Depression
Despair

Defining Characteristics[23]

Loss of urinary control typically associated with urinary urgency
Inability to reach toilet facility in time
Loss of recognition of sensation or signs of impending micturition

Expected Patient Outcomes & Nursing Interventions[3,6,23]

Restores continence, as evidenced by:

Regular, complete bladder emptying is achieved without intermittent urinary leakage

Access to toilet allows evacuation of urine during daytime and nighttime hours

- Assess patient's current voiding pattern.
- Assess factors associated with incontinent episodes, including environmental factors and patient's cognitive function and physical mobility.
- Assess other forms of urinary incontinence associated with functional incontinence.
- Institute a timed voiding schedule, patterned urge toileting response program, or other toileting schedule based on the patient's cognitive status, alertness, motivation, and physical abilities and bladder log data.[9,12]
- Alter environment to maximize access to toilet facilities. Provide bedside toilet facility or urinal. Provide toilet facility that may be reached with minimum number of steps and without necessity of using stairs. Provide patient with assistance choosing toilet device, as needed. Consider following criteria when choosing a toilet seat:

    Accessibility Device should be firmly anchored to floor with rubber grips. Toilet should have side arms to help support patient while sitting down. Height of chair should be adjustable to allow patient to place both feet and heels firmly on floor while using the device. Width of chair may be a constraint for obese patients.

    Convenience of cleaning Device should be easily disassembled to empty.

    Comfort As assessed by patient, padded seat may enhance comfort.

    Cost

- Begin prompted voiding program or patterned urge response toileting program, based on nursing assessment and data from bladder record or log.
- Teach patient to clean and empty device on routine basis; white vinegar or Urikleen is used to clean and deodorize receptacle.
- Teach patient to use incontinent containment devices or systems as needed to control urinary leakage between trips to toilet. (See Total Incontinence on p. 1587 and Stress Incontinence on p. 1583.)
- Provide telephone or intercom access for patient at the side of the commode.
- Help patient formulate plans for bladder management during outings. Outings should be determined in consultation with patient and significant others and may include trips to shops and restaurants or visits to friends and relatives. Accompany patient on one or more such outings, as feasible.

Maintains skin integrity, as evidenced by:

Skin exposed to urinary leakage remains without rash or lesions
Patient and family demonstrating adequate knowledge of care routine for skin affected by urinary leakage and indications for contacting physician concerning skin lesions

- Assess condition of patient's perineal skin.
- Assess strategies, including routine hygiene habits and products patient is using to protect perineal skin from irritation caused by urinary leakage.

- Provide skin care to areas exposed to urinary leakage using regular hygiene routine:

    Wash skin once daily with soap and water or specially formulated incontinence cleanser. Dry thoroughly using hair dryer at low or warm setting with fan at lowest speed.

    Use skin sealant or moisture barrier to protect skin between washings.

- Teach patient and family to perform skin care and to recognize common skin rashes, as well as indications for contacting health care professional regarding rashes, inflammation, or skin infection.

Principles and Rationale for Nursing Interventions

Strategies to regain continence among individuals with functional incontinence are designed to minimize or remove the cognitive, mobility, dexterity, or environmental factors that contribute to urinary leakage. When functional incontinence coexists with other forms of incontinence, management strategies for functional deficits are combined with strategies to overcome urge, reflex, or stress incontinence or urinary retention.

A timed voiding schedule, patterned urge response toileting program, or related programs overcome leakage by assisting the individual to reestablish an acceptable pattern of toileting, thus reducing incontinent episodes. These programs are based on individualized assessments of patients according to their cognitive and physical abilities in addition to the function of their lower urinary systems.[9,12]

Providing a toilet that is easily accessible minimizes impaired physical mobility. A nighttime toilet seat precludes the necessity of the patient attempting to awaken sufficiently and walk to the bathroom.[3] A telephone or intercom system at the commode allows the patient to contact others in the home or other helpers, if needed.[6,23]

Provision of plans for bladder management during outings allows patients to engage in anticipatory management of a problem and increases their confidence as they seek to increase social contacts. Accompanying patients on a trial outing may increase confidence for continued social activities and provides added support, while newly learned strategies for bladder control are attempted.

Recurrent urinary leakage threatens to impair the integrity of affected skin. Use of an appropriate skin care regimen provides routine cleaning, thorough drying, and moisture barriers that help protect integumentary integrity. (See Total Incontinence on p. 1587.)

■ REFLEX INCONTINENCE

Reflex incontinence is the state in which an individual experiences an involuntary loss of urine, occurring at somewhat predictable intervals when a specific bladder volume is reached.

Reflex incontinence is distinguished from urge incontinence by the absence of sensations and differing etiology. The diagnosis probably arises from the term *reflex incontinence* used by the International Continence Society[19] to denote incontinence caused by neurologic abnormality. This form of incontinence arises from complete spinal cord injury or abnormality occurring below the pons but above sacral segments 2 to 4.

Establishment of the diagnosis reflex incontinence requires the presence of a known neurologic deficit and documentation of bladder contraction (often described as *spastic*) in the absence of sensations.[23] Since the underlying abnormality is an unstable detrusor muscle, the value of establishing unique nursing diagnoses for each form of instability incontinence remains controversial.

Related Factors[3,29]

Neurologic abnormalities
    Complete spinal cord injury above sacral micturition center
    Cerebellar ataxia
    Amyotrophic lateral sclerosis
    Multiple sclerosis
    Spinovascular disease
    Spinal cord tumor
    Myelomeningocele (greatest in first years of life)
Autonomic dysreflexia
Neuropathic sphincter: detrusor sphincter dyssynergia
Urinary retention
Obstructive uropathy
    Urinary tract infection
    Trabeculation of bladder with poor bladder wall compliance
    Bladder diverticula
    Hydronephrosis
    Upper urinary tract deterioration
    Renal insufficiency

Defining Characteristics[23]

Uncontrolled urinary leakage associated with detrusor muscle instability and absent sensations of urgency
Absent sensations of bladder filling
Detrusor sphincter dyssynergia and intermittent urinary stream

Expected Patient Outcomes & Nursing Interventions[17]

Restores continence, as evidenced by:

Maintaining continence between catheterizations
Dry at night
Successful use of urinary containment device or system

Prevents urinary tract infection, as evidenced by:

No symptoms of urinary tract infection
Sterile urine in urine culture
- Assess patient's current urinary elimination pattern and incidence of incontinence.
- Determine stimuli that cause bladder emptying in addition to reaching a certain intravesical volume.

- Assess for presence of diaphoresis, dizziness, or palpitations with voiding. (See Chapter 12 on p. 988.)
- Monitor patient's current fluid intake (amount and time).
- Begin clean intermittent catheterization program with appropriate autonomic drugs (propantheline or oxybutynin) or spasmolytic drugs (flavoxate or dicyclomine) under physician's direction:
    Teach catheterization using clean, rather than sterile, technique unless latter is specified by physician.
    Teach patient to wash hands.
    Use clean or sterile catheter; water-soluble lubricant is necessary for men and advisable for women.
    May wash perineum with soap and water or a prepackaged towelette.
    Lubricate catheter and gently insert into urethra; bladder is drained completely. Teach patient to withdraw catheter slowly to ensure adequate evacuation of urine.
    Pinch catheter on removal from urethra to prevent spillage of urine.
    Wash catheter immediately with cold tap water and lather with warm, soapy water. Rinse thoroughly.
    Store catheters in clean, dry container suitable for carrying in purse or pocket. Catheters are never stored in any solution because of infection risk.
- Establish catheterization schedule in accordance with patient's schedule, approximately every 4 to 6 hours as needed during waking hours. Sleep is not typically interrupted for intermittent catheterization.
- Teach patient and family members catheterization procedure as feasible.
- Teach the patient to maintain an adequate intake of fluids (30 ml/kg of body weight).
- Monitor patient for side effects of medications: dry mouth, blurred vision, dizziness, weakness, or tachycardia if cardiac disease is present. Consult physician concerning altering pharmacologic regimen if incontinent episodes occur between catheterizations.
- Teach patient signs of urinary tract infection: sudden change in continence between catheterizations, fever, flank pain, hematuria, or change in character or odor of urinary output.
- If clean intermittent schedule is not feasible or successful, use urinary containment devices.
- Institute a reflex voiding program with containment of urine by a condom catheter for the male who is unable or unwilling to perform self-intermittent catheterization. Teach the male and his family to select and apply a condom catheter with the following features:
    Availability in appropriate size
    Adequate comfort, as perceived by patient
    Adequate drainage, including resistance to twisting at distal end
    Adherence to penis by inherent adhesive, adhesive straps, or external straps, forming a watertight seal without creating a tourniquet effect

- Teach the patient and family to select an appropriate leg bag for urinary drainage and storage. The leg bag should have the following features:

    Nonrubberized straps attached to the drainage bag *to prevent skin irritation.*

    A cloth pouch or cloth backing *to minimize skin irritation against the leg.*

    Adequate volume with properties that minimize bulging under clothing.

    A drainage spout that can be opened and closed with one hand using minimal fine motor movements of the finger.

    An antireflux, proximal opening preventing reflux of urine from drainage bag to condom catheter.

    Durable, flexible tubing connecting the condom catheter and leg bag.

- Teach the patient and family to regularly inspect the penile skin, with every change of the condom catheter and to inform the nurse or physician when skin integrity is altered.

- Teach patient and significant others to apply device as feasible and to care for drainage system.

- Use other urinary containment devices (pads, incontinent briefs), as indicated. (See Total Incontinence on p. 1587.)

- Insert a temporary indwelling Foley catheter, as directed, when skin integrity is compromised. Reinstitute a reflex voiding program after the penile skin is healed, and reinforce instruction concerning skin care.

- Insert a long-term indwelling or suprapubic catheter, as directed, when alternative management strategies are proven unfeasible. Choose a Foley catheter constructed of a cystocompatible, hydrophilic material that has the lowest feasible friction coefficient.

- Choose appropriate drainage system for daytime and nighttime use. Daytime system should be reasonably concealed in clothing and comfortable against leg or thigh. Cloth sleeve is best for drainage bag. Nighttime drainage system should contain a minimum of 2000 ml.

- Teach patient to clean drainage bags regularly with vinegar and water solution.

- Maintain adequate fluid intake. Fluid intake control is not indicated when indwelling Foley catheter is used.

- Consult physician if patient is incontinent around catheter. Consider use of drugs to decrease detrusor muscle instability before increasing size of Foley catheter.

- Do not overfill catheter balloon.

- Teach patient and family indications for contacting health care professional concerning indwelling Foley catheter use (signs of urinary tract infection, untoward drug reactions, decreasing urinary output).

- Teach patient and family to assess catheter daily to ensure adequate drainage.

- Change the catheter as needed, approximately every 30 days.

Principles and Rationale for Nursing Interventions

The goals of management of reflex incontinence are the restoration of continence and prevention of urinary tract infection and associated complications. Bladder training is typically not feasible in these patients. The neurologic abnormality underlying reflex incontinence is centered in the spinal reflex arcs.[23] Attempts at cortical retraining are rarely successful.

Autonomic or spasmolytic drugs are used to convert the bladder to a low-pressure storage vesicle that can be regularly emptied through a clean intermittent catheterization (CIC) program. Medications are closely monitored for side effects and may have to be altered periodically because of development of tolerance or untoward effects. The rates of infection and upper urinary tract abnormality associated with this strategy are minimal compared to patients who experience chronic urinary retention.[17]

Patients who fail to respond adequately to pharmacologic management of reflex incontinence may undergo augmentation cystoplasty to enhance bladder capacity and ablate potentially dangerous high-pressure contractions. Augmentation cystoplasty is the surgical enlargement of the bladder, using a segment of detubularized small or large bowel that has been isolated from the fecal stream. An alternative approach is to use a portion of the fundus of the stomach. The reconstructed bladder is then catheterized on a routine basis, while the need for chronic administration of antispasmodic medications is avoided.[15]

A significant reason for failure of a pharmacologic-CIC program is noncompliance. Compliance to the regimen may be maximized by carefully tailoring the catheterizations around the patient's daily schedule. Teaching others in the patient's environment to catheterize provides the patient with other resources for catheterization, if needed.

Quadriplegic males who are unable to perform intermittent catheterization or paraplegic males who refuse to perform catheterization may be managed by a reflex-voiding program. In this case the bladder is allowed to fill until it contracts and the urinary leakage is contained by a condom catheter connected to a leg bag. Because reflex incontinence is typically accompanied by detrusor sphincter dyssynergia, a reduction in bladder outlet resistance is often required to prevent chronic urinary retention and upper urinary tract distress. Several strategies are employed to reduce the obstruction associated with dyssynergia. An α-blocking medication, such as doxazosin (Cardura) or terazosin (Hytrin) may be used to reduce bladder outlet resistance at the bladder neck, proximal urethra, and rhabdosphincter. A surgical sphincterotomy is the surgical incision of the membranous urethra via a transurethral approach. A technique for implanting a urethral stint (wire mesh or spiral device) also reduces obstruction by preventing complete closure of the striated sphincter mechanism.[3,13] This technique for management is limited to males because no acceptable condom device exists for female patients.

The long-term indwelling catheter is considered a last resort for patients with reflex incontinence. Long-term catheter drainage is associated with significant urinary tract complications, including infection, upper tract dilation and deterioration, and renal insufficiency. Complications associated with the catheter may be minimized with careful care of the system. The choice of catheter material is important. Inert or hydrophilic materials are purported to reduce urethral irritation. Choosing a catheter with a large internal lumen relative to the external French size will minimize the likelihood of the catheter becoming clogged with urinary sediment. Choosing an appropriate drainage system allows optimum patient comfort and prevents urinary stasis caused by filling of an inadequately sized bag.

Bacteriuria is inevitable in the presence of a long-term indwelling Foley catheter. A suprapubic cystostomy site may be chosen by the physician instead of urethral catheterization in an attempt to create a cleaner insertion site and prevent complications associated with infection. The goal of care is not prevention of bacteriuria; rather, care is aimed at preventing symptomatic urinary tract infections and serious related urologic conditions.[36] Long-term use of prophylactic antibiotics are not indicated because resistance will develop, requiring the use of intravenous antiinfective agents when symptomatic urinary tract infections occur. Maintenance of adequate fluid intake assists in the prevention of serious urinary tract infections by flushing the urinary system of sediment. Maintaining a patent catheter through regular assessment of urinary drainage and routine changes, as well as use of an adequately sized drainage bag, also prevents stasis. Routine cleansing of the drainage bag may help prevent serious urinary tract infection by preventing bacterial overgrowth and colonization of the bladder.

Silver alloy coated catheters have been shown to reduce the presence of bacteriuria after relatively short-term use (6 days), and they may play a role in the prevention of symptomatic urinary tract infection among those managed by long-term urethral catheterization.[27] Further investigation is needed before this catheter material can be recommended among patients with reflex incontinence.

Incontinence around the Foley catheter may indicate a catheter that is no longer patent or persistent detrusor muscle instability. Increasing the catheter size is not indicated unless routine clogging of the catheter is a known problem. Consulting the physician concerning use of a drug to decrease detrusor instability may be adequate to prevent incontinence. Increasing the size of the retention balloon is contraindicated, since this is associated with irritation of the bladder outlet and may lead to exacerbation of detrusor instability.[3]

■ STRESS INCONTINENCE

■ Stress incontinence is the state in which an individual experiences a urine loss of less than 50 ml, occurring with increased abdominal pressure.

This nursing diagnosis arises from descriptions of stress incontinence or stress urinary incontinence in which urinary leakage is associated with physical exertion.[14,19,36,37] The International Continence Society[15] defines stress incontinence as a symptom or sign. The *symptom* of stress incontinence is the patient's subjective report of urinary leakage on physical exertion; the *sign* of stress incontinence is the objective confirmation of the symptom in a clinical or laboratory setting. *Genuine stress incontinence* is a urodynamically proved condition in which urinary leakage occurs when intravesical (bladder) pressure exceeds urethral closure pressure in the absence of a detrusor muscle contraction.

The limitation of stress incontinence to volumes less than 50 ml is an attempt to differentiate stress incontinence from total incontinence. The use of volume as a distinction to differentiate these conditions is certainly vulnerable to criticism. A better differentiation could be made by recognizing the difficulty of distinguishing incontinence by symptoms such as the magnitude of urinary leakage. Other classification systems avoid this problem by distinguishing stress urinary incontinence from extraurethral (continuous or constant) incontinence. Under such a system, stress incontinence would be defined as the leakage of urine on physical exertion caused by increased abdominal pressure, whereas extraurethral incontinence would be defined as the leakage of urine that occurs when the normal sphincteric mechanism is bypassed. Unfortunately, under the current schema, overlapping related factors and defining characteristics will be noted between stress incontinence and total incontinence.

Related Factors[2,14,22,33,37]

Forms of pelvic relaxation
  Cystocele
  Rectocele
  Enterocele
  Urethral hypermobility
  Uterine prolapse
Risk factors of urethral hypermobility
  Family history of SUI
  Multiple vaginal deliveries
  Aging and menopause
  Peripheral neuropathies
  Trauma to pelvic support structures
  Iatrogenic pelvic floor denervation
Obesity
Chronic cough
Smoking
Frequent straining or heavy exercise including long distance running
Gravid uterus
Sphincteric incompetence
  Trauma to sphincteric mechanism
  Iatrogenic trauma to sphincteric mechanism
    Multiple anti-incontinence procedures
    Radical prostatectomy
    Transurethral prostatectomy (rare)

Congenital sphincteric incompetence
  Myelomeningocele
  Spina bifida
  Sacral agenesis
  Spinal dysraphism
Urinary frequency
Urinary urgency
Urge incontinence
Functional incontinence
Nocturia

Defining Characteristics[19,23]

Reported urinary leakage associated with physical exertion (increased abdominal pressure)

Observed urinary leakage associated with increased abdominal pressure

Urinary leakage when urodynamically assessed bladder pressure exceeds urethral pressure in absence of detrusor contraction

Expected Patient Outcomes & Nursing Interventions

Contains continence, as evidenced by:

No longer perceiving urinary leakage as uncontrollable problem

- Determine causes of incontinence and any association with coughing, laughing, sneezing, abdominal strain.
- Assess urgency associated with incontinence. Determine if element of urge incontinence is related, and identify stressors that produce these symptoms. (See Urge Incontinence on p. 1585.)
- Assess severity of incontinence and frequency that urinary leakage requires a change of clothing.
- Determine frequency of voiding, if patient is nocturic, and how often desire to void interrupts sleep each night.
- Monitor patient's current fluid intake pattern (volume and time).
- Assess coping strategies, including drugs or mechanical devices, patient currently employs to cope with urinary leakage.
- Assess risk factors for this patient (e.g., number of vaginal deliveries, status of estrogen production or replacement, relation to climacteric, previous surgical procedures, conditions related to peripheral neuropathies).
- Provide patient with incontinent containment device or system. Absorbent pads are usually sufficient. Pad is evaluated on the basis of following criteria:
  - *Absorbency* Devices with Superabsorbents are typically the most absorbent of all pads; often a less absorbent device is adequate in cases of mild to moderate leakage.
  - *Wetness protection* Outer waterproof lining should protect clothing from urinary leakage.
  - *Size* Pads should be easily concealed in clothing.
  - *Comfort* This is assessed by patient.

- Teach female patient to do pelvic muscle exercises to strengthen circumvaginal muscles (CVMs) through resistive and endurance maneuvers.[14] Instruct patient to:
  - Empty bladder.
  - Lie down in comfortable position with knees elevated 20 degrees.
  - Relax completely.
  - Tighten CVMs with abdominal and thigh muscles relaxed. Patient will need help isolating the CVMs. Ask patient to visualize vagina and contract only those muscles that press against pubic bone as if they were stopping the urinary stream.
  - Tighten muscles quickly and hold for 10 seconds. Relax completely for 10 seconds and repeat procedure.
  - Begin with 10 repetitions and increase regimen to 35 to 50 repetitions daily; advise patient to increase repetitions in increments of five until goal is attained.
- Supplement a pelvic muscle exercise regimen with electrostimulation of the pelvic floor muscles in the female who fails to adequately respond to exercises only.[9]
- Teach the female to use weighted vaginal cones as an alternative or supplement to pelvic muscle exercises.
- Provide female patient with appropriate pessary device in consultation with or under direction of physician; teach patient care of pessary device, including appropriate hygiene and necessity of regular follow-up to change device, as indicated.
- Administer sympathomimetic medications (pseudoephedrine), as directed.
- Inform patient of availability of surgical options to correct stress incontinence, as indicated, and encourage patient to speak with appropriate health care professional.

Principles and Rationale for Nursing Interventions

Conservative treatment for stress incontinence is typically recommended for a mild to moderate disorder. Stress incontinence is not typically associated with serious urologic complications. It is important to remember that the treatment of stress incontinence is based on the patient's perceptions of the condition as a significant social or hygienic problem. Providing a patient with a suitable pad to contain incontinence may be an acceptable solution for the condition, whereas other persons will seek more definitive solutions.

Kegel[18] is credited for originating an exercise regimen to strengthen the pelvic floor muscles to control stress incontinence in women. The exercises are designed to strengthen the striated portion of the sphincteric mechanisms and may play a role in alleviation of pelvic descent caused by muscle weakness. Balloon devices have been used, but their contribution to the success of exercise remains unclear.

The success of a pelvic floor exercise may be enhanced by the use of electrostimulation therapy. Electrostimulation therapy uses a transcutaneous or transvaginal route to apply a nonpainful, low-voltage current to the pelvic floor muscles, causing contraction. The application of multiple stimulations passively exercises these muscles, while providing biofeedback for the individual who has difficulty isolating and contracting the correct muscles.[9] Weighted vaginal cones also provide an alternative to pelvic floor exercises. These devices are placed in the vagina, requiring contraction of the circumvaginal muscles to remain in place.[1]

The pessary device alleviates stress incontinence by mechanically alleviating pelvic descent and loss of anatomic relationships of the urethrovesical unit. Voiding is not obstructed when the pessary is placed correctly, and adequate care prevents common hygienic problems associated with use of a pessary.[4,14]

Alpha-sympathomimetic medications are available in several over-the-counter preparations. Such drugs are effective in cases of stress incontinence because they increase tone at the smooth muscle component of the sphincteric mechanism. In addition, sympathomimetics may contribute to sphincteric closure through a vascular effect at the urethral submucosa.[16]

Many patients with more severe urinary leakage may undergo surgical correction of stress incontinence. Evaluation of a patient for surgical repair is done by a urologist or gynecologist and includes urodynamic assessment. (See Chapter 12 on p. 988 for a description of the care of patients undergoing urethral suspension procedures.)

URGE INCONTINENCE

Urge incontinence is the state in which an individual experiences involuntary passage of urine, occurring soon after a strong sense of urgency to void.

Urge incontinence arises from the International Continence Society's (ICS) designation. The ICS subdivides the concept into two forms of urge incontinence. *Motor* urge incontinence is associated with detrusor muscle instability; *sensory* urgency is associated with hypersensitivity (irritative) disorders of the bladder. (See Chapter 12 on p. 988.) These may represent similar or distinct conditions.

The physiologic mechanism underlying urge incontinence is detrusor muscle instability. Nonetheless, cognitive, functional, and logistic components of the patient and environment influence whether incontinence occurs. A patient who is alert, ambulatory, and familiar with the environment may be able to prevent urinary leakage by use of the pelvic floor muscles until a toilet is reached. A person who is confused, immobile, or unfamiliar with the location of a nearby toilet is more likely to experience incontinence. Thus, the diagnosis urge incontinence is not mutually exclusive of functional incontinence.

Related Factors[14,23,28,37]

Neurologic disease/trauma
    Cerebrovascular accident
    Brain tumor
    Parkinsonism

Alzheimer's disease
    Multiple sclerosis
    Incomplete suprasacral spinal cord injury
    Closed head injury
Bladder outlet obstruction
    Prostatic enlargement
        Benign prostatic hyperplasia
        Prostatic adenocarcinoma
        Prostatitis
        Bladder neck hypertrophy
        Bladder neck contracture
        Bladder neck dyssynergia
    Irritative bladder disorders
        Cystitis
            Bacterial
            Viral
            Fungal
            Parasitic
            Chemotherapy-induced
            Radiotherapy-induced
        Bladder wall tumor
        Bladder calculi
Stress incontinence
Age (childhood or elderly)
Altered thought processes
Altered state of mobility
Unfamiliar environment
    Lack of knowledge of toilet facilities
    Toilet facilities unavailable
    Lack of access to toilet
Anxiety
Impaired physical mobility
Impaired verbal communication
Sleep pattern disturbance related to nocturia

Defining Characteristics[23]

Urinary leakage associated with marked sensation of urge to void
Inability to reach toilet in time
Urinary urgency
Urinary frequency (voids more often than every 2 hours)
Nocturia (awakened by desire to void more than once per night)

Expected Patient Outcomes & Nursing Interventions[23,31]

Restores urinary continence, as evidenced by:

Symptoms of urge incontinence are absent
Symptoms of urinary urgency and urinary frequency remain present, but incontinent episodes are absent
Patient and family describing goals and process of timed voiding schedule with fluid intake control
Patient and family demonstrating adequate knowledge of continence containment device
Patient reporting dryness between intermittent catheterizations

Foley catheter in place; patient reporting no leakage around catheter

Patient having rapid and adequate access to toilet facilities in hospital, extended care, and/or home environment

- Assess related factors that predispose toward urge incontinence: neurologic disease or trauma, bladder outlet obstruction, irritative bladder disorders, stress incontinence.
- Determine if patient is in high-risk age group for condition.
- Assess associated related factors for urge incontinence: physical or cognitive impairment, environmental alterations.
- Assess patient's access to toilet facilities and approximate transit time to nearest toilet facility, considering the patient's physical mobility limitations, if any.
- Determine patient's current daytime urinary elimination patterns (frequency of urination, number of incontinent episodes per day).
- Ask if patient experiences nocturia, enuresis, or incontinence before reaching toilet.
- Check patient's current fluid intake pattern (volume and time).
- Determine specific circumstances that patient and family identify as predisposing toward urge incontinence.
- Assess current coping strategies, including drugs or medical treatments, patient uses to deal with urge incontinence.
- Have patient maintain timed voiding schedule of approximately every 2 to 3 hours during the day. Schedule must be individualized in consultation with patient and family. Progress to every 3 to 4 hours as feasible.
- Teach patient to stop, and rapidly contract the pelvic muscles for a period of 2 to 6 seconds when precipitous episode of urgency occurs. Advise the patient to repeat this maneuver until the urgency subsides, and to promptly move to the bathroom and urinate. Warn the elderly patient to avoid rushing to the bathroom since this increases the risk of falling.
- Consider administration of anticholinergic drugs (propantheline or oxybutynin) or spasmolytic drugs (flavoxate or dicyclomine) under physicians' direction to increase functional bladder capacity if urinary frequency and urge incontinence persist despite timed voiding schedule with fluid intake control.
- Institute bladder drill-bladder retraining therapy regimen in consultation with physician. Instruct the patient to postpone urination for 1½ hours during waking hours even if incontinence occurs in the interim. As continence is attained for this period, increase increment between voidings by ½ hour until a goal of 3 to 4 hours is reached. Negotiation of goals concerning bladder drill therapy must occur in conjunction with patient and family.
- Institute electrostimulation therapy in consultation with the physician using a transcutaneous, transvaginal, or transrectal route. Combine electrostimulation with bladder drill therapy, timed voiding schedules, as indicated.

- If attempts at timed voiding and fluid control schedules and bladder drill therapy fail, consult physician concerning institution of significant pharmacologic relaxation of the detrusor muscle with intermittent catheterization schedule.
- Begin clean intermittent catheterization program and teach patient and family members as soon as feasible. Catheterization should be accomplished approximately every 4 to 6 hours. Sleep patterns are not usually interrupted for catheterization. (See Reflex Incontinence.)
- Monitor patient for side effects of autonomic or spasmolytic drugs (blurred vision, constipation, dry mouth, weakness, tachycardia in presence of existing cardiac disease or acute confusion or nightmares, particularly in elderly patients).
- If attempts to control urge incontinence fail, consult physician concerning use of indwelling Foley catheter.
- Alter patient's environment in following ways to promote restoration of continence:

  Provide portable urinal as feasible.

  Assess home environment for access to toilet facility. Climbing stairs to the toilet is not feasible for patients with limited mobility.

  Provide for bedside toilet facility for nocturic voiding needs. Because of nighttime awakening, urinal or bedside commode is needed for patients with limited physical mobility or potential altered cognition.

  Allow patient to sit up to use toilet whenever possible; bedpans or continent briefs should be employed as a final resort rather than for convenience.

Prevents urinary tract infections, as evidenced by:

No symptoms of urinary tract infection being present
Urine cultures showing sterile urine

- Assess patient for history of urinary tract infections, their frequency, and any association with fever or hematuria.
- Assess coping strategies, including pharmacologic agents, patient currently uses to deal with infections.
- Determine if patient thinks that bladder is completely emptied and if patient uses specific strategies (e.g., double voiding, self–intermittent catheterization) *to ensure complete bladder emptying.*
- Assess efficiency of bladder emptying by maintaining accurate record of fluid intake and urinary output.
- Measure postvoiding residuals at least three times using straight catheter or ultrasound assessment within 5 minutes of voiding.
- Encourage adequate fluid intake.

Principles and Rationale for Nursing Interventions

The overriding goal of treating any patient with altered urinary elimination patterns is the prevention of incontinence and the assurance of complete, regular bladder emptying. A timed voiding schedule is used in an attempt to prevent urinary leakage precipitated by bladder filling to a threshold volume. Oral fluid control is used to ensure adequate intake and encourage maximum urinary output while the patient is awake, maximally mobile, and engaged in activities of daily living. Fluid intake is severely restricted just before bedtime in an attempt to minimize altered sleep patterns caused by nocturia.

Autonomic or spasmolytic drugs are used to increase functional bladder capacity and decrease urinary frequency.[11] They are adjunct measures to the timed voiding and fluid control schedule and should not be used as a substitute. Urinary residuals may increase with these agents, and assessment of postvoiding residual is essential.

Bladder drill therapy is a strategy designed to eliminate detrusor muscle instability or bladder hypersensitivity through behavioral means. The patient is taught to postpone urination for increasingly longer periods until an optimum routine of urinary frequency (every 3 to 4 hours) during waking hours is attained. Sleep patterns are not interrupted for bladder therapy regimens. Success of such a program is optimized by intensive support of persons undergoing bladder drill therapy. Goals for therapy should be determined by both patient and nurse. It is probably best to begin with a relatively modest goal of voiding every 1½ hours and working toward a 3- to 4-hour interval between voiding at ½-hour increments.[14,20,38]

Pharmacologic relaxation of the bladder can be attained by careful use of autonomic or spasmolytic drugs.[16] The goal of pharmacologic therapy is to decrease detrusor contractions significantly and convert the bladder to a low-compliance storage compartment for urine suitable for routine emptying using catheterization. Bladder evacuation through clean intermittent catheterization is employed to ensure regular, complete vesicle emptying. This strategy is typically used if the patient fails other means of therapy because of significant urinary retention or persistent incontinence.

An indwelling Foley catheter is used when conservative management, as well as surgical options in selected patients, have failed and the incontinence continues to be a significant health and hygiene problem as perceived by the patient and/or family.[21] (See Urinary Retention on p. 1589.)

Control of the environment is needed to maximize the chances of success of a fluid control and timed voiding program. Accessibility of toilet facilities is essential for the patient to establish a reasonable voiding schedule that does not unduly interfere with other activities of daily living. It is important to remember that the goal is control of incontinence; a timed voiding and fluid control program is a coping strategy and not a curative measure for urge incontinence.

Prevention of urinary tract infection and associated urologic abnormalities is accomplished by ensuring that the patient completely empties the bladder on a regular schedule. Persistent residual urine is a significant risk factor for recurrent urinary tract infections with their associated complications. (See Chapters 11 and 12 on pp. 923 and 988.)

■ TOTAL INCONTINENCE

■ Total incontinence is the state in which an individual experiences a continuous and unpredictable loss of urine.

Total incontinence is partly analogous to extraurethral incontinence, as described by the International Continence Society (ICS).[15] and to severe genuine stress incontinence.

Total incontinence is caused by urinary ectopia or a fistulous tract through which urine leaks, bypassing the normal sphincteric mechanism. Because of the limited definition of stress incontinence to volumes of 50 ml or less, the diagnosis total incontinence also applies to cases of severe stress incontinence caused by intrinsic sphincter deficiency.

Related Factors[3,22,23]

Urinary fistula
  Vesicovaginal
  Ureterovaginal
  Urethrovaginal
  Urethrocutaneous
Urinary ectopia
  Ectopic ureter that bypasses sphincteric mechanism
  Bladder exstrophy
  Urethral duplication
Surgically created stomas
  Ileal conduit
  Sigmoid conduit
  Ureterostomy
  Pyelostomy
  Vesicostomy
Intrinsic sphincter deficiency
Iatrogenic
  Multiple anti-incontinence procedures
  Y-V plasty
Trauma to sphincteric mechanism
Congenital sphincteric incompetence
  Epispadias
  Absent urethra (associated with cloacal deformity)
  Spina bifida
  Myelomeningocele
  Sacral agenesis
  Spinal dysraphism
Urinary tract infection
Functional incontinence

Defining Characteristics

Continuous urinary leakage imposed on otherwise normal voiding pattern
Continuous urinary leakage with failure of urinary storage
Unawareness of incontinence
Refractory to pharmacologic or behavioral treatment

Expected Patient Outcomes & Nursing Interventions

Contains continence, as evidenced by:

Urinary leakage around continent pad, continent brief, or brief being absent

Urinary leakage from condom catheter system being absent
Urinary leakage from urinary pouch system being absent

- Determine when incontinence occurs and if patient is ever dry.
- Assess conditions (if any) that make leakage more or less severe.
- Determine if leakage is ever associated with sensation of urgency.
- Assess patient's normal voiding patterns. Determine if continuous urinary leakage occurs in addition to "regular" voiding pattern or if incontinence is severe enough to have replaced micturition.
- Determine origin of urinary leakage: urethra, vagina, or other opening.
- Assess whether urinary tract infections are associated with leakage and whether hematuria or fever is present.
- Provide patient with urinary containment device or system to cope with incontinence. Evaluate products using following criteria:

  Absorbency
  Ease of application, use
  Ability to conceal in clothing
  Comfort
  Patient's desires, preferences
  Cost

- Consider following devices:

  Pads should adhere to the patient's underclothing and remain well concealed in clothing. Pads should have water-resistant backing to prevent leaking through device onto clothing. Absorption may be relatively limited; products containing Superabsorbents hold maximum amount.

  Adult briefs combine a pad with a brief specifically designed to hold pad in place. Absorbency is typically greater than with pads. Application of system may be more difficult than with pads, particularly in patients with limited mobility. Certain devices are equipped with panel that opens in front, using Velcro strips for patients confined to wheelchair. System should be easily concealed in clothing and have outward appearance of normal underclothing. Briefs should be constructed of breathable material with comfort comparable to regular undergarments.

  Condom catheters. (See Reflex Incontinence on p. 1580.)

  Adult continent briefs are typically reserved for particularly severe cases of incontinence or for persons confined to bed. Devices are very absorbent and relatively easy to apply, but they are difficult to conceal in clothing and often are considered uncomfortable to wear. Patient acceptance of continent briefs is often problematic because of social stigma attached to "wearing diapers."

  Urinary pouching system is option of choice for patients with total incontinence caused by surgical diversion. This system requires enterostomal therapy (ET) nurse to design and place pouch for urinary containment. System provides watertight drainage device connected to a drainage bag so that absorbency is not an issue. System may be more difficult to apply than other prepackaged devices. Device should be relatively simple to conceal under clothing and comfortable. Patient acceptance is typically high because of interaction with the ET nurse. (See Chapter 12 on p. 988.)

- Consult physician concerning definitive plan for repairing fistulous tract, implanting artificial urinary sphincter device, or removing ectopic urinary segment.

Maintains skin integrity, as evidenced by:

Skin rashes, lesions, inflammation, and infection being absent
Patient and family accurately describing routine for providing skin care to areas exposed to constant urinary leakage
Patient and family accurately describing indications for contacting health care professional concerning loss of skin integrity

- Assess condition of patient's perineal skin.
- Assess strategies, including routine hygiene habits, and products patient is currently using to protect perineal skin from irritation caused by urinary leakage.
- Provide skin care to areas exposed to urinary leakage using regular hygiene routine:

  Wash skin once daily with soap and water or specially formulated incontinence cleanser. Dry thoroughly using hair dryer at low or warm setting with fan at lowest speed.

  Use skin sealant or moisture barrier to protect skin between washings.

- Teach patient and family to perform skin care and to recognize common skin rashes, as well as indications for contacting health care professional regarding rashes, inflammation, or skin infections.

Principles and Rationale for Nursing Interventions

Because the normal sphincteric mechanism is bypassed or ablated, total incontinence is refractory to routine management with treatment modalities such as timed voiding, fluid control, bladder drill, physiotherapy, or pharmacologic manipulation. Urinary containment devices are the immediate treatment of choice. For certain patients who are suitable surgical candidates, extraurethral incontinence is resolved by surgical closure of a fistulous tract or resection of an ectopic urinary structure. For others who are not surgical candidates or for whom a urinary diversion has been accomplished as a lifesaving measure, urinary containment is a permanent management strategy.

Intrinsic sphincter deficiency may be managed by a suburethral sling, implantation of an artificial urinary sphincter, or injection of a glutaraldehyde cross linked (GAX) collagen into the submucosa of the urethra. Refer to Chapter 12 on p. 988 for the nursing care related to these procedures.

Skin care is essential for the patient with total incontinence. The goal of skin care is to prevent loss of integrity. Routine cleaning is followed by careful and thorough drying. Skin sealants or moisture barriers form a protective barrier to protect the integument from urine; sealants with an alcohol base are not used on a patient who does not have intact skin because the solution will cause severe discomfort.[5]

URINARY RETENTION

Urinary retention is the state in which the individual experiences incomplete emptying of the bladder.

Two factors contribute to urinary retention: deficient detrusor muscle, strength and bladder outlet obstruction. Urinary retention may manifest as an acute state requiring immediate intervention or as a chronic condition. The symptom of urinary retention is not necessarily harmful to the individual. A person requires treatment for urinary retention when potentially harmful sequelae of the condition, such as urinary tract infection and upper tract dilation, threaten to compromise renal function.

Related Factors[7,14,37]

Bladder outlet obstruction
  Prostatic enlargement
    Benign prostatic hyperplasia
    Prostatic cancer
    Prostatitis
  Bladder neck hypertrophy
  Bladder neck dyssynergia
  Bladder neck contracture
  Urethral stricture
  Female urethral distortion
  Detrusor sphincter dyssynergia
  Urethral trauma
Deficient detrusor function
  Chronic overdistention
    Infrequent voiding
    Sensory paralytic bladder
      Diabetes mellitus
      Incomplete spinal cord injury
  Pelvic trauma
  Sacral spinal cord injury
  Cauda equina injury
  Cauda equina syndrome
  Tabes dorsalis
  Polio and post-polio syndrome
  Multiple sclerosis
  Herpes zoster
  Cannabis ingestion
  Constipation/fecal impaction
  Prolonged bed rest
  Hysterical conversions
  Drugs
    Propantheline
    Oxybutynin
    Methantheline
    Flavoxate
    Dicyclomine
    Ganglion-blocking agents
    Tricylic antidepressants
    Phenothiazines
    Antiparkinsonian agents
    Calcium channel blockers
Instability incontinence (related to bladder obstruction)
Urinary tract infections
Pyelonephritis
Bladder overdistention
Bladder trabeculation
Hydronephrosis
Upper urinary tract deterioration
Renal insufficiency

Defining Characteristics[23]

Urinary frequency
Small voided volumes
Intermittent or poor urinary stream
Nocturia
Overflow incontinence
Postvoiding dribble
Absence of micturition with suprapubic pain or pressure
Postvoiding residual greater than 25% of total bladder volume

Expected Patient Outcomes & Nursing Interventions

Resolves acute urinary voiding as evidenced by:

- Relief of urinary retention by employing straight urethral catheterization or introduction of indwelling catheter as directed.
- Institution of intermittent catheterization or maintenance of indwelling catheter as appropriate. (See Reflex Incontinence on p. 1580.)

Resolves urinary retention, as evidenced by:

Urinary frequency and nocturia being absent
Overflow incontinence being absent
Postvoiding residual is less than 25% of total bladder volume

- Assess patient's current diurnal voiding patterns.
- Assess quality of patient's voided stream.
- Determine patient's awareness of feelings of incomplete emptying.
- Assess maneuvers (if any) patient is using to cope with urinary retention. Determine if patient strains or uses Credé's maneuver to assist voiding.
- Teach patient to double void to enhance complete bladder emptying. Patient should void normally, then wait on the toilet for approximately 5 minutes and attempt to void again. Use of abdominal straining may be used to enhance bladder evacuation.

- Teach patient to void using a timed schedule. Patient should void every 3 to 4 hours when awake regardless of absence of desire to urinate. Sleep patterns are not typically interrupted for timed voiding schedule.
- Consult physician concerning use of bethanechol chloride to stimulate detrusor muscle contractility for patients with deficient detrusor function or terazosin or doxazosin for patients with increased sphincteric resistance.

Establishes regular, complete bladder emptying using mechanical means to manage urinary retention, as evidenced by:

Postvoiding residual being less than 25% of total bladder volume

Overflow incontinence is absent

- Teach patient and family members to perform intermittent catheterization. (See Reflex Incontinence on p. 1580.)
- Teach patient to perform intermittent catheterization after micturition. Teach patient to keep diary or log of voided volume versus volume catheterized, and provide parameters for returning to physician for alteration of catheterization schedule as needed.
- Teach patient to maintain long-term indwelling catheter. (See Reflex Incontinence on p. 1580.)

Prevents urinary tract infection, as evidenced by:

Urine cultures being negative

Symptoms of urinary tract infections being absent

- Assess for presence of current urinary tract infections.
- Determine if constipation is present and if patient has routine bowel program.
- Assess strategies, including medically prescribed ones, patient uses to manage urinary tract infections.
- Teach patient to completely empty bladder on regular basis.
- Provide patient with bowel program, including dietary manipulation (increased fluid intake with dietary fiber and bulk), stool softeners, and/or enemas in consultation with physician.
- Consult physician concerning use of long-term antibiotic prophylaxis for patients with chronic urinary retention as appropriate.

Principles and Rationale for Nursing Interventions

Acute urinary retention represents an immediate threat to the patient experiencing the condition. Urethral or suprapubic catheterization is used to relieve immediate bladder overdistention. Severe suprapubic pain and pressure sensations arise because of bladder overdistention. Following relief of immediate urinary retention, the nurse clarifies causative factors of voiding insufficiency and institutes a care plan to prevent recurrent acute urinary retention and manage chronic incomplete bladder emptying.

Timed voiding and double voiding are attempts to maximize the individual's ability to empty the bladder. *Double voiding* attempts to allow a brief resting period followed by an attempt to empty remaining urine through a second bladder contraction. *Timed voiding* is a preventive strategy as well as treatment modality for urinary retention. Chronic bladder overdistention is avoided by retraining the patient to void at regular intervals. The strategy is most effective among patients with moderate to severe bladder sensory deficit and minimum to mild motor deficit.

Bethanechol chloride is designed to increase bladder contractility by action at the neuromuscular junctions of the detrusor muscle. Terazosin or doxazosin are designed to decrease sphincteric resistance to urinary outflow by antagonistic action at the bladder neck and urethral smooth muscle. These drugs may assist in bladder evacuation among patients with deficient detrusor function or bladder outlet obstruction caused by bladder neck smooth muscle overactivity.

The goal of intermittent catheterization or indwelling catheterization for patients experiencing urinary retention is to ensure regular, complete bladder emptying, thus preventing the complications associated with the condition. Urinary tract infection still is a prominent complication, and these strategies are used primarily when more definitive methodologies prove inadequate.[14]

The likelihood of urinary tract infection is enhanced by urinary stasis and subsequent ischemia of the bladder wall. Regular, complete bladder emptying through intermittent catheterization is one strategy to prevent this condition.[17] Prevention of constipation also may help in the prevention of urinary tract infection. Bacteriuria is inevitable in the presence of a long-term indwelling catheter; this strategy is primarily used as a temporary measure to relieve urinary retention unless other strategies have failed to resolve the condition.

References

Colonic constipation, perceived constipation, constipation

1. Battle E, Hanan C: Evaluation of a dietary regimen for chronic constipation: report of a pilot study, *J Gerontol Nurs* 6(9):527, 1980.
2. Clark J, Queener S, Burke-Karb V, editors: *Pharmacological basis of nursing practice*, ed 2, St Louis, 1986, Mosby.
3. Ellickson EB: Bowel management plan for the homebound elderly, *J Gerontol Nurs* 14:16, 1988.
4. Georges JM, Heitkemper MM: Dietary fiber and distressing gastrointestinal symptoms in midlife women, *Nurs Res* 43(6):357, 1994.
5. Kim MJ, McFarland GK, McLane AM, editors: *Classification of nursing diagnoses: proceedings of the fifth national conference*, St Louis, 1984, Mosby.
6. Kim MJ, McFarland GK, McLane AM: *Pocket guide to nursing diagnoses*, ed 6, St Louis, 1995, Mosby.
7. McCloskey JC, Bulechek GM: Bowel irrigation. In *Nursing interventions classification (NIC)*, p 151, St Louis, 1996, Mosby.
8. McCloskey JC, Bulechek GM: Constipation/impaction management. In McCloskey JC, Bulechek GM, editors, *Nursing interventions classification (NIC)*, p 184, St Louis, 1996, Mosby.
9. McLane AM: *Classification of nursing diagnoses: proceedings of the seventh conference*, St Louis, 1987, Mosby.
10. McLane AM, McShane RE: Bowel management. In Bulechek GM, McCloskey JC, editors: *Nursing interventions: essential nursing treatments*, ed 2, p 73, St Louis, 1992, Mosby.
11. McLane AM, McShane RE: Constipation. In Maas M, Buckwalter KC, Hardy M, editors: *Nursing diagnoses and interventions for the elderly*, p 147, Redwood City, CA, 1991, Addison-Wesley.

12. McShane RE, McLane AM: Constipation: consensual and empirical validation, *Nurs Clin North Am* 20:801, 1985.

13. McShane RE, McLane AM: Constipation: impact of etiological factors, *J Gerontol Nurs* 14:31, 1988.

14. Mitchell D: The effect of patient-controlled analgesia on bowel habits. In Larson PJ, editor: *Symptom management proceedings,* p 82, San Francisco, 1992, University of California, San Francisco School of Nursing.

15. Moore L, et al: Therapeutic regimen used to prevent/reduce gas pain following cesarean section. In Larson PJ, editor: *Symptom management proceedings,* p 82, San Francisco, 1992, University of California, San Francisco School of Nursing.

16. Shannon ML, Moore L, Richard P, Vacca G: Effects of rocking on post-op GI motility after abdominal hysterectomy. In Larson PJ, editor: *Symptom management proceedings,* p 65, San Francisco, 1994, University of California, San Francisco School of Nursing.

17. Yakabowich M: Prescribe with care: the role of laxatives in treatment of constipation, *J Gerontol Nurs* 16(7):4, 1990.

Diarrhea

1. Georges JM, Heitkemper MM: Stressors, stress arousal, and functional bowel distress in midlife women. In Larson PJ, editor: *Symptom management proceedings,* p 84, San Francisco, 1994, University of California, San Francisco School of Nursing.

2. Georges JM, Heitkemper MM: Dietary fiber intake and distressing gastrointestinal symptoms in postmenopausal women. In Larson PJ, editor: *Symptom management proceedings,* p 119, San Francisco, 1992, University of California, San Francisco School of Nursing.

3. Kim MJ, McFarland GK, McLane AM: *Pocket guide to nursing diagnoses* St Louis, 1995, Mosby.

4. McCloskey JC, Bulechek GM: Diarrhea management. In *Nursing interventions classification (NIC),* p 205, St Louis, 1996, Mosby.

5. Snape WM, editor: *Pathogenesis of functional bowel disease,* New York, 1989. Plenum Medical Book Co.

6. Wadle K: Diarrhea. In Maas M, Buckwalter KC, Hardy M, editors: *Nursing diagnosis and interventions for the elderly,* p 159, Redwood City, CA, 1991, Addison-Wesley.

Bowel incontinence

1. Kim MJ, McFarland GK, McLane AM: *Pocket guide to nursing diagnoses,* St Louis, 1995, Mosby.

2. Maas M, Specht J: Bowel incontinence. In Maas M, Buckwalter KC, Hardy M, editors: *Nursing diagnoses and interventions for the elderly,* p 169, Redwood City, CA, 1991, Addison-Wesley.

3. McCloskey JC, Bulechek GM: Bowel incontinence care. In *Nursing interventions classification (NIC),* p 149, St Louis, 1996, Mosby.

4. McLane AM, McShane RE: Bowel management. In Bulechek GM, McCloskey JC, editors: *Nursing interventions: essential nursing treatments,* ed 2, p 73, St Louis, 1992, Mosby.

Altered urinary elimination; functional incontinence; reflex incontinence; stress incontinence, urge incontinence, total incontinence, urinary retention

1. Agency for Health Care Policy and Research: *Clinical practice guideline: urinary incontinence in adults,* Department of Health and Human Services, Rockville, MD, 1992, The Agency.

2. Anderson RS: A neurogenic element to urinary genuine stress incontinence, *Br J Obstet Gynaecol* 91:41, 1984.

3. Benta S et al: *Rehabilitation nursing: a core curriculum,* Evanston, Ill, 1987, Rehabilitation Nursing Institute.

4. Bhatia NN, Bergman A, Guning JE; Urodynamic effects of a vaginal pessary in women with stress urinary incontinence, *Am J Obstet Gynecol* 147:876, 1983.

5. Broadwell DC, Jackson BS: *Principles of ostomy care,* St Louis, 1982, Mosby.

6. Brocklehurst JC: *Urology in the elderly,* London, 1984, Churchill Livingstone.

7. Burton TA: Urinary retention following cannabis ingestion, *JAMA* 242:351, 1979.

8. Castleden CM, Duffin HM, McGrowther CW: Dementia and locomotor problems associated with incontinence. Paper presented at the International Continence Society Meeting, Bristol, Eng, Sept 1987.

9. Colling J et al: Patterned urge response toileting for urinary incontinence. In Funk SG, et al, editors: *Key aspects of elder care: managing falls, incontinence and cognitive impairment,* p 169, New York, 1992, Springer.

10. Dougherty MC, Bishop KR: *Circumvaginal (CVM) muscle exercise instruction* Gainesville, 1987, University of Florida.

11. Dougherty MC et al: Effect of exercise on the circumvaginal muscles (CVM), *Neurourol Urodynamics* 6:189, 1987.

12. Faller N: *Toilet training people with mental retardation.* In Jeter K, Faller N, Norton C, editors: *Nursing for continence,* Philadelphia, 1990, Saunders.

13. Gray ML: *Genitourinary disorders,* St Louis, 1992, Mosby.

14. Gray ML, Dougherty MC: Urinary incontinence—pathophysiology and treatment, *J Enterostomal Ther* 14:152, 1987.

15. Gray M et al: *Management of urinary incontinence.* In Doughty D, editor: *Urinary and fecal incontinence: nursing management,* St Louis, 1991, Mosby.

16. Horsley JA, Crane J, Reynolds MA: *Clean intermittent catheterization: CURN project.* New York, 1982, Grune & Stratton.

17. Howe SM, Bates P: The cranberry juice cure: fact or fiction: *AUAA J* 8:13, 1987.

18. Hurst JW: *Medicine for the practicing physician,* ed 2, Boston, 1988, Butterworth.

19. International Continence Society: *Standardization of terminology of lower urinary tract function.* Glasgow, UK, 1984, Department of Physics and Bioengineering.

20. Jarvis GJ, Millar DR: Controlled bladder drill for detrusor instability, *Br Med J* 281:1322, 1980.

21. Kegel A: Progressive resistance exercises in the functional restoration of the perineal muscles, *Am J Obstet Gynecol* 56:238, 1948.

22. Kelalis PP, King LR, Belman AB, editors: *Clinical Pediatric Urology,* ed 3, Philadelphia, 1992, Saunders.

23. Kim MJ, McFarland GK, McLane AM: *Pocket Guide to Nursing Diagnoses,* ed 6, St Louis, 1995, Mosby.

24. Krane RJ, Siroky MB, editors: *Clinical Neuro-urology,* ed 2, Boston, 1992, Little-Brown.

25. Lapides J et al: Clean intermittent self catheterization in the treatment of urinary tract disease, *J Urol* 107:458, 1972.

26. Lepor, H and the multicenter study group: Long term efficacy and safety of doxazosin for the treatment of benign prostatic hypertrophy, *J Urol* 153:273A, 1995.

27. Liedberg H, Lundberg T: Silver alloy coated catheters reduce catheter-associated bacteriuria, *Br J Urol* 65:379, 1990.

28. Mundy AR: The unstable bladder, *Urol Clin North Am* 12:317, 1985.

29. Mundy AR, Stephenson TP, Wein AJ: *Urodynamics: principles, practice and application,* London, 1984, Churchill Livingstone.

30. Pearson BD, Larson JM: Urine control for elders: Non-invasive strategies. In Funk SG, Tornquist EM, Champagne MT, Weise RA, editors: *Key aspects of elder care:* managing falls, incontinence and cognitive impairment, p 154, New York, 1992, Springer.

31. *Physician's desk reference,* Oradell, NJ, 1992, Medical Economics.

32. Recommended daily allowances: RDA for fluids, The Academy, ed 9, Washington, DC, 1980.

33. Snooks SJ et al: Perineal nerve damage in genuine stress incontinence, *Br J Urol* 57:422, 1985.

34. Sorenson KC, Luckman J: *Basic nursing,* ed 4, Philadelphia, 1987, Saunders.

35. Stamey TA: *Pathogenesis and treatment of urinary tract infections,* Baltimore, 1980, Williams & Wilkins.

36. Walsh PC, Retik AB, Stamey TA, Vaughan ED: *Campbell's Urology,* ed 6, Philadelphia, 1992, Saunders.

37. Wheatley JK: Causes and treatment of bladder incontinence, *Compr Ther* 9:27, 1983.

38. Wyman JF, Fantl JA: Bladder training in ambulatory care management of urinary incontinence, *Urol Nurs* 11:11, 1991.

IV

FUNCTIONAL HEALTH PATTERN

Activity-Exercise

ACTIVITY INTOLERANCE

Activity intolerance is a state in which an individual has insufficient physiologic or psychologic energy to endure or complete required or desired daily activities.[20]

The definitions for activity intolerance proposed by other authors contribute to further understanding of the concept. Campbell's definition[2] is presented in terms of the degree of activity that can be tolerated, i.e., minimum, mild, and moderate activity tolerance. Her definitions are as follows:

Minimum activity tolerance: the inability to tolerate any physical activity without the presence of discomforts . . . Mild activity tolerance: the ability to tolerate only a very limited amount of physical activity without the presence of discomforts . . . Moderate activity tolerance: the ability to tolerate a moderate, but not a full day of physical activity without the presence of discomfort.

Gordon[9] defines activity intolerance in terms of "abnormal responses to energy-consuming body movements involved in required or desired daily activities." Four levels of endurance are specified that, when used with the diagnostic label, describe an individual's response to specific activities. Gordon supports using activity intolerance, when appropriate, "in describing the etiology for problems such as self-care deficit, perceived sexual dysfunction, impaired home maintenance management, or social isolation." Randell[21] expresses concern that this is an inconsistency in the diagnostic process that should be examined carefully.

Activity intolerance is a diagnosis that is frequently made in critical care[12] and acute care[13] settings, as well as in long-term care,[15] ambulatory care,[6] home care,[22] and rehabilitation[10,11] settings. Assessment data indicating that a patient may be experiencing activity intolerance may be as vague as a single report that the patient feels tired after taking a shower or as obvious as a report that the patient is experiencing dysrhythmia, dyspnea, or profuse diaphoresis after walking up a flight of stairs.

The diagnostic label of activity intolerance implies inability to engage in and endure a required or desired physical activity as a result of functional, structural, or situational limitations. Physical activity encompasses all activity that requires the expenditure of energy. *Functional* limitations include those factors reflecting altered or impaired physiologic functioning. The energy expenditure required to perform the activity may be more than the individual has to expend. *Structural* limitations that can lead to activity intolerance are associated with an impairment or alteration of the anatomic structure. The extent of the structural impairment or alteration influences the degree to which the individual's mobility is restricted and the consequent effect on his ability to tolerate activity. *Situational* limitations that can alter an individual's tolerance for activity include factors relevant to the person's cognitive and emotional status and environment.

The diagnosis of activity intolerance is made in relation to a specified etiology or related factor. The related factor can be a functional, structural, or situational limitation that an individual experiences.

Related Factors[1,7,17,20,22]

Functional limitations
    Generalized weakness
    Decreased mobility or immobility
    Imbalance between oxygen supply and demand
    Obesity
    Pain
Structural limitation
    Decreased mobility or immobility
Situational limitation
    Lack of knowledge
    Lack of motivation
    Deconditioning (related to lifestyle)
    Lack of support
    Climate extremes

Defining Characteristics*

Decrease in activity (self-care, exercise, leisure)
Avoidance of activity
Verbal report of fatigue or weakness
Cardiovascular response to activity
    Bradycardia
    Inappropriate tachycardia
    Dysrhythmia

---

*References 1, 3, 5, 7, 17, 20.

Decrease in pulse strength
Inappropirate increases or decreases in blood pressure
Respiratory response to activity
Dyspnea
Tachypnea
Decrease in rate
Irregular rhythm
Skin in response to activity
Pallor, cyanosis, flushing
Profuse diaphoresis
Dry with strenuous activity
Posture
Drooping of shoulders or head
Decrease in muscle tone and strength
Equilibrium
Ataxia
Dizziness, vertigo
Syncope
Emotional status
Lack of interest in activity
Fearful of activity

Expected Patient Outcomes & Nursing Interventions[1,6,16,17,19]

Participate in activities that enhance physiologic well-being, as evidence by:

Balance between oxygen supply and demand
Absence of weakness and fatigue during or after engaging in activity
Verbal report of tolerance to activities

- Assess patient's past and present activity pattern.
    Determine past activities (self-care, exercise, and leisure) engaged in; intensity, duration, and frequency of each activity; and how these activities were tolerated.
    Determine present activities and how these are tolerated.
- Assess physical impediments.
    Determine if any physical impediments restrict participation in particular activities.
    Determine if any physical impediments prevent active participation in activities.
- Assess physiologic status.
    Determine if there is any change in physiologic status when engaging in activity.
    Cardiovascular response: note heart rate and rhythm; pulse strength; blood pressure.
    Respirator response: note rate, depth, and rhythm of respirations.
    Skin: note color, signs, temperature, moistness.
    Posture: note signs of muscle fatigue.
    Equilibrium: note gait, fine and gross movements.
- Assess emotional status.
    Determine if there is any change in emotional status before or when engaging in activity.
    Determine if patient is fearful of harming himself.

- Provide patient information about activities in which to participate.
- Assist patient in interpretation of activity/exercise prescription.
- Seek consultation with physician, exercise physiologist, and occupational and physical therapists as necessary.
- Assist patient in identifying factors that reduce activity tolerance (inadequate sleep, medication, treatments, environmental conditions).
- Engage immobile patients in passive exercise regimen.
- Assist patient with structural limitations to adapt self-care, exercise, and leisure activities to meet needs.
- Provide assistance to patient as needed, encouraging independence in performing activities.
- Encourage patient to engage in self-care, exercise, and leisure activities that can be tolerated.
- Guide patient in increasing activity within therapeutic limits.

Develop activity and rest pattern supporting increased tolerance of activity, as evidenced by:

Adherence to a schedule that promotes increased activity without increasing weakness, fatigue, and untoward physiologic responses to the activity.

- Discuss with patient usual activity/rest pattern; suggest ways to modify an ineffective pattern.
- Discuss the importance of increasing activity tolerance.
- Encourage patient to participate in planning daily rest periods and activity periods.
- Adjust medication and treatment schedule to support adequate rest.
- Teach patient to monitor response to activity and to alter activity when signs and symptoms of anoxia or excessive fatigue are present.
- Encourage patient to increase active participation gradually in self-care, exercise, and leisure activities.
- Encourage patient to adhere to activity/rest schedule that best promotes increase in activity tolerance.

Use support of family, friends, and health care providers in adjusting an activity and rest pattern to meet need fo activity, as evidenced by:

The description of the role of significant others in revising and implementing the activity and rest schedule

- Provide patient and significant others with information about importance of establishing therapeutic activity/rest pattern.
- Review schedule of daily activities of significant others and identify with them how it can be altered to support fulfillment of patient's needs.
- Encourage patient and significant others to participate in planning mutually agreeable daily schedule of activity/rest periods.
- Facilitate expression of patient and significant others' concerns regarding proposed schedule.

- Identify support available from health care providers if need arises to revise or alter schedule.
- Encourage family and friends to support patient in efforts to meet need for activity.

Principles and Rationale for Nursing Interventions

The initial nursing assessment provides the opportunity to collect data relevant to an individual's ability to engage in activity and his response to activity. The identification of factors contributing to an inability to tolerate activities (the related factors) and the presence of signs and symptoms that reflect this inability (the defining characteristics) lead to a nursing diagnosis of activity intolerance.

In the preceding section, expected patient outcomes and nursing interventions supporting achievement of the outcomes were specified. Although the outcomes and interventions are presented in general terms, it is assumed that these will be adapted and expanded according to the needs of each individual. The general physiologic and emotional status of the individual, as well as the optimum therapeutic level of activity that should be attained, must be a primary consideration in planning nursing care.

An activity/exercise prescription must be tailored to each patient's needs and abilities. The data gathered in the assessment phase of the nursing process and the consequent identification of the outcome should be validated with the patient. In reviewing the patient's past and present activity pattern, as well as the patient's physiologic and emotional status related to participation in activity and exercise, information should be shared to assist the patient in identifying activities that will enhance physiologic well-being. The patient should understand the importance of engaging in regular activity and exercise. When developing a schedule of activities and exercise with the patient, the nurse should explain the recommended intensity, duration, and frequency of various activities and exercise routines.

To ensure a patient's adherence to a recommended activity/exercise pattern, it is important that the pattern can be integrated into the patient's life-style. The patient should be assisted in developing and implementing an activity/rest schedule that supports an increased tolerance of activity. The schedule should incorporate the patient's requirements for medications and treatments, as well as participation in self-care and leisure activities. The patient should be taught to monitor responses to activity and to adjust the activity/execise schedule as needed.

The patient's own life-style incorporates the life-styles of family, friends, and significant others. It may be necessary for family members to alter or revise their daily activities to support a therapeutic activity/rest schedule for the patient. Support of family and friends can be essential in assisting the patient to adhere to an activity/rest pattern that will promote optimum participation in therapeutic activities and exercise.

■ RISK FOR ACTIVITY INTOLERANCE

Risk for activity intolerance is a state in which an individual is at risk of experiencing insufficient physiologic or psychologic energy to endure or complete required or desired daily activities.[20]

Yura and Walsh[23] define the human need for activity as "a behavior or action requiring an expenditure of energy by the person with volition and intent." The need is further described as one that contributes to a person's survival. The potential inability to tolerate activity can threaten a person's well-being.

Definitions of the diagnosis "Risk for Activity Intolerance" address the presence of risk factors in distinguishing this diagnosis from that of "Activity Intolerance." This diagnosis can be viewed as an indication that a person is at risk for developing physiologic or psychologic deficits that will hinder participation in an expected or desired activity.[2] Gordon[9] refers to the diagnosis as "a useful category to describe the presence of risk factors for abnormal response to energy-consuming activities."

A person's health history should provide clues to determine whether the risk for activity intolerance is present. Reviewing the person's usual life-style and current physiologic and psychologic status through a thorough health assessment is essential to identify risk factors. Patients with cardiovascular, respiratory, musculoskeletal, and neurologic alterations are at risk for experiencing activity intolerance.[5,14] Treatments for a particular physical alteration may make a patient more vulnerable to activity intolerance, for example, prolonged bed rest. Therefore ongoing assessment is critical and should focus on changes in a patient's level of activity, as well as on the patient's response to activity in terms of cardiovascular and respiratory changes and feelings of fatigue and weakness.

Risk Factors[3,14,18,20]

History of previous intolerance to activity
Fatigue, weakness
Sedentary life-style
Climate extremes
Deconditioned status (prolonged bed rest, inactivity)
Presence of chronic or progressive disease (e.g., chronic obstructive pulmonary disease, multiple sclerosis, coronary artery disease, arthritis, and depression)
Presence of circulatory or respiratory problems
More than 15% overweight
Pain
Inexperience with activity
Expresses concern about ability to perform the activity
Expresses lack of interest in engaging in activity/exercise
Refuses to participate in prescribed activities

Expected Patient Outcomes & Nursing Interventions[16,18,19]

Participate in activities that promote optimum well-being, as evidenced by:

Daily performance of recommended self-care, exercise, and leisure activities

- Assess patient's past and present activity pattern.
- Assess type, intensity, duration, and frequency of each patient activity.
- Determine physiologic response to activity.
- Determine psychologic response to activity.
- Assess risk factors for potential activity intolerance.
- Provide patient with information about desired or required daily activities.
- Assist patient in selecting activities that are enjoyable and can be integrated into life-style.
- Assist patient in identifying risk factors that reduce activity tolerance.
- Encourage patient to participate in activities that promote an increase in activity tolerance within therapeutic limits.
- Identify organized activities and exercise programs in which patient might want to participate.
- Encourage family and significant others to support patient and to participate in activities and exercise programs with patient.

Appreciate the need to participate in required and desired activities, as evidenced by:

Specifying the benefits of engaging in activity and identifying factors that could inhibit activity tolerance

- Review benefits of regularly engaging in activities that promote physical and psychologic well-being, as well as factors that could inhibit activity tolerance.
- Assist the patient in developing a realistic plan that includes self-care, exercise, and leisure activities.
- Encourage the patient to plan activities with persons who can support participation in activities that will enhance well-being.

Principles and Rationale for Nursing Intervention

The person who is at risk for experiencing an inability to tolerate activity requires support and guidance in choosing activities that will promote optimum well-being. The patient's physiologic and psychologic response to particular activities must be taken into consideration when developing an appropriate plan for the patient's participation in required or desired activities.

The patient should be given information that will assist in identifying those activities that are therapeutic and enjoyable and within the patient's physiologic capabilities. Information about factors that might interfere with the patient's ability to tolerate activity can help the patient to make changes that will promote activity tolerance. If the patient lacks the motivation to participate in required or desired activities on a regular basis, support can be elicited from significant others and through organized activity or exercise programs.

▪ FATIGUE

Fatigue is an overwhelming sense of exhaustion and decreased capacity for physical and mental work, regardless of adequate sleep or rest.

Fatigue is a universal phenomenon—one of the least understood and most neglected symptoms. A subjectively experienced feeling of discomfort, fatigue may be a symptom of excessive physical activity, emotional stress, lack of sleep, or pathologic disease processes, among others.[4,18,19,22] Indeed, the causes of fatigue have been identified as physical, mental, environmental, emotional, physiologic, and pathologic factors.[9,13,19] Although acute fatigue is thought to protect against overwork or exhaustion, a homeostatic function for chronic fatigue has not been identified.[21] Furthermore, chronic prolonged fatigue interferes with activities of daily living, impairs functional status, and decreases quality of life.[1] Chronic fatigue persists over time, lasting for more than 1 month, and is characterized as constant or recurrent.[21]

Fatigue is differentiated from tiredness; tiredness is a temporary state caused by transient factors, such as an increase in work or a lack of sleep, and is relieved by rest or sleep.[17] Fatigue is much more pervasive and subjective and does not disappear with rest and sleep—it is often present on awakening. Fatigue is different from activity intolerance; activity intolerance is decreased or reversed by progressive endurance, whereas fatigue often may not be reversed to achieve a previous level of functioning.

Fatigue has been associated with the accumulation of metabolites, such as lactic acid; changes in energy or energy substrate patterns, such as in cachexia or fever; disorders in neurotransmission; treatments, such as surgery, radiation therapy, or chemotherapy; and patterns of chronic diseases, such as cancer, arthritis, and emphysema.[2,4,5,11,26] In fact, prolonged stress that leads to depletion of body reserves has been proposed as a major cause of fatigue in the person with cancer;[1] the model seems applicable to individuals with chronic anxiety, depression, or a variety of other situations, as well. In addition, environmental factors such as noise, temperature, and stages of the life cycle, such as pregnancy and old age, have been associated with fatigue.[13,14,23] It seems likely that several factors may interact to produce fatigue in all of these situations.[19] The specific mechanisms that underlie fatigue are unknown.[19] Despite the acknowledged prevalence of fatigue, research studies that determine correlates, causes, consequences, and effective treatments for fatigue have been limited. Further investigation of the fatigue experience is needed.[10,21]

Related Factors*

Altered body chemistry (e.g., medications, drug withdrawal)
Overwhelming psychologic or emotional demands
Increased energy requirements to perform activities of daily living (ADLs)
Excessive social role demands
States of discomfort
Decreased metabolic energy production

Defining Characteristics[6, 11,12,17,25]

Verbalization of fatigue/lack of energy
Inability to maintain usual routines
Perceived need for additional energy to accomplish routine tasks
Lethargy or listlessness
Emotional lability or irritability
Impaired ability to concentrate
Disinterest in surroundings/introspection
Decreased performance
Accident proneness
Decreased libido
Increase in physical complaints

Expected Patient Outcomes & Nursing Interventions[7-9,16,19,21]

Have sufficient energy to engage in ADLs and fulfill role demands or adapt to decreased energy levels, as evidenced by:

Successful independent completion of ADLs or seeking assistance for incomplete ADLs
Verbalized improvement in mental outlook
Ability to concentrate
Participation in regular exercise program
Engaging in scheduled rest and sleep
Injury-free status

- Assess patterns of family; identify correlates of fatigue; *planning for energy conservation involves identification of energy-depleting factors and energy requirements of common ADLs.*
- Ensure that patient has complete physical workup *to identify and treat physical and mental causes.*
- Assist patient to establish a daily activities plan for effective energy use based upon identification of tasks/activities that require more effort; patient's most productive hours of day; specific tasks that patient is unable to perform; support systems and resources available; priorities for activities or roles valued by the patient; measures to conserve energy and to use energy more effectively; need for rest between activities.

*References 2, 3, 5, 7, 11, 12, 19, 21, 25.

- *With careful planning to maintain energy resources and prevent energy depletion, the patient can still participate in valued activities, while delegating less valued or more energy-consuming tasks to supportive others.*
- Consult with physiatrist or physical therapist to develop incremental physical exercise program; engage in regular exercise; *aerobic exercise stimulates the body's endurance energy systems and improves functional capacity.*
- Enhance patient's ability to sleep by means of mild sedatives, warm bath, massage, and quiet environment; allow for uninterrupted periods of sleep; *adequate amounts of undisturbed sleep are necessary to replace energy stores.*
- Assess nutritional habits and alter those that contribute to fatigue; *high-quality nutrition supplies basic materials essential to energy production.*
- Administer treatments or medications to relieve other discomforts (e.g., pain, nausea, itching); *unmanaged contributory symptoms may exacerbate fatigue and/or decrease tolerance to fatigue.*
- Evaluate new or added stressors (e.g., new baby, ill family member, financial burdens, multiple competing demands); *prolonged stress may lead to depletion of body reserves and cause fatigue.*
- Provide supportive listening for irretrievable functional losses; *supportive listening can decrease the anxiety and anguish that accompany loss and can facilitate adaptation.*

Experience reduction or resolution of fatigue, as evidenced by:

Absence or reduction of defining characteristics

- Monitor regularly the level of fatigue, contributing factors, and degree of adaptation to fatigue; *progress toward goals is facilitated by ongoing evaluation of the effectiveness of interventions and by periodic revisions as indicated in the plan of care.*

Principles and Rationale for Nursing Interventions

Interventions for management of fatigue begin with the identification of factors that cause or contribute to fatigue. If fatigue is a new symptom, physical and psychiatric illnesses should be ruled out. Treatable factors, such as sleep pattern disturbance, depression, situational stress, hypothyroidism, or iron-deficiency anemia, should be corrected. Unmanaged symptoms, such as pain, nausea, and anxiety, that exacerbate fatigue should be controlled. Patients at high risk for fatigue, such as those beginning chemotherapy or radiation therapy, should be taught about potential fatigue, and a plan for prevention and treatment should be established.[11] Because extreme fatigue is closely related to the performance of valued roles and the concept of self as independent and capable, it may have profound effects on the quality of life; therefore it assumes an important priority in nursing management.

Three guiding principles basic to nursing interventions for fatigue are energy conservation, effective energy use, and energy restoration.[1,19] Useful strategies are prioritizing, planning, and pacing.

Energy conservation involves identification of energy-depleting factors and energy requirements for common daily activities[18] With the assistance of the nurse, the patient and family should be encouraged to develop an activity/rest program that permits the patient to identify and carry out priority activities and to delegate less valued or more fatiguing roles and activities. The plan should include specific rest periods spaced between energy-depleting pursuits to prevent loss of energy reserves.

Effective energy use focuses on the maintenance of present abilities, strength, and energy reserves.[19] A daily activity plan should schedule more strenuous activities during the patient's most productive and peak energy times of the day. Patients should be encouraged to pace activities; however, they need to continue doing as much as they are capable of doing. Progressive decreases in activity levels can lead to permanent decreases in functional ability.

Energy restoration encompasses activities that maintain and restore strength, including good nutrition, adequate rest and sleep, stress management, and a progressive physical exercise program. Aerobic exercise stimulates the body's endurance energy systems, improves functional capacity, and reduces fatigue of cancer patients receiving chemotherapy.[15] In addition, a walking exercise program has been reported to decrease fatigue in women in treatment for breast cancer.[16] A specific exercise prescription, developed in consultation with a physiatrist or physical therapist, should be based on the patient's physical status, activity tolerance, and personal goals.[9] Adequate, undisturbed sleep to replace energy stores, and high-quality nutrition to supply material for energy production, are also essential to prevent or treat fatigue.

Because fatigue is a subjective experience, the effectiveness of nursing interventions is best evaluated by the patient by means of self-report. Several self-report measures, such as the Rhoten Fatigue Scale[24] and the Piper Fatigue Scale[20] have been shown to measure fatigue effectively. Undiminished fatigue requires reassessment and revisions in the plan of care, as indicated. Diminished fatigue and increased vigor attest to successful interventions and contribute to improved quality of life.

◼ IMPAIRED PHYSICAL MOBILITY

Impaired physical mobility is the state in which the individual experiences a limitation of ability for independent physical movement.[9]

The nursing diagnosis of Impaired Physical mobility is one of the most frequent and most important that nurses encounter in practice. Impaired physical mobility is found in conjunction with numerous medical-surgical conditions.

In addition, this nursing diagnosis can occur in conjunction with psychiatric diagnoses and as a result of prescribed medical-surgical treatments. Impaired physical mobility affects patients across the life span in a variety of health care settings.[4,8,11,13,14]

The three elements that are necessary for mobility include the ability to move, the motivation to move, and an unrestrictive environment in which to move.[3] *Impaired physical mobility* should not be used to describe complete immobility. Instead, *risk of disuse syndrome* is the appropriate diagnosis to select when there is complete immobility.

Related Factors/Risk Factors[2,5,7,9,10]

Intolerance to activity
Decreased strength or endurance
Pain or discomfort
Perceptual or cognitive impairment
Neuromuscular impairment
Musculoskeletal impairment
Depression
Severe anxiety
External device (casts, splints, traction, braces, intravenous tubing, cardiac monitors, ventilators)
Trauma
Surgical procedure
Nonfunctioning or missing limbs
Advanced age
Mechanical/medical protocol restrictions

Defining Characteristics[2,5,7,9,10]

Inability to move purposefully within physical environment (e.g., bed mobility)
Inability to transfer
Inability to ambulate
Reluctance or refusal to attempt movement
Limited range of motion
Decreased muscle strength, control, and/or mass
Impaired coordination
Imposed restrictions of movement

Expected Patient Outcomes & Nursing Interventions[1,6,12,15]

Demonstrate measures to increase mobility, as evidenced by:

The performance of progressive mobilization, the performance of functional activities, and the use of appropriate transfer techniques
- Provide for progressive mobilization.
- Assist the patient to progress from active range of motion exercises to functional activities, as indicated, *because the use of such approaches will improve the functional abilities of the patient.*
- Teach transfer techniques.

Demonstrate maximum range of motion in all joints, as evidenced by:

The maintenance of range of motion and muscle mass and strength in unaffected limbs at the patient's usual level and the maintenance of joint mobility in affected limbs

- Teach patient to perform active range of motion exercises on unaffected limbs at least four times a day *to increase muscle mass, tone, and strength.*
- Perform passive range of motion exercises on affected limbs at least four times a day *to improve joint mobility.*

Demonstrate the use of adaptive devices to increase mobility, as evidenced by:

The patient properly using whatever adaptive devices are appropriate for use in his or her particular situation

- Teach and observe proper use of appropriate adaptive devices: crutches, walkers, wheelchairs, prostheses, slings, Ace bandages *to significantly improve mobility and independent functioning.*
- Teach and observe use of appropriate adaptive equipment to enhance use of arms.

Use safety measures to minimize high risk for injury, as evidenced by:

The patient's compliance with whatever safety precautions are appropriate in his or her particular situation

- Teach and observe safety precautions, such as protecting areas of decreased sensation from extremes of heat and cold, instructing patients confined to wheelchairs to shift position and lift up buttocks every 15 minutes, and instructing patients with decreased perception of lower extremity to check where limb is placed when changing positions *to decrease the possibility of physical dangers associated with impaired physical mobility.*

Participate in a plan for integrating the mobility impairment into established life-style patterns, as evidenced by:

The patient's active participation in discussions about and positive responses to possible alternatives and modifications necessary in his or her life-style patterns

- Explore the patient's perceptions of mobility impairment in regards to his or her previous life-style patterns, the possibility of resuming previous patterns, and his or her willingness to accept limitations.
- Discuss alternatives (i.e., substitutions or modifications) for activities that are not achievable (either temporarily or permanently) *to enhance patient's sense of control and his or her actual control.*
- Identify resources, special equipment, devices, and environmental modifications necessary to permit patient functioning despite physical limitations.

Identify and utilize institutional or community resources to manage altered mobility, as evidenced by:

The patient's acceptance of and use of whatever support services are appropriate in his or her particular situation

- Provide patient with information about available resources.
- Facilitate access to available resources by means of printed materials, telephone contacts, introductions, or written referral.
- Mobilize resources existing within the patient's support network.
- Refer to support services according to need; physical therapy, occupational therapy, and social services *to assist the patient to achieve the highest level of independence possible.*

Principles and Rationale for Nursing Interventions[1,6,12,15]

The rationale for the specified nursing interventions corresponding to the expected patient outcome, the patient will demonstrate measures to increase mobility, is that these interventions promote the development of increasingly independent movement, utilizing an approach marked by progressive activity. The patient becomes able to assume increasing responsibility for his or her own functional activities.

The rationale for the specified nursing interventions corresponding to the expected patient outcome, the patient will demonstrate maximum range of motion in all joints, is that these interventions promote the maintenance of functioning in unaffected limbs and promote the improvement of joint mobility in affected limbs. Both of these factors are important in regaining or retaining the highest possible level of functioning.

The rationale for the specified nursing interventions corresponding to the expected patient outcome, the patient will demonstrate the use of adaptive devices to increase mobility, is that these interventions promote maximal independence by teaching the patient to make effective use of a variety of pieces of equipment (those that are appropriate to the individual). The use of such equipment can be viewed as extending the patient's abilities.

The rationale for the specified nursing interventions corresponding to the expected patient outcome, the patient will utilize safety measures to minimize high risk for injury, is that these interventions assist the patient in protecting himself or herself from injuries that can typically occur concomitant with decreased mobility. The likelihood of impaired physical mobility becoming a cause for other nursing diagnoses is thereby decreased.

The rationale for the specified nursing interventions corresponding to the expected patient outcome, the patient will participate in a plan for integrating the mobility impairment into established lifestyle patterns, is that these interventions promote patient adaptation to changes in mobility status. By encouraging exploration of perceptions, and by providing informational support, the patient's sense of control and his or her actual control is enhanced.

The rationale for the specified nursing interventions corresponding to the expected patient outcome, the patient will identify and utilize institutional or community resources to manage altered mobility, is that these interventions assist the patient in becoming aware of support that is available and in learning how to use the support to his or her advantage, fostering patient independence and self-responsibility.

RISK FOR DISUSE SYNDROME

Risk for disuse syndrome is the state in which an individual is at risk for deterioration of body systems as the result of prescribed or unavoidable inactivity.

This diagnosis provides the focus for the cluster of potential physiologic and psychosocial alterations that may result from musculoskeletal inactivity. For example, the patient with a spinal cord injury is at high risk for impaired skin integrity, ineffective airway clearance, impaired physical mobility, self-care deficits, ineffective individual coping, and impaired social interactions. Risk for Disuse Syndrome encompasses all of these, permitting the nurse to plan a more comprehensive, appropriate approach to care rather than separating the interventions that should occur simultaneously[9]

The goal of nursing intervention is to prevent the deterioration of bodily functions and systems that may result from inactivity in order to avoid permanent complications and loss of function. Patient inactivity may be prescribed—as in the case of bed rest following myocardial infarction or following threatened spontaneous abortion—or it may be unavoidable, e.g., skeletal traction or mechanical ventilation.

The physiologic and psychosocial alterations inherent in Risk for Disuse Syndrome can have a dramatic and negative effect on a healthy individual's ability to function and an even more injurious effect on an already ill or debilitated person.

Prolonged musculoskeletal inactivity results in negative or deleterious effects on every body system, as well as on the patient's psychosocial equilibrium.[1-5,11,12,16] Studies have shown that enforced bed rest, even with young, healthy individuals for short periods, can cause distorted sensations and bodily discomforts, loss of muscle strength, and cardiovascular symptoms[3,5,7,14] Patients who are elderly and/or debilitated are at even greater risk. Complications from immobility, which have been considered defining characteristics for disuse syndrome, include pressure ulcers, constipation, stasis of pulmonary secretions, thrombosis, urinary tract infection/retention, decreased strength/endurance, orthostatic hypotension, decreased range of motion, disorientation, body image disturbance, and powerlessness.[6,9]

Nursing interventions to *prevent* the development of disuse syndrome in a high-risk individuals include nursing interventions that are consistent with those used to *treat* Impaired Physical Mobility. (See nursing interventions for Impaired Physical Mobility in this text.) The expected outcome of maintaining normal functioning of all body systems is similar for both diagnoses.

Risk Factors

Altered level of consciousness
Paralysis
Mechanical immobilization
Prescribed immobilization
Severe pain

Expected Patient Outcomes & Nursing Interventions*

Does not experience disuse syndrome, as evidenced by:

Maintenance of normal function of all body systems, as well as maintenance of psychosocial equilibrium

- Assess, document, and monitor patient's risk factors for effects of immobilization on body systems; *progress toward goals is facilitated by accurate identification of risk factors and ongoing evaluation of the effectiveness of interventions.*
- Plan and implement (as the patient's condition warrants) a progressive program to maximize musculoskeletal activity and cardiovascular function:
  Consult with physiatrist or physical therapist, as appropriate.
  Implement passive and active range of motion exercises; instruct patient in isometric exercises and use of idle body parts; *the pumping action of contracting muscles promotes venous return. Isotonic, isometric, and passive muscle exercises stretch muscle fibers and also help maintain cardiac work capacity.*
  If appropriate, place patient on kinetic treatment table or tilt table *to maintain motion, circulation, and orthostatic equilibrium and to provide stress on long bones to reduce demineralization.*
  Implement a pain management protocol, if necessary, *to allow patient to move comfortably and exercise enough in bed to achieve therapeutic goals.*
  Consult with physician regarding prophylactic use of anticoagulants *to prevent thrombus formation by decreasing clotting factors.*
  Teach patient to move in bed without increasing intrathoracic pressure *to decrease cardiac workload.*
  Frequently turn and position patient *to prevent contractures.*

---

*References 1, 2, 8, 10, 12-15.

- Plan and implement a program to prevent respiratory complications:

  Assess lungs frequently and promote cough and deep breathing *to mobilize secretions and prevent atelectasis.* Increase fluid intake *to liquify secretions.*

  Teach use of incentive spirometer *to promote chest expansion, more complete inflation of alveoli, and better gas exchange.*

- Plan and implement a program to maintain integument and to prevent skin breakdown:

  Assess skin frequently; monitor for possible breakdown or abrasions related to traction or other devices; *early identification of skin problems allows early intervention to limit damage.*

  Assess need for air or fluid flotation bed or provide convoluted foam mattress *to decrease pressure and increase circulation to skin.*

  Ensure that patient receives excellent hygiene: skin, hair, and mouth care.

  Encourage and assist patient to change position frequently; avoid shearing motions; *prevention of pressure ulcers requires prevention of prolonged pressure and maintenance of intact, clean, dry skin.*

- Plan and implement a program to maintain nutrition and elimination:

  Optimize nutrition and fluid status *to maintain adequate balance; prevent muscle and skin breakdown; promote normal bladder and bowel elimination.*

  Assess need for stool softener or bulk laxative and administer, as needed per physician's order *to increase bowel peristalsis and maintain regular, soft formed stool.*

- Plan and implement a program to maintain psychosocial equilibrium:

  Assess and maximize available support resources *to facilitate meeting emotional needs and stimulate intellectual faculties.*

  Ensure that patient has clock, calendar, radio, and television to assist in reality orientation.

  Provide frequent interactions *to maintain sensory stimulation and reality orientation.*

  Provide opportunities for patient participation in decisions regarding care *to restore a feeling of control over the environment.*

Principles and Rationale for Nursing Interventions*

The overall goal of nursing interventions is to prevent the development of disuse syndrome. Attaining this goal involves planning and implementing a progressive program to maximize musculoskeletal activity within the limits of the patient's disease state, physical condition, and/or therapeutic prescription for inactivity. Because many of the body's usual functions either maintain mobility or are main-

---

*References 3-5, 8, 9, 11, 16.

tained by mobility, inactivity has adverse consequences for functional capacities. No matter how restrictive the condition, the patient's capabilities should be identified, maintained, and developed.

Active participation in activities of daily living (ADLs), such as bathing, eating, dressing, and turning, provides exercise for muscles and joints. As muscles contract, they increase venous return to the heart, stimulating circulation to all body tissues and decreasing clotting factors. A plan for periodic activity and rest should include active range of motion exercises, if possible, and passive exercises by the nurse or physical therapist if the patient is incapable of performing active exercises.

Helping the patient out of bed at regular intervals, to sit or stand, provides stress on long bones, prevents demineralization, and facilitates maintenance of orthostatic mechanisms. A Stryker frame, tilt table, or kinetic treatment table may be used when the patient cannot get out of bed. Respiratory complications from inactivity may be prevented by coughing and deep breathing exercises, chest physical therapy, and use of incentive spirometer to improve airway clearance, lung expansion, and gas exchange. Good hydration helps to liquify secretions for easier removal.

Principles of pressure ulcer prevention include reduction of prolonged pressure on soft tissues, prevention of friction and shearing forces, positive nitrogen balance via good nutritional intake, and maintenance of clean, dry skin. Frequent turning, to relieve pressure, and inspection of pressure points are important in prevention and early detection of skin problems.

Psychosocial equilibrium is also threatened by enforced inactivity as social interaction is decreased, with resulting loss of intellectual stimulation, role function, and even orientation. Disturbances in self-concept, feelings of powerlessness, and ineffective coping may become evident. Maintaining control over decision-making may help to restore an immobilized patient's perception of control over the environment. Frequent socialization with others may facilitate reality orientation. Individuals who experience Risk for Disuse Syndrome will benefit from a comprehensive, personalized plan to identify and prevent the particular complications of inactivity that threaten their health.

▌ SELF-CARE DEFICIT

(Bathing/hygiene; dressing/grooming; feeding, toileting)

Bathing/hygiene self-care deficit is the state in which an individual experiences an impaired ability to perform or complete bathing and hygiene activities.

Dressing/grooming self-care deficit is the state in which an individual experiences an impaired ability to perform or complete dressing and grooming activities.

Feeding self-care deficit is the state in which an individual experiences an impaired ability to perform or complete feeding activities.

Toileting self-care deficit is the state in which in individual experiences an impaired ability to perform or complete toileting activities.[9]

The impaired ability to perform self-care may be temporary or permanent. It occurs as a result of decreased motor of cognitive/perceptual function. These in turn may be related to a physiologic or psychologic health problem. In some instances, physical restraint, such as being in a cast to treat a bone fracture, impairs self-care. The ability to perform these activities independently provides the individual with a sense of control, which contributes to a healthy self-concept.

These activities of daily living (bathing/hygiene, dressing/grooming, feeding, toileting) are learned and become habitual, usually having a certain pattern or sequence. They are principally affected by the functional health status of the individual, but social and situational factors also play a part. The functional health status has three components that are assessed in determining the diagnosis of self-care deficit: the age-related biologic status, developmental task status, and disease (if present) and its treatment.

Age-related factors that may affect basic self-care are most often portrayed in elderly persons. Developmental task assessment relates to maturational factors, including knowledge, skill, and motivation. Pathologic states caused by trauma or disease may alter structure and function and thus compromise self-care ability in all age groups. The treatment may also impose limitations (e.g., being in a cast for a fracture, restricted by bed rest). Being functionally dependent, i.e., requiring assistance from others in the activities of bathing/hygiene, dressing/grooming, feeding, and toileting, affects the individual's morale, self-esteem, and sense of dignity. These are human needs that contribute to the quality of life. Functional dependency provides the basis for establishing eligibility for long-term care services and is a measure of the success of those services. Functional dependency is a central ingredient of geriatric assessment (see Table IV-6).

Related Factors[2,7,9,10]

Intolerance to activity
Decreased strength and endurance
Pain, discomfort
Perceptual or cognitive impairment
Neuromuscular impairment
Musculoskeletal impairment
Depression, severe anxiety

Defining Characteristics

Bathing/Hygiene

Inability to wash body or body parts
Inability to obtain or get to water source
Inability to regulate temperature or flow

Dressing/Grooming

Impaired ability to put on or take off necessary items of clothing
Impaired ability to obtain or replace articles of clothing
Impaired ability to fasten clothing
Inability to maintain appearance at satisfactory level

Feeding

Inability to bring food from receptacle to mouth
Inability to cut food

Toileting

Unable to get to toilet or commode
Unable to sit on or rise from toilet or commode
Unable to manipulate clothing for toileting
Unable to carry out proper toilet hygiene
Unable to flush toilet or empty commode

Research validating the characteristics of Self-Care Deficit has been reported by Chang[3] and Doughtery et al.[5] Finch et al[6] reported on a new method to measure the type and extent of dependency in ADLs. Daly et al[4] reported on a review of computerized care plans in a long-term care facility. A total of 214 nursing diagnoses were recorded on 29 care plans with 36 of them being different diagnoses. Twenty-six listed Self-Care Deficit: Bathing/Hygiene and 25 were Self-Care Deficit: Dressing/Grooming. Self-Care Deficit: Feeding and Self-Care Deficit: Toileting were also included.

Expected Patient Outcomes & Nursing Interventions[2,7,9,10]

*For all four self-care deficits:

Achieves or maintains as much situational control as physically and cognitively capable, as evidenced by:

Stating realistic appraisal of own strengths and limitations
Verbal participation in plan of care
Discussing and expressing feelings concerning limitations and
    progress
  • Monitor and discuss changes in situation with patient; discuss how and what activities can be performed; *giving the*

---

*The above expected patient outcomes and nursing interventions with accompanying rationale are applicable to each of the self-care deficits with modifications for the specific activity. For example, situational control, completion of task, and avoidance of complications are desirable patient outcomes for all activities, and the nursing interventions, with modifications for the specific activity, are applicable.

 TABLE IV-6 Classification of Functional Levels of Self-Care*

Level	Behavioral Indicator
0	*Independent:* no help or oversight needed; able to initiate and complete activity for self
1	*Supervision:* minimal assistance, oversight, encouragement, reminders, cueing
2	*Limited assistance:* highly involved in activity; needs some physical assistance from others
3	*Extensive assistance:* contribution to activity is minor; needs extensive physical assistance from others
4	*Total dependence:* does not participate in activity; total care by caregivers

*The scale is a modification of functional levels from minimum data set for nursing facility resident assessment. Use of this scale to indicate level of independence or dependence further defines functional deficit and guides nursing intervention. Self-care deficits exist for levels 1 through 4.[1]

patient the opportunity to take an active part in the assessment and plan of care acknowledges patient rights and increases self-esteem.

- Plan care and validate conclusions with patient; *adds to sense of situational control necessary for morale.*
- Discuss changes in condition with patient; *knowing that changes (good or bad) are shared with others improves the patient's sense of trust and security.*
- Inform patient about anticipated effects of therapy; *invites patient participation in plan of care.*
- Assist in relating concerns to physician; *overcoming reluctance or hesitancy in addressing physician and having concerns made known contribute to security and improve self-care options.*
- Discuss daily routine with patient *to allow the patient an opportunity to have a voice in scheduling and sequencing activities.*
- Consult with patient in making choices about his or her treatment *to allow an opportunity for expressing preferences.*
- Evaluate outcomes of care with patient; *shared evaluation is a natural outcome of the shared decision-making process and is the patient's right.*

Self-care is completed with participation of patient to fullest extent, as evidenced by:

Satisfactory fulfillment of basic human needs for cleanliness, grooming, nutrition, and toileting
Expressions of satisfaction with mastery of skill

- Provide prescribed treatment for underlying disease conditions or disruptive symptoms, such as pain, *to decrease effects of impairment on self-care performance.*
- Encourage or allow patient to do as much as possible for himself or herself *to support and help restore independence.*
- Initiate exercises *to strengthen weakened limbs and improve balance and dexterity.*
- Provide help, supervision, and teaching, as necessary, *to improve self-care.*
- Explore the use of assistive devices *that can help the patient become more self-sufficient.*
- Monitor interest and motivation for an increasing level of participation in care; offer cues and encouragement *to support the patient's readiness to relearn or participate in a skill.*
- Make changes in the environment (moving furniture and placing objects within reach) *to improve the patient's opportunity for self-care.*
- For discharge planning, assess factors in home and work setting that support or hinder self-care; *physical arrangements (stairs, narrow traffic ways, clutter, and access to transportation) can influence self-care activities.*

Complications are avoided, as evidenced by:

Absence of or minimal signs or symptoms of
    Powerlessness (perceived)

Lack of situational control with decreased self-esteem
Sense of worthlessness
Physical harm
Deterioration of abilities

- Evaluate success of above nursing interventions designed *to increase behavioral, cognitive, and decisional control.*
- Evaluate risks and take safety precautions *to minimize physical hazards and prevent injury.*
- Monitor self-care activities to determine energy expenditure and tolerance level *to decrease fatigue, reduce frustration, and enhance compliance.*
- Increase level of support resources, if necessary, *to decrease or reduce rate of further disability and maintain patient involvement.*

Bathing and hygiene activities are completed independently or with assistance, as evidenced by:

Clean body, hair, nails, teeth
No offensive odors
Expressions of satisfaction with resulting accomplishment

- Provide teaching, supervision, and assistance, as necessary; offer praise and encouragement *as reinforcement and reward; cleanliness adds to self-esteem.*
- Provide bath at time desirable to patient and afford maximum privacy *to encourage more active participation.*
- Use tub or shower, if possible; seat in chair for safety; place equipment within easy reach; check water temperature; place call bell within reach *as measures to increase safety.*

Dressing and grooming activities are completed independently or with assistance, as evidenced by:

Being appropriately clothed
Neat in appearance
Positive expressions

- Provide loose-fitting clothing with simple fasteners; give ample time to complete dressing *to decrease frustration and to improve likelihood of success.*
- Monitor dressing and grooming activity (combing hair, applying makeup, or shaving), and offer assistance, as necessary, *to ensure satisfactory completion of task so that patient's appearance is neat and clean (increases self-esteem).*

Feeding activity is satisfactorily completed independently or with assistance, as evidenced by:

Adequate intake of food and drink
Maintaining appropriate weight
Expressing interest in overcoming feeding limitations

- Consider cognitive or perceptual dysfunctions, oral-motor impairment, or ability to control arms and hands when prescribing intervention, selection of assistive devices, utensils, or choice and preparation of food and drink *to facilitate independence and safety.*
- Monitor feeding activity at each meal *to determine progress, identify problems, and offer reinforcement.*

- In concert with patient or family identify food preferences, preferred time for eating, preferred place, and with whom *to provide as nearly customary pattern as possible.*
- Provide ample time for eating, cut up food, as necessary, arrange utensils within reach, and place patient in comfortable position for eating and swallowing *to decrease frustration, to aid patient in chewing and swallowing, and to reduce risk of choking or aspiration.*
- Have suction equipment available for emergencies.

Toileting activity is completed independently or with assistance, as evidenced by:

Adequate intake and output
Satisfactory management of toileting and cleaning

- Monitor toileting activity; provide supervision and assistance, as needed, *to determine progress, to identify problems, and to offer praise and encouragement in self-care.*
- Identify pattern, or help to establish program of urination and defecation; respond promptly to patient's request for assistance *to help achieve control and avoid "accidents."*
- Provide privacy when toileting; be nonjudgmental in case of incontinence *to avoid patient embarrassment resulting in patient withholding need to toilet.*
- Provide assistive devices, if needed; raised commode and grab bars. Have call bell within reach; have adequate assistance in lifting and transferring patient *to avoid risk of falling and accidental physical harm.*
- Assist patient with cleaning and rearranging clothes, as necessary, *to ensure cleanliness, comfort, and neat appearance.*

Principles and Rationale for Nursing Interventions[2,7,8,9,10]

Lack of ability to perform the necessary activities of daily living independently prolongs a patient's stay in an acute care facility. *Functional dependency* in the elderly is a major contributing factor to placement in long-term care facilities. Changes in the health status, particularly long-lasting musculoskeletal and perceptual/cognitive impairment, are the bases for formation of self-care deficits. However, independence in self-care can be influenced by factors and resources in the environment, and these should be assessed. Such factors and resources include not only assistive devices, but also household arrangements and access to transportation, shops, and professional services. Social support systems, including family, friends, and neighbors, should be evaluated, as should the possibility of home care. At the same time the nurse should be aware that these resources also generate demands on the individual (e.g., when, where, and how long it will take to eat, bathe, and dress). The patient and family should be involved in this appraisal.

The primary goal is that the basic human needs be met. Requiring assistance from others in these activities affects the individual's morale, self-esteem, and sense of dignity. The loss of the ability to perform a functional task and the loss of respect,

threatened or real, that may accompany that loss may have a devastating effect on the sense of self of the individual. One expects to be in control of one's simplest functions and of the appropriateness of the time and place of their occurrence; when this control is lost, one is ashamed of oneself. A personal judgment of failure is made and the ego is threatened; it is even more telling when one's failure is witnessed by others. Lack of participation in activities of daily living and verbal responses indicating lack of control over activities and outcomes, associated with negative affective responses (withdrawal, pessimism, submissiveness, undifferentiated anger), indicate the diagnosis of powerlessness.[8]

The interventions of the nurse or caregiver and her attitudes are essential in determining the responses and outcomes of self-care deficits in body functions. The perception of situational control is a key variable for the morale of the individual.[9] The outcome will also be affected by the specific nature of the deficit and whether it is temporary or long term. For example, individuals who are temporarily restrained by intravenous tubing and have to be fed by others may feel uncomfortable and prefer not to eat. On the other hand, the sudden traumatic deficits of accident-related quadriplegia and the progressive deficits that sometimes accompany growing older present more serious problems that may eventually threaten the ego.

■ DIVERSIONAL ACTIVITY DEFICIT

Diversional activity deficit is the state in which an individual experiences decreased stimulation from, interest in, or engagement in recreational or leisure activities. It is a personally defined dissatisfaction with a lack of sufficient leisure time recreational activities.

Diversional deficits occur at two ends of a continuum of activity. At one end are those persons with too much time on their hands and not enough to do. In those persons, a deficit in diversional activity often is manifested by reports of boredom because usual forms of activity are interrupted by illness, disability, or life changes. Boredom is especially prevalent in patients whose illnesses extend for a long time, those who are hospitalized or otherwise institutionalized, those who spend many hours in health treatment situations, or those who are homebound.

At the other end of the continuum from boredom is the frustration of insufficient time for leisure activities. Persons who have too many demands in their lives have little or no time that is free from obligations. Such persons are also prone to diversional activity deficits and appear in health care situations with stress-related illnesses.

While the nursing diagnosis, Diversional Activity deficit, has had little empirical study in nursing, increasingly its importance is being acknowledged, especially as a phenomenon in gerontologic populations.[14] At present, studies of the related concepts of leisure, recreation, and personal activities are helpful in understanding the significance of this diagnosis.

Diversion encompasses those activities that are recreational and are pursued during leisure time for the purpose of personal amusement or satisfaction. Leisure is the time that is free from obligations. Recreational or leisure activities are significant factors in studies of quality of life, meaningful living strategies, self-care, caregiving, and loneliness. Rodgers,[16] in her study of loneliness, found that recreational activities were cited most frequently as missed by hospitalized subjects.

The value of recreational activities has been cited in several studies related to quality and meaning of life. Diversional activities such as walking, dancing, singing, and reading, have been identified as components of health-related self-care activities in middle-aged women.[6] Satisfaction in relaxing and having fun was part of a pattern of "sustaining myself" identified by older widows living alone.[12] With examples of painting, baking, reading, quilt-making, elderly women illustrated a pattern of "working hard and staying active" as important to successful aging.[11] Similarly, 10% of Burbank's older adult subjects reported activities such as bingo, fishing, hobbies, crafts, and travel, as being important to meaning in life.[4]

Diversional activities have particular value in long-term care situations. Aller and Van Ess Coeling found that residents of long-term care facilities valued recreational activities.[1] Likewise, Daley, studying women's strategies for living in nursing homes, found "keeping active" to be a theme. Personal activities included, among others, watching TV, reading newspapers and books, parties, music programs, games, current events discussions and exercise classes.[5]

When there is lack of time for personal recreational activities people identify it as a problem. This problem is a recurrent theme found in research on care giving, for example. Sayles-Cross found caregivers' social lives restricted and they were held back from doing what they wanted to do.[18] In Krach and Brooks' research, of the 760 caregivers, 52% reported that caregiving responsibilities interfered with leisure activities.[9] Beach's caregiver subjects reported no time for self and cessation of personal activities, such as ceramics and hobbies.[2] Frustration and sacrifice of self were also part of a theme in Boykin and Winland-Brown's study of caregivers.[3] The personal meaning of diversional activity and the importance of deficits are areas needing further study. It has been suggested that this phenomenon be studied qualitatively so that the meaning of diversional activities can be found.[10]

The need to individualize diversional activities has been illustrated by Ragsdale's study of the quality of life of hospitalized persons with AIDS.[3] Six management styles were identified in this population, one of which was the "timekeeper," who made many references to being bored and spending time waiting for things to happen. Persons like this would benefit from diversional activities, while persons with other management styles may have less need for such activities.

What one does with leisure time is closely linked to self-expression and with past activities. Fun and personal satisfaction are the usual outcomes of diversional activities. Zoerink emphasized the importance of past play experiences on the formation of attitudes toward leisure.[20] Ross found that elderly persons were more satisfied with individualized recreation.[16] Vogel and Mercier advocated diversional activities in nursing homes that were part of the individual's interest and not just the focus of a particular group.[19] It is imperative that nurses consider the individuality of patients when assessing and developing interventions for patients' diversional activity deficits. Too often, patients are given few options, or they are given the standard list of options for activities. Television is often used as the answer to each bored patient's needs. When diversional activities are available (such as in long-term care facilities where regular recreational programs are scheduled), some patients choose not to participate because the scheduled programs are not meaningful to them. Patients who do not take advantage of available options may still have diversional deficits.

Some persons are better than others at devising leisure activities for themselves. Jongbloed and Morgan[7] in their study of leisure activities after stroke, found that persons who had a large variety of interests before illness were better able to continue an activity after illness than those who had limited variety to begin with. Nurses need to be alert to preillness patterns of diversional activities to adequately assess this problem and to plan interventions.

Related Factors[8,14,17]

Time factors
   Problematic time management
   Excess obligations on time
   Decrease in obligated time (increase in available unobligated time)
   Major life change (e.g., retirement, children leaving home, long-term illness)
Environmental factors
   Home-based patients: limited finances, lack of transportation, social isolation, fear of crime
   Treatment center—based patients: space constraints, lack of resources, unfamiliarity with routines or expectations
Functional abilities
   Impaired mobility
   Activity intolerance
   Impaired senses or pain
   Impaired cardiopulmonary functions
   Fatigue
   Depression or lack of motivation
   Loneliness
   Apathy
   Maturational factors (e.g., child—no toys)
Interest in activities
   Lack of exposure or orientation to diversional activities
   Lack of knowledge of options
   Personal preference at odds with available options

Defining Characteristics[8,14,17]

Little or no unobligated time or increase in amount of unobligated time

No pattern of leisure activities
Preillness leisure activities impossible since illness
No postillness substitute activities defined
Unavailability of resources for identified leisure activities
Confined space
Perception of impossibility of leisure activities
Perception of time passing slowly
Statement of desire for something to do
Statement of boredom
Daytime napping (seemingly unwarranted)
Disinterest in television viewing
Energy level sufficient for recreational activities but no participation in such activities
Restlessness
Flat affect
Frequent yawning
Hostility
Inattentiveness
Overeating or decreased eating
Refusal to attend planned recreation programs
Selective attendance at planned recreation programs

Expected Patient Outcomes & Nursing Interventions

Describe usual pattern of diversional activities, as evidenced by:

Indicating time free from obligations
Listing activities that are self-chosen
Relating the what, where, when, and how of diversional activities
- Assess usual activity routines before illness: *the usual pattern is a baseline for planning.*
    Amount of unobligated time
    Leisure activities: type, amount, and resources used
    Knowledge of recreational options
- For persons with excessive stress and little unobligated time, suggest that they record their schedule of activities for 1 week; *recording will help show time patterns.*

Identify changes in ability to engage in usual diversional activities, *or* identify problems perceived with usual pattern of activities, as evidenced by:

Realistically listing changes in situation
Comparing present situation to past
- Assess usual activity routines since illness, hospitalization, or life change:
    Amount of unobligated time
    Leisure activities: type, amount, and resources used
    Degree of confinement
    Energy level (sufficient for diversional activities?)
    Desire for activity
    Mental status
Patient's report of present situation will reveal accuracy and personal meaning of perceived changes.

Choose one usual diversional activity to continue, *and/or* identify usual diversional activity that may be adapted to new constraints, *and/or* identify new diversional activity that may be started, as evidenced by:

Making a personal choice
Seeing possibilities of continuation of activity within constraints, *or* is able to see old activity in new light, *or* lists other interests that could be tried
Using a problem-solving approach to changed situation
- Whenever possible, encourage patient to continue with these activities that were meaningful to him or her; *personal satisfaction will come with meaningful activities.*
- Encourage creativity in choices; *more possibilities will emerge.*
- Help person with busy schedule to prioritize activities.
- Encourage patient to identify activity; avoid suggestions unless patient unable to think of possibilities; *the desire to please the nurse may preclude true choice.*
- If necessary, prompt patient thinking with suggestions of categories of activities, e.g., music, games, arts, crafts, physical exercise, toys, reading, writing, change of scene, change of routine, companionship, video programs, talking, productive chores (sorting, cleaning, etc.).
- *Remember that diversional activities should be personally meaningful.*
- Focus on the positive more than negative ("You can do this " rather than "You can't do that").
- Orient patient to options available within the system, e.g., recreational therapy programs.
- After patient makes choice, if appropriate, validate with medical team patient capabilities to engage in chosen activity, *for realistic planning.*

Satisfactorily engage in chosen diversional activity, as evidenced by:

Listing resources needed for chosen activity
Identifying means to obtain needed resources
Engaging in chosen diversional activity
Expressing satisfaction with chosen activity
- Maintain emphasis on personal choice; *this promotes patient control and minimizes nurse assumptions.*
- Consider what can be obtained within the system, what could be provided by family and friends, what are vital to activity, and what can be adapted from available options; *be creative.*
- If necessary, teach time management or stress management strategies; *these may be needed by overly stressed patients.*
- Support patient in chosen activity.
- Adapt environment as necessary.
- Provide positive feedback.
- Evaluate patient's perception of chosen activity.
- Allow for change of plans if activity is unsatisfactory; *creative options do not always work as anticipated.*

Principles and Rationale for Nursing Interventions

Because diversional activities have meaning, purpose, and value for the individual, the determination of a deficit in those activities is highly personal. The amount of time spent idly and the point at which boredom occurs vary greatly. Therefore, to study diversion and diagnose a deficit in this area, a patient's own preillness or pre–life change schedule of activities must be a baseline for comparison with the postillness or post–life change schedule.

To maintain the personal meaning of a new or adapted diversional activity, the nurse must avoid planning the activity for the patient; rather, interventions should be geared to assisting the patient to identify a meaningful activity. Often patients in hospitals cannot think of alternative activities, nor do they consider the possibility of developing new methods of expression. The social structure of hospitals is such that patients have little say in establishing routines. Their world becomes small and detail oriented. In these cases the nurse can educate patients as to the possibilities for change in the routine. A focus on the positive possibilities rather than on the negative aspects of their situation will allow for more creativity in choosing a diversional activity. This same focus on the positive options should be applied in interventions with homebound patients who have an excess of unobligated time and with persons who have diversional deficits because of schedules with too little unobligated time.

Creativity is another principle guiding nursing intervention. Possibilities for diversional activities are as numerous as the creative mind allows. Creativity means considering options beyond the common three: reading, watching television, and doing crossword puzzles. The creative mind sees ways to adapt resources to meet diversional needs. For the immobilized patient who misses a daily workout in the gym, exercises that can be done in bed, such as squeezing a rubber ball, may be a welcomed diversional activity. Children's toys can be adapted to adult needs. Introducing two bored patients gives each of them companionship. The list is limited only by the confines of the imagination.

▌IMPAIRED HOME MAINTENANCE MANAGEMENT

▌ Impaired home maintenance management is the inability to independently maintain a safe, growth-promoting immediate environment.

The overall nursing goal for impaired home maintenance management is to enable the patient to continue living at home as long as it is safe and desirable. High-risk populations include physically and mentally disabled patients, dependent children, acutely ill patients in the home, the frail elderly, chronically ill patients, substance abusers, and the medically indigent. Adaptation of the home for health care is also relevant to this diagnosis. The recent trend in the increased complexity of home care has placed additional demands on patients and families to adapt their homes to facilitate high-tech durable medical equipment.[7]

To facilitate discharge and effective long-term care, and when planning discharge, nurses in the hospital need to look beyond the identified patient to assess the family, home environment, and access to resources. Whether this is an acutely ill, chronically ill, newly disabled, or terminally ill person who is going home, the family will be the principal caregivers. Ideally, planning is done before the patient is discharged to train the patient and caregivers in the techniques of patient care, to adapt the home as a workplace to provide necessary nursing care and to identify availability of community resources. The social roles of family members may also need to be permanently adapted to compensate for patient disability or susceptibility caused by illness. Success or failure of home placement may also hinge on the structural characteristics of the dwelling and the supports available in the community for both family respite and professional services.[13] The case manager/home care nurse works as a part of the multidisciplinary team to assist the family and patient to coordinate services and to adapt their home and roles to allow maximum independence for the disabled member.[2]

Related Factors[8]

Individual and family characteristics
  Disabled by acute illness, injury, or congenital anomaly
  Chronic debilitating disease
  Impaired sensory functioning
  Impaired cognitive or emotional functioning
  Change in family composition
Insufficient knowledge
  Lack of socialization (role model and/or emigration)
  Unfamiliarity with neighborhood resources
  Lack of training in adaptation of home maintenance skills
Insufficient family organization and planning
Insufficient finances or insurance
Dysfunctional grieving
Inadequate social support system
  Insufficient amount
  Insufficient quality
  Impaired family member
Inadequate dwelling and/or furnishings
  Overcrowding
  Lack of adaptation of home structure or furnishings
  Structural defects including lack of heat, water, electricity
  Lack of equipment or aids for home care
Inadequate community resources
  Insufficient community environmental sanitation or control
    of environmental contaminants or pollutants
  Lack of community professional and paraprofessional home
    care services

Defining Characteristics[3,8,7,10]

Subjective (Stated by Patient or Household Member)

Expresses difficulty in maintaining the home in a comfortable,
  safe, and hygienic manner

Expresses difficulty in supporting personal growth of family members

Requests assistance with home maintenance management

Describes outstanding debts or financial crises that impede home maintenance management

Expresses ignorance in how to provide environment conducive for patient care

Expresses exhaustion or inability to keep up the home

Discusses dissatisfaction with dwelling because of overcrowding or lack of personal space

Complains that furnishings are inadequate to maintain order or support healthful living patterns

Shows nurse defects in structure or utilities and expresses inability to have them repaired

Expresses lack of knowledge about community resources

Expresses that environmental factors negatively affect ability to maintain the home

Expresses frustration that known resources are unavailable or insufficient in community

Requests assistance in working with durable medical equipment

Objective (Observed by Nurse)

Presence of disease or disability necessitating adaptation of home maintenance

Lack of knowledge of caregiver

Overtaxed family members

Inadequate support system

Apparent lack of economic resources

Disorganized home

Knowledge of home maintenance inconsistent with current environment

Home lacking personal items and attempts at decoration

Presence of indoor pets that are not housebroken

Disorderly surroundings

Unavailable cooking utensils, linen, or clothes because of insufficient supply or being unwashed

Accumulation of dirt, food waste, or hygienic waste

Offensive odors

Inadequate lighting

Inappropriate household temperature and/or insufficient ventilation

Presence of vermin or rodents

Repeated hygienic disorders, infestations, or infections

Lack of necessary equipment or aids

Overcrowding for available space

Presence of structural barriers

Unrepaired defects in structure or utilities

Characteristics of neighborhood making it difficult for effective home maintenance

Neighborhood unsafe for professionals/paraprofessionals to visit home

Inadequate or contaminated water or sewage supply

Inability of caregiver to operate durable medical equipment

Expected Patient Outcomes & Nursing Interventions

Participate in appropriate discharge planning, as evidenced by:

Identification of needs and a feasible discharge plan
- Document discharge plan after assessing needs with patient and family.
- Teach patient and family as appropriate.
- Identify appropriate referrals using multidisciplinary team.
- Establish realistic plan for home management involving patient and family members.
- Plan and coordinate a smooth transition from inpatient to home.

Identify factors perceived as making it difficult to maintain home, as evidenced by:

Home maintenance defined as a health problem

Each member stating personal standard of home maintenance

Each member contributing identification of factors that impede home maintenance

Family verbalizing financial constraints
- Ask each member to identify how the home is different now and how long they think it has been unsatisfactory.
- Systematically identify factors that impede meeting household standard.
- Have members state what factors in the home affect their health and in what way.
- Compare patient's perceptions with nurse's observations. Share nurse's observations.
- Increase family awareness of changed capabilities of members.

Recognize what daily maintenance can be realistically performed, as evidenced by:

Current roles that are stated and possible role changes that are discussed

Hygienic factors that are differentiated
- Discuss what each member now does and how often. Discuss possible role changes.
- Differentiate factors that are esthetic from ones that negatively affect health.
- Listen nonjudgmentally to realities of home situation.
- Assist family to realign roles and expectations for household maintenance standards congruent with increased patient dependency.

Use current support system and participate in developing plan to supplement family resources, as evidenced by:

Patient sharing perception of support system and its strengths and weaknesses

Need for outside help being defined

Patient who states what resources are available after nurse shares knowledge of available resources

Nurse and patient developing plan of care
- Identify members of current support system and assess their capabilities.
- Discuss community resources for daily home maintenance.
- Mutually develop plan of care to increase supports consistent with family values.
- Assist families to seek outside assistance for respite; they may be reluctant to meet ongoing caregiver needs.

Use community resources in efficient, appropriate manner, as evidenced by:

Contact with resources being initiated
Deficits in support being compensated
Support system members using nursing services appropriately
- Initiate referrals for supplementation of daily home maintenance.
- Investigate community resources for long-term maintenance.
- Review with support system members how to use nurse as continuing resources.
- Increase family awareness of community resources and appropriate utilization.

Adapt the home and/or lifestyle to promote maximum health and safety, as evidenced by:

Unsafe objects being removed
Patient relating change to improvement of health status
Patient participating as able in performance of activities of daily living and home maintenance
Patient remaining at home as long as feasible and desirable
Universal precautions being used appropriately
- Discuss specific lifestyle and home changes that will promote health.
- Discuss rearranging furnishings for cleaning and safety.
- Reinforce changes by discussing positive impact. Praise attempts at adaptation.
- Review with family plan to respond to emergencies.
- Assist family to complete home safety assessment and follow up on deficits found.
- Teach family universal precautions.
- Assist family members to adapt to physical demands associated with caregiving.

Repair structural defects, as evidenced by:

Patient stating relationship between defects and maintaining healthy, safe home
Patient and family seeking help from community resources for repair of and financial help in eliminating structural defects
Observation of repairs being made
- Discuss relationship of defects to health.
- Discuss possible disease caused by defects.
- Investigate alternative ways to have repairs made within financial capabilities of family.
- Support attempts to obtain repairs.
- Refer to assistance with utility payments.

Obtain and appropriately use equipment facilitating home maintenance, as evidenced by:

Equipment and supplies being obtained
Equipment being used appropriately
Patient verbalizing how to obtain future supplies and how to arrange for repair of equipment
- Determine equipment and supplies needed, identify sources, and obtain.
- Teach appropriate use and maintenance of equipment.
- Review means of maintaining sufficient supplies.

Manage home maintenance adequately, as evidenced by:

Additional support being obtained
Client and household members mutually determining standard of cleanliness for home
Family maximally participating in home maintenance
Family discussing roles in maintaining cleaner, safer environment
Patient and family expressing satisfaction with home situation
Clean, safe, growth-promoting environment being achieved
- Arrange for additional support regularly or periodically for caregiver respite.
- Have caregiver and family establish mutually agreeable standard of cleanliness and order that is safe.
- Teach caregiver to support maximum independence of patient.
- Observe for increased level of health secondary to cleaner home environment. When observed, compliment on changes.
- Facilitate collaboration among family members.

Increase awareness of impact of neighborhood on home maintenance, as evidenced by:

Patient verbalizing factors negatively affecting home maintenance
Patient identifying neighborhood improvement resources: at least one family member participates
Patient and family verbalizing factors that would lead to changing residence
- Identify factors in community that negatively affect client's ability to maintain home.
- Identify local resources that work to promote changes. Encourage family participation.
- Assist family to assess safety of neighborhood and periodically consider their housing options.
- Assess dangers of neighborhood for visiting by professionals/paraprofessionals.

Principles and Rationale for Nursing Interventions

Impaired home maintenance management is rarely the reason a patient seeks nursing care in the home. However, in the nursing assessment of the patient, family, support system, dwelling, and community the nurse may identify current home maintenance management as a barrier to either healthful living or to providing nursing care.[1,14] Necessary adaptations of the structure or furnishings for home care may be missing. Aids that could increase the patient's independence may be lacking. Intervention for this diagnosis may take precedence over others to create a workplace for safe care or to prevent injury to the patient or family. The home maintenance practices and facilities may be adequate for a family with healthy members but may be hazardous for a patient.

Impaired home maintenance management may also be secondary to other nursing diagnoses or even a sign of their presence. For example, one objective sign of dysfunctional grieving is failing to participate in home maintenance tasks until the home is unsafe or unhygienic. Other diagnoses in which impaired home maintenance management may be a sign are altered parenting and ineffective individual or family coping. Impaired home maintenance may also be part of the cause of another nursing diagnosis, such as risk for injury, especially the subcategories of risk for poisoning (if garbage is not removed or food is stored under unsafe conditions), or risk for trauma (if necessary home repairs are not done).[7]

Several excellent tools developed for the assessment of the family and the home environment are printed in the community health literature.[4,6,11,14] Laferrier[9] describes a tool that assesses the family for hospice care using Orem's self-care nursing framework and also includes the collection of environmental data. Gordon[5] includes an assessment guide that addresses the nursing diagnosis of impaired home maintenance management in her text.

When assessing for the nursing diagnosis of impaired home maintenance management, the nurse must consider the individual, family, dwelling, and the community. The key observation is of the dwelling itself and its organization, cleanliness, and safety for both daily living and patient care. Observation for signs of provision for personal growth and individuality of family members is also necessary. The following parameters should be considered:

1. What is the individual patient's physical or mental status? Is there a disease or disability present that may impede home maintenance?
2. Are there any cultural barriers that impede home maintenance management?
3. What is the home situation?
    a. Type of housing unit
    b. Location of housing unit
    c. Condition of housing unit
    d. Number of occupants in unit
4. What is the patient's standard of home maintenance?
5. What is the patient's perception of ability to maintain the home?
6. What support system is available, and what are its capabilities?
7. What community resources are available to enable the patient to remain in the home situation?
8. Are financial resources adequate to maintain the home?
9. What equipment is needed to facilitate adaptation?
10. Are there structural deficits or barriers that make home maintenance difficult?
11. What effect does the neighborhood or community have on the patient's ability to maintain the home? Is the neighborhood safe for visiting by professionals?

A safe, hygienic environment that offers social and physical stimulation for personal growth and development is the baseline sought for each identified patient. Failure to achieve this goal is associated with an imbalance in compensation by the patient, family, and/or community or with a deficit in the dwelling or in the surround environment. The dwelling may be unsuitable for the patient and family, may be in need of adaptation, or may be situated in a community that is unsafe or unhealthy for the patient.

Support may also be the case manager, home care nurse, or other professionals in the community, who provide social stimulation and refer the patient to appropriate resources. People are often unaware of community services until they have a need for them. The consumer movement and health education campaigns by local, state, and federal governments, as well as professional organizations, have increased the public's knowledge of health practices and of resources available in their communities. Many communities have homemaker services, extended payment plans for winter heating bills, institutional temporary respite care for the disabled, and other programs to assist families to maintain disabled members at home.

The community also contributes to the quality of the life of its residents through its environmental, health, and sanitation programs. This support is especially important to community members who are disabled or sick. For instance, no matter how well the person maintains and adapts the home, if the building codes are not enforced and if pest control is not done on a community-wide basis, the home will not be hygienic or safe. In addition, disabled people may be especially susceptible to pollutants that the general population can tolerate. An example is a person with emphysema living where there is smog.[13]

Lack of knowledge of community resources was mentioned previously. A person may also be unaware of how to maintain a safe, hygienic home or how to provide a growth-stimulating environment because of developmental status, impaired cognitive functioning, or lack of role models. A young person with few social supports may not have the necessary experience in caring for a dwelling to keep it clean or to control pests. Another person may not know that a baby has poor internal temperature control and needs extra warmth in cold weather. Alternatively, elderly persons may not realize their declining ability to sense cold and may fail to keep themselves warm enough at night.

Impaired cognitive functioning is a problem for both mentally retarded adults and patients with organic brain dysfunctions. The health care trend of deinstitutionalization may have led to their placement in the community without the supports and training they need for home maintenance management. However, many programs demonstrate how these patients can learn to care for themselves and their homes through training and continuing support in halfway houses, group homes, or foster homes.

DYSFUNCTIONAL VENTILATORY WEANING RESPONSE

Dysfunctional ventilatory weaning response is a state in which a patient's inability to adjust to lowered levels of mechanical ventilatory support interrupts and prolongs the weaning process.[22]

Most patients who require the initial use of mechanical ventilatory support have rapidly reversible ventilatory problems and are successfully weaned from the ventilator within a few days. However, patients with severe, complicated acute or chronic lung disease, with multisystem extrapulmonary disease, or with neuromuscular disease may require long-term mechanical ventilation. These patients experience problems that interfere with the weaning process.[10,12,14,15,27]

The term "dysfunctional ventilatory weaning response" (DVWR) refers to a temporary state in which a patient lacks readiness to mobilize the necessary physical and emotional resources for adjusting to lowered levels of mechanical ventilatory support.[18,19] Physiologic, psychologic, environmental, and equipment problems contribute to the patient's inability to tolerate lowered levels of ventilatory support.[9] Signs and symptoms that are defining characteristics of dysfunctional ventilatory weaning response are categorized as mild, moderate, and severe.[13,18,19]

Related Factors*

Ineffective airway clearance
Respiratory muscle fatigue
Multisystem disease
Neuromuscular chronic disability
Cardiac failure
Acute or chronic lung disease
Electrolyte disorders (e.g., hypophosphatemia)
Anemia
Sleep pattern disturbance
Malnutrition (less than or more than body requirements)
Drug therapy
Obesity
Infection
Uncontrolled pain or discomfort
Uncontrolled episodic energy demands or problems
Inappropriate pacing of diminished ventilatory support
History of ventilatory dependence greater than 1 week
History of multiple unsuccessful weaning attempts
Inability to effectively communicate
Adverse environment (e.g., noisy, overly active)
Negative events in patient's room
Moderate to severe anxiety
State anxiety
Low nurse-patient ratio
Extended absence of nurse from bedside
Unfamiliar nursing staff
Lack of trust in nurse
Decreased motivation
Terminal illness
Inadequate information about role in weaning process
Perception of futility regarding own ability to be weaned
Fear
Clinical depression or prolonged depressed state
Hopelessness
Powerlessness
Decreased self-esteem

Defining Characteristics[22]

Mild
   Restlessness
   Slight increased respiratory rate from baseline
   Responses to lowered levels of mechanical ventilator support may include conveying increased need for oxygen, experiencing breathing discomfort, complaining of fatigue, feeling warm, questioning about possible machine malfunction, and exhibiting undue concentration on breathing
Moderate
   Responses to lowered levels of mechanical ventilatory support include slight increase from baseline blood pressure, slight increase from baseline heart rate, and baseline increase in respiratory rate
   Hypervigilance in activities
   Inability to respond to coaching
   Inability to cooperate
   Apprehension
   Diaphoresis
   Eye widening ("wide-eyed" look)
   Decreased air entry on auscultation
   Color changes (e.g., pale, with slight cyanosis)
   Slight respiratory accessory muscle use
Severe
   Responses to lowered levels of mechanical ventilatory support include agitation, deterioration in arterial blood gases from current baseline, increase from baseline blood pressure, increase from baseline heart rate, and significant increase in respiratory rate from baseline
   Profuse diaphoresis
   Full respiratory accessory muscle use
   Shallow, gasping breaths
   Paradoxical abdominal breathing
   Discoordinated breathing with the ventilator
   Decreased level of consciousness
   Adventitious breath sounds, audible airway secretion
   Cyanois

Expected Patient Outcomes & Nursing Interventions†

Tolerate lowered levels of mechanical ventilation, as evidenced by:

Demonstrating ability to convey and receive information
Maintaining baseline clinical status (e.g., vital signs, cardiac rhythm, laboratory values, mentation)
Conveying comfortable and relaxed appearance (e.g., absence of irritability, restlessness, agitation, or fatigue)
   • Based on individual assessment, establish an effective communication system (e.g., lip reading, head nods, writ-

---

ing, sign language, alphabet or communication board, and talking tracheostomy) *to reduce potential patient frustration and anxiety, to minimize negative aspects of mechanical ventilation, and to maximize patient's sense of control and energy conservation.*

- Monitor for presence of altered thought process (e.g., fluctuations in concentration, attention, or orientation) before initiating weaning process and throughout weaning process; collaborate with patient's medical team to search for and treat underlying cause (e.g., fever, infection, drug therapy, fluid overload) *to optimize likelihood of successful weaning.*
- Repeat information until patient conveys understanding of explanations.
- Allow patient sufficient time to respond to information and explanations.
- Before initiating weaning:
    "Know" the patient (e.g., usual mannerisms; past respiratory history, including reactions to previous weaning attempts).
    Collaborate with multidisciplinary team to clarify whether underlying need for ventilation is resolved *to determine weaning readiness.*
    Obtain baseline vital signs, including temperature, and report abnormal findings to physician.
    Determine current pulmonary status (e.g., lung sounds; respiratory rate; color; secretions; oxygen saturation, when available; and chest x-ray examination).
    Conduct baseline physical assessment (e.g., cardiac rhythm and rate, hemodynamic response, renal function, fluid and electrolyte balance, and bowel function).
    Determine a position of comfort that allows fullest expansion of lungs, *keeping in mind that upright position allows optimal gas exchange.*
    Conduct pain assessment.
- Collaborate with multidisciplinary team to minimize unnecessary invasive procedures immediately before or during weaning process *to reduce potential for nosocomial infections and complications.*
- Determine patient's baseline mental status, using pre-established criteria that can be shared with other caregivers who will be working with the patient.
- Collaborate with multidisciplinary team to determine surveillance parameters that must be continuously reviewed throughout the weaning process (e.g., oxygen saturation, heart and respiratory rate, color, signs of hypoxemia, and hypercapnia).
- Collaborate with patient's physician or pharmacist regarding drug therapy that may cause CNS depression *to ensure that the patient does not receive medication that interferes with ventilatory drive.*
- Collaborate with physician regarding use of methylxanthines *to facilitate bronchodilation and to increase diaphragm contractility.*
- Collaborate with multidisciplinary team to reduce ventilatory support in small increments, such as one parameter *to

maximize physiologic tolerance and to minimize potential for psychologic sense of failure.*
- Collaborate with multidisciplinary team regarding the best method for weaning patient (e.g., SIMV, CPAP, T-tube) *to maximize physiologic tolerance.*
- Prepare physical environment for potential cardiopulmonary arrest (e.g., suction equipment, Ambu-bag, defibrilator) *to ensure early intervention in the event of emergency.*
- Inform patient and family regarding emergency plans *to prevent undue anxiety and to build trust in health care team.*
- Use coaching during weaning process, based on previous agreement with patient (e.g., reminding patient about correct breathing during episodes of shortness of breath) *to promote patient's control of breathing.*
- Collaborate with resources, such as psychiatric consultation/liaison clinical nurse specialist for individualized stress management techniques (e.g., relaxation, imagery, and music) during weaning *to maximize potential for decreased heart and respiratory rates and to promote increased oxygen saturation.*
- Create a therapeutic weaning environment by controlling and minimizing noise and activity level in patient's bedside area, providing privacy, allowing for scheduled rest times *to decrease patient's apprehension and tension.*
- Based on individual assessment, use family as a supportive resource *to minimize patient's anxiety and fears.*
- Prepare family for a supportive role in weaning process by:
    Providing information about the unit environment (e.g., alarms, monitoring equipment, and nurse call system)
    Providing information about the weaning plan
    Introducing all caregivers and explaining their roles in the weaning process
    Inviting family to share issues of concern
    Offering suggestions for appropriate conversation
    Negotiating visiting times
    Clarifying family's role as supportive resource
- Promote effective management of acute and chronic pain. Incorporate adequate periods of rest throughout the weaning process.
- During weaning trials, observe (e.g., every 5 minutes for 15 minutes and then every 15 minutes until stable) for signs of respiratory muscle fatigue:
    Increased respiratory rate, minute ventilation, hypercarbia, with associated respiratory acidosis
    Altered breathing pattern (i.e., dyspnea, tachypnea, tidal volume, abdominal paradox, or asynchrony), and increased discomfort

Adhere to the weaning plan, as evidenced by:

Participating with primary nurse or registered nurse case manager in implementation of weaning plan and ongoing regimen

Communicating self-observations and concerns throughout the weaning process

- Assess the patient's cognitive ability (e.g., attention, concentration, short-term memory) to understand and remember information about the weaning process and plan.
- Obtain information from patient and family about patient's usual responses to anxiety-producing situations during illness, as well as during health.
- Obtain information about patient's past ability to cope with increased anxiety *to identify coping problems and to reinforce coping strengths.*
- Evaluate for behaviors indicative of psychologic dependence on ventilator (e.g., anticipatory anxiety, expressions of fear of dying, and tuning out or blocking discussion of weaning).
- Based on individual assessment and collaboration with the patient and the multidisciplinary team, consider use of a formal written weaning contract, mapping, or critical pathway that includes:

  Identification of specific goals

  Timing of weaning interventions

  Expectations regarding adherence to activity or exercise protocols

  Patient's participation in self-care activities

  Role of patient and individual team members in achieving weaning goals

  Schedule for reevaluating, renegotiating, and revising the weaning plan

- Provide patient and caregivers with a copy of the formal written plan, and include a copy in patient's chart *to ensure consistency and adherence to the weaning plan.*
- Use clear and direct communication (e.g., short and simple sentences) to convey plans for the weaning process. Negotiate the weaning process with patient *to facilitate patient's control in decision-making regarding weaning plan.*
- Ensure that patient has a primary nurse or registered nurse case manager who collaborates on a consistent basis with the patient and family, as well as the multidisciplinary team (e.g., pulmonary clinical nurse specialist, psychiatric consultation/liaison clinical nurse specialist, pulmonologist, respiratory therapist, physical therapist, occupational therapist, dietitian, speech pathologist, chaplain, and social worker), as well as the patient and family *to facilitate successful integration of treatment approaches and evaluation of interventions.*
- Ensure that all caregivers provide consistent explanations about weaning and actual implementation and consistency in daily routines *to promote trust in staff.*
- Provide information on a consistent basis about progress in reassuring manner *to convey recognition of successful weaning and to minimize unnecessary anxiety.*
- Use positive reinforcers (e.g., crossing out criteria that have been met on patient's copy of weaning plan and placing gold stars on patient's calendar) *to convey recognition of patient's achievements and success.*
- Encourage expression of thoughts and feelings about perceptions of the weaning process.

- Encourage patient to convey perceptions of physiologic changes (e.g., breathing patterns, recognition of breathing difficulties, or presence of secretions) *to promote self-monitoring.*
- Use touch, such as a pat on the shoulder, *to convey support and encouragement of patient's progress and endeavors.*
- Promote active decision making throughout weaning process in the setting of realistic, attainable goals for patient's participation with self-care activities (e.g., personal hygiene, grooming, bathing, toileting) *to increase sense of personal control and to decrease stress.*

Principles and Rationale for Nursing Interventions

Resolution of DVWR is dependent on the patient being able to tolerate lowered levels of mechanical ventilation. Nursing interventions before and during the weaning process that strengthen the patient's physiologic and psychologic preparedness increase the likelihood of successful weaning. The development of an individualized communication system for the patient facilitates the patient's participation with the family and the health care team, and it serves to minimize negative aspects of mechanical ventilation. Nursing interventions that incorporate a working knowledge of the patient's usual behaviors and mannerisms, previous weaning attempts, and current pulmonary status contribute to the patient's maintaining baseline status. The patient's ability to oxygenate depends on interventions that create a therapeutic weaning environment, use the family as a resource, and provide close observation for indicators of respiratory and muscle fatigue. As a result the patient conveys a comfortable and relaxed appearance.

The patient's ability to adhere to the weaning plan as an active participant, who communicates self-observations and concerns throughout the weaning process, is an important outcome for the resolution of DVWR. Interventions that increase the patient's sense of control and facilitate the patient's decision making regarding the weaning plan contribute to this outcome. A formal written weaning contract, mapping, or critical pathway that is developed in collaboration with the patient and the multidisciplinary team ensures consistency and adherence to the weaning plan. The designation of a primary nurse or a registered nurse case manager for the patient facilitates a successful integration of treatment approaches and evaluation of interventions.

▌ INABILITY TO SUSTAIN SPONTANEOUS VENTILATION

The inability to sustain spontaneous ventilation (ISSV) is a response pattern of decreased energy reserves in which a patient is unable to maintain adequate breathing to support life.[18]

People who are at risk for ISSV are usually admitted to critical care units. Patients who have undergone major, complicated surgical procedures, patients with acute traumatic conditions, and patients with acute exacerbation of a chronic respiratory disease present with severe physiologic abnormalities. These categories of patients with hypermetabolic energy needs or depletion of energy reserves are unable to sustain the workload of spontaneous breathing.[2,5,6,19] For example, the postoperative patient with surgery for a ruptured aorta, the cachectic patient with chronic obstructive pulmonary disease, the patient with a head injury, and the obese patient with a thoracotomy are at risk for ISSV.

The determination of ISSV is based on deterioration of arterial blood gases, the increased work of breathing, and decreasing energy. Patient behaviors, such as increased restlessness, increased use of accessory muscles, and compromised ability to cooperate, are outward manifestations of ISSV. Other characteristics if ISSV, such as cardiac disrhythmias and decreased SaO_2 are recognized through the interpretation of findings from monitoring equipment.[6,7]

Related Factors*

Anemia

Infection

Increased metabolic requirements to resist nosocomial infections.

Hypothermia

Electrolyte imbalance

Left ventricular dysfunction

Increased intrathoracic pressure

Pulmonary edema

Atelectasis

Carbohydrate overfeeding

Abdominal distention (e.g., bowel, obesity)

Uncontrolled pain

Activity greater than available energy

Respiratory muscle fatigue

Defining Characteristics†

Dyspnea

Tachypnea

Increased restlessness

Increased use of accessory muscles

Decreased spontaneous tidal volume

Increased heart rate

Cardiac dysrhythmias

Apprehension

Compromised ability to cooperate

Decreased SaO_2

Decreased PO_2

Increased PCO_2

Increased metabolic rate

Expected Patient Outcomes & Nursing Interventions‡

Sustain spontaneous ventilation, as evidenced by:

Oxygenation of tissues (e.g., arterial-alveolar gradient <350, pH 7.35 to 7.45, PO_2 >60, PCO_2 <50, SaO_2 >90)

Increased level of consciousness with associated, purposeful, or nonpurposeful movement

Demonstrating synchronous use of respiratory muscles

- Conduct a thorough baseline physical assessment, and use family and medical records as resources for obtaining medical history *to identify organs at risk because of altered oxygenation.*
- Observe for presence of diaphragm or respiratory muscle fatigue, increased respiratory rate, minute ventilation, and hypercarbia with respiratory acidosis *to reevaluate adequacy of oxygen therapy parameters.*
- Call patient by preferred name, introduce self, and give brief explanation of purpose for being with patient during each patient contact *to decrease patient anxiety associated with unfamiliar environment.*
- Ensure that patient has a primary nurse *to coordinate multidisciplinary care and to monitor progress toward goals.*
- Check for correct initial placement of endotracheal tube and monitor placement according to unit protocols *to maximize air entry and to maintain placement.*
- Collaborate with the multidisciplinary team to determine ventilation parameters (e.g., FlO_2, mode of ventilatory assistance, tidal volume frequency) *to ensure adequate oxygenation and to prevent ventilator-induced complications.*
- Collaborate with multidisciplinary team to develop a suction protocol that incorporates parameters for hyperoxygeneration, hyperinflation, and length of stabilization period between suction catheter passes *to maximize tissue oxygenation and to prevent complications.*
- Initiate passive or active exercise (e.g., turning, postural drainage, range of motion exercises, induced coughing, and deep breathing) *to mobilize secretions.*
- Remove secretions *to reduce airway resistance;* use sterile technique *to minimize exposure to infectious agents.*
- Monitor hemodynamic status (e.g., cardiac rate, rhythm, pulmonary artery pressure, and pulmonary wedge pressure) *to detect decreased cardiac output caused by increased thoracic pressure.*
- Collaborate with the multidisciplinary team to determine timing and appropriateness for increasing ventilatory assistance, until patient exhibits no spontaneous breathing effort *to allow adequate diaphragmatic rest and to prevent diaphragm muscle fatigue.*
- Observe for indicators of airway resistance that can reduce the work of breathing (e.g., endotracheal tube size, mechanical ventilator system or node, or uncoordinated efforts of the patient with the machine); share observations with physician.

---

*References 2, 4-8, 10-14, 19.
†References 3-7, 12, 16-18, 21.

‡References 1-3, 5-15, 17, 19-23.

- Position patient upright or supine, based on individual tolerance, *to enhance full lung expansion and to improve cardiac output.*
- Observe breathing pattern (e.g., dyspnea, tachypnea, tidal volume, abdominal paradox or asynchrony, and patient's level of comfort) *to determine work of breathing.*
- Use negative inspiratory pressure, positive expiratory pressure, and tidal volume as parameters to regulate activity *to prevent diaphragm fatigue, injury, and atrophy.*
- Establish a schedule for muscle reconditioning:
    Collaborate with physician and respiratory therapy to determine timing and appropriateness of mechanically assisted muscle training (e.g., pressure support, intermittent mechanical ventilation, and inspiratory resistive training) *to maximize respiratory muscle strength.*
    Collaborate with physical therapist and physician to determine a schedule for graded manual diaphragmatic muscle exercises, incorporating principles of overload, specificity, and reversibility *to maximize diaphragm endurance.*
- Collaborate with physician regarding use of methylxanthines *to facilitate bronchodilation and to increase diaphragm contractility.*

Meet metabolic energy requirements, as evidenced by:

Maintaining nutritional intake equal to calculated requirements for nutrition

Demonstrating absence of infection

Tolerating progressive increase in activity

- Evaluate for factors that contribute to increased energy expenditure (e.g., white blood cell count with or without fever, renal function, fluid status, acid-base disturbances, hepatic function, gastric bleeding, and bowel function) *to formulate a comprehensive multidisciplinary plan of care.*
- Collaborate with dietitian and physician to maintain adequate nutrition (e.g., 25 to 35 kcal/kg with appropriate carbohydrate, fat, and protein) *to maximize energy resources and to prevent increased carbon dioxide production.*
- Monitor daily weight and intake and output.
- Monitor bowel function (e.g., constipation or diarrhea) *to prevent complications, such as ileus, skin breakdown, and dehydration.*
- Monitor levels of serum phosphate, potassium, calcium, and magnesium; collaborate with physician, dietitian, or pharmacist to provide replacement therapy, as necessary, *to maintain respiratory muscle strength.*
- Observe for subtle signs of systemic or local infection (e.g., increased white blood cell count, hypothermia or hyperthermia, redness, or swelling); report findings to physician or pharmacist *to conserve energy expenditure through early treatment.*
- Minimize patient's exposure to infection by:
    Providing frequent oral hygiene (e.g., alternate endotracheal tube side, brush teeth, and swab patient's mouth)

    Teaching family to report their own exposure to possible infection or illness
    Emphasizing to multidisciplinary team the importance of universal precautions
    Monitoring the sterility of equipment in conjunction with respiratory therapy, infection control, and decontamination services
- Strive to develop a therapeutic alliance (e.g., use calm, low voice; provide simple explanations; encourage family visitation) *to foster patient's cooperation with and participation in progressive activity plan.*
- Monitor patient's response to movement *to establish baseline tolerance and to observe for progress.*
- Establish a regular schedule for muscle reconditioning; incorporate adequate rest periods.
- Schedule rest periods that are congruent with patient's circadian rhythm *to facilitate adequate rapid eye movement (REM) sleep.*
- Evaluate rest and activity schedule on a daily basis; revise according to patient's tolerance.

Principles and Rationale for Nursing Interventions

Nursing interventions to resolve the patient's inability to sustain spontaneous ventilation begin with an assessment of the patient's ability to oxygenate and to maintain energy requirements. The primary nurse plays a pivotal role in the development of a multidisciplinary plan of care and in observation of the patient's progress toward sustaining spontaneous ventilation. Nursing strategies that maximize the patient's oxygenation of tissues, while minimizing unintended workload, contribute to maintenance of respiratory muscle strength needed for unassisted breathing.

Nursing interventions to facilitate the patient's meeting metabolic energy requirements include a nutritional assessment for replacement of cellular nutrients. Conservation of energy expenditure is managed by minimizing the patient's exposure to infection from family, staff, and equipment. The development of a therapeutic alliance with the patient contributes to the patient's ability to cooperate with and to participate in the progressive activity plan.

■ INEFFECTIVE AIRWAY CLEARANCE[8]

Ineffective airway clearance is a state in which an individual is unable to clear secretions or obstructions from the respiratory tract to maintain airway patency.

Related Factors

Decreased energy and fatigue

Tracheobronchial

Infection

Obstruction

Secretion

Perceptual/cognitive impairment

Trauma

Defining Characteristics

Abnormal breath sounds—rales (crackles), rhonchi (wheezes)

Changes in rate or depth of respiration

Tachypnea

Cough, effective or ineffective, with or without sputum

Cyanosis

Dyspnea

Fever

Expected Patient Outcomes & Nursing Interventions[1,4,8,10-12]

Maintain patent airways, as evidenced by:

Clear breath sounds

Fewer or less tenacious secretions

Dyspnea absent or decreased

- Auscultate lungs for rhonchi, crackles, or wheezing.
- Monitor respiratory patterns for rate, depth, and ease of breathing.
- Assess characteristics of secretions for quantity, color, consistency, and odor.
- Monitor blood gases for hypoxia and hypercapnia.
- When patient has an obstructed airway, assess patient's ability to talk; apply Heimlich maneuver as needed.
- Teach patient and family effective coughing techniques.
- Encourage patient to change positions every few hours and ambulate when possible.
- Encourage 3-4 liters fluids daily if not contraindicated.
- Remove secretions by suctioning airway as needed.
- Position patient in proper body alignment for optimal breathing pattern (head of bed up 45 degrees; if tolerated, 90 degrees).
- If patient has unilateral lung disease, alternate semi-Fowler's position with a lateral position with unaffected lung in a dependent position ("good lung down"). (This position is contraindicated for patients with pulmonary abscess, hemorrhage, or interstitial emphysema.)[12]
- Administer oxygen as ordered.
- Administer bronchodilators as ordered.
- Administer corticosteroids and anti-infective agents, as ordered.
- Avoid suppressing cough reflex unless cough is frequent and nonproductive.
- Assist patient with oral hygiene, as needed.

Communicate knowledge of self-care, as evidenced by:

Patient and family explaining reason for ineffective airway clearance

Actions to avoid ineffective airway clearance

Medications and treatments for home use

Plan for follow-up care

- Assess what patient and family need to learn.
- Provide information concerning:

  How to prevent recurrence of airway obstruction

  How to perform diaphragmatic and pursed-lip breathing

  Purpose of drugs taken at home, frequency of administration, and side effects

  Smoking cessation

  Eating balanced meals with adequate fluids

  Performing bronchial hygiene and productive coughing techniques

  Changing daily activities to decrease oxygen demands

  Plans for follow-up

Principles and Rationale for Nursing Interventions[1,4,8,10-12]

Assessment interventions begin with auscultating the patient's lungs for crackles (rales), rhonchi, and wheezes to determine airway patency. The rate and depth and use of accessory muscles are assessed to determine the work of breathing. The nurse observes color, consistency, and amount of sputum because pulmonary irritants or infections often cause an increased mucus production. Changes in the color or consistency of sputum may indicate the presence of an infection, e.g., sputum that becomes thinner and changes from yellow or green to white may indicate improvement, whereas increased amounts of sputum that change from white to yellow or green may indicate a pulmonary infection.

When the cause of upper airway obstruction is the tongue or a foreign object, the patient requires immediate care to clear the obstruction. When a *foreign body* is suspected, the nurse determines if the patient can speak to distinguish an occluded airway from another condition, such as myocardial infarction. The person with an occluded airway will be unable to speak. To dislodge the obstruction, the nurse uses the *Heimlich maneuver;* four quick back blows to the patient between the scapula followed by abdominal thrusts. To deliver the abdominal thrusts, the nurse stands behind the patient and places both hands at the patient's diaphragm, grabs the right fist with the left hand, and gives a sudden, strong upward thrust against the abdomen. This pressure compresses the lungs, forcing the object into the mouth to clear the airway. This procedure can be done with the patient supine and the nurse kneeling astride and facing the patient. The nurse places the heel of one hand just above the umbilicus and places the other hand atop the first. A quick upward thrust is delivered against the abdomen to dislodge the object. The back blows and abdominal thrust are continued until the obstruction is relieved or until advanced life support is available. The airway is suctioned to remove excess secretions.

Ineffective airway clearance related to laryngospasm occurs most frequently in infants and children. It requires prompt care also but is placed in order of priority after obstruction by foreign object or tongue. Initially, the airway is opened using the head tilt with forward displacement of the mandible. An oropharyngeal airway is inserted followed by artificial ventilation by mouth-to-mouth means or inflation bag. A medical treatment of laryngospasm is administration of a paralytic drug followed by orotracheal intubation. If this action is inadequate, and if the patient is unconscious, the nurse, in collaboration with the physician, inserts an esophageal obturator airway. An emergency tracheostomy is performed by a physician as a last resort to open the airway. Once the airway is opened, the patient is placed in an upright position and encouraged to breathe deeply. Humidified oxygen is given as ordered.

When the cause of lower airway obstruction is edema or excessive mucus and secretion production, the airways are cleared by effective coughing. The patient is instructed to sit up as high as possible to facilitate chest expansion. Then the patient inhales slowly and deeply to dilate airways and force air behind the mucus and secretions. The patient exhales forcibly until the cough reflex is stimulated. Endotracheal stimulation is used to produce coughing when the patient is too weak to cough. Coughing is necessary but requires work that can fatigue the patient. The nurse determines the frequency of coughing needed by patients to clear the airways but not to tire them unnecessarily. Along with coughing, postural drainage is recommended to allow gravity to drain secretions from segmental bronchi. Percussion and vibration are used to dislodge pulmonary secretions. The patient who is obese, has unstable vital signs, or has extreme dyspnea may not be able to tolerate postural drainage. Positioning the patient so that the unaffected lung is down or dependent allows better ventilation and perfusion of that lung by means of gravity and hydrostatic pressure.[12]

Increasing fluids orally and/or parenterally helps minimize mucosal drying and increase ciliary action to move secretions.[4] Humidified oxygen prevents drying of mucous membranes and provides needed supplemental oxygen for cell metabolism. Bronchodilators are given to relax the bronchial smooth muscles that surround the bronchi to increase their diameter thereby decreasing the work of breathing. Corticosteroids are given to reduce the edema caused by inflammation. Antiinfectives reduce infection of the pulmonary system.

To maintain comfort, the nurse encourages frequent oral and nasal hygiene for the patient who has a productive cough. The patient should blow the nose gently to remove mucus. Nostrils may be cleaned with moistened cotton-tipped applicators. Since coughing can cause fatigue and can interfere with sleep, the patient needs planned rest periods of at least 1 hour. After receiving treatments for airway clearance and medications, the patient can be encouraged to sleep. A dyspneic, apprehensive patient may need to talk with the nurse about fears and anxieties related to breathing.

∎ INEFFECTIVE BREATHING PATTERN[8]

Ineffective breathing pattern is a state in which an individual's inhalation and/or exhalation pattern does not enable adequate ventilation.

Related Factors

Neuromuscular impairments
Pain
Musculoskeletal impairment
Perception or cognitive impairment
Anxiety
Decreased energy and fatigue
Inflammatory process
Decreased lung expansion
Tracheobronchial obstruction

Defining Characteristics

Dyspnea
Shortness of breath
Tachypnea
Fremitus
Abnormal arterial blood gas levels
Cyanosis
Cough
Nasal flaring
Respiratory depth changes
Assumption of three-point position
Pursed-lip breathing and prolonged expiratory phase
Increased anteroposterior diameter
Use of accessory muscles
Altered chest excursion

Expected Patient Outcomes & Nursing Interventions[1,3,4,6-12]

Respiratory pattern is effective without tiring patient, as evidenced by:

Respiratory rate within normal limits
Tidal volume optimal for patient
Pao_2 >60 mm Hg
$Paco_2$ normal for patient
Mild to absent dyspnea

- Monitor respiratory rate, depth, and ease of respiration.
- Observe for use of accessory muscles, abdominal breathing, nasal flaring, retractions, irritability, confusion, or lethargy.
- Auscultate breathing sounds for decreased or absent sounds, crackles, and wheezes.
- Monitor patient's oxygen saturation and arterial blood gases for hypoxia.
- Observe sputum for color, odor, and volume.
- Determine degree of dyspnea by counting number of words the patient can say between breaths.
- Monitor the patient's tidal volume for a decrease.
- Review chest x-rays that indicate severity of skeletal and lung impairment.
- Assess emotional response that may alter breathing, i.e., anxiety.
- Assess patient for pain that may result in hypoventilation.
- If patient has unilateral lung disease, position in semi-Fowler's alternated with side lying with the unaffected lung in a dependent position ("good lung down") unless patient has pulmonary abscess, hemorrhage, or interstitial emphysema.

- Encourage patient to cough, splinting chest as necessary.
- Assist patient with weak or paralyzed intercostal or abdominal muscles to cough effectively by splinting intercostal muscles or applying upward pressure just below the diaphragm.
- Supervise use of respiratory, diaphragmatic stimulator rocking bed, and iron lung when neuromuscular problems are diagnosed.
- Medicate with analgesics without depressing respirations.
- Assist patient to use relaxation techniques.
- Teach pursed lip breathing.
- Encourage use of blow bottles or incentive spirometry.
- Teach use of abdominal breathing exercises.

Communicate knowledge of self-care, as evidenced by:

Patient and family explaining:

Reasons for ineffective breathing

Medication and treatment for home use

Plan for follow-up care

- Assess what patient and family need to know.
- Review reasons for ineffective breathing patterns.
- Make referral for ventilatory equipment to be used in the home.
- Review reasons for medications and treatments ordered for home use.
- Review plan for follow-up care.

Principles and Rationale for Nursing Interventions[1,3,4,6-12]

Assessment interventions begin with counting the respiratory rate and observing the depth and difficulty the patient is having to breathe. Observing the thorax for symmetry may indicate a breathing pattern problem. An increase in the work of breathing may be recognized by contraction of accessory muscles (e.g., trapezius), flaring of nostrils, retraction of the chest, or a change in behavior that may indicate hypoxia (e.g., confusion, lethargy, irritability). When rhonchi are found on auscultation, they indicate secretions in the airways that can alter the breathing pattern. Hypoxia can also be identified by monitoring oxygen saturation and arterial blood gases. Observing changes in the patient's sputum may be useful to evaluate therapeutic interventions. Sputum that becomes thinner and changes from yellow or green to white may indicate improvement, whereas increased amounts of sputum that change from white to yellow or green may indicate a pulmonary infection. The number of words a patient can say between breaths is an indirect way to determine dyspnea; an expected average is 8 to 10 words between breaths. As the dyspnea becomes worse, the patient is able to say fewer words between breaths. Measuring the tidal volume indicates the amount of air that the patient moves in and out of the lungs with each breath; an ineffective breathing pattern may decrease the tidal volume. Chest x-ray examinations show the extent of the lung and thorax involvement that contribute to an altered breathing pattern such as pleural effusion or fractured ribs. Pain, stress, or anxiety may impair breathing patterns and need to be assessed so that treatment can be instituted.

Therapeutic interventions begin with positioning of the patient for optimal diaphragmatic excursion. Positioning the patient so that the unaffected lung is down or dependent allows better ventilation and perfusion of that lung by means of gravity and hydrostatic pressure.[12] Coughing is beneficial, but the patient's thorax may need to be splinted when pain or weak muscles are experienced. Medicating the patient, as ordered, for pain 20 to 30 minutes before coughing, turning, or chest physiotherapy is helpful to improve ventilation. The patient with weak thoracic muscles may benefit from splinting of the intercostal muscles or from firm pressure just below the diaphragm to assist with coughing. Often mechanical devices such as ventilators are needed to maintain ventilation. Relaxation techniques improve ventilation when the patient is anxious. Fatigue associated with coughing can be reduced by abdominal strengthening exercises and controlled coughing techniques when support is provided to muscles of expiration. By using blow bottles or incentive spirometry, the patient is encouraged to deep breathe. Pursed lip breathing forces client to breathe more slowly and deeply and prolongs expiration to increase exhalation of carbon dioxide. Many patients benefit from using abdominal exercises to decrease the work of breathing.

Finally, the patient and family require instruction about how to prevent the ineffective breathing pattern from recurring. Also, they need to know how to use ventilatory equipment, the purpose and side effects of medications prescribed, and the plans for follow-up care. They need to be well informed so that they can carry out the plan of care after discharge.

◼ IMPAIRED GAS EXCHANGE[8]

Impaired gas exchange is a state in which an individual experiences an imbalance between oxygen uptake and carbon dioxide elimination at the alveolar-capillary membrane gas exchange area.

Related Factors

Altered oxygen supply

Alveolar-capillary membrane changes

Altered blood flow

Altered oxygen-carrying capacity of blood

Defining Characteristics

Confusion

Somnolence

Restlessness

Irritability

Inability to move secretions

Hypercapnia

Hypoxia

Polycythemia (a compensatory mechanism)

Increased anterior-posterior diameter of chest
Tachycardia, dysrhythmias
Anxiety
Dyspnea
Cyanosis
Decreased mental acuity
Tachypnea
Widened alveolar-arterial gradient
Three-point position
Pursed-lip breathing with prolonged expiratory phase

Expected Patient Outcomes & Nursing Interventions*

Maintain adequate oxygenation as evidenced by:

Po_2: 80-95 mm Hg (lower for patient with chronic obstructive pulmonary disease)
Pco_2: 35-45 mm Hg (higher for patient with COPD)
O_2 saturation: 95%-99%
Hemoglobin: 12-14 g/dl (women)
Hemoglobin: 14-16 g/dl (men)
Respiratory rate: 12-20/min
Performing activities of daily living without becoming short of breath

- Monitor respiratory rate, depth, and effort, including use of accessory muscles, nasal flaring, and thoracic or abdominal breathing.
- Auscultate breath sounds for rhonchi, crackles, and wheezes.
- Assess patient's behavior and mental status for restlessness, agitation, confusion, and lethargy.
- Monitor oxygen saturation continually via pulse oximeter for hypoxia and, when available, arterial blood gases for hypoxia and hypercapnia.
- Monitor complete blood count for decreases in hemoglobin and hematocrit.
- Observe patient's skin color for paleness or cyanosis.
- Note number of words patient can say between breaths at rest and during activity.
- Position patient for maximal ventilation and perfusion. If client has unilateral lung disease, alternate semi-Fowler's position with lateral position with unaffected lung dependent ("good lung down"). (This method is contraindicated when patients have pulmonary abscess, hemorrhage, or interstitial emphysema.) If patient has bilateral lung disease, position patient on either side or semi-Fowler's position supine, changing position every few hours.
- Encourage patient to deep breath and cough or use incentive spirometry every few hours while awake.
- Suction the airways when coughing is ineffective.
- Teach patient pursed lip breathing.
- Pace activities to patient's tolerance.
- Use sedation cautiously so that respirations are not depressed.
- Administer humidified oxygen as ordered.
- Administer packed cells as ordered.
- Administer medications as ordered (e.g., bronchodilators, diuretics, corticosteroids, antibiotics, anticoagulants).

Communicate knowledge of self-care, as evidenced by:

The patient and family explaining:
   Reasons for impaired gas exchange
   Medication and treatment for home use
   Plan for follow-up care
- Assess what patient and family need to know.
- Provide information about pursed-lip breathing and diaphragmatic breathing.
- Discover reason for impaired gas exchange, and discuss how to prevent it in the future.
- Know actions, side effects, dosage, and frequency of administration of all medications ordered by physician.
- Plan referral for ventilatory equipment to be used in the home.
- Alter daily activities, as necessary, to decrease oxygen demand.

Principles and Rationale for Nursing Interventions*

Assessment interventions begin with monitoring the rate and depth of respiration, and use of accessory muscles to determine the work of breathing. The lungs are auscultated for adventitious sounds such as crackles (rales) indicating fluid in alveoli, rhonchi indicating secretions in bronchi, or wheezes indicating narrowed airways. Decreased or absent breath sounds may indicate collapsed alveoli. Changes in mental status may indicate hypoxia created by a lack of oxygen to brain cells. Pulse oximeter provides continuous oxygen saturation to monitor hypoxia. Arterial blood gases are monitored to evaluate the exchange of gases between the alveoli and pulmonary capillaries. Hemoglobin and hematocrit values determine if the patient has anemia that may decrease the oxygen-carrying capacity. Anemia or hypoxia may contribute to pale skin color. Cyanosis is a late sign of hypoxia. The number of words a patient can speak between breaths is an indirect way to determine dyspnea that may indicate hypoxia: an average is 8 to 10 words between breaths. As the dyspnea develops, the patient is able to say fewer words between breaths.

Therapeutic interventions include positioning. Positioning the patient in a semi-Fowler's position allows gravity to move the abdominal contents away from the diaphragm to facilitate breathing. Positioning the patient so that the unaffected lung is down or dependent improves ventilation and perfusion of that lung by means of gravity and hydrostatic pressure.[12] Coughing and deep breathing clear the airways of secretions; suctioning can be performed when coughing is not possible or effective. The work of breathing can be reduced by pursed-lip breathing. The patient should be encouraged to pace activities to personal

---

*References 1-3, 5, 8, 10-12.

tolerance to avoid increasing the oxygen demand. Sedation is used with caution with these patients so that the drive for respiration is not depressed. Humidified oxygen is administered as ordered to improve gas exchange and reduce the work of breathing. Packed cells may be given when anemia impairs gas exchange. Medications are given to facilitate breathing: bronchodilators to relax bronchial smooth muscle and increase the size of bronchi, diuretics to remove excessive fluid from alveoli that impair gas exchange, corticosteroids to reduce inflammation of airways, antibiotics to treat infections, and anticoagulants to prevent thrombi when pulmonary embolism impairs gas exchange.

Before discharge the patient and family need instruction on how to prevent impaired gas exchange in the future. Also, they must know how to use ventilatory equipment, the purpose and side effects of medications prescribed, and the plans for follow-up care. They need to discuss how to alter their life-styles, as needed, because of chronic gas exchange impairment.

■ DECREASED CARDIAC OUTPUT[8]

Decreased cardiac output is a state in which the blood pumped by an individual's heart is sufficiently reduced to the extent that it is inadequate to meet the needs of the body's tissues.[8]

Related Factors

Mechanical
    Alteration in preload
    Alteration in afterload
    Alteration in inotropic changes in heart
Electrical
    Alteration in rate
    Alteration in rhythm
    Alteration in conduction
Structural

Defining Characteristics

Variations in hemodynamic readings
Dysrhythmias; ECG changes
Fatigue
Jugular vein distention[R]
Cyanosis; pallor of skin and mucous membranes
Oliguria, anuria
Decreased peripheral pulses
Cold, clammy skin
Crackles[L]
Dyspnea[L]
Change in mental status[R]
Syncope[R]
Vertigo[R]
Edema, dependent[R]
Shortness of breath[L]

Cough[L]
Frothy sputum[L]
Abnormal heart sounds (e.g., gallop rhythm)[L]
Weakness
Liver engorgement and tenderness[R]
Ascites[R]
Tachycardia
Angina

Expected Patient Outcomes & Nursing Interventions[1,8,10]

Maintain adequate cardiac output, as evidenced by:

Normal sinus rhythm
Heart rate within 20 beats of normal
Blood pressure upper limits:
    140 mm Hg systolic
    90 mm Hg diastolic
    30 to 40 mm Hg pulse pressure
Absence of angina
Urinary output at least 30 ml per hour
Skin warm, dry
Peripheral pulses present and strong (normal for patient)

- Assess heart rate and blood pressure because they are indicators of cardiac output.
- Listen to heart sounds—rate, rhythm, S3 and S4, rub, onset of new systolic murmur.
- Observe for chest pain noting location, severity, radiation, quality, duration, and factors that precipitate and relieve the pain.
- Auscultate lungs for crackles that may indicate fluid in the pulmonary capillaries.
- Monitor cardiac rhythm continuously for changes.
- Weight patient daily.
- Monitor arterial blood gases.
- Assess mental status for confusion, dizziness.
- Monitor cardiac enzymes.
- Monitor electrolyte values (especially potassium).
- Titrate inotropic and vasoactive medication within defined parameters as ordered.
- Measure fluid intake and urine output.
- Administer oxygen, as ordered.
- Administer pain medications as ordered.
- Administer plasma volume expanders, as ordered; adjust flow rate according to pulmonary artery pressures and pulmonary capillary wedge pressures.
- Administer diuretics, as ordered.
- Administer thrombolytic therapy, as ordered.
- Monitor intraaortic balloon pump, as indicated.
- Restrict fluids, as ordered.
- Maintain bed rest with head of bed elevated 30 degrees and restrict activities, as indicated.

[R]Occurs with right ventricular failure
[L]Occurs with left ventricular failure

- Maintain a quiet environment and reduced stimuli.
- Assist with self-care or perform activities to decrease cardiac workload.
- Serve smaller meals of low sodium and low cholesterol foods.
- Increase activity level, as indicated, by clinical status (e.g., blood pressure, heart rate).
- Schedule rest periods between activities.
- Encourage deep breathing and coughing during activities.

Communicate knowledge of self-care, as evidenced by:

The patient and family explaining:
  Reasons for decreased cardiac output and how to prevent it
  Dietary alterations
  Exercise program
  Stress management activities
  Medication uses and side effects
  Plan for follow-up care
  - Assess patient's current knowledge and provide information, as needed.
  - Provide information concerning:
    Prevention of recurrence
    Risk factors to avoid
    Pathophysiology of illness
    Medication uses, side effects, and frequency of administration
    Stress management techniques
    Physical activity program
    Dietary alterations
    Guidelines for resuming sexual relations
    Guidelines for returning to work

Principles and Rationale for Nursing Interventions[1,8]

Cardiac output is the amount of blood ejected from the left ventricle each minute and normally ranges from 4 to 8 L. Cardiac output is a function of the stroke volume (amount of blood ejected per contraction) and the heart rate (number of contractions per minute).

The care varies with the acuity of the problem. To restore cardiac output, the causative condition must be corrected. Assessment data the nurse collects to meet this goal include the following:
  Auscultating the heart
  Measuring the heart rate and blood pressure
  Palpating pulses
  Identifying the rhythm of the heart through the ECG pattern
  Measuring the pressures of the right atria, pulmonary artery, and pulmonary capillary wedge through a pulmonary artery catheter
  Measuring cardiac output and urinary output
  Measuring daily body weight to detect fluid gain or loss

The nurse is aware of laboratory data, including electrolytes, cardiac enzymes, arterial blood gases, hemoglobin, and hematocrit. Under physician orders the nurse administers medications to maintain cardiac output and monitors the therapeutic effects and side effects of these drugs. When preload is reduced because of decreased volume, the nurse administers intravenous fluids, as ordered. Per physician orders, medications are administered to maintain the delicate balance to stimulate the heart without increasing its workload and maintain adequate perfusion of the body.

An intraaortic balloon is inserted by the physician to increase oxygen supply to the myocardium, decrease left ventricular work, and improve cardiac output. Assessment of the patient with balloon pump therapy includes monitoring heart rate, mean arterial pressure, pulmonary capillary wedge pressure, heart rhythm and regularity, urine output, skin color, peripheral perfusion, and mental status.

To reduce the workload on the patient's heart, the nurse intervenes to meet physical and psychologic needs. Oxygen is provided, as ordered, to ensure an adequate supply for the myocardium. Pain medication is given based on protocol for comfort, as needed. Morphine is a preferred drug because it not only relieves pain, but also provides peripheral vasodilation to reduce venous return. Diuretics and vasodilators are given to reduce systemic vascular resistance. The patient is asked to reduce physical activity by resting in bed in a semi-Fowler's or Fowler's position or in a chair. This position also reduces the patient's work of breathing, thereby decreasing the workload of the heart. Hygiene activities are performed for the patient. Specific times of rest are planned throughout the day. As the patient improves, a progressive activity schedule is implemented. The physician may prescribe stool softeners to prevent straining during defecation. The diet is changed, as needed. Frequently caffeine and sodium are restricted. Small meals require less work by the heart.

To meet psychologic needs, the nurse attempts to reduce the patient's stress and anxiety. A quiet, pleasant environment relieves stress. The patient is encouraged to discuss feelings and is given as much information as possible. Relaxation techniques are taught to reduce tension (see Ineffective Individual Coping on p. 1739).

To achieve awareness of learning needs, the nurse first assesses what the patient and family already know. They need to know what caused the decrease in cardiac output and how to avoid its recurrence. The patient and family will need to know actions and side effects of medications. Lifestyle changes will require regular exercise of at least 30 minutes three times a week. Dietary alterations are needed to restrict sodium or cholesterol. It is important to consider the patient's cultural food preferences when adapting dietary alterations to fit the lifestyle. When obesity is a problem, the patient needs to understand that extra weight increases the heart's workload. Smoking adds a burden to the heart by causing vasoconstriction.

ALTERED TISSUE PERFUSION (SPECIFY TYPE) (RENAL, CEREBRAL, CARDIOPULMONARY, GASTROINTESTINAL, PERIPHERAL)[8]

Altered tissue perfusion is a state in which an individual experiences a decrease in nutrition and oxygenation at the cellular level due to a deficit in capillary blood supply.

Related Factors

Interruption of flow, arterial
Interruption of flow, venous
Exchange problems
Hypervolemia
Hypovolemia

Defining Characteristics

Skin temperature: cold extremities
Skin color
  Dependent, blue or purple
Pale on elevation, and color does not return on lowering leg
Diminished arterial pulsations
Skin quality: shining
Lack of lanugo
Round scars covered with atrophied skin
Gangrene
Slow-growing, dry, thick, brittle nails
Claudication
Blood pressure changes in extremities
Bruits
Slow healing of lesions
Renal
  Edema
  Decreased urinary output
  Hypertension
Cerebral
  Decrease in consciousness
  Restlessness
  Altered thought processes
  Memory loss
Cardiopulmonary
  Low systolic and diastolic blood pressure readings
  Cold, clammy skin
  Slow capillary filing
  Tachycardia
  Angina
  Tachypnea
Gastrointestinal
  Pain
  Abdominal distention
  Positive guaiac findings of stool
  Nausea or vomiting
  Thirst
  Melena
Peripheral
  Edema
  Pain
  Numbness, tingling
  Muscle weakness
  Diminished sensitivity to pressure, temperature, and tissue trauma

Expected Patient Outcomes & Nursing Interventions[1,8,10]

Maintain tissue perfusion and cellular oxygenation, as evidenced by:

All pulses palpable
Extremities warm and normal color
Vital signs normal for patient
Bowel sounds present
1500 to 3000 ml output daily, or equivalent to intake
Alert with recent memory normal
Hemoglobin (g/dl)
  Men: 15.5 ± 1.1
  Women: 13.7 ± 1.0
Partial thromboplastin time: 25-39 seconds (usually stated to be within 10 seconds of control)
Arterial blood gases
  pH:7.35-7.45
  Po_2: 80-95 mm Hg
  Pco_2 35-45 mm Hg
  O_2 sat: 95%-99%

- Assess all pulses to determine the extent of tissue perfusion.

Peripheral assessment for inadequate peripheral tissue perfusion

- Assess skin color and temperature: inadequately perfused tissue will appear pale and feel cool to the touch.
- Assess the capillary refill that is slowed when circulation is impaired.
- Inspect extremities for edema and measure circumference of extremities; a thrombus or emboli may impede circulation, causing fluid to move from the intravascular to the interstitial spaces.
- Auscultate for systolic or continuous bruits below obstruction in extremities.
- Note characteristics of pain with or without activity.
- Monitor clotting time *to prevent bleeding*.
- Monitor hemoglobin and hematocrit *to detect blood loss and anemia*.

Cerebral assessment for inadequate perfusion to the brain

- Assess level of consciousness of memory.
- Assess motor and sensory changes.
- Note reports of dizziness or headache.

Cardiac assessment for inadequate perfusion of the myocardium

- Assess baseline arterial blood gases, electrolytes, blood urea nitrogen/creatinine, and cardiac enzymes.

- Monitor cardiac rhythm for dysrhythmias.
- Note complaints of chest pain/angina.

Gastrointestinal assessment for inadequate perfusion of the gastrointestinal system

- Auscultate bowel sounds.
- Measure abdominal girth to detect edema.
- Note complaints of nausea, vomiting, and abdominal pain.

Renal assessment for inadequate perfusion of the kidneys

- Measure urine output because oliguria may be an early sign of decreased perfusion.
- Monitor for elevated levels of the following:
  - Blood urea
  - Nitrogen/creatinine
  - Proteinuria
  - Specific gravity
  - Serum electrolytes
- Assess mentation, which may decrease as the blood urea, nitrogen/creatinine levels rise.
- Monitor blood pressure for elevations from a decreased glomerular filtration rate.
- Administer medication, as ordered (vasodilators, anticoagulants, antilipemics, and papaverine) *to promote circulation.*
- Perform assistive/active range of motion exercises (Buerger and Buerger-Allen); venous impairments respond to elevation of the legs; arterial impairments response to supine or lowered positions.
- Encourage early ambulation to promote circulation.
- Discourage sitting or standing for long periods of time; wearing constrictive clothing; crossing legs, impairing circulation.
- Apply antithromboembolic hose or Ace bandages.
- Use heating pads and hot water bottles cautiously because ischemia may decrease sensitivity.
- Encourage patient to quit smoking because nicotine causes vasoconstriction.
- Provide air mattress, sheep skin, or cradle.
- Elevate head of bed and maintain head in midline position.
- Administer medication, as ordered (e.g., corticosteroids, diuretics).
- When patient is confused, provide a safe environment.
- Administer antidysrhythmics, as ordered.
- Caution patient against straining during any activity because straining increases workload of the heart (e.g., straining at stool or sitting up without assistance).
- Administer oxygen, as ordered, to improve oxygenation to the myocardium.
- Maintain gastric and intestinal decompression.
- Provide small, easily digested foods, when tolerated.
- Encourage rest after meals.
- Measure urine output.
- Weigh daily; a change in weight of one pound may represent 500 ml of fluid.
- Administer dopamine, as ordered, to improve renal perfusion.

- Administer corticosteroids, as ordered.
- Provide dietary restriction, as indicated, (e.g., reduced sodium, and protein).

Communicate knowledge of self-care

- Assess what patient and family need to know.
- Provide information concerning:
  - Changes required in activities of daily living
  - Maintaining reduction in metabolic needs
  - Assessing skin and peripheral circulation daily
  - Purpose, frequency of administration, and side effects of medication
  - Safety needs for patients taking anticoagulants
  - Providing balanced diet
  - Taking action to prevent recurrence of altered tissue perfusion
  - Plans for rehabilitation

Principles and Rationale for Nursing Interventions[1,8]

Therapeutic interventions to maintain tissue perfusion are based on the cause of the alteration. Elevation of the affected extremity is appropriate when venous circulation is altered because this position uses gravity to facilitate return of blood toward the heart. Likewise, elevating both legs is helpful when the patient has hypovolemic shock to facilitate blood flow from the lower extremities to the trunk. Conversely, arterial circulation is hindered by prolonged elevation of lower extremities because the normal flow of arterial blood is downward. The flat position is best for long periods. The patient needs a firm bed to prevent hip flexion allowed on a soft mattress. Flexion of the hip may compromise circulation of the legs. The patient must also select chairs carefully. The knees must not be bent at more than a 90-degree angle, and the popliteal space must not press against the chair seat. Active and passive exercises, as well as walking stimulate blood flow to the legs. External pressure on the legs is reduced by not crossing the legs, not wearing tight clothing on the legs, and not sitting for long periods. Drug administration may include heparin or warfarin (coumadin) as prophylaxis against blood clotting, per physician's order. Vasodilators are given, as ordered by physician, for arterial spasm and to improve general circulation. Cellular oxygenation is promoted by maintaining tissue perfusion. In acute conditions, however, supplemental oxygen may be ordered. Anemia needs to be treated per physician's order to maximize oxygen transport.

Cellular metabolic needs are reduced by alternating periods of rest and activity. The patient needs to protect affected extremities from trauma and infection, which increase metabolic needs. Extremities need to be warm without becoming overheated. To accomplish this, heating pads, time spent in hot tubs, and exercise must be used in moderation. Fear, worry, and anxiety can increase the metabolic needs of tissue. To the extent possible, the patient needs to use stress reduction strategies to prevent detrimental physical effects of these psychologic states.

To achieve awareness of learning needs, the nurse discusses with the patient and family the actions needed to maintain tissue perfusion and decrease metabolic demands. Activities of daily living may need to be changed. The need for rehabilitation also will vary depending on the site and extent of altered perfusion. Safety needs to be emphasized for the patient taking anticoagulants. This includes watching for signs of bleeding from the gums, rectum, and skin. The patient and family should be informed about the anticoagulation properties of aspirin and cautioned against using it in combination with other anticoagulants. A well-balanced diet is important to provide sufficient glucose for adenosine triphosphate formation. Family members need to discuss action required to prevent recurrence of this problem. This may include smoking cessation, dietary alterations, stress reduction strategies, and exercise programs.

■ DYSREFLEXIA

Dysreflexia (autonomic dysreflexia) is a state in which a person with a spinal cord injury at the seventh thoracic vertebra (T7) or above experiences or is at risk for a life-threatening uninhibited response of the nervous system to a noxious stimulus.

Autonomic dysreflexia was first described in 1917 and continues to be a problem in the care of patients with spinal cord injuries and those undergoing rehabilitation.

Related Factors*

Bladder distention or spasm
Catheter insertion or irrigation
Obstructed catheter
Bowel distention
Bowel stimulation
Traction of viscera during surgery
Manipulation of perineum
Sexual stimulation or intercourse
Cystometric examination or cystogram
Uterine contractions

Defining Characteristics*

Paroxysmal hypertension (sudden periodic elevated blood pressure with systolic pressure greater than 140 mm Hg and diastolic greater than 90 mm Hg)
Bradycardia or tachycardia (pulse rate less than 60 or more than 100 beats/minute)
Diaphoresis (above injury)
Patchy erythema (above injury)
Pallor (below injury)
Headache (diffuse pain in different portions of head and not confined to any nerve distribution area)

Chilling (shivering accompanied by sensation of coldness or pallor of skin)
Conjunctival congestion (excessive amount of blood or tissue fluid in conjunctiva)
Horner's syndrome (contraction of pupil, partial ptosis of eyelid, enophthalmos, and sometimes loss of sweating over affected side of face; caused by paralysis of cervical sympathetic nerve trunk)
Paresthesia (abnormal sensation, e.g., numbness, prickling, tingling; increased sensitivity)
Pilomotor reflex (gooseflesh formation when skin is cooled)
Blurred vision
Chest pain and cardiac irregularities
Metallic taste in mouth
Nasal congestion
Nausea

Expected Patient Outcomes & Nursing Interventions

Learns to prevent frequent episodes of autonomic dysreflexia

- Assist patient in learning to carry out hygiene maintenance regimens: good bowel and bladder care, prevention of pressure sores, avoiding falls, burns, or other injuries, and selection of proper shoes and clothing.

Assists with identification of symptoms and causes, if necessary

- Teach patient to identify an episode early; patient knows when to seek further assistance from health care professional and understands that many health care professionals may be unfamiliar with the syndrome.
- Instruct patient to direct care and explain interventions to staff, if necessary.
- Arrange for patient to wear Medic-Alert bracelet.

Experiences fewer and less severe episodes of dysreflexia, as evidenced by:

Blood pressure and heart rate returning to normal
Usual bowel and bladder elimination patterns being maintained
Headache subsiding
Patient participating in avoiding or minimizing bowel and bladder distention
Patient recognizing symptoms and notifying health care professional

- Develop awareness for signs and symptoms of dysreflexia and ensure that other staff and patients are aware of symptoms and precipitating factors.
- Assess patient for history of previous attacks of dysreflexia and possible causes.
- Assess and monitor bowel and bladder elimination patterns to prevent distention.
- Observe urinary catheters for kinks and obstructions; ensure patency and change catheter if unable to attain patency with irrigation.

---

*Adapted from North American Nursing Diagnosis Association, 1995.

- Check cautiously for fecal impaction, if necessary, and relieve promptly with suppository or enema. If ordered, numb anal area and 1 inch into rectum first.
- Minimize manipulation and stimulation when performing procedures involving bladder and bowel.
- Be aware that early symptoms can include sudden pounding headache, sweating, and blotching of skin of face and thorax.
- If symptoms occur, stop any procedure being performed, notify physician immediately, and prepare to assist with treatment.
- Monitor blood pressure and pulse continuously until symptoms subside.
- Administer antihypertensive or α-adrenergic blockers, as ordered.
- Elevate head of bed and lower patient's legs to counteract hypertension with orthostatic hypotension in attempt to reduce headache.
- Remove all support hose or binders to promote venous pooling and decrease venous return, decreasing blood pressure.
- Reassure patient and take measures to promote comfort.
- Instruct patient about syndrome so that awareness is developed about possible causes and early symptoms experienced.
- Arrange for patient to wear Medic-Alert bracelet.

Principles and Rationale for Nursing Interventions[2,4,5]

Autonomic dysreflexia results most frequently from distention of pelvic viscera (bladder, colon, rectum) and less frequently from manipulation of the renal pelvis and intestines during surgery, uterine contractions during labor, skin stimulation, and other proprioceptive stimuli below the level of the lesion. Sensory impulses from pelvic viscera reach the spinal cord by way of pelvic parasympathetic, hypogastric, and pudendal nerves, and cutaneous sensations enter through peripheral and dorsal nerve roots. These afferent impulses ascend along spinothalamic tracts and dorsal columns. At segmental levels these impulses may cause reflex motor response. With reflex motor outflow through neurons in the lateral horns, sensory impulses may cause vasoconstriction below the level of the spinal cord lesion (in the splanchnic vascular bed, kidney, skin, legs), with resultant elevation of the blood pressure, pilomotor spasm, and sweating.[4]

■ RISK FOR PERIPHERAL NEUROVASCULAR DYSFUNCTION

■ Risk for peripheral neurovascular dysfunction is a state in which an individual is at risk for experiencing a disruption in circulation, motion, or sensation of an extremity.[7]

Peripheral neurovascular dysfunction may occur when an individual has interrupted blood flow to an extremity, which may eventually lead to tissue ischemia, muscle damage, and nerve damage. Examples of physical conditions that can lead to peripheral neurovascular dysfunction include arterial insufficiency, venous insufficiency, and compartment syndrome. These are discussed in the following section.

An interruption in arterial blood flow prevents tissue from receiving adequate oxygen and nutrients, which results in arterial insufficiency. Neurologic changes can occur within hours after arterial occlusion occurs.[2] The incidence of peripheral arterial disease is unknown, but it is usually found in men over age 45 years and in postmenopausal women.[6] On the other hand, venous insufficiency may occur from thrombus formation secondary to stasis of blood flow, hypercoagulability, or endothelial injury. Patients at risk for thrombophlebitis include those who undergo surgical procedures, trauma, immobility, use of oral contraceptives, pregnancy, heart failure, and severe infections.[6]

Compartment syndrome is another complication that can lead to neurovascular dysfunction. It occurs as a result of limited space occupied by bone, blood vessels, nerves, muscles, and soft tissues.[8] When an injury (e.g., fracture, frostbite, burn) occurs that results in swelling, there may be no room for edema within the muscle group. Thus blood flow is interrupted, leading to ischemia, muscle damage, nerve damage, and eventually necrosis.[1] The incidence of this condition is unknown.

Risk Factors

Fractures
Mechanical compression (e.g., tourniquet, cast, brace, restraint, and dressing)
Trauma
Acute compartment syndrome
Crush syndrome
Frostbite or snakebite
Orthopedic surgery
Immobilization
Burns
Arterial occlusion
Venous occlusion

Defining Characteristics

Pain (out of proportion to the injury)
Pallor
Cool, mottled skin
Decreased pulses
Paresthesia (burning or tingling)
Numbness or lessening sensation
Paralysis
Weakness
Edema
Increased intracompartment pressure

Expected Patient Outcomes & Nursing Interventions

Neurovascular status distal to the problem/injury remains intact, as evidenced by:

Pinkish hue to skin
Absence of edema
Rapid capillary refill
Warm skin temperature
Strong peripheral pulses
Absence of pain
Normal sensation and movement of all digits

- Assess circulatory and neurologic status in the extremity distal to the problem/injury; compare bilaterally and simultaneously; *early detection of circulatory and neurologic abnormalities is necessary to prevent loss of function.*

Peripheral Vascular Assessment

Inspect skin color for pallor, cyanosis, or mottled discoloration; *skin is an excellent indicator of cardiovascular status.*

Inspect for the presence and severity of edema by observing for swelling accompanied by taut and shining skin in the extremity. *Edema is a manifestation of excess fluid in the tissues.*

If edema is present, describe if it is pitting or nonpitting by applying pressure with fingers; if it is dependent or unilateral; and the severity of the edema with the following scale.[11]

    0 = none
    +1 = trace
    +2 = moderate
    +3 = deep
    +4 = very deep

Elevate the extremity to heart level; *elevating an extremity promotes arterial flow and venous return thus reducing edema.*[5]

Perform passive or active ROM to all joints in the affected extremity; *muscle contraction increases venous return, keeps joints supple, and prevents contractures.*

- Assess capillary refill time by compressing nailbeds or surrounding tissue and by observing the return of usual color; *capillary refill time is an indicator of arterial perfusion and should occur within 1 to 2 seconds.*

- Monitor intracompartment pressures (as appropriate) at prescribed intervals; depending on the device and the compartment, pressures greater than 8 to 10 are considered elevated and may cause compromised function.[3,5,10]

- Assess the skin temperature using the back of the fingers; *skin temperature is an indictor of arterial perfusion.*

- Palpate peripheral pulses for quality; pulses are evaluated with the following scale:[2]

0 = absent
1 = diminished

2 = normal
3 = full or increased
4 = bounding

- Make an "X" with an ink pen or permanent marker over pulses that are difficult to palpate.

- Auscultate peripheral pulses with Doppler ultrasound device if pulses are difficult to evaluate; *an ultrasonic Doppler device magnifies sound over pulse points to assist in assessing peripheral pulses.*

Peripheral Neurologic Assessment

Assess for pain (character, location, intensity) at rest and with passive stretching of the muscle group.

Have patient rate pain on a scale of 0 to 10 with 0 being "no pain" and 10 being "extreme pain"; *pain on passive stretch of the muscle passing through the compartment or pain out of proportion to what is anticipated for the type of problem or injury may be an indication of compartment syndrome.*

With patient's eyes closed or head turned, assess for sensation in the extremities; *the presence of paresthesia (burning or tingling sensations), numbness, or lessened sensibility to touch may be the result of increased pressure, stretching, or lacerated nerves.*

Determine the patient's ability to move appendages distal to the problem or injury (all fingers or all toes should be assessed); *decreasing ability to perform active movements is indicative of increasing pressure, stretched, or lacerated nerves.*

Record the above assessments on a flowsheet or other appropriate documentation tool; *a flowsheet provides at a glance determination of changes in the neurovascular status.*

Patient and/or significant other will recognize and report signs and symptoms of neurovascular compromise

- Teach patient and/or significant other signs and symptoms of neurovascular compromise (as previously described); *the patient is often the first to detect subtle changes that can lead to early detection of neurovascular compromises.*

- Provide patient and/or significant other with verbal, as well as written, instructions for assessing neurovascular status; *learning is enhanced by both verbal and written instruction.*

- The physician should be notified immediately of abnormal neurovascular findings; *prompt treatment of circulatory and neurologic problems can result in a decreased disability or in an absence of permanent disability.*

Principles and Rationale for Nursing Interventions

The following expected patient outcomes are derived from collecting assessment data: pinkish hue of skin, absence of edema, rapid capillary refill, warm skin temperature, strong peripheral pulses, absence of pain, normal sensation and movement, and the ability to recognize and report signs and symptoms of neurovascular compromise.[11]

An inspection of skin color should be made distal to the problem or injury and bilaterally to compare the affected extremity with the unaffected extremity. In individuals with lighter skin, a light to dark pinkish tone is normally found. An underlying pinkish red tone is normally found in the individual with darker skin. When assessing the individual with darker skin, inspect the lighter-colored areas such as palms of the hand, soles of the feet, and nailbeds.[12] A pale or blanched coloration may indicate an insufficient arterial blood supply, whereas a dusky, blue, cyanotic, or mottled discoloration may indicate inadequate venous return.[9]

Edema often results as a physiologic response to injury or surgical procedures. As edema accumulates in the inelastic tissue of a muscle group, increased pressure is exerted on arteries, nerves, and muscle tissue. Histamine is released as the muscles become ischemic from interrupted blood supply, and it triggers dilation of the capillaries and results in more edema in the muscle compartment. Muscle damage begins within 2 to 4 hours after the blood supply is decreased.[1] Doubtful return of blood flow results following 6 to 8 hours of ischemia.[9] Nerve damage starts within 30 minutes, with irreversible nerve damage taking place within 12 hours.[1] Therefore inspecting for the presence and severity of edema is vital.

As edema is detected and assessed, the nurse intervenes by elevating the extremity above the level of the heart. This intervention promotes circulation and increases venous return to the heart. Periodically, the extremity should be lowered so that proximal joints can be placed through range of motion (ROM) exercises. Performing passive or active range of motion exercises to the affected extremity distal to the injury will also increase circulation and venous return. In addition, these exercises will keep the joints supple and prevent contractures.[5] All joints in the affected extremity should be exercised in accordance with the patient's tolerance level.

One method of assessing peripheral circulation is to apply tactile pressure to the nailbed or surrounding tissue until blanching occurs. Capillary refill time is determined by the speed with which the blood or usual color returns to tissue. A brisk return (1 to 2 seconds) is normal.[9] Prolonged capillary refill time suggests inadequate arterial blood supply. On the other hand, an immediate capillary refill may be abnormal in local venous congestion, thus suggesting inadequate venous return.[9]

Compartment syndrome develops when increased pressure within the semirigid fascia surrounding muscle groups compromise nerve, blood vessel, and muscle function.[3] Measurement of direct intracompartment pressure is used to confirm compartment syndrome. Pressure readings are also used to monitor the patient's condition.[10]

Further circulatory assessment includes determining skin temperature of the affected and unaffected extremities. The back of the fingers should be used because they are more sensitive to temperature than the palmed surface of the fingers.[6] The skin should be warm or the same temperature as the unaffected extremity. Cool, mottled skin with a decreased or absent pulse may indicate arterial insufficiency, while hot skin temperature may indicate inadequate venous return. However, temperature of the skin is the least reliable indication of vascular compromise.[9]

Peripheral pulses distal to the problem or injury should also be checked bilaterally on the affected and unaffected extremities to rule out compromise of arterial blood flow. Pulses should be equally strong bilaterally. Pulses may be present even with damaged arterial structures.[9] However, arterial occlusion or laceration will result in decreased or absent pulses.

Pressure on the nerve endings may cause extraordinary pain. This manifestation results from increased blood, chemical irritants, cellular substances, or debris. The nurse assesses for pain while the patient is at rest and on passive stretching of the muscles in the affected extremity. Pain elicited on passive muscle stretching is caused by tissue ischemia and may be a sign of compartment syndrome. Although pain is a frequent occurrence with orthopedic and other related problems or injuries, pain that is not proportional to what is anticipated or that escalates after stabilization may signal the advent of compartment syndrome. Pressure being exerted on the nerve causes pain, numbness, and finally, paralysis.[4]

Numbness, burning, tingling, weakness, or inability to move muscles indicates peripheral nerves are compressed, stretched, or lacerated.[9] Assessing sensation and movement of the affected extremity in comparison to the unaffected extremity reveals information specific to peripheral neurologic functioning. While assessing sensation, the patient's eyes should be closed or the face turned away from the examiner. Having the patient tell the nurse where he or she is being touched, rather than asking the patient if sensation is present, will provide a more accurate and meaningful assessment. Next, the patient is asked to describe the sensation to determine if burning, tingling, numbness, or lessening sensibility to touch is being experienced.

By astute neurovascular assessment, the nurse can detect early signs and symptoms of neurovascular compromise. Preexisting conditions, such as impairment from a stroke or neurologic or circulatory deficits as a result of diabetes, should be taken into account as part of a thorough, individualized assessment. For accurate comparisons, assessments are made with the affected and unaffected extremity, bilaterally and simultaneously, when possible. An alert, oriented, and cooperative patient will greatly assist in an accurate neurologic assessment. Although not as informative, responses to painful stimuli in the unresponsive patient can be observed. Nursing interventions should be implemented once abnormalities are recognized. Additionally, the physician should be notified immediately of abnormal neurovascular findings. Therefore the nurse's role in early detection and appropriate interventions in response to peripheral neurovascular dysfunction is vital in avoiding or lessening permanent disabilities.

ALTERED GROWTH AND DEVELOPMENT

Altered growth and development is a state in which an individual demonstrates deviations in norms from his or her age group.

The development process is continuous and dynamic throughout the entire life span. While genetic endowment defines the parameters of growth and development, environmental factors modulate the expression of that potential.[34] The extent to which each person realizes his or her biologic potential is determined by the interrelation of many factors. The study of altered growth and development encompasses the physical, cognitive, psychosocial, and spiritual aspects of a person. Causative factors of altered growth and development fall into four broad categories: heredity, including genetic and metabolic abnormalities; problems that occur during pregnancy or in the perinatal period; acquired diseases; and environmental and behavioral problems.[4,7,8,14] The dysfunction that causes altered growth and development can occur before a child's birth, during delivery, or after birth. For instance, an infant who is normal at birth can later develop a dysfunction as a result of maladaptive family relationships or other harmful environmental conditions. Developmental disabilities, defined by the Rehabilitation, Comprehensive Services and Developmental Disabilities Amendments of 1978 (P.L. 95-602), are frequently the focus of this nursing diagnosis. These are severe, lifelong, disabling conditions that interfere with a person's ability to function in society and complete his developmental tasks. These conditions are acquired prior to a person's 22nd birthday and are the result of a mental and/or physical impairment. The nursing diagnosis of Altered Growth and Development can be identified in patients who have a broad spectrum of medical diagnoses and conditions. This nursing diagnosis describes a deviation from accepted norms in both quality and quantity of maturational changes.

Related Factors*

Problems Occurring During Pregnancy and Perinatal Period

Maternal chronic or acute disease during prenatal period
Inadequate prenatal care
Maternal age
Exposure to teratogens
Fetal distress
Prolonged or precipitous labor
Interruption of oxygen intrapartally
Prematurity
Low birthweight
Asphyxia in neonatal period
Low Apgar score

*References 3, 4, 7, 14, 25, 34.

Birth injury
Significant blood loss
Suboptimal infant-parent attachment
Difficult infant temperature
Trauma: physical, chemical, infection, radiation, immunologic, psychologic, or emotional
Malnutrition: maternal

Heredity

Congenital defect(s)
Genetic abnormality
Familial history: mental retardation, genetic disorders

Acquired Disease

Kernicterus
Metabolic disorder
Neonatal disease
Neonatal infection
Chronic illness
Malnutrition: infant
Trauma, injury
Infectious disease

Environmental and Behavioral Problems

Inadequate caretaking
Substance abuse
Poor support system
Disadvantaged social environment: poverty, homelessness
Separation from significant others
Lack of stimulation in the environment
Overstimulation from the environment

Defining Characteristics[4,19]

Impaired physical growth
Cognitive development inappropriate for age
Impaired sensory function
Delayed, altered, or compromised development of motor skills
Abnormal movement patterns
Abnormal neurologic function
Abnormal muscle tone
Decreased coordination
Decreased balance
Unable to perform appropriately in activities of daily living
Deficient in modulating behavior
Delayed, altered, or compromised development of receptive and/or expressive communication skills
Deficient in following instructions
Delayed, altered, or compromised development of social skills
Impaired ability to interact with others
Limitation in ability for self-direction
Limited capacity for independent living
Limited capacity for economic self-sufficiency

Expected Patient Outcomes and Nursing Interventions

Patient will have growth and development monitored regularly, as evidenced by:

Detection of developmental delays and initiation of the interventions aimed at maximizing potential for development and minimizing secondary problems

- Assess anthropometrics (weight, length or height, and head circumference if less than 2 years of age).
- Engage in "development surveillance:" continuous, skillful observation of children during any child health encounter, soliciting input from parents, teachers, and others who have contact with the child; utilize screening tools to confirm suspicions of delay.[8,11]
- Refer for further testing and treatment. Gross and fine motor, cognitive, language, and social development, as well as health, physical growth, family dynamics, and environmental factors are assessed in a comprehensive developmental evaluation.

Family will demonstrate increased knowledge, confidence, and competence as caregivers, as evidenced by:

Successful incorporation of all therapy and treatments into the daily routine of the family

Setting realistic goals which are based on the child's strengths and abilities as well as the family's needs and aspirations[10]

Decreasing dependence on professional caregivers[2,10]

- Evaluate family's knowledge about condition and its management; family must be confident and competent in use of necessary equipment, in administration of medications, and in performing medical procedures.
- Demonstrate care.
- Clarify terminology and share information on a continuous basis, in a supportive and unbiased fashion.[1,28]

Patient will have access to and use all necessary health services, as evidenced by:

The maintenance of optimal health and the absence of secondary disabilities

- Promote safety and maintenance of health and wellness.
- Teach developmentally appropriate injury prevention.
- Assist family in accessing primary physicians and dentists who are familiar with the special health care needs of individuals with altered growth and development throughout the life span. These patients may be more vulnerable to nutritional deficits, obesity, dehydration, constipation, skin breakdown, and upper respiratory tract infection. Other special health concerns may exist related to specific disabilities (i.e., thyroid and cardiac disease are often present in patients with Down Syndrome).[21]

Patient and family will demonstrate successful management of difficulties relating to activities of daily living, as evidenced by:

The patient eventually attaining the highest possible degree of independence in self-care

- Assist family in dealing with difficulties in behavior, feeding, sleeping, bathing, dressing, and toileting; family dynamics, family coping strategies, family's group and individual goals, and practical limitations of the situation will need to be considered in problem solving.[27,35]

Patient will engage in comprehensive, developmentally appropriate education and habilitative interventions, as evidenced by:

Physical, occupational, and speech therapy as warranted

Use of prescribed adaptive equipment, prosthetic or orthotic devices

- Work collaboratively with family and interdisciplinary team to identify and meet health, psychologic, social, educational, and emotional needs; identify community resources.
- Assist family in gaining access to needed professional services, equipment, and financial resources.[35]

Family will achieve a positive adaptation as evidenced by[1,17-19,24,29]

Integration of individual with altered growth and development into the family

Successfully meeting the needs of all family members

Decreased anxiety and increased confidence

Increased ability to discuss fears and concerns and to deal constructively with emotions

Demonstrating resilience, or the ability to rebound successfully from a stressful event[9,18,22]

Utilization of cognitive and behavioral strategies to resolve or adapt to stressful situations

- Support family through crisis of diagnosis and later critical periods; offer anticipatory guidance.
- Establish a caring, trusting relationship with the patient and family, demonstrate professional competence and commitment to the patient's care.[23]
- Encourage expression of feelings and fears, validate as normal emotional reaction to illness, recognizing problematic reaction and referring to appropriate professional; remain accepting and non-judgmental.[16]
- Advocate for the rights and needs of family; help family develop advocacy skills.
- Support positive family relationships, encourage cohesiveness.
- Recognize family's strengths and skills.
- Encourage awareness of siblings' needs; determine meaning of illness to sibling(s), offer support group, encourage communication within the family including verbalization of fears, questions, concerns by sibling(s).[12]

- Celebrate family's accomplishments and successes in caring for their child.[5]
- Encourage maintenance of a hopeful outlook.[24]

To the extent determined by the his/her abilities, patient will achieve positive adaptation to disability, as evidenced by:[15,31]

Achievement of therapeutic goals
Behavior indicating positive self-concept
Increased understanding of disability and treatment
Involvement in management of own care

- Reinforce positive behaviors and adaptation to illness, recognizing adaptation is not static and continues throughout development.
- Encourage communication of questions and concerns, share information about disability and its impact.
- Encourage normalization of activities.
- Educate on health-related issues such as nutrition, exercise, physiologic functions, and sexuality to help the patient maintain optimal health and to facilitate early recognition of health problems.[27]

The family will successfully adapt to the changing needs of the individual with altered growth and development throughout his/her life span, as evidenced by:[21,31]

Family's ability to anticipate and cope with transition periods

- Provide anticipatory guidance in recognizing changing needs as patient ages.
- Assist family in dealing with transition issues such as: entering school; physical changes; adolescent sexuality and need for independence; increased involvement with peergroup and changing relationships with peers; completion of school and need for alternative support systems; prevocational and vocational training; learning skills for independent living; movement out of family home; employment; guardianship; geriatric care.
- Prepare parents for the possibility of revisiting feelings of disappointment and grief as they experience life cycle transitions and again mourn for the loss of their "ideal" child.[6]

Principles and Rationale for Nursing Interventions

There are three major areas of nursing intervention for patients with altered growth and development: (1) those involving education or nursing functions related to the ongoing health needs of the patient; (2) those involving coordination of services with other professionals; and (3) those relating to the provision of family support. Nursing interventions may fall anywhere on a continuum from assisting parents to become skilled observers of their children's development to managing and coordinating a complex network of services.[5,11,20] All interventions should be family-centered, recognizing the family's ultimate responsibility for making decisions about care, and supporting the family's

role as the primary and constant caregiver, educator, and advocate.[1,5,28] The privacy and confidentiality of the family must always be respected.[10] It is important to be aware of the unique significance to the family of racial, cultural, ethnic, spiritual, and socio-economic variables, respecting the diversity of families and not making assumptions about how a family will behave based on stereotypes.[17,28] Working in partnership with the family and acknowledging their expertise, the nurse acts as a consultant to the family in assessing needs, setting goals and priorities, planning care, identifying and mobilizing resources, and evaluating outcomes. The nurse encourages the building, maintenance, and utilization of the family's personal social support network and refers to and encourages the use of family-to-family support as these have been found to enhance a family's ability to cope.[10,26,28] Assisting the family in obtaining respite and day care services may also help to decrease the impact of caring for a child with special needs.[13,35] According to Ray and Ritchie, the extent to which caregiving is burdensome is related to the caregiving and management tasks that the family must perform as well as the restrictions on family activities created by the caregiving needs. They found that as the degree of burden increased, the situation became more stressful.[24] Clearly, one of the goals of any intervention should be to help alleviate the burden associated with caregiving.

Nursing interventions may take place at any stage in the family's process of adapting to the disability. Each family has a unique way of adapting to the stress of a long-term disability. Although some families adapt poorly and become dysfunctional, others function at a high level and make a positive adjustment.[9,13,22,32,33] Assisting the family as they adapt to the emotional challenges and lifestyle changes brought about by a disability is an important aspect of the nursing role in the diagnosis Altered Growth and Development. The nurse has the ongoing responsibility to assist all family members in understanding and coping with the unique and changing needs at various stages of development of the individual with Altered Growth and Development.[17] By helping families to identify and utilize their existing strengths, and gain the knowledge and skills that are necessary to meet the needs of their child, the nurse enhances the family's ability to manage the demands that impinge upon them, thus empowering the family and strengthening family functioning.[10]

References

Activity intolerance; Risk for activity intolerance

1. American Association of Critical-Care Nurses: *Outcome standards for nursing care of the critically ill,* Laguna Niguel, CA, 1990, The Association.
2. Campbell C: *Nursing diagnosis and intervention in nursing practice,* New York, 1978, Wiley.
3. Carrieri VK, Lindsey AM, West CM, editors: *Pathophysiological phenomena in nursing: human responses to illness,* Philadelphia, 1986, Saunders.
4. Chyun D, Ford CF, Yursha-Johnston M: Silent myocardial ischemia, *Focus Crit Care* 18(4):295, 1991.
5. Creason NS: Operational and conceptual definition tool development in nursing diagnosis validation research. In Carroll-Johnson RM, Paquette M, editors: *Classification of nursing diagnosis: proceedings of the tenth conference,* Philadelphia, 1994, Lippincott.

6. Fukuda N: Outcome standards for the client with chronic congestive heart failure, *J Cardiovasc Nurs* 4(3):59, 1990.
7. Glick OJ, Swanson EA: Motor performance correlates of functional dependence in long-term care residents, *Nurs Res* 44(1):4, 1995.
8. Gordon M: High-risk nursing diagnosis in critical care. In Carroll-Johnson RM, Paquette M, editors: *Classification of nursing diagnoses: proceedings of the tenth conference,* Philadelphia, 1994, Lippincott.
9. Gordon M: *Nursing diagnosis: process and application,* St Louis, 1994, Mosby.
10. Gordon M: Report of an RNF study to determine which nursing diagnoses have high frequency and high treatment priority in rehabilitation nursing, part I, *Rehabil Nurs Res* 4(1):3-10, 1995.
11. Gordon M: Report of an RNF study to determine which nursing diagnoses have high frequency and high treatment priority in rehabilitation nursing, part II, *Rehabil Nurs Res* 4(2):38, 1995.
12. Greenlee KK: The effects of implementation of an operational definition and guidelines for the formulation of nursing diagnoses in a critical care setting. In Carroll-Johnson RM, editor: *Classification of nursing diagnoses: proceedings of the ninth conference,* Philadelphia, 1991, Lippincott.
13. Henning M: Comparison of nursing diagnostic statements using a functional health pattern and a health history/body systems format. In Carroll-Johnson RM, editor: *Classification of nursing diagnoses: proceedings of the ninth conference,* Philadelphia, 1991, Lippincott.
14. Hwu, Y-J: The impact of chronic illness on patients, *Rehabil Nurs* 20(4):221, 1995.
15. Matheny ML, Wolff LM: Critical dimensions of chronic care, *J Cardiovasc Nurs* 4(3):71, 1990.
16. McCloskey JC, Bulechek GM: *Nursing interventions classification (NIC),* ed 2, St Louis, 1996, Mosby.
17. McFarlane EA: Activity intolerance. In McFarland GK, McFarlane EA: *Nursing diagnosis and intervention: planning for patient care,* ed 2, St Louis, 1993, Mosby.
18. McFarlane EA: Potential activity intolerance. In McFarland GK, McFarlane EA: *Nursing diagnosis and intervention: planning for patient care,* ed 2, St Louis, 1993, Mosby.
19. Neuberger GB et al: Determinants of exercise and aerobic fitness in outpatients with arthritis, *Nurs Res* 43(1):11, 1994.
20. North American Nursing Diagnosis Association: *Nursing diagnoses: definitions and classification, 1995-1996,* Philadelphia, 1994, NANDA.
21. Randell BP: Signs and symptoms, etiologies, diagnostic labels: what do we mean and where do we want to go? In Carroll-Johnson RM, editor: *Classification of nursing diagnoses: proceedings of the ninth conference,* Philadelphia, 1991, Lippincott.
22. Tack BB, Gilliss CL: Nurse-monitored cardiac recovery: a description of the first 8 weeks, *Heart Lung* 19(5): 491, 1990.
23. Yura H, Walsh MB: *The nursing process: assessing, planning, implementing, evaluating,* ed 5, Norwalk, Conn, 1988, Appleton & Lange.

Fatigue

1. Aistars J: Fatigue in the cancer patient: a conceptual approach to a clinical problem, *Oncol Nurs Forum* 14(6):25, 1987.
2. Belza BL et al: Correlates of fatigue in older adults with rheumatoid arthritis, *Nurs Res* 42:93, 1993.
3. Blesch KA et al: Correlates of fatigue in people with breast or lung cancer, *Oncol Nurs Forum* 18(1):81, 1991.
4. Douris PC: The effect of isokinetic exercise on the relationship between blood lactate and muscle fatigue, *J Orthop Sports Phys Ther* 17(1):31, 1993.
5. Gift AG, Pugh LC: Dyspnea and fatigue, *Adv Clin Nurs Res* 28:373, 1993.
6. Green D et al: A comparison of patient-reported side effects among three chemotherapy regimens for breast cancer, *Cancer Prac* 2(1):57, 1994.
7. Grindel CG: Fatigue and nutrition, *Med Surg Nurs* 3(6):475, 1994.
8. Held JL: Managing fatigue, *Nursing* 24(2):26, 1994.
9. Holder-Powell HM, Jones DA: Fatigue and muscular activity: a review, *Physiotherapy* 76(11):672, 1990.
10. Irvine DM, Vincent L, Bubela N, Thompson L, Graydon J: A critical appraisal of the research literature investigating fatigue in the individual with cancer, *Cancer Nurs* 14(4):188, 1991.
11. Irvine DM et al: The prevalence and correlates of fatigue in patients receiving treatment with chemotherapy and radiotherapy: a comparison with the fatigue experienced by healthy individuals, *Cancer Nurs* 17(5):367, 1994.
12. Kim MJ, McFarland GK, McLane, AM: *Pocket guide to nursing diagnoses,* ed 6, St Louis, 1995, Mosby.
13. Lee KA et al: Fatigue as a response to environmental demands in women's lives, *Image: J Nurs Scholarship* 26(2):149, 1994.
14. Lee KA, DeJoseph JF: Sleep disturbances, vitality, and fatigue among a select group of employed childbearing women, *Birth: Iss Perinatal Care Educ* 19(4):208, 1992.
15. MacVicar MG, Winningham ML, Nickel JL: Effects of aerobic interval training on cancer patients' functional capacity, *Nurs Res* 38:346, 1989.
16. Mock V et al: A nursing rehabilitation program for women with breast cancer receiving adjuvant chemotherapy, *Oncol Nurs Forum,* 21(5):899, 1994.
17. Morris ML: Tiredness and fatigue. In Norris CM, editor: *Concept clarification in nursing,* Rockville MD, 1982, Aspen.
18. Piper BF, Lindsey AM, Dodd MJ: Fatigue mechanisms in cancer patients: developing nursing theory, *Oncol Nurs Forum* 14(6):17, 1987.
19. Piper BF: Fatigue. In: Carrieri-Kohlman V, Lindsey AM, West CM: *Pathophysiological phenomena in nursing: human responses to illness,* p 279, ed 2, Philadelphia, 1993, Saunders.
20. Piper BF et al: The development of an instrument to measure the subjective dimension of fatigue. In Funk SG et al, editors: *Key aspects of comfort—management of pain, fatigue, and nausea,* p 199, New York, 1989.
21. Potempa KM: Chronic fatigue, *Ann Rev Nurs Res* 11:57, 1993.
22. Puffer JC, McShane JM: Depression and chronic fatigue in athletes, *Clin Sports Med* 11(2):327, 1992.
23. Pugh LC, Milligan R: A framework for the study of childbearing fatigue, *Adv Nurs Sci* 15(4):60, 1993.
24. Rhoten D: Fatigue and the postsurgical patient, In Norris CM, editor: *Concept clarification in nursing,* Rockville MD, 1982, Aspen.
25. Voith AM, Frank AM, Pegg JS: Nursing diagnosis: fatigue. In Carroll-Johnson RM, editor: *Classification of nursing diagnoses: proceedings of the eighth conference,* Philadelphia, 1988, Lippincott.
26. Winningham ML et al: Fatigue and the cancer experience: the state of the knowledge, *Oncol Nurs Forum* 21:23, 1994.

Impaired physical mobility

1. Craven RF, Hirnle CJ: Body mechanics and mobility. In Craven RF, Hirnle CJ, editors: *Fundamentals of nursing: human health and function,* Philadelphia, 1992, Lippincott.
2. Creason NS: Toward a model of clinical validation of nursing diagnoses: developing conceptual and operational definitions of impaired physical mobility. In Carroll-Johnson RM, editor: *Classification of nursing diagnoses: proceedings of the Ninth Conference,* Philadelphia, 1991, Lippincott.
3. Edlund BJ: Activity-sleep assessment. In Bellack JP, Edlund BJ, editors: *Nursing diagnosis and assessment,* ed 2, Boston, 1992, Jones & Bartlett.
4. Gordon M: Report of an RNF study to determine which nursing diagnoses have high frequency and high treatment priority in rehabilitation nursing, Part 1, *Rehabil Nurs Res* 4(1):3, 1995.
5. Johnson PA, Stone MA, Larson AM, Hromek CA: Applying nursing diagnosis and nursing process to activities of daily living and mobility, *Geriatric Nurs* 13(1):25, 1992.
6. Loeper JM: Positioning. In Bulechek GM, McCloskey JC, editors: *Nursing interventions: essential nursing treatments,* ed 2, Philadelphia, 1992, Saunders.
7. Mehmert PA, Delaney CW: Validating impaired physical mobility, *Nurs Diagn* 2(4):143, 1991.
8. Mobily PR, Kelley LS: Iatrogenesis in the elderly: factors of immobility, *J Gerontol Nurs* 17(9):5, 1991.
9. North American Nursing Diagnosis Association: *NANDA nursing diagnoses: definitions and classification, 1995-1996,* Philadelphia, 1994, The Association.
10. Ouellet LL, Rush KL: A synthesis of selected literature on mobility: a basis for studying impaired mobility, *Nurs Diagn* 3(2):72, 1992.
11. Pierce L et al: Frequently selected nursing diagnoses for the rehabilitation client with stroke, *Rehabil Nurs* 20(3):138, 1995.
12. Potter PA, Perry AG: Mobility and immobility. In Potter PA, Perry AG, editors: *Fundamentals of nursing: concepts, process, and practice,* ed 3, St Louis, 1993, Mosby.

13. Rantz M, Vinz-Miller T, Matson S: Nursing diagnoses in long-term care: a longitudinal perspective for strategic planning, *Nurs Diagn* 6(2):57, 1995.
14. Sawin KJ, Heard L: Nursing diagnoses used most frequently in rehabilitation nursing practice, *Rehabil Nurs* 17(5):256, 1992.
15. Taylor C, Lillis C, LeMone P: Activity. In Taylor C, Lillis C, LeMone P, editors: *Fundamentals of nursing: the art and science of nursing care,* ed 2, Philadelphia, 1993, Lippincott.

Risk for disuse syndrome

1. Blocker WP Jr: Maintaining functional independence by mobilizing the aged, *Geriatrics* 47(1):42, 1992.
2. Braden BJ, Bryant R: Innovations to prevent and treat pressure sores, *Geriatric Nurs* 11:182, 1990.
3. Buschbacher, RM: Deconditioning, conditioning, and the benefits of exercise. In Braddom RL, editor: *Physical Medicine & Rehabilitation,* Philadelphia, 1996, Saunders.
4. Corcoran PJ: Use it or lose it—the hazards of bed rest and inactivity, *West J Med* 154(5):536, 1991.
5. Dittmer DK, Teasell R: Complications of immobilization and bed rest. Part I: Musculoskeletal and cardiovascular complications, *Can Fam Physician* 39:1428, 1993.
6. Esposito MC, Tracey C, McCourt A: Nursing diagnosis: potential for disuse syndrome. In Carroll-Johnson RM, editor: *Classification of nursing diagnoses: proceedings of the eighth conference,* Philadelphia, 1988, Lippincott.
7. Guyton AC, Hall JE: *Textbook of medical physiology,* ed 9, Philadelphia , 1994, Saunders.
8. Kosiak M: Prevention and rehabilitation of pressure ulcers, *Decubitus* 4(2):60, 1991.
9. McFarland GK, McLane FA; *Nursing diagnosis and intervention: planning for patient care,* ed 2, St Louis, 1993, Mosby.
10. Miller, CA; *Nursing care of older adults: theory and practice,* ed 2, Philadelphia, 1995, Lippincott.
11. Mobily PR, Kelley LS: Iatrogenesis in the elderly: factors of immobility, *J Gerontol Nurs* 17(9):5, 1991.
12. Olson E et al: The hazards of immobility, *Am J Nurs* 67:780, 1967.
13. Schilke JM: Slowing the aging process with physical activity, *J Gerontol Nurs* 17(6):4, 1991.
14. Shekleton ME: Impaired physical mobility. In Shekleton M, Litwack K, editors: *Critical care nursing of the surgical patient,* Philadelphia, 1991, Saunders.
15. Staas WE Jr, Cioschi HM: Pressure sores: a multifaceted approach to prevention and treatment. In *Rehabilitation medicine: adding life to years* [Special Issue], *West J Med* 154:539, 1991.
16. Teasell R, Dittmer DK: Complications of immobilization and bed rest. Part 2: Other complications, *Can Fam Physician* 39:1440, 1993.

Self-care deficit

1. Boondas J: Nursing home resident assessment classification and focused care, *Nurs Health Care* 12:308, 1991.
2. Carpenito LJ: *Handbook of nursing diagnosis,* ed 6, Philadelphia , 1995, Lippincott.
3. Chang BL: Validity of concepts for selected nursing diagnoses, *Clin Nurs Res* 3:183, 1995.
4. Daley JM, Maas M, Buckwalter K: Use of standardized nursing diagnoses and interventions in long-term care, *J Gerontol Nurs* 21(8):29, 1995.
5. Dougherty CM, Jankin JK, Lunney MR, Whitley GG: Conceptual and research-based validation of nursing diagnoses: 1950-1993, *Nurs Diagn* 4:156, 1993.
6. Finch M, Kane RL, Philp I: Developing a new metric for ADLs, *J Geriatrics Soc* 43:877, 1995.
7. McFarland GK, McFarlane, EA: *Nursing diagnosis & intervention: planning for patient care,* St Louis, 1993, Mosby.
8. Miller JM: *Coping with chronic illness: overcoming powerlessness,* Philadelphia, 1992, Davis
9. North American Nursing Diagnosis Association: *Nursing diagnoses: Definitions and classification 1997-1998,* Philadelphia, 1996, NANDA.
10. Sparks SM, Taylor CM: *Nursing diagnosis reference manual,* Springhouse PA, 1995, Springhouse.

Diversional activity deficit

1. Aller LJ, Van Ess Coeling H: Quality of life: Its meaning to the long-term care resident, *J Gerontol Nurs* 21(2):20, 1995.
2. Beach DL: Gerontological caregiving analysis of family experience, *J Gerontol Nurs* 19(12):35, 1993.
3. Boykin A, Winland-Brown J: The dark side of caring challenges of caregiving, *J Gerontol Nurs* 21(5):13, 1995.
4. Burbank PM: An exploratory study: assessing the meaning in life among older adult clients, *J Gerontol Nurs* 18(9):19, 1992.
5. Daley OE: Women's strategies for living in a nursing home, *J Gerontol Nurs* 19(9):5, 1993.
6. Hartweg DL: Self-care actions of healthy middle-aged women to promote well-being, *Nurs Res* 42(4):221, 1993.
7. Jongbloed L, Morgan D: An investigation of involvement in leisure activities after a stroke, *Am J Occup Ther* 45(5):420, 1991.
8. Kim MJ, McFarland GK, McLane AM: *Pocket Guide to Nursing Diagnoses,* ed 6, St Louis, 1995, Mosby.
9. Krach P, Brooks JA: Identifying the responsibilities and needs of working adults who are primary caregivers, *J Gerontol Nurs* 21(10):41, 1995.
10. Krefting L, Krefting D: Leisure activities after a stroke: an ethnographic approach, *Am J Occup Ther* 45(5):439, 1991.
11. Laferriere RH, Hamel-Bissell BP: Successful aging of oldest old women in the northeast kingdom of Vermont, *Image* 26(4):319, 1994.
12. Porter EJ: Older widows' experience of living alone at home, *Image* 26(1):19, 1994.
13. Ragsdale D, Kotarba JA, Morrow JR: Quality of life of hospitalized persons with AIDS, *Image* 24(4)259, 1992.
14. Rantz M: Diversional activity deficit. In Maas M, Buckwalter KC, Hardy M, editors; *Nursing diagnoses and interventions for the elderly,* p 299, Redwood City, CA, 1991, Addison-Wesley Nursing.
15. Rodgers BL: Loneliness: easing the pain of the hospitalized elderly, *J Gerontol Nurs* 15(8):16, 1989.
16. Ros M: Time-use in later life, *J Adv Nurs* 15(2):394, 1990.
17. Rubenfeld MG; Diversional activity deficit. In McFarland GK, McFarlane EA: *Nursing diagnosis and intervention: planning for patient care,* ed 2, St Louis, 1993, Mosby.
18. Sayles-Cross S: Perceptions of familial caregivers of elder adults, *Image* 25(2):88, 1993.
19. Vogel CH, Mercier J: The effect of institutionalization on nursing home populations, *J Gerontol Nurs* 17(3):30, 1991.
20. Zoerink DA: Attitudes toward leisure: persons with congenital orthopedic disabilities versus able-bodied persons, *J Rehabil* 54(2):60, 1988.

Impaired home maintenance management

1. American Nurses Association: *A conceptual model of community health nursing,* Washington, DC, 1986, ANA.
2. Bower K: *Case management by nurses.* Washington DC, 1992, American Nurses Publishing.
3. Carpenito, L: *Nursing diagnosis: application to clinical practice,* ed 6, Philadelphia, 1995, JB Lippincott.
4. Clemen-Stone S, Eigsti D, McGuire S: *Comprehensive community health nursing: family, aggregate and community practice,* ed 4, St Louis, 1995, Mosby.
5. Gordon M: *Nursing diagnosis,* ed 3, St Louis, 1991, Mosby.
6. Greif J, Golden B: *AIDS care at home: a guide for caregivers, loved ones and people with AIDS,* New York, 1994, Wiley.
7. Jaffe M, Skidmore-Roth, L: *Home health nursing care plans,* St Louis, 1993, Mosby.
8. Kim M, McFarland GK, McLane A: *Pocket guide to nursing diagnoses,* ed 6, St Louis, 1995, Mosby.
9. Laferriere RH: Orem's theory in practice: hospice nursing care. *Home Healthcare Nurse* 13(5):50, 1995.
10. Lentz J, Meyer, E: The dirty house, *Nurse Outlook* 27(9):590, 1979.
11. Marrelli TM, Hillard LS: *Home care and clinical paths: Effective care planning across the continuum,* St Louis, 1996, Mosby.
12. Rankin SH, Stallings KDP: *Patient education: issues, education, practice,* Philadelphia, 1995, Lippincott.
13. Smith CM, Maurer F: *Community health nursing: Theory and practice,* Philadelphia, 1995, Saunders.
14. Stanhope M, Knollmueller R: Handbook of community and home health nursing: tools for assessment, intervention and education, *ed 2,* St Louis, 1996, Mosby.

Dysfunctional ventilatory weaning response

1. Acosta F; Biofeedback and progressive relaxation in weaning the anxious patient from the ventilator: a brief report, *Heart Lung* 17(3):299, 1988.

2. Bridges EJ: Transition from ventilatory support; knowing when the patient is ready to wean, *Crit Care Nurs Q* 15(1):14, 1992.

3. Burns SM: Preventing diaphragm fatigue in the ventilated patient, *Dimensions Crit Care Nurs* 10(1):13, 1991.

4. Burns SM et al: Weaning from long-term mechanical ventilation. (Review), *Am J Crit Care* 4(1):4, 1995.

5. Connolly MA, Shekleton ME: Communicating with ventilator dependent patients, *Dimensions Crit Care Nurs* 10(2):115, 1991.

6. Dougherty CM: Surveillance. In Bulechek GM, McCloskey JC: *Nursing interventions: essential nursing treatments,* ed 2, Philadelphia, 1992, Saunders.

7. Gracey DR et al: Outcomes of patients admitted to a chronic ventilator-dependent unit in an acute care hospital, *Mayo Clin Proc* 67:131, 1992.

8. Gries ML, Fernsler J: Patient perceptions of the mechanical ventilation experience, *Focus Crit Care* 15(2):52, 1988.

9. Grossbach-Landis I: Successful weaning of ventilator-dependent patients, *Top Clin Nurs* 2(3):45, 1980.

10. Henneman EA; The art and science of weaning from mechanical ventilation, *Focus Crit Care* 18(6):490, 1991.

11. Holliday JE, Hyers TM: The reduction of weaning time from mechanical ventilation using tidal volume and relaxation biofeedback, *Am Rev Resp Dis* 141:1214, 1990.

12. Jackson NC: Pulmonary rehabilitation for mechanically ventilated patients, *Crit Care Clin North Am* 3(4):591, 1991.

13. Jenny J, Logan J: Analyzing expert nursing practice to develop a new nursing diagnosis dysfunctional ventilatory weaning response. In Carroll-Johnson RM, ed: *Classification of nursing diagnoses, proceedings of the ninth conference,* Philadelphia, 1990, Lippincott.

14. Knebel AR: Weaning from mechanical ventilation: current controversies, *Heart Lung* 20(4):321, 1991.

15. Knebel AR: When weaning from mechanical ventilation fails, *Am J Crit Care* 1(3):19, 1992.

16. Knebel AR et al: Weaning from mechanical ventilation: Concept development, *Am J Crit Care* 3(6):416, 1994.

17. Knipper JS, Alpen MA: Ventilatory support. In Bulecheck GM, McCloskey JC: *Nursing interventions: essential nursing treatments,* ed 2, Philadelphia, 1991, Saunders.

18. Logan J, Jenny J: Deriving a new nursing diagnosis through qualitative research: dysfunctional ventilatory weaning response: *Nurs Diagn* 1(1):37, 1990.

19. Logan J, Jenny J: Interventions for the nursing diagnosis dysfunctional ventilatory weaning response: a qualitative study. In Carroll-Johnson RM, ed: *Classification of nursing diagnoses, proceedings of the ninth conference,* Philadelphia, 1990, Lippincott.

20. McFarland GK, Wasli EL, Gerety EK: *Nursing diagnoses and process in psychiatric mental health nursing,* ed 2, Philadelphia, 1992, Lippincott.

21. Morganroth ML et al: Criteria for weaning from prolonged mechanical ventilation, *Arch Intern Med* 144:1012, 1984.

22. North American Nursing Diagnosis Association: *Nursing Diagnoses: Definitions and Classification 1995-1996,* Philadelphia, 1994, NANDA.

23. Radwin LE: Conceptualizations of decision making in nursing: Analytic models and "knowing the patient," *Nurs Diagn* 6(1):16, 1995.

24. Riggio RE et al: Psychological issues in the care of critically-ill respirator patients: differential perceptions of patients, relatives, and staff, *Psychol Rep* 51:363, 1982.

25. Shapiro BA, Peruzzi WT: Changing practices in ventilator management: A review of the literature and suggested clinical correlations, *Surgery* 117(2):121, 1995.

26. Spector N: Nutritional support of the ventilator dependent patient, *Nurs Clin North Am* 24(2): 407, 1989.

27. Thompson KS et al: Building a critical path for ventilator dependency, *Am J Nurs* 91(7):28, 1991.

28. Urden LD, Davie JK, Thelan LA: Pulmonary therapeutic management. In *Essentials of Critical Care Nursing,* St Louis, 1992, Mosby.

Inability to sustain spontaneous ventilation

1. Aldrich TK et al: Weaning from mechanical ventilation: adjunctive use of inspiratory muscle resistive training, *Crit Care Med* 17(2):143, 1989.

2. Benotti PN, Bistrian B: Metabolic and nutritional aspects of weaning from mechanical ventilation, *Crit Care Med* 17(2):181, 1989.

3. Bersten AD et al: Additional work of breathing imposed by endotracheal tubes, breathing circuits, and intensive care ventilators, *Crit Care Med* 17(7):671, 1989.

4. Burns SM: Preventing diaphragm fatigue in the ventilated patient, *Dimensions Crit Care Nurs* 10(1):13, 1991.

5. Cohen CA et al: Clinical manifestations of inspiratory muscle fatigue, *Am J Med* 73:308, 1982.

6. Grossbach-Landis I: Successful weaning of ventilator-dependent patients, *Top Clin Nurs* 2(3):45, 1980.

7. Hanneman SKG et al: Weaning from short term mechanical ventilation: a review, *Am J Crit Care* 3(6):421, 1994.

8. Henneman EA: The art and science of weaning from mechanical ventilation, *Focus Crit Care* 18(6):490, 1991.

9. Henneman EA, Lee JL, Cohen JI: Collaboration a concept analysis, *J Advanced Nurs* 21:103, 1995.

10. Kigin CM: Breathing exercises for the medical patient: the art and the science, *Phys Ther* 70(11):700, 1990.

11. Knebel A, Strider VC, Wood, C: The art and science of caring for ventilator-assisted patients, *Crit Care Nurs Clin North Am* 6(4):819, 1994.

12. Knebel AR: Weaning from mechanical ventilation: current controversies, *Heart Lung* 20(4):321, 1991.

13. Knipper JS, Alpen MA: Ventilatory support. In Bulechek GM, McCloskey JC: *Nursing interventions: essential nursing treatments,* ed 2, Philadelphia, 1992, Saunders.

14. Lookinland S, Appel PL: Hemodynamic and oxygen transport changes following endotracheal suctioning in trauma patients, *Nurs Res* 40(3):133, 1991.

15. McFarland GK, Wasli EL, Gerety EK: *Nursing diagnoses and process in psychiatric mental health nursing,* ed 2, Philadelphia, 1992, Lippincott.

16. Montenegro HD: Complications of mechanical ventilation, *Resp Ther* 14(5):20, 1984.

17. Nelson DM: Interventions related to respiratory care, *Nurs Clin North Am* 27(2):301, 1992.

18. North American Nursing Diagnosis Association: *Nursing Diagnoses: Definitions and Classification 1995-1996,* Philadelphia, 1994, NANDA.

19. Shapiro BA, Peruzzi WT: Changing practices in ventilator management: a review of the literature and suggested clinical correlations, *Surgery* 117(2):121, 1995.

20. Spector N: Nutritional support of the ventilator dependent patient, *Nurs Clin North Am* 24(2):407, 1989.

21. Tobin MJ: What should the clinician do when a patient fights the ventilator? *Resp Care* 36(5):395, 1991.

22. Urden LD, Davie JK, Thelan LA: Pulmonary therapeutic management. In *Essentials of Critical Care Nursing,* St Louis, 1992, Mosby.

23. Weilitz PB: New modes of mechanical ventilation, *Crit Care Nurs Clin North Am* 1(4):689, 1989.

Ineffective airway clearance; Ineffective breathing pattern; Impaired gas exchange; Decreased cardiac output; Altered tissue perfusion

1. Ackley BJ, Ladwig GB: *Nursing diagnosis handbook: a guide to planning care,* ed 2, St Louis, 1995, Mosby.

2. Ahrens T: Changing perspectives in the assessment of oxygenation, *Crit Care Nurs* 13:78, 1993.

3. American Thoracic Society: Standards of nursing care for adult patients with pulmonary dysfunction, *Am Rev Respir Dis* 143:231, 1991.

4. Carroll P: Safe suctioning prn, *RN* 57(5) 32, 1994.

5. Epstein CD, Henning RJ: Oxygen transport variables in the identification and treatment of tissue hypoxia, *Heart Lung* 22:328, 1993.

6. Fishman AP: Pulmonary rehabilitation research, *Resp Crit Care Med* 149:825, 1994.

7. Gift A, Moore T, Soeken K: Relaxation to reduce dyspnea and anxiety in COPD patients, *Nurs Res* 41(4):242, 1992.

9. Kim MJ et al: Inspiratory muscle training in patients with chronic obstructive pulmonary diagnosis, *Nurs Res* 42:356, 1993.

8. Kim MJ, McFarland GK, McLane AM: *Pocket guide to nursing diagnoses,* ed 6, St Louis, 1995, Mosby.

10. Thompson JM, Wilson SF: *Health assessment for nursing practice,* St Louis, 1996, Mosby.

11. Wilson SF, Thompson JM: *Respiratory Disorders*, St Louis, 1990, Mosby.
12. Yeaw P: Good lung down, *Am J Nurs* 92(3):27, 1992.

Dysreflexia

1. Ackley BV, Ladwig GB: *Nursing diagnosis handbook: a guide to planning care*, St Louis, 1993, Mosby.
2. Dunn KL: Autonomic dysreflexia, *J Cardiovasc Nurs* 5(4):57, 1991.
3. Guttman L, Whitteridge D: Effects of bladder retention on autonomic mechanisms after spinal cord injuries, *Brain* 70:361, 1947.
4. Head H, Riddoch G: The automatic bladder, excessive sweating and some other reflex conditions in gross injuries of the spinal cord. *Brain* 40:188, 1917.
5. Kewalramani LS: Autonomic dysreflexia in a traumatic myelopathy, *Am J Phys Med* 59:1, 1980.
6. Kurnick NB: Autonomic hyperreflexia and its control in patients with spinal cord lesions, *Ann Intern Med* 44:678, 1956.
7. Lindan R et al: Incidence and clinical features of autonomic dysreflexia in patients with spinal cord injury, *Paraplegia* 18:285, 1980.
8. Mathias CJ et al: Plasma catecholamines during paroxysmal neurogenic hypertension in quadriplegic man, *Circ Res* 39:204, 1976.
9. Naftchi NE et al: Hypertensive crisis in quadriplegic patients, *Circulation* 57:336, 1978.
10. Neiderpruem MS: Autonomic dysreflexia, *Rehabil Nurs* 9:29, 1984.

Risk for peripheral neurovascular dysfunction

1. Andrews LW: Neurovascular assessment, *Adv Clin Care* 5(6):5, 1990.
2. Blank CA, Irwin GH: Peripheral vascular disorders: assessment and interventions, *Nurs Clin North Am* 25(4):777, 1990.
3. Cheney P: Early management and physiologic changes in crush syndrome, *Crit Care Nurs Q* 17(2):62, 1994.
4. Farrell J: *Illustrated guide to orthopedic nursing*, Philadelphia, 1986, Lippincott.
5. Fecht-Gramley ME: Recognizing compartment syndrome, *Am J Nurs* 94(10):41, 1994.
6. Ignatavicius DD, Workman ML, Mishler MA: *Medical-surgical nursing: a nursing process approach*, pp 938, 1920, Philadelphia, 1995, Saunders.
7. North American Nursing Diagnosis Association, *NANDA proposed new nursing diagnoses*, 1994, 10th national conference on classifications of nursing diagnoses, Nashville, TN, NANDA.
8. Slye DA: Orthopedic complications: compartment syndrome, fat embolism syndrome, and venous thromboembolism, *Nurs Clin North Am* 26(1):113, 1991.
9. Slye DA, Theis LM: *An introduction to orthopaedic nursing: an orientation module*, Pitman, NJ, 1991, Jannetti.
10. Stuart MJ, Karaharja TK, Howe WB: Acute compartment syndrome: recognizing the progressive signs and symptoms, *Physician Sports Med* 22(3):91, 1994.
11. Taylor C, Lillis C, LeMone P: *Fundamentals of nursing: art and science of nursing care*, p 434, Philadelphia, 1993, Lippincott.
12. Weber J: *Nurses' handbook of health assessment*, p 45, Philadelphia, 1992, Lippincott.

Altered growth and development

1. Ahmann E: Family centered care: shifting orientation, *Pediatr Nurs* 20:113, 1994.
2. Ahmann E: Family-centered care: the time has come, *Pediatr Nurs* 20:52, 1994.
3. Allen MC: The high-risk infant, *Pediatr Clin North Am* 40:479, 1993.
4. Batshaw ML, Perret YM: *Children with disabilities: a medical primer*, ed 3, Baltimore, 1992, Brookes.
5. Bond N, Phillips P, Rollins JA: Family-centered care at home for families with children who are technology dependent, *Pediatr Nurs* 20:123, 1994.
6. Clubb RL: Chronic sorrow: adaptation patterns of parents with chronically ill children, *Pediatr Nurs* 17:461, 1991.
7. Crocker AC, Nelson RP: mental retardation. In Levine MD, Carey WB, Crocker AC, editors: *Developmental behavioral pediatrics*, Philadelphia, 1992, Saunders.
8. Curry DM, Duby JC: Developmental surveillance by pediatric nurses, *Pediatr Nurs* 20;40, 1994.

9. Danielson CB, Hamel-Bissell B, Winstead-Fry P: *Families, health, and illness: perspectives on coping and intervention*, St Louis, 1993, Mosby.
10. Dunst CJ, Trivette CM, Deal AG, editors: *Supporting and strengthening families volume 1: methods, strategies, and practices*, Cambridge, MA 1994, Brookline Books.
11. Dworkin PH: British-American recommendations for developmental monitoring: the role of surveillance, *Pediatr* 84:1000, 1989.
12. Faux SA: Siblings of children with chronic physical and cognitive disabilities, *J Pediatr Nurs* 8:305, 1993.
13. Fleming J et al: Impact on the family of children who are technology dependent and cared for in the home, *Pediatr Nurs* 20:379, 1994.
14. Foye HR, Sulkes SB: Developmental and behavioral pediatrics. In Berhman RE, Kliegman RM, editors: *Nelson essentials of pediatrics*, ed 2, Philadelphia, 1994, Saunders.
15. Hamilton B, Vessey J: Pediatric discharge planning, *Pediatr Nurs* 18:475, 1992.
16. Johnston CE, Marder LR: Parenting the child with a chronic condition; an emotional experience, *Pediatr Nurs* 20:611, 1994.
17. Konstantareas MM, Homatidis S: Effects of developmental disorder on parents: theoretical and applied considerations, *Psychiatr Clin North Am* 14:183, 1991.
18. McCubbin MA, McCubbin HI: Families coping with illness: the resiliency model of family stress, adjustment, and adaptation. In Danielson CB, Hamel-Bissel B, Winstead-Fry P: *Families, health, and illness: perspectives on coping and intervention*, St Louis, 1993, Mosby.
19. Morse JS: An overview of developmental disabilities nursing. In Roth SP, Morse JS: *A life-span approach to nursing care for individuals with developmental disabilities*, Baltimore, 1994, Brookes.
20. Nehring W: The nurse whose specialty is developmental disabilities, *Pediatr Nurs* 20:78, 1994.
21. O'Brien DR: Health maintenance and promotion in adults. In Roth SP, Morse JS: *A life-span approach to nursing care for individuals with developmental disabilities*, Baltimore, 1994, Brookes.
22. Patterson JM: Promoting resilience in families experiencing stress, *Pediatr Clin North Am* 42:47, 1995.
23. Patterson JM, Jernell J, Loenard BJ, Titus JC: Caring for medically fragile children at home: the parent-professional relationship, *J Pediatr Nurs* 9:98, 1994.
24. Ray LD, Ritchie JA: Caring for chronically ill children at home: factors that influence parents coping, *J Pediatr Nurs* 8:217, 1993.
25. Russell FF, Free TA; The nurse's role in habilitation. In Roth SP, Morse JS: *A life-span approach to nursing care for individuals with developmental disabilities*, Baltimore, 1994, Brookes.
26. Santelli B, Turnbull AP, Marquis JG, Lerner EP: Parent to parent programs: a unique form of mutual support, *Infants Young Children* 8:48, 1995.
27. Selekman J: Pediatric rehabilitation: from concepts to practice, *Pediatr Nurs* 17:11, 1991.
28. Shelton TL, Stepanek JS: *Family-entered care for children needing specialized health and developmental services*, Bethesda, MD, 1994, ACCH.
29. Snowden AW, Cameron S, Dunham K: Relationship between stress, coping resources, and satisfaction with family functioning in families of children with disabilities, *Can J Nurs Res* 23:63, 1994.
30. Steadham CI: Health maintenance and promotion: infancy through adolescence. In Roth SP, Morse JS, editors: *A life-span approach to nursing care for individuals with developmental disabilities*, Baltimore, 1994, Brookes.
31. Steadham CI: Role of professional nurses in the field of developmental disabilities, *Mental Retardation* 31:179, 1993.
32. Tengue BR et al: "High-tech" home care for children with chronic health conditions: a pilot study, *J Pediatr Nurs* 8:226, 1993.
33. Thomas GH, Thomas B, Trachtenberg SW: Growing up with Patricia, *Pediatr Clin North Am* 40:675, 1993.
34. Uauy R, Mena P, Warshaw JB: Growth and metabolic adaptation of the fetus and newborn. In Oski FA et al, editors: *Principles and practice of pediatrics*, ed 2, Philadelphia, 1994, Lippincott.
35. Youngblut JM, Brennan PF, Stewart LA: Families with medically fragile children: an exploratory study, *Pediatr Nurs* 20:463, 1994.

Sleep-Rest

■ SLEEP PATTERN DISTURBANCE

Sleep pattern disturbance is a state in which disruption of sleep time causes discomfort or interferes with an individual's desired life activities.

Sleep has been identified as a basic human need.[11] Bahr[2] states, "The phenomenon of sleep has the potential for relieving an individual of stress and responsibility when a break is needed to recharge the person's spirit, mind, and body; or, it can remain maddeningly aloof when it is needed the most." Henderson[5] has described the inability to rest and sleep as "one of the causes, as well as one of the accompaniments, of disease."

Sleep is a complex physiologic phenomenon influenced by pathophysiologic, physical, psychologic, environmental, and maturational factors. Sleep patterns are highly individual, and their natural pattern should be assessed for each individual. The cyclic pattern of sleep stages for rapid eye movement (REM) and non-REM sleep and the circadian rhythmic synchronization of sleep are influenced by chronic and acute illness, stress, age, pain, medications, hospitalization, sensory overload and deprivation, and lifestyle disruptions. Because of this complexity, the nursing management of the patient with a diagnosis of sleep pattern disturbance requires a holistic approach.

Related Factors[3,6]

Major categories
  Fragmented sleep
  Circadian desynchronization
Pathologic factors
  Impaired oxygen transport
    Cardiopulmonary disease
    Peripheral arteriosclerosis
  Impaired bowel or bladder elimination
  Impaired metabolism
    Hyperthyroidism
    Hepatic disorders
  Sleep apnea
Physical factors
  Immobility imposed by traction, casts, or restraints
  Inadequate physical exercise
  Pain
  Pregnancy

Psychologic factors
  Stress
  Anxiety
  Fear
  Depression
  Psychiatric disorders
  Lifestyle disruptions
Environmental factors
  Hospitalization
  Unfamiliar or uncomfortable sleep environment
  Rapid time zone change (jet lag)
  Frequent changes in sleep schedule
  Medications/drugs (e.g., tranquilizers, barbiturates, monoamine oxidase inhibitors, amphetamines, hypnotics, antidepressants, antihypertensives, sedatives, anesthetics, steroids, decongestants, caffeine, alcohol)
Maturational factor: age

Defining Characteristics

Verbal complaints of difficulty in falling asleep
Awakening earlier or later than desired
Interrupted sleep
Verbal complaints of not feeling well rested
Changes in behavior and performance
  Increasing irritability
  Restlessness
  Disorientation
  Lethargy
  Listlessness
Physical signs
  Mild, fleeting nystagmus
  Slight hand tremor
  Ptosis of eyelid
  Expressionless face
Thick speech with mispronunciation and incorrect words
Dark circles under eyes
Frequent yawning
Changes in posture
Related to fragmented sleep:
  Decreased sleep time occurring in one block of time
  Daytime sleepiness
  Fatigue

Sleep deprivation
  Less than one-half normal total sleep time
  Decreased slow-wave or REM sleep
Frequent awakenings
Decreased arousal threshold
Agitation or mood alteration
Related to circadian desynchronization:
  Sleep out of synchronization with biologic rhythms, resulting in sleeping during daytime and awakening at night
  Anxiety and restlessness
  Decreased arousal threshold

Expected Patient Outcomes & Nursing Interventions

Patient and family express understanding of factors contributing to altered sleep pattern and contribute to the individualized plan of care to promote sleep

- Educate patient and significant others about sleep and rest and rest needs and about factors that contribute to sleep pattern disturbances (e.g., pain, fear, stress, immobility, decreased activity, impaired oxygen transport, pregnancy, urinary frequency, medication, unfamiliar environment; see related factors.)
- Facilitate patient expression of emotional factors that may be interfering with normal sleep.
- Offer emotional support and continuity of care providers.
- Assess normal sleep pattern and any history of sleep disturbance or illness that may affect sleep.
- Facilitate patient's normal bedtime rituals.
- Assess sedative/hypnotic use or abuse.
- Promote normal sleep activity and pattern while hospitalized.
- Assess sleep effectiveness by asking patient how sleep in hospital compares to that at home.
- Limit liquids in evening.
- Schedule diuretics in AM and early PM.
- Do not schedule routine procedures at night.
- Promote comfort, relaxation, and a sense of well-being; relieve pain.
- Eliminate stressful situations before bedtime; use of stress relaxation techniques may be helpful.
- White noise may promote greater depth and quality of sleep.[7]
- Minimize awakenings; allow for at least 90-minute sleep cycles. Continually assess need to awaken patient, particularly at night; distinguish between essential and nonessential nursing tasks.
- Organize nursing care to allow for maximum amount of uninterrupted sleep while ensuring close monitoring of patient's condition.

- Assist patient to maintain normal day/night cycles by decreasing lighting, noise, and sensory stimulation at night.

Total sleep time and pattern approximates normal for patient, as evidenced by:

Minimal awakenings
Feeling rested
Absence of daytime sleepiness
Absence of signs of sleep deprivation

- Monitor physiologic parameters without awakening patient whenever possible.
- Inform patient about when you will awaken him during the night so as not to startle patient.
- Coordinate awakenings with other departments (e.g., respiratory therapy, laboratory, radiology).
- Minimize noise, particularly related to staff and equipment.
- Reduce level of environmental stimuli that may cause sensory overload.
- Plan nap times to assist in equilibrating normal sleep time; early morning naps may be beneficial in promoting REM sleep.[8]
- Be aware of effects of commonly used medications on sleep, since many sedative and hypnotic medications decreased REM sleep. Do not withhold sedative and analgesic medications; rather, use drugs that minimally disrupt sleep to complement comfort measures, reducing dosages gradually as medication becomes no longer necessary. Diuretics may interrupt sleep by increasing number of awakenings and should not be scheduled near bedtime.
- Offer milk in evening to promote sleep.
- Assess for signs of sleep deprivation (e.g., confusion, hallucinations, delusions, restlessness, combativeness, paranoia, irritability, and decreased judgment. Be aware that best treatment for sleep deprivation is prevention.
- Document amount of uninterrupted sleep and time awake per shift in hospitalized patients.
- Promote staff attitude that sleep is essential and should be encouraged. Assess unit for sleep-reducing stimuli and work to reduce them.
- Encourage moderate and how-intensity exercise *to promote sleep.*
- Be aware that cardiac dysrhythmias can be precipitated because of decreased arousal threshold secondary to desynchronization.
- If desynchronization occurs, plan for resynchronization by maintaining constancy in day/night pattern for at least 3 days (may require 5 to 12 days to reacclimatize). Plan for activities during day to stimulate wakefulness, and use comfort measures (position of comfort, warm blankets, back rub, etc.) *to promote sleep at night.* During resynchronization, fatigue, malaise, and decreased ability to perform tasks typically are found.[6]
- Administer hypnotics, as ordered, and monitor their effectiveness.

Principles and Rationale for Nursing Interventions

Sleep occurs in two distinct stages, REM and non-REM, as determined by the electroencephalogram (EEG), electro-oculogram (EOG), and electromyogram (EMG). In addition, non-REM sleep has four stages. Stage 1 is a transitional stage between sleep and wakefulness. During stage 2 the individual becomes progressively more relaxed. A young adult typically spends 50% to 60% of total sleep time in non-REM stages 1 and 2. Non-REM stages 3 and 4 are characterized by slow-frequency delta waves on the EEG and differentiated by the relative percentage of these waves. Non-REM stages 3 and 4, the deeper stages of sleep, comprise approximately 20% of total sleep time. These are the restorative stages of sleep during which much protein synthesis and energy conservation occurs.

During REM sleep, or paradoxic sleep, there are bursts of eye movements seen on the EOG. The large muscles of the body become functionally paralyzed. EEG activity increases so that there is a resemblance to the waking state. REM sleep comprises 20% to 25% of the total sleep time and is the stage during which the individual is most difficult to awaken. The many functions of sleep are only theorized by researchers in the field.

Sleep is cyclic. At its onset the individual normally progresses through repetitive cycles, beginning with non-REM stages 1 through 4 and then back again to stage 2. From stage 2, REM sleep is entered. Stage 2 is then reentered and the cycle repeats. These cycles occur at approximately 90-minute intervals, so that four or five cycles are normally completed in the sleep period.

Illness can decrease the amount, quality, and consistency of sleep. Sleep is often interrupted or fragmented, altering the normal stages and cycles and producing dysfunctional sleep. With frequent interruptions the patient spends more time in the transitional stages (non-REM 1 and 2) and less time in the deeper stages of sleep (non-REM 3 and 4, REM). Thus, total sleep time and/or selective deprivation of the deeper stages of sleep can occur.[8]

Sleep is normally synchronized with the circadian rhythm; thus, sleep normally occurs at the low phase of the circadian cycle. Sleep that is desynchronized is rated as poor in quality. Irritability, restlessness, daytime hypersomnolence, fatigue, depression, anxiety, and decreased accuracy of task performance are characteristic effects of desynchronized sleep.[6] Barbiturates, sedatives/hypnotics, and analgesic medications may add to sleep disorders by promoting the lighter stages of sleep (non-REM 2) and/or further decreasing non-REM stages 3 and 4 and REM sleep. Knowledge of the effects of these drugs on sleep will assist the nurse to use them more effectively in patient care.

References

1. American Nurses' Association: *Social policy statement*, Kansas City, MO, 1980, ANA.
2. Bahr R: Sleep-wake patterns in the aged, *J Gerontol Nurs* 9:534, 1983.
3. Carpenito LJ: *Nursing diagnosis: application to clinical practice*, Philadelphia, 1987, Lippincott.
4. Henderson V: *Basic principles of nursing care*, New York, 1969, Macmillan.
5. Miller J: *Coping with chronic illness: overcoming powerlessness*, Philadelphia, 1984, Davis.
6. Sanford S: Sleep and the cardiac patient, *Cardiovasc Nurs* 19(5):19, 1983.
7. Williamson J: The effects of ocean sounds on sleep after CABG surgery, *Am J Crit Care* 1:91, 1992.
8. Yura H, Walsh MB: *Human needs and the nursing process*, New York, 1978, Appleton-Century-Crofts.

VI

Cognitive-Perceptual

■ PAIN

Pain is a state in which an individual experiences and reports the presence of severe discomfort or an uncomfortable sensation.

The diagnostic category of pain concerns the phenomenon of pain and the nurse's role as a patient advocate in its management. Pain is an abstract concept; it is an invisible yet complex personal experience. Pain is defined by the International Association for the Study of Pain as "an unpleasant sensory and emotional experience associated with actual or potential tissue damage or described in terms of such a damage."[5]

Even in similar situations, the pain experience varies from individual to individual and includes sensory and affective components. Pain is aggravated by anxiety and fear. It is described in terms of both the sensation of pain and the distress or degree of suffering that an individual experiences. Feldman[14] describes the total pain response as being "determined by such factors as threshold, tolerance, attention to pain, action of pain relievers, counter irritation measures (such as heat or cold), summation, expectations, and perceptions." These factors help determine an individual's perception of pain, response to the pain, effectiveness of the pain control measures, and tendency to report pain.

McCaffery[27] defines pain as "whatever the experiencing person says it is, existing whenever he says it does." Pain means different things to different people. An individual may have difficulty describing the pain to others because pain is a personal experience. Pain expression can be influenced by gender and cultural norms. Although the results of studies examining ethnic differences in the report and tolerance of pain are mixed, northern European caucasian groups are more often reported to have a higher tolerance than other racial or ethnic groups. Men may also report less pain than women regardless of ancestry.[13] Individuals with chronic pain may learn to live with their pain. Therefore, pain expression is not always an accurate indication of pain.

Pain is further described according to its duration. *Acute pain* is intense and has an end point. It provides a warning to the individual of actual or potential tissue damage and resolves when healing occurs. *Chronic pain* is often characterized as lasting longer than 6 months. The pain can be either continuous or intermittent and as intense as acute pain. Chronic pain does not serve as a warning of tissue damage (see Chronic Pain on p. 1640).

This discussion provides an overview of the pain phenomenon to address pain's wide spectrum. It emphasizes the nurse's independent and collaborative roles in pain management.

Related Factors*

Injuring agents
   Biologic
      Disease
      Inflammation
      Ischemia
   Chemical
      Cytotoxic agents
      Electrolyte imbalance
      Endocrine dysfunction
      Noxious agents
   Physical
      Trauma
      Temperature extremes
   Psychologic
      Anxiety
      Distress
      Fear
      Stress
      Tension

Defining Characteristics†

Communication (verbal or coded) of pain descriptor
Guarding, protective behavior
Hands placed over painful area
Autonomic response (with acute pain only); may have periods
   of physiologic adaptation and potential for shock:
      Diaphoresis
      Pallor
      Changes in blood pressure (accentuated in patients with
         hypovolemia and unstable hemodynamics), pulse rate,
         stroke volume, respiratory rate and depth, muscle tone

---

*References 7, 17, 18, 21, 23, 28, 30, 32-34, 37.
†References 1, 9, 18, 20, 21, 35, 37.

Dry mouth

Pupillary dilation

Distraction behavior (moaning, crying, pacing, seeking out other people, or activities, restlessless)

Change in appetite

Weight change

Fatigue

Preoccupation with pain

Self-focusing

Shortened attention span

Altered time perception

Impaired thought processes

Facial mask of pain (eyes lack luster, "beaten look," fixed or scattered movement, grimace)

May or may not verbalize:

Pain descriptors (may deny them)

Fear, anxiety, anger, helplessness, depression, hopelessness, suicidal thoughts

Hope that pain will end

Frustration at lack of treatment

Increased irritability, feelings of being a burden, feelings of guilt, anger at others

Does not verbalize anger at caretakers when dependent

Disturbed sleep pattern with difficulty falling asleep; awakens from sleep because of pain

Inability to continue previous activities

Social isolation

Discontinues or reduces employment

Financially dependent on external sources if pain prolonged

Expected Patient Outcomes & Nursing Interventions*

Verbalizes information about the pain experience:

- Assess patient's pain status, incorporating the following information:

    Nurse and patient have perceptions of pain based on past experiences, cultural influences, and other factors.

    Patient may assume that nurse is aware of how patient is experiencing pain so may not readily offer information about it.

    Patients will provide honest information if they know that this information will be used to help control their pain. People need reassurance that their complaints of pain are believed and that the nurse will continue to provide control interventions.

    Patients may not offer information about pain experience because of desire to be a "good patient" or if a positive relationship has not been established with the health care provider(s).

    Meaning of pain for each patient influences that person's response to pain.

Patient's belief about his or her ability to control pain influences the person's emotional response to pain.

Pain can cause fatigue; therefore a complete pain assessment is not always practical. Eliciting information on changes since the last pain assessment may help conserve the patient's energy.

- Incorporate the following factors in the assessment of the patient's pain status:

    Location/characteristics

    Onset/duration

    Frequency

    Intensity, using 0 to 10 scale: 0, no pain; 10, worst pain possible

    Quality

    Precipitating factors

    Effective pain control measures

    Ineffective pain control measures

    Desired interventions

    Pain expression style (stoic, verbal, crying, moaning)

    Movement (guarding, favoring posture)

    Muscle tone

    Emotional distress

    Impact on quality of life

    Effect of pain on daily activities

    Activities affected or eliminated because of pain

    Effect on sleep/awake pattern

    Effect on energy level

    Effect on sexual activity

    Effect on relations with others

    Effect on feelings of self-worth

    Use of health care system

- Perception of ability to control pain

    Typical coping response for stress or pain

    Pressure of psychiatric disorders such as depression, anxiety, or psychosis

    Attitude toward and use of opiod, anxiolytic, or other medications, including any history of substance abuse

Identifies strategies that eliminate or control pain, as evidenced by:

Demonstrating ability to differentiate between strategies that are effective and ineffective

Applying previous strategies that have controlled the pain

Using a variety of pain control strategies

- Explore strategies that have been successful in past.
- Identify strategies that patient values as essential for pain reduction.
- Assess patient's willingness to incorporate nonpharmaceutical pain control measures.
- Instruct patient on pain reduction strategies as pain experience dictates (for short attention span in acute pain, give brief explanations; for chronic pain, provide more detail).
- Administer medication per physician's orders and protocol using appropriate delivery system.

    Monitor effectiveness at frequent intervals.

---

*References 1-4, 6, 7, 10-12, 14, 16, 20, 22-29, 31-39.

Graphically record pain assessment data.

Provide physician with evidence of need to change medication.

Provide or instruct patient in importance of regular doses around the clock as well as "as needed" doses.

- Intervene at onset of pain, before pain becomes severe.
- Implement remaining strategies for this patient goal, as indicated by patient condition and pain status.

Position for comfort.

Encourage attention to proper posture and alignment.

Immobilize or rest affected area.

Relieve pressure areas with turning or pressure-reduction devices such as air-fluidized support systems.

Provide distraction.

Suggest and instruct patient in relaxation techniques, short, simple techniques with nurse directing for acute pain; more complex techniques for chronic pain; use patient's memory of a peaceful event.

Help patient use imagery to the extent he or she is able to concentrate; use image patient has actually experienced; one at a time and employ all senses.

Employ hypnotic strategies:

Blocking awareness of pain

Substitution of painful feeling

Displacement of pain sensation

Use electrical counter stimulation: pressure, massage, vibration, heat/cold, external analgesics, transcutaneous nerve stimulation (TENS).

Provide music therapy: easy listening, or patient preference.

Pace activities and plan activities ahead of time.

Provide touch, especially for infants, or for disoriented or unresponsive patients.

- Control environmental factors that influence pain: room temperature, lighting, noise.
- Provide supportive environment.
- Give positive suggestions regarding feelings of comfort.
- Determine realistic pain control goals with patient.
- Attempt interventions several times before judging success.
- Assess which pain reduction strategies patient finds helpful.
- Use several pain reduction strategies.

Identifies and reduces activities that precipitate or enhance pain:

- Help patient to identify activities that may enhance or precipitate pain.
- Discuss strategies to prevent or reduce precipitation or enhancement of pain (e.g., fear, fatigue, or lack of knowledge).
- Discuss strategies to avoid these activities within patient's lifestyle.
- Encourage family members to help patient prevent precipitation of painful event.
- Encourage patient to keep daily log to help identify other activities that precipitate or enhance pain.

Incorporate interventions to reduce or eliminate pain, as evidenced by:

Using pain control strategies appropriately

Attention span returning to or approaching pre-pain status

Reduction or absence of guarding, protective behavior

Verbalizing increased control over pain

Social and family interactions approaching pre-pain status

Incorporating lifestyle modifications

Using community resources or referrals appropriately

Fatigue being controlled

Returning sleep pattern toward normal or adapts to changes in sleep pattern

Activity returning toward normal or modifying activity to control pain

- Assess patient's ability to implement interventions into present lifestyle.
- Discuss lifestyle modifications that may be necessary.
- Assess patient's desire and ability to change these aspects of his or her life.
- Help patient identify measures to implement lifestyle modifications.
- Provide referrals or information on community resources.

Sets realistic goals, as evidenced by:

Goals realistic for pain experience

Setting priorities for achievement of goals

Identifying short-term achievable goals and implementing goal progression after accurate evaluation of previous goal attainment

Moving toward resumption of previous lifestyle or modifying lifestyle according to limitations imposed by pain experience

Ability to control or reduce fatigue, anxiety, and depression

- Assess patient's ability to realistically project impact of pain in all areas of life.
- Encourage patient to set priorities and plan ahead.
- Ask patient to identify one or two realistic goals to achieve each day.
- Discuss progress in goal attainment.
- Teach patient that realistic goal setting can aid in reducing fatigue, anxiety, and depression.
- Instruct patient in goal setting to normalize lifestyle and place pain on periphery of life.

Verbalizes positive feelings about self, as evidenced by:

Building on personal strengths

Reentering family, society, and work activities at level consistent with pain experience

Life no longer revolving around pain experience

Verbalizing increased control over self

Incorporating effective coping strategies

- Assess patient's perception of his or her progress in goal attainment.
- If patient is unable to return to work, help identify meaningful ways to fill time and promote positive feelings of self-worth during free hours.

- Provide patient with positive reinforcement for activities focused away from pain.
- Assist patient in developing normalizing strategies for activities encountered in daily life.
- Educate patient on community resources for prevention or reduction of problems related to job retraining, financial assistance, etc.
- Inform patient of importance of maintaining communication with all health professionals.
- Assess need for referrals for family or individual counseling, financial needs, or sexual concerns.
- Encourage gradual reentry into family, society, and work activities; set realistic goals for reentry.
- Provide positive reinforcement for achievements.
- Discuss patient and family feelings regarding role changes.
- Assess patient's ability to identify strengths and weaknesses and to build on strengths.

Principles and Rationale for Nursing Interventions

Nursing interventions are derived from information elicited during pain assessment. The information may or may not give clues to the source of the pain. Knowing the etiology is helpful, but not essential in selecting appropriate nursing interventions. Barriers to effective pain management include both nurse and physician knowledge and the time and cooperation of patients and their families.[15]

At times the nurse may be able to modify or act directly on the factors that cause pain. At other times, however, the cause is unknown. The expected patient outcomes are appropriate for any individual in pain, but the emphasis may differ for patients in acute or chronic pain. The interventions are directed at achieving the expected patient outcomes and are not specific for either acute or chronic pain.

The pain assessment includes both subjective and objective data. The depth of the assessment varies according to the individual's pain status, the situation, and setting. The frequency of the assessments varies according to individual needs. The data can be recorded on a flowsheet or a graph to identify trends. Some patients are able to assist in monitoring their pain and keeping a diary of their pain experience. The nurse assesses children according to their developmental level and their understanding of the meaning of their pain.

To treat pain effectively, the patient (and nurse) must be able to identify strategies that eliminate or control pain. Strategies that were effective in the past may be continued or adapted for the current situation, for example, breathing techniques to aid in relaxation for a woman who has had Lamaze preparation before childbirth. Medications to manage pain are individualized to the patient. The simplest dosage schedules and the least invasive pain management modalities should be used first. The cost of drugs and technologies to the patient should be considered when selecting pain control strategies. Optional pain relief should be the goal when prescribing analgesics. How an indi-

vidual copes with pain is usually enduring. The nurse should help the patient identify the style of pain coping he or she typically uses. This may help the individual understand why some strategies are more effective. Additional interventions can be tried and evaluated. The patient should be instructed to use several strategies to obtain better pain control.

A pain assessment flowsheet or a diary of pain kept by the patient will help to identify activities that precipitate or enhance pain. Nursing care should be planned when the patient feels the pain is best controlled. A subjective pain rating scale is helpful. A daily log will help patients identify pain-producing activities. The nurse and family can help the patient evaluate the significance of these activities to determine if they can be modified or eliminated.

Realistic goal setting is important for both acute and chronic pain. The goals related to acute pain have a shorter deadline. All goals should be realistic for the individual and measurable. The nurse and patient should mutually determine the goals and evaluate goal achievement regularly. Goals should be progressed as healing occurs and/or the patient begins to adjust to the pain. Goal progression is an essential component of coping with the chronic pain.

Research in the area of pain experience and analgesic administration for general medical and surgical inpatients has shown that patients continue to have pain despite treatment and that analgesic doses ordered are inadequate.* Pain affects all aspects of an individual's existence. There may be deterioration of relationships with significant others, resulting in social isolation and loss of support systems. Many feelings can occur as an individual attempts to cope with acute or chronic pain. Patients can be anxious, depressed, and angry all at the same time. Pain disrupts basic life activities that are essential for positive feelings about self. If the patient is able to perceive control over the pain and focus on aspects of life other than pain, a more positive view of self will prevail.

■ CHRONIC PAIN

Chronic pain is a state in which an individual experiences pain that continues for more than 6 months in duration. Chronic pain frequently is divided into two categories: chronic nonmalignant pain and chronic malignant pain.

Chronic nonmalignant pain is pain that persists after tissue damage has healed or in the absence of evident tissue damage.

Chronic malignant pain may be associated with a disease or injury but has continued beyond the normal healing time. The pain may be caused by progressive or destructive disease processes, such as cancer or arthritis. Even though a cause is not identified, the pain still exists. Individuals with chronic pain may not show outward evidence of pain. Health care professionals should ask about pain, and the patient's self-report should be the primary source of assessment.[13]

---

*References 1, 8, 15, 17, 25-28.

Chronic pain can be continuous or intermittent and can be as intense as acute pain. Habituation of the autonomic response occurs so that the fight-or-flight response is no longer present. Chronic pain does not serve as a warning of tissue danger. In rheumatoid arthritis, for example, joint pain may still be present when the disease process is no longer active because of the structural damage that has already occurred in the joint. The reason for some forms of chronic pain may not be known. Chronic pain does not necessarily serve a purpose. Fortin (in Kim et al[14]) provides a vivid description of the effects of chronic pain.

Eventually the debilitating effects of the chronic pain experience and loss of coping reserves alters the individual's perceptions, personality and social functioning. As the person changes, the environment to which he responds changes; that is, personal variability in pain sensation and psychophysiologic responses become intrinsically woven into the situational milieu. Problems of altered self-esteem, social identity, changes in roles and social interaction, and the responses that feed back into the problem, depression, anxiety, and irritability become integral to the chronic pain experience.

Fortin suggests a beginning model for viewing chronic pain. Acute pain has traditionally been viewed from a sensory-reactive model that does not encompass the chronic pain experience. Fortin uses the gate control theory to depict the psychophysiologic aspects of pain and describes the psychosocial aspects using an interactional approach. Viewing these models together, Fortin has reformulated a model for describing chronic pain and defines the model as (Kim et al[14]):

An integrated pattern of sensory, sentience and interactive components. Sensory refers to the quality and intensity of the pain sensation. Sentience refers to the motivational and affective qualities of the experience. Interactive refers to the simultaneous interaction between the individual and the environment. It is suggested that in the experience of chronic pain, these forces act collectively to repattern the person and the environment in a transactional process.

Related Factors[3,11,17,21]

Chronic physical/psychosocial disability
Lack of support systems
Fear about addiction
Fatigue
Lack of knowledge about pain control measures
Poor self-concept
Inflammation
Overactivity or inactivity
Helplessness/hopelessness
Overweight
Medication dependence

Defining Characteristics

Verbal report or observed evidence of pain experienced for more than 6 months
Guarding, protective movements

Change in appetite or weight
Facial mask (of pain)
Fatigue
Fear of reinjury
Physical and social withdrawal
Altered ability to continue previous activities
Helplessness/hopelessness
Preoccupation with pain
Self-focusing
Shortened attention span
Altered time perception
Impaired thought processes

Expected Patient Outcomes & Nursing Interventions*

Verbalizes information about pain experience

- Assess patient's pain status (see Pain on p. 1637).
- Incorporate factors in assessment of patient's pain status (see Pain on p. 1637).

Identifies strategies that control pain

- See Pain.
- Implement remaining strategies for this patient goal as indicated by patient condition and pain status.
  Provide therapeutic positioning.
  Encourage attention to proper posture and alignment.
  Rest affected area.
  Provide distraction.
  Instruct patient in relaxation techniques or guided imagery.
  Use hypnosis and biofeedback.
  Provide music therapy, play therapy, activity therapy.
  Use counterstimulation: pressure, massage, vibration, heat/cold, external analgesics, transcutaneous electrical nerve stimulator (TENS).
  Pace activities and plan activities ahead of time.
  Provide touch.
- Determine realistic pain control goals with patient.
- Provide supportive environment.
- Identify emotional responses from patient.
- Assess which pain reduction strategies patient finds helpful.
- Use several pain reduction strategies.
- Attempt interventions several times before judging success.
- Include patient and family education about pain and its management.

Identifies activities that enhance pain

- Help patient to identify activities that may enhance pain or precipitate pain (disease-related, treatment-related, environment).

---

*References 1, 2, 4-10, 12-20, 22-28, 30.

- Discuss strategies to reduce enhancement of pain (e.g., fear, fatigue, or lack of knowledge).
- Discuss strategies to avoid these activities within patient's lifestyle.
- Encourage family members to help patient prevent enhancing painful event.
- Encourage patient to keep daily log to monitor changes in pain and to help identify other activities that enhance pain.
- Encourage patient to report to health care professional development of new pain or changes in his or her pain.

Incorporate interventions to reduce pain

- See Pain on p. 1637.

Sets realistic goals

- Assess patient's ability to realistically project impact of pain in all areas of life.
- Teach patient to discriminate between pain that is normal and pain that is abnormal.
- Enpower patient to take active role in pain control.
- Encourage patient to set priorities and plan ahead.
- Ask patient to identify one or two realistic goals to achieve each day.
- Discuss progress in goal attainment.
- Teach patient that realistic goal setting can aid in reducing fatigue, anxiety, and depression.
- Instruct patient in goal setting to normalize lifestyle and place pain on periphery of life.
- Use quota-setting principles for achieving exercise goals when behavioral barriers exist.

Verbalizes positive feelings about self

- Assess patient's perception of progress toward goal attainment.
- If the patient is unable to return to work, help identify meaningful ways to fill time and promote positive feelings of self-worth.
- Reinforce behaviors that decrease the risk of medical, social, and financial problems.
- Provide patient with positive reinforcement for activities focused away from pain.
- Assist patient in developing normalizing strategies for activities encountered in daily life.
- Educate patient on community resources for prevention or reduction of problems related to job retraining and financial assistance.
- Inform patient of importance of maintaining communications with all health professionals.
- Assess need for referrals for family or individual counseling, financial needs, or sexual concerns.
- Encourage gradual reentry into family, society, and work activities; set realistic goals for reentry.
- Assist patient in effective transition to retirement if work is no longer a realistic option.
- Use support groups.
- Provide positive reinforcement for achievements.

- Discuss patient and family feelings regarding role changes.
- Assess patient's ability to identify strengths and weaknesses and to build on strengths.
- Explore the losses associated with illness and pain.
- Implement appropriate activity/exercise plan for physical condition.
- Assess feelings regarding pain, suffering, and spiritual well-being.
- Provide for spiritual interventions (e.g., counseling, prayer, and rituals).
- Discuss feelings about death and dying, pain relief, grief, and hope in the context of advancing disease.
- Encourage open communication between patient and family.
- Help patient and family understand effects of pain experience on each family member (e.g., spouse, children).
- Reinforce each person's role in helping the patient cope with the pain experience.

Avoid use of life-threatening unproven remedies, as evidenced by:

Identifying dangers of life-threatening, unproven remedies

Verbalizes knowledge of resources to assist in identification of unproven remedies

Seeking support to avoid using life-threatening, unproven remedies

Maintaining contact with health care system

- Inform patient and family about identification of unproven remedies.
- Instruct patient in dangers of unproven remedies; they can be life-threatening, expensive, and can serve as a substitute for ongoing health care.
- Assist patient in exploring feelings regarding unproven remedies.
- Counsel patient in determining how to respond to individuals who suggest unproven remedies.
- Provide patient with community resources to assist in identification of unproven remedies.
- Do not remove unharmful unproven remedies from patient (patient may have faith in this remedy not found in other treatments).

Maintain weight or move toward normal weight index for height and frame, as evidenced by:

Incorporating strategies for weight gain or weight loss

Using resources within family, community, and health care agency as warranted

Adjusting weight to identified goal

- Instruct patient about effects of pain on nutrition and influence of proper nutrition on health status.
- Instruct patient on need for balanced diet to maintain ideal weight for height and frame.
- Obtain dietitian referral.
- Assess motivation toward obtaining proper nutrition and achievement of ideal weight.
- If underweight for height and frame, refer to Altered nutrition: less than body requirements on p. 1546.

- If overweight for height and frame, refer to Altered nutrition: more than body requirements.

Principles and Rationale for Nursing Interventions

To determine which interventions should be incorporated into the nursing care plan, the nurse must first consider the pain assessment information and relate this to current knowledge derived from pain theories. Clinicians should be aware of common pain syndromes as this prompt recognition can hasten treatment and minimize the morbidity of unrelieved pain. The pain assessment information may or may not give clues to the source of pain. Knowing the related factors is helpful in selecting appropriate interventions. Because pain is a subjective experience perceived by the individual, the mainstay of pain assessment is the patient's self-report. The frequency of assessment is individualized but must be ongoing. Pain should be assessed at regular intervals after starting the treatment plan, with each new report of pain, and at suitable intervals after pharmacologic or nonpharmacologic interventions.[13]

To treat pain, the patient must be able to identify strategies that are effective in controlling pain. Any previously used interventions that were effective in controlling this pain should be continued. The nurse should consider the patient's willingness to participate, ability to participate, preferred support of significant others for method, and contraindications when selecting a pain relief strategy. Interventions unfamiliar to the patient should also be attempted and assessed using a subjective rating scale. Using more than one intervention may provide better pain control.

Activities that intensify pain should be identified. By keeping a daily diary of activities and pain ratings, the patient may be able to identify variations in pain and occurrences of new pain. Once activities that intensify pain are identified, methods to modify or reduce the activity can be explored. The importance of the activity to the individual should be addressed. If the activity has little meaning or value, the patient may readily avoid it, but interventions are needed to maintain the activity if it is meaningful to the person.

Throughout the pain management process, realistic goal setting is important. The individual in chronic pain must make an active decision to participate in the pain management plan. Goals should be mutually determined by the patient and nurse. Goals should be measurable and achievable. After achievement, another goal is identified. Goal progression continues until the final outcome is reached. Frequently a multidisciplinary team is working with the patient in chronic pain. All team members should be aware of established goals so that all goals are consistent in working toward the final outcome and the health care regimens required for goal attainment remain realistic.

The patient may acquire a positive view of self as he or she perceives control over pain and is able to focus on aspects of life other than pain. At this point, nonpain behaviors are reinforced. The patient focuses on relationships with family, friends, work, society, and God. The individual takes self-responsibility for pain management and learns to use the health care system appropriately.

The use of unproven remedies poses a special problem for persons with chronic pain. Individuals need to feel comfortable discussing their use of unproven remedies. The nurse can provide comfort by remaining nonjudgmental. The nurse needs to provide information about the expense of some forms of unproven remedies and that some forms may be life threatening. The patient can then make informed decisions. It can be easy to reject current health care when pain relief is not found and an unproven remedy proclaims pain relief abilities.

Weight problems frequently occur when chronic pain is present. Many patients find that loss of appetite occurs during severe episodes of pain. Weight loss can occur also as a consequence of disease such as cancer. If a patient has decreased mobility, yet appetite is unchanged, he or she is at risk of gaining weight. Interventions for weight problems should be implemented as early as possible.

Chronic pain is multidimensional. It affects every aspect of life and the significant individuals in the person's life. Interventions are geared toward improving the quality of life through pain control.

▎ SENSORY/PERCEPTUAL ALTERATIONS (SPECIFY) (VISUAL, AUDITORY, KINESTHETIC, GUSTATORY, TACTILE, OLFACTORY)

Sensory/perceptual alteration (visual, auditory, kinesthetic, gustatory, tactile, olfactory) is a state in which an individual experiences a change in the amount or patterning of incoming stimuli accompanied by a diminished, exaggerated, distorted, or impaired response to such stimuli.

Understanding the definition of sensory/perceptual alteration is enhanced by viewing and defining the concept of perception. The following definition is stated as a serial order of emergent behaviors. This technique is described as a method for defining abstract concepts.

An individual with physiologic, psychologic, and sociocultural sets who has certain assumptions, motivations, and expectations encounters a concrete situation.

Stimuli bombard one or more of the sense organs. Categories of senses:

Exteroreceptors (distance senses)
1. Vision
2. Audition

Proprioceptors (near senses)
1. Tactile sense
2. Taste (gustatory)
3. Smell (olfactory)

Interoceptors (deep senses)
1. Kinesthetic (muscle, bone, joint sense)
2. Vestibular (sense of balance)
3. Visceral (hollow organ sense)

Sense organs transduce the stimuli (transduction is the sensory transformation of raw stimulus data into informational messages/nerve impulses).

Nerve impulses are relayed to the brain and reticular activating system (RAS), which creates an arousal state.

Impulses are automatically forwarded, or impulses are selected, reorganized, and modified based on perceptual set, past experience, present needs, and future goals and then forwarded (transformation).

Meaningful impulses are integrated, and a percept is formed.

The resulting percept may have a direct or indirect effect on subsequent emotions and behavior.

An alteration in sensory perception occurs when an interruption occurs at or during one or more of the steps set forth in the operational definition. The extent and severity of the alteration depend on the point or points of interruption and the causal nature of the interruption. The classification of related factors also spells out persons at risk for an alteration in sensory perception.

Related Factors[6]

Altered environments (excessive or insufficient stimuli)

Therapeutically restricted (isolation, intensive care, bed rest, traction, continuing illness, incubator)

Socially restricted (institutionalization, homebound, aging, chronic illness, dying, infant deprivation)

Stigmatized (mentally ill, retarded, handicapped)

Bereaved

Altered sensory reception, transmission, or integration

Neurologic disease, trauma, or deficit

Altered state of sense organs

Inability to communicate, understand, speak, or respond

Sleep deprivation

Pain

Chemical alteration

Endogenous (electrolyte imbalance, elevated blood urea nitrogen, elevated ammonia, hypoxia)

Exogenous (central nervous system stimulants/depressants, mind-altering drugs)

Extreme anxiety or panic (narrowed perceptual fields caused by anxiety)

Defining Characteristics[1,3,6,9]

Changes in thought processes
    Disorientation in time, place, or person
    Disordered sequencing in thought, time, or events
    Altered abstraction or conceptualization
    Change in problem-solving abilities
    Bizarre thinking
    Hallucinations
    Hypersuggestibility
Changes in attention span
    Diminished concentration
    Daydreaming

Restlessness
Increased distractibility
Inability to follow flow of conversation
Emotional lability
    Rapid mood swings
    Exaggerated responses
    Ambivalence
    Apathy
    Flat affect
    Emotional detachment
    Anger
    Depression
    Fear
    Irritability
    Anxiety
Changes in routine patterns or habits
    Change in behavior pattern
    Change in response to stimuli
    Altered communication patterns
    Change in sleeping patterns
    Altered eating habits
Changes in sensory capabilities
    Vision
        Diminished visual capacity
        Visual distortion
        Photosensitivity
    Audition
        Hypersensitivity/hyposensitivity
        Auditory distortion
        Distortion of verbal messages
    Tactile sense
        Hyperesthesias/hypoesthesias
        Inability to tell nature of object by touch
    Taste
        Increased taste sensitivity
        Diminished sense of taste
        Altered taste sense
        Loss of appetite
    Smell
        Diminished sense of smell
        Hypersensitivity to odor
        Distortion of odor
    Kinesthetic sense
        Motor incoordination
        Inability to tell where body parts are located
        Paralysis
        Muscular weakness, flaccidity, rigidity
        Surgical joint replacement
    Vestibular sense
        Diminished sense of balance
    Visceral sense
        Feelings of emptiness, hollowness
Presence of any of related factors associated with diagnosis
Changes in percept characteristics
    Distortion of color, hue, intensity, light, or size
    Distortion of environment
    Growth of inanimate objects

Failure to notice stimuli
Disregard of normally "important" percepts

Expected Patient Outcomes & Nursing Interventions

Prevention

Identifies related risk factors, as evidenced by:

Stating related factors
Recognizing self-risk profile

- Assess patient for risks and potential risks for alteration (see related factors); present risk profile to patient when possible.

Identify risk reduction methods, as evidenced by:

Stated or demonstrated use of strategies for reduction or elimination of identified risk factors

- Provide strategies for reduction or elimination of identified related factors (e.g., altering sleep pattern to reduce sleep deprivation; altering drug habits; rearranging environment).

Identifies stimuli needed for daily functioning, as evidenced by:

Stating source, type, amount, and patterns of usual daily stimulation
Recounting lifestyle and role patterns

- Explore source, type, amount, and patterns of stimuli needed by patient for optimum functioning.

Identify methods for maintaining adequate stimuli in environment, as evidenced by:

Verbalizing or demonstrating use for strategies for maintaining or altering environment
Listing changes planned for or already made

- Provide strategies for maintaining adequate amounts of meaningful stimuli in identified therapeutically or socially restricted environments (e.g., introducing pattern and structure in environment, orienting features, noise control, presence of familiar objects and persons).

Acute Care*

No injury sustained, as evidenced by:

No physical or reported signs of injury

- Maintain safety precautions (bed rails up; bed lowered; sharp objects out of reach; call bell in reach).

Decrease in or elimination of defining characteristics, as evidenced by:

Increased ability to test reality
Orientation to person, place, and time
Absence of hallucinations and delusions

Stabilization of emotions
Increased participation in care
Appropriate verbal feedback
Appropriate responses to environment
Absence of bizarre behavior
Increased decision-making and problem-solving abilities
Lowered anxiety levels

- Restore sensory/perceptual function by implementing following interventions:
  Assess stimuli present in environment: intensity, quantity, quality, repetitiveness, movement, change, novelty, incongruity, clarity, ambiguity.
- Alter environmental factors to increase meaningful stimuli and decrease extraneous stimuli:
  Use orienting features (e.g., clocks, calendars, windows, name tags, favorite objects).
- Maintain verbal contact, eye contact, and touch.
- Reduce unnecessary traffic, personnel, and noise.
- Structure routines.
- Structure input by giving clear, concise explanations of surroundings, treatments, and procedures.
- Allow frequent short visits by significant others.
- Orienting to reality:
  Address by name; introduce self frequently and regularly; state time and place.
- Explain and allow participation, when possible, in all tasks and treatments.
- Interpret sights, sounds, and smells present in environment.
- Explain routines and policies.
- Obtain feedback or perception of events and objects; clarify misperceptions.
- Assist in clarifying reality (see Altered Thought Processes on p. 1651 for more detailed intervention with hallucinations, delusions).

Chronic Care†

Oriented to surroundings, as evidenced by:

Orientation to person, time, and place
Recollections of past and present events
Verbalization of future plans
Absence of confusion

- Use reality orientation techniques:
  Address by name; orient to time.
  Point out surroundings; identify self.
  Structure input with concrete, concise explanations.
  Maintain eye contact.
  Reinforce behavior that is reality oriented (e.g., responding to meaningful comments).
- Provide meaningful stimuli and reduce extraneous stimuli in environment:
  Keep clocks and calendars in view; make use of windows and outdoors.

*References 1, 2, 5, 7, 8, 10-12.

†References 1, 4, 5, 7, 9, 11.

Observe holidays and significant occasions.
Provide structured routines.
Place familiar objects in plain sight.
Structure experiences that make use of all senses.

Increase appropriate social interaction, as evidenced by:

Appropriate response to questions and cues
Initiation of interaction
Increase in interaction time
Increase in meaningful interaction
Verbalization about social events, time spent with others, and future plans

- Arrange physical environment to encourage interaction (open spaces; circles instead of rows); increase mobility with wheelchairs, walkers, and carts.
- Encourage exploration of surroundings; encourage verbalization of experiences, desires, and thoughts.
- Set up interactions with others in structural settings with defined purpose.
- Encourage reminiscence.
- Encourage decision making.
- Use small group sessions to widen interaction.

Principles and Rationale for Nursing Interventions

Perceptual adequacy and accuracy are necessary prerequisites to enable nurses and patients to engage in mutual goal setting and exploration of means for goal achievement.

The nursing diagnostic category Sensory/Perceptual Alterations on p. 1643 is an encompassing one. Alterations range from mild to severe; manifestations can be acute or chronic; age of affected persons ranges from infancy to old age. Thus many specific nursing interventions depend on individual patient characteristics, identified related factors for a particular patient, and defining characteristics for the patient.

Nursing care is divided into three major modes: prevention, acute care, and chronic care. *Prevention* requires careful assessment of the patient's environment for risk factors. Patient education plays a major role. Once a pattern of defining characteristics appears and a diagnosis of sensory/perceptual alteration is made, the alteration may be classified as acute or chronic.

Acute alterations tend to be abrupt in onset and temporary in nature. The degree of alteration is usually severe and dramatic in presentation of defining characteristics (e.g., sudden confusion and disorientation, rapid large mood swings, bizarre behavior). Causes for acute alterations include trauma, drug intoxication, sudden sensory loss (blindness, deafness), acute pain, panic, and placement in intensive care units or recovery rooms.

Chronic alterations are progressive in onset and are subject to recurrence because of the long-term or permanent nature of the related factors. The degree of alteration may range from mild to severe, and defining characteristics may be subtle and ambiguous. When chronic alterations are left untreated, defining characteristics become more clear-cut and overt. Causes for chronic alterations typically include socially restricted environ-

ments (e.g., nursing homes, children's homes, prisons), declining sensory equipment, neurologic disease, chronic pain, prolonged immobility, social isolation, and chronic illness.

In all cases the ultimate goal is to promote, maintain, and restore optimum contact with reality. Nursing interventions are aimed at preventing, reducing, or eliminating related factors and defining characteristics.

▌ UNILATERAL NEGLECT

Unilateral neglect is a state in which an individual is perceptually unaware of and inattentive to one side of the body.

Associated with brain damage on the contralateral side, most often right cerebral hemisphere lesions (e.g., cerebrovascular accidents[10]), unilateral neglect is frequently accompanied by hemiplegia, hemiparesis, or hemianopia.[4,5]

The patient typically fails to complete one side of drawings, dress or groom the affected side of the body, or eat food from one half of a tray and may not respond to commands from someone standing in the unattended space.[2,5,12] In more severe forms patients may not realize that they are paralyzed or may not recognize their own limbs on the affected side.[2,11]

Although manifestations of unilateral neglect tend to be most pronounced in the first few weeks following the cerebral damage, some deficits may persist for months or years.[1,7] Symptoms tend to resolve slowly and may complicate patient rehabilitation.[9,10] Certainly the behavior of patients with unilateral neglect presents a challenge for nursing management.

Related Factors[1,2,5,6]

Effects of disturbed perceptual abilities, e.g., hemianopia
One-sided blindness
Neurologic illness or trauma

Defining Characteristics[5,6,10,12]

Consistent inattention to stimuli on affected side
Inadequate self-care
Absence of positioning or safety precautions in regard to affected side
Does not look toward affected side
Leaves food on plate on affected side

Expected Patient Outcomes & Nursing Interventions*

Realistic awareness of perceptual deficit, as evidenced by:

Verbalization of realistic estimation of degree of deficit
Does not ignore or underestimate

- Explain to patient that one side is being neglected; explain cause and mechanisms: repeat, as needed; encourage pa-

---

*References 2, 3, 5, 8, 11, 12.

tient to share perceptions; provide realistic feedback; *the nurse can assist the patient to understand and acknowledge the condition by encouraging the patient to share perceptions and by providing realistic feedback.*

Protection from injury; accidents prevented or minimized, as demonstrated by:

Absence of physical or reported evidence of injury.

- Provide safe environment; regularly orient patient to environment; remove excess furniture and equipment; provide good lighting; place call bell and frequently used objects on unaffected side within easy reach; keep side rail up on affected side; *structuring the environment to decrease hazards is essential to safety.*
- Supervise or assist to transfer and ambulate *to ensure protection from injury for the affected side;* protect neglected side during activities; teach patient to assume this responsibility; teach patient to check position of limbs on affected side to prevent unfelt trauma.
- Note perceptual deficit on patient record and in patient's room to inform caregivers; *continuity of safe care is enhanced when all caregivers are aware of the patient's perceptual deficits.*

Adequate knowledge and skill in adaptive coping strategies, as evidenced by:

Responses to verbal or visual cues to decrease neglect of affected side
Compensation for perceptual loss
Scanning and protection of affected side
Increased participation and independence in ADLs
Verbalization of progress in regard to perceptual deficit

- *Initially,* arrange environment within patient's perceptual field *in order to assist compensation for perceptual deficit* (e.g., place frequently used items on unaffected side).
- *After initial stress, to promote conscious attention to neglected side:*
    Place frequently used items on affected side.
    Position patient so affected side is in view.
    Talk to patient from affected side.
- Spend time with patient manipulating affected side and encouraging patient to use it.
    Have patient handle ignored limbs with unaffected side.
    Increase stimulation to affected side by touching, or massage with scented lotion.
    Use visual and verbal communication regarding limb placement on affected side.
    Verbal, visual, and tactile cues to decrease neglect of the affected side are effective in enhancing perceptual functioning.
- Teach patient to scan affected side; place clock or some frequently used item on side of deficit *to help establish pattern of scanning.*
- Use "cueing" to affected side *to increase awareness of that side:*
    Mark red line in margin of books on affected side.
    Attach small bells to limbs of affected side.

- Place food tray toward unaffected side; teach patient to rotate plate periodically.
- Encourage patient to perform activities of daily living (ADLs) (e.g., toothbrushing in front of mirror). Supervise and give feedback. *Activities that direct attention to the neglected side can increase awareness and use of that side.*
- Decrease confusing stimuli:
    Avoid relocation.
    Maintain constancy of caregivers and consistent routine for self-care.
    Explain procedures and treatment well in advance.
    An established plan of care by consistent caregivers can decrease distortions in perception and subsequent disorientation.
- Include family in rehabilitation process *so that they understand, support, and can continue it in home environment.*

Reduction or resolution of deficit or adaptation to deficit, as evidenced by:

Absence or reduction of defining characteristics of unilateral neglect.

- Assess regularly for degree of deficit, contributing factors, and adaptation to deficit; *progress toward goals is facilitated by ongoing evaluation of the effectiveness of intervention and by periodic revisions in the rehabilitation plan.*

Principles and Rationale for Nursing Intervention

Initially, nursing management for the patient with unilateral neglect is oriented toward provision of safety and assistance in developing a realistic awareness of the perceptual deficit. Structuring the environment to decrease hazards is essential for the patient who typically ignores or underestimates the disability during this period.[2,12] An established plan of care and assistance with ADLs by consistent caregivers can do much to decrease the confusion and disorientation that results from distortions in perception.[5] The nurse can assist the patient to understand and acknowledge the condition by encouraging the patient to share perceptions and by providing realistic feedback in response.

Active rehabilitation focuses on decreasing the deficit and increasing the patient's ability to manage self-care. This is accomplished by helping the patient organize and interpret experiences and the environment. Verbal and visual cues to decrease neglect of the affected side have demonstrated effectiveness in enhancing perceptual functioning.[3,9,11] An environment that provides the high levels of meaningful sensory stimulation is also effective.[5] Specific activities that involve assisting the patient to direct attention to the affected side can improve functional performance in activities of daily living.[9] Involvement of the family in the rehabilitation process facilitates their understanding and support in both hospital and home environments.[4]

◾ KNOWLEDGE DEFICIT (SPECIFY)

◾ Knowledge deficit is a state in which specific information is lacking.

Knowledge deficit occurs frequently, usually for one of four reasons:

1. The patient may have entered a new health condition (e.g., pregnancy), may be undergoing newly prescribed treatments or diagnostic tests, may be taking new medications, or may be beginning a new developmental phase (e.g., adolescence, parenthood, old age). If one has not experienced these states before or learned about them from others in the culture, knowledge deficit is possible.

2. Some patients may not have access to information or know where to seek it; others may have providers who are not interested in teaching them or who cannot be understood because of cultural or language differences. This lack of an open, information-flowing relationship with a provider often causes the patient to misinterpret information or to forget it because of disuse or lack of reinforcement for correct use.

3. Temporary or permanent deficits in ability to learn often have a physiologic base and may preclude removal of knowledge deficits through instructional means. High blood urea nitrogen concentration, low oxygenation of the blood, chemical substances (e.g., alcohol, drugs), brain damage from trauma or cerebrovascular accident, mental retardation, or to a lesser extent fatigue are examples, as are limitations caused by immature developmental stage.

4. Lack of motivation to learn, often accompanied by anxiety and coupled with lack of adherence to a health care regimen, is another typical reason for knowledge deficit.

Several cautions are in order. It should not be assumed that a patient has a knowledge deficit if one or more of these four conditions is present; adequate assessment to establish that there is a knowledge deficit is necessary. Also, the diagnosis requires specificity of which knowledge elements are absent, and their interaction with other cognitive elements. For example, research on causes of delay in seeking treatment for heart attack shows that some people do not experience the classic symptoms; therefore, some patients do not recognize their symptoms as being cardiac in origin. Similarly, a study of women trying to self-diagnose preterm labor found that even if they are knowledgable about symptoms, women can become confused when there is no symptom pattern, or if primagravidas, they have no prior experience for comparison of the symptoms. Thus, not only must factual knowledge accurately describe the variation in symptoms, people need to learn how to monitor and interpret bodily feelings.

The standard by which to judge the adequacy of knowledge (and thus absence of a deficit) is changing rapidly as more self-management is required, not only to assist those with chronic illness, but also to contain health care costs in general and to maintain patients in their normal social settings. Sometimes knowledge deficit is defined by a legal standard, as in informed consent. It also must be noted that knowledge is the lowest level of cognitive learning—recalling or remembering information as opposed to applying and synthesizing information in problem solving. In general, it has been found that removal of knowledge deficits is insufficient for most significant health behavior changes. Attitudinal change, a higher level of understanding, and practiced behavioral sequences with adequate reinforcement are necessary. Much health teaching is still knowledge-oriented, probably because it is much easier to teach information than it is to change behavior.

Related Factors

Need to make sense of life-threatening diseases

Underdeveloped or inappropriate cognitive level

Low level of formal education, including illiteracy

Lack of orientation to future

Lack of emotional stability in patient, family, or environment, often linked to chaotic or irresponsible behavior

Inadequate economic resources

Irrational beliefs

Lack of belief in efficacy of treatment

Denial regarding diagnosis and/or need to learn

Ineffective coping regarding diagnosis or treatment

Inadequate self-confidence to carry out specific action (self-efficacy)

Self-defeating attitudes: frustration, confusion

Impaired practitioner/patient communication

Depression and excessive anxiety

Fantasies that one is immune from harm; denial of need for knowledge

Altered locus of control

Social isolation restricting sources of information

Lack of awareness by health care providers of body of knowledge important to patients

Lack of appropriate cultural focus in available information

For patients on ongoing regimen, past experiences and learning, including misinformation

New stressor in patient's life

Impairment of neurologic and perceptual functioning; abnormal physiology regarding blood oxygenation or clearance of waste products from body; impaired thinking caused by drugs and/or alcohol

Lack of exposure

Decreased motivation to learn

Inability to recall

Anger and hostility

Withdrawal

Misinterpretation of information

Inability to see or hear

Need to follow new, complex treatment

Insufficient maturation to understand

In community, lack of access to information, self-defeating attitudes, lack of a custom, or lack of open communication between health care providers and patients

Defining Characteristics

Verbalization of problem, which can point out lack of knowledge or perception of inability to cope

Inaccurate or no follow-through of instructions

Inadequate performance of test or task

Occurrence of preventable and undesired event (e.g., premature readmission)

Inability to make decision about own care

Not seeking needed services

Infant or child not meeting developmental norms because of actions of caregiver

Living with a health problem, below level of potential well-being

Overdependence on others for self-care

Request for information

Inability to repeat and comprehend correctly information taught

Inability to demonstrate correctly skills previously taught

Inability to care for self after discharge

Verbalization of inaccurate information

Failure to adhere

Development of complications or exacerbations

Multiple hospitalizations for the same problem

Social support provides an opportunity for patients to clarify their situation and obtain new information. It also helps in development of a cognitive schema, or way of conceptualizing their situation, and ways of coping that they had not considered. Teaching is not only a focused intervention to deal with a particular knowledge deficit. It is also an integral part of the everyday provider/patient relationship, with the goal of making patients independent regarding health in their natural environments.

Patient education usually cannot assist with development of basic learning skills. In this day of required self-management, however, it is important to help patients become as independent as possible in recognizing and resolving their own knowledge deficits. The questioning, discussing, application, and feedback approach is most likely to develop not only knowledge but greater satisfaction, improved problem-solving, and more complete learning.

Increasingly, summaries of research studies of the outcomes of interventions are available that include in their goals the alleviation of knowledge deficits, and the clinical outcomes that can follow. The results of these studies provide a guide for how successful interventions should be: (1) Devine[1]: psychoeducational interventions with adult surgical patients produced small to moderate-sized beneficial effects on recovery, postoperative pain, and psychological distress; (2) Hirano, Laurent, and Lorig[4]: patient education interventions produce improvement in symptoms of arthritis 15%-30% above the 20%-50% improvement attainable with medical care; (3) Meyer and Mark[6]: psychosocial interventions intended to improve the quality of life of adults with cancer found moderate effects on emotional and functional adjustment, and treatment- and disease-related symptoms. Each of these sets of interventions addressed knowledge deficits along with other learning and psychological needs.

Expected Patient Outcomes & Nursing Interventions

Acquire and use adequate knowledge, skill, and self-confidence to support needed health care decisions and activities satisfactory to patient, including procedures, medications, when to seek care, and use of appropriate community resources, as evidenced by:

Having adequate knowledge to carry out health care regimen

Explaining how and why to take action or perform skill

Using knowledge to lessen discomfort and side effects

Describing why decision was made

Having accurate expectations of likely outcomes of health care actions

- Check that communities and institutions provide freely available information through reading materials, hotlines, mass media, health fairs at work sites and schools, etc.
- At every provider/patient interaction, assess for knowledge deficit.
- Talk to patient's significant other to obtain evidence of knowledge deficit.
- Use patient's theories about his or her illness as a starting point for teaching, and continually seek patient's perceptions.
- During interactions, check frequently to see if patient understands.
- See if patient accepts diagnosis.
- Simplify information to conform to patient's terms, thought patterns, and daily routines.
- Set clear learning goals with patient.
- Be accessible to patient when he or she has a question; this may require new structures of care (e.g., a diabetes education center).
- Demonstrate to patient and family how to use information.
- Reinforce correct use of information, and ensure that others in patient's natural environment do the same.
- Teach patient how to set up system of cues in the environment to remember health actions.
- Teach patient how to rehearse mentally and physically, when possible, a necessary health action.
- Teach patient how to use rewards for positive health behaviors.
- Call patient to remind him or her; show support, and see if he or she has questions.
- Make certain patient is actively involved in decisions about own care.
- Provide opportunities for patient to gain sense of control over illness.
- Offer peer support network and opportunity for patient to watch others successfully mastering health care problems.
- Ask patient if he or she is satisfied with care.

- Use practice of knowledge and skill, perhaps with role playing, until patient feels confident and has met the standard.
- Use special teaching approaches to deal with neurologic learning deficits.
- After procedure, offer opportunity for reflection about what happened.
- Provide instruction in multiple modalities (visual, experimental, written, discussion) so that patient will remember it in various ways.
- Provide materials for patient to take so that he or she can review and use the new knowledge.
- Provide motivators by appealing to patient's interests and future uses of new knowledge, allowing patient to identify what is most important.

Acquire knowledge and become competent in how to guide own and others' development in area of health, in how to carry out health care activities necessary to well-being, and in how to cope adequately with health stresses, as evidenced by:

Monitoring body and mental health state for signs and symptoms of illness

Acting on basis of realistic expectations in guiding development of self and others

Describing how to use verified health knowledge in daily living

Moving ahead to take health actions when satisfied they are worthwhile including programs for self-management of disease and symptoms

Making participatory decisions with health care provider

Decrease in symptoms and indicators of disease state, and increase in indicators of health and well-being

Knowing where to obtain sources of health care information efficiently and doing so when needed

Describing problem-solving process to deal successfully with injury, threatening diagnosis, or persistent symptom

Describing how action met personal standards of adequate coping

Developing sense of mastery and self-efficacy regarding particular health behavior

Avoiding overreactions, feelings of helplessness and depression caused by inadequate knowledge and skill

- Teach with a questioning, discussion, application of knowledge, and feedback approach.
- Teach patient and family to use self-care protocols and instructional packages when appropriate.
- Teach patient how to find and use sources of knowledge and social support in the community.
- If available, help patient learn to use computerized monitoring systems (e.g., those providing diabetic persons with running summary of food and medication requirements met for the day).
- Contract with patient.
- Build on patient's developmental and learning level: this may require assistance with transferring and integrating knowledge into his or her life.

- Use like individuals as models of appropriate knowledge and motivation.
- Use culturally relevant instruction.
- Provide assists for those with sensory or psychomotor limitations, such as books with large print for visually impaired patients.
- Provide environment conducive to concentration and learning.

Principles and Rationale for Nursing Interventions

Essentially all evidence of knowledge deficit is more or less indirect. With assessment, the nurse sets up situations in which the quality of the inference obtained from verbalizations or behaviors is as strong and direct as possible: ask the patient directly or set up an unobtrusive test. Because most meaningful health behaviors require knowledge, motivation, and skill, it is important in the assessment to seek evidence in each of these areas to obtain as complete a diagnosis as possible. This means data gathered must be both objective, to determine adequacy of present knowledge and behaviors, and subjective, which is the source of crucial information about the patient's motivation, sense of self-efficacy, frame of reference, and cognitive schemata.

A diagnosis of knowledge deficit means the evidence gathered does not meet the standard of adequate knowledge. However, the nurse must be certain that the standard is justified and that the nurse intends to provide an opportunity for the patient to learn.

In general, nursing goals include helping the patient attain the knowledge and skills needed through the teaching and learning process. This includes assessing readiness, planning realistic goals, developing a teaching plan using appropriate multiple verbal, behavioral, and audiovisual instructional strategies, and evaluation of learning and reteaching when necessary.[8]

Active involvement of the patient is essential, as is practice of the thoughts and behaviors to be learned. For many, psychologic support and follow-up are important, along with a feeling of personal reward, sometimes developed through a contract with the provider, and involvement of the family. Instruction provides models for behavior, cues for correct responses, corrective feedback, and problem-solving strategies.

Learning in health care settings as they exist at present has many constraints for adequate knowledge and skill development. This has occurred in part because what was reimbursed and therefore rewarded were medical procedures, not adapted patients. At the same time it is clearly possible to alter delivery of care so that teaching and learning are expected and rewarded components of care and consistent over sufficient periods so that complex learning can occur. Diabetes education and detection centers and oncology centers are examples of these new organizations of services in which education and learning are central. Also, examples of tools used for assessment can be found in various sources, such as assessment of patient knowledge of arthritis and its self-management, assessment of self-efficacy among college students in correct use of condoms, or assessment of self-efficacy of battered women in dealing with their situation. Self-efficacy involves not only knowing what to do but also having confidence that one can do it in various stressful situations. Tools that measure knowledge can be used at the beginning of the nursing process to assess patient knowledge and need to learn and at the end to evaluate patient knowledge after an appropriate intervention. It should be noted that very few knowledge evaluation tools have been tested for their ability to measure the domain of knowledge in question (validity and reliability).

ALTERED THOUGHT PROCESSES

Altered thought processes is a state in which an individual experiences a disruption in cognitive operations and activities.

As nursing diagnoses, altered thought processes and sensory/perceptual alterations are closely aligned. Many of the defining characteristics and nursing interventions are similar. This is to be expected because perception and thought are both higher-order cognitive processes. Because the two processes are internal and highly interrelated, an alteration in either process is likely to produce an alteration in the other. (See Sensory/Perceptual Alterations.)

Carpenito[4] makes a distinction between the two diagnoses on the basis of cause. She states that sensory/perceptual alterations result from environmental, sensory, physical, or motor alterations. Altered thought processes are seen as stemming from personality and mental disorders. This may serve as a viable distinction, although it should be noted that both diagnoses share some common ground (e.g., chemical alteration). Based on this distinction, Carpenito[4] offers the following definition of altered thought processes: "A state in which an individual experiences a disruption in such mental activities as conscious thought, reality orientation, problem-solving, judgment, and comprehension related to coping."

A disruption in thought processes, whether in the area of comprehension, judgment, memory, problem solving, or other aspects, creates a disruption in the way one perceives reality. Thus one's thinking processes become nonreality-based, the critical defining characteristic for this nursing diagnosis. Additional defining characteristics assist in the evaluation of the severity of nonreality-based thinking and the extent of altered thought processes.

Related Factors[4,5,14,15]

Physiologic changes
Biochemical changes
Genetic predispositions
Psychologic conflicts
Impaired judgment
Ineffective coping
Loss of memory
Sleep deprivation
Substance abuse
Mental disorders and illnesses

Defining Characteristics[4,13,14,15]

Disruption of thinking process
　Disorientation in time, place, person, circumstances, or events
　Disordered sequencing of thought
　Impaired ability to think abstractly
　Impaired ability to solve problems and make decisions
　Impaired reasoning ability
　Impaired ability to grasp ideas
　Impaired ability to calculate
　Concretizing of ideas
Memory disruption
　Memory deficit
　Changes in remote, recent, and immediate memory
　Confabulation
Changes in attention span
　Distractibility
　Difficulty concentrating
　Inability to follow flow of conversation
Emotional changes
　Feelings of worthlessness
　Extreme sadness
　Mistrust
　Guilt
　Anxiety
　Lability
　Exaggerated response
　Fear of others, of losing control, of falling apart
　Decreased or shallow affect
　Apathy
Inaccurate interpretation of stimuli
　Hallucinations
　Delusions
　Ideas of reference
　Obsessions
Changes in routine patterns and habits
　Altered sleep pattern
　Insomnia
　Too much sleep
　Change in grooming habits
　Change in eating habits
　Change in motor activity: repetition, agitation
　Hypervigilance
　Inappropriate social behavior
Bizarre thinking, as noted by language use
　Inappropriate use of global pronouns and global adjectives
　Evidence of automatic thinking: universal "you know," assumption that listener knows omitted details
　Circumstantiality: inability to get to the point

Lack of verbal distinction between thoughts, feelings, and actions

Use of indirect statements, extensive use of modifiers and qualifiers

Overgeneralization

Imputing intentions to others

Loose connection of ideas

Use of neologisms

Expected Patient Outcomes & Nursing Interventions*

Safety maintained (no injury to self or others), as evidenced by:

Lack of reported or observed injury

Absence or decrease in violent response

Absence or decrease in suicidal behavior

Ability to control own behavior

- Maintain patient safety.
- Prevent suicide and aggression.
- Assess for suicide potential (history, plans for self-harm, verbalization of desire to die, disposal of possessions, viewing self in past tense).
- Institute suicide precautions, as indicated.
- Assess potential for aggressive behavior.
- Identify early signs of aggressive behavior.
- Remove environmental factors that contribute to aggression.
- Promote individual control:
    Set limits on destructive behavior.
    Encourage verbalization and safe acting-out behaviors, within limits.
    Allow choice within constraint.
    Use seclusion if indicated.
- Help patient set limits on own behavior.
    Substitute verbalizations and physical activity for behavioral acting out.
    Set incremental goals.
    Recall and repeat successful ways of coping.

Anxiety and stress reduced, as evidenced by:

Verbal statements that indicate that patient feels less anxious

Physical signs of stress and anxiety decreased or absent

- Approach in calm, nurturing manner:
    Use calm, level voice, lower tone, familiar terms.
    Avoid sudden movements, compose facial expression.
- Provide physical and emotional structure, as needed:
Physical structure. Environment is altered to provide for safety and comfort.
Emotional structure. A prediction of feelings and occurrences and an imaging of situations that evoke safety and comfort exists.

*References 1, 2, 4, 8-12, 15-18.

Interpretation of reality is realistic and constructive, as evidenced by:

Clearer, more well-rounded verbalizations (decrease in generalizations, deletions, nominalistic statements, distortions of control, and distortions of intent)

Orientation to environment, self, time, and space

Decrease in or absence of delusions or hallucinations

Increased signs of problem solving and abstract reasoning abilities

- Explore patient's representation of reality by analyzing language behavior:
    Listen intently to patient's verbal and nonverbal communication.
    Analyze communication for generalization and distortions.
- Assist patient in clarifying representation of reality:
    Clarify generalizations ("Nobody pays any attention to what I say." Clarify who, specifically. Ask, "What, specifically, do you say?") Elicit deletions in communication ("I am scared." Scared about what?) Clarify nominalistic statements. Change statements of event into statements of process ("I hate my relationship with my wife." Explore "relating" as a process versus "relationship" as an event.) Challenge distortions of control ("Steve makes me act up." Repeat statement with emphasis on "Steve makes?" Explore how that is possible.) Challenge distortions that impute intentions to others ("The doctor hates me." Analyze basis for statement: "What was said or done that makes you feel your doctor hates you?")
- Use reality orientation where indicated:
    Orient to person, time, and place.
    Use direct terminology, clear sentence structure. Avoid generalization. Use terms that help patient maintain individuality (e.g., "I" instead of "we"). Avoid vagueness, asides, and whispered comments. Have patient focus on real things and people.

Ability to relate with others in a positive manner is increased, as evidenced by:

Functioning as a group member (expressing thoughts and feelings: making wants and needs known to group, using group responses as guide to monitoring behavior)

Increasing interaction with others

Observation of appropriate interaction process

- Provide group process situations that allow patients to experience relating in a controlled setting.
- Encourage validation of thoughts and feelings.
- Encourage patient to ask for wants and to express feelings.
- Help patient examine the effect of patient's behavior on others.
- Help patient recognize use of and need for personal space and distance.

Assumes responsibility for self-care, as evidenced by:

Contributions to treatment plan
Follow-through on assumed responsibility
Seeking increased responsibility for self-activities and behavior
Increase in self-monitoring

- Provide opportunity for patient to contribute to own treatment plan.
- Encourage acceptance of responsibility for actions and interactions.
- Encourage acceptance of responsibility for seeking help, following treatment plans, and changing behaviors.

Principles and Rationale for Nursing Interventions

The goal of nursing intervention for patients with altered thought processes is to improve the individual's ability to define and communicate reality. This goal is achieved primarily through a patient/nurse dyadic interaction or small group process. Such encounters frequently occur in, but need not be limited to, mental health care settings. Nursing intervention strategies are aimed at reducing or eliminating related factors and/or defining characteristics.

Thought and language are closely tied and interrelated.[7] Therefore it is logical to assume that altered thought processes are reflected in the patient's language behavior. The nursing interventions are based on this link between cognitive processes and language.

Paradoxically, the same cognitive processes that allow survival, growth, and change can also block growth, inhibit change, and produce limitations in living. Through the cognitive processes (thought, perception, memory, judgment) the patient creates his or her own unique representation or model of reality. That model is bounded by physical, social, and physiologic factors that make each representation unique.

Three major mechanisms are used in a person's model making: generalization, deletion, and distortion.[1] *Generalization* is the process by which elements from an experience structure themselves to represent a category; the experience is an example of this category. For example, one generalizes from the experience of being cut that knives are sharp and must be used with care. This is a useful and necessary coping skill. If, however, one were to refuse to use knives at all or even to have knives in the house as a result of being cut, the generalization has become limiting.

Deletion is a process of selective attention to certain parts of an experience (e.g., the ability to read while the television is on). Deletion allows one to manage the world and not be overwhelmed. However, one can also use deletion in ways that are limiting (e.g., not hearing compliments about accomplishments; hearing only criticism).

Distortion is a process of experience shifting. It allows one to interpret experience under a different set of circumstances or to project an experience into the future (e.g., fantasizing). Distortion can also be limiting if experiences are shifted in a limiting fashion (e.g., compliments about accomplishments might be heard but shifted to mean that the person giving the compliment must want something).

These three mechanisms work together to create a person's model of reality. An altered cognitive process disrupts or distorts this model. These alterations can be detected by viewing the individual's model of reality, as expressed symbolically in language behavior. Exploration of the patient's use of generalization, deletion, and distortion can clarify his or her reality model. Limiting uses of generalization, deletion, and distortion can then be challenged. This allows patients to broaden their models of reality.

■ ACUTE CONFUSION

Acute confusion is the abrupt onset of a cluster of global, transient changes and disturbances in attention, cognition, psychomotor activity, level of consciousness, and or sleep/wake cycle.[18]

Acute confusion refers to an acute organic mental disorder commonly seen in the elderly and medically ill and characterized by disorganized thinking, global cognitive impairment, and attentional difficulties.[15] Frequently described in the literature by such terms as delirium, encephalopathy, acute brain syndrome, toxic psychosis, postoperative delirium, and nocturnal delirium or "sundowning,"[1,13,30] Acute confusion results from multifactorial causes that are physiologic, environmental, or psychosocial in nature. This syndrome is usually transitory and fluctuating, affecting brain functioning until the underlying medical problem is treated. Medical conditions contributing to acute confusion include brain trauma and disease, organ failure, infections, systemic diseases affecting the brain, toxic states from illicit substances or prescribed medications, withdrawal from alcohol and other addictive substances, endocrine disorders, and metabolic disorders, among other myriad causes.[9,12,13,28] Severe psychosocial stress, relocation, immobilization, and sensory deprivation or overload are also risk factors for acute confusion.[14,15] Classical clinical presentation of acute confusion includes sudden onset, waxing and waning of symptoms, and quick resolution of cognitive impairment and behavioral problems after organic causes are treated. Vulnerable groups of patients include the elderly, especially those with prior cognitive impairment, advanced age, and fracture;[25] persons with compromised brain function from disease or trauma; the chronically medically ill; patients treated with multiple medications; and individuals with alcohol and substance abuse problems.[2,8]

Acute confusion is frequently underdetected in the medically ill and elderly and may mimic many psychiatric disorders in presentation.[11] For example, it is common to misdiagnose acute confusion in a patient with depression if the person is quietly confused and hypoalert.[5] An agitated patient may appear manic or delusional when acute confusion related to an untreated organic problem is the correct diagnosis. Acute confusion is also easily misidentified as dementia or chronic confusion, but differs in onset, that is, abrupt onset in acute confusion versus an insidious progression of cognitive impairment in chronic confusion.[9] A common prototype of cognitive problems seen in hospitalized patients is the demented individual with superimposed delirium.[14]

Since acute confusion is frequently unrecognized in patients or presents in a confusing clinical pattern, early assessment and treatment is thus imperative in order to facilitate rapid medical treatment and appropriate nursing care. Common negative outcomes associated with acute confusion include increased length of hospital stay, increased comorbidities such as falls and other injuries, increased disruptive behaviors that increase the intensity of nursing care required, and use of restraints, and increased mortality in the elderly.*

Related Factors†

Advanced age (over 60 years)
Dementia
Alcohol abuse
Drug abuse
Precipitating organic factors
  Intoxication from medically prescribed medications
  Polypharmacy
  Monotherapy with corticosteroids, benzodiazepines, anticholinergics, digoxin, antihypertensives, narcotic analgesics, histamine-2-receptor blockers, psychotropics
  Intoxication from street drugs
  Intoxication from alcohol
  Withdrawal from alcohol
  Infections (including sepsis, AIDS)
  Electrolyte abnormalities
  Hypoxia
  Organ failure (e.g., renal and hepatic)
  Acute pain
  Altered body temperature
  Elimination problems (fecal impaction, urinary retention)
  Sleep deprivation
  Trauma (including burns)
Recent surgical procedure (e.g., cardiac surgery)
Injury from physical agents (e.g., hypothermia, heat stroke)
Recent relocation (especially in the elderly)
Immobilization
Sensory deprivation or overload (e.g., isolation, excessive noise)

Defining Characteristics[2,7,14]

Fluctuation in cognition (e.g., global cognitive impairment)
Fluctuation in sleep/wake cycle (e.g., insomnia, hypersomnia)

Fluctuation in level of consciousness (e.g., hyperalert or hypoalert)
Attentional changes (inability to maintain concentration)
Fluctuation in psychomotor activity (e.g., increased agitation, restlessness, or slowing)
Misperceptions
Hallucinations (especially visual)
Poorly organized delusions
Lack of motivation to initiate and/or follow through with goal-directed or purposeful behavior

Expected Patient Outcomes and Nursing Interventions‡

Appropriate level of psychomotor activity as evidenced by:

Decreased risk of injury to self or others
Decreased agitation level
Decreased slowing or lethargy
- Assess for causes of inappropriate activity level:
    Monitor laboratory data for acute electrolyte imbalances, abnormal hepatic and renal function *for early detection of organ failure,* and infection (especially urinary tract infection and pneumonia in the elderly.
    Monitor vital signs *to identify infection (febrile states), increased autonomic irritability related to withdrawal syndromes (especially withdrawal from alcohol, benzodizepines, or narcotic analgesics); increased intracranial pressure; level of oxygenation; and pain level. These conditions contribute to agitation and acute confusion.*
    Monitor fluid intake. *Dehydration causes electrolyte disturbances and may exacerbate cognitive problems.*
    Monitor therapeutic medication records and therapeutic drug levels (e.g., digoxin, phenytoin, lithium) *to assess for early toxicity.*
    Assess for elimination problems (e.g., urinary retention, fecal impaction) *especially in the demented elderly who may not be able to communicate distress.*
    Assess level of pain especially in the elderly postoperative patient, and utilize appropriate interventions for pain control. *A demented patient may be unable to reliably request pain medication or use a patient-controlled analgesia pump (PCA) appropriately due to waxing and waning of acute confusion.*
- Maintain a safe environment to reduce risk of injury.
    Place patient in room close to nurses' station whenever possible and check frequently. *Patients with acute confusion are frequently impulsive with global cognitive deficits that fluctuate widely. Increased surveillance will facilitate early assessment and treatment of organic problems, as well as decrease risk of injury.*

---

*References 8, 9, 13, 21, 28, 33.
†References 3, 4, 7, 14, 16, 19, 24, 27, 28, 30, 31.
‡References 3, 6, 10, 11, 15, 17, 20, 22, 23, 26, 29, 32.

Restrict patient's access to essential intravenous lines, endotracheal tubing, oxygen nasal prongs, and other equipment by frequently orienting patient, restricting access by concealment when appropriate, and offering patient an alternative object to hold or pull (e.g., wash cloth, safe toy).

Use soft limb or hard restraints sparingly and only on a time-limited basis *to protect patient from falls and self-injury, such as extubating self.*

Administer high-potency neuroleptic medication as ordered by physician (e.g., haloperidol), and minimize use of benzodiazepines *since they may worsen acute confusion.*
Use only in alcohol and sedative-hypnotic withdrawal.

Improved cognitive functioning as evidenced by:

Increased attention and concentration
Improved orientation
Increased recent and remote memory
Increased ability to follow commands and process new information

- Assess cognitive status on admission to the hospital and every shift (orientation, attention and concentration, memory, thought processes) *to obtain baseline information.*
    Obtain collateral information from care providers, family, and medical records *to ascertain patient's baseline cognitive functioning.*
    Use bedside mental status questions or mental status questionnaires such as Folstein's Mini-Mental State Examination (MMSE) or Pfeiffer's Short Portable Mental Status Questionnaire (SPMSQ).
- Reorient patient frequently to surroundings, routines, date and time, reason for hospitalization, and names of care providers *as short-term memory is impaired in acute confusion and disorientation will increase anxiety.*
- Use visual cues for orientation: signs in the room, signs on door, clocks, and calendars, instructional signs at bedside, (e.g., "Call nurse. Do not get out of bed alone.").
- Modify the environment to decrease incidence of sensory-perceptual alterations:
    Avoid lighting that contributes to shadows.
    Provide sensory aides (e.g., corrective lenses, hearing aids).
    Avoid overstimulation or sensory isolation.
    Maintain comfortable room temperature.
- Maintain consistent care providers *in order to provide consistency and decrease anxiety.*
- Communicate with patient in brief, simple, concrete language *as abstract thinking is impaired in acute confusion.*

Improved sleep-wake cycle as evidenced by:

Ability to rest and sleep.
Normal sleep/wake patterns are maintained.

- Assess for sleep deprivation.
- Maintain sleep/wake cycles (e.g., curtains open during the day to increase light, lights off at night to promote sleep).

- Allow for rest periods during the day *to decrease fatigue and overstimulation.*
- Establish a schedule for patient to promote normal sleep/wake cycles and rest periods.
- Continue familiar bedtime routines whenever possible.

Principles and Rationale for Nursing Interventions

Nursing interventions for Acute Confusion focus on early assessment of risk factors and ongoing communication to the medical team about physical factors assessed to be contributory to transient, global cognitive impairment. Timely medical treatment and prevention of comorbidities are thus facilitated, along with increased costs and acuity of nursing care. Ongoing interdisciplinary collaboration between clinicians about cognitive assessment of the patient will increase consistency and appropriateness of interventions. For example, patient teaching cannot occur effectively if the individual is unable to maintain attention and concentration due to undiagnosed, untreated acute confusion.

The importance of supportive care in acute confusion cannot be overemphasized. Agitation, misperceptions, and disorientation create anxiety and a sense of threat to the patient. Interventions that focus on anxiety reduction and correction of environmental irritants will be most helpful to the patient experiencing acute confusion. Non-threatening, non-confrontational reality orientation and frequent contact with the confused individual will reduce anxiety and allow for ongoing monitoring of mental status.

Patients and family members should be reminded that acute confusion is a transitory, treatable, organic mental disorder. While symptoms are frightening and disruptive, a return to baseline functioning is a realistic expected outcome following medical treatment of underlying causes. Discharge planning should include a review of multifactorial risk factors and defining characteristics of acute confusion to allow for prevention as well as early assessment of the syndrome by family or community providers.

■ CHRONIC CONFUSION

■ Chronic Confusion is an irreversible, long-standing, and/or progressive deterioration of intellect and personality characterized by decreased ability to interpret environmental stimuli, decreased capacity for intellectual thought processes, and manifested by disturbances of memory, orientation, and behavior.

Chronic confusional states, also referred to as dementia, are irreversible as the result of a degenerative type of cerebral pathology.[1,3,19] Elderly individuals experiencing such disease processes generally demonstrate a long and steady deterioration in functional and intellectual abilities as well as a kaleidoscope of behavioral changes. Dementia (chronic confusion) affects approximately 10%-45% of the U.S. population over age 65; those that are 85 and older have a greater incidence of a dementia diagnosis.[20] The cost of health care for the individual with dementia is greater, associated with an extended length of acute care stay, and requirements for more resources to provide for the special care needs of this population.[16] Approaching care planning often requires the participation of a multidisciplinary team with the nurse coordinating care to meet patient needs in a consistent and efficient manner.[6]

The individual labeled as confused often displays a behavioral inconsistency with the environment. Response to environmental stimuli, problem-solving ability, and capacity to follow complex instruction is compromised. A confused patient often spends his/her time in a solitary activity, does nothing or exhibits disruptive behavior that may include wandering, resisting care, and agitation. Many patients are unable to communicate their needs. The dementia patient requires increased time and supervision to provide for their safety and well-being. Management and the provision of care for these individuals can present an overwhelming challenge.[2,5,17]

Related Factors

Alzheimer's disease
Dementia of the Alzheimer's type
AIDS-related dementia
Multi-infarct dementia
Cerebral vascular accident
Korsakoff's psychosis
Head injury

Defining Characteristics[1-21]

Clinical evidence of organic impairment
Progressive or long-standing cognitive impairment
Altered interpretation of stimuli
Altered response to stimuli
No change in consciousness
Impaired memory (short term, long term)
Impaired orientation to person, time and/or place
Impaired ability for abstraction and conceptualization
Altered personality
Impaired socialization
Depression

Expected Patient Outcomes & Nursing Interventions

The patient will be able to function in a structured environment, as evidenced by:

Establishing a consistent daily routine and environment that will enable the patient to compensate for inability to plan activities
- Post a written daily routine for patient to follow. *Written directions or schedules provide additional cues to the chronically confused individual who retains the ability to read.*[1,18]

- Provide a consistent caregiver(s). *Patients will experience increased security when cared for by people they recognize.*[5,16]
- Provide a daily time for small group activity that is valued by patient, such as music, art, reminiscence group, selected television program, Bible therapy. *Planned activities are beneficial if they are pleasurable and incorporate the patient's culture, habits, values, manners, preferences, and occupation.*[8,10,12]
- Place meaningful possessions (photographs, mementos, favorite furniture) in the patient's environment. *Familiar belongings promote a sense of security.*[16]
- Avoid change in room environment, such as reassignment of patient's room, rearrangement of furniture or items, holiday decoration. *Frequent environment change may produce conflicting cues.*[4]

Ensuring that the patient has optimal sensory input to enable them to participate within the environment
- Make provision for optimal sensory input (eye glasses are clean, hearing aid is functional, absence of cerumen impaction): *The cognitively impaired individual is at risk for misinterpretation of environment when sensory input is not accurate.*[1,4]
- Provide adequate nonglare lighting. *Visual perceptions may be altered by glare or shadows.*[4]
- Eliminate unnecessary environmental stimuli (excessive noise level, multiple conversation/activity, violent/aggressive movies or television programs): *Disturbing visual images or loud noise can precipitate a catastrophic reaction.*[14]

Providing opportunities for meaningful communication and socialization
- Provide opportunity for one-to-one conversation with caregiver(s). *Providing sufficient time for interacting with patient reinforces socialization skill and a sense of self-worth.*[9]
- Maintain eye contact, smile and present a pleasant affect when interacting with the patient. *Verbal and nonverbal communications are important in establishing a relationship with a cognitively impaired person.*[18]
- Encourage continued interaction with a pet (allow pet to remain with patient, allow pet to visit patient if an inpatient, or provide access to animal-assisted therapy). *Pets provide links to the past, encourage conversation, and provide a pleasurable activity option.*[16]

The patient will demonstrate no increase in episodes of behavioral disturbance, as evidenced by:

Identification of situations and/or circumstances that precipitate the individual's episodes of behavioral disturbance
- Initiate use of an observational instrument to document episodes and context of incidents of behavioral disturbance. *Documentation of behavior over time provides data to identify precursors to behavioral events.*[4]
- Educate caregiver/staff to possible "triggers" and appropriate response (i.e., time-out, rest, distraction) to behav-

ioral disturbance. *Early intervention may prevent or modify a behavioral disturbance.*[11]

- Communicate new or relevant client information to other staff who see the patient. *Communication among staff is vital to the provision of continuity of care to the cognitively impaired client.*[18]

Implement strategies to decrease incidents of behavioral disturbance

- Maintain a level of environmental stimuli below the individual's "trigger" threshold. *Dysfunctional behavior occurs if stress levels exceed the individual's tolerance.*[18]
- Communicate using simple one-step commands. *Complex sequenced instructions are overwhelming to the cognitively impaired individual.*[15,18]
- Allow sufficient time for completion of directed task. *Sensory input/communication is slowly interpreted by the individual with dementia.*[18]

Principles and Rationale for Nursing Interventions

The cognitively impaired individual is able to experience optimal function in a supportive, structured environment. The physical setting and staff contribute to the milieu that makes up the patient's environment. The staff must interact with the patient using a positive approach and communication skills that demonstrate a high regard for the individual. Consistency in daily routine and caregivers (staff) play an important part in successful care delivery for this population. The provision of items familiar to the individual (i.e., photographs, furniture, special possessions) will support a sense of belonging and comfort. Controlling the bombardment of external stimuli (i.e., noise level, traffic activity, disturbing visual images) that affects the milieu is critical. Activities must be selected based on the unique needs and interests of the patient.

It is important to establish a historical behavior baseline through interviewing the family and/or caregiver. Environmental change, such as admission to an inpatient setting, may precipitate episodes of problematic behavior for individuals with cognitive impairment. It may be necessary to initiate a monitor that utilizes systematic observation of episodes of behavioral disturbance over a twenty-four to thirty-six hour period. All staff must be alert to subtle changes that may effect patient response and record incidents accurately. The staff and family members may benefit from reviewing results of the behavior monitor and the opportunity to validate their own experiences. This discussion may provide opportunities for family and/or caregiver education.

▌ IMPAIRED ENVIRONMENTAL INTERPRETATION SYNDROME

▌ Impaired Environmental Interpretation Syndrome is a consistent lack of orientation to person, time, or circumstances over more than 3-6 months, necessitating a protective environment.

This population requires increased time and supervision to provide for their safety and well-being. The confused person displays a behavioral inconsistency with the immediate environment. His/her response to environmental stimuli, problem-solving ability, and capacity to follow complex instruction is compromised. The person may not be aware of the change in his/her behavior or may not recognize that they are no longer participating in usual activities. They often spend their time in a solitary activity, do nothing, or engage in behaviors such as pacing or wandering. The degree of cognitive impairment is moderate to severe and usually necessitates admission or placement in an alternative living situation. Individuals are not able to live alone. Management and the cost of care for these individuals are significant and often present an overwhelming burden for caregivers.[2,5,13] Continuity of care issues are usually ongoing and require a number of resources to provide for the special needs of this population.[13] This nursing diagnosis is similar to the nursing diagnosis Chronic Confusion on p. 1655.

Related Factors

Dementia (Alzheimer's' disease, multi-infarct dementia, Pick's disease, AIDS dementia)
Parkinson's disease
Huntington's disease
Depression
Alcoholism

Defining Characteristics[1-14]

Consistent disorientation in known and unknown environments
Chronic confusional states
Loss of occupation or social functioning from memory decline
Inability to follow simple directions/instructions
Inability to reason
Inability to concentrate
Slowness in responding to questions

Expected Patient Outcomes & Nursing Interventions

The patient will be able to function in a structured environment, as evidenced by:

Structuring the environment to support the individual in their ability to interact within that milieu

- Establish a consistent daily routine schedule. *Patients compensate for inability to plan activities by developing a daily routine that becomes automatic.*[8]
- Provide a consistent caregiver/staff member. *Patients will experience increased security when cared for by people they recognize.*[12]
- Approach and communicate with the patient in a positive manner. *Verbal and nonverbal communication are important in establishing a relationship with a person who is cognitively impaired.*[14]

- Provide opportunity for one-to-one conversation with caregiver(s). *Providing sufficient time for interacting with patient reinforces socialization skill and a sense of self-worth.*[10]
- Ensure optimal sensory input (eye glasses are clean, hearing aid is functional, absence of cerumen impaction). *The cognitively impaired individual is at risk for misinterpretation of environment when sensory input is not accurate.*[1,2]
- Provide adequate nonglare lighting. *Visual perceptions may be altered by glare or shadows.*[4]
- Eliminate unnecessary environmental stimuli (excessive noise level, multiple conversation/activity, violent/aggressive movies or television programs). *Disturbing visual images or loud noise can precipitate a catastrophic reaction.*[11]
- Place meaningful possessions (e.g., photographs, furniture, special possessions) in the patient's environment. *Familiar belongings promote a sense of security.*[12]
- Avoid change in room environment (e.g., reassignment of patient's room, rearrangement of furniture or items, holiday decoration). *Frequent environment change may produce conflicting cues.*[4]
- Provide a daily time for small group activity that is valued by patient (e.g., music, art, reminiscence group, selected television program, Bible therapy). *Planned activities are beneficial if they are pleasurable and incorporate the patient's culture, habits, values, manners, preferences, and occupation.*[6,8,9]

Principles and Rationale for Nursing Interventions

The cognitively impaired individual is often overwhelmed and has difficulty processing an accurate interpretation of their surroundings. Sensory impairment, if not corrected, may contribute to the individual's misinterpretation of environmental stimuli. Reports by caregiver, family, or friends of missing or broken glasses, hearing aids, or dentures must be noted and attempts made to repair or replace item(s). Referrals to appropriate disciplines (i.e., physical therapy, occupational therapy, audiology, optometry, psychology) may be necessary to assist the individual patient to compensate for sensory deficits).[1]

The person will achieve an optimum level of function in a supportive, structured environment. The physical setting and caregiver/staff contribute to the milieu that makes up the person's environment. Controlling the bombardment of external stimuli (i.e., noise level, traffic activity, disturbing visual images) that affects the milieu is critical. The provision of items familiar to the individual (e.g., photographs, furniture, special possessions) will support a sense of belonging and comfort. Consistency in daily routine and caregivers (staff) play an important part in successful care delivery for this population. Change or interruption of the sleep-wake pattern and/or environment may result in overstimulation and problematic behaviors. Environmental changes include circumstances such as

relocation, rearrangement of furniture, changing pictures/accessories, daylight savings time, holiday activities, change in caregiver, or an altered daily schedule. The focus of treatment is to provide an environment that remains consistent and promotes optimal interaction of the person with his or her surroundings.

▮ IMPAIRED MEMORY

Impaired Memory is a state in which an individual experiences the inability to remember or recall bits of information or behavioral skills. Impaired memory may be attributed to pathophysiologic or situational causes that are either temporary or permanent.

Deficits in memory and ability to learn new materials are common sequelae to conditions affecting the integrity and functioning of the brain as a vital organ. Impaired Memory is an early neuropsychologic cognitive problem often accompanied by sensory deficits, headaches, dizziness, pain, and affective/behavioral disturbances.[1] Impaired memory is frequently a temporary disability and represents part of a larger constellation of global cognitive impairments seen in chronic brain and neurologic disorders, acute confusional states, traumatic brain injury, and iatrogenic conditions such as electroconvulsive therapy or brain surgery.[1,3,5,15,18]

For patients suffering from traumatic brain injury, impaired memory develops within a hierarchy of injury severity meaning that the nature of cognitive impairment is additive and dependent upon level of injury.[1] Deficits in core functions such as attentional skills, and speed of information processing interfere with the individual's ability to acquire new information and organize stimuli into meaningful patterns consistent with normal cognition.[14] Within this context, impaired memory rarely occurs in isolation from other cognitive deficits. An exception would be transient global amnesia which is thought to be largely vascular in origin.[8]

Related Factors*

Traumatic brain injury (e.g., closed head injury)
Transient global amnesia
Post-concussion syndrome
Delirium (acute confusion)
Dementia (chronic confusion)
Cerebral vascular accident
Post-traumatic amnesia
Retrograde amnesia
Cerebral anoxia
Seizure disorder
Herpes simplex encephalitis
Limbic encephalitis
Wernicke-Korsakoff syndrome

*References 2, 5, 6, 8, 12, 15, 16, 18, 23.

Electroconvulsive therapy
Brain surgical lesions

Defining Characteristics[1,9,14,16]

Observed or reported experiences of forgetting
Inability to learn or retain new skills or information
Inability to perform a previously learned skill
Inability to recall factual information
Inability to recall recent or past events
Inability to perform a behavior at a scheduled time
Short and immediate-term memory deficits

Expected Patient Outcomes and Nursing Interventions*

Acknowledges memory impairment and shows awareness of limitations as evidenced by:

Verbalization about memory deficits and impact on functioning
Accepts feedback about memory errors
Able to self-monitor memory lapses
Cooperates with memory assessment and testing
  Testing of *recent* memory, for example, three word recall after five minutes, ascertaining hospital room number or location
  Testing of *remote* memory, for example, place of birth, significant dates, names of past presidents
  • Encourage verbalization about memory deficits *in order to decrease anxiety about impairment and unknown outcomes.*
  • Provide information about cognitive rehabilitation and expected course of recovery *as severity of traumatic brain injury will influence type and length of memory deficits.*
  • Assist with realistic goal-setting for self during convalescence.
  • Acknowledge emotional distress and provide encouragement. *Early stress management may help prepare the patient for emotional responses associated with return of functional activities.*

Participates in activities of daily living and utilizes environmental cues to assist memory and orientation as evidenced by:

Using adaptive coping strategies to assist memory
Attends to environmental routines and activities of daily living appropriate to level of functioning
  • Assist with problem-solving strategies to cope with memory deficits.
    Use simple, concrete (versus abstract) communication.
    Use repetition techniques (e.g., provide explanations, instructions, and introductions repeatedly).
    Avoid giving explanations or instructions ahead of time.

Use structured, one-to-one approach *to minimize over-stimulation.*
    Use clocks and calendars.
    Do not dispute confabulated responses, but provide reality orientation.
    Reorient throughout the day.
    Emphasize familiar skills *to pair new learning with old learning and maximize memory during new tasks.*
  • Teach augmentation of impaired memory with memory aids.
    Teach use of a recording system, such as a notebook at the bedside for written entries and reminders.
    Post a calendar in the room.
    Place signs in room to aid memory (e.g., "Do not get out of bed alone. Use call light to call nurse.").
    Provide simple instruction sheets at the bedside.
    Use multiple modalities, especially multisensory stimuli to aid memory retention (e.g., visual, auditory, kinesthetic, etc.).
  • Maintain daily care routines and schedule *to decrease confusion and disorientation and maintain consistency.*
    Post daily schedule in room.
    Promote regular rest periods.
    Provide consistent caregivers whenever possible.
    Wear name tag and remind patient frequently of caregiver's identity and purpose of interaction.
    Keep belongings and call light in same location.
    Use familiar objects in room to augment memory and assist with orientation to surroundings (e.g., locating own room).

Principles and Rationale for Nursing Interventions

Nursing interventions for the nursing diagnosis of Impaired Memory focus on supporting the patient who experiences a temporary period of disability and teaching memory augmentation strategies to maximize participation in the environment and to promote independent functioning. A multidisciplinary approach by caregivers is essential during the rehabilitation period and should include family members and other supportive persons.

Emotional lability and global cognitive dysfunction related to physiologic disturbances often interfere with new learning and memory retraining. The nurse should assess regularly for fluid and electrolyte imbalances, level of oxygenation, pain response, infection, fever, responses to medications, and other factors that may contribute to delirium or an acute confusional state caused by physical factors. The extent and location of traumatic brain injury will also influence the degree of memory impairment and mental status changes present. Family members will need support and teaching about physical causes for behavior changes and memory impairment in their loved one in order to have realistic expectations during convalescence.

Memory loss and inability to learn new materials can lead to increased anxiety and disorientation. Assessment of level of

---

*References 6, 7, 10, 13, 17, 20.

anxiety should be done on an ongoing basis. Interventions to promote a calm, consistent environment should be implemented, including attention to degree of noise and other stimuli, room temperature, number of caregivers, schedules, and routines to minimize catastrophic reactions and disorientation.

Further specialized memory retraining strategies have been discussed in the literature* and should occur after careful physical as well as neuropsychological evaluation of the patient by consultants. Hierarchical progression from simple to more complex learning will maximize memory retention. Neuropsychological testing is frequently indicated as another early intervention to determine level of impairment and realistic guideposts toward resumption of normal functioning.

■ DECISIONAL CONFLICT (SPECIFY)

Decisional conflict is a state of uncertainty about courses of action to be taken when choice among competing actions involves risk, loss, or challenge to personal life values. (Specify means identifying the focus of conflict, e.g., choices regarding health, family relationships, career, finances, or other life events.)[7,8]

Decision making involves making a choice among alternative courses of action after judging the relative effectiveness and desirability of each alternative. Although theorists disagree about the way individuals make or should make judgments and decisions, many agree that expectations and values are essential inputs into decision making.[10] Expectations are beliefs or subjective judgments about the likelihood of the consequences or outcomes of a course of action. Values are preferences for or the relative desirability of those outcomes.

Generally, individuals are more likely to choose an alternative that makes desirable outcomes likely and undesirable outcomes unlikely. Unfortunately, many important decisions are likely to produce desirable and undesirable outcomes. Moreover, the desirable outcomes occur partly with one alternative and partly with another. Therefore no single alternative will meet all our objectives and every alternative poses a risk of undesirable outcomes. These difficult decisions have been referred to as choice dilemmas or conflicted decisions.[13] They are characterized by difficulty in identifying good alternatives, risks or uncertainty of outcomes, high stakes in terms of potential gains and losses, and the need to make value tradeoffs in selecting a course of action. Janis[4] describes decisional conflict as "the simultaneous opposing tendencies within the individual to accept and reject a given course of action."

Patients experiencing a choice dilemma may demonstrate symptoms of hesitation, vacillation, or feelings of uncertainty about the course of action to take. They may express concern about the undesirable consequences of the choice facing them and question their personal values in their deliberation. Delayed decision making is a common response to difficult decision making. The patient may be self-focused and manifest

physiologic signs of distress such as increased muscle tension, heart rate, and restlessness. For some decisions, autonomic indicators of stress increase as subjects move toward a decision and gradually return to the level of the resting state after the decision is made.[4]

Subjectively, patients may express feelings of distress. Responses vary according to the degree of conflict inherent in the decision. A low degree of conflict may be attractive and stimulating; a moderate degree of conflict may produce defensiveness; and a high degree of conflict may bring about hypervigilance and panic.[13] The intensity of stress symptoms depend, in part, on the perceived magnitude of losses anticipated from whatever choice is made and on the magnitude of anticipated regret over the positive aspects of rejected options.

Other clinical, personal, and environmental factors exacerbate the perceived difficulty.[3,12] Cognitive functioning may be impaired by organic brain disease, psychiatric disorders, or extreme anxiety, making even simple decisions difficult. Inexperience with decision making or lack of information may contribute to the unclear or unrealistic perceptions about courses of action and consequences, thereby magnifying the conflict. Hesitation in making a decision may also be influenced by a person's lack of knowledge or skill to implement the decision once it is made. Social factors also influence the conflict experienced. The patient may lack the requisite social support to implement the decision. Alternatively, the person's support network may interfere with the decision-making process, by interjecting alternative views. Health professionals can contribute to the difficulty by imposing their values and belief systems or by assuming control over decision making.

Related Factors[7]

Knowledge deficit (lack of relevant information)
Identified consequences equally desirable/undesirable
Conflicting or unclear values and beliefs
Lack of experience
Lack of problem-solving skills
Indecisive behavior pattern
Support system deficit
Interference in decision-making process
Perceived threat to value system

Defining Characteristics[7]

Expressed or unexpressed distress about choices available
Verbalization of undesirable consequences of alternatives being considered
Vacillation between alternative choices
Delayed decision making
Self-focusing
Physical signs of stress or tension (increased heart rate, increased muscle tension, restlessness)
Questioning personal values and beliefs while attempting to make decision
Expresses concern about inadequate knowledge base to make choice

---

*References 4, 10, 11, 17, 19, 21, 22, 24.

Expected Patient Outcomes & Nursing Intervention*

Makes and takes action on an informed decision that is consistent with personal values, as evidenced by:

Becoming informed and basing decisions on this information
Selecting a course of action consistent with values
Implementing decision

- Aid patient in clarifying goals, alternatives, and potential consequences; *Lack of information or clarity in these items leads to decisional conflict.*
- Help the patient clarify the likelihood of potential consequences; realign unrealistic expectations; *distortion in expectations often increases conflict (e.g., anticipating a negative consequence when the likelihood is extremely low) or regret (anticipating a positive consequence when the likelihood is extremely low).*
- With the patient, clarify the desirability of possible consequences and their priority; *unclear values contribute to decisional conflict.*[9,16]
- Identify value tradeoffs implicit in making choices; *having to make tradeoffs often contributes to conflict; knowing what makes the decision difficult helps in its resolution.*
- Facilitate alternative selection consistent with personal values; *this increases satisfaction with the decision and the likelihood that the patient will follow through on the choice.*
- Teach and reinforce self-help skills required to implement the choice; *individuals have difficulty translating preferences into permanent behavior change without the resources necessary to do so.*

Principles and Rationale for Nursing Interventions

Patients experience less decisional conflict when they make a decision that is informed, consistent with personal values, and behaviorally implemented.[8] Informed decision making means patients are aware of alternatives open to them and have pared alternatives down to those that are viable to implement. Patients also need to be informed of possible consequences. Their expectations of consequences must be realistic. By realigning distorted expectations to ones that are consistent with current knowledge, nurses will minimize conflict or regret experienced by the patient. For example, patients often experience distress from anticipating a negative consequence whose likelihood they believe is quite high, when in actuality it is extremely low. Alternatively, regret can be minimized by altering patients' high expectations of positive consequences, when the likelihood is extremely low. Patients also need to be aware of the relative importance or value they hold for each of the conse-

quences. By clarifying values and the implicit tradeoffs the patients must make when choosing among alternatives, they will have greater insight into what makes their decisions difficult. Moreover, a choice that is consistent with personal values (and not those important to others) increases the likelihood that patients will stick with their choices. Finally, patients often fail to translate preferences into permanent behavior change because they lack the requisite knowledge, skills, and motivation to implement the decision. Nurses are in a position to assist the patient to develop the self-help skills necessary to follow through on a decision.

▮ DECREASED INTRACRANIAL ADAPTIVE CAPACITY

Decreased intracranial adaptive capacity is a clinical state in which intracranial fluid dynamic mechanisms that normally compensate for increases in intracranial volumes are compromised, resulting in repeated disproportionate increases in intracranial pressure (ICP) in response to a variety of noxious and non-noxious stimuli.

Related Factors

Brain injuries
Sustained increase in ICP $\geq$10-15 mm Hg
Decreased cerebral perfusion pressures $\leq$50-60 mm Hg
Systemic hypotension with intracranial hypertension

Defining Characteristics

Repeated increases in ICP of greater than 10 mm Hg for more than 5 minutes following any of a variety of external stimuli
Disproportionate increase in ICP following single environmental or nursing maneuver stimulus
Elevated P2 ICP waveform
Volume pressure test variations (Volume-pressure ratio >2, pressure = volume index <10)
Baseline ICP $\geq$10 mm Hg
Wide amplitude waveform

Expected Patient Outcomes and Nursing Interventions

Intracranial pressure within normal limits (4-15 mm Hg or 50-200 mm H₂O) as evidenced by spontaneous eye opening; orientation to time, place, and person; and motor function intact

- Monitor changes in ICP waveforms.
- Monitor cerebral perfusion pressure (CPP) for normal values between 80-100 mm Hg.
- Assess pupil size and reactivity.
- Monitor patient's orientation.
- Assess purposeful and non-purposeful movement comparing left and right sides.

- Monitor arterial blood gases for hypercarbia and hypoxia.
- Monitor temperature for elevations.
- Monitor blood glucose for hypoglycemia.
- Observe for seizure activity.
- Observe for restlessness to correct cause (e.g., hypoxia, full bladder from kinked urinary catheter) or initiate sedation as ordered.
- Monitor fluid balance and monitor for weight gain.
- Monitor effects of hemodilution or hemoconcentration on electrolytes and hematologic laboratory values.
- Elevate head of the bed 30 degrees.
- Keep head in neutral position.
- Pace nursing care activities such as bed bath, linen change, range of motion to allow rest periods after each. Omit nursing procedures unless essential.
- Reduce external stimuli such as radio, television, noises from walls, voices of staff and visitors.
- Keep room lights dim.
- Administer oxygen as ordered to prevent hypoxia.
- Hyperventilate patient as ordered to prevent hypercarbia.
- Suction airway as little as possible; monitor ICP when suctioning. Limit suctioning to 2 passes of 10 seconds each.
- Maintain body temperature with decreased bed linens and hypothermia blanket.
- Administer medications as ordered including diuretics, corticosteroids, antipyretics, neuromuscular blocking, barbiturates, anticonvulsants, antihypertensives, vasopressors.

Significant others will verbalize their needs for support and information

- Encourage significant others to verbalize their feelings about the patient's condition.
- Make referral to counselor, pastor, social worker, physician, or advocate as needed to meet significant others' needs.
- Provide information about the patient's condition at a level they can understand.

Principles and Rationale for Nursing Interventions

Intracranial pressure monitoring provides wave forms that indicate pressures within the brain. An elevated P2 waveform may indicate actions are needed as ordered to reduce intracranial pressure.

Cerebral perfusion pressure (CPP) is calculated by subtracting the mean intracranial pressure (MICP) from the mean arterial pressure (MAP); CPP = MAP − MICP. The cerebral vessels normally have autoregulation, the ability to adapt or maintain constant-rate perfusion pressures despite changes in arterial blood pressure and intracranial pressure. When these adaptive capacities are inadequate due to cerebral edema, the intracranial pressure rises. Normal range for cerebral perfusion is 50-150 mm Hg, with the optimal CPP being 80-90 mm Hg.

Autoregulation fails when the CPP falls below 50 mm Hg. Antihypertensives and vasopressors may be given as needed to adjust the mean arterial pressure to maintain cerebral perfusion pressure.

As pressure rises in the brain, the patient's level of consciousness declines. Consciousness is assessed by determining the client's orientation to time, place, and person. When this is not possible due to reduced consciousness, then consciousness is assessed by the amount and kind of stimulation required to get a response from the patient. These responses, in increasing order of severity, may be withdrawal from pain, flexion to pain, abnormal flexion, or abnormal extension. Abnormal flexion (decorticate posturing) with arms adducted and flexed in response to stimulation indicates high intracerebral pressure in the diencephalon. As the pressure in the cranium increases, and pushes downward, the patient's posturing may change to abnormal extension (decerebrate posturing) which indicates increased pressure in the midbrain and pons.

Pupillary changes of dilation and non-reactivity may indicate increased pressure on the oculomotor nerve (cranial nerve III) that controls pupillary size and reactivity.

The Monro-Kellie hypothesis states that when one of the three contents of the brain increases (brain tissue, cerebrospinal fluid, and blood), the other two must decrease in size or volume to adapt to the expansion of the third. Hypercarbia ($PaCO_2$ >45 mm Hg) acts as a cerebral vasodilator, increasing cerebral blood flow and intracranial pressure. Every increase of 1 mm Hg $PaCO_2$ causes a 2%-3% increase in cerebral blood flow.[1] Hypoxemia also causes cerebral vasodilation when the PaO_2 falls below 50 mm Hg, creating lactic acidosis which results in vasodilation. Thus, hyperventilating the patient decreases $PaCO_2$ and vasoconstricts cerebral vessels allowing more room in the brain for expansion. This rationale supports the therapeutic interventions for administering oxygen to maintain PaO_2 within normal limits and hyperventilating the patient to maintain $PaCO_2$ about 30 mm Hg. Another intervention that can alter the carbon dioxide and oxygen is suctioning of the airway. Endotracheal or tracheal suctioning can cause hypoxia by removing oxygen from the trachea while removing secretions. Conversely if airway suctioning is not performed when needed, the patient's $PaCO_2$ may increase to cause hypercarbia. Suction is performed when needed, but should be limited to two passes each no longer than 10 seconds.[5]

Fever, pain, agitation, external stimuli seizures, and nursing activities such as bath, linen change, range of motion exercises, or position changes may increase cerebral metabolic rate of oxygen and therefore, the oxygen demand. When this increased oxygen demand is not met by appropriate oxygen supply, then cerebral ischemia may result in increasing intracranial pressure. The head of the bed is elevated to facilitate venous return from the brain to the systemic circulation. Head alignment prevents occlusion of the jugular veins and improves venous return. Anticonvulsants and barbiturates are given to reduce muscle contraction to reduce metabolic need for oxygen. Antipyretics are given to maintain normothermia. Hypothermia should be accomplished slowly with acetaminophen, tepid water bath, or hypothermia blanket to avoid shivering which increases intracranial pressure. Chlorpromazine (Thorazine) can be given to control shivering. Neuromuscular blocking agents such as pancuronium (Pavulon) or vecuronium (Norcuron) are given to chemically paralyze the patient to decrease metabolic need for oxygen and facilitate mechanical ventilation. Neuromuscular blocking agents are always given with sedation such as diazepam (Valium) or morphine to reduce sensation of the motor paralysis.[1-6]

Serum glucose levels must be monitored to ensure the brain has sufficient glucose for cellular metabolism and to prevent formation of lactic acidosis. Intravenous sources of glucose may be necessary.

Monitor fluid balance and weight to detect gains; a change of 1 kg equals 1 liter of fluid. Gain of fluid or weight gain may indicate syndrome of inappropriate antidiuretic hormone (SIADH) caused by an excess of antidiuretic hormone. This may result from trauma to the pituitary or hypothalamus. The additional fluid contributes to the increased intracranial pressure and can be treated with diuretics. Additionally this increase in fluid creates dilution of plasma, resulting in lower laboratory values for electrolytes and hematologic measures.

Medications are given to reduce intracranial pressure. Diuretics such as mannitol (Osmitrol) or furosemide (Lasix) are given to reduce blood volume which subsequently reduces cerebral edema. Corticosteroids such as dexamethasone (Decadron) or methylprednisolone (Solu-Medrol) are given to reduce the inflammatory response by stabilizing cell membranes and capillary endothelium. Histamine receptor antagonists such as cimetidine (Tagamet) or ranitidine (Zantac) are given to counteract gastric irritation induced by corticosteroids and to prevent stress ulcers from high levels of cortisol.

When an intraventricular catheter is used to monitor intracranial pressures, it also can be used to withdraw cerebrospinal fluid as ordered to reduce ICP. This method is usually performed when more conservative measures have failed.

The patient's family and significant others need information and support during their time of waiting. Encourage them to verbalize their feeling and fears. They need information about the patient's status and what they can do to help the patient. Monitor the patient's ICP when the family is present to determine the effects of the visit. Some visitors may increase the patient's ICP, while others may decrease it.

References

Pain

1. Acute Pain Management Guideline Panel: *Acute pain management: operative or medical procedures and trauma,* AHCPR Pub. No. 92-0032, Rockville, Maryland, 1992, Agency for Health Care Policy and Research, Public Health Service, U.S. Department of Health and Human Services.
2. American Pain Society: *Principles of analgesic use in the treatment of acute pain and chronic cancer pain,* Skokie, IL, 1992, American Pain Society.
3. Bachiocco V, Morselli AM, Carli G: Self control expectancy and post-surgical pain: relationships to previous pain, behavior in past pain, familial pain tolerance models, and personality, *J Pain Symptom Management* 8:4, 1993.
4. Bailey LM: Music therapy in pain management, *J Pain Symptom Management* 1:25, 1986.
5. Bonica JJ: The need for a taxonomy of pain, *Pain* 6:247, 1979.
6. Bonica JJ, Ventagridda V, editors: *Advances in pain research and therapy,* vol 2, New York, 1979, Raven Press.
7. Bourbannais F: Pain assessment: development of a tool for the nurse and the patient, *J Adv Nurs* 6:277, 1981.
8. Brockopp DY, Warden S, Colclough G, Brockopp GW: Nursing knowledge: acute postoperative pain management in the elderly, *J Geront Nurs* 19:31, 1993.
9. Carrol-Johnson RM, editor: *Classification of nursing diagnoses: proceedings of the eighth conference,* Philadelphia, 1989, Lippincott.
10. Chapman RO, Turner JA: Psychological control of acute pain in medical settings, *J Pain Symptom Management* 1:9, 1986.
11. Copp LH, editor: *Perspectives on pain,* Edinburgh, 1985, Churchill Livingstone.
12. Cotanch PH, Harrison M, Roberts J: Hypnosis as an intervention for pain control, *Nurs Clin North Am* 22:699, 1987.
13. Faucett J, Gordon N, Levine J: Differences in postoperative pain severity among four ethnic groups, *J Pain Symptom Management* 9:6, 1994.
14. Feldman HR: Psychological differentiation and the phenomenon of pain, *Adv Nurs Sci* 50:50, 1984.
15. Ferrell BR, Eberts MT, McCaffery M, Grant M: Clinical decision making and pain, *Cancer Nurs* 14:6, 1991.
16. Fordyce W: *Behavioral methods for chronic pain and illness,* St Louis, 1976, Mosby.
17. Gujol MC: A survey of pain assessment and management practices among critical care nurses, *Am J Crit Care* 3:2, 1994.
18. Guyton AC: *Textbook of medical physiology,* ed 8, 1991, Saunders.
19. Hendler NH, Long DM, Wise TN, editors: *Diagnosis and treatment of chronic pain,* Boston, 1982, John Wright/PSG.
20. Infante MC, Mooney NE: Interactive aspects of pain assessment, *Orthop Nurs* 6:31, 1987.
21. Jacox A: *Pain, a source book for nurses and other health professionals,* Boston, 1977, Little, Brown.
22. Lipton S, editor: *Persistent pain: modern methods of treatment,* New York, 1980, Grune & Stratton.
23. Lutz WJ: Helping hospitalized children and their parents cope with painful procedures, *J Pediatr Nurs* 1:24, 1986.
24. Mastrovito RC: Psychogenic pain, *Am J Nurs* 74:514, 1974.
25. Maxam-Moore VA, Wilkie DJ, Woods SL: Analgesics for cardiac surgery patients in critical care: describing current practice, *Am J Crit Care* 3:1, 1994.
26. McCaffery M: Nursing approaches to non-pharmacological pain control, *Int J Nurs Studies* 27:1, 1990.
27. McCaffery M: *Nursing management of the patient with pain,* Philadelphia, 1979, Lippincott.
28. McCaffery M, Beebe H: *Pain: clinical manual for nursing practice,* Philadelphia, 1989, Lippincott.
29. McCloskey JC, Bulechek GM, editors: *Iowa intervention project, nursing interventions classification (NIC),* St Louis, 1992, Mosby.
30. Meinhart NT, McCaffery M: *Pain: a nursing approach to assessment and analysis,* Norwalk, CT, 1983, Appleton-Century-Crofts.
31. Mooney NE: Pain management in the orthopaedic patient, *Nurs Clin North Am* 26:73, 1991.
32. Ng LKY, Bonica JJ, editors: *Pain discomfort and humanitarian care: proceedings of the national conference,* New York, 1980, Elsevier/North Holland.
33. NIH Consensus Development Conference: The integrated approach to the management of pain, *J Pain Symptom Management* 2(1):35, 1987.
34. North American Nursing Diagnosis Association: *Taxonomy I: revised 1990,* St Louis, 1990, NANDA.
35. Paice JA: Unraveling the mystery of pain, *Oncol Nurs Forum* 18:843, 1991.
36. Pomerleau OF, Brady JP, editors: *Behavioral medicine: theory and practice,* Baltimore, 1979, Williams & Wilkins.
37. Porth C, editor: *Pathophysiology: concepts of altered health states,* ed 4, Philadelphia, 1994.
38. Talbert RL: Pharmacotherapeutic modification of the stress response: analgesics, *Crit Care Q* 7:27, 1985.
39. Wright SM: The use of therapeutic touch in the management of pain, *Nurs Clin North Am* 22:705, 1987.

40. Zabrowski M: Cultural components in response to pain. *J Soc Iss* 8:16, 1952.

Chronic pain

1. American Pain Society: *Principles of analgesic use in the treatment of acute pain and chronic pain and chronic cancer pain,* Skokie, Ill, 1992, American Pain Society.
2. Bonica JJ, editor: *The management of pain,* Philadelphia, 1990, Lea & Febiger.
3. Carroll-Johnson RM, editor: *Classification of nursing diagnoses: proceedings of the eighth conference,* Philadelphia, 1989, Lippincott.
4. Copp LA, editor: *Perspectives on pain,* Edinburgh, 1985, Churchill Livingstone.
5. Cotanch PH, Harrison M, Roberts J: Hypnosis as an intervention for pain control, *Nurs Clin North Am* 22:699, 1987.
6. Davis GE: Measurement of the chronic pain experience: development of an instrument, *Res Nurs Health* 12:221, 1989.
7. Degner L, Barkwell D: Nonanalgesic approaches to pain control, *Cancer Nurs* 3:27, 1991.
8. Ferrell BR, Dean G: The meaning of cancer pain, *Semin Oncol Nurs* 11:1, 1995.
9. Ferrell BR et al: Pain management at home: struggle, comfort, mission, *Cancer Nurs* 16:3, 1993.
10. Fordyce W: *Behavior methods for chronic pain and illness,* St Louis, 1976, Mobsy.
11. Gordon M: *Manual of nursing diagnoses,* St Louis, 1991, Mosby.
12. Hendler NH, Long DM, Wise TN, editors: *Diagnosis and treatment of chronic pain,* Boston, 1982, John Wright/PSG.
13. Jacox A et al: *Management of cancer pain, clinical practice guidelines No. 94-0592,* Rockville, MD, Agency for Health Care Policy and Research, US Department of Health & Human Services, Public Health Services, March 1984.
14. Kim MH, McFarland GK, McLane AM, editors: *Classification of nursing diagnoses: proceedings of the fifth national conference,* St Louis, 1984, Mosby.
15. Lamb SL, Barbaro NM: Neurosurgical approaches to the management of chronic pain syndromes, *Orthop Nurs* 6:23, 1987.
16. McCaffery M, Beebe H: *Pain: clinical manual for nursing practice,* Philadelphia, 1989, Lippincott.
17. McCloskey JC, Balechek GM: *Nursing interventions classification (NIC),* St Louis, 1992, Mosby.
18. McLane A, editor: *Classification of nursing diagnoses: proceedings of the seventh conference,* St Louis, 1987, Mosby.
19. Meinhart NT, McCaffery M: *Pain: a nursing approach to assessment and analysis,* Norwalk, CT, 1983, Appleton-Century-Crofts.
20. NIH Consensus Development Conference: The integrated approach to the management of pain, *J Pain Symptom Management* 2(1):35, 1987.
21. North American Nursing Diagnosis Association: *Taxonomy I: revised 1990,* St Louis, 1990, NANDA.
22. Paice JA: Unraveling the mystery of pain, *Oncol Nurs Forum* 18:5, 1991.
23. Stack J, Faut-Callahan M: Pain management, *Nurs Clin North Am* 26:2, 1991.
24. Snelling J: The effect of chronic pain on the family unit, *J Nurs Res* 11:3, 1994.
25. Spross JA, McGuire DB, Schmidt RM: Oncology Nursing Society Position Paper on Cancer Pain, Parts I, II, III, *Oncol Nurs Forum* 17:4, 1990.
26. Taylor AG: Chronic pain: a guide to nursing intervention applied, *Nurs Res* 1:1, 1988.
27. Wallace KG, Hays J: Nursing management of chronic pain, *J Neurosurg Nurs* 14:185, 1982.
28. Wright SM: The use of therapeutic touch in the management of pain, *Nurs Clin North Am* 22:705, 1987.
29. Zabrowski M: Cultural components in response to pain, *J Soc Iss* 8:16, 1952.
30. Zimmerman L et al: Effects of music in patients who had chronic cancer pain, *Western J Nurs Res* 19:543, 1989.

Sensory/Perceptual alterations (specify)

1. Carpenito L: *Nursing diagnosis: application to clinical practice,* ed 6, Philadelphia, 1995, Lippincott.
2. Carpenito LJ: *Handbook of nursing diagnosis,* ed 6, Philadelphia, 1995, Lippincott.
3. Carrol-Johnson R: *Classification of Nursing Diagnoses: proceedings of the eighth conference,* Philadelphia, 1989, Lippincott.
4. Cook E, Thigpen R: Identification and management of cognitive and perceptual deficits in the rehabilitation patient, *Rehabil Nurs* 18(5):310, 1993.
5. Cox HC et al: *Clinical applications of nursing diagnosis,* ed 2, Baltimore, 1993, Williams & Wilkins.
6. Kim M, McFarland G, McLane A: *Pocket guide to nursing diagnosis,* ed 6, St Louis, 1995, Mosby.
7. McFarland G, McFarlane E: *Nursing diagnosis and intervention,* ed 2, St Louis, 1993, Mosby.
8. Peduzzi T, editor: Alterations in sensory perception: nursing implications, *Top Clin Nurs* 6(4):7, 1985.
9. Perreault J: Assessing for perceptual clarity: closing the gap between theory and practice, *Rehabil Nurs* 10(3):28, 1985.
10. Sparks SM, Taylor C: *Nursing diagnosis reference manual,* Springhouse, 1991, Springhouse, PA.
11. Toglia J: Generalization of treatment: a multicontext approach to cognitive perceptual impairments in adults with brain injury, *Am J Occup Ther* 45:505, 1990.
12. Wyness M: Perceptual dysfunction: nursing assessment and management, *J Neurosurg Nurs* 17(2):105, 1985.

Unilateral neglect

1. Baggerly J: Sensory perceptual problems following stroke, *Nurs Clin North Am* 26(4):997, 1991.
2. Booth K: The neglect syndrome, *J Neurosurg Nurs* 14:38, 1982.
3. Butter CM, Kirsch N: Combined and separate effects of eye patching and visual stimulation on unilateral neglect following stroke, *Arch Phys Med Rehabil* 73:1133, 1992.
4. Hickey JV: *The clinical practice of neurological and neurosurgical nursing,* ed 3, Philadelphia, 1992, Lippincott.
5. Kalbach LR: Unilateral neglect: mechanisms and nursing care, *J Neurosci Nurs* 23:125, 1991.
6. Kim MJ, McFarland GK, McLane AM: *Pocket guide to nursing diagnoses,* ed 6, St Louis, 1995, Mosby.
7. Kinsella G et al: Analysis of the syndrome of unilateral neglect, *Cortex* 29(1):135, 1993.
8. Mattingley JB et al: To see or not to see: the effects of visible and invisible cues on line bisection judgements in unilateral neglect, *Neuropsychologia* 31(11):1201, 1993.
9. Robertson IH et al: Sustained attention training for unilateral neglect: theoretical and rehabilitation implications, *J Clin Exp Neuropsychol* 17(3):416, 1995.
10. Rubio KB, Van Deusen J: Relation of perceptual and body image dysfunction to activities of daily living of persons after stroke, *Am J Occup Ther* 49(6):551, 1995.
11. Warren M: A Hierachical model for evaluation and treatment of visual perceptual dysfunction in adult acquired brain injury, Parts 1 & 2, *Am J Occup Ther* 47(1):42, 1993.
12. Wyness MA: Perceptual dysfunction: nursing assessment and management, *J Neurosurg Nurs* 17:105, 1985.

Knowledge deficit

1. Devine EC: Effects of psychoeducational care for adult surgical patients: a meta-analysis of 191 studies, *Patient Educ Couns* 19:129, 1992.
2. Dracup K et al: Causes of delay in seeking treatment for heart attack symptoms, *Soc Sci Med* 40:379, 1995.
3. Edworthy SM, Devins GM, Watson MM: The arthritis knowledge questionnaire, *Arthritis Rheum* 5:590, 1995.
4. Hirano PC, Laurent DD, Lorig K: Arthritis patient education studies, 1987-1991: a review of the literature, *Patient Educ Couns* 24:9, 1994.
5. Joffe A, Radius SM: Self-efficacy and intent to use condoms among entering college freshmen, *J Adoles Health* 14:262, 1993.
6. Meyer TJ, Mark MM: Effects of psychosocial interventions with adult cancer patients: a meta-analysis of randomized experiments, *Health Psychol* 14:101, 1995.
7. Patterson ET et al: Symptoms of preterm labor and self-diagnostic confusion, *Nurs Res* 41:367, 1992.
8. Redman BK: *Practice of patient education,* ed 8, St Louis, 1996, Mosby.

9. Varvara FF, Palmer M: Promotion of adaptation in battered women: a self-efficacy approach, *J Am Acad Nurs Practitioners* 5:264, 1993.

Altered thought processes

1. Bandler R, Grindler J: *The structure of magic,* Palo Alto, CA, 1975, Science and Behavior Books.
2. Burgener S, Chiverton P: Conceptualizing psychological wellbeing in cognitively-impaired older persons, *Image,* 24(3):209, 1992.
3. Carpenito LJ: *Handbook of nursing diagnosis,* ed 6, Philadelphia, 1995, Lippincott.
4. Carpenito L: *Nursing diagnoses: application to clinical practice,* ed 6, Philadelphia, 1995, Lippincott.
5. Carrol-Johnson R: *Classification of nursing diagnoses: proceedings of the eighth conference,* Philadelphia, 1989, Lippincott.
6. Carrol-Johnson R, Paquette M: *Classification of nursing diagnoses: proceedings of the tenth conference,* Philadelphia, 1993, Lippincott.
7. Chomsky N: *Language and mind,* New York, 1968, Harcourt-Brace-Jovanovich.
8. Cox HC et al: *Clinical applications of nursing diagnosis,* ed 2, Baltimore, 1993, Williams and Wilkins.
9. Foreman M: Acute confusion in the elderly, *Ann Rev Nurs Res* 2:3, 1993.
10. Haber et al: *Comprehensive psychiatric nursing,* ed 4, St Louis, 1992, Mosby.
11. Hall GR: Alterations in thought process, *J Gerontol Nurs* 14(3):30, 1988.
12. Hall GR: This hospital patient has Alzheimer's, *Am J Nurs* 91(10):44, 1991.
13. Hurley ME, editor: *Classification of nursing diagnoses: proceedings of the sixth conference,* St Louis, 1986, Mosby.
14. Kim M, McFarland G, McLane A: *Pocket guide to nursing diagnoses,* ed 6, St Louis, 1995, Mosby.
15. McFarland G, McFarlane E: *Nursing diagnosis and intervention,* ed 2, St Louis, 1993, Mosby.
16. Murphy GE: A conceptual framework for the choice of interventions in cognitive therapy, *Cognitive Ther Res* 9(2):127, 1985.
17. Paiva Z: Sundown syndrome: calming the agitated patient, *RN* 53(7):46, 1990.
18. Sparks SM, Taylor C: *Nursing diagnosis reference manual,* Springhouse, 1991, Springhouse, PA.

Acute confusion

1. Beck CK, Heacock P, Rapp CG, Shue V: Cognitive impairment in the elderly, *Nurs Clin North Am* 28(2):335, 1993.
2. Byrne EJ: *Confusional states in older people,* Boston, 1994, Little, Brown.
3. Clark S: Psychiatric and mental health concerns in the patient with sepsis, *Crit Care Nurs Clin North Am* 6(2):389, 1994.
4. Dyer CB, Ashton CM, Teasdale TA: Postoperative delirium: a review of 80 primary data-collection studies, *Arch Intern Med* 155:461, 1995.
5. Farrell KR, Ganzini L: Misdiagnosing delirium as depression in medically ill elderly patients, *Arch Intern Med* 155:2459, 1995.
6. Folstein MF et al: Mini-mental state: a practical guide for grading the cognitive state of patients for clinicians, *J Psychiatr Res* 12:189, 1975.
7. Foreman MD: Acute confusion in the elderly, *Ann Rev Nurs Res* 11:3, 1993.
8. Foreman MD: Diagnostic dilemma: cognitive impairment in the elderly, *J Gerontol Nurs* 18(9):5, 1992.
9. Foreman MD: Diagnostic dilemma: Confusion in the hospitalized elderly: incidence, onset, and associated factors, *Res Nurs Health* 12:21, 1989.
10. Geary SM: Intensive care unit psychosis revisited: understanding and managing delirium in the critical care setting, *Crit Care Nurs Q* 17(1):51, 1994.
11. Inaba-Roland KE, Maricle RM: Assessing delirium in the acute care setting, *Heart Lung* 21(1):48, 1992.
12. Inouye SK et al: A predictive model for delirium in hospitalized elderly medical patients based on admission characteristics, *Ann Intern Med* 119:474, 1993.
13. Lipowski ZJ: Update on delirium, *Psychiatr Clin North Am* 15(2):335, 1992.
14. Lipowski ZJ: *Delirium: acute confusional states,* New York, 1990, Oxford University Press.

15. Matthiesen V, Silvertsen L, Foreman MD, Cronin-Stubbs D: Acute confusion: nursing intervention in older patients, *Orthop Nurs* 13(2):21, 1994.
16. Mentes JC: A nursing protocol to assess causes of delirium: identifying delirium in nursing home residents, *J Gerontol Nurs* 21(2):26, 1995.
17. Minarik PA: Cognitive assessment of the cardiovascular patient in the acute care setting, *J Cardiovasc Nurs* 9(4):36, 1995.
18. North American Nursing Diagnosis Association: *Nursing diagnoses: definitions and classification 1995-1996,* Philadelphia, 1994, NANDA.
19. Palmieri DT: Clearing up the confusional adverse effects of medications in the elderly, *J Gerontol Nurs* 17(10):32, 1991.
20. Pfeiffer E: A short portable mental status questionnaire for the assessment of organic brain deficit in elderly patients, *J Am Geriatr Soc* 23:433, 1975.
21. Pompei et al: Detecting delirium among hospitalized patients, *Arch Intern Med* 155:301, 1995.
22. Rabins PV: Psychosocial and management aspects of delirium, *Int Psychogeriatr* 3(2):319, 1991.
23. Rummans TA, Evans JM, Krahn LE, Fleming KC: Delirium in elderly patients: evaluation and management, *Mayo Clin Proc* 70:989, 1995.
24. Sanders KM et al: Delirium during intra-aortic balloon pump therapy: incidence and management, *Psychosom* 33:35, 1992.
25. Schor JD et al: Risk factors for delirium in the hospitalized elderly, *JAMA* 267(6):827, 1992.
26. Stanley M: Ensuring a safe ICU stay for your confused elderly patient, *Dimen Crit Care Nurs* 10(2):62-67, 1991.
27. Stewart RB, Hale WE: Acute confusional states in older adults and the role of polypharmacy, *Ann Rev Health,* 13:415, 1992.
28. Sullivan-Marx EM: Delirium and physical restraint in the hospitalized elderly, *Image* 26(4):295, 1994.
29. Tess MM: Acute confusional states in critically ill patients: a review, *J Neurosci Nurs* 23(6):398, 1991.
30. Tune LE: Postoperative delirium, *Int Psychogeriatr* 3(2):325, 1991.
31. Tune LE, Carr S, Hoag E, Cooper T: Anticholinergic effects of drugs commonly prescribed for the elderly: potential means for assessing risk of delirium, *Am J Psychiatr* 149:1393, 1992.
32. Wolanin MO, Phillips LRF: *Confusion: prevention and care,* St Louis, 1981, Mosby.
33. Yeaw EMJ, Abbate JH: Identification of confusion among the elderly in an acute care setting, *Clin Nurs Spec* 7(4):192, 1993.

Chronic confusion

1. Abraham IL et al: Multidisciplinary assessment of patients with Alzheimer's disease, *Nurs Clin North Am* 29(1):113, 1994.
2. Armstrong-Esther CA, Browne KD, McAfee JG: Elderly patients: still clean and sitting quietly, *J Adv Nurs* 19:264, 1994.
3. Barry PP: Medical evaluation of the demented patient, *Med Clin North Am* 78(4):779, 1994.
4. Beck CK, Shue VM: Interventions for treating disruptive behavior in demented elderly people, *Nurs Clin North Am* 29(1):143, 1994.
5. Bowie P, Mountain G: Using direct observation to record the behavior of long-stay patients with dementia, *Int J Geriatr Psychiatry* 8:857, 1993.
6. Daly JM, Maas M, Buckwalter K: Use of standardized nursing diagnosis and interventions in long-term care, *J Gerontol Nurs* 21(8):29, 1995.
7. Fisher JE, Fink CM, Loomis CC: Frequency and management difficulty of behavioral problems among dementia patients in long-term care facilities, *Clin Gerontol* 13(1):3, 1993.
8. Forbes SJ: Spirituality, aging and the community-dwelling caregiver and care recipient, *Geriatr Nurs* 15(6):296, 1994.
9. Goldsmith SM, Hoeffer B, Rader J: Problematic wandering behavior in the cognitively impaired elderly, *J Psychosoc Nurs* 33(2):6, 1995.
10. Hall GR: Caring for people with Alzheimer's disease using the conceptual model of progressively lowered stress threshold in the clinical setting, *Nurs Clin North Am* 29(1):129, 1994.
11. Harvath TA, Patsdaughter CA, Bumbalo JA, McCann MK: Dementia related behaviors in Alzheimer's disease and AIDS, *J Psychosoc Nurs* 33(1):35, 1995.
12. Khovzam HR: Bible study: A treatment in elderly patients with Alzheimer's disease, *Clin Gerontol* 15(2):71, 1994.

13. Loewenstein DA: Neuropsychological assessment in Alzheimer's disease, *Med Clin North Am* 78(4):789, 1994.
14. Nelson J: The influence of environmental factors in incidents of disruptive behavior, *J Gerontol Nurs* 21(5):19, 1995.
15. Rader J, Doan J, Schwab M: How to decrease wandering, a form of agenda behavior, *Geriatr Nurs* 64(4):196, 1985.
16. Rantz MJ, McShane RE: Nursing interventions for chronically confused nursing home residents, *Geriatr Nurs* 16(1):22, 1995.
17. Shedd PP, Kobokovich LJ, Slattery MJ: Confused patients in the acute care setting: prevalence, interventions, and outcomes, *J Gerontol Nurs* 21(4):5, 1995.
18. Stolley JM et al: Managing the care of patients with irreversible dementia during hospitalization for comorbidities, *Nurs Clin North Am* 28(4):767, 1993.
19. Ugarriza DN, Gray T: Alzheimer's disease: nursing interventions for clients and caretakers, *J Psychosoc Nurs* 31(10):7, 1993.
20. U.S. Bureau of the Census: Projection estimated from March 1987 Current Population Survey, Washington DC, 1987, US Government Printing Office.
21. Webber PA, Fox P, Burnette D: Living alone with Alzheimer's disease: effects on health and social service utilization patterns, *Gerontol* 34(1):8, 1994.

Impaired environmental interpretation syndrome
1. Abraham IL et al: Multidisciplinary assessment of patients with Alzheimer's disease, *Nurs Clin North Am* 29(1):113, 1994.
2. Armstrong-Esther CA, Browne KD, McAfee JG: Elderly patients: still clean and sitting quietly, *J Adv Nurs* 19:264, 1994.
3. Barry PP: Medical evaluation of the demented patient, *Med Clin North Am* 78(4):779, 1994.
4. Beck CK, Shue VM: Interventions for treating disruptive behavior in demented elderly people, *Nurs Clin North Am* 29(1):143, 1994.
5. Bowie P, Mountain G: Using direct observation to record the behavior of long-stay patients with dementia, *Int J Geriatr Psychiatry* 8:857, 1993.
6. Forbes EJ: Spirituality, aging and the community-dwelling caregiver and care recipient, *Geriatr Nurs* 15(6):296, 1994.
7. Goldsmith SM, Hoeffer B, Rader J: Problematic wandering behavior in the cognitively impaired elderly, *J Psychosoc Nurs* 33(2):6, 1995.
8. Hall GR: Caring for people with Alzheimer's disease using the conceptual model of progressively lowered stress threshold in the clinical setting, *Nurs Clin North Am* 29(1):129, 1994.
9. Khovzam HR: Bible study: A treatment in elderly patients with Alzheimer's disease, *Clin Gerontol* 15(2):71, 1994.
10. Loewenstein DA: Neuropsychological assessment in Alzheimer's disease, *Med Clin North Am* 78(4):789, 1994.
11. Nelson J: The influence of environmental factors in incidents of disruptive behavior, *J Gerontol Nurs* 21(5):19, 1995.
12. Rantz MJ, McShane RE: Nursing interventions for chronically confused nursing home residents, *Geriatr Nurs* 16(1):22, 1995.
13. Shedd PP, Kobokovich LJ, Slattery MJ: Confused patients in the acute care setting: prevalence, interventions, and outcomes, *J Gerontol Nurs* 21(4):5, 1995.
14. Stolley JM et al: Managing the care of patients with irreversible dementia during hospitalization for comorbidities, *Nurs Clin North Am* 28(4):767, 1993.

Impaired memory
1. Alves WM: Natural history of post-concussive signs and symptoms, *Phys Med Rehabil* 6(1):21, 1992.
2. Bauer RM, Tobias B, Valenstein E: Amnesic disorders. In Heilman KM, Valenstein E, editors: *Clinical neuropsychology,* ed 3, New York, 1993, Oxford University Press.
3. Bell DS: Impairment of memory. In Bell DS: *Medico-legal assessment of head injury,* Springfield, Illinois, 1992, Charles C. Thomas.
4. Benedict RH, Wechsler F: Evaluation of memory retraining in head-injured adults, *J Head Trauma Rehabil* 7:84, 1992.
5. Brown GG et al: Modeling the immediate free recall impairment of patients with surgical repair of anterior communicating artery aneurysm, *Neuropsychol* 9(1):27, 1995.
6. Cicerone KD: Psychological management of post-concussive disorders, *Phys Med Rehabil* 6(1):129, 1992.
7. Cromwell SL, Phillips LR: Forgetfulness in elders: strategies for protective caregiving, *Geriatr Nurs* 16(2):55, 1995.

8. Foote AW: Transient global amnesia, *J Neurosci Nurs* 21(1):14, 1989.
9. Gasquoine PG: Learning in post-traumatic amnesia following extremely severe closed head injury, *Brain Injury* 5(2):169, 1991.
10. Hanak M: *Rehabilitation nursing for the neurological patient,* New York, 1992, Springer.
11. Harrell M, Parente F, Bellingrath EG, Lisicia KA: *Cognitive rehabilitation of memory: a practical guide,* Gaithersburg, MD, 1992, Aspen.
12. Harrington DE, Malec J, Cicerone K, Katz HT: Current perceptions of rehabilitation professional toward mild traumatic brain injury, *Arch Phys Med Rehabil* 74(6):579, 1993.
13. Haslam C et al: Post-coma disturbance and post-traumatic amnesia as nonlinear predictors of cognitive outcome following severe closed head injury: findings from the Westmead head injury project, *Brain Injury* 8(6):519, 1994.
14. Leininger BE, Kreutzer JS: Neuropsychological outcome of adults with mild traumatic brain injury: implications for clinical practice and research, *Phys Med Rehabil* 6(1):169, 1992.
15. McIlhiney MC et al: Autobiographical memory and mood: effects of electroconvulsive therapy, *Neuropsychol* 9(4):501, 1995.
16. North American Nursing Diagnosis Association: *Nursing diagnoses: definitions and classification 1995-1996,* Philadelphia, 1994, NANDA.
17. Paulanka BJ, Griffin LS: Behavioral responses of memory impaired clients to selected nursing interventions, *Phys Occup Ther Geriatr* 12(1):65, 1993.
18. Rosenthal M: Mild traumatic brain injury syndrome, *Ann Emerg Med* 22(6):1048, 1993.
19. Semenza C, Sgaramella TM: Production of proper names: a clinical case study of phonemic cuing, *Memory* 1:265, 1993.
20. Slater MC: Alterations in thought process. In Snyder M: *A guide to neurological and neurosurgical nursing,* Albany, NY, 1991, Delmar.
21. Thoene AIT, Glisky EL: Learning of name-face associations in memory impaired patients: a comparison of different training procedures, *J Int Neuropsychol Soc* 1(1):29, 1995.
22. Toglia JP: Generalization of treatment: a multicontext approach to cognitive impairment in adults with brain injury, *Am J Occup Ther* 45(6):505, 1993.
23. Welte PO: Indices of verbal learning and memory deficits after right hemisphere stroke, *Arch Phys Med Rehabil* 74(6):631, 1993.
24. Wilson B: Recovery and compensatory strategies in head injured memory impaired people several years after insult, *J Neurol Neurosurg Psychiatr* 55:177, 1992.

Decisional conflict
1. Barry MJ et al: Patient reactions to a program designed to facilitate patient participation in treatment decisions for benign prostatic hyperplasia: pilot results, *Med Care,* 3:765, 1995.
2. Clancy C, Cebul R, Williams S: Guiding individual decisions: a randomized, controlled trial of decision analysis, *Am J Med* 84:283, 1988.
3. Fitten LJ, Waite MS: Impact of medical hospitalization on treatment decision making capacity in the elderly, *Arch Intern Med* 150:1717, 1990.
4. Janis IL, Mann L: *Decision making,* New York, 1977, Free Press.
5. Kaufman DH: An interview guide for helping children make healthcare decisions, *Pediatr Nurs* 11:365, 1985.
6. Llewellyn-Thomas HA: Patient's health-care decision making: a framework for descriptive and experimental investigations, *Med Decis Making* 15:101, 1995.
7. North American Nursing Diagnosis Association, *Taxonomy I: revised, 1990, with official nursing diagnoses,* St Louis, 1990, NANDA.
8. O'Connor AM: Validation of a decisional conflict scale, *Med Decis Making,* 15:25, 1995.
9. Pender NJ, Pender AR: *Health promotion in nursing practice,* ed 2, p 159, Norwalk, Conn, 1987 Appleton-Lange.
10. Pitz GF, Sachs NJ: Judgement and decision: theory and application, *Ann Rev Psychiatr* 35:139, 1984.
11. Rothert ML, Talarczyk GJ: Patient compliance and the decision making process of clinicians and patients, *J Compliance Health Care* 2:55, 1987.
12. Scott D: Anxiety, critical thinking and information processing during and after breast biopsy, *Nurs Res* 32:24, 1983.
13. Sjoberg L: To smoke or not to smoke: conflict or lack of differentiation? In Humphreys P, Svenson O, Vari A, editors: *Analyzing and aiding decision processes,* New York, 1983, North-Holland.

14. Slimmer LW, Brown RT: Parent's decision making process in medication administration for control of hyperactivity, *J Sch Health* 55:221, 1985.
15. Sox HC et al: *Medical decision making,* Boston 1988, Butterworths.
16. Wilberding JZ: Values clarification. In Bulecheck GM, McLoskey JC, editors: *Nursing interventions: treatments for nursing diagnoses,* p 173, Philadelphia, 1985, Saunders.

Decreased intracranial adaptive capacity

1. King M: Closed head injury. In Mins BC, editor: *Case studies in critical care nursing,* Baltimore, 1990, William & Wilkins.
2. Lipe HP, Mitchell PH: Positioning the patient with intracranial pressure: how turning and head rotation affect the internal jugular vein, *Heart Lung* 9:1031, 1980.
3. Mitchell PH, Ozuna J, Lipe HP: Moving the patient in bed: effects of turning and range of motion on intracranial pressure, *Nurs Res* 30:212, 1981.
4. Parsons LC, Wilson MM: Cerebrovascular status of severe closed head injured patients following passive position changes, *Nurs Res* 33:68, 1984.
5. Rudy EB et al: Endotracheal suctioning in adults with head injury, *Heart Lung* 20(6):667, 1991.
6. Snyder M: Relation of nursing activities to increases in intracranial pressure, *J Adv Nurs* 8:273, 1983.

▮ FEAR

Fear is the feeling of dread related to an identifiable source that an individual validates.

Fear is a primary emotion aroused by a person's perception of a real external threat along with a desire to flee.[3] Fear is a patient-expressed dread of the presence of a recognized, usually external, threat or danger to limb, autonomy, self-image, or community with others.[17] Fear can be viewed as a protective response preparing the person for fight or flight to cope with a danger; that is, it can be viewed as a warning against actually present danger and lead to immediate action.[3] Physiologic reactions to fear include increased heart rate, blood pressure, and respiration; urinary frequency and urgency; dilated pupils; and dry mouth. Neurochemical processes that give rise to different fears are being researched in animals and will lay the "groundwork for deciphering the relative contributions of various brain systems to inordinate fear in humans."[6, p. 101]

Related Factors[7,12,14-17]

Definable, specific danger
Abrupt or intense stimuli that increase rapidly or lack regularity
Environmental stimuli
Life-threatening illness
Sensory impairment
Undesirable outcome of therapy or medical procedure
Novel objects or situations
Unfamiliar diagnostic tests, procedures, and/or conditions
Discharge to unfamiliar setting
Natural danger (e.g., sudden noise, loss of physical support, height, and pain)
Powerful unmet needs
Learned response as by means of conditioning or identification
Language barrier
Impending threatening or difficult role change
Sudden touch or proximity of people or animals
Separation from familiar people
Lack of social support in threatening situations
Threatening behavior of others
Ridicule

Defining Characteristics[7,13,15,16]

Differentiated emotional response to definable specific danger
Diaphoresis
Increased muscle tension
Pupil dilation
Increased respiratory and heart rates
Crying
Irritability
Increased tension
Apprehension
Frightened
Fearful
Scared
Terrified; panic
Ability to identify object of fear
Concentration on danger
Increased alertness
Fight behavior (aggression)
Flight behavior (withdrawal)
Questioning
Reassurance seeking behavior
Goal-directed behavior facilitated (during mild or moderate fear)

Expected Patient Outcomes & Nursing Interventions[1, 2, 4, 5, 7, 9, 11, 14-17]

Experience absence or reduced fear, as evidenced by:

Absence of or less diaphoresis, muscle tension, irritability, apprehension, fright, fight or flight behavior, and questioning
Normal heart and respiratory rate
Absence of pupil dilation
Verbalizations by patient about experiencing less fear
Good sleep

- Determine presence and level of fear (e.g., can use instrument such as the Fear Survey Schedule).[8] *Keep in mind that patients tend to overpredict fear and exaggerate it retrospectively.*[10]
- Assist patient to recognize signs and symptoms of fear using indirect and open-ended questions.
- Help patient to identify danger that is causing fear by using indirect and open-ended questions.

- Encourage patient to verbalize feelings *to decrease intensity and duration of emotional response.*
- Provide emotional support and calm, soothing environment *to facilitate emotional coping.*
- Have patient record both episodes of fear and blocks of time when not feeling fearful. *Focusing only on fearful episodes may emphasize such experiences at the expense of episodes when fear is not experienced.*[10]
- Assist patient in identifying major response pattern to danger (fight or flight) *to help patient develop self-understanding of response pattern.*
- Encourage verbalization, when timing is appropriate, about:

  Perception of what is happening and degree of danger
  Perception of ability to cope with danger
  Questions about outcome of diagnoses and treatment
- Help patient use most appropriate coping strategies to deal with fear:

  Facilitate realistic perception of danger
  Use strategies to avoid or work around danger
  Develop alternative resources and goals
  Engage patient in problem solving to cope with danger
- Help patient identify strengths and adaptive skills *to cope with perceived danger and emotional responses.*
- Provide (at the level of patient understanding) factual and theoretical information about patient's illness and treatment *to facilitate understanding by the patient of his or her health status and treatment.*
- Engage in stimulus exposure or systematic desensitization, progressive muscle relaxation, visual imagery, and thought-stopping technique *to reduce and eliminate fear and related emotions.*
- Ask patient to predict experience of fear before exposure to feared event and compare with actual fear experienced in order to identify discrepancies and give the patient a chance to use this information.[10]
- Refer for spiritual counseling or assistance from social worker.
- Avoid situations that could aggravate the fear and related feelings; give careful explanations about what is to happen to patient in the health care setting *to decrease threat from planned procedures and treatment course.*
- Involve family and friends in patient's care.
- Encourage family and friends to offer patient emotional support.

Principles and Rationale for Nursing Interventions

The nursing diagnosis of fear is formulated from a synthesis of data that are collected by means of clinical assessment. Assessment parameters for consideration for fear include the following:

Identify and observe for definable specific dangers.
What behavioral and physiologic changes indicating fear are present?

How does the patient perceive the danger and describe the discomfort?
Identify maladaptive or adaptive coping responses to fear.
What strategies has the patient used to cope with past fear?
What resources are available to deal with the fear?

Determination of the diagnosis of fear is based on the presentation of a set of cluster of defining characteristics. The defining characteristics manifested by a client are useful in determining the nursing diagnosis. Not all characteristics need be present at a given time. To complete the nursing diagnosis, the nurse then adds, when possible, the identified related factor, to the diagnostic label of fear. An example is fear related to unfamiliar medical procedure.

◼ ANXIETY

Anxiety is a vague, uneasy feeling; the source is often nonspecific or unknown to an individual.[8]

Pratt states that "anxiety is an emotional state which is subjectively experienced as unpleasant or threatening. Symptoms include changes in mood (e.g., apprehension and fear) and cognitions (e.g., thoughts of impending mishap), and is generally accompanied by physiological and behavioral changes such as palpitations, sweating, and hypervigilance. Unlike other psychiatric disorders, anxiety is a normal emotion serving as a useful arousal response to threatening or stressful stimuli. However, it becomes pathological when the response to the perceived stimuli becomes overexaggerated, irrational, and disruptive and hence interferes with a person's ability to function normally."[16, p. 150]

Two types of anxiety are state and trait anxiety.[19] *State* anxiety is a transitory condition varying in intensity and fluctuating over time. *Trait* anxiety is a stable personality characteristic that predisposes a person's response and intensity in reaction to stress (i.e., anxiety proneness). When a person has a relatively high level of trait anxiety, he or she will tend to perceive a greater danger in situations that threaten the self than do persons who have lower levels of trait anxiety and who, consequently, respond with higher levels of state anxiety.

Capabilities are increased in mild and moderate anxiety; capabilities and structures are paralyzed or overworked in severe or extreme anxiety.[1] Observational capacity is increased in mild anxiety, whereas in moderate anxiety the perceptual field is somewhat narrowed, and attention is directed to the situation of concern. In severe anxiety, attention is focused on scattered detail; in extreme anxiety the detailed focus is blown out of proportion or the speed of focusing on scattered details is increased. In mild anxiety the person is aware, is alert, and perceives connections among the elements of a situation. In moderate anxiety the person does not notice peripheral details. In severe and extreme anxiety the person displays dissociating tendencies, failing to notice what goes on in a situation. In mild and moderate anxiety the person can learn, "i.e., is able to observe, describe, analyze, formulate meanings and relations, validate with another person, test, integrate, use the learning product."[1] In severe and extreme anxiety, learning is diminished and the person seeks to reduce the discomfort of anxiety.

One model of anxiety identifies predisposing factors—genetic endowment; present needs, thoughts, feelings, and resources; and past experiences—that affect the actual internal or external stimuli the person then cognitively evaluates as a threat.[20] Threats to physical integrity (physiologic disability) and threats to self-system (self-concept) are the two major groups of precipitating stressors.[20] The central nervous system is aroused and anxiety is felt. The sympathetic reaction appears to prepare the body for a flight-or-fight reaction in most persons. With perception of the threat in the cortex, the sympathetic branch of the autonomic nervous system is stimulated and the adrenal glands are activated. Epinephrine is released. Blood flows to the central nervous system, muscle, and heart from the stomach and intestines. The heart beats faster, blood pressure rises, breathing becomes more rapid, and blood glucose levels increase. Physiologic changes can also result in such manifestations as anorexia, urinary urgency, shifts in temperature, and changes in menstrual flow. "In considering the neuroanatomical basis of anxiety it is therefore important to take into account the anxiogenic stimulus that is presented, how this may be interpreted prior to making a response and also how other factors such as previously learned experiences influence the response."[16, p. 152]

Related Factors*

Acute or chronic illness
Terminal illness or potential death
Diminished sensory capabilities
Diminished functional capabilities
Anticipated operation
Possible adverse parts of treatment plan
Anticipated discomfort or pain
Perceived or actual threat to physical safety
Uncertainty about own health
Unmet needs
Perceived or actual threat to core or to essence of personality
Perceived or actual threat to self-concept or self-esteem
Perceived or actual threat to goal achievement
Unconscious conflict
Arousal of both positive and negative evaluative thoughts
Interpersonal transmission or contagion
Empathic linkage with significant other
Perceived or actual threat to personal security pattern
Adverse interpersonal relationships
Perceived, actual, or anticipated disapproval by significant others
Perceived or actual threat to meaningful interpersonal relationship or patterns and belonging
Adverse influences (especially in childhood)
   Absence of love from significant other(s)
   Absence of respect from significant other(s)

Criticism by significant other(s)
Rejection by significant other(s)
Disapproval by other person(s)
Situational or maturational crises
Array of psychosocial stressors (e.g., change, losses)
Perceived or actual failure of adaptive coping skills
Perceived or actual change in role functioning
Perceived or actual threat to stable environment
Minimal previous exposures to health care setting
Invasion of privacy in health care setting
Impending hospitalization
Inadequate knowledge about illness and treatment
Perceived or actual change in socioeconomic status
Environmental stressors (e.g., housing problems, transportation difficulties, depressed economy, unemployment)
Perceived or actual threat to value system, beliefs, or ideals

Defining Characteristics†

Mild anxiety

Mild, vague, diffuse, objectless, apprehensive, anxious response to threat
Mild, vague, diffuse, objectless, apprehensive, anxious response to threat to personality core
Tension-relieving behaviors
   Lip-chewing
   Finger-tapping
   Foot-shuffling
   Nail-biting
Restlessness
Irritability
Belittling others
Misunderstandings
Slight discomfort or tension
Slight uneasiness
Increased alertness
Increased awareness and perception
Attention seeking
Repetitive questioning
Enhanced problem-solving ability
Increased learning
Increased involvement in activities approved by others (especially during childhood)

Moderate anxiety

Moderate, vague, diffuse, objectless, apprehensive, anxious response to threat
Moderate, vague, diffuse, objectless, apprehensive, anxious response to threat to personality core
Increased muscle tension
   Trembling
   Hand tremors
   Facial tension

---

*References 7-9, 11, 12, 18, 23-25.

†References 1, 7, 8, 9, 12, 13, 22-25.

Increased heart rate
Increased respiratory rate
Urinary frequency
Urinary urgency
Diaphoresis
Sleeplessness
Change in voice pitch
Voice tremors
Somatic complaints
Shakiness
Keyed up
Worrying
Moderate uneasiness
Increased verbalizations
Moderate feeling of diffuseness
Slightly lowered self-esteem
Slight sense of worthlessness
Moderate discomfort or tension
Pacing
Increased alertness
Increased learning
Selective inattention
Increasing concentration on problem situation
Narrowing of perceptual field
Increased concentration on sensory data relevant to problem
Moderate sense of isolation
Increasingly engaging in activities that elicit approval from significant others (especially during childhood)

Severe anxiety

Severe, vague, diffuse, objectless, apprehensive, anxious response to threat
Severe, vague, diffuse, objectless, apprehensive, anxious response to threat to personality core
Tachycardia
Hyperventilation
Urinary frequency
Urinary urgency
Nausea
Dizziness
Headache
Insomnia
Uncertainty
Severe uneasiness
Jitters
Severe worry
Sense of impending doom
Painful sense of helplessness and inadequacy
Moderate feeling of powerlessness
Moderate sense of worthlessness
Difficult or inappropriate verbalizations
Severe feeling of diffuseness
Dissociation of anxious feelings from self
Moderately low self-esteem
Denial of existence of uncomfortable feelings
Severe discomfort, distress, and tension

Purposeless activity
Reduced range of perception
  Inability to concentrate
  Focus on scattered or small details
  Selective inattention
  Inability to see connections between events or details
Lack of clear comprehension of immediate situation
Inability to learn
Severe feeling of being in hostile environment
Severe sense of isolation
Ineffective functioning

Extreme anxiety (panic)

Extremely severe, vague, diffuse, objectless, apprehensive, anxious response to threat
Extremely severe, vague, diffuse, objectless, apprehensive, anxious response to threat to personality core
Dilated pupils
Pallor
Vomiting
Sleeplessness
Severe shakiness
Feeling of personality disintegration
Extremely severe discomfort and tension
Extreme feeling of diffuseness
Extreme uncertainty
Extremely severe uneasiness
Inability to communicate
Unintelligible communication
Extreme sense of helplessness and inadequacy
Severe worthlessness
Severe powerlessness
Severely lowered self-esteem
Severe hyperactivity
Immobility
Disruption of perceptual field
Distortion of unrealistic perception of situation
Enlargement of detail
Inability to learn
Extreme feeling of isolation
Extreme sense of being in a hostile environment

Expected Patient Outcomes & Nursing Interventions*

Experience reduced anxiety, as evidenced by:

Absence or reduction in defining characteristics indicating presence of anxiety
- Develop constructive, positive, interpersonal relationship with patient:
  Be empathetic.
  Convey unconditional positive regard.
  Be congruent.

---

*References 3-8, 10, 13-15, 17, 21.

- Remain calm *so as not to increase patient's anxiety:*
    Avoid reciprocal anxiety.
    Recognize own anxiety.
    Develop control over own responses.
- Determine signs and symptoms (defining characteristics) indicating presence of anxiety; *this will assist in determining level of anxiety present.* Tools such as the Anxiety Symptoms and Beliefs Scale assess level of anxiety-related sensations.[6,21]
- Observe for perceived or actual threats *to develop some understanding about the patient's experience of anxiety:*
    Personal security pattern
    Core or essence of personality
    Self-concept
    Value system, beliefs, or ideals
    Fear *(Anxiety sensitivity can be present, which is a fear stemming from beliefs that sensations present in anxiety lead to harmful social, somatic, or psychological consequences.[21])*
- Listen to patient's description of state of discomfort.
- Identify maladaptive and adaptive current responses to anxiety.
- Identify strategies used by patient in past to cope with anxiety: *these can often be useful in coping with current anxiety.*
- Determine strengths and resources that are available to cope with current anxiety: problem-solving skills, decision-making skills, significant others, religion, professional assistance, recreational activities, hobbies.
- For patient with severe or extreme anxiety:
    Avoid asking patient to make decisions.
    Avoid probing for cause of anxiety.
    Avoid interpreting behavior or confrontation; *it is essential to lower anxiety when patient is at the severe or extreme level.*
    Use comfort measures (e.g., warm bath and restful environment).
    Keep in calm, nonstimulating milieu; remove any stress or threat; limit contact with other anxious patients.
    Use short, simple sentences.
    Use calm, firm tone of voice.
    Administer tranquilizers or sedatives, as prescribed.
    Observe for and institute needed protective measures.
    Use nonverbal behavior (e.g., quiet physical presence or touch) to offer reassurance.
- Intervene early *to prevent escalation of anxiety to severe or extreme levels.*
- In collaboration with psychiatrist, administer medications (e.g., benzodiazepines, buspirone):
    - Refer to therapist for systematic desensitization, biofeedback, or psychotherapy; *these therapies can be useful in decreasing experiences of severe or extreme anxiety.*
    - Refer to self-help programs.
    - Use active listening skills.

- Facilitate patient's participation in recreational and diversional activities *because these activities can be aimed at decreasing anxiety:*
    Sedative music *(In certain circumstances the use of earphones may enhance the effects of music.[2])*
    Group singing or instrumental groups
    Simple games
    Housekeeping chores
    Grooming activities
    Routine tasks
    Walking or jogging
    Simple, concrete tasks
    Swimming
- Facilitate patient's participation in exercise (e.g., walking, jogging, swimming). *Exercise reduces anxiety. Aerobic exercise has a greater effect in reducing state anxiety. Length of exercise (16 weeks or longer) has greater effect in reducing trait anxiety. Duration of exercise (at least 21 minutes) has been shown to reduce both trait and state anxiety.[15]*
- Encourage ventilation of feelings when patient is ready; permit crying.
- Offer brief and clear information about experiences during hospitalization; *this can prevent anxiety.*
- Use therapeutic touch, if appropriate, or relaxation therapy because these have been found to reduce anxiety.
- Convey attitude that there is hope and that a constructive resolution can be found.
- Prevent further escalation of anxiety *by avoiding threats, indifference, rejection, judgmental attitude, impatience, unrealistic demands, insincerity, and focusing on patient's weaknesses because these can increase feelings of insecurity and anxiety.*
- During short-term hospitalization, offer additional support and assistance in dealing with anxiety on admission, on the fifth day, and on notification of discharge.
- Mutually develop daily schedule of activities, incorporating patient's strengths, abilities, preferences, and goals.

Recognize anxiety, develop insight, and use adaptive coping strategies, as evidenced by:

Verbalizing recognition of anxiety in self
Describing situations in which anxiety is increased
Using strategies to reduce own anxiety
Using mild anxiety for personal growth and change
- If anxiety is at mild or moderate levels, help patient to:
    Recognize presence of anxiety by providing feedback on characteristics indicating anxiety and by asking questions: "Are you uncomfortable right now?"
    Explore similarity between present and past experiences; ask questions: "Have you felt like this before? What was happening to you then? What did you do to reduce your discomfort?"
    Identify thoughts or expectations before becoming anxious.
    Identify relationship between anxiety and consequent adaptive or maladaptive responses.

Clarify nature of threat to self.

Develop adaptive strategies to prevent escalation of anxiety.

Problem-solve.

Evaluate results of strategies used.

Implement alternatives for unsuccessful results.

- Reduce any secondary gains from maladaptive strategies used in coping with anxiety.
- Permit patient to set pace in solving problems.
- Reduce negative expectations.
- Facilitate development of constructive and optimistic view of existence, especially if patient's view is distorted.
- Facilitate choice of effective, objective environmental interventions to cope with anxiety; this is important especially *if patient is already optimistic, open to new experiences, and flexible.*
- Encourage participation in new interests and hobbies.
- After establishing relationship with patient and after extreme or severe anxiety has been reduced:

  Encourage social activities despite reluctance and fears.

  Attend activities with patient initially; permit patient to leave if anxiety is greatly increased; gradually encourage attendance independent of staff support.
- Use role playing to deal with anxiety-provoking situations; with children, try role-play strategies using puppets, dolls, or other playthings, art, or play requiring large motor activities.
- Teach patient to:

  Recognize constructive aspects of mild or moderate anxiety in learning, growth, and movement toward self-actualization. Provide patient education pamphlets about anxiety.

  Recognize personal characteristics that indicate presence of anxiety.

  Recognize causes and management strategies for anxiety.

  Examine current goals and beliefs in relation to what is actually happening.

  Observe self and monitor management of own anxiety.

  Develop assertive communication skills.

  Develop problem-solving and decision-making skills.

  Practice cognitive coping skills.

  Use progressive muscle relaxation.

  Increase repertoire of strategies to reduce anxiety (e.g., talking or being in presence of someone; simple, concrete tasks; walking; noncompetitive sports; professional assistance; listening to soothing music; meditating; prayer; performing deep breathing exercises and relaxation exercises).

  Engage in progressive muscle relaxation.

Principles and Rationale for Nursing Interventions[26]

Anxiety varies among persons in its intensity, depending on severity of threat, perception by the person, previous and current coping skills, and success or failure of the person's efforts to cope with the feelings of discomfort experienced in anxiety. Coping mechanisms can be either adaptive or maladaptive. Disturbed or maladaptive coping strategies include inability to make choices, rigidity and repetition, alienation, withdrawal, conflict, extreme denial, distortion of awareness of the situation, acting out, depression, moderate to severe aggression, somatizing, and seeking secondary gains. Adaptive strategies or dealing with anxiety include learning more about the confronting situation, problem solving, increasing self-understanding, and seeking and engaging in constructive outlets for emotions.

In anxiety the security pattern (the foundation on which the patient distinguishes himself or herself from the environment) is threatened. These threats can be directed toward anything the patient holds essential to that central core or security pattern: a threat to physical safety; the ability to meet physiologic needs; or the ability to meet higher-level needs (e.g., self-esteem, belonging, meaning, freedom, patriotism, or goal achievement).

For the patient with severe and extreme anxiety, an important expected patient outcome is the reduction of anxiety. Develop a constructive, positive interpersonal relationship with the patient. Assess the level of anxiety and evaluate the patient for maladaptive coping patterns. Nursing interventions are tailored to provide reassurance to the patient in a calm, nonthreatening environment.

At a moderate or low level of anxiety the patient can be assisted in recognizing anxiety in self, in gaining insight into the anxiety, and in developing constructive strategies to cope with the anxiety. A number of nursing interventions described in the literature are useful in reducing a patient's anxiety (e.g., visitation by a familiar person while in a postanesthesia care unit; preoperative teaching; anxiety management group; exposure therapy; cognitive therapy; cognitive restructuring; pharmacologic treatment; prediction and rehearsal; exercise[19] progressive relaxation;[26] assertive behavior training; biofeedback; supportive, educative counseling; and guided imagery.[26]

RISK FOR LONELINESS

A subjective state in which an individual is at risk for having a vague, unpleasant experience and/or unwanted experience related to a need for more quality social relationships.[4,9]

Loneliness has been described as a vague, empty, uncomfortable feeling that individuals try to avoid.[4] It is a subjective emotional state that is identified when a person expresses a discrepancy between desired and available relationships.[23] Weiss,[24] an early reseacher of loneliness, described two theories responsible for loneliness—the situational theory and the characterology theory. The situational theory describes a lack of relationships as the cause for loneliness. The characterology theory describes certain personality traits such as shyness, low self-esteem, and excessive dependency on another as causes for loneliness. When a person lacks relationships, it may be a deficit of either quantity (number of relationships) or quality.[19]

Yet, it is the quality deficit or lack of meaningful relationships that is most often associated with loneliness.[9] Loneliness may exist for varying lengths of time.[25] Transient loneliness occurs occasionally for a short period. Chronic loneliness may last more than 2 consecutive years. Situational loneliness occurs concurrently with a major stressful life event. It is important for nurses to identify patients who are at risk for loneliness because loneliness has been associated with an increased potential for illness[15] and serious chronic health problems across the life span, such as depression, alcoholism, and suicide.[4]

Risk Factors

Social isolation
Decreased number of social contacts[24]
Decreased quality of social relationships[24]
Lack of social supports[22]
Fear of rejection
Immobility
Lack of transportation
Chronic illnesses that restrict activity and social interactions (i.e., AIDS, chronic mental illness, alcoholism, chronic obstructive pulmonary disorder, cancer, rheumatic diseases)*
Situation in which one has difficulty acting in accordance with own ethical reasoning and feelings[11]
Visually impaired elderly[2]
Hearing impaired elderly[3]
Homeless individuals[15,18]
Fearful, life-threatening conditions
Older adults[23]
Spiritual distress
Loss of close relationships[23]

Defining Characteristics

Verbalizes desire to have more social contacts
Verbalizes desire to have more meaningful relationships
Expresses vague, empty, unpleasant, unhappy, sad feelings[4]
Describes self as not part of a group[4]
Describes inability to discuss fears, anxieties, and uncertainties openly with others[10]
Distancing from others and preoccupation with self

Expected Patient Outcomes & Nursing Interventions

Achieve and maintain meaningful social relationships as evidenced by:

Demonstrating effective ways to learn to meet and interact with others
Verbalizing presence of meaningful social relationships
Verbalizing comfort in being with self and others

---

*References 4, 5, 7, 9-11, 16, 20, 22.

Demonstrating ability to develop supportive networks
Interacting effectively with family members or significant others
Interacting effectively with others within the community
Verbalizing fears, anxieties, and concerns with appropriate others

- Display a genuine concern for the patient as a person. *A caring relationship will promote trust and help establish an appropriate working environment.*[8]
- Be aware that loneliness may be disguised or expressed in physical or psychological forms.[8] *A careful assessment is needed to determine a correct nursing diagnosis and plan appropriate interventions.*
- Provide the patient with ample opportunities to describe, interpret, and validate feelings of loneliness[8] *so appropriate interventions can be planned.*
- Encourage the patient to recall how loneliness was successfully dealt with in the past[8,11]; *successful past experiences with loneliness may be applied to the current situation.*
- Assist patient in determining emotional and social needs and who within the patient's network can best meet those needs; *specific needs must be matched with available resources.*[6]
- Assess size and satisfaction with current support networks *to determine adequacy.*
- Encourage discussion of network expectations *to help patient determine whether patient's expectations are realistic.*[2]
- Help patient to expand network beyond that of a few individuals.[2] *This will increase the likelihood that a supportive person will be available when needed.*
- Encourage the patient to assertively communicate his/her needs to the support network.[2] *The network must perceive a need before it can mobilize to assist the individual.*
- Assist the elderly patient to increase and use networks beyond calling on adult children to meet all needs; *this will help prevent "burn-out" of the children.*[6]
- Encourage (if not already doing so) patient to serve as a support person for others. *Providing support to others may increase self-esteem by feeling needed and decreasing loneliness.*[6]
- Promote *meaningful* activities, such as reading; beginning a new hobby; caring for a pet; watching television; church/synagogue services; involvement in organizations; volunteer work with the elderly, youth, or homeless, or in such places as hospitals, nursing homes, schools, libraries, or relief agencies.[11,23] *The activity must hold significance for the individual or loneliness may only be accentuated rather than alleviated.*
- Stress the importance of *future* thinking and planning of activities or events. *Dwelling on the past may magnify feelings of current loneliness.*
- Inform patient that often loneliness is increased at night.[11] *Being aware of this increased occurrence may allow the patient to plan activities specifically for the evening hours.*

- Encourage the use of music, such as listening, playing in a group, or attending a music program; *to increase socialization, and promote relaxation.*[18]
- Teach stress management strategies and relaxation techniques. *This may help to decrease the need for extensive and active relaxation networks.*
- Teach positive coping skills. *A sense of hopefulness can be promoted, which is necessary for effective coping, gaining a sense of control, and promoting quality of life.*[20]
- Encourage the patient to select a story, poem, song, or picture that best expresses his/her feelings. *This can be useful in helping personalize loneliness and facilitate communicating thoughts and feelings to others.*[4]
- Involve the patient in keeping a journal. *This may be helpful in identifying repeating themes or patterns of loneliness.*[4]
- Assist the patient to identify and diminish barriers that may restrict social contact, such as transportation, communication, financial constraints, or aesthetic problems (e.g., body odors, dental problems, deformities, bowel or bladder incontinence).

Principles and Rationale for Nursing Interventions

Loneliness is a subjective state. Therefore individuals can identify their feelings and degree of loneliness, and can often determine how to reduce or alleviate the causes of loneliness.[8,11] The nurse must realize that being alone does not cause loneliness.[24] It is rather the lack of desired relationships that results in loneliness. Superficial relationships or indiscriminate socializing may in fact exacerbate loneliness because it can emphasize that which is missing in one's life.[24]

The degree of loneliness has been inversely related to the size of one's supportive network.[9] Yet, others suggest that networks are made up of quality rather than quantity of relationships.[6,9,24] Support networks need to be sufficient in size to provide for the individual's needs, share supportive care, help prevent overuse of any one person, and that in crisis situations a support person is available.[6] Because different types of supportive networks serve specific functions, an individual's specific needs must be closely matched with available resources.

Adult children are often the major support system for their elderly parents and relatives. It is important to increase the scope and quality of the older person's network to decrease overdependence on the supportive person(s), which may lead to burn-out.[6]

Supportive networks also provide emotional and social support, allow for the expression of caring and comfort, and provide an avenue for relaxation and coping.[2] Encouraging the individual to become part of networks for others can improve self-satisfaction and self-esteem. By becoming involved in meaningful relationships, feelings of loneliness may be reduced or alleviated. Research findings support that as satisfaction with networks increases, feelings of loneliness and depression decrease.[9] The need for relaxation or the need for someone to help the lonely individual relax was indicated in a study by Barron and associates[2] as a major factor associated with loneliness. Loneliness was associated with greater network dissatisfaction related to a need for caring and relaxation. Social support provides not only emotional support but also furnishes an avenue for expressing comfort and caring and to share thoughts and feelings.[1,2] However, if expectations for benefits from networks are unrealistically high and are not met, a sense of dissatisfaction will likely amplify feelings of loneliness.

Effective coping can assist the individual to gain control of his or her life and foster a sense of hopefulness.[20] Walton et al.[23] found that hopelessness was associated with increased loneliness in older adults. Conversely, decreased loneliness was found to be associated with a stronger sense of spiritual well-being.[23]

Music can be used to improve social skills and enhance one's ability to interact more comfortably with others. Music then provides an opportunity for the individual to establish relationships with those who have similar musical preferences.[18] Penden[18] suggests that listening to music can decrease feelings of loneliness and isolation. Music may also foster a sense of well-being and allow patients to come together in a meaningful activity.[18]

The nurses can play an active role in assisting the patient in dealing with loneliness whether it be chronic or situational in nature. Assisting the patient to actively participate in the care will increase the likelihood of positive outcomes.

■ HOPELESSNESS

Hopelessness is the subjective state in which an individual sees limited or no alternatives or personal choices available and is unable to mobilize energy on own behalf.

The inability to mobilize energy, or state of inactivity, that occurs in hopelessness results in dependence on others and a concomitant lowering of self-esteem. Some authors describe a relationship between hopelessness and goal attainment.[3,7] Motivation (action) to achieve a goal is related to the individual's perception of the probability of attaining the goal and the perceived significance of the goal. When experiencing hopelessness, the individual believes that the future holds little promise and that plans will not achieve goals. A passive acceptance of the future and inability to determine personal goals result.

Hopelessness may evolve from powerlessness, a perception that one's behavior cannot affect an outcome. The perception of inability to achieve outcomes through personal actions results in helplessness. The individual who feels helpless is hesitant to initiate actions and develops negative expectations for the future. Inability to cope with the present and the belief that the future will not improve result in hopelessness.

Related Factors[5,7,10-12]

Prolonged restriction of activity resulting in isolation
Deteriorating physiologic condition

Deteriorating mental condition
Terminal illness
Sudden event disruptive to life pattern
Long-term stress
Abandonment
Perceived significant loss (e.g., loved one, youth, influence, opportunity)
Belief that stress, event, or illness is uncontrollable
Loss of belief in transcendent values or God
Series of failures to reach desired goal
Persistent cognitive errors (i.e., negative ideas of self, world, and future)
Lifestyle of helplessness

Defining Characteristics*

Passivity
Decreased verbalization
Apathy
Verbal cues indicating despondency
Lack of initiative or motivation
Decreased response to stimuli
Nonverbal cues of withdrawal from others (e.g., turning away from speaker, closing eyes)
Decreased appetite
Increased or decreased sleep
Fatigue or lethargy
Lack of participation in self-care
Verbalization of low self-esteem
Verbalization of lack of control over self and environment
Isolating self from others
Inability to identify specific feelings
Expressions of psychologic discomfort (e.g., tenseness, irritability, sensation of lump in throat)
Expressed loss of gratification from roles or relationships
Absence of sense of continuity between past, present, and future
Verbal or nonverbal expressions of negative future expectations
Lack of personal goals
Impaired decision making

Expected Patient Outcomes & Nursing Interventions[7-9,13,14]

Maintain adequate self-care, as evidenced by:

Implementing self-care activities
Recognizing unmet need
Selecting appropriate self-care activity
- Assist patient in assuming responsibility for selection and implementation of self-care activities through teaching and support; *activity level affects internal sense of hopefulness.*

*References 4, 5, 7, 8, 11, 13.

- Implement self-care activities to meet needs patient is unable to meet.
- Involve significant others in selection and implementation of self-care activities; *hope depends on interaction with significant others.*
- Provide positive reinforcement for successful attempts at self-care; *rewards encourage repetition of behaviors.*

Establish support system, as evidenced by:

Maintaining sustaining relationships
Visiting with significant others
Accepting assistance from others, when appropriate
- Build trust through consistency and reliability; *hope thrives in an atmosphere of trust.*
- Designate same staff, as possible, to work with patient; *for some patients, professionals are their only source of support.*
- Furnish opportunities for patient to spend time with others; gradually increase amount of time and number of persons; *the nurse can serve as the vehicle through which the patient negotiates a broader support system.*
- Identify options for increasing support system for patient.

Develop realistic self-esteem, as evidenced by:

Expressing positive self-statements
Identifying strengths and abilities
Verbalizing feelings of adequacy
- Convey unconditional positive regard; *development of self-esteem depends on repetitive positive interactions with others.*
- Assist patient to identify strengths and abilities; *identification of strengths positively influences the patient's self-esteem.*
- Assist patient to develop skills that contribute to mastery of the environment; *a positive self-esteem enables a person to seek out a new environment or deal with his or her existing environment constructively.*
- Encourage patient to carry out roles and responsibilities that reinforce positive feelings; *hopelessness is based on present opportunities for success.*

Verbalize feeling of hopefulness, as evidenced by:

Verbalizing future expectations
Verbalizing feelings of adequacy
- Observe for suicidal intent; *a negative attitude toward the future is a strong indicator of suicidal intent.*
- Encourage expression of feelings through communication; *hopelessness is abated by expression of feelings.*
- Assist patient to recognize and describe feelings of hopelessness.
- Assist patient to identify reason for living by focusing on concrete ideas and feelings.
- Assist patient to direct thoughts beyond the present to the future; *a sense of the possible and of the future is a critical element of hope.*

Control or influence self and environment, as evidenced by:

Participating in or making health care decisions

Setting realistic goals

Using problem-solving skills

- Provide opportunity for patient input into health care decisions; *patient input into care results in a sense of responsibility for outcome.*
- Teach patient to distinguish between controllable and uncontrollable events; *hopelessness is characterized by a perception of loss of control over present events and future outcomes.*
- Demonstrate and teach problem-solving skills; *control over self and environment is enhanced through expanding problem-solving capacity.*
- Assist patient to evaluate performance realistically.

Principles and Rationale for Nursing Interventions[1,3,5,7,14]

Hope is an expectation of achieving a goal. A hopeful patient believes that there is a way out and that changes can be managed with help.[4] Hopefulness has been positively correlated with health status and quality of life, even in chronic or terminal illness. In addition, hopefulness is influenced by others. Therefore the concept of hopefulness is pertinent to the practice of nursing (i.e., a nurse can affect health care outcomes through positively influencing a patient's hopefulness).

Tools are available for assessment of hope.[4,12] Nursing interventions designed to facilitate the patient's ability to identify a variety of alternatives, mobilize energy and resources, determine personal goals, and initiate effective actions to meet goals will overcome feelings of hopelessness.

A patient's hopelessness can be abated by involvement in his or her self- or health care. Activity level affects the patient's internal sense of hopefulness. In a multinational validation study of the nursing diagnosis of hopelessness, the diagnostic content validation (DCV) model was used. In this model, defining characteristics with ratios of 0.80 or greater are labeled as critical. In this study the DCV ratio for the defining characteristic of lack of involvement in care for the nursing diagnosis of hopelessness was greater than 0.80.[13] Therefore nursing interventions to assist a patient to maintain adequate self-care focus on assisting, supporting, and reinforcing the patient's efforts to perform self-care, implementing self-care activities that the patient is unable to perform, and involving significant others in self-care activities.

A person's hope depends on interaction with significant others[3] and thrives in an atmosphere of trust. The nurse must assess the adequacy of the patient's social support system and whether it functions in a positive or negative manner.[8] For some patients, health care professionals are the only source of support. The nurse may be the vehicle through which the patient negotiates a broader support system. Therefore nursing interventions to assist the patient to establish a support system focus on building trust, assigning consistent staff, identifying with the patient options for increasing support, and providing opportunities for spending time with others.

A patient's hopelessness can also be abated by enhancement of self-esteem (the estimate an individual places on himself or herself). Development of self-esteem depends on repetitive, positive interactions with significant others. A positive self-esteem enables a person to seek and deal with environmental experiences constructively.[6] Hopefulness is based on present opportunities for and memories of successes.[4] Nursing interventions that assist the patient to develop realistic self-esteem focus on conveying unconditional, positive regard, assisting the patient to identify strengths and develop skills that contribute to mastery of the environment, and encouraging the patient to carry out roles and responsibilities that reinforce positive feelings.

Verbal cues have been identified as a defining characteristic of hopelessness since the North American Nursing Diagnosis Association accepted this nursing diagnosis in 1987. In an international validation study on the nursing diagnosis of hopelessness, verbal cues met the criterion (DCV ratio of equal or greater than 0.80) for a critical characteristic in two of the six participating countries. The mean DCV ratio of 0.765 for verbal cues for all participating countries approached the criterion for designation as critical.[13] The presence of verbal cues is also critical in terms of need for nursing intervention because a negative attitude toward the future has been determined to be a strong indicator of suicidal intent.[9] Therefore nursing interventions to assist a patient to verbalize feelings of hopefulness focus on assisting the patient to identify reasons for living and to direct thoughts beyond the present; the nurse must observe the patient for suicidal intent, encourage expression of feelings, and help the patient to recognize and describe feelings of hopelessness.

A patient's hopelessness can be further abated by control over self and the environment.[9] Common manifestations of hopelessness include a perception of loss of control over future outcomes and passive acceptance of the futility of planning to achieve goals. Perception of control or influence over self and the environment is enhanced by expanding coping ability and problem-solving capacity, as well as by a sense of cognitive mastery.[10] Critical elements of hope include a sense of the possible, anticipation, achieving goals and freedom, as opposed to a sense of entrapment.[9] Therefore nursing interventions that assist the patient to control or influence self and the environment focus on providing opportunities for patient input into health care decisions. These interventions teach the patient to distinguish between controllable and uncontrollable events; enhance problem-solving skills; help the patient evaluate performance realistically, develop realistic goals; and provide positive reinforcement for success in problem solving, coping, and control.

■ POWERLESSNESS

Powerlessness is the patient's perception that his or her action will not significantly affect an outcome; it is a perceived lack of control over a current situation or immediate happening.[8]

McFarland, Leonard, and Morris[10] define power as the generalized capacity or potential to get others to do something one wants them to do, which they would not ordinarily do otherwise. Although power can be abused, these authors point out that power has a positive aspect and exists within the context of interpersonal relationships. "The feeling of possessing some form of personal power, the sense that one is to a degree the creator of one's own life, is essential to the sense of self."[9] Antecedents for power include personal self-confidence, involvement of two or more persons, power perceived as good, possession of power skills (respect, concern, communication skills), and possession of at least one of the bases of power.[7]

One can identify five bases for personal social power[4]:

Expert power—based on skill or knowledge

Reward power—based on ability to give positive rewards to others

Referent power—based on the personal characteristics with which another person identifies

Legitimate power—based on the right to be influential over others

Coercive power—based on the ability to administer punishment

Powerlessness can be situationally determined and related to locus of control; it can be a long-term tendency to perceive situations in a certain way.[11]

"The focal stimulus for powerlessness will be the immediate situation impinging on the person's sense of control. Illness is often that focus stimulus."[3] A sense of powerlessness arises from an individual's belief that outside forces, such as chance, govern what happens in life and that personal resources are not available to influence the consequences of a person's own actions or give control over a person's situation. The degree of perceived powerlessness can be influenced by the importance of a desired outcome, the person's expectation for being in control, or the person's expectation that his or her actions can make a difference in the outcome.

Related Factors*

Authoritarian health care team behavior

Stripping of personal possessions
Excessive surveillance
Assault on privacy
Lack of individualization
Castelike separation from persons in authority
Misuse of rewards and punishment
Monopoly of scarce or strategic resources
Misuse of power or authority
Controlled conditions of negotiation
Blocking of resources

Sociocultural factors

Lack of parental role model
Parental influences and parenting styles

Perception of authority figures as distant or unapproachable
Excessive threatening experiences
Unsupportive environment
Unequal power among or between persons (e.g., battering relationship)
Peer influence
Repeated interpersonal failures and problems
Actual or potential loss of significant other
Presence of stigma

Altered health status

Altered state of physical wellness
Physiologic lack of control
Frustration in obtaining adequate pain relief[5]
Dependence on chemical substances
Physical immobility
Loss of functional ability
Alterations in mental status
Weak ego identity

Cognitive perceptual factors

Altered attention span
Negative self-esteem
Lack of knowledge
Lack of ability to participate in decision making
Lack of belief in ability to do a task or engage in a behavior

Environmental factors

Lack of available or accessible personal resources
Lack of ability to reward a favor
Lack of ability to extort a concession or do without
Belief in lack of control over resources
Disturbing experiences in relation to institutions
Hostile environment
Negative experiences before admission to health care facilities
Hospitalization
Threatening, unfamiliar technology
Unpredictable environment
Alterations in schedule
Overwhelming stressors

Developmental factors

Delay or distortion in accomplishing development tasks
Developmental changes
Loss of independent role
Loss of autonomy

Defining Characteristics†

Verbal expression of having no control or influence over the situation or outcome
Verbalization of feelings of loss of control
Verbal expression of having no control over self-care

---

*References 3, 5, 8, 9, 11-13, 15, 17-19.

†References 2, 3, 8, 13, 15-17, 19.

Feelings of depression
Passivity
Resignation
Anxiety
Inappropriate aggression
Aimlessness
Resentment
Expression of feelings of inadequacy
Rationalization of failure
Projection of blame on others and environment
Lack of knowledge about own illness
Not willing to seek information about care
Few plans to use health care services
Doubts about role performance
Frustration about inability to perform previously mastered activities
Fears about alienation from caregivers
Overdependence on others
Asking many questions or no questions
Loss of control over environment
Loss of control over self-functioning and personal behavior
Inappropriate, immature coping abilities for development stage
Inability to influence others
Preference for immediate rewards over long-term goals
Sleeplessness
Withdrawal from activities
Wandering

Expected Patient Outcomes & Nursing Interventions[1,6,8,17]

Influence outcomes in current situations, as evidenced by:

Verbalization of ability to control or influence situation and outcomes
Verbalization of feelings of powerfulness and adequacy
Knowledge about control-relevant situation
Adequate role-functioning and coping skills
Goal-directed behavior
Expression of hope
Involvement in decision making
Working toward long-term goals

- Monitor patient's powerlessness by asking these questions:
    Are perceived abilities to influence personal outcome present?
    Are there verbal expressions of:
        Having no control or influence over situation or outcome?
        Feelings of loss of control and powerlessness?
    Does the patient experience characteristics such as lack of decision making? Lack of knowledge about illness and treatment? Withdrawal?
    Are environmental factors, staff behaviors, or other related factors present that can lead to a sense of powerlessness (e.g., excessive surveillance, assault on privacy, lack of individualization)?

Does patient believe he or she has ability to accomplish given task?
Baseline data are essential for developing an individualized plan of care.

- Make change within institutions or residential settings:
    Determine organizational barriers to patient empowerment.
    Decrease surveillance of patient unless essential for safety.
    Minimize rules and regulations; permit patient input in his or her development.
    Enhance individuality and autonomy.
    Increase patient control over rewards.
    Preserve privacy; increase territorial rights.
    Allow patient to wear own clothes.
    Prevent a castelike separation between staff and patients.
    Vary setting and routine of daily activities based on patient input. *It is important to develop a sense of partnership among health care providers, the patient, and the patient's significant others.*
    Do not block patient's attainment and use of resources (within limits of safety).
    Do not use coercion.
    Support patient's efforts to increase resources.
    Decrease dependency on staff; encourage independent behavior.
    Maintain patient's sense of dignity; permit exploration of environment.
    Be less directive and overprotective.
    Foster personal powerfulness by putting bedside stand, call light, telephone, etc., within reach.
    Promote active involvement in appropriate decision making in activities of daily living.
    Involve patient in other decision-making opportunities and planning own care.
    Provide patient with positive and predictable events (e.g., group experiences).
    Provide opportunities for engagement in meaningful activities.
    Provide opportunities for family to participate in care.
These environmental changes help patient maximize the patient's ability to control events and decrease the sense of powerlessness.
- Help patient reduce feelings of powerlessness:
    Build trusting relationship.
    Be consistent and dependable.
    Use active listening.
    Encourage verbalization about feelings and concerns about feelings of powerlessness.
- Help patient recognize and describe powerlessness; identify the behavior with patient.
- Help patient separate controllable from uncontrollable events.
- Help patient identify personal preferences, wants, feelings, values, and attitudes.

- Help patient set realistic goals.
- Teach patient to problem solve and try out alternative coping strategies.
- Help patient identify and use strengths and potential; identify improvement in condition.
- Help patient improve self-esteem *because this can help patient feel capable in exerting more influence.*
- Provide situations in which patient can succeed and experience control.
- Assess patient's perception and knowledge of treatment program, encouraging expression of views before giving information.
- Assess internal versus external locus of control before patient teaching.
- *For those with internal locus of control,* provide information that gives patient a sense of control, using different strategies of content presentation.
- *For those with external locus of control,* provide structured approaches, teach in small increments, and involve in determining readiness for learning.
- Help patient seek and master relevant health information.
- Provide needed information.
- Encourage patient to ask questions; reinforce right to ask questions.
- Help patient use health care personnel.
- Restore energy imbalance.
- Allow patient to assume more complicated decision making when ready.
- Provide positive reinforcement and acknowledgement for active participation in appropriately selected therapeutic modalities, such as sensitivity training, behavior modification, brief psychotherapy, encounter groups, and community action programs, or by using interventions, such as altering perception of life situation; using behavioral rehearsal and role playing, rewarding manifestations of internality, challenging external locus of control-oriented verbalizations, examining possible outcomes of alternative approaches, and teaching assertive communication skills.
- Facilitate improvement in life circumstances: returning to work, constructive interactions with significant other, successful therapy experiences, constructive family interactions, and role models.
- Involve significant others, alerting them to importance of their reactions to the patient.
- Refer for family therapy as appropriate.
- Refer to self-help groups as appropriate.

Principles and Rationale for Nursing Interventions

A patient with a high *internal* locus of control perceives that his or her life and circumstances are controlled primarily by self-determined activity, actions, and characteristics. A patient with a high *external* locus of control, on the other hand, perceives his life and circumstances to be primarily controlled by external events (e.g., fate, chance, luck, powerful people, or unpre-

dictability caused by the complexity of situations). Increased external locus of control reflects a sense of helplessness[14] and a general expectancy of powerlessness. Most person's locus of control is somewhere in the middle of this continuum.[18]

Powerlessness can cause difficulty in learning control-relevant information. It is important to involve the patient in making decisions about content to be included in patient teaching programs. Because locus of control can influence the patient's ability to use control-relevant information,[14] the degree of powerlessness needs to be assessed before patient teaching. Provide information that gives patients with an internal locus of control, a sense of control, using different strategies of content presentation. For those with an external locus of control, the nurse should provide structured approaches, teach in small increments, and involve them in determining what aspects of health care they are ready to learn.

A patient's powerlessness can be diminished by power rebuilding, augmenting, or improving power resources—physical strength, psychologic stamina, support networks, self-concept, energy, knowledge, motivation, and a belief system (hope). Effective coping strategies must be preserved, augmented, and developed. Effective coping strategies result in a decrease in uncomfortable feelings, generation of hope, enhancement of self-esteem, maintenance of positive interpersonal relationships, and maintenance of or improvement in the state of coping.

SELF-ESTEEM DISTURBANCE; SITUATIONAL LOW SELF-ESTEEM; CHRONIC LOW SELF-ESTEEM

Self-esteem disturbance is the direct or indirect expression of negative self-evaluation and/or feelings about one's competence, social acceptability, and/or physical attractiveness.[25,28]

Situational low self-esteem is a negative self-evaluation and negative feelings about the self that develop in response to a loss or change in an individual who previously had a positive self-evaluation.[25]

Chronic low self-esteem is a long-standing negative self-evaluation for feelings about the self or about the individual's capabilities.[25]

Self-esteem disturbance is a disruption in self-estimation, including self-worth, self-approval, self-confidence, and self-respect. The person with low self-esteem has trouble incorporating constructive information for maintaining a positive self-concept.[28] Self-esteem is a "subjective and enduring sense of realistic self-approval. It reflects how the individual views and values the self at the most fundamental level of psychological experiencing, . . . a central component of personality that affects and is affected by almost any psychological difficulty."[1, p. 4] Self-esteem is the evaluative component of self-concept. Although the terms "self-concept" and "self-esteem" are often used interchangeably, "self-esteem is viewed as one of the many components of the self concept."[31, p. 189] Self-concept has been defined "as a complex and multifaceted knowledge structure that consists of a stable and enduring collection of images, beliefs, and attitudes about the self."[30, p. 406] Variables that influence a person's self-concept and that can produce tension and stress, resulting in subsequent anxiety and eventual disorganization of a person's self-concept, are physical and personality characteristics present at birth, family and environmental factors, emotional/social/cultural interactive experiences, and any psychologic difficulty.

Coopersmith[7] identifies four major factors that contribute to self-esteem development in children: (1) others' perceived value of the child, as evidenced by attention and affection; (2) the child's pattern of coping with negative criticisms; (3) successful experiences; and (4) the child's own definition of failure or success. The development of self-esteem is influenced by the number of repetitive, positive experiences encountered in interactions with significant others in the environment. Parental relationships and the reflected appraisal the child receives from parents are important, as are the appraisals the child receives from others that are perceived as significant (e.g., teachers and older siblings). Symmetrical interactions—friendships—become increasingly important to adolescents, whose self-esteem is influenced by their friends' evaluations.[15,28]

A person's overall evaluation of self can result from the "tendency to consistently cope with or avoid that which one fears."[1] Persons with high self-esteem feel significant and confident and capable of achieving desired goals, whereas those with lowered self-esteem may be less confident. People with high self-esteem confront rather than retreat from challenges. They demonstrate the ability to learn from failures, as well as successes. They convey respect for themselves and others.[4]

Related Factors*

Perception of ill health
Health problems
Chronic illness
Inability to adjust to body function alterations
Inability to adjust to body structure losses
Cognitive perceptual difficulties
Depression
Early loss of parent or significant other
Traumatic developmental experiences
Excessive ridicule by others
Inadequate early parenting
Inadequate positive feedback
Parental alcoholism or family dysfunction
Parents' negative perception of *their* own competence and
   self-esteem
Multiple stressors encountered over limited time
Unresolved emotionally traumatic experiences
Difficulty accepting positive feedback
Unrealistic self-expectations
Negative interpretations of life events (e.g., assuming guilt)

*References 2, 3, 5, 8, 9, 11-13, 16-18, 22, 23, 28.

Inadequate knowledge to cope with life stressors
Lack of problem-solving skills
Repeated negative interpersonal experiences with significant others (e.g., spouse, partner, or children)
Spouse abuse or elder abuse
Inadequate social support
Lack of close relationship with significant others
Lack of supportive experiences outside home
External locus of control

Situational low self-esteem

Major Loss

Loss of body part, function, or process
Loss of significant other
Loss of job, work, or role
Loss of pet
Loss of material goods
Loss of reputation

Major Life Change or Stress

Divorce or marriage
Prison term
Addition or loss of family member
Failure in school
Financial burden
Promotion or demotion
Adolescent adjustments
Sexual difficulties
Hospitalization
Occupational change
Incongruence between behavior and values

Environmental Factors

Disasters
Poverty
Change in living conditions or residence
Discrimination
Acculturation

Chronic Low Self-Esteem

Chronic medical condition that impacts on self-care abilities
   or life patterns
Chronic mental disorder
Chronic, severe pain
Familial dysfunction
Significant early loss
Abuse, neglect, or abandonment
Loss of self-control
External locus of control
Institutionalization (e.g., especially in a setting with minimal opportunity for self-control)
Learned helplessness
Long-standing, pernicious, nebulous-fixated life response
Insular lifestyle pattern
Maladroit survival patterns
Perceived low status (social or economic)

Defining Characteristics*

Lack of eye contact

Slouched or drooping posture

Decrease in sexual relationship and drive

Lack of motivation to assume responsibilities for self-care

Lack of attention to appearance

Behavioral problems

Feelings of inferiority, inadequacy, failure, defeatism, disappointment, or worthlessness

Projection of past failures into the future

Decrease in motivation and spontaneous behavior

Difficulty with reality testing

Timidity

Feelings of self-deprecation, inadequacy, and self-dislike

Deprecative, negative comments about self

Self-accusation

Self-blame

Preoccupation with self

Overattention to shortcomings or deficiencies

Frequent rumination over past problems

Expressions of shame or guilt

Unassertiveness

Avoidance of self-disclosure; assumption of passive, non-participatory roles

Perception of minimum strengths and assets, with refusal to accept positive feedback

Hypersensitivity to criticism

Denial of past and present successes and accomplishments

Lack of confidence in one-to-one or group interactions

Fear of handling change or taking risks

Hesitancy to ask for help

Inability to communicate own needs and concerns

Inability to confront and overcome difficulties

Projection of blame or responsibility

Inability to face new situations

Evaluation of self as unable to deal with situations

Denial of problem

Rationalization of failure

Lack of initiative in problem solving

Verbalization of difficulty in coping with tasks

Hostility, laughs at or ridicules others

Attitude of superiority

Grandiose

Reluctance to engage in social interactions

Withdrawal from activities and interpersonal-social relationships

Difficulties in school

Lack of participation in therapy

Situational low self-esteem

Feelings of helplessness or uselessness

Expressions of shame or guilt

Episodic negative self-appraisal

Self-negative verbalization

Indecisiveness

Difficulty in making decisions

Chronic low self-esteem

Self-destructive behavior

Expressions of shame and guilt

Ruminations about past problems

Preoccupation with self and shortcomings

Withdrawal

Nonassertiveness and passivity

Long-standing, low self-evaluations

Self-negating verbalizations

Self-evaluation of inability to deal with situations

Rationalizing away positive feedback

Exaggeration of negative feedback

Overconformance

Seeks excessive reassurance

Hesitation about trying new things and situations

Indecisiveness

Lack of follow-through

Lack of success

Frequent lack of success in work or other life events

Alienation from community resource network

Expected Patient Outcomes & Nursing Interventions†

Achieve and maintain a constructive level of self-esteem, as evidenced by:

Improvement in personal appearance

Expressing appropriate mood

Increase in self-worth, self-respect, self-approval, and self-confidence

Engaging in positive talk about self

Identifying and using existing strengths, assets, and successes

Using strategies that can promote and maintain positive level of self-esteem

Recognizing value of and using various treatment modalities

Engaging in age-appropriate activities

Interacting with family, friends, and neighbors

Taking initiative for new learning tasks

Demonstrating adequate involvement in relevant job performance

Expressing satisfaction with own achievements

Expressing satisfaction with functional ability in preferred life roles

- Demonstrate recognition of patient as a worthwhile, trusted human being by conveying genuine interest and concern.

---

*References 1, 7, 13, 22, 25, 28.

†References 3, 5, 6, 9, 13, 14, 18-24, 26, 29, 32-34.

- Monitor patient for eye contact, posture, self-care, evidence of self-neglect, and indecision.
- Evaluate and monitor the following: patient's self-description; negative feelings about self; likes and dislikes about self; strengths and weaknesses; past and current events leading to positive self-feelings or negative self-feelings; any changes planned for self; any life situations that patient does not perceive as having the power to change; perceptions of how others view patient; perceptions of ability to get along with others; feelings about self in social situations with large gatherings. *Findings from evaluation and monitoring are used to design appropriate strategies for individual enhancement of the patient's self-esteem.*
- Avoid conveying judgmental attitudes or criticism or belittling patient's feelings, actions, or ideas *to minimize reinforcement of patient's low self-esteem.*
- Maintain therapeutic environment that will foster patient's level of self-esteem. *Emphasis should be on helping patient recognize that self-respect is first related to the ability to respect self and then to respect and understand others.*
- Assist patient in expressing positive statements about self and eliminating self-derogatory statements:
    Listen to statements.
    Help patient to reappraise statements cognitively and to make more positive statements.
- Assist patient to examine maladaptive responses to threat to self-esteem (e.g., physical aggression, sexual acting out, substance abuse, high-risk behavior, and violence.
- Provide opportunities for patients with substance abuse to discuss positive role models (Betty Ford, John Lucas) who have struggled with similar problems to achieve recovery, *to lessen the stigma of illness associated with decreased self-esteem.*[10]
- Encourage patient to identify and describe previous hopes and aspirations that may have been "buried." *"Rekindled dreams can foster renewed hope and self-esteem."*[10 p 24]
- Encourage patient to accept responsibility for personal opinions and behavior and to evaluate their outcome in relation to options available.
- Encourage patient to identify disappointment and dissatisfactions. In turn, have patient develop constructive problem-solving steps, with action behaviors and realistic timeframes and goals *to lessen or correct these problem areas successfully.* Encourage patient to use this same approach when confronted with future problems.
- Offer supportive, positive, and genuine comments and feedback to patient, when appropriate; focus on specific changes in behavior and appearance when making these statements; offer positive reinforcers for actual achievements; avoid false praise.
- Assist patient to recognize the fallacies associated with "having to be perfect" to feel good; *it is important for patient to realize that he or she is as worthwhile as anyone else despite imperfections.*

- Emphasize the importance of thinking positively by teaching patient to examine and monitor own negative thoughts of self and to practice positive self-talk: "I can achieve that goal."
- Teach patient to avoid illogical thoughts that precipitate low self-esteem: thinking the worst will always happen; thinking something is a total failure; believing that a bad experience will repeat itself; focusing on negative details.
- Suggest that patient keep a journal to use as a tool to enhance thought stopping of negative thoughts and concomitant events and feelings; teach patient to generate and to record positive thoughts about self at these times.
- Have patient describe current and past successes and accomplishments *to reinforce recognition of coping skills and to foster a sense of achievement.*
- Encourage patient's recognition of current strengths, assets, and potential *to draw on these resources in dealing with new life demands.*
- Teach patient assertive techniques and communication skills: use of "I" statements; conveying clear expectations of others; using negotiation as viable tactic; using body posture, facial expression, and tone of voice consistent with verbal communication; remaining firm, yet gentle and unyielding, when appropriate; teach patient to value and accept sincere compliments; *use of assertive communication skills will assist patient in meeting own needs while preserving the integrity of others.*
- Teach patient good personal grooming skills and health habits.
- Encourage good body posture and expression of pleasant affect.
- Encourage patient to identify and participate in satisfying and rewarding experience *to enhance self-worth.*
- Encourage patient to initiate activities and to develop new interpersonal and social skills in which patient will be reasonably successful *to minimize failure and decreased self-confidence.*
- Assist patient to establish reasonable goals for self.
- Encourage patients with physical disabilities to participate in fitness programs that are designed for people with disabilities. *"This environment allows them to interact with persons with similar interests and to experience positive interactions."*[17, p 823]
- Explore with patient additional skills needed for personal competency (e.g., success at job).
- Encourage patient to reward self for personal achievements.
- Facilitate patient's participation in treatment modalities that emphasize mutual support, acceptance, and concern for others (e.g., social skills, stress management, health management, and group or family therapy) *to decrease sense of aloneness in experiencing fears and failures.*
- Encourage abused women to enroll in abused women's support groups; *women's support groups can enhance abused women's self-esteem by: (1) providing knowledge about theories of violence and reducing sense of*

personal responsibility for the abuse; (2) replacing negative verbalizations of self-image with positive ones; and (3) recognizing the women's strengths and accomplishments.

- Encourage women to participate self-esteem enhancing therapies such as women's issues groups.[26]
- Increase opportunities to gain social support, especially for patients with chronic conditions, such as multiple sclerosis. *Social support and love can contribute to the maintenance of self-esteem.*
- Use group therapy, including support groups to work with patients who experience similar problems *to focus realistically on their problems, diminish isolation, provide realistic support and reinforcement from other members, strengthen coping patterns, provide feedback information about the environment, and improve the patient's overall self-esteem.*
- Promote structured life review reminiscence (for elderly patients) that focuses on positive recollections and discussions of the past.
- Provide opportunities for children from dysfunctional families (e.g., families with parental substance abuse) to: (1) obtain age-appropriate appraisals for their abilities on important dimensions, such as age-appropriate level of responsibility; (2) obtain feedback and information that does not disconfirm the child's existing self-perception, *making certain that the person providing the feedback is viewed as credible by the child;* spend time engaging in activities or in an environment where the children can feel good about themselves.
- Refer for mental health services such as family therapy, when appropriate. *Families benefit from opportunities to learn how their roles enhance the patient's self-esteem and how they may unwittingly contribute to the patient's self-esteem disturbance.*
- Review appropriate social activities with patient.
- Assist patient in becoming aware of effect of constructive social experiences in building self-esteem; increase social opportunities for interactions and opportunities to gain social support, especially for patients with chronic conditions.

(For patient with situational low self-esteem) improve and maintain constructive level of self-esteem:

- Explore with patient the reason for loss, stress, or environmental factors causing low self-esteem.
- Have patient describe recollections of previous sense of positive self-esteem *to provide hope for a return to sense of constructive level of self-esteem.*
- Use psychoeducational groups for populations such as depressed women *to teach information about self-esteem and to foster the development of specific strategies for improving self-esteem.*[18]
- Teach patient to develop strategies for coping with loss, stress, or environmental factors causing low self-esteem (e.g., problem-solving) *to increase patient's awareness of*

the relationship between effective coping strategies and increased self-esteem.
- Help the patient to focus on overall strengths and capabilities, as well as the loss or alteration that has contributed to the low self-esteem. *This focus can help the client to mobilize a constructive coping repertoire.*
- See also Self-Esteem Disturbance on p. 1680.

(For Patient With Chronic Low Self-Esteem) Improve and Maintain Constructive Level of Self-Esteem:

- Conduct an assessment that includes evaluation of factors, such as substance abuse, physical abuse, and/or depression, that affect the patient's self-esteem.
- Help patient to identify lifestyle patterns that contribute to positive or negative self-esteem.
- Teach patient strategies to increase self-confidence, such as developing and expressing own opinions about specific issues, engaging in hobbies.
- Encourage patient to plan for change in small increments. *Small successes augment one's self-esteem.*
- Help patient to enhance decision-making skills *to increase perception and belief of ability to have control over own life.*
- Convey genuine concern and willingness to help patient and family obtain help.
- Help patient in identifying family and community resources for improving self-esteem. *Social support contributes to an individual's improved self-esteem and the perception of an increased sense of control.*
- Help family to recognize the possibility that client's improvement might be slow; *it is important for family and caregivers to have realistic expectations.*
- Collaborate with interdisciplinary colleagues for assistance in referrals for resources such as treatment for substance abuse, need for domestic violence shelter.
- Initiate referrals to mental health professional if indicated.
- See also Self-Esteem Disturbance on p. 1680.

Principles and Rationale for Nursing Interventions

Low self-esteem is caused by repeated negative experiences and attacks on self-worth, self-respect, self-confidence, and self-appraisal systems.

All people have a need to esteem or value themselves. Positive values about self help persons seek and deal with their environmental experiences constructively. A person with a low value of self tends to perceive environmental stimuli as negative and threatening. In turn, the ability to deal with environmental experiences positively is disrupted in an effort to ward off further threats to an already damaged self-esteem. Positive self-esteem can be a powerful resource in enabling a patient to participate in care, engage confidently in interpersonal communications, gain accurate feedback from others, and enhance the ability to cope successfully in role demands.

The patient with a self-esteem disturbance can feel worthless and unable to cope with daily stressors or achieve desired outcomes for self.[22] Thus it is important to provide a supportive but reality-oriented environment in which a patient can engage in a variety of activities and therapies that allow for successful and constructive experiences to aid in the development of a positive self-esteem. Nursing interventions for patients with situational low self-esteem focus on helping the patient to recognize problems and situational factors that contribute to these problems. Subsequent interventions support the patient's efforts for effective coping with or adaptation to problematic areas.[22] The nurse should recognize that progress for patients with chronic low self-esteem will be in small increments. Initial nursing interventions for this population focus on helping the patient to maintain and to avoid additional threats to existing self-esteem. Referrals to a mental health professional for further evaluation and treatment may be necessary.[22]

BODY IMAGE DISTURBANCE

Body image disturbance is the disruption in an individual's perception or appraisal of his or her own body image.

The formation of body image, the mental image of one's body, is influenced by visual perceptions of self and others, as well as developmental, cognitive, and affective processes. Body image, a dynamic process that is closely related to the development of self-concept, also includes perceptions of others' opinions, as well as appraisals of the individual's appearance, body functions, beliefs, and values. An individual's body image is influenced by cultural beliefs and values. Reality-based, as well as fantasy-directed, perceptions and appraisals contribute to the formation of body image.[1,3,6,8,18]

Body image disturbance refers to difficulties experienced in the perception or appraisal of a person's own appearance or body functions, as well as difficulties with the accompanying beliefs and values. Events that can potentially result in a body image disturbance include normal developmental changes, medical conditions and interventions, mutilative surgery or injury, psychosis, and congenital or hereditary conditions.

Related Factors*

Prolonged or chronic illness
Acute physical trauma
Loss of body part(s)
Progressive deformities
Disfigurement of body or body surface
Change in body function or structure
Inability to adjust to normal developmental body changes
Mental disorders (e.g., eating disorders—anorexia nervosa, bulimia nervosa), body dysmorphic, schizophrenia
Treatment side effects (e.g., chemotherapy, radiation therapy)

Medication side effects (e.g., steroids)
Cognitive and perceptual distortions
Poor self-concept
Identification with others whose bodies are ideal
Rigid ideals about appearance and body function
Inadequate knowledge about social norms related to appearance
Peer criticism or ostracism
Family and cultural attitudes
Social and cultural attitudes toward physical disfigurement

Defining Characteristics†

Verbalization about difficulties accepting loss or change in body function or structure
Verbalization about difficulties adjusting to limitations of body change
Refusal to acknowledge recognition of physical limitations
Negative feelings about body
Feelings of helplessness, hopelessness regarding body change
Preoccupation with change in body image or lost part
Negation of awareness of reality of body change
Avoidance of looking at or touching body part
Denial of change in body boundaries (e.g., the stroke patient who is unaware of paralysis despite efforts to make patient conscious of his or her condition)
Change in ability to estimate spatial relationship of body to environment
Hiding or overexposing body part
Feelings of grandiosity about physical size and strength
Overemphasis on past strength, function, or appearance
Overestimation or underestimation of body size
Feelings of depersonalization or estrangement
Depersonalization of part or loss by use of impersonal pronouns
Incorporation of environmental objects into body boundary (e.g., ventilator equipment seen as part of body)
Overt or covert grieving
Personalization of part or loss by name
Fear of rejection by others
Change in social functioning
Disruption in activities of daily living
Change in life-style

Expected Patient Outcomes & Nursing Interventions‡

Experience reintegration of body image, as evidenced by:

Conveying positive expression of acceptance of body change
Learning to compensate for anatomic alterations
- Encourage description of patient's perception of body image *to promote patient's understanding and accepting of*

---

*References 1-3, 7, 8, 10, 11, 14-16, 18.

†References 1, 2, 7, 8, 10, 15, 17.
‡References 2-7, 9, 12, 14, 15.

reality of current situation and to obtain data to formulate an individualized plan of care, by asking questions that explore:

    Aspects of body that are pleasing or not pleasing

    Perception of body changes in relation to perceived social norms

    Integration of changes in body function or structure

    Impact on patient of attitudes and feelings of significant others

- Explore origins of patient's perceptions or appraisal of body image as negative (as in past experiences with significant others).
- Encourage verbalization and exploration of feelings regarding the impact of missing body part of change in body image on ability to assume ADLs (family, work, social relationships).
- Encourage verbalization of feelings of concern, anger, anxiety, loss, and fear over changes in body image *to facilitate normal grieving process.*
- Encourage patient to look at, touch, and explore affected area; ask patient to verbalize feelings after doing this.
- Help patient to describe how overt body changes will be discussed with others.
- Be nonjudgmental.
- Prepare patient for possible experiences that might be encountered as consequence of physical limitations *to assist in adaptation to body changes.*
- Offer physical assistance, as needed (e.g., stoma care), when patient is unable to care for self.
- Encourage self-care activities, such as personal grooming and altering clothing *to promote perception of positive body image.*
- Assist patient to set specific self-care goals, such as exercise program *to strengthen weakened muscles.*
- Stress that certain physical characteristics of a person cannot be changed; emphasize the importance of learning to recognize own unique positive strengths, *to help patient achieve acceptance and a realistic appraisal of present physical self.*
- Use a buddy system of pairing "new" patients with patients who have progressed in their recovery and rehabilitation *to encourage mutual sharing of experiences and problem solving.*
- Assist significant others to understand potential impact of patient's limitations *to minimize ineffective denial and to promote family support.*
- Convey recognition of rehabilitation accomplishments *to instill hope for further gains and to promote optimism for the future.*

Reintegrate ego functions and boundaries, as evidenced by:

    Ability to discriminate between environmental stimuli and internal stimuli

    Maximizing use of remaining strengths

Resuming previous activities of daily living and lifestyle to extent that is realistically possible

- Encourage patient to verbalize feelings and anxieties over distorted perceptions of reality, *to facilitate discrimination between real and unreal environmental and internal stimuli.*
- Engage patient in reality-oriented activities.
- Encourage patient to participate in all treatment modalities (pharmacologic therapy, individual or group therapies); discuss therapeutic benefits of these modalities.
- When patient has regained control of ego boundaries, encourage discussion and evaluation of possible precipitant of disturbance in body boundaries.
- Encourage patient to list strengths.
- Have patient describe perceptions of strengths, potentials, availability of social and community resources.
- Teach patient techniques and strategies for improving body image (e.g., how to dress, apply makeup, perform exercises to improve physical tone, and use cosmetic devices).
- Help patient determine the appropriate use of cosmetic services, hairpieces, wigs, and prostheses after disfiguring surgery or treatments.
- Acknowledge and give positive reinforcement whenever patient attempts to improve personal body image (e.g., improved hygiene, wearing makeup, wearing new clothes, wearing cosmetic devices after disfiguring surgery or treatment).
- Encourage participation in activities that promote increased use of body musculature (e.g., athletic games, dancing, structured exercise programs) *to enhance ego functioning for strengthening body image.*
- Offer supportive counseling *to facilitate a more rapid adjustment to change.*
- Determine need for mental health referral for evaluation for psychotherapy or antidepressant medication.
- Facilitate contact with others who have successfully adjusted to similar difficulties (people with an ostomy, laryngectomy, or mastectomy) *to convey assurance and hope for successful reintegration.*
- Encourage use of support services or reference groups in the community (e.g., self-help groups, Reach to Recovery, Voices Restored).
- Encourage patient to resume normal social activities as soon as possible, without hiding or overexposing changed body area.

Principles and Rationale for Nursing Interventions

Readjustment of body image is a gradual process that may require a period of time to complete resolution of the disturbance. The development of individualized nursing interventions for the patient with body image disturbance is based on an accurate assessment of the nature of the threat to the patient's body function and structure and the meaning the patient attaches to this threat. The more central the change is to a person's sense of self, the greater the potential for difficulties in body image. Knowledge of the patient's coping abilities and supportive resources is essential. Self-esteem is preserved when the patient is encouraged to use remaining skills and to develop strategies for adjusting to changes in body image. Resources and services that can preserve appearance or aid in adjusting to a physical limitation, foster successful coping, and reduce body image disturbances. Social support and knowledge about community resources augment coping skills.

■ RISK FOR SELF-MUTILATION

■ Risk for self-mutilation is a state in which an individual is at risk to perform a deliberate act on the self with the intent to injure, not kill, which produces immediate tissue damage to the body.

Self-mutilation includes an array of behaviors: self-biting; self-scratching; self-hitting; hair pulling; eye enucleation; facial-skinning; and amputation of limbs, breasts, or genitals.[3,14] The underlying dynamics and meanings of these behaviors are multiply determined and complex. Self-mutilating behavior occurs in patients with a variety of diagnoses. Self-mutilation is reported in patients with personality disorders, such as narcissitic and antisocial personality disorder, and is a diagnostic criterion for borderline personality. Self-mutilation may also occur in psychiatric diagnoses of obsessive-compulsive disorders and certain psychoses, as well as in mental retardation and organic conditions.[3,9]

Self-mutilation can be correlated with childhood experiences of sexual or physical abuse and with stormy or violent family interactions. Loss of a parent (divorce or death) or mental illness in family members, especially alcoholism, is also correlated with self-mutilation in adults.[3,10] Feelings reported by patients preceding self-mutilation most commonly include tension; anxiety; self-anger; powerlessness; numbing; and overwhelming guilt, loneliness, and boredom. The reason most often offered for these behaviors is to regain control over racing thoughts, fluctuating emotions, and unstable environments.[3]

Risk Factors*

Groups at risk:
 Patients with borderline personality disorder
 Patients in psychotic state
 Emotionally disturbed or battered children
 Mentally retarded and autistic children
 Patients with a history of self-injury
 Patients with history of physical, emotional, or sexual abuse
 Inability to cope with increased tension
 Feelings of depression, rejection, self-hatred, separation anxiety, guilt, and depersonalization

 Fluctuating emotions
 Command hallucinations
 Need for sensory stimuli
 Parental emotional deprivation
 Dysfunctional family
 Inability to control impulses

Expected Patient Outcomes & Nursing Interventions†

Express feelings appropriately, as evidenced by:
 Naming feelings being experienced
 Managing anxiety
 Matching expression of feeling state to person and context
 • Build trust through consistency and reliability.
 • Designate same staff as much as possible to work with patient.
 • Create nonthreatening environment; *a sense of being safe in the environment and with people enhances ability to express feelings.*
 • Assist patient to label feeling state.
 • Assist patient to identify situations that precipitate feeling states.
 • Support use of appropriate defense mechanisms and expression of feelings *to reduce acting-out behaviors.*
 • Instruct patient in the use of relaxation techniques *to reduce anxiety level.*

Experience fewer episodes of impulsive behavior, as evidenced by:
 Using resources effectively to reduce stress
 Identifying consequences of behavior
 Using problem-solving skills
 • Assist patient to identify perceived stressors.
 • Assist patient to replace faulty interpretations of perceived stressors with reality-based interpretations.
 • Explore with patient past successes in reducing stress *to capitalize use of patient's strengths.*
 • Collaborate with patient in developing a plan to reduce stress; *an increase in stressors can precipitate self-mutilation.*
 • Instruct patient on stress reduction techniques and assertive skills.
 • Set limits on inappropriate behavior; *setting limits is helpful in differentiating appropriate behavior from inappropriate behavior.*
 • Demonstrate and teach problem-solving skills.
 • Assist patient to identify advantages and disadvantages of alternatives for behavior.
 • Teach patient to evaluate behavior. *Increasing the patient's ability to problem solve and think through consequences expands the range of behavioral responses.*

*References 2, 3, 5, 6, 9, 13.

†References 1, 4, 6-8, 10, 12, 14, 15.

Interact positively with family, as evidenced by:

Making positive self-statements
Demonstrating self-differentiation
Reporting satisfaction from interactions with family

- Convey unconditional positive regard.
- Facilitate an environment that will increase self-esteem.
- Assist patient in identifying positive attributes of self; *identification of strengths and repetitive positive interactions with others and the environment influence the patient's self-estimate.*
- Engage patient in values clarification, self-appraisal, and identification of ideal self *to develop a clearer sense of self-identity.*
- Point out situations in which patient overidentifies with others.
- Ascertain the extent to which the patient's self-perception is affected by his or her dysfunctional family.
- Demonstrate interpersonal skills through role play.
- Assist patient to identify positive responses from others.
- Encourage patient to carry out familial roles and responsibilities that reinforce positive feeling and interaction *to support success in and satisfaction from interaction in family.*
- Explore with patient strategies to enhance family interaction (e.g., family therapy *to decrease stressors or threats to self*).

Principles and Rationale for Nursing Interventions

Self-mutilation is a patient behavior commonly encountered by nurses because it occurs in a number of psychiatric, medical, and organic diagnoses. Although the determinants and meanings of self-mutilation are multidetermined and complex in meaning, nursing interventions based on reported causes and interpretations of the behavior can reduce a patient's risk for self-mutilation.

A patient's risk for self-mutilation can be lessened by appropriate expression of feelings. Self-mutilation is preceded by feelings of anger, depression, self-hatred, and anxiety that mount steadily.[3] These feelings are often accompanied by a desire for immediate relief of tension regardless of results. Self-mutilation attempts to regulate anxiety and affect in the absence of more healthy and constructive strategies.[4] Therefore nursing interventions that assist a patient to verbalize feelings and manage anxiety reduce the potential for self-mutilation.[1,3,14]

Reasons commonly offered by patients for self-mutilating include an urge to release tension and a need to control irresistible urges.[3] Self-mutilation is often impulsive behavior reflective of an inability to delay gratification with a lack of concern for immediate consequences. The actuality of or potential for impulsive behavior can be reduced through nursing interventions that assist the patient to reduce stress, lessen the disruptive impact of behavior on self and others, use constructive behavior, and improve problem-solving skills.[1,3,4,8,15]

Correlation exists between self-mutilation and disrupted or dysfunctional family relationships.[3,11] Early childhood experiences of the self-mutilator often include conflict, violence, and abuse from mother-father or parent-child relationships, as well as mental illness or loss of a parent.[4,5,10,12] These experiences result in low self-esteem, lack of self-differentiation, and ineffective interpersonal skills.

Nursing interventions that assist the patient to raise self-esteem focus on conveying unconditional positive regard, identifying strengths, and developing skills that contribute to mastery of the environment. Nursing interventions that enable a patient to develop a clearer sense of self-identity and improve interpersonal relationships include clarification of values, broadening of perceptual field, mastery of roles and responsibilities, and improvement of interpersonal skills.[1,4,6,7,8,13]

■ PERSONAL IDENTITY DISTURBANCE

Personal identity disturbance is the inability of a person to experience an acceptable and coherent integration of sense of self and values within the context of personal, situational, and environmental stressors.[1,7,12]

Personal identity, a component of one's self-concept is a dynamic social product that refers to an individual's subjective recognition of personal characteristics, feelings, values, beliefs, and goals.[4,7] This subjective recognition serves as a reference point for evaluation of personal, situational, and environmental reality.

Personal identity formation is a life-long process that begins in early infancy when the child begins to differentiate self from the environment and culminates in old age.[17] It is influenced by an individual's developmental needs, capabilities, consistent role models, identifications, and successful ego defenses. It is through personal identity that a person recognizes what belongs to self. If this process of differentiation does not occur (e.g., if a pathologic symbiotic relationship exists between the child and mother from which the child never learns or experiences separateness and autonomy from the mother), the person's ego becomes fused or undifferentiated. The person then loses a sense of coherent self with a resultant inability to actualize abilities. There are accompanying feelings of confusion and indecisiveness.[3] A chronically ill older adult who perceives the loss of autonomy and fears separation and loneliness may relinquish individual identity for a "merged identity," and "long to be engulfed by the caring partner."[17, p. 9] Characteristics of a mature relationship include the ability to temporarily merge one's identity to respond to the needs of the other, "and then to separate and fulfill an individual identity."[17, p. 9]

Related Factors*

Chronic illness
Being adopted
Pathologic symbiotic relationship with significant other

---

*References 2, 6-9, 11-13, 15, 17.

Dysfunctional, abusive family life during childhood
Parental deprivation
Unexpected ending of a fused relationship (e.g., divorce)
Inappropriate or negative role model
Identification with inappropriate or inadequate person
Faulty resolution of sexual conflicts
Negative social influence (e.g., education, propaganda)
Unemployment
Sexually atypical employment
Nonsupportive social structure (e.g., interpersonal networks, group relationships)
Homelessness

Defining Characteristics*

Feelings of confusion
Conflicting emotions about own role and future goals
Uncertainty and indecision about career
Uncertainty about values (e.g., moral issues, religious affiliation)
Conflicting emotions about sexual identity or sexual preference
Withdrawal (e.g., psychologic, physical, social)
Depression
Clinging, dependent behavior
Inability to articulate feelings
Overwhelmed by excessive feelings
Denial of significance of prior traumatic interpersonal events
Embellishment of past and present experiences
Pathologic fabrication of medical and/or social identity
Verbal, future-oriented fantasizing
Fear of making changes (e.g., education, career goals)
Indecisiveness or inability to make decisions (e.g., occupation, friendships)
Indecisiveness about sense of self, purpose, and direction in life (e.g., "Who am I?")

Expected Patient Outcomes & Nursing Interventions†

Develops and maintains a positive integrated sense of self and values, as evidenced by:

Describing positive attributes about self
Verbalizing acceptance of sexual identity and preference and conveying understanding of consequences associated with decisions regarding sexual preference
Responding to personal, situational, and environmental stressors without experiencing disintegration of self-identity
Demonstrating problem-solving skills and strategies that promote and maintain integration of personal identity

---

*References 1, 4, 5, 7, 9, 11, 15.
†References 2, 3, 6-8, 10-12, 14, 16, 17.

- Provide a therapeutic, nonjudgmental environment for discussion of concerns.
- Establish a therapeutic alliance *to encourage patient to verbalize concerns and anxieties regarding personal identity.*
- Evaluate the need for a mental health referral for the individual or family.
- Collaborate with physician regarding the need for judicious use of neuroleptics for patients with a psychosis-based identity disturbance.
- Encourage patient to verbalize anxieties concerning sexual identity and preference *to facilitate patient's gaining a healthy sense of self.*
- Have patient explore meanings of being male or female; assist patient to recognize that sexuality is only one component of personal identity.
- Emphasize that decisions associated with sexual identity and preferences are personal choices.
- Encourage patient to explore positive and negative consequences related to these choices.
- Help patient to differentiate between adaptive and maladaptive behaviors associated with sexuality.
- Teach patient principles of normal growth and development *to facilitate patient's recognition of stressors that are associated with normal developmental phases.*
- Encourage participation in peer group activities *to increase personal competency in meaningful interpersonal relationships.*
- Based on individual assessment:
    Have patient keep a daily written record of thoughts and feelings *to promote autonomy by providing opportunity for ongoing view of self that is not solely dependent on outside feedback.*
    Have patient draw pictures and write stories about self and family *to elicit information that might be overlooked or disconfirmed.*
    Collaborate with patient in developing an agreed on written treatment contract *to encourage patient responsibility in the development of problem-solving skills and strategies.*
    Use contingency contracting (rewards or negative reinforcement) *to help the patient develop improved coping skills for maintaining integration of personal identity.*

Principles and Rationale for Nursing Interventions

Providing a therapeutic, nonjudgmental environment assists the patient to openly express feelings about self-identity. Teaching coping skills and providing opportunities for taking personal responsibility for one's own behavior in successful situations increase self-confidence. Personal identity disturbances can be associated with normal developmental stressors such as an adolescent who wonders, "What direction is my life taking"? or an adult in midlife who becomes concerned with a perceived lack of accomplishments. Although many of these developmental stressors are resolved within the normal course of events, an individual may become overly anxious or may become overtly psychotic; then the problem's resolution requires intervention by a mental health professional for the patient and/or family. It is important to recognize the role that antipsychotics can play in shaping the patient's beliefs about self.[7]

References

Fear

1. Barker E: Brain tumor: frightening diagnosis, nursing challenge, *RN* 53:46, 1990.
2. Grainger R: Conquering fears and phobias, *AJN* 91:15, 1991.
3. Hodiamont P: How normal are anxiety and fear? *Int J Soc Psychiatry* 37:43, 1991.
4. Joiner G, Kolodychuk G: Neoplastic cardiac tamponade, *Crit Care Nurs* 11:50, 1991.
5. Jones P, Jakob D: Nursing diagnosis: differentiating fear and anxiety, *Nurs Papers* 13:20, 1981.
6. Kalin NH: The neurobiology of fear, *Sci Am* 94-101, May, 1993.
7. Kim M, McFarland G, McLane A: *Pocket guide to nursing diagnoses,* ed 6, St Louis, 1995, Mosby.
8. Klieger DM: The non-standardization of the Fear Survey Schedule. *J Behav Ther Exp Psychiatry* 23:81, 1992.
9. Luttrell P: Care of the pediatric near-drowning victim, *Clin North Am* 3:293, 1991.
10. Marks M, deSilva P: The match/mismatch model of fear: empirical status and clinical implications, *Behav Res Ther* 32:759, 1994.
11. McConnell J: Fear. In McFarland G, Thomas M: *Psychiatric mental health nursing: application of the nursing process,* Philadelphia, 1991, JB Lippincott.
12. Mock V: Fear. In McFarland G, McFarlane E: *Nursing diagnoses and interventions: planning for patient care,* ed 3, St Louis, 1997, Mosby.
13. Taylor-Loughran AE, O'Brien ME, LaChapelle R, Rangel S: Defining characteristics of the nursing diagnoses fear and anxiety: a validation study, *Appl Nurs Res* 2:178, 1989.
14. Teplitz L: Nursing diagnoses for automatic implantable cardioverter defibrillation patients, *DCCN* 10:188, 1991.
15. Whitley GG: Concept analysis of fear, *Nurs Diag* 3:155, 1992.
16. Whitley GG: Expert validation and differentiation of the nursing diagnoses, anxiety and fear, *Nurs Diag* 5:143, 1994.
17. Yocom C: *The differentiation of fear and anxiety.* In Kim MJ, McFarland G, McLane A, editors: *Classification of nursing diagnoses: proceedings of the fifth national conference,* St Louis, 1984, Mosby.

Anxiety

1. Burd S, Marshall M, editors: *Some clinical approaches to psychiatric nursing,* New York, 1966, Macmillan.
2. Cirina A: Effects of sedative music on patient preoperative anxiety, *Today's OR Nurse* 16:15-18, 1994.
3. Danton W, Altrocchi J, Antonuccio D, Basta R: Nondrug treatment of anxiety, *Am Fam Phys* January, 1994, p. 161.
4. Fernandez F, Levy J, Lachar B, Small G: The management of depression and anxiety in the elderly, *J Clin Psychiatry* 56(suppl 2):20, 1995.
5. Gagne D, Toye R: The effects of therapeutic touch and relaxation therapy in reducing anxiety, *Arch Psych Nurs* 8:184, 1994.
6. Kenardy J, Evans L, Oei T: The latent structure of anxiety symptoms in anxiety disorders, *Am J Psychiatry* 149:1058, 1992.
7. Kim J, McFarland G, McLane A, editors: *Classification of nursing diagnoses: proceedings of the fifth national conference,* St Louis, 1984, Mosby.
8. Kim M, McFarland G, McLane A: *Pocket guide to nursing diagnoses,* ed 6, St Louis, 1995, Mosby.
9. Mackinnon A, et al: A latent trait analysis of an inventory designed to detect symptoms of anxiety and depression using an elderly community sample. *Psychol Med* 24:977, 1994.
10. Markovitz P: Treatment of anxiety in the elderly, *J Clin Psychiatry* 54:64, 1993.
11. Martin L, Fleming K, Evans J: Recognition and management of anxiety and depression in elderly patients, *Mayo Clinic Proc* 70:999, 1995.
12. May R: *The meaning of anxiety,* New York, 1979, Pocket Books.
13. Meldman M, McFarland G, Johnson E: *The problem oriented psychiatric index and treatment plans,* St Louis, 1976, Mosby.
14. Perley N: *Anxiety.* In Roy C, editor: *Introduction to nursing: an adaptation model,* Englewood Cliffs, NJ, 1984, Prentice-Hall.
15. Petruzzello S, et al: A meta analysis on the anxiety reducing effects of acute and chronic exercise, *Sports Med* 11:143, 1991.
16. Pratt J: The neuroanatomical basis of anxiety, *Pharmacol Ther* 55:149, 1992.
17. Robinson L: Stress and anxiety, *Nurs Clin North Am* 25:935, 1990.
18. Smith S: Assessing and treating anxiety in elderly persons, *Psychiatric Services* 46:36, 1995.
19. Spielberger CD: Anxiety and behavior, New York, 1966, Academic Press.
20. Stuart G, Sundeen S: *Principles and practice of psychiatric nursing,* ed 5, St Louis, 1991, Mosby.
21. Taylor S: Anxiety sensitivity: theoretical perspectives and recent findings, *Behav Res Ther* 33:243, 1995.
22. Wake M, Fehring R: Multinational validation of anxiety, hopelessness, and ineffective airway clearance, *Nurs Diagn* 2:57, 1991.
23. Weiss K: Management of anxiety and depression syndromes in the elderly, *J Clin Psychiatry* 55 (suppl2):5, 1994.
24. Whitley G: Anxiety defining the diagnosis, *J Psychosoc Nurs* 27:7, 1989.
25. Whitley G: *Anxiety.* In McFarland G, Thomas M: *Psychiatric mental health nursing,* Philadelphia, 1991, Lippincott.
26. Williams D: Anxiety, *Adv Clin Care* 6:5, 1991.

Risk for loneliness

1. Astrom G, Jansson L, NorBerg A, Hallberg IR: Experienced nurses' narratives of their being in ethically difficult care situations, *Cancer Nurs* 16:179, 1993.
2. Barron CR et al: Marital status, social support, and loneliness in visually impaired elderly people, *J Adv Nurs* 19:272, 1994.
3. Chen H: Hearing in the elderly: relation of hearing loss, loneliness, and self-esteem, *J Gerontol Nurs* 20:22, 1994.
4. Davis BD: Loneliness in children and adolescents, *Iss Comprehensive Pediatric Nurs* 13:59, 1990.
5. Drew N: Combating the social isolation of chronic mental illness, *J Psychosocial Nursing Mental Health Services* 29:14, 1991.
6. Foxall MJ et al: Low-vision elders: living arrangements, loneliness, and social support, *J Gerontol Nurs* 20:6, 1994.
7. Hochberger JM, Fisher-James L: A discharge group for chronically mentally ill: easing the way, *J Psychosocial Nursing Mental Health Services* 30:25, 1992.
8. Holt-Ashley M: Loneliness as a nursing diagnosis in bone marrow transplantation patients, *Dimensions Oncol Nurs* 11:16, 1988.
9. Keele-Card G, Foxall MJ, Barron CR: Loneliness, depression, and social support of patients with COPD and their spouses, *Public Health Nursing* 10:245, 1993.
10. Laryea M, Gien L: The impact of HIV-positive diagnosis on the individual, Part 1: Stigma, rejection, and loneliness, *Clin Nurs Res* 2:245, 1993.
11. Lee H, Coenen A, Heim K: Island living: the experience of loneliness in a psychiatric hospital, *Appl Nurs Res* 7:7, 1994.
12. Mahon NE, Yarcheski A: Alternate explanations of loneliness in adolescents: a replication and extension study, *Nurs Res* 41:151, 1992.
13. Mahon NE, Yarcheski A, Yarcheski TJ: Differences in social support and loneliness in adolescents according to developmental stage and gender, *Public Health Nursing* 11:361, 1994.
14. Mahon NE, Yarcheski A, Yarcheski TJ: Health consequences of loneliness in adolescents, *Res Nurs Health* 16:22, 1993.
15. Malloy C, Christ MA: The homeless: social isolates, *J Community Health Nursing* 7:25, 1990.
16. O'Brien ME, Pheifer WG: Physical and psychosocial nursing care for patients with HIV infections, *Nurs Clin North Am* 28:303, 1993.
17. Page RM, Allen O, Moore L, Hewitt C: Co-occurrence of substance use and loneliness as a risk factor for adolescent hopelessness, *J School Health* 63:104, 1993.

18. Peden AR: Music: making the connection with persons who are homeless, *J Psychosocial Nurs Mental Health Services* 31:17, 1993.
19. Perlman D, Pepau LA: Toward a social psychology of loneliness. In Gilman R, Duck S, editors: *Personal relationships in disorder,* New York, 1981, Academic Press.
20. Perry GR: Loneliness and coping among tertiary-level adult cancer patients in the home, *Cancer Nurs* 13:293, 1990.
21. Ricci MS: Aloneness in tenuous self-states, *Perspect Psychiatric Care* 27:7, 1991.
22. Samuelsson A, Ahlmen M, Sullivan M: The rheumatic patient's early needs and expectations, *Patient Educ Couns* 20:77, 1993.
23. Walton CG, Shultz CM, Beck CM, Walls RC: Psychological correlates of loneliness in the older adult, *Arch Psychiatric Nurs* 5:165, 1991.
24. Weiss RS: Loneliness: the experience of emotional and social isolation, Cambridge, Mass, 1973, Massachusetts Institute of Technology.
25. Young JL: Loneliness, depression, and cognitive therapy: theory and application. In Peplau LA, Perlman D, editors: *Loneliness: a sourcebook of current theory, research and therapy,* New York, 1982, Wiley.

Hopelessness

1. American Nurses Association: *Statement on psychiatric-mental health nursing practice and standards of psychiatric-mental health nursing practice,* Washington, DC, 1994, American Nurses Publishing.
2. Bulechek G, McCloskey J: *Nursing interventions: essential nursing treatments,* Philadelphia, 1992, Saunders.
3. Carpenito L: *Nursing diagnosis: application to clinical practice,* Philadelphia, 1992, JB Lippincott.
4. Herth K: Development and refinement of an instrument to measure home, *Sch Inq Nurs Pract* 5:39, 1991.
5. Kim M, McFarland G, McLane A: *Pocket guide to nursing diagnosis,* ed 5, St Louis, 1993, Mosby.
6. Maslow A: *Motivation and personality,* New York, 1954, Harper.
7. McFarland G, Wasli E, Gerety E: *Nursing diagnoses and process in psychiatric-mental health nursing,* ed 2, Philadelphia, 1992, JB Lippincott.
8. Perakyla A: Hope work in the care of seriously ill patients, *Qual Health Res* 1:407, 1991.
9. Range L, Penton S: Hope, hopelessness and suicidality in college students, *Psychol Rep* 75:456, 1994.
10. Rickelman B, Houfek J: Toward an interactional model of suicidal behaviors: cognitive rigidity, attributional style, stress, hopelessness and depression, *Arch Psychol Nurs* 9:158, 1995.
11. Rifai A et al: Hopelessness in suicide attempters after acute treatment of major depression in late life, *Am J Psychol* 151:1687, 1994.
12. Thackston-Hawkins L, Compton W, Kelly D: Correlates of hopelessness on the MMPI-2, *Psychol Rep* 75:1071, 1994.
13. Wake M, Fehring R, Fadden T: Multination validation of anxiety, hopelessness and ineffective airway clearance, *J Nurs Diagn* 2:57, 1991.
14. Wake M, Miller J: Treating hopelessness: nursing strategies from six countries, *Clin Nurs Res* 1:347, 1992.

Powerlessness

1. Arakelian M: An assessment and nursing application of the concept of locus of control, *Adv Nurs Sci* 3:25, 1980.
2. Boeing MH, Mongera CO: Powerlessness in critical care patients, *Dimens Crit Care Nurs* 8:274, 1989.
3. Buck MH: *The personal self.* In Roy C, Andrews HA, editors: *Roy adaptation model: the definitive statement,* Norwalk, Conn, 1991, Appleton & Lange.
4. Cartwright D, editor: *Studies in social power,* Ann Arbor, Mich, 1959, The University of Michigan Press.
5. Clements S, Cummings S: Helplessness and powerlessness: caring for clients in pain, *Holistic Nurs Pract* 6:76, 1991.
6. Herth K: Powerlessness. In McFarland GK, McFarland EA: *Nursing diagnoses and interventions: planning for patient care,* ed 3, St Louis, 1997, Mosby.
7. Hokanson HJ: Power: a concept analysis. *J Adv Nurs* 16:754, 1991.
8. Kim MJ, McFarland GK, McLane A: *Pocket guide to nursing diagnoses,* ed 6, St Louis, 1995, Mosby.
9. Mack JE: Power, powerlessness, and empowerment in psychotherapy, *Psychiatry* 57:178, 1994.

10. McFarland GK, Leonard H, Morris M: *Nursing leadership and management: contemporary strategies,* New York, 1984, Wiley.
11. Miller J; *Coping with chronic illness: overcoming powerlessness,* ed 2, Philadelphia, 1991, Davis.
12. Nystrom AE, Segesten KM: On sources of powerlessness in nursing home life, *J Adv Nurs* 19:124, 1994.
13. Roberts SL, White BS: *Powerlessness and personal control model applied to the myocardial infarction patient* 5:84, 1990.
14. Rotter J: Generalized expectancies for internal versus external control of reinforcement, *Psychol Monogr Gen Appl* 80:1, 1966.
15. Roy C: *Introduction to nursing: an adaptation model,* Englewood Cliffs, NJ, 1984, Simon & Schuster.
16. Schorr JA, Farnham RC, Ervin SM: Health patterns in aging women as expanding consciousness, *Adv Nurs Sci* 13:52, 1991.
17. Seeman M: Alienation studies, *Annu Rev Sociol* 1:91, 1975.
18. Walding MF: Pain, anxiety and powerlessness, *J Adv Nurs* 16:388, 1991.
19. White BS, Roberts SL: Nursing management of high permeability pulmonary edema, *Intens Care Nurs* 7:11, 1991.

Self-esteem disturbance

1. Bednar RL, Wells MG, Peterson SR: *Self-esteem: paradoxes and innovations in clinical theory and practice,* Washington, DC, 1989, American Psychological Association.
2. Bisagni GM, Eckenrode J: The role of work identity in women's adjustment to divorce, *Am J Orthopsychiatry* 64:574, 1995.
3. Borelli MD, DeLuca E: Physical health promotion in psychiatric day treatment, *J Psychosoc Nurs Ment Health Serv* 31:15, 1993.
4. Brooks RB: Children at risk: fostering resilience and hope, *Am J Orthopsychiatry,* 64:545, 1994.
5. Brown GW, Bifulco A, Veiel HO, Andrews B: Self esteem and depression. II. Social correlates of self-esteem. *Soc Psychiatry Psychiat Epidemiol* 25:225, 1990.
6. Caley JC, McFarland GK, Gerety EK. Self esteem, chronic low. In Kim MJ, McFarland GK, McLane AM: *Pocket guide to nursing diagnoses,* ed 6, 1995, St Louis, Mosby.
7. Coopersmith S: *The antecedents of self-esteem,* San Francisco, 1967, Freeman.
8. Cornwell C, Schmitt M: Perceived health status, self-esteem and body image in women with rheumatoid arthritis or systemic lupus erythematosus, *Res Nurs Health* 13:99, 1990.
9. Foote AW, et al: Hope, self-esteem and social support in persons with multiple sclerosis, *J Neuroscience Nurs* 22:155, 1990.
10. Francis R, Franklin J, Borg L: Psychodynamics. In Galanter M, Kleber HD, editors: *The American Psychiatric Press textbook of substance abuse treatment,* Washington, DC, 1994, American Psychiatric Press.
11. Goodman SH, et al: Locus of control and self-esteem in depressed, low-income African-American women, *Community Ment Health J* 30:259, 1994.
12. King GA, et al. Self-evaluation and self-concept of adolescents with physical disabilities, *Am J Occup Ther* 47:132, 1993.
13. Klose P, Tinius T: Confidence builders: a self-esteem group at an inpatient psychiatric hospital, *J Psychosoc Nurs Ment Health Serv* 30:5, 1992.
14. Kurek-Ovshinsky C: Group psychotherapy in an acute inpatient setting: techniques that nourish self-esteem, *Issues Ment Health Nurs* 12:81, 1991.
15. Lackovic-Grgin K, Dekovic M: The contribution of significant others to adolescents' self esteem, *Adolescence* 25:839, 1990.
16. Lamm B, Dungan JM, Hiromoto B: Long-term lifestyle management, *Clin Nurse Specialist* 5:182, 1991.
17. Magill-Evans JE: Self-esteem of persons with cerebral palsy: from adolescence to adulthood, *Am J Occup Ther* 45:819, 1991.
18. Maynard C: Psychoeducational approach to depression in women, *J Psychosoc Nurs Ment Health Serv* 31:9, 1993.
19. McFarland GK, Caley JC, Gerety EK. Self esteem, situational low. In Kim MJ, McFarland GK, McLane AM: *Pocket guide to nursing diagnoses,* ed 6, St Louis, 1995, Mosby.
20. McFarland GK, Gerety EK: Self esteem disturbance. In Kim MJ, McFarland GK, McLane AM: *Pocket guide to nursing diagnoses,* ed 6, St Louis, 1995, Mosby.

21. McFarland GK, Wasli EL, Gerety EK: *Nursing diagnoses and process in psychiatric mental health nursing,* ed 2, Philadelphia, 1992, JB Lippincott.

22. Miller JF: Enhancing self-esteem. In Miller JF: *Coping with chronic illness: overcoming powerlessness,* ed 2, Philadelphia, 1992, FA Davis.

23. Norris J: Nursing intervention for self-esteem disturbances. *Nurs Diag* 3:48, 1992.

24. Norris J, Kunes-Connell M: A multimodal approach to validation and refinement of an existing nursing diagnosis, *Arch Psychiatric Nurs* 2:103, 1988.

25. North American Nursing Diagnosis Association: *NANDA Nursing Diagnoses: Definitions and classification 1995-1996,* Philadelphia, 1994, NANDA.

26. Prehn RA, Thomas P: Does it make a difference? The effect of a women's issues group on female psychiatric inpatients, *J Psychosoc Nurs Ment Health Serv* 28:34, 1990.

27. Rosen I: Self-esteem as a factor in social and domestic violence, *Br J Psychiatry* 158:18, 1991.

28. Rugel RP: *Dealing with the problem of low self-esteem: common characteristics and treatment in individual, marital/family and group psychotherapy,* Springfield, Ill, 1995, Charles C Thomas.

29. Snyder M: *Independent nursing interventions,* ed 2, Albany, New York, 1992, Delmar Publishers.

30. Stein KF: The organizational properties of the self-concept and instability of affect, *Res Nurs Health* 18:405, 1995.

31. Stein KF: Schema model of the self-concept, *Image J Nurs Scholarship* 27:187, 1995.

32. Stevens-Ratchford RG: The effect of life review reminiscence activities on depression and self-esteem in older adults. *Am J Occup Ther* 47:413, 1993.

33. Walsh A, Walsh PA: Love, self-esteem, and multiple sclerosis, *Soc Sci Med* 29(7):793, 1989.

34. Yalom ID: *The theory and practice of group psychotherapy,* ed 4, New York, 1995, Basic Books.

Body image disturbance

1. Austin J, Champion V, Tzeng O: Cross-cultural relationships between self-concept and body image in high school-age boys, *Arch Psychiatr Nurs* 3:234, 1989.

2. Brand P: Coping with a chronic disease: the role of the mind and spirit, *Patient Educ Counsel* 26:107, 1995.

3. Cohen A: Body image in the person with a stoma, *J Enterostomal Ther* 18:68, 1991.

4. Dewis M: Spinal cord injured adolescents and young adults: the meaning of body changes, *J Adv Nurs,* 14:389, 1989.

5. French J, Phillips J: Shattered images: recovery for the SCI client, *Rehabil Nurs* 16:134, 1991.

6. Helman CG: The body image in health and disease: exploring patients' maps of body and self, *Patient Educ Counsel* 26:169, 1995.

7. Horne R, Van Vactor J, Emerson S: Disturbed body image in patients with eating disorders, *Am J Psychiatry* 148:2, 1991.

8. Laufer M: Body image, sexuality and the psychotic core, *Int J Psychoanal* 72:63, 1991.

9. McFarland G, Wasli E, Gerety E: *Nursing diagnoses and process in psychiatric mental health nursing,* ed 2, Philadelphia, 1992, JB Lippincott.

10. NANDA: *Nursing diagnoses: definitions and classification, 1995-1996.* Philadelphia, 1994, North American Nursing Diagnosis Association.

11. Neatherlin J, Brillhart B: Body image in preoperative and postoperative lumbar laminectomy patients, *J Neurosci Nurs* 27:43, 1995.

12. Olson B, Ustanko L, Warner S: The patient in a halo brace: striving for normalcy in body image and self-concept, *Orthopaedic Nurs* 10:44, 1991.

13. Popkess-Vawter S: Assessment of positive and negative body image in normal weight and overweight females. In Carroll-Johnson R, editor: *Classification of nursing diagnoses: proceedings of the 8th conference.* Philadelphia, 1989, JB Lippincott.

14. Rosen JC, Reiter J, Orosan P: Cognitive-behavioral body image therapy for body dysmorphic disorder, *J Consulting Clin Psychology* 63:263, 1995.

15. Salter M: What are the differences in body image between patients with a conventional stoma compared with those who have had a conventional stoma followed by a continent pouch? *J Adv Nurs* 17:841, 1992.

16. Utz S, Hammer J, Whitmire V, Grass S: Perceptions of body image and health status in persons with mitral valve prolapse, *Image: J Nurs Scholarship* 22:18, 1990.

17. Weir AM, et al: Bell's palsy: the effect on self-image, mood state and social activity, *Clin Rehabil* 9:121, 1995.

18. Williamson M: The nursing diagnosis of body image disturbance in adolescents dissatisfied with their physical characteristics, *Holistic Nurs Pract* 1:52, 1987.

Risk for self-mutilation

1. Anderson M: Clients with altered impulse control. In McFarland G, Thomas M: *Psychiatric mental health nursing practice: application of the nursing process,* Philadelphia, 1991, JB Lippincott.

2. Emerson J, Walker E: Self-injurious behavior in people with a mental handicap, *Nurs Times* 86:43, 1990.

3. Favazza A: *Bodies under siege: self-mutilation in culture and psychiatry,* Baltimore, 1993, Johns Hopkins Press.

4. Godfrey M: Clients with personality disorders. In McFarland G, Thomas M: *Psychiatric mental health nursing: application of the nursing process,* Philadelphia, 1991, JB Lippincott.

5. Jacobson A, Herald C: The relevance of childhood sexual abuse to adult psychiatric in-patient care, *Hosp Commun Psychol* 41:154, 1990.

6. Kim M, McFarland G, McLane A: *A pocket guide to nursing diagnosis,* ed 5, St Louis, 1993, Mosby.

7. McCloskey J, Bulechek G: *Nursing interventions classification,* St Louis, 1992, Mosby.

8. McFarland G, Wasli E, Gerety E: *Nursing diagnosis and process in psychiatric mental health nursing,* ed 2, Philadelphia, 1992, JB Lippincott.

9. Oldham J: *Personality disorders: new perspectives on diagnostic validity,* Washington, DC, 1991, American Psychiatric Press.

10. Rose S, Peabody C, Stratigeas B: Undetected abuse among intensive case management clients, *Hosp Commun Psychol* 42:499, 1991.

11. Russ M, et al: Subtypes of self-injurious patients with borderline personality disorder, *Am J Psychol* 150:1869, 1993.

12. Sabo A, et al: Changes in self-destructiveness of borderline patients in psychotherapy, *J Nerv Ment Dis* 183(6):370, 1995.

13. Sansone R, Sansone L, Wiederman M: The prevalence of trauma and its relationship to borderline personality symptoms and self-destructive behaviors in a primary care setting, *Arch Fam Med* 4:439, 1995.

14. Sebree R, Popkess-Vawter S: Self-injury concept formation: nursing diagnosis development, *Perspec Psychol Care* 27:27, 1991.

15. Shearer S: Phenomenology of self-injury among inpatient women with borderline personality disorder, *J Nerv Ment Diseases* 182:524, 1994.

Personal identity disturbance

1. American Psychiatric Association: *Diagnostic and statistical manual of mental disorders,* ed 4, Washington, DC, 1994, American Psychiatric Association.

2. Anderson G, Ross CA: Strategies for working with a patient who has multiple personality disorder, *Arch Psychiatric Nurs* 2:236, 1988.

3. Bohlander JR: Differentiation of self: an examination of the concept, *Issues Ment Health Nurs* 16:165, 1995.

4. Breakwell GM: *Coping with threatened identities,* New York, 1987, Methuen.

5. Cohen CR, Chartrand JM, Jowdy DP: Relationships between career indecision subtypes and ego identity development, *J Counsel Psychol* 42:440, 1995.

6. Dyckoff D, Goldstein L, Schacht-Levine L: The investigation of behavioral contracting in patients with borderline personality disorder, *J Am Psychiat Nurs Assoc* 2:71, 1996.

7. Gara MA, Rosenberg S, Cohen BD: Personal identity and the schizophrenic process: an integration, *Psychiatry* 50:267, 1987.

8. Haber J: A family systems model for divorce and the loss of self, *Arch Psychiatric Nurs* 4:228, 1990.

9. Hauser ST, et al: Paths of adolescent ego development: links with family life and individual adjustment, *Psychiatr Clin North Am* 13:489, 1990.

10. McFarland GK, Wasli EL, Gerety EK: *Nursing diagnoses and process in psychiatric mental health nursing,* ed 2, Philadelphia, 1992, JB Lippincott.

11. Plassmann R. Munchausen syndromes and factitious diseases, *Psychother Psychosom* 62:7, 1994.

12. Robertson SM: Self-concept disturbance (personal identity disturbance, self-esteem disturbance, body image disturbance, role performance disturbance). In McFarland GK, Thomas MD, editors: *Psychiatric mental health nursing,* Philadelphia, 1991, JB Lippincott.

13. Rosenberg BE, Horner TM: Birthparent romances and identity formation in adopted children, *Am J Orthopsychiat* 61:70, 1991.

14. Sebastian L: Promoting object constancy: writing as a nursing intervention, *J Psychosoc Nurs Ment Health Serv* 1:21, 1991.

15. Snow DA: Identity: work among the homeless, *Am J Sociology* 92:1336, 1987.

16. Snyder M: *Independent nursing interventions,* ed 2, Albany, New York, 1992, Delmar Publishers.

17. Warren MT: Maintaining identity in elderly couples with chronic illness, *J Psychol Soc Nurs Ment Health Serv* 30:9, 1992.

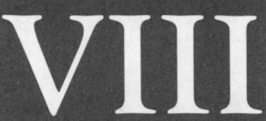

Role-Relationship

■ ANTICIPATORY GRIEVING

■ Anticipatory grieving is the initiation of the process of grieving in anticipation of a potential impending significant loss.

Anticipatory grieving is a multidimensional process that includes grieving in anticipation of a potential impending significant loss embedded in possible grieving for past, present, and future losses.[10,18] The significant impending loss may be, for example, the potential death of a significant person with a terminal illness, the potential loss of a limb in surgery, the potential loss of a friend who is planning to move away, or anticipation of one's own impending death.[14,18] The perceived potential of a significant loss forces an individual to begin to deal with the consequences of the loss before the actual loss occurs.[3] Anticipatory grieving can help a person adjust to the actual loss, and it can have a beneficial effect on bereavement outcome[11,18,20]; however, anticipatory grieving may be dysfunctional for an individual or family, depending on the manner in which it is experienced and responded to by others in the environment.[5,13,21]

Related Factors*

Perceived potential loss of significant person
Perceived potential loss of significant animal
Perceived potential loss of prized material possessions(s)
Perceived potential loss of body part(s) or function(s)
Perceived potential loss of physiopsychosocial well-being
Perceived potential loss of social role
Perceived potential developmental or role-transition loss(es)
Perceived impending death of self
Perceived potential loss of dreams for the future
Perceived potential loss of future life-style

Defining Characteristics[1,3,11,18,20]

Denial of potential loss, e.g., shock, disbelief, avoiding focusing on loss
Symptoms of somatic distress may include:
 Decreased muscular power
 Feeling of emptiness in stomach

Tightness in throat
Shortness of breath
Sighing
Perspiration
Lack of energy
Changes in eating habits, e.g., increased or decreased appetite
Internal preoccupation
Disinterest or difficulty in carrying out activities of daily living
Anger, hostility, or irritability toward others
Guilt, e.g.; self-accusation of negligence
Sorrow/weeping
Feelings of loss and loneliness
Emotional distance from others
Sense of unreality
Alterations in sleep patterns
Social isolation and inhibition
Ambivalence
Altered communication patterns, e.g., pressured speech, reduced communication
Psychomotor retardation
Restlessness with inability to engage in organized activities
Altered libido
Hope for preventing loss
Decreased acceleration of grieving, increased defense mechanisms as death or loss approaches
Realization or resolution of impending death or loss

Expected Patient Outcomes & Nursing Interventions†

Participate in constructive anticipatory grief work, as evidenced by:

Discussing thoughts and feelings related to anticipated loss
Verbalizing information needs
Using appropriate resources (e.g., friends, clergy, support groups, legal consultants, Social Security representatives)
Maintaining constructive interpersonal relationships
Meeting ongoing care needs
Verbalizing perception of ability to exist in the future without significant person or valued object

---

*References 1, 4, 7, 11-13, 14, 16, 22, 23.

†References 1-4, 6-9, 12, 13, 16, 19, 20.

Making realistic plans for dealing with future without significant person or valued object
- Encourage description of perceptions of potential loss.
- Encourage verbalization of fears and concerns.
- Determine:
  - Length of time since learning potential loss
  - Past experience with loss, illness, and death, as well as problem solving and coping skills used; *past adaptation to loss influences current adaptation*
  - Cultural beliefs *because they influence the manner in which people express grief and adapt to an impending loss*
  - Spiritual beliefs. *Past problem-solving abilities, and personal beliefs influence current and future coping*
  - Socioeconomic background
  - Educational preparation
  - Current sources of social support (family, friends, church)
  - Disruptions in current life-style related to anticipated loss (finances, living arrangements, transportation)
- Assess for indications of suicidal ideation or intent.
- Recognize that patient and significant others may differ in stage of grieving they are experiencing.
- Acknowledge to patient and significant others that pattern of their past relationships with each other will be similar to their relationships as they experience anticipated loss.
- During stage of shock and disbelief:
  - Provide quiet environment.
  - Allow for constructive use of denial. *Recognize that denial and other similar mental mechanisms serve to increase the patient's or significant others' tolerance for potential overwhelming stress.*
  - Avoid reinforcement of pathologic denial.
  - Avoid confronting patient or significant others when they are experiencing distorted perceptions.
  - Provide opportunity for expression of emotions.
  - Provide assurance that it is normal to experience intense feelings and reactions.
  - Avoid defensive and judgmental responses to criticisms of health care providers.
  - Do not encourage use of antianxiety medications. *Anxiolytics may interfere with the process of constructive grief work.*
  - Do not force decisions.
  - Enlist support from others (e.g., family, friends, clergy).
- During stage of developing awareness of potential loss:
  - Encourage expression of feelings with relatives and friends, *keeping in mind that cultural patterns influence expression of feelings.*
  - Facilitate contact with nursing staff and other health team members to correct misinformation about cause of loss.
  - Facilitate exploration of available options.
  - Support verbalizations about possible body image changes.

Offer hope for ability to cope with anticipated loss.
Encourage and teach good health habits.
Provide information on supportive and informational groups for patient and/or family.
Encourage persons experiencing similar anticipated losses to consider spending time together to share mutual fears, feelings, and concerns. *Based on individual evaluation, initiate referral to formal support group to facilitate successful closure and to reduce potential for dysfunctional grieving.*
Evaluate need for referral to resources (e.g., Social Security representatives, legal consultants, support groups).
- During stage of developing awareness of potential loss of significant other:
  - Provide significant others with ongoing information of patient's diagnosis, prognosis, and plan of care *to decrease their feelings of uncertainty and anxiety.*
  - Encourage significant others to describe their desires and information needs in caring for patient.
  - Facilitate significant other's assistance with patient's physical care *to reduce feelings of helplessness and to decrease potential for future regret.*
  - Facilitate flexible visiting hours and include younger children when appropriate.
  - Help patient and significant others to share mutual fears, concerns, plans, and hopes with each other.
  - Based on individual assessment, suggest the use of letter writing, audio or video taping *to provide encouragement for the patient when family and friends are unable to be physically present; the terminally ill patient can also use these forms of communication as a "legacy" for significant others, e.g., grandchildren, infants.*
  - Offer hope to patient and significant others that they will have quality time together.
  - Help significant others to understand the patient's verbalization of anger should not be perceived as personal attacks.
  - Encourage significant others to maintain their own self-care needs for rest, sleep, nutrition, leisure activities, and time away from patient.
  - Facilitate patient's and significant others' discussion of final arrangements (e.g., funeral services, burial wishes, organ donation, desire for autopsy).
  - Teach patient and significant others to recognize and trust decisions that "feel" right to them in relation to their coping with impending losses.
- During period of mourning for anticipated loss:
  - Help patient accept reality of impending loss.
  - Provide information as sought *to minimize feelings of uncertainty and anxiety.*
  - Allow patient to talk freely about anticipated loss. *There may be an increased preoccupation with the anticipated loss and an increased need to talk with others about the meaning of the potential loss.*
  - Encourage expression of feelings (e.g., crying).

Facilitate discussion of both negative and positive aspects of anticipated loss.

Foster environment in which loss can be experienced within spiritual context.

Provide guidance regarding availability of community resources.

- During period of mourning before death of loved one:

Promote discussion of what to expect when death occurs *to decrease fear and anxiety about the unknown.*

Encourage significant others and patient to share their wishes about family members being present with patient at death. Avoid judgmental responses to choices made.

Help significant others to accept that choosing to be absent at death does not indicate a lack of love or caring for patient.

Discuss indicators of impending death as appropriate.

Provide comforting measures for patient; encourage significant others to assist if they wish.

Encourage significant others to maintain verbal communication and touch with their loved one, even though patient may not respond *to facilitate successful closure of the relationship.*

Provide as much privacy as possible for significant others to be alone or with patient when death is imminent.

Principles and Rationale for Nursing Interventions

The perception of an anticipated loss is subjective. The individual's perception of an anticipated loss is influenced by a variety of factors that include past problem-solving abilities, previous experience with loss and illness, socioeconomic background, educational preparation, and cultural and spiritual beliefs.

Behaviors of shock and disbelief in anticipatory grieving are indicative of the individual's need for protection from the intensity of the painful feelings evoked by the potential loss. Denial is a normal and common coping response at this time.

Developing awareness of the potential loss is characterized by feelings of anxiety and helplessness. Feelings of hopelessness are also accompanied by hope that the loss can be averted. Expressions of anger and guilt may be directed inward or toward other family or to health care providers. Cultural patterns influence the expression of feelings during this time.

As the reality of the impending loss becomes more evident, there may be an increased preoccupation with the personal experience of the anticipated loss and an increased need to talk with others about the meaning of the loss.

◼ DYSFUNCTIONAL GRIEVING

Dysfunctional grieving represents a distortion of normal grieving. Dysfunctional grieving is characterized by delayed, distorted, prolonged or excessive emotional responses to a loss.[14,15]

Normal grieving, the process by which a person adapts to a significant loss, is viewed as a self-limiting response of suffering that varies in length from a few months to several years. The process of restructuring a new life and achieving personal reorganization after a significant loss includes emotional emancipation from the significant loss and readjustment to an environment without the lost object or significant other.[7,11,22] The person with dysfunctional grieving has not been able to experience the process of normal grieving.

Related Factors*

Perceived or actual loss of significant person, animal, or prized possession(s)

Perceived or actual loss of health

Perceived or actual loss of body part(s) or function(s)

Perceived or actual developmental or role-transition loss(es)

Perceived or actual loss of social role(s)

Perceived or actual lack of social support network

Perceived vulnerability to loss

Dysfunctional grieving process of parents

Multiple previous or concurrent losses

History of delayed or dysfunctional grief reactions

Preexisting poor self-image

Unresolved guilt and ambivalence

Sudden, untimely, unexpected death or loss e.g., pregnancy, loved one

Chronic physical or mental illness or significant other

Socially unspeakable loss

Social negation of loss

Overidentification with deceased person

Difficulty or inability to freely express feelings

Postponement of grief reactions

Protracted anticipatory grief

Secondary gain from others to maintain grieving

Uncertainty of loss

Defining Characteristics†

Delayed emotional reactions
    Denial of impact of loss
    Inability to deal with excessive ambivalence
Arrested grieving without movement toward resolution
    Maladaptive denial of loss
    Inability to relinquish feelings of sadness
    Repression of expression of joy or humor
    Somatizations, e.g., choking sensation, breathing attacks
    Vague somatic complaints
    Verbalization of role distress, e.g., inadequate parenting
    Decreased participation in religious or ritual activities
Prolonged grieving beyond expected time or cultural norms
    Developmental regression, e.g., unusual dependency

---

*References 1, 4, 5, 7-17, 19, 21.
†References 1, 3, 6, 7, 10, 12, 14, 21, 22.

Refusal to follow therapies for treatment of chronic physical or mental illness

Low self-esteem

Prolonged difficulty keeping up with usual activities

Severe feelings of loss of identity

Prolonged loss of interest in and planning for future

Feeling or behaving as if the loss occurred yesterday

Unabated searching behavior or yearning for lost person or object

Excessive, distorted, exaggerated emotional reactions and/or behaviors

Labile affect

Symptoms or behaviors similar to deceased's last illness

Extreme anger or hostility

Excessive self-blame or self-reproach

Overwhelming or prolonged guilt

Protracted apathy

Irrational despair, severe hopelessness

Severe depression

Engaging in self-detrimental activities

Suicidal thoughts and fantasies

False sense of euphoria

Expansive, adventurous overactivity without conveying sense of loss

Intense separation anxiety

Prolonged panic attacks

Prolonged difficulty keeping up with usual activities

Radical life-style changes

Refusal to remove material possessions of deceased

Expected Patient Outcomes & Nursing Interventions*

Experience resolution of dysfunctional grieving, as evidenced by:

Acknowledging reality of the loss

Demonstrating emotional responses that are congruent with personal and cultural context in which loss occurred

Participating in recommended treatment modalities

Identifying alternate plans for meeting goals that were significant before the loss

Resuming or developing new social relationships and making new emotional investments

- Avoid imposing a normative standard for manifestation and resolution of grief. *There is no specific "timetable" for successful resolution of a loss.*
- Monitor patient's perception of current adaptation, responses from significant others, social network, life experiences, and past problem-solving and coping skills *to determine patient's actual and potential coping strengths and deficits.*
- Evaluate influence of denial on patient's participation with recommended treatments.

- Assess possible needs met by denial *to avoid inadvertent reinforcement of secondary gains.*
- Observe for responses by health care providers that may be reinforcing maladaptive denial.
- Point out reality in nonthreatening manner without arguing with patient or significant others.
- Present patient with increasing facts.
- Defer teaching related to adaptation to loss until patient demonstrates decrease in denial.
- Monitor for suicidal ideation *to determine need for mental health referral for evaluation of need for antidepressant medication, psychotherapy, or admission to inpatient psychiatric unit for treatment.*
- Clarify and offer missing factual information *to facilitate corrections of distorted perceptions.*
- Provide opportunity for patient to describe experiences that preceded current loss *to increase patient's awareness of thoughts and feelings associated with actual loss.*
- Encourage description of current and anticipated problems related to loss.
- Point out universality of need for normal grieving.
- Facilitate constructive working through of expression of feelings *to decrease indirect expression of grief through behavioral problems or physical illness.*
- Facilitate contact with people who can openly express feelings.
- Assist patient to reality test feelings of guilt *to minimize irrational guilt.*
- Promote therapeutic use of humor *to encourage patient to experience laughter and joy without feeling guilt.*
- Encourage patient to talk and reminisce about loss *to facilitate exploration of feelings of hurt, anger, and disappointment.*
- Convey unconditional acceptance of patient's communication of behaviors and feelings that may be viewed as socially or culturally unacceptable *to prevent grief stagnation and fixation on loss.*
- Facilitate review of positive and negative aspects of loss *to decrease ambivalence.*
- Evaluate need for referral to resources, e.g., brief psychotherapy, support groups, family therapy, spiritual counselor.
- Promote patient's recognition of past and present strengths that can be used for coping with current loss.
- Promote description of additional potential strategies for coping with current loss.
- Encourage description of future expectations.
- Offer hope for successful adaptation to loss.
- Facilitate contact with others who have successfully adapted to similar loss *to provide visible proof that grief can be resolved.*
- Provide guidance about available community resources, e.g., assertiveness training, continuing education, driver education.
- Promote coordination of resources *to help patient develop new skills, make readjustments in life-style, and make new emotional investments.*

---

*References 1, 2, 4-6, 10, 11, 16, 18, 20, 23.

Principles and Rationale for Nursing Interventions

Expressions of grief are influenced by cultural, social, economic, and spiritual factors, the nature and number of previous losses, the person's previous resolution of loss through the normal grieving process, as well as the context in which the loss occurred.[12] Postponement of emotional responses to a loss may occur when an individual initially has to deal with difficult tasks, feels compelled to maintain a facade of "good behavior," or helps to maintain the morale of others immediately after a loss.[15] Denial, an attempt to minimize the anxiety-producing effects from a loss, can contribute to a patient's lack of acknowledgement of the loss and delayed emotional reactions. Assessment for suicidal ideation and intent is important to determine the need for a mental health referral to evaluate the need for antidepressant medication, psychotherapy, or admission for inpatient psychiatric treatment. Referral to and coordination of mental health and or community resources facilitate the patient's resuming and/or developing new social relationships and emotional investments. The resolution of dysfunctional grieving allows the patient to place the past in its proper perspective. Development of new coping strategies assists the patient to find meaning in the present and to make life-style adjustments in an environment without the lost object or significant other.[2,7,12,22]

■ ALTERED ROLE PERFORMANCE

Altered role performance is a disruption in the way an individual perceives and/or performs his or her role.

Problems associated with role functioning include role insufficiency, role distance, interrole conflict, intrarole conflict, role failure, and ineffective role transition.[1,15,16,17,20]

Role[1,15,16,17,19] is the basic unit of function in society, and it involves a set of expectations about how one person in a particular role expresses instrumental and expressive behaviors. When an individual demonstrates adaptive instrumental (goal-oriented actions) and expressive (feelings/attitudes about a role) behaviors that are congruent with social expectations, the individual is exhibiting *role mastery.*

Role insufficiency occurs whenever an individual has difficulty in the cognizance and/or performance of a role or of the sentiments and goals associated with the role behavior as perceived by the self or by significant others.[11]

Role distance implies that an individual demonstrates both instrumental (goal-oriented actions) and expressive (feelings/attitudes) behaviors appropriate to a specific role, but the behaviors demonstrated differ from those behaviors that are generally prescribed for the role.[2,15,16]

Interrole conflict occurs when the individual demonstrates instrumental (goal-oriented actions) and expressive (feelings/attitudes) behaviors that are incompatible with the expected behaviors for one or more roles in which the individual is performing.[2,15,16]

Intrarole conflict occurs when the individual demonstrates instrumental (goal-oriented actions) and/or expressive (feelings/attitudes) behaviors that are incompatible with the expected behaviors of the role as a result of incompatible expectations from one or more persons in the environment.

Role failure occurs when there is a lack of ineffective instrumental behaviors and/or an absence of or inadequate expression of feelings.[2,15,16]

Ineffective role transition occurs when ineffective instrumental (goal-oriented actions) behaviors but adaptive expressive (feelings/attitudes) behaviors are exhibited as a result of lack of knowledge or lack of a role model.[2,15,16]

Each of these role-functioning problems can develop in relation to developmental transitions (e.g., moving from adulthood to old age), situational transitions (e.g., the addition of a family member), and health-illness transitions (e.g., going from a well state to an acute or chronic illness state).

Roles and role performance can be examined from both a functionalist and an interactionist perspective. Functionalists view roles as somewhat fixed in society and see roles as reinforced by positive or negative reinforcements from others. Interactionists view society as providing the framework within which the person interacts with others, interprets behavior, and then constructs his or her role response. Social action and role performance are not only learned responses, but also serve as a source for one's organization and interpretation of environmental cues.[6,7] Overall, an understanding of roles, role performance, and alterations in role performance is important. Nurse theorists emphasize this importance: distorted perceptions of roles can, for example, affect the outcome of health care.[3,4,19,20,23]

Related Factors*

Absence of significant role models

Cognitive difficulties

Changes in values and beliefs

Inadequate role socialization

Perceptual difficulties

Mental illness (e.g., schizophrenia, borderline personality disorder)

Developmental transitions

Negative self-perception

Negative role spillover from multiple roles[22]

Situational transitions

Cultural discrepancies

Health-illness transition

Conflicting demands of multiple roles[21]

Physical limitations

Incompatible prescribed behaviors from two or more roles

Major disruptions in life-style (e.g., loss of job/income)

Abuse (e.g., rape)

Inadequate knowledge

Lack of opportunity to practice role

*References 6, 7, 14-16, 18, 19.

Threat to self-concept
Incompatible role expectation from others
Excessive family caregiving demands[5]
Community problems (e.g., lack of resources)

Defining Characteristics[6,7,11-16,19]

Role failure
Role distance
Interrole conflict
Intrarole conflict
Role insufficiency
Ineffective role transition
Ineffective expressive (feelings/attitudes) behaviors
Absence of adaptive expressive (feelings/attitudes) behaviors
Dysfunctional grieving
Feelings of powerlessness, severe anger, severe anxiety, depression, withdrawal
Discomfort with role
Dislike of role
Belittling or derogatory comments about role
Lack of motivation for role
Ambivalence about role
Ineffective instrumental (goal-oriented actions) behaviors
Change in self-perception of role
Change in others' perception of role performance
Change in usual patterns of responsibility
Behaviors that contradict others' expectation of role performance
Inability to meet social expectations
Failure to perform prescribed behavior
Behaviors that contradict self-expectation of role performance
Confusion about personal values and goals
Verbalizations of inadequate role performance

Expected Patient Outcomes & Nursing Interventions*

Develop role mastery, as evidenced by:

Demonstrating stable pattern of mastery of role
Expressing positive acceptance of new role
Verbalizing understanding of appropriate cognitive, instrumental, and expressive behaviors associated with role
Describing impact new role will have in assuming other role behaviors
Demonstrating use of various role supplementation strategies, with resultant ability to perform role without difficulty
Demonstrating problem-solving skills and strategies for promoting and maintaining mastery of newly acquired role and possible future roles
Exhibiting adaptive instrumental/expressive behaviors in coping with role change/transition

---

*References 1, 2, 3, 8, 9, 10, 11, 12, 14-16.

Demonstrating integration of instrumental/expressive role behaviors
- Determine type of role-functioning problem patient is experiencing: role insufficiency, role distance, interrole conflict, intrarole conflict, role failure, or ineffective role transition.
- Determine transitions that may be predisposing patient to problems with role functioning: developmental, situational, or health-illness transition.
- Encourage patient to verbalize feelings, concerns, fears, and anxieties associated with assuming a particular role.
- Help patient to assess impact of new role on ability to assume present or future roles.
- Once type of role-functioning problem has been identified, use:
  Role clarification *to teach patient what role entails in terms of behavior, sentiments, costs, rewards, and positive and negative reinforcement by significant others.*
  Role taking *to help patient imaginatively assume position or point of view of another person taking on new role.*
  Role modeling *to help patient enact and play out new role so that he or she can understand and emulate intricacies of behavior associated with new role.*
  Role rehearsal *to help patient fantasize, imagine, and mentally enact how encounter might take place and how new role might evolve and develop.*
  Reference groups *to expose patient to other individuals or groups who have successfully assumed mastery of new role.*
- Provide therapeutic environment that allows for opportunities to learn and practice new role behaviors.
- Give patient feedback regarding failure to assume or perform expected role behaviors *to facilitate the learning of new behaviors.*
- Identify and provide appropriate role models *for patient to learn role expectations.*
- Assist patient to obtain necessary knowledge and skills for role performance.
- Have patient use role play *to practice newly acquired role behaviors.*
- Assist patient to resolve role conflicts.
- Convey recognition of approximations of expected role performance *to reinforce learning of new behaviors.*
- Be nonjudgmental *so that patient can freely engage in learning and trying out role.*
- Identify and support strengths and capabilities related to adequate role performance *to foster patient's self-awareness of abilities and self-efficacy and to support and enhance patient's belief in own self-worth.*
- Encourage self-monitoring of changes in role behavior.

Principles and Rationale for Nursing Interventions[3,7,10-12]

In formulating appropriate intervention strategies for altered role performance, the nurse assesses the type of role disturbance and the patient's perception of self; e.g., Is the patient satisfied with present role performance? What would the patient like to change? What are the perceived consequences of this change? Because role performance is partly learned, learning experiences that include opportunities to practice the new role should be made available to the patient. Empathy and a supportive environment assist the patient in making maximum behavioral changes. Positive reinforcement of adaptive expressive and instrumental behaviors is important. Family and community resources should be assessed. When appropriate, these resources should be used to help the patient with role mastery.

■ SOCIAL ISOLATION

Social isolation is aloneness experienced by an individual and perceived as imposed by others or self and as a negative or threatened state.

Social isolation also can be defined as the state in which the individual has a need or desire for contact with others but is unable to make that contact because of physiologic, biologic, or sociocultural factors.[3] Social isolation is a negative state of aloneness.

Human relationships are important to mental and physical well-being. Social isolation, the lack of human companionship, death or absence of parents in early childhood, sudden loss of love, and chronic human loneliness are significant contributors to premature death and abnormal human functioning.[11,12]

To realize the consequences of social isolation, it is important to understand relevant personality theory. A number of personality theorists—Adler, Freud, Horney, Sullivan, Erikson, and Fromm—contributed to an understanding of this diagnosis. Sullivan developed the interpersonal theory of personality. He believed that an individual cannot exist apart from relationships with other people.[12]

Social isolation can be a result of faulty development in the life span. The psychologic ramifications are multiple. If an individual does not learn to cope with the stress and anxieties of life in a healthy manner, he or she may end up with grave psychologic difficulties.

Often it is difficult to completely separate biologically related factors of isolation from psychologic ones because a biologic cause can lead an individual to exhibit psychologic manifestations of isolation. Conversely, a psychologic cause can lead to a biologic outcome. Moreover, sociocultural causes of social isolation overlap the psychologic and biologic causative factors.

Social isolation is a subjective experience and therefore should be validated with the patient before a diagnosis is made.

Related Factors[9,10,12]

Psychologic
    Emotional illness (extreme anxiety, depression, paranoia, phobias, psychosis)
    Inability to engage in satisfying personal relationships
    Delay in accomplishing developmental tasks
    Immature interests
    Obesity, anorexia, bulimia
    Drug or alcohol addiction
    Alterations in physical appearance
Physiologic
    Altered state of wellness
    Drug or alcohol addiction
    Obesity, anorexia, bulimia
    Cancer
    Hospitalization or terminal illness
    Physical handicaps (paraplegia, amputation, arthritis, hemiplegia)
    Incontinence (embarrassment, odor)
    Sensory loss
    Nervous system alteration
Sociocultural
    Death of significant other
    Divorce
    Extreme poverty
    Hospitalization
    Living alone
    Moving into another culture
    Alternative life-styles
    Loss of usual means of transportation
    Unaccepted social values
    Inadequate personal resources
    Single parent

Defining Characteristics[3,8]

Absence of supportive significant other(s): family, friends, group
Sad, dull affect
Inappropriate or immature interests and activities for developmental age or stage
Incommunicative
Withdrawn
No eye contact
Preoccupation with own thoughts; repetitive, meaningless actions
Projects hostility in voice and behavior
Seeks to be alone or exists in subculture
Evidence of physical and/or mental handicap or altered state of wellness

Expected Patient Outcomes[1,8,9,11-14] & Nursing Interventions[3,7,8,13]

Acknowledge state of social isolation and verbalize a desire and willingness to be involved with others, as evidenced by:

Expressing feelings associated with social isolation
Expressing a desire to interact with caregivers in a positive way
Participating in group activities and appropriately functioning as part of a group

Stating a plan to participate in social activity

- Explore patient's perception of social isolation.
- Assess specific causes of social isolation through the use of a social history and physical assessment.
- Initiate a trusting nurse/patient relationship.
- Spend time with the patient engaged in active listening, maintaining eye contact, and when appropriate, using touch as a means of contact and comfort. (On an inpatient unit spend at least 15 minutes per shift involved in conversation with the patient.)
- Explore and help the patient identify available specific activities, groups, social outlets that promote social interaction.
- Positively reinforce active involvement with others. (On an inpatient unit, encourage attendance and participation in groups, social outings, social interaction at meal time or leisure time.)
- Arrange with patient for specific periods of planned socially interactive diversionary activity. Whether this is active or passive recreation depends on the patient's physical condition (e.g., cards, sports).
- Provide immediate and honest feedback about patient's behavior, especially withdrawn or alienating behaviors.
- Involve patient and family or significant other in setting goals and planning care.
- Give recognition and positive reinforcement for self-initiated and self-directed attendance at activities.
- Provide educational opportunities for patient and family to enhance knowledge about needs and to facilitate skill development (e.g., social skills, assertiveness, communication, reading material).

Identify factors that contribute to state of social isolation, as evidenced by:

Verbalizing fears, limitations, and barriers that he or she possess that inhibit social interaction

Verbalizing feelings of loneliness and concerns about low self-esteem

Verbally identifying the nature and extent of social isolation

Exploring expectations of self and others within past and future relations

Recognizing need for intimacy

Communicating knowledge of disease process and understanding of present situation

Expressing feelings about lack of supportive relationships

Identifying areas of skill or resources development necessary for establishing new relationships

Acknowledging physical and/or sensory impairment as a possible limitation to social intervention

- Explore patient's perception of social isolation.
- Assess specific causes of social isolation through the use of a social history and physical assessment.
- Initiate a trusting nurse/patient relationship.
- Spend time with the patient engaged in active listening, maintaining eye contact, and when appropriate, using

touch as a means of contact and comfort. (On an inpatient unit spend at least 15 mintues per shift involved in conversation with the patient.)

- Explore and help the patient identify specific activities, groups, social outlets available to him or her that promote social interaction.
- Provide educational opportunities for patient and family to enhance knowledge about needs and to facilitate skill development (e.g., social skills, assertiveness, communication, reading material).
- Identify resources available to the patient, and refer the patient and family when necessary (e.g., agencies, financial planning, transportation, social service people).

Verbalize and demonstrate way to promote meaningful relationships, as evidenced by:

Actively participating in activities on inpatient unit

Approaching others to socialize

Developing a plan to join a social peer group or activity on a regular basis

Interacting with family or significant others

Setting realistic goals and identifying realistic time schedules for achieving goals

Using resources available through an agency (social service, home health care, psychology services, self-improvement classes) to establish realistic plan for the future

- Initiate a trusting nurse/patient relationship.
- Spend time with the patient engaged in active listening, maintaining eye contact, and when appropriate, using touch as a means of contact and comfort. (On an inpatient unit spend at least 15 minutes per shift involved in conversation with the patient.)
- Explore and help the patient identify specific activities, groups, social outlets available to him or her that promote social interaction.
- Positively reinforce active involvement with others. (On an inpatient unit, encourage attendance and participation in groups, social outings, social interaction at meal time or leisure time.)
- Arrange with patient for specific periods of planning socially interactive diversionary activity. Whether this is active or passive recreation depends on the patient's physical condition (e.g., cards, sports).
- Provide immediate and honest feedback about patient's behavior, especially withdrawn or alienating behaviors.
- Involve patient and family or significant other in setting goals and planning care.
- Give recognition and positive reinforcement for self-initiated and self-directed attendance at activities.
- Provide educational opportunities for patient and family to enhance knowledge about needs and to facilitate skill development (e.g., social skills, assertiveness, communication, reading material).
- Explore available volunteer activities.

Identify activities that provide diversion and stimulate interest as well as enhance self-esteem, as evidenced by:

Being actively involved with others

Expressing increased feelings of comfort with involvement

Identifying factors that have contributed to his or her success

Recovering from negative feelings associated with social isolation

Participating daily in a meaningful diversionary activity (exercise, education, self-help group, interest group)

Achieving expected self of wellness

- Spend time with the patient engaged in active listening, maintaining eye contact, and when appropriate, using touch as a means of contact and comfort. (On an inpatient unit spend at least 15 minutes per shift involved in conversation with the patient.)
- Explore and help the patient identify specific activities, groups, social outlets available to him or her that promote social interaction.
- Positively reinforce active involvement with others. (On an inpatient unit, encourage attendance and participation in groups, social outings, social interaction at meal time or leisure time.)
- Arrange with patient for specific periods of planned socially interactive diversionary activity. Whether this is active or passive recreation depends on the patient's physical condition (e.g., cards, sports).
- Provide immediate and honest feedback about patient's behavior, especially withdrawn or alienating behaviors.
- Involve patient and family or significant other in setting goals and planning care.
- Give recognition and positive reinforcement for self-initiated and self-directed attendance at activities.
- Provide educational opportunities for patient and family to enhance knowledge about needs and to facilitate skill development (e.g., social skills, assertiveness, communication, reading material).
- Identify resources available to the patient, and refer the patient and family when necessary (e.g., agencies, financial planning, transportation, social service people).
- Explore available volunteer activities.

Principles and Rationale for Nursing Interventions

The information of effective human relationships affects the health and well-being of all patients.[6] Therefore it is essential that the nurse assess carefully the patient's social history when limitations or barriers are found in the ability to form relationships with others. Because social isolation is a subjective state, all inferences made regarding a person's feelings of aloneness must be validated.[3] The nurse must possess skilled interview and communication techniques to effectively help patients identify and overcome social isolation.

It is important for the nurse to discuss any feelings of loneliness that the patient expresses. Loneliness is the result of unmet intimacy needs.[2] After a therapeutic nurse/patient relationship is established, these feelings can be discussed and ways of meeting intimacy needs explored. To do this effectively, nurses must accept and deal with any of their own feelings of loneliness. Possible causes of social isolation must be explored with the patient in an open, direct, and supportive manner. Problem-solving techniques should be discussed and taught to the patient, with the ultimate decision-making process focusing on the patient to promote behavioral change.[12] Follow-up care is absolutely necessary for the patient's continued support and accomplishment of the outcomes desired.

Isolated older persons pose a complex problem for nursing care because the likelihood that they will seek assistance depends on several factors.[11] A painful physical disorder that cannot be ignored is more likely to lead the individual to seek help. Second, the more isolated older or mentally impaired persons are, the less likely they are to seek help. Third, the social support resource must be familiar and acceptable to the person. Last, unsuccessful, uncaring, or inappropriate experiences with the social resources will discourage older or mentally impaired persons from seeking future contact.[1]

The elderly and mentally impaired persons often lack the social skills to find supports and use referral services. It is important to increase the patient's awareness of appropriate resources that best meet his or her needs. The nurse can help develop adequate communication and assertiveness skills to facilitate the use of available social resources to decrease social isolation. Encouraging these people to accept the need for a broader support system can be challenging. The nurse must establish mutual respect and trust to promote continued self-esteem and openness to outside resources. Family members can often assist in this process.[12] The patient, however, must be encouraged to make his or her own decisions to maintain pride and self-respect, unless the patient is cognitively incapable of making appropriate decisions. Peer groups and other social organizations close to the patient can also help increase awareness of and openness to social support resources.

Cultural differences also affect the social isolation of the elderly and mentally impaired. Separation from their extended family, low expectations of service providers, language differences from those of the larger population, limited education, language deficits, and noncitizen status are other barriers that contribute to lack of knowledge of social service resources. The nurse must assess for the presence of these barriers and find ways to promote social interaction.

The chronically mentally disabled elderly face long-standing isolators, including broken family relationships and community ties, limited social coping skills, limited education, and limited employability.[11] These patients need complex multidisciplinary intervention guided by the nurse.

■ IMPAIRED SOCIAL INTERACTION

Impaired social interaction is the state in which an individual participates in an insufficient or excessive quantity or ineffective quality of social change.

A person exhibiting impaired social interactive behavior may have a personality impairment, may have been environmentally deprived, may be developmentally disabled, or may be physically impaired. The related factors are similar to those for the nursing diagnosis *social isolation,* but the behavior exhibited in impaired social interaction might be considered less severe in psychiatric terms.

Children who are physically separated from parents often have difficulty in forming attachments to others in their adult life.[1,5,6,10] Severe adult depression, dependency, psychosis (social isolation), various adjustment disorders (impaired social interaction), and suicide all have been frequently reported among individuals who suffer early parental loss.

Any way in which a child finds to cope may become a permanent characteristic in the child's adult personality. The maladaptive child may learn to cope by using irrational means. Alternately, the child may learn to cope normally by using rational means in a home where there is security, trust, love, respect, tolerance, and warmth.[5,6] The person who is likely to become adjustment disordered is one who has experienced the culturally determined difficulties in an accentuated form, primarily through childhood experience.[4]

Physical deprivation and/or physical ailments can cause social isolation, pathologic disorders, and impaired social interaction in individuals. Physical deprivation can be viewed as removal of an individual from social supports, e.g., loss of parents, institutionalization, and loss of physical functioning.

Related Factors[1,2,7,11]

Knowledge/skill deficit about ways to enhance mutuality
Communication barriers
Low self-concept
Absence of available significant others or peers
Limited physical mobility
Therapeutic isolation
Sociocultural dissonance
Altered thought processes
Inappropriate social behavior
Chemical addiction
Chronic illness
Mental retardation
Altered physical appearance
Poor impulse control
Attention-deficit disorder
Severe anxiety

Defining Characteristics[2,7,9,11]

Verbalized or observed discomfort in social situations
Verbalized or observed inability to receive or communicate satisfying sense of belonging, caring, interest, or shared history
Observed use of unsuccessful social interaction behaviors
Dysfunctional interaction with peers, family, and/or others (care givers)
Family report of change of style or pattern of interaction
Delusional thinking

Sensory and perceptual alterations, including auditory, visual, or tactile hallucinations
Inability to care for self

Expected Patient Outcomes[2,3,7,9-11] & Nursing Interventions

Acknowledge the existence of an impairment in the social interaction and verbalize a desire to diminish the impairment, as evidenced by:

Verbalizing thoughts and feelings related to existing inability to form close interpersonal relationships with others
Verbalizing a desire to interact within a peer group
Verbalizing knowledge of rejection by others (if it exists) and identifying ways to cope
Verbalizing with others (care givers, if inpatient) the nature of previous and/or current relationships exploring patterns of communication and behavior that enhance and inhibit relationships
Verbalizing feelings and needs for positive, appropriate social interaction

- Explain care-related activities clearly, answering questions as accurately as possible.
- Use an interpreter when necessary.
- Involve patient and family or significant other in planning care, and encourage patient's participation in self-care on a continuing basis.
- Assist patient in identifying and using effective social-interaction behaviors (e.g., increased eye contact, using people's names when appropriate, asking questions).
- Provide non-care-related time with the patient (inpatient unit) to encourage social interaction. Start with one-to-one interaction, and build up to group as the patient's skills indicate.
- Give positive reinforcement for appropriate and effective interaction behaviors (verbal and nonverbal).
- Explore feelings related to interaction with others including fears, anxieties, insecurities, needs, and wishes.
- Assist patient in the interpretation of his or her behaviors when interacting with others including distortions, automatic thoughts, and assumptions.
- Assist in the development of interactive skills by the techniques of modeling, education, role play, and direct, honest, immediate feedback.

Identify factors that contribute to inability to interact socially and develop a plan to improve social interaction, as evidenced by:

Patient and/or family providing information concerning medical background
Patient and/or family providing information concerning social history
Maintaining orientation to time, place, and person
Demonstrating understanding of care-related instructions (e.g., medications, physical limitations)
Patient and family actively participating in planning and implementation of prescribed therapies

Identifying behavioral goals for change

Participating in skill development specific to areas of deficit

Identifying effective coping techniques to deal with particular impairment (e.g., sociocultural differences, neurologic disorders, mental retardation, anxiety)

Remaining reality based

Developing alternate means of communication if sensory impairment is present

Demonstrating problem-solving ability

- Use an interpreter when necessary.
- Involve patient and family or significant others in planning care, and encourage patient's participation in self-care on a continuing basis.
- If delusions and/or hallucinations occur, do not focus on them; provide patient with reality-based information, and reassure patient of his or her safety.
- Give positive reinforcement for appropriate and effective interaction behaviors (verbal and nonverbal).
- Assist in finding referral sources of community support systems (if indicated), such as social services, financial counseling, home health care, mental health care, self-help groups.
- Assess for preexisting mental health problem(s) that may be reduced by the use of psychotropic medication or psychotherapy.
- Explore feelings related to interaction with others including fears, anxieties, insecurities, needs, and wishes.
- Assist patient in the interpretation of his or her behaviors when interacting with others including distortions, automatic thoughts and assumptions.
- Assist in the development of interactive skills by the techniques of modeling, education, role play, and direct, honest, immediate feedback.
- Educate patient and family (if indicated) on the use and side effects of psychoactive medications, as well as other symptom management strategies.

Interact with peers, family members, and society in an appropriate and satisfying manner, as evidenced by:

Seeking out others for social interaction

Demonstrating effective social interaction skills in both one-to-one and group settings

Using resources outside of normal sociocultural group as necessary

Demonstrating independent social interactions

Verbalizing and demonstrating improved self-esteem

Engaging in social activities without feeling anxious or embarrassed

- Involve patient and family or significant other in planning care, and encourage patient's participation in self-care on a continuing basis.
- Provide non-care-related time with the patient (inpatient unit) to encourage social interactions. Start with the one-to-one interaction, and build up to group as the patient's skills indicate.

- Give positive reinforcement for appropriate and effective interaction behaviors (verbal and nonverbal).
- Assist in finding referral sources or community support systems (if indicated), such as social services, financial counseling, home health care, mental health care, self-help groups.
- Assess for preexisting mental health problem(s) that may be reduced by the use of psychotropic medication or psychotherapy.
- Explore feelings related to interaction with others, including fears, anxieties, insecurities, needs, and wishes.
- Assist patient in the interpretation of his or her behaviors when interacting with others, including distortions, automatic thoughts and assumptions.
- Assist in the development of interactive skills by the techniques of modeling, education, role play, and direct, honest, immediate feedback.

Principles and Rationale for Nursing Interventions

A major cause of impaired social interaction is the inability to communicate effectively. This inability can be caused partly by feelings of inadequacy. Another cause is mental impairment. The nurse must be attuned to a patient's feelings of inadequacy or the extent of mental impairment. This is often difficult because people exhibit their inadequacies by different and varying forms of communication, e.g., overtalkativeness, silence, anger, or hostility.

Nursing interventions for this patient are similar to interventions for a socially isolated individual; however, one must keep in mind that the person who is interactively impaired may not be as severely impaired as one who is socially isolated. This means that the nurse has a better base from which to begin.

Often, social impairment is not perceived by the patient as a problem for himself or herself. The nurse needs to establish a trusting relationship to deal with the issues with the patient, the family, and friends.

Possible causal factors related to impaired social interaction must be explored with the patient in an open, direct, and supportive manner. Problem-solving techniques should be discussed and taught to the patient, with the ultimate decision-making process focusing on the patient to promote behavioral change. Follow-up care is absolutely necessary for the patient's continued support and accomplishment of the outcomes desired.

■ RELOCATION STRESS SYNDROME

Relocation stress syndrome includes physiologic and psychosocial disturbances related to transfer from one environment to another.

Relocation is a life event that creates change and stress for many individuals. Moves from one environment to another often result in adjustment difficulties as the person reorients to new surroundings and establishes attachments with others in a different setting. Relocation stress syndrome may occur in response to relocation to a retirement center, admission to a nursing home, hospitalization, hospital discharge, foster home placement or discharge for a child, geographic moves and immigration into another culture.*

The individual's ability to adapt to changes in his or her social and physical environment is influenced by personal coping skills, the quality of social support, the person's perception of events, and the presence or absence of supportive strategies before, during, and after the relocation event. For example, elderly persons' adjustments to relocation are affected by their perceived understanding of control over the transfer events, the predictability of stressors, their decisional control over some aspect of the posttransfer environment, and the amount of preparation before the move.[1,22,30]

Relocation stress syndrome in the hospitalized patient may appear shortly after relocation from the home or hospital to a nursing home.[16,25] It can also occur following a transfer from the intensive care unit to a step-down unit or general care ward,[31] after other intrahospital moves or deinstitutionalization.[8,24]

Common manifestations of relocation stress syndrome include anxiety about resettlement task and grieving responses for multiple losses.[2] In patients who have been institutionalized for a long time, the relocation experience may lead to increased aggression, anger, and fear.[15,24,32] In some elderly, increased anxiety and morbidity *are* related to moves.[21] In children, relocation stress may appear as developmental regression, social withdrawal, negativism, psychosomatic complaints, detachment, or angry protest.[7,14,26]

Related Factors†

Sudden, unanticipated move
Little or no preparation for the impending move
Forced move
Repeated relocation
Lack of adequate support system
Hospital admission or discharge
Admission to a nursing home
Transfer between hospital wards
Transfer between facilities
Job transfers with geographic moves
Cross-cultural migration

Defining Characteristics‡

Sleep disturbance
Change in eating habits
Increased confusion (elderly)

Alienation
Anger
Anxiety
Depression
Feelings of displacement
Increased aggression
Loneliness
Loss of identity
Powerlessness
Sense of abandonment
Social withdrawal
Uncertainty
Unfavorable comparison of posttransfer and pretransfer environment or staff
Verbalization of concern and distress about move
Performance problems in school (child or adolescent)
Regressed behaviors
Lack of acculturation behaviors

Expected Patient Outcomes & Nursing Interventions

Adjust to relocation, as evidenced by:

Decreased anxiety and grieving
Establishing new relationships
Participating in activities in the new setting
Verbalizing acceptance of changed environment

- Build relationship with patient *to foster trust, security, and support during a time of many losses.*
- Orient patient to new staff, equipment, and environment *to decrease uncertainty and anxiety.*
- Allow patient to control some aspects of the posttransfer environment (e.g., privacy, room decorations) *to increase control and autonomy.*
- Arrange for consistent caregivers and daily care routines *to facilitate continuity and predictability for the patient.*
- Teach family interventions to support the patient after relocation.
- Acknowledge patient's feelings of loss and anxiety related to relocation.
- Assist patient in identifying strengths and resources *to increase coping and problem solving in new environment.*
- Assess patient for dysfunctional grieving responses.
- Support patient in formulating realistic goals for self in the new setting *to promote a sense of mastery and to enhance self-esteem.*

Principles and Rationale for Nursing Interventions

Providing a supportive, structured, predictable environment for the patient decreases anxiety and the sense of disruption associated with relocation. The nurse should manage the milieu to minimize unnecessary changes and environmental stressors during the posttransfer adaptation period. Orienting the patient to a new environment should include describing changes in

---

*References 2, 7, 11, 14, 20, 28, 30.
†References 1, 2, 5, 6, 9, 10, 12, 18-20, 22, 29, 31, 32, 35.
‡References 1-4, 7, 8, 13, 17, 23, 25, 27, 28, 33, 34.

staff, staffing patterns, equipment, and activities. Allowing the patient to participate in decision making and to control some aspects of the new environment will decrease the patient's sense of powerlessness. Assessment of the patient's adjustment should continue long after the relocation event because anxiety and dysfunctional grieving may interfere with the individual's ability to learn new behaviors and coping skills required in the new setting.

■ ALTERED FAMILY PROCESSES

Altered family processes is the state in which a family who normally functions effectively experiences a dysfunction.

The family has been described as a "human group with significant emotional bonds."[8] Functions of the family include the following.[12]

Reproduction
Socialization (education of the young)
Protection and safety
Economic security (provision of food and shelter)
Conferral of roles
Social contact
Sexual fulfillment
Conferral of status
Belongingness, love, and affection
Physiologic needs
Recreation
Religious needs

In disturbed families several factors apparently cluster at the same time. "A combination of events produce symptomatic behavior in one or more members of a given family.[5]

Characteristics of a functional family include the following[10,12]:

Homeostatic balance is maintained, along with flexibility.
The family is able to adapt to external (environmental) and internal (developmental) stress or changes.
Levels of authority are not blurred; family hierarchy is fair and clear.
Emotional contact is maintained between family members and across generations.
Emotional problems are viewed as a product of the family as a whole, not blamed entirely on one family member.
Overcloseness (fusion-enmeshment) is avoided.
Distance (disengagement) is avoided or not used to solve problems.
Problems between two family members (spouses, spouse and child, children) are resolved by the two people. A third person is not involved to take sides or become triangulated.
Individual differences are encouraged to promote growth.
Preservation of a positive emotional climate is encouraged.
Children have age-appropriate expectations and responsibility within the family; parents negotiate openly with their children for age-appropriate privileges.
Each spouse functions within his or her respective role, and spouses maintain a balance of effective expres-

sion, rational thought, caretaking, object orientation, and relationship focus.

Altered family process can be viewed as the lack of one or more of these characteristics.

Related Factors[2,7,13]

Situation transition and/or crises
　Poverty
　Disaster
　Divorce
　Relocation
　Unemployment
　Economic crisis
　Change in family roles
　Conflict
　Breach of trust between members
　Social deviance by family member
Development transition and/or crises
　Birth of infant with defect
　Loss of family member
　Gain of new family member
Pathophysiologic factors
　Illness of a family member
　　Discomforts related to illness symptoms
　　Change in member's ability to function
　　Time-consuming treatments
　　Disabling treatments
　　Expensive treatments
　　Psychiatric illness
　　Hospitalization
　Trauma
　　Surgery
　　Loss of body parts or function

Defining Characteristics[2,7,13]

Family system unable or unwilling to meet physical needs of its members
Family system unable or unwilling to meet emotional needs of its members
Family system unable or unwilling to meet spiritual needs of its members
Parents do not demonstrate respect for each other's view on childbearing practices
Parents do not respect children's age-appropriate abilities
Inability to express or accept wide range of feelings
Inability to express or accept feelings of members
Family unable to meet security needs of its members
Inability of family members to relate to each other for mutual growth and maturation
Family uninvolved in community activities
Inability to accept help appropriately
Rigidity in function, rules, and roles
Family does not demonstrate respect for individuality and autonomy of its members

Family unable to adapt to change and deal with traumatic experience constructively

Family fails to accomplish current and past developmental tasks

Ineffective family decision-making process

Family enmeshment

Family disengagement

Fixed triangulation

Blurred hierarchical system

Members use distance to maintain homeostasis

Use of member scapegoating

Spouses do not maintain balance in relationship

Failure to send and receive clear messages

Inappropriate boundary maintenance

Inappropriate or poorly communicated family rules, rituals, or symbols

Impaired communication

Unexamined family myths

Inappropriate level and directions of energy

Physical, sexual, or verbal abuse

Expected Patient Outcomes* & Nursing Interventions†

Develop and practice positive communication among family members, as evidenced by:

Family members sharing feelings and thoughts related to illness, crises, traumas experienced in the family and expressing how these events affected the family individuality and as a whole

Family members working to resolve conflict among members and developing a respectful tolerance for individual coping needs

Family members verbalizing a desire to work together to resolve issues or conflicts

- Create a supportive environment that provides safety, protects privacy, supports trust, and promotes comfort of the family unit and of individual members.
- Provide regular contacts with the family, especially at time of crisis.
- Assess family's structural, behavioral, and interactive patterns including boundaries, developmental stages, coping skills, role expectations, overt and covert rules, and energy output.
- Engage family members in the problem-solving process including setting realistic goals, identifying clear behavioral objectives to be met, and anticipating possible barriers to crisis/conflict resolution.
- Expedite communication within the family to allow members to express their feelings about the present situation or past situation.
- Reinforce, positively, exhibition of adaptive family behaviors.

- If the crisis involves hospitalization, provide for the physical and emotional comfort of the family throughout the hospitalization. Provide liberal visitation, orientation to important areas of the unit/hospital, adequate space for family privacy, overnights as appropriate, and emotional support as indicated.
- Ascertain the religious and cultural background of the family.
- Arrange for and participate in family conferences (including the identified patient) to teach family members how to apply what is learned and engage in problem solving about how to work through potential problems that may arise after discharge and to develop a discharge plan that may involve referral to community supports. Ensure privacy for these conferences.
- In the community setting assume appropriate role(s) when interviewing with families in crisis. Consider among the following: support, education, guidance, role modeling, monitoring, facilitating, advocacy, and referral.

Exhibit an ability to positively negotiate issues, solve problems, or make decisions as a family or between individual family members, as evidenced by:

Family members identifying goals consistent with role relationships and that focus on crisis/conflict resolution

Family members verbalizing personal values that are involved in the negotiation process without judgment

Family members exhibiting an ability to ask or accept help appropriately either from others in the family or from outside support resources

Family members anticipating inhibiting factors and developing strategies for coping with them

- Create a supportive environment that provides safety, protects privacy, supports trust, and promotes comfort of the family unit and of individual members.
- Provide regular contacts with the family, especially at time of crisis.
- Assess family's structural, behavioral, and interactive patterns including boundaries, developmental stages, coping skills, role expectations, overt and covert rules, and energy output.
- Engage family members in the problem-solving process including setting realistic goals, identifying clear behavioral objectives to be met, and anticipating possible barriers to crisis/conflict resolution.
- Initiate involvement of additional formal and informal supports to assist the family to move toward crisis/conflict resolution (i.e., teaching stress reduction and coping skills, engaging extended family if authorized to do so). Referral to family therapy (if indicated), social support agencies, self-help groups, financial advisors, church-affiliated supports as appropriate.
- Expedite communication within the family to allow members to express their feelings about the present situation or past situation.

---

*References 1-3, 5-8, 14, 15.

†References 1-3, 5, 9, 11, 12, 14, 15.

- Reinforce, positively, exhibition of adaptive family behaviors.
- If the crisis involves hospitalization, provide for the physical and emotional comfort of the family throughout the hospitalization. Provide liberal visitation, orientation to important areas of the unit/hospital, adequate space for family privacy, overnights as appropriate, and emotional support as indicated.
- Ascertain the religious and cultural background of the family.
- Provide the family and the identified patient basic information about the nature of the illness, answer questions, and discuss strategies for managing symptoms.
- Arrange for and participate in family conferences (including the identified patient) to teach family members how to apply what is learned and engage in problem solving about how to work through potential problems that may arise after discharge and to develop a discharge plan that may involve referral to community supports. Ensure privacy for these conferences.
- In the community setting assume appropriate role(s) when interviewing with families in crisis. Consider among the following: support, education, guidance, role modeling, monitoring, facilitating, advocacy, and referral.

Exhibit an ability to adapt to external or internal change, as evidenced by:

Family members dealing constructively with crisis

Family members accomplishing individual developmental tasks

- Create a supportive environment that provides safety, protects privacy, supports trust, and promotes comfort of the family unit and of individual members.
- Provide regular contacts with the family, especially at time of crisis.
- Assess family's structural, behavioral, and interactive patterns including boundaries, developmental stages, coping skills, role expectations, overt and covert rules, and energy output.
- Engage family members in the problem-solving process including setting realistic goals, identifying clear behavioral objectives to be met, and anticipating possible barriers to crisis/conflict resolution.
- Initiate involvement of additional formal and informal supports to assist the family to move toward crisis/conflict resolution (i.e., teaching stress reduction and coping skills, engaging extended family if authorized to do so). Referral to family therapy (if indicated), social support agencies, self-help groups, financial advisors, church affiliated supports as appropriate.
- Expedite communication within the family to allow members to express their feelings about the present situation or past situation.
- Ascertain the religious and cultural background of the family.

- In the community setting assume appropriate role(s) when interviewing with families in crisis. Consider among the following: support, education, guidance, role modeling, monitoring, facilitating, advocacy, and referral.

Resolution of issues leads to family members' achievement of a new state of equilibrium with enhanced coping and problem-solving skills, as evidenced by:

Family members directing energy toward crisis resolution

Family members experiencing mutual support and a sense of cohesion

Family members meeting basic emotional and physical needs of one another in appropriate ways that do not confuse boundaries

- Provide regular contacts with the family, especially at time of crisis.
- Engage family members in the problem-solving process including setting realistic goals, identifying clear behavioral objectives to be met, and anticipating possible barriers to crisis/conflict resolution.
- Initiate involvement of additional formal and informal supports to assist the family to move toward crisis/conflict resolution (i.e., teaching stress reduction and coping skills, engaging extended family if authorized to do so). Referral to family therapy (if indicated), social support agencies, self-help groups, financial advisors, church-affiliated supports as appropriate.
- Expedite communication within the family to allow members to express their feelings about the present situation or past situation.
- Reinforce, positively, exhibition of adaptive family behaviors.
- Provide the family and the identified patient basic information about the nature of the illness, answer questions, and discuss strategies for managing symptoms.
- Arrange for and participate in family conferences (including the identified patient) to teach family members how to apply what is learned and engage in problem solving about how to work through potential problems that may arise after discharge and to develop a discharge plan that may involve referral to community supports. Ensure privacy for these conferences.
- In the community setting assume appropriate role(s) when interviewing with families in crisis. Consider among the following: support, education, guidance, role modeling, monitoring, facilitating, advocacy, and referral.
- Assist the family to identify problems and establish goals for crisis/conflict resolution.

Nurture and growth promoted within the family unit as a whole and for individual members, as evidenced by:

Family members clarifying roles within the family and between members

Family members openly discussing and coming to an agreement concerning rules and boundaries

Family members demonstrating emotional bonding and offering support to each other when indicated

Family members identifying mutual interest

Family members experiencing enhanced understanding and support for one another

- Create a supportive environment that provides safety, protects privacy, supports trust, and promotes comfort of the family unit and of individual members.
- Provide regular contacts with the family, especially at time of crisis.
- Assess family's structural, behavioral, and interactive patterns including boundaries, developmental stages, coping skills, role expectations, overt and covert rules, and energy output.
- Engage family members in the problem-solving process including setting realistic goals, identifying clear behavioral objectives to be met, and anticipating possible barriers to crisis/conflict resolution.
- Expedite communication within the family to allow members to express their feelings about the present situation or past situation.
- Reinforce, positively, exhibition of adaptive family behaviors.
- If the crisis involves hospitalization, provide for the physical and emotional comfort of the family throughout the hospitalization. Provide liberal visitation, orientation to important areas of the unit/hospital, adequate space for family privacy, overnights as appropriate, and emotional support as indicated.
- Provide the family and the identified patient basic information about the nature of the illness, answer questions, and discuss strategies for managing symptoms.
- Arrange for and participate in family conferences (including the identified patient) to teach family members how to apply what is learned and engage in problem solving about how to work through potential problems that may arise after discharge and to develop a discharge plan that may involve referral to community supports. Ensure privacy for these conferences.
- Assist the family to identify problems and establish goals for crisis/conflict resolution.

Principles and Rationale for Nursing Interventions*

Assessment of the family may be difficult because often not all members are available to interact with the nurse. It is of utmost importance that nurses provide early intervention for families at risk because altered family processes, e.g., relationship problems and communication barriers, can be prevented. The nurse

*References 2, 3, 5, 12, 14, 15.

should become attuned to the family's environment so that she or he can exchange information with the family system. Three major categories for family assessment are described in the Calgary Family Assessment Model: structural, developmental, and functional.

Structural: who is in the family and what is the connection among household members versus those outside the family

    Internal structure

        Family composition

        Rank order

        Subsystem (delineated by generation, gender, interest, or function)

        Boundary (defines who participates and how)

    External structure

        Culture

        Religion

        Social class status and mobility

        Environment

        Extended family

    Effective tool (genogram)

Developmental: how this family came to be at this stage in its developmental life cycle

    Developmental stage family is in

    Tasks requiring completion during this developmental stage

Functional: details of how individuals actually behave in relation to one another

    Instrumental functioning (routine, mechanical activities of daily living)

    Expressive functioning

    Emotional communication

    Verbal communication

    Nonverbal communication

    Circular communication

    Problem solving

    Roles

    Control

    Beliefs

    Alliances/coalitions

Facilitating change within the family system is the primary goal in family work; thus a thorough knowledge of change theory is essential.[5] The role of nursing in the care of families also includes teaching and helping families to develop adaptive skills. For example, careful family assessment is necessary to intervene effectively when the crisis is a chronically ill individual in the family. Family roles must be revised and strengths and weaknesses identified. Dysfunctional coping mechanisms must be replaced with effective ones. Family members can be supportive of one another by communicating needs and by adapting roles to meet reciprocal physical, emotional, spiritual, and mutual respect needs.

The nurse can help the family identify and work toward mutual goals by becoming involved with the family from the onset of the health care situation. For instance, if the family is dealing with painful news, the nurse can acknowledge that the news is unfavorable, encourage and listen to angry or distraught family members, recognize the need to discharge feelings, and facilitate the family's awareness of the nurse's ability to assist in identifying coping strategies. Regular patient/nurse interactions, particularly at crisis times, are necessary to reinforce stress-reducing techniques and problem-solving efforts. When the nurse offers choices, this can help the family satisfy the important need for control over what is happening. The nurse can often assist best by being the liaison among other health care professionals involved in the care of the family. Later, helping the family examine realistic approaches or expectations of the situation provides structure despite the disequilibrium being experienced.

The process of review of the negative experience can help the family sort out what has happened and help them verbalize fears. Guilt feelings may surface and can be dealt with realistically at this time.

Family participation in the care of an ill family member helps meet the needs of closeness, love, sharing, and order in their lives. Separation is extremely threatening and causes pain and anxiety. Even small tasks can be of great comfort to the hospitalized member and the other family members. Family members should be given the opportunity to participate whenever hospitalization occurs.

Preparation for resuming family interactions after a crisis must be made and ongoing follow-up provided. Families lacking nursing support after having received it before flounder and may again become ineffective. Follow-up at 1, 3, and 6 months helps them make the transition to independent role relationships within the family system and provides a time for evaluating the coping mechanisms they are using.

Another important nursing role is to provide family therapy by a qualified family therapist, who has usually had additional education in this area, or intervention that helps clients solve problems now and in future crisis. This involves identifying how the family obtains and uses information from the environment.[5] Evaluating the family's ability to seek and use help gives clues to the ability of the family to resolve problems. Dysfunctional families do little or no negotiating when problem solving. The family's cognitive capacity—their ability to appraise a situation realistically and competently and their own capabilities in relation to it—depends on their openness and their respect for each other's unique capabilities.[5,15] The nurse must help the family adapt to change, deal with the crisis constructively, accomplish developmental tasks, readjust roles to accommodate situational and developmental crises, and use problem-solving techniques. If difficulty is observed with either the family's or the individual's ability to function in the family system when the problem is an acting-out adolescent, a member with anorexia, a young person with bulimia, or a violent or sexually abusing member, family therapy is indicated and referral to a qualified family therapist necessary. A family unable to negotiate rules effectively or demonstrating continued enmeshment, disengagement, fixed triangulation, use of distance to maintain homeostasis, or scapegoating also needs family therapy.

ALTERED FAMILY PROCESSES: ALCOHOLISM

The state in which the psychosocial, spiritual, and physiologic functions of the family unit are chronically disorganized, leading to conflict, denial of problems, resistance to change, ineffective problem solving, and a series of self-perpetuating crises.

Alcoholism is a family disease that establishes unhealthy patterns of behavior. The four general rules that operate in the alcoholic family are rigidity, silence, denial, and isolation. These "rules" often continue to operate from one generation to the next, even though active drinking may no longer be in the system.[2]

To survive the rules of the family, individual members often adapt by taking on various roles that are extensions of the family rules. This provides some stability and can divert attention away from the drinking family member. The roles are as follows:[2,5]

- **The hero:** Portrays an image of self-confidence but feels inadequate; achieves success in school or work to make the family look good.
- **The scapegoat:** Diverts attention away from problems of alcoholism by acting out the family anger; gets into trouble or gets inappropriately blamed.
- **The lost one:** Tries not to attract attention and withdraws from the family; loses self in reading, television, or other activities; learns to deal with family pain by developing dysfunctional eating patterns; avoids others by hiding out; avoids making waves and draws attention by nonpresence.
- **The family mascot or clown:** Often the youngest in the family, reacts to stress by providing comic relief; lessens attention in the family by joking, being funny and cute; may have trouble assuming responsibilities as individual matures.
- **The placater:** Tries to reduce conflict in the family by making things better and smoothing things over.
- **The enabler:** Prevents the alcoholic from experiencing the consequences of his/her alcoholic behavior.

These descriptions are generalizations; in reality, the roles often become blended. In exploring relationships and communication patterns, it is important for the nurse to assist the family in identifying their roles and the impact on family processes.[7]

Alcoholic families often have experiences of trauma such as verbal or physical altercations between members. A state of shock is a typical reaction to an episode of trauma and is characterized by both physical and emotional responses. Physical responses at the time of the event include initial breath holding, uneven breathing, tachycardia, increase in blood pressure, vacant-appearing eyes, loss of color in the face, and skin that is cool to the touch. On the emotional level, the person becomes numb and simply shuts down. After the shock stage is a rebound stage wherein the individual attempts to return to the preshock state. Suppressed emotions begin to be felt, and the person needs to talk about the event. The next stage is the resolution stage in which the person resolves the feelings they experienced. The person learns and grows from the catastrophic event. These normal responses to shock do not occur effectively in an alcoholic family because of the rule of silence. No one talks about the incident and they act as if nothing happened. The individual is left to deal with his or her feeling in any way possible including memory loss. The individual may dissociate themselves from the event as if it happened to someone else. The person then enters a chronic shock state that continues until these issues are resolved. The nurse must be aware of this phenomenon when interacting with family members.

Family members may not be ready to talk about the issue at the same time. It is likely that the members have extremely different perceptions of the same traumatic event. When the event is unresolved, the person may reexperience both the physical and emotional characteristics of a shock victim during a family discussion, e.g., rapid heartbeat, breath holding or uneven breathing, look of blankness, coldness. The release of intense and deep emotions discharges the energy that releases the family member from the effects of chronic shock. This is often evidenced by crying, sobbing, screaming in anger, rage, or fear. The individual experiences a sense of release and often expresses a feeling of freedom. Resolution occurs when the shock event loses its power over the person and has been integrated into his or her life experience. Knowing the sequence to resolution of the shock experience is important when caring for alcoholic families. It is important to understand that recovery is a process and not an event, and the nurse's interactions may occur at any time along the continuum of recovery.[3,5]

Related Factors[4]

Abuse of alcohol
Family history of alcoholism, resistance to treatment
Inadequate coping skills
Genetic predisposition
Addictive personality
Lack of problem-solving skills
Biochemical influences

Defining Characteristics[4]

Major

Feelings

Decreases self-esteem or sense of worthlessness
Anger or suppressed rage
Frustration
Powerlessness
Anxiety
Tension
Distress
Insecurity
Repressed emotions
Responsibility for alcoholic's behavior
Lingering resentment
Shame or embarrassment

Hurt
Unhappiness
Guilt
Emotional isolation and loneliness
Vulnerability
Mistrust
Hopelessness
Rejection

Roles and Relationships

Deterioration in family relationships or disturbed family dynamics
Ineffective spouse communication or marital problems
Altered role function or disruption of family roles
Inconsistent parenting or low perception of parental support
Family denial
Intimacy dysfunction
Chronic family problems
Closed communication systems

Behaviors

Expression of anger inappropriately
Difficulty with intimate relationships
Loss of control of drinking
Impaired communication
Inefective problem-solving skills
Enabling alcoholic to maintain drinking
Inability to meet emotional needs of its members
Manipulation
Dependency
Criticizing
Alcohol abuse
Broken promises
Rationalization or denial of problems
Refusal to get help or inability to accept and receive help appropriately
Blaming
Inadequate understanding or knowledge of alcoholism

Minor

Feelings

Being different from other people
Depression
Hostility
Fear
Emotional control by others
Confusion
Dissatisfaction
Loss
Misunderstood
Abandonment
Confused love and pity
Moodiness
Failure
Being unloved
Lack of identity

Roles and Relationships

Triangulating family relationships

Reduced ability of family members to relate to each other for mutual growth and maturation

Lack of skills necessary for relationships

Lack of cohesiveness

Disrupted family rituals

Family unable to meet security needs of its members

Family does not demonstrate respect for individuality and autonomy of its members

Pattern of rejection

Economic problems

Neglected obligations

Behaviors

Inability to meet spiritual needs of its members

Inability to express or accept wide range of feelings

Orientation toward tension relief rather than achievement of goals

Family special occasions are alcohol centered

Escalating conflict

Lying

Contradictory, paradoxic communication

Lack of dealing with conflict

Harsh self-judgment

Isolation

Nicotine addiction

Difficulty having fun

Self-blaming

Unresolved grief

Controlling communication and power struggles

Inability to adapt to change

Immaturity

Stress-related illnesses

Inability to deal with traumatic experiences constructively

Seeking approval and affirmation

Lack of reliability

Disturbances in academic performance in children

Disturbances in concentration

Chaos

Sustance abuse other than alcohol

Failure to accomplish current or past developmental tasks or difficulty with life-cycle transitions

Verbal abuse of spouse or parent

Agitation

Diminished physical contact

Expected Family Outcomes & Nursing Interventions[1,3,5,6,8]

Family develops insights into the association of alcoholism and role relationships, communication processes, and coping mechanisms as evidenced by:

Expediting communication within the family to share feelings and thoughts related to the impact of the alcoholic member on the family group and as individuals

Understanding information about the characteristics and causes of alcoholism and correcting misinformation

The role of the nurse is in:

Facilitating family members in discussing and positively reinforcing adaptive coping skills in one another, and realizing that they must first help themselves by changing their own personal response

Reinforcing that family members are not responsible for the person's drinking

Assisting family members in identifying their role in enabling the alcoholic member to continue their drinking, e.g., making excuses, putting to bed, bailing out of jail, and discussion of strategies to avoid enabling behaviors

Encouraging the family to discuss that which has been covert in the past, e.g., avoidance, silence, denial, ignoring, distancing self, isolation or overt, e.g., threats, hiding alcohol or car keys, crying, rigidity

Giving examples of confusing, contradictory, and paradoxic communication, as well as broken promises that have contributed to lack of trust, consistency, predictability, and reliability

Assisting family members in expressing anger in an appropriate manner and encouraging their willingness to support the alcoholic person to obtain necessary treatment

Informing the family that the person is responsible for his/her drinking behavior and that family attempts to control the drinking prevents the person from suffering the consequences of their drinking behavior

Identifying strategies to positively change role patterns and coping mechanisms while supporting other family members to do the same

Supporting the family to understand that focusing on their behavior will remove the alcoholic from the center of attention and all family roles will be challenged

Encouraging the family to commit to continued family communication sessions and to create appropriate action plans based on the development of new insights related to role relationships, communication processes, and coping skills

The family can be assisted to create conditions that facilitates the alcoholic family member to enter into a treatment program as evidenced by:

Verbalizing recognition and acknowledgment by the family members that alcoholism is a family problem

Committing to seek and implement appropriate interventions

The role of the nurse is in:

Supporting the family members in deciding to enable the drinking member to enter into a treatment program by determining/initiating appropriate action plans, e.g., changes in household responsibilities, contact with treatment program, child care services

Guiding the family to locate and access child care services to facilitate the initiation and continuation of treatment since this is often a barrier to staying in treatment

Supporting the family in seeking help from and accepting assistance from competent professional caregivers and counselors including AL-ANON, Alcoholics Anonymous, and self-help groups, e.g., ACOA (Adult Children of Alcoholics)

Principles and Rationale for Nursing Interventions

Facilitating insight and appropriate problem solving is the primary role of the nurse in caring for alcoholic families. The nurse can assist the family members to recognize their feelings and thoughts and engage in discussions about their role to enhance insight. Encouraging the verbalization of thoughts and feelings is the first step of recovery. The nurse must also be aware that family members are often reluctant or unwilling to talk about issues. When only one of the family members is ready to deal with and resolve issues, it is important to be cognizant that the other family members may inhibit the willing person. The nurse must reinforce the idea that it is possible for the willing member to move toward recovery, even when other family members decline to participate.

In addition to interacting with the family, the nurse needs to support them in facilitating the entrance of the alcoholic person into a treatment program. Referral of family members to AL-ANON or ACOA can also facilitate their recovery. Families often benefit and are receptive to family therapy that can be provided in either an outpatient or residential setting. The nurse's role is to inform the family and explore the options they are ready to accept.

■ CAREGIVER ROLE STRAIN

■ Caregiver role strain is a caregiver's experienced difficulty in performing the caregiving role.

Caregiver role strain is conceptualized as an objective burden (regarding the activities of daily living/independent activities of daily living (ADL/IADL) tasks of caregiving) and a subjective burden (regarding the caregiver's response to the circumstances of the role).[9,13] Caregiver role strain tends to focus primarily on the subjective portion of burden.

The individual caregiver is most often female, usually a spouse, daughter, or daughter-in-law. Caregivers often assume their roles following an unexpected crisis and without any previous experience.[6]

Caregivers are involved with many roles and competing demands for their time, energy, and resources. Self-care needs of the caregiver are often neglected because of care demands. The caregiver seldom recognizes the association between the psychologic, psychosocial, and medical limitations of the stress of caregiving. Factors that may influence caregiver role strain are a negative relationship between the caregiver and care receiver, length of time and/or experience in the caregiving role, a decrease in the cognitive status of the care receiver, and unpredictable care receiver behavior.[4,13]

Related Factors[1-21]

Illness severity of care receiver
  Caregiver not developmentally ready for caregiving role
Increased care needs of care receiver
  Developmental delay or retardation of the care receiver or caregiver
Addiction or codependency of caregiver and care receiver
Premature birth/congenital defect of care receiver
  Marginal family adaptation or dysfunction before caregiving situation
Caregiver health impairment
  Marginal coping patterns of caregiver
Discharge of family member with significant home care needs
  Past history of poor relationship between caregiver and care receiver
Unpredictable illness course or instability in the care receiver's health
  Care receiver exhibits deviant, bizarre behavior
Psychologic or cognitive problems in the care receiver

Defining Characteristics[1-21]

Feeling exhausted
Increased emotional lability
Inability to complete caregiving tasks
Preoccupation with care routine
Declining health status
Family conflict
Withdrawal from social support
Feeling depressed
Change in leisure activities
Feeling loss of usual or expected relationship with care receiver
Sleep pattern disturbance
Increased stress or nervousness

Expected Patient Outcomes & Nursing Interventions

The caregiver will state appropriate informal or formal resources, as evidenced by:

Listing and describing such formal resources as the public health nurse, day care, respite care, hospice, and informal resources, such as church groups, social clubs, or neighbors
  • Review caregiver's knowledge of available resources; *competency level of the caregiver can be enhanced by increasing his or her knowledge base of resources available and teaching basic caregiving skills.*[20]
  • Establish financial eligibility to obtain community resources.
  • Determine caregiver's and care receiver's willingness to accept resource support.
  • Evaluate current family network.
  • Assist in referral process, as appropriate.

The caregiver will use stress reduction strategies, as evidenced by:

Verbalizing that stress is reduced and that stress reduction techniques are incorporated into daily routine.

- Establish a pattern of "timeout" from caregiver role.
- Provide information and access to relaxation tapes, guided imagery exercises, meditation and biofeedback techniques; *modalities must be selected appropriately to meet the unique individual needs of the caregiver.*
- Teach time management strategies.
- Encourage involvement in church and in social activities.
- Provide information, and refer caregivers to community support groups, *opportunities for caregivers with varied levels of experience to network/share information may be valuable.*[3,5,7,15,18]
- Provide time for active listening to caregiver's concerns.
- Validate caregiver's feelings of role strain.
- Encourage consistent health monitoring for caregiver.
- Monitor for caregiver depression.

The caregiver is able to verbalize change in role expectations, as evidenced by:

Prioritizing role demands and experiencing less role strain

- Examine usual roles within the family system; compare past, present, and future relationships within the unit, *a positive relationship between caregiver and care receiver correlates with less role strain.*[2]
- Identify the various roles in which the caregiver engages.
- Assist the caregiver to negotiate roles with other family members.
- Educate the family about the process of caregiving; *the competency level of the caregiver can be enhanced by increasing his or her knowledge base and skill level.*[3,17,18]
- Assist family members in dealing with the disengaged member and with the changes of status within the family unit.
- Acknowledge and validate the caregiver role; *caregivers want to be acknowledged and appreciated.*[1,3]

Principles and Rationale for Nursing Interventions

Communities have a myriad of services to offer the caregiver; however, the task of learning how to access the system, the specific resources available, and which agencies are appropriate for an individual situation is overwhelming to the uninitiated. Caregivers perceive the lack of information and the lack of coordinated services as stressors.[6] Because caregivers often come to the role with little or no experience, they frequently express guilt or uncertainty about their performance.[5] The competency level of the caregiver can be enhanced by increasing his or her knowledge base of resources available and by teaching basic caregiving skills.[20]

There is a tendency among caregivers to neglect self-care activities and to experience an increased level of stress. Self-care neglect can translate into aggravated health problems, increased somatic complaints, or depression. The caregiver seldom recognizes the association between the psychologic, psychosocial, and medical limitations and the stress of caregiving. The nurse is instrumental in monitoring the caregiver for changes in his or her health status and in referring that person to appropriate health care services.

The many roles and competing demands for the caregiver's time, resources, and energy are presumed to be associated with high levels of stress and burden.[19] Caregivers often try to be all things to all people as they attempt to fulfill their roles at the same level of performance as they did before they assumed the caregiving role. Assistance and reassurance in establishing priorities and in establishing realistic time management strategies are critical to alleviate some of the perceived strain. Once the tasks of caregiving are identified, they can be negotiated with other informal caregivers or met by incorporating other resources into the plan of care.

▮ RISK FOR CAREGIVER ROLE STRAIN

▮ High risk for caregiver role strain is a caregiver's risk for experiencing difficulty in performing the caregiving role.

Because of rising health care costs, the provision of ongoing health care is shifting from formal inpatient settings to home care. It is often necessary for individuals without previous caregiving experience to assume responsibility of care for or manage the care of another person. Situations (factors) leading to the assumption of the role of caregiving could include an unexpected medical event involving a family member or the realization that an individual is no longer able to maintain an independent life-style.[4] Assessment and identification of risk factors associated with caregiver role strain, appropriate intervention, and evaluation can prevent actual caregiver role strain.[7]

Risk Factors[1-21]

Severity of illness of care receiver
Addiction or codependency of care receiver or caregiver
Premature birth or congenital defect of care receiver
Caregiver health impairment
Discharge of family member with significant home care needs
Unpredictable illness course or instability in the care receiver's health
Psychologic or cognitive problems in the care receiver
Family or caregiver isolation
Caregiver's competing role commitments
Inadequate physical environment for providing care
Caregiver not developmentally ready for role
Developmental delay or retardation of the caregiver or care receiver
Marginal family adaptation or dysfunction before caregiving situation
Marginal coping patterns of caregiver

Past history of poor relationship between caregiver and care receiver

Care receiver exhibits deviant, bizarre behavior

Incontinence in the care receiver

Presence of abuse or violence

Duration of caregiving required

Inexperience of caregiving

Complexity and/or amount of ADL/IADL tasks

Presence of situational stressors

Patient Care Outcomes & Nursing Interventions

The caregiver will identify appropriate community resources and how to access them, as evidenced by:

Verbalizing resources for specific care needs

- Discuss range and availability of community resources appropiate for both present and future needs; *a plan for use of appropriate resources needs to be identified to diminish inappropriate decisions.*[20]
- Discuss financial eligibility requirements for resources.
- Evaluate willingness of caregiver to accept resource support.
- Discuss and evaluate circumstances in which resources might be incorporated into the care regimen. *Competency level of the caregiver can be enhanced by increasing his or her knowledge base of resources available and teaching basic caregiving skills.*[17,20]
- Evaluate family and social support network.
- Discuss and provide information about appropriate support groups.[20]
- Encourage caregiver to participate in a support group; *opportunities for caregivers with varied levels of experience to network/share information may be valuable.*

The caregiver will identify existing strengths and weaknesses in family dynamics as evidenced by:

Identification of potential stressors

- Identifying the family relationship between caregiver and care receiver. *A positive relationship between caregiver and care receiver correlates with less role strain.*[2]
- Identify past methods of coping with crisis.
- Offer family or individual therapy for resolution of conflict and unresolved issues.

Principles and Rationale for Nursing Interventions

When a new caregiving situation arises or when a stable one changes, there is a need to reexamine available resources within the informal support network and within the community. The caregiver may initially require a consultant to assist in obtaining health care information to meet the needs of the care receiver, to access community resources, and to select appropriate services.[15] If the caregiver is unable to acknowledge the need or is unwilling to accept assistance with the caregiving role, is is difficult for the caregiver to use resources. Early identification and intervention of those factors predictive of burden can lessen the perception of caregiver role strain.

The nurse will assist the caregiver in identifying the existing strength and weaknesses of the current family system. The relationship among family members, particularly between the caregiver and the care receiver, is predictive of increased risk for role strain.[2] Families and individuals may discover that psychotherapy is helpful in working through unresolved issues or in learning more effective conflict management techniques.

■ IMPAIRED VERBAL COMMUNICATION

Impaired verbal communication is the state in which an individual experiences a decreased or absent ability to use or understand language in human interaction.

Communication is a dynamic, complex, continuous series of reciprocal events through which messages are exchanged, primarily to produce a response from a person or a group. Communication includes all modes of behavior used by a person, consciously or unconsciously, to affect another person. Thus communication is an integral part of interpersonal relationships. The types and quality of relationships, as well as what happens to a person in the environment, are determined to a large extent by communication.[9] A person's communication pattern is the particular sequence of communication behaviors practiced over time by that person. All persons experiencing emotional disorders encounter problems in interpersonal relationships. Communication and interpersonal relationship difficulties can also be related to physical condition, mechanical impairments, age-related stages, or cultural differences.

Successful communication is characterized by the following elements:[3,5,6,8-12]

Both the sender and receiver have the physical ability to receive, analyze, and send messages.

The relationship between the sender and receiver is considered in all components of the communication process.

Selective attention is given to appropriate input.

Both the digital/verbal and the analogic/nonverbal forms of communication are used.

The sender selects and organizes words to best describe the intended meaning of the message.

The sender or receiver have similar meanings for words.

All channels of nonverbal communication are synchronized.

Nonverbal behavior is consistent with verbal communication.

The message sent is appropriate to the context.

The message is complete, i.e., not overloaded with or insufficient in information.

The timing of the message is appropriate to its content and the context.

The receiver listens actively.

The sender and receiver agree on the punctuation of a communication sequence.

Feedback is requested and accepted.

Feedback is relevant to the persons and context, clearly stated, and appropriately timed.

The sender is able to correct the information or message.

Both the sender and receiver assume responsibility for their communication.

Concordant information is established between the sender and receiver.

Both the sender and receiver attain confirmation and gratification.

Related Factors[6]

Decrease in circulation to the brain
Physical barrier, e.g., intubation
Anatomic defect, e.g., cleft palate
Physical condition(s), e.g., brain tumor
Mechanical impairment(s)
Developmental or age-related stage(s)
Severe psychosocial stressor
Mental disorder
Moderate to severe depression
Extreme anger
Severe anxiety or panic
Significant impairment of perception
Unrealistic or inadequate self-concept
Faulty communication skills
Cultural differences

Defining Characteristics[6]

Disorientation
Too little or too much attention to stimuli
Stuttering
Inability to speak dominant language
Inability or reluctance to speak
Disregard for speaker
Reliance on nonverbal communication
Inability to organize words
Inability to find words
Inappropriate selection of words
Use of unfamiliar words
Message inappropriate to context
Excessive or insufficient verbiage
Ill-timed message
Absent or inappropriate feedback
Discordant information
Disconfirmation
Absence of gratification
Inability or reluctance to express feelings
Withdrawal from interaction
Unrestrained or inappropriate emotional expression

Imaginary or false perceptions
Incongruent communication styles

Expected Patient Outcomes & Nursing Interventions*

Attend to appropriate input, as evidenced by:

Being oriented to person, place, and time
Selecting and responding to relevant stimuli
Demonstrating accurate perception and absence or control of physical symptoms

- Reduce or increase environmental stimuli. *Perception and interpretation of communication is based on stimuli within the perceptual field.*
- Teach patient to identify and focus on relevant stimuli. *A person can focus consciously on only a few of the many stimuli available.*
- Assist in corection of faulty perception. *Reception and selection of appropriate stimuli depend on an individual's perception.*
- Encourage patient to seek assistance in correcting, modifying, or preventing physical conditions that interfere with communication. *Physical conditions can interfere with the ability to receive and process sensory input or generate output.*

Send concise understandable messages, as evidenced by:

Demonstrating absence of speech impediments
Selecting and organizing words appropriate to receiver and context
Speaking dominant language
Using effective communication techniques
Using appropriate amount of verbiage
Expressing feelings appropriately

- Use facilitative communication techniques in interacting with patient (e.g., reflection, focusing, validation). *The nurse promotes further communication and role models through use of these techniques.*
- Point out discrepancies in message sent and context within which it is sent. *Connection between message and context is explained, and perception is corrected.*
- Teach and support patient's use of appropriate communication techniques and assertive skills. *Use of effective communication techniques and assertive skills communicates sensitivity to the rights and feelings of persons involved and contributes to mutually agreed outcomes.*
- Assist patient in increasing or modifying language skills. *Words that describe intended meaning and that the other person understands must be selected.*
- Teach and encourage expression of feelings. *Appropriate expression of feelings facilitates communication.*

---

*References 1, 2, 4-8, 12.

Send congruent nonverbal and verbal communication, as evidenced by:

Expressing congruent nonverbal behaviors

Expressing congruent verbal and nonverbal behaviors

Balancing use of verbal and nonverbal behaviors

- Point out discrepancies in verbal and nonverbal behavior. *Clear communication requires congruity of verbal and nonverbal messages, as well as consistency in meaning of nonverbal behaviors.*

Send and receive feedback, as evidenced by:

Listening actively

Examining effects of behavior on others

Asking for and receiving feedback

Sending feedback to others

- Describe, demonstrate, and encourage use of active listening skills. *Listening communicates concern, interest, or acceptance.*
- Increase awareness of effects of behavior and strengths and limitations in communicating with others. *Awareness of impact on another provides opportunity for modification or correction of behavior.*
- Assist and encourage patient efforts to accept positive and negative feedback. *Feedback regulates communication by stimulating modification or correction.*
- *Request patient to ask for feedback when communicating with others.*

Experience gratification from communication, as evidenced by:

Reporting satisfaction from communication

Reporting sense of high self-esteem

Reporting or showing willingness to assume responsibility for communication

Sending and receiving confirmation when communicating

- Assist patient in mastering tasks appropriate for age or developmental level. *Communication involves learning a series of progressive tasks over time.*
- Encourage interaction with others.
- Teach and encourage use of stress reduction techniques. *Excessive stress can result in impaired communication.*
- Increase self-esteem.
- Help patient develop understanding of dynamics of relationships. *Communication occurs within the context of relationships, all variables of which impact on the process of communication.*
- Demonstrate and support responsibility for communication. *In successful communication both sender and receiver accept responsibility for communication.*

Principles and Rationale for Nursing Interventions

The overall goal for the patient with impaired verbal communication is to reduce or resolve impaired verbal communication. Expected patient outcomes include the following:

Attend to appropriate input.

Transmit clear, concise, understandable messages.

Use congruent analogue/nonverbal and digital/verbal communication.

Send and receive feedback.

Experience gratification from communication.

The nurse/patient relationship provides the vehicle for nursing care and is the major tool of the psychiatric mental health nurse. The effectiveness of this relationship depends on the strength of the communication process.[12] Therefore it is essential for the nurse to become more aware of the complexity of the communication process. Communication has no beginning or end. The events in communication are in dynamic interaction.

The nurse ascertains a patient's pattern of communication through analysis of clinical data acquired from history taking, interaction, and observation. The objective in assessing the communication pattern is to obtain data about how, when, where, what, and with whom the patient communicates. Specific details assessed include the components of the communication process, the variables affecting the communication process, and the characteristics manifested.

To generate and communicate a message, stimuli from the interior or exterior environment are received, selected, organized, and interpreted. At any given time, numerous stimuli are present, except for rare circumstances such as solitary confinement. A person responds to input evaluated as relevant. Selection of and response to stimuli are influenced by such factors as physical condition, experience, values, and emotional state. When any one or more of these factors produce distortion, omission, or falsification of stimuli, perception is limited and impaired verbal communication may result.[3,9] Therefore nursing interventions that assist the patient to attend to appropriate stimuli focus on manipulation of the environment to provide adequate stimuli, assisting the patient in identification of relevant stimuli and correction of faulty perception, as well as obtaining assistance in correction, modification, or prevention of physical conditions that hinder communication.[8,12]

A message, the translation of ideas, purpose, and intention, must be sent in language that the other can understand and that describes the intended meaning and must be conveyed using a style and specific skills that enhance the communication process.[12] A person who uses effective communication and assertive skills is sensitive to the feelings and rights of self and others, is able to negotiate, is firm but gentle, and accepts workable outcomes.[8] Communication style is effective when words and actions reflect the inner experience of self and awareness of the needs and feelings of the other and are appropriate to the context.[11] Expressing feelings enhances communication by enabling another to know about us and what we are experiencing. Therefore nursing interventions that help a patient transmit clear, concise, understandable messages focus on use of effective communication techniques and assertive skills, appropriate language skills, feeling expression, and congruence of message and context.

Verbal communication is the representation of concepts, ideas, and items by signs or symbols organized into a language.

Successful verbal communication depends on selection of words that best describe the intended meaning and are understood by the other. Nonverbal communication is any form of communication that does not use words, such as body movements, facial expressions, proxemics, touch, and the use of cultural artifacts. Nonverbal communication is as effective and important as verbal communication. In some instances the nonverbal message predominates the words spoken.[5,10] Validity and effectiveness of communication require congruity of verbal and nonverbal communication, as well as consistency of the nonverbal behaviors. Therefore nursing interventions that assist the patient to send congruent nonverbal and verbal communication focus on pointing out and correcting discrepancies in nonverbal and verbal behaviors.[8]

Feedback is information received about the other's reaction to the message sent. Helpful feedback is clearly stated, relevant to the persons and context, and appropriately timed. Feedback processes provide information to the person about the effects of the behavior and promote modification or correction. Understanding and agreement between communicators are thereby facilitated.[9,10] Nursing interventions therefore that assist the patient to send and receive feedback focus on use of listening skills, examining effects of behavior, awareness of strengths and limitations in communication, and acceptance of feedback.

Communication involves learning a series of progressive tasks over time. Mastery of age or developmental level communication tasks contributes to success in and gratification from interpersonal relationships and interactions.[9] Gratification from communication also results when feedback from the receiver indicates mutual understanding and appreciation of the message sent. Reactions to feedback that disagreement exists vary, but in general, the stronger the person's self-concept, the better disagreement is tolerated.[10] Communication and resulting level of gratification are affected by stress.[12] Successful communication with a person experiencing stress requires recognition of the existence and source of the stress and reduction of the stress. Therefore nursing interventions to assist a patient to experience gratification from communication focus on mastering age or developmental level communication tasks, understanding dynamics of relationships, encouraging interaction, increasing self-esteem, supporting responsibility for communication, and reducing stress.

▌ RISK FOR VIOLENCE: SELF-DIRECTED OR DIRECTED AT OTHERS

▌ High risk for violence: self-directed or directed at others is the state in which an individual experiences behaviors that can be physically harmful either to the self or to others.

The causes of human violence are complex and remain unclear. By definition the term *violence* means an act of destructiveness. Violence is not an emotion. Violence can be viewed as a result of several psychologic (emotional), biologic, or sociologic influences. No one theory explaining these influences is more valid than the other. Moreover, a combination of theories is often used to explain the cause of violent behavior because the potential for violent behavior should be assessed on an individual basis.

Risk Factors[3,4,9,12]

Psychologic

History of assaultive behavior
Physical abuse in the family
Panic states
Antisocial behavior
Drug or alcohol abuse
Depression
Delusions
Hallucinations
Inability to verbalize feelings
Increase in stressors within short time
Physical immobility
Poor impulse control
Real or perceived threat to self
Fear of the unknown
Perception of self as worthless or hopeless
Minimum tolerance to anxiety or stress
Proneness to action rather than words
Inability to remember all or part of recent or past events
Disconnected thoughts
Disorientation to time, place, and person
Fear of self or others
Response to catastrophic event
Suspicion of others
Misperceived messages from others
Response to dysfunctional family through developmental stages
Dysfunctional communication patterns

Physiologic/Biologic

Dementia
Mental retardation
Organic brain syndrome
Temporal lobe epilepsy
Toxic reaction to medication
Toxic reaction to alcohol
Viral encephalopathy
Hormonal imbalance
Alteration in biochemical functioning leading to depression or manic-depressive illness
Physical trauma (results of accidents or battering)

Sociocultural

Environmental controls
Response to dysfunctional family
Dysfunctional communication pattern
Possession of destructive means, e.g., guns available

Defining Characteristics[3,4,9,12]

Body language
  Clenched fists
  Clenched jaw
  Rigid posture
  Tautness indicating intense effort to control
  Agitation
  Increased motor activity
  Pacing
Hostile, threatening verbalization
Self-destructive behavior resulting in minimum injury
Provocative behavior
  Argumentative
  Dissatisfied
  Overreactive
Repetition of verbalizing, e.g., continued complaints, requests, demands
Surface appearance of overcontrol, inhibition
Staring eye contact or avoidance of eye contact

Expected Patient Outcomes & Nursing Interventions[4-6,9,11,12]

Verbalize a lessened desire for exhibiting specific aggressive behavior and decreased feelings of anger and hostility, as evidenced by:

Verbalizing specific sources of anger, frustration, or rage
Describing their current level of stress tolerance
Demonstrating a desire to control aggressive behavior
Identifying and demonstrating appropriate aids to decrease anger and hostility (physical exercise, visual imagery, relaxation techniques, appropriate verbal expressions of feelings, taking medication when indicated)
Exhibiting a knowledge of physiologic or chemical causes of alterations in behavior (if appropriate)
Recognizing perceptual distortions that result from intense anger, rage, or hostility
  • Provide trusting relationship with the patient to help the patient feel more comfortable by being honest, clear, and concise during interaction.
  • Provide close supervision, and watch for early signs of agitation or increasing anxiety, such as increased motor activity and unreasonable requests or demands.
  • Make short-term contracts with the patient that he or she will not harm herself or himself during a specific time period. Continue negotiating until there is no evidence of suicidal ideation.
  • Set limits on the patient's behavior, acknowledge and understand the patient's feelings, and invite conversation about his or her feelings.
  • Encourage alternatives to violent outburst, e.g., physical expenditure of energy, by exercise, unit jobs (if inpatient), games, cleaning, discussion.
  • Take the patient's feelings seriously.

  • Administer and monitor effectiveness of medications prescribed to control aggressive behavior.
  • Discuss reason and plan for safety and protective measures with family and significant other.
  • Use positive reinforcement for no violent or suicidal behavior.

Demonstrate self-control, as evidenced by:

Having relaxed body and muscles and no redness in the face
Maintaining eye contact when communicating without a threatening stance or look
Verbalizing rationally and calmy precipitating factors to the incidents that cause anger
Verbalizing feelings of hopelessness, loneliness, and decreased self-esteem
Demonstrating and verbalizing alternatives to violent, aggressive behavior
Reporting feelings of losing control to others
Allowing trusted people (staff, family, friends) to approach boundaries of personal space
Demonstrating an understanding of rationale for limit setting or seclusion, if required
  • Provide close supervision, and watch for early signs of agitation or increasing anxiety, such as increased motor activity and unreasonable requests or demands.
  • If the patient is in an inpatient unit as a result of a suicide attempt, remove from the patient's environment anything that could be used to inflict further self-injury (e.g., razor blade, belts, glass objects, pills).
  • Make short-term contracts with the patient that he or she will not harm herself or himself during a specific time period. Continue negotiating until there is no evidence of suicidal ideation.
  • Set limits on the patient's behavior, acknowledge and understand the patient's feelings, and invite conversations about his or her feelings.
  • Encourage alternative to violent outbursts, e.g., physical expenditure of energy, by exercise, unit jobs (if inpatient), games, cleaning, discussion.
  • Administer and monitor effectiveness of medications prescribed to control aggressive behavior and help patient remain calm.
  • Establish a structured routine, and aid patient in following it.
  • Assess sleep pattern, and establish a regular routine to combat sleep deprivation.
  • Use short, declarative sentences when speaking to a patient who may be out of control. Speak in a firm, but not threatening, tone of voice.
  • Refer the patient for appropriate assistance from a nurse therapist, psychiatrist, alcohol rehabilitation counselor, drug counselor, psychologist, social worker, etc.
  • Provide patient and family with telephone numbers and other information about crisis centers, hot lines, counselors, etc.

Use learned adaptive coping mechanisms in conflict situations or when feeling self-destructive, as evidenced by:

Demonstrating a knowledge of alternative ways to deal with aggressive feelings toward self and/or others

Demonstrating the ability to maintain self-control

Verbalizing feelings when self-esteem is threatened

Demonstrating ability to use thought processes rather than a physical response to feelings of anger or low self-esteem

Demonstrating an understanding of violence and what is socially acceptable versus unacceptable and incorporating this into own value system

Identifying verbally and demonstrating constructive ways to increase own value system

Identifying verbally and demonstrating constructive ways to increase sense of power

Identifying supportive persons(s) or groups in the community

Verbalizing the need for help from individuals who are appropriately prepared to assist (support groups, staff on inpatient units, social service workers, mental health workers)

Maintaining normal sleep-wake cycle

- Provide trusting relationship with the patient to help the patient feel more comfortable by being honest, clear, and concise during interaction.
- Provide close supervision, and watch for early signs of agitation or increasing anxiety, such as increased motor activity and unreasonable requests or demands.
- Make short-term contracts with the patient that he or she will not harm herself or himself during a specific time period. Continue negotiating until there is no evidence of suicidal ideation.
- Set limits on the patient's behavior, acknowledge and understand the patient's feelings, and invite conversation about his or her feelings.
- Encourage alternatives to violent outbursts, e.g., physical expenditure of energy, by exercise, unit jobs (if inpatient), games, cleaning, discussion.
- Take the patient's feelings seriously.
- Administer and monitor effectiveness of medications prescribed to control aggressive behavior and help patient remain calm.
- Establish a daily routine, and aid patient in following it.
- Assess sleep pattern, and establish a regular routine to combat sleep deprivation.
- Discuss reason and plan for safety and protective measures with family or significant other.
- Refer the patient for appropriate assistance from a nurse therapist, psychiatrist, alcohol rehabilitation counselor, drug counselor, psychologist, social worker, etc.
- Provide patient and family with telephone numbers and other information about crisis centers, hot lines, counselors, etc.

Display no overt or covert dangerous behaviors, as evidenced by:

Avoiding injuring or harming self

Avoiding injuring or harming others

Verbalizing increased feelings of self-esteem

Expressing feelings in a nonviolent and nondestructive manner

Remaining calm in a secure environment

Verbalizing feelings of anger and hostility rather than acting out physically

Actively participating in the prescribed treatment regimen (medications, support groups, individual therapy, hospitalization when indicated)

Verbalizing a knowledge of the supports available and demonstrating an ability to use them when needed

- Provide close supervision, and watch for early signs of agitation or increasing anxiety, such as increased motor activity and/or unreasonable requests or demands.
- If the patient is in an inpatient unit as a result of a suicide attempt, remove from the patient's environment anything that could be used to inflict further self-injury (e.g., razor blades, belts, glass objects, pills).
- Make short-term contracts with the patient that he or she will not harm herself or himself during a specific time period. Continue negotiating until there is no evidence of suicidal ideation.
- Set limits on the patient's behavior, acknowledge and understand the patient's feelings, and invite conversation about his or her feelings.
- Encourage alternatives to violent outbursts, e.g., physical expenditure of energy, by exercise, unit jobs (if inpatient), games, cleaning, discussion.
- Acknowledge that you are aware of patient's potentially violent behavior.
- Administer and monitor effectiveness of medications prescribed to control aggressive behavior and remain calm.
- Establish a structured daily routine, and aid patient in following it.
- Discuss reason and plan for safety and protective measures with family or significant other.
- Refer the patient for appropriate assistance from a nurse therapist, psychiatrist, alcohol rehabilitation counselor, drug counselor, psychologist, social worker, etc.
- Provide patient and family with telephone numbers and other information about crisis centers, hot lines, counselors, etc.
- Use positive reinforcement for no violent or suicidal behavior.

Principles and Rationale for Nursing Interventions

The nurse must provide controls to prevent violent behavior. Setting limits, seclusion, and restraints (chemical and physical, which are not often used today) are all methods of controlling behavior if the patient loses control.[11,14] The nurse must understand that the potentially violent patient often has low self-esteem, may be lonely, and may feel hopeless. Thus it is of utmost importance to establish trust and rapport by approaching calmly and allowing personal space.[6] Helping the patient think and talk about his or her problems can correct distorted perceptions and ideas. The violent, threatening patient fails and believes violence is the sole exit from his or her "stress-bound box of life." The patient is unable to perceive any alternatives other than violence. Complex, long-term supportive or deterrent measures may be required.

Because fear is a possible source for violent behavior, the nurse must help eliminate the patient's fear. One way to decrease fear is to discuss it and try to find ways to eliminate or deal with it. The nurse can also help to control the environment by minimizing noise and traffic (by other patients or visitors) and by carefully explaining procedures that require equipment or medication.[11,14]

A person who commits a violent act frequently has tremendous feelings of guilt and remorse. Those family members or staff who witnessed or were victims of the violent behavior also need to verbalize their feelings, fear, and anger. How a person sees and interprets the surrounding world is crucial to the future eruption of violent behavior.[2]

The nurse must encourage and allow verbal expressions of anger. The key to prevention of violent aggression is finding out what precipitates feeling of anger, frustration, or rage.[6] Then, after careful discussion, the nurse and patient can find ways to decrease or eliminate the related factors and develop alternative coping mechanisms. Encouraging physical expenditure of energy by exercise, unit jobs, games, or discussion helps decrease anxiety and increase self-esteem.

Parents who feel aggressive tendencies toward their child must learn to deal consistently with their feelings and retain control.[6] Teaching the parents stress reduction techniques and realistic expectations of their child by discussing growth and development in detail helps them recognize and deal with frustrations in child rearing. Also, finding acceptable alternate coping mechanisms for those frustrating times is essential in preventing aggressive violence. This must be done on an individual basis for each parent. Trust is again essential to work effectively toward changing behavior.

Nurses who work with abusive families must first work through their own feelings and be nonjudgmental and accepting of the family members as persons. The nurse must be able to use confrontation when necessary. Parents who abuse their children generally have not received the love or nurturing they needed as children and actually lack a basic trust in people. Their basic needs have not been met. Consequently the parents place unrealistic expectations on the child; the child cannot meet these expectations and in turn becomes neglected or abused. The parent is looking for gratification of needs from the child instead of the reverse—providing the child with those needs. The role of the nurse is to provide support and education for the parents to understand themselves, motivation for behavioral change, and strategies for interacting effectively with others. Parent modeling is equally important for abusive adults. Lay therapists who go into the home and provide a warm parent model for the abusing parent help reduce the tendency for future abuse and neglect. Intensive work with a nurse, psychiatric clinical nurse specialist, psychotherapist, case worker, and lay therapist is required for any hope of changing behavior.

The cause of spouse abuse is similar to that for child abuse. Each spouse may have a tremendous amount of unmet needs, and violence occurs when spouses fail to meet each other's needs. The victim of this abuse must understand that the behavior might not change until the violent person seeks help. The victim may need to get out of the situation. This is a long process and requires maximum support from the nurse.

References

Anticipatory grieving

1. Allan J, Hall B: Between diagnosis and death: the case for studying grief before death, *Arch Psychiatric Nurs* 2:30, 1988.
2. Carson VB: Losses and endings in the nurse-client relationship. In Arnold E, Boggs KU: *Interpersonal relationships: professional communication skills for nurses,* Philadelphia, 1995, WB Saunders.
3. Curry L, Stone J: The grief process: a preparation for death, *Clin Nurse Spec* 5:17, 1991.
4. Drysdale AE, Nelson CF, Wineman NM: Families need help too: group treatment for families of nursing home residents, *Clin Nurs Spec* 7:130, 1993.
5. Engel G: *Psychological development in health and disease,* Philadelphia, 1968, WB Saunders.
6. Gerety E: Grieving, anticipatory grieving, dysfunctional grieving. In McFarland GK, Thomas MD: *Psychiatric mental health nursing,* Philadelphia, 1991, JB Lippincott.
7. Glass BC: *The role of the nurse in advanced practice in bereavement care* 7:62, 1993.
8. Hampe S: Needs of the grieving spouse in a hospital setting, *Nurs Res* 24:113, 1975.
9. Kerr RB: Meanings adult daughters attach to a parent's death, *West J Nurs Res* 16:347, 1994.
10. Kubler-Ross E: *On death and dying,* New York, 1969, Macmillan.
11. Lev E: Dealing with loss: concerns of patients and families in a hospice setting, *Clin Nurse Spec* 5:87, 191.
12. Liken MA, Collins CE: Grieving: facilitating the process for demential caregivers, *J Psychosoc Nurs Ment Health Serv* 31:21, 1993.
13. Lindemann E: Symptomatology and management of acute grief, *Am J Psychiatry* 101:141-148, 1944.
14. McCain NL, Gramling LF: Living with dying: coping with HIV disease, *Issues Ment Health Nurs* 13:271, 1992.
15. McClement SE, Degner LF: Expert nursing behaviors in the care of the dying adult in the intensive care unit, *Heart Lung* 24:408, 1995.
16. McFarland G, Wasli E, Gerety E: *Nursing diagnoses and process in psychiatric mental health nursing,* ed 2, Philadelphia, 1992, JB Lippincott.
17. NANDA: *Nursing diagnoses: definitions & classification, 1995-1996,* Philadelphia, 1994, North American Nursing Diagnosis Association.
18. Rando T: A comprehensive analysis of anticipatory grief: perspectives, processes, promises, and problems. In Rando T: *Anticipatory grief,* Lexington, Mass, 1986, Lexington Books.
19. Rando T: Understanding and facilitating anticipatory grief in the loved ones of the dying. In Rando T, *Anticipatory grief,* Lexington, 1986, Lexington Books.
20. Worden J: *Grief counseling and grief therapy,* ed 2, New York, 1991, Springer.

Dysfunctional grieving

1. Almeida CM: Grief among parents of children wtih diabetes, *Diabetes Educ* 21:530, 1995.
2. Browning MA: Depression, suicide, and bereavement. In Hogstel MO, editor, *Geropsychiatric Nursing,* ed 2, St Louis, 1995, Mosby.
3. Cowles KV, Rodgers BL: The concept of grief: a foundation for nursing research and practice, *Res Nurs Health* 14:119, 1991.
4. Covington SN, Theut SK: Reactions to perinatal loss: a qualitative analysis of the national maternal and infant health survey, *Am J Orthopsychiatry* 63:215, 1993.
5. Curry LC, Stone JG: Moving on: recovering from the death of a spouse, *Clin Nurs Spec* 6:180, 1992.
6. Demi AS, Gilbert CM: Relationship of parental grief to sibling grief, *Arch Psychiatr Nurs,* 1:385, 1987.
7. Gerety EK: Grieving, anticipatory grieving, dysfunctional grieving. In McFarland GK, Thomas MD: *Psychiatric mental health nursing,* Philadelphia, 1991, JB Lippincott.

8. Herth K: Relationship of hope, coping styles, concurrent losses, and setting to grief resolution in the elderly widow(er), *Res Nurs Health* 13:109, 1990.
9. Horowitz M, Wilner N, Marmare C: Pathological grief and the activation of latent and self images, *Am J Psychiatry* 137:1157, 1980.
10. Houseman C, Pheifer WG: Potential for unresolved grief in survivors of persons with AIDS, *Arch Psychiatr Nurs* 3:86, 1989.
11. Johnson SE: *After a child dies: counseling bereaved families,* New York, 1987, Springer Publishing.
12. Kerr RB: Meanings adult daughters attach to a parent's death, *West J Nurs Res* 16:347, 1994.
13. Lasker JN, Toedter LG: Acute versus chronic grief: the case of pregnancy loss, *Am J Orthopsychiatr* 61 (4):510, 1991.
14. Lin SX, Lasker JN: Patterns of grief reaction after pregnancy loss, *Am J Orthopsychiatry* 66:262, 1996.
15. Lindemann E: Symptomatology and management of acute grief, *Am J Psychiatry* 101:141, 1944.
16. Mireault GC, Bond LA: Parental death in childhood: perceived vulnerability, and adult depression and anxiety, *Am J Orthopsychiatry* 62:517, 1992.
17. NANDA: *Nursing diagnoses: definitions & classification,* 1995-1996, Philadelphia, 1994, North American Nursing Diagnosis Association.
18. Ness DE, Pfeffer CR: Sequelae of bereavement resulting from suicide. *Am J Psychiatry* 147:279, 1990.
19. Saler L, Skolnick N: Childhood parental death and depression in adulthood: roles of surviving parent and family environment, *Am J Orthopsychiatry* 62:504, 1992.
20. Smith BJ et al: Exploring widows' experiences after the suicide of their spouse, *J Psychosoc Nurs Ment Health Serv* 10, 1995.
21. Wood A, Seymour LM: Psychodynamic group therapy for older adults: the life experiences group, *J Psychosoc Nurs Ment Health Serv* 32:19, 1994.
22. Worden JW: *Grief counseling & grief therapy,* ed 2, New York, 1991, Springer Publishing.
23. Zisook S, Schuchter SR: Depression through the first year after the death of a spouse, *Am J Psychiatry* 148:10, 1991.

Altered role performance
1. Akinsanya JA, Roy C: *The Roy adaptation model in action,* London, 1994, Macmillan Press.
2. Andrews H: Overview of the role function mode. In Andrews H, Roy C: *The Roy adaptation model: the definitive statement,* Norwalk, Conn, 1991, Appleton & Lange.
3. Andrews HA, Roy C: *Essentials of the Roy adaptation model,* Norwalk, Conn, 1986, Appleton-Century Crofts.
4. Andrews HA, Roy C: *The Roy adaptation model: the definitive statement,* Norwalk, Conn, 1991, Appleton & Lange.
5. Burns C, Archbold P, Stewart B, Shelton K: New diagnosis: caregiver role strain, *Nurs Diag* 4:70-76, 1993.
6. Hardy M, Conway M: *Role theory perspectives for health professionals,* Norwalk, Conn, 1988, Appleton & Lange.
7. Hardy M, Hardy W: Role stress and role strain. In Hardy M, Conway M: *Role theory: perspectives for health professionals,* Norwalk, Conn, 1988, Appleton & Lange.
8. Kim M, McFarland GK, McLane A: *Pocket guide to nursing diagnoses,* ed 6, St Louis, 1995, Mosby.
9. Kim M, Moritz D: *Classification of nursing diagnoses: proceedings of the third and fourth national conferences,* New York, 1982, McGraw-Hill.
10. McFarland GK, Wasli EL, Gerety EK: *Nursing diagnoses and process in psychiatric mental health nursing,* ed 2, Philadelphia, 1992, JB Lippincott.
11. Meleis A: Role insufficiency and role supplementation: a conceptual framework, *Nurs Res* 24:264-271, 1975.
12. Moorhead SA: Role supplementation. In Bulecheck GM, McCloskey JC: *Nursing interventions: treatment for nursing diagnosis,* Philadelphia, 1985, WB Saunders.
13. North American Nursing Diagnoses Association: *Nursing diagnosis: definitions and classification, 1995-1996,* Philadelphia, 1994, NANDA.
14. Nuwayhid K: Role function: theory and development. In Roy C: *Introduction to nursing: an adaptation model,* Englewood Cliffs, NJ, 1984, Prentice Hall.
15. Nuwayhid K: Role transition, distance, and conflict. In Andrews H, Roy C: *The Roy adaptation model: the definitive statement,* Norwalk, Conn, 1991, Appleton & Lange.
16. Nuwayhid K: Role transition, distance and conflict. In Roy C: *Introduction to nursing: an adaptation model,* Englewood Cliffs, NJ, 1984, Prentice Hall.
17. Randell B, Tedrow MP, Van Landingham J: *Adaptation nursing: the Roy conceptual model applied,* St Louis, 1982, Mosby.
18. Robertson SM: Self-concept disturbance: role performance disturbance. In McFarland GK, Thomas MD: *Psychiatric mental health nursing,* Philadelphia, 1991, JB Lippincott.
19. Roy C: *Introduction to nursing: an adaptation model,* Englewood Cliffs, NJ, 1984, Prentice-Hall.
20. Roy C, Roberts S: *Theory construction in nursing: an adaptation model,* Englewood Cliffs, NJ, 1981, Prentice-Hall.
21. Spitze G, Logan JR, Joseph G, Lee E: Middle generation roles and the well-being of men and women, *J Gerontol* 49:107-116, 1994.
22. Stephens MAP, Franks MM: Spillover between daughters' roles as caregiver and wife: interferences or enhancement? *J Gerontol* 50B:9-17, 1995.
23. Temple A, Fawdry K: King's theory of goal attainment, resolving filial caregiver role strain. *J Gerontol Nurs* 8:11-15, 1992.

Social isolation
1. Barth R: *Social and cognitive treatment of children and adolescents,* San Francisco, 1986, Jossey-Bass.
2. Bowlby J: *Attachment and loss,* vol 1, *Attachment,* New York, 1969, Basic Books.
3. Carpenito LJ: *Nursing diagnosis: application to clinical practice,* ed 4, Philadelphia, 1991, JB Lippincott.
4. Drew N: Combating the social isolation of chronic mental illness, *J Psychosoc Nurs* 29:14-17, 1991.
5. Elsen J, Blegen M: Social isolation. In Mass M, Buckwalter K, Hardy M, editors: *Nursing diagnosis and interventions for the elderly,* ed 5, Redwood City, Calif, 1991, Addison Wesley Nursing.
6. Horney K: *Neurotic personality of our times,* New York, 1937, WW Norton.
7. Horney K: *Our inner conflicts,* New York, 1945, WW Norton.
8. Kim M, McFarland GK, McLane A: *Pocket guide to nursing diagnoses,* ed 4, St Louis, 1991, Mosby.
9. McFarland GK, Wasli EL, Gerety EA: *Nursing diagnosis and process in psychiatric mental health nursing,* ed 2, Philadelphia, 1992, JB Lippincott.
10. Murray RB, Huelskoetter MMW: *Psychiatric/mental nursing: giving emotional care,* ed 3, Norwalk, 1991, Appleton & Lange.

Impaired social interaction
1. Bowlby J: *Attachment and loss,* vol 1, *Attachment* New York, 1969, Basic Books.
2. Gordon M: *Nursing diagnosis: process and application,* ed 3, St Louis, 1994, Mosby.
3. Haber J et al: *Comprehensive psychiatric nursing,* ed 4, St Louis, 1992, Mosby.
4. Horney K: *Neurotic personality of our times,* New York, 1937, WW Norton.
5. Kaplan H: *The comprehensive textbook of psychiatry,* ed 6, Baltimore, 1995, Williams & Wilkins.
6. Kaplan H, Sadock B: *Synopsis of psychiatry—behavioral science—clinical psychiatry,* ed 7, Baltimore, 1994, Williams & Wilkins.
7. Kim M, McFarland G, McLane A: *Pocket guide to nursing diagnoses,* ed 4, St Louis, 1991, Mosby.
8. Rawlins PR, Williams SR, Beck CM: *Mental health-psychiatric nursing,* ed 3, St Louis, 1993, Mosby.
9. Stuart G, Sundeen S: *Principles and practice of psychiatric nursing,* ed 5, St Louis, 1995, Mosby.
10. Taylor CM: *Essentials of psychiatric nursing,* ed 14, St Louis, 1994, Mosby.
11. Taylor C, Sparks S: *Nursing diagnosis cards,* ed 6, Springhouse, Pa, 1991, Springhouse.
12. Park D, Vandenberg B: The influence of separation orientation on life satisfaction in the elderly, *Int J Aging Hum Dev* 39:177-87, 1994.
13. Stuart GW, Sundeen SJ: *Principles and practice of psychiatric nursing,* ed 5, St Louis, 1995, Mosby.

14. Taylor C, Sparks S: *Nursing diagnosis cards,* ed 6, Springhouse, Pa, 1991, Springhouse.
15. Wilson HS, Kneisl CR: *Psychiatric nursing,* ed 4, Redwood City, Calif, 1992, Addison-Wesley.

Relocation stress syndrome

1. Armer JM: Elderly relocation to a congregate setting: factors influencing adjustment, *Issues Ment Health Nurs* 14:157, 1993.
2. Aroian KJ: A model of psychological adaptation to migration and resettlement, *Nurs Res* 39:5-10, 1990.
3. Bashir MR: Issues of immigration for the health and adjustment of young people, *J Pediatr Child Health* 29(suppl 2):S42-S45, 1993.
4. Beiser M, Edward RG: Mental health of immigrants and refugees, *New Dir Ment Health Serv* 20:73-86, 1994.
5. Belcher TL: Program transition from sheltered workshop to community-based endeavors, *Psychol Rep* 74(3 pt. 1):1058, 1994.
6. Dimond M, McCance K, King K: Forced residential relocation—its impact on the well-being of older adults, *West J Nurs Res* 9:445-464, 1987.
7. Eagle RS: The separation experience in children in long-term care: theory, research, and implications for practice, *Am J Orthopsychiatry* 64:421-434, 1995.
8. Esier SV, Grob MC: Patient outcomes after transfer within a psychiatric hospital, *Hosp Community Psychiatry* 43:803-806, 1992.
9. Everard K, Rowles GD, High DM: Nursing home changes: toward a decision-making model, *Gerontologist* 34:520-527, 1994.
10. Gil AG, Vega WA, Dimas JM: Acculturative stress and personal adjustment among hispanic adolescent boys, *J Commun Psychol* 22:43-54, 1994.
11. Hertz DG: Bio-psycho-social consequences of migration stress: a multidimensional approach, *Isr J Psychiatry Relat Sci* 30:204-212, 1993.
12. Hobbs MS: A study of the characteristics and needs of people transferred from acute hospitals to nursing homes, *Med J Aust* 159:385-388, 1993.
13. Holzapfel SK, Schoch CP, Dodman JB, Grant MM: Responses of nursing home residents to intrainstitutional relocation, *Geriatr Nurs* 13:192-195, 1992.
14. Horwitz SM, Simms MD, Farrington R: Impact of developmental problems on young children's exits from foster care, *J Behav Pediatr* 15:105-110, 1994.
15. Jones EM: Interhospital relocation of long-stay psychiatric patients: a prospective study, *Acta Psychiatr Scand* 83:214-216, 1991.
16. LeFroy RB, Davey M, Hyndman J, Hobbs MS: A study of the characteristics and needs of people transferred from acute hospitals to nursing homes, *Med J Aust* 159:385-388, 1993.
17. Lindesay J, Macdonald A, Stark I: *Delirium in the elderly,* Oxford, England, 1990, Oxford University Press.
18. Lipson JG: The health and adjustment of Iranian immigrants, *West J Nurs Res* 14:10-24, 1992.
19. Magwaza AS: Migration and psychological status in South African black migrant children, *J Gent Psychol* 155:283-288, 1994.
20. Mikhail ML: Psychological responses to relocation to a nursing home, *J Gerontol Nurs* 18:35-39, 1992.
21. Mirotznik J, Lombardi TG: The impact of intrainstitutional relocation on morbidity in an acute care setting, *Gerontology* 35:217-224, 1995.
22. O'Conner BP, Vallerand RJ: Motivation, self-determination, and person-environment fit as predictors of psychological adjustment among nursing home residents, *Psychol Aging* 9:1891-1894, 1994.
23. Oleson M: Application of Moos and Schaefer's (1986) model to nursing care of elderly persons relocating to a nursing home, *J Adv Nurs* 18:479-485, 1993.
24. Osborne OH et al: Forced relocation of hospitalized psychiatric patients, *Arch Psychiatr Nurs* 4:221-227, 1990.
25. Patterson BJ: The process of social support: adjusting to life in a nursing home, *J Adv Nurs* 21:682-689, 1995.
26. Penzerro RM, Lein L: Burning their bridges: disordered attachment and foster care discharge, *Child Welfare* 74:351-366, 1995.
27. Porter EJ, Clinton JF: Adjusting to the nursing home, *West J Nurs Res* 14:464-481, 1992.
28. Puskar KR, Dvorsak KG: Relocating stress in adolescents: helping teenagers cope with a moving dilemma, *Pediatr Nurs* 17:295-298, 1991.
29. Puskar KR, Martsolf DS: Adolescent geographic relocation, *Issues Ment Health Nurs* 15:471-481, 1994.
30. Reinardy JR: Decisional control in moving to a nursing home: postadmission adjustment and well-being, *Geronotologist* 32:96-103, 1992.
31. Schactman M: Transfer stress in patients after myocardial infarction, *Focus Crit Care* 14:34-37, 1987.
32. Thomas MD et al: Intrahospital relocation of psychiatric patients and effects on aggression, *Arch Psychiatr Nurs* 4:154-160, 1990.
33. Vercruysse NJ, Chandler LA: Coping strategies used by adolescents in dealing with family relocation overseas, *J Adolesc* 15:67-82, 1992.
34. Wamboldt FS, Steinglass P, Kaplan De-Nour A: Coping within couples: adjustment two years after forced geographic relocation, *Fam Process* 30:347-361, 1991.
35. Wells DA: Management of early postdischarge adjustment reaction following psychiatric hospitalization, *Hosp Commun Psychiatr* 43:803-806, 1992.

Altered family processes

1. Cohen D: A primary care checklist for effective family management, *Med Clin North Am* 78:795, 1994.
2. Gordon M: *Nursing diagnosis: process and applications,* ed 3, St Louis, 1994, Mosby.
3. Haber J et al: Comprehensive psychiatric nursing, ed 4, St Louis, 1992, Mosby.
4. Hammens M: Domestic violence: facing the epidemic, *Nurse Week* 5:6-8, 1993.
5. Hogarth C: Families and family therapy. In Johnson B, editor: *Psychiatric-mental health nursing adaption and growth,* ed 3, Philadelphia, 1993, JB Lippincott.
6. Kansas Child Abuse Prevention Council (KCAPC): *A guide about child abuse and neglect,* Wichita, Kansas, 1992, National Committee for Prevention of Child Abuse and Parents Anonymous, Inc.
7. Kim M, McFarland GK, McLane A: *Pocket guide to nursing diagnoses* ed 4, St Louis, 1991, Mosby.
8. Leavitt MB: *Families at risk: nursing assessment and strategies for the family at risk,* Philadelphia, 1982, JB Lippincott.
9. Minuchin S, Fishman HC: *Family therapy techniques,* Cambridge, Mass, 1981, Harvard University Press.
10. Munuchin S: *Families and family therapy,* Cambridge, Mass, 1979, Harvard University Press.
11. Satir U: *Conjoint family therapy,* Palo Alto, Calif, 1964, Science & Behavior Books.
12. Schuster CS, Ashurn SS: *The process of human development: a holistic approach,* Boston, 1980, Little, Brown.
13. Taylor C, Sparks S: *Nursing diagnosis cards,* ed 6, Springhouse, Pa, 1991, Springhouse Publishing.
14. Townsend M: *Psychiatric mental health nursing: concepts of care,* Philadelphia, 1993, FA Davis.
15. Wilson HS, Kneisl CR: *Psychiatric nursing,* ed 4, Redwood City, Calif, 1992, Addison-Wesley.

Altered family processes: alcoholism

1. Beare PG, Myers JL: *Adult health nursing,* St Louis, Mosby, 1994.
2. Graham AV, Berolzheimer N, Burge S: Alcohol abuse: a family disease, *Primary Care* 20:121-129, 1993.
3. Grisham K, Estes N: Dynamics of alcoholic families. In Estes N, Heinemann ME, editors: *Alcoholism: development, consequences and interventions,* St Louis, 1992, Mosby.
4. Kim MJ, McFarland GK, McLane AM: *Pocket guide to nursing diagnosis,* St Louis, 1995, Mosby.
5. Kritsberg W: The adult children of alcoholics syndrome, New York, 1985, Bantam Books.
6. McCloskey JC, Belecheck GM: *Nusing interventions classification (NIC),* St Louis, 1992, Mosby.
7. Navarra T: Enabling behavior: the tender trap, *Am J Nurs* 95:50-52, 1995.
8. Salinas RC, O'Farrell TJ, Jones WC, Cutter HS: Services for families of alcoholics: a national survey of Veterans Affairs treatment programs, *J Stud Alcohol* 52:541, 1991.
9. Wright LM, Leahey M: *Nurses and families: a guide to family assessment and intervention,* Philadelphia, 1988, FA Davis.

Caregiver role strain

1. Anderson CS et al: A population-based assessment of the impact and burden of caregiving for long-term stroke survivors, *Stroke* 26:843-849, 1995.
2. Archbold PG et al: Mutuality and preparedness as predictors of caregiver role strain, *Res Nurs Health* 13:375-384, 1990.
3. Browning JS, Schwirian PM: Spousal caregivers' burden: impact of care recipient health problems and mental status, *J Gerontol Nurs* 20:17-22, 1994.
4. Burns C et al: New diagnosis: caregiver role strain, *Nurs Diagn* 4:70-75, 1993.
5. Cossete S, Levesque L, Laurin L: Informal and formal support for caregivers of a demented relative: Do gender and kinship make a difference? *Res Nurs Health* 18:437-451, 1995.
6. Decker SD, Young E: Self-perceived needs of primary caregivers of home-hospice clients, *J Community Health Nurs* 8:147-154, 1991.
7. Farran CJ, Keane-Hagerty E: Interventions for caregivers of persons with dementia: educational support groups and Alzheimer's association support groups, *Appl Nurs Res* 7:112-117, 1994.
8. Folkman S et al: Caregiver burden in HIV-positive and HIV-negative partners of men with aids, *J Consult Clin Psychol* 62:746-756, 1994.
9. Fredman L, Daly MP, Lazur AM: Burden among white and black caregivers to elderly adults, *J Gerontol* 50B:S110-S118, 1995.
10. Hadjistavropoulos T et al: Neuropsychological deficits, caregivers' perception of deficits and caregiver burden, *J Am Geriatr Soc* 42:308-314, 1994.
11. Heller T, Factor A: Aging family caregivers: support resources and changes in burden and placement desire, *Am Assoc Mental Retard* 98:417-426, 1993.
12. Homer AC, Gilleard CJ: The effects of inpatient respite care on elderly patients and their careers, *Age Aging* 23:274-276, 1994.
13. Jones SL, Roth D, Jones PK: Effect of demographic and behavioral variables on burden of caregivers of chronic mentally ill persons, *Psychiatric Services* 46:141-145, 1995.
14. Karmilovich SE: Burden and stress associated with spousal caregiving for individuals with heart failure, *Prog Cardiovasc Nurs* 9:33-38, 1994.
15. Keady J, Nolan M: A stitch in time. Facilitating proactive interventions with dementia caregivers: the role of community practitioners, *J Psychiatr Ment Health Nurs* 2:33-40, 1995.
16. Loukissa DA: Family burden in chronic mental illness: a review of research studies, *J Adv Nurs* 21:248-255, 1995.
17. O'Neill G, Ross MM: Burden of care; an important concept for nurses, *Health Care Women Int* 12:111-121, 1991.
18. Robinson K, Yates K: Effects of two caregiver-training programs on burden and attitude toward help, *Arch Psych Nurs* 8:312-319, 1994.
19. Siegel K et al: Caregiver burden and unmet patients needs, *Cancer* 68:1131-1140, 1991.
20. Siegel K et al: The relationship of spousal caregiver burden to patient disease and treatment-related conditions, *Ann Oncol* 2:511-516, 1991.
21. Thompson EH et al: Social support and caregiving burden in family caregivers of frail elders, *J Gerontol* 48:S245-S254, 1993.

Risk for caregiver role strain

1. Anderson CS et al: A population-based assessment of the impact and burden of caregiving for long-term stroke survivors, *Stroke* 26:843-849, 1995.
2. Archbold PG et al: Mutuality and preparedness as predictors of caregiver role strain, *Res Nurs Health* 13:375-384, 1990.
3. Browning JS, Schwirian PM: Spousal caregivers' burden: impact of care recipient health problems and mental status, *J Gerontol Nurs* 20:17-22, 1994.
4. Burns C et al: New diagnosis: caregiver role strain, *Nurs Diagn* 4:70-75, 1993.
5. Cossete S, Levesque L, Laurin L: Informal and formal support for caregivers of a demented relative: Do gender and kinship make a difference? *Res Nurs Health* 18:437-451, 1995.
6. Decker SD, Young E: Self-perceived needs of primary caregivers of home-hospice clients, *J Community Health Nurs* 8:147-154, 1991.
7. Farran CJ, Keane-Hagerty E: Interventions for caregivers of persons with dementia: educational support groups and Alzheimer's association support groups, *Appl Nurs Res* 7:112-117, 1994.

8. Folkman S et al: Caregiver burden in HIV-positive and HIV-negative partners of men with AIDS. *J Consult Clin Psychol* 62:746-756, 1994.
9. Fredman L, Daly MP, Lazur AM: Burden among white and black caregivers to elderly adults, *J Gerontol* 50B:S110-S118, 1995.
10. Hadjistavropoulos T et al: Neuropsychological deficits, caregivers' perception of deficits and caregiver burden, *J Ann Gerontol Soc* 42:308-314, 1994.
11. Heller T, Factor A: Aging family caregivers: support resources and changes in burden and placement desire, *Am Assoc Mental Retardation* 98:417-426, 1993.
12. Homer AC, Gilleard CJ: The effect of inpatient respite care on elderly patients and their carers, *Age Aging* 23:274-276, 1994.
13. Jones SL, Roth D, Jones PK: Effect of demographic and behavioral variables on burden of caregivers of chronic mentally ill persons, *Psychiatr Serv* 46:141-145, 1995.
14. Karmilovich SE: Burden and stress associated with spousal caregiving for individuals with heart failure, *Prog Cardiovasc Nurs* 9:33-38, 1994.
15. Keady J, Nolan M: A stitch in time. Facilitating proactive interventions with dementia caregivers: the role of community practitioners, *J Psychiatr Mental Health Nurs* 2:33-40, 1995.
16. Loukissa DA: Family burden in chronic mental illness: a review of research studies, *J Adv Nurs* 21:248-255, 1995.
17. O'Neill G, Ross MM: Burden of care: an important concept for nurses, *Health Care Women Int* 12:111-121, 1991.
18. Robinson K, Yates K: Effects of two caregiver-training programs on burden and attitude toward help, *Arch Psychiatr Nurs* 8:312-319, 1994.
19. Siegel K et al: Caregiver burden and unmet patients needs, *Cancer* 68:1131-1140, 1991.
20. Siegel K et al: The relationship of spousal caregiver burden to patient disease and treatment-related conditions, *Ann Oncol* 2:511-516, 1991.
21. Thompson EH et al: Social support and caregiving burden in family caregivers of frail elders, *J Gerontol* 48:S245-S254, 1993.

Impaired verbal communication

1. Adkins E: Nursing care of clients with impaired communication, *Rehabil Nurs* 16:74-77, 1992.
2. Boss B: Managing communication disorders in stroke, *Nurs Clin North Am* 26:985-990, 1991.
3. Brunner J: *Beyond the information given,* New York, 1973, WW Norton.
4. Buckwalter K, Cusack D, Kruckeberg T, Shoemaker A: Family involvement with communication-impaired residents in long-term care settings, *Appl Nurs Res* 4:77-83, 1991.
5. Crowther D: Metacommunications: a missed opportunity, *J Psychosoc Nurs Ment Health Serv* 29:13-16, 1991.
6. Kim M, McFarland G, McLane A: *Pocket guide to nursing diagnoses,* ed 5, St Louis, 1993, Mosby.
7. McCloskey J, Bulechek G: *Nursing interventions classification (NIC),* St Louis, 1992, Mosby.
8. McFarland G, Wasli E, Gerety E: *Nursing diagnoses and process in psychiatric mental health nursing,* ed 2, Philadelphia, 1992, JB Lippincott.
9. Palmer J, Yantis P: *Survey of communication disorders,* Baltimore, 1990, Williams & Wilkins.
10. Ruesch J, Bateson G: *Communication: the social matrix of psychiatry,* New York, 1987, WW Norton.
11. Satir V: *Peoplemaking* Palo Alto, Calif, 1972, Science & Behavior Books.
12. Stuart G, Sundeen S: *Pocket guide: psychiatric nursing,* ed 2, St Louis, 1991, Mosby.

Risk for violence: self directed or directed at others

1. Apperson LJ, Mulvey EP, Lidz CW: Short-term clinical prediction of assaultive behavior: artifacts of research methods, *Am J Psychiatry* 150:1374, 1993.
2. Aldarondo E, Strauss MA: Screening for physical violence in couple therapy: methodological, practical and ethical considerations, *Fam Process* 33:425, 1994.
3. Carpenito LJ: *Handbook of nursing diagnosis,* ed 6, Philadelphia, 1995, JB Lippincott.
4. Carpenito LJ: *Nursing diagnosis: application to clinical practice,* ed 4, Philadelphia, 1991, JB Lippincott.

5. Dollard J et al: *Frustration and aggression,* New Haven, Conn, 1939, Yale University Press.
6. Ellich BA: Prevention of violence, *Primary care* 20:277, 1993.
7. Evans LK, Strumpf NE, Williams CC: Limiting use of physical restraints: a prerequisite for independent functioning. In Calkins E, Ford A, Katz P, editors: *The practice of geriatrics,* ed 2, Philadelphia, 1992, WB Saunders.
8. Fawcett J: *Dynamics of violence,* Chicago, 1972, American Medical Association.
9. Kim M, McFarland G, McLane A: *Pocket guide to nursing diagnoses,* ed 4, St Louis, 1991, Mosby.
10. Quinn C: The four A's of restraint reduction: attitude, assessment, anticipation, avoidance, *Orthop Nurs* 13:11-19, 1994.
11. Stuart GW, Sundeen SJ: *Principles and practices of psychiatric nursing,* ed 4, St Louis, 1991, Mosby.
12. Taylor C, Sparks S: *Nursing diagnosis cards,* ed 6, Springhouse, Pa, 1991, Springhouse.
13. Townsend MC: *Nursing diagnosis in psychiatric nursing,* ed 3, Philadelphia, 1994, FA Davis.
14. Wilson M: Seclusion practice in psychiatric nursing, *Nurs Stan* 7:28-30, 1993.

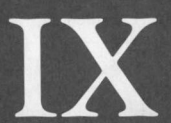

Sexuality-Reproductive

▪ ALTERED SEXUALITY PATTERNS

Altered sexuality patterns are states in which an individual expresses concern regarding his or her sexuality.

An altered sexuality pattern is one in which the individual expresses concern regarding sexuality because of actual or perceived difficulties, limitations, or changes in sexual behavior. This is contrasted with the nursing diagnosis of sexual dysfunction, in which the individual experiences a change in actual function that is viewed as unsatisfying, unrewarding, or inadequate. The focus of altered sexuality patterns is with the individual's concern about sexuality, which may or may not be associated with changes in sexual function (dysfunction).

Related Factors

Knowledge/skill deficit about alternative responses to health-related transitions, altered body function or structure, or illness or medical treatment
Lack of privacy
Lack of significant other
Ineffective or absent role models
Conflicts with experience orientation or variant preferences
Fear of pregnancy or of acquiring sexually transmitted disease
Impaired relationship with significant other
Body image disturbances

Defining Characteristics

Reported difficulties, limitations, or changes in sexual behaviors or activities
Impaired expression of one's sexuality
Expression of fear of potential limitations of sexual performance

Expected Patient Outcomes & Nursing Interventions

Altered sexual patterns
Identify misinformation and areas of knowledge (personal and otherwise) that contribute to concerns over sexuality, as evidenced by:
Recognizing how internal thoughts about sexual performance reduces erection
Recognizing how the connection of strict critical parental attitudes have influenced daughter's avoidance of sexual experiences

No longer fearing sexual practices during phases of pregnancy
- Assess the fears, expectation, doubts, and information basis for the sexual concerns expressed.
- Evaluate the context in which the specific experience concern has arisen; pay particular attention to relationship changes or habits, work disruption, use of drugs and alcohol.
- Explore sexual practices, fears associated with pregnancy and sexually transmitted diseases.
- Evaluate sexual information, and provide information that can alter misperceptions/perceptions.
- Explore issues related to physical setting or environment where sexual activities are usually performed, including attention to visual and auditory factors, privacy, furniture, comfort, and ambience that may be distracting or undesirable.

Make cognitive, behavioral, and interpersonal changes that enhance sexual confidence and reduce concerns over sexuality, as evidenced by:
Expressing satisfaction with sexuality and sexual experiences
Removing self from exploitive partner
Stopping shame-producing ideas regarding natural bodily functions
- Assist in trying behavioral, interpersonal changes that are thought to enhance sexual satisfaction and counteract sexual concern.

Principles and Rationale for Nursing Interventions

The focus of the nursing interventions is to assist the patient to identify the source of concerns that result in an altered sexuality pattern and to remediate problems by clarifying misconceptions and learning correct information. (See interventions for Sexual Dysfunction for appropriate rationales.)

▪ SEXUAL DYSFUNCTION

Sexual dysfunction is the state in which an individual experiences a change in sexual function that is viewed as unsatisfying, unrewarding, or inadequate.

Causes of dysfunctional sexual response patterns can be primarily psychogenic, organic, or secondary to illness, secondary to psychologic disorders, or stress. The identification of disruption in one of the three phases (orgasm phase disorders, excitement phase disorders, desire phase disorders) is critical when considering focused sex therapy interventions.[8] Self-report of sexual problems [2,8] is insufficient evidence of actual dysfunctional sexual response patterns. When dysfunctional sexual response patterns are not in evidence, self-reports of sexual problems and dissatisfaction most often have causal roots in psychiatric disorders or relationship problems rather than primary dysfunctional sexual responses. Situational sexual response systems, avoidance and phobic responses, and situational inhibition are most often sexual problems not associated with medical problems.[2,8,9,12]

As a general rule, a primary sexual symptom that has "always" been present is more likely to be psychogenic than a secondary disorder that occurs after a period of good functioning, especially in the absence of trauma or stress.[2,8,9]

Organic causes should be suspected in a person whose sexual functioning has been normal for a significant period, especially when there is deterioration of ejaculatory functions or orgasm becomes delayed.[2]

Sexual disorders frequently associated with organic causes are as follows.[8,9,11]

Impotence
Dyspareunia
Vaginismus
Unconsummated marriage
Low or absent libido
Secondary anorgasmia in males and females
Secondary premature ejaculation
Secondary retarded ejaculation

Sexual dysfunction can be a disruption of extreme variation in sexual behavior. It is defined further by an identifiable disturbance of a phase in the sexual response pattern and excessive pain and phobic avoidance of sex (both simple and panic). Sexual dysfunction, as an extreme variation of sexual behavior, is defined by the object, animate or inanimate, required for sexual arousal and release; its habitual use; and a disregard to the rights, damage, pain, fear, and sensitivities when the object is animate.[1,15]

Estimates of prevalence of sexual dysfunction of phases among the general population are:[1,15]

Sexual Dysfunction	Men	Women
Erectile disorder	4%-9%	—
Female arousal, dyspareunia, vaginismus	—	Not available
Hypoactive desire	16%	34%
Orgasmic disorder	4%-10%	4%-9%
Premature ejaculation	36%-38%	—

Sexual dysfunction as an extreme variation of sexual behavior, often called *sexual deviations*, by virtue of its long-standing and habitual characteristics, is most often psychogenic with roots in psychic conflict and early conditioning. The behavior

(e.g., voyeurism, exhibitionism, pedophilia) often brings the individual in conflict with the law; or family members are implicated, as in incest, when the child comes to the attention of the health professional.[1,15]

The prevalence of perpetrators is not known. What is known from the reports about pedophiles is that, on average, pedophiles target 150 male victims; those with female victims target, on average, 20, and exhibitionists and voyeurs average 429 to 513 victims. These figures demonstrate the highly repeatable nature of sexual deviations in an individual perpetrator.[1,15]

A framework of categorizing the broad nursing diagnoses of sexual dysfunction into subdiagnoses is used here. Each subdiagnostic category is described separately with regard to the related factors and some defining characteristics. Because multiple subdiagnoses can be made, it is important to make a differential diagnosis.

Related Factors[1-17]/Risk Factors

Biopsychosocial alteration of sexuality
    Ineffectual or absent role models
    Physical abuse
    Psychosocial abuse (e.g., harmful relationships)
    Vulnerability
    Misinformation or lack of knowledge
    Values conflict
    Lack of privacy
    Lack of significant other
Altered body structure or function: pregnancy, recent childbirth, drugs, surgery, anomalies, disease process, trauma, radiation
Possible lowered hormonal functioning as a process of aging, compensating fear of failing sexual prowess
Transitory life experience (e.g., loss of spouse, loss of self-esteem)
Organic brain disease
Complex and severe psychologic disorders with primary character disorder; disturbed social relations
    Marked cognitive set justifying object choice and behavior, claiming it is nonharmful to immature individuals
    History of victimization as child (sexual, physical)
    Primary social networks and family that overlooks, condones indirectly, or supports behavior
Sexual trauma: rape, sexual exploitation (chronic, delayed, silent)

Concern about Sexual Functioning without Disruption of Sexual Response Pattern (Secondary to Organic and/or Psychosocial Causes)

Common organic factors
    Pregnancy, childbirth
    Mild infections of genitourinary tract and genitals (epididymitis, trichomoniasis)
    Disease states (heart attack, back surgery)
    Drugs or medication
Common psychosocial causes

Unrealistic expectations of self and others
Inadequate sexual techniques and poor communications
Religious beliefs or cultural taboos
Diminished interest and attachment to present sexual object
Preoccupation with demanding and/or stressful activity
Disruption and/or lack of comfort and privacy
Lack of desired sex object (e.g., isolation imposed because of travel, imprisonment)
Age changes (e.g., in appearance, social functioning)
More serious psychologic disorders (obsessional disorders, affective disorders, psychotic disorders)
More serious, complex relationship issues (pathologic spouse, parental transference problems, incompatible marriage)

Pain (Pre- and Post-Orgasm/Ejaculatory Phase)

Organic causes
Genital muscle spasm
Infection in urinary tract (prostatitis, vesiculitis, herpes)
Painful gynecologic conditions (pelvic inflammatory disease, endometriosis, hymenal remnants, ovarian pathology, ectopic pregnancy, lower bowel disease, herpes)
Conditioned, voluntary painful spasm of perineal muscles of internal reproductive organs; secondary to psychologic problems, can range from minor to severe; neurosis and relationship problems

Function Pain/Disgust (Dyspareunia)

Organic causes (Pain is more often organic than psychogenic; therefore organic causes must be ruled out.)
Psychogenic causes (There are usually complex and moderate to severe intrapsychic and relationship problems. Pain provides defense against pleasure.)
Hypochondriacreaction to hormonal shifts
Pain: hysterical, depression syndrome
Intractable schizophrenia
Functional genital muscle spasm
Brutal sexual assault; intercourse; foreign object

Phobic Avoidance of Sexual Experience (Simple/Complex)

Associated with panic disorders (hypothesized to panic threshold, as if alarm is on; overreacts to hazards and separations)
Simple sexual phobia (conditioning and neurotic conflicts)
Sexual trauma (rape, sexual exploitation, sex stress situations)

Paraphilias

Extreme variation of sexual behavior and object of sexual arousal without regard for welfare of object; nonhuman objects, suffering or humiliation of oneself or another, children or nonconsenting person(s)
Pedophile—object; infant, child, adolescent (both genders)
Rapist—object: female, male
Sexual arousal dependent on inanimate objects, parts of body, animals, or particular ritualized acts; causes conflict within subject or with partner or society at large

Most common are:
Fetishism (article of women's clothing)
Transvestism (cross dressing)
Frotteurism (rubbing against another)
Exhibitionism (displaying genitals in public)
Others:
Telephone scatology (lewdness)
Necrophilia (corpse)
Partialism (body parts)
Zoophilia (animals)
Coprophilia (feces)
Klismaphilia (enemas)
Urophilia (urine)
Other variations of sexual behavior, act dominated:
Sexual masochism (hypoxyphilia: sexual arousal through partial strangulation; beatings; etc.)
Sexual sadism (whipping, beating another)
Voyeurism (peeping)

Gender Identity Disorders

Nonacceptance of biologically determined sexuality; nonacceptance of socially determined sex role

Ego-Dystonic Homosexuality

Conflict over preference for sexual gratification from same-sex partner

Defining Characteristics

Verbalization of sexual problem/concern
Alterations in achieving perceived sex role
Actual or perceived limitation imposed by disease and/or therapy
Conflicts involving values
Alteration in achieving sexual satisfaction
Inability to achieve desired satisfaction
Seeking of confirmation of desirability
Alteration in relationship with significant other
Change of interest in self and others
Concern about sexual functioning without disruption of sexual response pattern (secondary to organic and/or psychosocial causes)
Concern over sexual functioning because of sudden minor alterations in responsiveness (e.g., time it takes to achieve sexual satisfaction)
Questions regarding sexual practices (e.g., amount, exertion, should erection be encouraged)
Confusion, anxiety toward expression of sexual drive
Confusion over intensity of response
Concern over adequacy in meeting sexual desire of partner
Confusion over object of sexual arousal (same for male and female)
Disruption of sexual response pattern: orgasm/ejaculation phase
Men
Premature ejaculation (inadequate control of ejaculation reflex)

Retarded ejaculation (delayed or absent)
  Partial retarded ejaculation; inhibition of emission phase only; no pleasure
  Women
    Inhibited orgasm (delayed or absent orgasm, missed orgasm)
    Insufficient stimulation
Disruption of sexual response pattern: excitement phase
  Men
    Impotence
    Disturbance of sexual pleasure
    Diminished excitement
  Women
    Vaginal dryness
    Painful coitus
    Disturbance of sexual pleasure
Disruption of sexual response pattern: desire phase
  Total loss of desire
  Loss of desire in specific situations only
  Chronic, low sexual desire
Pain (pre- and post-orgasm/ejaculatory phase)
  Pain before sex (prevents entry or ejaculation)
  Perineal pain (muscle spasm)
  Vaginal spasms after penis has entered
  Postorgasmic uterine spasms
Functional pain (dyspareunia)
  Pain on entry (deep thrusting)
  Vaginismus
Phobic avoidance of sexual experience (simple/complex)
  Phobic avoidance of sexual experience and sexual arousal
Extreme variations of sexual behavior and object of sexual arousal without regard for the welfare of object
  Pedophile
    Expression of primary sexual interest in infant, child, and/or adolescent by an adult male or female
    Hypersexual activity with underaged persons
    Compulsion for involvement with immature sex object
    Focusing on one object at a time or on a group of children
    Involvement in pornography purchases and/or production
    Prefers to be alone (however, can be involved in work activities that either provide contact with immature individuals or time to pursue sexual activities with immature individuals or time to pursue sexual activities with one underaged person)
    Uses bribes, coercion, and intimidation with object
    Potentially violent; potentially homicidal
    Marriage of convenience (cover); or marriage to have access to child
    May be in clandestine social relationships with other pedophiles
    More males than females as perpetrators
    History of legal confrontation for involvement with immature individuals
    Intelligence often average to above average
  Rapist
    Requires absolute control of the object

Uses force
Inflicts physical abuse; can result in murder
Justifies actions
Blames victim
Expresses high level of psychologic abuse (displays disqualifying degrading behavior)
Requires power, control, and/or aggression for sexual arousal
Experiences disruption of excitement phase with impotence and disruption frequently
Experiences orgasm phase with partial ejaculation frequently

Expected Patient Outcomes & Nursing Interventions[4,5,12,17]

Psychosocial

Openly appraises values and cultural practices that can interfere with personal sexual responsivity, as evidenced by:

Clarifying issues regarding the incest taboo
Recognizing appropriate interpersonal transactions that govern sexual exchanges
Recognizing the boundaries of violence and coercion between sexual partners

- As part of the comprehensive evaluation process (including assessment of the orgasm-ejaculation phase, excitement phase, and desire phase), focus on values and practices associated with sex role, sexual practices, and power within the sexual partner relationship. Note value and cultural conflicts that can interfere with satisfying, nonexploitive, noncoercive, age-appropriate sexual experiences. This can be done with individuals, with couples, and within the context of groups.
- Elicit cognitive/behavioral criteria that are used to justify self-limiting or exploitive, coercive acts; encourage the individual to challenge these criteria (NOTE: This step follows from the values-cultural assessment).
- If nurse is in doubt of this process and is unfamiliar with his or her own values, make a referral to nurse or specialist in the area of sexual dysfunctions and value clarification procedures or to a clinical specialist in psychiatric-mental-health nursing.

Does not adhere to beliefs and attitudes that inhibit or disrupt noncoercive, consensual sex and personal sex response patterns and phases, as evidenced by:

Appraising self positively with regard to sexual response, activities
Clarifying and reducing: fears; nonfunctional guilt; anger or sense of inferiority over sexual prowess and bodily features

- Use cognitive-behavioral approaches: reframing; thought stopping; this requires training in self-monitoring of internal processes, such as internal dialogue, imaging, and sensory experiences.

- Elicit beliefs regarding sexual performance and adequacy; explore relationship of these thoughts to inhibition and dissatisfaction with sexual experiences.

Identify and reduce interpersonal conflicts with sex partner (age-appropriate, noncoercive), as evidenced by:

Opening up communication with partner to reduce interpersonal conflicts that are carried over to the sexual experience

- With couple, assess and work through barriers to communication; use exercises that emphasize communication and comfort with each other rather than the culmination of the sexual act.
- Delay this (sexual intercourse) demand if marital conflicts are severe; refer for counseling before trying any specific strategies to enhance sexual enjoyment; these activities require that the couple trust each other because of the openness required; unresolved marital conflicts that go beyond the sexual experience should be lessened before focused sex therapy is attempted; this is basic regardless of the origins of the sexual dysfunction.

Alter shifts in attitudes and expectations of self and others that reduce sexual satisfaction and functioning, as evidenced by:

Not expecting supreme sexual satisfaction with every encounter
Finding pleasure in holding and caressing
Not criticizing partner

- Provide focused counseling on how expectations detract from the communication process; this requires the individual to recognize that expectations should be replaced with open requests and negotiation; this is done with individual and with couple.
- Individually or in a group, work through unconscious hostility to opposite sex, guilt regarding sexual pleasure.

Reduce anxiety or anger associated with past conflicted relationships and traumas that have an impact on present relationship and sexual functioning, as evidenced by:

Not confusing present partner with past negative interpersonal experiences
Recognizing anxiety associated with past threatening event and beginning to relax and share concern with partner

- Provide focused counseling identifying and resolving past conflicted relationships and traumas.

Use internal psychic resources to enhance erotic experiences, as evidenced by:

Using kinesthetic focusing
Reducing dissociation from the sexual act by linking traumagenic or guilt-associated cues associated with sexual arousal

- Provide focused counseling on past negative relationships and traumatic events that have affected sexual expression; this requires the individual to explore how his or her sex-

uality was affected and how this impact carries over into the present situation.

- Provide training with regard to images that either increase sensory experiences or decrease them; work with reducing reliance on imagery and moving more into kinesthetic awareness, thus combating dissociation.
- If movement toward kinesthetic involvement is met with increase anxiety, assess for basis of anxiety (e.g., past trauma, strong beliefs that attach fear and anxiety to pleasurable states, or feelings of loss control).
- Reinforce prescribed sensation—enhancing exercises with self and partner.
- Assist in exploring means of intensifying sensations.
- In severely blocked individuals, refer to sex therapist for biofeedback and to counseling for psychologic problems.

Openly discuss sexual experiences with partner to increase sexual satisfaction for both, as evidenced by:

Comfortably exploring body zones with partner and communicating pleasurable sensations
Asking partner to shift position to increase comfort and ease during the sex act
Making it clear what is arousing and sustaining of sexual arousal to partner

- Provide education about techniques to increase communication and sexual techniques.

Separate out thoughts, fears, and misinformation that link sexual dysfunctions with organic illness, limitation, and changes (reduces stress secondary to both reversible and irreversible organic states), as evidenced by:

Recognizing the physical changes associated with heart condition
Separating out sense of bodily change because of loss of limb from sexual desirability and functioning

- Educate regarding physical illness, illness process, and treatment interventions.
- Provide accurate information regarding the temporary disruption of sexual activities caused by organic impairment.
- Provide information necessary to enhance sexual functioning, despite organic impairment (educational materials, counseling, and focused exercises).

Organic factors

Understand organic issues or illness states' impact on sexual functioning (phases of sexual response), as evidenced by:

Understanding the relationship of antidepressant to sexual arousal phase
Understanding the loss of penile sensation caused by spinal cord injury
Working through with partner alterations in sexual functioning caused by illness state and treatment responses

- Provide focused counseling on the impact of the organic issues (chronic or temporary) and their influence on the phases of sexual functioning; this should be done with the couple, as well as the individual; it can be an opportunity for positive sex education for both.

Participate in educational and counseling activities that inform and provide strategies to reduce stress of organic factors affecting sexual functioning (reversible and irreversible), as evidenced by:

Demonstrating knowledge of the influence of prescribed drugs on sexual functioning through discussion and adjustment with sexual partner.

Understanding the methods of penile implant and methods of addressing sexual activities with sexual partner through open communication

- Do focused assessment and counseling with the individual and the couple regarding their relationship and their past sexual practices and what alteration may be present with current functioning.
- Identify and address attitudes that impede acceptance of changes.
- Provide information that is lacking, and deal with values, personal expectation, and possible grief surrounding losses.
- Counsel and educate patient and sex partner regarding prosthetics, implants, or techniques; group work can be helpful for individual, as well as couples.
- Assess that disease process is under control, and carefully review drugs and other interventions as to their influence on sexual responsivity.
- Increase the identification and participation in activities that give pleasure to the couple and the individual in lieu of sexual activity.
- Refer to differential diagnosis of simple and complex phobic responses to sexual activity.

Follow regimen to reduce organic source of pain or pain caused by psychologic problems including sexual trauma, as evidenced by:

Following pain medication regimen to reduce pain during intercourse

Following strategies to reduce painful voluntary muscle response caused by psychologic problems

- Educate in carrying out necessary medical interventions to reduce underlying disease process.
- Follow pain reduction regimen.
- Teach relaxation of muscles involved in sexual act to reduce pain.

Aggressive dominance factors (pedophile/rapist)

Acknowledge offense behavior, as evidenced by:

Identifying victims

Acknowledging the force and coercion used against the victim

Detailing all aspects of assault

- Report sexual misconduct to the authorities.
- Refer to experienced counselor: confront behavior and its impact on others; drug intervention; individual/family counseling; hypnotherapy; age regression; concerted effort to have perpetrator identify with victim; management of secondary psychiatric problems; specific strategies to reduce reliance and arousal potential of fantasies, objects, and acts.

Follow the regimen to prevent relapse into sexually exploitive behavior, as evidenced by:

Maintaining regular meetings to offender-monitoring group

Challenging, as well as identifying, rationalization for deviant behavior, such as staying with young children when court has ordered not to be in the house

- Teach self-monitoring of thoughts and ideas that justify sexually acting out.
- Assign to 12-step program directed toward sexual addiction and addiction to violence and coercion.

Follow regimen that reduces reliance on object or act for sexual arousal that is deviant, as evidenced by:

Using methods that reduce fantasies with deviant object or act that result in sexual arousal

Self-monitoring rationalization to engage in deviant sexual behavior

- Provide focused behavioral treatment, aversive conditioning of deviant sexual fantasies and sexual arousal to nonappropriate sexual objects/behaviors such as children or violent acts.

Develop nonexploitive patterns of sexual expression, as evidenced by:

Developing age-appropriate sexual interests

Unlinking aggressive, exploitive ideation from sexual expression

- Provide focused behavioral treatment to enhance positive sexual expression.
- Enhance positive regard for victims and their rights; under special conditions, confrontation with victims might be useful in raising the consciousness about the harm inflicted.
- Assist in the development of socially positive outlets for creative energies, e.g., activity in self-help groups where the individual takes on the responsibility of helping another offender stop his or her behavior.

Gender identity disorders

Clarify values and cultural determinants that intensify dissatisfaction with gender identity or sexual orientation, as evidenced by:

Exploring values toward male/female orientation; toward heterosexual

- Examine own personal beliefs and values surrounding people who are in conflict over their gender identity and their sexual orientation to like sex.

- For gender identity disorder refer to specialist for evaluation and treatment; this may take the form of counseling to negotiate acceptance of deep-seated conflicts regarding gender orientation, or in rare situations, may be resolved by sex change surgery.
- Ego-dystonic homosexual, that is, a person who believes he or she is homosexual, is in distress, and requires counseling; this must be carried out by a nonjudgmental individual who is willing to work with the person, allowing him or her to arrive at his or her own decision.

Evaluate personal sexual development and its relationship to gender identity and sexual orientation, as evidenced by:

Exploring sex role development, orientation to sexual functions, genital orientation, friendships, and interpersonal relationships.

Not being conflicted about gender identity or sexual orientation

- Provide focused counseling on personal sexual development, attitudes, and fantasies that impede acceptance of gender or sexual orientation.

Use nondestructive resources for reducing conflict regarding gender identity or sexual orientation, as evidenced by:

Using counseling for resolution of conflict over gender and sexual orientation concerns

Participating in self-help groups

- Provide counseling and education regarding behavior and relationships, regardless of identity issues or sexual orientation.
- Explore issues of intimacy and attachment (NOTE: Sexual problems can reflect more basic problems in relating to others).
- Group work with individuals exploring similar confusion can be helpful.
- Help seek out a network of friends with whom these concerns can be shared without being rejected; this must be done carefully.

Develop healthy, nonexploitive, nonconflictual orientation and expression of gender identity and sexual orientation, as evidenced by:

Practicing safe sex methods

Refraining from degrading or harmful sex practices

- Follow strategies just listed for previous expected patient outcomes.

Principles and Rationale for Nursing Interventions[2-14,17]

When a behavioral matrix such as sexual functioning becomes a problem, the characteristics of the problem must be understood by the objective evidence, as well as the subjective data. The closer the objective evidence coincides with a definitive etiology, the more apt the specific intervention will be.

The following sequence of data illustrates decisions in the evaluation of defining characteristics and in terms of broad considerations or related factors.

Does the patient have a disruption of sexual response patterns? (Sexual Dysfunction on p. 1726)

If normal functioning present, consider psychiatric diagnosis. If no psychiatric problems exist, provide education and reassurance. (Altered Sexual Patterns on p. 1726)

If psychiatric diagnosis made, differentiate problems, then provide appropriate psychiatric treatment (or refer).

If abnormal functioning present, diagnosis: organic or psychogenic.

If organic, make medical diagnosis. Is it a treatable medical problem that will result in correction, or is it nontreatable? If treatable, consider sexual rehabilitation, counseling, penile implant.

If psychogenic, check etiology. If it is a major psychologic cause, consider long-term therapy. If it is a minor and moderate psychologic cause, consider sex therapy.

If sexual problem is secondary to other psychiatric disorder (e.g., stress, depression, panic disorder, severe marital disorder, substance abuse, major mental or emotional illness), consider appropriate psychiatric treatment.

Sexual dysfunction as a diagnosis provides a broad spectrum of general data with a broad array of related factors. When these factors are considered, second- and third-order levels of assessment are required for specifying the particular type of sexual dysfunction and its relationship to important biopsychosocial parameters. In addition, particular types of intervention must be evaluated as to their impact physically, psychologically, and interpersonally. Assessment and differential diagnosis, as well as specialized-assessment diagnostic skill are necessary given the complexity of the functional disorder. Collaboration with other professionals, as well as the nurse's specialized expertise, is required both for differential diagnostic activities and for particular intervention modes.

Concern about Sexual Functioning

When the related factor is organic, nursing care focuses on educating the client and counseling about misconceptions that provoke anxiety and depression. Because sexual functioning most often involves a partner, nursing intervention is also directed at the appropriate partner.

For example, consider a husband recovering from a mild heart attack. The husband and wife are hesitant to resume their sexual relationship for fear the husband will have a heart attack. Sexual desire is present, as are sexual arousal and orgasmic experiences. For these people a causal connection between the energy expended in the sexual act and heart attack has been determined. Information and experience in monitoring exertion with concomitant signs (pulse rate, chest pain) become important for the husband. This is usually done through gradual increments in physical activity. Involvement of the wife provides experience for her, as well as an opportunity for them to open up communication between them. Unrealistic expectations can be revealed and countered. In addition, the couple can become comfortable exploring, relaxing, and finding less strenuous methods for enjoying their sexual relationship.

When the related factors are psychologic and secondary to organic causes, education and counseling are the primary interventions. This is particularly true when the problems are minor. Severity of the primary psychologic and relationship problems is determined in part by assessment of the psychologic makeup of the person and/or couple and the critical interactional components of the relationship.

Some medical interventions greatly alter body structure, as well as impinge on the physiology of penile erection and erotic responses; therefore special attention must be paid to the process of the patient gaining acceptance of the body image changes. Partners need support and counseling during periods of adjustment.

Vaginal dryness that impedes the enhancement of sexual excitement may be related to estrogen deficiency, most often associated with menopause. When hormonal replacement is contraindicated or not desire, lubricants can greatly reduce the problem.[10,13] Nursing care is influenced according to whether the medical problem is reversible. With reversible problems, nursing care supports the patient and partner until the reestablishment of sexual functioning. If the medical problem is irreversible, rehabilitative efforts and counseling are the modes of intervention.

Removing a sexual complaint can escalate anxiety by exposing other human demands of relating (e.g., commitment, intimacy). Problems in these personal areas are masked through many symptoms of dysfunction. The symptoms may be viewed as defenses for the individual. At times in complex relationship problems the partner with the complaint may be a foil for the more severe psychologic problems of the nonsymptomatic partner. When the symptom is removed, there is an imbalance in the relationship, and the partner's underlying psychologic difficulties are revealed.

In general, the nurse should determine if the disorder has an organic or a psychogenic cause. If there is doubt, the nurse should refer for more specialized evaluation. If organic and psychogenic causes are established, as well as their primary and secondary relationships, the nurse uses one of the following nursing interventions most appropriate to the causes and the level of sexual behavior issues: education, general counseling around personal and relationship issues, focused exercises to alter cognitive sets and physical behavior that impede sexual and erotic behaviors, and inclusion of the partner.

RAPE-TRAUMA SYNDROME; RAPE TRAUMA: COMPOUND REACTION; RAPE TRAUMA: SILENT REACTION

Rape-trauma syndrome is forced, violent sexual penetration against the victim's will and consent. The trauma syndrome that develops from this attack or attempted attack includes an acute phase, or disorganization of the victim's life-style, and a long-term process of life-style reorganization.

Rape trauma syndrome is the acute and long-term psychosocial process of reintegration that occurs as an aftermath of forcible rape or attempted forcible rape.[4] The syndrome is influenced by the type of rape activity; forcible, nonconsenting, sexual exploitation, or sex-stress situation. The legal definition of rape varies from state to state; however, the issues generally addressed include lack of consent, force or threat of force, and sexual penetration. The clinical definition of rape trauma—the focus of this nursing diagnosis—is the stress response pattern of the victim after forced, nonconsenting sexual activity. The rape trauma syndrome of somatic, cognitive, psychologic, and behavioral symptoms is an active stress reaction to a life-threatening situation.[1,9]

The trauma to the victim results from that person being confronted with the life-threatening and highly stressful situation of rape and sexual abuse. The crisis or reaction that results is in the service of self-preservation. It is the nucleus around which an adaptive pattern may be noted.*

What is traumatizing to a rape victim (in all types of rape) is that her life is in jeopardy and she is helpless in the situation. Forcible rape, an act forced on a victim (usually female) by an assailant (usually male), is viewed as an act of violence expressing power, aggression, conquest, degradation, anger, hatred, and contempt.[8,15] Hilberman[13] characterizes rape as the "ultimate violation of the self, short of homicide, with the invasion of one's inner and most private space, as well as loss of autonomy and control." Hilberman argues that it is the person's self, not an orifice, that has been invaded and that the core meaning of rape is the same for a virgin, a housewife, a lesbian, and a prostitute.

A study of motivational intent of the offender indicates that rape behavior involves a hierarchy of life issues such as power, anger, and sexuality. On the basis of clinical data on 133 convicted rapists and 92 adult victims, Groth et al.[8] viewed rape as complex and multidetermined, and they addressed issues of hostility (anger) and control (power) more than passion (sexuality). Subdivisions of these categories include the power-assertive rapist, who perceives rape as a means of expressing his virility and dominance; the power-reassurance rapist, who uses the act of rape to resolve doubts about his sexual adequacy; the anger-retaliation rapist, who seeks revenge by degrading and humiliating women; and the anger-excitation rapist, who derives sexual excitement from inflicting pain and punishing his victim. In pair or group rape the motive of seeking male camaraderie has been suggested, and the motive of a sense of entitlement to sexual services has been observed in data on father-daughter incest,[12] wife rape, and date situations.[19]

Analysis of the dynamics and method of operation of the rapist helps to explain what specific aspects have terrorized and victimized the person. Style of attack has been found to contain characteristics classified as *blitz*, in which the victim is quickly subdued and propelled into the assault,[6] *con*, in which the victim is approached verbally and then betrayed and assaulted,[6]

---

*References 1-6, 8, 9, 13, 14, 16, 17.

and *surprise,* in which the rapist waits and targets a victim or sneaks up on and surprises her.[6]

Sexual Exploitation

Rape trauma syndrome falls within the general category of sexual traumas. Two additional sexual traumas were identified in the study in which rape trauma syndrome was reported.[15,17] A differential diagnosis needs to be made regarding the additional two sexual traumas.

A second group of sexual assault victims, most of whom were children and young adolescents, were categorized as *accessory-to-sex victims*. In this type of sexual assault, victims are *pressured into sexual activity by a person or persons who stand in a power position over them through age or authority*. Victims are unable to make a responsible decision of consent because of their level of personality of cognitive development or their learned rules of behavior. The emotional reaction of the victim results from being pressured into sexual activity and from the tension to keep the activity secret. The offender gains access to the victim in several ways: offering material rewards (candy, money); offering psychologic rewards (attention, interest, affection); or misrepresenting moral standards ("It's okay to do this—your mother and I do it").[5]

This trauma syndrome is often characterized by a gradual social and psychologic withdrawal from usual life activities. This withdrawal is most apt to occur when the sexual activity is repeated with the same person over an extended time. Physical symptoms of trauma may be evidenced through changes in motor behavior and signs of infection. Such overall signs and symptoms are especially prominent when the victim has been pressured into secrecy by the offender. The burden of carrying the secret creates considerable tension, and the victim feels constantly on guard to maintain the secret.[5]

Sex-Stress Situation

A third group of sexual trauma situations results from a sexual encounter in which *both parties initially consent to sexual activity (date rape)*. The person for whom the sexual situation produces the most anxiety usually brings the situation to the attention of the nurse. The situation usually includes two consenting people for whom something "goes wrong" during the sexual activity; or there may be anxiety about the results of the sexual activity (pregnancy, infection, disease).[3]

Related Factors

Rape Trauma Syndrome: Nonconsenting Forcible Rape

1. Type of rape (e.g., Blitz, con, surprise)
   Force/threat (e.g., gun, knife)
   Damage/physical
2. Age
3. Demand for cognitive/behavioral assimilation of experience (how the process proceeds)
   Surprise
   Death threat
   Physical penetration
   Physical injury

Immobilization
Attributions for cause of rape
Self-appraisal of response to rapist or victim, mastery
Stored sounds, smells, images, sensations
4. Major coping behaviors employed to handle assault
5. Demand for cognitive/behavioral assimilation of disclosing experience to others
   Response of judicial/police system
   Response of immediate social support system
6. Prior psychosocial issues
   Prior victimization
   Prior stress experiences
   Social network response
   Major coping behaviors

Rape Trauma Syndrome: Compound Reaction

Factors 1 to 6 with particular emphasis on:
Major defenses and coping mechanisms used to handle the exploitation
Characteristics of social support system
   Excessive blame
   Excessive worry, reinforcement of victim role
   Amount of physical violence
   Coping mechanism to master rape
   Quality of support system
   Older age of victims
Prior psychosocial issues
   Attachment to perpetrator
   Degree of political, personal, and financial power of victimizer over victim
   Chronic history of abuse, self-deprecation
   Limited sense of alternatives
   Limited psychologic capacities
   Socialization (delayed labeling of experience[s] as rape because of prevailing sense of social milieu holding victim responsible, deserving and provoking sexual abuse)
   Primary use of dissociative and avoidant defenses and coping behaviors during time of sexual exploitation and through disclosure process, plus perception of self vis-à-vis social support system, seem most important

Rape Trauma Syndrome: Delayed Reaction

Factors 1 to 6 with particular emphasis on dissociative defenses and avoidant coping behavior
Factors contributing to compound reaction also contribute to delayed reaction

Rape Trauma Syndrome: Silent Reaction

Type of rape (particular attention to the threat/fear of violence used to control and the distortion of sense of self, sense of right, wrong, responsibility, perpetrated)
Disclosure
   Confrontation by self/others of sexual exploitation
   Police/judicial proceedings
   Immediate social support system
   Peer and school reaction

Demand for cognitive/behavioral assimilation of experience
(how process proceeds)
Betrayal
Sorting out responsibility
Dealing and subtle threats, coercion, distortion
Blurring of aggressive/sexual impulses
Stress reaction to disclosure
Stored sounds, smells, images, sensations
Major coping mechanisms employed to handle exploitation
Prior psychosocial issues; prior victimization
Fears retaliation
Denies importance of rape to avoid deeper personal reactions:
shame, guilt
Attachment to offender before abuse
Psychologic problems
Source of powerlessness
Socialization; woman to bear humiliation alone
Use of defense; dissociation of affect from memory of rape

Defining Characteristics

Somatic reactions
Physical trauma: cuts and bruises on neck, throat, breasts,
thighs, legs, arms
Physical trauma to genitals
Gastrointestinal irritability
Stomach pains
Nausea
Change in appetite
Skeletal muscle tension, headaches, fatigue
Sleep disturbance reactions
Genitourinary disturbances
Vaginal discharges
Rectal bleeding
Burning on urination
Itching
Psychologic/behavioral reactions
Disturbance of mood: depressed, anxious
Cognitive disruption: confusion, failure of memory, indeci-
siveness
Self-appraisal: fear, embarrassment, humiliation, self-blame
Fear of violence toward self and others
Desire for revenge
Intrusive thoughts, nightmares, daymares
Replication of the victimization
Thoughts of the rape
Mastery dreams of overcoming assailant
Phobic reactions
Avoidance of sex
Avoidance of people
Avoidance of crowds
Avoidance of being alone
More severe psychologic reactions
Ideas of reference
Psychotic states
Severe acting out

Dysfunctional coping
Alcohol, drugs
Promiscuity, prostitution
Suicidal behavior, homicidal behavior
Self-blame, low self-esteem
Restrictive and avoidance behaviors
Fear that something is wrong with sexual organs
Social reactions
Dependence on others
Work or school failure, withdrawal
Avoidance of close or family relationship; social isolation
Disruption of couple's relationship
Social stigmatization
Constant moves to deal with anxiety and fear
Additional aspects
When patient presents herself as psychotic or sexually
promiscuous, has psychosomatic complaints, avoids sex-
ual relationships, or has sudden social withdrawal and
alcohol and drug abuse, evaluation should be done to
rule out sexual trauma diagnoses. These major behavioral deviations often mask sexual trauma, either because
prior psychiatric problems are exacerbated by trauma or
because these other syndromes defend against sexual
event.
There is also a group of victims who do not reveal to others
that they have been raped (silent reaction). This population
appears different from those with delayed reactions in that
total event is not dissociated and repressed; rather, there is
memory of event, but emotional reaction and its assimilation are not addressed, nor is event disclosed to others.
Characteristics associated with silent reaction
Marked anxiety in personal interviews with long periods
of silence, blocking of associations, minor stuttering,
and physical distress
Reported extreme irritability or actual avoidance of relationships with men
History of extreme change in sexual behavior
History of sudden onset of phobic reactions: fear of being
alone, going outside, being inside alone
Persistent loss of self-confidence and self-esteem; self-
blame
Suspiciousness
Frequent dreams of violence and nightmares

Expected Patient Outcomes & Nursing Interventions[1,2,7]

Rape trauma syndrome

**Demonstrate reduction in immediate negative reaction
to rape experience and disclosure, as evidenced by:**

Experiencing return of normal sleep pattern
Experiencing reduction of intrusive recollection of the rape ex-
perience
Experiencing reduction in generalized autonomic arousal
• Provide safety.

- Provide effective, considerate physical examination, necessary prescriptions and repair of injuries.
- Assist individual in establishing close relationship with safe person to provide for catharsis, with attention to correction of distorted premises regarding self-blame.
- Assist individual in establishing self-control over person and decisions.
- Assist individual in establishing a safe, supportive social network.
- Counsel regarding stress response images, sounds, smells, or sensations that provoke anxiety.
- Teach methods of relaxation, if possible.
- Counsel immediate family, spouse, or partner about rape trauma syndrome and manifestations of symptoms of trauma.
- Orient the individual and family to the criminal justice system.
- Ensure careful preservation of evidence; carefully document the physical and emotional status of the individual.
- Assign to a rape crisis worker, as well as to needed follow-up visits after emergency visit.
- Counsel regarding exacerbation of earlier crisis symptoms with prolonged investigative procedures and court appearances.
- Counsel immediate family, spouse, or partner as to their own reactions regarding the rape and the symptoms of the victim; evaluate them for traumatic response.
- Gain permission for and explain any photographic procedures used to document injury.

Return to positive psychologic functioning, as evidenced by:

Exhibiting positive self-regard

Having no self-blame

Having reasonable trust in relationships

Having physical and psychologic energy to learn

Having intact memory and recalling event without undue anxiety

Having regulated mood

Having appropriate affective expression

Demonstrating consistent self-protective strategies

- Provide counseling and focused therapy for prolonged anxiety reaction associated with specific flashback phenomena and for reframing of disruptive belief patterns. This can be done individually, with family and couples, and in groups especially focused on recovery from rape.
- Provide counseling for couples where conflict and restriction in sexual activity occur; the support groups that exist for the victim, as well as for the partner, are available and helpful.
- Provide careful examination and follow-up on physical injuries and symptoms.
- Provide counseling around follow-up for sexually transmitted diseases; this factor may contribute to the prolongation of symptoms and disruption in intimate relationships.

Return to social functioning, as evidenced by:

Returning to work successfully

Experiencing intact family relationships

Being comfortable with sex role and sexual functioning

Engaging friends and making new friends

- Assist in reinstating life plan, counseling focuses on beliefs and attitudes that change or challenge in the sense that life plans can be carried out after the rape.
- Assist in developing a reasonable sense of safety and caution in strange situations, at night, and with people.
- Assist in being comfortable in social situations.
- Assist and refer, if necessary, for gaining comfort in sexual relationships.
- Assist in not avoiding the rape experience because of undue fear and anxiety when recollecting the events; group work with victims and helping victims can aid with the recovery.
- Counsel family, friends, and victim regarding the event and in the reestablishment of life goals.

Principles and Rationale for Nursing Interventions

In the acute phase of rape trauma syndrome there is a great deal of disorganization in the victim's life-style. This disorganization is evidenced as follows.[1-6,9]

In *impact reactions* one of two styles of reaction is generally noted: the expressed style, in which feelings of fear, anger, and anxiety are shown through such behavior as crying, sobbing, smiling, restlessness, and tenseness, or the controlled style, in which feelings are masked or hidden and a calm, composed, or subdued affect is noted.[4]

In the first several weeks after a rape the following acute *somatic manifestations* may be evident:

Physical trauma, which includes general soreness and bruising (e.g., throat, neck, breasts, thighs, legs, arms)

Skeletal muscle tension, which includes tension headaches and fatigue, as well as sleep pattern disturbances and complaints of hyperalertness, feeling edgy and nervous

Gastrointestinal irritability, which includes stomach pains, appetite disruption, and nausea

Genitourinary disturbance, which includes gynecologic symptoms of vaginal discharge, itching, burning on urination, and generalized pain; also, symptoms from sexual penetration of the mouth and rectum

A wide gamut of *emotional reactions* may be expressed and include fear, humiliation, embarrassment, anger, revenge, and self-blame. Fear of physical violence and death is usually the primary effect experienced during the rape.

The long-term process of reorganization is the second phase of the rape trauma syndrome. Although the time of onset varies from victim to victim, this phase often begins several weeks after the assault or identification of the rape. Various factors affect the coping behavior of victims, e.g., ego strength, social network support, and the way people treat them as victims.[1,4]

The following characteristics are noted:

Motor activity: There generally is an increase in motor activity, especially changing residence and taking trips. Victims also turn for support to family members not necessarily seen daily, as well as to friends, associates, and colleagues.

Dreams and nightmares. Intrusive thoughts of the rape break into the victim's conscious mind, as well as during sleep (nightmares). Three types of nightmares may be reported: replications of the state of victimization and helplessness; symbolic dreams, which include a theme from the rape; and mastery dreams, in which the victim is powerful in assuming control. Nonmastery dreams dominate until the victim is recovered.

Traumatophobia. Fears and phobias are common characteristics after rape. The phobia develops as a defensive reaction to the circumstances of the rape. Some common phobias include fear of indoors, fear of outdoors, fear of being alone, fear of crowds, fear of people behind them, and sexual fears.

The nursing care of the rape trauma victim is based on four models of nursing intervention: biologic, social, cognitive-behavioral, and psychologic.[14,15]

Biologic Model of Intervention

During the acute phase after the assault, the nurse should carefully review any somatic alteration in the body system such as the following: circulatory system (flushing, perspiration, feeling hot or cold, headaches); respiratory system (breathing style, sighing respirations, rapid breathing, dizziness); gastrointestinal system (abdominal pain, nausea, lack of appetite, constipation); genitourinary system (urinary frequency, interference with sexual functioning).

On the follow-up it is essential for the nurse to document carefully the nature and intensity of the symptoms over a 24-hour period. The somatic side effects of any medication prescribed need to be distinguished from the somatic aftereffects of the assault. For example, the nausea and vomiting from antipregnancy medication should significantly decrease when the medicine is stopped. It is important to check if nausea is from an emotional reaction to thinking about the rape. Similarly, itching and vaginal discharge may be a result of the heavy dose of antibiotics and should decrease on completion of the medication. A careful note should be made that the patient is taking the correct amount prescribed. Physical symptoms after 5 days should be carefully investigated, since the therapeutic regimen of medication is usually completed by then. Minor tranquilizers and sleeping medication should not be routinely prescribed without a careful assessment of the patient's needs.

The victim should have a gynecologic and medical follow-up appointment after she completes her first menstrual period after the assault. All victims, male and female, should have a blood test for hepatitis B virus, HIV, and syphilis and a culture for sexually transmitted diseases taken during a 4- to 6-week follow-up visit. The referral and follow-up is a primary nursing intervention and may be made to either a nurse practitioner or physician.

Social Model of Intervention

This nursing intervention makes explicit use of the victim's social network. The goal of using family and friends of the victim is to strengthen the victim's self-confidence to help her resume a normal style of living. Whether the victim chooses to tell family and friends about the rape is not the point, but rather that the victim seeks support from the network.

The victim is encouraged to resume a normal style of activity according to her ability to pace the activities. The longer a victim avoids a normal activity such as school or work, the greater the difficulty in trying to return to it.

An important nursing intervention is to encourage the victim to seek out understanding people to talk to about any concerns. The victim often has specific decisions to make and seeks advice about issues such as whether to press charges against the rapist, whether to quit work, or how to tell people about the incident. It is important for the victim to have an active involvement with a social network and environment to resume a somewhat normal life-style. Repairing estranged family and social relationships is encouraged to provide the victim with additional emotional support during this time.

Cognitive-Behavioral Model of Intervention

The focus of the cognitive-behavioral model is on the belief patterns the victim holds regarding rape and sexual assault, as well as on desensitizing the person to the behavior that results from the assault, specifically the phobic reactions. Identifying the belief patterns (why the victim thinks the rape occurred) provides the nurse with a measurement of the victim's attribution of blame. For example, if the victim believes women are raped because of the way they dress, she will need to be educated as to the myths about rape. If the victim believes that rapists stalk victims and therefore anyone may become a victim, attention can be placed on increasing safety tactics for the prevention of invasion from predators.

One goal of this intervention is to deflate the fears, stresses, and anxieties the victim experiences after the assault and to help inflate the victim' own self-esteem and self-confidence in dealing with the world again. The victim has the potential to reach her previous level of adaptive functioning and to strengthen capabilities to feel secure again.

The nursing intervention is aimed at desensitizing the victim to the memory of the rape. Talking about the painful parts gives the victim psychologic control over the memory and strips it of its power to distress the victim. The victim is encouraged to master her fears, i.e., to think back over the very frightening situation with support from the nurse and friends. Gradually, this method desensitizes the victim so that the thoughts can gradually enter the mind without the terrifying reactions. This technique may be used with the physical setting or other circumstances of the assault.

As the nurse talks with a victim, it is essential to help the victim make psychologic connections between the symptoms and the rape trauma. Although repression may be a protective process it absorbs valuable psychic energy necessary for the victim to settle the crisis.

A common fear of victims and their families is that the offender will retaliate in some manner or that he will try to harm the victim in some other way. If concrete data exist that the offender is harassing the victim, the police can be notified to help in the matter. In some cases the victim is threatened by the defendant's family, and in such cases the judge may be explicit in condemning such behavior and in stating the sanctions for the assailant if such behavior continues. Retaliative behavior can be quite frightening to the victim.

Psychologic Model of Intervention

During the acute phase the nurse should carefully review mental functioning in terms of impaired attention, poor concentration, poor memory, changes in outlook, and future planning; and emotional reaction in terms of irritability, mood changes, dream disturbance, and changes in relationships with family and friends.

Talking with the victim during the impact phase, or as close as possible to the actual time of the rape, is essential to help repair the emotional damage inflicted on the victim. This intervention also attempts to minimize the psychologic aftereffects of the rape by providing emotional support of a nonjudgmental nature. Talking with the victim helps to establish an alliance and provides an opportunity for assessing the impact of the assault on the victim's reactions.

The overwhelming impulse of the victim is to avoid dealing with the experience. In such situations the nurse encourages the victim to talk about the rape and supports any fearful reaction by saying that the fear is a natural reaction to the danger to which the victim was exposed.

Talking about the assault and bearing the accompanying distressing feelings are essential steps in the total process of settling the crisis and mastering the experience. The treatment goals for the victim are to reestablish a normal style of living and to restore a sense of equilibrium. This means the victim must come to terms intellectually and viscerally by acknowledging the impact of the rape on her life and incorporating it as a stressful memory in the total life experience. The meaning of the assault must be talked about and thought about. The feelings, which may be accompanied by various physical and emotional manifestations, must be experienced. In this way the victim can diminish the painful impact of the experience.

References

Sexual dysfunction
1. Abel GG et al: Self-reported sex crimes of nonincarceted paraphiliacs. *J Interpersonal Violence* 2:3-25, 1987.
2. American Psychiatric Association: *Diagnostic and statistical manual of mental disorders*, ed 4, Washington, DC, 1994, American Psychiatric Association Press.
3. Burgess AW et al: *Child molestation: assessing impact in multiple victims*, Part I, Orlando, Fla. 1987, Grune & Stratton.
4. Burgess AW, editor: *Child pornography and sex rings*, Lexington, Mass, 1984, Lexington Books.
5. Fagan PJ, Schmidt Jr CW: Psychosexual disorders. In Stoudemire, A, editor: *Clinical Psychiatry for medical students*, ed 2, Philadelphia, 1994, JB Lippincott.
6. Finkelhor D: *Child sexual abuse*, New York, 1984, The Free Press.
7. Groth AN: *Men who rape: the psychology of the offender*, New York, 1979, Plenum Press.
8. Kaplan HS: Psychosexual dysfunctions. In Michels R, et al, editors: *Psychiatry*, Philadelphia, 1991, JB Lippincott.
9. Kaplan HS: *Sexual aversion, sexual phobias, and panic disorders*, New York, 1987, Brunner/Mazel.
10. Kaplan HS: *The evaluation of sexual disorders: psychological and medical aspects*, New York, 1983, Brunner/Mazel.
11. Langevin R: Sexual anomalies and the brain. In Marshall WL, Laws DR, Barbaree HE: *Handbook of sexual assault: issues, theories, and treatment of the offender*, New York, 1990, Plenum Press.
12. Masters WS, Johnson VE: *Human sexual inadequacy*, Boston, 1970, Little, Brown.
13. Meyer J, Schmidt C, Wise T, editors: *Clinical management of sexual disorders*, Baltimore, 1983, Williams & Wilkins.
14. Murphy WD, Schwartz ED: Paraphilias. In Soudemire A, editor: *Clinical psychiatry for medical students*, ed 2, Philadelphia, 1994, JB Lippincott.
15. Quinsey VL, Rice ME, Harris GT; *Actuarial prediction of sexual recidivism, J Interpersonal Violence* 10:85-106, 1995.
16. Spector HP, Carey MP: Incidence and prevalence of the sexual dysfunctions; a critical review of impirical literature, *Arch sex Behav* 19:389-408, 1990.
17. Zimmerman ML et al: *Art and group work: interventions for multiple victims of child molestation*, Part II, Orlando Fla, 1987, Grune & Stratton.

Rape-trauma syndrome; rape trauma: compound reaction; rape trauma: silent reaction
1. Burgess AW, Hartman CR: Rape trauma and posttraumatic stress disorder. In McBride A Barron, Austin JK:: *Psychiatric-mental health nursing: integrating the behavioral and biological sciences*, Philadelphia, 1995, WB Saunders.
2. Burgess AW, Holmstrom LL: Rape: sexual disruption and recovery, *Am J Orthopsychiatry* 49:648, 1979.
3. Burgess AW, Holmstrom LL: *Rape: crisis and recovery*, Bowies, Md, 1979, Brady.
4. Burgess AW, Holmstrom LL: Coping behavior and the rape victim, *Am J Psychiatry* 133:413, 1976.
5. Burgess AW, Holmstrom LL: Sexual trauma of children and adolescents: pressure, sex and secrecy, *Nurs Clin North Am* 10:551, 1975.
6. Burgess AW, Holmstrom LL: Rape trauma syndrome, *Am J Psychiatry,* 131:981, 1974.
7. Foa E, Kozak M: Emotional processing of fear: exposure to corrective information, *Psychol Bull* 99:20-35, 1986.
8. Groth AN, Burgess AW, Holmstrom LL: Rape: power, anger and sexuality, *Am J Psychiatry* 134:1239, 1977.
9. Hartman CR, Burgess AW; Information processing of trauma: case application of a model, *J Interpersonal Violence* 3:443-457, 1988.
10. Hazelwood RR: *A behavioral interview of the rape victim*, FBI Bulletin.
11. Hazelwood RR, Rboussin R, Warren JI: Serial rape: correlates of increased aggression and the relationship of offender pleasure to victim resistance, *J Interpersonal Violence* 4:65-78, 1989.
12. Herman J, Hirschman L: Families at risk for father-daughter incest, *Am J Psychiatry* 138:967, 1981.
13. Hilberman E: *The rape victim*, Washington DC, 1976, American Psychiatric Association.
14. Holmstrom LL, Burgess AW: Assessing trauma in the rape victim, *Am J Nurs* 75:1288, 1975.
15. Holmstrom LL, Burgess AW: Sexual behavior of assailants during reported rape, *Arch Sex Behav* 9:427, 1980.
16. Kilpatrick DG, Edmunds CN, Seymour A: *Rape in America*, Arlington, Va, 1992, National Victim Center.
17. Kilpatrick DG, Resick H, Veronen LJ: Effects of a rape—experience longitudinal study, *J Social Issues* 37:105-120, 1981.
18. Russell DEH: *Rape in marriage*, New York, 1982, Macmillan.
19. Ullman SE, Siegel JM: The role of victim-offender relationship in women's sexual assault experiences: Poster, International Society for Traumatic Stress Studies, Los Angeles, October, 1992.
20. Willis CE, Wrightsman LS: Effects of victim gaze behavior and prior relationship on rape culpability attributions, *J Interpersonal Violence* 10:367-377, 1995.

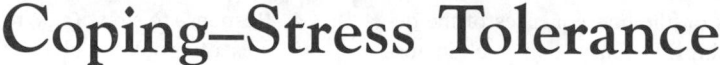

Coping–Stress Tolerance

■ INEFFECTIVE INDIVIDUAL COPING

Ineffective individual coping is the impairment of adaptive behaviors and problem-solving abilities of a person in meeting life's demands and roles.

An integrated model of stress and coping by Rahe[63,64] is presented as an overall framework the nurse can use to assist in integrating the numerous concepts and basic knowledge about the person operating in a complex body system and in a complex environment. Then the chapter presents a view of the person as a self-regulating system in which coping is one of the processes. Finally a transactional system in with coping and cognitive appraisal mediates between the environment and stress encounters is described and outcomes presented.

A skilled, sensitive, thoughtful, caring clinician can perceive the effectiveness of coping efforts as maladaptive or ineffective. Too often one says, "Denial is bad; that illness is the consequence of poor coping; just look at it objectively; put your mind to it; prayer does no good." Browne et al[15] encourages the continued research of coping by nurses. Problems in studying coping are noted by McHaffie.[49] The theories and studies of stress and coping invite further study and application to practice.

The Stress and Coping Model by Rahe[63,64] identifies six steps in processing stress.

Step 1: Life Events

Some changes demand immediate attention by the individual; others seemingly go unnoticed. Forty-two life change events and estimates of the amount of change required have been identified and studied since 1967. Most recently the Recent Life Changes Questionnaire (RLCQ) was rescaled,[64] with death of a spouse ranking first, divorce second, serious personal injury or illness fifth, and change in health or behavior of family member fourteenth. Important factors that vary the perception of an event are past experiences (loss of a pet, loneliness of a latch key child); one's support system (captain of football team, homeless and no friends); constitutional factors (learning disabled, deafness); and demographic characteristics (economically disadvantaged, inability to read, being female, a foreigner, older person).

Step 2: Psychological Defenses

Perceiving the life-change event(s) as threatening evokes a defense. The perception of the event itself may be distorted. ("My buddy died"); but the death of the other 25 people is only briefly mentioned and in awareness. The awareness of the event may be blocked. ("I can't remember anything . . . only a tiny bit.") The response to the threatening event may be distorted. ("I cried and cried;" when he/she was immobilized for a long period of time.) Thus the protective function of psychologic defense mechanisms, or mental mechanisms, becomes apparent.

Valillant[81] divides psychologic defenses into four groups: psychotic defenses (denial of external reality, distortion, delusional projection), immature defenses (projection, passive aggression, acting-out, fantasy), intermediate defenses (dissociation, displacement, repression, reaction formation, intellectualization), and mature defenses (suppression, sublimation, altruism). Bond[11] identified four defense styles using the Defense Style Questionnaire and found maladaptive defenses grouped as (1) withdrawal, regression, acting-out, inhibition, passive-aggression, projection; (2) omnipotence, splitting, primitive idealization; and (3) reaction formation, pseudoaltruism.

No treatment or therapy is required for mature defenses; short-term use of immature and intermediate defenses in situations of overwhelming stress is expected. Psychoanalysis or psychotherapy is used with varying degrees of success for treatment of immature and intermediate defenses. Psychotic defenses are more amenable to treatment with medication to stabilize the central nervous system first followed by psychotherapy. Examples include the administration of antipsychotics to schizophrenics and the detoxification of delirium for the alcoholic. Distortion of reality can be lessened by manipulating the external environment, for example, providing sensory stimulation for the elderly bedridden, the paraplegic, or the infant in intensive care.

Denial may be an effective mechanism, particularly when faced with severe anxiety and conflicts.[44,67,68] Patients dealing with their illness and treatment and perceiving the fear of death, loss, increasing dependency, or self-vulnerability may consciously suppress such thoughts or unconsciously repress them. The effect of the use of denial can be positive if it allows time for adjustment to fact, or if it permits personal functioning without worrying about disability or death. Noncompliance may be a negative consequence of denial. Outcomes of continued noncompliance are increased morbidity for the person and increased disruption of the patient-doctor, patient-nurse relationships.

The defense mechanism is evoked to preserve the self. However, the perception of a self depends on being in relationship to another. Benjamin[8] contends that the determination of a defense as maladaptive depends on the consequences of the defense, particularly to relationships. Defenses that result in hostile behavior or unfriendliness or that do not promote attachment are maladaptive.

Step 3: Psychophysiologic Responsivity

Rahe[63,64] states that the responses to stress on the person may be either within or outside his or her awareness. Changes in mood, increased tenseness of muscles, and headache may occur. More subtle changes such as an increase in blood pressure, a decrease in blood glucose, and an increase in serum lipids, are also occurring.

Increased heart rate, quickened breathing, visual acuity, muscle tension, focus of attention on specific tasks, dry mouth, urinary frequency, and various gastrointestinal symptoms are experienced when a threat is perceived and the autonomic nervous system responds. The central nervous system also acts. For example, the frontal lobe acts to evaluate and control emotions and conduct; the thalamus serves as a connector for sensations; and the hypothalamus contains the pleasure-fear response.

Interrelationships among the autonomic and central nervous systems and the nerve cell based on biochemical reactions create changes leading to excessive amounts or deficits in the neurotransmitters. These chemical messages are associated with anxiety and stress. Either an excess or deficit in the neurotransmitters contributes to the development of symptoms or illness. For example, hypertension or obesity is related to dopamine, a loss of appetite or depression to norepinephrine, increased sedation or hostility to serotonin, psychophysiologic complaints or manic behavior to acetylcholine, impaired recent memory or epilepsy to GABA, and auditory hallucinations or anorexia nervosa to endorphins.[7,18,75,84]

Step 4: Response Reduction

The person seeks to manage the threat or the recent life event and the symptom or response that is produced. One's attention is generally directed to the most uncomfortable sensation. Rahe[64] divides the ways an individual manages into four categories:

1. Social supports (e.g., experiencing the care, concern of family, spouse, a nurse)
2. Health-sustaining habits:
   * Diet (e.g., eating a diet with an abundance of vegetables, fruits, and fiber)
   * Relaxation (e.g., using exercise programs to promote relaxation or sleep)
   * Exercise (e.g., maintaining aerobic fitness and lowering of heart rate and blood pressure through vigorous, regular exercise)
   * Pace (e.g., using one's energy supply gradually to avoid depletion when climbing a hill or doing household tasks)
   * Medication (e.g., short-term relief of anxiety following a severe loss or disaster with an anxiolytic or hypnotic, allowing the person to return to full functioning)

3. Life satisfactions (e.g., participation in creative activities found in work, in family life, in nature, in the arts, in humor, and in religion)
4. Response to stress (e.g., using the coping styles or strategies of problem solving, seeking help from others, of looking for a basis for hope or comfort). (Further description of cognitive and emotion focused coping strategies follows the discussion of the Stress and Coping Model)

People have been assisted in coping through psychotherapeutic interventions and skills training. Some formalized approaches are brief psychotherapies,[80] crisis intervention,[3] relapse prevention,[48] stress inoculation training (SIT),[51] and cognitive therapy.[50]

Step 5: Illness Behavior

Symptoms that cannot be managed become the symptom(s) that cause a person to seek medical attention. Rahe[63,64] describes the associated behaviors as recognition of symptom, believing in the physician as a helpful person, adaption of the sick role, which implies following a treatment plan, seeking medical help, and altering work and/or other activities.

Step 6: Illness Measure

The last step represents the disease as identified by the physician and recorded in the medical record.[63,64] The person will have experienced diagnostic testing and undergone many treatments. Many people do not develop an illness. They manage the stress effectively. Others are overwhelmed by an event(s), may have poor coping techniques and limited coping strategies, and few personal or external resources. An illness develops or a person experiences a series of illnesses.

Leventhal and Nerenz have proposed a *self-regulating system* as a response to illness.[45] The system has three stages or processes with feedback loops.

Input stage (interpretation process). The registering of input from a stimulus through the sense organs to the central nervous system begins the interpretation process. Memory is stimulated and used to develop a cognitive encoding of the stimulus or a schema. Some stimuli arouse powerful emotional schemata, which overwhelm the concrete, factual features of the stimulus. The concrete, affective, and conceptual memories activated result in interpretations of the stimulus/experience/illness. The schema involves symptoms, labels, interpretations, time lines, attributed causes, and expectations. An objective informational system is developed along with a distress or emotional system.

Coping stage (planning and executing processes). The interpretations of the stimulus/experience/illness are crucial to the coping stage. Plans and actions are made to deal with the emotional reactions and with the objective features of the stress/experience/illness. Memories of past symptoms, meanings, time involved, explanations, and outcomes affect the strategies generated and then implemented. It appears important to perceive self as able to cope and have support of others. The distress or emotional system dominates the objective-informational system. When plans and actions are being taken, a pain demands attention before understanding why it is being experienced.

Experiencing pain or hearing the word *cancer* is replete with meanings for a person. Enduring discomfort in a hospital setting is quite different from being in a one-bedroom apartment on the third floor or from having significant family members and professionals quickly available. Also, time is a consideration, e.g., "Will I have to be on a diet for 6 months . . . or the rest of my life?" A person can rationalize a fever as, "All I need is an antibiotic," in an effort to explain symptoms or acknowledge their existence. "Where did I put the pills the doctor gave me for my last cold . . . they will work this time," reflects a belief in things that worked in the past and may again despite professional opinions to the contrary. The outcome of the event/illness varies, e.g., "It was an accident, and it will never happen again." Future plans may need to be changed, as, "I'll never ski, but I can. . . ." It is important for a person to perceive self as able to cope. Having self-esteem affects the plans and actions envisioned. Seeing in one's mind the image of self as coping is vital. Watching another person model desired behaviors and actions and having the support of others also are related to effective coping.

Monitoring stage (appraisal and evaluation processes). The outcomes of the actions taken are compared with the goals set. Feedback obtained regarding emotional states is foremost when the coping process is governed by automatic process of the emotional system. Assistance may be needed, because the information gathered or interpreted may be incomplete, not related to the situation, inaccurate, and/or conflictual. Informational system data are easier for the person to appraise. Achieving a representation of the stimuli/event/illness, and of the self as able to act results in a more stable state. An unstable, self-regulating system demonstrates behaviors characterized by inconsistency, unevenness, purposelessness, distress, unhappiness, and threats.

Another conceptualization describes a transactional system[25,43] to explain how the person and environment interact. This further expands particularly Steps 1, 2, and 4 of the Stress and Coping model.

"Coping 'refers' to the person's cognitive and behavioral efforts to manage (reduce, minimize, master or tolerate) the internal and external demands of the person-environment transaction that is appraised as taxing or exceeding the persons' resources."[25] Regulation of the emotions and management of the person-environment are the two functions of coping in this model.

Coping is the result of appraisals made by the person. A primary appraisal evaluates the negative and positive effects on the self, one's goals or values, and commitments. In addition, a determination of possible actions is done, which is a secondary appraisal. The appraisals result in ideas that serve to guide the strategies developed, i.e., What threat is it to the self? What is the meaning? What can be predicted? What is the degree of control for the individual?

The coping strategies are divided into problem-focused and emotion-focused groups. Problem-focused strategies include confrontation, information seeking, direct actions, and seeking help from others. These strategies function to determine or alter the consequences of stimulus/event/illness or the cognitive actions and/or functioning. Emotion-focused strategies serve to regulate the emotions.

The immediate and long-term effects of the patient's appraisal and coping processes are the outcomes. Effects can be demonstrated (1) by observing feeling states (satisfaction, pleasure, disgust, anger), noting appraisal process (active versus avoiding) and (2) by monitoring coping. Long-term effects are noted as an increase or decrease in social functioning, in psychologic well-being, and in the presence of various illnesses.

Conceptualization of the process of coping used by children is under study. The variable of constantly changing developmental levels complicates investigations. Also, the dependency on the caregiver(s), as a major factor in the process of coping, must be considered.

For children there is no consensus of a common list of defenses or coping mechanisms, although there is agreement that age, sex, and cognitive and ego development affect coping of children. Sorensen[76] has grouped children's coping efforts into three domains: cognitive behavior, cognitive-intrapsychic, and interpersonal. In the cognitive-behavior domain, the more frequent occupying responses were in submission/endurance, problem solving, emotional expression, distraction, and behavioral reframing. In the cognitive-intrapsychic domain, coping categories were emotional/sensory, thought reframing, and analyzing/intellectualizing. In the interpersonal domain the categories of mother and others were the focus of coping efforts. Stress arose from relationships; the child experienced stress about friends, school, brothers and sisters, and disappointments.

In the last few years, nursing researchers have examined age and gender differences and changes in stressors and coping strategies of children.[70] Another study focused on the coping methods of rural adolescents.[62] Ritchie[66] studied the effects of cancer on psychosocial development of adolescents. The areas more affected were self-concept and self-esteem; both were lowered. Another study focused on coping strategies of children dealing with medical procedures.[83] Better distress ratings and appropriate behaviors were found in children adjusting to stressors rather than attempting to change the conditions.

Related Factors*

Relationship Impairments/Changes

Loss of loved one
Change in school
Divorce, separation
Birth, abortion
Change of health of family member
Marriage

---

*References 4, 22, 30-33, 35, 36, 39, 40, 42, 56-59, 60, 63, 64.

Physical/Psychologic Impairment/Change

Major illness, injury
Threat, impending death
Pain
Sexual, physical, or emotional abuse
Autonomic or central nervous system deficits
Hormonal changes, menopause
Immunologic deficits
Memory loss
Sensory/perceptual impairment (e.g., blindness, deafness)
Personality disorders
High anxiety level
Conflict arising from incompatible motives and goals

Impaired Self-Efficacy/Self-Concept

Powerlessness
Impaired competency
Lack of reason to live
Failure to feel valued by others
Personal achievement
Lack of optimism
Degree of hardiness
Life-style change

Situational/Contextual Impairment/Change

Major disasters (e.g., war, nature)
Lack of adequate resources (e.g., financial)
Sociocultural stressors
Retirement
Major purchases (e.g., home)
Vacation, holidays
Loss of job
Overload/daily hassles
Multiple repetitive stressors over time
Treatments for illness
Diagnostic testing
Exhaustion of available treatments
Lack of social support
Lack of time

Inaccurate Appraisal of Stress/Event/Illness

Inability to make valid appraisal of situation
Inability to redefine or interpret threat correctly
Inability to identify skills, knowledge, and abilities to cope with threat
Lack of clear, realistic goals or outcomes
Unresolved memories of past threats or negative experiences
Premature cognitive appraisal as noted in stereotypical behavior ("I always do it this way.")

Inadequate Response Repertoire

Difficulty in expressing feelings
Use of behavior destructive to self or others
Inability to seek out or to learn new skills and knowledge
Inability to deal with tangible consequences of stress/event/illness

Increasing emotional responsiveness or lack of objective responsiveness
Defensive avoidance of dealing with threatening situations
Lack of assertive behaviors
Impaired communication skills
Lack of palliative skills
Inability to seek out and use a social support system
All are affected by age, race, gender, ethnicity, culture.*

Inappropriate Deployment of Coping Resources

Inability to develop alternative goals, plans, actions, and rewards
Lack of ability to transfer knowledge and skills to actual problem resolution
Giving up hope and spiritual values
Social withdrawal
Difficulty in using problem-solving skills and decision-making skills
Concerns and/or fears about initiating action
Lack of supportive social network

Defining Characteristics†

Presence of a "Bad Event", Disease, Stress-related Illness, Stress Reaction, or Physiologic Disturbance

Diabetes
Hypertension
Cancer
Drug abuse or dependence
Catastrophic event
Increased anxiety
Headache, stomach pain, back pain
Frequent colds
Accident proneness

Presence of Impairment in Work/Social Functioning

Overdependence on others
Nonproductive life-style
Nonperformance of activities of daily living
Lack of functioning in usual social roles
Poor parenting
Refusal or rejection of help

Disruption in Relationship(s)

Detachment from usual social supports
Inappropriate aggressiveness

Presence of Individual Characteristics

High anxiety
Lack of planning for future
Pessimism
Dissatisfaction with life

---

*References 16, 23, 54, 69, 71, 72.
†References 7, 12, 24, 25, 31, 32, 36, 43, 45, 51, 53, 63, 64, 79, 81.

Inflexibility
Self-focus and strong feelings
Worrying
High anxiety or increased psychological distress

Presence of Defensive Patterns

Hypervigilance
Avoidance
Denial
Dissociation
Blaming
Taking no responsibility
Continuous mourning for the lost or longing for the past
Psychotic defenses

Expected Patient Outcomes & Nursing Interventions*

Acknowledge the presence/help of nurse as part of support system to assist in process of coping, as evidenced by:

Recognizing nurse
Describing event or problem to nurse
Interacting with nurse
Listening to comments from nurse
- Provide 1:1 nurse/patient relationship times.
- Use supportive techniques.

Has beginning appraisal of stress/illness, as evidenced by:

Describing event as to who, what, when, where, how, why
Relating time sequences
Identifying beliefs about what should be or should not be
Describing role of significant others
- Explore perception of the event by encouraging full description.
- Raise questions; encourage data gathering; and promote attitude of openness to new information.

Make accurate appraisal of emotional reactions to stress/illness, as evidenced by:

Describing what is feared; what is threatening to self
Describing feelings experienced
Relating feelings to event/illness
Using new facts to redefine threat or fears
- Give empathetic responses to expressions of feelings to encourage acceptance of these feelings in self.
- Elicit what patient fears or what causes anger or depression.
- Give feedback about behavior observed and feelings expressed.
- Assist in identifying feelings with names that are acceptable and understandable to patient.

- Assist in developing ideas about relationship of patient's emotional and consequent thought patterns and behaviors.
- Provide factual information about threatening stimulus.

Make accurate objective appraisal of the stress/illness, as evidenced by:

Identifying various sources of stress
Using facts to redefine misinformation
- Provide preparatory information to patients undergoing new procedures and experiences.
    Describe sounds, smells, tastes, and appearances.
    Explain causes of sensations.
    Give information about how long pain, procedure, or treatment will last.
- Avoid evaluative statements when providing information.
- Work through unresolved memories of events; use image-based reconstruction.
- Encourage medical, social work, legal, and other consultation to assist in interpretations.
- Give patient conceptual model for understanding event or treatment regimen.

Use coping responses for emotional reactions to stress/illness, as evidenced by:

Expressing feelings appropriately
Experiencing decreased emotional responsiveness
Experiencing increased objectivity and ability to problem solve
Communicating needs and plans
Identifying way to reduce anxiety, aggression, depression
Demonstrating no behavior destructive to self or others
- Assist patient in reduction of anxiety by use of distraction, recreational, and diversional activities, as well as working through feelings of anxiety.
- Foster constructive outlets for anger and hostility by teaching warning signs of outbursts, ways to gain self-control, and ways to express anger appropriately.
- Assist patient to work through denial or other defensive avoidance and hypervigilance, which may impede decision making.
- Encourage attitude of realistic hope as way to deal with feelings of helplessness.
- Teach relaxation techniques.
- Teach effect of negative self-reflections and derogatory ideas on emotional reactions.
- Foster expression feelings through open communication.
- Encourage socialization and social support.
- Use music therapy.

Use coping resources for the objective features of the stress/illness, as evidenced by:

Talking with others about stress/illness and joining mutual support group
Using problem-solving skills
Finding personal meaning for event
- Assist in identifying and making changes in health behaviors that are necessary because of stress/illness.

*References 2, 5, 6, 8, 9, 10, 13-15, 19, 20, 25, 27-29, 34, 37, 38, 41, 43, 45, 46, 47, 51, 52, 61, 73, 75, 77, 78, 82.

- Serve as role model and/or social support when helping patient perform activities of daily living.
- Teach patient skill involving problem solving, decision making, assertive communication, goal setting, evaluation, study, palliative coping, and relaxation.
- Assist in identifying coping responses patient is using and other possible ones.
- Engage patient in role rehearsal and mental imagery for active social role participation.
- Teach patient to monitor self for noneffective thoughts about self or maladaptive behaviors.
- Explore past situations in which effective coping behaviors were demonstrated.
- Assist in biofeedback by giving information about pulse and blood pressure as patient uses relaxation technique.
- Provide constructive tasks to perform and ignore responses that are nonproductive and interfering.

Deploy coping resources, as evidenced by:

Having alternative goals, plans, actions, and rewards

Using knowledge and skills leaned in past or in training sessions to achieve problem resolution

Using support system and/or developing own supportive network

Using hope and spiritual values

Using problem-solving and decision-making skills

Initiating action

Using cognitive cues to indicate appropriate actions

Demonstrating appropriate use of others, including professional persons

- Provide practice and use in real situations.
- Confront patient about impaired judgment when appropriate.
- Assist patient in determining reasonable goals.
- Provide feedback to patient, and assist in eliciting feedback from others.
- Assist patient to develop cues for self to indicate whether he or she is reacting automatically or objectively.
- Discuss importance of locus of control in maintaining sense of self-effectiveness.

Evaluate impact of coping response, as evidenced by:

Identify current productive life-style

Identifying view of self as performing useful social roles

Seeking ways to assist others

- Teach evaluation process as an ongoing appraisal (1) of the threats or situation being encountered; (2) of perception of self as coping successfully or failing; (3) of the adequate use of resources within self and those available; and (4) of desired outcomes.

Principles and Rationale for Nursing Interventions

Research on interventions to manage stress supports the importance of assessing the population receiving the interventions, of assessing the situational variables, and of providing information, modeling, and behavior-cognitive techniques to improve problem- and/or emotion-focused coping.

Some strategies designed to encompass both emotional and informational aspects are presented. Stress inoculation training is based on cognitive theory and involves three phases: conceptualization; skills acquisition; application, follow-through, and rehearsal.[51] Patients are assisted in analysis of their stress-related problems to understand the relationships among feelings, thoughts, and behavior. Automatic thoughts and feelings are disclosed. Patients then are taught several coping techniques, which generally include relaxation training, problem-solving training, cognitive restructuring, and guided self-dialogue. Finally, the therapist provides opportunities to practice the skills using imaginal and behavioral rehearsal, as well as the real-life situations.

The following studies are a sampling of the literature that illustrates the use, effectiveness, and value of interventions to enhance the coping processes of a person.

Assessment of stressors and coping techniques of specific populations/groups:

    Cancer and chemotherapy outpatients[22]

    Chronic obstructive pulmonary disease[57]

    Multiple sclerosis[59]

    Experiencing diagnostic exercise stress testing[35]

    Incest survivors[21]

    Breast biopsy[58]

    Breast cancer[42]

    Eating disorders[79]

    Periodontal surgeries[5]

    Cardiac catheterization[6]

    Pregnancy[2]

    Caregivers of persons with AIDS[26]

    Spouses or significant other of multiple sclerosis patients[30]

    Family care givers in hospice home care[33]

Providing information, modeling:

    Preparation for invasive medical procedure[46]

    Unplanned hospitalization for child and parent[52]

    Cardiac catheterization[20]

Skill training

    Prosocial coping to youth[9]

    Coping skill training to schizophrenics[13]

    Coaching skills in coping promotion to parents[10]

    Social skills to alcoholics[55]

    Techniques for auditory hallucinations[27]

    Cognitive behavior skills to women with premenstrual symptoms[37]

Programs for specific groups:

    Elderly in nursing homes[14]

    Low-birth-weight children[1,65]

    Management of dyspnea[17]

■ DEFENSIVE COPING

Defensive coping is the state in which an individual experiences a falsely positive self-evaluation based on a self-protective pattern that defends against underlying perceived threats to positive self-regard.

A defensive reaction is one in which the individual responds to stressors by demonstrating behaviors indicative of an unrealistic or falsely positive self-evaluation. This type of reaction serves to defend against perceived threats to emotional safety and security. Coping strategies may be classified as *problem-focused* (aimed at managing the perceived problem or situation) or as *emotion-focused* (directed toward managing the emotional distress and the threat to self that the event represents).[5,11] Emotion-focused coping happens when individuals have cognitively appraised the event as one that is either not responsive to problem-solving or requires more resources or abilities than the person perceives himself or herself to have.[5,11]

Emotion-focused coping involves the use of ego defense mechanisms, unconsciously called into use whenever the ego determines to protect itself against unpleasant or unwanted feelings, threats, or anxieties. When these defense mechanisms are successful in protecting the self-image, preventing feelings of shame, fear, and despair or when they effectively control anxiety, the ego's use of protective defenses is reinforced, and the ego learns to protect itself in the same way when encountering the next similar or similarly perceived stressor.[5,11]

All persons unconsciously use defense mechanisms to greater or lesser degrees; research has indicated that an individual's preference of specific defense mechanisms may be present from birth.[3] One mode is not necessarily preferable to another, (the efficacy and desirability needing to be determined for each individual) and context.[3,10,16] It is increasingly understood that a person's culture profoundly influences both appraisal of events and what are seen to be appropriate defense mechanisms and coping behaviors.[1,2,7,10,13]

The diagnosis of defensive coping is made when the individual struggles to reach a state of psychic equilibrium and unsuccessfully resolves the crisis by developing an unrealistically positive sense of self-esteem, interfering with his or her ability to take in and process information from the environment for problem-solving, role fulfillment, and reciprocal, interpersonal relationships.[5,12] The resultant behaviors are not perceived as socially acceptable by others, and the response of others to the individual may further stimulate the development of more socially aggressive maladaptive behaviors. Any number of combinations of the defining characteristics can be manifested by the individual who experiences defensive coping. Generally, the individual denies any obvious problems or weaknesses (denial) and blames others for personal shortcomings (projection). Failures are rationalized, and hypersensitivity to the slightest criticism (which questions the rationalization)[16] tends to affect interpersonal communications. Subsequent difficulties ensue as a superior attitude, intellectualization, and ridicule of others (reaction formation) erode existing relationships and prohibit the establishment of new ones.[5,12]

Related Factors

Repeated negative past experiences
Cognitive/perceptual difficulties
Excessive ridicule by others
Unresolved emotionally traumatic experiences
Multiple stressors
Negative interpretation of life events
Inadequate coping strategies
Inadequate social relationships
Psychiatric disorders
Lack of realistic goals for self
Lack of insight into behavior
Learned family behavior pattern
Victim of abusive/dysfunctional parents (e.g., alcholic family syndrome)

Defining Characteristics

Denial (of obvious problems/weaknesses)
Projection (of blame/responsibility)
Rationalization of failures
Defensiveness; hypersensitivity to slight criticism
Grandiosity
Superior attitude toward others
Difficulty establishing or maintaining relationships
Hostile laughter or ridicule of others
Difficulty in reality-testing perceptions
Lack of follow-through or participation in treatment or therapy
Intellectualization
Seeking special attention or privilege
Attention-seeking behavior
Refuses or rejects assistance from others
Domineering, authoritative
Autocratic management style
Exaggerated self-importance
Avoidance of intimacy
Difficulty in accepting praise
Criticizes readily
Aggressiveness: "bullies" others
Haughty
Abject self-righteousness
Perceived omnipotence

Expected Patient Outcomes & Nursing Interventions

Experience increased feelings of security and worthiness, as evidenced by:

Decreasing verbalizations of anxiety, fear, shame
Stating an understanding of origins and the functioning of defensive coping behaviors

- Establish therapeutic alliance *to reduce sense of threat and anxiety and to preserve the patient's integrity as behaviors and feelings are examined.*[5,12,13]
- Consider cultural expressions and values *to facilitate a culturally responsive and mutually acceptable treatment plan.*[1,2,6]
- Assess self-concept and the underlying reasons for behavior *to understand the purpose and protective function the defense serves and to judge the appropriateness of intervening.*[5,11,12]

- Explore patient's past experiences with similar situations and problems *to determine cognitive appraisal and the personal meaning influencing usual patterns of coping and defending.*[1,11]

Experience decreased feelings of defensiveness and use of maladaptive defense mechanisms, as evidenced by:

Demonstrating realistic appraisal of personal strengths, needs
Acknowledging responsibility for own feelings and behaviors
Demonstrating respect for others in interpersonal relationships
Using feedback to modify cognitions and behaviors
Accepting praise without criticizing own or others' efforts
Fulfilling role or situational obligations
Seeking and participating in required assistance or therapy
Using reality-based problem solving

- Let patient know you understand that coping behavior to date represents his/her best efforts *to maintain self-esteem and decrease feelings of failure.*[4]
- Respect and support reality-based aspects of defenses *to provide a secure base from which the patient can begin to identify unwanted feelings and behavioral alternatives.*[5,12,16]
- Negotiate with the patient the particular behaviors they desire to change *to respect his/her right to be involved in decision making and to enhance appraisals of self-efficacy.*[5,12,15]
- Provide information about coping and defense mechanisms and assist patient to relate this knowledge to their personal situation *to decrease feelings of shame and help them understand the universality of defenses and the protective function their behavior serves.*[4,5,8]
- Assist patient in detailing past situations in which he or she demonstrated change and used effective strategies in response to stressors *to encourage considering the possibility of changing his or her current models of response and to enhance his or her perceptions of his or her strengths and coping skills.*[5,12,16]
- Be aware of personal responses to patient *to facilitate maintenance of a neutral, nonjudgmental approach.*[2,5,9,12]
- Teach assertive behavior techniques *to replace aggressive behaviors.*[12]
- Encourage patient to keep a journal of situations in which he or she notes increased anxiety or discomfort, subsequent behavior, and the response the behavior elicit from others *to assist the patient to more objectively evaluate the efficacy of current methods of coping.*[8]
- Provide patient with immediate feedback about problematic behaviors *to assist in reality testing.*[16]
- Gently clarify distortions in thinking *to help the patient separate personal feelings from the reality of the situation.*[4,5,14,16]
- Use role-playing techniques *to model appropriate interactions and provide a safe palce to try out new communication skills.*[5,14]

- Support the patient as the meaning of the situation, feelings about the event, the actions required, and the desired goals and options for response, are explored.[5,12]

Principles and Rationale for Nursing Interventions

The focus of nursing interventions for defensive coping is to assist patients to understand the origins of their behavior and to work through them so that positive interrelationships can be established and maintained with others.[5,12,16] The nurse must keep foremost in mind that the function, cultural relevance and the situational appropriateness of defense strategies needs to be individually determined before deciding to intervene.[5,7,8,16] Interventions which reduce the patient's perception of threat and the attendent negative emotions, while increasing the fragile self's perception of its abilities, are most likely to preserve the patient's integrity and assist him or her to consider moving outside his or her defended but distorted reality.[5,12,16] Socially acceptable behaviors are promoted that result in positive feedback and therefore become self-perpetuating as secondary gains for inappropriate behavior are removed.[12]

INEFFECTIVE DENIAL

Ineffective denial is the unconscious attempt of an individual to disavow the knowledge or impact of a problem that can threaten or jeopardize his or her health.

Coping adequately and effectively with health problems and their potential or actual consequences is an ongoing process involving the interplay of several factors. One key factor is the interpretation of the event or illness and the perceived consequences for the individual. The actual threat of an illness may not be matched by a reality-based perception and interpretation by the patient. What may be a threatening, anxiety-provoking illness to one person may not necessarily be so for another person. Previous coping skills, self-confidence, and ability to deal with emotions constitute a second set of factors. A history of successful previous coping, effective coping skills, a positive self-concept, and the ability to deal constructively with the emotions created by a stressor such as illness all mitigate the response to illness. Finally, the environment, including social resources, is critically important in shaping a patient's coping response to a major illness. When this overall adaptive coping process falters and becomes less effective, or the stressors become increasingly threatening, ineffective coping responses may come into play. Among these is ineffective denial.

Denial is a defense mechanism in which a person avoids acknowledging a threatening situation or a loss. For example, "one of the most difficult aspects of treatment for alcoholism or other drug dependence is overcoming denial . . . They commonly believe that they do not have a problem with alcohol or other drugs, even in the face of overwhelming evidence to the contrary."[22, p. 463] The situation is unconsciously changed to something different, thereby reducing the pain or anxiety resulting from reality.[21] Reality can be distorted in varying degrees depending on the type of denial (i.e., denial of "information, threat, personal relevance, urgency, vulnerability/responsibility, affect and affect relevance").[12, p. 188] Denial serves as a buffer to the pain of reality.[21] Denial can be defined as the repudiation of an illness or its impact. It is often an initial reaction to threatening health status information,[8] occurring most frequently when the person has no way to reduce the threat effectively and quickly.[13]

Denial can facilitate coping behavior; it enables the person to cope with a threat or loss or death anxiety related to terminal illness and to cope with intolerable feelings of anxiety, pain, fear, rage, or sadness.[8] Denial can be valuable in coping, if it does not keep the person from adjusting to the situation.[21] In certain illnesses (e.g., patients with heart disease) denial may have a bimodal effect: denial is associated with less behavioral dysfunction and better survival during surgery and in the immediate postoperative period, while denial is associated with decreased compliance and increased morbidity in the long term. With strong levels of denial, patients may inappropriately ignore life-threatening signs and symptoms; they rarely seek medical advice and follow it.[24]

There may be several measurable aspects to denial, as for example in heart transplantation patients. One form of denial—denial related to emotional responsiveness—may imply poorer prognosis for heart transplantation. Another form of denial—denial emphasizing the physical or the physiologic threat—may be more closely related to survival from heart surgery or intensive care.[10] The Illness Behavior Denial Scale[10] is recommended for clinical use to measure denial. Other scales to measure denial are available (e.g., the Alcoholism Denial Assessment Tool [ADAT]).[23]

Ineffective denial is manifested in maladaptive coping behaviors, such as rejecting facts and refusing essential medical treatment.[9,15,20] These patients often delay medical attention, do not admit to negative consequences of their current illnesses, do not accept loss of body parts or function, and are often self-absorbed.

Related Factors[11,18]

Fear of consequences of health problem (e.g, treatment, pain, death, or stigma)
Fear of hospitalization
Perception of being healthy despite contrary diagnostic findings
Sense of invincibility
Overwhelming stressors
Overwhelming feelings (anxiety, anger, depression)
Severe aggression
Authoritarian manner
Chronic avoidance pattern
Negative past experiences
Learned response pattern
Lack of knowledge
Inadequate coping skills
Lack of social support network
Personal or family value system and beliefs
Lack of adequate resources (money)
Cultural factors

Defining Characteristics[11]

No perception of personal relevance and consequences of signs or symptoms
Minimization of consequences of illness
Perception of being healthy despite contrary findings
Minimization of known loss of body function or part
Avoidance of acceptance of loss of body part or function
Rejection of facts in face of known anger to health
Minimization of signs or symptoms
Displacement of source of symptoms
Delay in seeking medical attention
Failure to admit fear of invalidism or death
Refusal of medical attention
Displacement of fear of impact of health problems
Display of inappropriate affect
Blaming others for distressing facts
Self-absorption
Refusal to master adaptive skills to illness
Refusal to master adaptive skills to therapeutic regimen
Persistent noncompliance
Changes in interpersonal relationships
Changes in daily life-style patterns (escape behaviors)

Expected Patient Outcomes & Nursing Interventions*

Seek and accept appropriate treatment for health problems, or palliative care as evidenced by:

Seeking medical attention
Being compliant with medical treatment regimen
Verbalizing understanding of health problem and consequences
Exhibiting appropriate and emotional responses to significance of health problem
Coping adequately and realistically with health problem
Experiencing an improved health status
Coping with terminal illness and impending death
- Assess presence of denial:
  Ask questions such as "Tell me why you think you are here and about your present health condition?"
  Give the patient the chance to either deny the illness or acknowledge a degree of concern.
- Assess level of knowledge about illness, personal beliefs and values, and perceptions of situation *because it is important to determine the role such factors play in behavior manifested and to diagnose denial accurately.*
- Assess seriousness of situation and whether continuation of denial will be harmful to patient's life or well-being; *in certain illnesses, such as acute myocardial infarction, delays caused by denial can be life threatening.*

*References 1, 4-7, 9, 11, 13-19, 21, 24.

- Assess patient's level of denial, dynamics involved in the denial, and readiness to accept reality of situation; *it is important to reduce threatening information if the patient is experiencing a high level of denial, unless the patient is in a life-threatening situation and immediate action is required. If denial is not interfering with patient's care and treatment, it may have a therapeutic role for the patient.*
- Determine level of patient's fear and other emotions.
- Decrease fears, such as fear of hospitalization.
- Stress successful outcomes of others as a result of hospitalization and treatment.
- Allow patient to have control over aspects of the treatment regimen.
- Encourage significant others to be supportive.
- Assess support system.
- Assess level of knowledge about subject and consequences of health problem. *Too much information given to a patient at one time may lead to the patient's withdrawal. It is useful to provide information in such a way so that the patient understands it will help him/her gain control.*
- Determine cultural and personal values related to health care or specific problem.
- Assess and use patient's previous coping strategies and patterns.
- Be accessible to patient *to encourage open communication.*
- Be aware of own response to denial *to ensure therapeutic interactions with patient.*
- Agree only with parts of statements that are true *to avoid reinforcing denial.*
- Ensure patient and family have all appropriate information and objective appraisal regarding diagnoses, treatment, and consequences.
- Reduce myths and misconceptions.
- Provide supportive atmosphere for patient, without becoming angry or blaming patient for denial.
- Do not intervene when denial is at a low level, does not interfere with functioning, and appears temporary *because denial can serve as a protective function and can be adaptive.*
- Do not use direct confrontation *because it can increase anxiety and the need for denial.*
- Provide for a supportive team member to meet and discuss diagnosis with patient (e.g., social worker, counselor, clinical nurse specialist).
- Develop with family and other caregivers a timetable for introduction of reality.
- Encourage trusted family member or close friend to talk gently but openly with patient regarding need for treatment.
- Assist patient in developing awareness of usual cognitive and emotional responses to health problem.
- Gradually point out behaviors exhibited by patient that contradict the reality of the situation.
- Graduallly point out potential loss or risk associated with illness and treatment *to avoid increasing patient's anxiety.*

- In collaboration with other disciplines, involve family system, when appropriate, in confronting patient with denial about chemical dependence.[22]
- Convey a sense of realistic hope; *describing the successful health outcomes of others with similar health problems may lessen threat to patient, reduce anxiety, and decrease the need for denial.*
- Provide adequate reassurance.
- Incorporate cultural patterns and resources into intervention strategies.
- Refer to supportive self-help groups.
- Refer for pyschotherapy, *which may be indicated in severe and prolonged denial.*
- For patients with terminal illness and facing impending death:
    Support patient's use of denial as a coping strategy.
    Assist staff in resolving personal conflict that can arise from patient's use of denial as a coping mechanism.

Principles and Rationale for Nursing Interventions

The nurse needs to conduct a thorough assessment to intervene in denial to avoid destroying the patient's defense mechanisms. Assessment of family members is imperative to identify the extent to which they support the denial. The nurse needs to intervene in denial at an appropriate level, based on urgency of the situation. Also, the nurse must ensure that the staff and other caregivers are aware of cultural differences.

IMPAIRED ADJUSTMENT

Impaired adjustment is the inability to adapt to the stressful and problematic aspects associated with a change in health status. The inability to adapt can extend to nonadherence to recommended therapeutic regimens.[9] The patient may be unable to incorporate health/illness behavior into the repetoire of daily living.[5]

The individual with impaired adjustment may experience difficulty handling responsibilities and fulfilling personal needs and goals as well. The inability to modify attitudes and behaviors after a change in health status interferes with an individual's initiating and maintaining constructive relationships with family, peers, and society.

Related Factors*

Loss of previous physical and/or mental abilities
Fluctuations of exacerbation and remission of illness
Disability requiring change in life-style
Impaired cognition

---

*References 1, 5, 9, 11, 12, 14-16, 18, 19, 21.

Progression of disabiilty, despite adherence to recommended regimen

Sensory overload

Loss of self-esteem

Altered locus of control

Incomplete grieving

Treatment side effects, discomforts, and risks

Complexity of health regimen

Amount of changes required

Lack of direct access for obtaining care

Lack of confidence in health care providers

Dissatisfaction with health care system

Increased confinement and social isolation

Perceived beliefs of others

Alteration in self-care, family, and/or work roles

Significant others alternating between overprotection and rejection

Inadequate support systems

Inadequate, dwindling financial resources

Uncertainty, lack of predictability of future

Inability to achieve career goals

Defining Characteristics[15,19]

Verbalization of nonacceptance of health status change

Extended period of shock, disbelief, or anger regarding health status change

Nonexistent or unsuccessful ability to be involved in problem solving or goal setting

Lack of adherence to recommended therapeutic regimens

Lack of movement toward independence

Lack of future-oriented thinking

Expected Patient Outcomes & Nursing Interventions*

Resolve feelings of loss related to change in health status, as evidenced by:

Acknowledging losses that accompany change in health status

- Promote therapeutic alliance with patient *to encourage ongoing expression of feelings of distress related to changes.*
- Provide opportunity for expression of fear of disease and death *to evaluate for distorted perceptions.*
- Avoid trivialization of patient's fright and distress.
- Encourage patient and family to share mutual feelings and perceptions of loss, including impact of change in health status on social life of patient and family.
- Recognize influence of premorbid personality and past coping mechanisms on patient's current adaptation.
- Avoid conveying blame to patient for current health problems.

---

*References 2-14, 16-18, 20-25.

Modify life-style to experience maximum control and self-sufficiency within limitations imposed by changed health status, as evidenced by:

Verbalizing recognition of influence of self-care practices on own health care outcomes.

Refocusing attention to address other aspects and concerns in life, besides health status change

- Provide factual information regarding disability, treatment, and prognosis *based on assessment of patient's identification of learning needs and readiness.*
- Recognize influence of age of onset, previous family functioning, and severity of illness on patient's and family's understanding of impact of illness.
- Teach patient and family to differentiate between denial of *presence* of change in health status and denial of *possible limitations.*
- Assist patient to identify previous coping behaviors and support systems used for past problem solving *to mobilize hope for coping with current situation.*
- Collaborate with patient to develop individually tailored health care regimen *using observations from assessment of patient behaviors indicative of external versus internal locus of control and high versus low hardiness to maximize patient's potential for successful adaptation.*
- Assess for possible correlation between perceived beliefs of family and patient's willingness to participate in plan of care.
- Teach family to elicit *patient's* perceptions of difficulties as opposed to *the family's* possible intrepretations and explanations.
- Recognize influence of role disruption that might be experienced (e.g., occupational, family, sexual).
- Assist patient and family to explore positive aspects associated with management of change in health status, (e.g., increase in mutual family support, recognition of family strengths).
- Explore patient's perceptions of how changed health status and treatment will affect life-style.
- Encourage identification of current remaining personal strengths and intact roles.
- Support patient's use of personal and/or formal spiritual beliefs.
- Encourage patient and family communication that is not related to patient's health problems (e.g., current events, family activities, hobbies, recreational plans) *to avoid making health problem a focal point of interaction.*

Assume responsibility for using personal and social resources to assist in ongoing health management, as evidenced by:

Seeking help from and accepting assistance from competent caregivers

Demonstrating self-care practices that are within prescribed regimen

Making plans for future that are congruent with change in health status

Using available community resources and support networks so as to engage in maximally independent and constructive lifestyle.

- Collaborate with health team in the development of strategies to control and manage patient's health status change.
- Teach patient negotiating strategies for discussing decision-making issues with health care providers.
- Facilitate compromise when patient's identified goals differ from goals developed by health care providers.
- Recognize influence of cultural factors on patient's participation with health care system and compliance with treatments.
- *Promote patient's maintaining a sense of control* by encouraging patient to:

    Make decisions related to specific aspects of care.

    Evaluate treatments and therapies in terms of patient's goals.

    Share observations of status and progress with caregivers.

    Assume accountability for select aspects of care (e.g., active range of motion, tracheostomy and colostomy care).

- Collaborate with patient to identify factors that interfere with adhering to recommended health regimen.
- Provide referrals, as appropriate, to patient education groups (e.g., medication), patient/family support groups led by health professional(s).
- Include family, as well as the patient, in discussion of planned health care regimen, and assess for possible correlation between extent of family's willingness to support patient's changed life-style and patient's ability to adapt to change in health status.
- Use cognitive behavioral interventions for patients who convey feelings of extreme helplessness *to facilitate achievement of a more realistic perception of assets and limitations associated with disability.*
- Promote patient's engaging in self-monitoring activities (e.g., blood pressure, diet, rest, activity patterns) *to strengthen self-directed modification in life-style.*
- Convey recognition of patient's self-help tips and strategies (e.g., home remedies that work, improvising needed equipment in the home to avoid unnecessary financial expenditures).
- Assist patient to develop plan for stress management (e.g., relaxation exercises, use of imagery).
- Assist patient to examine: own values and beliefs; perceptions of family, caregivers, and society to change in health status; current physical and mental well-being; and availability of resources to assist with physical or mental limitations.
- Assist patient to develop realistic goals and plans for self, within context of factors just listed.
- Collaborate with patient to develop health care regimen that can be incorporated within work setting.
- Inform patient about generic medications and discount stores for obtaining supplies and equipment, and help pa-

tient to differentiate between essential and less necessary equipment to maintain health regimen *to minimize financial expenditures.*

- Encourage patient and family to explore social resources (e.g., Medicare, Medicaid, Crippled Children's Programs, Social Security Disability Insurance).
- Encourage patient to capitalize on social support from relatives, friends, and colleagues in work setting.
- Refer patient and family to self-help organizations and support groups for assistance with ongoing informational needs, advocacy issues, and current developments in treatment and research.

Principles and Rationale for Nursing Interventions

The patient who experiences a change in health status faces losses that range from mild to severe. Successful adjustment to these changes includes an acknowledgement of and appropriate grieving for losses that are a part of the health change. The patient's family, as well as the patient, must grieve.[14] Interventions that incorporate recognition of the frightening or destructive aspects of the change in health status for the patient and family contribute to resolution of the intensity of the feelings of loss and promote a redirecting of attention to other rewarding aspects in life.[8,13,22,25]

Nursing interventions should be designed to encourage patients to evaluate the effectiveness of therapies and treatments and to actively participate in the ongoing decision-making aspects of their health care management. Such interventions can significantly influence patients' perceptions of their ability to experience maximum control and self-sufficiency.[10]

Successful development and implementation of plans for stress management and adherence to a health care regimen that can be incorporated within the work setting are indicators of the patient's ability to use personal resources. Patients who experience a change in health status frequently need formalized help from community resources, in addition to the help provided by the health team. Self-help and support groups can foster mutual encouragement and empathy, as well as a sense of belonging and support, in coping with the stigmatizing that occurs with certain health problems.[6,14,16]

▎ POSTTRAUMA RESPONSE

Posttrauma response is the state of an individual experiencing a sustained, painful response to an unexpected, extraordinary life event(s).

Posttrauma response (PTR) is characterized by a range of emotional responses, from fear and anger to flashbacks and emotional numbing. PTR affects combat veterans, as well as victims and survivors of rape, childhood sexual and/or physical abuse, kidnapping, accidents, natural and man-made disasters, and any experience that may pose a threat to one's emotional and/or physical survival or that of loved ones.[1]

PTR is a process with acute and long-term phases.[3] In the acute phase the individual may experience shock and disbelief followed by intense fear and anxiety. Some victims are highly emotive, whereas others appear calm and subdued, giving the impression of coping well. In the long-term phase, which begins within a few days to several months after the traumatic event, the individual may have flashbacks (revisualizations of the traumatic scene that seem real),[4,5] intrusive thoughts, and nightmares in which the event is reenacted. Victims may be preoccupied with the traumatic event and may have difficulty concentrating on work or other matters of daily living. Some remain in denial about the event and develop emotional numbing, which may lead to total amnesia for the event.[1,6,7]

Those who survive disasters in which others die or are seriously injured may feel helpless, feel guilty for being spared, and ashamed that they did not do enough to save others. In their efforts to cope with these feelings, some patients with PTR abuse drugs and/or alcohol, which may aggravate the symptoms. Interpersonal relationships are impaired, and the victim becomes increasingly alienated from pretrauma activities and commitments.

Related Factors[1,4-7,9]

Disasters (e.g., flood, fire, earthquake)
Participation in combat
Rape
Assault
Childhood sexual and/or physical abuse
Torture
Kidnapping
Catastrophic illness
Accidents
Preexisting emotional disorders (e.g., depression)
Previous experience of trauma
Interpersonal isolation
Limited community supports

Defining Characteristics[1-10,13,15]

Flashbacks of traumatic event triggered by visual, auditory, and olfactory stimuli
Nightmares
Intrusive thoughts
Impaired concentration, memory, and cognition
Emotional numbing, including amnesia for and confusion about event
Denial of impact of trauma
Generalized fear and anxiety about possibility of trauma recurring, as well as nonrelated experiences
Guilt
Impaired interpersonal relationships
Social withdrawal
Impaired occupational functioning
Withdrawal from activities and commitments
Alcohol and drug abuse
Helplessness
Hopelessness

More common in children and adolescents:
Posttraumatic play and reenactment
Impaired time orientation for traumatic event and related events
Limited view of future
Fear of dying young

Expected Patient Outcomes & Nursing Interventions

Resolve physiologic changes suffered in trauma, as evidenced by:

Following medical regimen
Using prescribed medications responsibly
Becoming involved in rehabilitative services
- Provide prescribed medical treatment and nursing care. *Patient's physical recovery is essential to resolution of emotional conflicts.*
- Allow patient to focus on recovery and rehabilitation of physical health while medical status remains compromised. *Forcing emotional issues may increase patient's anxiety and fears.*
- Increase patient's responsibility for activities of daily living (ADLs) as physical tolerance permits. *Recovery is promoted by self-care activities.*
- Discuss with patient and family that as physical recovery progresses, more extreme emotional responses may occur. *Resolution of physical injuries shifts focus to emotional impact of trauma.*

Adapt to altered body image, as evidenced by:

Verbalizing feelings about physical injuries
Accepting limitations of physical injuries through involvement in appropriate exercise and activities
Enhancing self-care through use of services for disabled persons
Seeking assistance from professionals and significant others
- Encourage verbalization of feelings about self-image, and physical limitations (e.g., loss, inadequacy, decreased self-esteem). *Acknowledging feelings is the first step to incorporating body image changes.*
- Discourage patient from using feelings about trauma as an excuse to avoid responsibility for ADLs and life goals, while providing empathic responses for the feelings. *Painful emotions can be tolerated and understood while expecting responsible self-care.*
- Make referrals to community and professional services available to assist trauma survivors (e.g., Compassionate Friends, Victim's Assistance). *Using available resources can enhance the patient's feeling of support and hope for recovery.*

Achieve restored cognitive abilities, as evidenced by:

Not experiencing flashbacks, nightmares, and intrusive thoughts
Concentrating on and conversing about varied topics and interests

Performing ADLs and work-related tasks smoothly
Appearing less anxious when discussing trauma

- Encourage patient to talk about traumatic event, helping him sort out facts from distortions. *Feelings of self-blame, guilt, and shame can be mitigated by an accurate perception of the individual's behavior and response during the traumatic event.*
- Accept patient's fears associated with thoughts and revisualizations of traumatic scene, acknowledging how real these thoughts seem. *Respecting the patient's need to describe painful and graphic details of trauma will assist in accepting and integrating the experience into his life.*
- Teach relaxation techniques and introduce patient to calming activities to employ when anxious (e.g., progressive relaxation, imagery, listening to soothing music). *Self-calming activities will assist patient in achieving control and perspective on intrusive thoughts and flashbacks.*
- Encourage structured time and ADL rituals throughout the day to reduce opportunity for intrusive thoughts. *Developing meaningful activities and habits will assist in the reduction of cognitive impairments.*

Experience improved interpersonal relationships, as evidenced by:

Interacting daily with family and significant others
Verbalizing need for support and desire to help others
Becoming increasingly involved in work activities and with colleagues

- Arrange family meetings while patient is hospitalized to discuss how family can provide support and assistance. *Family, significant friends, and colleagues should be encouraged to interact with patient despite his or her initial withdrawal. They can provide immediate and ongoing support to the patient.*
- Encourage involvement in unit and outpatient activities, work, and hobbies. *Interacting with others around structured activities can minimize the awkwardness of social, interpersonal contacts.*
- Schedule frequent one-to-one contacts to encourage patient to discuss fears about interpersonal relationships. *Talking to a concerned, trusted nurse can assist the patient to overcome interpersonal anxieties.*
- Discuss with significant others the meaning of patient's withdrawal from interpersonal contact; empathize with their pain and confusion while encouraging them to maintain involvement with patient. *Loved ones and colleagues may feel awkward and helpless and need reassurance that their efforts to support patient will eventually succeed.*

Integrate emotional impact of trauma into an adaptive response, as evidenced by:

Abstaining from drugs and alcohol
Resolving feelings of guilt, shame, and loss
Expressing hope for the future

Renewing involvement in religious or spiritual growth activities

- Refer for individual or group psychotherapy and evaluation for psychoactive drug treatment. *More intensive psychotherapeutic intervention is necessary for many PTS victims to assist in the ongoing resolution of the crisis and aftermath of trauma.*
- Refer to Alcoholics Anonymous and Narcotics Anonymous. *The structure and support of AA and NA programs can greatly enhance the patient's ability to abstain from alcohol and drugs and to develop supportive relationships with others in recovery.*
- Arrange for assistance from employer, clergy, and social organizations to help patient return to pretrauma activities and responsibilities. *A multipronged approach in which the assistance of people from the entire spectrum of the patient's life is enlisted will facilitate recovery and resolution of the trauma and assist the patient to develop a new level of functioning in his life.*

Principles and Rationale for Nursing Interventions

Before the victim of PTR can work through the emotional reactions to the trauma, he must be assisted to a state of physiologic equilibrium. Denial is a healthy, necessary, and expected reaction in the initial posttrauma period and should not be discouraged.[6] The patient will focus energies on following the necessary medical regimen to recover from injuries sustained and begin to assess the long-term physical impairment. Rushing in to explore the patient's feelings about the trauma may only contribute to the use of pathologic denial and impair future emotional adjustment. The nurse must be sensitive to the patient's cues of readiness to discuss feelings, realizing that each person has a different ability to be emotionally expressive.

Flashbacks, nightmares, and intrusive thoughts are the most disturbing symptoms of PTR. The patient needs the opportunity to describe the traumatic event in detail, even if it involves an increase in anxiety. Providing a safe, trusting environment in which the patient can talk will permit gradual acceptance of the impact of the trauma. The patient can then begin to integrate feelings about the trauma into his lifestyle. As new coping strategies are learned, the patient will not limit activities and responsibilities. Relaxation techniques and other self-calming measures increase a sense of control and decrease fears.[5,7]

Most who suffer from PTR will benefit from supportive psychotherapy, usually focused on the traumatic event and conducted over 6 to 12 sessions.[6] Some patients with a preexisting mental health disorder may need ongoing, insight-oriented psychotherapy to help them integrate the complex emotions about the trauma with other life problems. Victim support groups help the patient learn new ways of coping, feel less isolated, and feel more useful to others with similar struggles. The family and significant others of the PTR patient are also victims in that they often feel helpless to respond. Being sensitive to their frustration, as well as giving information, will help them maintain the emotional support and attentiveness that the loved one needs. If the patient has an established support network, he will benefit from regular contact with them. The patient who has been socially isolated and estranged from family will need encouragement to seek out support groups that are safe and non-threatening. Interpersonal contact provides a healing effect on the victim that advances recovery and return to all areas of life.

In despair, the PTR patient may turn to drugs and alcohol to medicate against overwhelming anxiety and disturbing thoughts. The patient needs to understand how substance abuse can aggravate symptoms so that he can choose safer, drug-free ways of coping. Involvement in AA, NA, and Al-Anon for the family provides support, information, and encouragement to deal with the drug's effect on the patient's life and the family. Appropriate psychoactive drugs, prescribed by a specialist and administered judiciously, will help the patient tolerate anxiety and will assist in the control of flashbacks while discouraging dependence on the medication.[11,12,14]

FAMILY COPING: POTENTIAL FOR GROWTH

Family coping: potential for growth is the effective managing of adaptive tasks by a family member who is involved with the patient's health challenge and who is now exhibiting desire and readiness for enhanced health and growth in regard to self and in relation to the patient. The family member's basic needs are being met sufficiently, and other adaptive tasks are being addressed effectively. This allows the emergence of these self-actualizing goals.[4]

The family's ability to manage effectively the adaptive tasks required by an altered health status in one of its members may be viewed as a coping response indicating the potential for movement to a different stage of development or growth. In turn, the types of family coping behaviors may significantly influence the family's ability to function during times of stress.[14] Internal coping strategies are the ways in which members of the family use resources within the family system to handle stress. External strategies are the active behaviors used by the family to acquire outside resources.[8] Readiness for enhanced understanding of the roles and contributions of each family member and acceptance of the required changes resulting from the challenge suggest that the family can use problem-solving techniques to deal with the current situational stresses and to devise preventive measures to maintain the family system's stability.

Research into the effects of stress on family systems indicates that many of the concepts of individual coping and stress theories also apply. Family coping differs, however, in that several persons at various developmental stages participate in the process.[2] Perception of the event, role relations, expectations, value orientation, and situational support are concepts that can be applied in family assessment during crises. These concepts form a construct relating to family constellations, which can be assessed separately from the coping strategies usually used.[9] Nine family tasks related to the ability to cope with stress have been identified.[10]

Owning up to the stress situation
Redefining the family identity
Referring to successful past coping strategies
Exploring alternative solutions
Organizing responses
Attempting new responses
Reaching decisions by consensus
Responding to the outcomes of the decisions
Performing family self-evaluation

One model of family adjustment and adaptation to stress suggests that the three factors of demands on the family, family resources, and the family's perspective of the situation interact in successive phases of adjustment, restructuring, and consolidation. This produces an outcome that is indicative of the family's ability to cope productively.[16] Thus a situation that produces stress within the family system offers an opportunity to strengthen the family and produce growth instead of compromising or disabling the family's ability to cope.[13]

Related Factors[3,4,11,15,19]

Basic needs of family/individual members sufficiently gratified
Adaptive tasks related to situation effectively addressed
Goals relating to self-actualization of family/individual members surfacing
Role relationships support positive family communication and adaptive patterns
Family developmental stages
  Courtship
  Marriage
  Childbirth and young children
  Middle marriage and school-aged children
  Children leaving home
  Retirement and old age
Situational crises
  Illness of family member—nature, severity, stigma
  Changes in situational supports (e.g., job, friends, extended family, natural disaster)
Family structure and process
  Nature of boundaries between members
  Openness of communication process in family
  Patient's role in family
  Conflict resolution patterns

Defining Characteristics[3,4,11,15,19]

Requests assistance to recognize sources and signs of stress
Attempts to describe growth impact of situation on values, priorities, goals, or relationships
Moves toward health-promoting and enriching life-style that supports and monitors maturational processes
Audits and negotiates treatment programs
Chooses experiences that optimize wellness
Expresses interest in contacting others experiencing similar situations

Indicates that basic needs for all family members are being met in a timely fashion

Recovery or stabilization of family member with health problem is seen

Expected Family Member(s) Outcomes & Nursing Interventions*

Actualize growth potential of situation, as evidenced by:

Verbalizing changes in family roles/relationships

Verbalizing changes in individual attitudes, values, goals

Choosing new individual/family goals

Choosing new strategies to meet goals

Choosing experiences that foster growth

- Assist family to identify changes in family dynamics resulting from situation.
- Assist family to identify changes in individual family members resulting from situation.
- Discuss goals and experiences that maximize growth potential with family/individual members.
- Provide information as needed to enable family/individual members to develop new goals and methods of achieving them.
- Facilitate development of new methods of goal attainment.
- Collaborate with family members in planning and implementing life-style changes.

Develop strategies for coping with behavior of family members other than patient, as evidenced by:

Identifying situations and ways in which transfer of learning may occur

Reporting usefulness of transfer of learning to other situations

- Assist family members to discuss ways in which they may transfer learning from the strategies used with patient to other family members.
- Assist family members to identify situations in which transfer of learning may be appropriate.

Develop broader base of support, as evidenced by:

Verbalizing interest in contacting others experiencing similar situations

Contacting additional persons or groups when referred

Developing additional relationships for physical or emotional support

Maintaining contact with additional sources

- Identify individual or family readiness to accept support from additional sources.
- Assist family members to identify type(s) of support needed.
- Inform family members of appropriate health care and community resources.

*References 2, 4, 5, 7, 9, 15, 18, 20.

- Teach strategies to access and maximize community resources.
- Refer individual or family to appropriate resources.
- Initiate contact, if necessary.
- Follow up to ensure sustained contact and appropriateness of assistance.

Principles and Rationale for Nursing Interventions

Facilitating the family's potential for growth begins with an assessment of the changes that have resulted from the situation produced by a health challenge to one of its members. These changes may be seen in the dynamics of the family as roles and relationships are altered and new patterns of interaction are required or in the attitudes, values and goals of the individual family members.[17] Discussions with individual family members and the family as a whole provide validation that the family system has been changed as a result of the current situation and that new goals and strategies are appropriate. The use of teaching strategies to provide new information about goals, alternative methods of achieving them, and support for attempting new behaviors recognizes that the family members are ready for problem-solving activities and learning.[7,15]

Supporting the family's efforts to develop its own expanded base of both physical and emotional resources reinforces the potential for growth as the family moves toward decreased dependency on health care professionals. Referrals to appropriate community services and appropriate follow-up contacts ensure the family's ability to continue moving toward its goals.

■ INEFFECTIVE FAMILY COPING: COMPROMISED

Ineffective family coping: compromised is insufficient, ineffective, or compromised support, comfort, assistance, or encouragement, usually by a supportive primary person (family member, close friend). The patient may need this to manage or master adaptive tasks related to his or her health challenge.

When a family demonstrates an inability to maintain its usual patterns of functioning as a result of internal or external stressors, its coping abilities are said to be compromised. These behaviors may take the form of insufficient or ineffective support, comfort, assistance, or encouragement to the identified patient by the primary significant person(s) in the family constellation. Such behaviors are usually the result of inadequate physical, psychologic, cognitive, or behavioral resources.[7,11]

Whereas functional families allow for individual views, experiences, and values during stress situations, families whose abilities to cope are compromised appear to require more conformity to expected behavior and become less tolerant in response to the situation.[1] Boundaries between the family and outside social systems become less permeable, and coalitions form between family members.[9] The focus of much of the anxiety and fear in a family with compromised coping skills centers on a need to find a cause or learn the rules that will provide guidance for appropriate behavior in the situation.[1] In many instances, particularly when the family has dealt with a chronic illness or a member with a long-term disability, the resources needed to continue to function have been depleted.[18]

Related Factors[7,11,14,15]

Inadequate or incorrect information or understanding by family member(s)
Temporary preoccupation by significant family member(s)
    Inability to cope with own emotional conflict
    Inability to perceive needs of identified patient
    Inability to act effectively to meet needs of identified patient
Role changes resulting in temporary family disorganization
Concurrent situational or developmental crises
Limited support received from identified patient
Prolonged illness or disability that exhausts coping abilities
Economic problems (inflation, unemployment, lack of insurance)
Unrealistic expectations of significant family member(s) by identified patient
Unrealistic expectations of identified patient by significant family member(s)
Lack of mutual decision-making skills
Rigid or inappropriate boundaries within family
Inversion of normal power hierarchies
Coalitions of family members

Defining Characteristics[7,11,13,14]

Concern or complaint by patient about response(s) of family member(s)
Family member(s):
    Verbalize fear, anxiety, and/or anger
    Verbalize inadequate understanding or knowledge base
    Engage in destructive bickering
    Make direct or subtle appeal for help
        Assistance with communication
        Permission to express feelings
        Permission to leave bedside of patient
        Reassurance that illness is not his or her fault
    Unable to make decision together
    Refuse to assist with patient's care
    Attempt assistive or supportive behaviors with ineffective results
    Display absence of verbal or nonverbal interaction
    Display disproportionate protective behavior
    Tend to interfere with necessary nursing or medical interventions
    Display sudden outburst of emotions without apparent cause or show emotional lability
    Form coalitions
    Describe preoccupation with personal reaction to situation

    Display protective behavior disproportionate to patient's abilities or need for autonomy
    Verbalize concern with own unmet needs

Expected Family Member(s)/Significant Other(s) Outcomes & Nursing Interventions*

Develop adequate understanding of health challenge, as evidenced by:

Verbalizing need for more information or clearer understanding
Demonstrating that the information given is understood
Discussing changes in patient and family as a result of health challenge
- Provide adequate and correct information to patient and family.
- Discuss "sick role" with patient and family.
- Encourage family to have realistic perception based on accurate information.
- Discuss usual reactions to health challenges (e.g., anxiety, dependency, depression).
- Monitor areas in which knowledge or understanding is inadequate in relation to situation.
- Encourage patient and family member(s) to discuss expectations of each other in situation.
- Provide coordination of services through a case manager.

Experience increasing comfort, as evidenced by:

Experiencing decreased levels of anxiety
Verbalizing that the environment is supportive
Verbalizing feelings to health care professionals and other family members
- Maintain as much privacy as possible.
- Provide alternative to patient's room for family discussions.
- Encourage patient and family members to verbalize feelings (e.g., loss, guilt, anger, relief).
- Provide opportunities for patient to discuss need for support with family members.
- Use communication techniques to confirm legitimacy of both positive and negative feelings, e.g., reflecting feelings ("You seem frightened"), presenting reality ("Many people feel angry in situations like this").

Cope with changes in family structure and dynamics, as evidenced by:

Identifying changes in family roles and dynamics
Recognizing roles needed to maintain family integrity
Assuming new roles as necessary to maintain family integrity
Participating effectively in care of patient
- Assist family to assess situation, including both strengths and weaknesses.
- Assist family to identify changes in relationships.
- Assist family members to recognize role changes needed to maintain family integrity.

---

*References 2, 4, 11, 15, 17, 20.

- Assist family members to assume new roles as needed.
- Involve family members in care of patient as much as possible.
- Encourage family members to seek additional sources of help in adjusting to changes in family processes: friends, clergy, other professional health care providers.
- Refer family member to appropriate additional sources for help in adjusting to changes in family processes.

Principles and Rationale for Nursing Interventions

Most families may be viewed as healthy, but in need of temporary support. Interventions should be aimed at promoting family competence. Many of the interventions appropriate for helping the family whose coping skills are compromised center on providing sufficient information. Validation of feelings and perceptions of the situation can relieve anxiety to the extent that the learning of new coping strategies may be effective.[18] The nurse should provide information about the extent of the illness of a family member and the probable long-range effects on both the individual and the family system. This information can aid in developing realistic expectations about the positive and negative changes that must occur to maintain functioning. Both supportive and informational family education is essential in helping a family that is experiencing ineffective coping. Family growth can be promoted through fostering a sense of "family" within an educational climate.[6] Encouragement to use sources outside the family may be appropriate to preserve the supportive capacity of family members in assuming new roles over time.

▌ INEFFECTIVE FAMILY COPING: DISABLING

Ineffective family coping: disabling is the behavior of a significant person (family member, other primary person) that disables his or her capacities and the patient's capacities to address effectively tasks essential to either person's adaptation to the health challenge.

The coping abilities of a family may be diagnosed as disabling when the behaviors of individual family members or of the family system become destructive in response to either internal or external stressors.[1] Behavior of a significant family member that interferes with the abilities of the identified patient and/or other family members to adapt effectively to the health challenge may also be considered disabling to the family system.[11]

Related Factors*

Significant person with chronically unexpressed feelings (e.g., guilt, anxiety, hostility, despair)

---

*References 1, 7, 11, 13, 14, 19.

Dissonant discrepancy of coping styles used to deal with adaptive tasks
Highly ambivalent family relationships
Arbitrary handling of family's resistance to treatment (tends to solidify defensiveness as it fails to deal adequately with underlying anxiety)
High-risk individual(s) or family
Characteristics of parent(s)
   Single
   Adolescent
   Abusive
   Emotionally disturbed
   Substance abuser
   Terminally ill
   Acute disability or accident
Unwanted characteristics or handicaps of child
   Of unwanted pregnancy
   Of undesired sex
   With undesired characteristics
   Physically handicapped
   Mentally handicapped
   Hyperactive
   Terminally ill
Separation from nuclear family
Lack of extended family
Inadequate knowledge base or incorrect information
Economic problems (inflation, unemployment)
Change in composition of family unit
History of ineffective relationships (e.g., abusive with parents)
Lack of mutual decision-making skills
Rigid or inappropriate boundaries within family
Inversion of normal power hierarchies
Coalitions of family members
Maturational
   Low self-esteem
   Physical and emotional adolescent changes
   Birth of a sibling
   Retirement
   Failure to progress in school
   Inability of a parent to maintain independence (requires assistance with transportation, ADLs, finances)
   Any condition that challenges one's ability for self-care or for fulfilling role responsibilities

Defining Characteristics[7,11,13]

Abusive or neglectful care of patient (in regard to basic human needs, illness treatment)
Distortion of reality (in regard to patient's health problem, including extreme denial about its existence or severity)
Intolerance
Rejection
Abandonment
Desertion
Psychosomatic tendency
Taking on illness signs of patient

Decisions and actions by family that are detrimental to economic or social well-being of family members

Unresolved emotions, especially agitation, depression, aggression, hostility

Impaired restructuring of meaningful life for self as result of impaired individualization; prolonged overconcern for patient

Abusive or neglectful relationships with other family members

Patient's development of helpless, inactive dependence

Verbalization of abuse by family member(s)

Presence of any serious symptom(s) over protracted period

Communication processes within family that are negative, blaming, critical, often concrete in thinking, and poor in affective expressions—role deficiencies and reversals, permeable generational boundaries, disengagement, enmeshment

Expected Family Member(s)/Significant Other(s) Outcomes & Nursing Interventions*

Demonstrate accurate understanding of conflict in coping style, as evidenced by:

Verbalizing perceptions of coping styles and areas of conflict

Identifying alternative coping behaviors that may minimize conflict

- Assist family member(s) to verbalize own perceptions of individual coping styles and areas of conflict.
- Identify areas of conflict in coping styles among family members.
- Assist family member(s) to identify alternative coping behaviors that minimize conflict.

Develop alternative coping strategies, as evidenced by:

Incorporating alternative coping behaviors in adapting to health challenge

Continuing to use positive coping strategies in stressful situations

- Assist family member(s) to focus on present feelings and behaviors.
- Clarify communications among family members.
- Emphasize positive aspects of present coping strategies.
- Assist family member(s) to practice alternative coping behaviors through relabeling, role playing, contracting, etc.
- Monitor coping strategies of family members.
- Reinforce positive use of new coping strategies.

Improve level of complementarity in role relationships, as evidenced by:

Verbalizing individual needs and expectations of family relationships

Identifying strengths and weaknesses in adapting to health challenge

Discussing complementary nature of strengths, needs, and expectations of relationships

Identifying areas where needs and expectations are not being met leading to feelings of powerlessness

Identifying strategies to aid in developing complementary role relationships that can overcome feelings of powerlessness

Incorporating alternative strategies in relationships

- Assist family member(s) to verbalize needs and expectations of relationships.
- Assist family member(s) to discuss where individual strengths, needs, and expectations complement each other.
- Assist family member(s) to identify needs and expectations not being met.
- Assist family member(s) to identify strategies to develop complementary role relationships in adapting to changes in patient's physical and mental status.
- Assist family member(s) to practice new strategies.
- Reinforce positive strategies and improved complementarity in role relationships.

Develop adequate understanding of health challenge, as evidenced by:

Verbalizing need for more information or clearer understanding

Demonstrating that the information given is understood

Discussing changes in patient and family as a result of health challenge

- Provide adequate and correct information to patient and family.
- Discuss "sick role" with patient and family.
- Encourage family to develop more realistic expectations.
- Discuss usual reactions to health challenges.
- Monitor areas in which knowledge or understanding is inadequate.
- Encourage family to discuss expectations of each other.

Principles and Rationale for Nursing Interventions

An understanding of the ways each family member is attempting to cope with the stressors created by any given situation is essential to introducing change in the family system.[8] Members of a disabled family are usually experiencing sufficient anxiety to restrict their ability to view the behavior of others realistically. Thus one of the first goals must be helping the family as individuals or as a group to focus on how the current situation is affecting the identified patient and each member.[13] As various attempts to cope are identified, the patient and family members begin to identify the areas of conflict.

Once coping strategies have been identified and the areas of conflict assessed, the patient and other family members can be introduced to other behaviors that will decrease the potential for conflict within the family structure.[19] A psychoeducational approach has been suggested in which a cognitive basis for behavior is presented for understanding the behavior of family members. This approach allows the family to develop a framework from which to view the behavior of its members and to

---

*References 2, 9-11, 13, 17, 18, 20.

establish realistic goals for changes in coping strategies.[19] In family in identifying the role expectations of each other and to assess strengths and weaknesses in fulfilling the required roles in a functional family.[9]

The need for accurate information has consistently been demonstrated in nursing studies.[18] Once the disabling level of anxiety has been reduced, the patient and significant others should be given sufficient information about the nature and course of the health challenge to aid in the restructuring of role relationships and the developing of alternative coping strategies. Information given through structured progress reports and conferences with interdisciplinary team members can enable the reconstruction of the family unit and provide a focus for developing plans for change.[12]

References

Ineffective individual coping

1. Achenbach TM et al: Nine-year outcome of the Vermont intervention program for low birth weight infants, *Pediatrics* 91:45-55, 1993.
2. Affonso DD et al: Cognitive adaptation to stressful events during pregnancy and postpartum: development and testing of the CASE instrument, *Nurs Res* 43:338-343, 1994.
3. Aguilera DC: *Crisis intervention: theory and methodology,* ed 7, St Louis, 1994, Mosby.
4. Aldwin CM: *Stress, coping & development: an integrative perspective,* New York, 1994, Guilford Press.
5. Baume RM, Croog SH, Nalbandian J: Pain perception, coping strategies, and stress management among periodontal patients with repeated surgeries, *Percept Mot Skills* 80:307-319, 1995.
6. Beckerman A, Grossman D, Marquez L: Cardiac catheterization: the patient's perspective, *Heart Lung* 24:213-219, 1995.
7. Benes F: Alterations in coticolimbic circuitry may be linked to schizophrenia, *Psychiatric Times* April 12-13, 1990.
8. Benjamin LS: Good defenses make good neighbors. In Conte HR, Plutchik R, editors: *Ego defenses: theory and measurement,* New York, 1995, J Wiley & Sons.
9. Blechman EA, Dumas JE, Prinz RJ: Prosocial coping by youth exposed to violence, *J Child Adolesc Group Therapy* 4:205-227, 1994.
10. Blount RI et al: Making the system work: training pediatric oncology patients to cope & their parents to coach them during BMA/LP procedures, *Behav Modif* 18:6-31, 1994.
11. Bond M: The development & properties of the Defense Style Questionnaire. In Conte HR, Plutchik R, editors: *Ego defenses: theory and measurement,* New York, 1995, J Wiley & Sons.
12. Borkeovec TD: The nature, function and origins of worry. In Davey CL, Tallis F, editor: *Worrying: perspective in theory, assessment and treatment,* New York, 1994, J Wiley & Sons.
13. Bradshaw WH: Coping-skills training versus a problem-solving approach with schizophrenic patients, *Hosp Community Pyschiatry* 44:1102-1104, 1993.
14. Bordy CM, Simel VL: *Strategies for therapy with the elderly: living with hope and meaning,* New York, 1993, Springer.
15. Browne GB et al: Methodological challenges in coping and adaptation research, *Can J Nurs Res* 26:89-96, 1994.
16. Burke M, Flaherty MJ: Coping strategies and health status of elderly arthritic women, *J Adv Nurs* 18:7-13, 1993.
17. Carrieri-Kohlman V et al: Desensitization and guided mastery: treatment approaches for the management of dyspnea, *Heart Lung* 22:226-234, 1993.
18. Cohen S: *The chemical brain: the neurochemistry of addictive disorders,* Irvine, Calif, 1988, The Care Institute.
19. Cooper C: Psychiatric stress debriefing: alleviating the impact of patient suicide and assault, *J Psychosoc Nurs Ment Health Serv* 33:21-25, 1995.
20. Davis TMA et al: Undergoing cardiac catheterization: the effects of informational preparation and coping style on patient anxiety during the procedure, *Heart Lung* 23:140-150, 1994.

21. DiPalma LM: Patterns of coping and characteristics of high-functioning incest survivors, *Arch Psychiatr Nurs* 8:82-90, 1994.
22. Dodd MJ, Dibble SL, Thomas ML: Predictors of concerns and coping strategies of cancer chemotherapy outpatients, *Appl Nurs Res* 6:2-7, 1993.
23. Dwevdi KN: Coping with unhappy children who are from ethnic minorities. In Varma V, editor: *Coping with unhappy children,* New York, 1993, Cassell.
24. Evans DM, Dunn NJ: Alcohol expectancies, coping responses & self-efficacy judgments: a replication and extension of Copper's et al's 1988 study in a college sample, *J Stud Alcohol* 56:186-193, 1995.
25. Folkman S et al: Dynamics of a stressful encounter: cognitive appraisal, coping and encounter outcomes, *J Pers Soc Psychol* 50:992-1003, 1986.
26. Folkman S, Chesney MA, Christopher-Richards A: Stress and coping in caregiving partners of men with AIDS, *Psychiatr Clin North Am* 17:35-53, 1994.
27. Frederick J, Cotanch P: Self-help techniques for auditory hallucinations, *Issues Ment Health Nurs* 16:213-224, 1995.
28. Freeman A, Dattilio FM, editors: *Cognitive-behavioral strategies in crisis intervention,* New York, 1994, Guilford Press.
29. Good M: Relaxation techniques for surgical patients, *Am J Nurs* 95:39-43, 1995.
30. Gulick EE: Coping among spouses or significant others of persons with multiple sclerosis, *Nurs Res* 44:220-225, 1995.
31. Holahan CJ, Moos RH: Life stresses and mental health: advances in conceptualizing stress resistance. In Avison WR, Gotlib IH, editors: *Stress and mental health: contemporary issues and prospects for the future,* New York, 1994, Plenum Press.
32. Holahan CJ, Moos RH: Life stressors, personal and social resources, & depression: a 4-year structural model, *J Abnorm Psychol* 100:31-38, 1991.
33. Hull MM: Coping strategies of family caregivers in hospice home care, *Oncol Nurs Forum* 19:1179-1187, 1992.
34. Jacobson G: Identifying and responding to children's stressful experiences, *Pediatr Nurs* 21:391-394, 1995.
35. Johnson JA: Appraisal, moods, and coping among individuals experiencing diagnostic exercise stress testing, *Res Nurs Health* 17:441-448, 1994.
36. Kim MJ, McFarland GK, McLane AM: *Pocket guide to nursing diagnoses,* ed 6, St Louis, 1995, Mosby.
37. Kirkby RJ: Changes in premenstrual symptoms and irrational thinking following cognitive-behavioral coping skills training, *J Consult Clin Psychol* 62:1026-1032, 1994.
38. Kumasaka LMKB, Dungan JM: Nursing strategy for initial emotional response to cancer diagnosis, *Cancer Nurs* 16:296-303, 1993.
39. LaMontagne LL et al: Psychophysiological response of parents to pediatric critical care stress, *Clin Nurs Res* 3:104-118, 1994.
40. Langer: *Mindfulness,* New York, 1989, Addison-Wesley.
41. Larson DG: *The helper's journey,* Champaign, Ill, 1993, Research Press.
42. Lauver D, Tak Y: Optimism and coping with a breast cancer symptom, *Nurs Res* 44:202-207, 1995.
43. Lazarus RS, Folkman S: *Stress, appraisal and coping,* New York, 1984, Springer.
44. Levenson JL: Psychosocial interventions in chronic medical illness: an overview of outcome research, *Gen Hosp Psychiatry* 14S:43-49, 1992.
45. Leventhal H, Nerenz DR: A model for stress research with some applications for control of stress disorder. In Meichenbaum D, Jarenko ME, editors: *Stress reduction and prevention,* New York, 1983, Plenum.
46. Ludwick-Rosenthal R, Neufeld R: Preparation for undergoing an invasive medical procedure: interacting effects of information and coping style, *J Consult Clin Psychol* 61:156-164, 1993.
47. Manion J: Understanding the seven stages of change, *Am J Nurs* 95:41-43, 1995.
48. Marlatt GA, Gordon JR, editors: *Relapse prevention: maintenance strategies in the treatment of addictive behaviors,* New York, 1985, Guilford Press.
49. McHaffie HE: The assessment of coping, *Clin Nurs Res* 1:67-69, 1992.

50. McKay M, Davis M, Fannign P: *Thoughts and feelings: the art of cognitive stress intervention,* Richmond, Calif, 1981, New Harbinger.
51. Meichenbaum D, Fitzpatrick D: Constructivist narrative perspective on stress and coping: stress inoculation applications. In Goldberger I, Breznitz S, editors: *Handbook of stress: theoretical and clinical aspects,* ed 2, New York, 1993, Free Press.
52. Melnyk BM: Coping with unplanned childhood hospitalization: effects of informational interventions on mothers and children, *Nurs Res* 43:50-55, 1994.
53. Mikulincer M: *Human learned helplessness: a coping perspective,* New York, 1994, Plenum Press.
54. Miller SM et al: Effects of coping style on psychological reactions of low income, minority women to colposcopy, *J Reprod Med* 39:711-718, 1994.
55. Monti PM, Gulliver SB, Myers MG: Social skills training for alcoholics: assessment and treatment, *Alcohol Alcohol* 29:627-637, 1994.
56. Moos RH, Schaeffer JA: Coping resources and processes: current concepts and measures. In Goldberger L, Breznitz S, editors: *Handbook of stress: theoretical & clinical aspects,* ed 2, New York, 1993, Free Press.
57. Narsavage GL, Weaver TE: Physiological status, coping, and hardiness as predictors of outcomes in chronic obstructive pulmonary disease, *Nurs Res* 43:90-94, 1994.
58. Northouse LL et al: Emotional distress reported by women and husbands prior to a breast biopsy, *Nurse Res* 44:196-201, 1995.
59. O'Brien MT: Multiple sclerosis: the relationship among self-esteem, social support, and coping behavior, *Appl Nurs Res* 6:54-63, 1993.
60. Palinkas LA, Browner D: Effects of prolonged isolation in extreme environments on stress, coping and depression, *J Appl Soc Psychol* 25:557-576, 1995.
61. Palmer S, Dryden W: *Counseling for stress problems,* London, 1995, Sage.
62. Puskar KR, Lamb JM, Bartolovic M: Examining the common stressors and coping methods of rural adolescents, *Nurs Pract* 18:50-53, 1993.
63. Rahe RH: Acute versus chronic post-traumatic stress disorder, *Integr Physiol Behav Sci* 28:46-56, 1993.
64. Rahe RH: Stress and psychiatry. In Kaplan HI, Sadock BJ, editors: *Comprehensive textbook of psychiatry,* vol 2, ed 6, Baltimore, Williams & Wilkins, 1995.
65. Ramey CT et al: Infant health and development program for low birth weight premature infants: program elements, family participation, and child intelligence, *Pediatrics* 9:454-465, 1992.
66. Ritchie MA: Psychosocial functioning of adolescents with cancer: a developmental perspective, *Oncol Nurs Forum* 19:1497-1501, 1992.
67. Robinson KR: Denial: an adaptive response, *Dimens Crit Care Nurs* 12:102-106, 1993.
68. Russell GC: The role of denial in clinical practice, *J Adv Nurs* 18:938-940, 1993.
69. Ryan-Wenger NM, Copland SG: Coping strategies used by black school age children from low-income families, *J Pediatr Nurs* 9:33-40, 1994.
70. Sharrer VW, Ryan-Wenger MN: A longitudinal study of age and gender differences of stressors and coping: strategies in school-aged children, *J Pediatr Health Care* 9:123-130, 1995.
71. Sharts-Hopko NC: Birth in the Japanese context, *J Obstet Gynecol Neonatal Nurs* 24:343-351, 1995.
72. Shea S et al: Predisposing factors for severe uncontrolled hypertension in an inner city minority population, *N Engl J Med* 327:776-781, 1992.
73. Smith BJ et al: Exploring widows' experiences after the suicide of their spouse, *J Psychosoc Nurs Ment Health Serv* 33:10-15, 1995.
74. Snow DL, Kline ML: Preventive interventions in the workplace to reduce negative psychiatric consequences of work and family stress. In Mazure CM, editor: *Does stress cause psychiatric illness?* Washington, DC, 1995, Am Psychiatric Press.
75. Snyder S: Drug and neurotransmittor receptors—new perspectives with clinical relevance, *JAMA* 261:3126-3129, 1989.
76. Sorensen ES: *Children's stress and coping: a family perspective,* New York, 1993, Guilford Press.
77. Spiegel D: Facilitating emotional coping during treatment, *Cancer* 66(Suppl 6):1422-1426, Sept. 15, 1990.
78. Steefel L: The World Trade Center disaster: healing the unseen wounds, *J Psychosoc Nurs Ment Health Serv* 31:5-7, 1993.
79. Troop NA et al: Ways of coping in women with eating disorders, *J Nerv Ment Dis* 182:535-540, 1994.
80. Ursano RJ, Silberman EK: Psychodynamic and supportive psychotherapy. In Hales SR, Yudofsky SC, Talbot JA, editors: *Textbook of psychiatry,* Washington, DC, 1994, American Psychiatric Press.
81. Vaillant GE: Ego mechanisms of defense: a guide for clinicians and research, Washington, DC, 1992, American Psychiatric Press.
82. Weaver PL et al: Adult survivors of childhood sexual abuse: survivor's disclosure and nurse therapist's response, *J Psychosoc Nurs Ment Health Serv* 32:19-25, 1994.
83. Weiss JR, McCabe MA, Dennig MD: Primary and secondary control among children undergoing medical procedures: adjustment as a function of coping style, *J Consult Clin Psychol* 62:324-332, 1994.
84. Wolf S: Some thoughts on the language of cognitive research, *Integr Physiol Behav Sci* 2:267-268, 1991.

Defensive coping

1. Antai-Otong D, editor: *Psychiatric nursing: biological and behavioral concepts,* Philadelphia, 1995, WB Saunders.
2. Campinha-Bacote J: Cultural competence in psychiatric mental health nursing, *Nurs Clin North Am* 29:1, 1994.
3. Cooper SH: Recent contributions to the theory of defense mechanisms: a comparative view, *J Am Psychoanal Assoc* 37:865, 1989.
4. Cox HC, et al: *Clinical applications of nursing diagnosis: adult, child, women's, psychiatric, gerontic and home health considerations,* ed 2, Philadelphia, 1993, FA Davis.
5. Fitch ML, O'Brien-Pallas L: Defensive coping. In McFarland GK, Thomas, MD, editors: *Psychiatric mental health nursing: application of the nursing process,* Philadelphia, 1991, JB Lippincott.
6. Foster SW: The pragmatics of culture: the rhetoric of difference in psychiatric nursing, *Arch Psychiatr Nurs* 4:292, 1990.
7. Friedmann ML: Evaluation of the congruence model with rehabilitating substance abusers, *Int J Nurs Stud* 3:97, 1994.
8. Johnston NE: Cognitive therapy. In Baumann AO, Johnstone NE, Antai-Otong D, editors: *Decision making in psychiatric and psychosocial nursing,* St Louis, 1990, Mosby.
9. Kahn DL, Steeves RH, Benoliel JQ: Nurses' views of the coping of patients, *Soc Sci Med* 38:1423, 1994.
10. Kettles AM: Catharsis: an investigation of its meaning and nature, *J Adv Nurs* 20:368, 1994.
11. Lazarus RS: Coping theory and research: past, present, and future, *Psychosomatic Med* 55:234, 1993.
12. McFarland GK, Wasli EL, Gerety EK: *Nursing diagnosis and process in psychiatric mental health nursing,* ed 2, Philadelphia, 1992, JB Lippincott.
13. Outlaw FH: Stress and coping: the influence of racism on the cognitive appraisal processing of African Americans, *Issues Ment Health Nurs* 14:399, 1993.
14. Reeder DM: Cognitive therapy of anger management: theoretical and practical considerations, *Arch Psychiatr Nurs* 5:147, 1991.
15. Savage P: Patient assessment in psychiatric nursing, *J Adv Nurs* 16:311, 1991.
16. Wilson HS, Kneisl CR: *Psychiatric nursing,* ed 4, Redwood City, Calif, 1995, Addison-Wesley.

Ineffective denial

1. Amodeo M: Treating the late life alcoholic: guidelines for working through denial, integrating individual, family, and group approaches, *J Geriatr Psychiatry* 23:91, 1990.
2. Breznitz S, editor: *The denial of stress,* New York, 1985, International Universities Press.
3. Breznitz S: The seven kinds of denial. In Spielberger C, Sarason I, Defares P, editors: *Stress and anxiety,* Washington, DC, 1988, Hemisphere.
4. Burgess D: Denial and terminal illness, *Am J Hosp Palliat Care,* March/April: 46, 1994.
5. Cockrell K: The wounded healer, *Indiana Med* 84:348, 1991.
6. Connor SR: Denial in terminal illness: to intervene or not to intervene, *Hospice J* 8:1, 1992.
7. Cook EA: Understanding your patient's denial, *Nursing '94* 24:66, 1994.

8. Croyle R, Ditto P: Illness cognition and behavior: an experimental approach, *J Behav Med* 13:31, 1990.
9. Gleeson B: After myocardial infarction: how to teach a patient in denial, *Nursing '91* 21:48, 1991.
10. Hackett TP, Cassem NH: Development of a quantitative rating scale to assess denial, *J Psychosom Res* 18:93, 1974.
11. Kim M, McFarland GK, McLane A: *Pocket guide to nursing diagnoses,* ed 6, St Louis, 1995, Mosby.
12. Langer KG: Depression and denial in psychotherapy of persons with disabilities, *Am J Psychother* 48:181, 1994.
13. Lazarus R: The costs and benefits of denial. In Breznitz S, editor: *The denial of stress,* New York, 1983, International Universities Press.
14. Miller H: Addiction in a coworker: getting past the denial, *Am J Nurs* 90:72, 1990.
15. Miller L: Psychotic denial of pregnancy: phenomenology and clinical management, *Hosp Community Psychiatry* 41:1233, 1990.
16. Murray M, Neilson L: Denial: coping or cop-out? *Can Nurse* February, pp 33-35, 1994.
17. Perkinson L: A tangle of denial. *J Psychosoc Nurs Ment Health Serv* 32:47, 1994.
18. Robinson K: Denial in myocardial infarction patients, *Crit Care Nurs* 10:138, 1990.
19. Robinson KR: Denial: an adaptive response, *Dimens Crit Care Nurs* 12:102, 1993.
20. Vaillant G: Theoretical hierarchy of adaptive ego mechanisms, *Arch Gen Psychiatry* 24:107, 1971.
21. Westwell J, Forchuk C: Denial: buffer and barrier, *Can Nurs* 85(9):16, 1989.
22. White R, LeVan D, McDuff D: Helping the patient in denial: the role of the family in intervention, *Md Med J* 44:462, 1995.
23. Wing DM, Hansen H, Martin B: The alcoholism denial assessment tool (ADAT) *Md Med J* 3:228, 1994.
24. Young L et al: Denial in heart transplant candidates, *Psychother Psychosom* 55:141, 1991.

Impaired adjustment

1. Belgrave FZ: Psychosocial predictors of adjustment to disability in African Americans, *J Rehabil* 57:57, 1991.
2. Burckhardt CS: Coping strategies of the chronically ill, *Nurs Clin North Am* 22:543, 1987.
3. Call JG, Davis LL: The effect of hardiness on coping strategies and adjustment to illness in chronically ill individuals, *Appl Nurs Res* 2:187, 1989.
4. Charonko CV: Cultural influences in "noncompliant" behavior and decision making, *Holist Nurs Pract* 6:73, 1992.
5. Connelly CE: An empirical study of a model of self-care in chronic illness, *Clin Nurse Spec* 7:247, 1993.
6. Connelly CE, Dilonardo JD: Self-care issues with chronically ill psychotic clients, *Perspect Psychiatr Care* 29:31, 1993.
7. Degazon CE: Coping, diabetes, and the older African-American, *Nurs Outlook* 43:254, 1995.
8. Donnelly GF: Chronicity: concept and reality. *Holist Nurs Pract* 8:1, 1993.
9. Ebersole P, Hess P: *Toward healthy aging,* ed 4, St Louis, 1994, Mosby.
10. Forsyth GL, Delaney KD, Gresham ML: Vying for a winning position: management style of the chronically ill, *Res Nurs Health* 7:181, 1984.
11. Guimon J: The use of group progams to improve medication compliance in patients with chronic disease, *Patient Educ Couns* 26:189, 1995.
12. Handron DS: Denial and serious chronic illness—a personal perspective, *Perspect Psychiatr Care* 29:29, 1993.
13. Heim E: Coping-based intervention strategies, *Patient Educ Couns* 26:145, 1995.
14. Kerson TS, Kerson LA: *Understanding chronic illness: the medical and psychosocial dimension of nine diseases,* New York, 1985, Free Press.
15. Kim MJ, McFarland GK, McLane AM: *Pocket guide to nursing diagnoses,* ed 6, St Louis, 1995, Mosby.
16. Lamm B, Dungan JM, Hiromoto B: Long-term lifestyle management, *Clin Nurse Special* 5:182, 1991.

17. Lowry BJ: Psychological stress, denial and myocardial infarction outcomes, *Image: J Nurs Sch* 23:51, 1991.
18. Moser D, Dracup K: Psychosocial recovery from a cardiac event: the influence of perceived control, *Heart Lung* 24:273, 1995.
19. NANDA: *Nursing diagnoses: Definitions and classification, 1995-1996,* Philadelphia, 1994, North American Nursing Diagnosis Association.
20. Piringer P, Agana-Defensor R, Mullen NM, Lee L: A model for the development and implementation of a patient support group in a medical-surgical setting, *Holist Nurse Pract* 8:16, 1993.
21. Rancour P: Guided imagery: healing when curing is out of the question, *Perspect Psychiatr Care* 27:30, 1991.
22. Schaefer KM: Women living in paradox: loss and discovery in chronic illness, *Holist Nurs Pract* 9:63, 1995.
23. Snyder M: Independent nursing interventions, ed 2, Albany, NY, 1992, Delmar Publishers.
24. Swanson B, Cronin-Stubbs D, Sheldon JA: The impact of psychosocial factors on adapting to physical disability: a review of the research literature, *Rehabil Nurs* 14:64, 1989.
25. Winterhalter JG: Group support for families during the acute phase of rehabilitation, *Holist Nurs Pract* 6:23, 1992.

Posttrauma response

1. Americna Psychological Association: *Diagnostic and statistical manual of mental disorders DSM IV.* Washington, DC, 1994, The Association.
2. Armsworth M, Holaday M: The effects of psychological trauma on children and adolescents, *J Counsel Dev* 72:49-56, September/October 1993.
3. Breslau N, Davis G, Andreski P: Risk factors for PTSD-related traumatic event: a prospective analysis, *Am J Psychiatry* 154:4, 1995.
4. Burgess A, Holstrom L: Rape trauma syndrome, *Am J Psychiatry* 131:981, 1974.
5. Foa E, Riggs D, Gershuny B: Arousal, numbing, and intrusion: symptoms structure of PTSD following assault, *Am J Psychiatry* 152:1, 1995.
6. Horowitz M: *Stress-response syndromes,* New York, 1976, Jason Aronson.
7. Kulka R et al: *Trauma and the Vietnam war generation,* New York, 1990, Brunner Mazel.
8. Lee L et al: A 50 year prospective study of the psychological sequelae of WWII combat veterans, *Am J Psychiatry* 152:4, 1995.
9. McCann L, Pearlman L: *Psychological trauma and the adult survivor,* New York, 1990, Bruner Mazel.
10. Schwartz E, Perry B: The post-traumatic response in children and adolescents, *Psychiatr Clin North Am* 17:2, 1994.
11. Southwick S et al: Psychobiologic research in posttraumatic stress disorder, *Psychiatr Clin North Am* 17:2, 1994.
12. Sutherland S, Davidson J: Pharmacotherapy for posttraumatic stress disorder, *Psychiatr Clin North Am* 17:2, 1994.
13. Terr L: Chowchilla revisited: the effects of psychic trauma four years after a school bus kidnapping, *Am J Psychiatry* 140:1543, 1983.
14. Vander Kolk B, Fisler R: The biological basis of posttraumatic stress, *Psychiatr Clin North Am* 17:2, 1994.
15. Weisman G: Adolescent PTSD and developmental consequences of crack dealing, *Am J Orthopsychiatry* 63:553, 1993.

Family coping: potential for growth: ineffective family coping: compromised; ineffective family coping: disabling

1. Alexrod J, Geismar L, Ross R: Families of chronically mentally ill patients: Their structure, coping resources and tolerance for deviant behavior, *Health Soc Work* 19:271, 1994.
2. Birenbaum LK: Measurement of family coping, *J Pediatr Oncol* 8:39, 1991.
3. Block K, Brandt T, Magyary D: A nursing assessment standard for early intervention: Family coping, *J Pediatr Nurs* 10:28, 1995.
4. Bowers JE: Coping, family, potential for growth. In McFarland GK, Thomas MD: *Psychiatric mental health nursing: application of the nursing process,* Philadelphia, 1991, JB Lippincott.
5. Brandt P: Coping/stress tolerance. In *Children with special health care needs: Guidelines for specialty practice,* Unpublished manual, Seattle, WA, 1990, University of Washington.

6. Butcher LA: A family-focused perspective on chronic illness, *Rehabil Nurs* 19:70, 194.

7. Carpenito LJ: *Nursing diagnosis: application to clinical practice,* ed 4, Philadelphia, 1992, JB Lippincott.

8. Dietz-Omar MA: Family coping: a comparison of stepfamilies and traditional nuclear families during pregnancy, *Appl Nurs Res* 4:31, 1991.

9. Fawcett CS: *Family psychiatric nursing,* St Louis, 1993, Mosby.

10. Kaslow FW, editor: *The international book of family therapy,* New York, 1982, Brunner/Mazel.

11. Kim MJ, McFarland GK, McLane AM: *Pocket guide to nursing diagnoses,* ed 6, St Louis, 1995, Mosby.

12. Knafl KA, Deatrick JA: Family management style: concept analysis and development, *J Pediatr Nurs* 5:4, 1990.

13. Koller PA: Family needs and coping strategies during illness crisis, *Am Assoc Clin Nurs* 2:338, 1991.

14. Lewis FM, Hammond MA, Woods NF: The family's functioning with newly diagnosed breast cancer in the mother: the development of an explanatory model, *J Behav Med* 16:351, 1993.

15. Lipman TH: Assessing family strengths to guide plans of care using Hymovich's framework, *J Pediatr Nurs* 4:186, 1989.

16. McCubbin HI, Thompson A, editors: *Family assessment for research and practice,* Madison, Wis, 1987, University of Wisconsin, Madison.

17. Minuchin S, Fishman HC: *Family therapy techniques,* Cambridge, Mass, 1981, Harvard University Press.

18. Reeder JM: Family perception: a key to intervention, *AACN Clin Iss* 2:188, 1991.

19. Stetz KM, Lewis FM, Houck GM: Family goals as indicants of adaptation during chronic illness, *Public Health Nurs* 11:385, 1994.

20. Tunali B, Power TG: Creating satisfaction: a psychological perspective on stress and coping in families of handicapped children, *J Child Psychiatry* 34:945, 1993.

XI

FUNCTIONAL HEALTH PATTERN

Value-Belief

SPIRITUAL DISTRESS (DISTRESS OF HUMAN SPIRIT)

Spiritual distress (distress of the human spirit) is a disruption in the life principle that pervades a person's entire being and integrates and transcends one's biologic and psychosocial nature.

Tubesing[15] believes that all stress-related illness is fundamentally a spiritual disorder, "often growing from a conflict of values, beliefs and goals" and that differences in stress levels may be determined by the answers persons give to a series of spiritual questions. Assessment and research tools developed to measure one or more aspects of spirituality were reviewed by Ellerhorst-Ryan[3] and include Hess' Spiritual Needs Survey, Stoll's Guidelines for Spiritual Assessment, Spiritual Needs of Patients Questionnaire, Spiritual Well-Being Scale, Moberg's Indexes of Spiritual Well-Being, The Patient Spiritual Coping Interview, and Intrinsic Religious Motivation Scale. The reviewer identified the need for additional research tools and more refinement of existing measures.

Historically, nurses interested in spirituality investigated the extent to which nurses assessed patients' spiritual needs and incorporated spiritual care in their practice. Although it remains a continuing concern,[14] the focus has shifted from the nurse as caregiver to patients' needs and families' concerns in the spiritual realm. Reed's review[14] of extant knowledge of spirituality and mental health in older adults is an excellent resource for nurses working with the elderly. Holistic nurse practitioners have shown a renewed interest in spirituality, and some have placed it at the forefront of their practice.[10]

Validation of defining characteristics of nursing diagnoses continues to be a priority in the profession. Weatherall and Creason[16] used a content analysis of nursing literature and patient data to validate the defining characteristics of spiritual distress. Three NANDA defining characteristics (questions meaning of suffering, verbalizes concern about relationship with deity, and verbalizes inner conflict about beliefs) and two other characteristics (hopelessness and cues having to do with relationships with others) were supported by patient data and nursing literature. Small sample size limited the generalizability of the study.

Related Factors

Separation from religious and cultural ties
Challenged belief and value systems
Sense of meaninglessness or purposelessness
Remoteness from God
Disrupted spiritual trust
Moral or ethical nature of therapy
Sense of guilt and shame
Intense suffering
Unresolved feelings about death
Anger toward God

Defining Characteristics

Expresses concern with meaning of life or death or any belief system*
Verbalizes inner conflict about beliefs
Verbalizes concern about relationship with deity
Questions meaning of suffering
Questions meaning for own existence
Questions moral or ethical implications of therapeutic regimen
Expresses anger toward God
Displaces anger toward religious representatives
Seeks spiritual assistance
Unable to participate in usual religious practices
Experiences alteration of behavior or mood evidenced by anger, crying withdrawal, preoccupation, anxiety, hostility, apathy, etc.
Experiences nightmares or sleep disturbance
Gallows humor
Loss or separation from God and/or institutionalized religion[11]
Experience of evil or disillusionment[11]
Sense of failing God: The recognition of one's own sinfulness[11]
Lack of reconciliation with God[11]
A perceived loneliness of spirit[11]

---

*Critical defining characteristic.

Expected Patient Outcomes & Nursing Interventions

Experience sense of harmonious connectedness to religious and/or cultural ties, as evidenced by:

Verbalizing positive relationships with members of cultural/ religious group

Having availability of religious and/or cultural resources

Achieving high score on the JARL Spiritual Well-being Scale and/or low score on loneliness scale[6,12]

- Take time to listen and be open to patient's expression of loneliness and type of relationship to religious and cultural groups.
- Discuss and assess patient's religious and cultural background.
- Refer to spiritual and/or cultural advisor of patient's choice *to help alleviate spiritual distress.*
- Provide contact with people with similar cultural background, especially those people who have coped with similar situations *to provide a role model for coping.*
- Prepare patient for religious and cultural rituals of choice.
- Provide an environment conducive to the patient's culture and/or religion; e.g., provide religious/cultural articles and objects, prayer pamphlets, and audiotapes of spiritual and cultural prayers and songs.
- Provide time for personal reflection, meditation, and/or prayer (if patient expresses that need).
- Share appropriate readings that convey a message of hope *in dealing with loneliness and doubt, if patient is open and ready.*
- Express to patient that the feeling of loneliness is normal.

Freely express beliefs and values, as evidenced by:

Delineating short- and long-term goals

Making plans to meet goals

Completing value clarification

- Assist with value clarification *to help patient deal with challenged or unclear belief and value system.*
- Have patient get in touch with self through use of meditation, reflection, and/or prayer.
- Have patient make list of what is important and how much time is spent on things that are important and not important.
- Delineate long-term and short-term goals.
- Plan short-term tasks to meet short-term goals.
- Suggest that patient imagine self asking God, a friend, or an inner advisor to help clarify doubts and to ask what that person should do and be.
- Have patient act on advice from inner advisor.
- Provide opportunity for patient to meet with spiritual advisor *to help achieve peace of mind.*

Experience sense of meaning and purpose in life, illness, and suffering, as evidenced by:

Making positive statements on purpose in and satisfaction with life

Scoring high (40 to 60) on Existential Well-Being (EWB) scale[4] of Spiritual Well-Being (SWB) index

Participating in activities that are directed toward helping other people

- Be available to listen to and be empathetic to patient's feelings *to help patient feel comfortable with expressing those feelings.*
- Use religious and/or other readings that describe others who have found meaning in difficult situations.
- Help patient to put problems into a wider perspective.
- Have patient select and write down positive labels for each stressor of life.
- Aid patient in replacing negative thoughts and labels with positive ones *to help a person be less depressed and discouraged.*
- Help patients find in illness a means to grow and develop depth in understanding life.
- Help patient take risks and make commitment to something or someone.
- Help patient to do some type of volunteer activity, even something as simple as writing letters to a lonely person.

Experience relief from and/or accept suffering, as evidenced by:

Sharing feelings of relief and/or ability to endure and expressions of comfort and peace.

- Assure patient that nurse will be available *to support patient in times of suffering.*
- If comfortable to do so, offer to pray with patient in times of suffering *to help patient cope.*
- Refer to or provide a spiritual advisor or pastoral minister who is experienced in spiritual healing.
- Provide time with family, friends, and/or significant others.

Achieve relief of anger toward God, self, and/or others, as evidenced by:

Expressing understanding or acceptance of God's will

Scoring high (40 to 60) on Religious Well-Being (RWB) scale of SWB index

Feeling that God and others love and accept them for who they are

- Develop trust with patient by listening and by being present and responsive to patient's needs.
- Mention to patient that anger toward God and others is a normal (or common) part of the process of healing past hurts.
- Help patient to get in touch with feelings of anger.
- Help patient share feelings of anger with self or trusting friend *to obtain a perspective on the anger.*
- Problem solve ways to properly express and relieve anger.
- Use prayer, reflection, and/or imagery to heal past hurts.

Achieve closeness with God/supreme being, as evidenced by:

Praying and/or meditating

Gaining satisfaction with prayer

Scoring high (40 to 60) on RWB scale of SWB index[4]

- Express that God accepts and loves people for who they are.
- Encourage patient to adopt attitude of gratitude *for getting deeper insights into life.*
- Be present and available to patient.
- Offer to obtain for patient religious articles that could aid prayer or other religious activities.
- Teach simple quieting and relaxation skills so patient can relax and experience the presence of God.
- Offer to pray with patient *to increase relationship with God.*
- Suggest the need to find God's presence in self and others.
- Remind patient that many people have experienced remoteness from God (give appropriate examples of people in religious stories and writings).
- Refer to clergy.

Achieve sense of forgiveness (and decreased sense of guilt), as evidenced by:

Sharing past hurts and guilt
Accepting forgiveness from God and others
Sensing God's and other's love

- Be open and present when patient is willing to share past hurts and guilts.
- Suggest the use of reflection and personal journals to analyze and understand past hurts.
- Teach patient the use of centering prayer and healing of memories.
- Have patients imagine themselves sharing with a loving God/supreme being, and/or friend their painful memories and hurts, asking God and/or friend *to take the hurt away, heal them, and allow them to be filled with love.*
- Refer to clergy *to assist in dealing with guilt.*

Express decreased fear of and/or acceptance of death, as evidenced by:

Imaging and talking about death without undue anxiety

- Be open, present, and empathetic to patient's feelings about death.
- Support patient's beliefs of an afterlife in the presence of a loving God/supreme being.
- Have patient visualize own death while relaxing and meditating; include in the image being in the presence of God and friends and family who have died *to help resolve fears about death and to help prepare for death.*
- Refer patient to clergy or other spiritual advisor for religious rites.
- Refer patient to religious writings that support concept of afterlife.

Principles and Rationale for Nursing Interventions

Interest in the human spirit as a nursing phenomenon has increased. Efforts have been made to clarify the concept and

to delineate means to enable spirituality.[2] Common nursing interventions to enable the spirit and to unfold the harmonious interconnectedness of the person with self, others, the environment, and God/supreme being include presence, trust, surrendering, prayer, silence, meditation, imaging, scripture reading, touch, and referring to clergy or spiritual advisors. Reed[13] determined that arranging a visit with clergy, allowing time for personal prayer, talking with patient about beliefs, and providing time for family were the most commonly preferred spiritually related nursing interventions by nonterminally ill and terminally ill hospitalized patients. In a sense, providing an environment conducive to the patient's spiritual needs and talking with the patient about beliefs and concerns are primary spiritual interventions from the patient's perspective. Reed's study indicated that the clergy and family, rather than the nurse, are viewed as the primary spiritual providers.

Because separation from religious and cultural ties is a factor contributing to spiritual distress, interventions that enhance or provide contact with a religion or culture may help alleviate the problem. The first step in this intervention entails taking time to listen to the patient's expression of feelings and to assess the patient's religious and cultural background. The subsequent interventions are directed toward providing people (spiritual advisors and/or cultural representatives), religious and cultural objects, and resources for religious and cultural rituals. Providing a personal contact with a cultural representative who has coped with a similar problem could help the patient identify with the representative and provide a role model for coping. Helping a person to pray if he or she desires to do so and providing readings that convey a message of hope can help to decrease feelings of separation from religion and cultural ties and subsequent loneliness.

Another contributing factor to spiritual distress is having a challenged or unclear belief and value system. This is especially so when a person is suffering or is having a moral/ethical conflict. Helping a person to clarify his or her beliefs and values could help in this situation. Value clarification is one method designed for that purpose. These interventions provide a simple method of value clarification that includes relaxation and imagery from the perspective of the patient's faith system. A patient who does not believe in God can bring problems to an imaginative friend. Advice from a spiritual advisor who is from the person's faith could also bring peace of mind.

A typical symptom of spiritual distress is struggling with meaning and purpose of life and questioning the meaning and purpose of suffering and illness. A nurse is often present and available when that happens. Assisting a patient in that situation begins with helping the patient feel comfortable with expressing those feelings. Once patients articulate their doubts and feelings to another person, they can see their problem more clearly and put the problem into better perspective. Meditation, reflection, and prayer can help a person get in touch with his or her feelings and provide a sense of calm. Providing examples of other people who were able to find meaning and purpose under diverse conditions could provide hope, inspiration, and examples of how to cope with life's difficulties. Other cognitive techniques, such as refuting negative thoughts and looking for positive aspects of diversity (e.g., growth in understanding life), help a person be less depressed and discouraged because people often feel the way they think. Finally, volunteer activity and helping other people can help clear the mind of problems, provide perspective, and help to transcend everyday existence.

Because suffering is often associated with a depressed spirit and a questioning of meaning and purpose, helping a person to cope with the suffering or to decrease the suffering could help to lift the spirit. Just the presence of another individual can help a person cope with suffering. Nurses can convey to a person who is suffering that they will be available when needed. Gently touching a person who is suffering can also convey a message of support in a nonverbal way. For many people who suffer, prayer is a way of coping. Helping a person to pray in a form acceptable to the patient is important. Bringing in significant others to pray with the patient and using imagery to enhance the prayer are other ways of showing individuals that they are not alone in their suffering.

Typical symptoms of spiritual distress also may include anger with and alienation from God, self, and others. The interventions in this case are designed to decrease or to understand the feeling of anger. Other interventions can help the patient to develop and increase a relationship with God and thereby decrease the sense of alienation. The first steps in helping the patient to cope with anger are to develop a trusting relationship and to convey the message that anger is a normal or typical response. If the patient realizes that anger is a common feeling and that God is accepting of that anger, the patient might not have as much guilt. Sharing the anger with another individual helps the patient obtain a perspective on the anger. Problem-solving ways to express and to relieve the anger in an acceptable way are positive actions that help channel the anger. Prayer and imagery processes often can be used to heal past hurts that were the initial reason for the anger and alienation. Part of the process of healing life's past hurts and decreasing the anger is helping the patient to realize that one can grow and learn from adversity.

Increasing a relationship with God is often accomplished through prayer. Some people who are spiritually depressed, however, are unable to pray. For them, some type of passive prayer process might be needed. Having patients just let the presence of God be with them without trying to think or say anything is a way of passive prayer. Helping them to pray by providing religious objects and a quiet atmosphere or by actually praying with them could be helpful for those having difficulty praying. Providing stories of holy people who also had difficulty praying at times encourages patients, provides an example, and helps them to understand that they are not the only ones who feel that way. Referral to a spiritual advisor of a patient's choice might be appropriate at this time.

Obviously a person's faith system must be considered for any interventions. A patient who does not believe in God/supreme being could benefit from techniques not religiously oriented (e.g., relaxation; meditation on life; quieting and uplifting music; allowing patient to express and share feelings, values, and beliefs in a nonjudgmental way).

Although the lack of reconciliation and the feelings of guilt from past hurts and transgressions are defining characteristics

of spiritual distress, they could also be related factors. The sense of guilt and hurt can weigh a person down and depress the spirit. Experiencing a sense of forgiveness can relieve these feelings. Sharing past hurts and guilts with another person is one common way of reconciling life's transgressions and getting a perspective on them. Many faith systems have special rituals for dealing with guilt. A spiritual advisor of the patient's faith system could be of help. Reflective prayer and journaling are also effective ways to help a person get a perspective and understanding of past hurts. For patients who have a belief in God, sharing past hurts and memories in a prayer and imagery process (guided by a nurse or spiritual advisor comfortable in this process) could bring a sense of healing and forgiveness.

Unresolved feelings about death and the fear of death could also distress the spirit. Many faith systems have beliefs about death and afterlife that could be comforting to a patient. Supporting and reinforcing these beliefs are important. Referring to a spiritual advisor of the patient's choice is appropriate, especially for religious rites. Having patients visualize their own death while they are in a relaxed or meditative state can help resolve fears about death and prepare for death. Patients should be comforted if they are able to visualize their death in the presence of a loving God/supreme being or friends and family members who have died. The nurse's assurance of his or her presence is important for those who do not have a belief in an afterlife.

POTENTIAL FOR ENHANCED SPIRITUAL WELL-BEING

Spiritual well-being is the process of an individual's developing or unfolding of mystery through harmonious interconnectedness that springs from inner strengths.

Health care events may strengthen one's belief in God or a higher power. Such events have been referred to as core spiritual experiences. Historically, spirituality has been a part of modern nursing beginning with Nightingale.[7] She viewed nursing as a search for truth and a discovery of God's laws of healing with their proper application. Hearing a person's life story marks the beginning of a comprehensive spiritual assessment. Assessment guides may be used to supplement a careful interview but do not replace listening to another tell a life story. Recognition and response to spiritual concerns require a sensitivity to the ways in which spirituality is experienced and expressed. Knowing a patient, that is, a moral knowing, as described by Jenny and Logan,[4] is a prerequisite to using knowledge to individualize care.

Defining Characteristics[6]

Inner strengths
A sense of awareness, self-consciousness, sacred source, unifying force, inner core, and transcendence
Unfolding mystery
One's experience about life's purpose and meaning, mystery, uncertainty, and struggles
Harmonious interconnectedness

Relatedness, connectedness, harmony with self, others, higher power or God, and the environment

Expected Outcomes & Nursing Interventions

Interact with nurse and others to form caring connections, attachments, and relationships as evidenced by:

- Expresses desire to find meaning and purpose in health care events
- Tells life story in response to interviewer's questions
- Identifies potential barriers to developing closer relationships to family and friends
- Expresses spiritual concerns with respect to threat to health and life

  Listen and pay attention to patient's life story.

  Provide materials to keep a journal of life experience.

  Assist a patient with identification and description of sacred rituals. Sacred rituals are "ways of connecting with the sacred life force."[2]

  Help patient develop a plan for communicating more openly with family and friends.

Develop and implement plan for enhanced spiritual well-being as evidenced by:

- Expresses feelings about illness and death
- Expresses feelings of hope for the future
- Sets aside time for prayer, meditation, and other religious rituals
- Sees spiritual advisor on a regular basis
- Confronts end-of-life issues with family and friends

  Be open to expressions of anger and loneliness.

  Help patient uncover the meaning of hope.

  Provide information about spiritual resources, a list of spiritual advisors, chapel, etc.

  Offer a patient the gift of rest, a quiet time in a healing space.

  Help patient discover ways to evaluate ongoing spiritual growth.

Principles and Rationale for Nursing Interventions

Spirituality is an essential component of health. Belief in God or a higher power helps individuals deal with threats to health and life. The role of the nurse in providing spiritual care goes beyond referring patients to clergy. Listening, being present, and paying attention are cited as ways of helping patients with expressions of their spirituality and spiritual needs. "Paying attention" has been described as the essence of true spirituality and is an essential element of many different spiritual practices. Some of these practices include centering, meditation, prayer, bodywork/movement/sensing/, rest/waiting/leisure, ritual, and play.[2] A health crisis or other life crisis may precipitate a patient's search for meaning and purpose in life and provide an opportunity for spiritual growth. Being open to expres-

sions of feelings enables a patient to hear what is being felt and may provide the nurse with a clue as to how help may be given. Talking with patients about their beliefs and concerns; providing time for prayer, meditation, and family visits; helping patients and families to find reasons for hope; and praying with patients/families have been identified as spiritual interventions.

References

Spiritual distress (distress of human spirit)
1. Bauer T, Barron CR: Nursing interventions for spiritual care: preferences of the community-based elderly, *J Holist Nurs* 13:268, 1995.
2. Burkhardt MA, Nagai-Jacobson MG: Reawakening spirit in clinical practice, *J Holist Nurs* 12:9, 1994.
3. Ellerhorst-Ryan JM: Measuring aspects of spirituality. In Frank-Stromberg M, editor: *Instruments for clinical nursing research*, Norwalk, Conn, 1988, Appleton & Lange.
4. Ellison CW: Spiritual well-being: conceptualization and measurement, *J Psychol Theol* 11:30, 1983.
5. Fryback PB: Health for people with a terminal diagnosis, *Nursing Sci Q* 6:147, 1993.
6. Hungelmann J et al: Development of the JAREL Spiritual well-being scale. In Carroll-Johnson RM, editor: *Classification of nursing diagnosis: proceedings of the eighth conference*, Philadelphia, 1989, JB Lippincott.
7. Kaye J, Robinson KM: Spirituality among caregivers, *Image J Nurs Sch* 26:218, 1994.
8. Macrae J: Nightingale's spiritual philosophy and its significance for modern nursing, *Image J Nurs Sch* 27:8, 1995.
9. McCloskey JC, Bulechek GM: Spiritual support. In *Nursing interventions classification (NIC)*, St Louis, 1996, Mosby.
10. Nagal-Jacobson MG, Burkhardt MA: Spirituality: cornerstone of holistic nursing practice, *Holist Nurs Pract* 3:18, 1989.
11. O'Brien ME: The need for spiritual integrity. In Yura H, Walsh MB, editors: *Human needs and the nursing process*, Norwalk, Conn, 1982, Appleton-Century-Crofts.
12. Peplau L, Perlman D, editors: *Loneliness: a sourcebook of current theory, research and therapy*, New York, 1983, John Wiley & Sons.
13. Reed PG: Preferences for spiritually related nursing interventions among terminally ill and nonterminally ill hospitalized adults and well adults, *Appl Nurs Res* 4:122, 1991.
14. Reed PG: Spirituality and mental health in older adults: extant knowledge of for nursing, *Fam Community Health* 14:14, 1991.
15. Tubesing DA: Stress, spiritual outlook and health, *Specialized Pastoral Care J* 3:17, 1980.
16. Weatherall J, Creason NS: Validation of the nursing diagnosis, spiritual distress. In McLane AM, editor: *Classification of nursing diagnoses: proceedings of the seventh conference*, St Louis, 1987, Mosby.

Potential for enhanced spiritual well-being
1. Bauer T, Barron CR: Nursing interventions for spiritual care: preferences of the community-based elderly, *J Holist Nurs* 13:268, 1995.
2. Burkhardt MA, Nagai-Jacobson MG: Reawakening spirit in clinical practice, *J Holist Nurs* 12:9, 1994.
3. Fryback PB: Health for people with a terminal diagnosis, *Nurs Sci Q* 6:147, 1993.
4. Jenny J, Logan J: Knowing the patient: one aspect of clinical knowledge, *Image J Nurs Sch* 24:254, 1992.
5. Kaye J, Robinson KM: Spirituality among caregivers, *Image J Nurs Sch* 26:218, 1994.
6. Kim MJ, McFarland GK, McLane AM: *Pocket guide to nursing diagnoses*, ed 6, St Louis, 1995, Mosby.
7. Macrae J: Nightingale's spiritual philosophy and its significance for modern nursing, *Image J Nurs Sch* 27:8, 1995.
8. McCloskey JC, Bulechek GM: Spiritual support. In *Nursing interventions classification (NIC)*, St Louis, 1996, Mosby.
9. Reed PG: Preferences for spiritually related nursing interventions among terminally ill and nonterminally ill hospitalized adults and well adults, *Appl Nurs Res* 4:122, 1991.

Conversion Factors to International System of Units (SI Units)

Conversion Factors (SI Units)

Component	Normal Range in Units as Customarily Reported	Conversion Factor	Normal Range in SI Units, Molecular Units, International Units, or Decimal Fractions
Biochemical Components of Blood*			
Acetoacetic acid (S)	0.2-1.0 mg/dl	98	19.6-98.0 μmol/L
Acetone (S)	0.3-2.0 mg/dl	172	51.6-344.0 μmol/L
Albumin (S)	3.2-4.5 g/dl	10	32-45 g/L
Ammonia (P)	20-120 μg/dl	0.588	11.7-70.5 μmol/L
Amylase (S)	60-160 Somogyi units/dl	1.85	111-296 U/L
Base, total (S)	145-160 mEq/L	1	145-160 mmol/L
Bicarbonate (P)	21-28 mEq/L	1	21-28 mmol/L
Bile acids (S)	0.3-3.0 mg/dl	10	3-30 mg/L
		2.547	0.8-7.6 μmol/L
Bilirubin, direct (S)	Up to 0.3 mg/dl	17.1	Up to 5.1 μmol/L
Bilirubin, indirect (S)	0.1-1.0 mg/dl	17.1	1.7-17.1 μmol/L
Blood gases (B)			
P_{CO_2} arterial	35-40 mm Hg	0.133	4.66-5.32 kPa
P_{O_2} arterial	95-100 mm Hg	0.133	12.64-13.30 kPa
Calcium (S)	8.5-10.5 mg/dl	0.25	2.1-2.6 mmol/L
Chloride (S)	95-103 mEq/L	1	95-103 mmol/L
Creatine (S)	0.1-0.4 mg/dl	76.3	7.6-30.5 μmol/L
Creatinine (S)	0.6-1.2 mg/dl	88.4	53-106 μmol/L
Creatinine clearance (P)	107-139 mL/min	0.0167	1.78-2.32 mL/s
Fatty acids (total) (S)	8-20 mg/dl	0.01	0.08-2.00 mg/L
Fibrinogen (P)	200-400 mg/dl	0.01	2.00-4.00 g/L
Gamma globulin (S)	0.5-1.6 g/dl	10	5-16 g/L
Globulins (total) (S)	2.3-3.5 g/dl	10	23-35 g/L
Glucose (fasting) (S)	70-110 mg/dl	0.055	3.85-6.05 mmol/L
Insulin (radioimmunoassay) (P)	4-24 μIU/ml	0.0417	0.17-1.00 μg/L
	0.20-0.84 μg/L	172.2	35-145 pmol/L
Iodine, BEI (S)	3.5-6.5 μg/dl	0.079	0.28-0.51 μmol/L
Iodine, PBI (S)	4.0-8.0 μg/dl	0.079	0.32-0.63 μmol/L
Iron, total (S)	60-150 μg/dl	0.179	11-27 μmol/L
Iron-binding capacity (S)	300-360 μg/dl	0.179	54-64 μmol/L
17-Ketosteroids (P)	25-125 μg/dl	0.01	0.25-1.25 mg/L
Lactic dehydrogenase (S)	80-120 units at 30° C	0.48	38-62 U/L at 30° C
	Lactate → pyruvate		
	100-190 U/L at 37° C	1	100-190 U/L at 37° C
Lipase (S)	0-1.5 U/ml (Cherry-Crandall)	278	0-417 U/L

From Tilkian, S.M., Conover, M.B., and Tilkian, A.G.: Clinical implications of laboratory tests, ed 5, St Louis, 1996, Mosby.
*This is a selected (not a complete) list of biochemical components. The ranges listed may differ from those accepted in some laboratories and are shown to illustrate the conversion factor and the method of expression in SI molecular units. For a more complete listing, see Henry, J.B., editor: Todd-Sanford-Davidsohn clinical diagnosis and management by laboratory methods, ed. 16, Philadelphia, W.B. Saunders Co.

Conversion Factors (SI Units)—cont'd

Component	Normal Range in Units as Customarily Reported	Conversion Factor	Normal Range in SI Units, Molecular Units, International Units, or Decimal Fractions
Lipids (total) (S)	400-800 mg/dl	0.01	4.00-8.00 g/L
Cholesterol	150-250 mg/dl	0.026	3.9-6.5 mmol/L
Triglycerides	75-165 mg/dl	0.0114	0.85-1.89 mmol/L
Phospholipids	150-380 mg/dl	0.01	1.50-380 g/L
Free fatty acids	9.0-15.0 mM/L	1	9.0-15.0 mmol/L
Nonprotein nitrogen (S)	20-35 mg/dl	0.714	14.3-25.0 mmol/L
Phosphatase (P)			
Acid (units/dl)	Cherry-Crandall	2.77	0-5.5 U/L
	King-Armstrong	1.77	0-5.5 U/L
	Bodansky	5.37	0-5.5 U/L
Alkaline (units/dl)	King-Armstrong	1.77	30-120 U/L
	Bodansky	5.37	30-120 U/L
	Bessey-Lowry-Brock	16.67	30-120 U/L
Phosphorus, inorganic (S)	3.0-4.5 mg/dl	0.323	0.97-1.45 mmol/L
Potassium (P)	3.8-5.0 mEq/L	1	3.8-5.0 mmol/L
Proteins, total (S)	6.0-7.8 g/dl	10	60-78 g/L
Albumin	3.2-4.5 g/dl	10	32-45 g/L
Globulin	2.3-3.5 g/dl	10	23-35 g/L
Sodium (P)	136-142 mEq/L	1	136-142 mmol/L
Testosterone: Male (S)	300-1,200 ng/dl	0.035	10.5-42.0 nmol/L
Female	30-95 ng/dl	0.035	1.0-3.3 nmol/L
Thyroid tests (S)			
Thyroxine (T_4)	4-11 μg/dl	12.87	51-142 nmol/L
T_4 expressed as iodine	3.2-7.2 μg/dl	79.0	253-569 nmol/L
T_3 resin uptake	25%-38% relative uptake	0.01	0.25%-0.38% relative uptake
TSH (S)	10 μU/mL	1	$<10^{-3}$ IU/L
Urea nitrogen (S)	8-23 mg/dl	0.357	2.9-8.2 mmol/L
Uric acid (S)	2-6 mg/dl	59.5	0.120-0.360 mmol/L
Vitamin B_{12} (S)	160-950 pg/mL	0.74	118-703 pmol/L
Hematology Values*			
Red cell volume (male)	25-35 mL/kg body weight	0.001	0.025-0.035 L/kg body weight
Hematocrit	40%-50%	0.01	0.40-0.50
Hemoglobin	13.5-18.0 g/dl	10	135-180 g/L
Hemoglobin	13.5-18.0 g/dl	0.155	2.09-2.79 mmol/L
RBC count	$4.5\text{-}6 \times 10^6/\mu L$	1	$4.6\text{-}6 \times 10^{12}/L$
WBC count	$4.5\text{-}10 \times 10^3/\mu L$	1	$4.5\text{-}10 \times 10^9/L$
Mean corpuscular volume	80-96 μm³	1	80-96 fL

*The International Committee for Standardization in Hematology recommends that the numbers remain the same but that the units change, so that hemoglobin is expressed as grams per deciliter (g/dl) even though other measurements are expressed as units per liter (U/L).

General Index

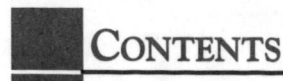

CONTENTS